3rd Edition

TEXTBOOK OF
Gastrointestinal
Radiology

Richard M. Gore, MD
Professor of Radiology
Northwestern University Feinberg School of Medicine
Chief, Gastrointestinal Radiology Section
Evanston Northwestern Healthcare
Evanston, Illinois

Marc S. Levine, MD
Professor of Radiology
Advisory Dean
University of Pennsylvania School of Medicine
Chief, Gastrointestinal Radiology Section
University of Pennsylvania Medical Center
Philadelphia, Pennsylvania

VOLUME **1**

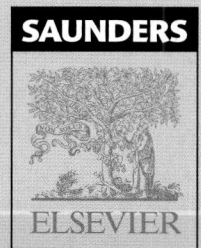

SAUNDERS

ELSEVIER

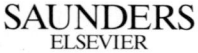

1600 John F. Kennedy Blvd.
Ste. 1800
Philadelphia, PA 19103-2899

TEXTBOOK OF GASTROINTESTINAL RADIOLOGY

Copyright © 2008, 2000, 1994 by Saunders, an imprint of Elsevier Inc.

Set ISBN: 978-1-4160-2332-6
Volume 1 Part No. 9996008037
Volume 2 Part No. 9996007553

Library of Congress Cataloging-in-Publication Data

Textbook of gastrointestinal radiology/[edited by] Richard M. Gore,
    Marc S. Levine.—3rd ed.
        p. ; cm.
    Includes bibliographical references and index.
    ISBN-10 : 1-4160-2332-1   ISBN-13: 978-1-4160-2332-6
    1. Gastrointestinal system—Radiography. I. Gore, Richard M.
II. Levine, Marc S.
    [DNLM: 1. Gastrointestinal Diseases—diagnosis. 2. Diagnostic
Imaging—methods. 3. Digestive System—pathology. WI 141 T355 2008]
    RC804. R6T46—2007   616.3'307572—dc22   2006030686

Acquisitions Editor: Rebecca Schmidt Gaertner
Developmental Editor: Jean Nevius
Publishing Services Manager: Linda Van Pelt
Project Managers: Joan Nikelsky, Melanie Johnstone
Design Direction: Ellen Zanolle

Printed in China

Last digit is the print number: 9 8 7 6 5 4 3 2

Contributors

SECTION EDITOR

STEPHEN E. RUBESIN, MD
Professor of Radiology, University of Pennsylvania School of
Medicine; Radiologist, Hospital of the University of
Pennsylvania, Philadelphia, Pennsylvania

SAMUEL NATHAN ADLER, MD
Chief, Department of Gastroenterology, Bikur Holim
Hospital, Jerusalem, Israel

STEPHEN R. BAKER, MD, MPHIL
Professor and Chairman, Department of Radiology, UMDJ
New Jersey Medical School; Chief, Department of Radiology,
The University Hospital, Newark, New Jersey

APARNA BALACHANDRAN, MD
Assistant Professor, Department of Radiology, Division of
Diagnostic Imaging, University of Texas MD Anderson
Cancer Center, Houston, Texas

DENNIS M. BALFE, MD
Professor of Radiology, Department of Diagnostic Radiology,
Washington University in St. Louis School of Medicine;
Radiologist, Department of Diagnostic Radiology, Barnes-
Jewish Hospital, St. Louis, Missouri

EMIL J. BALTHAZAR, MD
Professor Emeritus, Department of Radiology, New York
University School of Medicine; Attending Consultant,
Department of Radiology, Bellevue Hospital, New York,
New York

STUART A. BARNARD, MB, BS, MA, MRCS, FRCR
Radiologist, Department of Radiology, Middlemore Hospital,
Auckland, New Zealand

CLIVE BARTRAM, MD, FRCS, FRCP, FRCR
Honorary Professor of Gastrointestinal Radiology, School of
Medicine, Imperial College Faculty of Medicine, London;
Emeritus Consultant, Department of Radiology, St. Mark's
Hospital, Harrow, United Kingdom

GENEVIEVE L. BENNETT, MD
Assistant Professor of Radiology, Department of Radiology,
Abdominal Imaging Division, New York University School
of Medicine, Bellevue Hospital Medical Center, New York,
New York

JONATHAN W. BERLIN, MD, MBA
Associate Professor of Radiology, Northwestern University
Feinberg School of Medicine, Evanston; Radiologist, Body
Imaging Section, Evanston Northwestern Healthcare,
Evanston; Lecturer, Department of Radiology, Rosalind
Franklin University of Medicine and Science, North Chicago,
Illinois

GEORGE S. BISSETT III, MD
Professor of Radiology and Pediatrics, Vice Chairman,
Department of Radiology, Duke University School of
Medicine, Durham, North Carolina

PEYMAN BORGHEI, MD
Visiting Research Scholar, Department of Diagnostic
Radiology, University of California Irvine Medical Center,
Orange, California

JAMES L. BUCK, MD
Professor, Department of Diagnostic Radiology, University of
Kentucky College of Medicine, Lexington, Kentucky

CARINA L. BUTLER, MD
Assistant Professor, Department of Diagnostic Radiology,
University of Kentucky College of Medicine, University
of Kentucky Chandler Medical Center, Lexington, Kentucky

MARC A. CAMACHO, MD, MS
Chief, Emergency Radiology, Department of Radiology, Beth
Israel Deaconess Medical Center, Boston, Massachusetts.
Formerly: Assistant Professor, Department of Radiology,
Virginia Commonwealth University College of Medicine;
Chief, Emergency Radiology, Department of Radiology,
Virginia Commonwealth University Health System, Medical
College of Virginia Hospital, Richmond, Virginia

DINA F. CAROLINE, MD, PHD
Professor, Department of Radiology, Temple University
School of Medicine, Temple University Hospital,
Philadelphia, Pennsylvania

CAROLINE W. T. CARRICO, MD
Assistant Clinical Professor, Departments of Radiology and
Pediatrics, Duke University School of Medicine, Durham,
North Carolina

RICHARD I. CHEN, MD
Assistant Professor, Department of Interventional Radiology,
Northwestern University Feinberg School of Medicine;
Medical Director, Department of Interventional Radiology,
Northwestern Memorial Hospital, Chicago, Illinois

BYUNG IHN CHOI, MD
Professor of Radiology, Department of Radiology, Seoul
National University College of Medicine, Seoul National
University Hospital, Seoul, Republic of Korea

HOWARD B. CHRISMAN, MD
Associate Professor, Department of Radiology, Northwestern
University Feinberg School of Medicine, Northwestern
Memorial Hospital, Chicago, Illinois

PETER L. COOPERBERG, MDCM, FRCPC, FACR
Professor and Vice Chairman, Department of Radiology,
University of British Columbia Faculty of Medicine, St. Paul's
Hospital, Vancouver, British Columbia, Canada

ABRAHAM H. DACHMAN, MD
Professor, Director of Fellowship Programs, Department of
Radiology, University of Chicago Pritzker School of
Medicine, Chicago, Illinois

SUSAN DELANEY, MD, FRCPC
Lecturer, Department of Radiology, Dalhousie University
Faculty of Medicine, Halifax; Staff Radiologist, Department
of Radiology, Dartmouth General Hospital, Dartmouth,
Nova Scotia, Canada

GERALD D. DODD III, MD
Professor and Chairman, Department of Radiology,
University of Texas School of Medicine at San Antonio,
University Hospital System, San Antonio, Texas

RONALD L. EISENBERG, MD
Department of Radiology, Beth Israel Deaconess, Harvard
Medical School, Boston, Massachusetts. *Formerly*: Clinical
Professor of Radiology, University of California, San
Francisco, School of Medicine, San Francisco; University of
California, Davis, School of Medicine, Davis, California

SUKRU MEHMET ERTURK, MD, PHD
Lecturer in Radiology, Harvard Medical School; Research
Fellow, Department of Radiology, Brigham and Women's
Hospital, Boston, Massachusetts; Radiologist, Department of
Radiology, Sisli Etfal Training and Research Hospital,
Istanbul, Turkey

SANDRA K. FERNBACH, MD
Professor of Radiology, Northwestern University Feinberg
School of Medicine, Chicago; Pediatric Radiologist,
Department of Radiology, Evanston Northwestern
Healthcare, Evanston, Illinois

JULIA R. FIELDING, MD
Associate Professor, Director of Abdominal Imaging,
Department of Radiology, University of North Carolina
Medical Center, Chapel Hill, North Carolina

ELLIOT K. FISHMAN, MD
Professor of Radiology and Oncology, Johns Hopkins
University School of Medicine; Attending Radiologist,
Department of Radiology, Johns Hopkins Hospital,
Baltimore, Maryland

FRANS-THOMAS FORK, MD, PHD
Associate Professor of Radiology, Department of Clinical
Sciences/Medical Radiology, Lund University Faculty of
Medicine; Consultant Radiologist, Department of Radiology,
Malmo University Hospital, Malmo, Sweden

MARTIN C. FREUND, MD
Associate Professor, Department of Radiology, Medical
University Innsbruck, Innsbruck, Austria

ANN S. FULCHER, MD
Professor and Chairman, Department of Radiology, Virginia
Commonwealth University School of Medicine, Medical
College of Virginia Hospitals and Physicians, Richmond,
Virginia

EMMA E. FURTH, MD
Professor of Pathology and Laboratory Medicine,
Department of Pathology, University of Pennsylvania School
of Medicine, Hospital of the University of Pennsylvania,
Philadelphia, Pennsylvania

HELENA GABRIEL, MD
Associate Professor, Department of Radiology, Northwestern
University Feinberg School of Medicine; Director, Division of
Ultrasound, Department of Radiology, Northwestern
Memorial Hospital, Chicago, Illinois

ANA MARIA GACA, MD
Clinical Associate, Department of Radiology, Duke University
Medical Center, Durham, North Carolina

GABRIELA GAYER, MD
Senior Lecturer, Department of Radiology, Sackler Faculty of
Medicine, Tel Aviv University, Tel Aviv; Chief, CT Division,
Department of Diagnostic Imaging, Assaf Harofeh Medical
Center, Ramat-Gan, Israel

GARY G. GHAHREMANI, MD, FACR
Clinical Professor of Radiology, Department of Radiology,
University of California, San Diego, School of Medicine, La
Jolla, California; Emeritus Professor of Radiology,
Northwestern University Feinberg School of Medicine,
Chicago, Illinois

SETH N. GLICK, MD
Clinical Professor of Radiology, Department of Radiology,
University of Pennsylvania School of Medicine, Philadelphia,
Pennsylvania

MARGARET D. GORE, MD
Assistant Professor, Department of Radiology, Northwestern
University Feinberg School of Medicine, Senior Attending
Radiologist, Department of Radiology, Evanston
Northwestern Healthcare, Evanston, Illinois

RICHARD M. GORE, MD
Professor of Radiology, Northwestern University Feinberg School of Medicine; Chief, Gastrointestinal Radiology Section, Evanston Northwestern Healthcare, Evanston, Illinois

NICHOLAS C. GOURTSOYIANNIS, MD
Professor, Department of Radiology, University of Crete Medical School; Chairman, Department of Radiology, University Hospital of Heraklion, Heraklion, Crete, Greece

DAVID HAHN, MD
Assistant Professor, Department of Radiology, Northwestern University Feinberg School of Medicine, Chicago; Section Chief, Department of Interventional Radiology; Director, ENH Endovascular Lab, Evanston Northwestern Healthcare, Evanston, Illinois

ROBERT A. HALVORSEN, MD, FACR
Professor, Department of Radiology, Division of Abdominal Imaging, Virginia Commonwealth University School of Medicine; Staff Radiologist, Medical College of Virginia Hospitals, Richmond, Virginia

NANCY A. HAMMOND, MD
Assistant Professor, Department of Radiology, Northwestern University Feinberg School of Medicine, Northwestern Memorial Hospital, Chicago, Illinois

MARJORIE HERTZ, MD
Professor Emeritus, Department of Radiology, Sackler Faculty of Medicine, Tel Aviv University, Tel Aviv; Attending Staff Radiologist, Department of Diagnostic Imaging, Sheba Medical Center, Maccabim, Israel

FREDERICK L. HOFF, MD
Associate Professor, Department of Radiology, Northwestern University Feinberg School of Medicine; Staff Radiologist, Department of Diagnostic Radiology, Northwestern Memorial Hospital, Chicago, Illinois

CAROLINE L. HOLLINGSWORTH, MD, MPH
Assistant Professor, Department of Radiology, Division of Pediatric Radiology, Duke University School of Medicine, Durham, North Carolina

KAREN M. HORTON, MD
Associate Professor, The Russell H. Morgan Department of Radiology and Radiological Sciences, Johns Hopkins University School of Medicine, Baltimore, Maryland

JILL E. JACOBS, MD
Associate Professor of Radiology, New York University School of Medicine; Chief of Cardiac Imaging, Department of Radiology, New York University Medical Center, New York, New York

WERNER R. JASCHKE, MD, PHD
Professor and Chairman, Department of Radiology, Medical University Innsbruck, Innsbruck, Austria

BRUCE R. JAVORS, MD
Professor of Clinical Radiology, Department of Radiology, New York Medical College, Valhalla; Chairman, Department of Radiology, St. Vincent's Hospital–Manhattan, New York, New York

BRONWYN JONES, MD, FRACP, FRCR
Professor of Radiology, The Russell H. Morgan Department of Radiology and Radiological Sciences, Johns Hopkins University School of Medicine; Radiologist, Department of Radiology; Director, Johns Hopkins Swallowing Center, Johns Hopkins Hospital, Baltimore, Maryland; Editor-in-Chief, *Dysphagia,* Springer Publishers, New York, New York

MANNUDEEP K. KALRA, MD
Clinical Fellow, Department of Radiology, Harvard Medical School/Massachusetts General Hospital, Boston, Massachusetts

ANA L. KEPPKE, MD
Radiology Resident, Department of Radiology, Advocate Illinois Masonic Medical Center, Chicago, Illinois

STANLEY TAESON KIM, MD
Instructor, Department of Radiology, Northwestern University Feinberg School of Medicine; Interventional Radiologist, Department of Radiology, Northwestern Memorial Hospital; Interventional Radiologist, Department of Medical Imaging, Children's Memorial Hospital, Chicago, Illinois

MICHAEL L. KOCHMAN, MD, FACP
Professor of Medicine, Department of Medicine, Gastroenterology Division, University of Pennsylvania School of Medicine, Hospital of the University of Pennsylvania, Philadelphia, Pennsylvania

JOHN C. LAPPAS, MD
Professor, Department of Radiology, Indiana University School of Medicine; Chief of Abdominal Imaging, Indiana University Medical Center/Clarian Health, Wishard Memorial Hospital, Indianapolis, Indiana

THOMAS C. LAUENSTEIN, MD
Assistant Professor, Department of Radiology, Emory University School of Medicine, Emory University Hospital, Atlanta, Georgia

IGOR LAUFER, MD
Professor of Radiology, Department of Radiology, University of Pennsylvania School of Medicine; Staff, Gastrointestinal Radiology Section, Hospital of the University of Pennsylvania, Philadelphia, Pennsylvania

JEONG MIN LEE, MD
Associate Professor, Department of Radiology, Seoul National University College of Medicine, Seoul National University Hospital, Seoul, South Korea

KANG HOON LEE, MD
Staff Radiologist, Body Imaging Section, Department of
Radiology, University of North Carolina Medical Center,
Chapel Hill, North Carolina

MARC S. LEVINE, MD
Professor of Radiology, Advisory Dean, University of
Pennsylvania School of Medicine; Chief, Gastrointestinal
Radiology Section, University of Pennsylvania Medical
Center, Philadelphia, Pennsylvania

RUSSELL N. LOW, MD
Medical Director, Sharp and Children's MRI Center,
Department of Radiology, Sharp Memorial Hospital, San
Diego, California

MICHAEL MACARI, MD
Associate Professor, Section Chief, Department of Radiology,
New York University School of Medicine; Tish Hospital,
New York, New York

ROBERT L. MACCARTY, MD, FACR
Professor, Department of Radiology, Mayo Clinic College of
Medicine; Consultant, Mayo Clinic, Mayo Foundation,
Rochester, Minnesota

DEAN D. T. MAGLINTE, MD, FACR
Professor, Department of Radiology, Indiana University
School of Medicine; Attending Radiologist, Indiana
University Medical Center, Indianapolis, Indiana

CHARLES S. MARN, MD
Associate Professor of Radiology and Gastroenterology,
Medical College of Wisconsin; Chief, Gastrointestinal
Radiology, Department of Radiology, Froedtert Memorial
Lutheran Hospital, Milwaukee, Wisconsin

GABRIELE MASSELLI, MD
Staff Radiologist, Consultant, Abdominal and Pelvic MRI,
Radiology Department, Umberto I Hospital, La Sapienza
University, Rome, Italy

ALAN H. MAURER, MD
Professor of Radiology and Internal Medicine, Department
of Radiology, Temple University School of Medicine; Director
of Nuclear Medicine, Department of Radiology, Temple
University Hospital, Philadelphia, Pennsylvania

JOSEPH PATRICK MAZZIE, DO
Chief Resident, Department of Radiology, St. Vincent's
Hospital and Medical Center, New York, New York

ALEC J. MEGIBOW, MD, MPH, FACR
Professor, Department of Radiology, New York University
School of Medicine, New York, New York

UDAY K. MEHTA, MD
Assistant Professor of Radiology, Department of Radiology,
Northwestern University Feinberg School of Medicine;
Diagnostic Radiologist, Evanston Hospital, Evanston, Illinois

JAMES M. MESSMER, MD, MED
Professor, Senior Associate Dean for Medical Education,
Department of Radiology, Virginia Commonwealth
University School of Medicine, Richmond, Virginia

MORTON A. MEYERS, MD, FACR, FACG
Distinguished Professor, Departments of Radiology and
Internal Medicine, Stony Brook School of Medicine, Stony
Brook, New York

FRANK H. MILLER, MD
Professor, Department of Radiology, Northwestern University
Feinberg School of Medicine; Director, Body Imaging Section
and Fellowship, Chief, Gastrointestinal Radiology,
Northwestern Memorial Hospital, Chicago, Illinois

KOENRAAD J. MORTELE, MD
Associate Professor, Department of Radiology, Harvard
Medical School; Associate Director, Division of Abdominal
Imaging and Intervention; Director, Abdominal and Pelvic
MRI, CME, Department of Radiology, Brigham and Women's
Hospital, Boston, Massachusetts

KAREN A. MOURTZIKOS, MD
Assistant Professor, Department of Radiology, Division of
Nuclear Medicine, New York University School of Medicine,
New York, New York

SARAVANAN NAMASIVAYAM, MD, DNB, DHA*
Research Fellow, Department of Radiology, Division of
Abdominal Imaging and Intervention, Harvard University/
Massachusetts General Hospital, Boston, Massachusetts
*Deceased

VAMSI R. NARRA, MD, FRCR
Associate Professor of Radiology, Co-Chief, Body MRI, Co-
Director, Body MRI Fellowship, Mallinckrodt Institute of
Radiology, Washington University in St. Louis School of
Medicine; Chief, Clinical Operations, Barnes-Jewish West
County Hospital, St. Louis, Missouri

RENDON C. NELSON, MD
Professor and Vice-Chair, Department of Radiology, Duke
University School of Medicine, Durham, North Carolina

ALBERT A. NEMCEK, JR., MD
Professor, Department of Radiology, Northwestern University
Feinberg School of Medicine; Attending Staff, Department of
Radiology, Northwestern Memorial Hospital, Chicago, Illinois

GERALDINE MOGAVERO NEWMARK, MD
Assistant Professor, Department of Radiology, Northwestern
University Feinberg School of Medicine; Chief, Section of
Body Imaging, Department of Radiology, Evanston
Northwestern Healthcare, Evanston, Illinois

PAUL NIKOLAIDIS, MD
Associate Professor of Radiology, Department of Radiology,
Northwestern University Feinberg School of Medicine;
Chicago, Illinois

DAVID J. OTT, MD
Professor of Radiology, Department of Radiologic Sciences, Wake Forest University School of Medicine; Staff Radiologist, Section of Abdominal Imaging, Wake Forest University Baptist Medical Center, Winston-Salem, North Carolina

NICKOLAS PAPANIKOLAOU, PHD
Biomedical Engineer, Research Associate, Department of Radiology, University of Crete Medical School, Heraklion, Crete, Greece

ERIK K. PAULSON, MD
Professor, Department of Radiology, Duke University School of Medicine; Chief, Abdominal Imaging Division, Department of Radiology, Duke University Medical Center, Durham, North Carolina

F. SCOTT PERELES, MD
Salinas Valley Radiologists, Director, Magnetic Resonance Imaging, Coastal Valley Imaging, Salinas, California

CHRISTINE M. PETERSON, MD
Clinical Instructor, Mallinckrodt Institute of Radiology, Washington University in St. Louis School of Medicine, St. Louis, Missouri

VIKRAM A. RAO, MD
Instructor of Radiology, Department of Radiology, Northwestern University Feinberg School of Medicine, Chicago; Staff Radiologist, Evanston Northwestern Healthcare, Evanston, Illinois

RICHARD D. REDVANLY, MD
Radiologist, MR Body Imaging Section, Charlotte Radiology, Charlotte, North Carolina

PABLO R. ROS, MD, MPH
Professor of Radiology, Department of Radiology, Harvard Medical School; Executive Vice Chair, Department of Radiology, Brigham and Women's Hospital; Chief, Department of Radiology, Dana Farber Cancer Institute, Boston, Massachusetts

SANJAY SAINI, MD
Professor of Radiology, Harvard Medical School; Vice Chairman, Department of Radiology, Massachusetts General Hospital, Boston, Massachusetts

RIAD SALEM, MD, MBA
Associate Professor, Department of Radiology, Northwestern University Feinberg School of Medicine; Director of Interventional Oncology, Department of Radiology, Northwestern Memorial Hospital, Chicago, Illinois

KUMARESAN SANDRASEGARAN, MD
Assistant Professor, Department of Radiology, Indiana University School of Medicine, Indianapolis, Indiana

KENT T. SATO, MD
Assistant Professor, Department of Interventional Radiology, Northwestern University Feinberg School of Medicine, Chicago, Illinois

CHRISTOPHER D. SCHEIREY, MD
Clinical Instructor, Department of Diagnostic Radiology, Tufts University School of Medicine, Boston; Staff Radiologist, Department of Diagnostic Radiology, Lahey Clinic Medical Center, Burlington, Massachusetts

FRANCIS J. SCHOLZ, MD
Clinical Professor, Department of Radiology, Tufts University School of Medicine, Boston; Radiologist, Department of Diagnostic Radiology, Lahey Clinic Medical Center, Burlington, Massachusetts

ALI SHIRKHODA, MD
Clinical Professor of Radiology, Department of Radiology, University of California, Irvine, Irvine, California; Clinical Professor of Radiology, Department of Radiology, Wayne State University School of Medicine, Detroit; Director, Division of Diagnostic Imaging, William Beaumont Hospital, Royal Oak, Michigan

PAUL M. SILVERMAN, MD
Department of Radiology, Division of Diagnostic Imaging, MD Anderson Medical Center, Houston, Texas

STUART G. SILVERMAN, MD
Professor, Department of Radiology, Harvard Medical School; Director, Abdominal Imaging and Intervention, Director, CT scan, Director, Cross-sectional Imaging Service, Department of Radiology, Brigham and Women's Hospital, Boston, Massachusetts

JOVITAS SKUCAS, MD
Professor Emeritus, Department of Imaging Science, University of Rochester School of Medicine and Dentistry; Attending Radiologist, Department of Imaging Science, Strong Memorial Hospital, Rochester, New York

WILLIAM C. SMALL, MD, PHD
Associate Professor, Director of Abdominal Imaging, Department of Radiology, Emory University School of Medicine, Atlanta, Georgia

CLAIRE H. SMITH, MD, FACR
Professor, Rush Medical College; Senior Attending Radiologist, Section Director, Gastrointestinal Radiology, Department of Diagnostic Radiology and Nuclear Medicine, Rush University Medical Center, Chicago, Illinois

ROBERT H. SMITH, MD
Director, Department of Vascular and Interventional Radiology, Roper St. Francis Healthcare, Charleston, South Carolina

SAT SOMERS, MBCHB, FRCPC, FFRRCSI
Professor, Department of Radiology, Michael G. DeGroote School of Medicine, McMaster University Faculty of Health Sciences, Hamilton, Ontario, Canada

ALLISON L. SUMMERS, MD
Instructor in Radiology, Department of Radiology, Northwestern University Feinberg School of Medicine, Northwestern Memorial Hospital, Chicago, Illinois

RAJEEV SURI, MD
Assistant Professor, Department of Radiology, University of Texas School of Medicine at San Antonio; Associate Director, Radiology Residency Program, University of Texas Health Sciences Center at San Antonio; Interim Section Chief, Department of Interventional Radiology, University Hospital System; Director, Department of Interventional Radiology, Audie L. Murphy Veterans Affairs Medical Center, San Antonio, Texas

RICHARD A. SZUCS, MD
Clinical Assistant Professor of Radiology, Virginia Commonwealth University School of Medicine; Chairman, Department of Radiology, Bon Secours St. Mary's Hospital, Richmond, Virginia

MARK TALAMONTI, MD
Associate Professor, Chairman, Department of Surgery, Northwestern University Feinberg School of Medicine, Evanston Northwestern Healthcare, Chicago, Illinois

ANDREW J. TAYLOR, MD
Professor of Radiology, Department of Radiology, University of Wisconsin School of Medicine and Public Health, Chief of Gastrointestinal Radiology, University of Wisconsin Hospital and Clinics, Madison, Wisconsin

RUEDI F. THOENI, MD
Professor, Department of Radiology, University of California, San Francisco, School of Medicine; Chief, Department of Abdominal Imaging, San Francisco General Hospital; Staff Radiologist, Moffitt-Long Hospital, San Francisco, California

WILLIAM MOREAU THOMPSON, MD
Professor, Department of Radiology, Duke University School of Medicine, Durham, North Carolina

RANISTA TONGDEE, MD
Clinical Fellow, Department of Body MR Imaging, Mallinckrodt Institute of Radiology, St. Louis, Missouri; Instructor in Radiology, Department of Diagnostic Radiology, Abdominal Section, Siriraj Hospital, Bangkok, Thailand

MITCHELL E. TUBLIN, MD
Associate Professor, Department of Radiology, University of Pittsburgh School of Medicine; Chief, Ultrasound Section, Department of Radiology Abdominal Imaging, University of Pittsburgh Medical Center, University of Pittsburgh Hospital, Pittsburgh, Pennsylvania

MARY ANN TURNER, MD
Professor, Department of Radiology, Virginia Commonwealth University School of Medicine; Director, Gastrointestinal Radiology, Virginia Commonwealth University Medical Center, Richmond, Virginia

SEAN M. TUTTON, MD, FSIR
Associate Professor, Department of Radiology, Medical College of Wisconsin, Milwaukee, Wisconsin

ROBERT L. VOGELZANG, MD
Professor, Department of Radiology, Northwestern University Feinberg School of Medicine; Chief of Interventional Radiology, Department of Radiology, Northwestern Memorial Hospital, Chicago, Illinois

PATRICK M. VOS, MD
Clinical Instructor, Department of Radiology, University of British Columbia Faculty of Medicine; Hospital Staff, Department of Radiology, St. Paul's Hospital, Vancouver, British Columbia, Canada

DAPHNA WEINSTEIN, MD
Surgeon, Surgery B, Assaf-Harofeh Medical Center, Zrifin, Ramat-Hasharon, Israel

NOEL N. WILLIAMS, MD
Director, Bariatric Surgery Program, Department of Gastrointestinal Surgery, Hospital of the University of Pennsylvania, Philadelphia, Pennsylvania

STEPHANIE R. WILSON, MD
Department of Diagnostic Imaging, Foothills Medical Center; Professor of Radiology, University of Calgary, Calgary, Alberta, Canada. *Formerly*: Professor of Diagnostic Imaging, University of Toronto; Head, Section of Ultrasound, Department of Medical Imaging, Toronto General Hospital, Toronto, Ontario, Canada

ELLEN L. WOLF, MD
Professor of Clinical Radiology, Albert Einstein College of Medicine; Chief of Gastrointestinal Radiology, Department of Radiology, Montefiore Medical Center, Bronx, New York

VAHID YAGHMAI, MD, MS
Associate Professor, Department of Radiology, Northwestern University Feinberg School of Medicine; Medical Director of CT, Department of Radiology, Northwestern Memorial Hospital, Chicago, Illinois

SILAJA YITTA, MD
Resident, Department of Radiology, New York University Medical Center, New York, New York

RIVKA ZISSIN, MD
Senior Lecturer, Department of Radiology, Sackler Faculty of Medicine, Tel Aviv University, Tel Aviv; Head, CT Unit, Department of Diagnostic Imaging, Meir Medical Center, Kochav Yair, Israel

Preface

Since the publication in 1994 of the first edition of *Textbook of Gastrointestinal Radiology*, much has changed in our discipline. Technological advances have dramatically improved the capabilities of computed tomography (CT), magnetic resonance imaging (MRI), ultrasonography, fluoroscopy, and positron emission tomography (PET) for abdominal and pelvic imaging. CT has evolved from a single-detector row to multidetector rows that permit isotropic volumetric imaging, greatly expanding the clinical utility of this imaging technique. Multidetector CT has become the gold standard for evaluating the acute abdomen, as well as most abdominal and pelvic infectious, inflammatory, neoplastic, ischemic, vascular, and hemorrhagic disorders. CT colonography, CT enterography, and CT enteroclysis are now well-established methods for evaluating the colon and small bowel. CT angiography and venography are currently the preferred means for noninvasively evaluating the splanchnic circulation.

Innovations in software and hardware technology, such as faster pulse sequences, the development of parallel imaging, and improved coil design, have encouraged the growth of MRI. Magnetic resonance cholangiopancreatography (MRCP) has largely replaced diagnostic endoscopic retrograde cholangiopancreatography (ERCP), and at many institutions, MRI also has been increasingly performed as the primary staging examination for hepatic and pancreatic malignancies. MR angiography and venography also are widely used to assess the patency of abdominal and pelvic blood vessels, as well as for tumor invasion of these vessels.

The usefulness of abdominal ultrasound examination has been enhanced by the increasing application of color and power Doppler techniques and harmonic imaging, improvements in high-resolution transducers with greater fields of view, and identification of wider indications for the use of ultrasound contrast agents.

Digital radiography and digital fluoroscopy have dramatically altered the practice of gastrointestinal fluoroscopic procedures and barium studies, and the dissemination of picture archiving and communication systems (PACS) in most radiologic departments has transformed the abdominal radiologist's workday.

PET/CT has emerged as one of the most exciting applications of new technology in gastrointestinal radiology. Both functional and anatomic data can now be provided in a single image. This technique has gained wide acceptance for the initial staging and follow-up evaluation of primary colorectal and esophageal neoplasms and for the detection of lymph node and hepatic malignancies from other primary tumors.

To keep pace with these technological and scientific advances, every chapter of the third edition has been updated and revised. In addition, several chapters have been added (and a few were deleted), and nearly one third of the chapters have new authors to provide their topics with fresh insight and perspective.

Throughout this new edition, we have taken great care to maintain the fundamental goals of the first two editions for providing complete and up-to-date coverage of the state of the art in gastrointestinal radiology in a practical and usable form. As in the first two editions, our basic organizing principle is the integration of rapidly changing information, common sense, and good judgment in an orderly and useful approach for radiologic diagnosis and treatment. To this end, the text contains sections on general radiologic principles for evaluating the hollow viscera and solid organs and for performing and applying specific imaging and therapeutic techniques. Other sections present the clinical, radiologic, and pathologic aspects of disease in the various gastrointestinal organs. The chapters in these sections are designed to illustrate and integrate the spectrum of abnormalities seen with all diagnostic modalities available to the radiologist, including conventional radiography, barium studies, cholangiography, multidetector CT, ultrasonography, MRI, PET, PET/CT, and angiography. To make the book even more user friendly, the contributing authors have worked diligently—as have we—to eliminate redundancies and produce a shorter, more compact text. With the addition of color graphics and images, the book's format has been redesigned to facilitate reading and review.

Once again, we have been able to assemble an outstanding group of internationally recognized and renowned authors for the third edition. Their time, effort, cooperation, and expertise are greatly appreciated. As editors, we have tried to strike a balance between uniformity of style and individuality of author contributions, so that each contributor is able to speak in his or her own unique voice.

We hope that the collective efforts of the authors of the 130 chapters, as well as our own, have accomplished our goal of providing students and practitioners of gastrointestinal radiology with a valuable educational resource that is clear, interesting, and enjoyable to read.

Richard M. Gore, MD
Marc S. Levine, MD

Contents

VOLUME 1

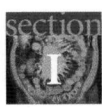

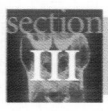

Pharynx   STEPHEN E. RUBESIN, SECTION EDITOR

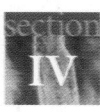

Esophagus

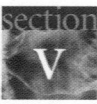

Stomach and Duodenum

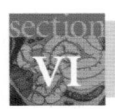

Small Bowel   STEPHEN E. RUBESIN, SECTION EDITOR

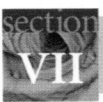

Colon

VOLUME 2

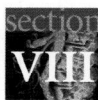

General Radiologic Principles for Imaging and Intervention of the Solid Viscera

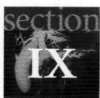

Gallbladder and Biliary Tract

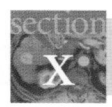

Liver

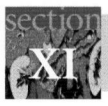

Pancreas

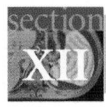

Spleen

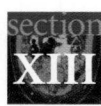

XIII   Peritoneal Cavity

XIV   Pediatric Disease

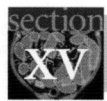

Common Clinical Problems

DVD Contents

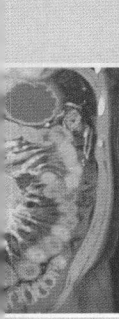

General Radiologic Principles

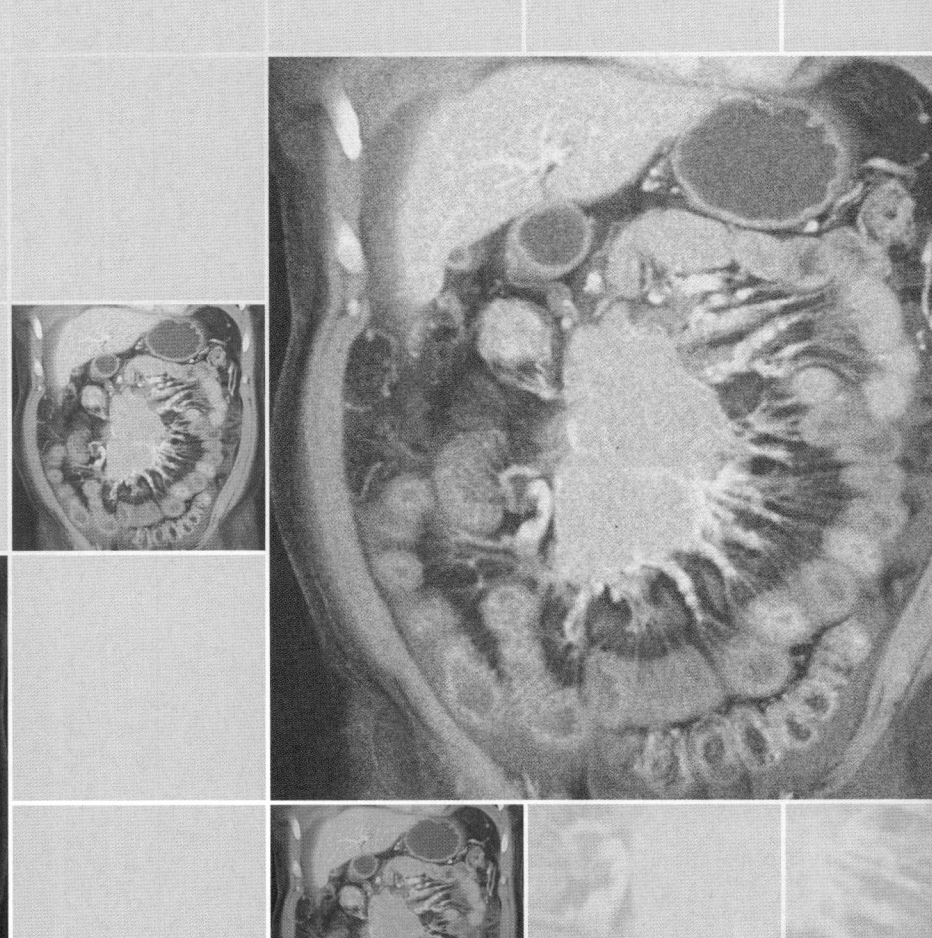

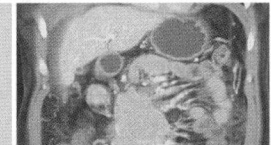

Imaging Contrast Agents

Jovitas Skucas, MD

Contrast agents used for medical imaging can be classified into four groups: (1) intravascular contrast agents for CT and angiography; (2) intraluminal agents for gastrointestinal tract studies; (3) contrast agents for cholangiography; and (4) contrast agents for MRI. These various types of contrast agents are discussed separately in the following sections.

INTRAVASCULAR CONTRAST AGENTS

Iodinated Water-Soluble Contrast Agents

Basic Properties

All current intravascular contrast agents (except contrast agents for MRI) utilize iodine for x-ray absorption. Sodium iodide would be an ideal contrast agent, but its toxicity and iodism preclude its use. The development of complex delivery molecules represents an attempt to deliver the greatest iodine concentration to blood vessels or other structures with the least possible toxicity. Water-soluble intravascular contrast agents can be classified into three groups: (1) ionic, high-osmolality agents, which have five times the osmolality of blood; (2) nonionic, low-osmolality agents, which have about twice the osmolality of blood; and (3) isotonic agents, which are nonionic dimers. Basic structures and physicochemical characteristics of available contrast agents are not covered here but are discussed in other publications.[1,2]

At the x-ray energies used for CT, the mass attenuation coefficient for iodine is considerably greater than that of the surrounding soft tissues and blood. After intravascular injection of iodinated contrast agents, initial CT images reveal aortic and major arterial enhancement, followed by a capillary or parenchymal "blush" and eventual venous opacification. The rate of injection of contrast agents and the timing of subsequent CT scans determine which structures enhance on individual images. Multidetector-row CT (MDCT) scanners require faster injection rates than earlier CT scanners because of shorter scanning times. As a result, faster injection rates of more concentrated contrast agents are necessary and viscosity achieves a more dominant role. Various techniques of intravascular contrast agent administration are discussed elsewhere in the text.

Ionic Contrast Agents

Acetylation of aminotriiodobenzoic acid and other structural changes led to the development of ionic contrast agents. These agents are formulated as salts, consisting of a cation and an anion. Two commonly used cations are sodium and meglumine. The anion portion of the molecule consists of a benzene ring containing iodine substituted at positions 2, 4, and 6 and a number of other side chains. These side chains determine water solubility and indirectly affect toxicity. The benzene ring can be viewed as a scaffold for attaching iodine and side chains.

When the molecule dissociates, three iodine atoms are available for every two particles in solution, for a ratio of 1.5:1.

Further refinements of ionic contrast media include attachment of two monomer triiodinated benzene rings at one of the side groups. Such a dimer, containing two benzene rings, each with three iodine atoms and one cation particle, has six iodine atoms per two particles, for a ratio of 3:1.

Ionic contrast agents are hypertonic at the concentrations used for vascular opacification; considerable effort has therefore been spent in an attempt to decrease their osmolality. In general, the viscosity of the sodium salt is less than that of the corresponding meglumine salt but the sodium salt tends to be more toxic. Toxicity and viscosity limitations encountered during intra-arterial injections of these contrast agents are not as relevant for the intravenous injections used with CT.

Nonionic Contrast Agents

If the carboxyl group in position 1 on the benzene ring is replaced with a stable side group, the molecule no longer dissociates in solution, so that each particle in solution has three iodine atoms, or a ratio of 3:1. A dimer structure can also be achieved by linking two triiodobenzoic acid molecules (ioxaglic acid), formulated as a meglumine-sodium salt, another contrast agent with a ratio of 3:1. A contrast agent (iodixanol) with a ratio of 6:1 has also been developed and is often called iso-osmolar.

Various manufacturers have taken different approaches to the type of side chains used with both ionic and nonionic contrast agents. As a result, these compounds differ in their viscosities and other properties. The interaction with other molecules also differs between ionic and nonionic agents and is affected by the type of side branches present. Within limits for each group of contrast agents, however, viscosity varies directly with iodine concentration.

Commercial contrast agents also contain chelating agents (most often calcium edetate disodium) to chelate impurities and buffering agents to achieve an acceptable pH. Their action is more important during manufacture of these contrast agents than during their clinical use.

The American College of Radiology has published criteria for clinical scenarios in which nonionic contrast agents are preferred,[3] although this issue is not relevant for many practices in which nonionic contrast agents are used almost exclusively. The nonionic agents also are associated with less patient discomfort and thus result in less motion artifact, an evident advantage, especially with complex examinations such as three-dimensional reconstruction.

Pharmacokinetics

After bolus intravascular injection, initial plasma iodine concentration is determined by the iodine concentration and volume of the administered contrast agent. Both ionic and nonionic contrast agents are eventually distributed throughout the extravascular, extracellular space; intravascular and extravascular equilibrium is achieved within 10 minutes after intravascular injection. These contrast agents are excreted primarily by renal glomerular filtration. After injection, relative plasma iodine concentration in a particular vessel depends on dilution by blood, extravascular diffusion, and renal excretion; the first factor is most important during arterial

and venous phase imaging, with extravascular diffusion playing a larger role during parenchymal phase imaging. In theory, a contrast agent can be designed to have fast or slow extravascular diffusion and rapid or slow renal clearance; an ideal blood pool agent should have slow extravascular diffusion. In practice, nonionic contrast agents achieve greater initial peak vascular enhancement than ionic agents of equivalent iodine dose but subsequent blood iodine concentrations and parenchymal opacification are similar for the two types of agents (except renal visualization). Both ionic and nonionic agents have similar extravascular diffusion rates. It is only in the design of contrast agents for MRI that considerable variation in diffusion and renal clearance is achieved, thus leading to a specific contrast agent for a specific application. Extensive literature is available on relative time-dependent blood iodine concentrations and renal excretion of various contrast agents.

Dynamic CT after single-bolus injection of contrast agents relies on enhancement of vascular structures above baseline. Correct arterial phase timing is obtained either by the use of an initial test dose or automatic bolus tracking. One milligram of iodine per gram of tissue corresponds to an increase of 30 Hounsfield units (HU), which is about the limit for detection. In general, it is desirable to have a sufficient iodine concentration in the vascular structures of interest to elevate these structures up to 100 HU above baseline. With such enhancement, major vessel thrombi are detected and vascular fistulas and related conditions can be evaluated. Whether early dynamic scanning (arterial phase) is superior to portal venous phase or even delayed scanning after contrast equilibration depends on the organ in question and the information being sought. For the liver, these arterial and portal phase time windows are roughly 20 to 30 seconds. Such short time intervals are readily achieved with MDCT.

A typical CT examination consists of a precontrast scan, followed by scanning after the initial bolus reaches the structure of interest. A relatively large-caliber venous catheter and a power injector provide reproducible injection rates, recognizing that prediction of bolus arrival is somewhat empirical because other factors, such as decreased cardiac output, can prolong vascular flow times.

Intravascular contrast agents cross the placenta, are excreted in breast milk, and affect fetal and infant thyroid function. If feasible, alternate studies should therefore be considered during pregnancy. Breast feeding should be stopped for 1 to 2 days after contrast agent injection.

Acute Adverse Reactions

Only a brief summary of contrast reactions and their therapy is provided here. More detailed information is available from publications by the American College of Radiology and European Society of Urogenital Radiology.[3,4]

Iodinated contrast agents are contraindicated in patients with hyperthyroidism. Also, iodinated contrast agents should be avoided for 2 months before thyroid isotope imaging or radioactive thyroid therapy.[4]

Types of Reactions

Acute reactions vary from minor effects to severe or life-threatening. Sensations of warmth, nausea, and vomiting appear to be a direct side effect of these agents. Mild changes in blood pressure or mild wheezing may be self limited or may progress to more severe reactions. An arbitrary but useful grading of contrast reactions includes mild, moderate, severe, and fatal. Compilations of reactions to ionic contrast agents from the 1970s and 1980s found the risk of severe reactions to be 1 in 1000 to 1 in 4000 across the studies. The types of reactions are similar with ionic and nonionic contrast agents. In general, the risk of adverse reactions is directly related to contrast osmolality, so that fewer reactions occur with nonionic agents than with ionic agents. Although the risk of severe adverse reactions is lower with nonionic contrast agents,[5] deaths have occurred with both ionic and nonionic agents.

Urticaria and other more severe contrast reactions do not represent classic antigen-antibody reactions but are secondary to histamine or serotonin release induced directly by the contrast agent. Contrast agents may also activate the complement system, which acts as a host defense and is related to coagulation abnormalities and bradykinin release. Overall, only a minority of unpredictable reactions mimic IgE hypersensitivity and are probably secondary to an antigen-antibody reaction.

Some reactions are disease specific. In the presence of a pheochromocytoma, intravenous contrast agents may cause massive release of catecholamines and acute hypertension. The sudden onset of such hypertension should suggest an underlying pheochromocytoma.

Over a prolonged period of time, bottled hyperosmolar contrast agents can leach allergens from rubber stoppers. As a rule, contrast-containing vials and bottles should be stored in an upright position.

Premedication

The specific allergen responsible for sensitization to iodinated contrast agents is unknown. It is difficult to prove that iodine is indeed responsible for hypersensitive contrast reactions, a common assumption. A myosin protein rather than iodine is believed to be the allergen responsible for such reactions in shellfish. Rather than asking about iodine allergies, a more appropriate question appears to be whether drug allergies are present. In many patients, the specific cause of an adverse reaction is not sought, and the reaction is simply labeled as *allergic, hypersensitive,* or *anaphylactic.*

There are no reliable blood tests that detect those patients who are allergic to contrast media. Risk factors associated with a high frequency of contrast reactions include asthma and a history of prior reactions to contrast agents. Yet even these are unpredictable and a patient manifesting a severe reaction may have had prior intravascular contrast with no adverse reaction. Although patients with urticaria-like reactions have increased plasma levels of prekallikrein and α_2-macroglobulin and lower levels of C1-esterase inhibitor, the predictive value of these findings is limited because of normal variation.[6] Pretesting with a small dose of contrast agent was in vogue several decades ago but has been abandoned because these tests have little or no clinical value. Acute reactions can develop even after intravenous administration of less than 1 mL of these contrast agents.

In a multi-institutional study involving ionic contrast agents, pretreatment with 32 mg of methylprednisolone 12 hours and 2 hours before administration of the contrast agent significantly decreased the frequency of adverse reactions.[7]

With this two-dose regimen of corticosteroids, the number of adverse reactions in patients receiving ionic contrast agents was comparable to that with nonionic agents and no pretreatment. Premedication should also be considered for patients who have had previous reactions to these contrast agents. At our institution, we currently recommend that patients who have had clinically significant reactions to intravenous contrast agents in the past receive pretreatment with the following regimen: (1) 50 mg of oral prednisone every 12 hours for a total of three doses, with the last dose given approximately 1 hour before the examination; and (2) 25 to 50 mg of oral diphenhydramine (Benadryl) 2 hours before the examination.

The prevalence of seizures after intravenous administration of water-soluble contrast agents is higher in patients with brain metastases, possibly because the capillaries in brain metastases do not exhibit normal blood-brain barrier integrity and are permeable to these agents. It has therefore been suggested that these patients be premedicated with 5 mg of intravenous diazepam before contrast administration to decrease the risk of seizures.[8]

Treatment of Reactions

Any physician injecting a contrast agent intravascularly can expect to encounter a broad spectrum of reactions (ranging from mild to severe) and must be prepared to deal with these reactions. In general, mild reactions such as flushing or urticaria require no treatment, and most of these reactions resolve spontaneously. Similarly, nausea and vomiting require only general support and observation. If symptoms occur before all the contrast agent has been administered, either the rate of injection should be slowed or the injection postponed until the symptoms have resolved.

Early intravenous access should be established. The catheter used for contrast injection should be kept in place, ensuring intravascular access until the possibility of a reaction has passed. With progressive hypotension, it may also become increasingly difficult to cannulate a peripheral vein.

Moderate urticaria developing in the absence of other significant symptoms can be treated with 25 to 50 mg of diphenhydramine, given orally or injected. With more severe urticaria, it may be appropriate to administer a histamine receptor antagonist such as cimetidine (Tagamet) (300 mg injected slowly [diluted] intravenously). For severe urticaria, epinephrine (0.1 to 0.3 mL [1:1000]) should be given subcutaneously, unless contraindicated. If needed, the dose can be repeated in 15 minutes. Epinephrine should be used with caution in elderly patients who have underlying cardiovascular disease; electrocardiographic monitoring should be considered for these patients.

Severe reactions such as severe bronchospasm, convulsions, or significant cardiopulmonary reactions require prompt and vigorous therapy. Bronchospasm and laryngeal edema generally respond to subcutaneous epinephrine. If needed, the epinephrine dose can be repeated. Diphenhydramine and corticosteroids, such as hydrocortisone, 100 to 300 mg intravenously, are also often employed. Oxygen should be administered by mask or nasal cannula. β-Agonist inhalers alone may be successful in patients with mild bronchospasm or can be used in conjunction with aminophylline therapy. With refractory bronchospasm, aminophylline (250 to 400 mg diluted in dextrose and water) can be administered intravenously over a 10- to 20-minute period. Aminophylline should be used with caution because it may exacerbate coexisting hypotension. Tracheal intubation should be considered early in the course of these symptoms, because later, severe laryngeal edema may make intubation difficult, if not impossible.

Because therapy of hypotension in settings of tachycardia and bradycardia is different, the pulse rate should be monitored. A pulse may not be palpable in a hypotensive patient; cardiac auscultation or electrocardiographic monitoring may be necessary.

Hypotension in the absence of other major signs of an anaphylactic reaction should initially be treated with oxygen, leg elevation, and rapid administration of intravenous fluids. Epinephrine should be considered, recognizing that fluid therapy alone is often sufficient and avoids potential cardiac complications of epinephrine. Although subcutaneous epinephrine injections are adequate for mild-to-moderate reactions, intravenous administration is needed for moderate-to-severe hypotension. For intravenous administration, epinephrine should be diluted to 1:10,000, and 1.0 to 3.0 mL should be administered slowly. The dose can be repeated in 15 minutes. The rate of injection can also be titrated to achieve a desired result. A vasopressor agent such as dopamine, 2 to 5 µg/kg/min, can be added to sustain blood pressure. For unresponsive hypotension, other agents are available for treatment of underlying shock. A histamine receptor antagonist such as cimetidine (300 mg in dextrose and water infused slowly) can be added. Diphenhydramine (25 to 50 mg) can also be injected intravenously. Corticosteroids are also often employed, with a typical dose of hydrocortisone being 500 mg intravenously. Corticosteroids probably have no immediate effect on a reaction; their main use is to decrease delayed reactions.

It has been proposed that severe hypotension can be corrected with vigorous hydration alone.[9] Such therapy avoids complications encountered with epinephrine. On the other hand, overhydration of patients with possible underlying cardiovascular and renal disease also carries a risk. Thus, initiation of therapy by adequate hydration may be reasonable, but appropriate pharmacologic therapy should be instituted without delay.[10]

Hypotension in the presence of bradycardia should suggest a vasovagal reaction. Some patients respond to being placed in a Trendelenburg position. Hypotension in these patients should be treated with rapid intravenous infusion of isotonic saline. Oxygen should also be administered. Bradycardia can be treated with atropine (0.5 to 1.0 mg intravenously), with the dose repeated every 5 minutes to a maximal total dose of 3.0 mg.

Some patients are receiving long-term therapy with β-blocking agents such as propranolol. A contrast reaction in these patients can be confusing because even in a setting of anaphylactic shock, β-blocker–induced bradycardia can persist. Intravenous glucagon (1.0 mg or more) may be useful for treating this bradycardia.[11] Dopamine is also effective. The usual doses of epinephrine employed may not be effective in reversing such hypotension.

Emergency cardiopulmonary resuscitation is necessary for cardiovascular collapse. Refractory seizures are treated with intravenous diazepam, phenobarbital, or both.

Contrast extravasation is treated by extremity elevation, warm or cold compresses, and, if extensive, a plastic surgery consultation. Injection of hyaluronidase (an enzyme that breaks down interstitial barriers) into the extravasation site is advocated by some investigators,[12] but its impact on tissue healing is uncertain.

The previous outline is meant only to be a general guide for treatment. All reactions should be individualized. The suggested doses are those for an average-sized adult.

Contrast-Induced Renal Failure

The pathogenesis of contrast-induced nephrotoxicity is incompletely understood, but a number of intrinsic renal events lead to renal medullary ischemia, often exacerbated by a reduced intravascular volume.[13] Direct cytotoxicity, oxidative tissue damage, and apoptosis are thought to be contributing factors. Nephrotoxicity manifests as a *significant* rise in serum creatinine from baseline. Various authors have different definitions of *significant*, with the European Society of Urogenital Radiology Guidelines using a creatinine rise of more than 25% or 44 µmol/L (0.5 mg/dL) within 3 days.[4] A transient nonoliguric decrease in renal function lasting up to 2 weeks is more common than the more ominous oliguric manifestation of nephrotoxicity requiring hemodialysis.

Risk factors include preexisting renal insufficiency, diabetes, dehydration, cardiovascular disease, advanced age, myeloma, hypertension, and hyperuricemia. Patients at greatest risk for developing acute renal failure are diabetics with preexisting renal insufficiency. Caution is also necessary in patients receiving treatment with drugs causing nephrotoxicity, including nonsteroidal anti-inflammatory agents, aminoglycosides, cyclosporine, and sulfonamides.

In diabetics with underlying cardiovascular or renal insufficiency, metformin (Glucophage), a biguanide antihyperglycemic agent, is associated with lactic acidosis and resultant high mortality after intravenous contrast administration. This association appears to be indirect and is probably related to underlying renal insufficiency, but enough patients taking metformin and receiving intravenous contrast have developed lactic acidosis to prompt the U.S. Food and Drug Administration to issue a warning that metformin should be discontinued for 48 hours after intravenous contrast administration and reinstated only if renal function remains normal. Adequate hydration should be maintained.

Because iodinated contrast agents are not protein bound (except for cholangiographic agents), they are dialyzable. In patients on hemodialysis, additional hemodialysis sessions therefore are generally unnecessary.

The most important preventive measure is to ensure that the patient is well hydrated. If intravenous hydration is necessary, there is evidence suggesting that the use of sodium bicarbonate hydration is superior to sodium chloride.[14] Other guidelines include the use of a low-osmolar contrast agent, the withholding of nephrotoxic drugs for at least 24 hours, and the use of alternate imaging techniques in high-risk patients. The osmotic diuretic mannitol does not provide any benefit; in fact, the loop diuretic furosemide exacerbates renal dysfunction.[3] Currently, it is probably safe to assume that diuretics do not offer any protective effect; anecdotal evidence even suggests that diuretics should be stopped before performing a contrast study.[15]

Several studies suggest that N-acetylcysteine (an antioxidant given orally) decreases the risk of contrast-induced renal toxicity,[16,17] although others have questioned the renal benefit of this agent.[18] Many studies have involved coronary angiography and differ in methodology from contrast CT or have included critically ill patients. In either case, a number of institutions have adopted the use of prophylactic *N*-acetylcysteine. The role for theophylline is less well established.

Hemodialysis after intravenous contrast administration in patients with preexisting renal failure is not thought to be warranted. On the other hand, hemofiltration has resulted in a smaller rise in creatinine in patients with chronic renal failure than in controls.[19] The complexity and cost of hemofiltration limit its use to select patients.

Iodinated Oil

Intra-arterial iodized poppy seed oil (Ethiodol or Lipiodol) is used as a CT diagnostic agent for detection of liver tumors, especially hepatocellular carcinoma. Often used as a gold standard, it detects more tumors than other imaging modalities. Nevertheless, study of explanted livers reveals that pretransplantation iodized oil CT tumor sensitivity is still rather low. Also, one should keep in mind that iodized oil is retained by some benign tumors, even hemangiomas. Ethiodol is also a chemoembolization ingredient injected into tumor-feeding arteries. It acts as a chemotherapeutic agent carrier and, because of its high viscosity, is a temporary embolizing material that prolongs contact between the chemotherapeutic agent and the tumor. Because Ethiodol remains within areas of tumor neovascularity much longer than in normal liver parenchyma, it also acts as a tumor marker. Occasionally, Ethiodol is injected during percutaneous radiofrequency ablation of hepatocellular carcinomas[20] because it aids in CT delineation of the extent of coagulation necrosis. Despite its many uses, intra-arterial iodized oil is considerably more popular in the Far East than in the West.

Other Contrast Agents

Several reports describe the use of gadolinium-based contrast agents for CT in patients with renal insufficiency or prior severe reactions to iodinated contrast agents. Gadopentetate dimeglumine (Gd-DTPA) containing only one gadolinium ion has pharmacokinetic properties similar to those of iodinated agents containing three to six iodine atoms. Nevertheless, the toxicity of gadolinium agents (at doses achieving equivalent x-ray stopping power) is greater than that of nonionic iodinated agents.[21] This is in contrast to the lower gadolinium doses used for MRI, which are insufficient for useful x-ray contrast but have negligible nephrotoxicity.[3] The European Society of Urogenital Radiology takes the position that gadolinium-based contrast agents are more nephrotoxic than iodinated contrast agents in equivalent x-ray attenuation doses.[4]

Carbon dioxide is a viable angiographic contrast agent for certain digital vascular indications in the abdomen. It has also been used to guide vascular interventional procedures. Carbon dioxide displaces blood, forms a gaseous column, and is cleared by the lungs.

Apart from MRI, viable abdominal reticuloendothelial contrast agents have eluded clinical development. The first such agent, thorium dioxide (Thorotrast), which was used until the 1950s, has left a painful and tragic legacy. Iodinated oily emulsions accumulate in the liver, spleen, bone marrow, and, to a lesser degree, other organs long enough to permit CT, but these agents have been abandoned because of their high

toxicity and low specificity. Colloidal iodine or emulsified perfluorocytlbromide particles are also incorporated in reticuloendothelial cells, but the latter agent has lost favor since the 1980s.

Liposomes are taken up by the reticuloendothelial system, and considerable effort has been devoted to encapsulating water-soluble iodinated contrast agents inside liposomes. Research activity peaked in the 1990s, but despite occasional more recent papers, pronounced adverse reactions limit the use of liposomal CT contrast agents. Most current reticuloendothelial contrast research has focused on agents used in MRI (see later discussion in this chapter).

CONTRAST AGENTS FOR GASTROINTESTINAL STUDIES

Barium Sulfate

Physical Characteristics

Barium sulfate is a white crystalline powder with a molecular weight of 233 daltons. Because of its high specific gravity (4.5), patients tend to comment that a cup of barium is inordinately "heavy." The terms *thick* and *thin* should be used only when referring to viscosity and not to signify radiodensity, which results from many factors.

Although barium sulfate itself is inert and does not support bacterial growth, some additives are organic. When a container is opened or reconstituted with tap water, the suspension should be refrigerated if it is to be kept overnight. Although many commercial formulations contain preservatives, bacterial contamination can and does occur.

Certain commercial formulations are advertised as being applicable throughout the gastrointestinal tract. Invariably they represent a compromise. The gastrointestinal tract varies in pH, composition of mucus, and type of mucosa, and optimal coating in one part does not mean that a similar coating can be expected in another. Coating the mucosa with barium or simply opacifying the lumen requires different barium formulations.[22] The large-particle, high-density barium suspensions designed for double-contrast use should not simply be diluted and used for single-contrast studies. Ingesting such a diluted suspension causes rapid sedimentation of barium particles, with the nondependent lumen containing little barium; lesions here can be missed. Products designed primarily for single-contrast examinations, on the other hand, can be diluted considerably before any settling occurs mainly because they contain relatively small size barium particles.

Pharyngography

Pharyngeal radiography was already established in the 1960s when cineradiography became popular for evaluating patients with dysphagia. Although conventional or digital radiography produces high anatomic resolution, dynamic swallowing is best assessed either with videofluoroscopy or cineradiography. Such a pharyngogram (commonly called a modified barium swallow) permits evaluation of both oropharyngeal anatomy and function using contrast agents of varying consistencies.

After patients have suffered strokes, the risk of aspiration during feeding can be assessed on pharyngography by using barium suspensions and barium-coated food items of varying density and viscosity. Contrast consistencies for these examinations can range from barium-coated crackers to a viscosity approaching that of water. To improve patient acceptance of this procedure, investigators have developed their own contrast agents, including a honey-thick barium and a barium pudding.[23] Anatomic detail is best evaluated with high-density barium products such as the 250% w/v suspensions designed for double-contrast upper gastrointestinal tract examinations. Fistulas are also best evaluated with these high-density barium suspensions. A barium paste can also be used to study anatomy, but the high viscosity of the paste limits its application in the detection of fistulas. The volume of barium used for pharyngography should be individualized. In patients with suspected aspiration, for example, a small barium bolus of only several milliliters is initially swallowed; if no aspiration is detected, the bolus size is gradually increased.

Because the oropharynx handles high- and low-viscosity liquids differently, pharyngeal function should be evaluated with both high- and low-viscosity barium suspensions.[24] The low-viscosity suspension should have a viscosity approaching that of water, while the high-viscosity suspension should have a viscosity similar to that of a thick milkshake. It should be emphasized that some high-density barium products for double-contrast examinations are relatively fluid and therefore cannot be used as high-viscosity preparations.

Upper Gastrointestinal Tract Radiography

A complete examination of the esophagus consists of single-contrast, double-contrast, and mucosal relief views as well as fluoroscopic evaluation of motility. Normal esophageal tonicity causes the lumen to collapse after a primary peristaltic wave has passed. The study should therefore be performed with reasonable dispatch, regardless of the technique used. Previous reports have suggested that a cold barium suspension or an acidified suspension may be useful for reproducing symptoms in some patients,[25] but acidified bariums are rarely employed.

Sufficient air is introduced into the esophagus for a double-contrast study in some patients with poor esophageal motility or those with gastroesophageal reflux. In most patients, however, an additional negative contrast agent (a gas-producing tablet or powder or liquid effervescent agent) is required to obtain adequate distention of the esophagus and stomach for double-contrast views of these structures. These effervescent agents contain sodium bicarbonate and an acid (usually tartaric acid or citric acid), which form carbon dioxide gas in the presence of a liquid. About 400 to 500 mL of gas is necessary to achieve adequate esophageal and gastric distention. One technique is to have the patient drink first one and then another liquid effervescent solution, followed immediately by 60 to 120 mL of the barium suspension. The two effervescent agents distend the esophagus by releasing carbon dioxide, and barium then coats the esophageal mucosa.

The high-density, low-viscosity barium products designed for the stomach and duodenum also coat the esophagus well. Visualization of the esophagus is impaired, however, if the barium is ingested before the effervescent agents. Conversely, the quality of mucosal coating in the stomach is improved if the barium suspension is given first. The sequence of ingestion should therefore be tailored to the patient's symptoms:

if esophageal disease is suspected, the effervescent agents are given first, but if gastroduodenal disease is suspected, the barium suspension is given first.

Esophageal varices tend to be more prominent and are easier to detect if the esophageal lumen is collapsed. Although high-density, low-viscosity barium products can demonstrate large esophageal varices, commercially available barium pastes are the product of choice. Some pastes are so viscous that they tend to flow in a coherent bolus; these pastes should be diluted with water until the viscosity is similar to that of honey.

In patients with acute dysphagia caused by an acute esophageal food impaction, an esophagogram can be therapeutic. With the patient upright, the weight of the barium column can dislodge impacted food in the esophagus, so that it passes into the stomach. In such patients, effervescent agents may also be used to increase intraluminal esophageal pressure and facilitate passage of the impacted food into the stomach. Nevertheless, these techniques should be performed with care to avoid esophageal perforation. Glucagon has also been proposed to help relieve spasm,[26] although it is not clear whether pharmacoradiology has a significant role in acute dysphagia.

Commercial barium sulfate tablets with a diameter of 12.5 mm are useful for the evaluation of subtle esophageal strictures. The patient should swallow these tablets with the table at least in a 45-degree upright position, and 60 mL or more of water should be ingested with the tablets.[27] Normal tablet transit time through the esophagus is less than 20 seconds. These tablets contain 650 mg of barium sulfate plus additives and dissolve either in the esophagus or in the stomach (Fig. 1-1). Relatively fresh tablets should be used, because older tablets take longer to dissolve.[28] Some investigators have even proposed that barium tablets be administered on a routine basis during chest radiography, because retention of tablets in the esophagus on chest radiographs may indicate the presence of structural or functional abnormalities in the esophagus.[29]

In patients with suspected esophageal perforation, evaluation of the esophagus with a water-soluble contrast agent may fail to detect subtle extravasation from the esophagus. It is therefore recommended that the examination immediately be repeated with a higher density barium suspension to allow visualization of more subtle leaks that could be missed with the water-soluble contrast agent.[30] When a leak is present, residual barium in the mediastinum does not result in clinically detectable mediastinitis and does not interfere with subsequent radiographic evaluation.[31]

High-density, low-viscosity barium preparations specifically designed for the upper gastrointestinal tract produce the best double-contrast results. A volume of 60 to 120 mL of a 250% w/v suspension is generally sufficient. A good barium formulation should result in routine visualization of the areae gastricae in the stomach. Small cancers, ulcers, gastritis, and duodenitis should also be readily detectable on a high-quality double-contrast examination.

After appropriate double contrast gastric views have been obtained, a lower density barium suspension is ingested for subsequent single-contrast evaluation. For this part of the examination, barium suspensions varying from 35% to 80% w/v are used. Various external compression paddles are available and are helpful for obtaining mucosal relief views of the stomach and duodenum.

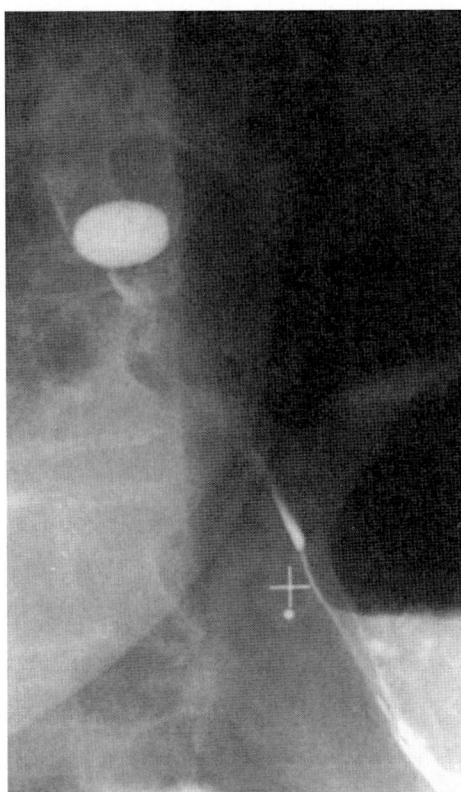

Figure 1-1. Barium sulfate tablet proximal to a stricture. A previous esophagogram suggested narrowing at this site, and the tablet confirms this finding. (From Schabel SI, Skucas J: Esophageal obstruction following administration of "aged" barium sulfate tablets—a warning. Radiology 122:835-836, 1977.)

Small Bowel Studies

A number of techniques have been developed to evaluate the small bowel, including conventional antegrade examinations, enteroclysis, retrograde ileography, peroral pneumocolon and, most recently, abdominal CT. The type of examination that should be performed depends on the clinical indication. Specific contrast agents have been developed for each type of study.

An antegrade examination (small bowel series) is the simplest and traditional way of studying the small bowel. Serial radiographs of the small bowel are taken with manual palpation after the patient ingests the barium suspension. An appropriate barium should not flocculate or precipitate during transit through the small intestine. A 40% to 60% w/v barium suspension is typically employed; a total volume of 500 to 800 mL of barium is usually ingested for this examination. This barium does not coat the mucosa; visualization instead is obtained primarily by filling of the lumen with the barium suspension.

Contraindications to an antegrade small bowel barium study include suspected colonic obstruction or bowel perforation. Small bowel obstruction is not a contraindication, however, because barium proximal to the obstruction remains in suspension and barium inspissation does not occur. With small bowel obstruction, an antegrade study with barium

therefore poses no risk to the patient and can not only detect the site of obstruction but also suggest an etiology.

With enteroclysis (small bowel enema), the contrast agent is injected through steerable catheters directly into the small bowel, bypassing the flow-limiting function of the pylorus. The barium suspension can be infused by gravity, hand-held syringes, or an infusion pump. Typical infusion rates range from 75 to 100 mL/min, but flow rates should be individualized for each patient. Infusion rates that are too low may permit excessive small bowel peristalsis, while infusion rates that are too high may cause overdistention, resulting in atonia with inadequate progression of barium through the small bowel.

It is debatable whether single-contrast or double-contrast enteroclysis yields better results.[32,33] For the double-contrast portion of the examination, most American investigators advocate a 0.5% or greater solution of methylcellulose in water. Methylcellulose helps propel the barium suspension ahead of it. Alternatively, water can be used as the second contrast agent, but water tends to wash off barium adhering to the mucosa. The total volume of the two contrast agents is tailored for each examination; up to 2 L may be required. The contrast agents are instilled until a lesion is detected or contrast material reaches the right colon. If needed, glucagon may be administered to produce hypotonia.

In Europe and Japan, air is more commonly used as the second contrast agent for enteroclysis to achieve a double-contrast effect. In general, air produces considerably more radiographic contrast than methylcellulose. On the other hand, air tends to percolate through barium-filled loops of small bowel rather than propelling the barium ahead of it; this phenomenon can result in numerous air bubbles. Nevertheless, some investigators believe that better diagnostic results are achieved with air, even in patients with inflammatory bowel disease.[34]

Several "tubeless" enteroclysis techniques have been described. One simple method is to perform a conventional antegrade small bowel study and then to administer effervescent agent when barium approaches the cecum. Efflux of gas is facilitated by turning the patient into the prone position and placing the table in a 20- to 40-degree Trendelenburg position,[35] often resulting in a double-contrast study of the small bowel. A novel tubeless double-contrast small bowel technique employs effervescent granules and tablets coated with an acid-resistant acrylic lacquer that allows gas to be released directly into the small bowel lumen.[36]

Barium formulations specifically designed for enteroclysis provide the best results and are commercially available. For single-contrast studies, a barium suspension with a specific gravity of about 1.25 (equivalent to approximately 35% w/v) is typically used. For double-contrast studies, a 50% to 95% w/v barium suspension is employed.

Retrograde ileography consists initially of a single-contrast barium enema, followed by continued infusion of barium in a retrograde fashion into the ileum. Because flow rates are controlled by the examiner, the ileum can be readily studied without overlapping proximal small bowel loops obscuring the area of interest. Barium is instilled until the small bowel loops in question have been filled. Premedication with glucagon decreases patient discomfort and also relaxes the ileocecal valve. If there is concern about a redundant sigmoid colon obscuring pelvic loops of ileum, the barium enema can be followed by a saline enema; the saline solution pushes barium ahead of it, resulting in a see-through effect for better visualization of these ileal loops. A 20% to 25% w/v barium suspension is typically used for retrograde ileography.

It is not unusual to obtain a double-contrast study of the terminal ileum during a double-contrast barium enema, especially if glucagon is used to relax the ileocecal valve. Such an examination is particularly useful for patients with suspected ileal Crohn's disease or malignant gynecologic tumors involving the distal ileum.

A peroral pneumocolon, consisting of both antegrade and retrograde components, is designed to evaluate the distal ileum or right colon. A conventional antegrade small bowel examination is initially performed. When barium has filled the terminal ileum and right colon, air is instilled through the rectum via a small catheter and refluxed into the right colon and distal small bowel for double-contrast views of the terminal ileum or cecum and ascending colon.[37] This study can also be combined with enteroclysis. Routine use of a hypotonic agent appears helpful.[33]

Barium Enemas

The techniques for both single-contrast and double-contrast barium enemas are well established. Numerous studies have compared the relative accuracy of single-contrast versus double-contrast barium enemas. Some radiologists prefer to perform single-contrast studies in elderly or debilitated patients, but double-contrast studies can be performed in many of these patients.

Both dry and liquid barium formulations are commercially available. If dry, prefilled barium enema bags are used, the amount of water added and degree of subsequent shaking to achieve an appropriate liquid suspension should be standardized. The level marking inscribed on the enema bag should not be used to gauge the amount of water needed; resulting dilutions tend to be erratic. Liquid barium-filled enema bags should be kept on their sides, because considerable settling can occur if bags are stored for some time before use.

A 12% to 25% w/v barium suspension is commonly used for single-contrast barium enemas. The main requirement of the barium suspension is that it neither flocculates nor settles during the examination. Because the sedimentation rate depends in part on the amount and type of additives present, some products that are well suspended at higher concentrations settle readily when diluted. If there is doubt about a commercial product's sedimentation rate, a radiograph obtained with a horizontal x-ray beam should reveal any settling tendencies.

Double-contrast barium enema suspensions should consist of relatively high barium concentrations but still be sufficiently fluid to flow readily through enema tubing. Of necessity, their viscosity is greater than that of the lower concentration barium formulations designed for single-contrast studies. Resultant mucosal coating should be uniform without undue artifacts, and the barium suspension should not dry out while the examination is in progress. These barium formulations are generally in the range of 60% to 120% w/v (an 85% w/v is commonly used).

Even with properly prepared barium suspensions, subsequent mucosal coating can vary from one practice to another because of variations in the hardness of the local water and the type of water used (distilled water vs. cold or hot tap water). Manufacturers sell premixed liquid formulations to avoid these variations. The barium suspension is simply poured into the enema bag without further dilution.

Some radiologists utilize colonic lavage for cleansing of the colon before performing a double-contrast barium enema. Such lavage invariably results in water retention, however, and a subsequent dilution of the barium suspension. The barium manufacturers recognize this problem and therefore market two different barium preparations; the barium suspension designed to be used after colonic lavage has a slightly higher specific gravity.

Tumors may be difficult to detect in portions of the colon (especially the sigmoid colon) involved by severe diverticulosis. In such cases, the area of the colon in question can be further studied if the double-contrast barium enema is followed by a methylcellulose enema.[38]

Water-Soluble Contrast Agents

Indications

Water-soluble organic iodine compounds designed for the gastrointestinal tract were introduced in the 1950s. Since that time, there has been continuing controversy about the role of these agents and their relative merits. Water-soluble contrast agents do not coat the gastrointestinal mucosa; rather, they provide visualization of the bowel by passive filling of the intestinal lumen.

For most gastrointestinal examinations, experienced radiologists prefer barium as the contrast agent. Some surgeons, however, are still taught by their seniors of the purported dangers of barium and insist on the use of water-soluble contrast agents, ignoring their limitations. Reasons cited for the use of these agents include stimulation of peristalsis in postoperative patients and the safety of these agents when a gastrointestinal perforation is present.

Water-soluble contrast agents are indicated if an acute intestinal perforation is suspected. The examination generally confirms or excludes a perforation, recognizing that small, subtle perforations can be missed. Similarly, walled-off perforations or a perforation in an area of spasm can be difficult to detect. In such cases, barium can be safely administered because extravasated barium will be confined to a sealed-off extraluminal collection and the greater radiographic visibility of barium yields more information than that obtained with water-soluble contrast agents. When water-soluble contrast agents fail to detect a leak, the examination should therefore be completed with barium to evaluate for a chronic or loculated perforation that could otherwise be missed. If there is clinical concern about a free perforation into the peritoneal cavity, however, water-soluble contrast agents are preferred.

Meconium ileus and meconium plug syndrome can sometimes be treated with an iodinated water-soluble contrast enema. Ionic contrast agents are preferred, and the patient should be well hydrated.

Some surgeons treat postoperative adynamic ileus using oral ionic contrast agents. Data on the value of this approach are limited. Hypertonic fluid that accumulates proximal to a site of mechanical obstruction also may draw fluid into the bowel, resulting in even further distention.

Contrast Agents

In general, a 60% or higher solution of ionic contrast agents is needed to achieve adequate radiographic opacification of the gastrointestinal tract. This results in an iodine concentration of 282 to 292 mg/mL and an osmolality of about 1500 mOsm/kg (approximately five times that of serum) for the more commonly used commercial products. Because of this hyperosmolarity, fluid is drawn into the bowel lumen and diarrhea is common after the use of these agents. Because ionic contrast agents stimulate intestinal peristalsis, they also result in more rapid visualization of the distal small bowel than can be achieved with barium sulfate. The advantage of a shorter examination, however, should be balanced against the decreased radiographic contrast obtained with these agents. In general, intraluminal dilution leads to progressively worse visualization of the mid and distal small bowel.

Some commercial ionic contrast agents designed for oral use, such as the diatrizoate meglumine preparations Gastrografin and oral Hypaque, contain flavoring agents. Such contrast agents are preferred to their nonflavored counterparts, which are designed primarily for intravenous use.

Nonionic contrast agents with an iodine concentration of approximately 300 mg/mL have an osmolality of 600 to 710 mOsm/kg, which is less than half that of ionic agents. Ideally, one of the nonionic agents should be used when a water-soluble contrast agent is indicated for evaluation of the gastrointestinal tract and, for specific reasons, ionic contrast agents need to be avoided.[39] For example, if a perforation into the pleural or peritoneal cavity is suspected in patients at high risk for aspiration, nonionic contrast agents appear to be safer than their ionic counterparts. At the same time, it should be recognized that small or subtle areas of perforation are better defined with barium than with water-soluble contrast agents. In routine studies of the gastrointestinal tract in infants and children in whom perforation was not at issue, a study comparing iohexol and barium concluded that barium is the preferred contrast agent.[40]

Negative Contrast Agents

Air is by far the least expensive negative contrast agent for performing double-contrast studies of the gastrointestinal tract. Excellent double-contrast views of the esophagus can be obtained if the patient swallows air together with the barium preparation.

One commercial preparation incorporated carbon dioxide directly into the barium suspension; when the patient drank this "bubbly barium," carbon dioxide was released into the esophagus and stomach. The effect was similar to that of drinking a bottle of club soda, but this product never gained widespread acceptance.

Effervescent tablets, granules, and powders are commercially available. These products produce carbon dioxide on contact with water, and most are satisfactory for achieving adequate distention of the stomach and duodenum. Nevertheless, there is considerable variation in the dissolution time of these agents. Most commercial effervescent powders and granules are supplied in single-dose packages. In clinical use, the patient places the effervescent agent in his or her mouth and uses a small amount of water to wash it down. The barium suspension is then immediately ingested. This technique generally produces satisfactory double-contrast views of the esophagus, stomach, and duodenum.

Liquid effervescent agents (consisting of separate acid and base solutions) can be prepared locally by a hospital pharmacy. The acid portion is usually citric or tartaric acid, and the base portion is sodium bicarbonate. A dose of 12 to 15 mL is satisfactory for most patients.

Some authors advocate carbon dioxide in place of air for double-contrast barium enemas and CT colonography, arguing that carbon dioxide is absorbed faster and causes less patient discomfort than air,[41] but others disagree.[42] Whether carbon dioxide or air is used probably does not influence the quality of the examination, but there is less colonic distention with carbon dioxide than with air.[43]

Some double-contrast preparations result in the formation of excessive gas bubbles. An antifoam agent should be added empirically if bubbles are encountered on a regular basis. Although many commercial barium preparations already include an antifoam agent, the dose of this agent is not always sufficient. A commonly used antifoam agent is dimethyl polysiloxane (simethicone); addition of 1.5 mL of simethicone (equivalent to 100 mg) is often adequate to eliminate bubbles.

Contrast Agents for Gastrointestinal Computed Tomography

The term *double-contrast abdominal CT* is used by some to signify the use of both intravenous and oral contrast agents; this is a misuse of the traditional connotation of "double contrast" and is best avoided to prevent confusion.

Full-strength barium preparations should not be diluted to the low concentrations needed for CT. The barium particles settle out after ingestion of such a dilute suspension, leading to inhomogeneous opacification of the bowel lumen. As a result, the uppermost part of a bowel loop may not contain enough barium for visualization while excess barium in the dependent portion of the loop results in streak artifacts.

Stable but low-concentration barium formulations designed for CT are commercially available, with most of the brand names ending in *CAT*. These CT barium products contain small particles that resist settling. Additives also prevent barium sedimentation. At the low barium concentrations used, barium particles do not coat the mucosa but simply provide lumen opacification.

An esophagus opacified by a contrast agent aids in evaluating the mediastinum during chest CT. The low-concentration CT agents used for the rest of the gastrointestinal tract do not adhere to the esophagus long enough to provide adequate opacification; one option is to have the patient drink small sips of a conventional CT contrast agent before each scan. A more convenient approach is to use a high-viscosity, low-concentration barium paste that provides prolonged coating of the esophageal mucosa for better visualization of the esophagus on CT.[44]

The traditional method for opacifying the stomach and small bowel is to have the patient drink approximately 500 mL of a dilute CT contrast agent several hours before the examination, with a similar amount ingested immediately before scanning. Ideally, such an agent should differentiate bowel from surrounding structures without introducing artifacts. The choice between a dilute iodine solution or barium suspension is a matter of personal preference. A 1% to 3% w/v barium sulfate suspension or 2% to 5% solution of Gastrografin or similar iodinated agent is typically employed. One refinement is the use of a 2% barium suspension for jejunal opacification and a slightly lower concentration for pelvic structures. With slower CT scanners, an iodine solution produces fewer streak artifacts than barium, but streak artifacts are not an issue with multislice CT scanners. Commercial barium suspensions tend to taste better than iodine solutions, a factor that becomes important when performing CT on children or nausea-prone cancer patients. The taste of iodinated contrast agents can be masked by adding sugar and various fruit extracts or flavored juices such as Kool-Aid.[45] At the dilutions used, iodinated solutions are hypo-osmolar yet some patients still develop diarrhea. Because of the low concentration of iodine, nonionic contrast agents do not have any significant advantage over ionic agents when used for abdominal CT.

With suspected pelvic disease, a contrast agent should be ingested the evening before the examination. Even if full-strength Gastrografin is ingested, overnight dilution in the bowel lumen is sufficient to eliminate most streak artifacts. In fact, better rectosigmoid opacification is obtained after ingesting a full-strength iodinated contrast agent than a dilute barium suspension, probably because of hyperperistalsis induced by the iodinated agent. Nevertheless, identifying fluid-filled colonic loops is less of a problem than identifying fluid-filled small bowel loops on abdominal CT.

CT enteroclysis consists of bowel intubation with an enteroclysis catheter and instilling the bowel with an iodinated contrast agent, dilute barium suspension, or methylcellulose before the CT scan is performed. It remains unclear whether a positive contrast agent or water-density contrast agent is superior for CT enteroclysis, but the use of an intravenous contrast agent facilitates detection of bowel lesions by opacifying the intestinal mucosa. Negative oral contrast agents designed specifically for CT enteroclysis are also becoming available. With MDCT and coronal reconstruction becoming more readily available, retained bowel fluid often provides an adequate bowel marker, especially in patients with dilated bowel.

Helical CT enterography can be used to assess the extent of Crohn's disease[46]; adequate bowel opacification is achieved by using a larger than usual volume (1600 mL) of a 2% flavored barium suspension. Another approach is to inject barium through an enteroclysis catheter.[47,48]

A dilute contrast enema can be administered if colonic distention is needed. If the imaging study is performed to evaluate a rectal lesion, a high-viscosity, low-volume barium paste may suffice; a paste mixture of approximately 100 mL of a 3.6% w/v carboxymethylcellulose and 2% w/v barium sulfate has been proposed in this clinical setting.[49]

A basic question, especially with MDCT, is whether intraluminal, water-density, or fat-density contrast or even gas is superior to a positive contrast agent. With maximal intensity projection images of vascular structures, positive bowel contrast creates artifacts. When an intravenous contrast agent is used for bowel wall enhancement, positive intraluminal contrast can also obscure subtle lesions. As a result, MDCT studies are increasingly performed with oral water-density or even negative contrast agents. Ingested water is usually adequate for gastric and duodenal distention, but ingested water usually does not provide adequate distention of the distal small bowel

because of absorption from the intestinal lumen. For this reason, a carboxymethylcellulose or polyethylene glycol solution is sometimes used to prevent absorption and improve small bowel distention (compared with water). A preliminary study of simethicone-coated cellulose (SonoRx; Bracco Diagnostics, Princeton, NJ), developed for oral use in upper abdominal ultrasonography, found that this solution has no significant advantage over oral water for abdominal CT.[50]

In the past, a number of fat-density products (including mineral oil, corn oil, milk, and even a paraffin emulsion) have been proposed for abdominal CT, but these agents have had limited application.

Residual bowel gas often serves as an intestinal marker, especially in the colon. If a nasogastric tube is in place, air can also be injected into the stomach and small bowel. If excessive amounts of gas are present, imaging with slightly wider window settings than usual may be helpful.

Two-dimensional colonography and three-dimensional virtual colonoscopy require colonic distention with a contrast agent; air is typically used, but carbon dioxide is resorbed more quickly and appears to cause less patient discomfort during this examination.

Adverse Reactions

Barium Sulfate

Barium sulfate is poorly soluble in water. The constipating tendency of barium products is well known to most radiologists. Through judicious use of additives, this side effect is minimized in most present-day formulations, but barium impaction in the colon is still occasionally reported.[51]

Aspiration of small amounts of commercial barium formulations is of little clinical significance. Most aspirated barium is cleared from the trachea and major bronchi within several hours, but some barium is retained in the interstitium and in macrophages. This residual barium is generally not visible on radiographs. Alveolarization of barium, however, can result in prolonged retention. If aspiration is suspected on clinical grounds, barium rather than one of the ionic contrast agents is preferred. In this setting, some radiologists prefer to use nonionic contrast agents, but the advantages of nonionic agents versus barium are not clear.

Hypersensitivity reactions to barium are rare but have been reported during both upper gastrointestinal tract examinations and barium enemas.[52] Although barium sulfate is inert, commercial formulations contain numerous known and proprietary additives.[53] These include stabilizing, flavoring, coating, and viscosity-varying agents ranging from natural flavors and gums (e.g., lemon, pectin, and guar) to synthetic products (e.g., various methylcellulose solutions). Older radiologists are familiar with chocolate-flavored barium products that are no longer used because of a frequent patient allergy to chocolate. Anaphylaxis to carboxymethylcellulose has been described.[54] The role of effervescent agents in these reactions is speculative. Methylparaben and similar compounds used as preservatives can induce hypersensitivity reactions, but barium manufacturers have replaced them in most commercial barium products with more innocuous preservatives.

Reactions appear to be more common during double-contrast than single-contrast studies. Most reactions are mild, consisting of urticaria or pruritus, but erythema multiforme, respiratory complications, anaphylaxis, gastrointestinal angioedema, and even death have been reported. Patients with asthma and severe food allergies appear to be at slightly increased risk for developing these reactions, but to put this problem in perspective, the average radiologist will not encounter a hypersensitivity reaction to a barium product in a lifetime of practice.

The etiology of hypersensitivity reactions during most barium studies is unknown. In general, the incriminating agent is not sought, and no testing is performed in patients who develop reactions.

Esophageal perforation and spillage of barium into the mediastinum result in an inflammatory reaction, with barium persisting in the mediastinum for prolonged periods of time. Such prior extravasation can often be recognized radiographically by the presence of dense linear radiopacities in the mediastinum, but no solid evidence exists that sequelae are more severe than with water-soluble contrast agents.

Most perforations associated with barium enema studies occur in the rectum and are not immediately detected by fluoroscopy. Rectal perforations tend to result from the injudicious insufflation of an enema balloon. A United Kingdom survey of barium enemas during a 3-year period revealed a complication rate of 1 in 9,000 and a death rate of 1 in 57,000.[55] Only 10% of patients (3/30) with a bowel perforation died, but the mortality was 56% (9/16) in patients who developed a cardiac arrhythmia.

Spillage of barium into the peritoneal cavity can be secondary to a preexisting lesion that has perforated. Nevertheless, perforations may rarely occur during barium studies, including barium enemas, enteroclysis, and even upper gastrointestinal tract examinations. When perforation occurs, leukocytes are initially drawn into the peritoneal cavity together with an outpouring of fluid. Profound hypovolemia develops if massive amounts of fluid accumulate in the peritoneal cavity. Bacterial contamination can lead to overwhelming sepsis and shock within hours.

Immediate management of barium peritonitis includes infusion of large volumes of intravenous fluid. Antibiotics are administered because of associated bacterial contamination. Most patients undergo early surgery, with an attempt made to evacuate barium from the peritoneal cavity. Invariably, barium crystals embedded on the peritoneal surface resist dislodgement. Attempts to remove barium particles with a wet sponge simply induce diffuse peritoneal bleeding.

Barium crystals in the peritoneal cavity subsequently incite an inflammatory reaction and, eventually, these crystals become coated by a fibrin membrane with extensive fibrosis and an intense granulomatous reaction. Dense fibrosis can involve adjacent structures and, depending on location, can eventually lead to intestinal or even ureteral obstruction. Perirectal fibrosis can also narrow the lumen of the rectosigmoid colon, even mimicking colonic carcinoma. Residual barium is identified either by conventional radiography or CT. There is no evidence to suggest that extraluminal barium in the soft tissues is carcinogenic (Fig. 1-2).

Barium can intravasate into systemic veins and the portal venous system.[56,57] Intravasation of barium into the vena cava has also been described in a patient with a duodenal ulcer; CT revealed barium in the lungs, liver, and spleen in this

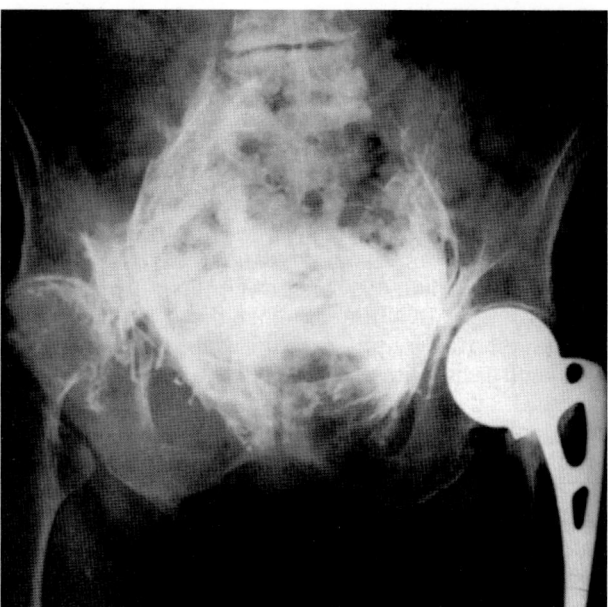

Figure 1-2. Prior colon perforation during barium enema. Barium crystals are encased by dense adhesions that also involve the bowel. (From Miler RE, Skucas J: Radiographic Contrast Agents. Gaithersburg, MD, Aspen, 1977, p 137.)

patient.[58] Barium intravasation is associated with a mortality rate of greater than 50%.

Water-Soluble Contrast Agents

The risk of sensitivity reactions to iodinated contrast agents is considerably less when these agents are administered orally rather than by intravascular injection. In young children and adults with hypovolemia, however, introduction of large volumes of a hypertonic agent into the gastrointestinal tract can result in hypovolemia, shock, and even death. In this setting, adequate intravascular fluid replacement and use of a nonionic contrast agent should therefore be considered.

If aspiration or a tracheoesophageal fistula is suspected, hyperosmolar ionic contrast agents are contraindicated because they may cause pneumonia and even life-threatening pulmonary edema. Nonionic agents are reasonable substitutes.[39] In most adults, however, barium sulfate is the preferred contrast agent of choice for patients with possible esophageal-airway fistulas.

Other Contrast Agents

Reactions can occur even before a contrast agent is instilled. In the past, the latex used in enema balloons was implicated in some early reactions during barium enema examinations.[59] As a result, a major manufacturer of barium sulfate products in the United States recalled all enema tips containing natural latex balloons in 1990.

The offending antigen in latex is believed to be a water-soluble protein that is heat stable. It is found on the surface of cured latex and probably is a contaminant of natural latex when it is obtained from the *Hevea brasiliensis* tree. In sensitive individuals, contact with the skin leads to urticaria but contact with mucous membranes can result in severe anaphylactic reactions.[60] Currently, nonlatex and synthetic latex products are available.

CONTRAST AGENTS FOR CHOLANGIOGRAPHY

With normal renal function, only about 1% of administered ionic or nonionic contrast agents undergo hepatic excretion, an insufficient dose for visualization of the bile ducts on CT. In a setting of renal failure, however, it is not unusual to opacify the gallbladder even with conventional radiography.

Cholecystography using oral cholecystographic agents has been supplanted by other imaging modalities and is currently performed only for limited indications. Several commercial cholecystographic agents are available. To ensure oral absorption, they manifest both hydrophilic and lipophilic properties; in the blood, these agents are bound to albumin and, theoretically, should have high toxicity, but in actual practice, adverse reactions are uncommon. These agents undergo enterohepatic circulation, and delayed reactions are occasionally encountered.

Intravenous cholangiographic agents undergo hepatocyte uptake and biliary excretion by active transport. They are excreted either unchanged or after conjugation with glucuronic acid. These hepatocyte-specific liver contrast agents consist of triiodobenzene compounds that, by means of benzene ring substitutions, have had their hydrophilicity decreased to the point that they can now pass through membranes. Iodipamide meglumine (Cholografin) is the only such agent available in the United States. Most of the injected contrast agent is bound to albumin; biliary visualization is generally evident about 15 minutes after intravenous administration. One might assume that because cholangiographic agents undergo hepatocyte uptake they would make useful liver contrast agents for CT; in actual practice, however, hepatocyte uptake is too slow and excretion too fast for them to serve this function.

Toxicity and allergic reactions are greater with iodipamide than with more typical intravascular contrast agents. Nephrotoxicity is dose dependent. In part because of this toxicity, cholangiography has been supplanted by other imaging techniques, including MRI and direct cholangiopancreatography, in which the bile ducts are visualized by percutaneous transhepatic cholangiography, an endoscopic retrograde approach, or administration of contrast agent via a surgically placed tube.

Direct cholangiography is generally performed with "full strength" contrast concentrations (about 300 mg iodine/mL). A high iodine concentration is advantageous when searching for subtle bile duct leaks. Also, when injecting contrast material proximal to an obstruction, a high iodine concentration allows for dilution by residual bile. When searching for bile duct stones, however, dilution of the contrast agent with an equal volume of water increases detection of stones, because subtle stones can be missed in bile ducts that are densely opacified. Overinjection of contrast material should be avoided during direct cholangiography. In the United States, syringe injection is common; but in Europe, a drip infusion technique is more popular. The study should be terminated if the pancreatic duct begins to opacify, because acute pancreatitis is a recognized complication of this procedure.

Earlier studies suggested that meglumine salts of ionic contrast agents result in less bile duct epithelial damage than corresponding sodium salts; the use of nonionic contrast agents makes this a moot point.

The indications for CT cholangiography are still evolving. CT cholecystography is performed 10 to 12 hours after oral administration of a cholecystographic contrast agent (iopanoic acid). Another approach is slow infusion of a cholangiographic contrast agent, resulting in biliary images superior to those obtained with conventional intravenous cholangiography. The major intrahepatic ducts are visualized in most individuals. Preliminary evidence suggests that CT cholangiography is better than MR cholangiopancreatography (MRCP) for visualizing small bile duct stones. However, this technique is not useful in jaundiced patients, because insufficient contrast material is excreted into bile ducts.

MRCP is a noninvasive imaging technique for visualizing biliary and pancreatic ducts that has evolved as an alternative to diagnostic endoscopic retrograde cholangiopancreatography and diagnostic percutaneous cholangiography. Two MR approaches are feasible: an intravenous contrast-assisted technique and a technique without contrast, using heavily T2-weighted images to render nonflowing fluid hyperintense. The former approach entails the use of primarily hepatobiliary MR agents (discussed in the next section); contrast-containing bile is hyperintense on T1-weighted imaging sequences. A limitation of this procedure is that reasonable hepatocyte function is required to achieve an adequate concentration of contrast agent in the bile ducts for imaging purposes. The latter technique, simply called MRCP, has no such limitations and has become the primary imaging study for visualizing the bile ducts.

CONTRAST AGENTS FOR MAGNETIC RESONANCE IMAGING

Intravascular Contrast Agents

The term *contrast agent* has a different meaning in MRI than is usually applied to barium sulfate or iodinated agents. Contrast agents for MRI are not visualized directly; rather, their primary function is to alter water proton relaxation times. Although MRI contrast agents are more complex and serve a more varied function than CT contrast agents, they are used for the same primary purpose—to improve lesion detection and characterization by increasing contrast tissue signal intensity differences due to varying effects on tissue proton relaxation. These differences vary with time and depend on the degree of vascularity of the lesion. Much of the current research on contrast agents for MRI focuses on improving the specificity of these agents.

Contrast agents used in MRI are often classified by their metal component. A more useful classification, however, is based on the distribution of these agents, recognizing that there is some overlap between categories; many of these agents are initially blood-pool agents, but subsequent distribution depends on their molecular configuration, as follows:
1. Conventional gadolinium chelates (extracellular agents)
2. Macrophage-monocytic, phagocytic (reticuloendothelial) agents
3. Primarily hepatobiliary agents (intracellular agents)
4. Primarily blood-pool agents

All currently available contrast agents used for MRI shorten tissue TI and T2 relaxation times. The paramagnetic gadolinium and manganese contrast agents primarily shorten T1 relaxation time, thus increasing signal intensity (enhancement) of normal parenchyma on T1-weighted images. The superparamagnetic iron oxides primarily shorten T2 relaxation time, thus decreasing signal intensity on T2-weighted images and, depending on the sequences used, increasing signal intensity on T1-weighted images. These metal ions are chelated to other structures, such as DTPA, to reduce their toxicity.

Gadolinium chelates are the most frequently used vascular MRI contrast agents. These mostly hydrophilic compounds are chelated to "mask" the toxic gadolinium ion. Their biodistribution and perfusion-related characteristics are similar to those of iodine-containing contrast agents. To take full advantage of these MRI contrast agents, dynamic imaging must be performed shortly after contrast injection (arterial to portal venous phases); these agents later equilibrate with the extracellular space, so that lesions become isointense to hepatic parenchyma on delayed views. Detection of liver tumors with these agents depends on differences in blood flow between the tumor and adjacent normal tissue. More recently, these agents have been used for MR angiography as a substitute for abdominal digital subtraction angiography. Image processing allows separation of arteries and veins.

At recommended doses, gadolinium chelates have a lower rate of adverse reactions than iodinated contrast agents but anaphylactic reactions and even cardiopulmonary arrest can occur. The risk factors for reactions are not well defined but appear to be similar to those for iodinated contrast agents. Unlike iodine-related reactions, however, gadolinium-related reactions tend to be delayed, at times occurring 1 hour or more after contrast administration. These agents are excreted by glomerular filtration and, in the usual doses, nephrotoxicity is uncommon. In patients on hemodialysis, about 80% of the gadolinium is dialyzed after the first dialysis and essentially all of the gadolinium is dialyzed after the fourth dialysis; a normal dose has therefore been used in hemodialysis patients.

Gadolinium agents exhibit poor water relaxivity at higher magnetic fields (>4T). Undoubtedly, new MR agents will be developed for use with high field strength magnets.

Larger superparamagnetic iron oxide (SPIO) particles are taken up by the reticuloendothelial system (RES), resulting in decreased parenchymal enhancement of the liver and spleen on T2-weighted images. Uptake is also present in lymph nodes and bone marrow. Ferumoxide (Endorem; Guerbet, Aulney-Sous-Bois, France) is a SPIO agent consisting of a colloidal mixture of ferrous and ferric oxide. Tissues lacking RES cells, such as metastases, have little or no signal loss and therefore appear hyperintense compared with the hypointense normal RES-containing liver or spleen parenchyma. Not only are known tumors better visualized, but compared with unenhanced MR sequences, more tumors are detected. This advantage is limited, however, because some well-differentiated neoplasms contain RES cells and thus take up iron oxide particles. These SPIO-induced changes vary among tumors, potentially enabling tissue characterization of different tumors. Nevertheless, imaging interpretation with these compounds is complex; some of the particles are ultrasmall, and T1-weighted gradient echo sequences result in imaging patterns similar to those with gadolinium chelates and ultrasmall SPIO particles.

Reticuloendothelial agents have a longer intravascular half-life than gadolinium chelates. A prolonged scanning window is available once these particles are within the RES; eventually, free iron is used in normal iron metabolism. The role of these contrast agents in clinical imaging is not yet clearly defined. Disadvantages include prolonged scanning times and a higher false-positive rate.

Several hepatobiliary specific paramagnetic contrast agents such as Gd-EOB-DTPA (Eovist; Schering, Berlin) and Gd-BOPTA (MultiHance; Bracco, Milan) are initially extracellular and then undergo hepatocyte uptake. Early dynamic perfusion imaging is similar to that with conventional gadolinium chelates, but this can be followed by delayed hepatic imaging; each phase yields different information. Image interpretation differs from conventional gadolinium scans; thus, with Gd-BOPTA, a hepatocellular carcinoma shows early peripheral enhancement but parenchymal phase images reveal an isointense or even hypointense tumor.[61]

Hepatobiliary agents are eliminated by both biliary and renal pathways. Eovist achieves greater liver enhancement than MultiHance and has a biliary excretion rate of about 50% of the injected dose, and a delayed biliary phase is evident. MultiHance exhibits a T1 relaxation time about double that of conventional gadolinium agents, probably secondary to binding to albumin, which decreases extravascular leakage. Only a small percentage of these agents is taken up by hepatocytes, but this uptake has a prolonged effect on liver signal intensity.

Mn-DPDP (Teslascan; Nycomed, Oslo) dissociates partly in plasma, with free manganese taken up by hepatocytes and other tissues, including the pancreas. Nondissociated Mn-DPDP is eventually eliminated by the kidneys. It is often considered to be a hepatobiliary specific paramagnetic contrast agent having an effect lasting for several hours, thus permitting delayed imaging. Mn-DPDP is injected by slow intravenous infusion, so that dynamic imaging is not feasible. This agent selectively enhances both normal liver parenchyma and hepatocyte-containing tumors such as focal nodular hyperplasia, regenerative nodules, and hepatocellular adenomas and carcinomas on T1-weighted images but shows little or no enhancement of metastases, cysts, and hemangiomas. Mn-DPDP differentiates hepatocellular carcinomas from metastases, with non–hepatocyte-origin metastases becoming more conspicuous due to increased signal from the surrounding normal liver parenchyma. One exception is metastatic neuroendocrine tumors that occasionally enhance with Mn-DPDP. One possible use is MR-guided thermal tumor ablation, in which prolonged tumor visualization is beneficial[62]; Mn-DPDP identifies more focal tumors both in cirrhotic and noncirrhotic livers than are detected on precontrast images. It also appears to be useful for defining intrahepatic biliary anatomic variants in pretransplantation liver lobe donors. Because Mn-DPDP does not differentiate benign and malignant liver tumors, its diagnostic impact is not yet clear.

Manganese is excreted in bile, but excretion is inhibited by biliary stasis. Its use is contraindicated in patients with severe liver failure. The overall safety of Mn-DPDP appears to be similar to that of other hepatocyte gadolinium products.

Ultrasmall superparamagnetic iron oxide (USPIO) particles, unlike most MRI contrast agents, usually shorten both T1 and T2 relaxation times. Initially conceived as MR lymphographic agents, they currently are used primarily as blood-pool agents. They have a blood half-life measured in hours. One disadvantage is superimposition of arteries and veins, although image processing techniques such as subtraction and phase contrast can differentiate these structures. USPIO contrast agents appear to be useful for differentiating highly vascular lesions such as hemangiomas from solid neoplasms. Also, their prolonged reduction of intravascular T1 values makes these agents useful for MR angiographic interventional procedures without need for repeat contrast injections. Their relaxation time increases at lower field strengths, and they are therefore suitable for use in open magnets.

Iron oxide particles less than 10 nm pass through capillaries and are eventually cleared by the liver, spleen, bone marrow, and lymph node reticuloendothelial cells, resulting in homogeneous signal loss in these structures. Such agents can therefore potentially identify lymph node metastases independent of nodal size, because normal nodes lose signal intensity but nodes (or regions of nodes) containing metastases do not take up these particles.[63]

A separate group of blood-pool contrast agents consists of gadolinium-based products bound to albumin, dextran, or other similar large molecules (also called macromolecular MRI contrast agents); imaging using Gd-BOPTA has already been mentioned. Even biodegradable polymeric coatings are feasible.[64] Tight albumin binding prolongs blood-pool time. The clinical role of these agents presumably will be similar to that of the USPIO agents.

MRI contrast agents may also be used in combination (also known as double-contrast MRI). For example, more information is obtained about a focal tumor by combining the perfusion data of a gadolinium chelate with the RES data of an SPIO agent than it is possible to obtain with a single agent alone. This combined use of contrast agents remains experimental.

Gastrointestinal Contrast Agents

An oral MR bowel contrast agent can identify the bowel lumen and it differentiates normal bowel wall from an abnormal process. Bowel distention may be obtained by injecting the contrast agent via a nasojejunal catheter or having the patient drink a large quantity of fluid, often with variable results.

Oral MRI contrast agents are classified either as positive contrast agents, which predominantly shorten T1 relaxation time and increase MR signal intensity on T1-weighted images, or as negative contrast agents, which either shorten T2 relaxation time and decrease signal intensity or simply lack hydrogen protons and water density contrast. Positive contrast agents consist of various iron, manganese, and gadolinium paramagnetic compounds; they are useful for detecting sinus tracts; on the other hand, they can mask intraluminal contents, so that visualization of the bowel wall is more difficult.

A distinction between positive and negative contrast agents is not absolute, and some agents change properties both with dilution and the MR sequence used. Gadolinium is a positive contrast agent and shortens T1 relaxation in the small bowel, but when concentrated in the colon, it acts as a negative contrast agent. Ferric ammonium citrate is hyperintense on both T1- and T2-weighted images at concentrations of less than 45 mg/mL[65]; at higher concentrations, however, bowel loops become hypointense on T2-weighted images. A more relevant issue is whether such contrast improves lesion detection; current results are not clear.[66]

A dilute barium sulfate suspension is a useful negative agent. Perfluorocarbons lack hydrogen protons and do not produce an MR signal either on T1- or T2-weighted images, but their role as oral agents is not established. Of course, air and water are also MRI contrast agents. Nonabsorbable water-density agents are similar to those used for CT (discussed earlier).

Positive contrast agents accentuate motion artifacts. Although contrast artifacts are more pronounced with negative agents, such agents are better for evaluating bowel wall abnormalities. Antiperistaltic pharmacologic agents are employed by some; these agents reduce motion artifacts even with a high-field strength unit.

MR colonography is performed using water, a gadolinium solution, or a barium suspension as the luminal contrast agent. Evaluation can include surface-rendered virtual endoscopic endoluminal views, orthogonal sections in three planes, and water-sensitive images.[67]

References

1. Krause W, Schneider PW: Chemistry of X-Ray Contrast Agents. In: Topics in Current Chemistry. Heidelberg, Springer-Verlag, 2002, vol 222.
2. Swanson DP, Chilton HM, Thrall JH: Pharmaceuticals in Medical Imaging. New York, Macmillan, 1990.
3. American College of Radiology: Manual on Contrast Media, 4th ed. Reston, VA, ACR, 1998.
4. European Society of Urogenital Radiology: Guidelines on Contrast Media, 2004, version 4.0. Available at www.esur.org.
5. Lawrence V, Matthai W, Hartmaier S: Comparative safety of high-osmolality and low-osmolality radiographic contrast agents: Report of a multidisciplinary working group. Invest Radiol 27:2-28, 1992.
6. Mikkonen R, Aronen HJ, Kivisaari L, et al: Plasma levels of prekallikrein, alpha-2-macroglobulin and C1-esterase inhibitor in patients with urticarial reaction to contrast media. Acta Radiol 38:466-473, 1997.
7. Lasser EC, Berry CC, Talner LB, et al: Pretreatment with corticosteroids to alleviate reactions to intravenous contrast material. N Engl J Med 317:845-849, 1987.
8. Pagani JJ, Hayman LA, Bigelow RH, et al: Diazepam prophylaxis of contrast media-induced seizures during computed tomography of patients with brain metastases. AJNR 4:67-72, 1983.
9. van Sonnenberg E, Neff CC, Pfister RC: Life-threatening hypotensive reactions to contrast media administration: Comparison of pharmacologic and fluid therapy. Radiology 162:15-19, 1987.
10. Addlestone RB, Roach AC: Pharmacologic treatment of contrast media reactions [Letter]. Radiology 165:876, 1987.
11. Zaloga GP, Delacey W, Holmboe E, et al: Glucagon reversal of hypotension in a case of anaphylactoid shock. Ann Intern Med 105:65-66, 1986.
12. Cochran ST, Bomyea K, Kahn M: Treatment of iodinated contrast material extravasation with hyaluronidase. Acad Radiol 9(Suppl 2):S544-S546, 2002.
13. Gleedon TG, Bulugahapitiya S: Contrast-induced nephropathy [Review]. AJR 183:1673-1689, 2004.
14. Merten GJ, Burgess WP, Gray LV, et al: Prevention of contrast-induced nephropathy with sodium bicarbonate: A randomized trial. JAMA 291:2328-2334, 2004.
15. Kramer BK, Kamerl M, Schweda F, Schreiber M: A primer in radiocontrast-induced nephropathy. Nephrol Dial Transplant 14:2830-2834, 1999.
16. Tepel M, van der Giet M, Schwarzfeld C, et al: Prevention of radiographic-contrast-agent–induced reductions in renal function by acetylcysteine. N Engl J Med 343:180-184, 2000.
17. Briguori C, Colombo A, Violante A, et al: Standard vs. double dose of N-acetylcysteine to prevent contrast agent associated nephrotoxicity. Eur Heart J 25:206-211, 2004.
18. Goldenberg I, Shechter M, Matetzky S, et al: Oral acetylcysteine as an adjunct to saline hydration for the prevention of contrast-induced nephropathy following coronary angiography: A randomized control trial and review of the current literature. Eur Heart J 25:212-218, 2004.

19. Marenzi G, Marana I, Lauri G, et al: The prevention of radiocontrast-agent–induced nephropathy by hemofiltration. N Engl J Med 349:1333-1340, 2003.

20. Kurokohchi K, Masaki T, Miyauchi Y, et al: Efficacy of combination therapies of percutaneous or laparoscopic ethanol-lipiodol injection and radiofrequency ablation. Int J Oncol 25:1737-1743, 2004.

21. Nyman U, Elmståhl B, Leander P, et al: Gadolinium contrast media for DSA in azotemia. Acta Radiol 9(Suppl 2):S528-S530, 2002.

22. Skucas J: Barium sulfate: Clinical application. In Skucas J (ed): Radiographic Contrast Agents, 2nd ed. Rockville, MD, Aspen, 1989, pp 14-17.

23. Chen HS, Wang TG, Chang YC, et al: [Barium-pudding: a new medium for videofluoroscopic examination] [Chinese]. J Formos Med Assoc 93:S156-160, 1994.

24. Dantas RO, Dodds WJ, Massey BT, et al: The effect of high- vs low-density barium preparations on the quantitative features of swallowing. Am J Roentgenol 153:1191-1195, 1989.

25. Jones B, Donner MW: Examination of the patient with dysphagia. Radiology 167:319-326, 1988.

26. Kaszar-Seibert DJ, Korn WT, Bindman DJ, et al: Treatment of acute esophageal food impaction with a combination of glucagon, effervescent agent, and water. Am J Roentgenol 154:533-534, 1990.

27. Gallo SH, McClave SA, Makk LJ, Looney SW: Standardization of clinical criteria required for use of the 12.5 millimeter barium tablet in evaluating esophageal luminal patency. Gastrointest Endosc 44:181-184, 1996.

28. Schabel SI, Skucas J: Esophageal obstruction following administration of "aged" barium sulfate tablets—a warning. Radiology 122:835-836, 1977.

29. Ghahremani GG, Weingardt JP, Curtin KR, Yaghmai V: Detection of occult esophageal narrowing with a barium tablet during chest radiography. Clin Imag 20:184-190, 1996.

30. Buecker A, Wein BB, Neuerburg JM, Guenther RW: Esophageal perforation: Comparison of use of aqueous and barium-containing contrast media. Radiology 202:683-686, 1997.

31. Gollub MJ, Bains MS: Barium sulfate: A new (old) contrast agent for diagnosis of postoperative esophageal leaks. Radiology 202:360-362, 1997.

32. Taverne PP, van der Jagt EJ: Small-bowel radiography: A prospective comparative study of three techniques in 200 patients. ROFO 143:293-297, 1985.

33. Nolan DJ, Traill ZC: The current role of the barium examination of the small intestine. Clin Radiol 52:809-820, 1997.

34. Geyer L, Reisinger W: Air or methylcellulose as a double contrast medium in x-ray studies of the small intestine? Radiol Diagn (Berl) 31:359-363, 1990.

35. Phillips JK, Scott RL, Nicell DT: The magic tilt method of tubeless enteroclysis: A modification to the gas-enhanced barium small-bowel examination. Am J Roentgenol 166:358-359, 1996.

36. Klein HM, Gunther RW: Double contrast small bowel follow-through with an acid-resistant effervescent agent. Invest Radiol 28:581-585, 1993.

37. Fitzgerald EJ, Thompson GT, Sommers SS, et al: Pneumocolon as an aid to small-bowel studies. Clin Radiol 36:633-637, 1985.

38. Olsson R, Adnerhill I, Bjorkdahl P, et al: Addition of methylcellulose enema to double contrast barium imaging of sigmoid diverticulosis. Acta Radiol 38:73-75, 1997.

39. Ginai AZ: Barium sulfate versus water-soluble, low-osmolarity contrast medium in esophageal examinations [Letter]. Radiology 205:287-288, 1997.

40. Cohen MD, Towbin R, Baker S, et al: Comparison of iohexol with barium in gastrointestinal studies of infants and children. AJR 156:345-350, 1991.

41. Robson NK, Lloyd M, Regan F: The use of carbon dioxide as an insufflation agent in barium enema—does it have a role? Br J Radiol 66:197-198, 1993.

42. Skovgaard N, Sloth C, von Benzon E, Jensen GS: The role of carbon dioxide and atmospheric air in double contrast barium enema. Abdom Imag 20:436-439, 1995.

43. Scullion DA, Wetton CW, Davies C, et al: The use of air or CO_2 as insufflation agents for double contrast barium enema (DCBE): Is there a qualitative difference? Clin Radiol 50:558-561, 1995.

44. Noda Y, Ogawa Y, Nishioka A, et al: New barium paste mixture for helical (slip-ring) CT evaluation of the esophagus. J Comput Assist Tomogr 20:773-776, 1996.

45. Quagliano PV, Austin RF Jr: Oral contrast agents for CT: A taste test survey. J Comput Assist Tomogr 21:720-722, 1997.

46. Raptopoulos V, Schwartz RK, McNicholas MM, et al: Multiplanar helical CT enterography in patients with Crohn's disease. AJR 169:1545-1550, 1997.

47. Pecher G, Kloeppel R, Thiele J: CT enteroclysis of small bowel [Abstract]. Radiology 201(P):496, 1996.

48. Bender GN, Timmons JH, Willard WC, Carter J: Computed tomography enteroclysis: One methodology. Invest Radiol 31:43-49, 1996.

49. Ogawa Y, Noda Y, Nishioka A, et al: New barium paste mixture for helical (slip-ring) CT evaluation of rectal carcinoma. J Comput Assist Tomogr 21:398-401, 1997.

50. Sahani DV, Jhaveri KS, D'Souza RV, et al: Evaluation of simethicone-coated cellulose as a negative oral contrast agent for abdominal CT. Acad Radiol 10:491-496, 2003.

51. McDonnell WM, Jung F: Images in clinical medicine: Barium impaction in the sigmoid colon. N Engl J Med 337:1278, 1997.

52. Janower ML: Hypersensitivity reactions after barium studies of the upper and lower gastrointestinal tract. Radiology 161:139-140, 1986.

53. Skucas J: Anaphylactoid reactions with gastrointestinal contrast media. AJR 168:962-964, 1997.

54. Muroi N, Nishibori M, Fujii T, et al: Anaphylaxis from the carboxymethylcellulose component of barium sulfate suspension. N Engl J Med 337:1275-1277, 1997.

55. Blakeborough A, Sheridan MB, Chapman AH: Complications of barium enema examinations: A survey of UK Consultant Radiologists 1992 to 1994. Clin Radiol 52:142-148, 1997.

56. Zalev AH: Venous barium embolization, a rare, potentially fatal complication of barium enema: 2 case reports. Can Assoc Radiol J 48:323-326, 1997.

57. Murphy KD, Poster RB, Marx WH, et al: Upper gastrointestinal examination complicated by venous intravasation and portal vein thrombosis. AJR 169:501-503, 1997.

58. Vitellas KM, Stone JA, Bennett WF, Mueller CF: The hyperdense liver and spleen: A CT manifestation of barium embolization through a duodenocaval fistula [Letter]. AJR 169:915-916, 1997.

59. Ownby DR, Tomlanovich M, Sammons N, et al: Anaphylaxis associated with latex allergy during barium enema examinations. AJR 156:903-908, 1991.

60. Sondheimer JM, Pearlman DS, Bailey WC: Systemic anaphylaxis during rectal manometry with a latex balloon. Am J Gastroenterol 84:975-977, 1989.

61. Manfredi R, Maresca G, Baron RL, et al: Delayed MR imaging of hepatocellular carcinoma enhanced by gadobenate dimeglumine (Gd-BOPTA). J Magn Reson Imaging 9:704-710, 1999.

62. Joarder R, de Jode M, Lamb GA, Gedroyc WM: The value of MnDPDP enhancement during MR guided laser interstitial thermoablation of liver tumors. J Magn Reson Imaging 13:37-41, 2001.

63. Harisinghani MG, Dixon WT, Saksena MA, et al: MR lymphangiography: Imaging strategies to optimize the imaging of lymph nodes with ferumoxtran-10. Radiographics 24:867-878, 2004.

64. Wen X, Jackson EF, Price RE, et al: Synthesis and characterization of poly(L-glutamic acid) gadolinium chelate: A new biodegradable MRI contrast agent. Bioconjugate Chem 15:1408-1415, 2004.

65. Broglia L, Tortora A, Maccioni F, et al: [Optimization of dosage and exam technique in the use of oral contrast media in magnetic resonance] [Italian]. Radiol Med 97:365-370, 1999.

66. Malcolm PN, Brown JJ, Hahn PF, et al: The clinical value of ferric ammonium citrate: A positive oral contrast agent for T1-weighted MR imaging of the upper abdomen. J Magn Reson Imaging 12:702-707, 2000.

67. Luboldt W, Bauerfeind P, Wildermuth S, et al: Colonic masses: Detection with MR colonography. Radiology 216:383-388, 2000.

Pharmacoradiology

Jovitas Skucas, MD

VASOCONSTRICTORS	Neostigmine
VASODILATORS	Erythromycin
HYPOTONIC GASTROINTESTINAL AGENTS	**MIXED ACTION AGENTS**
Glucagon	Morphine
Anticholinergic Agents	Cholecystokinin
HYPERTONIC GASTROINTESTINAL AGENTS	Ceruletide
Metoclopramide	**DRUGS AFFECTING THE BILIARY TRACT AND PANCREAS**
Domperidone	
Cisapride	

This chapter discusses pharmacologic agents of actual or potential use in gastrointestinal radiology, including those that have an intravascular effect (vasoconstrictors and vasodilators), those that modify gut motility, and those that affect bile flow. A discussion of experimental agents and agents designed for molecular imaging is beyond the scope of this chapter.

From a radiologist's viewpoint, most gut motility agents can be divided into those that increase gastrointestinal tonicity and motility and those that decrease these functions. Some agents have different effects on different parts of the gastrointestinal tract; they are discussed separately in the section on mixed action agents.

One exception to this classification is famotidine, which suppresses gastric secretions. A preliminary report suggests that famotidine may be useful prior to performing upper gastrointestinal barium studies; decreased gastric secretions improved the quality of these examinations.[1]

Bowel tonicity is not the same as peristalsis. In general, however, pharmacologic agents that increase bowel tonicity also result in increased peristalsis. For example, agents inducing gastric hypertonia tend to result in faster gastric emptying, and hypertonic small bowel agents result in faster small bowel transit. Conversely, hypotonic agents have the opposite effect.

VASOCONSTRICTORS

The primary use of vasoactive drugs in abdominal imaging is to alter blood flow in a way designed to increase diagnostic accuracy. Some drugs aid in delivering chemotherapeutic agents to neoplasms. All of these drugs must have acceptable side effects.

Vasoconstrictors aid primarily in detecting and characterizing neoplasms. These agents cause constriction of normal blood vessels but have little, if any, effect on malignant vessels.

Epinephrine, an adrenergic hormone, stimulates both α and β receptors and, depending on the specific innervation, results either in vasoconstriction or vasodilation. Initially used in renal arteriography, epinephrine decreases contrast opacification of normal renal parenchyma, and thereby accentuates the vasculature of renal cell carcinomas. Limitations for the use of epinephrine include a variable dose response and the ability of some inflammatory neovascularity to respond in a manner similar to that of neoplastic neovascularity. Hepatic and splenic arterial injection of epinephrine results in spasm of these vessels but little constriction of normal hepatic, gastric, duodenal, and pancreatic small vessels. Normal mesenteric vessels also do not respond appreciably to epinephrine. Propranolol, however, does block β-adrenergic vasodilation and, when used in conjunction with epinephrine, results in mesenteric vasoconstriction.

Norepinephrine has similar α-receptor stimulation as epinephrine but lacks β-receptor stimulation. It has been less well studied for use in imaging than epinephrine.

Of considerable interest in patients with pheochromocytomas is the increase in epinephrine or norepinephrine levels that occurs after contrast agent injection; it therefore is prudent to premedicate these patients with α- and β-adrenoceptor antagonists to control symptoms and prevent an adrenergic crisis, although this may not be necessary with some of the nonionic contrast agents.

Angiotensin, a hormone, is a potent vasoconstrictor acting directly on normal smooth muscle in vessels. Like epinephrine, it tends to enhance visualization of malignant neoplasms by a selective increase in tumor blood flow.

In pharmacologic doses, vasopressin constricts normal splanchnic vessels (including capillaries), thus decreasing portal blood flow. This agent has little effect, however, on hepatic arterial flow. Transcatheter vasopressin infusion can therefore be used to control gastrointestinal bleeding in some patients.

Secretin increases pancreatic blood flow. At times, selective venous sampling after intra-arterial injection of secretin aids in detecting gastrinomas.

Bombesin, a gut peptide, releases endogenous gastrin, which activates gastric mucosal sensory neurons. In turn, this increases gastric mucosal blood flow and therefore protects the mucosa from damage. Somatostatin negates this bombesin-induced gastric protection. Although bombesin is not employed in radiologic practice, the somatostatin analog octreotide has been used for treatment of esophageal and gastric variceal bleeding. Neuroendocrine tumors of the gut also contain somatostatin receptors; somatostatin analogs are therefore useful for diagnosis and radiotherapy of these tumors.

VASODILATORS

Vasodilators increase blood flow in a selective vascular bed. Their effect differs in normal and neoplastic vessels, but they are less suitable than vasoconstrictors for visualizing small neoplasms, because increased vascularity in normal vessels tends to obscure small tumors. A high-caloric meal is occasionally helpful for accentuating the superior mesenteric artery and portal vein.

Tolazoline, a synthetic vasodilator, facilitates angiographic visualization of small vessels. Direct injection into the mesenteric artery leads to improved venous opacification. Its effect on visualization of neoplasms is mixed. Whether tolazoline has a role in intra-arterial provocative mesenteric angiography to identify lower gastrointestinal bleeding is not clear.[2] Infusion therapy with tolazoline and heparin have been used to treat nonocclusive mesenteric ischemia.[3]

Bradykinin injected into the superior mesenteric artery improves portal vein visualization.

Acetylcholine, a parasympathetic hormone, is a vasodilator previously used to evaluate renal artery stenosis. Dopamine is a potent renal artery dilator similar to acetylcholine; it has also been studied in renal vessels. A preliminary report suggested that dopamine decreases contrast-induced nephrotoxicity, but other investigators found that it can have a deleterious effect on the kidneys.[4]

Prostaglandins have variable vascular effects, depending on their chemical composition and specific use. Prostaglandin E_1 has a similar effect on the splanchnic vasculature as acetylcholine and tolazoline, resulting in increased portal venous blood flow. Superior mesenteric artery injection of prostaglandin E_1 during CT hepatic arteriography therefore results in increased conspicuity between hepatocellular carcinoma nodules and the surrounding parenchyma.[5] The use of prostaglandin E_1 during CT hepatic arteriography also helps reduce the number of pseudolesions around the gallbladder bed.[6] Preliminary work suggests that prostaglandin E_1 may also decrease contrast-induced nephropathy, but this agent is associated with a number of side effects and its role in imaging studies is not clear. Prostaglandin $F_{2\alpha}$ dilates normal colonic vessels but causes vasoconstriction of inflammatory and neoplastic vessels in the colon.

Prostaglandin therapy is used in neonates with cyanotic congenital heart disease. Persistent, often asymptomatic gastric distention, detected on abdominal radiographs, is a complication of prostaglandin therapy. The distention usually resolves after cessation of therapy. This condition may superficially resemble pyloric stenosis, but imaging studies show gastric mucosal thickening and distal antral and pyloric elongation without muscular wall thickening.

Papaverine is a vasodilator of both large and small vessels. Similar to other vasodilators, it improves portal vein visualization during mesenteric angiography. It is not degraded in a single pass through the liver, however, and repeated injections can lead to systemic hypotension.

HYPOTONIC GASTROINTESTINAL AGENTS

Bowel hypotonia is helpful in a number of radiologic settings. For example, a spasmolytic agent can be used to dilate a segment of spastic colon mimicking a benign or malignant stricture. Similarly, polyps and diverticula in the small bowel can be detected more readily if the bowel is dilated and atonic. Spasmolytic pharmacologic agents can be classified as hormonal agents (glucagon is the classic example) and anticholinergic agents. Agents that have been evaluated for use in the gastrointestinal tract include morphine, propantheline bromide (Pro-Banthine), atropine, and related compounds. Some of these agents were abandoned, however, after recognition of their toxicity and undesirable side effects.

Glucagon

Human glucagon is a single-chain polypeptide containing 29 amino acid residues and having a molecular weight of 3485 daltons. Glucagon is generated by α cells in the islets of Langerhans. In some species, glucagon is also produced in the stomach; whether any gastric glucagon is produced in humans is controversial. The amino acid sequence of glucagon in animals ranges from one similar to humans to others with completely different sequences. Identical amino acid sequences are found in humans, pigs, and cattle, an important consideration when glucagon was obtained from animal pancreatic tissue. This became a moot issue, however, when a synthetic glucagon analog was developed.

Glucagon is a hormone having substantial metabolic influence on a number of organs. It binds at specific receptor cell membranes in target organs. In the liver, it stimulates glucose output and hepatic ketogenesis. Glucagon lyses adipose tissue and leads to a reduction of circulating cholesterol and triglyceride levels. It stimulates insulin release and appears to be involved in liver regeneration, where its full role is not clear. Glucagon increases blood flow to the kidneys. It also has specific effects on the adrenal glands and heart.

Glucagon is a relatively potent spasmolytic agent in smooth muscle, and it is this spasmolytic action that accounts for the extensive use of glucagon in gastrointestinal radiology.

Table 2-1
Spasmolytic Effect of Intravenous Glucagon: Average Duration (in Minutes) of Atonicity

Location and Response	Glucagon Dose (mg)			
	0.25	0.5	1.0	2.0
Stomach	4.9	8.7	10.1	15.1
Duodenal bulb	7.5	10.1	12.5	16.7
Duodenum	7.8	10.1	12.5	16.1
Proximal small bowel	8.3	9.4	13.7	19.7
Distal small bowel	8.6	9.4	14.0	19.7

Adapted from Miller RE, Chernish SM, Brunelle RL, et al: Double-blind radiographic study of dose response to intravenous glucagon for hypotonic duodenography. Radiology 127:55-59, 1978, with permission.

Pharmacologic doses are employed. Smooth muscle in different portions of the gastrointestinal tract varies in its sensitivity to glucagon (Table 2-1). For example, 0.1 mg of glucagon administered intravenously is sufficient to induce gastroduodenal hypotonia in most adults,[7] but such a small dose is inadequate for achieving colonic hypotonia, when a dose up to 10 times greater may be required.

Intravascular glucagon is also a vasodilator. As a result, it improves portal vein visualization during mesenteric arteriography. Nevertheless, glucagon has been replaced by other vasodilators because of its propensity to cause nausea and vomiting at the doses required for vasodilation.

Glucagon is degraded by gastric secretions and is therefore ineffective when given orally. Although glucagon is generally administered intravenously, an intranasal route is effective and well tolerated and holds promise for future use.[8]

Effect on Gastrointestinal Tract

Acute esophageal obstruction due to food impaction is common and is often related to an underlying stricture or spasm. Spasmolytic drugs have been suggested if spasm is suspected, but in a multicenter, double-blind study of glucagon and diazepam, no significant difference in disimpaction rates were found for spasmolytic agents versus a placebo.[9] Effervescent agents have also been used with varying success for treatment of esophageal food impactions.

The major advantage of glucagon over anticholinergic agents in inducing hypotonicity of the upper gastrointestinal tract is its lack of side effects. In the United States, glucagon is generally used to induce gastrointestinal hypotonia; in other countries, an anticholinergic agent, scopolamine butylbromide (Buscopan), is more often employed. Although anticholinergic agents are less expensive than glucagon, the price ratio of glucagon to Buscopan fluctuates considerably throughout the world.

Glucagon decreases mean pressures in both the stomach and duodenum.[10] Earlier studies have suggested that anticholinergic agents are better than glucagon for obtaining optimal mucosal coating of the stomach and duodenum with barium, presumably because anticholinergics decrease gastric secretions while glucagon has no effect on gastric secretions. In actual practice, however, Buscopan and glucagon produce comparable distention of the stomach and duodenum and

comparable mucosa coating. A more fundamental question is whether glucagon-induced gastric and duodenal hypotonia improves one's ability to detect lesions in these structures. At least one study found that the diagnostic quality with and without glucagon does not differ significantly.[11] Many radiologists in the United States do not routinely use a hypotonic agent when performing double-contrast upper gastrointestinal studies.

In enteroclysis, barium is instilled until a lesion is detected, a site of obstruction is reached, or the terminal ileum is filled. Glucagon is helpful, if it is deemed desirable to slow barium through the small bowel, such as when a suspicious region is identified. In general, 0.25 mg of glucagon given intravenously produces adequate hypotonia for a leisurely study of the area in question. Alternatively, small bowel distention can be achieved by increasing the injection rate of barium to induce hypotonia.

Glucagon has a relaxant effect on the ileocecal valve, so that barium can reflux more easily into the distal small bowel. If retrograde ileography is being performed because of suspected disease in the distal ileum, glucagon should therefore be routinely administered. Anticholinergics have little effect, however, on the ileocecal valve.

Glucagon may have a role in radiologic therapy of meconium ileus and the ileal plug syndrome.[12]

In select patients, a peroral pneumocolon examination allows double contrast study of the terminal ileum and right colon. Barium is introduced either via a conventional small bowel follow-through study or an enteroclysis approach and air is then insufflated into the colon via an enema tip. Because glucagon relaxes the ileocecal valve, it enables air to reflux more easily into the terminal ileum for double-contrast views of this region.

Colonic hypotonia can be achieved by injecting 2 mg of glucagon intramuscularly. Hypotonia begins within several minutes and lasts about 15 minutes. Hypotonia can also be achieved with 0.25 to 0.5 mg of glucagon given intravenously, although some patients require up to 1.0 mg; the onset of hypotonia with an intravenous injection is almost immediate and lasts approximately 10 minutes. In general, the smaller intravenous dose is used because of cost considerations. In infants and children, an intravenous dose of 0.8 to 1.25 µg/kg has been recommended.[13]

The use of glucagon for barium enema examinations varies considerably among radiologic practices. Glucagon is more commonly employed in hospitalized, elderly, and ill patients. In some practices, glucagon is routinely employed for double-contrast barium enemas but is used more selectively for single-contrast barium enemas. In an outpatient setting, many radiologists use glucagon when a patient has painful spasm, when visualized spasm interferes with the diagnostic aspects of the study, or when a patient is unable to retain the barium. Glucagon decreases both the extent and severity of colonic spasm during a barium enema, so these patients are more comfortable during the examination.

Few studies have evaluated whether the use of glucagon increases the accuracy of double-contrast barium enemas. One prospective double-blind crossover study comparing glucagon with placebo found that both the sensitivity and specificity of the double-contrast barium enema improved after glucagon but that the results were not statistically significant.[14,15] The authors therefore recommended that glucagon be reserved only for patients who have considerable discomfort during the examination, colonic spasm, difficulty retaining the enema, or suspected colitis or diverticulitis. Other investigators found that glucagon actually degrades the examination by promoting reflux of air into the small bowel,[16] but these findings have been questioned.[17]

Occasionally, colonic spasm persists despite the use of intravenous glucagon. It has been my empirical observation that patients with long-standing diabetes have more glucagon-resistant colonic spasm than nondiabetic patients, but the reason for this decreased response in diabetics is not known. At times, refilling the colon with low-density barium several minutes after a failed double-contrast barium enema can result in markedly decreased spasm, enabling the study to be completed.[18]

Reduction of Intussusceptions

Because of its spasmolytic effect and relaxant effect on the ileocecal valve, it has been suggested that glucagon may have a role in reduction of ileocolic intussusceptions. A number of reports have described intussusception reduction after administration of glucagon, but such empirical use does not necessarily indicate that the reduction of these intussusceptions can be attributed to glucagon; even a second or third attempt at reduction is known to improve the overall success rate. Other controlled studies have found similar success rates for intussusception reduction with and without glucagon.

Glucagon in Computed Tomography

Despite glucagon's diverse effects on the liver, it does not appear to influence hepatic CT enhancement.

Both glucagon and somatostatin have been used to decrease motion artifacts when using older scanners with prolonged examination times. Motion artifacts are less of an issue with multidetector CT scanners. Nevertheless, the ability to maintain bowel distention with a hypotonic agent may aid in gastric and bowel wall evaluation.

Although some studies have suggested that glucagon before CT colonography does not improve colonic distention,[19,20] others have found that an antispasmotic agent is useful for maintaining colonic hypotonia during air insufflation and scanning. Spasm that develops during CT colonography can also be decreased by the judicious use of glucagon.

Glucagon in Ultrasound

Occasionally it is helpful to induce bowel atonia in abdominal ultrasound. At times, a sonic window to the biliary tract can be obtained by filling the stomach with fluid and inducing hypotonia of surrounding gastrointestinal structures.[21]

Glucagon in Magnetic Resonance Imaging

Glucagon is currently little used in MRI, although it may have a role if both oral MRI contrasts agents and bowel distention are employed. In one study, intravenous glucagon allowed excellent visualization of normal bowel loops and bowel wall thickening.[22] Glucagon can also help eliminate "ghost" images of positive-contrast opacified bowel.

Contraindications and Side Effects

A myth continues to persist that glucagon should not be given to diabetic patients. It should be pointed out that glucagon is used to treat hypoglycemic reactions in diabetic patients. On the other hand, in the setting of hyperglycemia and ketoacidosis, a temporary additional glucose elevation induced by glucagon is of little clinical significance. The diabetic patient can safely receive glucagon whenever its use is clinically indicated for imaging studies.

Side effects of glucagon are less than those with atropine or propantheline. In one study, the side effects with glucagon were comparable to those seen with a placebo. The prevalence of nausea and vomiting after intravenous injection of glucagon is dose dependent.[23] When given intravenously, slow injection of glucagon decreases this side effect.

Contraindications to glucagon include prior sensitivity to glucagon and a known or suspected pheochromocytoma or insulinoma. Anaphylactic reactions have also been described with the use of glucagon. A rash, periorbital edema, erythema multiforme, respiratory distress, and hypotension have been reported. Glucagon is a naturally occurring polypeptide and in pure form should not result in hypersensitivity reactions. Previously, commercial glucagon contained bovine or porcine insulins, protoinsulins, other nonglucagon protein contaminants, and preservatives, and any of these could be associated with a hypersensitivity reaction. Currently, however, genetically engineered glucagon is associated with very few anaphylactic reactions.

Glucagon can induce release of catecholamines from a pheochromocytoma, resulting in the sudden onset of life-threatening hypertension.

Glucagon can stimulate insulin release from an insulinoma, resulting in severe hypoglycemia; this condition is treated with glucose.

Anticholinergic Agents

Anticholinergic agents as a group are effective in tissues having receptors supplied by cholinergic postganglionic autonomic nerves. These agents block the effect of acetylcholine liberated from nerve endings. Their action on tonicity and motility is similar to that of glucagon, but, unlike glucagon, these agents also reduce secretions. Current evidence suggests that the latter effect is irrelevant for imaging studies.

Anticholinergic agents have been used for the treatment of peptic ulcer disease in conjunction with antacids and histamine receptor antagonists, but data about the effectiveness of this approach are inconclusive and controversial. These agents may also play a role in the therapy for irritable bowel syndrome and have been used as supplemental therapy for decreasing smooth muscle spasm in patients with biliary and ureteral colic; the results of this approach are also inconsistent.

Useful Agents

Anticholinergic agents reduce gastrointestinal tract motility and secretions, decrease tonicity in the urinary tract, and also have a hypotonic effect on the bile ducts. These agents decrease salivary and bronchial secretions, dilate the pupils, and increase the heart rate; the duration of action and specific effects on various target organs depend on the specific agent and dose.

The most widely known anticholinergic agent is atropine sulfate. This agent is available in tablets and as a parenteral injectable liquid. Senior radiologists in North America may still remember the anticholinergic agent, propantheline bromide (ProBanthine), which was in vogue in the 1960s and early 1970s as a gastrointestinal hypotonic agent. Since then, however, it has been supplanted by other agents.

In many countries, the short-acting anticholinergic agent scopolamine butylbromide (Buscopan) is the agent most often employed, but this agent is not available in the United States. It is administered intravenously, a common dose being 20 mg before an upper gastrointestinal examination. Its hypotonic effect lasts for 15 to 20 minutes. Among other indications, Buscopan is useful in CT and MRI for evaluating patients with suspected gastric carcinoma.[24] One study found that Buscopan improves colonic distention during CT colonography compared with controls; the authors therefore recommended that it be used routinely for this procedure.[25]

Scopolamine butylbromide inhibits contraction of the sphincter of Oddi and is therefore thought to facilitate pancreaticobiliary intubation during endoscopic cholangiopancreatography. This agent probably does not induce gastroesophageal reflux, nor does it have any significant effect on the visualization of hiatal hernias.[26]

Pirenzepine, an antimuscarinic drug, shows promise as a hypotonic agent without the adverse effects of scopolamine. Although other anticholinergic agents are available, their side effects and longer action limit their application in gastrointestinal radiology. Thus, scopolamine hydrobromide is available but is not often used in radiologic examinations because of untoward side effects.

Oral hyoscyamine sulfate is a potential hypotonic agent[27] that has similar actions and contraindications as atropine and other anticholinergic agents.[28] One study found that hyoscyamine provided no benefit when used as pain premedication during a barium enema.[29]

Complications

Buscopan can result in blurred vision.[30] In patients predisposed to glaucoma, increased intraocular pressure induced by anticholinergic drugs may precipitate an acute attack. Although most patients with a history of glaucoma have chronic glaucoma, a patient may have acute angle-closure glaucoma and not be aware of it. Acute glaucoma should be suspected if eye pain or loss of vision develop after administration of an anticholinergic agent.

Because of their effect on the autonomic nervous system, anticholinergic agents can also lead to urinary retention. This complication is exacerbated in patients with prostatic hypertrophy or other conditions predisposing to urinary retention.

Allergic reactions to anticholinergic agents are uncommon.

HYPERTONIC GASTROINTESTINAL AGENTS

In some patients, the rate of gastric emptying is increased if the volume of administered barium is increased. A cold barium suspension is not only better tolerated but also leads to more rapid gastric emptying. Faster small bowel transit can be achieved by adding a hyperosmolar product to the barium suspension. In the past, a small amount of diatrizoate meglumine (Gastrografin) was often added to oral barium suspensions to facilitate small bowel transit, but this practice is rare today.

High-osmolality sorbitol added to oral CT contrast agents will accelerate opacification of bowel. For this reason, some manufacturers add sorbitol to their barium sulfate products.

Metoclopramide

Metoclopramide (Maxolon) is an antiemetic agent used to treat diabetic gastroparesis. Its primary effects on the gastrointestinal tract are increased gastric peristalsis, pyloric relaxation, and increased small bowel peristalsis. However, metoclopramide has no major effect on the colon. This agent appears to decrease gastric secretions but has little effect on mucosal coating with barium. A typical dose is 10 to 20 mg given parenterally or orally. It is a relatively safe drug, but extrapyramidal side effects such as acute dystonia and tardive dyskinesia occasionally develop.[31]

Oral metoclopramide reduces small bowel transit time. It can be given shortly before the small bowel study or up to 90 minutes before the examination.[32] Orally administered metoclopramide before CT improves opacification of the ileum and ascending and transverse colon but not the more proximal bowel. A combination of ceruletide and metoclopramide also facilitates visualization of the ileum,[33] because longitudinal contractions and foreshortening of ileal loops tend to elevate the ileum out of the pelvis.

Metoclopramide also appears to be useful for visualizing the pancreas in abdominal ultrasound.[34] Its primary benefit is decreased gastric and duodenal gas artifacts.

Domperidone

Domperidone, a potent dopamine antagonist, increases gastric emptying and accelerates small bowel transit. Its effect on the small bowel appears to be less than that of metoclopramide; a study comparing intravenous domperidone (8 mg) and intravenous metoclopramide (10 mg) found that metoclopramide resulted in significantly faster small bowel transit, but no significant difference was found in examination quality.[35]

Cisapride

Cisapride is a prokinetic substance that increases antral contractility, enhancing gastric emptying and promoting small bowel peristalsis.[36] This agent also enhances lower esophageal sphincter tone and is a relatively potent esophageal motor stimulator. It has been proposed as an agent for treating diabetics with gastroparesis and as an anti–gastroesophageal reflux agent. Cisapride has had limited application in gastrointestinal radiology, and its use has been discontinued in the United States because of associated cardiac arrhythmias and even death.[37]

Neostigmine

Neostigmine methylsulfate (Prostigmin) is a cholinesterase inhibitor that increases gastric and small bowel peristalsis, leading to more rapid gastric emptying and shorter small bowel transit time. This agent promotes peristalsis when intestinal activity is depressed by cholinergic stimulation. It is useful for the treatment of Ogilvie's syndrome[38] but is contraindicated in patients with mechanical bowel obstruction and adynamic ileus.[39] The use of neostigmine has occasionally led to colon perforation.

Erythromycin

Erythromycin improves gastric motility and promotes gastric emptying. It is used in patients with postoperative gastric dilatation and diabetic gastroparesis but has had little application in gastrointestinal radiology.

MIXED ACTION AGENTS

Morphine

Senior radiologists undoubtedly remember using morphine sulfate for hypotonic duodenography, a procedure relegated to history. Currently, morphine has a role in nuclear medicine and a possible role in magnetic resonance cholangiopancreatography (MRCP) (see later).

Cholecystokinin

Cholecystokinin, a peptide hormone, has a myriad of functions; it induces gallbladder contraction and increases bowel peristalsis, resulting in faster small bowel transit. It also regulates pancreatic enzyme secretion, inhibits gastric acid secretion, affects satiety signaling, and acts as a neurotransmitter. The secretion of cholecystokinin is impaired in patients with celiac disease and bulimia nervosa. Untreated patients with celiac disease have low postprandial cholecystokinin levels. This agent is overexpressed in certain neuroendocrine tumors.

In general, only the carboxy-terminal octapeptide of cholecystokinin is used; this fragment is more potent than the entire molecule.

Ceruletide

Ceruletide is a synthetic compound similar to cholecystokinin in its pharmacologic actions; it delays gastric emptying, increases contraction of the gallbladder, and causes hypoperistalsis of the duodenum and hyperperistalsis of the jejunum, ileum, and colon. Ceruletide reverses bowel aperistalsis induced by drugs acting on enteric neural or smooth muscle.

In the early 1980s, ceruletide appeared to be a promising agent for increasing small bowel peristalsis and shortening the duration of small bowel barium studies but radiologists subsequently lost interest in this agent. When given intravenously, ceruletide induces nausea, vomiting, and abdominal cramps. A dose of 0.25 to 0.3 μg/kg is typically used to accelerate small bowel transit. Whether this shorter small bowel transit time leads to a better small bowel study is debatable; pronounced intestinal contractions tend to obscure anatomic detail, particularly in the distal ileum.

Because ceruletide induces gastric hypotonia, it should not be administered before substantial amounts of barium have reached the jejunum. Such gastric stasis can be overcome by administration of metoclopramide.[33]

DRUGS AFFECTING THE BILIARY TRACT AND PANCREAS

Bile flow into the duodenum is regulated both by bile production in the liver and gallbladder tonicity; drugs affecting only the gallbladder are considered in this section.

Inhibition of gallbladder contractions can be achieved by glucagon, atropine and other cholinergic drugs, somatostatin, calcium channel antagonists, and other less-studied agents. Gallbladder contractions are also inhibited in patients with obesity, diabetes mellitus, celiac disease, and autonomic neuropathy. Conversely, gallbladder contraction is stimulated by cholecystokinin, ceruletide, motilin, prostigmine, erythromycin, and possibly cisapride and cholestyramine.

Glucagon relaxes the gallbladder. Glucagon also decreases mean systolic and diastolic pressures in the papilla of Vater,[10] but these effects of glucagon have little clinical utility for biliary imaging studies. In patients with persistent narrowing of the distal common bile duct at or near the sphincter of Oddi, the use of glucagon can sometimes aid in differentiating tumor or an impacted stone from spasm. In most patients, however, the judicious use of fluoroscopy is adequate for this purpose.

The use of intravenous glucagon improves visualization of the bile ducts during MRCP.[40] Because incomplete visualization of the bile ducts often leads to a repeat study or even an invasive procedure such as ERCP, the routine of glucagon for MRCP seems warranted.

Although earlier studies suggested that glucagon improves the quality of operative cholangiography, a double-blind prospective study did not support this finding.[41] The use of fentanyl during surgery is associated with spasm of the sphincter of Oddi, and glucagon may also have a role in these patients.

Hypotonic agents are commonly employed to induce duodenal hypotonia and facilitate cannulation of the ampulla during endoscopic retrograde cholangiopancreatography (ERCP). In the United States, glucagon is used almost exclusively for this purpose, but in other countries one of the anticholinergic drugs is more often employed.

The combined use of neostigmine and morphine has been proposed as a provocative test in hepatobiliary scintigraphy for evaluating sphincter of Oddi dyskinesia in postcholecystectomy patients.[42]

Morphine may have a role in MRCP; intravenous morphine constricts the sphincter of Oddi, thus distending the biliary and pancreatic ducts.[5] As a result, morphine may improve visualization of the biliary ducts in patients with primary sclerosing cholangitis. An interval of 10 to 20 minutes between morphine injection and imaging appears reasonable.[43]

Cholecystokinin's effect on the gallbladder has been used to increase radiographic contrast during oral cholecystography; this agent also is useful for evaluating gallbladder function. Gallbladder ejection fraction is typically determined with hepatobiliary scintigraphy and less often with ultrasonography. If needed, MRCP with infusion of a cholecystokinin derivative (sincalide) can also be used as an alternate method for determining gallbladder ejection fraction.

A provocative test using sincalide to identify patients with acalculous cholecystitis who are likely to benefit from cholecystectomy has not achieved general clinical acceptance. Cholecystokinin relaxes the sphincter of Oddi and appears to facilitate passage of bile duct stones. On the other hand, a cholecystokinin receptor antagonist provides pain relief in patients with biliary colic.[44] Interestingly, cholecystokinin does not have its usual inhibitory effect on the sphincter of Oddi after a cholecystectomy.[45] Cholecystokinin is also useful as a diagnostic test of pancreatic function.

Ceruletide has an effect on the gallbladder similar to that of cholecystokinin or a fatty meal.[46] In patients with recurrent symptoms after cholecystectomy, an ultrasonographically detected increase in extrahepatic bile duct dilation after ceruletide injection should suggest dysfunction of the sphincter of Oddi.[47]

Secretin is used less often for MRCP than glucagon; its specific role is not yet clear.

The cholecystokinin/secretin pancreatic exocrine function test is used to detect pancreatic exocrine insufficiency but does not differentiate between chronic pancreatitis and pancreatic carcinoma. MRI can also evaluate pancreatic exocrine function by measuring duodenal filling after stimulation with secretin.[48] Secretin improves pancreatic duct visualization and aids in detecting abnormalities during MRCP.[49] Pancreas divisum and other abnormalities are more readily detected after secretin, potentially obviating the need for ERCP. MRCP is best performed within 5 minutes after secretin injection.[50] Secretin-augmented MRCP and MR perfusion are also useful for detecting graft dysfunction after pancreatic transplants.[51]

Analysis of duodenal aspirations of pancreatic juice after cholecystokinin-octapeptide stimulation will enable detection of pancreatic insufficiency in patients with chronic pancreatitis, but the analogous secretin test is more commonly performed.

References

1. Tanioka H, Araki T, Sasaki Y, et al: Famotidine for gastric radiography. Radiat Med 11:12-16, 1993.
2. Ryan JM, Key SM, Dumbleton SA, Smith TP: Nonlocalized lower gastrointestinal bleeding: Provocative bleeding studies with intraarterial tPA, heparin, and tolazoline. J Vasc Intervent Radiol 12:1273-1277, 2001.
3. Huwer H, Winning J, Straub U, et al: Clinically diagnosed nonocclusive mesenteric ischemia after cardiopulmonary bypass: Retrospective study. Vascular 12:114-120, 2004.
4. Chamsuddin AA, Kowalik KJ, Bjarnason H, et al: Using a dopamine type 1A receptor agonist in high-risk patients to ameliorate contrast-associated nephropathy. AJR 179:591-596, 2002.
5. Yamagami T, Nakamura T, Iida S, et al: Effects of prostaglandin E(1) injection through the superior mesenteric artery on the hemodynamics of hepatocellular carcinoma. AJR 178:349-352, 2002.
6. Yamagami T, Nakamura T, Sato O, et al: Value of intraarterial prostaglandin E(1) injection during CT hepatic arteriography. AJR 177:115-119, 2001.
7. Miller RE, Chernish SM, Brunelle RL, et al: Double-blind radiographic study of dose response to intravenous glucagon for hypotonic duodenography. Radiology 127:55-59, 1978.
8. Pacchioni M, Orena C, Panizza P, et al: The hypotonic effect of intranasal and intravenous glucagon in gastrointestinal radiology. Abdom Imaging 20:44-46, 1995.
9. Tibbling L, Bjorkhoel A, Jansson E, Stenkvist M: Effect of spasmolytic drugs on esophageal foreign bodies. Dysphagia 10:126-127 1995.
10. Takemoto T, Okia K, Tada M, et al: Glucagon in digestive endoscopy—its usefulness for premedication. In Picazo J (ed): Glucagon in 1987. Lancaster, England, MTP Press, 1987, pp 55-66.
11. Rothe AJ, Young JWR, Keramati B: The value of glucagon in routine barium investigations of the gastrointestinal tract. Invest Radiol 22:786-791, 1987.
12. Mandell GA, Teplick SK: Glucagon—its application to childhood gastrointestinal radiology. Gastrointest Radiol 7:7-13, 1982.
13. Ratcliffe JF: Glucagon in barium examinations in infants and children: Special reference to dosage. Br J Radiol 53:860-862, 1980.
14. Thoeni RF, Vandeman F, Wall SD: Effect of glucagon on the diagnostic accuracy of double-contrast barium enema examinations. AJR 142:111-114, 1984.
15. Thoeni RFL: Importance of sample size for statistical significance [Letter]. AJR 143:924, 1984.
16. Stone EE, Conte FA: Glucagon-induced small bowel air reflux: Degrading effects on double-contrast colon examinations. Gastrointest Radiol 13:212-214, 1988.
17. Maglinte DDT, Chernish SM: Glucagon-induced small bowel air reflux: Degrading effects on double-contrast colon examination [Letter]. Gastrointest Radiol 14:85-87, 1989.
18. Levine MS, Gasparaitis AE: Barium filling for glucagon-resistant spasm on double-contrast barium enema examinations. Radiology 160:264-265, 1986.
19. Yee J, Hung RK, Akerkar GA, Wall SD: The usefulness of glucagon hydrochloride for colonic distention in CT colonography. AJR 173:169-172, 1999.
20. Morrin MM, Farrell RJ, Keogan MT, et al: CT colonography: Colonic distention improved by dual positioning but not intravenous glucagon. Eur Radiol 12:525-530, 2002.
21. Op den Orth JO: Sonography of the pancreatic head aided by water and glucagon. Radiographics 7:85-100, 1987.
22. Low RN, Francis IR: MR imaging of the gastrointestinal tract with IV gadolinium and diluted barium oral contrast media compared with unenhanced MR imaging and CT. AJR 169:1051-1059, 1997.
23. Chernish SM, Maglinte DDT: Glucagon: Common untoward reactions—review and recommendations. Radiology 177:145-146, 1990.
24. Sohn KM, Lee JM, Lee SY, et al: Comparing MR imaging and CT in the staging of gastric carcinoma. AJR 174:1551-1557, 2000.
25. Taylor SA, Halligan S, Goh V, et al: Optimizing colonic distention for multi-detector row CT colonography: Effect of hyoscine butylbromide and rectal balloon catheter. Radiology 229:99-108, 2003.
26. McLoughlin RF, Mathieson JR, Chipperfield PM, et al: Effect of hyoscine butylbromide on gastroesophageal reflux in barium studies of the upper gastrointestinal tract. Can Assoc Radiol J 45:452-454, 1994.
27. Bova JG, Jurdi RA, Bennett WF. Antispasmodic drugs to reduce discomfort and colonic spasm during barium enemas: Comparison of oral hyoscyamine, I.V. glucagon, and no drug. AJR 161:965-968, 1993.
28. Skucas J: The use of antispasmotic drugs during barium enemas. AJR 162:1323-1325, 1994.
29. Bova JG, Bhattacharjee N, Jurdi R, Bennett WF: Comparison of no medication, placebo, and hyoscyamine for reducing pain during a barium enema. AJR 172:1285-1287, 1999.
30. Goei R, Nix M, Kessels AH, et al: Use of antispasmodic drugs in double contrast barium enema examination: Glucagon or buscopan? Clin Radiol 50:553-557, 1995.
31. Cory DA: Adverse reaction to metoclopramide during enteroclysis [Letter]. AJR 163:480, 1994.
32. Paul N, Rawlinson J, Keir M: The use of metoclopramide for the small bowel meal examination: Pre-procedural versus peri-procedural oral administration. Br J Radiol 69:1130-1133, 1996.
33. Weidenmaier W, Friedrich JM, Schif A, et al: Medikamentöse Beeinflussung der fractionierten Dünndarmdoppelkontrastdarstellung. ROFO 152:137-141, 1990.
34. duCret RP, Jackson VP, Rees C, et al: Pancreatic sonography: Enhancement by metoclopramide. AJR 146:341-343, 1986.
35. Morewood DJW, Whitehouse GH: A comparison of three methods for performing barium follow-through studies of the small intestine. Br J Radiol 59:971-973, 1986.
36. Degryse H, De Schepper A, Verlinden M: A double-blind fluoroscopic study of cisapride on gastrointestinal motility in patients with functional dyspepsia. Scand J Gastroenterol (Suppl) 195:1-4, 1993.
37. Wysowski DK, Corken A, Gallo-Torres H, et al: Postmarketing reports of QT prolongation and ventricular arrhythmia in association with cisapride and Food and Drug Administration regulatory actions. Am J Gastroenterol 96:1698-1703, 2001.
38. Fazel A, Verne GN: New solutions to an old problem: Acute colonic pseudo-obstruction. J Clin Gastroenterol 39:17-20, 2005.
39. St John PH, Radcliffe AG: Contraindication for the use of neostigmine in colonic pseudo-obstruction [Letter]. Br J Surg 84:1481-1482, 1997.
40. Dalal PU, Howlett DC, Sallomi DF, et al: Does intravenous glucagon improve common bile duct visualisation during magnetic resonance cholangiopancreatography? Results in 42 patients. Eur J Radiol 49:258-261, 2004.
41. Cofer JB, Barnett RM, Major GR, et al: Effect of intravenous glucagon on intraoperative cholangiography. South Med J 81:455-456, 1988.
42. Madacsy L, Velosy B, Lonovics J, et al: Evaluation of results of the prostigmine-morphine test with quantitative hepatobiliary scintigraphy: A new method for the diagnosis of sphincter of Oddi dyskinesia. Eur J Nucl Med 22:227-232, 1995.

43. Silva AC, Friese JL, Hara AK, Liu PT: MR cholangiopancreatography: Improved ductal distention with intravenous morphine administration. Radiographics 24:677-687, 2004.

44. Malesci A, Pezzilli R, D'Amato M, Rovati L: CCK-1 receptor blockade for treatment of biliary colic: a pilot study. Aliment Pharmacol Ther 18:333-337, 2003.

45. Luman W, Williams AJ, Pryde A, et al: Influence of cholecystectomy on sphincter of Oddi motility. Gut 41:371-374, 1997.

46. Muraca M, Cianci V, Vilei MT, et al: Ultrasonic evaluation of gallbladder emptying with ceruletide. Ital J Gastroenterol 28:38-39, 1996.

47. Wehrmann T, Aharonoff H, Dietrich CF, et al: [Do ultrasound parameters allow diagnosis of biliary sphincter of Oddi dysfunction?] [German]. Z Gastroenterol 35:449-457, 1997.

48. Heverhagen JT, Muller D, Battmann A, et al: MR hydrometry to assess exocrine function of the pancreas: Initial results of noninvasive quantification of secretion. Radiology 218:61-67, 2001.

49. Monill J, Pernas J, Clavero J, et al: Pancreatic duct after pancreato-duodenectomy: Morphologic and functional evaluation with secretin-stimulated MR pancreatography. AJR 183:1267-1274, 2004.

50. Fukukura Y, Fujiyoshi F, Sasaki M, Nakajo M: Pancreatic duct: Morphologic evaluation with MR cholangiopancreatography after secretin stimulation. Radiology 222:674-680, 2002.

51. Heverhagen JT, Wagner HJ, Ebel H, et al: Pancreatic transplants: Noninvasive evaluation with secretin-augmented MR pancreatography and MR perfusion measurements—preliminary results. Radiology 233:273-280, 2004.

Barium Studies: Single Contrast

David J. Ott, MD

DIAGNOSTIC PRINCIPLES	**UPPER GASTROINTESTINAL SERIES**
EQUIPMENT	**SMALL BOWEL**
BARIUM SUSPENSIONS	**ENTEROCLYSIS**
QUALITY CONTROLS	**BARIUM ENEMA**
ESOPHAGOGRAM	

Since the 1980s, advances in cross-sectional imaging and endoscopy have led to a gradual but steady decline in the number of barium studies performed in the United States.[1] Nevertheless, single-contrast barium examinations are still performed and are most appropriate in elderly or debilitated patients who are unable to cooperate fully for a double-contrast study.[2,3] The purpose of this chapter is to review the various technical and interpretive aspects of single-contrast studies.

DIAGNOSTIC PRINCIPLES

Depending on the organ examined, single-contrast techniques may include observation of function (e.g., the pharynx and esophagus for motility), compression imaging, full-column distention, mucosal relief views, and limited air-contrast images (e.g., the duodenal bulb).[4-6] Compression imaging and the use of compression during fluoroscopy are critical components of the single-contrast examination. Small lesions (e.g., small ulcers or polypoid neoplasms) are often visible only when the barium pool is thinned or displaced by compression. The barium suspension must also be adequately diluted if abnormalities (especially small lesions) are to be detected.

Full-column distention of a particular gastrointestinal viscus is ideal for showing focal areas of narrowing, large neoplasms, and tangentially projecting lesions such as ulcers or diverticula. Multiple full-column views of barium-filled organs in various projections are best for depicting large ulcers and bulky tumors. On the other hand, many small lesions will not be visible on full-column views unless they are viewed in profile. In such cases, mucosal techniques are required to supplement the barium-filled views.

EQUIPMENT

Fluoroscopic equipment has evolved dramatically with the transition from film-cassette–based radiography to digital imaging and viewing on PACS workstations.[7-10] Regardless of the imaging technology, single-contrast examinations can be performed on conventional or remote-control fluoroscopic equipment.[7] The ability to obtain optimal compression views is a major prerequisite of any well-designed fluoroscope. Compression can be performed manually or with a variety of hand-held devices on a conventional machine; alternatively, the compression cone on the spot image device can be used for compression.

On remote-control equipment, compression is easily performed with a vertical movable device incorporated into the machine, and is facilitated by the ability to angle the x-ray tube. All fluoroscopic studies performed in my department are on remote control digital fluoroscopes. The digital machines that we use (Siemens; Erlangen, Germany) have an excellent compression device that allows graded compression as well as tube angulation with compression. Several different compression cones are available; a gently rounded, pyramidal plastic device is used primarily for upper gastrointestinal, small bowel, and colonic studies. This allows large areas of the abdomen to be compressed and imaged. With digital fluoroscopes, compression can also be obtained using the "zoom" features of the equipment.

BARIUM SUSPENSIONS

Numerous barium products are available commercially; a number are formulated for specific purposes (e.g., the double-contrast barium enema), whereas others can be used for a variety of examinations.[11,12] Barium suspensions for single-contrast studies should be well suspended and of moderate density (50% to 100% w/v) when not diluted; the optimal density of the barium suspension depends on the type of examination, the equipment, the recording method (i.e., film-based vs. digital), and the desired kilovoltage. The ideal kilovoltage also depends on a variety of factors, including the need to obtain adequate penetration of the barium column without degradation of the image. Barium suspensions used for single-contrast examinations should exhibit good coating properties to ensure adequate visualization on mucosal relief views, double-contrast views of the duodenal bulb, and post-evacuation radiographs of the colon.

The optimal densities of barium suspensions for single-contrast examinations of the gastrointestinal tract depend on the organ being examined and the type of examination that is being performed. For example, the esophagogram requires an undiluted, moderately dense barium suspension that can provide full-column and mucosal relief imaging; a high-density barium suspension or paste may also be needed for optimal mucosal coating. A similar barium suspension can be used for the upper gastrointestinal examination in which compression views, mucosal relief views, and limited double-contrast views are required. A standard peroral small bowel examination can be performed with the same barium suspension used for the upper gastrointestinal series. A single-contrast enteroclysis study requires a 15% to 20% w/v barium suspension, although somewhat denser solutions have been recommended.[13,14] For the single-contrast barium enema, a 15% to 20% w/v barium suspension is generally recommended, because this is the optimal suspension for obtaining compression views of the colon.

QUALITY CONTROLS

Quality control for single-contrast examinations requires balancing barium density, kilovoltage, and width of the barium column to provide translucency of the barium-filled bowel. This permits radiographic penetration of the barium suspension to ensure visualization of lesions that may be hidden by the barium-filled viscus.[2,5,6] Sufficient penetration of the barium column is achieved if skeletal shadows are visible through the barium column. Visibility of bone shadows through the barium column indicates that small filling defects will also be seen, which is particularly important for detection of colonic polyps.

Another quality control consideration, especially during the barium enema and small bowel examinations, is the ability to see through two overlapping loops of bowel.[2,15] On some barium enema studies, a tortuous sigmoid colon may prevent separation of overlapping loops, even with compression and the ability to obtain angled images. Also, overlapping small bowel loops within the pelvis may compromise the fluoroscopist's ability to detect abnormalities in the distal ileum. In such cases, visualization of pelvic loops of small bowel and colon can be improved by placing the patient in a prone position while he or she lies on some type of bolster.[16]

ESOPHAGOGRAM

A routine esophagogram may include fluoroscopic observation of the esophagus supplemented by motion recordings, double-contrast imaging, full-column technique, and mucosal relief views.[17,18] Full-column (barium-filled views) and mucosal relief views constitute the single-contrast phase of the examination. Motion recordings can be used to document pharyngeal function and esophageal motility using analog or digital videotape or rapid sequence solid-state recordings built into modern digital fluoroscopes.[7-10]

Depending on the imaging options of the fluoroscopic equipment, obtaining partial or full-length views of the esophagus distended with barium is the basis of the full-column technique. These images of the barium-filled esophagus allow detection of esophageal carcinoma (Fig. 3-1) and of the common abnormalities at the gastroesophageal junction, including hiatal hernias, peptic strictures, and lower esophageal rings.[17] Lower esophageal rings are best visualized on prone views of the barium-distended lower esophagus, especially if supplemented by the use of a solid bolus such as a marshmallow or barium tablet.[17-19]

Full-column images of the esophagus are usually obtained with the patient on the fluoroscopic table in the prone, right anterior oblique position (a bolster may be used to increase intra-abdominal pressure). Esophageal peristalsis is inhibited by rapid swallowing of barium, allowing the esophagus to fully distend. Multiple images of the esophagus at all levels should be obtained; these images may be full-length views of the entire esophagus or smaller images exposed at different levels, depending on the imaging options available.

Maximal distention of the esophagogastric region is required for optimal detection of hiatal hernias and lower

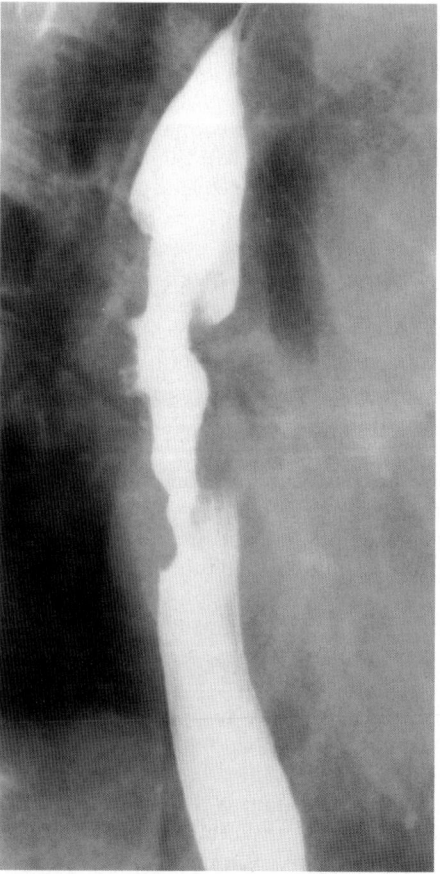

Figure 3-1. Annular carcinoma of the midesophagus. The lesion is well shown on the full-column portion of the barium esophagram.

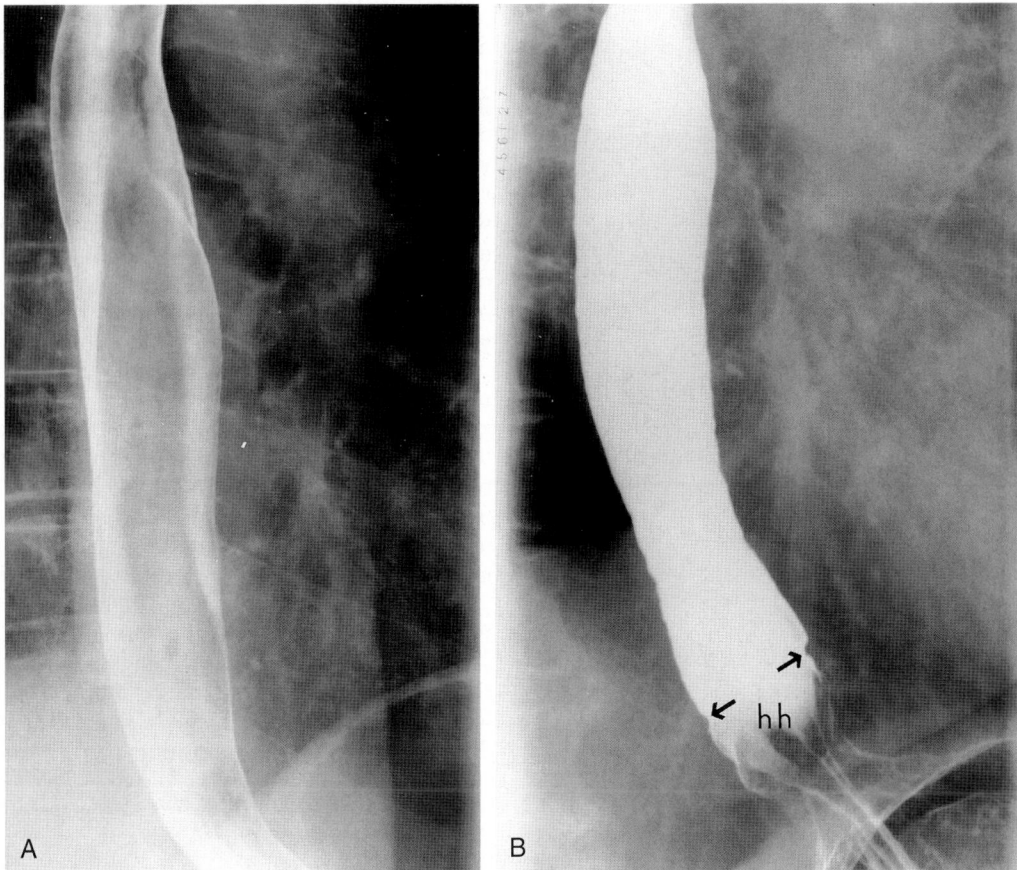

Figure 3-2. Hiatal hernia and lower esophageal ring seen only on prone single-contrast esophagogram. A. Upright double-contrast view of the esophagus shows no abnormalities. **B.** Prone full-column view of the esophagogastric region in the same patient shows a hiatal hernia (hh) and a widely patent lower esophageal mucosal ring (*arrows*).

esophageal rings (Fig. 3-2).[17,19] Rapid ingestion of the barium suspension followed by deep inspiration (and a Valsalva maneuver) promotes maximal distention of the gastroesophageal junction. Fluoroscopic observation will ensure optimal distention of the lower esophagus and maximize visualization of lesions seen as transient findings during swallowing.

The full-column views are complemented by mucosal relief views of the collapsed esophagus with the esophageal folds coated by the barium suspension.[18] This technique provides excellent views of the esophageal mucosa. A high-density barium suspension (such as that used for the double-contrast upper gastrointestinal examination) is ideal for this purpose. The patient takes one or several swallows of the high-density barium suspension with imaging of the collapsed esophageal folds coated with barium.

Mucosal relief views can demonstrate thickening and irregularity of esophageal folds; small esophageal neoplasms and reflux or infectious esophagitis may be detected with this technique (Fig. 3-3). Although the diagnosis of infectious esophagitis can be suggested on mucosal relief views, it may not be possible to determine the type of infection causing the esophagitis. Double-contrast views of the esophagus better demonstrate discrete erosions or larger ulcers, which are more specific for viral or human immunodeficiency virus infection.[20]

The single-contrast mucosal relief technique is also best for detecting esophageal varices.[18,21] The patient takes several swallows of the barium suspension, which coats the lower esophagus, and is then asked not to swallow to inhibit peristalsis. Intermittent fluoroscopic observation is performed for several minutes to visualize the submucosal varices as they become more distended. Various drugs such as atropine can be given to enhance variceal filling by inducing esophageal relaxation.

Fluoroscopic observation is an integral part of the radiographic evaluation of the esophagus and is usually adequate to assess esophageal function.[4,18] Motion recording methods greatly aid in evaluating oropharyngeal swallowing disorders because of the rapid events that occur with deglutition and may also be used to assess esophageal motility. The patient is asked to take multiple, separate single swallows of barium. Each swallow must be viewed completely; rapid swallowing causes reflex inhibition of esophageal peristalsis. With the use of single swallows, the esophagogram is an excellent technique for evaluating esophageal motility.[4]

UPPER GASTROINTESTINAL SERIES

The single-contrast upper gastrointestinal series is a complex examination requiring abdominal compression, fluoroscopic observation, the use of multiple techniques, and limited air-contrast views of the stomach and duodenum.[6,22] The esophagus, stomach, and duodenum are examined routinely using a combination of these techniques. The examination can be

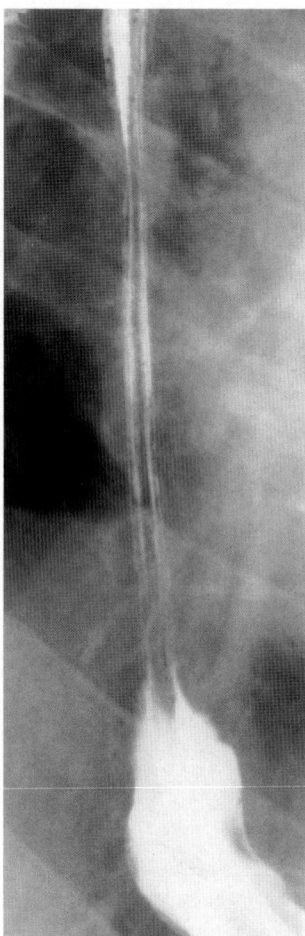

Figure 3-3. Reflux esophagitis on mucosal relief view of the esophagus. Mucosal relief view from single-contrast esophagogram shows crenulated, irregular folds in the distal esophagus, suggesting esophagitis. Reflux esophagitis was confirmed at endoscopy.

performed quickly, and it can be tolerated by patients who are immobile or unable to cooperate fully.

The examination starts with the table upright. The patient ingests several swallows of the barium suspension. Compression of the stomach below the ribs is then performed manually or with a compression device, depending on the fluoroscopic equipment. During compression imaging, the rugal folds of the stomach should be clearly seen. Compression also allows assessment of the pliability of the gastric wall and detection of focal areas of rigidity secondary to tumor or scarring. The barium-filled duodenal bulb can also be examined by compression at this time (or later in the examination).

Without additional ingestion of barium suspension, the table is lowered to the horizontal position. Mucosal relief views of the stomach are then obtained, first with the patient in a supine position and then after the patient turns into a prone position. These views supplement the upright compression views and may show small polyps, erosions, or ulcers that are obscured by further barium filling of the stomach (Fig. 3-4).[23-25]

With the patient in the prone, right anterior oblique position, the esophagus is examined using the same fluoroscopic and imaging techniques described previously (see section on Esophagogram). The duodenal bulb usually fills with barium in this position. Images of the barium-filled gastric antrum, duodenal bulb, and remaining duodenum are obtained. Prone compression imaging of the distal stomach and duodenal bulb can be achieved at this time using an inflatable balloon paddle placed beneath the patient; this maneuver allows detection of anterior wall lesions in the antrum and duodenal bulb (Fig. 3-5).[22]

With the patient in the supine left posterior oblique position, air in the stomach rises into the gastric antrum and duodenal bulb and double-contrast images of these areas are obtained (Fig. 3-6). Compression can be used to displace the barium suspension, separate the antroduodenal structures,

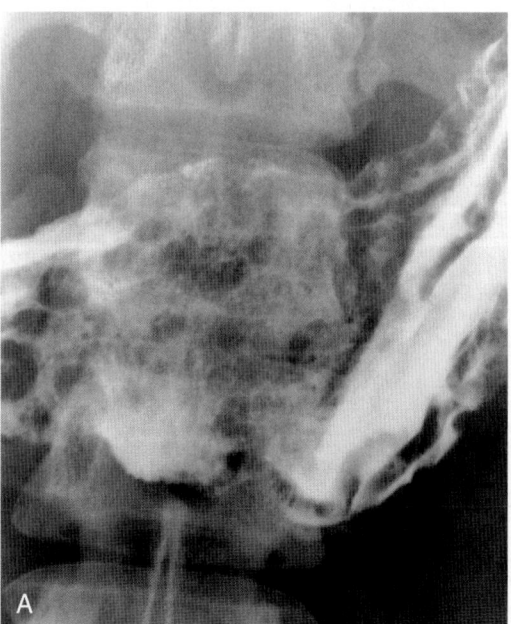
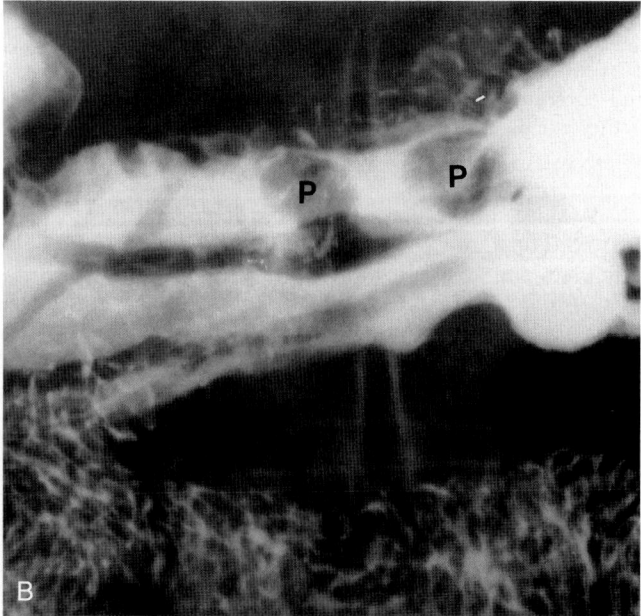

Figure 3-4. Recumbent compression views for detecting lesions in the stomach. A. Compression view of the gastric antrum shows antral erosions as multiple tiny nodules containing punctate collections of barium. **B.** In another patient, compression view of the antrum shows several small polyps (P) as filling defects in the barium pool. The findings in **A** and **B** were not well shown on double-contrast views but were confirmed at endoscopy.

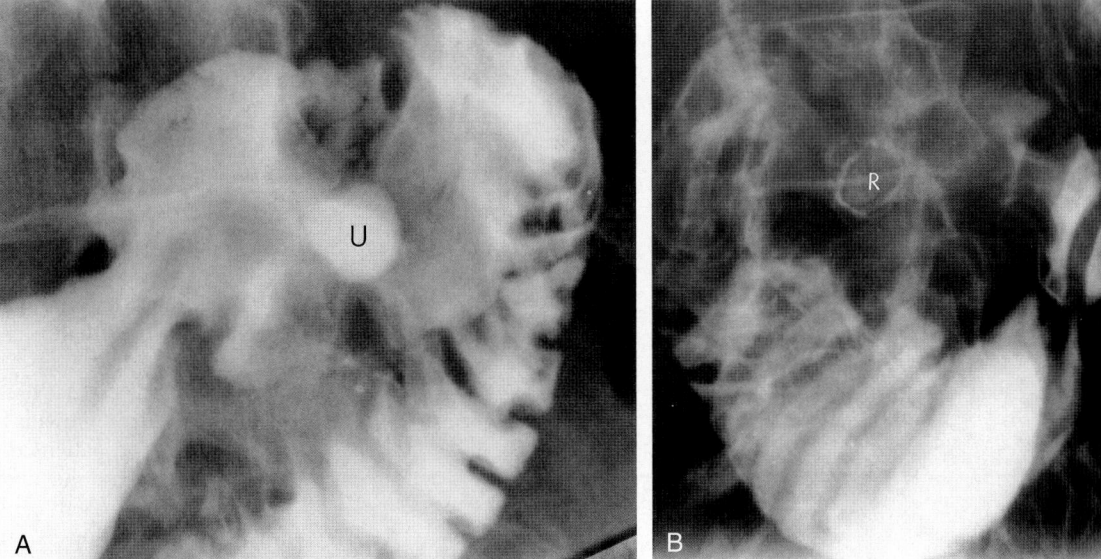

Figure 3-5. Prone compression view of the duodenal bulb for detecting an anterior wall ulcer. A. Prone view of the duodenal bulb (a balloon paddle compression device was used) shows an anterior wall ulcer (U) with surrounding edema. **B.** Supine oblique air-contrast view of the duodenal bulb in the same patient shows a ring shadow (R) due to barium coating the rim of the unfilled anterior wall ulcer crater.

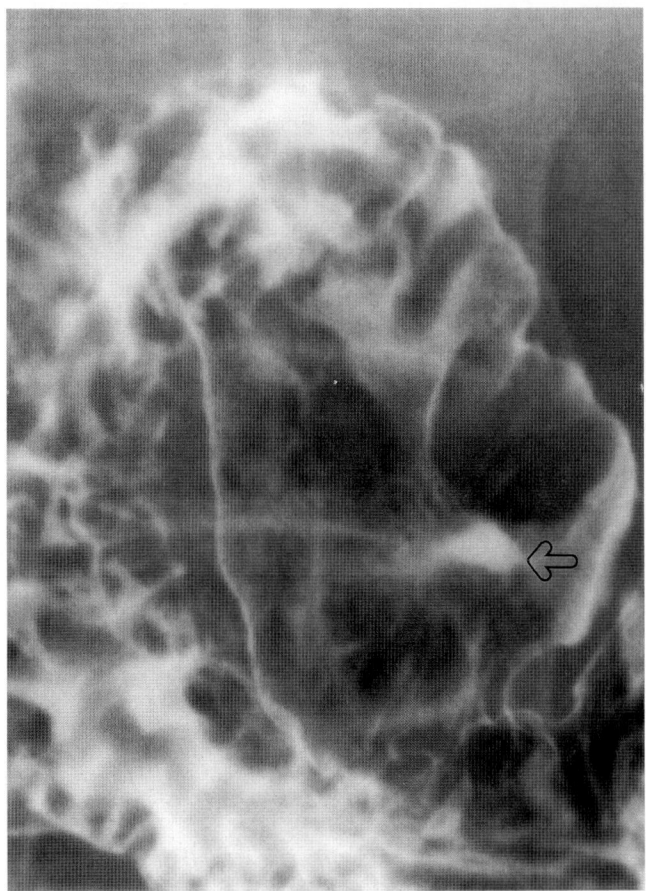

Figure 3-6. Posterior wall duodenal ulcer on air-contrast view of the bulb. Supine oblique air-contrast view of the duodenal bulb with compression shows a small posterior wall ulcer (*arrow*), emphasizing the importance of obtaining limited double-contrast views as part of a thorough "single-contrast" upper gastrointestinal examination.

and improve distention with air. The fluoroscopic portion of the examination is completed at this time.

After the fluoroscopic examination is completed, overhead radiographs of the barium-filled stomach and duodenum can be obtained by the technologist, who may use fluoroscopy for optimal positioning of the stomach and duodenum for each radiograph. On remote-control devices, these views can be obtained during the fluoroscopic examination. A standard set of images includes views of the stomach and duodenum with the patient in prone, supine, right anterior oblique, and right lateral positions.

SMALL BOWEL

The small bowel can be examined by peroral techniques, by enteroclysis, or in a retrograde manner via an ostomy or reflux from the colon.[13,14,16] The peroral study may be performed after a single-contrast upper gastrointestinal series or as a separate examination. Careful fluoroscopic compression of all small bowel loops is crucial to ensure an accurate examination.

A large volume (at least 500 mL) of barium suspension is used for the peroral examination; this volume of barium promotes gastric emptying, accelerates small bowel transit, and allows optimal distention of small bowel loops. Filling of the entire small bowel is best achieved if the patient ingests additional barium suspension after the stomach has emptied. Careful compression is then applied to separate individual small bowel loops for fluoroscopic inspection and imaging.

The following method for the peroral small bowel examination is recommended. The patient initially ingests a minimum of 500 mL of a well-suspended barium suspension, which can be the same product used for the single-contrast upper gastrointestinal examination. Prone large images of the small intestine are taken at timed intervals (e.g., 15 minutes, 30 minutes, 1 hour, 2 hours) until the barium suspension fills

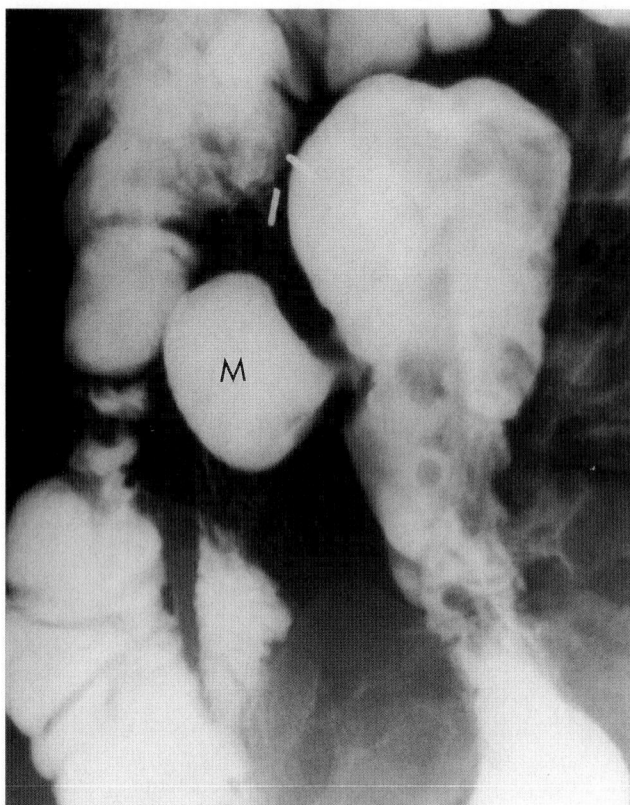

Figure 3-7. Compression spot image of the small bowel for detecting Meckel's diverticulum. Peroral small bowel examination was performed in a patient with gastrointestinal bleeding. Compression spot image of the right lower quadrant shows a Meckel diverticulum (M) as the cause of the patient's bleeding. The diverticulum was removed at surgery.

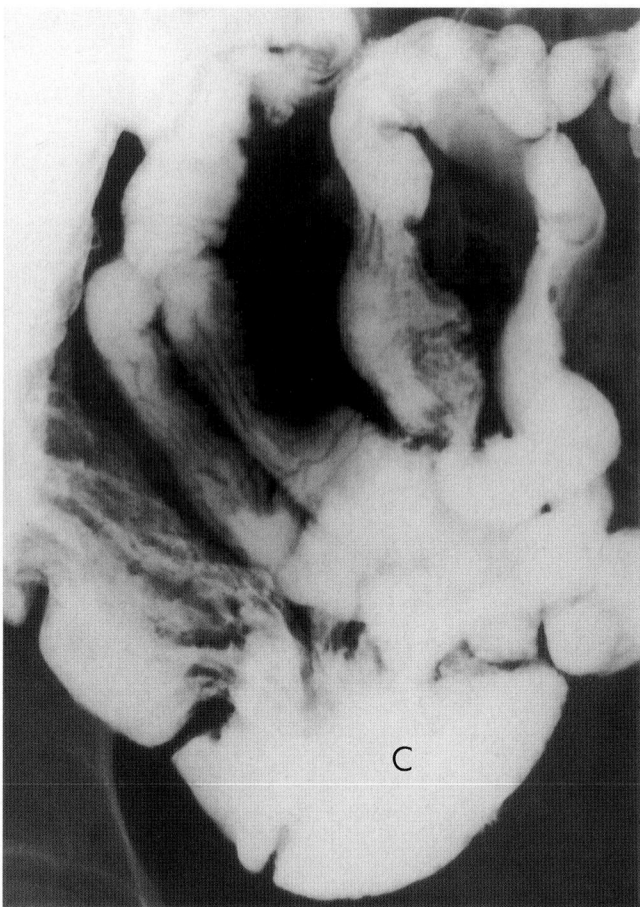

Figure 3-8. Peroral small bowel examination in a posthysterectomy patient with pelvic small bowel loops lying deep within the pelvis. Prone image of the pelvis with a bolster placed beneath the patient and x-ray tube angulation clearly shows the cecum (C) and ileocecal junction. Note how pelvic loops of ileum are well separated and visualized.

the right side of the colon. Depending on the barium product used, transit time through the small bowel is typically 60 to 90 minutes in most patients. If the stomach is kept full of barium, transit time is shortened and small bowel distention is improved during the study.

Fluoroscopic compression and imaging should be performed at various times during the examination. Compression of all loops and appropriate imaging of the entire small bowel should be performed to optimize detection of lesions (Fig. 3-7). When the barium suspension has reached the colon, compression imaging of the distal small bowel and terminal ileum is carefully performed. Placing the patient in both oblique positions will also better separate laterally located loops of small bowel and minimize overlap. The terminal ileum is best visualized with the patient in a supine position or turned slightly to the left; compression is used to displace adjacent loops of small bowel for a better view of the terminal ileum.

Clear delineation of pelvic loops of small intestine, which are often overlapped, is not always possible, but several maneuvers may be performed to improved visualization of these loops.[16] First, the patient should be told not to void during the examination because a full bladder elevates pelvic loops, enabling better visualization. A similar effect may be achieved by instilling air into the rectum. Respiratory maneuvers may also displace bowel loops from the pelvis. Finally, the patient can be placed in the prone position (head down)

with a bolster placed beneath the lower abdomen and pelvis; this maneuver displaces pelvic small bowel loops superiorly, and, if available, tube angulation can further separate these loops (Fig. 3-8).

ENTEROCLYSIS

An intubation small bowel study (i.e., enteroclysis) is performed via a tube placed into the duodenum or jejunum.[14,16,26] Several enteroclysis tubes are available commercially. The route of intubation can be via the mouth or the nose, with each having advantages and drawbacks. When single-contrast enteroclysis is performed, jejunal intubation is preferred to prevent duodenogastric reflux and vomiting of the barium suspension.

Approximately 800 mL of a 15% to 20% w/v barium suspension is placed in an enema bag, which is hung on an adjustable vertical stand or IV pole. Water-soluble contrast material (60 mL) is added to stimulate intestinal peristalsis and shorten the length of the examination.[11,12,16] The barium suspension is allowed to flow through the tube by gravity, and the rate of flow (80 to 120 mL/min) can be regulated by adjusting the height of the enema bag. If the barium suspension flows too slowly, adequate distention is not achieved. Conversely, a rapid

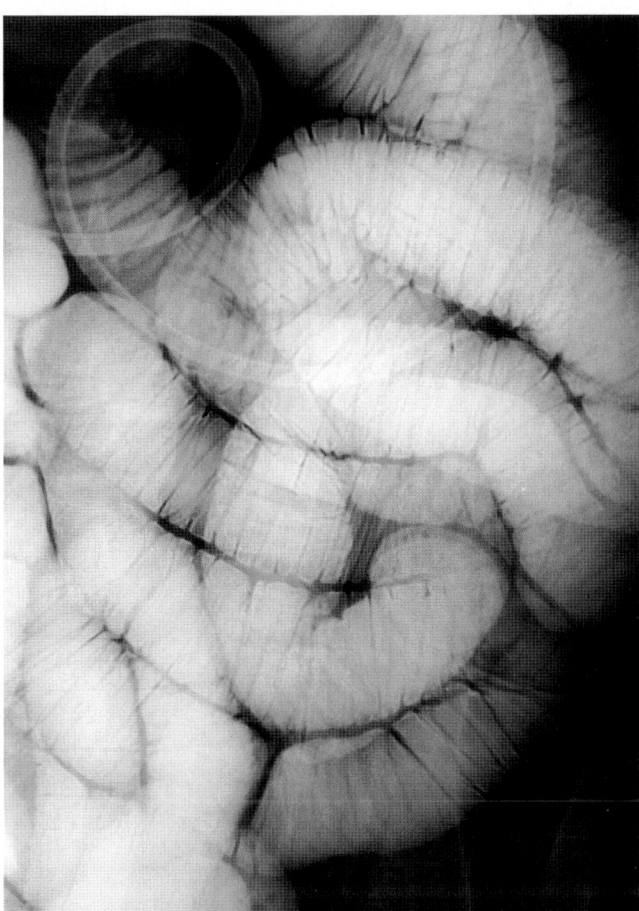

Figure 3-9. Single-contrast enteroclysis. Normal small bowel loops are well distended with the valvulae conniventes in a parallel arrangement. The use of a dilute barium suspension permits a "see-through" effect for visualization of overlapping loops of small bowel.

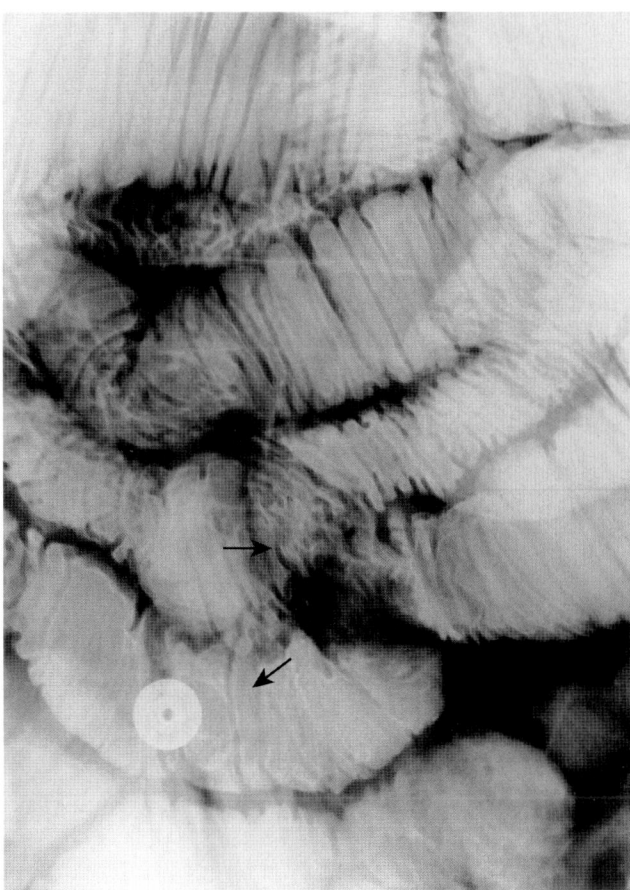

Figure 3-10. Nonobstructing adhesions on single-contrast enteroclysis with compression. Compression view of the mid small bowel shows focal nonobstructing adhesions (*arrows*) with angulation of the affected bowel and an inability to separate adjacent loops.

flow rate may cause reflex paralysis of the small intestine with slow transit and excessive duodenogastric reflux. Initially, the enema bag is placed about 2 ft above the table; the bag can be raised or lowered during the examination to adjust the flow rate for optimal distention of small bowel loops (Fig. 3-9).

The examination is performed under fluoroscopic guidance with the patient in a supine position. Careful compression spot images of all loops of small intestine are obtained under fluoroscopic guidance as bowel segments become fully distended with barium to better depict subtle abnormalities (Fig. 3-10). When the entire small intestine has been opacified, overhead radiographs or digital images of the small bowel are also obtained; the patient can be placed in a prone position to aid in separating small bowel loops, and the tube can be removed before or after the final images are obtained.

BARIUM ENEMA

For single-contrast examination of the colon, fluoroscopic observation, careful compression imaging, and knowledge of appropriate technical factors allows detection of a variety of lesions in the barium-filled colon.[15,27] The single-contrast barium enema is less accurate than the double-contrast examination for detection of small polypoid lesions and for evaluation of inflammatory bowel disease.[2,15,28] However, the examination can be performed quickly and is usually a better choice for examining patients who are immobile, elderly, or incontinent.[2,3]

Preparation of the large bowel is the most important requisite for obtaining an accurate single- or double-contrast barium enema.[27,29] In a well-cleansed colon, diagnosis of neoplasms, including small polyps, is easier and more reliable. Conversely, the presence of stool invariably limits detection of polyps and is the most common cause of errors during interpretation of the barium enema images.[27,29]

A variety of colon-cleansing protocols can be used to obtain a thoroughly clean colon in the vast majority of patients.[27,29] One recommended bowel preparation regimen includes (1) a 24-hour clear liquid diet; (2) one glass of water hourly the day before the examination; (3) a saline cathartic such as magnesium citrate at 4:00 PM the day before the examination; (4) 60 mL of a flavored castor oil or other irritant cathartic at 8:00 PM the day before the examination; and (5) an optional 1500 mL tap water cleansing enema the morning of the barium enema examination, although the need for a water enema is controversial.[30] If a tap water enema is administered, the patient needs to wait at least 30 minutes before the single-contrast barium enema is performed to avoid excess fluid in the colon, which may further dilute the barium suspension and degrade the quality of the study.[27,29,31]

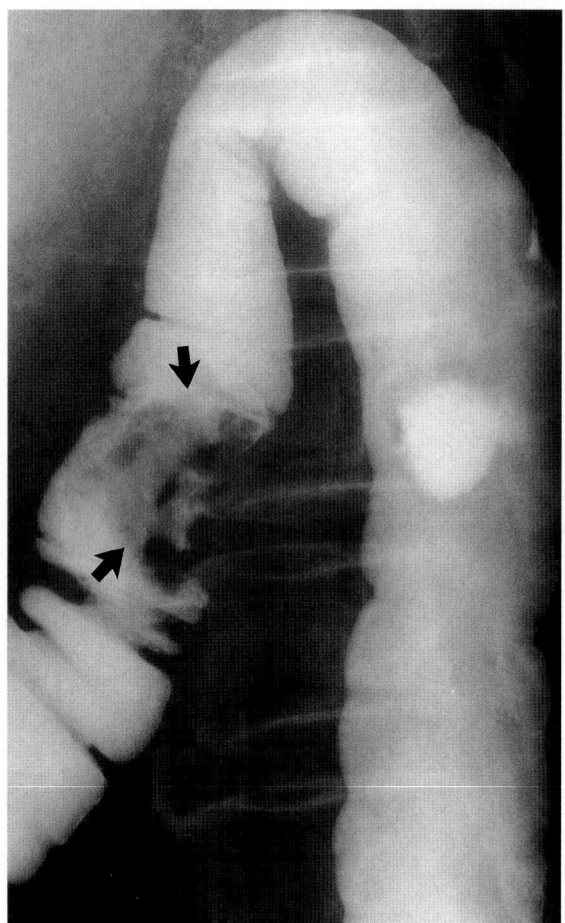

Figure 3-11. Colonic carcinoma on single-contrast barium enema. Oblique compression spot image of the splenic flexure shows a polypoid, ulcerated carcinoma (*arrows*) of the distal transverse colon. Careful patient positioning and the use of compression are critical components of this examination.

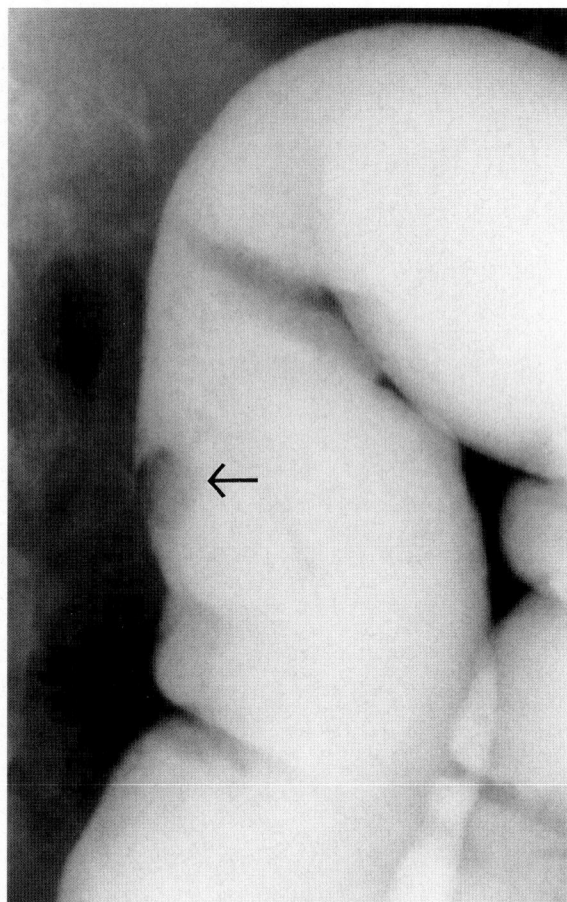

Figure 3-12. Small colonic polyp on compression spot image from a single-contrast barium enema. Oblique compression spot image of the splenic flexure shows an 8-mm colonic polyp (*arrow*). The small polyp was not seen on other images of the same area when compression was not applied.

A thorough examination protocol must be followed to ensure an accurate single-contrast barium enema.[2,15,27] All portions of the colon must be imaged and seen well without overlapping segments, preferably on several views, to increase the fluoroscopist's confidence that suspected lesions are real. Careful fluoroscopy and compression spot imaging of the entire colon (except the rectum) must be performed to demonstrate abnormalities (Fig. 3-11). Depending on the equipment used, overhead radiographs may be obtained to provide additional views of the colon.

The most important part of the single-contrast barium enema examination is compression spot imaging under fluoroscopic guidance.[15,27] The barium-filled colon is wide in caliber and will obscure and prevent detection of small filling defects. Compression is applied to further narrow the barium column, ensuring that small lesions are surrounded by less barium suspension and thus are more easily visualized (Fig. 3-12).

The following technique can be used for performing a thorough single-contrast barium enema.[27] After insertion of a rectal tip, the patient is placed in the left posterior oblique position, the flow of barium suspension is started slowly, and a spot image of the rectosigmoid region is obtained while distention is minimal; because the rectum cannot be com-

pressed, this early image allows smaller lesions to be detected more easily. The rectosigmoid region is again imaged when fully distended. An appropriate number of views are obtained to demonstrate the sigmoid colon without overlapping loops. The entire colon is then opacified to the cecum, avoiding ileal reflux, if possible. Compression spot images of the remaining segments of colon are then obtained. Typically, 8 to 10 spot images are required. After the fluoroscopic examination has been completed, overhead radiographs are obtained; however, when using a remote-control fluoroscope with conventional radiographs or digital imaging, these images are taken during the fluoroscopic portion of the examination. A suggested sequence of larger images includes (1) a left lateral view of the rectum; (2) prone and supine views of the colon; (3) supine left and right anterior oblique views of the colon; and (4) a prone angled view of the rectosigmoid colon.

A postevacuation radiograph is often obtained at the conclusion of a single-contrast barium enema; however, this additional image may slow throughput of patients through the fluoroscopic suite, and this view may be of limited diagnostic value. In some cases, however, the postevacuation radiograph may show that a filling defect seen on earlier barium-filled views persists or disappears, thereby indicating whether this finding was caused by a true polyp or residual stool (Fig. 3-13).

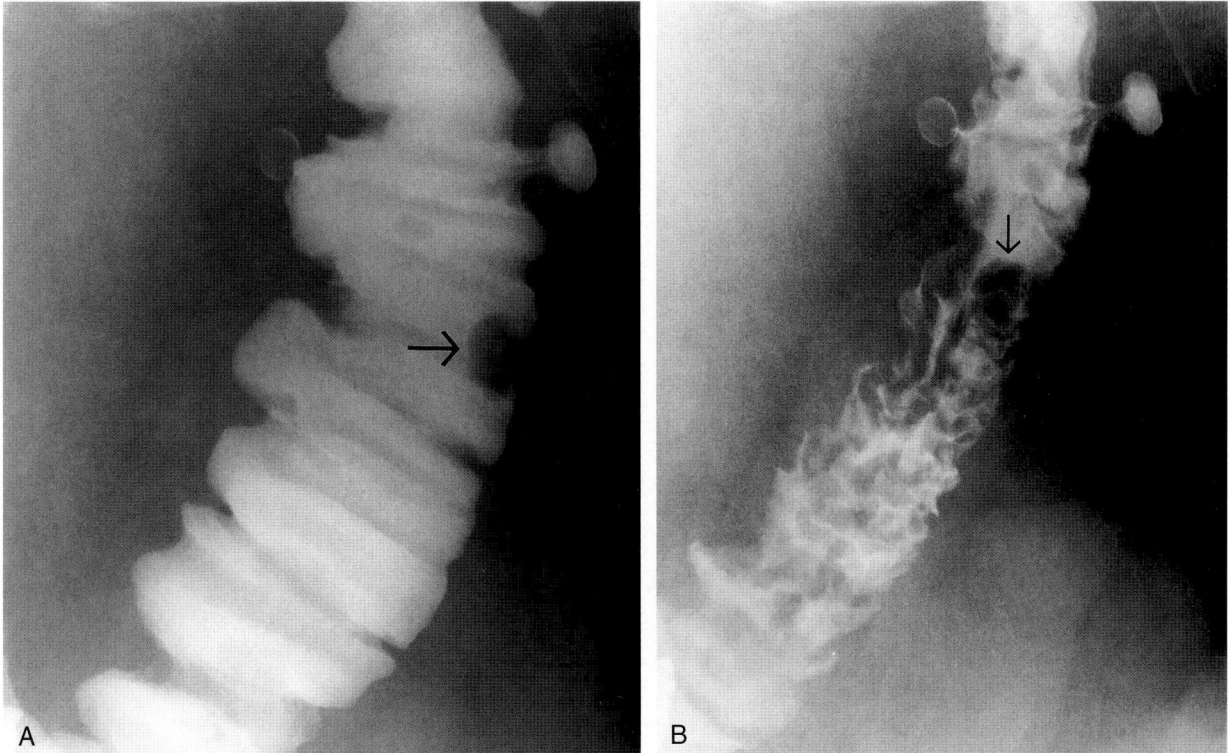

Figure 3-13. Value of postevacuation radiographs for detecting colonic polyps. A. Compression spot image shows a small (less than 1 cm) "filling defect" (*arrow*) in the descending colon on a single-contrast barium enema. Diverticula are also present in this region. The filling defect was not clearly present on other views. **B.** Postevacuation compression spot image of the descending colon (notice the location of the previously seen diverticula) again shows this small filling defect (*arrow*), indicating that it is a true polyp. A small adenoma was removed at colonoscopy.

References

1. Ott DJ, Gelfand DW: The future of barium radiology. Br J Radiol 70:S171-S176, 1997.
2. Gelfand DW, Chen YM, Ott DJ: Detection of colonic polyps on single-contrast barium enema study: Emphasis on the elderly. Radiology 164:333-337, 1987.
3. Frederick MG, Ott DJ, Gelfand DW, et al: Gastrointestinal fluoroscopy in difficult patients. Appl Radiol 26:12-22, 1997.
4. Ott DJ, Chen YM, Hewson EG, et al: Esophageal motility: Assessment with synchronous video tape fluoroscopy and manometry. Radiology 173:419-422, 1989.
5. Gelfand DW, Ott DJ, Chen MYM: Compression filming with high-density barium suspensions. Abdom Imaging 18:320-322, 1993.
6. Gelfand DW: The multiphasic upper gastrointestinal examination. Radiol Clin North Am 32:1067-1081, 1994.
7. Gelfand DW: Fluoroscopic equipment. In Ott DJ, Gelfand DW, Chen MYM (eds): Manual of Gastrointestinal Fluoroscopy—Performance of Procedures. Springfield, IL, Charles C Thomas, 1996, pp 15-23.
8. Levine MS, Laufer I: The gastrointestinal tract: Dos and don'ts of digital imaging. Radiology 207:311-316, 1998.
9. Taylor AJ: Impact of digital spot imaging in gastrointestinal fluoroscopy. AJR 173:1065-1069, 1999.
10. Chawla S, Levine MS, Laufer I, et al: Gastrointestinal imaging: A systems analysis comparing digital and conventional techniques. AJR 172:1279-1284, 1999.
11. Gelfand DW: Gastrointestinal contrast materials. In Ott DJ, Gelfand DW, Chen MYM (eds): Manual of Gastrointestinal Fluoroscopy—Performance of Procedures. Springfield, IL, Charles C Thomas, 1996, pp 3-14.
12. Skucas J: Contrast media. In Gore RM, Levine MS (eds): Textbook of Gastrointestinal Radiology, 2nd ed. Philadelphia, WB Saunders, 2000, pp 2-14.
13. Davidson JC, Einstein DM, Herts BR, et al: Comparison of two barium suspensions for dedicated small-bowel series. AJR 172:379-382, 1999.
14. Ott DJ, Chen YM, Gelfand DW, et al: Detailed per-oral small bowel examination vs. enteroclysis. Radiology 155:29-34, 1985.
15. Ott DJ, Gelfand DW: How to improve the efficacy of the barium enema examination. AJR 160:491-495, 1993.
16. Chen MYM, Gelfand DW: Small bowel. In Ott DJ, Gelfand DW, Chen MYM (eds): Manual of Gastrointestinal Fluoroscopy—Performance of Procedures. Springfield, IL, Charles C Thomas, 1996, pp 69-90.
17. Chen YM, Ott DJ, Gelfand DW, Munitz HA: Multiphasic examination of the esophagogastric region for strictures, rings, and hiatal hernias: Evaluation of the individual techniques. Gastrointest Radiol 10:311-316, 1985.
18. Ott DJ: Pharynx and esophagus. In Ott DJ, Gelfand DW, Chen MYM (eds): Manual of Gastrointestinal Fluoroscopy—Performance of Procedures. Springfield, IL, Charles C Thomas, 1996, pp 24-51.
19. Smith DF, Ott DJ, Gelfand DW, Chen MYM: Lower esophageal mucosal ring: Correlation of referred symptoms with radiographic findings using a marshmallow bolus. AJR 171:1361-1365, 1998.
20. Levine MS: Radiology of esophagitis: A pattern approach. Radiology 179:1-7, 1991.
21. Levine MS: Varices. In Gore RM, Levine MS (eds): Textbook of Gastrointestinal Radiology, 2nd ed. Philadelphia, WB Saunders, 2000, pp 452-463.
22. Gelfand DW: Stomach and duodenum. In Ott DJ, Gelfand DW, Chen MYM (eds): Manual of Gastrointestinal Fluoroscopy—Performance of Procedures. Springfield, IL, Charles C Thomas, 1996, pp 52-68.
23. Gelfand DW, Dale WJ, Ott DJ, et al: The radiologic detection of duodenal ulcers: Effects of examiner variability, ulcer size and location, and technique. AJR 145:551-553, 1985.
24. Gelfand DW, Chen YM, Ott DJ: Multiphasic examinations of the stomach: Efficacy of individual techniques and combinations of techniques in detecting 153 lesions. Radiology 162:829-834, 1987.
25. Gelfand DW, Ott DJ, Chen MYM: Radiologic evaluation of gastritis and duodenitis. AJR 173:357-361, 1999.
26. Herlinger H, Maglinte DDT, Yao T: Enteroclysis—technique and variations. In Herlinger H, Maglinte DDT, Birnbaum BA (eds): Clinical Imaging of the Small Intestine, 2nd ed. New York, Springer, 1999, pp 95-123.

27. Ott DJ: Large bowel. In Ott DJ, Gelfand DW, Chen MYM (eds): Manual of Gastrointestinal Fluoroscopy—Performance of Procedures. Springfield, IL, Charles C Thomas, 1996, pp 91-119.

28. Ott DJ: Accuracy of double-contrast barium enema in diagnosing colorectal polyps and cancer. Semin Roentgenol 35:333-341, 2000.

29. Gelfand DW, Chen MYM, Ott DJ: Preparing the colon for the barium enema examination. Radiology 178:609-613, 1991.

30. Hageman MJHH, Goei R: Cleansing enema prior to double-contrast barium enema examination: Is it necessary? Radiology 187:109-112, 1993.

31. Freimanis MG: Interval between cleansing enema and barium examination of the colon. Gastrointest Radiol 14:83-84, 1989.

Barium Studies: Principles of Double-Contrast Diagnosis

Igor Laufer, MD • Marc S. Levine, MD

PERFORMANCE	Dependent and Nondependent Surfaces
Mucosal Coating	Protrusions
Distention	Depressed Lesions
Projection	Barium Pool
INTERPRETATION	**ARTIFACTS**

Although barium studies once reigned supreme in the arena of morphologic diagnosis in the gastrointestinal tract, these responsibilities are now shared with endoscopy and cross-sectional imaging techniques.[1] As would be expected, the development of alternative imaging methods has led to improvements in barium studies, with particular emphasis on double-contrast techniques as a viable choice for the diagnosis of mucosal lesions in the gastrointestinal tract.[2]

In general terms, barium studies can demonstrate the mucosal surface in three different ways:

1. Mucosal relief views are obtained with a small amount of barium, just sufficient to demonstrate the mucosal folds (Fig. 4-1A). These views are particularly useful for showing abnormalities that affect the folds, such as esophageal varices or the mucosal lesions associated with inflammatory bowel disease.
2. Barium filling is achieved with a larger volume of low-density barium (Fig. 4-1B). These views are important for showing contour abnormalities, strictures, and large polypoid filling defects.
3. Double-contrast views are obtained after the mucosal surface has been coated with a thin layer of high-density barium and the viscus has been distended with air (Fig. 4-1C). These views are essential for showing subtle mucosal lesions, such as the early changes of various inflammatory and neoplastic diseases.

Although these three types of views are incorporated to varying degrees in both single- and double-contrast examinations, single-contrast studies tend to rely more heavily on diagnostic fluoroscopy, mucosal relief, and barium filling.[3] In contrast, double-contrast techniques emphasize the inter-pretation of double-contrast radiographs supplemented by barium filling and mucosal relief.

In the past, there was considerable controversy about the relative virtues of single-contrast and double-contrast techniques.[4,5] Currently, however, most authors believe that double-contrast techniques provide superior mucosal detail and allow earlier detection of subtle lesions and that double-contrast technique should routinely be used when barium studies are performed on patients who are young enough and healthy enough to undergo this form of examination. This chapter discusses the principles that must be understood for the proper performance and interpretation of double-contrast studies.[6] These principles are illustrated with examples drawn throughout the gastrointestinal tract. The principles applicable to single-contrast examinations are discussed in Chapter 3.

PERFORMANCE

The yield of diagnostic information from double-contrast studies can be maximized only with meticulous attention to the technical aspects of the examination. The major principles of performance include mucosal coating, distention, and projection.

Mucosal Coating

The diagnostic quality of double-contrast studies depends on the quality of mucosal coating. In the absence of good coating, lesions can be missed or patchy coating can be mistaken for a lesion. Good mucosal coating requires optimal interaction

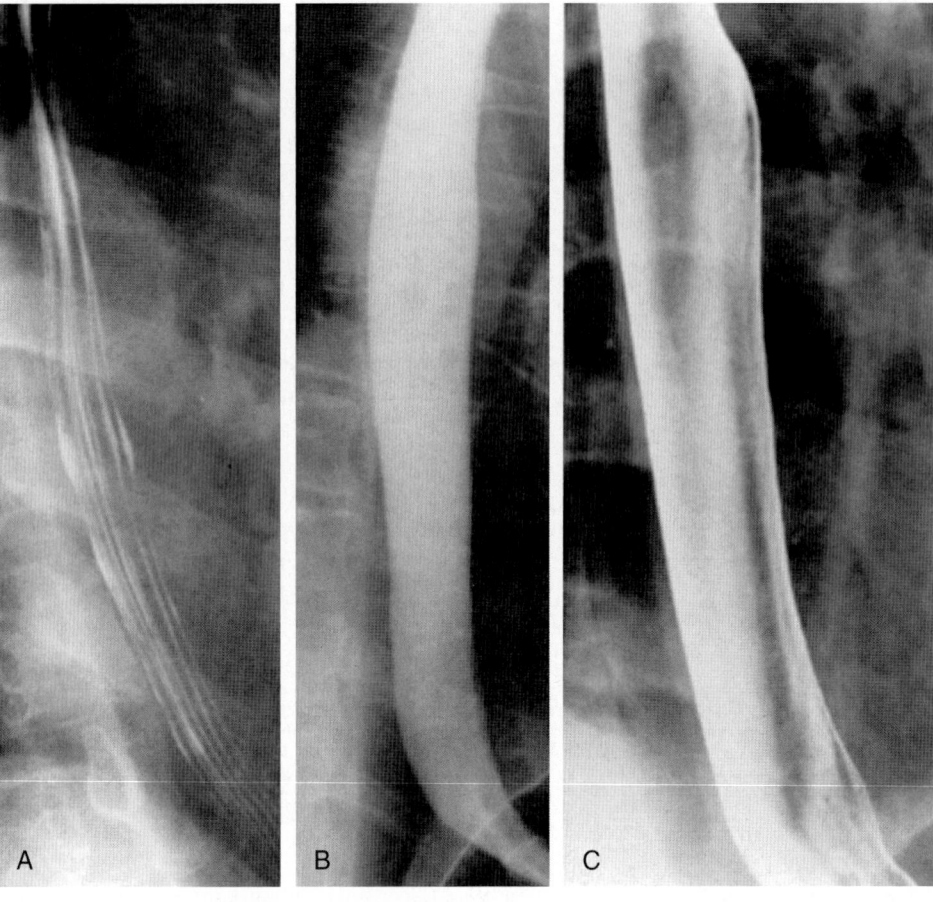

Figure 4-1. **Approaches to the gastrointestinal tract as illustrated in the esophagus. A.** Mucosal relief view. With the esophagus collapsed and coated, the normal longitudinal folds are seen. **B.** Barium filling view. With the patient in the prone position and with continuous drinking, the barium-filled esophagus is demonstrated. **C.** Double-contrast view. With the patient in the upright position, the smooth, featureless surface of the esophagus is seen.

between the barium suspension and the mucosal surface. An appropriate barium suspension must be chosen; it must be prepared properly,[7] and the mucosal surface must be clean enough to receive the barium coating. Even when mucosal coating is only slightly impaired, extensive abnormalities can be missed (Fig. 4-2).

Distention

Normal mucosal folds are soft and pliable and are therefore effaced with moderate distention. The optimal degree of distention is that which just effaces the normal mucosal folds. Inadequate distention may conceal lesions, but overdistention can also obscure lesions such as shallow ulcers. Varying degrees of distention may therefore be required for optimal visualization of complex or subtle lesions. Overdistention may accentuate areas of rigidity, whereas partial collapse may accentuate abnormalities of the mucosal folds. The final diagnosis represents a synthesis of the information obtained with these various views (Fig. 4-3).

Projection

An adequate number of views should be obtained, so that each loop of bowel is projected free of overlapping loops. Ideally, each segment of bowel should also be demonstrated in profile. In practice, however, these goals cannot always be achieved. It is therefore important to develop the habit of looking through overlapping loops of bowel and to be able to recognize

abnormalities that are viewed en face as well as in profile. This is particularly important for recognition of short, annular lesions in the colon, because it may be difficult to demonstrate every bend in profile (Fig. 4-4).

INTERPRETATION

After every effort is made to obtain excellent images, it is important to extract all the diagnostic information that is available on these images. The interpretation of double-contrast studies differs substantially from the interpretation of single-contrast studies.

Dependent and Nondependent Surfaces

The distinction between the dependent and nondependent surfaces must be clearly understood. The nondependent surface has a thin coating of barium because all the free barium falls onto the dependent surface. The dependent surface, therefore, has a thicker coating of barium, and a barium pool or puddle accumulates in any depression or concavity. The usual double-contrast image obtained with a vertical beam results in superimposition of the dependent and nondependent surfaces and any barium pool that might be present. The distinction between these surfaces is more clearly demonstrated on horizontal beam radiographs (Fig. 4-5).

Lesions in the gastrointestinal tract can generally be classified as protruded or depressed, and their appearance

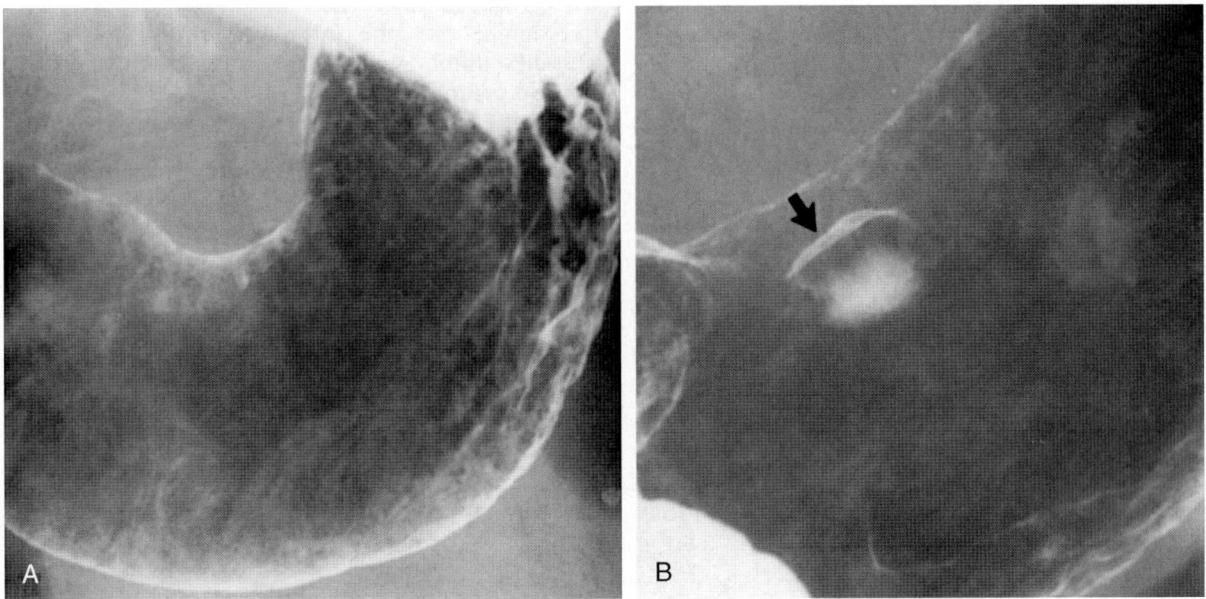

Figure 4-2. Risk of suboptimal coating. A. On the initial radiograph, an ulcer crater is barely recognizable along the lesser curvature. **B.** With additional rotation and improved coating, the large ulcer crater (*arrow*) is clearly seen.

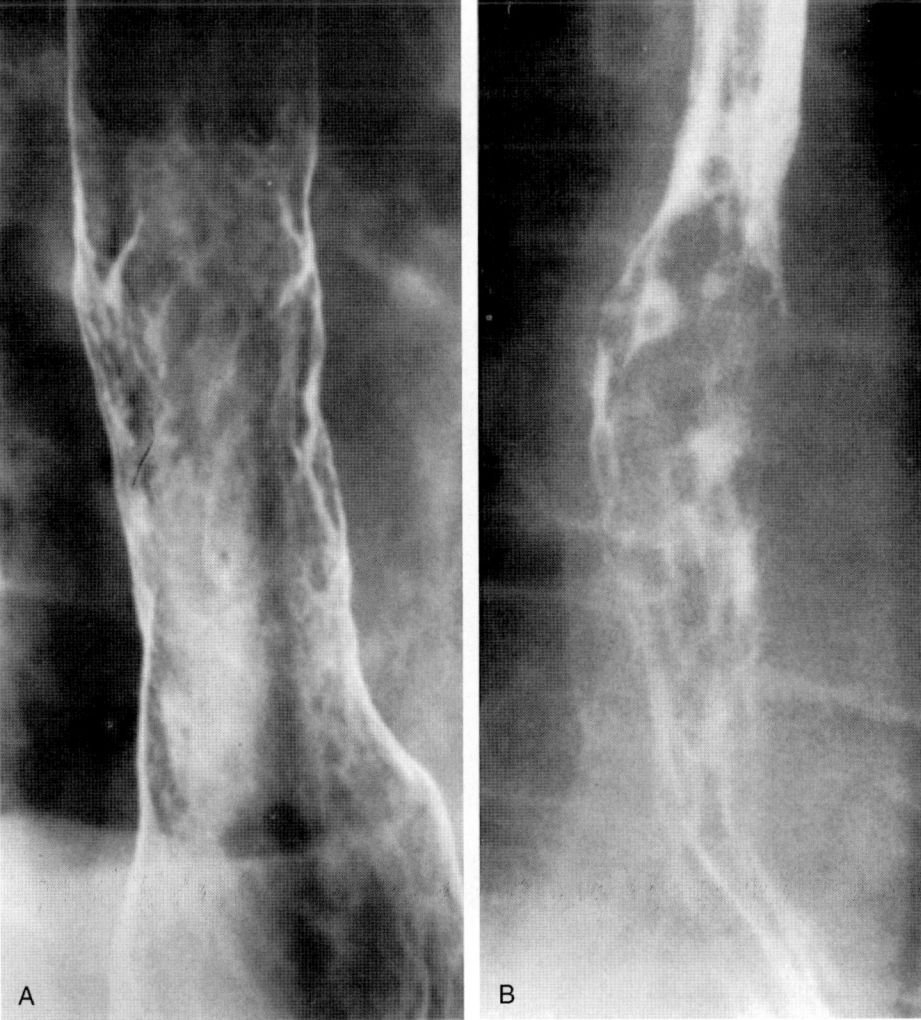

Figure 4-3. Adenocarcinoma in Barrett's esophagus. A. Double-contrast view shows ulceration and slight rigidity of the contour. **B.** Mucosal relief view shows the polypoid nature of the lesion. (From Laufer I, Levine MS [eds]: Double Contrast Gastrointestinal Radiology, 2nd ed. Philadelphia, WB Saunders, 1992.)

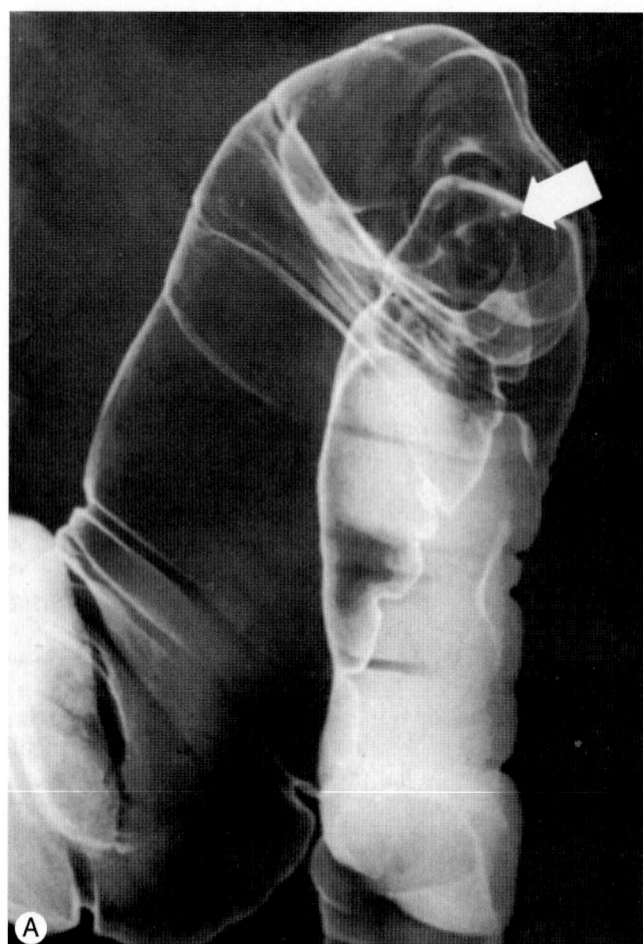

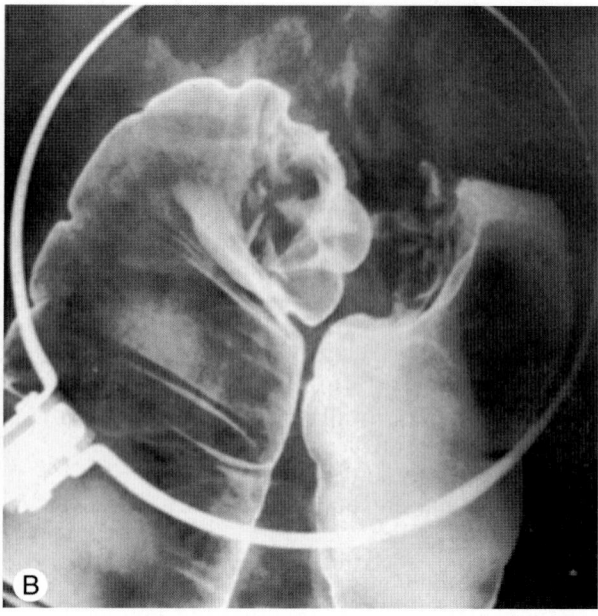

Figure 4-4. Annular carcinoma seen en face and in profile. **A.** The irregularity of the lumen seen end on (*arrow*) is the result of an annular carcinoma. **B.** Carcinoma is confirmed on the appropriate oblique projection showing the lesion in profile. (From Laufer I, Levine MS [eds]: Double Contrast Gastrointestinal Radiology, 2nd ed. Philadelphia, WB Saunders, 1992.)

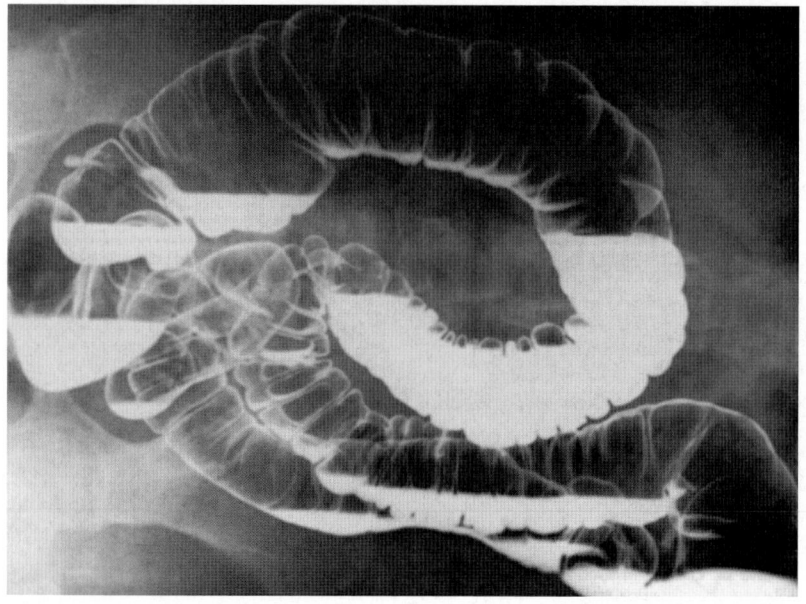

Figure 4-5. Dependent and nondependent surfaces. The distinction between the dependent and the nondependent surfaces is clearly shown on this horizontal beam radiograph of the colon. The nondependent surface has a thin coating of barium, whereas the dependent surface contains the barium pool.

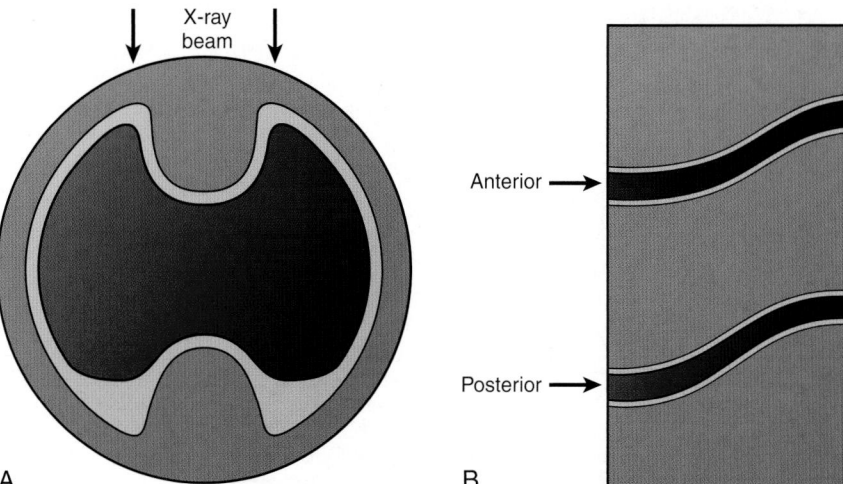

Figure 4-6. Principles underlying the appearance of protrusions. A and **B.** Diagrammatic representations of the appearance of a rugal fold on the anterior and posterior walls of the stomach. (From Laufer I, Levine MS [eds]: Double Contrast Gastrointestinal Radiology, 2nd ed. Philadelphia, WB Saunders, 1992.)

depends on whether they are located on the dependent or nondependent surface. Their appearance can also be affected or even masked by the barium pool.

Protrusions

Protrusions into the lumen of a hollow viscus can be normal structures such as mucosal folds or pathologic lesions such as polypoid tumors. The radiographic principles underlying the appearance of protrusions are illustrated in Figure 4-6, which represents a cross section through the stomach with rugal folds on the anterior and posterior walls. With the patient

in the supine position, the posterior wall is dependent and the anterior wall is nondependent.

A protrusion on the dependent surface displaces barium from the barium pool and is therefore seen as a radiolucent filling defect. A protrusion on the nondependent surface is coated with barium, and the x-ray beam catches the edges of the protrusion, which are then "etched in white." Figure 4-7 illustrates the different appearances of a lesion when it is located on the dependent surface and then on the nondependent surface.

In general, the density of the etching depends on the thickness of the lesion, so that the etching of a slightly protruded

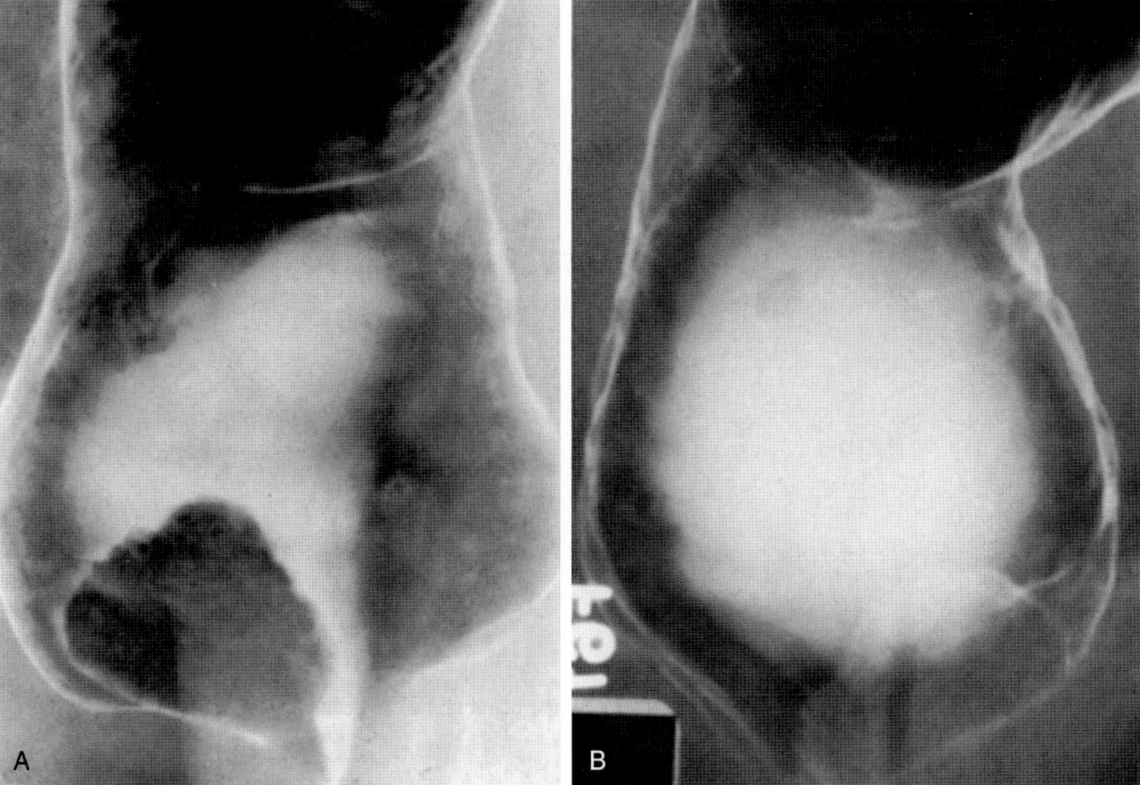

Figure 4-7. Effect of position on the appearance of a rectal carcinoma. A. With the patient in the supine position there is a lobulated filling defect in the distal rectum. The plaquelike carcinoma is therefore on the posterior wall. **B.** With the patient turned to the prone position, the carcinoma is now etched in white because it is on the nondependent surface.

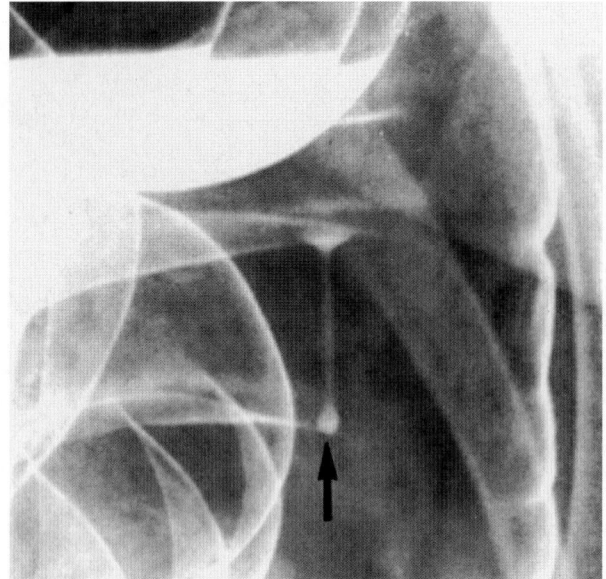

Figure 4-8. The stalactite phenomenon. Radiograph of the colon with the patient in the upright position shows a long droplet of barium (*arrow*) hanging from a haustral fold. (From Laufer I, Levine MS [eds]: Double Contrast Gastrointestinal Radiology, 2nd ed. Philadelphia, WB Saunders, 1992.)

or plaquelike lesion may be extremely faint. Such lesions are best demonstrated on the dependent surface in the presence of a shallow barium pool. Flow technique is particularly valuable for detecting these lesions.[8]

Several other appearances are associated with protruded lesions. The stalactite phenomenon represents a droplet of barium hanging from a protrusion on the nondependent surface (Fig. 4-8).[9] These barium droplets can be differentiated from ulcers because they are almost always associated with protrusions on the nondependent surface and disappear as the droplet falls away. Nevertheless, it is important to recognize these stalactites, because they may be the only clue to the presence of a protruded lesion on the nondependent surface.[10]

The "bowler hat" sign may be seen with either a polypoid lesion or a diverticulum. With a polyp, however, the dome of the hat points inward toward the long axis of the bowel, whereas with a diverticulum, the dome of the hat points outward (Fig. 4-9).[11] The "Mexican hat" sign represents a pedunculated polyp hanging from the nondependent surface. The outer ring represents the head of the polyp, and the inner ring represents the stalk seen end on through the head (Fig. 4-10).

Depressed Lesions

Depressed lesions are lesions that extend beyond the normal contour of the bowel, such as ulcers or diverticula. When located on the dependent surface, they trap barium and are therefore seen as focal barium collections (Fig. 4-11A). When located on the nondependent surface, they empty of barium. If there is adequate coating of the sides of a depressed lesion, however, it can be recognized as a ring shadow (Fig. 4-11B and C). In patients with colonic diverticulosis, the appearance of these lesions therefore depends on their location in the bowel; diverticula on the dependent surface tend to fill

with barium, whereas diverticula on the nondependent surface usually appear as ring shadows (Fig. 4-12).

This concept is particularly important for the recognition of anterior wall duodenal ulcers. With the patient in the supine or supine left posterior oblique position, the ulcer may be manifested by a ring shadow or crescent due to barium coating the rim of the unfilled, nondependent ulcer crater (see Fig. 4-11B). When the patient is placed in the prone position, however, the ulcer fills with barium (see Fig. 4-11C).

Barium Pool

The barium pool is the paint of the radiologic artist. The double-contrast examination, in essence, represents a manipulation of the barium pool to coat the entire mucosal surface. At the same time, the barium pool may compromise the study in a variety of ways (Fig. 4-13). It can cover over and submerge a lesion on the dependent surface. Even a small barium pool on the dependent surface can also obscure the etching of a lesion on the nondependent surface (Fig. 4-14). Finally, the barium pool in an overlapping loop of bowel can obscure lesions in the loop of interest.

In general terms, lesions on the dependent surface are best demonstrated with an extremely shallow barium pool. Recognition of lesions on the nondependent surface requires that the barium pool on the dependent surface be entirely eliminated. These varying requirements can be met by the use of flow technique (Fig. 4-15).[8] As the patient is turned under fluoroscopic control, the flow of the barium pool across the dependent surface is observed. In this way, shallow lesions can be demonstrated on the dependent surface, and as the barium pool flows away, lesions can also be seen on the nondependent surface. The concept of flow technique is important for demonstrating subtle lesions and avoiding diagnostic error.

ARTIFACTS

Many of the artifactual appearances associated with double-contrast studies are obvious to the radiologist.[12] These artifacts include findings caused by barium precipitation (Fig. 4-16A), patchy mucosal coating, and extraneous debris. However, some artifacts may be confusing because they closely resemble pathologic states.

In the colon, some barium suspensions may crack or flake, producing an appearance suggestive of inflammatory bowel disease (Fig. 4-16B). In some patients, there may be inadequate distention for separating the anterior and posterior walls. The area of apposition, also known as "kissing" artifact, is outlined and may resemble a mass lesion (Fig. 4-17A). In other patients, kissing artifact is produced by extrinsic compression (Fig. 4-17B), causing the anterior and posterior walls to appose. In such cases, the appropriate projection should be obtained to identify an extrinsic mass compressing the lumen.

Because the air-filled bowel is transradiant, structures in front of or behind the bowel may be projected over the bowel, so that they simulate lesions arising from the bowel. It is particularly important to recognize the true nature of barium-filled diverticula and calcified structures overlying the bowel and not to mistake them for polypoid or ulcerated lesions (Fig. 4-18). Other double-contrast artifacts are discussed in chapters dealing with specific organs.

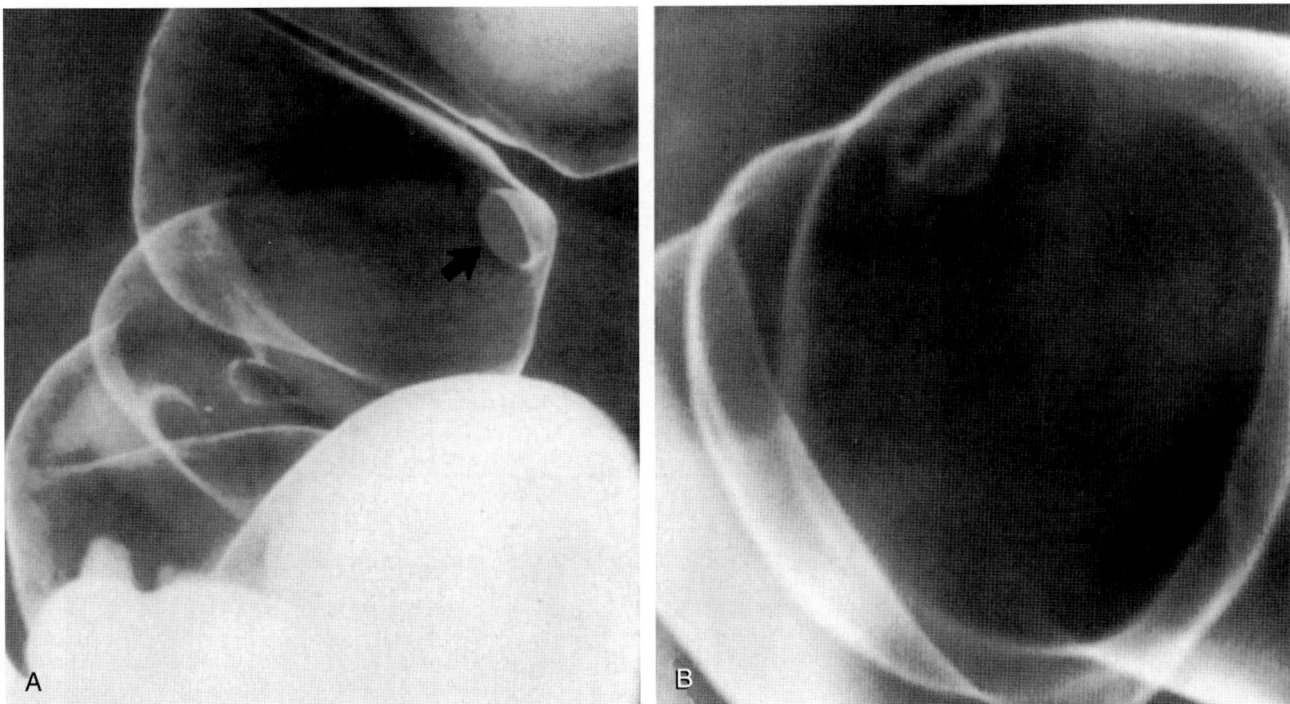

Figure 4-9. Bowler hat: diverticulum or polyp? A. When the dome of the hat (*arrow*) points away from the axis of the bowel, it is a diverticulum. **B.** When the dome of the hat points toward the lumen of the bowel, it is a polyp. (From Laufer I, Levine MS [eds]: Double Contrast Gastrointestinal Radiology, 2nd ed. Philadelphia, WB Saunders, 1992.)

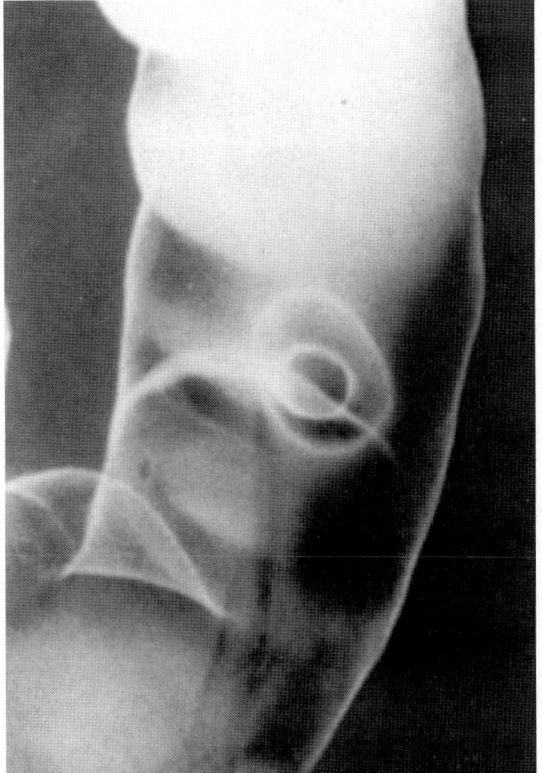

Figure 4-10. The Mexican hat sign. Typical appearance of pedunculated polyp seen end on. The outer ring represents the head of the polyp, and the inner ring represents the stalk.

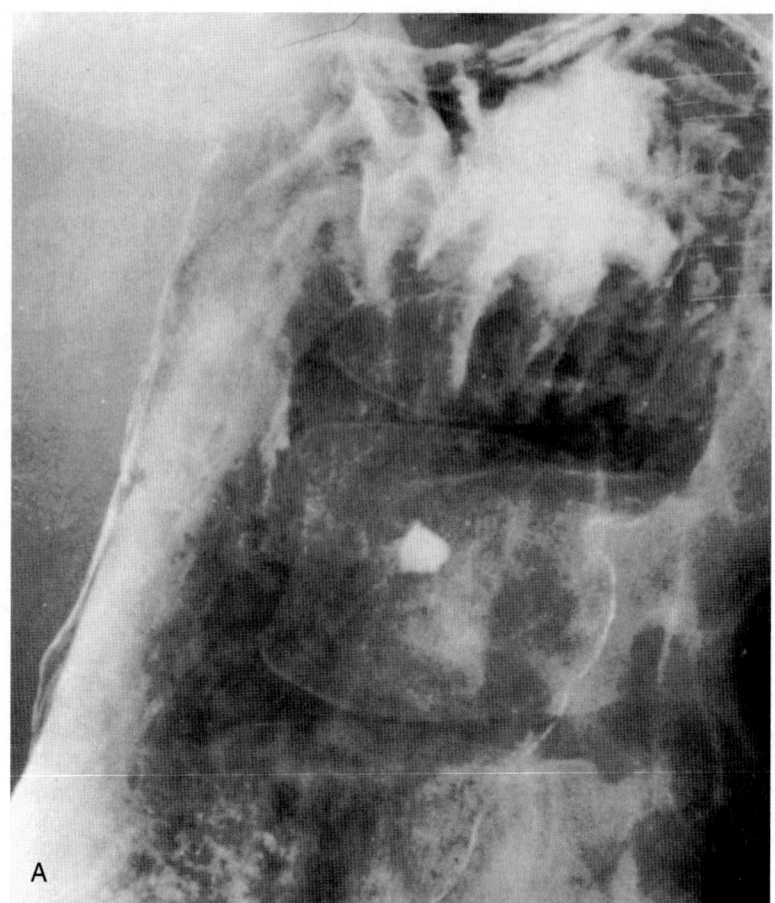

Figure 4-11. **Depressed lesions. A.** Dependent wall ulcer. Radiograph of the stomach in the right posterior oblique projection shows a high ulcer on the lesser curvature. **B.** Anterior wall ulcer. Spot image in the left posterior oblique projection shows a ring shadow (*arrow*) representing the ulcer crater on the anterior wall of a deformed duodenal bulb. **C.** With the patient in the prone position, the ring shadow fills with barium (*arrow*), indicating an anterior wall duodenal ulcer. (From Laufer I, Levine MS [eds]: Double Contrast Gastrointestinal Radiology, 2nd ed. Philadelphia, WB Saunders, 1992.)

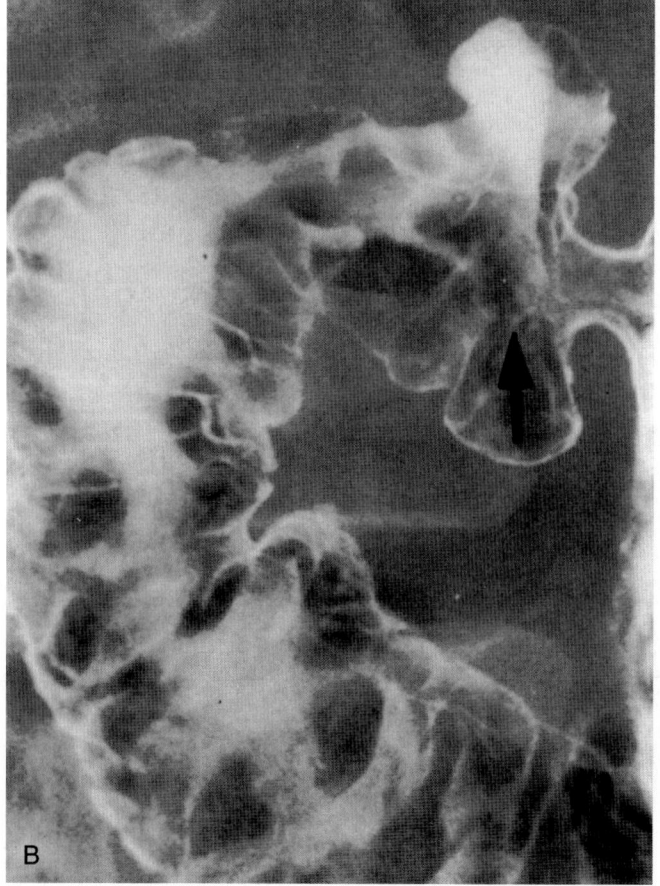

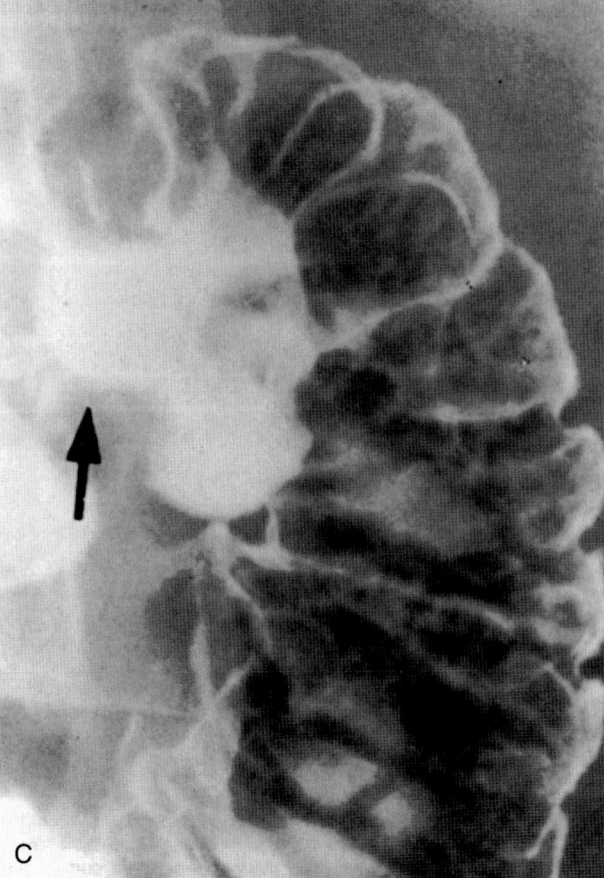

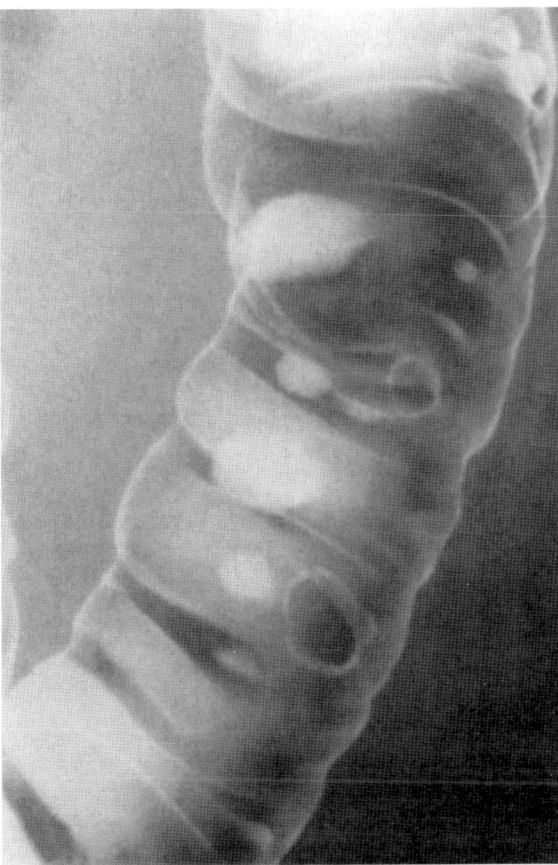

Figure 4-12. Depressed lesions on the dependent and nondependent surfaces. In a segment of colonic diverticulosis, barium-filled diverticula are on the dependent surface whereas unfilled diverticula on the nondependent surface are seen as ring shadows.

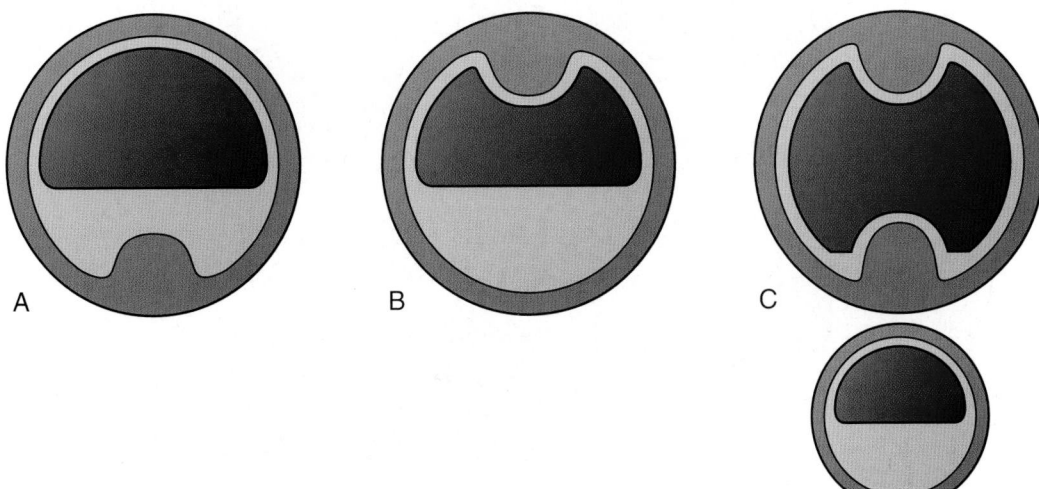

Figure 4-13. Diagrammatic representation of the hazards of the barium pool. A. The barium pool obscures the lesion on the dependent surface. **B.** The barium pool obscures the fine white etching of the lesion on the nondependent surface. **C.** The barium pool in an overlapping loop of bowel may obscure a lesion on either the dependent or the nondependent surface. (**A** and **B** from Laufer I, Levine MS [eds]: Double Contrast Gastrointestinal Radiology, 2nd ed. Philadelphia, WB Saunders, 1992.)

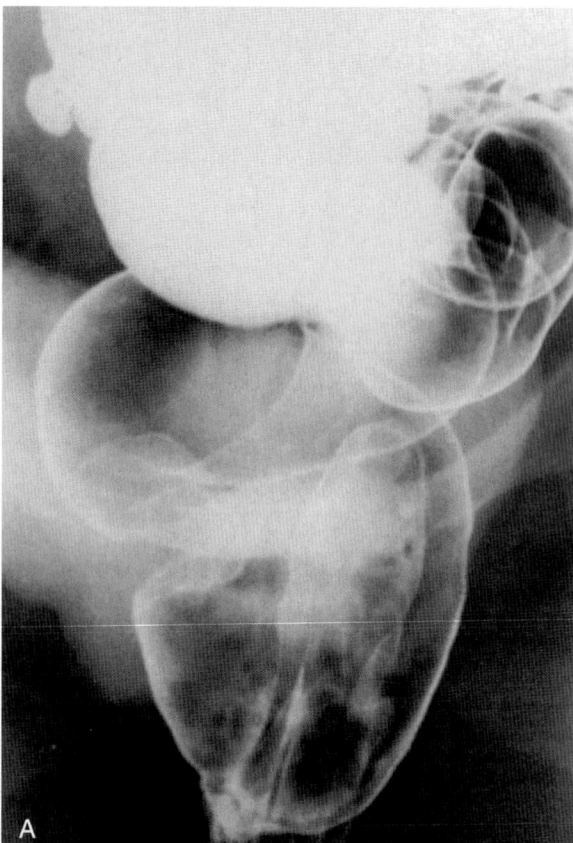

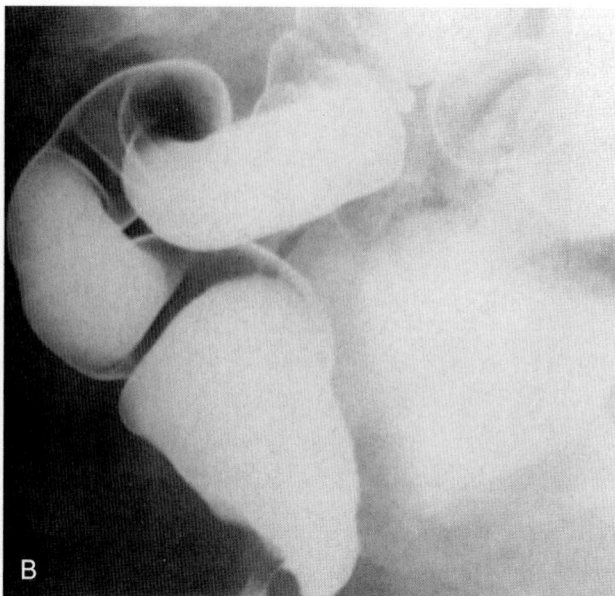

Figure 4-14. Barium pool obscuring a lesion on the nondependent surface. A. In the frontal projection, a polypoid carcinoma is seen along the right lateral wall of the rectum. **B.** In the left lateral projection, the rectal carcinoma is on the nondependent surface (the right lateral wall) of the rectum and its outline is obscured by the barium pool on the dependent surface (the left lateral wall).

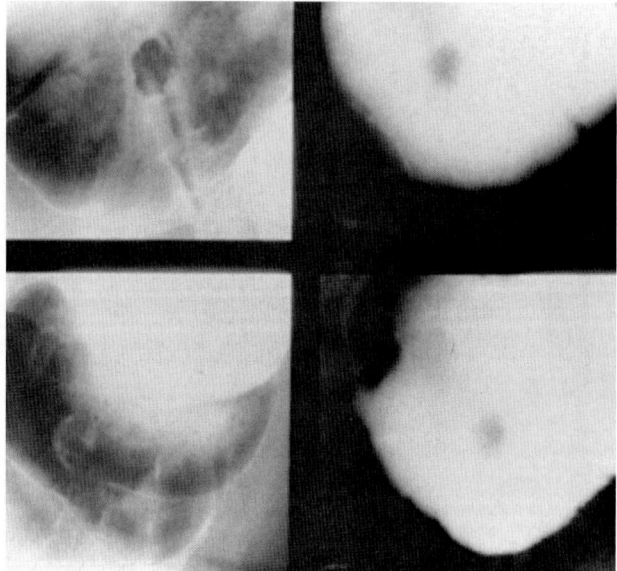

Figure 4-15. Flow technique. There is a 1-cm sessile polyp in the cecum. Its appearance varies as barium flows across the dependent surface of the cecum.

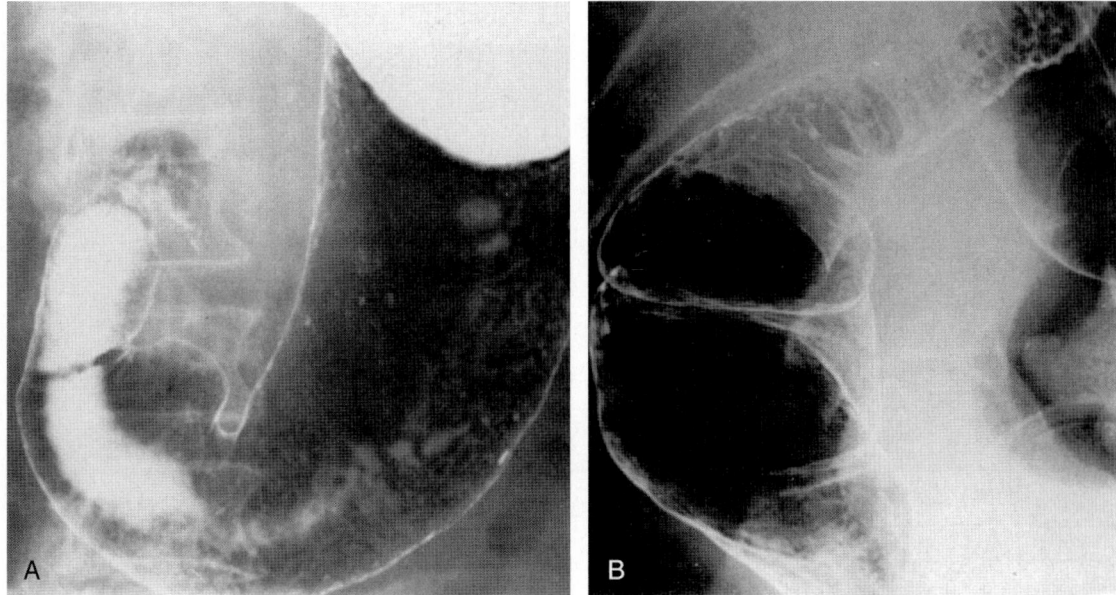

Figure 4-16. Double-contrast artifacts. A. Barium precipitates are recognized as sharp, dense barium collections on the mucosal surface. **B.** Flaking of the barium suspension simulates inflammatory bowel disease. (**B** from Laufer I: Air contrast studies of the colon in inflammatory bowel disease. Crit Rev Diagn Imaging 9:421-447, 1977. Copyright CRC Press, Inc., Boca Raton, FL.)

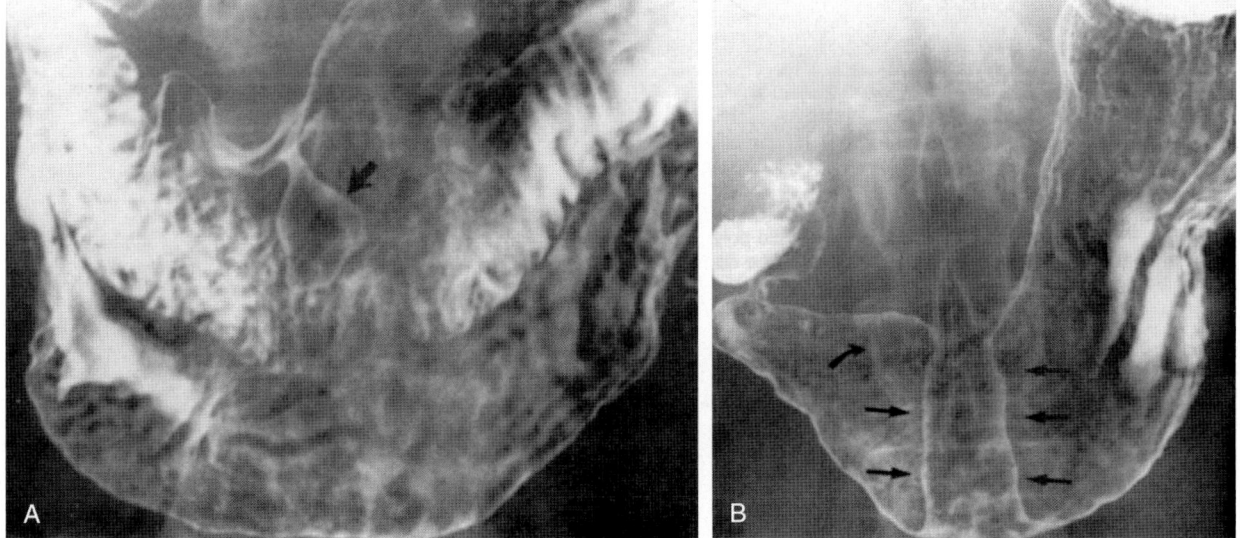

Figure 4-17. Kissing artifact. A. A kissing artifact is seen near the lesser curvature of the stomach, simulating a polypoid lesion (*arrow*). **B.** This kissing artifact results from compression of the stomach by the abdominal aorta (*arrows*). The *curved arrow* indicates calcification in the wall of the aorta.

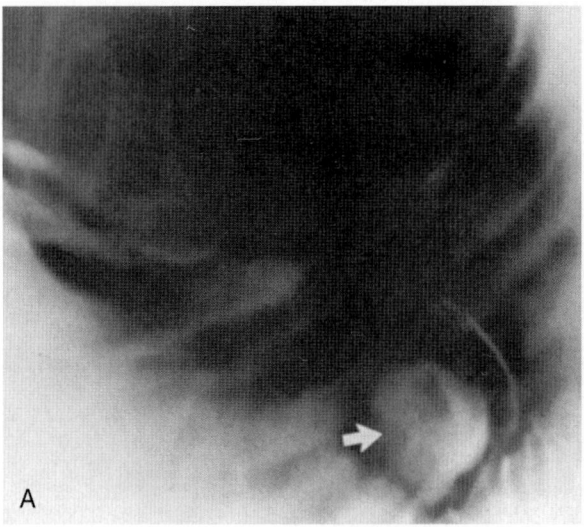 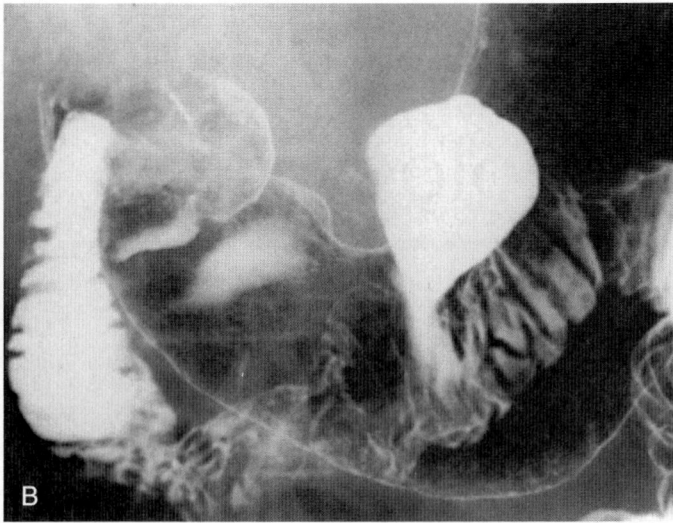

Figure 4-18. Duodenal diverticulum simulating a gastric ulcer. A. Compression radiograph of the stomach shows a large barium collection (*arrow*) suggestive of a gastric ulcer. **B.** Supine double-contrast radiograph shows that the barium-filled structure is a large diverticulum arising from the fourth portion of the duodenum.

References

1. Gelfand DW, Ott DJ, Chen YM: Decreasing numbers of gastrointestinal studies: Report of data from 69 radiologic practices. AJR 148:1133-1136, 1987.
2. Young JW, Ginthner TP, Keramati B: The competitive barium meal. Clin Radiol 36:43-46, 1985.
3. Dekker W, Op den Orth JO: Biphasic radiologic examination and endoscopy of the upper gastrointestinal tract: A comparative study. J Clin Gastroenterol 10:461-465, 1988.
4. Gelfand DW, Chen YM, Ott DJ: Multiphasic examinations of the stomach: Efficacy of individual techniques and combinations of techniques in detecting 153 lesions. Radiology 162:829-834, 1987.
5. Gelfand DW, Ott DJ: Single vs. double-contrast gastrointestinal studies: Critical analysis of reported statistics. AJR 137:523-528, 1981.
6. Laufer I, Kressel HY: Principles of double contrast diagnosis. In Laufer I, Levine MS (eds): Double Contrast Gastrointestinal Radiology, 2nd ed. Philadelphia, WB Saunders, 1992, pp 9-54.
7. Miller RE: Recipes for gastrointestinal examinations. AJR 137:1285-1286, 1981.
8. Kikuchi Y, Levine MS, Laufer I, et al: Value of flow technique for double-contrast examination of the stomach. AJR 147:1183-1184, 1986.
9. Op den Orth JO, Ploem S: The stalactite phenomenon in double contrast studies of the stomach. Radiology 117:523-525, 1975.
10. Aronchick J, Laufer I, Glick S: Barium stalactites: Observations on their nature and significance. Radiology 149:588-591, 1983.
11. Miller WT Jr, Levine MS, Rubesin SE, et al: Bowler-hat sign: A simple principle for differentiating polyps from diverticula. Radiology 173:615-617, 1989.
12. Gohel VK, Kressel HY, Laufer I: Double contrast artifacts. Gastrointest Radiol 3:139-146, 1978.

Pictorial Glossary of Double-Contrast Radiology

Stephen E. Rubesin, MD

SURFACE PATTERNS

Villous Pattern

Reticular Pattern

Granularity

Nodularity

Shaggy

Cobblestoning

FOLD PATTERNS

Striae

Web

"Coil Spring" Sign

Radiating Folds

Polypoid Folds

Serpentine (Serpiginous) Folds

"Stack of Coins" Appearance

Tethering

Pleating

PROTRUDING LESIONS

Filling Defect

Contour Defect

Polyp

Plaque

Carpet Lesion

Ulcerated Mass

Annular Lesion

Saddle Lesion

Submucosal Mass

Target Lesion

Pliability

Extrinsic Mass Effect

DEPRESSED LESIONS

Erosion

Aphthoid Ulcer

Ulcer Niche (Crater)

Linear Ulcer/Linear Erosion

"Collar Button" Ulcer

Exoenteric Mass

Tracking

CONTOUR ABNORMALITIES

Tapering

Linitis Plastica

String Sign

Thumbprinting

Sacculation

Spiculation

Angulation

Careful use of descriptive terms aids in radiologic analysis of perceived abnormalities. By describing the radiographic characteristics of a lesion, a radiologist can localize the lesion to the mucosa, bowel wall, or tissue extrinsic to bowel. This radiographic description, in conjunction with the site and size of the lesion, the age of the patient, and the clinical history, enables the radiologist to make a specific diagnosis or formulate a graded differential diagnosis of the most likely possibilities. In addition, precise use of descriptive terms enhances communication between the radiologist and the clinician. A radiologist should be able to describe an abnormality so that the person reading or listening to the radiographic report can visualize the lesion without looking at the images.

This chapter is a pictorial glossary that visually defines common descriptive terms in gastrointestinal radiology. The terms are divided according to whether they refer to mucosal lesions, wall (i.e., "submucosal," "intramural," or "extramucosal") lesions, or extrinsic lesions.

SURFACE PATTERNS

Villous Pattern

The villi of the small intestine are at the radiographic limits of resolution. Some villi may be seen if the mucosa is well coated and slightly magnified. This *villous pattern* is manifested as barely perceptible radiolucencies surrounded by barium in the interstices between villi (Fig. 5-1).

Reticular Pattern

Reticular means netlike (Fig. 5-2). This net is formed by barium in the interstices of normal columnar mucosa such as the areae gastricae of the stomach (see Fig. 5-2A) or in the interstices of a mucosal lesion such as a carpet lesion. The intervening radiolucent mucosa may be round, ovoid, or polygonal. A reticular pattern typically occurs in abnormalities arising in columnar mucosa. For example, a reticular pattern is seen in the columnar metaplasia of Barrett's esophagus or in a colonic urticarial pattern (see Fig. 5-2B).

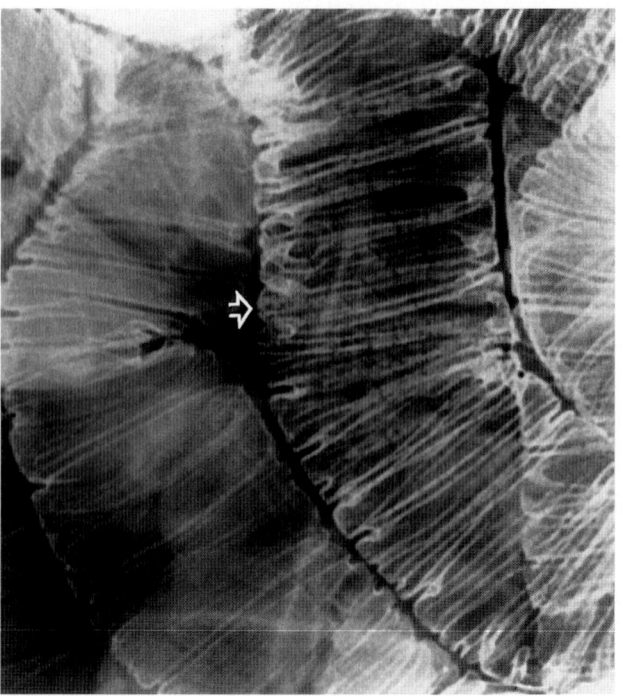

Figure 5-1. Villous pattern. Normal small bowel mucosa. Multiple punctate radiolucencies are seen in the small bowel mucosa (*arrow*). In some loops of small intestine, the villous pattern is not seen.

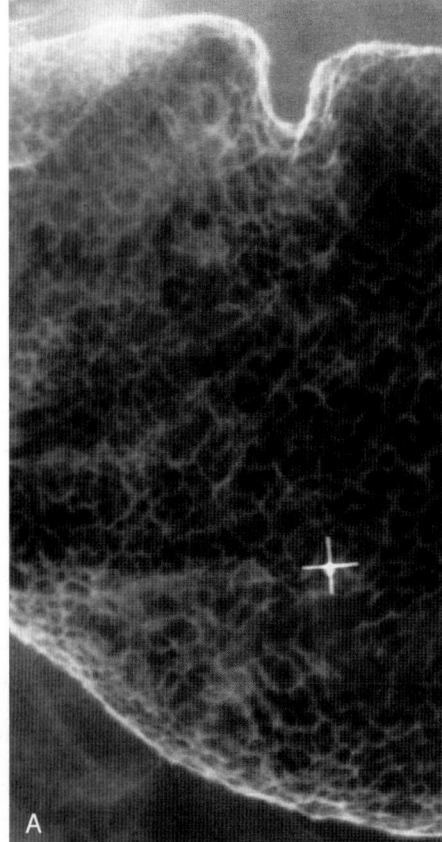

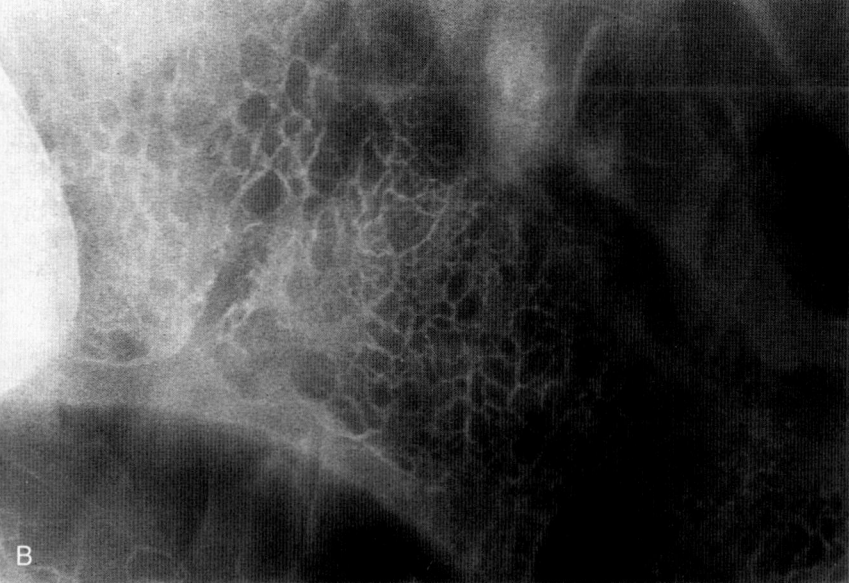

Figure 5-2. Reticular pattern. A. Areae gastricae. In general, columnar mucosa in the gastrointestinal tract is divided into islands of tissue surrounded by shallow grooves. This pattern is best exemplified in the areae gastricae of the stomach. The areae gastricae are seen as well-circumscribed, polygonal radiolucencies surrounded by barium-filled grooves. **B.** Urticarial pattern in the colon. When colonic mucosa is slightly elevated by edema and/or mild inflammation, the colonic surface may assume a reticular pattern. Barium etches sharply polygonal epithelial islands. This has been termed an *urticarial pattern* because it was first described in colonic urticaria. However, any disease that causes mild edema, inflammation, or ischemia of the mucosa may cause the columnar mucosa of the colon to assume an urticarial pattern, including ischemia caused by obstruction or adynamic ileus or inflammation due to viral infections. (**B** from Rubesin SE, Saul SH, Laufer I, et al: Carpet lesions of the colon. RadioGraphics 5:537-552, 1985.)

Granularity

Granularity implies subtle elevation of the mucosal surface seen en face as small radiolucencies in the shallow barium pool or as punctate dots of barium between lucencies (Fig. 5-3). The "granules" are barely perceptible elevations with indistinct borders, as if salt had been sprinkled on a plate. Granularity implies mucosa elevated by edema, inflammatory exudate, or tumor. Barium flocculated on an inflamed mucosal surface can mimic a granular mucosa.

Nodularity

Mucosal nodules are relatively well-circumscribed elevations seen en face as round to ovoid radiolucencies in the barium pool or as small rings etched in white (Fig. 5-4). In profile, nodules are seen as small hemispheric or sharp-edged elevations of the contour. Nodules may arise in the mucosa itself, the lamina propria, or the adjacent submucosa. If a mucosal nodule involves a bowel fold, especially the rugae of the stomach or the valvulae conniventes of the small bowel, the fold is eccentrically enlarged. Submucosal nodules involving a bowel fold, seen en face, symmetrically splay the parallel surfaces of the fold. Mucosal nodularity may be described as fine or coarse. The distinction between fine nodularity and mucosal granularity is somewhat arbitrary, although mucosal nodules are generally larger and more discrete than granules.

Shaggy

Shaggy describes such severe mucosal disease that it is difficult to distinguish ulcerated mucosa from sloughed epithelium and inflammatory detritus (Fig. 5-5). In profile, the contour is jagged. En face, numerous lines reflect barium filling the interstices between ulcerated mucosa and debris. Shaggy is frequently used to describe the radiographic findings in severe *Candida* esophagitis (see Fig. 5-5) and ulcerative colitis.

Cobblestoning

Transverse and longitudinal fissuring of the mucosal surface with extension of knifelike clefts into the submucosa and muscularis propria results in *cobblestoning*, typically seen in Crohn's disease (Fig. 5-6). The cobblestones appear as a carpet of nodules on the luminal surface. The cobblestones represent residual tissue between the transverse and longitudinal clefts.

FOLD PATTERNS

The folds in the gastrointestinal tract are composed of mucosa (epithelium, lamina propria, and muscularis mucosae) and submucosa. When a radiograph demonstrates enlarged or nodular folds, the process therefore involves the mucosal or submucosal layers, or both. A desmoplastic process involving the serosa or adventitia of the bowel or the adjacent mesenteric or omental fat can secondarily pull on the bowel wall, so that the smooth mucosal surface is thrown into an abnormal fold pattern.

Striae

When a viscus is less than fully distended, transverse striations may be seen perpendicular to the longitudinal axis of

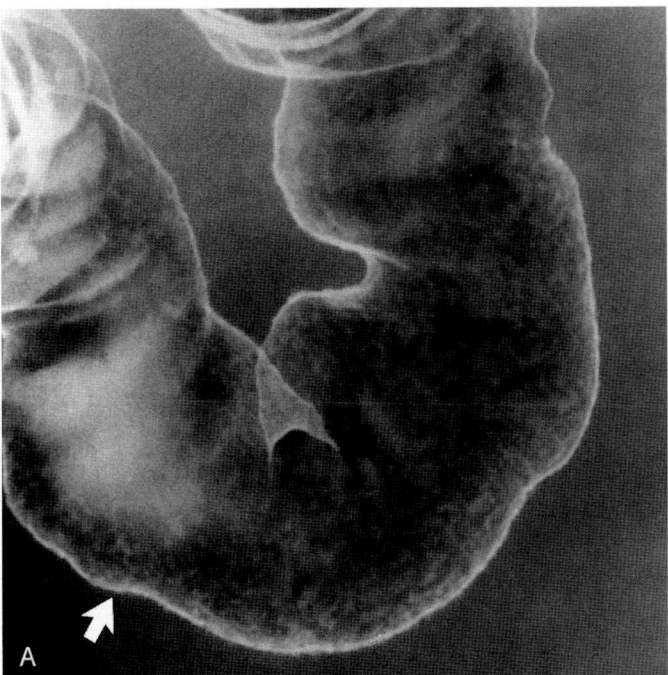
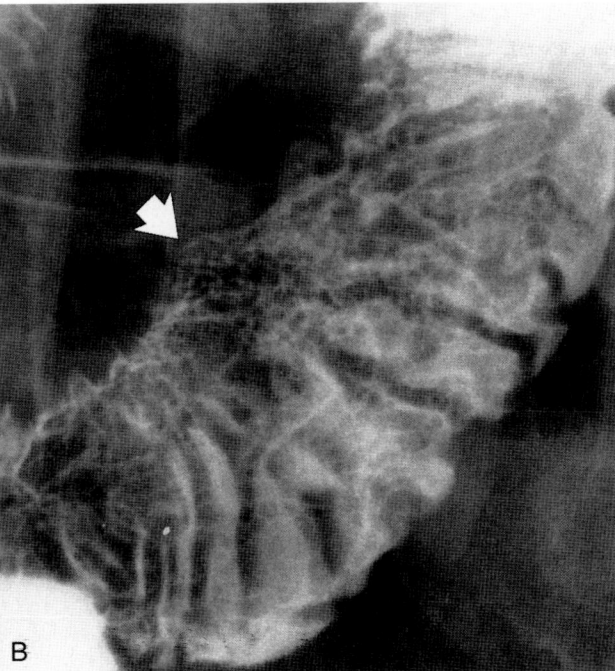

Figure 5-3. Granularity. A. Ulcerative colitis. Numerous punctate dots of barium lie between radiolucent islands of mucosa (representative area identified by *arrow*). The colonic contour is slightly irregular as well. The interhaustral folds are absent. **B.** Crohn's disease. Mucosal granularity (*arrow*) is seen along the mesenteric border of the ileum. The granular mucosa represents fusion and clubbing of villi and/or edema and inflammatory changes in the lamina propria that widen villi. The distinction between fine nodularity and granularity is arbitrary. (**A** from Rubesin SE: Gallery of double-contrast terminology. Gastroenterol Clin North Am 24:259-288, 1995; **B** from Rubesin SE, Bronner M: Radiologic-pathologic concepts in Crohn's disease. In Herlinger H, Megibow AJ [eds]: Advances in Gastrointestinal Radiology. Chicago, Mosby-Year Book, 1991, vol 1, pp 27-55.)

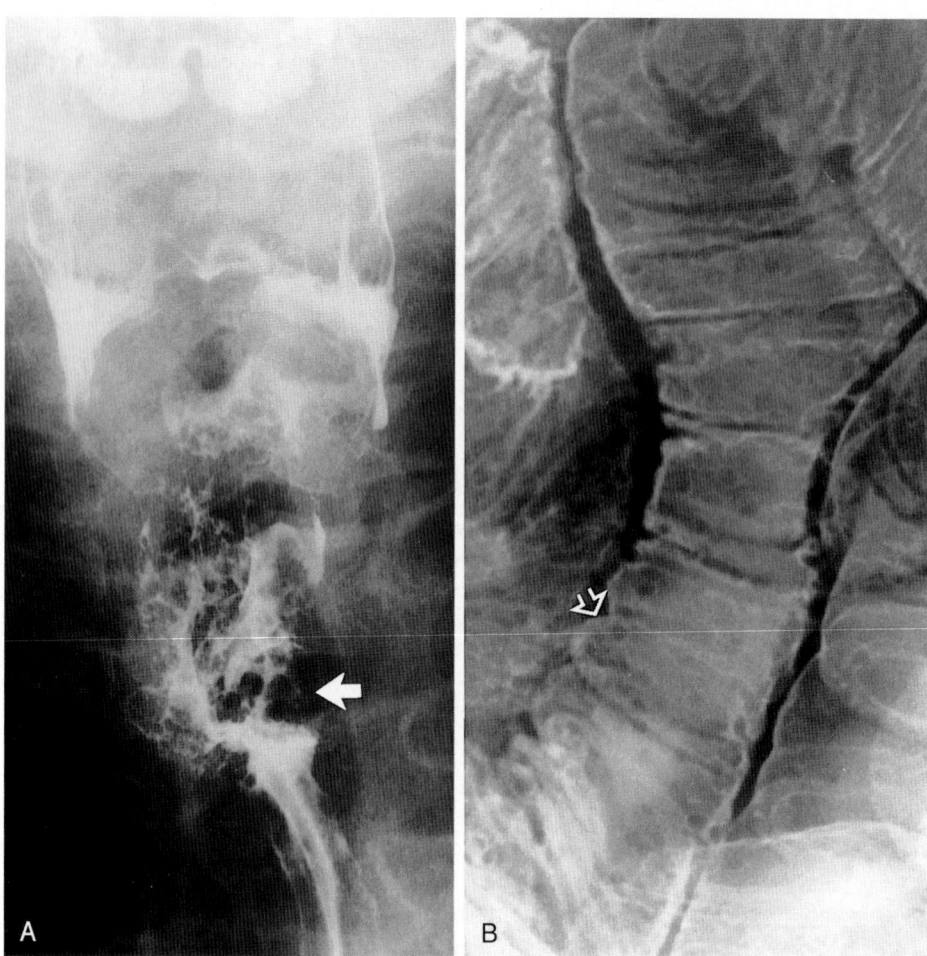

Figure 5-4. Nodularity. A. Squamous cell carcinoma of the postcricoid region. The lumen is expanded by numerous radiolucent nodules of varying size and shape seen as filling defects in the barium pool (representative area identified by *arrow*). **B.** Lymphoid hyperplasia of the small bowel. Multiple subtle, well-circumscribed, round, radiolucent filling defects, many etched in white (*arrow*), carpet the surface of the small bowel. Note separation of these small nodules by normal mucosa. In profile, nodules are seen as hemispheric radiolucencies or ring shadows. This patient had hypogammaglobulinemia associated with diffuse lymphoid hyperplasia of the small bowel.

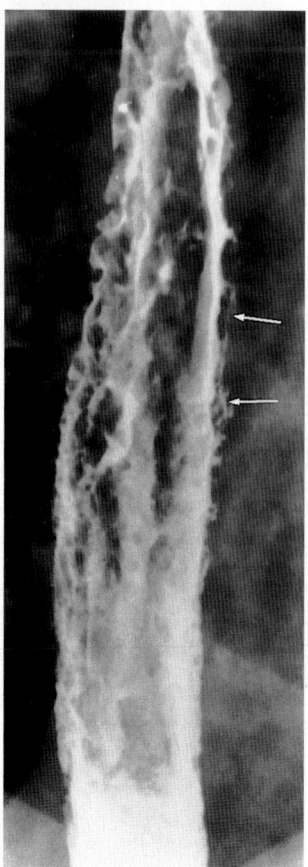

Figure 5-5. Shaggy. *Candida* esophagitis. The mucosal contour is markedly irregular or shaggy. Barium appears to be beneath the mucosal surface (*arrows*). In reality, this barium is trapped between sloughed epithelial debris and the ulcerated mucosa. En face, there are numerous variable-sized plaques. (From Rubesin SE, Levine MS, Laufer I: Odynophagia. In Thompson WM [ed]: Common Problems in Gastrointestinal Radiology. Chicago, Year Book Medical, 1989, pp 108-117.)

the bowel. Examples of this phenomenon include the "feline esophagus" (Fig. 5-7A), gastric striae (Fig. 5-7B), and innominate grooves of the colon.

Web

A *web* is a thin band of mucosa (with or without submucosa) that traverses a variable portion of the intestinal lumen. Webs vary from small shelflike lesions to hemispheric bars and circumferential rings (Fig. 5-8). Webs may be normal variants or the sequelae of inflammatory disease.

"Coil Spring" Sign

If barium is forced between one loop of bowel intussuscepting into another loop, the barium may coat the mucosal folds of the outer loop. The result is the radiographic appearance of concentric rings of barium said to resemble a coil spring (Fig. 5-9).

Radiating Folds

Folds that radiate to a focal site guide the radiologist's eye toward gastrointestinal lesions. Radiographic analysis of the radiating folds aids in differential diagnosis. Smooth folds radiating to a mucosal lesion indicate an active inflammatory process or scarring (Fig. 5-10A). Lobulated, pointed, or clubbed

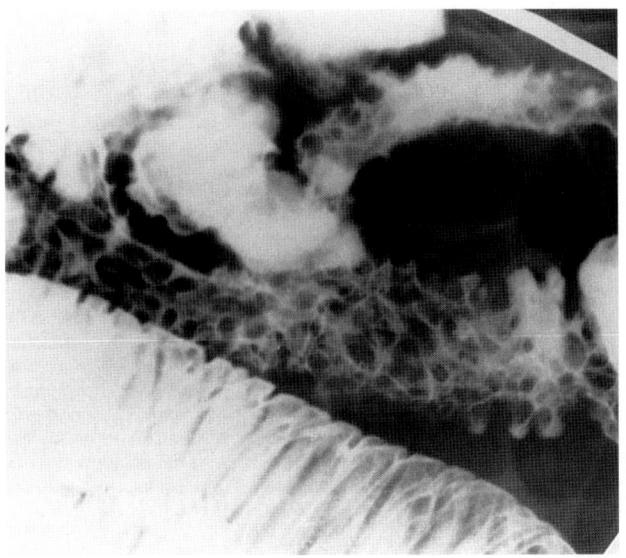

Figure 5-6. Cobblestoning. Crohn's disease involving the small intestine. Multiple round, ovoid, or polygonal radiolucencies are surrounded by barium-filled transverse and longitudinal fissures. This is also termed the *ulceronodular pattern* of Crohn's disease. The "cobblestones" represent the mildly inflamed residual mucosa and submucosa between the knifelike clefts. Narrowing of the bowel lumen reflects a transmural inflammatory reaction and bowel wall thickening. (From Rubesin SE, Laufer I, Dinsmore B: Radiologic investigation of inflammatory bowel disease. In MacDermott RP, Stenson WF [eds]: Inflammatory Bowel Disease. New York, Elsevier Science, 1992, pp 453-492.)

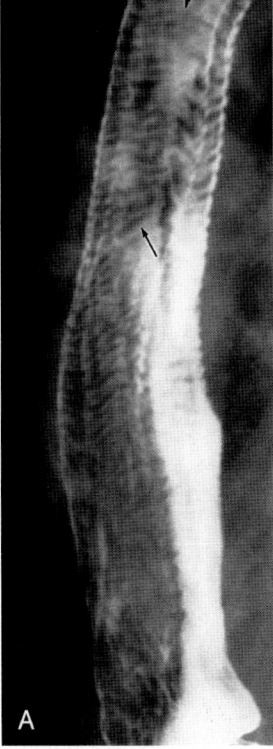
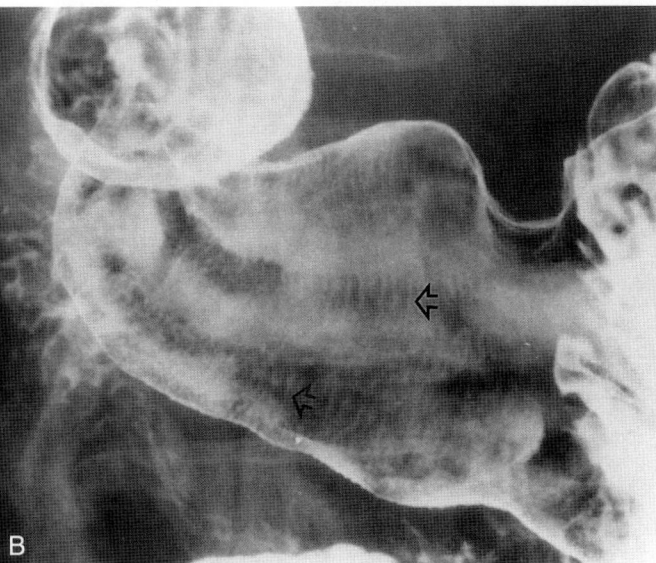

Figure 5-7. Striae. A. Feline esophagus. Fine, barium-etched, thin transverse striations (*arrows*) cross the entire luminal diameter of the esophagus. Note that the esophagus is slightly collapsed proximally. The striations are due to contractions of the muscularis mucosae. This pattern has been termed *feline esophagus* or esophageal *shiver*. The feline esophagus is often associated with gastroesophageal reflux. **B.** Gastric striae. Fine, barium-etched striae (*arrow*) perpendicularly cross the longitudinal axis of a slightly contracted gastric antrum. The striae are probably due to contraction of the muscularis mucosae and have been described in patients with biopsy specimens showing normal mucosa or antral gastritis. (**B** from Rubesin SE: Gallery of double-contrast terminology. Gastroenterol Clin North Am 24:259-288, 1995.)

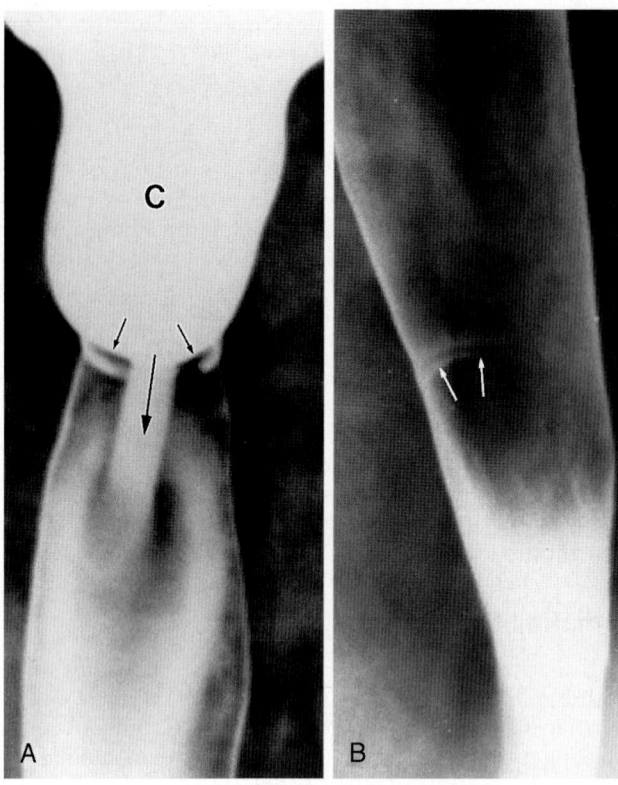

Figure 5-8. **Web. A.** Cervical esophageal web. A thin, radiolucent bar (*short arrows*) crosses the cervical esophagus. Obstruction is implied by dilatation of the proximal cervical esophagus (C) and a spurt of barium through the web (a jet phenomenon) (*long arrow*). **B.** Web in distal esophagus. A thin, radiolucent bar (*arrows*) is etched in white and crosses part of the circumference of the distal esophagus. Distal esophageal webs are usually related to gastroesophageal reflux disease. (**A** from Laufer I, Levine MS [eds]: Double Contrast Gastrointestinal Radiology, 2nd ed. Philadelphia, WB Saunders, 1992.)

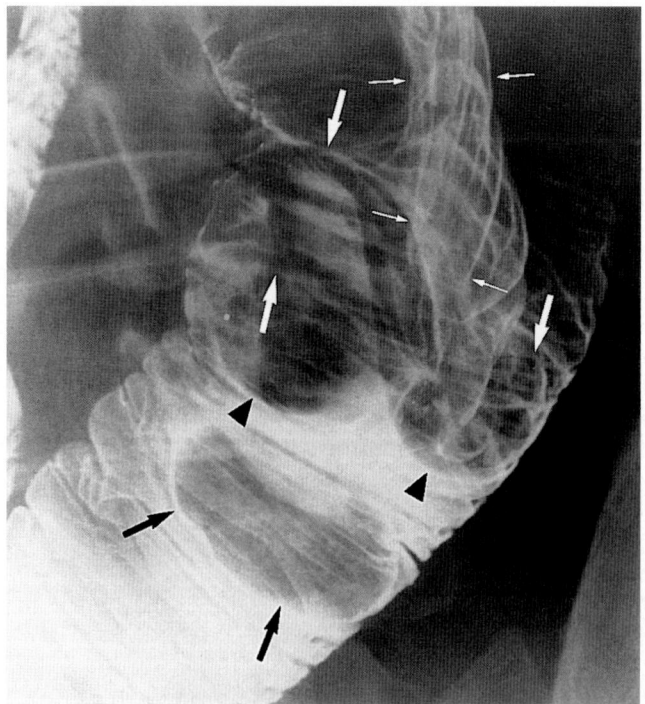

Figure 5-9. **"Coil spring" sign.** Metastatic melanoma causing intussusception of the small bowel. Barium refluxes in a retrograde direction into the space between the prolapsing loop of the intussusception (intussusceptum) and the outer loop (intussuscipiens). The parallel folds of the coil spring (*large white arrows*) are identified. The intussusceptum is seen as a radiolucency (*arrowheads*) within the intussuscipiens. The lumen of the intussusceptum is narrow (*small white arrows*). The lead point of the intussusceptum is a polypoid mass (*black arrows*).

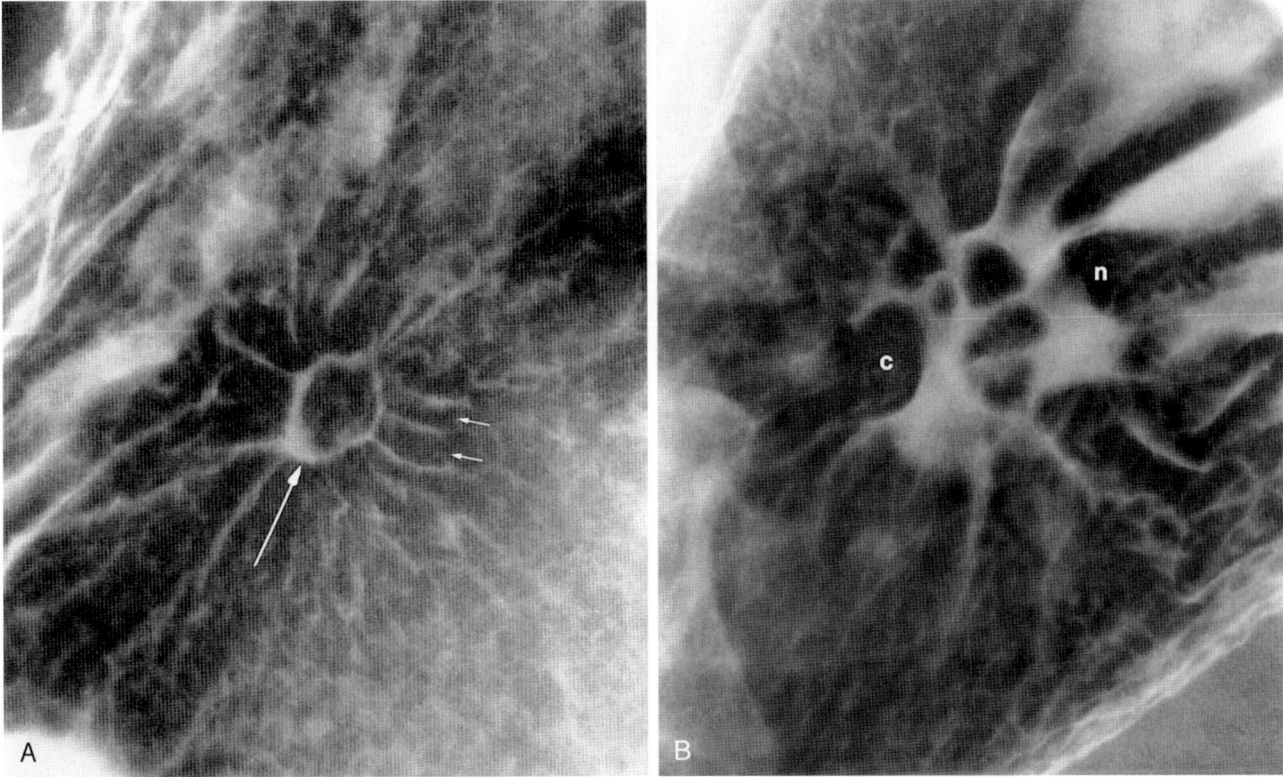

Figure 5-10. Radiating folds. A. Benign gastric ulcer. Smooth, straight folds (*short arrows*) radiate toward the barium-etched rim of the ulcer (*long arrow*). **B.** Adenocarcinoma of the stomach. Abnormal folds radiate toward the center of the lesion. The folds are club shaped (c) and nodular (n). Note the nodular mucosa in the center of the ulcer crater.

radiating folds indicate the presence of a malignant or severe inflammatory process (Fig. 5-10B).

Polypoid Folds

Enlarged folds with a lobulated contour may appear *polypoid* (Fig. 5-11). Diseases that cause polypoid folds originate in the mucosa and submucosa and may also produce distinct polyps.

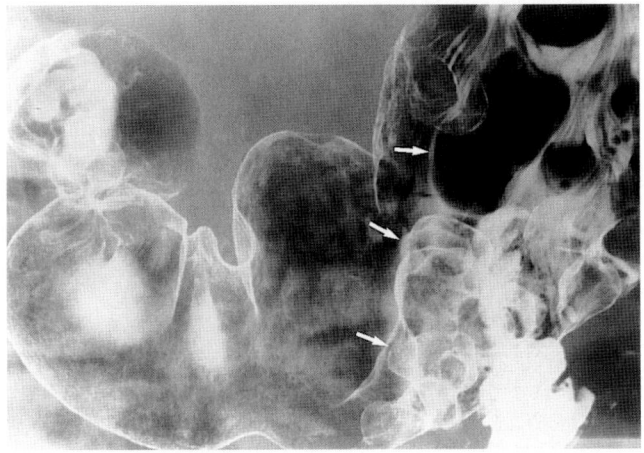

Figure 5-11. Polypoid folds. Large lobulated folds (*arrows*) are present along the greater curvature of the stomach. These thickened folds were caused by *Helicobacter pylori* gastritis.

Serpentine (Serpiginous) Folds

Serpentine (snakelike) and *serpiginous* (from the Latin, meaning "to creep") folds are sinuous or wavy and are often aligned parallel to the longitudinal axis of the bowel. Serpentine folds are seen in mucosal and submucosal inflammatory or vascular processes (Fig. 5-12), especially varices.

"Stack of Coins" Appearance

Smooth, straight, enlarged folds perpendicular to the longitudinal axis of the small bowel resemble a *stack of coins* (Fig. 5-13). This appearance usually indicates submucosal edema or hemorrhage and, rarely, infiltrating tumor. Causes of submucosal hemorrhage include trauma, ischemia, radiation damage, and a bleeding diathesis resulting from anticoagulants, hemophilia, and thrombocytopenic purpura.

Tethering

Mucosal folds may be pulled toward an extrinsic process, resulting in *tethering* of the folds (Fig. 5-14).

Pleating

If an extrinsic desmoplastic process extends into the bowel wall, the overlying mucosa may be thrown into thin folds, termed *pleating* (Fig. 5-15). In the colon, this finding suggests

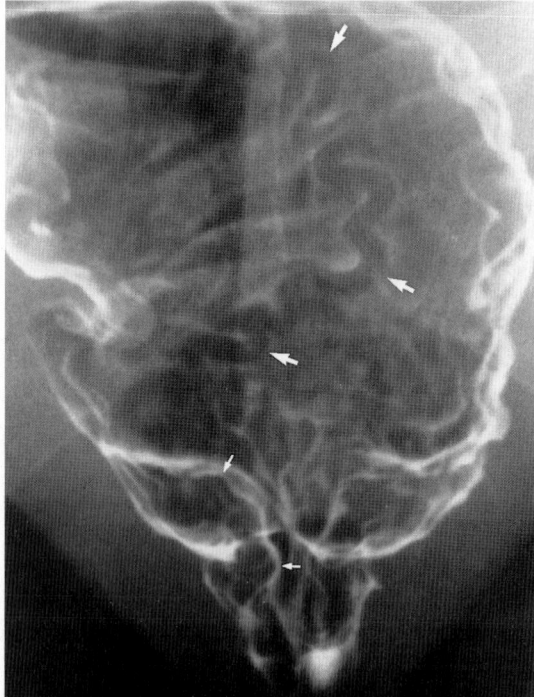

Figure 5-12. Serpentine (serpiginous) folds. Rectal varices. A sinuous radiolucent rectal fold (*large arrows*) is etched in white by barium. In the partially collapsed distal rectum, barium-etched varices create undulating lines (*small arrows*) in an abnormal location.

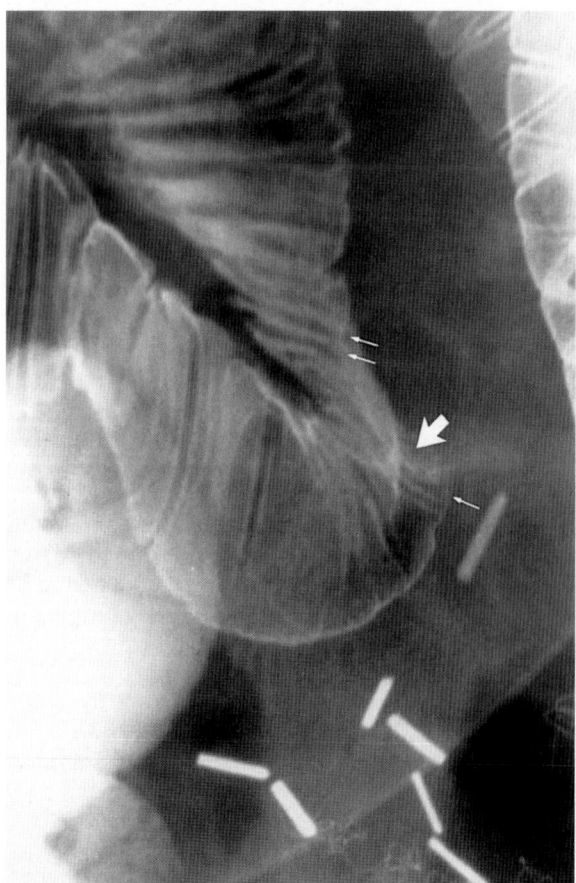

Figure 5-14. Tethering of mucosal folds. Postoperative adhesions involving the pelvic ileum. Smooth mucosal folds (*thin arrows*) are pulled toward an adhesive band. Note narrowing of the lumen and angulation of the bowel contour at the site of adhesion (*thick arrow*).

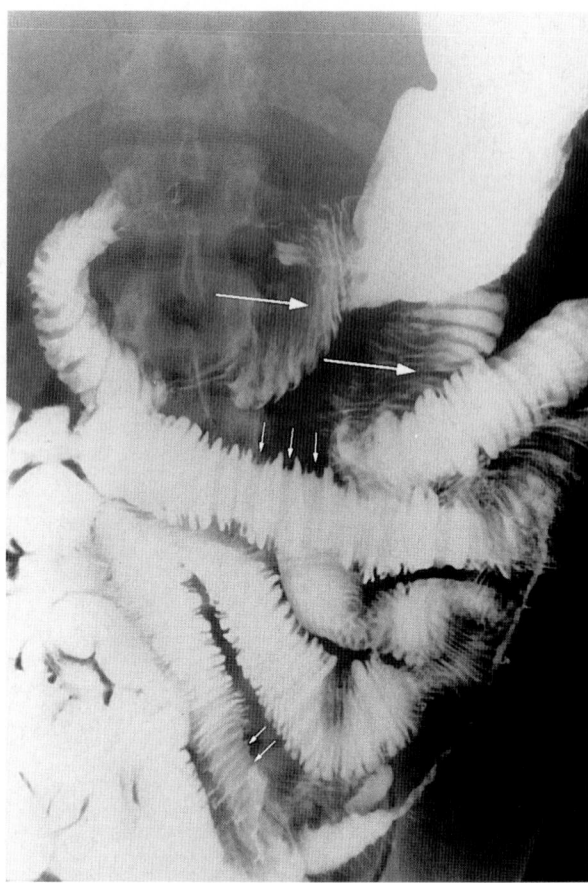

Figure 5-13. "Stack of coins" appearance. Small bowel ischemia caused by pancreatic carcinoma infiltrating mesenteric vessels. Enlarged, smooth, straight, parallel folds (*short arrows*) in the jejunum resemble a stack of coins or a picket fence. Also note the extrinsic mass impression of the enlarged head and body of the pancreas on the duodenum and first loop of jejunum (*long arrows*).

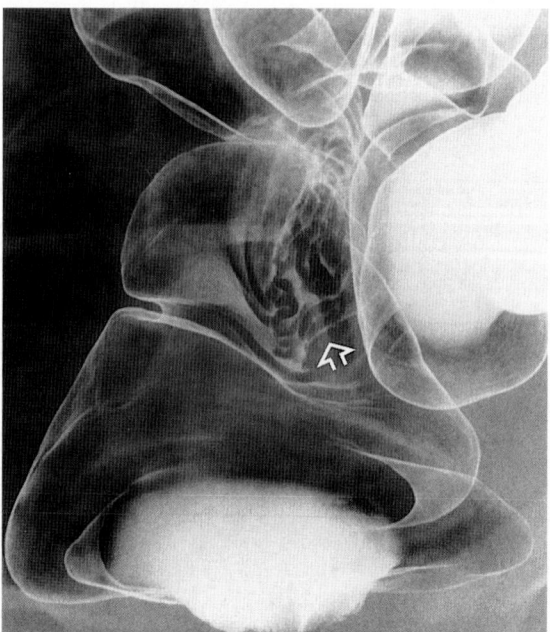

Figure 5-15. Pleating of the mucosa. Endometriosis involving the recto-sigmoid junction. The colonic mucosa is thrown into sinuous folds (*arrow*) by a desmoplastic process in the serosa and muscular layers.

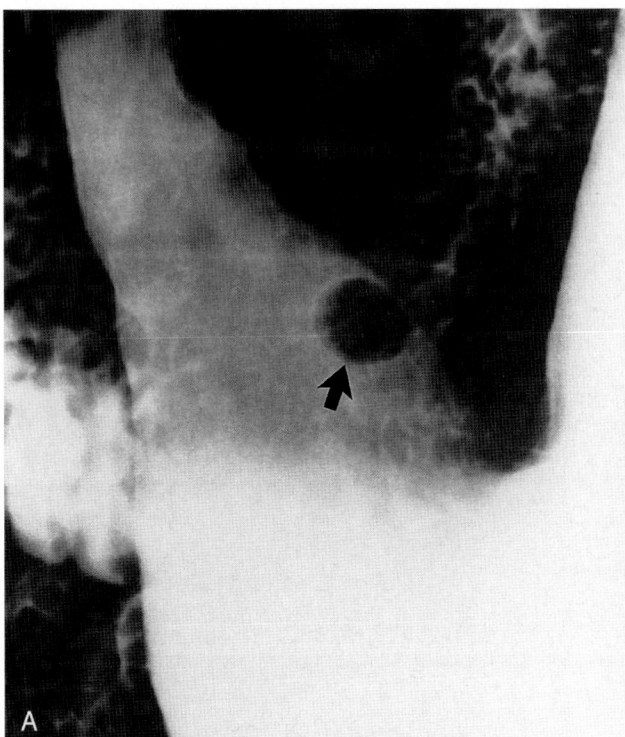
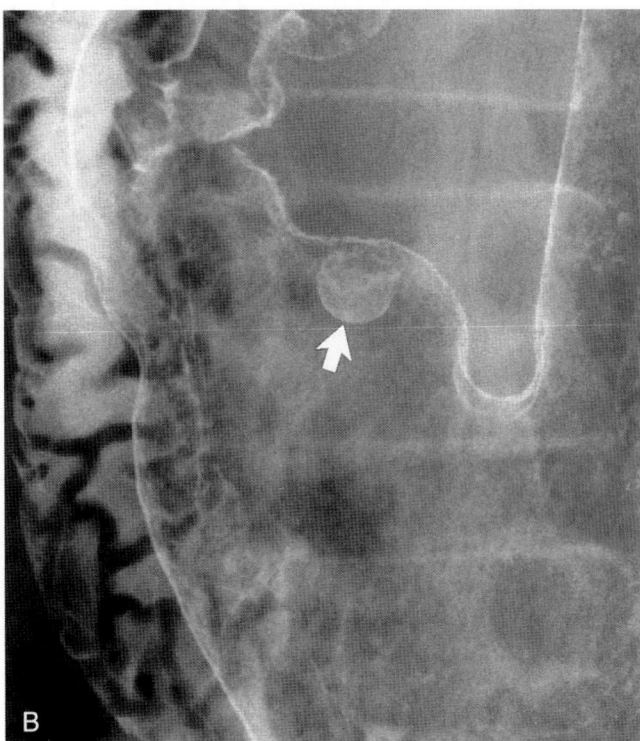

Figure 5-16. Filling defect. A. Hyperplastic polyp in the gastric antrum. A filling defect (*arrow*) is seen in the barium pool. **B.** The same polyp is seen in air contrast as a round, increased radiodensity etched in white (*arrow*). In **B**, the polyp is not described as a "filling defect."

endometriosis or intraperitoneal metastases involving the serosal surface.

PROTRUDING LESIONS

Filling Defect

A *filling defect* is a radiolucency in the barium pool caused by displacement of the barium by a protruding lesion (Fig. 5-16).

Contour Defect

A *contour defect* is a disruption of the expected luminal contour by a sessile lesion protruding into the gastrointestinal lumen (Fig. 5-17). A contour defect is not, in itself, a sign of malignancy. However, because the size of the contour defect is related to the size of the lesion, the larger the contour defect, the greater the likelihood of malignancy.

Polyp

A *polyp* is a protrusion from a mucous membrane. *Polyp* is not a histologically definitive term and does not imply adenomatous (dysplastic) change. In general, the height of a polyp is comparable to its width but a polyp is relatively tall in comparison to a mucosal plaque. Polyps may be seen as radiolucent filling defects on the dependent surface or may be etched in white on the nondependent surface (Fig. 5-18). They have many shapes and many radiographic appearances, depending on whether they are small or large, sessile or pedunculated, and smooth or nodular (see Fig. 5-18) (see Chapter 4).

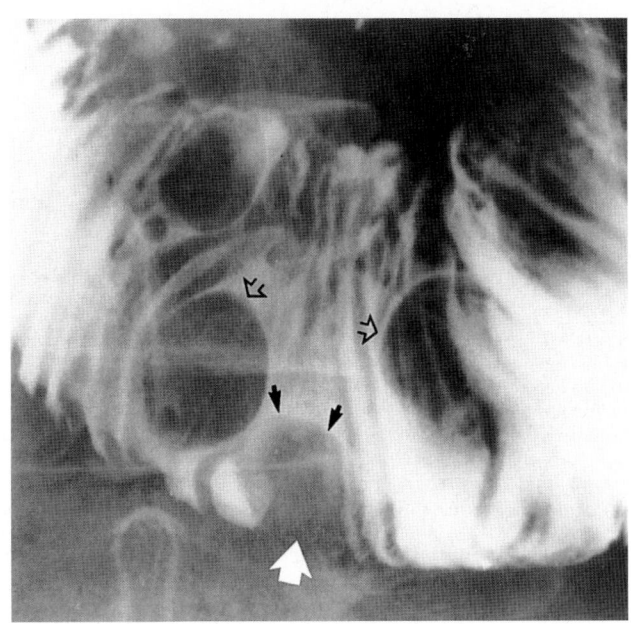

Figure 5-17. Contour defect. Metastatic melanoma in the small intestine. A contour defect (*white arrow*) is seen as loss of the expected normal contour of the bowel. The contour of the lumen is pushed toward the center of the bowel loop. In this case, a submucosal metastasis is seen in profile (*black arrows*). Other metastases are seen en face as smooth-surfaced, ovoid filling defects (*open arrows*) in the barium pool.

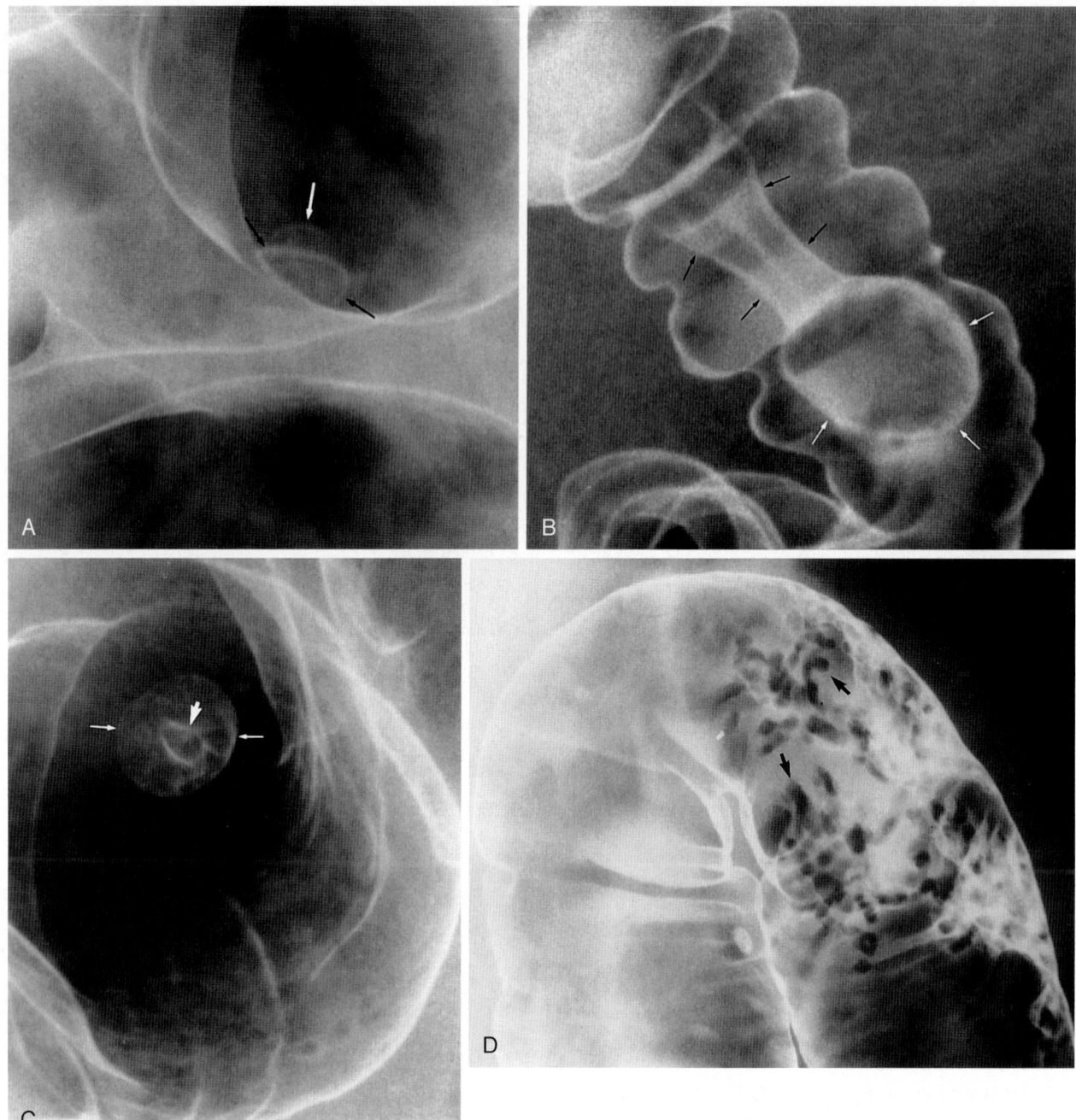

Figure 5-18. Polyp. A. "Bowler hat" polyp. Barium may be trapped between the edge of the polyp and the intestinal lumen as the polyp is pulled against the adjacent wall by its stalk. If the surface and edge of the polyp are at the proper radiographic angle, the polyp appears similar to an English bowler hat. The ring (*black arrows*) of the polyp is the junction of the polyp and mucosal surface. The dome (*white arrow*) of the polyp points toward the longitudinal axis of the lumen. **B.** Pedunculated polyp. When a pedunculated polyp is seen in profile, the pedicle of the polyp appears as parallel barium-etched lines (*black arrows*) or as a tubular radiolucency in the barium pool. The head of the polyp (*white arrows*) is seen as a round or ovoid filling defect in the barium pool or is etched in white. **C.** "Mexican hat" polyp. If a pedunculated polyp is seen en face, the pedicle appears as a ring shadow (*thick arrow*) central to the larger ring shadow of the head of the polyp (*thin arrows*). These concentric ring shadows have been termed the *sombrero* or *Mexican hat* sign. **D.** Filiform polyp. A filiform polyp is a tubular or branched polyp, often with a clubbed head. Filiform polyps imply that there has been prior inflammatory disease involving the mucosal surface of the bowel. When residual inflamed, hyperplastic, or reparative tissue protrudes into the lumen, the resulting projections appear filiform. In this patient with quiescent Crohn's disease, numerous filiform polyps (*arrows*) are seen in the splenic flexure of the colon. (**A** from Miller WT, Levine MS, Rubesin SE, et al: Bowler-hat sign: A simple principle for differentiating polyps from diverticula. Radiology 173:615-617, 1989.)

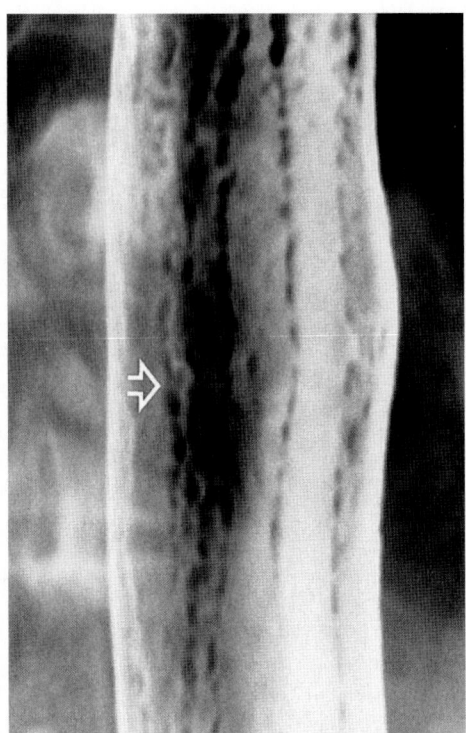

Figure 5-19. Plaque. *Candida* esophagitis. Small, well-circumscribed radiolucencies etched in white (*arrow*) are aligned longitudinally along the esophageal mucosa. Note the normal intervening esophageal mucosa. (From Rubesin SE, Levine MS, Laufer I: Odynophagia. In Thompson WM [ed]: Common Problems in Gastrointestinal Radiology. Chicago, Year Book Medical, 1989, pp 108-117.)

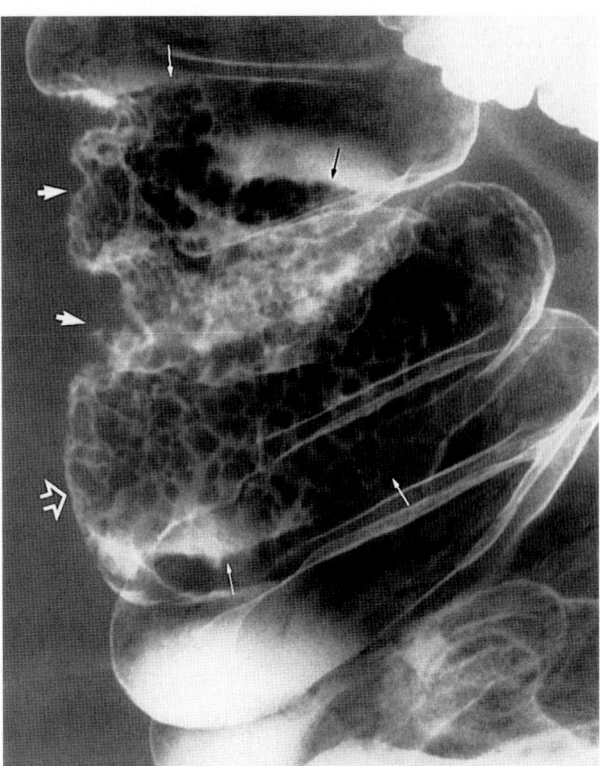

Figure 5-20. Carpet lesion. Tubulovillous adenoma with carcinoma. A focal reticular network of barium lines crosses the lumen of the ascending colon (*thin arrows*). The contour of the colon is relatively maintained in one region (*open arrow*). In an area in which carcinoma is present, the contour is indented and angulated (*thick arrows*).

Plaque

A *plaque* is a shallow surface elevation much broader than it is high. Plaques are so distinct that their margins are etched in white by barium trapped at the edges of the plaque and the adjacent mucosa (Fig. 5-19). Plaques may vary greatly in size, from the small plaques of *Candida* esophagitis to plaquelike tumors.

Carpet Lesion

Carpet lesions are focal, flat, well-circumscribed surface elevations. En face, the margin of the lesion is etched in white by barium (Fig. 5-20). When barium fills the interstices of the lesion, multiple small, polygonal radiolucent filling defects are seen surrounded by barium. In profile, the contour may be finely spiculated or nodular. The most characteristic carpet lesions are flat colonic adenomas.

Ulcerated Mass

Lesions that have both depressed and elevated components are typically *ulcerated masses* of either mucosal or submucosal origin (Fig. 5-21).

Annular Lesion

Lesions that extend circumferentially around the bowel lumen are termed *annular*. Circumferential spread around the lumen implies that the neoplastic or inflammatory process has spread

at least into the submucosa. Annular configurations are seen in benign strictures caused by ischemia, radiation therapy, or diverticulitis or in malignancies such as primary tumors or metastases (Fig. 5-22).

Saddle Lesion

A focal mass that is just beginning to encircle but is still predominantly on one wall may resemble a saddle and is described as a *saddle* or semiannular lesion (Fig. 5-23).

Submucosal Mass

The term *submucosal mass* refers to lesions arising in the submucosa and muscularis propria. These are typically benign or malignant tumors of smooth muscle, fat, or neural origin. Because the lesions arise in either submucosa or muscularis propria, they have also been referred to as *intramural* or *extramucosal*. The overlying mucosa is stretched and may be ulcerated.

In profile, a smooth-surfaced mass is seen forming right angles to the luminal contour (Fig. 5-24). En face, barium trapped in the abrupt margins results in a well-defined tumor. Central ulcers are seen in about half of all submucosal masses (see Fig. 5-24B). Small submucosal masses involving a fold symmetrically splay the edges of the fold. Although the radiographic findings are distinctive for large lesions, small (0.5 to 2.0 cm) submucosal masses may be difficult to distinguish from mucosal polyps.

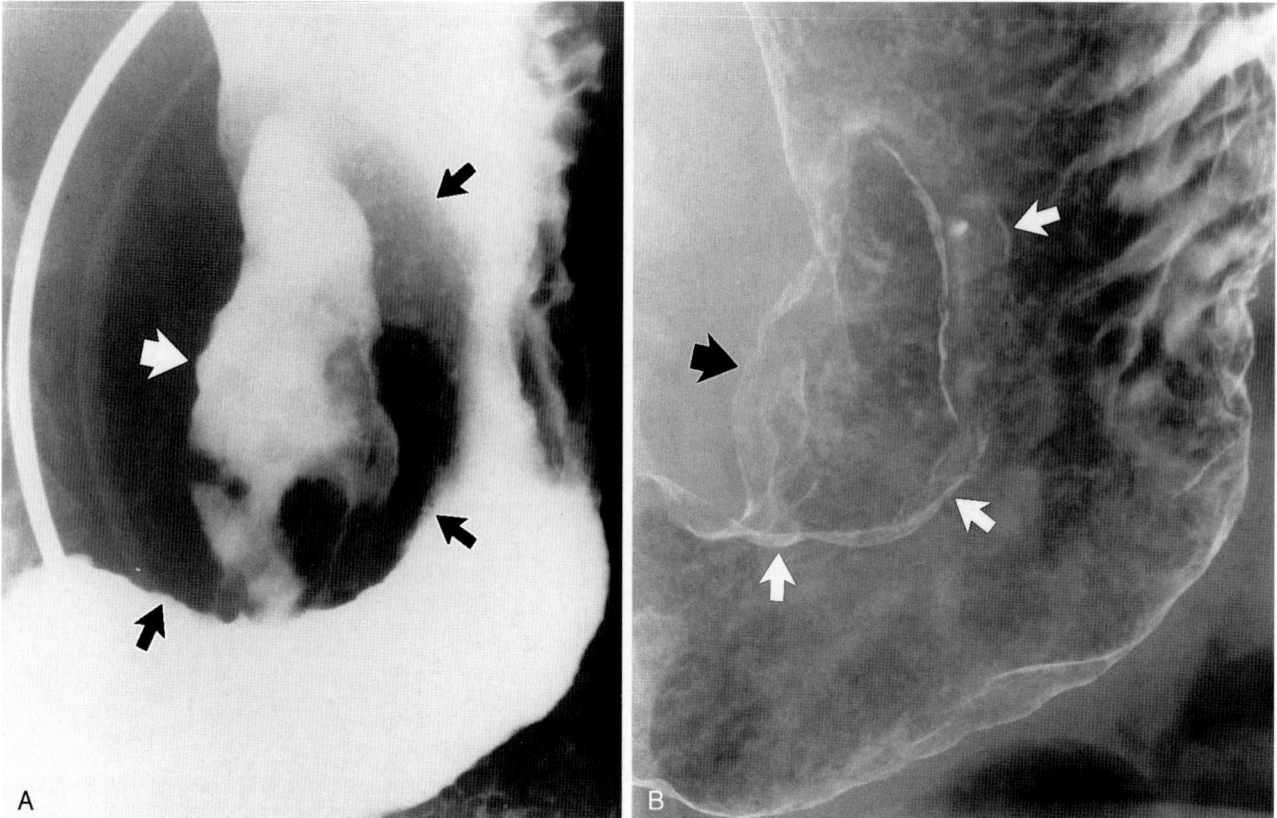

Figure 5-21. Ulcerated mass. A. Adenocarcinoma involving the lesser curvature of the stomach. A single-contrast compression view of the lesser curvature shows an ulcerated mass as an irregular barium collection (*white arrow*) within a radiolucent mass (*black arrows*) protruding into the gastric lumen. **B.** With air contrast, barium has spilled from the ulcer crater and etched the mass (shown in **A**). The rim of the mass is seen en face as a curved increased radiodensity etched in white (*white arrows*). The irregular contour of the lesser curvature represents the ulcer seen in profile (*black arrow*).

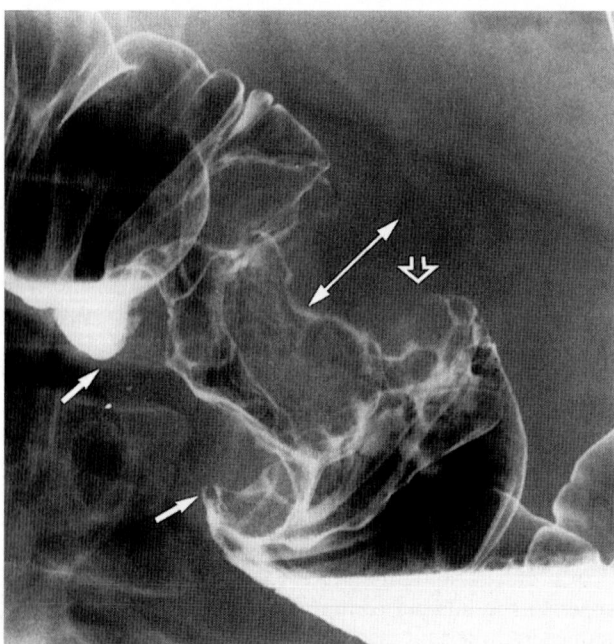

Figure 5-22. Annular lesion. Adenocarcinoma of the transverse colon. A focal annular lesion with abrupt, shelflike margins (*short arrows*) and nodular mucosa (*open arrow*) is seen on this erect view. The large amount of luminal narrowing (*double-ended arrow*) means that the tumor has spread at least into the muscularis propria. An annular cancer of the colon has a 90% chance of serosal extension and a 50% chance of lymph node metastases. (From Rubesin SE: Gallery of double-contrast terminology. Gastroenterol Clin North Am 24:259-288, 1995.)

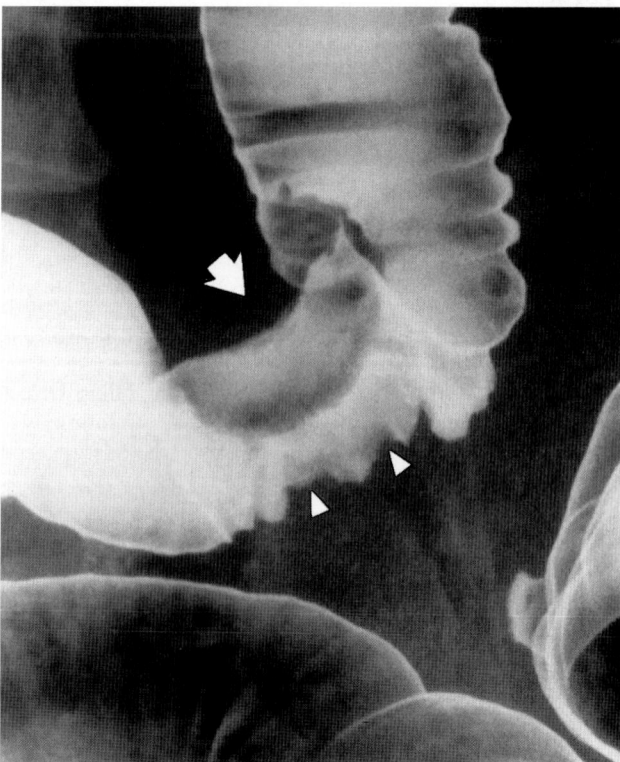

Figure 5-23. Saddle lesion. A polypoid carcinoma (*arrow*) has begun to spread circumferentially around the bowel wall (*arrowheads*), resulting in a "saddle-like" appearance. (From Rubesin SE: Gallery of double-contrast terminology. Gastroenterol Clin North Am 24:259-288, 1995.)

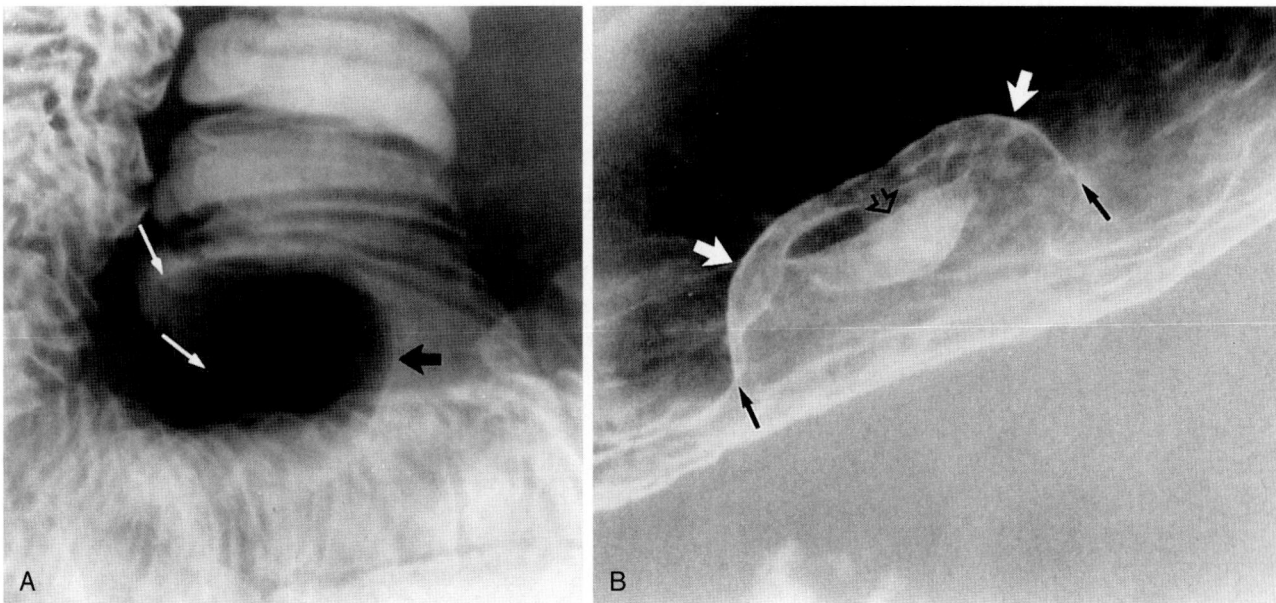

Figure 5-24. Submucosal mass. A. Lipoma of the small intestine. A smooth-surfaced polypoid mass (*black arrow*) projects into the lumen of the mid small bowel. Note the abrupt angulation (*white arrows*) of the tumor margins and adjacent normal mucosa. **B.** Metastatic melanoma on the greater curvature of the stomach. A smooth-surfaced mass is etched in white (*white arrows*). The mass forms right angles with the adjacent mucosa (*black arrows*). A pool of barium fills a central ulcer (*open arrow*). (From Rubesin SE: Gallery of double-contrast terminology. Gastroenterol Clin North Am 24:259-288, 1995.)

Target Lesion

A *target lesion* or *"bull's-eye" lesion* is a mass with a central ulcer crater (Fig. 5-25). Target lesions are typically ulcerated submucosal masses caused by primary tumors such as gastro-

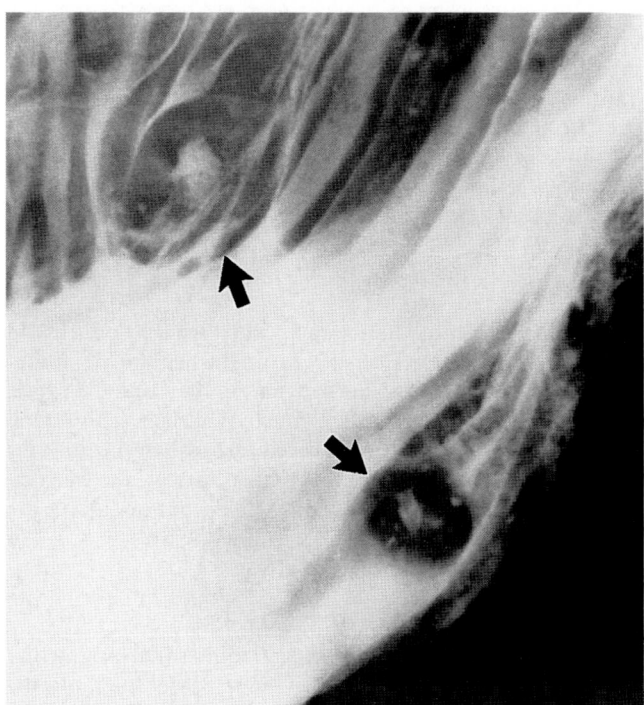

Figure 5-25. Target lesion. Disseminated lymphoma involving the stomach. Ovoid, well-circumscribed masses that are 2 cm in diameter (*arrows*) with small, central barium collections are seen along the greater curvature of the gastric body. (From Rubesin SE, Gilchrist AM, Bronner M, et al: Non-Hodgkin lymphoma of the small intestine. RadioGraphics 10:985-998, 1990.)

intestinal stromal tumors or by malignant tumors, especially metastatic melanoma, Kaposi's sarcoma, and disseminated lymphoma.

Pliability

Change or lack of change in the size and shape of a lesion is a clue to its composition (Fig. 5-26). Lesions that change in size or shape depending on the amount of luminal distention or manual compression are often composed of fat, fluid, or blood.

Extrinsic Mass Effect

Masses arising outside the gastrointestinal tract or gastrointestinal processes extending outside the luminal contour may indent the adjacent bowel wall. In profile, an extrinsic mass impression appears as a broad-based indentation with shallow angles to the contour (Fig. 5-27). En face, an extrinsic mass may appear as an ill-defined area of increased density in the air-filled lumen (see Fig. 5-27B). If imaged obliquely, an extrinsic mass effect may appear as a line.

DEPRESSED LESIONS

Erosion

An *erosion* is a defect in the mucosa that does not extend beneath the muscularis mucosae. Erosions are characterized by a small central barium collection and a surrounding radiolucent mound of edema (Fig. 5-28). The radiographic appearance is similar to that of aphthoid ulcers seen throughout the gastrointestinal tract. In some cases there is no known cause for erosive gastritis, but in most patients the condition is due to ingestion of aspirin or other nonsteroidal antiinflammatory drugs, viral infection, or alcohol ingestion.

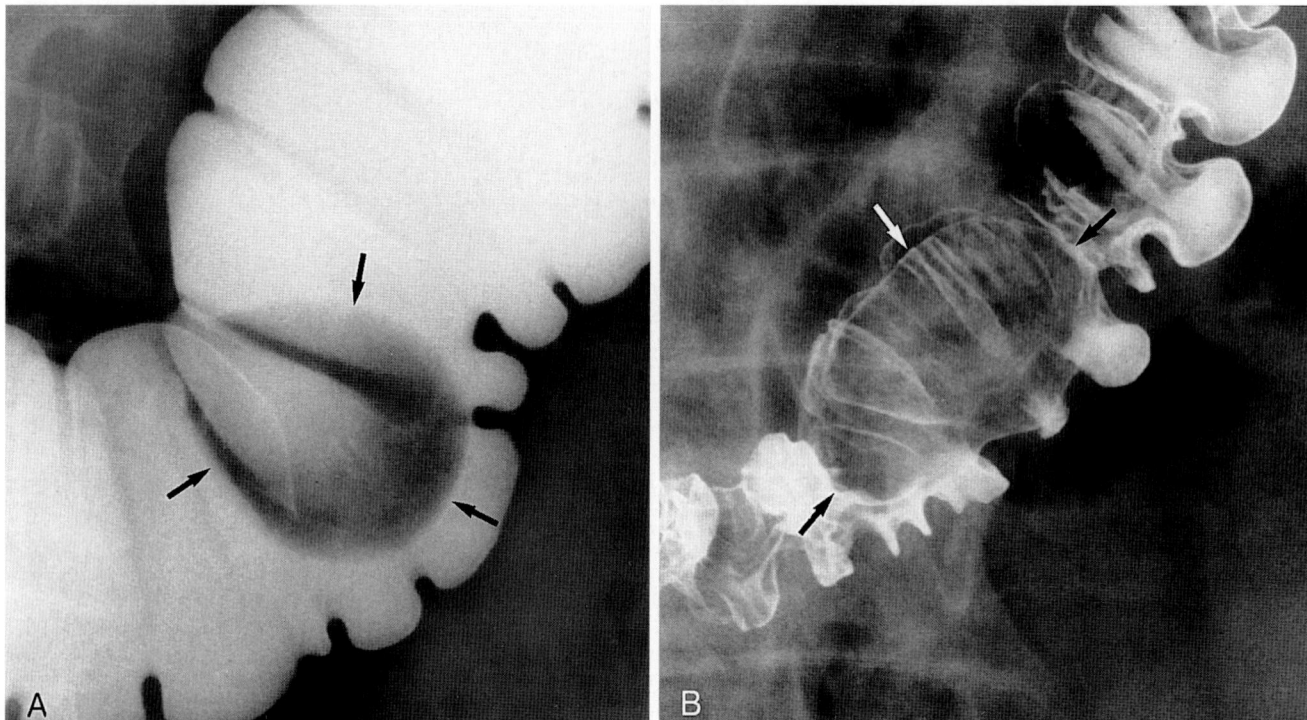

Figure 5-26. Pliability. A. Lipoma of the colon. A pear-shaped, smooth-surfaced filling defect (*arrows*) is seen in the barium column. **B.** A postevacuation radiograph shows that the polypoid mass has elongated (*arrows*) to conform to the collapsed lumen. These are classic findings of a colonic lipoma.

These erosions have also been termed *complete* or *varioliform* erosions (resembling smallpox). In some patients, only the barium collection is seen, termed an *incomplete erosion.*

Aphthoid Ulcer

An *aphthoid ulcer* is a small ulcer occurring on a mucous membrane. This is a nonspecific pathologic term derived from the Greek root *aphthai,* which meant "to set on fire" or "to inflame," and originally referred to the oral lesions of thrush, which are raised white plaques. The term was later used by the Greeks to refer to small ulcers on mucous membranes of the mouth ("canker sores"). *Aphthoid* means "resembling aphthae." *Aphthous* means "related to aphthae." Radiologists use the terms *aphthoid ulcer* and *aphthous ulcer* interchangeably, but the preferred term is *aphthoid ulcer.* The most common causes of aphthoid ulcers are Crohn's disease, viral infections, varioliform erosions, and amebiasis (Fig. 5-29). Erosions related to nonsteroidal anti-inflammatory agents may appear identical to aphthoid ulcers.

Ulcer Niche (Crater)

The term *niche* or *crater* refers to the defect or hole in the mucosal surface, representing an ulcer. The niche may be visualized in profile as a projection of barium extending beyond the luminal contour. Alternatively, the niche may be seen en face as a barium collection or the edges of the crater may be etched in white (Fig. 5-30).

Linear Ulcer/Linear Erosion

Ulcers of the gastrointestinal tract need not be round or ovoid. *Linear ulcers* are not infrequently seen (Fig. 5-31) and have a variety of causes, especially Crohn's disease (see Fig. 5-31B), trauma resulting from intubation or vomiting, or the toxic effects of drugs such as aspirin and other nonsteroidal anti-inflammatory agents (see Fig. 5-31A). Linear erosions in the stomach are almost always related to the use of nonsteroidal anti-inflammatory agents.

"Collar Button" Ulcer

Collar button ulcers are ulcers with a narrow neck and a broad base (Fig. 5-32). These ulcers are formed when the inflammatory process spreads in the soft fat of the lamina propria and submucosa, parallel to the mucosal surface. This lateral extension gives the ulcer a relatively broad base in the submucosa and a narrow neck as it passes through the mucosa. In the colon, common causes of collar button ulcers are amebiasis, ulcerative colitis, and Crohn's disease.

Exoenteric Mass

Exoenteric masses are masses of gastrointestinal origin that extend predominantly outside the bowel rather than into the lumen of the bowel. They often extend into the mesentery or omentum. These lesions may cavitate, with the cavity extending outside the expected contour of the bowel (Fig. 5-33). The most common neoplastic exoenteric masses include lymphoma, metastatic melanoma, and gastrointestinal stromal tumors.

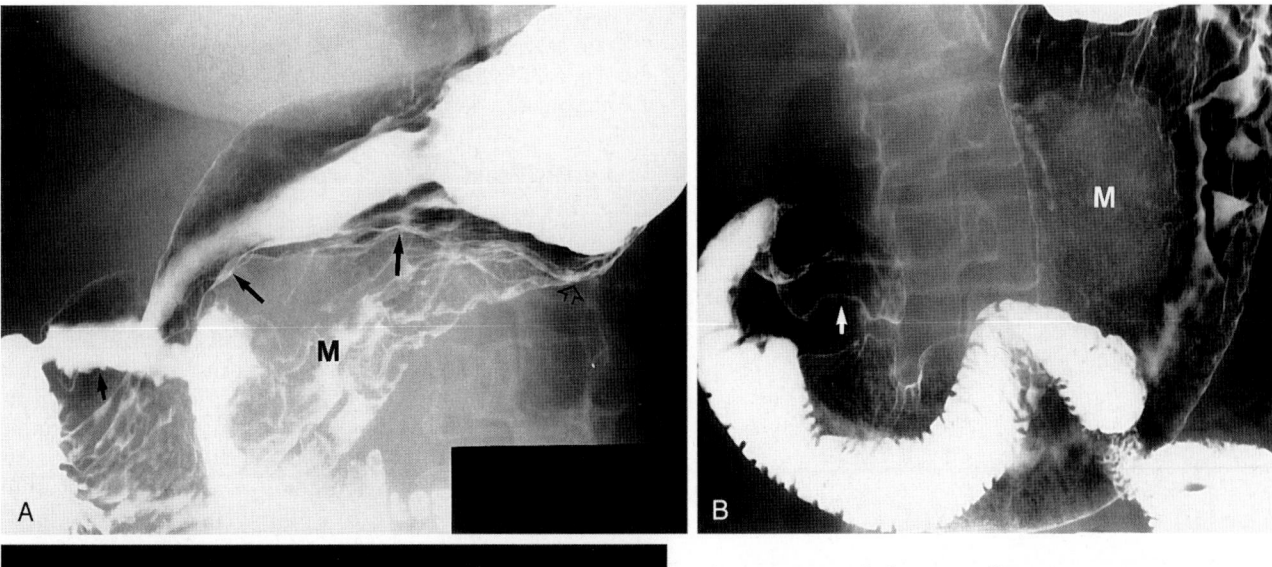

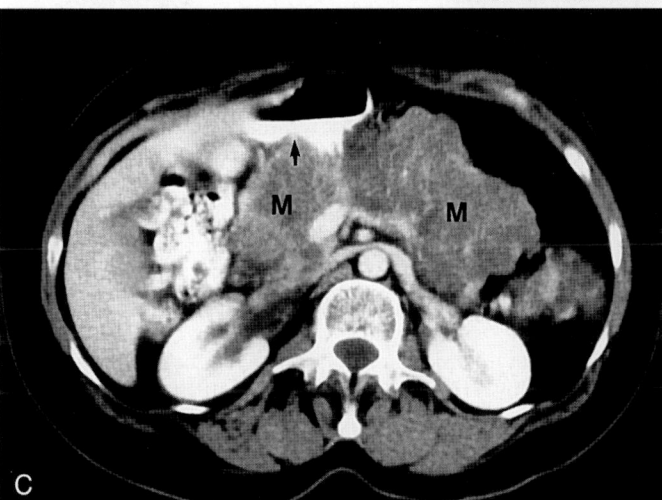

Figure 5-27. Extrinsic mass effect. A. An extrinsic mass is manifested in profile by a broad-based line crossing the partially compressed lumen of the posterior wall of the stomach (*long arrows*) and duodenum (*short arrow*). The indentation forms a shallow angle with the gastric contour (*open arrow*). There is increased density in the part of the stomach (M) where air in the gastric lumen is displaced by the soft tissue mass. **B.** En face, the extrinsic mass (M) appears as an ill-defined area of increased density in the stomach. A duodenal impression is manifested by inbowing of the luminal contour (*arrow*). **C.** CT performed after the upper gastrointestinal series shows an extrinsic mass compressing the stomach. Diffuse enlargement of the pancreas results from a low-attenuation, lobulated mass (M) showing focal linear areas of contrast enhancement. The posterior wall of the gastric antrum is indented (*arrow*) by the pancreatic mass and later proved to be a diffuse microcystic adenoma in a patient with unsuspected von Hippel-Lindau disease. (From Rubesin SE: Gallery of double-contrast terminology. Gastroenterol Clin North Am 24:259-288, 1995.)

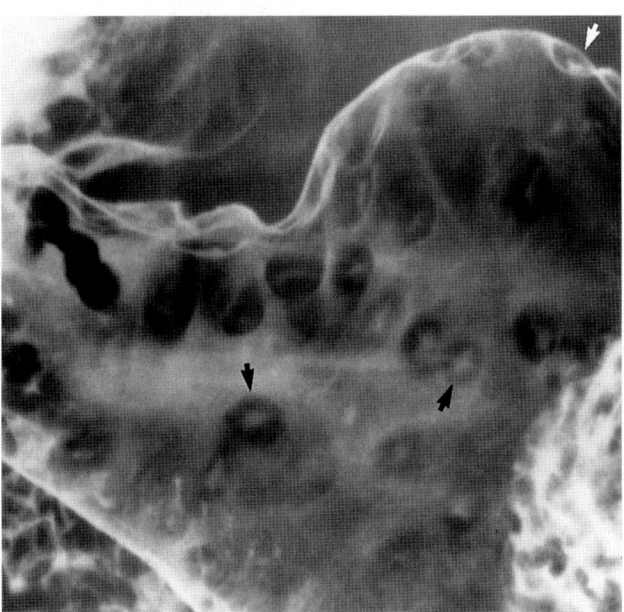

Figure 5-28. Erosions. Numerous linear and ovoid collections of barium (*arrows*) are surrounded by radiolucent halos of edema. This erosive gastritis was due to aspirin use.

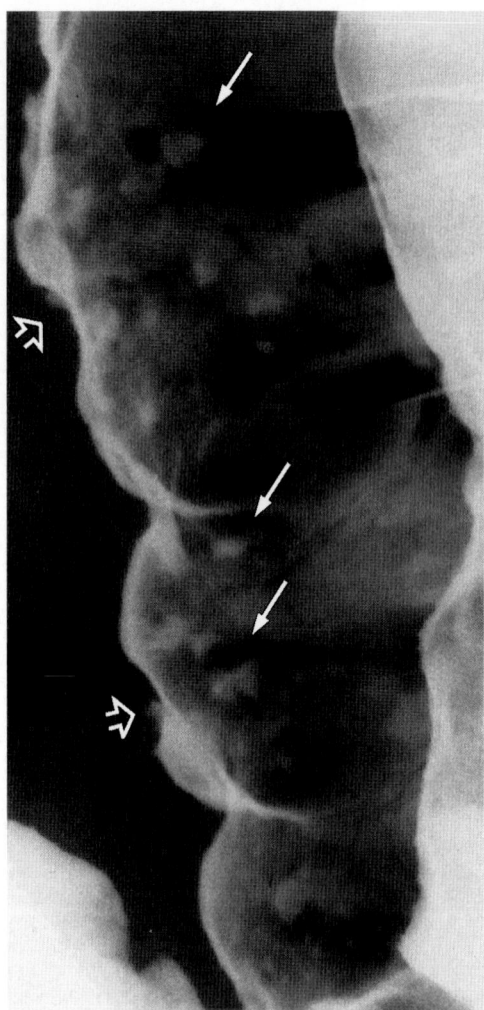

Figure 5-29. Aphthoid ulcers. Crohn's disease involving the splenic flexure of the colon. Numerous aphthoid ulcers are seen en face as punctate barium collections surrounded by radiolucent halos of edema (*solid arrows*). In profile, small ulcers are seen within edematous mounds of mucosa (*open arrows*).

Tracking

Linear collections of contrast medium within the bowel wall are termed *intramural tracks*. Linear collections of contrast medium outside the expected confines of the bowel are referred to as *extramural tracks*. Intramural tracks frequently course perpendicular to the longitudinal axis of the bowel (Fig. 5-34). Extramural tracks caused by diverticulitis often spread longitudinally in the pericolic fat. Tracks associated with radiation damage, trauma, Crohn's disease, or iatrogenic perforation may spread in any direction.

CONTOUR ABNORMALITIES

Tapering

A shallow, smooth-surfaced, gradual narrowing of the contour of the bowel reflects a desmoplastic disease in the mucosa and submucosa that *tapers* the lumen. Tapering is usually due to benign scarring from chronic inflammatory disease (Fig. 5-35). Occasionally, a neoplasm infiltrating the submucosa may incite a desmoplastic reaction that causes tapering.

Linitis Plastica

Linitis plastica refers to diffuse narrowing and loss of pliability of a gastrointestinal organ. The linitis pattern is most commonly seen in scirrhous carcinoma of the stomach (Fig. 5-36). This type of cancer is also seen in the colon, especially in patients with chronic ulcerative colitis. Both inflammatory and neoplastic processes, however, can result in a linitis appearance. For example, linitis plastica of the stomach may be due to caustic ingestion or metastatic breast carcinoma. Because these infiltrative processes are primarily in a submucosal location, endoscopic biopsy specimens and brushings may be negative.

String Sign

The term *string sign* is used when severe narrowing of a bowel loop causes the lumen to resemble a string. This term is especially applied in Crohn's disease when severe narrowing is caused by edema, spasm, inflammation, or fibrosis (Fig. 5-37). Narrowing, therefore, may not reflect the true luminal diameter because of this component of spasm.

Thumbprinting

Submucosal hemorrhage or severe edema occurs to a greater degree along the mesenteric border of the small bowel and is manifested radiographically by *thumbprinting* (Fig. 5-38).

Sacculation

Sacculation refers to broad-based outpouchings of the bowel wall. Relatively normal bowel wall may appear sacculated between folds radiating toward a neoplastic or a desmoplastic process. This form of sacculation occurs on the bowel wall opposite the mesenteric changes of Crohn's disease (Fig. 5-39A), ischemia, or diverticulitis. These sacculations do not extend beyond the expected contour of the bowel. A bowel wall weakened by atrophy or fibrosis of the muscularis propria may also appear sacculated, especially in scleroderma (Fig. 5-39B). Sacculation related to weakening extends beyond the usual contour of the bowel.

Spiculation

A desmosplastic process extrinsic to the bowel, resulting from either inflammatory or neoplastic disease, may extend into the serosa or muscularis propria and pull the luminal contour into spikelike points, termed *spiculation* (Fig. 5-40).

Angulation

Gross *angulation* of the bowel may occur when an extrinsic desmoplastic process tethers the bowel wall (Fig. 5-41).

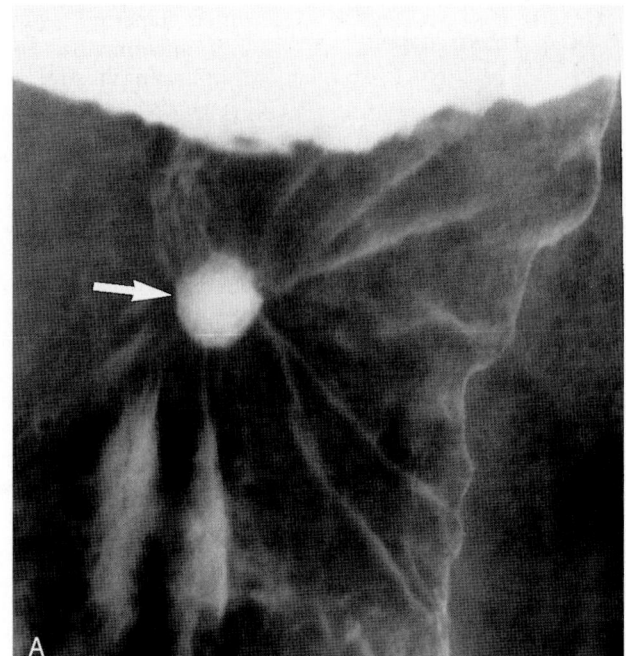

Figure 5-30. Ulcer niche (crater). A. Benign gastric ulcer. The ulcer niche (crater) is seen as a focal barium collection (*arrow*). The benign nature of the lesion is indicated by smooth folds that radiate to the ulcer's margin and the lack of surrounding mass effect or mucosal nodularity. **B.** Benign gastric ulcer. In another patient the ulcer crater is seen en face as a hemispheric ring shadow etched in white by barium (*arrows*). **C.** As the patient is turned, the ulcer projects outside the expected contour of the lesser curvature. The ulcer crater is now seen as a hemispheric line (*arrows*) extending beyond the lesser curvature of the stomach.

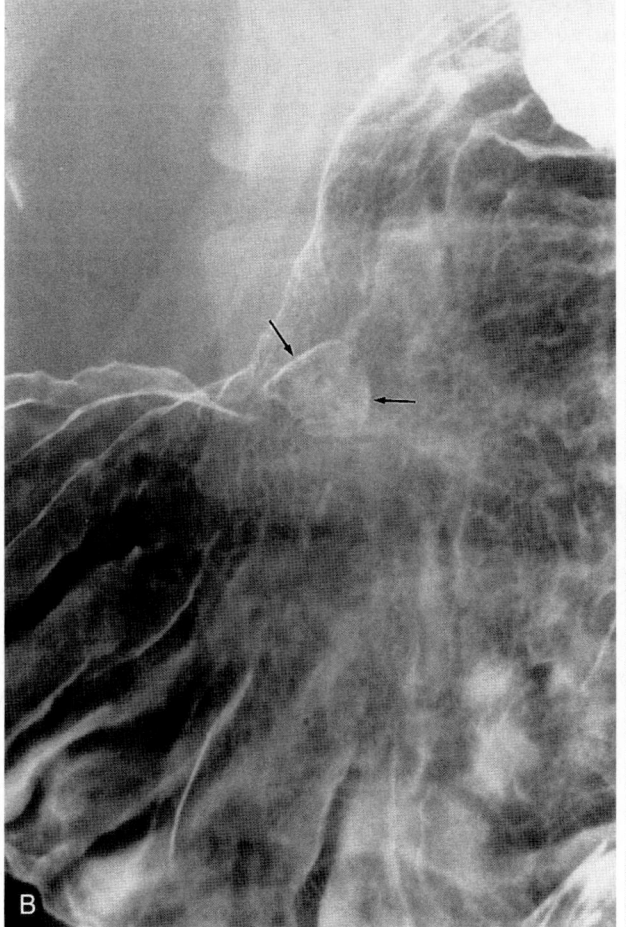

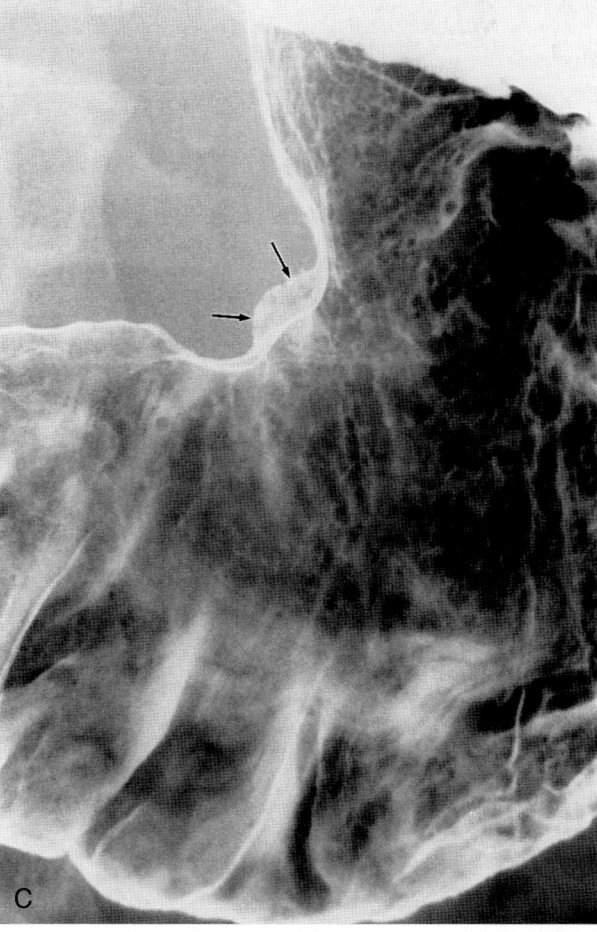

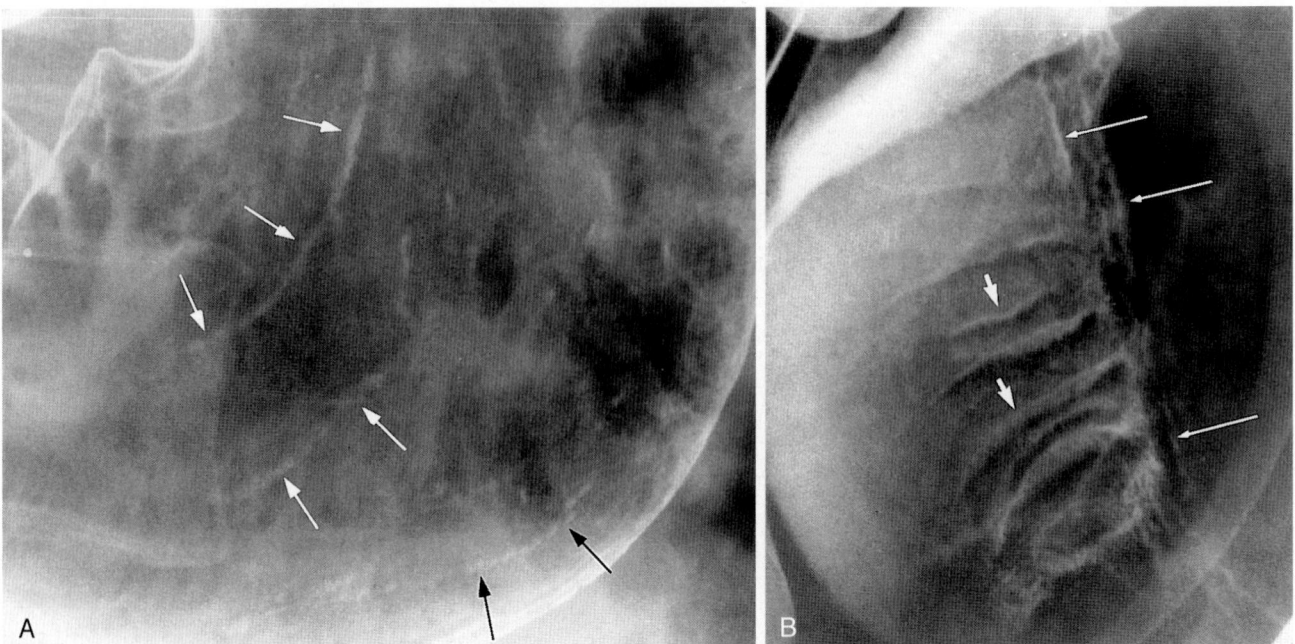

Figure 5-31. Linear ulcers. A. Ibuprofen-induced gastric ulceration. Long, linear collections of barium (*arrows*) are seen in the proximal gastric antrum. **B.** Crohn's disease involving the small bowel. Linear ulcers are seen as irregular barium collections (*long arrows*) along the mesenteric border of the ileum. Note the folds (*short arrows*) radiating toward these mesenteric border ulcers. (**B** from Rubesin SE, Bronner M: Radiologic-pathologic concepts in Crohn's disease. In Herlinger H, Megibow AJ [eds]: Advances in Gastrointestinal Radiology. Chicago, Mosby–Year Book, 1991, vol 1, pp 27-55.)

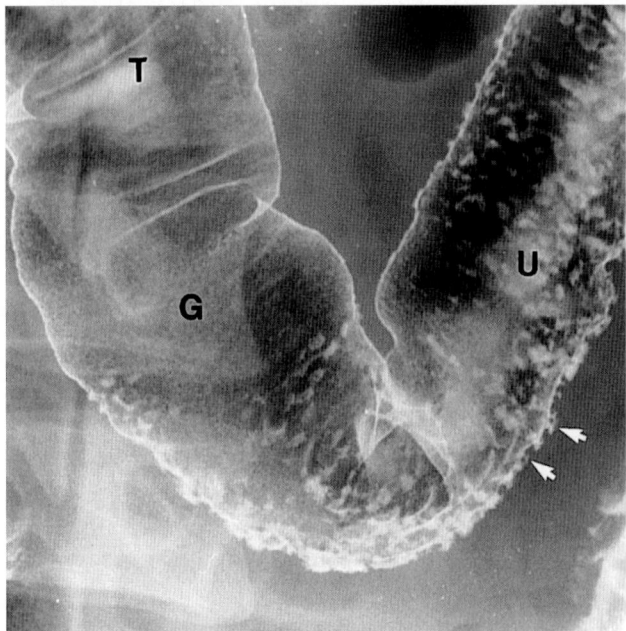

Figure 5-32. "Collar button" ulcers. The spectrum of inflammatory changes in ulcerative colitis. In the proximal transverse colon (T), there is relatively smooth mucosa. This progresses to a granular pattern (G). Distally, there is superficial ulceration (U). When the superficial ulcers penetrate the mucosa, lateral spread of inflammation in the submucosa results in collar button ulcers (*arrows*). (From Rubesin SE, Laufer I, Dinsmore B: Radiologic investigation of inflammatory bowel disease. In MacDermott RP, Stenson WF, [eds]: Inflammatory Bowel Disease. New York, Elsevier Science, 1992, pp 453-492.)

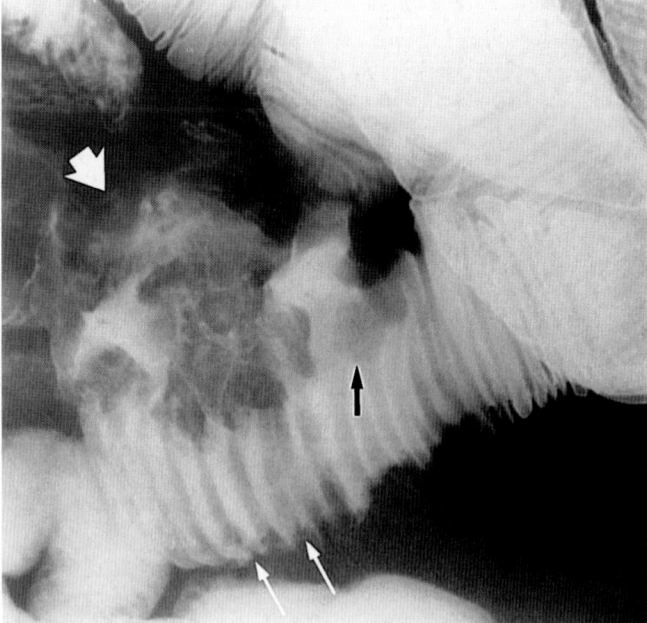

Figure 5-33. Exoenteric mass. Primary lymphoma of the small intestine. A large barium-filled excavation (*thick white arrow*) projects from the mesenteric border of the small bowel. Note other radiographic findings of primary small bowel lymphoma, including thickened, nodular folds (*thin white arrows*) and mucosal nodularity (*black arrow*).

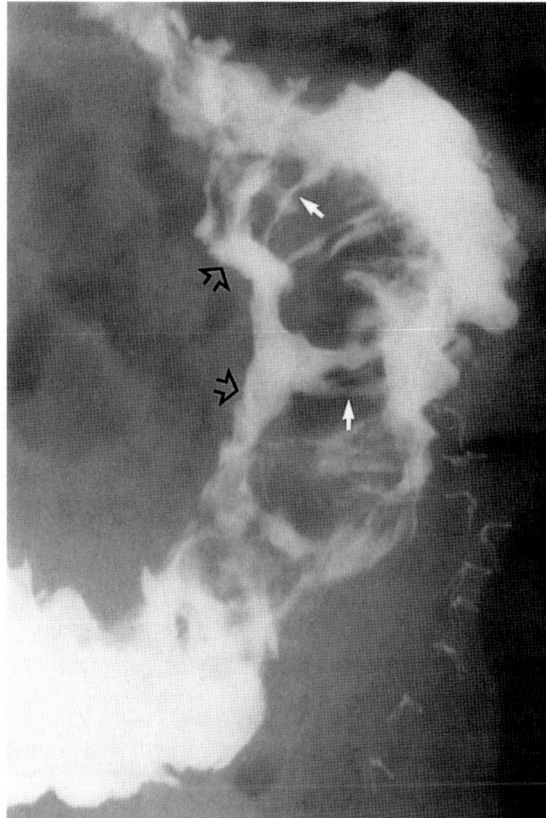

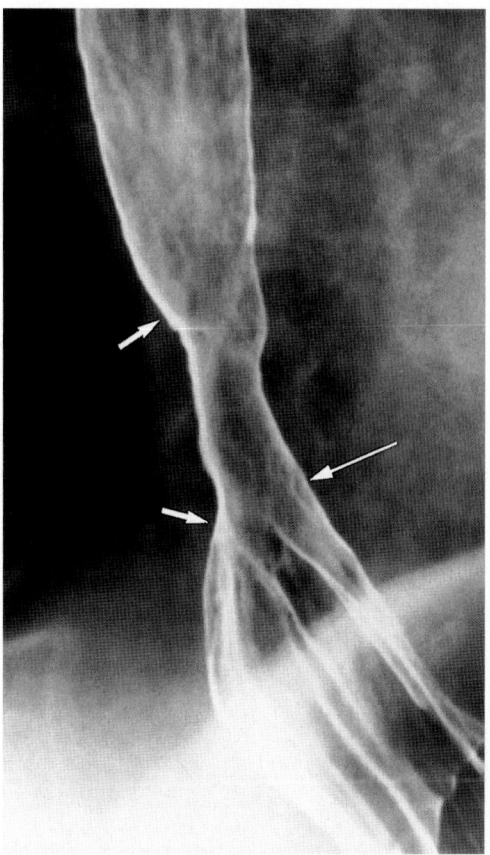

Figure 5-34. Tracking. Crohn's disease involving the descending colon. Numerous intramural tracks (*white arrows*) extend from the colonic lumen into the pericolic space. The intramural tracks course perpendicular to the lumen through the muscularis propria. A large, linear, extramural barium collection (an extramural track) (*open arrows*) lies in the pericolic fat parallel to the lumen.

Figure 5-35. Tapering. Benign reflux-induced stricture in distal esophagus. A circumferential narrowing of the distal esophagus has a smooth, tapered contour (*small arrows*) and relatively smooth mucosa. The hiatal hernia and esophagogastric junction (*long arrow*) lie above the diaphragm in this erect image, implying that there is shortening of the esophagus as a result of scarring. (From Low VHS, Rubesin SE: Contrast evaluation of the pharynx and esophagus. Radiol Clin North Am 31:1265-1291, 1993.)

Figure 5-36. Linitis plastica. Adenocarcinoma of the stomach. The fundus and body of the stomach are diffusely narrowed. The luminal contour is altered by nodular, broad-based indentations (*arrows*), but the mucosa is relatively smooth. These findings indicate the submucosal location of the bulk of the infiltrating tumor.

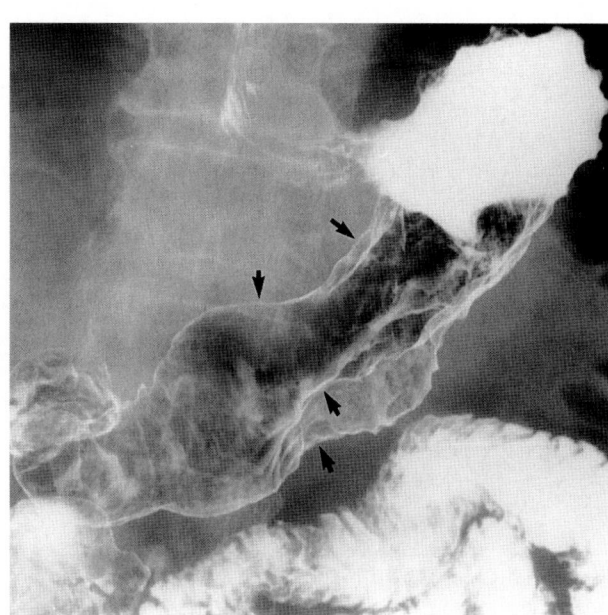

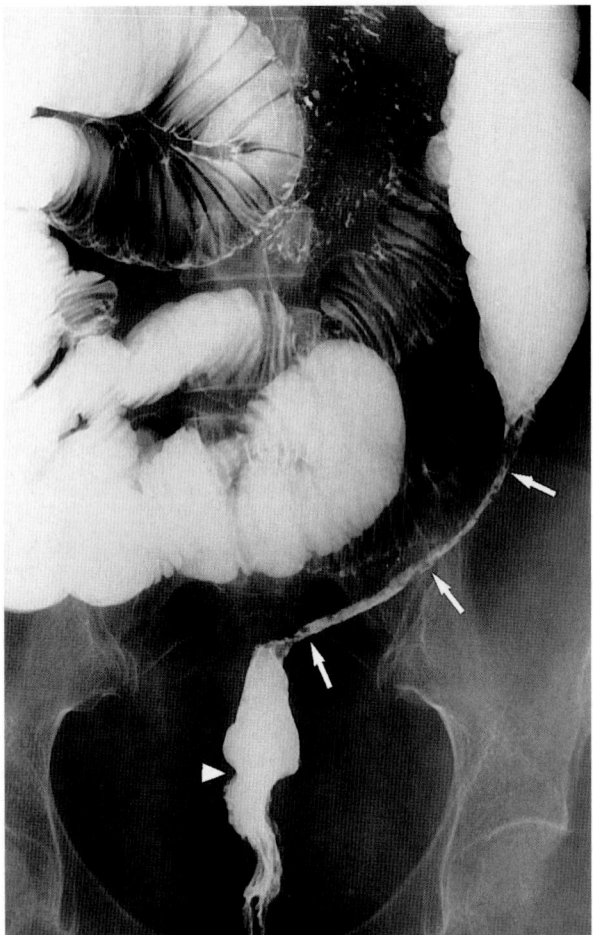

Figure 5-37. String sign. Recurrent Crohn's disease involving the neoterminal ileum. Diffuse narrowing (*arrows*) of the neoterminal ileum is seen proximal to an ileorectal anastomosis (*arrowhead*).

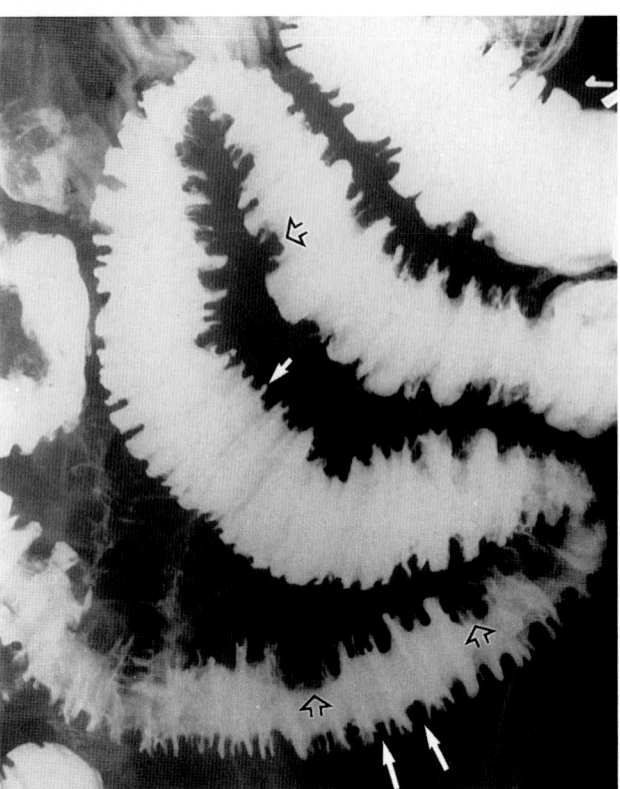

Figure 5-38. Thumbprinting. Polypoid projections (*open arrows*) are seen along the mesenteric border of the ileum. Note the abrupt angulation of the protrusions and smooth surfaces, radiographic findings typical of submucosal lesions. This thumbprinting reflects submucosal hemorrhage in a patient with small bowel vasculitis. Also note the smooth, straight, parallel folds (*long white arrows*)—the stack of coins appearance—and interspace spikes (*short white arrow*).

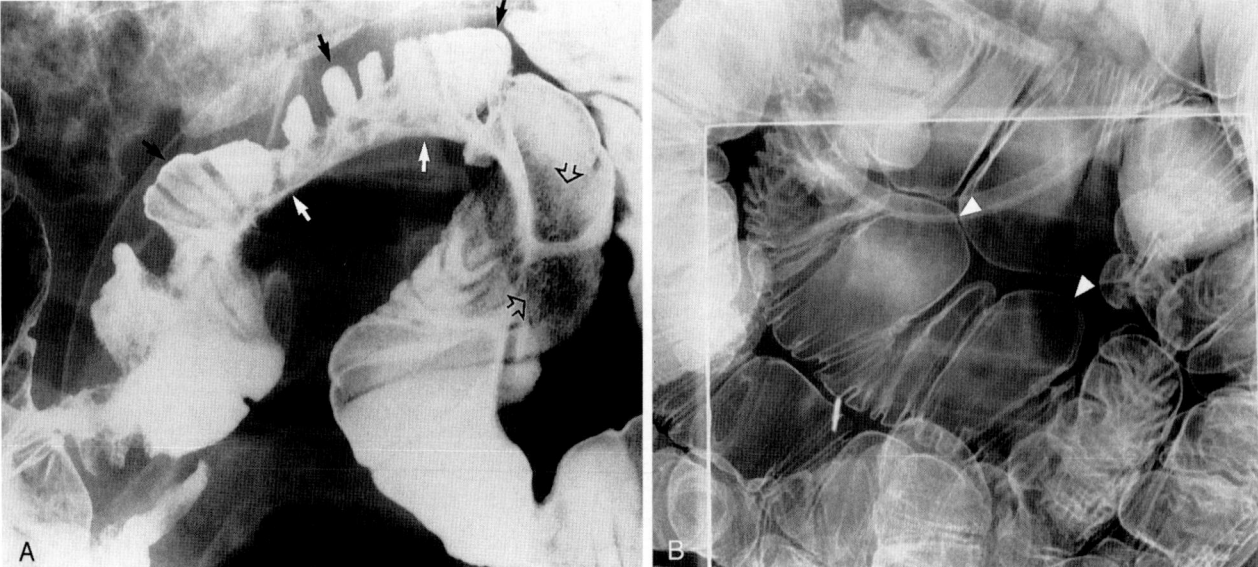

Figure 5-39. Sacculation. A. Crohn's disease involving the terminal ileum. The ileal contour is sacculated (*black arrows*) opposite a longitudinal ulcer (*white arrows*) on the mesenteric border. Note folds radiating toward the mesenteric border ulcer. Also note a reticular or granular mucosa (*open arrows*), reflecting mild mucosal changes. **B.** Scleroderma involving the small intestine. Large broad-based sacculations (*arrowheads*) protrude from the expected contour of the mesenteric border of the small bowel. (**A** courtesy of Henrik DeGryse, MD, Antwerp, Belgium.)

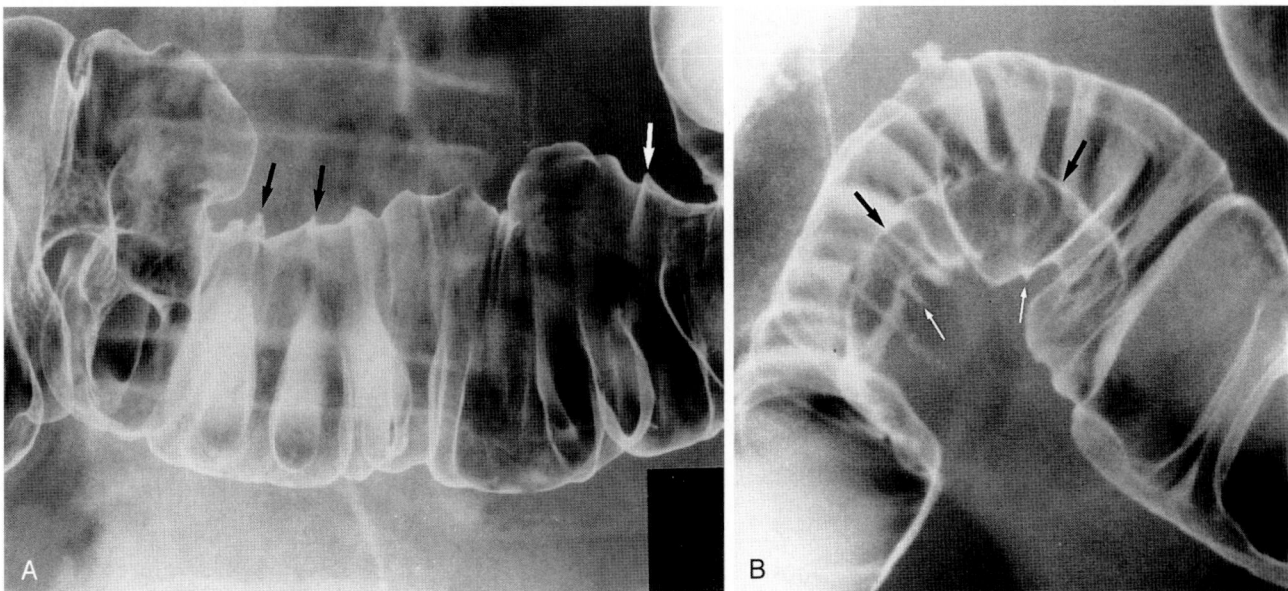

Figure 5-40. Spiculation. A. Omental metastases from breast carcinoma extend to the transverse colon. The superior border of the transverse colon is spiculated (*arrows*). **B.** Endometriosis involving the sigmoid colon. The contour of the inferior border of the sigmoid colon is spiculated (*white arrows*). A smooth-surfaced "submucosal" mass (*black arrows*) is seen, reflecting deep extension of endometrial tissue into the muscularis propria with resulting muscular hyperplasia. (From Rubesin SE: Gallery of double-contrast terminology. Gastroenterol Clin North Am 24:259-288, 1995.)

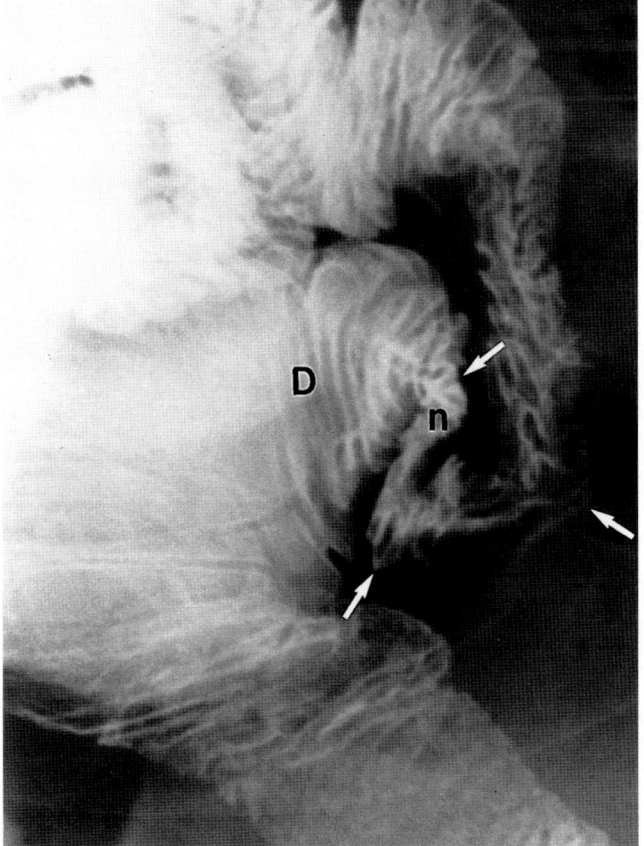

Figure 5-41. Angulation of bowel loops. Adhesions involving the pelvic ileum. The small bowel is abruptly angulated (*arrows*) in several locations. Note narrowing of the lumen distal to the obstruction (n) and dilatation of the lumen (D) proximal to the angulation. The mucosa is intact.

Ultrasonography of the Hollow Viscera

Stephanie R. Wilson, MD

TECHNIQUE

NORMAL GUT

ABNORMAL GUT

Mural Thickening

Mural Masses

Perienteric Evaluation

PERITONEAL, MESENTERIC, AND OMENTAL ABNORMALITIES

The significant artifact arising from gas in the lumen of the gastrointestinal tract has led many investigators to ignore the hollow viscera when performing routine abdominal ultrasonography. This is regrettable because ultrasonography is an excellent means of assessing a wide variety of gastrointestinal tract diseases, notably those that produce mural abnormality (either gut wall thickening or gut wall masses) and abnormality of the adjacent soft tissues, including the peritoneum, mesentery, omentum, and solid organs. Although mucosal abnormalities and small mass lesions are beneath its spatial resolution, ultrasonography, like CT, excels in demonstrating the nonmucosal aspects of gastrointestinal tract disease and in detecting extraintestinal complications.

In some patients, ultrasonography is performed specifically to detect gastrointestinal tract disease and characterize its nature and extent. In other patients, a gastrointestinal abnormality may be detected on sonograms performed for nonspecific reasons, such as evaluation of a palpable abdominal mass or abdominal pain. In addition, gut-related disease may be an occasional incidental observation on ultrasonography. In all instances, recognition of the gastrointestinal origin of a sonographic finding should lead to appropriate further investigation.

TECHNIQUE

Abdominal sonograms are ideally performed after an overnight fast to minimize luminal gas and fluid content. Oral or rectal fluid is not routinely administered, although reports describe the use of oral contrast agents for optimizing assessment of the gut as well as the retroperitoneum.[1] Routine survey of the peritoneal cavity should be performed with a transducer that visualizes both deep (e.g., gastroesophageal junction) and more superficial (e.g., small bowel loops) structures. The

region of interest must be assessed within the focal zone of the transducer; therefore, transducers with short focal zones or variable focusing are best. Suspicious gut loops should then receive detailed analysis using graded compression ultrasonography (Fig. 6-1), a technique popularized by Julien Puylaert for patients with suspected appendicitis.[2] Gradually-increasing pressure is applied to the region of interest. Normal loops of intestine are displaced or compressed, whereas abnormally thickened or obstructed loops are noncompressible and are trapped between the transducer anteriorly and the body wall musculature posteriorly. This optimizes visualiza-

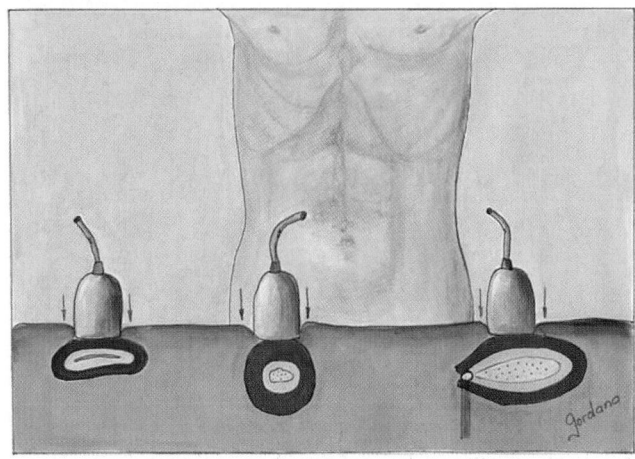

Figure 6-1. Compression ultrasonography, schematic depiction. Normal gut is compressible. Abnormally thickened gut or an obstructed segment (e.g., acute appendicitis) is noncompressible. (Modified from Puylaert JBCM, in Wilson SR: Gastrointestinal tract sonography. In Rumack C, Wilson SR, Charboneau JW [eds]: Diagnostic Ultrasound, 3rd ed. St. Louis, Elsevier Mosby, 2005, pp 269-320.)

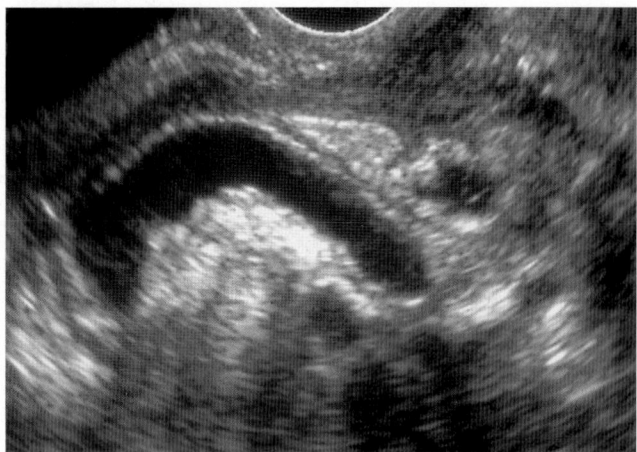

Figure 6-2. Transvaginal ultrasonography: appendicitis. A blind-ended tubular structure with a fluid-distended lumen is shown in a woman with acute appendicitis. The appendix could not be seen on the suprapubic scan because of its location deep in the pelvis. (From Wilson SR: Gastrointestinal tract sonography. In Rumack C, Wilson SR, Charboneau JW [eds]: Diagnostic Ultrasound, 3rd ed. St. Louis, Elsevier Mosby, 2005, pp 269-320.)

tion of the region of interest without annoying interference from luminal gas. In patients with peritoneal irritation or localized abdominal pain, it is important to use gentle, continuous graded compression because rapid or jerky movements of the transducer result in a nondiagnostic study and an unhappy patient.

In women with unexplained pelvic pain, mass, or fever, particularly those in the childbearing years, transvaginal scans are performed routinely if regular abdominal and pelvic sonograms are negative. Both appendicitis (Fig. 6-2) and diverticulitis (Fig. 6-3) may involve gut deep in the true pelvis that is more optimally detected with the transvaginal approach. Transvaginal, transanal, and transperineal scans can also be used for evaluation of perianal inflammatory disease and fistulas.

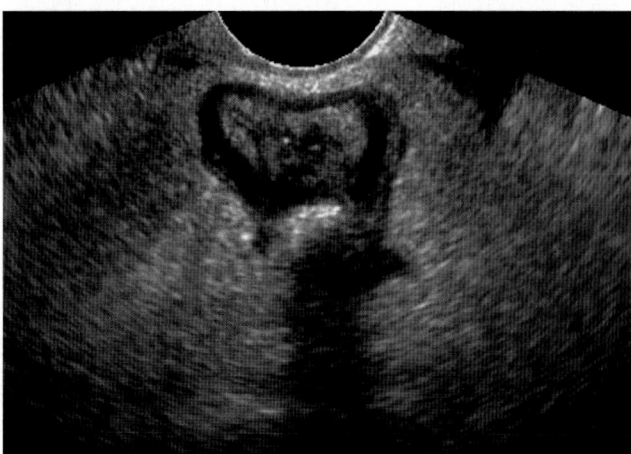

Figure 6-3. Transvaginal ultrasonography: diverticulitis. A middle-aged woman presented with pelvic pain and fever and was believed to have pelvic inflammatory disease. The uterus and ovaries were normal. Deep in the pelvic pouch there is a thick-walled loop of bowel. An acutely inflamed diverticulum shows as a bright echogenic air-containing focus projecting beyond the margin of the abnormal gut. The inflamed surrounding fat is echogenic and prominent.

NORMAL GUT

The normal gut is a long, hollow tube comprising multiple concentric layers. On ultrasonography, these layers are seen as five alternating echogenic and hypoechoic rings that correspond to the histologic layers from the lumen outward as follows[3]:
1. Echogenic: luminal content–mucous membrane interface
2. Hypoechoic: deep mucosa including muscularis mucosae
3. Echogenic: submucosa and submucosa/muscularis propria interface
4. Hypoechoic: muscularis propria
5. Echogenic: serosa or adventitia and muscularis propria/serosa interface

The patient's habitus, the scan quality, and the transducer frequency all affect the delineation of the gut wall layers. Their appearance and identification on longitudinal and cross-sectional ultrasonography is specific and is referred to as *the gut signature* (Fig. 6-4).

Both the location and the morphology of the gut are helpful in determining the portion of the gut studied. The segments of the gastrointestinal tract that, by virtue of their peritoneal attachments, are relatively fixed in location are easiest to identify. Therefore, the gastroesophageal junction, antral-pyloric part of the stomach, duodenum, terminal ileum, ascending colon, descending colon, and rectum can usually be identified. The remainder of the gastrointestinal tract is localized by inference with somewhat less accuracy.

Identified morphologic features, such as gastric rugae, valvulae conniventes (Fig. 6-5), colonic haustra (Fig. 6-6), and appendices epiploicae, are all helpful localizers. However, these tend to be visualized more frequently in patients with an abnormally fluid-filled gastrointestinal tract or ascites than in the normal fasting patient.[4]

The normal thickness of the gut wall is 3 to 5 mm, varying with luminal distention. The stomach wall in the fasting patient may normally appear somewhat thicker. In a fasting patient, the gastrointestinal content is usually quite minimal, although variable amounts of fluid and particulate material may be seen throughout the bowel. Peristaltic activity is frequently observed in the small bowel and the stomach and may be a useful sonographic observation. The presence of gut activity is particularly helpful in determining whether a sonographically identified "collection" represents a fluid-filled hollow viscus or a true collection such as an abscess, hematoma, or seroma. It is also helpful to assess peristaltic activity in patients with suspected mechanical bowel obstruction where the activity not only is increased but also may show abnormal to-and-fro directional movement. Decreased peristaltic activity associated with paralytic ileus is much harder to appreciate on a sonogram, although a local ileus with associated focal fluid-filled loops may be readily seen.

ABNORMAL GUT

Detection of a gut abnormality, either gut wall thickening or a gut wall mass (Fig. 6-7), should prompt thorough assessment of both the bowel and the surrounding soft tissue. In cases of gut wall thickening, documentation should include the location, length, and number of involved segments; preservation or destruction of the normal gut wall layers; symmetrical or

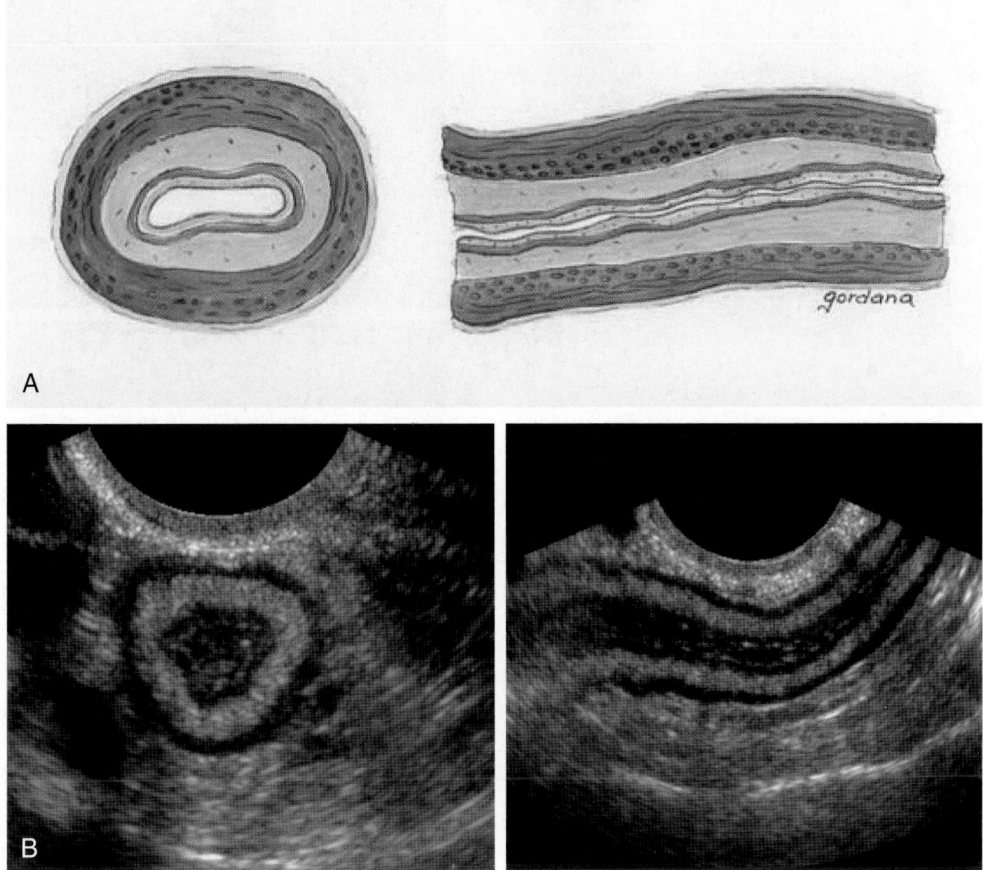

Figure 6-4. Normal gut signature: terminal ileum. Schematic (**A**) and corresponding sonograms (**B**) in a patient with mild gut thickening from Crohn's disease. *Blue layers,* representing the muscle, are black or hypoechoic on the sonogram. *Yellow layers,* representing the submucosa and the superficial mucosa, are hyperechoic. (From Wilson SR: Gastrointestinal tract sonography. In Rumack C, Wilson SR, Charboneau JW [eds]: Diagnostic Ultrasound, 3rd ed. St. Louis, Elsevier Mosby, 2005, pp 269-320.)

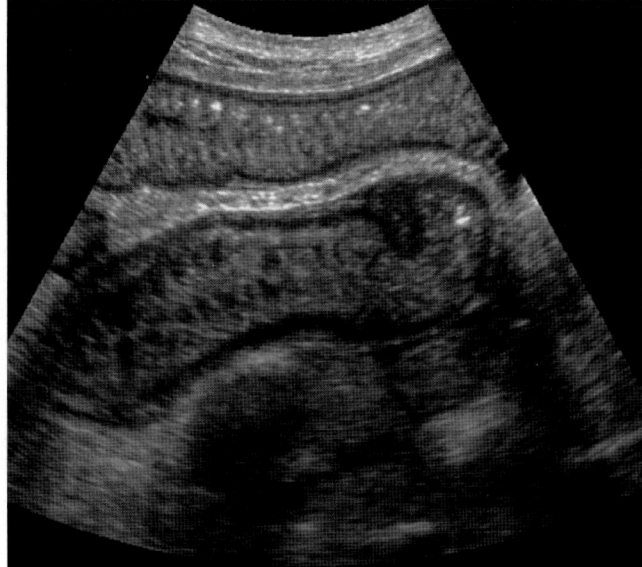

Figure 6-5. Valvulae conniventes. Visualization of mildly edematous valvulae conniventes indicates the small bowel origin of this loop of gut. (From Wilson SR: Gastrointestinal tract sonography. In Rumack C, Wilson SR, Charboneau JW [eds]: Diagnostic Ultrasound, 3rd ed. St. Louis, Elsevier Mosby, 2005, pp 269-320.)

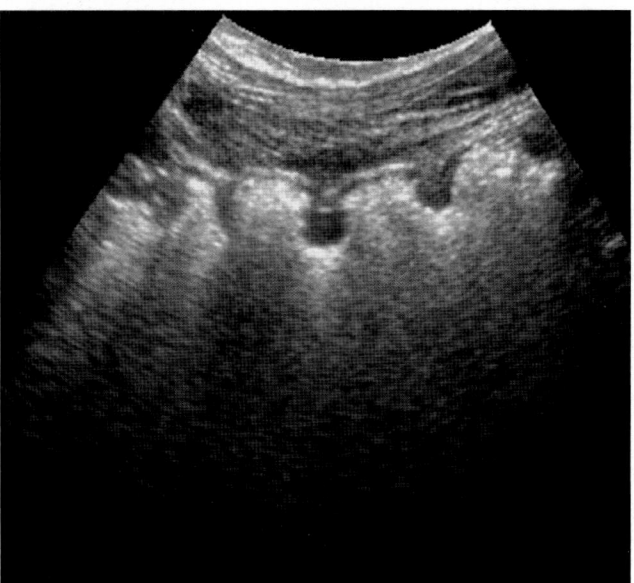

Figure 6-6. Colonic haustra. Long-axis sonogram of the ascending colon demonstrates the normal haustral pattern. In this instance the anterior wall of the gut only shows the haustral pattern as luminal air hides the posterior wall.

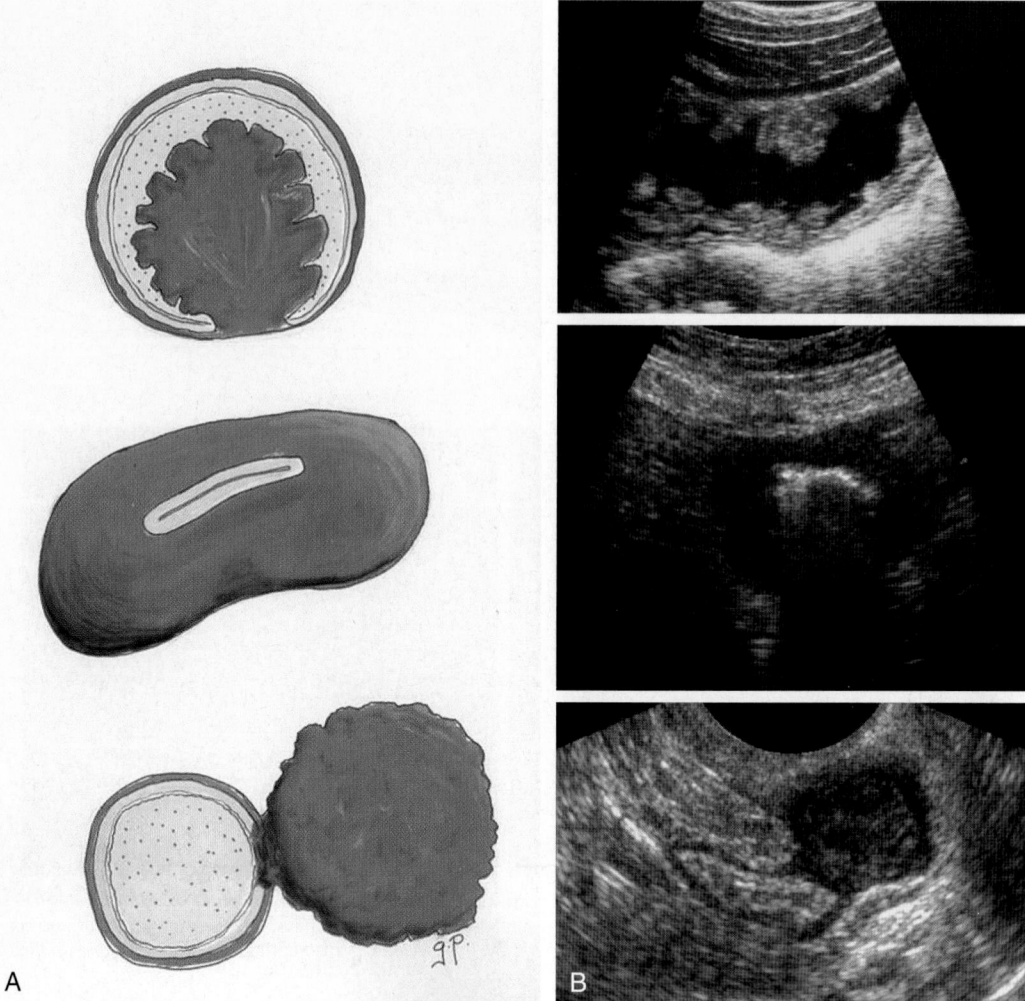

Figure 6-7. Gut wall pathology. Schematic of ultrasonographic appearances (**A**) with ultrasonographic equivalents (**B**). *Top,* Intraluminal mass. Inflammatory pseudopolyp on sonogram. *Middle,* Pseudokidney sign with symmetrical wall thickening and wall layer destruction. Carcinoma of the colon on sonogram. *Bottom,* Exophytic mass. Serosal implant is evident on visceral peritoneum of the gut on sonogram. (From Wilson SR: The bowel wall looks thickened: What does that mean? Categorical course in diagnostic radiology: Findings at US—what do they mean. Paper presented at the annual meeting of the Radiological Society of North America, Dec. 5, 2003, Chicago.)

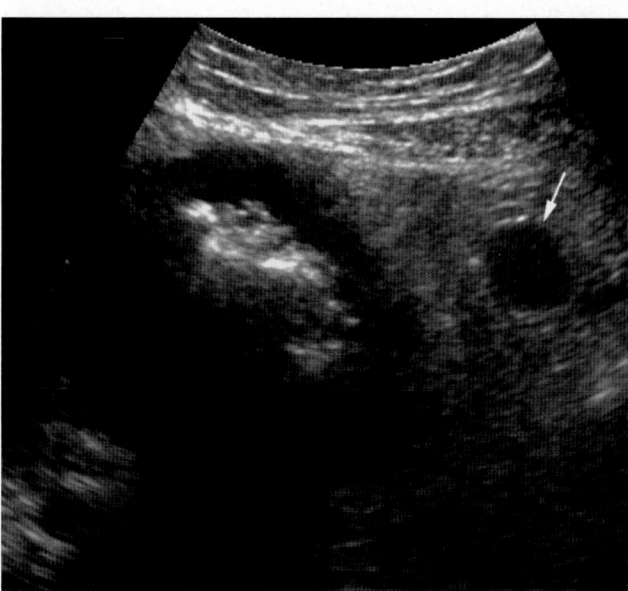

Figure 6-8. Pseudokidney sign of gastric carcinoma. The lumen of the gut is seen as a central bright echogenic region. The infiltrated stomach wall is very hypoechoic with complete loss of stratification. There is surrounding infiltrated echogenic fat and also a round lymph node. (From Wilson SR: Gastrointestinal tract sonography. In Rumack C, Wilson SR, Charboneau JW [eds]: Diagnostic Ultrasound, 3rd ed. St. Louis, Elsevier Mosby, 2005, pp 269-320.)

asymmetrical pattern; and the appearance of the external gut surface.[5] A mural mass should also be assessed for ulceration and mass morphology.

Mural Thickening

The "pseudokidney" or "target" sign is the familiar sonographic abnormality seen with gut wall thickening, with the central echogenicity representing the lumen of the gut and the hypoechoic rim representing the thickened gut wall (Fig. 6-8).[6,7] Malignant thickening is most often focal, is frequently asymmetrical, and is without preservation of gut wall stratification (Fig. 6-9). Benign thickening is more often diffuse, is usually symmetrical, and maintains some preservation of the gut wall

layers. Gut wall thickening is the dominant feature of inflammatory bowel disease, and Crohn's disease is certainly the most frequent example of benign thickening seen on ultrasonography (Fig. 6-10). Ultrasonography has shown sensitivity and specificity in the detection and assessment of Crohn's disease,[8] and the activity of disease is predicted by both color Doppler imaging (Fig. 6-11) and, more recently, contrast-enhanced ultrasonography (Fig. 6-12), which is able to grade the inflammatory activity and predict patients on whom treatment modifications may be made.[9,10] Most inflammatory conditions and also neoplasms will show increased vascularity on state-of-the-art ultrasound equipment.

Sonographic features of gut wall thickening are not always specific, and the clinical picture should be considered in

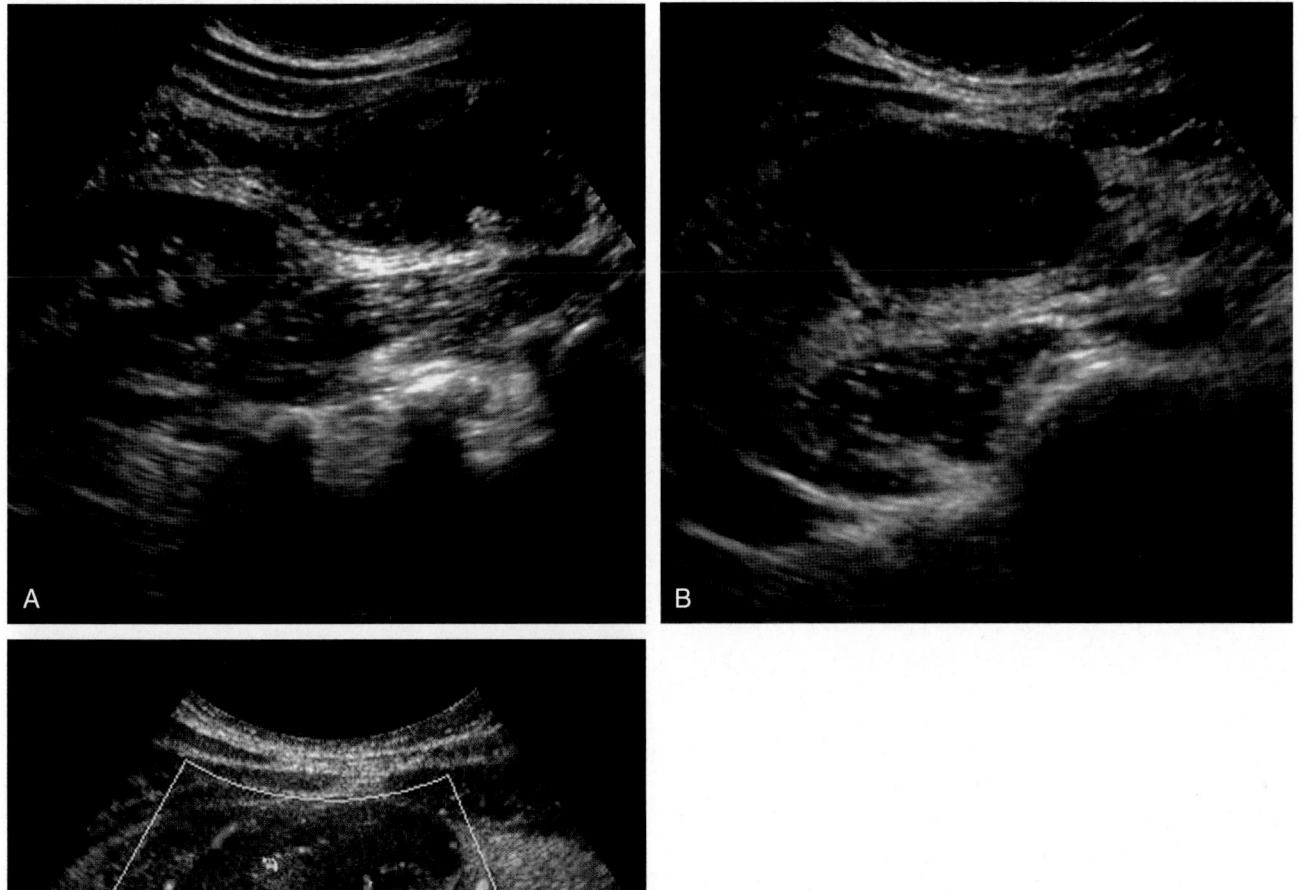

Figure 6-9. Malignant neoplasm of the bowel. A. Longitudinal view of the ascending colon shows an abrupt transition from normal bowel to a focal expansive hypoechoic mass in the region of the cecum. **B.** Transverse image through the mass shows total wall layer destruction by the hypoechoic mass. **C.** Color Doppler image shows vascularity within the mass.

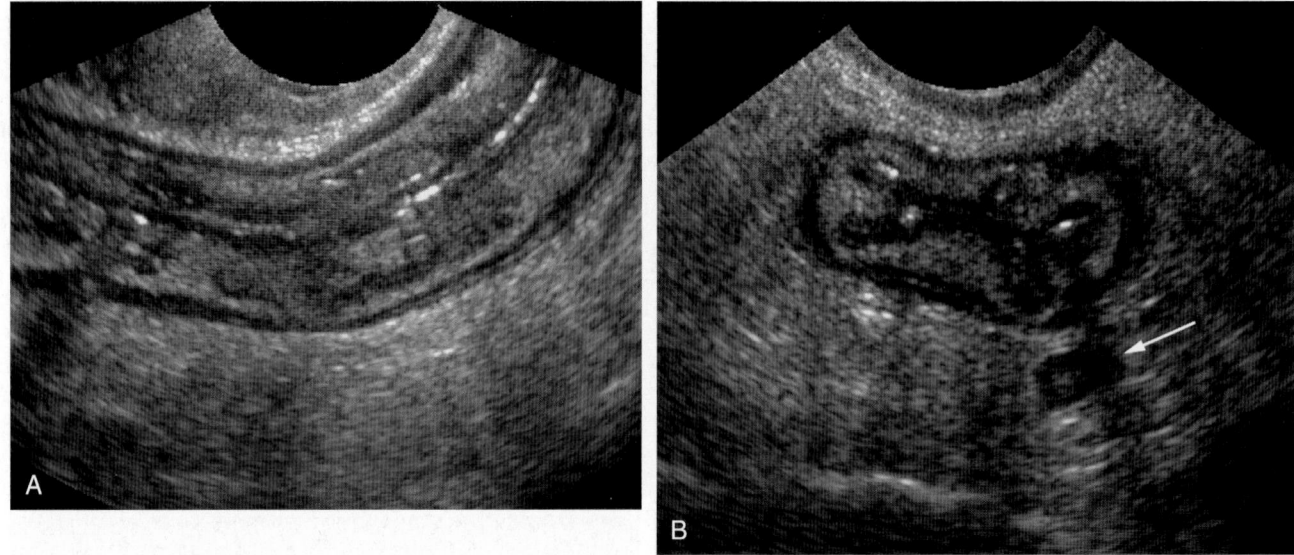

Figure 6-10. Inflammatory thickening of the gut: Crohn's disease. A. Long axis. **B.** Cross section. Sonograms show a uniformly thickened loop of terminal ileum. Stratification of the normal gut wall layers is partially preserved. An *arrow* marks a perienteric lymph node. (From Wilson SR: Gastrointestinal tract sonography. In Rumack C, Wilson SR, Charboneau JW [eds]: Diagnostic Ultrasound, 3rd ed. St. Louis, Elsevier Mosby, 2005, pp 269-320.)

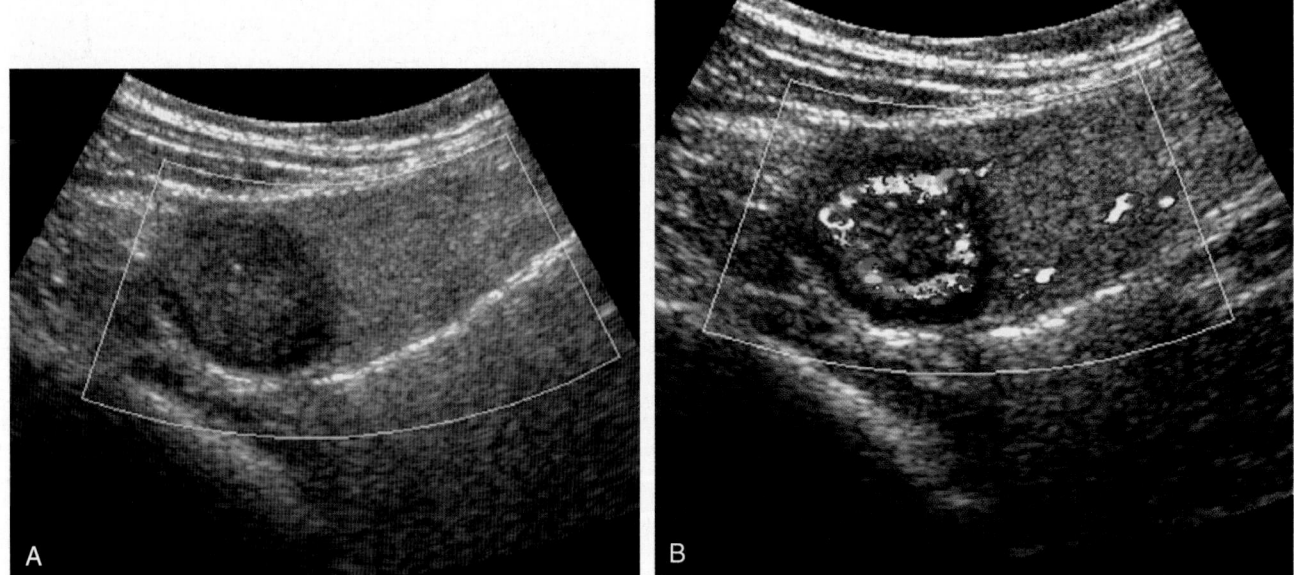

Figure 6-11. Contribution of color Doppler imaging to the evaluation of gut pathology. A. Cross-sectional sonogram of the terminal ileum shows mural wall thickening. Adjacent is echogenic inflammatory fat. **B.** The addition of color Doppler imaging shows hyperemia of both the gut wall and the adjacent fat.

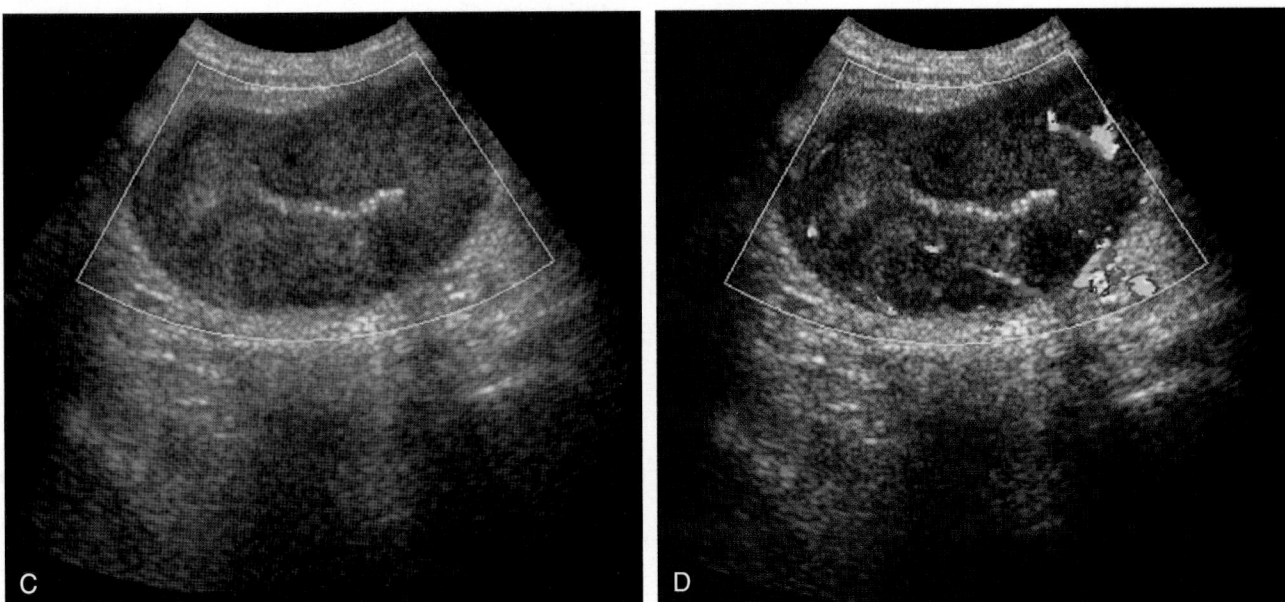

Figure 6-11 *Cont'd.* **C.** Cross-sectional view of the ascending colon shows a pseudokidney sign from adenocarcinoma. **D.** The addition of color Doppler imaging shows lesional vascularity, validating that this as a true observation. (From Wilson SR: Gastrointestinal tract sonography. In Rumack C, Wilson SR, Charboneau JW [eds]: Diagnostic Ultrasound, 3rd ed. St. Louis, Elsevier Mosby, 2005, pp 269-320.)

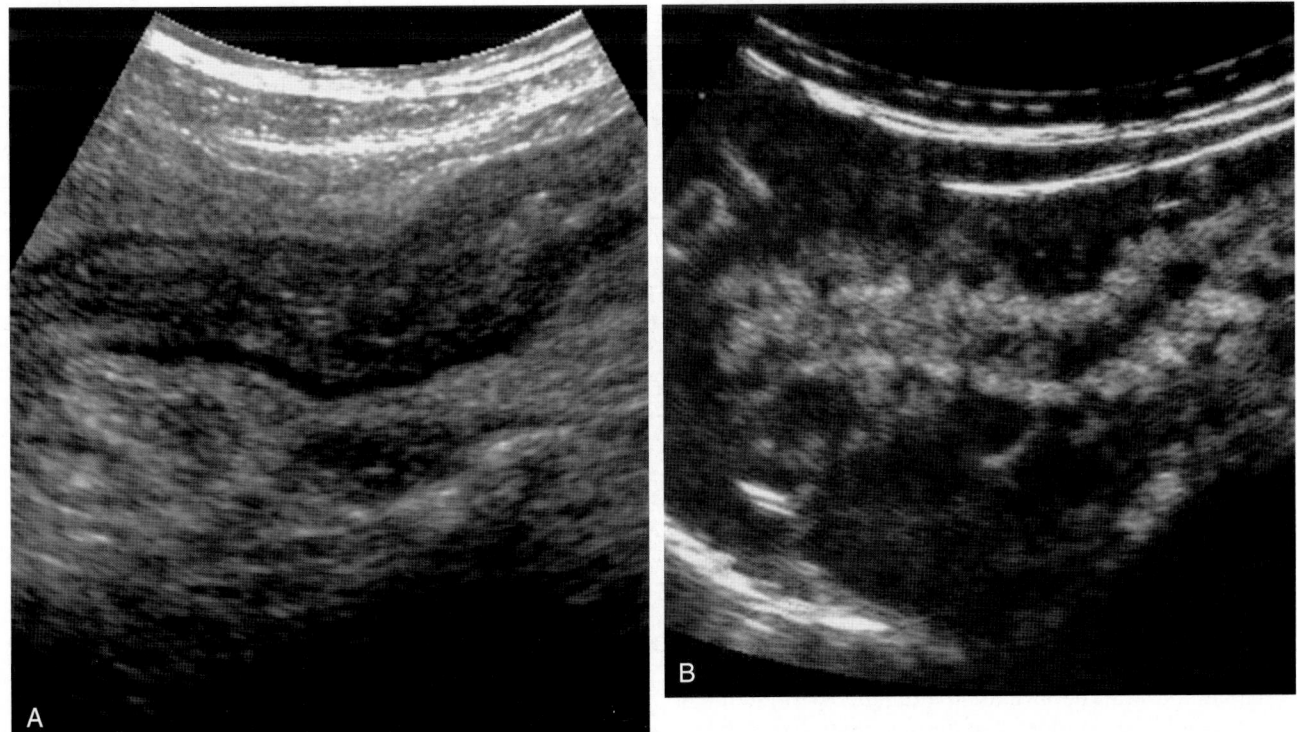

Figure 6-12. Contrast-enhanced ultrasonography of the bowel wall in a patient with Crohn's exacerbation. A. Longitudinal sonogram shows thickening of the wall of the terminal ileum with layer preservation. **B.** Arterial phase contrast-enhanced ultrasound evaluation performed with a second-generation contrast agent, Definity (Bristol-Myers Squibb, Billerica, MA), shows enhancement of the entire wall consistent with active inflammation.

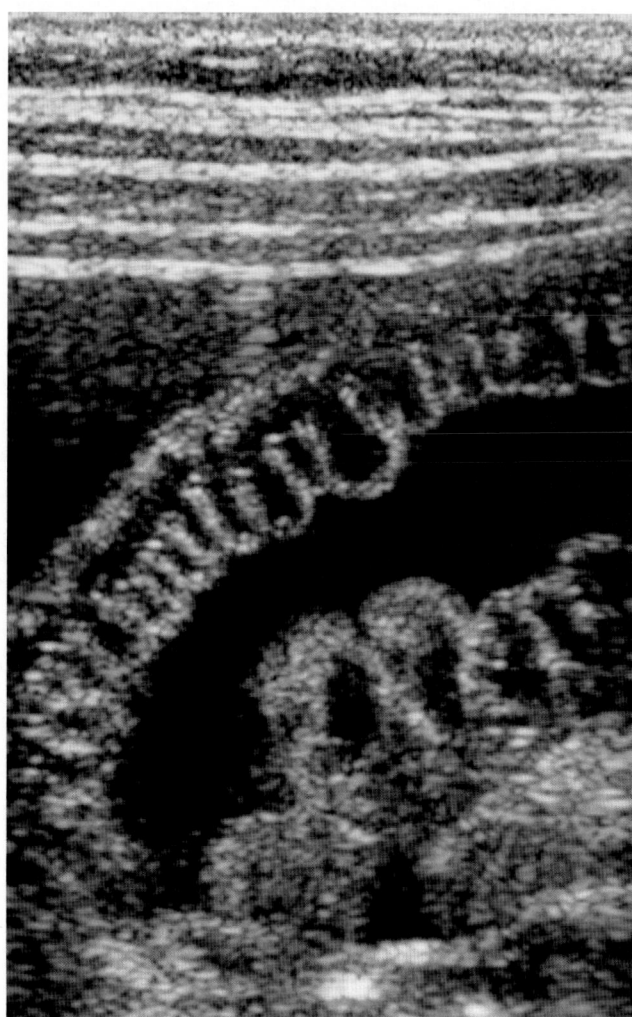

Figure 6-13. Edematous valvulae conniventes. This appearance is usually encountered in patients with vasculitis or venous thrombosis. (From Wilson SR: Gastrointestinal tract sonography. In Rumack C, Wilson SR, Charboneau JW [eds]: Diagnostic Ultrasound, 3rd ed. St. Louis, Elsevier Mosby, 2005, pp 269-320.)

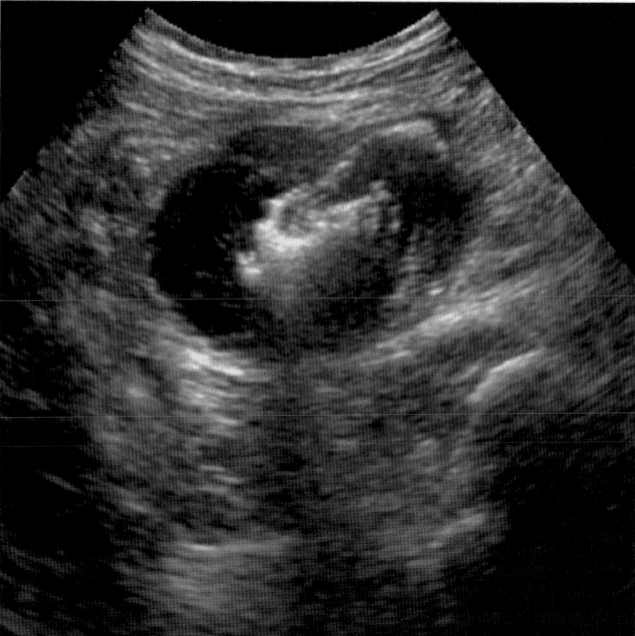

Figure 6-14. Lymphoma of the cecum suggests a pseudokidney morphology. The gut wall is thickened and extremely hypoechoic consistent with this diagnosis.

conjunction with the sonographic abnormalities. Pathologic considerations for thickened gut include inflammatory (see Fig. 6-10), neoplastic (see Figs. 6-8 and 6-9), and edematous (Fig. 6-13) diseases of the gut wall.[11,12]

Mural Masses

Intramural masses affecting the gastrointestinal tract are frequently solid or complex. If these masses are large, their origin may not always be obvious. Accordingly, gastrointestinal tumors should be considered if intraperitoneal or appropriately positioned retroperitoneal masses are identified that do not arise from the abdominal solid organs. With ulceration, pockets of gas are often seen within the mass, and their typical bright echogenicity with distal ring-down artifact is helpful in localizing the origin of the abnormality to the gastrointestinal tract. Pathologic considerations for gut wall masses include lymphoma (Fig. 6-14), mesenchymal tumors

(Fig. 6-15), gut metastases, and adenocarcinoma with local tumor extension. Smooth muscle tumors and lymphomas are the most commonly encountered causes of this sonographic morphology. Their sonographic detection is usually relatively easy because these tumors are often large at the time of presentation. In addition, both of these tumors have highly suggestive sonographic features. The tendency of smooth muscle tumors to undergo central necrosis frequently results in complex masses with both cystic and solid components (Fig. 6-15). This morphology is virtually pathognomonic.[13] Lymphoma typically is strikingly hypoechoic and may suggest a cyst or fluid collection sonographically (see Fig. 6-14).[14]

Perienteric Evaluation

All evaluations of the gut should include evaluation of the surrounding and regional soft tissues. The fat and the lymph nodes are the areas deserving focused study. Inflammatory disorders, notably Crohn's disease, appendicitis, and diverticulitis, are often associated with edema of the perienteric fat (Fig. 6-16) and fibrofatty proliferation of the mesentery. These both appear as echogenic masslike areas on sonograms and are often the most easily appreciated abnormalities on patients with gut disease on ultrasonography, similar to CT. Mesenteric adenopathy shows as round or oval soft tissue structures within the perienteric soft tissues that maintain integrity in perpendicular planes (Fig. 6-17). A phlegmon shows as a focal hypoechoic area within a region of inflamed fat (Fig. 6-18), and abscess shows as an actual fluid collection that may show gas particles as bright echogenic foci with distal dirty shadowing. Similarly, neoplasm is suggested if metastases or tumor invasion are shown.

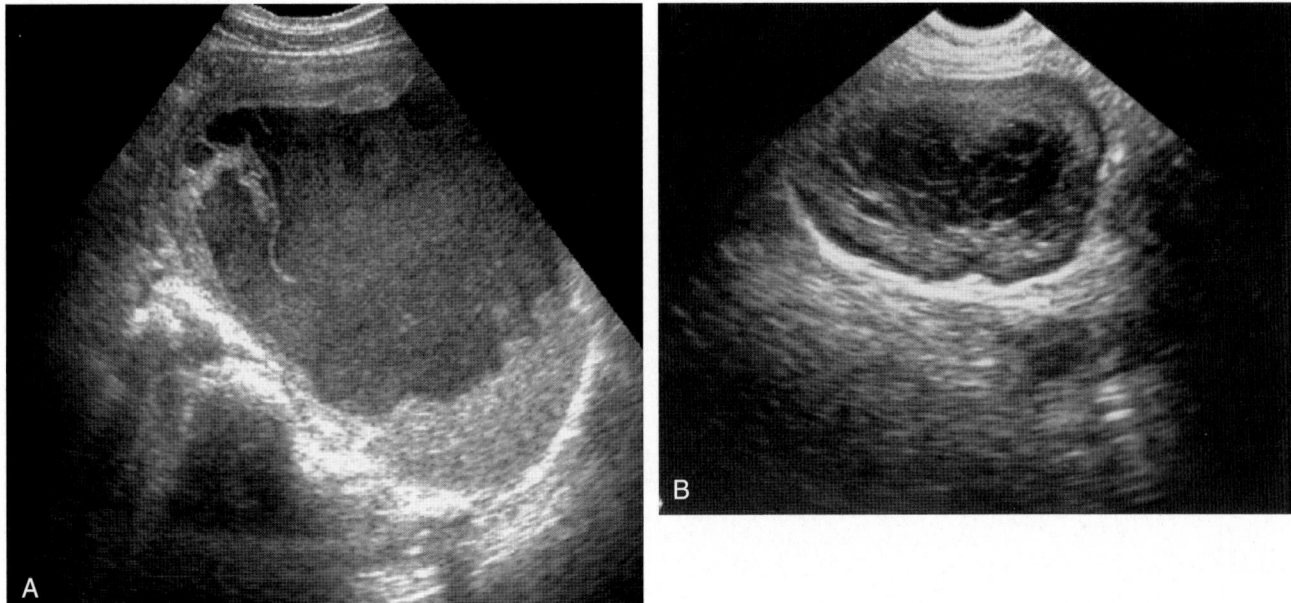

Figure 6-15. Gastrointestinal stromal tumors. A and **B.** GISTs in two patients show as intraperitoneal masses with a highly complex nature typical of this pathologic process. (From Wilson SR: Gastrointestinal tract sonography. In Rumack C, Wilson SR, Charboneau JW [eds]: Diagnostic Ultrasound, 3rd ed. St. Louis, Elsevier Mosby, 2005, pp 269-320.)

PERITONEAL, MESENTERIC, AND OMENTAL ABNORMALITIES

Ultrasound is highly sensitive to the detection of tiny volumes of peritoneal fluid, and the sonographic appearance of the fluid provides rough qualitative information as well. The presence of particles and strands within the fluid has some association with the presence of blood, inflammatory, and neoplastic cells. Peritoneal abnormalities, such as primary or secondary tumors, require a meticulous attention to technique with a prior knowledge of the most likely location for abnormalities to be detected. To this end, the pelvic peritoneal pouch in women is optimally assessed with a transvaginal approach. Visualization of peritoneal implants (Fig. 6-19) and omental cakes is enhanced by the presence of intraperitoneal fluid. Detection of neoplastic invasion and of metastatic adenopathy is related to the size of the tumor deposits.

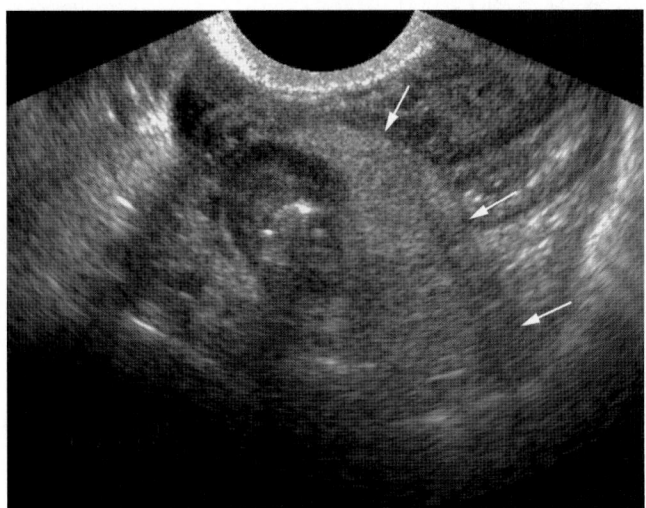

Figure 6-16. Inflamed fat. Inflamed fat is present in axial view of the terminal ileum in this patient with Crohn's ileitis. The fat manifests as a focal echogenic mass effect on the mesenteric border of the thickened bowel.

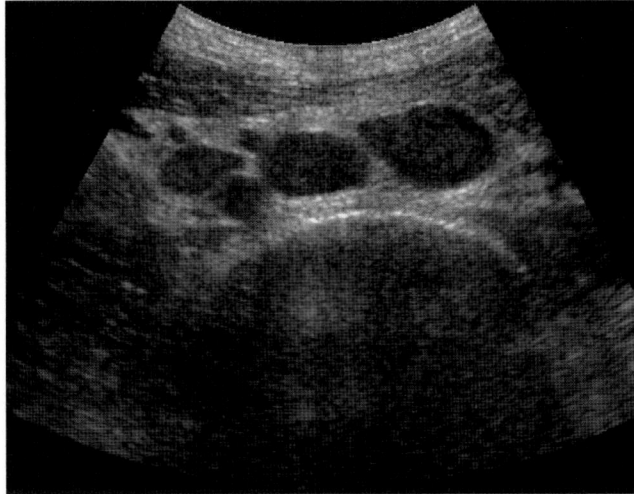

Figure 6-17. Lymph nodes. Lymph nodes are shown in the mesentery of the small bowel in a patient with Crohn's disease. They are round or oval structures that maintain their integrity in perpendicular planes. (From Wilson SR: Gastrointestinal tract sonography. In Rumack C, Wilson SR, Charboneau JW [eds]: Diagnostic Ultrasound, 3rd ed. St. Louis, Elsevier Mosby, 2005, pp 269-320.)

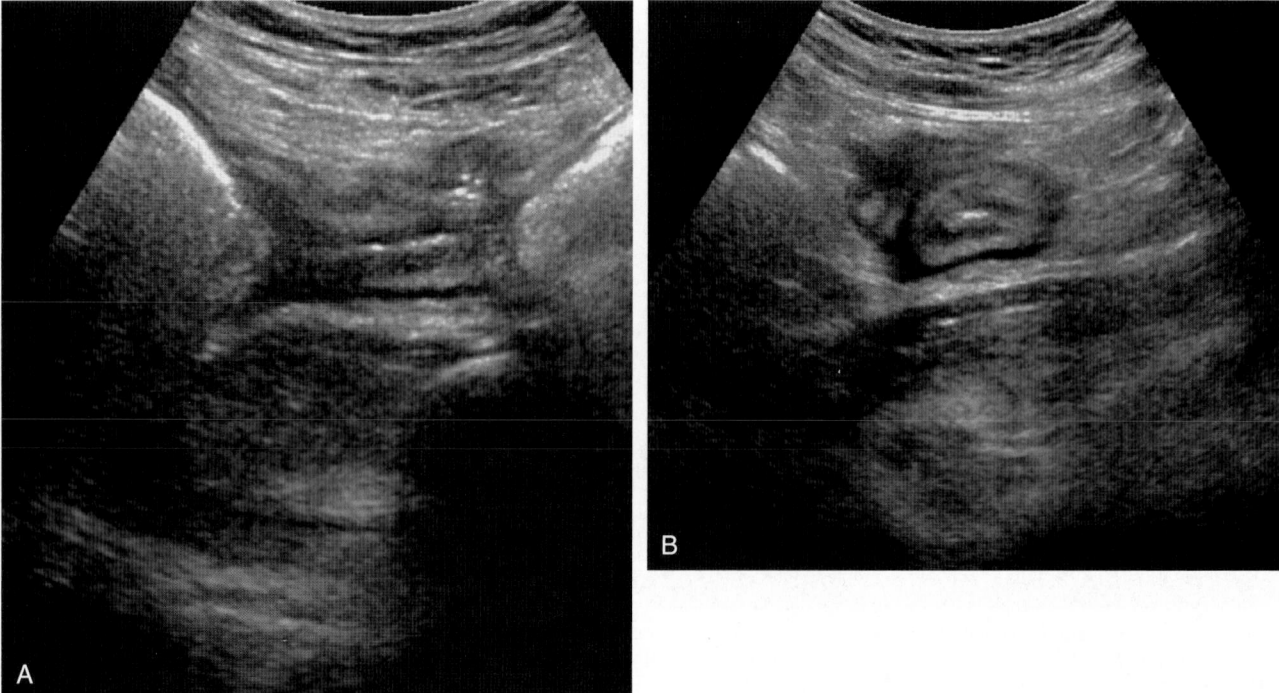

Figure 6-18. Phlegmon associated with Crohn's disease in a patient with exacerbation of symptoms. A. Long-axis scan of the terminal ileum shows a short thick-walled segment of gut with a stricture. The luminal surfaces are in apposition and appear as an echogenic central line. At either end of the stricture, the bowel lumen is dilated and air filled, appearing echogenic. **B.** Axial image of the strictured segment shows a focal hypoechoic and tender phlegmon within the surrounding inflammatory fat.

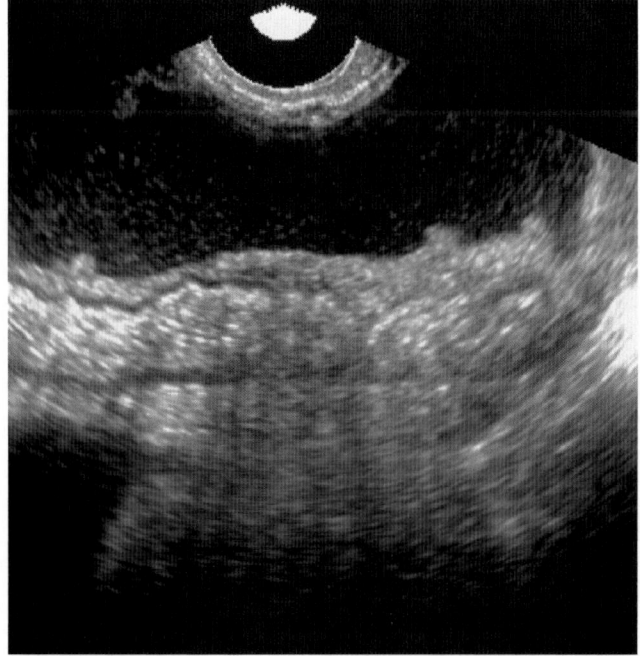

Figure 6-19. Transvaginal ultrasonography: ovarian carcinoma. Visceral peritoneal implants from ovarian carcinoma are seen on the surface of the ileum. There is mildly particulate ascites.

References

1. Muradali D, Burns PN, Pron G, et al: Improved retroperitoneal and gastrointestinal sonography using oral contrast agents in a porcine model. AJR 171:475-481, 1998.
2. Puylaert JBCM: Acute appendicitis: US evaluation using graded compression. Radiology 158:355-360, 1986.
3. Heyder N, Kaarmann H, Giedl J: Experimental investigations into the possibility of differentiating early from invasive carcinoma of the stomach by means of ultrasound. Endoscopy 19:228-232, 1987.
4. Fleischer AC, Muhletaler CA, James AE Jr: Sonographic assessment of the bowel wall. AJR 136:887-891, 1981.
5. Wilson SR: Gastrointestinal tract sonography. In Rumack C, Wilson SR, Charboneau JW (eds): Diagnostic Ultrasound, 3rd ed. St. Louis, Elsevier Mosby, 2005, pp 269-320.
6. Lutz H, Petzoldt R: Ultrasonic patterns of space occupying lesions of the stomach and intestine. Ultrasound Med Biol 2:129-131, 1976.
7. Bluth EL, Merritt CRB, Sullivan MA: Ultrasonic evaluation of the stomach, small bowel, and colon. Radiology 133:677-680, 1979.
8. Parente F, Greco S, Molteni M, et al: Imaging inflammatory bowel disease using bowel ultrasound. Eur J Gastroenterol Hepatol 17:283-291, 2005.
9. Pauls S, Gabelmann A, Schmidt SA, et al: Evaluating bowel wall vascularity in Crohn's disease: A comparison of dynamic MRI and wideband harmonic contrast-enhanced low MI ultrasound. Eur Radiol 16:2410-2417, 2006.
10. Robotti D, Cammarota T, Debani P, et al: Activity of Crohn's disease: Value of color-power-Doppler and contrast-enhanced ultrasonography. Abdom Imaging 29:648-652, 2004.
11. De Pascale A, Garofalo G, Perna M, et al: Contrast-enhanced ultrasonography in Crohn's disease. Radiol Med (Torino) 111:539-550, 2006.
12. Downey DB, Wilson SR: Pseudomembranous colitis: Sonographic features. Radiology 180:61-64, 1991.
13. Lassau N, Lamuraglia M, Chami L, et al: Gastrointestinal stromal tumors treated with imatinib: Monitoring response with contrast-enhanced sonography. AJR Am J Roentgenol 187:1267-1273, 2006.
14. Di Raimondo F, Caruso L, Bonanno G, et al: Is endoscopic ultrasound clinically useful for follow-up of gastric lymphoma? Ann Oncol 18:351-356, 2007.

Multidetector-Row Computed Tomography of the Gastrointestinal Tract: Principles of Interpretation

Richard M. Gore, MD

Multidetector-row CT (MDCT) has become the premier imaging technique for evaluating luminal, mural, and mesenteric abnormalities of the gastrointestinal tract. With MDCT technology, imaging data can be acquired with near isotropic voxels that allow for high-quality and clinically useful volume imaging. The CT data can be viewed in any plane and 3D techniques can be used to effectively and graphically display large data sets in a user-friendly format that is understandable to referring physicians.[1-3]

LUMEN OPACIFICATION

Proper distention and marking of the bowel lumen are vital in detecting mural thickening and excluding mural masses and mesenteric and omental pathology. There are a number of methods available to accomplish this goal, and the choice depends upon the clinical setting.

In the emergent setting in which bowel obstruction or intestinal ischemia is suspected, the intrinsic secretions within the gut are usually sufficient to highlight the lumen. Orally administered contrast may be vomited and may remain in the stomach due to absent or diminished gastrointestinal motility.

As part of a general survey examination of patients with no localizing signs or symptoms, a study performed with positive luminal is often obtained. As a caveat, the assessment of mural and mucosal enhancement of the gut will be compromised with the positive contrast. Additionally, positive intraluminal contrast will interfere with CT angiography and some 3D techniques.

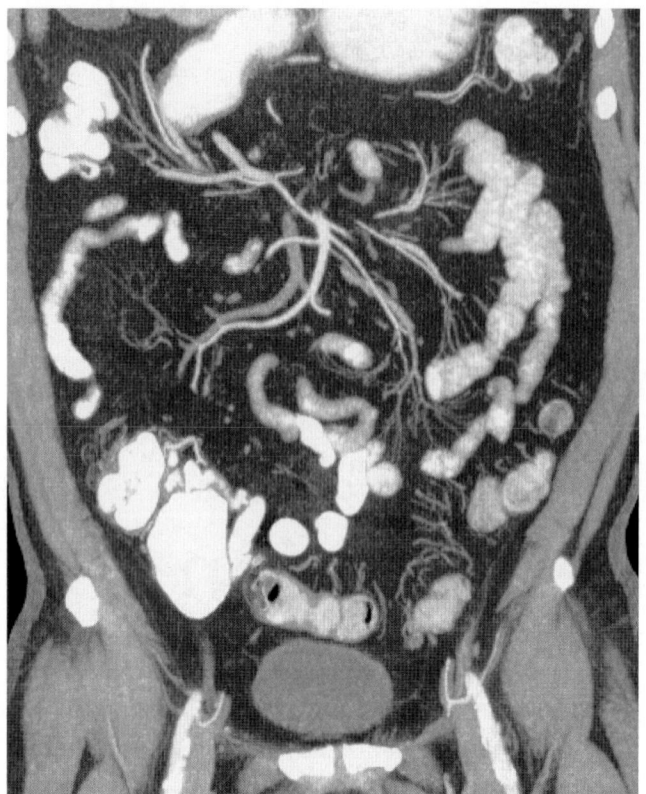

Figure 7-1. Positive contrast opacification. Positive contrast within the lumen of the gut does provide lumen distention and helps differentiate collapsed bowel from masses, adenopathy, and abscesses. In this obese individual, the mesenteric vessels are well depicted.

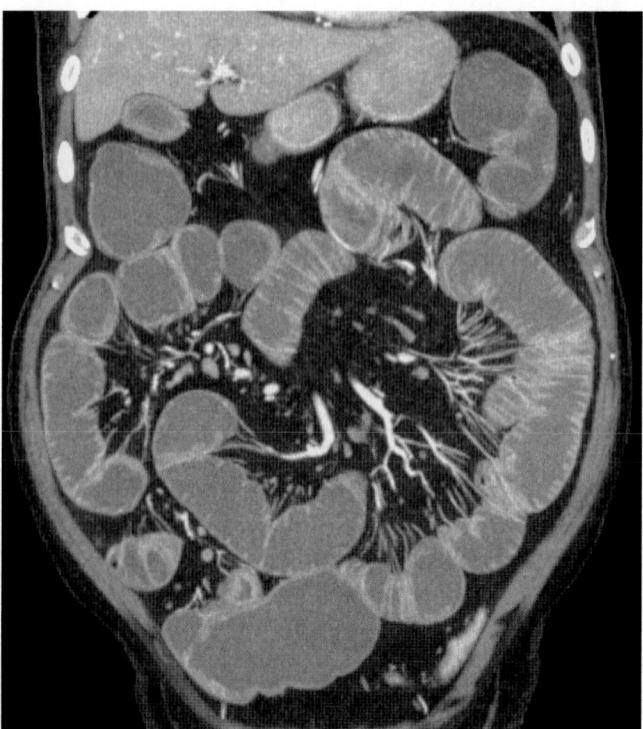

Figure 7-2. Neutral contrast opacification. Neutral contrast not only distends the lumen but also provides for easier evaluation of mural enhancement and the mesenteric vessels.

Air or carbon dioxide as intraluminal contrast agents are used in the setting of CT gastrography and colonography.

Positive Contrast Agents

Positive contrast opacification (Fig. 7-1) of the gut is accomplished by giving either 1% to 2% barium suspensions or 2% to 3% solutions of iodinated water-soluble agents. The low percentage of barium requires commercial preparations made specifically for CT, in which additives are used to ensure that the barium remains in suspension

In most patients, contrast material will reach the distal ileum within 45 minutes after initiation of drinking. Prolonged transit times are to be anticipated. Some common conditions altering the transit time include recent postoperative status, serum electrolyte disturbances, collagen-vascular diseases (e.g., scleroderma), hypothyroidism, and intestinal obstruction. Conversely, patients who are hyperthyroid, who have syndromes with associated increased intestinal motility (e.g., carcinoid, islet cell tumor), or who have infections (e.g., cryptosporidiosis, giardiasis) will display a significantly accelerated intestinal transit time.

The choice between oral barium suspensions and water-soluble agents is dictated by the experience and preference of the radiologist. Water-soluble agents should be used exclusively for patients with abdominal trauma or suspected perforated viscus, those who have a high likelihood of immediate surgery, and as an aid in percutaneous CT biopsy or other interventional procedures.

Neutral Contrast Agents

Neutral contrast agents (Fig. 7-2) have several advantages over positive contrast agents for evaluating mucosal, mural, and serosal pathology.[4-9] They allow excellent depiction of mural enhancement of the gut without the algorithm undershoot or overshoot that accompanies intraluminal high density positive contrast and low density gas. Neutral contrast agents also facilitate the performance of CT angiography and other three dimensional techniques. Neutral contrast agents include water, milk, a 0.1% solution of barium (Volumen E-Z-EM; Lake Success, NY), and water with mannitol or polyethylene glycol.

Orally administered water or Volumen can easily be administered orally to enhance the evaluation of gastric, duodenal, and small bowel pathology. These agents also are helpful when performing CT angiography for staging and preoperative evaluation of hepatic, biliary, and pancreatic malignancies.

Gas Contrast

Gaseous distention of the stomach is important when evaluating mucosal and mural pathology. It has been used with great success in CT gastrography for the diagnosis and staging of upper gastrointestinal malignancies.[10-12]

For CT colonography (Fig. 7-3), either room air or carbon dioxide is insufflated per rectum. Adequate gaseous distention of the colon is very important for image interpretation because a significant lesion may be obscured in a collapsed segment of colon.[13-17] A complete discussion of this technique is presented in Chapter 57.

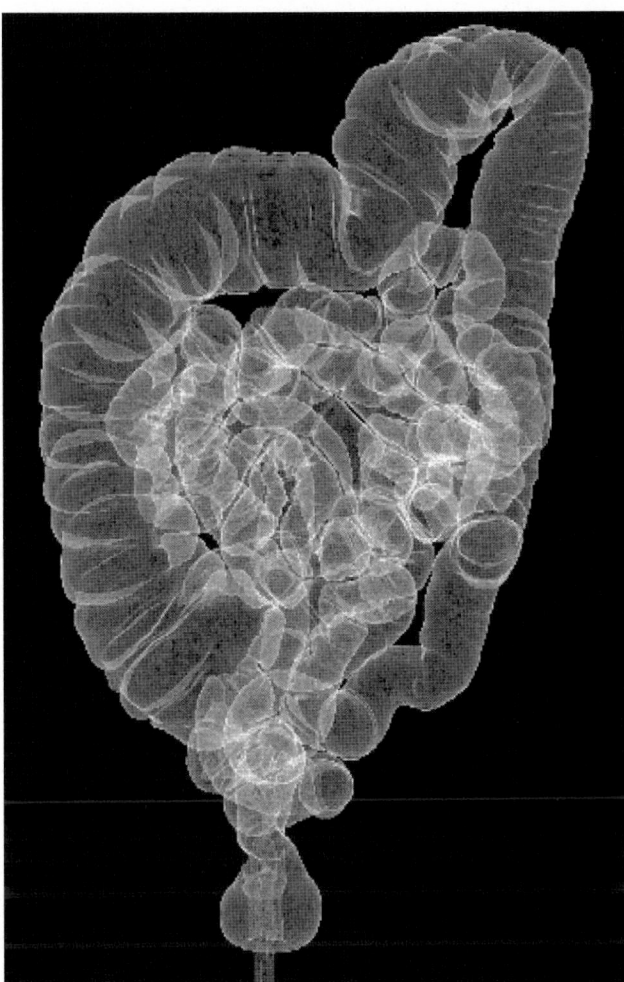

Figure 7-3. Gas opacification. Distention of the lumen of the gut is an important part of CT colonography.

VASCULAR OPACIFICATION

Opacification of the blood vessels is essential for complete evaluation of inflammatory, infectious, neoplastic, vascular and traumatic diseases of the gastrointestinal tract. Obviously, this cannot be performed in all clinical settings (e.g., poor renal function, poor venous access). For general diagnostic cases, 100 to 150 mL (depending on concentration) of nonionic contrast is administered at a rate of 3 mL/s with a power injector. If CT angiography or other 3D techniques are to be performed, the rate is increased to 5 mL/s.

One of the advantages of MDCT is that multiple data sets can be acquired with a single bolus of contrast. The following is a list of possible imaging times that may be used when imaging the abdomen and pelvis: unenhanced, early arterial phase (20 seconds), late arterial-enteric phase (40 seconds), portal venous phase (70-90 seconds), equilibrium phase (210 seconds), delayed phase (15-20 minutes).

For general survey abdominal imaging, obtaining scans during the portal venous phase is adequate. When assessing the viability of bowel, searching for a source of gastrointestinal hemorrhage, evaluating the cirrhotic liver, and searching for hypervascular metastases, it is useful to obtain noncontrast scans as well as scans during the later hepatic arterial phase

and portal venous phase. When performing CT angiography, scans should be obtained during the early arterial phase. The enteric phase corresponds to the late arterial phase and has been found useful in evaluating Crohn's disease activity.

NORMAL BOWEL WALL

Virtually all pathology of the bowel wall results in mural thickening, which is often accompanied by changes in the density of the bowel wall due to edema, hemorrhage, tumor, fat, or gas. One of the most common pitfalls in interpreting CT examinations of the gut is confusing an insufficiently distended loop of bowel for pathologic thickening or mistaking a poorly opacified bowel loop for an abdominal mass. Techniques for achieving lumen distention were presented in the prior section.

Esophagus

The esophagus (Fig. 7-4) has a length of 23 to 25 cm in the average adult. The wall of the distended esophagus is 3 mm in thickness. The cervical esophagus lies posterior to the trachea in the midline. It may normally bulge into the posterior aspect of the trachea because of the limited space of the neck.

At the level of the thoracic inlet, the esophagus courses to the left of the midline and then lies adjacent to the left main stem bronchus and pericardium of the left atrium in the mid thorax. More distally, the esophagus lies anterior to the descending aorta to the left of the midline as it enters the esophageal hiatus of the diaphragm. Normally, the thoracic esophagus should not indent the trachea, and there should

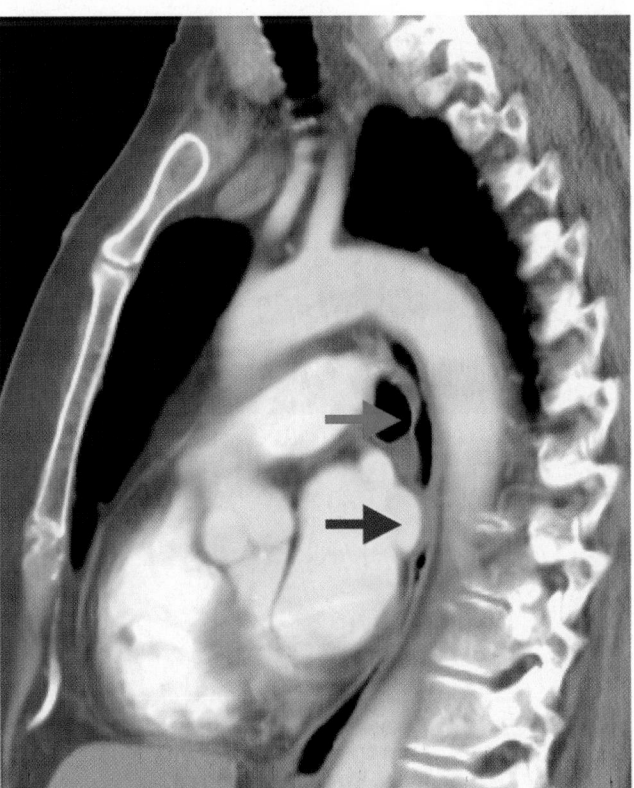

Figure 7-4. Normal esophagus. On this sagittal, reformatted image of the thorax, the normal esophagus is depicted as a thin-walled tubular structure. Note that it courses posterior to the left main stem bronchus (*red arrow*) and the left atrial appendage (*black arrow*).

be a triangle of fat between the aorta, spine, and esophagus distally. In patients with invasive esophageal carcinoma, the trachea is bowed along its posterior aspect by the esophageal tumor. More distally, invasive esophageal neoplasms obliterate the triangle of fat.

Contrast-enhanced examinations should show uniform mural enhancement of the esophagus without mural stratification.

Stomach

The stomach is a functionally and anatomically dynamic organ, and its appearance depends upon the degree of luminal distention and gastric location (Fig. 7-5). For the well-distended, nondependent gastric fundus and body, a wall thickness of up to 5 mm is considered normal.[18] The mural thickness of the antrum however is affected by anatomic and functional factors that make it normally thicker than other portions of the stomach. The gastric smooth muscle, particularly the circular layer, is thicker and denser in the antrum compared to more proximal portions of the stomach. Periodic concentric and eccentric antral contractions, as seen fluoroscopically, also contribute to apparent mural thickening of the stomach.

When the normal stomach is distended with neutral contrast, enhancement of the mucosa may be seen, highlighted against the lower attenuation mucosa and muscularis propria.

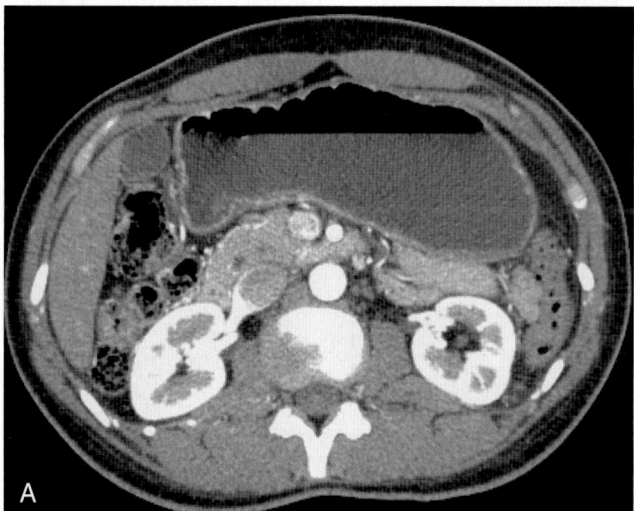

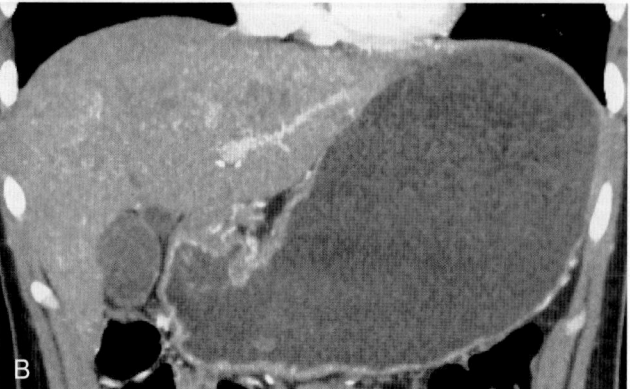

Figure 7-5. Normal stomach. Axial (**A**) and coronal reformatted (**B**) images show a thin gastric wall. Often, the antrum is slightly thicker than the more proximal stomach.

Up to one quarter of patients show linear submucosal low attenuation or mural stratification in the antrum on contrast enhanced MDCT examination. This may be in part due to deposition of fat in the submucosa.

Small Bowel

The normal small bowel is approximately 22 feet long and is suspended by a root that measures 6 to 9 inches and courses from the level of the ligament of Treitz caudal to the level of the ileocecal valve. As with conventional barium small bowel examinations, the valvulae conniventes are more prominent in the jejunum than ileum. The normal small bowel wall (Fig. 7-6) measures between 1 and 2 mm when the lumen is well distended with positive, neutral, or air contrast media. When collapsed, the normal mural thickness of the small bowel measures between 2 and 3 mm.

When scanning patients during the enteric phase (40 seconds following contrast injection) collapsed bowel segments have greater attenuation than distended bowel segments. Also the jejunum has greater attenuation than the ileum. Because collapsed small bowel loops have increased attenuation that is similar to that of inflamed bowel loops, secondary findings of infectious or inflammatory small bowel disease (e.g., engorged vasa rectae, creeping fat of the mesentery, enlarged lymph nodes) should be considered.

Colon

The thickness of the colon wall as imaged on MDCT depends on the degree of distention. Fecal contents, fluid, colonic redundancy and muscular hypertrophy (myochosis) make accurate determination of true colonic wall thickness difficult. The normal colon wall (see Fig. 7-6) is normally less than 4 mm thick with proper distention. The normal wall is typically homogeneous in attenuation. With obesity becoming increasingly prevalent, submucosal fat is being identified in otherwise normal patients throughout the gut but particularly in the colon.

BOWEL WALL: PATHOLOGIC CHANGES

Mural thickening is the pathologic hallmark of gastrointestinal disease. When evaluating the abnormal gut the following features should be carefully analyzed: mural attenuation and enhancement patterns (Table 7-1); the degree of mural thickening (Table 7-2); the symmetry of bowel wall thickening (Table 7-3); and the length of the diseased segment (Table 7-4). Wittenberg and Harisinghani and colleagues[19,20] described a classification system for the abnormal bowel wall as depicted on MDCT (Fig. 7-7).

White Attenuation Pattern

When the diseased segment of gut demonstrates contrast enhancement (Fig. 7-8A) to a degree equal to or greater than that of venous opacification on the same scan, this indicates abnormal enhancement. Avid mural contrast enhancement is probably related to vasodilation and/or injury to intramural vessels with interstitial leakage of the contrast medium.

This pattern of enhancement is seen most commonly in patients with acute inflammatory and infectious bowel disease

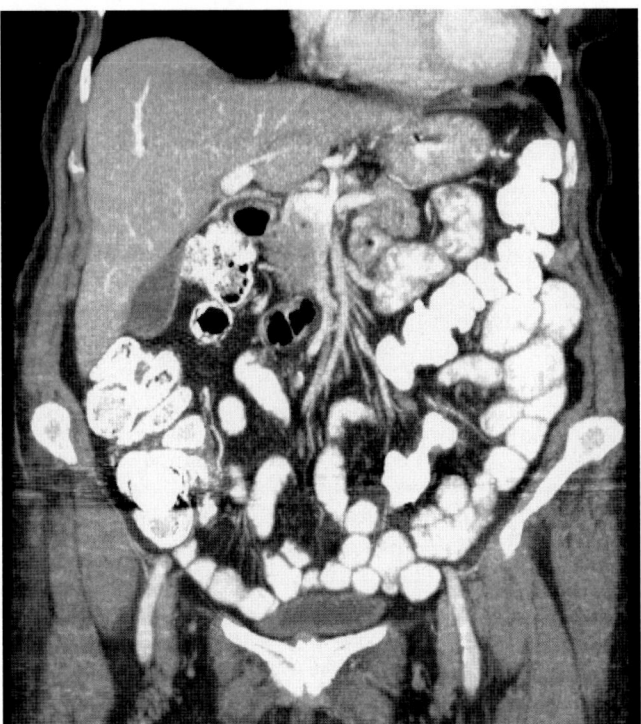

Figure 7-6. Normal small bowel and colon. Coronal reformatted image shows nice distention of the small bowel and colon by positive contrast. The high-density intraluminal material does limit assessment of the enhancement of the bowel wall.

Table 7-1
Patterns of Attenuation

I. *Homogeneous*
  A. Common
    1. Submucosal hemorrhage
    2. Lymphoma
    3. Small adenocarcinoma
  B. Uncommon
    1. Infarcted bowel
    2. Pitfalls related to residual fluid
    3. Chronic Crohn's disease
    4. Chronic radiation injury

II. *Heterogeneous*
  A. Stratified attenuation
    1. Common
      a. Ischemia
      b. Infectious enterocolitis
      c. Crohn's disease, ulcerative colitis
      d. Vasculitis, lupus, Henoch-Schönlein purpura
      e. Radiation
      f. Bowel edema related to cirrhosis or low-protein state
    2. Uncommon
      a. Infiltrating scirrhous carcinoma (usually stomach or rectum)
      b. Residual fluid and contrast material
      c. Submucosal fat deposition
      d. Pneumatosis
  B. Mixed attenuation, common
    1. Large adenocarcinoma
    2. Gastrointestinal stromal tumor
    3. Mucinous adenocarcinoma

From Macari M, Balthazar EJ: CT of bowel wall: Significance and pitfalls of interpretation. AJR 176:1105-1116, 2001; Appendix 1, p 1115.

Table 7-2
Degree of Mural Thickening

I. *Mild Thickening (<2 cm)*
  A. Common
    1. Infectious enterocolitis
    2. Ulcerative colitis
    3. Crohn's disease
    4. Radiation injury
    5. Ischemia
    6. Bowel edema in cirrhosis
    7. Submucosal hemorrhage
  B. Uncommon
    1. Adenocarcinoma
    2. Lymphoma

II. *Marked Thickening (>2 cm)*
  A. Common
    1. Adenocarcinoma, gastrointestinal stromal tumor, metastases, lymphoma
    2. Severe colitis
    3. Systemic lupus erythematosus
  B. Uncommon
    1. Crohn's disease, tuberculosis, histoplasmosis, cytomegalovirus
    2. Submucosal hemorrhage

From Macari M, Balthazar EJ: CT of bowel wall: Significance and pitfalls of interpretation. AJR 176:1105-1116, 2001; Appendix 2, p 1116.

reflecting the hyperemic and hypervascular state found with acute inflammation and infection.

Vascular disorders such as shock bowel also may manifest with the white attenuation pattern. The increased vascular permeability and slowed perfusion that accompanies hypoperfusion permits the interstitial leakage of molecules of contrast material. Delayed venous drainage and altered vascular permeability are also responsible for this sign in patients with bowel ischemia.

On non–contrast-enhanced scans, intramural hemorrhage (Fig. 7-8B) will produce a hyperdense bowel wall.

Gray Attenuation Pattern

In this pattern, thickened bowel wall (Fig. 7-9) shows little enhancement and a homogeneous attenuation comparable with that of enhanced muscle. This pattern should only be diagnosed if the intravascular contrast levels are adequate.

Table 7-3
Symmetry of Mural Thickening

I. *Symmetric*
  A. Infections of the small and large bowel
  B. Ulcerative colitis
  C. Crohn's disease
  D. Radiation injury
  E. Ischemia
  F. Bowel edema in cirrhosis
  G. Lymphoma
  H. Submucosal hemorrhage

II. *Asymmetric*
  A. Adenocarcinoma
  B. Gastrointestinal stromal tumor

From Macari M, Balthazar EJ: CT of bowel wall: Significance and pitfalls of interpretation. AJR 176:1105-1116, 2001; Appendix 3, p 1116.

Table 7-4
Length of Mural Thickening

I. *Focal (<10 cm)*
  A. Common
    1. Diverticulitis, appendicitis
    2. Adenocarcinoma
  B. Uncommon
    1. Lymphoma
    2. Tuberculosis
    3. Crohn's disease

II. *Segmental (10-30 cm)*
  A. Common
    1. Lymphoma
    2. Crohn's disease
    3. Infectious ileitis
    4. Radiation
    5. Submucosal hemorrhage
    6. Ischemia
  B. Uncommon: systemic lupus erythematosus

III. *Diffuse*
  A. Common
    1. Ulcerative colitis
    2. Infectious enterocolitis
    3. Edema from low protein and cirrhosis
    4. Systemic lupus erythematosus
  B. Uncommon: ischemia

From Macari M, Balthazar EJ: CT of bowel wall: Significance and pitfalls of interpretation. AJR 176:1105-1116, 2001; Appendix 4, p 1116.

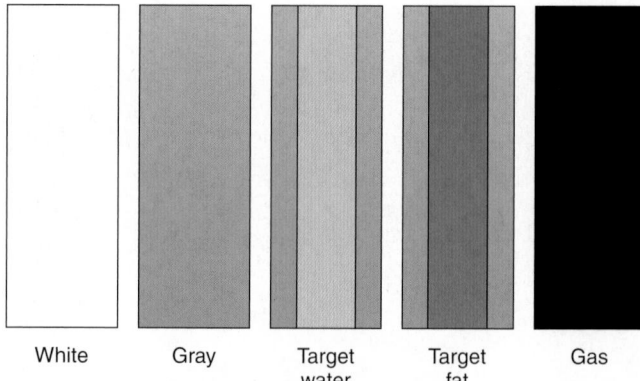

Figure 7-7. Classification scheme for mural thickening of the gastrointestinal tract.

Malignancy should be suspected in thickened segments of gut that show minimal enhancement and do not exhibit mural stratification.

Adenocarcinomas of the gastrointestinal tract usually show the uniform, gray-enhancement pattern unless there are focal regions of necrosis. Lymphomas usually show a greater degree of wall thickening and are homogeneous in attenuation as well. Gastrointestinal stromal tumors and metastases often cause mural thickening but are typically inhomogeneous in attenuation.

In patients with Crohn's disease the presence of a thick, nonenhancing segment suggests the fibrotic-cicatrizing stage of the disease.

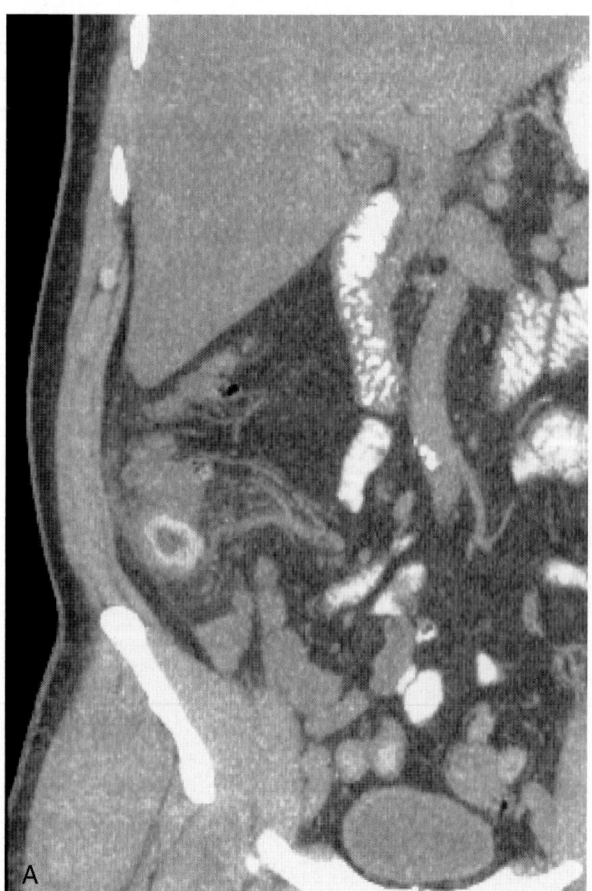

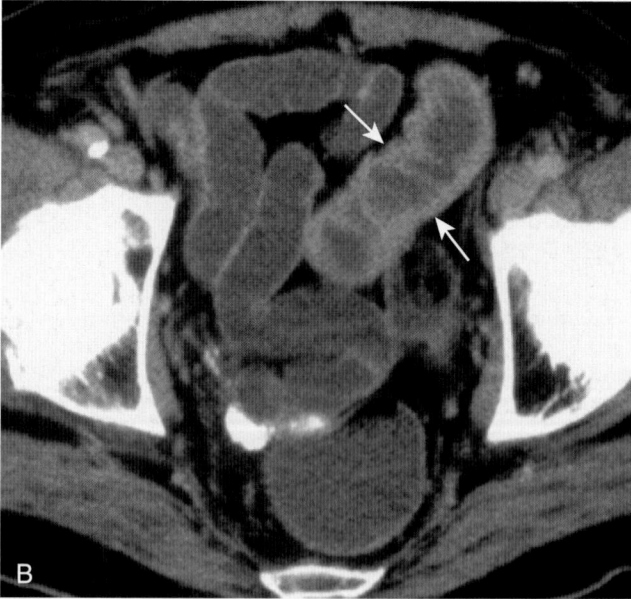

Figure 7-8. White enhancement pattern. A. Coronal reformatted image shows a uniformly, densely enhancing distal ileal loop due to active Crohn's disease. There is disproportionate fat stranding surrounding this inflamed loop. Note the engorged vasa rectae. This pattern is seen in patients with acute inflammatory bowel disease and shock bowel. **B.** On unenhanced scans, a hyperdense bowel wall (*arrows*) can be seen with intramural hemorrhage. A thickened segment of ileum is identified in this patient with systemic lupus erythematosus.

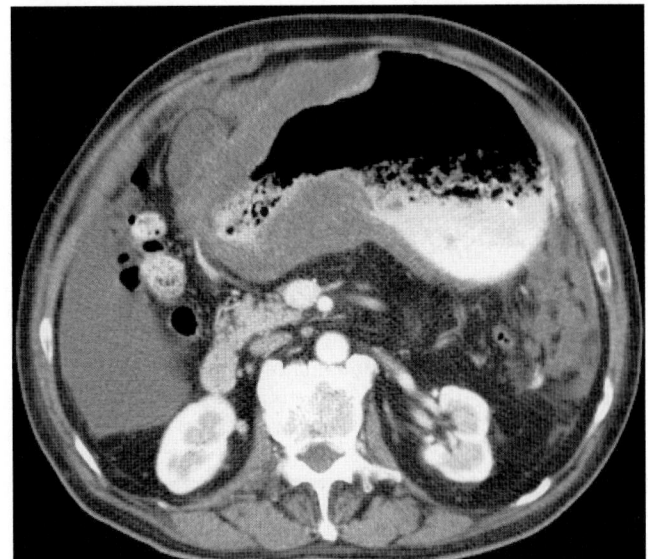

Figure 7-9. Gray enhancement pattern. The thickened wall of the gastric antrum in this patient with adenocarcinoma of the stomach shows uniform, gray enhancement. Malignancies do not typically demonstrate mural stratification.

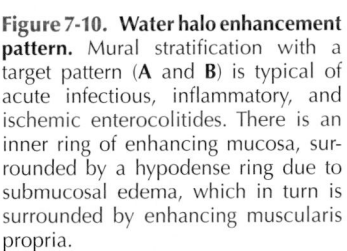

Figure 7-10. Water halo enhancement pattern. Mural stratification with a target pattern (**A** and **B**) is typical of acute infectious, inflammatory, and ischemic enterocolitides. There is an inner ring of enhancing mucosa, surrounded by a hypodense ring due to submucosal edema, which in turn is surrounded by enhancing muscularis propria.

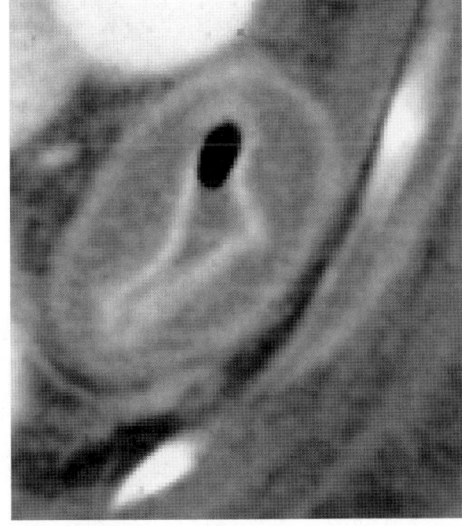

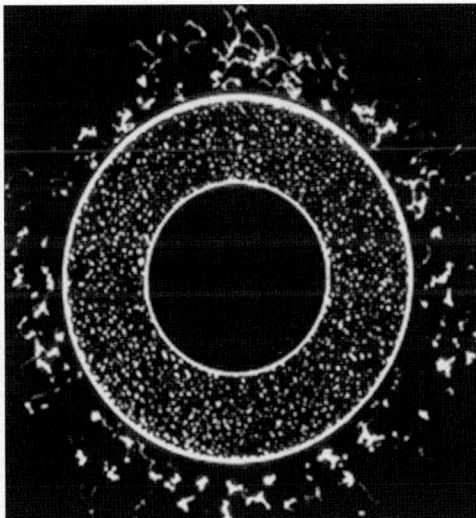

Water Halo Pattern

The water halo pattern (Fig. 7-10) is the most commonly seen in patients with active infectious, inflammatory, ischemic disorders of the gastrointestinal tract. The bowel, when viewed in the axial plane, has a target or "bull's-eye" appearance. An enhancing central higher density mucosal layer is surrounded by a water density submucosa that in turn is surrounded by a higher density muscularis propria.

Fat Halo Pattern

Fat in the submucosa (Fig. 7-11) of the gut produces the fat halo pattern. It has lower attenuation than the grayer tone of the water halo sign. When visualized in the small bowel, chronic Crohn's disease should be suspected. In the colon, the fat halo sign is seen in patients with chronic ulcerative colitis and Crohn's disease. Rapid accumulation of submucosal fat has also been reported in patients undergoing cytoreductive surgery for lymphoproliferative and myeloproliferative disorders and graft-versus-host disease.

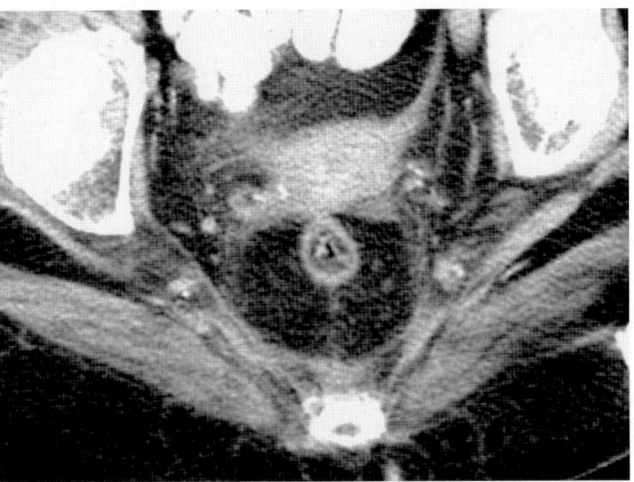

Figure 7-11. Fat halo enhancement pattern. In this patient with chronic ulcerative colitis, fat is present within the submucosa. The lumen of the rectum is narrow and there is an increase in the presacral space due to fatty deposition.

Submucosal fat deposition in the stomach, duodenum, small bowel, and colon is now understood to be a fairly common, benign finding in obese individuals.

Black Attenuation Pattern

Pneumatosis (Fig. 7-12) of the gut should always be considered as part of an acute injury to the gut: ischemic, infectious, or traumatic. Any disease process that compromises the integrity of the mucosa can introduce intramural gas. The presence of intramural gas can herald an abdominal catastrophe and must be viewed with suspicion. It can be seen as a benign process in patients with pneumatosis cystoides intestinalis, scleroderma, or other connective tissue disease that weakens

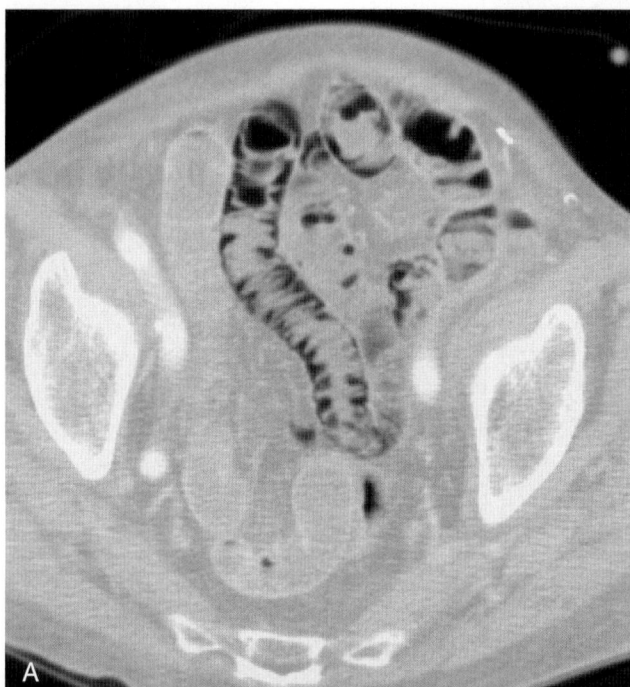

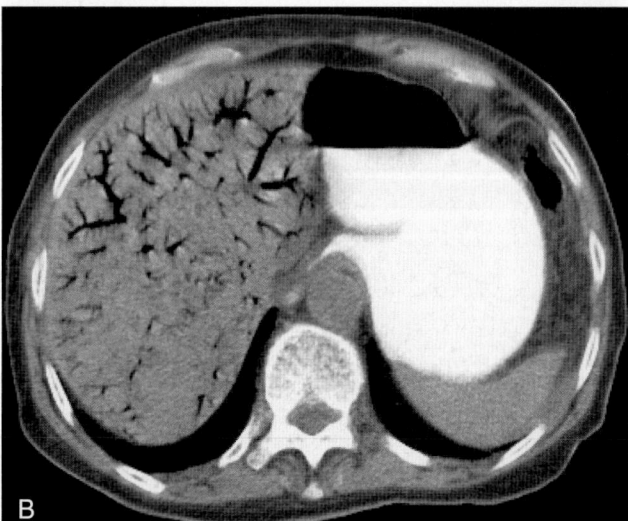

Figure 7-12. Black enhancement pattern. A. Scan of the pelvis displayed with lung windows shows intramural gas with ischemic necrosis of a segment of ileum. **B.** CT of the liver of this patient shows extensive portal venous gas.

the integrity of the bowel wall and in the setting of enteral catheters.

It is important not only to detect small intramural collections of gas but to avoid confusing them with pseudo-pneumatosis. Gas bubbles can cling to the mucosa in the dependent portion of the bowel wall and do not always seek nondependency. Also, gas bubbles in the colon may become trapped between fecal debris and mucosa.

MESENTERIC AND OMENTAL FAT PATHOLOGY

Careful evaluation of the attenuation, vascularity, and lymph nodes of the fat within the subperitoneal spaces surrounding the gut provides important information about the pathology in the adjacent bowel segment. There are six abdominal mesenteries: small bowel mesentery, transverse mesocolon, sigmoid mesocolon, ascending mesocolon, descending mesocolon, and mesoappendix. There are two omenta: the lesser and greater omentum. They may be involved by any number of ischemic, infectious, inflammatory, trauma, and malignant disorders.

Blood Vessels

When a thickened segment of gut (Fig. 7-13) is supplied by engorged blood vessels (vasa rectae), the pathology most likely is infectious or inflammatory. In the small bowel, mural thickening can be seen in Crohn's disease and lymphoma. If the vasa rectae supplying the affected segment are engorged

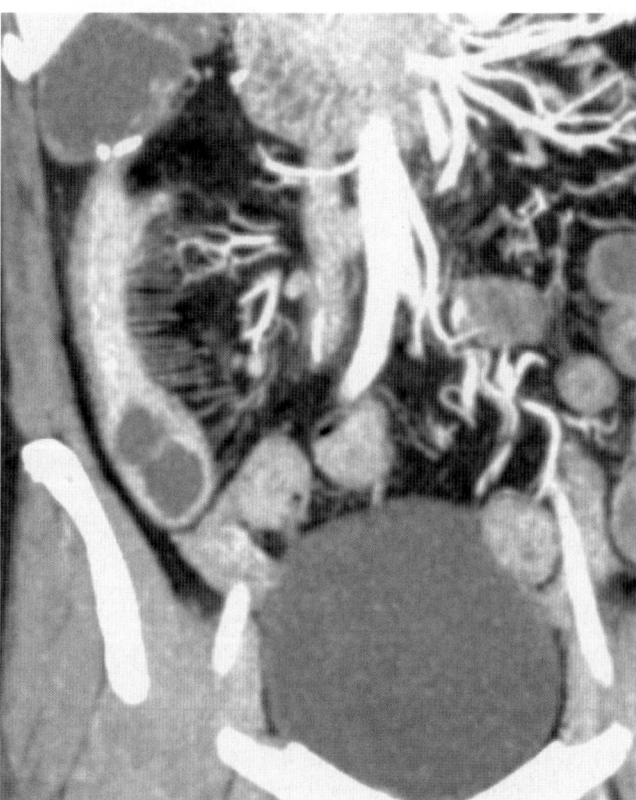

Figure 7-13. Engorged vasa rectae. There is engorgement of the vasa rectae of the ileocolic mesentery in this patient with Crohn's disease: the so-called comb sign. Infectious and inflammatory enterocolitides tend to be more vascular than malignancies.

(the comb sign), then the disease is most likely Crohn's disease. Similarly in a patient with mural thickening of the sigmoid colon, the presence of engorged vasa rectae (the caterpillar sign) is more suggestive of the diagnosis of diverticulitis as opposed to colon cancer.

Serosal and Subperitoneal Fat Density

Comparing the degree of fat stranding surrounding an abnormal segment of gut and the associated mural thickening is an important clue to diagnosing patients with the acute abdomen. Inflammatory condition such as appendicitis, diverticulitis, epiploic appendagitis (Fig. 7-14), and omental infarction are associated with disproportionate fat stranding. In other words, the amount of fat stranding is greater than the degree of mural thickening.[21]

In patients with small bowel obstruction, engorged vasa rectae supplying the obstructed segment is a finding that can be seen in closed loop obstruction and in patients with venous compromise.

"Creeping fat of the mesentery" is a common finding in patients with Crohn's disease. This abnormal fat often demonstrates prominent lymph nodes and engorged vasa rectae (see Chapter 45) and causes separation of bowel loops. Carcinoids tumors of the small bowel induce an intense desmoplastic reaction, creating a retractile appearance on CT.

Neoplasms also produce changes in the subperitoneal fat of the adjacent mesentery or omentum. Tumor invasion into the pericolic fat results in more sharply defined and thicker dense strands than those found with inflammation and infection. Spikelike densities correlate with pathologic findings of tumor extension through the serosa into perienteric fat.

Lymph Nodes

The evaluation of mesenteric and omental lymph nodes (Fig. 7-15) is an important part of assessing abnormal bowel pathology. As a general rule, when lymph node size is disproportionately greater than the mesenteric or omental inflammatory response, a malignancy should be considered.

In patients with mural thickening of the sigmoid colon, differentiating colon carcinoma from diverticulitis is a common clinical problem. Patients with carcinoma often have large lymph nodes in the sigmoid mesocolon, have a greater degree of mural thickening, and tend to have acute, irregular, and eccentric margins. Diverticulitis produces disproportionate fat stranding, the length of involvement is longer, and lymph nodes are typically normal in size.

Patients with Crohn's disease will often have mildly enlarged lymph nodes in the mesentery adjacent to the involved segment of gut. Gastrointestinal infections and mesenteric adenitis often produce mildly enlarged lymph nodes as well. The adenopathy, however, is less impressive than that found in patients with lymphoma.

The attenuation of the lymph nodes can also help narrow the differential diagnosis. A fat containing lymph node can

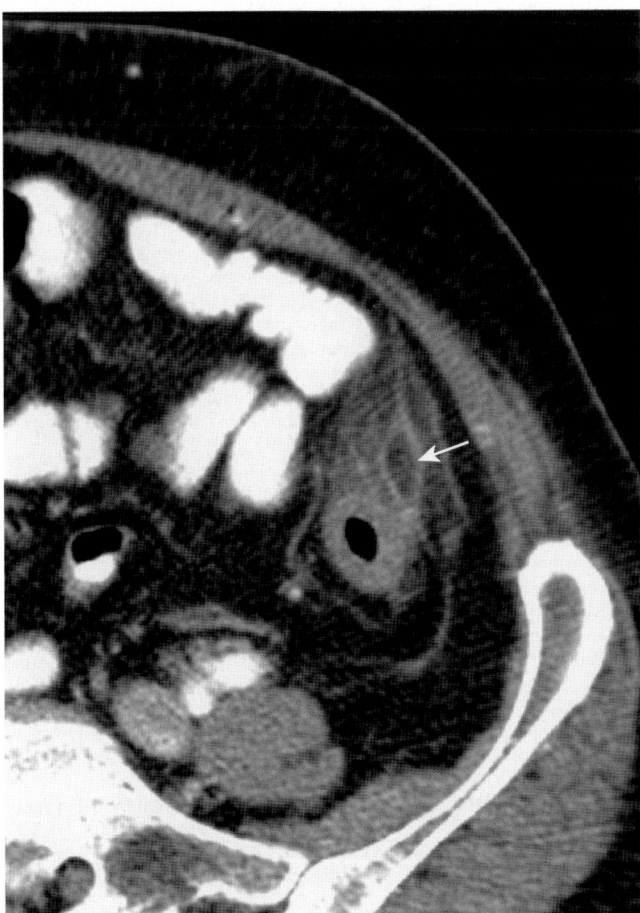

Figure 7-14. Disproportionate fat stranding: Epiploic appendagitis. There is an inflamed-ischemic epiploic appendage (*arrow*) adjacent to a slightly thickened segment of descending colon. Note the stranding in the adjacent fat.

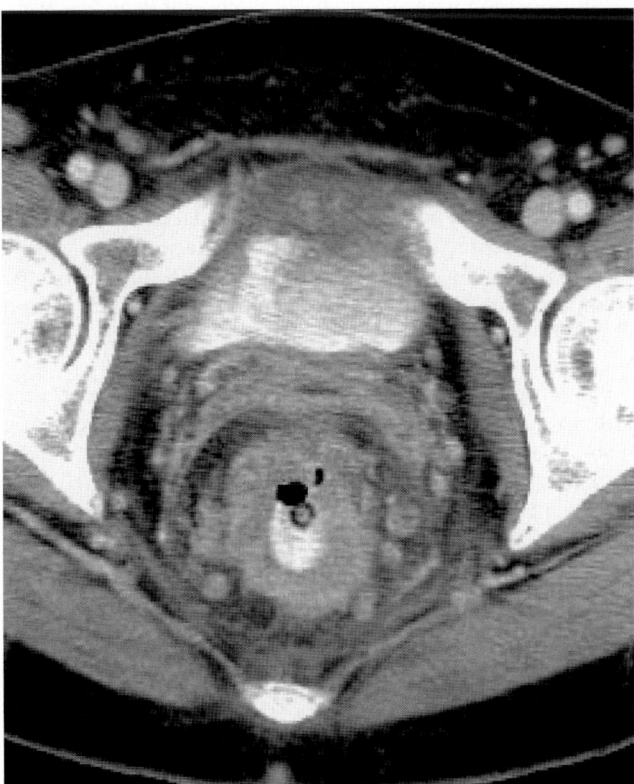

Figure 7-15. Adenopathy. Enlarged lymph nodes are identified in the mesorectal fat in this patient with a thickened rectal wall due to adenocarcinoma. The presence of adenopathy favors a malignant as opposed to a benign cause of the bowel wall thickening.

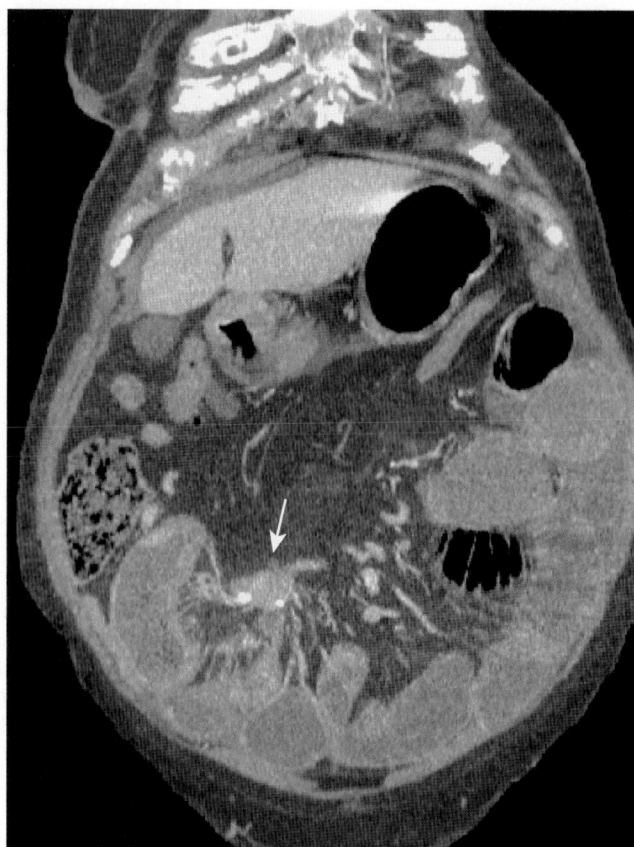

Figure 7-16. Calcifications. Mesenteric calcifications are identified in the ileocolic mesentery in this patient with an obstructing ileal carcinoid (*arrow*). Note the increased stranding of the mesentery due to the desmoplasia induced by the vasoactive peptides secreted by these tumors.

be seen in patients with sprue and giant cavitary lymph node syndrome. If the low attenuation lymph node demonstrates a rim of contrast enhancement or calcifications, infections such tuberculosis, other mycobacterial infections, and histoplasmosis should be considered. Mucinous tumors of the colon may also produce low attenuation metastatic lymph nodes. In patients with AIDS, high-attenuation lymph nodes suggest the diagnosis of Kaposi's sarcoma.

Carcinomas of the stomach, small bowel, and colon may only infiltrate a lymph node without necessarily increasing it size. Accordingly, any normal sized lymph nodes, especially if three or more in number, near a gastrointestinal tract malignancy must be viewed with suspicion. Local lymph nodes associated with carcinoid tumors may calcify.

Calcifications

Omental and mesenteric calcifications can develop in a number of benign and malignant disorders of the abdomen and pelvis.

Carcinoid tumor (Fig. 7-16) often presents with a calcified mass in the mesentery associated with tethering of adjacent

small bowel loops. The vasoactive peptides secreted by these tumors cause a local desmoplastic reaction with retraction of the mesentery, kinking of the adjacent loops, and mural thickening. Foci of mesenteric and omental calcifications can also be seen in patients with metastatic mucinous ovarian and gastrointestinal tract neoplasms.

References

1. Nishino M, Kubo T, Kataoka ML, et al: Coronal reformations of the chest on 64-row multi-detector row CT: Evaluation of image quality in comparison with 16-, 8- and 4-row multi-detector row CT. Eur J Radiol 59:231-238, 2006

2. Macari M, Balthazar EJ: CT of bowel wall thickening: Significance and pitfalls of interpretation. AJR 176:1105-1116, 2001.

3. Megibow AJ, Babb JS, Hecht EM, et al: Evaluation of bowel distention and bowel wall appearance by using neutral oral contrast agent for multi-detector row CT. Radiology 238:87-95, 2006.

4. Arslan H, Etlik O, Kayan M, et al: Peroral CT enterography with lactulose solution: Preliminary observations. AJR 185:1173-1179, 2005.

5. Gollub MJ: Multidetector computed tomography enteroclysis of patients with small bowel obstruction: A volume-rendered "surgical perspective." J Comput Assist Tomogr 29:401-407, 2005.

6. Bodily KD, Fletcher JG, Solem CA, et al: Crohn disease: Mural attenuation and thickness at contrast-enhanced CT enterography—Correlation with endoscopic and histologic findings of inflammation. Radiology 238: 505-516, 2006.

7. Hong SS, Kim AY, Byun JH, et al: MDCT of small-bowel disease: Value of 3D imaging. AJR 187:1212-1221, 2006.

8. Boudiaf M, Jaff A, Soyer P, et al: Small-bowel diseases: Prospective evaluation of multi-detector row helical CT enteroclysis in 107 consecutive patients. Radiology 233:338-344, 2004.

9. Kim JH, Eun HW, Goo DE, et al: Imaging of various gastric lesions with 2D MPR and CT gastrography performed with multidetector CT. RadioGraphics 26:1101-1116, 2006.

10. Umeoka S, Koyama T, Togashi K, et al: Esophageal cancer: Evaluation with triple-phase dynamic CT—Initial experience. Radiology 239:777-783, 2006.

11. Hur J, Park MS, Lee JH, et al: Diagnostic accuracy of multidetector row computed tomography in T and N staging of gastric cancer with histopathologic correlation. J Comput Assist Tomogr 30:372-377, 2006.

12. Beer AJ, Wieder HA, Lordick F, et al: Adenocarcinomas of esophagogastric junction: Multi-detector row CT to evaluate early response to neoadjuvant chemotherapy. Radiology 239:472-480, 2006.

13. Shi R, Schraedley-Desmond P, Napel S, et al: CT colonography: Influence of 3D viewing and polyp candidate features on interpretation with computer-aided detection. Radiology 239:768-776, 2006.

14. Ash L, Baker ME, O'Malley CM Jr, et al: Colonic abnormalities on CT in adult hospitalized patients with *Clostridium difficile* colitis: Prevalence and significance of findings. AJR 186:1393-1400, 2006.

15. Taylor SA, Halligan S, Slater A, et al: Comparison of radiologists' confidence in excluding significant colorectal neoplasia with multidetector-row CT colonography compared with double contrast barium enema. Br J Radiol 79:208-215, 2006.

16. Johnson KT, Johnson CD, Fletcher JG, et al: CT colonography using 360-degree virtual dissection: A feasibility study. AJR 186:90-95, 2006.

17. Macari M, Bini EJ: CT colonography: Where have we been and where are we going? Radiology 237:819-833, 2005.

18. Pickhardt PJ, Asher DB: Wall thickening of the gastric antrum as a normal finding: Multidetector CT with cadaveric comparison. AJR 181:973-979, 2003.

19. Wittenberg J, Harisinghani MG, Jhaveri K, et al: Algorithmic approach to CT diagnosis of the abnormal bowel wall. RadioGraphics 22:1093-1107, 2002.

20. Harisinghani MG, Wittenberg J, Lee W, et al: Bowel wall fat halo sign in patients without intestinal disease. AJR 181:781-784, 2003.

21. Pereira JM, Sirlin CB, Pinto PS, et al: Disproportionate fat stranding: A helpful CT sign in patients with acute abdominal pain. RadioGraphics 24:703-717, 2004.

Magnetic Resonance Imaging of the Hollow Viscera

Russell N. Low, MD

MAGNETIC RESONANCE IMAGING OF GASTROINTESTINAL TRACT—PROTOCOLS	**CLINICAL APPLICATIONS**
COIL SELECTION	Inflammatory Bowel Disease
PATIENT PREPARATION AND INTRALUMINAL CONTRAST MATERIAL	Infectious Bowel Diseases
ROUTES OF CONTRAST AGENT ADMINISTRATION	Ischemic Bowel Disease
	Gastrointestinal Malignancy
	SUMMARY

Magnetic resonance imaging of the gastrointestinal tract takes advantage of the inherent outstanding soft tissue contrast of MRI to provide excellent depiction of inflammatory, infectious, ischemic, and neoplastic gastrointestinal diseases. By combining fast imaging pulse sequences with intraluminal and intravenous contrast agents MRI can show the normal and diseased bowel wall as well as adjacent inflammatory and neoplastic changes involving the mesentery, peritoneum, and omentum.[1-5]

Imaging the gastrointestinal tract presents significant challenges that can be met with current MRI techniques. In the past, slower MR pulse sequences required several minutes to acquire, resulting in degraded image quality due to bowel peristalsis and respiratory motion. Current high-field MRI represents a confluence of hardware and software development that has resulted in fast MRI obtained in a few seconds. Breath-hold precontrast and dynamic breath-hold contrast-enhanced MRI of the abdomen and pelvis can be easily performed with outstanding image quality.

Extracellular intravenous MR contrast agents are relatively inexpensive and have a long track record of safety and efficacy for evaluating abdominal diseases. Intraluminal contrast agents can be administered using "off the shelf" agents or commercially available oral contrast material.

MAGNETIC RESONANCE IMAGING OF THE GASTROINTESTINAL TRACT—PROTOCOLS

In MRI of the gastrointestinal tract rapid breath-hold acquisitions are used to minimize motion artifact. Each MR imager has available pulse sequences that can be optimized for MRI of the gastrointestinal tract. Although they are called by different acronyms, similar pulse sequences and image types are available on scanners from all the major MR imager manufacturers. The specific pulse sequence parameters, however, will be vendor specific.

For a general evaluation of the gastrointestinal tract I utilize breath-hold single-shot rapid acquisition with relaxation enhancement (RARE) imaging in the axial and coronal planes.[1-3] This pulse sequence is known by a number of different acronyms, including single-shot fast spin-echo (SSFSE), single-shot turbo spin-echo (SSTSE), and half-Fourier acquisition single-shot turbo spin-echo (HASTE). These single-slice images are breathing-independent and are thus insensitive to respiratory or peristaltic motion. They provide heavily T2-weighted images and an excellent overall abdominal and pelvic survey. Water-soluble intraluminal contrast material demonstrates high signal intensity, whereas the bowel wall is depicted as a thin line of intermediate signal intensity surrounding the bowel contents. Intestinal mural thickening is depicted on single-shot RARE images when the bowel wall measures more than 3 mm. The single-shot images are obtained without fat suppression.

Fat-suppressed T2-weighted fast spin-echo images can be obtained as an optional sequence to distinguish intestinal mural edema from fibrosis. This can help differentiate an acute inflammatory process with mural thickening from a thickened wall due to a chronic fibrotic stricture. An acute inflammatory stricture will show high signal intensity edema in the thickened bowel wall, whereas the thickened fibrotic wall of a chronic stricture will demonstrate low signal intensity. Fat-suppressed T2-wighted images may be obtained with breath-holding or with respiratory triggering. I do not routinely acquire these images but will add them to the MR protocol to characterize an acute versus chronic stricture.

After the intravenous injection of gadolinium, two sets of axial fat-suppressed gradient-echo MR images are obtained through the abdomen and pelvis.[4] One may use 2D or 3D gradient-echo imaging. The 2D gradient-echo images use a thicker slice thickness of 8 to 10 mm but are typically sharper and have a greater range of contrast than the 3D gradient-echo images. The 3D images have a thinner slice thickness and provide more efficient coverage of the abdomen and pelvis. A typical slice thickness for the 3D images is 4 to 6 mm. Some 3D acquisitions incorporate a fixed or variable slice overlap.

Water-soluble intraluminal contrast material demonstrates low signal intensity on the fat-suppressed, gadolinium-enhanced gradient-echo MR images. The bowel wall is shown as the rings or lines surrounding the bowel lumen. The thickness of the normal bowel wall measures less than 3 mm. The normal bowel wall will show gadolinium enhancement equal to or less than the liver parenchyma. Abnormal mural thickening or enhancement can be evaluated as signs of inflammatory or neoplastic intestinal disease.

Important features of the optimized gadolinium-enhanced MR image include (1) fat suppression, (2) image homogeneity, (3) high in-plane resolution, and (4) breath-hold imaging. In practice I often combine early dynamic 3D gradient-echo imaging with delayed 2D gradient-echo imaging. The delayed 2D gradient-echo images are often most useful for depicting intestinal mural disease and adjacent disease of the peritoneum, showing excellent image sharpness and contrast conspicuity. Coronal and sagittal 3D or 2D gradient-echo images are obained before obtaining the delayed 2D gradient-echo images.

This rapid MR examination of the gastrointestinal tract can be performed in 20 to 25 minutes. Breath-hold single-shot RARE images in the axial and coronal plane are followed by fat-suppressed gadolinium-enhanced 3D and 2D gradient-echo MRI. Specific imaging parameters are listed in Table 8-1.

Another sequence that is commonly used for gastrointestinal tract imaging is balanced steady-state free precession (SSFP) sequences.[6] The image contrast is determined by $T2^*/T1$ properties depending heavily on repetition time. The speed and relative motion insensitivity of acquisition are useful features for gastrointestinal imaging. On the balanced SSFP images water-soluble intraluminal contrast material, blood, bile, ascites, and urine will all demonstrate high signal intensity.

Vendor acronyms for this pulse sequence include balanced turbo field-echo (b-TFE), fast imaging employing steady-state acquisition (FIESTA), and true fast imaging with steady-state precession (true FISP). The balanced SSFP images show excellent homogeneity of luminal signal and visualization of the bowel wall. Compared with 3D gradient-echo images, the balanced SSFP images are less sensitive to motion artifact but show increased sensitivity to chemical shift and susceptibility artifact.

COIL SELECTION

Coil selection will depend on availability of surface coils for a specific MR imager. Using the large body coil can provide excellent results with the most homogeneous images and the most extensive anatomic coverage. Dedicated surface coils with larger areas of anatomic coverage are becoming available. I typically require 48-cm coverage in the craniocaudal direction when imaging the abdomen and pelvis. There are now several surface coils available that provide this extensive coverage. Image homogeneity should not be sacrificed when using a dedicated surface coil. Inhomogeneous images can create problems when assessing subtle gastrointestinal tract or peritoneal disease. Some form of intensity correction algorithm should be utilized to maximize the homogeneity of the images. Ultimately, phased-array surface coils combined with parallel imaging should provide optimal signal and speed of image acquisition.

PATIENT PREPARATION AND INTRALUMINAL CONTRAST MATERIAL

All patients are asked not to eat or drink for 4 hours before their MR appointment. If rectal water is to be administered, patients administer a Fleet's enema before the examination. If more thorough bowel cleansing is desired, patients are also asked to have a clear liquid diet starting for 12 hours before the MR examination and to orally take four bisacodyl tablets the evening before their appointment.

The use of intraluminal contrast material is an essential element of the MRI protocol for gastrointestinal tract imaging.[4,7-16] Oral and/or rectal contrast material will distend the stomach, small intestine, and colon, improving the depiction of inflammatory or neoplastic mural disease. Subtle mural thickening can be easily masked by collapsed segments of bowel. Alternatively, incompletely distended bowel can mimic diseased bowel with apparent mural thickening that will disappear when the bowel is adequately distended. In addiion, well-distended bowel facilitates the depiction of adjacent peritoneal, serosal, or omental tumor.

In our experience, a biphasic intraluminal contrast agent is optimal for gastrointestinal tract imaging (Fig. 8-1). Water is the classic biphasic MR intraluminal agent, showing high signal intensity on T2-weighted images and low signal intensity on T1-weighted images. On fat-suppressed gadolinium-enhanced T1-weighted spoiled gradient-echo images the water-soluble contrast material is low in signal intensity. This depicts the normal bowel wall as a thin, linear, mildly enhancing structure surrounding the dark bowel lumen. Water can be used as an oral contrast agent. However, because water is absorbed through the small intestinal wall, its use as an oral agent for MRI often results in unpredictable distention of the distal small bowel. For this reason, water-soluble contrast agents that are iso-osmolar are preferred because the ingested contrast will remain in the intestinal tract. In my practice I have used a number of different intraluminal agents for MRI. All of the agents produce a biphasic appearance on MR images. They are readily available and relatively inexpensive. Other commercially available oral agents for MRI containing iron oxides and manganese have been described but are not currently used in my practice.[14-16]

Dilute barium sulfate (ReadiCat 2; E-Z-EM Inc, Lake Success, NY) is composed of 98% water and 2% barium and other additives. On MR images, dilute barium sulfate has a biphasic appearance with low signal on T1-weighted images and a high signal on T2-weighted images. ReadiCat2 is commonly used for helical CT scans of the abdomen and pelvis.

Table 8-1
Protocol for Gastrointestinal Magnetic Resonance Imaging

Field Strength	1.5 T					
Gradients	30 MT/m, 150 MT/m/s					
Plane	Coronal	Axial	Axial	Axial	Coronal	Axial
Sequence	SSTSE	SSTSE	Resp Trig TSE	Gad 3D GE	Gad 3D GE	HiRes 2D GE
Anatomy	A & P	A & P	A & P	A & P	A & P	A & P
Scan time	20 s	18.6 s	3:28 min	22 s	19 s	22 s
No. of packages	1	2	2	3	1	3
Geometry						
Coil	Q body	Q body	Q body	Q body	Q body	Q body
FOV	460	375	375	375	465	375
RFOV	95	80	80	80	85	70
Foldover suppression	Yes	No	No	No	Yes	No
Matrix scan	256	256	256	240	240	304
Matrix reconstruction	256	512	512	512	256	512
Scan percentage	80	80	80	80	80	90
SENSE	No	No	No	No	No	No
Over-contiguous	No	No	No	Yes	Yes	No
No. of stacks	1	2	2	3	1	3
No. of slices	25	24	30	50	50	16
Slice thickness	8	7	7	3 over-contig.	4 over-contig.	10
Slice gap	1	3	1	—	—	0
Slice orientation	Cor	Trans.	Trans.	Trans.	Cor	Trans.
Foldover direction	RL	AP	AP	AP	RL	AP
No. of chunks	1	2	2	1	1	1
No. of REST slabs	0	0	2	2	2	2
REST type	—	—	Parallel	Parallel	Free	Parallel
REST thickness	—	—	60	60	60	60
REST position	—	—	Head	Feet	—	Head
REST orientation	—	—	SI	SI	Free	SI
Patient position	Head	Head	Head	Head	Head	Head
Patient orientation	Supine	Supine	Supine	Supine	Supine	Supine
Contrast						
Scan mode	M2D	M2D	MS	3D	3D	MS
Scan technique	SE	SE	SE	FFE	FFE	FFE
Contrast enhancement	No	No	No	Yes	Yes	Yes
Fast imaging mode	TSE	TSE	TSE	TFE	TFE	None
Single shot	Yes	Yes	No	Multi	Multi	No
TFE factor	90	90	24	30	30	—
Number of echoes	1	1	1	1	1	1
Partial echo	No	No	No	No	No	No
TE	80	80	70	Shortest	Shortest	Shortest
Flip angle	90	90	90	10	10	70
TR	Shortest	Shortest	1600	Shortest	Shortest	Shortest
Halfscan	Yes	Yes	No	No	No	Yes
Halfscan factor	0.65	0.65	No	No	No	0.65
Water fat shift (pixels)	Max.	Max.	Max.	0.35 user-defined	0.35 user-defined	Max
TSE factor	90	90	24	—	—	—
TSE ultrashort	Yes	Yes	No	—	—	—
Shim	Auto	Auto	Auto	Auto	Auto	Auto
SPIR	No	No	Yes	Yes	Yes	No
ProSet	No	No	No	No	No	Water select
ProSet pulse type	—	—	—	—	—	121
Respiratory compensation	Breath-hold	Breath-hold	Trigger	Breath-hold	Breath-hold	Breath-hold
Max slices / breath hold	25	24	—	50	50	16
Flow compensation	No	No	No	No	No	No
NSA	1	1	2	1	1	1
Notes						
Parameter notes	Mobitrack; 25 slices; single breath-hold	Mobitrack; 2 stations; 24 slices per station; 1 breath-hold per station; 48 images total	Mobitrack; 2 stations; 24 slices per station; resp. trig.; 48 images total	Mobitrack; 3 stations; 50 slices per station; 1 breath-hold per station; 150 images total	Single breath-hold; 50 slices	Mobitrack; 3 stations; 16 slices per station; 1 breath-hold (16 images per breath-hold); 48 images total

SSTSE, single-shot turbo spin-echo; TSE, turbo spin-echo; GAD, gadolinium; GE, gradient-echo; A & P, anterior and posterior; FOV, field of view; RFOV, receiver field of view; SENSE, sensitivity encoding; REST, regional saturation technique; SE, spin-echo; FFE, fast field echo; TFE, turbo field echo; TE, echo time; TR, repetition time; SPIR, spectral presaturation by inversion recovery; NSA, number of signal averages; Cor, coronal; SI, signal intensity.

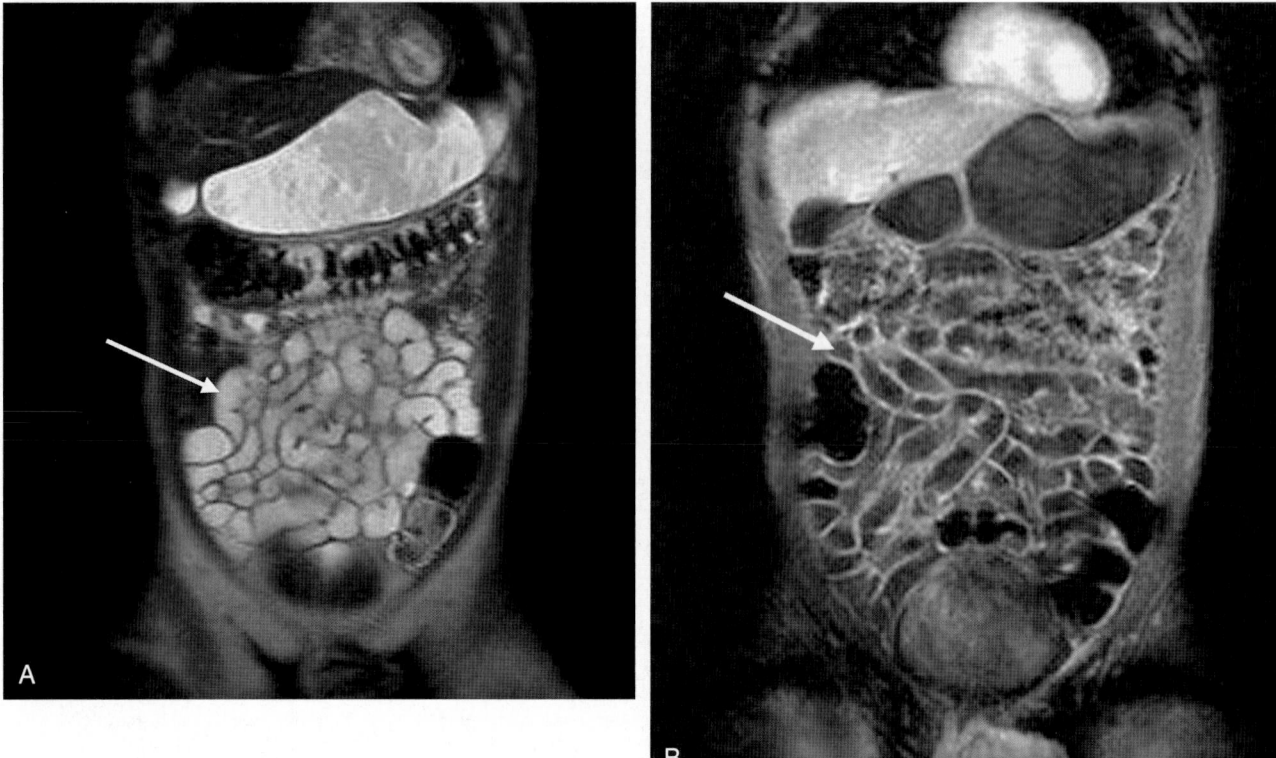

Figure 8-1. Oral contrast material. Coronal single-shot turbo spin-echo (SSTSE) (**A**) and gadolinium-enhanced 3D gradient-echo MR images (**B**) were obtained after oral administration of 1.5 L Metamucil mixed with water. The water-soluble intraluminal contrast material demonstrates high signal intensity on the T2-weighted SSTSE images (*arrow* in **A**) and low signal intensity on the T1-weighted 3D gradient-echo images (*arrow* in **B**).

Dilute barium sulfate will remain within the intestines and is very effective in distending the small bowel and colon. Patients ingest three to four of the 450-mL bottles of the dilute barium starting 1 hour before the MR examination.[4,5,7]

Psyllium fiber mixed with water is another water-soluble contrast agent that produces a biphasic appearance on MR T1-wieghted and T2-weighted images (see Fig. 8-1).[8,9] Metamucil (Proctor & Gamble Co., Cincinnati, OH) is composed of psyllium fiber with orange flavoring. It is a dietary fiber supplement that can be purchased off the shelf. Its active ingredient is psyllium husk, a natural plant fiber with a high percentage of soluble fiber. Because the Metamucil is orange flavored it is typically preferred by patients and better tolerated than dilute barium sulfate. A total dose of 0.8 mg/kg Metamucil is mixed in 1.0 to 1.5 L of water. I mix a half scoop of Metamucil per 8-oz glass of water and have patients ingest four to five glasses over 1 hour before the examination. To improve filling of the distal small bowel I have patients drink two of the glasses of Metamucil at home before leaving for their appointment. Unlike the ReadiCat2, some of the water in the Metamucil is absorbed in the small intestine and will be excreted by the kidney.

Mannitol 2.5% mixed with 2% locust bean gum has been proposed as an effective iso-osmolar water-soluble oral agent for MRI.[10,11] Mannitol is a white, crystalline, water-soluble, slightly sweet alcohol, $C_6H_8(OH)_6$, used as a dietary supplement and dietetic sweetener. Mannitol comes in 500-mL bags mixed to a concentration of 20%. One and one-half liters of 2.5% mannitol can be prepared by mixing 187.5 mL of 20% mannitol with enough tap water to achieve a volume of 1.5 L.

Three grams of the locust bean gum (2%) is added to the 1.5 L of mannitol solution to slow down the transit time through the intestinal tract. Locust bean gum, also called carob bean gum and carubin, is extracted from the seed of the carob tree. It is used in ice cream, cultured dairy products, and cream cheese. The locust bean gum has been reported to decrease the diarrhea produced by orally ingested mannitol. The 1.5 L of 2.5% mannitol solution with locust bean gum is ingested over 1 hour before the MR examination. Sorbitol 2% can be used as an alternative to mannitol.[10]

Polyethylene glycol (PEG) 2% is a water-soluble, waxy solid substance. Solutions of polyethylene glycol (PEG-ES) are used to cleanse the bowel before a gastrointestinal examination or surgery. It works by causing diarrhea. Solutions of polyethylene glycol have been used as an oral agent for gastrointestinal tract MRI and as the intraluminal agent for the patient undergoing MR enteroclysis.[12,13]

Rectal water can be administered to distend the rectum and colon. I administer 500 to 1000 mL of tap water through a balloon-tipped barium enema catheter. Slow administration will help to maximize the amount of fluid tolerated by the patient. The balloon at the tip of the catheter should be filled with water to avoid the susceptibility artifact caused by air in the balloon.

ROUTES OF CONTRAST AGENT ADMINISTRATION

Intraluminal contrast material can be administered orally with patients drinking 1 to 1.5 L of contrast material over 1 hour before the examination. Alternatively, contrast agents may be administered via a nasojejunal tube, as has been described for CT and MR enteroclysis. The enteroclysis technique has the advantage of more controlled and consistent small bowel distention but obviously requires nasojejunal intubation.[17-19] Oral administration or intraluminal contrast material is effective in cooperative patients and can be combined with rectally administered water for simultaneous evaluation of the small bowel and colon.

CLINICAL APPLICATIONS

Inflammatory Bowel Disease

Crohn's Disease

Magnetic resonance imaging provides many unique advantages when evaluating the mural changes of Crohn's disease.[20-29] Distending the bowel lumen with water-soluble contrast material improves visualization of the diseased bowel wall in patients with active Crohn's disease. MRI assesses mural changes, the degree and pattern of enhancement, and the presence of adjacent mesenteric inflammation. Helical CT is equally effective in assessing bowel wall thickening but is more limited in its assessment of mural enhancement. The degree of bowel wall enhancement is much more conspicuous on gadolinium-enhanced MRI than multidetector CT. This marked enhancement of inflamed bowel segments on 2D or 3D gadolinium-enhanced MRI facilitates detection of subtle Crohn's disease. A wall thickness greater than 3 mm is abnormal in a well-distended segment of bowel. Bowel wall thickening can be assessed on single-shot RARE images or fat-suppressed gadolinium-enhanced images.

Crohn's Disease Activity

Determining the activity of Crohn's disease has important clinical implications affecting selection of appropriate treatment options. Patients with recurrent abdominal pain due to active Crohn's disease require treatment. However, patients commonly present with symptoms that may be unrelated to reactivation of their Crohn's disease. This latter group of patients requires entirely different management. The activity of Crohn's disease may be determined from clinical parameters, including the Crohn's Disease Activity Index, an assessment of acute phase reactants (white blood cell count, erythrocyte sedimentation rate, C-reactive protein, and orosomucoids), or clinical symptoms and physical findings. In practice, these clinical parameters may be misleading or inconclusive. The results of endoscopy and imaging studies can play an important role in determining the activity and extent of Crohn's disease.

The activity of Crohn's disease can be assessed by a number of different MRI parameters, including degree of bowel wall enhancement, the pattern of enhancement, the thickness and length of the involved diseased segment, and the presence of edema in the bowel wall on T2-weighted images. Perienteric changes including enhancing lymph nodes, infiltration of mesenteric fat, and increased mesenteric vascularity can also reflect active Crohn's disease.[7,21,22,28,29]

DEGREE OF BOWEL WALL ENHANCEMENT

The degree of mural enhancement with intravascular gadolinium correlates with the activity of Crohn's disease.[7] Enhancement of the thickened bowel wall can be assessed on the first set of gadolinium-enhanced images by comparing bowel wall enhancement to the liver and intravascular gadolinium. The normal bowel wall enhances less than the liver parenchyma. Mural enhancement of thickened bowel greater than the liver is abnormal, and mural enhancement equal to intravascular gadolinium is markedly abnormal. In chronic inactive Crohn's disease the thickened bowel wall will show no or only mild enhancement (Fig. 8-2). Chronic fibrotic strictures produce mural thickening with minimal enhancement. Active Crohn's disease shows moderate to marked bowel wall enhancement (Fig. 8-3). In cases with a stratified pattern

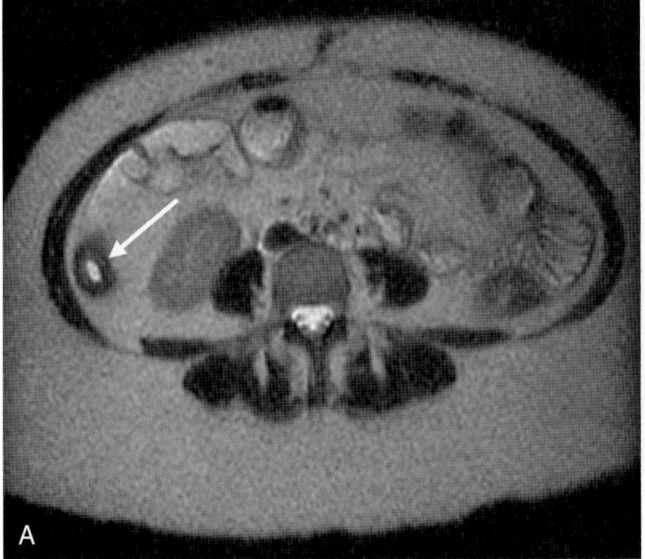
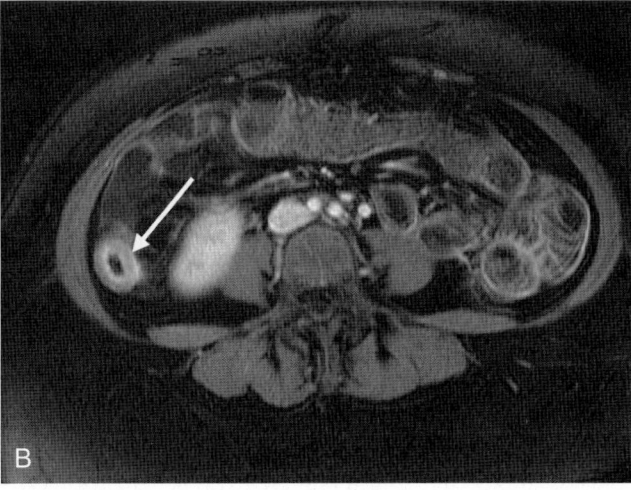

Figure 8-2. Inactive Crohn's disease. Axial single-shot fast spin-echo image (**A**) shows distal ileum with mural thickening (*arrow*). Note the low signal intensity of the thickening bowel wall. Immediate postinjection gadolinium-enhanced spoiled gradient-echo image (**B**) shows minimal enhancement of the thickened bowel wall. Absence of perienteric inflammation and stranding is also noted. Findings correlate with inactive Crohn's disease, which was confirmed at endoscopy.

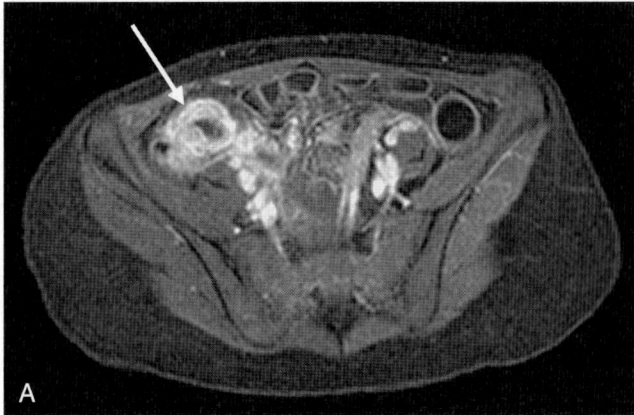

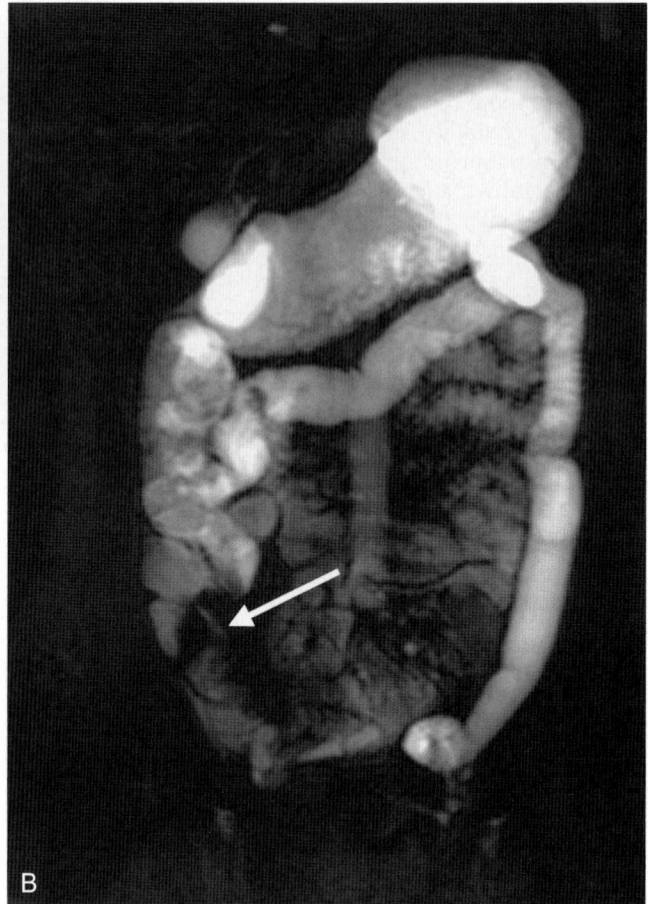

Figure 8-3. Active Crohn's disease with marked mural enhancement. Axial gadolinium-enhanced 3D gradient-echo image (**A**) shows an abnormal terminal ileum (*arrow*) with moderate mural thickening and marked enhancement. The degree of enhancement indicates active Crohn's disease. Coronal MR hydrogram (**B**) shows a stricture (*arrow*) of the terminal ileum.

of enhancement, the mucosa should show moderate to marked enhancement.

PATTERN OF BOWEL WALL ENHANCEMENT

A stratified pattern of mural enhancement indicates active Crohn's inflammation (Fig. 8-4).[22] There is marked mucosal and serosal enhancement with an intervening nonenhancing layer representing an edematous submucosa. In one study this stratified pattern of mural enhancement was present in 7 of 24 bowel segments with active Crohn's disease and in no segments with inactive disease.[22] Full thickness or diffuse enhancement of the thickened bowel wall also indicates active Crohn's disease if there is moderate to marked mural enhancement. Diffuse mural enhancement is the most common pattern of enhancement observed in active Crohn's disease. Mild diffuse enhancement can be seen in bowel segments with inactive Crohn's disease.

T2-WEIGHTED APPEARANCE OF THE BOWEL WALL

On T2-weighted images, active Crohn's disease shows high signal in the thickened bowel wall, indicating mural edema and inflammation.[28] Chronic inactive Crohn's disease will show less intense signal in the thickened bowel wall usually equal to or less than muscle. A fibrotic stricture can show very low mural signal similar to the psoas muscle. Fat-suppressed T2-weighted images are most useful in assessing the signal intensity of diseased segments of gut. Single-shot RARE images are useful for showing the segments of bowel but are less sensitive to the presence of bowel wall edema.

BOWEL WALL THICKNESS

In general, segments of bowel with active Crohn's disease show greater mural thickness than those segments with inactive disease.[7,22,28] This assessment is affected by the degree of luminal distention. In one study the mean thickness of segments with active Crohn's disease was 6.7 mm compared with 3.3 mm for segments with inactive disease. However, significant overlap exists between the mural thickness of the active and inactive groups.[22] Fibrotic strictures without active inflammation may show a moderately thickened bowel wall. In these cases, absence of moderate or marked mural enhancement will help to characterize this as a chronic process without active inflammation.[7]

MESENTERIC STRANDING

Infiltration of the adjacent mesentery and "whiskering" of the bowel wall are indirect indications of active Crohn's disease (see Fig. 8-4). This finding may be depicted on single-shot RARE images, true FISP images, or fat-suppressed, gadolinium-enhanced gradient-echo images as linear signal or enhancement extending from the inflamed bowel into the adjacent small bowel or colonic mesentery.[21,22]

INCREASED MESENTERIC VASCULARITY

Increased prominence of the size and/or number of mesenteric vessels and vasa rectae can be an indication of active inflammation. In one study, increased mesenteric vascularity was present in 18 of 23 patients with active disease and 3 of 7 patients with inactive disease.[22]

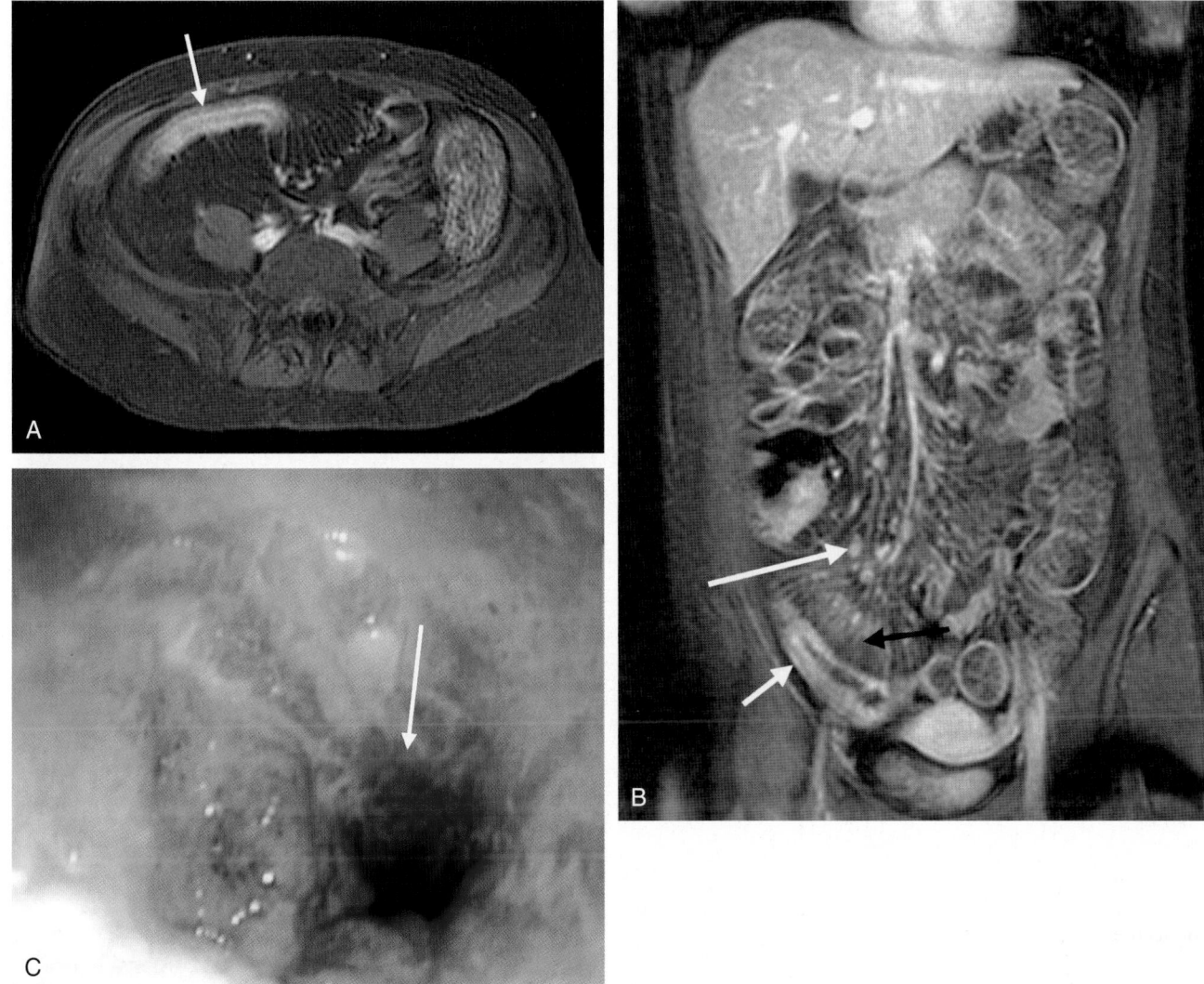

Figure 8-4. Active Crohn's disease with layered pattern of enhancement. Immediate axial gadolinium-enhanced 3D gradient-echo image (**A**) shows an abnormally thickened terminal ileum (*arrow*) with a layered pattern of enhancement. Coronal gadolinium-enhanced 3D gradient-echo image (**B**) confirms the diseased terminal ileum (*short white arrow*) and shows associated findings of acute Crohn's disease including enhancing mesenteric lymph nodes (*long white arrow*) and mesenteric stranding (*black arrow*). Endoscopic view (**C**) of the terminal ileum confirms active Crohn's disease with mucosal inflammation (*arrow*).

ENHANCEMENT OF MESENTERIC LYMPH NODES

Gadolinium enhancement of mesenteric lymph nodes is another strong indicator of active Crohn's disease (see Fig. 8-4).[21] When comparing nodal signal intensity with that of adjacent fat, an enhancement ratio of 1.3 has been found to be a sensitive marker for active Crohn's disease. Mesenteric lymph nodes in patients with inactive Crohn's disease will not show significant enhancement.

COMPLICATIONS OF CROHN'S DISEASE

Perienteric complications of Crohn's disease include abscess or phlegmon formation and fistulas. Abscesses are depicted on MR images as extraintestinal fluid collections with a surrounding thick enhancing abscess wall.[7] After administration of water-soluble intraluminal contrast material, the fluid content of an abscess may be difficult to distinguish from bowel contents on T1- or T2-weighted images. However, on fat-suppressed gadolinium-enhanced MR images, the thick, enhancing abscess wall is easy to identify. The marked degree

of enhancement of the abscess wall with gadolinium often makes the abscess easier to detect on MR images than on helical CT scans with iodinated contrast material (Fig. 8-5).

The development of fistulas in Crohn's disease is a common complication presenting as abnormal connections between the diseased bowel and other organs or the skin. Enteroenteric fistulas occur between segments of bowel whereas enterocutaneous fistulas occur between diseased bowel and the skin surface. Enterovesicle and enterovaginal fistulas are common complications of pelvic Crohn's disease.

On MRI, Crohn's fistulas are depicted as fluid- or air-containing tracts on fat-suppressed T2-weighted images or as enhancing tracts on fat-suppressed gadolinium-enhanced gradient-echo MR images.[27] High-resolution surface coil images with thin-section short tau inversion recovery (STIR) images or gadolinium-enhanced 3D gradient-echo images are most useful to depict the fistulous communication. The accurate depiction of Crohn's fistulas is important in selecting patients for anti–tumor necrosis factor (TNF) therapy.

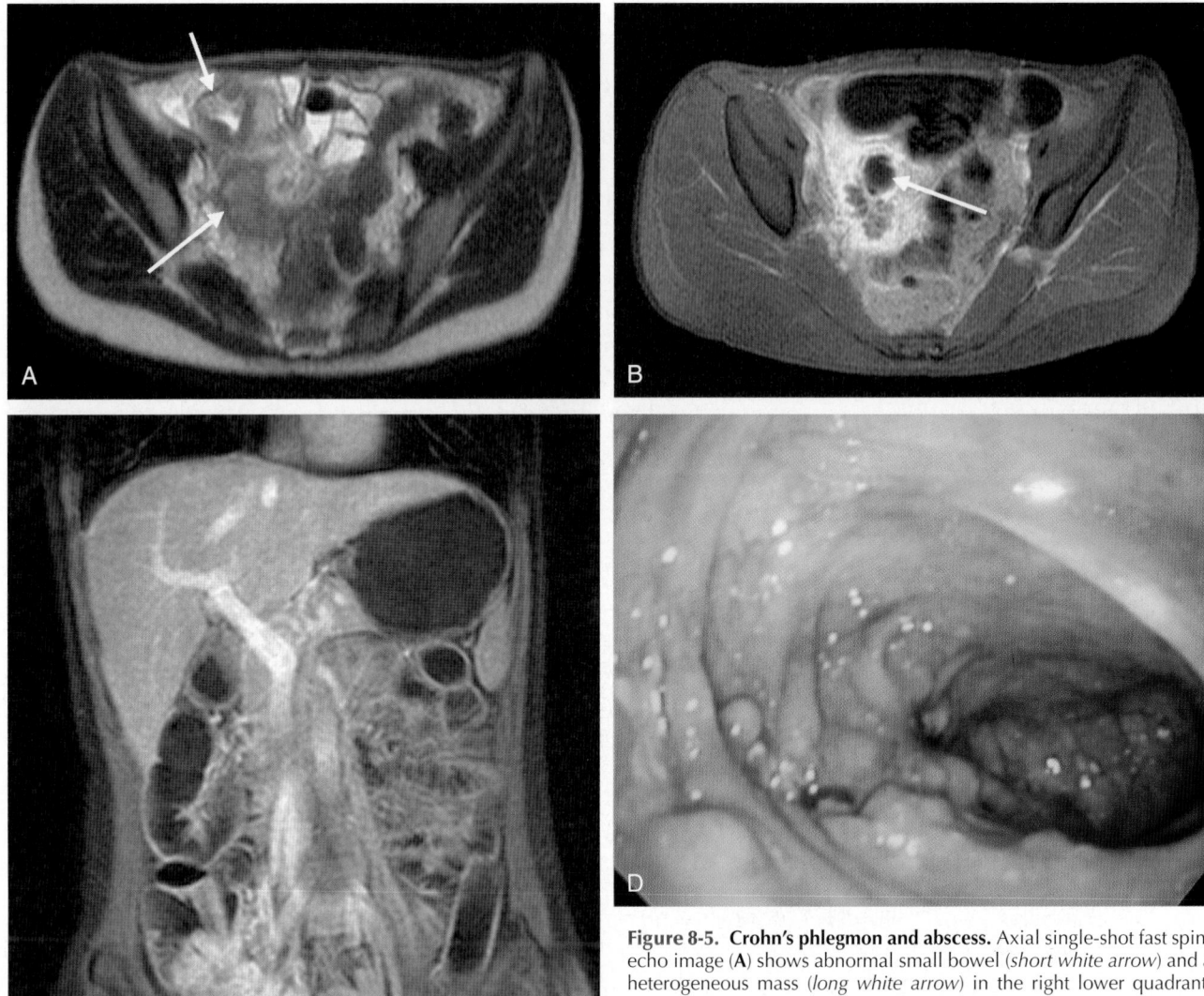

Figure 8-5. Crohn's phlegmon and abscess. Axial single-shot fast spin-echo image (**A**) shows abnormal small bowel (*short white arrow*) and a heterogeneous mass (*long white arrow*) in the right lower quadrant. Axial gadolinium-enhanced spoiled gradient-echo image (**B**) depicts a markedly enhancing phlegmon and central nonenhancing abscess (*arrow*). Coronal gadolinium-enhanced spoiled gradient-echo image (**C**) confirms the thickened and enhancing terminal ileum (*arrow*). Endoscopic view (**D**) of the terminal ileum shows a nodular inflamed mucosa. Biopsy confirmed active inflammation of Crohn's disease.

Infliximab (Remicade) blocks the immune system's overproduction of a protein (TNF-α), with subsequent reduction in draining enterocutaneous and rectovaginal fistulas.

Perirectal and perianal complications of Crohn's disease include fistulas and abscess formation. Surface coil images of the rectum can be obtained using thin-section images angled perpendicular and parallel to the rectum and perianal area. Fat-suppressed STIR images and thin-section 3D gadolinium-enhanced images are particularly useful to evaluate this anatomic region. Fistulous tracts will be depicted as high signal linear tracts on the STIR images or as linear enhancing tracts extending between diseased bowel and adjacent structures on 2D or 3D gadolinium-enhanced images. An abscess will be shown as a pericolonic or perirectal fluid collection with an enhancing abscess wall. Surrounding inflammation will show similar enhancement with intravenous gadolinium.

Ulcerative Colitis

Ulcerative colitis presents on MRI with colonic mural thickening and enhancement.[30] Unlike Crohn's disease, which can be discontinuous with skip areas, ulcerative colitis is a continuous, circumferential, and confluent process that always begins in the distal colon and rectum and progresses proximally. Although the inflammation of ulcerative colitis usually involves only the mucosa and submucosa, on MRI the entire colonic wall is thickened and shows abnormal enhancement. There is the potential that with higher-resolution MRI combined with rapid and earlier dynamic imaging it may be possible to distinguish the superficial inflammatory changes of ulcerative colitis from the transmural inflammation of Crohn's disease. With current techniques, Crohn's disease with pancolitis has a very similar appearance to ulcerative colitis on MRI.

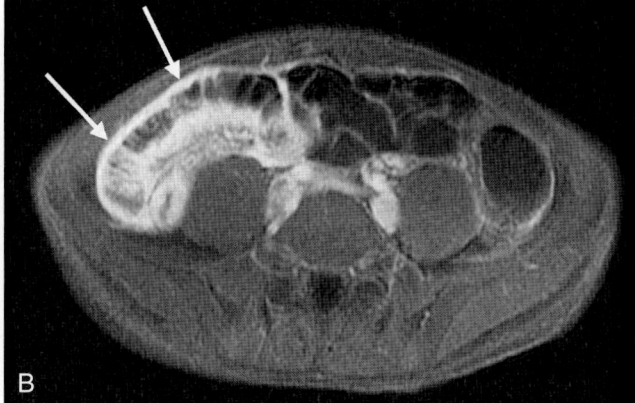

Figure 8-6. Infectious ileitis. Helical CT scan (**A**) through the midabdomen is unremarkable. Gadolinium-enhanced fat-suppressed spoiled gradient-echo MR image (**B**) with oral contrast material shows abnormally thickened and enhancing ileum (*arrows*) in the right side of the abdomen. After the MRI examination the patient was treated for an infectious ileitis and had a good clinical response.

Infectious Bowel Diseases

Bacterial, viral, or parasitic organisms can infect the stomach, small intestine, and colon. Infectious enteritis or colitis will cause mural thickening and enhancement that are indistinguishable from inflammatory bowel disease. The infectious disease may be focal or may involve long segments of the small intestine or colon. Associated infiltration of the peri-intestinal fat is depicted as linear strands extending from the diseased bowel into the adjacent mesenteric fat on single-shot RARE and fat-suppressed gadolinium-enhanced images. In the acute phase there is marked mural enhancement of the diseased small bowel or colon (Fig. 8-6). Complications including peri-intestinal abscess or phlegmon are depicted on MR images as adjacent fluid collections with an enhancing abscess wall or as soft tissue inflammatory masses.

On MRI, pseudomembranous colitis is depicted as marked colonic mural thickening and gadolinium enhancement. The descending and sigmoid colon is typically involved in pseudomembranous colitis. The degree of mural thickening can be quite marked, and the disease typically involves long segments of the colon. The marked mural thickening can help to distinguish pseudomembranous colitis from other forms of infectious colitis.

Ischemic Bowel Disease

Acute or chronic mesenteric ischemia results from insufficient blood supply through the mesenteric circulation to the gut. Chronic mesenteric ischemia develops slowly as a late stage complication of atherosclerotic disease. It causes classic "intestinal angina" with postprandial abdominal discomfort. Acute mesenteric ischemia results from a sudden decrease in mesenteric blood flow and is potentially life-threatening.

Gadolinium-enhanced 3D MR angiography can be combined with anatomic images of the abdomen and pelvis.[31-35] This approach allows direct visualization of the mesenteric arteries and assesses the small bowel and colon for secondary mural changes of mesenteric ischemia. In my experience, it is more common to see the secondary bowel wall changes with mural thickening and altered enhancement. In patients with acute arterial insufficiency, there will be diminished or absent enhancement within the thickened segments of ischemic

bowel (Fig. 8-7). Mural stratification with mucosal and serosal enhancement is identified, but there is decreased enhancement of the intervening submucosa and muscularis layers. In the nonacute setting, the pattern of enhancement is variable, depending on the degree of revascularization, fibrosis, or tissue necrosis. In my experience the findings on MRI can resolve very rapidly after spontaneous revascularization of the ischemic segment of bowel. An assessment of the degree of mural enhancement should be based on the first arterial phase set of images. On delayed images, the diseased bowel wall may enhance due to leaking, damaged capillaries.

The MRI protocol I use for patients with suspected ischemic bowel includes administration of oral and or rectal contrast material before the examination. Axial and coronal single-shot RARE images are performed through the abdomen and pelvis, followed by 3D gadolinium-enhanced MR angiography of the abdominal aorta and mesenteric arteries. Delayed fat-suppressed gadolinium-enhanced images are then obtained in the axial and coronal planes. This comprehensive MRI evaluation can be performed fairly quickly using breath-hold anatomic and MR angiographic techniques.

Gastrointestinal Malignancy

Stomach

Gastric Cancer

Magnetic resonance imaging provides an elegant means of imaging gastric cancer.[36-41] The depth of tumor penetration into the gastric wall can be accurately assessed with high-resolution T2-weighted and gadolinium-enhanced MRI. Maximal distention of the gastric lumen with water-soluble oral contrast is essential to optimize depiction of mural thickening or mass. Negative intraluminal agents on fat-suppressed, gadolinium-enhanced T1-weighted images are desirable, because the dark lumen will help to highlight the adjacent bowel wall and mural tumors. Large volumes of water or other oral agents should be ingested immediately before scanning. Pharmacologic agents can be administered to decrease peristalsis but are not essential.

Thin-section breath-hold T2-weighted single-shot RARE images (SSTSE, SSFSE, HASTE) combined with fat-suppressed

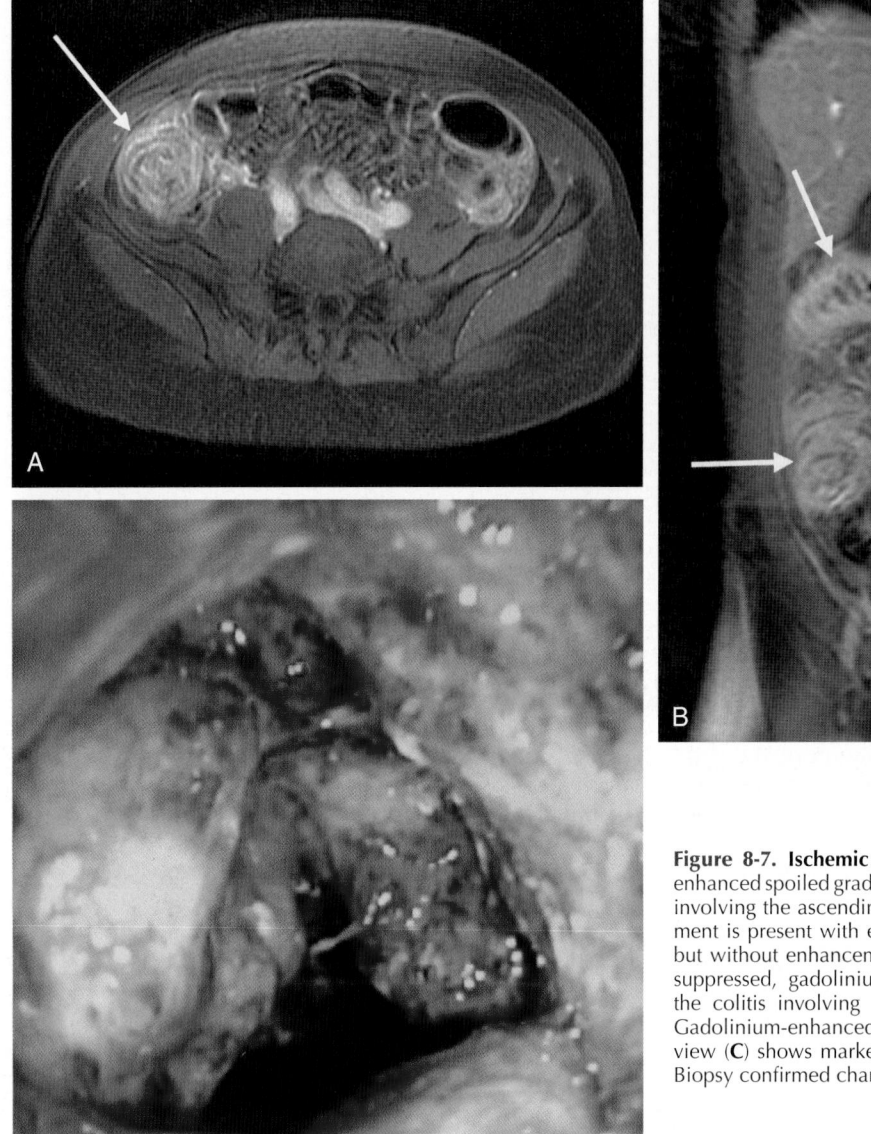

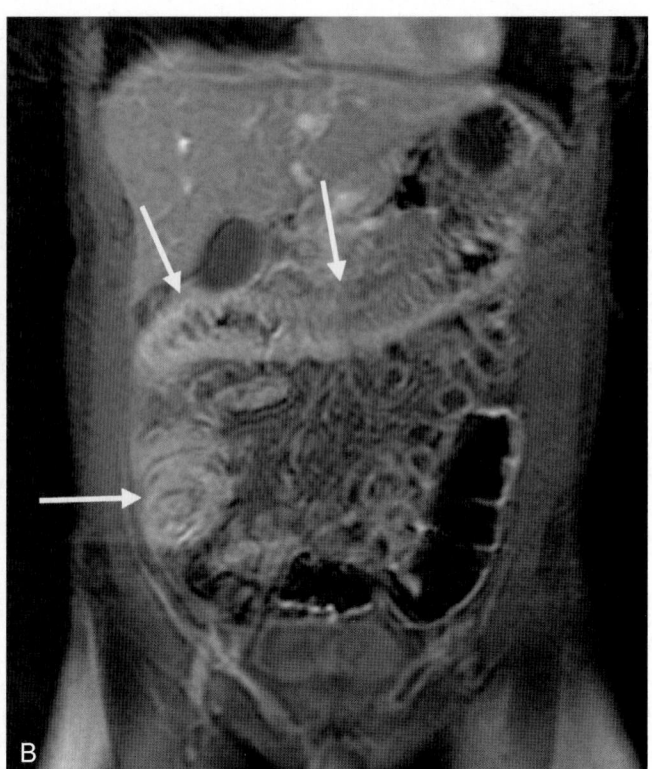

Figure 8-7. Ischemic colitis. Axial (**A**) fat-suppressed, gadolinium-enhanced spoiled gradient-echo image shows colonic mural thickening involving the ascending colon (*arrow*). A layered pattern of enhancement is present with enhancement of the mucosa and bowel serosa, but without enhancement of the muscularis propria. Coronal (**B**) fat-suppressed, gadolinium-enhanced image shows the distribution of the colitis involving the ascending and transverse colon (*arrows*). Gadolinium-enhanced MRA (not shown) was normal. Endoscopic view (**C**) shows markedly abnormal mucosa in the ascending colon. Biopsy confirmed changes of ischemic colitis.

gadolinium-enhanced 3D gradient-echo imaging is most effective for depicting the transmural tumor extension used for tumor staging. The wall of the normal, well-distended stomach is depicted on unenhanced T1, T2, and SSFSE images as a thin, uniform hypointense line typically measuring 2 to 3 mm in thickness. Prominent gastric rugal folds can increase the apparent thickness of the stomach wall. On dynamic gadolinium-enhanced images and delayed equilibrium phase images the stomach wall will show only mild, uniform, and homogeneous enhancement.

Gastric cancers will be depicted on MR images as areas of focal mural thickening (Fig. 8-8) or as mural masses. Superficial gastric cancer may initially not be visible on cross-sectional imaging. As these lesions grow, they manifest as areas of focal mural thickening and eventually as a gastric mass. On dynamic gadolinium-enhanced MRI, gastric cancers show more enhancement than the adjacent normal gastric wall. The presence of focal gastric mural thickening with a

pattern of rapid enhancement is suggestive of gastric cancer. Linitis plastica appears as a nondistensible stomach with a thickened, enhancing wall.

Transmural tumor invasion by a T3 or T4 tumor is indicated by disruption of this low signal intensity band overlying the mural tumor, tumor nodule, or enhancing tumor mass extending from the gastric wall into the surrounding perigastric fat.

Nodal metastases are best shown on fat-suppressed T2-weighted images or diffusion-weighted imaging (DWI) using a B value of 500 s/mm². In our experience, DWI is the most sensitive sequence for depicting lymphadenopathy. Liver metastases are best shown on T1-weighted and T2-weighted imaging and dynamic gadolinium-enhanced imaging. Peritoneal metastases commonly occur with gastrointestinal malignancies and are best visualized on delayed fat-suppressed gadolinium-enhanced images. Osseous metastases can be visualized as high signal intensity lesions on fat-suppressed

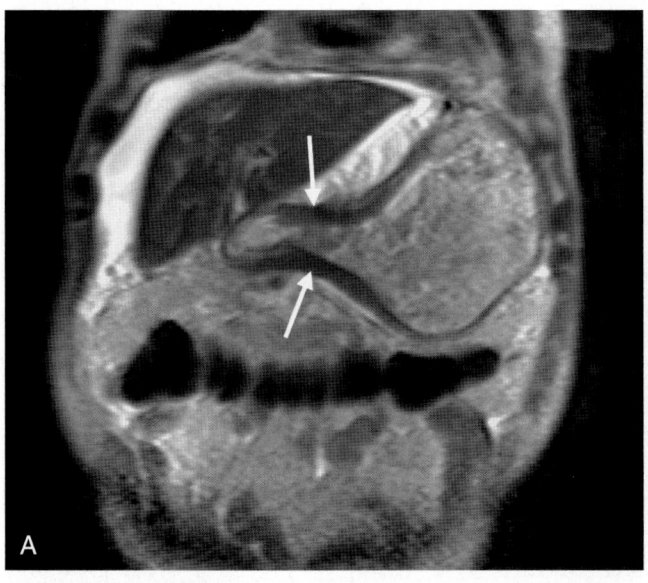
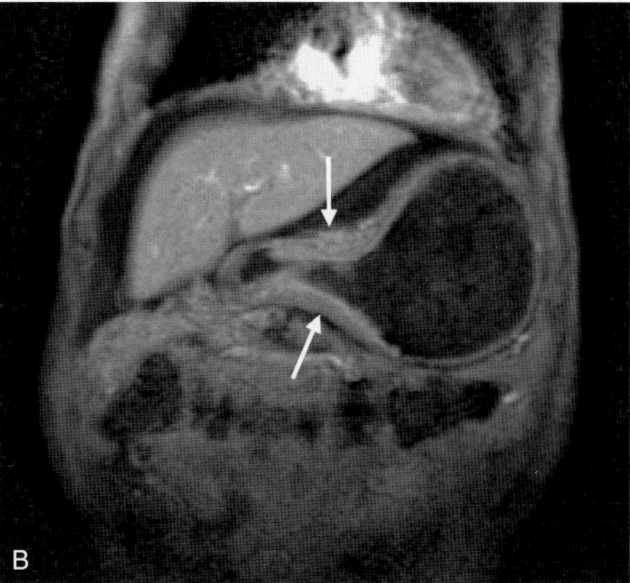

Figure 8-8. Gastric cancer. Coronal single-shot turbo spin-echo image (**A**) and gadolinium-enhanced 3D gradient-echo image (**B**) demonstrate moderate mural thickening of the distal gastric body and antrum (*arrows*). Ascites is also present. Note the distention of the gastric lumen with water facilitating depiction of the mural thickening. Gastric cancer was confirmed at endoscopy and biopsy.

T2-weighted images or as enhancing lesions on fat-suppressed gadolinium-enhanced images.

Small Intestine

Small Intestinal Cancer

Cancer arising in the small intestine is an uncommon malignancy, accounting for 2% of gastrointestinal cancers.[42-44] Bowel distention is essential for MRI of small intestinal cancer. Intraluminal contrast can be administered orally with any of the oral contrast agents described earlier. Alternatively, small bowel enteroclysis may be performed with intraluminal contrast material infused through a nasojejunal tube providing maximal small bowel distention. On breath-hold single-shot RARE and fat-suppressed gadolinium-enhanced imaging small bowel cancers will be depicted as areas of small intestinal mural thickening and masses. Because of their late clinical presentation, small bowel tumors are typically large tumor masses. Associated small bowel obstruction is indicated by distended loops of fluid-filled small bowel proximal to the obstructing mass.

Semelka and colleagues described the appearance of small bowel tumors on MRI,[43] noting that small bowel tumors are isointense to small bowel on T1-weighted images. Malignant tumors showed moderate heterogeneous enhancement greater than adjacent normal bowel on gadolinium-enhanced spoiled gradient-echo imaging. Unenhanced T1-weighted and fat-suppressed, gadolinium-enhanced imaging are best for depicting tumor extent.

Colon and Rectum

Techniques for Magnetic Resonance Imaging of Colorectal Cancer

The role of MRI for preoperative staging of colorectal cancer is well established and has been described in multiple studies.[45-61]

Different techniques have been proposed for MRI of colorectal cancer.[46-54] Endorectal coil or phased-array surface coils have been employed to increase spatial resolution while maintaining adequate signal-to-noise ratio.[54-56] Some authors have advocated using positive or negative intraluminal contrast agents administered rectally to distend the rectosigmoid colon.[58-60]

In addition to the routine MRI examination of the abdomen and pelvis described earlier, specific imaging sequences are used in the patient with colorectal cancer to assess local tumor extent and regional or distant metastases.

THIN-SECTION, HIGH-RESOLUTION ANGLED T2-WEIGHTED TURBO SPIN-ECHO MAGNETIC RESONANCE IMAGING

High-resolution phased-array surface coil images of the rectal or colon cancer are performed using thin-section T2-weighted turbo spin-echo images oriented perpendicular and parallel to the cancer (Fig. 8-9).[46-48] These angled T2-weighted images are generally prescribed from the sagittal T2-weighted images of the pelvis. Specific parameters for my rectal cancer MR protocol are shown in Table 8-2. These angled T2-weighted

Table 8-2
Angled T2-Weighted Imaging of Rectal Cancer

Sequence: 2D turbo spin-echo
Plane: oblique (angled perpendicular and parallel to tumor)
Repetition time (TR): 3263 (shortest)
Echo time (TE): 85
NSA: 6
Field of view: 20 to 22 cm
Matrix: 512 × 256
Echo train length: 28
Slice thickness: 4 mm with 0.5-mm gap
No. of slices: 24
90% Receiver field of view
Sense: 2
Time: 2:56
Coil: phased-array surface coil

NSA, number of signal averages; sense, sensitivity encoding.

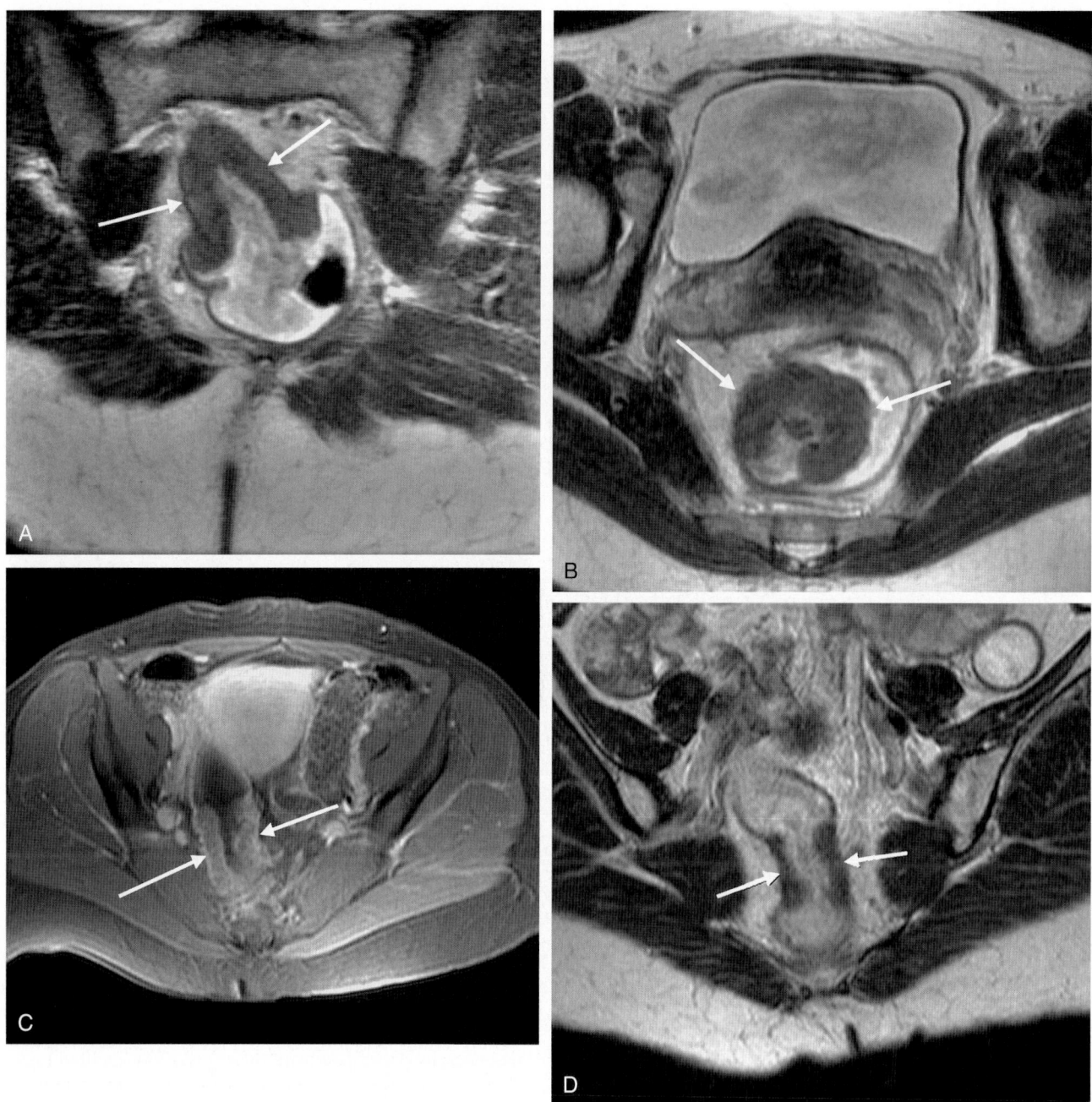

Figure 8-9. Rectal cancer. Coronal (**A**) and axial (**B**) surface coil T2-weighted MR images angled parallel and perpendicular to rectal cancer depict a T3 rectal cancer (*arrows*) with extramural tumor extension. Axial gadolinium-enhanced spoiled gradient-echo image (**C**) shows the irregular rectal mass (*arrows*). Follow-up MR image (**D**) obtained after chemotherapy shows response to treatment with marked decrease in the rectal cancer (*arrows*).

images use a smaller field of view (FOV) and 3- to 4-mm slice thickness for detailed high-resolution imaging of the rectal cancer. Higher signal averages combined with the phased-array surface coils are utilized to maintain image signal-to-noise-ratio. The thin-section images are most useful for tumor staging, determining the depth of tumor penetration into the wall of the rectum or colon. The muscularis propria is easily depicted as a thin, low signal intensity linear structure. Disruption of the muscularis propria by tumor is evidence of stage T3 cancer with transmural tumor extension.

DIFFUSION-WEIGHTED MAGNETIC RESONANCE IMAGING

Diffusion-weighted MRI can also be used to evaluate colorectal cancers. Gastrointestinal tract cancers show marked hyperintensity on diffusion-weighted images, improving their conspicuity (see Fig. 8-9).[62] Diffusion-weighted images are also very useful for nodal staging of colon and rectal cancer.[63] Small perirectal and pericolonic nodal metastases are markedly hyperintense on diffusion-weighted images, facilitating their detection (Fig. 8-10). I typically use a B value of 500 for extrahepatic DWI. With a B value of 500, anatomic landmarks

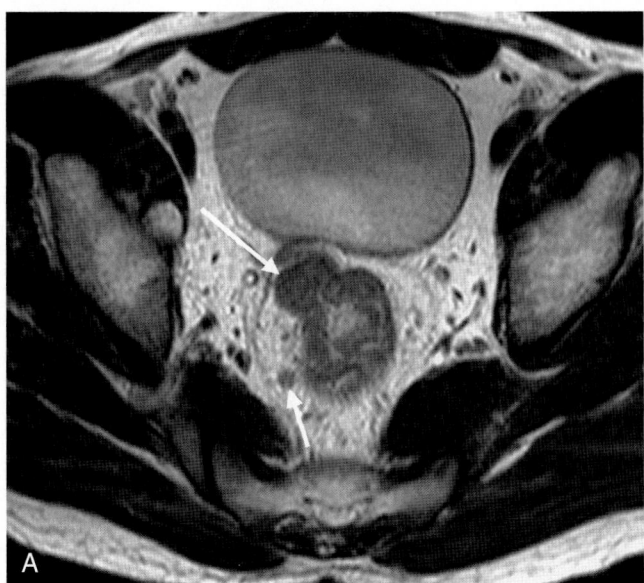

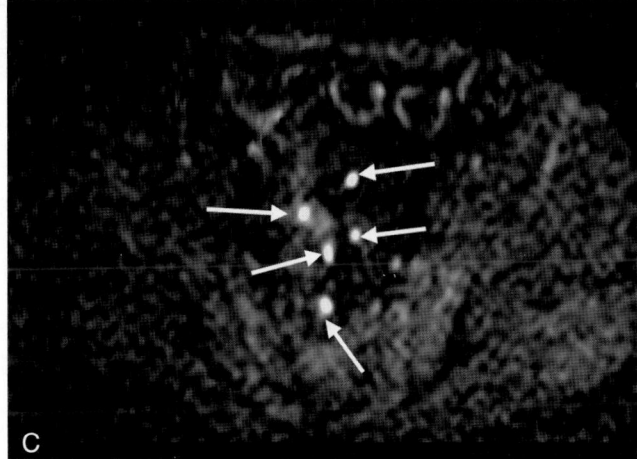

Figure 8-10. Rectal cancer. Angled T2-weighted image (**A**) depicts a T3 rectal cancer (*arrow*). Diffusion-weighted B500 image (**B**) shows marked hyperintensity of the rectal cancer (*long arrow*) and perirectal lymph node (*short arrow*). Diffusion-weighted B500 image at an adjacent level (**C**) shows multiple markedly hyperintense nodal metastases (*arrows*). Findings indicated a stage III T3N1M0 rectal cancer.

are still visible whereas most intestinal fluid and ascites is suppressed. Specific MRI parameters for DWI are shown in Table 8-3.

Magnetic Resonance Staging of Colorectal Cancer

Preoperative MRI of colon and rectal cancer effectively determines local tumor extension, nodal metastases, and distant abdominal metastases.[46-54] These three features form the basis of TNM staging. The overall MR staging accuracy for rectal cancer has ranged from 67% to 100%.[45]

Table 8-3
Diffusion-Weighted Imaging of Colorectal Cancer

Sequence: single-shot spin-echo EPI
Plane: axial
Repetition time (TR): 2700
Echo time (TE): 58
NSA: 2
Matrix: 256 × 128
B value: 500
7 mm, skip 1 mm
No. of slices: 24
Sense: 2
Time: 20 s
Coil: phased-array surface coil

EPI, echo planar imaging; NSA, number of signal averages; sense, sensitivity encoding.

The information from preoperative MRI is used to direct patient management. Rectal cancers in which MRI reveals stage III cancers with transmural tumor extension (T3 or T4) or stage IV cancers with nodal metastases undergo preoperative radiation therapy. After radiation therapy, follow-up MRI documents a reduction in tumor volume, resulting in improved chance for successful surgical resection (see Fig. 8-9). In this scenario the information from preoperative MRI is critical in directing management decisions in the patient with colorectal cancer.

LOCAL TUMOR EXTENSION

Tumor staging determines the depth of mural penetration by the colon or rectal cancer. Tis indicates carcinoma in situ, T1 tumors invade the submucosa, T2 tumors invade the muscularis propria, T3 tumors extend through the muscularis propria onto the subserosa or nonperitonealized pericolic or perirectal tissues, and T4 tumors directly invade adjacent organs or structures.

The most challenging assessment is to distinguish T2 from borderline T3 cancers. Peritumoral fibrosis extending into the perirectal fat in a T2 tumor can be difficult to distinguish from early transmural extension from a T3 tumor. On the other hand, nodular soft tissue extending through the disrupted rectal wall into the surrounding tissues confidently predicts a T3 or T4 cancer.

NODAL METASTASES

Node staging is based on the presence or absence of local or regional nodal metastases. Although MRI can depict lymph nodes 2 to 3 mm in diameter (see Fig. 8-10), the MR assessment of nodal metastases remains limited to an evaluation of the size and number of lymph nodes. Morphologic criteria for evaluating of lymph nodes pose obvious limitations. Microscopic metastases in normal-sized lymph nodes cannot be detected, and enlarged inflammatory lymph nodes cannot be distinguished from nodal metastases. Accuracy rates for detection of nodal metastases vary between 39% and 95%.[45] The use of ultrasmall superparamagnetic iron oxide (USPIO) contrast agents for depicting lymph node metastases has shown promise in early reports. The iron particles are phagocytosed by macrophages and taken up by the reticuloendothelial system. Normal lymph nodes will contain macrophages with iron particles and will show loss of signal on gradient-echo MR images due to susceptibility effect. Tumor deposits within lymph nodes will displace the reticuloendothelial system and will show areas of increased signal due to less uptake of the USPIO.

DISTANT METASTASES

Metastasis staging is based on the presence or absence of distant metastases to the liver, the peritoneum (Fig. 8-11),

mesentery, omentum, bowel serosa, lymph nodes, osseous structures, and lungs.

Circumferential Resection Margin and the Mesorectal Fascia

Whereas TNM staging provides important information, it is actually more important to determine the circumferential tumor-free resection margin, which is the distance between the rectal tumor and the surrounding mesorectal fascia.[60,61] This tumor-free resection margin can be accurately and consistently predicted on high-resolution phased-array surface coil MR images.

The mesorectal fascia encloses the mesorectum, an anatomic unit that is composed of the rectum, perirectal fat, superior hemorrhoidal vessels, nerves, and lymphatics. At surgery, patients undergo total mesorectal excision with en bloc resection of the rectal cancer and surrounding tissues enclosed within the mesorectal fascia. This technique has resulted in a decrease in local tumor recurrence. With mesorectal excision, surgical failure resulting in local tumor recurrence is most often due to incomplete removal of the lateral spread of tumor with microscopically positive resection margins.

Based on the MR assessment of the circumferential resection margin, patients can be categorized and treated according to their risk of local recurrence. Superficial tumors may

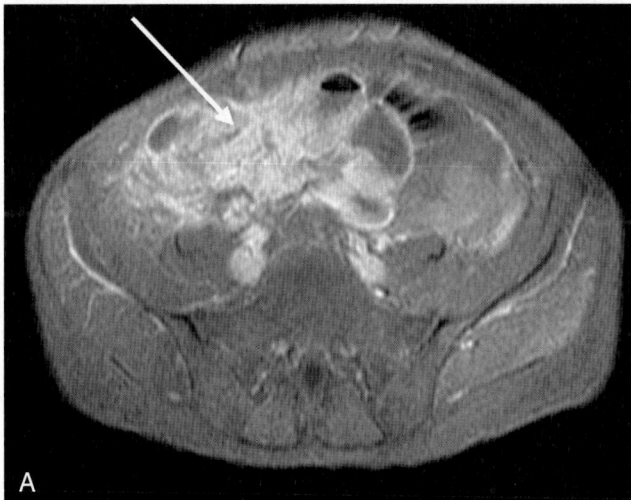

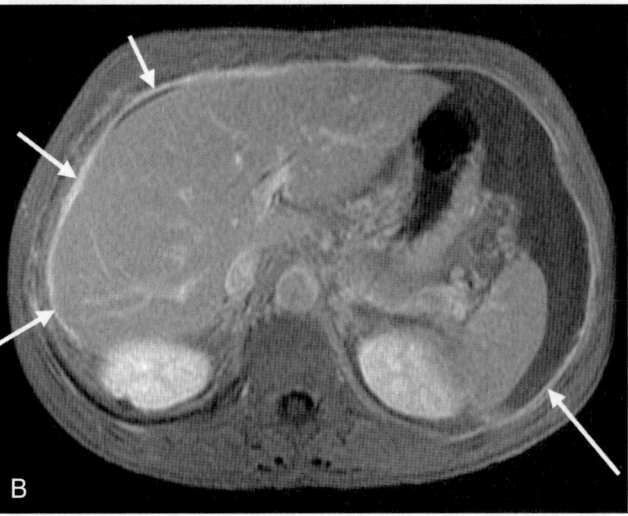

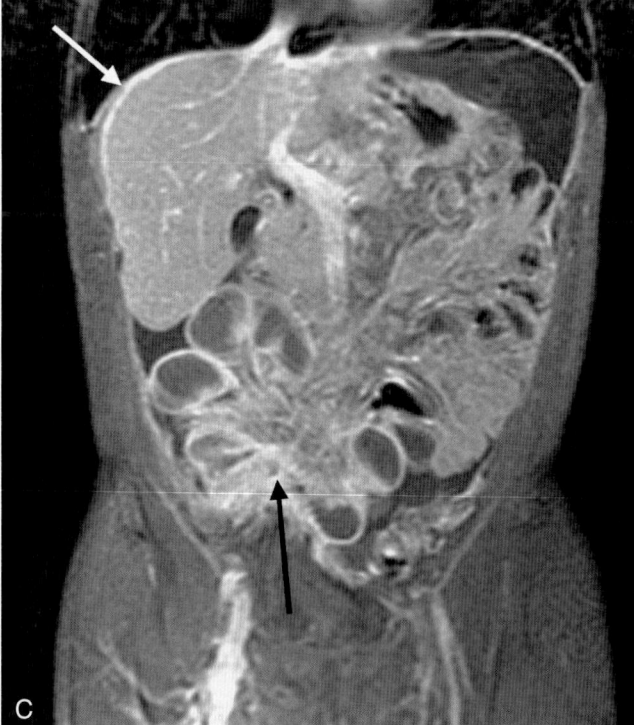

Figure 8-11. Metastatic colon cancer. Axial gadolinium-enhanced spoiled gradient-echo image (**A**) shows a heterogeneous enhancing mass (*arrow*) in the right lower quadrant. Axial gadolinium-enhanced image (**B**) through the upper abdomen depicts enhancing right subphrenic peritoneal metastases (*short arrows*) and left subphrenic peritoneal metastases (*long arrow*). Coronal gadolinium-enhanced spoiled gradient-echo image (**C**) shows the mass in the right lower quadrant (*black arrow*) with associated bowel obstruction. Right subphrenic peritoneal metastases (*white arrow*) are confirmed. MR findings indicated a stage IV colon cancer with bowel obstruction and peritoneal metastases.

be treated with surgery alone. Operable T3 cancers with a wide circumferential resection margin are treated with a short course of radiation therapy followed by mesorectal excision. Patients with locally advanced cancer in whom the tumor approaches or involves the resection margin are at greater risk for recurrence and will benefit from a more extended course of radiation therapy and chemotherapy, followed by surgical resection.

In a study of 76 patients with rectal cancer, Beets-Tan and associates evaluated the MR assessment of the circumferential resection margin compared with histopathology.[60] They noted that two observers correctly predicted a 0-mm resection margin in 12 of 12 patients with T4 cancers. In 29 patients with histologic resection margins of 10 mm or less, the two MR observers correctly predicted a 10-mm resection margin in 27 and 28 patients. In a study of 98 patients with rectal cancer, Brown and coworkers reported a 92% agreement between MRI and histologic findings for predicting the circumferential resection margin.[47]

Locally advanced rectal cancers extend beyond the mesorectal fascia to invade surrounding structures and organs. High-resolution surface coil MRI is more accurate than helical CT for depicting invasion of adjacent structures by advanced rectal cancers. In one study of 26 patients, MRI had a 97% sensitivity and 98% specificity for local invasion compared with 70% and 85% for helical CT.[61]

SUMMARY

Magnetic resonance imaging offers unique advantages for evaluating inflammatory, infectious, ischemic, and malignant diseases of the gastrointestinal tract. By combining readily available intraluminal and intravenous contrast agents with fast MR techniques, the wall of the stomach, small intestine, colon, and rectum can be reliably imaged. The inherent high contrast resolution of MRI allows confident depiction of mural disease as areas of wall thickening and abnormal enhancement. MRI of the gastrointestinal tract is a robust and versatile technique that can be applied to a wide variety of benign and malignant gastrointestinal diseases.

References

1. Regan F, Beall DP, Bohlman ME, et al: Fast MR imaging and the detection of small-bowel obstruction. AJR 170:1465-1469, 1988.
2. Lee JKT, Marcos HB, Semelka RC: MR Imaging of the small bowel using the HASTE sequence. AJR 170:1457-1463, 1998.
3. Marcos HB, Semelka RC, Noone TC, et al: MRI of normal and abnormal duodenum using Half-Fourier Single-Shot RARE and gadolinium-enhanced spoiled gradient echo sequences. Magn Reson Imaging 17:869-880, 1999.
4. Low RN, Francis IR: MR imaging of the gastrointestinal tract with IV gadolinium and diluted barium oral contrast media compared with unenhanced MR imaging and CT. AJR 169:1051-1059, 1997.
5. Low RN, Semelka RC, Worawattanakul S, et al: Extrahepatic abdominal imaging in patients with malignancy: Comparison of MR imaging and helical CT, with subsequent surgical correlation. Radiology 210:625-632, 1999.
6. Gourtsoyiannis N, Papanikolaou N, Grammatikakis J, et al: MR imaging of the small bowel with a true-FISP sequence after enteroclysis with water solution. Invest Radiol 35:707-711, 2000.
7. Low RN, Sebrechts CP, Politoske DA, et al: Crohn disease with endoscopic correlation: Single-shot fast spin-echo and gadolinium-enhanced fat-suppressed spoiled gradient-echo MR imaging. Radiology 222:652-660, 2002.
8. Patak MA, Froehlich JM, von Weymarn C, et al: Cook Book for MR-Small Bowel Imaging. 2004. Available at http://www.ksw.ch/kliniken/downloads/magnetres_cookbook.pdf.
9. Froehlich JM, Patak MA, von Weymarn C, et al: Small bowel motility assessment with magnetic resonance imaging. J Magn Reson Imaging 21:370-375, 2005.
10. Ajaj W, Goehd SC, Schneemann H, et al: Oral contrast agents for small bowel MRI: Comparison of different additives to optimize bowel distension. Eur Radiol 14:458-464, 2004.
11. Ajaj W, Goehde SC, Schneemann H, et al: Dose optimization of mannitol solution for small bowel distension in MRI. J Magn Reson Imaging 20:648-653, 2004.
12. Sood RS, Joubert I, Franklin H, et al: Small bowel MRI: Comparison of a polyethylene glycol preparation and water as oral contrast media. J Magn Reson Imaging 15:401-408, 2002.
13. Laghi A, Carbone L, Catalano C, et al: Polyethylene glycol solution as an oral contrast agent for MR imaging of the small bowel. AJR 177:1333-1334, 2001.
14. Johnson WK, Stoupis C, Torres GM, et al: Superparamagnetic iron oxide (SPIO) as an oral contrast agent in gastrointestinal (GI) magnetic resonance imaging (MRI): Comparison with state-of-the-art computed tomography (CT). Magn Reson Imaging 14:43-49, 2001.
15. Wiarda BM, Kuipers EJ, Heitbrink MA, et al: MR enteroclysis of inflammatory small-bowel diseases. AJR Am J Roentgenol 187:522-531, 2006.
16. Maccioni F, Viscido A, Marini M, Caprilli R: MRI evaluation of Crohn's disease of the small and large bowel with the use of negative superparamagnetic oral contrast agents. Abdom Imaging 27:384-393, 2002.
17. Gourtsoyiannis NC, Grammatikakis J, Papamastorakis G, et al: Imaging of small intestinal Crohn's disease: Comparison between MR enteroclysis and conventional enteroclysis. Eur Radiol 16:1915-1925, 2006.
18. Gourtsoyiannis N, Papanikolaou N, Grammatikakis J, et al: MR enteroclysis protocol optimization: Comparison between 3D FLASH with fat saturation after intravenous gadolinium injection and true FISP sequences. Eur Radiol 11:908-913, 2001.
19. Masselli G, Casciani E, Polettini E, et al: Assessment of Crohn's disease in the small bowel: Prospective comparison of magnetic resonance enteroclysis with conventional enteroclysis. Eur Radiol 16:2817-2827, 2006.
20. Prassopoulos P, Papanikolaou N, Grammatikakis J, et al: MR enteroclysis imaging of Crohn disease. RadioGraphics 21(Spec No):S161-S172, 2001.
21. Gourtsoyiannis N, Papanikolaou N, Grammatikakis J, et al: Assessment of Crohn's disease activity in the small bowel with MR and conventional enteroclysis: Preliminary results. Eur Radiol 14:1017-1024, 2004.
22. Rottgen R, Herzog H, Lopez-Haninnen E, et al: Bowel wall enhancement in magnetic resonance colonography for assessing activity in Crohn's disease. Clin Imaging 30:27-31, 2006.
23. Low RN, Francis IR, Politoske D, Bennett M: Crohn's disease evaluation: Comparison of contrast-enhanced MR imaging and single phase helical CT scanning. J Magn Reson Imaging 11:127-135, 1999.
24. Kettritz U, Isaacs K, Warshauer DM, Semelka RC: Crohn's disease: Pilot study comparing MRI of the abdomen with clinical evaluation. J Clin Gastroenterol 21:249-253, 1995.
25. Maccioni F, Bruni A, Viscido A, et al: MR imaging in patients with Crohn's disease: Value of T2- versus T1-weighted gadolinium-enhanced MR sequences with use of an oral superparamagnetic contrast agent. Radiology 238:517-530, 2006.
26. Laghi A, Borrelli O, Paolantonio P, et al: Contrast enhanced magnetic resonance imaging of the terminal ileum in children with Crohn's disease. Gut 52:393-397, 2003.
27. Maccioni F, Colaiacomo MC, Stasolla A, et al: Value of MRI performed with phased-array coil in the diagnosis and pre-operative classification of perianal and anal fistulas. Radiol Med (Torino) 104:58-67, 2002.
28. Maccioni F, Viscido A, Broglia L, et al: Evaluation of Crohn disease activity with magnetic resonance imaging. Abdom Imaging 25:219-228, 2000.
29. Horsthuis K, Lavini C, Stoker J: MRI in Crohn's disease. J Magn Reson Imaging 22:1-12, 2005.
30. Nozue T, Kobayashi A, Takagi Y, et al: Assessment of disease activity and extent by magnetic resonance imaging in ulcerative colitis. Pediatr Int 42:285-288, 2000.
31. Chow LC, Chan FP, Li KP: A comprehensive approach to MR imaging of mesenteric ischemia. Abdom Imaging 27:507-516, 2002.
32. Rha SE, Ha HK, Lee SH, et al: CT and MR imaging findings of bowel ischemia from various primary causes. Radiographics 20:29-42, 2000.
33. Baden JG, Racy DJ, Grist TM: Contrast-enhanced three-dimensional magnetic resonance angiography of the mesenteric vasculature. J Magn Reson Imaging 10:369-375, 1999.

34. Debatin JF: MR quantification of flow in abdominal vessels. Abdom Imaging 23:485-495, 1998.

35. Lauenstein TC, Ajaj W, Narin B, et al: MR Imaging of apparent small-bowel perfusion for diagnosing mesenteric ischemia: Feasibility study. Radiology 234:569-575, 2005.

36. American Cancer Society: What are the key statistics about stomach cancer. Available at 2005.http://www.cancer.org/docroot/CRI/content/CRI_2_4_1X_What_are_the_key_statistics_for_stomach_cancer_4.

37. Yamada I, Saito N, Takeshita K, et al: Early gastric carcinoma: Evaluation with high-spatial-resolution MR imaging in vitro. Radiology 220:115-121, 2001.

38. Kim AY, Han JK, Seong CK, et al: MRI in staging advanced gastric cancer: Is it useful compared with spiral CT? J Comput Assist Tomogr 24:389-394, 2000.

39. Sohn KM, Lee JM, Lee SY, et al: Comparing MR imaging and CT in the staging of gastric carcinoma. AJR 174:1551-1557, 2000.

40. Oi H, Matsushita M, Murakami T, Nakamura H: Dynamic MR imaging for extraserosal invasion of advanced gastric cancer. Abdom Imaging 22:35-40, 1997.

41. Motohara T, Semelka RC: MRI in staging of gastric cancer. Abdom Imaging 27:376-383, 2002.

42. American Cancer Society: Cancer Facts and Figures 2007. Atlanta, American Cancer Society, 2007. Available online at cancer.org.

43. De Franco A, Celi G, Restaino G, et al: Imaging of small bowel tumors. Rays 27:35-50, 2002.

44. Semelka RC, John G, Kelekis NL, et al: Small bowel neoplastic disease: Demonstration by MRI. J Magn Reson Imaging 6:855-860, 1996.

45. Levine MS, Rubesin SE, Pantongrag-Brown L, et al: Non-Hodgkin's lymphoma of the gastrointestinal tract: Radiographic findings. AJR 168:165-172, 1997.

46. Beets-Tan RGH, Beets GL: Rectal cancer: Review with emphasis on MR Imaging. Radiology 232:335-346, 2004.

47. Brown G, Richards CJ, Bourne MW, et al: Morphologic predictors of lymph node status in rectal cancer with use of high-spatial-resolution MR imaging with histopathologic comparison. Radiology 227:371-377, 2003.

48. Brown G, Richards CJ, Newcombe RG, et al: Rectal carcinoma: Thin-section MR imaging for staging in 28 patients. Radiology 211:215-222, 1999.

49. Kim NK, Kim MJ, Yun SH, et al: Comparative study of transrectal ultra-sonography, pelvic computerized tomography, and magnetic resonance imaging in preoperative staging of rectal cancer. Dis Colon Rectum 42:770-775, 1999.

50. Wallengren NO, Holtas S, Andren-Sandberg A, et al: Rectal carcinoma: Double-contrast MR imaging for preoperative staging. Radiology 215:108-114, 2000.

51. Brown G, Radcliffe AG, Newcombe RG, et al: Preoperative assessment of prognostic factors in rectal cancer using high-resolution magnetic resonance imaging. Br J Surg 90:355-364, 2003.

52. Matsuoka H, Nakamura A, Masaki T, et al: A prospective comparison between multidetector-row computed tomography and magnetic resonance imaging in the preoperative evaluation of rectal carcinoma. Am J Surg 185:556-559, 2003.

53. Gagliardi G, Bayar S, Smith R, Salem RR: Preoperative staging of rectal cancer using magnetic resonance imaging with external phase-arrayed coils. Arch Surg 137:447-451, 2002.

54. Chun HK, Choi D, Kim MJ, et al: Preoperative staging of rectal cancer: Comparison of 3-T high-field MRI and endorectal sonography. AJR Am J Roentgenol 187:1557-1562, 2006.

55. Hunerbein M, Pegios W, Rau B, et al: Prospective comparison of endorectal ultrasound, three-dimensional endorectal ultrasound, and endorectal MRI in the preoperative evaluation of rectal tumors: Preliminary results. Surg Endosc 14:1005-1009, 2000.

56. Matsuoka H, Nakamura A, Masaki T, et al: Comparison between endorectal coil and pelvic phased-array coil magnetic resonance imaging in patients with anorectal tumor. Am J Surg 185:328-332, 2003.

57. Maldjian C, Smith R, Kilger A, et al: Endorectal surface coil MR imaging as a staging technique for rectal carcinoma: A comparison study to rectal endosonography. Abdom Imaging 25:75-80, 2000.

58. Maier AG, Kersting-Sommerhoff B, Reeders JW, et al: Staging of rectal cancer by double-contrast MR imaging using the rectally administered superparamagnetic iron oxide contrast agent ferristene and IV gadodiamide injection: Results of a multicenter phase II trial. J Magn Reson Imaging 12:651-660, 2000.

59. Low RN, McCue M, Barone R, et al: MR staging of primary colorectal carcinoma: Comparison to surgical and histopathologic findings. Abdom Imaging 28:784-793, 2003.

60. Low RN: MRI of colorectal cancer. Abdom Imaging 27:418-424, 2002.

61. Beets-Tan RGH, Beets GL, Vliegen RFA, et al: Accuracy of magnetic resonance imaging in prediction of tumor free resection margin in rectal cancer surgery. Lancet 357:497-504, 2001.

62. Allen SD, Padhani AR, Dzik-Jurasz AS, et al: Rectal carcinoma: MRI with histologic correlation before and after chemoradiation therapy. AJR Am J Roentgenol 188:442-451, 2007.

63. Engelen SM, Beets GL, Beets-Tan RG: Role of preoperative local and distant staging in rectal cancer. Onkologie 30(3):141-145, 2007.

Positron Emission Tomography/Computed Tomography of the Hollow Viscera

Karen A. Mourtzikos, MD

Positron emission tomography (PET) is a scintigraphic imaging modality that utilizes annihilation photons from positron-emitting radionuclides injected into patients to visualize and characterize metabolic processes in vivo. PET yields physiologic information based on altered tissue metabolism, and semiquantitative analysis may be used to reflect the actual amounts of tracer in regions of interest. The advent of PET/CT allows for the fusion of this metabolic information with anatomic images to improve localization and increase accuracy.[1] The modality has numerous indications, including cardiac and brain imaging, but it is applied predominantly in oncology. PET provides multiple advantages in cancer patient management, including (1) diagnosing disease before structural changes become detectable with anatomic imaging techniques, potentially improving prognosis; (2) identifying distant, occult metastases that may affect the course of treatment; and (3) monitoring response to a given regimen and providing early feedback on its efficacy.

IMAGING CONSIDERATIONS

Although many physiologic processes in the body depend on glucose, tumors demonstrate accelerated glucose metabolism.[2] The primary radionuclide administered in current clinical practice is 2-(fluorine-18) fluoro-2-deoxy-D-glucose (FDG), which acts as a glucose analog and mimics the natural substrate. FDG is structurally similar to glucose and gains entry into the cell via Glut-1 transporters, which are often overexpressed in cancer cells,[3] and is subsequently recognized and phosphorylated by hexokinase. However, FDG-6-phosphate is not analogous to glucose-6-phosphate and cannot be further utilized by the cell. Therefore, the radionuclide effectively becomes trapped and emits photons that are imaged by the PET camera. In this manner, a metabolic map is created demonstrating a relative range of activity with more intense uptake in tissue with increased glucose demands and thus greater accumulation of FDG, such as in malignancy. A neoplasm is not the only biologic process that may require an increased glucose supply. Inflammation and infection may also show higher accumulation of FDG, although these are considered relatively benign processes.

Imaging is predicated on the production of positrons in the nucleus, which occurs when a proton in the nucleus is transformed into a neutron and a positron. The positron has the same mass as the electron but has a positive charge of exactly the same magnitude as the negative charge of the electron. Positron emission occurs when a positron reaches thermal energy and combines with an electron.

Their mass converts into energy in the form of γ-rays, and two γ-rays with 511 keV of energy emitted 180 degrees to each other must be produced to conserve both momentum and energy.

Detection of these paired 511 keV γ-rays forms the basis for imaging with PET.

PATIENT PREPARATION AND SCANNING

FDG PET/CT is based on glucose metabolism and accumulation of the radiopharmaceutical. Accordingly, the patient must be in a metabolic state that will maximize the target-to-background ratio as well as limit competitors for FDG uptake. Before scanning, patients must fast for at least 4 hours, and only water is permissible during this period. Any additional glucose in the bloodstream will far exceed the amount of glucose administered in the form of FDG, which will not only alter the distribution of uptake but also trigger an insulin response and drive the FDG into skeletal muscle.

Diabetic patients must be screened before the day of the study to ensure appropriate glucose management and that any insulin administered by the patient to control blood sugar is done so that its peak occurs before FDG injection. Blood glucose levels must be below 150 to 200 mg/dL at the time of radiopharmaceutical administration in all patients.

The usual calculated dose of FDG is 0.22 mCi/kg for whole-body studies in adults and is given as an intravenous bolus with a normal saline flush. The patient then rests quietly for 45 minutes before imaging. During this uptake phase, talking and movement should be kept to a minimum to limit FDG accumulation in muscle. Oral contrast, if used, should be glucose-free, low-density barium (1.3%)[4] and should be given in two divided doses, one before injection and the second after the uptake phase is completed, again to minimize muscular concentration of FDG.

The CT portion of the study is performed first using a protocol that adjusts the mA based on information regarding the area of the body currently being scanned. Whole-body images are acquired from the base of the skull to the mid femurs to fuse with the whole-body PET scan. The intravenous use of a contrast agent is not currently universal because imaging artifacts in the PET may result from the application of the attenuation correction algorithm, which is derived from the CT data. High-density objects, including intravenous or oral contrast, may degrade the quality of the PET by creating

foci of increased activity after processing.[5] Recall that the PET images are created by photons escaping the body and hitting the detectors. Understandably, more photons from the periphery of the body will be able to do so in comparison with those emitted in the center of the body.

The CT scan is employed as an applied attenuation correction algorithm to increase counts centrally and to correct for disproportionally high counts from the periphery or from less dense organs such as the lungs. Therefore, objects identified as high density on CT, that is, those that may cause increased attenuation, are essentially overcorrected. A delay between intravenous contrast agent administration and CT may decrease such artifacts because the contrast agent will have dispersed.[6] Most of these artifacts have limited negative impact on examination quality because the fusion images assist in anatomic localization of the source of increased uptake. Ultimately, because the contrast bolus/timing is not optimized for any one region of the body, intravenous contrast in PET/CT is used to enhance anatomic landmarks and increase accuracy of lesion location.

Semiquantitative analysis of FDG uptake may be performed using the standardized uptake value (SUV)[7] or SUV formula, which is defined as:

$$SUV = (mCi/mL \text{ [decay corrected] in tissue})/(mCi \text{ of tracer injected in the patient/body weight in grams})$$

PET/CT software performs this calculation, which is corrected for body weight and height, and displays the SUV for a designated region of interest. Ongoing research strives to establish SUV guidelines for detection of malignancy, as a pretreatment prognostic indicator, and especially as a measure of response to therapy.

ARTIFACTS

Artifacts in the PET scan are primarily created by differences in patient positioning between CT acquisition and PET acquisition. Although the images are fused, the CT and the PET are not acquired concomitantly. As mentioned previously, the CT is obtained first and differences in breathing patterns between the two studies can cause misregistration and mislocalization. In regard to the abdomen, these factors are primarily limited to the borders of the abdominal organs with the lungs. For example, a lesion in the dome of the liver may appear to localize in the lung owing to deep respiration during the PET acquisition. Using the nonattenuation correction images may be useful in clarifying the location of misregistered and mislocalized lesions.

ESOPHAGUS

Physiologic distribution of FDG in the esophagus is minimal and usually less than the level of activity in the mediastinum or liver and without significant focal areas of uptake. Variants are primarily related to esophageal resection and subsequent altered motility and musculature. PET/CT is useful in the evaluation of esophageal malignancy and has applications in TNM classification staging.

Imaging Characteristics

Focally increased FDG activity in the esophagus, which is greater than the level of uptake in the liver and fuses to an

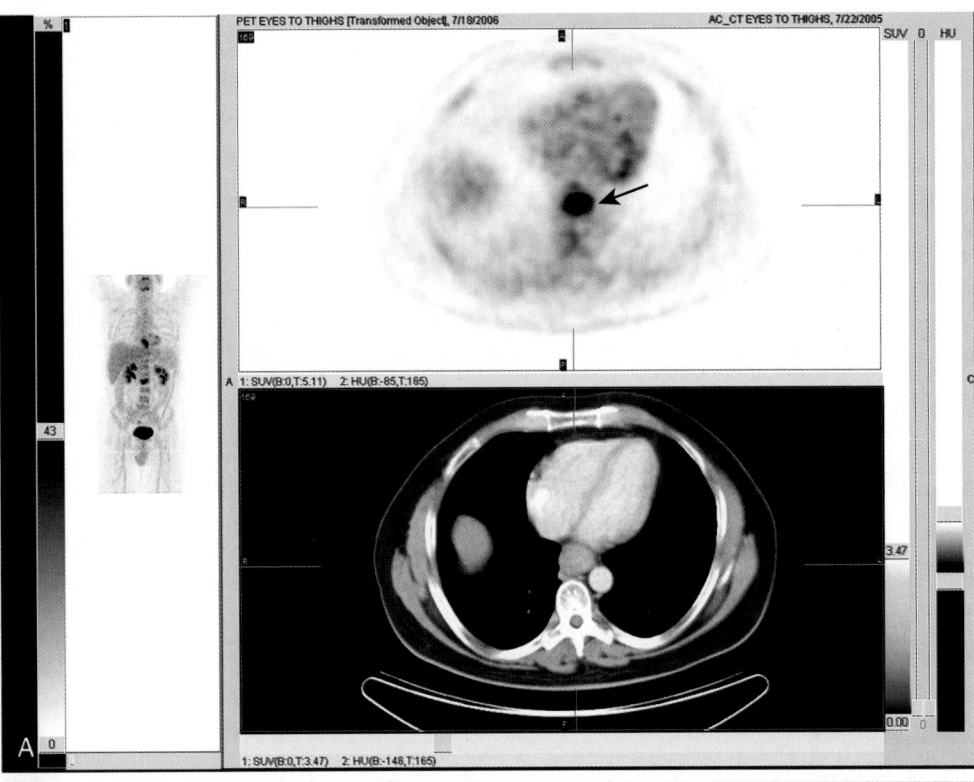

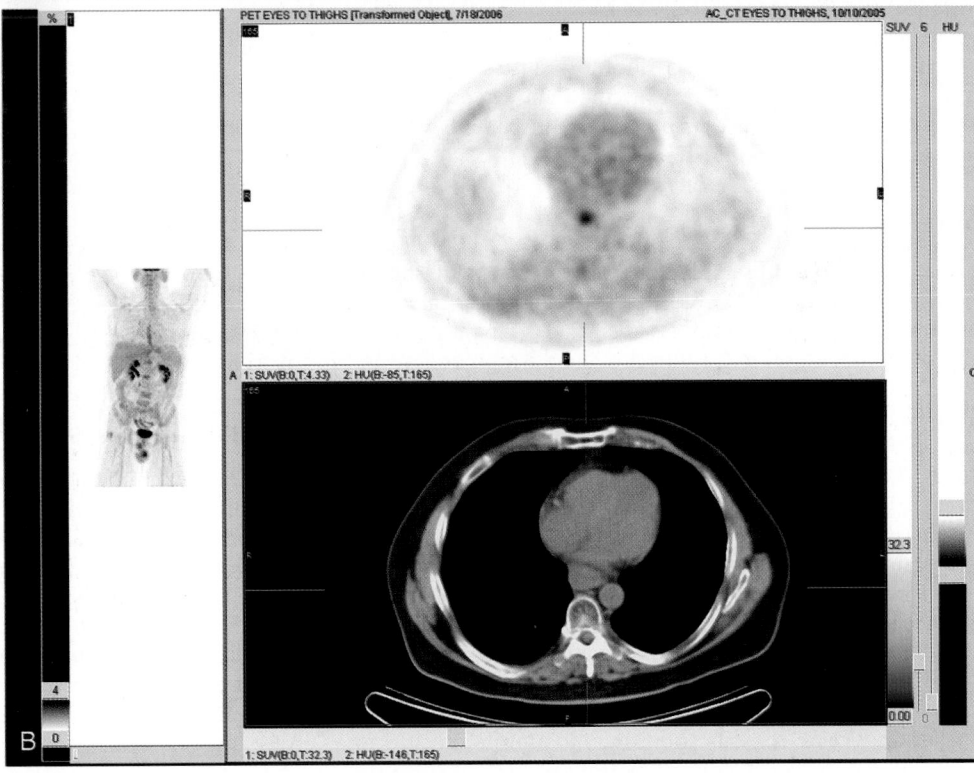

Figure 9-1. Esophageal cancer: PET/CT features. A. Scan obtained before therapy shows intensely increased FDG activity (*arrow*) identified in the esophagus, fusing to the thickened area on the CT, consistent with the patient's known malignancy. **B.** Repeat imaging after radiation therapy demonstrates a dramatic response with a decrease in the extent of metabolically active tumor as well as in the SUV from 10.9 to 4.3.

abnormality on the CT, is suggestive of malignancy (Fig. 9-1). In the absence of anatomic abnormality, focally intense uptake still raises concern for neoplasm. Necrotic portions of the tumor will appear photopenic. As discussed earlier, postoperative alteration of metabolism may be difficult to differentiate from recurrence. In this setting, serial scans in 6 to 8 weeks or at up to 3-month intervals could be useful in further characterizing such findings and in documenting stability of FDG uptake to exclude the possibility of malignancy.

Staging

T Staging

Both adenocarcinoma and squamous cell carcinoma of the esophagus are FDG avid. PET detects primary tumors with higher sensitivity than CT, 95% to 100% versus 81% to 92%, respectively, as shown in multiple studies.[8-15] False-negative results, however, are secondary to small tumor volume and well-differentiated tumors, which tend to be less FDG avid.

Inflammation, such as from reflux esophagitis or radiation, may mimic focal uptake of active malignancy and contribute to false-negative findings.

PET/CT has the resolution to detect tumors that extend to the submucosa but in general is unable to distinguish those involving only the mucosa.[16] Currently, no clear relationship exists between SUV uptake and tumor depth.[15,17] In addition, the level of FDG uptake is similar in adenocarcinomas and squamous cell carcinomas and cannot be reliably differentiated using SUV measurements.[17]

N Staging

Survival in esophageal cancer is related to the extent of lymph node involvement[18] so that accurate N staging is critical to both the treatment plan as well as to the overall prognosis. Although endoscopic ultrasonography (EUS) is more accurate than CT in the evaluation of locoregional lymph node involvement, both modalities are limited in detection of disease in normal-size lymph nodes. A study comparing the sensitivity, specificity, and accuracy of PET with CT and histopathologic results from lymph node dissection demonstrated that PET has the same specificity (94%-97%) as CT but significantly greater sensitivity (52% vs. 15%) and accuracy (84% vs. 77%).[19] EUS, however, is significantly more sensitive than PET in the detection of regional lymph node involvement (81% vs. 33%) but less specific (67% vs. 89%).[15] The combination of EUS and CT is more sensitive than PET but, again, less specific.[20] Overall, for N classification staging, PET, EUS, and CT are less sensitive and specific than extensive lymph node dissection, which remains routine in patients who are considered surgical candidates.

M Staging

Distant metastatic disease precludes patients from surgery with curative intent, in favor of palliative, nonsurgical management. PET is demonstratively superior to CT in the detection of distant metastases in the lung, liver, and lymph nodes.[8-11,21] A prospective study showed the sensitivity and specificity of PET in the detection of distant disease to be 74% and 92% in comparison to 41% and 83% for CT and 42% and 94% for EUS.[21] In general, PET tends to upstage disease; however, because of the potential for false-positive or false-negative findings, histologic confirmation of metastatic disease should be obtained before confirmation of staging, which could deny a patient potentially curative treatment. Fortunately, PET/CT can facilitate this process by indicating the area of most increased FDG activity in relation to anatomic landmarks, thus ensuring appropriate biopsy of the lesion in question.

In staging of esophageal cancer using the tumor-node-metastasis (TNM) classification, the most profound impact of PET/CT is in the detection of distant metastatic disease and in the direction of biopsy to the anatomic site that may be sampled with minimally invasive procedures. This information can spare the patient unnecessary staging procedures as well as the morbidity of therapies that are inappropriate for advanced disease.

Prognosis

The level of FDG uptake in tumor at presentation has been found to be predictive of overall prognosis, and an SUV greater than 7.0 prognosticates a poorer outcome than in patients with less FDG uptake.[17] Furthermore, PET evidence of metastatic disease, local or distant, also indicates overall survival.[21]

Response to Therapy

FDG-PET has been evaluated to determine its ability to predict tumor response to initial therapy or overall response to neoadjuvant therapy, in comparison to multidetector CT and EUS. A study that examined patients who underwent FDG-PET before and 14 days after the induction of neoadjuvant chemotherapy demonstrated that PET was able to predict responders, those whose tumor length and wall thickness decreased by more than 50% at 3 months after completion of treatment by endoscopy and conventional imaging, with a sensitivity of 93% and a specificity of 95% when the FDG uptake decreased by 35%.[22] The 2-year disease-free survival of patients after induction therapy and esophagectomy was 38%, and overall survival was 63% when the SUV of the tumor decreased less than 60% between the initial study and the post-therapy scan. Those values increase to 67% disease-free survival and 89% survival when the SUV change was greater than 60%.[23] Overall, a decrease in FDG activity in the tumor is identified in response to therapy, with no change or even an increase in accumulation of radiopharmaceutical in less effective treatment.

Recurrence

In esophageal cancer, early detection of tumor recurrence can facilitate therapy with the goal of extending disease-free survival or even of curative intent. Conventional anatomic imaging faces the challenge of differentiating recurrence from post-therapy changes, such as scarring and inflammation. Increased metabolic activity indicating viable tumor may be identified on FDG-PET before visible structural alterations on anatomic imaging. Again, the ability to determine increased uptake allows PET a high degree of accuracy in the detection of recurrent disease.[14]

Benign Processes

Most benign processes in the esophagus demonstrate either decreased FDG accumulation or a linear pattern of uptake. Inflammation from gastroesophageal reflux disease or esophagitis is usually diffuse and involves an extended segment of the esophagus, often without a discrete focus of activity. Radiation changes may also demonstrate a similar pattern but tend to decrease in intensity over time. Coronal images are useful in this setting to fully visualize the extent of uptake and to confirm a linear pattern without discrete foci.

STOMACH

Imaging Characteristics

Uptake of FDG in the stomach may be diffusely increased and depends on the use of oral contrast media as well as on the distention of the gastric walls. Although there may be elements of heterogeneity, in general a physiologic pattern of activity has few or no discrete foci fusing to the gastric walls. Increased activity may be seen at the gastroesophageal junction and in the absence of CT abnormality is also likely to be physiologic

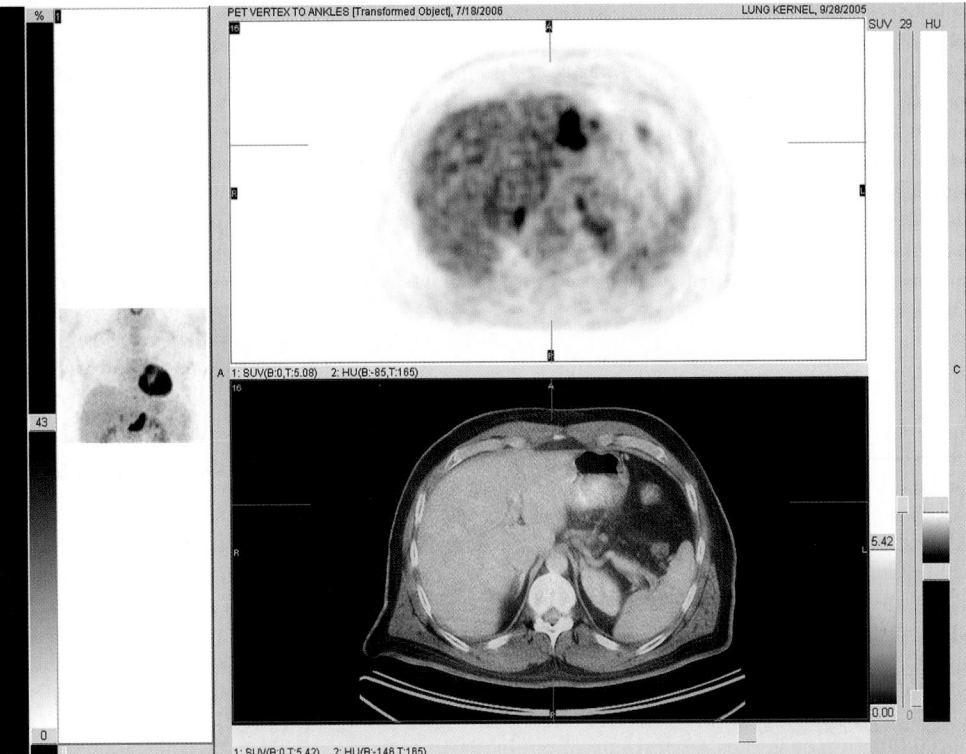

Figure 9-2. Gastric lymphoma and bilateral adrenal metastases. PET/CT shows an FDG-avid mass involving the lesser curvature of the stomach and bilateral adrenal foci consistent with lymphoma.

and secondary to normal muscular contraction of the lower esophageal sphincter. An analysis of the pattern of gastric uptake suggests that in patients without a history of esophagogastric disease, a gastroesophageal SUV maximum of less than 4 is less likely to represent neoplasm. If the SUV is greater than 4, further evaluation with endoscopy may be indicated.[24]

PET has corresponding levels of uptake (Fig. 9-2) in lymphoma of the stomach, with a higher SUV associated with high-grade malignancy and a lower SUV consistent with low-grade tumors. Similarly, high-grade gastric gastrointestinal stromal tumors (GISTs) are FDG avid and PET/CT can be used to follow treatment and detect recurrence. The use of PET/CT in the evaluation and staging of gastric cancer is not clearly established, but studies indicate there may be an evolving role for this imaging modality.

Staging

T Staging

Studies have demonstrated sensitivity of 93%[25] to 94%[26] for PET in the detection of gastric cancer, which is similar to the sensitivity of CT. False-negative results are again related to small tumor size and histopathologic type. A significant difference in sensitivity has been shown in PET's ability to identify early gastric cancer (63%) as opposed to advanced gastric cancer (98%).[26] Furthermore, a higher mean SUV (7.7)[26] is associated with the tubular adenocarcinoma type of malignancy. Decreased FDG activity is seen in mucinous and signet ring cell tumors (SUV mean 4.2),[26] which is a function of both the minimal glucose metabolism of mucin as well as the nominal expression of Glut-1 transporters on the cell membrane surface of mucinous and signet ring cell tumors.[27] Physiologic background FDG activity in the stomach may obscure these tumor types.

N Staging

In the detection of local lymph node involvement, PET demonstrates a lower sensitivity than CT (56% vs. 78%)[26] but a higher specificity (92% vs. 62%).[26] The overall accuracy of PET and CT in the detection of malignancy in local and distant lymph nodes is not significantly different. PET faces a challenge in distinguishing between N0 and N1 disease due to the intense uptake from the primary malignancy, which may obscure FDG accumulation in discrete lymph nodes adjacent to the tumor. In addition, studies suggest a correlation between the FDG avidity of the primary tumor and the likelihood of lymph node involvement; the higher the SUV, the more likely the presence of metastases to lymph nodes.[26,28]

M Staging

PET has shown a low sensitivity in comparison with CT in patients with peritoneal dissemination,[25,29] possibly owing to the diffuse distribution of malignant cells within fibrotic changes, which does not permit adequate accumulation of detectable FDG. Overall, PET may be useful in locating metastases in the liver, lungs, and lymph nodes but is less so in identifying osseous metastases and peritoneal carcinomatosis,[30] in which spatial resolution becomes a limiting factor.

Detection of Recurrence

A small study that used FDG-PET to examine patients with suspected gastric cancer recurrence after surgery demonstrated a sensitivity of 70%, a specificity of 69%, a positive predictive value of 78%, and a negative predictive value of 60%[31] in the detection of recurrent disease. In addition, the investigators found a longer survival in patients with a negative PET scan (21.9 ± 19.0 months) versus those with a positive PET scan (9.2 ± 8.2 months).[31]

Benign Processes

Inflammatory conditions, including gastritis, subclinical infection with *Helicobacter pylori,* and chemotherapy toxicity, usually demonstrate diffusely increased uptake that fuses to the wall without focal abnormality on a CT scan. Clinical correlation is important in stratifying the differential diagnosis in that the pattern of radiopharmaceutical distribution and the SUV do not preclude infiltrative malignant processes. Hiatal hernias may also demonstrate increased FDG activity but are distinguishable from the esophagus by CT comparison.

SMALL BOWEL

Imaging Considerations

Mildly increased FDG activity, less than that in the liver, is often seen in the small bowel, secondary to accumulation of the radiotracer in the smooth muscle, and less often as a result of metabolically active mucosa or swallowed secretions.[32] If the involved segment of small bowel is very short, it may appear focal. Otherwise, correlation with the CT images should demonstrate the portion of intestine demonstrating increased metabolic activity.

More intense activity may be identified in the gastroduodenal junction or in the ileocecal valve, both likely physiologic due to increased muscle activity in these regions. Again, confirmation of the absence of anatomic abnormality on the CT scan lends greater confidence in the benign nature of this uptake.

Malignancies

Lymphoma may arise in or secondarily involve the small intestine and demonstrates FDG avidity according to its grade. High-grade lymphoma has a higher SUV, and low-grade disease has a lower SUV. FDG-PET is useful in the diagnosis, staging, restaging, and evaluation of response to treatment in lymphoma, including that in the small bowel.

Melanoma is one of the most FDG-avid tumors and is often imaged using PET/CT. Case reports indicate the utility of this imaging modality in the detection of previously unsuspected metastases in the small intestine.

Carcinoid of the small bowel is not especially FDG avid, and other radiopharmaceuticals including carbon-11–labeled serotonin precursor 5-HTP and levodopa show promising signs of future use in PET of these tumors.

Metastatic lesions to the small intestine are common, and their ability to be imaged using FDG-PET is predicated on the avidity of the primary tumor. For example, ovarian cancer, with the exception of mucinous histology, is FDG avid and, therefore, ovarian metastases to the small bowel are visualized on PET/CT.

Benign Processes

Benign tumors of the small intestine including adenomas, leiomyomas, and lipomas are in general not FDG avid and are likely indistinguishable from the background physiologic uptake in the bowel.

Infectious and inflammatory processes demonstrate increased radiopharmaceutical uptake, and the potential differential diagnosis includes abscess, inflammatory bowel disease, or tuberculosis. Clinical history and radiographic or endoscopic correlation are crucial to pinpointing the cause of benign focal or diffuse uptake.

COLON

Physiologic distribution of radiopharmaceuticals in the colon can range from minimal, barely discernable from the background, to extensive and diffuse and is a function of smooth muscle uptake as well as swallowed secretions or excretion and accumulation of FDG within the contents of the colon.[32]

Diagnosis and Staging of Colorectal Cancer

In patients with known or suspected primary disease, FDG-PET identified all primary lesions (Fig. 9-3). In addition, PET and CT were comparable in sensitivity (29%) of local lymph node involvement but FDG-PET is superior to CT for detecting hepatic metastases. Currently, the role of PET/CT in preoperative staging (Fig. 9-4) is still debated except in high-risk patients for whom unnecessary surgery can be avoided with the detection of metastatic disease.[33-35]

Detection of Precancerous Polyps

Adenomatous polyps are often detected incidentally on whole-body images acquired for other indications, with a sensitivity of 24%. The typical lesion size range that may be visualized by the PET/CT camera is 5 to 30 mm. If the lesion is larger than 13 mm, the positivity rate increases to 90%. Although PET is not recommended for detection or screening for precancerous or malignant neoplasms, identification of focal colon uptake requires follow-up and may warrant colonoscopy for further evaluation.[36]

Detection of Recurrence

The use of CT in detection of recurrence has an overall accuracy of 25% to 73% and may miss up to 7% of hepatic metastases. In addition, CT may underestimate the number of hepatic lobes involved in up to 33% of patients. Further challenges lie in visualizing all metastases to the peritoneum, mesentery, and lymph nodes, as well as in differentiating postoperative changes from recurrence, which is often equivocal. Of the patients with negative CT, up to 50% will have nonresectable lesions at laparotomy. PET demonstrates an overall sensitivity of 90% and specificity greater than 70% in the diagnosis of recurrence. It is able to use metabolic information to distinguish scar from local recurrence with more than 90% accuracy. In a study of 76 patients, the accuracy of CT in recurrence detection was 65% versus 95% for PET.[37] In the setting of rising serum carcinoembryonic antigen after resection of the primary tumor with no abnormalities on conventional work-up, FDG-PET has a sensitivity of 93% to 100% and a specificity up to 92%. In addition, PET demonstrated tumor in two thirds of patients with this clinical presentation.[38,39]

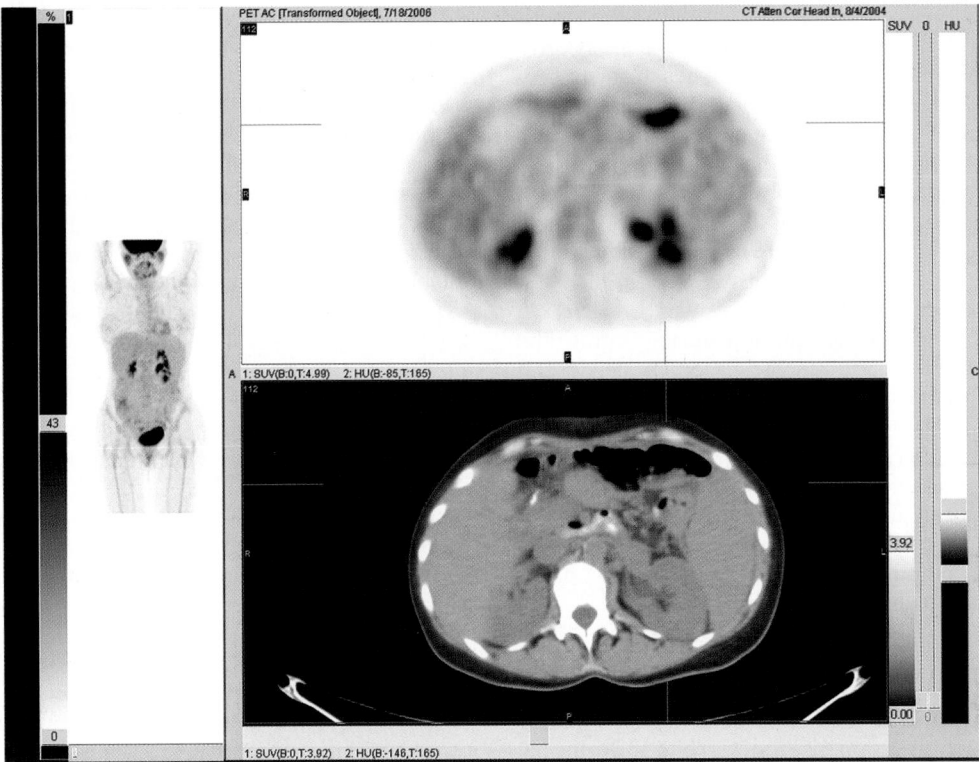

Figure 9-3. Primary colon adenocarcinoma. Increased radiopharmaceutical uptake seen fusing to colonic thickening in the splenic flexure, consistent with malignancy.

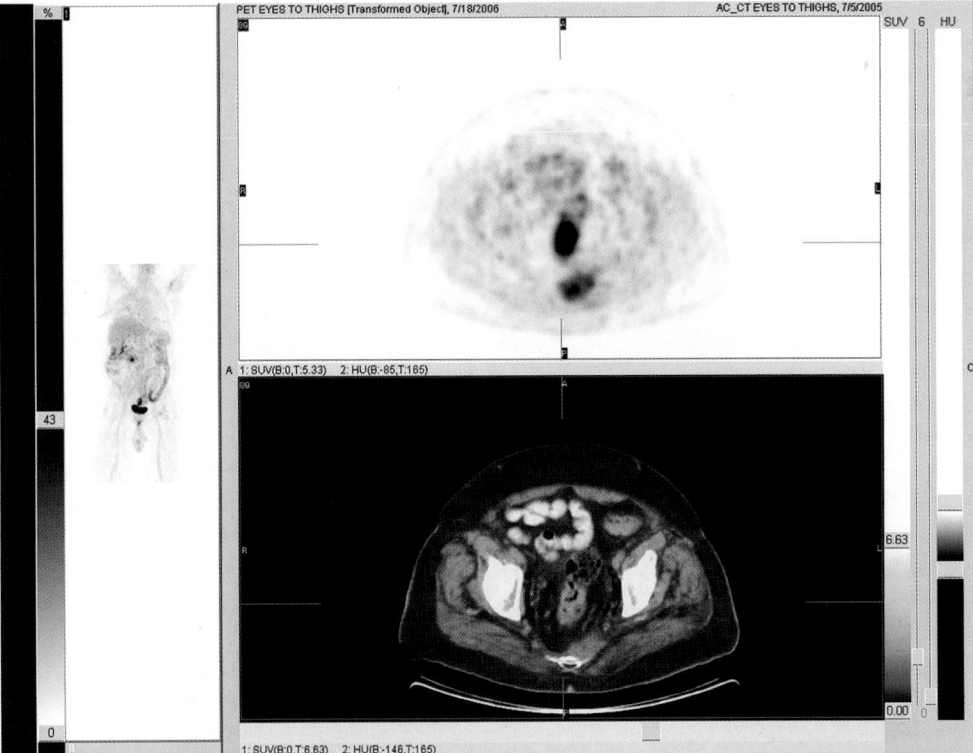

Figure 9-4. Mucinous adenocarcinoma of the colon: PET/CT features. Atypical presentation of mucinous adenocarcinoma of the sigmoid colon with metastasis to the sacrum. Mucinous adenocarcinomas are typically less FDG avid.

Detection of Metastases

In the evaluation of hepatic metastases a meta-analysis comparing noninvasive imaging for detection of hepatic metastasis from colorectal (Fig. 9-5), gastric, and esophageal cancers demonstrated that, at equivalent specificity of 85%, FDG-PET had sensitivity of 90% in comparison with that of MRI at 76%, CT at 72%, and ultrasonography at 55%.[40] Comparison of sensitivity and specificity of FDG-PET and CT for detection of recurrence or metastatic disease by particular anatomic locations finds that PET is more sensitive except in the lung, where the two were equivalent, likely secondary to decreased resolution on PET due to lung motion during acquisition. The largest discrepancy occurs in the abdomen, pelvis, and retroperitoneum where one third of PET-positive lesions were negative by CT. PET was also more specific than CT in all sites except the retroperitoneum, but these differences were smaller than those seen in sensitivity.[39] Therefore, overall, FDG-PET is useful in distinguishing local recurrence from postoperative changes, identifying hepatic metastases, classifying indeterminate pulmonary nodules, demonstrating nodal involvement, and providing a whole-body study.

Monitoring Treatment Response

In the clinical scenario of decreased FDG uptake without immediate decrease in lesion size on CT either during or after therapy, this finding indicates response to treatment. Radiation therapy presents challenges in the form of immediate post-treatment inflammation, but FDG-PET can assess residual tumor versus scarring[41] based on the pattern of uptake as well as on the degree of metabolic activity. Postirradiation-type changes are generally diffuse and nonfocal in contra-distinction to viable tumor, which is more focal and more intense. Delay of post-therapy PET to 6 or more weeks after irradiation increases specificity.

PET/CT is also useful in determining response to chemotherapy both during treatment to predict response as well as after completion to evaluate for residual viable tumor. Patients with hepatic metastases had PET/CT prediction of response to 5 weeks of fluorouracil therapy based on pretreatment FDG uptake as well as during therapy.[42] Current research strives to establish more definitive guidelines for prediction of response to preoperative chemoradiotherapy using specific SUVs.

Limitations of PET/CT in Colorectal Cancer

Partial volume averaging, necrotic lesions with thin visible rim, or mucinous adenocarcinoma may cause false-negative results. The last is most likely a function of the relative hypocellularity of mucinous tumors as well as the minimal glucose metabolism of mucin.

Inflammation caused by treatment or other causes such as inflammatory bowel disease (Fig. 9-6) is a frequent cause of false-positive findings. Also, infection, recent incisions, and biopsy or colostomy sites may show focally increased FDG activity that is of concern for malignancy. Obtaining an accurate history from the patient or referring clinician, including procedure dates, is imperative.

PET/CT is useful in the diagnosis (incidental), staging, restaging, and evaluation for recurrence, metastases, and treatment response of colorectal carcinoma. Although false-positive and false-negative results may challenge the application of this modality, appropriate clinical information may assist in limiting these confounding factors.[43,44]

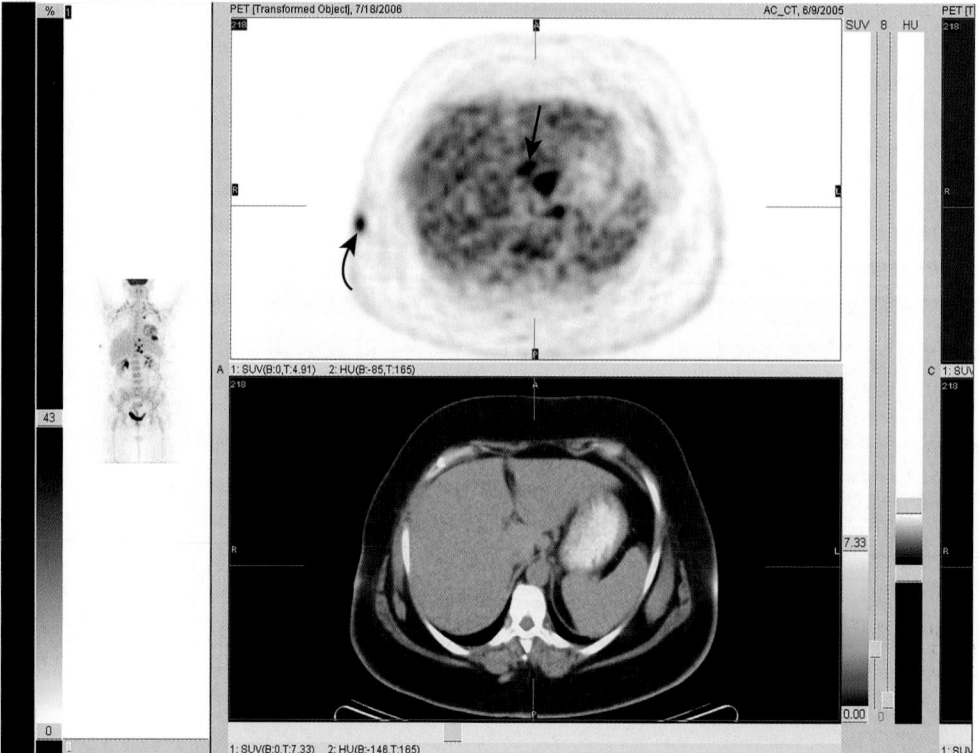

Figure 9-5. Metastases from colon adenocarcinoma. Multiple FDG-avid lymph nodes and a soft tissue nodule seen in the right flank (*curved arrow*) consistent with metastatic disease. Note the small focus of increased activity in the left lobe of the liver (*straight arrow*), also consistent with early metastatic disease.

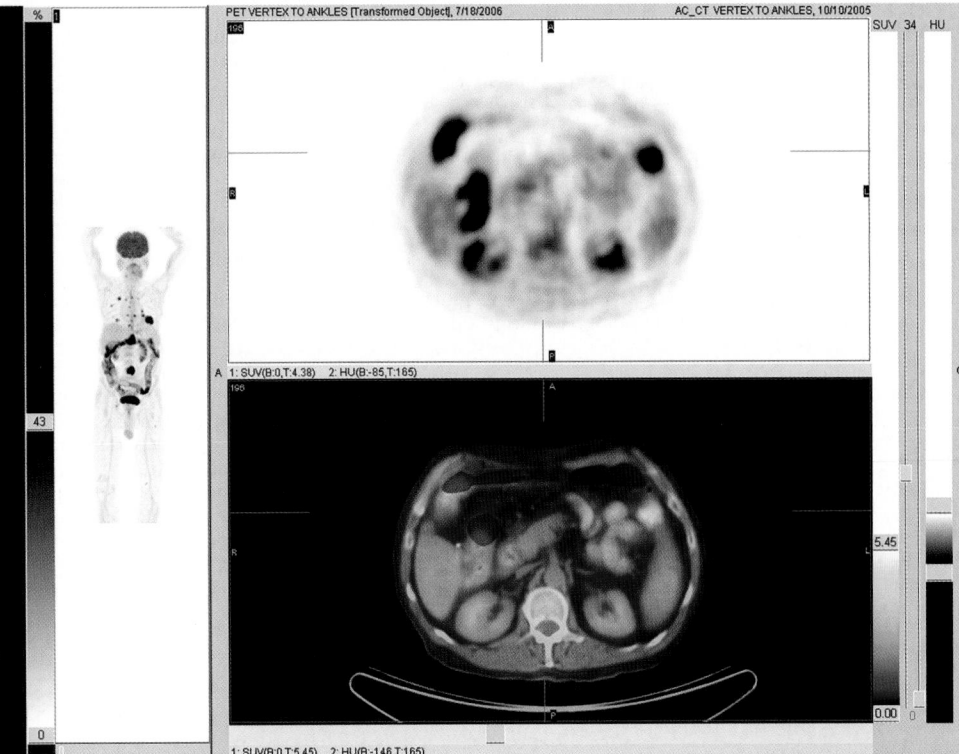

Figure 9-6. Crohn's disease: PET/CT finding. Intensely increased FDG activity in multiple segments of the colon consistent with enteritis in a patient on chemotherapy.

References

1. Blodgett TM, Meltzer CC, Townsend DW: PET/CT: Form and function. Radiology 242:360-385, 2007.
2. Warburg O: The Metabolism of Tumors. New York, Richard R Smith, 1931, pp 129-169.
3. Wong TZ, Paulson EK, Nelson RC, et al: Practical approach to diagnostic CT combined with PET. AJR Am J Roentgenol 188:622-629, 2007.
4. Cohade C, Osman M, Nakamoto Y, et al: Initial experience with oral contrast in PET/CT: Phantom and clinical studies. J Nucl Med 44:412-416, 2003.
5. Antoch G, Freudenberg LS, Egelhof T, et al: Focal tracer uptake: A potential artifact in contrast-enhanced dual-modality PET/CT scans. J Nucl Med 43:1339-1342, 2002.
6. Antoch G, Freudenberg LS, Stattaus T, et al: Whole-body positron emission tomography-CT: Optimized CT using oral and IV contrast materials. AJR 179:1555-1560, 2002.
7. Gregoire V, Haustermans K, Geets X, et al: PET-based treatment planning in radiotherapy: A new standard? J Nucl Med 48(Suppl 1):68S-77S, 2007.
8. Flanagan FL, Dehdashti F, Siegel BA, et al: Staging of esophageal cancer with ^{18}F-fluorodeoxyglucose positron emission tomography. AJR 168: 417-424, 1997.
9. Block MI, Patterson GA, Sundaresan RS, et al: Improvement in staging of esophageal cancer with the addition of positron emission tomography. Ann Thorac Surg 64:770-776, 1997; discussion 776-777.
10. Kole AC, Plukker JT, Nieweg OE, Vaalburg W: Positron emission tomography for staging of oesophageal and gastroesophageal malignancy. Br J Cancer 78:521-527, 1998.
11. Dam HQ, Manzone TM, Sagar VV: Evolving role of (18)F-fluoro-deoxyglucose positron emission tomography in the management of esophageal carcinoma. Surg Oncol Clin N Am 15:733-749, 2006.
12. Plukker JT, van Westreenen HL: Staging in oesophageal cancer. Best Pract Res Clin Gastroenterol 20:877-891, 2006.
13. McAteer D, Wallis F, Couper G, et al: Evaluation of ^{18}F-FDG positron emission tomography in gastric and oesophageal carcinoma. Br J Radiol 72:525-529, 1999.
14. Yeung HW, Macapinlac HA, Mazumdar M, et al: FDG-PET in esophageal cancer: Incremental value over computed tomography. Clin Positron Imaging 2:255-260, 1999.
15. Flamen P, Lerut A, Van Cutsem E, et al: Utility of positron emission tomography for the staging of patients with potentially operable esophageal carcinoma. J Clin Oncol 18:3202-3210, 2000.
16. Himeno S, Yasuda S, Shimada H, et al: Evaluation of esophageal cancer by positron emission tomography. Jpn J Clin Oncol 32:340-346, 2002.
17. Fukunaga T, Okazumi S, Koide Y, et al: Evaluation of esophageal cancers using fluorine-18-fluorodeoxyglucose PET. J Nucl Med 39:1002-1007, 1998.
18. Lerut T, Coosemans W, Decker G, et al: Cancer of the esophagus and gastro-esophageal junction: Potentially curative therapies. Surg Oncol 10:113-122, 2001.
19. Kim K, Park SJ, Kim BT, et al: Evaluation of lymph node metastases in squamous cell carcinoma of the esophagus with positron emission tomography. Ann Thorac Surg 71:290-294, 2001.
20. Lerut T, Flamen P, Ectors N, et al: Histopathologic validation of lymph node staging with FDG-PET scan in cancer of the esophagus and gastroesophageal junction: A prospective study based on primary surgery with extensive lymphadenectomy. Ann Surg 232:743-752, 2000.
21. Luketich JD, Friedman DM, Weigel TL, et al: Evaluation of distant metastases in esophageal cancer: 100 consecutive positron emission tomography scans. Ann Thorac Surg 68:1133-1136, 1999; discussion 1136-1137.
22. Weber WA, Ott K, Becker K, et al: Prediction of response to preoperative chemotherapy in adenocarcinomas of the esophagogastric junction by metabolic imaging. J Clin Oncol 19:3058-3065, 2001.
23. Downey RJ, Akhurst T, Ilson D, et al: Whole-body [18]FDG-PET and the response of esophageal cancer to induction therapy: Results of a prospective trial. J Clin Oncol 21:428-432, 2003.
24. Salaun PY, Grewal RK, Dodamane I, et al: An analysis of the ^{18}F-FDG uptake pattern in the stomach. J Nucl Med 46:48-51, 2005.
25. Yeung HW, Macapinlac H, Karpeh M, et al: Accuracy of FDG-PET in gastric cancer: Preliminary experience. Clin Positron Imaging 1:213-221, 1998.
26. Chen J, Cheong JH, Yun MJ, et al: Improvement in preoperative staging of gastric adenocarcinoma with positron emission tomography. Cancer 103:2383-2390, 2005.
27. Kawamura T, Kusakabe T, Sugino T, et al: Expression of glucose transporter-1 in human gastric carcinoma: Association with tumor aggressiveness, metastasis, and patient survival. Cancer 92:634-641, 2001.

28. Mochiki E, Kuwano H, Katoh H, et al: Evaluation of ^{18}F-2-deoxy-2-fluoro-D-glucose positron emission tomography for gastric cancer. World J Surg 28:247-253, 2004.

29. Jadvar H, Tatlidil R, Garcia AA, Conti PS: Evaluation of recurrent gastric malignancy with (F-18)-FDG positron emission tomography. Clin Radiol 58:215-221, 2003.

30. Yoshioka T, Yamaguchi K, Kubota K, et al: Evaluation of ^{18}F-FDG PET in patients with a metastatic or recurrent gastric cancer. J Nucl Med 44:690-699, 2003.

31. De Potter T, Flamen P, Van Cutsem E, et al: Whole-body PET with FDG for the diagnosis of recurrent gastric cancer. Eur J Nucl Med Mol Imaging 29:525-529, 2002.

32. Endo K, Oriuchi N, Higuchi T, et al: PET and PET/CT using 18F-FDG in the diagnosis and management of cancer patients. Int J Clin Oncol 11:286-296, 2006.

33. Abdel-Nabi H, Doerr RJ, Lamonica DM, et al: Staging of primary colorectal carcinomas with fluorine-18 fluorodeoxyglucose whole-body PET: Correlation with histopathologic and CT findings. Radiology 206:755-760, 1998.

34. Mukai M, Sadahiro S, Yasuda S, et al: Preoperative evaluation by whole-body ^{18}F-fluorodeoxyglucose positron emission tomography in patients with primary colorectal cancer. Oncol Rep 7:85-87, 2000.

35. Kantorova I, Lipska L, Belohlavek O, et al: Routine (18)F-FDG PET preoperative staging of colorectal cancer: Comparison with conventional staging and its impact on treatment decision making. J Nucl Med 44:1784-1788, 2003.

36. Yasuda S, Fujii H, Nakahara T, et al: 18F-FDG PET detection of colonic adenomas. J Nucl Med 42:989-992, 2001.

37. Schiepers C, Penninckx F, De Vadder N, et al: Contribution of PET in the diagnosis of recurrent colorectal cancer: Comparison with conventional imaging. Eur J Surg Oncol 21:517-522, 1995.

38. Flanagan FL, Dehdashti F, Ogunbiyi OA, et al: Utility of FDG-PET for investigating unexplained plasma CEA elevation in patients with colorectal cancer. Ann Surg 227:319-323, 1998.

39. Kuehl H, Veit P, Rosenbaum SJ, et al: Can PET/CT replace separate diagnostic CT for cancer imaging? Optimizing CT protocols for imaging cancers of the chest and abdomen. J Nucl Med 48(Suppl 1):45S-57S, 2007.

40. Kinkel K, Lu Y, Both M, et al: Detection of hepatic metastases from cancers of the gastrointestinal tract by using noninvasive imaging methods (US, CT, MR imaging, PET): A meta-analysis. Radiology 224:748-756, 2002.

41. Haberkorn U, Strauss LG, Dimitrakopoulou A, et al: PET studies of fluorodeoxyglucose metabolism in patients with recurrent colorectal tumors receiving radiotherapy. J Nucl Med 32:1485-1490, 1991.

42. Findlay M, Young H, Cunningham D, et al: Noninvasive monitoring of tumor metabolism using fluorodeoxyglucose and positron emission tomography in colorectal cancer liver metastases: Correlation with tumor response to fluorouracil. J Clin Oncol 14:700-708, 1996.

43. Tsukamoto E, Ochi S: PET/CT today: System and its impact on cancer diagnosis. Ann Nucl Med 20:255-267, 2006.

44. Veit-Haibach P, Kuehle CA, Beyer T, et al: Diagnostic accuracy of colorectal cancer staging with whole-body PET/CT colonography. JAMA 296:2590-2600, 2006.

Angiography and Interventional Radiology of the Hollow Viscera

Stanley Taeson Kim, MD • Albert A. Nemcek, Jr., MD • Robert L. Vogelzang, MD

Over the past 2 decades the applications of angiography and interventional radiology in hollow abdominal viscera have dramatically changed.[1,2] Multidetector CT (MDCT) angiography and MR angiography have replaced much of the diagnostic angiography that had been performed for investigating mesenteric ischemia, diagnosing abdominal masses, and detecting gastrointestinal tract bleeding sites.[3-7] Interventional applications in the gastrointestinal tract, however, have dramatically increased. In this chapter, new developments in angiography and interventional radiology of the hollow viscera are addressed.

PREPARATION OF PATIENTS

Certain preprocedural steps can enhance the diagnostic quality of a visceral angiogram. For elective studies, a standard bowel cleansing should be considered to more clearly delineate vessels and pathologic findings. Intravenous glucagon (1.0 mg) given at the time of the procedure helps reduce the effects of bowel motion, particularly in studies utilizing digital subtraction.

A Foley catheter is useful in studies of the inferior mesenteric artery because a contrast agent filling the bladder can obscure its branches. It also increases the patient's comfort and helps prevent unnecessary delays during long examinations.

Unless contraindicated, we routinely premedicate patients undergoing visceral angiography with fentanyl (Sublimaze) and midazolam (Versed) in an attempt to achieve the analgesic, anxiolytic, and amnestic effects of these combined agents while maintaining the patient's ability to cooperate. All patients have intraprocedural monitoring of pulse, electrocardiogram, arterial oxygenation (via a pulse oximeter), and blood pressure.

TECHNICAL FACTORS

Vascular Access

In general, the femoral arterial route of catheterization is used for abdominal aortography as well as selective visceral angiography; the safety and ease of this approach are well established. Brachial or axillary access may be used in cases of difficult femoral access or when there is a need to advance a catheter more deeply into a vessel that has a steep caudad course.

Catheter Selection

Our catheter of choice for celiac and superior mesenteric arteriography is a simple angled visceral hook with a single side hole; for inferior mesenteric arteriography we prefer a catheter with a short curved tip. For most indications, 5-Fr catheters are used to minimize puncture site complications. An angiographic sheath with a check flow valve is placed if multiple catheter exchanges are anticipated.

Advances in guidewire and catheter technology have made subselective catheterization of visceral vessels easier. These include the development of flexible, hydrophilic torque-control guidewires and of catheters that have low coefficients of friction that allow them to more readily follow wires around complex or tight curves.

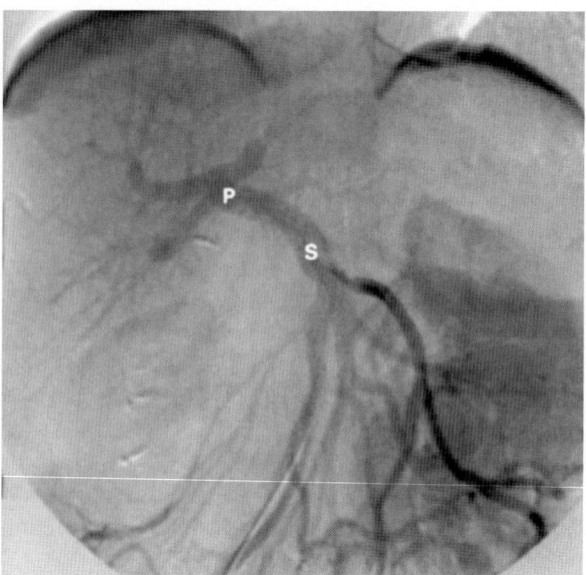

Figure 10-1. Arterial portography obtained during digital subtraction angiography. Excellent opacification of the mesenteric and portal venous system is achieved after superior mesenteric arterial injection. S, superior mesenteric vein; P, portal vein.

Equipment

Digital subtraction angiography (DSA) is the preferred technique for visceral angiography (Fig. 10-1). In addition, digital image processing features greatly facilitate the guidance of complex vascular catheterizations and interventions.

ANGIOGRAPHY OF THE MAJOR VISCERAL VESSELS

Visceral angiography begins with injection of the aorta or one of the three major visceral vessels: the celiac artery, the superior mesenteric artery (SMA), or the inferior mesenteric artery (IMA). Aortic injection is usually limited to situations that pose a risk for selective catheterization: suspicion of severe narrowing or occlusion of one or more of the origins of the major visceral vessels, especially in patients with clinical evidence of intestinal ischemia or those with severe aortic atherosclerosis.

The order of examination of the visceral vessels depends on the clinical situation. Thus, in gastrointestinal bleeding, angiography should begin with the vessel most likely to be bleeding based on clinical history and the results of prior diagnostic studies. It is critical to not limit the study excessively. Again, using the example of gastrointestinal bleeding, a patient who has clear clinical and endoscopic evidence for acute hemorrhage into the colon may nonetheless have a bleeding source in the celiac territory.

Selective catheterization of the visceral arteries can be performed as an initial step or after aortography. The celiac artery generally arises from the aorta anteriorly, at the middle T12 or upper L1 vertebral level. The SMA originates slightly caudal to the celiac trunk. Generally, 7 to 10 mL/s of contrast medium is injected into these arteries, for a total of 35 to 60 mL; the rate is based on test injections. Certain clinical situations require alteration in these rates and volumes. For example, when evaluation of the mesenteric and portal venous systems is important, particularly in patients with portal hypertension, higher rates and volumes are needed (e.g., 8 to 10 mL/s for a total of 80 to 100 mL). For the IMA, which usually arises to the left of midline from the abdominal aorta at the lower aspect of the L3 vertebral body, injection at a rate of 3 to 4 mL/s for a total of 12 to 16 mL is generally appropriate. Injection rates are proportionately decreased for mesenteric branches.

ARTERIAL ANATOMY OF SPECIFIC SEGMENTS OF THE GUT

The vascular anatomy of the hollow abdominal viscera is quite complex. We have utilized a number of excellent general references in preparing this chapter; the reader is referred to these for more detailed discussions of angiographic and gross anatomy and of the embryologic basis for many of the observed anatomic variations.

Esophagus

From a practical standpoint, only the distal esophageal arterial supply is important for angiographers. The gastroesophageal junction is a reasonably common site of arterial hemorrhage potentially treatable by embolization or vasopressin infusion. This region is typically supplied by branches of the left gastric artery (discussed later) or the left inferior phrenic artery (Figs. 10-2 and 10-3).

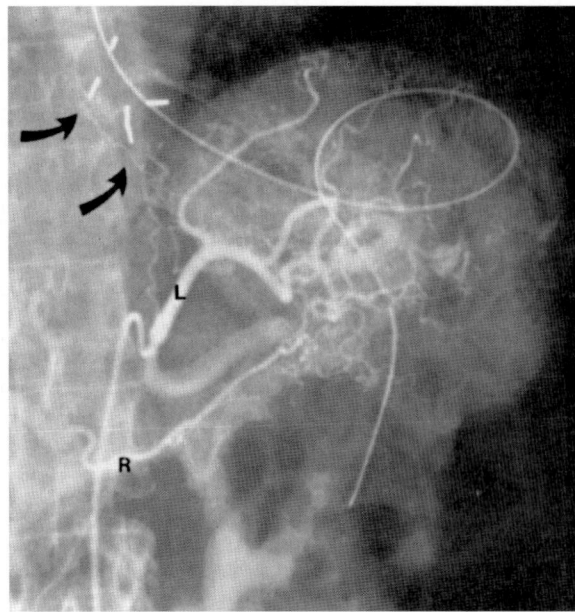

Figure 10-3. Selective left gastric artery injection. L, left gastric artery; R, right gastric artery (filling retrograde via the left gastric branches); *arrows,* branches of the left gastric artery supplying the lower esophagus.

Catheterization of the upper and middle portions of the esophagus is difficult but fortunately rarely necessary. The cervical esophagus typically receives its arterial supply from the inferior thyroid arteries (branches of the subclavian arteries), with predominant supply from the right. Subclavian, common carotid, or aortic branches may also supply this segment. The thoracic esophageal arteries arise either directly from the aorta or as branches of the intercostal or bronchial arteries. Esophageal arteries anastomose along the length of the esophagus.

Stomach

The stomach has two major vascular arcades, one along the lesser curve formed by the right and left gastric arteries and the other along the greater curve consisting of the right and left gastro-omental (gastroepiploic) arteries.

The left gastric artery (Figs. 10-4 through 10-6; see also Figs. 10-2 and 10-3) usually arises as one of the three major branches of the celiac trunk, originating anywhere from the orifice of the trunk to the hepatic-splenic bifurcation. In 2% to 6% of patients, this vessel arises separately from the aorta.[1,2]

A replaced or accessory left hepatic artery arises from the left gastric artery in 20% to 30% of cases.[1,2] This has important clinical implications in patients for whom embolization or infusion therapy of hepatic or gastric arteries is anticipated. When this variant is present, the relative blood supply to the stomach and liver can vary, so that minimal supply to either may be present. In about 5% of cases, one or both inferior phrenic arteries arise from the left gastric trunk; this association is much higher when the left gastric artery arises as a separate aortic branch. The importance of this variant is emphasized by the reported association of hypertension and cardiac arrhythmias with vasopressin infusion into the phrenic artery. Accessory left gastric arteries are common.[1,2]

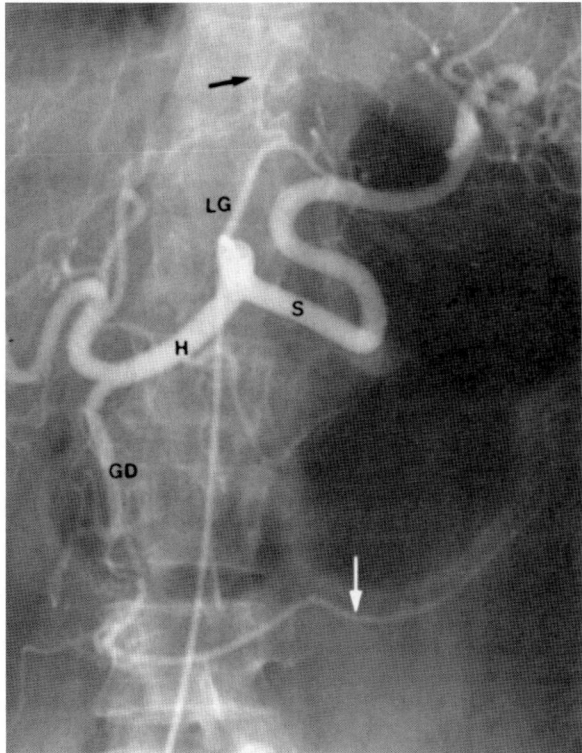

Figure 10-2. Celiac arteriogram. LG, left gastric artery; H, common hepatic artery; S, splenic artery; GD, gastroduodenal artery; *black arrow,* branches of the left gastric artery supplying the lower esophagus; *white arrow,* right gastro-omental artery.

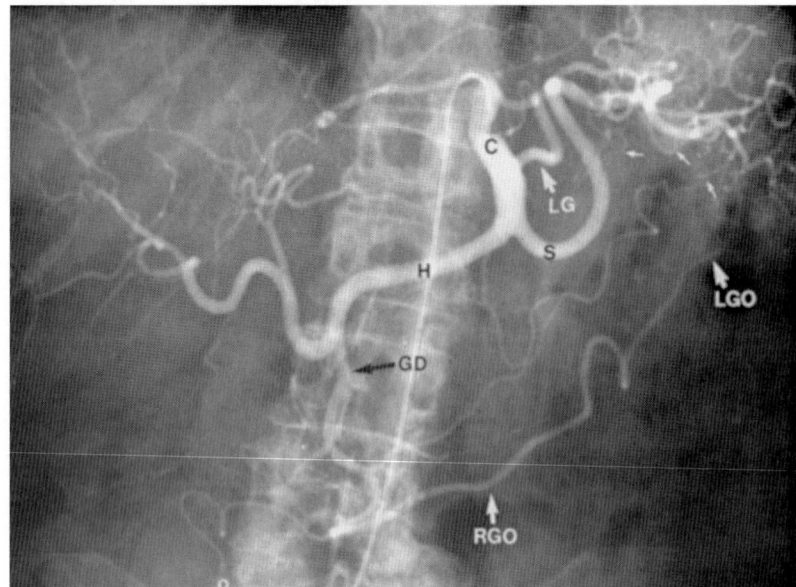

Figure 10-4. Celiac arteriogram. A well-formed gastro-omental anastomosis is present. C, celiac artery; LG, left gastric artery; GD, gastroduodenal artery; RGO, right gastro-omental artery; LGO, left gastro-omental artery; S, splenic artery; H, common hepatic artery; *small white arrows*, short gastric branches.

Because most gastric angiography is performed for gastrointestinal bleeding and the left gastric arterial ramifications account for about 85% of gastric hemorrhage, this is clearly an important vessel for subselective catheterization. Unfortunately, whereas the celiac artery is most readily catheterized with a caudally directed catheter, the course of the left gastric artery is cephalad. This may make selective catheterization difficult. A number of articles and texts detail methods that facilitate catheterization of this sometimes elusive vessel. The basic principle of these methods is initial selection of the celiac artery with a catheter that has a caudally directed tip, followed by intraceliac exchange for, conversion to, or coaxial insertion of a catheter with a tip that points upward.[1,2]

The right gastric artery arises at or distal to the common hepatic artery bifurcation, usually from the proper hepatic (57%) but occasionally from left (17%) or right hepatic (2%) branches or at the origin or proximal portion of the gastroduodenal artery (10%). It has generally been considered an

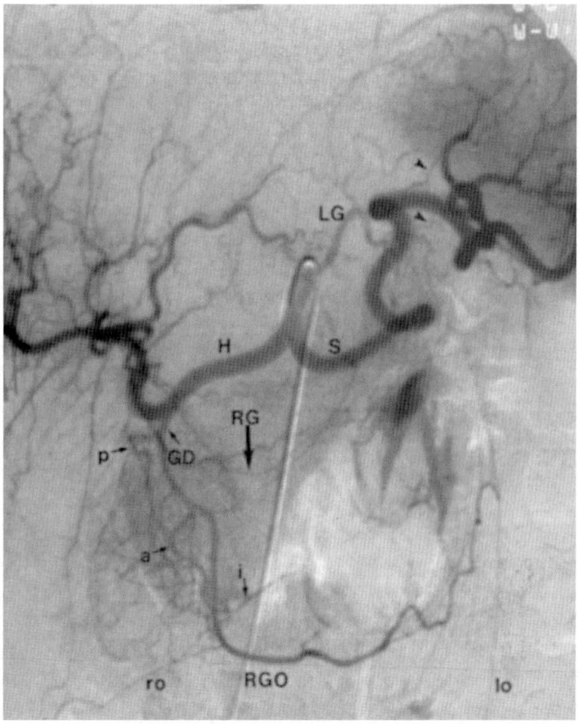

Figure 10-5. Celiac arteriogram. LG, left gastric artery; GD, gastroduodenal artery; S, splenic artery; H, common hepatic artery; RGO, right gastro-omental artery (the left gastro-omental artery is not well opacified); p, posterior superior pancreaticoduodenal branch; a, anterosuperior pancreaticoduodenal branch; i, inferior pancreaticoduodenal branch (filling retrograde via the pancreaticoduodenal arcades); ro, right omental branch; lo, left omental branch; *arrowheads*, short gastric branches.

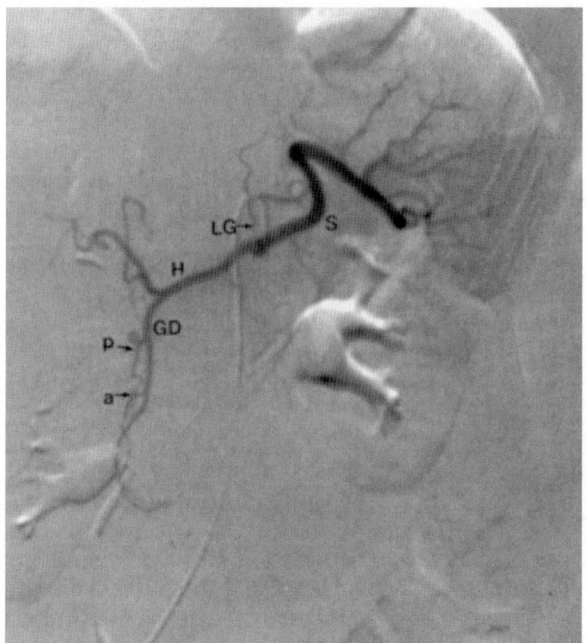

Figure 10-6. Early arterial phase, celiac arteriogram. LG, left gastric artery; S, splenic artery; H, common hepatic artery; GD, gastroduodenal artery; p, posterior superior pancreaticoduodenal branch; a, anterior superior pancreaticoduodenal branch.

unimportant vessel for arteriographers along with the cystic and falciform arteries; however, these small vessels are found to be of increasing concern with the evolution of transarterial chemoembolization and arterial brachytherapy. Because the right gastric and cystic arteries have variable origins, these vessels increase the possibility of nontarget embolization with subsequent tissue necrosis and/or inflammation (i.e., mucosal ulceration, cholecystitis, and skin necrosis).[1,2]

The right gastro-omental (gastroepiploic) artery (see Figs. 10-2, 10-4, and 10-5) is typically the larger of the two gastro-omental vessels. It is the terminal branch of the gastroduodenal artery. The left gastro-omental (gastroepiploic) artery (see Fig. 10-4) arises from the splenic artery or in conjunction with its inferior splenic branch. The gastro-omental arteries anastomose in a well-formed arcade along the greater curve of the stomach in 65% to 75% of cases; in most other instances, an anastomosis is still present but not as well developed. In slightly fewer than half of individuals, a parallel anastomotic arcade called the arc of Barkow is present in the greater omentum, joining right and left omental arteries (see Figs. 10-4 and 10-5), branches (respectively) of the right and left gastro-omental arteries.[1,2]

The supply from the gastric and gastro-omental arcades is supplemented by other branches. A variable number of short gastric arteries (see Figs. 10-4 and 10-5) supply the fundus and the superior aspect of the greater curve of the stomach, arising most often from splenic hilar vessels. In 36% to 60% of individuals, a posterior gastric artery arises from the main splenic artery to supply the posterior wall of the stomach and parts of the fundus and gastroesophageal junction. The pyloric region typically receives part of its supply via branches of the gastroduodenal artery.[1,2]

Small Bowel

Much of the blood supply to the duodenum is via a series of freely anastomosing vessels: the anterior and posterior pancreaticoduodenal arcades provide a rich source of collaterals for the duodenum and head of the pancreas and between the celiac artery and the SMA. These arcades (usually dual) form a continuous loop along the descending and transverse duodenum and the pancreatic head. The superior origin of this complex is usually dual, with both branches arising from the gastroduodenal artery and the posterior arcade typically arising more cephalad than the anterior (Fig. 10-7; see also Figs. 10-5 and 10-6). The inferior origin is most often a single trunk (see Figs. 10-5 and 10-7), usually arising from the SMA or its first or second jejunal branch.

Other sources of duodenal perfusion are branches of the right gastro-omental artery, the supraduodenal artery (which has many possible origins including the hepatic artery, the gastroduodenal artery, the posterior pancreaticoduodenal arcade, and the right gastric artery), and smaller gastroduodenal branches.

In addition to the pancreaticoduodenal arcades, another potential collateral route between the celiac and the superior mesenteric territories is the arc of Buhler, which represents persistence of an embryologic anastomosis between the celiac and the superior mesenteric trunks.

The jejunum and ileum are supplied primarily by multiple branches arising from the left side of the SMA (Figs. 10-8 and 10-9); the level of the ileocolic artery origin is a good general indicator of the division between jejunal and ileal

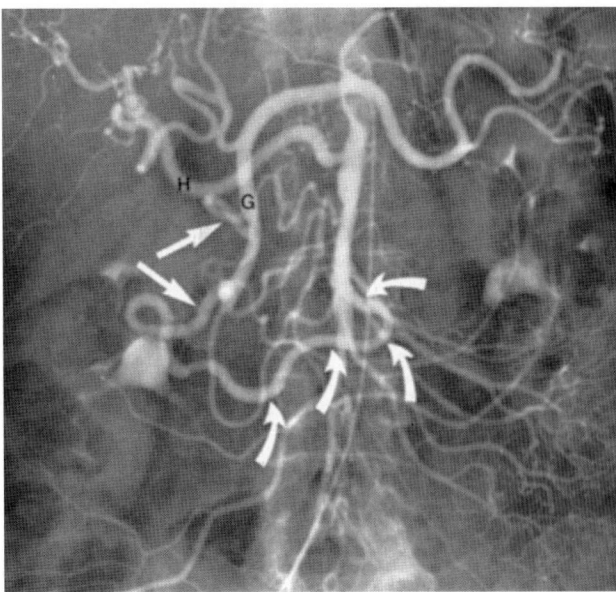

Figure 10-7. Superior mesenteric arteriogram. Enlarged pancreaticoduodenal arcades provide collaterals to the celiac territory in a patient with occlusion of the proximal celiac artery. Inferior pancreaticoduodenal branch (*curved arrows*) arises from the superior mesenteric artery and anastomoses with superior pancreaticoduodenal branches (*straight arrows*) to reconstitute the gastroduodenal artery (G). H, replaced right hepatic artery arising from the superior mesenteric artery.

territories. The distal ileum also receives blood from the ileocolic artery (discussed later). An extensive network of vascular arcades connects the jejunal and ileal branches; along the mesenteric border of the small bowel the distal arcades give rise to multiple straight vasa recta that enter the bowel wall. The number of arcades increases, and the length of the vasa recta decreases more distally in the small bowel; these anatomic factors must be considered when performing small bowel embolization.

An important anatomic variant is a persistent vitelline artery, indicating the presence of a Meckel diverticulum. This vessel has a characteristic appearance: a relatively long vessel arising in the ileal region, without anastomoses to other ileal branches and with a network of irregular small distal branches (Fig. 10-10). A Meckel diverticulum may also be supplied by ileal branches without a well-defined vitelline artery, although this is less common. A dense mucosal stain at the tip of the diverticulum suggests the presence of ectopic gastric mucosa.

Colon and Rectum

The right colon and transverse colon are usually supplied by the SMA. Classically, this supply is described and diagrammed as consisting of three main branches arising independently from the SMA: the ileocolic, the right colic, and the middle colic arteries. Although the ileocolic is a constant vessel, a true right colic artery (arising independently from the SMA) is uncommon and the middle colic "artery" is frequently variable in extent and branching pattern, consisting of one or more of five distinct vessels. The discrepancy between the classic description of three main independent branches and the most common situation in which there are two independent branches has given rise to some confusion and has caused the termination of the SMA to be labeled as the "ileocolic artery" on angiograms in various anatomic texts. It should be

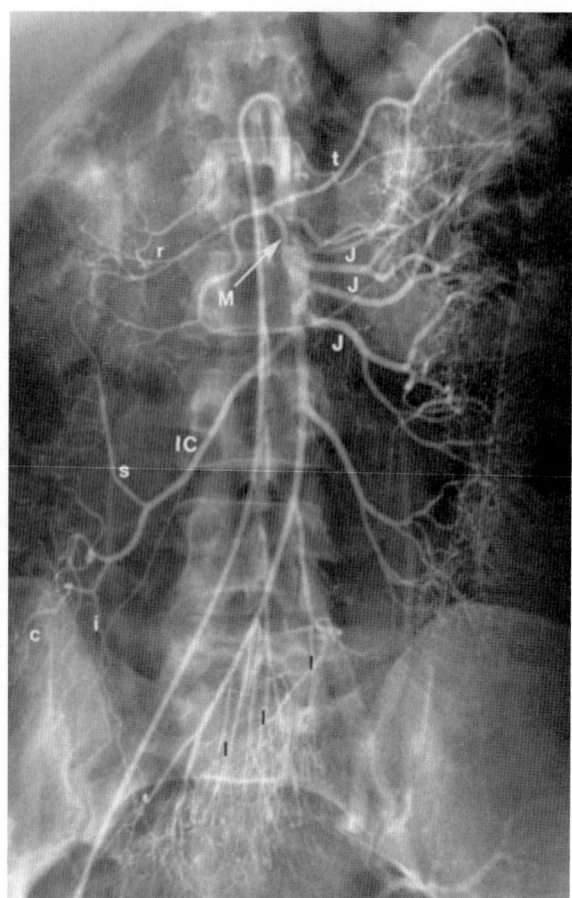

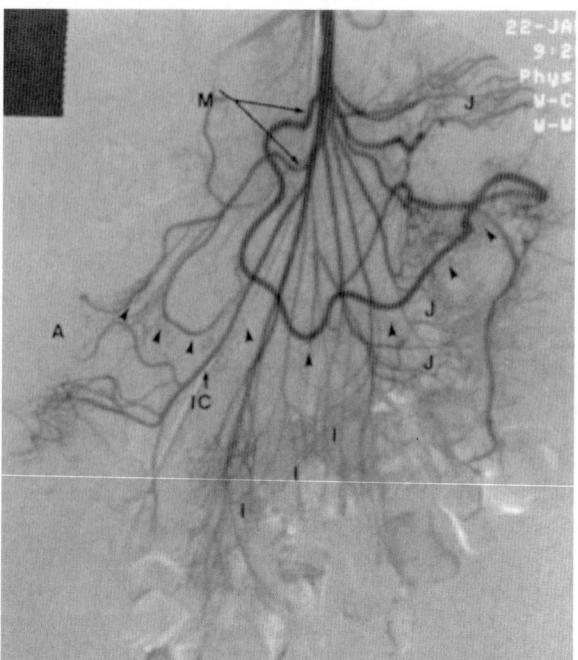

Figure 10-9. Superior mesenteric arteriogram. The middle colic territory (*arrowheads*) is supplied by two anastomosing superior mesenteric branches (M, *arrows*), one of which supplies the right colonic flexure and the other the mid to distal transverse colon. No discrete right colic artery to the ascending colon is present. IC, ileocolic artery; J, jejunal branches; I, ileal branches; A, position of ascending colon.

Figure 10-8. Superior mesenteric arteriogram. J, jejunal branches; I, ileal branches; IC, ileocolic artery; s, superior colic branch of the ileocolic artery, supplying the ascending colon and anastomosing with branches of the middle colic artery; c, cecal branches of the ileocolic artery; i, ileal branch of the ileocolic artery, anastomosing with terminal branches of the main superior mesenteric trunk; M, middle colic artery, with branches to the right colonic flexure (r) and the transverse colon (t).

emphasized that the SMA termination is not a colic artery: its branches supply the ileum, and its final terminus joins the ileal branch of the ileocolic artery in a vascular arcade at the ileocecal junction.

The ileocolic artery (see Figs. 10-8 and 10-9) supplies the transition between the small bowel and the colon, with branches to the terminal ileum, the cecum, the ascending

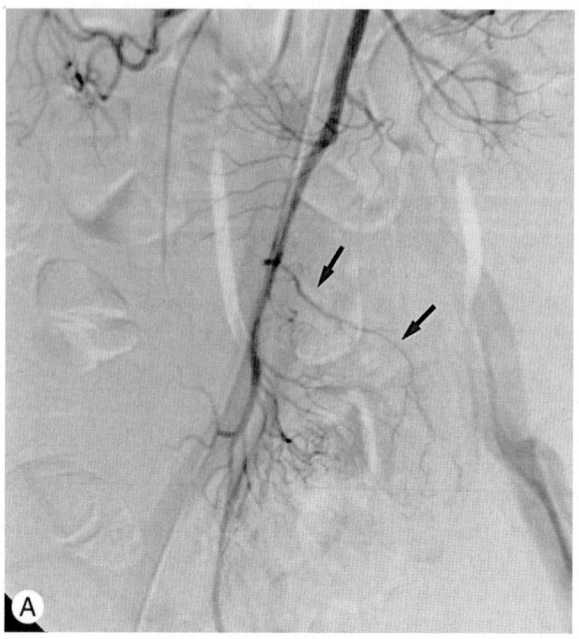

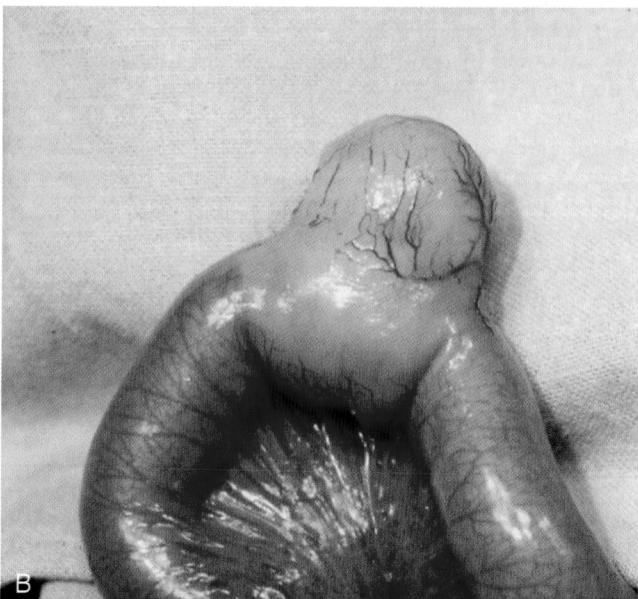

Figure 10-10. Persistent vitelline artery and Meckel's diverticulum. A. Selective superior mesenteric angiogram in a patient with recurrent gastrointestinal hemorrhage shows a characteristic elongated artery (*arrows*) without anastomoses to adjacent ileal vessels. More proximal vessels show an abrupt change in direction relative to this vessel, reflecting intussusception (inversion) of the Meckel diverticulum. **B.** Surgical specimen of an inverted Meckel's diverticulum.

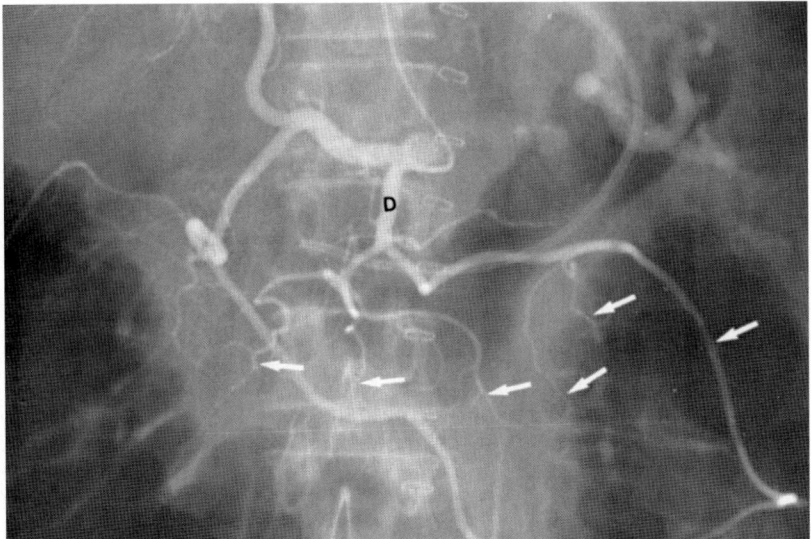

Figure 10-11. Variant middle colic supply. Celiac injection reveals an enlarged dorsal pancreatic artery (D), from which branches (*arrows*) arise that course to the middle colic territory and the transverse mesocolon.

colon, and the appendix. It is the last branch arising from the right side of the superior mesenteric trunk, and its constancy makes it a very important angiographic landmark. Most often, it consists of a main stem branching into two cecal branches distally, with anastomotic branches arising along the main stem. A nearly constant branch of the ileocolic artery is the superior colic, which anastomoses with the next colic artery arising from the SMA, whether the right colic or part of the middle colic complex.

The designation "right colic artery" should apply only to an independent branch arising directly from the superior mesenteric trunk that supplies the middle portion of the ascending colon. The midportion of the ascending colon is usually supplied via an arcade formed between the ileocolic artery and the middle colic system.

The middle colic artery has been classically described as the major proximal branch of the SMA that supplies the right colonic flexure and transverse colon. A true middle colic artery is actually seen in slightly fewer than half of patients cases. In other instances, variant arteries or combinations of these arteries supply the vascular territory between the ileocolic or right colic artery and the left colic artery; a single vessel is present 75% of the time (see Figs. 10-8 and 10-9).[1,2]

The middle colic artery or accessory arteries to the middle colic territory can arise from the celiac, splenic, hepatic, or pancreatic arteries (especially the dorsal pancreatic artery) (Fig. 10-11). Thus, angiography of the entire colon may require injection of the celiac artery or its branches.

In unusual situations, portions of the blood supply to the colon can arise directly from the aorta between the origins of the SMA and IMA. In two publications, such a variant has been called the "middle mesenteric artery," although in one the artery supplied the distal transverse and proximal descending colon and in the other the artery supplied the entire proximal colon up to and including the splenic flexure.

The IMA (Figs. 10-12 through 10-15) most often supplies the left colonic flexure, the descending colon, the sigmoid colon, and the upper rectum. However, the boundary between the parts of the colon supplied by the SMA and by the IMA can be variable—proximal or distal to the splenic flexure. The IMA terminates in two superior rectal (hemorrhoidal) branches (see Figs. 10-12 and 10-13). It gives off branches from

its left side. The first is the left colic artery (see Figs. 10-12, 10-14, and 10-15), which courses toward the splenic flexure. Its branches anastomose with branches of the middle colic territory (see Figs. 10-12 and 10-15). The left colic artery is frequently absent if there is an accessory left colic vessel arising as a portion of the middle colic supply. Other branches arise from the left colic artery or the IMA trunk proximal to the superior rectal arteries to supply the descending and sigmoid colon and the upper rectum. A colosigmoid artery or branch

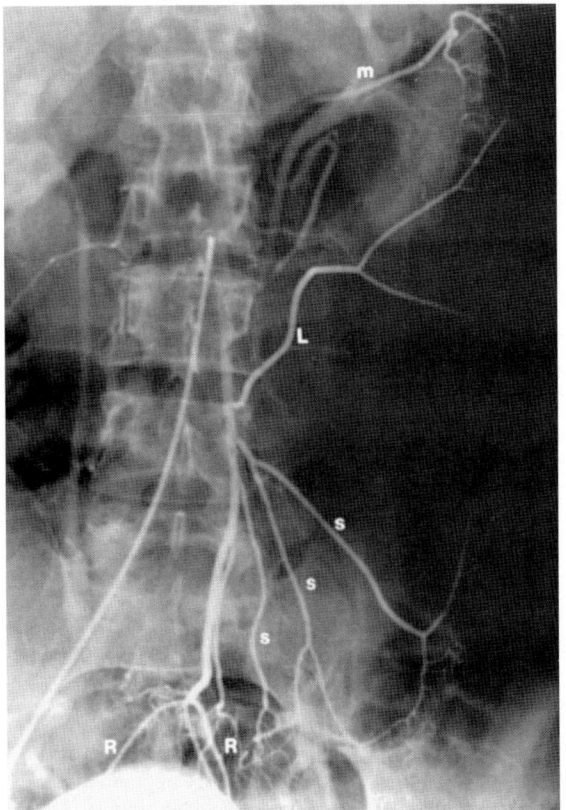

Figure 10-12. Inferior mesenteric arteriogram. L, left colic artery; s, sigmoid branches; R, superior rectal (hemorrhoidal) arteries; m, partial filling of the middle colic territory via the marginal artery.

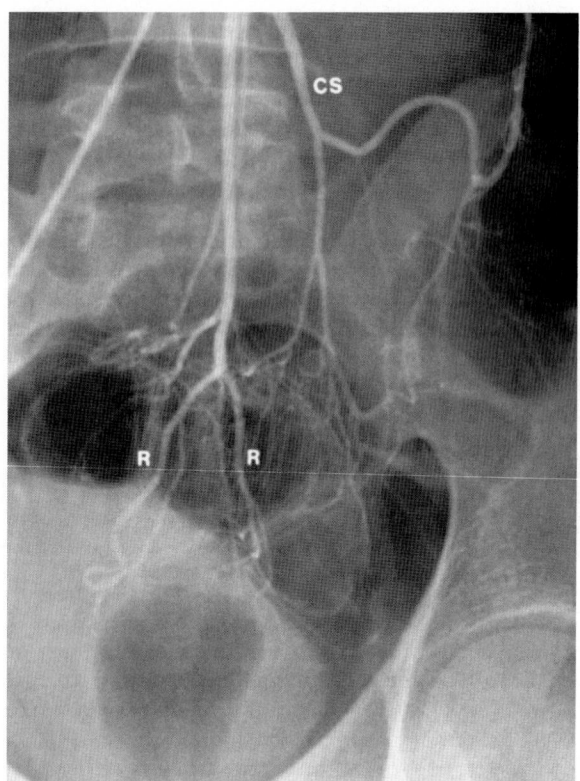

Figure 10-13. Caudal branches of inferior mesenteric trunk. CS, colosigmoid trunk; R, superior rectal (hemorrhoidal) arteries.

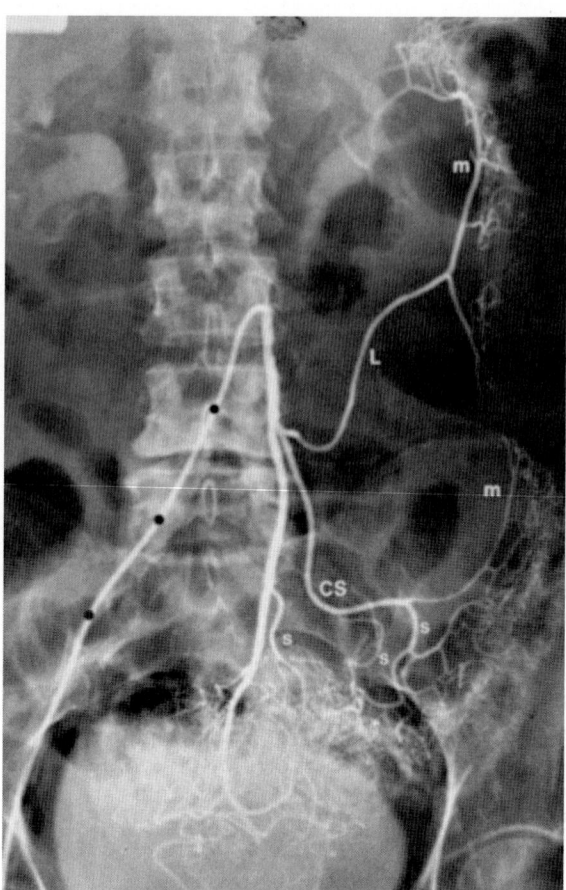

Figure 10-14. Inferior mesenteric arteriogram. L, left colic artery; CS, colosigmoid branch; s, sigmoid branches; m, marginal artery; *black dots,* selective catheter.

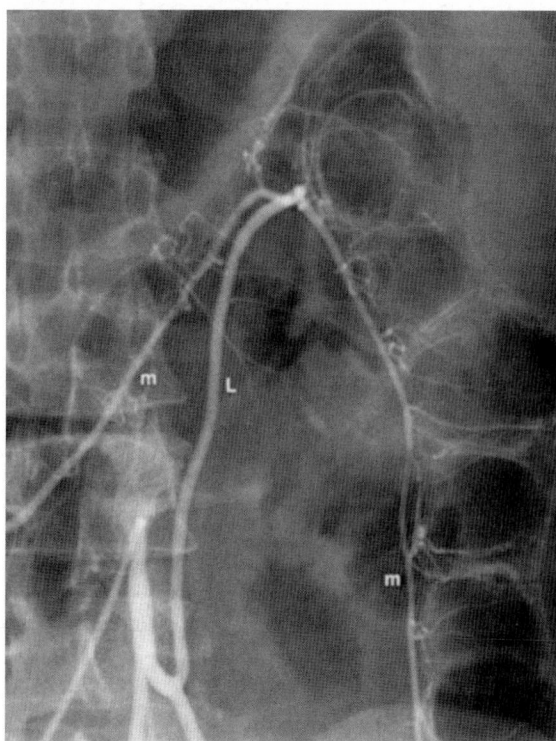

Figure 10-15. Inferior mesenteric injection. The left colic artery (L) ascends toward the left colonic flexure, and the marginal artery (m) is opacified in a continuous fashion from the transverse colon to the descending colon.

(see Figs. 10-13 and 10-14) can usually be identified as a large dominant vessel supplying the transition between the descending colon and the sigmoid.

The marginal artery of Drummond (Figs. 10-16 and 10-17; also see Figs. 10-12, 10-14, and 10-15) designates a vascular arcade that runs along the mesenteric border of the colon, where it gives off its nutrient vessels. Defined in this way, the major colic arteries can parallel the marginal artery or constitute part of it: the paracolic arcade can be considered part of the generalized system of paraintestinal arcades present throughout the abdominal gastrointestinal tract. An enlarged marginal artery frequently provides a collateral pathway between the SMA and the IMA territories (see Figs. 10-16 and 10-17). The marginal artery is not always reliably complete along its entire length. Griffith's point, for example, represents a watershed area of a potentially poor anastomotic connection between the SMA territory and the marginal artery of the descending colon at the splenic flexure; it is an area susceptible to ischemic injury when its marginal artery is poorly developed. The arc of Riolan refers to a more central anastomotic loop that lies within the mesentery, joining IMA and SMA territories. The term *meandering mesenteric artery* has also been used. This actually represents an enlarged and tortuous left colic artery (see Figs. 10-16 and 10-17) acting as part of a collateral pathway.

The more distal rectum is supplied by branches of the internal iliac territory: the middle rectal and inferior rectal

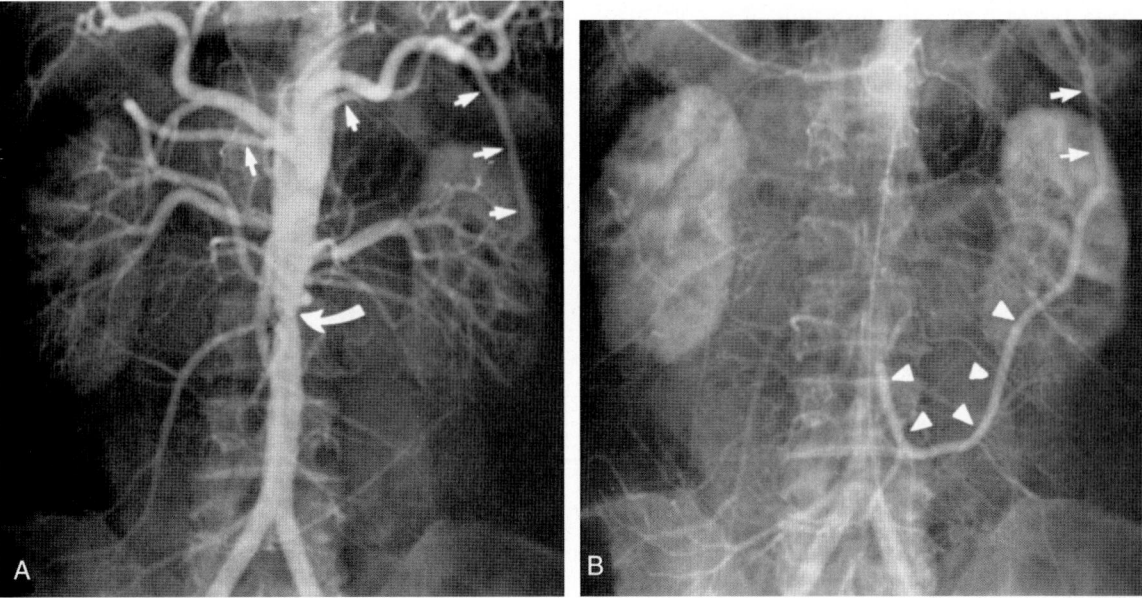

Figure 10-16. Collateral blood supply of the colon. Early (**A**) and delayed (**B**) radiographs from an abdominal aortogram show a dilated marginal artery fed by the middle colic artery, which courses along the transverse and proximal descending colon (*straight arrows*) and reconstitutes the inferior mesenteric artery via the left colic artery (*arrowheads* in **B**). Stenosis of the abdominal aorta is present between the origins of the superior and the inferior mesenteric arteries (*curved arrow* in **A**) and may contribute to diminished flow at the origin of the inferior mesenteric artery.

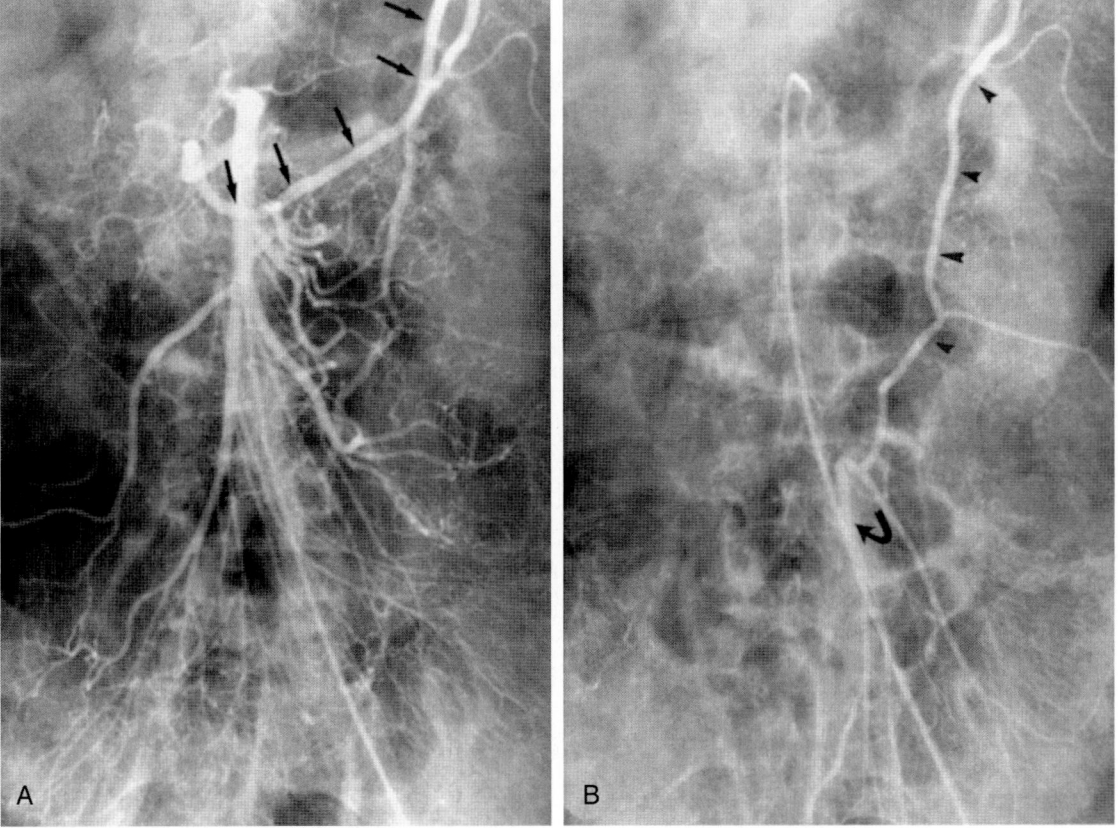

Figure 10-17. Collateral blood supply of the colon. Early (**A**) and delayed (**B**) radiographs from a superior mesenteric arteriogram demonstrate an enlarged marginal artery arising from the middle colic in **A** (*arrows*). In **B** the marginal artery fills the left colic artery (*arrowheads*) in a retrograde fashion, allowing reconstitution of the inferior mesenteric trunk (*curved arrow*). The dilated, tortuous collateral pathway has been called a meandering mesenteric artery.

arteries. As is the case with the most proximal portion of the gut, angiography of this region is infrequently performed. Collateralization via the rectal arteries between the IMA and the internal iliac system can become important in occlusive disease of the aorta and common iliac arteries.

Venous Anatomy

The mesenteric venous system is studied for two main indications: (1) evaluation of the patency of the mesenteric veins in the setting of suspected acute mesenteric ischemia and (2) evaluation of the patency and direction of flow in the mesenteric, splenic, and portal veins and potential collateral pathways in portal hypertension. As noted earlier, in patients with portal hypertension, large flow rates and volumes of contrast medium are needed for optimal visualization of these vessels, and DSA may be useful in cooperative patients. Tolazoline (Priscoline), a vasodilator that acts directly on smooth muscle, injected into the SMA improves visualization of the mesenteric and portal veins. We dilute 25 mg in 10 mL of normal saline solution and inject it slowly for 2 minutes; contrast medium injection and filming begin immediately after drug administration.

The most important gastric vein is the left gastric, or coronary, vein, which courses along the lesser curve of the stomach and joins the splenic/portal venous system at variable sites. It is a frequent pathway for portosystemic collateralization in portal hypertension and splenoportal collateralization in splenic vein occlusion. Gastro-omental and short gastric veins

parallel their respective arteries and can be important collateral pathways as well. The superior mesenteric and inferior mesenteric veins run to the right of and parallel to, and drain the respective territories of, the SMA and IMA. The superior mesenteric vein (see Fig. 10-1) joins the splenic vein behind the pancreatic neck to form the portal vein; the inferior mesenteric vein (Fig. 10-18) can join either the splenic or the superior mesenteric vein or their confluence.

VASCULAR DIAGNOSIS AND INTERVENTION IN THE GASTROINTESTINAL TRACT

Primary Vascular Pathology

Atherosclerotic involvement of the visceral arteries is common, and the angiographic appearance is typical of atherosclerosis in other locations: irregular plaque formation, eccentric or concentric stenosis, and occlusion. Visceral artery stenoses can also occur in other primary vascular disorders, including fibromuscular dysplasia, Takayasu's arteritis, and Behçet's disease, or as the result of response to extrinsic agents such as ergot preparations. It has been stated that in cases of celiac or SMA fibromuscular dysplasia, the classic "string of beads" appearance of this entity is less common than a tubular stenosis.

Although visceral artery aneurysms most commonly involve the splenic and hepatic arteries, they can occur in any of the mesenteric arteries. Causes of such aneurysms include arteriosclerosis, medial degeneration, infection (particularly common in the SMA territory), inflammation (particularly pancreatitis), dissection, connective tissue disorders, vasculitides such as polyarteritis nodosa (which involves the gastrointestinal tract in about 50% of cases) (Fig. 10-19), intravenous drug abuse, trauma, and other more unusual conditions. Many are discovered during work-up for gastrointestinal and intraperitoneal hemorrhage. Aneurysms of the gastrointestinal tract vasculature may also thrombose and, as a result, present

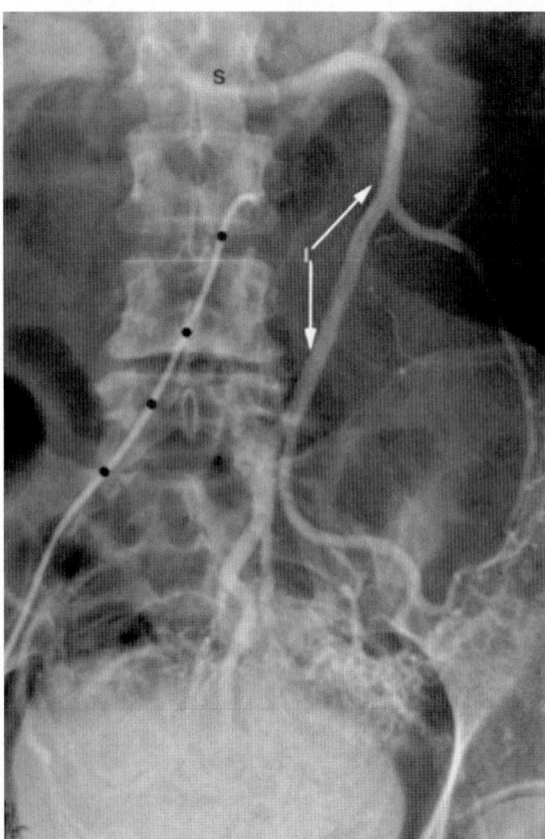

Figure 10-18. Venous phase of inferior mesenteric artery injection. The inferior mesenteric vein (I) joins the splenic vein (S). *Black dots,* catheter placed selectively into the inferior mesenteric artery.

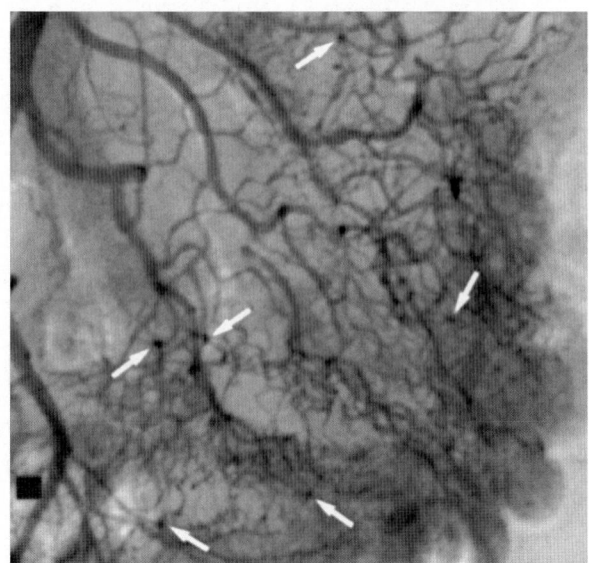

Figure 10-19. Polyarteritis nodosa. Multiple small aneurysms, some of which are indicated by *arrows,* arise from superior mesenteric branches in a patient with polyarteritis nodosa.

with mesenteric ischemia. Therapy for visceral aneurysms has traditionally been surgical, but, more recently, catheter embolization has been used successfully.[8-13]

Aneurysms of the superior mesenteric vein have also been described. Congenital, traumatic, and inflammatory causes have been proposed. Although rare, they may cause abdominal pain, gastrointestinal bleeding, or compression of adjacent structures.

Arteriovenous malformations, characterized by dilated, tortuous feeding arteries, capillary blush, and prominent venous drainage, can occur throughout the gastrointestinal tract. Thought to be developmental in origin, they are often seen in younger adults or children. They can be an elusive cause of gastrointestinal hemorrhage, often discovered only on angiographic work-up for the same. MDCT has proven useful in the depiction of some of these vascular malformations.

Vascular malformations of the gastrointestinal tract may also occur in association with systemic disorders such as pseudoxanthoma elasticum, hereditary hemorrhagic telangiectasia, and Klippel-Trenaunay-Weber syndrome. Pseudoxanthoma elasticum is a hereditary, autosomal recessive disorder of connective tissue that involves systemic abnormalities of elastic fibers. Patients display characteristic ocular and cutaneous lesions. Cardiovascular manifestations occur because of fragmentation, degeneration, and calcification of the arterial elastic laminae and premature atherosclerosis. A variety of splanchnic angiographic abnormalities have been described, including angiomatous malformations, vascular tortuosity, segments of vascular narrowing and occlusion, and small aneurysms. Upper gastrointestinal tract bleeding is common and probably results from submucosal vascular degeneration and inability of the abnormal vessels to constrict at sites adjacent to areas of erosion and hemorrhage. Embolization has been used to treat hemorrhage in this disorder.[8-14]

Patients with hereditary hemorrhagic telangiectasia (Osler-Weber-Rendu disease) have multiple systemic vascular lesions involving the skin, mucous membranes, and gut. Abnormalities on abdominal visceral angiography include tangled masses of tortuous vessels with early venous filling, direct arteriovenous fistulas, arterial aneurysms, localized venous dilatations, and small focal accumulations of contrast medium representing angiomas that are visualized during the arterial phase of injection of the contrast medium. Thin, fragile walls are characteristic of these vascular lesions and help explain their propensity to bleed; recurrent gastrointestinal hemorrhage is common.

Arteriovenous fistulas of the mesenteric vessels can be congenital or can result from penetrating trauma or from prior abdominal surgery. Successful transcatheter embolization of fistulas involving main mesenteric trunks or branches has been described.

Tumors

Although rarely used in the primary diagnosis of tumors of the gastrointestinal tract, angiography will occasionally detect neoplasms as incidental abnormalities or as the cause of active or occult gastrointestinal bleeding. Gastrointestinal stromal tumors are common neoplasms of the upper gastrointestinal tract and small bowel that have a tendency to bleed. They are typically hypervascular and well defined on angiography (Fig. 10-20); venous shunting is common in gastrointestinal stromal tumors of the small bowel but not typical of those in the stomach. Carcinoid tumors elicit a fibrotic response in the adjacent mesentery that is reflected in a characteristic angiographic appearance of stellate crowding, kinking, and an irregular contour of mesenteric branches. The neoplasm itself is hypovascular but can cause smooth arterial narrowings and occlusions. Venous drainage is typically via multiple collaterals. As might be expected, other processes resulting in mesenteric fibrosis may give a similar appearance.

Adenocarcinomas of the small bowel tend to show signs of encasement without tumor vascularity; in the colon, lesions may be hypervascular. Adenomatous polyps of the colon are

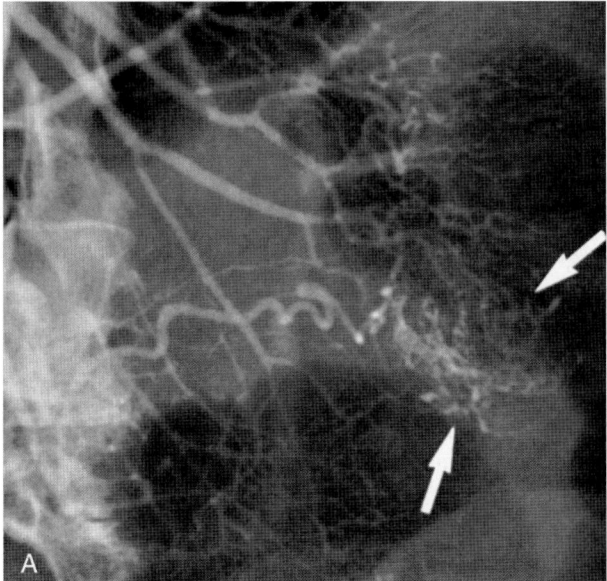 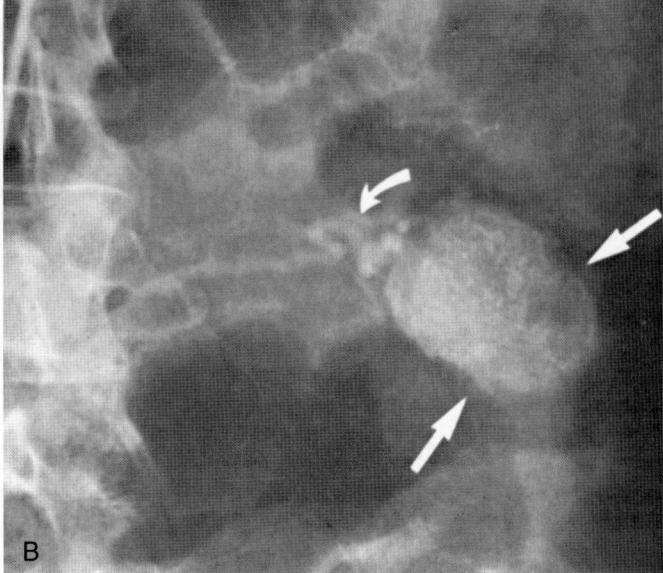

Figure 10-20. Superior mesenteric arteriography in a patient with intermittent arterial bleeding. A. Increased vascularity (*arrows*) is noted in a portion of the jejunum in the arterial phase. **B.** In the late arterial phase, a well-defined tumor stain (*straight arrows*) is noted, with a dilated early draining vein (*curved arrow*). Diagnosis: gastrointestinal stromal tumor.

hypovascular in most instances, whereas villous adenomas tend to be vascular lesions, with enlarged feeding arteries and draining veins and contrast staining in the parenchymal phase.

Other primary and metastatic upper gastrointestinal tract tumors, depending on their pathology, may demonstrate non-specific signs of neoplasia, including neovascularity, vascular encasement, vascular displacement and stretching, and arteriovenous shunting.

Inflammatory Disorders

Angiography is seldom used in the work-up of inflammatory lesions such as ulcerative colitis, Crohn's disease, or diverticulitis. Acute inflammation usually produces nonspecific findings: increased vascularity with enlargement of feeding arteries, dense capillary blush of the bowel wall, and enlargement and sometimes early opacification of draining veins. In the colon, these findings overlap with those found in early ischemic colitis and may even be normal in the postprandial state. As Crohn's disease progresses, arterial occlusions, irre-gular arterial narrowing, and hypovascularity may develop in the involved segment.

Angiodysplasia of the Colon

Angiodysplasia (vascular ectasia) of the colon is a vascular disorder that usually affects the right colon in elderly individuals. It has a number of characteristic angiographic features, which depend on the stage and size of the lesion: intense and prolonged opacification of a dilated and tortuous mural colonic vein (the earliest sign), vascular "tufts" (small, densely staining clusters of vessels), tortuous feeding (Fig. 10-21). To ensure that the early opacification of the draining vein is not simply the result of prolonged arterial injection, it helps to limit the duration of injection of contrast medium to 4 seconds or less.

Although the exact cause is unknown, angiodysplasia may be the result of a degenerative process in which intermittent intramural venous obstruction leads to venous dilatation and, later, to direct arteriovenous communication. There is an association of colonic vascular ectasia and aortic stenosis.

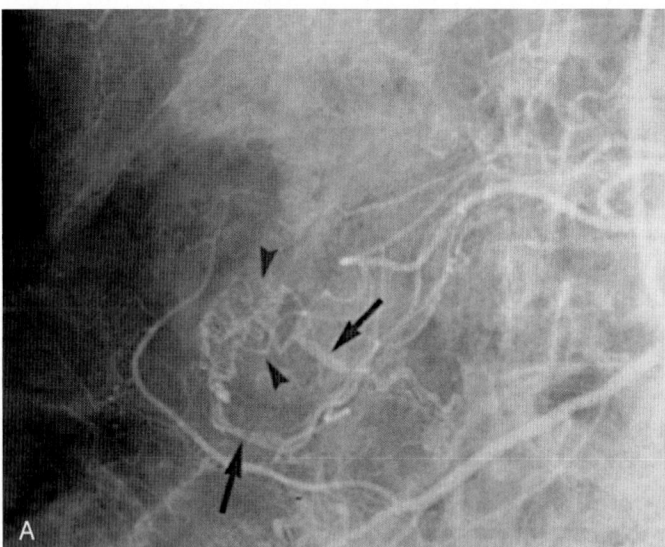

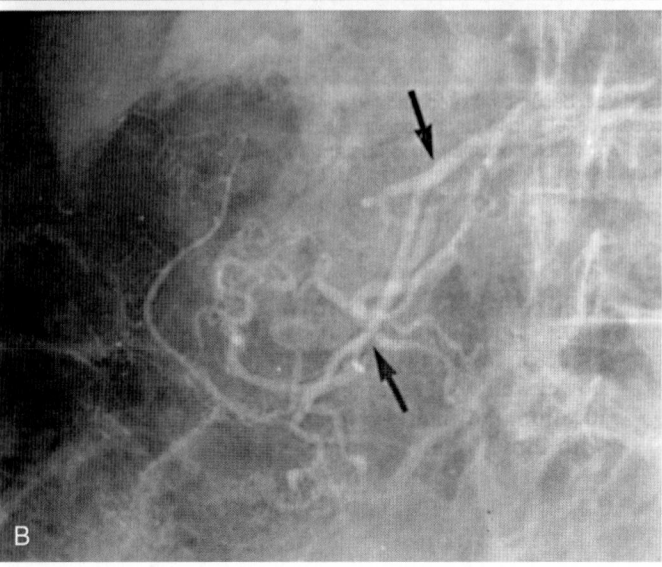

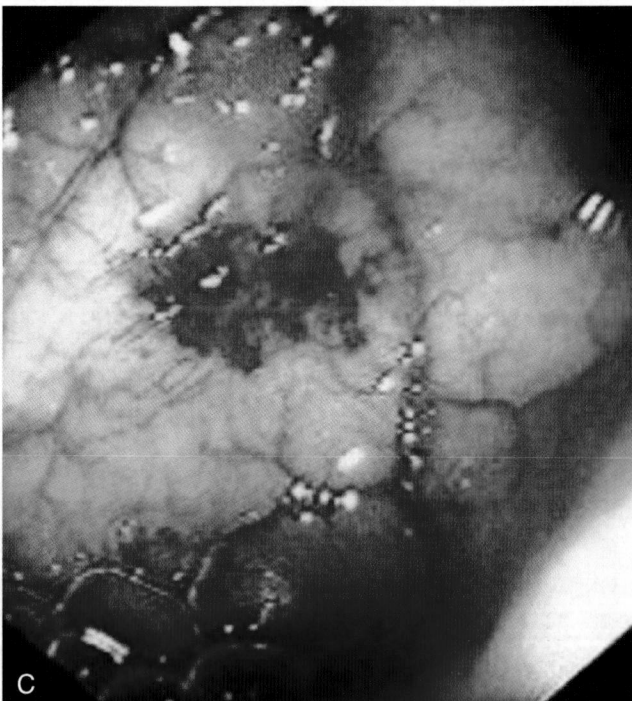

Figure 10-21. Angiodysplasia of the right colon. A. Angiogram in a patient with intermittent lower gastrointestinal hemorrhage demonstrates a vascular tuft (*arrowheads*) and paired vessels (*arrows*) indicating early draining veins adjacent to colonic arterial branches. **B.** Prominent draining veins (*arrows*) are opacified later in the angiogram. **C.** Colonoscopic view demonstrates an abnormal tuft of vessels in the right colon in a patient with gastrointestinal hemorrhage.

Miscellaneous Vascular Disorders

The effects of radiation therapy on the mesenteric vasculature depend on the time course relative to such therapy. In the subacute phase, a hyperemic "blush" associated with early venous drainage has been described, correlating with an inflammatory response. In the more chronic setting, radiation enteritis may produce obliterative findings, with irregular stenoses or occlusions of mesenteric branches, as well as findings related to shortening of bowel length, including tortuosity and vascular crowding.

Abnormalities of bowel position, although not typically diagnosed by angiography, may also be picked up in the angiographic work-up of abdominal symptoms. Findings in conditions such as intussusception, internal hernias, and volvulus include unusual displacement of vessels, abrupt angulation and overlapping of branches, and abrupt changes in vessel caliber.

ACUTE MESENTERIC ISCHEMIA

Clinical and Angiographic Features

Multidetector CT has become the major imaging method for assessing patients with acute abdominal pain. Because it can evaluate the bowel wall, the surrounding mesentery, and major vascular structures, MDCT can often suggest the presence of mesenteric ischemia or infarction and depict the thrombus if it is sufficiently large and central. Angiography provides detailed anatomic and etiologic information necessary for the urgent management of mesenteric ischemia and, in addition, allows initiation of selective transcatheter therapy when appropriate.

Lateral abdominal aortography reveals the status of the proximal mesenteric vessels and should be the initial step in angiographic evaluation of mesenteric ischemia. If the proximal portion of the SMA is patent, selective arteriography of this vessel is performed for a detailed study of the superior mesenteric trunk and its branches and of the mesenteric venous drainage. Acute mesenteric ischemia is primarily a disorder of the SMA territory, and selective celiac and inferior mesenteric injections are not usually necessary. However, these further studies can provide information about the presence and extent of collateral supply to the superior mesenteric territory, particularly when the chronicity of a superior mesenteric occlusion is questioned. These additional angiograms can also be considered if clinical data strongly suggest involvement of the stomach, the duodenum, or the segment of colon supplied by the IMA.

Major causes of acute mesenteric ischemia are SMA thrombosis or embolism, mesenteric venous thrombosis, and the nonocclusive form of ischemia. Vasculitis, aortic or mesenteric arterial dissection, trauma, bowel strangulation, and other disorders are less common causes of mesenteric ischemia. Involvement of all or most of the SMA territory typically produces severe and life-threatening mesenteric ischemia. Focal ischemia can result from more limited or segmental forms of the previously mentioned causes and has less severe clinical manifestations.[15-20]

SMA occlusion (Figs. 10-22 through 10-25) with embolism is more common than thrombosis. The angiographic distinction between these two entities can be difficult. Multiple filling defects, tracking of contrast medium at the lateral aspects

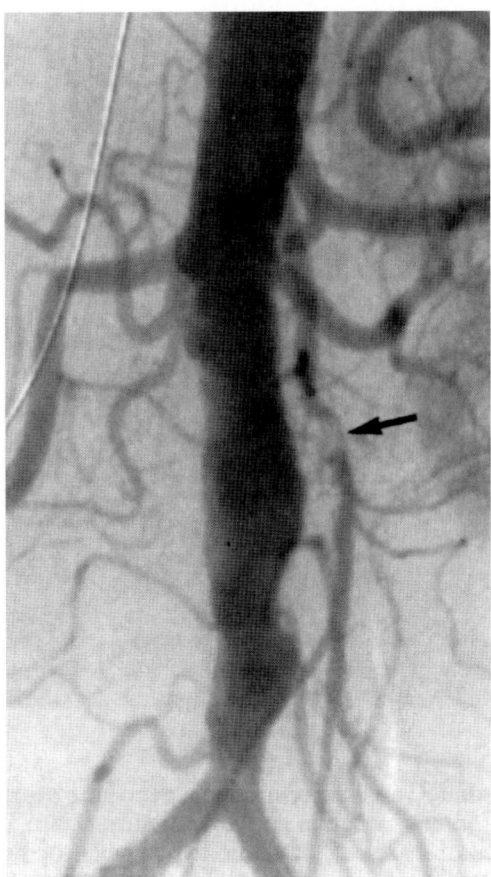

Figure 10-22. Superior mesenteric embolus. A nearly occlusive filling defect (*arrow*) is present in the main superior mesenteric artery trunk, with tracking of contrast medium around it and patency of the more distal superior mesenteric artery.

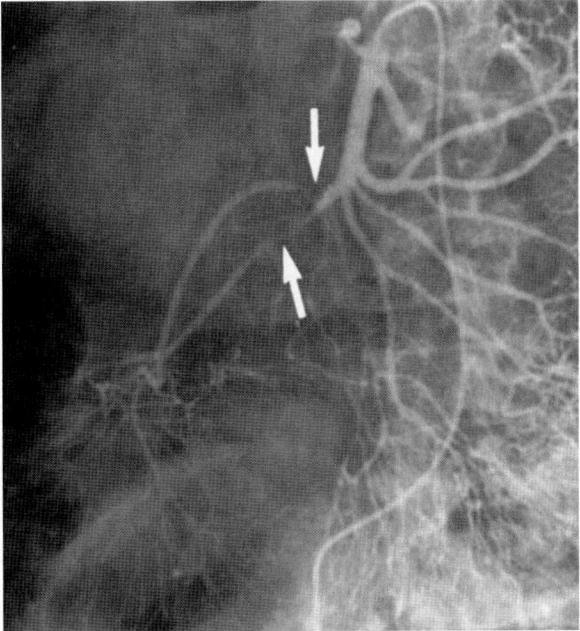

Figure 10-23. Superior mesenteric emboli. Multiple filling defects (*arrows*) are present in the superior mesenteric artery branches in a patient with atrial fibrillation.

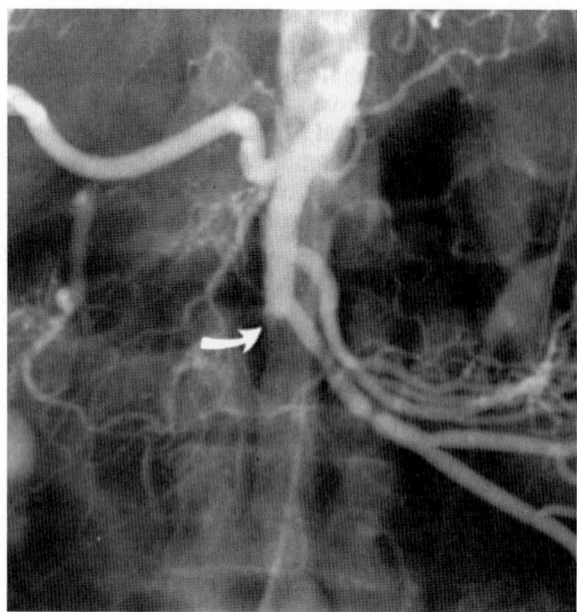

Figure 10-24. Superior mesenteric embolus. Abrupt occlusion (*arrow*) of the superior mesenteric trunk is present distal to jejunal branches in a patient with atrial fibrillation.

of a filling defect, and convex menisci protruding into the opacified vascular lumen suggest emboli. Emboli also tend to lodge at vascular branch points, generally more distally than occlusive thrombus, which typically forms in the vicinity of a preexistent atherosclerotic stenosis of the proximal SMA. At times, however, emboli can lodge at proximal stenoses, or an embolus can initiate more proximal or distal propagation of thrombus. Extramesenteric emboli are common in cases of embolic mesenteric ischemia.[15-20]

Mesenteric venous thrombosis accounts for up to 10% to 20% of cases of acute mesenteric ischemia. Causes of this

disorder include bowel obstruction, hypercoagulable states, portal hypertension, abdominal inflammatory disease, previous surgery (particularly splenectomy), and trauma. Often, no predisposing condition is identified. Patients may present with less severe illness than in other forms of acute mesenteric ischemia; recognition that major venous occlusion does not always result in ischemia has increased as more cases of mesenteric venous thrombosis are identified with the use of cross-sectional imaging. MDCT has excellent sensitivity for the diagnosis. However, angiographic recognition remains important as part of the favored algorithm for acute mesenteric ischemia. On superior mesenteric arteriography, slowing of arterial flow is noted, with prolonged staining of the bowel wall and of smaller mesenteric arterial branches. Arterial vasoconstriction may be present. Normal mesenteric veins either fail to opacify or show filling defects; venous collaterals may be visualized.[15-20]

Anatomic vascular obstruction need not be present for mesenteric ischemia and infarction to occur. Diminished cardiac output, systemic hypotension or hypovolemia, and certain pharmacologic agents—particularly digitalis—can result in severely diminished intestinal blood flow, presumably mediated by vasoconstriction of the mesenteric arteries. Nonocclusive mesenteric ischemia (see Fig. 10-25) accounts for a substantial proportion of cases of acute mesenteric ischemia. On angiography, intense vasospasm is characteristic. Spasm is frequently irregular or segmental, with more severe areas of narrowing often seen at the origins of arterial branches. Regular and diffuse spasm can also occur. Contrast medium flows sluggishly through mesenteric vessels, causing delayed opacification of peripheral and mural branches. In this regard, the findings are similar to those of mesenteric venous thrombosis, although normal veins eventually fill in most cases of nonocclusive ischemia. Increased reflux of contrast medium into the aorta can also be seen, reflecting increased impedance to mesenteric flow. In practice, this finding is

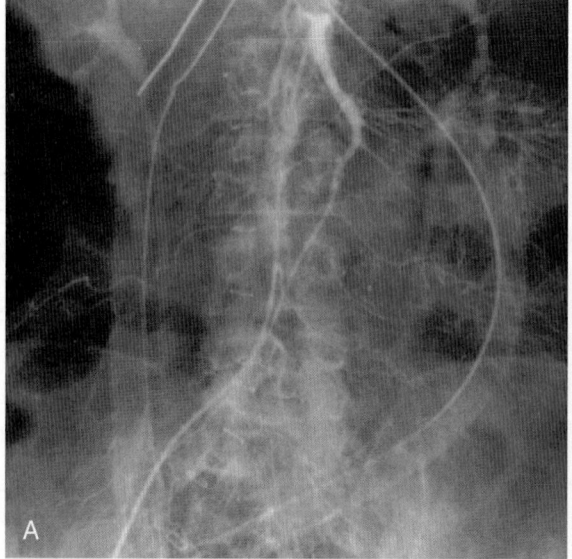

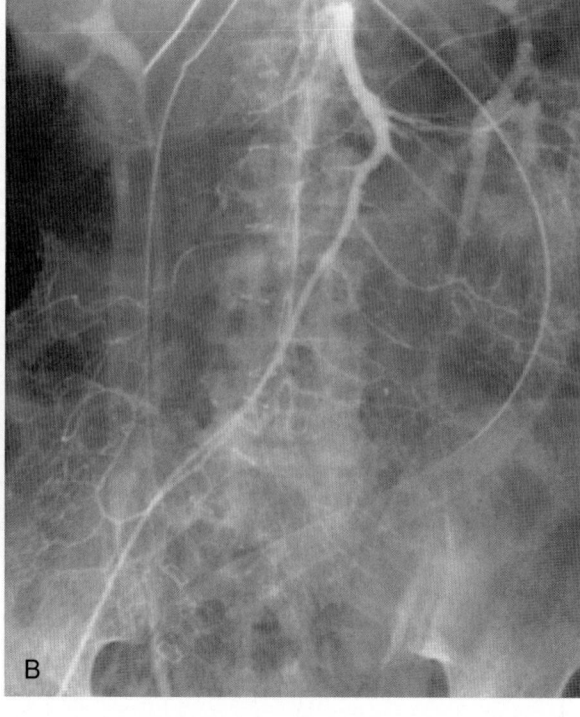

Figure 10-25. Nonocclusive mesenteric ischemia. A. Diffuse mesenteric arterial spasm is present, with poor filling of smaller arterial branches. **B.** Improvement in the spasm is noted after initiation of intra-arterial papaverine infusion.

usually judged subjectively, although more objective and quantitative means of assessing superior mesenteric flow based on aortic reflux have been described.

Despite improved methods of diagnosis and therapy for acute mesenteric ischemia, this disorder continues to be associated with a high mortality rate. In the late 1970s, Boley and colleagues described their "aggressive approach" to acute mesenteric ischemia that remains the standard of care. Although about half of the patients presenting with the full syndrome of acute mesenteric ischemia still die, this approach represents a distinct improvement compared with earlier controlled studies that showed only 10% to 30% survival; in addition, the aggressive approach may allow more bowel to be salvaged in those who have survived. Key features of this approach include maintenance of a high level of suspicion for the disorder, followed by prompt diagnosis and therapy utilizing emergency angiography.[15-20]

Another feature of the aggressive algorithm is the selective infusion of vasodilators (see Fig. 10-25) into the SMA, the rationale being that vasospasm is associated with acute mesenteric ischemia, not only the nonocclusive variety but occlusive forms as well. When mesenteric angiography has revealed vasospasm or arterial occlusion, a test dose of a vasodilator should be given.

Thrombolytic Therapy for Mesenteric Vascular Occlusion

In most instances of acute mesenteric ischemia (Figs. 10-26 and 10-27) with major vascular occlusion, the rapid deterioration of bowel status with time and the need to resect in-

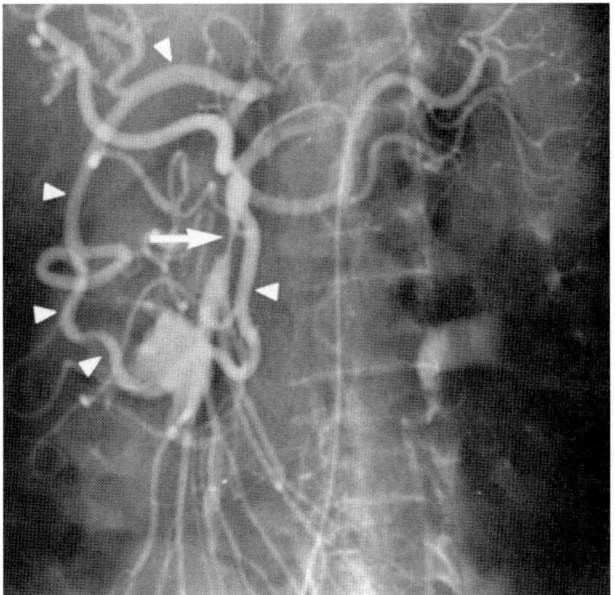

Figure 10-26. Chronic mesenteric ischemia. Superior mesenteric arteriogram of a 62-year-old woman with intermittent episodes of abdominal pain reveals a severe superior mesenteric artery stenosis (*arrow*). There is filling of the celiac territory via an enlarged pancreaticoduodenal arcade (*arrowheads*) (the inferior pancreaticoduodenal artery arises from the superior mesenteric artery proximal to the stenosis). The presence of the collateral flow attests to the occlusion of the celiac origin, as also noted with lateral aortography. Symptomatic relief occurred after patch angioplasty of the superior mesenteric artery and aorta-to-celiac artery bypass with autologous vein.

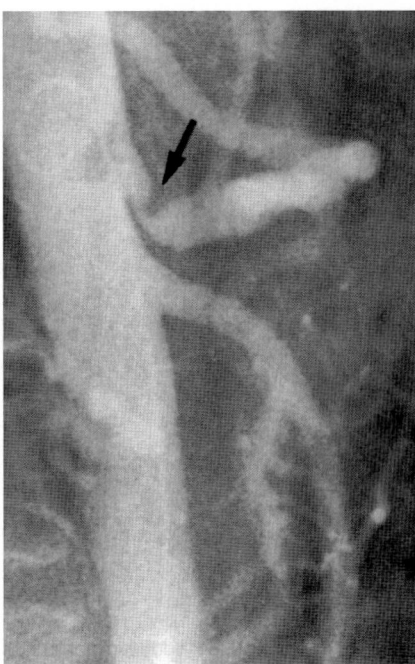

Figure 10-27. Celiac artery compression (*arrow*). Typical appearance shown by a lateral aortogram.

farcted bowel mandate prompt surgical therapy. However, a number of case reports suggest a potential role for transcatheter thrombolytic therapy or (via a transhepatic route) mechanical thrombectomy in selected cases of recent mesenteric vascular occlusion, either alone or, as with vasodilator therapy, as part of a combined treatment approach. Candidates for this therapy (Fig. 10-28) have included patients deemed unlikely to survive major surgery because of coexistent disease, those with minor or partial vascular occlusions or mild symptoms (who, it could be argued, might need only observation, conservative therapy, and possibly anticoagulation), those with extensive portal/mesenteric venous thrombosis precluding surgical thrombectomy or bypass, and those who develop occlusion of mesenteric arterial grafts. The presence of peritoneal signs suggesting bowel necrosis is considered a contraindication to thrombolytic therapy alone.

The following section has been conceived as a response to the question of why radiologists might place needles or catheters into or through portions of the gastrointestinal tract.

Inadvertent Catheterization of the Bowel

The first topic relates not to a specific indication but to a complication that has been described in the setting of a variety of abdominal interventions, specifically unintentional puncture of and placement of tubes into (Fig. 10-29) or through bowel. The underlying principle of management (and one that is reiterated later) is that, given intrinsically normal bowel with no distal obstruction, intestinal contents will flow preferentially along the intestinal lumen. When inadvertent catheterization occurs, handling of the complication should include drainage of any adjacent infected fluid. Antibiotics, bowel rest, and extended catheter drainage (to allow an organized tract to form) should permit safe catheter withdrawal; at this point, the site of perforation should seal readily due to muscular contraction of the bowel wall.

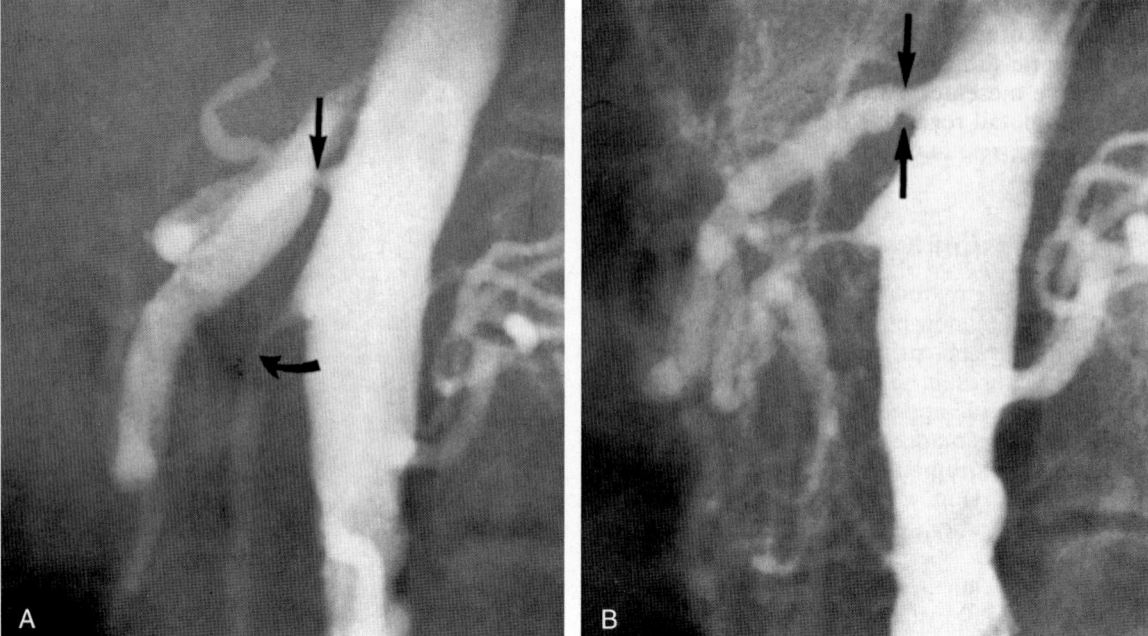

Figure 10-28. Balloon angioplasty. A. Lateral aortography shows severe narrowing of the celiac (*straight arrow*) and superior mesenteric (*curved arrow*) arteries in a patient with symptoms of chronic mesenteric ischemia. **B.** Improved patency of the celiac artery (*arrows*) is noted after balloon angioplasty. The superior mesenteric stenosis could not be catheterized; despite this, there was symptomatic improvement. The case also illustrates a possible complication of this procedure: catheterization via a left axillary puncture site was necessary for celiac angioplasty, and the patient developed a large axillary pseudoaneurysm with a left upper extremity neurologic deficit.

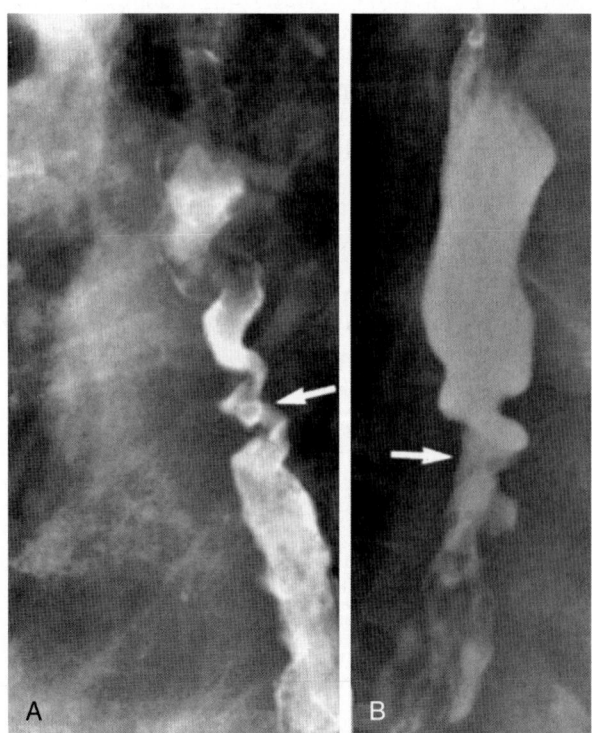

Figure 10-29. Dilatation of a benign esophageal stricture. Predilatation (**A**) and postdilatation (**B**) images. Endoscopic dilatation was first attempted but proved difficult in this elderly patient. A steerable wire was manipulated through the stenosis under fluoroscopic guidance. After dilatation of the stricture (*arrow*) to 15 mm, symptomatic improvement was noted.

Transenteric Biopsy and Fluid Aspiration

Frequently, bowel is interposed along potential paths for percutaneous diagnostic aspiration of fluid collections or biopsy of masses. Transgression of bowel in such cases as well as during therapeutic drainage can sometimes be avoided by the use of injection of physiologic saline solution or carbon dioxide to displace structures. Nevertheless, avoidance of bowel is not always possible. Because the aspirating needle passes through a colonized space, with increasing bacterial counts the more distal the segment of the gastrointestinal tract, the potential for contamination must be acknowledged: either confounding of culture results in fluid aspiration or leakage of contaminated contents along the path of the needle. The former instance may be aided by Gram stain of fluid, because a contaminated sample will tend not to have a cellular response. With regard to the latter, considerable clinical and laboratory experience seems to indicate that transgression of the bowel wall with fine needles rarely leads to clinically evident infectious complications. As with any interventional procedure, the risks of bowel puncture should be balanced against the risks of alternate methods of diagnosis and the need to obtain a pathologic or microbiologic diagnosis. Although it seems prudent to choose an approach that avoids bowel, particularly colon, and although it seems reasonable to avoid larger cutting needles if bowel must be punctured, the need to pass a needle through bowel does not in itself constitute a contraindication to needle aspiration. Possible exceptions would include passage through an obstructed loop or through bowel in an immunosuppressed patient, although little hard data exist in these settings.

Puncture of Bowel to Confirm Identity

At times, unopacified bowel loops may mimic abnormal fluid collections; conversely, collapsed loops may mimic masses (e.g., in the case of afferent loops in patients with a history of gastrointestinal malignancy). Percutaneous puncture of such indeterminate structures with thin needles and injection of water-soluble contrast medium can be invaluable in guiding further diagnosis and therapy. Contrast medium is injected through one of the needles as it is withdrawn; if bowel has been crossed, the needles can be withdrawn and another path chosen.

Drainage of Fluid Collections Shielded by Bowel

Taking the concept of transenteric diagnostic aspiration (Figs. 10-30 through 10-33) a step farther, and mimicking traditional surgical therapy (e.g., pseudocystogastrostomy) to some extent, transenteric drainage of infected or inflammatory fluid

collections has been proposed. This has been an area of particular interest in the setting of pancreatitis, which is often associated with lesser sac collections unapproachable for percutaneous drainage except through the stomach. Although the approach is controversial, its advocates argue that it can help avoid spillage of pancreatic enzymes around the drainage site and prevent formation of pancreaticocutaneous fistulas. Along the same lines, there is growing favorable experience with transrectal drainage of pelvic collections, either by standard catheter placement or by "one-step" complete aspiration. This approach offers increased patient comfort and possibly decreased complications compared with the more standard transgluteal drainage route.

Diagnostic Biopsy of Bowel Masses

Several investigators have found sonographic and fluoroscopic (via barium studies) biopsy of pathologic processes directly

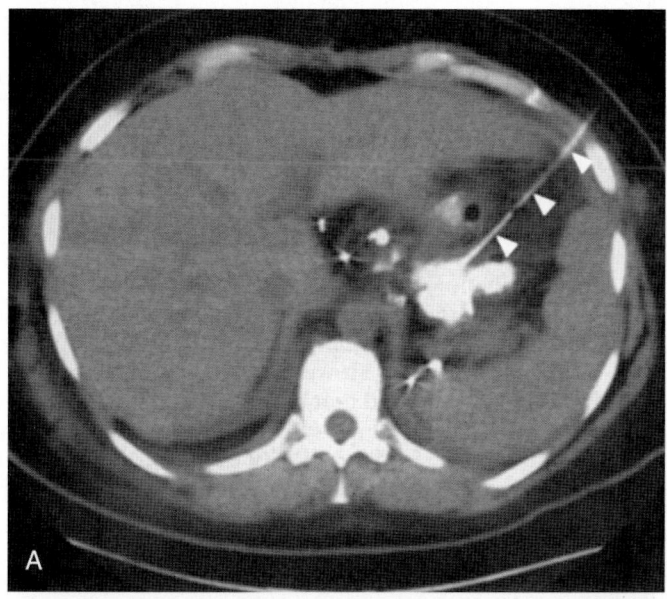

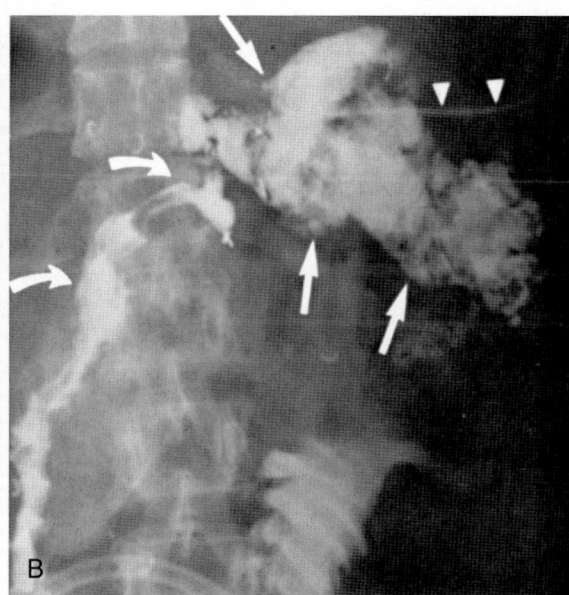

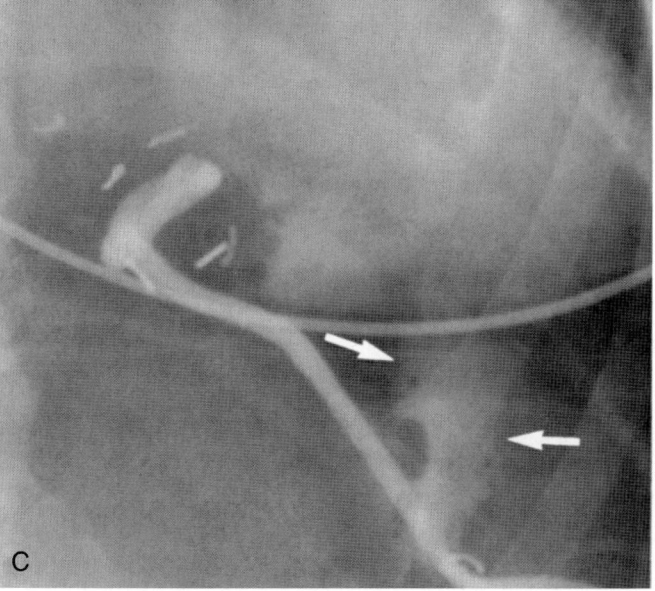

Figure 10-30. Abscess drainage. Images of a patient with a history of lye-induced esophageal and gastric injury in whom a colonic interposition and coloenteric anastomosis were carried out. **A.** After the patient presented with fever and nausea, a left upper quadrant abscess was drained under CT guidance. A drainage catheter (*arrowheads*) enters an abscess cavity containing contrast medium. **B.** Sinogram obtained via drainage catheter (*arrowheads*) shows an irregular abscess cavity (*straight arrows*) that communicates with the bowel (*curved arrows*). **C.** After 8 weeks of catheter drainage, contrast medium injection results in spill (*arrows*) along the tract to collect on the skin surface; there was no filling of bowel. The catheter was removed without recurrence of earlier symptoms.

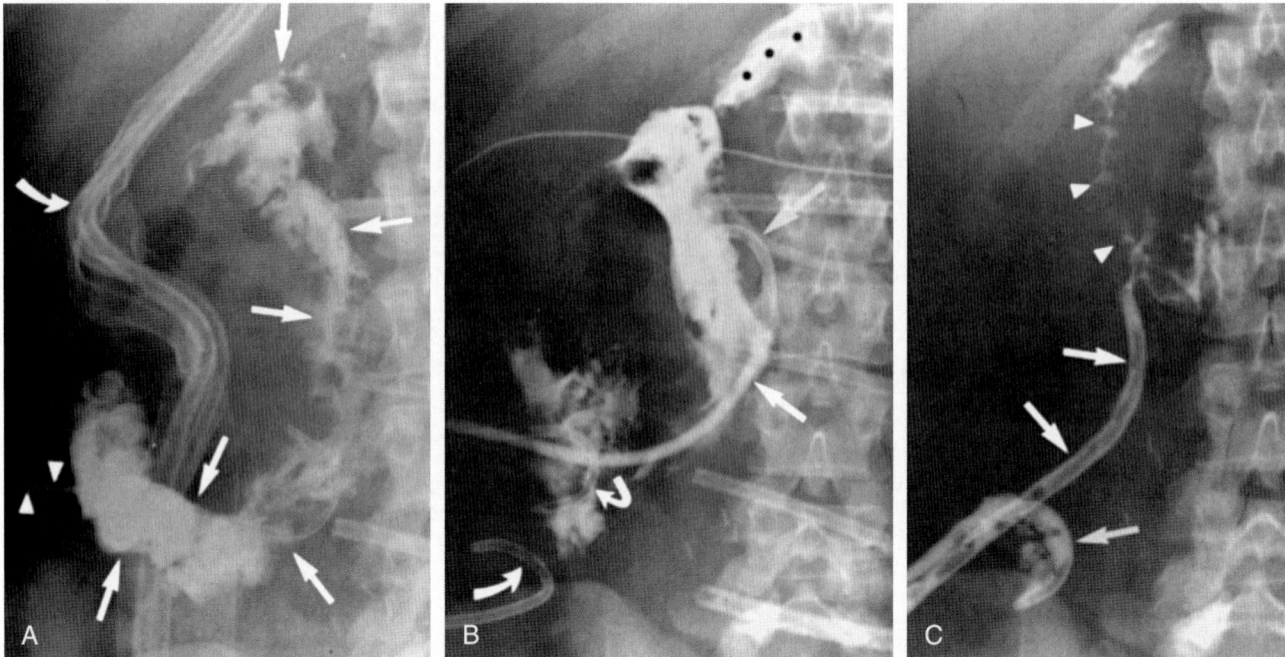

Figure 10-31. Abscess drainage: multiple catheters. Bowel injury was discovered at laparotomy in a patient who had abdominal trauma. **A.** Sinogram obtained immediately after abscess drainage. The drainage catheter (*arrowheads*) enters an irregular cavity (*straight arrows*); no filling of bowel is noted on initial injection. *Curved arrow,* surgical drain. **B.** Ten days later, three drainage catheters have been placed, two in the lower portion of the abscess cavity (*curved arrows*) and one in its cephalad aspect (*straight arrow*). Filling of bowel (*black dots*) is now apparent. **C.** Three months later, the abscess cavity has almost completely collapsed, but a fistula to the bowel (*arrowheads*) is still present. Two catheters remain in place (*arrows*). With continued drainage, the fistula eventually closed and the catheters were removed.

involving the bowel wall both effective and safe. Indications for this approach include (1) lesions yielding no diagnostic tissue via endoscopic biopsy (a common problem with submucosal lesions); (2) lesions in patients who are poor candidates for endoscopy or open exploration; (3) lesions that because of their location are not accessible endoscopically; and (4) lesions that, if proved malignant, will obviate the need for further investigation or change in therapy.[21,22]

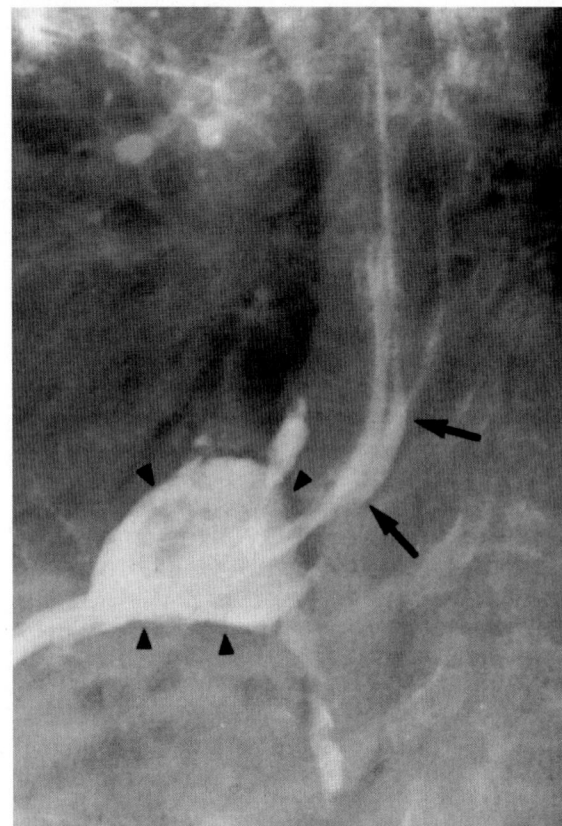

Figure 10-32. Percutaneous drainage of an esophageal leak. Sinogram performed after CT-guided drainage of a juxtapleural fluid collection (*arrowheads*) shows communication with the esophagus (*arrows*).

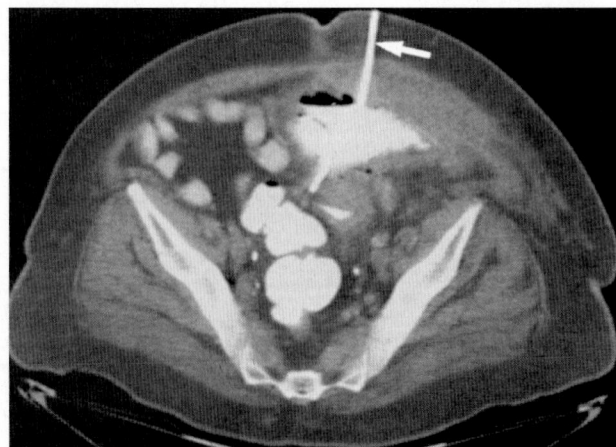

Figure 10-33. Percutaneous drainage of a diverticular abscess. A drain (*arrow*) courses through the anterior abdominal wall and enters the abscess, which has been opacified with contrast medium. The patient underwent a single-stage surgical resection after successful abscess drainage.

Enteric Puncture for Diagnostic or Therapeutic Access

An uncommon but potentially very useful application of transenteric access is to allow diagnostic or therapeutic access to various structures.

One example of this is access to gastrointestinal tract strictures difficult to reach via nasoenteric or rectal approaches. Another novel approach involved placement of a percutaneous cecostomy tube to allow diagnostic and therapeutic endoscopy of the small bowel in a patient who was bleeding from ileal angiodysplasia.

Transenteric access to the biliary tree can be used in cases in which a choledochojejunostomy or hepaticojejunostomy has been performed previously. Advantages of the approach are that it allows repeated access to the biliary tree without the need to traverse liver parenchyma, that it gives a mechanical advantage in cases in which multiple sites of disease need to be treated (e.g., sclerosing cholangitis), and that it allows easier access when the biliary tree is nondilated. Surgical techniques anticipating these advantages have been designed to allow easier access to the relevant bowel loop. Initially, this consisted of a formal jejunostomy or so-called Hutson loop. Although access to the bowel was guaranteed, problems with skin excoriation due to leakage of bile or mucus developed. Subcutaneous tacking of the jejunal loop was another option, but this was plagued by subcutaneous inflammation in the early postoperative period and by peristomal hernias later on. Consequently, the favored approach at this time is subparietal tacking of the loop, the site of which can be marked with surgical clips.

Puncture is generally performed with fluoroscopic guidance (by identification of the gas within the loop), although opacification could potentially be obtained with manipulation of a nasoenteric tube.

Enteral Access for Bowel Decompression

Whereas percutaneous gastrostomy is most frequently used to provide a route for enteral alimentation, it can also serve as an effective means of decompressing the bowel in patients with chronic intestinal obstruction and symptoms of nausea and vomiting, eliminating most of complications associated with long-term nasogastric intubation. However, this subset of patients may present unique technical problems, mainly the result of more limited access to the stomach due to diffuse peritoneal carcinomatosis, adhesions from prior radiation or surgical therapy, or ascites. Gastrostomy has also been used to provide symptomatic relief in a patient with gastroparesis or delay in gastric emptying in the absence of a fixed anatomic obstruction.

Direct percutaneous small bowel catheterization has also been used to treat symptoms of enteric obstruction or stasis in instances in which gastric decompression alone would not suffice. Such situations usually require surgery, but percutaneous management can be considered an alternative in patients who are poor surgical candidates. Maneuvers designed to distend or fix the bowel are often not possible, nor are they likely to be necessary because significant intrinsic distention of bowel is present. Acute palliation and long-term prevention of recurrence of closed-loop obstruction in a patient with metastatic colon carcinoma have been described. Symptoms of blind or afferent loop stasis have also been relieved by this

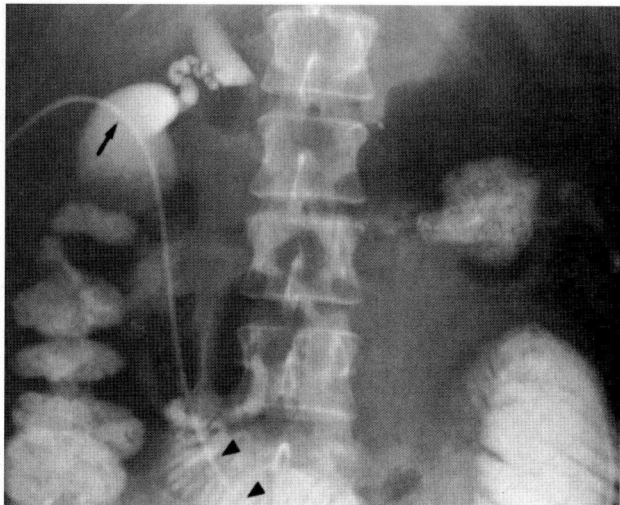

Figure 10-34. Percutaneous cholecystostomy. A patient with pancreatic carcinoma, after Roux-en-Y cholecystojejunostomy and gastrojejunostomy, who developed abdominal pain, elevated serum bilirubin level, and septicemia. CT revealed a dilated afferent bowel loop anastomosed to the gallbladder. Percutaneous cholecystostomy with passage of a catheter via the gallbladder (*arrow*) and into the jejunal loop (*arrowheads*) resulted in improvement of symptoms.

method. An alternative approach in afferent loop syndromes has been percutaneous management: a drainage tube can be passed percutaneously into the liver or gallbladder and through the biliary tree into the affected bowel limb (Fig. 10-34). A possible benefit of this route is simultaneous drainage of the biliary tree, because these patients may have associated biliary stasis or cholangitis. The occurrence of delayed septic shock in one patient in whom transhepatic treatment of an afferent loop was performed suggests that placement of a separate biliary drain may be advisable. In appropriate circumstances, feeding tubes have been placed via a transhepatic biliary route. It is important in such cases to infuse feeding solutions through a tube placed well beyond the native or postsurgical biliary-enteric junction.

In nonobstructive colonic distention, the cecum is usually the most severely involved segment. This finding demonstrates the Laplace law, in which the portion of colon with the greatest diameter (the cecum) responds first with further distention once intraluminal pressure begins to increase. *Cecal ileus* refers to the situation in which cecal distention develops out of proportion to that of the remainder of the colon. These patients have a mobile cecum suspended on a mesentery. When the patient is in the supine position, the cecum can rotate anteriorly, leading to progressive distention.

Massive colonic distention, when left untreated, may lead to colonic perforation, ischemia, peritonitis, and death. Once massive distention (≥9 cm) of the cecum occurs, the risk of perforation seems less related to the absolute degree of distention than to the duration of distention. Therefore, early recognition of and therapy for this condition is critical.

The initial treatment of nonobstructive colonic distention is conservative and includes placement of a nasogastric tube, withholding of oral intake, and treatment of underlying metabolic and other medical disorders. If the distention fails to improve, colonoscopy and colonic decompression tube placement should be attempted; a fluoroscopic approach to

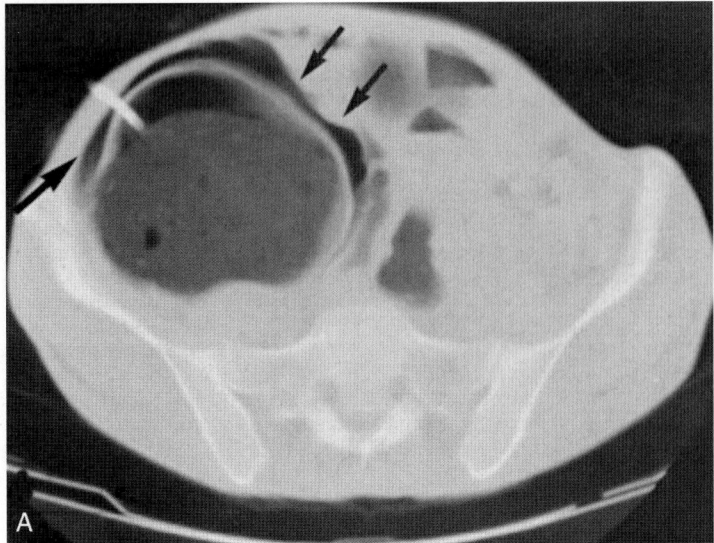

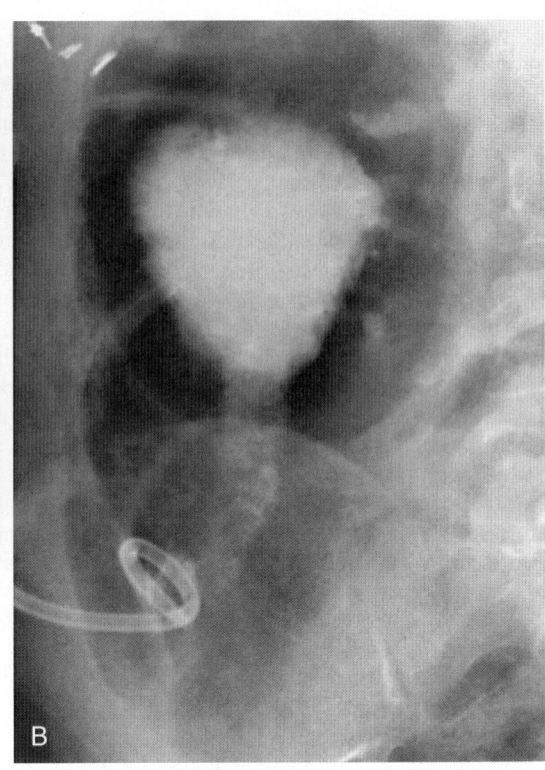

Figure 10-35. Percutaneous cecostomy. A transperitoneal approach was used. **A.** CT scan. **B.** Abdominal plain film. Air (*arrows* in **A**) was introduced into the peritoneal cavity during the procedure.

decompression using a coaxial, steerable system for intubation has been described. These methods may prove ineffective because of thick retained stool. Distention may recur after initial colonoscopic success.

After unsuccessful colonoscopic decompression, surgical cecostomy has been the next therapeutic approach. However, surgery in these patients, who are often seriously ill, can be risky. Consequently, a number of investigators have attempted percutaneous decompression of the massively dilated but unobstructed cecum. Successful decompression has been achieved with both simple aspiration and drainage tube placement. Reports of percutaneous decompression of the mechanically obstructed colon have also appeared.

A variety of approaches (Fig. 10-35), methods, and tube sizes have been used for percutaneous cecostomy. Usually, fluoroscopy provides sufficient guidance, although CT may be helpful if there are questions about the approach. Both the trocar and the Seldinger methods of tube placement are feasible for these patients. Although further experience with percutaneous cecostomy is necessary to fully assess risks and to evaluate optimal technique and indications, this procedure is an alternative method of colonic decompression in severely ill and debilitated patients. As an aside, cecostomy has also been used to treat fecal incontinence in children by allowing antegrade cleansing enemas to be administered.[23-25]

Enteral Access for Alimentation

The last, but most common and important indication for radiologic enteric access is for nutritional support. The majority of such procedures are percutaneous gastrostomies and gastrojejunostomies, but percutaneous jejunostomy and duodenostomy have been used in increasing numbers.[26-31]

In the short term, nasoenteric tubes can be used quite effectively for alimentation. However, longer-term use is associated with a variety of problems. Such tubes are uncomfortable and often psychologically untenable for patients. Additionally, they predispose the patient to gastroesophageal reflux, esophagitis, and stricture formation. Also, the luminal diameter of most nasoenteric tubes is small, predisposing them to occlusion.

Total parenteral nutrition is another option for feeding patients. It is particularly useful for patients who are unable to assimilate enteric nutrients or who require bowel rest. As a general method for alimentation, however, it has disadvantages compared with the enteral route. It is more costly than the enteral alternative. Over the long term, it is associated with several complications including small bowel atrophy, abnormalities of hepatic function, and electrolyte disturbances. The need for prolonged venous access also places the patient at high risk for development of venous thromboses and stenoses.

Enteral access, on the other hand, is associated with few complications once it is established, and it is less expensive than total parenteral nutrition. Thus, enteral alimentation is indicated in patients with longer-term nutritional requirements who, because of mechanical, functional, or psychologic disorders, are unable to meet their nutritional needs without assistance but who are still able to assimilate enterically administered nutrients.

In the past, gastrostomy tubes were placed surgically. However, many patients who require gastrostomy tubes are poor operative risks because of malnutrition, debilitation, and coexistent illnesses. Gastrostomy has increasingly been performed using less invasive techniques, including radiologic, endoscopic (percutaneous endoscopic gastrostomy), and laparoscopic methods. Although each method has certain advantages and disadvantages, there has been little randomized prospective comparison among them. Indeed, as much as in any area of interventional radiology, local referral patterns, politics, and local expertise may result in widely variable patterns of practice among institutions.

Several other differences exist among the techniques. Radiologic gastrostomy or gastrojejunostomy appears to be less costly than the surgical alternative, does not require general anesthesia, and has less associated postprocedural ileus. The endoscopic method does not require exposure to ionizing radiation and can be performed easily and rapidly at the bedside. Although bedside placement using ultrasonography or portable fluoroscopy is possible, it is rarely performed. Endoscopic placement may be difficult or impossible when there is obstruction or high-grade narrowing of the esophagus or pharynx, leaving imaging-guided placement as the only feasible nonoperative alternative. Imaging guidance may also be critical in delineating and avoiding interposed structures (e.g., the colon) between the anterior abdominal wall and the stomach. In patients prone to aspiration, imaging guidance is usually preferable because endoscopy may require heavy sedation and may be a lengthy procedure if tube placement into the jejunum is required. Tubes placed under imaging guidance seem less likely to give rise to stomal wound infections than those inserted endoscopically. The endoscope must pass through the contaminated oral cavity rather than the scrubbed anterior abdominal wall. Finally, endoscopic placement does offer the possibility of biopsy and other diagnostic methods when these are relevant.

Percutaneous gastrostomy can be performed by a variety of methods. Before the procedure, the patient should be given nothing by mouth for at least 12 hours to minimize risks of aspiration and peritoneal leakage. Usually, prophylactic antibiotics are not necessary. Only mild sedation combined with local anesthesia at the puncture site is usually required, although general anesthesia offers advantages in infants and younger children.

An entry site is chosen in the anterior left upper quadrant, which allows direct puncture of the stomach with no transgression of bowel, liver, or vascular structures. Preprocedural ultrasonography or CT provides delineation of these structures (Fig. 10-36). Ultrasound is quickly and easily performed in the fluoroscopy suite and is often used routinely to demarcate a safe "window" on the skin surface. Another helpful adjunct in patients who have no obstruction or altered enteric motility is the administration of oral contrast medium the night before the examination, which provides good opacification of the colon at the time of the procedure.

One potential hazard of percutaneous gastrostomy is injury to the inferior epigastric artery, which lies at the junction of the medial two thirds and lateral third of the rectus abdominis. Therefore, skin puncture should be made at a site lateral to this muscle or close to the midline of the abdomen, depending on the position of the stomach. A subcostal puncture site usually provides good access to the stomach, is more comfortable for the patient, and avoids pleural and pulmonary complications.

Gastric distention makes it easier to pierce the gastric wall, which tends to invaginate and move away from the puncture needle. Distention also helps bring the stomach closer to the anterior abdominal wall and displace any interposed bowel. Distention is provided by insufflation of the stomach with several hundred milliliters of room air administered via a previously placed nasogastric tube. If a nasogastric tube cannot be placed, the stomach can be punctured with a Seldinger needle and air can be injected through its lumen. Another means of providing distention is the oral administration of

effervescent granules that produce carbon dioxide. Intravenous glucagon (1.0 mg in adults, 0.14 mg/kg in children) can be used to augment these measures by diminishing gastric peristalsis and decreasing passage of air through the pylorus. If fluoroscopic puncture proves difficult because of interposed structures or variant anatomy, inability to pass a nasogastric tube, or inability to tolerate gastric distention, cross-sectional imaging can also be used for guidance (see Fig. 10-36).

One other option for providing distention is intragastric inflation of a latex balloon attached to the end of a nasogastric tube. The balloon is inflated with diluted contrast medium or with air, providing an easily visualized and stable target for fluoroscopically or sonographically guided puncture. Bursting of the balloon confirms intragastric positioning of the needle tip. Although this device can be difficult for some patients to tolerate and is usually unnecessary, it may be helpful when simple insufflation is unsuccessful in providing gastric distention, as occurs in patients with a partial gastrectomy.

The anterior wall of the stomach is usually punctured in its middle third toward the side of the greater curvature (Fig. 10-37). The greater and lesser curvatures should be

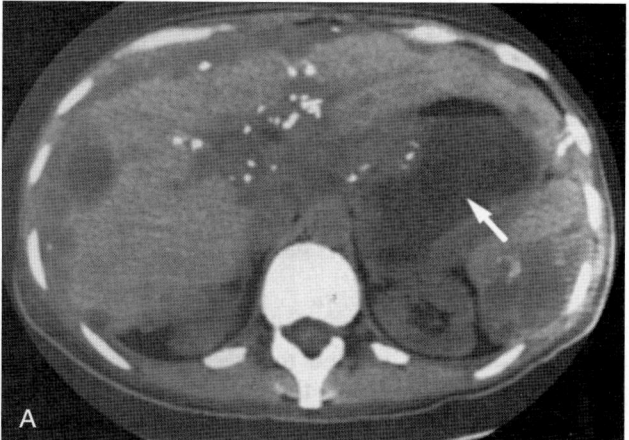

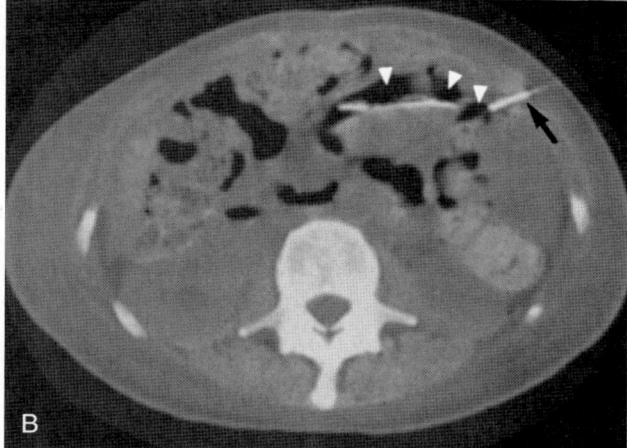

Figure 10-36. CT-guided percutaneous gastrostomy. A. CT of the upper abdomen in a patient with pseudomyxoma peritonei attributable to ovarian carcinoma shows the stomach (*arrow*) surrounded by adjacent organs and peritoneal metastases. **B.** At a more caudal level, a safe window to the stomach is present. Percutaneous gastrostomy was successfully performed under CT guidance. *Arrowheads,* gastric lumen; *arrow,* initial puncture needle.

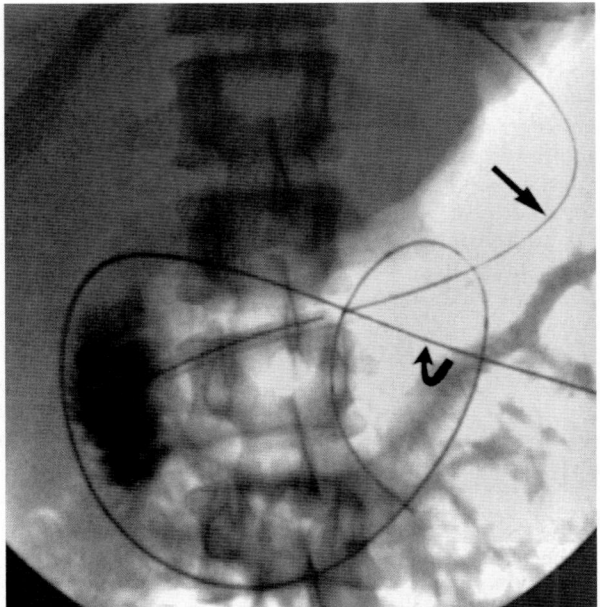

Figure 10-37. Fluoroscopically guided percutaneous gastrostomy. The midbody of the gas-filled stomach has been punctured at the site of the curved arrow with an 18-gauge Seldinger needle. It is angulated toward the pylorus, and a wire has been manipulated into the proximal jejunum. A gastrojejunostomy tube was subsequently placed. *Straight arrow* indicates the nasogastric tube used for insufflation of air.

avoided because the larger vascular arcades of the stomach are located in these regions. Lateral fluoroscopy is used to access the proximity of the anterior gastric wall to the skin surface. If initial or delayed small bowel catheterization is anticipated, a "downhill" puncture angled toward the pyloric region makes manipulations of the guidewire and catheter easier. Too great an angle, however, makes tract dilatation and catheter exchange difficult. If the tube is being placed for decompressive purposes only, it can be angled somewhat more vertically and toward the gastric fundus. Once the gastric wall is indented by the puncture needle, a short vigorous thrust is used to pierce its muscular layers.

Final catheter placement can be achieved by a variety of methods. One is the Seldinger technique and its variants, in which initial puncture is made with an 18- to 22-gauge Seldinger needle or a small sheathed needle. A wire is passed through the sheath or cannula, and successive guidewire and catheter exchange is used to place a final gastrostomy tube. Techniques using a trocar, an instrument consisting of a catheter or sheath mounted on the puncture needle, have also been successfully employed in placing gastrostomy tubes. The trocar technique allows larger and softer tubes to be inserted at the time of the initial procedure and requires fewer catheter and wire exchanges, each of which may result in loss of gastric access. Initial puncture, however, may be difficult and risky with trocars, which are usually larger devices.

When the Seldinger technique is used, a peel-away sheath may facilitate insertion if catheter exchange is difficult or if placement of a soft catheter or catheter without an end hole is desired. In addition, removal of the peel-away sheath may correct any gastric wall invagination that has occurred. During passage of catheters or dilators, the stabilizing guidewire has a free end within the gastrointestinal tract and must not be

displaced out of the gastric lumen. A method of preventing this problem in children has been described: the free end of the wire is secured and pulled from the stomach to the mouth by a wire basket or snare, allowing stable control of both ends of the wire in a manner analogous to that of endoscopic methods. In general, however, these maneuvers are unnecessary.

The use of fixation devices as an adjunct to percutaneous gastrostomy has generated some controversy. These devices are fasteners that can be placed through a small needle to affix the anterior gastric wall to the anterior abdominal wall at one or more sites. Advocates of these devices cite a number of potential advantages, including reduced intraperitoneal leakage of gastric contents, facilitation of guidewire and catheter exchange and immediate placement of large catheters, increased safety in patients expected to have difficulty with track maturation (e.g., patients on corticosteroid therapy), easy reinsertion in cases of early catheter dislodgment (of greater concern in uncooperative patients), and possible tamponade of gastric hemorrhage induced at the gastrostomy site. Theoretical disadvantages of gastric fixation are interference with gastric peristalsis and excessive traction on the gastric wall resulting in pressure necrosis, bleeding, infection, or catheter dislodgment. Problems related to excessive traction are not unique to the use of fixation devices. Other potential disadvantages that can be obviated by careful technique include anchor misplacement into the peritoneal cavity and difficulty with tube passage immediately adjacent to the anchor. Most of the controversy, however, has resulted from extensive clinical and laboratory experience with percutaneous gastrostomy accomplished without fixation devices, which suggests that the procedure can be performed easily, safely, and less expensively in most instances without their use. No large prospective comparisons have yet been made.[26-31]

Massive ascites is generally considered a contraindication to percutaneous gastrostomy. Large quantities of peritoneal fluid make gastric puncture difficult and can lead to tube dislodgment, gastropexy breakdown, peritonitis, and skin breakdown. However, gastrostomies have been safely placed and managed in patients with smaller amounts of ascites via a combination of gastropexy, preprocedural paracentesis, and regular postprocedural paracentesis to allow the enterostomy track to mature.

Another area of controversy is the final position of the tube. Some practitioners prefer that the tube be manipulated into the proximal jejunum at the time of the initial procedure. This method allows immediate catheter feeding, diminishes the risks of gastroesophageal reflux and aspiration of gastric contents, and provides additional insurance against catheter dislodgment. Other practitioners have maintained that routine gastrojejunostomy is not indicated, and they have reserved jejunal placement for patients who are prone to reflux or aspiration, have impaired gastric motility, or have partial gastric obstruction. Scintigraphy has been reported to be helpful in determining whether a patient can safely tolerate a gastrostomy tube without risk of reflux and aspiration. Even if the tube is left in the stomach initially, subsequent conversion to a gastrojejunostomy tube can usually be accomplished without difficulty, so long as the original angle of puncture is toward the pylorus. If not, a stiff sheath can frequently be used to redirect the tube, although in cases of severe unfavorable angulation, a new access site may be the best approach.

A large variety of tubes have been used for percutaneous gastrostomy, including simple Cope loop catheters, Foley catheters, and catheters specially designed for percutaneous gastrostomy and gastrojejunostomy. Catheter sizes usually range from about 12 to 20 French. Because of its ease of insertion, the Cope loop is preferred by many investigators, except in patients who require gastrojejunostomy.

Altered gastric anatomy due to prior surgery, although it may preclude percutaneous gastrostomy in some instances, should not be considered an absolute contraindication. However, a full understanding of the postsurgical anatomy is important. Generally, gastrostomy can be performed with minor modifications of standard methods such as longer needles and craniocaudal fluoroscopy. Other techniques reported to be helpful in this setting include gastric balloon support and the use of a transhepatic catheter route guided by CT.

Potential complications of percutaneous gastrostomy include catheter dislodgment, pericatheter leakage, peritonitis, sepsis, pain, hemorrhage, inadvertent puncture of other organs, pulmonary aspiration, subcutaneous inflammation, and wound infection. Although patients should be observed carefully after percutaneous gastrostomy for signs of complications, it should be noted that a number of postprocedural radiologic findings are common and should not by themselves cause alarm or prompt laparotomy. These radiologic findings include pneumoperitoneum and small abdominal wall and gastric hematomas. Subcutaneous emphysema, gastric pneumatosis, free or loculated intraperitoneal fluid (Fig. 10-38), and pneumoperitoneum that increases in volume are uncommon and should be viewed with more concern.

Long-term care of percutaneous gastrostomy catheters include keeping the catheter entry site clean and maintaining tube patency after feeding with injection of saline solution. A tract between the abdominal wall and the gastric lumen is usually well established in about 7 days, and exchange of an occluded tube or replacement of a recently dislodged tube after this time is generally easy. If the tube is inadvertently removed at an earlier time, an attempt can be made to re-catheterize the tract, but it is less likely to be successful. As noted earlier, one possible advantage to using gastric fixation devices is that it facilitates tube replacement or repeated puncture of the stomach in this early period. If pericatheter leakage is noted, the problem may respond to replacement of the tube with one slightly larger. Delayed pericatheter hemorrhage, presumably attributable to erosion into an adjacent vessel, has been described. Successful tamponade and long-term control of the bleeding can be achieved with gentle traction by a Foley catheter against the gastric wall. Another delayed complication, occurring from days to months after gastrostomy placement, is perforation of the gastrointestinal tract by the tube. Perforations can be managed with nonsurgical means including tube replacement, antibiotic therapy, drainage of associated abscesses, and gastric compression.

Direct percutaneous catheterization of the small bowel has been performed much less often than percutaneous gastrostomy. The procedure is made difficult by the mobility and compliance of small bowel loops as well as by the difficulty associated with providing and maintaining their distention. Although fluoroscopic guidance has been used in many cases, CT and ultrasonography have also proved useful in localization and puncture of small bowel.[32]

Indications for percutaneous jejunostomy include the need for prolonged enteric feeding in patients in whom a gastrostomy by percutaneous or endoscopic route is not possible. This can occur, for example, when a large hiatal hernia is present or in postsurgical patients after a gastric pull-up procedure or after a partial gastrectomy with a small and high-positioned gastric remnant. Other potential indications include chronic aspiration, gastric outlet or duodenal obstruction, recurrent dislodgment of previously placed gastrostomies or retrograde gastrojejunostomy dislodgment back into the stomach, or premature dislodgment of a jejunostomy.

Adequate distention of the jejunum is an important facet of the procedure. Transnasal or transoral intubation of the small bowel can provide access for small bowel distention with air, contrast medium, or supportive balloons. Direct fine needle puncture and air insufflation into the left upper quadrant can also be used to identify the jejunum.[32]

References

1. Kessel D, Robertson I: Interventional Radiology. London, Churchill Livingstone, 2005.
2. Wicke L: Atlas of Radiologic Anatomy, 7th ed. Philadelphia, Saunders, 2004.
3. Wintersperger BJ, Nikolaou K, Becker CR: Multidetector-row CT angiography of the aorta and visceral arteries. Semin Ultrasound CT MR. 25:25-40, 2004.
4. Hellinger JC: Evaluating mesenteric ischemia with multidetector-row CT angiography. Tech Vasc Interv Radiol 7:160-166, 2004.
5. Chicoskie C, Tello R: Gadolinium-enhanced MDCT angiography of the abdomen: Feasibility and limitations. AJR 184:1821-1828, 2005.
6. Vosshenrich R, Fischer U: Contrast-enhanced MR angiography of abdominal vessels: Is there still a role for angiography? Eur Radiol 12:218-230, 2002.
7. Laissy JP, Trillaud H, Douek P: MR angiography: Noninvasive vascular imaging of the abdomen. Abdom Imaging 27:488-506, 2002.
8. Haage P, Krings T, Schmitz-Rode T: Nontraumatic vascular emergencies: Imaging and intervention in acute venous occlusion. Eur Radiol 12: 2627-2643, 2002.

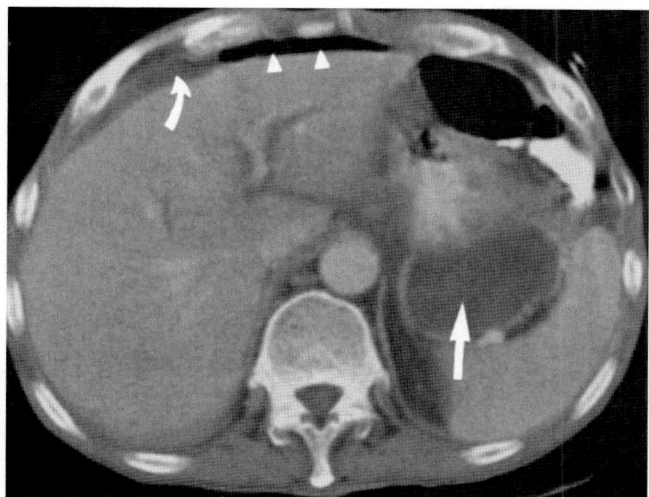

Figure 10-38. Percutaneous gastrostomy: complication. CT scan obtained 3 days after percutaneous gastrostomy. Although pneumoperitoneum (*arrowheads*) is often seen in the absence of clinically apparent complications, findings of loculated (*straight arrow*) and free (*curved arrow*) intraperitoneal fluid are atypical and are cause for concern. Peritoneal spillage in this case resulted from intraperitoneal positioning of a side hole of the gastrostomy tube. The patient required surgical treatment.

9. Sachdev U, Baril DT, Ellozy SH, et al: Management of aneurysms involving branches of the celiac and superior mesenteric arteries: A comparison of surgical and endovascular therapy. J Vasc Surg 44:718-724, 2006.

10. Connell JM, Han DC: Celiac artery aneurysms: A case report and review of the literature. Am Surg 72:746-749, 2006.

11. Chang SH, Lien WC, Liu YP, et al: Isolated superior mesenteric artery dissection in a patient without risk factors or aortic dissection. Am J Emerg Med 24:385-387, 2006.

12. Ozaki T, Kimura M, Yoshimura N, et al: Endovascular treatment of spontaneous isolated dissecting aneurysm of the superior mesenteric artery using stent-assisted coil embolization. Cardiovasc Intervent Radiol 29:435-437, 2006.

13. Kobayashi M, Morishita S, Okabayashi T, et al: Preoperative assessment of vascular anatomy of inferior mesenteric artery by volume-rendered 3D-CT for laparoscopic lymph node dissection with left colic artery preservation in lower sigmoid and rectal cancer. World J Gastroenterol 12:553-555, 2006.

14. Saikia N, Talukdar R, Mazumder S, et al: Polyarteritis nodosa presenting as massive upper gastrointestinal hemorrhage. Gastrointest Endosc 63:868-870, 2006.

15. Strate LL: Lower GI bleeding: Epidemiology and diagnosis. Gastroenterol Clin North Am 34:643-664, 2005.

16. Gray BH, Sullivan TM: Mesenteric Vascular Disease. Curr Treat Options Cardiovasc Med 3:195-206, 2001.

17. Haage P, Krings T, Schmitz-Rode T: Nontraumatic vascular emergencies: Imaging and intervention in acute venous occlusion. Eur Radiol 12:2627-2643, 2002.

18. Horton KM, Talamini MA, Fishman EK: Median arcuate ligament syndrome: Evaluation with CT angiography. RadioGraphics 25:1177-1182, 2005.

19. Strate LL: Lower GI bleeding: Epidemiology and diagnosis. Gastroenterol Clin North Am 34:643-664, 2005.

20. Siersema PD: Therapeutic esophageal interventions for dysphagia and bleeding. Curr Opin Gastroenterol 22:442-447, 2006.

21. Christie NA, Patel AN, Landreneau RJ: Esophageal palliation—photodynamic therapy/stents/brachytherapy. Surg Clin North Am 85:569-582, 2005

22. Mitton D, Ackroyd R: Oesophageal stenting. Scand J Gastroenterol 40:1-14, 2005.

23. Gillman LM, Latosinsky S: Anterograde colonic stent placement via a cecostomy tube site. Can J Gastroenterol 20:425-426, 2006.

24. Stefanidis D, Brown K, Nazario H, et al: Safety and efficacy of metallic stents in the management of colorectal obstruction. JSLS 9:454-459, 2005.

25. Lynch CR, Jones RG, Hilden K, et al: Percutaneous endoscopic cecostomy in adults: A case series. Gastrointest Endosc 64:279-282, 2006.

26. Burke DT, El Shami A, Heinle E, et al: Comparison of gastrostomy tube replacement verification using air insufflation versus Gastrografin. Arch Phys Med Rehabil 87:1530-1533, 2006.

27. Chio A, Galletti R, Finocchiaro C, et al: Percutaneous radiological gastrostomy: A safe and effective method of nutritional tube placement in advanced ALS. J Neurol Neurosurg Psychiatry 75:645-647, 2004.

28. Desport JC, Mabrouk T, Bouillet P, et al: Complications and survival following radiologically and endoscopically guided gastrostomy in patients with amyotrophic lateral sclerosis. Amyotroph Lateral Scler Other Motor Neuron Disord 6:88-93, 2005.

29. Shaw AS, Ampong MA, Rio A, et al: Entristar skin-level gastrostomy tube: Primary placement with radiologic guidance in patients with amyotrophic lateral sclerosis. Radiology 233:392-399, 2004.

30. Thornton FJ, Varghese JC, Haslam PJ, et al: Percutaneous gastrostomy in patients who fail or are unsuitable for endoscopic gastrostomy. Cardiovasc Intervent Radiol 23:279-284, 2000.

31. Wollman B, D'Agostino HB: Percutaneous radiologic and endoscopic gastrostomy: A 3-year institutional analysis of procedure performance. AJR 169:1551-1553, 1997.

32. Ross AS, Semrad C, Alverdy J, et al: Use of double-balloon enteroscopy to perform PEG in the excluded stomach after Roux-en-Y gastric bypass. Gastrointest Endosc 64:797-800, 2006.

Abdominal Computed Tomographic Angiography

Vahid Yaghmai, MD

Computed tomographic angiography (CTA) revolutionized vascular imaging when vessels smaller than 1 mm in diameter were imaged with single-slice spiral CT.[1-5] However, because of the small volume of coverage and limitations in the speed of image processing, CTA did not become widely utilized until the introduction of multidetector CT (MDCT) in 1998.[6-8] With the advent of MDCT, temporal and spatial resolution of the scanners significantly improved.[9,10] Gantry rotation times of 0.33 to 0.5 second with slice thickness of 0.5 to 0.75 mm are now available on most MDCT scanners.

The details of this technology are beyond the scope of this chapter and are discussed in Chapters 7 and 69. Briefly, there are several parallel detectors along the z-axis with multiple channels of data (currently up to 64) allowing significant improvement in z-axis resolution. This allows isotropic resolution for most vascular applications with images obtained during a single short breath-hold. The result has been elimination of the tradeoff between spatial resolution (z-axis) and scanning range, a significant limitation of single-detector spiral CT.[11,12] Hence, a significant benefit has been a paradigm shift from single-slice to volumetric data acquisition. This, in turn, has made imaging of different vascular phases with a single-contrast bolus a reality.[7]

Other than its limited invasiveness, advantages of CTA include lower cost as well as the ability to potentially reduce the total volume of contrast material administered. With the fastest scanners currently available (16- and 64-slice), abdominal CTA can be obtained with as little as 50 mL of contrast material with the use of saline flush.[13,14] This requires meticulous attention to the timing of contrast bolus, which is discussed later in this chapter. In evaluation of life-threatening vascular disease such as traumatic aortic injury or pulmo-

nary embolus, CTA has a clear advantage because of short acquisition times.[15]

An important advantage of CTA over catheter angiography is its ability to examine the vessel wall as well as its lumen. The adjacent organs can also be evaluated (e.g., staging of pancreatic adenocarcinoma). Another advantage of CTA is the ability to evaluate a vessel in projections that cannot be obtained with conventional techniques.

Increased utility of CT has led to significant increase in radiation exposure and concerns about its effect.[16] CT currently accounts for approximately 75% of the total radiation dose delivered by medical imaging.[17] Development of automatic tube current modulation software that is now available on all advanced MDCT systems has been a positive side effect of this awareness. Tube current modulation automatically adjusts the current during scanning to decrease the amount of radiation in anatomic regions that do not require higher current (e.g., lung bases or above the iliac crest) while maintaining image quality.[16] In the appropriate setting, abdominal CTA may be performed with reduced kV setting to decrease radiation to the patient and to improve signal-to-noise ratio.[18]

TECHNICAL CONSIDERATIONS

Until the introduction of latest generation of 16- and 64-slice CT scanners, improvement in spatial resolution came at the cost of temporal resolution. Now, with faster gantry rotation time (0.33-0.5 second) and increase in the number of detector rows, isotropic voxel acquisition independent of the length of coverage is possible. The new CT scanners utilize very complex spiral cone beam reconstruction algorithms instead of the filtered back projection mathematical reconstruction algorithm that was used in older scanners. These mathematical reconstruction algorithms are a byproduct of significant advances in computer technology. A combination of all these advances has made isotropic scanning of the abdominal aorta and its branches in a single breath-hold a clinical reality.[7,12,19]

With shortened acquisition times of the multislice scanners, optimizing and maximizing vascular enhancement has become more challenging.[20,21] CTA requires excellent contrast enhancement of the targeted vessels. A good quality CT angiogram requires arterial density value of greater than 200 HU.[22,23] This should be achieved rapidly, and the peak should coincide with the acquisition interval. It is, therefore, crucial to time the contrast bolus correctly. However, rapid administration of contrast material shortens the plateau phase of contrast enhancement, thus creating further challenge for correct timing of the study.[20,21,24] For most abdominal CTA applications, an injection rate of 4 to 5 mL/s yields optimal vascular enhancement.

To achieve rapid intravenous administration of contrast material excellent intravenous access (18 or 20 gauge) and a dual-head power injector are required. A saline bolus via a dual-head injector after contrast agent administration prolongs and improves arterial enhancement and also decreases the amount of contrast agent required by using the residual contrast in the tubing and the patient's arm veins and superior vena cava.[14,25,26]

There are several factors that affect time to peak from the start of contrast bolus. These include the iodine content of contrast material, injection rate, and patient's cardiac status.[20,21,25,27] A faster injection rate, for example, can achieve a higher density in the targeted vessel and results in a higher quality CT angiogram. It also separates the arterial from portal venous phase and, hence, results in excellent image quality without cross-contamination by different phases.[20] Contrast material with higher iodine concentration improves vascular enhancement, if all other parameters are held constant.[20,28] Because several factors affect time-to-peak enhancement in the aorta, fixed timing delay for image acquisition is not advised.

All modern CT scanners provide software for calculating the optimal time for the start of scanning after administration of a test bolus—"test bolus injection" (Fig. 11-1A)—or allow automatic image acquisition once a preset Hounsfield unit threshold in the target vessel has been reached—"bolus triggering" (Fig. 11-1B). An important consideration with the 16- and 64-slice scanners is the possibility of "outrunning" the contrast bolus in patients with low cardiac output or in cases that require long z-axis coverage (e.g., combination of extremity and abdominal CTA); to overcome this issue, one can slow down the scanner by increasing the gantry rotation time and slowing the table speed.[29,30]

As discussed previously, the new multislice scanners in combination with dual-head injectors allow marked decrease in the amount of contrast used for routine CTA. However, the total volume of contrast agent administered for a routine abdominal CT (usually 150 mL of 300 mg/mL concentration of contrast material) should not change if solid organs, such as liver, are evaluated in conjunction with CTA. Lowering the total volume of contrast agent may potentially reduce the sensitivity of lesion detection.[12,28]

Many authors have reported the use of gadolinium chelates for CTA in patients who have diminished renal function.[31-34]

ROI	Peak (HU)	Times to peak(s)	Sample (HU) at 18.0 s
1	147.3	18.0	147.3

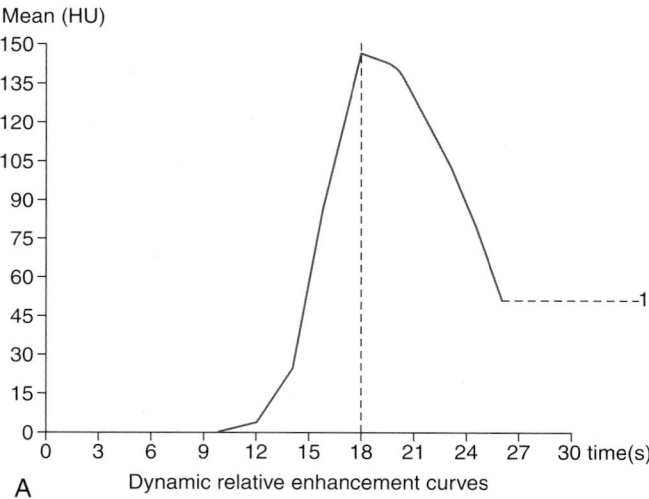

A   Dynamic relative enhancement curves

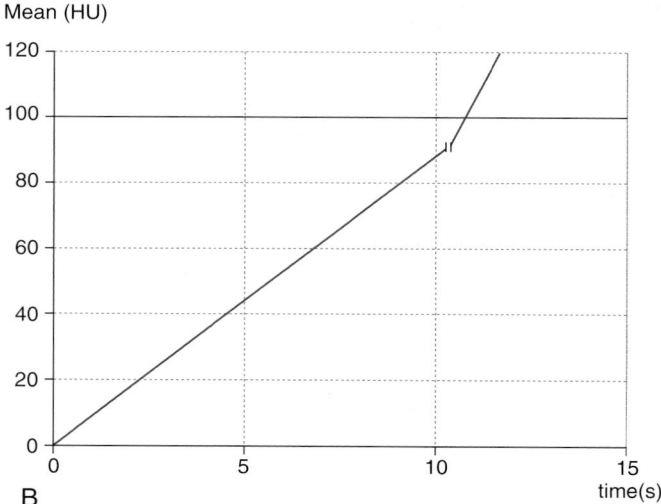

B

Figure 11-1. Contrast bolus monitoring methods. A. Test bolus injection technique. With this technique a small bolus of contrast material (usually 15-20 mL) is administered followed by a saline chase of similar volume. Time to peak is calculated after acquisition of several images with the region of interest placed on the target vessel. **B.** Bolus triggering technique. A region of interest is placed on the target vessel and injection of contrast material is started. After reaching the preset threshold (100 HU in this case), the scanner automatically instructs the patient to hold his or her breath and image acquisition takes place automatically. With the bolus triggering technique, less contrast material is used because a test bolus is not needed.

Although gadolinium is radiodense and may be used as a contrast agent with radiography, many gadolinium-based products have higher osmolality than iodine-based contrast media and are, therefore, potentially more nephrotoxic. More importantly, there have been several reports of nephrogenic systemic fibrosis leading to serious physical disability in patients with end-stage renal disease receiving gadolinium-containing contrast agents.[35,36]

IMAGE PROCESSING

Thinner slice acquisition with CTA has resulted in significant increase in the number of images acquired. Hence, "data overload" has been a direct side effect of isotropic and near isotropic scanning. CTA of the abdominal aorta and its branches on the newest scanners generates over 1000 images.[37] As the volume of data significantly increases, the processing power of many of the current image processing workstations is pushed to its limits. The strain on the fiberoptic networks and image processing workstations has become a significant challenge for many institutions that have installed the fastest CT scanners. Workflow and image transfer issues are significant by products of CTA that are beyond the scope of this discussion but an important issue to consider when one upgrades to the latest CT technology.

Postprocessing of the source data not only improves visualization of the vascular structures and their relationship to the adjacent organs but also decreases the number of slices needed for the review of the dataset.[38,39] Images can be processed on the scanner or a freestanding image processing workstation. Thicker slices may be produced for review of the axial images on the picture archiving and communications system (PACS).[40] Volume rendering, maximum intensity projection (MIP) rendering, or multiplanar reconstructions are routinely utilized to display large datasets.[7,41] The volume-rendering technique uses attenuation thresholds to create volumetric display of data and allows visualization of different tissue types by simply changing threshold settings. MIP rendering does not provide spatial depth but improves visualization of smaller vessels. Most institutions, including mine, routinely use a combination of the MIP and volume-rendered display of data for CTA, because these are complementary. Although volume rendering is useful for the display of soft tissues and 3D relationships, MIP provides a more detailed view of the vessels within the slab of data and is less operator dependent.[41]

ANATOMY

The major branches of the abdominal aorta are readily visible on both single-slice CT and CTA. However, to appreciate vascular disease thin sections with sufficient contrast enhancement are required. The typical branching of celiac artery to the common hepatic, left gastric, and splenic arteries can routinely be appreciated on CTA. The smaller branches arising from the common hepatic artery may also be evaluated by CTA if thin slices are acquired and contrast enhancement is optimized by bolus timing or tracking techniques. The superior mesenteric artery and its branching are also easily evaluated by CTA. A significant portion of patients studied with CTA demonstrate variations in the branching of abdominal aorta.[42-45]

The renal arteries arise at approximately the L1-2 level caudal to the origin of the superior mesenteric artery and cephalad to the origin of the inferior mesenteric artery. In approximately 28% of cases there are multiple renal arteries.[46]

The venous structures in the abdomen can also be evaluated by CTA. However, timing of scanning will be different depending on the venous structure imaged. Renal veins will rapidly enhance as they return blood to the inferior vena cava. This in combination with unopacified blood from the lower extremities can create a pseudothrombus in the inferior vena cava. For optimal imaging of the portal vein delays of 65 seconds after the start of contrast medium administration are needed. Therefore, to obtain CTA and CT portography one has to scan the abdomen successively with the newest multichannel scanners because these scanners in combination with rapid administration of contrast material allow complete separation of the arterial and venous phases of hepatic enhancement. This separation of phases is more difficult with single- and four-slice MDCT owing to lower temporal and spatial resolution. With the latest 16- and 64-channel scanners, early and late arterial enhancement of the liver can be separately imaged.

The portal vein arises from the confluence of the superior mesenteric and splenic veins and branches into right and left branches at the hepatic hilum. The right portal vein divides into anterior and posterior branches. The left portal vein defines the boundaries of the segments II, III, IVa, and IVb. When portal hypertension is present, numerous venous collaterals may be visible on MIP and volume-rendered images. The inferior mesenteric vein can be followed parallel to the course of superior mesenteric vein in the lower abdomen, coursing anterior to the left renal vein and draining into the splenic vein.

Anatomic variations of the major branches of the abdominal aorta, the inferior vena cava, the portal vein, and the renal veins are common and visible on CTA. For example, an accessory hepatic vein may be seen between segments V and VI. Single retroaortic or duplicated left renal veins are seen in 2.5% and 9% of population, respectively. CTA allows accurate mapping of these variants.[42,47,48] Assessment for these variations is essential when evaluating for hepatic segmentectomy, Whipple procedure, hepatic or renal donor assessment, or bowel resection. This is discussed in detail later in this chapter.

CLINICAL APPLICATIONS

Common abdominal applications of CTA include evaluation of the abdominal aorta, preoperative and postoperative assessment for renal and liver transplantation, preoperative planning for hepatic segmentectomy and pancreatic surgery, mesenteric ischemia, and gastrointestinal hemorrhage. Other applications include planning for cholecystectomy and splenectomy as well as assessment for renal arterial disease in evaluation of hypertension. The protocols for each application should be individually tailored to optimize imaging of the targeted vascular structures. For example, planning a Whipple procedure should include both arterial and portal venous phase images.

Aortic Dissection and Aneurysm

MDCT has revolutionized imaging of the abdominal aorta due to its excellent spatial resolution and the advantages over DCA that were described in the previous sections. Because of these advantages, CTA is usually the preferred imaging modality for evaluation of the abdominal aorta in both the acute and nonemergent settings.[9,10,49,50]

Aortic Dissection

CTA allows accurate depiction of intimal separation from the adventitia and its extension into branch vessels. The site

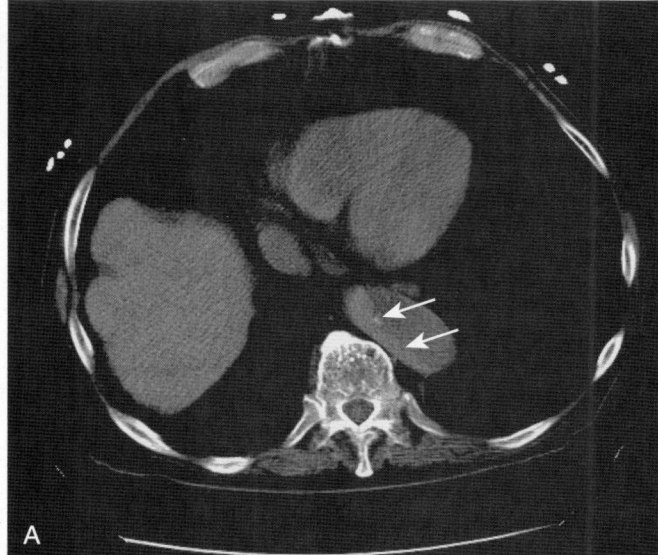

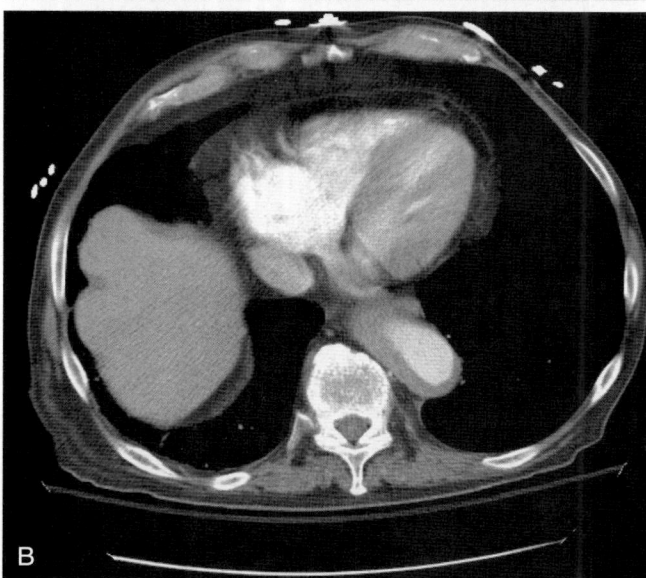

Figure 11-2. Intramural hematoma. A. Unenhanced image of the upper abdomen shows hyperattenuating aortic intramural hematoma (*arrows*). **B.** Enhanced image of the upper abdomen shows thrombus in the aortic wall that may be mistaken with chronic aortic thrombus or periaortic fluid.

of intimal tear and its extension determine prognosis. Most institutions use the Stanford classification to assess prognosis because type A dissections (involving the ascending aorta) require surgical management but type B dissections (confined to the descending aorta) are often managed conservatively.

Full assessment of aortic dissection by CTA requires an unenhanced CT followed by a contrast-enhanced CT. The unenhanced CT is useful for detection of dense intramural hematoma that may be mistaken for chronic thrombus on the enhanced images (Fig. 11-2). On the enhanced images, extension of the intimal flap to the aortic side branches and perfusion of organs affected by dissection should be assessed. Although quite variable, the true lumen is usually anterior to the false lumen in the upper abdominal aorta. At the level

of renal arteries, the false lumen usually supplies the left renal artery. The false lumen can also be distinguished from the true lumen by its larger diameter that also shows lower attenuation if images are acquired during peak arterial enhancement. If there are iatrogenic or spontaneous fenestrations of the intima, the false lumen may show similar enhancement as the true lumen (Fig. 11-3). Complications of aortic dissection include hemorrhage, hypoperfusion of the involved organs, and aneurysm formation.

Aortic Aneurysm

An abdominal aortic aneurysm (AAA) is a fusiform or focal saccular dilatation, usually of the infrarenal portion of aorta, greater than 4 cm in external anteroposterior diameter.[51] About 90% of abdominal aortic aneurysms are infrarenal and the majority limited to the abdominal aorta, but extension to the common iliac arteries does occur. Accessory renal arteries may arise from an infrarenal aneurysm, thus affecting management. Around 10% of aneurysms are juxtarenal, involving main renal arteries, or suprarenal, involving the celiac or superior mesenteric arteries. Suprarenal and infrarenal aortic aneurysms together form a dumbbell configuration.

Aortic aneurysms are frequent in the elder population and can be a cause of sudden death if ruptured.[52] The prevalence of AAA is estimated at 1.5% of the population older than the age of 50 and 5% to 8% percent of men older than the age of 65.[53,54] Because rupture of an aortic aneurysm can be catastrophic, aggressive screening and treatment has been advocated.[55] An untreated AAA greater than 5 cm in diameter has a 20% likelihood of rupture in 5 years.[56]

Ultrasonography has been advocated as the imaging modality of choice for AAA screening.[57,58] However, it has several shortcomings, including variability in transverse dimensions of the aneurysm, limitations in aneurysm neck assessment, and limited visualization of luminal thrombus.[59] Thus, CTA is obtained for confirming diagnosis, characterizing the aneurysm, and preoperative planning.[60,61]

Currently, there are two accepted methods of treatment for AAA: open surgical repair and endovascular approach.[52] Open surgical repair is associated with significant risk, including 6% to 10% mortality, which is commonly caused by myocardial infarction.[54,62,63] Endovascular aneurysm repair (EVAR) is a relatively new technique that was first described by Parodi and colleagues in 1991.[64] This method excludes the aneurysm by traversing it with a stent/graft and thus reducing pressure on the aortic wall.[65] The results of this less invasive treatment have been excellent with fewer complications and more rapid recovery.[66,67]

Preoperative assessment of the aorta is preferably performed with multislice CTA, because accurate measurement of the diameter of the aneurysm, its length, and its relation to major vessels (e.g., renal arteries) is essential.[68-70] For EVAR planning, diameter and angle of the aneurysm neck as well as its relation to the renal arteries is evaluated. Additionally, the amount of luminal clot may affect treatment. Three-dimensional evaluation of the aneurysm is particularly helpful for treatment planning (Fig. 11-4).[71] CTA provides useful information regarding femoral access sites and aortic accessibility.[70] Orthogonal measurements of the aneurysm using a center line provide accurate measurements for preoperative planning. CTA has been shown to be extremely accurate in

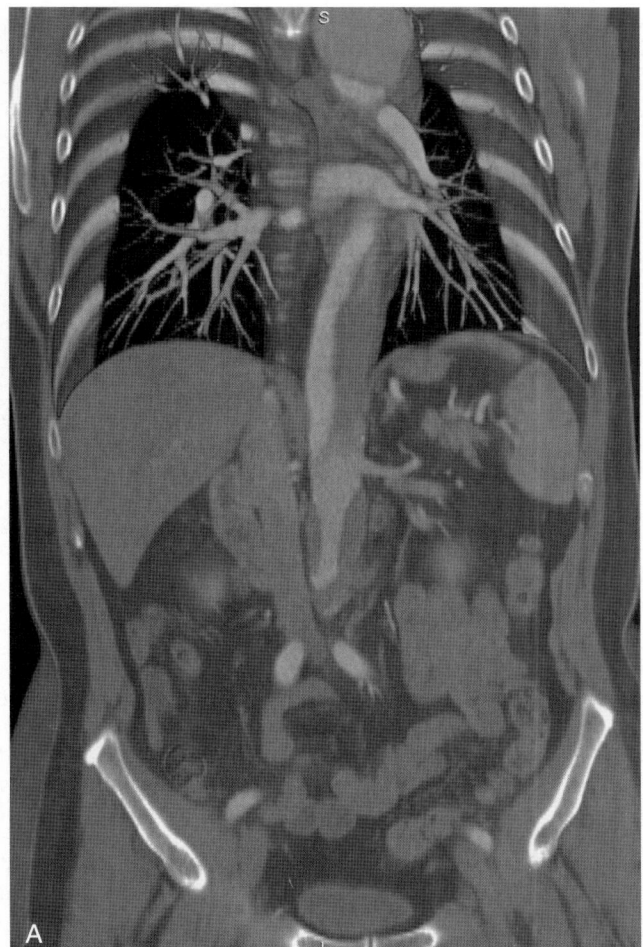

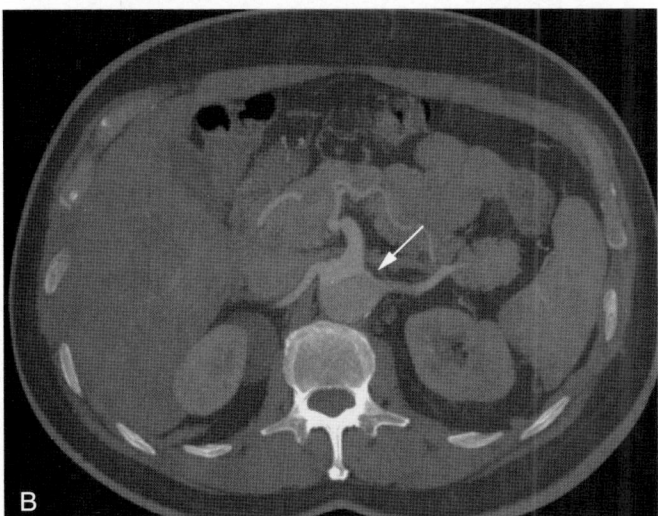

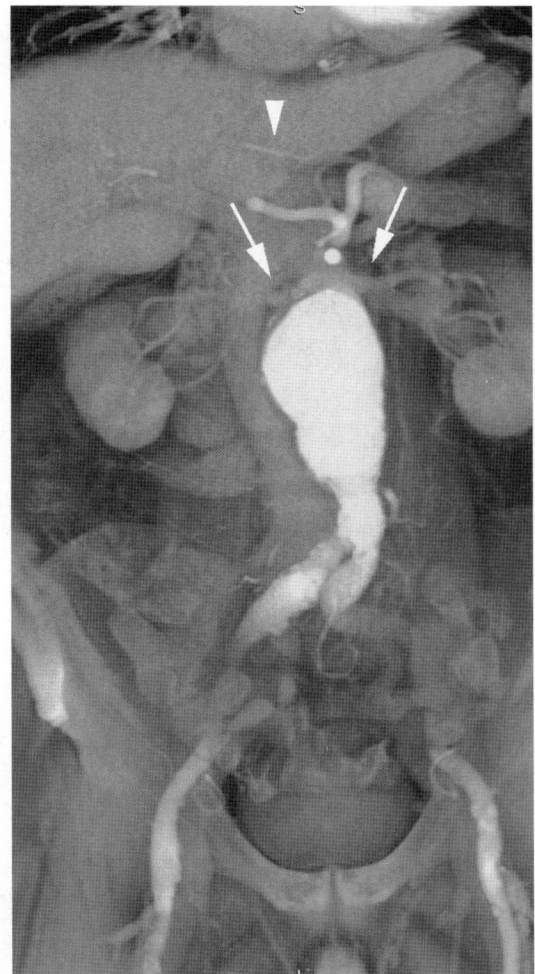

Figure 11-4. Infrarenal abdominal aortic aneurysm. Volume-rendered image shows relation of the aneurysm neck to the renal arteries (*arrows*). The distance from the renal arteries using vessel analysis software and centerline measurements should be calculated before EVAR. Incidentally noted is a replaced left hepatic artery arising from the left gastric artery (*arrowhead*).

Figure 11-3. Type A aortic dissection. A. Volume-rendered image. The false lumen has a larger diameter and lower density. Note higher density of the contrast material in the distal portion of the false lumen due to fenestration in the intima that is better seen on the transverse image. **B.** Maximum intensity projection image shows the left renal artery being supplied by the false lumen. Intimal dehiscence (*arrow*) allows perfusion of the left kidney.

measuring vessel lengths, diameters, and angles, as well as in assessing for occlusive disease and calcification.[72]

Patients treated with EVAR undergo frequent imaging by CTA to monitor for endoleak, stent migration or fracture, as well as stability of aneurysm size (Fig. 11-5).[73] Increase in the diameter of an aneurysm is associated with endoleak. Evaluation of an endoleak requires imaging with unenhanced CT as well as imaging during arterial and venous phases of contrast enhancement (Fig. 11-6). Unenhanced images are used to detect artifact from calcification or embolization material that may mimic endoleak on the enhanced images. Venous phase images have been shown to enhance detection rate of endoleaks. In type I endoleak there is a leak in the proximal or distal end of the graft. Type II endoleaks are caused by the retrograde flow from aortic side branches, commonly the inferior mesenteric or lumbar arteries. Type III endoleaks are related to separation of the graft components and require immediate treatment. Type IV endoleaks have been associated with leakage through the graft pores and are usually transient.

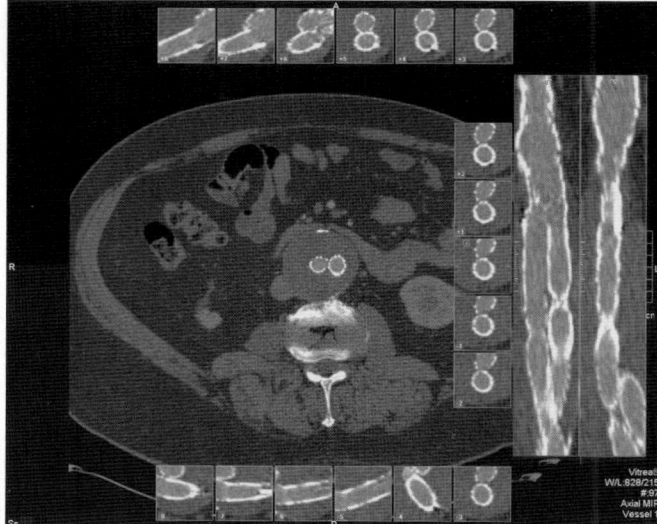

Figure 11-5. Endovascular stent graft. Orthogonal images allow assessment of the stent lumen.

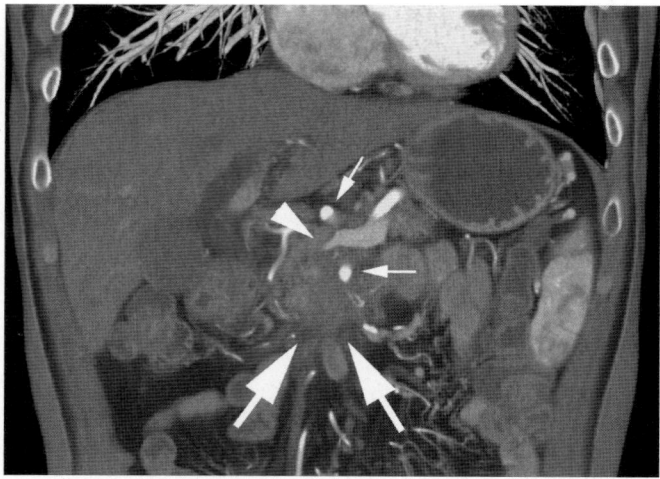

Figure 11-7. CT angiogram for the staging of pancreatic carcinoma. Large infiltrating pancreatic mass (*large arrows*) is encasing the superior mesenteric and common hepatic arteries (*small arrows*) and occludes the splenic vein (*arrowhead*). Note perigastric collateral veins.

Pancreatic Imaging

Staging of pancreatic cancer with multiphasic CT is now the standard of care in many institutions.[74] It requires arterial, parenchymal, and portal venous phase images to evaluate both the solid organs and the mesentery (Fig. 11-7).[75-77] Addition of a noncontrast phase allows detection of parenchymal and vascular calcifications. Neutral oral contrast agents help distend the bowel and improve visualization of the bowel wall. Positive oral contrast agents (e.g., iodine based agents) obscure vascular detail and should be avoided in all abdominal CTA.

Although curved multiplanar reformats of the pancreas improve visualization of the parenchyma and pancreatic duct, MIP and volume-rendered images are needed for vascular analysis (Fig. 11-8).[78,79] The newest generation of scanners allows rapid multiplanar and MIP images to be generated by

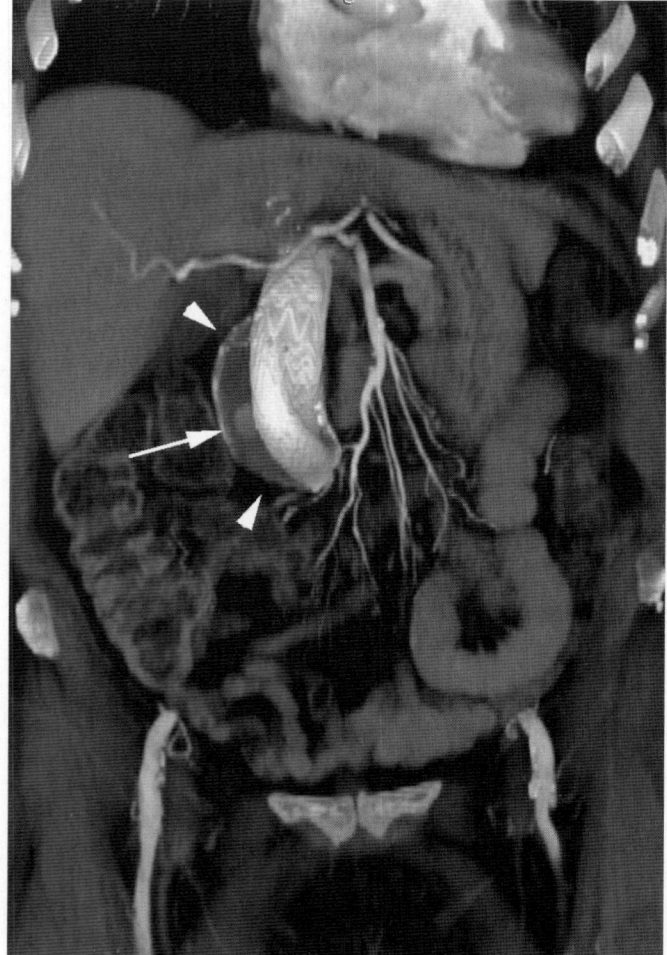

Figure 11-6. Stent graft placement for abdominal aortic aneurysm. There is opacification of the excluded portion of the abdominal aortic aneurysm (*arrowheads*) by a type II endoleak (*arrow*). The endoleak may be better visualized during the venous phase of the study.

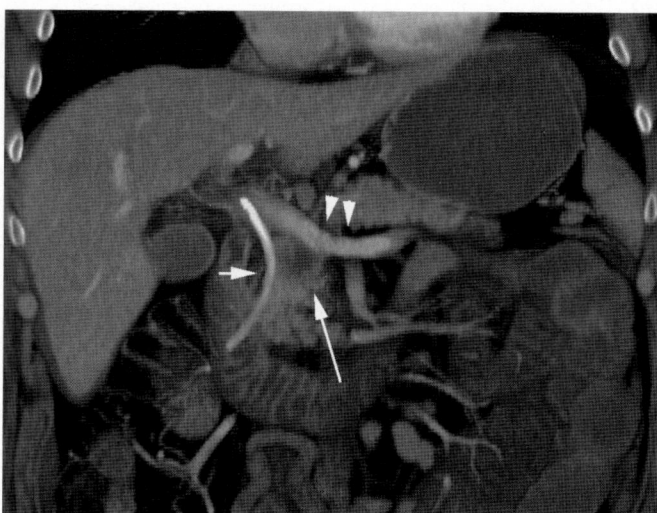

Figure 11-8. Volume-rendered image of pancreatic carcinoma (*long arrow*) with involvement of the portal vein. Note irregularity and subtle narrowing of the portal vein (*arrowheads*). Biliary stent in place (*short arrow*).

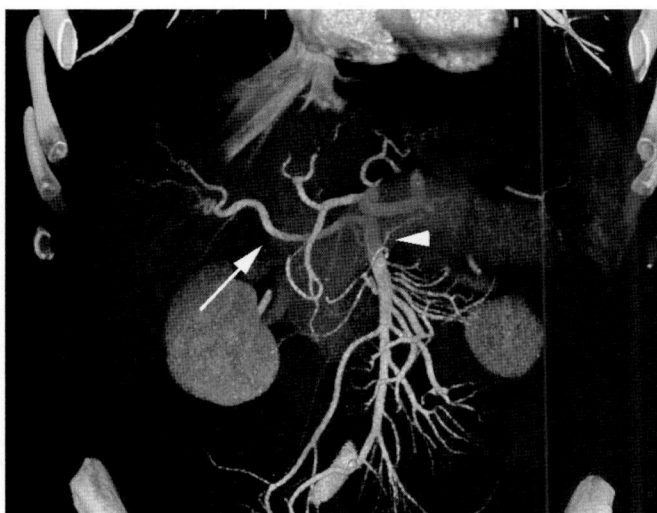

Figure 11-9. CT angiogram performed for staging of pancreatic head carcinoma shows replaced right hepatic artery (*arrow*) arising from the superior mesenteric artery (*arrowhead*).

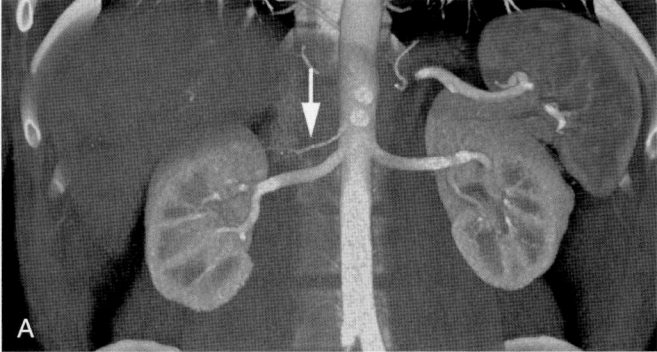

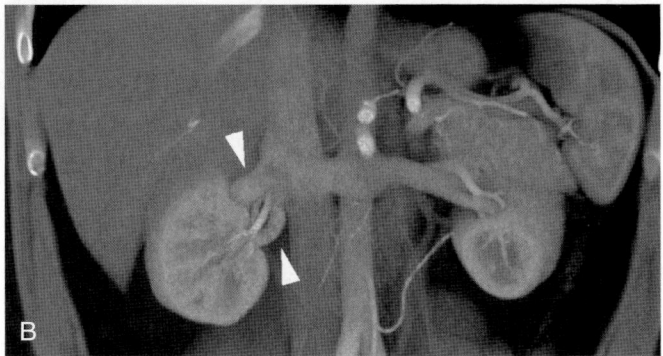

Figure 11-10. CT angiogram for evaluation of potential renal donor. **A.** There is a small accessory right renal artery (*arrow*). **B.** There are also two right renal veins (*arrowheads*).

the scanner, thus obviating the need for routine data transfer to a PACS workstation.

Staging of the pancreatic carcinoma has been discussed in detail in Chapter 100. Because of the frequent variations of vascular anatomy that can affect the surgical approach, close evaluation of the anatomic variants in addition to tumor encasement of the adjacent vasculature is essential. For example, presence of a replaced right hepatic artery originating from the superior mesenteric artery can significantly alter the planning for a Whipple procedure because this vessel traverses posterior to the pancreatic head (Fig. 11-9).

Renal Imaging

CTA is routinely used in preoperative planning for nephrectomy, diagnosing renal artery stenosis, and evaluating ureteropelvic junction obstruction.[80-82] It has been shown to be extremely accurate for the assessment of renal artery stenosis as well as other renal vascular pathologies. Although MR angiography (MRA) may be the initial study of choice in patients with reduced renal function, CTA and MRA are equally accurate for the assessment of significant renal artery stenosis.[83] CTA is the imaging technique of choice for the evaluation of potential renal donors.[84] Its role is to assess vascular anatomy and to evaluate for renal pathology (Fig. 11-10). A comprehensive examination includes noncontrast images to evaluate for renal calculi and vascular calcification, an arterial phase to detect vascular anatomic variants and anomalies, a nephrographic phase to detect renal parenchymal abnormalities, and an excretory phase to evaluate the collecting systems and ureters.[48,81,85,86] Coronal thin-slab MIP images are useful for optimal visualization of the renal arteries.[87] However, because MIP images do not provide spatial depth, volume-rendered images are also beneficial (Fig. 11-11).

It is feasible to scan the renal vasculature with 50 mL of nonionic iodinated contrast material and saline chase using a dual injector on a 16- or 64-slice CT with excellent results.[14] However, to improve opacification of the ureters, saline bolus or diuretics may be beneficial.[88]

Liver Imaging

Vascular complications are a significant contributor to morbidity after hepatic surgery. The hepatic surgeon greatly benefits from vascular mapping of the liver when planning tumor resection, laparoscopic surgery, or transplantation (Fig. 11-12). Until recently, catheter angiography was the standard diagnostic

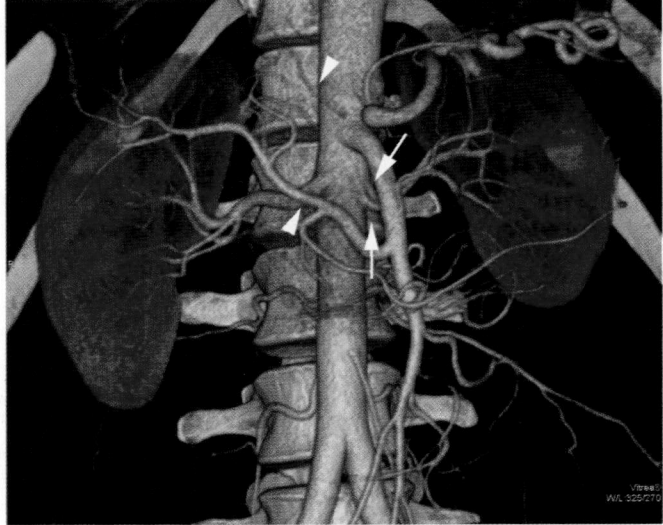

Figure 11-11. Volume-rendered images of a CT angiogram performed for renal donor evaluation. There are two left renal arteries (*arrows*). Also, note the replaced common hepatic artery arising from the superior mesenteric artery as well as a small accessory left hepatic artery arising directly from the aorta (*arrowheads*).

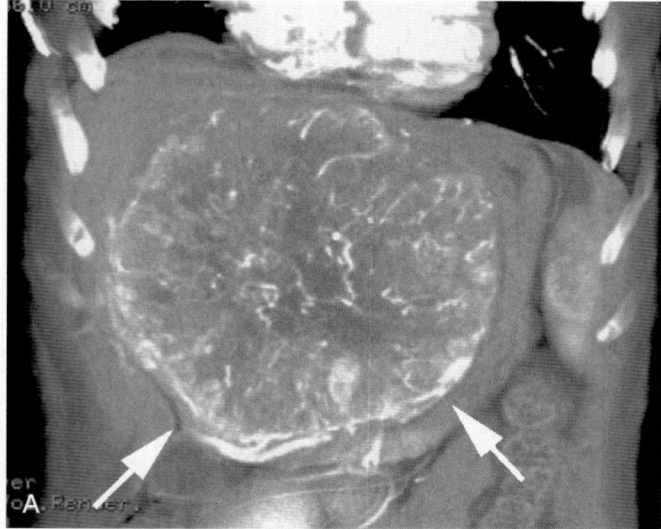

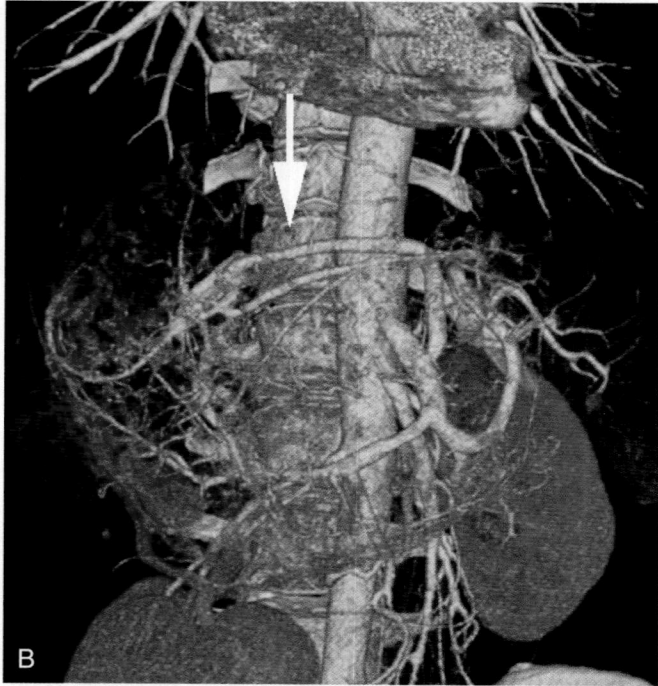

Figure 11-12. Patient with metastatic hemangiopericytoma evaluated for resection. A. A large very vascular hepatic mass (*arrows*) displacing the stomach. **B.** The mass is supplied by a replaced left hepatic artery (*arrow*) arising from the left gastric artery. Accurate vascular mapping resulted in uneventful resection of the mass.

method for preoperative planning of hepatic surgery. However, its associated morbidity and suboptimal visualization of the venous structures have made CT angiography the new standard in many institutions. CT angiography provides exquisite hepatic vascular detail and allows evaluation of the liver parenchyma and other organs.[42,43]

When planning any type of hepatic surgery, knowledge of the vascular anatomy variation is essential. Accessory and aberrant hepatic venous and arterial branches are common and easily visualized by CTA.[42] CTA has been shown to be as effective as catheter angiography in planning of selective hepatic arterial infusion of chemotherapy.[44]

Mesenteric Vasculature

CTA allows excellent visualization of the mesenteric vasculature (Fig. 11-13).[89] Aneurysms, thrombosis, stenosis, dissection, and inflammatory processes affecting the mesenteric vasculature have been evaluated by MDCT. CTA is a robust method for evaluation of acute as well as chronic bowel ischemia (Fig. 11-14). However, owing to high temporal resolution, it may be necessary to scan the region of interest twice because a "pure" arterial phase does not allow evaluation of the venous structures. This is necessary because incomplete enhancement of the mesenteric venous branches during late arterial phase may mimic thrombosis.

Compression of the celiac axis by the median arcuate ligament is referred to as median arcuate ligament syndrome and may cause abdominal angina (Fig. 11-15). Additionally, this entity has been reported to predispose patients who have undergone orthotopic liver transplantation to develop hepatic artery thrombosis. Although surgical treatment can lead to clinical improvement in symptomatic patients, the importance of celiac artery compression in asymptomatic patients is not established. If median arcuate ligament syndrome is suspected, imaging should be obtained during full inspiration to avoid artifactual stenosis.[90,91] Celiac and mesenteric stenoses are best visualized by sagittal thin-slab MIP or volume-rendered images (Fig. 11-16). However, a thin-slab

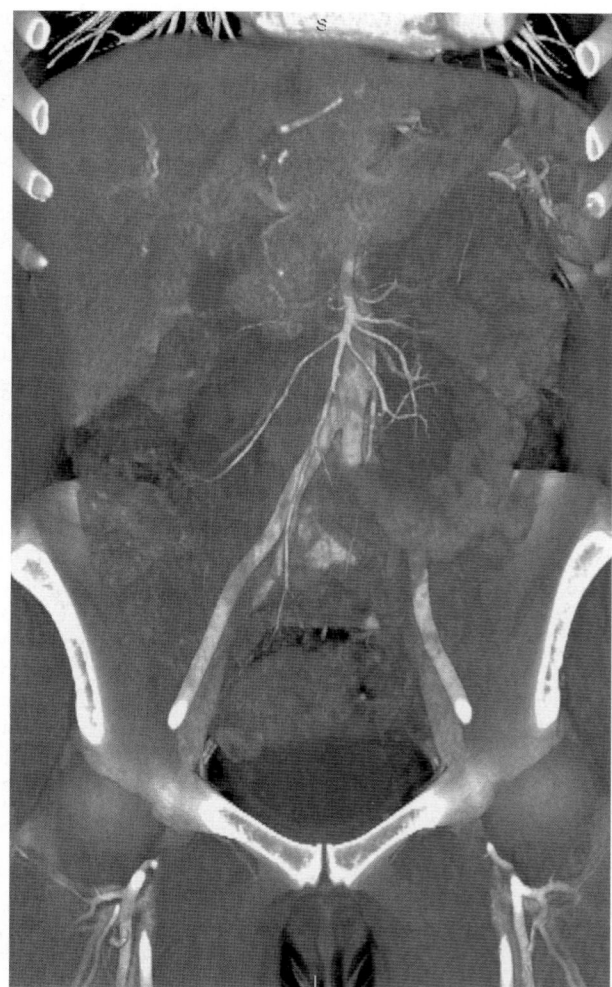

Figure 11-13. CT angiogram of the mesenteric vessels.

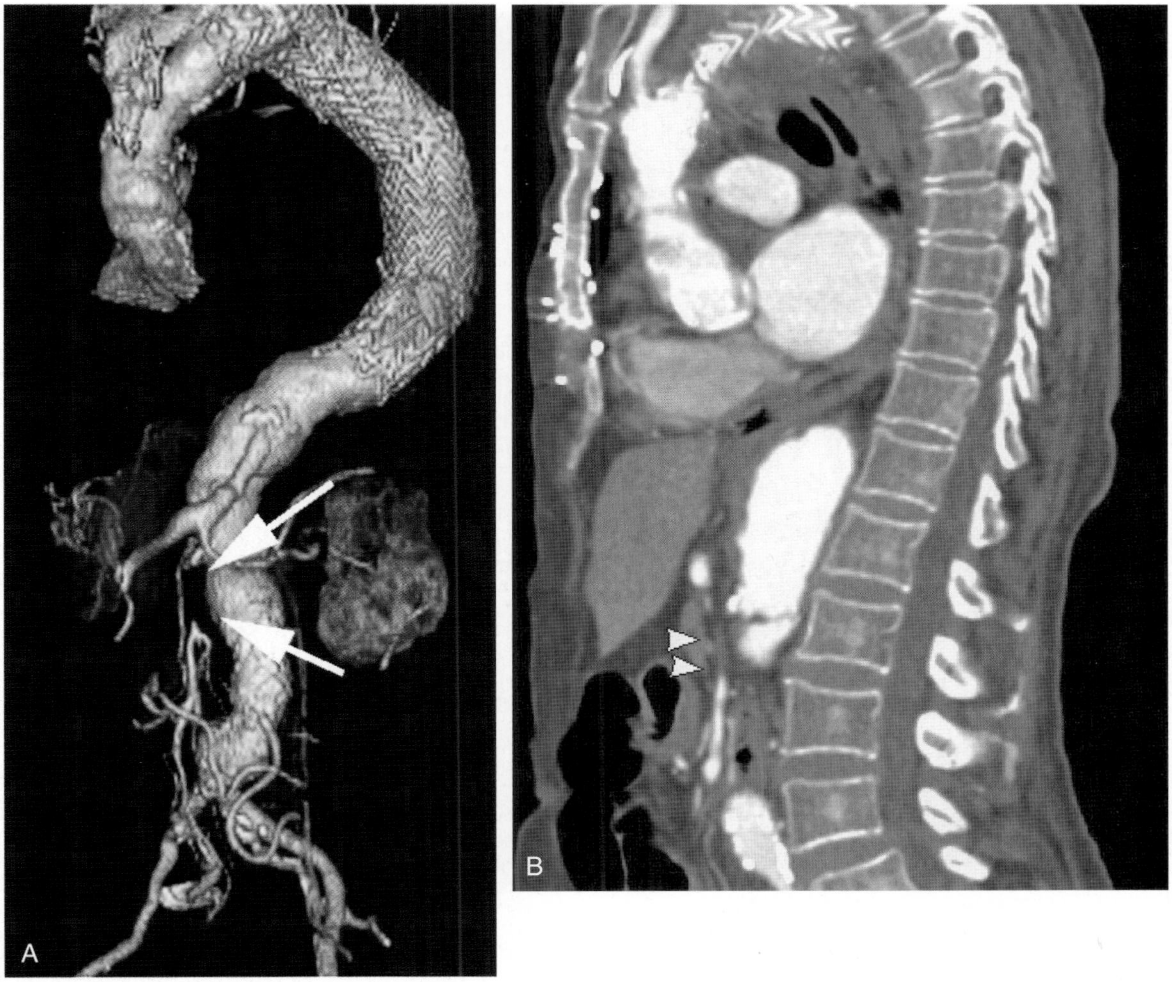

Figure 11-14. Occlusive thrombus in the superior mesenteric artery. A. Volume rendering shows defect in the superior mesenteric artery (*arrows*). Note aortic stent graft. **B.** Sagittal reformatted image better demonstrates the occlusive thrombus (*arrowheads*) in the superior mesenteric artery.

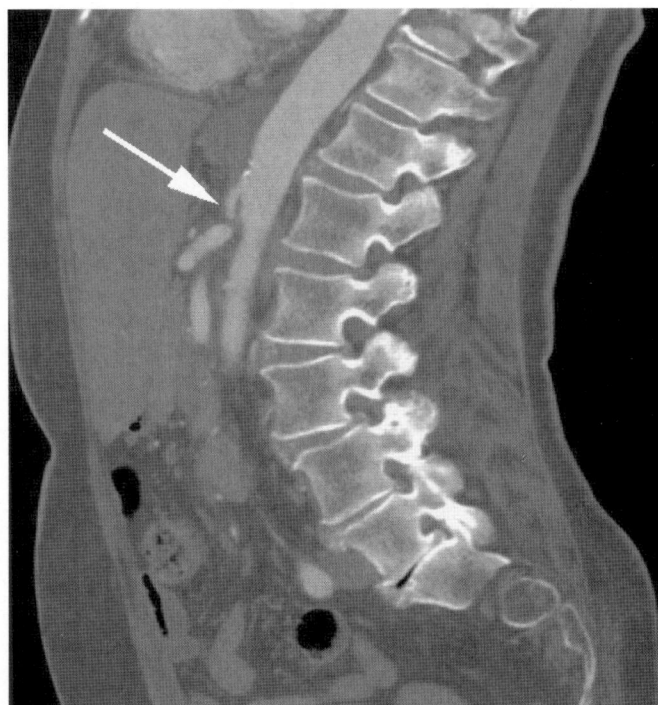

Figure 11-15. Compression of the celiac artery by the median arcuate ligament (*arrow*).

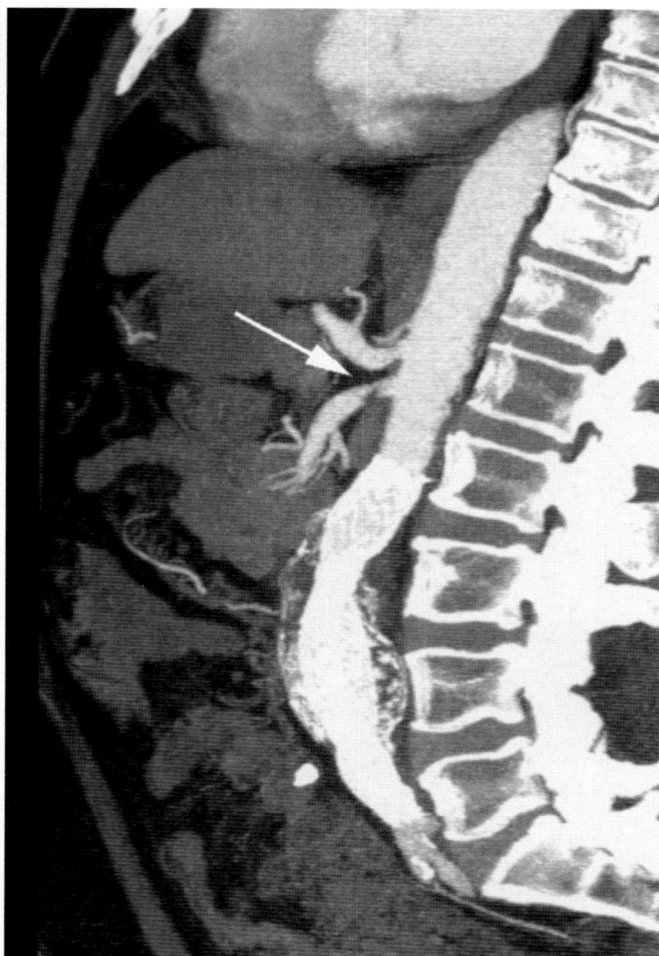

Figure 11-16. Thrombus in the superior mesenteric artery (*arrow*) in a patient with acute abdominal pain.

coronal MIP image also provides an excellent overview of the mesenteric vascular structures as well as the bowel loops.[92] The use of neutral oral contrast agents is important when evaluating the mesentery to improve visualization of the bowel mucosa.

Acute mesenteric ischemia is a life-threatening event that may be caused by a variety of causes. These include embolic phenomenon, severe hypoperfusion, thrombosis of stenotic vessels, dissection, hypercoagulable states, and vasculitis. As discussed previously, diagnosis of mesenteric venous thrombosis requires delayed images to avoid early-phase incomplete enhancement. Unenhanced images are also beneficial because they may show a hyperdense thrombus.[7,93]

When evaluating for mesenteric vascular pathology, close attention to the morphology of the bowel is important, because thickened bowel loops with pneumatosis or altered enhancement (either hyper- or hypoenhancement of the affected bowel) are signs of ischemia.

SUMMARY

Computed tomographic angiography is the byproduct of rapid advances in CT technology and has replaced catheter angiography in many institutions. Both image acquisition

and processing techniques can significantly affect diagnostic image quality. A thorough knowledge of the scanner hardware and contrast optimization methods is, therefore, essential.

References

1. Rubin GD, Dake MD, Napel SA, et al: Three-dimensional spiral CT angiography of the abdomen: Initial clinical experience. Radiology 186:147-152, 1993.
2. Adachi H, Ino T, Mizuhara A, et al: Assessment of aortic disease using three-dimensional CT angiography. J Card Surg 9:673-678, 1994.
3. Napel S, Marks MP, Rubin GD, et al: CT angiography with spiral CT and maximum intensity projection. Radiology 185:607-610, 1992.
4. Dillon EH, van Leeuwen MS, Fernandez MA, et al: Spiral CT angiography. AJR 160:1273-1278, 1993.
5. Galanski M, Prokop M, Chavan A, et al: Renal arterial stenoses: Spiral CT angiography. Radiology 189:185-192, 1993.
6. Rydberg J, Buckwalker KA, Caldemeyer KS, et al: Multisection CT: Scanning techniques and clinical applications. RadioGraphics 20: 1787-1806, 2000.
7. Fishman EK: From the RSNA Refresher Courses: CT Angiography: Clinical applications in the abdomen. Radiographics 21:3S-16S, 2001.
8. Lawler LP, Fishman EK: Three-dimensional CT angiography with multidetector CT data: Study optimization, protocol design, and clinical applications in the abdomen. Crit Rev Comput Tomogr 43:77-141, 2002.
9. Rubin GD: MDCT imaging of the aorta and peripheral vessels. Eur J Radiol 45(Suppl 1):S42-S49, 2003.
10. Rubin GD, Shiau MC, Leung AN, et al: Aorta and iliac arteries: Single versus multiple detector-row helical CT angiography. Radiology 215: 670-676, 2000.
11. Vrtiska TJ, Fletcher JG, McCollough CH: State-of-the-art imaging with 64-channel multidetector CT angiography. Perspect Vasc Surg Endovasc Ther 17:3-8, 2005.
12. Saini S: Multi-detector row CT: Principles and practice for abdominal applications. Radiology 233:323-327, 2004.
13. Schoellnast H, Tillich M, Deutschmann MJ, et al: Aortoiliac enhancement during computed tomography angiography with reduced contrast material dose and saline solution flush: Influence on magnitude and uniformity of the contrast column. Invest Radiol 39:20-26, 2004.
14. Utsunomiya D, Awai K, Tamura Y, et al: 16-MDCT aortography with a low-dose contrast material protocol. AJR 186:374-378, 2006.
15. Anderson SW, Lucey BC, Varghese JC, et al: Sixty-four multi-detector row computed tomography in multitrauma patient imaging: Early experience. Curr Probl Diagn Radiol 35:188-198, 2006.
16. Kalra MK, Maher MM, Toth TL, et al: Strategies for CT radiation dose optimization. Radiology 230:619-628, 2004.
17. Mettler FA Jr., Wiest PW, Locken JA, et al: CT scanning: Patterns of use and dose. J Radiol Prot 20:353-359, 2004.
18. Wintersperger B, Jakobs T, Herzog P, et al: Aorto-iliac multidetector-row CT angiography with low kV settings: Improved vessel enhancement and simultaneous reduction of radiation dose. Eur Radiol 15:334-341, 2005.
19. Brink JA: Contrast optimization and scan timing for single and multidetector-row computed tomography. J Comput Assist Tomogr 27(Suppl 1):S3-S8, 2003.
20. Bae KT: Peak contrast enhancement in CT and MR angiography: When does it occur and why? Pharmacokinetic study in a porcine model. Radiology 227:809-816, 2003.
21. Bae KT, Tran HQ, Heiken JP: Uniform vascular contrast enhancement and reduced contrast medium volume achieved by using exponentially decelerated contrast material injection method. Radiology 231:732-736, 2004.
22. Macari M, Israel GM, Berman P, et al: Infrarenal abdominal aortic aneurysms at multi-detector row CT angiography: Intravascular enhancement without a timing acquisition. Radiology 220:519-523, 2001.
23. Johnson PT, Fishman EK: IV contrast selection for MDCT: Current thoughts and practice. AJR 186:406-415, 2006.
24. Kim MJ, Chung YE, Kim KW, et al: Variation of the time to aortic enhancement of fixed-duration versus fixed-rate injection protocols. AJR 186:185-192, 2006.
25. Fleischmann D: Use of high concentration contrast media: Principles and rationale—vascular district. Eur J Radiol 45(Suppl 1):S88-S93, 2003.
26. Hittmair K, Fleischmann D: Accuracy of predicting and controlling time-

dependent aortic enhancement from a test bolus injection. J Comput Assist Tomogr 25:287-294, 2001.

27. Fleischmann D, Rubin GD, Bankier AA, et al: Improved uniformity of aortic enhancement with customized contrast medium injection protocols at CT angiography. Radiology 214:363-371, 2000.

28. Furuta A, Ito K, Fujita T, et al: Hepatic enhancement in multiphasic contrast-enhanced MDCT: Comparison of high- and low-iodine-concentration contrast medium in same patients with chronic liver disease. AJR 183:157-162, 2004.

29. Fleischmann D, Hallett RL, Rubin GD: CT angiography of peripheral arterial disease. J Vasc Intervent Radiol 17:3-26, 2006.

30. Fleischmann D, Rubin GD: Quantification of intravenously administered contrast medium transit through the peripheral arteries: Implications for CT angiography. Radiology 236:1076-1082, 2005.

31. Karcaaltincaba M, Foley WD: Gadolinium-enhanced multidetector CT angiography of the thoracoabdominal aorta. J Comput Assist Tomogr 26:875-878, 2002.

32. Pena CS, Kaufman JA, Geller SC, et al: Gadopentetate dimeglumine: A possible alternative contrast agent for CT angiography of the aorta. J Comput Assist Tomogr 23:23-24, 1999.

33. Chicoskie C, Tello R: Gadolinium-enhanced MDCT angiography of the abdomen: Feasibility and limitations. AJR 184:1821-1828, 2005.

34. Wicky S, Greenfield A, Fan CM, et al: Aortoiliac gadolinium-enhanced CT angiography: Improved results with a 16-detector row scanner compared with a four-detector row scanner. J Vasc Intervent Radiol 15:947-954, 2004.

35. Grobner T: Gadolinium—a specific trigger for the development of nephrogenic fibrosing dermopathy and nephrogenic systemic fibrosis? Nephrol Dial Transplant 21:1104-1108, 2006.

36. Thomsen HS: Nephrogenic systemic fibrosis: A serious late adverse reaction to gadodiamide. Eur Radiol 16:2619-2621, 2006.

37. Rubin GD: Data explosion: The challenge of multidetector-row CT. Eur J Radiol 36:74-80, 2000.

38. Yaghmai V, Nikolaidis P, Hammond NA, et al: Multidetector-row computed tomography diagnosis of small bowel obstruction: Can coronal reformations replace axial images? Emerg Radiol 13:69-72, 2006.

39. Cody DD: AAPM/RSNA physics tutorial for residents: Topics in CT: Image processing in CT. Radiographics 22:1255-1268, 2002.

40. Prokop M: General principles of MDCT. Eur J Radiol 45(Suppl 1):S4-S10, 2003.

41. Fishman EK, Ney DR, Heath DG, et al: Volume rendering versus maximum intensity projection in CT angiography: What works best, when, and why. RadioGraphics 26:905-922, 2006.

42. Sahani D, Mehta A, Blake M, et al: Preoperative hepatic vascular evaluation with CT and MR angiography: Implications for surgery. RadioGraphics 24:1367-1380, 2004.

43. Sahani D, Saini S, Pena C, et al: Using multidetector CT for preoperative vascular evaluation of liver neoplasms: Technique and results. AJR 179:53-59, 2002.

44. Sahani DV, Krishnamurthy SK, Kalva S, et al: Multidetector-row computed tomography angiography for planning intra-arterial chemotherapy pump placement in patients with colorectal metastases to the liver. J Comput Assist Tomogr 28:478-484, 2004.

45. Winter TC 3rd, Nghiem HV, Freeny PC, et al: Hepatic arterial anatomy in transplantation candidates: Evaluation with three-dimensional CT arteriography. Radiology 195:363-370, 1995.

46. Pollak R, Prusak BF, Mozes MF: Anatomic abnormalities of cadaver kidneys procured for purposes of transplantation. Am Surg 52:233-235, 1986.

47. Kawamoto S, Montgomery RA, Lawler LP, et al: Multidetector CT angiography for preoperative evaluation of living laparoscopic kidney donors. AJR 180:1633-1638, 2003.

48. Raman SS, Pojchamarnwiputh S, Muangsomboon K, et al: Utility of 16-MDCT angiography for comprehensive preoperative vascular evaluation of laparoscopic renal donors. AJR 186:1630-1638, 2006.

49. Stueckle CA, Haegele KF, Jendreck M, et al: Multislice computed tomography angiography of the abdominal arteries: Comparison between computed tomography angiography and digital subtraction angiography findings in 52 cases. Australas Radiol 48:142-147, 2004.

50. Romano M, Mainenti PP, Imbriaco M, et al: Multidetector row CT angiography of the abdominal aorta and lower extremities in patients with peripheral arterial occlusive disease: Diagnostic accuracy and interobserver agreement. Eur J Radiol 50:303-308, 2004.

51. Lederle FA, Wilson SE, Johnson GR, et al: Design of the abdominal aortic Aneurysm Detection and Management Study. ADAM VA Cooperative Study Group. J Vasc Surg 20:296-303, 1994.

52. Daly KJ, Torella F, Ashleigh R, et al: Screening, diagnosis and advances in aortic aneurysm surgery. Gerontology 50:349-359, 2004.

53. Scott RA, Vardulaki KA, Walker NM, et al: The long-term benefits of a single scan for abdominal aortic aneurysm (AAA) at age 65. Eur J Vasc Endovasc Surg 21:535-540, 2001.

54. Ashton HA, Buxton MJ, Day NE, et al: The Multicentre Aneurysm Screening Study (MASS) into the effect of abdominal aortic aneurysm screening on mortality in men: A randomised controlled trial. Lancet 360:1531-1539, 2002.

55. Health service costs and quality of life for early elective surgery or ultrasonographic surveillance for small abdominal aortic aneurysms. UK Small Aneurysm Trial Participants. Lancet 352:1656-1660, 1998.

56. Guirguis EM, Barber GG: The natural history of abdominal aortic aneurysms. Am J Surg 162:481-483, 1991.

57. Powell JT, Brady AR: Detection, management, and prospects for the medical treatment of small abdominal aortic aneurysms. Arterioscler Thromb Vasc Biol 24:241-245, 2004.

58. Longo C, Upchurch GR: Abdominal aortic aneurysm screening: Recommendations and controversies. Vasc Endovascular Surg 39:213-219, 2005.

59. Ellis M, Powell JT, Greenhalgh RM: Limitations of ultrasonography in surveillance of small abdominal aortic aneurysms. Br J Surg 78:614-616, 1991.

60. Ouriel K, Srivastava SD, Sarac TP, et al: Disparate outcome after endovascular treatment of small versus large abdominal aortic aneurysm. J Vasc Surg 37:1206-1212, 2003.

61. Ng CS, Watson CJ, Palmer CR, et al: Evaluation of early abdomino-pelvic computed tomography in patients with acute abdominal pain of unknown cause: Prospective randomised study. BMJ 325:1387, 2002.

62. Brady AR, Fowkes FG, Greenhalgh RM, et al: Risk factors for post-operative death following elective surgical repair of abdominal aortic aneurysm: Results from the UK Small Aneurysm Trial. On behalf of the UK Small Aneurysm Trial participants. Br J Surg 87:742-749, 2000.

63. Benoit AG, Campbell BI, Tanner JR, et al: Risk factors and prevalence of perioperative cognitive dysfunction in abdominal aneurysm patients. J Vasc Surg 42:884-890, 2005.

64. Parodi JC, Palmaz JC, Barone HD: Transfemoral intraluminal graft implantation for abdominal aortic aneurysms. Ann Vasc Surg 5:491-499, 1991.

65. Vignali C, Cioni R, Neri E, et al: Endoluminal treatment of abdominal aortic aneurysms. Abdominal Imaging 26:461-468, 2001.

66. Blankensteijn JD, de Jong SE, Prinssen M, et al: Two-year outcomes after conventional or endovascular repair of abdominal aortic aneurysms. N Engl J Med 352:2398-2405, 2005.

67. Buth J, van Marrewijk CJ, Harris PL, et al: Outcome of endovascular abdominal aortic aneurysm repair in patients with conditions considered unfit for an open procedure: A report on the EUROSTAR experience. J Vasc Surg 35:211-221, 2002.

68. Qanadli SD, Mesurolle B, Coggia M, et al: Abdominal aortic aneurysm: Pretherapy assessment with dual-slice helical CT angiography. AJR 174:181-187, 2000.

69. Resch T, Ivancev K, Lindh M, et al: Abdominal aortic aneurysm morphology in candidates for endovascular repair evaluated with spiral computed tomography and digital subtraction angiography. J Endovasc Surg 6:227-232, 1999.

70. Morasch MD: Percutaneous thoracic and abdominal aortic aneurysm repair. Ann Vasc Surg 19:585-589, 2005.

71. White RA, Donayre CE, Walot I, et al: Preliminary clinical outcome and imaging criterion for endovascular prosthesis development in high-risk patients who have aortoiliac and traumatic arterial lesions. J Vasc Surg 24:556-569; discussion 569-571, 1996.

72. Armerding MD, Rubin GD, Beaulieu CF, et al: Aortic aneurysmal disease: Assessment of stent-graft treatment-CT versus conventional angiography. Radiology 215:138-146, 2000.

73. Golzarian J, Valenti D: Endoleakage after endovascular treatment of abdominal aortic aneurysms: Diagnosis, significance and treatment. Eur Radiol 16:2849-2857, 2006.

74. Brugel M, Link TM, Rummeny EJ, et al: Assessment of vascular invasion in pancreatic head cancer with multislice spiral CT: Value of multiplanar reconstructions. Eur Radiol 14:1188-1195, 2004.

75. Foley WD, Mallisee TA, Hohenwalter MD, et al: Multiphase hepatic CT with a multirow detector CT scanner. AJR 175:679-685, 2000.

76. Foley WD: Special focus session: Multidetector CT: Abdominal visceral imaging. Radiographics 22:701-719, 2002.

77. Fletcher JG, Wiersema MJ, Farrell MA, et al: Pancreatic malignancy: Value of arterial, pancreatic, and hepatic phase imaging with multidetector row CT. Radiology 229:81-90, 2003.

78. Nino-Murcia M, Jeffrey RB Jr., Beaulieu CF, et al: Multidetector CT of the pancreas and bile duct system: Value of curved planar reformations. AJR 176:689-693, 2001.

79. Vargas R, Nino-Murcia M, Trueblood W, et al: MDCT in pancreatic adenocarcinoma: Prediction of vascular invasion and resectability using a multiphasic technique with curved planar reformations. AJR 182:419-425, 2004.

80. Rouviere O, Lyonnet D, Berger P, et al: Ureteropelvic junction obstruction: Use of helical CT for preoperative assessment: Comparison with intraarterial angiography. Radiology 213:668-673, 1999.

81. Urban BA, Ratner LE, Fishman EK: Three-dimensional volume-rendered CT angiography of the renal arteries and veins: Normal anatomy, variants, and clinical applications. RadioGraphics 21:373-386, 2001.

82. Kaatee R, Beek FJ, de Lange EE, et al: Renal artery stenosis: Detection and quantification with spiral CT angiography versus optimized digital subtraction angiography. Radiology 205:121-127, 1997.

83. Willmann JK, Wildermuth S, Pfammatter T, et al: Aortoiliac and renal arteries: Prospective intraindividual comparison of contrast-enhanced three-dimensional MR angiography and multi-detector row CT angiography. Radiology 226:798-811, 2003.

84. Tsuda K, Murakami T, Kim T, et al: Helical CT angiography of living renal donors: Comparison with 3D Fourier transformation phase contrast MRA. J Comput Assist Tomogr 22:186-193, 1998.

85. Patil UD, Ragavan A, Nadaraj, et al: Helical CT angiography in evaluation of live kidney donors. Nephrol Dial Transplant 16:1900-1904, 2001.

86. Kim JK, Park SY, Kim H, et al: Living donor kidneys: Usefulness of multidetector row CT for comprehensive evaluation. Radiology 229:869-876, 2003.

87. Kim JK, Kim JH, Bae SJ, et al: CT angiography for evaluation of living renal donors: Comparison of four reconstruction methods. AJR 183:471-477, 2004.

88. Noroozian M, Cohan RH, Caoili EM, et al: Multislice CT urography: State of the art. Br J Radiol 77(Suppl 1):S74-S86, 2004.

89. Laghi A, Iannaccone R, Catalano C, et al: Multislice spiral computed tomography angiography of mesenteric arteries. Lancet 358:638-639, 2001.

90. Lee VS, Morgan JN, Tan AG, et al: Celiac artery compression by the median arcuate ligament: A pitfall of end-expiratory MR imaging. Radiology 228:437-442, 2003.

91. Horton KM, Talamini MA, Fishman EK: Median arcuate ligament syndrome: Evaluation with CT angiography. RadioGraphics 25:1177-1182, 2005.

92. Kirkpatrick IDC, Kroeker MA, Greenberg HM: Biphasic CT with mesenteric CT angiography in the evaluation of acute mesenteric ischemia: Initial experience. Radiology 229:91-98, 2003.

93. Bradbury MS, Kavanagh PV, Bechtold RE, et al: Mesenteric venous thrombosis: Diagnosis and noninvasive imaging. RadioGraphics 22:527-541, 2002.

Magnetic Resonance Angiography of the Mesenteric Vasculature

Ranista Tongdee, MD • Vamsi R. Narra, MD, FRCR

Magnetic resonance angiography (MRA) is a noninvasive vascular imaging technique that is being used with increasing frequency as an alternate to conventional catheter angiography. Initially, time-of-flight (TOF) and phase-contrast (PC) MRA were the main means of evaluating the visceral vasculature, primarily the renal arteries. Advances in MR technology facilitated the implementation of three-dimensional contrast-enhanced MRA, which significantly expanded the role of MRA in imaging of the abdomen. Not only is contrast-enhanced MRA useful for anatomic assessment of the visceral arteries and veins, but when combined with phase-contrast MRA, these techniques also can provide physiologic information, which is particularly useful in the evaluation of mesenteric ischemia.

In this chapter, we briefly discuss the various MR angiographic techniques with emphasis on contrast-enhanced MRA (CE MRA). This chapter also presents an approach to evaluation of visceral vasculature with MRA, including patient preparation, imaging protocols, and image postprocessing techniques. The various clinical applications of MRA in the abdomen are also illustrated.

MAGNETIC RESONANCE ANGIOGRAPHIC TECHNIQUES

Time-of-flight (TOF) is the oldest MRA technique for evaluation of vasculature. This technique exploits blood motion to visualize vascular structures directly without the use of intravenous contrast material. It is performed using a gradient refocused sequence in which the stationary tissues are saturated, producing low background signal intensity. In contrast, blood moving into the imaging volume is unsaturated with full longitudinal magnetization. As a result, when blood is excited it gives a bright signal compared with the stationary, saturated background tissues. There are limitations with TOF technique; it is time consuming and requires patient co-operation. Long acquisition times limit its use during a breath-hold. In addition, this technique is susceptible to in-plane saturation and phase dispersion, preventing application of TOF for routine evaluation of the visceral vasculature. TOF is still applicable in certain areas when evaluating the mesenteric vasculature. These include evaluation of large vessels such as abdominal aorta, proximal portions of celiac and superior mesenteric arteries, large venous structures such as the inferior vena cava (IVC), portal vein, superior mesenteric vein, portosystemic collaterals, and so on.[1,2] Diseased vessels or small size arteries such as the proper hepatic artery, gastroduodenal artery, and branches of superior mesenteric arteries cannot be well evaluated with this technique.[3,4] The direction of portal venous blood flow can be assessed using TOF technique by simply applying a saturation band over the portal vein.

Phase-contrast (PC) technique utilizes phase shifts of the flowing protons in the vascular structures to create MRA images. Phase shifts of stationary tissues are compensated by using a bipolar gradient. Two imaging acquisitions are performed in which the first has positive bipolar gradient and the second has negative bipolar gradient. The data from these two acquisitions are subtracted in k space to eliminate phase shift induced by other sequence parameters. The net effect is an image of flowing spins. The amount of phase difference that remains after subtraction is proportional to the velocity of the moving spins. The flow sensitivity can be adjusted by setting the velocity encoding value (Venc). Venc determines the highest and lowest detectable velocities encoded by a phase-contrast sequence. For example, Venc = 100 cm/s is ideal for a phase-contrast MRA with a measurable range of flow velocities of ±100 cm/s. PC MRA allows functional assessment of mesenteric circulation and has been shown to be helpful for diagnosing mesenteric ischemia.[5-7] The information from phase-contrast measurements can be processed into either magnitude (bright-blood and anatomic) images or phase-contrast (velocity) images. A major disadvantage of the phase-contrast technique is long acquisition times requiring patient cooperation. This technique is not used as a primary imaging tool for anatomic assessment of visceral arteries or the portal system.

Balanced steady-state free precession (b-SSFP) is a rapid imaging technique that provides a very high signal-to-noise ratio with T2*/T1-weighted image contrast. The different T2*/T1 ratios of blood and surrounding tissue are beneficial for angiographic imaging.[8] This technique is not flow dependent so that venous structures demonstrate as bright a signal intensity as arterial structures. Clotted blood is low in signal intensity, depending on the clotting stage and composition of blood products. b-SSFP is best suited for morphologic imaging of the vessels. It allows rough anatomic visualization of adjacent tissues, such as mural thrombus and the vascular wall, which may not be optimally evaluated when using a CE MRA sequence alone. The drawback of this technique is the banding artifacts caused by magnetic field inhomogeneity. One solution to this problem is to use a very short repetition time (TR) to eliminate the artifacts from the regions of interest. Given the high signal-to-noise ratio of b-SSFP sequences, bright signal intensity of fat can obscure anatomic structures. In such circumstances, effective fat suppression can be used to improve the image quality.

Three-dimensional (3D) CE MRA is an excellent technique for anatomic evaluation of the abdominal arterial and venous structures. The image contrast is based on the differences in the T1 relaxation time of blood and the surrounding tissues. Gadolinium chelate is administered to significantly shorten the T1 relaxation time of blood, and T1-weighted images are obtained with 3D spoiled gradient-echo technique (3D SPGR/ 3D FLASH [fast low-angle shot]) using very short echo times

(TE) and repetition times (TR) in combination with a relatively high excitation flip angle (25 to 40 degrees). The other imaging parameters are detailed later in the chapter.

Contrast Material Dosage, Injection Rate, and Timing Considerations

Appropriate timing of contrast material injection is critical in obtaining good arterial phase CE MRA images without significant venous contamination. The volume of contrast material, chasing saline solution, delivery rate, and scan delay time need to be optimized to enhance image quality.

The arterial and venous enhancement pattern after bolus contrast injection is shown in Figure 12-1.[9] To achieve excellent image contrast and signal-to-noise ratio, the imaging sequences have to be timed such that the acquisition of central portion of k space (low-frequency data lines) corresponds with the plateau phase of maximum concentration of contrast material in the vessels of interest. If the central portion of k space is filled before the peak of the contrast concentration, severe "ringing" or "banding" artifacts result (Fig. 12-2). On the other hand, images acquired too late are usually corrupted by venous contamination. Injection rate and duration of injection also have a significant effect on the pattern of arterial enhancement. Faster injection rate leads to sharper arterial peak and higher maximum arterial signal intensity. In contrast, arterial peak would be lower and broader with the slower injection rate.[9] Contrary to the arterial enhancement pattern, the degree of venous enhancement does not vary substantially with the injection rate but depends mostly on the total dose of contrast material. Thus, a larger amount of contrast material would produce better vascular contrast when performing gadolinium-enhanced portography or venography.[10] The time to peak for venous enhancement is longer with a slower injection rate, and image acquisition should be delayed proportionally to obtain the best contrast enhancement of the venous structures.

In its infancy, CE MRA images were acquired as non–breath-hold sequence with the acquisition times of 3 to 5 minutes. Accordingly, the gadolinium chelate was infused at

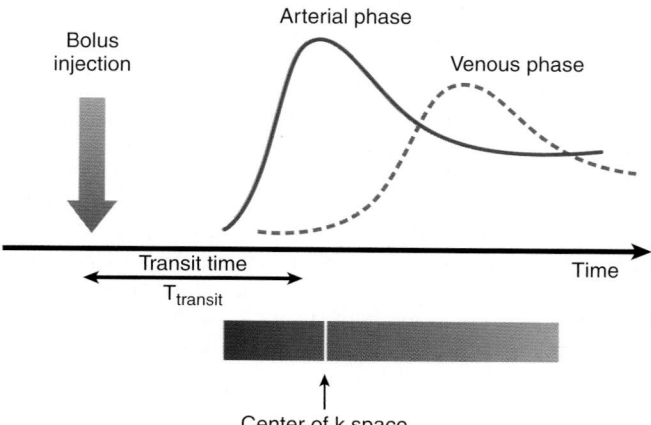

Figure 12-1. Line diagram depicting arterial and venous enhancement pattern after a bolus injection. To achieve the best MR angiographic quality without venous contamination, the data at the center of the k space should be acquired during the peak arterial enhancement before opacification of the venous structures.

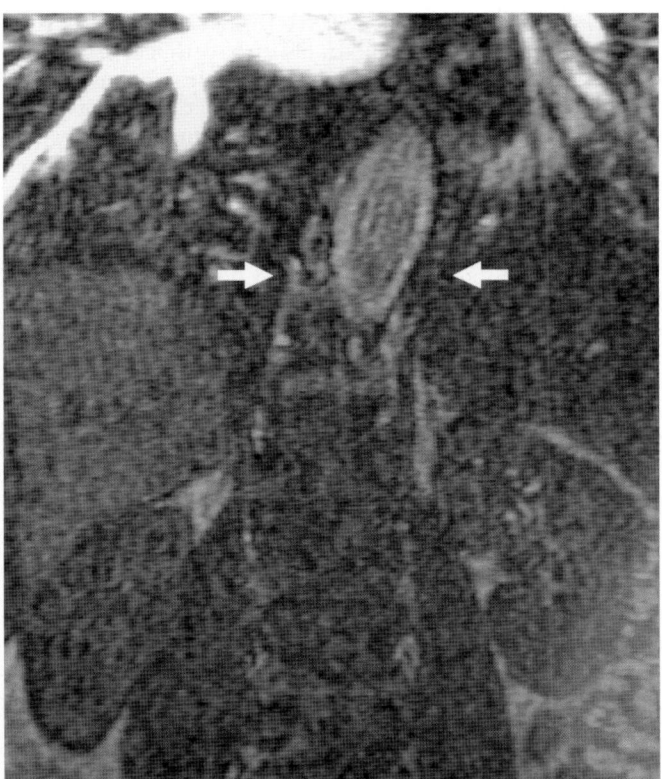

Figure 12-2. Ringing or banding artifact. This artifact (*arrows*) occurs when the central portion of the k space is filled before the peak of the contrast concentration, and there is contrast in the vessel when the periphery of the k space is acquired.

a slow, uniform rate over the entire scan duration to prolong the window of preferential arterial to venous enhancement.[11] Presently, high-speed gradient MR systems and improvement in sequences permit much shorter acquisition times, typically less than 25 seconds. This allows data acquisition during the first pass of contrast material and in a single breath-hold. The rapid bolus injection with automatic MR-compatible power injectors is preferred.

The dosage of contrast used for performing abdominal MR angiography usually varies from a single dose to triple dose (0.1 to 0.3 mmol/kg).[12-17] Although some studies have shown that single-dose CE MRA is sufficient for diagnostic assessment of the aorta and its major branches,[13-15] others report that image quality, vessel delineation, and confidence in diagnosis is improved with the use of higher dose (double dose[16,17] or triple dose[12]). With regard to injection rate, a faster injection allows greater degree of preferential arterial to venous enhancement.[9] Additionally, the interval between arterial and venous peaks tends to be longer with higher injection rate.[10] Hence, the venous contamination can be diminished by using a high-rate injection protocol. For mesenteric MRA, we use a double dose (0.2 mmol/kg) of contrast material, injected at the rate of 2 to 3 mL/s, followed by 15 to 20 mL normal saline flush at the same rate.

Bolus Timing Methods

Because the image quality of CE MRA depends primarily on the distribution and concentration of gadolinium during the acquisition of the center of k space, the proper timing is paramount to achieving a good MRA image, particularly when using fast imaging techniques. There are several ways to synchronize the arterial peak enhancement with the center of k space data acquisition.

The "best guess" technique is the simplest timing method performed by using an estimated contrast travel time from the injection site to the vascular structure of interest. The variation in contrast travel time depends on age, sex, injection site, injection rate, and other clinical parameters, such as cardiac output status and vascular anatomy. Generally, the estimated contrast travel time from an antecubital vein to the abdominal aorta is approximately 15 seconds in a healthy young patient and 20 to 25 seconds in a healthy elderly patient. In patients with decreased cardiac output or a large aortic aneurysm, the estimated contrast travel time may vary widely from 25 to 50 seconds.[18]

The test bolus technique is a more precise timing method performed by injecting a small amount of contrast material (1 to 2 mL) followed by a normal saline flush (10 to 20 mL) at the same injection rate as in the planned contrast-enhanced MR angiography study. The vascular structure of interest is imaged with a timing bolus acquisition (single-slice fast 2D gradient-echo sequence) acquired at a rate of one image every second. The time to peak of contrast enhancement is determined visually or by drawing a region-of-interest over the vessel. The scan delay time is calculated as follows when using a sequential (linear) order of k-space acquisition in the 3D MRA sequence:

$$\text{Imaging delay time or scan delay} = (\text{time to peak of}$$
$$\text{contrast enhancement}) + (\text{injection duration time}/2) -$$
$$(\text{time to center of k space})$$

If a centrically reordered k-space acquisition sequence is used, the estimated scan delay is equal to the time to peak of contrast enhancement. This is a robust and reliable technique that offers the advantage of ensuring adequate intravenous. The drawback of this technique is that there is no guarantee that the imaging bolus will behave identical to the test bolus because of the differences in total volume of injection especially in the setting of poor cardiac function.

Automatic triggering technique (SmartPrep; GE Medical Systems) is another technique to optimize the imaging delay time by automatically synchronizing bolus arrival and the image acquisition. In this technique, a tracker volume is placed over the desired vascular structure, typically at a level slightly proximal to the area of interest. The signal level of the tracker volume is serially obtained using a tracker sequence during the contrast injection. When the signal intensity reaches a threshold value (usually 2 to 3 SD or 15% to 30% above the mean signal level), the 3D MRA sequence (3D SPGR sequence with centric reordering of k space) is triggered. Generally, there is a 4- to 5-second delay between the detection of the bolus and the start of 3D acquisition, which allows the contrast agent to reach its peak level and gives the patient time to suspend respiration. This method ensures that peak arterial and central k-space data acquisition occur simultaneously.[19] A disadvantage of this technique is that if the size of the tracker volume (approximately $2 \times 2 \times 2.5$ cm) is larger than the arterial structure of interest and there is overlap of an adjacent vascular structure, misting of contrast can occur.

Magnetic resonance fluoroscopy (CARE bolus, Siemens Medical Solutions) is a fluoroscopic triggering technique. Similar to the automatic triggering technique, the entire volume of contrast is injected. With the use of a fast 2D gradient-echo technique rapid images are acquired in real time over the vessel of interest. As the contrast agent arrives within the vessel of interest, the 3D MRA sequence is triggered by the operator. The operator-triggered approach has some advantages. For example, in evaluation of cases with asymmetrical flow patterns, in cases where there is displacement of the monitoring plane due to patient motion, an experienced operator can adapt and initiate the triggering accordingly.[20]

MESENTERIC CONTRAST-ENHANCED MAGNETIC RESONANCE ANGIOGRAPHY PROTOCOL

No special preparation for the scan is required. Some believe that a mesenteric MRA is better performed post prandial because there is increased splanchnic circulation.[16] After the patient is positioned supine on the table and centered for the midabdomen, the basic imaging protocol for mesenteric MRA generally starts with the multiplane scout images of the abdomen. Coronal and axial true fast-imaging with steady-state precession (true FISP; balanced SSFP) images of the abdomen are acquired to provide anatomic assessment of the outer wall of the vessel and as an additional set of localizers to position the subsequent test bolus and 3D MRA slab. Precontrast 3D MRA sequence is performed in the coronal plane using the shortest possible TR to shorten the acquisition time. TE should be short enough to eliminate dephasing artifact and to minimize $T2^*$ effects. Appropriated flip angle is in between 25 and 60 degrees. The thickness of slabs and sections varies depending on the patient so that the entire mesenteric vasculature is imaged. A slice thickness of 1 to 1.5 mm after interpolation is preferred. If using a test bolus technique, a timing bolus sequence (TurboFLASH sequences: acquisition speed = 1 image/s) of the abdominal aorta is performed in sagittal plane using a test injection of gadolinium chelate (1 to 2 mL injected at 2 to 3 mL/s). If there is an aortic aneurysm, the estimated contrast arrival time should be timed to include the distal part of aneurysm. After administration of contrast (0.1 to 0.2 mmol/kg at 2 to 3 mL/s) at appropriated delay time (as calculated or automatically trigger) followed by saline flush solution of 15 to 20 mL at the same rate, two imaging sets are consecutively acquired post contrast. The imaging time for each sequence should range between 20 and 25 seconds to encompass a single breath-hold.

IMAGE POSTPROCESSING AND DISPLAY

Three-dimensional CE MRA produces a contiguous volume of image data so that it can be easily reformatted in any desired plane or reconstructed using various 3D reconstruction algorithms for better demonstration of targeted vessels.

Subtraction is a simple postprocessing technique that allows elimination of the background tissue signal such as fat. Postcontrast images are subtracted from the precontrast images, resulting in a new subtracted dataset. The subtracted dataset can be further postprocessed using the techniques described below.

Multiplanar reformat (MPR) is the reconstruction of images in an arbitrary orientation such as orthogonal, oblique, or curved planes. This method allows the viewer to slide through a given volume in any plane in real time. Reformatted slices remain thin and eliminate overlapping structures and unfolding tortuous vessels. The reformatted images often better demonstrate and provide additional diagnostic information. This is particularly true in the evaluation of complex anatomic structures or areas that are traditionally difficult to evaluate on axial source images (Fig. 12-3).

Maximum intensity projection (MIP) is the projection of pixels with highest intensity onto an arbitrarily oriented plane. MIP images have an aspect similar to that of conventional angiograms and are commonly used for angiographic display because the vascular signal is much greater than the background signal. The image data can be reconstructed in either full-volumetric MIP or subvolumetric MIP, in which only a small portion of the slab is reconstructed. The thickness of the slab and the desired viewing plane can be adjusted. A drawback of MIP images is the lack of depth information so that the objects lying in the same projection plane of high intensity structures cannot be visualized.[21] For example, the stationary tissues that have greater signal intensity than the vascular structures, such as fat, hemorrhage, or metallic susceptibility artifact, can lead to mapping of these nonvascular structures to the projection image and cause a discontinuity in vessel signal, potentially mimicking stenosis or occlusion.[22] On the other hand, eccentrically located stenoses may remain undetected.[23] Careful evaluations with multiple angle projections as well as subvolumetric MIP reconstruction technique can help minimize the chance of diagnostic errors incurred by full-volumetric MIP images. Given the potential pitfalls, MIP images should be used as a roadmap while the source images and MPR are preferably used for definitive diagnosis (Figs. 12-4A and B; see Fig. 12-12A).[17,22,24]

Shaded surface display (SSD) is the three-dimensional display of surface from a series of contiguous slices using variable threshold settings. The 3D objects can be rotated and

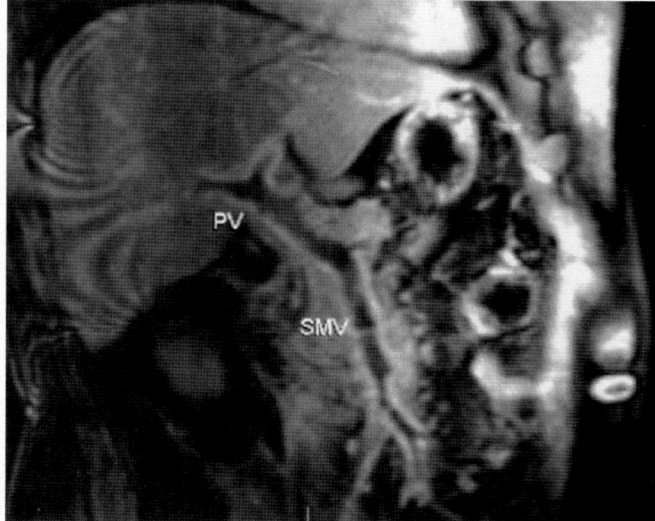

Figure 12-3. Portal vein and superior mesenteric vein thrombosis. Curved multiplanar reformatted contrast-enhanced MR portogram demonstrates extensive thrombus in the portal vein (PV) and the superior mesenteric vein (SMV).

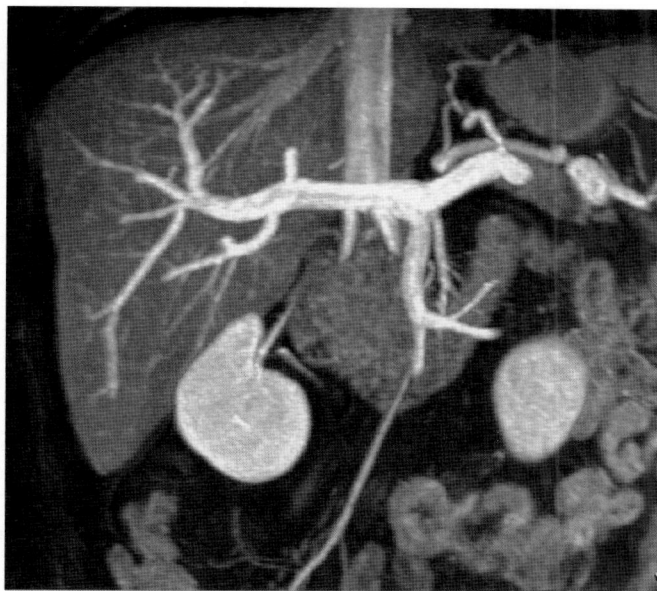

Figure 12-13. Normal contrast-enhanced portal venography. Coronal subvolumetric MIP reconstruction of the 3D contrast-enhanced MR portography demonstrates normal opacification of the portal vein, splenic vein, and superior mesenteric veins.

invasion of the portal vein (Figs. 12-13 and 12-14).[49] The principle of CE MR portography is to image a high concentration of contrast material circulating in the portal venous system. Boeve and associates[50] found that optimal portal venous enhancement occurs approximately 30 seconds after the maximum arterial enhancement. In our practice, three to four 3D MRA datasets are obtained after the intravenous injection of gadolinium. The first dataset is acquired during the arterial phase and can be used as a mask for image subtraction. One or two contrast-enhanced 3D MR portograms are then created by reconstructing images of the portal phase

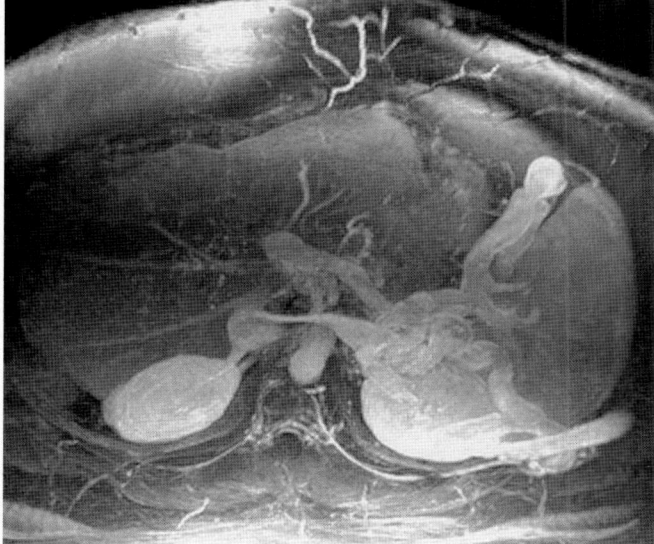

Figure 12-14. Portal hypertension with spontaneous splenorenal shunt. Portal hypertension is well depicted on this axial projection MIP image.

with MIP display. Subtraction can be used to eliminate arterial flow from obscuring portal venous anatomy.[51]

The major limitation of CE MR portography is its inability to provide hemodynamic data regarding flow direction in portal venous system. Portal venous flow direction can be assessed by using PC MR angiography or 2D gradient-echo time of flight sequences. In this technique, a saturation band is placed across the proximal aspect of the portal vein, with another saturation band placed transversely above the hepatic dome to eliminate signal within the hepatic artery. In normal hepatopetal flow, the distal portal vein beyond the first saturation band should lose the signal intensity. Bright signal intensity beyond the first saturation band indicates abnormal hepatofugal flow.[52]

Diseases of the Inferior Vena Cava

Two-dimensional time-of-flight technique with a superior traveling saturation band to suppress the arterial signal can be used to demonstrate iliac veins and the inferior vena cava (Fig. 12-15). Many prior studies[53-56] have shown high accuracy and high sensitivity of time-of-flight MRA in detecting thrombosis in the abdominal and pelvic vessels. 3D CE MR venography is also a sensitive technique of evaluating the IVC. Venous structures are better delineated by giving a double dose of contrast material. This technique permits higher spatial resolution images with short acquisition times and enables differentiation of bland thrombus from tumor thrombus based on enhancement profiles. Additionally, 3D data can be reconstructed into any desired plane to achieve the best anatomic delineation.

MAGNETIC RESONANCE ANGIOGRAPHY PITFALLS

MRA has several potential pitfalls. Some result from improper scan technique. For example, inappropriate positioning of the imaging volume may simulate vascular occlusion by eliminating the structures from the imaging volume. Banding or ringing artifact results from suboptimal timing when the center of k-space data is acquired before the peak of contrast enhancement. This can result in a dark signal with the vessel and can mimic dissection or occlusion of the vessel.

Some MRA pitfalls result from subtraction and reconstruction techniques. For instance, an aneurysm with mural thrombus may be misinterpreted as a normal vessel because MIP images only depict the opacified lumen. Additionally, MIP may cause either overestimation or underestimation of stenosis owing to partial volume effects or poor spatial resolution. Because MIP is generated by projecting only the pixel with the highest attenuation along a ray projected through the dataset, the signal intensity within the volume-averaged pixels may simply be below the MIP threshold and be erroneously excluded from the final image, resulting in an overestimation of the stenosis. On the other hand, if the stenotic segment extends equally into two pixels, the signal intensity would be averaged over the two pixels and each pixel would appear in the MIP image as part of the lumen, resulting in underestimation of the stenosis.[57-59] Metallic artifacts from vascular stents or surgical clips may obscure the adjacent vascular structures and simulate stenosis. However, most MRA interpretation pitfalls can be avoided by reviewing the source images.

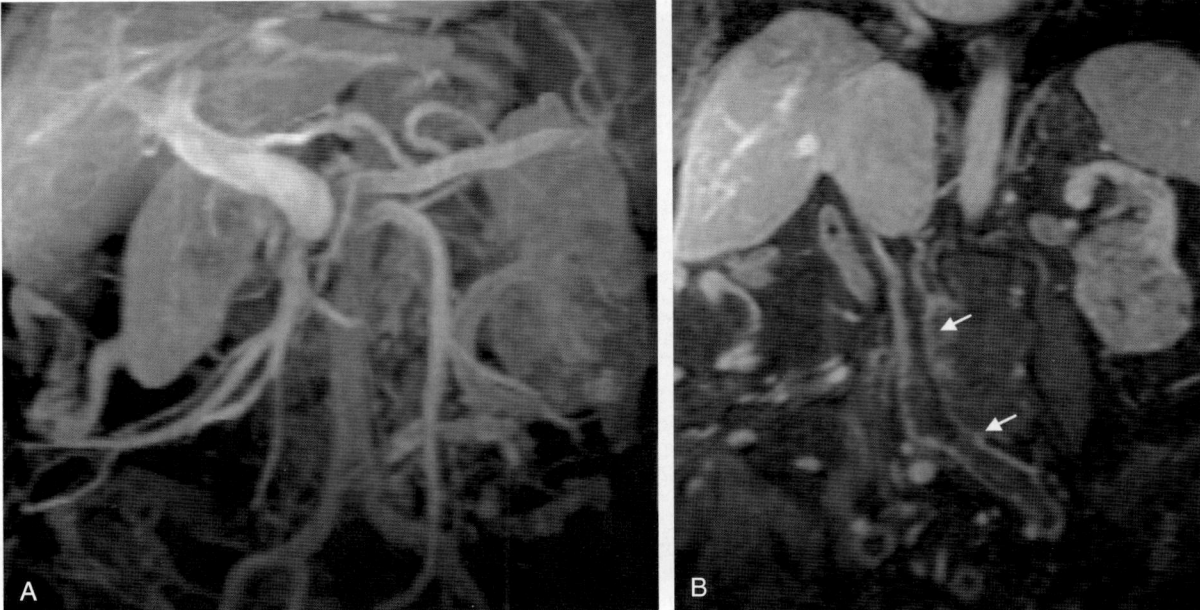

Figure 12-15. Inferior vena cava and iliac vein thrombosis. Coronal full volumetric MIP reconstruction (**A**) of contrast-enhanced MR venography demonstrates nonopacification of the inferior vena cava. Coronal oblique multiplanar reformatted image (**B**) reveals an extensive thrombus within the inferior vena cava and left iliac veins (*arrows*).

SUMMARY

Magnetic resonance angiography provides a superb, noninvasive means of evaluating visceral vessels because of its ability to provide high resolution images within short imaging time. Different MR techniques offer complementary information. b-SSFP can provide rough anatomic detail both within and outside the vascular lumen without gadolinium administration. The time-of-flight technique can still be used for venous evaluation in conjunction to contrast-enhanced images. Phase-contrast sequences allow flow quantification within vessels. The combination of these techniques permits anatomic and functional evaluation of the visceral vasculature. Knowledge of the advantages, disadvantages, and the potential pitfalls and artifacts of each MRA technique is important when performing and interpreting visceral MRA.

References

1. Shih MC, Hagspiel KD: CTA and MRA in mesenteric ischemia. Part 1: Role in diagnosis and differential diagnosis. AJR 188:452-461, 2007.
2. Suto Y, Ohuchi Y, Kimura T, et al: Three-dimensional black blood MR angiography of the liver during breath-holding: A comparison with two-dimensional time-of-flight MR angiography. Acta Radiol 35:131-134, 1994.
3. Finn JP, Edelman RR, Jenkins RL, et al: Liver transplantation: MR angiography with surgical validation. Radiology 179:265-269, 1991.
4. Lewis WD, Finn JP, Jenkins RL, et al: Use of magnetic resonance angiography in the pretransplant evaluation of portal vein pathology. Transplantation 56:64-68, 1993.
5. Burkart DJ, Johnson CD, Reading CC, et al: MR measurements of mesenteric venous flow: Prospective evaluation in healthy volunteers and patients with suspected chronic mesenteric ischemia. Radiology 194:801-806, 1995.
6. Shih MC, Angle JF, Leung DA, et al: CTA and MRA in mesenteric ischemia. Part 2: Normal findings and complications after surgical and endovascular treatment. AJR 188:462-471, 2007.
7. Li KC, Whitney WS, McDonnell CH, et al: Chronic mesenteric ischemia: Evaluation with phase-contrast cine-MR imaging. Radiology 190:175-179, 1994.
8. Scheffler K, Lehnhardt S: Principles and applications of balanced SSFP techniques. Eur Radiol 13:2409-2418, 2003.
9. Strouse PJ, Prince MR, Chenevert TL: Effect of the rate of gadopentetate dimeglumine administration on abdominal vascular and soft-tissue MR imaging enhancement patterns. Radiology 201:809-816, 1996.
10. Mitsuzaki K, Yamashita Y, Ogata I, et al: Optimal protocol for injection of contrast material at MR angiography: Study of healthy volunteers. Radiology 213:913-918, 1999.
11. Prince MR, Yucel EK, Kaufman JA, et al: Dynamic gadolinium-enhanced three-dimensional abdominal MR arteriography. J MRI 3:877-881, 1993.
12. Krinsky GA, Reuss PM, Lee VS, et al: Thoracic aorta: Comparison of single-dose breath-hold and double-dose non-breath-hold gadolinium-enhanced three-dimensional MR angiography. AJR 173:145-150, 1999.
13. Lentschig MG, Reimer P, Rausch-Lentschig UL, et al: Breath-hold gadolinium-enhanced MR angiography of the major vessels at 1.0 T: Dose-response findings and angiographic correlation. Radiology 208:353-357, 1998.
14. Kroencke TJ, Wasser MN, Pattynama PMT, et al: Gadobenate dimeglumine-enhanced MR angiography of the abdominal aorta and renal arteries. AJR 179:1573-1582, 2002.
15. Shetty AN, Bis KG, Vrachliotis TG, et al: Contrast-enhanced 3D MRA with centric ordering in k space: A preliminary clinical experience in imaging the abdominal aorta and renal and peripheral arterial vasculature. J Magn Reson Imaging 8:603-615, 1998.
16. Prince MR, Grist TM, Debatin JF: 3D Contrast MR Angiography, 2nd ed. Berlin, Springer-Verlag, 1999.
17. Thurnher SA, Capelastegui A, Del Olmo FH, et al: Safety and effectiveness of single- versus triple-dose Gadodiamide injection–enhanced MR angiography of the abdomen: A phase III double-blind multicenter study. Radiology 219:137-146, 2001.
18. Maki JH, Chenevert TL, Prince MR: Contrast-enhanced MR angiography. Abdom Imaging 23:469-484, 1998.
19. Foo TK, Saranathan M, Prince MR, Chenevert TL: Automated detection of bolus arrival and initiation of data acquisition in fast, three-dimensional, gadolinium-enhanced MR angiography. Radiology 203:275-280, 1997.
20. Riederer SJ, Bernstein MA, Breen JF, et al: Three-dimensional contrast-enhanced MR angiography with real-time fluoroscopic triggering: Design specifications and technical reliability in 330 patient studies. Radiology 215:584-593, 2000.

21. Calhoun PS, Kuszyk BS, Heath DG, et al: Three-dimensional volume rendering of spiral CT data: Theory and method. RadioGraphics 19: 745-764, 1999.

22. Saloner D: MRA: Principles and display. In Higgins CB, Hricak J, Jelms CA (eds): Magnetic Resonance Imaging of the Body. Philadelphia, Lippincott-Raven, 1997, pp 1345-1368.

23. Hany TF, Schmidt M, Davis CP, et al: Diagnostic impact of four postprocessing techniques in evaluating contrast-enhanced three-dimensional MR angiography. AJR 170:907-912, 1998.

24. Anderson C, Saloner D, Tsuruda J, et al: Artifacts in maximum intensity projection display of MR angiograms. AJR 154:623-629, 1990.

25. Lauffer RB, Parmelee DJ, Dunham SU, et al: MS-325: Albumin-targeted contrast agent for MR angiography. Radiology 207:529-538, 1998.

26. Parmelee DJ, Walovitch RC, Ouellet JS, et al: Preclinical evaluation of the pharmacokinetics, biodistribution, and elimination of MS-325, a blood pool agent for magnetic resonance imaging. Invest Radiol 32:741-747, 1997.

27. Grist TM, Korosec FR, Peters DC, et al: Steady-state and dynamic MR angiography with MS-325: Initial experience in humans. Radiology 207:539-544, 1998.

28. Sharafuddin MJ, Stolpen AH, Dang YM, et al: Comparison of MS-325 and Gadodiamide-enhanced MR venography of iliocaval veins. J Vasc Interv Radiol 13:1021-1027, 2002.

29. Cunningham CG, Reilly LM, Stoney R: Chronic visceral ischemia. Surg Clin North Am 72:231-244, 1992.

30. Hagspiel KD, Leung DA, Angle JF, et al: MR angiography of the mesenteric vasculature. Radiol Clin North Am 40:867-886, 2002.

31. Silva JA, White CJ, Collins TJ, et al: Endovascular therapy for chronic mesenteric ischemia. J Am Coll Cardiol 47:944-950, 2006.

32. Meaney JF: Non-invasive evaluation of the visceral arteries with magnetic resonance angiography. Eur Radiol 9:1267-1276, 1999.

33. Meaney JF, Prince MR, Nostrant TT, et al: Gadolinium-enhanced MR angiography of visceral arteries in patients with suspected chronic mesenteric ischemia. J Magn Reson Imaging 7:171-176, 1997.

34. Shirkhoda A, Konez O, Shetty AN, et al: Mesenteric circulation: Three-dimensional MR angiography with a gadolinium-enhanced multiecho gradient-echo technique. Radiology 202:257-261, 1997.

35. Gaa J, Laub G, Edelmann RR, et al: First clinical results of ultrafast, contrast-enhanced 2-phase 3D magnetic resonance angiography technique for imaging visceral abdominal arteries and veins. Invest Radiol 35:111-117, 2000.

36. Szilagyi DE, Rian RL, Elliott JP, et al: The celiac artery compression syndrome: Does it exist? Surgery 72:849-863, 1972.

37. Bron KM, Redman HC: Splanchnic artery stenosis and occlusion: Incidence, arteriographic and clinical manifestations. Radiology 92:323-328, 1969.

38. Reilly LM, Ammar AD, Stoney RJ, et al: Late results following operative repair for celiac artery compression syndrome. J Vasc Surg 2:79-91, 1985.

39. Lee VS, Morgan JN, Tan AG, et al: Celiac artery compression by the median arcuate ligament: A pitfall of end-expiratory MR imaging. Radiology 228:437-442, 2003.

40. Solis MM, Ranval TJ, McFarland DR, et al: Surgical treatment of superior mesenteric artery dissecting aneurysm and simultaneous celiac artery compression. Ann Vasc Surg 7:457-462, 1993.

41. Carr SC, Pearce WH, Vogelzang RL: Current management of visceral artery aneurysms. Surgery 120:627-634, 1996.

42. Takeda J, Matsunaga N, Sakamoto I: Spontaneous dissection of the celiac and hepatic arteries treated by transcatheter embolisation. AJR 165:1288-1289, 1995.

43. Laissy JP, Trillaud J, Douek P: MR angiography: Noninvasive vascular imaging of the abdomen. Abdom Imaging 27:488-506, 2002.

44. Zelenock GB, Stanley JC: Splanchnic artery aneurysms. In Rutherford RB (ed): Vascular Surgery, 5th ed. Philadelphia, WB Saunders, 2000, pp 1369-1382.

45. Shanley CJ, Shah NL, Messina LM: Common splanchnic artery aneurysms: Splenic, hepatic, and celiac. Ann Vasc Surg 10:315-322, 1996.

46. Grego FG, Lepidi S, Ragazzi R, et al: Visceral artery aneurysms: A single center experience. Cardiovasc Surg 11:19-25, 2003.

47. Ishigami K, Zhang Y, Rayhill S, et al: Does variant hepatic artery anatomy in a liver transplant recipient increase the risk of hepatic artery complications after transplantation? AJR 183:1577-1584, 2004.

48. Sahani D, Souza RD, Kadavigere R, et al: Evaluation of living liver transplant donors: Method for precise anatomic definition by using a dedicated contrast-enhanced MR imaging protocol. RadioGraphics 24:957-967, 2004.

49. Rodgers PM, Ward J, Baudouin CJ, et al: Dynamic contrast-enhanced MR imaging of the portal venous system: Comparison with x-ray angiography. Radiology 191:741-745, 1994.

50. Boeve WJ, Sluiter WJ, Kamman RL: Optimization of scan timing in abdominal breathhold contrast-enhanced MRA: An empirical guideline. Magn Reson Imaging 19:193-200, 2001.

51. Lee MW, Lee JM, Lee JY, et al: Preoperative evaluation of the hepatic vascular anatomy in living liver donors: Comparison of CT angiography and MR angiography. J Magn Reson Imaging 24:1081-1087, 2006.

52. Leyendecker JR, Brown JJ: Practical Guide to Abdominal & Pelvic MRI. Philadelphia, Lippincott Williams & Wilkins, 2004.

53. Laissy JP, Cinqualbre A, Loshkajian A, et al: Assessment of deep venous thrombosis in the lower limbs and pelvis: MR venography versus duplex Doppler sonography. AJR 167:971-975, 1996.

54. Arrive L, Menu Y, Dessarts I, et al: Diagnosis of abdominal venous thrombosis by means of spin-echo and gradient-echo MR imaging: Analysis with receiver operating characteristic curves. Radiology 181: 661-668, 1991.

55. Evans JA, Sostman HD, Knelson MH: Detection of deep venous thrombosis: Prospective comparison of MR imaging with contrast venography. AJR 161:131-135, 1993.

56. Salvador SJ, Otero RR, Salvador BL: Puerperal ovarian vein thrombosis: Evaluation with CT, US, and MR imaging. Radiology 167:637-639, 1988.

57. Turski P: Sources of variability in measuring carotid stenosis on time-resolved contrast-enhanced MR angiograms. AJNR 23:178-179, 2002.

58. Mallouhi A, Schocke M, Judmaier W, et al: MR Angiography of renal arteries: Comparison of volume rendering and maximum intensity projection algorithms. Radiology 223:509-516, 2002.

59. Kim JC, Kim CD, Jang MH, et al: Can magnetic resonance angiogram be a reliable alternative for donor evaluation for laparoscopic nephrectomy? Clin Transplant 21:126-135, 2007.

Endoscopic Ultrasound

Richard M. Gore, MD

Endoscopic ultrasound (EUS) combines features of endoscopy and ultrasound to provide information about the mucosa, submucosa, muscularis propria, serosa, and surrounding tissues and lymph nodes of the gut. High-frequency sound waves are transmitted from the transducer at the tip of the echoendoscope to the target tissue. With the development of linear-array echoendoscopes and the incorporation of color flow and Doppler data, the utility of this technique has expanded.[1-5]

INSTRUMENTATION

Two types of echoendoscopes are employed during EUS. These scopes have become lighter and smaller and provide better image resolution. To eliminate air artifacts, both probes employ acoustic coupling with the target structure by filling a small latex balloon covering the transducer with deaerated water or by placing 300 to 500 mL of water into the intestinal lumen.[3]

Radial Echoendoscopes

Radial instruments use a built-in mechanical or electronic rotating transducer that is rotated in a 360-degree arc by a motor mounted in the proximal portion of the endoscope. This produces a radial ultrasonic image that is perpendicular to the long axis of the endoscope. Endoscopic images can be obtained simultaneously, but the angle of view is 80 degrees oblique to the image obtained with the standard forward-viewing endoscope. Current radial endoscopes have the capability to switch from frequencies of 5 to 20 MHz to optimize depth of penetration and image resolution. The higher frequencies provided superb mural imaging but only provide 2 cm of tissue penetration. The lower frequencies have a depth of penetration of 8 cm and are useful for imaging extramural

pathology. The radial echoendoscope is limited because it cannot follow the needle path during fine-needle aspiration.[3]

Linear Echoendoscopes

This instrument uses an electronic curved-array transducer mounted in front of the optical lens of an oblique viewing endoscope (Fig. 13-1). It generates a 100- to 180-degree linear sector scan that is parallel to the long axis of the scope and is oriented at an angle of 90 degrees to the radial anatomy. Linear echoendoscopes can generate color flow and Doppler images and have a frequency range of 5 to 10 MHz. This is the probe

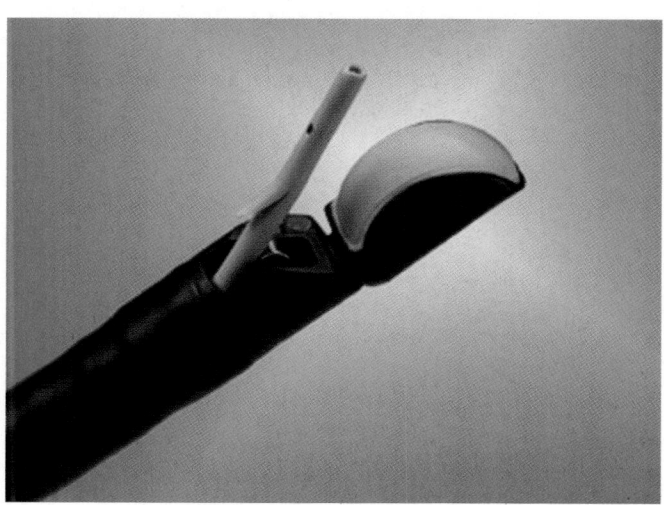

Figure 13-1. Sonoendoscope. Linear echoendoscopes use an electronic curved array transducer mounted in front of the optical lens of an oblique viewing endoscope.

used when performing fine-needle aspiration because the needle can be tracked in its entirety from exiting the biopsy channel to entering and aspirating the target lesion.[3]

FINE-NEEDLE ASPIRATION

Endoscopic ultrasound-guided fine-needle aspiration has become an important tool in the diagnosis and staging of gastrointestinal malignancies. Typically, a 22-gauge needle is employed, but a 19-gauge needle may be more appropriate for biopsy of smooth muscle tumors.[3,6]

The needle course and biopsy technique depend on three factors: the size and consistency of the target lesion, the proximity of surrounding blood vessels, and the consistency of the gastrointestinal wall.[1] The needle is advanced through the biopsy channel and is monitored with real-time sonography as it advances into the lesion (Fig. 13-2).

NORMAL APPEARANCE OF THE GUT

Five layers are visualized in the normal gut wall on EUS (Fig. 13-3). The inner layer is hyperechoic and corresponds to the mucosa. The next layer is hypoechoic and constitutes the muscularis mucosae. The third layer is hyperechoic and represents the submucosa. The fourth layer is hypoechoic and is composed of the muscularis propria. The fifth, or outer, layer includes the subserosa, serosa, and fat. The circular and longitudinal muscle of the muscularis propria can sometimes be distinguished so that seven mural layers may be visible.[1-3]

INDICATIONS

Esophagus

Endoscopic ultrasound is uniquely suitable for the staging of esophageal cancer because it is the only imaging modality that

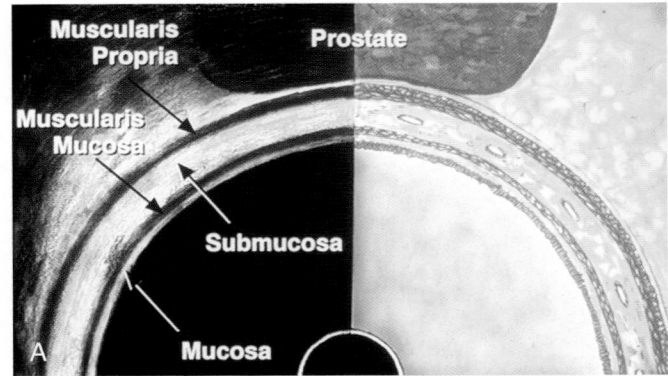
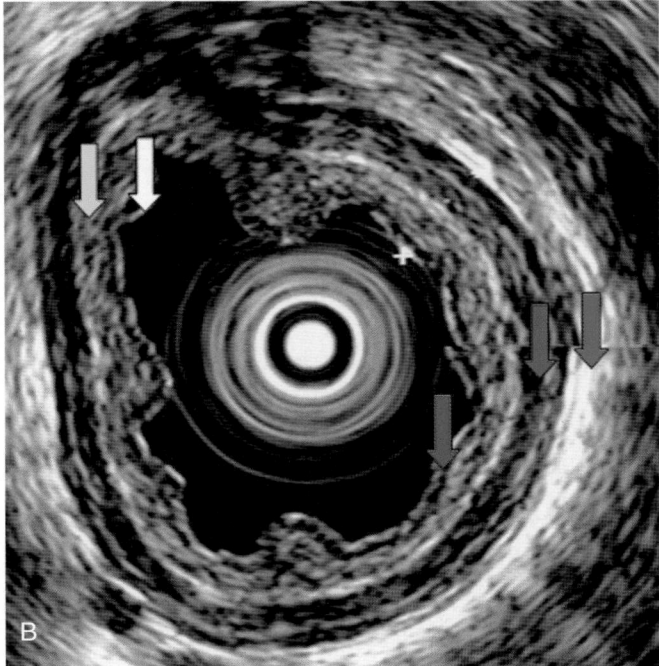

Figure 13-3. Endosonographic appearance of normal gut. A. Transrectal ultrasound shows normal mural stratification with an echogenic inner ring (mucosa), surrounded by a hypoechoic ring (muscularis mucosa), which is surrounded by another echogenic ring (submucosa), which is surrounded by a hypoechoic ring (muscularis propria), which is surrounded by an outer echogenic ring (serosal fat). **B.** These layers are also present on this endosonogram of the normal stomach. *White arrow,* mucosa; *red arrow,* muscularis propria; *yellow arrow,* submucosa; *blue arrow,* muscularis propria; *green arrow,* serosa.

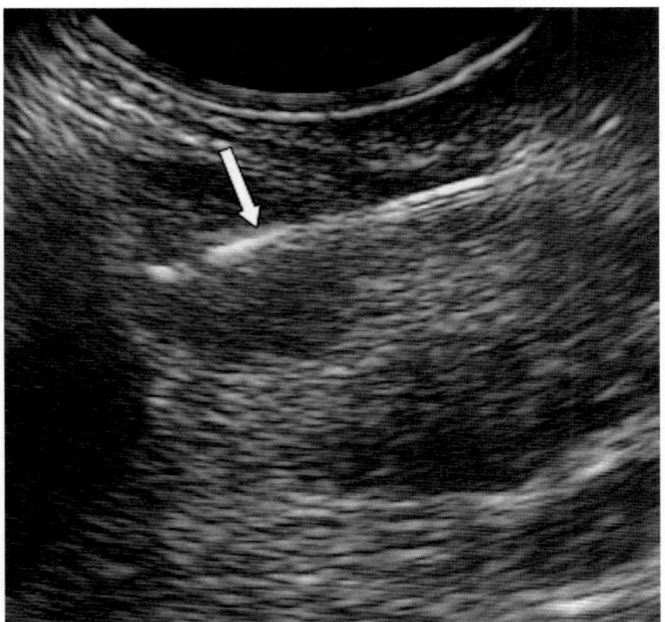

Figure 13-2. Endosonographic directed biopsy of pancreatic mass. The *arrow* points to the echogenic needle within the mass.

can reliably depict the layers of the esophageal wall (Fig. 13-4). EUS-guided fine-needle aspiration has further enhanced the diagnostic accuracy of nodal staging.[6,7] EUS is used in conjunction with multidetector computed tomography (MDCT) in assessing the respectability of esophageal tumors. EUS tumor-staging accuracy ranges from 73% to 92% whereas the accuracy of nodal staging ranges from 50% to 90%.[8] EUS and MDCT are used to select patients for palliative therapy or neoadjuvant therapy.[9]

EUS can also detect submucosal invasion, high-grade dysplasia, and carcinoma in situ in patients with Barrett's esophagus.[10] By showing absence of deep invasion, EUS can select patients who may benefit from mucosectomy or ablation rather than the standard esophagectomy.[11]

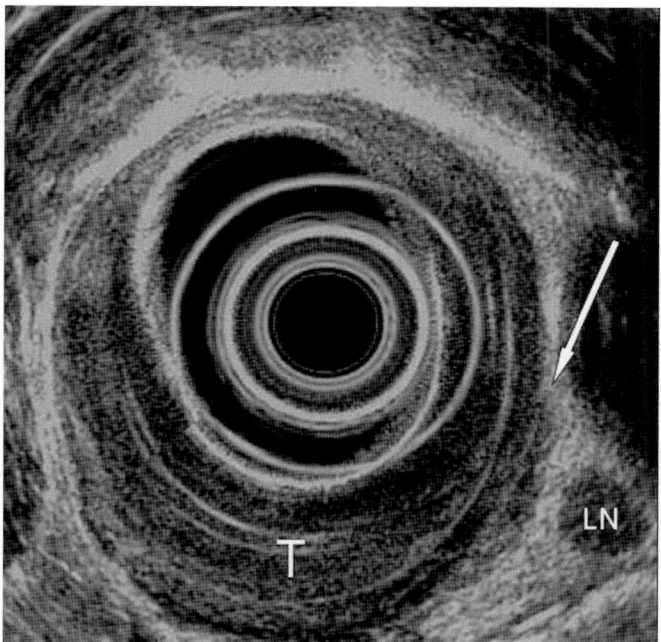

Figure 13-4. Stage T3N1 esophageal cancer. The tumor (T) is confined by the muscularis propria except where the *arrow* shows invasion of the adjacent fat. LN, hypoechoic, spherical metastatic lymph node.

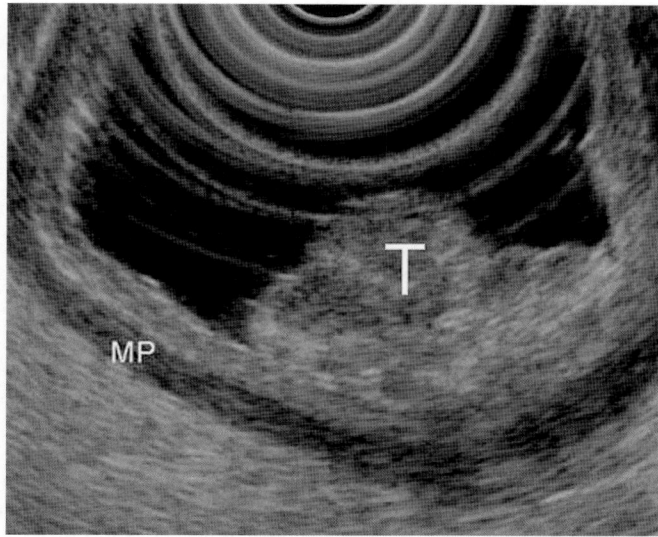

Figure 13-5. Stage T1N0 gastric cancer. The tumor (T) is confined by the submucosa and does not extend into the muscularis propria (MP). No adenopathy is present.

Benign mural tumors such as fibromas, hemangiomas, cysts, leiomyomas, and lipomas can also be evaluated by EUS. This technique is very useful in identifying the layer of origin of these tumors.

In patients with cirrhosis and portal hypertension, EUS has proven useful in depicting the vascular anatomy of the distal esophagus and proximal stomach. By employing echoendoscopic and Doppler guidance, sclerosant can be directly injected into perforating veins that appear as anechoic communicating channels between submucosal and paraesophageal collaterals.

Stomach

Endoscopic ultrasound is a well-established technique in the staging of gastric adenocarcinoma (Fig. 13-5) and lymphoma, in characterizing submucosal masses, and in evaluating the cause of thick gastric folds. The normal gastric wall is 3 to 4 mm thick, and it increases in the antrum.

On EUS, gastric cancer appears as a diffuse mural thickening that is either hypoechoic or heterogeneous in tissue texture. EUS can identify early gastric cancer involving the mucosa and superficial submucosa, and these patients may by treated nonoperatively with removal of the tumor by endoscopic mucosal resection.[12-15]

EUS is approximately 80% accurate for tumor staging and 70% accurate for nodal staging of all gastric cancers.[16-18] Inflammation and fibrosis frequently accompany ulcerating tumors, and there is a tendency to overstage these neoplasms. Linitis plastica produces hypoechoic or inhomogeneous mural thickening of the stomach (Fig. 13-6).

Gastric lymphoma manifests as hypoechoic infiltration of the deep mucosa and submucosa. Metastatic lymph nodes have the same echogenicity as the primary mass.[19,20]

Rectum

Endoscopic ultrasound has an important role in the staging of rectal cancer (Figs. 13-7 and 13-8), having an accuracy of 80% to 85% for tumor stage and 70% to 80% for nodal stage.[21-24] The accuracy of EUS decreases after radiation therapy because of inflammatory and fibrotic changes in the perirectal fat and peritumor edema. EUS can also detect local recurrences as small as 5 mm. The EUS staging of rectal cancer is discussed more fully in Chapter 63. EUS is also useful for localizing intramural rectal carcinoids.

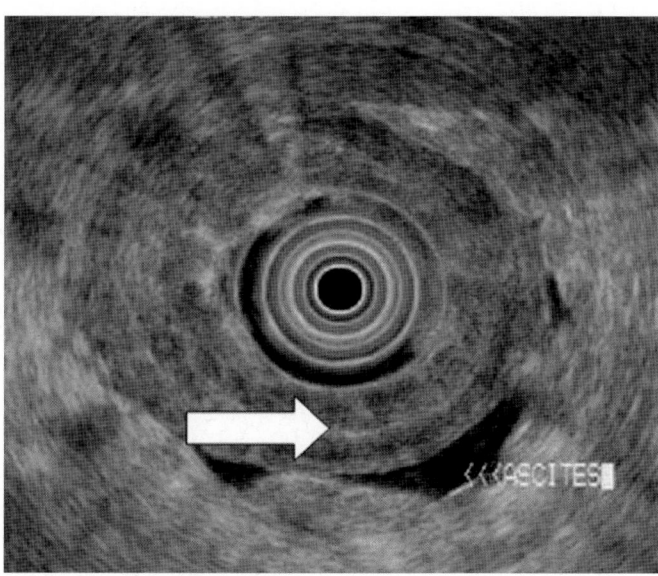

Figure 13-6. Linitis plastica. The tumor (*arrow*) produces diffusely hypoechoic and inhomogeneous mural thickening of the stomach. The presence of ascites is suggestive of peritoneal tumor spread.

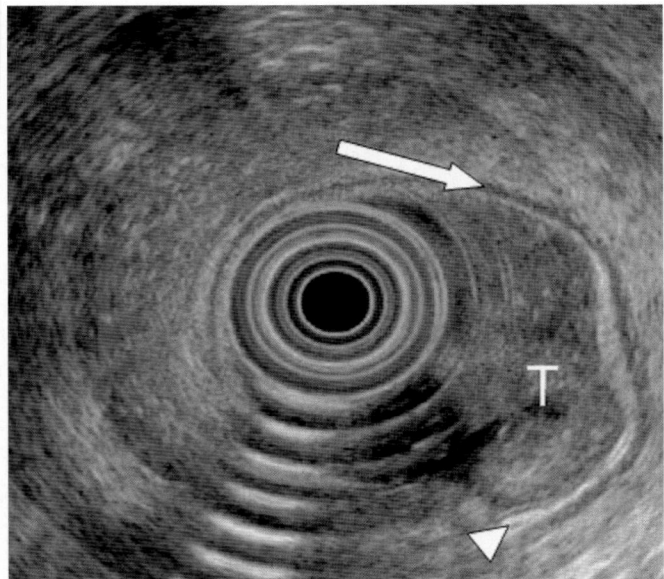

Figure 13-7. T1N0 rectal cancer. The tumor (T) invades into the submucosa (*arrowhead*) but not the muscularis propria (*arrow*). No adenopathy is present.

Pancreas

EUS is usually performed when a suspicious lesion is identified on MDCT or MRI. EUS remains the most sensitive and specific method of identifying benign and malignant pancreatic lesions.[25]

Pancreatic pseudocysts on EUS are typically anechoic and may have a smooth thin or thick wall. EUS can provide imaging guidance for drainage of these cysts. Chronic pancreatitis manifests as a gland with a lobulated contour, ductal dilation (>3 mm in the head, >2 mm in the body, and >1 mm in the tail), heterogeneous and increased echogenicity, hyperechoic foci due to calcification, and hypoechoic foci if there are areas with active acute inflammation and edema.[26]

Improvements in MDCT, MRCP, and MR technology have led to the detection of a large number of cystic pancreatic masses. The differentiation between benign, premalignant, and malignant cysts is difficult, and EUS provides exquisite images of the cyst and its relationship to the pancreatic duct and can guide fine-needle aspiration of the cyst fluid for analysis.[27-29]

Serous cystadenomas may show septations and calcifications seen on MDCT. The cyst fluid shows low viscosity, low carcinoembryonic antigen (CEA), low CA19-9, negative cytology, and negative mucin stain and is strongly positive for periodic acid–Schiff stain owing to the abundance of glycogen.[27-29]

Mucinous cystic neoplasms (Fig. 13-9), which range from benign cystadenomas to malignant cystadenocarcinomas, are cystic and often have internal septations. The cysts are lined with mucin-secreting columar cells that stain strongly positive for mucin, and the fluid has high viscosity and CEA levels.

On EUS, intraductal papillary mucinous tumors present as dilation of the pancreatic duct and side branches with filling defects due to mucin. There is communication of the cystic areas with side branches. The cyst fluid has little cellular material.[25,29-32]

EUS is the most sensitive means of diagnosing pancreatic adenocarcinoma (Fig. 13-10). With fine-needle aspiration, EUS can provide a histologic diagnosis and evaluate the status of regional lymph node involvement. MDCT and MRI are superior in staging regional and distant metastatic disease. Sonographically, adenocarcinoma presents as a hypoechoic irregular mass with or without hypoechoic, spherically shaped hypoechoic lymph nodes.[29-31]

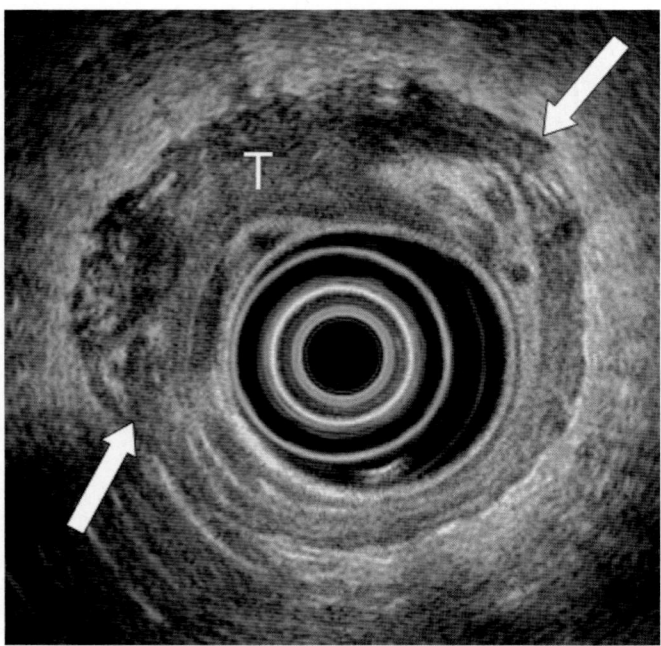

Figure 13-8. T3N0 rectal cancer. The hypoechoic tumor (T) invades (*arrows*) the echogenic mesorectal fat. No adenopathy is present.

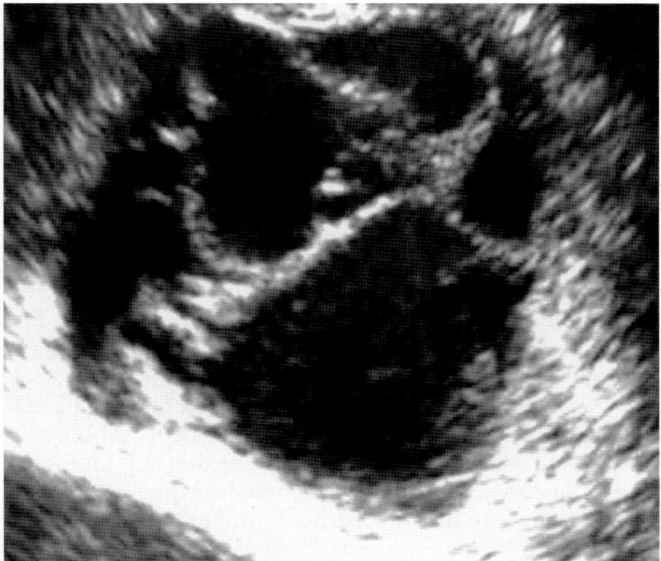

Figure 13-9. Mucinous cystadenoma of pancreas. Multiple septations are present in this cystic lesion of the pancreatic head that stained for mucin on aspiration.

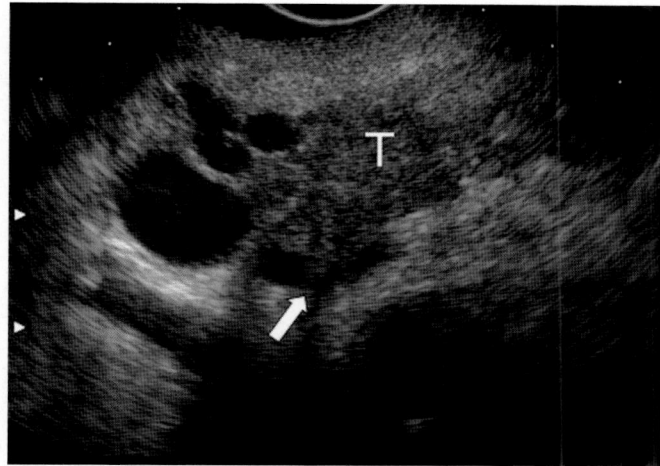

Figure 13-10. Adenocarcinoma of pancreas. This hypoechoic tumor invades (*arrow*) the splenic vein/portal vein confluence.

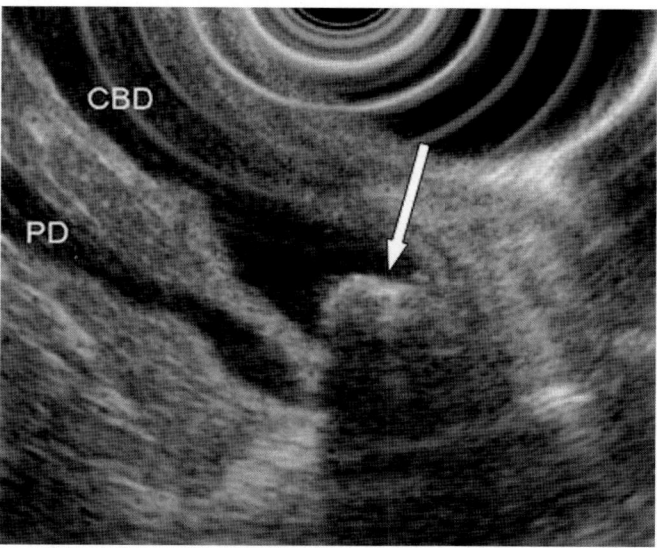

Figure 13-11. Choledocholithiasis. A shadowing stone is identified in the distal common bile duct (CBD), which is dilated. The pancreatic duct (PD) is also dilated.

Biliary Tract Disease

There are three major applications of EUS in the evaluation of biliary tract disorders: staging cholangiocarcinoma, detecting choledocholithiasis, and evaluating biliary strictures. EUS is more accurate than CT for local staging of cholangiocarcinomas, and intraductal ultrasonography can improve the staging of T1 tumors and distinguish between benign and malignant biliary strictures.[32-35]

EUS can also diagnosis common bile duct stones (Fig. 13-11), but magnetic resonance cholangiopancreatography is usually the first imaging modality employed because it is noninvasive.[36]

References

1. Jones DB: Role of endoscopic ultrasound in staging upper gastrointestinal cancers. ANZ J Surg 77:166-172, 2007.
2. Ingram M, Arregui ME: Endoscopic ultrasonography. Surg Clin North Am 84:1035-1059, 2004.
3. Roesch T: Endoscopic ultrasonography: Equipment and technique. Gastrointest Endosc Clin North Am 15:13-31, 2005.
4. Tsutsui A, Okamura S, Muguruma N, et al: Three-dimensional reconstruction of endosonographic images of gastric lesions: Preliminary experience. J Clin Ultrasound 33:112-118, 2005.
5. Fusaroli P, Caletti G: Endoscopic ultrasonography: Current clinical role. Eur J Gastroenterol Hepatol 17:293-301, 2005.
6. Oh YS, Early DS, Azar RR: Clinical applications of endoscopic ultrasound to oncology. Oncology 68:526-537, 2005.
7. Sreenarasimhaiah J: The emerging role of endoscopic ultrasonography in cancer staging. Am J Med Sci 329:247-258, 2005.
8. Klapman J, Chang KJ, Wiersema M, et al: Endoscopic ultrasound-guided fine-needle aspiration biopsy in esophageal cancer. Endoscopy 37:381-385, 2005.
9. DeWitt J, Kesler K, Brooks JA, et al: Endoscopic ultrasound for esophageal and gastroesophageal junction cancer: Impact of increased use of primary neoadjuvant therapy on preoperative locoregional staging accuracy. Dis Esophagus 18:21-27, 2005.
10. Savoy AD, Wallace MB. EUS in the management of the patient with dysplasia in Barrett's esophagus. J Clin Gastroenterol 39:263-267, 2005.
11. Yasuda K, Kamaguchi M, Morikawa J: Role of endoscopic ultrasonography in the diagnosis of early esophageal carcinoma. Gastrointest Endosc Clin North Am 15:83-92, 2005.
12. Weber WA, Ott K: Imaging of esophageal and gastric cancer. Semin Oncol 31:530-541, 2004.
13. Abdalla EK, Pisters PW: Staging and preoperative evaluation of upper gastrointestinal malignancies. Semin Oncol 31:513-529, 2004.
14. Ishigami S, Toshinaka H, Sakamoto F, et al: Preoperative assessment of the depth of early gastric cancer invasion by transabdominal ultrasound sonography: A comparison with endoscopic ultrasound sonography. Hepatogastroenterology 51:1202-1205, 2004.
15. Bhandari S, Shim CS, Kim JH, et al: Usefulness of three-dimensional, multidetector row CT (virtual gastroscopy and multiplanar reconstruction) in the evaluation of gastric cancer: A comparison with conventional endoscopy, EUS, and histopathology. Gastrointest Endosc 59:619-626, 2004.
16. Gore RM: Upper gastrointestinal tract tumours: Diagnosis and staging strategies. Cancer Imaging 5:95-98, 2005.
17. Tamerisa R, Irisawa A, Bhutani MS: Endoscopic ultrasound in the diagnosis, staging, and management of gastrointestinal and adjacent malignancies. Med Clin North Am 89:139-158, 2005.
18. Abdalla EK, Pisters PW: Staging and preoperative evaluation of upper gastrointestinal malignancies. Semin Oncol 31:513-529, 2005.
19. Arantes V, Logrono R, Faruqi S, et al: Endoscopic sonographically guided fine-needle aspiration yield in submucosal tumors of the gastrointestinal tract. J Ultrasound Med 23:1141-1150, 2005.
20. Ishigami S, Toshinaka H, Sakamoto F, et al: Preoperative assessment of the depth of early gastric cancer invasion by transabdominal ultrasound sonography: A comparison with endoscopic ultrasound sonography. Hepatogastroenterology 51:1202-1205, 2004.
21. Bhutani MS: Recent developments in the role of endoscopic ultrasonography in diseases of the colon and rectum. Curr Opin Gastroenterol 23:67-73, 2007.
22. Kobayashi K, Katsumata T, Yoshizawa S, et al: Indications of endoscopic polypectomy for rectal carcinoid tumors and clinical usefulness of endoscopic ultrasonography. Dis Colon Rectum 48:285-291, 2005.
23. Sasaki Y, Niwa Y, Hirooka Y, et al: The use of endoscopic ultrasound-guided fine-needle aspiration for investigation of submucosal and extrinsic masses of the colon and rectum. Endoscopy 37:154-160, 2005.
24. Santoro GA, Fortling B: The advantages of volume rendering in three-dimensional endosonography of the anorectum. Dis Colon Rectum 50:359-368, 2007.
25. Tox U, Hackenberg R, Stelzer A, et al: Endosonographic diagnosis of solid pancreatic tumors: A retrospective analysis from a tertiary referral center. Z Gastroenterol 45:307-312, 2007.
26. Moparty B, Brugge WR: Approach to pancreatic cystic lesions. Curr Gastroenterol Rep 9:130-135, 2007.
27. Sahani DV, Kadavigere R, Saokar A, et al: Cystic pancreatic lesions: A simple imaging-based classification system for guiding management. RadioGraphics 25:1471-1484, 2005.
28. Kim YH, Saini S, Sahani D, et al: Imaging diagnosis of cystic pancreatic lesions: Pseudocyst versus nonpseudocyst. RadioGraphics 25:671-685, 2005.

29. Levy MJ, Smyrk TC, Reddy RP, et al: Endoscopic ultrasound-guided Tru-Cut biopsy of the cyst wall for diagnosing cystic pancreatic tumors. Clin Gastroenterol Hepatol 3:974-979, 2005.
30. Levy MJ, Wiersema MJ: Pancreatic neoplasms. Gastrointest Endosc Clin North Am 15:117- 142, 2005.
31. Sole M, Iglesias C, Fernandez-Esparrach G, et al: Fine-needle aspiration cytology of intraductal papillary mucinous tumors of the pancreas. Cancer 105:298-303, 2005.
32. Varadarajulu S, Eloubeidi MA: The role of endoscopic ultrasonography in the evaluation of pancreatico-biliary cancer. Gastrointest Endosc Clin North Am15:497-511, 2005.
33. Brugge WR: Endoscopic techniques to diagnose and manage biliary tumors. J Clin Oncol 23:4561-4565, 2005.
34. Palazzo L, O'Toole D: Biliary stones including acute biliary pancreatitis. Gastrointest Endosc Clin North Am 15:63-82, 2005.
35. Fusaroli P, Caletti G: Endoscopic ultrasonography. Endoscopy 37:1-7, 2005.
36. Bories E, Pesenti C, Caillol F, et al: Transgastric endoscopic ultra-sonography-guided biliary drainage: Results of a pilot study. Endoscopy 39:287-291, 2007.

Gastrointestinal Scintigraphy

Alan H. Maurer, MD

The advantages of scintigraphy for studying gastrointestinal tract function have remained the same since the ingestion of a radiolabeled meal to measure gastric emptying was first proposed. In contrast to invasive manometric methods, scintigraphy is simple to perform, does not disturb normal physiology, and permits accurate quantification of bulk transit of solids and liquids throughout the entire gastrointestinal tract. Compared with other radiologic methods, scintigraphy involves low radiation exposure, is easily quantifiable, and uses commonly ingested foods rather than barium. This chapter discusses gastrointestinal scintigraphy as it applies to functional studies of the esophagus, stomach, small bowel, and colon.

Although any conventional gamma camera can be used for imaging, functional imaging studies are best performed with cameras that have a large field of view to image the entire chest for esophageal transit studies or the entire abdomen for gastroenterocolic transit studies. The two radioisotopes used most frequently are technetium-99m (^{99m}Tc) and indium-111 (^{111}In). To simultaneously image solid and liquids, the camera and collimator should be able to image the energies of ^{111}In (273 keV) and ^{99m}Tc (140 keV). The final form in which the radioisotope is administered depends on the study to be performed. For upper gastrointestinal transit studies, ^{99m}Tc is usually given as the radiopharmaceutical ^{99m}Tc sulfur colloid (^{99m}Tc-SC). ^{99m}Tc-SC has a short radioactive decay (half-life = 6 hours) and, when cooked, is physically bound to certain foods and is nonabsorbable, resulting in low radiation exposure. ^{111}In diethylenetriaminepentaacetic acid (DTPA) is usually given suspended in liquid and is also stable and nonabsorbable. With a longer half-life (72 hours), ^{111}In-DTPA is used to image transit that requires several days, such as colonic transit. Because oral ^{111}In-DTPA is not approved for routine clinical use in the United States, a special radiopharmaceutical license may be required for this agent.

ESOPHAGEAL TRANSIT STUDIES

The choice of diagnostic imaging studies for evaluating patients with suspected esophageal dysmotility depends on the presenting symptoms. If dysphagia is present, a barium swallow or endoscopy is initially performed to exclude an anatomic lesion. If anatomic studies are not diagnostic, manometry is performed. Studies have shown that manometry, however, provides only an indirect measure of peristalsis because the pressure waves recorded do not always correlate with the force applied aborally to a solid bolus at a given level of the esophagus. It can also be argued that the presence of a manometric tube itself can affect normal physiology. More importantly, quantification of the volume of retained solids or liquids is not possible.

Esophageal transit scintigraphy (ETS) is a noninvasive, quantitative method of assessing esophageal motility. As many as 50% of patients with dysphagia who have normal manometry and barium examinations are found to have esophageal dysmotility on scintigraphy. Early studies reported a high sensitivity for detecting esophageal dysmotility, but later studies reported a lower sensitivity, especially for disorders with intact peristalsis but high-amplitude contractions or isolated elevation of lower esophageal sphincter (LES) pressures.[1,2] More recent studies confirm a high sensitivity for detecting a wide range of esophageal motility disorders.[3,4]

The widespread use of ETS is limited, however, by lack of a standardized method for performing ETS. The simplest measure of transit is the esophageal transit time (ETT) required for ^{99m}Tc-DTPA in water to traverse the esophagus. ETT is reproducible, with a normal range of 6 to 15 seconds.[2,5] Dynamic images are recorded and examined visually on computer playback. Regional esophageal transit can be analyzed by dividing the esophagus into upper, middle, and distal thirds; time-activity curves (similar to manometric tracings) are then

generated for each third (Fig. 14-1). A composite image can be generated to summarize the regional data in a single image, but it is also important to review the cinescintigraphic images as a movie to detect abnormal peristaltic contractions or reflux.[6]

In addition to analyzing regional transit, the total count remaining in the esophagus after multiple swallows is obtained to quantify esophageal emptying. After the initial swallow, the subject performs dry swallows every 30 seconds for 10 minutes. An esophageal region of interest comprising the entire esophagus is defined for computer analysis. The counts in the esophagus (E_t) are plotted as a percentage of maximal counts (E_{max}): % esophageal emptying = $E_{max} - E_t/E_{max}$. Normally, there is no significant activity remaining in the esophagus after 10 minutes (Fig. 14-2). Primary esophageal motility disorders are associated with different patterns of esophageal emptying (Fig. 14-3).

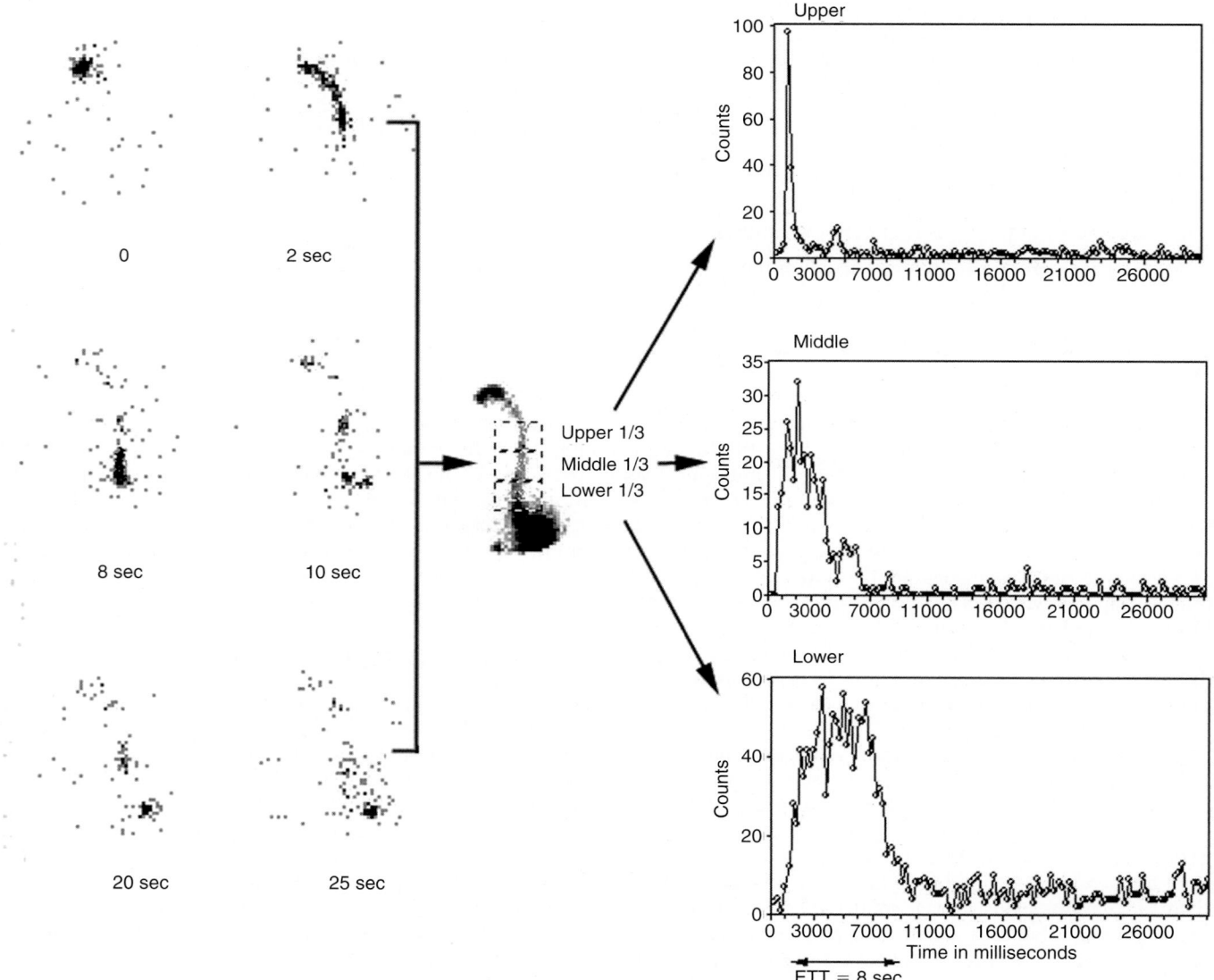

Figure 14-1. Normal esophageal transit images (single swallow). Dynamic images (*left*, 0-25 seconds) demonstrate normal bolus transit through the esophagus. A composite image is produced by summing all the images from the initial 30 seconds (*center*). Regions of interest (*dotted lines*) that define the upper, middle, and lower thirds of the esophagus are shown. Time-activity curves (*right*) show the counts recorded in each region as the bolus progresses down the esophagus. Esophageal transit time (ETT) (8 seconds) is measured, using the leading and trailing edges of the esophageal activity curves.

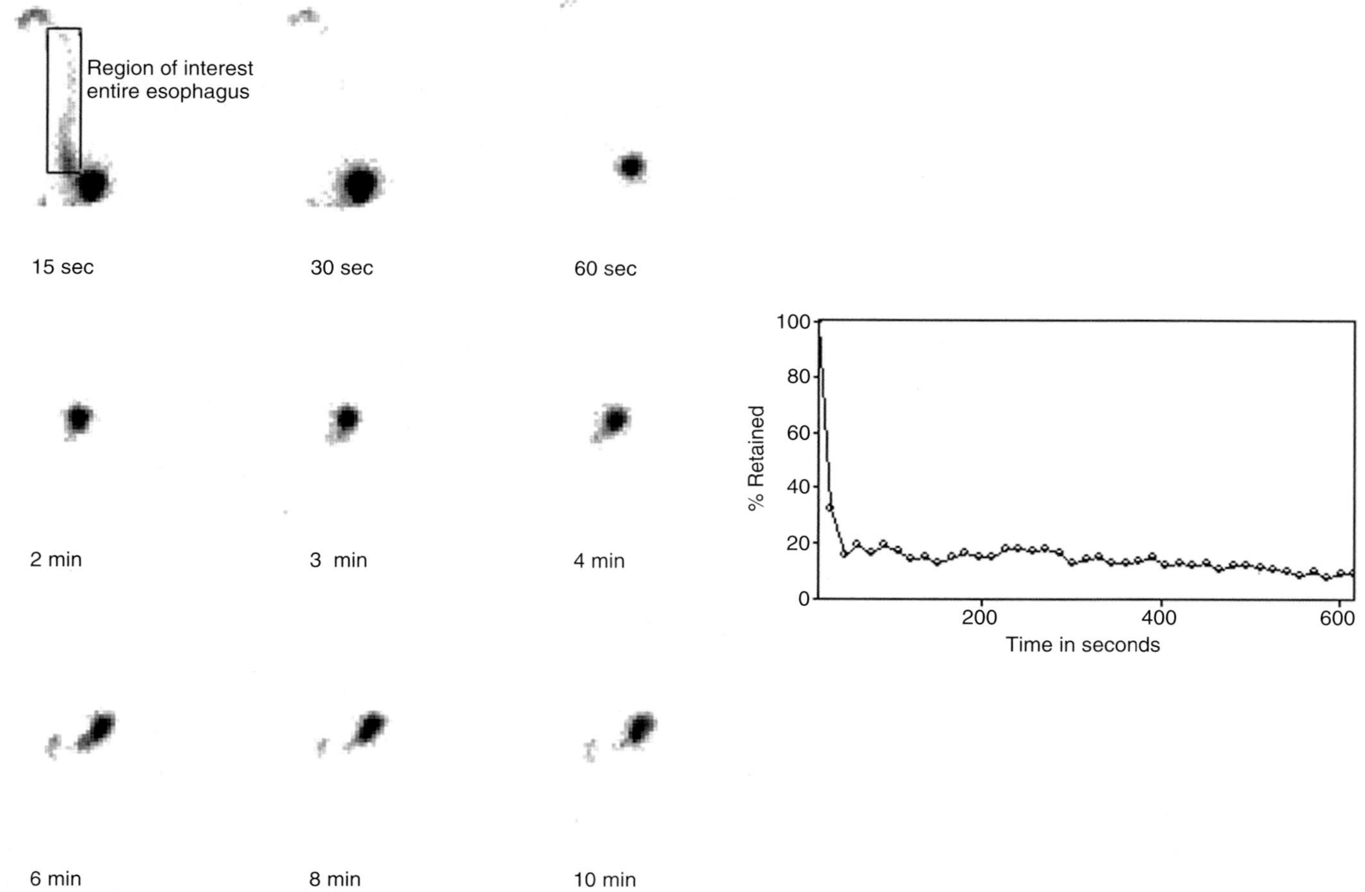

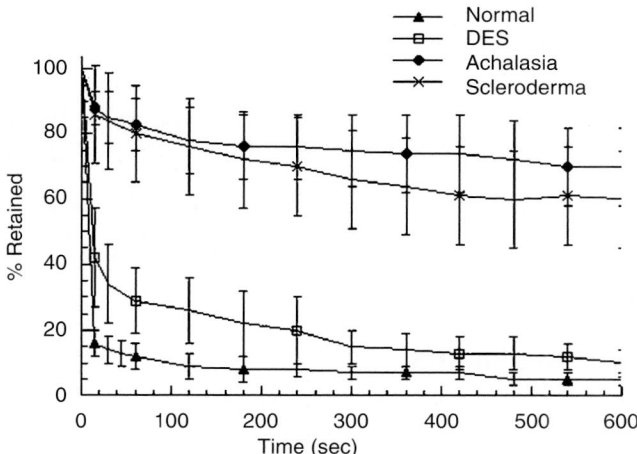

Region of interest
entire esophagus

15 sec   30 sec   60 sec

2 min   3 min   4 min

6 min   8 min   10 min

% Retained — Time in seconds

Figure 14-2. Normal esophageal emptying (multiple swallows). Images at 15 seconds per image are shown (*left*). A region of interest (*box*) is drawn over the entire esophagus. From this region, a time activity curve (*right*) is generated, showing the percent of activity retained in the esophagus at each time. The amount of activity retained after multiple swallows can be used to diagnose various primary esophageal motility disorders (see Fig. 14-3) or to follow therapeutic interventions.

Normal
DES
Achalasia
Scleroderma

% Retained — Time (sec)

Figure 14-3. Esophageal emptying for various primary esophageal motility disorders. The mean data for normal subjects are shown in comparison to the mean data for diffuse esophageal spasm (DES), achalasia, and scleroderma.

Nonspecific esophageal motility disorders are characterized by one or more minor manometric abnormalities. There have been conflicting results about the sensitivity of ETS for nonspecific esophageal motility disorders, with some studies showing low sensitivity (42% to 56%) for this common motility disorder.[7,8] The use of a more viscous, semisolid bolus or an increased number of swallows, however, can increase the sensitivity of ETS.[9] It has been shown that as many as five separate swallows are needed to achieve maximal sensitivity for detection of esophageal dysmotility. The use of multiple swallows (up to six) has also been proposed to optimize ETS.[10] One study that compared ETS (using supine and upright swallows) to manometry and videoesophagography found that these tests have similar sensitivities for detecting a variety of esophageal motor disorders. Specific criteria for diagnosing primary esophageal motor disorders can be established by visual assessment of a cinescintigraphic liquid bolus transit combined with measurement of ETT and global esophageal retention (Table 14-1).[3]

Although the role of ETS for diagnosing esophageal disorders remains controversial, its ability to quantify esophageal emptying is valuable for assessing the response to therapy, particularly in patients with achalasia.[11,12] This ability to objectively quantify the response to therapy remains one of the most useful applications of ETS. ETS and videofluoroscopy

Table 14-1
Diagnostic Criteria for Radionuclide Esophageal Transit Scintigraphy

Disorder	Visual Bolus Analysis from Cineradiography	Esophageal Transit Time	Esophageal Retention at 10 Minutes
Normal	Normal antegrade bolus transit through upper, middle, and lower third of the esophagus with normal relaxation of the lower esophageal sphincter	<14 seconds	<18%
Nonspecific esophageal motility disorder	Any localized abnormal retrograde/antegrade bolus movement	>14 seconds	>18%
Isolated lower esophageal sphincter dysfunction	Normal bolus transit in upper and middle esophagus with delayed transit localized at gastroesophageal junction	>14 seconds	Usually <18%; may see mild retention <30%
Scleroderma	Marked delay in bolus transit; may be localized to distal esophagus	>30 seconds	>30% with marked improvement in upright position vs. supine
Diffuse esophageal spasm	Repetitive retrograde/antegrade contractions throughout the esophagus	>14 seconds	Normal or mild retention; <30%
Achalasia	Marked delay in bolus transit throughout esophagus; may progress normally in upper esophagus from oropharyngeal force	>30 seconds	>50%; no improvement in upright position

Modified from Parkman HP, Maurer AH, Caroline DF, et al: Optimal evaluation of patients with nonobstructive esophageal dysphagia: Manometry, scintigraphy, or videoesophagography? Dig Dis Sci 41:1355-1368, 1996.

remain complementary; optimal sensitivity for detecting esophageal dysmotility (especially achalasia) is achieved when both techniques are employed.[13]

GASTROESOPHAGEAL REFLUX AND PULMONARY ASPIRATION

Adult Studies

Multiple factors have been implicated in the pathogenesis of gastroesophageal reflux (GER), including (1) transient relaxations or decreased resting pressure of the LES; (2) increased gastric acidity; (3) abnormal esophageal clearance and defense mechanisms; and (4) delayed gastric emptying. Indirect methods for diagnosing GER include barium fluoroscopy or evaluation of symptomatic response to intraesophageal acid (the Bernstein test). Studies such as 24-hour esophageal pH monitoring are designed to detect acid in the distal esophagus. GER scintigraphy was developed in adults both to document and quantify the volume of reflux.

To perform GER scintigraphy, adults drink 300 µCi of ^{99m}Tc-SC suspended in 150 mL of orange juice mixed with 0.1 N HCl. The patient is imaged supine under a gamma camera, and an abdominal binder is used to increase abdominal pressures in 20-mm increments up to 100 mm Hg. Computer images are recorded for 30 seconds at each level of binder pressure.

In normal individuals, no reflux is seen. In patients with reflux, activity is visualized in the esophagus (Fig. 14-4). Esophageal activity seen on the first image may be secondary to reflux or abnormal esophageal transit. Because abnormal esophageal transit and GER are often present in the same patient, it is best to perform both studies together. GER can be identified during review of a multiswallow esophageal emptying study even when the abdominal binder pressure study is negative.[14]

Quantification of GER can be helpful and is calculated using the following formula:

$$R = E_p - E_b/G_o \times 100\%,$$

where R represents the GER index expressed as a percentage, E_p represents the esophageal counts at abdominal pressure p, E_b represents the background counts, and G_o represents the gastric counts at the beginning of the study. The mean reflux index for patients with symptomatic GER is 11.7 ± 1.8%, compared with 2.7 ± 0.3% for normal controls. Early studies (which used a normal upper limit of 4%) detected reflux in 90% of patients with confirmed reflux and in only 10% of controls. The low measured counts (up to 4%) detected in normals are due to "scatter" counts from the adjacent gastric fundus. However, later studies have not consistently confirmed high sensitivity.

Patients may have visually obvious reflux but reflux indices of less than 4%. This is due to the need to correct for depth and attenuation of counts in the esophagus. GER scintigraphy has been shown to be complementary to 24-hour esophageal pH monitoring for evaluating the volume of reflux during reflux episodes, which are underestimated by esophageal pH monitoring.[15,16] As with ETS, GER scintigraphy appears to be most useful when there is a need to quantify the volume of reflux and changes in response to medical or surgical treatment. A gastric emptying scintigraphic study may also be useful for evaluating patients with GER who can benefit from a prokinetic agent, because delayed GER is found in approximately 30% of patients using a 4-hour gastric emptying study.[17]

Attempts have been made to image pulmonary aspiration of gastric contents in adults. Insufficient data are available, however, to evaluate the role of scintigraphy for detecting aspiration in adults.

Pediatric Studies

In children, the "milk scan" is used to evaluate esophageal transit, GER, gastric emptying, and pulmonary aspiration. Previous studies that compared scintigraphy with simultaneous esophageal pH monitoring reported a sensitivity and specificity of 79% and 93%, respectively. In a more recent study, scintigraphy revealed an incidence of reflux ranging from 20% to 40% in children 1 to 6 years of age.[18]

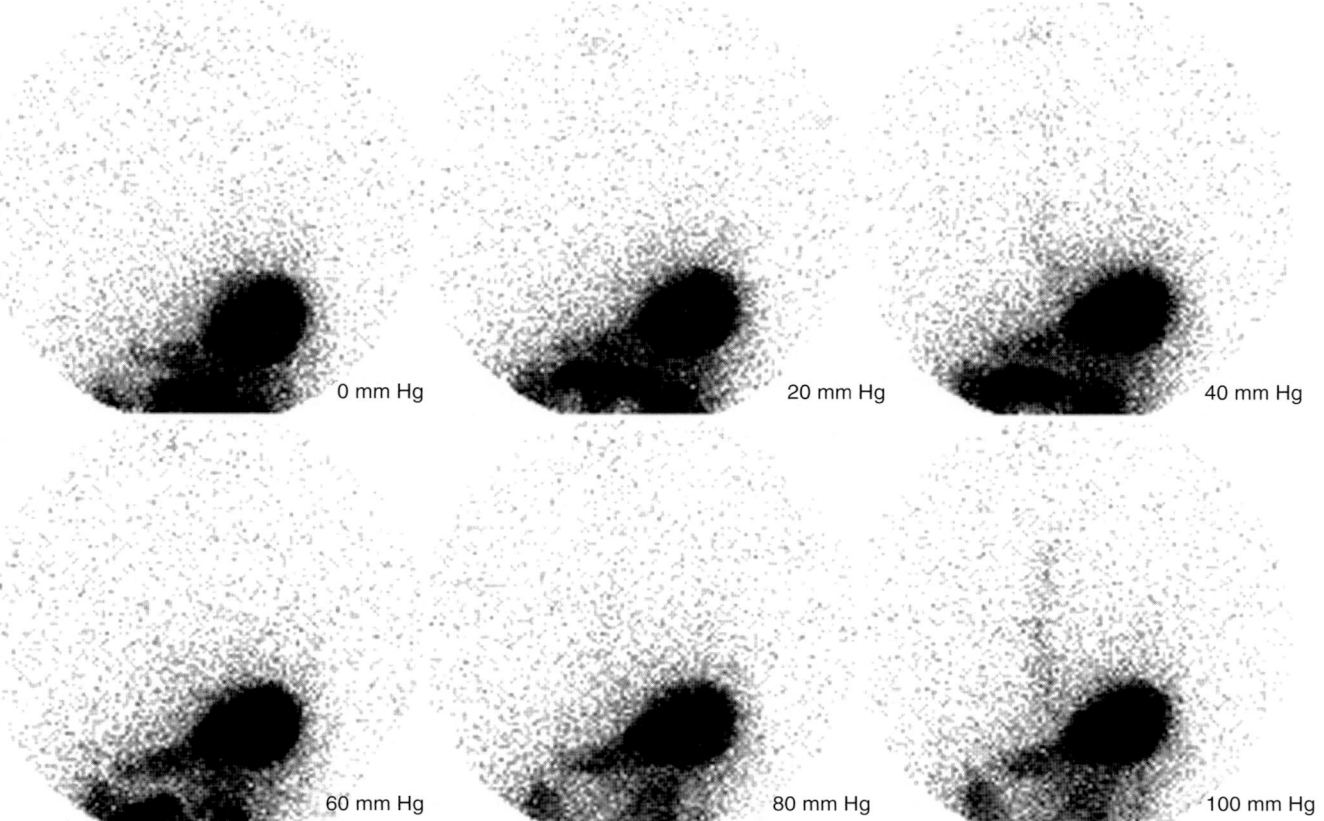

Figure 14-4. Gastroesophageal reflux scintigraphy. Serial images are acquired while increasing abdominal binder pressure is applied. At 0 and 20 mm Hg pressure, no reflux is seen. Mild reflux is seen at 40 mm Hg, and more marked reflux is seen at 100 mm Hg pressure.

^{99m}Tc-SC is mixed with the child's usual volume of milk, formula, apple juice, or glucose water and is given at the time of routine feeding. Images are recorded after the feeding is completed. A high-sensitivity collimator is recommended to increase counting efficiency. Initial swallowing curves can be recorded to evaluate esophageal transit. With the patient lying supine on the camera, posterior images of the chest and abdomen are obtained for at least 60 minutes.[19] Visual review of computer-enhanced cinescintigraphic images increases sensitivity for detecting small volumes of reflux. Time-activity curves are helpful for documenting the frequency of reflux and delayed esophageal clearance and for improving the reproducibility of the readings.[20] Rapid imaging (10 to 20 seconds/image) is important because transient reflux can rapidly dissipate. Delayed images at 1, 2, and 24 hours can be acquired to detect pulmonary aspiration. Pulmonary aspiration is documented with this method in 35% to 55% of children with severe pulmonary disease.[21]

GASTRIC EMPTYING

Solid-Liquid Gastric Emptying Studies

Patients referred for gastric emptying studies often do not have well-defined gastrointestinal symptoms but rather present with complaints of dyspepsia (symptoms thought to originate in the upper gastrointestinal tract). Gastroparesis (delayed gastric emptying) is usually associated with upper gastrointestinal symptoms, including nausea (92%), vomiting (84%), abdominal fullness or distention (75%), and early satiety (60%). In 50% of patients, no cause is found, and the dyspepsia is classified either as idiopathic, essential, or functional (i.e., nonulcer dyspepsia).[22] Patients with dyspepsia are often classified into subgroups based on the predominant symptoms and whether they are reflux-like, ulcer-like, or dysmotility-like, because the treatment is symptom guided. Gastric acid secretion inhibitors are recommended for ulcer-like dyspepsia, and prokinetics are used for dysmotility-like dyspepsia. A functional gastric emptying study is indicated for patients with dyspepsia after an anatomic cause has been excluded. A gastric emptying study may also be indicated in the absence of gastric symptoms for patients with severe GER disease not responding to acid suppressants, for identification of a "pan-motility" gastrointestinal disorder, or for evaluating diabetics with poor glycemic control. The purpose of performing a gastric emptying study is to identify those patients with delayed gastric emptying who will benefit from prokinetic agents for relief of symptoms.[23]

The use of a radiolabeled meal has become the gold standard for measuring gastric emptying. Once the solid or liquid phase of a meal is radiolabeled, the counts measured by the scintigraphy camera are directly proportional to the volume of meal remaining independent of any geometric assumptions needed for estimating volume with other imaging modalities.

Understanding the separate roles of the gastric fundus and antrum for gastric emptying has become increasingly important in analyzing gastric emptying studies. Normally, solid foods are temporarily stored in the fundus until slow, sustained contractions transfer solids to the antrum. This early segregation of solids in the fundus is usually apparent on the initial images of a gastric emptying study (Fig. 14-5). A persistent transverse band is commonly found to separate the fundus from the antrum. Solids then move from the posteriorly located fundus to the more anteriorly located antrum, causing an increase in measured counts as these solids move closer to the camera positioned in front of the patient (see Fig. 14-5). After solids have reached the antrum, peristaltic contractions work by a process called trituration, in which solids are mixed with gastric digestive juices and ground into 1- to 2-mm particles, which are then able to pass through the pylorus. The contractile activity of the antrum is controlled by a pacemaker located high on the greater curvature at the boundary between the fundus and antrum. The time required to complete trituration (so that solid particles can then empty from the stomach) is commonly referred to as the lag phase.

Emptying of liquids is controlled by a sustained pressure gradient generated by the gastric fundus. Ingested liquids require no trituration and are distributed rapidly throughout the stomach, then emptying monoexponentially. Liquid gastric emptying studies by themselves are of little clinical value because liquid emptying is usually not abnormal until gastroparesis is far advanced.[24] In contrast, solid-phase studies usually reveal delayed gastric emptying much earlier than liquids. Nevertheless, liquid studies may occasionally be useful for patients who are unable to tolerate solid meals. In such cases, an abnormal liquid emptying study indicates that significant gastroparesis must be present.

Normal values for a variety of meals, including meats, porridge, pancakes, eggs, and chemical resins, have been reported. For any test meal, the stability of the radioisotope bound to the solid phase must be established to ensure that the radioisotope does not dissociate in gastric juices. When ^{99m}Tc-SC is injected into a live chicken, it is phagocytosed by the Kupffer cells of the liver, resulting in an intracellularly bound radiolabeled food. Such a meal is the "gold standard" to which all other radiolabeled solid foods have been compared, but this is impractical. Instead, most solid food gastric emptying studies are performed with ^{99m}Tc-SC–labeled eggs because of the ease of preparation and high stability of this meal.

A large multicenter study has established normal values for a commercially available egg substitute (EggBeaters) using 0.5 mCi of ^{99m}Tc-SC, 120 g of egg, 2 slices of white wheat bread, 30 g of strawberry jam, and 120 mL of water (255 kcal; 24% protein, 2% fat, 72% carbohydrate, and 2% fiber).[25] The 1-hour, 2-hour, and 4-hour values for the percentage of the meal retained are very similar to a simpler meal consisting of two large eggs, two pieces of white toast, and 300 mL of water (282 kcal; 22% fat, 32% protein, and 46% carbohydrate).[26] With either of these egg meals, gastric emptying is abnormal if greater that 50% of the meal is retained at 2 hours or greater than 10% at 4 hours.

Normal values must be established not only for the meal but also for the method used for image acquisition and processing. Gastric emptying is dependent on body position, smoking, gender, phase of the menstrual cycle, and the time of day that the test is performed.[27-29] Medications such as pro-

kinetic agents, antisecretory drugs, gastric acid suppressants, and narcotics can also affect gastric emptying.

The patient is requested to consume the meal within 10 minutes. Immediately after eating the meal, the patient is ideally imaged in the upright position or, if necessary, in the supine position. It should be recognized, however, that gastric emptying can be significantly delayed in the supine position.[30]

Attenuation correction is needed for accurate measurement of the lag phase for solids. Correction using a geometric mean [anterior counts (A) × posterior counts (P)]$^{1/2}$ is most commonly used. This correction results in only a 3% to 4% variation in counts for the depths typically encountered. When necessary, a single left anterior oblique view can be used.[31]

Computer regions of interest corresponding to the stomach are defined in order to analyze gastric counts. Because of its 6-hour half-life, ^{99m}Tc counts must also be corrected for radioactive decay. After attenuation and decay correction, the percentage of activity remaining in the stomach is normalized to 100% for maximal gastric counts and then plotted for all times.

The simplest approach for interpreting gastric emptying data has been to report the time to 50% emptying of the meal ($T_{1/2}$) or to use the percentage of emptying measured at fixed times after meal ingestion. Until recently, gastric emptying studies were often performed only up to 2 hours after meal ingestion. However, recent studies have shown that the percentage retained at 4 hours is most reproducible[32] and that 4-hour studies detect a higher frequency of patients with abnormal gastric emptying.[26]

Numerous studies have confirmed the presence of an early lag phase, followed by an emptying phase during which the stomach expels solids at a characteristic rate.[33-35] To completely characterize all phases of gastric emptying, it is best to fit the data to a mathematic function known as a modified power exponential[36] given by the following equation:

$$y(t) = 1 - [1 - \exp(-kt)]^\beta,$$

where y(t) is the percentage of gastric activity remaining at time t; k is the slope of the exponential portion of the curve; and β is the y intercept. The lag phase (ln [β/k]) corresponds to the time of peak activity in the antrum, which physically corresponds to maximal filling of the antrum just before the triturated and suspended solids begin to empty at the same uniform rate (k) as liquids.

SPECIALIZED TESTS OF GASTRIC EMPTYING

Delayed gastric emptying is found in 30% to 70% of patients with diabetes or functional dyspepsia.[37] It is increasingly recognized that special studies are needed to more completely evaluate normal and abnormal gastric peristalsis, including fundal and antral motor function, fundic relaxation, visceral hypersensitivity, asynchronous antroduodenal coordination, and gastric dysrhythmias.[38-40]

Bicompartmental (Fundal-Antral) Gastric Emptying Studies

Because scintigraphy easily permits analysis of the intragastric distribution of a test meal between the gastric fundus and

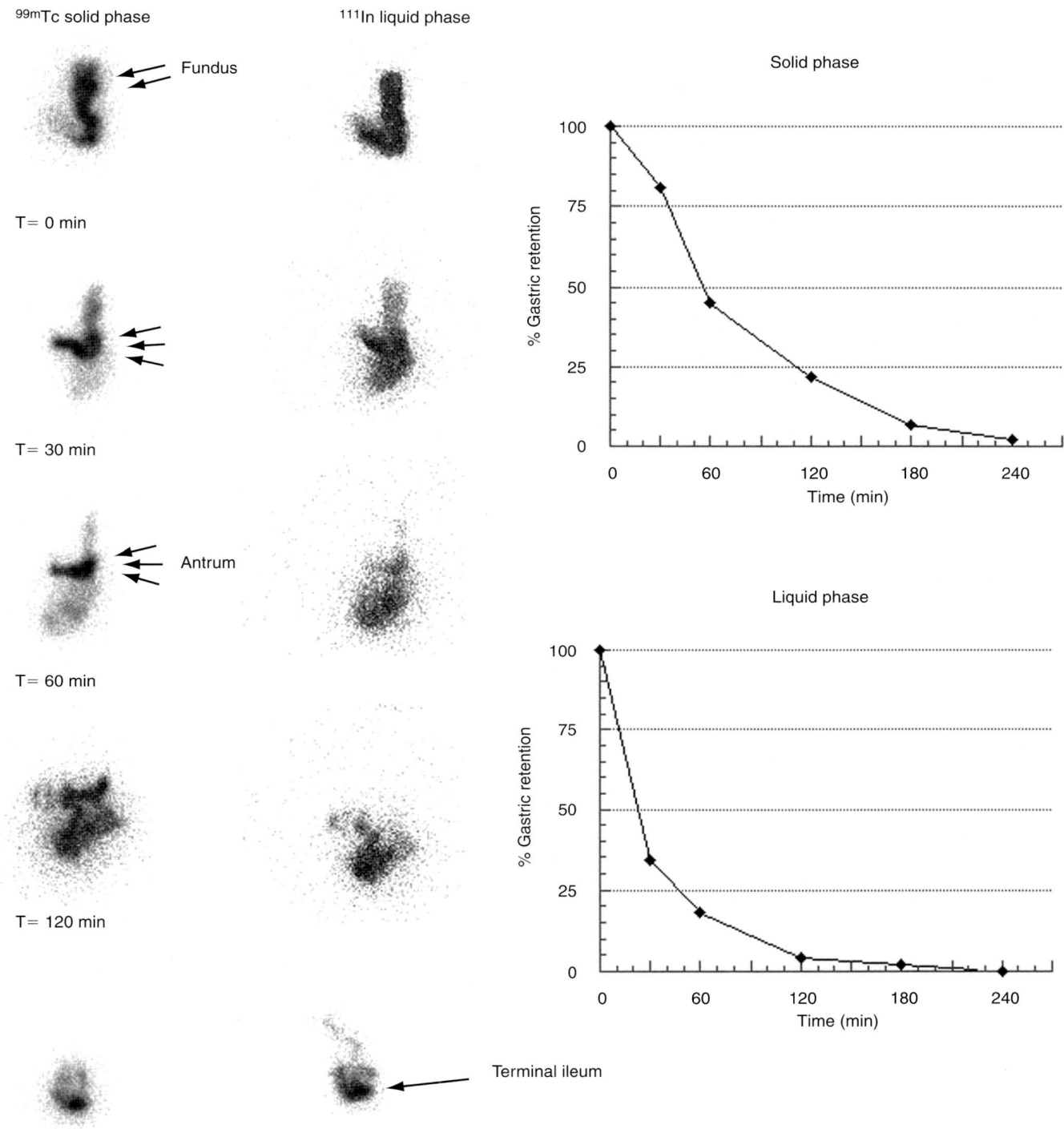

Figure 14-5. Normal dual-isotope, solid-liquid gastric emptying study (only anterior views shown). These images demonstrate early rapid distribution of liquids throughout the stomach (t = 0 min). In contrast, the initial preferential localization of solids is the fundus (*double arrows*). With time, solids move distally into the antrum (*triple arrows*). The solid emptying curve is sigmoidal because of the early lag phase for solids. The liquid emptying curve is monoexponential. When images are acquired for 4 to 6 hours, build-up of activity is seen in the terminal ileum (*large single arrow*), which can be used to assess small bowel transit.

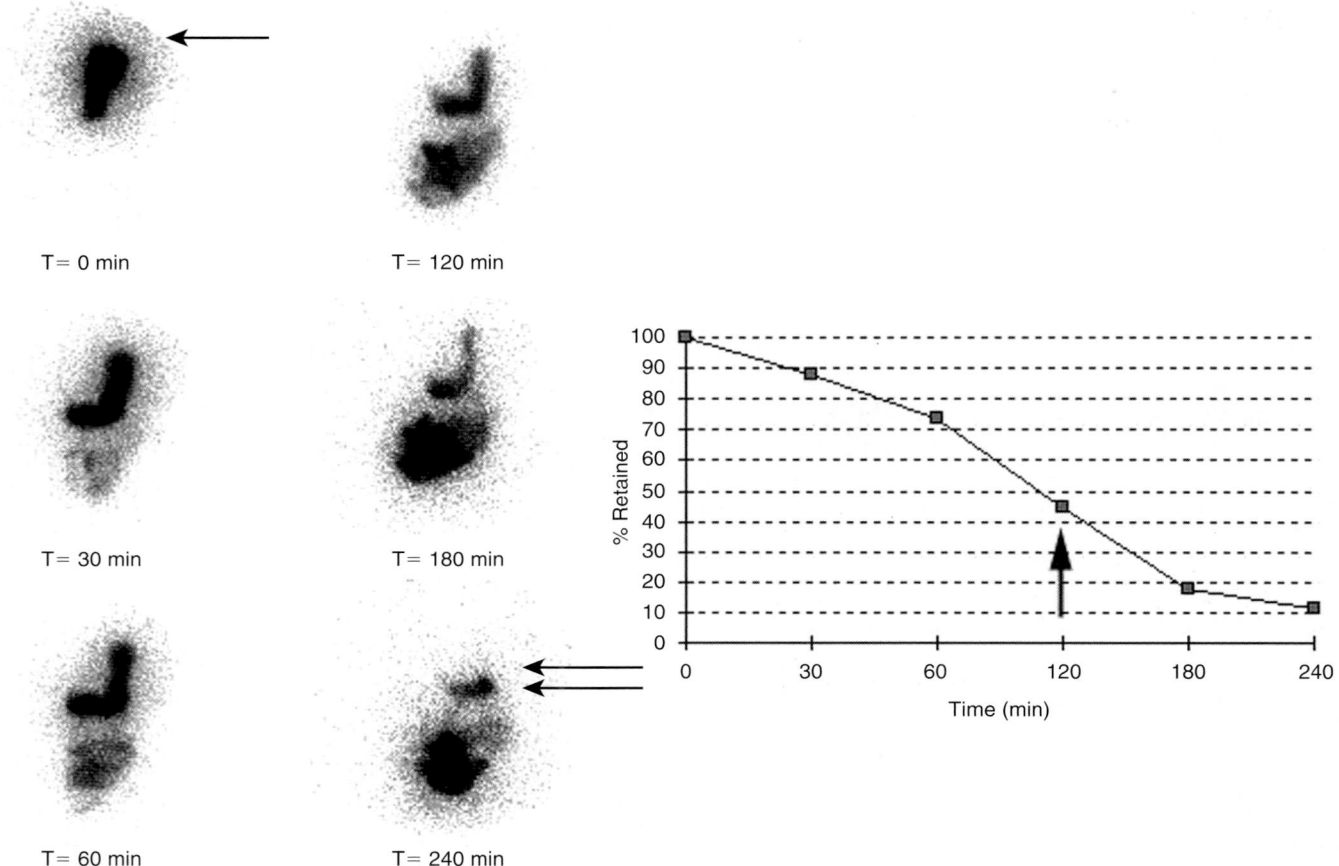

Figure 14-6. Normal gastric emptying at 2 hours, but abnormal gastric emptying at 4 hours (solid phase, only anterior views shown). Patients may have borderline or even normal values for gastric emptying at 2 hours (less than 50% retained for the two whole-egg meal), as in this case. However, there is abnormal gastric retention at 4 hours (14%). These patients typically show normal fundal filling and emptying (*single arrows*) with late retention of solids in the antrum (*double arrows*).

antrum, it is ideal for measuring both regional and total gastric emptying. Studies have shown an association between symptoms of nausea, early satiety, abdominal distention, and acid reflux with proximal gastric retention, whereas vomiting is associated more with delayed distal gastric emptying. Evaluation of fundal and antral gastric emptying on scintigraphy and quantification of regional emptying can be helpful for explaining dyspeptic symptoms, especially when total gastric emptying values are normal.[41,42] Regional analysis of gastric emptying should therefore be included as a part of the routine interpretation of gastric emptying scintigraphy studies (Figs. 14-6 and 14-7).

Antral Contraction Scintigraphy

Methods for analyzing gastric emptying data have also been introduced that permit analysis of the frequency and amplitude of antral contractions. Normal antral contractions occur at a rate of three per minute (Fig. 14-8). The ability to measure both the frequency and strength of antral contractions has increased our understanding of normal and abnormal gastric emptying. In diabetic gastroparesis, gastric emptying is delayed not only because of retention of food in the fundus but also because of decreased strength of antral contractions, which occur at a higher frequency.[43] The majority of patients

with gastroparesis are women, with an 82% female predominance in one large study.[44] Differences in normal male and female gastric emptying have been shown to be secondary to the amplitude rather than the frequency of antral contractions. The use of scintigraphy to measure the amplitude of antral contractions has shown that woman have lower amplitude contractions (not associated with higher progesterone) during the luteal (late) phase of the menstrual cycle.[45]

Fundal Accommodation Studies

Fundal relaxation (accommodation) is a well-established physiologic response that allows the stomach to increased intragastric volume without increasing intragastric pressure. The barostat is the current reference method for assessing fundal accommodation, although this technique has been criticized as invasive and nonphysiologic.[46] Nutrient- or water-loading tests have also been used to assess gastric filling capacity and sensation (visceral hypersensitivity).

Because intravenously administered ^{99m}Tc pertechnetate accumulates in the gastric mucosa, 3D SPECT volumetric imaging of the outer wall of the stomach can be performed. This has been validated as a noninvasive method for measuring gastric volumes before and at any time after meals (Fig. 14-9).[47,48] It is also possible to simultaneously assess the

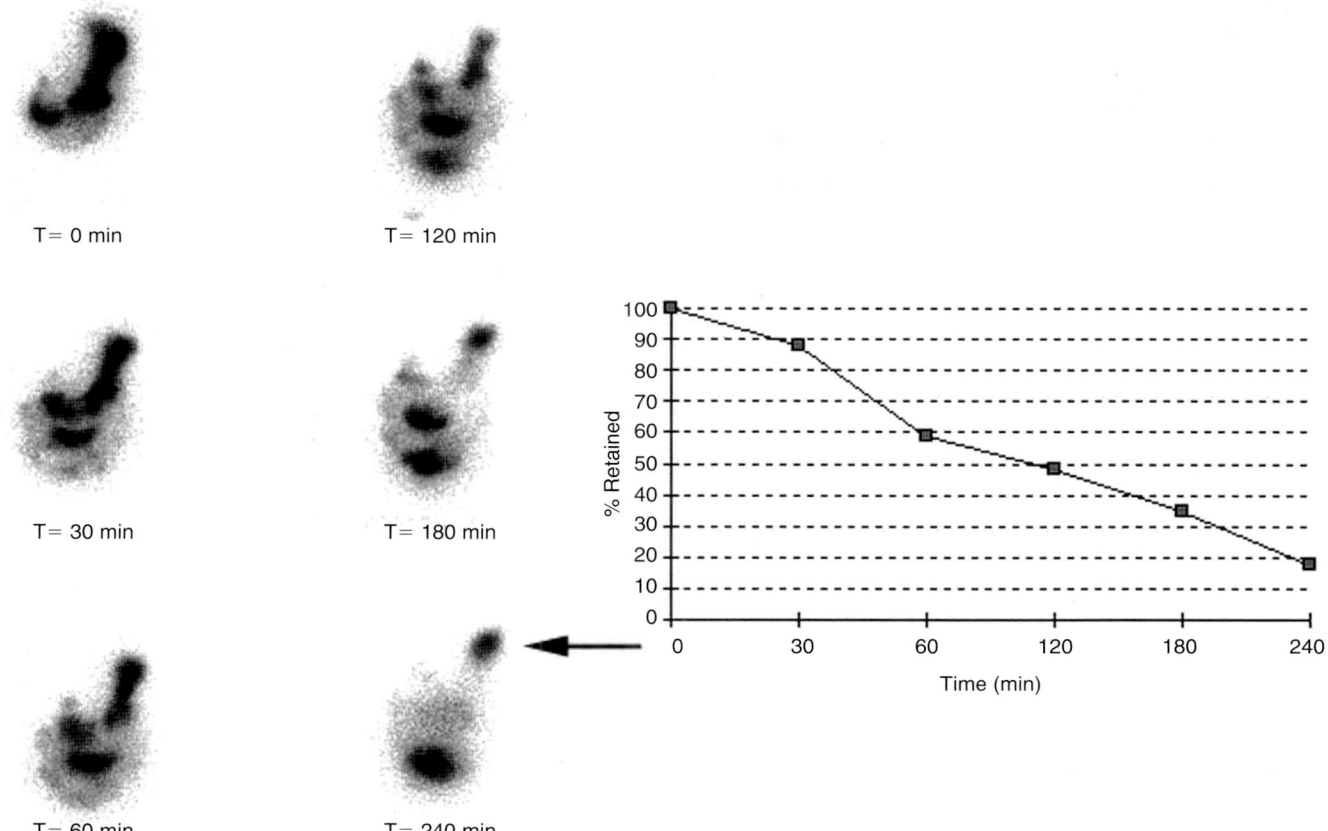

Figure 14-7. Localized fundal retention (solid phase, only anterior views shown). This patient with idiopathic gastroparesis has persistent fundal retention (*arrow*) with failure of solids to progress into the antrum. Compare this emptying pattern to the pattern in another patient in whom the fundus empties normally (see Fig. 14-6).

relationship of liquid or solid meal emptying and gastric accommodation. Studies have shown that maximal gastric volume change (mean = 185%) occurs immediately after ingestion of a meal and persists despite relatively rapid emptying of the meal.[49]

It is expected that these new methods to measure gastric accommodation will be of clinical value, especially for studying patients with dyspepsia and normal gastric emptying and may help direct medical therapy.

Pediatric Gastric Emptying Studies

Delayed gastric emptying may be suspected in infants younger than 2 years of age who have vomiting, abdominal pain, or early satiety. In infants, gastric emptying scintigraphy is usually combined with evaluation of GER, using milk or formula feeds containing ^{99m}Tc-SC. The normal values for gastric emptying of various meals in infants have not been established because of a lack of normal control studies. However, gastric retention of 40% to 70% at 1 hour has been reported.[50]

INTESTINAL TRANSIT STUDIES

Symptoms related to colonic dysmotility usually include abdominal pain, constipation, and diarrhea. In many cases, dyspeptic symptoms overlap, so that it is difficult to determine if the site of origin is the upper or lower gastrointestinal

tract or both. It is now recommended that gastrointestinal transit studies be used to localize the potential site of disease and guide therapy.[51] Because of the need to evaluate motility throughout the gastrointestinal tract, gastroenterocolic or whole-gut transit (combined gastric emptying and small bowel and colon transit) scintigraphy has been developed.

Small Bowel Transit Studies

Measurement of small bowel transit (SBT) is difficult because the input of a meal into the small intestine depends on gastric emptying, and small intestinal chyme is spread out over a large distance as it progresses toward the colon. There is no simple peristaltic pattern. Antegrade and retrograde movements of chyme occur, with some areas progressing rapidly and others more slowly. Although this process is irregular, it results in a net progression of chyme toward the colon.

Analogous to lactulose breath testing, the simplest scintigraphic approach for measuring SBT is to measure orocecal transit time. Precise definition of the initial arrival of activity in the cecum requires frequent imaging (every 10 to 15 minutes) (Fig. 14-10). Hydrogen breath testing correlates well with scintigraphy. In one study, orocecal transit time was 56 ± 4 minutes for lactulose breath testing and 43 ± 4 minutes for simultaneously performed scintigraphy. However, lactulose significantly accelerates orocecal transit. Without lactulose, the scintigraphic orocecal transit time was 231 ± 37 minutes.[52]

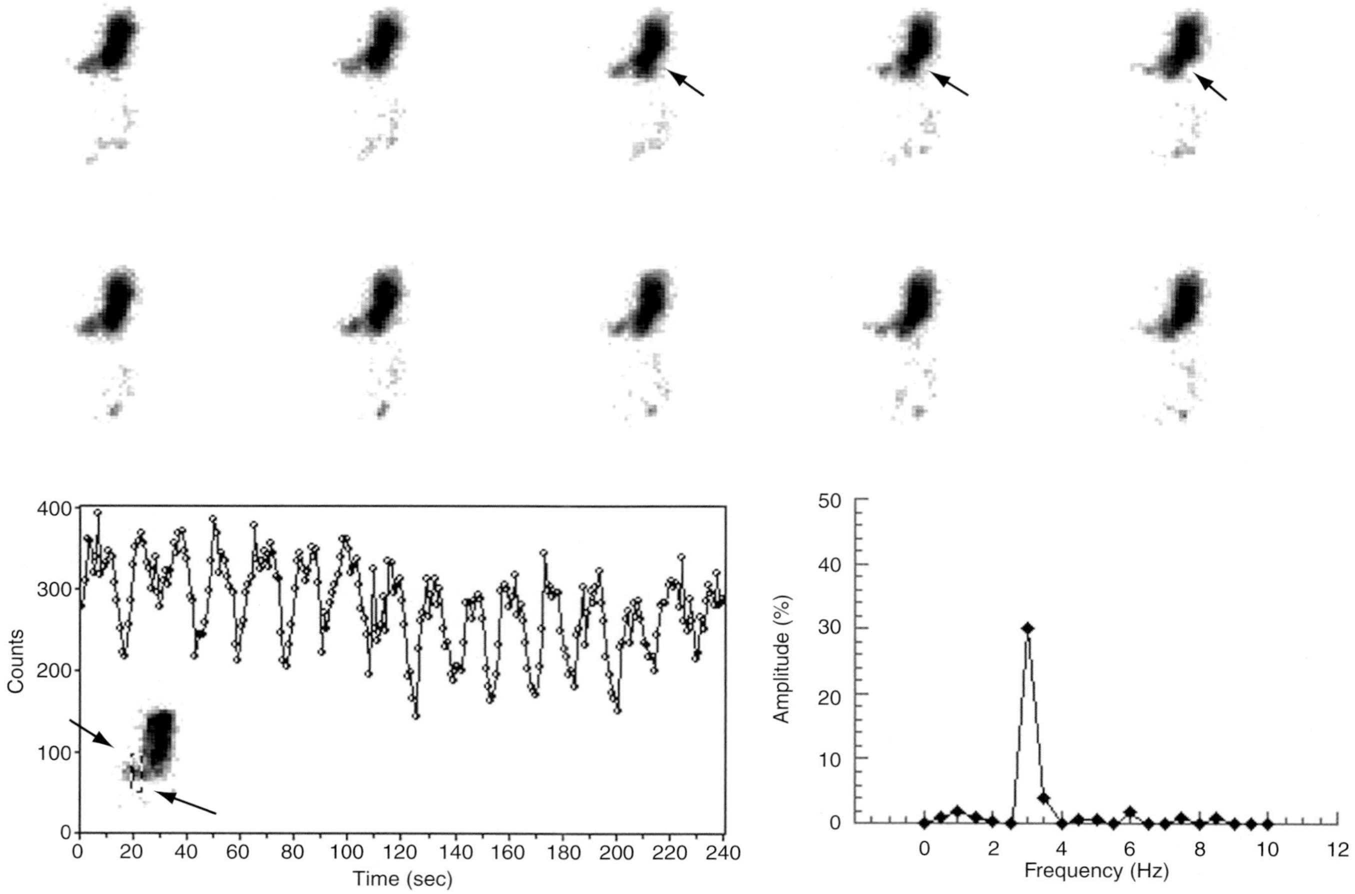

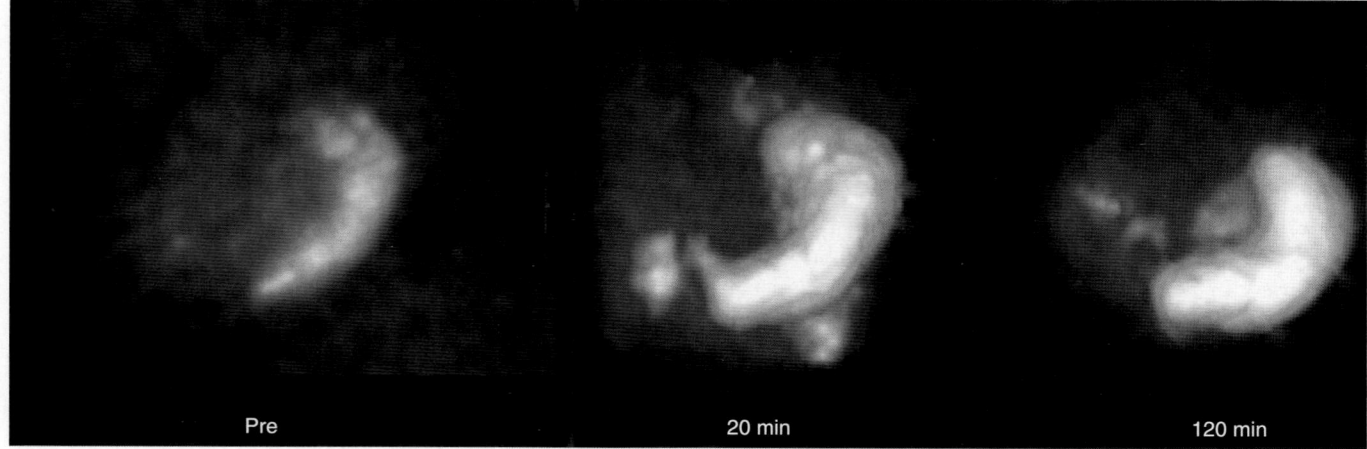

Figure 14-8. Scintigraphic analysis of antral contractions. To characterize the amplitude and frequency of antral contractions (*single arrows*) images of the stomach are acquired rapidly at one second per frame. By placing a region of interest over the antrum, a time activity curve of the counts in the region yields a recording of antral contractions (*paired arrows*). Fourier analysis is then used to measure both the amplitude and frequency of antral contractions. In this example, the graph (*lower right inset*) shows a normal antral frequency of 3 Hz.

Figure 14-9. SPECT 3D volume study. These 3D volumetric images demonstrate the contracted state of the stomach before a gastric emptying meal. At 20 minutes there is a marked increase in the volume of the gastric fundus (accommodation). Gastric dilatation persists to 4 hours despite normal gastric emptying of solids.

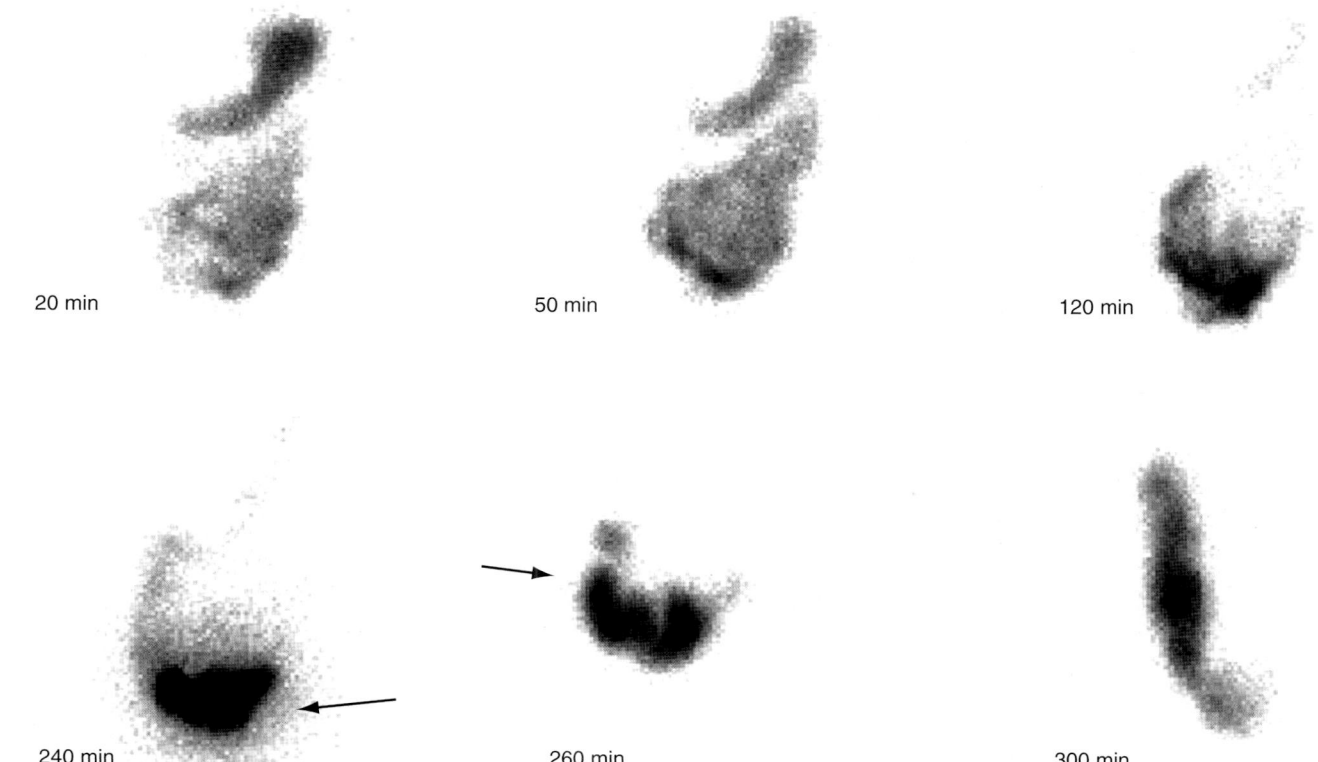

Figure 14-10. Normal small bowel transit (liquid phase, only anterior views shown). Sequential images of the liquid phase of a gastric emptying meal are shown. Over time, a diffuse small bowel activity pattern demonstrates focal accumulation of activity in the terminal ileum, which acts as a temporary reservoir (*long arrow*) for intestinal chyme that subsequently enters the cecum-ascending colon (*short arrow*), with progressive filling of the ascending colon by 5 hours.

Scintigraphic measurements of SBT do not attempt to characterize complex temporal or spatial peristaltic small bowel patterns but rather use measurement of bulk volume movement of activity distally into the terminal ileum or proximal colon.[53,54] Rapid peristalsis and transit occurs in the duodenum and jejunum and slows in the ileum. It has been observed that isotope collects in a well-defined region of the pelvis proximal to the ileocolic junction before passing into the colon. This buildup of activity in the distal small bowel occurs because the terminal ileum functions as a reservoir for chyme that subsequently passes into the colon.[55] This ileal reservoir can be identified as an area of increased counts before visualization of the cecum or ascending colon (see Figs. 14-5 and 14-10).

The rate of isotope accumulation in the terminal ileum can be used as an index of small bowel motility.[56] A simple index of SBT is obtained by determining the percentage of administered activity that has accumulated in the terminal ileum 6 hours after ingestion of a meal. When ^{111}In-DTPA in water is given with the two-egg gastric emptying study, normal small bowel transit is present when more than 40% of administered activity has progressed into the terminal ileum and/or cecum and ascending colon at 6 hours.[57] Others use a measure of proximal colonic filling.[58]

Colonic Transit Studies

Therapy for patients with chronic constipation depends on whether there is slow colonic transit, pelvic floor dysfunction, and functional or irritable bowel syndrome. Motor function of the colon can be studied using manometric and myoelectric devices. However, these techniques are inconsistent, are difficult to use, and have limited recording sites. Imaging of colonic transit can also be performed using serial abdominal radiographs and radiopaque markers. The markers are ingested with a meal, and serial radiographs are obtained to monitor the number of markers in various segments of the colon. Such markers are nonphysiologic compared with intestinal chyme, and intracolonic localization of the markers can be difficult because of limited anatomic landmarks of the colon on abdominal radiographs. Nevertheless, these colonic transit studies have been shown to correlate well with scintigraphic measurement of colonic transit.[59,60]

^{111}In-DTPA is an ideal agent for colon transit scintigraphy. It is a nonabsorbable agent that has a long half-life, permitting imaging over a period of several days. To quantify colonic transit, a geometric center (GC) has been defined for measuring the progression of colonic activity.[61] The GC is calculated by dividing the colon into anatomic regions with separate numerical values, including: (1) the cecum-ascending colon;

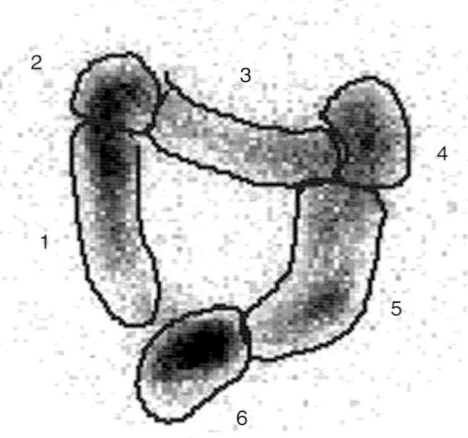

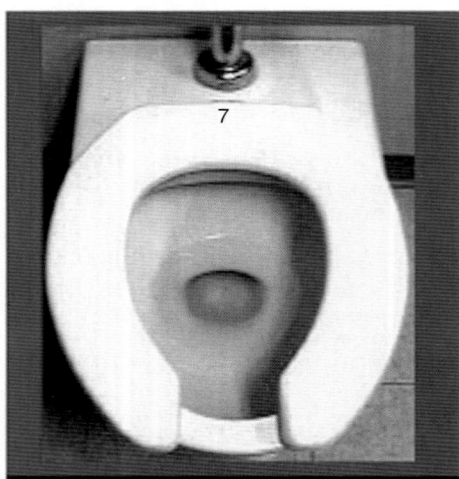

Figure 14-11. Geometric center colonic transit analysis. To calculate the geometric center of colonic transit, regions of interest (ROIs) (1 to 6) are defined for the colon to obtain a numerical value for the location of the radiotracer as it passes through the colon and is then excreted (ROI 7).

(2) the hepatic flexure; (3) the transverse colon; (4) the splenic flexure; (5) the descending colon; (6) the rectosigmoid colon; and (7) excreted stool. The GC is a weighted average of the counts in each region (Fig. 14-11). A low GC (1 to 2) indicates that the center of activity is in the proximal colon, and a higher GC (5 to 7) indicates that it has progressed to the left side of the colon or has been eliminated in the stool. With this approach, a single numerical value can be used to measure transit of activity through the colon.

Two methods that use oral ^{111}In-DTPA to measure colonic transit are in use. One from the Mayo Clinic requires preparation of a resin-coated capsule designed to dissolve at a pH between 7.2 and 7.4 in the environment of the ileum (pH = 7.4).[62] A simpler alternate method from Temple University requires administration of ^{111}In-DTPA as part of a

standard solid-liquid gastric emptying scintigraphy study.[56] Using the solid-liquid meal, the normal mean GC values (± 1 SD) are 4.6 ± 1.5 at 24 hours, 6.1 ± 1.0 at 48 hours, and 6.6 ± 0.19 at 72 hours.

In practice, the colon should be imaged at 24 and 48 hours. If the GC at 48 hours is less than 4.1 (proximal to the splenic flexure), no further imaging is needed because colonic transit is delayed. If the GC is greater than 4.1 but less than 6.4, an image should be obtained at 72 hours to exclude functional outlet obstruction. Three patterns of slow colonic transit have been recognized, including (1) generalized slow transit with diffuse retention throughout the length of the colon; (2) marked right-sided retention proximal to the splenic flexure (colonic inertia); and (3) retention in the rectosigmoid (functional rectosigmoid obstruction) (Fig. 14-12).[63] In patients with diarrhea, accelerated colonic transit can be confirmed by a GC greater than 6.1 (at or beyond the rectosigmoid) at 24 hours.

Whole-Gut Transit Studies

Whole-gut transit scintigraphy (WGTS) combines measurement of gastric emptying with small bowel and colonic transit after administration of a dual-isotope solid-liquid meal. These studies are helpful for evaluating patients whose symptoms cannot be classified either as having an upper or lower gastrointestinal tract origin or for evaluating patients in whom a functional rather an organic cause of slow transit is suspected. Patients with diarrhea-predominant irritable bowel syndrome have shorter small bowel transit and rapid colonic filling, whereas constipated patients have slower small bowel transit and delayed colonic filling.[54] In one study, 40% of patients referred for upper gastrointestinal symptoms, constipation, or diarrhea were found to have an organic cause of symptoms, but the remaining 60% had a functional cause.[64] Colonic transit tends to be prolonged in patients with organic disease, whereas it may be normal in patients with functional constipation. In a study evaluating the clinical utility of WGTS at Temple University, organic disease was found in many patients originally suspected of having a functional disorder; the initial diagnosis was changed in 45% of patients, and management was changed in 67%.[57]

WGTS appears to be most helpful for evaluating patients with constipation. Many patients with severe idiopathic constipation have prominent upper gastrointestinal symptoms. It is important to exclude significant upper gastrointestinal dysmotility in such patients before surgery because a subtotal colectomy may not correct their symptoms.[65] A colectomy should be performed only if abnormal transit is confined to the colon. In a study of patients with severe idiopathic constipation who had upper gastrointestinal symptoms, many were found to have abnormal gastric emptying and small bowel transit as well as delayed colonic transit.[66] The presence of abnormal gastric emptying combined with abnormal small bowel and colonic transit should suggest a diagnosis of chronic idiopathic intestinal pseudo-obstruction.

Normal   Generalized   Functional obstruction   Colonic inertia

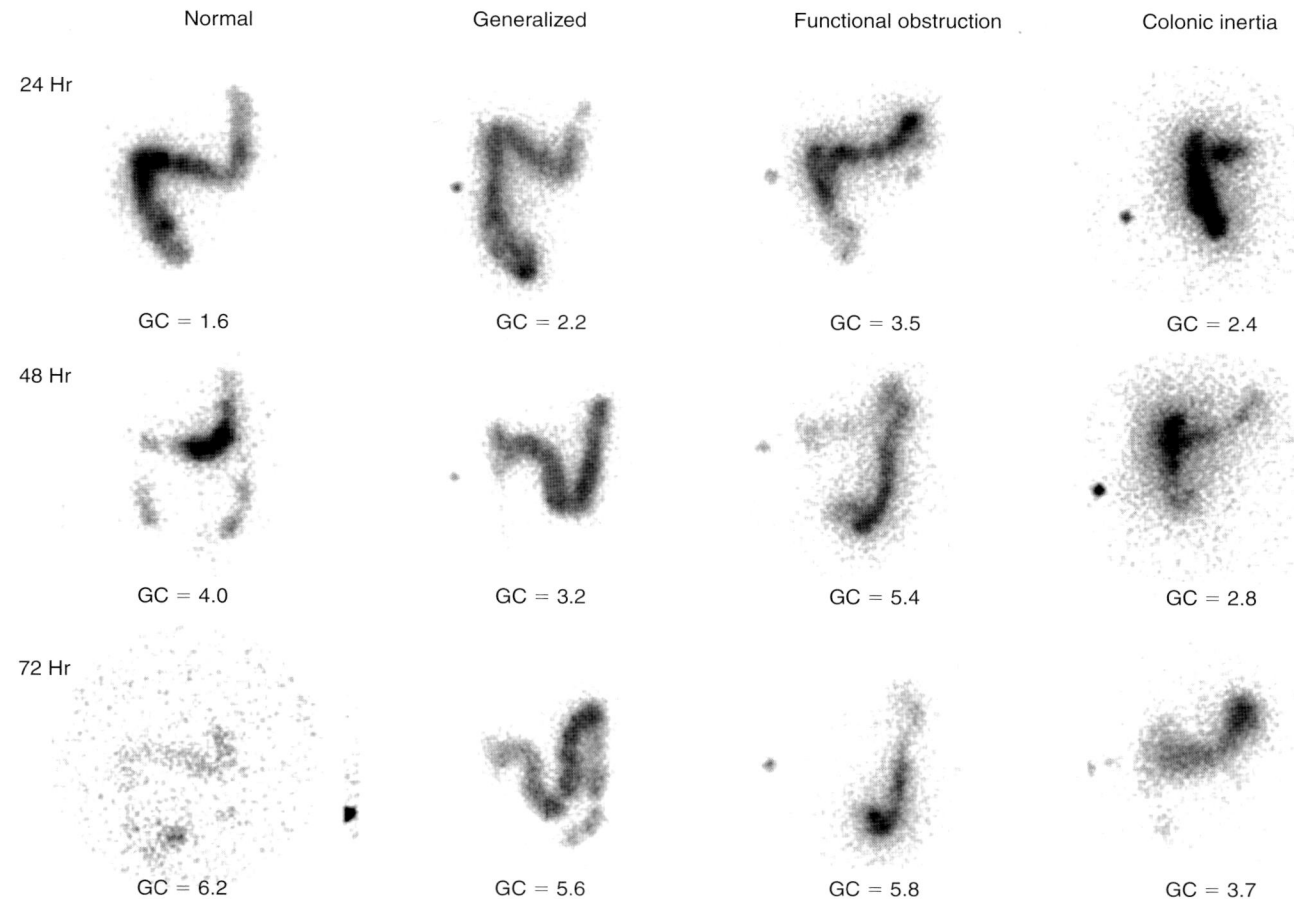

24 Hr

GC = 1.6   GC = 2.2   GC = 3.5   GC = 2.4

48 Hr

GC = 4.0   GC = 3.2   GC = 5.4   GC = 2.8

72 Hr

GC = 6.2   GC = 5.6   GC = 5.8   GC = 3.7

Figure 14-12. Normal and abnormal colonic transit patterns. Normal colonic transit shows activity predominantly in the right colon at 24 hours, with near-complete emptying at 72 hours. Generalized slow colonic transit shows a diffuse pattern of retention at 72 hours. Functional rectosigmoid outlet obstruction shows normal progression from the right colon to the left, but with retention in the rectosigmoid at 72 hours. Colonic inertia shows failure of activity to progress beyond the splenic flexure at 48 and 72 hours. GC, geometric center.

References

1. Drane WE, Johnson DA, Hagan DP, et al: "Nutcracker" esophagus: diagnosis with radionuclide esophageal scintigraphy versus manometry. Radiology 163:33-37, 1987.
2. Holloway RH, Lange RC, Plankey MW, et al: Detection of esophageal motor disorders by radionuclide transit studies: a reappraisal. Dig Dis Sci 34:905-912, 1989.
3. Parkman HP, Maurer AH, Caroline DF, et al: Optimal evaluation of patients with nonobstructive esophageal dysphagia. Manometry, scintigraphy, or videoesophagography? Dig Dis Sci 41:1355-1368, 1996.
4. Taillefer R, Jadliwalla M, Pellerin E, et al: Radionuclide esophageal transit study in detection of esophageal motor dysfunction: comparison with motility studies (manometry). J Nucl Med 31:1921-1926, 1990.
5. Jorgensen F, Hesse B, Tromholt N, et al: Esophageal scintigraphy: reproducibility and normal ranges. J Nucl Med 33:2106-2109, 1992.
6. Klein H: Esophageal transit scintigraphy. Sem Nuc Med 25:306-317, 1995.
7. Iascone C, Di Giulio E, Maffi C, et al: Use of radioisotopic esophageal transit in the assessment of patients with symptoms of reflux and non-specific esophageal motor disorders. Dis Esoph 17:218-222, 2004.
8. Mughal MM, Marples M, Bancewicz J: Scintigraphic assessment of oesophageal motility: what does it show and how reliable is it? Gut 27:946-953, 1986.
9. Bestetti A, Carola F, Conciato L, et al: Esophageal scintigraphy with a semisolid meal to evaluate esophageal dysmotility in systemic sclerosis and Raynaud's phenomenon. J Nucl Med 40:77-84, 1999.
10. Tatsch K: Multiple swallow test for quantitative and qualitative evaluation of esophageal motility disorders. J Nucl Med 32:1365-1370, 1991.
11. Robertson CS, Hardy JG, Atkinson M: Quantitative assessment of the response to therapy in achalasia of the cardia. Gut 30:768-773, 1989.
12. Wong RK, Maydonovitch C, Garcia JE, et al: The effect of terbutaline sulfate, nitroglycerin, and aminophylline on lower esophageal sphincter pressure and radionuclide esophageal emptying in patients with achalasia. J Clinical Gastroenterol 9:386-389, 1987.
13. Stacher G, Schima W, Bergmann H, et al: Sensitivity of radionuclide bolus transport and videofluoroscopic studies compared with manometry in the detection of achalasia. Am J Gastroenterol 89:1484-1488, 1994.
14. Kochan P, Maurer A, Parkman H, et al: Clinical role of esophageal and gastroesophageal reflux scintigraphy. J Nucl Med 43:162P, 2002.
15. Madan K, Ahuja V, Gupta SD, et al: Impact of 24-h esophageal pH monitoring on the diagnosis of gastroesophageal reflux disease: defining the gold standard. J Gastroenterol Hepatol 20:30-37, 2005.
16. Shay SS, Johnson LF, Richter JE: Acid reflux: a review, emphasizing detection by impedance, manometry, and scintigraphy, and the impact on acid clearing pathophysiology as well as interpreting the pH record. Dig Dis Sci 48:1-9, 2003.
17. Buckles DC, Sarosiek I, McMillin C, et al: Delayed gastric emptying in gastroesophageal reflux disease: reassessment with new methods and symptomatic correlations. Am J Med Sci 327:1-4, 2004.
18. Thomas EJ, Kumar R, Dasan JB, et al: Prevalence of silent gastroesophageal reflux in association with recurrent lower respiratory tract infections. Clin Nucl Med 28:476-479, 2003.
19. Reyhan M, Yapar AF, Aydin M, et al: Gastroesophageal scintigraphy in children: a comparison of posterior and anterior imaging. Ann Nucl Med 19:17-21, 2005.
20. Caglar M, Volkan B, Alpar R: Reliability of radionuclide gastroesophageal reflux studies using visual and time-activity curve analysis: inter-observer

and intra-observer variation and description of minimum detectable reflux. Nucl Med Communications 24:421-428, 2003.

21. Thomas EJ, Kumar R, Dasan JB, et al: Gastroesophageal reflux in asthmatic children not responding to asthma medication: a scintigraphic study in 126 patients with correlation between scintigraphic and clinical findings of reflux. Clin Imaging 27:333-336, 2003.

22. Fisher R, Parkman H: Current concepts: management of nonulcer dyspepsia. N Engl J Med 339:1376-1381, 1998.

23. Feldman M, Smith HJ: Effect of cisapride on gastric emptying of indigestible solids in patients with gastroparesis diabeticorum. Gastroenterology 92:171-174, 1987.

24. Couturier O, Bodet-Milin C, Querellou S, et al: Gastric scintigraphy with a liquid-solid radiolabelled meal: performances of solid and liquid parameters. Nucl Med Communications 25:1143-1150, 2004.

25. Tougas G, Eaker EY, Abell TL, et al: Assessment of gastric emptying using a low fat meal: establishment of international control values. Am J Gastroenterol 95:1456-1462, 2000.

26. Guo JP, Maurer AH, Fisher RS, et al: Extending gastric emptying scintigraphy from two to four hours detects more patients with gastroparesis. Dig Dis Sci 46:24-29, 2001.

27. Datz F, Christian P, Moore J: Gender-related differences in gastric emptying. J Nucl Med 28:1204-1207, 1987.

28. Gill R, Murphy P, Hooper H, et al: Effect of the menstrual cycle on gastric emptying. Digestion 36:168-174, 1987.

29. Knight LC, Parkman HP, Brown KL, et al: Delayed gastric emptying and decreased antral contractility in normal premenopausal women compared with men. Am J Gastroenterol 92:968-975, 1997.

30. Moore JG, Datz FL, Greenberg CE, et al: Effect of body posture on radionuclide measurements of gastric emptying. Dig Dis Sci 33:1592-1595, 1988.

31. Maurer AH, Knight LC, Vitti RA, et al: Geometric mean vs left anterior oblique attenuation correction: Effect on half emptying time, lag phase, and rate of gastric emptying. J Nucl Med 32, 1991.

32. Cremonini F, Delgado-Aros S, Talley NJ: Functional dyspepsia: Drugs for new (and old) therapeutic targets. Best Pract Res Clin Gastroenterol 18:717-733, 2004.

33. Camilleri M, Malagelada JR, Brown ML, et al: Relation between antral motility and gastric emptying of solids and liquids in humans. Am J Physiol 245:G580-G585, 1985.

34. Collins PJ, Horowitz M, Chatterton BE: Proximal, distal and total stomach emptying of a digestible solid meal in normal subjects. Br J Radiol 61: 12-18, 1988.

35. Urbain JL, Siegel JA, Charkes ND, et al: The two-component stomach: Effects of meal particle size on fundal and antral emptying. Eur J Nucl Med 15:254-259, 1989.

36. Siegel JA, Urbain JL, Adler LP, et al: Biphasic nature of gastric emptying. Gut 29:85-89, 1988.

37. Thumshirn M: Pathophysiology of functional dyspepsia. Gut 51(Suppl 1): 63-66, 2002.

38. Delgado-Aros S, Camilleri M, Cremonini F, et al: Contributions of gastric volumes and gastric emptying to meal size and postmeal symptoms in functional dyspepsia. Gastroenterology 127:1685-1694, 2004.

39. Sarnelli G, Caenepeel P, Geypens B, et al: Symptoms associated with impaired gastric emptying of solids and liquids in functional dyspepsia. Am J Gastroenterol 98:783-788, 2003.

40. Scott A, Kellow J, Shuter B, et al: Intragastric distribution and gastric emptying of solids and liquids in functional dyspepsia. Dig Dis Sci 38:2247-2254, 1993.

41. Gonlachanvit S, Aronchick R, Kantor S, et al: Regional gastric emptying abnormalities in nonulcer dyspepsia and gastroesophageal reflux disease. Am J Gastroenterol 95:2452-2453, 2000.

42. Piessevaux H, Tack J, Walrand S, et al: Intragastric distribution of a standardized meal in health and functional dyspepsia: Correlation with specific symptoms. Neurogastroenterol Motil 15:447-455, 2003.

43. Urbain JL, Vekemans MC, Bouillon R, et al: Characterization of gastric antral motility disturbances in diabetes using the scintigraphic technique. J Nucl Med 34:576-581, 1993.

44. Soykan I, Sivri B, Sarosiek I, et al: Demography, clinical characteristics, psychological profiles, treatment and long-term follow-up of patients with gastroparesis. Dig Dis Sci 43:2398-2404, 1998.

45. Knight LC, Parkman HP, Miller MA, et al: Delayed gastric emptying in normal women is associated with decreased antral contractility. Am J Gastroenterol 92:968-975, 1997.

46. Gregersen H, Frieling T: Function and dyspepsia: A start of a new friendship. Neurogastroenterol Motil 16:271-273, 2004.

47. Bouras E, Delgado-Aros S, Camilleri M, et al: SPECT imaging of the stomach: Comparison with barostat and effects of sex, age, body mass index, and fundoplication. Gut 51:781-786, 2002.

48. Kuiken S, Samson M, Camilleri M, et al: Development of a test to measure gastric accommodation in humans. Am J Physiol 277:G1217-G1221, 1999.

49. Simonian H, Maurer A, Knight L, et al: Simultaneous assessment of gastric accommodation and emptying: Studies with liquid and solid meals. J Nucl Med 45:1155-1160, 2004.

50. Heyman S: Gastric emptying in children. J Nucl Med 39:865-869, 1998.

51. Lin H, Prather C, Fisher R, et al: Measurement of gastrointestinal transit. Dig Dis Sci 50:989-1004, 2005.

52. Miller MA, Parkman HP, Urbain JL, et al: Comparison of scintigraphy and lactulose breath hydrogen test for assessment of orocecal transit: Lactulose accelerates small bowel transit. Dig Dis Sci 42:10-18, 1997.

53. Graff J, Brinch K, Madsen JL: Simplified scintigraphic methods for measuring gastrointestinal transit times. Clin Physiol 20:262-266, 2000.

54. Read NW, Al-Janabi MN, Holgate AM, et al: Simultaneous measurement of gastric emptying, small bowel residence and colonic filling of a solid meal by the use of the gamma camera. Gut 27:300-308, 1986.

55. Phillips SF, Quigley EM, Kumar D, et al: Motility of the ileocolonic junction. Gut 29:390-406, 1988.

56. Krevsky B, Maurer AH, Niewiarowski T, et al: The effect of verapamil on human intestinal transit. Dig Dis Sci 37:919-924, 1992.

57. Bonapace ES, Maurer AH, Davidoff S, et al: Whole gut transit scintigraphy in the clinical evaluation of patients with upper and lower gastrointestinal symptoms. Am J Gastroenterol 95:2838-2847, 2000.

58. Prather CM, Camilleri M, Zinsmeister AR, et al: Tegaserod accelerates orocecal transit in patients with constipation-predominant irritable bowel syndrome. Gastroenterology 118:463-468, 2000.

59. Kanamalla U, Bromer M, Maurer A, et al: Comparison of colon transit scintigraphy and radiopaque markers in patients with constipation. J Nucl Med 42:129, 2001.

60. Proano M, Camilleri M, Phillips SF, et al: Transit of solids through the human colon: Regional quantification in the unprepared bowel. Am J Physiol 258:G856-G862, 1990.

61. Krevsky B, Malmud LS, D'Ercole F, et al: Colonic transit scintigraphy: A physiologic approach to the quantitative measurement of colonic transit in humans. Gastroenterology 91:1102-1112, 1986.

62. Camilleri M, Colemont LJ, Phillips SF, et al: Human gastric emptying and colonic filling of solids characterized by a new method. Am J Physiol 257: G284-G290, 1989.

63. Krevsky B, Maurer AH, Fisher RS: Patterns of colonic transit in chronic idiopathic constipation. Am J Gastroenterol 84:127-132, 1989.

64. Charles F, Camilleri M, Phillips SF, et al: Scintigraphy of the whole gut: Clinical evaluation of transit disorders. Mayo Clin Proc 70:113-118, 1995.

65. Kamm M, Hawley P, Lennard-Jones J: Outcome of colectomy for severe idiopathic constipation. Gut 29:969-973, 1988.

66. VanDerSijp JR, Kamm MA, Nightingale JM, et al: Disturbed gastric and small bowel transit in severe idiopathic constipation. Dig Dis Sci 38: 837-844, 1993.

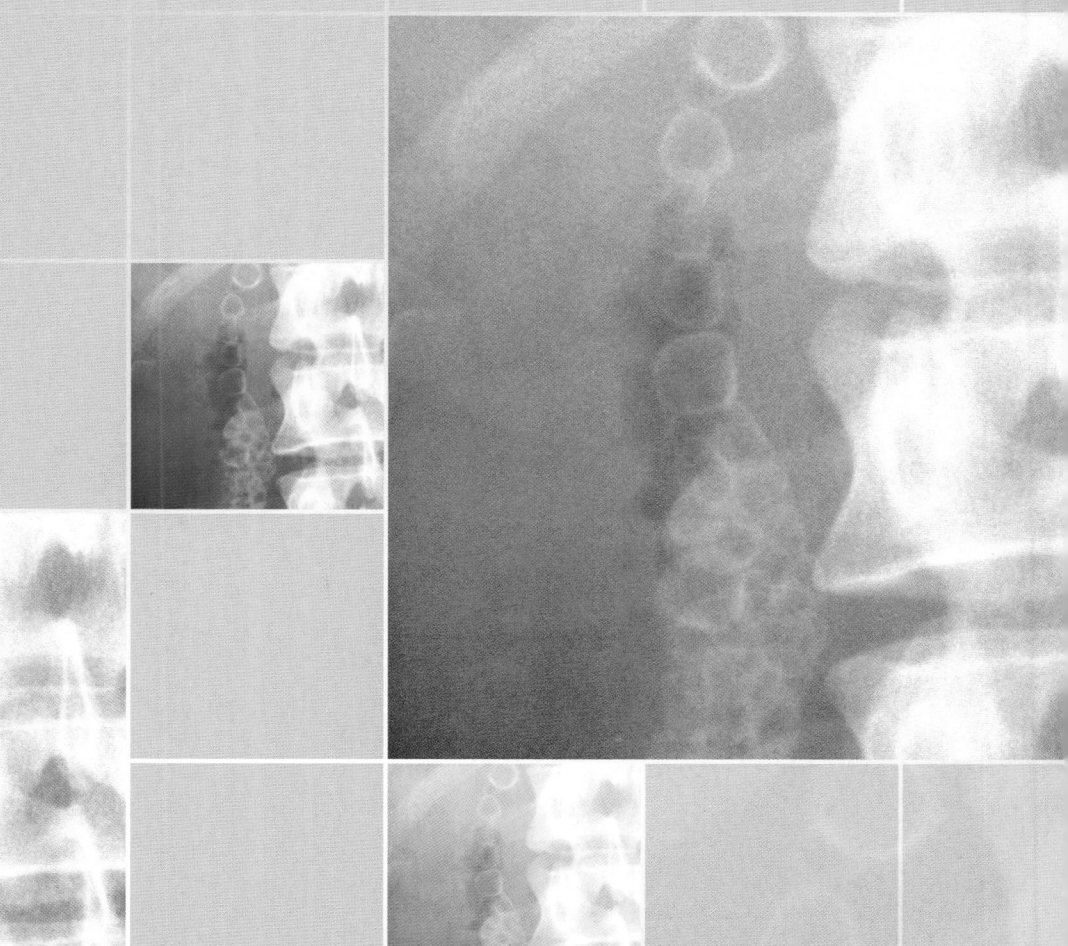

II

Abdominal Plain Radiographs

Abdomen: Normal Anatomy and Examination Techniques

William Moreau Thompson, MD

From the 1970s to 1990s, the abdominal radiograph traditionally served as the initial radiologic means of evaluating patients with suspected abdominal pathology. During the past two decades, however, CT has become the major imaging procedure in patients with suspected acute abdominal pathology.[1-3] When abdominal radiographs were obtained as a screening test, the diagnostic yield of this examination was low and most abnormalities that were detected were nonspecific.[4-6] In a review of 1780 screening abdominal radiographs, important abnormalities were found in only 10% of cases.[5] No clinically significant disease would have been missed if abdominal radiographs had been obtained only in patients with a strong clinical suspicion of disease and/or moderate to severe abdominal symptoms. Abdominal radiographs have the greatest value in patients in whom bowel obstruction or perforation, urinary calculi, or bowel ischemia is suggested on clinical grounds.[2,3,7-9] In patients with mild or nonspecific symptoms, however, abdominal radiographs have a low diagnostic yield. The major value of a normal abdominal series is the exclusion of bowel obstruction or free air secondary to bowel perforation.[7-9] Despite the increasing use of CT and the declining role of abdominal radiographs, this examination is still obtained in many patients, especially those who have undergone recent surgery and those who have some form of catheter, tube, or drain in the abdomen. Emergency department physicians may also order abdominal radiographs in patients with a low clinical suspicion of disease to ensure that a major abdominal disorder is not overlooked and to calm a concerned patient.

TECHNIQUE

Standard Projections

An anteroposterior radiograph taken with the patient in a supine position is the most common plain film examination of the abdomen (Fig. 15-1A). Whether one uses conventional film or digital techniques, the patient should be positioned comfortably on his or her back without rotation of the pelvis. Maximal relaxation of the abdominal musculature is important in reducing artifact caused by motion; this is facilitated by supporting and slightly flexing the patient's knees. The film or field of view for digital imaging should be positioned with

its lower edge at the symphysis pubis and the x-ray beam centered at the iliac crest. Both the lung bases and the symphysis pubis should be included on the radiograph. The exposure is made during expiration and should begin 1 to 2 seconds after respiration is suspended.[10]

Delineation of intra-abdominal soft tissues on abdominal radiographs depends on the inherent contrast provided by soft tissues, fat, and intraluminal gas. Subject contrast on the radiograph is caused by differential attenuation of the x-ray beam in the patient.[11] Most abdominal radiographs are taken using routine equipment exposed at low kV (60 to 75 kV), depending on the size of the patient.[10] A short exposure time is desirable to avoid motion unsharpness. Also, an increase in

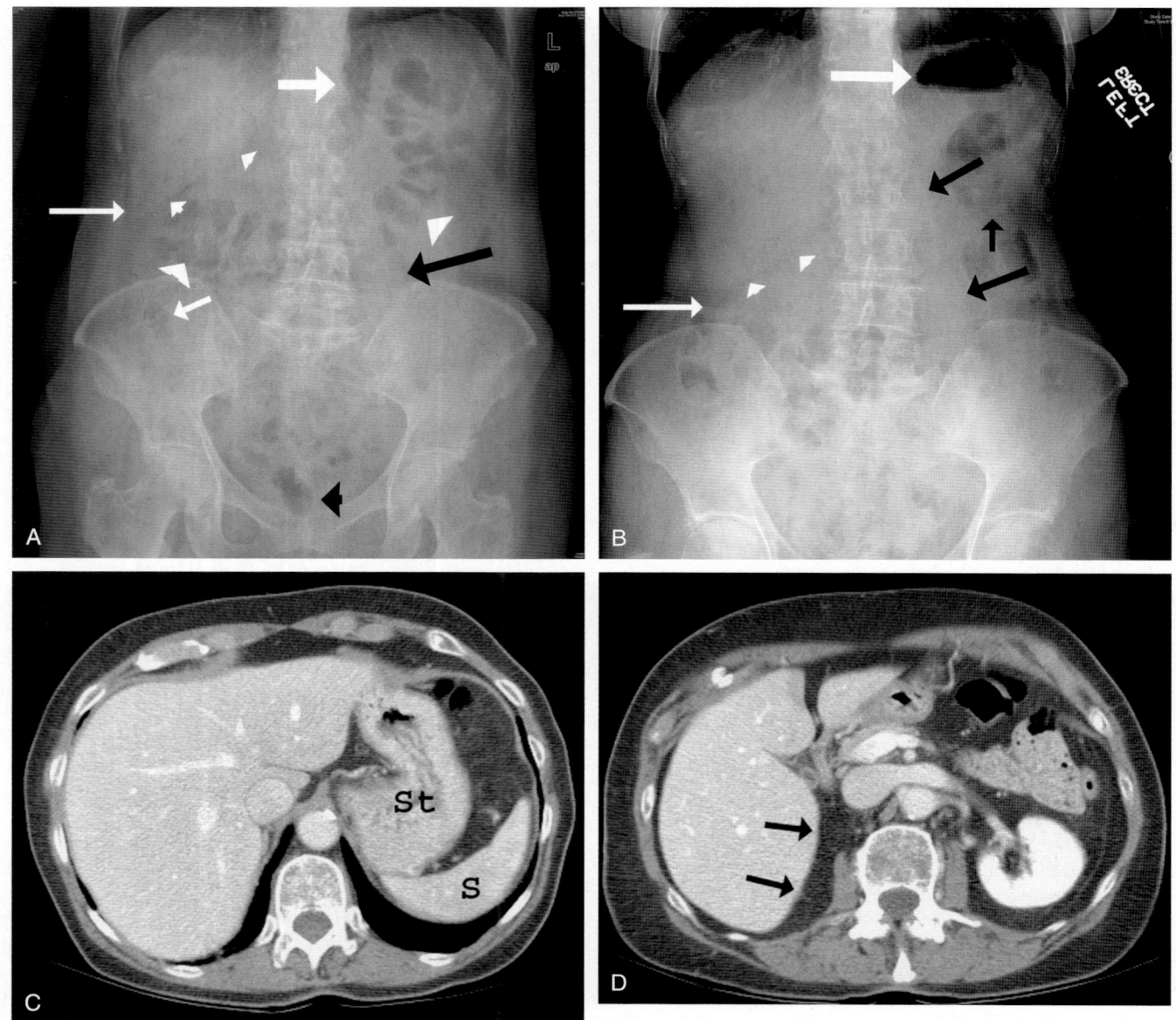

Figure 15-1. Normal supine and upright abdominal radiographs. A. Supine abdominal radiograph shows a normal bowel gas pattern with gas in the stomach (*large white arrow*), small bowel (*small white arrow*), colon (*large white arrowheads*), and rectum (*black arrowhead*). The hepatic angle (*long white arrow*) is outlined by extraperitoneal fat, and the posteromedial surface of the right lobe of the liver is outlined by perirenal fat (*small white arrowheads*). The left psoas muscle (*black arrow*) is also seen. **B.** Upright abdominal radiograph shows a normal air-fluid level in the stomach (*large white arrow*). Note the hepatic angle (*small white arrow*), posteromedial surface of the right lobe of the liver (*arrowheads*), left psoas muscle (*large black arrows*), and splenic tip (*small black arrow*). **C.** Axial CT of the upper abdomen shows fat outlining the wall of the stomach (St) and spleen (S). **D.** Another axial CT more caudad shows the posteromedial surface of the right lobe of the liver outlined by perirenal fat (*arrows*).

peak kilovoltage increases scattered radiation, which degrades soft tissue contrast. Thus, the lowest possible peak kilovoltage that can penetrate the patient and that has an acceptable exposure time should be used. With conventional films, a reciprocating (Potter-Bucky) grid and careful collimation are used to reduce scatter.[10] In males with reproductive potential, gonadal shielding should be used if the gonads lie within 5 cm of the primary beam and if such shielding does not compromise the clinical objectives of the examination.

Portable abdominal radiographs may be obtained in hospitalized, extremely ill patients; however, these radiographs are usually of lower quality than standard abdominal radiographs obtained in the radiology department. These patients are usually too ill to breath-hold, and most portable x-ray units have fixed milliampere settings, which may necessitate techniques of higher peak kilovoltage, resulting in reduced contrast. In addition, a stationary grid, rather than a Potter-Bucky grid, must be used to control scatter; and when these grids are poorly positioned, the image may be degraded secondary to grid cut-off. Whenever possible, abdominal radiographs should therefore be obtained using standard x-ray equipment in the radiology department.

Supplemental Projections

In addition to the standard anteroposterior supine view, other projections may help in specific clinical situations and are frequently obtained as part of a routine abdominal series. In patients with abdominal pain, upright posteroanterior abdominal or chest radiographs may be useful to facilitate detection of small amounts of free intraperitoneal air, small bowel obstruction, and unsuspected thoracic disease that is causing abdominal pain (Figs. 15-1B and 15-2).

An upright abdominal radiograph is often ordered on a routine basis, but some authors believe it does not contribute significant information in many patients. Mirvis and colleagues reviewed the emergency department radiographs of 252 patients, which included supine and upright abdominal radiographs as well as upright chest radiographs.[6] The upright abdominal radiographs did not contribute to the management of any patients with acute abdominal conditions in their series. The authors concluded that this view could be omitted to reduce the time and cost of the examination without sacrificing important diagnostic information. However, upright abdominal radiographs may be helpful in patients with suspected bowel obstruction who have a gasless abdomen on supine radiographs to further assess the appearance of gas and fluid in the small bowel (see Fig. 15-2A and B). Alternatively, this information could be obtained on abdominal radiographs taken with the patient in the lateral decubitus position. For extremely ill patients who cannot easily stand, a lateral decubitus view may be more helpful than a suboptimal upright radiograph.

Miller and Nelson showed that when a perforated viscus is suspected on clinical grounds, a specific sequence of exposures is most likely to demonstrate extraluminal gas.[12] The authors recommended that the patient be placed in the left-side-down position for at least 10 minutes before a left lateral decubitus view is obtained. This allows gas to rise and accumulate over the right margin of the liver and, occasionally, beneath the iliac crest. If the patient is unable to stand, an abdominal radiograph should be obtained with the patient in the left lateral decubitus

position with a horizontal beam, using a short exposure technique. This results in underpenetration of the abdominal viscera but good visualization of extraalimentary gas between the nondependent lateral abdominal wall and the liver (Fig. 15-3). If the patient is able to stand, the table is tilted upright and an upright posteroanterior chest radiograph is obtained. In one study, lateral chest radiographs were found to be superior to frontal radiographs in detecting subtle pneumoperitoneum.[13] Radiographs of the abdomen in upright and supine positions are also obtained to complete the "perforation series" (see Fig. 15-2C and D).[14] Even tiny amounts of free air can be detected with proper technique (see Fig. 15-2E). Some authors have reported that upright posteroanterior chest radiographs are more sensitive for detecting pneumoperitoneum than are upright abdominal radiographs.[12] This difference in sensitivity probably occurs because the x-ray beam is centered at the iliac crest on abdominal radiographs, so that it penetrates air beneath the diaphragm obliquely rather than tangentially, making small gas collections more difficult to detect. The higher exposure techniques required to penetrate the abdomen also result in excessive penetration at the lung interface, sometimes obscuring small collections of free intraperitoneal air. Nevertheless, most experts believe that upright and supine abdominal radiographs are a useful part of the abdominal series for detecting intra-abdominal disease in these patients.[14,15]

Additional projections such as prone, oblique, lateral, or coned views may be helpful in some clinical situations for better defining and localizing mass lesions, calcifications, or hernias. When distal colonic obstruction is suspected, prone abdominal radiographs are more helpful than supine radiographs because colonic gas occupies the more anterior transverse and sigmoid segments of the colon with the patient in the supine position (Fig. 15-4A, C, and D). As a result, a distal colonic obstruction may be difficult to distinguish from an ileus or pseudo-obstruction on supine and upright views of the abdomen. In this situation, a prone radiograph (Fig. 15-4B) or right lateral decubitus radiograph (Fig. 15-4E) may be useful, because abdominal radiographs in these positions allow gas to fill the rectosigmoid colon if no mechanical obstruction is present.[16]

NORMAL ANATOMY

Abdominal soft tissue planes and visceral surfaces are visible on abdominal radiographs because of the natural contrast created by surrounding fat. The best visualized interfaces are those that are smoothly marginated and oriented in a sagittal or transverse plane tangential to the incident x-ray beam. Familiarity with the location of abdominal organs and the most commonly visualized tissue planes is helpful in identifying normal anatomic structures and in recognizing and localizing pathologic processes.

PERITONEAL CAVITY

Liver

In the normal adult, the liver occupies the right upper quadrant of the abdomen. It measures 20 to 22 cm in its greatest transverse dimension and 15 to 17 cm in its greatest vertical dimension near its right lateral border.[17] There is considerable

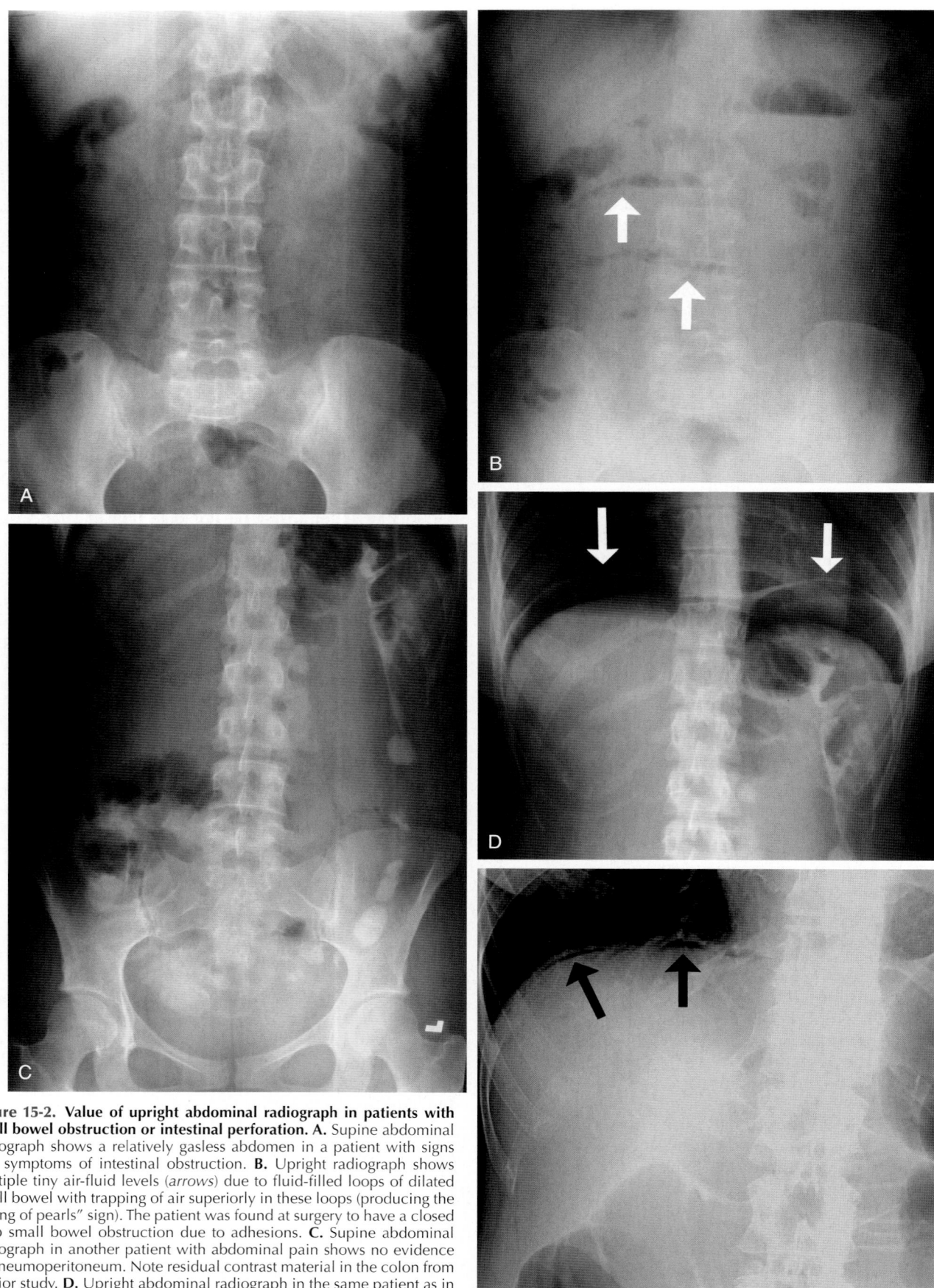

Figure 15-2. Value of upright abdominal radiograph in patients with small bowel obstruction or intestinal perforation. A. Supine abdominal radiograph shows a relatively gasless abdomen in a patient with signs and symptoms of intestinal obstruction. **B.** Upright radiograph shows multiple tiny air-fluid levels (*arrows*) due to fluid-filled loops of dilated small bowel with trapping of air superiorly in these loops (producing the "string of pearls" sign). The patient was found at surgery to have a closed loop small bowel obstruction due to adhesions. **C.** Supine abdominal radiograph in another patient with abdominal pain shows no evidence of pneumoperitoneum. Note residual contrast material in the colon from a prior study. **D.** Upright abdominal radiograph in the same patient as in **C** shows a large amount of free intraperitoneal air (*arrows*) beneath both hemidiaphragms. **E.** Upright radiograph in another patient shows a tiny amount of free air (*arrows*) between the liver and right hemidiaphragm.

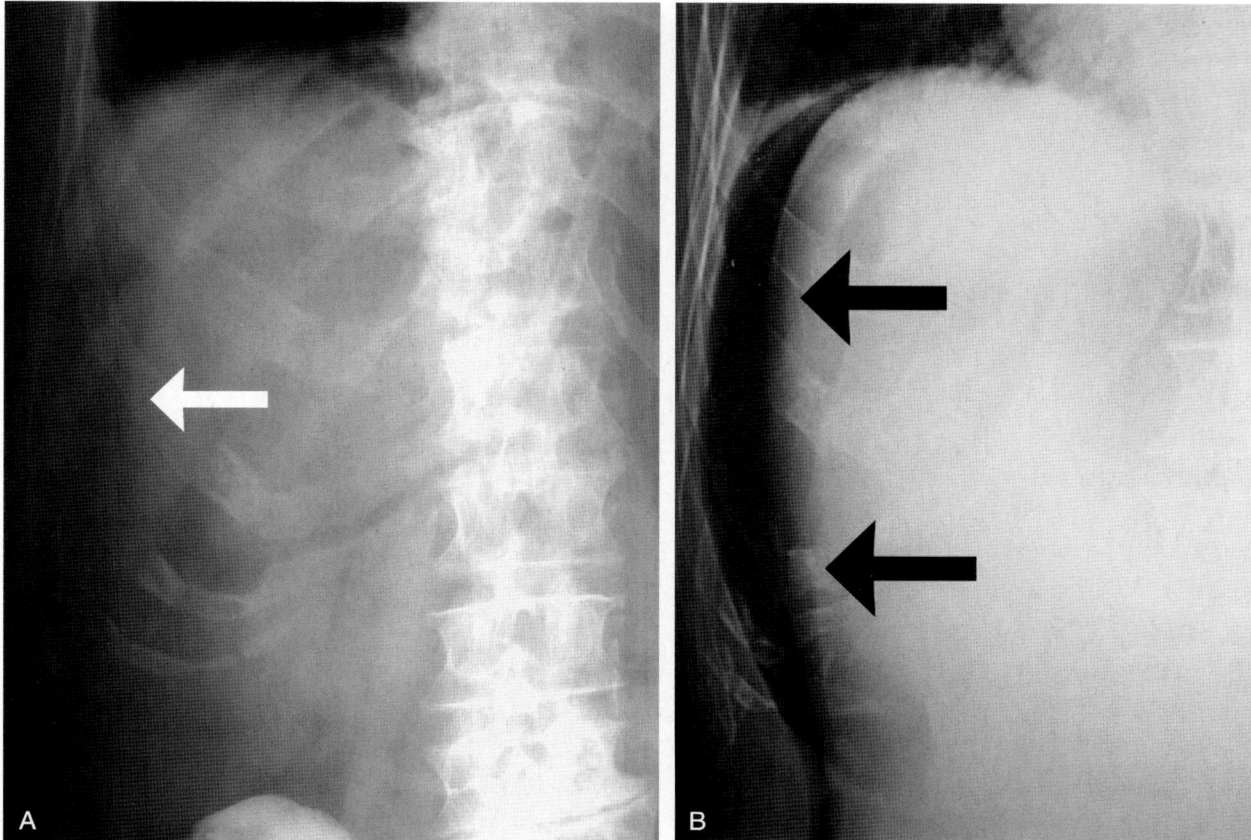

Figure 15-3. Value of left lateral decubitus radiograph of the abdomen in a patient with pneumoperitoneum. A. Coned-down view of the right upper quadrant from a supine abdominal radiograph shows a vague radiolucency in the right lateral portion of the abdomen (*arrow*) but no definite free intraperitoneal air. **B.** Coned-down view of the right upper quadrant from a left lateral decubitus radiograph shows obvious free intraperitoneal air (*arrows*) between the liver and right lateral abdominal wall.

variation in the normal shape of the liver.[18] With its most cephalad portion lying just beneath the dome of the right hemidiaphragm the superior aspect of the liver is commonly S-shaped or concave. The inferior edge is most commonly triangular, with its apex directed caudad toward the right lower quadrant. Between 4% and 14% of the population has a prominent inferior extension of the right lower lobe, the *Riedel lobe.* This lobe usually extends caudally below the iliac crest and does not by itself indicate hepatomegaly.

Although intraperitoneal fat is not always present around the liver, the right inferior edge of the liver (hepatic angle) is often visible on abdominal radiographs because it indents the extraperitoneal fat in the parietal peritoneum[18] (Fig. 15-5; see Fig. 15-1). This fat consists of posterior pararenal fat laterally and perirenal fat medially. The perirenal fat may outline not only the medial aspect of the hepatic angle but also the more cephalad portion of the posteromedial surface of the right lobe of the liver (see Fig. 15-1A). The hepatic angle may be obscured by effusions or blood that infiltrate the retroperitoneal fat or by ascites that displaces the liver edge away from the adjacent fat (Fig. 15-6).[19] The posterior edge of the liver is visible on abdominal radiographs (see Fig. 15-1), whereas the anterior and left lateral margins of the liver are not. Because it is the anterior margin of an enlarged liver that is palpated on physical examination, a discrepancy may arise between clinical and radiographic measurements of the liver.

On abdominal radiographs, hepatomegaly may be diagnosed by elevation of the right hemidiaphragm, visualization of the entire liver (not just a Riedel's lobe) extending into the lower abdomen, inferior displacement of the hepatic flexure of the colon, and lateral displacement of the lesser curvature of the stomach by an enlarged left lobe of the liver.[20]

Gallbladder

The gallbladder occupies a shallow fossa on the inferior surface of the liver between the right and left lobes and is not usually visualized on abdominal radiographs.[17] The gallbladder lies superior and lateral to the duodenal bulb and gastric antrum and superior to the proximal transverse colon. Occasionally, the fundus of the gallbladder may be visualized in normal patients if it indents the surrounding fat (Fig. 15-7; see Fig. 15-5A). Only about 15% of gallstones are sufficiently calcified to be seen on abdominal radiographs, so that the abdominal series is a poor screening study for gallbladder disease.

Spleen

The spleen occupies the left upper quadrant of the peritoneal cavity beneath the left tenth rib and hemidiaphragm postero-lateral to the gastric fundus (see Figs. 15-1B and 15-5).[21] The

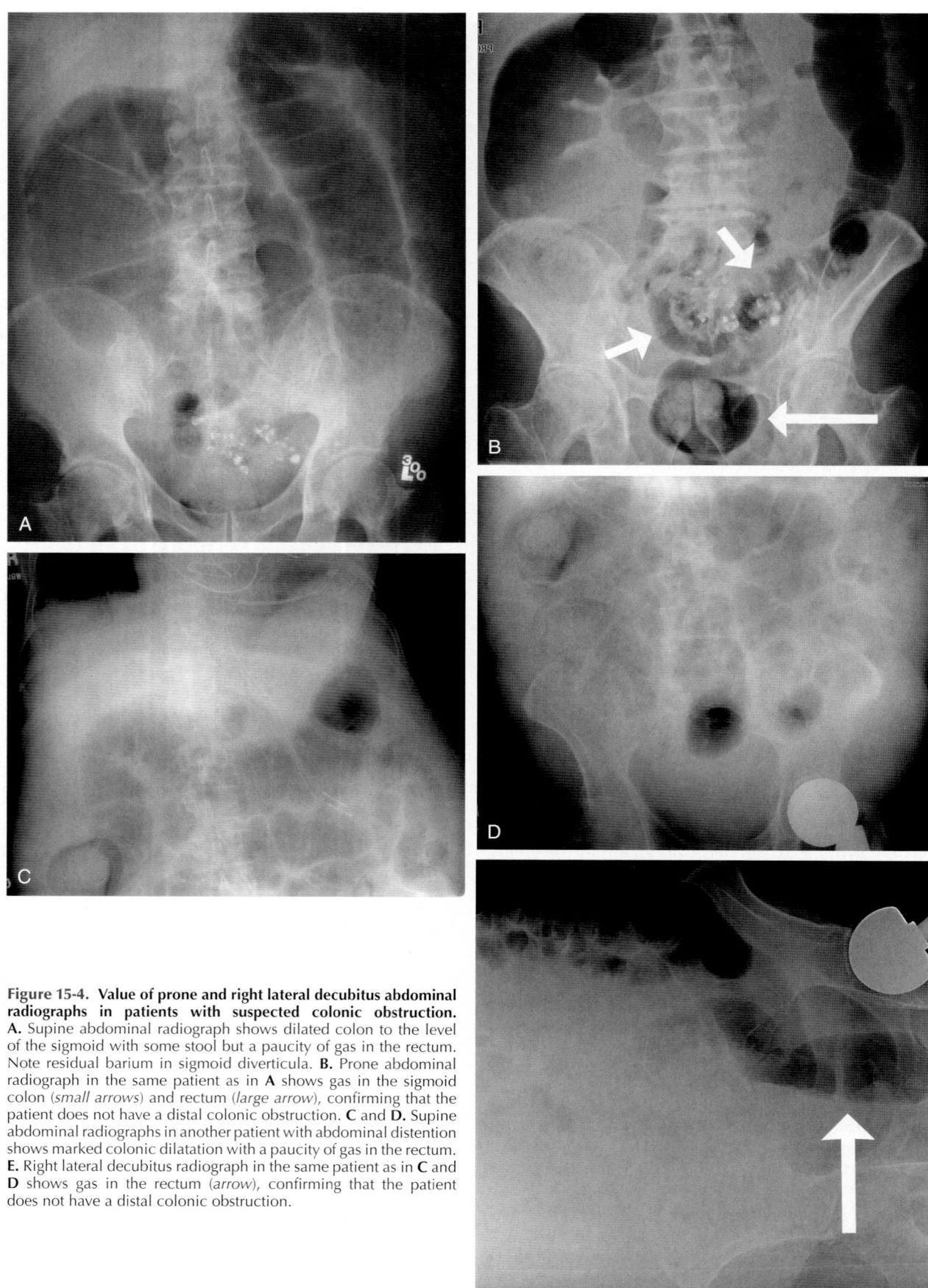

Figure 15-4. Value of prone and right lateral decubitus abdominal radiographs in patients with suspected colonic obstruction. **A.** Supine abdominal radiograph shows dilated colon to the level of the sigmoid with some stool but a paucity of gas in the rectum. Note residual barium in sigmoid diverticula. **B.** Prone abdominal radiograph in the same patient as in **A** shows gas in the sigmoid colon (*small arrows*) and rectum (*large arrow*), confirming that the patient does not have a distal colonic obstruction. **C** and **D.** Supine abdominal radiographs in another patient with abdominal distention shows marked colonic dilatation with a paucity of gas in the rectum. **E.** Right lateral decubitus radiograph in the same patient as in **C** and **D** shows gas in the rectum (*arrow*), confirming that the patient does not have a distal colonic obstruction.

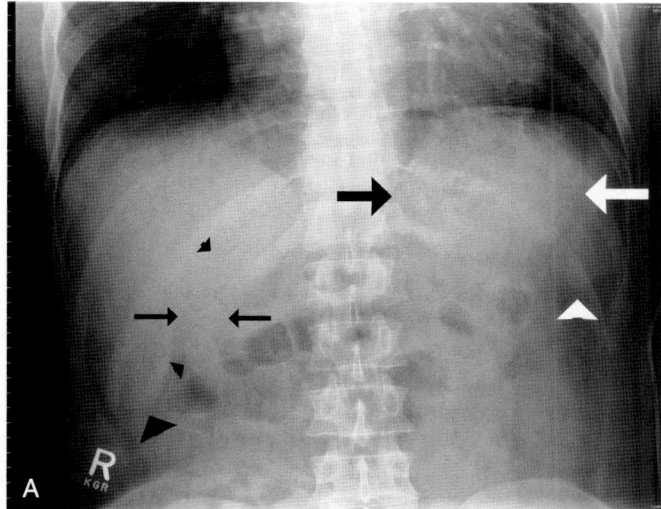

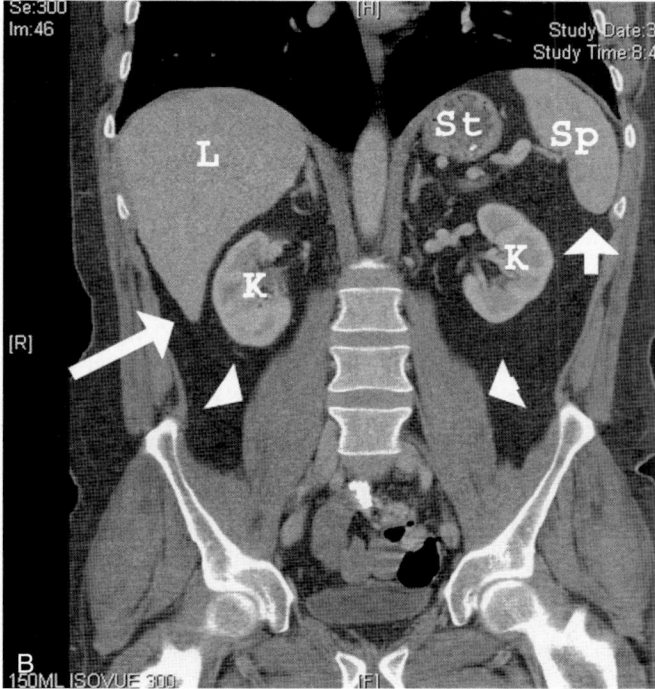

Figure 15-5. Gallbladder, liver, spleen, and stomach. A. Supine abdominal radiograph shows the gallbladder (*small black arrows*), hepatic angle (*large black arrowhead*), splenic tip (*white arrowhead*), and stomach (*large black and white arrows*). Note the partially visualized right kidney (*small black arrowheads*). **B.** Coronal CT of the abdomen shows the hepatic angle (*large arrow*) outlined by perirenal fat, splenic tip (*small arrow*), psoas muscles (*arrowheads*), and kidneys. L, liver; St, stomach; Sp, spleen; K, kidney.

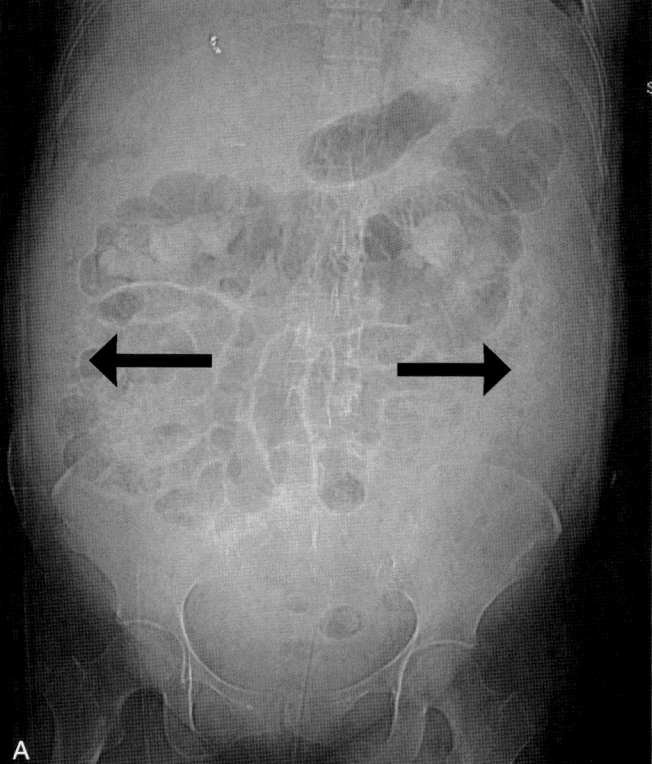

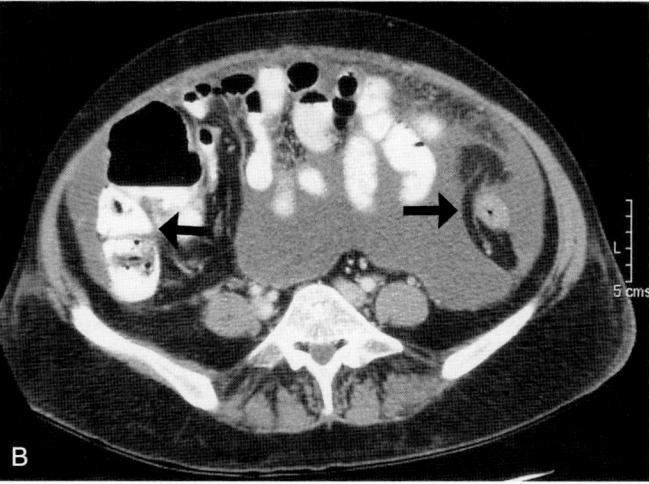

Figure 15-6. Intraperitoneal fluid (hemorrhage) in paracolic gutters. A. Supine abdominal radiograph in a patient with a traumatic liver laceration shows a large amount of fluid in both paracolic gutters (*arrows*) displacing bowel medially from the flank stripes. Also note loss of the hepatic angle normally outlined by extraperitoneal fat. The bleeding was controlled by embolization of the liver (note radiopaque coil overlying liver). **B.** Axial CT of the abdomen confirms the presence of ascitic fluid displacing adjacent bowel (*arrows*) from the paracolic gutters.

normal adult spleen measures 12 cm in length and 7 cm in width.[20] The lower edge of its inferolateral surface often indents extraperitoneal fat, and the lower medial aspect is adjacent to the left kidney and may be outlined by perirenal fat, enabling it to be visualized on abdominal radiographs (see Figs. 15-1B and C and 15-5). The bulk of the spleen, however, extends medially behind the stomach, where it is not visible on abdominal radiographs, so that splenomegaly cannot always be diagnosed on these radiographs. Nevertheless,

an enlarged spleen should be suspected when abdominal radiographs show elevation of the left hemidiaphragm, medial displacement of the gastric air bubble, or the splenic tip below the left costal margin.[20]

The most inferior surface of the spleen abuts the phrenicocolic ligament, a thick peritoneal fold that marks the anatomic splenic flexure of the colon. The left lateral pleural

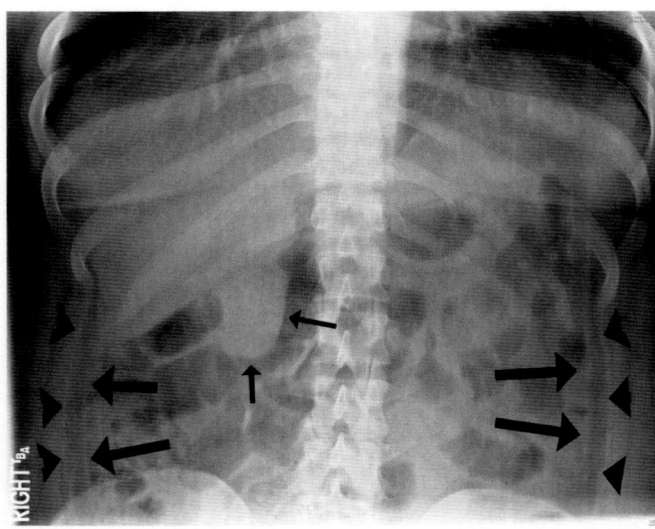

Figure 15-7. Paracolic gutters and lateral conal fascia. Coned-down view from supine abdominal radiograph shows the left and right paracolic gutters between the transversalis fascia (*arrowheads*) and the lateral conal fascia (*large arrows*). *Small arrows* denote the gallbladder.

recess may extend inferiorly along the lateral margin of the spleen to the splenic tip.[21]

Stomach

The stomach usually contains air and fluid, so that it can be recognized in the left upper quadrant by its characteristic location and by the configuration of its rugal folds (see Fig. 15-1A). When the patient is in the supine position, gas in the stomach rises to the anteriorly located antrum while fluid gravitates to the fundus. When the fluid-filled fundus is visible on abdominal radiographs, it can occasionally be mistaken for a soft tissue mass (see Fig. 15-5A). However, confusion may be eliminated by the use of upright radiographs, which allow gas to enter the gastric fundus (see Fig. 15-1B). The stomach is a valuable landmark for identifying space-occupying lesions in surrounding structures such as the spleen laterally, the liver medially, and the lesser sac and pancreas posteriorly (see Figs. 15-1B and C and 15-5).[17]

Small Intestine

The small bowel and its associated mesentery occupy the central portion of the peritoneal cavity.[17] Although transit time through the small bowel is sufficiently rapid to prevent swallowed air from accumulating in normal small bowel loops, these loops may be visible on abdominal radiographs when they contain small amounts of gas (see Fig. 15-1A). In contrast, large amounts of air and fluid in dilated small bowel indicate prolonged transit time due to mechanical obstruction or an adynamic ileus. Scattered gas and fluid within normal to minimally dilated small bowel loops may occur in a variety of normal or pathologic conditions, including gastroenteritis, pancreatitis, inflammatory bowel disease, and aerophagia. Unfortunately, considerable interobserver variation occurs in interpretation of small bowel gas. The term *nonspecific gas pattern* has been used to describe abdominal radiographs showing more than the average amount of small bowel gas

without a clear indication of bowel obstruction. However, this term is vague or even misleading and is not helpful to the referring physician and therefore should not be used. Instead, radiologists should provide a clear description of the radiographic findings and the most reasonable diagnostic considerations. The gas-filled small bowel is distinguished from the colon by its more central location, smaller caliber, and typical mucosal folds, the valvulae conniventes (see Fig. 15-1A). When visualized, the small bowel folds are usually thin and extend across the entire lumen of the bowel.

Colon

The adult colon usually contains some gas and fecal material and frames the abdomen, with the small bowel located more centrally. The more anterior transverse and sigmoid segments usually contain the greatest amount of gas when the patient is in the supine position. Unlike the valvulae conniventes of the small bowel, the colonic haustral folds are more widely spaced and usually do not cross the entire lumen[17] (see Fig. 15-1A). The caliber of the colon varies from 3 to 8 cm, with the largest diameter found in the cecum. Persistent cecal diameters of 9 to 10 cm or greater may indicate a risk of impending perforation from mechanical obstruction or ileus.[22]

The sigmoid and transverse colon are intraperitoneal structures that are suspended by the sigmoid mesentery and transverse mesocolon, respectively. Conversely, the ascending and descending colon and rectum are retroperitoneal structures, fixed to the posterior abdominal wall. In about 20% of the population, the cecum and a variable portion of the ascending colon have a persistent mesentery.[23] In such cases the cecum is mobile and its position is more anterior and medial than usual. Although most of these patients are asymptomatic, this anatomic variation predisposes to an ileus, cecal bascule, and cecal volvulus.[24] The sigmoid colon is an intraperitoneal structure, but sigmoid diverticula are frequently oriented toward the sigmoid mesentery, so that rupture of a diverticulum (with subsequent diverticulitis) usually results in the development of retroperitoneal gas rather than free intraperitoneal air.[23]

On upright abdominal radiographs, air-fluid levels in the bowel can be interpreted as a sign of bowel obstruction. However, air-fluid levels in both the small bowel and colon may occur in nonobstructive conditions and also in normal patients. Air-fluid levels are particularly common in the right side of the colon after cathartic preparation.[25]

Potential Intraperitoneal Spaces

The peritoneal reflections from the posterior abdominal wall over the viscera give rise to potential spaces in which blood, fluid, or pus may localize in the peritoneal cavity.[17] In the normal abdomen, these compartments are not directly visible on abdominal radiographs but their location can be inferred from the location of adjacent organs. The right subphrenic space is located between the right hemidiaphragm and the liver. It is above the superior reflection of the right coronary ligament and continuous around the lateral edge of the liver with the right subhepatic space. The anterior subhepatic space lies just above the transverse colon and mesocolon and anterior to the right kidney and duodenum. The posterior subhepatic space, *Morison's pouch*, continues posteriorly and superiorly to the inferior reflection of the coronary ligament. On abdominal radiographs, Morison's pouch overlies the superior pole of the right kidney.[17] This is the most dependent portion of the upper peritoneal cavity with the patient in the supine position, and it is a frequent site of abscess formation. The subhepatic space is continuous with the right paracolic gutter between the ascending colon and the properitoneal fat. The right paracolic gutter is deeper and wider than the left paracolic gutter. Fluid and abscesses are often visible here and can be recognized on abdominal radiographs by separation of the ascending and descending colon from the properitoneal fat (see Fig. 15-6). The left subphrenic space is separated from the right subphrenic space by the falciform ligament, which is a right midclavicular line structure in most patients. This space surrounds the left lobe of the liver and spleen and is limited inferiorly by the phrenicocolic ligament. Below the phrenicocolic ligament, the shallow left paracolic gutter extends inferiorly into the portion of the pelvis lateral to the descending colon (see Fig. 15-7).

The lesser sac of the peritoneal cavity is a potential space in the midabdomen, extending into the left upper quadrant. It is bounded superiorly by the left coronary ligament; posteriorly by the pancreas; anteriorly by the stomach, lesser omentum, and gastrocolic ligament; and inferiorly by the transverse colon and mesocolon[17] (Fig. 15-8). Its left lateral borders are formed by the gastrosplenic and splenorenal ligaments. The lesser sac opens into the right subhepatic space via the foramen of Winslow at a site just posterior and superior to the duodenal bulb, beneath the free margin of the hepatoduodenal ligament. Dodds and associates described the lesser sac as an area defined by placing the right hand over the epigastrium with the thumb extended over the midline toward the hilus of the liver and the fingers directed toward the hilum of the spleen.[26] The thumb represents the extension of the superior medial recess and the palm and fingers the main portion of

the lesser sac. Space-occupying lesions or fluid collections in the lesser sac may displace the transverse colon inferiorly and the stomach superiorly, anteriorly, laterally, or medially (see Fig. 15-8).

RETROPERITONEUM AND ABDOMINAL WALL

The anatomy of the retroperitoneal space has been well described by Meyers.[23] It is posterior to the parietal peritoneum and anterior to the transversalis fascia. The retroperitoneal space is divided into three distinct compartments: the perirenal space, the posterior pararenal space, and the anterior pararenal space.

Perirenal Space: Kidneys and Adrenal Glands

The kidneys, adrenal glands, and abundant fat are located within the left and right perirenal spaces, which are confined by the anterior and posterior layers of renal fascia. It is the perirenal fat that allows visualization of some or all the renal outlines on abdominal radiographs in most patients (see Fig. 15-5). On the other hand, the adrenal glands are small and not discernible unless they are calcified as a result of previous hemorrhage or granulomatous disease (Fig. 15-9). The upper half of the psoas muscle and the medial aspects of the hepatic and splenic angles are visualized on abdominal radiographs due to perirenal fat. Obliteration of the perirenal fat by inflammation, blood, or urine therefore obscures visualization of these structures. The medial perirenal space is continuous with the aorta and often fills with blood in patients with ruptured abdominal aortic aneurysms.[27] The anterior and posterior layers of perirenal fascia fuse laterally to form the lateroconal fascia, which continues laterally and ventrally to fuse with the parietal peritoneum along the lateral abdominal

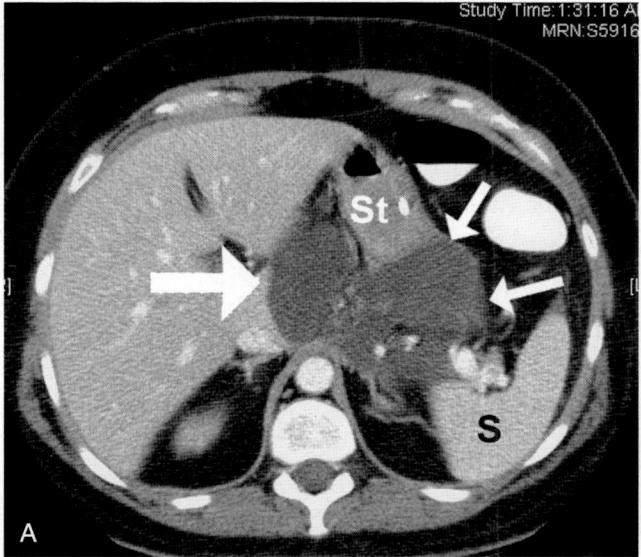
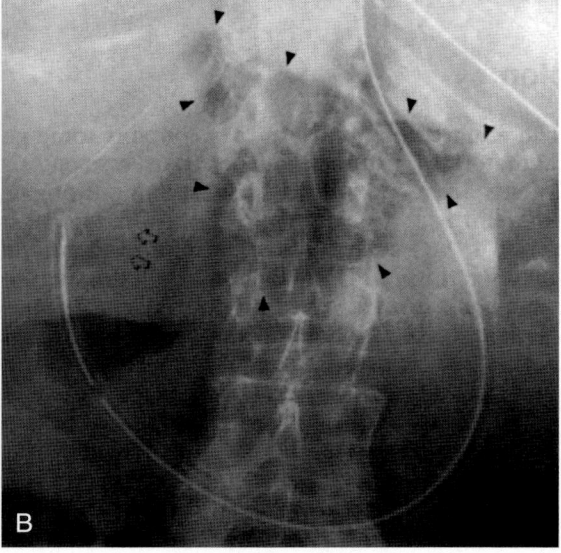

Figure 15-8. Lesser peritoneal sac. A. Axial CT of the abdomen in a patient with acute pancreatitis shows fluid posterior to the stomach in the lesser sac, extending into the superior medial recess (*large white arrow*). The fluid is contained on the left by the gastrosplenic ligament (*small arrows*). S, spleen. **B.** The boundaries of the lesser sac (*arrowheads*) are well delineated on a supine abdominal radiograph in another patient with gas in the lesser sac due to an abscess. The superior recess of the lesser sac extends toward the diaphragm just to the right of the spine. The foramen of Winslow is denoted by *open arrows*. A nasogastric tube is present in the stomach. (Courtesy of Susan M. Williams, MD, Omaha, NE.)

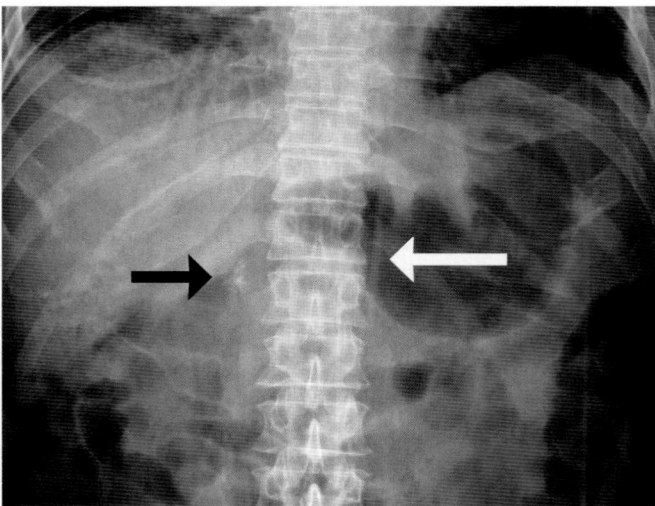

Figure 15-9. Diaphragmatic crus and calcified adrenal gland. Supine abdominal radiograph shows a calcified right adrenal gland (*black arrow*) and left diaphragmatic crus (*white arrow*). The right diaphragmatic crus is partially visualized just medial to the calcified right adrenal gland.

wall. In patients with abundant fat, the lateroconal fascia may be visible on abdominal radiographs as a thin line separating the posterior pararenal and anterior pararenal fat (Fig. 15-10).[28]

Posterior Pararenal Space

The posterior pararenal space is located posterior to the posterior perirenal and lateroconal fascia and it is anterior to the transversalis fascia lining the abdominal wall (see Figs. 15-7 and 15-10).[17] This space contains a variable amount of fat but no organs. Medially, the posterior pararenal space originates at the lateral margin of the psoas muscle and is not continuous across the midline. Laterally, the posterior pararenal fat extends around the flank, joining the properitoneal fat of the lateral abdominal wall to form the "flank stripe" (Fig. 15-11). The width of the flank stripe is variable and depends on body habitus. The posterior pararenal fat is continuous inferiorly with extraperitoneal fat in the pelvis.

Anterior Pararenal Space: Ascending and Descending Colon, Duodenum, and Pancreas

The anterior pararenal space, which lies anterior to the perirenal space and lateroconal fascia, contains the ascending and descending colon, retroperitoneal duodenum, and pancreas (see Fig. 15-10).[17] In most patients, the ascending and descending colon can be identified by intraluminal fecal material and gas medial to the flank stripes (see Fig. 15-1). Semisolid fecal material in the cecum and ascending colon often has a characteristic bubbly appearance. The retroperitoneal duodenum is usually not visible on abdominal radiographs unless it is filled with gas as a result of an ileus, proximal small bowel obstruction, or pancreatitis. The pancreas also is not visualized on abdominal radiographs because it has undulating, lobulated borders that are not outlined by fat. The normal location of the pancreas may be recognized on abdominal radiographs, however, if there is pancreatic calcification due to chronic pancreatitis (Fig. 15-12).

Psoas Muscle

The psoas muscle arises from the T12-L5 vertebrae and extends inferiorly to join the iliac muscle below the iliac crest. It continues as the iliopsoas muscle to the lesser trochanter.[17]

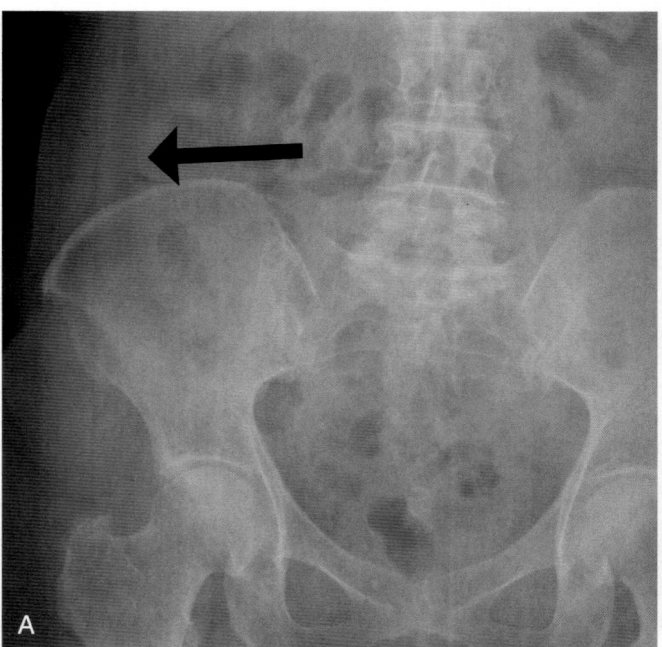
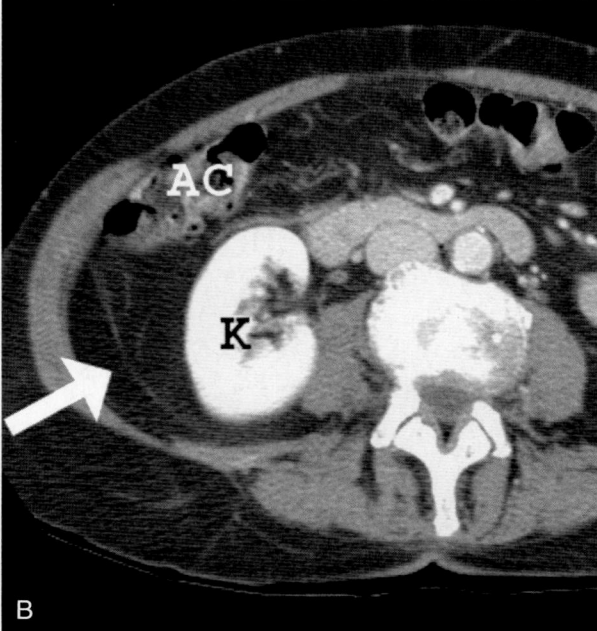

Figure 15-10. Lateroconal fascia. A. Supine abdominal radiograph shows the lateroconal fascia (*arrow*) along the paracolic gutter as a thin, white line extending from the liver tip to the right lower quadrant. **B.** Axial CT scan shows the lateroconal fascia (*arrow*), which is composed of the anterior and posterior layers of the perirenal fascia that fuse laterally. The ascending colon (AC) is contained within the anterior pararenal space. K, kidney.

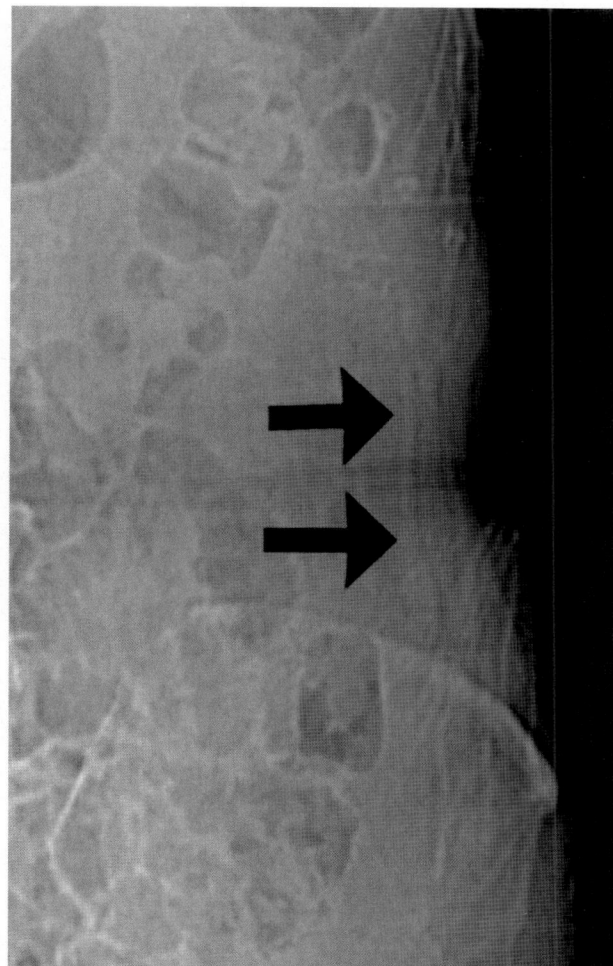

Figure 15-11. Flank stripe. Supine coned-down view of the left side of the abdomen shows the flank stripe (*arrows*) outlined by properitoneal fat just lateral to the descending colon. This fat is contiguous with the retroperitoneal fat in the posterior pararenal space. When there is no fluid in the left paracolic gutter, it is only a few millimeters in width.

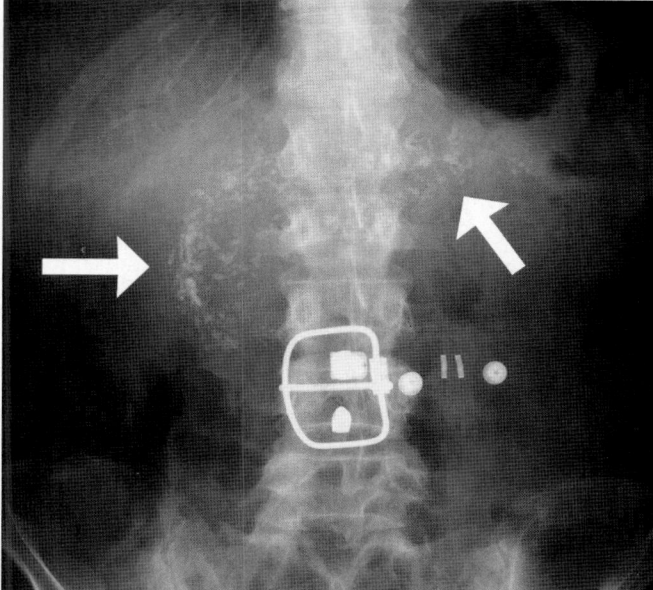

Figure 15-12. Pancreatic calcification. Supine abdominal radiograph shows multiple calcifications outlining the pancreas (*arrows*) due to chronic pancreatitis. The pancreas normally is not visible on abdominal radiographs.

tural scoliosis but also in those with a positional scoliosis, when muscle spasm causes contraction of the muscles in the flank. When there is a limited amount of retroperitoneal fat, the peritoneal cavity extends posteriorly, so that fluid-filled bowel loops may come to lie directly adjacent to the psoas muscle, obscuring its margin. Occasionally, the kidney may also cause segmental nonvisualization of the psoas muscle, particularly in patients with an enlarged spleen that displaces

Perirenal fat superiorly and posterior pararenal fat below the level of the kidneys outline the lateral margin of the psoas muscle. In about 75% of patients, the psoas muscle is seen to extend from the diaphragmatic crura to its junction with the iliac muscle (Fig. 15-13; see Fig. 15-1A and B).[29,30] Fluid in the adjacent retroperitoneal fat may cause obliteration of the margin of the psoas muscle. Loss of one or both shadows of the psoas muscle is a common finding on abdominal radiographs when there is a ruptured abdominal aortic aneurysm, with blood infiltrating the perirenal and posterior pararenal spaces.

The psoas muscle is optimally visualized when its lateral margin is straight and nearly parallel to the x-ray beam. Nonvisualization of the psoas margin on abdominal radiographs must be interpreted with caution. A lumbar scoliosis may result in nonvisualization of the psoas shadow.[30] Rotation of the spinal column causes the psoas muscle on the concave side of the spine to assume a more flattened, horizontal configuration. The margin is then more perpendicular to the incident x-ray, so that it may not be visible on abdominal radiographs. This phenomenon occurs not only in patients with a struc-

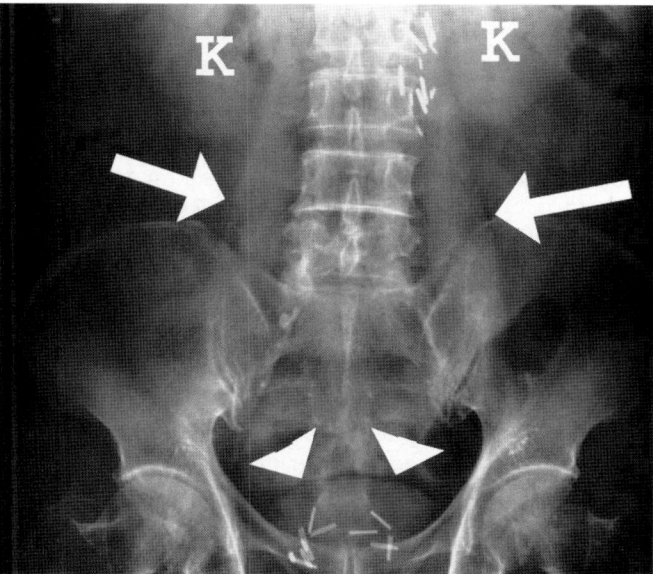

Figure 15-13. Psoas muscles. Supine abdominal radiograph shows both psoas muscles (*arrows*). The lateral margins of the psoas muscle extend inferiorly from the diaphragmatic crura to just below the iliac crest. The medial margins of the psoas muscles are also demonstrated. Note perivesical fat over the dome of the bladder (*arrowheads*). K, kidney.

the kidney medially.[30] Thus, retroperitoneal or intraperitoneal disease, scoliosis, or even normal variation can obscure the psoas margin.

Quadratus Lumborum Muscle

Lateral and parallel to the psoas muscle is the lateral margin of the quadratus lumborum muscle, often seen to extend to its origin at the iliac crest. The quadratus lumborum muscle is part of the posterior abdominal wall and lies dorsal to the transversalis fascia, which passes between it and the psoas muscle.[17] However, visualization of the quadratus lumborum muscle depends on the integrity of the posterior pararenal fat, which outlines its lateral margin.

Diaphragmatic Crura

The diaphragmatic crura may outline retroperitoneal fat that is continuous with the origin of the psoas muscle (see Fig. 15-9). The crura are best seen on abdominal radiographs when the x-ray beam is centered near the level of the diaphragm.[31] Occasionally, posterior pararenal fat continues superiorly beneath the diaphragm, simulating pneumoperitoneum. In such cases, a left lateral decubitus view should differentiate pneumoperitoneum from pararenal fat, because the lucency associated with fat is not affected by changes in patient position.

PELVIS

Delineation of the various muscles and visceral structures in the pelvis is highly variable and depends on a variety of factors, including the amount of extraperitoneal pelvic fat, bowel contents, the degree of bladder distention, the position of the patient, and body habitus. As a result, these structures are not always identified even in the absence of pelvic disease.

Piriformis Muscle

The piriformis muscle is in the superolateral posterior aspect of the pelvis.[17] Its inferior margin can be visualized as a smooth, convex interface passing from the sacrum to the greater sciatic foramen (Fig. 15-14). Just caudal to the piriformis muscle, the sciatic nerve passes out of the pelvis. Internal hernias can extend through the greater sciatic foramen into the buttocks; these hernias may contain bowel, bladder, or ureter.

Obturator Internus Muscle

The obturator internus muscle abuts the lateral pelvic sidewall and surrounds the greater portion of the obturator foramen.[17] It originates from the pubic ramus, ischium, and pelvic wall, and its tendon exits the pelvis at the lesser sciatic foramen just below the sacrospinous ligament. The obturator internus muscle may be identified on abdominal radiographs as a result of subperitoneal fat that surrounds it superiorly and ischiorectal fat that surrounds it inferiorly below the origin of the levator ani muscle (Fig. 15-15). The obturator canal is located at the superolateral aspect of the obturator foramen; this canal transmits the obturator vessels and nerve.[32] Hernias may occur at this site, particularly in elderly women (Fig. 15-16).

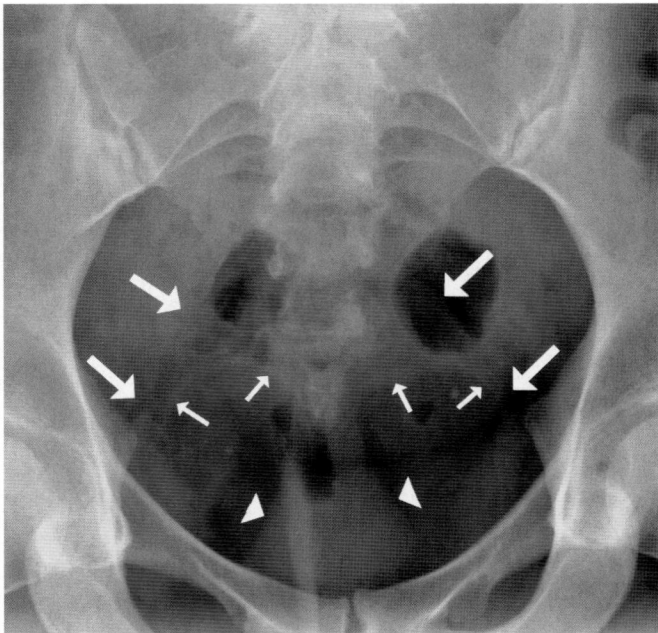

Figure 15-14. Piriformis muscle. Coned-down view of the pelvis from a supine abdominal radiograph shows the inferior margins of the piriformis muscles bilaterally (*large arrows*). Inferior to the piriformis muscles is the edge of the sacrospinous ligament and associated coccygeus muscles (*small arrows*) outlining the roof of the ischiorectal fossa. The perineum forms the medial boundary of the ischiorectal fossa (*arrowheads*).

These hernias often produce characteristic neuralgia in the thigh secondary to nerve compression.[32-34]

Sacrospinous Ligament and Coccygeus Muscle

The edge of the sacrospinous ligament and associated coccygeus muscle are outlined by underlying ischiorectal fat.[17] These structures are located just inferior to the piriformis muscle and may be seen as a smooth band arching from the tip of the sacrum to the ischial spine (see Fig. 15-14).

Ischiorectal Fossa

The left and right ischiorectal fossae are wedge-shaped subcutaneous fatty masses, with their bases at the perineum and their apices at the junction of the obturator internus and levator ani muscles.[17] They are often visible on abdominal radiographs (see Fig. 15-14).

Gluteus Maximus Muscle

The gluteus maximus muscle forms the posterior border of the ischiorectal fossa.[17] The medial edge of this muscle is outlined by subcutaneous fat, so that it often appears on abdominal radiographs as a smooth line extending inferiorly and laterally from the tip of the sacrum.

Pelvic Viscera

The superior and lateral aspects of the urinary bladder are outlined by perivesical fat (Fig. 15-17; see Fig. 15-13). The uterus may also be visible in the pelvis just above this fat,

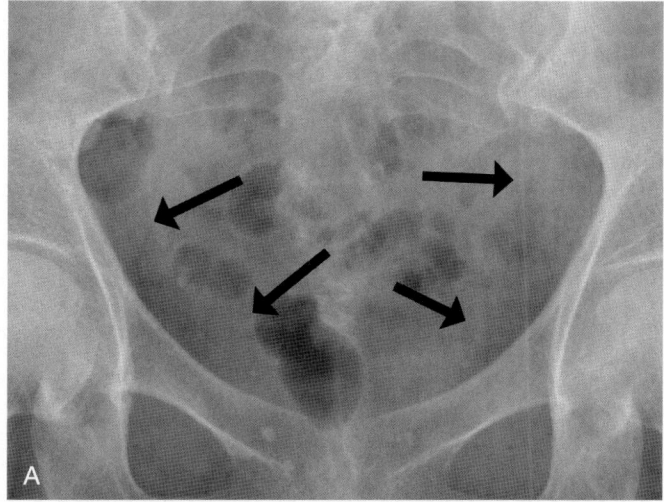

Figure 15-15. Obturator internus muscles. A. Coned-down view of the pelvis from a supine abdominal radiograph shows the obturator internus muscles (*arrows*). **B.** Axial CT of the pelvis shows the superior portion of the obturator internus muscles (*arrows*) outlined by extra-peritoneal fat. **C.** Axial CT more caudad shows the obturator internus muscles (*white arrows*) outlined by ischiorectal fat. The left and right ischiorectal fossae are bounded by the levator ani muscles (*black arrows*) and obturator internus muscles.

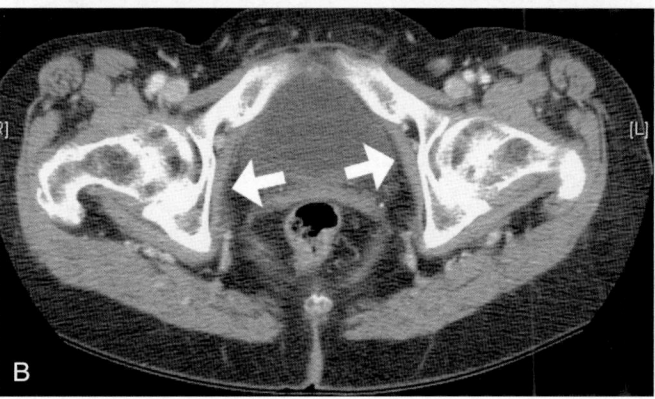
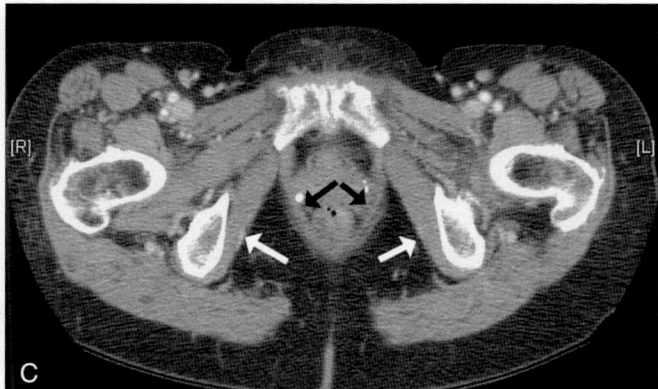

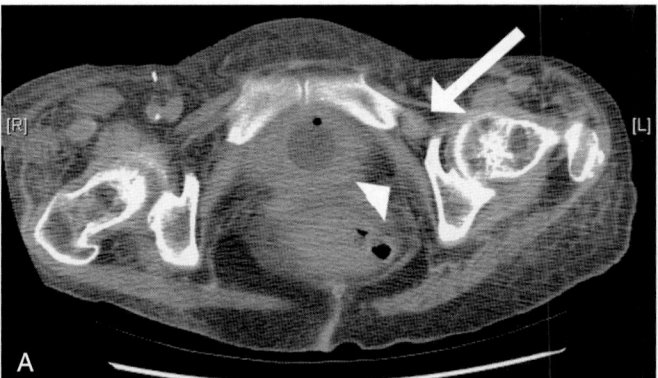
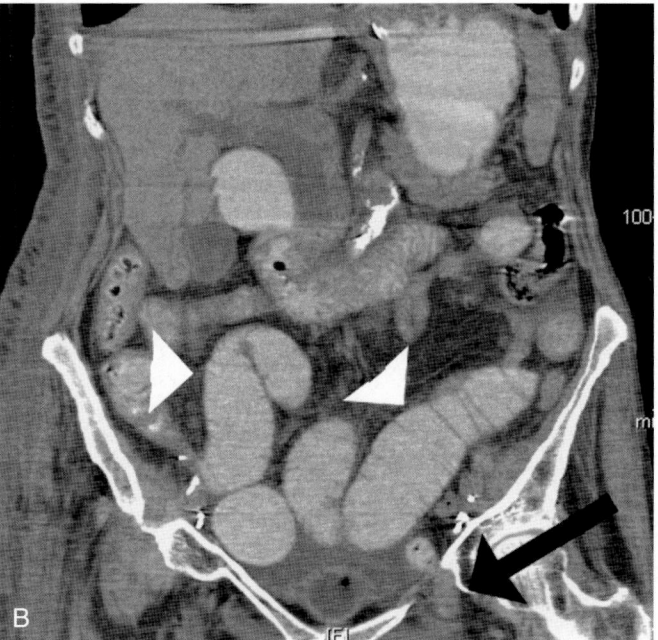

Figure 15-16. Obturator hernia causing small bowel obstruction. A. Axial CT of the pelvis in an elderly woman shows a left obturator hernia (*arrow*). Also note the left obturator internus muscle (*arrowhead*). **B.** Coronal CT of the pelvis shows the left obturator hernia (*arrow*) with dilated small bowel (*arrowheads*) proximal to the obstructing hernia.

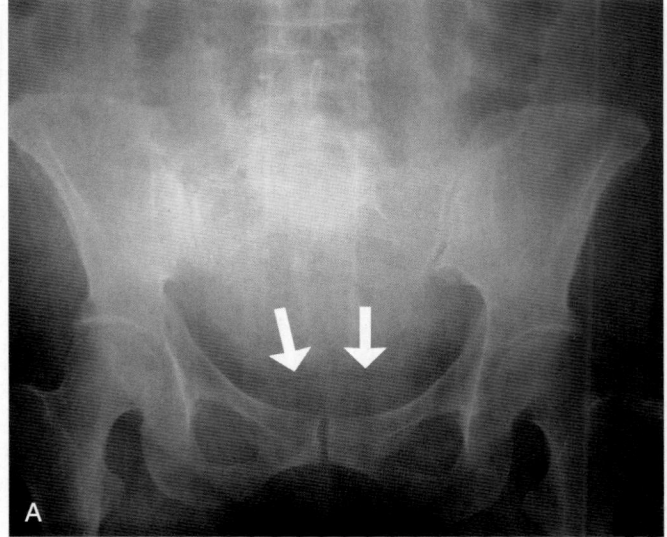

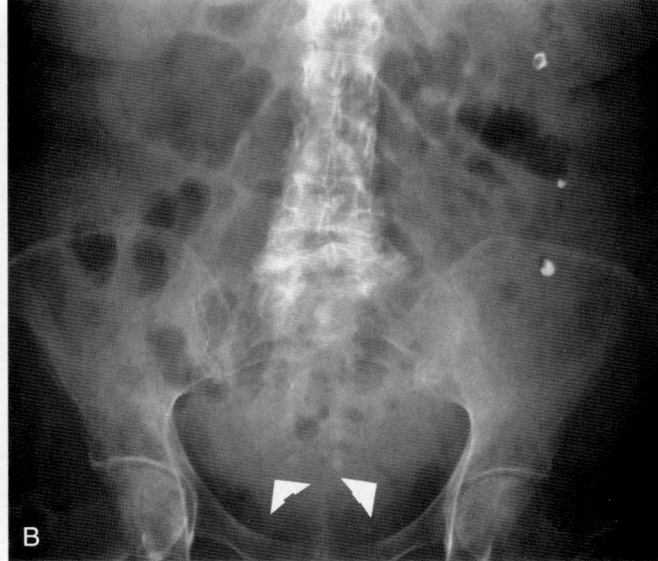

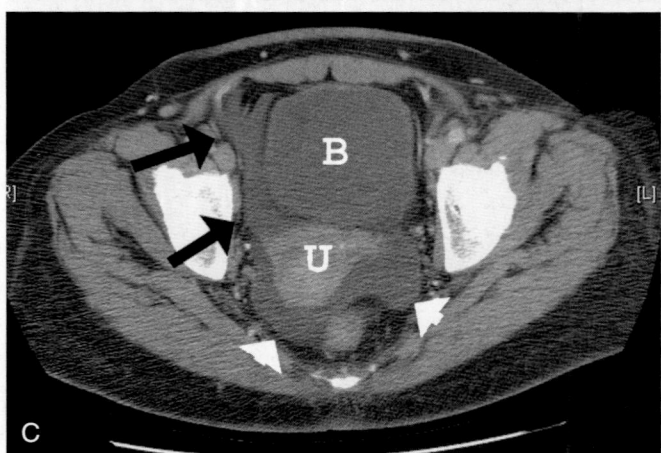

Figure 15-17. Ascites demarcated by perivesical fat. A. Coned-down view of pelvis from a supine abdominal radiograph shows evidence of ascites with increased density above the perivesical fat (*arrows*). Also note how the small bowel is displaced medially by ascitic fluid in the abdomen. **B.** Increased density is again seen in the paravesical spaces above the bladder on a supine abdominal radiograph in another patient with ascites. Note how the top of the bladder is outlined by perivesical fat (*arrowheads*). **C.** Axial CT of the pelvis in the same patient as in **B** confirms the presence of ascites (*black arrows*) around the bladder (B). Also note fluid (*arrowheads*) behind the bladder, surrounding the uterus (U).

particularly if the fundus is anteverted and indents the adjacent fat. This perivesical fat can be used to help identify fluid in the pelvis (see Fig. 15-17). Prostatic calculi will identify the position of the prostate gland, which is caudal to the urinary bladder and usually not seen on abdominal radiographs. Posterior to the bladder and uterus, the rectum can usually be recognized by the presence of intraluminal gas and stool (see Fig. 15-1).

Acknowledgment

The author would like to acknowledge and thank Susan M. Williams, MD, for being able to use parts of her excellent chapter 10 from the previous edition of this textbook.

References

1. Rosen MP, Sands DZ, Longmaid HE III, et al: Impact of abdominal CT on the management of patients presenting to the emergency department with acute abdominal pain. AJR 174:1391-1396, 2000.
2. Ahn SH, Mayo-Smith WW, Murphy BL, et al: Acute nontraumatic abdominal pain in adult patients: Abdominal radiography compared with CT evaluation. Radiology 225:159-164, 2002.
3. MacKersie AB, Lane MJ, Gerhardt RT, et al: Nontraumatic acute abdominal pain: Unenhanced helical CT compared with three-view acute abdominal series. Radiology 237:114-122, 2005.
4. Brewer RJ, Golden GT, Hitch DC, et al: Abdominal pain: An analysis of 1000 consecutive cases in a university hospital emergency room. Am Surg 131:219-224, 1976.
5. Eisenberg RL, Heineken P, Hedgcock MW, et al: Evaluation of plain abdominal radiographs in the diagnosis of abdominal pain. Ann Surg 197:464-469, 1983.
6. Mirvis SE, Young JWR, Keramati B, et al: Plain film evaluation of patients with abdominal pain: Are three radiographs necessary? AJR 147:501-503, 1986.
7. Eisenberg RL, Hedgcock MW: Preliminary radiograph for barium enema examination: Is it necessary? AJR 136:115-116, 1981.
8. Harned RK, Wolf GL, Williams SM: Preliminary abdominal films for gastrointestinal examinations: How efficacious? Gastrointest Radiol 5:343-347, 1980.
9. Schwab FJ, Glick SN, Teplick SK, et al: The barium enema scout film: Cost effectiveness and clinical efficacy. Radiology 160:619-622, 1986.
10. Ballinger PW: Merrill's Atlas of Radiographic Positions and Radiologic Procedures, vol 2, 9th ed. St. Louis, CV Mosby, 1999.
11. Curry TS, Dowdey JE, Murry RC: Christensen's Physics of Diagnostic Radiology, 4th ed. Philadelphia, Lea & Febiger, 1990.
12. Miller RE, Nelson SW: The roentgenologic demonstration of tiny amounts of free intraperitoneal gas: Experimental and clinical studies. AJR 112:574-585, 1971.
13. Woodring JH, Heiser J: Detection of pneumoperitoneum on chest radiographs: Comparison of upright lateral and posteroanterior projections. AJR 165:45-49, 1995.

14. Baker SR: Imaging pneumoperitoneum. Abdom Imaging 21:413-416, 1996.

15. Lappas JC, Reyes BL, Maglinte DD: Abdominal radiography findings in small-bowel obstruction: Relevance to triage for additional diagnostic imaging. AJR 176:167-174, 2001.

16. Laufer I: The left lateral view in the plain film assessment of abdominal distention. Radiology 119:265-269, 1976.

17. Gray H, Bannister LH (eds): Gray's Anatomy of the Human Body, 39th ed. St. Louis, Mosby, 2004.

18. Mould RF: An investigation of the variations in normal liver shape. Br J Radiol 45:586-590, 1972.

19. Bundrick TJ, Cho SR, Brewer WH: Ascites: Comparison of plain film radiographs with ultrasonograms. Radiology 152:503-506, 1984.

20. Riemenschneider PA, Whalen JP: The relative accuracy of estimation of enlargement of the liver and spleen by radiologic and clinical methods. AJR 94:462-468, 1965.

21. Dodds WJ, Taylor AJ, Erickson SJ, et al: Radiologic imaging of splenic anomalies. AJR 155:805-810, 1990.

22. Johnson CD, Rice RP, Kelvin FM, et al: The radiologic evaluation of gross cecal distension: Emphasis on cecal ileus. AJR 145:1211-1217, 1985.

23. Meyers MA: Dynamic Radiology of the Abdomen, 4th ed. New York, Springer-Verlag, 1994.

24. Weinstein M: Volvulus of the cecum and ascending colon. Am Surg 107:248-259, 1938.

25. Gammill SL, Nice CM: Air fluid levels: Their occurrence in normal patients and their role in the analysis of ileus. Surgery 71:771-780, 1972.

26. Dodds WJ, Foley WD, Lawson TL: Anatomy and imaging of the lesser peritoneal sac. AJR 144:567-575, 1985.

27. Loughran CF: A review of the plain abdominal radiograph in acute rupture of abdominal aortic aneurysms. Clin Radiol 37:383-387, 1986.

28 Whalen JP, Berne AS, Riemenschneider PA: The extraperitoneal perivisceral fat pad. Radiology 92:466-480, 1969.

29. Elkin M, Cohen G: Diagnostic value of the psoas shadow. Clin Radiol 13:210-217, 1962.

30. Williams SM, Harned RK, Hultman SA, et al: The psoas sign: A reevaluation. RadioGraphics 5:525-536, 1985.

31. Boyd DP: The anatomy and pathology of the subsplenic spaces. Surg Clin North Am 38:619-626, 1988.

32. Wechsler RJ, Kurtz AB, Needleman L, et al: Cross-sectional imaging of abdominal wall hernias. AJR 153:517-521, 1989.

33. Glicklich M, Eliasoph J: Incarcerated obturator hernia: Case diagnosed at barium enema fluoroscopy. Radiology 172:51-52, 1989.

34. Baker SR, Cho KC: The Abdominal Plain Film with Correlative Imaging, 2nd ed. Norwalk, CT, Appleton & Lange, 1999.

Gas and Soft Tissue Abnormalities

James M. Messmer, MD, MEd

The plain abdominal radiograph is one of the most commonly ordered radiographs in radiologic practice. Although the advent of ultrasound and CT has challenged its worth, plain abdominal radiography has the advantages of relatively low cost, ease of acquisition, and low level of necessary co-operation of the patient, which makes it extremely valuable as a simple diagnostic study to the trained and perceptive observer. The abdominal radiograph has also been called a *KUB,* signifying kidneys, ureters (which are not visible), and bladder. The term *flat plate of the abdomen* is dated and refers to a time when glass plates were used to produce images. Other terms include *plain film of the abdomen* and *abdominal plain film,* but with the widespread use of digital imaging and PACS for interpretation of the images, *plain abdominal radiograph* and *abdominal radiograph* have become the most appropriate terms.

A wealth of diagnostic information can be gained from correct interpretation of abdominal radiographs, and several excellent texts are available on the subject.[1-3] In this chapter, the discussion centers on abnormalities of gas and soft tissues that can be detected on these radiographs.

NORMAL BOWEL GAS PATTERNS

The intestinal tract of adults usually contains less than 200 mL of gas. Intestinal gas has three sources: swallowing of air, bacterial production, and diffusion from the blood. In the supine patient, gas rises and accumulates in the anteriorly placed segments of intestine, including the antrum and body of the stomach, transverse colon, and sigmoid colon. Gas is also frequently found in the rest of the colon, particularly the rectum. The radiographic evaluation of intestinal gas should include: (1) identification of the bowel segment containing the gas; (2) assessment of the caliber of the segment; (3) assessment of the most distal point of passage of the gas; and (4) evaluation of the mucosa outlined by the gas.

The normal bowel gas pattern is readily visible on supine abdominal radiographs (Fig. 16-1). The first collection of gas encountered from the top of the radiograph is usually in the antrum and body of the stomach. Gas may also be seen in the transverse colon immediately inferior to the stomach. Gas in the ascending and descending portions of the colon usually occupies the lateral margins of the peritoneal cavity. The

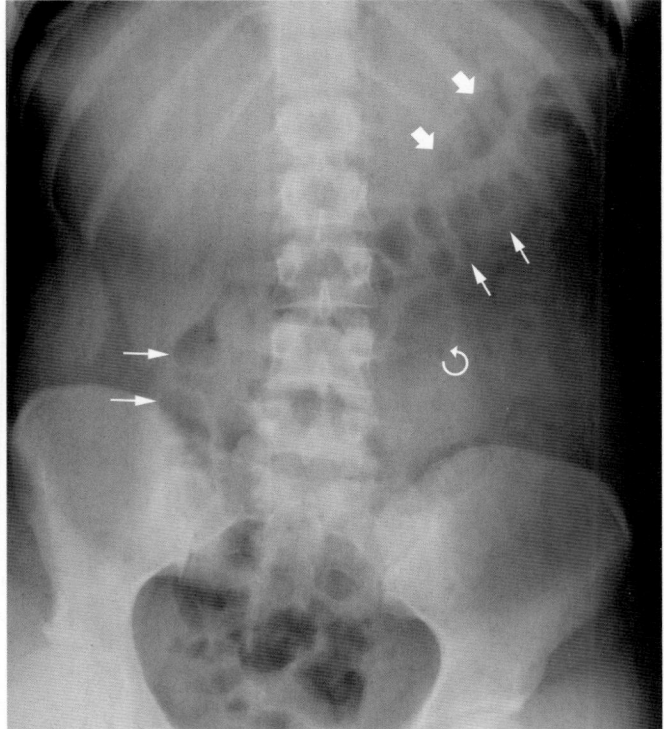

Figure 16-1. Normal bowel gas pattern. The most superior collection of intestinal gas is contained in the stomach (*large arrows*). Gas and stool outline the ascending and transverse colon (*small arrows*). Gas can also be seen in a portion of the small intestine (*curved arrow*).

sigmoid colon occupies the inferior aspect of the abdomen and is often recognized by its characteristic shape and haustra. Rectal gas occupies a midline position in the pelvis and generally extends to the level of the pubic symphysis. The gas-filled small intestine tends to occupy the central portion of the abdomen and has a smaller caliber than the colon.

Although the location of intestinal gas is helpful in differentiating colon from small bowel, recognition of mucosal features is also important. Haustra of the colon tend to be 2 to 3 mm wide and occur at intervals of 1 cm, whereas the plicae circulares or circular folds of the small bowel, are 1 to 2 mm wide and occur at intervals of 1 mm. Occasionally the differentiation of colon from small bowel is difficult without a positive contrast study. In general, the small bowel is less than 3 cm in diameter and the colon is less than 5 cm in diameter.

Intestinal gas should be considered a natural contrast agent in the interpretation of abdominal radiographs. When the patient is in the supine position, the gastric antrum and body tend to distend with air. A long, narrowed segment of air-filled stomach may indicate a diffuse infiltrating process such as linitis plastica. Gastric ulcerations and malignant masses are also occasionally visible (Fig. 16-2A). In the colon, a narrowed lumen associated with lack of haustra or nodular mucosa may be seen in patients with granulomatous or ulcerative colitis. Thickening of the haustra and annular colonic carcinomas may also be visible (Fig. 16-2B).

ABNORMAL BOWEL GAS PATTERNS

Gastric Outlet Obstruction

Recognition of gastric outlet obstruction on abdominal radiographs depends on the degree of distention of the stomach by air or fluid. The duration of obstruction, the position of the patient, and the frequency of emesis also affect the radiographic appearance. The dilated, air-filled stomach is usually recognized without difficulty because of its characteristic shape and location. Occasionally, however, a massively dilated, fluid-filled stomach can mimic the appearance of ascites or hepatomegaly. Displacement of the transverse colon inferiorly and the characteristic contour of the soft tissue density should help establish that the stomach is dilated. Furthermore, a small amount of air is almost always present within the stomach, so that an upright radiograph of the chest or right lateral

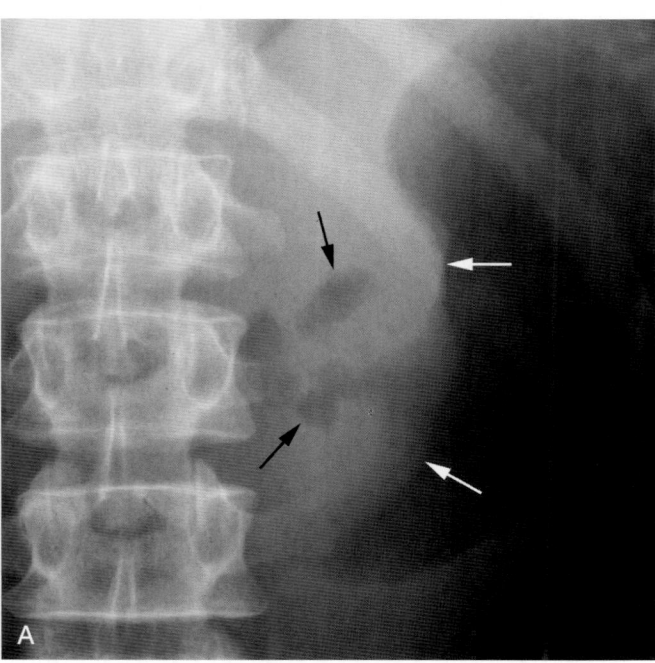

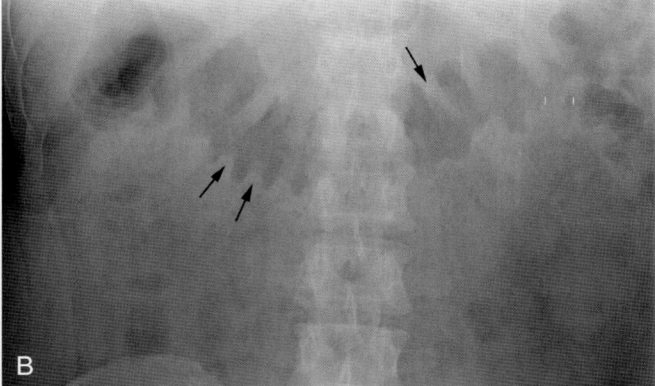

Figure 16-2. Abnormal bowel contours. A. Gas in the stomach outlines a mass (*white arrows*) on the lesser curvature with an irregular collection of central gas (*black arrows*), representing a large benign ulcer with surrounding edema. **B.** Air in the transverse colon outlines thickened haustrations (*arrows*). (**A** courtesy of Timothy J. Cole, MD, Richmond, VA.)

decubitus radiograph should confirm the gastric location of the fluid.

The antrum or pyloric region is the usual site of gastric outlet obstruction. The most common causes of obstruction include edema and spasm resulting from an acute pyloric channel ulcer and antral scarring caused by previous ulcers. Other causes include scirrhous gastric carcinomas and scarring from previous ingestion of a caustic substance.

Not all patients with gastric distention have a mechanical obstruction. Metabolic or drug-induced alterations of gastric peristalsis may cause the stomach to become dilated. Gastric atony may also occur in patients with chronic diabetes (i.e., gastroparesis diabeticorum) and is almost always associated with evidence of peripheral neuropathy.[4] Other causes of gastric dilatation include morphine and other atropine-like drugs, uremia, hypokalemia, porphyria, lead poisoning, and previous truncal vagotomy. Pancreatitis or gastritis may also result in reflex gastric atony, and general anesthesia may occasionally cause marked gastric dilatation.

Patients with obstructive lesions in the duodenum may also present with gastric outlet obstruction. The duodenum may be filled with fluid, so that it is not readily visible on supine radiographs. Left lateral decubitus views of the abdomen may allow air to enter the dilated duodenum, indicating that the obstruction is distal to the pylorus. Contrast studies are often performed to confirm the presence of gastric outlet obstruction, so that the duodenum must be examined if the stomach appears normal.

Adynamic Ileus

The term *adynamic ileus* refers to dilated bowel, usually small intestine, in the absence of mechanical obstruction. It is used synonymously with the terms *paralytic ileus* and *nonobstruc-* *tive ileus*. Other authors prefer the term *nonspecific bowel gas pattern*. A more specific term, *postoperative ileus*, is limited to patients who have undergone recent surgical procedures (Fig. 16-3). All of these terms refer to a state of absent or decreased intestinal peristalsis, which allows swallowed air to accumulate in dilated small intestine.[5] The presence of colonic gas may be helpful in distinguishing this condition from a mechanical small bowel obstruction. An adynamic ileus may result from a variety of causes, including electrolyte imbalances, sepsis, generalized peritonitis, blunt abdominal trauma, and infiltration of the mesentery by tumor.[6]

Small Bowel Obstruction

Small bowel obstruction is often difficult to diagnose on abdominal radiographs. The duration of obstruction, the frequency of emesis, and the use of nasogastric suction may affect the radiographic appearance. False-positive and false-negative rates of 20% have been reported in the diagnosis of intestinal obstruction based solely on the radiographic findings.[7] The diagnostic sensitivity can be increased by correlating the radiographs with the presence or absence of bowel sounds. Sequential radiographs over 12 to 24 hours may be helpful in demonstrating an evolving obstructive pattern.

When the small intestine becomes completely obstructed, accumulation of swallowed air and intestinal secretions causes proximal dilatation of bowel. Normal peristalsis and colonic contractions progressively eliminate intestinal contents distal to the site of obstruction within 12 to 24 hours. Abdominal radiographs may reveal dilated small bowel loops, usually measuring greater than 3 cm in diameter (allowing for magnification), with little, if any, gas seen distally in the colon.

Air-fluid levels are often present in patients with small bowel obstruction. In his classic work on the acute abdomen,

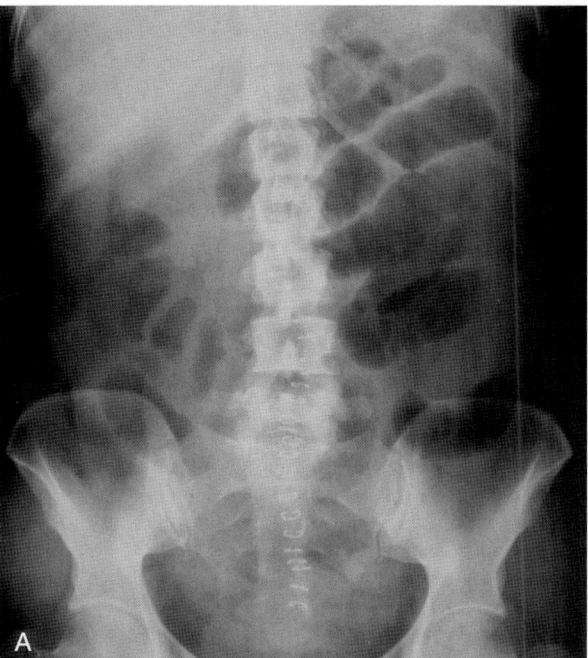 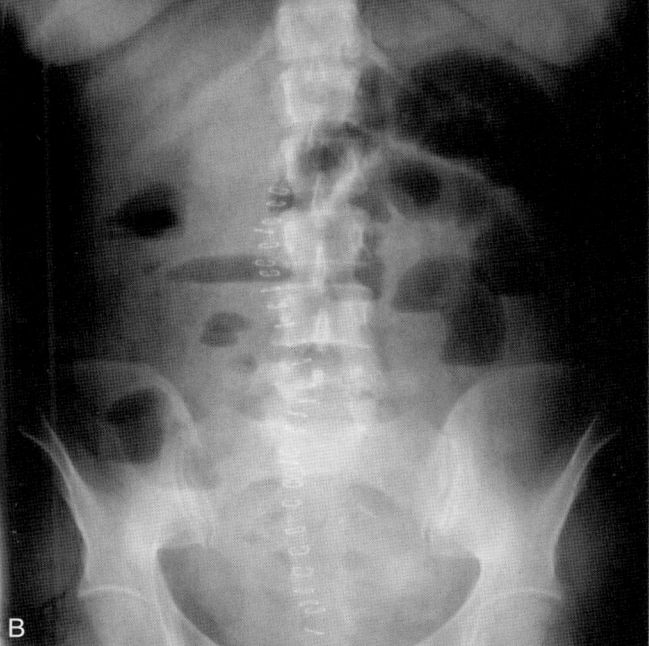

Figure 16-3. Postoperative ileus. A. Supine radiograph in a postoperative patient with absent bowel sounds shows multiple loops of mildly dilated small bowel in the abdomen. **B.** Upright radiograph shows differential air-fluid levels. This finding may be seen with an adynamic ileus or obstruction. (Note skin staples from recent abdominal surgery.)

Frimann-Dahl[8] stated that the presence of air-fluid levels at two different levels in the same segment of bowel indicated a hyperperistaltic small intestine and was therefore a sign of obstruction. Subsequent investigators have found that differential air-fluid levels may be present in any tubular structure filled with air and fluid that can be altered with changes in the patient's position. Thus, air-fluid levels should be recognized as a nonspecific finding that can accompany an adynamic ileus or mechanical obstruction.

The degree of small bowel dilatation tends to be greater in patients with true mechanical obstruction than in those with an adynamic ileus. As the loops fill with air, they may assume a "stepladder" configuration. Occasionally, air may be resorbed through the intestinal wall, producing a "gasless" abdomen. Small amounts of air trapped between the plicae circulares on upright abdominal radiographs may also produce an appearance that has been likened to a string of beads or pearls (Fig. 16-4). This radiographic finding is seldom seen in adynamic ileus and should therefore suggest mechanical obstruction.

Most small bowel obstructions are caused by postoperative adhesions. Such adhesions may occur as early as 1 week after surgery, but more typically the surgery is remote in time. Although most patients are knowledgeable about their own surgical history, they may not recall having undergone laparoscopy or surgical procedures during childhood. In the absence of a surgical history, an obstructing hernia should be suspected. Ninety-five percent of such hernias are external (i.e., inguinal, femoral, umbilical, or incisional). The presence of air-filled bowel below the pubic ramus should suggest the possibility of an obstructing inguinal hernia. Internal hernias such as paraduodenal or mesenteric hernias are an uncommon cause of intestinal obstruction and are rarely suspected on

abdominal radiographs. Other less common causes of small bowel obstruction include tumors of the small bowel, ectopic gallstones, acute appendicitis, and, occasionally, intestinal parasites or food.[9-13]

It may not be possible to distinguish mechanical obstruction from adynamic ileus on the basis of a single set of abdominal radiographs. If immediate surgery is not contemplated, further radiographic work-up with contrast studies may be indicated. This topic is discussed in detail in Chapter 50. In general, barium studies are helpful for determining the presence, site, and cause of obstruction when abdominal radiographs suggest a low-grade or partial small bowel obstruction. When higher grades of small bowel obstruction are suspected, however, CT is the best test for determining the site and cause of obstruction. Combining multidetector CT with positive or negative intraluminal contrast agents allows for 3D imaging that has dramatically improved the evaluation of patients with small bowel obstruction.[14]

Colonic Obstruction

More than 50% of colonic obstructions are caused by primary adenocarcinomas of the colon.[15,16] The obstruction usually occurs in the sigmoid colon, where the bowel tends to have a narrower caliber and the stool is more solid. Conversely, carcinomas of the cecum and ascending colon are less likely to cause obstruction because of the wider caliber of the bowel and more liquid character of the stool.

Colonic obstruction is typically manifested on abdominal radiographs by dilated, gas-filled loops of colon proximal to the site of obstruction and a paucity or absence of gas in the distal colon and rectum (Fig. 16-5A). Air-fluid levels may be seen on upright or decubitus views (Fig. 16-5B). A single-

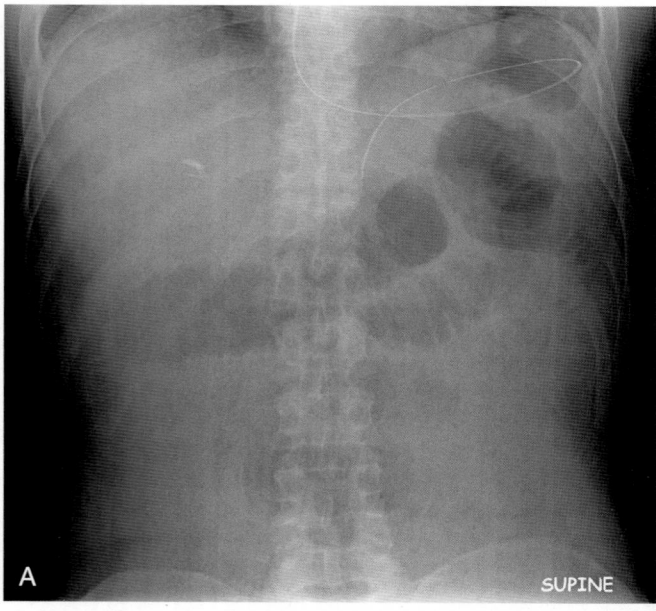

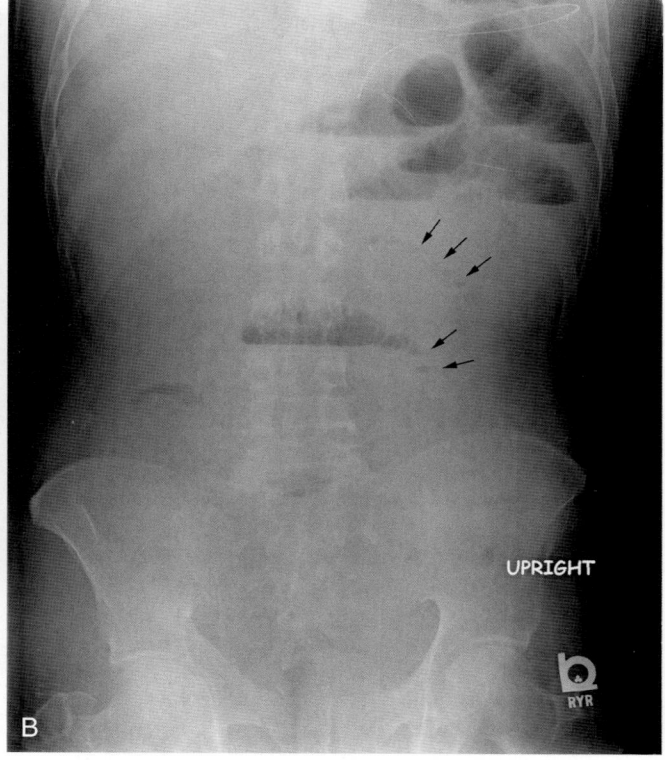

Figure 16-4. Small bowel obstruction. A. Supine radiograph demonstrates dilated small bowel. **B.** Upright radiograph demonstrates multiple air-fluid levels. Small amounts of gas trapped between the plicae circulares in the left mid abdomen (*arrows*) produce the "string of pearls" sign.

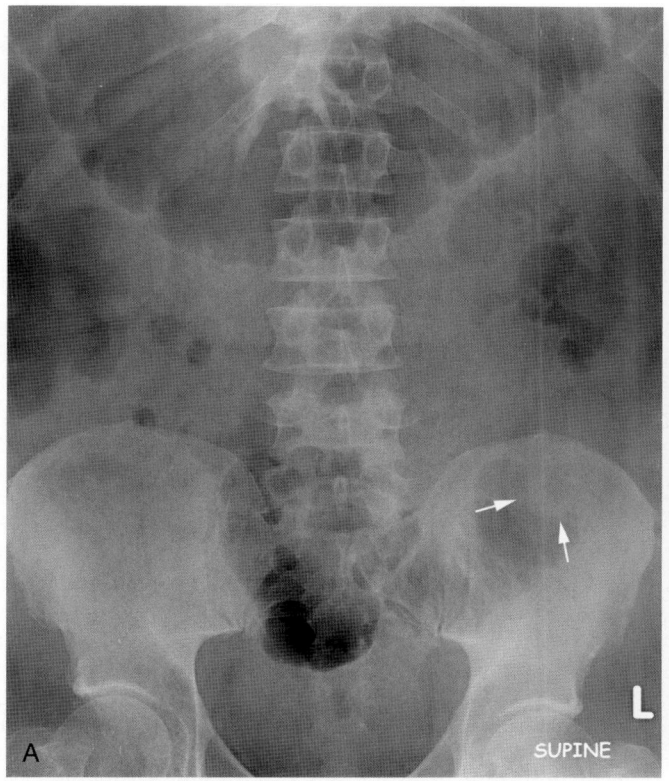

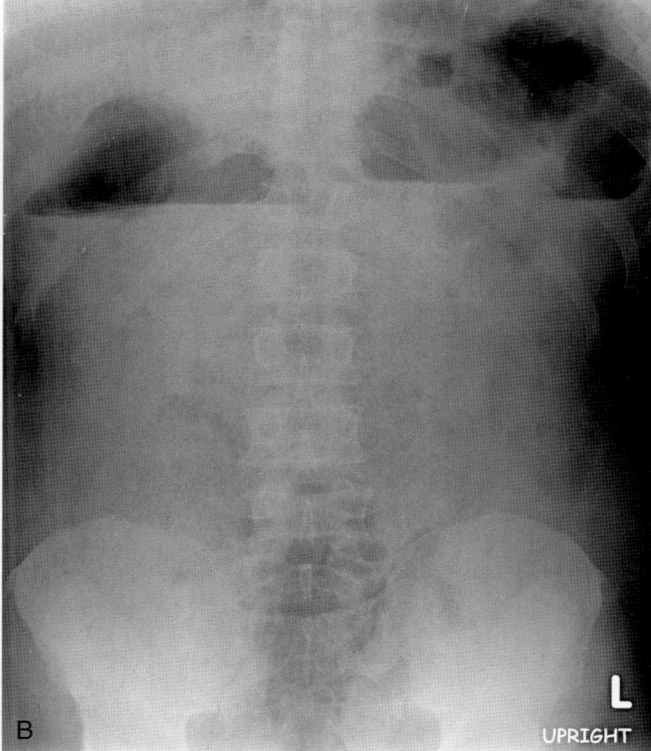

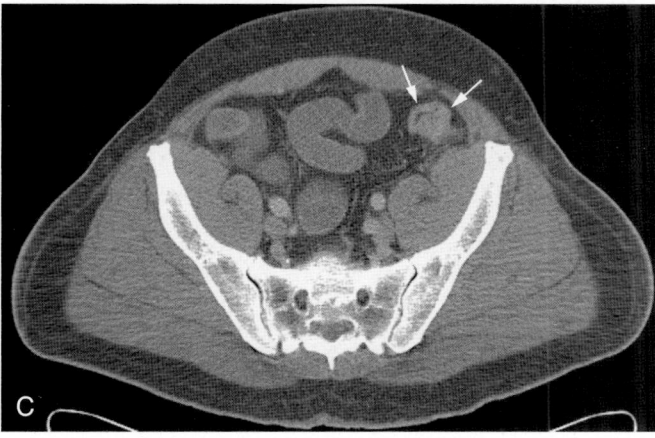

Figure 16-5. Colonic obstruction resulting from colonic carcinoma. **A.** Supine radiograph shows dilated colon with a soft tissue mass in the sigmoid (*arrows*). **B.** Upright radiograph shows air-fluid levels in the colon. **C.** CT scan confirms sigmoid colon cancer (*arrows*).

contrast barium enema or CT scan may be performed to confirm the presence of obstruction and determine its cause (Fig. 16-5C). In patients with a competent ileocecal valve, the colon (particularly the cecum) may become markedly dilated and little, if any, gas may be seen in the small bowel. As the cecal diameter increases, the risk of perforation also increases. In various series, colonic perforations have been reported in as many as 7% of all large bowel obstructions and 2% of obstructing colonic carcinomas.[17-19] Perforations tend to occur at the site of obstruction but may also result from ischemic change more proximally in the dilated colon or cecum.[20]

An incompetent ileocecal valve allows gas to reflux proximally into the small bowel, so that the radiographic findings can mimic a small bowel obstruction. A close search for colonic gas is therefore required. A right lateral decubitus view may be used to facilitate passage of gas distally into the descending colon and rectosigmoid. The distinction between colonic obstruction and small bowel obstruction has important diagnostic implications because orally administered barium may inspissate above an unsuspected colonic obstruction. A single-contrast barium enema or water-soluble contrast enema should therefore be considered in any patient with apparent obstruction of the distal small bowel on abdominal radiographs to rule out an underlying colonic obstruction. CT may also reveal the obstructing lesion (see Fig. 16-5C). If an obstructing carcinoma is encountered in the colon, the fluoroscopist should try to minimize reflux of barium above the level of the tumor.

Colonic Ileus

Acute colonic pseudo-obstruction was first described in 1948 by Ogilvie,[21] who postulated that progressive colonic dilatation was caused by interruption of sympathetic innervation with unopposed parasympathetic innervation of the colon. The most common clinical presentation is acute abdominal distention, usually occurring within 10 days of the onset of the precipitating pathologic process. Intra-abdominal inflammation, alcoholism, cardiac disease, burns, retroperitoneal disease, trauma, and normal pregnancy with spontaneous delivery or cesarean section have all been described as precipitating causes.[22-25]

Abdominal radiographs may demonstrate marked colonic distention, which is usually confined to the cecum, ascending colon, and transverse colon. Occasionally, however, gas may extend to the level of the sigmoid colon. The underlying clinical condition and rapid onset of colonic distention usually suggest the diagnosis of colonic pseudo-obstruction, but a limited contrast enema may be performed to rule out obstructing lesions in the colon.

Prediction of impending perforation of the cecum, as judged by cecal diameter, is fraught with difficulty. Although some authors have indicated that a cecal diameter of 9 to 12 cm suggests impending perforation, cecal diameters of 15 to 20 cm are commonly observed in patients who recover spontaneously.[24,26-28] When portable technique is used in obese patients who have an anteriorly placed cecum, marked radiographic magnification may occur. Radiographs obtained with the patient in prone or decubitus positions should lessen the effect of magnification. Serial radiographs showing a change in cecal diameter at 12- to 24-hour intervals may be more helpful than a single radiograph showing a dilated cecum. Intravenous neostigmine is considered the best initial treatment.[29,30] Prolonged cecal distention beyond 2 to 3 days should prompt colonoscopic or surgical decompression.[31] The presence of intramural gas in the region of the dilated cecum should strongly suggest infarction and impending perforation.

Closed Loop Obstruction

A closed loop obstruction refers to a segment of bowel that is obstructed at two points. These obstructions usually involve the small bowel and are caused by adhesions, internal hernias, or volvulus. The findings on abdominal radiographs are often nonspecific. Occasionally the dilated, air-filled segment of bowel may assume a "coffee bean" configuration. Persistence of such an air-filled loop on sequential radiographs over several days should suggest the possibility of a closed loop obstruction. Vascular compromise may lead to edema and thickening or effacement of the plicae circulares. If the obstructed segment becomes filled with fluid, a rounded soft tissue density outlined by intra-abdominal fat may appear as a pseudotumor. The clinical presentation may lead to the correct diagnosis in these patients. Intermittent, crampy abdominal pain that is replaced by steady, unrelenting pain suggests vascular compromise. Nevertheless, a definitive diagnosis of a closed loop obstruction can be made only at surgery.

Volvulus

Any segment of intestine that has a mesenteric attachment has the potential to undergo a volvulus. Some patients may have intermittent intestinal twists associated with recurrent episodes of abdominal pain or emesis. If the twist is greater than 360 degrees, it is unlikely to resolve spontaneously. In some cases, air and intestinal contents may enter the twisted

segment of bowel, producing abdominal distention and pain. The risk of vascular compromise in the twisted segment is more important than the mechanical effects of the volvulus. Severe vascular compromise may result in necrosis and perforation of bowel, causing sepsis and even death. Gastric volvulus is discussed in Chapter 38. Colonic volvulus may involve different segments of the colon, as discussed in the following sections.

Sigmoid Colon

Sixty to 75 percent of cases of colonic volvulus involve the sigmoid colon. Overall, sigmoid volvulus accounts for 1% to 2% of all cases of intestinal obstruction in the United States.[32,33] In some areas of South America and Africa, the incidence of this type of volvulus is extraordinarily high, reportedly because of a high-fiber diet and the resultant large, bulky stools, which produce a chronically dilated, elongated sigmoid colon. The incidence of sigmoid volvulus also appears to be increased in people living at higher altitudes in South America and Africa. In the United States, sigmoid volvulus tends to occur in elderly men and residents of nursing homes and mental hospitals, in whom chronic constipation and obtundation from medication are predisposing factors for gaseous distention of the sigmoid colon.

Patients with sigmoid volvulus may present with abdominal pain and distention resulting from colonic obstruction. Obstipation and vomiting are also common findings. The symptoms are usually acute, but they may have a gradual onset in some patients.

Findings on abdominal radiographs are diagnostic of sigmoid volvulus in 75% of patients with this condition. The classic radiographic appearance consists of a dilated loop of sigmoid colon that has an inverted-U configuration and absent haustra. Extension of the sigmoid colon above the transverse colon can be helpful in distinguishing volvulus from simple colonic dilatation.[34] The bowel may be located in the midline, or it may be directed toward the right or left upper quadrants, where it can elevate the hemidiaphragm (Fig. 16-6). Because sigmoid volvulus represents a closed loop obstruction, there is usually a considerable amount of gas in the more proximal colon and even in the small intestine. The apposed inner walls of the sigmoid colon may occasionally form a dense white line that points toward the pelvis. Absence of rectal gas is also an important finding. Prone or decubitus views should facilitate passage of gas into the rectum and exclude the diagnosis of sigmoid volvulus.

A contrast enema may occasionally be required in patients with suspected sigmoid volvulus. A low-pressure barium enema performed without inflation of a rectal balloon should demonstrate smooth, tapered narrowing, or "beaking," at the rectosigmoid junction. After decompression and stabilization of the patient, a follow-up barium enema should be performed to rule out an underlying colonic neoplasm.

Transverse Colon

Volvulus of the transverse colon is an uncommon condition, accounting for about 4% of all cases of colonic volvulus in the United States.[33] As with sigmoid volvulus, elongation of the transverse mesocolon and close approximation of the hepatic and splenic flexures may allow the transverse colon to rotate.

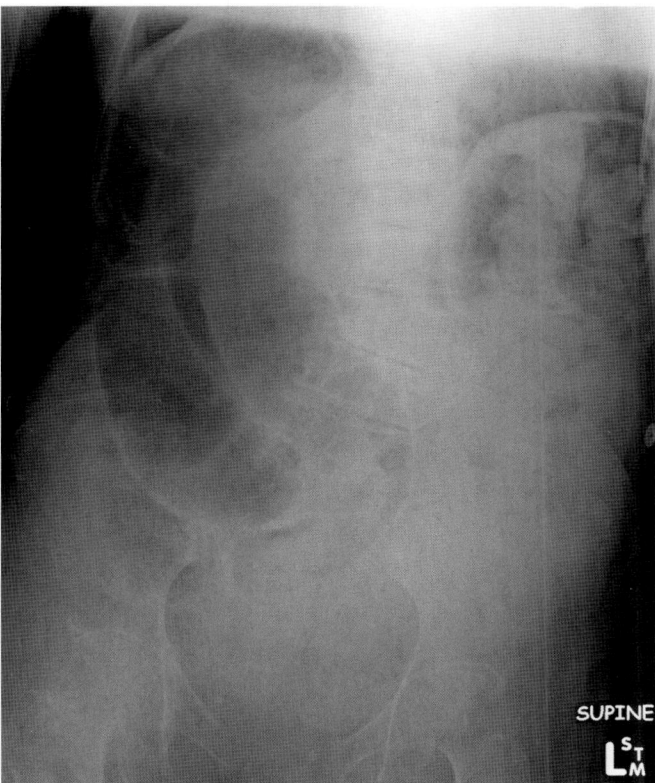

SUPINE

L S T
  M

Figure 16-6. Sigmoid volvulus. Supine abdominal radiograph in a patient with sigmoid volvulus shows the characteristic loop of dilated sigmoid colon with no gas seen in the rectum.

Failure of normal fixation of the mesentery may lead to increased mobility of the ascending colon and hepatic flexure, predisposing the patient to volvulus of the transverse colon.[35,36] Compression of the duodenojejunal junction at the root of the mesentery may cause severe vomiting. Mortality rates in these patients have been as high as 33%.[37]

Abdominal radiographs are usually not helpful in patients with volvulus of the transverse colon and may erroneously suggest sigmoid volvulus. A barium enema can confirm the diagnosis if it demonstrates the typical beaking at the level of the transverse colon. The presence of two air-fluid levels can often be seen in the dilated transverse colon and is helpful in distinguishing volvulus of the transverse colon from cecal volvulus.

Splenic Flexure of the Colon

The least common site for a colonic volvulus is the splenic flexure. Postoperative adhesions, chronic constipation, and congenital or postsurgical absence of the normal peritoneal attachments may predispose patients to this uncommon condition.[38-41] Abdominal radiographs may suggest the diagnosis of volvulus of the splenic flexure, but as with volvulus of the transverse colon a barium enema is often needed to confirm the diagnosis. Abdominal radiographs may reveal a dilated, featureless, air-filled loop of bowel in the left upper quadrant that is separate from the stomach, with air-fluid levels in the transverse colon and cecum.

Cecum

The term *cecal volvulus* refers to a condition caused by a rotational twist of the right colon on its axis associated with folding of the right colon, so that the cecum is located in the midabdomen or left upper quadrant. Cecal volvulus can occur only when the right colon is incompletely fused to the posterior parietal peritoneum, an embryologic variant present in 10% to 37% of normal adults.[42,43] There can also be metachronous bowel volvuli.[44] The term *cecal volvulus* is actually a misnomer because the twist is distal to the ileocecal valve. Cecal volvulus is less common than sigmoid volvulus, accounting for 2% to 3% of all colonic obstructions and about one third of all cases of colonic volvulus.

The findings on abdominal radiographs are diagnostic of cecal volvulus in about 75% of patients with this condition. Abdominal radiographs typically reveal a dilated, air-filled cecum in an ectopic location, usually with the cecal apex in the left upper quadrant (Fig. 16-7A). The medially placed ileocecal valve may produce a soft tissue indentation, so that the gas-filled cecum has the appearance of a coffee bean or kidney (Fig. 16-7B). Usually, little gas is seen distally in the colon. If the ileocecal valve is incompetent, refluxed gas in the small bowel may erroneously suggest a small bowel obstruction and obscure the diagnosis. A contrast enema shows typical beaking at the point of the volvulus in the midascending colon. The diagnosis can also be made with CT.[45] Cecal volvulus is likely to occur in a variety of settings, including colonoscopy, barium enema, obstructive lesions in the distal colon, and pregnancy.[46-48]

In 1938, Weinstein described a condition known as *cecal bascule,* which involved folding of the right colon without twisting, so that the cecum occupied a position in the midabdomen.[49] The term *bascule* is derived from *bascula,* the Latin word for "scale."[1] The point at which the ascending colon is folded represents the fulcrum of the scale. This entity also requires a loosely attached right colon.[50] The concept of a cecal bascule was challenged by Johnson and colleagues,[29] who believed that these patients have a focal adynamic ileus of the cecum. Twenty percent of their patients had cecal perforation. They emphasized that the duration of cecal distention was more important than cecal diameter in predicting impending perforation. Whether cecal bascule represents an actual anatomic folding of the right colon or an adynamic ileus is not as important as the recognition of a dilated, ectopically located cecum as a source of symptoms and potential perforation.

APPENDICITIS

The development of acute appendicitis requires obliteration of the appendiceal lumen, usually by a concretion that may be visible on abdominal radiographs. The concretion has been called a fecalith or coprolith, but the preferred term is *appendicolith.* This concretion forms around a nidus such as a piece of vegetable matter. Inspissated feces and calcium salts may adhere to this nidus, so that it eventually reaches a size that occludes the appendiceal lumen. Accumulation of mucus proximal to the obstruction may distend the appendix, causing infection, ischemia, and subsequent perforation.

Acute appendicitis is a common cause of abdominal pain. Some investigators believe that abdominal radiographs have little value in patients with suspected appendicitis.[51,52] Nevertheless, such radiographs are frequently obtained as the first

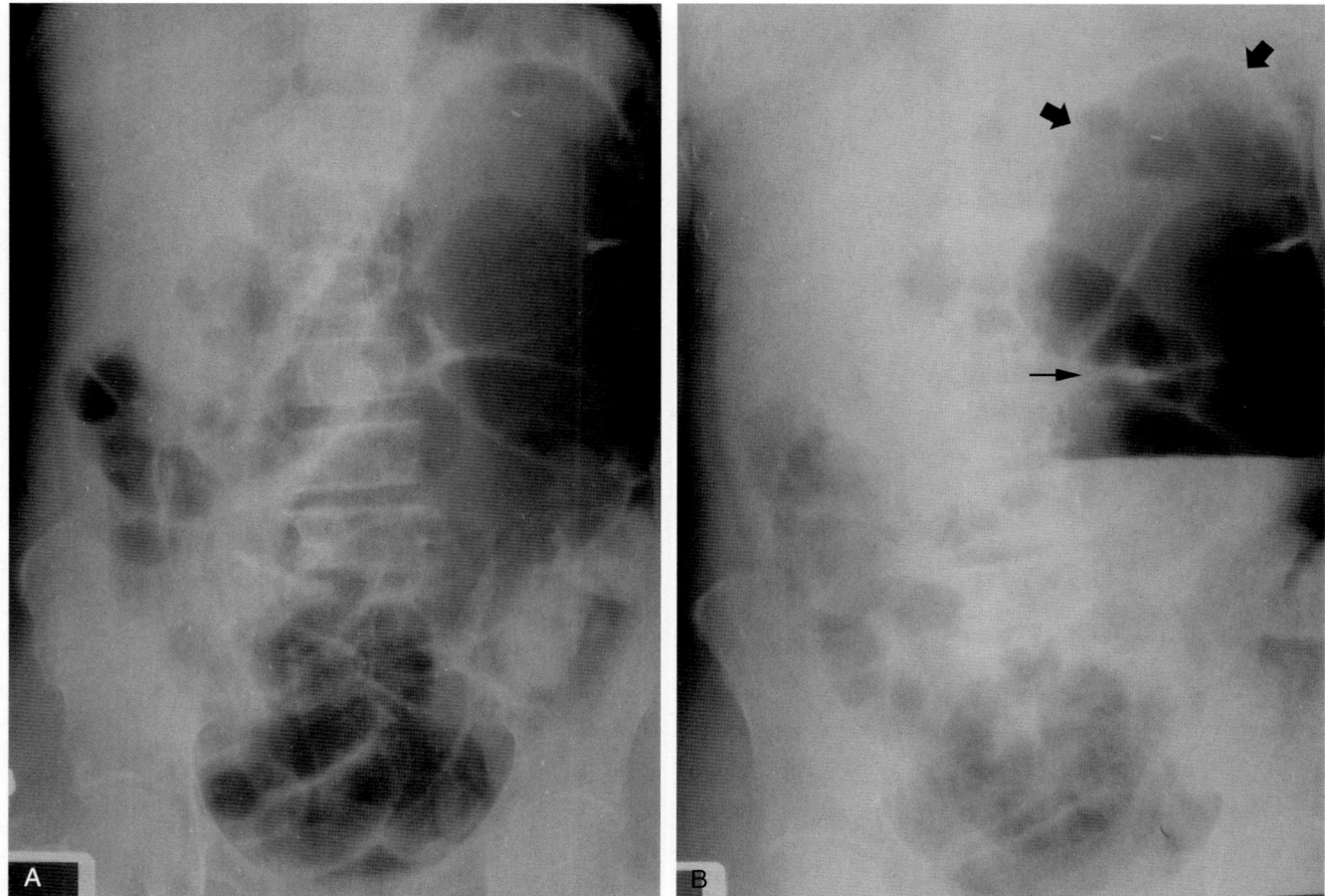

Figure 16-7. Cecal volvulus. A. Supine abdominal radiograph shows a markedly dilated viscus in the left upper quadrant, representing the obstructed cecum. Note multiple loops of dilated small bowel. **B.** Upright radiograph shows the caput of the cecum (*thick arrows*) and the ileocecal valve (*thin arrow*) with a single air-fluid level in the dilated cecum.

imaging study in these patients. Signs of appendicitis on abdominal radiographs include the following:

1. *Appendicolith.* The appearance of an appendicolith is the single most helpful finding on abdominal radiographs. Appendicoliths are found in about 10% of patients with acute appendicitis. They typically appear as round or oval calcified densities and are frequently laminated (Fig. 16-8). Appendicoliths usually range from 1 to 2 cm but may be as large as 4 cm.[53-56] They are usually located in the right lower quadrant but can also be located in the pelvis, right upper quadrant, or left upper quadrant. The presence of an appendicolith has important clinical implications because it often indicates appendicitis complicated by perforation and abscess formation.

2. *Abnormal bowel gas pattern.* About 25% of patients with appendicitis have an abnormal bowel gas pattern—most commonly an adynamic ileus but occasionally a partial or even complete small bowel obstruction.[57] An adynamic ileus occurs as a response to focal inflammation and may be localized to the right lower quadrant. Air-fluid levels in the jejunum have also been described in up to 50% of cases.[58] A dilated transverse colon may also be seen as an early sign of appendiceal perforation.[59] A mechanical obstruction

may occur if the terminal ileum is compressed by the appendix or is bound by adhesive bands.

3. *Abnormal cecum and ascending colon.* Local inflammation and edema may cause thickening of the cecal wall and widening of the haustra. A cecal air-fluid level may also be present on upright or decubitus radiographs, but this finding is transient and nonspecific.

4. *Extraluminal soft tissue mass.* A soft tissue mass can be found in up to one third of patients with perforation. It may be caused by a combination of edema, fluid, and fluid-filled loops of small bowel in the right lower quadrant. The presence of mottled gas within the soft tissue mass indicates an abscess.

5. *Gas in the appendix.* This sign has been described as one of acute appendicitis, even though the pathophysiology of the disease would more likely result in an absence of gas.[60] Most often, an air-filled appendix is a normal finding, simply reflecting the position of the appendix in relation to the cecum.[61] An ascending retrocecal appendix is more likely to contain gas.

6. *Free intraperitoneal air.* A ruptured appendix may rarely lead to the development of a small amount of free intraperitoneal air. The obstructed appendiceal lumen prevents larger collections of gas from escaping

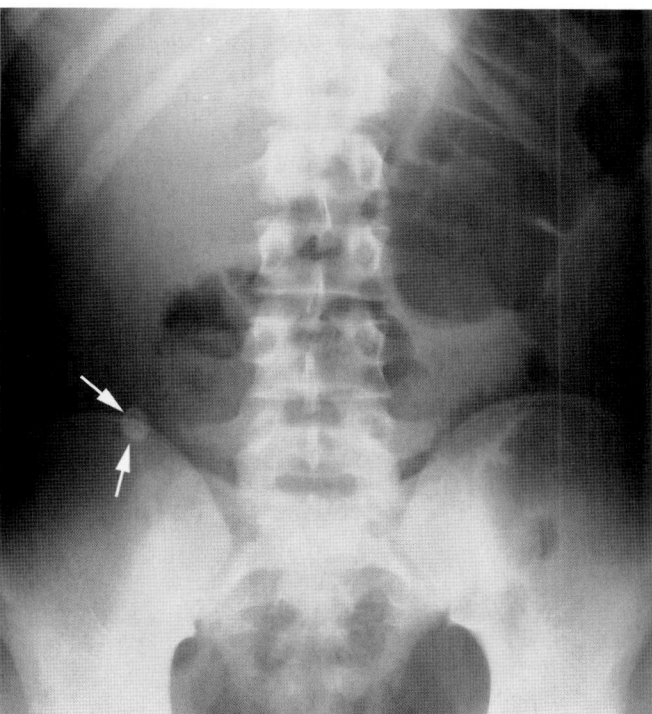

Figure 16-8. Acute appendicitis with partial small bowel obstruction. Supine radiograph shows a paucity of small bowel in the right lower quadrant with a laminated appendicolith (*arrows*).

into the peritoneal cavity, except in the case of a ruptured gas-containing abscess.[62,63]

7. *Obliteration of normal fat planes.* Inflammation and edema may alter the water content of surrounding fat and obscure the normal fat planes of the psoas muscle, obturator muscle, or properitoneal flank stripe. This finding is nonspecific and is usually associated with other signs of appendicitis on abdominal radiographs.

8. *Scoliosis of the lumbar spine.* Some patients with appendicitis may develop lumbar scoliosis as a result of splinting. This finding is nonspecific, however, and can be related to positioning of the patient.

Surgeons have long believed that false-negative laparotomies are acceptable in some patients with right lower quadrant pain because of the serious, potentially life-threatening complications of untreated acute appendicitis. Cross-sectional imaging techniques such as ultrasound and CT have shown significant promise in improving the preoperative work-up of patients with suspected appendicitis (see Chapter 60).

TOXIC MEGACOLON

Toxic megacolon, or toxic dilatation of the colon, may be diagnosed on the basis of a dilated colon on abdominal radiographs in a patient with fever, tachycardia, and hypotension. Toxic megacolon is traditionally associated with ulcerative colitis, but it can occur in patients with granulomatous colitis, amebiasis, cholera, pseudomembranous colitis, cytomegaloviral colitis, and ischemic colitis. Toxic megacolon develops in 5% to 10% of patients with ulcerative colitis but in only 2% to 4% of patients with granulomatous colitis.[64-67] The duration of the underlying disease has no relationship to the develop-

ment of toxic megacolon. In fact, 70% of patients with toxic megacolon develop this complication during their first episode of colitis.

When toxic megacolon is suspected on clinical grounds, assessment must be made not only of the degree of bowel dilatation but also of the appearance of the colonic mucosa outlined by air and the presence or absence of free intraperitoneal air. In general, the transverse and ascending portions of the colon tend to dilate, but this tendency is a reflection more of their anterior position within the abdomen or their underlying capacity to dilate than of a predisposition to disease.[68] Although magnification may be a factor in obese patients, the upper normal limit for the transverse colonic diameter is about 6 cm. In toxic megacolon, the diameter of the transverse colon ranges from 6 to 15 cm.[69] A nodular mucosa may be readily visible in the dilated transverse colon (Fig. 16-9).[70] Colonic perforation occurs in 30% to 50% of cases and is associated with a high mortality rate.[66,71] Thus, a delay in the diagnosis of toxic megacolon on abdominal radiographs may have disastrous consequences for these patients. The presence of increased amounts of gas in the small intestine in patients with severe colitis has been associated with an increased likelihood of developing toxic megacolon.[72]

The diagnosis of toxic megacolon is made by use of a combination of the clinical and radiographic findings, so that a contrast enema does not need to be performed in these patients. Although some patients with toxic megacolon have undergone barium enema examinations without complications, most authors believe that contrast enemas are contraindicated in patients suspected of having this condition

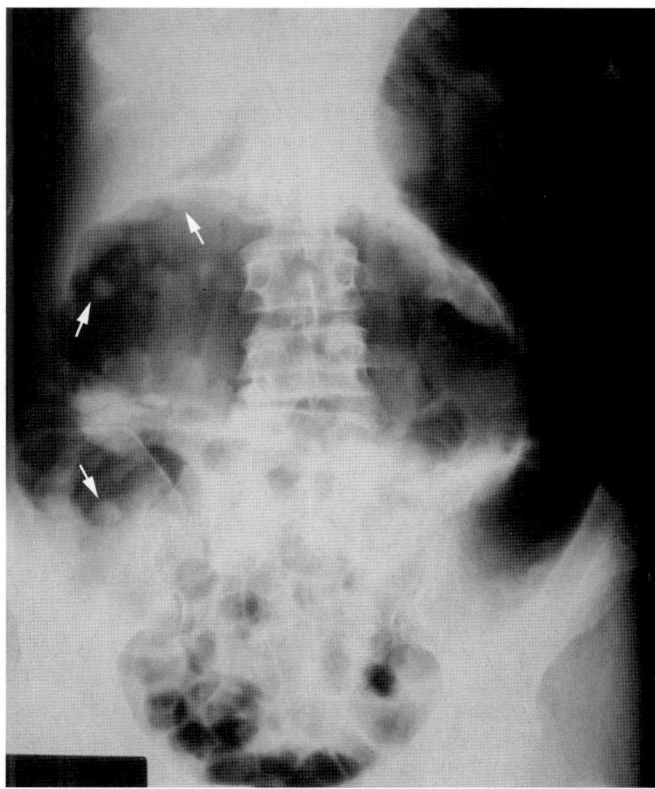

Figure 16-9. Toxic megacolon. There is marked colonic distention in a patient with ulcerative colitis and toxic megacolon. Note the nodular mucosal contour (*arrows*) in the transverse colon.

because of the risk of perforation.[73] CT is valuable in depicting diffuse colitis and in detecting life-threatening abdominal complications.[74]

PNEUMOPERITONEUM

The presence of intraperitoneal air in acutely ill patients is an important radiographic observation that usually indicates bowel perforation. Classic experimental studies by Miller and Nelson showed that as little as 1 mL of air can be detected below the right hemidiaphragm on properly exposed upright chest radiographs.[75] These investigators emphasized the importance of placing the patient in the left lateral decubitus position for 15 to 20 minutes before obtaining a radiograph with the patient in an upright position to maximize the possibility of detecting small amounts of free air. Radiographs obtained in mid-inspiration or mid-expiration are even more likely to reveal tiny amounts of free air.[76] Chest radiographs obtained with the patient in an upright position are ideal for demonstrating free air because the x-ray beam strikes the hemidiaphragms tangentially at their highest point. Although a posteroanterior view is usually obtained, a lateral view of the chest may be even more sensitive.[77] As sensitive as the upright chest radiograph is, CT of the abdomen has been shown to be more sensitive in detecting small amounts of free air in acute trauma.[78]

In contrast, upright abdominal radiographs result in an oblique view of the hemidiaphragms that may obscure free air because the x-ray beam is centered more inferiorly. Left lateral decubitus views of the abdomen are sensitive for detecting small amounts of free air interposed between the free edge of the liver and the lateral wall of the peritoneal cavity. Care should be taken to include the upper abdomen because air rises to the highest point in the abdomen, which frequently is beneath the lower ribs. Alternatively, the highest point may be the lower abdomen in very obese patients. Radiographs obtained with the patient in the right lateral decubitus posi-

tion can also be helpful, but gas in the stomach or colon may obscure small amounts of free air. A cross-table lateral view of the abdomen with the patient in a supine position may demonstrate free air in individuals who are physically unable to roll onto their sides. As demonstrated with other radiographic positions, CT is more sensitive in detecting free air than left lateral decubitus radiographs.[79]

All of these horizontal beam views are based on the principle that air rises to the highest point in the peritoneal cavity. If for various reasons, however, horizontal beam views cannot be obtained, the radiologist must be able to recognize the presence of intraperitoneal air on supine abdominal radiographs.[80] The following signs have been described:

1. *Serosal or Rigler's sign.* Normally, gas outlines only the luminal side of the bowel. Gas on both sides of the bowel, however, may outline the bowel wall as a thin, linear stripe (Fig. 16-10A). Since its original description by Rigler in 1941, this sign has been recognized as an important finding of pneumoperitoneum, although a moderate amount of free air must be present.[81] Overlapping loops of dilated small bowel in the midabdomen can mimic this sign, so it is helpful to evaluate the periphery of the radiograph. Air trapped between loops of bowel may have a characteristic triangular configuration (Fig. 16-10B).

2. *Increased lucency in the right upper quadrant.* Air accumulating superiorly in the free space between the anterior aspect of the liver and the abdominal wall may cause increased lucency in the right upper quadrant (Fig. 16-11A). Depending on the habitus of the patient, the lateral border of the air collection may be linear. Small collections of air may be seen as subtle rounded lucencies overlying the liver.[82]

3. *Visualization of the undersurface of the diaphragm.* Air may be trapped anteriorly in the cupola of the diaphragm, permitting visualization of the undersurface of the central portion of the diaphragm

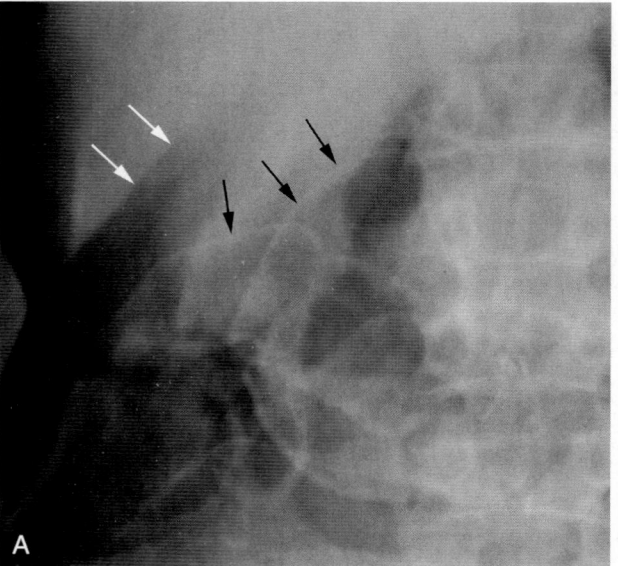
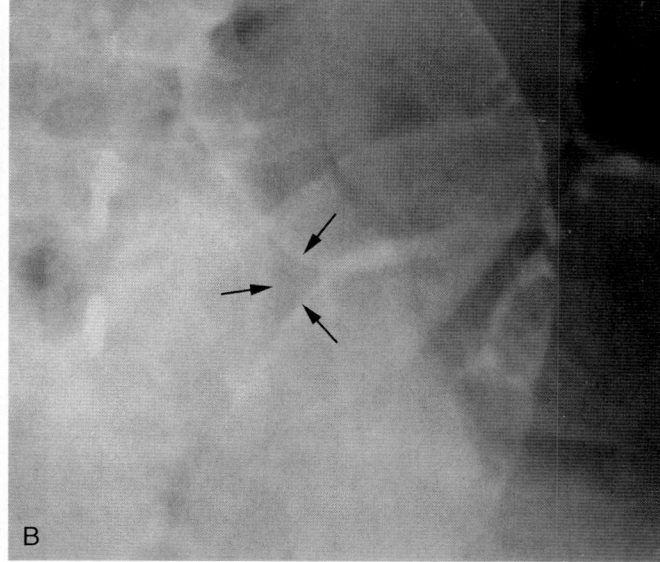

Figure 16-10. Pneumoperitoneum with Rigler's sign. A. A close-up view of the right upper quadrant in a patient with massive pneumoperitoneum shows a sharp liver edge (*white arrows*) with air outlining both sides of the bowel wall (*black arrows*). **B.** Air trapped between adjacent loops of bowel may have a characteristic triangular configuration (*arrows*).

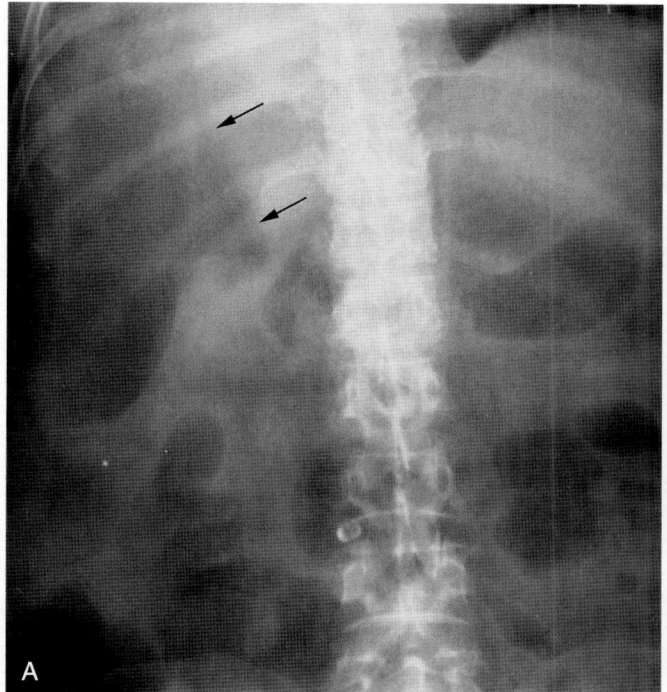

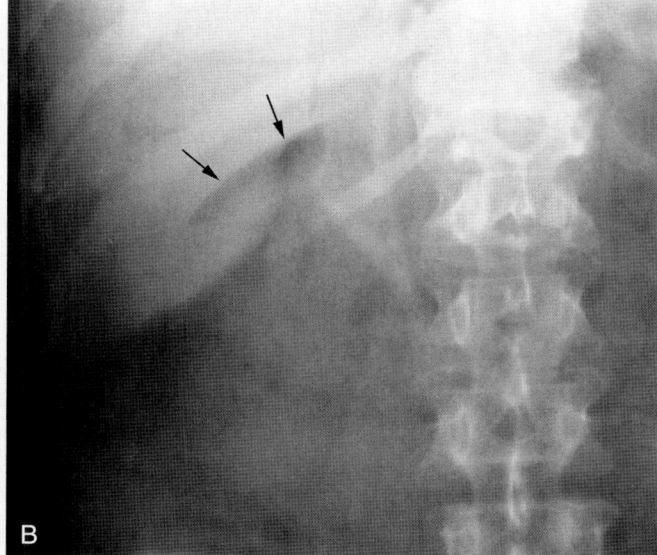

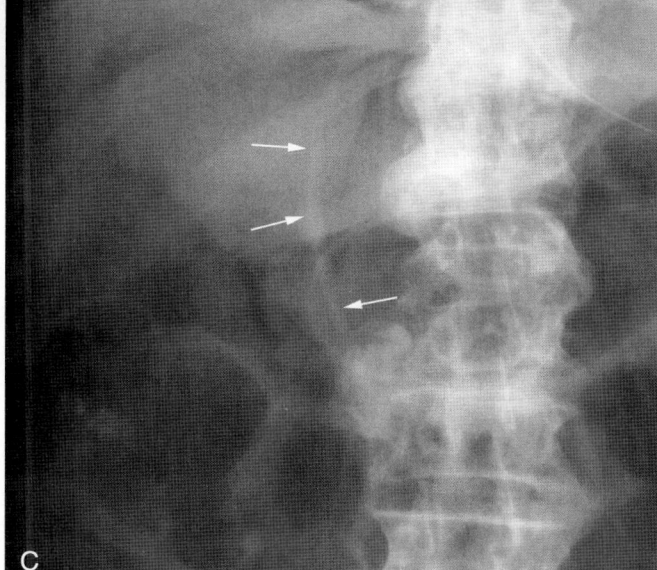

Figure 16-11. Other signs of pneumoperitoneum on supine abdominal radiographs. A. Increased radiolucency is seen in the right upper quadrant (*arrows*). This finding is due to air interposed between the anterior abdominal wall and the liver. **B.** Air collecting in Morison's pouch outlines the inferior border of the liver (*arrows*). **C.** Air outlines the falciform ligament (*arrows*).

or of the diaphragmatic muscle slips laterally. These signs depend on the amount of air present and on the orientation of the diaphragm.[83,84]

4. *Air in Morison's pouch (posterior hepatorenal space).* Morison's pouch is an intraperitoneal recess that is bounded anteriorly by the liver and posteriorly by the right kidney. In the supine position, fluid may gravitate to this space. Air escaping from a perforated viscus may become loculated in this space because of surrounding inflammation. Air in Morison's pouch is characterized radiographically by a linear or triangular collection of gas in the right upper quadrant outside the expected location of the bowel (Fig. 16-11B).[85-87] The gallbladder may also be visualized.[88]

5. *Outline of the normal peritoneal ligaments.* With larger amounts of free air, the falciform ligament and extrahepatic segment of the ligamentum teres in the upper abdomen (Fig. 16-11C), the lateral umbilical ligaments (inverted-V sign) in the lower abdomen, and the urachus may occasionally be visualized.[89-92]

6. *"Football" sign.* Originally described by Miller in infants, this sign results from a large amount of free air filling the oval-shaped peritoneal cavity, mimicking an American football.[93] This sign has limited value in adults.

7. *Air in the lesser sac of the peritoneal cavity.* Intraperitoneal air may occasionally enter the foramen of Winslow and become loculated in the lesser sac. This gas may be manifested by an ill-defined lucency above the lesser curvature of the stomach.[94]

The presence of pneumoperitoneum does not always indicate an acute abdominal emergency. Various causes of free air are listed in Table 16-1.

Table 16-1
Causes of Pneumoperitoneum

Bowel
Perforation of benign ulcer
Perforation of neoplasm
Perforation of appendix
Jejunal diverticulitis
Diverticulitis of sigmoid colon
Pneumatosis cystoides intestinalis
Foreign body perforation

Trauma
Abdominal surgery
Anastomotic leak
Peritoneal tap
Endoscopy or biopsy
Penetrating injury
Percutaneous endoscopic gastrostomy

Female Genital Tract
Rubin test
Sexual intercourse or cunnilingus
Pelvic examination
Athletic activities such as water-skiing

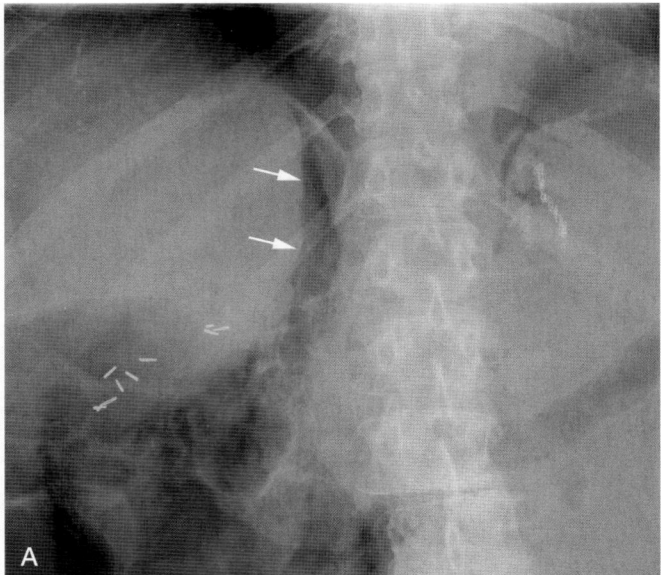

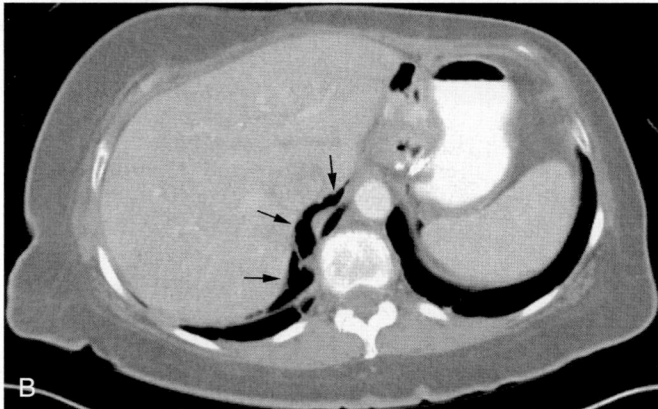

Figure 16-12. Retroperitoneal air in a patient with retroperitoneal perforation after endoscopy. A. The retroperitoneal air is manifested by linear gas collections (*arrows*) dissecting along the right margin of the psoas muscle in the upper retroperitoneum. **B.** CT confirms retroperitoneal location of the air (*arrows*). (Courtesy of Laura R. Carucci, MD, Richmond, VA.)

PNEUMORETROPERITONEUM

Gas that enters the retroperitoneal spaces can usually be easily distinguished from intraperitoneal gas. Because retroperitoneal gas is bound by fascial planes, it collects in a linear fashion along the margins of the psoas muscle, the renal outlines, and the medial undersurface of the hemidiaphragms (Fig. 16-12). Meyers has described the various pathways that retroperitoneal gas can travel.[95] The retroperitoneal portions of the intestines, such as the duodenum, ascending and descending colon, and rectum, can serve as sources. In patients with sigmoid diverticulitis, gas can extend laterally along the left margin of the psoas muscle or, if the perforation involves the root of the sigmoid mesocolon, along both margins of the psoas muscle.

The location of the retroperitoneal gas may provide a clue to its site of origin. Gas escaping from duodenal perforations tends to be confined to the right anterior pararenal space. Gas may extend medially across the anterior aspect of the psoas muscle, sparing the lateral margin of the muscle. Less commonly, gas may enter the perirenal space and outline the right kidney. Duodenal ulcers, iatrogenic duodenal injuries, and blunt abdominal trauma can all result in perforation of the extraperitoneal portion of the duodenum.[96]

Gas from a rectal perforation may be limited to the perirectal space, or it may extend into both the anterior and the posterior retroperitoneal spaces and even rarely into the mediastinum.[97] Iatrogenic trauma is a common cause of rectal perforation. Radiologists must be aware of the potential risk of causing a rectal perforation when insufflating a balloon during barium enema examinations.[98]

PNEUMOBILIA

Gas in the bile ducts, or pneumobilia, is characterized radiographically by thin, branched, tubular areas of lucency in the central portion of the liver (Fig. 16-13). This central location can be explained by the flow of bile from the periphery of the liver toward the porta hepatis.

Pneumobilia almost always results from some type of communication between the bile duct and the intestine. One of its most common causes is surgical creation of a biliary-enteric fistula, such as a choledochojejunostomy or cholecystoenterostomy. A choledochoduodenal fistula secondary to a penetrating duodenal ulcer represents the most common nonsurgical communication between the common bile duct and the duodenum.[99] In contrast, a cholecystoduodenal fistula secondary to a gallstone that erodes into the duodenum represents the most common nonsurgical communication between the gallbladder and the duodenum. In some patients with a cholecystoduodenal fistula, a patent cystic duct may allow air to enter the intrahepatic biliary ducts.[100,101] If the ectopic gallstone is 2.5 cm or greater in diameter, it may obstruct the intestine, usually at or near the ileocecal valve, producing a "gallstone ileus." The classic triad (i.e., Rigler's triad) of air in the biliary tree, small bowel obstruction, and an ectopic gallstone is virtually diagnostic of gallstone ileus.[102] Anomalous insertions of the biliary tree, recent passage of

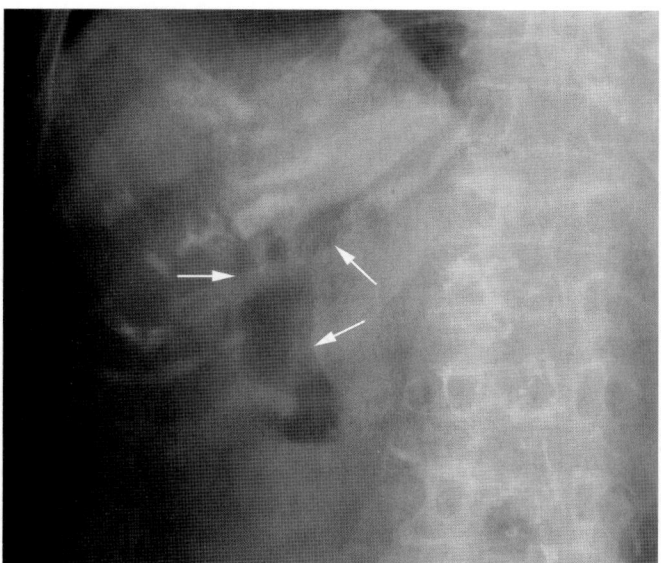

Figure 16-13. Pneumobilia. Air is seen in the biliary tree (*arrows*) in a patient who had a previous choledochojejunostomy.

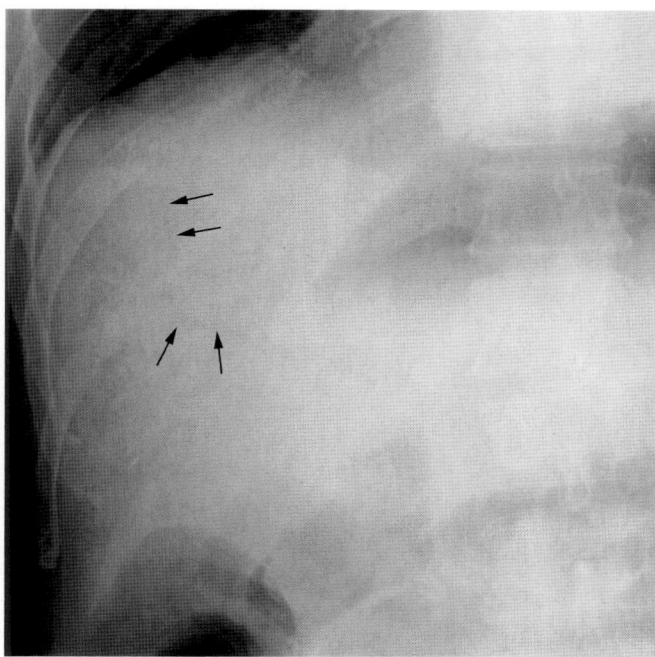

Figure 16-14. Portal venous gas. Tiny, branching gas collections (*arrows*) are seen extending toward the periphery of the liver.

a common duct stone, and infestation of the biliary tree by *Ascaris* organisms are other causes of pneumobilia.[103,104]

The radiographic appearance of pneumobilia is sufficiently characteristic to permit a confident diagnosis on the basis of abdominal radiographs. Occasionally, periportal fat or fat around the ligamentum teres hepatis may be manifested by faint lucency over the liver, but its appearance is different from that of pneumobilia.[105,106] The most important consideration in the differential diagnosis of pneumobilia is the presence of gas in the portal venous system.

PORTAL VENOUS GAS

The first report of portal venous gas in adults is attributed to Susman and Senturia in 1960.[107] This ominous radiographic finding is manifested by thin, branching, tubular areas of lucency that occupy the periphery of the liver and extend almost to the liver surface (Fig. 16-14). The peripheral location of the gas reflects the hepatopetal flow of blood in the portal venous system. In advanced cases, air can be seen outlining the more centrally located main portal vein, but this finding is less common. A left lateral decubitus radiograph of the abdomen may facilitate visualization of portal venous gas. Unless the gas has been introduced iatrogenically by vascular catheterization, the source of the gas is almost invariably the intestine. Intraluminal intestinal air can breach a damaged mucosa, enter the bloodstream, and eventually reach the portal venous system of the liver.

The most important cause of portal venous gas is intestinal ischemia or infarction. In adults, death often occurs shortly after portal venous gas has been observed.[108,109] The finding of portal venous gas should therefore lead to a careful search for gas in the wall of the bowel as a result of intestinal infarction.

Portal venous gas may occasionally have other benign causes. Dilatation of the stomach and of the small bowel may allow some air to enter the intestinal mucosa, eventually reaching the liver.[110] Double-contrast barium enemas and

colonoscopy performed on patients with inflammatory bowel disease or sigmoid diverticulitis have also resulted in nonfatal cases of portal venous gas.[111-115] Doppler ultrasound has been used to detect gas in the portal vein in the immediate postoperative period after liver transplantation.[116]

HEPATIC ARTERIAL GAS

Gas in the hepatic artery has been anecdotally reported in a patient in whom the hepatic artery was ligated for the treatment of an unresectable hepatic adenoma.[117] The smaller caliber of the hepatic artery and relative paucity of intrahepatic branches should differentiate this finding from portal venous gas. Hepatic arterial gas may be reported more frequently as the use of aggressive interventional radiographic techniques increases for the treatment of hepatic neoplasms.

INTRAMURAL GAS (PNEUMATOSIS)

Gas in the wall of the intestine, or pneumatosis, may be characterized by two radiographic patterns: a bubbly appearance or thin, linear streaks of gas.[118] The bubbly appearance of intramural gas is easily mimicked by fecal material within the colon. In patients with this form of pneumatosis, close inspection may reveal small bubbles of gas outside the confines of the bowel, leading to the correct diagnosis. In contrast, linear gas collections tend to be more readily apparent and should always be considered an important finding on abdominal radiographs, regardless of their location (Fig. 16-15). In combination with portal venous gas (see earlier section), linear gas collections in the intestinal wall are almost always a sign of bowel infarction in adult patients.[119] Other findings of bowel ischemia or infarction on abdominal radiographs include dilatation of bowel and nodular thickening or thumbprinting of the bowel wall. CT may also reveal characteristic

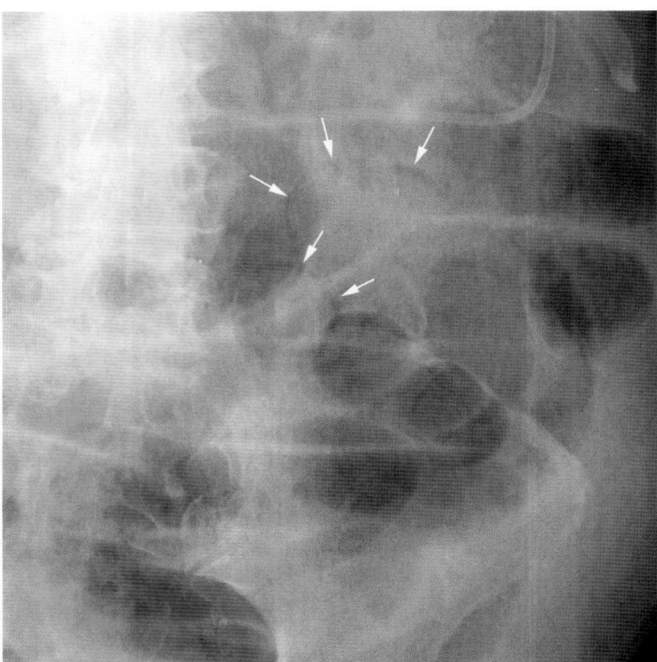

Figure 16-15. Infarcted bowel with intramural gas. Linear gas collections (*arrows*) are seen in the wall of several moderately dilated small bowel loops in a patient with bowel infarction.

findings in patients with bowel ischemia or infarction.[120,121] Pneumatosis is particularly well demonstrated by CT but does not always indicate infarction of the bowel unless the pneumatosis is associated with portomesenteric venous gas.[122] The linear pattern of pneumatosis identified on CT is more likely to be associated with transmural bowel infarction than the bubbly pattern.[123]

Air in the wall of the stomach is a focal form of pneumatosis. *Emphysematous gastritis* is the term used to describe the rare fulminant variant of phlegmonous gastritis that results from infection of the gastric wall. Hemolytic *Streptococcus* is the most commonly implicated organism.[124] Ingestion of caustic substances, gastroduodenal surgery, gastroenteritis, intubation injury, ulceration, and gastric outlet obstruction are other causes of air in the gastric wall.[125-127]

Pneumatosis cystoides coli is a rare, benign condition characterized by multiple gas-filled blebs or cysts in the wall of the colon. These cysts appear radiographically as grapelike clusters of gas, usually segmental in distribution (Fig. 16-16). The left colon tends to be involved more frequently than the right colon. These cystic collections may protrude into the bowel lumen, giving the colon a scalloped appearance on barium studies. The cysts tend to resolve spontaneously, but oxygen inhalation therapy has been used to facilitate resolution of these lesions.[128-130]

ABSCESSES

Although CT is the most definitive radiologic test for diagnosing an abscess, abdominal radiographs may also be helpful in these patients.[124,131,132] An abscess may be manifested by an extraluminal soft tissue mass that displaces adjacent bowel or by an extraluminal collection of gas. The most characteristic finding on abdominal radiographs is a localized, mottled,

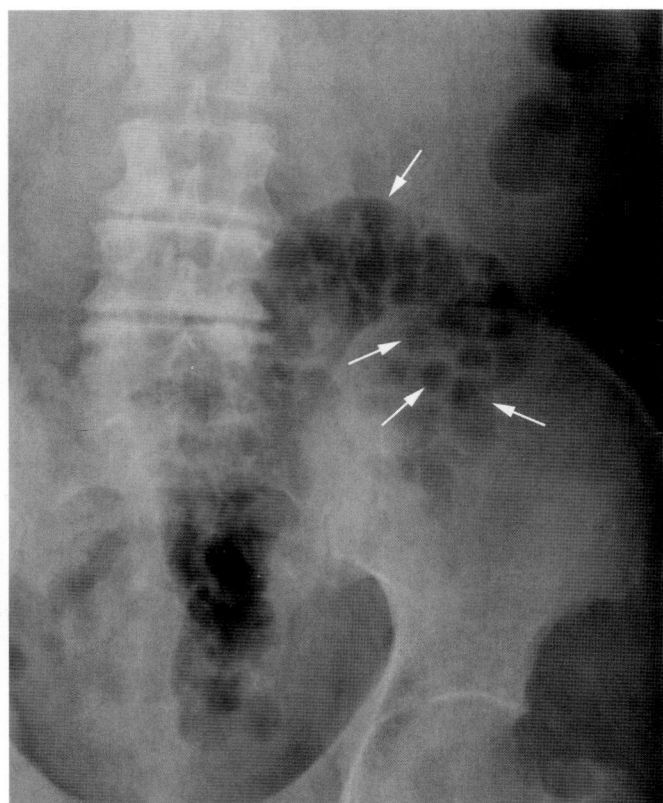

Figure 16-16. Pneumatosis cystoides coli. Multiple rounded, grapelike collections of gas (*arrows*) are seen in the wall of the sigmoid colon in a patient with benign pneumatosis cystoides coli.

or bubbly gas collection (Fig. 16-17). Other patients may have a single, rounded or oval collection of gas with an air-fluid level on horizontal beam views. Fecal material can mimic the appearance of a mottled collection of gas but usually is distinguished by its location within the colon. A gastric bezoar can also mimic an abscess.

Infections of any of the intra-abdominal or retroperitoneal structures can result in the production of gas. Correlation of a linear or bubbly gas collection with knowledge of anatomy is usually sufficient to localize the structure involved. The abdominal radiograph may be the initial study to suggest a gas-forming process, but CT is typically more helpful in assessing the extent of disease and the presence of surrounding pathology.[133]

NORMAL SOFT TISSUE STRUCTURES

The ability to discern the edge of intra-abdominal organs on abdominal radiographs obtained with the patient in a supine position depends on the differences in x-ray attenuation between water density, fat density, and air. Intraperitoneal and retroperitoneal fat are present in varying degrees in even the thinnest patients. The liver, spleen, kidneys, psoas muscles, and urinary bladder can often be readily demonstrated because of surrounding fat (Fig. 16-18). In patients with sufficient fat, the serosal surface of the stomach may also appear as a faint edge. This subtle radiographic observation should not be confused with the much more distinct appearance of the

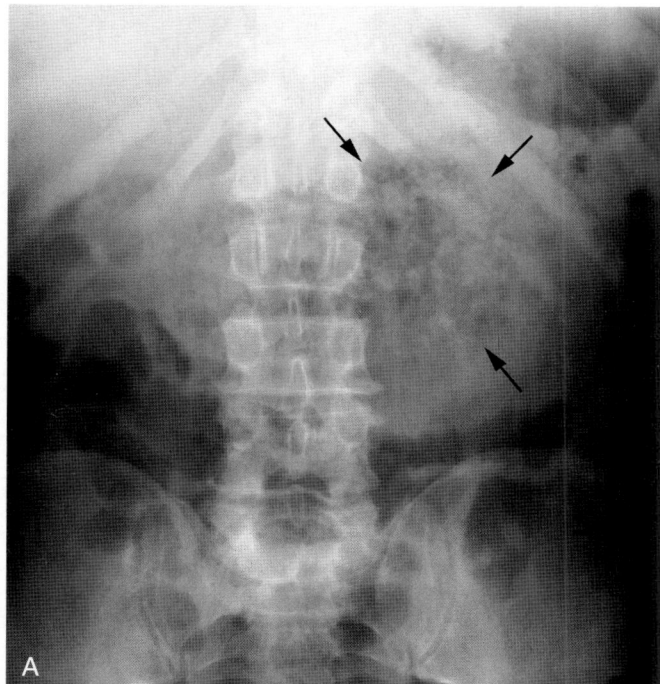

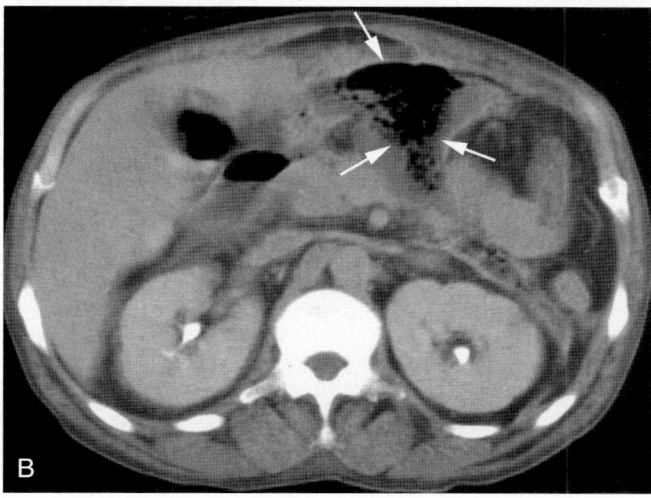

Figure 16-17. Lesser sac abscess secondary to pancreatitis. A. A mottled collection of gas (*arrows*) is present in the upper abdomen. **B.** CT shows gas and fluid (*arrows*) in the abscess cavity in a patient with pancreatitis.

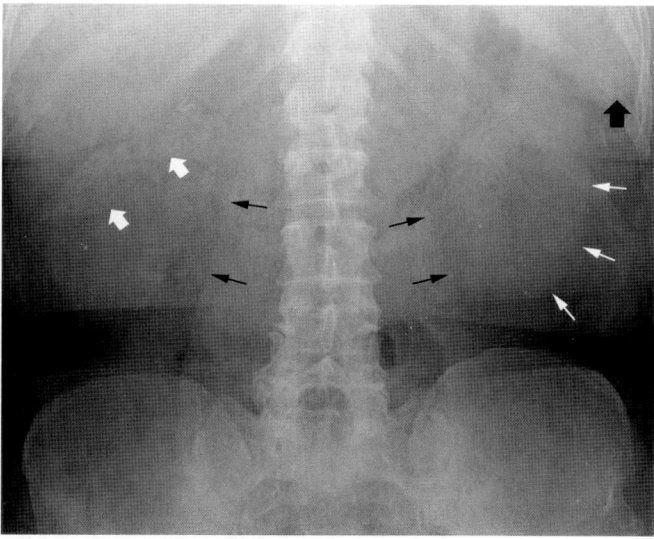

Figure 16-18. Normal soft tissue planes outlined by fat. The liver edge (*large white arrows*), left renal outline (*small white arrows*), margins of the psoas muscles (*small black arrows*), and splenic tip (*large black arrow*) can be identified.

serosa when it is outlined by air in patients with pneumoperitoneum. Fluid-filled loops of small and large bowel may also appear as tubular densities on a backdrop of abdominal fat. Recognition of organs is important because an abnormal contour or size of these organs may be the first indication of intra-abdominal disease.

SOFT TISSUE ABNORMALITIES

Liver

Liver size was estimated on abdominal radiographs by Pfahler as early as 1926.[134] Measurements of the liver from the upright abdominal radiograph have been found to be reliable in detecting hepatomegaly.[135] The inferior tip of the liver usually does not extend below the iliac crest, except in asthenic individuals. Generalized hepatic enlargement tends to displace the hepatic flexure and transverse colon inferiorly and the stomach to the left (Fig. 16-19). Other signs of hepatic enlargement include: (1) displacement of the inferior edge of the liver beyond the right margin of the psoas muscle; (2) displacement of the duodenal bulb below the L2 vertebral body or to the left of the midline; (3) inferior displacement of the right kidney; (4) enlargement or marked rounding of the hepatic angle; (5) elevation of the right hemidiaphragm with decreased motion on normal respiration; (6) inferior displacement of the gastric fundus away from the diaphragm with left lobe enlargement; and (7) anterior displacement of the duodenal bulb on lateral radiographs with caudate lobe enlargement.[136-139] A small liver may result in reversal of some of these findings, with the right kidney higher than the left, the stomach displaced upward and to the right, and the duodenal bulb displaced above the level of the right 12th rib.

Spleen

Brogdon and Cros found that the inferior tip of the spleen could be seen on abdominal radiographs in 44% of patients who had no evidence of splenomegaly.[140] Normally the superior margin of the spleen lies just beneath the left hemidiaphragm and its lateral edge approximates the lateral abdominal wall. As the spleen increases in size, its tip extends inferiorly below the 12th rib (Fig. 16-20). Displacement of the splenic flexure of the colon is an uncommon finding because the splenic flexure usually lies anterior to the spleen. Marked splenomegaly may also displace the stomach medially.

Kidneys

Because of surrounding fat, the renal outlines are visible on the majority of abdominal radiographs. Moel studied 100 men and 100 women between 20 and 49 years of age and found

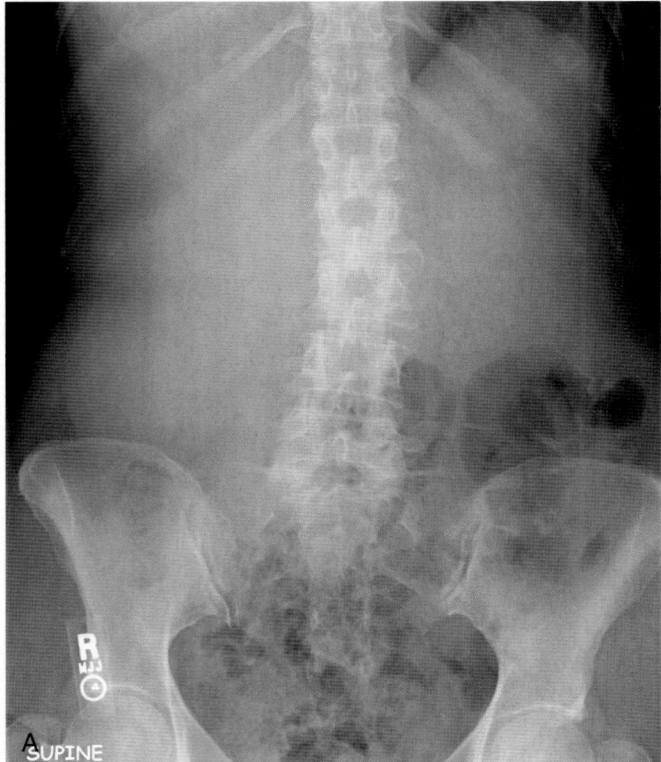

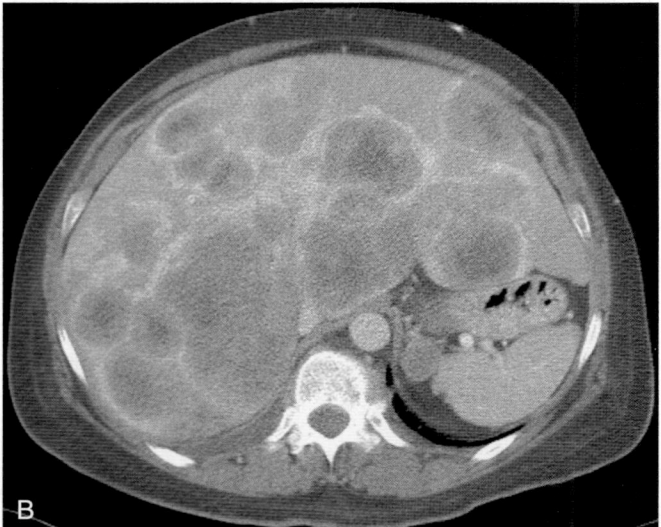

Figure 16-19. Hepatomegaly. A. Marked hepatic enlargement causes increased soft tissue density over the upper abdomen and displacement of bowel inferiorly. **B.** CT shows multiple large metastases throughout the liver.

that the average renal length on abdominal radiographs was 13.0 cm for men and 12.5 cm for women.[141] Estimates of renal size must also take into account the foreshortening of the kidney that occurs because of angulation of this structure in normal individuals. Because of its retroperitoneal location, an enlarged kidney does not displace intra-abdominal organs, except in extreme cases. Renal cysts or tumors that produce contour abnormalities in the kidney may be readily apparent.

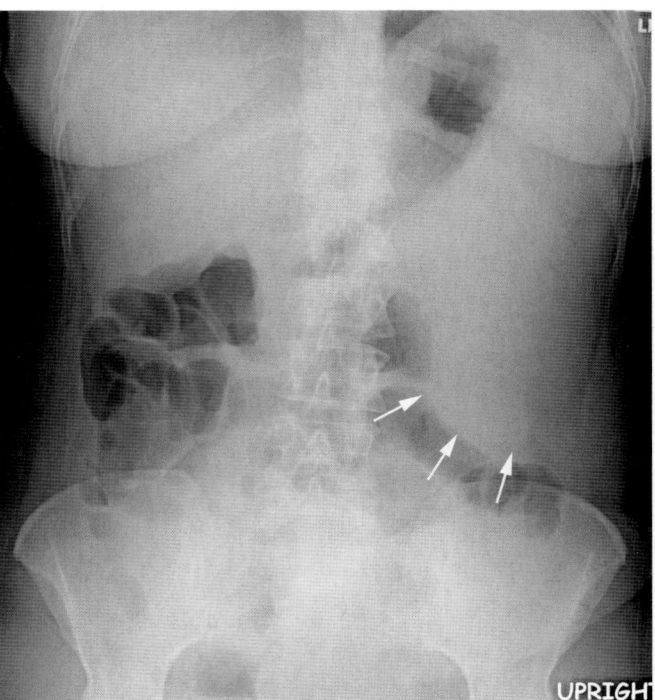

Figure 16-20. Splenomegaly. Supine abdominal radiograph demonstrates marked splenic enlargement (*arrows*) with displacement of bowel inferiorly.

Other Structures

Retroperitoneal fat and intraperitoneal fat that permit visualization of adjacent water-density organs are also helpful for evaluating contiguous pathologic processes in the abdomen. Surrounding inflammation may cause the fat to become edematous, so that it takes in more water and approximates soft tissue density, thus obliterating contiguous planes.

These changes are exemplified in patients with appendicitis. The normal margin of the psoas muscle and the properitoneal fat planes that demarcate the internal oblique, external oblique, and transversalis muscles of the abdomen may become obliterated. Although obliteration of these fat planes is an important sign of inflammation, it seldom occurs as an isolated finding, so that it should be interpreted with caution and in conjunction with other signs of abdominal disease.

Ascites

The widespread use of ultrasound and CT has lessened the emphasis placed on the findings of ascites on abdominal radiographs. It is still important to recognize these signs, however, because abdominal radiography is frequently one of the first imaging studies performed in patients with abdominal distention. In general, only large amounts of ascites can be identified on abdominal radiographs (Fig. 16-21). The following findings for ascites have been described:

1. *Obliteration of the inferior edge of the liver.* This sign can be extremely helpful (see Fig. 16-21A). Proper technique, in which low kilovoltage is used, is essential. The liver edge may be preserved in patients with

3. *Medial displacement of the lateral edge of the liver (Hellmer's sign).* This finding usually requires a large amount of ascites and is more common with malignant ascites than with cirrhosis, probably because the fat content of the cirrhotic liver approximates the density of ascites.[143]
4. *Fluid accumulation in the pelvis.* As the most inferior intraperitoneal recess, the pouch of Douglas, or cul de sac, readily accumulates intraperitoneal fluid. A distended bladder or rectum may impress centrally on this fluid, causing symmetrical bulges that have been described as "dog ears."
5. *Separation of bowel loops.* This sign is seldom an isolated finding and requires a large amount of ascites (see Fig. 16-21A). It can easily be mimicked by a disproportionately large amount of fluid and smaller amount of air in juxtaposed bowel loops.
6. *Centrally located bowel loops with bulging flanks.* With large amounts of ascites, the bowel loops may float to the highest central portion of the abdomen (see Fig. 16-21A).
7. *Ground-glass appearance.* This radiographic finding also requires large amounts of fluid and may erroneously be suggested by improper radiographic technique or marked obesity.

References

1. Baker SR, Cho KC: The Abdominal Plain Film with Correlative Imaging. East Norwalk, CT, Appleton & Lange, 1999.
2. McCort JJ (ed): Abdominal Radiology. Baltimore, Williams & Wilkins, 1981.
3. Welch JP: Bowel Obstruction: Differential Diagnosis and Clinical Management. Philadelphia, WB Saunders, 1990.
4. Goyal RK, Spiro HM: Gastrointestinal manifestations of diabetes mellitus. Med Clin North Am 55:1031-1040, 1971.
5. Seaman WB: Motor dysfunction of the gastrointestinal tract. AJR 116:235-248, 1972.
6. Cantor MO: Ileus. Am J Gastroenterol 47:461-484, 1967.
7. Tibblin S: Diagnosis of intestinal obstruction with special regard to plain roentgen examination of the abdomen. Acta Chir Scand 135:249-252, 1969.
8. Frimann-Dahl J: Roentgen findings in intestinal knots. Acta Radiol 23:22-33, 1942.
9. Holder LE, Schneider HJ: Spigelian hernias: Anatomy and roentgenographic manifestations. Radiology 112:309-313, 1974.
10. Spiers TC, Rosenbloom MB, Palayew MJ: Spigelian hernia: Plain film diagnosis. J Can Assoc Radiol 31:147-148, 1980.
11. Strauss S, Rubinstein ZJ, Shapiro Z: Food as a cause of small intestinal obstruction: A report of five cases without previous gastric surgery. Gastrointest Radiol 2:17-20, 1977.
12. Weissberg DL, Berk RN: Ascariasis of the gastrointestinal tract. Gastrointest Radiol 3:415-418, 1978.
13. Gupta S, Vaidya MP: Mechanical small bowel obstruction caused by acute appendicitis. Am Surg 35:670-674, 1969.
14. Gollub MJ: Multidetector computed tomography enteroclysis of patients with small bowel obstruction: A volume-rendered "surgical perspective." J Comput Assist Tomogr 29:401-407, 2005.
15. Welch CE, Ottinger LW, Welch JP: Manual of Lower Gastrointestinal Surgery. New York, Springer-Verlag, 1980.
16. Phillips RK, Hittinger R, Fry JS, et al: Malignant large bowel obstruction. Br J Surg 72:296-302, 1985.
17. Albers JH, Smith LL, Carter R: Perforation of the cecum. Ann Surg 143:251-255, 1956.
18. Crowder VH Jr, Cohn I Jr: Perforation in cancer of the colon and rectum. Dis Colon Rectum 10:415-420, 1967.
19. Glenn F, McSherry CK: Obstruction and perforation in colorectal cancer. Ann Surg 173:983-992, 1971.
20. Khan S, Pawlak SE, Eggenberger JC, et al: Acute colonic perforation associated with colorectal cancer. Am Surg 67:261-264, 2001.

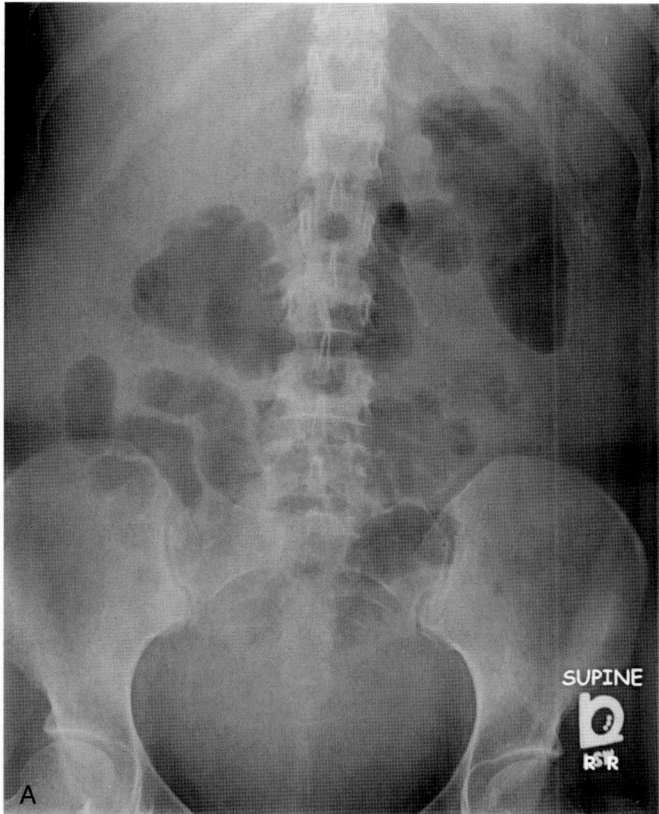
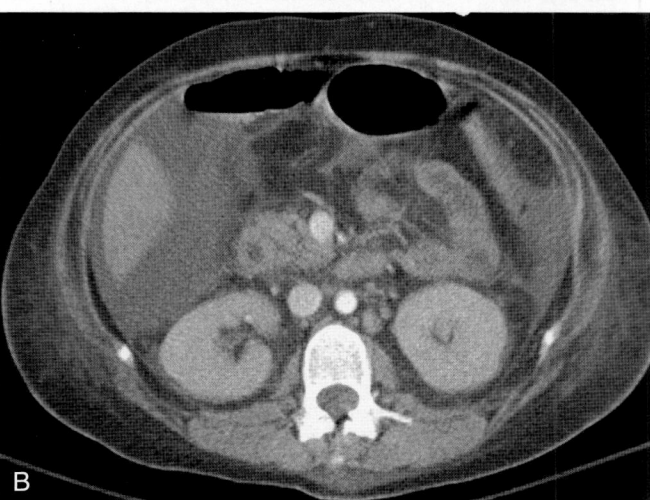

Figure 16-21. Ascites. A. The normal liver edge is obscured. The bowel loops are centrally located in the abdomen, and there is separation of bowel loops. **B.** CT confirms the presence of perihepatic ascites.

loculated ascites, and excessive feces in the hepatic flexure of the colon may falsely obliterate the liver edge.[142]

2. *Widening of the distance between the flank stripe and the ascending colon.* This distance is normally 2 to 3 mm, but it may increase as fluid fills the right paracolic gutter. This finding may be accentuated by placing the patient in a right lateral decubitus position for several minutes.

21. Ogilvie H: Large intestine colic due to sympathetic deprivation. BMJ 2:671-673, 1948.

22. Lescher TJ, Teegarden DK, Pruitt BA: Acute pseudo-obstruction of the colon in thermally injured patients. Dis Colon Rectum 21:618-622, 1978.

23. Caccese WJ, Bronzo RL, Wadler G, et al: Ogilvie's syndrome associated with herpes zoster infection. J Clin Gastroenterol 7:309-313, 1985.

24. Nanni C, Garbini A, Luchett P, et al: Ogilvie's syndrome (acute colonic pseudo-obstruction): review of the literature (October 1948 to March 1980) and report of four additional cases. Dis Colon Rectum 25: 157-166, 1982.

25. Ravo B, Pollane M, Ger R: Pseudo-obstruction of the colon following caesarean section: A review. Dis Colon Rectum 26:440-444, 1983.

26. Nakhgevany KB: Colonoscopic decompression of the colon in patients with Ogilvie's syndrome. Am J Surg 148:317-320, 1984.

27. Shirazi KK, Agha FP, Strodel WE, et al: Nonobstructive colonic dilation: Radiologic findings in 50 patients following colonoscopic treatment. J Can Assoc Radiol 35:116-119, 1984.

28. Strodel WE, Nostrant TT, Eckhauser FE, et al: Therapeutic and diagnostic colonoscopy in nonobstructive colonic dilatation. Ann Surg 197: 416-421, 1983.

29. Fazel A, Verne GN: New solutions to an old problem: Acute colonic pseudo-obstruction. J Clin Gastroenterol 39:17-20, 2005.

30. Saunders MD: Acute colonic pseudoobstruction. Curr Gastroenterol Rep 6:410-416, 2004.

31. Johnson CD, Rice RP, Kelvin FM, et al: The radiological evaluation of gross cecal distensions: Emphasis on cecal ileus. AJR 145:1211-1217, 1985.

32. Ballantyne GH: Review of sigmoid volvulus: Clinical patterns and pathogenesis. Dis Colon Rectum 25:823-830, 1982.

33. Ballantyne GH, Brandner MD, Beart RW Jr, et al: Volvulus of the colon: Incidence and mortality. Ann Surg 202:83-92, 1985.

34. Javors BR, Baker SR, Miller JA: The northern exposure sign: A newly described finding in sigmoid volvulus. AJR 173:571-574, 1999.

35. Newton NA, Reines HD: Transverse colon volvulus: Case reports and review. AJR 128:69-72, 1977.

36. Zinken LD, Katz LD, Rosin JD: Volvulus of the transverse colon: Report of a case and review of the literature. Dis Colon Rectum 22:492-496, 1979.

37. Kerry RL, Ransom HK: Volvulus of the colon: Etiology, diagnosis, and treatment. Arch Surg 99:215-222, 1963.

38. Ballantyne GH: Volvulus of the splenic flexure: Report of a case and review of the literature. Dis Colon Rectum 24:630-632, 1981.

39. Lantieri R, Teplick SK, Labell MJ: Splenic flexure volvulus: Two case reports and review. AJR 132:463-464, 1979.

40. Sachidananthan CK, Soehrer B: Volvulus of the splenic flexure of the colon: Report of a case and review of the literature. Dis Colon Rectum 15:466-469, 1972.

41. Mindelzun RE, Stone JM: Volvulus of the splenic flexure: Radiographic features. Radiology 181:221-223, 1991.

42. Young WS: Further radiological observations in caecal volvulus. Clin Radiol 31:479-483, 1980.

43. Anderson JR, Mills JOM: Cecal volvulus: A frequently missed diagnosis? Clin Radiol 35:65-69, 1985.

44. Yang SH, Lin JK, Lee RC, et al: Cecal volvulus: Report of seven cases and literature review. Zhonghua Yi Xue Za Zhi (Taipei) 63:482-486, 2000.

45. Moore CJ, Corl FM, Fishman EK: CT of cecal volvulus: Unraveling the image. AJR 177:95-98, 2001.

46. Anderson JR, Spence RA, Wilson BG, et al: Gangrenous cecal volvulus after colonoscopy. BMJ 286:439-440, 1983.

47. Hemingway AP: Cecal volvulus—a new twist to the barium enema. Br J Radiol 53:806-807, 1980.

48. Howard RS, Catto J: Cecal volvulus: A case for non-resectional therapy. Arch Surg 115:273-277, 1980.

49. Weinstein M: Volvulus of the cecum and ascending colon. Ann Surg 107:248-259, 1938.

50. Bobroff LM, Messinger NH, Subbarao K, et al: The cecal bascule. AJR 115:249-252, 1972.

51. Campbell JP, Gunn AA: Plain abdominal radiographs and acute abdominal pain. Br J Surg 75:554-556, 1988.

52. Olutola PS: Plain film radiographic diagnosis of acute appendicitis: An evaluation of the signs. Can Assoc Radiol J 39:254-256, 1988.

53. Nitecki S, Karmeli R, Sarr MG: Appendiceal calculi and fecaliths as indications for appendectomy. Surg Gynecol Obstet 171:185-188, 1990.

54. Faegenburg D: Fecaliths of the appendix: Incidence and significance. AJR 89:752-759, 1963.

55. Thomas SF: Appendiceal coproliths: Their surgical importance. Radiology 49:39-49, 1947.

56. Bunch GH, Adcock DF: Giant faceted calculus. Ann Surg 109:143-146, 1939.

57. Lewis FR, Holcroft JW, Boey J, et al: Appendicitis: A critical review of diagnosis and treatment in 1000 cases. Arch Surg 110:677-684, 1975.

58. Mowji PJ, Jones MD, Cohen AJ: Localized ileus of the proximal jejunum: A new sign for acute appendicitis. Gastrointest Radiol 14:173-175, 1989.

59. Hayden CK, Swischuk LE: Appendicitis with perforation: The dilated transverse colon sign. AJR 135:687-689, 1980.

60. Killen DA, Brooks DW Jr: Gas-filled appendix: A roentgen sign of acute appendicitis. Ann Surg 161:474-478, 1965.

61. Lim MS: Gas-filled appendix: Lack of diagnostic specificity. AJR 128: 209-210, 1977.

62. Farman J, Kassner EG, Dallemand S, et al: Pneumoperitoneum and appendicitis. Gastrointest Radiol 1:277-279, 1976.

63. McCort JJ: Extra-alimentary gas in perforated appendicitis: Report of six cases. AJR 77:647-651, 1977.

64. Greenstein AJ, Sachar DB, Gibas A, et al: Outcome of toxic dilatation in ulcerative colitis and Crohn's colitis. J Clin Gastroenterol 7:137-144, 1985.

65. Jalan KN, Sircus W, Card WI, et al: An experience of ulcerative colitis: I. Toxic dilatation in 55 cases. Gastroenterology 8:213-220, 1947.

66. Roys G, Kaplan MS, Juler GL: Surgical management of toxic megacolon. Am J Gastroenterol 68:161-166, 1977.

67. Katzka I, Katz S, Morris E: Management of toxic megacolon: The significance of early recognition in medical management. J Clin Gastroenterol 1:307-311, 1979.

68. Kramer P, Wittenberg J: Colonic gas distribution in toxic megacolon. Gastroenterology 80:433-437, 1981.

69. Norland CC, Kirsner JB: Toxic dilatation of the colon (toxic megacolon): Etiology, treatment and prognosis in 42 patients. Medicine (Baltimore) 48:229-250, 1969.

70. Halpert RD: Toxic dilatation of the colon. Radiol Clin North Am 25: 147-155, 1987.

71. Greenstein AJ, Aufses AH: Differences in pathogenesis, incidence and outcome of perforation in inflammatory bowel disease. Surg Gynecol Obstet 160:63-69, 1985.

72. Caprilli R, Vernia P, Latella G, et al: Early recognition of toxic megacolon. J Clin Gastroenterol 9:160-164, 1987.

73. Wolf BS, Marshak RH: Toxic segmental dilatation of the colon during the course of fulminating ulcerative colitis: Roentgen findings. AJR 82:985-995, 1959.

74. Imbriaco M, Balthazar EJ: Toxic megacolon: Role of CT evaluation and detection of complications. Clin Imaging 25:349-354, 2001.

75. Miller RE, Nelson SW: The roentgenological demonstration of tiny amounts of free intraperitoneal gas: Experimental and clinical studies. AJR 112:574-585, 1971.

76. Miller RE, Becker GJ, Slabaugh RA: Detection of pneumoperitoneum: Optimum body position and respiratory phase. AJR 135:487-490, 1980.

77. Woodring JH, Heiser MJ: Detection of pneumoperitoneum on chest radiographs: Comparison of upright lateral and posteroanterior projections. AJR 165:45-47, 1995.

78. Stapakis JC, Thickman D: Diagnosis of pneumoperitoneum: Abdominal CT vs. upright chest film. J Comput Assist Tomogr 16:713-716, 1992.

79. Earls JP, Dachman AH, Colon E, et al: Prevalence and duration of postoperative pneumoperitoneum: Sensitivity of CT vs. left lateral decubitus radiography. AJR 161:781-785, 1993.

80. Levine MS, Scheiner JD, Rubesin SE, et al: Diagnosis of pneumoperitoneum on supine abdominal radiographs. AJR 156:731-735, 1991.

81. Rigler LG: Spontaneous pneumoperitoneum: A roentgenologic sign found in supine position. Radiology 37:604-607, 1941.

82. Cho KC, Baker SR, Lum C, Javors BR: Pneumoperitoneum: New observations on plain films and CT scans [abstract]. In Selected Scientific Exhibits in Gastrointestinal Radiology: RSNA 1996. RadioGraphics 17(Suppl 2):1616-1620, 1997.

83. Mindelzun RE, McCort JJ: Cupola sign of pneumoperitoneum in the supine patient. Gastrointest Radiol 11:283-285, 1986.

84. Cho KC, Baker SR: Depiction of diaphragmatic muscle slips on supine plain radiographs: A sign of pneumoperitoneum. Radiology 203: 431-433, 1997.

85. Hajdu N, de Lacy G: The Rutherford Morison pouch: A characteristic appearance on abdominal radiographs. Br J Radiol 43:706-709, 1970.

86. Brill PW, Olson SR, Winchester P: Neonatal necrotizing enterocolitis: Air in Morison pouch. Radiology 174:469-471, 1990.

87. Menuck L, Siemers PT: Pneumoperitoneum: Importance of right upper quadrant features. AJR 127:753-756, 1976.
88. Radin R, Van Allan RJ, Rosen RS: The visible gallbladder: A plain film sign of pneumoperitoneum. AJR 167:69-70, 1996.
89. Jelaso DV, Schultz EH Jr: The urachus—an aid to the diagnosis of pneumoperitoneum. Radiology 92:295-296, 1969.
90. Weiner CI, Diaconis JN, Dennis JM: The "inverted V": A new sign of pneumoperitoneum. Radiology 107:47-48, 1973.
91. Cho KC, Baker SR: Air in the fissure for the ligamentum teres: New sign of intraperitoneal air on plain radiographs. Radiology 178:489-492, 1991.
92. Cho KC, Baker SR: Visualization of the extrahepatic segment of the ligamentum teres: A sign of free air on plain radiographs. Radiology 202:651-654, 1997.
93. Miller RE: Perforated viscus in infants: A new roentgen sign. Radiology 74:65-67, 1960.
94. Walker LA, Weens HS: Radiological observations on the lesser peritoneal sac. Radiology 80:727-737, 1963.
95. Meyers MA: Radiological features of the spread and localization of extraperitoneal gas and their relationship to its source: An anatomical approach. Radiology 111:17-26, 1974.
96. Walker CW, Purnell GL, Diner WC: Complications from extravasated retroperitoneal barium: Case report and review of the literature. Radiology 173:618-620, 1989.
97. Beerman PJ, Gelfand DW, Ott DJ: Pneumomediastinum after double-contrast barium enema examination: A sign of colonic perforation. AJR 136:197-198, 1981.
98. Peterson N, Rohrmann CA Jr, Lennard ES: Diagnosis and treatment of retroperitoneal perforation complicating double-contrast barium enema examination. Radiology 144:249-252, 1982.
99. Balthazar EJ, Gurkin S: Cholecystoenteric fistulas: Significance and radiographic diagnosis. Am J Gastroenterol 65:168-173, 1976.
100. Balthazar EJ, Schecter LS: Air in gallbladder: a frequent finding in gallstone ileus. AJR 131:219-222, 1978.
101. Ulreich S, Massi J: Recurrent gallstone ileus. AJR 133:921-923, 1979.
102. Rigler LG, Borman DN, Noble JF: Gallstone obstruction: Pathogenesis and roentgen manifestations. JAMA 117:1753-1759, 1941.
103. Cremin BJ: Biliary parasites. Br J Radiol 42:506-508, 1969.
104. Mindelzun R, McCort JJ: Hepatic and perihepatic radiolucencies. Radiol Clin North Am 18:221-238, 1980.
105. Govoni AF, Meyers MD: Pseudopneumobilia. Radiology 118:526, 1976.
106. Halber MD, Daffner RH: Fat in the intrahepatic fissure. AJR 132:842-843, 1979.
107. Susman N, Senturia HR: Gas embolization of the portal venous system. AJR 83:847-850, 1960.
108. Sisk PB: Gas in the portal venous system. Radiology 77:103-107, 1981.
109. McClandless RL: Portal vein gas: A grave prognostic sign. AJR 92:1162-1165, 1964.
110. Benson MD: Adult survival with intrahepatic portal venous gas secondary to acute gastric dilatation, with a review of portal venous gas. Clin Radiol 36:441-443, 1985.
111. Graham GA, Bernstein RB, Gronner AT: Gas in the portal and inferior mesenteric veins caused by diverticulitis of the sigmoid colon: Report of a case with survival. Radiology 114:601-602, 1975.
112. Stein MG, Cruez JV III, Hamlin JA: Portal venous air associated with barium enema. AJR 140:1171-1172, 1983.
113. Birnberg FA, Gore RM, Shragg B, et al: Hepatic portal venous gas: A benign finding in a patient with ulcerative colitis. J Clin Gastroenterol 5:89-91, 1983.
114. Sadler VK, Brennan RE, Madan V: Portal vein gas following air-contrast barium enema in granulomatous colitis: Report of a case. Gastrointest Radiol 4:163-164, 1979.
115. Haber I: Hepatic portal vein gas following colonoscopy in ulcerative colitis—report of a case. Acta Gastroenterol Belg 46:14-17, 1983.
116. Chezmar JL, Nelson RC, Bernardino ME: Portal venous gas after hepatic transplantation: Sonographic detection and clinical significance. AJR 153:1203-1205, 1989.
117. Marks WM, Filly RA: Computed tomographic demonstration of intra-arterial air following hepatic artery ligation. Radiology 132:665-666, 1979.
118. Pear BL: Pneumatosis intestinalis: A review. Radiology 207:13-19, 1998.
119. Tomchik FS, Wittenberg J, Ottinger LW: The roentgenographic spectrum of bowel infarction. Radiology 96:249-260, 1970.
120. Smerud MJ, Johnson CD, Stephens DH: Diagnosis of bowel infarction: A comparison of plain films and CT scans in 23 cases. AJR 154:99-103, 1990.
121. Lund EC, Han SY, Holley HC, et al: Intestinal ischemia: Comparison of plain radiographic and computed tomographic findings. RadioGraphics 8:1083-1108, 1988.
122. Kernagis LY, Levine MS, Jacobs JE: Pneumatosis intestinalis in patients with ischemia: Correlation of CT finding with viability of the bowel. AJR 180:733-736, 2003.
123. Wiesner W, Koenraad J, Mortele JN, et al: Pneumatosis intestinalis and portomesenteric venous gas in intestinal ischemia. AJR 177:1319-1323, 2003.
124. Zweig GJ, Yuk-Pui L, Srinantaswamy S, et al: Gas forming infections of the abdomen: plain film findings. Appl Radiol 19:37-42, 1990.
125. Shipman PJ, Drury P: Emphysematous gastritis: Case report and literature review. Australas Radiol 45:64-66, 2001.
126. Berens SV, Moskowitz H, Mellins HZ: Air within the wall of the stomach: Roentgen manifestations and a new roentgenographic sign. AJR 103:310-313, 1968.
127. Seaman WB, Fleming RJ: Intramural gastric emphysema. AJR 101:431-436, 1967.
128. Marshak RH, Lindner AE, Milano AM: Pneumatosis coli. Am J Gastroenterol 56:68-73, 1971.
129. Bloch C: The natural history of pneumatosis coli. Radiology 123:311-314, 1977.
130. Simons NM, Hyman KE, Divertie MB, et al: Pneumatosis cystoides intestinalis: Treatment with oxygen via close-fitting mask. JAMA 231:1354-1356, 1975.
131. Sands WW: Extraluminal localized gas vesicles: An aid in the diagnosis of abdominal abscesses from plain roentgenograms. AJR 74:195-203, 1955.
132. Rice RP, Masters SJ: Intraabdominal abscess. Semin Roentgenol 8:365-374, 1973.
133. Grayson DE, Abbott RM, Levy AD, et al: Emphysematous infections of the abdomen and pelvis: A pictorial review. RadioGraphics 22:543-561, 2002.
134. Pfahler GE: Measurement of the liver by means of roentgen rays based upon a study of 502 subjects. AJR 16:558-564, 1926.
135. Unal B, Bilgili E, Kocacikli S, et al: Simple evaluation of liver size on erect abdominal plain radiography. Clin Radiol 59:1132-1135, 2004.
136. Gelfand DW: The liver: Plain film diagnosis. Semin Roentgenol 10:177-185, 1975.
137. Chon H, Arger PH, Miller WT: Displacement of duodenum by an enlarged liver. AJR 119:85-88, 1987.
138. Kattan KR, Moskowitz M: Position of the duodenal bulb and liver size. AJR 119:78-84, 1973.
139. Whalen JP, Evans JA, Meyers MS: Vector principle in the differential diagnosis of abdominal masses: II. Right upper quadrant. AJR 115:318-333, 1972.
140. Brogdon BG, Cros NE: Observations on the "normal" spleen. Radiology 72:412-414, 1959.
141. Moel H: Size of the normal kidneys. Acta Radiol Diagn 46:640, 1956.
142. Proto AV, Lane EJ: Visualization of differences in soft tissue densities: The liver in ascites. Radiology 121:19-23, 1976.
143. Wixson D, Kazam E, Whalen JP: Displaced lateral surface of the liver (Hellmer's sign) secondary to an extraperitoneal fluid collection. AJR 127:679-682, 1976.

Abdominal Calcifications

Stephen R. Baker, MD

The abdomen is a closely packed space containing numerous conduits and organs related to each other in a complex spatial arrangement. Each of these structures is subject to a unique range of diseases, all having specific causes and characteristic manifestations. However, the spectrum of findings on abdominal radiographs is surprisingly limited. Important signs include displacement, enlargement, or atrophy of organs; distention of bowel; extraluminal gas; and calcification in parenchymal and supporting tissues. In many cases, the pattern of calcium deposition is the most informative and distinctive radiographic finding.

Calcification may occur in the wall of blood vessels or other conduits, the lumen of hollow structures, and the solid substance of viscera or neoplasms. Despite the variety of causes of abdominal calcification, a systematic evaluation of the morphologic features, location, and mobility of an abnormal opacity usually narrows the diagnostic considerations to just a few likely possibilities. In many instances, analysis of the appearance of an abdominal calcification on abdominal radiographs provides sufficient information for an unequivocal diagnosis without need for additional examinations. In other cases, careful assessment of the morphology, location, and mobility of an abdominal calcification helps focus the choice and sequence of subsequent imaging examinations.

PHYSIOLOGY

The precipitation of calcareous substances requires an alkaline medium and high local concentrations of ionic calcium. The term *metastatic calcification* refers to the deposition of calcium salts in normal tissues as the result of hypercalcemia and an elevated pH. Although the stomach and kidneys are the most frequent sites of metastatic calcification in the abdomen, the degree of parenchymal opacification in these organs is usually too faint to be detected on abdominal radiographs. The most common cause of radiographically detectable metastatic calcification is chronic renal failure with secondary hyperparathyroidism.[1] As a result of this pathologic process, diffuse opacification of the kidneys is often accompanied by osteomalacia or osteoporosis.

The term *dystrophic calcification* refers to a phenomenon, far more frequent than metastatic calcification, that occurs despite normal serum levels of calcium. Dystrophic calcification may be caused by trauma, ischemia, infarction, or other pathologic processes resulting in a predisposition to calcium deposition. In some tumors, the rapid breakdown of lipids releases fatty acids that bind calcium with particular avidity. Mucin-producing adenocarcinomas of the gastrointestinal tract possess a glycoprotein that is similar in chemical configuration to cartilage and shares with it an affinity for calcium aggregation.[2] Although some structures in the abdomen have a propensity for dystrophic calcification, the mechanisms and kinetics of calcium deposition have not been fully elucidated.

Some devitalized or degenerative tissues are also associated with new bone formation. However, ossification is less common than dystrophic calcification. Calcified osteoid may be found as an isolated finding, or it may coexist with adjacent areas of calcium deposition that lack the histologic structure of bone. In either case, local tissue damage appears to be the precipitating factor. Ossification may occur in ovarian or retroperitoneal teratomas (Fig. 17-1), abdominal scars, particularly after gastric surgery or suprapubic bladder catheterization, and, rarely, colonic and retroperitoneal neoplasms.

Papillary serous cystadenocarcinomas of the ovary often contains a distinctive form of calcification that is characterized by a psammomatous or cloudlike opacity attributable to intracellular deposition of calcium salts in the lesion (Fig. 17-2).[3] In contrast, dystrophic calcification associated with other metastatic tumors is caused by extracellular precipitation of calcium salts. Both psammomatous and dystrophic calcification may be manifested by amorphous, poorly outlined areas of increased density. With such a finding,

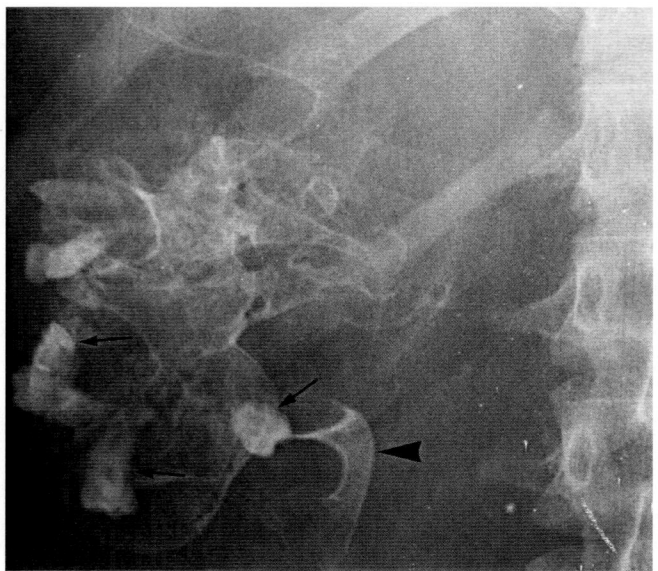

Figure 17-1. Retroperitoneal teratoma. Both teeth *(arrows)* and bone *(arrowhead)* are visualized. Note the cortex and trabecula in the disordered pattern of ossification.

the distribution pattern of calcified metastases may narrow the differential diagnosis, often leading to an unequivocal diagnosis.

MORPHOLOGY

The recognition of specific abdominal calcifications has been aided by the attribution of vivid, descriptive names to particular radiopacities. For example, a "staghorn calculus" is a large,

branching opacity in the renal pelvis. Such appellations are highly evocative and easily remembered; however, they do not help generate a differential diagnosis from among the many causes of abdominal calcification. Unfortunately, most surveys of abdominal calcification have relied primarily on such descriptive designations and have failed to emphasize diagnostic features that might help to organize the various opacities into categories with shared characteristics.

In this chapter, a logical scheme is presented for classifying almost all abdominal calcifications. They may be distinguished radiographically on the basis of various morphologic features, including contour, border, sharpness, marginal continuity, and internal architecture. Consideration of these features permits a grouping of calcifications into one of four classes: (1) concretions; (2) conduit wall calcification; (3) cystic calcification; and (4) solid mass calcification. In the following sections, the distinguishing features of each class are discussed in detail. Potential pitfalls and notable exceptions are also considered.

Concretions

Concretions are precipitates removed from solution in a liquid medium inside a vessel or hollow viscus. They often contain a central nidus, composed of an insoluble substance such as an inorganic foreign body, ingested vegetable matter, thrombus, or focal collection of pus and cellular debris. In pelvic veins and in the gastrointestinal and genitourinary tracts, concretions are likely to calcify. They can be brightly or faintly opaque; the radiographic density depends on the size of the opacity and the amount of calcium per unit volume. Concretions do not have a common shape. Biliary calculi are usually oval or rounded, whereas gallstones are often faceted (Fig. 17-3). Ureteral and pancreatic stones often have jagged edges, but in hollow viscera such as the urinary bladder and gallbladder, the concretions usually have smooth margins.

A sharply defined, continuous external margin is a unifying feature of concretions. Stones are almost always characterized

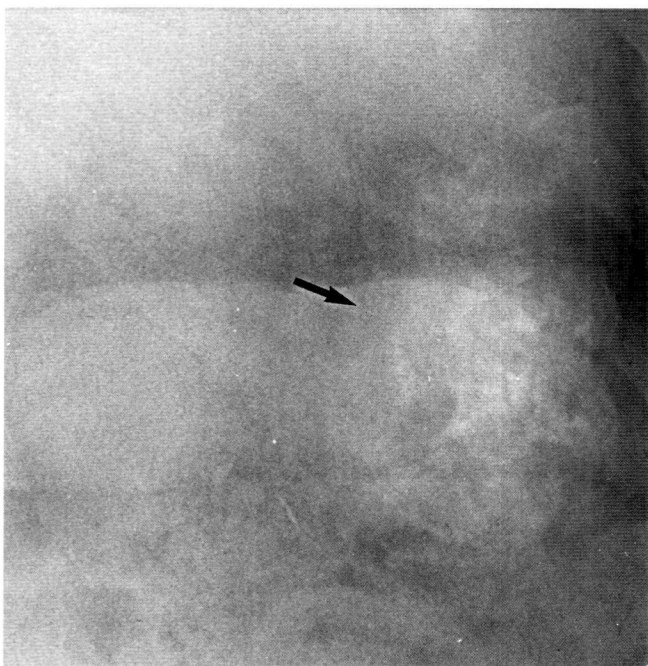

Figure 17-2. Ovarian papillary serous cystadenocarcinoma. Patches of psammomatous calcification *(arrow)* are seen in the left abdomen in an intraperitoneal metastasis.

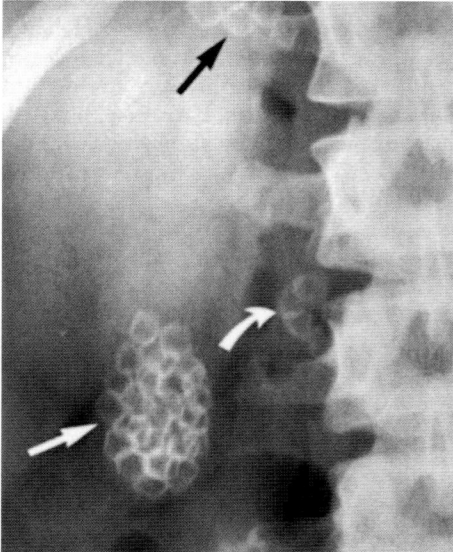

Figure 17-3. Biliary stones. Numerous stones are seen in the gallbladder *(straight white arrow)*, cystic duct *(black arrow)*, and common bile duct *(curved white arrow)*. Note how the stones have faceted margins.

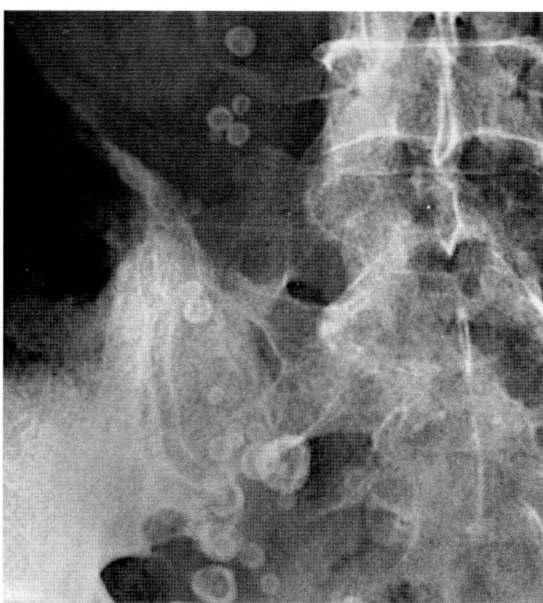

Figure 17-4. Ovarian vein phleboliths. Numerous phleboliths, each having a central lucency, are located within a dilated right ovarian vein.

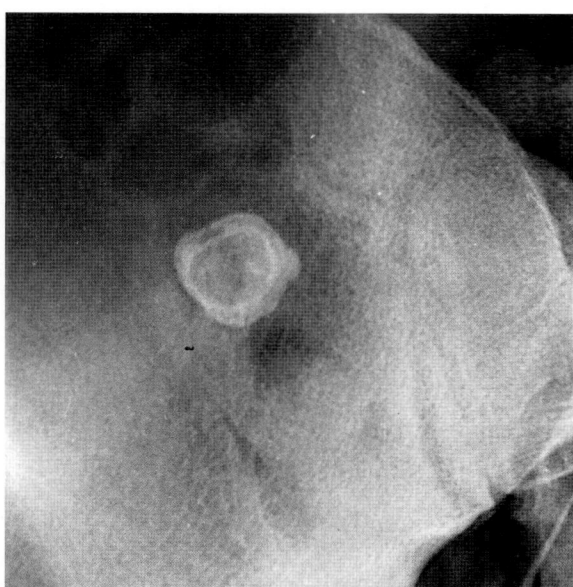

Figure 17-5. Lamellated appendicolith. Note the continuous margin of calcification, the parallel lamina, and a small medial bulge along the edge of this concretion.

by an uninterrupted edge of calcification throughout their entire perimeter, with no lucent gaps along the interface with the surrounding medium. This unique feature permits differentiation of small stones with radiolucent centers from calcified vessels seen on end. The circumferential opacification of the perimeter of large stones also helps distinguish them from calcified cysts.

Concretions may vary greatly in their internal architecture. A stone may be homogeneously dense, a pattern often encountered in urinary calculi, or it may contain a slightly eccentric area of lucency, an appearance typical of phleboliths (Fig. 17-4). Concentric laminations are characteristic of gallstones, bladder concretions, and appendicoliths (Fig. 17-5). Each of these various internal configurations has a certain predictability and uniformity. A central lucency is often present. Stones seldom have a mottled, speckled, or patchy appearance. The deposition of calcium on only one surface of the stone is extremely rare.

Unlike calcified solid lesions or cysts, which are pathologic tumefactions that distort or displace normal organs and supporting structures, stones tend to be confined within preexisting vessels or fluid-filled viscera. When multiple stones are present, they may outline the course of a hollow tube or the dimensions of a distensible reservoir. Concretions appearing outside expected anatomic locations are unusual; examples are multiple phleboliths in a hemangioma, ectopic gallstones in the distal small bowel, and appendicoliths from a ruptured appendix in the peritoneal cavity.

Conduit Wall Calcification

Conduits are fluid-conducting hollow tubes. In the abdomen, they include the ureter, urethra, vas deferens, pancreatic ducts, bile ducts, and vascular structures. The vast majority of conduit wall calcifications are located in the aorta and its branches. The tubular configuration characteristic of conduits

is readily appreciated if the calcification is extensive and circumferential. When the vessel is parallel to the radiographic beam, a ringlike density is often observed (Fig. 17-6). In contrast to calculi, conduit wall calcifications often have gaps in the opaque ring. Because calcification in conduit walls is not uniform, alternating radiopaque and radiolucent areas may be seen along the course of the vessel. Internal radiopacities are not a feature of conduit wall calcifications, so that the presence of central radiopaque areas brighter than the periphery of the agglomeration of a radiodensity should suggest another class of abdominal calcifications. Even when there is profuse mural calcification, the lateral walls of the conduit provide a longer path for the x-ray beam to traverse than either the anterior or posterior walls, so that they appear more opaque than the vessel wall oriented en face. As a result, a conduit wall calcification is usually manifested by parallel, linear opacities

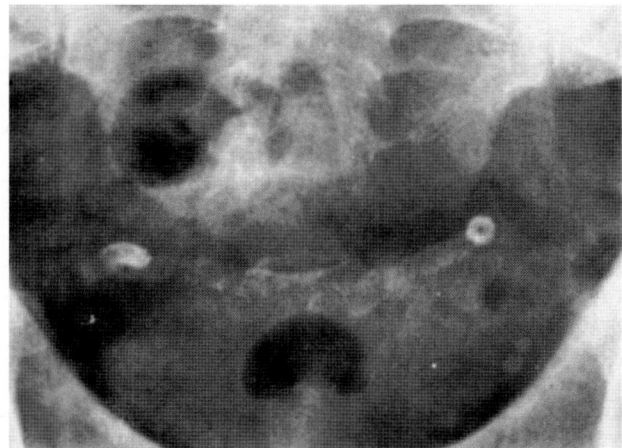

Figure 17-6. Conduit wall calcification in the vas deferens. Marginal opacities are seen en face and in profile.

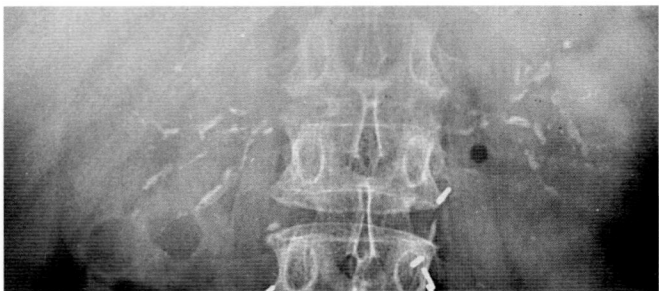

Figure 17-7. Calcification of the renal arteries and their intrarenal branches. These opacities have the typical configuration of conduit wall calcification.

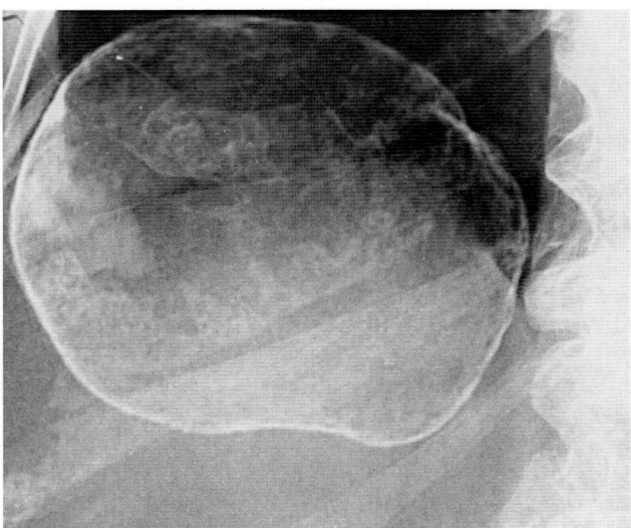

Figure 17-8. Large echinococcus cyst in the liver. Note how the calcified wall of the cyst is flattened inferiorly.

when the vessel is aligned along the course of the x-ray beam or by a circle of radiopacity when the beam is directed perpendicular to the course of the conduit. A marginal branching pattern may be observed at the bifurcation of the abdominal aorta or in the intrarenal arteries (Fig. 17-7). Calcification of narrow-caliber vessels occasionally produces a stringlike appearance. In the female pelvis, calcification of the uterine artery may be evident by a horizontal or slightly undulating linear opacity or by a series of curvilinear, stringlike densities.

Conduit wall calcification is clearly distinguishable only if deposition of calcium is extensive. A single fleck of calcification can simulate a small calculus or even a thin piece of cortical bone, particularly in the renal pelvis. Conversely, the lateral margin of the transverse process of a lumbar vertebra can mimic calcification in the renal artery. However, the lateral margin of the transverse process has a vertical orientation, whereas the renal artery is oriented horizontally (see Fig. 17-7).

Conduit wall calcification is usually found at the expected location of vessels. Thus, it is not seen at the lateral margin of the spleen or in other peripheral locations. As arteries become tortuous and dilated, however, their walls may eventually be displaced several centimeters or more from their expected location. Hence, the wall of a dilated, calcified aorta may be seen to overlie the midline, or even to lie to the right of the spine, on abdominal radiographs.

Cystic Calcification

Cystic calcification is characterized by the deposition of calcium in the wall of abnormal fluid-filled masses, a category encompassing true epithelial cysts, pseudocysts, and aneurysmally dilated arteries. Despite the diversity of cystic structures in the abdomen, cystic calcification exhibits remarkably uniform radiographic findings.

A cystic pattern of calcification is characterized by the presence of a smooth, arcuate rim of radiopacity in the wall of the cyst (Fig. 17-8). Although opacities may be present in both cysts and conduits, the calcified rims of nearly all cysts have a larger diameter than that of most conduits. Unlike stones, this calcified rim is often incomplete, and in many cases only a small section of the wall contains radiographically visible calcium. Moreover, morphologically uncomplicated cysts have only a single encircling wall, so that when calcified, they do not have a laminated appearance. Cysts need not be perfectly round; some can be compressed on one side, producing an ovoid configuration (see Fig. 17-8).

The configuration of cysts depends on their location. They may displace and distort adjacent structures, or they themselves may be displaced by nearby solid organs or vessels. Usually, the differentiation of cystic calcification from the diffuse opacification of solid masses is not difficult. Nevertheless, solid uterine leiomyomas may contain curvilinear calcifications at their margins, mimicking the appearance of cystic calcification.

Unlike concretions and conduit wall calcifications, which appear at expected locations, the cystic pattern of calcification may be found almost anywhere in the abdomen. Cystic calcification most commonly occurs in abdominal aortic aneurysms. It is usually associated with conduit wall calcification in contiguous sections of the aorta and in the common iliac arteries. Cystic calcification may also occur in aneurysms of the splenic artery in the left upper quadrant. Also, cystic calcification is encountered in a variety of urinary tract lesions, including aneurysms of the renal artery, echinococcus cysts, perirenal hematomas, multicystic kidneys, adrenal cysts, and renal carcinomas. Echinococcus cysts are the most common cause of cystic calcification in the liver, but a calcified gallbladder (i.e., a "porcelain" gallbladder) may occasionally produce similar findings.[1] Other causes of cystic calcification in the lower abdomen include mesenteric cysts, calcified appendiceal mucoceles, and calcified benign tumors of the ovary.

Solid Mass Calcification

Of all the classes of abdominal calcification, solid mass calcification includes the greatest variety of pathologic abnormalities. Solid masses may appear as mottled densities with scattered radiolucencies on a calcified background, an appearance typical of calcified mesenteric lymph nodes (Fig. 17-9). A whorled configuration with incomplete bands and arcs of calcification is a feature of uterine leiomyomas. Calcified leiomyomas may also be manifested by numerous flocculent densities superimposed on a radiolucent background. Solid calcifications share the unifying feature of a nongeometric inner architecture and an irregular, often incomplete margin.

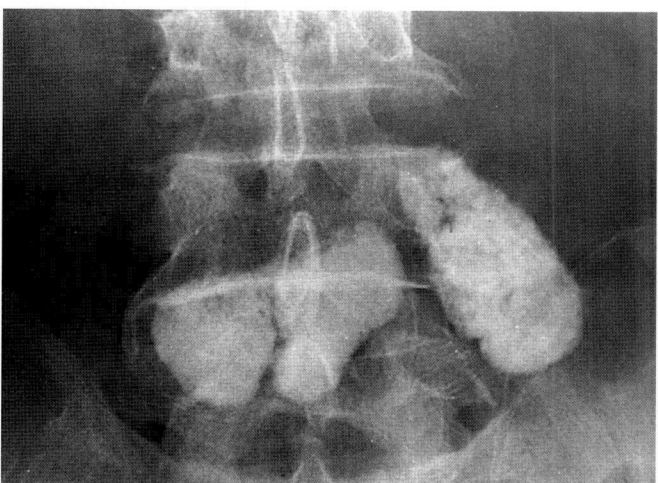

Figure 17-9. Calcified mesenteric nodes. Mottled interior and slightly irregular margins are typical of lymph node calcification.

Calcified solid masses can be located anywhere in the abdomen. Calcified mesenteric lymph nodes are usually found in middle-aged or elderly individuals who at one time in life were infected by tuberculosis even if they are now purified protein derivative negative and exhibit no other manifestations of the disease. They tend to be located in a broad arc along the course of the mesentery of the small bowel from the left upper quadrant to the right lower quadrant of the abdomen. Multiple calcified nodes are often present, and individual nodes may vary widely in diameter.

Uterine leiomyomas are the most common calcified solid masses in the female pelvis. Some patients have multiple leiomyomas that may become calcified as they grow to enormous sizes (Fig. 17-10). Although leiomyomas are usually located in the pelvis, they may occasionally be found almost anywhere in the abdomen (Fig. 17-11).

All other types of solid mass calcification are much less common than calcified mesenteric lymph nodes or calcified uterine leiomyomas. A solid pattern of calcification may occa-

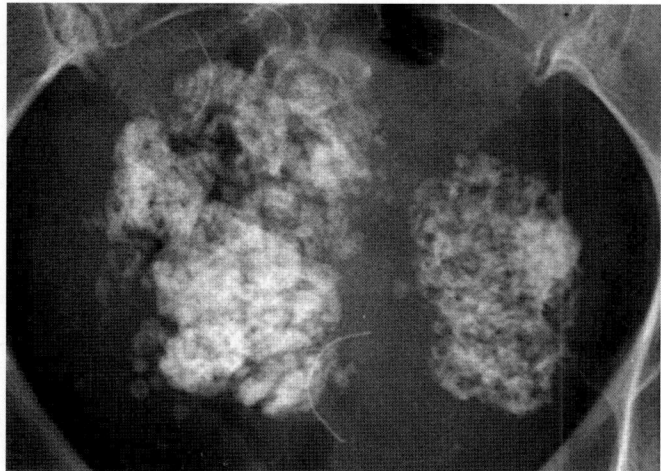

Figure 17-10. Calcified uterine leiomyomas. Two uterine fibroids are manifested by poorly defined, flocculent calcifications, admixed with irregular lucencies.

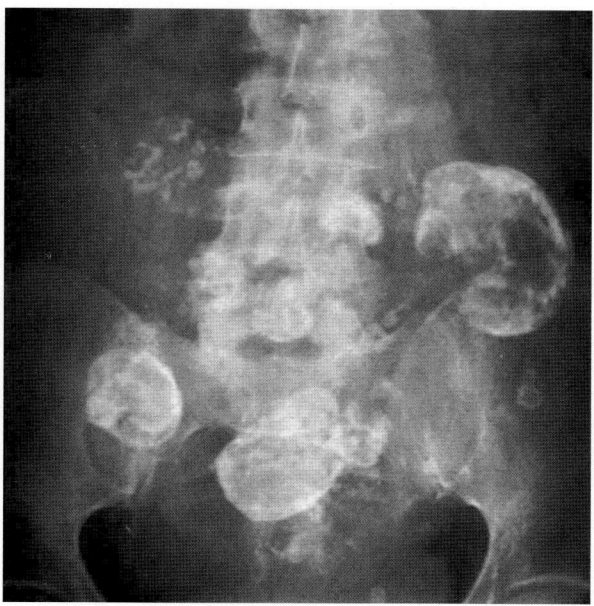

Figure 17-11. Multiple calcified leiomyomas. This patient has different patterns of calcification in leiomyomas extending from the pelvis to the midabdomen.

sionally be found in adenomas, hamartomas, and carcinomas of the kidney as well as in tuberculous and chronic pyogenic abscesses of the kidney. Calcified pancreatic masses are rare and are usually associated with benign or malignant cyst-adenomas. Small discretely outlined, calcified densities in the liver and spleen most often represent granulomas. In contra-distinction, poorly defined radiopaque areas in the liver should be considered an indication of calcified metastases from colonic carcinoma until proved otherwise.

Difficulty in Classification

This classification scheme can be applied broadly to determine the nature of most abdominal calcifications. However, some cannot be separated into one of the four classes. If the density is too faint to have a definite inner architecture or margin, morphologic analysis is not possible. In addition, if the calcification is extremely small, a concretion may be difficult to distinguish from a solid opacity. Other calcifications may have an appearance suggestive of more than one morphologic class. For example, a collection of pancreatic stones clustered together may resemble a solid mass, although the area of radiopacity actually represents innumerable intra-ductal concretions with irregular margins (Fig. 17-12). Thus, one must be aware of potential pitfalls in the classification of abdominal calcifications. Nevertheless, a specific abdominal calcification can usually be classified into one of the four morphologic categories with a reasonable degree of confidence.

LOCATION

The location of abdominal radiopacities also provides important clues about their identity. Most calcifications in the right upper quadrant are related to the gallbladder or right kidney. Gallstones are often multiple and are frequently laminated. Gallbladder wall calcification is much less common but can

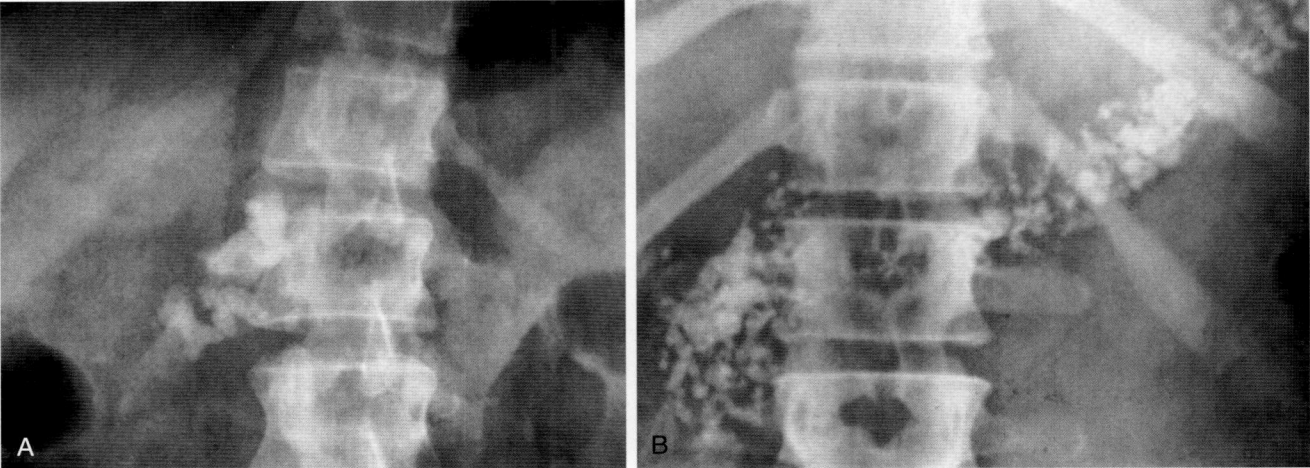

Figure 17-12. Two calcification patterns in pancreatic lithiasis. A. A conglomerate of stones filling larger ducts in the pancreatic head could be mistaken for calcification in conduits. **B.** Pancreatic stones can be seen throughout the pancreas. Each stone is located within a duct, but the cumulative appearance suggests diffuse acinar opacification.

be clearly recognized by its marginal arcuate configuration. A transverse orientation and conduit morphologic features indicate calcification of the renal artery. Stones in the renal pelvis and ureters have a range of specific appearances and are oriented along the course of the urinary tract.

In both upper quadrants, adrenal calcification may assume various forms, including the solid opacities of calcified granulomas and the eggshell calcification of cysts and pheochromocytomas. Multiple calcifications crossing the midline of the upper abdomen are characteristic of pancreatic lithiasis. Calcified mesenteric lymph nodes may also cross the midline but are usually situated more inferiorly, along an oblique path extending from the left midabdomen to the right lower quadrant.

Appendicoliths typically appear as a single or a tight grouping of several laminated calcifications in the right lower quadrant. However, the appendix may be located anywhere between the lower pelvis and the right upper quadrant, so that the diagnosis of an appendicolith should not be excluded simply because the concretion is found at a considerable distance from its expected location in the right iliac fossa.

In the lower abdomen and pelvis, calcifications that appear as concretions should arouse suspicion of ureteral calculi; however, a small ureteral stone is often difficult to distinguish from a phlebolith on a single radiograph. Reference should therefore be made to previous or subsequent radiographs. Calculi may move freely within the ureteral lumen, whereas pelvic phleboliths are fixed in position unless displaced by an enlarging extraperitoneal mass. Bladder stones are usually readily recognizable by their location and configuration. Because of their protean manifestations, however, calcified uterine leiomyomas may be confused with other calcified lesions in the pelvis, such as ovarian tumors and mesenteric lymph

nodes. Cystic teratomas of the ovary can frequently be recognized by the presence of teeth and bone, which are often accompanied by a large homogeneous lucency, indicating fat within the tumor.

MOBILITY

The movement of abdominal calcifications, either during a single examination or over a longer period, provides additional information that may lead to a specific diagnosis. Gravity, respiration, peristaltic activity, and growth of masses may all result in changes in location. Stones that are located in a fluid medium may undergo layering on abdominal radiographs obtained in upright or decubitus projections. Such manipulation of position may be helpful in the diagnosis of gallstones or of calculi in hydronephrotic sacs. Epiploic appendices that have become amputated or appendicoliths that lie free in the peritoneal cavity may exhibit a great range of movement on sequential radiographs. Whereas mesenteric nodes move slightly with positional changes, ovarian teratomas may move considerably as the bladder fills and empties (Fig. 17-13). Because of the effects of peristalsis, stones in the lumen of the gastrointestinal tract and pelvicaliceal system can migrate on successive radiographs. Consideration of this migration is particularly important in diagnosing ectopic gallstones and in differentiating distal ureteral calculi from stones in pelvic veins (Fig. 17-14). When images are obtained over a period of weeks or months, enlargement or shrinkage of abdominal masses may be recognized by the movement of calcifications or ossifications that lie within or adjacent to these lesions.

Even pelvic phleboliths can be displaced by hematomas or other masses.[4]

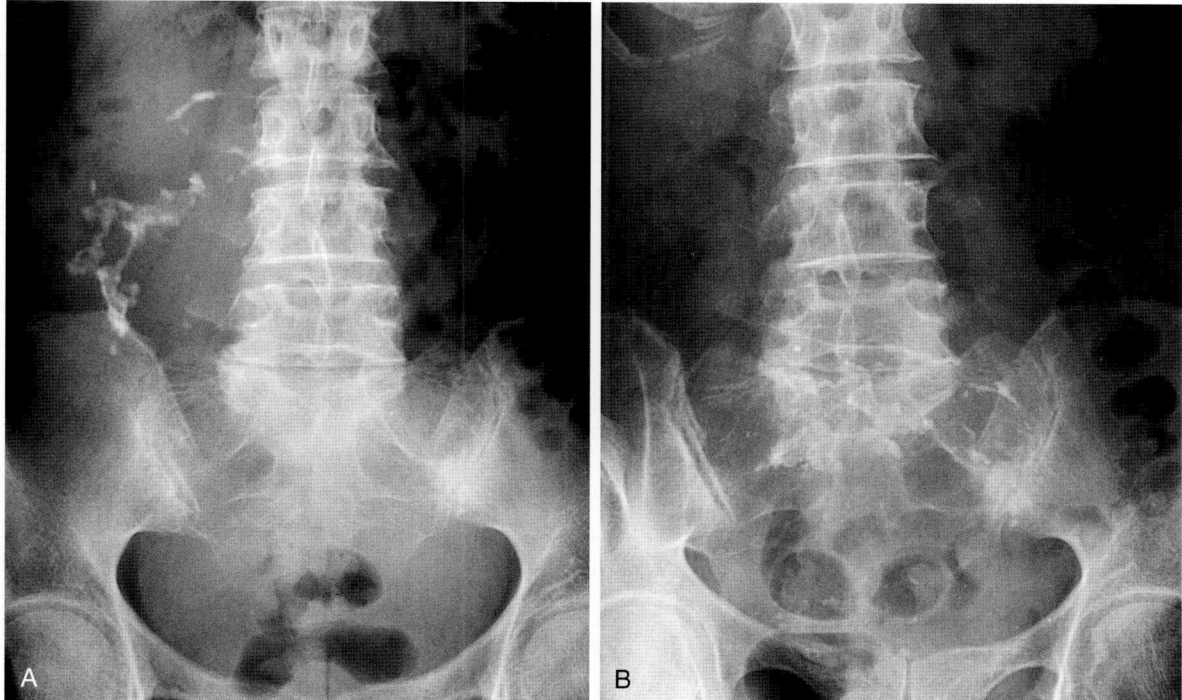

Figure 17-13. **Mobility of ovarian dermoid. A.** When the bladder is full, the tumor rises into the lower abdomen. **B.** When the bladder has been emptied, the calcified mass overlies the sacrum.

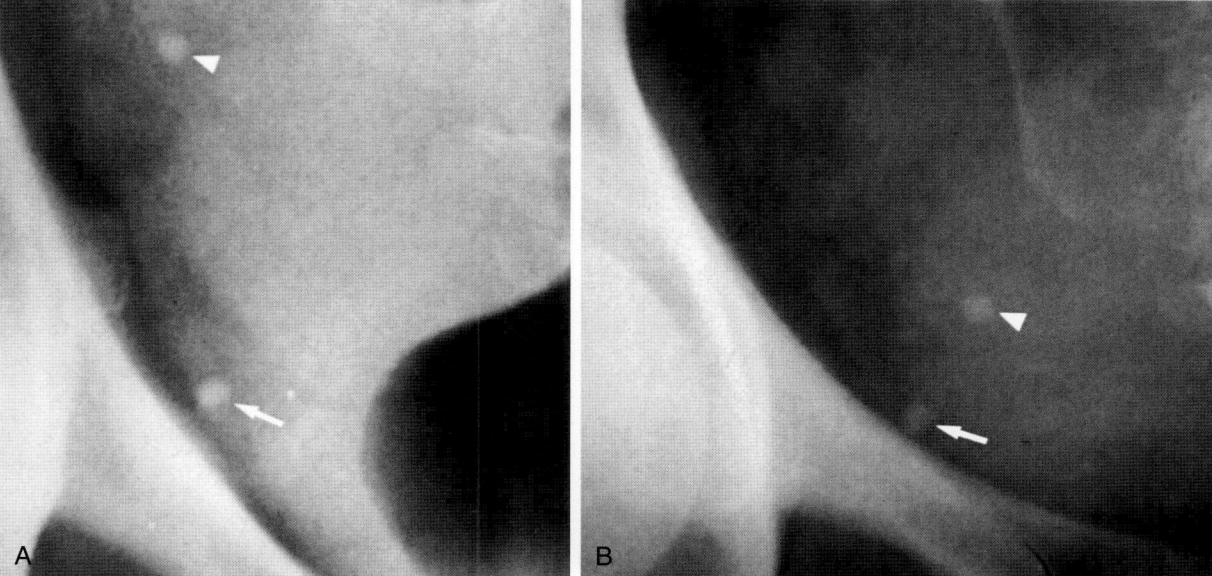

Figure 17-14. **Mobility of ureteral calculus. A.** A phlebolith (*arrow*) and a ureteral calculus (*arrowhead*) are morphologically identical on the initial abdominal radiograph. **B.** However, the venous stone (*arrow*) maintains a fixed position, whereas the ureteral stone (*arrowhead*) has migrated distally on a subsequent radiograph.

References

1. Hilbish TF, Bartter FC: Roentgen findings in abnormal deposition of calcium in tissues. AJR 87:1128-1129, 1962.
2. Kurturna P: A contribution to the problem of calcifications in malignant tumors: A case of late calcified retroperitoneal metastasis of an ovarian carcinoma. Neoplasma 11:633-642, 1964.
3. Widmann BF, Ostrum AW, Fried H: Practical aspects of calcification and ossification in the various body tissues. Radiology 30:598-609, 1938.
4. Steinbach HL: Identification of pelvic masses by phlebolith displacement. AJR 83:1063-1066, 1960.

III

Pharynx
STEPHEN E. RUBESIN
Section Editor

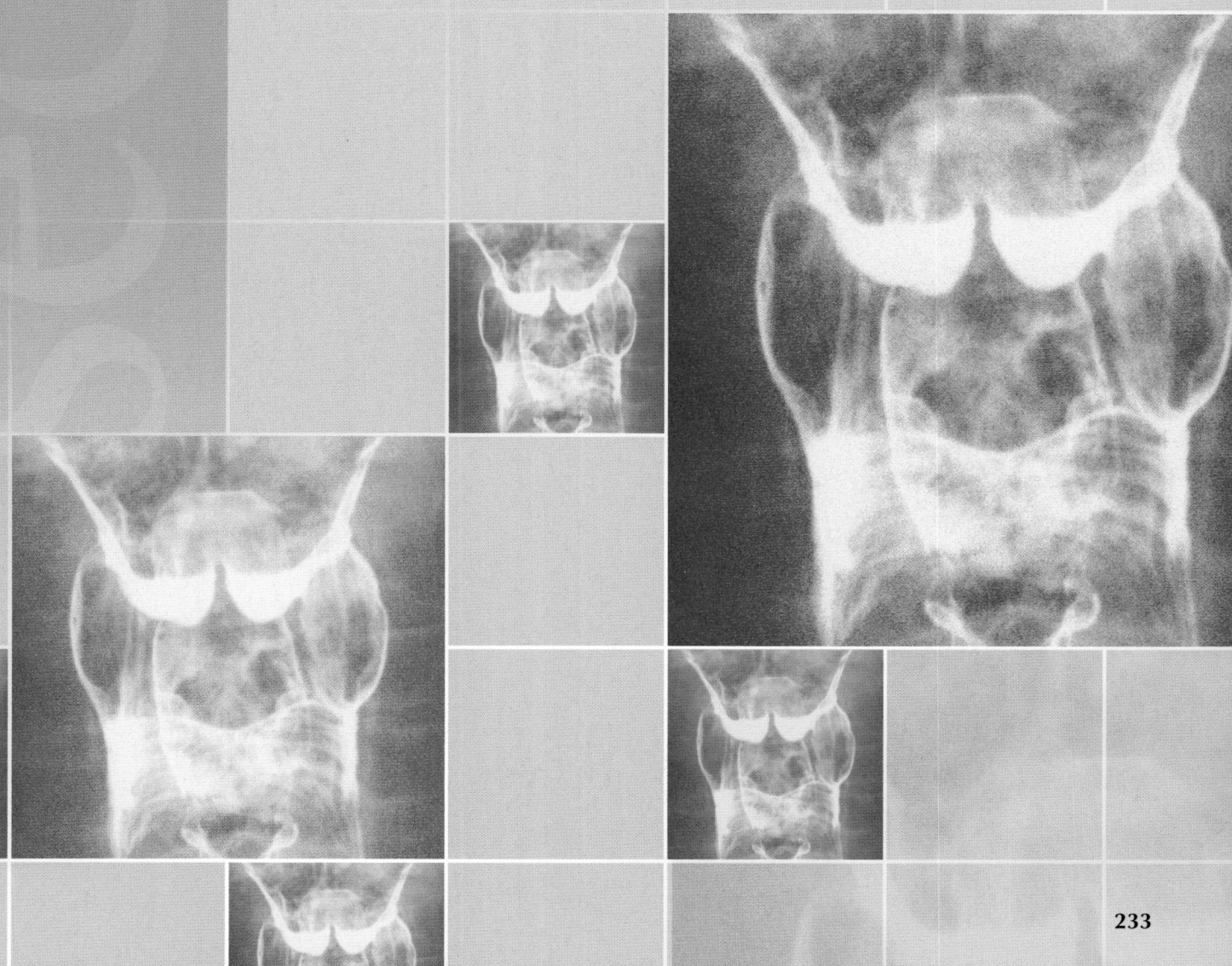

18

Pharynx: Normal Anatomy and Examination Techniques

Stephen E. Rubesin, MD

The pharynx is the crossroads of respiration, speech, and swallowing. During respiration, the pharynx is an active conduit for passage of air from the nasopharynx to the laryngeal aditus. During speech, the pharynx functions as a resonating chamber, changing size and shape to alter sounds. During swallowing, the pharynx directs the bolus into the esophagus and prevents the bolus from entering the tracheobronchial tree. Disorders of the pharynx may therefore be manifested by respiratory, speech, or swallowing dysfunction. Patients may complain of dysphagia, odynophagia, choking, or a feeling of a lump in the throat not associated with swallowing (a globus sensation). Soft palate insufficiency may be suggested by nasal regurgitation or a nasal voice quality. Recurrent pneumonia, asthma, chronic bronchitis, or coughing may indicate pharyngeal dysfunction. In this chapter the focus is on the anatomy of the pharynx as a basis for understanding both structural and motility disorders. The neurologic anatomy necessary for understanding motility disorders is presented in Chapter 19.

ANATOMY

Location

The pharynx is a funnel-shaped tube of skeletal muscle extending from the cranial base to the lower margin of the cricoid cartilage (Figs. 18-1 and 18-2A). The pharynx lies anterior to the vertebral bodies of the cervical spine, prevertebral

muscles, and loose connective tissue of the retropharyngeal space.[1] The pharynx is confined laterally by the muscles of the neck, the lateral portions of the hyoid bone and thyroid cartilage, and the carotid sheath (Fig. 18-2B).[2]

Divisions

The pharynx is arbitrarily divided into three parts: the nasopharynx (epipharynx), the oropharynx (mesopharynx), and the laryngopharynx (hypopharynx).[3] The nasopharynx is primarily a respiratory tract structure continuous anteriorly with the nasal cavity. The superior and posterior walls of the nasopharynx abut the basisphenoid and basilar part of the occipital bone. The nasopharynx is separated inferiorly from the oropharynx by the soft palate.

The oropharynx (Fig. 18-3) lies posterior to the oral cavity, extending from the soft palate to its arbitrary division from the hypopharynx at the level of the hyoid bone. Some anatomists divide the oropharynx from the hypopharynx at the level of the pharyngoepiglottic fold (Fig. 18-4), a mucosal fold overlying the stylopharyngeal muscle.[1] The base of the tongue forms the lower anterior wall of the oropharynx.

The hypopharynx lies behind and lateral to the larynx, extending from the level of the hyoid bone to the lower border of the cricopharyngeal muscle at the level of the inferior margin of the cricoid cartilage. These divisions are arbitrary because the soft palate and hyoid bone change position with phonation, swallowing, and respiration.

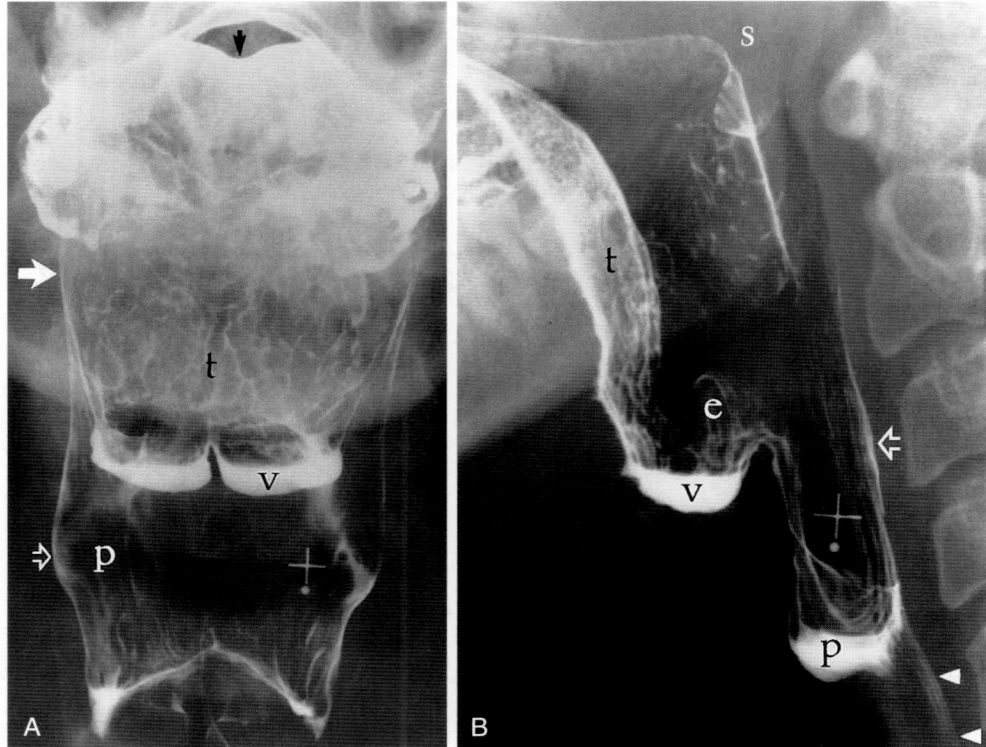

Figure 18-1. Basic structures of the normal pharynx. A. Double-contrast radiograph in the frontal view shows the contours of the superior surface of the tongue (*black arrow*), tonsillar fossa (right tonsillar fossa [*white arrow*]), valleculae (left vallecula [v]), and lateral wall (*open arrow*) of the piriform sinus (right piriform sinus [p]). The surface of the base of the tongue (t), seen en face, has a reticular appearance because of the underlying lingual tonsil. **B.** Double-contrast radiograph in the lateral view (during phonation) shows the contours of the soft palate (s), base of the tongue (t), epiglottis (e), valleculae (v), posterior pharyngeal wall (*arrow*), barium pooling in the lower piriform sinus (p), and collapsed region of the pharyngoesophageal segment (*arrowheads*). (**B** from Rubesin SE, Jones B, Donner MW: Contrast pharyngography: The importance of phonation. AJR 148:269-272, 1987. Copyright by American Roentgen Ray Society.)

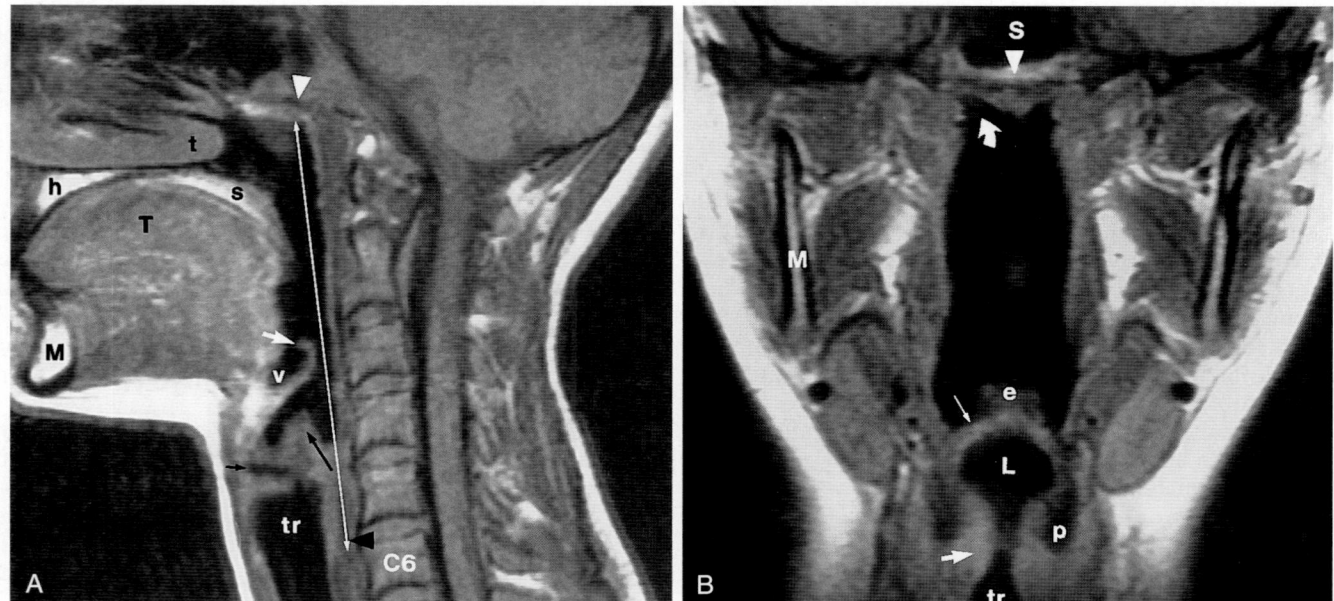

Figure 18-2. Location of the pharynx. A. Sagittal T1-weighted MR image of the head and neck shows the pharynx (*double arrow*) extending from the basisphenoid (*white arrowhead*) to the C6 vertebral body (C6) and pharyngoesophageal segment (*black arrowhead*). The pharynx is confined posteriorly by the cervical spine. The tongue (T) is apposed to the hard palate (h) and soft palate (s). The inferior turbinate (t), mandible in cross section (M), epiglottis (*white arrow*), vallecula (v), laryngeal ventricle (*small black arrow*), bulge of the arytenoid cartilages (*large black arrow*), and trachea (tr) are also shown. **B.** Coronal T1-weighted MR image of the neck shows the relationship of the pharynx to the basisphenoid (*arrowhead*) and sphenoidal sinus (S). The epiglottis (e), aryepiglottic folds (*thin white arrow*), and piriform sinus (p) are well depicted. The fossa of Rosenmüller (*curved arrow*), laryngeal vestibule (L), mandible (M), true vocal cord (*thick white arrow*), and trachea (tr) are also shown.

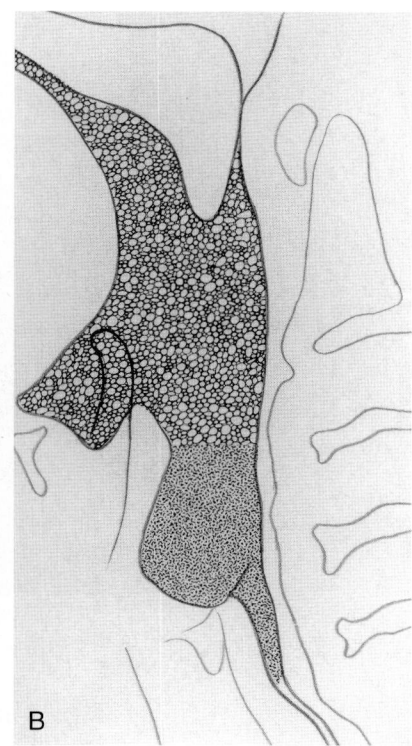

Figure 18-3. Divisions of the pharynx. Lateral double-contrast image of the pharynx (**A**) with its corresponding line drawing (**B**). The divisions of the pharynx involved in swallowing are the oropharynx (bubble pattern in **B**) and the hypopharynx (granular pattern in **B**). The oropharynx extends from the soft palate (S) to the level of the hyoid bone (h). The hypopharynx extends from the level of the hyoid bone to the inferior portion of the collapsed pharyngo-esophageal segment (*arrowhead*). The epiglottis (e) and aryepiglottic folds (*arrows*) span the oropharynx and hypopharynx. (From Rubesin SE, Jesserun J, Robertson D, et al: Lines of the pharynx. RadioGraphics 7:217-237, 1987.)

The oropharynx and hypopharynx are the divisions of the pharynx that participate in swallowing. The oropharynx and hypopharynx have four openings: the velopharyngeal portal superiorly between the nasopharynx and the oropharynx; the opening anteriorly to the oral cavity; the laryngeal aditus anteroinferiorly; and the opening into the esophagus postero-inferiorly.

Muscles

Oropharyngeal function depends on coordinated, sequential contraction of the extrinsic muscles of the pharynx, which arise from the skull base, neck, tongue, mandible, and hyoid bone, and the intrinsic skeletal muscles of the pharynx and larynx (Fig. 18-5 and Table 18-1).[3] The pharynx and larynx are suspended as a unit from the skull base, tongue, mandible, and hyoid bone. The suspensory muscles of the hyoid bone (the suprahyoid muscles) include the following (with their cranial nerve innervations in parentheses): from the tongue, mandible, or both, the anterior belly of the digastric muscle (V3), geniohyoid muscle (XII, via C1-2), hyoglossal muscle (XII), and mylohyoid muscle (V3); and from the skull base, the posterior belly of the digastric muscle (VII) and stylohyoid muscle (VII) (see Fig. 18-5).[4-9] The major function of the suprahyoid muscle group related to swallowing is to elevate and fix the hyoid bone, a motion that contributes to elevating and widening the pharynx and opening the pharyngoesophageal segment during passage of a bolus.

The soft palate is formed by an interweaving of muscles from the skull base (tensor veli palatini and levator veli palatini), tongue (palatoglossus muscle), and pharynx (palatopharyngeal muscle) (Figs. 18-6 and 18-7).[1,3,7] The musculus uvulae is the only intrinsic muscle of the soft palate.

The tendon of the tensor veli palatini (V) forms the fibrous skeleton of the anterior portion of the soft palate. This muscle depresses the anterior soft palate during swallowing. The levator veli palatini (X) suspends the midportion of the soft palate (see Figs. 18-6 and 18-7). During swallowing, the levator veli palatini pulls the mid-soft palate superiorly and posteriorly.[10] The palatopharyngeal muscle (X) depresses the posterior lateral part of the soft palate, elevates the pharynx, and constricts the faucial isthmus. The palatoglossus muscle (X) pulls the soft palate and tongue toward each other. The musculus uvulae (X) shortens, thickens, and elevates the uvula.

The thyrohyoid muscle (XII, via C1-2) courses from the hyoid bone to the thyroid cartilage (see Fig. 18-5). Its major function is approximation of the hyoid bone and thyroid cartilage, an action that is partly responsible for closing the laryngeal orifice. The thyroepiglottic and aryepiglottic muscles tilt the epiglottis inferiorly over the laryngeal aditus.[11] The infrahyoid depressors include the sternohyoid (C1-3), sternothyroid (C1-3), and omohyoid (C1-3) muscles.[8]

The muscular tube of the pharynx is surrounded by the buccopharyngeal fascia. The buccopharyngeal fascia is separated from the prevertebral muscles and fascia by the retropharyngeal space. The retropharyngeal space is an important site for the spread of malignant and inflammatory processes.

The muscular tube of the pharynx is formed by two layers: the inner longitudinal layer and the outer circular (constrictor) layer. The constrictor muscle layer (X) forms a ring that is incomplete anteriorly. The relationship of these muscles to the double-contrast appearance of the pharynx is illustrated in Figure 18-8. During swallowing, the constrictor muscles contract sequentially to propel the bolus into the esophagus.[12] Contraction of the superior constrictor muscle also apposes

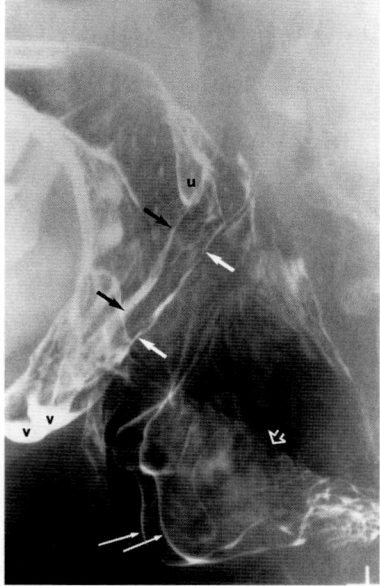

Figure 18-4. Pharyngoepiglottic folds. Spot image obtained in the lateral projection shows the paired pharyngoepiglottic folds (*thick arrows*) coursing as oblique lines across the lateral wall of the pharynx. The pharyngoepiglottic fold overlies the stylopharyngeal muscle, which extends from the styloid process to the posterior wall of the valleculae (v). The uvular tip (u) is seen. The anterior walls of the piriform sinuses (*thin arrows*) are well visualized. The mucosa overlying the muscular processes of the arytenoid cartilages (*open arrow*) is demonstrated. (Reprinted with permission from Rubesin SE, Glick SN: The tailored double-contrast pharyngogram. Crit Rev Diagn Imaging 28:133-179, 1988. Copyright CRC Press, Inc. Boca Raton, FL.)

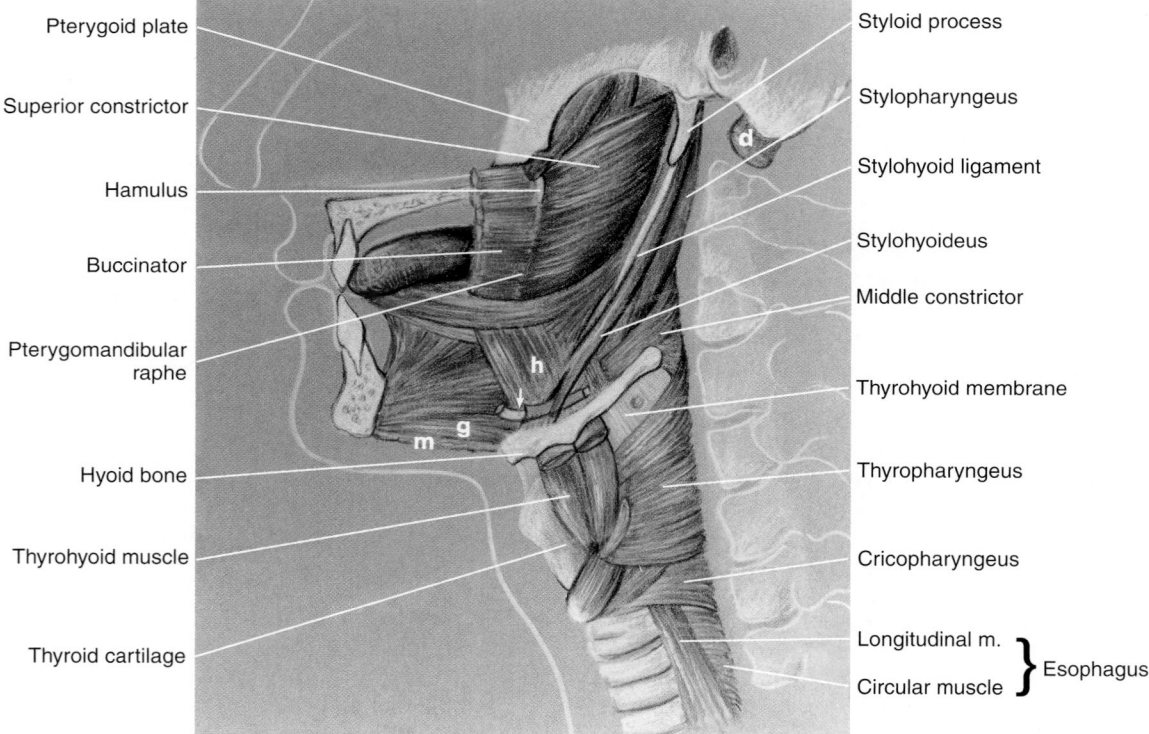

Figure 18-5. Lateral view of the muscles of the pharynx. The superficial muscles, nerves, arteries, and veins have been removed. The suspensory and constrictor muscles of the normal pharynx are demonstrated. The hyoid bone is suspended anteriorly by the geniohyoid muscle (g), mylohyoid muscle (m, cut in cross section), hyoglossus muscle (h), and anterior belly of the digastric muscle (resected). The tendon connecting the anterior and posterior belly of the digastric muscle is shown (*arrow*). The hyoid bone is suspended posteriorly by the stylohyoid ligament, stylohyoid muscle, and posterior belly of the digastric muscle (d) (resected). The thyrohyoid muscle and ligament suspend the thyroid cartilage from the hyoid bone. The overlying depressors of the hyoid bone, the omohyoid and sternohyoid muscles, have been resected. The constrictor muscles of the pharynx (superior, middle, and inferior) are incomplete anteriorly. The superior constrictor muscle originates at the pterygoid plate and hamulus, at the pterygomandibular raphe, and in the longitudinal muscles of the tongue; it inserts along the median raphe of the pharynx. The middle constrictor muscle originates on the greater and lesser horns of the hyoid bone and along the lower stylohyoid ligament; it inserts along the median raphe of the pharynx. The thyropharyngeal muscle (upper portion of the inferior constrictor muscle) originates from the oblique line of the thyroid cartilage; it inserts into the median raphe of the pharynx. The lower portion of the inferior constrictor muscle, the cricopharyngeal muscle, arises from the lateral surface of the cricoid cartilage, encircles the pharynx, and inserts on the opposite side of the cricoid cartilage. (Photographed directly from Rubesin S, Jesserun J, Robertson D, et al: Lines of the pharynx. Poster presented at the 71st Scientific Assembly and Annual Meeting, Radiological Society of North America, Chicago, 1985.)

Table 18–1

Tongue and Pharyngeal Motor Function

Function	Cranial Nerve	Muscle
Lip function	VII	Orbicularis oris, four others
Tongue function	VII	Lingualis, genioglossus, styloglossus, hyoglossus
Mastication	V3	Masseter, temporalis, lateral and medial pterygoid muscles
	VII	Buccinator
Eustachian tube opening	V3	Tensor veli palatini
	X	Salpingopharyngeus
Velopharyngeal portal closure		
Soft palate elevation	X	Levator veli palatini
Lateral portal closure	X	Superior constrictor
Hyoid elevation		
Larynx/pharynx elevation by extrinsic suprahyoid group	V3	Anterior belly digastric, mylohyoid muscle
	VII	Stylohyoid, posterior belly digastric
	XII	Geniohyoid, thyrohyoid muscles
Pharyngeal elevation by intrinsic muscles	IX	Stylopharyngeus
	IX, X	Palatopharyngeus, salpingopharyngeus
Epiglottic tilt		
Extrinsic muscles	V3, VII, XII	Suprahyoid group, thyrohyoid muscle
Intrinsic muscles	X	Aryepiglottic, thyroepiglottic muscles
Laryngeal vestibule closure	X	Thyroarytenoid, vocal cord muscles
Pharyngeal clearance	X	Superior, middle, inferior constrictor muscle
Upper esophageal sphincter opening	V3, VII, XII	Suprahyoid group
	IX, X	Intrinsic pharyngeal elevators
	X	Constrictor muscles
Hyoid depression after swallow	C1,2	Sternohyoid, omohyoid, sternothyroid muscles

From Rubesin SE, Stiles TD: Principles of performing a "modified barium swallow" examination. In Balfe DM, Levine MS (eds): RSNA Categorical Course in Diagnostic Radiology: Gastrointestinal. Oak Brook, IL, RSNA Publications, 1997, pp 7–19.

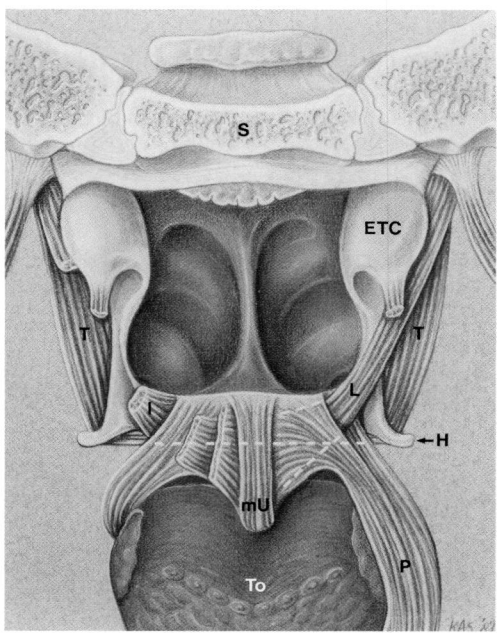

Figure 18-6. Muscles of the soft palate. The muscles forming the soft palate are viewed from behind, looking toward the tongue (To), nasal cavity, and sphenoid bone (S). The levator veli palatini (L) joins its partner (l) (partly resected in drawing) from the opposite side to form a sling, which supports the mid-soft palate. The tensor veli palatini (T) forms a tendon that hooks around the pterygoid hamulus (H) to join its partner from the other side, forming the fibrous skeleton of the anterior soft palate. The musculus uvulae (mU), palatopharyngeal muscle (P), and eustachian tube cartilage (ETC) are also shown. (From Rubesin SE, Rabischong P, Bilaniuk LT, et al: Contrast examination of the soft palate with cross sectional correlation. RadioGraphics 8:641-665, 1988.)

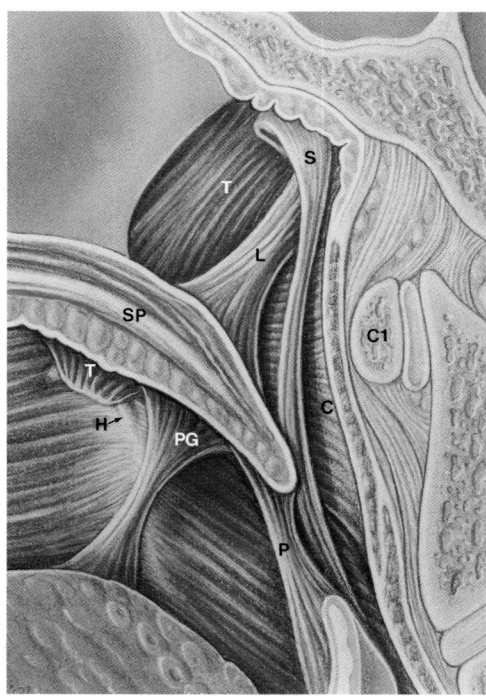

Figure 18-7. Muscles of the soft palate and tonsillar fossa. Drawing of the sagittal view of the nasopharynx and oropharynx after removal of the overlying mucosal layer. The levator veli palatini (L) pulls the midportion of the soft palate (SP) superiorly and posteriorly. The relationship between the tensor veli palatini (T) and the pterygoid hamulus (H) is shown. The palatoglossus muscle (PG) pulls the midtongue and mid-soft palate together. The salpingopharyngeal muscle (S) arises from the eustachian tube cartilage and forms the salpingopharyngeal fold. Also shown are the superior constrictor muscle (C) and the palatopharyngeal muscle (P). The anterior arch of the first cervical vertebra (C1) is shown.

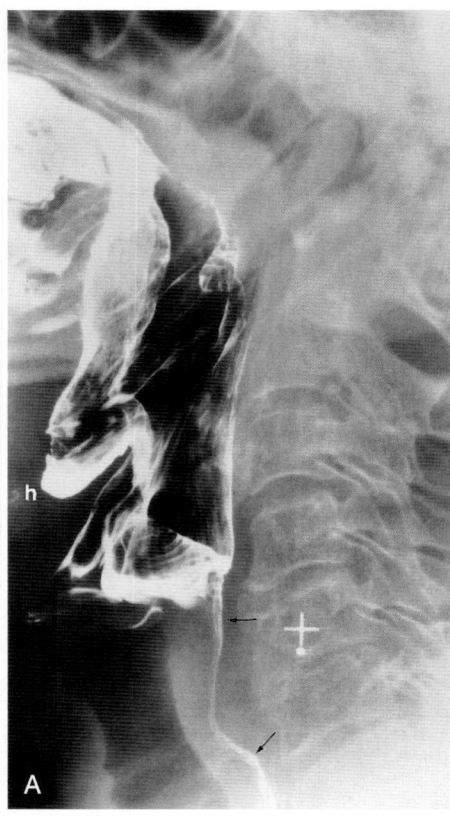
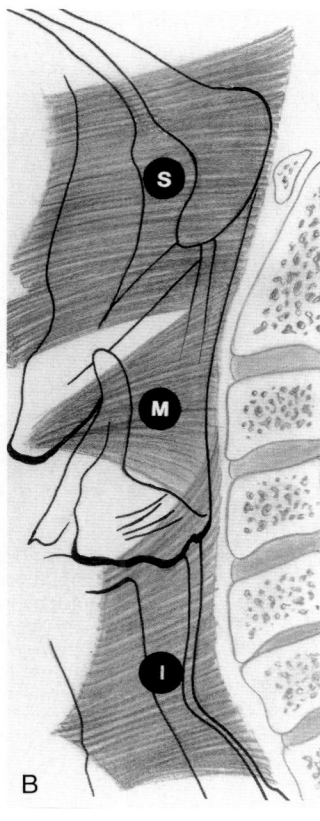

Figure 18-8. Constrictor muscle layer. Lateral radiograph obtained during phonation (**A**) and its corresponding anatomic drawing (**B**) show the relationship of the superior (S), middle (M), and inferior (I) constrictor muscles to the lateral view of the pharynx. The inferior border of the middle constrictor is at the level of the hyoid bone (h). A long segment of the lower hypopharynx (*arrows*) remains collapsed during phonation (and during suspended respiration). (From Rubesin SE, Jesserun J, Robertson D, et al: Lines of the pharynx. RadioGraphics 7:217-237, 1987.)

the lateral pharyngeal wall with the soft palate, closing the lateral portion of the velopharyngeal portal.[13-15]

During swallowing, the inner longitudinal muscle layer (see Figs. 18-5 through 18-7), which includes the stylopharyngeal muscle (IX), salpingopharyngeal muscle (X), and palatopharyngeal muscle (X), pulls the pharynx up and over the descending bolus of food.[16] The palatopharyngeal muscle also constricts the posterior portion of the pharynx, channeling the bolus into the hypopharynx and helping to prevent nasal regurgitation.

The double-contrast appearances and landmarks of the pharynx depend to a large extent on the inner longitudinal muscle layer.[3] Folds of mucosa are elevated into the pharyngeal lumen by the inner longitudinal layer of muscles. These muscular elevations are seen as the palatoglossal fold (anterior tonsillar pillar), palatopharyngeal fold (posterior tonsillar pillar) (Fig. 18-9), and pharyngoepiglottic fold (see Fig. 18-4).[1,3]

Basic Structures and Mucosal Surface Patterns

The shape of the pharynx is determined by the underlying musculature, the laryngeal cartilages, and the supporting skeleton (Fig. 18-10).[3] Although the nasopharynx is primarily a respiratory tract structure, certain nasopharyngeal structures participate in the act of swallowing. The eustachian tube connects the middle ear with the nasopharynx, allowing equilibration of air pressures on the internal and external aspects of the tympanic membrane during swallowing. During breathing, the eustachian tube is closed. The eustachian tube cartilage bulges into the lateral nasopharyngeal wall at the torus tubarius (Fig. 18-11).[17,18] A C-shaped prominence is

seen radiographically near the torus tubarius (Fig. 18-12).[19] The salpingopharyngeal fold overlying the salpingopharyngeal muscle courses inferiorly from the torus along the lateral pharyngeal wall to the level of the soft palate (Fig. 18-13).[20] The posterior nasopharyngeal wall has a variably nodular surface because of underlying adenoidal tissue.[21,22]

The oropharynx communicates anteriorly with the oral cavity. The vertical (pharyngeal) surface of the base of the tongue is variably nodular because of underlying lymphoid tissue of the lingual tonsil (see Fig. 18-13).[23] The median glossoepiglottic fold overlies the glossoepiglottic ligament, which courses from the base of the tongue to the epiglottis. The median glossoepiglottic fold divides the space between the tongue and the epiglottis into two sacs—the valleculae (Fig. 18-14). The lateral glossoepiglottic folds form the lateral walls of the valleculae. The pharyngoepiglottic folds course from the posterolateral portion of the valleculae into the lateral pharyngeal wall (Fig. 18-15).[1] These folds overlie the stylopharyngeal muscle and form the posterior lateral wall of the valleculae. The valleculae are spaces at rest but disappear during swallowing when the epiglottis inverts. The space behind the base of the tongue communicates freely with the remainder of the oropharynx after the epiglottis tilts.

The tonsillar fossa forms part of the lateral oropharyngeal wall. The tonsillar fossa is bounded anteriorly by the palatoglossal fold (anterior tonsillar pillar) (Figs. 18-16 and 18-17) and posteriorly by the palatopharyngeal fold (posterior tonsillar pillar) overlying the palatopharyngeal muscle (see Figs. 18-16 and 18-17).

The rounded epiglottic tip rises above the level of the valleculae.[24] The aryepiglottic folds connect the epiglottis

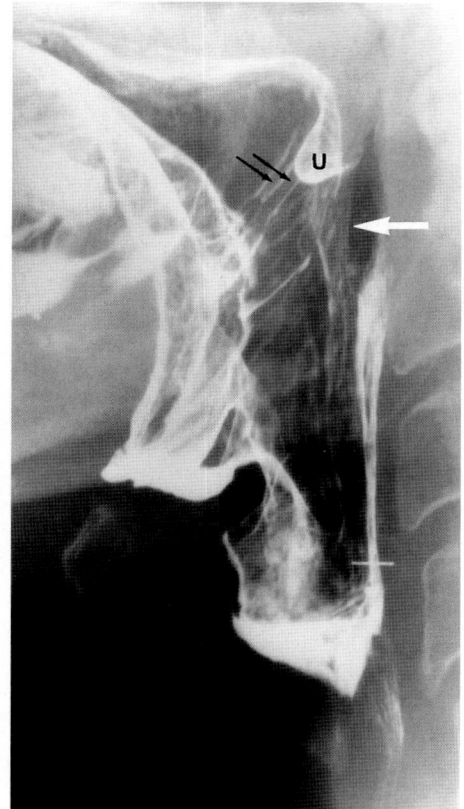

Figure 18-9. Palatopharyngeal folds. Lateral view of the pharynx shows the paired palatopharyngeal folds (posterior tonsillar pillars) (*white arrow*) coursing from the mid-soft palate to the lateral wall of the pharynx. The paired palatoglossal folds (*black arrows*) form the anterior tonsillar pillars. U, uvula. (From Rubesin SE, Jesserun J, Robertson D, et al: Lines of the pharynx. RadioGraphics 7:217-237, 1987.)

Figure 18-10. Relationship of the laryngeal cartilages to the double-contrast view of the pharynx. A and **B.** The laryngeal cartilages, including the epiglottis (e), thyroid cartilage (T), and cricoid cartilage (C), and the hyoid bone (h) are shown in relationship to the barium-coated pharynx. The thyrohyoid membrane (t) connects the hyoid bone to the thyroid cartilage. The junction of the ala of the thyroid cartilage and the thyrohyoid membrane (*white arrow*) is seen as a notch in the lateral wall of the hypopharynx on the double-contrast view (*black arrow*). (From Rubesin SE, Jesserun J, Robertson D, et al: Lines of the pharynx. RadioGraphics 7:217-237, 1987.)

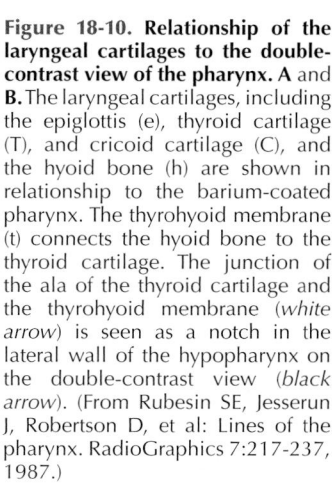

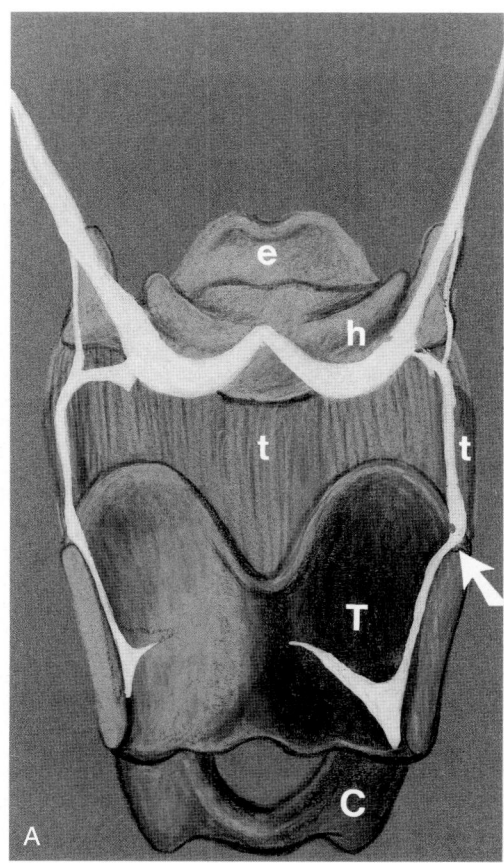

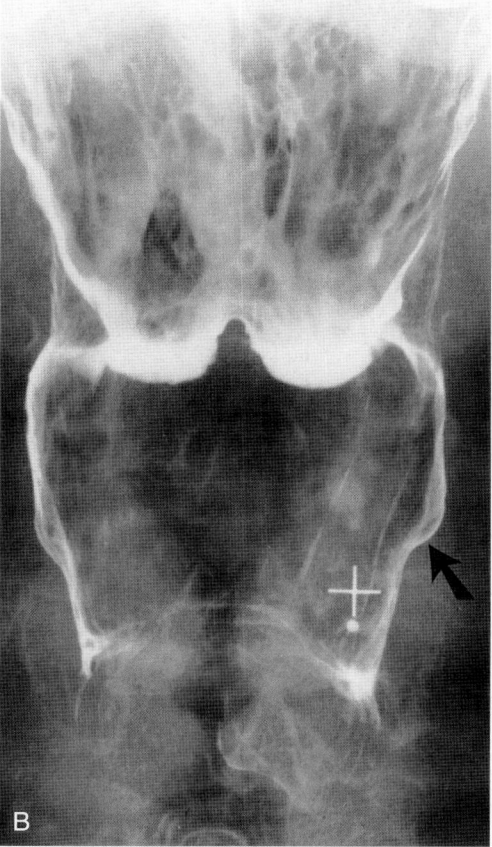

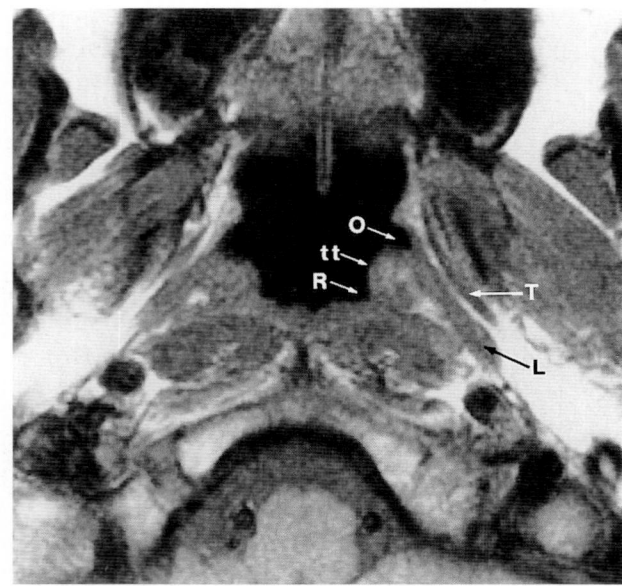

Figure 18-11. Nasopharynx. Axial T1-weighted MR image of naso-pharynx shows the relationship of the torus tubarius (tt) to the tensor veli palatini (T) and the levator veli palatini (L). The eustachian tube orifice (O) and fossa of Rosenmüller (R) are also shown. (From Rubesin SE, Rabischong P, Bilaniuk LT, et al: Contrast examination of the soft palate with cross sectional correlation. RadioGraphics 8:641-665, 1988.)

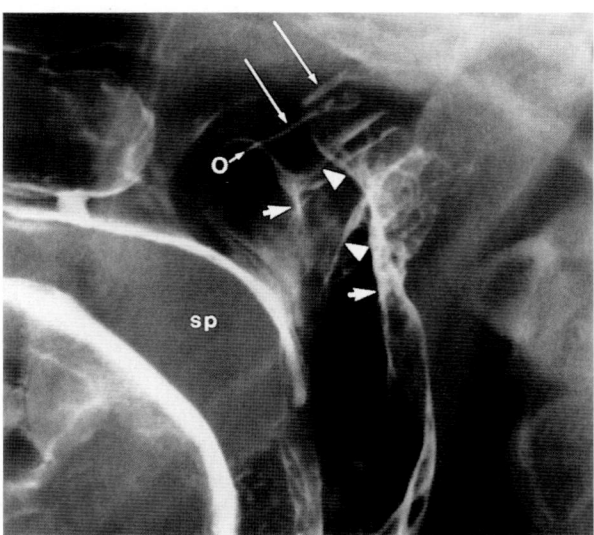

Figure 18-12. Lines of the nasopharynx. Lateral view of the nasopharynx after intranasal instillation of 1 mL of barium shows the paired, barium-filled eustachian tubes (*long arrows*). The orifice of one eustachian tube (O) is seen under the C-shaped slit of the torus tubarius. The paired salpingopharyngeal folds (*short arrows*) are seen. The levator veli palatini forms slight bulges in the lateral nasopharyngeal wall—the levator ridge. The inferior border of these bulges is marked with *arrowheads*. sp, soft palate. (From Rubesin SE, Rabischong P, Bilaniuk LT, et al: Contrast examination of the soft palate with cross sectional correlation. Radio-Graphics 8:641-665, 1988.)

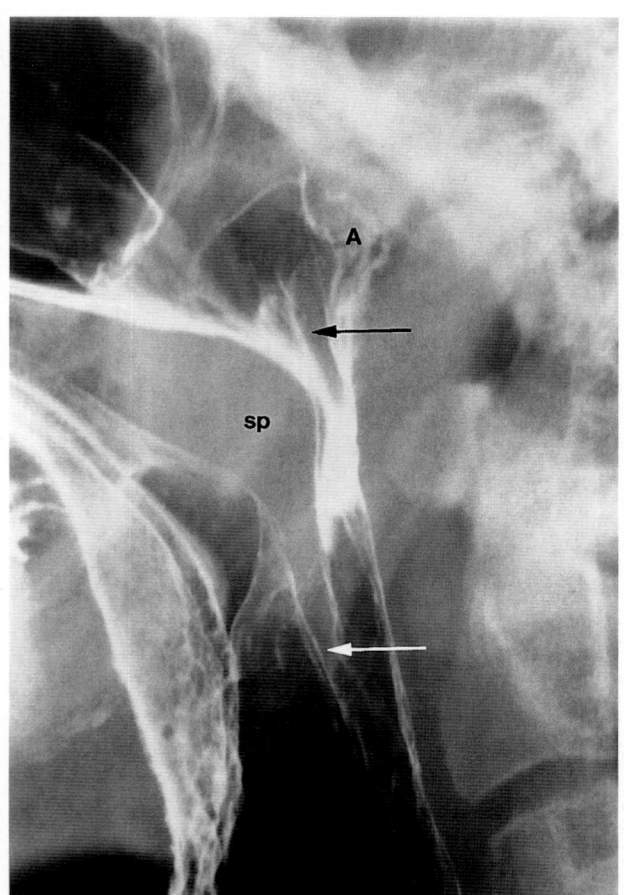

Figure 18-13. Salpingopharyngeal fold and adenoids. Lateral view of the nasopharynx during phonation after intranasal instillation of 1 mL of barium shows the salpingopharyngeal folds (*black arrow*). The posterior wall of the nasopharynx is slightly irregular because of the underlying adenoidal lymphoid tissue (A). The soft palate (sp) and palatopharyngeal fold (*white arrow*) are also demonstrated. The vertical surface of the tongue has a finely nodular appearance. (From Rubesin SE, Rabischong P, Bilaniuk LT, et al: Contrast examination of the soft palate with cross sectional correlation. RadioGraphics 8:641-665, 1988.)

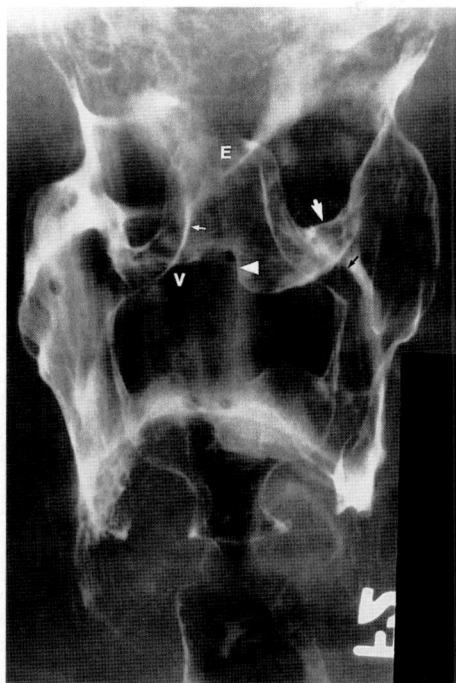

Figure 18-14. Frontal (supine) view of pharynx demonstrating the folds of the valleculae. The median glossoepiglottic fold (*arrowhead*) divides the retroglottic space into the two valleculae (right vallecula [V]). The pharyngoepiglottic folds (*large white arrow* identifies the left pharyngo-epiglottic fold) overlie the paired stylopharyngeal muscles and form part of the posterior wall of the valleculae. Also shown are the epiglottic tip (E) and aryepiglottic fold (*black arrow*). Barium coats the laryngeal surface of the epiglottis (*small white arrow*) as a result of laryngeal penetration.

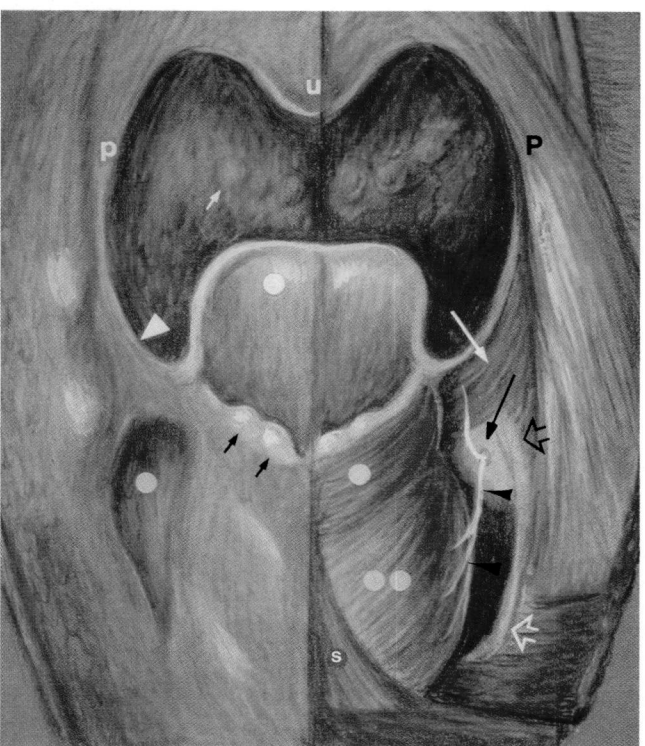

Figure 18-15. Posterior view of pharynx opened from behind. On the viewer's left, the mucosa has been left intact. The uvula (u), palato-pharyngeal fold (p), piriform sinus (*left dot*), and laryngeal surface of the epiglottis (*uppermost dot*) are seen en face. The pharyngoepiglottic fold (*white arrowhead*) separates the oropharynx from the hypopharynx. Bulges in the aryepiglottic fold overlie the cuneiform and corniculate cartilages (*short black arrows*). The circumvallate papillae (*short white arrow*) form a V-shaped protuberance along the base of the tongue. On the right side, the mucosa has been removed. The palatopharyngeal muscle (P) forms the palatopharyngeal fold. This muscle has been retracted laterally. The stylopharyngeal muscle (*long white arrow*) underlies the pharyngoepiglottic fold. The thyroid cartilage forms the lateral boundary of the pharynx. Its superior horn (*open black arrow*) and posterior border of the right lamina (*open white arrow*) form the lateral boundary of the piriform sinus. The thyrohyoid membrane (*long black arrow*) and the internal branch of the superior laryngeal nerve (*black arrowheads*) are identified. The transverse arytenoid muscle (*single dot on right*), posterior cricoarytenoid muscle (*two adjacent dots*), and suspensory ligament of the esophagus (s) are identified. (Photographed directly from Rubesin S, Jesserun J, Robertson D, et al: Lines of the pharynx. Poster presented at the 71st Scientific Assembly and Annual Meeting, Radiological Society of North America, Chicago, 1985.)

with the mucosa overlying the muscular processes of the arytenoid cartilages. Occasionally, round bulges are seen in the lower aryepiglottic folds, reflecting the small cuneiform and corniculate cartilages embedded in these folds.

The shape of the hypopharynx is created primarily by its relationship to the posteriorly protruding larynx (Fig. 18-18). Protrusion of the larynx into the pharynx creates two grooves in the anterior lateral hypopharynx—the piriform sinuses (recesses), pear-shaped structures that open posteriorly into the hypopharynx (Fig. 18-19; see also Figs. 18-4 and 18-18). Each piriform sinus is bounded medially by the aryepiglottic fold and mucosa overlying the muscular process of the arytenoid cartilage and laterally by the hyoid bone, thyrohyoid membrane, and thyroid cartilage.[1,3]

The lower end of the hypopharynx is collapsed, except during passage of a bolus. The posterior portion of the larynx (including the arytenoid cartilages, arytenoid muscles, and cricoid cartilage) protrudes deeply into the lower hypopharynx. The upper esophageal sphincter (formed predominantly by the cricopharyngeal muscle) is tonically contracted at rest, closing the pharyngoesophageal segment (see Fig. 18-1). As a result, the lower hypopharynx is markedly constricted in an anteroposterior direction and is often not appreciated on a frontal radiograph. The arcuate "lower border" of the hypopharynx seen on the frontal view reflects only the protrusion of the larynx into the hypopharynx (see Fig. 18-18).[3]

The squamous mucosa of the lateral and posterior pharyngeal walls is closely apposed to the longitudinally

striated inner longitudinal muscle layer and its aponeurosis. Only a thin tunica propria separates the epithelium from the muscle or the elastic tissue of the aponeurosis. On double-contrast views, longitudinally oriented lines may therefore be seen in the lateral and posterior pharyngeal walls, reflecting apposition of epithelium to muscle (Fig. 18-20A).[3]

Transversely oriented lines are seen on the anterior hypopharyngeal wall, where redundant squamous mucosa and submucosa overlie the muscular processes of the arytenoid cartilages and cricoid cartilage (Fig. 18-20B). Transverse lines and tissue bulging from the anterior hypopharyngeal wall have previously been described as a *postcricoid venous plexus*.[25] However, these radiographic findings are mainly due to redundant mucosa and submucosa on the anterior hypopharyngeal wall (Fig. 18-21).[3,26]

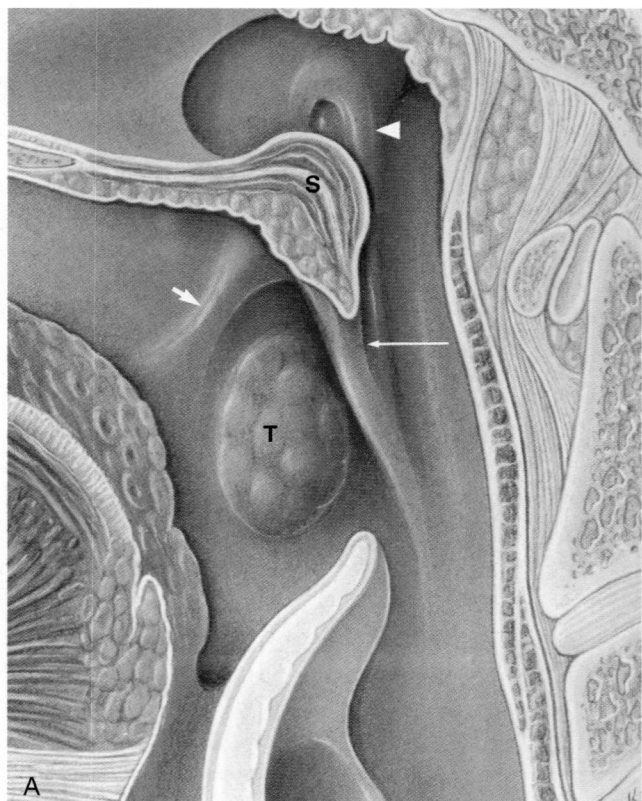
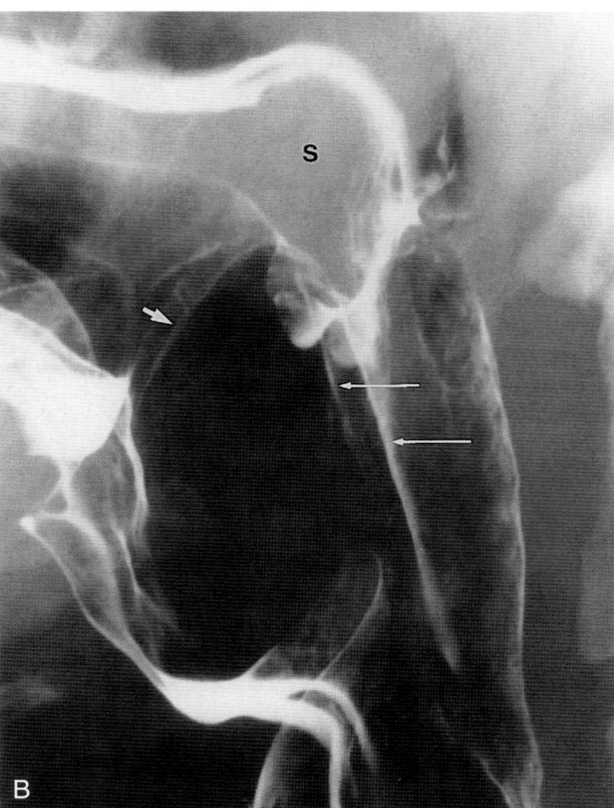

Figure 18-16. Tonsillar fossa. Lateral drawing (**A**) and its corresponding radiograph (**B**) demonstrate the tonsillar fossa during soft palate elevation by phonation. The palatine tonsil (T) is surrounded by the palatoglossal fold (anterior tonsillar pillar) (*short arrows*) and palatopharyngeal fold (posterior tonsillar pillar) (*long arrows*). The salpingopharyngeal fold is also shown (*arrowhead*). S, soft palate. (From Rubesin SE, Rabischong P, Bilaniuk LT, et al: Contrast examination of the soft palate with cross sectional correlation. RadioGraphics 8:641-665, 1988.)

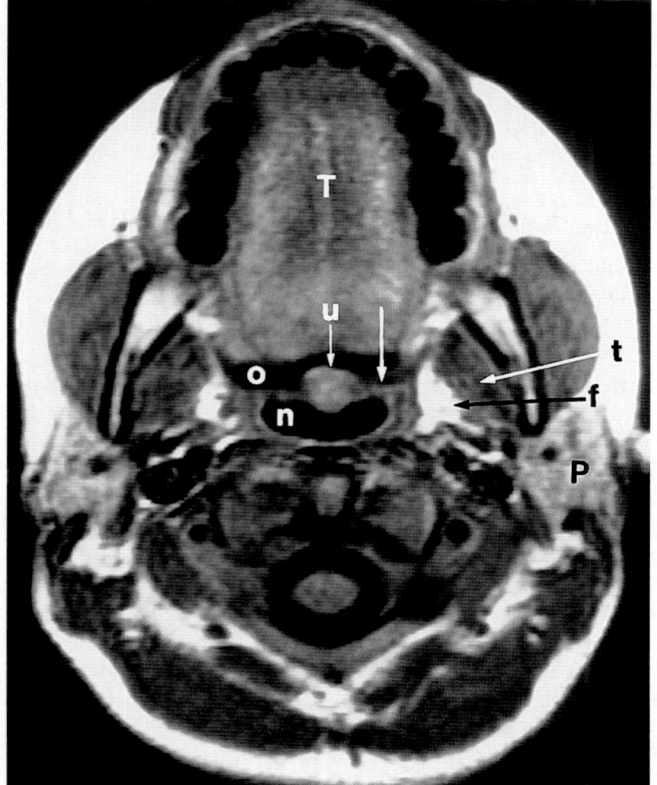

Figure 18-17. Palatopharyngeal fold. T1-weighted MR image of the pharynx shows the uvula (*white arrow*, u) and palatopharyngeal folds (*white arrow* identifies left palatopharyngeal fold) separating the oropharynx (o) from the nasopharynx (n). Parapharyngeal fat (*black arrow*, f) separates the pharynx from the masticator space, pterygoid muscle (*white arrow*, t), and parotid gland (P) posterolaterally. The region of the retromolar trigone is anterolateral to the parapharyngeal fat. T, tongue.

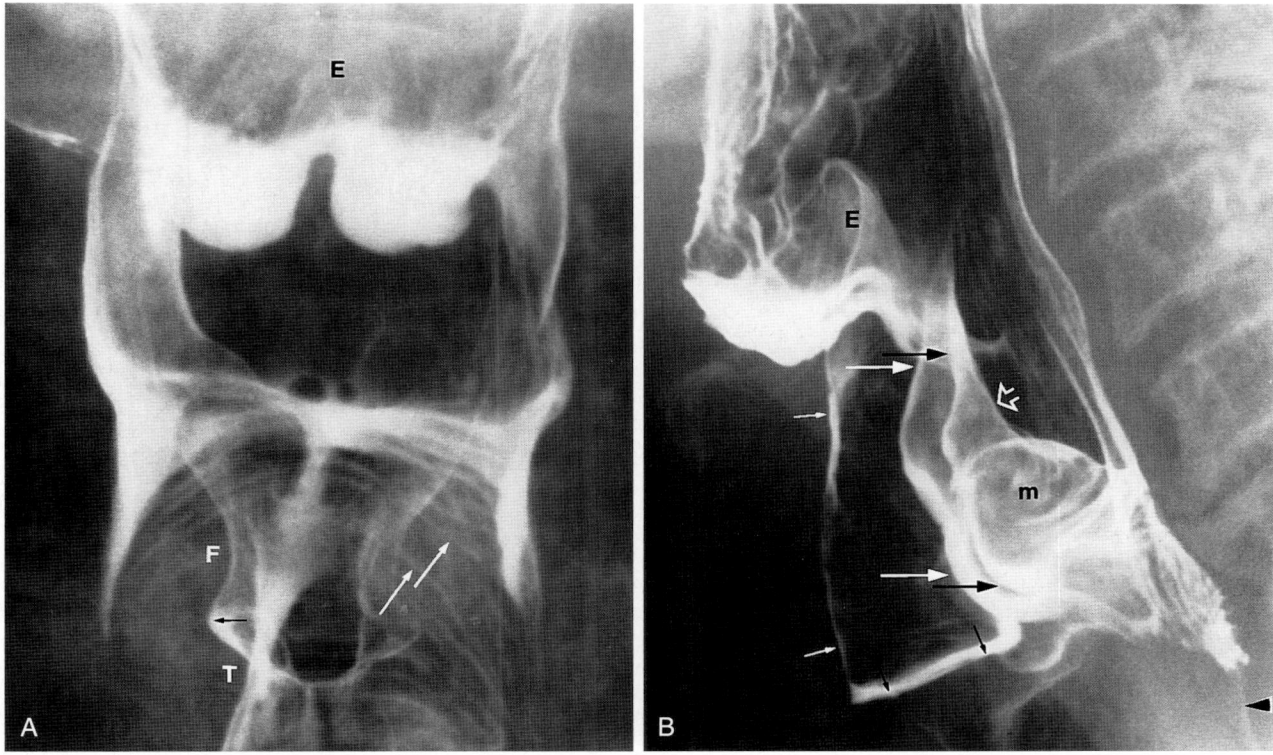

Figure 18-18. Relationship of larynx to pharynx. A. In a patient with laryngeal penetration, barium coats the false vocal cords (right false vocal cord, F), the true vocal cords (right true vocal cord, T), and the laryngeal ventricle (right laryngeal ventricle, *black arrow*). As the larynx protrudes into the mid-hypopharynx, arcuate lines (*white arrows*) are formed. E, epiglottis. **B.** The relationship of the barium-coated laryngeal vestibule (*small white arrows*) to the laryngeal ventricle (*small black arrows*) is shown. Note the angle of the laryngeal ventricle atop the true vocal cords. Note the tilt of the true vocal cords; the posterior portion of the cords is cranial to the anterior commissure. The anterior walls of the right piriform sinus (*large white arrows*) and left piriform sinus (*large black arrows*) are seen as anteriorly convex lines. The mucosa (m) overlying the muscular process of the arytenoid cartilages lies below the aryepiglottic fold (*open arrow*). The lower hypopharynx (*arrowhead*) is closed at rest. E, epiglottis. (**B** reprinted with permission from Rubesin SE, Glick SN: The tailored double-contrast pharyngogram. Crit Rev Diagn Imaging 28:133-179, 1988. Copyright CRC Press, Inc. Boca Raton, FL.)

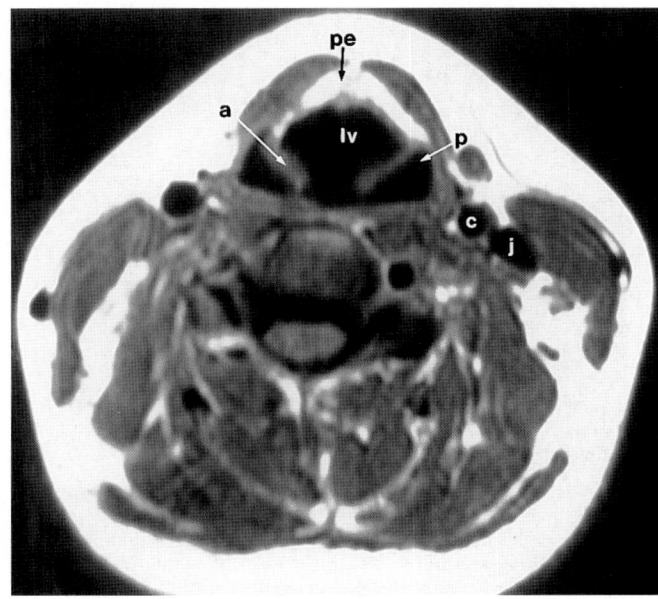

Figure 18-19. Aryepiglottic folds and piriform sinuses. Axial T1-weighted MR image of the hypopharynx shows the right aryepiglottic fold (a) forming the medial wall of piriform sinus (p, left piriform sinuses). The laryngeal vestibule (lv) is bounded posteriorly by the left and right aryepiglottic folds. The preepiglottic space (pe) has a high signal intensity because it is filled with fat. The carotid artery (c) and jugular vein (j) are identified.

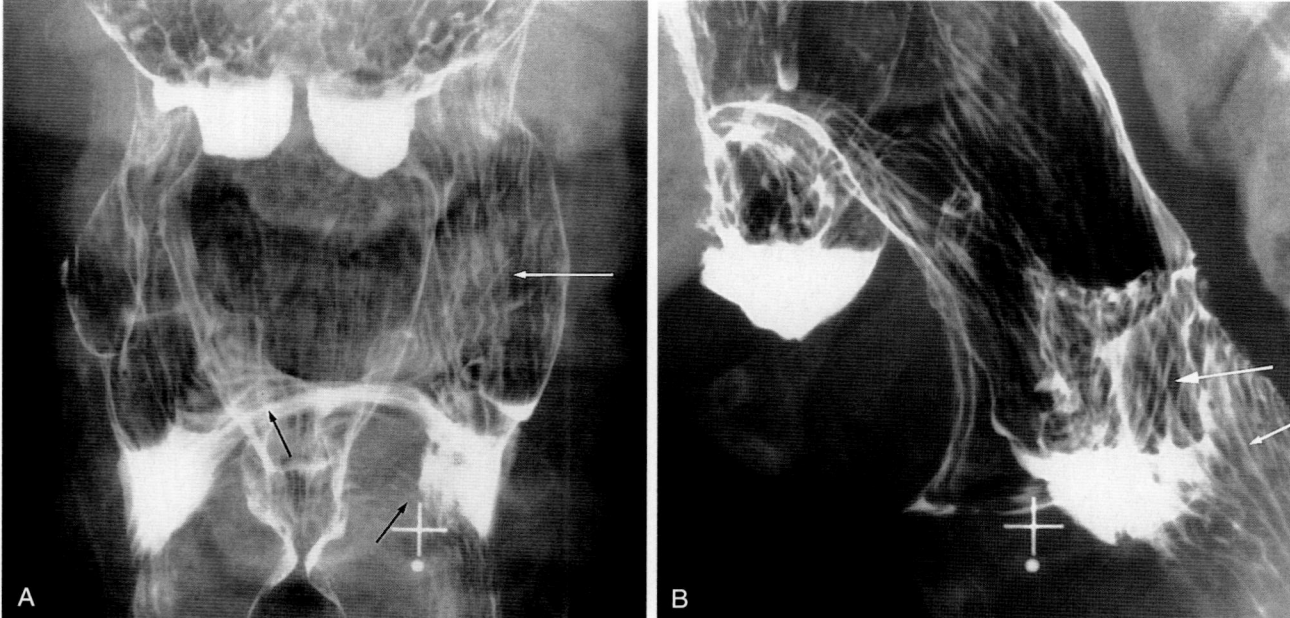

Figure 18-20. Lines of the pharynx. A. Longitudinally striated mucosa (*white arrow*) reflects close apposition of the squamous mucosa to the underlying longitudinal muscle layer of the pharynx. Arcuate lines of the anterior hypopharyngeal wall are identified (*black arrows*). **B.** Arcuate lines and transversely oriented lines overlying the muscular processes of the arytenoid cartilages (*large arrow*) and the lower hypopharynx (*small arrow*) reflect redundant mucosa in this region. (**B** reprinted with permission from Rubesin SE, Glick SN: The tailored double-contrast pharyngogram. Crit Rev Diagn Imaging 28:133-179, 1988. Copyright CRC Press, Inc. Boca Raton, FL.)

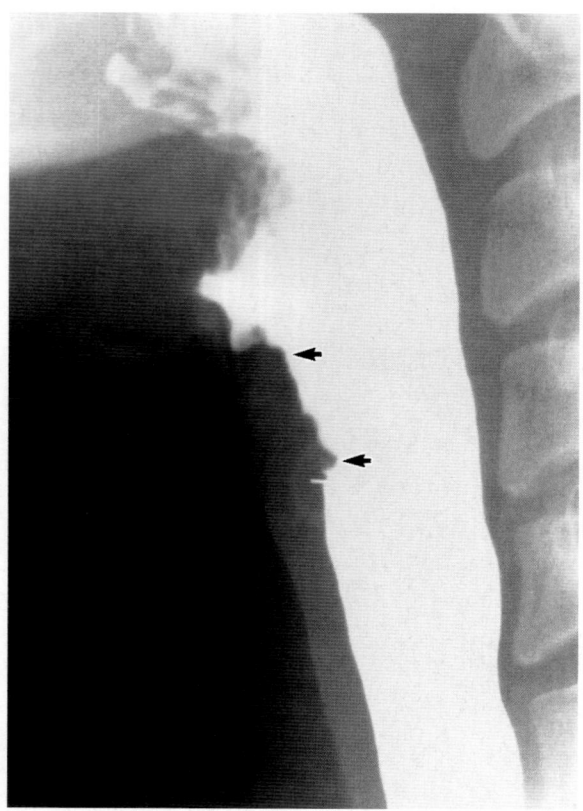

Figure 18-21. Postcricoid defect. During swallowing, redundant mucosa along the anterior wall of the distal hypopharynx may create an undulating or plaquelike contour (*arrows*). To rule out a subtle stricture, web, or infiltrating lesion, the radiologist must be certain this mucosal nodularity changes size and shape and flattens during swallowing.

PRINCIPLES OF TECHNIQUE

Preparation of Patients

High-density barium adheres to dry pharyngeal mucosa.[27] Despite continuous salivary secretion, the pharynx should therefore be made as dry as possible during the examination. As a result, patients are instructed not to eat or drink after midnight on the day of the examination.[9] In the morning, regular oral medications may be taken with small amounts of water, but insulin-dependent diabetics should not take their insulin on the morning of examination. Oral antacid medications impair barium coating and should also be avoided. If possible, the patient should refrain from activities that stimulate salivary secretion, such as sucking throat lozenges, smoking, or chewing gum.

Contrast examination of the pharynx may be dangerous in patients with suspected airway obstruction, especially in those with acute epiglottitis.[28,29] Lateral radiographs of the neck should therefore be obtained if airway obstruction is suspected (Fig. 18-22). Lateral radiographs are also obtained for suspected foreign body, fistula, abscess, perforation (Fig. 18-23), or a palpable neck mass.

Components of Routine Examination

Routine examination of the pharynx and esophagus includes (1) videofluoroscopy or DVD recording of the oral, pharyngeal, and esophageal phases of swallowing; (2) double-contrast spot images of the pharynx, esophagus, and gastric cardia; and (3) single-contrast and mucosal relief views of the esophagus (Table 18-2).[30-38] The examination is tailored to the patient's clinical history, symptoms, and initial fluoroscopic findings. The pharyngoesophagogram is an interactive study; if a

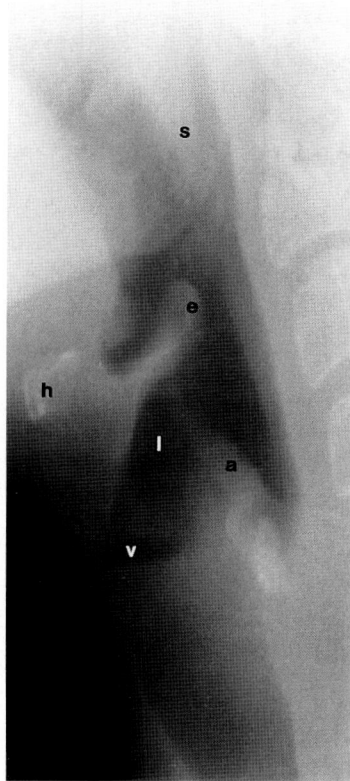

Figure 18-22. Lateral radiograph of normal pharynx. The soft palate (s), epiglottis (e), hyoid bone (h), laryngeal vestibule (l), laryngeal ventricle (v), and mucosa overlying the muscular process of the arytenoid cartilage (a) are shown.

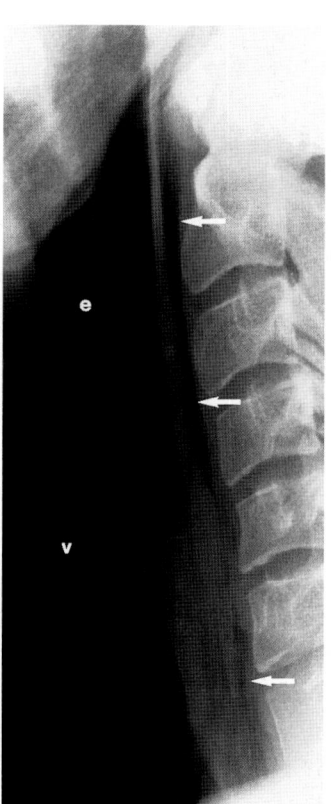

Figure 18-23. Neck pain after pharyngeal perforation by a taco chip. Lateral radiograph of the neck shows a large amount of retropharyngeal air (*arrows*). e, epiglottis; v, laryngeal ventricle.

motility disorder is the major radiographic finding, dynamic techniques (videofluoroscopy or DVD recording) are emphasized.[37] If a structural abnormality is the major radiographic finding, double-contrast spot images become more important. Both static and dynamic images are routinely obtained for the following reasons: (1) structural disorders often alter pharyngeal motility (Fig. 18-24); (2) structural features of motility disorders are often well demonstrated on static images; and (3) structural lesions and motility disorders may coexist.[38]

The oral and pharyngeal phases of swallowing should initially be evaluated if symptoms suggest an oral or pharyngeal disorder (see Table 18-2). If the clinical history and symptoms suggest thoracic esophageal disease, however, a double-contrast examination of the esophagus should first be performed, followed by examination of the oral and pharyngeal phases of swallowing (Table 18-3). The radiologist should remember that the subjective sensation of dysphagia often cannot be localized accurately and that esophageal lesions may cause referred dysphagia to the neck or suprasternal region.[39] Furthermore, patients may have an esophageal disorder that secondarily affects pharyngeal function or a disease that involves both the pharynx and the esophagus. Finally, some patients have more than one abnormality in the pharynx or esophagus, or both.

Table 18–2
Routine Pharyngoesophagogram for Respiratory or Pharyngeal Symptoms

View	Technique	Organ
Erect, left lateral	Videofluoroscopy, double contrast (R,P) (two films)	Mouth and pharynx
Erect, frontal	Videofluoroscopy, double contrast (R,V) (two films)	Pharynx
Obliques	Double contrast (V) (one film)	Pharynx
Effervescent Agent and Water		
Erect, LPO	Double contrast (two films)	Esophagus
Prone, RAO	Videofluoroscopy, single contrast (one film)	Esophagus
Right lateral	Double contrast	Gastric cardia

LPO, left posterior oblique with respect to table top; P, phonation; R, suspended respiration; RAO, right anterior oblique with respect to table top; V, modified Valsalva maneuver.

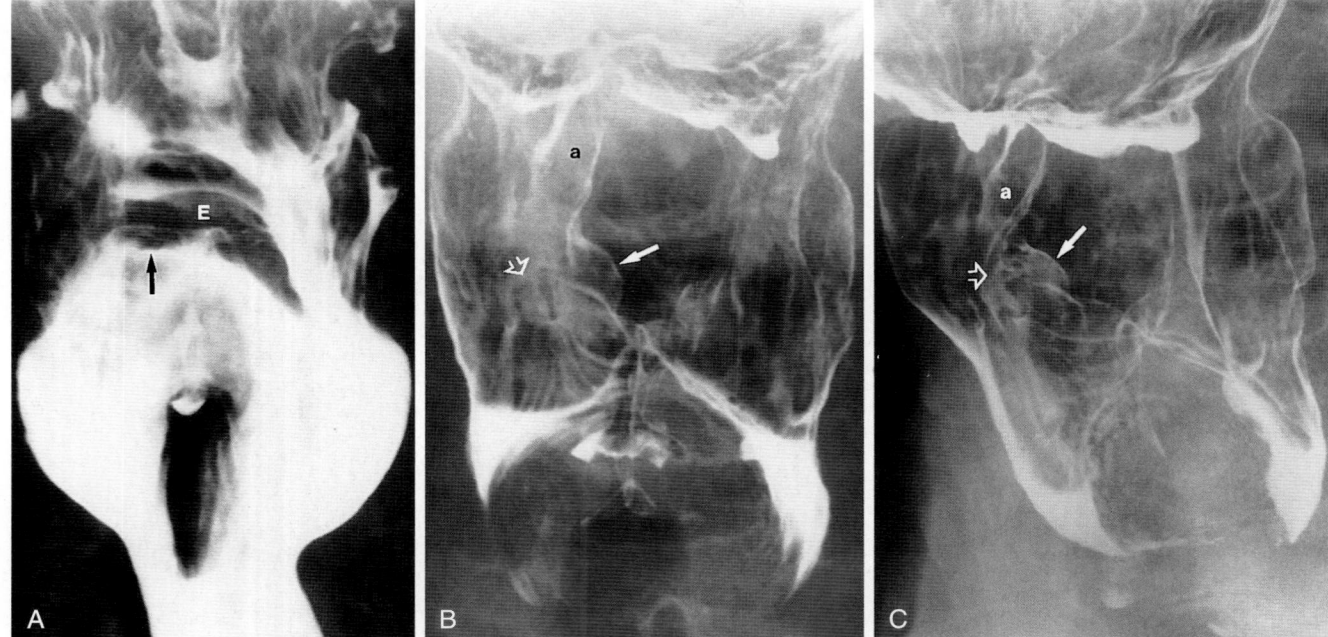

Figure 18-24. **Abnormal epiglottic tilt caused by squamous cell carcinoma involving right aryepiglottic fold and the mucosa overlying the arytenoid cartilage.** During swallowing, tilt of the epiglottis (E) is diminished on the right, as indicated by the *arrow* (**A**). Frontal (**B**) and slight right oblique (**C**) spot films show a small mass (*arrows*) and thickening of the aryepiglottic fold (a) and nodular mucosa (*open arrows*). A small squamous cell carcinoma was found to involve the aryepiglottic fold and mucosa overlying the right arytenoid process. (From Rubesin SE: Pharyngeal dysfunction. In Gore R [ed]: Syllabus for Categorical Course on Gastrointestinal Radiology. Reston, VA, American College of Radiology, 1991, pp 1-9.)

Double-Contrast Interpretation

The principles of double-contrast interpretation in studying the pharynx are the same as those in studying structures elsewhere in the gastrointestinal tract.[35] The double-contrast examination requires adequate mucosal coating, a sufficient number of projections, and varying degrees of luminal distention.

Table 18–3.
Routine Pharyngoesophagogram for Esophageal Symptoms

View	Technique	Organ
Effervescent Agent and Water		
Erect, LPO	Double contrast (two films)	Esophagus
Right lateral	Double contrast	Gastric cardia
Prone, RAO	Videofluoroscopy (2 to 5 swallows)	Esophagus
	Single contrast (one or two films)	Esophagus
	Mucosal relief (one film)	Esophagus
Erect, lateral	Videofluoroscopy, double contrast (R,P) (one film)	Pharynx
Erect, frontal	Videofluoroscopy, double contrast (R,V) (one film)	Pharynx

LPO, left posterior oblique with respect to table top; P, phonation; R, suspended respiration; RAO, right anterior oblique with respect to table top; V, modified Valsalva maneuver.

Mucosal Coating

Adequate mucosal coating depends primarily on two factors: dry pharyngeal mucosa and properly prepared high-density barium (250% weight/volume). If the barium is too thin, the barium is of insufficient radiodensity to outline the pharyngeal mucosa. If the barium is too thick, mucosal coating may be patchy or may obscure mucosal detail. Barium that is too viscous may be unable to wash and scrub the mucosa, resulting in artifactual strands of mucus. Several swallows of high-density barium may be needed in each projection to achieve uniform coating.

Projection

The lateral view best demonstrates the tonsillar fossa en face and the contours of the soft palate, base of the tongue, posterior pharyngeal wall, epiglottis, aryepiglottic folds, anterior hypopharyngeal wall, and region of the cricopharyngeal muscle in profile (Fig. 18-25; see also Figs. 18-1, 18-16, and 18-18). The lateral view is also crucial for evaluating penetration of barium into the laryngeal vestibule (Fig. 18-26). In contrast, the frontal view shows the surface of the tongue base en face and the contours of the median and lateral glossoepiglottic folds, tonsillar fossa, valleculae, and hypopharynx in profile (see Figs. 18-1, 18-14, and 18-18). Oblique views are valuable in some patients for demonstrating the obliquely oriented aryepiglottic folds, anterior walls of the piriform sinuses, and region of the pharyngoesophageal segment.[28,33,40] Spot images obtained in frontal and lateral projections are adequate for most examinations. If a portion of the pharynx

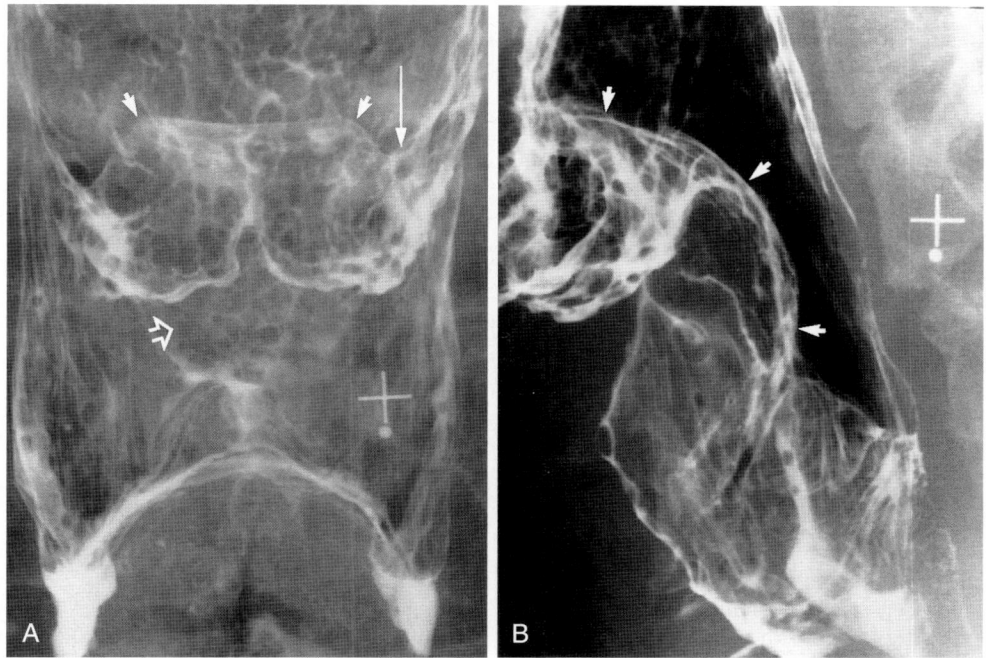

Figure 18-25. Effect of projection. A. Frontal view of pharynx shows subtle enlargement of the epiglottic tip (*small arrows*), elevation of the left pharyngoepiglottic fold (*long arrow*), and nodular mucosa overlying the region of the base of the tongue, extending below the valleculae into the region of the laryngeal vestibule (*open arrow*) and laryngeal surface of the epiglottis. **B.** Lateral view during phonation shows a markedly enlarged epiglottis and aryepiglottic folds (*arrows*). Supraglottic squamous cell carcinoma was confirmed at endoscopy and surgery. (**B** from Rubesin SE, Jones B, Donner MW: Contrast pharyngography: The importance of phonation. AJR 148:269-272, 1987. Copyright by American Roentgen Ray Society.)

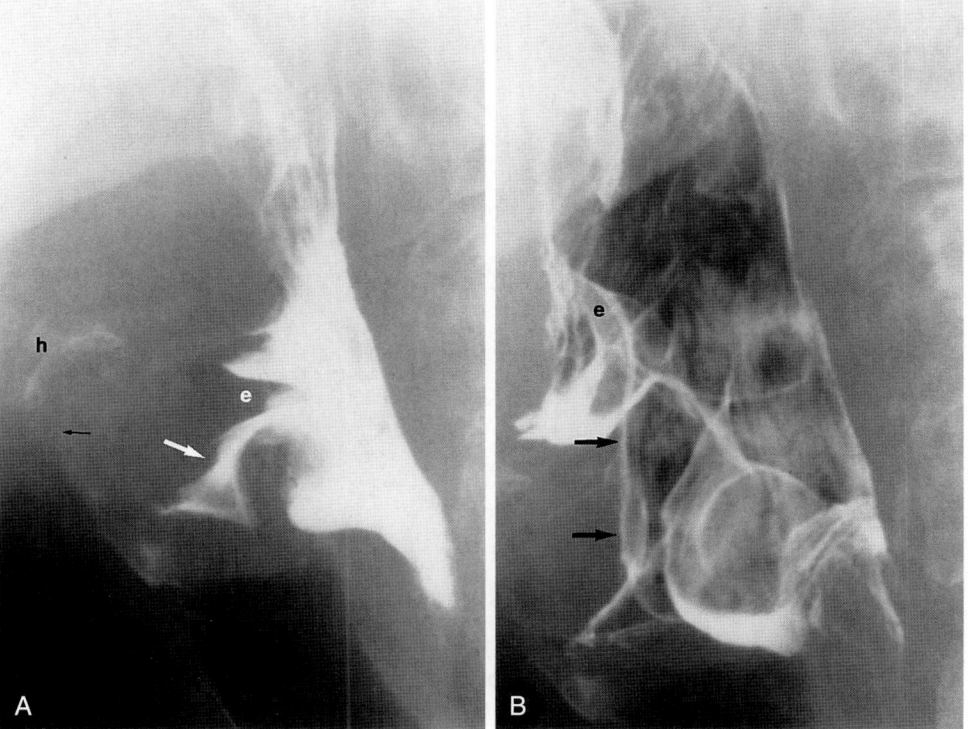

Figure 18-26. Laryngeal penetration. A. In an image obtained during swallowing, barium can be seen entering the laryngeal vestibule (*white arrow*). Note apposition of the hyoid bone (h) to the calcified edge of the thyroid cartilage (*black arrow*). **B.** Spot film obtained during phonation documents coating of the laryngeal vestibule with barium (*arrows*). e, epiglottis. (From Laufer I, Levine MS [eds]: Double Contrast Gastrointestinal Radiology, 2nd ed. Philadelphia, WB Saunders, 1992.)

is not well seen in frontal and lateral projections, however, the patient is turned and oblique views are obtained.

Distention

Adequate distention is important for the demonstration of mucosal surface and contour. The pharynx cannot be distended by the use of effervescent agents or tube insufflation, as in other regions of the gastrointestinal tract. Instead, pharyngeal distention is achieved with phonation (the long vowel sounds "eee" or "ooo") or some form of modified Valsalva maneuver (blowing against pursed or closed lips or whistling).[41,42]

Phonation with "eee" expands the pharynx, resulting in better visualization of the soft palate, tonsillar fossa, base of the tongue, valleculae, epiglottic tip, aryepiglottic folds, and mucosa overlying the muscular processes of the arytenoid cartilages on the lateral view (see Fig. 18-1).[41] The distal 2 cm of hypopharynx, however, remains collapsed during phonation because the pharyngoesophageal sphincter remains contracted and the larynx impresses on this region. In contrast, the distal 2 cm of the hypopharynx, pharyngoesophageal segment, and proximal cervical esophagus are optimally distended during swallowing and are therefore best visualized during the dynamic phase of the examination.

Pharyngeal distention on the frontal view is best obtained with a modified Valsalva procedure (Fig. 18-27). Alternately, the patient is asked to whistle or blow air out of the mouth (as if blowing out a candle) or to blow out against pursed lips. To optimize visualization of pharyngeal structures, the patient is positioned so that the mandible and hard palate are superimposed over the occiput. Flexion or extension of the neck, or protrusion or retraction of the tongue, may improve visualization of various anatomic structures such as the uvula, epiglottic tip, and lateral walls of the hypopharynx.

Motility Examination

DVD recording and videofluoroscopy are the best methods for studying pharyngeal motility.[26,30,31] Spot radiographs or rapid-sequence digital images are not adequate for detecting functional abnormalities. The dynamic portion of the pharyngoesophagogram focuses on patient posture and self-feeding; bolus holding; tongue motion; hyoid, laryngeal, and pharyngeal elevation; soft palate elevation; formation of Passavant's cushion; pharyngeal constrictor motion; epiglottic tilt; laryngeal penetration (see Fig. 18-26); and cricopharyngeal muscle activity.[26,30,31,43-45] An analysis of motility disorders is presented in Chapter 19.

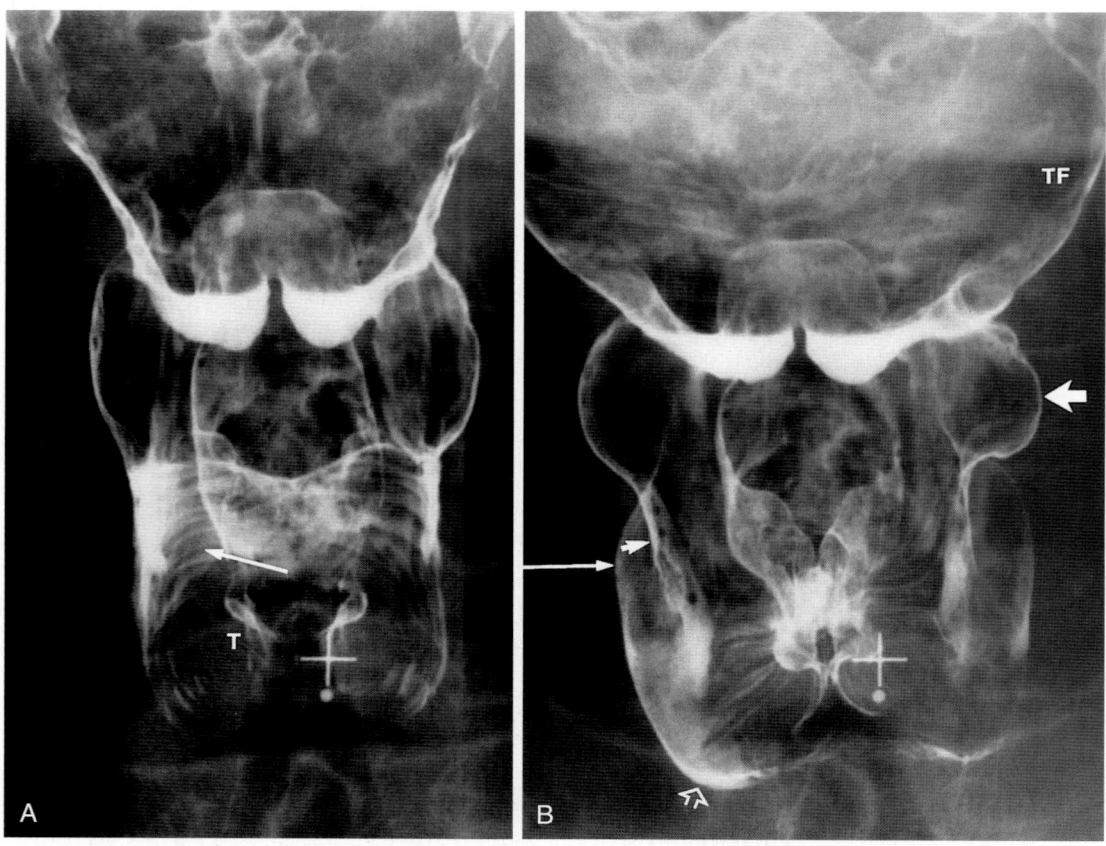

Figure 18-27. Modified Valsalva maneuver. A. During quiet inspiration, the right true cord identified by T and false vocal cords are open. The pharynx is mildly distended. Note arcuate lines in collapsed midhypopharynx (*arrow*). **B.** During a modified Valsalva maneuver, there is marked distention of the oral cavity and pharynx. Note ballooning of the left tonsillar fossae identified by TF. Lateral pharyngeal pouches (*left pouch is identified by short thick arrow*) protrude from the region of the thyrohyoid membrane. The lateral hypopharynx protrudes posterolaterally (*long thin arrow*) from the confines of the ala of the thyroid cartilage (*short thin arrow*). The lower hypopharynx, which was not apparent during inspiration, is now visible (*open arrow*). Protrusion of the lower hypopharynx is a sign of muscular weakness. (Reprinted with permission from Rubesin SE, Glick SN: The tailored double-contrast pharyngogram. Crit Rev Diagn Imaging 28:133-179, 1988. Copyright CRC Press, Inc. Boca Raton, FL.)

Choice of Contrast Agents

In general, the pharynx manipulates a cohesive bolus more readily than a liquid bolus.[9,46-48] Therefore, the pharyngeal phase of swallowing is usually safer with barium paste than with thick barium and safer with thick barium than with thin barium. We usually begin an examination with thick, high-density barium because this barium best demonstrates morphologic characteristics of the pharynx. High-density barium is more visible during review of dynamic images than thin barium. We then usually proceed to barium paste. If a motility disorder is seen during fluoroscopy, swallows of thin barium are videotaped in the lateral and frontal projections after double-contrast imaging of the pharynx and esophagus. Epiglottic motility is better assessed with thin barium because thick barium often obscures the epiglottic tip. Thin barium is also valuable because some patients show laryngeal penetration only with thin barium, not with thick barium or barium paste.

In general, the pharynx can manipulate small, nonphysiologic boluses (2 to 5 mL) more safely than larger physiologic boluses (8 to 10 mL).[9,49,50] If there are clinical signs of abnormal pharyngeal function, the patient should therefore be given small boluses first, then larger boluses. We routinely ask outpatients to "take a normal-sized swallow of barium."

For the patient who is massively aspirating barium, the clinical status of the patient determines the number of barium swallows deemed safe for the examination. If there is aspiration of barium to or below the carina, the examination should generally be discontinued. Even with massive aspiration, views of one swallow in the lateral projection and one swallow in the frontal projection are usually obtained. A suction apparatus should be available for prompt removal of barium that enters the distal trachea.

Position of the Patient

The patient is first examined in the upright lateral position—the best position for visualizing entry of barium into the laryngeal vestibule either during swallowing (penetration) or during normal breathing (aspiration). If unable to stand, the patient is strapped and seated in a "swallowing chair" or on the footboard of the fluoroscope in a lateral position. If unable to sit, the patient is placed on the fluoroscopic table in as lateral a position as possible. Dentures are left in place because denture removal may alter swallowing dynamics. If a portable or fixed C-arm fluoroscope is available, patients may be studied while they are confined to a wheelchair or lying on a stretcher.[51]

Therapeutic Examination

A "therapeutic" examination of the pharynx may be performed to employ modifications of swallowing that prevent or diminish laryngeal penetration and educate patients about their swallowing function.[50,52] This examination is usually performed in conjunction with a swallowing therapist from the department of rehabilitation medicine or speech pathology. During the therapeutic examination, various types of boluses, head positions, and breathing techniques are used to determine which foods can be safely swallowed. The swallowing team selects a technique based on a specific abnormality seen at fluoroscopy. Most strategies to improve swallowing are temporary measures, while a treatable cause of the swallowing problem is discovered or the patient recovers from a cerebrovascular accident, surgery, or radiation therapy.[9]

Compensatory Techniques

Compensatory techniques control bolus flow but do not improve swallowing physiology. Compensatory techniques include (1) changes in posture; (2) increased sensory input; and (3) alterations in food volume or consistency.[52] Eliminating food consistencies that are difficult to swallow is a short-term strategy that is used while a patient recovers from a swallowing disorder. Continuation of swallowing in a limited fashion may help improve muscular function and give the patient some pleasure, while not necessarily maintaining adequate hydration or nutrition. A patient needs 1500 to 2000 mL of fluid per day to maintain proper hydration. The therapist tests the patient's ability to manage barium boluses of progressively larger size and of varying viscosity. If a patient has reduced tongue motion, strength, or coordination, a thin liquid is easier to swallow. If premature spillage of the bolus from the oral cavity to the oropharynx is observed, a thick liquid or cohesive bolus (e.g., a barium paste or barium-impregnated pudding) may improve the timing between the oral and pharyngeal phases. A cohesive bolus may also decrease laryngeal penetration if there is poor timing between the oral and pharyngeal phases, abnormal epiglottic tilt, or abnormal glottic closure. Conversely, a thin liquid improves pharyngeal clearance if there is stasis in the piriform sinuses, thereby diminishing overflow aspiration. Although the use of thin liquids diminishes stasis, this practice results in decreased bolus control or laryngeal penetration in patients with abnormal epiglottic tilt or abnormal laryngeal closure. Thin liquids may also improve swallowing function in patients with isolated pharyngoesophageal segment dysfunction.

Postural techniques alter oral and pharyngeal relationships and redirect bolus flow. Commonly used head positions include chin-up, chin-down, and head rotation. When there is poor transfer of the bolus from the oral cavity to the oropharynx, the chin-up position causes gravity to help the bolus fall into the oropharynx. This position requires a relatively normal pharyngeal phase of swallowing to prevent laryngeal penetration.

The chin-down (chin-tuck) position is used for patients with premature spill, abnormal tongue push, or laryngeal penetration resulting from abnormal epiglottic tilt. If the bolus prematurely spills from the oral cavity, tucking the chin widens the valleculae, providing a space for the prematurely spilled bolus to pool rather than entering the laryngeal vestibule. The chin-tuck position also improves tongue push because the tongue is positioned more posteriorly. The chin-tuck position also narrows the laryngeal aditus by elevating the larynx and pharynx and tilting the epiglottis posteriorly, diminishing laryngeal vestibule penetration caused by abnormal epiglottic tilt. Finally, the chin-tuck position pulls the anterior wall of the pharyngoesophageal segment anteriorly, helping to improve clearance through a pharyngoesophageal segment that opens abnormally.

Rotating the head toward one side narrows the pharynx on that side and redirects the bolus toward the opposite swallowing channel. Head rotation is used for patients with unilateral pharyngeal paresis or asymmetrical epiglottic tilt to guide the bolus away from the weak side. The head is turned toward the side of weakness. Head rotation may be combined with the chin-tuck maneuver.

Therapeutic Techniques

Therapeutic techniques improve motion or strength of a structure or coordination of the timing of oral and pharyngeal events. Therapeutic techniques include (1) range of motion or muscle-strengthening exercises; (2) tactile stimulation; and (3) swallowing maneuvers.

Swallowing maneuvers include the supraglottic swallow, the super-supraglottic swallow, the Mendelsohn maneuver, and the effortful swallow. Such maneuvers require a patient with enough cognitive and physical ability to follow instructions for performing these examinations.

Both a supraglottic and a super-supraglottic swallow may be tried in patients who have laryngeal penetration because of abnormal timing between the oral and the pharyngeal phases of swallowing or abnormal closure of the laryngeal vestibule. In a supraglottic swallow, the patient takes a bolus into the mouth, takes a breath through the nose, consciously holds the breath, swallows, and then exhales or coughs. This sequence closes the true vocal cords before and during the swallow. Exhaling or coughing after the swallow helps to expel any part of the bolus that has entered the laryngeal vestibule. A super-supraglottic swallow is similar to a supraglottic swallow but employs a consciously "hard" breath hold, which closes the true vocal cords and tilts the arytenoids forward to help close the laryngeal aditus.

References

1. DuBrul EL: Sicher's Oral Anatomy, 7th ed. St. Louis, CV Mosby, 1980, pp 319-350.
2. Pernkopf E: Anatomy: vol 1, Head and Neck, 3rd ed. Baltimore, Urban & Schwarzenberg, 1989.
3. Rubesin SE, Jesserun J, Robertson D, et al: Lines of the pharynx. RadioGraphics 7:217-237, 1987.
4. Bosma JF, Donner MW, Tanako E, et al: Anatomy of the pharynx, pertinent to swallowing. Dysphagia 1:23-33, 1986.
5. Dodds WJ: The physiology of swallowing. Dysphagia 3:171-178, 1989.
6. Dodds WJ, Stewart ET, Logemann JA: Physiology and radiology of the normal oral and pharyngeal phases of swallowing. AJR 154:953-963, 1990.
7. Dickson DR: Anatomy of the normal velopharyngeal mechanism. Clin Plast Surg 2:235-248, 1975.
8. Sinclair DC: Muscles and fasciae. In Romanes GJ (ed): Cunningham's Textbook of Anatomy. London, Oxford University Press, 1972, pp 286-299.
9. Rubesin SE, Stiles TD: Principles of performing a "modified barium swallow" examination. In Balfe DM, Levine MS (eds): Categorical Course in Diagnostic Radiology: Gastrointestinal. Oak Brook, IL, RSNA Publications, 1997, pp 7-20.
10. Rubesin SE, Rabischong P, Bilaniuk LT, et al: Contrast examination of the soft palate with cross-sectional correlation. RadioGraphics 4:641-665, 1988.
11. Ekberg O, Nylander G: Anatomy and physiology. In Ekberg O (ed): Radiology of the Pharynx and Oesophagus. Berlin, Springer-Verlag, 2004, pp 1-14.
12. Doty RW, Bosma JF: An electromyographic analysis of reflex deglutition. J Neurophysiol 19:44-60, 1956.
13. Shprintzen RJ, McCall GN, Skolnick ML, et al: Selective movement of the lateral aspects of the pharyngeal walls during velopharyngeal closure for speech, blowing, and whistling in normals. Cleft Palate J 12:51-58, 1975.
14. Skolnick ML, McCall GN, Barnes M: The sphincteric mechanism of velopharyngeal closure. Cleft Palate J 10:286-305, 1973.
15. Skolnick ML: Videofluoroscopic examination of the velopharyngeal portal during phonation in lateral and base projections—a new technique for studying the mechanism of closure. Cleft Palate J 7:803-816, 1970.
16. Donner MW, Bosma JF, Robertson DL: Anatomy and physiology of the pharynx. Gastrointest Radiol 10:196-212, 1985.
17. Silver AJ, Sane P, Hilal SK: CT of the nasopharyngeal region: Normal and pathologic anatomy. Radiol Clin North Am 22:161-176, 1984.
18. Sobotta J, Figge FHJ: Atlas of Human Anatomy, vol 2. Baltimore, Urban & Schwarzenberg, 1977.
19. Rubesin SE: Pharyngeal morphology. In Ekberg O (ed): Radiology of the Pharynx and Oesophagus. Berlin, Springer-Verlag, 2004, pp 51-75.
20. McMyn JK: The anatomy of the salpingopharyngeus muscle. J Laryngol Otol 55:1-22, 1940.
21. Rubesin SE, Jones B, Donner MW: Radiology of the adult soft palate. Dysphagia 2:8-17, 1987.
22. Capitanio MA, Kirkpatrick JA: Nasopharyngeal lymphoid tissue: Roentgen observations in 257 children two years of age or less. Radiology 96:389-391, 1970.
23. Gromet M, Homer MJ, Carter BL: Lymphoid hyperplasia at the base of the tongue. Radiology 144:825-828, 1982.
24. Curtis DJ, Hudson T: Laryngotracheal aspiration: Analysis of specific neuromuscular factors. Radiology 149:517-522, 1983.
25. Pitman RG, Fraser GM: The post-cricoid impression of the esophagus. Clin Radiol 16:34-39, 1965.
26. Dodds WJ, Logemann JA, Stewart ET: Radiologic assessment of abnormal oral and pharyngeal phases of swallowing. AJR 154:965-974, 1990.
27. Rubesin SE, Ruiz CE, Levine MS: Principles of Performing a Barium Swallow. Lake Success, NY, E-Z-EM, 2003.
28. Balfe DM, Heiken JP: Contrast evaluation of structural lesions of the pharynx. Curr Probl Diagn Radiol 15:73-160, 1986.
29. Ott DJ, Gelfand DW: Gastrointestinal contrast agents: Indications, uses, risks. JAMA 249:2380-2384, 1984.
30. Jones B, Donner MW: Examination of the patient with dysphagia. Radiology 167:319-326, 1988.
31. Jones B, Kramer SS, Donner MW: Dynamic imaging of the pharynx. Gastrointest Radiol 10:213-224, 1985.
32. Levine MS, Rubesin SE: Radiologic investigation of dysphagia. AJR 154:1157-1163, 1990.
33. Rubesin SE, Glick SN: The tailored double-contrast pharyngogram. Crit Rev Diagn Imaging 28:133-179, 1988.
34. Ekberg O, Nylander G: Double contrast examination of the pharynx. Gastrointest Radiol 10:263-271, 1985.
35. Rubesin SE, Laufer I: Pictorial review: Principles of double contrast pharyngography. Dysphagia 6:170-178, 1991.
36. Logemann JA: Manual for the Videofluorographic Study of Swallowing, 2nd ed. Austin, TX, Pro-Ed, 1993.
37. Rubesin SE: Pharyngeal dysfunction. In Gore R (ed): Syllabus for Categorical Course on Gastrointestinal Radiology. Reston, VA, American College of Radiology, 1991, pp 1-9.
38. Rubesin SE: Pharynx. In Laufer I, Levine MS (eds): Double Contrast Gastrointestinal Radiology, 2nd ed. Philadelphia, WB Saunders, 1991, pp 73-105.
39. Jones B, Ravich WJ, Donner MW, et al: Pharyngoesophageal interrelationships: Observations and working concepts. Gastrointest Radiol 10:225-233, 1985.
40. Taylor AJ, Dodds WJ, Stewart ET: Pharynx: Value of oblique projections for radiographic examination. Radiology 178:59-61, 1991.
41. Rubesin SE, Jones B, Donner MW: Contrast pharyngography: The importance of phonation. AJR 148:269-272, 1987.
42. Jing BS: The pharynx and larynx: Roentgenographic technique. Semin Roentgenol 9:259-265, 1974.
43. Ekberg O: Posture of the head and pharyngeal swallow. Acta Radiol Diagn 1986:691-696.
44. Curtis DJ, Sepulveda GU: Epiglottic motion: Video recording of muscular dysfunction. Radiology 148:473-477, 1983.
45. Ekberg O, Sigurjonsson S: Movements of the epiglottis during deglutition: A cineradiographic study. Gastrointest Radiol 7:101-107, 1982.
46. Dantas RO, Dodds WJ, Massey BT, et al: The effect of high- vs. low-density barium preparations on the quantitative features of swallowing. AJR 153:1191-1195, 1989.
47. Curtis DJ, Cruess DF, Willgress ER: Abnormal solid bolus swallowing in the erect position. Dysphagia 2:46-49, 1987.
48. van Westen D, Ekberg O: Solid bolus swallowing in the radiologic evaluation of dysphagia. Acta Radiol 34:332-335, 1993.
49. Dodds WJ, Man KM, Cook IJ, et al: Influence of bolus volume on swallow-induced hyoid movement in normal subjects. AJR 150:1307-1309, 1988.
50. Logemann J: Anatomy and physiology of normal deglutition. In Logemann J (ed): Evaluation and Treatment of Swallowing Disorders. Austin, TX, Pro-Ed, 1983, pp 9-26.
51. Davis M, Palmer P, Kelsey C: Use of C-arm fluoroscope to examine patients with swallowing disorders. AJR 155:986-988, 1990.
52. Logemann JA: Rehabilitation of oropharyngeal swallowing disorders. Acta Otorhinolaryngol Belg 48:207-215, 1994.

Abnormalities of Pharyngeal Function

Bronwyn Jones, MD

ANALYSIS OF THE FUNCTIONAL ASPECTS OF SWALLOWING

In reviewing the examination of the pharynx and esophagus, the slow motion, reverse, and stop-frame capabilities of videofluoroscopy are essential. With these capabilities, the movement of individual structures can be analyzed, first in isolation and then in combination with other structures, including the tongue, palate, epiglottis, hyoid bone, larynx, and cricopharyngeus. Esophageal peristalsis should also be evaluated (Table 19-1), but discussion of this subject is beyond the scope of this chapter.

Familiarity with the anatomy, radiographic anatomy, and physiology of the pharynx and related structures is a necessity for abnormalities to be appreciated. Any lack of movement or abnormalities indicating compensation or decompensation must be noted.

Two important principles must be considered when reviewing pharyngeal studies:

1. *Dynamic imaging is vital.* Pharyngeal contraction occurs much faster than esophageal contraction (12-25 cm/second vs. 1-4 cm/second), which is why dynamic imaging is essential when examining the pharynx. In addition, a lesion such as a web or a ring may be visible on only 1 or 2 frames at 30 frames per second.
2. *The entire swallowing chain must be examined.* Such extensive examination is necessary because the level of symptoms is not a reliable indicator of the site of the abnormality.[1] Also, several lesions could be causing dysphagia, and esophageal disease may result in pharyngeal disease.[2]

Neurophysiologic Control of Swallowing

Swallowing involves the close cooperation of many muscles, six cranial nerves (trigeminal, facial, glossopharyngeal, vagus, spinal branch of accessory, and hypoglossal) and the first, second, and third cervical nerves (through the ansa cervicalis).

Table 19-1
Checklist When Reviewing Swallowing Studies

Head and Neck Posture
Swan neck or flexion at rest
Flexion during swallowing

Mouth-Tongue Coordination
Bolus transfer
Drooling
Loss of bolus in floor of mouth or cheek

Tongue
Atrophy, resection, or increased bulk
Bolus control
Abnormal or multiple movements

Hyoid Bone Motion
Original position
Elevation with swallowing

Tongue/Palate
Premature leakage

Palate/Posterior Pharyngeal Wall
Elevation with speech
Elevation and apposition to posterior pharyngeal wall with
    swallowing (Passavant's cushion)

Pharyngeal Stripping Wave
Wave normal, deeper than usual, absent, disordered
Cervical spine disease

Epiglottis
Tilt, asymmetry

Laryngeal Penetration
During, before, after swallowing
Contrast medium level extruded during swallow
Entry of contrast medium into trachea
Cough

Aspiration
Elevation of larynx
Closure of larynx
Cough

Cricopharyngeus
Opening completely and on time
Early closure

Esophagus
Normal motility
Emptying
Gastroesophageal reflux
Stricture or ring
Mucosal abnormality

Modified from Jones B, Gayler BW, Donner MW: Pharynx and cervical
esophagus. In Levine MS (ed): Radiology of the Esophagus.
Philadelphia, WB Saunders, 1989, pp 311-336.

Afferent sensory information is integrated in the "swallowing center" in the brain stem, and efferent signals originate in the motor ganglia of the cranial nerves; movements are then effected peripherally.[3-8]

The vagus nerve (CN X) supplies motor efferent fibers to all of the intrinsic pharyngeal muscles (constrictors, palatopharyngeus, and salpingopharyngeus), except the stylopharyngeus, which is supplied by the glossopharyngeal nerve (CN IX). The vagus nerve also supplies motor efferent fibers to all the palatal muscles, except the tensor veli palatini, which is supplied by the trigeminal nerve (CN V). The trigeminal

Table 19-2
Innervation of Muscles Used in Swallowing

Muscles	Nerve
All soft palate muscles (except tensor veli palatini)	CN X (CN V)
All pharyngeal muscles (except stylopharyngeus)	CN X (CN IX)
All laryngeal muscles (except cricothyroideus)	RLN (SLN)
All tongue muscles (except palatoglossus)	CN XII (CN X)
Suprahyoid muscles	CN V, CN VII
Infrahyoid muscles	Ansa cervicalis

CN, cranial nerve; RLN, recurrent laryngeal nerve; SLN, superior laryngeal nerve.

nerve also supplies the anterior digastricus and mylohyoideus. The facial nerve (CN VII) supplies the posterior digastricus and stylohyoideus. Although the vagus nerve carries the efferent fibers that innervate the striated pharyngeal musculature, most of these fibers probably emerge from the brain stem in the bulbar part of the accessory nerve (CN XI).

Pharyngeal branches of the glossopharyngeal and vagus nerves and rami of the sympathetic trunk and the superior cervical ganglion form a plexus in the connective tissue outside the constrictor muscles (the pharyngeal plexus). In this plexus, autonomic (parasympathetic and sympathetic) and afferent and efferent branchial fibers intermingle and branch into the muscles and the mucosal lining. Damage to this plexus can produce dysphagia.[9,10]

Pharyngeal sensation (including sensation of the tonsil and the postsulcal part of the tongue) appears to be mediated by the glossopharyngeal nerve. This nerve also supplies motor innervation to the stylopharyngeus and parasympathetic secretomotor fibers to the parotid gland. A summary of the innervation of the muscles involved in swallowing is presented in Table 19-2.

Functional Components of Swallowing

Oropharyngeal Phase

Tongue and Palate

Swallowing begins with the lips engulfing the bolus (Figs. 19-1 and 19-2). The bolus is then manipulated by the tongue and teeth until it is judged "swallowable." Two positions of the bolus preparatory to swallowing have been identified: the *tipper* type (in which the bolus is held in a midline groove of the tongue against the alveolar ridge) and the *dipper* type (in which the bolus is held anteriorly underneath the tongue in the floor of the mouth).[11]

The back of the tongue blade and the soft palate form a seal that prevents premature leakage into the pharynx before swallowing (see Figs. 19-1A and 19-2A). Weakness, atrophy, or resection of the tongue or soft palate can lead to aspiration before swallowing due to leakage of the bolus into the open, unprotected larynx. Viewed in the frontal position, unilateral leakage indicates decompensation on one side only.

As the bolus is propelled into the oropharynx by an upward backward movement of the tongue, the soft palate elevates to a right angle to appose the posterior pharyngeal wall, with

Figure 19-1. Line drawing of the normal swallow (lateral view). A. The bolus is held in the oral cavity by apposition of the soft palate and back of the tongue. **B.** As the bolus is presented to the oropharynx, the soft palate (*short arrow*) elevates to appose Passavant's cushion (*long arrow*) to prevent nasopharyngeal regurgitation. **C.** As the bolus passes through the pharynx, the beginning of the posterior pharyngeal stripping wave (*yellow arrow*) can be seen. The epiglottis (*black arrow*) is tilted to cover the laryngeal aditus, which is completely closed. **D.** As the bolus descends farther, the back of the tongue, soft palate, and pharyngeal stripping wave (*arrow*) continue to seal the nasopharyngeal inlet, the epiglottis remains tilted, and the larynx remains closed. The cricopharyngeus has opened completely to allow unimpeded bolus passage. **E.** As the bolus descends past the cricopharyngeal level, the tongue base begins to move forward and the soft palate begins to elevate. **F.** As the bolus passes into the thoracic esophagus, the tongue base moves forward, the epiglottis flips up, and the larynx returns to its resting, open position. (From Donner MW, Bosma JF, Robertson DL: Anatomy and physiology of the pharynx. Gastrointest Radiol 10:196-212, 1985, with kind permission from Springer Science and Business Media.)

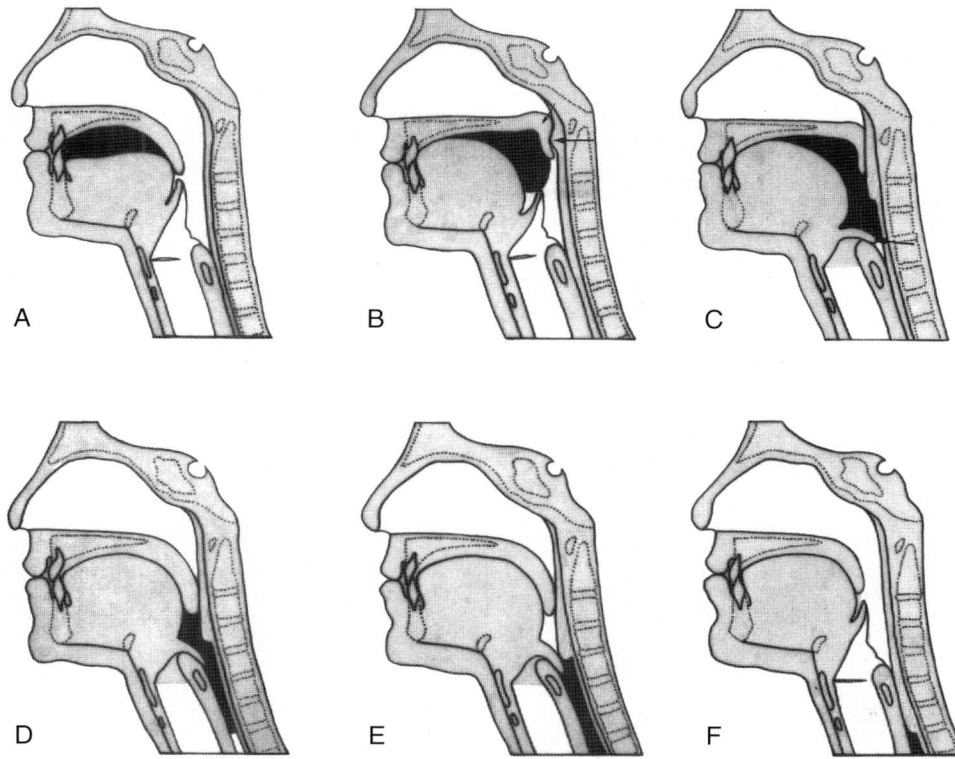

Passavant's cushion moving anteriorly to complete the seal of the palatopharyngeal isthmus. Passavant's cushion results from focal contraction of the upper fibers of the superior pharyngeal constrictor muscle of the pharynx (Fig. 19-3; see also Figs. 19-1B, 19-2B, 19-10A, 19-11A, and 19-11B). Tongue thrust (involving first the blade and then the base of the tongue), combined with pharyngeal constriction and intrabolus pressure, contributes to bolus compression and propulsion.

Pharynx

The constrictor stripping wave can be observed at the tail of the bolus in the lateral position as a progressive forward movement of the posterior pharyngeal wall (see Figs. 19-1C-F and 19-2C-E). In the frontal position, the wave can be appreciated as the lateral walls of the pharynx converge to the midline, completely obliterating the pharyngeal cavity behind the bolus. Unilateral weakness results in asymmetry on the frontal view; the contracting normal side can displace the bolus across to the atonic side, so that the bolus passes down the paralyzed side. The contracting normal side may be misinterpreted as a mass, whereas the abnormality is actually on the noncontracting, bulging side. Contraction of the constrictor muscles may be affected by intrinsic disease of the pharyngeal muscles (e.g., polymyositis), by neuromuscular disorders (e.g., amyotrophic lateral sclerosis, multiple sclerosis, or cerebrovascular accidents), or by local factors such as scarring, radiation, or cervical spine disease. Diseases that restrict laryngeal elevation (e.g., radiation or head and neck surgery) compound the problem. Large osteophytes in the cervical spine may hinder or prevent epiglottic tilt.[12]

Laryngeal Dynamics

Respiration is suspended during swallowing and resumes after swallowing. As the bolus enters the oropharynx, the larynx begins to elevate, moving upward and forward, and the true vocal cords, false vocal cords, and laryngeal vestibule close inferiorly to superiorly, with the vestibule closing last. Laryngeal elevation begins simultaneously with elevation of the hyoid bone but continues for a short time after the hyoid bone has reached its peak elevation. Laryngeal movement can be appreciated by observing the hyoid bone rising to appose the angle of the mandible. There is an excellent review of laryngeal dynamics by Curtis.[13] A direct correlation exists between hyoid bone excursion and bolus volume, with larger volumes producing more elevation.[14] Hyoid bone elevation may occur in one step (20%) or in two steps (80%), whereas descent occurs in one step, simultaneously with return of the epiglottis to the upright position.[15]

Epiglottic Tilt

Epiglottic tilt deflects food and liquid into the lateral food channels away from the larynx; and when completely inverted, the epiglottis covers the laryngeal aperture. In many people, this movement occurs in two steps: the first movement (to a horizontal position) is probably a passive one caused by elevation of the hyoid bone; the second movement (to complete inversion) is probably due to contraction of the thyroepiglotticus.[16] In a minority of people, the epiglottis fails to invert, tilting only to the horizontal or oblique position. In the frontal view, the completely inverted epiglottis produces

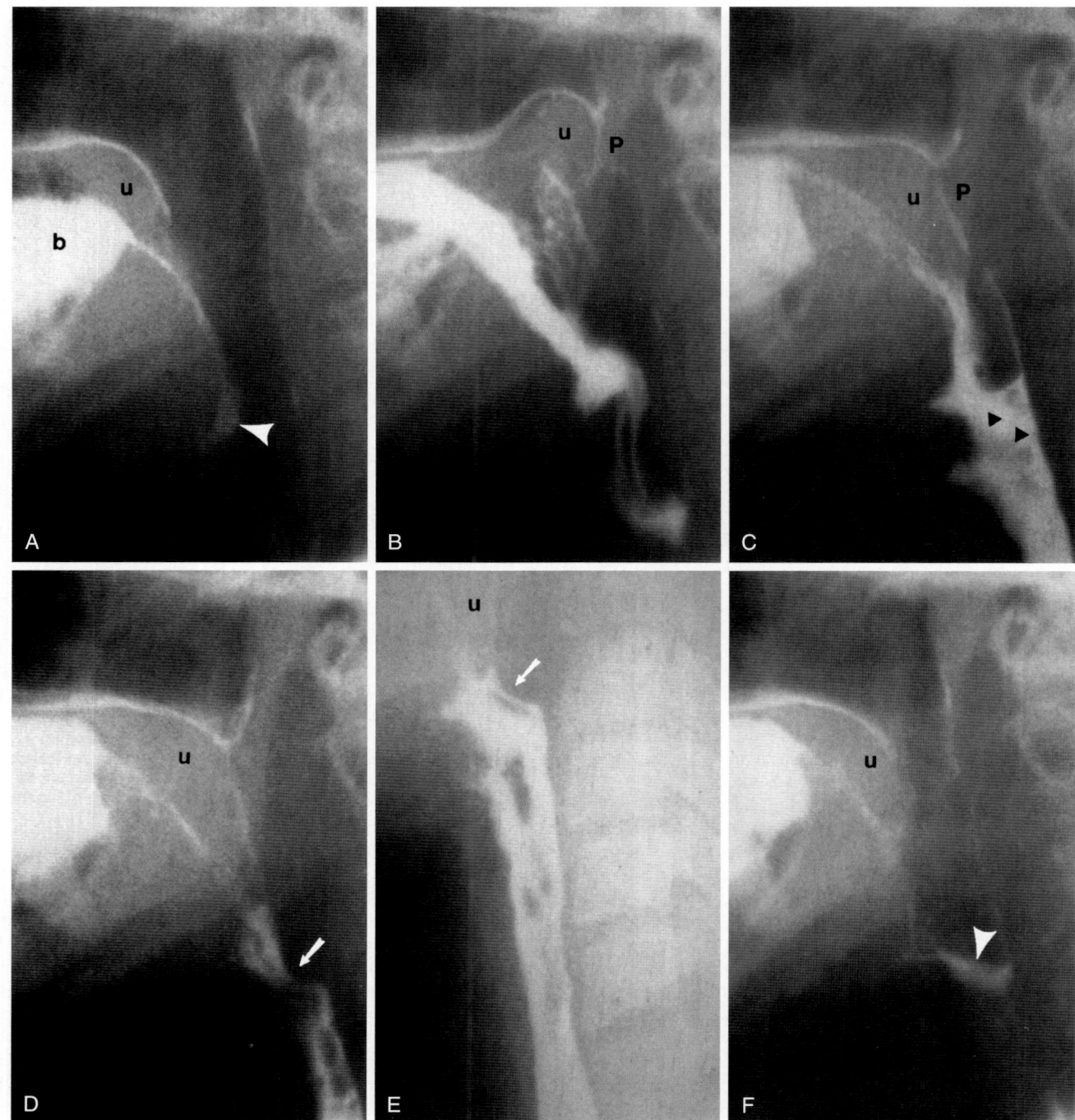

Figure 19-2.   The normal swallow. A to F. A series of stop-frame prints from a cinepharyngoesophagogram shows the normal swallow as it appears on the dynamic imaging study in the lateral position. The epiglottis (*arrowheads*) and stripping wave (*arrow*) are identified. Note that the superior and posterior surfaces of the soft palate have been coated by intranasal injection of barium. In **F,** the epiglottis is beginning to re-elevate but has not yet returned to its resting position. b, bolus; u, soft palate; p, Passavant's cushion.

a "sea gull"-shaped filling defect. Flow of the bolus into the lateral food channels may also produce a flow defect, simulating a mass.

Cricopharyngeal Opening

Pharyngeal constriction must be coordinated with cricopharyngeal relaxation and opening. The cricopharyngeus

must relax and open completely to allow unimpeded bolus passage.[17-32] Opening of the lumen at the pharyngoesophageal junction results from several actions: (1) cricopharyngeal relaxation; (2) superior and anterior movement of the larynx, resulting in traction on the anterior wall of the lumen; (3) pharyngeal constriction producing thrust; and (4) intrabolus pressure producing thrust. Thus, cricopharyngeal prominence is often observed in patients with pharyngeal paresis or

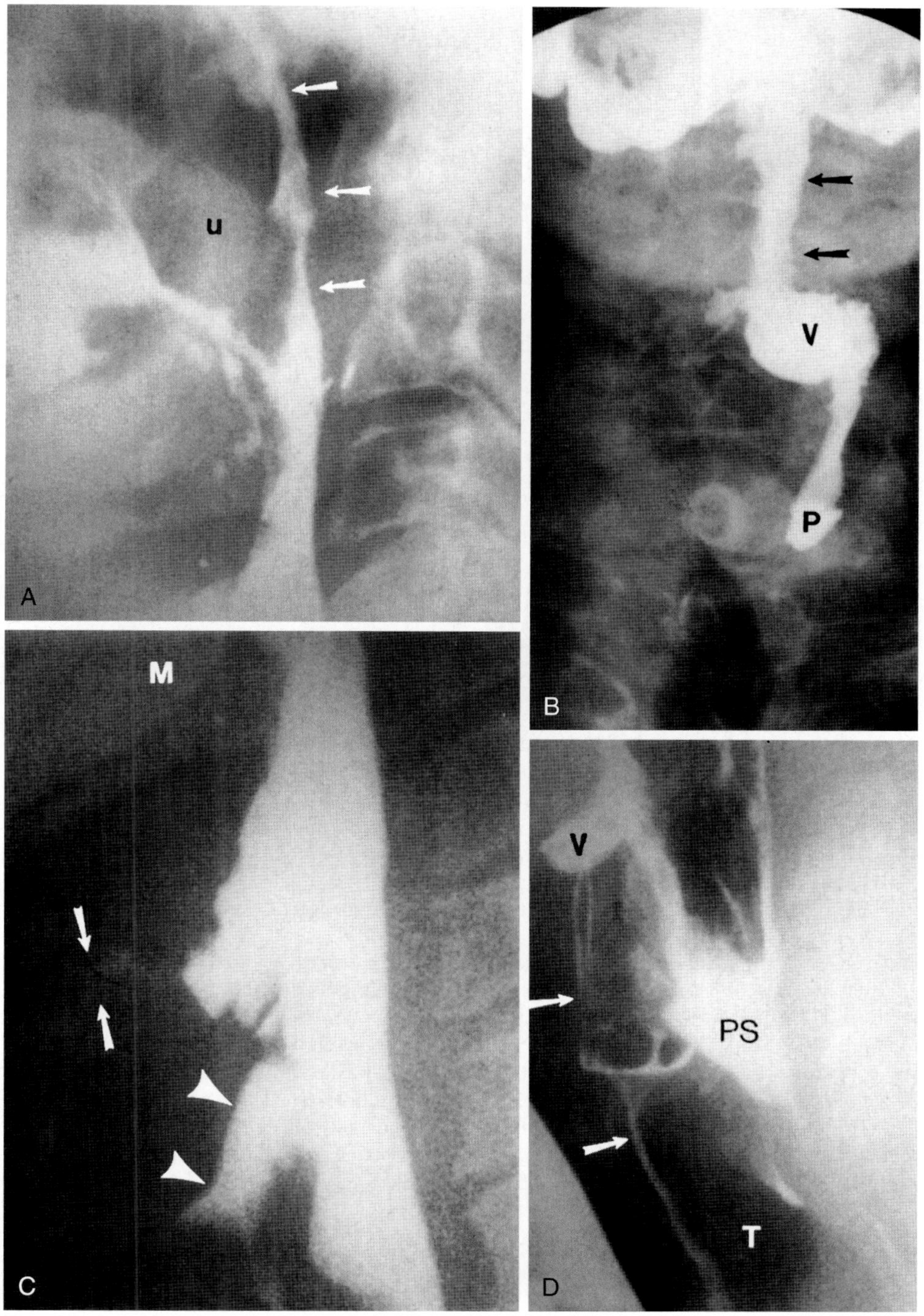

Figure 19-3. Multiple stop-frame prints from four different patients show multiple decompensations. A. Somewhat magnified view of the lateral oropharynx and nasopharynx demonstrates incomplete elevation of the soft palate (u) and marked nasopharyngeal regurgitation (*arrows*). **B.** There is unilateral leakage over the back of the tongue (*arrows*) into the left vallecula (V) and then into the piriform sinus (P). **C.** Lateral view shows marked laryngeal penetration into the widely open larynx (*arrowheads*) and incomplete elevation of the hyoid bone (*arrows*); normally, the hyoid elevates almost to the angle of the mandible (M). **D.** There is marked retention in the valleculae (V) and piriform sinuses (PS) after swallowing and overflow aspiration (*arrows*) into the larynx and trachea (T). (**B** from Jones B, Donner MW: Interpreting the study. In Jones B, Donner MW [eds]: Normal and Abnormal Swallowing: Imaging in Diagnosis and Therapy. New York, Springer-Verlag, 1991, p 60. With kind permission from Springer Science and Business Media.)

a frozen larynx. In such circumstances, the pharyngeal milieu, rather than the muscle itself, is abnormal.

Radiographically, one normally observes luminal opening, not cricopharyngeal relaxation; a radiographic report therefore should not comment on cricopharyngeal "relaxation" but only on "cricopharyngeal opening." *Cricopharyngeal achalasia* is a manometric term referring to complete failure of cricopharyngeal relaxation, an unusual entity. Other common conditions associated with cricopharyngeal prominence include Zenker's diverticulum, advanced age, gastroesophageal reflux,

and other esophageal motility disorders such as diffuse esophageal spasm and achalasia (Fig. 19-4).[2] The resulting luminal compromise may be minimal or marked. In severe cases, there may be a horizontal "bar." The luminal narrowing can be treated by endoscopic bougienage.

PREVENTION OF ASPIRATION

Many mechanisms protect the larynx from aspiration (Table 19-3; see Figs. 19-3 and 19-11). Laryngeal elevation and closure

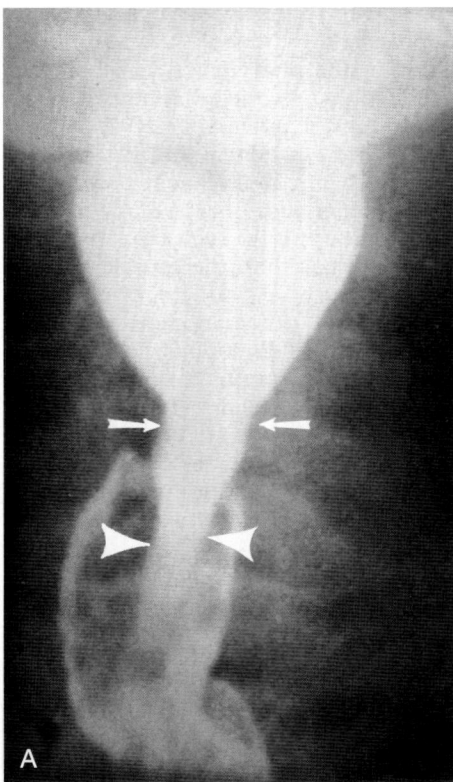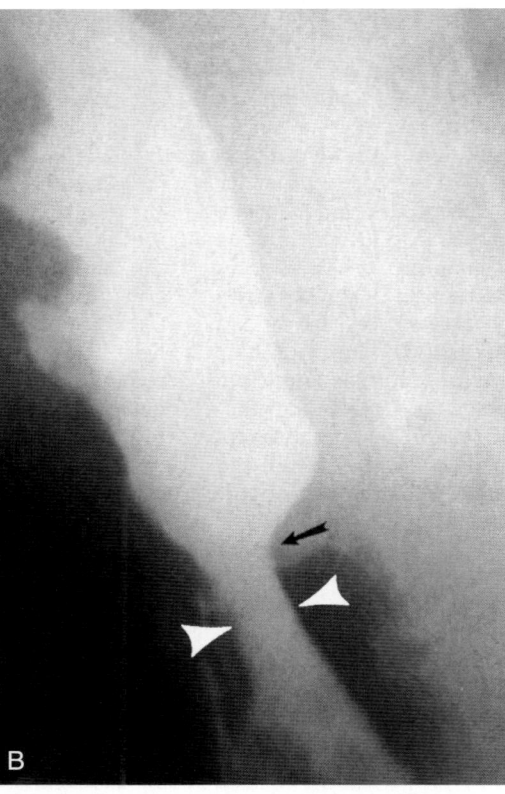

Figure 19-4. Cricopharyngeal prominence. Frontal (**A**) and lateral (**B**) radiographs show prominence of the cricopharyngeus (*arrows*). Note the jet effect below the narrowing (*arrowheads*), simulating a stenotic lesion, especially on the lateral view. The lumen of the cervical esophagus is actually dilated, because the patient had achalasia. (From Jones B, Donner MW, Rubesin SE, et al: Pharyngeal findings in 21 patients with achalasia of the esophagus. Dysphagia 2:87-92, 1987. With kind permission from Springer Science and Business Media.)

of the vocal folds, arytenoid cartilages, and laryngeal vestibule are as important as epiglottic tilt.[33] Thus, a frozen larynx can result in aspiration.

If aspiration is observed, all factors that prevent aspiration should be analyzed and the following questions asked. Does the epiglottis tilt, and does the larynx (hyoid bone) elevate adequately? Do the vocal folds and laryngeal vestibule close? It should also be noted when the aspiration is in relation to swallowing. Laryngeal penetration or aspiration through the vocal folds may occur during swallowing, before swallowing (premature leakage from the mouth), or after swallowing (overflow aspiration of a retained bolus in the pharynx, or regurgitated or refluxed material). The timing and causes of aspiration have potential therapeutic implications.

The important role that the mouth can play in aspiration was underestimated until two important studies highlighted the role of oral decompensation in aspiration.[34,35] Feinberg and Ekberg studied a group of 50 patients with known aspiration and found that aspiration was the result of oral decompensation in 23 patients, a combination of oral and pharyngeal decompensation in 17 patients, and pharyngeal decompensation alone in 10 patients.[34] The same authors studied oral decompensation in 75 patients who survived a near-fatal choking episode.[35] Abnormalities were found on videoradiography in 58 of these 75 patients. Oral stage dysfunction was the predominant finding in 32 patients, with pharyngeal abnormalities in 19 and pharyngoesophageal segment abnormalities in 28.

Another important observation is whether the aspirated material precipitates a cough; this observation needs to be conveyed to the referring physician in the radiologic report. Some patients with chronic aspiration are silent aspirators (presumably because of loss of laryngeal sensation). Bedside evaluation of these patients for aspiration is notoriously inaccurate. In fact, the "bedside evaluation" underestimates the possibility of aspiration in a substantial number of patients.[36-39]

ADAPTATION, COMPENSATION, AND DECOMPENSATION

The pharynx is an extremely flexible organ that must adapt to its various functions, including respiration, speech, and swallowing. In addition, the pharynx adapts to different stimuli, such as the size and consistency of the bolus and the temperature of ingested liquids and food, and the pharynx compensates when one of its parts is defective (Tables 19-4

Table 19-3
Airway Protection

Momentary suspension of respiration
Adduction of the true and false vocal folds
Inverting of the epiglottis
Constrictor contraction compressing the inverted epiglottis against the laryngeal aperture
Deflection of bolus away from the laryngeal vestibule into lateral food channels formed by the piriform sinuses
Elevation of the larynx
Closure of the laryngeal aperture (apposition of arytenoid masses)
Approximation of the thyroid cartilage to the hyoid bone
Coughing

Modified from Jones B, Gayler BW, Donner MW: Pharynx and cervical esophagus. In Levine MS (ed): Radiology of the Esophagus. Philadelphia, WB Saunders, 1989, pp 311-336.

Table 19-4
Pharyngeal Deficiency in Relation to Five Stages of Swallowing

Stage of Swallowing	Site of Deficiency	Signs of Compensation	Signs of Decompensation
1. Control of junction of mouth and pharynx (tongue/palate competence)	Tongue	Palate kinks to appose tongue (this is normal in the supine position)	Leakage into pharynx before swallowing
	Palate	Posterior aspect of tongue displaced upward	As above
2. Closure of palatopharyngeal isthmus (palate/constrictor muscle competence)	Palate	Greater convergence of pharyngeal wall by pharyngeal contraction (prominent Passavant's cushion)	Nasopharyngeal regurgitation
3. Compression of bolus	Constrictor	Tongue and larynx displaced posteriorly	Retention in valleculae and piriform sinuses after swallowing
	Tongue base	Excessive posterior retraction of tongue	As above
		Greater convergence of pharyngeal wall (prominent stripping wave)	
4. Closure of larynx	Intrinsic laryngeal muscles	Further displacement of larynx upward and forward	Laryngeal penetration
5. Opening of pharyngoesophageal segment	Cricopharyngeus	Head flexion	Overflow aspiration of retained bolus

and 19-5). The process of adjustment of normal swallowing to different stimuli is called *adaptation*.[40] The pharynx must adjust to the bolus, which may vary in volume, temperature, consistency, viscosity, and elasticity. The effect of different boluses can be seen on videofluoroscopy by watching the difference between a swallow of thin liquid barium and a swallow of the same volume of barium paste.[41]

Recently, the effect of a carbonated bolus on the physiology of the swallow was investigated.[42] Carbonated liquids reduced penetration/aspiration and pharyngeal retention, and pharyngeal transit time was shorter.

When signs of compensation are visible on dynamic studies, swallowing is already impaired.[40] Some types of compensation for impaired swallowing may be conscious and voluntary. For example, a patient may change the types of food eaten, perhaps omitting solid food and substituting puréed food, or may even restrict the diet to liquids only. Certain postures such as flexing the neck ("chin tuck") or turning the head may help a patient to swallow more effectively, reducing laryngeal penetration or aspiration and clearing any retained bolus.

Table 19-5
Common Abnormalities of Swallowing

Finding	Causes
Leakage	Weakness, atrophy, resection of tongue or soft palate
	Edentulous or missing teeth or ill-fitting dentures
Nasal regurgitation	Weakness, atrophy, or resection of soft palate or superior constrictor
Penetration or aspiration	Poor or absent epiglottic tilt
	Poor or absent elevation of larynx
	Poor or absent closure of larynx
Retention in valleculae or piriform sinuses	Poor or absent constriction
	Poor or absent tongue base retraction
	Relative obstruction such as prominent cricopharyngeus or web

Modified from Jones B, Gayler BW, Donner MW: Pharynx and cervical esophagus. In Levine MS (ed): Radiology of the Esophagus. Philadelphia, WB Saunders, 1989, pp 311-336.

Swallowing can be considered to have five distinct stages (see Table 19-4), each of which has a characteristic pattern of compensation and decompensation.[40] The five stages include:

1. Control of the junction of the mouth and pharynx (palatoglossal seal) (Fig. 19-5)
2. Closure of the palatopharyngeal isthmus (Fig. 19-6)
3. Compression of the bolus (Fig. 19-7)
4. Closure of the larynx (Fig. 19-8)
5. Opening of the pharyngoesophageal segment (Fig. 19-9)

During the first stage, for example, downward displacement of the soft palate may compensate for deficiencies of the tongue (resulting from atrophy, weakness, or surgical resection); conversely, upward displacement of the tongue may compensate for weakness of the soft palate (see Table 19-4 and Figs. 19-5 to 19-9 for compensation occurring during other stages of swallowing).

Another compensatory phenomenon is the development of a deeper pharyngeal stripping wave, which may be observed in the presence of a partially obstructing lesion in the cervical esophagus, such as a web or prominent cricopharyngeus.

Any radiographic findings of compensation must be communicated to the referring physician, so that the patient can be informed that swallowing is impaired and can be instructed to take additional care when eating or drinking quickly, for example, in a restaurant or in other social situations.

THE FUNCTIONAL ASPECTS OF ZENKER'S DIVERTICULUM

Zenker's diverticulum is a pulsion diverticulum located at the level of the pharyngoesophageal junction, the most common site being between the oblique and horizontal fibers of the cricopharyngeal muscle through a triangular area known as Killian's dehiscence (Fig. 19-10). It is a posterior diverticulum that may fill during or after swallowing, and, if large, it may flop to one side or the other, more often to the left. Once swallowing is completed, the diverticulum may empty back into the pharynx, filling the piriform sinuses. This often precipitates a second swallow, but it also places the patient at risk for overflow aspiration.

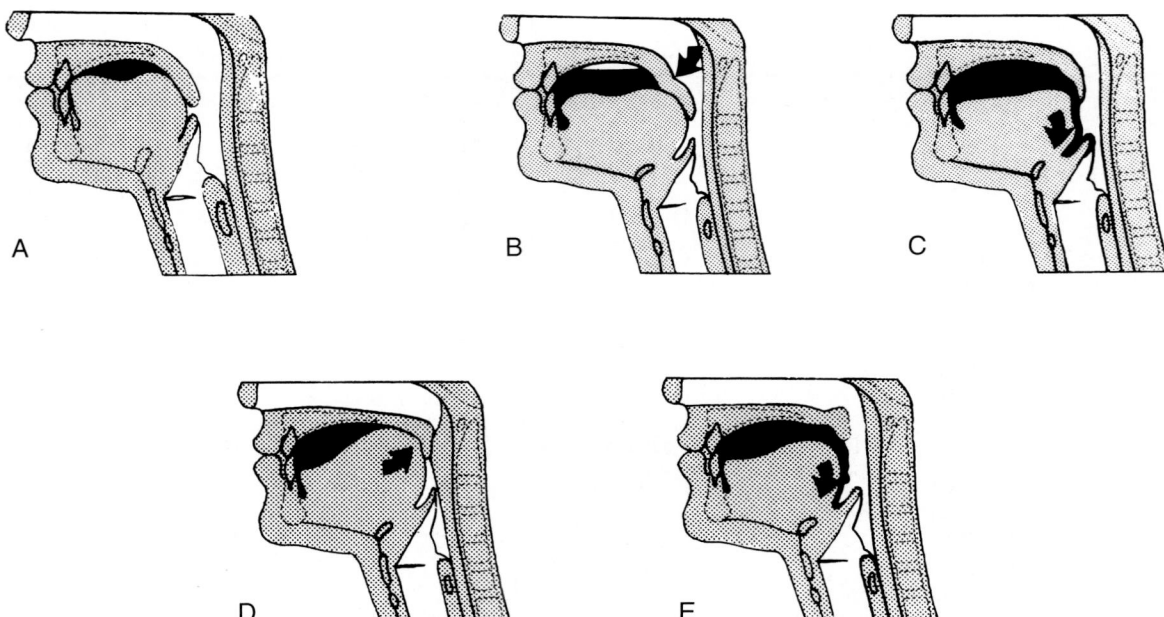

Figure 19-5. Control of the junction of the mouth and pharynx. A. Leakage from the back of the mouth is prevented in the normal patient when the soft palate abuts the posterior portion of the tongue. **B.** Deficiency of the tongue due to atrophy, weakness, incoordination, or postsurgical defect may be compensated by downward displacement of the palate (*arrow*), with the palate "kinking" to appose the tongue. **D.** Conversely, palatal deficiency is compensated by upward displacement of the tongue (*arrow*). Note that the bolus is held further forward in the mouth under these circumstances. **C** and **E.** Decompensation, in which there is premature leakage of oral contents into the pharynx (*arrow*), with the potential for overflow aspiration. (From Buchholz DW, Bosma JF, Donner MW: Adaptation, compensation, and decompensation of the pharyngeal swallow. Gastrointest Radiol 10:235-240, 1985, with kind permission from Springer Science and Business Media.)

The pathogenesis of Zenker's diverticulum remains unclear, although incoordination between pharyngeal contraction and cricopharyngeal opening may be a contributing factor.[43-46] Manometric and cineradiographic studies have demonstrated premature sphincter closure in some patients with Zenker's diverticulum. Other studies performed in patients with fully developed diverticula, however, have showed that the timing of pharyngeal contraction and cricopharyngeal relaxation may be normal.

Cook and colleagues demonstrated decreased compliance of the upper esophageal sphincter (UES) in a group of patients who had Zenker's diverticulum and in whom inadequate sphincter opening resulted in increased bolus pressure.[47-49] Shaw and associates subsequently demonstrated that with

cricopharyngeal myotomy and pouch ablation, the intrabolus pressure fell and full UES opening was restored.[50,51] Cook also observed structural abnormalities in muscle strips of the cricopharyngeus in 14 patients with Zenker's diverticulum.[52] They found type 1 fiber predominance and greater fiber size variability. The muscles also demonstrated fibroadipose tissue replacement and fiber degeneration. These studies suggest that decreased UES compliance may have a major role in the development of Zenker's diverticulum.

Gastroesophageal reflux may also contribute to the development of Zenker's diverticulum (Table 19-6).[52-55] In my experience with 36 patients with Zenker's diverticulum, all but one had free gastroesophageal reflux, segmental spasm, acid-induced spasm, hiatal hernia, or Schatzki's ring.

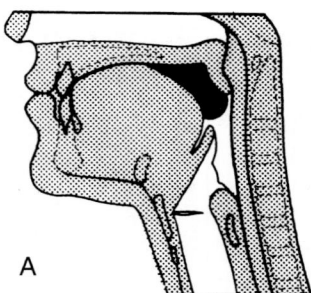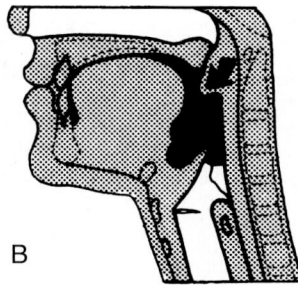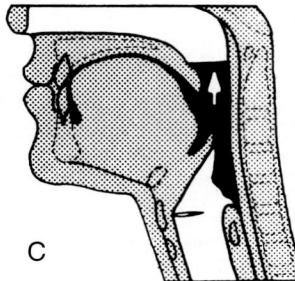

Figure 19-6. Closure of palatopharyngeal isthmus during swallowing. A. Normal closure, in which the soft palate has elevated to a right angle to abut Passavant's cushion. **B.** Deficiency of the pharyngeal palate may be compensated by increasing convergence of the pharyngeal constrictor muscles (*arrow*), resulting in a very prominent Passavant's cushion. **C.** Decompensation results in nasopharyngeal regurgitation though the palatopharyngeal isthmus (*arrow*). (From Buchholz DW, Bosma JF, Donner MW: Adaptation, compensation, and decompensation of the pharyngeal swallow. Gastrointest Radiol 10:235-240, 1985, with kind permission from Springer Science and Business Media.)

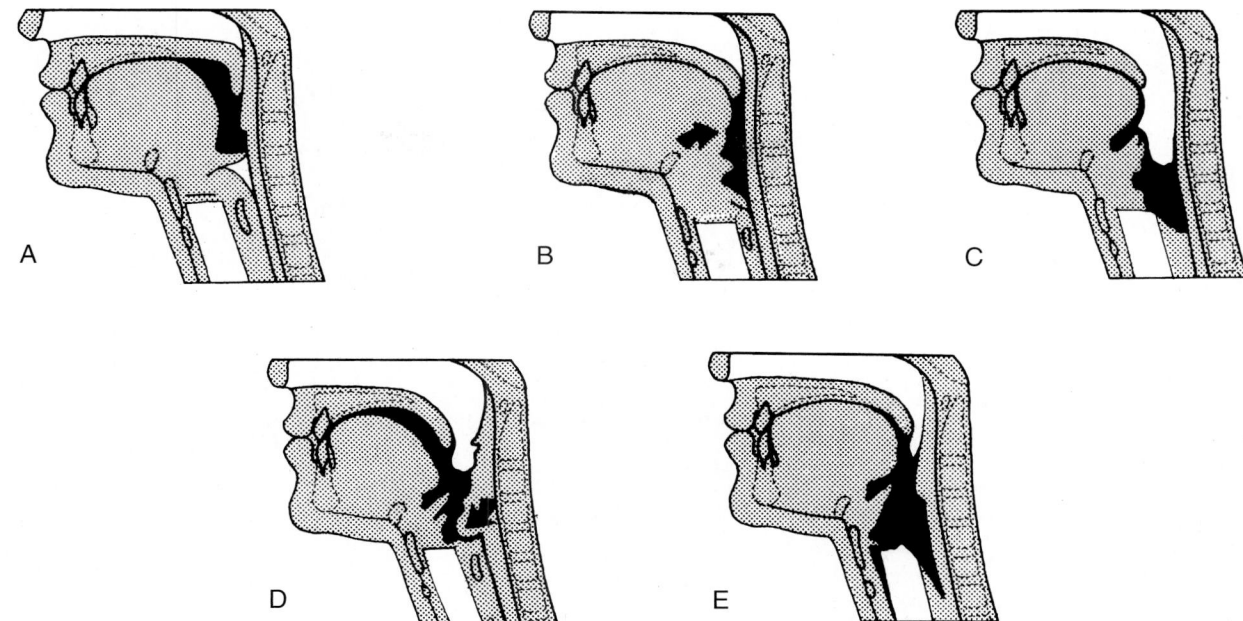

Figure 19-7. Compression of the bolus. A. Normal compression. **B.** Deficiency of the constrictor muscles may be compensated by increased upward and posterior displacement of the tongue and larynx (*arrow*). **D.** Deficiency of the tongue in bolus compression may be followed by more anterior displacement of the constrictor wall (*arrow*), resulting in a very prominent pharyngeal stripping wave. **C** and **E.** Decompensation due to inadequate bolus compression results in bolus retention in the valleculae and piriform sinuses after swallowing, with the potential for overflow aspiration. (From Buchholz DW, Bosma JF, Donner MW: Adaptation, compensation, and decompensation of the pharyngeal swallow. Gastrointest Radiol 10:235-240, 1985, with kind permission from Springer Science and Business Media.)

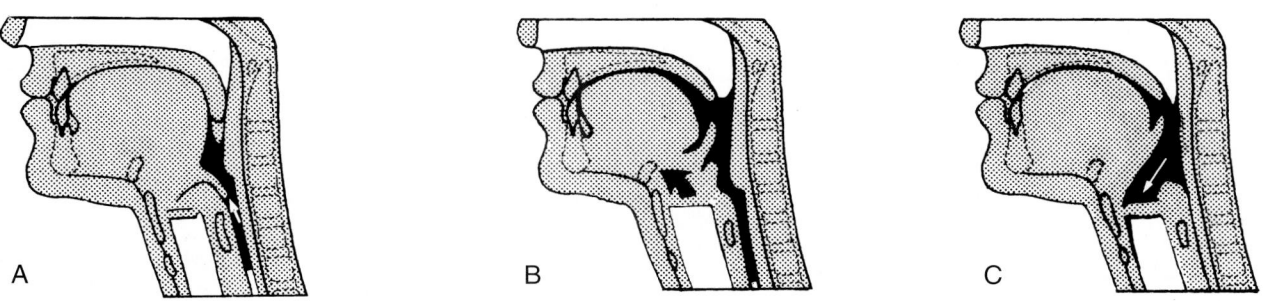

Figure 19-8. Closure of the larynx. A. The normal condition, in which the larynx is elevated and closed, and the epiglottis (*arrow*) is completely tilted down to cover the entrance to the laryngeal aditus. **B.** With deficiency of epiglottic tilting or glottic closure, there may be increased upward and anterior displacement of the larynx (*arrow*). Under these circumstances, the arytenoid masses may be enlarged as a sign of compensation (not illustrated). **C.** Failure of compensation results in penetration of bolus (*arrow*) into the laryngeal vestibule and even through the incompletely closed cords, with aspiration. (From Buchholz DW, Bosma JF, Donner MW: Adaptation, compensation, and decompensation of the pharyngeal swallow. Gastrointest Radiol 10:235-240, 1985, with kind permission from Springer Science and Business Media.)

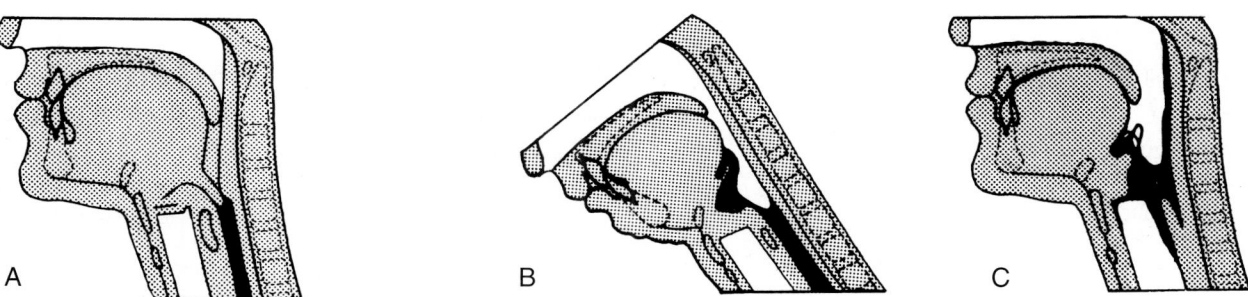

Figure 19-9. Opening of the pharyngoesophageal segment. A. Normal opening of pharyngoesophageal segment. **B.** Deficiency of upward laryngeal displacement (which contributes to opening of the pharyngoesophageal segment) results in flexion of the neck and/or forward thrusting of the jaw during swallowing. **C.** Failure of compensation results in poor pharyngoesophageal segment opening, with retention of the bolus in the piriform sinuses and the risk of overflow aspiration. (From Buchholz DW, Bosma JF, Donner MW: Adaptation, compensation, and decompensation of the pharyngeal swallow. Gastrointest Radiol 10:235-240, 1985, with kind permission from Springer Science and Business Media.)

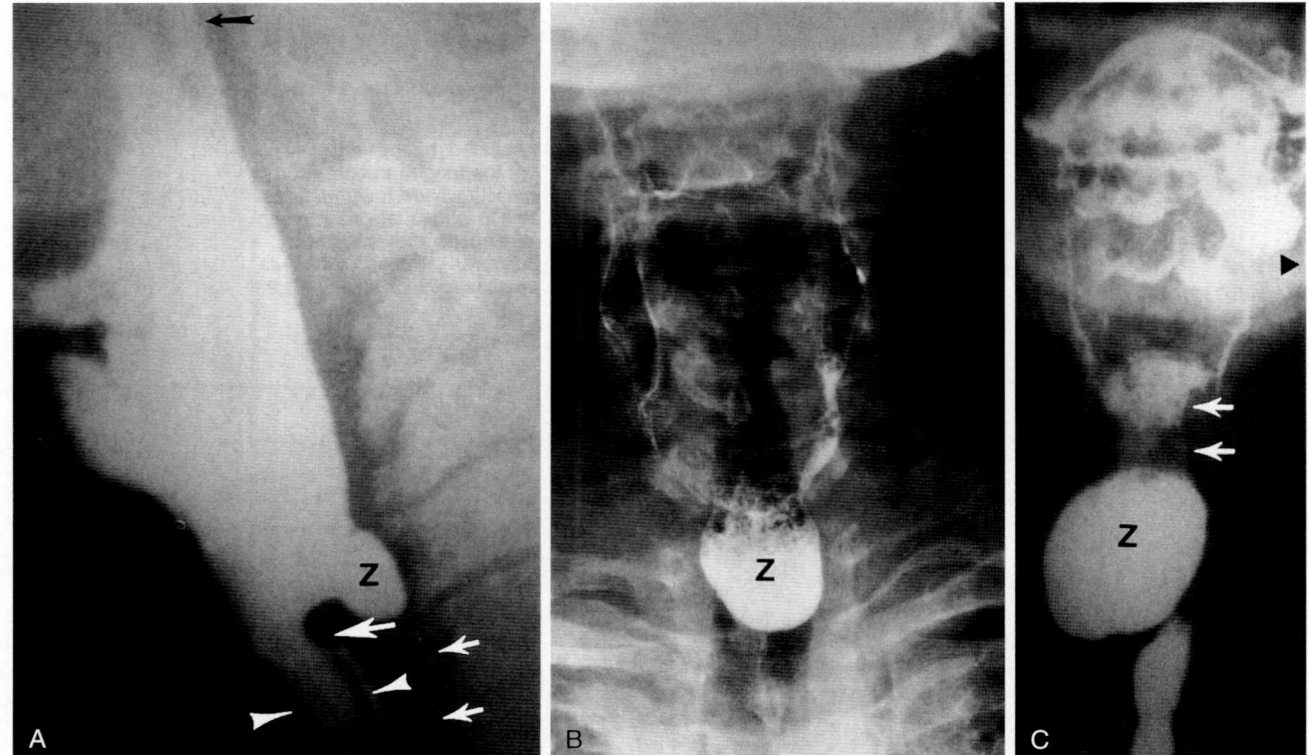

Figure 19-10. Zenker's diverticulum. A. Lateral view shows a small diverticulum (Z) above a very prominent cricopharyngeus (*large white arrow*) causing luminal narrowing of at least 50%, with a jet of barium (*arrowheads*) below it. The cervical esophageal lumen is actually abutting the spine (*small white arrows*). Also note nasopharyngeal regurgitation (*black arrow*) and marked degenerative changes in the cervical spine. **B.** After swallowing, Zenker's diverticulum (Z) remains filled. **C.** Frontal view in another patient shows emptying of the diverticulum (Z) back into the pharynx (*arrows*) after swallowing, placing this patient at risk for overflow aspiration. Note also the buccal pouch on the left side (*arrowhead*). (From Jones B, Donner MW [eds]: Normal and Abnormal Swallowing: Imaging in Diagnosis and Therapy. New York, Springer-Verlag, 1991. With kind permission from Springer Science and Business Media.)

Table 19-6
Remote Effects of Gastroesophageal Reflux

Pharynx
Pain
Lump or foreign body sensation ("globus")
Prominent cricopharyngeus
Asymmetry of contraction
Lateral pharyngeal pouches
Zenker's diverticulum

Larynx
Chronic cough
Pain and hoarseness
Laryngitis
Contact granuloma
Laryngeal ulcer
Laryngospasm
Laryngeal cancer

Lung
Aspiration pneumonia
Chronic lung disease
Asthma
Sleep apnea

Heart
Arrhythmias (tachycardia, bradycardia)
Swallow syncope

Radiologically, Zenker's diverticulum is usually associated with prominence of the cricopharyngeus or a cricopharyngeal bar. Esophageal disease may produce prominence of the cricopharyngeus (perhaps with decreased compliance), which in turn may raise intrapharyngeal (and intrabolus) pressure, necessitating more forceful contractions, with eventual bulging through a congenitally weak area.

Further studies are necessary (including those addressing the early developmental stages of Zenker's diverticulum) before the pathophysiology can be fully understood.

RELATIONSHIP OF ESOPHAGEAL DISTENTION TO THE CRICOPHARYNGEUS

Intraluminal foreign bodies lodged in the hypopharynx or upper esophagus may produce cricopharyngeal spasm.[56] In cats, it has been shown that stimulation of afferent receptors in the hypopharynx or upper cervical esophagus evokes reflex contraction and spasm in the cricopharyngeal muscle with an increase in intraluminal pressure in the sphincter segment. Similarly, esophageal distention by liquids or an intraluminal balloon in humans results in elevated pressure in the sphincter segment.[57-60]

RELATIONSHIP OF GASTROESOPHAGEAL REFLUX TO THE CRICOPHARYNGEUS

There are variable reports in the manometric literature as to whether acid bathing the esophagus produces a rise in pressure in the UES. In the 1970s, studies in human volunteers (using perfused catheters) reported elevated pressures in the sphincter segment after infusion of the esophagus with saline or acid.[61,62] The closer the infusion was to the UES, the greater the increase in pressure. In the 1990s, a study (using a modified sleeve sensor) compared UES pressures in normal persons and patients with esophagitis[63]; this study reported no UES response to acid reflux or acid perfusion. More recent manometric studies (using solid-state catheters) have shown many interactions among the lower esophageal sphincter, gastroesophageal reflux, intraesophageal pressure changes, and changes in pressure in the UES. Several new reflexes have been described, primarily by Shaker and coworkers[64-69]:

1. *UES contractile response to gastroesophageal reflux.* Shaker and coworkers compared UES pressure changes in normal controls and patients with reflux esophagitis[64]: most of the controls and patients with reflux esophagitis had a significant increase in UES pressures in response to reflux episodes.
2. *UES contractile response.* Mechanical stimulation of the pharynx in cats[65] and water stimulation in humans[66] results in an increase in UES resting tone. As little as 0.1 mL of water resulted in this reflex.
3. *Esophagoglottal closure reflex.* Esophageal distention during gastroesophageal reflux could overwhelm the UES with the potential for overflow aspiration. Recently, a reflex was described in both humans[67] and cats[68] in which esophageal distention resulted in reflex closure of the glottis.
4. *Pharyngoglottal adduction reflex.* Injection of minute amounts of water into the pharynx results in brief closure of the vocal folds. This is thought to be a protective maneuver to prevent aspiration.[69]

SWALLOWING-RELATED REFLEXES

Many cardiorespiratory reflexes are related to swallowing, resulting from laryngeal, pharyngeal, or esophageal stimulation. Examples include syncope, change in heart rate, apnea, and bronchoconstriction leading to asthma (Table 19-7).[70-74] A review of swallowing-related reflexes is referenced for further reading.[75]

FUNCTIONAL CHANGES AFTER IRRADIATION

The acute effects of radiation alone on pharyngeal function have not, to my knowledge, been studied radiographically. Within days or weeks, mucosal edema occurs. It is most marked over the arytenoid cartilages, although the epiglottis and posterior pharynx are also edematous. The mucosa becomes inflamed and friable, and lymphangiectasia develops. Endothelial vasculitis produces localized ischemia, which in the long term may result in fibrosis.[76]

The long-term effect of radiation on swallowing was studied by Ekberg and Nylander in a postoperative study of a group

Table 19-7
Type of Reflexes

Normal Reflexes	Abnormal Reflexes
Pharynx	*Cardiovascular*
Gagging	Bradycardia or hypotension,
Breathing	syncope or seizures
Swallowing	Tachycardia
Laryngeal closure	Hypertension
Respiratory suppression	Dysrhythmia
	Myocardial insufficiency
Larynx	*Respiratory*
Cough	Laryngospasm
Forced inspiration	Prolonged apnea
Laryngeal closure	Bronchospasm
Respiratory suppression	
Bronchoconstriction	
Secretion of mucus	
Arousal	
Esophagus	
Deglutitive inhibition of peristalsis	

of 13 patients with head and neck cancers who had received radiation therapy before tumor resection.[77] Abnormalities were present in 12 of the 13 patients and consisted of paresis of the constrictor muscle with bolus retention, laryngeal penetration, and cricopharyngeal incoordination. Interestingly, static films significantly underestimated the degree of decompensation whereas dynamic imaging revealed the true extent of the abnormalities.

Another more recent study reported the changes after intense chemoradiation in 29 patients with unresectable stage IV head and neck cancer.[78] Post-therapy studies were performed at 1 to 3 months and at 6 to 12 months. Post-therapy decompensations were common and included reduced epiglottic tilt, delayed swallow initiation, uncoordinated timing of bolus propulsion, and abnormal opening of the cricopharyngeus and closure of the larynx, resulting in aspiration during and after swallowing, which was typically "silent." Reduced base of tongue retraction and incomplete cricopharyngeal opening resulted in pooling of the bolus in the valleculae and piriform sinuses.

Postirradiation xerostomia often compounds swallowing difficulties. One study compared the findings in 15 cancer patients and 20 controls.[79] Patients with xerostomia took almost twice as long to chew a shortbread cookie, but the duration of swallowing was unaffected. For liquid barium and paste, timing measures were the same for controls and for patients with xerostomia.

AGING AND SWALLOWING

Swallowing in elderly persons is termed *presbyphagia*,[80] and it may be considered under two separate categories: (1) the effects of the normal aging process (primary presbyphagia) and (2) the effects on swallowing of other diseases that affect the elderly, such as cerebrovascular accidents and Parkinson's disease (secondary presbyphagia).

Prevalence studies have shown that the incidence of dysphagia is 12% to 20% in general hospitals and as high as 50% in nursing homes.[81] Although there is little loss of functioning motor neurons before 60 years of age, a striking and progressive depletion of functioning motor neurons occurs after this age, with subsequent deterioration of connective tissue, loss of elasticity, and atrophy of fat.[82] In the oropharynx, the suspensory ligaments of all structures become lax, resulting in premature leakage, low positioning of the hyoid, squaring of the valleculae, and expansion of the pharyngeal cavity.[83-86] Loss of pliability may also result in incomplete inversion of the epiglottis and incomplete closure of the larynx.[87] In one study, defective closure of the laryngeal vestibule with laryngeal penetration was found in 70 of 101 patients older than 80 years of age.[88] Thus, laryngeal penetration in the elderly may be normal.

The laryngeal epithelium appears to become less sensitive to aspirated material with increasing age, which may explain why silent aspiration can be a problem.[89] In addition, airway protection may be further compromised by medications for depression, anxiety, or Parkinson's disease.

One study found no significant change in the velocity of peristalsis with increasing age.[90] However, the oral and pharyngeal phases may become "uncoupled," resulting in delayed initiation of pharyngeal contraction and early cricopharyngeal closure.[84] With aging, there is also a decrease in the time the pharyngoesophageal segment remains opened to allow bolus passage.[84]

Borgstrom and Ekberg studied swallowing function in an asymptomatic group of 56 patients who ranged from 72 to 93 years of age.[91] Normal deglutition (as defined in younger persons) was found in only 16% of patients. Oral abnormalities were found in 63%, pharyngeal abnormalities in 25%, pharyngoesophageal segment abnormalities in 39%, and esophageal abnormalities in 36% of patients.

A discussion of other changes in esophageal motility that occur with increasing age is beyond the scope of this chapter.

NEUROLOGIC DISEASE AND THE PHARYNX

Neuromuscular disorders may cause dysphagia by affecting the afferent or efferent limbs of the swallowing reflex and by producing abnormalities at many levels, including the cerebral cortex, cranial nerve nuclei in the brain stem, cranial nerves themselves, pharyngeal plexus, neuromuscular junction, muscles, or sensory feedback mechanisms (Table 19-8).[91-94]

Dysphagia can be a minor or major symptom; occasionally, it may be the predominant or only complaint. For example, acute onset of dysphagia may signal a focal brain stem stroke, and chronic dysphagia may be the presenting symptom of an unrecognized neuromuscular disease such as amyotrophic lateral sclerosis. At the Johns Hopkins Swallowing Center, approximately 30% of patients have dysphagia in the setting of neuromuscular disease; dysphagia was the predominant or only symptom in 10% of these patients (Jones B: personal observation).

Bulbar and Pseudobulbar Palsy

Bulbar palsy implies dysfunction of the motor unit (i.e., a lower motor neuron and the muscle innervated by that lower motor neuron) and may involve cranial nerve nuclei, cranial nerves, the neuromuscular junction, or muscle. This kind of abnormality primarily affects the pharyngeal stage of swal-

Table 19-8
Common Neuromuscular Causes of Dysphagia

Brain and Brain Stem
Cerebrovascular accident
Multiple sclerosis
Amyotrophic lateral sclerosis (motor neuron disease)

Movement Disorders and Neurodegenerative Diseases
Parkinson's disease
Spinocerebellar degeneration
Olivopontocerebellar atrophy
Huntington's disease
Alzheimer's disease
Dystonia and dyskinesia

Infections
Poliomyelitis
Neurosyphilis
Encephalitis, meningitis

Myoneuronal Junction
Myasthenia gravis
Botulism
Eaton-Lambert syndrome

Muscle Disease
Dystrophy
Polymyositis, dermatomyositis
Ragged red fiber disease (mitochondrial myopathy)

Adapted from Buchholz D: Neurologic causes of dysphagia. Dysphagia 1:152-156, 1987.

lowing. Characteristic signs include atrophy, fasciculation, weakness, flaccidity, and decreased reflexes.

Pseudobulbar palsy affects the corticobulbar tract and therefore is an upper motor neuron abnormality causing weakness accompanied by spasticity, increased reflexes, and spastic dysarthria. Emotional lability is characteristic. Pseudobulbar palsy primarily affects the oral initiation phase of swallowing.

Formerly, it was thought that a unilateral abnormality of one corticobulbar tract did not produce a major swallowing deficit, because each corticobulbar tract supplies both sides of the brain stem with cortical input. Despite the supposed bilateral representation of swallowing, however, dysphagia occurs in 20% to 40% of patients with cerebrovascular accidents,[95-103] including those with "unilateral strokes." Robbins and Levine have challenged the theory of bilateral representation of swallowing.[104,105] These authors studied patients with unilateral cortical strokes (as diagnosed by CT) and compared swallowing abnormalities in the group with infarcts in the right cerebral cortex to swallowing abnormalities in the group with infarcts in the left cerebral cortex. Initiation of pharyngeal swallow was delayed in all patients. The left cortical stroke group, however, showed impaired oral stage function, difficulty initiating coordinated motor activity, and apraxia, whereas pharyngeal pooling, penetration, and aspiration were more prominent in patients with right cortical strokes. Studies with newer imaging modalities such as MRI are in progress to validate these observations. MRI, however, is not infallible and may be negative in patients with focal stroke.[106,107]

Wallenberg's syndrome is a cerebrovascular accident involving the medulla (lateral medullary infarction) in the distribution of the posterior inferior cerebellar artery. Traditional teaching stressed that the resulting pharyngeal paresis was unilateral, but two studies found that the deficit is, in fact, bilateral.[108,109] Lateral medullary infarction can also lead to aphagia.[110]

Amyotrophic Lateral Sclerosis (Lou Gehrig's Disease)

Amyotrophic lateral sclerosis, also known as motor neuron disease or Lou Gehrig's disease, can result in bulbar palsy, pseudobulbar palsy, or a combination of both. The disease may produce a wide spectrum of abnormal findings including muscle weakness and atrophy of the lips, tongue, palate, and pharyngeal constrictors with various degrees of retention of secretions.[94,111-115] Weakness of the intrinsic laryngeal muscles leads to airway penetration and aspiration. The tongue, hyoid, and larynx are weak and ptotic in the upright position. The patient will often compensate by holding the head and neck in a position of sustained extension ("swan neck") to help maintain the airway and facilitate swallowing.

Multiple Sclerosis

Corresponding to the course of the disease itself, swallowing impairment in multiple sclerosis is relapsing and remitting.[116-119] The radiographic appearance depends on the location and extent of the demyelinization process. Abnormalities may vary from difficulty initiating swallowing, to episodes of choking on liquids or sticking of solid particles. Sensory loss may compound the problem, and symptoms may be minimal or absent even in the presence of severe decompensation.

NEURODEGENERATIVE DISORDERS

Parkinson's disease is associated with dysphagia in as many as 50% of patients. Delayed initiation of swallowing and oral transfer problems predominate. The findings include lingual tremor or rocking, squeezing of the bolus between the tongue and palate, piecemeal deglutition, and hesitancy to propel the bolus into the pharynx.[120-123]

The esophagus may also be involved, with loss of the primary stripping wave. Whether this is an intrinsic esophageal motility problem or whether the peristaltic wave is absent because there is no pharyngeal contraction (i.e., no "message" to the esophagus) is unknown. Qualman and coworkers reported that patients with Parkinson's disease and achalasia had degeneration of the dorsal vagal motor nucleus.[124] The same study demonstrated that Lewy bodies, typically found in the vagal nucleus and substantia nigra in patients with Parkinson's disease, can be found in the esophageal myenteric plexus in patients with achalasia.

Huntington's disease,[125,126] progressive supranuclear palsy,[127-129] and Alzheimer's disease[130] may also produce dysphagia and feeding difficulties. The oropharyngeal findings simulate those of Parkinson's disease. Dementia, other cognitive problems, and uncontrolled movements may complicate feeding and rehabilitation.

Similarly, dystonia and dyskinesia may result in dysphagia or feeding difficulties due to involuntary localized muscle contractions.[131] In dystonia, the tonically contracted tongue, positioned in a tight mass in the back of the oral cavity,

produces a characteristic appearance, the "fisted tongue." To swallow, the patient tilts the head into extreme extension and "decants" the bolus into the pharynx by gravity.[131]

INFECTIONS

Viral infections of the nervous system may cause dysphagia.[92,93] For example, a patient with bulbar poliomyelitis can present with pharyngeal paralysis, aspiration, and disturbance of vasomotor control when motor neurons in the medullary reticular formation, especially those in or near the nucleus ambiguous, are involved. Acute bulbar poliomyelitis is now rare in countries with mass vaccination but is still seen in countries where vaccination is not widespread.

A "postpolio syndrome" has been described with symptoms of increasing weakness beginning 20 or more years after the acute attack of poliomyelitis; symptoms may include dysphagia.[132,133] In a minority of patients, the symptoms are progressive and this has been called "postpolio progressive muscle atrophy."

Buchholz and Jones reported 13 patients with a remote history of acute poliomyelitis and dysphagia.[134] Nine of the 13 patients reported progressive dysphagia. Constrictor weakness was found in 11 patients. Interestingly, esophageal dysfunction was found in 8 of the 13 patients. Subsequently, Jones and associates reviewed the dynamic imaging studies of 20 patients with dysphagia and a remote history of polio.[135] Multiple abnormalities were present in these patients, including atrophy of prevertebral soft tissues, pharyngeal paresis or paralysis with retention of the bolus after swallowing, incomplete or absent epiglottic tilt, laryngeal penetration or aspiration, luminal narrowing due to a prominent cricopharyngeus, palatal weakness, incomplete laryngeal closure, and poor or absent laryngeal elevation (Fig. 19-11).

Sonies and Dalakas evaluated 32 postpolio patients with videofluoroscopy and ultrasound; 18 of these patients did not report dysphagia.[136] Despite the lack of symptoms, all but one of the patients had abnormalities of oropharyngeal function of varying severity.

MYASTHENIA GRAVIS AND RELATED DISORDERS

Myasthenia gravis[137,138] and the Eaton-Lambert myasthenic-myopathic syndrome[139] are myoneural junction disorders with diminished release or inadequate binding of acetylcholine. In addition to ocular and proximal limb weakness, there may be dysphagia or choking characteristically appearing late in the day. Slowing of swallowing or decompensation after repetitive swallowing may suggest the diagnosis during dynamic studies.

The Eaton-Lambert myasthenic-myopathic syndrome (carcinomatous neuropathy) is most often seen with oat cell carcinoma of the lung but has also been reported in association with carcinoma of the breast, prostate, stomach, and rectum.[139] Diplopia, dysarthria, and dysphagia may accompany weakness of muscles of the trunk, pelvis, and shoulder girdle, the most common sites affected.

Botulism also affects transmission at the myoneuronal junction and may result in dysphagia.[92,93,140] Interestingly, botulinum toxin has been used to treat a variety of dystonias

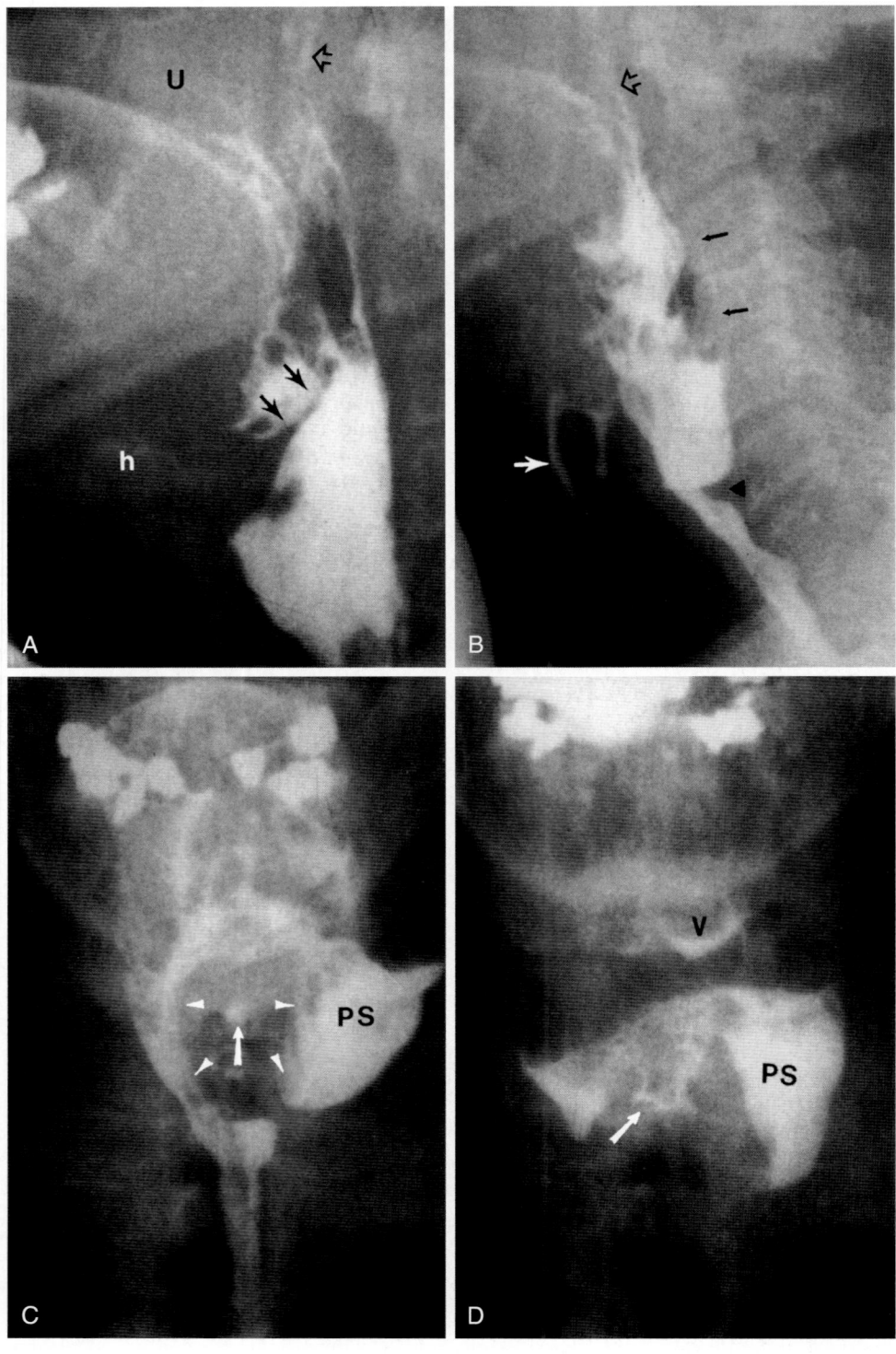

Figure 19-11. Postpolio dysphagia. A. Lateral view shows incomplete elevation of the soft palate (U) and minimal pharyngeal regurgitation (*open arrow*). Passavant's cushion is not evident. The bolus is past the epiglottis (*solid arrows*), which has remained almost completely upright, and there is incomplete elevation of the hyoid bone (h), which has not moved anteriorly. **B.** There is bulging of the pharynx, so that it is overlapping the cervical spine (*closed black arrows*) with laryngeal penetration (*white arrow*). There is prominence of the cricopharyngeus (*arrowhead*) and poor distention of the cervical esophagus below the cricopharyngeus. Also note nasopharyngeal regurgitation (*open black arrow*). **C.** Frontal view shows asymmetrical distention with the left piriform sinus (PS) bulging much more than the right due to pharyngeal constrictor weakness. There is a small amount of contrast agent in the laryngeal vestibule (*arrow*) and a moderate "pseudomass" effect due to a flow defect (*arrowheads*). **D.** After passage of the bolus, there is marked retention in the left piriform sinus (PS), which is larger than the right, and mild retention in the right piriform sinus. There is also asymmetrical retention in the vallecula on the left side (V). Contrast agent is also seen in the laryngeal vestibule and ventricle (*arrow*).

including torticollis; dysphagia may occur in a small number of patients as a side effect due to diffusion of the toxin into the soft tissues of the neck.[140]

FAMILIAL DYSAUTONOMIA (RILEY-DAY SYNDROME)

A characteristic finding in this syndrome is delayed cricopharyngeal relaxation with airway penetration.[141]

DISEASES OF THE MUSCLE

Diseases prominently affecting bulbar muscles may be due to inflammatory disease (polymyositis, dermatomyositis, sarcoidosis),[142-144] metabolic or endocrine disease (mitochondrial myopathy or ragged red fiber disease),[143,144] dysthyroid myopathy (hypothyroidism or hyperthyroidism), or muscular dystrophy.[145] They may also be caused by a prolonged course of corticosteroid medication. Muscular dystrophies affecting the pharynx include myotonic dystrophy (pharyngeal and esophageal motility disturbances),[145] Duchenne's muscular dystrophy, and oculopharyngeal dystrophy.[146-148] There is bilateral pharyngeal paresis with bolus retention; the cricopharyngeus may be prominent but closes with normal timing. The cervical esophagus may also be abnormal with diminished or absent peristalsis. The use of chilled barium accentuates the abnormalities in myotonic dystrophy.[149]

MEDICATIONS

Medications may cause localized pill-induced pharyngitis or esophagitis.[150] Medications may also induce or aggravate myasthenia gravis, dystonia, and myopathy or neuropathy.[151-163] More than 30 drugs in current clinical use may interfere with neuromuscular transmission, among them antibiotics such as neomycin, streptomycin, and certain tetracyclines and immunosuppressant agents such as adrenocorticotrophic hormone, prednisone, and azathioprine. Sedatives, antipsychotic drugs, and antidepressants may produce extrapyramidal symptoms and signs of muscle spasm or dystonia or may unmask a latent neuromuscular disease. Ideally, such drugs should be temporarily stopped for several days before a swallowing study. Tryptophan use has been associated with the development of an "eosinophilia-myalgia syndrome."[164-166] Studies suggest that this association is caused by a chemical constituent related to the specific manufacturing conditions at one company rather than to tryptophan itself.[166]

References

1. Edwards DAW: History and symptoms of esophageal disease of the esophagus. In Vantrappen G, Hellemans J (eds): Diseases of the Esophagus. New York, Springer-Verlag, 1972, pp 103-105.
2. Jones B, Ravich WJ, Donner MW, et al: Pharyngoesophageal interrelationships: Observations and working concepts. Gastrointest Radiol 10:225-233, 1985.
3. Bosma JF: Deglutition: Pharyngeal stage. Physiol Rev 37:275-300, 1957.
4. Miller AJ: Deglutition. Physiol Rev 62:129-184, 1982.
5. Donner MW, Bosma JF, Robertson DL: Anatomy and physiology of the pharynx. Gastrointest Radiol 10:196-212, 1985.
6. Miller AJ: Neurophysiological basis of swallowing. Dysphagia 1:91-100, 1986.
7. Miller AJ: Swallowing: Neurophysiologic control of the esophageal phase. Dysphagia 2:72-82, 1987.
8. Dodds WJ, Stewart ET, Logemann JA: Physiology and radiology of the normal oral and pharyngeal phases of swallowing. AJR 154:953-963, 1990.
9. Buchholz DW, Jones B, Ravich WJ: Dysphagia following anterior cervical fusion. Dysphagia 8:390(A), 1993.
10. Ekberg O, Bergqvist D, Takolander R, et al: Pharyngeal function after carotid endarterectomy. Dysphagia 4:151-154, 1989.
11. Dodds WJ, Taylor AJ, Stewart ET, et al: Tipper and dipper types of oral swallows. AJR 153:1197-1199, 1989.
12. Zerhouni EA, Bosma JF, Donner MW: Relationship of cervical spine disorders to dysphagia. Dysphagia 1:129-144, 1987.
13. Curtis DJ: Laryngeal dynamics. CRC Crit Rev Diagn Imaging 19:29-80, 1982.
14. Dodds WJ, Man KM, Cook IJ, et al: Influence of bolus volume on swallow-induced hyoid movement in normal subjects. AJR 150: 1307-1309, 1988.
15. Ekberg O: The normal movements of the hyoid bone during swallow. Invest Radiol 5:408-410, 1986.
16. Ekberg O, Sigurjonsson S: Movements of the epiglottis during deglutition: A cineradiographic study. Gastrointest Radiol 7:101-107, 1982.
17. Templeton RE, Kredel RA: Cricopharyngeal sphincter: Roentgenologic study. Laryngoscope 53:1-12, 1943.
18. Crichlow TVL: Cricopharyngeus in radiography and cineradiography. Br J Radiol 29:546-556, 1956.
19. Seaman WB: Cineroentgenographic observations of the cricopharyngeus. AJR 96:922-931, 1966.
20. Sokol EM, Heitman P, Wolfe BS, et al: Simultaneous cineradiographic and manometric study of the pharynx, hypopharynx, and cervical esophagus. Gastroenterology 51:960-974, 1966.
21. Seaman WB: Functional disorders of the pharyngoesophageal junction: Achalasia and chalasia. Radiol Clin North Am 7:113-119, 1969.
22. Palmer ED: Disorders of the cricopharyngeus muscle: A review. Gastroenterology 71:510-517, 1976.
23. Roed-Peterson K: The pharyngo-esophageal sphincter: A review of the literature. Dan Med Bull 26:275-281, 1979.
24. Ekberg O, Nylander B: Dysfunction of the cricopharyngeal muscle. Radiology 143:481-486, 1982.
25. Torres WE, Clements JL, Austin GE, et al: Cricopharyngeal muscle hypertrophy: Radiologic anatomic correlation. AJR 141:927-930, 1984.
26. Curtis DJ, Cruess DF, Berg T: The cricopharyngeal muscle: A video-recording review. AJR 142:497-500, 1984.
27. Kahrilas PJ, Dodds WJ, Dent J, et al: Upper esophageal sphincter function during deglutition. Gastroenterology 95:52-62, 1988.
28. Jacob P, Kahrilas PJ, Logemann JA, et al: Upper esophageal sphincter opening and modulation during swallowing. Gastroenterology 97: 1469-1478, 1989.
29. Olsson R, Ekberg O: Videomanometry of the pharynx in dysphagic patients with a posterior cricopharyngeal indentation. Acad Radiol 2:597-601, 1995.
30. Brady AP, Stevenson GW, Somers S, et al: Premature contraction of the cricopharyngeus: A new sign of gastroesophageal reflux disease. Abdom Imaging 20:225-229, 1995.
31. Ekberg O: Cricopharyngeal bar: Myth and reality. Abdom Imaging 20:179-180, 1995.
32. Halum SL, Merati AL, Kulpa JI, et al: Videofluoroscopic swallow studies in unilateral cricopharyngeal dysfunction. Laryngoscope 113:981-984, 2003.
33. Ekberg O, Hilderfors H: Defective closure of the laryngeal vestibule: Frequency of pulmonary complications. AJR 145:1159-1164, 1985.
34. Feinberg MJ, Ekberg O: Videofluoroscopy in elderly patients with aspiration: Importance of evaluating both oral and pharyngeal stages of deglutition. AJR 156:293-296, 1991.
35. Feinberg MJ, Ekberg O: Deglutition after near-fatal choking episode: Radiologic evaluation. Radiology 176:637-640, 1995.
36. Linden P, Siebens AA: Dysphagia: Predicting laryngeal penetration. Arch Phys Med Rehabil 64:281-284, 1983.
37. Linden P, Kuhlemeier KV, Patterson C: The probability of correctly predicting subglottic penetration from clinical observations. Dysphagia 8:170-179, 1993.
38. McCullough GH, Wertz RT, Rosenbek JC: Sensitivity and specificity of clinical/bedside examination signs for detecting aspiration in adults subsequent to stroke. J Commun Disord 34:55-72, 2001.
39. Ryu JS, Park SR, Choi KH: Prediction of laryngeal aspiration using voice analysis. Am J Phys Med Rehabil 83:753-757, 2004.
40. Buchholz DW, Bosma JF, Donner MW: Adaptation, compensation, and decompensation of the pharyngeal swallow. Gastrointest Radiol 10:235-240, 1985.
41. Dantas RO, Dodds WJ, Massey BT, Kern MK: The effect of high- vs low-density barium preparations on the quantitative features of swallowing. AJR 153:1191-1195, 1989.
42. Bulow M, Olsson R, Ekberg O: Videoradiographic analysis of how carbonated thin liquids and thickened liquids affect the physiology of swallowing in subjects with aspiration on thin liquids. Acta Radiol 44:366-372, 2003.
43. Dohlman G, Mattsson O: The role of the cricopharyngeal muscle in cases of hypopharyngeal diverticula. AJR 81:561-569, 1959.
44. Knuff TE, Benjamin SB, Castell DO: Pharyngoesophageal (Zenker's) diverticulum: A reappraisal. Gastroenterology 82:734-736, 1982.
45. Westrin KM, Ergun S, Carlsoo B. Zenker's diverticulum—a historical review and trends in therapy. Acta Otolaryngol 116:351-360, 1996.
46. van Overbeek JJ: Pathogenesis and methods of treatment of Zenker's diverticulum. Ann Otol Rhinol Laryngol 112:583-593, 2003.
47. Cook IJ, Gabb M, Panagopoulos V, et al: Zenker's diverticulum: A defect in upper esophageal sphincter compliance. Gastroenterology 96:A98, 1989.
48. Cook IJ, Blumbergs P, Cash K, et al: Zenker's diverticulum: Evidence for a restrictive cricopharyngeal myopathy. Gastroenterology 96:A98, 1989.

49. Cook IJ, Gabb M, Panagopoulos V, et al: Pharyngeal (Zenker's) diverticulum is a disorder of upper esophageal sphincter opening. Gastroenterology 103:1229-1235, 1992.

50. Shaw DW, Cook IJ, Simula ME, et al: Restoration of normal upper esophageal sphincter compliance following cricopharyngeal myotomy in patients with Zenker's diverticulum. Gastroenterology 95:A122, 1990.

51. Shaw DW, Cook IJ, Jamieson GG, et al: Influence of surgery on deglutitive upper oesophageal sphincter mechanics in Zenker's diverticulum. Gut 38:806-811, 1996.

52. Cook IJ, Blumbergs P, Cash K, et al: Structural abnormalities of the cricopharyngeus muscle in patients with pharyngeal (Zenker's) diverticulum. J Gastroenterol Hepatol 7:556-562, 1992.

53. Smiley TB, Caves PK, Porter DC: Relationship between posterior pharyngeal pouch and hiatus hernia. Thorax 25:725-731, 1970.

54. Delahunty JE, Margulies SE, Alonso UA, et al. The relationship of reflux esophagitis to pharyngeal pouch (Zenker's diverticulum). Laryngoscope 81:570-577, 1971.

55. Veenker EA, Anderson PE, Cohen JI: Cricopharyngeal spasm and Zenker's diverticulum. Head Neck 25:681-694, 2003.

56. Murakami Y, Fukuda H, Kirchner JA. The cricopharyngeus muscle. Acta Otolaryngol (Suppl) (Stockh) 311:1-19, 1972.

57. Creamer B, Schlegel J: Motor responses of the esophagus to distension. J Appl Physiol 10:498-504, 1957.

58. Enzmann DR, Harell GS, Zboralske FF: Upper esophageal responses to intraluminal distention in man. Gastroenterology 72:1292-1298, 1977.

59. Gerhardt DC, Shuck BS, Bordeaux RA, et al: Human upper esophageal sphincter: Response to volume, osmotic and acid stimuli. Gastroenterology 75:268-274, 1978.

60. Rosenberg SJ, Harris LD: A single physiologic mechanism for changing strength of both esophageal sphincters [abstract]. Gastroenterology 60:798, 1971.

61. Hunt PS, Connell AM, Smiley TB: The cricopharyngeal sphincter in gastric reflux. Gut 11:303-306, 1970.

62. Stanciu C, Bennett JR: Upper oesophageal sphincter yield pressure in normal subjects and in patients with gastroesophageal reflux. Thorax 29:459-462, 1974.

63. Vakil NB, Kahrilas PJ, Dodds WJ, Vanagunas A: Absence of an upper esophageal sphincter response to acid reflux. Gastroenterology 84:606-610, 1989.

64. Torrico S, Ren J, Sui Z, et al: Upper esophageal sphincter function during gastroesophageal reflux events. Gastroenterology 114:G3481, 1998.

65. Medda BK, Lang IM, Layman R, et al: Characterization and quantification of a pharyngo-UES contractile reflex in cats. Am J Physiol 267:G972-G983, 1994.

66. Shaker R, Ren J, Xie P, et al: Characterization of the pharyngo-UES contractile reflex in humans. Am J Physiol 273:G854-G858, 1997.

67. Shaker R, Ren J, Medda B, et al: Identification and characterization of the esophagoglottal closure reflex in a feline model. Am J Physiol 266:G147-G153, 1994.

68. Shaker R, Ren J, Kern M, Dodds WJ, et al: Mechanisms of airway protection and UES opening during belching. Am J Physiol 262:G621-G628, 1992.

69. Ren J, Shaker R, Dua K, et al: Glottal adduction response to pharyngeal water stimulation: Evidence for a pharyngoglottal closure reflex. Gastroenterology 106:A558, 1994.

70. Thach BT, Davies AM, Koenig JS, et al: Reflex induced apneas. In Issa FG, Suratt PM, Remmers JE (eds): Sleep and Respiration. New York, Wiley-Liss, 1990, pp 77-87.

71. Loughlin GM: Respiratory consequences of dysfunctional swallowing and aspiration. Dysphagia 3:126-130, 1989.

72. Levin B, Posner JB: Swallow syncope: Report of a case and review of the literature. Neurology (Minneap) 22:1086-1093, 1972.

73. Kalloo AN, Lewis JH, Maher K, et al: Swallowing: An unusual case of syncope. Dig Dis Sci 34:1117-1120, 1989.

74. Wright RA, Miller SA, Corsello BF: Acid-induced esophagobronchialcardiac reflexes in humans. Gastroenterology 99:71-73, 1990.

75. Cunningham ET Jr, Ravich WJ, Jones B, et al: Vagal reflexes referred from the upper aerodigestive tract: An infrequently recognized cause of common cardiorespiratory responses. Ann Intern Med 116:575-582, 1992.

76. Libshitz HI (ed): Diagnostic Roentgenology of Radiotherapy Change. Baltimore, Williams & Wilkins, 1979.

77. Ekberg O, Nylander G: Pharyngeal dysfunction after treatment for pharyngeal cancer with surgery and radiotherapy. Gastrointest Radiol 8:97-104, 1983.

78. Eisbruch A, Lyden T, Bradford CR, et al: Objective assessment of swallowing dysfunction and aspiration after radiation concurrent with chemotherapy for head-and-neck cancer. Int J Radiat Oncol Biol Phys 53:23-28, 2002.

79. Hamlet S, Faull J, Klein B, et al: Mastication and swallowing in patients with postirradiation xerostomia. Int J Radiat Oncol Biol Phys 37:789-796, 1997.

80. Kashima HK: Presbyphagia, introduction. In Goldstein JC, Kashima HK, Koopmann CF (eds): Geriatric Otorhinolaryngology. Toronto, BC Decker, 1989.

81. Groher ME, Bukatman R: The prevalence of swallowing disorders in two teaching hospitals. Dysphagia 1:3-6, 1986.

82. McComas AF, Lipton ARM, Sica REP: Motoneuron disease and aging. Lancet 2:1477-1480, 1973.

83. Baum BJ, Bodner L: Aging and oral motor function: Evidence for altered performance among older persons. J Dent Res 62:2-6, 1983.

84. Tracy JF, Logemann JA, Kahrilas PJ, et al: Preliminary observations on the effects of age on oropharyngeal deglutition. Dysphagia 4:90-94, 1989.

85. Ekberg O, Feinberg MJ: Altered swallowing function in elderly patients without dysphagia: Radiologic findings in 56 cases. AJR 156:1181-1184, 1991.

86. Shaker R, Dodds WJ, Hogan WJ, et al: Effect of aging on swallow induced lingual palatal closure pressure. Gastroenterology 96:A464, 1989.

87. Sonies BC, Stone M, Shawker T: Speech and swallowing in the elderly. Gerodontology 3:115-123, 1984.

88. Kahane JC: Postnatal development and aging of the human larynx. Semin Speech Lang 4:189-203, 1983.

89. Borgstrom PS, Ekberg O: Pharyngeal dysfunction in the elderly. J Med Imaging 2:74-81, 1988.

90. Pontoppidan H, Beecher HK: Progressive loss of protective reflexes in the airway with the advance of age. JAMA 174:2209-2213, 1960.

91. Borgstrom PS, Ekberg O: Speed of peristalsis in pharyngeal constrictor musculature: Correlations to age. Dysphagia 2:140-144, 1988.

92. Buchholz D: Neurologic causes of dysphagia. Dysphagia 1:152-156, 1987.

93. Kirshner S: Causes of neurogenic dysphagia. Dysphagia 3:184-188, 1989.

94. Silbiger ML, Pikheney R, Donner MW: Neuromuscular disorders affecting the pharynx: Cineradiographic analysis. Invest Radiol 2:442-448, 1967.

95. Veis SL, Logemann JA: Swallowing disorders in persons with cerebrovascular accident. Arch Phys Med Rehabil 66:372-375, 1985.

96. Gordon C, Hewer RL, Wade DT: Dysphagia in acute stroke. BMJ 295:411-414, 1987.

97. Paciaroni M, Mazzotta G, Corea F, et al: Dysphagia following stroke. Eur Neurol 51:162-167, 2004; Epub 2004.

98. Parker C, Power M, Hamdy S, et al: Awareness of dysphagia by patients following stroke predicts swallowing performance. Dysphagia 19:28-35, 2004.

99. Smithard DG: Swallowing and stroke: Neurological effects and recovery. Cerebrovasc Dis 4:1-8, 2002.

100. Martino R, Terrault N, Ezerzer F, et al: Dysphagia in a patient with lateral medullary syndrome: Insight into the central control of swallowing. Gastroenterology 121:420-426, 2001.

101. Mann G, Hankey GJ: Initial clinical and demographic predictors of swallowing impairment following acute stroke. Dysphagia 16:208-215, 2001.

102. Han TR, Paik NJ, Park JW: Quantifying swallowing function after stroke: A functional dysphagia scale based on videofluoroscopic studies. Arch Phys Med Rehabil 82:677-682, 2001.

103. Nilsson H, Ekberg O, Olsson R, et al: Dysphagia in stroke: A prospective study of quantitative aspects of swallowing in dysphagic patients. Dysphagia 13:32-38, 1988.

104. Robbins JA, Levine RL: Swallowing after unilateral stroke of the cerebral cortex: Preliminary experience. Dysphagia 3:11-17, 1988.

105. Robbins JA, Levine RL, Maser A, et al: Swallowing after unilateral stroke of the cerebral cortex. Arch Phys Med Rehabil 74:1295-1300, 1993.

106. Alberts MJ, Faulstich ME, Gray L: Stroke with negative brain magnetic resonance imaging. Stroke 23:663-667, 1992.

107. Buchholz DW: Clinically probable brain stem stroke presenting primarily as dysphagia and nonvisualized by MRI. Dysphagia 8:235-238, 1993.

108. Neumann S, Buchholz D, Wuttge-Hannig A, et al: Bilateral pharyngeal dysfunction after lateral medullary infarction (LMI). Dysphagia 9:263, 1994.

109. Neumann S, Buchholz D, Jones B, et al: Pharyngeal dysfunction after lateral medullary infarction is bilateral: Review of 15 additional cases. Dysphagia 10:136, 1995.

110. Buchholz D, Neumann S: Aphagia due to pharyngeal constrictor paresis from acute lateral medullary infarction. Dysphagia 14:187, 1999.

111. Garfinkle TJ, Kimmelman CP: Neurologic disorders: Amyotrophic lateral sclerosis, myasthenia gravis, multiple sclerosis and poliomyelitis. Am J Otolaryngol 3:204-212, 1982.

112. Kawai S, Tsukuda M, Mochimatsu I, et al: A study of the early stage of dysphagia in amyotrophic lateral sclerosis. Dysphagia 18:1-8, 2003.

113. Higo R, Tayama N, Watanabe T, et al: Videomanofluorometric study in amyotrophic lateral sclerosis. Laryngoscope 112:911-917, 2002.

114. Strand EA, Miller RM, Yorkston KM, et al: Management of oral-pharyngeal dysphagia symptoms in amyotrophic lateral sclerosis. Dysphagia 11:129-139, 1996.

115. Leighton SE, Burton MJ, Lund WS, et al: Swallowing in motor neuron disease. J R Soc Med 87:801-805, 1994.

116. Daly DD, Code CF, Anderson HA: Disturbances of swallowing and esophageal motility in patients with multiple sclerosis. Neurology 59:250-256, 1962.

117. Prosiegel M, Schelling A, Wagner-Sonntag E: Dysphagia and multiple sclerosis. Int MS J 11:22-31, 2004.

118. Wiesner W, Wetzel SG, Kappos L, et al: Swallowing abnormalities in multiple sclerosis: Correlation between videofluoroscopy and subjective symptoms. Eur Radiol 12:789-792, 2002; Epub 2001.

119. Daly DD, Code CF, Anderson HA: Disturbances of swallowing and esophageal motility in patients with multiple sclerosis. Neurology 59:250-256, 1962.

120. Lieberman AN, Horowitz L, Redmond P, et al: Dysphagia in Parkinson's disease. Am J Gastroenterol 74:157-160, 1980.

121. Nagaya M, Kachi T, Yamada T, et al: Videofluorographic study of swallowing in Parkinson's disease. Dysphagia 13:95-100, 1998.

122. Leopold NA, Kagel MC: Pharyngo-esophageal dysphagia in Parkinson's disease. Dysphagia 12:11-18, 1997.

123. Leopold NA, Kagel MC: Laryngeal deglutition movement in Parkinson's disease. Neurology 48:373-376, 1997.

124. Qualman SJ, Haupt HM, Yang P, et al: Esophageal Lewy bodies associated with ganglion cell loss in achalasia. Gastroenterology 87:848-856, 1984.

125. Leopold NA, Kagel MC: Dysphagia in Huntington's disease. Neurology 42:57-60, 1985.

126. Kagel MC, Leopold NA: Dysphagia in Huntington's disease: 16-year retrospective. Dysphagia 7:106-114, 1992.

127. Neumann S, Reich S, Buchholz D et al: Progressive supranuclear palsy (PSP): Characteristics of dysphagia in 14 patients. Dysphagia 11:164, 1996.

128. Johnston BT, Castell JA, Stumacher S, et al: Comparison of swallowing function in Parkinson's disease and progressive supranuclear palsy. Mov Disord 12:322-327, 1997.

129. Leopold NA, Kagel MC: Dysphagia in progressive supranuclear palsy: Radiologic features. Dysphagia 12:140-143, 1997.

130. Horner J, Alberts MJ, Dawson DV, et al: Swallowing in Alzheimer's disease. Alzheimer Dis Assoc Disord 8:177-189, 1994.

131. Bosma JF, Geoffrey VC, Thach BT, et al: A pattern of medication-induced persistent bulbar and cervical dystonia. Int J Orofacial Myology 8:5-18, 1982.

132. Dalakas MC, Elder G, Hallett M, et al: A long term follow-up study of patients with post-poliomyelitis neuromuscular symptoms. N Engl J Med 314:959-963, 1986.

133. Cashman NR, Maselli R, Wollmann RL, et al: Late denervation in patients with antecedent paralytic poliomyelitis. N Engl J Med 317:7-12, 1987.

134. Buchholz DW, Jones B: Dysphagia occurring after polio. Dysphagia 6:165-169, 1991.

135. Jones B, Buchholz DW, Ravich WJ, et al: Swallowing dysfunction in the post-polio syndrome: A cinefluorographic study. AJR 158:283-286, 1992.

136. Sonies BC, Dalakas MC: Dysphagia in patients with the post-polio syndrome. N Engl J Med 324:1162-1167, 1991.

137. Murray JP: Deglutition in myasthenia gravis. Br J Radiol 35:43-52, 1962.

138. Llabres M, Molina-Martinez FJ, Miralles F: Dysphagia as the sole manifestation of myasthenia gravis. Neurol Neurosurg Psychiatry 76:1297-1300, 2005.

139. Eaton LM, Lambert EH: Electromyography and electric stimulation of nerves and diseases of motor unit: Observations on myasthenia syndrome associated with malignant tumors. JAMA 163:1117-1124, 1957.

140. Jankovic J, Brin MF: Therapeutic uses of botulinum toxin. N Engl J Med 324:1186-1194, 1991.

141. Margulies SI, Bruint PW, Donner MW, et al: Familial dysautonomia: A cineradiographic study of the swallowing mechanism. Radiology 90:107-112, 1968.

142. Ertekin C, Secil Y, Yuceyar N, et al: Oropharyngeal dysphagia in polymyositis/dermatomyositis. Clin Neurol Neurosurg 107:32-37, 2004.

143. Rimington DS, Chambers ST, Parkin PJ, et al: Inclusion body myositis presenting solely as dysphagia. Neurology 43:1241-1243, 1993.

144. Buchholz DW, Neumann S, Ravich W, et al: Inclusion body myositis presenting as dysphagia: Report of 3 cases. Dysphagia 12:110, 1997.

145. Siegel CI, Hendrix TR, Harvey JC: The swallowing disorder in myotonia dystrophica. Gastroenterology 50:541-550, 1966.

146. Duranceau A, Jamieson G, Clemont RJ: Oropharyngeal dysphagia in patients with oculopharyngeal muscular dystrophy. Can J Surg 21: 326-329, 1978.

147. Castell JA, Castell DO, Duranceau CA, et al: Manometric characteristics of the pharynx, upper esophageal sphincter, esophagus, and lower esophageal sphincter in patients with oculopharyngeal muscular dystrophy. Dysphagia 10:22-26, 1995.

148. Perie S, Eymard B, Laccourreye L, et al: Dysphagia in oculopharyngeal muscular dystrophy: A series of 22 French cases. Neuromuscul Disord 7:S96-S99, 1997.

149. Bosma JF, Brodie DR: Cineradiographic demonstration of pharyngeal area myotonia in myotonic dystrophy patients. Radiology 92:104-109, 1969.

150. Kikendall JW, Friedman AC, Oyewole MA, et al: Pill-induced esophageal injury: Case reports and review of the medical literature. Dig Dis Sci 28:174-182, 1983.

151. Swift TR: Disorders of neuromuscular transmission other than myasthenia gravis. Muscle Nerve 4:334-353, 1981.

152. Miller CD, Oleshansky MA, Gibson KF, et al: Procainamide-induced myasthenia-like weakness and dysphagia. Ther Drug Monit 15:251-254, 1993.

153. McQuillen MP, Cantor HE, O'Rourke JR Jr: Myasthenic syndrome associated with antibiotics. Arch Neurol 18:402-415, 1968.

154. Pittinger CB, Eryase Y, Adamson R: Antibiotic induced paralysis. Anesth Analg 49:487-501, 1970.

155. Stewart JT: Reversible dysphagia associated with neuroleptic treatment. J Am Geriatr Soc 49:1260-1261, 2001.

156. Hhayashi T, Nishikawa T, Koga I, et al: Life-threatening dysphagia following prolonged neuroleptic therapy. Clin Neuropharmacol 20: 77-81, 1997.

157. Sokoloff LG, Pavlakovic R: Neuroleptic-induced dysphagia. Dysphagia 12:177-179, 1997.

158. Dantas RO, Nobre Souza MA: Dysphagia induced by chronic ingestion of benzodiazepine. Am J Gastroenterol 92:1194-1196, 1997.

159. Leopold NA: Dysphagia in drug-induced parkinsonism: A case report. Dysphagia 11:151-153, 1996.

160. Buchholz D, Jones B, Neumann S, et al: Benzodiazepine-induced pharyngeal dysphagia: Report of two probable cases. Dysphagia 10:142, 1995.

161. Buchholz DW: Oropharyngeal dysphagia due to iatrogenic neurological dysfunction. Dysphagia 10:248-254, 1995.

162. Hughes TA, Shone G, Lindsay G, et al: Severe dysphagia associated with major tranquilizer treatment. Postgrad Med J 70:581-583, 1994.

163. Bazemore PH, Tonkonogy J, Ananth R: Dysphagia in psychiatric patients: Clinical and videofluoroscopic study. Dysphagia 6:2-5, 1996.

164. Hertzman PA, Blevins WL, Mayer J, et al: Association of the eosinophilia-myalgia syndrome with the ingestion of tryptophan. N Engl J Med 322:869-873, 1990.

165. Dicker RM, James N, Cunha BA: The eosinophilia-myalgia syndrome with neuritis associated with L-tryptophan use. Ann Intern Med 112: 957-958, 1990.

166. Belongia EA, Hederg CW, Gleich GJ, et al: An investigation of the cause of the eosinophilia-myalgia syndrome associated with tryptophan use. N Engl J Med 323:357-365, 1990.

Structural Abnormalities of the Pharynx

Stephen E. Rubesin, MD

PHARYNGEAL POUCHES AND DIVERTICULA

Knowledge of the muscular anatomy and embryology of the pharynx allows a classification of pharyngeal outpouchings into five main categories[1]:
1. Lateral pharyngeal pouches and diverticula
2. Laryngocele
3. Branchial cleft cysts, branchial cleft fistulas, and branchial pouch sinuses
4. Zenker's diverticulum
5. Lateral cervical esophageal pouches and diverticula

Lateral Pharyngeal Pouches and Diverticula

The lateral pharyngeal wall may protrude beyond the normal expected contour of the pharynx in areas unsupported by muscle layers. The upper anterolateral pharyngeal wall is poorly supported in the region of the posterior and superior portion of the thyrohyoid membrane.[1] This region is bounded superiorly by the greater cornu of the hyoid bone, anteriorly by the thyrohyoid muscle, posteriorly by the superior cornu of the thyroid cartilage and stylopharyngeal muscle, and inferiorly by the ala of the thyroid cartilage.[2] This unsupported part of the thyrohyoid membrane is perforated by the superior laryngeal artery and vein and the internal laryngeal branch of the superior laryngeal nerve.[1]

Patients with lateral pharyngeal pouches usually have no symptoms. Approximately 5% of people with lateral pharyngeal pouches complain of dysphagia, choking, or regurgitation of undigested food.[3-5] Lateral pharyngeal pouches are extremely common, and the frequency of their occurrence increases with age.[1] The pouches are usually bilateral.

On frontal views during swallowing, pouches appear as transient, hemispheric, contrast-filled protrusions from the lateral hypopharyngeal wall, below the hyoid bone and above the calcified edge of the thyroid cartilage (Fig. 20-1). The junction of the ala of the thyroid cartilage and the thyrohyoid membrane is seen on frontal views as a notch in the lateral pharyngeal wall.[2] On double-contrast frontal views in which a modified Valsalva maneuver is performed, the pouches are seen as hemispheric, barium-coated protrusions above the "notch" in the lateral pharyngeal wall.[2] On lateral views, the pouches are seen as oval ring shadows (occasionally with an air-contrast level) below the hyoid bone at the level of the valleculae, just behind the epiglottic plate, along the anterior hypopharyngeal wall.[1,2] Barium that is retained in pouches during swallowing spills into the ipsilateral piriform sinus after the bolus passes. This delayed spill may result in dysphagia or a choking sensation because of overflow aspiration.[4-6]

In contrast, lateral pharyngeal diverticula are persistent protrusions of pharyngeal mucosa, usually through the thyrohyoid membrane or, rarely, through the tonsillar fossa.[1,2] The diverticula are lined by nonkeratinizing squamous epithelium surrounded by loose areolar connective tissue with many vascular spaces.[3] These protrusions are commonly found in people who have increased intrapharyngeal pressure (e.g., wind instrument players, glass blowers, and people with severe sneezing episodes). Clinical symptoms may include dysphagia, choking, cough, hoarseness, regurgitation of undigested food, or a painless neck mass.[1,3] Radiographically, the diverticula

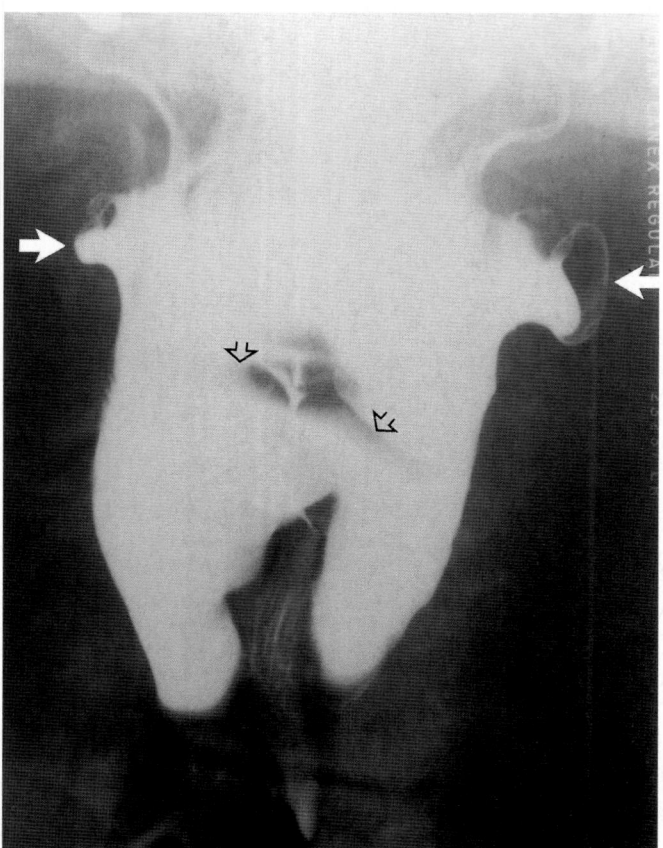

Figure 20-1. Lateral pharyngeal pouches. Frontal view of the pharynx during swallowing shows right and left lateral pharyngeal pouches (*white arrows*) protruding through the region of the thyrohyoid membrane. The epiglottis has slightly asymmetrical tilt (*open arrows*). (From Rubesin SE: Pharyngeal morphology. In Ekberg O [ed]: Radiology of the Pharynx and Oesophagus. Berlin, Springer, 2004, pp 51-77.)

are persistent, barium-filled sacs of various sizes connected to a bulging lateral hypopharyngeal wall by a narrow neck (Fig. 20-2). They are usually unilateral.

Laryngoceles

Lateral pharyngeal diverticula should not be confused with laryngoceles. A laryngocele is an abnormal saccular dilatation of the appendix of the laryngeal ventricle. The laryngocele is a protrusion of ciliated pseudostratified columnar epithelium and loose areolar connective tissue arising in the larynx.[7] In contrast, a pharyngeal diverticulum is a protrusion of nonkeratinizing squamous mucosa originating in the pharynx.

The appendix (saccule) of the laryngeal ventricle arises from the anterior end of the lateral recess of the laryngeal ventricle.[8] The appendix courses superiorly in the paralaryngeal space and is lateral to the false vocal cord and aryepiglottic fold, medial to the thyroid cartilage, and anterior to the pharynx. If saccular dilatation of the appendix is confined by the thyroid cartilage, it is termed an *internal laryngocele.* If the dilatation extends above the thyroid cartilage and through the thyrohyoid membrane, the sac is termed *external laryngocele.* A combination of internal and external laryngocele is termed a *mixed laryngocele.* Approximately 20% of these lesions are bilateral,[9] and 15% are associated with laryngeal neoplasms.[8,9]

Patients with laryngoceles and those with lateral pharyngeal diverticula have similar symptoms and physical findings. Most patients are asymptomatic and in the fifth to sixth decade of life.[7] Patients with external or mixed laryngoceles may have a compressible lateral neck mass. Patients with internal laryngoceles may complain of hoarseness, dysphagia, or choking. Laryngoceles are seen in patients with increased intralaryngeal pressure, such as glass blowers and wind instrument players.

Frontal radiographs in patients with an external laryngocele may show an air-filled sac above and lateral to the ala of the thyroid cartilage. Lateral radiographs may show the air-filled sac anterior to the epiglottic plate, in contrast to a lateral pharyngeal diverticulum, which lies posterior to the epiglottic plate.[1] External and internal laryngoceles do not fill with barium on pharyngograms. However, barium studies may reveal enlargement of the aryepiglottic fold with a smooth overlying mucosa.

Cross-sectional imaging of internal laryngoceles may demonstrate a mass filled with air, fluid, or both in the paralaryngeal space.[10] An external laryngocele appears as a mass that extends through the thyrohyoid membrane anterior to the jugular vein and carotid artery and medial to the sternocleidomastoid muscle (Fig. 20-3).[10] The density of the mass may be that of air, fluid, or soft tissue. Laryngoceles of soft tissue density are filled with mucus or infected secretions (laryngopyocele).

Branchial Cleft Cysts, Branchial Cleft Fistulas, and Branchial Pouch Sinuses

In the 4-week-old embryo, paired grooves appear on both sides of the neck region, leaving branchial ridges (arches) between them.[7,11] The grooves are called *branchial clefts* and are of ectodermal origin. Four outpouchings from the pharynx meet the branchial clefts. These pharyngeal outpouchings are of endodermal origin and are called *branchial pouches.* The

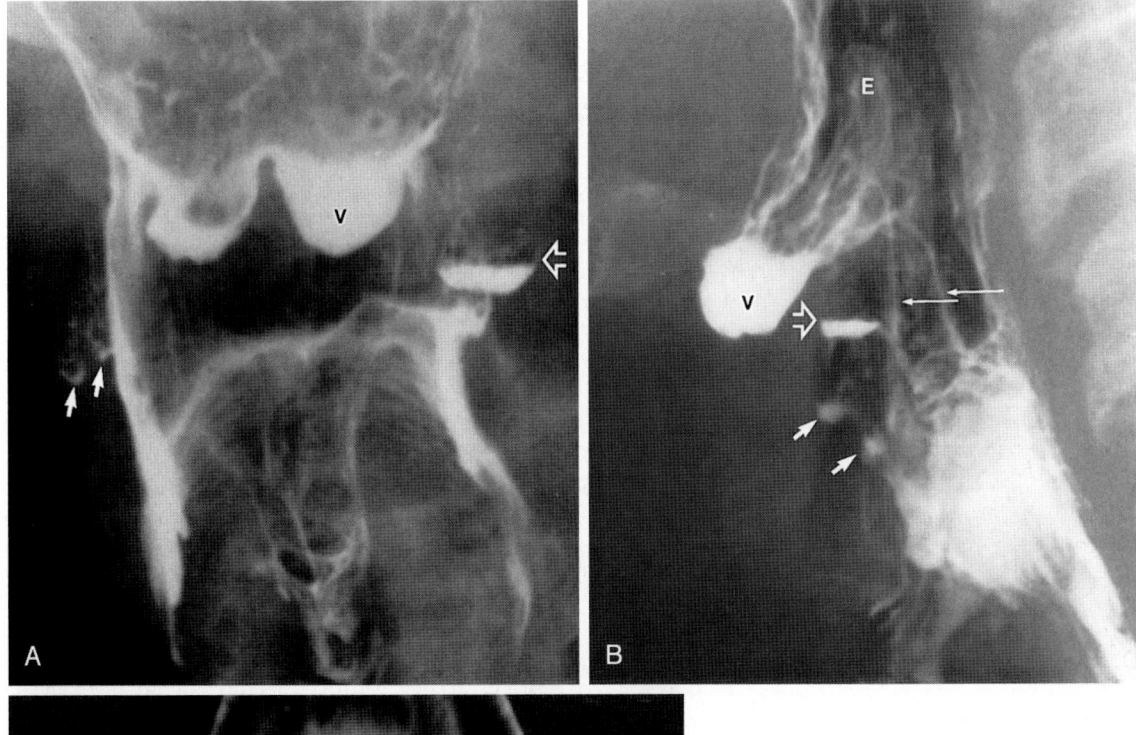

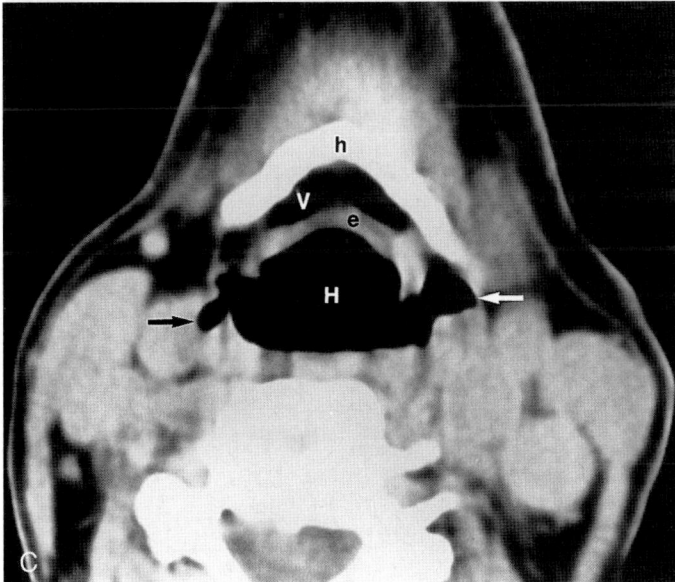

Figure 20-2. Lateral pharyngeal diverticula. A. Frontal view shows a round, saclike structure (*open arrow*) protruding from the left lateral pharyngeal wall. This lateral pharyngeal diverticulum contains an air-contrast level. A right lateral diverticulum is faintly seen as a bilobed structure (*solid arrows*). V, left vallecula. **B.** Lateral view shows that the left lateral pharyngeal diverticulum (*open arrow*) is behind and at the level of the vallecula (V). In this slightly tilted view, the bilobed right lateral pharyngeal diverticulum (*short arrows*) is faintly seen. *Long arrows* indicate the aryepiglottic folds. E, epiglottic tip. **C.** CT scan shows left and right lateral pharyngeal diverticula (*arrows*). e, epiglottis; H, hypopharynx; h, hyoid; V, right vallecula. (**A** and **B** modified from Rubesin SE, Glick SN: The tailored double-contrast pharyngogram. Crit Rev Diagn Imaging 28:133-179, 1988. Copyright CRC Press, Inc. Boca Raton, FL.)

first branchial cleft forms the external auditory meatus. The second branchial cleft forms the middle ear, eustachian tube, and floor of the tonsillar fossa. The third and fourth branchial pouches form the piriform sinus.[11] Persistence of either branchial pouches or clefts results in the formation of sinus tracts or cysts.

The most common branchial vestige is a cyst arising from the second branchial cleft. A second branchial cleft cyst is found at the level of the hyoid bone, deep to the sterno-cleidomastoid muscle.[7] Pathologically, a unilocular cyst is lined by keratinizing stratified squamous epithelium and is filled with desquamated keratinaceous debris. A zone of lymphoid tissue surrounds the epithelium.[7]

Patients with second branchial cleft cysts usually present between the ages of 10 and 40 years with a painless or fluc-tuant mass in the upper neck along the upper third of the anterior border of the sternocleidomastoid muscle.[12] When small, the cysts are anterior to the sternocleidomastoid muscle. When large, the cysts may extend posterior to the sterno-cleidomastoid muscle, displacing the carotid sheath.

Cross-sectional imaging of noninfected cysts may reveal a smooth, thin-walled mass with a homogeneous water core.[13] If infected, the wall of the branchial cleft cyst becomes thick-ened and may enhance with administration of intravenous contrast medium.[13] The second branchial cleft cyst may extend between the internal and external carotid arteries at a level superior to their bifurcation.[14] Rarely, branchial cleft cysts may communicate with the pharynx (branchial cleft fistulas), filling with barium during pharyngography.[1]

Branchial pouch sinuses or fistulas are tracts that extend from the pharynx and end blindly in the soft tissues of the neck (sinus) or extend to the skin (fistulas). These tracts

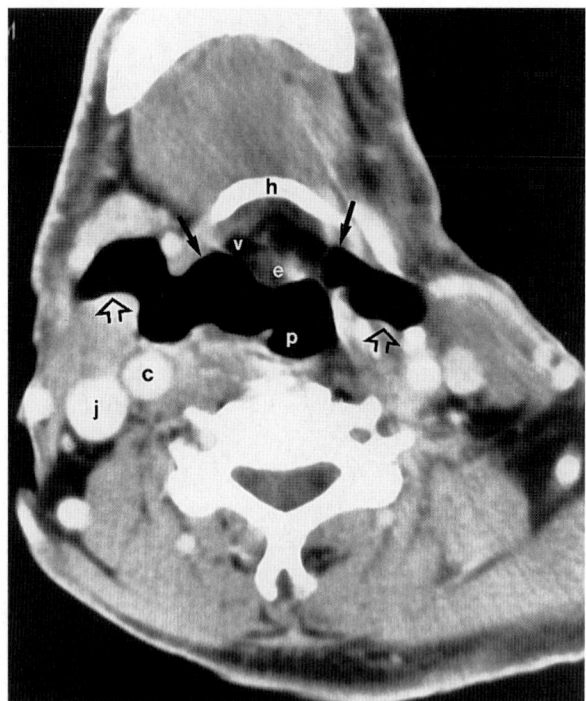

Figure 20-3. Right and left mixed laryngoceles. Axial CT scan at the level of the hyoid bone (h) shows air-filled sacs that extend through the thyrohyoid membrane and are anterior to the carotid artery (c) and jugular vein (j). The internal component (*solid arrows*) of the mixed laryngocele is in the paralaryngeal space. The external component (*open arrows*) of the laryngoceles is indicated. e, epiglottis; p, pharynx; v, right vallecula.

are lined by ciliated columnar epithelium. Branchial pouch sinuses arise from the tonsillar fossa (second pouch), the upper anterolateral piriform fossa (third pouch), or the lower anterolateral piriform sinus (fourth pouch). Many of these fistulas are present at birth[12] and communicate with the skin. Sinus tracts that end blindly are occasionally seen in adults. Radiographically, second branchial pouch vestiges appear as sinus tracts that arise from the tonsillar fossa and extend along the sternocleidomastoid muscle in the deep cervical fascia (Fig. 20-4).

Zenker's Diverticulum

Zenker's diverticulum (posterior hypopharyngeal diverticulum) is an acquired mucosal herniation through an area of anatomic weakness in the region of the cricopharyngeal muscle (Killian's dehiscence). The inferior constrictor muscle is composed of the thyropharyngeal and cricopharyngeal muscles. The thyropharyngeal muscle arises from the lateral ala of the thyroid cartilage; it courses laterally and posteriorly to merge with its counterpart from the opposite side in a raphe in the posterior pharyngeal wall. The cricopharyngeal muscle constitutes the lower portion of the inferior constrictor muscle, arising from the lateral cricoid cartilage to encircle the lowermost hypopharynx. The cricopharyngeal muscle has no midline raphe. No overlap of fibers exists between the thyropharyngeal and cricopharyngeal muscles. Considerable variation is found in the arrangement of the muscle bundles of the thyropharyngeal and cricopharyngeal muscles. Killian's dehiscence has been variably described as arising between the thyropharyngeal and cricopharyngeal muscles or between the

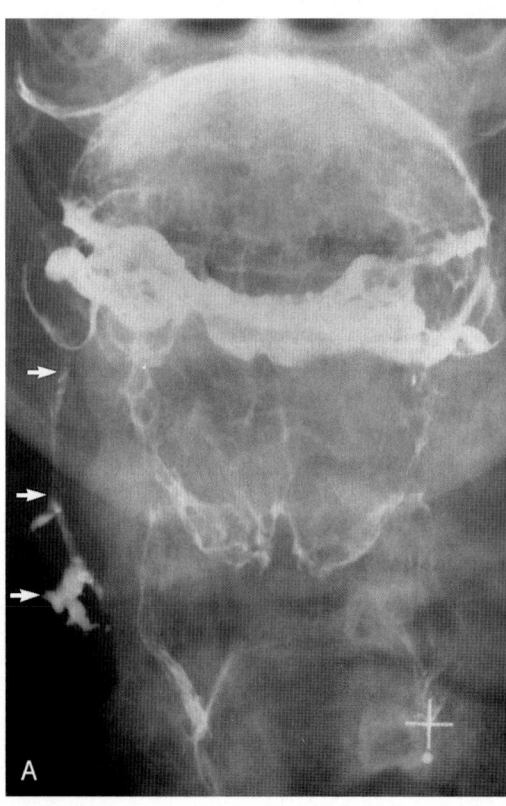

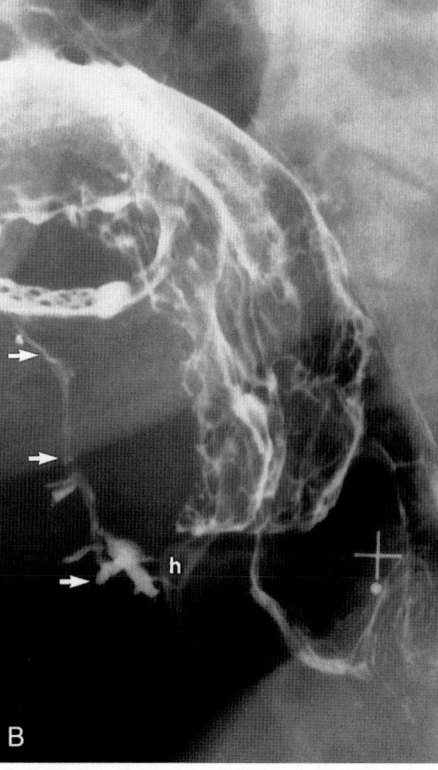

Figure 20-4. Second branchial pouch sinus. A. Frontal view shows a sinus tract (*arrows*) arising from the right lateral side of the oral cavity. **B.** Steep oblique view shows the sinus tract (*arrows*) arising from the region of the retromolar trigone just anterior to the tonsillar fossa and extending inferiorly toward the hyoid bone (h). (Reprinted with permission from Rubesin SE, Glick SN: The tailored double-contrast pharyngogram. Crit Rev Diagn Imaging 28:133-179, 1988. Copyright CRC Press, Inc. Boca Raton, FL.)

oblique and horizontal fibers of the cricopharyngeal muscle.[15,16] This area of weakness occurs in one third of patients.[17]

The pathogenesis of Zenker's diverticulum is as controversial as the muscular anatomy. Some radiographic and manometric studies have suggested that spasm with elevated pressure of the upper esophageal sphincter or incoordination and abnormal relaxation of the upper esophageal sphincter (achalasia) are contributing factors. However, other manometric studies have shown that (1) there is normal coordination between pharyngeal peristalsis and relaxation of the upper esophageal sphincter; (2) the upper esophageal sphincter relaxes completely during swallowing (i.e., there is no achalasia); and (3) the resting pressure of the upper esophageal sphincter is low (i.e., there is no spasm).[18,19] The relationship between gastroesophageal reflux disease and Zenker's diverticulum is also controversial. Almost all patients with Zenker's diverticulum have an associated hiatal hernia,[20,21] and many patients have radiographic evidence of gastroesophageal reflux, reflux esophagitis, or both. Whether gastroesophageal reflux predisposes patients with a large Killian dehiscence to the formation of Zenker's diverticulum is unknown.

Zenker's diverticulum is usually found in elderly patients who have dysphagia, regurgitation of undigested food, halitosis, choking, hoarseness, or a neck mass.[22] Some patients with Zenker's diverticulum are asymptomatic.

During swallowing, Zenker's diverticulum appears as a posterior bulging of the distal pharyngeal wall above an anteriorly protruding pharyngoesophageal segment (cricopharyngeal muscle) (Fig. 20-5). The neck of the Zenker's diverticulum can be very broad during swallowing. At rest,

the barium-filled diverticulum extends below the level of the cricopharyngeal muscle posterior to the proximal cervical esophagus (Fig. 20-6). After swallowing, barium in the diverticulum is regurgitated into the hypopharynx. In some patients, this regurgitation of barium results in overflow aspiration.

A true Zenker diverticulum may be confused with barium trapped above a cricopharyngeal muscle that has closed before the pharyngeal contraction wave has passed. This barium, trapped between downwardly progressing pharyngeal contraction and the cricopharyngeal muscle, is termed *pseudo-Zenker diverticulum* (Fig. 20-7). Barium may also be trapped above early closure of the upper cervical esophagus. Early closure of the cricopharyngeal muscle and upper cervical esophagus has been associated with gastroesophageal reflux disease.[23]

The complications of Zenker diverticulum include bronchitis, bronchiectasis, lung abscess, diverticulitis, ulceration, fistula formation, and carcinoma.[24] Any change in the character of dysphagia or bloody discharge in a patient known to have Zenker's diverticulum should suggest a complication.[25,26] On barium studies, irregularity of the contour of Zenker's diverticulum should suggest an inflammatory or neoplastic complication. Carcinoma arises in less than 1% of patients with Zenker's diverticulum,[26] but it is usually fatal.

Lateral Cervical Esophageal Pouches and Diverticula

The Killian-Jamieson space is a triangular area of weakness in the cervical esophagus just below the cricopharyngeal muscle. This space is bounded (1) superiorly by the inferior margin

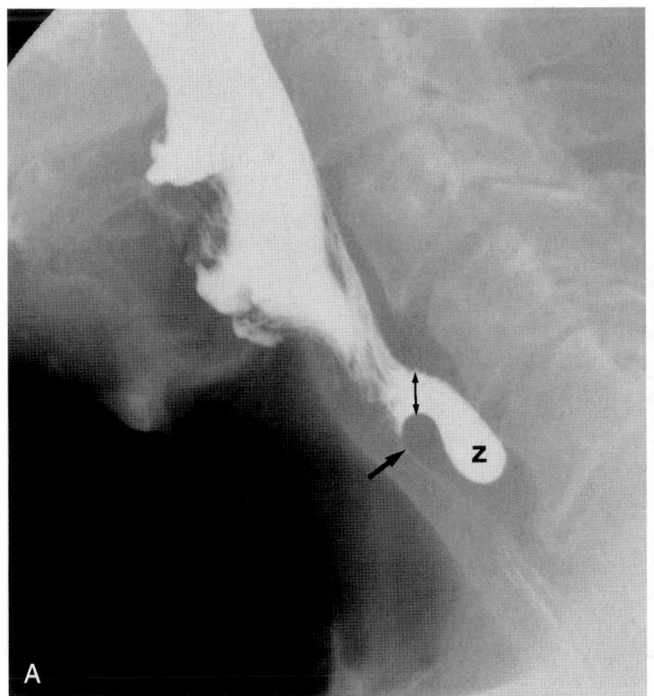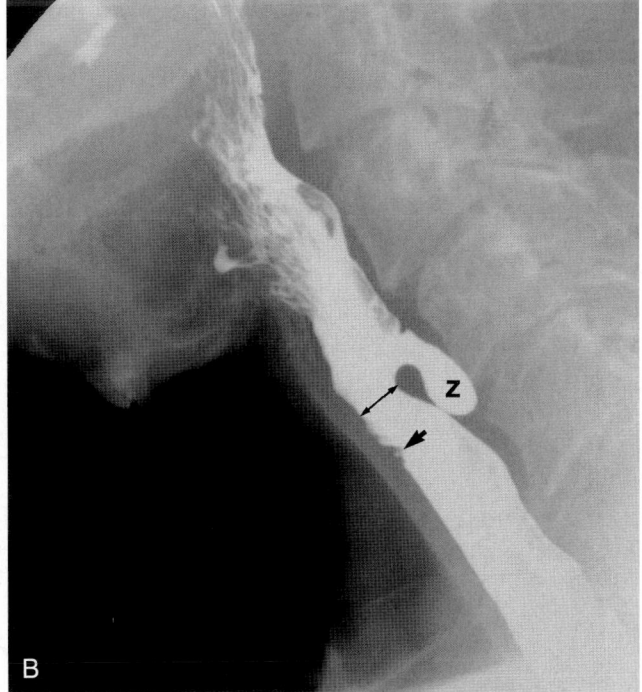

Figure 20-5. Zenker's diverticulum during swallowing. The relationship between the mouth of the Zenker diverticulum and the "prominent" cricopharyngeus is demonstrated. **A.** The bolus approaches the closed pharyngoesophageal segment, but barium has entered the mouth (*double arrow*) and lumen of the Zenker diverticulum (Z). The mouth of a Zenker diverticulum can be very broad, often larger than 1 cm. **B.** Most of the bolus has passed through the pharynx. The pharynx and larynx have continued to rise (about 3 mm), and the anterior wall of the trachea has been pulled forward slightly. The pharyngoesophageal segment is now open (*double arrow*). Redundant mucosa is seen in the postcricoid region (*arrow*). Opening of the pharyngoesophageal segment depends on elevation and anterior movement of the larynx as well as the pressure of the bolus due to gravity, tongue base thrust, and constrictor muscle contraction.

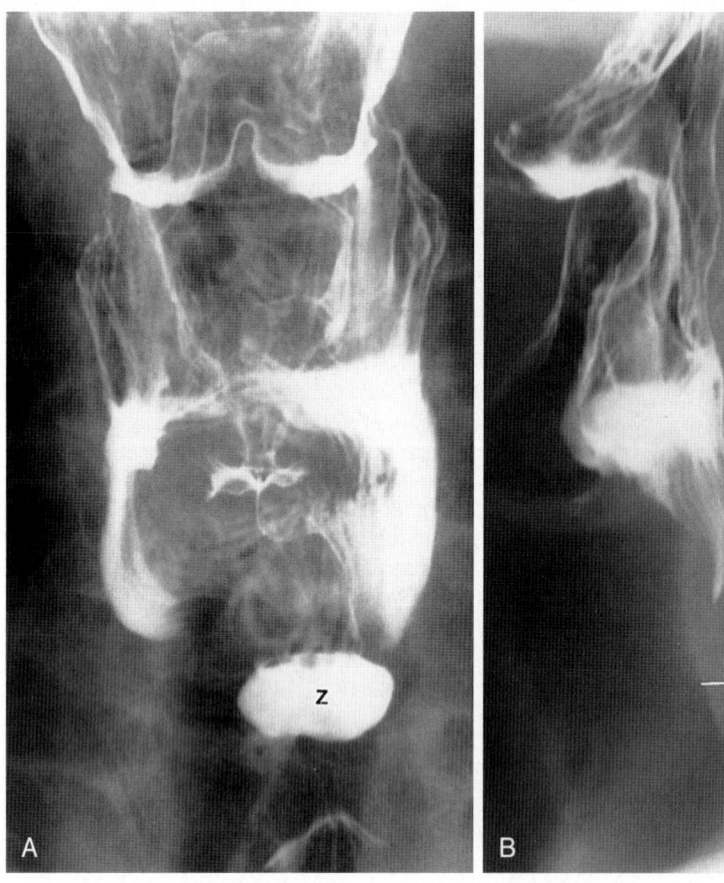
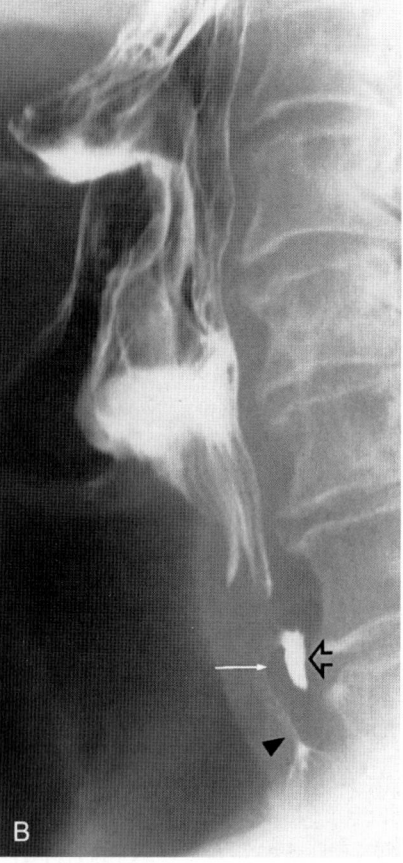

Figure 20-6. Small Zenker's diverticulum. **A.** Frontal view of the pharynx shows a barium-filled sac (Z) below the level of the hypopharynx. Neuromuscular weakness is indicated by barium stasis and ballooning of the lower hypopharynx. Barium also coats the vocal cords. **B.** In the lateral view, the Zenker diverticulum appears as a barium-filled sac (*open arrow*) posterior to the cervical esophagus (*arrowhead*). Note how flat the sac is in its anteroposterior dimension. Also note the prominent pharyngoesophageal segment (*solid arrow*).

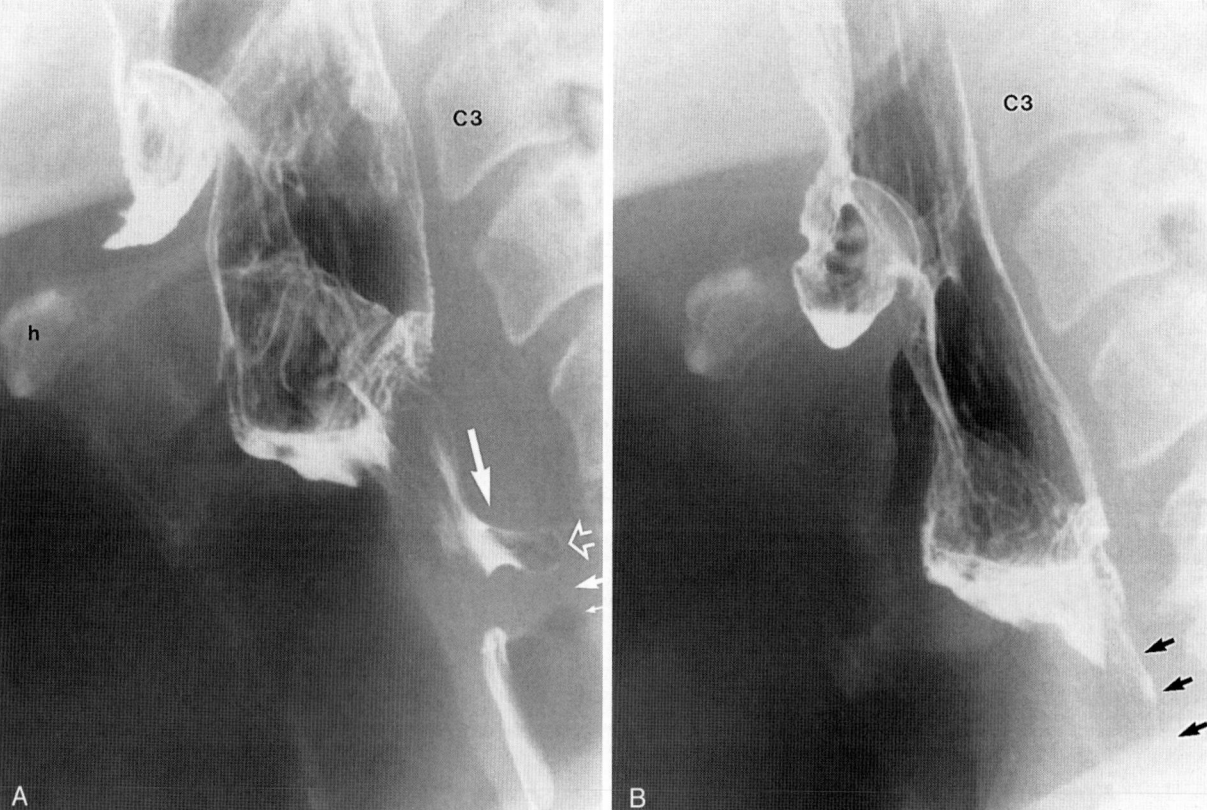

Figure 20-7. Pseudo-Zenker's diverticulum. Lateral view near the end of the swallow (**A**) is compared with a view taken during suspended respiration (**B**). **A.** A saclike collection of barium (pseudo-Zenker's diverticulum, *open arrow*) is trapped between the peristaltic wave (*large arrow* in **A**) and a prominent pharyngoesophageal segment ("cricopharyngeus") (*medium arrow* in **A**). Note, however, that the pseudo-Zenker diverticulum does not extend posteriorly beyond the expected contour of the cervical esophagus (*small arrow* in **A**). After the peristaltic wave has passed, during suspended respiration, the trapped barium has been cleared and the pseudo-Zenker diverticulum is not evident (*black arrows* in **B**). Note that the air-filled cervical esophagus is coated only on its anterior wall because the prominent cricopharyngeus prevents barium from contacting the posterior wall (*small arrow* in **A**). C3, third cervical vertebra. (From Laufer I, Levine MS [eds]: Double Contrast Gastrointestinal Radiology, 2nd ed. Philadelphia, WB Saunders, 1992.)

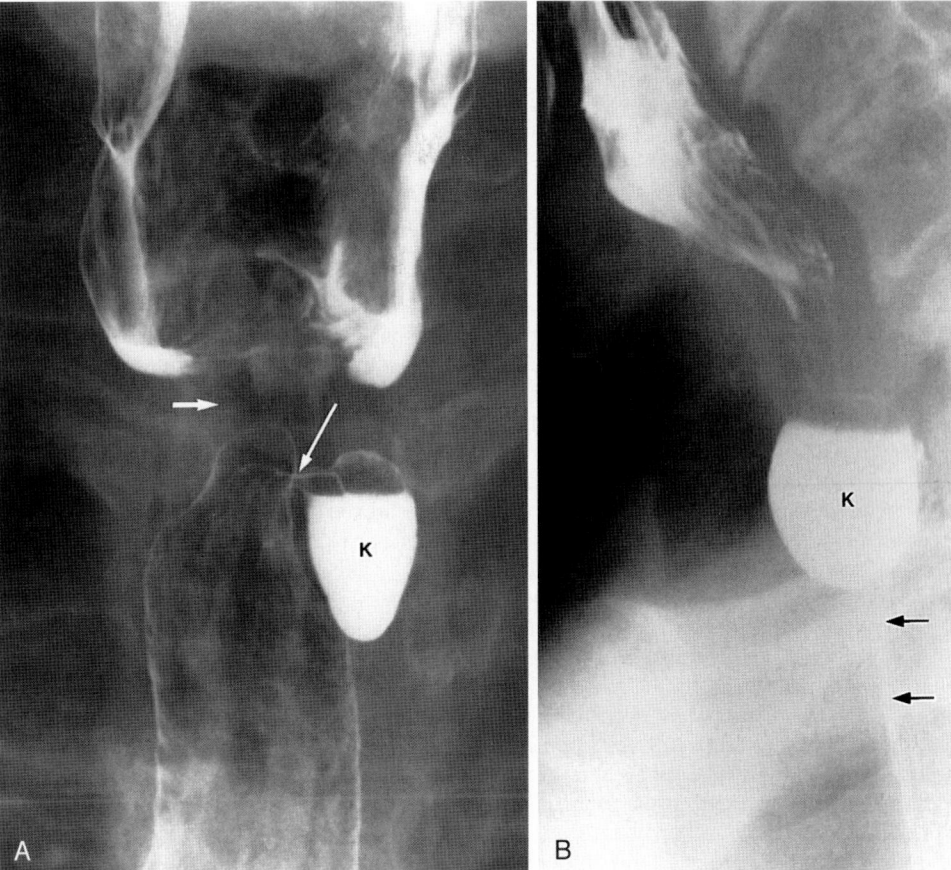

Figure 20-8. Killian-Jamieson diverticulum. A. Frontal view of the pharynx shows a barium-filled sac (K) to the left of the cervical esophagus. The neck of the diverticulum (*long arrow*) is below the level of the cricopharyngeal muscle (*short arrow*). **B.** Lateral view shows the diverticulum (K) protruding anterior to the course of the cervical esophagus (*arrows*). (From Rubesin SE: Pharynx. In Laufer I, Levine MS [eds]: Double Contrast Gastrointestinal Radiology, 2nd ed. Philadelphia, WB Saunders, 1992.)

of the cricopharyngeal muscle, (2) anteriorly by the inferior margin of the cricoid cartilage, and (3) inferomedially by the suspensory ligament of the esophagus originating from the posterior wall of the cricoid cartilage, just before the tendon forms the longitudinal muscle of the esophagus.[27]

Transient or persistent protrusions of the anterolateral cervical esophagus into the Killian-Jamieson space are termed *lateral cervical esophageal pouches* or *diverticula*, respectively. They are also known as *Killian-Jamieson pouches* or *Killian-Jamieson diverticula*. Most patients with Killian-Jamieson diverticula are asymptomatic, but some may complain of dysphagia or regurgitation.

These pouches and diverticula are relatively common and may be confused radiographically with Zenker's diverticulum. Killian-Jamieson diverticula can be bilateral or unilateral. If unilateral, the diverticula are usually found on the left side of the proximal cervical esophagus.[28] Radiographically, a small (3 to 20 mm in diameter), round to ovoid, smooth-surfaced outpouching is seen just below the level of the cricopharyngeal muscle (Figs. 20-8 and 20-9).[29] On frontal views, pouches appear as shallow, broad-based protrusions of the lateral upper esophageal wall that are filled late during swallowing and that empty after swallowing.[27] Diverticula appear as saccular protrusions that have narrow necks and do not empty as quickly after swallowing. On lateral views, the sac is anterior to the cervical esophagus below the level of the cricopharyngeal muscle.[22] In contrast, the neck of Zenker's diverticulum is on the posterior hypopharyngeal wall and the sac extends inferiorly behind the cervical esophagus.[22]

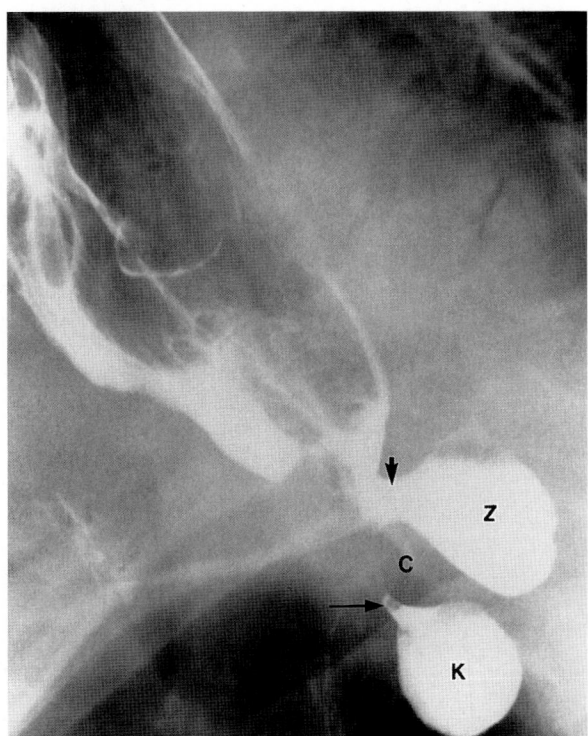

Figure 20-9. Simultaneous Zenker's diverticulum and Killian-Jamieson diverticulum. An oblique view of the pharynx shows Zenker's diverticulum (Z) with its opening (*short arrow*) above the prominent cricopharyngeus (C). The Killian-Jamieson diverticulum (K) has its opening (*long arrow*) below the prominent cricopharyngeus.

PHARYNGEAL AND CERVICAL ESOPHAGEAL WEBS

Webs are thin mucosal folds most frequently located along the anterior wall of the lower hypopharynx and proximal cervical esophagus. They are usually composed of normal epithelium and lamina propria.[29] Some webs show inflammatory changes.

The etiology and clinical significance of webs are controversial. Most patients with cervical esophageal webs are asymptomatic. The webs are seen as isolated findings in 3% to 8% of patients undergoing upper gastrointestinal barium studies.[30-34] In one autopsy series, 16% of patients had incidental cervical esophageal webs.[29]

Some pharyngeal and cervical esophageal webs are associated with diseases that cause inflammation and scarring, such as epidermolysis bullosa or benign mucous membrane pemphigoid. Several older northern European series showed an association of cervical esophageal webs, iron-deficiency anemia, and pharyngeal or esophageal carcinoma.[35,36] This association was termed *Plummer-Vinson syndrome* or *Paterson-Kelly syndrome*. In the United States, no strong association of cervical esophageal webs, iron-deficiency anemia, and pharyngoesophageal carcinoma has been found. Webs in the distal esophagus have been associated with gastroesophageal reflux disease.[31] Some cervical esophageal webs may also be associated with gastroesophageal reflux.[37]

Some webs are present in the valleculae or lower piriform sinus. These vallecular and piriform sinus webs are composed of mucosa, lamina propria, and underlying blood vessels. These webs are thought to be normal variants in the valleculae and piriform sinuses.[38]

Webs appear radiographically as 1- to 2-mm wide, shelflike filling defects along the anterior wall of the hypopharynx or cervical esophagus (Fig. 20-10). The webs protrude to various depths into the esophageal lumen. Webs may extend laterally, and a few extend circumferentially. Circumferential webs appear as ringlike shelves in the cervical esophagus. With severe luminal narrowing, dysphagia may result, especially in patients with circumferential cervical esophageal webs. Partial obstruction is suggested by a jet phenomenon[39,40] or by dilatation of the esophagus or pharynx proximal to the web (Fig. 20-10). A dynamic examination reveals a higher percentage of webs than do spot images alone.[30] Better demonstration of webs is also achieved with the use of large boluses of barium.[33]

Webs may be confused radiographically with redundant mucosa in the anterior wall of the hypopharynx at the level of the cricoid cartilage. This redundant mucosa has been termed the *postcricoid defect* and was previously attributed to a venous plexus in this region.[41] However, the postcricoid defect is probably related to redundancy of the mucosal and submucosal tissue in this area.[2]

Webs also should not be confused with a prominent cricopharyngeal muscle, which appears as a round, broad-based protrusion from the posterior pharyngeal wall at the level of the pharyngoesophageal segment.

INFLAMMATORY LESIONS OF THE PHARYNX

Although acute epiglottitis usually affects children between 3 and 6 years of age, it occasionally causes severe stridor and sore throat in adults.[42] Plain radiographic diagnosis of acute epiglottitis is important (even in adults) because manipulation of the tongue or pharynx may exacerbate edema and respiratory distress. Neck radiographs may show smooth enlargement of the epiglottis and aryepiglottic folds. Barium studies are

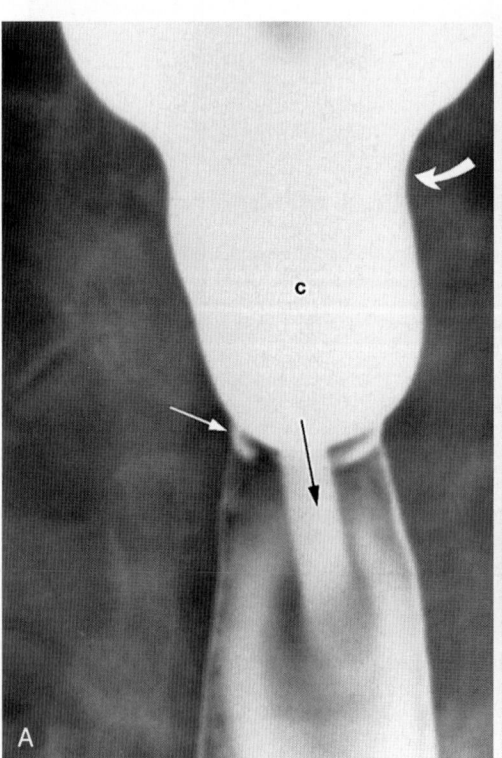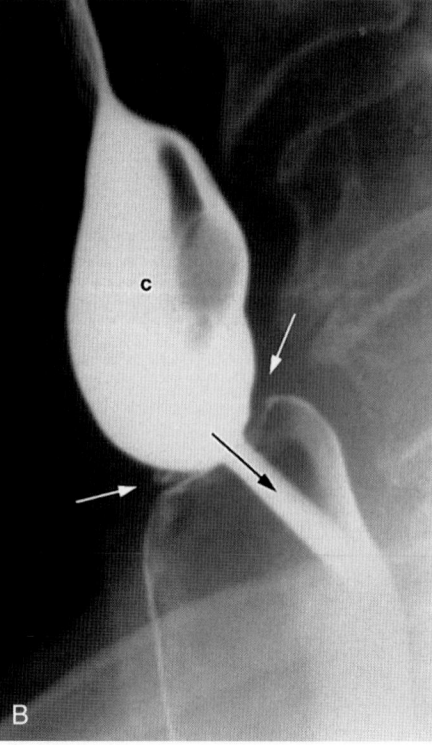

Figure 20-10. Partially obstructing cervical esophageal web. Frontal (**A**) and lateral (**B**) views show a circumferential, radiolucent ring (*straight white arrows*) in the proximal cervical esophagus. Partial obstruction is suggested by a jet phenomenon (*black arrows*), with barium spurting through the ring, and by mild dilatation of the proximal cervical esophagus (c). The level of the cricopharyngeus is identified (*curved arrow* in **A**). (From Rubesin SE: Pharynx. In Laufer I, Levine MS [eds]: Double Contrast Gastrointestinal Radiology, 2nd ed. Philadelphia, WB Saunders, 1992.)

contraindicated because they may exacerbate edema, triggering an acute respiratory arrest.[43]

Barium studies of the pharynx are usually of limited value in patients with *acute* sore throat due to viral, bacterial, or fungal infection.[43] Such patients usually demonstrate normal findings on pharyngograms or evidence of nonspecific lymphoid hyperplasia of the palatine or lingual tonsils (Figs. 20-11 and 20-12).

In immunosuppressed patients with acute dysphagia, barium studies are directed toward the esophagus to demonstrate the presence, site, and type of esophagitis. However, a double contrast examination of the pharynx may demonstrate the plaques of *Candida* pharyngitis or the ulcers of herpes pharyngitis, particularly in patients with AIDS (Fig. 20-13).[44]

In patients with *chronic* sore throat, barium studies may help to determine whether underlying gastroesophageal reflux and reflux esophagitis are present. Inflammatory disorders of the pharynx or gastroesophageal reflux can alter pharyngeal elevation, epiglottic tilt, or closure of the vocal cords and laryngeal vestibule. Inflammation-induced dysmotility may result in laryngeal penetration and stasis.

Some diseases with diffuse mucous membrane ulceration affect the pharynx. Pharyngeal inflammation and ulceration may be seen in patients with Behçet's syndrome, Stevens-Johnson syndrome, Reiter's syndrome, epidermolysis bullosa,[45,46] or bullous pemphigoid.[47] Most of these patients have recurrent aphthous stomatitis and oropharyngeal ulceration. With severe ulceration, amputation of the uvula and tip of the epiglottis may be observed radiographically.[47] Scarring may cause distortion of the pharyngeal contours. Severe ulceration with subsequent scarring may also be caused by lye ingestion (Fig. 20-14).[48]

Lymphoid Hyperplasia of the Lingual Tonsil

The lingual tonsil is an aggregate of 30 to 100 follicles along the pharyngeal surface of the tongue, extending from the circumvallate papillae to the root of the epiglottis.[49] This lymphoid tissue causes the normal surface of the base of the tongue to be divided into small nodules of varying size.

Hypertrophy of the lingual tonsil frequently occurs (1) after puberty; (2) as a compensatory response after tonsillectomy; or (3) as a nonspecific response to allergies or repeated infection.[49] Symptoms attributed to lymphoid hyperplasia of the lingual tonsil include throat discomfort, a globus sensation, and dysphagia. There are no criteria based on size for differentiating nodularity of the base of the tongue due to normal lingual tonsils from that resulting from reactive lymphoid hyperplasia. On frontal radiographs obtained in patients with lymphoid hyperplasia, multiple smooth, round or ovoid nodules are symmetrically distributed over the surface of the base of the tongue (see Fig. 20-11). On lateral radiographs, the base of the tongue may seem to protrude posteriorly. With severe lymphoid hyperplasia of the base of the tongue, the nodules may extend into the valleculae, along the lingual surface of the epiglottis, or even into the upper hypopharynx. Lymphoid hyperplasia can be coarsely nodular, asymmetrically distributed, or masslike. However, any asymmetrically distributed coarse nodularity or mass must be viewed with suspicion. The use of endoscopy and MRI may help to rule out malignancy.

FOREIGN BODY IMPACTION

A variety of foreign bodies may be become impacted in the pharynx. Tiny objects such as fragments of glass may become lodged in the interstices of the palatine tonsils. Larger swallowed objects may stick in the tips of the piriform sinuses at or just above the pharyngoesophageal segment (Fig. 20-15).[50]

BENIGN TUMORS OF THE PHARYNX

A wide variety of benign tumors occur in the pharynx.[7] Nonepithelial tumors arising from the supporting tissues of the pharynx are rare.[51,52] However, tumor-like cysts of various histologic types are not uncommonly seen in the pharynx.[53] The most common benign lesions are retention cysts of the valleculae or aryepiglottic folds.

Symptoms are related primarily to the location and to the polypoid or sessile nature of the lesion. Patients with benign tumors of the base of the tongue may be asymptomatic or may complain of throat irritation or dysphagia. Aryepiglottic fold nodules or mass lesions may cause dysphonia or respiratory symptoms such as stridor. Tumors of the epiglottis and aryepiglottic folds may also result in dysphagia, coughing, or choking because of laryngeal penetration. Rarely, pedunculated lesions (e.g., papillomas, lipomas,[54] and fibrovascular

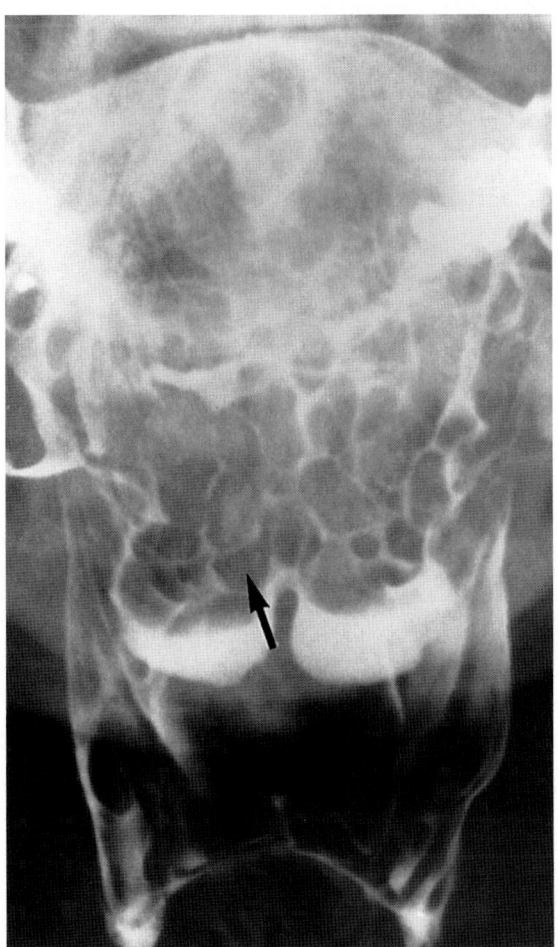

Figure 20-11. Lymphoid hyperplasia of the base of the tongue. Frontal view shows large, smooth-surfaced, round to ovoid nodules (*arrow*) symmetrically distributed over the surface of the base of the tongue.

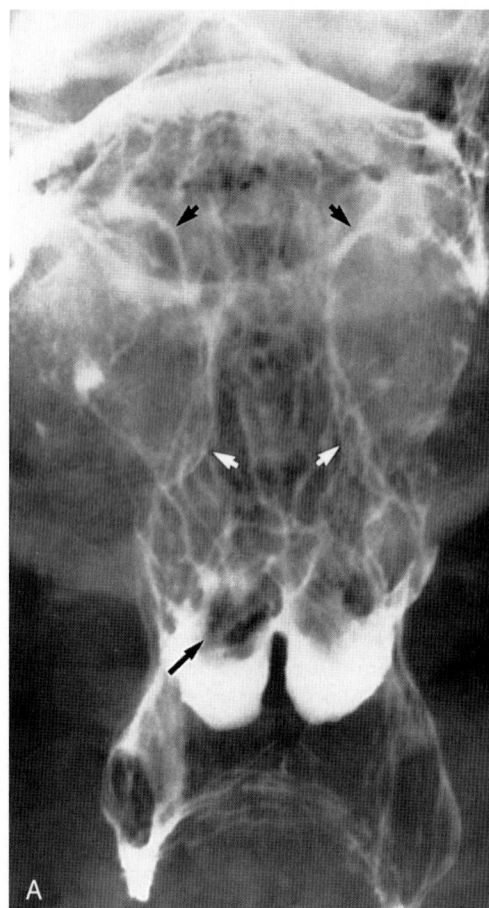
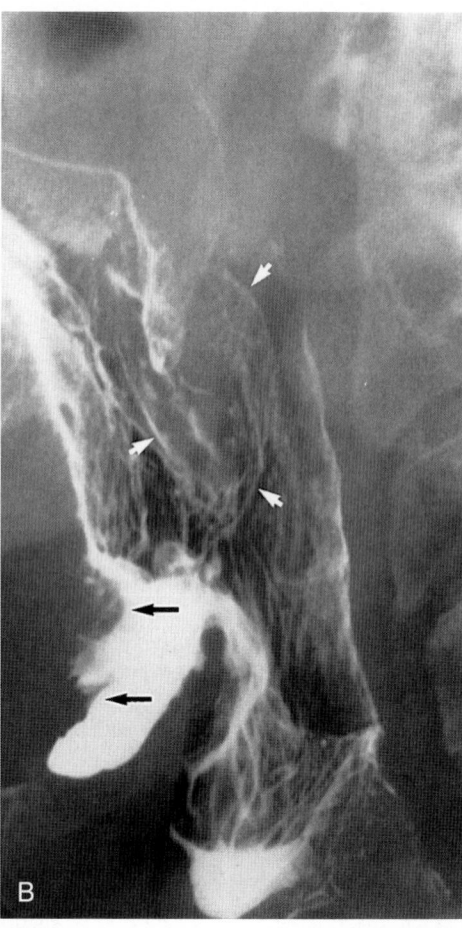

Figure 20-12. Lymphoid hyperplasia of the palatine tonsils and base of the tongue in a young patient with a chronic sore throat. Frontal (**A**) and lateral (**B**) views of the pharynx show moderate nodularity of the base of the tongue (*long arrows*) and bilateral, symmetrical enlargement of the palatine tonsils (*short arrows*).

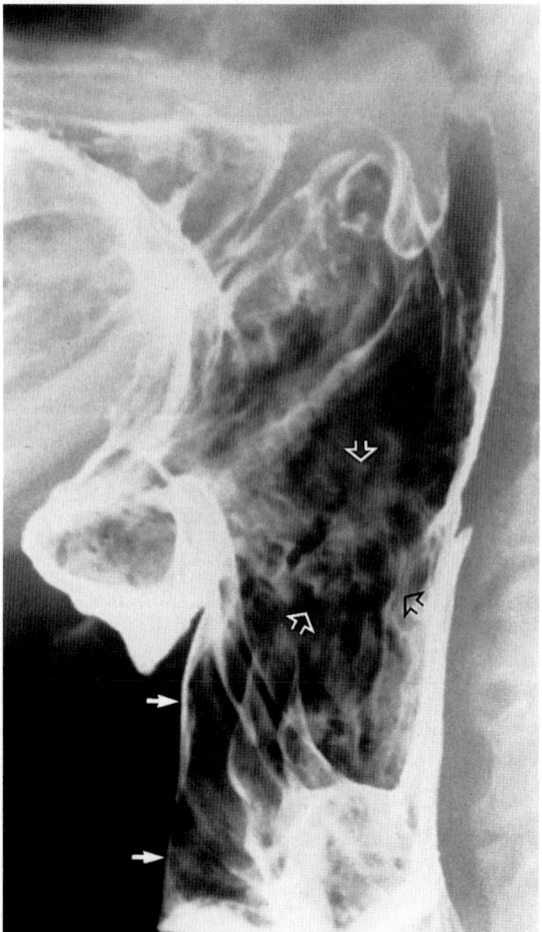

Figure 20-13. *Candida* pharyngitis. Lateral view of the pharynx shows well-circumscribed plaques (*open arrows*) at the level of the epiglottis. Note laryngeal vestibule penetration (*solid arrows*) resulting from abnormal pharyngeal motility associated with this inflammatory pharyngitis. (From Rubesin SE: Pharynx. In Laufer I, Levine MS [eds]: Double Contrast Gastrointestinal Radiology, 2nd ed. Philadelphia, WB Saunders, 1992.)

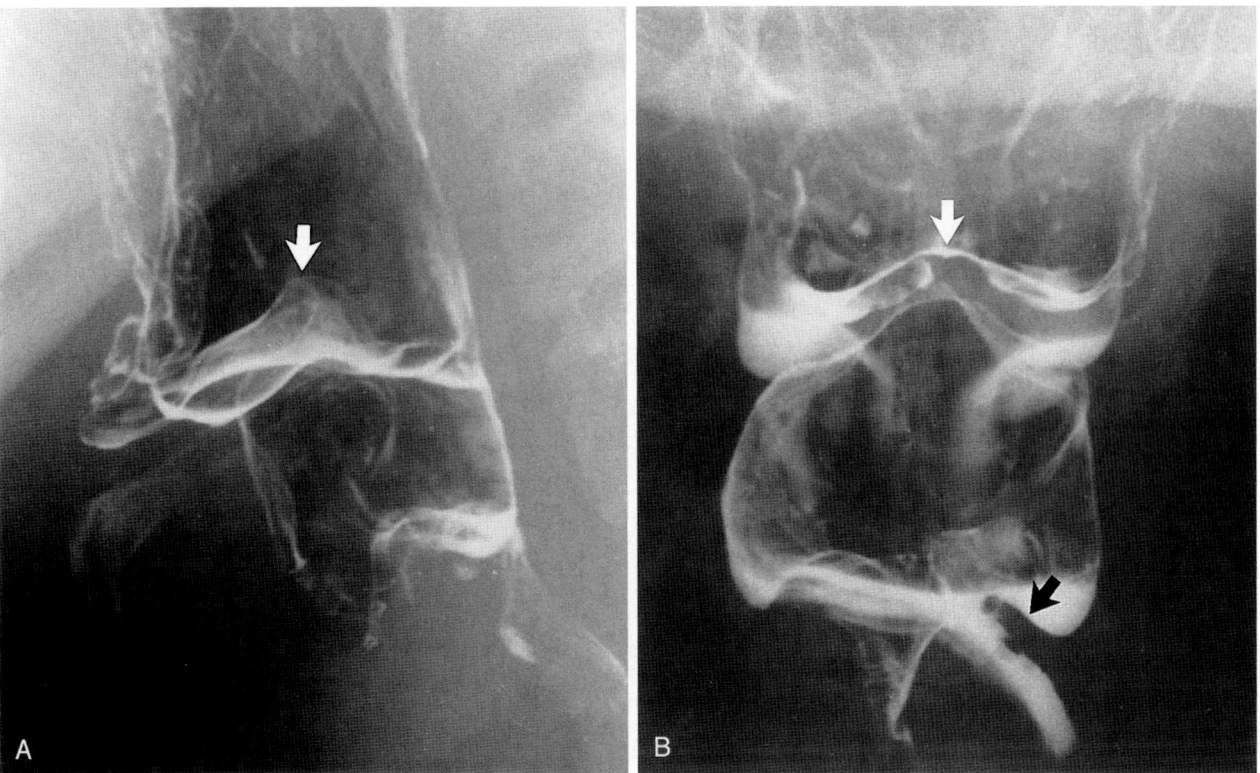

Figure 20-14. Scarring due to lye ingestion. A. On the lateral view, the tip of the epiglottis (*arrow*) appears truncated. **B.** On the frontal view, the epiglottis (*white arrow*) is located inferior to its normal position. A scar in the inferior portion of the left piriform sinus is seen as a fold of tissue (*black arrow*).

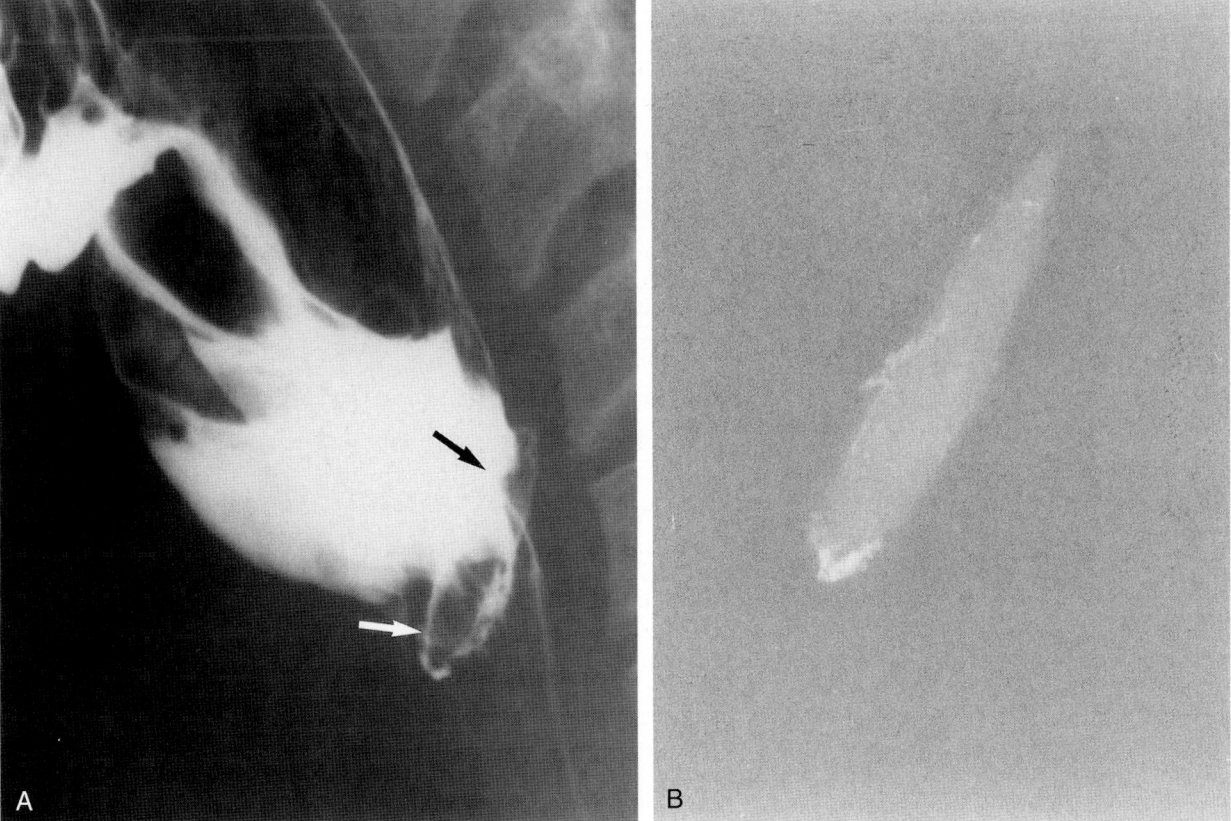

Figure 20-15. Foreign body impaction. A. Lateral view of the pharynx shows a long, ovoid radiolucency (*arrows*) in the barium pool of the lower hypopharynx, just above the closed pharyngoesophageal segment. **B.** Specimen radiograph shows an ovoid piece of fibrocartilage partly coated by barium. The patient had been eating chicken.

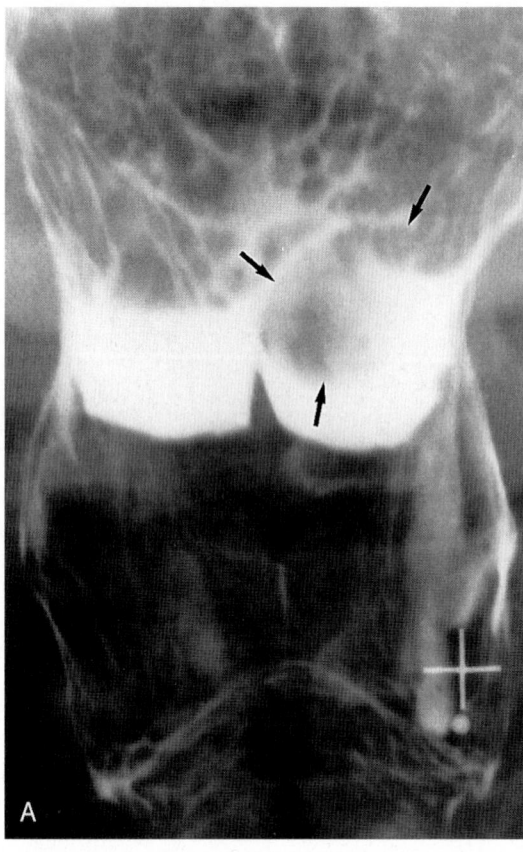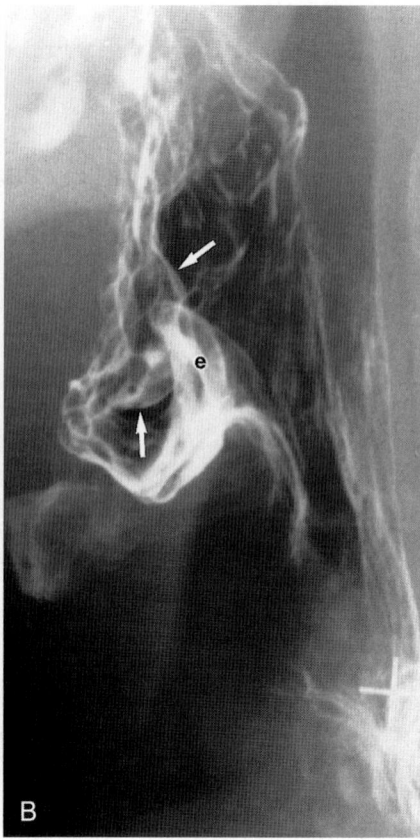

Figure 20-16. Retention cyst at the base of the tongue. A. Frontal view shows a faint, radiolucent filling defect in the barium pool (*arrows*) in the left vallecula. **B.** Lateral view shows a smooth-surfaced hemispheric mass (*arrows*) protruding posteriorly from the base of the tongue. The mass is partially obscured by the epiglottic tip (e). (From Rubesin SE, Laufer I: Pictorial review: principles of double contrast pharyngography. Dysphagia 6:170-178, 1991.)

polyps) may be coughed up into the mouth or may cause sudden death through asphyxiation.

Tumors of various histologic types tend to occur at specific locations in the pharynx. Retention cysts and granular cell tumors are the most common benign tumors of the base of the tongue (Fig. 20-16).[55] Ectopic thyroid tissue and thyroglossal duct cysts may occur at the tongue base but are rare. The tumor-like lesions that most commonly involve the aryepiglottic folds are retention cysts and saccular cysts. Retention cysts of the aryepiglottic folds are lined by squamous epithelium and filled with desquamated squamous debris (Fig. 20-17). In contrast, saccular cysts of the aryepiglottic folds arise from the mucus-secreting glands of the appendix of the laryngeal ventricle and are filled with mucoid secretions. True soft tissue tumors of the aryepiglottic folds, such as lipomas, neurofibromas, hamartomas,[52] granular cell tumors, and oncocytomas, are rare.[7] Laryngeal involvement in neurofibromatosis (von Recklinghausen's disease) is rare but most frequently involves the region of the arytenoid cartilage and aryepiglottic folds (Fig. 20-18).[56] Benign tumors arising from the minor mucoserous salivary glands are usually seen in the oropharynx in the region of the soft palate and base of the tongue. Benign cartilaginous tumors involving the pharynx (chondromas) usually arise from the posterior lamina of the cricoid cartilage.[57]

Regardless of its underlying histologic characteristics, a benign pharyngeal tumor usually appears radiographically as a smooth, round, sharply circumscribed mass en face and as a hemispheric line with abrupt angulation in profile (see Figs. 20-16 and 20-17).[43,55] Only rarely is a pedunculated, polypoid lesion (e.g., papilloma or fibrovascular polyp) seen. The benign nature of these lesions should be confirmed by

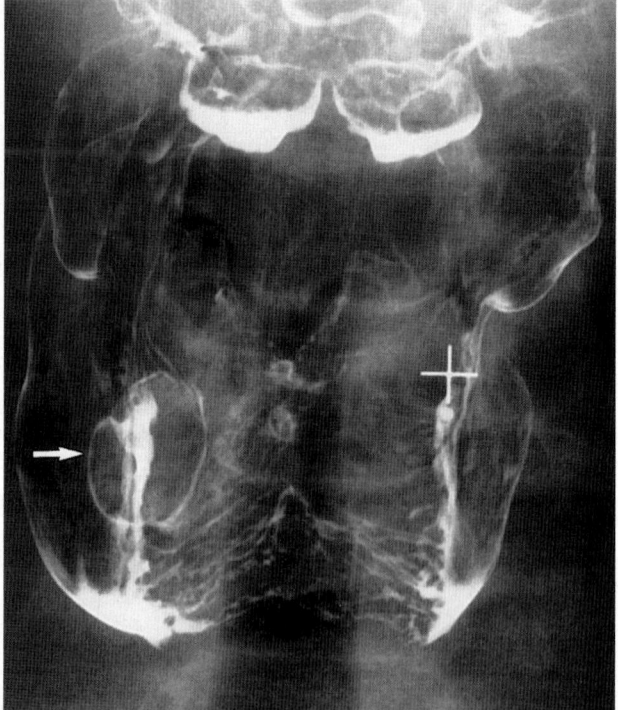

Figure 20-17. Retention cyst in the mucosa overlying the muscular process of the right arytenoid cartilage. A smooth-surfaced, well-circumscribed mass is seen in the region of the mucosa overlying the muscular process of the right arytenoid cartilage (*arrow*). This 2.5-cm mass was not detected on endoscopy. After a repeat endoscopic examination confirmed the presence of the lesion, surgery was performed and pathologic evaluation revealed a retention cyst lined by squamous epithelium. (Reprinted with permission from Rubesin SE, Glick SN: The tailored double-contrast pharyngogram. Crit Rev Diagn Imaging 28:133-179, 1988. Copyright CRC Press, Inc. Boca Raton, FL.)

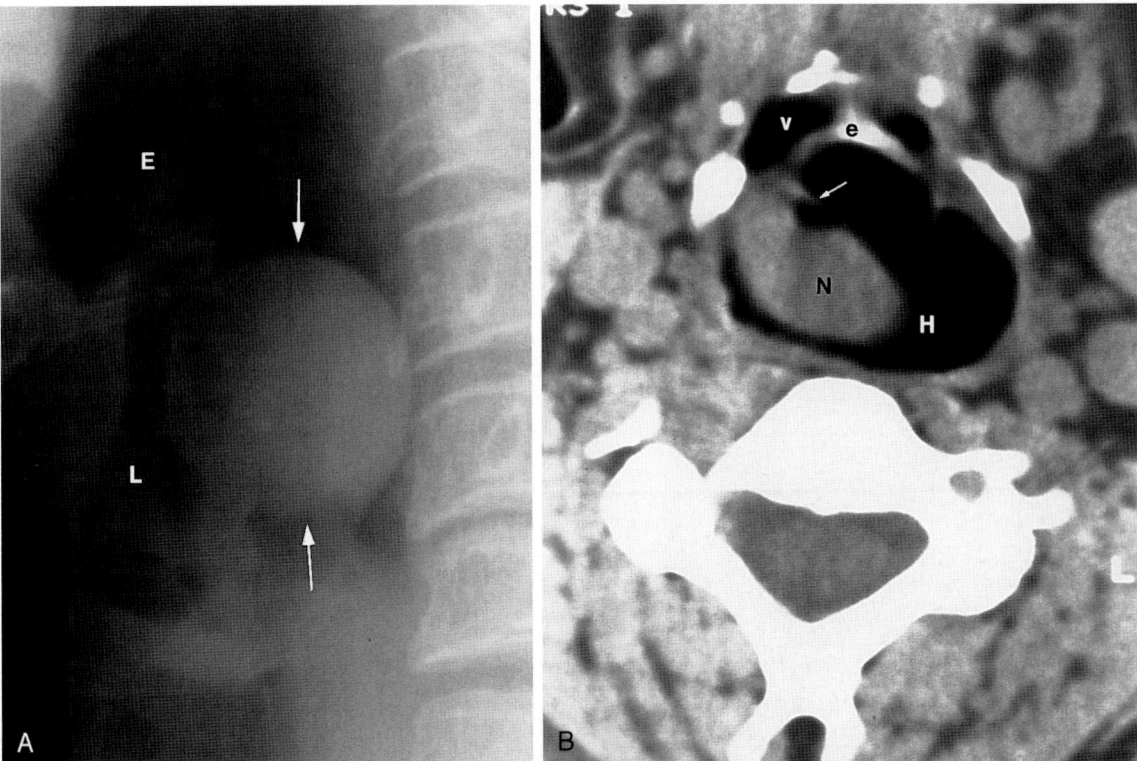

Figure 20-18. Neurofibroma of the right aryepiglottic fold. A 41-year-old man with known neurofibromatosis came to the emergency department complaining of work-related neck pain and mild inspiratory stridor. **A.** Lateral radiograph of the neck shows a smooth, well-circumscribed mass (*arrows*) in the region of the right aryepiglottic fold. E, epiglottis; L, laryngeal vestibule. **B.** CT scan shows a smooth-surfaced mass (N) protruding into the hypopharynx (H). *Arrow* indicates the uppermost portion of the aryepiglottic fold. e, epiglottis; v, right vallecula. (**A** from Rubesin SE, Laufer I: Pictorial review: Principles of double contrast pharyngography. Dysphagia 6:170-178, 1991.)

endoscopic examination. However, submucosal masses are sometimes missed at endoscopy.

MALIGNANT TUMORS OF THE PHARYNX

Radiologists should be as familiar with pharyngeal carcinoma as they are with esophageal carcinoma. Squamous cell carcinomas of the head and neck (e.g., tongue, pharynx, or larynx) constitute 5% of all cancers in the United States,[58] whereas esophageal carcinomas constitute only 1% of all cancers. The prognosis of pharyngeal cancer is better than that of esophageal cancer; the 5-year survival rate for pharyngeal cancer is 20% to 40%, whereas the 5-year survival rate for esophageal cancer is 5% to 10%.

The radiologist may be the first physician to suggest a diagnosis of pharyngeal carcinoma (Fig. 20-19). Some tumors may be detected during barium studies performed for other reasons. Patients with pharyngeal symptoms or a palpable neck mass may undergo pharyngoesophagography as the initial diagnostic examination. In patients with known pharyngeal cancer, a contrast examination is of value to assist in planning proper work-up and therapy. A barium examination can also be used to rule out a second primary lesion in the esophagus. Furthermore, the examination can detect co-existing structural lesions (e.g., a prominent cricopharyngeal muscle, Zenker's diverticulum, web, or stricture) that may be difficult to circumvent safely at endoscopy. Barium studies reveal the size, extent, and inferior limit of pharyngeal tumors and the degree of functional impairment. The barium examination can also show areas behind bulky tumors that are difficult to visualize by endoscopic examination.

Barium studies allow detection of more than 95% of structural lesions below the pharyngoesophageal fold.[59] These studies are especially valuable in areas of the pharynx that are difficult to evaluate by endoscopy (e.g., lower base of the tongue, valleculae, lower hypopharynx, and pharyngoesophageal segment).

Signs and Symptoms

The symptoms of pharyngeal carcinoma are nonspecific and usually of short duration (<4 months). They include sore throat, dysphagia, and odynophagia.[60] Choking or coughing may be due to laryngeal penetration during swallowing or aspiration of barium trapped in ulcerated tumors. Hoarseness occurs primarily in patients with laryngeal carcinoma, supraglottic carcinoma, or carcinoma of the medial piriform sinus infiltrating the arytenoid cartilage or cricoarytenoid joint. Referred earache may occur, especially when nasopharyngeal tumors block the eustachian tube.[60] Some patients are asymptomatic but present with a palpable neck mass. Most patients with squamous cell carcinoma are 50 to 70 years of age.[60,61] Almost all patients (>95%) are moderate to heavy abusers of alcohol and tobacco.[58]

Squamous Cell Carcinoma

Pathology

Squamous cell carcinomas represent 90% of malignant lesions involving the oropharynx and hypopharynx.[7,61,62] Most of these tumors are keratinizing squamous cell carcinomas.

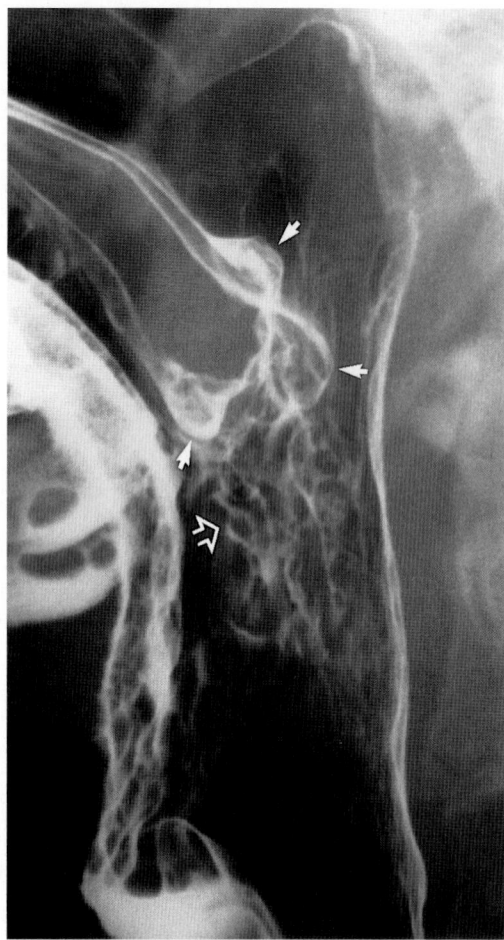

Figure 20-19. Unsuspected soft palate carcinoma. An 80-year-old patient with dementia underwent an upper gastrointestinal examination for epigastric pain. Nasal regurgitation was observed during the initial double-contrast swallow. Lateral spot image of the pharynx shows obliteration of the contour of the lower soft palate, which is replaced by a lobulated mass (*solid arrows*). Nodular mucosa in the tonsillar fossa (*open arrow*) indicates spread of the tumor into this region. (From Rubesin SE, Rabischong P, Bilaniuk LT, et al: Contrast examination of the soft palate with cross-sectional correlation. RadioGraphics 8:641-665, 1988.)

In general, they occur in two macroscopic forms: (1) exophytic tumors that spread over the mucosa and (2) infiltrative or ulcerative tumors that penetrate deeply into surrounding soft tissue, cartilage, and bone.[7] Multiple primary lesions of the oral cavity, pharynx, esophagus, and lung are seen in more than 20% of patients.[60] Because such a strong association exists between head and neck squamous cell carcinoma and esophageal carcinoma,[63,64] a major goal of a preoperative radiologic study is to rule out a synchronous primary esophageal cancer. Between 1% and 15% of patients with head and neck squamous cell carcinoma subsequently develop squamous cell carcinoma of the esophagus.[63-65]

Radiographic Findings

The radiographic findings of pharyngeal cancer include: (1) an intraluminal mass; (2) mucosal irregularity; and (3) impairment or loss of normal mobility or distensibility (Fig. 20-20).[43,66-69] An intraluminal mass may be manifested radiographically by obliteration of the normal luminal contour, by extra barium-coated lines protruding into the expected pharyngeal air column, by a focal area of increased radiopacity, or by a filling defect in the barium pool.[43,44,66,69] Mucosal irregularity may be seen as abnormal barium collections resulting from surface ulceration or as a lobulated, finely nodular, or granular surface texture.[66] Asymmetrical distensibility is seen as flattening of the pharyngeal contour due to fixation of structures by infiltrating tumor or due to an extrinsic mass impinging on the pharynx.[44,67,68]

Cross-sectional imaging studies are the examinations of choice for showing spread of tumor into the submucosa, intrinsic muscles, tissues extrinsic to the pharynx, and regional lymph nodes.[70-72] CT and MRI may occasionally reveal lesions (typically submucosal masses) that are not visible even with modern endoscopes.

Specific Sites

Nasopharynx

Squamous cell carcinoma is the most common histologic type of nasopharyngeal malignant tumor. Many nasopharyngeal squamous cell cancers are undifferentiated tumors, and many have a reactive lymphoid stroma. The risk factors, age of presentation, and histologic type are more varied than those of the typical squamous cell carcinoma of the oropharynx and hypopharynx. In addition to alcohol and smoking abuse, poor ventilation, nasal balms, ingested carcinogens, and upper respiratory viruses such as the Epstein-Barr virus have been implicated as causative factors.[7]

Nasopharyngeal squamous cell carcinoma occurs at a relatively young age, with 20% of patients being younger than 30 years old.[7] Approximately 50% of patients complain of hearing loss due to eustachian tube involvement. About half of these patients are asymptomatic and present with a neck mass caused by cervical nodal metastases. Other signs and symptoms include nasal obstruction, epistaxis, pain, headache, and damage to the fifth cranial nerve. The 5-year survival rate varies from 76% for patients with localized tumors to 10% to 20% for patients with cervical lymph node metastases.[73]

MRI is the method of choice for evaluating tumors of the nasopharynx.[74] The radiologist carefully searches for spread to the nasal cavity, sinuses, and cranial base, especially for cranial nerve involvement. Barium studies are used primarily to evaluate the symptoms of nasal regurgitation and voice changes due to soft palate insufficiency and to rule out a synchronous esophageal tumor (Fig. 20-21).

Palatine Tonsil

Squamous cell carcinoma of the palatine tonsil is the most common malignant tumor arising in the pharynx.[75] Well-differentiated tumors are usually exophytic and easily seen on barium studies (Fig. 20-22).[43] Poorly differentiated tumors are frequently of the ulcerative-infiltrative type and may be obscured on barium studies by the underlying nodular lymphoid tissue of the palatine tonsil.[44] Tonsillar tumors may spread to the soft palate, base of the tongue, and posterior pharyngeal wall. Approximately 50% of patients develop cervical nodal metastases.[43]

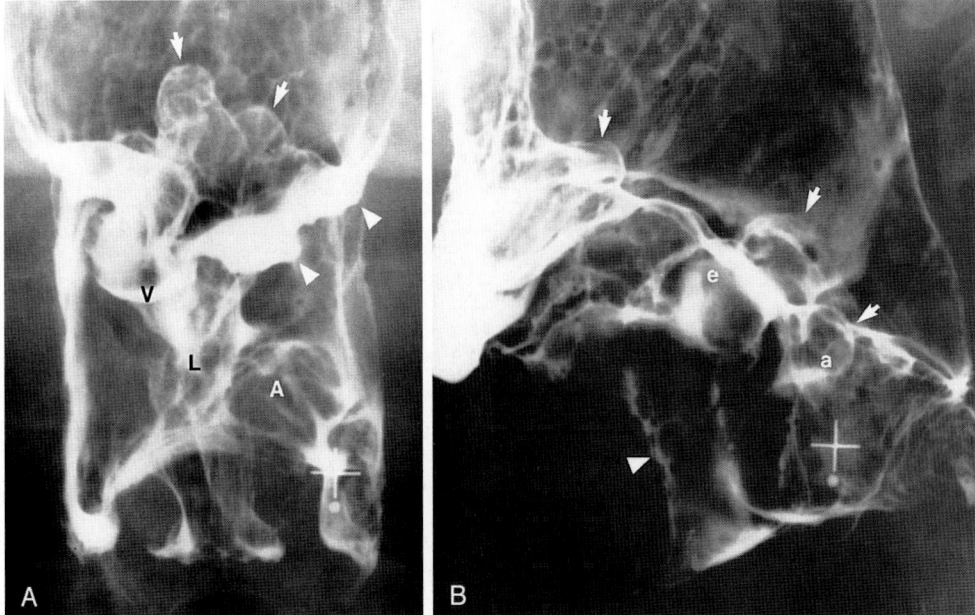

Figure 20-20. Radiographic findings in a patient with a large supraglottic pharyngeal carcinoma. A. On the frontal view, the normal contour of the epiglottis is obliterated and replaced by a lobulated mass (*white arrows*). The left vallecula is flattened and nodular (*arrowheads*). The right vallecula (V) is denoted for comparison. Nodularity is seen over the surface of the epiglottis, the laryngeal vestibule (L) (which has been coated by barium), and the mucosa overlying the muscular process of the left arytenoid cartilage (A). **B.** Lateral view shows loss of the normal contour of the epiglottis, with a huge lobulated mass (*arrows*) extending from the region of the epiglottis down the aryepiglottic folds (e) to the mucosa overlying the muscular process of the arytenoid cartilage (a). Barium coats the anterior wall of the laryngeal vestibule (*arrowhead*). This wall appears irregular in its proximal portion, a finding compatible with tumor infiltration. (Reprinted with permission from Rubesin SE, Glick SN: The tailored double-contrast pharyngogram. Crit Rev Diagn Imaging 28:133-179, 1988. Copyright CRC Press, Inc. Boca Raton, FL.)

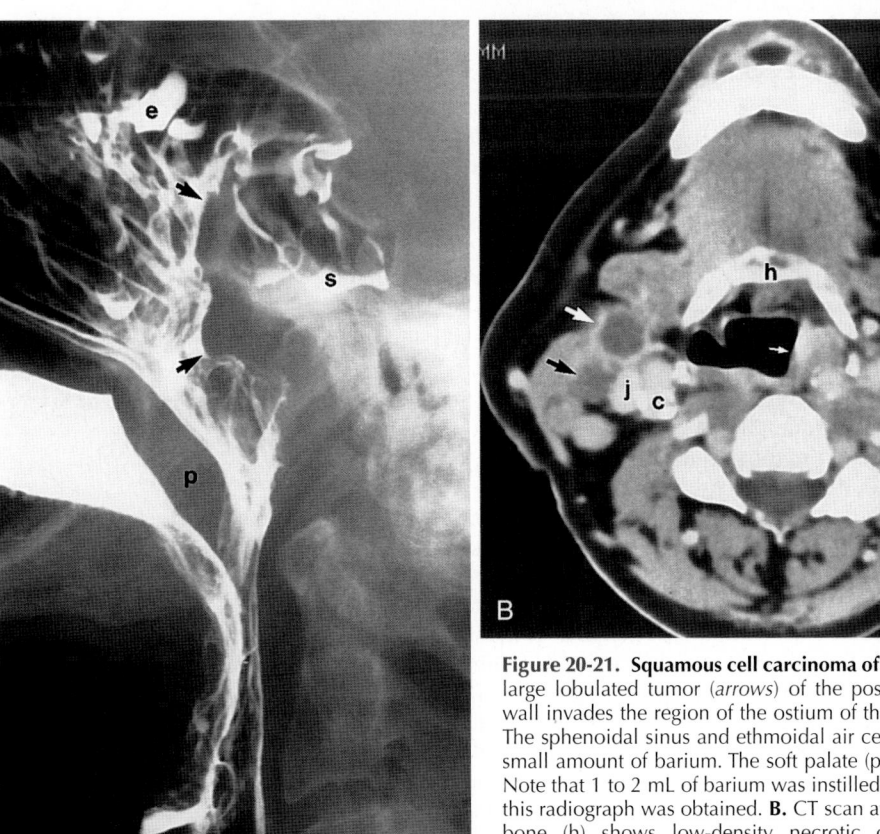

Figure 20-21. Squamous cell carcinoma of the nasopharynx. A. A large lobulated tumor (*arrows*) of the posterior nasopharyngeal wall invades the region of the ostium of the sphenoidal sinus (s). The sphenoidal sinus and ethmoidal air cells (e) are filled with a small amount of barium. The soft palate (p) is coated by barium. Note that 1 to 2 mL of barium was instilled into each naris before this radiograph was obtained. **B.** CT scan at the level of the hyoid bone (h) shows low-density necrotic cervical lymph node metastases (*large arrows*). The left lateral wall of the pharynx is flattened (*small arrow*). This flattening may have been caused by submucosal tumor infiltration. The calcified carotid artery (c) and jugular vein (j) are identified.

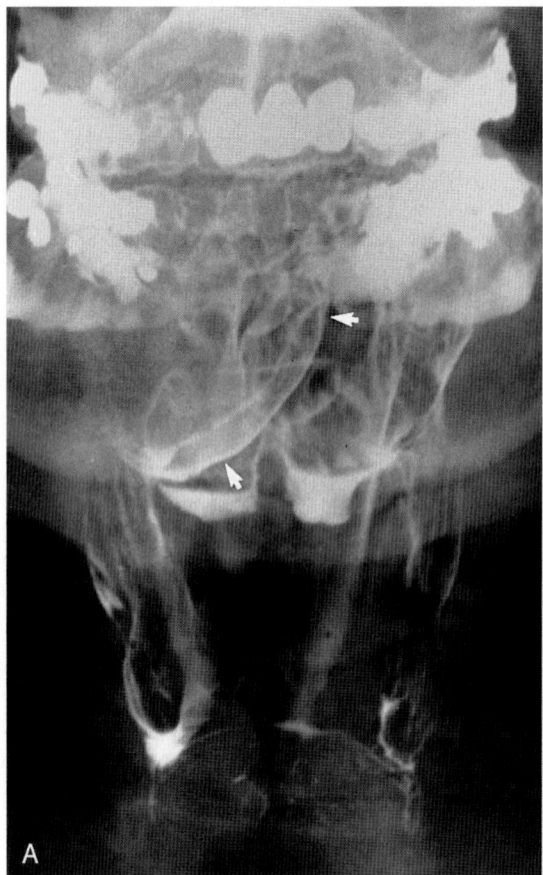
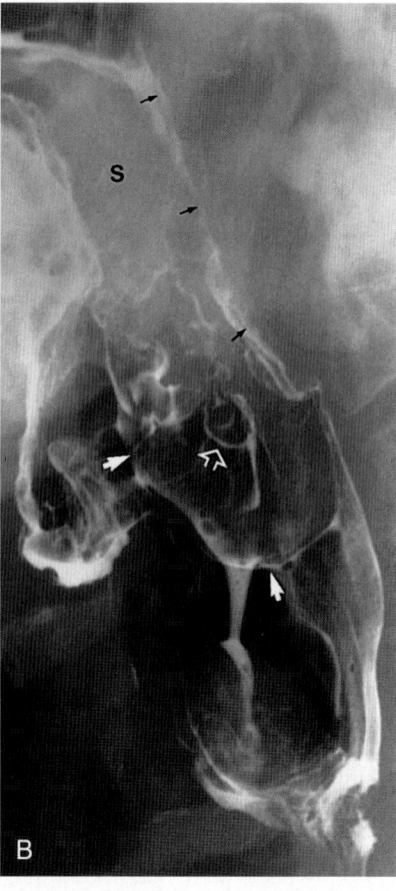

Figure 20-22. Squamous cell carcinoma of the right palatine tonsil. A. Frontal view shows a large polypoid mass (*arrows*) protruding into the oropharynx. The right lateral wall of the tonsillar fossa has been obliterated. **B.** Lateral view shows a large tonsillar fossa mass (*white arrows*) with a central ulcer (*open arrow*). Tumor infiltration of the posterior pharyngeal wall is manifested by enlargement of the soft tissue space in this region (*black arrows*). The soft palate (S) is also widened and has an irregular contour. (From Levine MS, Rubesin SE: Radiologic investigation of dysphagia. AJR 154:1157-1163, 1990, © by American Roentgen Ray Society.)

Base of the Tongue

Squamous cell carcinomas of the base of the tongue are poorly differentiated lesions that often present as advanced lesions with nodal metastases.[75-78] These tumors infiltrate deeply into the intrinsic and extrinsic muscles of the tongue. Lymph node metastases are seen ipsilaterally or contralaterally in more than 70% of patients. The 5-year survival rate is 20% to 40%.[61-76] Patients with small lesions are often asymptomatic but present as enlarged cervical nodes. Initial results of diagnostic endoscopy may be negative.[79] Small or predominantly submucosal lesions may be hidden in the valleculae or the recess between the tongue and the tonsil (glossotonsillar recess). Barium, MRI, or CT studies may be extremely helpful in detecting clinically occult lesions with nodal metastases.

Radiographically, an exophytic lesion appears as a polypoid mass projecting into the oropharyngeal airspace.[79,80] An ulcerated lesion appears as an irregular barium collection disrupting the expected contour of the base of the tongue. Nodules of tumor may spread to the palatine tonsil, valleculae, or pharyngoepiglottic fold. Occasionally, a deeply infiltrating, primarily submucosal lesion may be manifested by subtle, asymmetrical enlargement of the tongue base (Fig. 20-23). A small plaquelike or ulcerative lesion can easily be missed on barium or endoscopic studies but can be detected on MRI or CT studies.

Supraglottic Region

Squamous cell carcinomas that affect the epiglottis, aryepiglottic folds, mucosa overlying the arytenoid cartilages, false vocal cords, and laryngeal ventricles are defined as *supraglottic carcinomas*. These poorly differentiated or undifferentiated tumors spread rapidly to the entire supraglottic region and pre-epiglottic space.[43,81] Exophytic lesions are more common (Fig. 20-24).[67,82] Ulcerative lesions may deeply penetrate the tongue and valleculae and invade the pre-epiglottic space (Fig. 20-25).[67] These tumors may spread laterally to the pharyngoepiglottic folds and lateral pharyngeal walls. Only rarely do these tumors extend through the laryngeal ventricles into the true vocal cords. Cervical nodal metastases are seen in one third to one half of patients.[43,82] The 5-year survival rate is approximately 40%.

Piriform Sinus

Squamous cell carcinomas of the piriform sinuses are advanced lesions that spread quickly and metastasize widely.[66] Patients usually present with hoarseness or a neck mass.[66] Metastases to cervical lymph nodes are seen in 70% to 80% of patients.[43,75] The 5-year survival rate is 20% to 40%.[56,79] Tumors involving the medial wall of the piriform sinus (Fig. 20-26) have a slightly better prognosis than do lateral wall tumors.[60,83] Medial wall tumors infiltrate the aryepiglottic fold, arytenoid and cricoid cartilages, and paraglottic space, resulting in hoarseness.[66,84] Tumors involving the lateral wall infiltrate the thyrohyoid membrane, thyroid cartilage, and soft tissues of the neck, including the structures of the carotid sheath (Fig. 20-27).[43,84] Radiographically, an early lesion may appear as a subtle area of mucosal irregularity (Fig. 20-28). Advanced lesions are typically seen as bulky exophytic masses. Occasionally, infiltrative masses are seen.

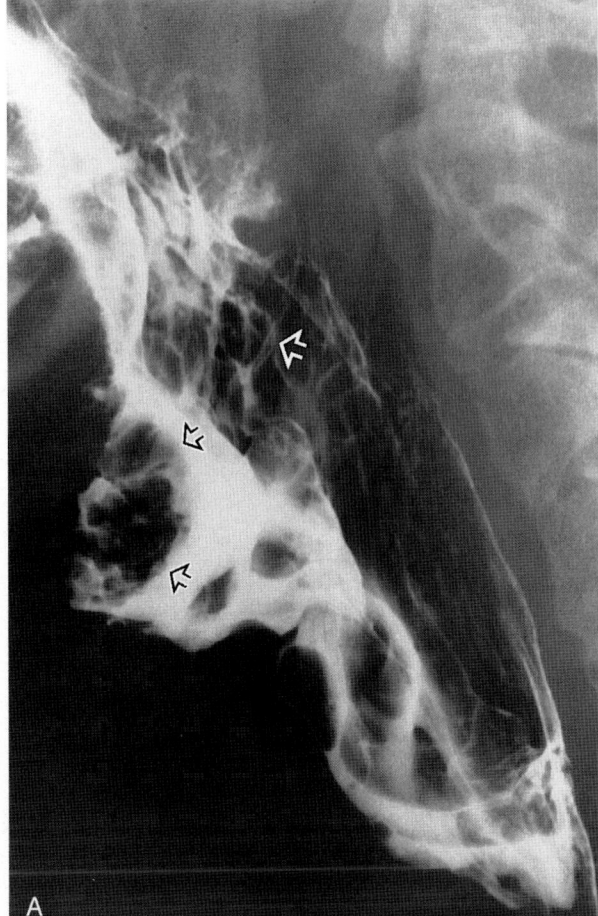

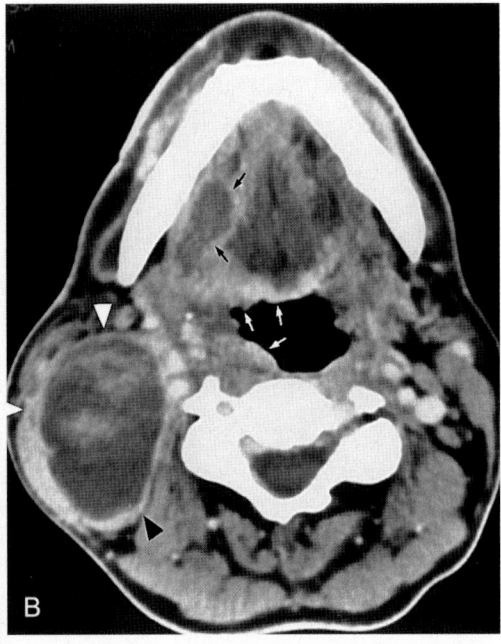

Figure 20-23. Deeply infiltrating squamous cell carcinoma of the base of the tongue. A. Lateral view of the pharynx shows a broad-based polypoid mass (*black arrows*). Tumor nodules also extend into the tonsillar fossa (*white arrow*). **B.** CT scan through the base of the tongue shows asymmetry of the tongue base and lateral pharyngeal wall (*white arrows*), with a peripherally enhanced mass also invading the sublingual space (*black arrows*). A large, centrally necrotic cervical lymph node metastasis (*arrowheads*) is identified.

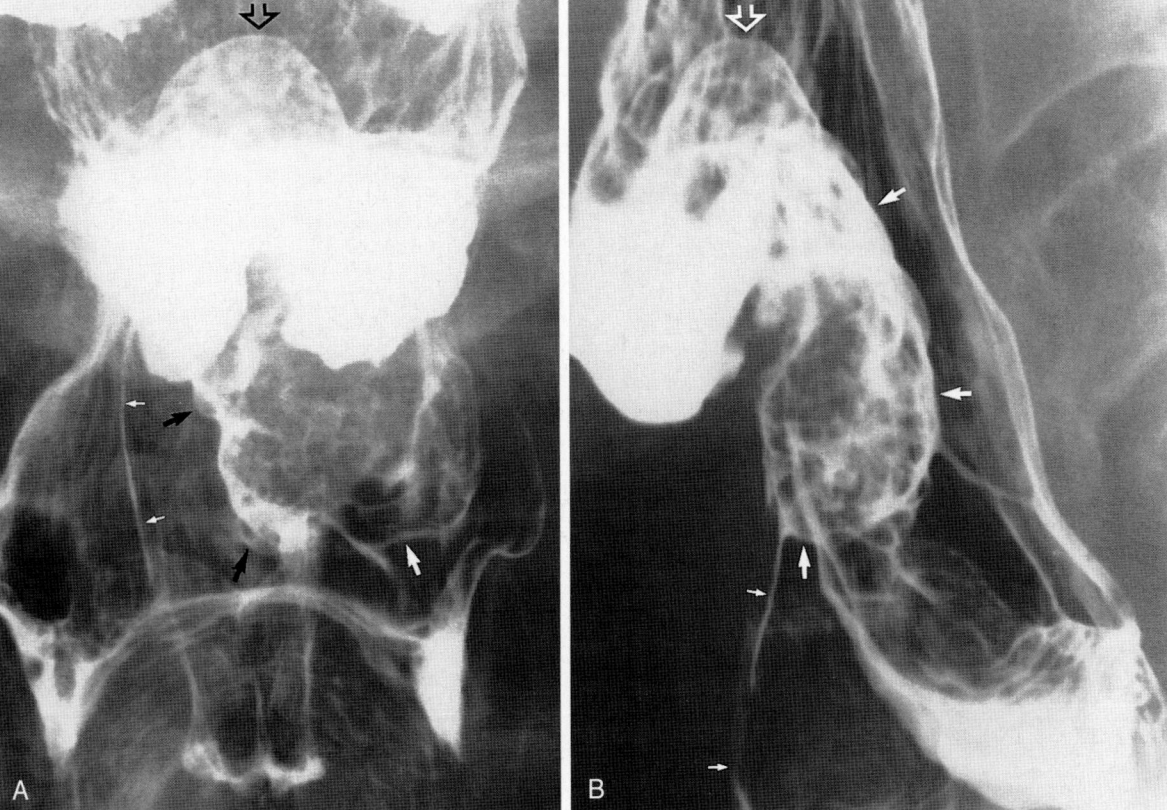

Figure 20-24. Polypoid squamous cell carcinoma of the epiglottis. A. Frontal view shows an enlarged, rounded epiglottic tip (*open arrow*) and an enlarged, nodular left aryepiglottic fold (*large solid arrows*). Note excessive pooling of barium in the valleculae. Laryngeal penetration has occurred, coating the laryngeal vestibule. This barium coating shows that the tumor has not spread to the lower right side of the epiglottis and right aryepiglottic fold (*small solid arrows*). **B.** Lateral view shows a bulbous, enlarged epiglottic tip (*open arrow*) and a large epiglottic mass (*large solid arrows*) extending down the aryepiglottic fold and along the anterior wall of the laryngeal vestibule. The lower portion of the laryngeal vestibule (*small solid arrows*) is not involved by tumor. (From Rubesin SE: Pharynx. In Laufer I, Levine MS [eds]: Double Contrast Gastrointestinal Radiology, 2nd ed. Philadelphia, WB Saunders, 1992.)

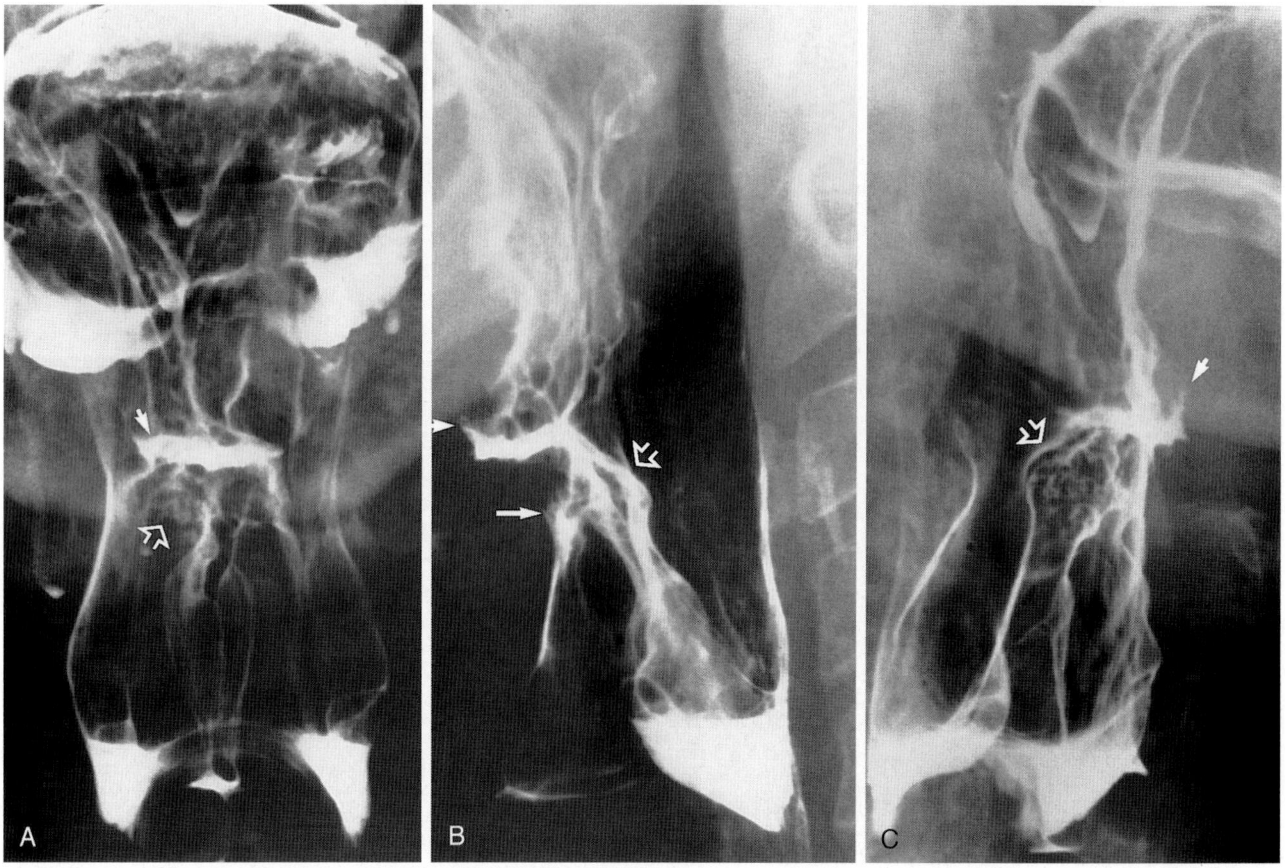

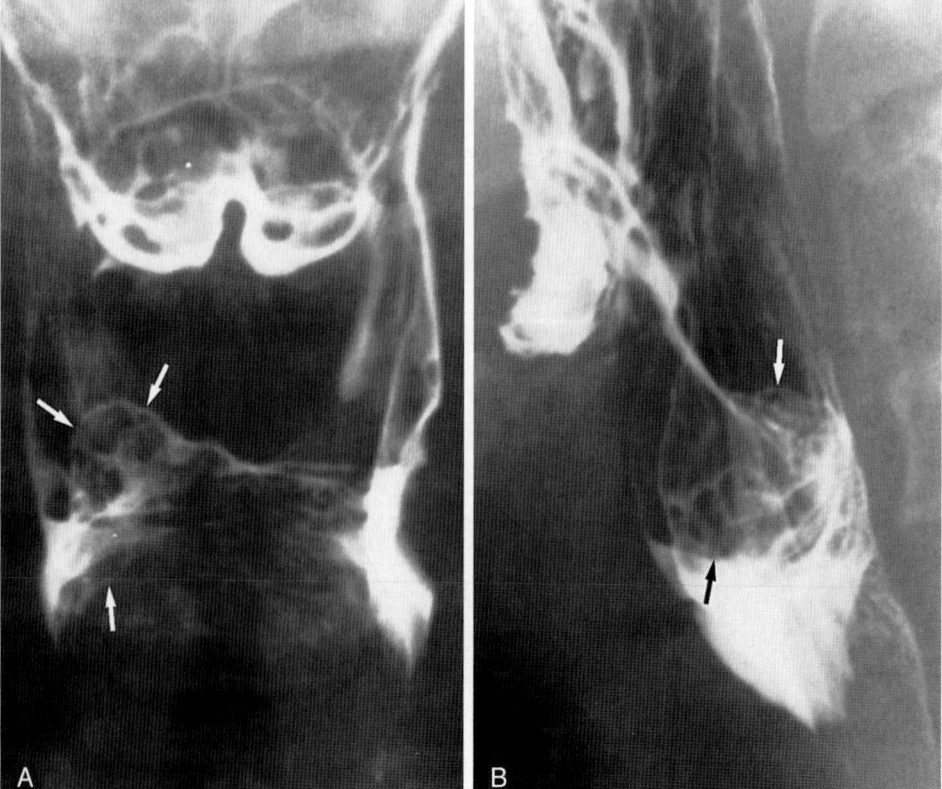

Figure 20-25. Ulcerative squamous cell carcinoma of the epiglottis and base of the tongue. Frontal (**A**), lateral (**B**), and left posterior oblique (**C**) views show that the epiglottic tip and median glossoepiglottic fold have been destroyed and are not visualized. The normal vallecular contour is not seen. Instead, an irregular barium collection is seen in the base of the tongue, with deep penetration into the contour of the tongue (*short solid arrows*). The tumor is manifest by finely nodular mucosa at the base of the tongue and in the upper right aryepiglottic fold (*open arrows*) as well as on the upper laryngeal surface of the residual epiglottis (*long solid arrow in* **B**).

Figure 20-26. Squamous cell carcinoma of the medial wall of the right piriform sinus. A. Frontal view of the pharynx shows a polypoid mass (*arrows*) involving the mucosa overlying the muscular process of the right arytenoid cartilage and medial wall of the right piriform sinus. **B.** Lateral view of the pharynx shows elevation and nodularity of the mucosa overlying the muscular process of the arytenoid cartilage (*white arrow*) and nodularity of the piriform sinus (*black arrow*) en face.

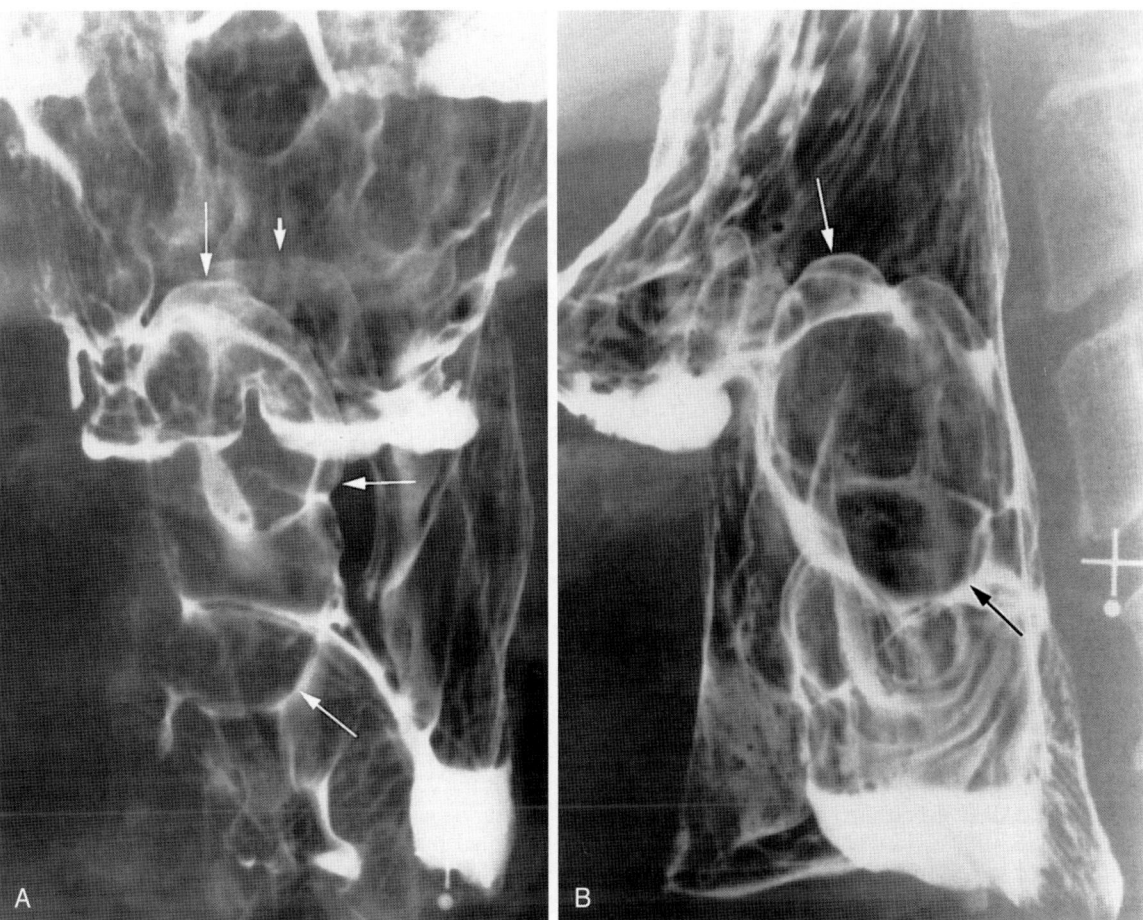

Figure 20-27. Squamous cell carcinoma of the lateral wall of the right piriform sinus. A. Frontal view shows obliteration of the right lateral wall of the piriform sinus. There is a large, polypoid mass (*long arrows*) protruding into the hypopharynx. The tip of the epiglottis (*short arrow*) is spared. **B.** Lateral view of the hypopharynx shows this large polypoid mass (*arrows*) en face. (Reprinted with permission from Rubesin SE, Glick SN: The tailored double-contrast pharyngogram. Crit Rev Diagn Imaging 28:133-179, 1988. Copyright CRC Press, Inc. Boca Raton, FL.)

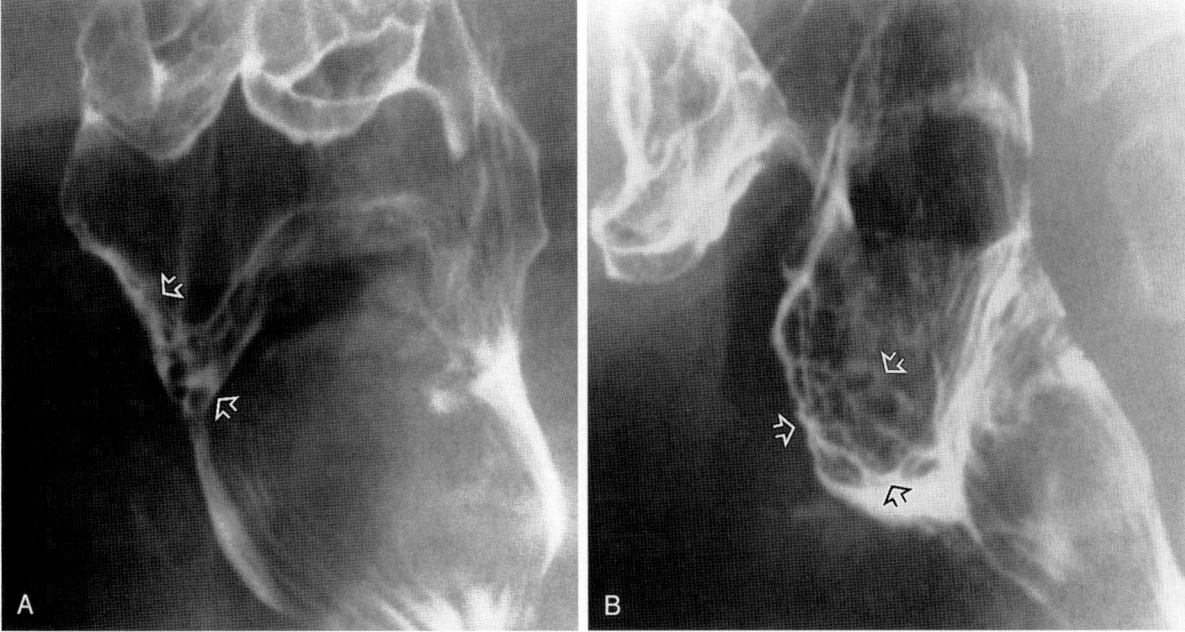

Figure 20-28. Early squamous cell carcinoma of the right piriform sinus extending into the submucosa. Slight right posterior oblique (**A**) and lateral (**B**) views of the pharynx show a flat area of nodular mucosa (*arrows*) along the lateral wall of the right piriform sinus. (From Levine MS, Rubesin SE, Ott DJ: Update on esophageal radiology. AJR 155:933-941, 1990, © by American Roentgen Ray Society.)

Posterior Pharyngeal Wall

Squamous cell carcinomas of the posterior pharyngeal wall are typically large, but some patients may present with a neck mass as the first clinical sign of tumor due to cervical lymphadenopathy.[43] These fungating lesions are usually greater than 5 cm in length (Fig. 20-29), often spreading vertically into the nasopharynx or cervical esophagus. Approximately 50% of patients have jugular or retropharyngeal lymphatic metastases, or both, at the time of diagnosis.[60] This form of pharyngeal cancer is the one most frequently associated with a synchronous or metachronous malignant lesion in the oral cavity, pharynx, or esophagus. The 5-year survival rate is approximately 20%.[60]

Postcricoid Area

Postcricoid squamous cell carcinomas are rare, except in Scandinavia.[66] In Scandinavia, primary postcricoid carcinomas may be associated with iron-deficiency anemia and cervical esophageal webs—the Plummer-Vinson syndrome. In the United States, however, only a rare association has been found between iron-deficiency anemia and malignant pharyngeal tumors. The pharyngoesophageal segment is more frequently involved by direct extension of squamous cell cancer of the piriform sinus, posterior pharyngeal wall, or cervical esophagus.[66] Radiographically, postcricoid carcinomas appear as annular, infiltrating lesions that may extend into the lower hypopharynx or cervical esophagus (Fig. 20-30).[43] These annular lesions are best detected while the pharyngoesophageal segment is fully distended with barium on videorecordings or rapid sequence spot images obtained during swallowing.

Lymphoma

Lymphomas of the pharynx represent approximately 10% of malignant pharyngeal tumors.[7,85] Almost all pharyngeal lymphomas are of the non-Hodgkin's type, arising from Waldeyer's ring (i.e., the adenoids, palatine tonsils, and lingual tonsil). Hodgkin's disease involving the pharynx is rare, despite the fact that Hodgkin's disease often begins in cervical lymph nodes.[86] Pharyngeal involvement occurs in only 1% to 2% of all patients with Hodgkin's disease, even those with disseminated tumor.

Most patients with pharyngeal lymphoma are in the fifth to sixth decade of life. Approximately 50% of patients have cervical lymphadenopathy as the initial clinical finding.[85] Cervical lymph nodes are involved in more than 60% of patients.[85] At the time of diagnosis, only 10% of patients have involvement of extranodal sites (lung and bones).[85] Approximately 50% of patients have symptoms related to local pharyngeal involvement, including nasal obstruction, earache, sore throat, or a lump in the throat.

The most frequent pharyngeal locations of lymphoma are the palatine tonsil (40% to 60% of patients),[7,85] nasopharynx (18% to 28%),[85,87] and base of the tongue (10%). Approximately 25% of tumors involve multiple sites. Bilateral involvement of the palatine tonsils occurs in 15% of pharyngeal lymphomas.[85] Lymphomas only rarely arise in the hypopharynx.

Pharyngeal lymphomas are manifested radiographically as lobulated masses involving the nasopharynx, palatine tonsil (Fig. 20-31), base of the tongue (Fig. 20-32), or a combination of these sites. The mucosal surface landmarks are frequently

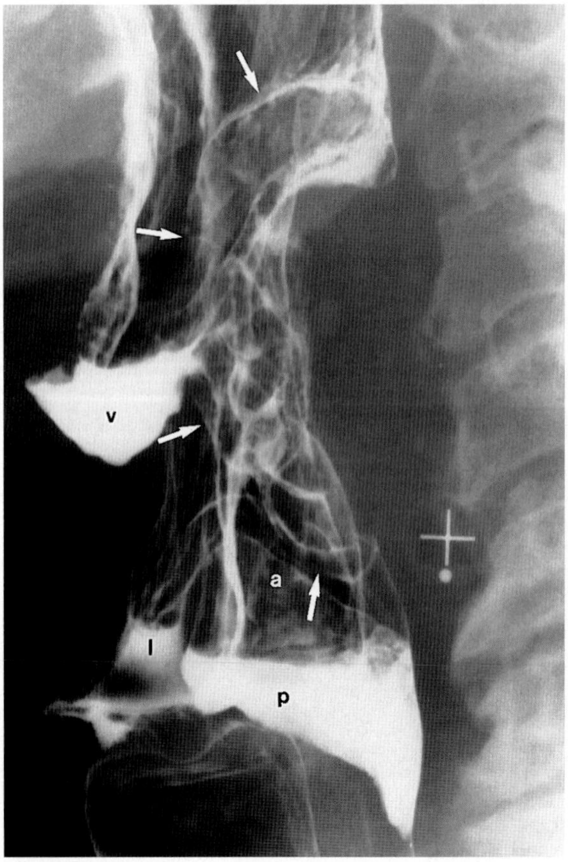

Figure 20-29. Squamous cell carcinoma of the posterior pharyngeal wall. Lateral spot image of the pharynx shows a large fungating mass (*arrows*) on the posterior pharyngeal wall, extending from the level of the uvula to the level of the muscular processes of the arytenoid cartilages (a). Note evidence of pharyngeal dysfunction with pooling of barium in the valleculae (v), piriform sinus (p), and laryngeal vestibule (l). (Reprinted with permission from Rubesin SE, Glick SN: The tailored double-contrast pharyngogram. Crit Rev Diagn Imaging 28:133-179, 1988. Copyright CRC Press, Inc. Boca Raton, FL.)

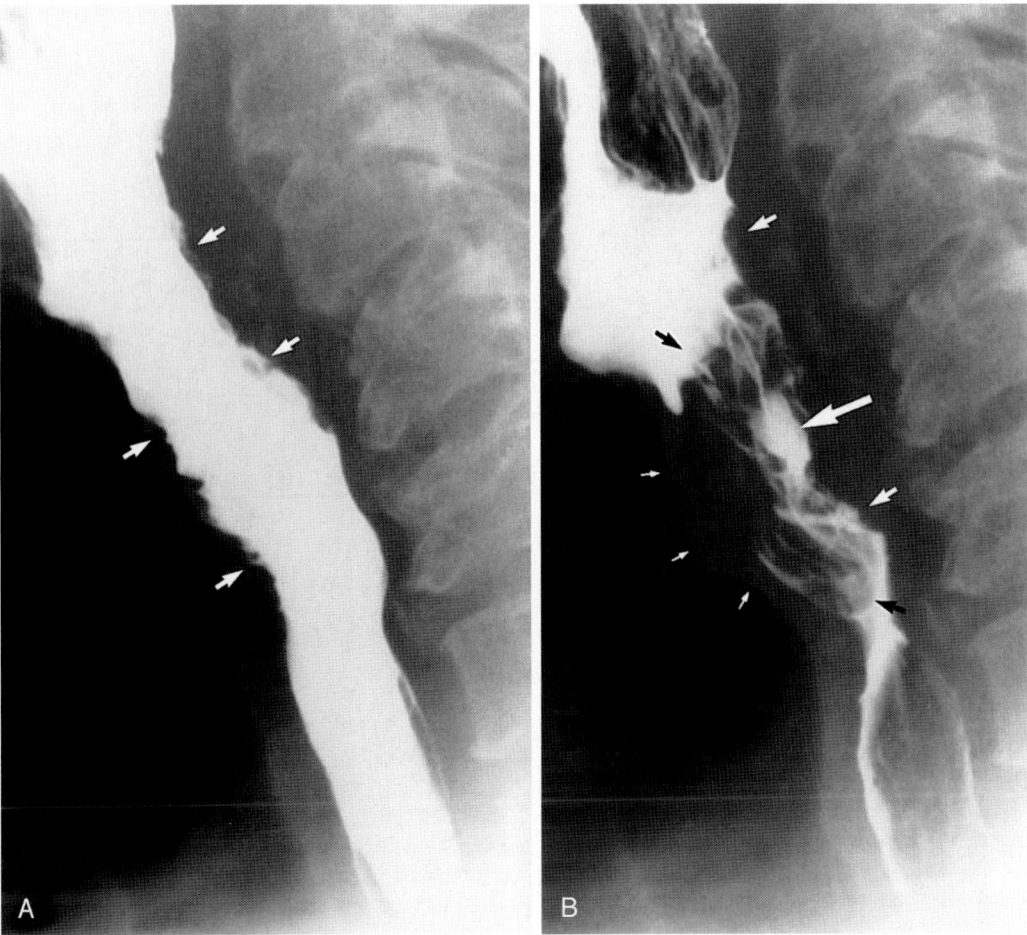

Figure 20-30. Squamous cell carcinoma of the postcricoid region. A. Lateral spot image obtained during swallowing shows a finely lobulated contour of the anterior and posterior walls of the pharyngoesophageal segment (*arrows*). **B.** Lateral spot image of the pharyngoesophageal segment during phonation shows an ulcerated mass. The central ulcer crater (*large white arrow*) is filled with barium. The mass is seen as a filling defect in the barium pool (*black arrows*) and as an irregular contour of the posterior pharyngeal wall (*medium white arrows*). The mass also causes a smooth, extrinsic impression on the posterior wall of the trachea (*small white arrows*).

obliterated by bulging submucosal masses (see Fig. 20-32).[7,22] Thus, the normal lymphoid follicular pattern of the base of the tongue or palatine tonsil may be effaced by these submucosal masses.

Rare Malignant Tumors

Carcinoma of the Minor Salivary Glands

Both benign and malignant tumors arise from the minor mucoserous salivary glands located deep to the epithelial layer of the pharynx. Minor salivary gland tumors constitute 20% of all salivary gland tumors and have diverse histologic features and a diverse clinical course (Fig. 20-33). Sixty-five to 88 percent of minor salivary gland tumors are malignant.[88,89] The most frequent malignant types are adenoid cystic carcinoma (35%), solid adenocarcinoma (22%) (Fig. 20-34), and mucoepidermoid carcinoma (16%).[88] By far the most common pharyngeal location of minor salivary gland tumors is the soft palate. Palatal salivary gland tumors are manifested clinically by painless masses near the junction of the hard and soft palate (see Fig. 20-33). Palatal salivary gland tumors spread to the tongue, submandibular gland, lingual

and hypoglossal nerves, and mandible. In contrast to squamous cell carcinoma, cervical metastases are relatively infrequent, occurring in approximately 25% of malignant lesions.[88] Adenoid cystic carcinoma has a particular propensity for perineural tumor spread.

Synovial Sarcoma

Synovial sarcomas of the pharynx are extremely rare. Most patients are 20 to 40 years of age and complain of a painless neck mass.[90] At initial diagnosis, synovial sarcomas appear radiographically as large, bulky tumors involving the larynx, pharynx, and soft tissues of the neck.[91]

Cartilaginous Tumors

Primary cartilaginous tumors of the pharynx are extremely rare. The pharynx may be invaded secondarily by cartilaginous tumors (chondroma, osteochondroma, and chondrosarcoma) arising in the larynx.[92] Cartilaginous tumors of the larynx are seen mainly in the fourth to sixth decade of life. Patients complain of hoarseness, poor voice, and dysphagia. Chondroid tumors usually arise from the cricoid cartilage.

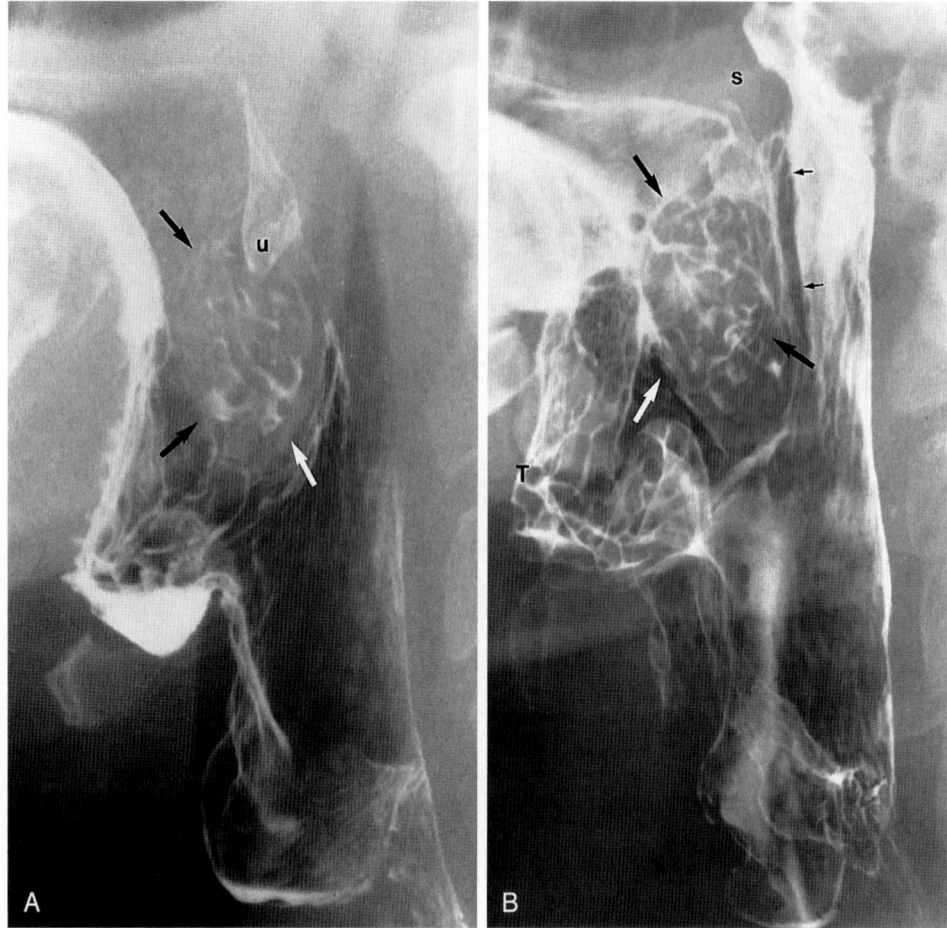

Figure 20-31. Lymphoma versus hyperplasia of the palatine tonsil. A. A large, lobulated palatine tonsil (*arrows*) is seen on a lateral view of the pharynx. In this elderly patient, the enlarged tonsil proved to be due to non-Hodgkin's lymphoma. u, uvula. **B.** A large, lobulated palatine tonsil (*long arrows*) is similar in appearance to the lymphoma in **A.** In this young patient with head trauma the enlarged tonsil was due to lymphoid hyperplasia. Note the associated lymphoid hyperplasia of the base of the tongue (T) and lingual surface of the epiglottis. Nasopharyngeal reflux outlines the posterior surface of the palatopharyngeal fold (*short arrows*) and posterior surface of the soft palate (s). Thus, tonsils that are enlarged and lobulated may be due to lymphoid hyperplasia of various causes or to infiltrating tumor.

Radiographically, a smooth-surfaced mass is usually seen in the posterior lamina of the cricoid cartilage, compressing and distorting the lower hypopharynx and pharyngoesophageal segment. Stippled calcification is seen in a central or peripheral location in more than 80% of patients.[7]

Kaposi's Sarcoma

Kaposi's sarcoma may arise anywhere in the gastrointestinal tract in patients with AIDS. Kaposi's sarcoma involving the pharynx may cause dysphagia or odynophagia.[93,94] Kaposi's sarcoma may be manifested radiographically by multiple small nodules or plaquelike lesions, small submucosal masses with or without central ulceration, or larger, bulky polypoid masses.[93,94]

PHARYNGEAL DAMAGE FROM RADIATION

Radiation therapy may be used as a primary or adjunctive form of treatment for pharyngeal tumors such as squamous cell carcinoma and lymphoma. The pharynx is included within the radiation portal during irradiation of tumors of the larynx and cervical lymph nodes. In the past, the pharynx was also included in the radiation portal during treatment of thyrotoxicosis or tuberculous lymphadenitis.[95]

Acute mucositis and edema occur early during the course of radiotherapy. Epithelial necrosis and ulceration result in a fibrinous exudate.[96-98] Submucosal inflammation also occurs early. Over time, the mucosa atrophies and submucosal fibrosis may occur.[98,99] The majority of chronic radiation damage results from vascular changes with thrombosis and fibrosis of capillaries and lymphatics and subintimal fibrosis and hyalinization of veins and arteries.[99,100] Vascular damage leads to atrophy of the skin and to fibrosis of subcutaneous tissues, submucosal tissues, and muscle.[100] The most frequent localization of persistent edema is in the glottis and mucosa overlying the arytenoid cartilages. Severe complications such as life-threatening osteomyelitis and chondronecrosis may occur.

Five to 10 days after initial radiotherapy, the patient may complain of local discomfort, hoarseness, dryness, dysphagia, or a lump in the throat. The peak occurrence of symptoms occurs near the end of the typical 6-week course of radiation treatment. Most symptoms gradually subside 2 to 6 weeks after cessation of radiotherapy.[97] However, a substantial number of patients have persistent symptoms. For example,

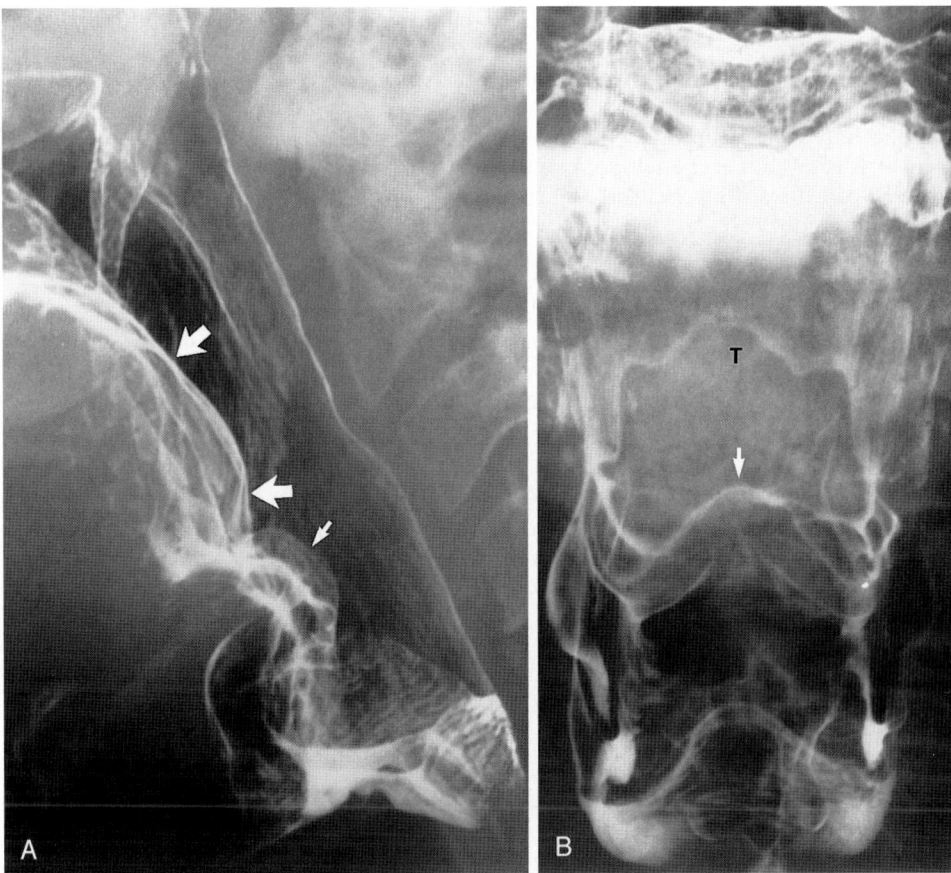

Figure 20-32. Lymphoma of the base of the tongue and epiglottic tip. A. Lateral view of the pharynx shows a large, lobulated mass involving the base of the tongue (*large arrows*) and tip of the epiglottis (*small arrow*). Note that the normal contours of the valleculae have been obliterated. **B.** Frontal view of the pharynx shows complete effacement of the normal lymphoid surface pattern of the base of the tongue (T). Loss of the contour of the valleculae is also seen. Laryngeal penetration has occurred, with barium coating both surfaces of the epiglottis. The epiglottic tip (*arrow*) is smoothly enlarged. The relative lack of mucosal irregularity suggests that this huge mass at the base of the tongue is due to infiltrating tumor in a primarily submucosal location. (From Rubesin SE, Laufer I: Pictorial review: Principles of double contrast pharyngography. Dysphagia 6:170-178, 1991.)

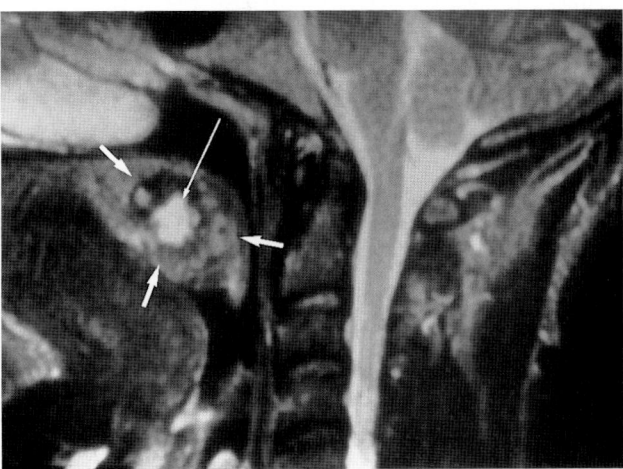

Figure 20-33. Pleomorphic adenoma of the soft palate on MR imaging. The midportion of the soft palate is markedly enlarged by a finely lobulated mass (*short arrows*) of mixed low and moderate signal intensity. On this T2-weighted image, the lobulated area of high signal intensity (*long arrow*) in the center of the mass is due to hemorrhage associated with a recent biopsy.

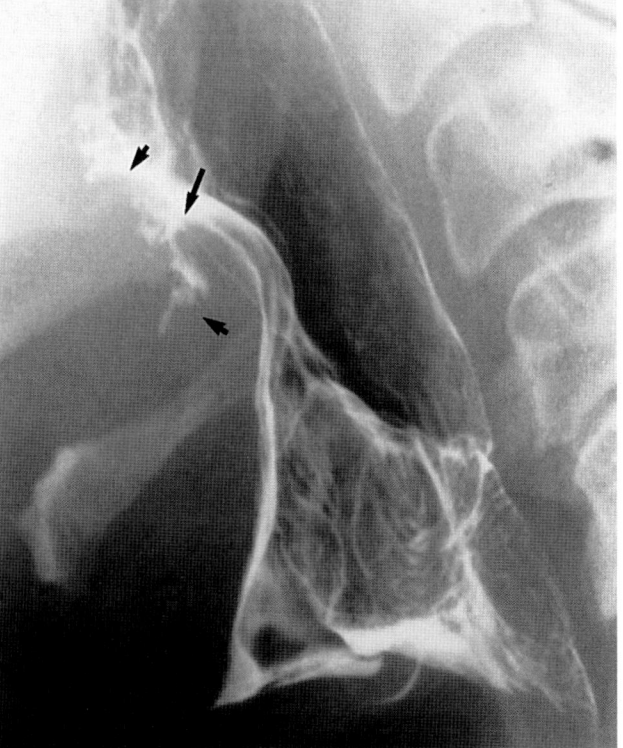

Figure 20-34. Adenocarcinoma of the minor salivary glands. The epiglottic tip (*long arrow*) is apposed to the base of the tongue, and its vallecular surface is ulcerated. The valleculae are obliterated and filled by lobulated tumor (*short arrows*) arising from the tongue base. This adenocarcinoma is radiographically indistinguishable from a typical squamous cell carcinoma of the base of the tongue. The tumor presumably arose in minor salivary gland tissue.

15% of patients have persistent edema after radiotherapy for carcinoma of the vocal cord.[101] If parotid or other salivary glands have been damaged, xerostomia may cause persistent dysphagia. Persistent edema may suggest a serious underlying complication such as persistent carcinoma or the development of osteomyelitis or chondronecrosis.[101-105] Approximately 50% of patients with persistent edema have recurrent or persistent tumor.[101]

The radiographic changes of radiation damage are seen in almost all patients after radiation therapy with or without surgery.[106] The most frequent dynamic findings are those of epiglottic and laryngeal vestibular dysfunction and pharyngeal paresis.[106] Spot images typically show that the epiglottis and aryepiglottic folds are diffusely and smoothly enlarged

(Fig. 20-35).[43,44,107,108] The valleculae may be flattened, and the mucosa overlying the muscular processes of the arytenoid cartilages may be elevated. Edema from radiation may be asymmetrical, especially in the region of the original tumor. Any surface irregularity on a postradiation pharyngogram should suggest the possibility of persistent cancer, although radiation-induced ulceration may produce identical radiographic findings (Fig. 20-36).[2,108] Soft tissue atrophy is observed in patients with chronic radiation damage (Fig. 20-37).

Cross-sectional imaging in the patient who has undergone radiation treatment is used for detection of recurrent tumor in lymph nodes or soft tissue.[72,98,109] Baseline studies after therapy are also helpful when patients are evaluated for recurrent tumor at a later date.

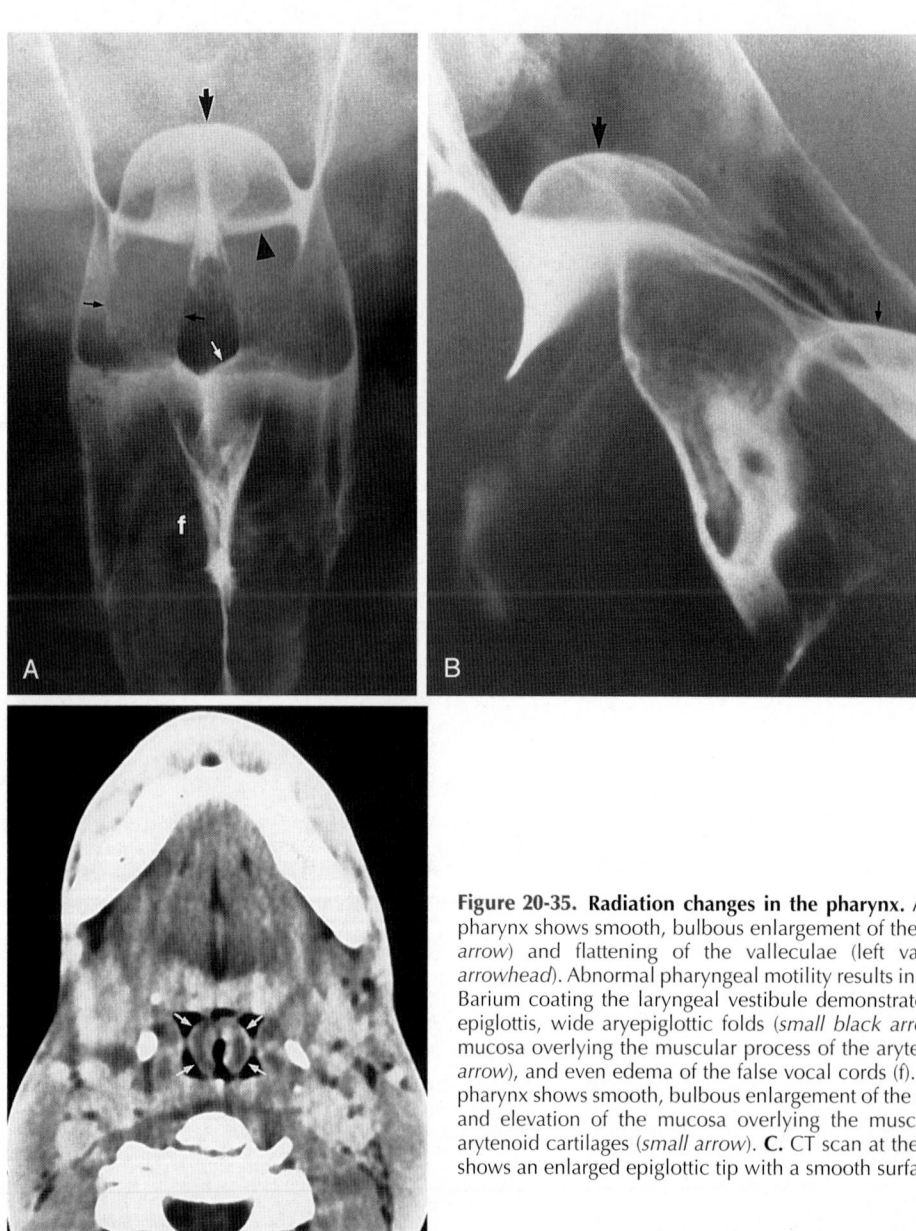

Figure 20-35. Radiation changes in the pharynx. A. Frontal view of the pharynx shows smooth, bulbous enlargement of the epiglottis (*large black arrow*) and flattening of the valleculae (left vallecula identified by *arrowhead*). Abnormal pharyngeal motility results in laryngeal penetration. Barium coating the laryngeal vestibule demonstrates enlargement of the epiglottis, wide aryepiglottic folds (*small black arrows*), elevation of the mucosa overlying the muscular process of the arytenoid cartilages (*white arrow*), and even edema of the false vocal cords (f). **B.** Lateral view of the pharynx shows smooth, bulbous enlargement of the epiglottis (*large arrow*) and elevation of the mucosa overlying the muscular processes of the arytenoid cartilages (*small arrow*). **C.** CT scan at the level of the epiglottis shows an enlarged epiglottic tip with a smooth surface (*arrows*).

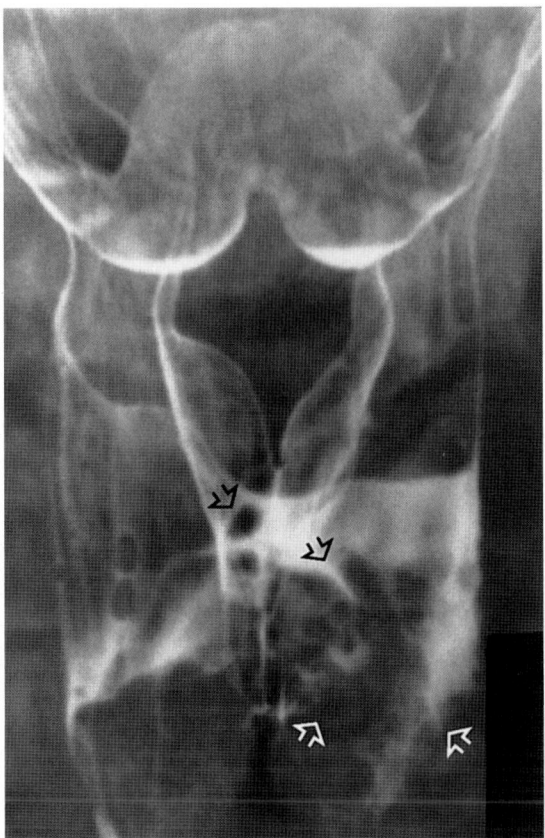

Figure 20-36. Radiation damage to the pharynx and recurrent squamous cell carcinoma in the piriform sinus. Frontal view shows the typical findings of radiation damage, with smooth enlargement of the epiglottis, flattening of the valleculae, laryngeal penetration (showing widening of the aryepiglottic folds), and elevation of the mucosa overlying the muscular process of the arytenoid cartilages. However, the lower contour of the left piriform sinus is irregular and a nodular mucosa (*arrows*) carpets the left piriform sinus. Endoscopic biopsy specimens revealed recurrent squamous cell carcinoma of the piriform sinus.

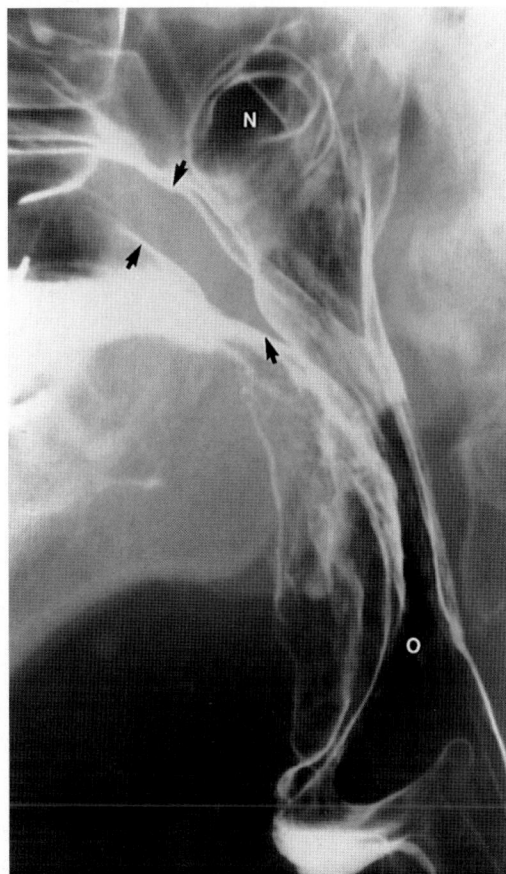

Figure 20-37. Atrophy after radiotherapy. This patient had two courses of radiotherapy for nasopharyngeal lymphoma, with recurrent tumor 10 and 20 years before this examination was performed. Lateral view of the nasopharynx (N) and oropharynx (O) shows barium coating the nasopharynx due to nasal regurgitation. The soft palate (*arrows*) is shortened and thinned, an indication of soft palate atrophy associated with radiotherapy. The nasal regurgitation is secondary to loss of soft palate function and volume.

POSTOPERATIVE PHARYNX

The radiologist frequently studies the pharynx in the early and remote postoperative periods, testing a patient's ability to swallow and looking for complications. Ideally, the surgeon provides a clear description of the postoperative anatomy to the radiologist and states what information needs to be obtained from the postoperative pharyngogram. In reality, the radiologist must be familiar with the numerous operations performed for a wide variety of pharyngeal tumors, Zenker's diverticulum, and "cricopharyngeal achalasia." The radiologist must also have a working knowledge of the spectrum of postoperative complications associated with these various operations (Table 20-1).[110]

Total Laryngectomy

Total laryngectomy is usually performed for advanced malignant tumors of the larynx, subglottic cancers, and small carcinomas of the low tongue base and for failed irradiation or voice-conserving surgery for laryngeal cancer.[111-113] Early glottic or supraglottic cancers are often treated by radiation therapy, endoscopic removal, or partial laryngectomy.[112,113]

Cancers of the piriform sinuses, lateral and posterior pharyngeal walls, and postcricoid region are treated by total laryngectomy with partial pharyngectomy or laryngopharyngectomy, depending on the degree of retropharyngeal invasion.

During total laryngectomy, the larynx is removed along with the thyroid, cricoid, epiglottic, and paired arytenoid cartilages. The hyoid bone may be removed or spared. Resection of the epiglottis, aryepiglottic folds, arytenoid cartilages, and anterior walls of the piriform sinuses results in creation of a large gap in the anterior wall of the hypopharynx. Total laryngectomy also disrupts most of the muscles of the pharynx. The suprahyoid muscles (mylohyoid, geniohyoid, hyoglossus, and stylohyoid) and infrahyoid muscles (thyrohyoid, sternohyoid, sternothyroid, and omohyoid) are transected. The thyropharyngeus and cricopharyngeus are detached from their lateral origins on the thyroid and cricoid cartilages, respectively. A permanent tracheostoma is necessary. In some patients, the ipsilateral thyroid gland and its accompanying parathyroid glands are excised.

The gap in the anterior wall of the pharynx is closed by approximating the residual pharyngeal mucosa. The constrictor muscles may be joined anteriorly as an additional

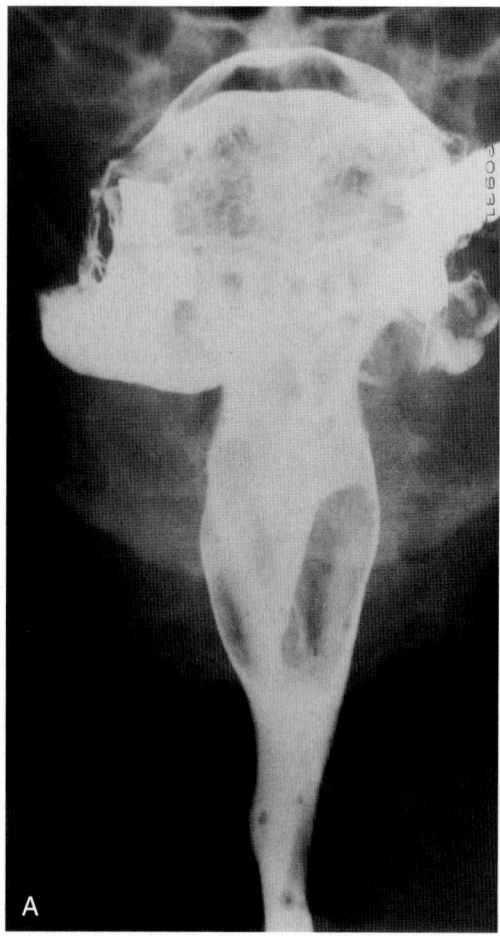
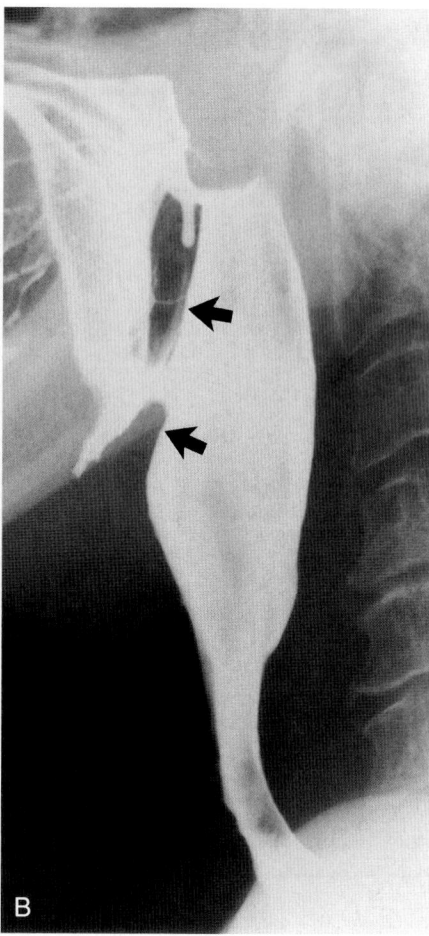

Figure 20-38. Total laryngectomy. A. Frontal view of the neopharynx shows a featureless tube that tapers distally. The tube is wider than 5 mm in each direction and the mucosa is smooth. The neopharyngeal tube is in the midline. **B.** Lateral view also shows a tubular structure that tapers inferiorly. Just behind the junction of the tongue and neopharyngeal tube, a tubular radiolucency (*arrows*) curves superiorly toward the lateral mid oropharyngeal wall. This is a pair of folds created surgically on each side of the lateral pharyngeal wall. Because these folds mimic the course of the epiglottis, they have been termed a *pseudoepiglottis*. The hyoid bone, valleculae, epiglottis, and piriform sinuses are missing. (From Rubesin SE, Eisele DW, Jones B: Pharyngography in the postoperative patient. In Jones B [ed]: Normal and Abnormal Swallowing. Imaging in Diagnosis and Therapy, 2nd ed. New York, Springer, 2003, pp 167-204.)

buttressing layer. A myocutaneous or free flap may be necessary to form the neopharyngeal tube if there is insufficient mucosa. A neck dissection may also be performed.

Radiographically, the normal neopharyngeal tube resembles an inverted cone with a smooth mucosal surface (Fig. 20-38).[111] On lateral views, the anterior wall of the neopharyngeal tube lies just below the skin of the neck and the posterior wall of the tube abuts the vertebral column. On frontal views, the tube lies within 0.5 cm of the midline.[114] The epiglottis, aryepiglottic folds, and "extrinsic mass" of the larynx on the hypopharynx are no longer present. The hyoid bone may also be absent. At the closure site of the base of the tongue and the anterior neopharyngeal tube, the contour may be angulated or sacculated. These postoperative sacculations at the tongue base are normal and resemble valleculae, hence the term *pseudovalleculae*. A fold of tissue courses from each posterolateral wall of the oropharynx to the new base of the tongue, superficially resembling an epiglottis, hence the term *pseudoepiglottis*.

The most common complication in the early postoperative period is formation of a pharyngocutaneous fistula, occurring in 6% to 21% of patients (see Table 20-1).[111,115-117] Fistulas develop at sites of mucosal closure, including the junction of the neopharyngeal tube with the tongue base, the anterior aspect of the neopharyngeal tube (Fig. 20-39), the margin of the flap (if one is used), and near the tracheal stoma. It is unknown if radiation therapy increases the risk of fistula formation.[117] Fistulas may end blindly in the subcutaneous

tissue or extend to the skin, and, rarely, may involve the carotid sheath. Most patients have signs of fistula formation within 10 to 14 days after surgery, including fever, wound erythema, swelling, and increased drainage from the wound.[118] Some patients with fistulas are asymptomatic. Most fistulas close spontaneously if feeding is delayed. The development of a fistula in the late postoperative period should suggest recurrent tumor. Radiographically, fistulas appear as contrast-filled tracks or collections arising from the anterior pharyngeal wall or base of the tongue.

Dysphagia is the most common symptom in the remote postoperative period. This symptom may be caused by benign strictures, a retracted thyropharyngeus/cricopharyngeus muscle, or recurrent tumor. Some patients have no symptoms because they compensate for luminal narrowing by changing their diet and chewing patterns. Radiographically, benign strictures have a smooth contour and mucosal surface. Long (>3 cm), symmetrical strictures involving a large portion of the neopharyngeal tube are usually the sequelae of radiation therapy or insufficient mucosa at the time of closure (Fig. 20-40).[111] Short (5 mm), weblike narrowings usually form at the upper or lower end of the closure line and are usually the sequelae of infection or fistula formation (Fig. 20-41).[111] Although some benign strictures have irregular contours, the presence of mucosal nodularity in the region of a stricture should suggest recurrent tumor. Deviation of the neopharyngeal tube from the midline is uncommon and should also suggest recurrent tumor.

Table 20-1
Common Postoperative Complications

	Voice-Sparing Procedure	Laryngectomy
Early Postoperative Period	Wound breakdown Fistula formation* Abscess (wound or fistula) Aspiration/pneumonia* Airway obstruction (edema) Hematoma Mediastinitis Thoracic duct or carotid injury from radical neck dissection	Wound breakdown* Fistula formation* Abscess (wound or fistula) Constrictor dysfunction* Tongue dysfunction (partial resection, immobility, rarely hypoglossal nerve damage)* Hematoma Mediastinitis Thoracic duct or carotid injury from radical neck dissection
Late Postoperative Period	Hoarseness Aspiration* Recurrent tumor* Laryngeal stenosis* Velopharyngeal incompetence* Failure of flap graft	Stricture* Constrictor dysfunction* Recurrent tumor* Stomal stenosis Stomal tumor recurrence Failure of flap graft or jejunal graft Hypothyroidism Hypoparathyroidism Abnormal vocalization*

*Pharyngography helpful in evaluation.
From Rubesin SE, Eisele DW, Jones B. Pharyngography in the postoperative patient. In Jones B (ed): Normal and Abnormal Swallowing. Imaging in Diagnosis and Therapy. New York, Springer, 2003, pp 167-203.

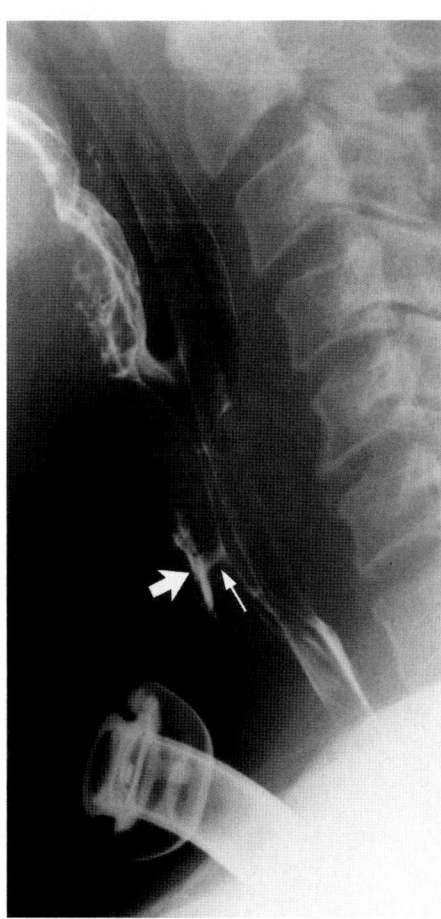

Figure 20-39. Leak after total laryngectomy. Lateral view of the neopharynx after the patient swallows water-soluble contrast shows a linear contrast collection (*thick arrow*) just anterior to the anterior wall of the neopharyngeal tube. The collection arises from a short track (*thin arrow*). A nasogastric tube is in place. (From Rubesin SE: Pharynx. In Levine MS, Rubesin SE, Laufer I [eds]: Double Contrast Gastrointestinal Radiology, 3rd ed. Philadelphia, WB Saunders, 2000, pp 61-89.)

After total laryngectomy, most of the muscles of the pharynx lose their normal bony or cartilaginous attachments and are partially or totally denervated. Dysphagia may result from abnormal muscular contraction. The thyropharyngeus and cricopharyngeus muscles, in particular, may not participate in a coordinated contraction wave with the spared superior constrictor muscle. Radiographically, abnormal inferior constrictor contraction is manifested by a smooth extrinsic mass impression on the posterior wall of the neopharyngeal tube (Fig. 20-42). Unlike recurrent tumor, this impression changes in size, shape, and position during swallowing. Stasis of barium and dilatation of the oropharynx above a "prominent cricopharyngeus" are clues that postoperative dysphagia may be related to abnormal muscular contraction.

Foreign bodies impactions often occur in the neopharyngeal tube. Patients with head and neck cancers frequently have poor dentition or have had teeth removed before radiotherapy. These patients may have difficulty chewing vegetables and meats. As a result, solid food may become lodged in normal areas of postoperative sacculation at the base of the tongue, in a neopharynx that contracts poorly, or above strictures (Fig. 20-43).

Recurrent squamous cell carcinoma usually develops within 2 years after laryngectomy.[118] Radiographically, recurrent tumor may be manifested by a large (>1.5 cm) mass with a nodular or ulcerated surface or as a stricture with an irregular contour and irregular mucosal surface.[2,110,119,120] The neopharynx may be deviated more than 1 cm from the midline, with narrowing of the neopharyngeal tube at the site of maximal deviation.[111]

The hypoglossal nerves that lie superficially on the hyoglossus muscle may be damaged during surgery.[121] Abnormal tongue motion may result from hypoglossal nerve damage, partial glossectomy, or postoperative scarring. Complications involving the tracheal stoma include stomal stenosis and recurrent tumor. Voice rehabilitation may be difficult because of a retracted cricopharyngeus, a malpositioned tracheoesophageal

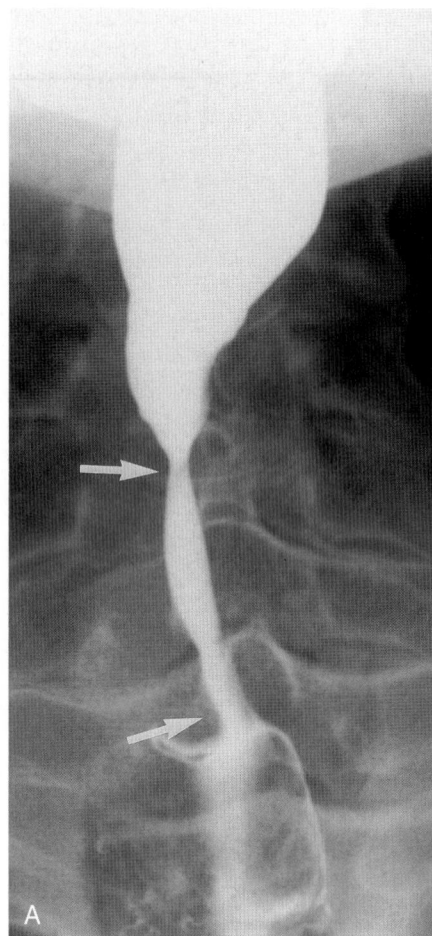
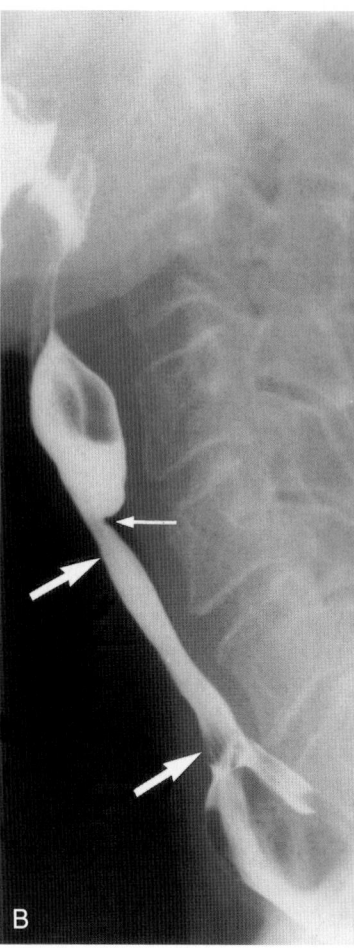

Figure 20-40. Stricture after total laryngectomy. Frontal (**A**) and lateral (**B**) views of the neck show diffuse narrowing of the neopharyngeal tube (*thick arrows*). An even tighter weblike area of narrowing (*thin arrow*) is seen proximally. Long strictures are usually attributed to radiation therapy or insufficient tissue to close the neopharynx. (From Rubesin SE: Pharynx. In Levine MS, Rubesin SE, Laufer I [eds]: Double Contrast Gastrointestinal Radiology, 3rd ed. Philadelphia, WB Saunders, 2000, pp 61-89.)

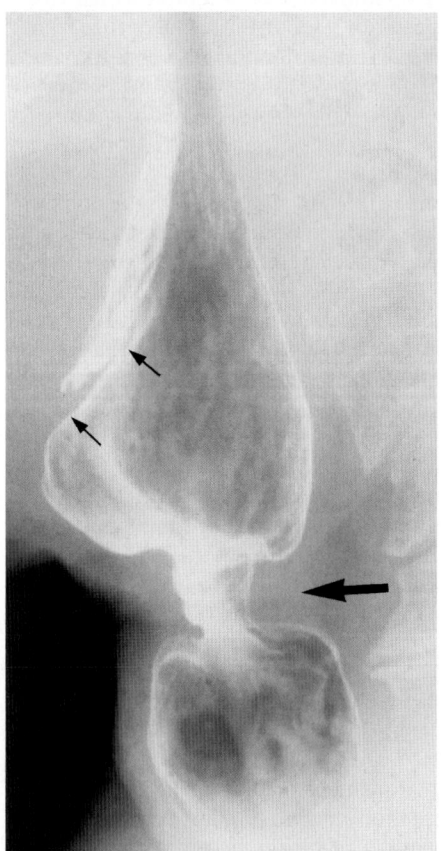

Figure 20-41. Short stricture after total laryngectomy. Lateral view shows a short, circumferential stricture (*thick arrow*) of the upper neopharyngeal tube. The anterior wall is undulating due to scarring. A pseudoepiglottis is identified (*thin arrows*).

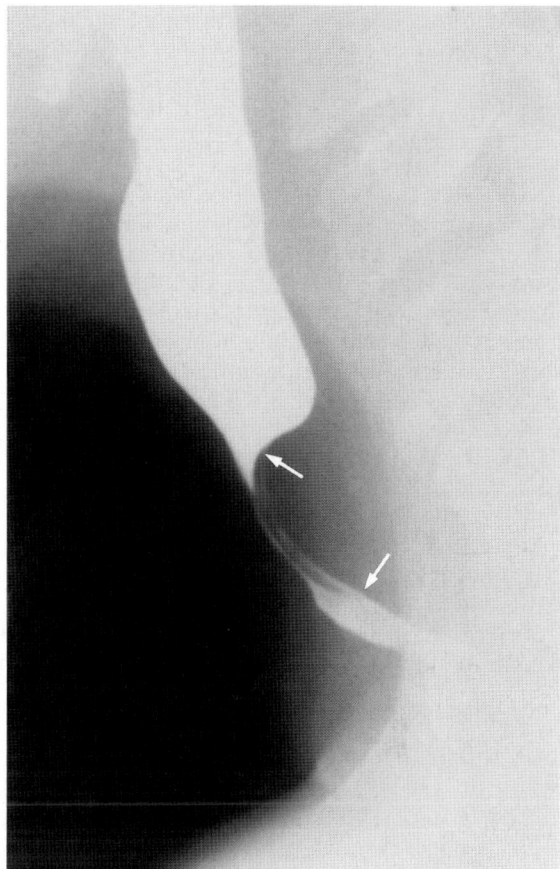

Figure 20-42. Incomplete opening of cricopharyngeus after total laryngectomy. Lateral view of the neck shows a smooth-surfaced protrusion (*arrows*) into the posterior wall of the lower neopharyngeal tube. During fluoroscopy, this indentation changed in size and shape due to "prominence" of the lower portion of the thyropharyngeus and cricopharyngeus.

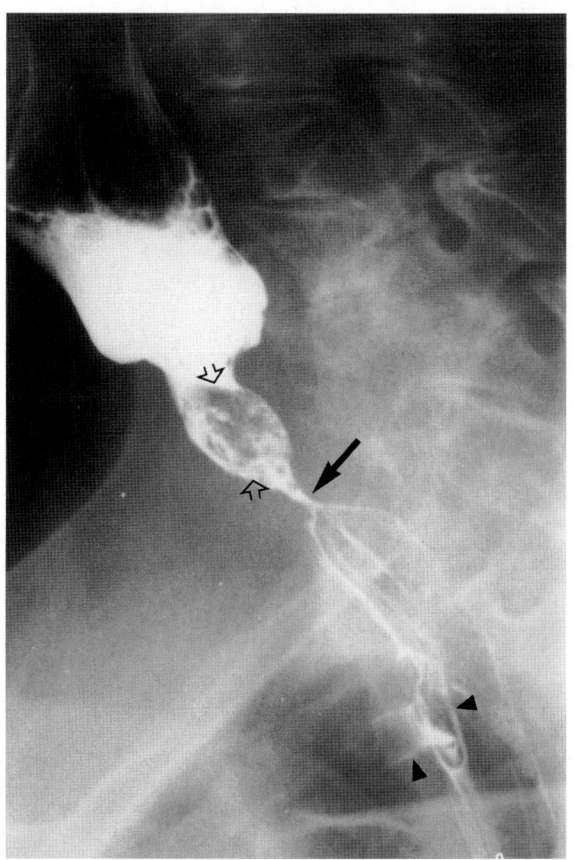

Figure 20-43. Foreign body impaction above stricture after total laryngectomy. Oblique view of the lower neck shows a 1-cm finely lobulated radiolucent filling defect (*open arrows*) in the lower neopharyngeal tube trapped above a 3-mm in length by 1- to 2-mm in diameter stricture (*large arrow*). This foreign body proved to be a piece of meat. A voice prosthesis is identified (*arrowheads*).

voice prosthesis, gastroesophageal reflux, or an esophageal motility disorder.

Pharyngolaryngectomy

Resection of the larynx and hypopharynx may be required if cancer involves the posterior pharyngeal wall, postcricoid region, or large portions of a piriform sinus. The gap between the oropharynx and cervical esophagus may be bridged by a free jejunal graft or by a gastric pull-through.[122,123] A defect in the anterolateral neopharyngeal wall may also be closed by a myocutaneous flap (pectoralis major or trapezius), a free flap (radial forearm), or cutaneous skin flap (thigh).[123,124]

Radiographically, flaps are atonic segments that form a portion of the walls of the pharynx. These flaps often protrude as masslike lesions into the expected lumen of the neopharynx. Complications of flaps include ischemic necrosis (Fig. 20-44) and leaks. Accumulation of hair and cutaneous debris on the luminal surface of a cutaneous flap (termed the *hirsute pharynx*) can cause mucosal nodularity and partial obstruction to the flow of liquids (Fig. 20-45).

In creating a jejunal free flap, a segment of proximal jejunum and its vascular arcade are autotransplanted into the neck and placed in a peristaltic direction. Jejunal contractions do not aid in bolus propulsion, however, as they occur at a slow rate of three per minute and are not coordinated with swallowing. Clearance of the bolus from jejunal grafts is accomplished by gravity and pressure generated by tongue base push.[125] Complications of jejunal free grafts include fistula formation and ischemia. A normal jejunal free flap radiographically appears as a tubular segment of bowel with thin valvulae conniventes. No acute narrowing, angulation, or tethering of the tube should be seen.

Esophageal Speech

Vocalization after total laryngectomy is accomplished by buccal, oropharyngeal, or esophageal speech or a voice prosthesis placed in a surgically created tracheoesophageal fistula. During esophageal speech, the patient swallows air into the esophagus, then expels the air through the cricopharyngeus into the neopharynx and oral cavity. The pharyngoesophageal segment narrowing varies in length and diameter during normal esophageal speech. Rapid change of configuration of the cricopharyngeus replaces the vibrations of the resected true vocal cords.

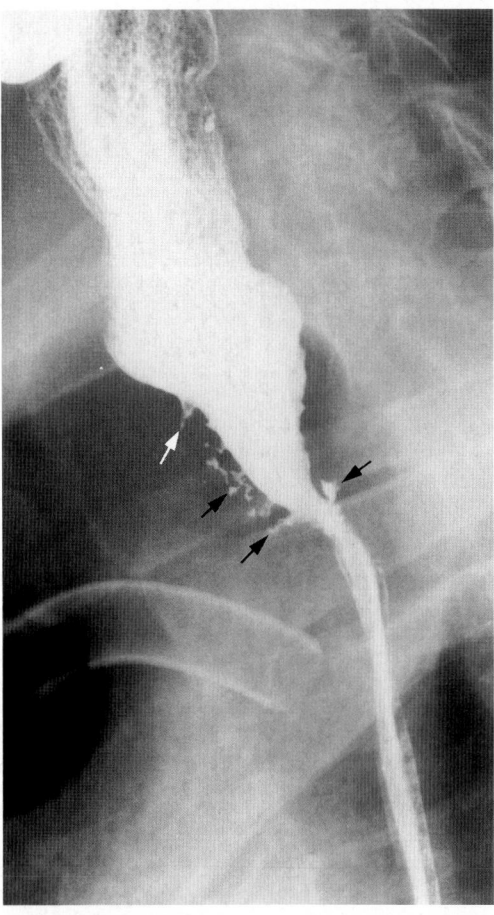

Figure 20-44. Partial breakdown of free flap. Oblique view shows numerous barium-filled tracks (*arrows*) extending into the interstices of the flap. (From Rubesin SE, Eisele DW, Jones B: Pharyngography in the postoperative patient. In Jones B [ed]: Normal and Abnormal Swallowing. Imaging in Diagnosis and Therapy, 2nd ed. New York, Springer, 2003, pp 167-204.)

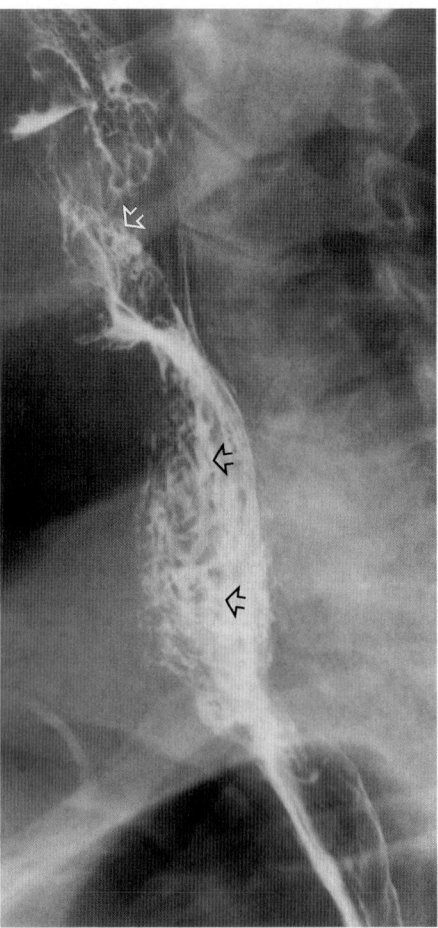

Figure 20-45. Hirsute neopharynx. Oblique view of the neck shows that the mucosa of the neopharynx is diffusely nodular (*arrows*) due to barium coating the skin and hair of this radial forearm flap. (From Rubesin SE, Eisele DW, Jones B: Pharyngography in the postoperative patient. In Jones B [ed]: Normal and Abnormal Swallowing. Imaging in Diagnosis and Therapy, 2nd ed. New York, Springer, 2003, pp 167-204.)

Pharyngoesophagography helps determine the causes of failure to attain esophageal speech.[126] Fixation and marked narrowing of the pharyngoesophageal segment may prevent esophageal speech.[127] Patients who have adequate quality of speech but diminished loudness may have a flaccid or strictured pharyngoesophageal segment.

Neck Dissection

A unilateral or bilateral neck dissection may be performed, depending on the initial location and size of the primary tumor and the presence of clinically or radiographically suspected lymph node metastases. The submandibular gland, internal jugular vein, spinal accessory nerve, hypoglossal nerve, external carotid artery, and sternocleidomastoid muscle may be preserved or resected.

A chylous collection may form in the left lower neck due to thoracic duct damage or in the right lower neck due to accessory duct damage. Damage or resection of the hypoglossal nerve may lead to tongue dysfunction. Shoulder dysfunction may result from damage or resection of the spinal accessory nerve supplying the trapezius muscle.[128]

Voice-Sparing Procedures

Horizontal (Supraglottic) Laryngectomy

During supraglottic laryngectomy, the epiglottis, aryepiglottic folds, and false vocal cords are removed. The thyroid cartilage is transected at the level of the laryngeal ventricle.[129] Voice is conserved, because the true vocal cords and arytenoid cartilages are spared. In some patients, one arytenoid cartilage and part of the medial wall of the piriform sinus on the side of the tumor are resected.[129] The hyoid bone may be spared or partially or fully resected. A cricopharyngeal myotomy may be performed.[130] The remaining portion of the thyroid cartilage and larynx are pulled up to the base of tongue (or hyoid if this structure is spared). The free anterior edge of the piriform sinus is pulled anteromedially, creating a fold superior to the vocal cord.[131,132]

Radiographically, the epiglottis and aryepiglottic folds are absent (Fig. 20-46). Barium penetrating the remaining larynx outlines the true vocal cords. On lateral views, the vocal cords lie just inferior to the tongue base. Barium etches the mucosa overlying the muscular processes of the arytenoid cartilages. The folds of the piriform sinus tissue that have been pulled

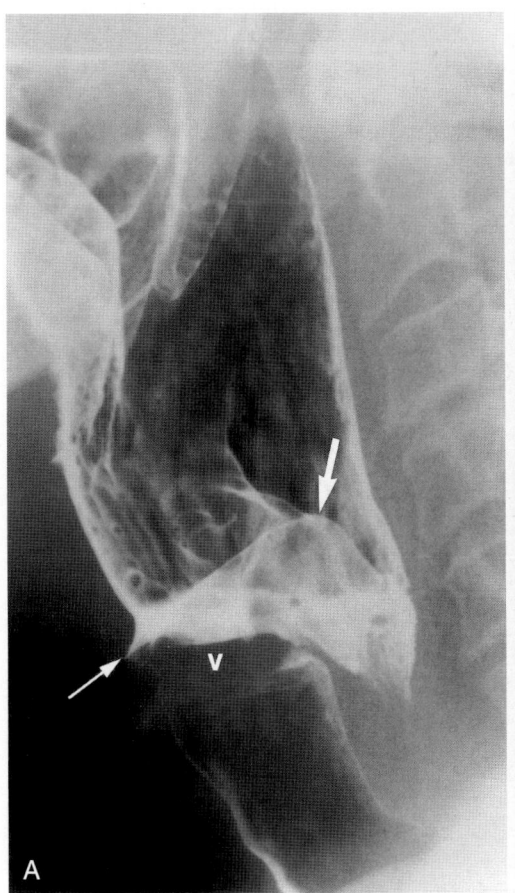 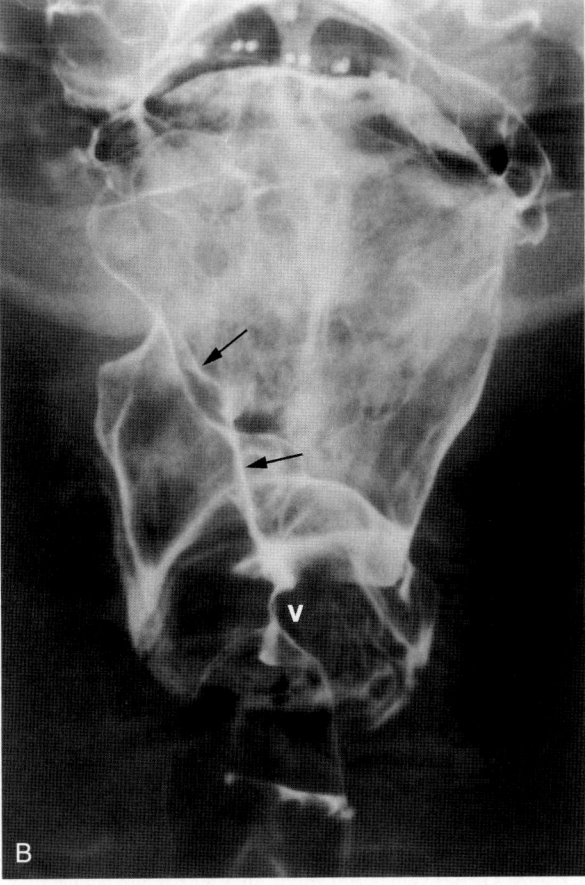

Figure 20-46. Horizontal (supraglottic) hemilaryngectomy. A. Lateral view shows that the anterior commissure (*thin arrow*) and true vocal cords (v), both coated by aspirated barium, are pulled up to the base of the tongue. The hyoid bone, valleculae, and epiglottis are missing. The mucosa overlying the muscular process of the arytenoid cartilages (*thick arrow*) is well seen and retracted superiorly. **B.** Frontal view shows the true vocal cords (left true vocal cord identified by v). The mucosa overlying the muscular processes of the arytenoid cartilages is asymmetrical. The anterior margin of the upper piriform sinus has been pulled medially to create a fold (*arrows*) above the ipsilateral true vocal cord. (From Rubesin SE, Eisele DW, Jones B: Pharyngography in the postoperative patient. In Jones B [ed]: Normal and Abnormal Swallowing. Imaging in Diagnosis and Therapy, 2nd ed. New York, Springer, 2003, pp 167-204.)

superior to the vocal cords are outlined by barium, termed *pseudocords*.[129] The mucosa at the junction between the tongue base and the true vocal cords may appear nodular. On frontal views, the barium-etched vocal cords and arytenoid cartilages are seen. If one arytenoid cartilage has been removed, the neolarynx appears asymmetrical. A concomitant neck dissection may result in ipsilateral flattening of the lateral pharyngeal wall.

Complications in the immediate postoperative period include aspiration, fistula formation, and airway obstruction due to postoperative edema. A Zenker diverticulum may develop (Fig. 20-47). Edema and fibrosis are manifested radiographically by smooth, symmetrical or asymmetrical enlargement of the mucosa overlying the muscular processes of the arytenoid cartilages. Fistulas develop in approximately 15% of patients.[132] The most common complications in the late postoperative period are aspiration in over 40% of patients and recurrent tumor in up to one third of patients.[129,133] Recurrent tumor is manifested radiographically by a focal mass with a nodular mucosal surface.

Vertical Partial Laryngectomy

Early glottic carcinomas may be treated by endoscopic surgery, radiotherapy, and open surgical procedures. Cancers of the anterior portion of the true vocal cords and anterior commissure can be treated by a variety of surgical procedures, including cordectomy, vertical partial laryngectomy, and vertical hemilaryngectomy.[134]

Cordectomy

Cancers localized to the true vocal cord or cancer with limited extension to the contralateral anterior commissure may be treated by cordectomy.[135] The vocal cord and internal perichondrium of the thyroid cartilage are resected.

Vertical Partial Laryngectomy

Vertical partial laryngectomy is used to treat glottic cancers with local extension to the arytenoid and floor of the laryngeal ventricle or cancers that occur after radiotherapy.[136] The cancerous vocal cord and approximately one third of the thyroid cartilage on the side of the tumor are resected.[137] The epiglottis is preserved, and its base is reattached. The false vocal fold on the side of the tumor may be reattached to the remaining ipsilateral thyroid cartilage.

Vertical Hemilaryngectomy

The true vocal cord, false vocal cord, arytenoid cartilage, and thyroid cartilage on the side of the tumor are resected. This procedure is often complicated by laryngeal stenosis and aspiration.

The radiographic findings associated with the various forms of vertical laryngectomy depend on the extent of surgery. If a cordectomy has been performed and no laryngeal penetration occurs, the pharynx may appear relatively normal.[138] If a complete vertical hemilaryngectomy has been performed,

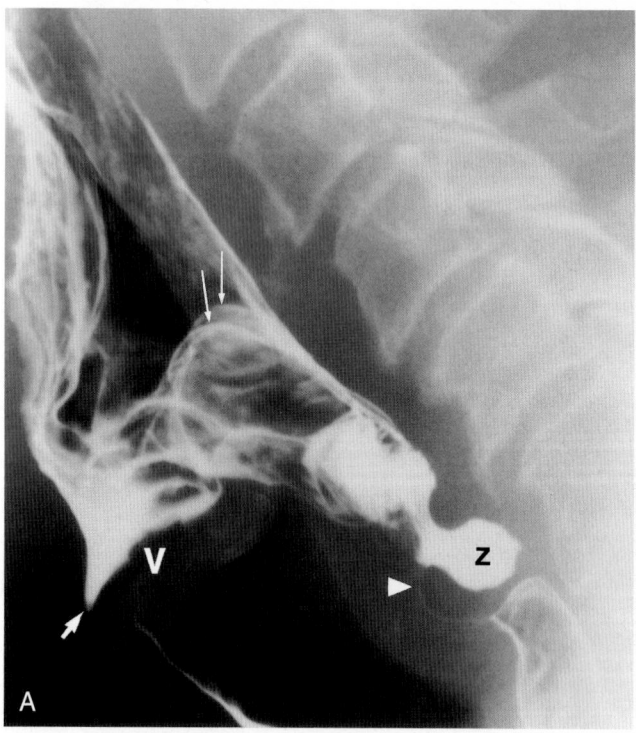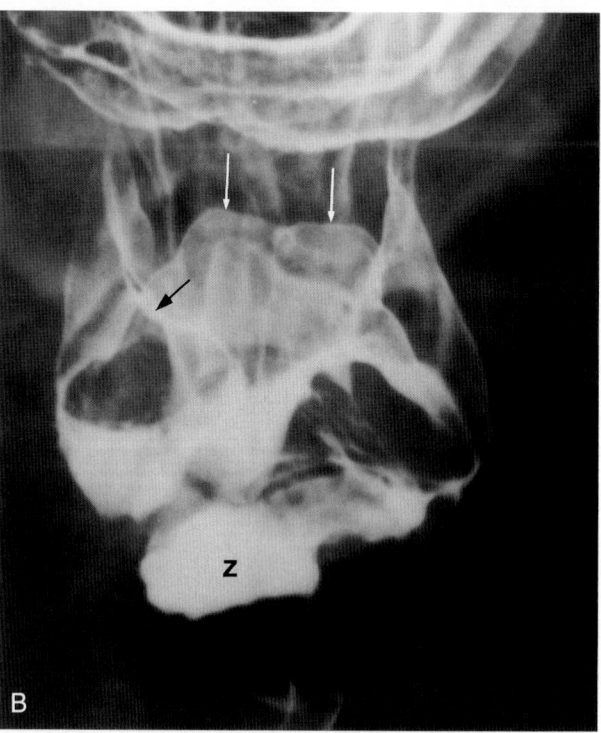

Figure 20-47. Zenker's diverticulum developing after horizontal hemilaryngectomy for epiglottic carcinoma. A. Lateral view of the pharynx shows that the hyoid bone, valleculae, epiglottis, and aryepiglottic folds are missing. Aspirated barium coats the true vocal cords (V) and anterior commissure (*short arrow*) that have been pulled up to the base of the tongue. The arytenoids (*long arrows*) are markedly elevated. The pharyngoesophageal segment is elevated, now opposite the anterior commissure. There also are a Zenker diverticulum (z) and "prominent" cricopharyngeal bar (*arrowhead*) that were not seen on preoperative images. **B.** Frontal view shows the prominent masslike arytenoids (*white arrows*). Folds of tissue arising from the lateral pharyngeal wall (right lateral fold identified by *black arrow*) have been pulled medially to cover the true vocal cords. The Zenker diverticulum is a 1.5-cm midline ovoid barium collection (z). (From Rubesin SE, Eisele DW, Jones B: Pharyngography in the postoperative patient. In Jones B [ed]: Normal and Abnormal Swallowing. Imaging in Diagnosis and Therapy, 2nd ed. New York, Springer, 2003, pp 167-204.)

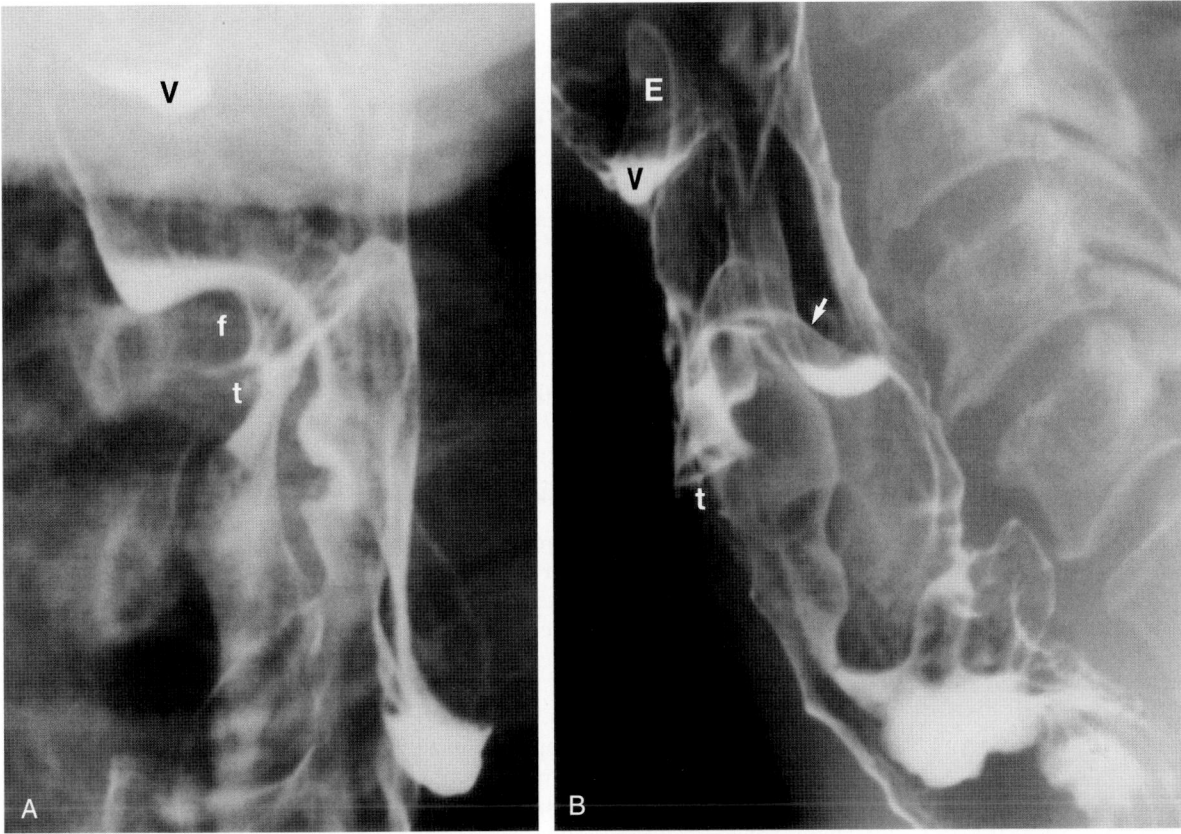

Figure 20-48. Vertical hemilaryngectomy. A. Frontal view shows that the right false (f) and right true (t) vocal cords remain. The presence of barium in the right vallecula (V) indicates that at least part of the epiglottis has been preserved. In contrast, the absence of the left vallecula indicates that the left side of the epiglottis has been resected. The left true and false vocal cords and left aryepiglottic fold are missing and have been resected. The remaining portion of the left side of the hypopharynx is dilated with barium stasis inferiorly in the pharyngoesophageal segment. **B.** Lateral view shows the epiglottic tip (E) and right vallecula (V). The anterior commissure is coated with aspirated barium, and one vocal cord (t) and arytenoid (*arrow*) remain. Kissing artifact is seen in the lower hypopharynx.

aspiration usually occurs. The true and false vocal cords and arytenoid that have been removed will be "missing" from the radiographs. The preserved contralateral true and false vocal cords will be etched by barium (Fig. 20-48).

A combination of endoscopy, cross-sectional imaging, and barium studies is helpful in the diagnosis of recurrent tumor.[138,139] Recurrent tumor may be manifested radiographically by narrowing and irregularity of the residual laryngeal vestibule or subglottic region. However, postoperative deformity due to edema or granulation tissue can mimic tumor recurrence.

Surgery for Tongue and Oropharyngeal Cancers

Glossectomy

Surgical approaches to the tongue depend on the size, location, and spread of the primary tumor.[140] Small lesions of the anterior tongue may be resected via a transoral approach. Larger lesions may require exposure via a mandibulotomy. Segmental mandibular resection is performed for lesions involving the mandible. Small lesions of the posterior tongue may be operated on via a transhyoid approach.

Large tumors of the posterior tongue may require near-total or total glossectomy. This procedure may include resec-

tion of tissue in the floor of the mouth, retromolar trigone, and lateral pharyngeal wall. A skin graft, tissue flap, or microvascular free flap can be used.[141] A concomitant cricopharyngeal myotomy may be performed as a "drainage" procedure. Approximately one third to one half of the tongue can be removed without significant swallowing disability.[142]

During a barium swallow, the radiologist evaluates collection and manipulation of the bolus by the residual tongue, stasis in the oral cavity, and premature spillage of the bolus into the hypopharynx. Abnormal tongue motion may reflect loss of tongue volume, adhesions, or damage to the hypoglossal nerve. A large proportion of the bolus may remain in the oral cavity. Abnormal elevation of the pharynx and larynx and abnormal epiglottic tilt may result from surgical transection of various suprahyoid muscles. Aspiration is detected in 10% to 33% of patients after total glossectomy.[143] Postoperative deformity of the tongue is the norm (Fig. 20-49) and is difficult to distinguish from recurrent tumor. The diagnosis of recurrent tumor is best made by a combination of direct visualization and cross-sectional imaging.

Malignant Oropharyngeal Lesions

Surgical approaches to the oropharynx include the transoral route, lip splitting with or without mandibulotomy, mandibulotomy, or a transcervical approach. A neck dissection is

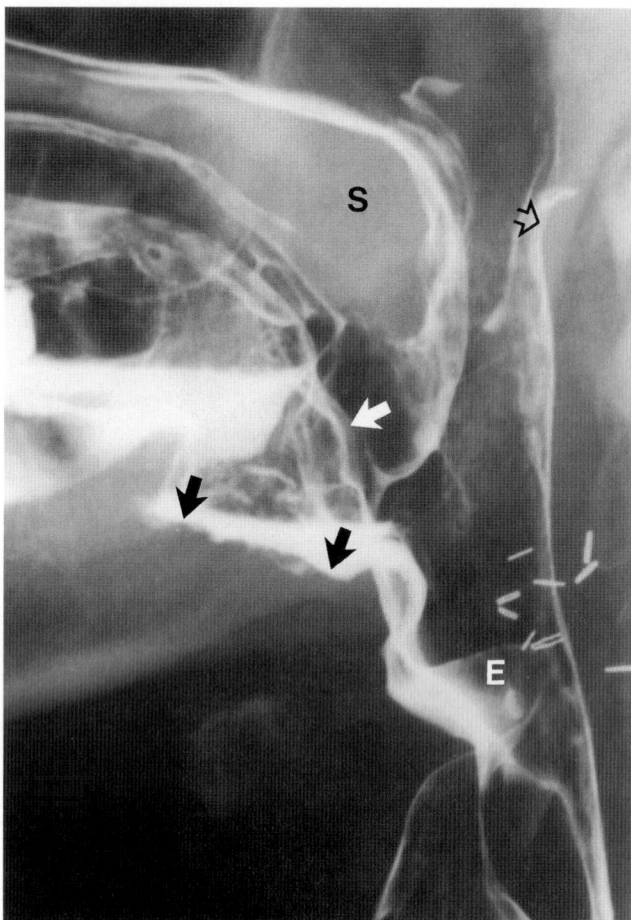

Figure 20-49. Partial glossectomy. A large barium-coated defect (*black arrows*) is seen at the tongue base. This defect and associated tongue dysfunction resulted in premature spill of the bolus into the oropharynx. The contralateral portion of the base of the tongue is intact (*white arrow*). It is impossible to determine whether there is recurrent tumor in the nodular tissue lining the tongue defect. Radiation-induced smooth-surfaced enlargement of the soft palate (S) and epiglottis (E) is seen. Nasal regurgitation results in barium coating the superior surface of the soft palate. Soft palate elevation is abnormal, as a gap remains between the soft palate and posterior pharyngeal wall despite phonation. Passavant's cushion (*open arrow*) is demonstrated. Abnormal soft palate elevation may have resulted from scarring related to surgery or prior radiation therapy. (From Rubesin SE, Eisele DW, Jones B: Pharyngography in the postoperative patient. In Jones B [ed]: Normal and Abnormal Swallowing. Imaging in Diagnosis and Therapy, 2nd ed. New York, Springer, 2003, pp 167-204.)

often concomitantly performed. Surgical defects may be filled with a skin grafts, myocutaneous flap, or free flap.[144]

Portions of the palate may be resected for primary squamous cell carcinoma, lymphoma, or minor salivary gland tumors or for contiguous tumors of the tonsil or retromolar trigone region secondarily invading the palate. Soft palate or tonsillar resection may result in hypernasal speech or nasal regurgitation. Partial palatectomy may also cause premature spillage of the bolus from the oral cavity into the oropharynx, resulting in poor timing of the swallow with subsequent laryngeal penetration. Postoperative defects in the palate may result in an oronasal or sinonasal fistula. Flap or graft breakdown may result in an orocutaneous or pharyngocutaneous fistula (Fig. 20-50). If the tongue base has been partially re-

moved or is fixed by adhesions, the patient may have difficulty chewing or swallowing.

Tracheostomy

Patients with a tracheostomy (with or without laryngectomy) may develop dysphagia or aspiration due to postoperative changes in the soft tissues of the neck, resulting in tethering of the trachea and pharynx with subsequent diminished laryngeal and pharyngeal elevation.[141,145] The presence of a tracheostomy may also result in poor coordination of laryngeal closure, with resultant aspiration during swallowing. A tracheostomy may also cause desensitization of the cough reflux.

Surgery for Zenker's Diverticulum and Pharyngeal Pouches

Various endoscopic and surgical procedures may be performed for treatment of Zenker's diverticulum. Some procedures alter the prominent cricopharyngeus, whereas others involve the diverticulum itself. The most successful procedure combines diverticulectomy with cricopharyngeal myotomy.

Endoscopic dilatation of the prominent cricopharyngeus has been performed,[146] but is often unsuccessful because the upper esophageal sphincter is not damaged enough to improve hypopharyngeal clearance and because the pouch is left intact. Surgical cricopharyngeal myotomy alone also has a poor success rate.[147]

Dohlman's procedure is an endoscopic procedure used in debilitated and elderly patients who are poor operative candidates.[148] The anterior lip of a specially designed endoscope is placed into the lumen of the pharyngoesophageal segment, and the posterior lip of the endoscope is inserted into the diverticulum.[149,150] The endoscopist then divides the posterior wall of the pharyngoesophageal segment between the lumen of the pharyngoesophageal segment/cervical esophagus and the lumen of the Zenker's diverticulum. The Zenker diverticulum is left intact, but the "prominent cricopharyngeus" is transected. On a postoperative pharyngogram, the Zenker diverticulum that remains intact should have less barium filling because there is improved drainage through an "opened" pharyngoesophageal segment. The barium-air level in the diverticulum should be lower in comparison to preoperative studies. The pharyngoesophageal segment should also open to a greater degree than was seen preoperatively.

Diverticulopexy is a surgical procedure performed in high-risk patients that avoids opening the pharynx. The apex of the Zenker diverticulum is suspended from the prevertebral fascia superior to the diverticulum.[151,152] A cricopharyngeal myotomy is performed. Although the diverticulum may partially fill during swallowing, it drains through the damaged cricopharyngeus, diminishing the risk of aspiration.

The most successful approach for treatment of Zenker's diverticulum is diverticulectomy with cricopharyngeal myotomy. An extended myotomy is performed, including division of the lowermost thyropharyngeus. The Zenker diverticulum is excised without removing the mucosa of the pharyngoesophageal segment.[151] During postoperative pharyngography, the Zenker diverticulum should not be seen. The pharyngoesophageal segment should open widely. In one series, however, 3 of 13 patients had a continued saclike outpouching at

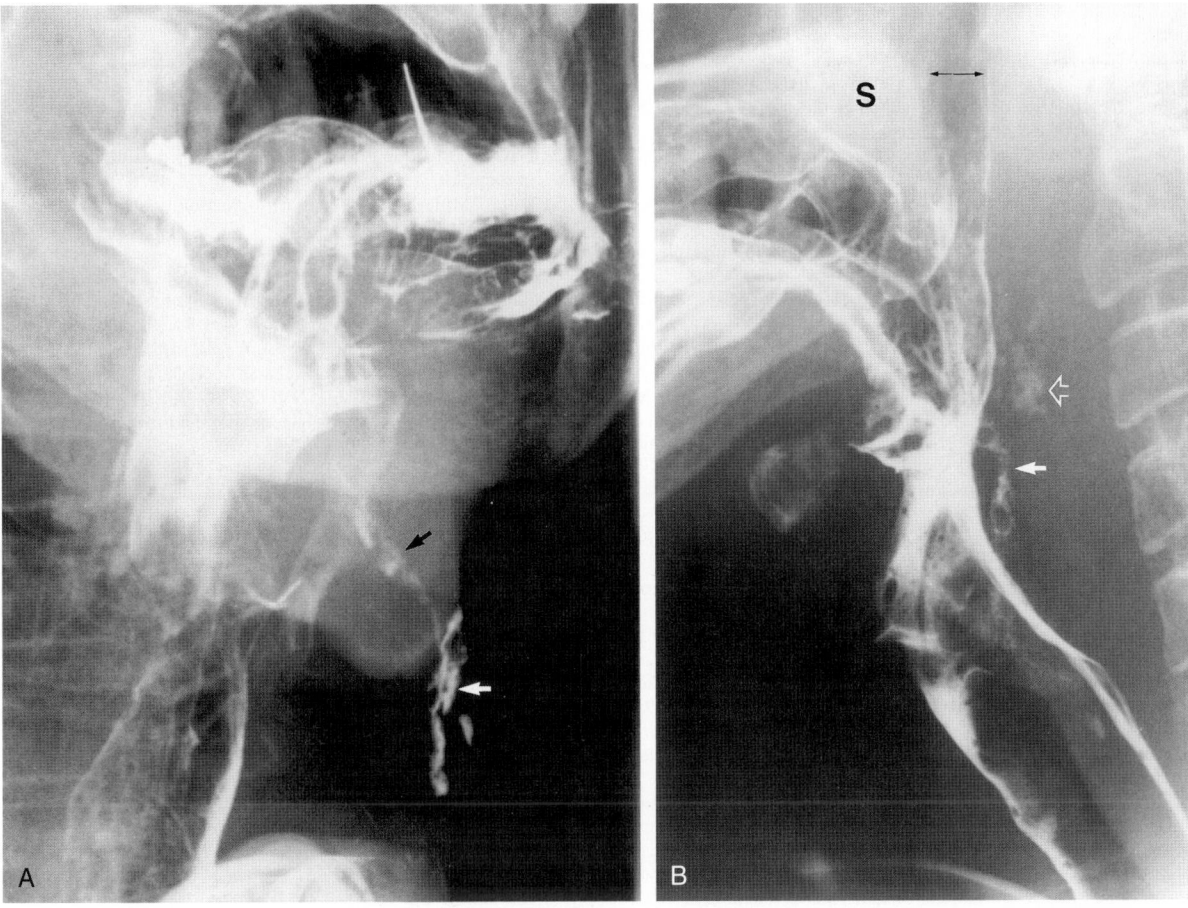

Figure 20-50. Fistula to the carotid sheath. A. Oblique view demonstrates a barium-filled track (*arrows*) extending inferiorly into the left neck.
B. Lateral view shows the barium-filled track (*arrows*) just below an area of calcification in the carotid artery (*open arrow*). Also note a gap between the soft palate (S) elevated during phonation and the posterior pharyngeal wall and a wide retropharyngeal space. Barium pours into the laryngeal vestibule. This patient was spitting up blood. At surgery, a fistula to the carotid sheath was found. (From Rubesin SE, Eisele DW, Jones B: Pharyngography in the postoperative patient. In Jones B [ed]: Normal and Abnormal Swallowing. Imaging in Diagnosis and Therapy, 2nd ed. New York, Springer, 2003, pp 167-204.)

the site of surgical excision.[153] Postoperative pharyngography may demonstrate unsuspected leaks as well as a characteristic beaklike postoperative deformity.[153]

Cricopharyngeal Myotomy

Cricopharyngeal myotomy is used as an isolated "drainage" procedure in patients with an abnormally functioning pharyngoesophageal segment due to a global pharyngeal motor disorder or Zenker diverticulum.[152,154] Cricopharyngeal myotomy facilitates drainage from a neuromuscularly impaired pharynx as does pyloroplasty in patients who develop abnormal gastric emptying due to vagotomy. Cricopharyngeal myotomy is not indicated in patients with globus symptoms alone.[152] Because the upper esophageal sphincter normally prevents reflux of esophageal contents into the pharynx, surgical destruction of the sphincter can sometimes lead to aspiration of esophageal contents into the lungs. The surgeon therefore balances the risk of aspiration due to pharyngeal stasis in an untreated patient with a neuromuscularly compromised pharynx with the risk of aspiration of esophageal contents from a cricopharyngeal myotomy. Given the operative risks of cricopharyngeal myotomy, some physicians are injecting botulinum toxin

into the cricopharyngeus as an alternative form of treatment for ameliorating symptoms.

After cricopharyngeal myotomy, pharyngography should demonstrate less stasis of barium in the hypopharynx. The cricopharyngeal bar should be absent, and there should be decreased or no luminal narrowing of the pharyngoesophageal segment in comparison to the preoperative pharyngogram. Complications include (1) incomplete myotomy manifested as a persistent cricopharyngeal bar; (2) fistula or abscess formation; and (3) vocal cord paralysis due to recurrent laryngeal nerve damage.

References

1. Bachman AL, Seaman WB, Macken KL: Lateral pharyngeal diverticula. Radiology 91:774-782, 1968.
2. Rubesin SE, Jessurun J, Robertson D, et al: Lines of the pharynx. RadioGraphics 7:217-237, 1987.
3. Norris CW: Pharyngoceles of the hypopharynx. Laryngoscope 89:1788-1807, 1979.
4. Curtis DJ, Cruess DF, Crain M, et al: Lateral pharyngeal outpouchings: A comparison of dysphagic and asymptomatic patients. Dysphagia 2:156-161, 1988.
5. Lindbichler F, Raith J, Uggowitzer M, et al: Aspiration resulting from lateral hypopharyngeal pouches. AJR 170:129-132, 1998.

6. Jones B: Common structural lesions. In Jones B (eds): Normal and Abnormal Swallowing: Imaging in Diagnosis and Therapy. New York, Springer-Verlag, 2003, pp 103-118.

7. Hyams VJ, Batsakis JG, Michaels L: Tumors of the upper respiratory tract and ear. In Atlas of Tumor Pathology, 2nd series, fascicle 25. Bethesda, MD, Armed Forces Institute of Pathology, 1988.

8. Lindell MM, Jing BS, Fischer EP, et al: Laryngocele. AJR 131:259-262, 1978.

9. Canalis RF, Maxwell DS, Hemenway WG: Laryngocele—an updated review. J Otolaryngol 6:191-199, 1977.

10. Glaser HS, Mauro MA, Aronberg DJ, et al: Computed tomography of laryngocele. AJR 140:549-552, 1983.

11. Maran AGD, Buchanan DR: Branchial cysts, sinuses and fistulae. Clin Otolaryngol 3:77-92, 1978.

12. Bhaskar SN, Bernier JL: Histogenesis of branchial cysts. Am J Pathol 35:407-414, 1959.

13. Som PM, Sacher M, Lanzieri CF, et al: Parenchymal cysts of the lower neck. Radiology 157:399-406, 1985.

14. Salazar JB, Duke RA, Ellis JV: Second branchial cleft cyst: Unusual location and a new CT diagnostic sign. AJR 145:965-966, 1985.

15. Perrott JW: Anatomical aspects of hypopharyngeal diverticula. Aust N Z J Surg 31:307-317, 1962.

16. Zaino C, Jacobson HG, Lepow H, et al: The pharyngoesophageal sphincter. Radiology 89:639-645, 1967.

17. Zaino C, Jacobson HG, Lepow H, et al: The Pharyngoesophageal Sphincter. Springfield, IL, Charles C Thomas, 1970.

18. Knuff TE, Benjamin SB, Castell DO: Pharyngoesophageal (Zenker's) diverticulum: A reappraisal. Gastroenterology 82:734-736, 1982.

19. Frieling T, Berges W, Lubke HJ, et al: Upper esophageal sphincter function in patients with Zenker's diverticulum. Dysphagia 3:90-92, 1988.

20. Smiley TB, Caves PK, Porter DC: Relationship between posterior pharyngeal pouch and hiatus hernia. Thorax 25:725-731, 1970.

21. Delahunty JE, Margulies SE, Alonso UA, et al: The relationship of reflux esophagitis to pharyngeal pouch (Zenker's diverticulum). Laryngoscope 81:570-577, 1971.

22. Rubesin SE: Pharynx. In Laufer I, Levine MS (eds): Double Contrast Gastrointestinal Radiology, 2nd ed. Philadelphia, WB Saunders, 1992, pp 73-105.

23. Brady AP, Stevenson GW, Somers S, et al: Premature contraction of the cricopharyngeus: New sign of gastroesophageal reflux disease. Abdom Imaging 20:225-229, 1995.

24. Shirazi KK, Daffner RH, Gaede JT: Ulcer occurring in Zenker's diverticulum. Gastrointest Radiol 2:117-118, 1977.

25. Nanson EM: Carcinoma in a long-standing pharyngeal diverticulum. Br J Surg 63:417-419, 1976.

26. Wychulis AR, Gunnulaugsson GH, Clagett OT: Carcinoma arising in pharyngoesophageal diverticulum. Surgery 66:976-979, 1969.

27. Ekberg O, Nylander G: Lateral diverticula from the pharyngoesophageal junction area. Radiology 146:117-122, 1983.

28. Rubesin SE, Levine MS: Killian-Jamieson diverticula: Radiographic findings in 16 patients. AJR 177:85-89, 2001.

29. Clements JL, Cox GW, Torres WE, et al: Cervical esophageal webs—a roentgen-anatomic correlation. AJR 121:221-231, 1974.

30. Nosher JL, Campbell WL, Seaman WB: The clinical significance of cervical esophageal and hypopharyngeal webs. Radiology 117:45-47, 1975.

31. Weaver JW, Kaude JV, Hamlin DJ: Webs of the lower esophagus: A complication of gastroesophageal reflux? AJR 142:289-292, 1984.

32. Seaman WB: The significance of webs in the hypopharynx and upper esophagus. Radiology 89:32-38, 1967.

33. Ekberg O: Cervical oesophageal webs in patients with dysphagia. Clin Radiol 32:633-641, 1981.

34. Ekberg O, Nylander G: Webs and web-like formations in the pharynx and cervical esophagus. Diagn Imaging 52:10-18, 1983.

35. Waldenström J, Kjeulberg SR: The roentgenological diagnosis of sideropenic dysphagia (Plummer-Vinson's syndrome). Acta Radiol 20:618-638, 1939.

36. McNab Jones RF: The Paterson-Brown-Kelly syndrome: Its relationship to iron deficiency and postcricoid carcinoma. J Laryngol Otol 71:529-561, 1961.

37. Gordon AR, Levine MS, Redfern RO, et al: Cervical esophageal webs: Association with gastroesophageal reflux. Abdom Imaging 26:574-577, 2001.

38. Ekberg O, Birch-Lensen M, Lindstrom C: Mucosal folds in the valleculae. Dysphagia 1:68-72, 1986.

39. Shauffer IA, Phillips HE, Sequeira J: The jet phenomenon: A manifestation of esophageal web. AJR 129:747-748, 1977.

40. Taylor AJ, Stewart ET, Dodds WJ: The esophageal jet phenomenon revisited. AJR 155:289-290, 1990.

41. Pitman RG, Fraser GM: The post-cricoid impression on the oesophagus. Clin Radiol 16:34-39, 1965.

42. Harris RD, Berdon WE, Baker DH: Roentgen diagnosis of acute epiglottis in the adult. J Can Assoc Radiol 21:270-272, 1970.

43. Balfe DM, Heiken JP: Contrast evaluation of structural lesions of the pharynx. Curr Probl Diagn Radiol 15:73-160, 1986.

44. Rubesin SE, Glick SN: The tailored double-contrast pharyngogram. Crit Rev Diagn Imaging 28:133-179, 1988.

45. Kabakian HA, Dahmash MS: Pharyngoesophageal manifestations of epidermolysis bullosa. Clin Radiol 29:91-94, 1978.

46. Agha FP, Francis IR, Ellis CN: Esophageal involvement in epidermolysis bullosa dystrophica: Clinical and roentgenographic manifestations. Gastrointest Radiol 8:111-117, 1983

47. Bosma JF, Gravkowski EA, Tryostad CW: Chronic ulcerative pharyngitis. Arch Otolaryngol 87:85-96, 1968.

48. Scott JC, Jones B, Eisele DW, et al: Caustic ingestion injuries of the upper aerodigestive tract. Laryngoscope 102:1-8, 1992.

49. Gromet M, Homer MJ, Carter BL: Lymphoid hyperplasia at the base of the tongue. Radiology 144:825-828, 1982.

50. Nayak SR, Kirtane MV, Shah AK, et al: Foreign bodies in the crico-pharyngeal region and oesophagus. J Postgrad Med 30:214-218, 1984.

51. Mansson T, Wilske J, Kindblom L-G: Lipoma of the hypopharynx: A case report and a review of the literature. J Laryngol Otol 92:1037-1043, 1978.

52. Patterson HC, Dickerson GR, Pilch BZ, et al: Hamartoma of the hypopharynx. Arch Otolaryngol 107:767-772, 1981.

53. Bachman AL: Benign, non-neoplastic conditions of the larynx and pharynx. Radiol Clin North Am 16:273-290, 1978.

54. DiBartolomeo JR, Olsen AR: Pedunculated lipoma of the epiglottis. Arch Otolaryngol 98:55-57, 1973.

55. Woodfield C, Levine MS, Rubesin SE, et al: Pharyngeal retention cysts: Radiographic findings in seven patients. AJR 184:793-796, 2005.

56. Chang-Lo M: Laryngeal involvement in Von Recklinghausen's disease. Laryngoscope 87:435-442, 1977.

57. Hyams VJ, Rabuzzi DD: Cartilaginous tumors of the larynx. Laryngoscope 80:755-767, 1970.

58. Decker J, Goldstein JC: Current concepts in otolaryngology: Risk factors in the head and neck cancer. N Engl J Med 306:1151-1155, 1982.

59. Semenkovich JW, Balfe DM, Weyman PJ, et al: Barium pharyngography: Comparison of single and double contrast. AJR 144:715-720, 1985.

60. Carpenter RJ III, DeSanto LW, Devine KD, et al: Cancer of the hypopharynx. Arch Otolaryngol 102:716-721, 1976.

61. Cunningham MP, Catlin D: Cancer of the pharyngeal wall. Cancer 20:1859-1866, 1967.

62. Dockerty MD, Parkhill EM, Dahlin DC, et al: Tumors of the Oral Cavity and Pharynx. Washington, DC, Armed Forces Institute of Pathology, 1968.

63. Goldstein HM, Zornoza J: Association of squamous cell carcinoma of the head and neck with cancer of the esophagus. AJR 131:791-794, 1978.

64. Thompson WM, Oddson TA, Kelvin F, et al: Synchronous and meta-chronous squamous cell carcinoma of the head, neck, and esophagus. Gastrointest Radiol 3:123-127, 1978.

65. Wagonfeld DJH, Harwood AR, Bryce EP, et al: Second primary respiratory tract malignant neoplasms in supraglottic carcinoma. Arch Otolaryngol 107:135-137, 1981.

66. Jing BS: Roentgen examination of the larynx and hypopharynx. Radiol Clin North Am 8:361-386, 1970.

67. Seaman WB: Contrast radiography in neoplastic disease of the larynx and pharynx. Semin Roentgenol 9:301-309, 1974.

68. Levine MS, Rubesin SE, Ott DJ: Update on esophageal radiology. AJR 155:933-941, 1990.

69. Rubesin SE, Laufer I: Pictorial review: Principles of double contrast pharyngography. Dysphagia 6:170-178, 1991.

70. Kassel E, Keller A, Kuchorczyk W: MRI of the floor of the mouth, tongue and orohypopharynx. Radiol Clin North Am 27:331-351, 1989.

71. Mancuso AA, Calcaterra TC, Hanafee WN: Computed tomography of the larynx. Radiol Clin North Am 16:195-208, 1978.

72. Som PM, Urken ML, Biller H, et al: Imaging the postoperative neck. Radiology 187:593-603, 1997.

73. Hoppe RT, Goffinet DR, Bagshaw MA: Carcinoma of the nasopharynx. Cancer 37:2605-2612, 1976.

74. Vogl T, Dresel S, Bilaniuk LT, et al: Tumors of the nasopharynx and adjacent areas: MR imaging with Gd-DTPA. AJNR 11:187-194, 1990.
75. Silver CE: Surgical management of neoplasms of the larynx, hypopharynx and cervical esophagus. Curr Probl Surg 14:2-69, 1977.
76. Frazell EL, Lucas JC: Cancer of the tongue: Report of the management of 1,554 patients. Cancer 15:1085-1099, 1962.
77. Barrs DM, DeSanto LW, O'Fallon WM: Squamous cell carcinoma of the tonsil and tongue-base region. Arch Otolaryngol 105:479-485, 1979.
78. Strong EW: Carcinoma of the tongue. Otolaryngol Clin North Am 12:107-114, 1979.
79. Jiminez JR: Roentgen examination of the oropharynx and oral cavity. Radiol Clin North Am 8:413-424, 1970.
80. Apter AJ, Levine MS, Glick SN: Carcinomas of the base of the tongue: Diagnosis using double-contrast radiography of the pharynx. Radiology 151:123-126, 1984.
81. Chung CK, Stryker JA, Abt AB, et al: Histologic grading in the clinical evaluation of laryngeal carcinoma. Arch Otolaryngol 106:623-624, 1980.
82. Kirchner JA, Owen JR: Five hundred cancers of the larynx and pyriform sinus: Results of treatment by radiation and surgery. Laryngoscope 87:1288-1303, 1977.
83. Zbaren P, Egger C: Growth patterns of piriform sinus carcinomas. Laryngoscope 107:511-518, 1997.
84. Johnson JT, Bacon GW, Meyers EN, et al: Medial vs. lateral wall pyriform sinus carcinomas: Implications for management of regional lymphatics. Head Neck 16:401-405, 1995.
85. Banfi A, Bonadonna G, Carnevali G, et al: Lymphoreticular sarcomas with primary involvement of Waldeyer's ring. Cancer 26:341-351, 1970.
86. Todd GB, Michaels L: Hodgkin's disease involving Waldeyer's lymphoid ring. Cancer 34:1769-1778, 1974.
87. Al-Saleem T, Harwick R, Robbins R, et al: Malignant lymphomas of the pharynx. Cancer 26:1383-1387, 1970.
88. Spiro RH, Koss LG, Hajdu SI, et al: Tumors of minor salivary origin. Cancer 31:117-129, 1973.
89. Conley J, Dingman DL: Adenoid cystic carcinoma in the head and neck (cylindroma). Arch Otolaryngol 100:81-90, 1974.
90. Krugman ME, Rosin HD, Toker C: Synovial sarcoma of the head and neck. Arch Otolaryngol 98:53-54, 1973.
91. Gatti WM, Strom CG, Orfei E: Synovial sarcoma of the laryngopharynx. Arch Otolaryngol 101:633-636, 1975.
92. Huizenga C, Balogh K: Cartilaginous tumors of the larynx. Cancer 26:201-210, 1970.
93. Emery CD, Wall S, Federle MP, et al: Pharyngeal Kaposi's sarcoma in patients with AIDS. AJR 147:919-922, 1986.
94. Wall S: Abdominal manifestations of AIDS. In Balfe DM, Levine MS (eds): RSNA Categorical Course in Diagnostic Radiology: Gastrointestinal 1997. Oak Brook, IL: RSNA Publications, 1997, pp 39-48.
95. Goolden AWG: Pharyngeal malignancy following irradiation of the neck [Abstract]. Br J Radiol 45:795, 1972.
96. Fajardo LF: Radiation-induced pathology of the alimentary tract. In Whitehead R (ed): Gastrointestinal and Oesophageal Pathology. Edinburgh, Churchill Livingstone, 1984, pp 813-814.
97. Chandler JR: Radiation fibrosis and necrosis of the larynx. Ann Otol Rhinol Laryngol 88:509-514, 1979.
98. Mukherji SK, Mancuso AA, Kotzur IM, et al: Radiologic appearance of the irradiated larynx. I. Expected changes. Radiology 193:141-148, 1994.
99. Goldman JL, Cheren RJ, Zak FG, et al: Histopathology of larynges and radical neck specimens in combined radiation and surgery for advanced carcinoma of the larynx and hypopharynx. Ann Otol 75:313-321, 1966.
100. Keene M, Harwood AR, Bryce DP, et al: Histopathological study of radionecrosis in laryngeal carcinoma. Laryngoscope 92:173-180, 1982.
101. Fu KK, Woodhouse RJ, Quivey JM, et al: The significance of laryngeal edema following radiotherapy of carcinoma of the vocal cord. Cancer 49:655-658, 1982.
102. Kagan AR, Calcaterra T, Ward P, et al: Significance of edema of the endolarynx following curative irradiation for carcinoma. AJR 120:169-172, 1974.
103. Larson DL, Lindberg RD, Lane E, et al: Major complications of radiotherapy in cancer of the oral cavity and oropharynx. A 10-year retrospective study. Am J Surg 146:531-536, 1983.
104. Goffinet DR, Eltringham FR, Glatstein E, et al: Carcinoma of the larynx: Results of radiation therapy in 213 patients. AJR 117:553-564, 1973.
105. Bedwinek JM, Shukovsky LJ, Fletcher GH, et al: Osteonecrosis in patients treated with definitive therapy for squamous cell carcinomas of the oral cavity and naso- and oropharynx. Radiology 119:665-667, 1976.
106. Ekberg O, Nylander G: Pharyngeal dysfunction after treatment for pharyngeal cancer with surgery and radiotherapy. Gastrointest Radiol 8:97-104, 1983.
107. Goldstein HM, Rogers LF, Fletcher GH, et al: Radiological manifestations of radiation-induced injury to the normal upper gastrointestinal tract. Radiology 117:135-140, 1975.
108. Quillen SP, Balfe DM, Glick SN: Pharyngography after head and neck irradiation: Differentiation of postirradiation edema from recurrent tumor. AJR 161:1205-1208, 1993.
109. Mukerji SK, Mancuso AA, Kotzur IM, et al: Radiologic appearance of the irradiated larynx. II. Primary site response. Radiology 193:149-154, 1994.
110. Rubesin SE, Eisele DW, Jones B: Pharyngography in the postoperative patient. In Jones B (ed): Normal and abnormal swallowing, 2nd ed. New York, Springer, 2003, pp 167-203.
111. Balfe DM, Koehler RE, Setzen M, et al: Barium examination of the esophagus after total laryngectomy. Radiology 143:501-508, 1982.
112. Wong F: Total Laryngectomy. In Bailey BJ (ed): Atlas of Head & Neck Surgery—Otolaryngology. Philadelphia, Lippincott-Raven, 1996, p 2000.
113. Gregor RT: Total laryngectomy. In Bleach N, Milford C, Van Hasselt A (eds): Operative Otorhinolaryngology. Oxford, Blackwell Science, 1997, pp 365-372.
114. Balfe DM: Imaging of the pharynx after surgical therapy. In Jones B, Donner MW (eds): Normal and Abnormal Swallowing. New York, Springer-Verlag, 1991, pp 147-171.
115. Moses BL, Eisele DW, Jones B: Radiologic assessment of the early postoperative total-laryngectomy patient. Laryngoscope 103:1157-1160, 1993.
116. Muller-Miny H, Eisele DW, Jones B: Dynamic radiographic imaging following total laryngectomy. Head Neck 15:342-347, 1993.
117. Hier M, Black MJ, Lafond G: Pharyngocutaneous fistulas after total laryngectomy: Incidence etiology and outcome analysis. J Otolaryngol 22:164-166, 1993.
118. DiSantis DJ, Balfe DM, Hayden RE, et al: The neck after total laryngectomy: CT study. Radiology 153:713-717, 1984.
119. Wippold FJ II, Balfe D: Imaging of the postoperative neck. In Gore RM, Levine MS, Laufer I: Textbook of Gastrointestinal Radiology. Philadelphia, WB Saunders, 1994, pp 277-290.
120. Quillen SP, Balfe DM, Glick SN: Pharyngography after head and neck irradiation: Differentiation of postirradiation edema from recurrent tumor. AJR 161:1205-1208, 1993.
121. Pernkopf E: Atlas of Topographical Applied Human Anatomy, Vol I, Head and Neck. Baltimore, Urban & Schwarzenberg, 1980, pp 231-339.
122. Stepnick DW, Hayden RE: Options for reconstruction of the pharyngo-esophageal defect. Otolaryngol Clin North Am 27:1151-1158, 1994.
123. Haughey BH: The jejunal free flap in oral cavity and pharyngeal reconstruction. Otolaryngol Clin North Am 27:1159-1170, 1994.
124. Wong F: Total pharyngolaryngectomy. In Bailey BJ (ed): Atlas of Head & Neck Surgery—Otolaryngology. Philadelphia, Lippincott-Raven, 1996, pp 206-209.
125. Wilson JA, Maran AG, Pryde A, et al: The function of free jejunal autografts in the pharyngoesophageal segment. J R Coll Surg Edinburgh 40:363-366, 1995.
126. Sloane PM, Griffin JM, O'Dwyer TP: Esophageal insufflation and videofluoroscopy for evaluation of esophageal speech in laryngectomy patients: Clinical implications. Radiology 181:433-437, 1991.
127. Gatenby RA, Rosenblum JS, Leonard CM, et al: Esophageal speech: Double contrast evaluation of the pharyngo-esophageal segment. Radiology 157:127-131, 1985.
128. Medina JE: Radical neck dissection. In Bailey BJ (ed): Atlas of Head & Neck Surgery—Otolaryngology. Philadelphia, Lippincott-Raven Publishers, 1996, pp 140-143.
129. Niemeyer JH, Balfe DM, Hayden RE: Neck evaluation with barium-enhanced radiographs and CT scans after supraglottic subtotal laryngectomy. Radiology 162:493-498, 1987.
130. Wong F: Supraglottic laryngectomy (horizontal hemilaryngectomy). In Bailey BJ (ed): Atlas of Head & Neck Surgery—Otolaryngology. Philadelphia, Lippincott-Raven Publishers, 1996, pp 190-193.
131. Gregor RT: Horizontal (supraglottic) laryngectomy. In Bleach N, Milford C, Van Hasselt A (eds): Operative Otorhinolaryngology. Oxford, Blackwell Science, 1997, pp 383-388.
132. Tabb HG, Druck NS, Thorton RS, et al: Supraglottic laryngectomy. South Med J 71:114-117, 1978.
133. Gregor RT, Oei SS, Baris G, et al: Supraglottic laryngectomy with neck dissection and post-operative radiation in the management of supraglottic laryngeal cancer. Am J Otolaryngol 17:316-321, 1996.

134. Roberson JB Jr, Fee WE Jr: Conservation surgery for laryngeal carcinoma. Ann Acad Med 20:656-664, 1991.

135. Rassekh CH: Laryngofissure and cordectomy. In Bailey BJ (ed): Atlas of Head & Neck Surgery—Otolaryngology. Philadelphia, Lippincott-Raven, 1996, pp 174-176.

136. Bailey BJ: Vertical partial laryngectomy. In Bailey BJ (ed): Atlas of Head & Neck Surgery—Otolaryngology. Philadelphia, Lippincott-Raven, 1996, pp 184-187.

137. Gopal HV, Fried MP: Vertical partial laryngectomy including the thyroid cartilage. In Bailey BJ (ed): Atlas of Head & Neck Surgery—Otolaryngology. Philadelphia: Lippincott-Raven, 1996, pp 176-179.

138. DiSantis DJ, Balfe DM, Koehler RE, et al: Barium examination of the pharynx after vertical hemilaryngectomy. AJR 141:335-339, 1983.

139. DiSantis DJ, Balfe DM, Hayden R: The neck after vertical hemilaryngectomy: Computed tomographic study. Radiology 151:683-687, 1984.

140. Johnson RC: Near total glossectomy. Total glossectomy. In Bailey BJ (ed): Atlas of Head & Neck Surgery—Otolaryngology. Philadelphia, Lippincott-Raven Publishers, 1996, pp 78-83.

141. Kronenberger MB, Meyers AD: Dysphagia following head and neck cancer surgery. Dysphagia 9:236-244, 1994.

142. Hirano M, Kuroiwa Y, Tanaka S, et al: Dysphagia following various degrees of surgical resection for oral cancer. Ann Otol Rhinol Laryngol 101:138-142, 1992.

143. Weber RS, Ohlms L, Bowman J, et al: Functional results after total or near-total glossectomy with laryngeal preservation. Arch Otolaryngol Head Neck Surg 117:512-516, 1991.

144. Waldron J: Surgery for malignant lesions of the oropharynx. In Bleach N, Milford C, Van Hasselt A (eds): Operative Otorhinolaryngology. Oxford, Blackwell Science, 1997, pp 357-362.

145. Nash M: Swallowing problems in the tracheotomized patient. Otolaryngol Clin North Am 21:701-709, 1988.

146. Ravich W, Neumann S, Jones B: Dilatation as treatment of pharyngoesophageal segment (PES) prominence with hypopharyngeal (Zenker's) diverticulum. Dysphagia 15:103, 2000.

147. Schmit PJ, Zuckerbraun L: Treatment of Zenker's diverticula by cricopharyngeus myotomy under local anesthesia. Am Surg 18:710-716, 1992.

148. Hadley JM, Ridley N, Djazaeri B, et al: The radiological appearances after endoscopic cricopharyngeal myotomy: Dohlman's procedure. Clin Radiol 52:613-615, 1997.

149. Dohlman G, Mattsson O: The endoscopic operation for hypopharyngeal diverticula: A roentgen cinematographic study. Arch Otolaryngol 71:744-752, 1960.

150. Collard JM, Otte JB, Kastens PJ: Endoscopic stapling technique of esophagodiverticulostomy for Zenker's diverticulum. Ann Thorac Surg 56:573-576, 1993.

151. Konowitz PM, Biller HF: Diverticulopexy and cricopharyngeal myotomy: Treatment for the high risk patient with a pharyngoesophageal (Zenker's) diverticulum. Otolaryngol Head Neck Surg 100:146-153, 1989.

152. McKenna A, Dedo HH: Cricopharyngeal myotomy: Indications and technique. Ann Otol Rhinol Laryngol 101:216-221, 1992.

153. Sydow BD, Levine MS, Rubesin SE, et al: Radiographic findings and complications after surgical or endoscopic repair of Zenker's diverticulum in 16 patients. AJR 177:1067-1071, 2001.

154. Overbeek JJM: Upper esophageal sphincterotomy in dysphagic patients with and without a diverticulum. Dysphagia 6:228-234, 1991.

IV

Esophagus

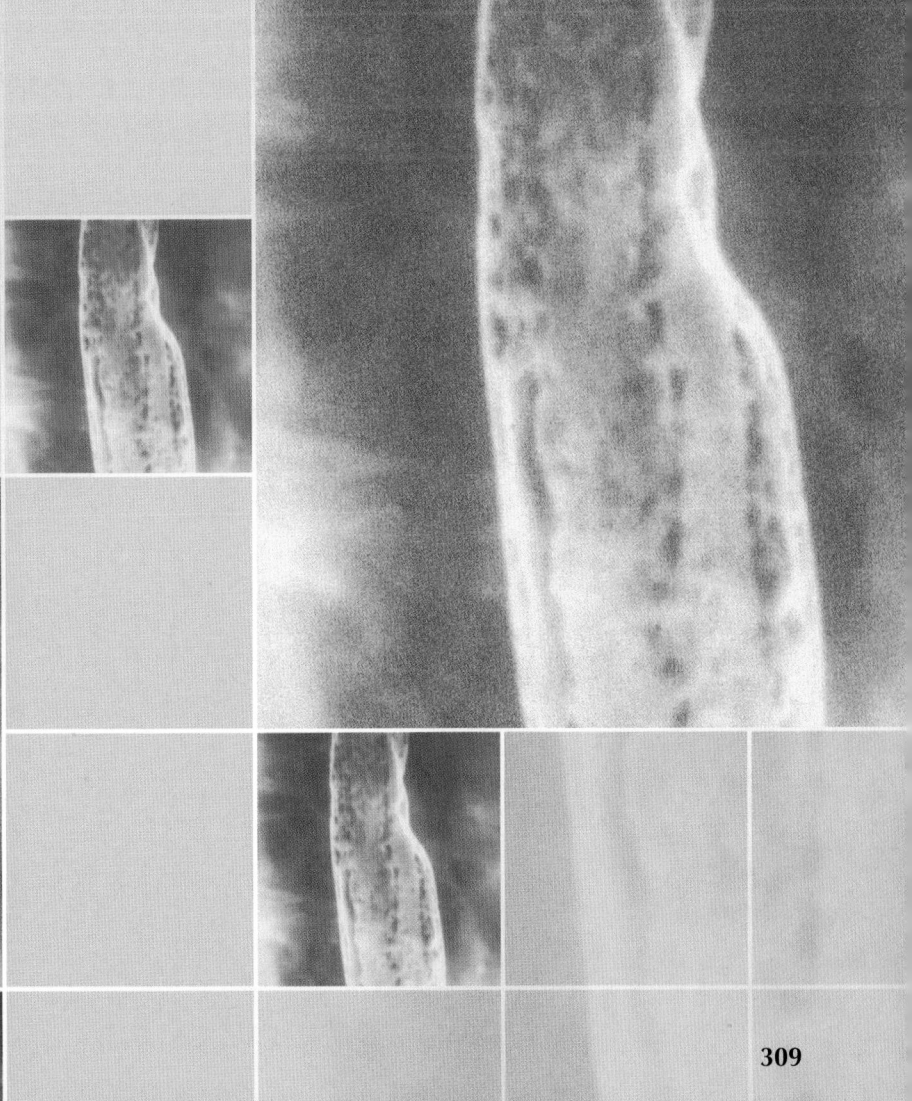

309

Barium Studies of the Upper Gastrointestinal Tract

Igor Laufer, MD • Marc S. Levine, MD

There are many ways to perform an upper gastrointestinal barium study. In Chapter 3, a technique was described that relies primarily on barium filling and mucosal relief. The method described in this chapter relies primarily on double contrast, although, in truth, it is a biphasic technique that combines the advantages of both single and double contrast. Individual practitioners undoubtedly develop their own particular routines and variations. Nevertheless, the techniques discussed in this chapter are representative of one approach for performing double-contrast upper gastrointestinal examinations.[1]

GENERAL PRINCIPLES

Double-contrast upper gastrointestinal studies are designed to coat the mucosal surface with a thin layer of high-density barium while the lumen is distended with gas. The routine examination should include the thoracic esophagus, stomach, and duodenum as far as the duodenojejunal junction. The examination should be performed quickly to maintain optimal mucosal coating and to prevent barium filling of the duodenum and small bowel from overlapping the stomach. It is not critical that each segment of the upper gastrointestinal tract be examined in anatomic sequence. For example, it may be preferable to examine the antrum, pylorus, and duodenum

before significant overlap has occurred. Similarly, when the pharynx needs to be evaluated, it may be preferable to perform this portion of the examination after the upper gastrointestinal study has been completed. The specific details of the examination should be tailored to the patient's presenting symptoms; the anatomic configuration of the esophagus, stomach and duodenum; and the specific abnormalities observed at fluoroscopy.

MATERIALS

Barium Suspensions

For the double-contrast examination, we use a high-density 250% w/v barium (E-Z-HD; E-Z-EM Company, Westbury, NY). The preparation of these barium suspensions is critical because slight deviations in concentration can impair the quality of mucosal coating and cause artifacts.[2]

Effervescent Agents

Various effervescent agents are available in powder, granular, or liquid form.[3] These agents release 300 to 400 mL of carbon dioxide on contact with fluid in the stomach.

Hypotonia

The use of a hypotonic agent to relax the stomach and duodenum results in a better examination and allows the examiner additional time to achieve optimal mucosal coating. In the United States, the only suitable hypotonic agent is glucagon; an injection of 0.1 mg intravenously usually produces transient hypotonia of the stomach. In some patients, this hypotonic effect may delay barium filling of the duodenum for several minutes. In other parts of the world, hyoscine *N*-butyl bromide (Buscopan) is frequently used to achieve gastrointestinal hypotonia.[4]

Radiography

The choice of a radiographic system represents a trade-off between resolution, contrast, and speed. In the past, we preferred a 400-speed system with a wide contrast scale to achieve a relatively uniform density over the entire radiograph. Spot radiographs were exposed at 105 kV(p). Currently, however, we routinely perform our studies with digital fluoroscopy and spot imaging.[5] The advantages of the digital system—better contrast resolution, shorter exposures, and faster examinations—more than compensate for the small decrease in spatial resolution. We interpret the images at

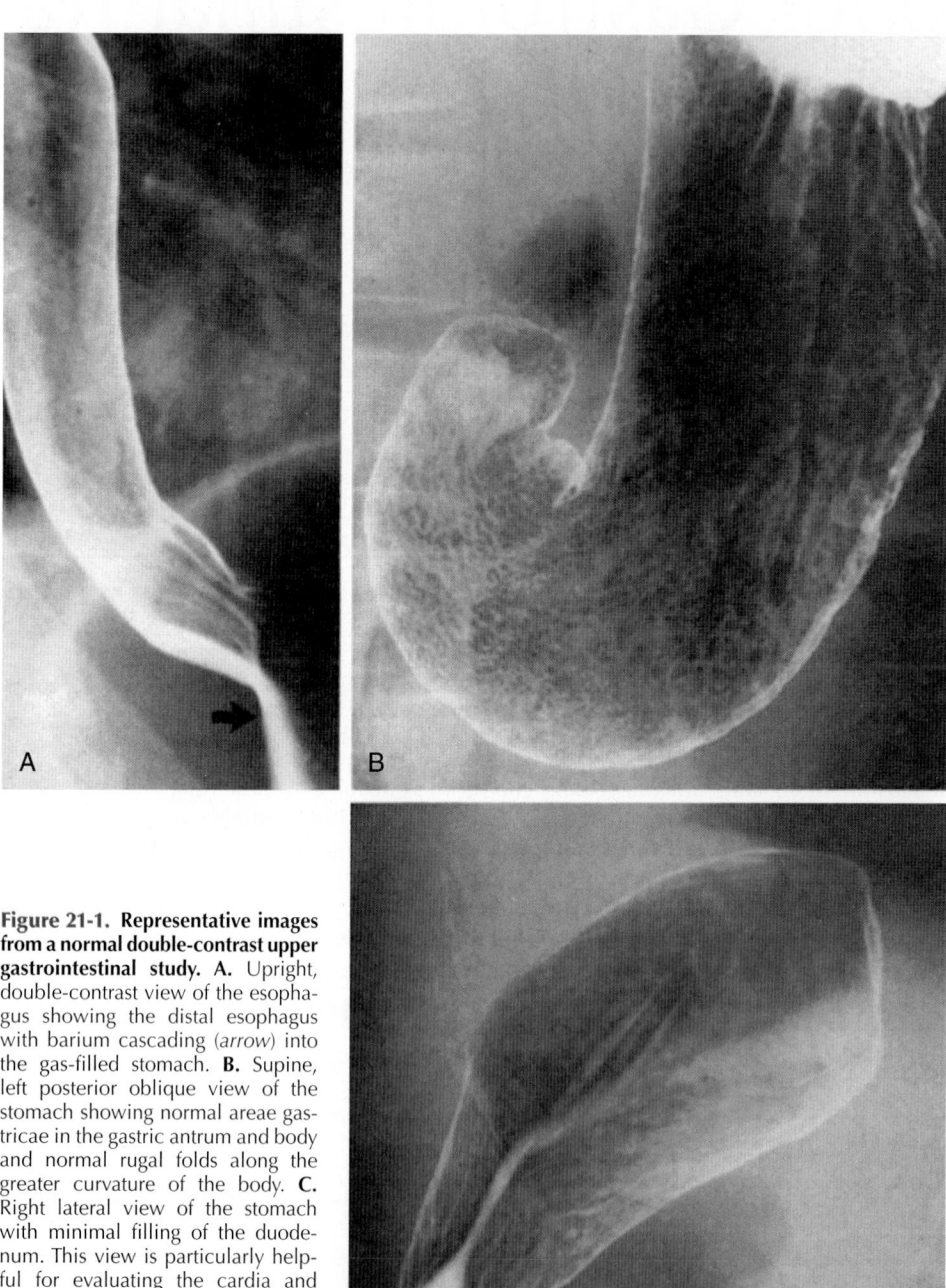

Figure 21-1. Representative images from a normal double-contrast upper gastrointestinal study. A. Upright, double-contrast view of the esophagus showing the distal esophagus with barium cascading (*arrow*) into the gas-filled stomach. **B.** Supine, left posterior oblique view of the stomach showing normal areae gastricae in the gastric antrum and body and normal rugal folds along the greater curvature of the body. **C.** Right lateral view of the stomach with minimal filling of the duodenum. This view is particularly helpful for evaluating the cardia and retrogastric region.

an electronic workstation,[6] with routine postprocessing of the images for optimal interpretation.[7] The studies are then archived on a central picture archiving and communications system, allowing easy electronic retrieval of prior examinations and eliminating the frustration of missing radiographs.

ROUTINE TECHNIQUE

Selected views from a normal double-contrast upper gastrointestinal study are shown in Figure 21-1. We begin with a short review of the patient's history and symptoms. In particular, we take special care to ask whether the patient has had any previous surgery and whether the patient is taking any ulcerogenic medications. The examination usually starts with an intravenous injection of 0.1 mg of glucagon. The patient then ingests the effervescent agent, followed by 10 mL of water to facilitate the release of carbon dioxide in the stomach. The patient then stands in the left posterior oblique position and is asked to gulp the contents of a cup containing 120 mL of high-density barium as rapidly as possible while double-contrast views of the esophagus are obtained in rapid succession. These views should include the distal esophagus and gastroesophageal junction. Barium is often seen cascading into the gas-filled stomach (see Fig. 21-1A).

After the esophagus has been examined, the table is lowered into the horizontal position and the patient is turned a full

circle to achieve adequate mucosal coating of all surfaces of the stomach. Supine, left posterior oblique, and right posterior oblique views of the gastric antrum and body are then obtained (see Fig. 21-1B). The patient is next placed in the recumbent, right side down position for a double-contrast view of the gastric cardia and fundus (see Fig. 21-1C). The patient is then placed in the semiupright, right posterior oblique position for a view of the high lesser curvature, upper body, and fundus (see Fig. 21-1D). The patient is next placed in the supine, left posterior oblique position for double-contrast views of the duodenal bulb and sweep (see Fig. 21-1E). Flow technique is then performed by slowly rotating the patient from side to side to manipulate a thin pool of barium over the dependent (posterior) gastric wall. Flow technique is extremely valuable for demonstrating shallow depressed or protruded lesions on the dependent surface (Fig. 21-2).[8]

After the double-contrast phase of the study has been completed, the patient is placed in a prone, right anterior oblique position to evaluate esophageal motility and obtain single-contrast views of the optimally distended thoracic esophagus. Prone and upright compression views of the barium-filled stomach and duodenum are then obtained. Finally, the fluoroscopist tests for spontaneous gastroesophageal reflux or reflux induced by a Valsalva maneuver to increase intra-abdominal pressure. Our routine double-contrast upper gastrointestinal study is summarized in Table 21-1.

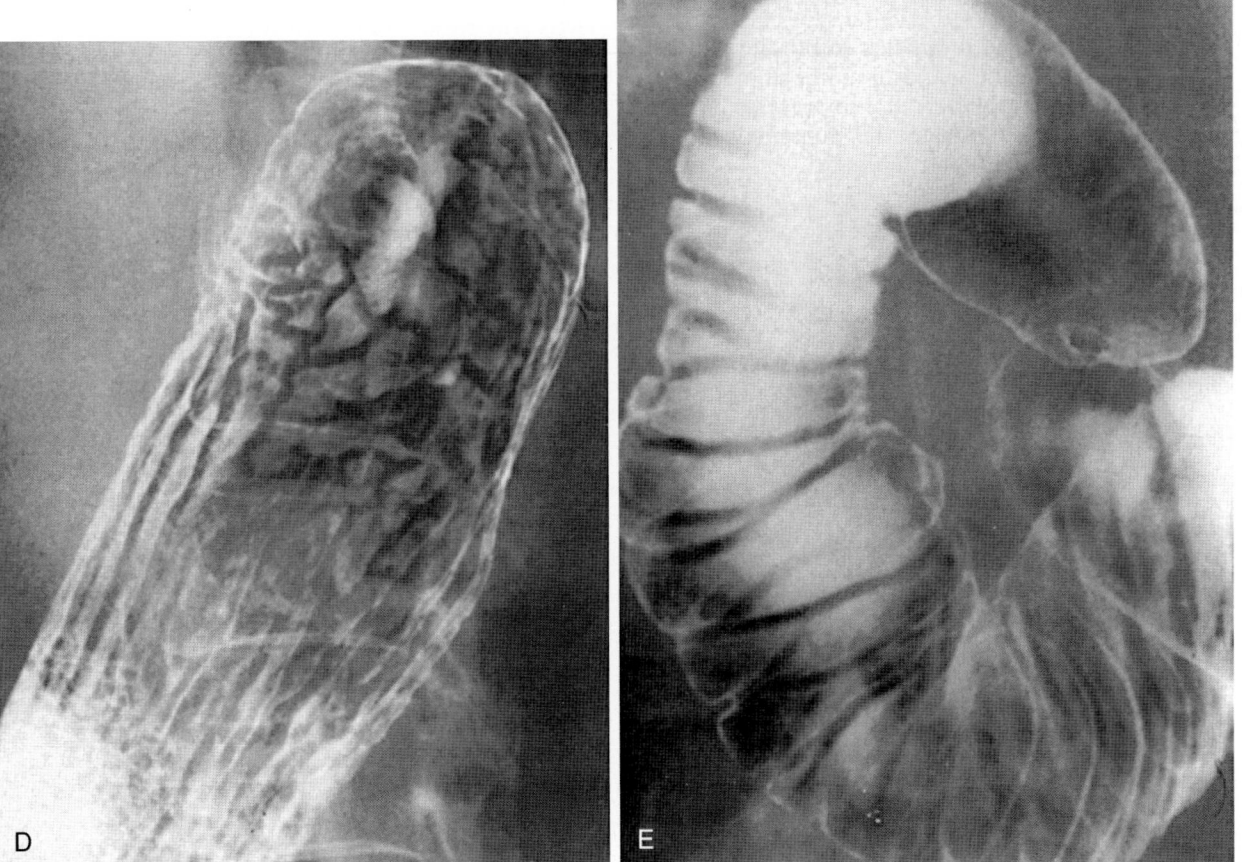

Figure 21-1. *Cont'd,* **D.** Semiupright, right posterior oblique view of high lesser curvature, upper body, and fundus. **E.** Supine, left posterior oblique view of the duodenum showing the smooth, featureless appearance of the bulb. (**D** and **E** from Laufer I, Levine MS [eds]: Double Contrast Gastrointestinal Radiology, 2nd ed. Philadelphia, WB Saunders, 1992.)

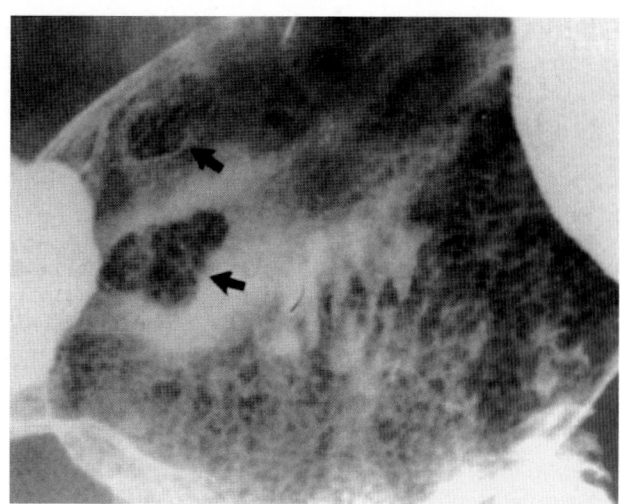

Figure 21-2. Flow technique. With barium flowing across the dependent surface of the stomach, two polypoid lesions (*arrows*) are identified on the posterior wall. This patient with AIDS had biopsy-proven Kaposi's sarcoma in the stomach.

ANATOMIC CONSIDERATIONS

Although the normal anatomy of the upper gastrointestinal tract is well known, several features that are particularly well demonstrated by double-contrast technique should be stressed.

Esophagus

The normal mucosal surface of the esophagus is smooth and featureless (Fig. 21-3A). With partial collapse of the esophagus, the normal longitudinal folds are seen (Fig. 21-3B). In some

Table 21-1
Routine Upper Gastrointestinal Technique: Double Contrast

Position	Purpose
Upright, LPO	Esophagus, double contrast
Supine, LPO	Stomach, antrum and body, double contrast
Supine	Stomach, antrum and body, double contrast
Supine, RPO	Stomach, antrum and body, double contrast
Right side down lateral	Stomach, cardia and fundus, double contrast
Supine, LPO	Antrum, pylorus, duodenal bulb and sweep, double contrast
Supine and supine oblique	Antrum and body, flow technique
Semiupright, RPO	Stomach, high lesser curvature and fundus, double contrast
Prone, RAO	Esophagus, function and barium filling
Prone or prone, RAO	Antrum and duodenum, compression
Upright	Stomach and duodenum, compression
Recumbent	Test for gastroesophageal reflux

LPO, left posterior oblique; RPO, right posterior oblique; RAO, right anterior oblique.

patients, fine transverse folds may also be observed in the body of the esophagus (Fig. 21-3C). These folds are thought to result from transient contraction of the longitudinally oriented muscularis mucosae and are often seen in patients with gastroesophageal reflux.[9] Occasionally, fine transverse folds may be detected as a normal variant in the upper thoracic esophagus at the junction of the striated and smooth muscle near the level of the aortic arch (Fig. 21-3D).[10] In older patients, small nodules may be seen on the mucosal surface of the esophagus due to glycogenic acanthosis, a common degenerative condition of no clinical significance (Fig. 21-4).[11]

The esophagus may be indented by normal extrinsic impressions from the aortic arch, left main bronchus, and heart (Fig. 21-5A). A smooth, gently sloping indentation may also be seen on the right posterolateral wall of the upper thoracic esophagus between the thoracic inlet and aortic arch in about 10% of patients (see Chapter 29).[12] This indentation represents a normal anatomic variant resulting from an unusually prominent right inferior supra-azygous recess of the mediastinum abutting the esophagus. This variation should not be mistaken for adenopathy or other masses in the mediastinum impinging on the esophagus.[12] In contrast, abnormal impressions may be caused by enlargement of normal structures such as the heart and aorta or by abnormal structures such as enlarged lymph nodes, mediastinal masses, or vertebral osteophytes (Fig. 21-5B).

Stomach

The mucosal surface of the stomach can be studied at several levels. The rugal fold pattern is best seen when the stomach is incompletely distended and is most prominent along the greater curvature of the gastric body (Fig. 21-6A). As the normal rugal folds are effaced, the finer mucosal pattern, the areae gastricae, can be visualized by double-contrast technique (see Fig. 21-1B) or by single-contrast technique with high-density barium and compression (see Fig. 21-6A).[13] This fine mucosal pattern can become distorted in patients with inflammatory or neoplastic lesions and also serves as a marker of the quality of mucosal coating. In some patients, fine transverse folds (striae) are seen as a normal variant in the gastric antrum (Fig. 21-6B) or as a sign of chronic antral gastritis.[14] In thin patients, the posterior wall of the stomach may be impressed by normal retrogastric structures that should not be mistaken for pathologic mass lesions (Fig. 21-6C).

The anatomy of the gastric cardia is particularly well shown on double-contrast studies. A variety of appearances may be seen, including a filling defect, radiating folds representing the cardiac rosette, and a hooding fold (Fig. 21-7).[15] In patients with ligamentous laxity and a small hiatal hernia, these anatomic landmarks may no longer be present. The cardiac rosette can also be distorted or obliterated in patients with tumors arising at the cardia (see Chapters 30 and 36).

Duodenum

The surface of the duodenal bulb is usually quite smooth. In some patients, double-contrast studies may reveal a fine, feathery or velvety surface in the bulb, probably representing a normal villous pattern in the duodenum (Fig. 21-8A).[16] In other patients, double-contrast studies may reveal small, angular filling defects near the base of the duodenal bulb,

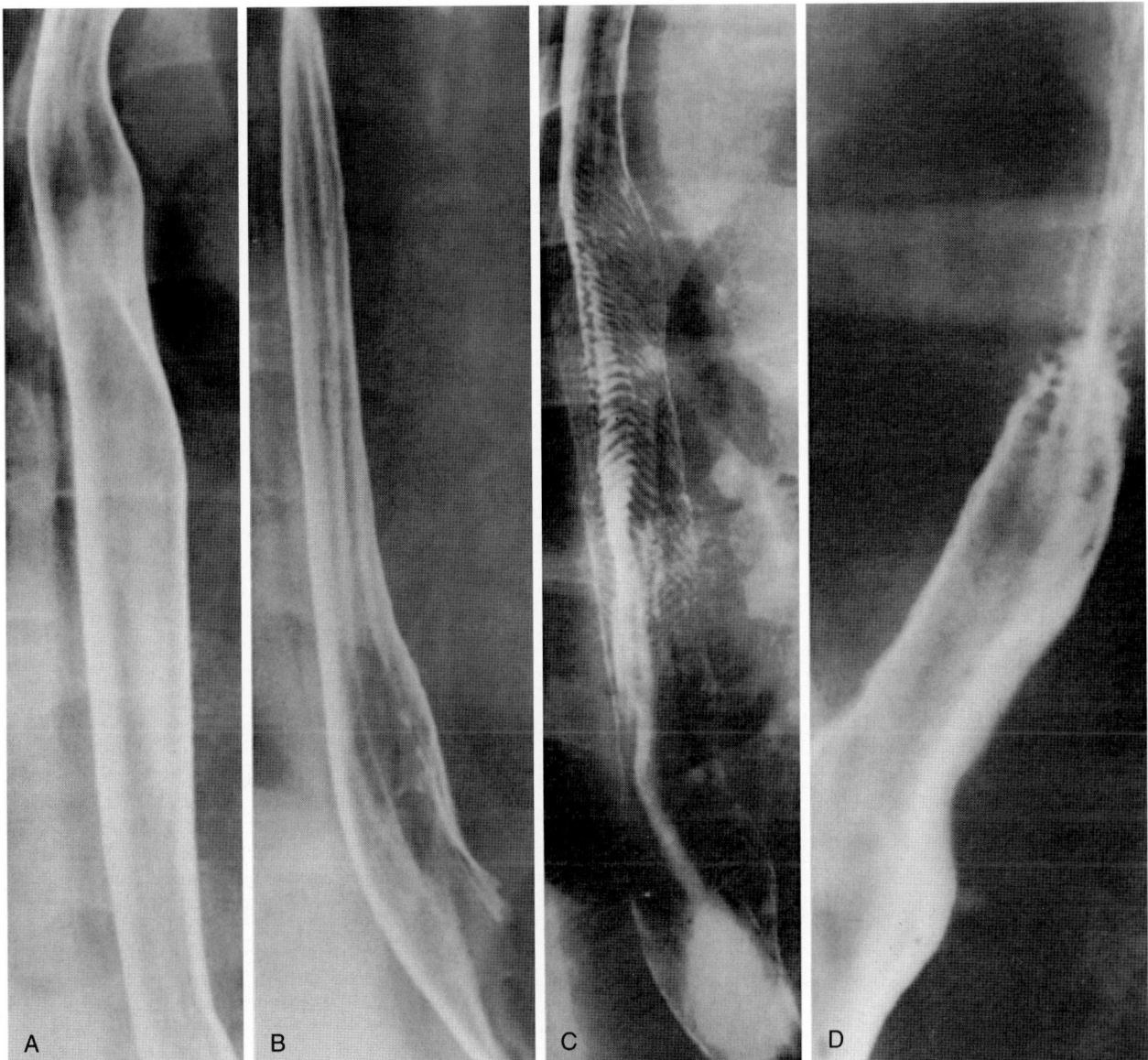

Figure 21-3. Normal esophagus. A. Double-contrast view. In the upright, left posterior oblique projection, the esophagus is thrown off the spine. Note the smooth, featureless appearance of the esophagus. **B.** Longitudinal folds. With the esophagus partially collapsed, the normal longitudinal folds are seen. **C.** Transverse folds. These transverse folds are thought to result from contraction of the longitudinally oriented muscularis mucosae and are often associated with gastroesophageal reflux. **D.** Spiculation of the upper esophagus due to focally prominent transverse folds. (**C** from Gohel VK, Edell SK, Laufer I, et al: Transverse folds in the human esophagus. Radiology 128:303-308, 1978.)

a finding characteristic of heterotopic gastric mucosa (Fig. 21-8B).[17] Still other patients may have a masslike filling defect with a central barium collection at the superior duodenal flexure (Fig. 21-8C). Although the appearance may resemble an ulcer with a surrounding mound of edema or even an ulcerated submucosal mass ("bull's-eye" lesion), this finding actually results from a normal anatomic variant in which there is an infolding of redundant mucosa at the superior duodenal flexure; it has been termed the *duodenal pseudolesion* or *flexural fallacy*.[18] Occasionally, the duodenal bulb contains tiny barium collections (Fig. 21-8D), representing normal pits in the duodenal mucosa that should not be mistaken for duodenal erosions.[19]

In the descending duodenum, the anatomy of the major papilla of Vater is particularly well demonstrated on double-contrast studies.[20] It is usually associated with a longitudinal fold as well as a hooding fold (Fig. 21-9A). The minor papilla is located on the anterior wall of the descending duodenum just proximal to the major papilla and is therefore best seen with the patient in the prone position (Fig. 21-9B).

VARIATIONS IN TECHNIQUE

Anterior Wall Lesions

The routine technique described previously is biased toward detecting lesions on the posterior (i.e., dependent) wall. Lesions on the anterior wall may be seen as ring shadows etched in white on radiographs obtained with the patient in the supine position. However, these lesions are best shown on compression views obtained with the patient in the prone position (Fig. 21-10). Double-contrast examination of the

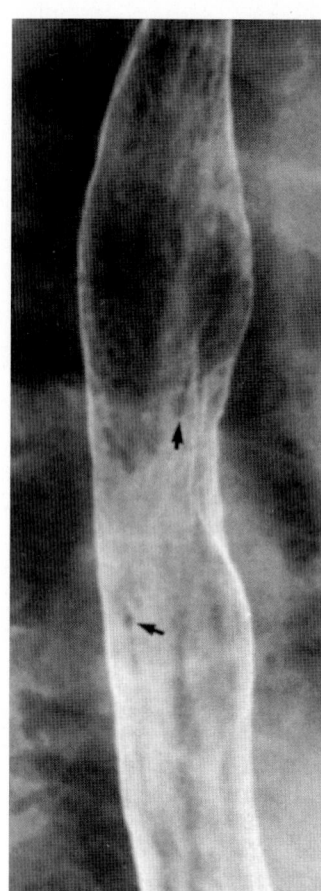

Figure 21-4. Glycogenic acanthosis. Small nodules (*arrows*) are seen on the mucosal surface of the midesophagus in an asymptomatic patient. These nodules result from a benign, degenerative condition known as glycogenic acanthosis.

Figure 21-5. Extrinsic impressions on the esophagus. A. Normal impressions. 1, aortic arch; 2, left main bronchus; 3, heart; 4, esophageal hiatus. **B.** Abnormal extrinsic impression on the posterior wall of the esophagus caused by a thoracic osteophyte.

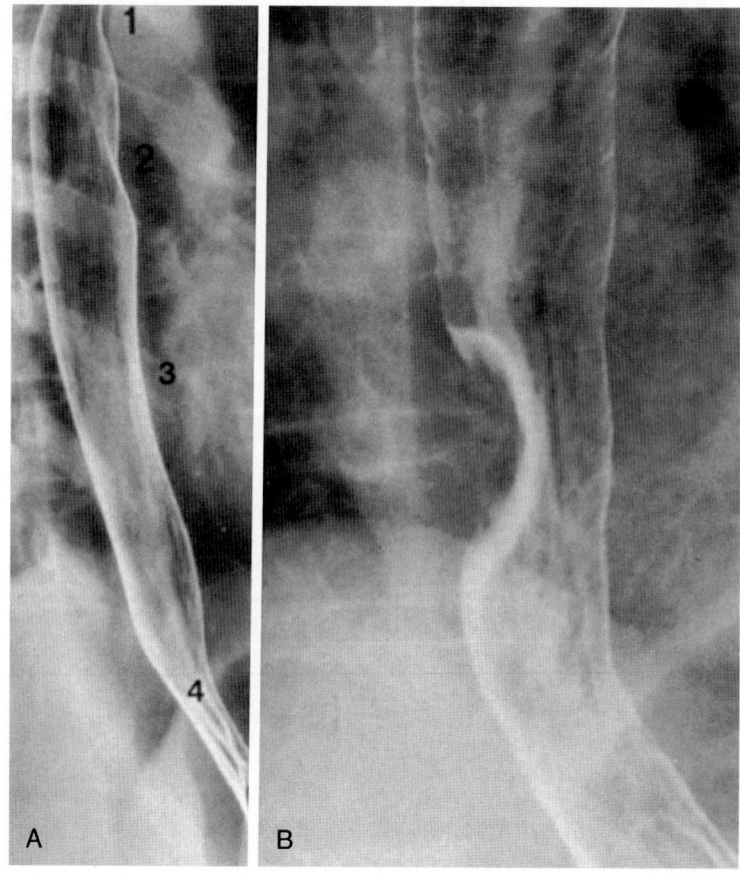

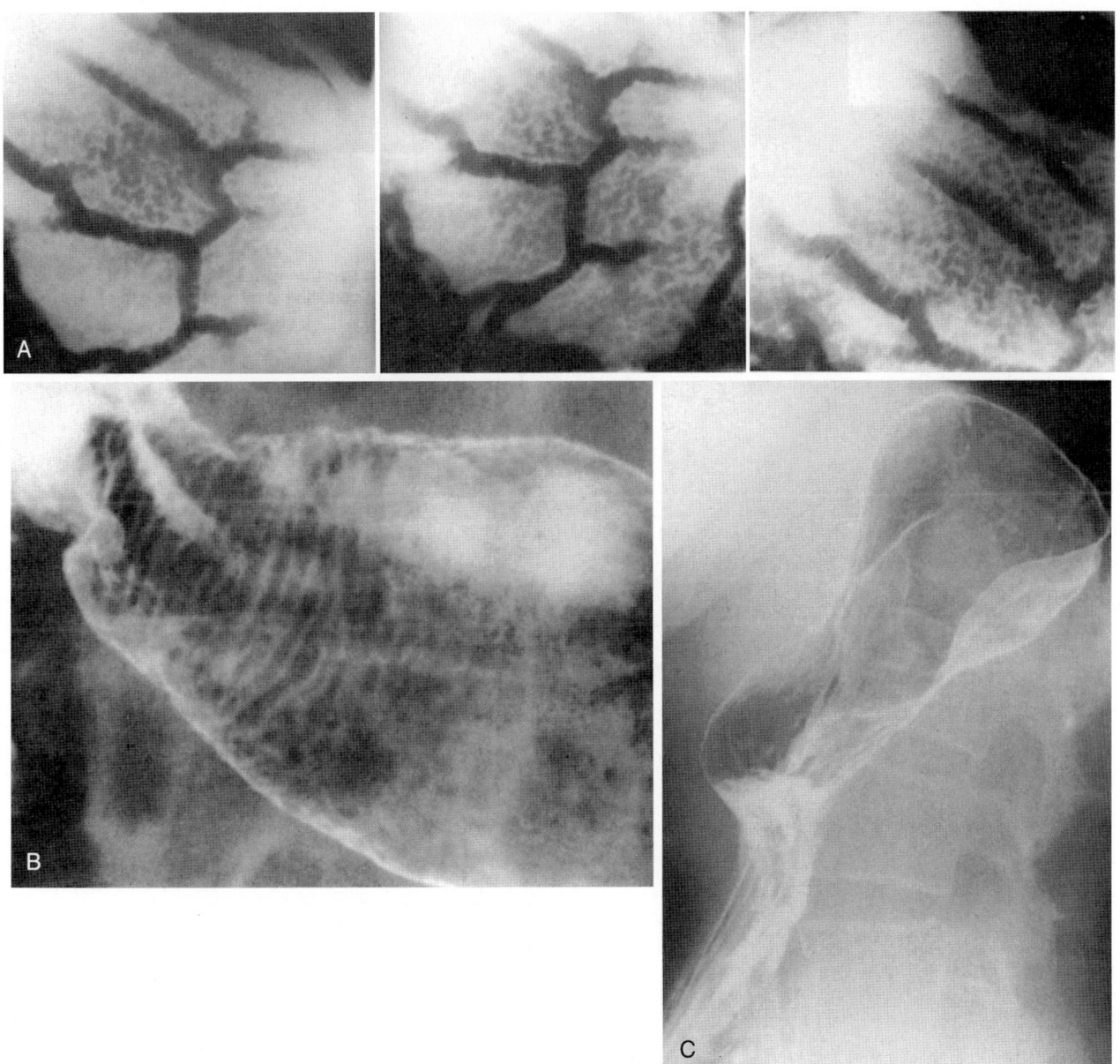

Figure 21-6. Normal surface patterns of the stomach. A. Prone compression views of the stomach with high-density barium show the rugal folds as branching, linear filling defects. Also note the fine reticular pattern of the areae gastricae. (See also Figure 21-1B.) **B.** Gastric striae in the distal antrum. Note the fine transverse folds traversing the distal antrum. **C.** Normal retrogastric impressions in a thin woman.

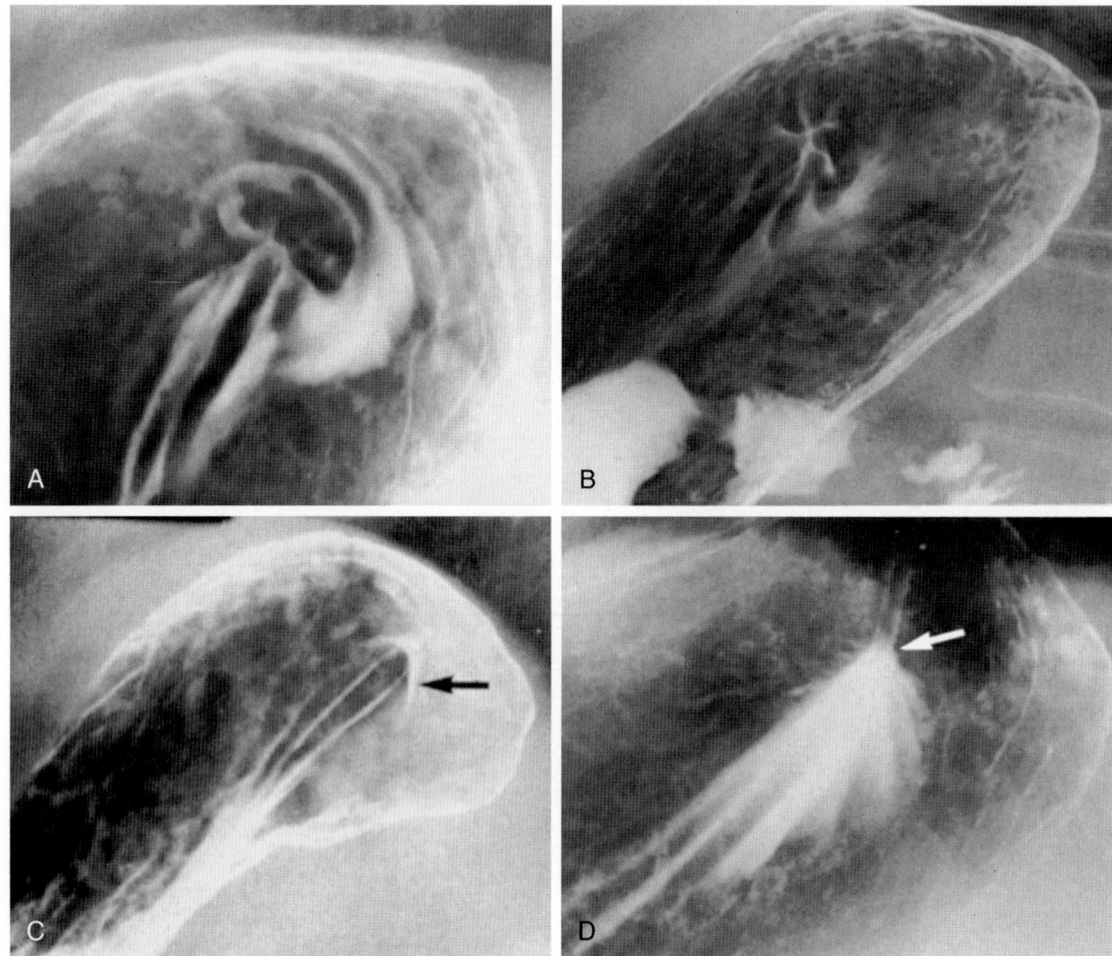

Figure 21-7. Normal cardia and its variations. A. Well-anchored cardia appears as a circular elevation with centrally radiating folds (the cardiac "rosette"). **B.** Stellate folds without the surrounding elevation caused by laxity of the ligamentous attachments. **C.** Further weakening of the ligaments with obliteration of the cardiac rosette. Note the crescentic line (*arrow*) crossing the area of the esophageal orifice. **D.** Severe ligamentous laxity with gastric folds in a small hiatal hernia converging superiorly (*arrow*) above the esophageal hiatus of the diaphragm. (From Laufer I, Levine MS [eds]: Double Contrast Gastrointestinal Radiology, 2nd ed. Philadelphia, WB Saunders, 1992.)

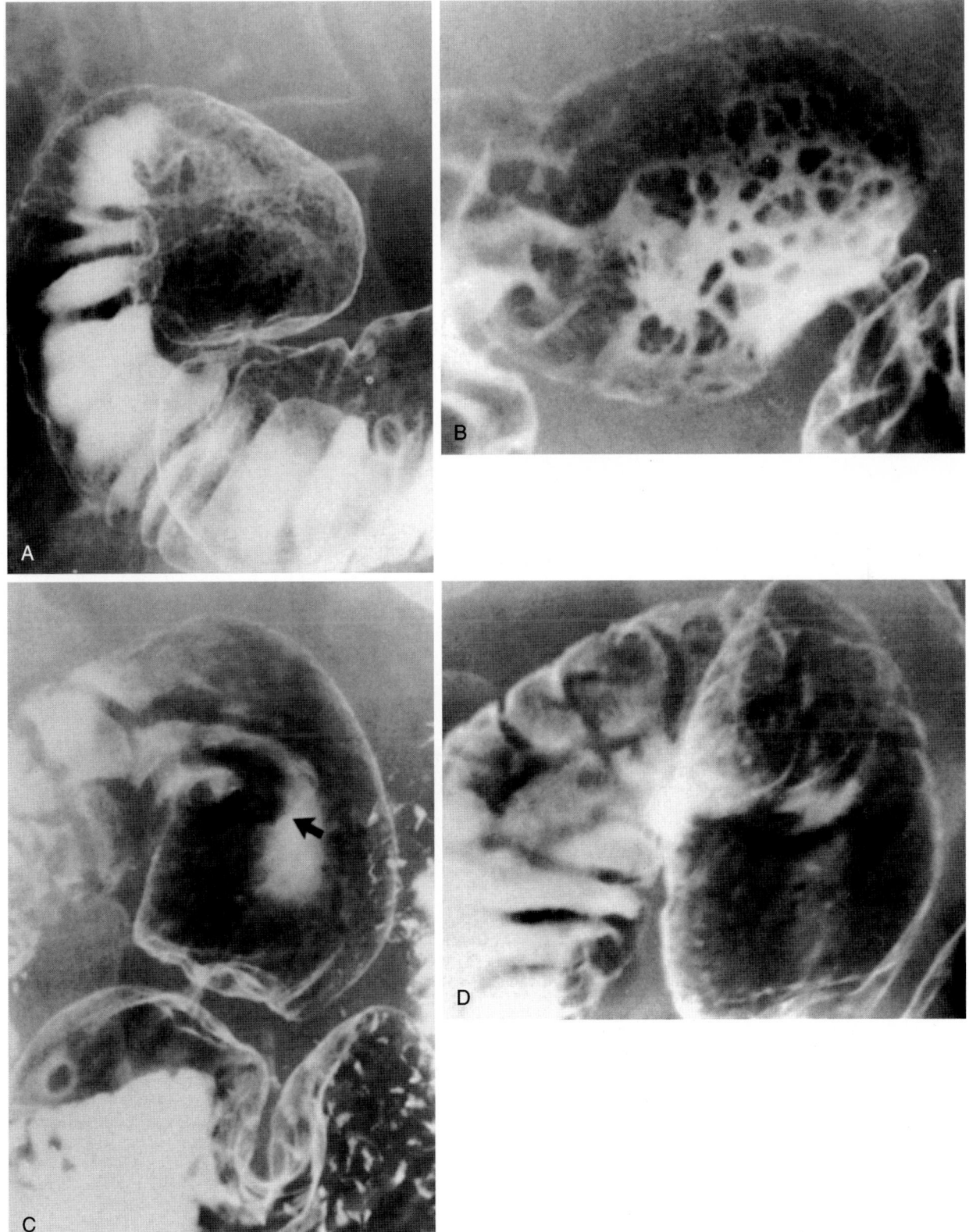

Figure 21-8. Normal surface patterns in the duodenum. A. A fine, velvety pattern is seen in the duodenal bulb. **B.** Angular filling defects represent heterotopic gastric mucosa in the duodenal bulb. **C.** The flexural pseudolesion (*arrow*) results from infolding of a heaped-up area of redundant mucosa at the superior duodenal flexure. **D.** Multiple punctate collections of barium in the duodenal bulb represent normal mucosal pits.

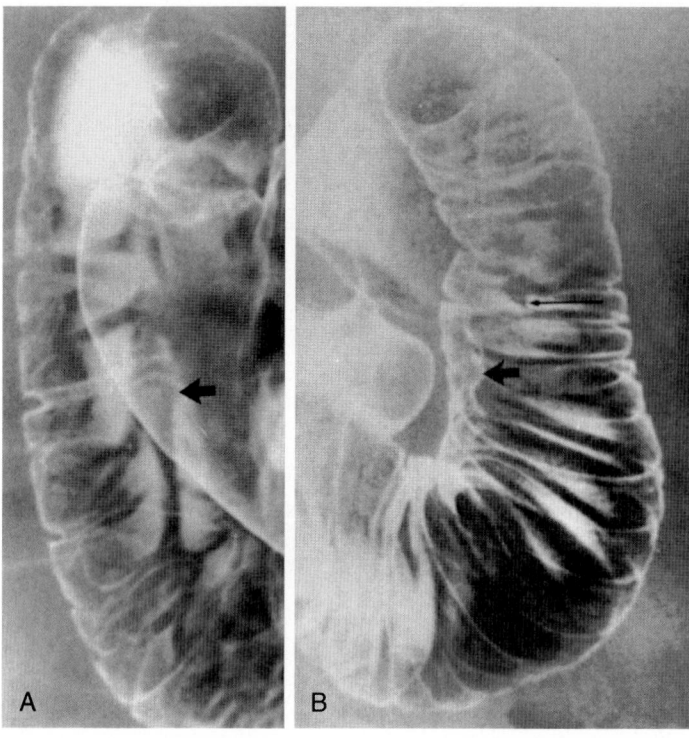

A

B

Figure 21-9. Descending duodenum. A. The descending duodenum is seen through the gas-filled antrum with the patient in the left posterior oblique position. Note the major papilla (*arrow*) and its associated folds. **B.** Prone view shows the major papilla (*short arrow*) on the medial wall of the descending duodenum, with the minor papilla (*long arrow*) seen anteriorly above this level. (**B** from Laufer I, Levine MS [ed]: Double Contrast Gastrointestinal Radiology, 2nd ed. Philadelphia, WB Saunders, 1992.)

Figure 21-10. Examination of the anterior wall of the stomach. The rugal folds on the anterior wall of the stomach are clearly seen with the patient in the prone position. The fundus is filled with gas. (From Laufer I, Levine MS [eds]: Double Contrast Gastrointestinal Radiology, 2nd ed. Philadelphia, WB Saunders, 1992.)

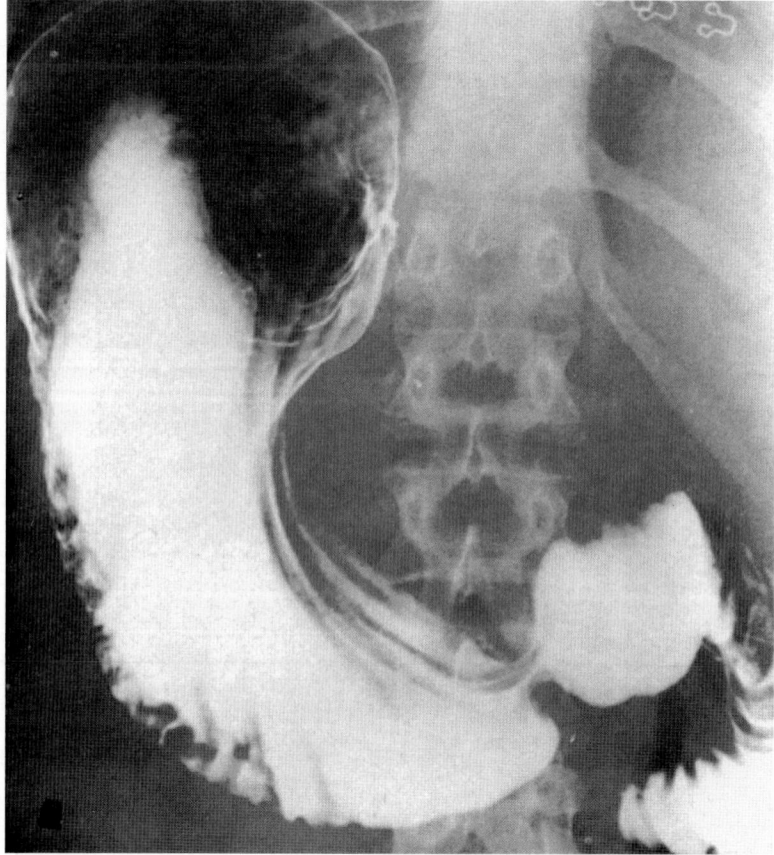

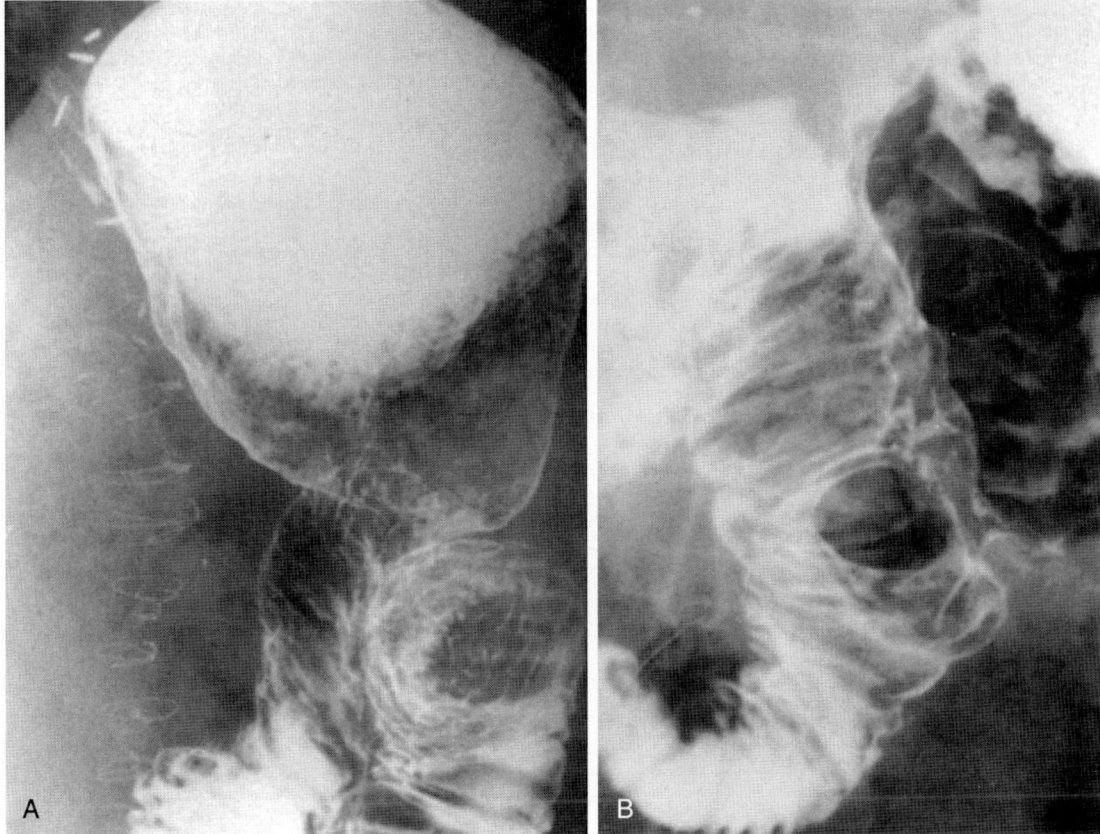

Figure 21-11. Postoperative stomach. A. Double-contrast view showing the normal postoperative appearance after a partial gastrectomy (Billroth II). **B.** Double-contrast view of the gastrojejunal anastomosis after a partial gastrectomy (Billroth II).

anterior wall of the stomach can also be performed with the patient in the prone position, turned slightly onto the left side with the head of the table lowered.[21] Similarly, the anterior wall of the duodenum can be studied by double contrast with the patient in the prone position (see Fig. 21-9B).

Possible Perforation

When a perforation of any portion of the gastrointestinal tract is suspected because of underlying disease, iatrogenic causes, or surgery, a water-soluble contrast agent such as diatrizoate meglumine and diatrizoate sodium (Gastroview; Mallinckrodt, Hazelwood, MO) should be used.[22] If no extravasation is demonstrated, the examination should be completed with barium because the better definition achieved with barium may reveal a small leak that cannot be detected with a water-soluble contrast agent.

After Gastric Resection

After gastric resection for ulcer disease or tumor, the examination must be modified to compensate for the absence of a pylorus (Fig. 21-11).[23] Important modifications include an increase in the dose of glucagon to at least 0.5 mg and a smaller dose of effervescent agent. In addition, the examination should not be started with the patient in the upright position, because rapid emptying of barium in this position may prevent adequate visualization of the gastric remnant. The details of the examination are discussed in Chapter 39.

Gastric Outlet Obstruction

When gastric outlet obstruction is suspected, the patient should initially be examined in the upright position to determine whether there is a fluid level in the stomach. If a fluid level is present, a single-contrast barium study should be performed to determine the site and nature of the obstruction.

Esophageal Varices

Esophageal varices are discussed in detail in Chapter 29. Esophageal varices are typically manifested by thickened, tortuous or serpiginous longitudinal folds and are best demonstrated with the patient in the recumbent position, with the esophageal mucosa coated and the esophagus relaxed.[24]

References

1. Levine MS, Rubesin SE, Herlinger H, et al: Double-contrast upper gastrointestinal examination: Technique and interpretation. Radiology 168:593-602, 1988.
2. Rubesin SE, Herlinger H: The effect of barium suspension viscosity on the delineation of areae gastricae. AJR 146:35-38, 1986.
3. Koehler RE, Weyman PJ, Stanley RJ, et al: Evaluation of three effervescent agents for double-contrast upper gastrointestinal radiography. Gastrointest Radiol 6:111-114, 1981.
4. Moeller G, Hughes JJ, Mangano FA, et al: Comparison of L-hyoscyamine, glucagon, and placebo for air-contrast upper gastrointestinal series. Gastrointest Radiol 17:195-198, 1992.
5. Kastan DJ, Ackerman LV, Feczko PJ: Digital gastrointestinal imaging: The effect of pixel size on detection of subtle mucosal abnormalities. Radiology 167:853-856, 1987.

6. Arenson RL, Chakraborty DP, Seshadri SB, et al: The digital imaging workstation. Radiology 176:303-315, 1990.

7. Levine MS, Laufer I: The gastrointestinal tract: Dos and don'ts of digital imaging (state of the art). Radiology 207:311-316, 1998.

8. Kikuchi Y, Levine MS, Laufer I, et al: Value of flow technique for double-contrast examination of the stomach. AJR 174:1183-1184, 1986.

9. Williams SM, Harned RK, Kaplan P, et al: Transverse striations of the esophagus: Association with gastroesophageal reflux. Radiology 146:25-27, 1983.

10. Levine MS, Low V, Laufer I, et al: Focal spiculation of the upper thoracic esophagus: A normal variant on double-contrast esophagography. Radiology 183:807-810, 1992.

11. Glick SN, Teplick SK, Goldstein J, et al: Glycogenic acanthosis of the esophagus. AJR 139:683-688, 1982.

12. Sam JW, Levine MS, Miller WT: The right inferior supraazygous recess: A cause of upper esophageal pseudomass on double-contrast esophagography. AJR 171:1583-1586, 1998.

13. Mackintosh CE, Kreel L: Anatomy and radiology of the areae gastricae. Gut 18:855-864, 1977.

14. Cho KC, Gold BM, Printz DA: Multiple transverse folds in the gastric antrum. Radiology 164:339-341, 1987.

15. Herlinger H, Grossman R, Laufer I, et al: The gastric cardia in double-contrast study: Its dynamic image. AJR 135:21-29, 1980.

16. Glick SN, Gohel VK, Laufer I: Mucosal surface patterns of the duodenal bulb. Radiology 150:317-322, 1984.

17. Langkemper R, Hoek AC, Dekker W, et al: Elevated lesions in the duodenal bulb caused by heterotopic gastric mucosa. Radiology 137:621-624, 1980.

18. Burrell M, Toffler R: Flexural pseudolesions of the duodenum. Radiology 120:313-315, 1976.

19. Bova JG, Kamath V, Tio FO, et al: The normal mucosal surface pattern of the duodenal bulb: Radiologic-histologic correlation. AJR 145:735-738, 1985.

20. Levine MS, Laufer I, Stevenson G: Duodenum. In Laufer I, Levine MS (eds): Double Contrast Gastrointestinal Radiology, 2nd ed. Philadelphia, WB Saunders, 1992, pp 321-361.

21. Goldsmith MR, Paul RE, Poplack WE, et al: Evaluation of routine double-contrast views of the anterior wall of the stomach. AJR 126:1159-1163, 1976.

22. Dodds WJ, Stewart ET, Vlymen WJ: Appropriate contrast media for evaluation of esophageal disruption. Radiology 144:439-441, 1982.

23. Op den Orth JO: The postoperative stomach. In Laufer I, Levine MS (eds): Double Contrast Gastrointestinal Radiology, 2nd ed. Philadelphia, WB Saunders, 1992, pp 287-320.

24. Cockerill EM, Miller RE, Chernish SM, et al: Optimal visualization of esophageal varices. AJR 126:512-523, 1976.

Motility Disorders of the Esophagus

David J. Ott, MD

Motility disorders of the esophagus are an important cause of esophageal complaints, especially when symptoms are not readily explained by a structural abnormality. An understanding of esophageal anatomy and physiology is required for proper radiographic evaluation of normal and abnormal esophageal function. In this chapter, first a review is provided of the normal anatomy and physiology of the esophagus and then a discussion is presented of the radiographic evaluation of esophageal function. Most of the chapter, is devoted to the various esophageal motility disorders, particularly the primary types. Radiologic efficacy in evaluating esophageal function in relation to esophageal manometry and clinical symptoms is also considered.

NORMAL ESOPHAGEAL ANATOMY

The esophagus is a muscular tube measuring 20 to 24 cm in length, composed of outer longitudinal and inner circular muscle fibers, and lined by stratified squamous epithelium.[1] Striated muscle predominates in the upper esophagus, with smooth muscle in the lower two thirds of the esophagus. The transition from striated to smooth muscle varies but usually occurs at the level of the aortic arch.[1,2] Although this transitional zone is not evident radiographically, certain motility disorders may selectively involve the smooth or striated muscle portions of the esophagus.

Opening and closing of the upper and lower ends of the esophagus are regulated by the upper esophageal sphincter (UES) and the lower esophageal sphincter (LES), respectively. The UES is located at the pharyngoesophageal junction and is formed primarily by the cricopharyngeal muscle, which is the horizontal portion of the inferior pharyngeal constrictor. The LES is not a distinct muscular entity but is defined manometrically as a high-pressure zone measuring 2 to 4 cm in length in the esophagogastric region.[1,3] This physiologic sphincter corresponds in location to the anatomic lower esophageal vestibule.[3,4]

NORMAL ESOPHAGEAL PHYSIOLOGY

In the resting state, the esophageal body is normally collapsed and the UES and LES are closed to prevent retrograde flow of esophageal and gastric contents.[1,5] The major function of the esophagus is the transport of solids and liquids from the oral cavity to the stomach. The chief mechanism of bolus transport is esophageal peristalsis, which is assisted by gravity in the upright position. However, radiographic and manometric evaluation of esophageal peristalsis is usually performed with the patient horizontal to eliminate the effects of gravity.

Primary esophageal peristalsis is initiated by swallowing. A rapid wave of inhibition, not apparent radiographically, is followed by a slower wave of contraction, which traverses the entire esophagus (Fig. 22-1). Relaxation of the UES occurs within 0.2 to 0.3 second of the initiation of swallowing, and relaxation of the LES occurs several seconds later.[1,5,6] The LES remains relaxed as the oncoming bolus approaches the distal esophagus, returning to its resting tone shortly after the bolus reaches the stomach. The primary peristaltic contraction wave propagates through the esophagus in 6 to 8 seconds.

Secondary peristalsis and nonperistaltic contractions are other types of esophageal functional activity.[1,6-9] Secondary peristalsis is similar to primary peristalsis, but it is initiated by local esophageal stimulation or distention. Once initiated, a secondary peristaltic contraction wave propagates aborally similar to primary peristalsis. In contrast, nonperistaltic or

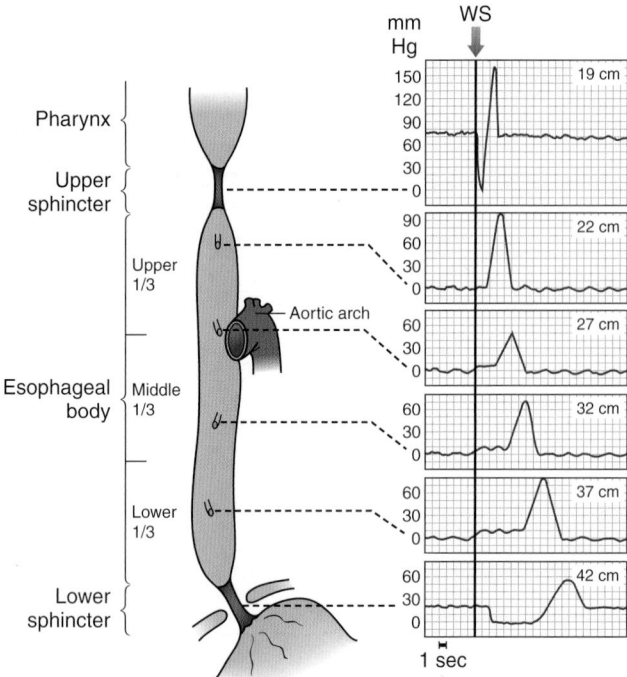

Figure 22-1. Manometric representation of normal esophageal peristalsis. Measurements are taken from multiple recording sites in the esophagus, including the upper esophageal sphincter (UES) and the lower esophageal sphincter (LES). After a wet swallow (WS), UES relaxation is followed almost immediately by prolonged LES relaxation. The primary peristaltic contraction wave is seen as an aborally progressing pressure peak. (From Dodds WJ: Esophagus-radiology. In Margulis AR, Burhenne HJ [eds]: Alimentary Tract Radiology, vol 1, 4th ed. St. Louis, CV Mosby, 1989, p 430.)

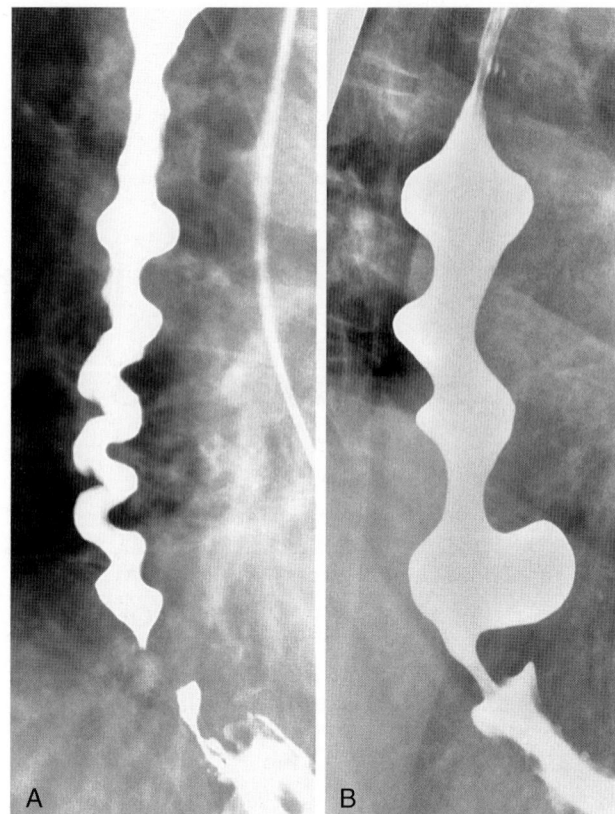

Figure 22-2. Nonperistaltic contractions in the esophagus. A. Barium study of an 89-year-old man with dysphagia but no chest pain. There is diffuse "curling" of the esophagus because of simultaneous nonperistaltic contractions. A nonspecific esophageal motility disorder was diagnosed on manometric examination. **B.** Another elderly man without esophageal symptoms has less severe simultaneous nonperistaltic contractions. (From Ott DJ: Radiologic evaluation of esophageal dysphagia. Curr Probl Diagn Radiol 17:1-33, 1988.)

tertiary contractions are not propagated aborally. They typically involve the smooth muscle segment of the esophagus and may occur spontaneously or during swallowing. Nonperistaltic contractions may be single or multiple, simultaneous or repetitive, and feeble or strong. Severe nonperistaltic contractions may narrow or obliterate the esophageal lumen, producing a characteristic appearance on barium studies (Fig. 22-2). Nonperistaltic contractions may be nonspecific, or they may be related to structural or motility disorders of the esophagus.

Individual variations in esophageal function are primarily related to aging. In young adults, the majority of "wet" swallows will initiate a complete peristaltic sequence, followed invariably by LES relaxation.[10] Nonperistaltic contractions are rare in this age group. However, older patients more often exhibit incomplete peristaltic sequences during swallowing, with occasional LES dysfunction and a higher prevalence and severity of nonperistaltic contractions.[10-13] The amplitude of peristalsis, as recorded manometrically, also decreases with age. Thus, mild functional disturbances of the esophagus that are observed in the elderly must be interpreted with caution and correlated with the clinical findings.

RADIOGRAPHIC EVALUATION

Radiographic evaluation of esophageal motility includes an examination of the esophageal body and both sphincters.[1,4,7-9,14] During swallowing, the UES relaxes and the pharyngoesopha-

geal segment opens in response to bolus distention. Abnormal relaxation or a persistent impression from the cricopharyngeal muscle may be observed in some patients.[8,14] These abnormalities are often associated with other signs of pharyngeal dysmotility, such as aspiration or stasis of barium within the pharyngeal recesses. Motion-recording techniques, using videotape or digital methods, facilitate evaluation of the pharynx and UES.

The fluoroscopic examination is adequate to evaluate esophageal motility, but motion-recording techniques may be used. The patient is placed in the prone right anterior oblique position and is instructed to take single swallows of barium. At least five barium swallows are required for adequate evaluation of esophageal peristalsis and LES relaxation.[4,7-9,15] Single swallows must be observed because a second swallow taken before completion of a primary contraction wave inhibits the propagating wave and may be mistaken for a peristaltic abnormality. Rapid, repetitive swallowing does not assess primary esophageal peristalsis but distends the esophagus maximally for structural evaluation (Fig. 22-3).

As barium is propelled into the esophagus through the relaxed UES, a normal primary peristaltic sequence is seen as an aboral contraction wave that obliterates the esophageal lumen and progressively strips the barium bolus from the esophagus (Fig. 22-4). The lumen-obliterating wave imparts

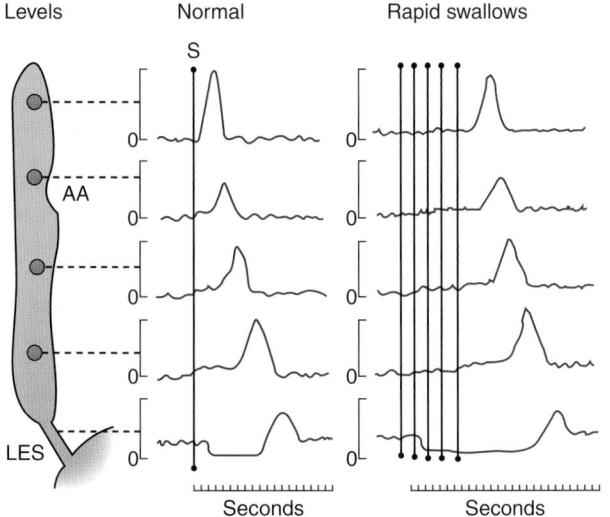

Figure 22-3. Manometric representation of normal esophageal peristalsis. Measurements are taken from multiple recording levels in the esophagus. Rapid swallows cause prolonged lower esophageal sphincter (LES) relaxation but do not generate a primary peristaltic sequence until the final swallow. AA, aortic arch; S, swallow.

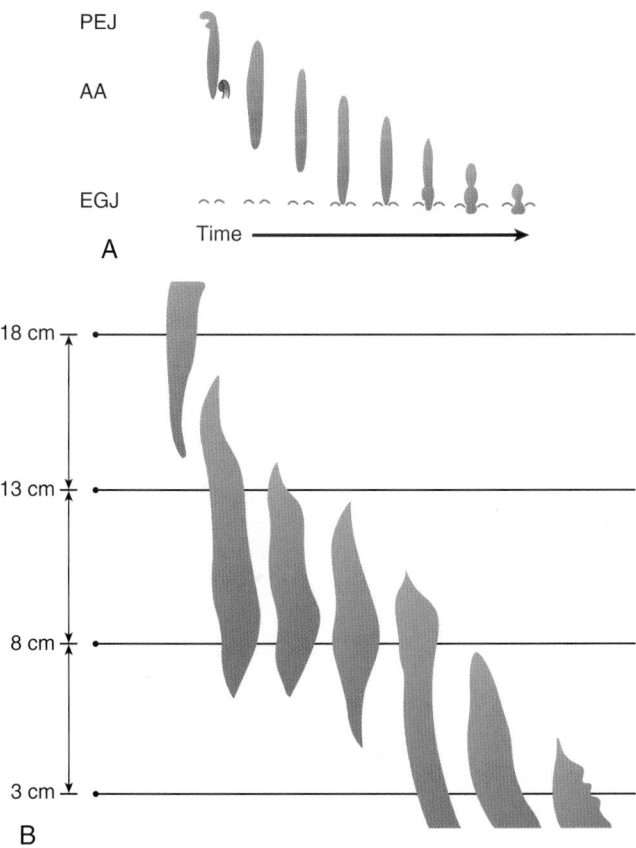

Figure 22-4. Normal primary peristalsis. A. Schematic representation of normal primary peristalsis with a lumen-obliterating contraction wave stripping all of the barium from the esophagus. AA, aortic arch; EGJ, esophagogastric junction; PEJ, pharyngoesophageal junction. **B.** Videotaped temporal tracings of a 5-mL barium bolus at 1-second intervals show normal primary peristalsis. The tapered tops of the barium column correspond to the peristaltic contraction wave seen during synchronous manometry. The numbers on the vertical axis represent the positions of the manometric catheter ports above the LES. (**A** from Ott DJ: Radiologic evaluation of esophageal dysphagia. Curr Probl Diagn Radiol 17:1-33, 1988; **B** from Ott DJ, Chen YM, Hewson EG, et al: Esophageal motility: Assessment with synchronous videotape fluoroscopy and manometry. Radiology 173:419-422, 1989.)

an inverted-V configuration to the top of the barium column, which corresponds to the peristaltic pressure peak seen at manometry. In younger individuals, the peristaltic contraction wave normally strips all of the barium from the esophagus. Occasionally, some proximal escape of barium occurs at the level of the aortic arch (Fig. 22-5). This proximal escape is caused by a low-amplitude pressure trough at the transition between the striated and smooth muscle portions of the esophagus, which prevents closure of the esophageal lumen and allows retrograde flow of barium.[2,6,16] Proximal escape increases with age and can mimic a peristaltic abnormality. True esophageal motility disorders may be manifested by weakened or absent primary peristalsis, nonperistaltic contractions, or associated structural abnormalities in the esophagus.

Radiographic examination of the LES requires evaluation of functional and structural abnormalities.[4,7-9] The LES relaxes shortly after swallowing, and the esophagogastric segment opens widely with bolus distention. In patients with achalasia,

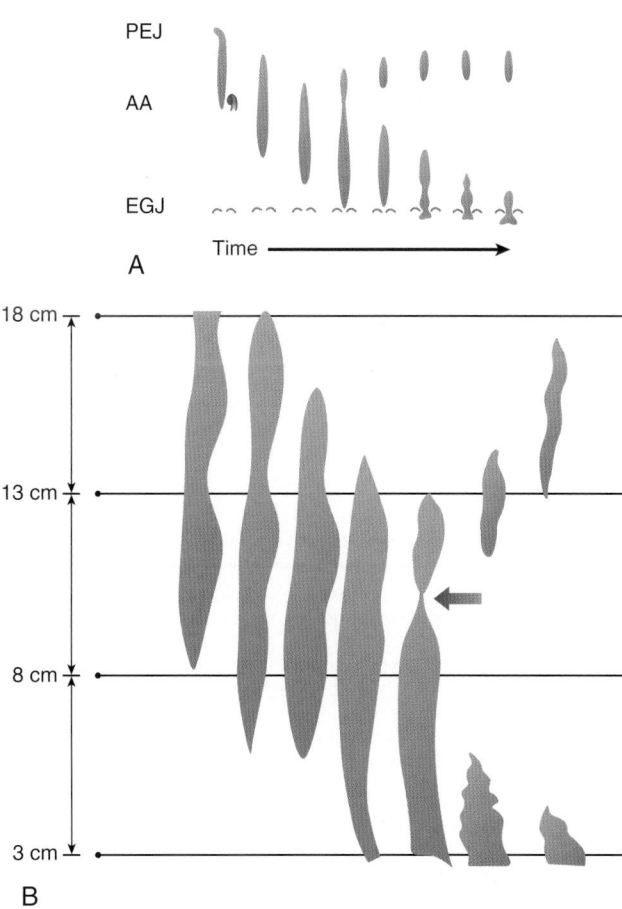

Figure 22-5. Proximal escape. A. Manometric representation shows normal primary peristalsis with proximal escape, as the contraction wave fails to obliterate the lumen completely at the level of the aortic arch (AA). Note that the peristaltic sequence continues aborally. EGJ, esophagogastric junction; PEJ, pharyngoesophageal junction. **B.** Videotaped temporal tracings of a 5-mL barium bolus at 1-second intervals show normal primary peristalsis associated with proximal escape (*arrow*). The lower esophagus is normally stripped of barium below the area of escape. The numbers on the vertical axis represent the positions of the manometric catheter ports above the LES. (**A** from Ott DJ: Radiologic evaluation of esophageal dysphagia. Curr Probl Diagn Radiol 17:1-33, 1988; **B** from Ott DJ, Chen YM, Hewson EG, et al: Esophageal motility: Assessment with synchronous videotape fluoroscopy and manometry. Radiology 173:419-422, 1989.)

incomplete relaxation of the LES produces a smooth, tapered appearance at the lower end of the esophagus because of failure of the esophagogastric junction to distend normally. Mucosal irregularity or nodularity of the esophagogastric region should suggest an inflammatory or neoplastic process, which may cause a secondary motility disorder of the esophagus.

ESOPHAGEAL MOTILITY DISORDERS

Esophageal motility disorders may be classified as primary or secondary types (Table 22-1).[1,5,7-9,17-19] In primary motility disorders, the esophagus is the main or only organ involved. Secondary esophageal motility disturbances result from a wide variety of systemic diseases or from physical or chemical injury of the esophagus. Current clinical classifications of esophageal motility disorders are based on manometric abnormalities and have been recategorized into the following groups: (1) inadequate LES relaxation (classic achalasia); (2) uncoordinated contraction (diffuse esophageal spasm); (3) hypercontraction (nutcracker esophagus; hypertensive LES); and (4) hypocontraction; the latter category would include previous terms such as *nonspecific esophageal motility disorder* and *presbyesophagus* and the manometric abnormalities seen in many of the secondary esophageal motility disorders.[17-19]

The newer clinical classifications provide a better description of the manometric changes observed and may help to direct therapeutic options but still do not clarify the etiology of these motility disorders. Also, many of the criteria used in this classification are based on quantitative manometric findings, which cannot be adequately evaluated on the radiologic examination. Consequently, the older classification will be used in this chapter; however, Table 22-1 also includes the corresponding newer manometric categories in parentheses.

Table 22-1
Classification of Esophageal Motility Disorders

Primary Motility Disorders (newer clinical categories)
Achalasia and variants (inadequate lower esophageal sphincter relaxation)
Diffuse esophageal spasm (uncoordinated contraction)
Nutcracker esophagus (hypercontraction)
Nonspecific esophageal motility disorder (hypocontraction)
Presbyesophagus (questionable entity—hypocontraction)
Hypertensive lower esophageal sphincter (hypercontraction)

Secondary Motility Disorders (many with hypocontraction)
Collagen-vascular disease
Chemical or physical agents
  Reflux esophagitis
  Caustic esophagitis
  Radiation therapy
Infectious causes
Diabetes mellitus
Alcoholism
Endocrine disease
Neuromuscular disorders
  Cerebrovascular disease
  Demyelinating disorders
  Chorea-related disorders
  Myasthenia gravis
  Muscular dystrophies
  Other rare causes
Idiopathic intestinal pseudo-obstruction

Primary Motility Disorders

Achalasia

Achalasia is characterized by aperistalsis and LES dysfunction.[7-9,17-20] The cause of achalasia is unknown, but histologic lesions have been found in the dorsal vagal nucleus, vagal trunks, and myenteric ganglia of the esophagus.[5,20,21] Ganglionic cells are decreased in number in achalasia, but a narrow aganglionic segment is not present, as in Hirschsprung's disease. Thus, achalasia appears to be a neurogenic disorder.

Achalasia is characterized by esophageal dilatation.[5,7-9,18-21] Some patients may develop a massively dilated esophagus, or megaesophagus, which is not specific for achalasia. Changes in smooth muscle are variable; both atrophy and hypertrophy have been described. Secondary stasis esophagitis is common and may be associated with ulceration. Achalasia may also be a precursor of esophageal carcinoma. The association with carcinoma varies, but in one large study, the risk of carcinoma was 9 to 28 times greater than that in the general population.[22]

Achalasia occurs equally in both genders and usually affects patients during the middle decades of life.[5,7,20,21] The typical clinical presentation is slowly progressive dysphagia for both solids and liquids. Painful swallowing and chest pain are less common. Weight loss often occurs in more severe cases. Regurgitation is a common finding, which can lead to pulmonary symptoms such as choking, coughing, aspiration, and pneumonia. If symptoms have a more rapid onset in older patients and are accompanied by chest pain or odynophagia, secondary achalasia due to malignancy is more likely.[7,20,23-25]

Achalasia is characterized manometrically by absence of primary peristalsis, elevated or normal resting LES pressures, and incomplete or absent LES relaxation (Fig. 22-6).[5,7,9,20] Other patients may have variants of achalasia with atypical manometric findings. A debated variant called *vigorous achalasia* is characterized by high-amplitude, simultaneous, and repetitive contractions.[20,26,27] These patients may present with chest pain and have less esophageal dilatation. Another controversial

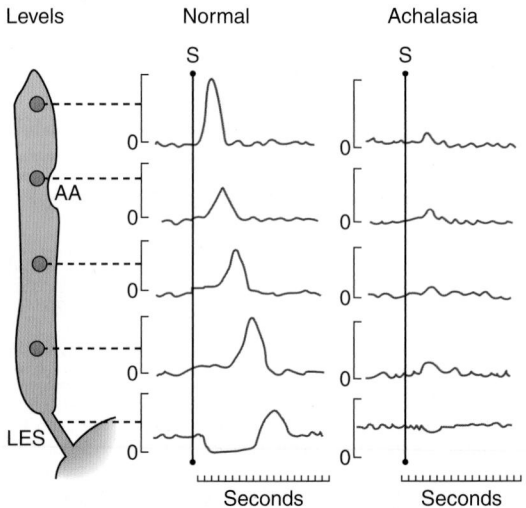

Figure 22-6. Manometric representation of normal peristalsis and achalasia. Measurements are taken from multiple recording levels in the esophagus. In this example of achalasia, peristalsis, and lower esophageal sphincter (LES) relaxation are absent, and LES pressure is elevated. AA, aortic arch; S, swallow.

variant, called *early achalasia,* is characterized by aperistalsis with normal LES relaxation.[28,29] Patients with this variant also have less esophageal dilatation and tend to be younger. Both of these variants may represent part of the spectrum of achalasia or, alternately, transitional motility disorders evolving toward classic achalasia.[30-33]

Radiographically, primary peristalsis is absent on all swallows observed.[1,5,7-9,20] Typically, the lower end of the esophagus has a smooth, tapered, beaklike appearance at the level of the esophageal hiatus (Fig. 22-7). This tapered appearance reflects LES dysfunction and failure of the barium bolus to distend the tonically contracted sphincter. Over time, the esophagus may become markedly dilated and tortuous, producing a sigmoid appearance. Some patients have retained food, secretions, and barium in the dilated esophagus (Fig. 22-8A). Advanced achalasia can sometimes be recognized on chest radiographs when massive esophageal dilatation is present (Fig. 22-8B). In vigorous achalasia, repetitive nonperistaltic contractions may be observed. Radiographic findings in early achalasia are similar to those of classic achalasia, but less esophageal dilatation is present.[29]

Achalasia must be differentiated from other causes of narrowing at the lower end of the esophagus (Table 22-2). Carcinoma of the esophagogastric region must be excluded.[7-9,20,23-25] Although most of these malignancies show mucosal irregularity or mass effect, carcinoma of the gastric cardia and other neoplasms may produce smooth, tapered narrowing of the lower esophagus and aperistalsis, simulating achalasia (i.e.,

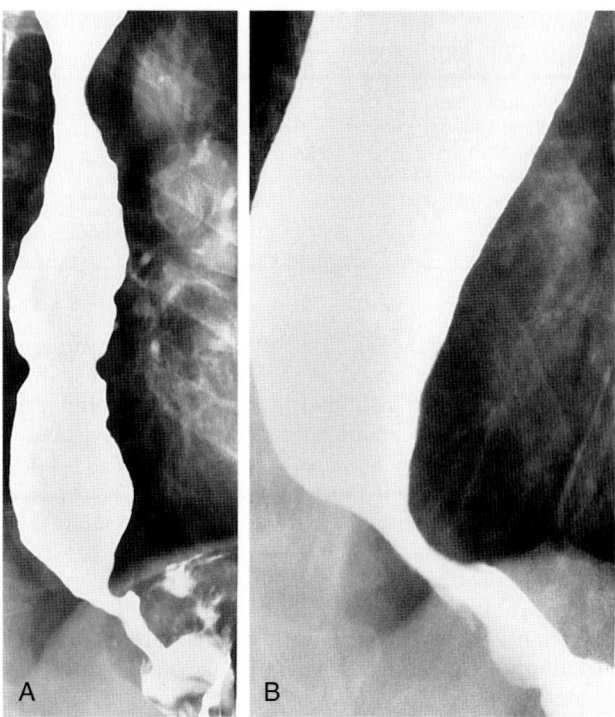

Figure 22-7. Achalasia. A. There is a dilated esophagus with smooth, tapered narrowing at the esophagogastric region. Esophageal aperistalsis was seen at fluoroscopy. **B.** Close-up view shows smooth, beaklike tapering at the lower end of the esophagus due to LES dysfunction.

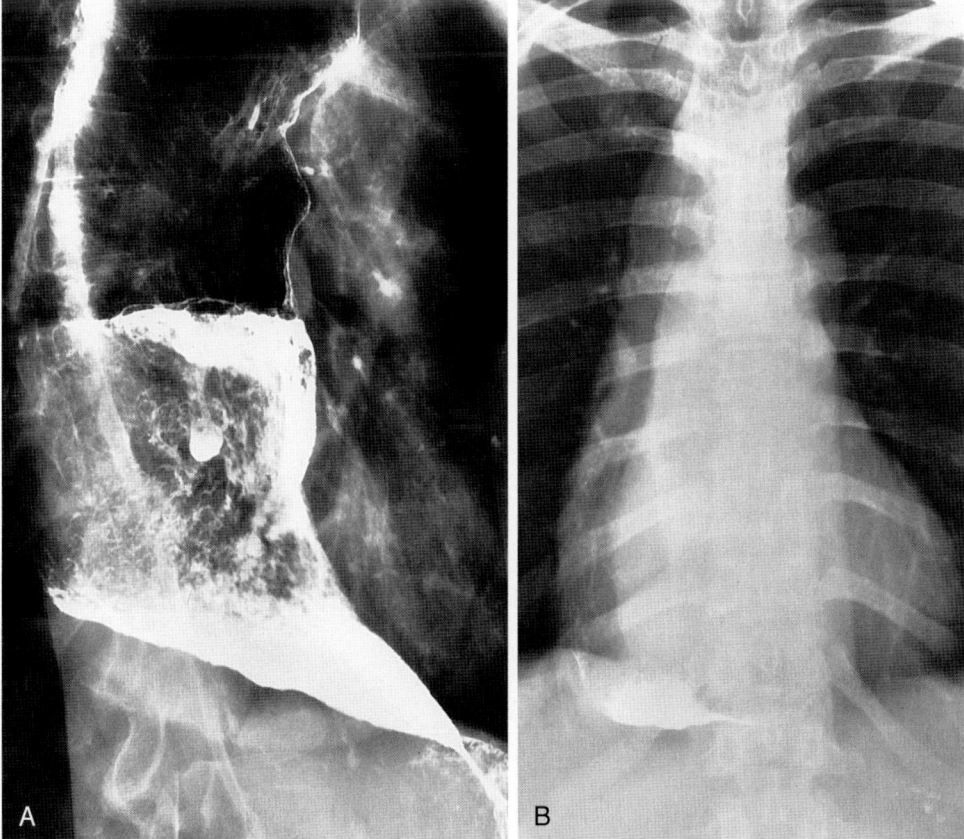

Figure 22-8. Advanced achalasia. A. There is a markedly dilated esophagus with retained secretions and food. **B.** A double contour of the right mediastinal border is seen in another patient with advanced achalasia. The outer border represents the dilated esophagus projecting beyond the shadows of the aorta and heart. A small amount of retained barium is present in the distal esophagus.

Table 22-2
Differential Diagnosis of Achalasia

Intrinsic neoplasms
Extrinsic neoplasms
Peptic stricture
Complicated scleroderma
Intestinal pseudo-obstruction
Chagas' disease
Postvagotomy effect

secondary achalasia) (Fig. 22-9). Peptic strictures are rarely associated with aperistalsis, and these patients almost always have hiatal hernias, a rare finding in achalasia.[34] Uncomplicated scleroderma can also be differentiated from achalasia, because it is characterized by a dilated esophagus with a patulous esophagogastric region. Occasionally, however, peptic strictures complicating scleroderma may produce an appearance resembling achalasia.

Achalasia is treated by pneumatic dilatation, laparoscopic myotomy, or botulinum toxin injection.[5,8,20,35-39] Radiographic evaluation of the esophagus immediately after pneumatic dilatation is helpful in detecting serious complications such as perforation.[20,36,40-44] After a Heller myotomy, a wide-mouthed outpouching or sacculation is typically present at the lower end of the esophagus (Fig. 22-10A). The treatment of achalasia may also be complicated by reflux esophagitis and subsequent peptic strictures (Fig. 22-10B); a "loose" fundoplication may be performed with a laparoscopic myotomy to prevent these complications.[20,36,37]

Radionuclide studies and timed barium swallows may aid the diagnosis and management of patients with achalasia.[20,28,29,45-48] Radionuclide transit and emptying studies are particularly helpful in quantitating esophageal retention before and after therapy. Timed barium swallows are simple to perform and provide results similar to those of radionuclide emptying studies.[45]

Diffuse Esophageal Spasm

Diffuse esophageal spasm (DES) is an uncommon motility disorder characterized by chest pain, which is often accompanied by dysphagia, and intermittently abnormal esophageal motility.[5,7-9,17,18,49] Although the cause of DES is unknown, a transition to other types of motility disorders has occasionally been described. DES, achalasia, and vigorous achalasia may be part of a spectrum of abnormal esophageal motility that is related to varying degrees of neurogenic damage.[17,18,30-33]

DES typically involves the smooth muscle portion of the esophagus. Pathologically, the esophageal musculature may be normal or markedly thickened because of hypertrophy.[50-52] However, some investigators have found that muscle thickening is rare in DES.[53,54] DES usually does not involve the LES, although transitional disorders may occur.[5,7,17,49]

The most common clinical presentation of DES is chest pain, often accompanied by dysphagia.[5,17,18,49,54] Radiation of pain to the shoulder or back may simulate angina and may even be relieved by nitroglycerin. The pain is often spontaneous and not related to swallowing, and it can worsen during emotional stress. Other patients with DES may have dysphagia

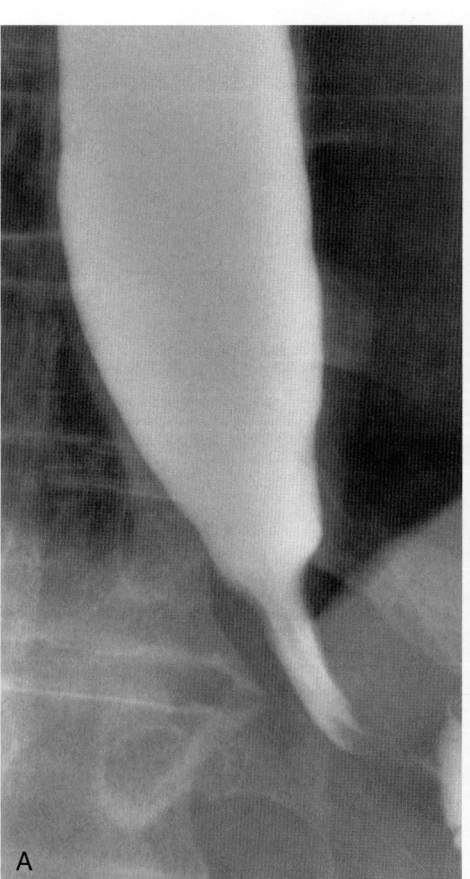 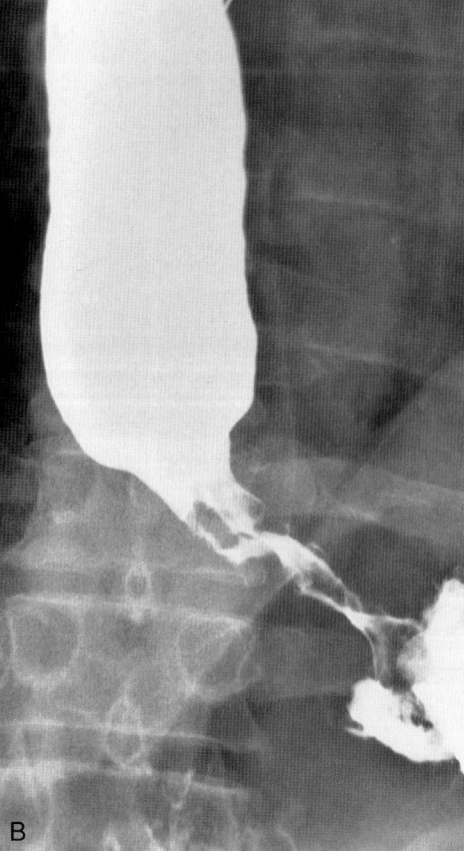

A   B

Figure 22-9. Secondary achalasia or pseudoachalasia. A. Smooth narrowing of the esophagogastric junction simulates achalasia. This patient had a scirrhous carcinoma of the proximal stomach invading the distal esophagus. **B.** Fluoroscopy in another patient revealed esophageal dilatation and aperistalsis. However, there is irregular tapering of the esophagogastric region due to gastric carcinoma. (**A** from Ott DJ: Radiologic evaluation of esophageal dysphagia. Curr Probl Diagn Radiol 17:1-33, 1988.)

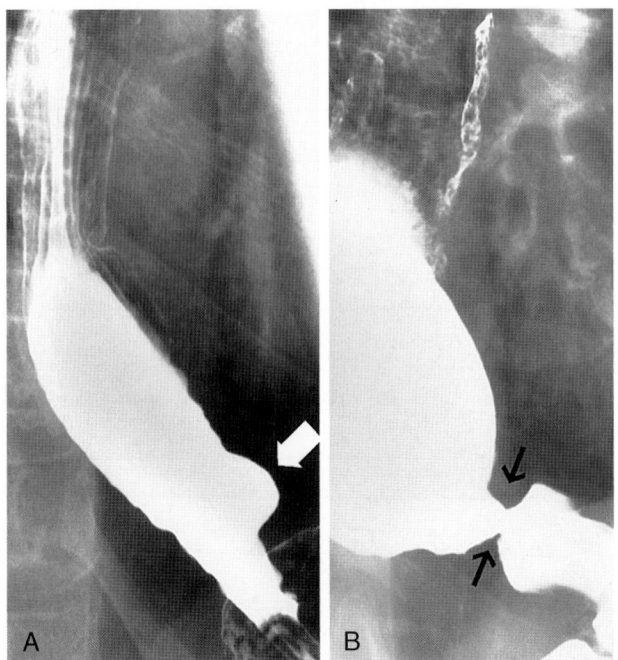

Figure 22-10. Complications of a Heller myotomy. A. A deformity (*arrow*) resembling a diverticulum is seen in this patient after a Heller myotomy for achalasia. **B.** A stricture (*arrows*) is present in the distal esophagus after a Heller myotomy in another patient with achalasia. The stricture was confirmed by endoscopy.

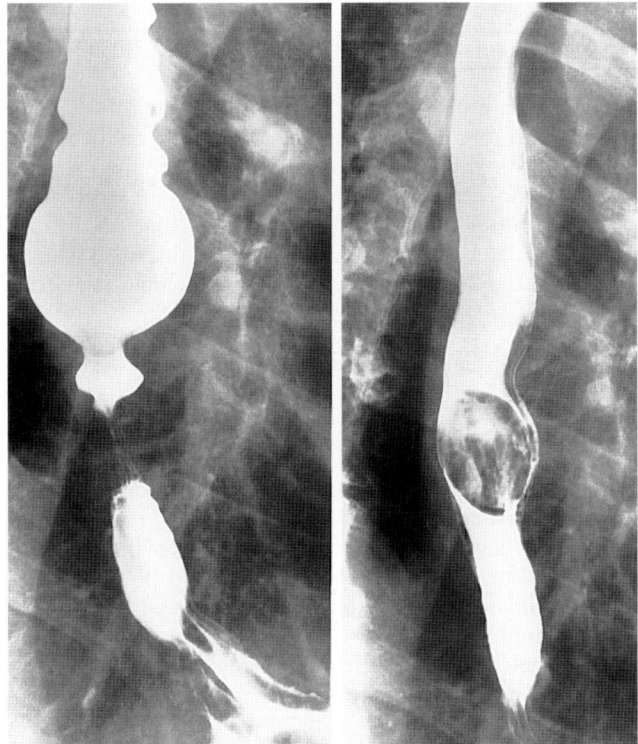

Figure 22-11. Diffuse esophageal spasm. This patient with diffuse esophageal spasm complained of acute odynophagia after ingestion of a hot dog. On the left, an obliterative contraction of the lower esophagus obscures the food bolus. On the right, another radiograph obtained moments later shows a piece of the hot dog. Endoscopic removal was required.

for solids or liquids without associated chest pain. Food impaction is a dramatic but unusual feature of DES (Fig. 22-11).

The major manometric criteria for DES are simultaneous contractions on more than 10% of wet swallows and intermittently normal primary peristalsis.[5,7,17,18] Associated findings include repetitive or prolonged-duration contractions, high-amplitude contractions, and frequent spontaneous contractions (Fig. 22-12). Some patients with DES have normal LES function, but others have incomplete LES relaxation during swallowing.[17,18,49]

The radiographic features of DES reflect the manometric findings.[1,7-9,49,54] Primary peristalsis is present in the cervical esophagus but intermittently absent in the thoracic esophagus. Nonperistaltic contractions affect the smooth muscle portion of the esophagus, replacing the disrupted primary wave (Fig. 22-13A). These contractions are often repetitive and simultaneous, and, if severe, they may compartmentalize the esophageal lumen, producing the classic "corkscrew" or "rosary bead" appearance (Fig. 22-13B). Coexisting pulsion diverticula may be present. Other patients have beaklike narrowing of the distal esophagus due to incomplete opening of the LES.[49]

Muscular thickening of the esophagus is uncommon in DES, but a wall thickness of 2 cm or more is occasionally seen (normal wall thickness is <4 mm).[50,51,53,54] Thickening of the esophageal wall is best estimated along the right border of the esophagus, where the wall is close to the pleural reflection line. Alternately, wall thickness can be measured directly by CT or endoscopic ultrasound.[51-53]

The radiographic findings in DES can be nonspecific, so that correlation with clinical symptoms and esophageal manometry is required. Also, neoplastic or inflammatory lesions involving the esophagogastric region may cause a secondary motility disorder that mimics DES. Similar radiographic findings are observed in other motility disorders and may sometimes occur in asymptomatic patients. Thus,

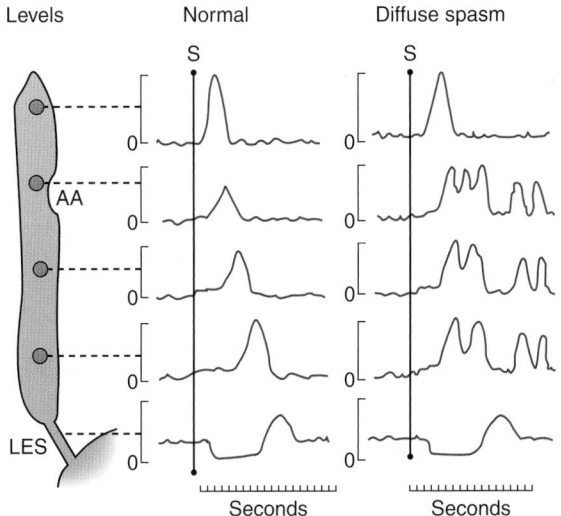

Figure 22-12. Manometric representation of normal peristalsis and diffuse esophageal spasm. Measurements are taken from multiple recording levels in the esophagus. Normal peristalsis is present in the upper esophagus, but it is replaced by simultaneous, repetitive contractions below the aortic arch (AA). Normal lower esophageal sphincter (LES) relaxation is seen. S, swallow.

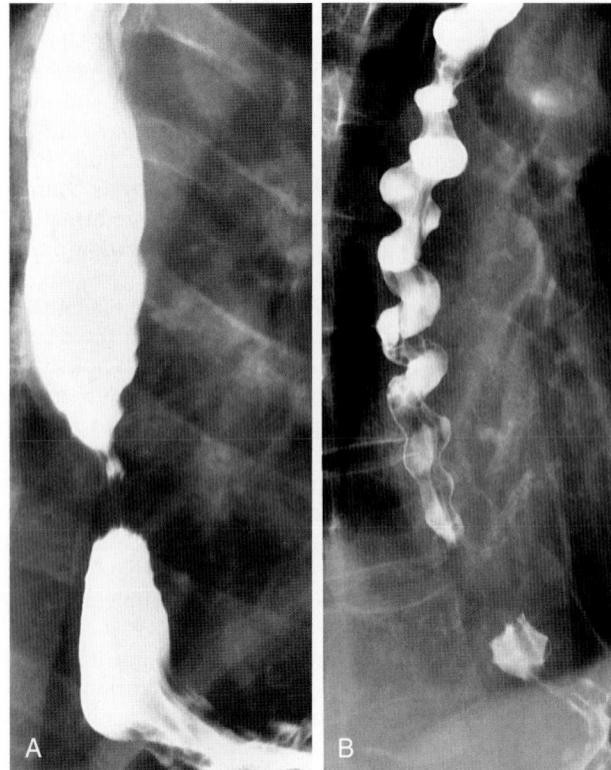

Figure 22-13. Diffuse esophageal spasm. A. This patient has diffuse esophageal spasm with intermittent disruption of primary peristalsis associated with focally obliterative simultaneous contractions. **B.** Another patient has the typical "corkscrew" or "rosary bead" appearance of diffuse esophageal spasm. Clinical and manometric correlations are required to confirm the diagnosis because this appearance is nonspecific, especially in the elderly. (From Levine MS, Rubesin SE, Ott DJ: Update on esophageal radiology. AJR 155:933-941, 1990, © by American Roentgen Ray Society.)

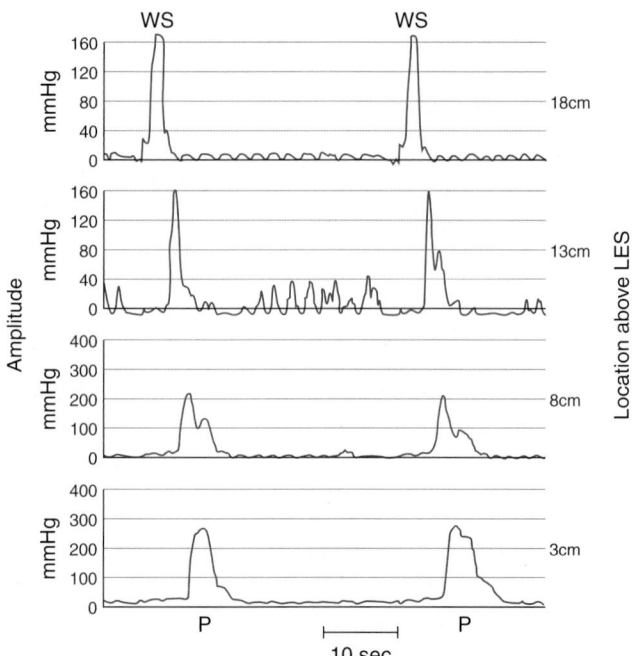

Figure 22-14. Manometric representation of nutcracker esophagus. This patient had a normal radiographic examination. There is normal peristalsis (P) manometrically with high-amplitude contractions (>200 mm Hg, lower two leads). Accentuated baseline activity in the 13-cm lead is cardiac artifact. LES, lower esophageal sphincter; WS, wet swallow. (Redrawn from Ott DJ, Richter JE, Chen YM, et al: Esophageal radiography and manometry: Correlation in 172 patients with dysphagia. AJR 149: 307-311, 1987, © by American Roentgen Ray Society.)

the diagnosis of DES is based on clinical, radiographic, and manometric findings.

Nutcracker Esophagus

Nutcracker esophagus is an esophageal motility disorder seen in some patients with chest pain or dysphagia.[5,7,17,18,55-57] Manometric examination shows normal peristalsis with distal contractions of abnormally high amplitude and prolonged duration. Nutcracker esophagus emerged as a potentially important motility disorder with the increasing referral of patients with noncardiac chest pain for esophageal manometry. However, debate has arisen over whether nutcracker esophagus is a motility disorder, a result of improved manometric instrumentation, or part of the normal spectrum of esophageal function.[5,17,18,55-61]

The specific manometric criteria for nutcracker esophagus include the presence of normal peristalsis with high-amplitude distal esophageal peristaltic contractions greater than 2 SD from normal and with prolonged duration of these contractions.[5,17,18] In our manometric laboratory, the normal mean distal esophageal amplitude is 100 ± 80 mm Hg (± 2 SD).[62] The diagnosis of nutcracker esophagus therefore requires peristaltic contractions with average amplitudes greater than 180 mm Hg (Fig. 22-14). The term *high-amplitude peristaltic*

esophageal contractions has also been used to describe this entity.

Nutcracker esophagus is a manometric diagnosis made in patients with appropriate symptoms. The radiographic examination is normal or reveals only nonspecific findings such as nonperistaltic contractions.[63,64] In addition, esophageal transit is normal, despite some controversy regarding the results of radionuclide studies in patients with this disorder.[65-69] Nutcracker esophagus is therefore not a radiologic diagnosis.

Nonspecific Esophageal Motility Disorder

Nonspecific esophageal motility disorder (NEMD) is a "catchall" category used in patients with motility disturbances that are unclassified.[5,7,17,18] Often, manometry reveals esophageal motility abnormalities that do not fit the criteria for specific motility disorders such as achalasia.[5,17,18,70,71] Patients with NEMD may have dysphagia or chest pain, but symptoms may be minimal or absent. These patients would now be classified as having hypocontraction abnormalities on manometric examination.[5,17,18]

Manometric abnormalities are mainly of the hypocontraction type and include intermittent absence of peristalsis on 20% or more of wet swallows, low-amplitude peristalsis, prolonged duration of peristalsis, repetitive or triple-peaked contractions, or incomplete LES relaxation (Fig. 22-15).[17,18,70] Radiographic findings may reflect these manometric abnormalities.[7-9] Disruption of primary peristalsis and nonperistaltic contractions are typically seen (Fig. 22-16). However, the radiographic examination is often normal in patients with

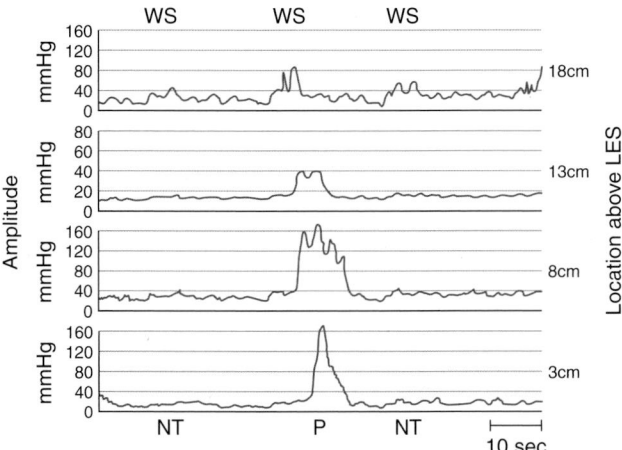

Figure 22-15. Manometric representation of nonspecific esophageal motility disorder. There is nontransmitted peristalsis (NT) in the lower leads and repetitive contractions during transmitted peristalsis (P). LES, lower esophageal sphincter; WS, wet swallow. (Redrawn from Ott DJ, Richter JE, Chen YM, et al: Esophageal radiography and manometry: Correlation in 172 patients with dysphagia. AJR 149:307-311, 1987, © by American Roentgen Ray Society.)

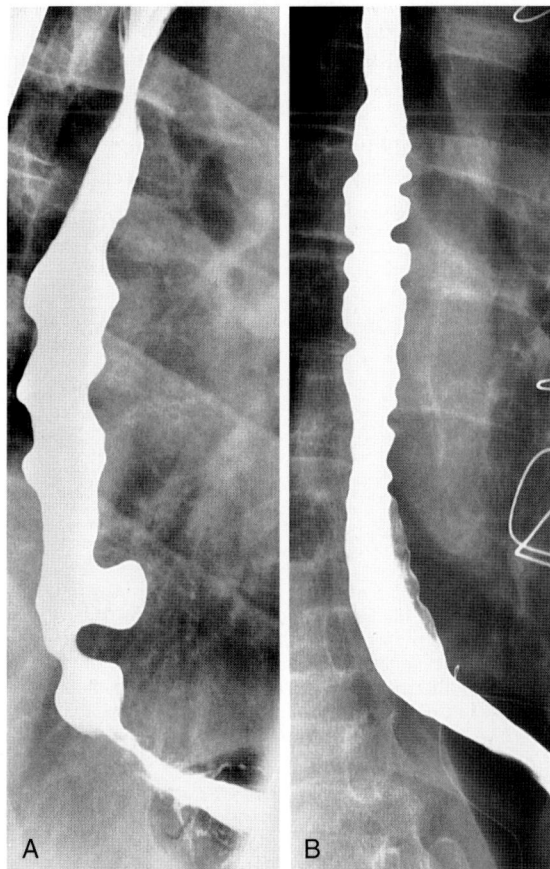

Figure 22-16. Nonspecific esophageal motility disorder. A. This asymptomatic patient had simultaneous nonperistaltic contractions. Primary peristalsis was disrupted intermittently at fluoroscopy. Nonspecific esophageal motility disorder was diagnosed by manometry. **B.** Multiple nonperistaltic contractions and disrupted primary peristalsis are seen in another patient with nonspecific esophageal motility disorder. Clinical and manometric correlations are needed to distinguish this appearance from that of diffuse esophageal spasm. (From Levine MS, Rubesin SE, Ott DJ: Update on esophageal radiology. AJR 155:933-941, 1990, © by American Roentgen Ray Society.)

NEMD who have only minor manometric abnormalities.[7-9] The nonspecific abnormalities identified radiographically may also overlap the findings seen in other motility disorders.

Presbyesophagus

Presbyesophagus has become a controversial entity.[7-9,11-14,72,73] As originally described, the term *presbyesophagus* referred to esophageal motility dysfunction associated with aging.[72,73] The major manometric criteria included decreased frequency of normal peristalsis, increased frequency of nonperistaltic contractions, and, less commonly, incomplete LES relaxation. These manometric changes are reflected by a wide spectrum of radiographic abnormalities. However, in early reports of presbyesophagus, many of the older patients had underlying neurologic disorders or diabetes, which could have accounted for their esophageal dysmotility. Later manometric studies in older patients have shown only minor changes in esophageal motility with aging.[11-13] Furthermore, many of the manometric criteria for presbyesophagus are similar to those for *NEMD*, which is the preferred radiologic term for esophageal dysfunction in these patients (*hypocontraction disorder* is the preferred manometric term).

Hypertensive Lower Esophageal Sphincter

Hypertensive LES was first described in patients with esophageal symptoms who had unusually high resting LES pressures.[5,17,18,74] Nearly all patients have chest pain, and many also have dysphagia. The reported manometric criteria have usually included a resting LES pressure greater than 40 mm Hg with normal LES relaxation and esophageal peristalsis. Results of radiographic evaluation, including radionuclide emptying studies, are usually normal.[74] Like nutcracker esophagus, hypertensive LES is a manometric diagnosis.

Secondary Motility Disorders

The causes of secondary esophageal motility disorders are numerous and varied (see Table 22-1).[1,7-9,17-19,75] The radiographic findings of these disorders are nonspecific and are often similar to those described for NEMD; also, many of these disorders would now be placed in the manometric category of hypocontraction abnormalities. Thus, clinical correlation is critical for the proper diagnosis of secondary esophageal motility disorders.

Collagen Vascular Diseases

Collagen vascular diseases have multisystemic involvement with immunologic and inflammatory changes in connective tissue. The esophagus may be affected by many of these collagen diseases, but it is most often involved by scleroderma, mixed connective tissue disease, dermatomyositis, and polymyositis.[17-19,75,76] Although these diseases produce similar manometric and radiologic abnormalities, diseases other than scleroderma may involve the striated muscle portion of the esophagus.

Scleroderma is characterized by fibrosis and degenerative changes in the skin, synovium, and parenchyma of multiple organs, including the esophagus. Esophageal involvement occurs in most patients with scleroderma, with the smooth

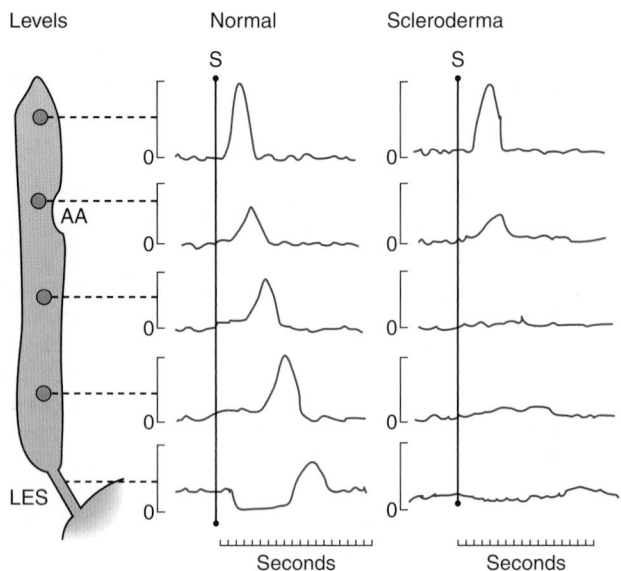

Figure 22-17. Manometric representation of normal peristalsis and scleroderma. Measurements are taken from multiple recording levels in the esophagus. Normal peristalsis is present in the upper esophagus with absence of peristalsis in the smooth muscle segment. The lower esophageal sphincter (LES) also shows low resting pressure. AA, aortic arch; S, swallow.

muscle segment and LES predominantly affected.[17-19,75-78] Because of LES incompetence, symptoms of gastroesophageal reflux are common, and dysphagia may result from abnormal motility, reflux esophagitis, or peptic strictures. Manometric features of scleroderma include decreased or absent resting LES pressure and weakened or absent peristalsis in the lower two thirds of the esophagus (Fig. 22-17).[17-19,75,76] These abnormalities are manifested radiographically by absent peristalsis in the smooth muscle portion of the esophagus, the presence of a hiatal hernia, and findings related to the development of reflux esophagitis and peptic strictures (Fig. 22-18).

Other Secondary Motility Disorders

A variety of conditions may be associated with motility disorders in the esophagus. Of the infectious causes, Chagas' disease has the most specific appearance.[5,17-19] It occurs primarily in South America and is caused by the protozoan *Trypanosoma cruzi*. The disease affects multiple organs, including the myenteric plexus of the gastrointestinal tract, and it produces esophageal abnormalities identical to those in achalasia.

A variety of metabolic and endocrine disorders may also affect esophageal motor function. In diabetic patients with peripheral neuropathy, manometric and radiographic abnormalities of the esophagus are common.[5,17-19] The most frequent radiologic findings include decreased primary peristalsis, increased nonperistaltic contractions, mild esophageal dilatation, and a hiatal hernia with gastroesophageal reflux. Esophageal dysmotility is also common in alcoholic patients, even in the absence of esophagitis and neuropathy. The functional abnormalities seen in the esophagus may be reversed by withdrawal of alcohol.[79]

Esophageal motility may also be affected by a variety of neuromuscular disorders, which can affect the pharynx and upper esophagus. Finally, idiopathic intestinal pseudo-

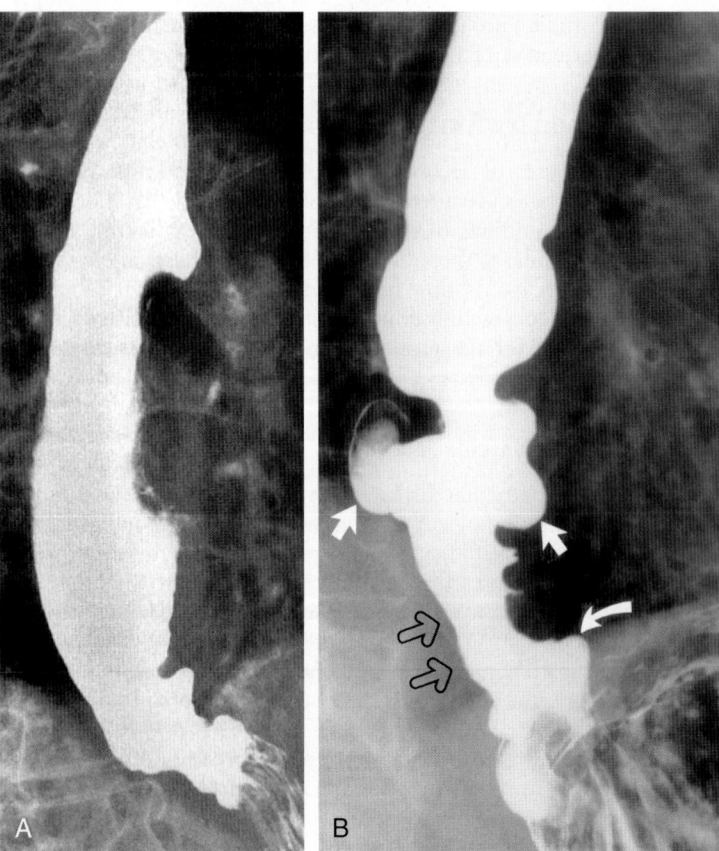

Figure 22-18. Esophageal involvement by scleroderma. A. This patient has a dilated esophagus and a patulous esophagogastric junction. There was aperistalsis at fluoroscopy. **B.** Another patient with scleroderma has developed a peptic stricture (*open arrows*) as a complication of reflux disease. Also note a small hiatal hernia (*curved arrow*) and sacculations (*straight arrows*) in the distal esophagus above the level of the stricture.

obstruction is a poorly understood syndrome associated with intermittent intestinal obstruction.[17-19] Various motility disorders throughout the bowel have been described in this syndrome. Most patients with intestinal pseudo-obstruction have abnormal esophageal motility with a radiographic appearance identical to that of achalasia.

RADIOLOGIC EFFICACY

The efficacy of radiologic evaluation of normal and abnormal esophageal motility depends on the quality of the examination performed and the types of motility disorders for which the patient is being evaluated.[7-9,15] Observation of multiple single swallows of barium is critical to the radiologic assessment of esophageal function if results are to correlate well with esophageal manometry.[5,15,80,81] The focus in this section is on a review of the radiologic efficacy in relation to manometry, on the types of primary motility disorders being evaluated, and on the clinical presentation of the patient.

Manometric Correlation

In one study, normal and abnormal esophageal motility were assessed by using synchronous videofluoroscopy and manometry. A total of 98 swallows was correlated (58 normal and 40 abnormal), and 96% agreement was found in establishing the correct status of primary peristalsis.[15] Segregating swallows into groups of five showed a 92% concordance and led to the recommendation of using five barium swallows to evaluate esophageal motility by fluoroscopy. If two or more of the five barium swallows were abnormal, the patient was considered to have a motility disorder. Radiologic specificity in that study was 95%, similar to that in other reports.[1,82]

Reported radiologic detection of esophageal motility disorders has been highly variable, depending primarily on the type of disorder being evaluated.[7-9,82] In retrospective studies, the radiologic sensitivity for those primary motility disorders amenable to fluoroscopic diagnosis has varied from 46% to 95%.[54,82] These studies have reported detection rates of about 95% for achalasia, 75% for DES, and 50% for NEMD. Nutcracker esophagus and hypertensive LES are not diagnosed radiographically, but their inclusion obviously lowers the overall radiologic sensitivity. Synchronous manometric and fluoroscopic investigations have suggested that observation of five barium swallows would improve radiologic detection of DES and NEMD.[15,81]

Clinical Considerations

Radiologic efficacy also depends on the clinical presentation of the patient.[83] Dysphagia and chest pain are the most common symptoms of esophageal motility disorders. However, the spectrum of motility disorders in patients with dysphagia is different from that in patients with chest pain.[84] Dysphagia is a more specific esophageal complaint that often results from structural or functional disorders of the esophagus. In a radiographic and manometric study of 172 patients with dysphagia, esophageal manometric findings were abnormal in 38% of the patients (66 of 172).[82] Achalasia was diagnosed in 29% (19 of 66) of those patients with abnormal manometric findings, and nutcracker esophagus was diagnosed in 18% (12 of 66) of the same group. Excluding the diagnosis of

nutcracker esophagus, the overall radiographic sensitivity in this group of patients with dysphagia was 69%.

Recurrent chest pain is a less specific indicator of esophageal motility disorders, and cardiac disease must first be excluded.[84-86] Only 10% to 15% of patients with chest pain are found to have an esophageal cause, which is usually structural disease or gastroesophageal reflux rather than a motility disorder. In a radiographic and manometric study of 170 patients with noncardiac chest pain, esophageal manometric findings were abnormal in 33% (56 of 170) of the patients.[87] Unlike patients with dysphagia, however, achalasia accounted for only 4% (2 of 56) of cases and nutcracker esophagus accounted for 29% (16 of 56) of cases. The overall radiographic sensitivity was only 36%. This lower figure presumably reflects a different spectrum of motility disorders occurring in patients with chest pain. In a more general population of individuals with chest pain, radiologic detection of abnormal motility would be detected radiographically in about only 1% to 2%.[88]

Before attributing dysphagia or chest pain to esophageal motility disorders, one should recognize that abnormal esophageal motility does not prove an esophageal origin of the symptom.[84-88] Most patients with dysphagia or chest pain and abnormal esophageal motility do not have complaints during routine manometric or radiologic examinations. Provocative testing by esophageal acid perfusion or drugs usually produces negative results in these patients. Prolonged ambulatory monitoring of esophageal function has also shown changing motility patterns in the same patient, raising questions about the value of brief temporal sampling of esophageal pressures during a routine manometric study.[89-92] Finally, the occasional observation of transitional motility disorders emphasizes the difficulty of correlating symptoms with abnormal esophageal function.

References

1. Dodds WJ: Esophagus-radiology. In Margulis AR, Burhenne HJ (eds): Alimentary Tract Radiology, vol 1, 4th ed. St. Louis, CV Mosby, 1989, pp 427-500.
2. Meyer GW, Austin RM, Brady CE III, et al: Muscle anatomy of the human esophagus. J Clin Gastroenterol 8:131-134, 1986.
3. Mittal RK, Balaban DH: The esophagogastric junction. N Engl J Med 336:924-932, 1997.
4. Ott DJ: Pharynx and esophagus. In Ott DJ, Gelfand DW, Chen MYM (eds): Manual of Gastrointestinal Fluoroscopy. Springfield, IL, Charles C Thomas, 1996, pp 24-51.
5. Clouse RE, Diamant NE: Esophageal motor and sensory function and motor disorders of the esophagus. In Feldman M, Friedman LS, Sleisenger MH (eds): Gastrointestinal and Liver Disease, vol 1, 7th ed. Philadelphia, Saunders, 2002, pp 561-598.
6. Goyal RK, Prasad M, Chang HY: Functional anatomy and physiology of swallowing and esophageal motility. In Castell DO, Richter JE (eds): The Esophagus, 4th ed. Philadelphia, Lippincott Williams & Wilkins, 2004, pp 1-36.
7. Ott DJ: Motility disorders of the esophagus. Radiol Clin North Am 32:1117-1134, 1994.
8. Levine MS, Rubesin SE: Radiology of the pharynx and esophagus. In Castell DO, Richter RE (eds): The Esophagus, 4th ed. Philadelphia, Lippincott Williams & Wilkins, 2004, pp 47-105.
9. Schima W, Eisenhuber E: Radiologic evaluation of esophageal function. In Ekberg O (ed): Radiology of the Pharynx and the Esophagus. Berlin, Springer, 2004, pp 109-125.
10. Ribeiro AC, Klingler PJ, Hinder RA, DeVault K: Esophageal manometry: A comparison of findings in younger and older patients. Am J Gastroenterol 93:706-710, 1998.
11. Grande L, Lacima G, Ros E, et al: Deterioration of esophageal motility with age: A manometric study of 79 healthy subjects. Am J Gastroenterol 94:1795-1801, 1999.

12. Shaker R, Lang IM: Effect of aging on the deglutitive oral, pharyngeal, and esophageal motor junction. Dysphagia 9:221-228, 1994.

13. Grishaw EK, Ott DJ, Frederick MG, et al: Functional abnormalities of the esophagus: A prospective analysis of radiographic findings relative to age and symptoms. AJR 167:719-723, 1996.

14. Ott DJ, Pikna LA: Clinical and videofluoroscopic evaluation of swallowing disorders. AJR 161:507-513, 1993.

15. Ott DJ, Chen YM, Hewson EG, et al: Esophageal motility: Assessment with synchronous video tape fluoroscopy and manometry. Radiology 173:419-422, 1989.

16. Clouse RE, Alrakawi A, Staiano A: Intersubject and interswallow variability in topography of esophageal motility. Dig Dis Sci 43:1978-1985, 1998.

17. Spechler SJ, Castell DO: Nonachalasia esophageal motility abnormalities. In Castell DO, Richter RE (eds): The Esophagus, 4th ed. Philadelphia, Lippincott Williams & Wilkins, 2004, pp 262-274.

18. Alrakawi A, Clouse RE: The changing use of esophageal manometry in clinical practice. Am J Gastroenterol 93:2359-2362, 1998.

19. Clouse RE, Staiano A, Alrakawi A, Haroian L: Application of topographical methods to clinical esophageal manometry. Am J Gastroenterol 95:2720-2730, 2000.

20. Richter RE: Achalasia. In Castell DO, Richter RE (eds): The Esophagus, 4th ed. Philadelphia, Lippincott Williams & Wilkins, 2004, pp 221-261.

21. Goldblum JR, Whyte RI, Orringer MB, et al: Achalasia—a morphologic study of 42 resected specimens. Am J Surg Pathol 18:327-337, 1994.

22. Sandler RS, Nyren O, Ekbom A, et al: The risk of esophageal cancer in patients with achalasia—a population-based study. JAMA 274:1359-1362, 1995.

23. Carter M, Deckmann RC, Smith RC, et al: Differentiation of achalasia from pseudoachalasia by computed tomography. Am J Gastroenterol 92:624-628, 1997.

24. Rosenzweig S, Traube M: The diagnosis and misdiagnosis of achalasia—a study of 25 consecutive patients. J Clin Gastroenterol 11:147-153, 1989.

25. Woodfield CA, Levine MS, Rubesin SE, et al: Diagnosis of primary versus secondary achalasia: Reassessment of clinical and radiographic criteria. AJR 175:727-731, 2000.

26. Goldenberg SP, Burrell M, Fette GG, et al: Classic and vigorous achalasia: A comparison of manometric, radiographic, and clinical findings. Gastroenterology 101:743-748, 1991.

27. Todorczuk JR, Aliperti G, Staiano A, et al: Reevaluation of manometric criteria for vigorous achalasia—is this a distinct clinical disorder? Dig Dis Sci 36:274-278, 1991.

28. Amaravadi R, Levine MS, Rubesin SE, et al: Achalasia with complete relaxation of lower esophageal sphincter: Radiographic-manometric correlation. Radiology 235:886-891, 2005.

29. Ott DJ, Richter JE, Chen YM, et al: Radiographic and manometric correlation in achalasia with apparent relaxation of the lower esophageal sphincter. Gastrointest Radiol 14:1-5, 1989.

30. Vaezi MF, Richter JE: Diagnosis and management of achalasia. Am J Gastroenterol 94:3406-3412, 1999.

31. Hirano I, Tatum RP, Shi G, et al: Manometric heterogeneity in patients with idiopathic achalasia. Gastroenterology 120:789-798, 2001.

32. Blam ME, Delfyett W, Levine MS, et al: Achalasia: A disease of varied and subtle symptoms that do not correlate with radiographic findings. Am J Gastroenterol 97:1916-1923, 2002.

33. Nayar DS, Khandwala F, Achkar E, et al: Esophageal manometry: Assessment of interpreter consistency. Clin Gastroenterol Hepatol 3:218-224, 2005.

34. Ott DJ, Hodge RG, Chen MYM, et al: Achalasia associated with hiatal hernia: Prevalence and potential implications. Abdom Imaging 18:7-9, 1993.

35. Katz PO, Gilbert J, Castell DO: Pneumatic dilatation is effective long-term treatment for achalasia. Dig Dis Sci 43:1973-1977, 1998.

36. Ott DJ, Pineau BC, Chen MY: Intervention on the esophagus. In Ekberg O (ed): Radiology of the Pharynx and the Esophagus. Berlin, Springer, 2004, pp 153-166.

37. Ackroyd R, Watson DI, Devitt PG, Jamieson GG: Laparoscopic cardiomyotomy and anterior partial fundoplication for achalasia. Surg Endosc 15:683-686, 2001.

38. West RL, Hirsch DP, Bartelsman JF, et al: Long term results of pneumatic dilation in achalasia followed for more than 5 years. Am J Gastroenterol 97:1346-1351, 2002.

39. Kolbasnik J, Waterfall WE, Fachnie B, et al: Long-term efficacy of botulinum toxin in classical achalasia: A prospective study. Am J Gastroenterol 94:3434-3439, 1999.

40. Metman E-H, Lagasse J-P, d'Alteroche L, et al: Risk factors for immediate complications after progressive pneumatic dilation for achalasia. Am J Gastroenterol 94:1179-1185, 1999.

41. Hui JM, Hunt DR, de Carle DJ, et al: Esophageal pneumatic dilation for postfundoplication dysphagia: Safety, efficacy, and predictors of outcome. Am J Gastroenterol 97:2986-2991, 2002.

42. Stark GA, Castell DO, Richter JE, et al: Prospective randomized comparison of Brown-McHardy and Microvasive balloon dilators in treatment of achalasia. Am J Gastroenterol 85:1322-1326, 1990.

43. Ott DJ, Donati D, Wu WC, et al: Radiographic evaluation of achalasia immediately after pneumatic dilatation with the Rigiflex dilator. Gastrointest Radiol 16:279-282, 1991.

44. Molina EG, Stollman N, Grauer L, et al: Conservative management of esophageal nontransmural tears after pneumatic dilation for achalasia. Am J Gastroenterol 91:15-18, 1995.

45. Vaezi MF, Baker ME, Achkar E, Richter JE: Timed barium oesophagram: Better predictor of long term success after pneumatic dilation in achalasia than symptom assessment. Gut 50:765-770, 2002.

46. Eckardt VF, Aignherr C, Bernhard G: Predictors of outcome in patients with achalasia treated by pneumatic dilation. Gastroenterology 103:1732-1738, 1992.

47. Wong RKH, Maydonovitch C: Utility of parameters measured during pneumatic dilation as predictors of successful dilation. Am J Gastroenterol 91:1126-1129, 1996.

48. Mariani G, Boni G, Barreca M, et al: Radionuclide gastroesophageal motor studies. J Nucl Med 45:1004-1028, 2004.

49. Prabhakar A, Levine MS, Rubesin S, et al: Relationship between diffuse esophageal spasm and lower esophageal sphincter dysfunction on barium studies and manometry in 14 patients. AJR 183:409-413, 2004.

50. Henderson RD, Ryder D, Marryatt G: Extended esophageal myotomy and short total fundoplication hernia repair in diffuse esophageal spasm: Five-year review in 34 patients. Ann Thorac Surg 43:25-31, 1987.

51. Mittal RK, Kassab G, Puckett JL, Liu J: Hypertrophy of the muscularis propria of the lower esophageal sphincter and the body of the esophagus in patients with primary motility disorders of the esophagus. Am J Gastroenterol 98:1705-1712, 2003.

52. Mittal RK, Liu J, Puckett JL, et al: Sensory and motor function of the esophagus: Lessons from ultrasound imaging. Gastroenterology 128:487-497, 2005.

53. Loebenberg MJ, Lewis JH, Fleischer DE, et al: Endoscopic ultrasound (EUS) for evaluating esophageal wall thickness (EWT) in esophageal motility disorders (EMD) [abstract]. Gastroenterology 94:A267, 1989.

54. Chen YM, Ott DJ, Hewson EG, et al: Diffuse esophageal spasm: Radiographic and manometric correlation. Radiology 170:807-810, 1989.

55. Mujica VR, Mudipalli RS, Rao SSC: Pathophysiology of chest pain in patients with nutcracker esophagus. Am J Gastroenterol 96:1371-1377, 2001.

56. Pilhall M, Borjesson M, Rolny P, Mannheimer C: Diagnosis of nutcracker esophagus, segmental or diffuse hypertensive patterns, and clinical characteristics. Dig Dis Sci 47:1381-1388, 2002.

57. Melzer E, Ron Y, Tiomni E, et al: Assessment of the esophageal wall by endoscopic ultrasonography in patients with nutcracker esophagus. Gastrointest Endosc 46:223-225, 1997.

58. Lacima G, Grande L, Pera M, et al: Utility of ambulatory 24-hour esophageal pH and motility monitoring in noncardiac chest pain: Report of 90 patients and review of the literature. Dig Dis Sci 48:952-961, 2003.

59. Valori RM: Nutcracker, neurosis, or sampling bias? Gut 31:736-737, 1990.

60. Nevens F, Janssens J, Piessens J, et al: Prospective study on prevalence of esophageal chest pain in patients referred on an elective basis to a cardiac unit for suspected myocardial ischemia. Dig Dis Sci 36:229-235, 1991.

61. Tack J, Janssens J: The esophagus and noncardiac chest pain. In Castell DO, Richter RE (eds): The Esophagus, 4th ed. Philadelphia, Lippincott Williams & Wilkins, 2004, pp 634-647.

62. Richter JE, Wu WC, Johns DN, et al: Esophageal manometry in 95 healthy adult volunteers. Dig Dis Sci 32:583-592, 1987.

63. Chobanian SJ, Curtis DJ, Benjamin SB, et al: Radiology of the nutcracker esophagus. J Clin Gastroenterol 8:230-232, 1986.

64. Ott DJ, Richter JE, Wu WC, et al: Radiologic and manometric correlation in "nutcracker esophagus." AJR 147:692-695, 1986.

65. Shah K, Morayati S, Freitas J, Maas L: "Nutcracker esophagus": A case of false-negative radionuclide esophageal transit study. South Med J 82:666, 1989.

66. De Caestecker JS, Blackwell JN, Adam RD, et al: Clinical value of radionuclide oesophageal transit measurement. Gut 27:659-666, 1986.

67. Holloway RH, Lange RC, Plankey MW, et al: Detection of esophageal motor disorders by radionuclide transit studies. Dig Dis Sci 34:905-912, 1989.
68. Drane WE, Johnson DA, Hagan DP, et al: "Nutcracker" esophagus: Diagnosis with radionuclide esophageal scintigraphy versus manometry. Radiology 163:33-37, 1987.
69. Richter JE, Wu WC, Ott DJ, et al: "Nutcracker" esophagus: Diagnosis with radionuclide esophageal scintigraphy versus manometry [letter]. Radiology 164:877-879, 1987.
70. Freeman J, Hila A, Castell DO: Esophageal manometry. In Castell DO, Richter RE (eds): The Esophagus, 4th ed. Philadelphia, Lippincott Williams & Wilkins, 2004, pp 115-134.
71. Hsu JJ, O'Connor MK, Kang YW, Kim CH: Nonspecific motor disorder of the esophagus: A real disorder or a manometric curiosity? Gastroenterology 104:1281-1284, 1993.
72. Ren J, Shaker R, Kusano M, et al: Effect of aging on the secondary esophageal peristalsis: Presbyesophagus revisited. Am J Physiol 268: G772-G779, 1995.
73. DeVault KR: Presbyesophagus: A reappraisal. Curr Gastroenterol Rep 4:193-199, 2002.
74. Waterman DC, Dalton CB, Ott DJ, et al: Hypertensive lower esophageal sphincter: What does it mean? J Clin Gastroenterol 11:139-146, 1989.
75. Wo JM: Esophageal involvement in systemic diseases. In Castell DO, Richter RE (eds): The Esophagus, 4th ed. Philadelphia, Lippincott Williams & Wilkins, 2004, pp 611-633.
76. Klein HA, Wald A, Graham TO, et al: Comparative studies of esophageal function in systemic sclerosis. Gastroenterology 102:1551-1556, 1992.
77. Wang SJ, Lan JL, Chen DY, et al: Solid-phase radionuclide esophageal transit in progressive systemic sclerosis. Hepatogastroenterology 49: 989-991, 2002.
78. Campbell WL, Schultz JC: Specificity and sensitivity of esophageal motor abnormality in systemic sclerosis (scleroderma) and related diseases: A cineradiographic study. Gastrointest Radiol 11:218-222, 1986.
79. Keshavarzian A, Iber FL, Ferguson Y: Esophageal manometry and radionuclide emptying in chronic alcoholics. Gastroenterology 92:651-657, 1987.
80. Kahrilas PJ, Dodds WJ, Hogan WJ: Effect of peristaltic dysfunction on esophageal volume clearance. Gastroenterology 94:73-80, 1988.
81. Hewson EG, Ott DJ, Dalton CB, et al: Manometry and radiology—complementary studies in the assessment of esophageal motility disorders. Gastroenterology 98:626-632, 1990.
82. Ott DJ, Richter JE, Chen YM, et al: Esophageal radiography and manometry: Correlation in 172 patients with dysphagia. AJR 149:307-311, 1987.
83. DiPalma JA, Meyer GW: A rational clinical approach to esophageal motor disorders. Dysphagia 2:97-108, 1987.
84. Katz PO, Dalton CB, Richter JE, et al: Esophageal testing of patients with noncardiac chest pain or dysphagia. Ann Intern Med 106:593-597, 1987.
85. Richter JE, Bradley LA, Castell DO: Esophageal chest pain: Current controversies in pathogenesis, diagnosis, and therapy. Ann Intern Med 110:66-78, 1989.
86. Battaglia E, Bassotti G, Buonafede G, et al: Noncardiac chest pain of esophageal origin in patients with and without coronary artery disease. Hepatogastroenterology 52:792-795, 2005.
87. Ott DJ, Abernethy WB, Chen MYM, et al: Radiologic evaluation of esophageal motility: results in 170 patients with chest pain. AJR 155: 983-985, 1990.
88. Levine MS, Rubesin SE, Ott DJ: Update on esophageal radiology. AJR 155:933-941, 1990.
89. Patti MG, Gorodner MV, Galvani C, et al: Spectrum of esophageal motility disorders: Implications for diagnosis and treatment. Arch Surg 140:442-448, 2005.
90. Orlando RC: Esophageal perception and noncardiac chest pain. Gastroenterol Clin North Am 33:25-33, 2004.
91. Hewson EG, Dalton CB, Richter JE: Comparison of esophageal manometry, provocative testing, and ambulatory monitoring in patients with unexplained chest pain. Dig Dis Sci 35:302-309, 1990.
92. Ghillebert G, Janssens J, Vantrappen G, et al: Ambulatory 24 hour intraoesophageal pH and pressure recording vs provocation tests in the diagnosis of chest pain of oesophageal origin. Gut 31:738-744, 1990.

Gastroesophageal Reflux Disease

Marc S. Levine, MD

Gastroesophageal reflux disease (GERD) is the most common inflammatory disease involving the esophagus. Fifteen to 20 percent of Americans experience heartburn on a weekly basis.[1,2] In the past, barium studies were advocated for patients with reflux symptoms primarily to show the presence of a hiatal hernia or gastroesophageal reflux, to detect complications such as deep ulcers or strictures, and to rule out other organic or motor abnormalities in the esophagus that can mimic reflux disease. By permitting a more detailed assessment of the esophageal mucosa, however, double-contrast radiographic techniques have made it possible to detect superficial ulceration and other changes of mild or moderate esophagitis before the development of deep ulcers or strictures. Double-contrast esophagography is also a useful screening examination for Barrett's esophagus to determine the need for endoscopy and biopsy in these patients. With double-contrast techniques, barium studies therefore have a major role in the evaluation of patients with suspected GERD.

REFLUX ESOPHAGITIS

Pathogenesis

Reflux esophagitis is thought to be a multifactorial process related to the frequency and duration of reflux episodes, the content of the refluxed material, and the intrinsic resistance of the esophageal mucosa.[3-8] Gastroesophageal reflux occurs when lower esophageal sphincter pressure is decreased or absent, so that the major barrier to reflux is lost.[3-5,9] In most patients, however, these reflux episodes are caused not by a sustained decrease in resting sphincter pressure but rather by transient relaxations of the lower esophageal sphincter that frequently occur at night.[6,10-12]

The severity of GERD depends not only on the frequency of reflux episodes but also on their duration. Because the duration of reflux is related to the efficacy of esophageal clearance by peristalsis, abnormal motility exacerbates reflux disease and increases the risk of developing esophagitis by prolonging exposure to the refluxed material.[4,5] As a result, esophageal involvement by scleroderma often leads to severe esophagitis resulting from absent peristalsis and extremely poor clearance of peptic acid from the esophagus after reflux has occurred. In one study, 60% of patients with scleroderma who underwent endoscopy had evidence of esophagitis.[13]

The severity of reflux disease also depends on the content of the refluxed material. Hydrochloric acid and pepsin are the noxious agents primarily responsible for injuring the esophageal mucosa. These agents appear to have a synergistic effect, so that reflux of acid and pepsin produces greater mucosal injury than reflux of acid alone.[14] The concentration of refluxed acid is another important determinant of the degree of mucosal injury. Patients with Zollinger-Ellison syndrome are therefore more likely to develop severe esophagitis or strictures resulting from reflux of highly acidic peptic juices into the esophagus.[15-17]

Finally, the severity of reflux esophagitis depends on the intrinsic resistance of the esophageal mucosa.[4-6,8] Because mucosal resistance and esophageal motor function deteriorate

337

with age, older patients are at greater risk for developing reflux esophagitis as a result of prolonged exposure of a susceptible mucosa to refluxed material in the esophagus.

Relationship between Hiatal Hernia, Gastroesophageal Reflux, and Reflux Esophagitis

Sliding hiatal hernias occur more frequently in elderly patients as a result of a degenerative process in which there is progressive weakening and laxity of the ligaments that anchor the gastroesophageal junction to the surrounding esophageal hiatus of the diaphragm.[4,18] There is considerable controversy about the relationship between a hiatal hernia and the subsequent development of gastroesophageal reflux or reflux esophagitis. Because most patients with clinically significant GERD have evidence of a hiatal hernia, it has been postulated that the presence of a hernia predisposes patients to the development of gastroesophageal reflux and reflux esophagitis.[19,20] Nevertheless, many patients with a hiatal hernia have no evidence of gastroesophageal reflux and many patients with gastroesophageal reflux have no evidence of a hernia.[21,22] Thus, intrinsic dysfunction of the lower esophageal sphincter is probably the major factor in the development of gastroesophageal reflux, independent of the anatomic location of the sphincter above or below the diaphragm.[3,5,21]

Although the presence of a sliding hiatal hernia is a poor predictor of GERD, most patients with severe reflux esophagitis or reflux-induced strictures (also known as *peptic strictures*) have hiatal hernias.[5,23,24] There is evidence that severe inflammation and scarring from reflux esophagitis cause longitudinal esophageal shortening that disrupts the ligaments surrounding the gastroesophageal junction and pulls the gastric fundus into the thorax.[25] Thus, the hiatal hernia may represent an effect rather than a cause of esophagitis in these patients.

Similarly, gastroesophageal reflux is a poor predictor of reflux esophagitis because reflux may be demonstrated in some asymptomatic individuals but not in others with proven reflux esophagitis.[4,5] Thus, the diagnosis of reflux esophagitis should be based not on the presence or absence of a hiatal hernia or gastroesophageal reflux but on specific morphologic evidence of inflammatory changes in the esophagus.

Clinical Findings

Patients with GERD classically present with heartburn (defined as retrosternal pain and burning that are worse after eating) and, less frequently, regurgitation.[3,26,27] Some patients may present with angina-like chest pain rather than heartburn. In one study, 43% of patients with chest pain of noncardiac origin were found to have GERD as the cause of their pain.[28] Others may present with epigastric pain or dyspepsia that is erroneously attributed to peptic ulcer disease.[29] Still others may have upper gastrointestinal bleeding with melena or guaiac-positive stool.[3] However, major hemorrhage from reflux esophagitis is extremely uncommon.

An association between GERD and pulmonary problems has been well documented. Abnormal reflux has been reported to occur in more than 80% of adult patients with asthma.[30] Such patients typically present with nocturnal coughing or wheezing, and they do not have an allergic component to their asthma.[26] It has been postulated that this condition is caused either by aspiration of refluxed acid into the airway or by vagally mediated bronchoconstriction resulting from reflux-induced irritation of the esophageal mucosa.[31] Esophagopharyngeal reflux of peptic acid may also cause pharyngitis or laryngitis, manifested by a globus sensation, chronic cough, or hoarseness.[26,32]

The perception of reflux symptoms depends on the duration of exposure to refluxed acid in the esophagus.[33] Nevertheless, the severity of symptoms correlates poorly with the severity of erosive esophagitis on endoscopy.[8] Some patients with marked reflux symptoms have normal endoscopic examinations, whereas others with unequivocal endoscopic evidence of erosive esophagitis are asymptomatic. It has therefore been postulated that the development of reflux symptoms is often related to esophageal visceral hypersensitivity and inappropriately heightened perception because of underlying neuronal dysfunction rather than the presence or degree of inflammation in the esophagus.[8,34]

The development of a peptic stricture is typically manifested by slowly progressive dysphagia for solids (followed by liquids) superimposed on a history of long-standing reflux symptoms.[35,36] Nevertheless, 25% of patients with peptic strictures present with dysphagia as the initial manifestation of their disease.[36] Associated weight loss is usually minimal because patients with peptic strictures modify their diets to compensate for their dysphagia. Thus, substantial weight loss should raise concern about the possibility of a malignant stricture (see Chapter 27).

Diagnosis

Patients with reflux symptoms may undergo a variety of clinical tests to determine whether the symptoms are esophageal in origin and whether there is objective evidence of gastroesophageal reflux or reflux esophagitis. Gastroesophageal reflux may be assessed by radiologic, scintigraphic, manometric, or esophageal pH-monitoring techniques. Esophagography or endoscopy is required to establish a diagnosis of reflux esophagitis. Barium studies are particularly useful for evaluating patients with GERD when surgical treatment is planned.[37]

Gastroesophageal Reflux

Spontaneous gastroesophageal reflux can be demonstrated on barium studies in only 20% to 35% of patients with reflux esophagitis.[5,24,38,39] Because gastroesophageal reflux often results from transient lower esophageal sphincter relaxations rather than a sustained decrease in sphincter tone, intermittent episodes of reflux are easily missed during the brief period of fluoroscopic observation. Some authors advocate the use of the water-siphon test to increase the radiographic sensitivity for reflux,[38] but others discourage the use of this physiologic technique for reflux because of its low specificity.[22,40] Furthermore, spontaneous gastroesophageal reflux can be demonstrated on barium studies in asymptomatic volunteers.[5] Thus, esophagography is neither a sensitive nor a specific technique for detecting gastroesophageal reflux.

Gastroesophageal scintigraphy is an alternative technique for detecting and quantifying gastroesophageal reflux (see Chapter 14).[41,42] Esophageal manometry can also be used to assess lower esophageal sphincter pressures, but many patients with normal resting sphincter pressures have intermittent gastroesophageal reflux resulting from transient relaxations of the lower esophageal sphincter.[10-12] Intraesophageal pH monitoring is thought to be the most accurate diagnostic test for gastroesophageal reflux,[43] but this test measures the acidity rather than the volume of refluxed material in the esophagus. Also, it has been shown that virtually all patients with massive reflux on barium studies (defined as reflux of barium to or above the thoracic inlet with the patient in a recumbent position) have pathologic acid reflux on 24-hour esophageal pH monitoring.[44] Patients with massive reflux on barium studies can therefore be further evaluated and treated for their reflux disease without need for pH monitoring.

Because the severity of GERD depends not only on the frequency of reflux episodes but also on their duration, esophageal clearance may be evaluated after reflux has occurred. Fluoroscopy, scintigraphy, intraesophageal pH monitoring, and manometry are various tests used to evaluate esophageal clearance or motility.[5,22,45,46]

Reflux Esophagitis

Conventional single-contrast esophagography has been considered to be an unreliable technique for detecting reflux esophagitis, with an overall sensitivity of only 50% to 75%.[47-50] With the use of double-contrast technique, however, the radiographic sensitivity approaches 90%.[48,50,51] A major advantage of double-contrast esophagography is that it permits a detailed assessment of the esophageal mucosa for superficial ulceration or other changes of mild or moderate esophagitis that cannot be detected with conventional barium studies. At the same time, single-contrast technique (with the patient in the prone position) is best for demonstrating areas of decreased distensibility in the distal esophagus as a result of strictures or rings.[52] A biphasic examination with upright double-contrast and prone single-contrast views of the esophagus therefore appears to be the best radiologic technique for evaluating patients with suspected reflux disease.

Endoscopy is generally advocated as the most definitive diagnostic test for reflux esophagitis. Various grading systems have been used to estimate the severity of esophagitis based on the endoscopic findings of erythema, friability, exudates, ulcers, and strictures.[53] Investigators have particularly focused on the importance of differentiating erosive esophagitis from nonerosive reflux disease.[54] Nevertheless, the use of endoscopy as the gold standard for reflux esophagitis is problematic because of controversies about the endoscopic definition of esophagitis and interobserver reliability.[55-57] In various studies, there was 50% or less agreement between the endoscopic and histologic findings of esophagitis.[58,59] Thus, endoscopy is by no means an infallible technique for detecting reflux esophagitis.

A definitive histologic diagnosis of reflux esophagitis can be made when endoscopic biopsy specimens reveal acute inflammatory changes with accumulation of neutrophils and eosinophils in the lamina propria. Basal cell hyperplasia of the squamous epithelium has also been recognized as an important sign of reflux disease, resulting from mucosal damage by refluxed acid and accelerated epithelial turnover in the esophagus.[60] Unfortunately, the histologic diagnosis of reflux esophagitis can be unreliable because of the patchy distribu-

tion of disease. In one study, 30% of patients with reflux symptoms had normal and abnormal biopsy specimens obtained from the same regions of the esophagus.[60] Some investigators have even questioned whether endoscopic biopsy specimens should be used as the gold standard for reflux esophagitis.[61]

Radiographic Findings

Abnormal Motility

Between 25% and 50% of patients with reflux esophagitis have abnormal esophageal motility on manometry, manifested by intermittently decreased or absent primary peristalsis in the middle or lower thirds of the thoracic esophagus.[4,62] In one study, this dysmotility was often observed on esophagography without evidence of nonperistaltic contractions,[63] whereas esophageal dysmotility in older patients is usually associated with multiple nonperistaltic contractions (the latter condition has been called "presbyesophagus").[64] The presence of intermittently weakened or absent primary peristalsis without nonperistaltic contractions on esophagography should therefore suggest underlying GERD, particularly in young patients.[63]

Much less frequently, esophageal aperistalsis may be the only radiographic finding in patients with reflux esophagitis.[65] In such cases, abnormal motility may be secondary to neuronal damage in Auerbach plexus caused by direct extension of the inflammatory process into the esophageal wall.[65] Conversely, preexisting esophageal dysmotility (such as that associated with scleroderma) may predispose patients to the development of reflux esophagitis by impairing clearance of refluxed peptic acid from the esophagus. In either case, the combination of abnormal motility and gastroesophageal reflux produces a vicious cycle, often leading to progressively severe esophagitis and stricture formation.[5]

Mucosal Nodularity

In the early stages of reflux esophagitis, mucosal edema and inflammation may be manifested on double-contrast images by a finely nodular or granular appearance in the distal third or half of the thoracic esophagus (Fig. 23-1).[59,66-68] In one study, mucosal granularity was the most frequent and reliable sign of reflux esophagitis on double-contrast esophagograms, with a specificity and positive predictive value of about 90%.[59] This granularity is characterized by poorly defined radiolucencies that fade peripherally into the adjacent mucosa. Less frequently, reflux esophagitis may be manifested by coarse nodularity of the mucosa. In almost all cases, this granularity or nodularity extends proximally from the gastroesophageal junction as a continuous area of disease.

More advanced reflux esophagitis may occasionally be associated with inflammatory exudates or pseudomembranes that resemble the plaquelike lesions of *Candida* esophagitis (Fig. 23-2),[69] but these patients usually present with reflux symptoms rather than odynophagia. A single, large pseudomembrane can also be mistaken for a plaquelike carcinoma, particularly an adenocarcinoma arising in Barrett's mucosa.[69] Pseudomembrane formation may be suggested, however, by the presence of other satellite lesions or by changes in the size or shape of the lesions at fluoroscopy. When the radiographic

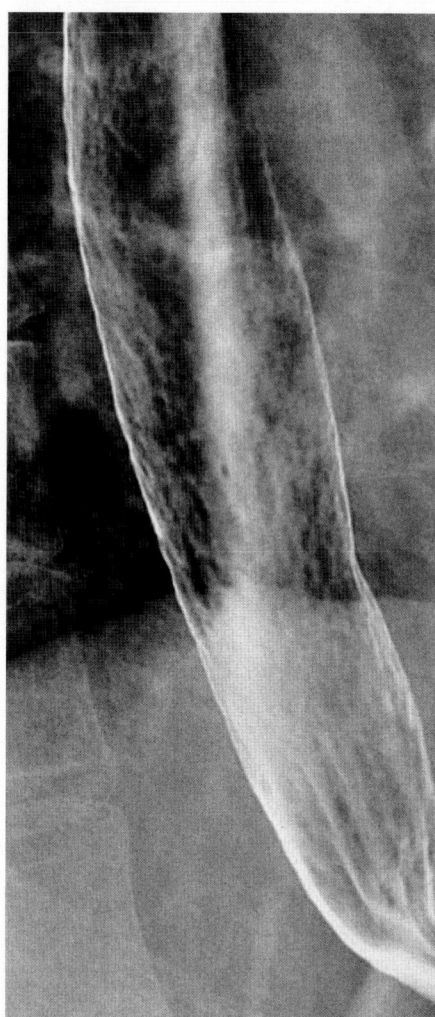

Figure 23-1. Reflux esophagitis with a granular mucosa. There is a finely nodular or granular appearance of the mucosa extending proximally from the gastroesophageal junction as a continuous area of disease. (From Levine MS, Rubesin SE: Diseases of the esophagus: Diagnosis with esophagography. Radiology 237:414-427, 2005.)

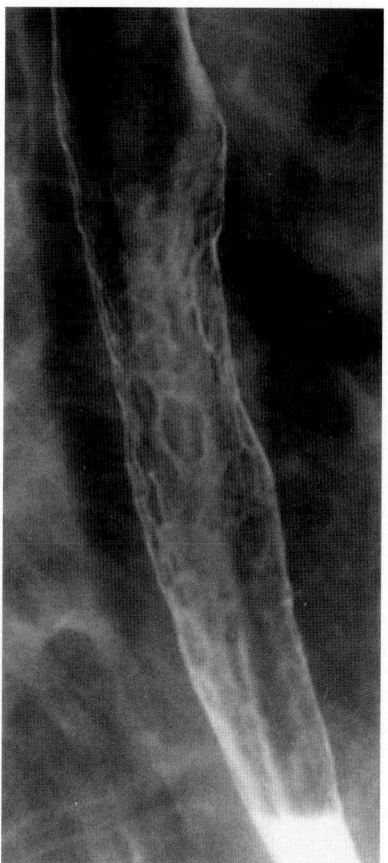

Figure 23-2. Reflux esophagitis with pseudomembranes. The pseudomembranes appear as discrete plaquelike defects that are indistinguishable from the plaques of candidiasis. (Courtesy of Howard Kessler, MD, Philadelphia, PA.)

findings are equivocal, endoscopy and biopsy should be performed for a definitive diagnosis.

Ulceration

Shallow ulcers and erosions associated with reflux esophagitis may appear on double-contrast images as one or more tiny collections of barium in the distal esophagus at or near the gastroesophageal junction (Fig. 23-3).[66,67,70] The ulcers can have a punctate, linear, stellate, or serpiginous configuration and are often associated with surrounding mounds of edematous mucosa, radiating folds, and puckering or sacculation of the adjacent esophageal wall (Fig. 23-4).[66,67,70,71] Some patients may have relatively diffuse ulceration of the distal third or even half of the thoracic esophagus. However, ulceration in reflux esophagitis tends to occur as a continuous area of disease extending proximally from the gastroesophageal junction, so that the presence of one or more ulcers in the upper or middle thirds of the esophagus with sparing of the distal third should suggest another cause for the patient's disease.

Reflux esophagitis may also be manifested by a solitary ulcer in the distal esophagus at or near the gastroesophageal junction.[72] These "marginal" ulcers may be recognized en face as discrete collections of barium (Fig. 23-5A) but are best visualized when the ulcers are projected in profile beyond the normal contour of the esophagus (Fig. 23-5B). In one study, about 70% of these solitary reflux-induced ulcers were found to be located on the posterior esophageal wall (see Fig. 23-5B).[72] Because gastroesophageal reflux often occurs during sleep, it has been postulated that patients who sleep primarily in the supine position are more likely to develop posterior wall ulcers as a result of prolonged exposure to refluxed acid that pools by gravity on the dependent or posterior esophageal wall, causing maximal injury in this location.[72]

In advanced reflux esophagitis, the esophagus may have a grossly irregular contour with serrated or spiculated margins, wall thickening, and decreased distensibility resulting from extensive ulceration, edema, and spasm (Fig. 23-6).[4,24,47,49] Occasionally, the narrowing and deformity associated with severe esophagitis can even mimic the appearance of an infiltrating carcinoma (Fig. 23-7). In such cases, endoscopy and biopsy should be performed for a definitive diagnosis.

Thickened Folds

In some patients with reflux esophagitis, submucosal edema and inflammation may lead to the development of thickened

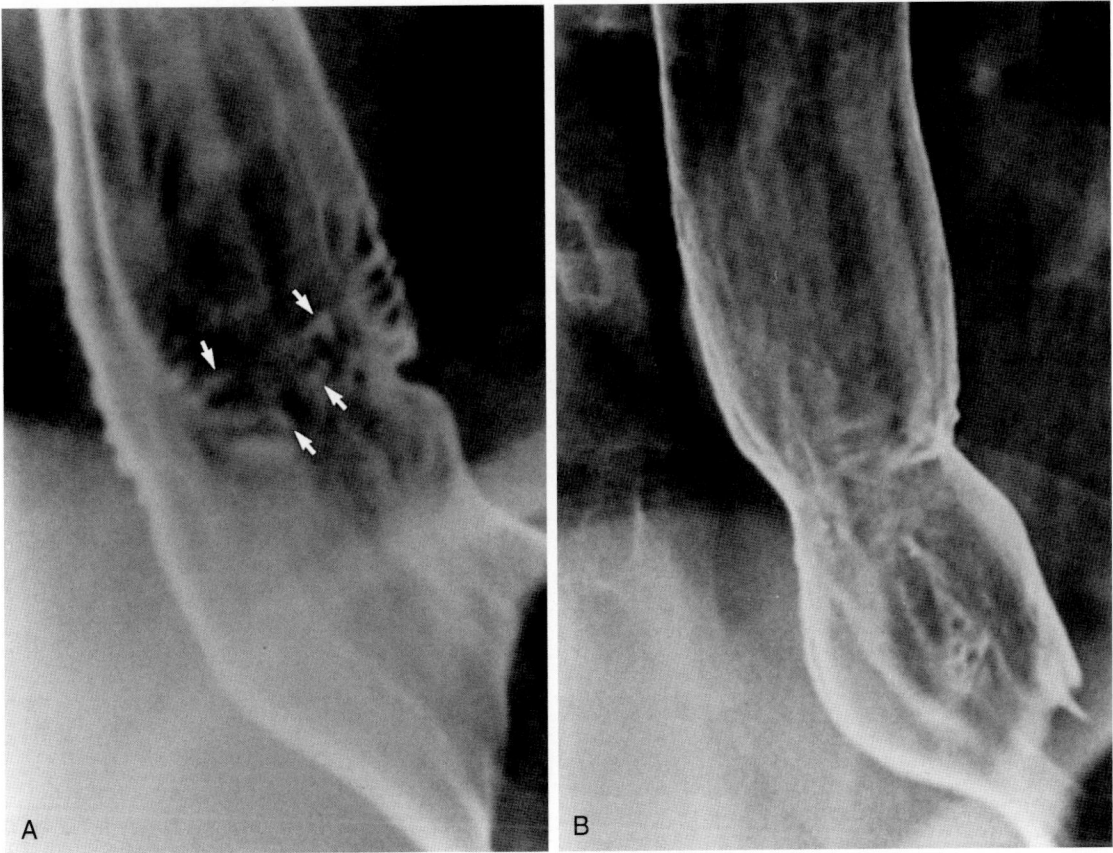

Figure 23-3. Reflux esophagitis with superficial ulceration. A. Multiple tiny ulcers (*arrows*) are seen en face in the distal esophagus near the gastroesophageal junction. Note radiating folds and puckering of the adjacent esophageal wall. **B.** Another patient has punctate and linear ulcers in the distal esophagus.

Figure 23-4. Reflux esophagitis with a linear ulcer. Note the radiolucent halo of edematous mucosa and folds radiating toward the ulcer (*arrow*) crater. (From Laufer I, Levine MS [eds]: Double Contrast Gastrointestinal Radiology, 2nd ed. Philadelphia, WB Saunders, 1992.)

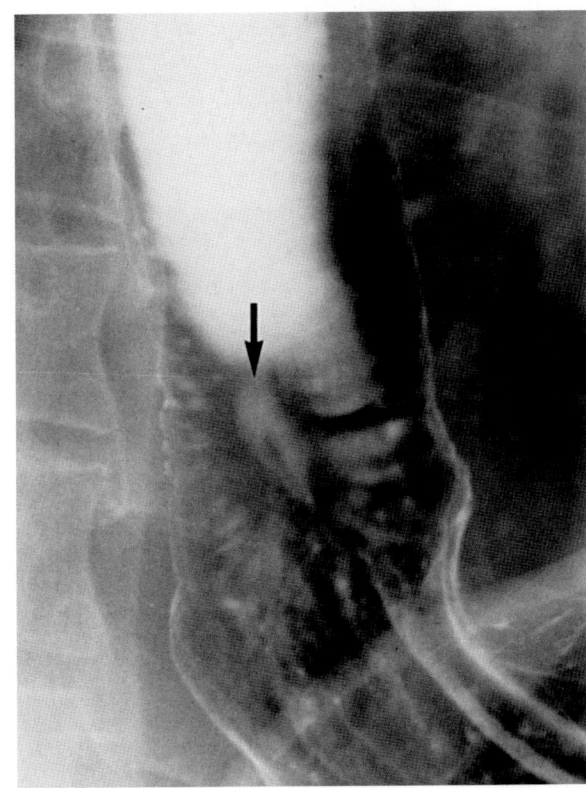

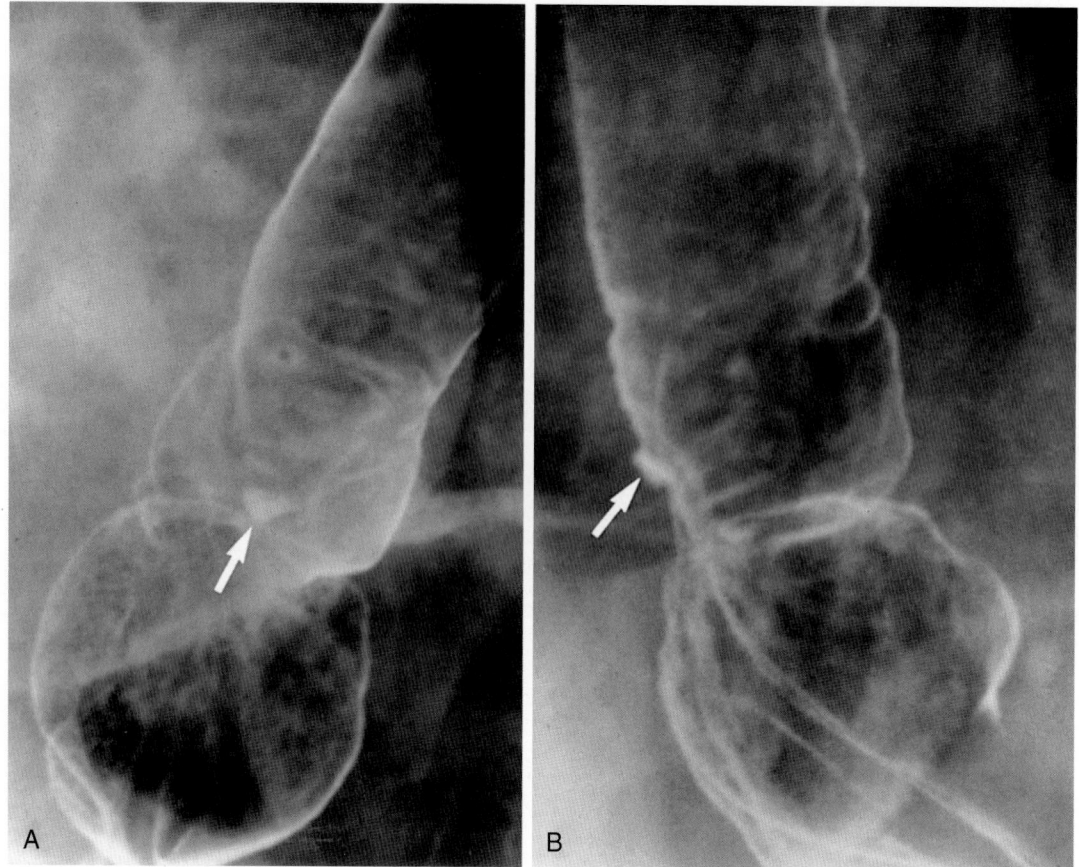

Figure 23-5. Reflux esophagitis with a discrete ulcer. This small ulcer (*arrows*) is seen both en face (**A**) and in profile (**B**) in the distal esophagus above a hiatal hernia. When viewed in profile (**B**), note how the ulcer is located on the right posterolateral wall of the distal esophagus. (From Laufer I, Levine MS [eds]: Double Contrast Gastrointestinal Radiology, 2nd ed. Philadelphia, WB Saunders, 1992.)

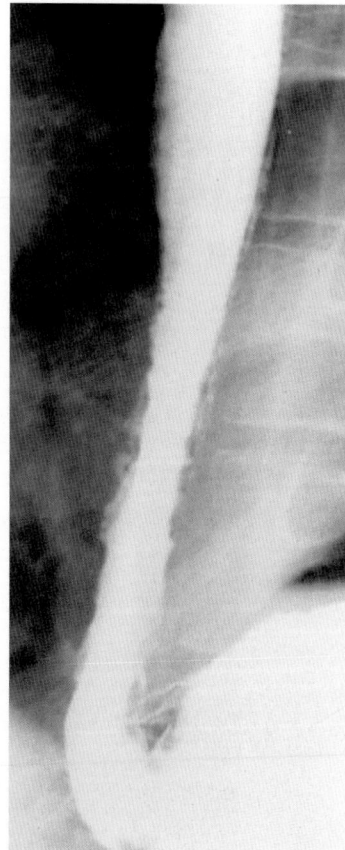

Figure 23-6. Advanced reflux esophagitis. There is decreased distensibility of the distal esophagus with an irregular, serrated esophageal contour due to extensive ulceration, edema, and spasm. (From Levine MS: Radiology of the Esophagus. Philadelphia, WB Saunders, 1989.)

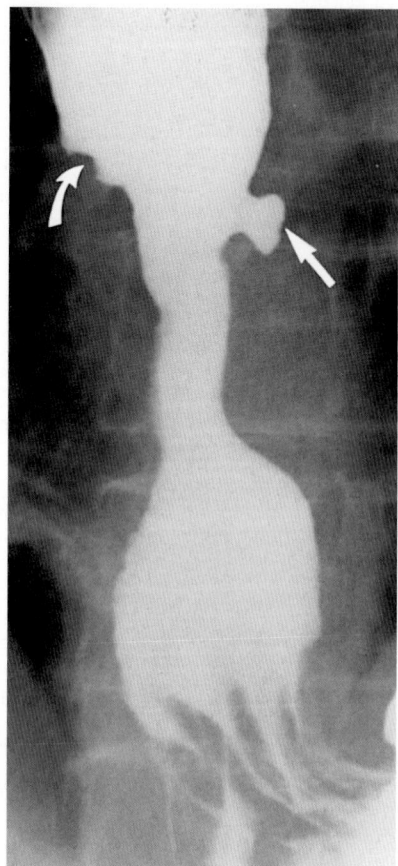

Figure 23-7. Reflux esophagitis with a deep ulcer (*straight arrow*). There is also asymmetric narrowing of the distal esophagus with a relatively abrupt cutoff (*curved arrow*) at the proximal border of the narrowed segment. These findings were caused by edema and spasm, but the possibility of malignant tumor cannot be excluded on this image. (From Levine MS: Radiology of the Esophagus. Philadelphia, WB Saunders, 1989.)

longitudinal folds (Fig. 23-8). Thickened folds are best seen on mucosal relief views of the collapsed or partially collapsed esophagus, in which folds wider than 3 mm are thought to be abnormal.[49,66] These thickened folds may have a smooth, nodular, scalloped, or crenulated appearance. Occasionally, they may be quite tortuous or serpiginous, mimicking the appearance of esophageal varices.[73]

Multiple transverse folds may also be found in patients with GERD (Fig. 23-9).[74,75] In the past, this appearance has been described as the "feline" esophagus because transverse esophageal folds are normally found in cats. These delicate transverse striations are only 1 to 2 mm wide and extend completely across the esophagus without interruption.[75] The folds occur as a transient phenomenon resulting from contraction of the longitudinally oriented muscularis mucosae,[76] so that they may be seen on only one of a number of spot images obtained during the radiologic examination (see Fig. 23-9). Although transverse folds are often observed in patients with gastroesophageal reflux, this finding alone does not indicate the presence of esophagitis.[75] Occasionally, however, thickening of these transverse folds may occur as a manifestation of esophagitis (Fig. 23-10).[66]

Inflammatory Esophagogastric Polyps

Other patients with reflux esophagitis may develop inflammatory esophagogastric polyps consisting of inflammatory and granulation tissue.[77-79] The polyps usually appear on barium studies as smooth, ovoid or club-shaped protuberances in the lower esophagus atop a single prominent mucosal fold that tapers distally at the gastroesophageal junction (Fig. 23-11).[77,78] Inflammatory esophagogastric polyps frequently straddle a hiatal hernia and may be associated with

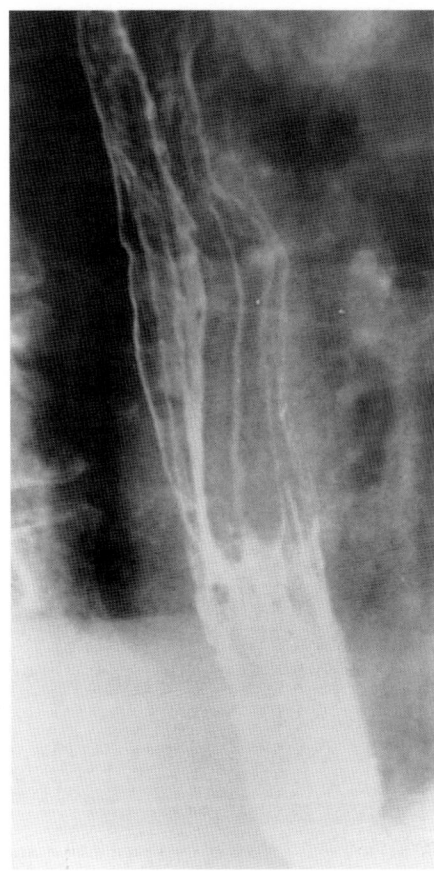

Figure 23-8. Reflux esophagitis with thickened longitudinal folds. (From Levine MS: Radiology of the Esophagus. Philadelphia, WB Saunders, 1989.)

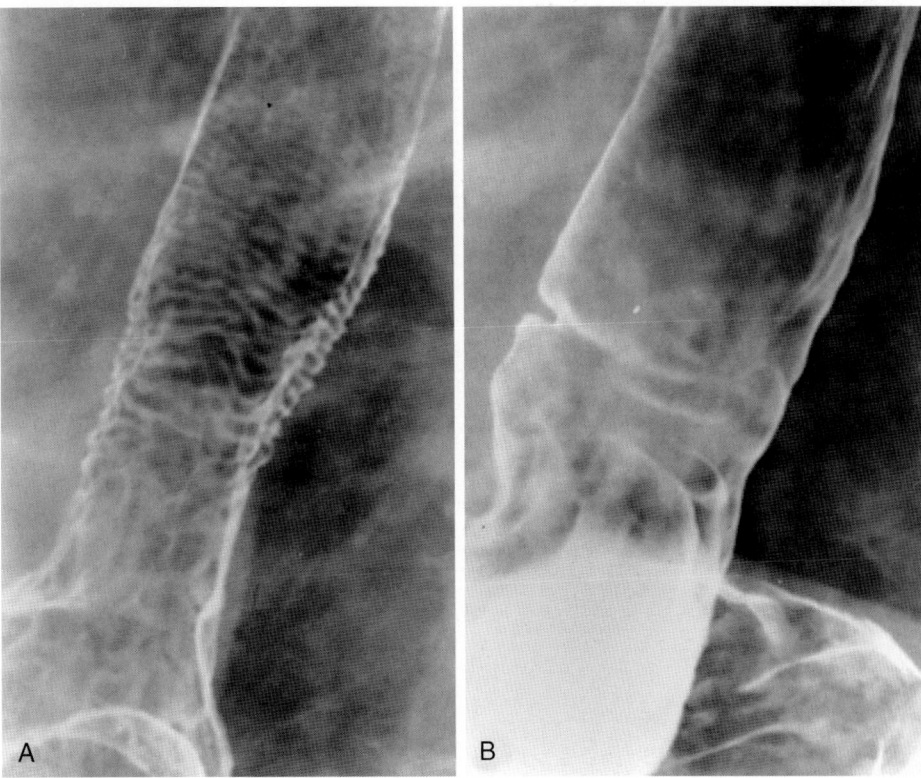

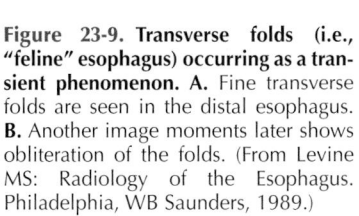

Figure 23-9. Transverse folds (i.e., "feline" esophagus) occurring as a transient phenomenon. A. Fine transverse folds are seen in the distal esophagus. **B.** Another image moments later shows obliteration of the folds. (From Levine MS: Radiology of the Esophagus. Philadelphia, WB Saunders, 1989.)

other radiographic evidence of reflux esophagitis. Because these lesions have no malignant potential, endoscopy is not warranted when typical inflammatory esophagogastric polyps are found on barium studies (see Fig. 23-11A).[78,79] If the lesions have a lobulated or irregular appearance (see Fig. 23-11B), however, endoscopy and biopsy should be performed to rule out malignant tumor.

Scarring and Strictures

Scarring from reflux esophagitis may be manifested by a variety of findings on esophagography. It is often possible to detect slight flattening or puckering of the esophageal wall, radiating folds, or both, in the absence of an actual stricture (Fig. 23-12). Asymmetric scarring from reflux esophagitis may also lead to focal outpouching or sacculation of the distal esophagus as a result of outward ballooning of the esophageal wall between areas of fibrosis (Fig. 23-13). These sacculations may resemble ulcer craters but can usually be differentiated from ulcers by their more rounded appearance and changeable configuration at fluoroscopy. Sacculations are particularly likely to develop in patients with scleroderma, presumably because of the severe esophagitis that occurs in these individuals. Much less frequently, patients with esophageal involvement by scleroderma may develop wide-mouthed outpouchings or sacculations in the absence of strictures as a result of asymmetric smooth muscle fibrosis and atrophy (Fig. 23-14).[80]

Scarring from reflux esophagitis may also be manifested by fixed transverse folds in the distal esophagus, producing a characteristic "stepladder" appearance resulting from pooling

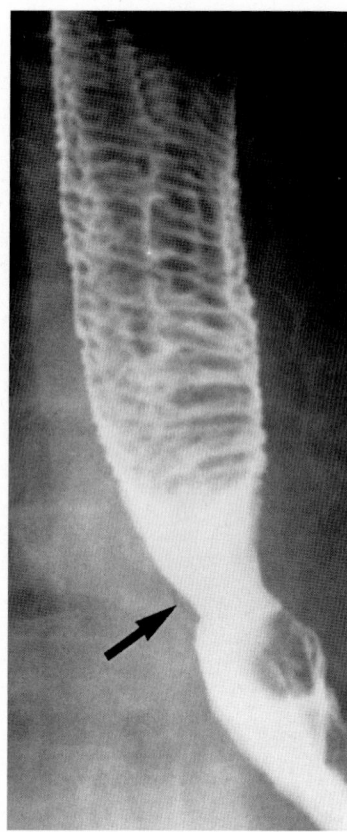

Figure 23-10. Reflux esophagitis with thickened transverse folds. There is also a peptic stricture (*arrow*) in the distal esophagus. (From Levine MS: Radiology of the Esophagus. Philadelphia, WB Saunders, 1989.)

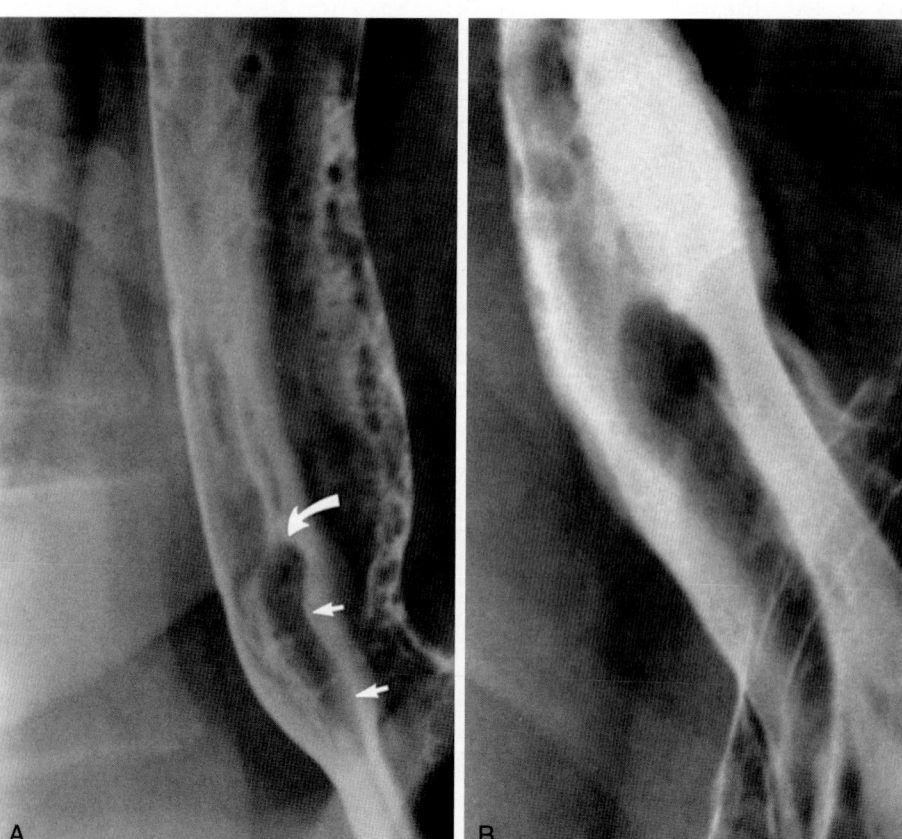

Figure 23-11. Inflammatory esophagogastric polyps. A. A prominent fold (*straight arrows*) is seen arising at the cardia and extending into the distal esophagus as a smooth, polypoid protuberance (*curved arrow*). This appearance is characteristic of inflammatory polyps. **B.** An inflammatory esophagogastric polyp is seen in the distal esophagus in another patient. This lesion is more lobulated than most inflammatory polyps, so that it cannot be differentiated from an adenomatous polyp or even an adenocarcinoma. (From Levine MS: Radiology of the Esophagus. Philadelphia, WB Saunders, 1989.)

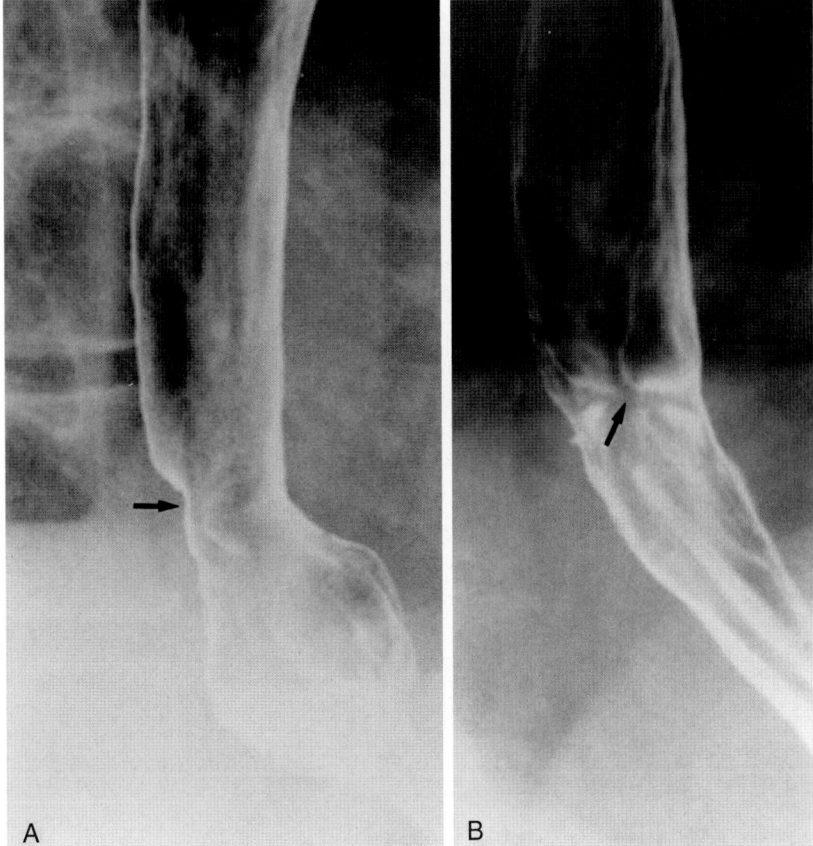

Figure 23-12. Mild peptic scarring in the distal esophagus. A. There is slight flattening and puckering of the distal esophagus (*arrow*) with radiating folds in this region as a result of scarring from reflux esophagitis. **B** In another patient, folds are seen radiating to a central scar (*arrow*).

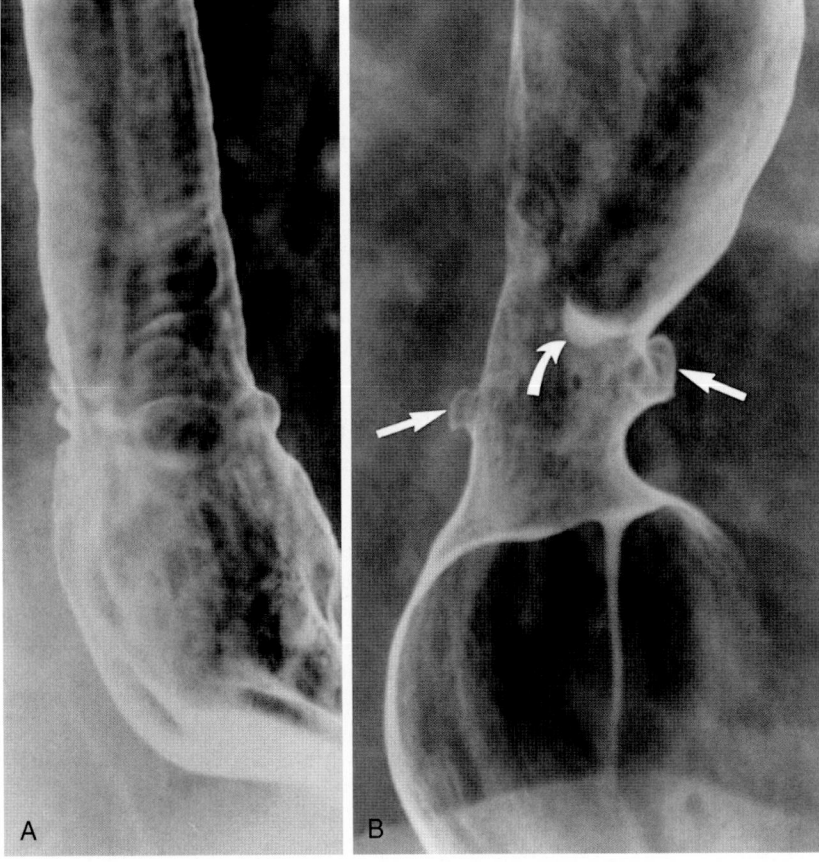

Figure 23-13. Scarring from reflux esophagitis with sacculations. A. There are sacculations and radiating folds in the distal esophagus without evidence of a stricture. **B.** In another patient with greater scarring, there is a peptic stricture with several large sacculations seen en face (*curved arrow*) and in profile (*straight arrows*) in the distal esophagus. (**A** from Levine MS, Goldstein HM: Fixed transverse folds in the esophagus: A sign of reflux esophagitis. AJR 143:275-278, 1984, © by American Roentgen Ray Society; **B** from Laufer I, Levine MS [eds]: Double Contrast Gastrointestinal Radiology, 2nd ed. Philadelphia, WB Saunders, 1992.)

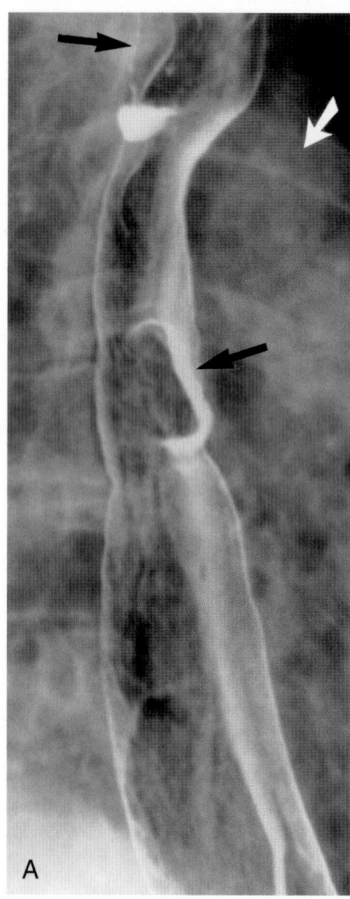
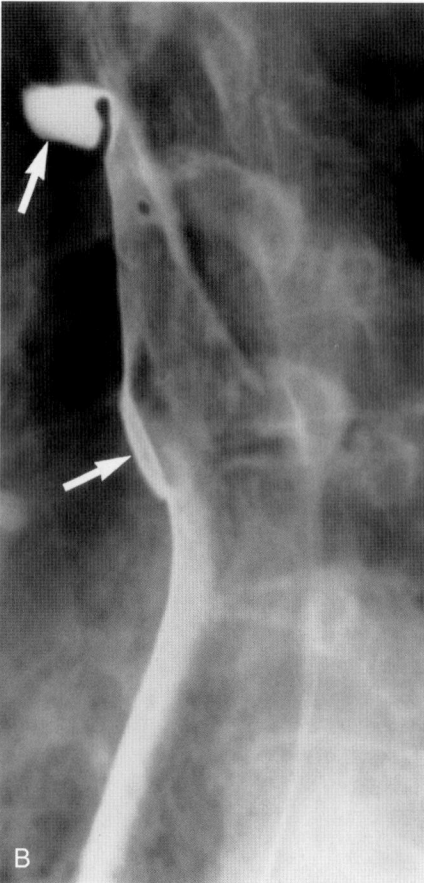

Figure 23-14. Wide-mouthed sacculations in scleroderma. A. Two large sacculations are seen en face (*black arrows*) in the upper and middle esophagus. Note how the upper sacculation extends superiorly just above the level of the aortic arch (*white arrow*). **B.** Additional view with the patient turned 90 degrees shows the sacculations in profile (*arrows*). (From Coggins CA, Levine MS, Kesack CD, et al: Wide-mouthed sacculations in the esophagus: A radiographic finding in scleroderma. AJR 176:953-954, 2001, © by American Roentgen Ray Society.)

of barium between the folds (Fig. 23-15).[71] These transverse folds are usually 2 to 5 mm wide and do not extend more than halfway across the esophagus. The folds tend to be relatively few in number, and they cannot be obliterated with esophageal distention. In most cases, there is other evidence of scarring from reflux esophagitis, and these transverse folds extend proximally a variable distance from the site of a distal stricture or scar. The folds probably represent areas of heaped-up or crinkled mucosa caused by simultaneous longitudinal scarring from reflux esophagitis. These fixed transverse folds should be distinguished from the thin transverse striations that are sometimes observed as a transient finding on double-contrast studies (see Fig. 23-9).[74,75]

Between 10% and 20% of patients with reflux esophagitis develop peptic strictures as a result of circumferential scarring of the distal esophagus.[50,81] Accurate radiographic diagnosis of these strictures requires continuous drinking of low-density barium in the prone position to distend the distal esophagus and optimally demonstrate mild or even moderate strictures that are not visible on upright double contrast images (Fig. 23-16). With careful biphasic technique, esophagography has a sensitivity of almost 95% in detecting peptic strictures and may occasionally reveal strictures that are missed at endoscopy.[82,83]

The vast majority of peptic strictures are located in the distal esophagus above a sliding hiatal hernia (Fig. 23-17). Because many patients with gastroesophageal reflux or mild reflux esophagitis do not have a concomitant hernia, it has been postulated that scarring from reflux esophagitis leads

not only to circumferential narrowing of the distal esophagus but also to longitudinal shortening and subsequent hernia formation.[3,23,25] Whatever the explanation, a hiatal hernia is found on barium studies in more than 95% of patients with peptic strictures.[23] When a hiatal hernia is not present in patients with distal esophageal strictures, the possibility of malignant tumor should therefore be considered as a possible cause of these strictures.

The classic appearance of a smooth, tapered area of concentric narrowing in the distal esophagus above a sliding hiatal hernia should be virtually pathognomonic of a peptic stricture (see Fig. 23-17A).[84] Many peptic strictures have an asymmetric appearance, however, with puckering, deformity, or sacculation of one wall of the stricture because of asymmetric scarring from reflux esophagitis (see Fig. 23-17B).[84] Other strictures may involve a longer segment of the distal esophagus and may have irregular margins because of associated reflux esophagitis (see Fig. 23-17C).[82]

The majority of peptic strictures range from 1 to 4 cm in length and from 0.2 to 2.0 cm in width.[82,85] These strictures rarely cause esophageal obstruction, but some patients may develop intermittent food impactions above the proximal end of the stricture.[36] As many as 40% of radiographically diagnosed peptic strictures, however, appear as ringlike areas of narrowing at the gastroesophageal junction with slightly tapered borders and a length of only 0.4 to 1 cm (Fig. 23-18).[85] Schatzki rings may produce similar radiographic findings, but they usually range from 2 to 4 mm in length and have more abrupt, symmetric borders (see Chapter 30).[86] Despite

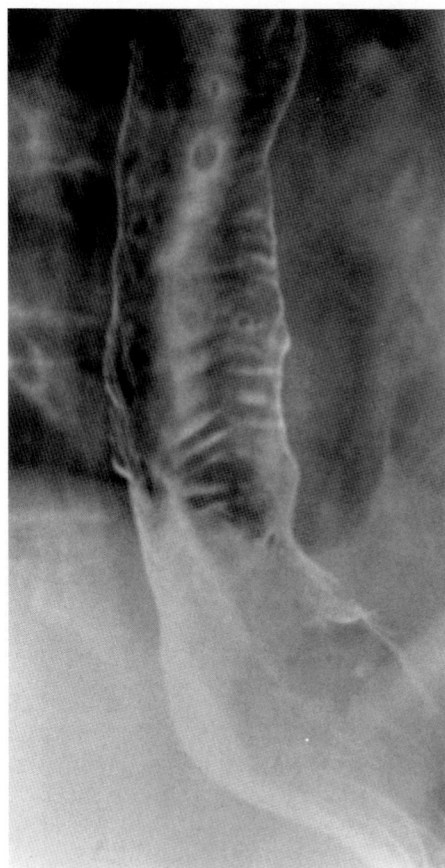

Figure 23-15. Fixed transverse folds in the esophagus. Multiple transverse folds in the distal esophagus produce a "stepladder" appearance due to longitudinal scarring from reflux esophagitis. (From Levine MS, Goldstein HM: Fixed transverse folds in the esophagus: A sign of reflux esophagitis. AJR 143:275-278, 1984, © by American Roentgen Ray Society.)

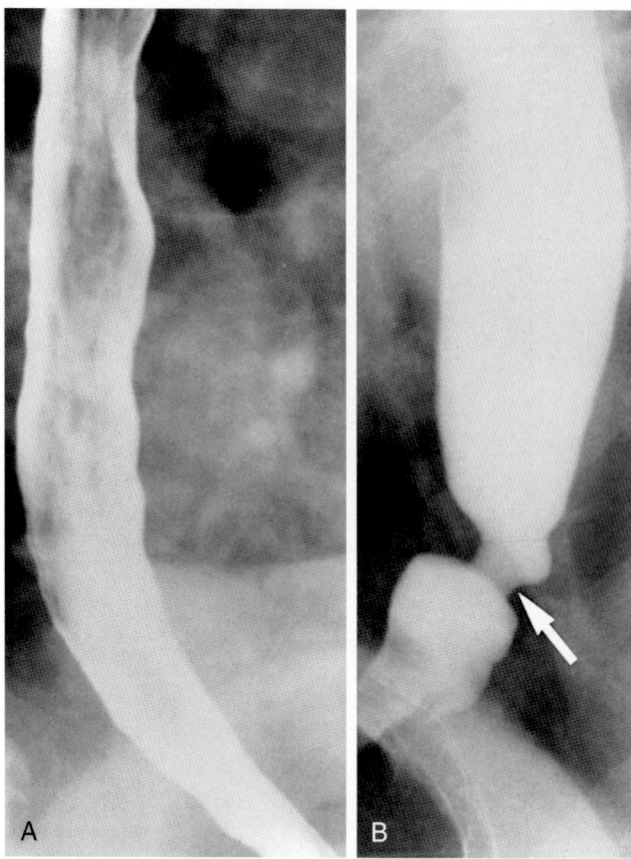

Figure 23-16. Peptic stricture seen only on prone single-contrast views of the esophagus. A. Double-contrast view with the patient upright shows no evidence of narrowing in the distal esophagus. B. Single-contrast view from the same examination with the patient prone reveals an unequivocal peptic stricture (arrow) above a hiatal hernia. Even in retrospect this short stricture was not visible on double-contrast images because of inadequate distention of this region.

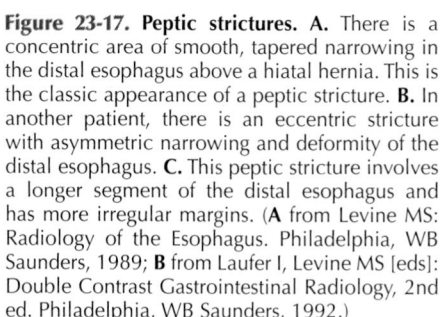

Figure 23-17. Peptic strictures. A. There is a concentric area of smooth, tapered narrowing in the distal esophagus above a hiatal hernia. This is the classic appearance of a peptic stricture. B. In another patient, there is an eccentric stricture with asymmetric narrowing and deformity of the distal esophagus. C. This peptic stricture involves a longer segment of the distal esophagus and has more irregular margins. (A from Levine MS: Radiology of the Esophagus. Philadelphia, WB Saunders, 1989; B from Laufer I, Levine MS [eds]: Double Contrast Gastrointestinal Radiology, 2nd ed. Philadelphia, WB Saunders, 1992.)

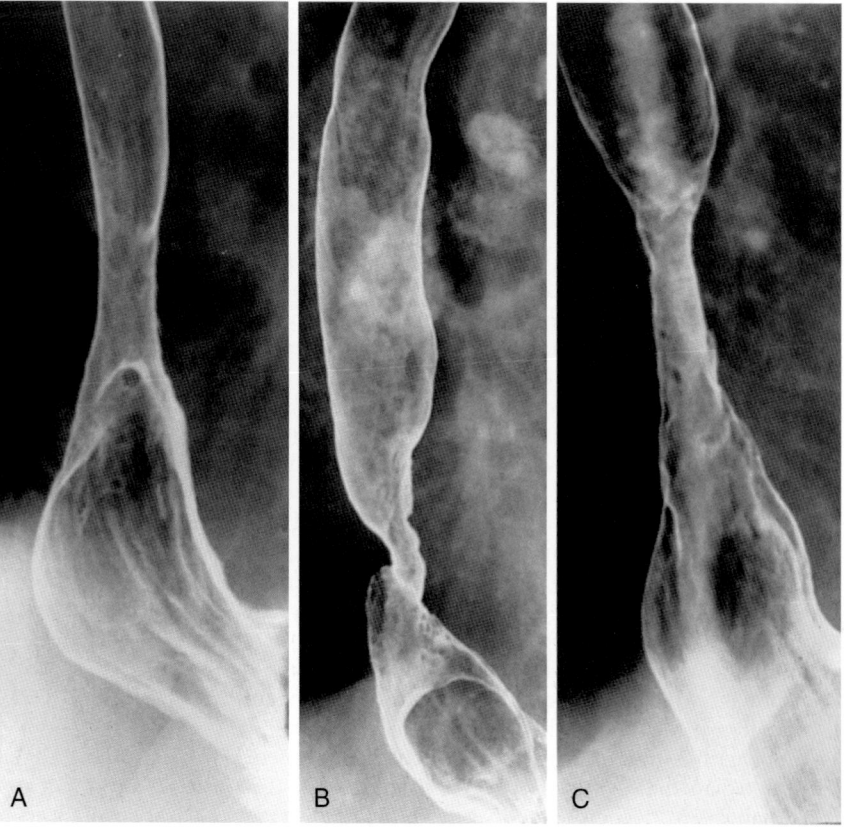

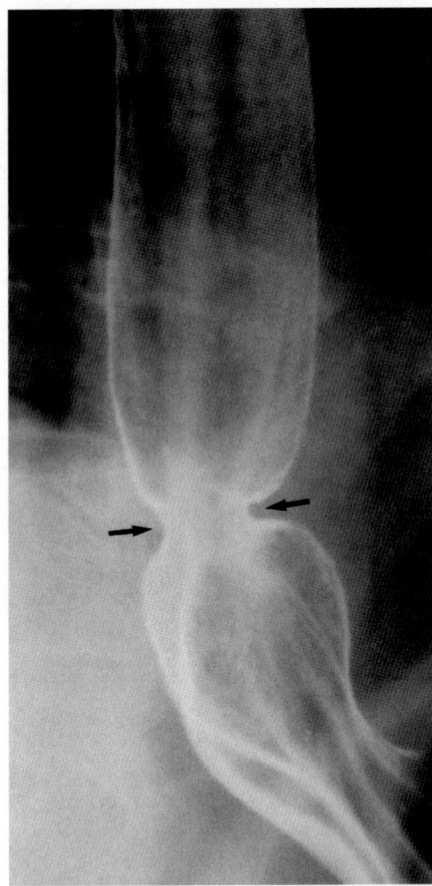

Figure 23-18. Ringlike peptic stricture. There is a ringlike stricture (*arrows*) in the distal esophagus above a hiatal hernia. Although this stricture could be mistaken for a Schatzki ring, it has a longer vertical height and more tapered borders than does a true Schatzki ring. (From Luedtke P, Levine MS, Rubesin SE, et al: Radiologic diagnosis of benign esophageal strictures: A pattern approach. RadioGraphics 23:897-909, 2003.)

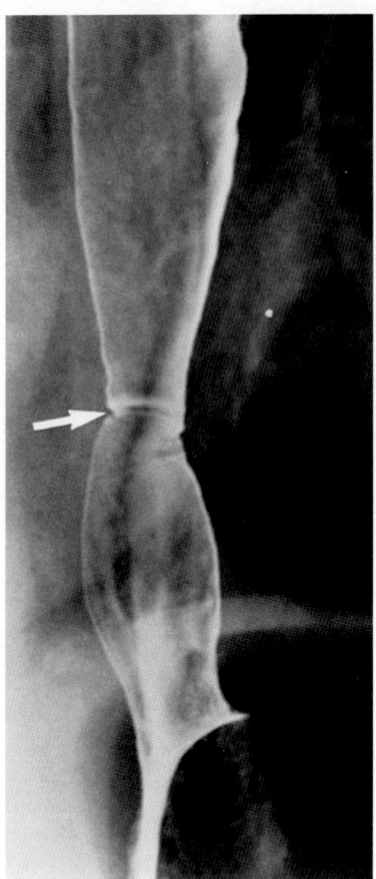

Figure 23-19. Peptic stricture with an associated web. The web (*arrow*) is located a greater distance from the gastroesophageal junction than expected for lower esophageal rings. (From Levine MS: Radiology of the Esophagus. Philadelphia, WB Saunders, 1989.)

these subtle distinctions, there probably is overlap between ringlike peptic strictures and Schatzki rings detected on barium studies or endoscopy.

Distal esophageal webs have also been recognized as a manifestation of scarring from reflux esophagitis.[87] The webs are almost always associated with peptic strictures, and they tend to occur at a discrete distance from the gastroesophageal junction, so that they can usually be differentiated from Schatzki rings by their more proximal location (Fig. 23-19). Some investigators have also found a significant association between cervical esophageal webs and gastroesophageal reflux,[88] possibly secondary to chronic injury from refluxed acid in the cervical esophagus.

Longer peptic strictures involving the distal third or half of the thoracic esophagus are relatively unusual. Such strictures may occur as a result of nasogastric intubation, protracted vomiting, bile reflux after partial or total gastrectomy, and Zollinger-Ellison syndrome (see Chapter 25).[15-17,35,89-92] Occasionally, patients with Zollinger-Ellison syndrome may even present with long strictures in the distal esophagus as the initial manifestation of their disease (Fig. 23-20).[15,16]

Esophageal intramural pseudodiverticula can sometimes be detected in the region of a peptic stricture (Fig. 23-21) (see Chapter 25).[93] The pseudodiverticula probably occur as

a sequela of chronic reflux esophagitis, but it is unclear why so few patients with esophagitis have this finding.

Many gastroenterologists believe that endoscopy and biopsy are required to rule out malignant tumor in all patients with radiographically diagnosed peptic strictures because of difficulty differentiating benign peptic strictures from infiltrating esophageal carcinomas on esophagography.[94-96] In a large retrospective study, however, no patients with unequivocally benign-appearing peptic strictures in the distal esophagus on double-contrast esophagograms were found to have malignant tumor on endoscopy,[84] so that endoscopy is not required to rule out esophageal cancer in these patients. If, however, the strictures have irregular contours, more abrupt margins, or other suspicious radiographic features, endoscopy and biopsy should be performed to rule out malignant tumor, particularly an adenocarcinoma arising in Barrett's esophagus (see Chapter 27).

Differential Diagnosis

Artifacts

A variety of technical artifacts may simulate the appearance of small ulcers on double-contrast esophagography.[66,97] When

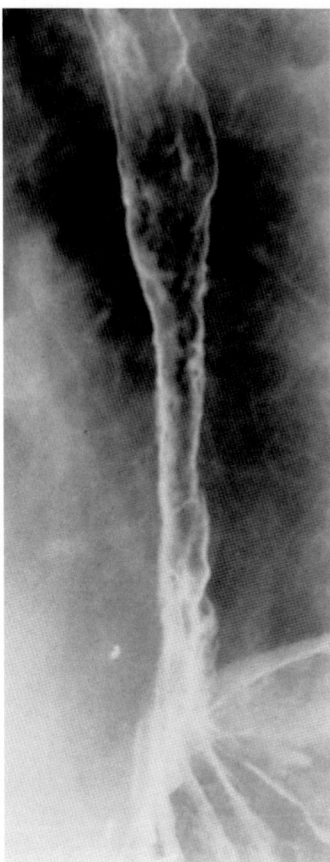

Figure 23-20. Long peptic stricture caused by Zollinger-Ellison syndrome. There is a long area of narrowing in the distal esophagus with extensive ulceration in the region of the stricture. The unusual length of the strictures in these patients is presumably related to the higher acidity of refluxed peptic contents in Zollinger-Ellison syndrome. (From Levine MS: Radiology of the Esophagus. Philadelphia, WB Saunders, 1989.)

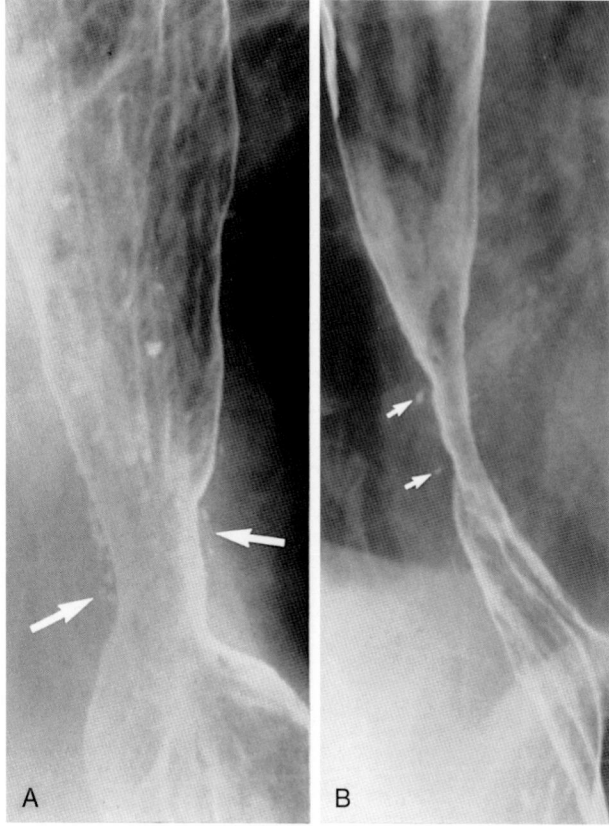

Figure 23-21. Peptic strictures with esophageal intramural pseudodiverticulosis. A. There is a mild peptic stricture in the distal esophagus with multiple intramural pseudodiverticula seen en face and in profile (*arrows*) in the region of the stricture. **B.** This patient has a more severe peptic stricture with several pseudodiverticula (*arrows*) adjacent to the stricture. Note how the pseudodiverticula seem to be floating outside the wall of the esophagus without apparent communication with the lumen. The latter feature is characteristic of these structures. (**A** from Levine MS: Radiology of the Esophagus. Philadelphia, WB Saunders, 1989.)

barium agents are improperly prepared, barium precipitates can be mistaken for numerous tiny ulcers (Fig. 23-22A). A similar appearance may also result from transient mucosal crinkling because of incomplete esophageal distention. Occasionally, an irregular Z line at the squamocolumnar junction may resemble a focal area of superficial ulceration. Even prominent interstitial lung markings or vascular shadows seen through the esophagus may create the erroneous impression of ulceration.

Apparent mucosal granularity or nodularity may be caused by undissolved effervescent agent, gas bubbles, or debris in the esophagus (Fig. 23-22B). As a result, the increased sensitivity of the double-contrast study has been compromised by the increased number of false-positive examinations with this technique.[48,50] If an artifact is suspected, however, additional double-contrast images should be obtained to demonstrate the transient nature of these findings.

Mucosal Nodularity

Glycogenic acanthosis should be the major consideration in the differential diagnosis of a nodular esophageal mucosa. This benign, degenerative condition is manifested on esophago-

graphy by multiple small, rounded nodules or plaques in the middle or distal third of the esophagus, so that it can resemble the nodular mucosa of reflux esophagitis (see Chapter 26).[98,99] The nodules of glycogenic acanthosis tend to be more well defined than those of reflux esophagitis, however, and are usually more prominent in the midesophagus than in the distal esophagus. The clinical history is also helpful because patients with glycogenic acanthosis are almost always asymptomatic.[98]

Candida esophagitis may occasionally produce a finely nodular or granular appearance in the esophagus, mimicking the appearance of reflux esophagitis (see Chapter 24). This form of *Candida* esophagitis has been observed more frequently in patients with AIDS.[100] Opportunistic esophagitis should be suggested by the typical history of odynophagia in an immunocompromised patient.

Rarely, superficial spreading carcinoma may produce a reticulonodular appearance of the mucosa, but the area of involvement is usually more localized than that in reflux esophagitis and the distal esophagus is often spared.[101] Finally, leukoplakia, squamous papillomatosis, and acanthosis nigricans are rare causes of mucosal nodularity in the esophagus, and the diagnosis is usually made unexpectedly at endoscopy or autopsy in these patients (see Chapter 26).

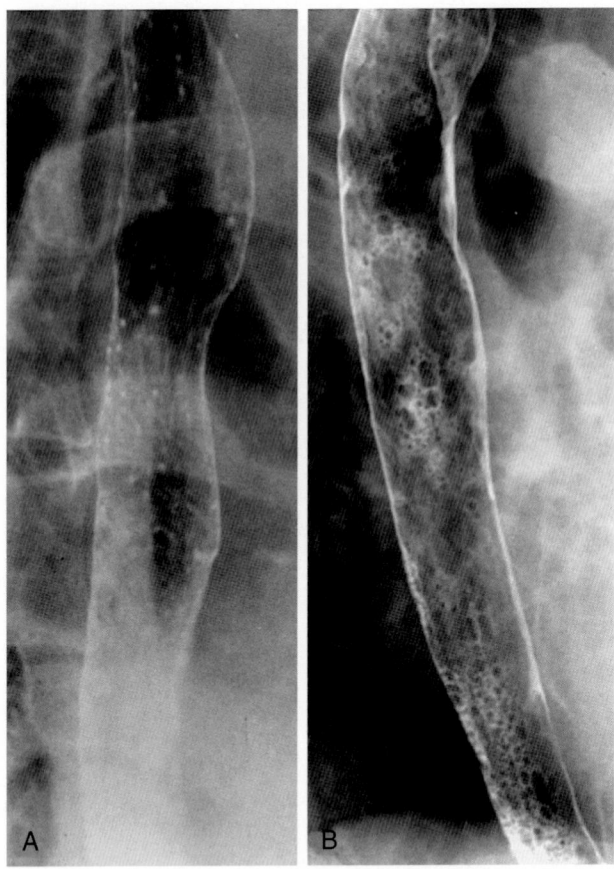

Figure 23-22. Double-contrast artifacts. A. Barium precipitates are present in the esophagus. These punctate collections of barium could be mistaken for tiny ulcers. **B.** In another patient, undissolved effervescent agent and gas bubbles in the esophagus cause apparent nodularity of the mucosa. If an artifact is suspected, additional double-contrast views should be obtained to demonstrate the transient nature of these findings. (**B** from Levine MS: Radiology of the Esophagus. Philadelphia, WB Saunders, 1989.)

Ulceration

Although reflux esophagitis is the most common cause of superficial ulceration in the esophagus, shallow ulcers and erosions may be caused by other types of esophagitis, including herpes esophagitis and drug-induced esophagitis.[102,103] In contrast to reflux esophagitis, herpes esophagitis and drug-induced esophagitis tend to involve the middle or upper third of the esophagus with distal esophageal sparing (see Chapters 24 and 25), and they are usually not associated with evidence of a hiatal hernia or gastroesophageal reflux. The correct diagnosis should also be suggested by a clinical history of acute odynophagia in patients who are immunocompromised or who are taking oral medications such as tetracycline and doxycycline.

Occasionally, esophageal involvement by Crohn's disease may be manifested on double-contrast esophagography by tiny "aphthoid" ulcers, mimicking the findings of reflux esophagitis.[104] Esophageal Crohn's disease is uncommon, however, and these patients almost always have evidence of advanced Crohn's disease in the small bowel or colon. More extensive ulceration may be caused by opportunistic infection, caustic ingestion, and mediastinal irradiation (see Chapters 24 and 25). In most cases, the correct diagnosis is suggested by the clinical history and presentation.

Thickened Folds

Thickened longitudinal folds in the esophagus may be caused by esophageal varices or by any inflammatory or neoplastic process that involves the submucosa. Although varices may occasionally resemble the thickened folds of esophagitis, they tend to be more tortuous or serpiginous and can usually be effaced to a greater degree or even obliterated by esophageal distention. Rarely, "varicoid" carcinomas can also be mistaken for esophagitis on a single image.[105] Because the folds are infiltrated by tumor, however, they are unaffected by esophageal peristalsis, respiration, and Valsalva maneuvers and cannot be substantially effaced by esophageal distention. As a result, these entities can usually be differentiated at fluoroscopy.

Scarring and Strictures

Fixed transverse folds in the esophagus as a result of scarring from reflux esophagitis should be distinguished not only from the delicate transverse striations of the feline esophagus but also from the broad transverse bands associated with non-peristaltic contractions. The horizontal collections of barium pooled between these fixed transverse folds should also not be mistaken for linear ulcers. The regularity and symmetry of these collections should suggest the correct diagnosis.

A smooth, tapered area of concentric narrowing above a hiatal hernia poses little diagnostic dilemma, but not all peptic strictures have this classic appearance. If suspicious radiographic features such as asymmetry, abrupt margins, and mucosal nodularity or ulceration are identified on the barium study (Fig. 23-23), endoscopy and biopsy should be performed to rule out an infiltrating carcinoma.

BARRETT'S ESOPHAGUS

Barrett's esophagus is an acquired condition in which there is progressive columnar metaplasia of the distal esophagus resulting from long-standing gastroesophageal reflux and reflux esophagitis.[106-110] The diagnosis of Barrett's esophagus has traditionally been reserved for patients who have endoscopic evidence of a columnar epithelial-lined esophagus extending more than 3 cm above the gastroesophageal junction with histopathologic findings of intestinal metaplasia on endoscopic biopsy specimens.[108] In various studies, the prevalence of Barrett's esophagus in patients with reflux esophagitis has ranged from 5% to 15%, with an overall prevalence of about 10%.[111-115] These figures may underestimate the true prevalence of Barrett's esophagus in the general population. In one study, the number of cases of Barrett's esophagus at autopsy was 20 times greater than the number of cases at endoscopy.[116] The findings in this study suggest that most cases of Barrett's esophagus remain undiagnosed because of the absence of esophageal symptoms. Nevertheless, Barrett's esophagus is being diagnosed with greater frequency as the number of patients who undergo endoscopy increases.

Despite its frequency, Barrett's esophagus would not be important if it were a benign entity. There is considerable evidence, however, that it is a premalignant condition associated with an increased risk of developing esophageal adenocarcinoma. These tumors evolve through a sequence of progressively severe epithelial dysplasia, eventually leading to the development of invasive carcinoma. In various studies, the prevalence of adenocarcinoma in patients with Barrett's

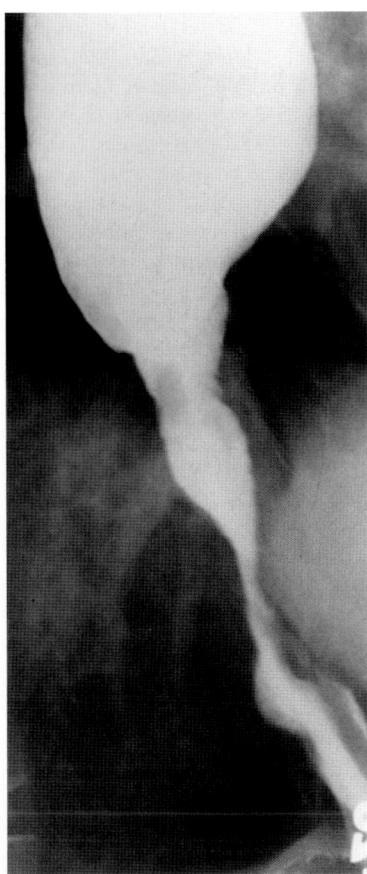

Figure 23-23. Esophageal carcinoma. There is a relatively long area of narrowing in the distal esophagus that could be mistaken for a benign peptic stricture. However, the asymmetric contour and relatively abrupt proximal borders of the narrowed segment should suggest the possibility of malignant tumor. (From Levine MS: Radiology of the Esophagus. Philadelphia, WB Saunders, 1989.)

As our understanding of Barrett's esophagus has evolved, investigators have developed revised histopathologic criteria for this condition in which patients are classified as having either "long-segment" (i.e., extending more than 3 cm from the gastroesophageal junction) or "short-segment" (i.e., extending 3 cm or less from the gastroesophageal junction) Barrett's esophagus based on the vertical extent of columnar metaplasia in the esophagus.[124] Short-segment Barrett's esophagus is even more common than long-segment Barrett's esophagus, with a reported prevalence of 10% to 15% at endoscopy.[125] Patients with short-segment Barrett's esophagus are more likely to develop dysplasia than the general population but less likely to develop dysplasia than those with long-segment Barrett's esophagus.[126,127] Although the cancer risk in these patients remains uncertain, some investigators believe that endoscopic surveillance is also warranted for patients with short-segment disease.[126-129]

Clinical Findings

The prevalence of Barrett's esophagus increases with age; the mean age is 55 to 60 years at the time of diagnosis.[130] This condition is more common in men than in women (2:1) and in whites than in blacks.[131] Affected individuals may present with reflux symptoms as a result of their underlying reflux disease, or they may present with dysphagia as a result of the development of strictures. However, as many as 40% of patients with Barrett's esophagus are asymptomatic.[120] Such patients may not seek medical attention until the development of a superimposed esophageal adenocarcinoma (see Chapter 27). When patients with Barrett's esophagus do have reflux symptoms, they are usually treated with proton pump inhibitors or, if necessary, a laparoscopic fundoplication. It should be recognized, however, that medical or even surgical treatment of the underlying reflux disease does not cause this Barrett's epithelium to regress, so that these individuals remain at risk for the development of esophageal adenocarcinoma even after a surgical fundoplication.[132]

Endoscopic and Histologic Findings

Long-segment Barrett's esophagus can be recognized at endoscopy by the presence of velvety, pinkish red columnar mucosa (often seen as islands or tongues) extending more than 3 cm above the lower esophageal sphincter or an endoscopically identified hiatal hernia.[108] Endoscopy is reported to have a sensitivity of greater than 90% in diagnosing Barrett's esophagus solely on the basis of the endoscopic findings.[133] Conversely, short-segment Barrett's esophagus is defined as endoscopically visualized columnar epithelium in the distal esophagus extending 3 cm or less above the gastroesophageal junction.[124]

In the past, the histopathologic criteria for Barrett's esophagus included the presence of columnar epithelium (including a junctional-type epithelium, a gastric fundic-type epithelium, and a specialized columnar epithelium or incomplete form of intestinal metaplasia) on endoscopic biopsy specimens more than 3 cm above the gastroesophageal junction.[134] Subsequently, however, investigators have focused on the importance of intestinal metaplasia on endoscopic biopsy specimens anywhere from the esophagus as the major prerequisite for the histopathologic diagnosis of Barrett's

esophagus has ranged from 2% to 46%, with an overall prevalence of about 10%.[113,117-119] It should be recognized that prevalence data tend to exaggerate the risk of cancer by failing to identify all patients with underlying Barrett's esophagus. This problem is exacerbated by the fact that as many as 40% of patients with Barrett's esophagus remain asymptomatic until the development of a superimposed adenocarcinoma.[120] Nevertheless, incidence data have shown that esophageal adenocarcinoma develops in about 0.5% of patients with Barrett's esophagus each year.[121]

Because of this increased cancer risk, the American College of Gastroenterology has recommended that patients with Barrett's esophagus undergo endoscopic surveillance at 2- to 3-year intervals to detect dysplastic changes before the development of overt cancer (see Chapter 27).[122] The cost-effectiveness of endoscopic surveillance of patients with known Barrett's esophagus is supported by a Markov model showing that it compares favorably to other widely accepted screening strategies for cancer.[123] On the other hand, endoscopic surveillance of patients with Barrett's esophagus has not yet been shown to improve the mortality from esophageal adenocarcinoma. Thus, many questions remain about the role of endoscopic surveillance and its ultimate value in patients with Barrett's esophagus.

esophagus.[124,135] This intestinal metaplasia is characterized histologically by goblet cells with acidic mucin and, in some cases, enterocyte differentiation with brush border formation. The revised definition for Barrett's esophagus is based on an emerging consensus that intestinal metaplasia represents the type of epithelium predisposing these individuals to esophageal adenocarcinoma.[135]

Radiographic Findings

Long-Segment Barrett's Esophagus

The classic radiologic features of long-segment Barrett's esophagus consist of a midesophageal stricture or ulcer, often associated with a sliding hiatal hernia or gastroesophageal reflux.[136-138] The unusually high location of these strictures or ulcers can be attributed to the fact that they often occur in the proximal zone of columnar metaplasia at or near the transposed squamocolumnar junction. The strictures may appear on barium studies as ringlike constrictions (Fig. 23-24A) or, less commonly, as tapered areas of narrowing (Fig. 23-24B) in the midesophagus.[136] Occasionally, early strictures may be recognized on double-contrast studies as subtle contour abnormalities with focal indentations or gently sloping con-

cavities of one wall.[139] Barrett's ulcers typically appear as relatively deep ulcer craters within the columnar mucosa, occurring at a considerable distance from the gastroesophageal junction (Fig. 23-25).[140] Because these findings are unusual in uncomplicated reflux disease, the presence of a midesophageal stricture or ulcer, particularly if associated with a hiatal hernia or gastroesophageal reflux, should be highly suggestive of Barrett's esophagus. However, studies have found that strictures are actually more common in the distal esophagus and that most cases do not fit the classic stereotype of a midesophageal stricture or ulcer.[141-144] Thus, esophagography is an inadequate screening examination for long-segment Barrett's esophagus when the diagnosis is made only in patients who have the classic radiologic features of this condition.

A reticular mucosal pattern has also been described as a relatively specific sign of long-segment Barrett's esophagus, particularly if located adjacent to a stricture.[142] This delicate reticular pattern is characterized radiographically by innumerable tiny, barium-filled grooves or crevices on the esophageal mucosa, resembling the areae gastricae pattern found on double-contrast studies of the stomach (Fig. 23-26). In most cases, there is an adjacent stricture in the midesophagus or, less commonly, distal esophagus, with the reticular pattern

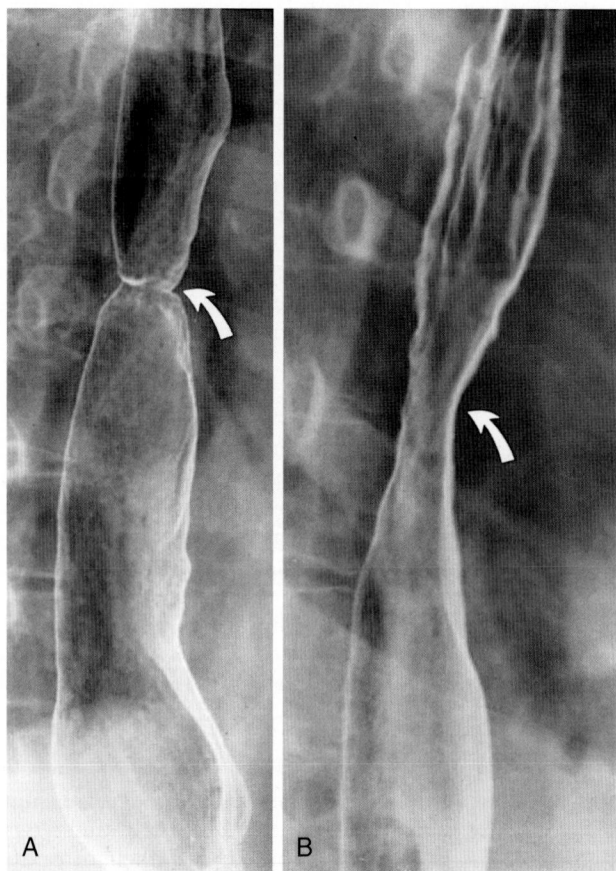

Figure 23-24. Barrett's esophagus with midesophageal strictures. A. There is a ringlike constriction (*arrow*) in the midesophagus. **B.** A smooth, tapered area of narrowing (*arrow*) is seen in the midesophagus. In the presence of a hiatal hernia and gastroesophageal reflux, a midesophageal stricture should be strongly suggestive of Barrett's esophagus. (From Levine MS: Radiology of the Esophagus. Philadelphia, WB Saunders, 1989.)

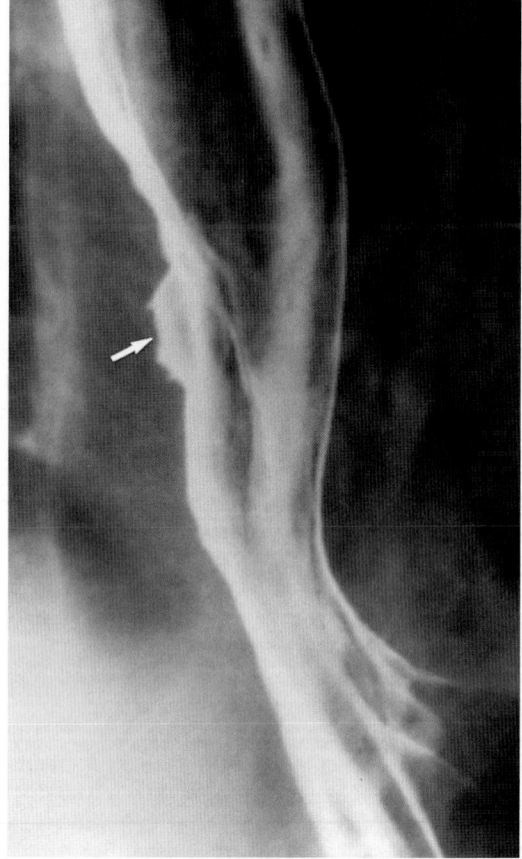

Figure 23-25. Barrett's esophagus with a high ulcer. There is a relatively deep ulcer crater (*arrow*) at a greater distance from the gastroesophageal junction than expected for uncomplicated reflux esophagitis. In the presence of a hiatal hernia and gastroesophageal reflux, a high ulcer should be strongly suggestive of Barrett's esophagus. (From Levine MS: Radiology of the Esophagus. Philadelphia, WB Saunders, 1989.)

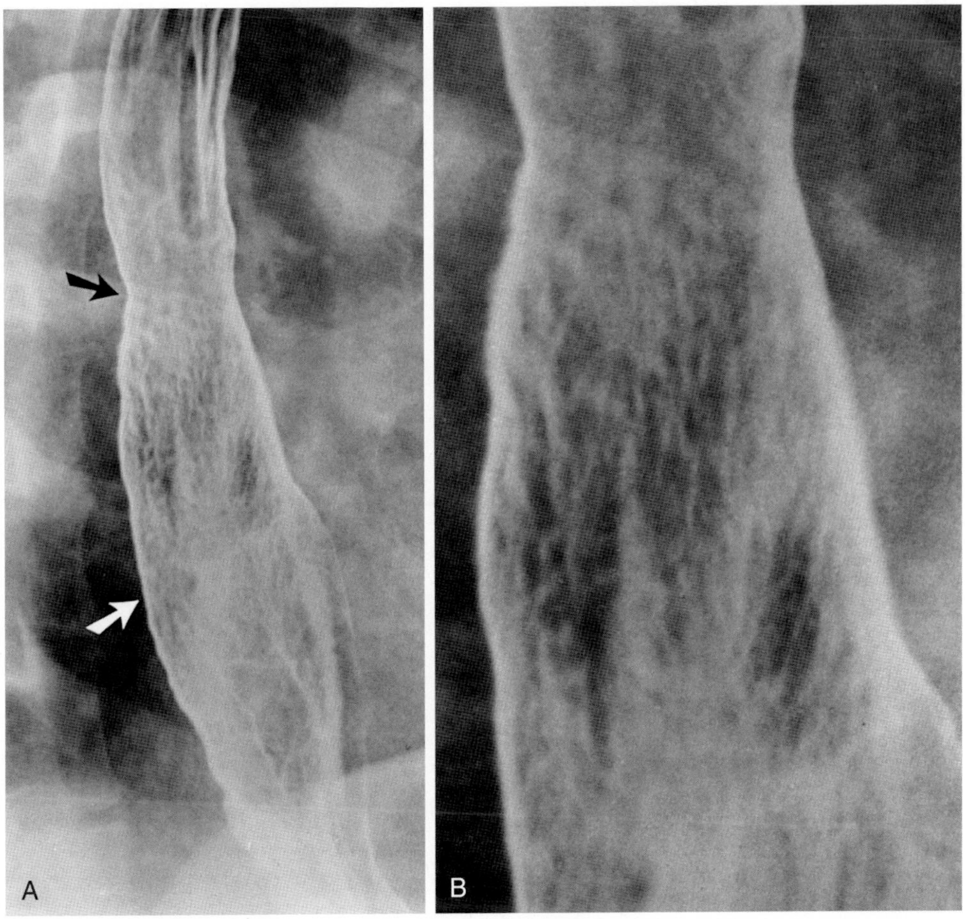

Figure 23-26. Barrett's esophagus with a reticular mucosal pattern. A. There is an early stricture (*black arrow*) in the midesophagus with a reticular pattern extending distally a considerable distance from the stricture (approximately to the level of the *white arrow*). **B.** A close-up view better delineates this delicate reticular pattern. (From Levine MS, Kressel HY, Caroline DF, et al: Barrett esophagus: Reticular pattern of the mucosa. Radiology 147:663-667, 1983.)

seen extending distally a short but variable distance from the stricture.[142] Occasionally, however, a reticular pattern of the mucosa may be observed as the only morphologic abnormality in Barrett's esophagus without evidence of strictures.[145] Whether or not a stricture is present, a reticular pattern should be highly suggestive of Barrett's esophagus, and endoscopy and biopsy should be performed for a definitive diagnosis. Nevertheless, this finding has been observed in only 5% to 30% of patients with Barrett's esophagus,[138,142-144,146] and its specificity has also been questioned.[147] Thus, most cases of long-segment Barrett's esophagus are missed on double-contrast esophagography if a reticular mucosal pattern is used as the primary radiologic criterion for diagnosing this condition.

Other morphologic findings of reflux disease, such as hiatal hernias, gastroesophageal reflux, reflux esophagitis, and peptic strictures, can be detected on double-contrast esophagograms in more than 95% of patients with long-segment Barrett's esophagus (Fig. 23-27),[137,138,141-144,146,148] but these findings frequently occur in patients with uncomplicated reflux disease. Thus, those findings that are relatively specific for Barrett's esophagus are not sensitive and those findings that are more sensitive are not specific. As a result, many investigators have traditionally believed that esophagography has limited value as a screening examination for Barrett's esophagus and that endoscopy and biopsy are required to diagnose this condition.

In 1988, Gilchrist and colleagues[149] introduced a novel approach for the diagnosis of long-segment Barrett's esopha-

gus on double-contrast esophagography by stratifying patients with reflux symptoms based on the following radiologic criteria: patients were classified at high risk if the images revealed the classic findings of a midesophageal stricture or ulcer or a reticular mucosal pattern; at moderate risk if the images revealed reflux esophagitis or a distal peptic stricture (because previous studies have shown that 10% of patients with reflux esophagitis and as many as 40% with peptic strictures have Barrett's esophagus[111-115,150]); and at low risk if the images revealed a normal-appearing esophagus. The vast majority of patients classified at high risk and approximately 15% classified at moderate risk for Barrett's esophagus on double-contrast esophagograms were found to have this condition. Conversely, less than 1% of patients classified at low risk for Barrett's esophagus because of the absence of esophagitis or strictures were found to have this condition. Thus, esophagitis or peptic scarring severe enough to cause Barrett's esophagus can almost always be detected on technically adequate double-contrast examinations.

On the basis of such data, the investigators concluded that patients who are found to be at high risk for Barrett's esophagus on double-contrast esophagograms because of a midesophageal stricture or ulcer or a reticular mucosal pattern should undergo endoscopy and biopsy for a definitive diagnosis.[149] A larger group of patients are found to be at moderate risk for Barrett's esophagus because of reflux esophagitis or peptic strictures in the distal esophagus, so that clinical judgment should be used regarding the decision for endoscopy in this group based on the severity of reflux

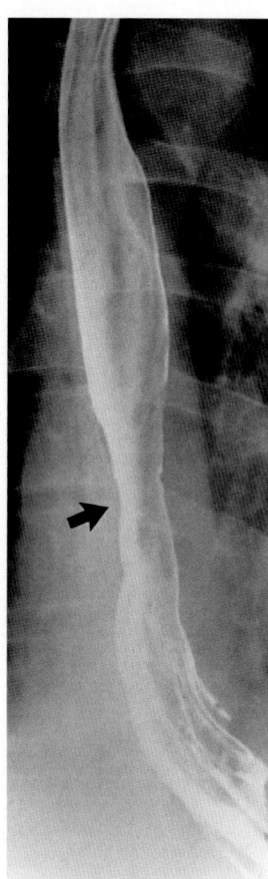

Figure 23-27. Barrett's esophagus with a distal stricture. There is a concentric area of narrowing (*arrow*) in the distal esophagus above a hiatal hernia. An ordinary peptic stricture without Barrett's esophagus could produce identical findings. (From Levine MS: Radiology of the Esophagus. Philadelphia, WB Saunders, 1989.)

symptoms, age, and overall health of the patient (i.e., whether they are reasonable candidates for endoscopic surveillance). However, most patients are found to be at low risk for Barrett's esophagus because of the absence of esophagitis or strictures and the risk of Barrett's esophagus is so low in this group that endoscopy does not appear to be warranted. Thus, the major value of double contrast esophagography is its ability to separate patients into these various risk groups for Barrett's esophagus to determine the relative need for endoscopy and biopsy.

Short-Segment Barrett's Esophagus

Although the radiographic features of long-segment Barrett's esophagus have been well documented, much less is known about the findings in short-segment Barrett's esophagus. In a study by Yamamoto and coworkers,[151] 70% of patients with short-segment Barrett's esophagus had morphologic evidence of esophagitis and/or peptic scarring or strictures in the distal esophagus on double-contrast esophagograms, but the remaining 30% had hiatal hernias or gastroesophageal reflux as the only radiographic findings. The absence of reflux esophagitis or peptic strictures on double-contrast studies therefore does not exclude the possibility of short-segment Barrett's esophagus. Thus, patients with short-segment Barrett's esopha-

gus are far more likely to have a normal-appearing esophagus on double-contrast esophagograms than those with long-segment disease. Nevertheless, the clinical importance of this observation remains uncertain because of the lower cancer risk of short-segment Barrett's esophagus compared with that associated with long-segment disease.[126,127]

In the study by Yamamoto and associates,[151] all of the patients with short-segment Barrett's esophagus had disease confined to the distal third of the esophagus on barium studies but the length of involvement of the distal esophagus by esophagitis or peptic scarring often extended more than 3 cm above the gastroesophageal junction, so that the diseased segment on esophagography does not necessarily correspond to the vertical extent of columnar metaplasia in the esophagus.

Differential Diagnosis

Uncomplicated peptic strictures are almost always located in the distal esophagus, so that the presence of a midesophageal stricture should strongly suggest the possibility of Barrett's esophagus, particularly if associated with a hiatal hernia and gastroesophageal reflux. Midesophageal strictures may also be caused by caustic ingestion (Fig. 23-28A); by mediastinal irradiation (Fig. 23-28B); by primary or metastatic tumors; and, rarely, by esophageal involvement by dermatologic disorders, such as epidermolysis bullosa dystrophica and benign

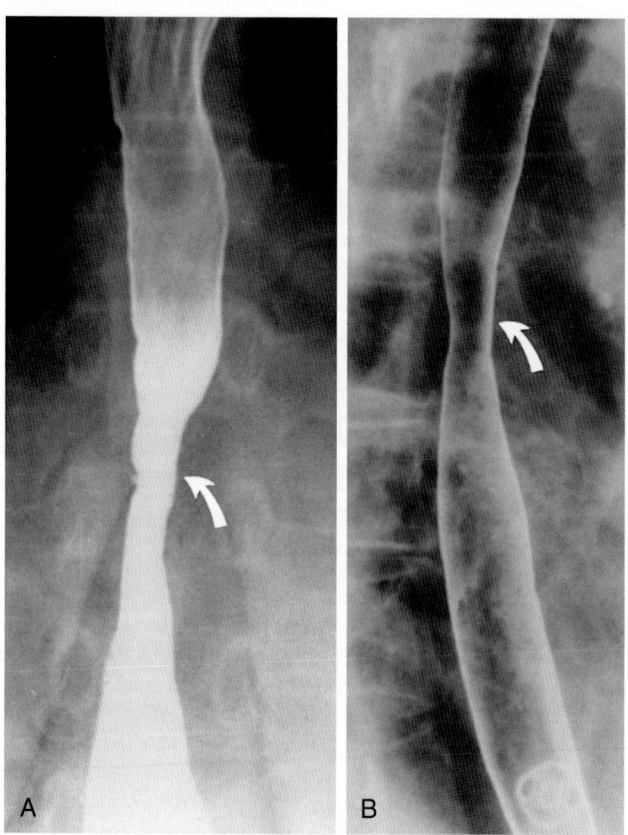

Figure 23-28. Other causes of midesophageal strictures. A. There is a segmental stricture (*arrow*) with shallow ulceration in the midesophagus due to prior lye ingestion. **B.** There is a smooth, tapered stricture (*arrow*) in the midesophagus due to mediastinal irradiation. (From Levine MS: Radiology of the Esophagus. Philadelphia, WB Saunders, 1989.)

mucous membrane pemphigoid. These conditions, however, can usually be differentiated from Barrett's esophagus by the clinical history and presentation.

The presence of a reticular mucosal pattern appears to be a relatively specific radiologic criterion for Barrett's esophagus, particularly if located adjacent to the distal aspect of a midesophageal stricture.[142] Although a reticulonodular appearance may occasionally be seen in patients with superficial spreading carcinoma, it is a rare entity that is not classically associated with strictures.[101] Shallow ulceration or mucosal irregularity resulting from reflux esophagitis might also conceivably produce a similar appearance. Reflux esophagitis usually occurs proximal to a peptic stricture, however, and it would be extremely unusual for an isolated area of esophagitis to occur at the distal aspect of a stricture. *Candida* esophagitis may also be manifested by mucosal nodularity, but the discrete plaquelike lesions of candidiasis can usually be differentiated from the reticular pattern of Barrett's mucosa.

References

1. Nebel OT, Fornes MF, Castell DO: Symptomatic gastroesophageal reflux: Incidence and precipitating factors. Dig Dis Sci 21:953-956, 1976.
2. Locke GR, Talley NJ, Fett SL, et al: Prevalence and clinical spectrum of gastroesophageal reflux: A population-based study in Olmsted County, Minnesota. Gastroenterology 112:1448-1456, 1997.
3. Behar J: Reflux esophagitis: Pathogenesis, diagnosis, and management. Arch Intern Med 136:560-566, 1976.
4. Dodds WJ: Current concepts of esophageal motor function: Clinical implications for radiology. AJR 128:549-561, 1977.
5. Dodds WJ, Hogan WJ, Helm JF, et al: Pathogenesis of reflux esophagitis. Gastroenterology 81:376-394, 1981.
6. Dodds WJ: The pathogenesis of gastroesophageal reflux disease. AJR 151:49-56, 1988.
7. Pope CE: Acid-reflux disorders. N Engl J Med 331:656-660, 1994.
8. Barlow WJ, Orlando RC: The pathogenesis of heartburn in nonerosive reflux disease: A unifying hypothesis. Gastroenterology 128:771-778, 2005.
9. Pope CE: Pathophysiology and diagnosis of reflux esophagitis. Gastroenterology 70:445-454, 1976.
10. Dodds WJ, Dent J, Hogan WJ, et al: Mechanisms of gastroesophageal reflux in patients with reflux esophagitis. N Engl J Med 307:1547-1552, 1982.
11. Schoeman MN, Tippett MD, Akkermans LMA, et al: Mechanisms of gastroesophageal reflux in ambulant healthy human subjects. Gastroenterology 108:83-91, 1995.
12. Mittal RK, Holloway RH, Penagini R, et al: Transient lower esophageal sphincter relaxation. Gastroenterology 109:601-610, 1995.
13. Zamost BJ, Hirschberg J, Ippoliti AF, et al: Esophagitis in scleroderma: Prevalence and risk factors. Gastroenterology 92:421-428, 1987.
14. Vaezi MF, Singh S, Richter JE: Role of acid and duodenogastric reflux in esophageal mucosal injury: A review of animal and human studies. Gastroenterology 108:1897-1907, 1995.
15. Dodds WJ, Dehn TG, Hogan WJ, et al: Severe peptic esophagitis in a patient with Zollinger-Ellison syndrome. AJR 113:237-240, 1971.
16. Smith HJ, Chapa HJ, Kilman WJ, et al: Zollinger-Ellison syndrome presenting as esophageal stricture. Gastrointest Radiol 4:349-351, 1979.
17. Agha FP: Esophageal involvement in Zollinger-Ellison syndrome. AJR 144:721-725, 1985.
18. Cohen S: The diagnosis and management of gastroesophageal reflux. Adv Intern Med 21:47-75, 1976.
19. Wright RA, Hurwitz AL: Relationship of hiatal hernia to endoscopically proved reflux esophagitis. Dig Dis Sci 24:311-313, 1979.
20. Ott DJ, Gelfand DW, Chen YM, et al: Predictive relationship of hiatal hernia to reflux esophagitis. Gastrointest Radiol 10:317-320, 1985.
21. Cohen S, Harris LD: Does hiatus hernia affect competence of the gastroesophageal sphincter? N Engl J Med 284:1053-1056, 1971.
22. Ellis FH: Current concepts: esophageal hiatal hernia. N Engl J Med 287:646-649, 1972.
23. Ho CS, Rodrigues PR: Lower esophageal strictures, benign or malignant? J Can Assoc Radiol 31:110-113, 1980.
24. Ott DJ, Dodds WJ, Wu WC, et al: Current status of radiology in evaluating for gastroesophageal reflux disease. J Clin Gastroenterol 4:365-375, 1982.
25. Paterson WG, Kolyn DM: Esophageal shortening induced by short-term intraluminal acid perfusion in opossum: A cause of hiatus hernia? Gastroenterology 107:1736-1740, 1994.
26. Rex DK: Gastroesophageal reflux disease in adults: Pathophysiology, diagnosis, and management. J Fam Pract 35:673-681, 1992.
27. DeVault KR, Castell DO: Guidelines for the diagnosis and treatment of gastroesophageal reflux disease. Arch Intern Med 155:2165-2172, 1995.
28. Lam HGT, Dekker W, Kan G, et al: Acute noncardiac chest pain in a coronary care unit. Gastroenterology 102:453-460, 1992.
29. Boyd EJS: The prevalence of esophagitis in patients with duodenal ulcer or ulcer-like dyspepsia. Am J Gastroenterol 91:1539-1542, 1996.
30. Sontag SJ, O'Connell S, Khandelwal S, et al: Most asthmatics have gastroesophageal reflux with or without bronchodilator therapy. Gastroenterology 99:613-620, 1990.
31. Hamilos DL: Gastroesophageal reflux and sinusitis in asthma. Clin Chest Med 16:683-697, 1995.
32. Deveney CW, Benner K, Cohen J: Gastroesophageal reflux and laryngeal disease. Arch Surg 128:1021-1027, 1993.
33. Weusten BLAM, Akkermans LMA, van Berge-Henegouwen GP, et al: Symptom perception in gastroesophageal reflux disease is dependent on spatiotemporal reflux characteristics. Gastroenterology 108:1739-1744, 1995.
34. Smith JL, Opekun AR, Larkai E, et al: Sensitivity of the esophageal mucosa to pH in gastroesophageal reflux disease. Gastroenterology 96:683-689, 1989.
35. Bennett JR: Oesophageal strictures. Clin Gastroenterol 7:555-569, 1978.
36. Marks RD, Richter JE: Peptic strictures of the esophagus. Am J Gastroenterol 88:1160-1172, 1993.
37. Canon CL, Morgan DE, Einstein DM, et al: Surgical approach to gastroesophageal reflux disease: What the radiologist needs to know. RadioGraphics 25:1485-1499, 2005.
38. Thompson JK, Koehler RE, Richter JE: Detection of gastroesophageal reflux: Value of barium studies compared with 24-hr pH monitoring. AJR 162:621-626, 1994.
39. Ott DJ: Gastroesophageal reflux: What is the role of barium studies? AJR 162:627-629, 1994.
40. Blumhagen JD, Christie DL: Gastroesophageal reflux in children: Evaluation of the water siphon test. Radiology 131:345-349, 1979.
41. Blumhagen JD, Rudd TG, Christie DL: Gastroesophageal reflux in children: Radionuclide gastroesophagography. AJR 135:1001-1004, 1980.
42. Malmud LS, Fisher RS: Gastroesophageal scintigraphy. Gastrointest Radiol 5:195-204, 1980.
43. Kahrilas PJ, Quigley EMM: Clinical esophageal pH recording: A technical review for practice guideline development. Gastroenterology 110:1982-1996, 1996.
44. Pan JJ, Levine MS, Redfern RO, et al: Gastroesophageal reflux: Comparison of barium studies with 24-h pH monitoring. Eur J Radiol 47:149-153, 2003.
45. Booth DJ, Kemmerer WT, Skinner DB: Acid clearing from the distal esophagus. Arch Surg 96:731-734, 1968.
46. Tolin RD, Malmud LS, Reilley J, et al: Esophageal scintigraphy to quantitate esophageal transit (quantitation of esophageal transit). Gastroenterology 76:1402-1408, 1979.
47. Ott DJ, Gelfand DW, Wu WC: Reflux esophagitis: Radiographic and endoscopic correlation. Radiology 130:583-588, 1979.
48. Koehler RE, Weyman PJ, Oakley HF: Single- and double-contrast techniques in esophagitis. AJR 135:15-19, 1980.
49. Ott DJ, Wu WC, Gelfand DW: Reflux esophagitis revisited: Prospective analysis of radiologic accuracy. Gastrointest Radiol 6:1-7, 1981.
50. Creteur V, Thoeni RF, Federle MP, et al: The role of single and double-contrast radiography in the diagnosis of reflux esophagitis. Radiology 147:71-75, 1983.
51. Graziani L, De Nigris E, Pesaresi A, et al: Reflux esophagitis: Radiologic-endoscopic correlation in 39 symptomatic cases. Gastrointest Radiol 8:1-6, 1983.
52. Chen YM, Ott DJ, Gelfand DW, et al: Multiphasic examination of the esophagogastric region for strictures, rings, and hiatal hernia: Evaluation of the individual techniques. Gastrointest Radiol 10:311-316, 1985.
53. Gibbs D: Endoscopy in the assessment of reflux oesophagitis. Clin Gastroenterol 5:135-142, 1976.
54. Fass R, Ofman JJ: Gastroesophageal reflux disease—should we adopt a new conceptual framework? Am J Gastroenterol 97:1901-1909, 2002.

55. Bytzere P, Havelund T, Hansen JM: Interobserver variation in the endoscopic diagnosis of reflux esophagitis. Scand J Gastroenterol 28:119-125, 1993.

56. Armstrong D, Bennett JR, Blum AL, et al: The endoscopic assessment of esophagitis: A progress report on observer agreement. Gastroenterology 111:85-92, 1996.

57. Lundell LR, Dent J, Bennett JR, et al: Endoscopic assessment of oesophagitis: Clinical and functional correlates and further validation of the Los Angeles classification. Gut 45:72-180, 1999.

58. Funch-Jensen P, Kock K, Christensen LA, et al: Microscopic appearance of the esophageal mucosa in a consecutive series of patients submitted to upper endoscopy: Correlation with gastroesophageal reflux symptoms and macroscopic findings. Scand J Gastroenterol 21:65-69, 1986.

59. Dibble C, Levine MS, Rubesin SE, et al: Detection of reflux esophagitis on double-contrast esophagrams and endoscopy using the histologic findings as the gold standard. Abdom Imaging 29:421-425, 2004.

60. Ismail-Beigi F, Horton PF, Pope CE: Histological consequences of gastroesophageal reflux. Gastroenterology 58:163-174, 1970.

61. Schindlbeck NE, Wiebecke B, Klauser AG, et al: Diagnostic value of histology in nonerosive gastroesophageal reflux disease. Gut 39:151-154, 1996.

62. Kahrilas PJ, Dodds WJ, Hogan WJ, et al: Esophageal peristaltic dysfunction in peptic esophagitis. Gastroenterology 91:897-904, 1986.

63. Campbell C, Levine MS, Rubesin SE, et al: Association between esophageal dysmotility and gastroesophageal reflux on barium studies. Eur J Radiol 59:88-92, 2006.

64. Zboralske FF, Amberg JR, Soergel KH: Presbyesophagus: Cineradiographic manifestations. Radiology 82:463-467, 1964.

65. Simeone JF, Burrell M, Toffler R, et al: Aperistalsis and esophagitis. Radiology 123:9-14, 1977.

66. Kressel HY, Glick SN, Laufer I, et al: Radiologic features of esophagitis. Gastrointest Radiol 6:103-108, 1981.

67. Laufer I: Radiology of esophagitis. Radiol Clin North Am 20:687-699, 1982.

68. Graziani L, Bearzi I, Romagnoli A, et al: Significance of diffuse granularity and nodularity of the esophageal mucosa at double-contrast radiography. Gastrointest Radiol 10:1-6, 1985.

69. Levine MS, Cajade AG, Herlinger H, et al: Pseudomembranes in reflux esophagitis. Radiology 159:43-45, 1986.

70. McDermott P, Wallers KJ, Holden R, et al: Double-contrast examination of the oesophagus: The radiological changes of peptic oesophagitis. Clin Radiol 33:259-264, 1982.

71. Levine MS, Goldstein HM: Fixed transverse folds in the esophagus: A sign of reflux esophagitis. AJR 143:275-278, 1984.

72. Hu C, Levine MS, Laufer I: Solitary ulcers in reflux esophagitis: Radiographic findings. Abdom Imaging 22:5-7, 1997.

73. Rabin M, Schmaman IB: Reflux oesophagitis resembling varices. S Afr Med J 55:293-295, 1979.

74. Gohel VK, Edell SL, Laufer I, et al: Transverse folds in the human esophagus. Radiology 128:303-308, 1978.

75. Williams SM, Harned RK, Kaplan P, et al: Transverse striations of the esophagus: Association with gastroesophageal reflux. Radiology 146:25-27, 1983.

76. Furth EE, Rubesin SE, Rose D: Feline esophagus. AJR 164:900, 1995.

77. Bleshman MH, Banner MP, Johnson RC, et al: The inflammatory esophagogastric polyp and fold. Radiology 128:589-593, 1978.

78. Ghahremani GG, Fisher MR, Rushovich AM: Prolapsing inflammatory pseudopolyp-fold complex of the oesophagogastric region. Eur J Radiol 4:47-51, 1984.

79. Styles RA, Gibb SP, Tarshis A, et al: Esophagogastric polyps: Radiographic and endoscopic findings. Radiology 154:307-311, 1985.

80. Coggins CA, Levine MS, Kesack CD, et al: Wide-mouthed sacculations in the esophagus: A radiographic finding in scleroderma. AJR 176:953-954, 2001.

81. Palmer ED: The hiatus hernia-esophagitis-esophageal stricture complex: Twenty-year prospective study. Am J Med 44:566-579, 1968.

82. Ott DJ, Gelfand DW, Lane TG, et al: Radiologic detection and spectrum of appearances of esophageal strictures. J Clin Gastroenterol 4:11-15, 1982.

83. Ott DJ, Chen YM, Wu WC, et al: Endoscopic sensitivity in the detection of esophageal strictures. J Clin Gastroenterol 7:121-125, 1985.

84. Luedtke P, Levine MS, Rubesin SE, et al: Radiologic diagnosis of benign esophageal strictures: A pattern approach. RadioGraphics 23:897-909, 2003.

85. Gupta S, Levine MS, Rubesin SE, et al: Usefulness of barium studies for differentiating benign and malignant strictures of the esophagus. AJR 180:737-744, 2003.

86. Schatzki R, Gary JE: Dysphagia due to a diaphragm-like localized narrowing in the lower esophagus ("lower esophageal ring"). AJR 70:911-922, 1953.

87. Weaver JW, Kaude JV, Hamlin DJ: Webs of the lower esophagus: A complication of gastroesophageal reflux? AJR 142:289-292, 1984.

88. Gordon AR, Levine MS, Redfern RO, et al: Cervical esophageal webs: Association with gastroesophageal reflux. Abdom Imaging 26:574-577, 2001.

89. Graham J, Barnes N, Rubenstein AS: The nasogastric tube as a cause of esophagitis and stricture. Am J Surg 98:116-119, 1959.

90. Waldman I, Berlin L: Strictures of the esophagus due to nasogastric intubation. Am J Roentgenol Radium Ther Nucl Med 94:321-324, 1965.

91. Banfield WJ, Hurwitz AL: Esophageal stricture associated with nasogastric intubation. Arch Intern Med 134:1083-1086, 1974.

92. Levine MS, Fisher AR, Rubesin SE, et al: Complications after total gastrectomy and esophagojejunostomy: Radiologic evaluation. AJR 157:1189-1194, 1991.

93. Levine MS, Moolten DN, Herlinger H, et al: Esophageal intramural pseudodiverticulosis: A reevaluation. AJR 147:1165-1170, 1986.

94. Marks RD, Richter JE: Peptic strictures of the esophagus. Am J Gastroenterol 88:1160-1173, 1993.

95. Castell DO, Katz PO: Approach to the patient with dysphagia and odynophagia. In Yamada T (ed): Textbook of Gastroenterology, 3rd ed. Philadelphia, Lippincott Williams & Wilkins, 1999, pp 683-693.

96. O'Connor JB, Richter JE: Esophageal strictures. In Castell DO, Richter JE (eds): The Esophagus, 3rd ed. Philadelphia, Lippincott Williams & Wilkins, 1999, pp 473-483.

97. Gohel VK, Kressel HY, Laufer I: Double contrast artifacts. Gastrointest Radiol 3:139-146, 1978.

98. Glick SN, Teplick SK, Goldstein J, et al: Glycogenic acanthosis of the esophagus. AJR 139:683-688, 1982.

99. Ghahremani GG, Rushovich AM: Glycogenic acanthosis of the esophagus: Radiographic and pathologic features. Gastrointest Radiol 9:93-98, 1984.

100. Levine MS, Woldenberg R, Herlinger H, et al: Opportunistic esophagitis in AIDS: Radiographic diagnosis. Radiology 165:815-820, 1987.

101. Itai Y, Kogure T, Okuyama Y, et al: Superficial esophageal carcinoma: Radiological findings in double-contrast studies. Radiology 126:597-601, 1978.

102. Levine MS, Laufer I, Kressel HY, et al: Herpes esophagitis. AJR 136:863-866, 1981.

103. Bova JG, Dutton NE, Goldstein HM, et al: Medication-induced esophagitis: Diagnosis by double-contrast esophagography. AJR 148:731-732, 1987.

104. DeGryse HR, De Schepper AM: Aphthoid esophageal ulcers in Crohn's disease of ileum and colon. Gastrointest Radiol 9:197-201, 1984.

105. Silver TM, Goldstein HM: Varicoid carcinoma of the esophagus. Am J Dig Dis 19:56-58, 1974.

106. Bozymski EM, Herlihy KH, Orlando RC: Barrett's esophagus. Ann Intern Med 97:103-107, 1982.

107. Sjogren RW, Johnson LF: Barrett's esophagus: A review. Am J Med 74:313-321, 1983.

108. Spechler SJ, Goyal RK: Barrett's esophagus. N Engl J Med 315:362-371, 1986.

109. Hassall E: Barrett's esophagus: Congenital or acquired? Am J Gastroenterol 88:819-824, 1993.

110. Spechler SJ: Barrett's esophagus. N Engl J Med 346:836-842, 2002.

111. Naef AP, Savary M, Ozello L: Columnar-lined lower esophagus: An acquired lesion with malignant predisposition. J Thorac Cardiovasc Surg 70:826-835, 1975.

112. Starnes VA, Adkins RB, Ballinger JF, et al: Barrett's esophagus: A surgical entity. Arch Surg 119:563-567, 1984.

113. Sarr MG, Hamilton SR, Marrone GC, et al: Barrett's esophagus: Its prevalence and association with adenocarcinoma in patients with symptoms of gastroesophageal reflux. Am J Surg 149:187-192, 1985.

114. Levine MS, Herman JB, Furth EE: Barrett's esophagus and esophageal adenocarcinoma: The scope of the problem. Abdom Imaging 20:291-298, 1995.

115. Shaheen N: Advances in Barrett's esophagus and esophageal adenocarcinoma. Gastroenterology 128:1554-1566, 2005.

116. Cameron AJ, Zinsmeister AR, Ballard DJ, et al: Prevalence of columnar-lined (Barrett's) esophagus: Comparison of population-based clinical and autopsy findings. Gastroenterology 99:918-922, 1990.

117. Reid BJ: Barrett's esophagus and esophageal adenocarcinoma. Gastroenterol Clin North Am 20:817-834, 1991.

118. Duhaylongsod FG, Wolfe WG: Barrett's esophagus and adenocarcinoma of the esophagus and gastroesophageal junction. J Thorac Cardiovasc Surg 102:36-42, 1991.

119. Li H, Walsh TN, Hennessy TPJ: Carcinoma arising in Barrett's esophagus. Surg Gynecol Obstet 175:167-172, 1992.

120. Lagergren J, Bergstrom R, Lindgren A, et al: Symptomatic gastroesophageal reflux as a risk factor for esophageal adenocarcinoma. N Engl J Med 340:825-831, 1999.

121. Shaheen NJ, Crosby MA, Bozymski EM, et al: Is there publication bias in the reporting of cancer risk for esophageal adenocarcinoma. Gastroenterology 119:333-338, 2000.

122. Sampliner RE: Practice Parameters Committee on the American College of Gastroenterology. Practice guidelines on the diagnosis, surveillance, and therapy of Barrett's esophagus. Am J Gastroenterol 93:1028-1032, 1998.

123. Gerson LB, Groeneveld PW, Triadafilopoulos G: Cost-effectiveness model of endoscopic screening and surveillance in patients with gastroesophageal reflux disease. Clin Gastroenterol Hepatol 2:868-879, 2004.

124. Sharma P, Morales TG, Sampliner RE: Short segment Barrett's esophagus—the need for standardization of the definition and of endoscopic criteria. Am J Gastroenterol 93:1033-1036, 1998.

125. Hirota WK, Loughney TM, Lazas DJ, et al: Specialized intestinal metaplasia, dysplasia, and cancer of the esophagus and esophagogastric junction: Prevalence and clinical data. Gastroenterology 116:277-285, 1999.

126. Sharma P, Morales TH, Bhattacharyya A, et al: Dysplasia in short-segment Barrett's esophagus: A prospective 3-year follow-up. Am J Gastroenterol 92:2012-2016, 1997.

127. Weston AP, Krmpotich PT, Cherian R, et al: Prospective long-term endoscopic and histological follow-up of short-segment Barrett's esophagus: Comparison with traditional long-segment Barrett's esophagus. Am J Gastroenterol 92:407-413, 1997.

128. Donahue D, Navab F: Significance of short-segment Barrett's esophagus. J Clin Gastroenterol 25:480-484, 1997.

129. Sharma P: Recent advances in Barrett's esophagus: Short-segment Barrett's esophagus and cardia intestinal metaplasia. Semin Gastrointest Dis 10:93-102, 1999.

130. Cameron AJ, Lomboy CT: Barrett's esophagus: Age, prevalence, and extent of columnar epithelium. Gastroenterology 103:1241-1245, 1992.

131. Wong A, Fitzgerald RC: Epidemiologic risk factors for Barrett's esophagus and associated adenocarcinoma. Clin Gastroenterol Hepatol 3:1-10, 2005.

132. Tran T, Spechler SJ, Richardson PE, et al: Fundoplication and the risk of esophageal cancer in gastroesophageal reflux disease: A Veterans Affairs cohort study. Am J Gastroenterol 100:1002-1008, 2005.

133. Winters C, Spurling TJ, Chobanian SJ, et al: Barrett's esophagus: A prevalent, occult complication of gastroesophageal reflux disease. Gastroenterology 92:118-124, 1987.

134. Paull A, Trier JS, Dalton D, et al: The histologic spectrum of Barrett's esophagus. N Engl J Med 295:476-480, 1976.

135. Weinstein WM, Ippoliti AF: The diagnosis of Barrett's esophagus: Goblets, goblets, goblets. Gastrointest Endosc 44:91-95, 1996.

136. Missakian MM, Carlson HC, Andersen HA: The roentgenologic features of the columnar epithelial-lined lower esophagus. AJR 99:212-217, 1967.

137. Robbins AH, Hermos JA, Schimmel EM, et al: The columnar-lined esophagus: Analysis of 26 cases. Radiology 123:1-7, 1977.

138. Chen YM, Gelfand DW, Ott DJ, et al: Barrett esophagus as an extension of severe esophagitis: Analysis of radiologic signs in 29 cases. AJR 145:275-281, 1985.

139. Glick SN: Barium studies in patients with Barrett's esophagus: Importance of focal areas of esophageal deformity. AJR 163:65-67, 1994.

140. Adler RH: The lower esophagus lined by columnar epithelium: Its association with hiatal hernia, ulcer, stricture, and tumor. J Thorac Cardiovasc Surg 45:13-34, 1963.

141. Robbins AH, Vincent ME, Saini M, et al: Revised radiologic concepts of the Barrett esophagus. Gastrointest Radiol 3:377-381, 1978.

142. Levine MS, Kressel HY, Caroline DF, et al: Barrett esophagus: Reticular pattern of the mucosa. Radiology 147:663-667, 1983.

143. Shapir J, DuBrow R, Frank P: Barrett oesophagus: Analysis of 19 cases. Br J Radiol 58:491-493, 1985.

144. Agha FP: Radiologic diagnosis of Barrett's esophagus: Critical analysis of 65 cases. Gastrointest Radiol 11:123-130, 1986.

145. Glick SN, Teplick SK, Amenta PS, et al: The radiologic diagnosis of Barrett esophagus: Importance of mucosal surface abnormalities on air-contrast barium studies. AJR 157:951-954, 1991.

146. Chernin MM, Amberg JR, Kogan FJ, et al: Efficacy of radiologic studies in the detection of Barrett esophagus. AJR 147:257-260, 1986.

147. Vincent ME, Robbins AH, Spechler SJ, et al: The reticular pattern as a radiographic sign of the Barrett esophagus: An assessment. Radiology 153:333-335, 1984.

148. Levine MS. Barrett esophagus: Update for radiologists. Abdom Imaging 30:133-141, 2005.

149. Gilchrist AM, Levine MS, Carr RF, et al: Barrett's esophagus: Diagnosis by double-contrast esophagography. AJR 150:97-102, 1988.

150. Spechler SJ, Sperber H, Doos WG, et al: The prevalence of Barrett's esophagus in patients with chronic peptic esophageal strictures. Dig Dis Sci 28:769-774, 1983.

151. Yamamoto AJ, Levine MS, Katzka DA, et al: Short-segment Barrett's esophagus: Findings on double-contrast esophagography in 20 patients. AJR 176:1173-1178, 2001.

Infectious Esophagitis

Marc S. Levine, MD

Because of the increased survival of immunocompromised patients with malignant neoplasms, organ transplants, and other debilitating diseases, infectious esophagitis has become an increasingly common problem in modern medical practice. *Candida albicans* is the usual offending organism, but herpes simplex virus and cytomegalovirus (CMV) have also been recognized with increased frequency as opportunistic esophageal invaders. The AIDS epidemic has led to the development of more fulminant forms of fungal and viral esophagitis (including human immunodeficiency virus [HIV] esophagitis), accentuating the need for early diagnosis and treatment of these patients.

CANDIDA ESOPHAGITIS

Pathogenesis

Candidiasis is the most common cause of infectious esophagitis. *C. albicans* is almost always the offending organism.[1,2] Because *C. albicans* is a commensal inhabitant of the pharynx, *Candida* esophagitis is presumably caused by downward spread of the fungus to the esophagus.[3] Clinically significant infection occurs primarily in patients who are immunocompromised because of underlying malignancy, debilitating illness, diabetes, or treatment with radiation, corticosteroids, or other cytotoxic agents.[2,4-7] *Candida* esophagitis is particularly prevalent in AIDS, occurring in 15% to 20% of patients with this disease.[6]

Local esophageal stasis is another factor that predisposes patients to the development of *Candida* esophagitis. Esophageal stasis may be due to mechanical obstruction resulting from achalasia or strictures or to physiologic obstruction resulting from scleroderma or other causes of weakened or absent esophageal peristalsis.[7,8] Delayed esophageal emptying in these patients permits the fungal organism to overgrow and colonize the esophagus with subsequent esophagitis.

Much less frequently, *Candida* esophagitis may develop in otherwise healthy individuals who have no underlying systemic or esophageal diseases.[9] The possibility of fungal infection should therefore not be excluded simply because the classic predisposing factors are not present in a particular patient.

Clinical Findings

Most patients with *Candida* esophagitis have acute onset of dysphagia or odynophagia, characterized by intense substernal pain or burning during swallowing.[1-4] In some cases, the pain may be so severe that these patients cannot even swallow their saliva. Others may have nonspecific findings (e.g., chest pain, epigastric pain, or upper gastrointestinal bleeding), or they may be asymptomatic.[1,2,5] Occasionally, patients with chronic *Candida* esophagitis may have persistent dysphagia because of the development of esophageal strictures.[10-12]

Despite the characteristic presentation, *Candida* esophagitis may be difficult to differentiate from viral esophagitis on clinical grounds. The presence of oropharyngeal candidiasis (i.e., thrush) is a helpful finding, but only 50% to 75% of patients with *Candida* esophagitis have fungal lesions in the oropharynx.[2,13] Other patients with thrush may have herpes or CMV esophagitis, so that the presence of oropharyngeal candidiasis does not preclude the possibility of viral esophagitis.[14]

The diagnosis of *Candida* esophagitis is further complicated by cases in which the esophagus is simultaneously colonized by fungal and viral organisms. Concomitant *Candida* and herpes esophagitis have been well documented at endoscopy.[2,15,16] In such cases, *Candida* esophagitis most likely occurs as a result of fungal superinfection of preexisting herpetic ulcers.[16]

Treatment of *Candida* esophagitis depends not only on the severity of infection but also on the degree to which the host's immune defenses are compromised. Patients who have a relatively normal immune system can be treated effectively with topical agents such as oral nystatin,[2] but immunocompromised patients require treatment with more potent antifungal agents such as fluconazole.[2,6,17] Affected individuals usually have a marked clinical response to antifungal therapy. In one study, however, recurrent *Candida* esophagitis occurred in 90% of successfully treated patients with AIDS, usually in less than 3 months.[18]

Endoscopic Findings

The characteristic endoscopic appearance of *Candida* esophagitis consists of patchy, white plaques covering a friable, erythematous mucosa.[1,2] In more advanced disease, the mucosa becomes ulcerated and necrotic with extensive pseudomembrane formation. The presence of budding yeast cells, hyphae, and pseudohyphae on endoscopic biopsy specimens with silver stain, periodic acid–Schiff stain, or Gram stain is diagnostic of *Candida* esophagitis.[1,2]

Radiographic Findings

The radiographic diagnosis of *Candida* esophagitis has been limited by the fact that it tends to be a superficial disease with mucosal abnormalities that are difficult to detect on conventional single-contrast barium studies. As a result, single-contrast esophagography has been considered an unreliable technique for diagnosing *Candida* esophagitis, with a reported sensitivity of less than 50%.[1,4,5,9] However, studies have shown that double-contrast esophagography has a sensitivity of about 90% in diagnosing *Candida* esophagitis.[7,19] The major advantage of this technique is its ability to demonstrate mucosal plaques that cannot easily be seen on single-contrast studies. Thus, only mild cases of *Candida* esophagitis are likely to be missed on double-contrast examinations.

Candida esophagitis is usually manifested on double-contrast images by discrete plaquelike lesions consisting of heaped-up areas of necrotic epithelial debris and actual colonies of *C. albicans* on the mucosa. The lesions tend to be longitudinally oriented, appearing en face as discrete, linear or irregular filling defects with normal intervening mucosa (Fig. 24-1).[7,14] The plaques are located predominantly in the upper esophagus, midesophagus, or both, occasionally having a focal distribution (Fig. 24-2). In the appropriate clinical setting, discrete plaquelike lesions should be highly suggestive of *Candida* esophagitis.

In other patients, *Candida* esophagitis may be manifested by a finely nodular or granular appearance because of tiny plaques on the mucosa (Fig. 24-3).[14,20] Some plaques may contain central umbilications that collect barium, mimicking the appearance of tiny ulcers caused by herpes esophagitis.[21] When larger plaques are present, the lesions may coalesce, producing a distinctive "snakeskin" appearance (Fig. 24-4).[19] Occasionally, submucosal edema and inflammation may result in thickened longitudinal folds, a nonspecific manifestation of esophagitis.[3] Thus, the classic radiographic features of *Candida* esophagitis are not present in all patients.

In severe candidiasis, the esophagus may have a grossly irregular or "shaggy" contour because of coalescent plaques and pseudomembranes with trapping of barium between these lesions (Fig. 24-5).[4,7,14,19,22] Some of the plaques and pseudomembranes may eventually slough, producing one or more deep ulcers superimposed on a background of diffuse plaque formation (see Fig. 24-5B). This fulminant form of candidiasis has been encountered primarily in patients with AIDS.[14] The possibility of AIDS should therefore be suspected when a shaggy esophagus is detected on barium studies, particularly in high-risk patients.

Candida esophagitis may occasionally produce other unusual radiographic findings. In some patients, barium may dissect beneath plaques or pseudomembranes, producing an intramural track or "double-barreled" esophagus.[22] A coalescent mass of heaped-up necrotic debris and fungal mycelia (i.e., a fungus ball) may be indistinguishable from a polypoid esophageal carcinoma.[23-25] Esophageal obstruction, perforation, and tracheoesophageal or aortoesophageal fistula formation are other rare but potentially life-threatening complications.[26-28]

Candida esophagitis usually responds quickly to antifungal therapy, but resolution of the radiographic findings sometimes lags behind the clinical recovery, so that follow-up barium studies may still be abnormal in patients who are asymptomatic.[24] The immediate effects of antifungal therapy should therefore be assessed primarily on clinical grounds.

Although *Candida* esophagitis is usually self-limited with proper treatment, occasional cases of stricture formation have been reported.[10-12] These strictures typically appear as long, tapered areas of esophageal narrowing (Fig. 24-6).[12] Fungal-induced strictures should be distinguished from pseudostrictures caused by esophageal spasm or the patient's inability to swallow an adequate bolus of barium. For this reason, a second examination may be necessary after treatment to determine if a true stricture is present.

Because of the effects of local esophageal stasis (see earlier section on Pathogenesis), patients with conditions such as achalasia and scleroderma are at increased risk for developing *Candida* esophagitis.[7,8] Such cases may be manifested on esophagography by tiny, nodular defects, polypoid folds, or a distinctive lacy appearance in the esophagus (Fig. 24-7).[8] Because of esophageal stasis in patients with achalasia or scleroderma, these individuals may also develop a "foamy" esophagus characterized by innumerable tiny, rounded bubbles that settle out along the top of the barium column, producing a layer of foam (Fig. 24-8).[29] It has been postulated that this finding results from extensive production of carbon dioxide by a yeast form of the organism.[29] Whatever the explanation, *Candida* esophagitis should be suspected when a foamy esophagus is detected on esophagography, particularly in patients with achalasia or scleroderma.

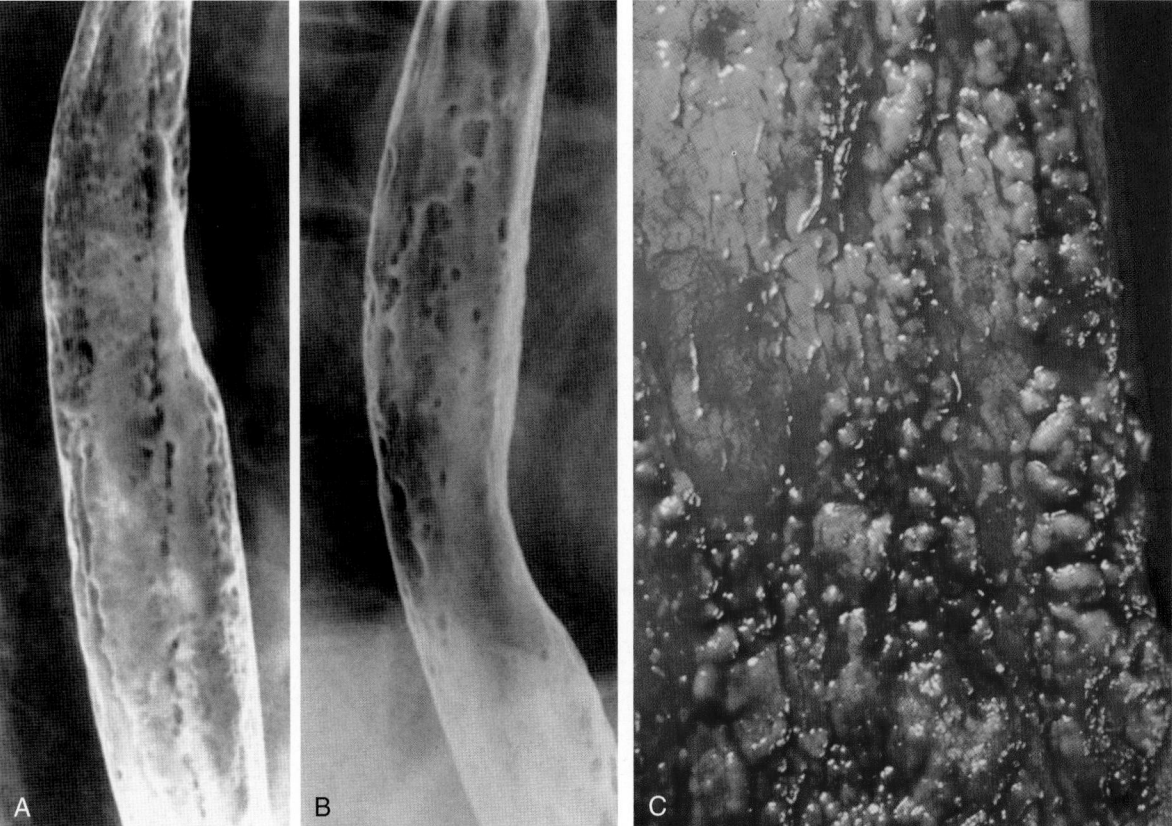

Figure 24-1. *Candida* **esophagitis with discrete plaques. A.** Multiple plaquelike lesions are present in the esophagus. The plaques have a characteristic appearance with discrete borders and a predominantly longitudinal orientation. **B.** In another patient, the plaques have a more irregular configuration. However, they are still seen as discrete lesions separated by normal mucosa. **C.** The gross specimen in another case shows how these plaquelike lesions represent heaped-up areas of necrotic epithelial debris and actual colonies of *C. albicans* on the mucosa. (**A** and **B** from Levine MS, Macones AJ, Laufer I: *Candida* esophagitis: Accuracy of radiographic diagnosis. Radiology 154:581-587, 1985.)

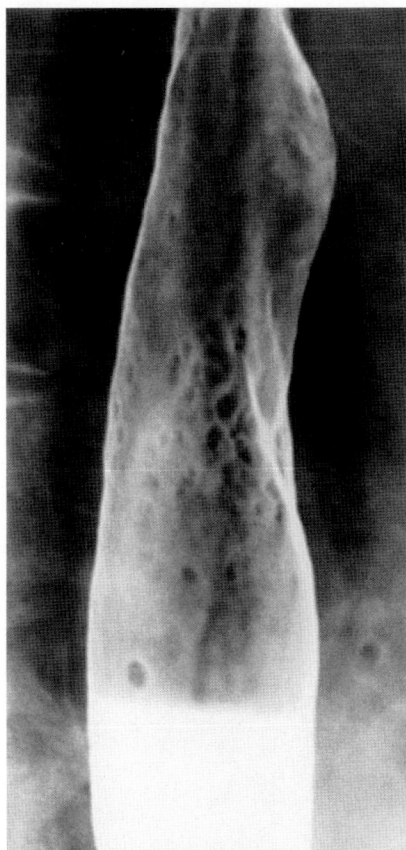

Figure 24-2. Localized *Candida* **esophagitis.** Discrete plaquelike lesions are clustered together in the midesophagus with normal-appearing mucosa above and below this level.

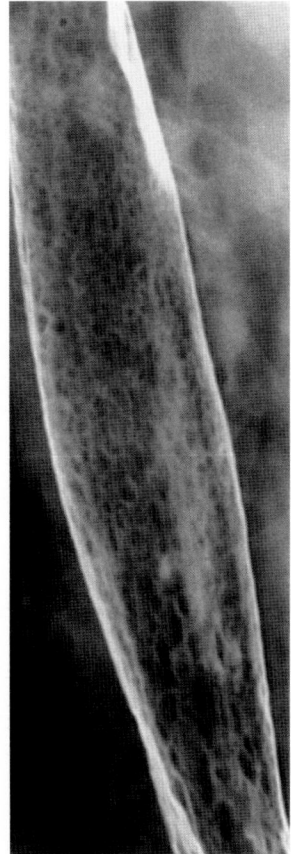

Figure 24-3. *Candida* **esophagitis with a granular mucosa.** This patient has innumerable tiny, nodular elevations in the esophagus rather than the typical plaquelike defects associated with candidiasis.

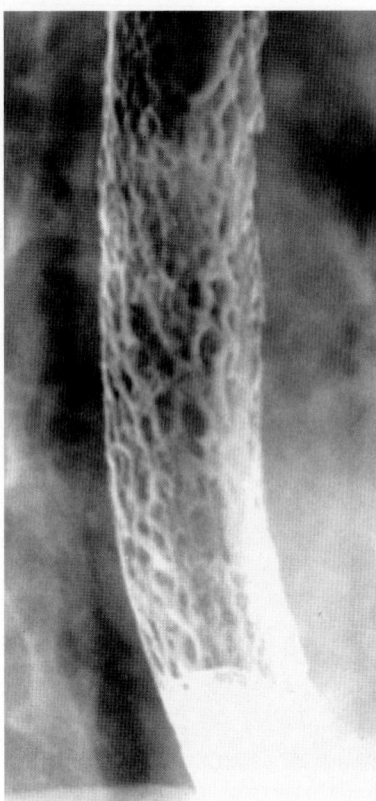

Figure 24-4. *Candida* **esophagitis with a cobblestone appearance.** There is confluent involvement of the mucosa by innumerable round, oval, and polygonal plaques. (From Levine MS: Radiology of the Esophagus. Philadelphia, WB Saunders, 1989.)

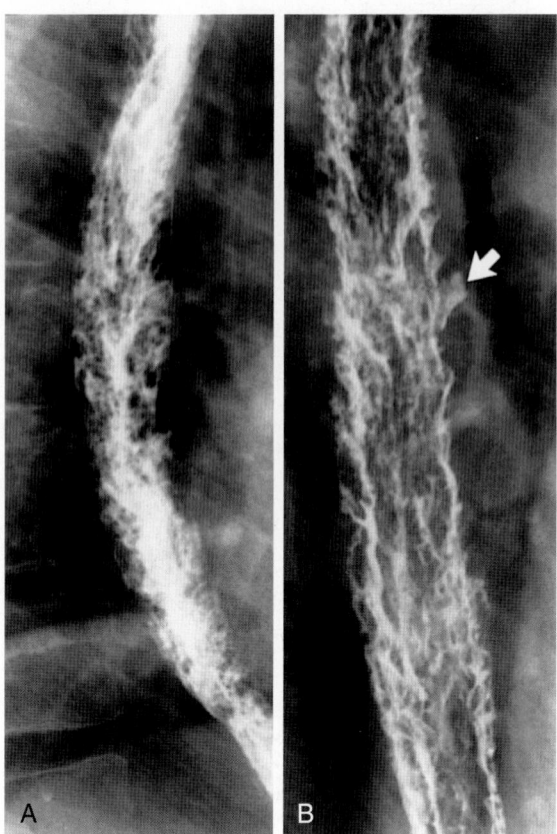

Figure 24-5. *Candida* **esophagitis with a shaggy esophagus. A** and **B.** The esophagus has a grossly irregular contour as a result of multiple plaques and pseudomembranes with trapping of barium between these lesions. In **B,** a deep area of ulceration (*arrow*) is also seen. Both patients had AIDS. (**A** from Levine MS: Radiology of the Esophagus. Philadelphia, WB Saunders, 1989; **B** from Levine MS, Woldenberg R, Herlinger H, et al: Opportunistic esophagitis in AIDS: Radiographic diagnosis. Radiology 165:815-820, 1987.)

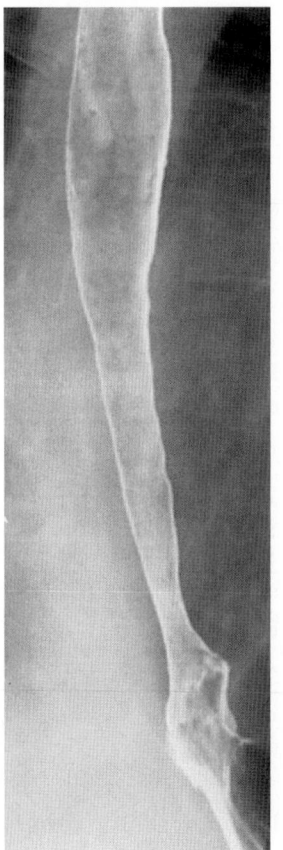

Figure 24-6. *Candida*-**induced esophageal stricture.** A long, tapered stricture is seen in the distal esophagus as a result of scarring from severe *Candida* esophagitis. (From Levine MS: Radiology of the Esophagus. Philadelphia, WB Saunders, 1989.)

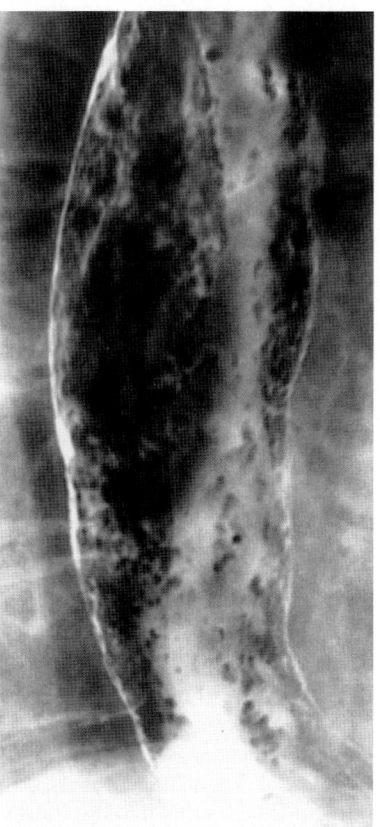

Figure 24-7. *Candida* **esophagitis in a patient with scleroderma.** Tiny, nodular defects in the esophagus could be mistaken for retained debris. The esophagus is dilated because of underlying involvement by scleroderma.

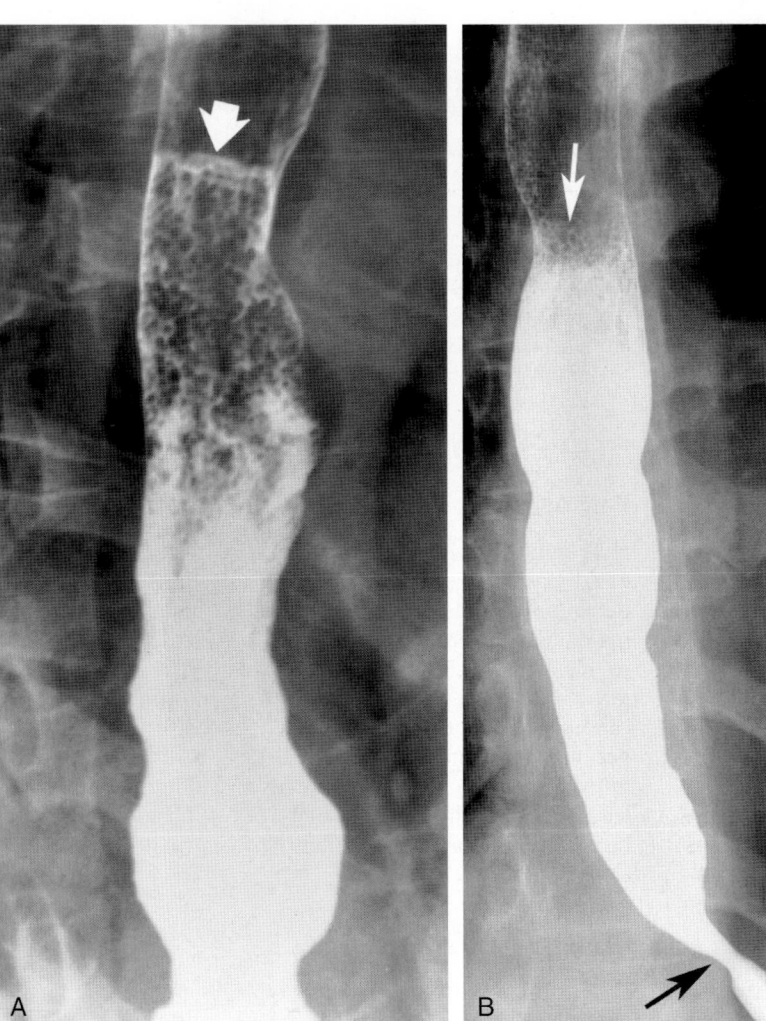

Figure 24-8. Candida esophagitis with a "foamy" esophagus in two patients with achalasia. A and **B.** In both cases, innumerable tiny, rounded bubbles are seen to settle out along the top of the barium column, producing a layer of foam (*white arrows*). In **B,** also note tapered narrowing of the distal esophagus (*black arrow*) due to underlying achalasia with incomplete opening of the lower esophageal sphincter.

Candida esophagitis is also known to be associated with esophageal intramural pseudodiverticulosis (see Chapter 25).[30-32] It has been postulated that the pseudodiverticula develop as a complication of fungal infection.[30] It is more widely believed, however, that the fungal organism is a secondary invader as a result of local stasis in these pseudodiverticula.[31,32]

Patients with defects in their cell-mediated immune response to *C. albicans* may have an unusual disease known as *chronic mucocutaneous candidiasis,* in which there is persistent fungal infection of the skin, mucous membranes, and nails.[33] Although uncommon, esophageal involvement may lead to chronic esophageal candidiasis.[33] In contrast to acute *Candida* esophagitis, this entity is characterized by chronic scarring and stricture formation in the esophagus.[33] The presence of a long esophageal stricture in patients with chronic mucocutaneous candidiasis should therefore suggest the possibility of esophageal involvement by this disease.

Differential Diagnosis

Mucosal plaques or nodules may also be caused by herpes esophagitis, reflux esophagitis, glycogenic acanthosis, and superficial spreading carcinoma.[20,34-39] Although herpes esophagitis is usually manifested by multiple small, discrete ulcers in the esophagus (see later section on Herpes Esophagitis), advanced herpetic infection may lead to the development of plaquelike lesions that are indistinguishable from those in *Candida* esophagitis (Fig. 24-9).[34,35]

Reflux esophagitis may also produce a nodular or granular appearance of the mucosa that resembles candidiasis (see Fig. 23-1).[20] However, the nodules of reflux esophagitis tend to have poorly defined borders that fade peripherally into the adjacent mucosa whereas the plaques of candidiasis have more discrete borders. The nodular mucosa of reflux esophagitis also occurs as a continuous area of disease extending proximally from the gastroesophageal junction, whereas *Candida* esophagitis often spares the distal esophagus. Rarely, severe reflux esophagitis may produce inflammatory exudates or pseudomembranes that are indistinguishable on double-contrast studies from the plaquelike lesions of candidiasis.[36]

Glycogenic acanthosis may also be manifested by discrete plaques or nodules, mimicking the appearance of *Candida* esophagitis (see Fig. 26-6).[37] However, the nodules of glycogenic acanthosis tend to have a more rounded appearance, whereas the plaques of candidiasis usually have a more linear configuration. The clinical history is also helpful for differentiating these conditions, because patients with glycogenic acanthosis are almost always asymptomatic.[37]

Superficial spreading carcinoma of the esophagus is characterized by focal nodularity of the mucosa that could be mistaken for a localized area of *Candida* esophagitis (see Fig. 27-4).[38,39] However, candidiasis usually produces discrete plaquelike lesions separated by segments of normal intervening mucosa, whereas the plaques or nodules of superficial spreading carcinoma tend to coalesce, producing a continuous area of disease.[38,39] Rarely an advanced, infiltrating carcinoma extending longitudinally in the wall can mimic the shaggy esophagus of candidiasis (Fig. 24-10).

Mucosal plaques may be simulated by technical artifacts on double-contrast studies, such as undissolved effervescent agent, air bubbles, and debris (Fig. 24-11).[20,40] When candi-

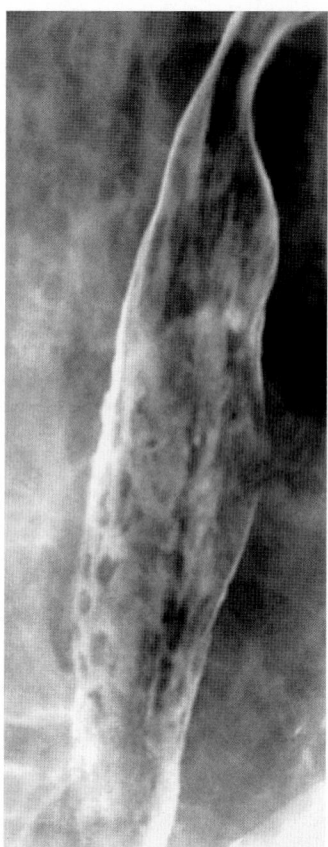

Figure 24-9. Herpes esophagitis. Multiple plaquelike lesions are seen in the midesophagus, mimicking the appearance of candidiasis. (From Levine MS, Laufer I, Kressel HY, et al: Herpes esophagitis. AJR 136: 863-866, 1981; © by American Roentgen Ray Society.)

diasis is suspected on clinical grounds, double-contrast images of the esophagus should be obtained before administration of an effervescent agent. Also, if the radiographic findings are equivocal, additional double-contrast images may be obtained to demonstrate the transient nature of these artifacts.

HERPES ESOPHAGITIS

Pathogenesis

Herpes simplex virus type 1, a DNA core virus, has been recognized as another common cause of infectious esophagitis in patients who are immunocompromised because of underlying malignant tumors, debilitating illness, AIDS, or treatment by irradiation, chemotherapy, or corticosteroids.[14,41-43] This infection should be suspected in the same clinical setting as candidiasis. Occasionally, however, herpes esophagitis may occur as an acute, self-limited disease in otherwise healthy individuals who have no underlying immunologic problems.[44-48] Thus, the diagnosis of herpes esophagitis should not be excluded because the patient has a normal immunologic status.

Clinical Findings

Patients with herpes esophagitis typically present with acute odynophagia, characterized by severe substernal chest pain

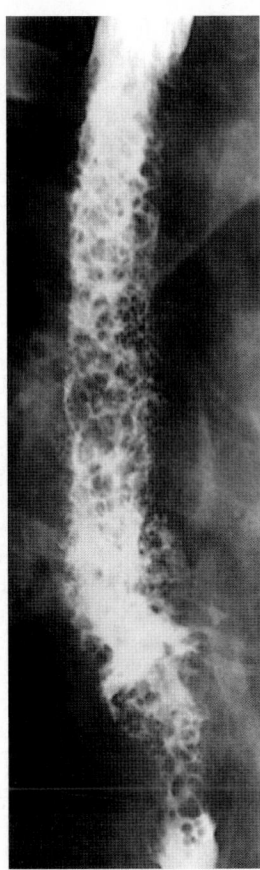

Figure 24-10. Advanced esophageal carcinoma. The esophagus has a grossly irregular or shaggy contour due to a highly invasive carcinoma extending longitudinally in the wall. (Courtesy of Hans Herlinger, MD, Philadelphia, PA.)

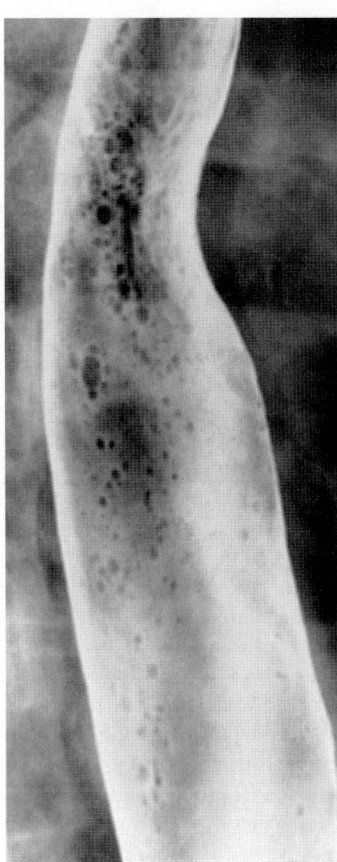

Figure 24-11. Undissolved effervescent agent and bubbles in the esophagus. Although this appearance could be mistaken for *Candida* esophagitis on a single radiograph, the transient nature of these artifacts can easily be confirmed by obtaining additional views.

during swallowing.[13,49] Other patients may have dysphagia, chest pain, and, less commonly, upper gastrointestinal bleeding.[50,51] In the appropriate clinical setting, the presence of herpetic lesions in the oropharynx should suggest a diagnosis of herpes esophagitis. Most patients do not have active infection of the oropharynx, however, so that the absence of oropharyngeal lesions does not preclude this diagnosis.[13,49] Furthermore, some patients with herpetic lesions in the oropharynx are found to have *Candida* esophagitis. It therefore can be extremely difficult to differentiate viral and fungal esophagitis on clinical grounds.

The natural history of herpes esophagitis is uncertain. In various autopsy series, it has been shown that immunocompromised hosts with herpes esophagitis may develop herpetic pneumonitis or even a disseminated herpetic infection.[43] However, most patients with herpes esophagitis recover spontaneously.[49,52,53] These individuals are usually treated effectively with analgesics and, if necessary, antiviral agents such as acyclovir or valacyclovir.[54] Although marked clinical improvement typically occurs within several days of treatment, it is unclear whether antiviral therapy substantially alters the course of this disease.

Otherwise healthy patients with herpes esophagitis have a characteristic clinical presentation. They typically are young men with a history of recent exposure to sexual partners with herpetic lesions on the lips or buccal mucosa.[45,47] Most of these patients have a 3- to 10-day influenza-like prodrome

characterized by fever, sore throat, upper respiratory tract infection, and myalgias.[44,45,47,48] This prodrome is followed by acute onset of odynophagia, which prompts the patient to seek medical attention. Despite the dramatic presentation, these patients almost always have an acute, self-limited illness with resolution of symptoms in less than 2 weeks.[44-47] As a result, they can be managed conservatively with analgesia and sedation.

Endoscopic Findings

Herpes esophagitis is initially manifested on endoscopy by esophageal blisters or vesicles that subsequently rupture to form discrete, punched-out ulcers on the mucosa.[43,52,53,55] With further progression, the ulcers may become covered by a fibrinous exudate or pseudomembranes.[43] Thus, early herpes esophagitis has a characteristic endoscopic appearance, whereas advanced herpes esophagitis may be indistinguishable from candidiasis. Whatever the stage of infection, the histologic or cytologic findings on endoscopic biopsy specimens or brushings from the esophagus are relatively specific for the herpesvirus group. The classic finding of Cowdry type A intranuclear inclusions in intact epithelial cells adjacent to ulcers is virtually pathognomonic of herpes.[43] The diagnosis of herpes esophagitis can also be confirmed by positive viral cultures from the esophagus or by direct immunofluorescent staining for the herpes simplex antigen.[2]

Radiographic Findings

Herpes esophagitis is usually manifested on double-contrast esophagograms by multiple small (<1 cm), superficial ulcers in the upper esophagus or midesophagus without plaque formation.[14,49,56-58] These ulcers are visible on double-contrast images in more than 50% of endoscopically proven cases.[58] The ulcers may have a punctate, linear, ringlike, or stellate configuration and are often surrounded by radiolucent mounds of edema (Fig. 24-12).[49] Although ulceration may occasionally be seen in advanced *Candida* esophagitis, the ulcers in these patients almost always occur on a background of diffuse plaque formation.[7,14] Thus, in the appropriate clinical setting, the presence of multiple small, discrete ulcers in the upper esophagus or midesophagus should be highly suggestive of herpes esophagitis. Nevertheless, endoscopy may be required for a definitive diagnosis if the radiographic findings are equivocal or if appropriate treatment with antiviral agents fails to produce an adequate clinical response in these patients.

More advanced herpes esophagitis may be associated with extensive ulceration, plaque formation, or a combination of ulcers and plaques in the esophagus (see Fig. 24-9).[34,35,49,56,58] Such cases may therefore be indistinguishable from advanced *Candida* esophagitis. Rarely, herpes esophagitis may be manifested by a giant ulcer with a surrounding mound of edema, mimicking the appearance of an ulcerated carcinoma.[58]

Herpes esophagitis in otherwise healthy patients is usually manifested on double-contrast esophagograms by innumerable tiny ulcers that tend to be clustered together in the midesophagus near the level of the left main bronchus (Fig. 24-13).[59,60] The small size of the ulcers may be related to an intact immune system that contains the herpetic infection and prevents the ulcers from enlarging. Whatever the explanation, the diagnosis of herpes esophagitis in otherwise healthy patients can usually be suggested on the basis of the clinical and radiographic findings.[60]

Differential Diagnosis

In the appropriate clinical setting, multiple small, discrete ulcers on an otherwise normal background mucosa should be virtually pathognomonic of viral esophagitis. Although most cases are caused by the herpes simplex virus, CMV may occasionally produce similar findings. However, CMV esophagitis is more commonly manifested by the development of one or more giant, flat ulcers in the esophagus (see next section on Cytomegalovirus Esophagitis). Oral medications such as doxycycline and tetracycline may cause a focal contact esophagitis, manifested by multiple shallow ulcers that are indistinguishable from those in herpes esophagitis (see Fig. 25-1).[61,62] The correct diagnosis should be suggested by a temporal relationship between ingestion of the offending medication and the onset of esophagitis. Reflux esophagitis is a common cause of ulceration, but it tends to involve the distal esophagus and is usually associated with a hiatal hernia or gastroesophageal reflux (see Fig. 23-3). Radiation esophagitis, caustic

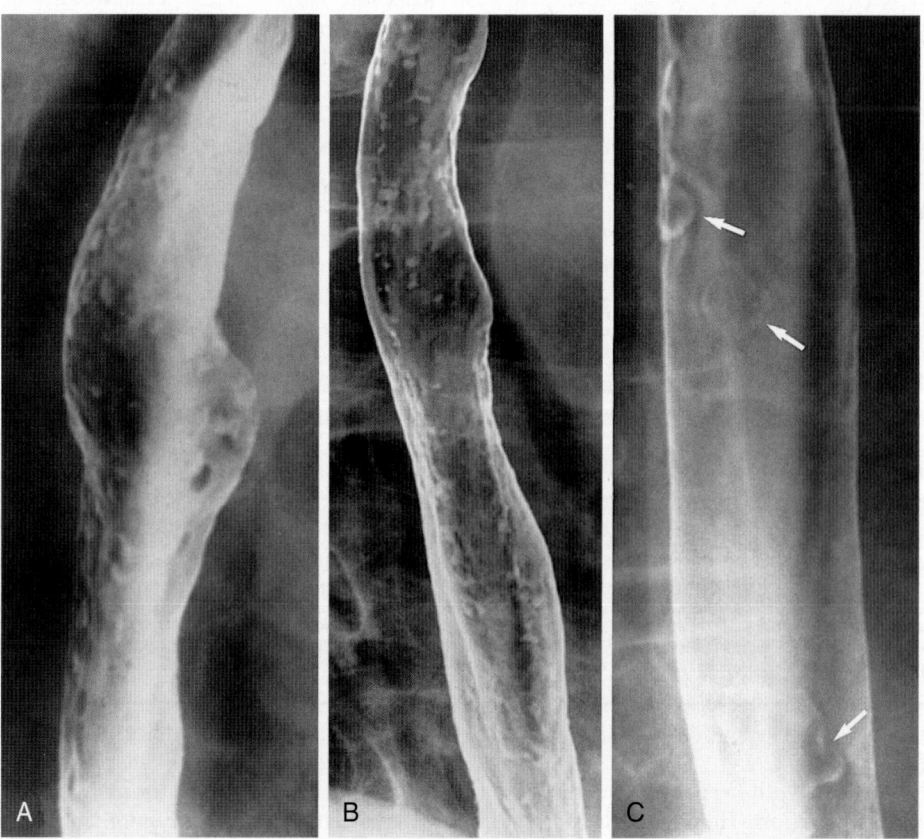

Figure 24-12. Herpes esophagitis with discrete ulcers. A and **B.** Multiple discrete, superficial ulcers are seen in the midesophagus. Many of the ulcers are surrounded by radiolucent mounds of edema. **C.** There are several widely separated ulcers (*arrows*) with a ringlike or stellate configuration. (**A** from Levine MS: Radiology of esophagitis: A pattern approach. Radiology 179:1-7, 1991. **B** courtesy of Harvey M. Goldstein, MD, San Antonio, TX.)

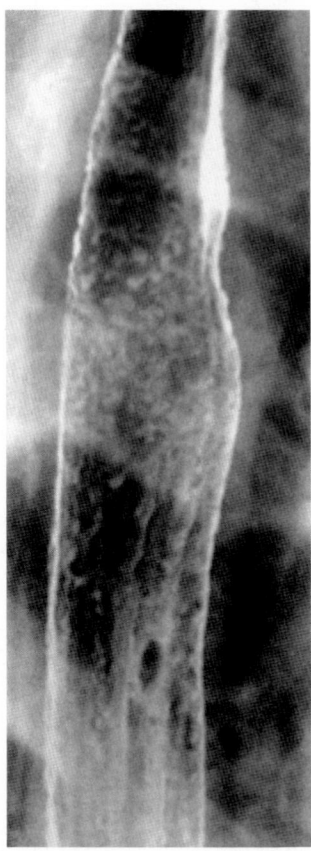

Figure 24-13. Herpes esophagitis in an otherwise healthy patient. Multiple punctate and linear areas of ulceration are seen in the midesophagus below the level of the left main bronchus. This appearance is characteristic of herpes esophagitis in immunocompetent patients. (From DeGaeta L, Levine MS, Guglielmi GE, et al: Herpes esophagitis in an otherwise healthy patient. AJR 144:1205-1206, 1985, © by American Roentgen Ray Society.)

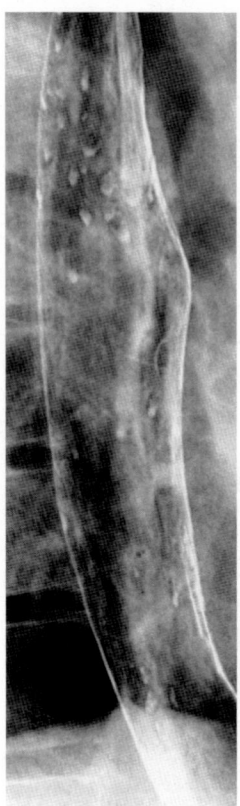

Figure 24-14. Cytomegalovirus esophagitis. Multiple discrete, superficial ulcers are seen in the midesophagus. Herpes esophagitis could produce identical radiographic findings. (From Levine MS: Radiology of the Esophagus. Philadelphia, WB Saunders, 1989.)

esophagitis, and, rarely, Crohn's disease involving the esophagus may cause superficial ulceration, but these entities can usually be differentiated from herpes esophagitis by the clinical history and presentation.

CYTOMEGALOVIRUS ESOPHAGITIS

CMV is another member of the herpesvirus group that has been recognized as a cause of infectious esophagitis in patients with AIDS.[63-65] For reasons that are unclear, however, CMV esophagitis rarely occurs in other immunocompromised patients. Affected individuals often present with severe odynophagia. Endoscopic examinations may demonstrate one or more ulcers in the esophagus. Characteristic features of CMV infection on endoscopic biopsy specimens include intranuclear inclusions and, in contrast to herpes simplex virus, small cytoplasmic inclusions in endothelial cells or fibroblasts at or near the base of the ulcers.[2,63,65] Endoscopic biopsy specimens, brushings, and viral cultures have a combined sensitivity of greater than 90% in detecting CMV esophagitis.[66,67] However, some investigators believe that endoscopic biopsy specimens are sufficient for the diagnosis of CMV without need for cytologic brushings or viral cultures from the esophagus because of a higher sensitivity and more rapid turnaround times.[68]

Radiographic Findings

CMV esophagitis may be manifested on esophagography by discrete, superficial ulcers that are indistinguishable from those in herpes esophagitis (Fig. 24-14).[63-65] More commonly, however, CMV esophagitis is associated with the development of one or more giant (>1 cm in size), flat ulcers in the midesophagus or distal esophagus.[14,63,64,69] These giant ulcers may be recognized in profile or en face as ovoid, elongated, or diamond-shaped collections of barium surrounded by a radiolucent rim of edematous mucosa (Fig. 24-15). Because herpetic ulcers rarely become this large, the presence of one or more giant esophageal ulcers should suggest the possibility of CMV esophagitis in patients with AIDS.

HIV has also been implicated as a cause of giant esophageal ulcers that are impossible to differentiate from CMV ulcers on radiographic criteria (see next section on Human Immunodeficiency Virus Esophagitis). Endoscopy is therefore required to distinguish these infections. If endoscopic biopsy specimens or brushings reveal the characteristic cytoplasmic inclusions of CMV or if viral cultures are positive for CMV, treatment can be initiated with potent antiviral agents, such as ganciclovir.[2,66] However, ganciclovir may cause severe bone marrow suppression with neutropenia, thrombocytopenia, or anemia.[2,70] Potentially toxic antiviral drugs should therefore be used only if cytopathologic confirmation of CMV is obtained.

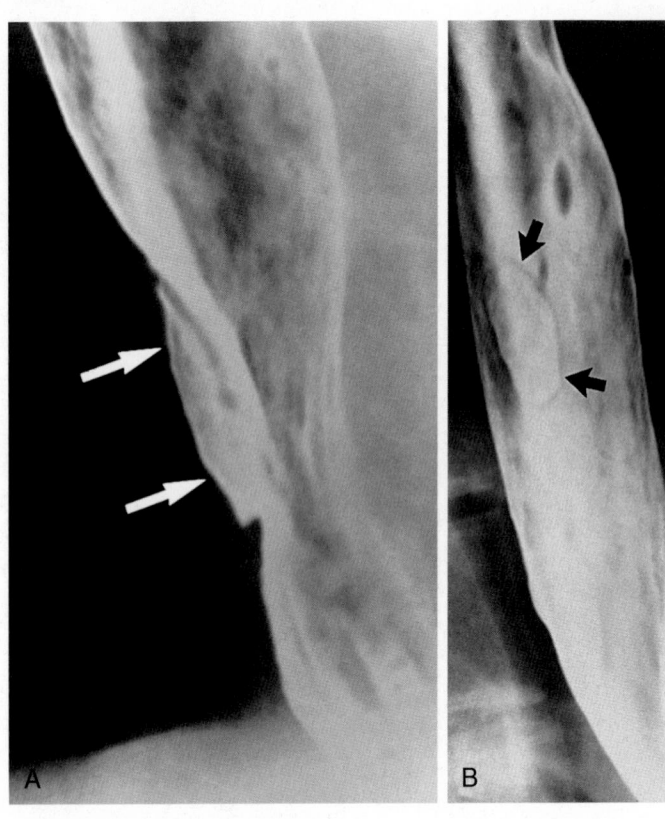

Figure 24-15. Cytomegalovirus esophagitis. A. A giant, relatively flat ulcer (*arrows*) is seen in profile in the distal esophagus. **B.** A large, ovoid ulcer (*arrows*) is seen en face in another patient. Note the thin radiolucent rim of edema surrounding the ulcer. Because herpetic ulcers rarely become this large, the presence of one or more giant esophageal ulcers should raise the possibility of cytomegalovirus esophagitis in patients with AIDS. (**A** courtesy of Sidney W. Nelson, MD, Seattle, WA; **B** courtesy of Kyunghee C. Cho, MD, Newark, NJ.)

HUMAN IMMUNODEFICIENCY VIRUS ESOPHAGITIS

A new clinical syndrome of odynophagia and giant esophageal ulcers has been recognized in patients with HIV infection.[71-78] Biopsy specimens, brushings, and cultures from the esophagus have failed to reveal any signs of the usual fungal or viral organisms associated with infectious esophagitis in patients with AIDS. Furthermore, electron microscopy of biopsy specimens from these ulcers has demonstrated viral particles with morphologic features of HIV infection, directly implicating HIV as the cause of the ulcers.[74] These HIV ulcers (also called *idiopathic ulcers*[76,77]) may develop in patients who have recently become HIV positive or in patients who have been HIV positive for extended periods and have had other clinical signs of AIDS.[2,73-76,78] Thus, giant esophageal ulcers may occur as a manifestation of acute or chronic HIV infection.

Clinical Findings

Patients with HIV ulcers in the esophagus typically present with acute onset of severe odynophagia or dysphagia.[72-76,78] The pain may be so intense that patients are unable to swallow their saliva. Occasionally, these patients may develop hematemesis or other signs of upper gastrointestinal bleeding.[71] The ulcers sometimes develop at or soon after the time of HIV seroconversion.[74] As part of this seroconversion syndrome, there may be associated ulcers in the oropharynx and soft palate or a characteristic maculopapular rash involving the face, trunk, and upper extremities.[72,73,76] In most cases, however, HIV ulcers in the esophagus occur after the patient has developed clinically overt AIDS with low CD4 counts.[2,78]

Candida, herpes, and CMV esophagitis are other common causes of odynophagia in HIV-positive patients, but the possibility of HIV esophagitis should be suspected if these individuals have the characteristic maculopapular rash or develop symptoms at or near the time of seroconversion. HIV can sometimes be confirmed as the cause of the ulcers by electron microscopy and in situ DNA hybridization.[74,76] Because these techniques are not widely available, however, HIV esophagitis has primarily been a diagnosis of exclusion when no cytopathologic changes of CMV or other opportunistic organisms are present on endoscopic biopsy specimens or brushings from the ulcers.[71,75,77,78]

Radiographic Findings

HIV esophagitis is usually manifested on esophagography by the development of one or more giant (>1 cm), flat ulcers in the midesophagus or distal esophagus, sometimes associated with small, satellite ulcers (Fig. 24-16).[75,78] The ulcers may appear in profile or en face as ovoid, elongated, or diamond-shaped collections of barium, often surrounded by a radiolucent rim of edema.[75,78] These HIV ulcers are therefore indistinguishable radiographically from CMV ulcers in the esophagus (see Fig. 24-15).[75,78] Data suggest that most giant esophageal ulcers in HIV-positive patients are caused by HIV rather than CMV.[78] In contrast to CMV ulcers, HIV ulcers in the esophagus may heal spontaneously or may respond to treatment with oral corticosteroids, but they do not require treatment with potentially toxic antiviral agents such as ganciclovir.[2,72-74,78,79] Endoscopic biopsy specimens, brushings, and viral cultures are therefore required to differentiate HIV

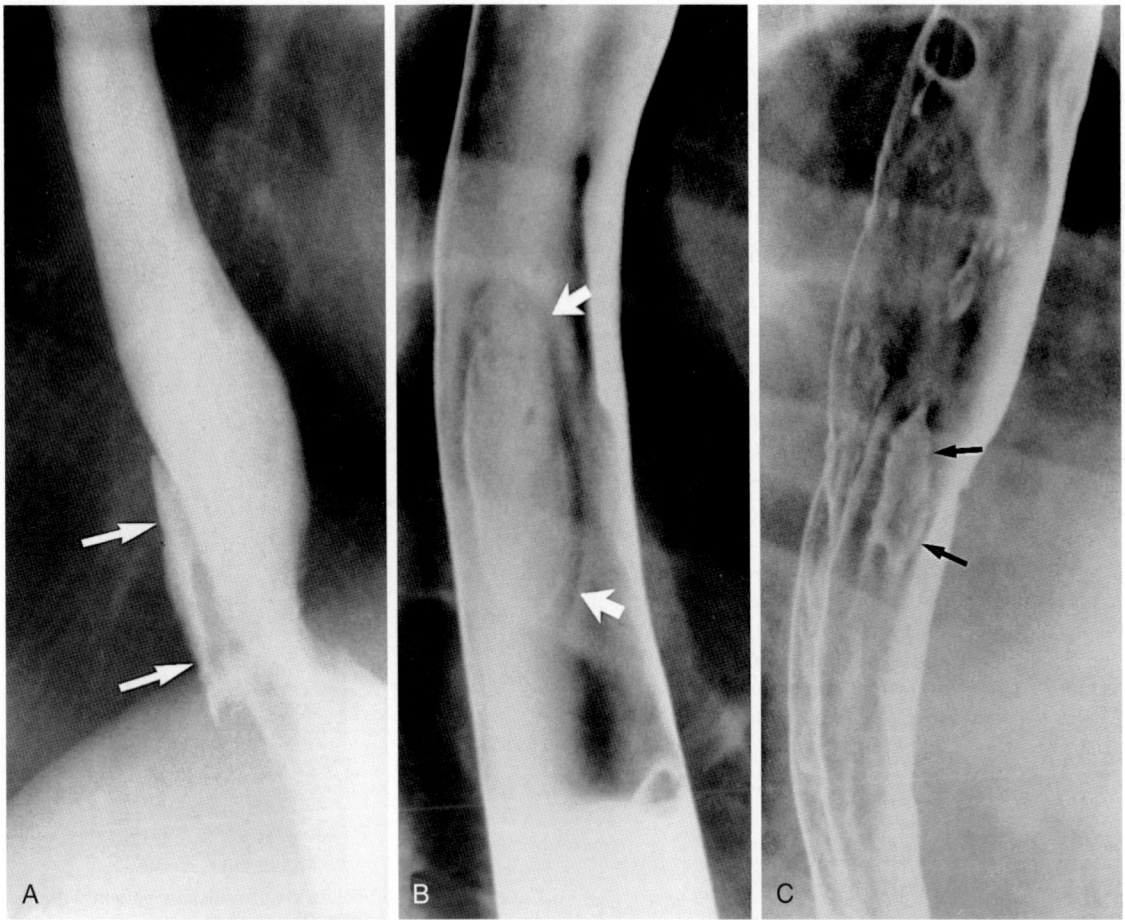

Figure 24-16. Human immunodeficiency virus (HIV) esophagitis. A. A giant, relatively flat ulcer (*arrows*) is seen in profile in the distal esophagus. This patient was HIV positive. **B.** In another HIV-positive patient, a large ovoid ulcer (*arrows*) is seen en face with a thin surrounding rim of edema. **C.** In a third patient, a diamond-shaped ulcer (*arrows*) is seen in the midesophagus with a cluster of small satellite ulcers. All three cases are indistinguishable from the cytomegalovirus ulcers illustrated in Figure 24-15. However, endoscopic biopsy specimens, brushings, and cultures were negative for cytomegalovirus in these patients. (From Levine MS, Loercher G, Katzka DA, et al: Giant, human immunodeficiency virus-related ulcers in the esophagus. Radiology 180:323-326, 1991.)

ulcers from CMV ulcers, so that appropriate treatment can be initiated in these patients.

Rarely, HIV esophagitis may be associated with the development of esophagoesophageal or esophagogastric fistulas or focal perforation into the mediastinum.[80] Tuberculous esophagitis can also be associated with intramural sinus tracks and fistulas, but these tracks and fistulas tend to be located more proximally in the esophagus in patients with tuberculosis (see next section on Tuberculosis).[81,82] Other causes of giant ulcers include nasogastric intubation, endoscopic sclerotherapy, caustic ingestion, and oral medications such as quinidine, potassium chloride, and nonsteroidal anti-inflammatory agents. The correct diagnosis is usually suggested by the clinical history and presentation. Thus, for all practical purposes, giant esophageal ulcers in HIV-positive patients are most likely caused by HIV or CMV.

TUBERCULOSIS

Esophageal involvement by tuberculosis is extremely uncommon. When it occurs, these patients usually have advanced tuberculosis in the lungs or mediastinum.[83,84] Both *Myco-*

bacterium tuberculosis and *Mycobacterium avium-intracellulare* have been implicated as causes of infectious esophagitis in patients with AIDS.[81,82]

Esophageal involvement is most frequently caused by adjacent tuberculous nodes in the mediastinum that compress or erode into the esophagus, causing narrowing, ulceration, or fistula formation.[81,84,85] In patients with active pulmonary tuberculosis, esophageal infection may also be caused by swallowed sputum containing the tubercle bacilli, particularly if there is a preexisting mucosal lesion or stricture in the esophagus. Rarely, hematogenous seeding of the esophagus may occur in patients with disseminated miliary tuberculosis.

Patients with tuberculous esophagitis may be asymptomatic, or they may present with dysphagia, odynophagia, or chest pain.[84] Although the clinical findings are nonspecific, the possibility of esophageal tuberculosis should be considered in patients with persistent dysphagia who have active pulmonary tuberculosis. In such cases, the diagnosis may be confirmed at endoscopy by the presence of tubercle bacilli or, rarely, caseating granulomas on endoscopic biopsy specimens or brushings from the esophagus.[86]

Radiographic Findings

Extrinsic esophageal involvement by tuberculous nodes in the mediastinum is usually manifested on esophagography by compression, displacement, or narrowing of the esophagus by an adjacent mediastinal mass.[83,85,86] These patients may also develop strictures or traction diverticula, most frequently at the level of the carina.[83,84] Occasionally, caseating nodes in the mediastinum may erode into the upper esophagus or mid-esophagus, producing superficial or deep areas of ulceration, longitudinal or transverse sinus tracks, or fistulas into the mediastinum or tracheobronchial tree (Fig. 24-17).[83-85] Sinus tracks and fistulas have been recognized as a prominent feature of tuberculous esophagitis in patients with AIDS (Fig. 24-18).[81,82] Similar findings may be demonstrated in patients with Crohn's disease, trauma, radiation, and esophageal carcinoma, but the presence of pulmonary or mediastinal tuberculosis should suggest the correct diagnosis, particularly in patients with AIDS.

Intrinsic tuberculous esophagitis occurs much less frequently and is characterized on barium studies by mucosal irregularity, ulcers, plaques, fistulas, and, eventually, strictures (Fig. 24-19).[83,86] Rarely, esophageal tuberculosis can lead to the development of an intramural abscess, seen on esophagography as a smooth submucosal mass and on CT as a well-marginated cystic mass with an enhancing rim in the

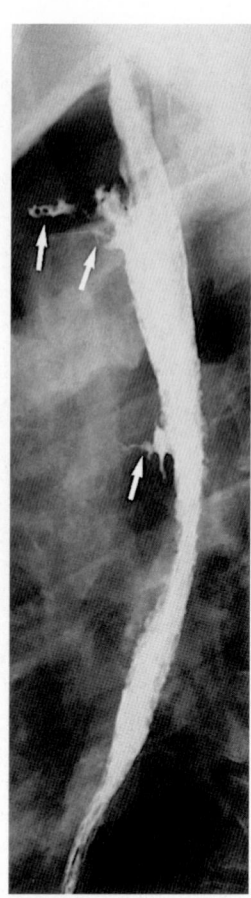

Figure 24-18. Tuberculous esophagitis in a patient with AIDS. There is diffuse esophagitis with several deep sinus tracks (*arrows*) extending anteriorly from the esophagus into the mediastinum. (From Goodman P, Pinero SS, Rance RM, et al: Mycobacterial esophagitis in AIDS. Gastrointest Radiol 14:103-105, 1989. With kind permission from Springer Science and Business Media.)

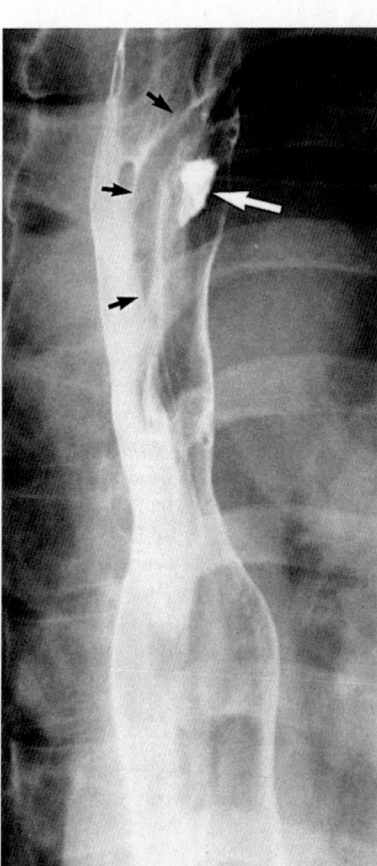

Figure 24-17. Tuberculous esophagitis. There is compression (*black arrows*) of the upper thoracic esophagus with associated ulceration (*white arrow*) due to caseating tuberculous nodes that have eroded into the esophagus. (Courtesy of Alan Grundy, MD, London, England.)

esophagus.[87] Tuberculous esophagitis may be indistinguishable from severe esophagitis resulting from caustic ingestion, radiation, or other causes.

ACTINOMYCOSIS

Actinomycosis is an indolent, suppurative infection caused by *Actinomyces israelii,* an anaerobic gram-positive bacterium. Rarely, this organism may cause severe esophagitis in patients with AIDS.[88] Esophageal actinomycosis may be manifested on esophagography by deep ulcers with multiple longitudinal and transverse fistulas and intramural tracks (Fig. 24-20).[88] Although tuberculous esophagitis may also cause ulceration and fistula formation (see earlier section on Tuberculosis), the presence of multiple intramural tracks parallel to the esophageal lumen should raise the possibility of esophageal actinomycosis in patients with AIDS.

OTHER INFECTIONS

Although infectious esophagitis is usually caused by fungal or viral organisms, other rare causes include *Staphylococcus, Streptococcus, Klebsiella, Blastomyces, Cryptosporidium, Torulopsis glabrata,* and *Lactobacillus acidophilus.*[89-94]

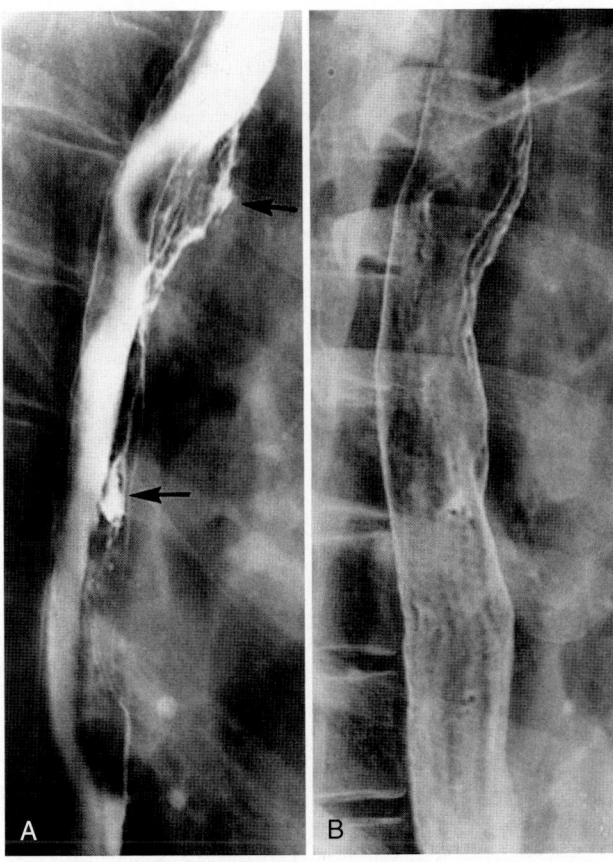

Figure 24-19. Tuberculous esophagitis. A. The initial esophagogram shows two areas of irregular ulceration (*arrows*) in the midesophagus due to proven tuberculous esophagitis. **B.** Another esophagogram after 6 months of antituberculous therapy shows healing of the ulcers. (From Savage PE, Grundy A: Oesophageal tuberculosis: An unusual cause of dysphagia. Br J Radiol 57:1153-1155, 1984.)

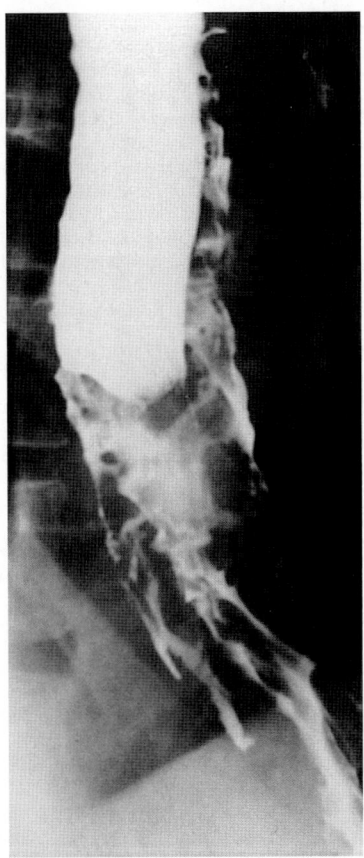

Figure 24-20. Esophageal actinomycosis. Multiple longitudinal and transverse intramural tracks and fistulas are seen in the distal esophagus due to actinomycosis involving the esophagus. This patient had AIDS. (Courtesy of Emil J. Balthazar, MD, New York, NY.)

References

1. Mathieson R, Dutta SK: *Candida* esophagitis. Dig Dis Sci 28:365-370, 1983.
2. Baehr PH, McDonald GB: Esophageal infections: Risk factors, presentation, diagnosis, and treatment. Gastroenterology 106:509-532, 1994.
3. Lewicki AM, Moore JP: Esophageal moniliasis. AJR 125:218-245, 1975.
4. Sheft DJ, Shrago G: Esophageal moniliasis: the spectrum of the disease. JAMA 213:1859-1862, 1970.
5. Eras P, Goldstein MJ, Sherlock P: *Candida* infection of the gastrointestinal tract. Medicine (Baltimore) 51:367-379, 1972.
6. Barbaro G, Barbarini G, Calderon W, et al: Fluconazole versus itraconazole for *Candida* esophagitis in acquired immunodeficiency syndrome. Gastroenterology 111:1169-1177, 1996.
7. Levine MS, Macones AJ, Laufer I: *Candida* esophagitis: Accuracy of radiographic diagnosis. Radiology 154:581-587, 1985.
8. Gefter WB, Laufer I, Edell S, et al: Candidiasis in the obstructed esophagus. Radiology 138:25-28, 1981.
9. Kodsi BE, Wickremesinghe PC, Kozinn PJ, et al: *Candida* esophagitis. Gastroenterology 71:715-719, 1976.
10. Ott DJ, Gelfand DW: Esophageal stricture secondary to candidiasis. Gastrointest Radiol 2:323-325, 1978.
11. Kelvin FM, Clark WM, Thompson WM, et al: Chronic esophageal stricture due to moniliasis. Br J Radiol 51:826-828, 1978.
12. Agha FP: Candidiasis-induced esophageal strictures. Gastrointest Radiol 9:283-286, 1984.
13. Friedman HM, Gluckman SJ: Infections of the esophagus. In Cohen S, Soloway RD (eds): Diseases of the Esophagus. New York, Churchill Livingstone, 1982, pp 277-286.
14. Levine MS, Woldenberg R, Herlinger H, et al: Opportunistic esophagitis in AIDS: radiographic diagnosis. Radiology 165:815-820, 1987.
15. Brayko CM, Kozavek RA, Sanowski RA, et al: Type I herpes simplex esophagitis with concomitant esophageal moniliasis. J Clin Gastroenterol 4:351-355, 1982.
16. Mirra SS, Bryan JA, Butz WC, et al: Concomitant herpes-monilial esophagitis: Case report with ultrastructural study. Hum Pathol 13:760-763, 1982.
17. Wilcox CM, Alexander LN, Clark WS, et al: Fluconazole compared with endoscopy for human immunodeficiency virus-infected patients with esophageal symptoms. Gastroenterology 110:1803-1809, 1996.
18. Laine L: The natural history of esophageal candidiasis after successful treatment in patients with AIDS. Gastroenterology 107:744-746, 1994.
19. Vahey TN, Maglinte DDT, Chernish SM: State-of-the-art barium examination in opportunistic esophagitis. Dig Dis Sci 31:1192-1195, 1986.
20. Kressel HY, Glick SN, Laufer I, et al: Radiologic features of esophagitis. Gastrointest Radiol 6:103-108, 1981.
21. Glick SN: Barium studies in patients with *Candida* esophagitis: Pseudo-ulcerations simulating viral esophagitis. AJR 163:349-352, 1994.
22. Gonzalez G: Esophageal moniliasis. AJR 113:233-236, 1971.
23. Ho CS, Cullen JB, Gray RR: An unusual manifestation of esophageal moniliasis. Radiology 123:287-288, 1977.
24. Roberts L, Gibbons R, Gibbons G, et al: Adult esophageal candidiasis: A radiographic spectrum. RadioGraphics 7:289-307, 1987.
25. Farman J, Tivitian A, Rosenthal LE, et al: Focal esophageal candidiasis in acquired immunodeficiency syndrome (AIDS). Gastrointest Radiol 11:213-217, 1986.
26. Obrecht WF, Richter JE, Olympio GA, et al: Tracheoesophageal fistula: A serious complication of infectious esophagitis. Gastroenterology 87:1174-1179, 1984.
27. Sehha S, Hazeghi K, Bajoghli M, et al: Oesophageal moniliasis causing fistula formation and lung abscess. Thorax 31:361-364, 1976.

28. Campero AA, Campbell GD: Complete oesophageal obstruction due to monilial infection. Aust N Z J Surg 43:244-246, 1973.
29. Sam JW, Levine MS, Rubesin SE, et al: The "foamy" esophagus: A radiographic sign of *Candida* esophagitis. AJR 174:999-1002, 2000.
30. Troupin RH: Intramural esophageal diverticulosis and moniliasis: A possible association. AJR 104:613-616, 1968.
31. Beauchamp JM, Nice CM, Belanger MA, et al: Esophageal intramural pseudodiverticulosis. Radiology 113:273-276, 1974.
32. Castillo S, Abvrashed A, Kimmelman J, et al: Diffuse intramural esophageal pseudodiverticulosis. Gastroenterology 72:541-545, 1977.
33. Rohrmann CA, Kidd R: Chronic mucocutaneous candidiasis: Radiologic abnormalities in the esophagus. AJR 130:473-476, 1978.
34. Meyers C, Durkin MG, Love L: Radiographic findings in herpetic esophagitis. Radiology 119:21-24, 1976.
35. Skucas J, Schrank WW, Meyer PC, et al: Herpes esophagitis: A case study by air-contrast esophagography. AJR 128:497-499, 1977.
36. Levine MS, Cajade AG, Herlinger H, et al: Pseudomembranes in reflux esophagitis. Radiology 159:43-45, 1986.
37. Glick SN, Teplick SK, Goldstein J, et al: Glycogenic acanthosis of the esophagus. AJR 139:683-688, 1982.
38. Itai Y, Kogure T, Okuyama Y, et al: Diffuse finely nodular lesions of the esophagus. AJR 128:563-566, 1977.
39. Itai Y, Kogure T, Okuyama Y, et al: Superficial esophageal carcinoma: Radiological findings in double-contrast studies. Radiology 126:597-601, 1978.
40. Gohel VK, Kressel HY, Laufer I: Double-contrast artifacts. Gastrointest Radiol 3:139-146, 1978.
41. Muller SA, Herrmann EC, Winkelmann RK: Herpes simplex infections in hematologic malignancies. Am J Med 52:102-114, 1972.
42. Weiden PL, Schuffler MD: Herpes esophagitis complicating Hodgkin's disease. Cancer 33:1100-1102, 1974.
43. Nash G, Ross JS: Herpetic esophagitis: A common cause of esophageal ulceration. Hum Pathol 5:339-345, 1974.
44. Depew WT, Prentice RS, Beck IT, et al: Herpes simplex ulcerative esophagitis in a healthy subject. Am J Gastroenterol 68:381-385, 1977.
45. Owensby LC, Stammer JL: Esophagitis associated with herpes simplex infection in an immunocompetent host. Gastroenterology 74:1305-1306, 1978.
46. Springer DJ, Da Costa LR, Beck IT: A syndrome of acute self-limiting ulcerative esophagitis in young adults probably due to herpes simplex virus. Dig Dis Sci 24:535-539, 1979.
47. Deshmukh M, Shah R, McCallum RW: Experience with herpes esophagitis in otherwise healthy patients. Am J Gastroenterol 79:173-176, 1984.
48. Desigan G, Schneider RP: Herpes simplex esophagitis in healthy adults. South Med J 78:1135-1137, 1985.
49. Levine MS, Laufer I, Kressel HY, et al: Herpes esophagitis. AJR 136:863-866, 1981.
50. Fishbein PG, Tuthill R, Kressel HY, et al: Herpes simplex esophagitis: A cause of upper gastrointestinal bleeding. Am J Dig Dis 24:540-544, 1979.
51. Rattner HM, Cooper DJ, Zaman MB: Severe bleeding from herpes esophagitis. Am J Gastroenterol 80:523-525, 1985.
52. Lightdale CJ, Wolf DJ, Marcucci RA, et al: Herpetic esophagitis in patients with cancer: Antemortem diagnosis by brush cytology. Cancer 39:243-246, 1977.
53. Lasser A: Herpes simplex virus esophagitis. Acta Cytol (Baltimore) 21:301-302, 1977.
54. Balfour HH: Antiviral drugs. N Engl J Med 340:1255-1268, 1999.
55. Klotz DA, Silverman L: Herpes virus esophagitis, consistent with herpes simplex, visualized endoscopically. Gastrointest Endosc 21:71-73, 1974.
56. Shortsleeve MJ, Gauvin GP, Gardner RC, et al: Herpetic esophagitis. Radiology 141:611-617, 1981.
57. Agha FP, Lee HH, Nostrant TT: Herpetic esophagitis: A diagnostic challenge in immunocompromised patients. Am J Gastroenterol 81:246-253, 1986.
58. Levine MS, Loevner LA, Saul SH, et al: Herpes esophagitis: Sensitivity of double-contrast esophagography. AJR 151:57-62, 1988.
59. DeGaeta L, Levine MS, Guglielmi GE, et al: Herpes esophagitis in an otherwise healthy patient. AJR 144:1205-1206, 1985.
60. Shortsleeve MJ, Levine MS: Herpes esophagitis in otherwise healthy patients: Clinical and radiographic findings. Radiology 182:859-861, 1992.
61. Creteur V, Laufer I, Kressel HY, et al: Drug-induced esophagitis detected by double-contrast radiography. Radiology 147:365-368, 1983.
62. Bova JG, Dutton NE, Goldstein HM, et al: Medication-induced esopha-
gitis: Diagnosis by double-contrast esophagography. AJR 148:731-732, 1987.
63. Balthazar EJ, Megibow AJ, Hulnick DH: Cytomegalovirus esophagitis and gastritis in AIDS. AJR 144:1201-1204, 1985.
64. Balthazar EJ, Megibow AJ, Hulnick D, et al: Cytomegalovirus esophagitis in AIDS: Radiographic features in 16 patients. AJR 149:919-923, 1987.
65. Teixidor HS, Honig CL, Norsoph E, et al: Cytomegalovirus infection of the alimentary canal: Radiologic findings with pathologic correlation. Radiology 163:317-323, 1987.
66. Wilcox CM, Diehl DL, Cello JP, et al: Cytomegalovirus esophagitis in patients with AIDS: A clinical, endoscopic, and pathologic correlation. Ann Intern Med 113:589-593, 1990.
67. Hackman RC, Wolford JL, Gleaves CA, et al: Recognition and rapid diagnosis of upper gastrointestinal cytomegalovirus infection in marrow transplant recipients: A comparison of seven virologic methods. Transplantation 57:231-237, 1994.
68. Wilcox CM, Rodgers W, Lazeny A: Prospective comparison of brush cytology, viral culture, and histology for the diagnosis of ulcerative esophagitis in AIDS. Clin Gastroenterol Hepatol 2:564-567, 2004.
69. Frager DH, Frager JD, Brandt LJ, et al: Gastrointestinal complications of AIDS: Radiologic features. Radiology 158:597-603, 1986.
70. Buhles WC, Mastre BJ, Tinker AJ, et al: Ganciclovir treatment of life- or sight-threatening cytomegalovirus infection: Experience in 314 immunocompromised patients. Rev Infect Dis 10(Suppl 3):495-506, 1988.
71. Kumar A, Posner G, Colby S, et al: Giant esophageal ulcers in AIDS-related complex. Gastrointest Endosc 34:153-154, 1988.
72. Bach MC, Valenti AJ, Howell DA, et al: Odynophagia from aphthous ulcers of the pharynx and esophagus in the acquired immunodeficiency syndrome (AIDS). Ann Intern Med 109:338-339, 1988.
73. Bach MC, Howell DA, Valenti AJ, et al: Aphthous ulceration of the gastrointestinal tract in patients with the acquired immunodeficiency syndrome (AIDS). Ann Intern Med 112:465-466, 1990.
74. Rabeneck L, Popovic M, Gartner S, et al: Acute HIV infection presenting with painful swallowing and esophageal ulcers. JAMA 263:2318-2324, 1990.
75. Levine MS, Loercher G, Katzka DA, et al: Giant, human immunodeficiency virus-related ulcers in the esophagus. Radiology 180:323-326, 1991.
76. Kotler DP, Reka S, Orenstein JM, et al: Chronic idiopathic esophageal ulceration in the acquired immunodeficiency syndrome: Characterization and treatment with corticosteroids. J Clin Gastroenterol 15:284-290, 1992.
77. Wilcox CM, Schwartz DA: Endoscopic characterization of idiopathic esophageal ulceration associated with human immunodeficiency virus infection. J Clin Gastroenterol 16:251-256, 1993.
78. Sor S, Levine MS, Kowalski TE, et al: Giant ulcers of the esophagus in patients with human immunodeficiency virus: Clinical, radiographic, and pathologic findings. Radiology 194:447-451, 1995.
79. Dretler RH, Rausher DB: Giant esophageal ulcer healed with steroid therapy in an AIDS patient. Rev Infect Dis 11:768-769, 1989.
80. Frager D, Kotler DP, Baer J: Idiopathic esophageal ulceration in the acquired immunodeficiency syndrome: Radiologic reappraisal in 10 patients. Abdom Imaging 19:2-5, 1994.
81. Goodman P, Pinero SS, Rance RM, et al: Mycobacterial esophagitis in AIDS. Gastrointest Radiol 14:103-105, 1989.
82. de Silva R, Stoopack PM, Raufman JP: Esophageal fistulas associated with mycobacterial infection in patients at risk for AIDS. Radiology 175:449-453, 1990.
83. Schneider R: Tuberculosis of the mediastinum. Gastrointest Radiol 1:143-145, 1976.
84. Williford ME, Thompson WM, Hamilton JD, et al: Esophageal tuberculosis: Findings on barium swallow and computed tomography. Gastrointest Radiol 8:119-124, 1983.
85. Ramakantan R, Shah P: Tuberculous fistulas of the pharynx and esophagus. Gastrointest Radiol 15:145-147, 1990.
86. Savage PE, Grundy A: Oesophageal tuberculosis: An unusual cause of dysphagia. Br J Radiol 57:1153-1155, 1984.
87. Kim HG: Esophageal tuberculosis manifesting as submucosal abscess. AJR 180:1482-1483, 2003.
88. Spencer GM, Roach D, Skucas J: Actinomycosis of the esophagus in a patient with AIDS: Findings on barium esophagograms. AJR 161:795-796, 1993.
89. Walsh TJ, Belitsos NJ, Hamilton SR: Bacterial esophagitis in immunocompromised patients. Arch Intern Med 146:1345-1348, 1986.
90. Miller JT, Slywka SW, Ellis JH: Staphylococcal esophagitis causing giant ulcers. Abdom Imaging 18:245-246, 1993.

91. McKenzie R, Khakoo R: Blastomycosis of the esophagus presenting with gastrointestinal bleeding. Gastroenterology 88:1271-1273, 1985.

92. Kazlow PG, Shah K, Benkov K, et al: Esophageal cryptosporidiosis in a child with acquired immune deficiency syndrome. Gastroenterology 91:1301-1303, 1986.

93. Bentlif PS, Widermann B: Esophagitis caused by *Torulopsis glabrata*. Am J Gastroenterol 71:395-397, 1979.

94. McManus JPA, Webb JN: A yeast-like infection of the esophagus caused by *Lactobacillus acidophilus*. Gastroenterology 68:583-586, 1975.

Other Esophagitides

Marc S. Levine, MD

DRUG-INDUCED ESOPHAGITIS

Since its original description in 1970,[1] drug-induced esophagitis has been recognized as a relatively common condition in today's pill-oriented society. The medications implicated most frequently include tetracycline, doxycycline, potassium chloride, quinidine, aspirin, other nonsteroidal anti-inflammatory drugs (NSAIDs), and alendronate sodium. These patients may have severe esophageal symptoms, but drug-induced esophagitis usually resolves rapidly after withdrawal of the offending agent. Conventional single-contrast barium studies have been of limited value in detecting mucosal abnormalities associated with drug-induced esophagitis. Double-contrast esophagography, however, appears to be a valuable technique for diagnosing this condition.

Pathogenesis

The type and degree of injury that occurs in drug-induced esophagitis depend not only on the specific properties of the offending medication but also on the manner in which it is taken. Many patients have a history of ingesting the medication with little or no water immediately before going to bed.[2-4] As a result, the tablets or capsules may become lodged in the midesophagus, where they are compressed by the adjacent aortic arch or left main bronchus.[2] Drug-induced esophagitis is therefore believed to represent a focal contact esophagitis with ulceration of the adjacent mucosa by the dissolving pills. Less frequently, prolonged retention of the medication may result from esophageal compression by an enlarged heart.[5] Occasionally, drug-induced esophagitis may occur in patients who have abnormal motility or preexisting strictures that delay transit of pills from the esophagus.[6,7]

Causative Agents

Tetracycline and Doxycycline

Tetracycline and doxycycline, two widely used antibiotics, account for about half the reported cases of drug-induced esophagitis.[2] Because these medications are given in the form of capsules that are relatively acidic, prolonged retention of the capsules in the upper esophagus or midesophagus may cause superficial ulceration of the adjacent mucosa.[2,8] Although doxycycline (pH 3.0) is slightly less acidic than tetracycline (pH 2.3), it dissolves more slowly and forms an adherent gel, presumably accounting for the high frequency of esophagitis in patients taking this agent.[9] Affected individuals almost never develop strictures, however, because the ulcers caused by tetracycline and doxycycline are so small and superficial that they rarely incite enough scarring and fibrosis to produce a stricture.[4]

Potassium Chloride

Potassium chloride tablets may produce a severe form of drug-induced esophagitis.[1,2,5,10-12] These patients often have mitral valvular disease with an enlarged left atrium compressing the distal esophagus, so that passage of the potassium chloride tablets is impeded at this level. Subsequent release of potassium chloride over a localized area of esophageal mucosa may cause severe chemical injury with focal ulceration and

stricture formation.[5,11,12] As a result, potassium supplements are sometimes given in liquid form to patients with known cardiomegaly to prevent this complication. Even liquid potassium, however, has been described as a cause of drug-induced esophagitis.[13]

Quinidine

Because oral quinidine is often given for cardiac arrhythmias, these patients may have associated cardiomegaly, with compression of the distal esophagus by an enlarged left atrium or ventricle. Retained quinidine above this level may have a corrosive effect on the adjacent mucosa, causing ulceration and strictures.[2,6,13] Patients who are receiving long-term quinidine therapy are more likely to develop strictures.[13]

Nonsteroidal Anti-inflammatory Drugs

Nonsteroidal anti-inflammatory drugs (NSAIDs) have been implicated with increasing frequency in the development of esophagitis. Major offending agents include aspirin, phenylbutazone, indomethacin (Indocin), ibuprofen (Motrin), naproxen (Naprosyn), piroxicam (Feldene), and sulindac (Clinoril).[2,14-19] These NSAIDs not only may cause a focal contact esophagitis but also may exacerbate preexisting esophagitis in patients with gastroesophageal reflux disease, increasing the risk of stricture formation.[15,16]

Alendronate

Alendronate sodium (Fosamax) is an aminobiphosphonate, a selective inhibitor of osteoclast-mediated bone resorption, that has been used with increasing frequency in the non-hormonal treatment of postmenopausal osteoporosis. Reports indicate that this agent is associated with the development of a severe form of ulcerative esophagitis and stricture formation in the distal esophagus.[20-23] The mechanism of injury in these patients is uncertain. Topical corrosive injury may be a contributing factor, but the high frequency of ulceration in the distal esophagus suggests that esophagitis may be related to a reflux-mediated process in these patients.[20]

Other Drugs

Other oral medications that have been implicated in the development of drug-induced esophagitis include emepronium bromide, ferrous sulfate, alprenolol chloride, ascorbic acid, theophylline, cromolyn sodium, and antibiotics such as clindamycin and lincomycin.[2,7,24-29]

Clinical Findings

Patients with drug-induced esophagitis typically present with odynophagia (painful swallowing) or unremitting chest pain that is accentuated by swallowing.[2] Others may present with signs of upper gastrointestinal bleeding.[7,19] Symptoms usually develop within several hours to days after taking the medication.[2] The symptoms of drug-induced esophagitis also tend to resolve rapidly after withdrawal of the offending agent, so that most patients are asymptomatic within 7 to 10 days after stopping the medication.[8] Occasionally, patients may have progressive dysphagia because of the development of strictures.[11,13,30]

Radiographic Findings

The radiographic findings in drug-induced esophagitis depend on the nature of the offending medication. Tetracycline, doxycycline, and, less commonly, other medications cause superficial ulceration in the esophagus without permanent sequelae. Double-contrast esophagography is a useful technique for detecting shallow ulcers that cannot easily be recognized on single-contrast studies. Affected patients may have a solitary ulcer (Fig. 25-1A), several discrete ulcers (Fig. 25-1B), or multiple small ulcers on a normal background mucosa (Fig. 25-1C).[4,31-33] The ulcers are usually clustered together in the midesophagus near the level of the aortic arch or left main bronchus. These ulcers may be recognized en face as punctate, linear, ovoid, stellate, or serpiginous collections of barium on the esophageal mucosa or in profile as shallow depressions (see Fig. 25-1).[4,31-33] There may be slight nodularity of the adjacent mucosa or thickening and distortion of adjacent folds. When esophageal ulcers are drug induced, a follow-up esophagogram 7 to 10 days after withdrawal of the offending agent may show dramatic healing of the lesions.[31]

Potassium chloride, quinidine, NSAIDs, and alendronate tend to produce a more severe esophagitis, sometimes associated with deep ulcers and strictures. Larger areas of ulceration are often caused by potassium chloride and quinidine, particularly in patients with cardiomegaly. Because of associated edema and inflammation, there may be considerable mass effect surrounding the ulcer, mimicking the appearance of an ulcerated carcinoma (Fig. 25-2A).[13,31,34] Subsequent healing of the ulcers may lead to the development of strictures, typically seen as segmental areas of concentric narrowing above the level of an enlarged left atrium (Fig. 25-2B).[5,12,13,18,30] Other patients may have giant, relatively flat ulcers that are several centimeters or more in length (Fig. 25-3A).[17] Healing of these ulcers may lead to the development of smooth, re-epithelialized depressions that can be mistaken for active ulcer craters (Fig. 25-3B).[17] Alendronate has been associated with the development of severe ulcerative esophagitis and stricture formation in the distal esophagus (Fig. 25-4).[20-22]

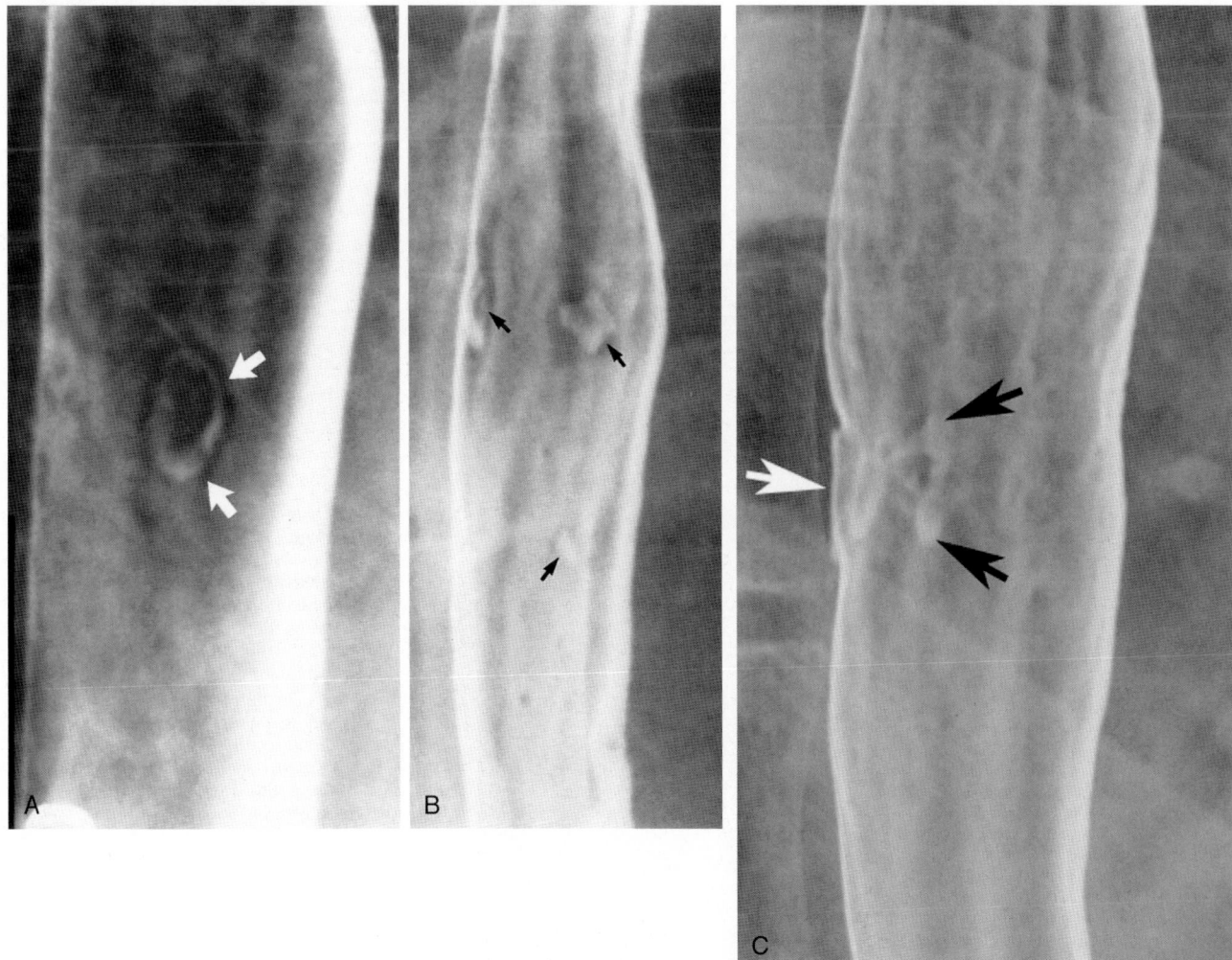

Figure 25-1. Drug-induced esophagitis with superficial ulcers. A. A solitary ringlike ulcer (*arrows*) is seen in the midesophagus. Note the thin, radiolucent halo of edematous mucosa surrounding the ulcer. **B.** Several discrete ulcers (*arrows*) are seen in the midesophagus on a normal background mucosa. The largest ulcer has a stellate configuration. **C.** This patient has a flat ulcer (*white arrow*) on the right lateral wall of the midesophagus with a cluster of small ulcers (*black arrows*) abutting the larger ulcer. The patient in **A** was taking doxycycline, the patient in **B** was taking tetracycline, and the patient in **C** was taking ibuprofen. (**A** and **B** from Levine MS: Radiology of the Esophagus. Philadelphia, WB Saunders, 1989.)

Figure 25-2. Spectrum of esophageal injury associated with potassium chloride ingestion. A. A giant ulcer (*white arrows*) is seen in the mid-esophagus with an associated area of mass effect (*black arrows*) due to a surrounding mound of edema. This lesion could be mistaken for an ulcerated carcinoma. **B.** A midesophageal stricture (*arrows*) is seen in another patient who had been taking slow-release potassium chloride tablets. The stricture has relatively tapered borders. (**B** from Levine MS: Radiology of the Esophagus. Philadelphia, WB Saunders, 1989.)

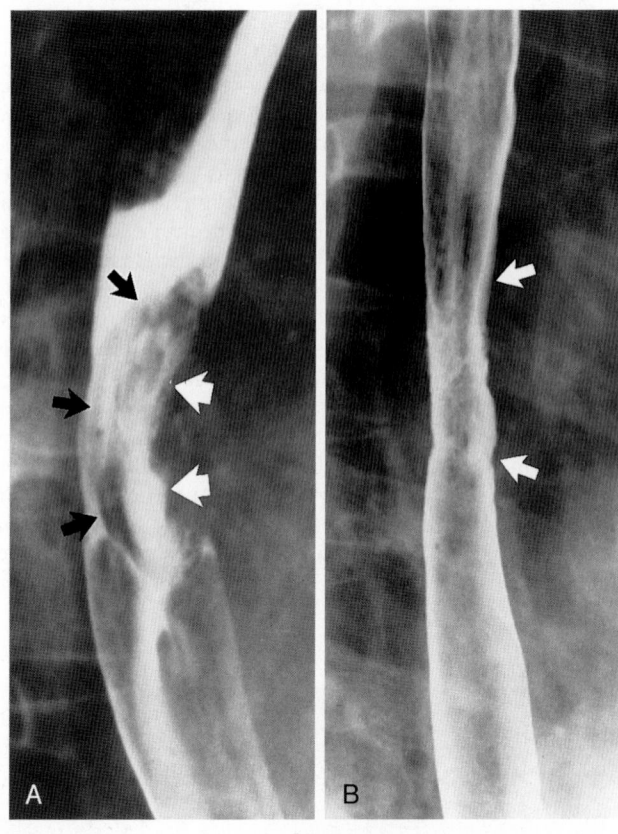

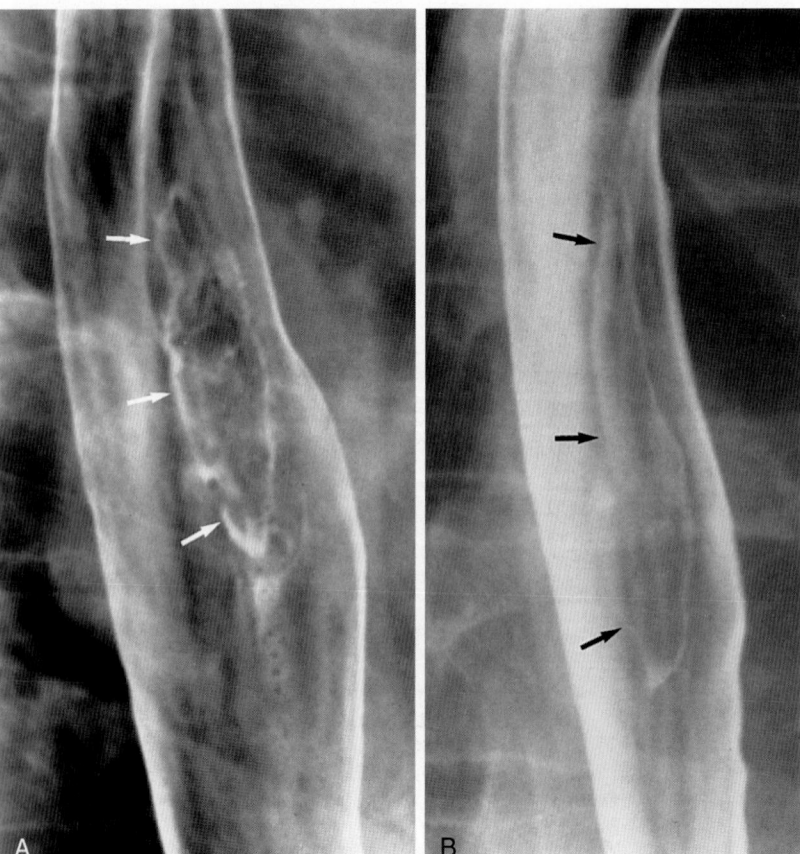

Figure 25-3. Drug-induced esophagitis with a giant esophageal ulcer. A. Initial double-contrast esophagogram shows a 7-cm-long, diamond-shaped ulcer (*arrows*) in the midesophagus below the level of the carina. The ulcer crater has irregular margins. This patient was taking sulindac (Clinoril), a nonsteroidal anti-inflammatory agent. **B.** Another esophagogram 6 months later shows a long, shallow depression with smooth borders (*arrows*) at the site of the previous ulcer. Endoscopy revealed that this was an ulcer scar with a re-epithelialized pit or depression. (From MS Levine, RD Rothstein, I Laufer: Giant esophageal ulcer due to Clinoril. AJR 156:955-956, 1991, © by American Roentgen Ray Society.)

AIDS (see Chapter 24).[38] However, these conditions can usually be differentiated by the clinical history and presentation.

Because drug-induced strictures are usually located at a considerable distance from the gastroesophageal junction, they must be differentiated from high esophageal strictures caused by Barrett's esophagus, mediastinal irradiation, caustic ingestion, eosinophilic esophagitis, and primary or metastatic tumors. However, the possibility of a drug-induced stricture should be suspected in patients with cardiomegaly who have a history of taking potassium chloride or quinidine.

RADIATION ESOPHAGITIS

Malignant tumors involving the lungs, mediastinum, or thoracic spine are often treated by high-dose, external-beam radiation to the chest. The major limiting factor with this form of treatment is esophageal damage by ionizing radiation. Total doses of 45 to 60 Gy may lead to severe esophagitis with irreversible damage and stricture formation.[39] Smaller doses (20 to 45 Gy) may cause a self-limited esophagitis without permanent sequelae. Most patients have clinical evidence of esophagitis shortly after the onset of radiation therapy, but barium studies are not usually performed during this period. Instead, esophagography has been used primarily to detect strictures or other signs of chronic radiation injury. Both the acute and the chronic forms of radiation esophagitis are considered in this chapter.

Pathogenesis

Experiments on laboratory animals have shown that high-dose radiation to the esophagus causes an acute, self-limited form of esophagitis within 1 to 3 weeks of the onset of radiation therapy.[40,41] Early postirradiation changes in humans appear to be comparable to those found in animal models. After the acute stage of radiation injury and subsequent epithelial repair, chronic radiation esophagitis is characterized by progressive submucosal scarring and fibrosis with the development of esophageal strictures 4 to 8 months after completion of radiation therapy at doses of 30 to 50 Gy.[42] If the radiation dose is more than 60 Gy, esophageal strictures may develop within 3 to 4 months.[42]

Clinical Findings

Most patients who receive mediastinal irradiation develop a self-limited esophagitis, manifested by acute onset of substernal burning, odynophagia, or dysphagia within 1 to 3 weeks after the onset of radiation therapy.[43] The symptoms usually subside within 24 to 48 hours but may occasionally persist for several weeks.[43] Because these patients are immunocompromised, the development of odynophagia may erroneously be attributed to opportunistic esophagitis. The correct diagnosis should be suggested, however, by the temporal relationship between the onset of radiation therapy and the onset of symptoms. When acute radiation esophagitis is suspected, these patients are usually treated empirically with viscous lidocaine and analgesics. As a result, radiologic or endoscopic examinations are not often performed in this setting.

Chronic radiation injury to the esophagus may cause dysphagia within several months after completion of radiation therapy. Dysphagia may result from abnormal esophageal

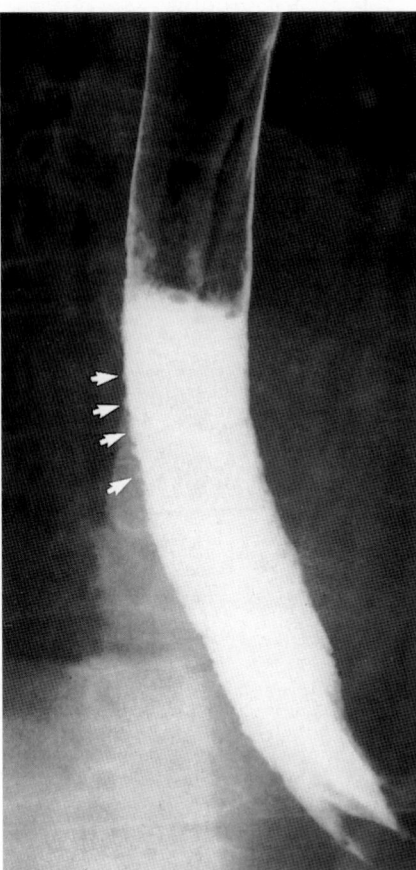

Figure 25-4. Alendronate-induced esophagitis. Multiple tiny ulcers (*arrows*) are seen in profile in the distal esophagus. This patient was taking alendronate (Fosamax) for the treatment of postmenopausal osteoporosis. (Courtesy of Barbara Sabinsky, MD, Stamford, CT.)

Differential Diagnosis

Herpes esophagitis is the major consideration in the differential diagnosis for discrete, superficial ulcers in the upper esophagus or midesophagus.[35] Although these viral ulcers may be indistinguishable from the ulcers of drug-induced esophagitis, the correct diagnosis can usually be suggested on the basis of the clinical history. Occasionally, however, herpes esophagitis may occur in otherwise healthy individuals who have no underlying immunologic problems (see Chapter 24).[36] Thus, the diagnosis of drug-induced esophagitis should be considered only when there is a definite temporal relationship between the ingestion of the offending medication and the onset of esophagitis.

Reflux esophagitis is a more common cause of superficial ulceration in the esophagus.[37] It would be extremely unusual, however, for patients with reflux esophagitis to have focal ulceration in the midesophagus with a normal-appearing mucosa below this level. Mediastinal irradiation and caustic ingestion are other causes of ulceration, but the correct diagnosis is usually suggested on clinical grounds. Crohn's disease may also be associated with shallow ulcers in the esophagus, but these patients usually have advanced Crohn's disease in the small bowel or colon (see later section on esophageal Crohn's disease). Finally, giant drug-induced ulcers may be indistinguishable from ulcerated carcinomas or from cytomegalovirus or human immunodeficiency virus ulcers in patients with motility or, less commonly, from the development of strictures.[39,42] Mild radiation strictures may be successfully dilated, but more severe strictures may necessitate feeding tube placement or other palliative measures. Occasionally, severe radiation injury may lead to life-threatening complications such as an esophageal-airway fistula or esophageal perforation. However, these unusual complications of radiation therapy almost always occur in an area of esophagus involved by tumor and rarely in normal irradiated tissue.[42,44]

Radiographic Findings

Although most patients with acute radiation esophagitis are treated empirically, barium studies are sometimes performed when the clinical diagnosis is uncertain. Acute radiation esophagitis may be manifested on double-contrast esophagography by a distinctive granular appearance of the mucosa and decreased distensibility resulting from edema and inflammation of the irradiated segment (Fig. 25-5).[45] In other cases, double-contrast esophagograms may reveal multiple small, discrete ulcers within a known radiation portal (Fig. 25-6).[41,45] With more severe disease, the esophagus may have a grossly irregular, serrated contour as a result of larger areas of ulceration and mucosal sloughing.

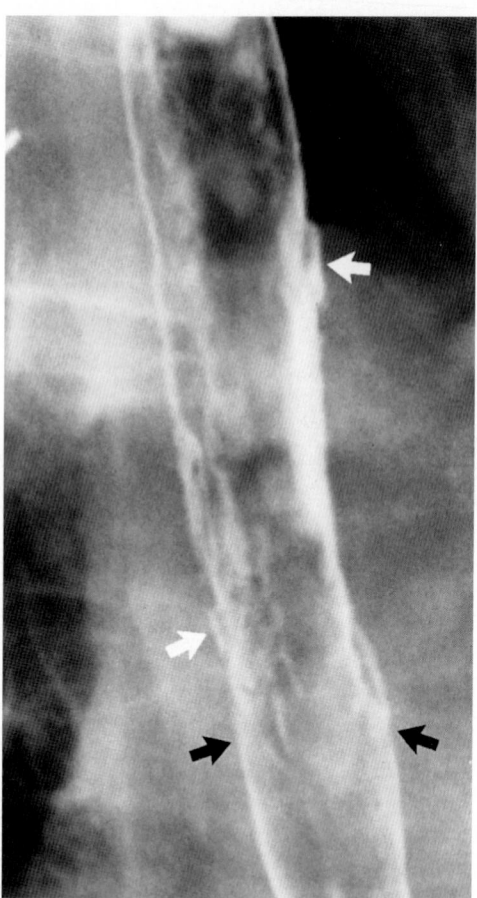

Figure 25-6. Acute radiation esophagitis. Multiple superficial ulcers are seen en face and in profile (*white arrows*) in the midesophagus. The area of ulceration has a relatively abrupt inferior demarcation (*black arrows*), which corresponds to the lower border of the radiation portal. This patient had undergone mediastinal irradiation for bronchogenic carcinoma several weeks earlier. (From Levine MS: Radiology of the Esophagus. Philadelphia, WB Saunders, 1989.)

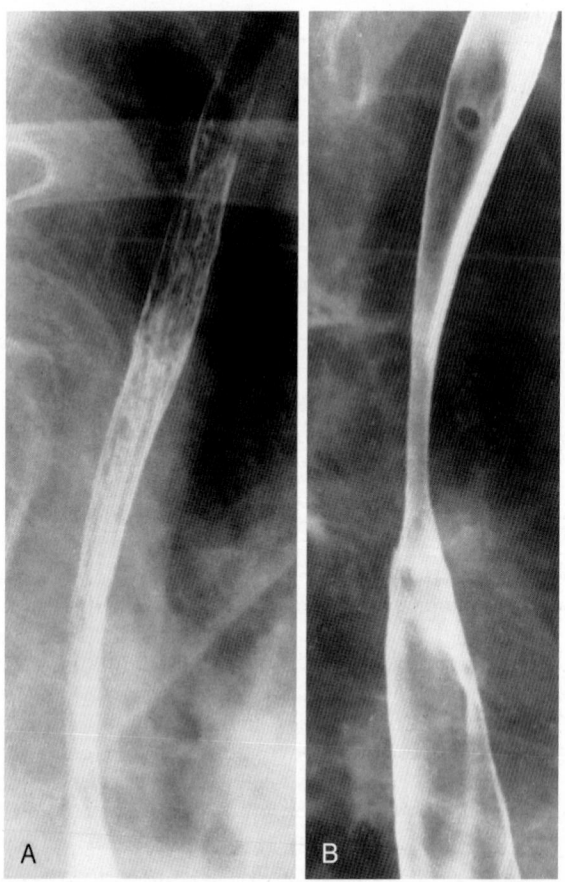

Figure 25-5. Acute radiation esophagitis with subsequent stricture formation. A. The mucosa has a granular appearance in the upper thoracic esophagus. Also note decreased distensibility of the irradiated segment. The patient presented with acute odynophagia 3 weeks after undergoing mediastinal irradiation for bronchogenic carcinoma. **B.** Another esophagogram 6 months later because of recurrent dysphagia shows a smooth, tapered stricture within the radiation portal.

After the acute phase of radiation injury, the most frequent finding on barium studies is abnormal esophageal motility, which usually develops 4 to 8 weeks after completion of radiation therapy.[39,42,46] This motor dysfunction is characterized by interruption of primary peristalsis at the superior border of the radiation portal, with numerous nonperistaltic contractions occurring distal to the point of disruption of the primary wave.[39,42,46] Less commonly, the irradiated segment may be totally aperistaltic.[42]

Radiation strictures in the esophagus usually develop 4 to 8 months after completion of radiation therapy.[39,42] Higher doses of radiation may shorten the interval for developing a stricture but have no effect on its length or caliber. The strictures typically appear as relatively smooth, tapered areas of narrowing in the upper esophagus or midesophagus within a preexisting radiation portal (see Fig. 25-5B).[39,42,44] Occasionally, there may be angulation or deformity of the stricture resulting from adherence of the narrowed segment to adjacent mediastinal structures.[39]

Chronic radiation esophagitis may also be manifested by the development of one or more ulcers, most frequently at the site of extrinsic compression of the esophagus by mediastinal lymphadenopathy or tumor.[42] These late-developing ulcers may be an ominous sign of impending fistula formation.

Tracheoesophageal and esophagobronchial fistulas are potentially life-threatening complications of mediastinal irradiation. The fistulas are usually caused by radiation necrosis, with erosion of tumor into the esophagus and adjacent airway.[44] The most frequent site of fistula formation is the left main bronchus, where it crosses the esophagus at the level of the fourth or fifth thoracic vertebra.[42] When an esophageal-airway fistula is suspected, the radiologic examination should be performed with barium sulfate because a water-soluble contrast agent may cause severe pulmonary edema if it enters the lungs via a fistula.[47]

Differential Diagnosis

When acute odynophagia or dysphagia develops several weeks after mediastinal irradiation, the major diagnostic considerations should be acute radiation esophagitis versus infectious esophagitis in an immunocompromised patient. If barium studies are performed, *Candida* esophagitis should be suggested by mucosal plaques whereas herpes esophagitis should be suggested by discrete, superficial ulcers without plaque formation.[35] In contrast, radiation esophagitis may be manifested by a granular appearance or by ulceration, but the area of involvement almost always conforms to a known radiation portal with a sharp demarcation at the inferior border of the portal (see Fig. 25-6).

Although many conditions should be considered in the differential diagnosis for an upper esophageal or midesophageal stricture,[48] the major diagnostic considerations after mediastinal irradiation for bronchogenic or other intrathoracic neoplasms should be a benign radiation stricture versus esophageal involvement by recurrent mediastinal tumor (see Chapter 28). A concentric area of smooth, tapered narrowing should favor the diagnosis of a radiation stricture, whereas irregular, eccentric narrowing with extrinsic mass effect should suggest malignant tumor. When the radiographic findings are equivocal, CT may be helpful for differentiating a radiation stricture from recurrent tumor in the mediastinum.

CAUSTIC ESOPHAGITIS

Caustic esophagitis did not become a serious medical problem in the United States until 1967, when concentrated liquid lye solutions were made commercially available to the American public for use as drain cleaners.[49] Because they could be swallowed rapidly, liquid corrosives exposed all surfaces of the upper gastrointestinal tract to potentially life-threatening caustic injury. Thus, caustic esophagitis became an important clinical entity. Endoscopy has generally been advocated as the best means of assessing the extent and severity of esophageal injury, but radiologic studies may also provide valuable information during both the acute and chronic stages of the disease.

Pathogenesis

Caustic injury to the esophagus may be caused by ingestion of alkali, acids, ammonium chloride, phenols, silver nitrate, and a variety of other common household products. Children usually ingest these corrosive substances accidentally, whereas adults take them intentionally to commit suicide. In either case, the degree of injury depends on the nature, concentration, and volume of the corrosive agent as well as the duration of tissue contact. In the United States, most patients with caustic esophagitis swallow some form of liquid lye (concentrated sodium hydroxide), which causes severe esophageal injury by liquefaction necrosis.[50,51] In contrast, ingested acids cause tissue damage by coagulative necrosis, forming a protective eschar that tends to limit further tissue penetration.[50,51] Nevertheless, acidic agents may produce severe esophagitis and strictures comparable to those caused by lye.[52]

Caustic esophagitis is characterized pathologically by three phases of injury: an acute necrotic phase, an ulceration-granulation phase, and a final phase of cicatrization and scarring.[53] The initial phase of acute cellular necrosis begins immediately after caustic ingestion. This acute phase usually lasts 1 to 4 days and is accompanied by an intense inflammatory reaction in the surrounding tissues.[53] The ulceration-granulation phase begins 3 to 5 days after caustic ingestion and is characterized by edema, ulceration, and sloughing of necrotic mucosa.[53] During the next 7 to 14 days, subsequent healing leads to the production of granulation tissue in areas of mucosal sloughing. The esophagus is thought to be weakest and therefore most vulnerable to perforation during this period. The final phase of cicatrization begins 3 to 4 weeks after caustic ingestion.[53] Depending on the degree of injury, this cicatrization process may lead to severe scarring and stricture formation in the esophagus.

Clinical Findings

Acute caustic esophagitis may be manifested by the rapid onset of intense odynophagia, chest pain, drooling, vomiting, or hematemesis.[50,51,53] Severe substernal pain, fever, and shock usually indicate esophageal perforation and mediastinitis.[50,51] Associated gastric perforation may lead to the development of peritonitis. If patients survive the acute illness, there may be a latent period of several weeks during which they are no longer symptomatic.[50,51,53] Subsequently, however, these patients may develop severe dysphagia resulting from progressive stricture formation 1 to 3 months after the initial injury.[50,51]

Diagnosis and Treatment

When caustic ingestion is suspected, examination of the mouth and oropharynx may reveal obvious tissue injury, with ulceration of the lingual, buccal, or pharyngeal mucosa. Liquid corrosives may be swallowed rapidly, however, so that caustic esophagitis often occurs without associated pharyngeal injury.[50,51,53] Direct visualization of the esophagus is therefore required to confirm this diagnosis. A limited radiographic study may be performed with a water-soluble contrast agent to detect an esophageal or gastric perforation or other signs of caustic injury. However, most authors advocate endoscopy within 24 hours of caustic ingestion (assuming that there are no clinical or radiographic signs of perforation) to assess the extent and severity of esophageal injury.[50,51,53]

Treatment of caustic esophagitis is generally aimed at preventing stricture formation. Some authors advocate early administration of corticosteroids and antibiotics to inhibit collagen formation and decrease the risk of infection.[54,55] Others believe that esophageal bougienage should be performed as early as 2 to 3 weeks after caustic ingestion. Despite these measures, 10% to 40% of patients with caustic esophagitis develop strictures.[51,56] Some may respond to periodic dilatations, but others eventually require an esophageal bypass operation, such as a jejunal or colonic interposition (see Chapter 31). When strictures develop after caustic ingestion, esophagography may be used to determine the degree and extent of stricture formation as well as the response to treatment. Patients with lye strictures are also thought to have a significantly increased risk of developing esophageal carcinoma 20 to 40 years after the initial caustic injury.[57,58] This subject is discussed in detail in Chapter 27.

Radiographic Findings

Chest and abdominal radiographs should be obtained routinely for patients who have ingested caustic agents. With severe esophageal injury, posteroanterior and lateral radiographs of the chest may demonstrate a dilated, gas-filled esophagus or, if esophageal perforation has occurred, mediastinal widening, pneumomediastinum, or pleural effusions.[59,60] Similarly, abdominal radiographs may demonstrate pneumoperitoneum or a localized gas-containing abscess resulting from gastric perforation.

When esophageal or gastric perforation is suspected in patients who have normal or equivocal chest and abdominal radiographs, a water-soluble contrast study should be performed to document the presence of a leak. Water-soluble contrast agents are used because barium in the mediastinum may cause mediastinal fibrosis and barium in the peritoneal cavity may cause severe peritonitis.[47] If there is no evidence of esophageal or gastric perforation, however, barium should be given for a more detailed examination.

Acute caustic esophagitis may be manifested on esophagography by abnormal esophageal motility with poor primary peristalsis, nonperistaltic contractions, diffuse esophageal spasm, or a dilated, atonic esophagus (Fig. 25-7).[59-62] Some authors believe that the latter finding indicates diffuse muscular necrosis and that it is an ominous sign of impending perforation.[59] Occasionally, the motor disturbance can mimic achalasia, with markedly elevated lower esophageal sphincter pressures.[63] These various motor abnormalities have been attributed to edema, inflammation, or destruction of ganglion cells in the Auerbach plexus.[61,63]

In other patients, acute caustic esophagitis may be manifested by multiple shallow, irregular ulcers (Fig. 25-8). With more severe caustic injury, the esophagus may be diffusely narrowed and may have a grossly irregular contour because of marked edema, spasm, and ulceration (Fig. 25-9).[52,59,60] Occasionally, contrast material may dissect beneath partially sloughed mucosal fragments, producing a double-barreled appearance, with linear or streaky collections in the esophageal wall.[59] Rarely, these intramural collections may remain visible on delayed radiographs after the lumen has emptied.[59]

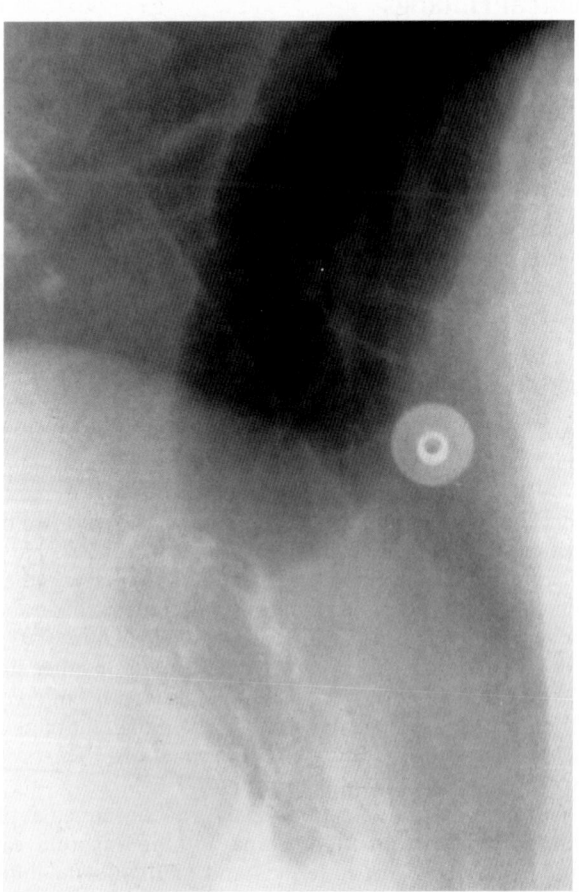

Figure 25-7. Acute caustic esophagitis with a dilated, atonic esophagus. There is a dilated, aperistaltic, gas-filled esophagus with a small amount of water-soluble contrast material in the stomach. This finding indicates a high risk of perforation.

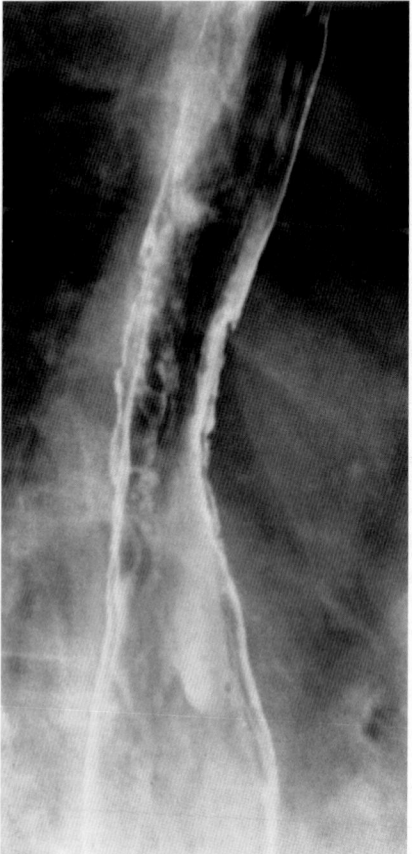

Figure 25-8. Acute caustic esophagitis. Multiple shallow, irregular ulcers are seen en face and in profile in the midesophagus. This patient had taken concentrated potassium hydroxide in a suicide attempt. (From Levine MS: Radiology of the Esophagus. Philadelphia, WB Saunders, 1989.)

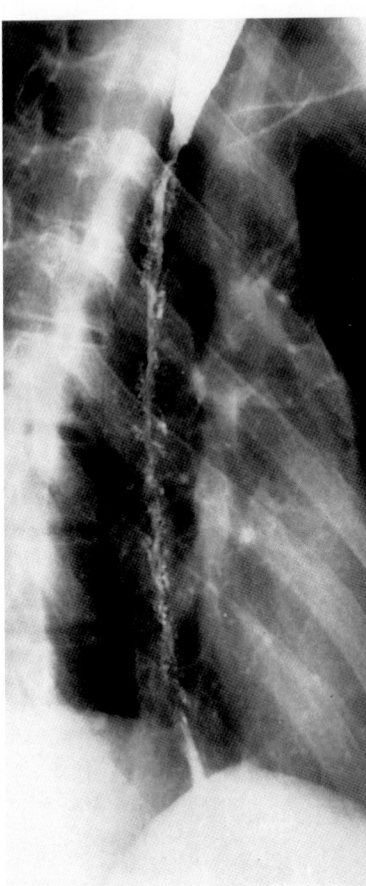

Figure 25-9. Severe caustic esophagitis. The thoracic esophagus is diffusely narrowed and has a grossly irregular contour with extensive ulceration because of ingestion of concentrated sodium hydroxide (liquid lye). (From Levine MS: Radiology of the Esophagus. Philadelphia, WB Saunders, 1989.)

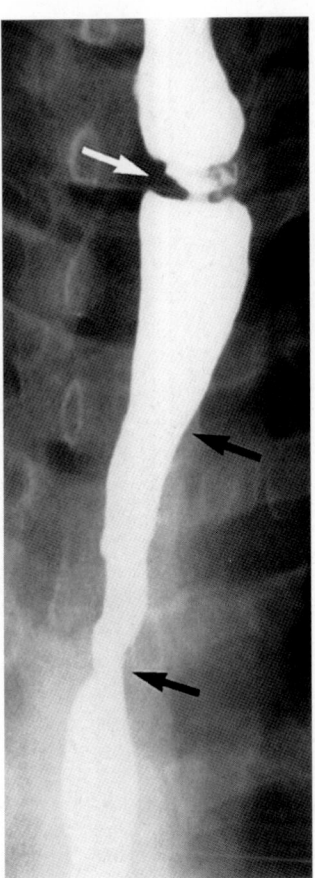

Figure 25-10. Lye strictures. A long, tapered stricture (*black arrows*) is seen in the upper thoracic esophagus. Another short, asymmetrical stricture (*white arrow*) is seen more proximally at the thoracic inlet. The presence of one or more segmental strictures in the cervical or thoracic esophagus is characteristic of caustic injury. (From Levine MS: Radiology of the Esophagus. Philadelphia, WB Saunders, 1989.)

Subsequent cicatrization and fibrosis may lead to the development of one or more segmental strictures in the esophagus 1 to 3 months after the acute injury. The strictures usually appear as relatively long areas of smooth, tapered narrowing in the upper esophagus or midesophagus (Fig. 25-10).[60] Some strictures may have an irregular contour or eccentric areas of sacculation because of asymmetrical scarring (see Fig. 25-10). With severe scarring, the entire thoracic esophagus may have a threadlike, filiform appearance (Fig. 25-11).[60] This finding should be highly suggestive of a caustic stricture because other conditions are rarely associated with such diffuse esophageal narrowing. When the esophagus is examined radiographically after caustic ingestion, the stomach should also be evaluated to determine whether associated gastric injury is present. This subject is discussed in detail in Chapter 34.

Differential Diagnosis

Acute caustic esophagitis may be difficult to differentiate from severe cases of reflux, infectious, drug-induced, or radiation esophagitis. However, reflux esophagitis tends to involve the distal esophagus, drug-induced esophagitis usually involves the midesophagus, and radiation esophagitis occurs within a preexisting radiation portal. In contrast, the site of caustic injury in the esophagus is unpredictable because these patients may have segmental or diffuse esophagitis involving the cervical or thoracic esophagus. Whatever the radiographic findings, the diagnosis of caustic esophagitis is usually apparent from the clinical history.

The classic finding of a long, tapered stricture in the cervical or thoracic esophagus should suggest prior caustic ingestion. However, localized caustic strictures in the upper esophagus or midesophagus may be indistinguishable from high esophageal strictures resulting from other causes, including Barrett's esophagus, mediastinal irradiation, oral medications, metastatic tumor, or, rarely, dermatologic diseases such as epidermolysis bullosa dystrophica and benign mucous membrane pemphigoid. When a lye stricture has irregular margins or relatively abrupt borders, differentiation from an infiltrating carcinoma may also be difficult. The ability to distinguish benign from malignant lesions is particularly important because of the increased risk of developing esophageal carcinoma in long-standing lye strictures (Fig. 25-12).[57,58] Thus, endoscopy and biopsy may be required for a definitive diagnosis.

IDIOPATHIC EOSINOPHILIC ESOPHAGITIS

Since its original description by Attwood and associates in 1993,[64] idiopathic eosinophilic esophagitis has been recognized

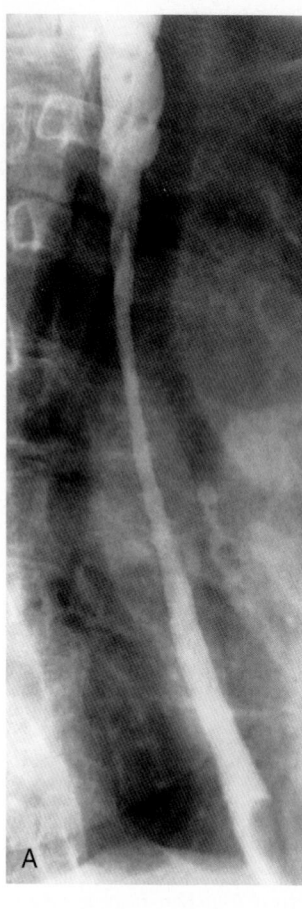

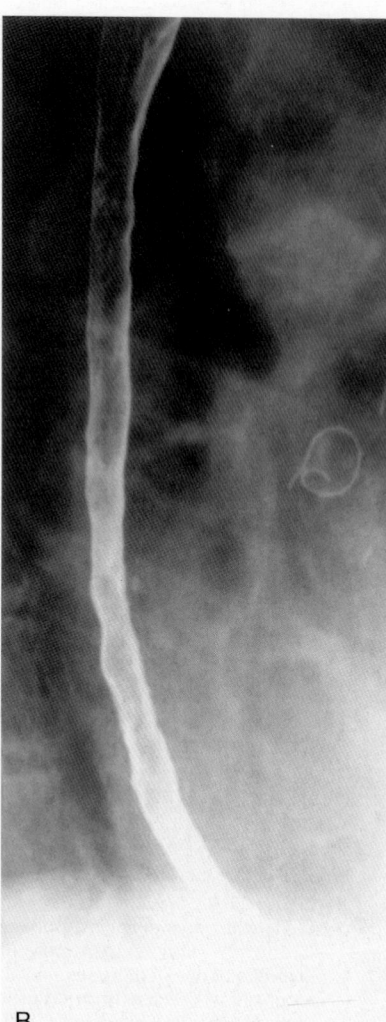

Figure 25-11. Advanced lye strictures. A and B. There is diffuse narrowing of the thoracic esophagus due to extensive scarring and fibrosis in two patients with lye strictures. This appearance should suggest caustic injury because other conditions are rarely associated with such severe esophageal narrowing. (**A** from Levine MS: Radiology of the Esophagus. Philadelphia, WB Saunders, 1989.)

as a chronic form of esophagitis in children and adults.[65-69] The diagnosis is established on pathologic grounds by an increased number of intraepithelial eosinophils (more than 20 per high power field) on endoscopic biopsy specimens from the esophagus.[64,67,68] The etiology is uncertain, but many investigators believe this condition develops as a result of an inflammatory response to ingested food allergens.[67-69] Idiopathic eosinophilic esophagitis tends to involve the muscular layers of the esophageal wall, sometimes resulting in the development of strictures.[70-72]

Clinical Findings

Most adults with idiopathic eosinophilic esophagitis are young men who present with long-standing dysphagia and recurrent food impactions.[67-69] These individuals classically have an atopic history (e.g., asthma, allergic rhinitis) and peripheral eosinophilia, sometimes associated with eosinophilic infiltration of the stomach and small bowel (i.e., eosinophilic gastroenteritis).[72,73] In a number of studies, however, the majority of patients did not have an atopic history, peripheral eosinophilia, or eosinophilic gastroenteritis.[69,74,75] It should therefore be recognized that idiopathic eosinophilic esophagitis

frequently occurs as an isolated condition in the absence of other allergic manifestations or gastrointestinal disease.

Based on the assumption that food allergens act as antigenic stimulation for eosinophilic inflammation of the esophagus, most patients are treated with antiallergy therapy, including oral corticosteroids, topical corticosteroids (e.g., swallowing metered doses of aerosolized corticosteroid preparations), and elemental diets (i.e., protein-free diets) with varying degrees of success.[76-78] Patients with strictures causing intractable dysphagia may undergo endoscopic dilatation procedures, but these individuals often have only transient relief of dysphagia, so multiple dilatations may be required.[69,79]

Radiographic Findings

Idiopathic eosinophilic esophagitis may be manifested on esophagography by the development of one or more segmental strictures in the upper esophagus, midesophagus, or, less commonly, distal esophagus.[70-73] Not infrequently, however, the strictures contain distinctive ringlike indentations, resulting in a so-called ringed esophagus (Fig. 25-13).[75] These ringlike indentations are characterized by multiple, closely spaced, concentric rings traversing the stricture.[75] Although

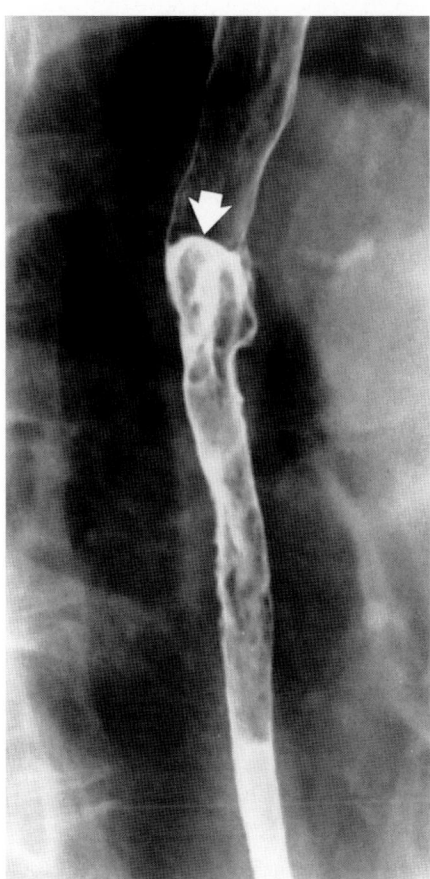

Figure 25-12. Esophageal carcinoma arising in a lye stricture. There is a long stricture in the thoracic esophagus due to caustic ingestion many years earlier. The irregular appearance and abrupt proximal border (*arrow*) of the narrowed segment are due to a superimposed carcinoma.

the pathogenesis is uncertain, such rings have been well documented at endoscopy.[69,80,81]

Other patients with idiopathic eosinophilic esophagitis may have diffuse esophageal narrowing, resulting in a "small-caliber" esophagus.[82] Paradoxically, these long segments of narrowing can be more difficult to recognize on barium studies than shorter segments of narrowing because of their long length, uniform luminal diameter, and smooth contour without obvious demarcations from adjacent normal-caliber esophagus. Despite the frequent subtlety of this finding, idiopathic eosinophilic esophagitis should be suspected when a small-caliber esophagus is detected on barium studies in the proper clinical setting.

Other patients may have abnormal motility, with an increased frequency of nonperistaltic contractions or even an achalasia-like syndrome.[72-83] Rarely, small, sessile eosinophilic polyps may be found in the esophagus.[70,71]

Differential Diagnosis

Upper esophageal or midesophageal strictures in idiopathic eosinophilic esophagitis cannot always be differentiated from high esophageal strictures caused by Barrett's esophagus, mediastinal irradiation, caustic ingestion, and metastatic tumor. The presence of an atopic history or peripheral eosinophilia, however, should suggest the correct diagnosis.

A ringed esophagus (i.e., an esophageal stricture associated with distinctive ringlike indentations) has also been described in patients with congenital esophageal stenosis (see Fig. 29-22). Such patients may have corrugated esophageal strictures with multiple concentric rings indistinguishable from those in idiopathic eosinophilic esophagitis.[84] Although congenital esophageal stenosis is usually not associated with an allergic history or peripheral eosinophilia, this condition also occurs in young men with long-standing dysphagia, and biopsy specimens from the esophagus may also reveal increased numbers of intraepithelial eosinophils.[84,85] Because of the similarities in the clinical, radiographic, and pathologic findings of these conditions, some of the reported patients with congenital esophageal stenosis may have had unrecognized idiopathic eosinophilic esophagitis as the cause of their symptoms.

The differential diagnosis of the ringed esophagus also includes fixed transverse folds in patients with strictures, but these folds generally are incomplete and further apart, producing a characteristic "stepladder" appearance.[86] The feline esophagus could also conceivably be mistaken for the ringed esophagus of idiopathic eosinophilic esophagitis, but these transverse striations occur as a transient phenomenon and are not associated with stricture formation.[87]

CROHN'S DISEASE

The esophagus is the least common site of involvement by Crohn's disease in the gastrointestinal tract. When the esophagus is involved, these patients almost always have associated disease in the small bowel or colon. As a result, esophageal lesions are usually found after a clinical diagnosis of Crohn's disease has been established. Occasionally, however, the onset of esophageal Crohn's disease coincides with the onset of disease in the small bowel or colon, so that these patients do not necessarily have known Crohn's disease when they seek medical attention. Rarely, isolated esophageal Crohn's disease may occur before the development of disease elsewhere in the gastrointestinal tract.[88]

A definitive diagnosis of esophageal Crohn's disease requires histologic confirmation, but endoscopic biopsy specimens often fail to reveal granulomas because of the superficial nature of the biopsies and the patchy distribution of the disease.[89,90] As a result, the absence of definitive histologic findings should not preclude a diagnosis of Crohn's disease if the clinical and radiographic findings suggest this condition.

Clinical Findings

Most patients with esophageal Crohn's disease have advanced Crohn's disease in the lower gastrointestinal tract, so that the clinical presentation is dominated by their ileocolitis. Nevertheless, esophageal Crohn's disease may cause dysphagia or, less commonly, odynophagia, chest pain, or upper gastrointestinal bleeding.[90-92] Because the esophagus is rarely involved by Crohn's disease as an isolated finding, the diagnosis should be considered only in patients with known Crohn's disease elsewhere in the gastrointestinal tract who develop dysphagia or other esophageal symptoms. When esophageal Crohn's disease is present, the clinical course may parallel that of the patient's ileal or colonic disease, with remission of both

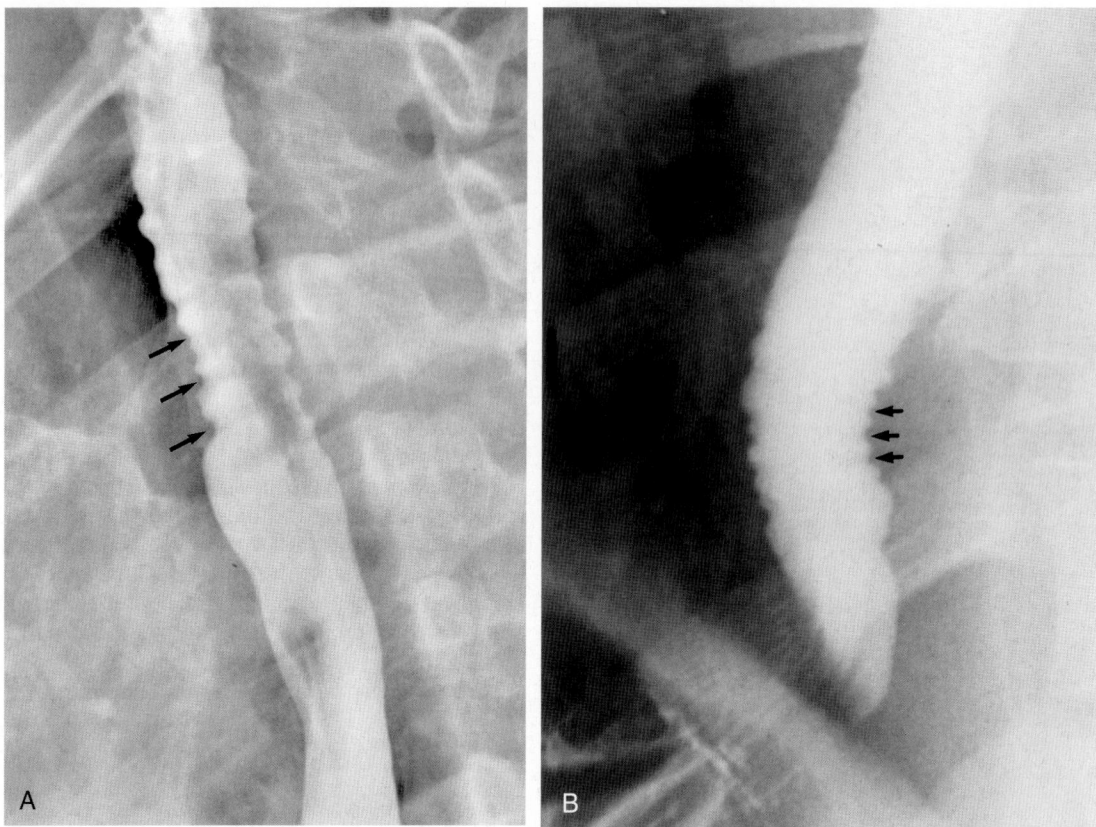

Figure 25-13. Eosinophilic esophagitis with a "ringed" esophagus. A. A moderately long stricture is seen in the upper thoracic esophagus, with multiple distinctive ringlike indentations (*arrows*) in the region of the stricture. **B.** In another patient, a mild stricture is seen in the distal esophagus with multiple ringlike constrictions (*arrows*) in the region of the stricture. Although these rings are characteristic of eosinophilic esophagitis, congenital esophageal stenosis could produce a similar appearance (see Chapter 29). (From Zimmerman SL, Levine MS, Rubesin SE, et al: Idiopathic eosinophilic esophagitis in adults: The ringed esophagus. Radiology 236:159-165, 2005.)

upper and lower gastrointestinal symptoms after medical treatment or ileocolectomy.[91]

Radiographic Findings

Although Crohn's disease primarily affects the small bowel or colon, esophageal involvement has been recognized with increased frequency on double-contrast esophagography. The major advantage of the double-contrast technique is its ability to detect aphthoid ulcers, which are seen on double-contrast examinations in about 3% of patients with granulomatous ileocolitis.[92] As in other portions of the gastrointestinal tract, these aphthoid ulcers appear as punctate, slitlike, or ringlike collections of barium surrounded by radiolucent halos of edematous mucosa (Fig. 25-14).[92-94] They are usually few in number and are sporadically distributed throughout the esophagus with intervening segments of normal mucosa (see Fig. 25-14A).[94] Occasionally, numerous aphthoid ulcers may be present in the esophagus (see Fig. 25-14B).

As the disease progresses, the size and number of ulcers may increase, producing localized or even diffuse esophagitis.[95] More advanced disease may be manifested by thickened folds, pseudomembranes, and, rarely, a "cobblestone" appearance.[91,95] Other patients may develop transverse or longitudinal intramural tracks (Fig. 25-15) or tracheoesophageal, esophagobronchial, esophagomediastinal, or esophagogastric fistulas.[91,95] Progressive scarring may also lead to the devel-

opment of strictures, most commonly in the distal third of the esophagus (Fig. 25-16).[91] Rarely, advanced esophageal Crohn's disease may be manifested by filiform polyposis of the esophagus, analogous to filiform polyposis of the colon in granulomatous colitis.[96]

Differential Diagnosis

The aphthoid ulcers of esophageal Crohn's disease may be indistinguishable from discrete, superficial ulcers associated with reflux, herpes, or drug-induced esophagitis. However, reflux esophagitis predominantly involves the distal esophagus and usually occurs in patients who have a history of reflux symptoms. Although herpetic ulcers may closely resemble aphthoid ulcers,[35] the correct diagnosis should be apparent in an immunocompromised patient with odynophagia. Drug-induced esophagitis may also be manifested by shallow ulcers, but they tend to be clustered in the region of the aortic arch or left main bronchus, and there is usually a recent history of ingesting oral medications such as tetracycline or doxycycline.[31-33] Thus, the clinical history and presentation are extremely helpful for differentiating these conditions.

More advanced esophageal Crohn's disease may be indistinguishable from other types of severe esophagitis. When intramural tracks or fistulas are present, the differential diagnosis includes radiation, trauma, malignant tumor, tuberculosis, and esophageal intramural pseudodiverticulosis.[97-99] Because

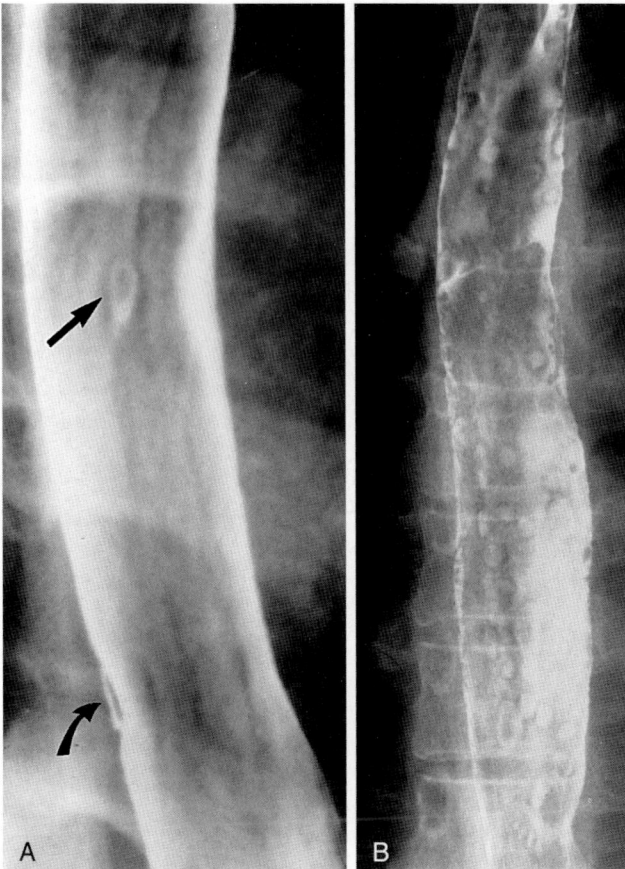

Figure 25-14. Esophageal Crohn's disease with aphthoid ulcers. A. Discrete, widely separated aphthoid ulcers are seen en face (*straight arrow*) and in profile (*curved arrow*) as a result of early esophageal involvement by Crohn's disease. **B.** This patient has more advanced Crohn's disease with multiple large aphthoid ulcers in the midesophagus and distal esophagus. The ulcers are surrounded by radiolucent mounds of edema. (**A** from Gohel V, Long BW, Richter G: Aphthous ulcers in the esophagus with Crohn colitis. AJR 137:872-873, 1981, © by American Roentgen Ray Society; **B** courtesy of Peter J. Feczko, MD, Royal Oak, MI.)

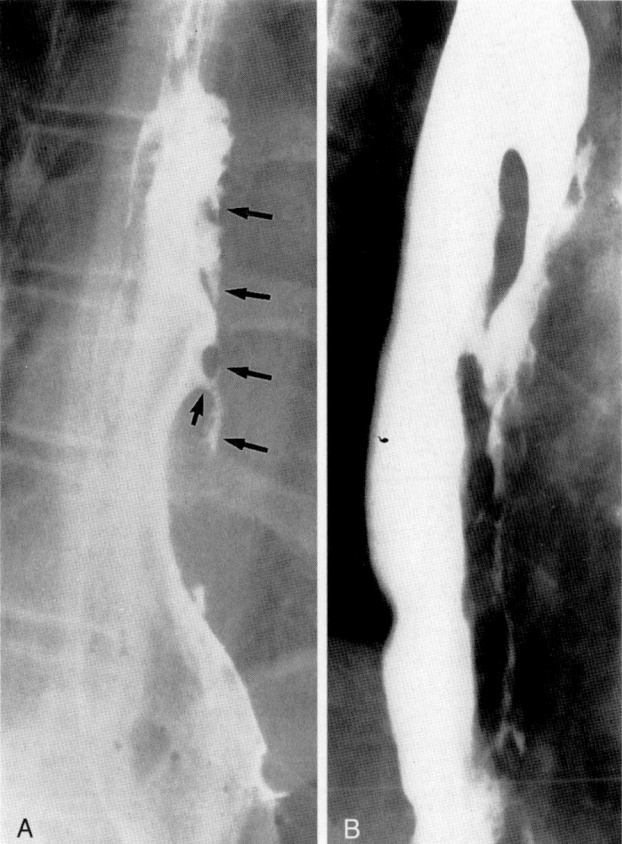

Figure 25-15. Esophageal Crohn's disease with intramural tracks. A. Longitudinal (*long arrows*) and transverse (*short arrow*) tracks are seen in the distal third of the esophagus due to transmural involvement by Crohn's disease. **B.** This patient has a "double-barreled" esophagus with a long intramural track as a result of advanced esophageal Crohn's disease. (**A** courtesy of Peter J. Feczko, MD, Royal Oak, MI; **B** courtesy of Francis J. Scholz, MD, Burlington, MA.)

esophageal Crohn's disease is much less common than other types of esophagitis, this diagnosis should be considered only in patients who have clinical or radiographic findings of Crohn's disease elsewhere in the gastrointestinal tract.

EPIDERMOLYSIS BULLOSA DYSTROPHICA

Epidermolysis bullosa is a rare hereditary skin disease in which minimal trauma causes separation of the epidermis and dermis with subsequent bulla formation. Two forms of the disease, epidermolysis bullosa simplex and epidermolysis bullosa dystrophica, have been described. In epidermolysis bullosa simplex, the bullae heal without scarring and the disease usually subsides at puberty. In contrast, epidermolysis bullosa dystrophica is a mutilating, potentially lethal condition manifested by progressive scarring and deformity throughout the body.[100] Epidermolysis bullosa dystrophica may be transmitted by autosomal dominant and autosomal recessive forms of inheritance. The autosomal dominant form involves only the skin, whereas the autosomal recessive form also involves mucous membranes in other squamous epithelium-lined organs such as the oropharynx, esophagus, and anus.[100]

Pathogenesis

In patients with epidermolysis bullosa dystrophica, solid food in the esophagus repeatedly traumatizes an already fragile mucosa, causing extensive bulla formation.[100,101] Some bullae rupture and heal without permanent sequelae, but others heal with severe scarring and stricture formation. Because these strictures further impede the passage of swallowed food, esophageal involvement may lead to a self-perpetuating cycle of blistering, scarring, and stenosis.[101]

Clinical Findings

Skin involvement by epidermolysis bullosa dystrophica may be recognized at or shortly after birth. Other findings include flexion contractures of the hands and feet, webbed digits (syndactyly), dystrophic or absent nails, microstomia, retarded epiphyseal development, and overconstriction of the shafts of long bones.[102] These deformities can be disabling or even fatal.

Although the esophagus is usually affected during the first decade of life, clinical signs of esophageal involvement may not be seen until puberty.[103] Affected individuals may present with intermittent dysphagia or odynophagia because of

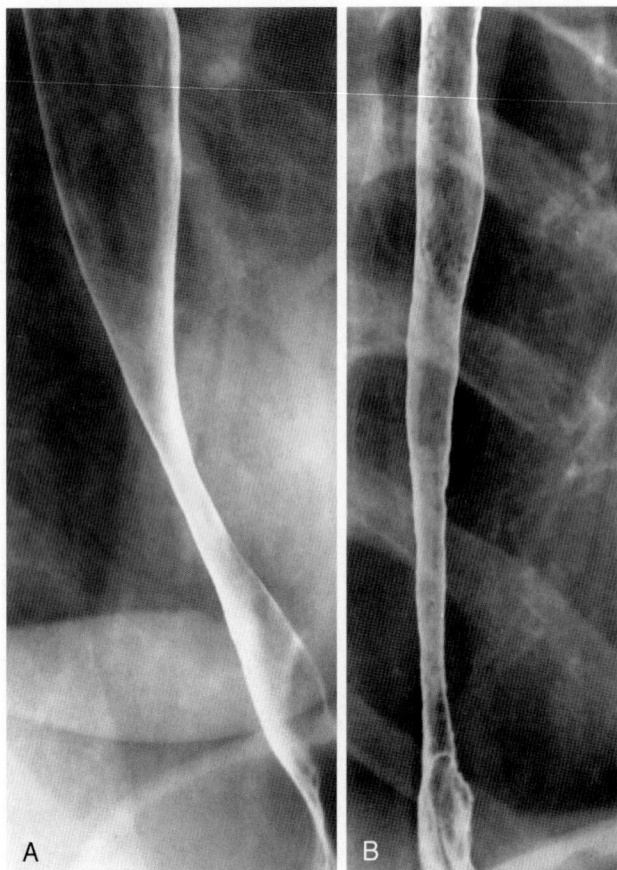

Figure 25-16. Esophageal Crohn's disease with strictures. A and B. Two patients have long strictures in the distal esophagus as a result of severe scarring from Crohn's disease. (**A** from Levine MS: Radiology of the Esophagus. Philadelphia, WB Saunders, 1989; **B** from Tishler JMA, Hellman CA: Crohn's disease of the esophagus. Can Assoc Radiol J 35:28-30, 1984, reprinted by permission of the publisher.)

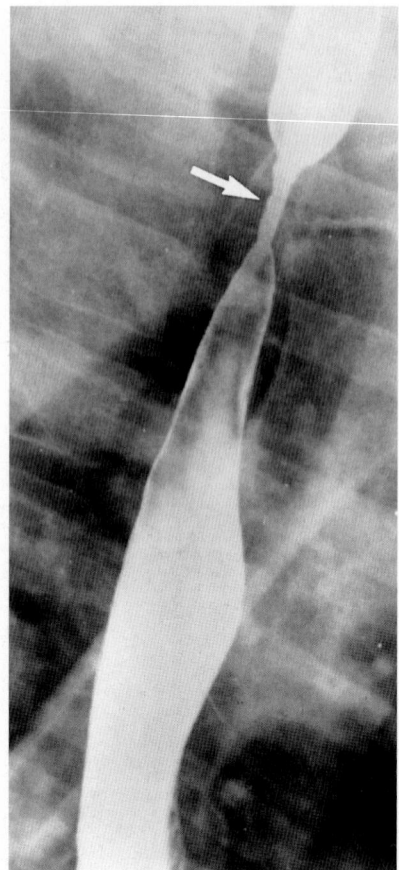

Figure 25-17. Epidermolysis bullosa dystrophica with a high esophageal stricture (*arrow*). (From Tishler JM, Han SY, Hellman CA: Esophageal involvement in epidermolysis bullosa dystrophica. AJR 141:1283-1286, 1983, © by American Roentgen Ray Society.)

recurrent bulla formation and healing.[103,104] Subsequently, they may develop severe dysphagia as a result of irreversible scarring and stricture formation.[101,103,104] Esophageal involvement should therefore be suspected in any patient with epidermolysis bullosa dystrophica who develops dysphagia or other esophageal symptoms.

Endoscopy should be avoided in patients with known or suspected epidermolysis bullosa dystrophica involving the esophagus because of the risk of further traumatizing an already fragile mucosa and causing bleeding, perforation, or further scarring and stenosis. Once strictures have developed, however, balloon dilatation or bougienage of the esophagus or, rarely, surgery may be required to alleviate symptoms.[100,104]

Radiographic Findings

Because of the risks associated with endoscopy, barium studies should be performed when esophageal involvement by epidermolysis bullosa dystrophica is suspected on clinical grounds. Early disease may be manifested on esophagography by abnormal motility, bullae, or ulcers.[103,105] Discrete bullae may be recognized as small, nodular filling defects in the esophagus, whereas extensive bulla formation may produce a diffusely serrated or spiculated esophageal contour.[103] Because of the reversible nature of the disease, these lesions may completely regress on follow-up examinations.

More advanced esophageal disease is characterized by scarring and stricture formation. The strictures tend to be located in the cervical or upper thoracic esophagus, appearing as concentric areas of segmental narrowing (Fig. 25-17).[103,105-107] These strictures may be difficult to differentiate from those caused by Barrett's esophagus, mediastinal irradiation, and caustic ingestion. Other patients with epidermolysis bullosa dystrophica may develop esophageal webs, most frequently in the cervical esophagus near the level of the cricopharyngeus.[103,106] Esophageal involvement by epidermolysis bullosa dystrophica should be suspected when high esophageal strictures or webs are seen on barium studies in children or young adults with other clinical signs of this disease.

PEMPHIGOID

Pemphigoid is a dermatologic disease characterized by chronic, recurrent bullous eruptions of the skin and mucous membranes. Two forms of pemphigoid, benign mucous membrane pemphigoid and bullous pemphigoid, have been described. Benign mucous membrane pemphigoid is much more likely to involve mucous membranes, however, so that esophageal abnormalities are primarily encountered in this form of the disease.

Clinical Findings

Benign mucous membrane pemphigoid usually occurs in middle-aged patients and is twice as common in women.[108] About 75% of patients have involvement of the oral mucosa and conjunctiva, 50% have skin involvement, and 5% to 10% have esophageal involvement.[108-110] The most severe complications of this disease occur in the eye, where conjunctival scarring causes corneal destruction and blindness in 25% of patients.[109] Thus, despite its name, benign mucous membrane pemphigoid should not be considered a benign condition.

Affected individuals usually present with dysphagia caused by edema, spasm, ulceration, or strictures.[108,110] Severe esophageal involvement may occasionally result in massive sloughing of mucosa, with subsequent expulsion of a hollow membranous cast from the patient's mouth.[111] When these patients initially develop dysphagia, systemic administration of corticosteroids may prevent further progression of esophageal disease and stricture formation. Once strictures have developed, however, one or more esophageal dilatation procedures are usually required to alleviate symptoms.[112]

Radiographic Findings

Although discrete bullae are rarely observed, barium studies may reveal superficial ulceration of the mucosa in the early stages of esophageal involvement by benign mucous membrane pemphigoid (Fig. 25-18).[108] Subsequent scarring may be manifested by the development of webs or strictures in the cervical or upper thoracic esophagus (Fig. 25-19) or, less commonly, the midthoracic or lower thoracic esophagus.[108,110,113,114] The strictures may be of variable length and are difficult to distinguish from those caused by Barrett's esophagus, mediastinal irradiation, and caustic ingestion. However, esophageal involvement by benign mucous membrane pemphigoid should be suspected in patients who have a history of bullous eruptions on the skin.

ERYTHEMA MULTIFORME MAJOR

Clinical Findings

Erythema multiforme is a hypersensitivity reaction characterized by a maculopapular or bullous rash that usually develops during the first three decades of life.[115] Erythema multiforme minor is confined to the skin, but erythema multiforme major also involves mucous membranes of the eyes, oropharynx, genitalia, or anus and, rarely, the tracheobronchial tree or esophagus.[115] Stevens-Johnson syndrome is a life-threatening form of esophageal multiforme major with associated constitutional symptoms.[116]

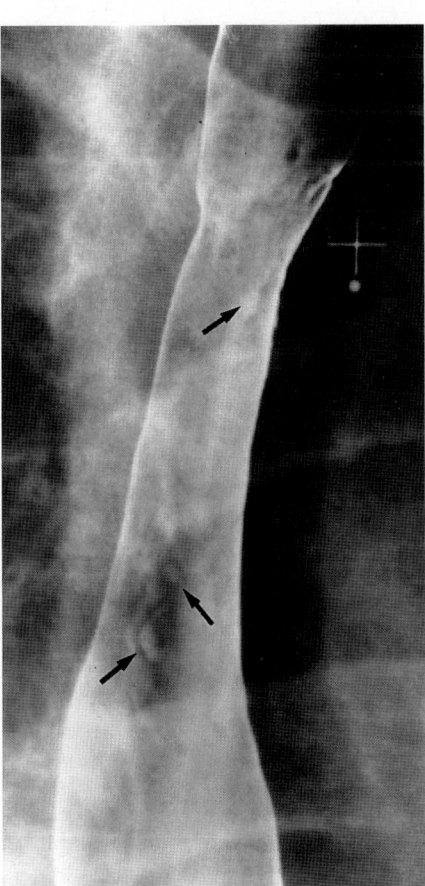

Figure 25-18. Benign mucous membrane pemphigoid with superficial ulceration. Multiple shallow ulcers (*arrows*) are seen in the midesophagus with decreased distensibility of this region. (Courtesy of Stephen E. Rubesin, MD, Philadelphia, PA.)

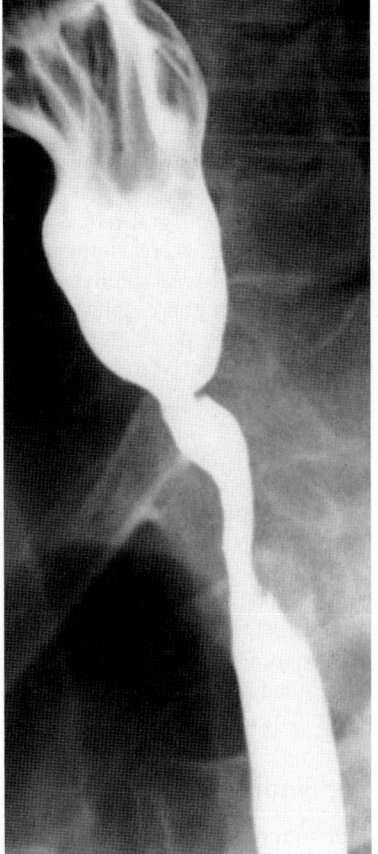

Figure 25-19. Benign mucous membrane pemphigoid with a high esophageal stricture. A long, asymmetrical stricture is seen in the cervical and upper thoracic esophagus. (Courtesy of John A. Bonavita, MD, Philadelphia, PA.)

Radiographic Findings

Esophageal involvement by erythema multiforme major is usually self-limited, but occasionally children or adolescents have been reported with dysphagia caused by esophageal strictures, predominantly in the upper esophagus or midesophagus.[116-118] Rarely, diffuse esophageal narrowing may be found on esophagography in children or adults with this condition.[119] Other more common causes of long esophageal strictures include mediastinal irradiation and caustic ingestion, but esophageal involvement by erythema multiforme major should be suspected in patients with characteristic mucocutaneous lesions. Epidermolysis bullosa dystrophica and benign mucous membrane pemphigoid may also be associated with the development of bullous lesions on the skin and esophageal strictures, but these patients usually have focal strictures or webs in the cervical or upper thoracic esophagus (see previous sections on epidermolysis bullosa dystrophica and pemphigoid).

NASOGASTRIC INTUBATION ESOPHAGITIS

Nasogastric intubation has been recognized as an unusual cause of esophagitis and stricture formation.[120,121] Most patients develop strictures only after repeated or prolonged nasogastric intubation. The strictures may progress rapidly after removal of the tube, causing severe dysphagia. When all causes of esophageal strictures are considered, nasogastric intubation is probably second only to caustic ingestion in terms of the length and severity of stricture formation.

Pathogenesis

The pathogenesis of esophageal injury is uncertain. Most patients who develop strictures have been intubated for 3 to 15 days.[121] Some investigators believe that esophagitis results from uncontrolled gastroesophageal reflux around the lower end of the nasogastric tube, whereas others believe that the tube occludes the lower esophageal sphincter, preventing clearance of refluxed acid from the esophagus after reflux has occurred.[122] It has also been postulated that the trauma of intubation or the irritant effect of the tube itself may cause a direct contact esophagitis.[123]

Clinical Findings

Most patients with esophageal injury develop symptoms several weeks to months after removal of the tube.[120,121] These patients may initially present with heartburn, substernal chest pain, or odynophagia resulting from esophagitis. Subsequently, they may develop severe dysphagia as a result of rapid stricture formation.[121] Despite the length and severity of the strictures, adequate relief from dysphagia may be obtained by periodic mechanical dilatation procedures.

Radiographic Findings

Nasogastric intubation esophagitis may be manifested by a long segment of extensive ulceration in the midesophagus and distal esophagus (Fig. 25-20).[123] Occasionally, large, flat ulcers in the distal esophagus are associated with considerable mass effect because of an adjacent mound of edema, mimick-

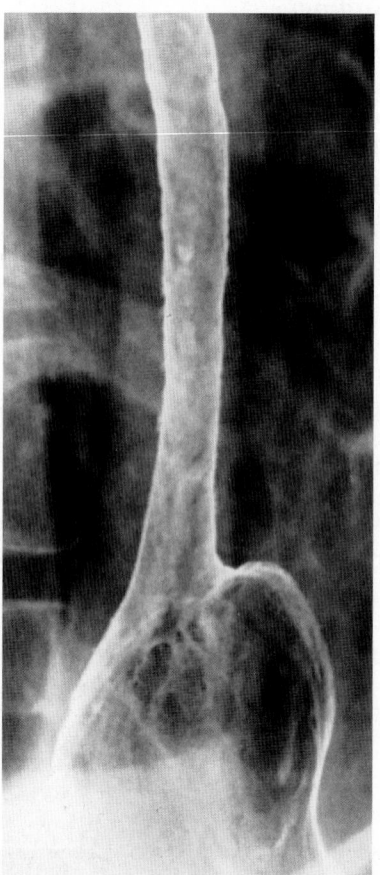

Figure 25-20. Severe esophagitis caused by nasogastric intubation. There are multiple areas of superficial ulceration and associated narrowing of the distal esophagus due to marked edema and spasm. A large hiatal hernia is also present. (From Levine MS: Radiology of the Esophagus. Philadelphia, WB Saunders, 1989.)

ing the appearance of an ulcerated esophageal carcinoma (Fig. 25-21). Subsequent stricture formation may be detected on esophagography 1 to 4 months after removal of the tube.[120,121] Initially, the strictures may appear as smooth, tapered areas of concentric narrowing in the distal esophagus that are indistinguishable from ordinary peptic strictures However, they tend to progress rapidly, increasing in length and severity within a relatively short period (Fig. 25-22). Because of the extent and severity of stricture formation, these patients may be suspected of ingesting caustic agents. The presence of an unusually long or rapidly progressive stricture in the distal esophagus, however, should suggest the possibility of prior nasogastric intubation.

ALKALINE REFLUX ESOPHAGITIS

Alkaline reflux esophagitis is an unusual condition caused by reflux of bile and pancreatic secretions into the esophagus after total or, less commonly, partial gastrectomy.[124] The development of esophagitis in these patients depends on the type of surgical reconstruction that is employed. Alkaline reflux esophagitis is a common complication of total gastrectomy and simple loop esophagojejunostomy but rarely occurs after a Roux-en-Y esophagojejunostomy.[125,126] Most surgeons therefore perform a Roux-en-Y reconstruction, placing the jejunojejunal anastomosis 40 cm or more distal to

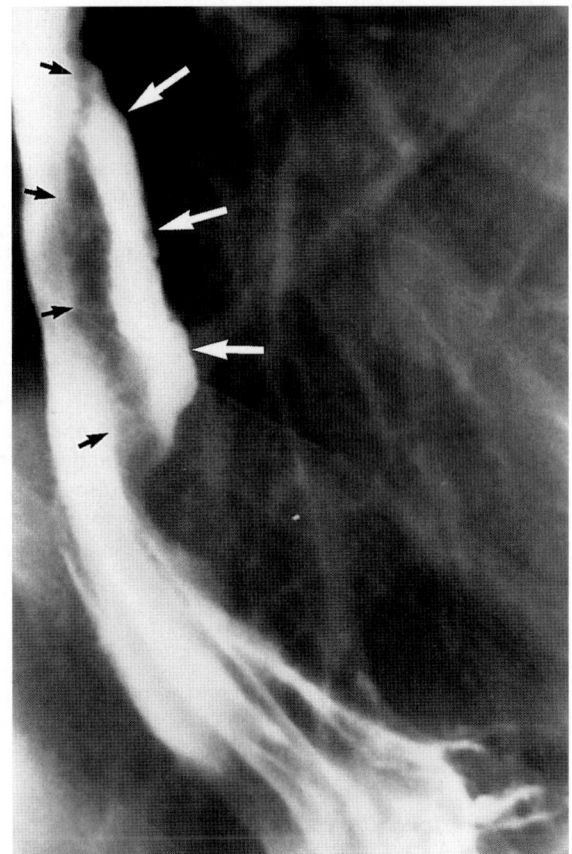

Figure 25-21. Giant esophageal ulcer caused by nasogastric intubation. A large, flat ulcer (*white arrows*) is seen in the distal esophagus; an associated area of mass effect (*black arrows*) is caused by an adjacent mound of edema. This appearance could be mistaken for that of an ulcerated esophageal carcinoma. (From Levine MS: Radiology of the Esophagus. Philadelphia, WB Saunders, 1989.)

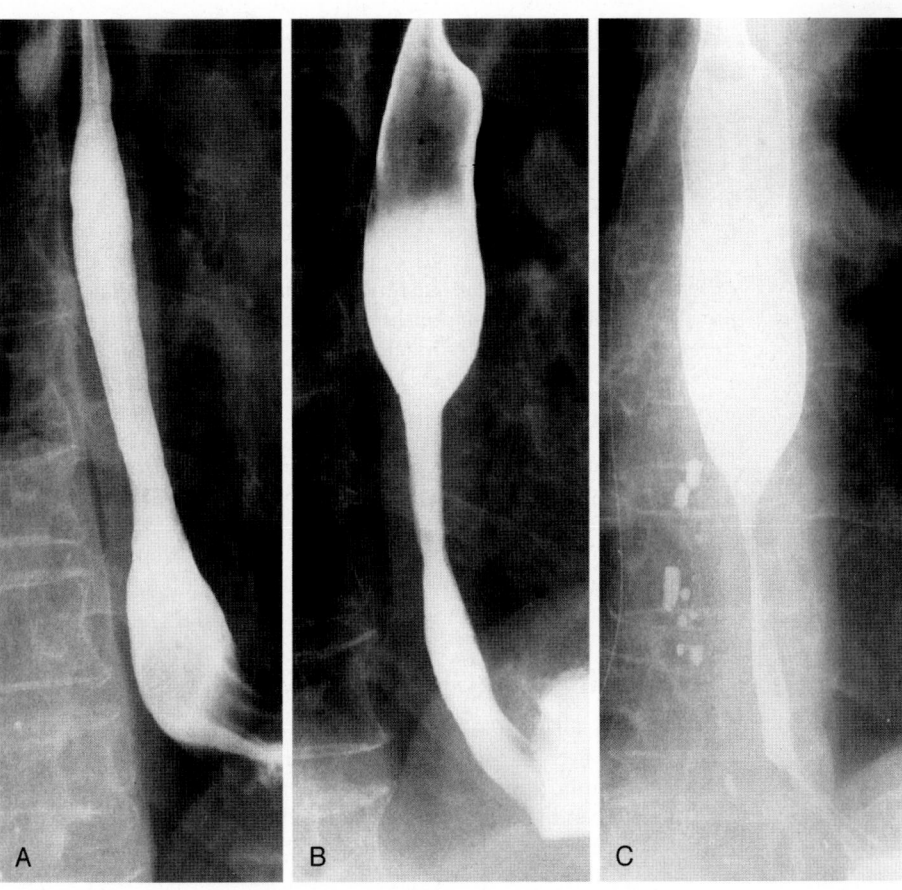

Figure 25-22. Rapidly progressive stricture caused by nasogastric intubation. **A.** Initial esophagogram shows moderately decreased distensibility of the distal esophagus shortly after removal of a nasogastric tube. **B.** Second esophagogram 3 weeks later shows rapid stricture formation with marked narrowing of the distal esophagus. **C.** Third esophagogram 6 weeks later shows further progression of the stricture. There is now evidence of esophageal obstruction. (Courtesy of Vijay Gohel, MD, Philadelphia, PA.)

the esophagojejunal anastomosis to prevent reflux of bile and pancreatic secretions into the esophagus. Nevertheless, alkaline reflux esophagitis has occasionally been documented in these patients, so that a Roux-en-Y reconstruction decreases the risk of esophagitis or strictures but does not completely eliminate these complications.[127] Some investigators have found that alkaline reflux esophagitis also predisposes to the development of Barrett's esophagus,[128,129] but the significance of this observation is doubtful because of the limited life expectancy of most patients who undergo esophagojejunostomy.

Clinical Findings

Alkaline reflux esophagitis may initially be manifested by retrosternal burning, chest pain, and regurgitation of bile.[125] These patients may then develop rapidly progressive dysphagia within several months after surgery because of stricture formation. In most cases, relief from dysphagia is obtained by mechanical dilatation of the stricture.

Radiographic Findings

Alkaline reflux esophagitis is characterized on esophagography by mucosal nodularity, thickened folds, and ulceration of the distal esophagus above the esophagojejunal anastomosis (Fig. 25-23).[130] Subsequent stricture formation may be

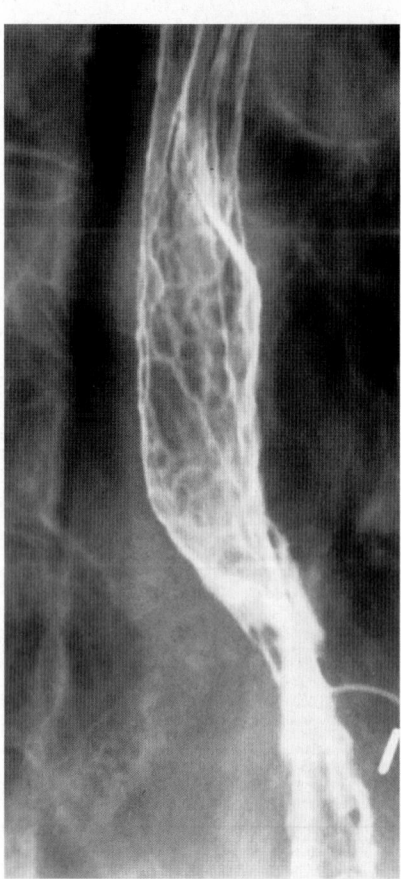

Figure 25-23. Alkaline reflux esophagitis. This patient has undergone a total gastrectomy and esophagojejunostomy. A nodular mucosa is seen in the distal esophagus above the anastomosis. (From Levine MS: Radiology of the Esophagus. Philadelphia, WB Saunders, 1989.)

detected as early as 1 to 3 months after surgery.[130] The strictures usually appear as smooth, tapered areas of narrowing in the distal esophagus, often extending a considerable distance above the anastomosis.[130] These strictures must be differentiated from benign anastomotic strictures or recurrent tumor involving the distal esophagus. However, anastomotic strictures usually appear as focal areas of symmetric narrowing at the esophagojejunal anastomosis, whereas recurrent tumor is manifested by more irregular esophageal narrowing, often associated with eccentric areas of mass effect.[130] Alkaline reflux strictures also tend to progress rapidly, increasing in length and severity within several months.[130] Most patients are intubated at the time of surgery, however, and nasogastric intubation may also lead to rapidly progressive stricture formation. Thus, alkaline reflux and nasogastric intubation may both contribute to the development of strictures in these patients.

ACUTE ALCOHOL-INDUCED ESOPHAGITIS

Alcohol abusers may occasionally develop an acute, transient esophagitis after an alcoholic binge.[131] The cause is uncertain, but heavy alcohol consumption appears to have an effect both on esophageal peristalsis and lower esophageal sphincter function. Several studies have shown that oral or intravenous ethanol in volunteers produces a reversible esophageal motor disturbance with impaired primary peristalsis and decreased lower esophageal sphincter pressures.[132,133] As a result, acute alcohol intoxication may cause increased gastroesophageal reflux with impaired clearance of refluxed peptic acid from the esophagus after reflux has occurred. Thus, alcohol-induced esophagitis may represent a self-limited form of reflux esophagitis.

Clinical Findings

Acute alcohol-induced esophagitis may be associated with abrupt onset of odynophagia, dysphagia, or hematemesis immediately after an alcoholic binge.[131] Marked clinical improvement occurs within 1 to 2 weeks after withdrawal of alcohol.[131] Although other conditions may have a similar presentation, the correct diagnosis is usually suggested by the temporal relationship between an alcoholic binge and the development of esophagitis.

Radiographic Findings

Acute alcohol-induced esophagitis is manifested radiographically by multiple areas of superficial ulceration in the distal third of the esophagus (Fig. 25-24).[131] Reflux esophagitis may produce identical radiographic findings. Nevertheless, the diagnosis should be suggested by the patient's recent drinking history.

CHRONIC GRAFT-VERSUS-HOST DISEASE

Transplantation of bone marrow from matched sibling donors has become an accepted treatment for patients with aplastic anemia, acute leukemia, and other hematologic malignancies. Depending on the underlying disease, these patients have 5-year survival rates of 60% to 80% after marrow transplantation.[134] However, 30% of long-term survivors develop chronic

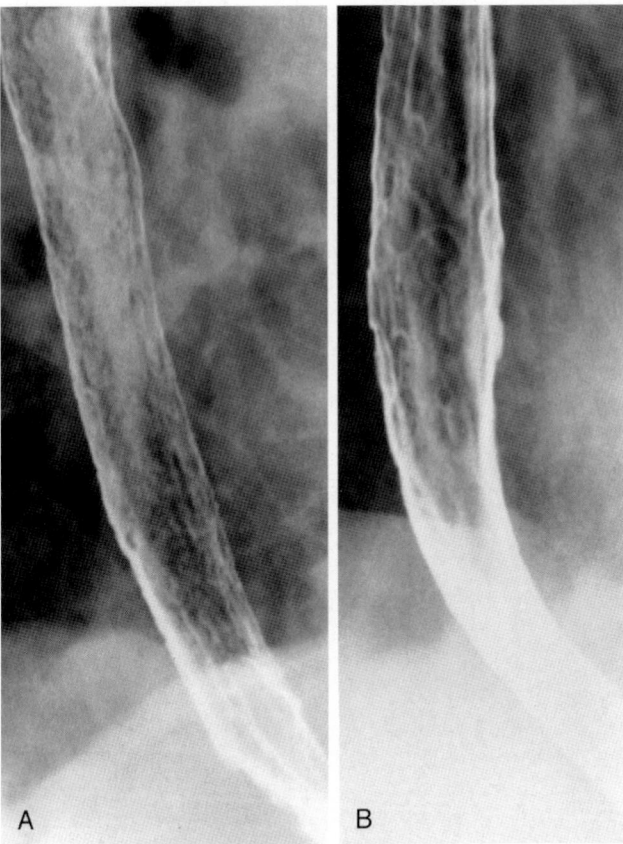

Figure 25-24. Acute alcohol-induced esophagitis. A and **B**. In both patients, multiple small, superficial ulcers are present in the midesophagus and distal esophagus. Reflux esophagitis could produce identical findings, but esophageal symptoms were precipitated by a recent alcoholic binge in both cases. (From O'Riordan D, Levine MS, Laufer I: Acute alcoholic esophagitis. Can Assoc Radiol J 37:54-55, 1986, reprinted by permission of the publisher.)

graft-versus-host disease within 3 to 12 months after undergoing this procedure.[135] The disease is an immunologic disorder in which immunocompetent donor lymphocytes react against antigenic differences in host tissues, causing severe tissue damage. The most frequently involved target organs are the skin and liver, but the eyes, mucous membranes, and gastrointestinal tract may also be affected.[134-136]

Esophageal involvement occurs in about 15% of patients with chronic graft-versus-host disease.[137] The immunologic process causes bulla formation, followed by desquamation and sloughing of esophageal mucosa and subsequent stricture formation.[137-139] The pathologic findings appear to be similar to those of epidermolysis bullosa dystrophica, benign mucous membrane pemphigoid, and other diseases associated with severe scarring and stricture formation in the esophagus.

Clinical Findings

Symptoms of esophageal involvement by chronic graft-versus-host disease include dysphagia, odynophagia, substernal chest pain, and weight loss.[135,137] Esophageal symptoms usually develop 3 to 12 months after marrow transplantation.[137] Infectious esophagitis may produce similar findings in this clinical setting.[140] Esophageal symptoms that occur within 1 to 8 weeks after transplantation are more likely to be caused by oppor-

tunistic infection, whereas symptoms that occur months to years after successful transplantation are more likely to be caused by chronic graft-versus-host disease.[137]

Radiographic Findings

In early esophageal involvement by chronic graft-versus-host disease, the esophagus may have an irregular, serrated contour resulting from mucosal desquamation and sloughing.[137] With the development of scarring, barium studies may demonstrate webs or strictures in the esophagus. Webs are usually found in the cervical esophagus near the level of the cricopharyngeus (Fig. 25-25A).[137] These lesions cannot be differentiated from idiopathic webs or those associated with other conditions, such as epidermolysis bullosa dystrophica and benign mucous membrane pemphigoid. Other patients may develop ringlike or smoothly tapered strictures in the upper esophagus, midesophagus, or, less commonly, distal esophagus (Fig. 25-25B).[135,137] The correct diagnosis should be suggested in patients who are known to have undergone marrow transplants.

GLUTARALDEHYDE-INDUCED ESOPHAGEAL INJURY

Glutaraldehyde is the agent most commonly used to disinfect endoscopic equipment. Outbreaks of hemorrhagic colitis in patients who underwent colonoscopy have been attributed to inadequate cleaning and rinsing of the endoscopic equipment with subsequent exposure of the colonic mucosa to residual glutaraldehyde.[141] A study on laboratory rats showed that glutaraldehyde also has a toxic effect on the esophagus, causing inflammation and segmental vasculitis.[142] Rarely,

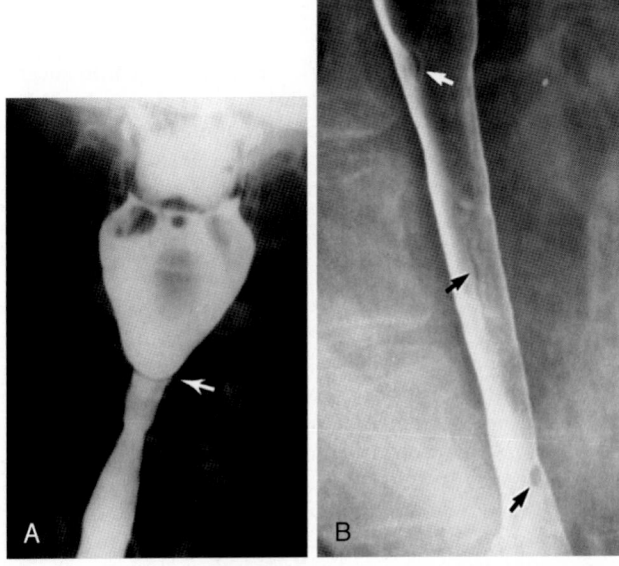

Figure 25-25. Chronic graft-versus-host disease with esophageal involvement. A. A web is seen en face (*arrow*) in the cervical esophagus. **B.** A long, tapered stricture is present in the distal esophagus in another patient. Nodular and linear filling defects (*arrows*) within the narrowed segment are due to mucosal desquamation and sloughing. (**A** from McDonald GB, Sullivan KM, Plumley TF: Radiographic features of esophageal involvement in chronic graft-vs.-host disease. AJR 142:501-506, 1984, © by American Roentgen Ray Society; **B** courtesy of Seth N. Glick, MD, Philadelphia, PA.)

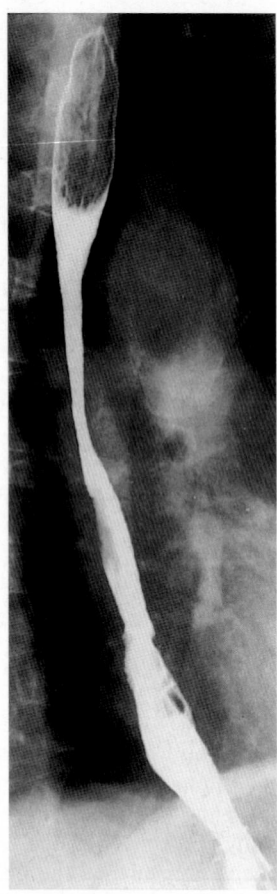

Figure 25-26. Glutaraldehyde-induced esophageal stricture. A long, tapered stricture is seen in the thoracic esophagus. This stricture developed 1 month after endoscopy, presumably because of exposure to residual glutaraldehyde on the endoscopic equipment. Scarring from caustic ingestion could produce identical radiographic findings.

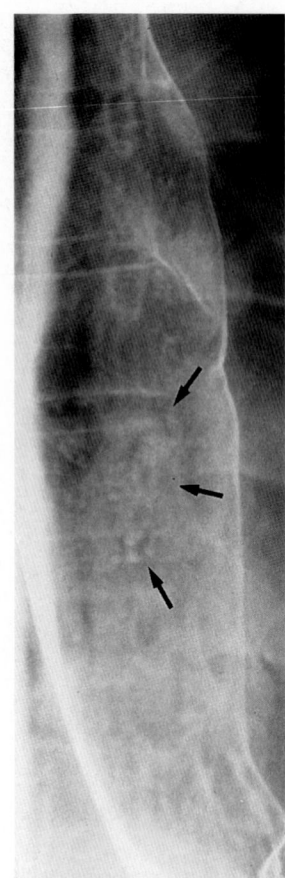

Figure 25-27. Behçet's disease with superficial ulceration. A cluster of tiny ulcers (*arrows*) is present in the midesophagus. Herpes esophagitis and drug-induced esophagitis are much more common causes of discrete ulcers in the midesophagus. (From Levine MS: Radiology of the Esophagus. Philadelphia, WB Saunders, 1989.)

esophageal strictures may develop in humans within several weeks of endoscopy, presumably because of exposure to glutaraldehyde-contaminated endoscopic equipment (Fig. 25-26).[142] Exposure to glutaraldehyde should therefore be considered as a possible cause of esophagitis and rapidly progressive esophageal strictures in these patients.

BEHÇET'S DISEASE

Behçet's disease was first described by Behçet in 1937 as the clinical triad of oral and genital ulceration and ocular inflammation. Behçet's disease is now recognized as a multisystem disorder characterized by a nonspecific vasculitis with resulting skin lesions, arthritis, colitis, thrombophlebitis, and, rarely, encephalitis.[143,144] In the gastrointestinal tract, Behçet's disease usually involves the colon, producing a localized or diffuse form of colitis in about 20% of patients.[143] Esophageal involvement has occasionally been reported.[144-149] Affected individuals may present with substernal chest pain, dysphagia, and, occasionally, hematemesis.[144,145] Double-contrast esophagography may reveal discrete, superficial ulcers in the midesophagus (Fig. 25-27), widespread esophagitis, or strictures.[144] Rarely, a single giant ulcer may be observed.[146] Because Behçet's disease is often treated with corticosteroids or other immunosuppressive agents, herpes esophagitis should be

suspected as a more likely cause of esophageal ulcers in these patients. Endoscopic brushings, biopsy specimens, and cultures are therefore required to differentiate this condition from viral esophagitis.

ESOPHAGEAL INTRAMURAL PSEUDODIVERTICULOSIS

When esophageal intramural pseudodiverticulosis was first described in 1960, it was thought that mucosal herniation through defects in the esophageal wall produced true intramural diverticula, analogous to Rokitansky-Aschoff sinuses in the gallbladder.[150] Since that time, however, the pathologic basis for these structures has been well elucidated. Although esophageal intramural pseudodiverticulosis is a relatively uncommon condition, it has received considerable attention in the radiologic literature because of its often spectacular appearance on barium studies.

Pathogenesis

The esophagus normally contains about 200 deep mucous glands that occur in longitudinal rows parallel to the long axis of the esophagus.[151] Within each gland, several short ducts converge to form a single main excretory duct that extends

2 to 5 mm through the esophageal wall, producing a small opening on the mucosa.[152] Pathologic studies have shown that esophageal intramural pseudodiverticula represent dilated excretory ducts of these deep mucous glands.[153-155]

Although the anatomic basis of these structures has been well delineated, the explanation for this ductal dilatation is unclear. One infectious organism, *Candida albicans*, has been cultured from the esophagus in 34% to 50% of patients.[151,156-158] It has therefore been postulated that *Candida* esophagitis predisposes to the development of esophageal intramural pseudodiverticulosis.[159] However, most investigators believe that the fungal organisms are secondary esophageal invaders and are not important causative factors in the development of this condition.[154,160-162]

Others have postulated that ductal dilatation results from plugging and obstruction of the ducts by thick, viscous mucus, inflammatory material, and desquamated epithelium.[152-154] In various series, 80% to 90% of patients with pseudodiverticulosis have had endoscopic or histologic evidence of inflammatory disease in the esophagus.[151,157] In one study, the majority of patients with this condition had associated scarring or strictures in the distal esophagus as a result of reflux esophagitis.[163] Thus, esophageal intramural pseudodiverticulosis is probably a sequela of chronic esophagitis, particularly reflux esophagitis, but it is unclear why so few patients with esophagitis develop this condition.

About 90% of patients with esophageal intramural pseudodiverticulosis have associated strictures.[151,156,157] It has therefore been suggested that increased intraluminal pressure or stasis above the stricture may cause ductal dilatation.[152] This theory is weakened, however, by the observation that the pseudodiverticula are often found below the level of the stricture.[151] Conversely, stricture formation could be caused by the development of microabscesses in the ducts, resulting in perforation, peridiverticulitis, and scarring.[162,164] This hypothesis would explain why there is often no other apparent cause for the development of esophageal strictures in these patients.

Clinical Findings

Esophageal intramural pseudodiverticulosis usually occurs in the elderly and is slightly more common in men.[151,156-158] About 20% of patients are diabetics, and 15% are alcoholics.[143,144] Most patients present with intermittent or slowly progressive dysphagia resulting from the high prevalence of associated strictures.[151,153,156,157,161,162] Treatment is usually directed toward the underlying stricture because the pseudodiverticula themselves rarely cause problems. Mechanical dilatation of strictures produces a dramatic clinical response in almost all patients.[162,164] The intramural pseudodiverticula may persist or disappear after treatment, but the fate of these structures has no relationship to the clinical course of the patient.

Radiographic Findings

Esophageal intramural pseudodiverticulosis is diagnosed in fewer than 1% of all patients who undergo radiologic examinations of the esophagus.[163] Failure to visualize the pseudodiverticula may result from ductal obstruction by inflammatory material or debris that prevents barium from entering the

ducts. Nevertheless, esophagography is more sensitive than endoscopy for detecting these lesions because the orifices of the dilated excretory ducts are extremely difficult to visualize at endoscopy.[156]

Esophageal intramural pseudodiverticulosis is classically manifested by innumerable, tiny (1- to 4-mm), flask-shaped outpouchings in longitudinal rows parallel to the long axis of the esophagus (Fig. 25-28).[151,153,156,157,160,164] Because the necks of the pseudodiverticula are 1 mm or less in diameter, incomplete filling may erroneously suggest lack of communication with the esophageal lumen.[163] The pseudodiverticula may occasionally be recognized on CT by marked thickening of the esophageal wall, diffuse irregularity of the lumen, and intramural gas collections corresponding to the pseudodiverticula.[165]

Bridging may sometimes occur between adjacent pseudodiverticula, resulting in discrete intramural tracks (Fig. 25-29).[156,157,160] In one study, intramural tracking was detected on esophagography in 50% of patients with esophageal intramural pseudodiverticulosis.[99] These tracks may vary from short, thin connections between two or more adjoining pseudodiverticula to long intramural collections of barium that parallel the lumen.[99] Occasionally, these long tracks can be mistaken for large ulcers or even extraluminal collections associated with an intramural esophageal dissection or perforation.[99]

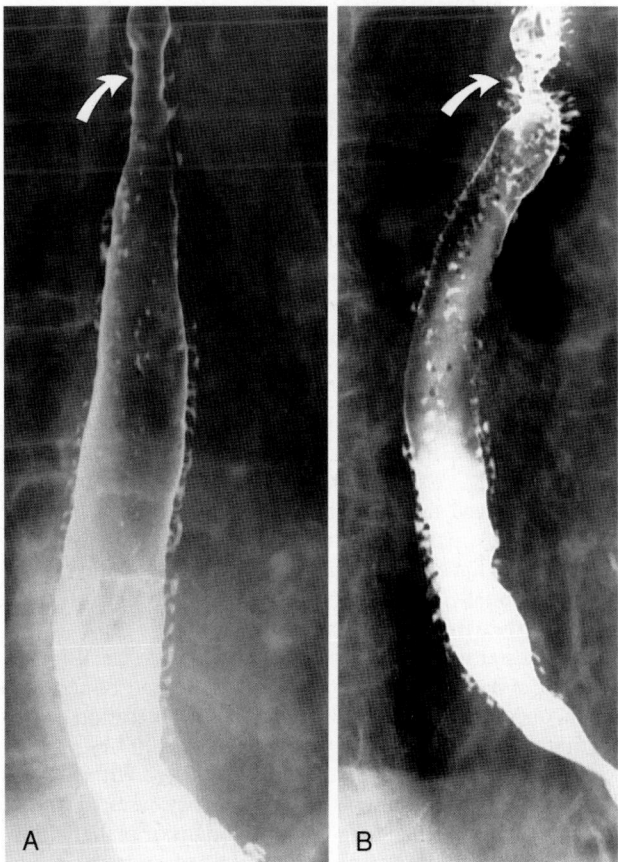

Figure 25-28. Esophageal intramural pseudodiverticulosis with high strictures. A and **B.** In both cases the pseudodiverticula appear as characteristic outpouchings in longitudinal rows parallel to the long axis of the esophagus. Associated strictures (*arrows*) are seen in the upper thoracic esophagus. (**B** from Levine MS: Radiology of the Esophagus. Philadelphia, WB Saunders, 1989.)

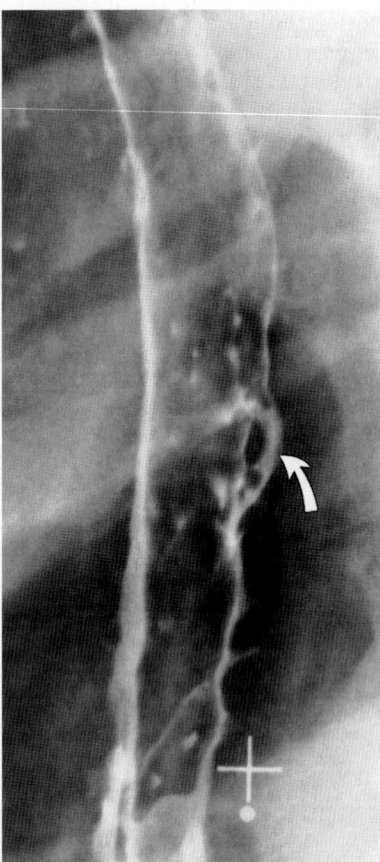

Figure 25-29. Esophageal intramural pseudodiverticulosis with an intramural track. This track (*arrow*) is caused by bridging of adjacent pseudodiverticula. Other pseudodiverticula seen en face could be mistaken for shallow ulcers. (Courtesy of Stephen E. Rubesin, MD, Philadelphia, PA.)

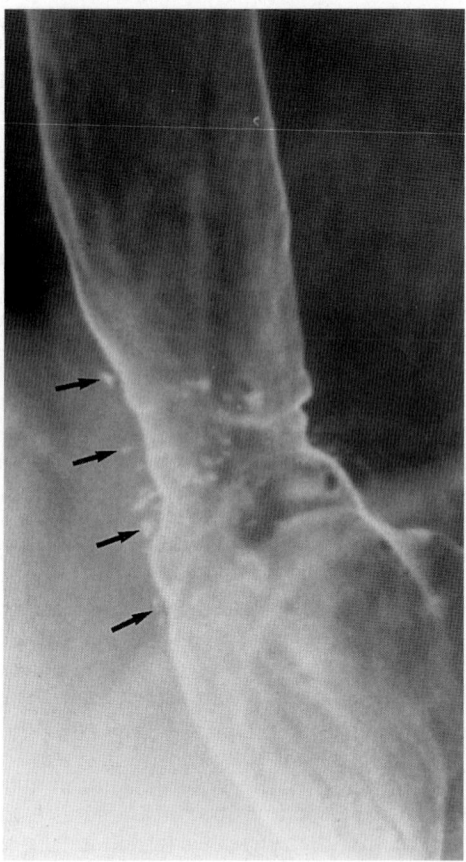

Figure 25-30. Esophageal intramural pseudodiverticulosis with a peptic stricture. When viewed en face, the pseudodiverticula could be mistaken for tiny ulcers. When viewed in profile, however, the pseudodiverticula (*arrows*) do not appear to communicate with the esophageal lumen. This characteristic feature helps differentiate these structures from ulcers. There also is narrowing and deformity of the distal esophagus due to an associated peptic stricture. (From Levine MS: Radiology of the Esophagus. Philadelphia, WB Saunders, 1989.)

Half the reported patients with esophageal intramural pseudodiverticulosis have diffuse disease, and half have segmental disease.[151,156,157] About 90% of patients have associated strictures, most frequently in the distal esophagus, with a focal cluster of pseudodiverticula in the region of a peptic stricture (Fig. 25-30).[163] Other patients may have segmental strictures in the upper or middle third of the esophagus (see Fig. 25-28).[151,156,157] In such cases, the pseudodiverticula often extend well above and below the level of the stricture.[156] Although most patients with esophageal intramural pseudodiverticulosis have esophagitis or strictures, pseudodiverticula may occasionally be observed in patients with an otherwise normal-appearing esophagus.[163]

Esophageal intramural pseudodiverticulosis has also been reported in patients with esophageal carcinoma.[166] Such cases could conceivably result from malignant degeneration of pre-existing peptic strictures in patients with Barrett's esophagus. Whatever the explanation, strictures associated with pseudodiverticulosis are not always benign, so that cases should be evaluated individually for radiographic signs of malignancy.

Rarely, perforation of an esophageal intramural pseudodiverticulum may result in diverticulitis with the development of a periesophageal inflammatory mass or abscess in the mediastinum.[167,168] Affected individuals may present with chest pain, fever, leukocytosis, or other signs of mediastinitis.[168] In such cases, esophagography may reveal localized extra-

vasation of contrast material into the mediastinum from the perforated pseudodiverticulum (Fig. 25-31).[168] CT may also reveal a periesophageal inflammatory mass with or without associated collections of gas.[167] In previously reported cases, the perforations have sealed off with parenteral nutrition and intravenous antibiotics.[167,168] Thus, esophageal perforation caused by ruptured pseudodiverticula may be more likely than other types of esophageal perforations to heal with conservative medical treatment.

Differential Diagnosis

The radiographic findings of esophageal intramural pseudodiverticulosis are virtually pathognomonic of this condition. Although pseudodiverticula can occasionally be confused with true diverticula, the latter structures are considerably larger and less numerous and should not pose a major diagnostic dilemma. When viewed en face, intramural pseudodiverticula are sometimes mistaken for tiny ulcers associated with various types of esophagitis. When viewed in profile, however, intramural pseudodiverticula have a typical flask-shaped configuration and often seem to be floating outside the esophageal wall without any apparent communication with the lumen, whereas true ulcers almost always communicate directly with

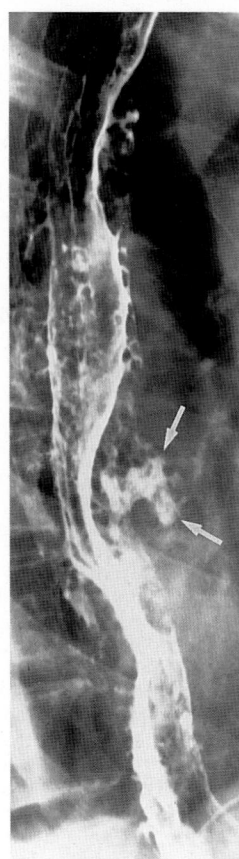

Figure 25-31. Esophageal intramural pseudodiverticulosis with associated diverticulitis. There is a large, irregular, extraluminal barium collection (*arrows*), presumably caused by a sealed-off perforation of a pseudodiverticulum. (Courtesy of Peter J. Feczko, MD, Royal Oak, MI.)

the lumen. The characteristic tangential appearance of the pseudodiverticula should therefore differentiate these structures from actual areas of ulceration.

References

1. Pemberton J: Oesophageal obstruction and ulceration caused by oral potassium therapy. Br Heart J 32:267-268, 1970.
2. Kikendall JW, Friedman AC, Oyewole MA, et al: Pill-induced esophageal injury: Case reports and review of the medical literature. Dig Dis Sci 28:174-182, 1983.
3. Evans KT, Roberts GM: Where do all the tablets go? Lancet 2:1237-1239, 1976.
4. Levine MS: Drug-induced disorders of the esophagus. Abdom Imaging 24:3-8, 1999.
5. Whitney B, Croxon R: Dysphagia caused by cardiac enlargement. Clin Radiol 23:147-152, 1972.
6. Mason SJ, O'Meara TF: Drug-induced esophagitis. J Clin Gastroenterol 3:115-120, 1981.
7. Walta DC, Giddens JD, Johnson LF, et al: Localized proximal esophagitis secondary to ascorbic acid ingestion and esophageal motor disorder. Gastroenterology 70:766-769, 1976.
8. Bokey L, Hugh TB: Oesophageal ulceration associated with doxycycline therapy. Med J Aust 1:236-237, 1975.
9. Crowson TD, Head LH, Ferrante WA: Esophageal ulcers associated with tetracycline therapy. JAMA 235:2747-2748, 1976.
10. Rosenthal T, Adar R, Militianu J, et al: Esophageal ulceration and oral potassium chloride ingestion. Chest 65:463-465, 1974.
11. Lubbe WF, Cadogan ES, Kannemeyer AHR: Oesophageal ulceration due to slow-release potassium in the presence of left atrial enlargement. N Z Med J 90:377-379, 1979.
12. Peters JL: Benign oesophageal stricture following oral potassium chloride therapy. Br J Surg 63:698-699, 1976.
13. Teplick JG, Teplick SK, Ominsky SH, et al: Esophagitis caused by oral medication. Radiology 134:23-25, 1980.
14. Heller SR, Fellows IW, Ogilvie AL, et al: Non-steroidal anti-inflammatory drugs and benign oesophageal stricture. BMJ 285:167-168, 1982.
15. Coates AG, Nostrand TT, Wilson JAP, et al: Esophagitis caused by non-steroidal antiinflammatory medication. South Med J 79:1094-1097, 1986.
16. Semble EL, Wu WC, Castell DO: Nonsteroidal antiinflammatory drugs and esophageal injury. Semin Arthritis Rheum 19:99-109, 1989.
17. Levine MS, Rothstein RD, Laufer I: Giant esophageal ulcer due to Clinoril. AJR 156:955-956, 1991.
18. Levine MS, Borislow SM, Rubesin SE, et al: Esophageal stricture caused by a Motrin tablet (ibuprofen). Abdom Imaging 19:6-7, 1994.
19. Sugawa C, Takekuma Y, Lucas CE, et al: Bleeding esophageal ulcers caused by NSAIDs. Surg Endosc 11:143-146, 1997.
20. de Groen PC, Lubbe DF, Hirsch LJ, et al: Esophagitis associated with the use of alendronate. N Engl J Med 335:1016-1021, 1996.
21. Colina RE, Smith M, Kikendall JW, et al: A new probable increasing cause of esophageal ulceration: Alendronate. Am J Gastroenterol 92:704-706, 1997.
22. Ryan JM, Kelsey P, Ryan BM, et al: Alendronate-induced esophagitis: Case report of a recently recognized form of severe esophagitis with esophageal stricture—radiographic features. AJR 206:389-391, 1998.
23. Lanza FL, Hunt RH, Thomson ABR, et al: Endoscopic comparison of esophageal and gastroduodenal effects of risedronate and alendronate in postmenopausal women. Gastroenterology 119:631-638, 2000.
24. Kavin H: Oesophageal ulceration due to emepronium bromide. Lancet 1:424-425, 1977.
25. Abbarah TR, Fredell JE, Ellenz GB: Ulceration by oral ferrous sulfate. JAMA 236:2320, 1976.
26. Stiris MG, Oyen D: Oesophagitis caused by oral ingestion of Aptin (alprenolol chloride) durettes. Eur J Radiol 2:38-40, 1982.
27. Enzenauer RW, Bass JW, McDonnell JT: Esophageal ulceration associated with oral theophylline. N Engl J Med 310:261, 1984.
28. Israel RH, Wood J: Esophagitis related to cromolyn. JAMA 242:2758-2759, 1979.
29. Sutton DR, Gosnold JK: Oesophageal ulceration due to clindamycin. BMJ 1:1598, 1977.
30. Bonavina L, DeMeester TR, McChesney L, et al: Drug-induced esophageal strictures. Ann Surg 206:173-183, 1987.
31. Creteur V, Laufer I, Kressel HY, et al: Drug-induced esophagitis detected by double contrast radiography. Radiology 147:365-368, 1983.
32. Agha FP, Wilson JAP, Nostrand TT: Medication-induced esophagitis. Gastrointest Radiol 11:7-11, 1986.
33. Bova JG, Dutton NE, Goldstein HM, et al: Medication-induced esophagitis: Diagnosis by double-contrast esophagography. AJR 148:731-732, 1987.
34. Ravich WJ, Kashima H, Donner MW: Drug-induced esophagitis simulating esophageal carcinoma. Dysphagia 1:13-18, 1986.
35. Levine MS, Laufer I, Kressel HY, et al: Herpes esophagitis. AJR 136:863-866, 1981.
36. Shortsleeve MJ, Levine MS: Herpes esophagitis in otherwise healthy patients: Clinical and radiographic findings. Radiology 182:859-861, 1992.
37. Kressel HY, Glick SN, Laufer I, et al: Radiologic features of esophagitis. Gastrointest Radiol 6:103-108, 1981.
38. Levine MS, Loercher G, Katzka DA, et al: Giant, human immunodeficiency virus–related ulcers in the esophagus. Radiology 180:323-326, 1991.
39. Goldstein HM, Rogers LF, Fletcher GH, et al: Radiological manifestations of radiation-induced injury to the normal upper gastrointestinal tract. Radiology 117:135-140, 1975.
40. Phillips TL, Ross G: Time-dose relationships in the mouse esophagus. Radiology 113:435-440, 1974.
41. Northway MG, Libshitz HI, West JJ, et al: The opossum as an animal model for studying radiation esophagitis. Radiology 131:731-735, 1979.
42. Lepke RA, Libshitz HI: Radiation-induced injury of the esophagus. Radiology 148:375-378, 1983.
43. Roswit B: Complications of radiation therapy: The alimentary tract. Semin Roentgenol 9:51-63, 1974.
44. Rubin P: The radiographic expression of radiotherapeutic injury: An overview. Semin Roentgenol 9:5-13, 1974.

45. Collazzo LA, Levine MS, Rubesin SE, et al: Acute radiation esophagitis: Radiographic findings. AJR 169:1067-1070, 1997.

46. DuBrow RA: Radiation changes in hollow viscera. Semin Roentgenol 28:344-362, 1994.

47. Dodds WJ, Stewart ET, Vlymen WJ: Appropriate contrast media for evaluation of esophageal disruption. Radiology 144:439-441, 1982.

48. Karasick S, Lev-Toaff AS: Esophageal strictures: Findings on barium radiographs. AJR 165:561-565, 1995.

49. Leape LL, Ashcraft KW, Scarpelli DG, et al: Hazard to health: Liquid lye. N Engl J Med 284:587-591, 1971.

50. Kirsh MM, Ritter F: Caustic ingestion and subsequent damage to the oropharyngeal and digestive passages. Ann Thorac Surg 21:74-82, 1976.

51. Goldman LP, Weigert JM: Corrosive substance ingestion: A review. Am J Gastroenterol 79:85-90, 1984.

52. Muhletaler CA, Gerlock AJ, de Soto L, et al: Acid corrosive esophagitis: Radiographic findings. AJR 134:1137-1140, 1980.

53. Citron BP, Pincus IJ, Geokas MC, et al: Chemical trauma of the esophagus and stomach. Surg Clin North Am 48:1303-1311, 1968.

54. Webb WR, Koutras P, Ecker RR: An evaluation of steroids and antibiotics in caustic burns of the esophagus. Ann Thorac Surg 9:95-102, 1970.

55. Cardona JC, Daly JF: Current management of corrosive esophagitis: An evaluation of results in 239 cases. Ann Otol 80:521-527, 1971.

56. Neimark S, Rogers AI: Chemical injury of the esophagus. In Berk JA (ed): Bockus Gastroenterology, 4th ed. Philadelphia, WB Saunders, 1985, pp 769-776.

57. Appelqvist P, Salmo M: Lye corrosion carcinoma of the esophagus: A review of 63 cases. Cancer 45:2655-2685, 1980.

58. Hopkins RA, Postlethwait RW: Caustic burns and carcinoma of the esophagus. Ann Surg 194:146-148, 1981.

59. Martel W: Radiologic features of esophagogastritis secondary to extremely caustic agents. Radiology 103:31-36, 1972.

60. Franken EA: Caustic damage of the gastrointestinal tract: Roentgen features. AJR 118:77-85, 1973.

61. Guelrud M, Arocha M: Motor function abnormalities in acute caustic esophagitis. J Clin Gastroenterol 2:247-250, 1980.

62. Dantas RO, Mamede RCM: Esophageal motility in patients with esophageal caustic injury. Am J Gastroenterol 91:1157-1161, 1996.

63. Moody FG, Garrett JM: Esophageal achalasia following lye ingestion. Ann Surg 170:775-784, 1969.

64. Attwood SE, Smyrk TC, DeMeester TR, et al: Esophageal eosinophilia with dysphagia: A distinct clinicopathologic syndrome. Dig Dis Sci 38:109-116, 1993.

65. Walsh SV, Antonioli DA, Goldman H, et al: Allergic esophagitis in children: A clinicopathological entity. Am J Surg Pathol 23:390-396, 1999.

66. Orenstein SR, Shalaby TM, Di Lorenzo C, et al: The spectrum of pediatric eosinophilic esophagitis beyond infancy: A clinical series of 30 children. Am J Gastroenterol 95:1422-1430, 2000.

67. Fox VL, Nurko S, Furuta GT: Eosinophilic esophagitis: It's not just kid's stuff. Gastrointest Endosc 56:260-270, 2002.

68. Markowitz JE, Liacouras CA: Eosinophilic esophagitis. Gastroenterol Clin North Am 32:949-966, 2003.

69. Croese J, Fairley SK, Masson JW, et al: Clinical and endoscopic features of eosinophilic esophagitis in adults. Gastrointest Endosc 58:516-522, 2003.

70. Picus D, Frank PH: Eosinophilic esophagitis. AJR 136:1001-1003, 1981.

71. Feczko PJ, Halpert RD, Zonca M: Radiographic abnormalities in eosinophilic esophagitis. Gastrointest Radiol 10:321-324, 1985.

72. Vitellas KM, Bennett WF, Bova JG, et al: Idiopathic eosinophilic esophagitis. Radiology 186:789-793, 1993.

73. Matzinger MA, Daneman A: Esophageal involvement in eosinophilic gastroenteritis. Pediatr Radiol 13:35-38, 1983.

74. Munitiz V, Martinez de Haro LF, Ortiz A, et al: Primary eosinophilic esophagitis. Dis Esoph 16:165-168, 2003.

75. Zimmerman SL, Levine MS, Rubesin SE, et al: Idiopathic eosinophilic esophagitis in adults: The ringed esophagus. 236:159-165, 2005.

76. Liacouras CA, Wenner WJ, Brown K, et al: Primary eosinophilic esophagitis in children: Successful treatment with oral corticosteroids. J Pediatr Gastroenterol Nutr 26:380-385, 1998.

77. Markowitz JE, Spergel JM, Ruchelli E, et al: Elemental diet is an effective treatment for eosinophilic esophagitis in children and adolescents. Am J Gastroenterol 98:777-782, 2003.

78. Arora AS, Perrault J, Smyrk TC: Topical corticosteroid treatment of dysphagia due to eosinophilic esophagitis in adults. Mayo Clin Proc 78:830-835, 2003.

79. Khan S, Orenstein SR, Di Lorenzo C, et al: Eosinophilic esophagitis: Strictures, impactions, dysphagia. Dig Dis Sci 48:22-29, 2003.

80. Bousvaros A, Antonioli DA, Winter HS: Ringed esophagus: An association with esophagitis. Am J Gastroenterol 87:1187-1190, 1992.

81. Siafakas CG, Ryan CK, Brown MR, et al: Multiple esophageal rings: An association with eosinophilic esophagitis. Am J Gastroenterol 95:1572-1575, 2000.

82. Vasilopoulos S, Murphy P, Auerbach A, et al: The small-caliber esophagus: An unappreciated cause of dysphagia for solids in patients with eosinophilic esophagitis. Gastrointest Endosc 55:99-106, 2002.

83. Landres RT, Kuster GGR, Strum WB: Eosinophilic esophagitis in a patient with vigorous achalasia. Gastroenterology 74:1298-1301, 1978.

84. Oh CH, Levine MS, Katzka DA, et al: Congenital esophageal stenosis in adults: Clinical and radiographic findings in seven patients. AJR 176:1179-1182, 2001.

85. Katzka DA, Levine MS, Ginsberg GG, et al: Congenital esophageal stenosis in adults. Am J Gastroenterol 95:32-36, 2000.

86. Levine MS, Goldstein HM: Fixed transverse folds in the esophagus: A sign of reflux esophagitis. AJR 143:275-278, 1984.

87. Gohel VK, Edell SL, Laufer I, et al: Transverse folds in the human esophagus. Radiology 128:303-308, 1978.

88. LiVolsi VA, Jaretzki A: Granulomatous esophagitis: A case of Crohn's disease limited to the esophagus. Gastroenterology 64:313-319, 1973.

89. Danzi JT, Farmer RG, Sullivan BH, et al: Endoscopic features of gastroduodenal Crohn's disease. Gastroenterology 70:9-13, 1976.

90. Weinstein T, Valderrama E, Pettei M, et al: Esophageal Crohn's disease: Medical management and correlation between clinical, endoscopic, and histologic features. Inflamm Bowel Dis 3:79-83, 1997.

91. Ghahremani GG, Gore RM, Breuer RI, et al: Esophageal manifestations of Crohn's disease. Gastrointest Radiol 7:199-203, 1982.

92. Tishler JMA, Helman CA: Crohn's disease of the esophagus. J Can Assoc Radiol 35:28-30, 1984.

93. Gohel V, Long BW, Richter G: Aphthoid ulcers in the esophagus with Crohn colitis. AJR 137:872-873, 1981.

94. Degryse HRM, De Schepper AM: Aphthoid esophageal ulcers in Crohn's disease of ileum and colon. Gastrointest Radiol 9:197-201, 1984.

95. Cynn WS, Chon H, Gureghian PA, et al: Crohn's disease of the esophagus. AJR 125:359-364, 1975.

96. Cockey BM, Jones B, Bayless TM, et al: Filiform polyps of the esophagus with inflammatory bowel disease. AJR 144:1207-1208, 1985.

97. Schneider R: Tuberculous esophagitis. Gastrointest Radiol 1:143-145, 1976.

98. Spalding AR, Burney DP, Richie RE: Acquired benign bronchoesophageal fistulas in the adult. Ann Thorac Surg 28:378-383, 1979.

99. Canon CL, Levine MS, Cherukuri R, et al: Intramural tracking: A feature of esophageal intramural pseudodiverticulosis. AJR 175:371-374, 2000.

100. Katz J, Gryboski JD, Rosenbaum HM, et al: Dysphagia in children with epidermolysis bullosa. Gastroenterology 52:259-262, 1967.

101. Nix TE, Christianson HB: Epidermolysis bullosa of the esophagus: Report of two cases and review of literature. South Med J 58:612-620, 1965.

102. Becker MH, Swinyard CA: Epidermolysis bullosa dystrophica in children: Radiologic manifestations. Radiology 90:124-128, 1968.

103. Agha FP, Francis IR, Ellis CN: Esophageal involvement in epidermolysis bullosa dystrophica: Clinical and roentgenographic manifestations. Gastrointest Radiol 8:111-117, 1983.

104. Schuman BM, Arciniegas E: The management of esophageal complications of epidermolysis bullosa. Am J Dig Dis 17:875-880, 1972.

105. Tishler JM, Han SY, Helman CA: Esophageal involvement in epidermolysis bullosa dystrophica. AJR 141:1283-1286, 1983.

106. Mauro MA, Parker LA, Hartley WS, et al: Epidermolysis bullosa: Radiographic findings in 16 cases. AJR 149:925-927, 1987.

107. Wong WL, Entwisle K, Pemberton J: Gastrointestinal manifestations in the Hallopeau-Siemens variant of recessive dystrophic epidermolysis bullosa. Br J Radiol 66:788-793, 1993.

108. Agha FP, Raji MR: Esophageal involvement in pemphigoid: Clinical and roentgen manifestations. Gastrointest Radiol 7:109-112, 1982.

109. Hardy KM, Perry HO, Pingree GC, et al: Benign mucous membrane pemphigoid. Arch Dermatol 104:467-475, 1971.

110. Al-kutoubi MA, Eliot C: Oesophageal involvement in benign mucous membrane pemphigoid. Clin Radiol 35:131-135, 1984.

111. Foroozan P, Enta T, Winship DH, et al: Loss and regeneration of esophageal mucosa in pemphigoid. Gastroenterology 52:548-558, 1967.

112. Soong C, Bynum TE: The endoscopic appearance of pemphigoid esophagitis. Gastrointest Endosc 19:17-18, 1972.

113. Karasick S, Mapp E, Karasick D: Esophageal involvement in benign mucous membrane pemphigoid. J Can Assoc Radiol 32:247-248, 1981.

114. Naylor MF, MacCarty RL, Rogers RS: Barium studies in esophageal cicatricial pemphigoid. Abdom Imaging 20:97-100, 1995.

115. Stampien TM, Schwartz RA: Erythema multiforme. Am Fam Physician 46:1171-1176, 1992.

116. Tan YM, Goh KL: Esophageal stricture as a late complication of Stevens-Johnson syndrome. Gastrointest Endosc 50:566-568, 1999.

117. Peters ME, Gourley G, Mann FA: Esophageal stricture and web secondary to Stevens-Johnson syndrome. Pediatr Radiol 13:290-291, 1983.

118. Howell CT, Mansberger JA, Parrish RA: Esophageal stricture secondary to Stevens-Johnson syndrome. J Pediatr Surg 22:994-995, 1987.

119. Carucci LR, Levine MS, Rubesin SE: Diffuse esophageal stricture caused by erythema multiforme major. AJR 180:749-750, 2003.

120. Waldman I, Berlin L: Stricture of the esophagus due to nasogastric intubation. AJR 94:321-324, 1965.

121. Banfield WJ, Hurwitz AL: Esophageal stricture associated with naso-gastric intubation. Arch Intern Med 134:1083-1086, 1974.

122. Nagler R, Spiro HM: Persistent gastroesophageal reflux induced during prolonged gastric intubation. N Engl J Med 269:495-500, 1963.

123. Balkany TJ, Baker BB, Bloustein PA, et al: Cervical esophagostomy in dogs: Endoscopic, radiographic, and histopathologic evaluation of esophagitis induced by feeding tubes. Ann Otol Rhinol Laryngol 86:1-6, 1977.

124. Salo JA, Kivilaakso E: Role of bile salts and trypsin in the pathogenesis of experimental alkaline esophagitis. Surgery 93:525-532, 1983.

125. Morrow D, Passaro ER: Alkaline reflux esophagitis after total gastrectomy. Am J Surg 132:287-290, 1976.

126. Sanchez RE, Gordon HE: Complications of total gastrectomy. Arch Surg 100:136-139, 1970.

127. Salo J, Kivilaakso E: Failure of long limb Roux-en-Y reconstruction to prevent alkaline reflux esophagitis after total gastrectomy. Endoscopy 22:65-67, 1990.

128. Meyer W, Vollmar F, Bar W: Barrett-esophagus following total gastrec-tomy. Endoscopy 2:121-126, 1979.

129. Sandvik AK, Halvorsen TB: Barrett's esophagus after total gastrectomy. J Clin Gastroenterol 10:587-588, 1988.

130. Levine MS, Fisher AR, Rubesin SE, et al: Complications after total gastrectomy and esophagojejunostomy: Radiologic evaluation. AJR 157:1189-1194, 1991.

131. O'Riordan D, Levine MS, Laufer I: Acute alcoholic esophagitis. J Can Assoc Radiol 37:54-55, 1986.

132. Hogan WJ, De Andrade SR, Winship DH: Ethanol-induced acute esophageal motor dysfunction. J Appl Physiol 32:755-760, 1972.

133. Kaufman SE, Kay MD: Induction of gastro-oesophageal reflux by alcohol. Gut 19:336-338, 1978.

134. McDonald GB, Shulman HM, Sullivan KM, et al: Intestinal and hepatic complications of human bone marrow transplantation: I. Gastro-enterology 90:460-477, 1986.

135. McDonald GB, Shulman HM, Sullivan KM, et al: Intestinal and hepatic complications of human bone marrow transplantation: II. Gastro-enterology 90:770-784, 1986.

136. Rosenberg HK, Serota FT, Hock P, et al: Radiographic features of gastrointestinal graft-vs.-host disease. Radiology 138:371-374, 1981.

137. McDonald GB, Sullivan KM, Plumley TF: Radiographic features of esophageal involvement in chronic graft-vs.-host disease. AJR 142:501-506, 1984.

138. McDonald GB, Sullivan KM, Schuffler MD, et al: Esophageal abnor-malities in chronic graft-vs.-host disease in humans. Gastroenterology 890:914-921, 1981.

139. Minocha A, Mandanas RA, Kida M, et al: Bullous esophagitis due to chronic graft-versus-host disease. Am J Gastroenterol 92:529-530, 1997.

140. McDonald GB, Sharma P, Hackman RC, et al: Esophageal infections in immunosuppressed patients after marrow transplantation. Gastro-enterology 88:1111-1117, 1985.

141. Dolce P, Gordeau M, April N, et al: Outbreak of glutaraldehyde-induced proctocolitis. Am J Infect Control 23:34-39, 1995.

142. Isserow JA, Kumar N, Goldschmidt MH, et al: Glutaraldehyde-induced esophageal injury: Histologic study of laboratory rats. Invest Radiol 33:730-733, 1998.

143. O'Duffy JD: Suggested criteria for diagnosis of Behçet's disease [abstract]. J Rheumatol 1:18, 1974.

144. Chung SY, Ha HK, Kim JH, et al: Radiologic findings of Behçet syndrome involving the gastrointestinal tract. RadioGraphics 21:911-926, 2001.

145. Kaplinsky N, Neumann G, Harzahav Y, et al: Esophageal ulceration in Behçet's syndrome. Gastrointest Endosc 23:160, 1977.

146. Lebwohl O, Forde KA, Berdon WE, et al: Ulcerative esophagitis and colitis in a pediatric patient with Behçet's syndrome. Am J Gastroenterol 68:550-555, 1977.

147. Mori S, Yoshihira A, Kawamura H, et al: Esophageal involvement in Behçet's disease. Am J Gastroenterol 78:548-553, 1983.

148. Yashiro K, Nagasako K, Hasegawa K, et al: Esophageal lesions in intestinal Behçet's disease. Endoscopy 18:57-60, 1986.

149. Anti M, Marra G, Rapaccini GL, et al: Esophageal involvement in Behçet's syndrome. J Clin Gastroenterol 8:514-519, 1986.

150. Mendl K, McKay JM, Tanner CH: Intramural diverticulosis of the oeso-phagus and Rokitansky-Aschoff sinuses in the gallbladder. Br J Radiol 33:496-501, 1960.

151. Cho SR, Sanders MM, Turner MA, et al: Esophageal intramural pseudo-diverticulosis. Gastrointest Radiol 6:9-16, 1981.

152. Hammon JW, Rice RP, Postlethwait RW, et al: Esophageal intramural diverticulosis. Ann Thorac Surg 17:260-267, 1974.

153. Wightman AJA, Wright EA: Intramural esophageal diverticulosis: A correlation of radiological and pathological findings. Br J Radiol 47:496-498, 1974.

154. Umlas J, Sakhuja R: The pathology of esophageal intramural pseudo-diverticulosis. Am J Clin Pathol 65:314-320, 1976.

155. Medeiros LJ, Doos WG, Balogh K: Esophageal intramural pseudo-diverticulosis: A report of two cases with analysis of similar, less extensive changes in "normal" autopsy esophagi. Hum Pathol 19:928-931, 1988.

156. Bruhlmann WF, Zollikofer CL, Maranta E, et al: Intramural pseudo-diverticulosis of the esophagus: Report of seven cases and literature review. Gastrointest Radiol 6:199-208, 1981.

157. Sabanathan S, Salama FD, Morgan WE: Oesophageal intramural pseudo-diverticulosis. Thorax 40:849-857, 1985.

158. Flora KD, Gordon MD, Lieberman D, et al: Esophageal intramural pseudodiverticulosis. Dig Dis 15:113-119, 1997.

159. Troupin RH: Intramural esophageal diverticulosis and moniliasis. AJR 104:613-616, 1968.

160. Boyd RM, Bogoch A, Greig JH, et al: Esophageal intramural pseudo-diverticulosis. Radiology 113:267-270, 1974.

161. Beauchamp JM, Nice CM, Belanger MA, et al: Esophageal intramural pseudodiverticulosis. Radiology 113:273-276, 1974.

162. Castillo S, Aburashed A, Kimmelman J, et al: Diffuse intramural esopha-geal pseudodiverticulosis. Gastroenterology 72:541-545, 1977.

163. Levine MS, Moolten DN, Herlinger H, et al: Esophageal intramural pseudodiverticulosis: A reevaluation. AJR 147:1165-1170, 1986.

164. Graham DY, Goyal RK, Sparkman J, et al: Diffuse intramural esophageal diverticulosis. Gastroenterology 68:781-785, 1975.

165. Pearlberg JL, Sandler MA, Madrazo BL: Computed tomographic features of esophageal intramural pseudodiverticulosis. Radiology 147:189-190, 1983.

166. Plavsic BM, Chen MYM, Gelfand DW, et al: Intramural pseudo-diverticulosis of the esophagus detected on barium esophagograms: Increased prevalence in patients with esophageal carcinoma. AJR 165:1381-1385, 1995.

167. Kim S, Choi C, Groskin SA: Esophageal intramural pseudodiverticulitis. Radiology 173:418-419, 1989.

168. Abrams LJ, Levine MS, Laufer I: Esophageal peridiverticulitis: An un-usual complication of esophageal intramural pseudodiverticulosis. Eur J Radiol 19:139-141, 1995.

Benign Tumors of the Esophagus

Marc S. Levine, MD

MUCOSAL LESIONS

Papilloma

Adenoma

Inflammatory Esophagogastric Polyp

Glycogenic Acanthosis

Leukoplakia

Acanthosis Nigricans

SUBMUCOSAL LESIONS

Leiomyoma

Leiomyomatosis and Idiopathic Muscular Hypertrophy

Fibrovascular Polyp

Granular Cell Tumor

Lipoma

Hemangioma

Hamartoma

Other Mesenchymal Tumors

Cysts

Benign tumors of the esophagus constitute only about 20% of all esophageal neoplasms.[1] Most are small lesions that cause no symptoms and have no malignant potential. As a result, they are usually discovered fortuitously on radiologic or endoscopic examinations. Occasionally, these lesions may cause dysphagia, bleeding, or other symptoms. In such cases, endoscopic or surgical removal may be required. Depending on the site of origin, benign tumors may be classified as mucosal or submucosal lesions, which have typical radiographic and endoscopic features.

MUCOSAL LESIONS

Papilloma

Squamous papillomas (or simply, papillomas) are uncommon benign tumors, accounting for less than 5% of all esophageal neoplasms.[2] The lesions consist histologically of a central fibrovascular core with multiple finger-like projections covered by hyperplastic squamous epithelium.[3] Although the cause of these papillomas is uncertain, the human papillomavirus[4] and chronic reflux esophagitis[5] have both been implicated in tumor pathogenesis.

All papillomas in the esophagus reported thus far have been benign lesions. However, malignant degeneration has been observed in experimentally induced esophageal papillomas in rats.[6] Malignant transformation has also been documented in papillomas arising in other sites such as the oral cavity, larynx, and uterine cervix.[7-9] In addition, benign papillomas may be confused on histologic examination with verrucous carcinoma, an uncommon form of squamous cell carcinoma.[10] Thus, some investigators believe that all papillomas in the esophagus should be resected because of the uncertain risk of malignant degeneration and potential confusion with verrucous carcinoma.[11]

Papillomas in the esophagus usually occur as solitary lesions, ranging from 0.5 to 1.5 cm. Most patients are asymptomatic, but dysphagia is an occasional finding.[3,11] Rarely, multiple papillomas may be present in the esophagus, a condition known as *esophageal papillomatosis*.[12-14]

Radiographic Findings

Papillomas are difficult to detect on conventional single-contrast esophagograms because of the small size of the lesions. In contrast, they can be recognized on double-contrast esophagograms as small (<1 cm), sessile polyps with a smooth or slightly lobulated contour (Fig. 26-1).[15] Because early esophageal cancers may also appear as small polypoid lesions, endoscopy should be performed to exclude an early carcinoma. Occasionally, larger papillomas may be manifested by lobulated intraluminal masses indistinguishable from more advanced esophageal carcinomas. Rarely, esophageal papillomas may have a bubbly appearance because of trapping of barium between the papillary fronds of the tumor (Fig. 26-2).[16]

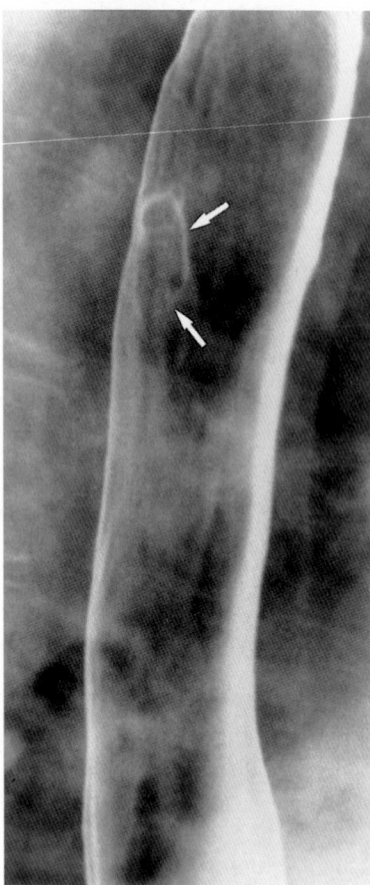

Figure 26-1. Papilloma. The lesion appears as a sessile, slightly lobulated polyp (*arrows*) in the midesophagus. An early esophageal carcinoma could produce similar findings.

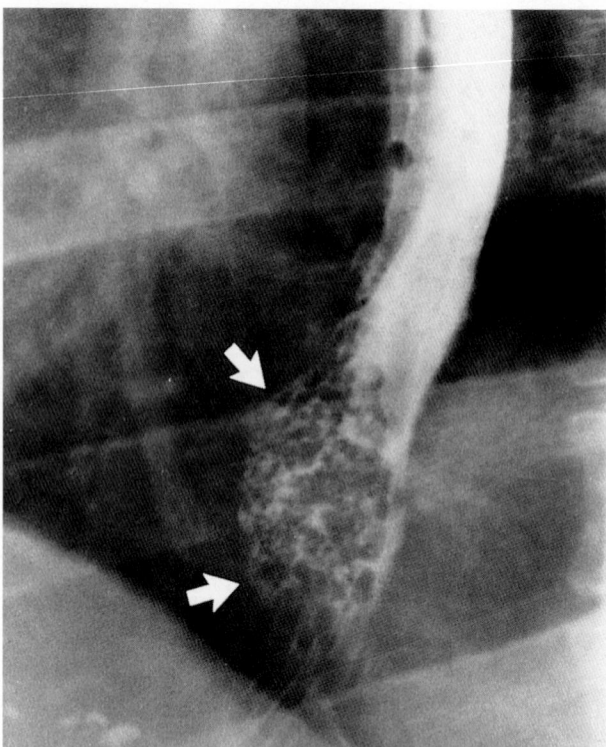

Figure 26-2. Giant esophageal papilloma. The lesion has a bubbly appearance (*arrows*) due to trapping of barium between the papillary fronds of the tumor. (From Walker JH: Giant papilloma of the thoracic esophagus. AJR 131:519-520, 1978, © by American Roentgen Ray Society.)

Multiple papillomas may be demonstrated on esophagography in patients with esophageal papillomatosis.[12-14] Despite its rarity, the diagnosis of papillomatosis should be suggested by the presence of multiple, discrete, wartlike excrescences on the esophageal mucosa (Fig. 26-3). Even when multiple papillomas are present, these lesions rarely cause esophageal obstruction.

Adenoma

Adenomas account for less than 1% of all benign esophageal neoplasms.[17] They are rarely found in the esophagus because it is lined by squamous rather than columnar epithelium. However, adenomas may develop in patients with Barrett's mucosa in the esophagus (see Chapter 27).[18,19] These adenomas are important because of the risk of malignant degeneration via an adenoma-carcinoma sequence similar to that found in the colon.[18,19] Esophageal adenomas should therefore be resected endoscopically or surgically whenever feasible.

Radiographic Findings

Esophageal adenomas may appear radiographically as sessile or pedunculated polyps in the esophagus (Fig. 26-4). Larger, more lobulated lesions have a greater likelihood of harboring adenocarcinoma. Most adenomas are located in the distal esophagus at or near the gastroesophageal junction.[17-19] As a result, they can be mistaken for inflammatory esophagogastric

polyps (see next section). Nodularity, lobulation, and the large size of the lesion should favor an adenoma or adenocarcinoma. When an adenoma is suggested on barium studies, endoscopy and biopsy should be performed for a definitive diagnosis.

Inflammatory Esophagogastric Polyp

Although inflammatory esophagogastric polyps are not neoplastic, they are included in this chapter because they are characterized by the presence of a polypoid protuberance in the distal esophagus near the gastroesophageal junction. An inflammatory esophagogastric polyp represents the bulbous tip of a thickened gastric fold extending into the distal esophagus from the gastric fundus.[20-24] The lesions are composed of inflammatory and granulation tissue, and they are thought to be a sequela of chronic reflux esophagitis (see Chapter 23).[21,22] As a result, these patients may have clinical signs of gastroesophageal reflux disease. Inflammatory esophagogastric polyps have no malignant potential, however, so that endoscopic resection is unwarranted.[24]

Radiographic Findings

Inflammatory esophagogastric polyps are usually manifested on barium studies by a single prominent mucosal fold that arises in the gastric fundus and extends into the distal esophagus as a smooth, ovoid or club-shaped protuberance (Fig. 26-5A).[20,23,24] The lesions frequently straddle a hiatal hernia and may be associated with other findings of reflux

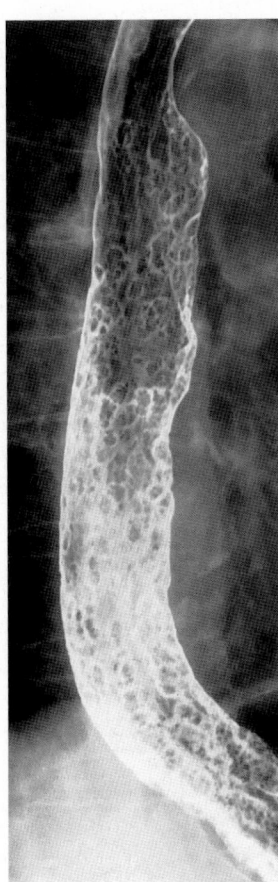

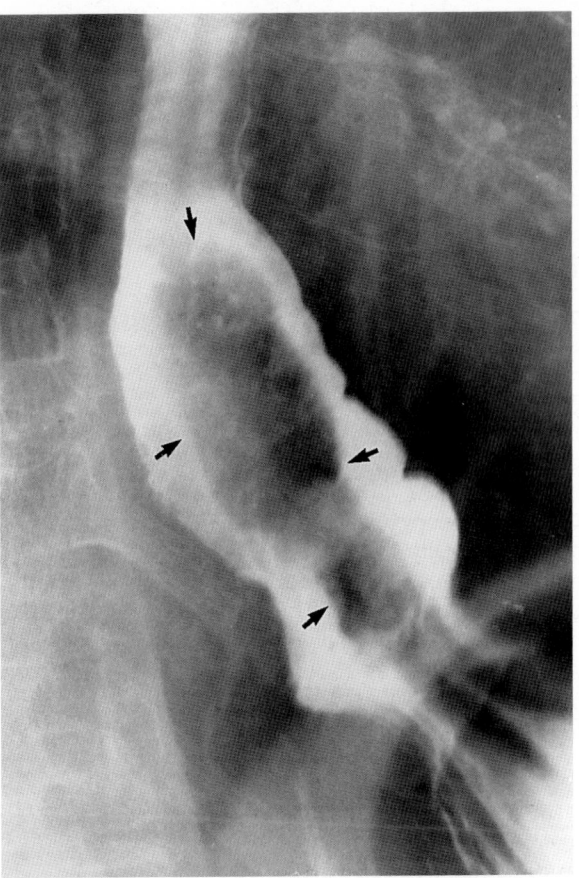

Figure 26-3. Esophageal papillomatosis. There are innumerable wartlike excrescences on the esophageal mucosa. Despite the dramatic radiographic appearance, this patient had no esophageal symptoms. (Courtesy of Harvey M. Goldstein, MD, San Antonio, TX.)

Figure 26-4. Adenomatous polyp in Barrett's esophagus. The polyp (*arrows*) originates at the gastroesophageal junction and extends into the distal esophagus above a hiatal hernia. Although this lesion could be mistaken for an inflammatory esophagogastric polyp, it is larger and more lobulated than most inflammatory polyps. The resected specimen contained a solitary focus of adenocarcinoma. (From Levine MS, Caroline D, Thompson JJ, et al: Adenocarcinoma of the esophagus: relationship to Barrett mucosa. Radiology 150:305-309, 1984.)

Figure 26-5. Inflammatory esophagogastric polyps. A. An inflammatory polyp is seen en face as a prominent fold (*straight arrows*) arising at the cardia and extending into the distal esophagus as a smooth, club-shaped mass (*curved arrow*). The radiographic findings are so characteristic that endoscopy is unwarranted. **B.** This inflammatory polyp has a more lobulated appearance (*arrows*), so that it cannot be differentiated from an adenomatous polyp or even an adenocarcinoma (see Fig. 26-4). (**B** from Levine MS: Radiology of the Esophagus. Philadelphia, WB Saunders, 1989.)

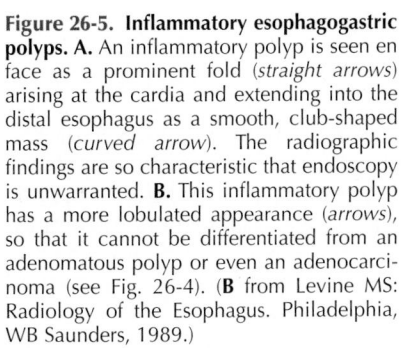

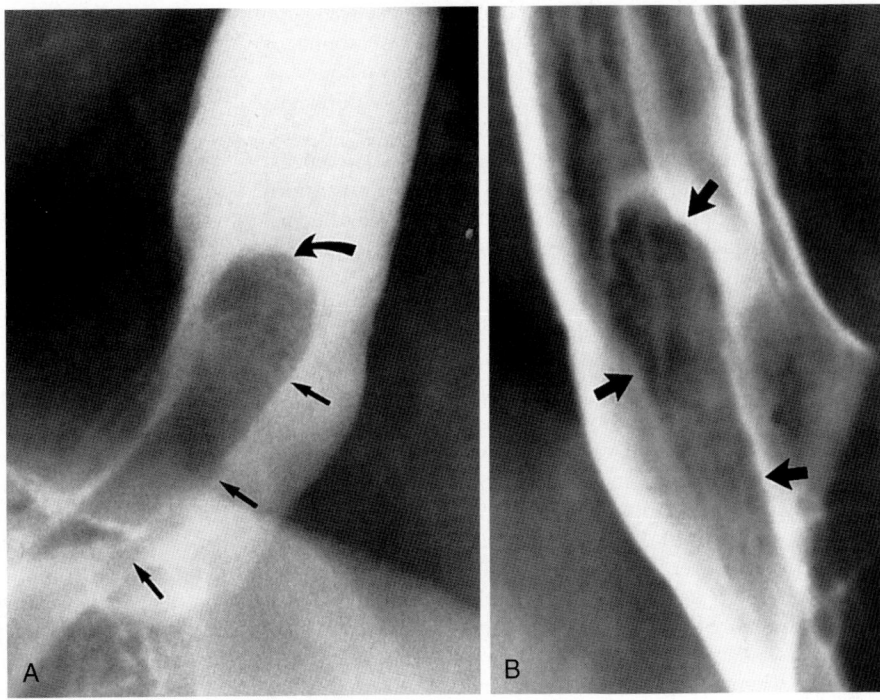

esophagitis. When the characteristic features of inflammatory esophagogastric polyps are present on esophagography, endoscopic confirmation is unnecessary. Occasionally, however, the polyps may have a more irregular, nodular, or lobulated appearance, so that a malignant lesion cannot be excluded (Fig. 26-5B).[23] In such cases, endoscopy and biopsy are required for a definitive diagnosis.

Glycogenic Acanthosis

Since its original description in 1970,[25] glycogenic acanthosis has been recognized as a benign condition of unknown cause in which there is accumulation of cytoplasmic glycogen in the squamous epithelium of the esophagus. Although glycogenic acanthosis is not considered to be neoplastic, it is included in this chapter because it is characterized by mucosal nodules or plaques. Glycogenic acanthosis is a common condition at endoscopy, with a prevalence of 3% to 15%.[26-28] The lesions are usually recognized as white mucosal plaques or nodules, ranging from 2 to 15 mm.[26,27] Glycogenic acanthosis is characterized histologically by hyperplasia of squamous epithelial cells resulting from increased cytoplasmic glycogen.[25,29] A definitive diagnosis is made by demonstrating the characteristic glycogen-rich epithelial cells on biopsy specimens stained with periodic acid–Schiff material.[25]

Glycogenic acanthosis seems to be a degenerative, age-related phenomenon, with the lesions first appearing when patients are in their 40s and 50s and becoming larger and more numerous in patients older than 60 years of age.[30] Glycogenic acanthosis rarely causes esophageal symptoms, and it is not associated with any known risk of malignant degeneration.[31] This condition is therefore almost always discovered as an incidental finding on radiologic or endoscopic examinations.

Radiographic Findings

Although the appearance of glycogenic acanthosis was not described on esophagography until 1981,[32] it has since been recognized as a frequent finding on double-contrast barium studies, occurring in up to 30% of patients.[30,31] Glycogenic acanthosis is usually manifested on double-contrast esophagograms by multiple small, rounded nodules or plaques in the middle or, less commonly, distal third of the esophagus (Fig. 26-6).[31] The lesions are more obvious in the midesophagus because this segment is best seen on double-contrast images, and the distal esophagus is often obscured by barium pooling in this region. The nodules are usually 1 to 3 mm, but occasional plaques may be as large as several centimeters.[31,32]

Differential Diagnosis

Although glycogenic acanthosis has little clinical significance, it should be distinguished from other causes of mucosal nodularity, such as superficial spreading carcinoma, esophageal papillomatosis, acanthosis nigricans, leukoplakia, and esophagitis. Because of the rarity of most of these conditions, the major consideration in the differential diagnosis, for all practical purposes, is esophagitis. In some patients, glycogenic acanthosis can be mistaken for the nodular mucosa of reflux esophagitis. However, the nodules of glycogenic acanthosis tend to be more well defined than those of reflux esophagitis and are more likely to occur in the midesophagus than in the distal esophagus. Other patients with glycogenic acanthosis may have discrete plaquelike defects, erroneously suggesting

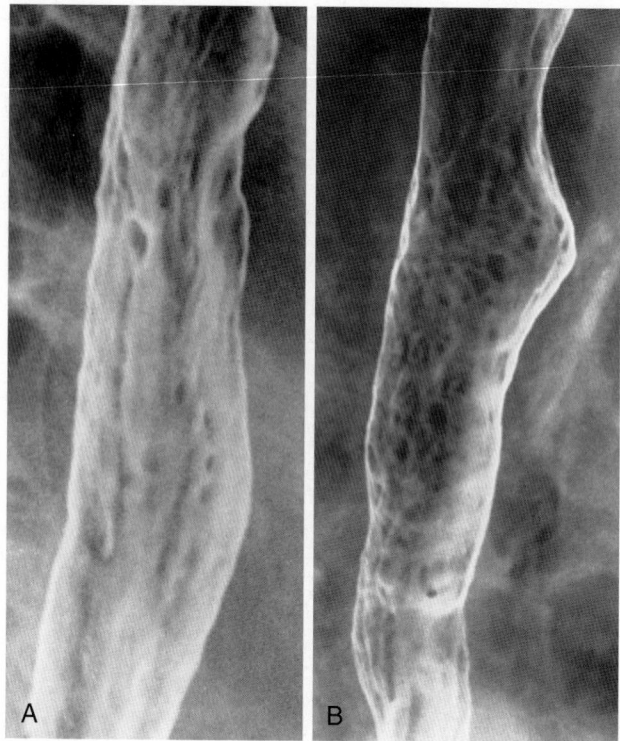

Figure 26-6. Glycogenic acanthosis. A and **B.** In both cases, this condition is manifested by multiple small plaques and nodules in the midesophagus. The lesions tend to have a rounded appearance. *Candida* esophagitis could produce similar findings, but patients with glycogenic acanthosis are almost always asymptomatic. (**A** from Levine MS, Macones AJ, Laufer I: *Candida* esophagitis: Accuracy of radiographic diagnosis. Radiology 154:581-587, 1985. **B** from Levine MS: Radiology of the Esophagus. Philadelphia, WB Saunders, 1989.)

a diagnosis of *Candida* esophagitis. However, the nodules of glycogenic acanthosis tend to have a more rounded appearance, whereas the plaques of candidiasis usually have a more linear configuration (see Chapter 24). The clinical history is also helpful because glycogenic acanthosis occurs in older people without esophageal symptoms, whereas *Candida* esophagitis typically occurs in immunocompromised patients with odynophagia. Thus, it is usually possible to distinguish glycogenic acanthosis from these various forms of esophagitis on clinical and radiographic grounds.

Leukoplakia

Oral leukoplakia is a relatively common condition characterized by white mucosal plaques that exhibit various combinations of hyperkeratosis, parakeratosis, epithelial dysplasia, and frank carcinoma on histologic examination. In contrast, leukoplakia rarely occurs in the esophagus,[33-35] and its malignant potential in this location is unknown. The few reported patients with esophageal leukoplakia have been asymptomatic.[33] Endoscopy may reveal discrete, slightly raised, white mucosal plaques less than 1 cm.[33] Rarely the lesions may be recognized on double-contrast esophagography as tiny nodules or plaques.[34,35] However, most asymptomatic patients with a nodular mucosa probably have glycogenic acanthosis.[31] Esophageal leukoplakia should therefore be considered a histologic rather than a radiologic diagnosis.

Acanthosis Nigricans

Acanthosis nigricans is a dermatologic disorder characterized by the triad of papillomatosis, pigmentation, and hyperkeratosis. Some patients have a malignant type of acanthosis nigricans associated with adenocarcinomas of the gastrointestinal tract, ovary, lung, or breast. Esophageal involvement has occasionally been reported in patients with the malignant form of the disease.[35,36] The esophageal lesions appear on barium studies as numerous tiny nodules on the esophageal mucosa.[35,36] Because this condition rarely involves the esophagus, the diagnosis should be suggested only in patients with known acanthosis nigricans involving the skin.

SUBMUCOSAL LESIONS

By definition, all submucosal lesions arising in the wall of the gastrointestinal tract are intramural. Not all intramural lesions are submucosal, however, because they can also arise from the muscularis propria or even the subserosa. Despite this distinction, the terms *submucosal* and *intramural* are used interchangeably in this text based on long-standing convention.

Leiomyoma

More than 50% of all benign esophageal tumors are leiomyomas.[2,37,38] These lesions consist histologically of intersecting bands of smooth muscle and fibrous tissue in a well-defined capsule. About 60% are located in the distal third of the esophagus, 30% in the middle third, and 10% in the proximal third.[39] Leiomyomas are less common above the level of the aortic arch because of the presence of striated rather than smooth muscle in this portion of the esophagus. These tumors usually appear grossly as discrete submucosal masses, ranging from 2 to 8 cm in size.[38] Occasionally, however, the lesions may have an exophytic, intraluminal, or circumferential pattern of growth. Giant leiomyomas as large as 20 cm have occasionally been reported.[40,41]

Most leiomyomas in the esophagus occur as solitary lesions, but multiple leiomyomas are present in 3% to 4% of patients.[42,43] Rarely, these tumors may be associated with uterine or vulvar leiomyomas, apparently on a familial basis.[44,45] Esophageal leiomyomas have also been documented in patients with hypertrophic osteoarthropathy, a condition characterized by clubbed fingers and toes, swollen joints, and subperiosteal new bone formation in the extremities.[46]

Clinical Findings

Most patients with leiomyomas in the esophagus are asymptomatic.[39] Even large masses significantly indenting the lumen may not produce symptoms. When these patients are symptomatic, they may present with intermittent, slowly worsening dysphagia or, less commonly, substernal discomfort, vomiting, or weight loss.[39,47] Unlike gastrointestinal stromal tumors in the stomach, esophageal leiomyomas rarely ulcerate, so that upper gastrointestinal bleeding is extremely uncommon.[47] Because of the slowly progressive nature of the lesions, symptoms may be present for several years before these patients seek medical attention.[39] Rarely, they may present with signs and symptoms of acute esophageal obstruction.[48] The treatment of choice for symptomatic patients is surgical enucleation of the tumor.[39] Occasionally, larger lesions may necessitate a more extensive esophageal resection.

Although leiomyomas are relatively common lesions in the esophagus, their malignant counterparts, leiomyosarcomas, are rare (see Chapter 28). Thus far, no case of malignant degeneration in an esophageal leiomyoma has been documented. In one series, esophageal leiomyomas were followed for 15 years without evidence of malignant transformation.[49] Because these tumors have little tendency to undergo sarcomatous degeneration, surgical removal of small leiomyomas in asymptomatic patients is probably unwarranted.

Radiographic Findings

Leiomyomas that grow exophytically away from the esophagus may be recognized on chest radiographs by the presence of a mediastinal mass.[50] Rarely, these tumors may contain amorphous or punctate areas of calcification.[51,52] In fact, the presence of a calcified esophageal mass should strongly suggest a leiomyoma because calcification almost never occurs in other benign or malignant tumors of the esophagus.[52] However, one case of a densely calcified esophageal leiomyosarcoma has been reported.[53]

Leiomyomas usually appear on barium studies as discrete submucosal masses, ranging from 2 to 8 cm in size (Figs. 26-7 and 26-8). These tumors have the classic features of intramural lesions elsewhere in the gastrointestinal tract.[54] When viewed en face, they appear as round or ovoid filling defects sharply outlined by barium on each side (see Fig. 26-8A).[38] When viewed in profile, the lesions have a smooth surface (etched in white on double-contrast images) and their upper and lower borders form right angles or slightly obtuse angles with the adjacent esophageal wall (see Figs. 26-7 and 26-8B). Occasionally, larger leiomyomas may substantially indent the lumen, causing the esophagus to appear narrowed in tangential projections but stretched and widened en face (see Fig. 26-8).[54] These tumors may continue to enlarge over a period of years,

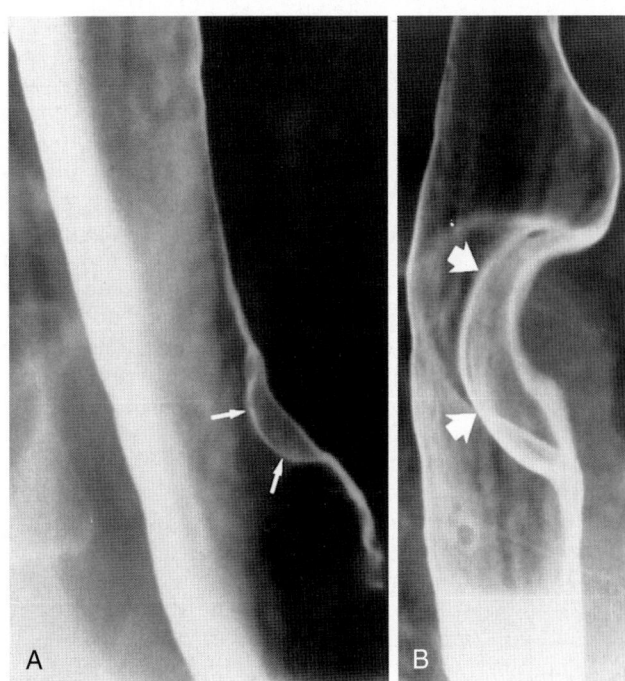

Figure 26-7. Esophageal leiomyomas. A and **B.** The lesions (*arrows*) have a smooth surface (*etched in white*) and slightly obtuse borders characteristic of submucosal masses.

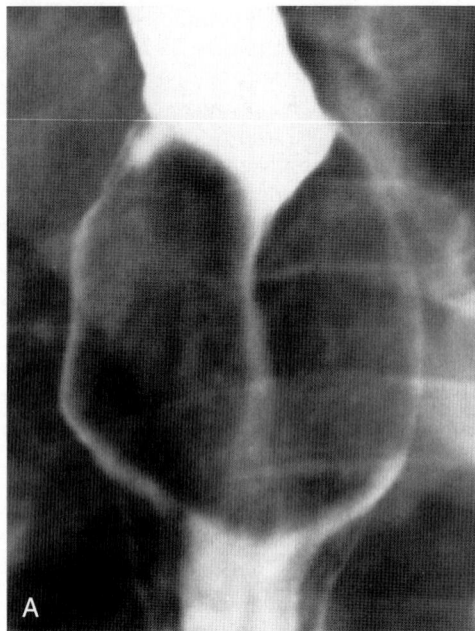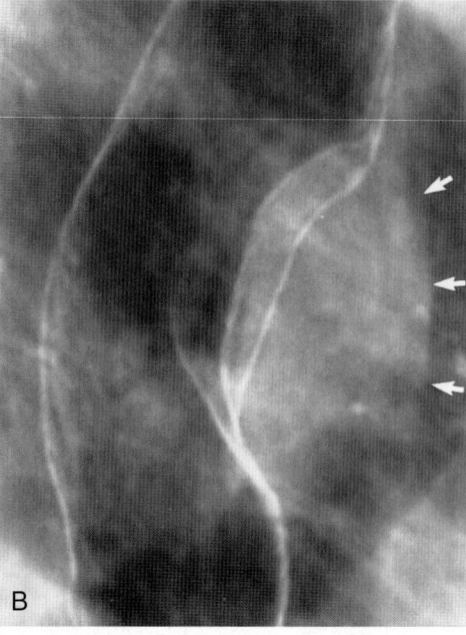

Figure 26-8. Esophageal leiomyoma. A. En face view shows a smooth, rounded filling defect in the esophagus, with splitting of barium around the lesion. The esophagus appears widened at this level. **B.** Tangential view reveals the characteristic features of a submucosal lesion. The outer margin of the leiomyoma is seen as a soft tissue shadow (*arrows*) abutting the lung. (Courtesy of Marc P. Banner, MD, Philadelphia, PA.)

but ulceration is rarely observed. Leiomyomas typically appear on CT as homogeneous soft tissue masses,[55] but differentiation from other esophageal tumors is difficult.

Although the vast majority of leiomyomas in the esophagus appear as solitary submucosal masses, esophagography may reveal multiple lesions[42,43] or even annular lesions with varying degrees of obstruction.[39] Occasionally, leiomyomas may be giant intraluminal masses that are attached to the upper thoracic or cervical esophagus by a long pedicle.[39,56] However, most pedunculated, intraluminal tumors in the esophagus contain a variety of other mesenchymal elements; these tumors have been classified together as fibrovascular polyps (see later section on Fibrovascular Polyp). Rarely, leiomyomas arising at or near the gastroesophageal junction may involve not only the distal esophagus but also the gastric cardia and fundus.[57]

Differential Diagnosis

Most submucosal masses in the esophagus are leiomyomas. However, other unusual intramural tumors such as granular cell tumors, lipomas, hemangiomas, fibromas, and neurofibromas, may produce identical radiographic findings (see later sections). Cystic lesions, such as congenital duplication cysts and acquired retention cysts, may also appear as submucosal masses on barium studies (see later section on Cysts). Even an isolated esophageal varix may resemble a submucosal tumor, but effacement or obliteration of the lesion by esophageal distention should suggest its vascular origin (see Chapter 29). When multiple submucosal masses are present in the esophagus, the differential diagnosis should include not only multiple leiomyomas but also esophageal retention cysts, Kaposi's sarcoma, and lymphomatous or leukemic infiltrates in the esophagus (see Chapter 28).

Leiomyomas should also be distinguished from extramural lesions that are extrinsically compressing or indenting the esophagus. When viewed in profile, extrinsic lesions tend to have more obtuse, gently sloping borders than intramural

lesions.[54] Another useful criterion for differentiating these lesions is the "spheroid" sign, which is based on the principle that the estimated center of the mass should lie outside the projected contour of the esophagus for extramural lesions but inside the projected contour for intramural lesions.[58] When the radiographic findings are equivocal, CT may be helpful for differentiating a submucosal tumor from a mediastinal mass compressing the esophagus.[55]

Leiomyomatosis and Idiopathic Muscular Hypertrophy

Esophageal leiomyomatosis is a rare, benign condition in which neoplastic proliferation of smooth muscle causes marked circumferential thickening of the esophageal wall, most commonly in the distal esophagus.[59-61] This condition is predominantly found in children and young adults who present with long-standing dysphagia.[61] Esophageal leiomyomatosis can occur sporadically, or it can occur on a familial basis with autosomal dominant inheritance.[62,63] In some cases, this condition is associated with more widespread visceral leiomyomatosis[64-66] or hereditary nephritis (Alport's syndrome).[62,63,65,67] Depending on the extent of the lesion, an esophagectomy or esophagogastrectomy is almost always curative.[59,63]

Idiopathic muscular hypertrophy of the esophagus is another condition that is closely related to esophageal leiomyomatosis.[68-71] Idiopathic muscular hypertrophy is characterized by non-neoplastic thickening of smooth muscle in the esophageal wall, possibly as a response to severe esophageal spasm. In contrast to patients with leiomyomatosis, these individuals usually remain asymptomatic or present with dysphagia during late adulthood.[69,71] Occasionally, however, patients with idiopathic muscular hypertrophy of the esophagus may have such severe dysphagia that an esophagectomy is required.

Radiographic Findings

Esophageal leiomyomatosis may be manifested on barium studies by smooth, tapered narrowing of the distal esophagus with decreased or absent esophageal peristalsis, mimicking the appearance of primary achalasia (Fig. 26-9A).[59,61,67] However, the narrowed segment tends to be longer than that in achalasia, and leiomyomatosis is sometimes associated with relatively symmetric paracardiac defects in the gastric fundus because of bulging of this thickened mass of muscle into the proximal stomach (see Fig. 26-9A).[61] CT may reveal marked circumferential thickening of the distal esophageal wall, resembling the findings of secondary achalasia resulting from metastatic tumor at the gastroesophageal junction (Figs. 26-9B and C).[61] However, leiomyomatosis usually occurs in children or adolescents with long-standing dysphagia,

whereas secondary achalasia occurs in older people with recent onset of dysphagia and weight loss.[72] Thus, despite its rarity, the diagnosis of esophageal leiomyomatosis can usually be suggested on the basis of the clinical and radiographic findings.

Idiopathic muscular hypertrophy of the esophagus may be manifested on esophagography by a corkscrew appearance with multiple lumen-obliterating, nonperistaltic contractions.[68-70] In other cases, this condition may produce an achalasia-like appearance with tapered narrowing of the distal esophagus and proximal dilatation on barium studies (Fig. 26-10A)[69,71] and marked circumferential thickening of the distal esophageal wall on CT (Fig. 26-10B).[69,71] The radiographic findings may therefore be indistinguishable from those of esophageal leiomyomatosis. However, patients with idiopathic muscular hypertrophy of the esophagus usually

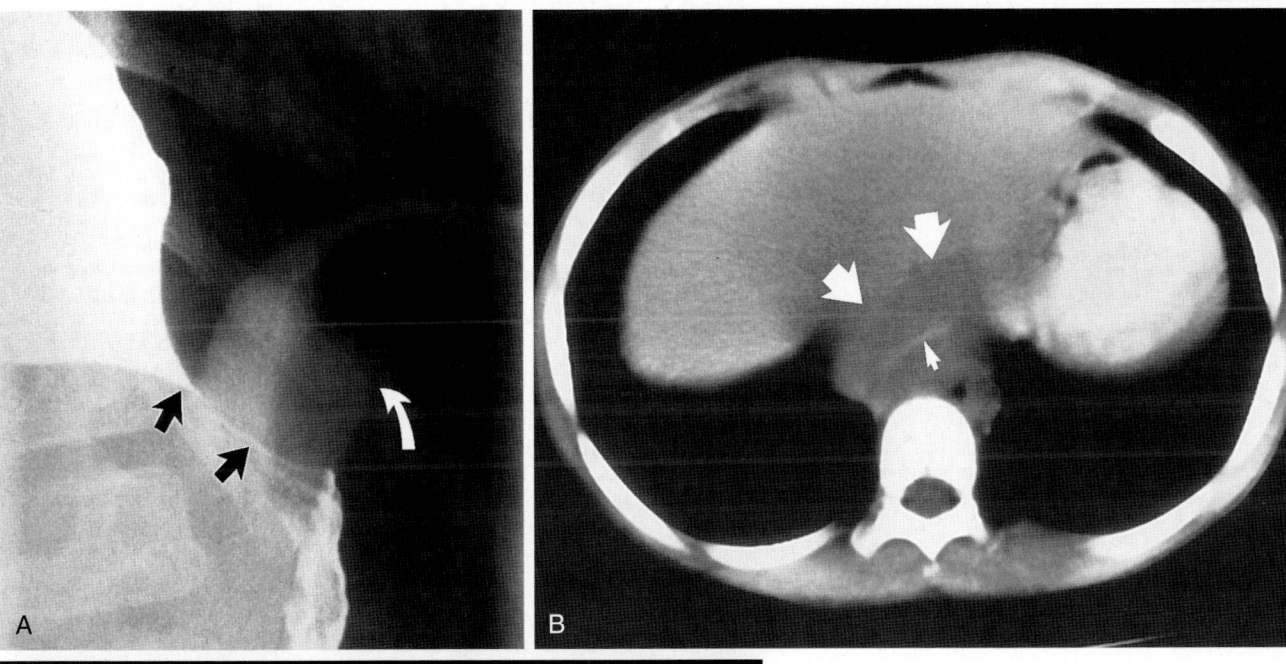

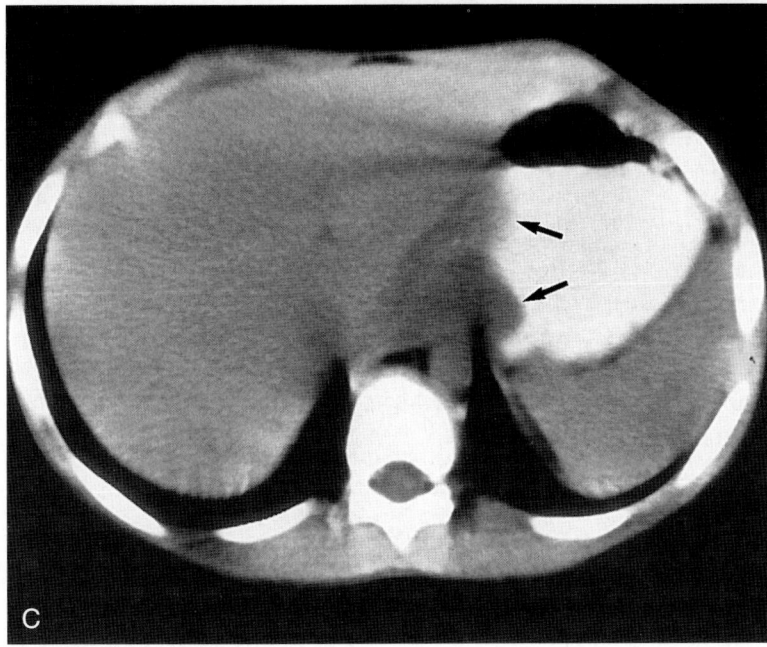

Figure 26-9. Esophageal leiomyomatosis. A. Barium study shows smooth, tapered narrowing of the distal esophagus (*black arrows*), resembling achalasia. However, the narrowed segment is longer than that typically seen in achalasia. Also, the thickened muscle is seen bulging into the gastric fundus as a soft tissue mass (*white arrow*). **B.** CT scan shows a mass of relatively low soft tissue attenuation (*large arrows*) surrounding the distal esophagus with a slitlike collection of contrast material (*small arrow*) in the compressed esophageal lumen. **C.** More caudad CT scan shows this thickened mass of muscle bulging into the gastric fundus (*arrows*) on both sides of the cardia. (From Levine MS, Buck JL, Pantongrag-Brown L, et al: Esophageal leiomyomatosis. Radiology 199:533-536, 1996.)

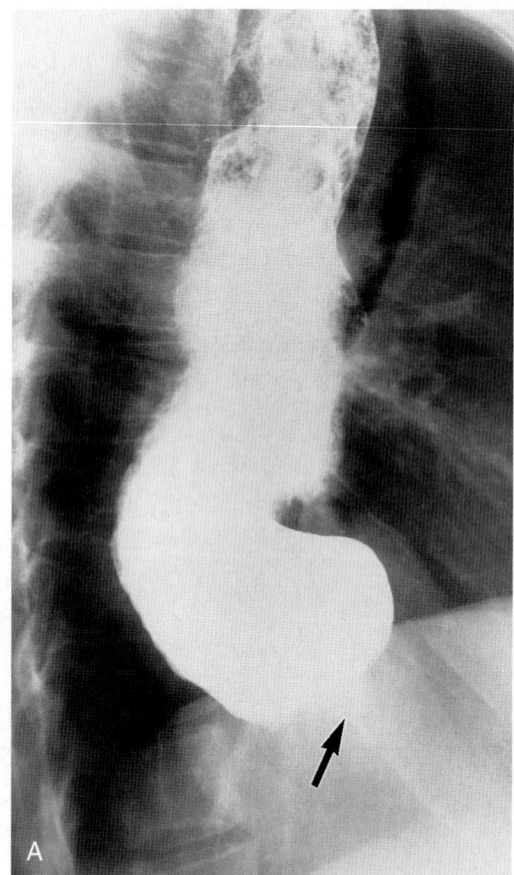

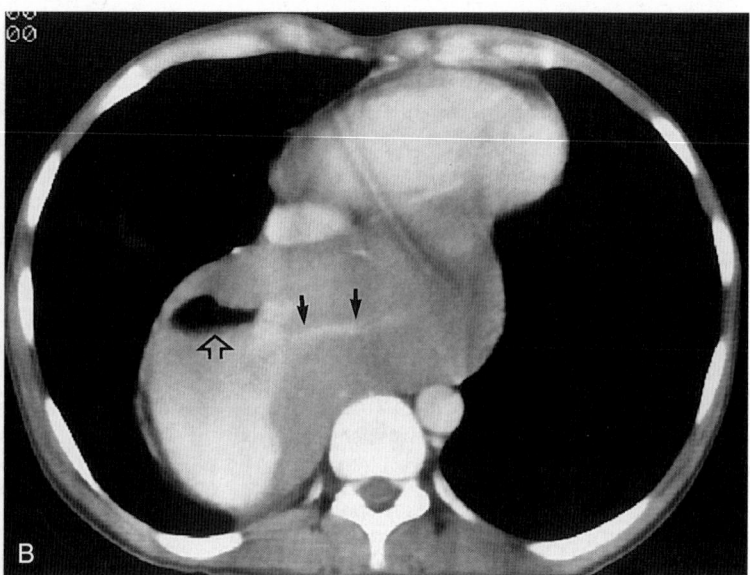

Figure 26-10. Idiopathic muscular hypertrophy of the esophagus. A. Barium study reveals a markedly dilated esophagus with relatively abrupt narrowing (*arrow*) near the gastroesophageal junction. **B.** CT scan near the level of the gastro-esophageal junction shows massive thickening of the distal esophageal wall and narrowing of the lumen (*closed arrows*). An air-contrast level (*open arrow*) is present in the dilated esophagus to the right. At surgery, there was a markedly thickened esophageal wall because of localized muscular hypertrophy without evidence of tumor. The radiographic findings in this case resemble those of esophageal leiomyomatosis shown in Figure 26-9. (Courtesy of Richard L. Baron, MD, Pittsburgh, PA.)

present later in life than those with leiomyomatosis, so that the clinical history is helpful for differentiating these conditions.

Fibrovascular Polyp

Fibrovascular polyps are rare, benign, tumor-like lesions characterized by the development of pedunculated, intra-luminal masses that can grow to gigantic sizes in the esopha-gus. The lesions consist histologically of varying amounts of fibrovascular and adipose tissue covered by normal squamous epithelium.[73-75] Depending on the predominant mesen-chymal components, these lesions have variously been called hamartomas, fibromas, lipomas, fibrolipomas, fibromyxomas, and fibroepithelial polyps.[76] More recently, however, they have all been classified together as *fibrovascular polyps*,[75,76] a term recommended by the World Health Organization in its histologic classification of tumors.[77]

Fibrovascular polyps almost always arise in the cervical esophagus near the level of the cricopharyngeus.[74-76] They probably originate in loose submucosal tissue in the cervical esophagus, gradually elongating over a period of years as they are dragged inferiorly into the middle or distal third of the esophagus by esophageal peristalsis until the intraluminal portion of the mass has attained gigantic proportions.[76] Occasionally, fibrovascular polyps can even prolapse through the cardia into the gastric fundus.[73] Regardless of the size of the polyp, its proximal end is almost always attached to the cervical esophagus by a discrete pedicle.[78]

Clinical Findings

Fibrovascular polyps most commonly occur in elderly men, who present with long-standing dysphagia that slowly pro-gresses over a period of years as the intraluminal portion of the polyp gradually enlarges.[79] Other patients may develop wheezing or inspiratory stridor because of compression of the adjacent trachea by the distended esophagus.[73,74,79] Occa-sionally, these individuals may have a spectacular clinical presentation with regurgitation of a fleshy mass into the pharynx or mouth.[73,75,76,78] Some distraught patients have even tried to bite off the lesion with their teeth or to remove it manually with their fingers. Aside from the bizarre clinical features of this entity, regurgitated fibrovascular polyps in the pharynx are potentially life-threatening because they have rarely been known to occlude the larynx, causing asphyxia and sudden death.[80]

Malignant degeneration of fibrovascular polyps is thought to be extremely rare. Nevertheless, removal of these lesions is recommended because of the progressive and eventually debilitating nature of the symptoms and the theoretical risk of asphyxia and sudden death. Small fibrovascular polyps may be resected endoscopically, but large tumors should be removed surgically because significant bleeding may occur when the stalk is transected.[79]

Radiographic Findings

Fibrovascular polyps can sometimes be recognized on chest radiographs by the presence of a right-sided superior media-

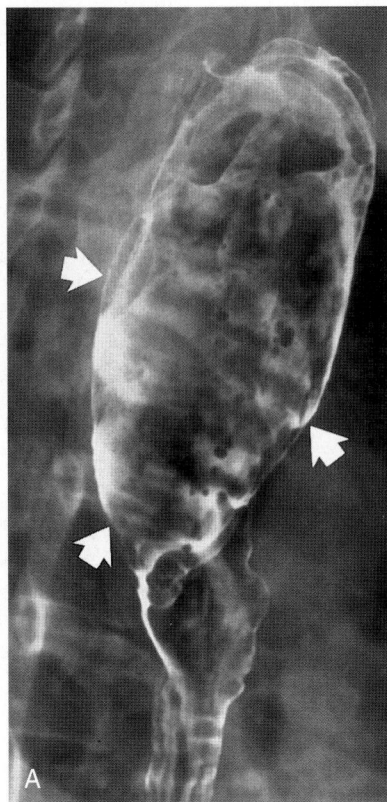
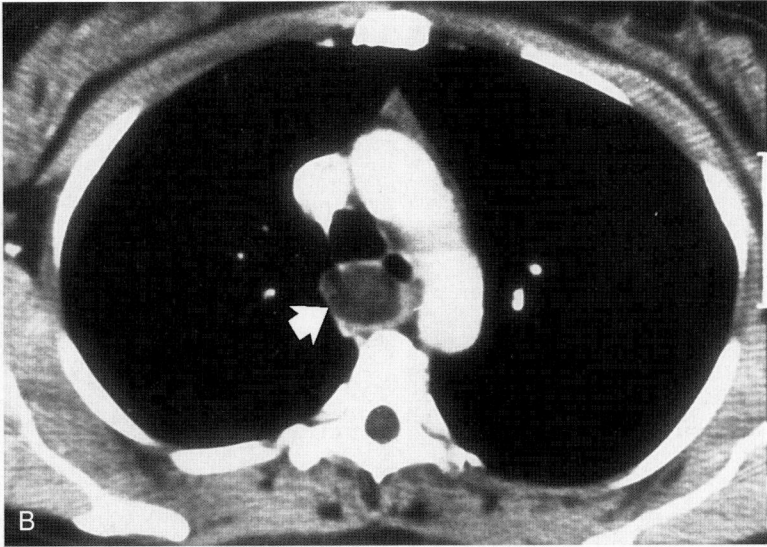

Figure 26-11. Fibrovascular polyp. A. Barium study shows a smooth, sausage-shaped mass (*arrows*) expanding the lumen of the upper thoracic esophagus. This lesion has the classic appearance of a fibrovascular polyp. **B.** CT scan shows an expansile mass (*arrow*) in the thoracic esophagus with a thin rim of contrast material surrounding the lesion, confirming its intraluminal location. The fat density of the polyp is due to an abundance of adipose tissue in this lesion. (From Levine MS, Buck JL, Pantongrag-Brown L, et al: Fibrovascular polyps of the esophagus: Clinical, radiographic, and pathologic findings in 16 patients. AJR 166:781-787, 1996, © by American Roentgen Ray Society.)

stinal mass, anterior tracheal bowing, or both.[79] The polyps usually appear on esophagography as smooth, expansile, sausage-shaped intraluminal masses that arise in the cervical esophagus and extend into the upper or middle third of the thoracic esophagus (Fig. 26-11A).[73,74,76,81] Occasionally, these lesions may show varying degrees of lobulation (Fig. 26-12A)[79] or they may extend into the distal esophagus or even the gastric fundus.[73,79] Although most fibrovascular polyps have a site of attachment in the cervical esophagus, it is often difficult to demonstrate a proximal pedicle on barium studies.[79]

Fibrovascular polyps containing an abundance of adipose tissue may appear on CT as fat-density lesions that expand the lumen of the esophagus, with a thin rim of contrast surrounding the polyp, confirming its intraluminal location (Fig. 26-11B).[79,82-84] Polyps containing equal amounts of adipose and fibrovascular tissue may appear as heterogeneous lesions with focal areas of fat density juxtaposed with areas of soft tissue density (Fig. 26-12B), and polyps containing an abundance of fibrovascular tissue may appear as areas of soft tissue density with a paucity of fat.[79] Thus, fibrovascular polyps may be manifested by a spectrum of findings on CT, depending on the amount of adipose and fibrovascular tissue in these lesions. Occasionally, a centrally located feeding artery within the polyp may show contrast enhancement on CT.[85]

Fibrovascular polyps containing an abundance of adipose tissue are characterized by high signal intensity on T1-weighted MRI.[83] Such polyps may be manifested on endoscopic sonography by increased echogenicity because of their high fat content.[75,86] However, these findings are not present in polyps containing a paucity of fat.

Differential Diagnosis

Despite their size, fibrovascular polyps are sometimes difficult to diagnose on barium studies. These lesions can be mistaken for giant, coalescent air bubbles, extrinsic masses compressing the esophagus, or other polypoid intraluminal tumors such as spindle cell carcinomas or primary malignant melanomas of the esophagus (particularly if the polyps are lobulated) (see Chapter 28). When fibrovascular polyps contain an abundance of adipose tissue, the typical findings on CT or MRI should suggest the correct diagnosis.

Granular Cell Tumor

Since its original description by Abrikossoff in 1926, granular cell myoblastoma has been recognized as a rare benign tumor that predominantly involves the skin, tongue, breast, and subcutaneous tissues.[87,88] Abrikossoff believed that these tumors had a myogenic origin, but pathologic data suggest that they have a neural derivation, arising from Schwann cells.[89] The term *granular cell myoblastoma* is therefore a misnomer, and the lesions have been more correctly described as *granular cell tumors*.[90-92] Histologically, these lesions consist of sheets of polygonal tumor cells containing an eosinophilic-staining granular cytoplasm.[90,92] The tumors are covered by hyperplastic but otherwise normal squamous epithelium. About 7% of granular cell tumors are located in the gastrointestinal tract, and one third of these lesions are located in the esophagus.[88,91]

Most granular cell tumors in the esophagus occur as solitary lesions, ranging from 0.5 to 2.0 cm in size.[90] Lesions

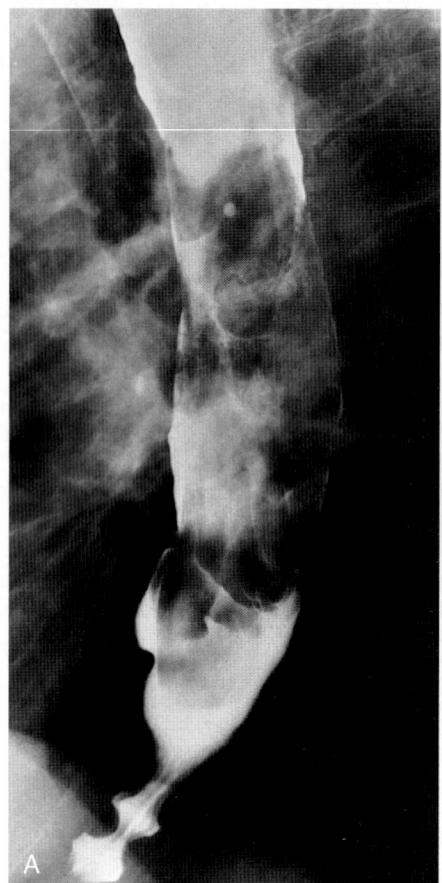
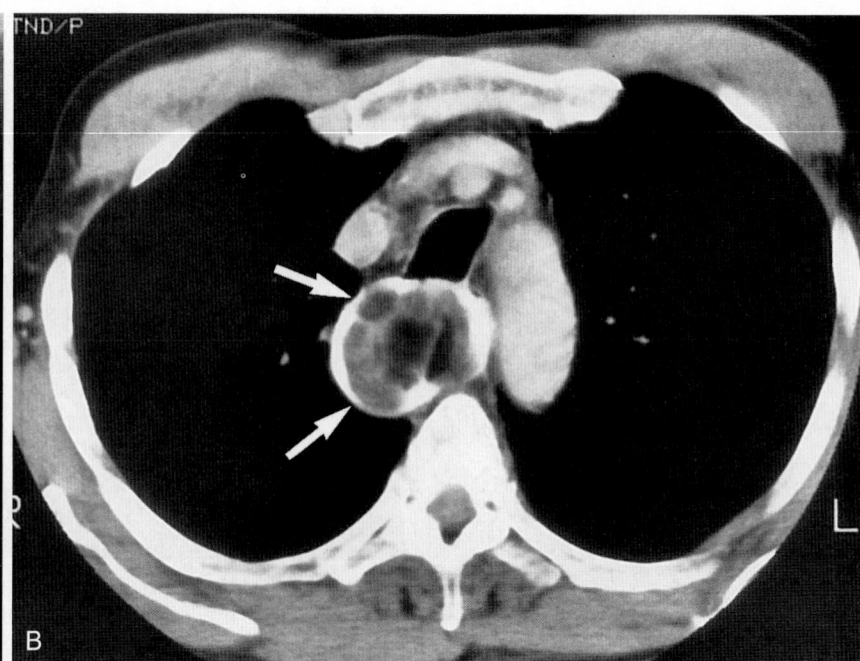

Figure 26-12. Fibrovascular polyp. A. Barium study shows an expansile mass extending into the distal thoracic esophagus. In contrast to the polyp in Figure 26-11A, this lesion has a lobulated contour, so that it could be mistaken for a malignant esophageal tumor. **B.** CT scan also shows an expansile mass (*arrows*) in the esophagus with intraluminal contrast material surrounding the lesion. In this case, note the heterogeneous appearance of the polyp with areas of fat juxtaposed with areas of soft tissue density. (From Levine MS, Buck JL, Pantongrag-Brown L, et al: Fibrovascular polyps of the esophagus: Clinical, radiographic, and pathologic findings in 16 patients. AJR 166:781-787, 1996, © by American Roentgen Ray Society.)

less than 1 cm are usually detected as incidental findings at autopsy, but larger lesions may cause dysphagia.[90,92,93] The treatment of choice for symptomatic patients with granular cell tumors is local excision because these lesions virtually never recur after endoscopic or surgical removal.[88,90-93] In contrast, asymptomatic patients with granular cell tumors found by endoscopic biopsy probably do not require surgery because of the negligible risk of malignant degeneration.[93,94] Occasionally, the findings on endoscopic biopsy specimens can be mistaken for squamous cell carcinoma as a result of pseudo-epitheliomatous hyperplasia of the overlying squamous mucosa.[90,92,94]

Radiographic Findings

Granular cell tumors usually appear on esophagography as small, round or oval submucosal masses in the distal or, less commonly, middle third of the esophagus (Fig. 26-13).[90,92] Because of their typical submucosal appearance, they are most often mistaken for leiomyomas.[90] Occasionally, granular cell tumors arising at the gastric cardia may be manifested by a polypoid or submucosal mass that distorts or obliterates the normal anatomic landmarks of this region.[92] Rarely, multiple granular cell tumors may be present in the esophagus or stomach (Fig. 26-14).[93,95]

Lipoma

The esophagus is the least common site of involvement by lipomas in the gastrointestinal tract. These tumors may appear on esophagography as discrete submucosal masses (Fig. 26-15) or, more commonly, as pedunculated, intraluminal masses.[96-99] Rarely, pedunculated lipomas in the upper esophagus can be regurgitated into the pharynx, causing asphyxia and sudden death.[98] Lipomas in the esophagus may be diagnosed preoperatively by their characteristic fat density on CT scans.[100]

Hemangioma

The esophagus is the least common site of involvement by vascular tumors in the gastrointestinal tract. Rarely, multiple esophageal hemangiomas may be found in patients with Osler-Weber-Rendu disease, a hereditary disorder characterized by multiple telangiectases of the face, lips, and mucous membranes.[101] However, most vascular tumors in the esophagus are solitary cavernous hemangiomas.[102] These highly vascular lesions may occasionally ulcerate, causing massive hematemesis and fatal exsanguination.[102] Esophageal hemangiomas usually appear on barium studies as smooth or slightly lobulated submucosal masses that are indistinguishable from other, more common benign intramural tumors.[103] Because of the risk of significant bleeding, the treatment of choice is surgical enucleation of the lesion.[102,103]

Hamartoma

Esophageal hamartomas are rare, benign tumors characterized histologically by metaplastic respiratory epithelium and

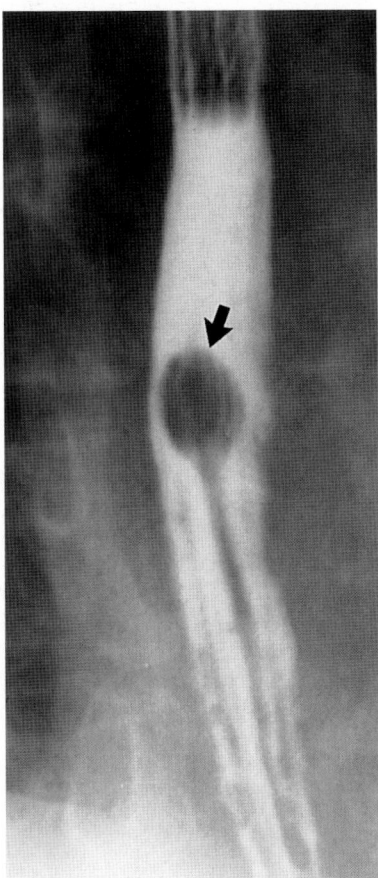

Figure 26-13. Granular cell tumor. A smooth submucosal mass (*arrow*) is seen in the midesophagus. This lesion cannot be differentiated from other, more common submucosal lesions in the esophagus, such as leiomyomas. (From Levine MS: Radiology of the Esophagus. Philadelphia, WB Saunders, 1989.)

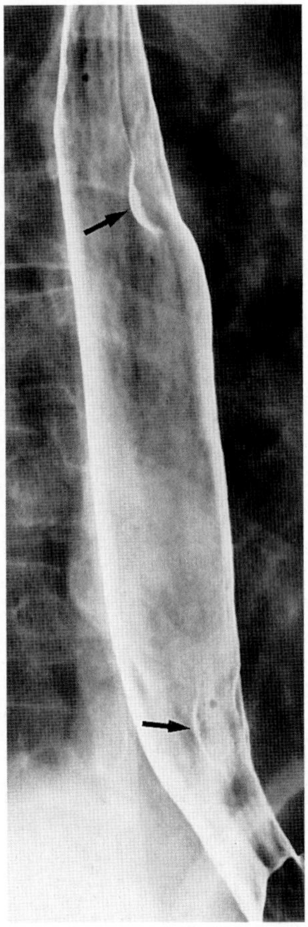

Figure 26-14. Multiple granular cell tumors. The lesions are seen as discrete submucosal masses (*arrows*) in the middle and distal thirds of the esophagus. This patient had additional granular cell tumors in the stomach. (From Levine MS: Radiology of the Esophagus. Philadelphia, WB Saunders, 1989.)

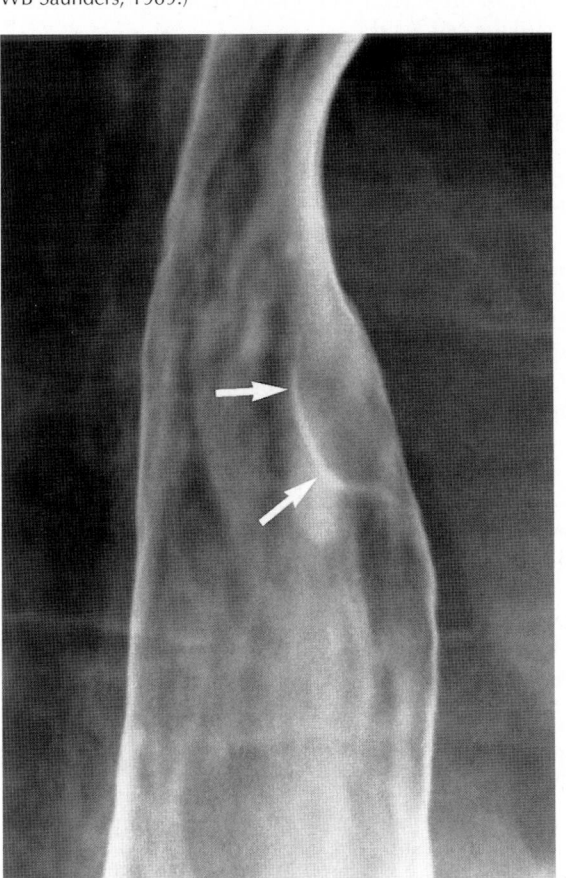

Figure 26-15. Esophageal lipoma. This patient has a discrete submucosal mass (*arrows*) that is indistinguishable from other, more common intramural tumors. (From Levine MS: Radiology of the Esophagus. Philadelphia, WB Saunders, 1989.)

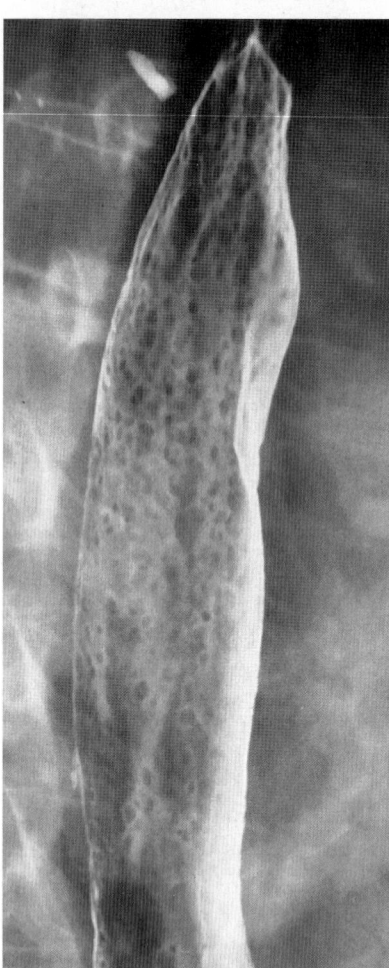

Figure 26-16. Cowden's disease with multiple hamartomatous polyps in the esophagus. The lesions appear as tiny, nodular elevations on the mucosa. (Courtesy of Stephen W. Trenkner, MD, Minneapolis, MN.)

islets of cartilage in a fibrous stroma.[104,105] These tumors usually appear on esophagography as pedunculated, intraluminal masses that are indistinguishable from fibrovascular polyps.[104] Rarely, multiple esophageal hamartomas may be found in patients with Cowden's disease or multiple hamartoma syndrome, an autosomal dominant, hereditary disorder characterized by multiple hamartomatous malformations of ectodermal, mesodermal, and endodermal layers as well as benign or malignant tumors of the skin, breast, gastrointestinal tract, and thyroid.[106,107] Esophageal involvement may be manifested by innumerable tiny, hamartomatous polyps in the esophagus, producing a diffusely nodular mucosa on double-contrast images (Fig. 26-16).[106,107] When the esophagus is involved by this disease, widespread polyposis of the gastrointestinal tract is usually present. Cowden's disease should be distinguished from other polyposis syndromes, however, which almost never involve the esophagus.

Other Mesenchymal Tumors

Other rare mesenchymal tumors in the esophagus include fibromas, neurofibromas, and myxofibromas.[47] These lesions usually appear on barium studies as discrete intramural masses that are indistinguishable from leiomyomas. When mesen-

chymal tumors contain a substantial amount of fibrovascular or adipose tissue, they can slowly elongate, forming pedunculated, intraluminal masses. Because the latter tumors have characteristic clinical, radiographic, and pathologic findings, they have been classified together as fibrovascular polyps (see earlier section on Fibrovascular Polyp).

Cysts

Duplication Cyst

Esophageal duplication cysts comprise about 20% of all gastrointestinal tract duplications.[108] These cysts result from abnormal embryologic development in which nests of cells are sequestered from the primitive foregut.[109] The lesions may be classified either as cystic duplications or, less commonly, as tubular duplications. About 60% are located in the lower half of the posterior mediastinum, often projecting to the right of the distal esophagus.[108] Although most duplication cysts are noncommunicating, tubular duplications occasionally may communicate directly with the esophageal lumen. Histologically, duplication cysts contain a mucosa, submucosa, and muscularis propria and are lined by ciliated columnar or cuboidal epithelium.[109] In about 40% of cases, ectopic gastric mucosa is found in the lining of the cyst wall.[108] Esophageal duplication cysts may be detected as an isolated finding, but some lesions are associated with vertebral anomalies, esophageal atresia, or other congenital anomalies.[108]

Most adults with esophageal duplication cysts are asymptomatic, but symptoms may occasionally be caused by obstruction, bleeding, or infection of the cyst.[110,111] Bleeding or perforation is more likely to occur when ectopic gastric mucosa is present in the cyst wall.[108]

Radiographic Findings

Esophageal duplication cysts can sometimes be recognized on chest radiographs by the presence of a right lower mediastinal mass. Chest radiographs may occasionally reveal associated vertebral anomalies in these patients.[108] The cysts usually appear on esophagography as discrete submucosal masses that are indistinguishable from solid intramural tumors (Fig. 26-17). Rarely, communicating duplications may be manifested by tubular, branching outpouchings from the esophagus as a result of filling of these structures with barium (Fig. 26-18).[112]

Cross-sectional imaging studies can sometimes aid in the diagnosis of esophageal duplication cysts. Because these cysts are fluid-filled structures, they typically have homogeneous low attenuation on CT scans and high signal intensity on T2-weighted MR images (Fig. 26-19).[113,114] Endoscopic ultrasound may reveal a smooth, spherical or, less commonly, tubular structure with a hyperechoic inner mucosa layer and a hypoechoic outer muscular layer.[115] Technetium Tc 99m pertechnetate scintigraphy may help to confirm the diagnosis of an esophageal duplication cyst containing ectopic gastric mucosa.[108]

Retention Cyst

Acquired esophageal cysts are much less common than congenital duplication cysts. They probably result from abnormal dilatation of columnar epithelium-lined mucous glands in

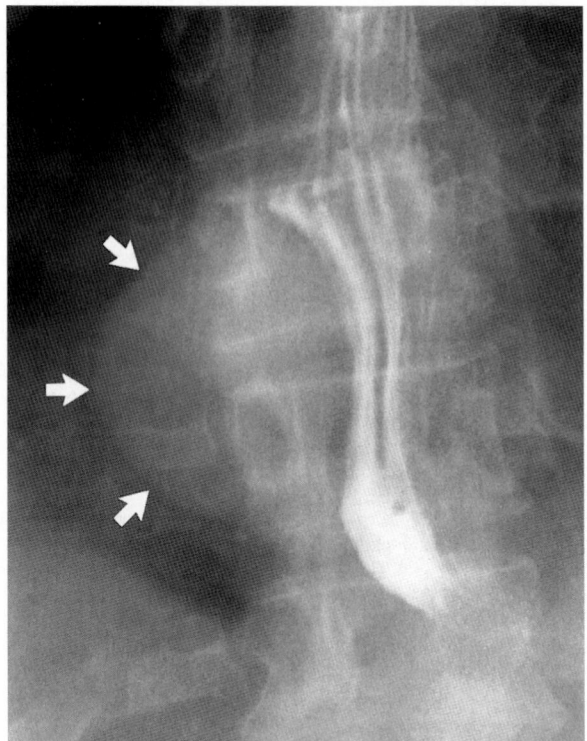

Figure 26-17. Duplication cyst. There is a large submucosal mass in the distal esophagus. The lateral border of the cyst (*arrows*) is readily visible where it abuts the right lung. Duplication cysts typically occur in this location. (From Levine MS: Radiology of the Esophagus. Philadelphia, WB Saunders, 1989.)

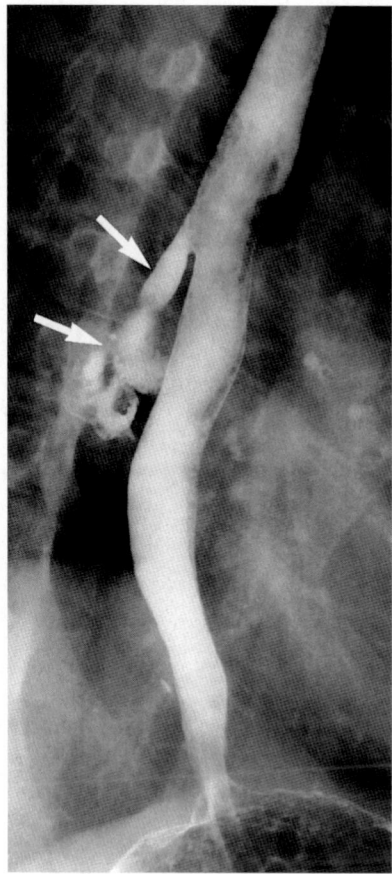

Figure 26-18. Duplication cyst. Barium study shows the rare communicating form of duplication cyst as a tubular, branching outpouching (*arrows*) from the midesophagus. (Courtesy of Marie Latour, MD, Philadelphia, PA.)

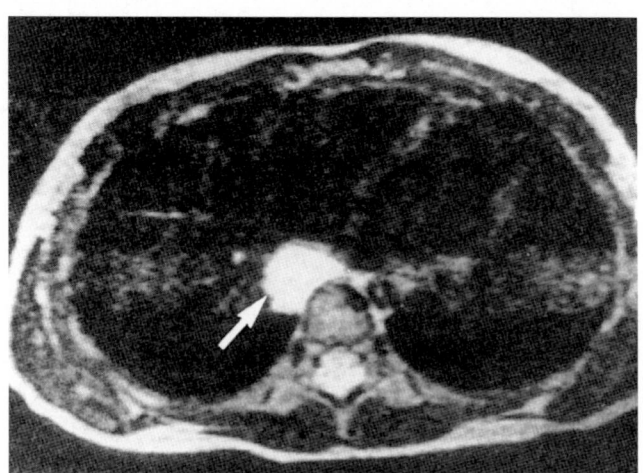

Figure 26-19. Duplication cyst. Axial T2-weighted MR image shows a fluid-filled, cystic mass (*arrow*) with high signal intensity in the right side of the mediastinum. (From Rafal RB, Markisz JA: Magnetic resonance imaging of an esophageal duplication cyst. Am J Gastroenterol 86:1809-1811, 1991, reprinted with permission from the American College of Gastroenterology.)

the submucosa and are therefore called *esophageal retention cysts* or *mucoceles*.[116-119] Histologically, these cysts are lined by nonciliated, columnar or cuboidal epithelium.[118] The pathogenesis of these lesions is uncertain, but it has been postulated that submucosal glands in the esophagus may become cystically dilated because of mechanical obstruction of the excretory ducts by mucus plugs or abnormally viscous mucus.[116,117] This entity has sometimes been described as esophagitis cystica, but *esophageal retention cyst* is a more appropriate descriptive term because only minimal inflammatory change may be present in these lesions.[116,117]

Esophageal retention cysts may appear on barium studies as solitary or, more commonly, multiple submucosal masses in the distal esophagus (Fig. 26-20).[116,117,119] As a result, the lesions cannot be distinguished radiographically from other submucosal tumors. These patients are usually asymptomatic, however, so that most esophageal retention cysts are discovered as incidental findings at autopsy.[116]

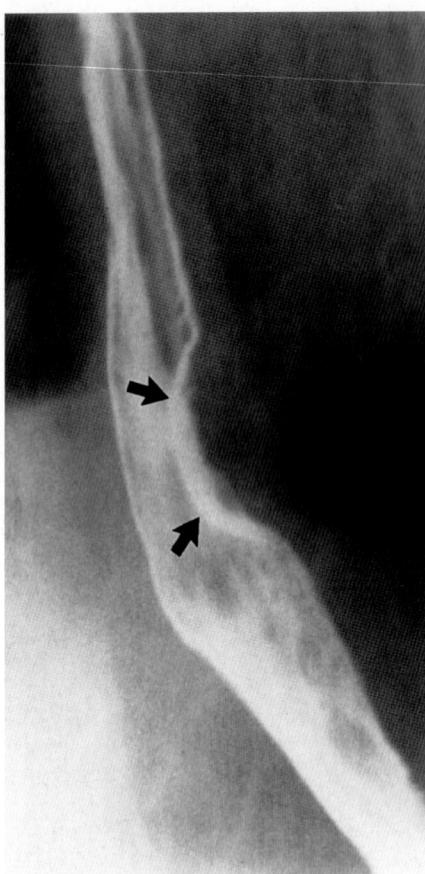

Figure 26-20. Esophageal retention cyst. The lesion is seen as a discrete submucosal mass (*arrows*) that is indistinguishable from other intramural lesions. (From Levine MS: Radiology of the Esophagus. Philadelphia, WB Saunders, 1989.)

References

1. Ming SC: Tumors of the esophagus and stomach. In Atlas of Tumor Pathology, fascicle 7. Washington, DC, Armed Forces Institute of Pathology, 1973, pp 16-23.
2. Plachta A: Benign tumors of the esophagus: Review of literature and report of 99 cases. Am J Gastroenterol 38:639-652, 1962.
3. Miller BJ, Murphy F, Lukie BE: Squamous cell papilloma of esophagus. Can J Surg 21:538-540, 1978.
4. Politoske EJ: Squamous papilloma of the esophagus associated with human papillomavirus. Gastroenterology 102:668-673, 1992.
5. Carr NJ, Monihan JM, Sobin LH: Squamous cell papilloma of the esophagus: A clinicopathologic and follow-up study of 25 cases. Am J Gastroenterol 89:245-248, 1994.
6. Napalkov NP, Pozharisski KM: Morphogenesis of experimental tumors of the esophagus. J Natl Cancer Inst 42:927-933, 1969.
7. Samitz MH, Ackerman AB, Lantis LR: Squamous cell carcinoma arising at the site of oral florid papillomatosis. Arch Dermatol 96:286-290, 1967.
8. Toso G: Epithelial papillomas-benign or malignant? Laryngoscope 81:1524-1531, 1971.
9. Gilbert EF, Palladino A: Squamous papillomas of the uterine cervix: Review of the literature and report of a giant papillary carcinoma. Am J Clin Pathol 46:115-121, 1966.
10. Minielly JA, Harrison EG, Fontana RS, et al: Verrucous squamous cell carcinoma of the esophagus. Cancer 20:2078-2087, 1967.
11. Zeabart LE, Fabian J, Nord HJ: Squamous papilloma of the esophagus: A report of 3 cases. Gastrointest Endosc 25:18-20, 1979.
12. Nuwayhid NS, Ballard ET, Cotton R: Esophageal papillomatosis. Ann Otol Rhinol Laryngol 86:623-625, 1977.
13. Waterfall WE, Somers S, Desa DJ: Benign oesophageal papillomatosis. J Clin Pathol 31:111-115, 1978.
14. Sandvik AK, Aase S, Kveberg KH, et al: Papillomatosis of the esophagus. J Clin Gastroenterol 22:35-37, 1996.
15. Montesi A, Alessandro P, Graziani L, et al: Small benign tumors of the esophagus: Radiological diagnosis with double-contrast examination. Gastrointest Radiol 8:207-212, 1983.
16. Walker JH: Giant papilloma of the thoracic esophagus. AJR 131:519-520, 1978.
17. Spin FP: Adenomas of the esophagus: A case report and review of the literature. Gastrointest Endosc 20:26-27, 1973.
18. McDonald GB, Brand DL, Thorning DR: Multiple adenomatous neoplasms arising in columnar-lined (Barrett's) esophagus. Gastroenterology 72:1317-1321, 1977.
19. Levine MS, Caroline D, Thompson JJ, et al: Adenocarcinoma of the esophagus: Relationship to Barrett mucosa. Radiology 150:305-309, 1984.
20. Bleshman MH, Banner MP, Johnson RC, et al: The inflammatory esophagogastric polyp and fold. Radiology 128:589-593, 1978.
21. Staples DC, Knodell RG, Johnson LF: Inflammatory pseudotumor of the esophagus. Gastrointest Endosc 24:175-176, 1978.
22. Jones TB, Heller RM, Kirchner SG, et al: Inflammatory esophagogastric polyp in children. AJR 133:314-316, 1979.
23. Styles RA, Gibb SP, Tarshis A, et al: Esophagogastric polyps: Radiographic and endoscopic findings. Radiology 154:307-311, 1985.
24. Ghahremani GG, Fisher MR, Rushovich AM: Prolapsing inflammatory pseudopolyp-fold complex of the oesophagogastric region. Eur J Radiol 4:47-51, 1984.
25. Rywlin AM, Ortega R: Glycogenic acanthosis of the esophagus. Arch Pathol 90:439-443, 1970.
26. Bender MD, Allison J, Cuartas F, et al: Glycogenic acanthosis of the esophagus: A form of benign epithelial hyperplasia. Gastroenterology 65:373-380, 1973.
27. Stern Z, Sharon P, Ligumsky M, et al: Glycogenic acanthosis of the esophagus: A benign but confusing endoscopic lesion. Am J Gastroenterol 74:261-263, 1980.
28. Vadva MD, Triadafilopoulos G: Glycogenic acanthosis of the esophagus and gastroesophageal reflux. J Clin Gastroenterol 17:79-83, 1993.
29. Rose D, Furth EE, Rubesin SE: Glycogenic acanthosis. AJR 164:96, 1995.
30. Ghahremani GG, Rushovich AM: Glycogenic acanthosis of the esophagus: Radiographic and pathologic features. Gastrointest Radiol 9:93-98, 1984.
31. Glick SN, Teplick SK, Goldstein J, et al: Glycogenic acanthosis of the esophagus. AJR 139:683-688, 1982.
32. Berliner L, Redmond P, Horowitz L, et al: Glycogen plaques (glycogenic acanthosis) of the esophagus. Radiology 141:607-610, 1981.
33. Herschman BR, Uppaputhangkule V, Maas L, et al: Esophageal leukoplakia: A rare entity. JAMA 239:2021, 1978.
34. Graziani L, Bearzi I, Romagnoli A, et al: Significance of diffuse granularity and nodularity of the esophageal mucosa at double-contrast radiography. Gastrointest Radiol 10:1-6, 1985.
35. Itai Y, Kogure T, Okuyama Y, et al: Diffuse finely nodular lesions of the esophagus. AJR 128:563-566, 1977.
36. Itai Y, Kogure T, Okuyama Y, et al: Radiological manifestations of oesophageal involvement in acanthosis nigricans. Br J Radiol 49:592-593, 1976.
37. Attah EB, Hajdu SI: Benign and malignant tumors of the esophagus at autopsy. J Thorac Cardiovasc Surg 5:396-404, 1968.
38. Goldstein HM, Zornoza J, Hopens T: Intrinsic diseases of the adult esophagus: Benign and malignant tumors. Semin Roentgenol 16:183-197, 1981.
39. Seremetis MG, Lyons WS, DeGuzman VC, et al: Leiomyomata of the esophagus: An analysis of 838 cases. Cancer 38:2166-2177, 1976.
40. Tsuzuki T, Kakegawa T, Arimori M, et al: Giant leiomyoma of the esophagus and cardia weighing more than 1,000 grams. Chest 60:396-399, 1971.
41. Barriero F, Seco JL, Molina J, et al: Giant esophageal leiomyoma with secondary megaesophagus. Surgery 7:436-439, 1976.
42. Godard JE, McCranie D: Multiple leiomyomas of the esophagus. AJR 117:259-262, 1973.
43. Shaffer HA: Multiple leiomyomas of the esophagus. Radiology 118:29-34, 1976.
44. Wahlen T, Astedt B: Familial occurrence of coexisting leiomyomas of vulva and oesophagus. Acta Obstet Gynecol Scand 44:197-203, 1965.
45. Schapiro RL, Sandrock AR: Esophagogastric and vulvar leiomyomatosis: A new radiologic syndrome. J Can Assoc Radiol 24:184-187, 1973.
46. Ullal SR: Hypertrophic osteoarthropathy and leiomyoma of the esophagus. Am J Surg 123:356-358, 1972.

47. Totten RS, Stout AP, Humphreys GH, et al: Benign tumors and cysts of the esophagus. J Thorac Surg 25:606-622, 1953.

48. Rubin RA, Lichtenstein GR, Morris JB: Acute esophageal obstruction: A unique presentation of a giant intramural esophageal leiomyoma. Am J Gastroenterol 87:1669-1671, 1992.

49. Glanz I, Grunebaum M: The radiological approach to leiomyoma of the oesophagus with a long-term follow-up. Clin Radiol 28:197-200, 1977.

50. Griff LC, Cooper J: Leiomyoma of the esophagus presenting as a mediastinal mass. AJR 101:472-481, 1967.

51. Gutman E: Posterior mediastinal calcification due to esophageal leiomyoma. Gastroenterology 63:665-666, 1972.

52. Ghahremani GG, Meyers MA, Port RB: Calcified primary tumors of the gastrointestinal tract. Gastrointest Radiol 2:331-339, 1978.

53. Itai Y, Shimazu H: Leiomyosarcoma of the oesophagus with dense calcification. Br J Radiol 51:469-471, 1978.

54. Schatzki R, Hawes LE: The roentgenological appearance of extramucosal tumors of the esophagus: Analysis of intramural extramucosal lesions of the gastrointestinal tract in general. AJR 48:1-15, 1942.

55. Megibow AJ, Balthazar EJ, Hulnick DH, et al: CT evaluation of gastrointestinal leiomyomas and leiomyosarcomas. AJR 144:727-731, 1985.

56. Orchard JL, Peternel WW, Arena S: Remarkably large, benign esophageal tumor: Difficulties in diagnosis. Dig Dis 22:266-269, 1977.

57. Schnug GE: Leiomyoma of the cardioesophageal junction. Arch Surg 65:342-346, 1952.

58. Stein LA, Margulis AR: The spheroid sign: A new sign for accurate differentiation of intramural from extramural masses. AJR 123:420-426, 1975.

59. Fernandes JP, Mascarenhas MJ, daCosta JC, et al: Diffuse leiomyomatosis of the esophagus: A case report and review of the literature. Am J Dig Dis 20:684-690, 1975.

60. Kabuto T, Taniguchi K, Iwanaga T, et al: Diffuse leiomyomatosis of the esophagus. Dig Dis Sci 25:388-391, 1980.

61. Levine MS, Buck JL, Pantongrag-Brown L, et al: Esophageal leiomyomatosis. Radiology 199:533-536, 1996.

62. Cochat P, Guibaud P, Garcia Torres R, et al: Diffuse leiomyomatosis in Alport syndrome. J Pediatr 133:339-343, 1988.

63. Lonsdale RN, Roberts PF, Vaughan R, et al: Familial oesophageal leiomyomatosis and nephropathy. Histopathology 20:127-133, 1992.

64. Rosen RM: Familial multiple upper gastrointestinal leiomyoma. Am J Gastroenterol 85:303-305, 1990.

65. Lerone M, Dodero P, Romeo G, et al: Leiomyomatosis of oesophagus, congenital cataracts and hematuria: Report of a case with rectal involvement. Pediatr Radiol 21:578-579, 1991.

66. Faber K, Jones MA, Spratt D, et al: Vulvar leiomyomatosis in a patient with esophagogastric leiomyomatosis: Review of the syndrome. Gynecol Oncol 41:929-994, 1991.

67. Rabushka LS, Fishman EK, Kuhlman JE, et al: Diffuse esophageal leiomyomatosis in a patient with Alport syndrome: CT demonstration. Radiology 179:176-178, 1991.

68. Johnstone AS: Diffuse spasm and diffuse muscle hypertrophy of lower oesophagus. Br J Radiol 32:723-725, 1960.

69. Demian SD, Vargas-Cortes F: Idiopathic muscular hypertrophy of the esophagus: Post-mortem incidental finding in six cases and review of the literature. Chest 73:288-292, 1978.

70. Zeller R, McLelland R, Meyers B, et al: Idiopathic muscular hypertrophy of the esophagus: A case report. Gastrointest Radiol 4:121-125, 1979.

71. Agostini S, Grimaud JC, Salducci J, et al: Idiopathic muscular hypertrophy of the esophagus: CT features. J Comput Assist Tomogr 12:1041-1043, 1988.

72. Tucker HJ, Snape WJ, Cohen SC: Achalasia secondary to carcinoma: Manometric and clinical features. Ann Intern Med 89:315-318, 1978.

73. Burrell M, Toffler R: Fibrovascular polyp of the esophagus. Am J Dig Dis 18:714-718, 1973.

74. Lolley D, Razzuk MA, Urschel HC: Giant fibrovascular polyp of the esophagus. Ann Thorac Surg 22:383-385, 1976.

75. Avezzano EA, Fleischer DE, Merida MA, et al: Giant fibrovascular polyps of the esophagus. Am J Gastroenterol 85:299-302, 1990.

76. Patel J, Kieffer RW, Martin M, et al: Giant fibrovascular polyp of the esophagus. Gastroenterology 87:953-956, 1984.

77. Watanabe H, Jass JR, Sobin LH: World Health Organization: Histological Typing of Oesophageal and Gastric Tumours, 2nd ed. Berlin, Springer-Verlag, 1990.

78. Timmons B, Sedwitz JL, Oller DW: Benign fibrovascular polyp of the esophagus. South Med J 84:1370-1372, 1991.

79. Levine MS, Buck JL, Pantongrag-Brown L, et al: Fibrovascular polyps of the esophagus: Clinical, radiographic, and pathologic findings in 16 patients. AJR 166:781-787, 1996.

80. Cochet B, Hohl P, Sans M, et al: Asphyxia caused by laryngeal impaction of an esophageal polyp. Arch Otolaryngol 106:176-178, 1980.

81. Carter MM, Kulkarni MV: Giant fibrovascular polyp of the esophagus. Gastrointest Radiol 9:301-303, 1984.

82. Walters NA, Coral A: Fibrovascular polyp of the oesophagus: The appearances on computed tomography. Br J Radiol 61:641-643, 1988.

83. Whitman GJ, Borkowski GP: Giant fibrovascular polyp of the esophagus: CT and MR findings. AJR 152:518-520, 1989.

84. LeBlanc J, Carrier G, Ferland S, et al: Fibrovascular polyp of the esophagus with computed tomographic and pathological correlation. Can Assoc Radiol J 41:87-89, 1990.

85. Kim TS, Song SY, Han J, et al: Giant fibrovascular polyp of the esophagus: CT findings. Abdom Imaging 20:653-655, 2005.

86. Lawrence SP, Larsen BR, Stacy CC, et al: Echoendosonographic and histologic correlation of a fibrovascular polyp of the esophagus. Gastrointest Endosc 40:81-84, 1994.

87. Paskin DL, Hall JD, Cookson PJ: Granular cell myoblastoma: A comprehensive review of 15 years experience. Ann Surg 175:501-504, 1972.

88. Lack EE, Worsham GF, Callihan MD, et al: Granular cell tumor: A clinicopathologic study of 110 patients. J Surg Oncol 13:301-306, 1980.

89. Fisher ER, Wechsler H: Granular cell myoblastoma—a misnomer: Electron microscopic and histochemical evidence concerning its Schwann cell derivation and nature (granular cell schwannoma). Cancer 15:936-954, 1962.

90. Gershwind ME, Chiat H, Addei KA, et al: Granular cell tumors of the esophagus. Gastrointest Radiol 2:327-330, 1978.

91. Johnston J, Helwig EB: Granular cell tumors of the gastrointestinal tract and perianal region: A study of 74 cases. Dig Dis Sci 26:807-816, 1981.

92. Rubesin SE, Herlinger H, Sigal H: Granular cell tumors of the esophagus. Gastrointest Radiol 10:11-15, 1985.

93. Orlowska J, Pachlewski J, Gugulski A, et al: A conservative approach to granular cell tumors of the esophagus: Four case reports and literature review. Am J Gastroenterol 88:311-315, 1993.

94. Subramanyam K, Shannon CR, Patterson M, et al: Granular cell myoblastoma of the esophagus. J Clin Gastroenterol 6:113-118, 1984.

95. Radin DR, Zelner R, Ray MJ, et al: Multiple granular cell tumors of the skin and gastrointestinal tract. AJR 147:1305-1307, 1986.

96. Kinnear JS: Report of case of intramural lipoma of the oesophagus. Br J Surg 42:439, 1955.

97. Nora PF: Lipoma of the esophagus. Am J Surg 108:353-356, 1964.

98. Allen MS, Talbot WH: Sudden death due to regurgitation of a pedunculated esophageal lipoma. J Thorac Cardiovasc Surg 54:756-758, 1967.

99. Liliequist B, Wiberg A: Pedunculated tumours of the oesophagus: Two cases of lipoma. Acta Radiol Diagn (Stockh) 15:383-392, 1974.

100. Gandini G, Andreis M, Avataneo T, et al: A case of esophageal lipoma diagnosed by computed tomography. Diagn Radiol 10:55-60, 1985.

101. Loughry RW: Hemangiomas of the esophagus. Rocky Mt Med J 68:37-39, 1971.

102. Grimes OF: Cavernous hemangioma of the esophagus. Dis Chest 48:384, 1965.

103. Govoni AF: Hemangiomas of the esophagus. Gastrointest Radiol 7:113-117, 1982.

104. Dieter RA, Riker WL, Holinger P: Pedunculated esophageal hamartoma in a child. J Thorac Cardiovasc Surg 59:851-854, 1970.

105. Shah B, Unger L, Heimlich HJ: Hamartomatous polyp of the esophagus. Arch Surg 110:326-328, 1975.

106. Hauser H, Ody B, Plojoux O, et al: Radiological findings in multiple hamartoma syndrome (Cowden disease): A report of three cases. Radiology 137:317-323, 1980.

107. Chen YM, Ott DJ, Wu WC, et al: Cowden's disease: A case report and literature review. Gastrointest Radiol 12:325-329, 1987.

108. Macpherson RI: Gastrointestinal tract duplications: Clinical, pathologic, etiologic, and radiologic considerations. RadioGraphics 13:1063-1080, 1993.

109. Vithespongse P, Blank S: Ciliated epithelial esophageal cyst. Am J Gastroenterol 56:436-440, 1971.

110. Gatzinsky P, Fasth S, Hansson G: Intramural oesophageal cyst with massive mediastinal bleeding. Scand J Thorac Cardiovasc Surg 12:143-145, 1978.

111. Whitaker JA, Deffenbaugh LD, Cooke AR: Esophageal duplication cyst. Am J Gastroenterol 73:329-332, 1980.

112. Erdozain JC, Lizasoain J, Martin-de-Argila C, et al: Esophagus duplication in a young adult. Am J Gastroenterol 90:663-665, 1995.

113. Bondestam S, Salo JA, Salonen OLM, et al: Imaging of congenital esophageal cysts in adults. Gastrointest Radiol 15:279-281, 1990.

114. Rafal RB, Markisz JA: Magnetic resonance imaging of an esophageal duplication cyst. Am J Gastroenterol 86:1809-1811, 1991.

115. Geller A, Wang KK, Dimagno EP: Diagnosis of foregut duplication cysts by endoscopic ultrasonography. Gastroenterology 109:838-842, 1995.

116. Voirol MW, Welsh RA, Genet EF: Esophagitis cystica. Am J Gastroenterol 59:446-453, 1973.

117. Farman J, Rosen Y, Dallemand S, et al: Esophagitis cystica: Lower esophageal retention cysts. AJR 128:495-496, 1977.

118. Edgin R, Mekhjian HS: Esophageal retention cyst: Unusual cause for dysphagia. J Clin Gastroenterol 3:57-59, 1981.

119. Hover AR, Brady CE, Williams JR, et al: Multiple retention cysts of the lower esophagus. J Clin Gastroenterol 4:209-212, 1982.

Carcinoma of the Esophagus

Marc S. Levine, MD • Robert A. Halvorsen, MD

Esophageal carcinoma constitutes only about 1% of all cancers and 7% of cancers in the gastrointestinal tract.[1] Nevertheless, it is a deadly disease, with an overall 5-year survival rate of only about 15%.[2] At one time, most malignant tumors of the esophagus were thought to be squamous cell carcinomas, but adenocarcinomas arising in Barrett's esophagus have increased dramatically in incidence since the 1970s. Because of important differences between these tumors, the chapter is divided into separate sections on squamous cell carcinoma and adenocarcinoma of the esophagus.

SQUAMOUS CELL CARCINOMA

Epidemiology

Esophageal carcinoma is predominantly a disease of elderly men, with a male-to-female ratio of nearly 4:1 and a peak incidence between 65 and 74 years of age.[2] The development of squamous cell carcinoma of the esophagus is a multifactorial process associated with a variety of risk factors, including tobacco and alcohol consumption, obesity, nutritional deficiencies, exposure to various environmental carcinogens, and geographic location.

Two of the major risk factors for the development of esophageal cancer in the United States are tobacco and alcohol consumption.[3,4] Tobacco and alcohol appear to have a synergistic effect, so that people who smoke and drink have even higher rates of esophageal cancer.[5] Although tobacco smoke is known to contain a variety of carcinogens, the development of esophageal carcinoma in alcoholics may be related to other factors, such as poor health and nutritional deficiencies. Obesity also has been recognized as an important risk factor for the development of esophageal cancer.[4,6]

Squamous cell carcinoma of the esophagus has striking geographic variations, with the highest incidences reported in an Asian esophageal cancer belt stretching from eastern Turkey and northern Iran to India and northern China.[7] A high incidence has also been reported in South Africa and France. These regional variations in the frequency of esophageal cancer have been attributed primarily to environmental rather than hereditary factors. Dietary habits in particular have been implicated, because people living in areas with a high incidence of esophageal cancer often have diets high in starch and low in fresh fruits and vegetables.[7] Other environmental factors may also have a role in cancer pathogenesis. For example, nitrosamines and other nitroso compounds are potent

417

carcinogens that occur in high concentration in the food and water supply of parts of northern China.[8] Epidemiologic studies in China and South Africa have shown that these areas also have unusually low levels of molybdenum in the soil.[9,10] Because molybdenum is required for the metabolism of nitrite to ammonia, low levels of molybdenum in the soil could lead to accumulation of nitrites and potentially carcinogenic nitrosamines in plants consumed by humans. The high prevalence of esophageal cancer in parts of Saudi Arabia has been attributed to contamination of drinking water by impurities such as petroleum oils.[11] Other substances such as tannin, betel leaves, and asbestos fibers have also been implicated in the development of esophageal cancer.[12-14]

Attention has also been focused on the potential role of human papillomavirus in the pathogenesis of esophageal cancer, particularly in high-risk areas such as China and South Africa. In studies from China, human papillomavirus has been isolated by in situ hybridization techniques in 25% to 50% of esophageal cancer specimens.[15,16] These data suggest that human papillomavirus may be an important contributing factor in the development of esophageal cancer.

Predisposing Conditions

Conditions that are thought to predispose patients to the development of squamous cell carcinoma of the esophagus include achalasia, lye strictures, head and neck tumors, celiac disease, Plummer-Vinson syndrome, radiation, and tylosis. Because of the increased risk of developing esophageal cancer, periodic surveillance has often been advocated for patients with these conditions.

Achalasia

Achalasia is thought to be a premalignant condition associated with an increased risk of developing esophageal carcinoma. In various studies, the prevalence of esophageal cancer in patients with long-standing achalasia has ranged from 2% to 8%.[17-19] Malignant degeneration presumably occurs as a result of chronic stasis esophagitis caused by retained food and debris in a dilated, obstructed esophagus.[17-20] Most patients have had achalasia for at least 20 years before the development of cancer.[17,19,20] Unfortunately, a neoplastic lesion growing inside a massively dilated esophagus may not cause symptoms until it is an advanced, unresectable tumor.[19,21] As a result, some authors believe that patients with long-standing achalasia should undergo annual surveillance with barium studies or endoscopy to detect developing cancers at the earliest possible stage.[17,20,21] However, one study failed to show an increased cancer risk in these patients.[22] Thus, not all investigators accept the need for surveillance.

Lye Strictures

Patients with chronic lye strictures have an increased risk of developing esophageal carcinoma. In various studies, the prevalence of cancer has ranged from 2% to 16%.[23,24] Although the pathogenesis is uncertain, it has been postulated that chronic inflammation and scarring from caustic esophagitis predispose these patients to the development of esophageal carcinoma. The average latent period between the ingestion of lye and the development of cancer is 40 to 45 years.[25,26]

These patients usually seek medical attention for recurrent or suddenly worsening dysphagia many years after lye ingestion. Carcinomas arising in lye strictures have a better prognosis than most esophageal cancers, with 5-year survival rates of 8% to 33%.[25] This more favorable prognosis may be related to the presence of dense scar tissue surrounding the tumor, which prevents early invasion of adjacent mediastinal structures.[25,26] Some investigators advocate periodic surveillance of patients with long-standing lye strictures, but these individuals are often in socioeconomic groups least likely to be compliant with surveillance programs.

Head and Neck Tumors

Patients with primary squamous cell carcinomas of the oral cavity, pharynx, and larynx have a significantly increased risk of developing separate primary esophageal carcinomas. In various studies, 2% to 8% of patients with head and neck tumors who underwent endoscopic surveillance were found to have synchronous esophageal cancers.[27-29] This association has been attributed to common predisposing factors, primarily smoking and drinking, because exposure to tobacco and alcohol considerably increases the risk of squamous cell carcinoma in both areas.[30] Radiologic or endoscopic evaluation of the esophagus has therefore been advocated in the initial work-up of all patients with head and neck tumors. Many of these synchronous esophageal cancers are small, asymptomatic lesions, so screening examinations may detect such tumors at an early stage, when they are potentially curable.[29] Discovery of an advanced lesion in the esophagus is also important, because radical head and neck surgery may no longer be appropriate in these patients. The risk of developing subsequent metachronous esophageal carcinomas is also considerably increased in patients with head and neck tumors. Some form of ongoing surveillance is therefore required to detect metachronous esophageal lesions.

Celiac Disease

Celiac disease (nontropical sprue) is thought to be associated with an increased risk of developing esophageal carcinoma.[31,32] The pathogenesis of cancer in these patients is uncertain, but it has been postulated that absorption of carcinogens occurs through an atrophic jejunal mucosa due to advanced celiac disease.[32] Most patients have long-standing disease; malabsorption is present for an average of 35 years before the development of cancer.[31] Some investigators therefore advocate radiologic or endoscopic surveillance of the esophagus in these patients.

Plummer-Vinson Syndrome

Plummer-Vinson, or Paterson-Kelly, syndrome is characterized by iron-deficiency anemia, glossitis, postcricoid webs, and dysphagia.[33] This syndrome has been described primarily in women of Scandinavian origin. The prevalence of hypopharyngeal or esophageal carcinoma in Plummer-Vinson syndrome has ranged from 4% to 16%.[33,34] Almost all such cancers are associated with postcricoid webs.[33] Radiologic or endoscopic examinations are therefore required to differentiate webs from superimposed hypopharyngeal or esophageal carcinomas in these patients.

Radiation

Esophageal cancer is a rare complication of chronic radiation injury to the esophagus. Most cases have occurred in the cervical or upper thoracic esophagus after radiation doses of 20 to 50 Gy to the mediastinum or neck.[35,36] In one study, women who received radiation therapy for carcinoma of the breast were found to have an increased risk of esophageal carcinoma.[37] In general, however, the average latent period between radiation therapy and the development of cancer is about 30 years.[36] It is therefore difficult to prove that these lesions are not coincidental cancers arising in a previously irradiated area.

Tylosis

Tylosis (Howel-Evans syndrome) is an extremely rare, hereditary, autosomal dominant disorder characterized by hyperkeratosis of the palms and soles, with thickening and fissuring of the skin. This disorder is associated with an extraordinarily high risk of developing esophageal cancer.[38-40] In one study, 95% of patients with tylosis had esophageal cancer by age 65 years.[39] Most of these patients are found to have advanced, unresectable tumors at the time of clinical presentation. However, asymptomatic individuals with tylosis may have hyperkeratotic esophageal plaques containing foci of dysplasia, intramucosal carcinoma, or invasive carcinoma.[40] Thus, periodic surveillance of asymptomatic family members has been advocated to detect premalignant lesions before the development of overt carcinoma. Because of the high likelihood of developing esophageal cancer, a prophylactic esophagectomy may sometimes be justified in these individuals.

Pathology

Gross Features

Squamous cell carcinomas of the esophagus may appear grossly as infiltrating, polypoid, ulcerative, or superficial spreading lesions. Infiltrating lesions, the most common type, cause irregular narrowing and constriction of the lumen. Polypoid lesions are lobulated or fungating masses that protrude into the lumen. Primary ulcerative lesions are relatively flat masses in which the bulk of the tumor is necrotic and ulcerated. Less frequently, superficial spreading lesions may extend longitudinally in the wall without invading beyond the mucosa or submucosa. Patients with superficial spreading carcinomas tend to have a better prognosis than those with other, more invasive forms of esophageal cancer.

Histologic Features

About 50% of esophageal cancers are squamous cell carcinomas, and the remaining 50% are adenocarcinomas arising in Barrett mucosa.[41] Other, less common malignant tumors of the esophagus are discussed in Chapter 28.

At the time of clinical presentation, most squamous cell carcinomas of the esophagus are advanced lesions that have already invaded regional lymph nodes or other local or distant structures. As a result, affected individuals have a dismal prognosis, with overall 5-year survival rates of only about 15%.[2] In contrast, early esophageal cancers are relatively curable lesions, with 5-year survival rates of more than 90%.[42,43] According to the Japanese Society for Esophageal Diseases, early esophageal cancer is defined histologically as cancer limited to the mucosa or submucosa without lymph node involvement.[44] Many of these cases have been reported in the Chinese literature as a result of mass screening of the adult population because of the high incidence of esophageal cancer in that country.[8,45]

Considerable confusion exists in the literature regarding the terminology for "early" cancer. *Early esophageal cancer*, *superficial esophageal cancer*, and *small esophageal cancer* are terms that have been used interchangeably to describe malignant esophageal tumors diagnosed at an early stage. However, these lesions should not be considered synonymous, because they have different histopathologic features that dramatically alter the prognosis of this disease. According to the Japanese Society for Esophageal Diseases, superficial esophageal cancer is also confined to the mucosa or submucosa, but, unlike patients with early esophageal cancer, patients with superficial disease may have lymph node metastases.[44] *Small esophageal cancer* is a term used to describe tumors less than 3.5 cm, regardless of the depth of invasion or the presence or absence of lymph node metastases.[46,47] Previous studies have shown that the 5-year survival for esophageal cancer decreases markedly when regional lymph nodes are involved by tumor.[48,49] Thus, some superficial or small esophageal cancers may be early lesions histologically whereas others may have invaded regional lymph nodes, with a prognosis comparable to that of advanced esophageal cancer.[47,49]

Distribution

Squamous cell carcinomas of the esophagus tend to be located in the upper, middle, or, less commonly, distal third of the esophagus.[48,50] Unlike adenocarcinomas arising in Barrett mucosa, squamous cell carcinomas of the distal esophagus almost never invade the stomach, and there is usually a discrete segment of normal esophagus between the tumor and the gastric cardia.

Routes of Spread

Esophageal carcinoma may invade local, regional, or distant structures by various pathways, including direct extension, lymphatic spread, and hematogenous metastases.

Direct Extension

Because the esophagus lacks a serosa and is attached to neighboring structures by only a loose adventitia, there is no anatomic barrier to prevent rapid spread of tumor into the adjacent mediastinum. As a result, esophageal cancer has a marked tendency to invade contiguous structures in the neck or chest, such as the thyroid, larynx, trachea, bronchi (usually the left main bronchus), aorta, thoracic duct, lung, pericardium, and diaphragm.[48,50] The tracheobronchial tree is a particularly common site of involvement; tracheoesophageal or esophagobronchial fistulas develop in 5% to 10% of all patients with esophageal cancer.[51,52] Rarely, aortoesophageal fistulas or even esophagopericardial fistulas may occur as a terminal complication of esophageal cancer due to aortic or pericardial invasion by tumor.[53,54]

Lymphatic Spread

Lymphatic metastases are found in up to 75% of patients with esophageal cancer.[55] Because the esophagus contains a rich network of interconnecting lymphatic channels, lymphatic spread from esophageal cancer is unpredictable, with "jump" metastases to lymph nodes in the neck or mediastinum often occurring in the absence of segmental lymph node involvement.[55,56] Submucosal esophageal lymphatics also communicate subdiaphragmatically with paracardiac, lesser curvature, and celiac nodes in the upper abdomen; these nodal groups are involved by tumor in 25% to 50% of patients with esophageal cancer.[55,56] Although tumors in the distal esophagus are more likely to metastasize to the abdomen, lymphatic spread of cancers in the upper or midesophagus can also result in metastases to celiac or other abdominal lymph nodes.[55]

Discrete lymphatic metastases or satellite nodules are found in the esophagus at autopsy in about 50% of patients with esophageal cancer.[55] These lesions should be distinguished pathologically from rare double primary carcinomas of the esophagus.[57,58] However, it may be impossible to determine whether two discrete lesions represent synchronous primary tumors or a single cancer with lymphatic dissemination.

Between 2% and 15% of patients dying of esophageal cancer have gastric metastases at autopsy.[59] These lesions probably result from tumor emboli that seed the gastric fundus via submucosal esophageal lymphatics extending subdiaphragmatically to the stomach.[59,60] In such cases, the primary esophageal cancer may be located a considerable distance from the gastroesophageal junction, with a normal esophageal segment below the lesion.

Hematogenous Metastases

Hematogenous, or blood-borne, metastases are often found in patients with advanced esophageal carcinoma. The most common sites of metastases are the lungs, liver, adrenals, kidneys, pancreas, peritoneum, and bones.

Clinical Aspects

Most patients with esophageal cancer develop dysphagia only when the lumen of the esophagus has been reduced by 50% to 75% of its normal circumference.[48,50] By that time, malignant invasion of periesophageal lymph nodes or surrounding mediastinal structures has usually occurred.[48] As a result, most patients have advanced, unresectable tumors at the time of diagnosis. Occasionally, however, patients do experience dysphagia while the tumor is at an early stage.[46,61-63] It is therefore possible to detect early esophageal cancer in some patients who are symptomatic.

Dysphagia is by far the most common complaint in patients with advanced esophageal cancer.[48] Dysphagia is usually present for a period of 2 to 4 months before these patients seek medical attention.[48] Some patients can accurately localize the level of obstruction, but others may have a sensation of blockage referred to the thoracic inlet or even the pharynx by a cancer arising in the middle or lower thoracic esophagus.[50] The esophagus should therefore be carefully evaluated in all patients with unexplained pharyngeal dysphagia to rule out an esophageal cancer below the subjective site of obstruction.

Patients with esophageal cancer may also present with odynophagia if the tumor is ulcerated or with substernal chest pain unrelated to swallowing if the tumor has invaded the mediastinum, so that unremitting chest pain is a poor prognostic sign.[50] Other common symptoms include anorexia and weight loss, which are present in up to 75% of cases.[2] Some patients may present with guaiac-positive stool or iron-deficiency anemia due to occult bleeding from the friable surface of the tumor.[48] However, frank hematemesis is uncommon.[64,65] Rarely, fatal hemorrhage may be caused by an aortoesophageal fistula.[66,67] The latter patients may have minimal hematemesis before the sudden development of massive hemorrhage, shock, and death.

Other patients with esophageal cancer may develop hoarseness due to direct extension of tumor into the larynx or involvement of the recurrent laryngeal nerve.[48] Recurrent aspiration may lead to a chronic cough. However, the presence of a paroxysmal cough on swallowing should suggest the development of a malignant tracheoesophageal or esophagobronchial fistula. Rarely, patients with esophageal cancer may have anorexia, weight loss, or other signs of widespread malignancy without experiencing dysphagia, so localizing esophageal symptoms are not always present.[50]

Endoscopic Findings

When multiple biopsy specimens are obtained, endoscopy has an overall sensitivity of nearly 100% in the diagnosis of esophageal carcinoma.[2,68,69] Brush cytology is also helpful when the esophageal lumen is so compromised by tumor that adequate biopsy specimens cannot be obtained. Detection of suspicious lesions on barium studies should therefore lead to early endoscopy and biopsy for a definitive diagnosis.

Radiographic Findings

Early Esophageal Cancer

Double-contrast esophagography has been widely advocated as the best radiologic technique for diagnosing early esophageal cancer. Unfortunately, the increased sensitivity of this technique has resulted in a lower specificity, as more subtle abnormalities are suspected of representing cancer.[46] Nevertheless, it is probably best to accept a certain percentage of false-positive findings to avoid missing early tumors. When a lesion is detected on barium studies, endoscopy and biopsy should therefore be performed to confirm the presence of carcinoma.

Early esophageal cancers classically appear on double-contrast esophagograms as small, protruded lesions less than 3.5 cm in diameter.[46,61,63,70,71] They may be plaquelike lesions (often with central ulceration) (Fig. 27-1) or small, sessile polyps with a smooth or slightly lobulated contour (Fig. 27-2). Other early cancers may be superficial or depressed lesions, causing focal irregularity, nodularity, or ulceration of the mucosa (Fig. 27-3).[72-74] When a lesion is detected on double-contrast studies, multiple projections should be obtained to determine its appearance both en face and in profile (see Fig. 27-1).

Although most early esophageal cancers appear as focal lesions, superficial spreading carcinomas may be manifested

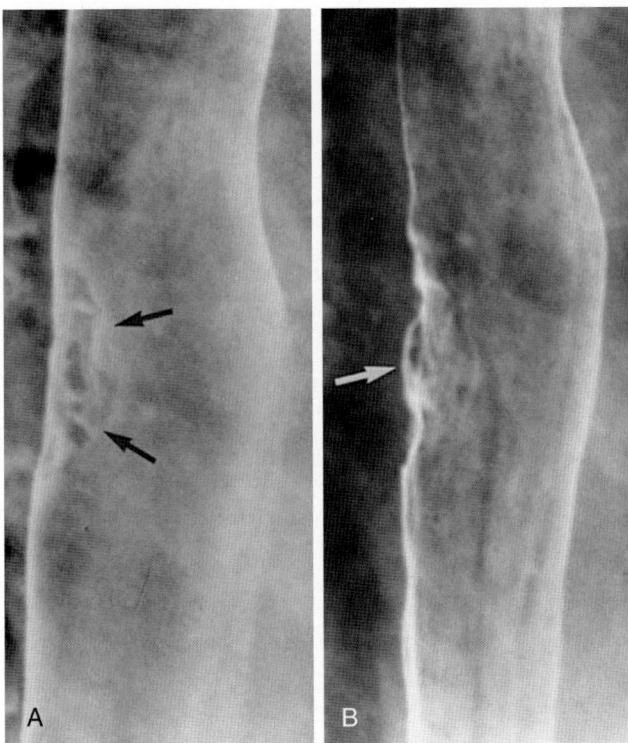

Figure 27-1. Early esophageal cancer. A. En face view from a double-contrast esophagogram shows a poorly defined lesion (*arrows*) in the midesophagus. **B.** However, a tangential view reveals a characteristic plaquelike lesion containing a central area of ulceration (*arrow*). (From Laufer I, Levine MS [eds]: Double Contrast Gastrointestinal Radiology, 2nd ed. Philadelphia, WB Saunders, 1992.)

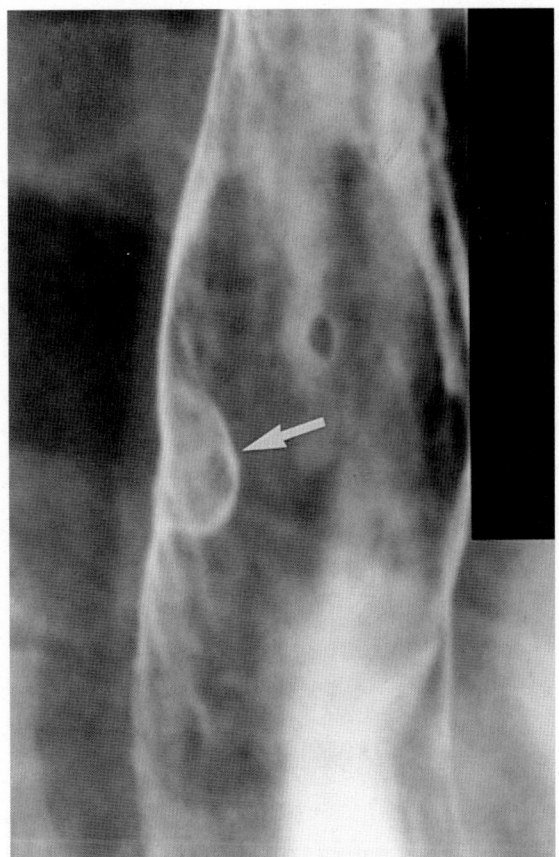

Figure 27-2. Early esophageal cancer. The lesion appears radiographically as a small, sessile polyp (*arrow*) in the midesophagus. (Courtesy of Seth N. Glick, MD, Philadelphia, PA.)

by tiny, poorly defined nodules or plaques, producing a confluent area of nodularity or granularity of the mucosa (Fig. 27-4).[63,72-75] Some superficial spreading carcinomas may be localized lesions, whereas others may involve a considerable segment of the esophagus.

Early esophageal cancers are generally thought to be small lesions, but some early cancers may appear on barium studies as relatively large intraluminal mass greater than 3.5 cm in diameter (Fig. 27-5).[63,76] Such lesions may be indistinguishable from advanced carcinomas. Thus, early esophageal cancers are not necessarily small cancers, because they may undergo considerable intraluminal or intramural growth and still be classified histologically as early lesions.

Advanced Carcinoma

Chest Radiographs

Nearly half of all patients with advanced esophageal cancers have abnormal chest radiographs.[77] The most common findings include mediastinal widening; a hilar, retrohilar, or retrocardiac mass; anterior tracheal bowing; a widened retrotracheal stripe; and an air-fluid level in the esophagus (Fig. 27-6).[77-79] Anterior bowing of the trachea or thickening of the retrotracheal stripe beyond 3 mm in width may result from lymphatic infiltration or direct invasion of the retrotracheal area by tumor.[78,79] Distally, obstructing cancers may be recognized by an air-fluid level in the esophagus. However,

esophageal obstruction from achalasia or other causes may also be manifested by anterior tracheal bowing or an esophageal air-fluid level.

Barium Studies

Double-contrast esophagography is often performed on patients with dysphagia to rule out carcinoma or other abnormalities in the esophagus. Some gastroenterologists believe endoscopy is required for all patients with negative esophagograms to find tumors that are missed on barium studies. In a large series of patients with esophageal cancer, however, the lesion was detected on double-contrast esophagograms in 98% of cases and malignant tumor was diagnosed or suspected on the basis of the radiographic findings in 96%.[80] An argument could be made that a high sensitivity is achieved in the radiographic diagnosis of esophageal cancer only by exposing an inordinate number of patients to unnecessary endoscopy. In the previous study, however, endoscopy was recommended to rule out malignant tumor in only about 1% of all patients who underwent double-contrast examinations.[80] Similarly, in other series, endoscopy has failed to reveal any cases of esophageal carcinoma that were missed on double-contrast esophagograms.[81,82] Thus, endoscopy is not routinely warranted in patients who have normal findings on barium studies.

Advanced esophageal carcinomas may appear on barium studies as infiltrating, polypoid, ulcerative, or varicoid lesions

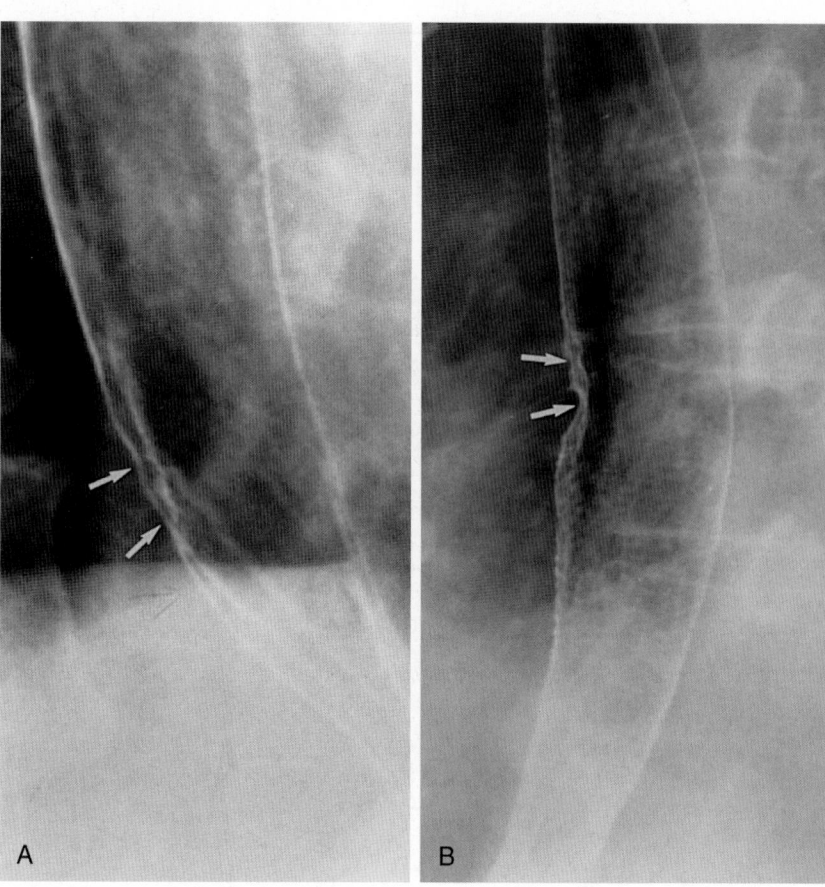

Figure 27-3. Two examples of early esophageal cancer. A and **B.** In both cases there is focal irregularity and puckering of one wall of the esophagus (*arrows*) without a discrete mass. (**A** courtesy of Akiyoshi Yamada, MD, Tokyo, Japan.)

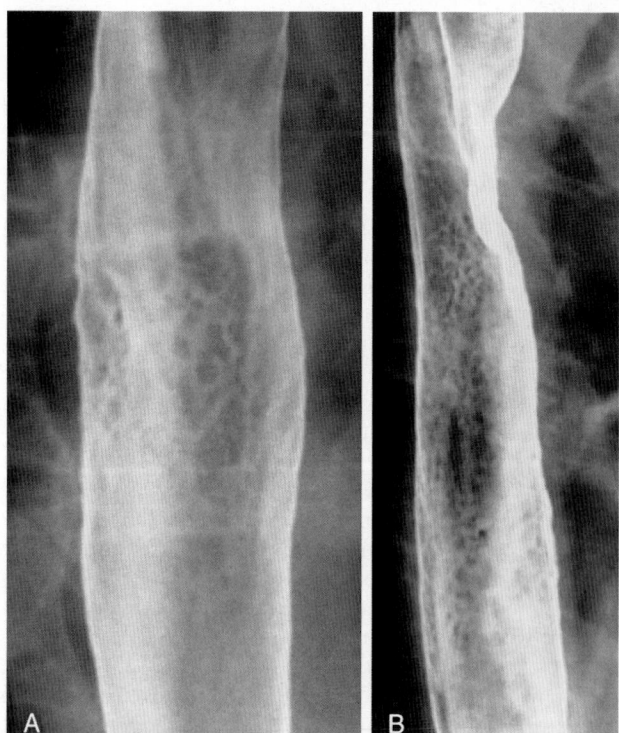

Figure 27-4. Superficial spreading carcinoma. A. There is focal nodularity in the midesophagus as a result of tiny, coalescent nodules and plaques. **B.** In another patient with a more extensive lesion there is diffuse granularity of the mucosa. (**A** from Levine MS: Radiology of the Esophagus. Philadelphia, WB Saunders, 1989.)

(Fig. 27-7).[83-86] However, many esophageal cancers have mixed morphologic features, so that there is considerable overlap in the classification of these tumors.

Infiltrating esophageal carcinomas are characterized by irregular narrowing and constriction of the lumen associated with a nodular or ulcerated mucosa and abrupt, well-defined proximal and distal borders (see Fig. 27-7A). Occasionally, these cancers have shelflike, overhanging borders, producing true annular lesions (Fig. 27-8A).[83] However, other infiltrating lesions have more gradual, tapered borders, occasionally mimicking the appearance of benign strictures (Fig. 27-8B).[84] Infiltrating lesions may eventually cause partial or even complete esophageal obstruction, with proximal dilatation and minimal or no emptying of barium into the stomach.

Polypoid carcinomas appear as lobulated or fungating intraluminal masses, usually larger than 3.5 cm (see Fig. 27-7B).[83-85] They often contain areas of ulceration due to necrosis of tumor. Bulky lesions may eventually cause luminal encroachment and obstruction. However, squamous cell carcinomas are not generally polypoid, so other malignant tumors such as spindle cell carcinoma should be considered in these patients (see Chapter 28).

Primary ulcerative carcinomas are those in which the bulk of the tumor mass is replaced by ulceration. When viewed in profile, these lesions appear as well-defined meniscoid ulcers, with a thick radiolucent rim of tumor surrounding the ulcer (see Fig. 27-7C).[85,87] As in the stomach, this rim of tumor may be obscured when the lesions are detected en face. Multiple projections should therefore be obtained to demonstrate these lesions in profile.

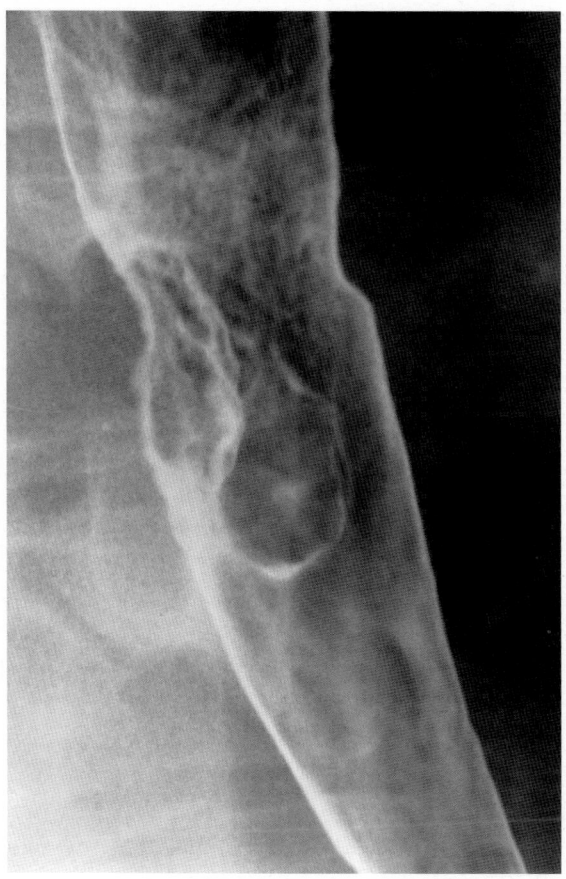

Figure 27-5. Early esophageal cancer. This lesion appears as a relatively large polypoid mass indistinguishable from an advanced carcinoma. (From Levine MS: Radiology of the Esophagus. Philadelphia, WB Saunders, 1989.)

Varicoid carcinomas are those in which submucosal spread of tumor results in thickened, tortuous, or serpiginous longitudinal folds, mimicking the appearance of esophageal varices (see Fig. 27-7D).[88-90] However, these entities can usually be differentiated at fluoroscopy (see later section on Differential Diagnosis). Although varicoid carcinomas are uncommon, submucosal extension of tumor not infrequently produces a focal varicoid pattern adjacent to an obvious squamous cell carcinoma. In one study, a varicoid pattern was seen on esophagography in 40% of patients with esophageal cancer.[91]

Mediastinal involvement by advanced esophageal carcinoma can also be recognized on barium studies. Lymphatic spread of tumor to paratracheal, subcarinal, or paraesophageal lymph nodes may lead to extrinsic compression or displacement of the esophagus, often at a considerable distance from the primary lesion (Fig. 27-9). Mediastinal lymphadenopathy is usually characterized by a smooth, extrinsic esophageal impression with gently sloping, obtuse borders. This finding almost always indicates an advanced, unresectable lesion.

Lymphatic metastases from esophageal cancer may be manifested by discrete implants adjacent to or remote from the primary lesion. These metastases may appear on barium studies as small polypoid, plaquelike, or ulcerated lesions separated from the main tumor by normal intervening mucosa (Fig. 27-10).[92] Although most of these satellite lesions represent lymphatic metastases from the original cancer, the possibility of two primary carcinomas (double primaries) should be considered when the lesions are separated by an unusually long segment of normal mucosa.[57]

Squamous cell metastases to the stomach usually appear on barium studies as solitary, large submucosal masses in the gastric fundus.[59,60] These lesions often contain areas of ulceration, so that they may resemble ulcerated gastrointestinal

Figure 27-6. Advanced esophageal carcinoma with abnormal chest radiographs. A. Posteroanterior chest radiograph shows widening of the superior mediastinum on the right (*arrows*). **B.** Lateral radiograph shows increased soft tissue density in the retrotracheal space with slight anterior bowing of the trachea (*straight arrow*) by an advanced esophageal cancer in this region. Also note thickening of the retrotracheal stripe inferiorly (*curved arrow*) due to direct invasion of this area by tumor. (Courtesy of Wallace T. Miller, MD, Philadelphia, PA.)

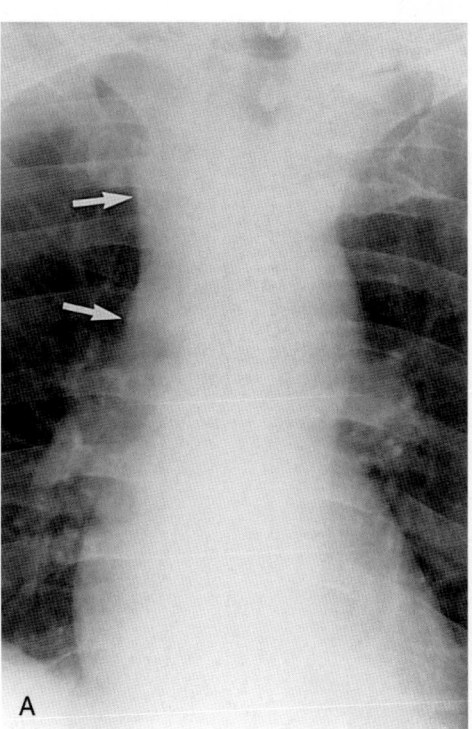
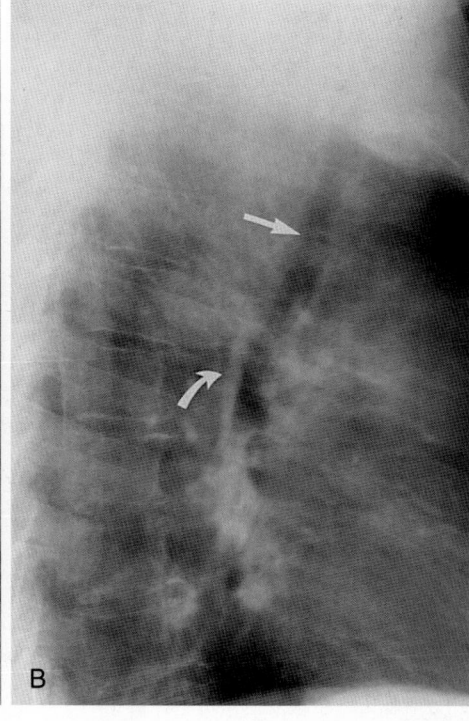

A   B

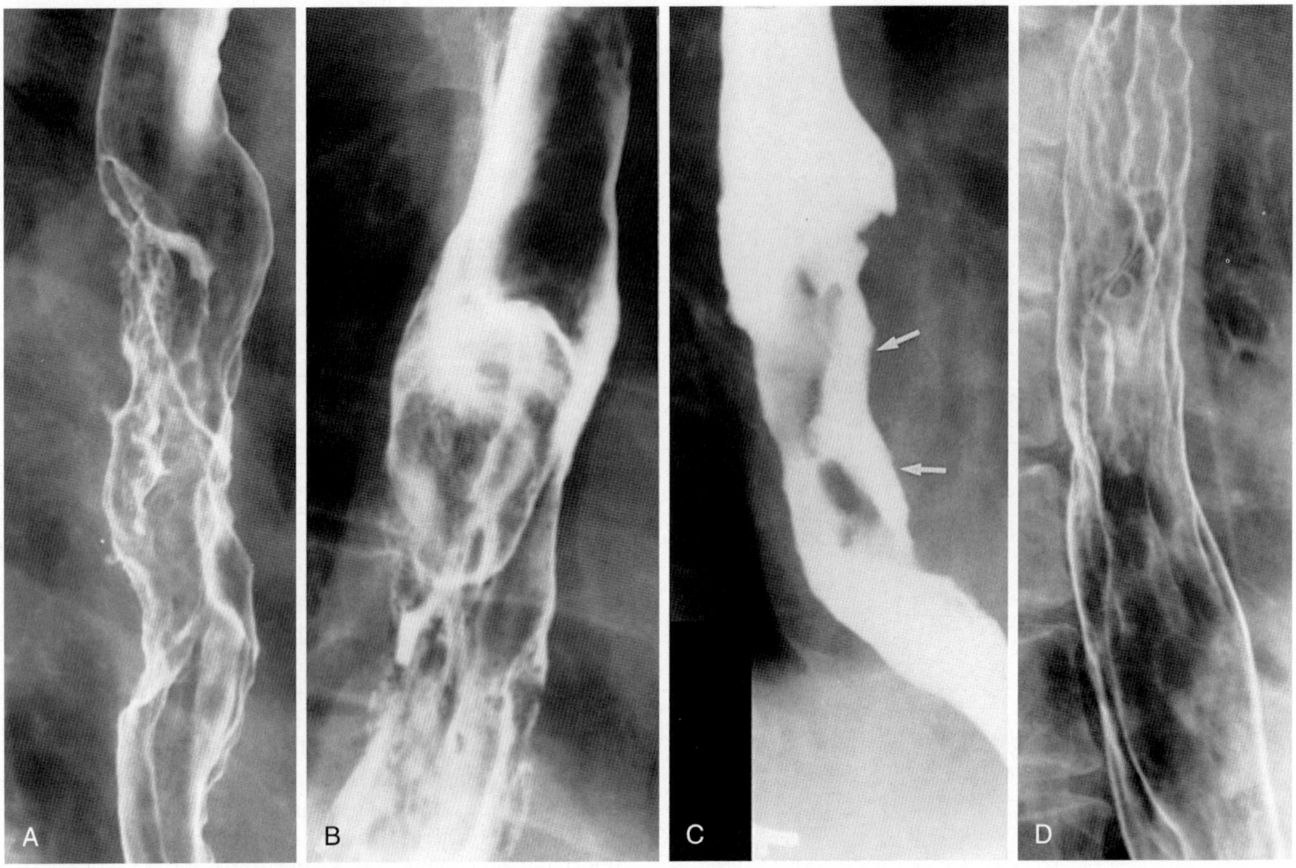

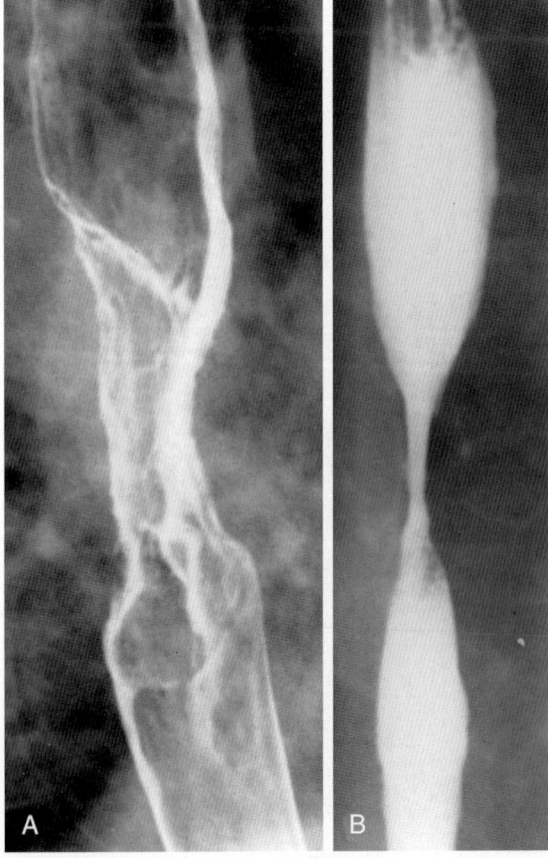

Figure 27-7. Advanced esophageal carcinoma: patterns of tumor. A. Infiltrating lesion. **B.** Polypoid lesion. **C.** Ulcerative lesion with a large, meniscoid ulcer (*arrows*) and a radiolucent rim of tumor. **D.** Varicoid lesion with thickened, tortuous folds in the midesophagus due to submucosal spread of tumor. (**A** to **C** from Levine MS: Radiology of the Esophagus. Philadelphia, WB Saunders, 1989; **D** courtesy of Akiyoshi Yamada, MD, Tokyo, Japan.)

Figure 27-8. Other forms of infiltrative esophageal carcinoma. A. This lesion has an annular appearance with shelflike proximal and distal borders. **B.** In another patient, the cancer is manifested by a relatively smooth, tapered area of narrowing that could be mistaken for a benign stricture. (From Levine MS: Radiology of the Esophagus. Philadelphia, WB Saunders, 1989.)

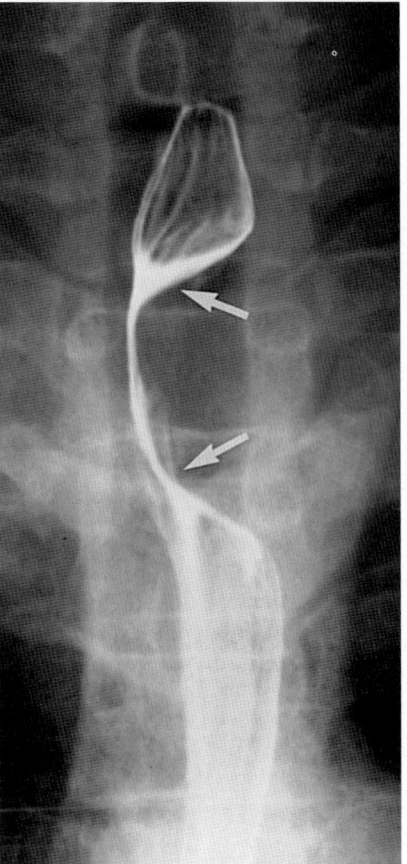

Figure 27-9. Advanced esophageal carcinoma with mediastinal adenopathy. There is a smooth, extrinsic area of mass effect on the left lateral wall of the upper thoracic esophagus (*arrows*) by mediastinal adenopathy from a distal esophageal cancer that is not shown on this image. (From Levine MS: Radiology of the Esophagus. Philadelphia, WB Saunders, 1989.)

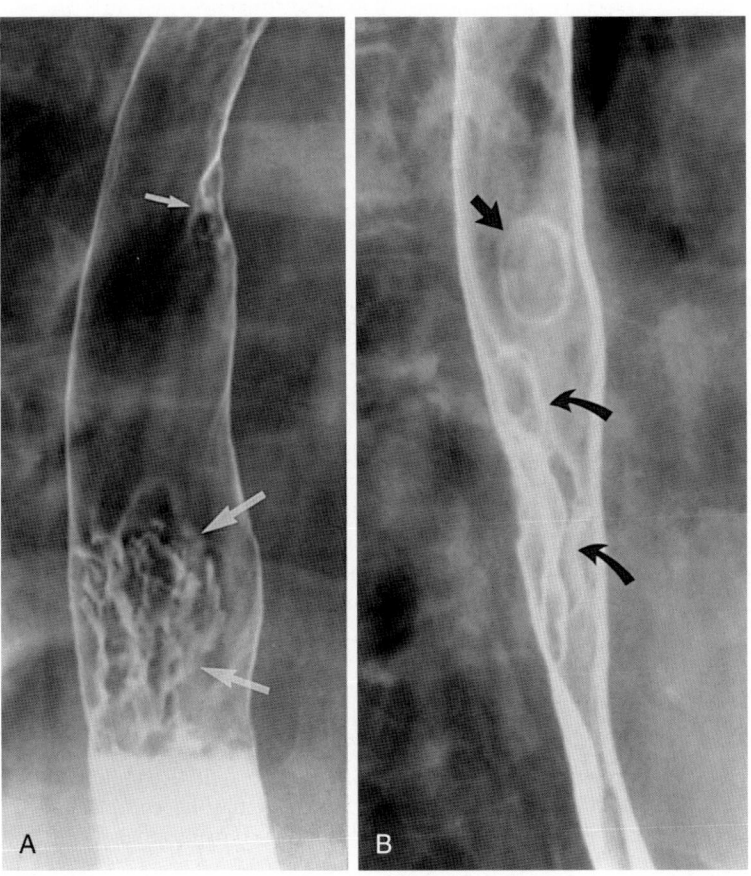

Figure 27-10. Two examples of advanced esophageal carcinoma with discrete lymphatic metastases. A. This patient has a large, ulcerated cancer (*large arrows*) in the midesophagus with a discrete metastatic implant (*small arrow*) separated from the main lesion by normal intervening mucosa. The implant appears as a plaquelike lesion. B. In another patient, a polypoid carcinoma (*curved arrows*) is present in the midesophagus with a discrete submucosal implant (*straight arrow*) more proximally.

stromal tumors (Fig. 27-11). Less frequently, they can be mistaken for primary gastric carcinomas.[93] Because the appropriate treatment for esophageal cancer depends on the stage of the tumor, the gastric cardia and fundus should be carefully examined radiographically in all patients with esophageal cancer to rule out unsuspected metastases to the stomach.

Five to 10 percent of patients with esophageal cancer develop esophageal airway fistulas (Fig. 27-12).[51,52] This complication frequently occurs after radiation therapy, probably as a result of radiation-induced tumor necrosis. Most such fistulas involve the trachea or left main bronchus.[52] Occasionally, however, a locally aggressive esophageal cancer may lead to the development of a necrotic, tumor-containing cavity in the mediastinum or lung that communicates directly with the esophagus (Fig. 27-13). When an esophageal airway fistula is suspected, the esophagogram should be performed with barium rather than water-soluble contrast agents because the latter agents are hyperosmolar and may draw fluid into the lungs if a fistula is present, causing severe pulmonary edema.

Esophageal airway fistulas are usually recognized on esophagography by the presence of barium in the bronchi or distal trachea. In many cases, the origin of the fistulous track is identified within an obvious, infiltrating carcinoma (see Fig. 27-12B). Once barium has entered the trachea or left main bronchus, however, it can be coughed up into the proximal trachea or larynx, so that delayed overhead radiographs may erroneously suggest tracheobronchial aspiration. When an esophageal airway fistula is suspected, the initial swallow should therefore be performed in a lateral projection with a videorecording of the hypopharynx to differentiate a fistula from aspiration.

Rarely, patients with advanced esophageal cancer may develop esophagopericardial fistulas, manifested by pneumopericardium on chest radiographs or CT.[54] In such cases, esophagography with water-soluble contrast agents may de-

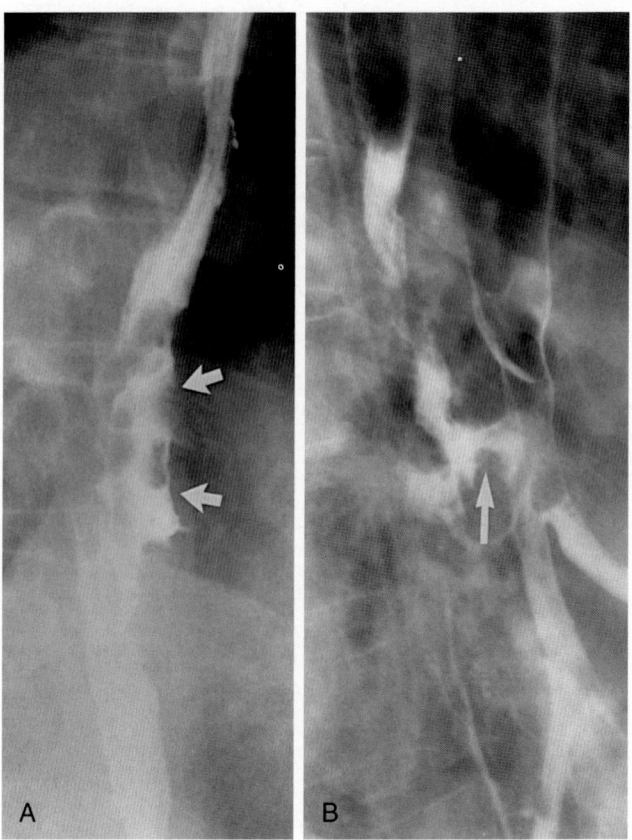

Figure 27-12. Advanced esophageal carcinoma with a tracheoesophageal fistula. A. An ulcerative esophageal carcinoma (*arrows*) is present in the midesophagus. **B.** A second esophagram 4 months after radiation therapy shows partial regression of the tumor with the development of a tracheoesophageal fistula (*arrow*). (From Levine MS: Radiology of the Esophagus. Philadelphia, WB Saunders, 1989.)

monstrate esophageal perforation at the site of the tumor, with contrast material entering the pericardial sac.

Associated Conditions

Achalasia

Esophageal carcinomas arising in patients with achalasia usually appear on barium studies as polypoid masses in the middle or, less commonly, distal third of the esophagus (Fig. 27-14).[17,21] Because these lesions often develop in a massively dilated esophagus, they can reach enormous sizes, producing bulky intraluminal masses that have a fungating or "cauliflower" appearance.[21] Nevertheless, the lesions may be obscured by retained fluid and debris in a dilated, partially obstructed esophagus.[19-21] Careful esophageal lavage with a soft rubber catheter may therefore be required to cleanse the esophagus before performing the radiologic examination.

Lye Strictures

The development of a lye cancer may be manifested on barium studies by increasing stenosis, mass effect, nodularity, or ulceration within a preexisting lye stricture (Fig. 27-15). The underlying strictures are often located in the region of the tracheal bifurcation, so lye cancers may be complicated by the development of tracheoesophageal or esophagobronchial

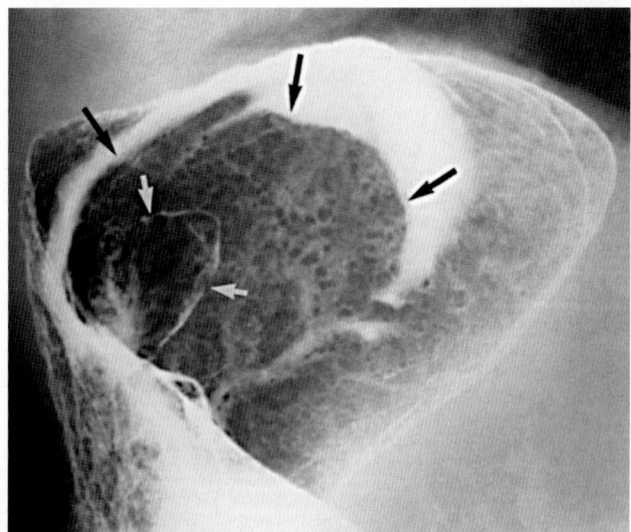

Figure 27-11. Advanced esophageal carcinoma with a squamous cell metastasis to the stomach. There is a giant submucosal mass (*black arrows*) in the gastric fundus, containing a triangular area of central ulceration (*white arrows*). A malignant gastrointestinal stromal tumor could produce similar findings. (From Glick SN, Teplick SK, Levine MS: Squamous cell metastases to the gastric cardia. Gastrointest Radiol 10:339-344, 1985. With kind permission from Springer Science and Business Media.)

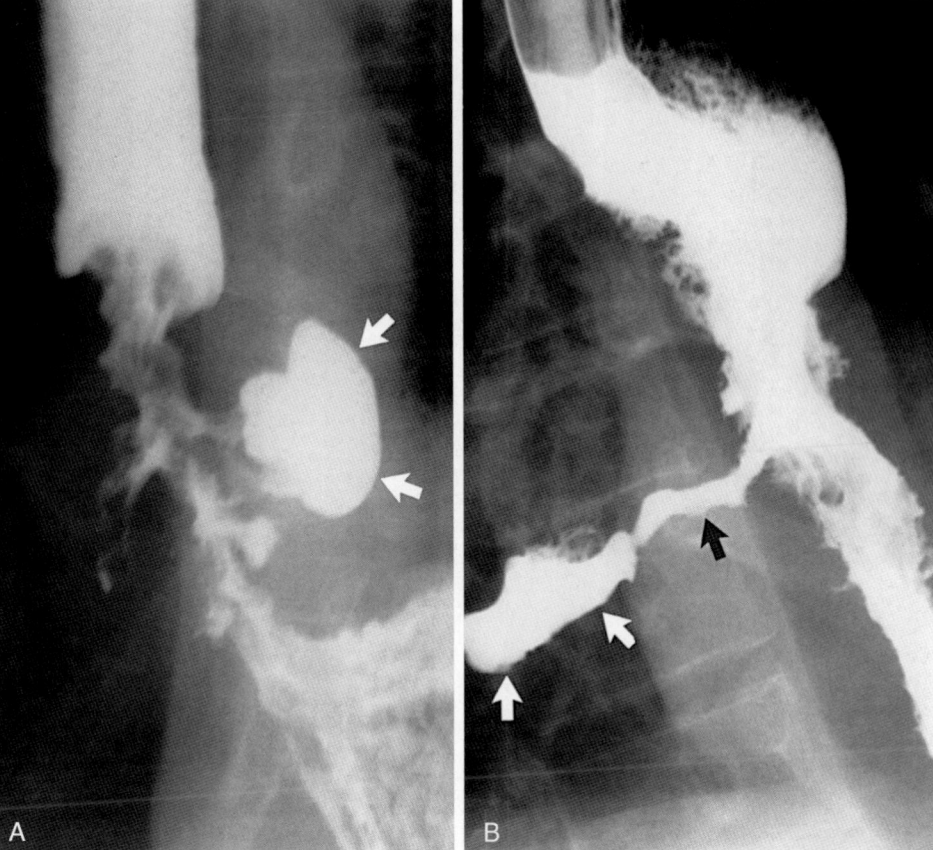

Figure 27-13. Advanced esophageal carcinoma with fistulas to the mediastinum and lung. In these two cases there is direct communication between the cancer and necrotic, tumor-containing cavities (*arrows*) in the mediastinum (A) and the right lung (B). (From Levine MS: Radiology of the Esophagus. Philadelphia, WB Saunders, 1989.)

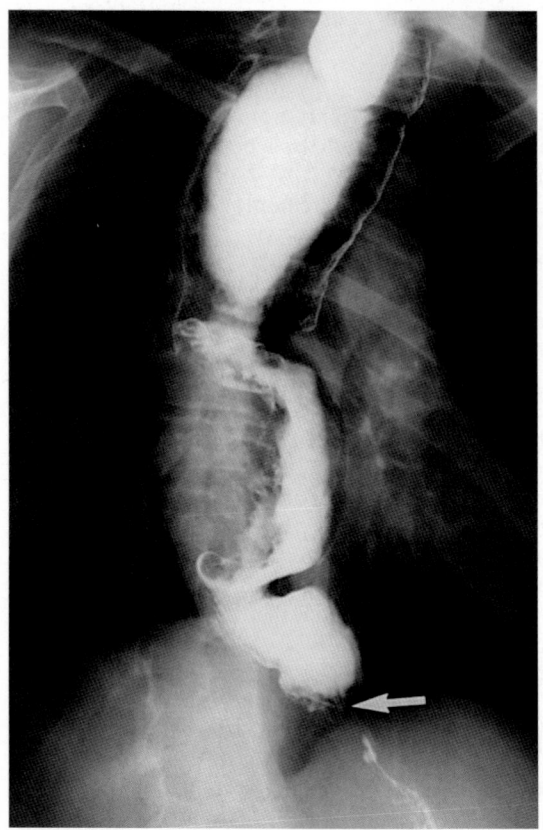

Figure 27-14. Advanced esophageal carcinoma associated with achalasia. There is a large, fungating mass in the midesophagus in a patient with long-standing achalasia. Note beaklike narrowing (*arrow*) of the distal esophagus due to incomplete opening of the lower esophageal sphincter. (From Levine MS: Radiology of the Esophagus. Philadelphia, WB Saunders, 1989.)

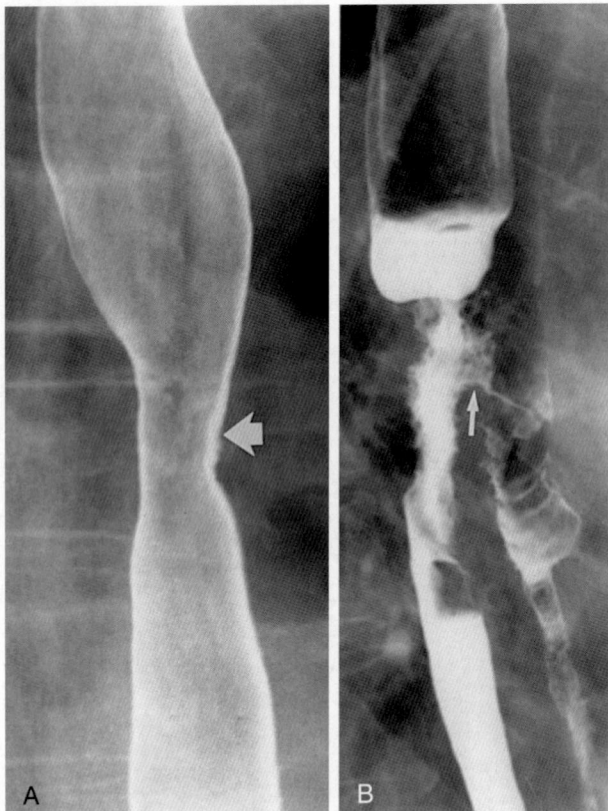

Figure 27-15. Advanced esophageal carcinoma arising in a lye stricture. A. Initial double-contrast esophagogram shows a focal stricture (*arrow*) in the midesophagus due to previous lye ingestion. Note superficial ulceration and nodularity of the mucosa in the region of the stricture. The patient refused surgery at this time. **B.** Another study 2 years later shows an advanced, infiltrating carcinoma at the site of the previous stricture, with an esophagobronchial fistula (*arrow*). (From Levine MS: Radiology of the Esophagus. Philadelphia, WB Saunders, 1989.)

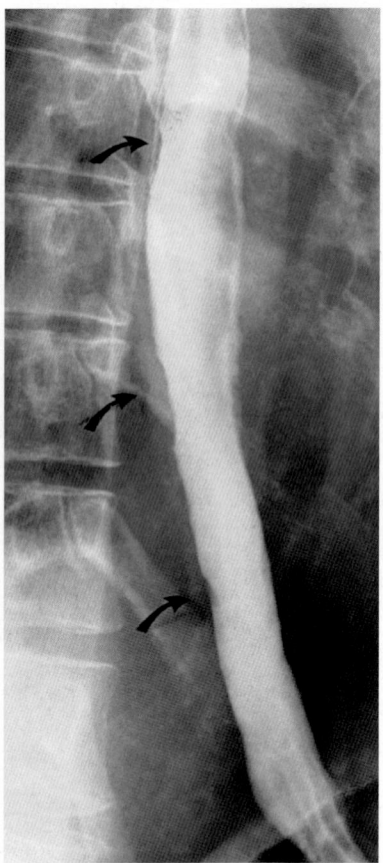

Figure 27-16. Tylosis with hyperkeratotic plaques. There are multiple discrete plaques (*arrows*) in the midesophagus and the distal esophagus. These lesions were found to be hyperkeratotic plaques in a patient with long-standing tylosis. (From Munyer TP, Margulis AR: Tylosis. AJR 136:1026-1027, 1981. © by American Roentgen Ray Society.)

fistulas (see Fig. 27-15B).[25] Any change in the appearance of a chronic lye stricture should therefore be evaluated by endoscopy with multiple biopsy specimens and brushings to rule out a superimposed carcinoma.

Tylosis

When patients with tylosis develop esophageal symptoms, they usually have advanced esophageal carcinomas, manifested on barium studies by annular, infiltrating, or plaque-like lesions.[40] Occasionally, however, asymptomatic patients with tylosis may have discrete hyperkeratotic plaques containing one or more foci of dysplasia or intramucosal carcinoma.[40] These lesions may appear on esophagograms as large, well-defined plaques with normal intervening mucosa (Fig. 27-16).[40]

ADENOCARCINOMA

Primary esophageal adenocarcinomas are almost always found to arise in the setting of Barrett's esophagus. In the past, such tumors were thought to be rare lesions, accounting for less than 5% of all esophageal cancers.[94-96] However, many of these adenocarcinomas involving the gastroesophageal junction or gastric fundus were incorrectly classified as primary gastric carcinomas secondarily invading the lower

end of the esophagus.[94,95] Apart from difficulties in tumor classification, the incidence of esophageal adenocarcinoma in white men has increased by 300% to 500% in the past 30 years.[41,97-99] Currently, adenocarcinomas are thought to constitute at least 50% of all esophageal cancers.[41] Nevertheless, many questions remain about the risk of malignant degeneration in Barrett's esophagus and the long-term management of patients with this condition.

Epidemiology and Pathogenesis

Considerable attention has been focused on the relationship between esophageal adenocarcinoma and the columnar epithelium–lined esophagus, or Barrett's esophagus. In various studies, 90% to 100% of all primary esophageal adenocarcinomas have been found to arise on a background of Barrett's mucosa.[100-102] Thus, adenocarcinoma of the esophagus is not only more common than had previously been recognized but the vast majority of these tumors also appear to result from malignant degeneration in Barrett's esophagus.

Barrett's Esophagus

Barrett's esophagus is a well-recognized condition in which there is progressive columnar metaplasia of the distal esophagus due to long-standing gastroesophageal reflux and reflux esophagitis.[102-106] In various studies, the prevalence of Barrett's esophagus in patients with reflux esophagitis has ranged from 5% to 15%, with an overall prevalence of about 10%.[107-110] The clinical and radiologic aspects of Barrett's esophagus are presented in Chapter 23.

Various types of columnar epithelium have been described in Barrett's esophagus, including a junctional-type epithelium, a gastric fundic-type epithelium, and an intestinal-type or specialized columnar epithelium.[111,112] It is currently believed, however, that intestinal metaplasia is the major prerequisite for a pathologic diagnosis of Barrett's esophagus.[113] This intestinal metaplasia is characterized histologically by goblet cells with acidic mucin and, in some cases, enterocyte differentiation with brush border formation. The revised definition of Barrett's esophagus is based on an emerging consensus that intestinal metaplasia represents the type of epithelium that usually predisposes these patients to esophageal adenocarcinoma.[113,114]

Investigators have also developed histopathologic criteria for Barrett's esophagus in which patients are classified as having either "long-segment" disease (i.e., extending more than 3 cm from the gastroesophageal junction) or "short-segment" disease (i.e., extending 3 cm or less from the gastroesophageal junction) based on the vertical extent of columnar metaplasia in the esophagus.[115] Short-segment Barrett's esophagus is even more common than long-segment Barrett's esophagus, with a reported prevalence of 10% to 15% at endoscopy.[114]

Risk of Adenocarcinoma

The risk of malignant degeneration in Barrett's esophagus can be assessed by prevalence or incidence data. In various series, the prevalence of adenocarcinoma in patients with Barrett's esophagus has ranged from 2% to 46%, with an overall prevalence of about 10%.[101,105,107,108,116,117] However, prevalence data tend to exaggerate the risk of cancer, because many patients with Barrett's esophagus remain asymptomatic until the development of a superimposed carcinoma. Incidence data therefore provide more realistic estimates of the risk of malignant transformation in Barrett's mucosa. In various prospective studies, it has been shown that the incidence of adenocarcinoma in patients with Barrett's esophagus is approximately 30 to 40 times greater than that in the general population.[118,119] Incidence data have also shown that adenocarcinoma develops in about 0.5% of patients with Barrett's esophagus each year.[120]

Dysplasia-Carcinoma Sequence

Pathologic data strongly suggest that esophageal adenocarcinoma in Barrett's esophagus evolves through a sequence of progressively severe epithelial dysplasia in areas of preexisting columnar metaplasia (usually intestinal metaplasia).[121-124] These dysplastic changes can be detected on endoscopic biopsy specimens obtained from Barrett's esophagus. Dysplasia may occur in all types of Barrett's mucosa but is most likely to occur in areas of intestinal metaplasia.[113,114] Dysplastic changes are classified as either low grade or high grade on the basis of the histologic findings; high-grade dysplasia may subsequently progress to invasive adenocarcinoma. In various studies, the prevalence of high-grade dysplasia in patients with esophageal adenocarcinoma has ranged from 68% to 100%.[105,116] Studies have also shown progression to cancer

in 22% of patients with high-grade dysplasia in Barrett's esophagus within 7 years.[2]

When Barrett's esophagus is stratified into short-segment and long-segment disease, it has been found that patients with short-segment disease are more likely to develop dysplasia than the general population but are less likely to develop dysplasia than patients with long-segment disease.[125,126] Esophageal adenocarcinoma has also been found to develop in patients with short-segment disease.[125,127,128] Additional studies are needed, however, to better elucidate the cancer risk in these patients.

Surveillance and Management of Barrett's Esophagus

Because of the increased cancer risk, many investigators advocate endoscopic surveillance of patients with known Barrett's esophagus to detect dysplastic changes, so that the patient can be treated before the development of overt carcinoma.[2,100,103-105,121-124] Endoscopic biopsy specimens are generally recommended from all four quadrants of the lower esophagus at 1- to 2-cm intervals starting at the gastroesophageal junction.[2] In patients with nondysplastic Barrett's esophagus, the American Gastroenterological Association recommends surveillance endoscopy at 5-year intervals, depending on the patient's health.[2] In patients with low-grade dysplasia, endoscopy is recommended at 1- to 2-year intervals because of an increased but uncertain risk of developing cancer.[2] Because of the much higher risk of developing cancer in patients with high-grade dysplasia, however, such individuals may proceed to definitive treatment with a surgical esophagogastrectomy.[2] Patients with high-grade dysplasia can also be managed by photoablation or endoscopic mucosal resection, which are minimally invasive therapeutic alternatives associated with lower morbidity and mortality rates than open surgery.[129,130] Alternatively, patients with high-grade dysplasia may undergo intensive endoscopic surveillance at 3- to 6-month intervals if they wish to avoid definitive treatment until the diagnosis of cancer is made.[2]

Despite these recommendations, there is continued controversy about whether endoscopic surveillance of patients with Barrett's esophagus is a cost-effective approach for detecting esophageal adenocarcinoma because of the low incidence of neoplasia and the high cost of endoscopy.[118,131] So far, endoscopic surveillance of patients with Barrett's esophagus also has not been shown to improve the mortality from esophageal adenocarcinoma.[132] Thus, many questions remain about the role of endoscopic surveillance and its ultimate value in patients with Barrett's esophagus.

Attention has also been focused on the role of DNA flow cytometry and cellular genetics analysis to determine which patients with Barrett's esophagus are at greatest risk for the development of adenocarcinoma. Some investigators have shown that a subset of patients with Barrett's esophagus have genomic instability with aneuploid populations of cells, predisposing to neoplastic transformation.[133] In various studies, the findings on DNA flow cytometry have correlated directly with the presence of high-grade dysplasia or invasive carcinoma on endoscopic biopsy specimens.[133,134] Thus, flow cytometry represents another potential diagnostic tool for surveillance of Barrett's esophagus.

Much less frequently, the development of cancer in Barrett's esophagus may result from an adenoma-carcinoma sequence similar to that found in the colon. Benign adenomatous polyps have occasionally been documented in Barrett's mucosa with or without focal areas of invasive adenocarcinoma.[101,135,136] Because malignant degeneration of these adenomas represents another potential pathway for the development of adenocarcinoma, endoscopic resection of adenomatous polyps in Barrett's esophagus may decrease the risk of cancer.

Relationship between Scleroderma, Barrett's Esophagus, and Adenocarcinoma

Scleroderma, a connective tissue disease characterized by smooth muscle atrophy and fibrosis, affects the esophagus in about 75% of patients. Esophageal involvement is usually characterized by a patulous, incompetent lower esophageal sphincter and absent esophageal peristalsis with poor clearance of refluxed peptic acid from the esophagus once reflux has occurred. As a result, patients with scleroderma often have reflux esophagitis. Because of the severity of esophagitis, these individuals have an even greater risk of developing Barrett's esophagus than other patients with reflux disease. In one study, 37% of those with scleroderma who underwent endoscopy for reflux symptoms had biopsy-proven Barrett's esophagus.[137] Because Barrett's esophagus predisposes to esophageal adenocarcinoma, patients with scleroderma also appear to have an increased risk of developing esophageal cancer.[137,138] Thus, scleroderma should indirectly be considered to be a premalignant condition in the esophagus.

Pathology

Gross Features

Adenocarcinomas arising in Barrett's mucosa appear grossly as infiltrating, polypoid, ulcerative, or varicoid lesions. These tumors tend to be located in the distal or, less commonly, middle third of the esophagus.[101,102,139] Unlike squamous cell carcinomas, adenocarcinomas of the distal esophagus frequently spread subdiaphragmatically to involve the gastric cardia or fundus.[101,102,112,139] In fact, studies have shown that adenocarcinomas arising in Barrett's esophagus account for up to 50% of all adenocarcinomas involving the gastroesophageal junction.[101,102,139] The remaining lesions are primary carcinomas of the gastric cardia or fundus invading the esophagus. Whether they arise in the esophagus or in the stomach, these tumors have similar morphologic features in terms of pattern of growth, degree of differentiation, and depth of invasion.[140] However, it is important to ascertain whether the cancer has arisen in Barrett's esophagus, because it may be necessary to resect not only the primary tumor but also all residual Barrett's mucosa. Detection of malignant tumor at the cardia should therefore lead to a careful search for Barrett's epithelium in the esophagus.

Histologic Features

At the time of diagnosis, most adenocarcinomas in Barrett's esophagus are advanced, unresectable tumors. Occasionally, however, early, potentially curable lesions may be detected by radiologic or endoscopic surveillance of patients with known Barrett's esophagus or such lesions may be detected fortuitously in patients who undergo barium studies or endoscopy because of their underlying reflux disease.[63,123,141]

Routes of Spread

Like squamous cell carcinoma, esophageal adenocarcinoma invades local, regional, or distant structures via direct extension, lymphatic spread, or hematogenous metastases. Unlike squamous cell carcinoma, however, adenocarcinoma in Barrett's esophagus has a marked tendency to invade the proximal stomach; involvement of the gastric cardia or fundus occurs in 35% to 50% of cases.[101,102,139]

Clinical Aspects

Barrett's esophagus is predominantly a disease of elderly white men, with a male:female ratio of 3:1 and a mean age about 65 years at the time of diagnosis, although there has been a significant increase in the incidence of these tumors in younger patients between 45 and 65 years of age.[2]

Patients with esophageal adenocarcinoma usually present with recent onset of dysphagia and weight loss.[104,105,120,116] Other findings include upper gastrointestinal bleeding, odynophagia, and chest pain.[116] Because of their underlying reflux disease, some patients may have long-standing reflux symptoms before the development of cancer.[104] By the time these individuals develop dysphagia, however, they almost always have advanced, unresectable tumors. As a result, patients with advanced esophageal adenocarcinomas have a poor prognosis, with overall 5-year survival rates of less than 20%.[2,142]

Most patients with early adenocarcinomas in Barrett's esophagus are asymptomatic, but some may present with melena, guaiac-positive stool, or iron-deficiency anemia resulting from low-grade bleeding from the friable surface of the tumor.[63] Others may seek medical attention because of their underlying reflux disease, so that early cancers may be detected as fortuitous findings in patients presenting with reflux symptoms.[63]

Radiographic Findings

Early Adenocarcinoma

Like squamous cell carcinomas, early adenocarcinomas in Barrett's esophagus may appear on double-contrast esophagograms as plaquelike lesions or as flat, sessile polyps.[63] Sessile or pedunculated polyps in the distal esophagus may also represent adenomatous polyps in Barrett's mucosa with or without foci of invasive carcinoma (Fig. 27-17).[101,136] In patients with peptic strictures, the earliest manifestation of a developing adenocarcinoma may be a localized area of flattening or stiffening in one wall of the stricture (Fig. 27-18).[63,101,102] Other patients may have superficial spreading cancers, manifested by confluent nodularity or granularity of the mucosa without a discrete lesion.[63] Although early adenocarcinomas are classically small lesions, some patients may have relatively larger polypoid masses that are indistinguishable radiographically from advanced esophageal carcinomas.[63]

Advanced Adenocarcinoma

Advanced esophageal adenocarcinomas usually appear on barium studies as infiltrating lesions with irregular luminal narrowing, nodularity or ulceration of the mucosa, and abrupt, asymmetrical borders (Fig. 27-19A).[101,102,139] In general, these lesions cannot be distinguished radiographically

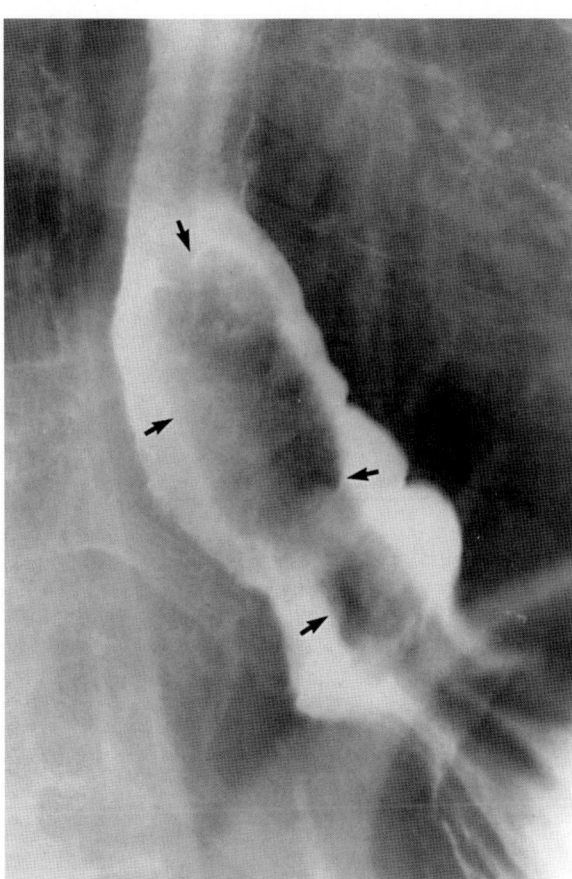

Figure 27-17. Early adenocarcinoma in Barrett's esophagus. There is a large, pedunculated polyp (*arrows*) in the distal esophagus. Pathologic examination of the resected specimen revealed an adenomatous polyp with a solitary focus of adenocarcinoma. (From Levine MS, Caroline D, Thompson JJ, et al: Adenocarcinoma of the esophagus: Relationship to Barrett mucosa. Radiology 150:305-309, 1984.)

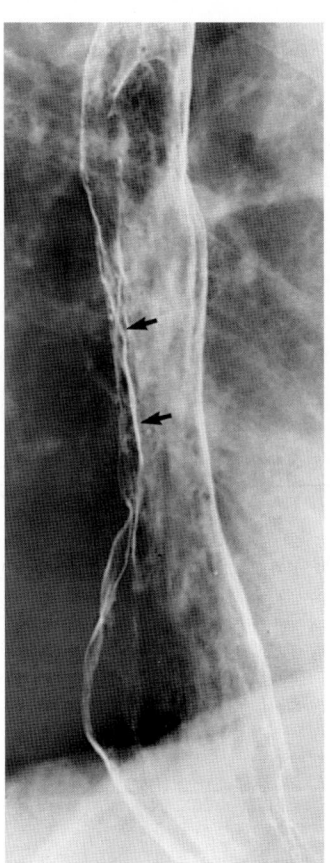

Figure 27-18. Early adenocarcinoma in Barrett's esophagus. There is a relatively long peptic stricture in the distal esophagus with slight flattening and stiffening of one wall of the stricture (*arrows*). Surgery revealed an intramucosal adenocarcinoma arising in Barrett's esophagus. (From Levine MS, Caroline D, Thompson JJ, et al: Adenocarcinoma of the esophagus: Relationship to Barrett mucosa. Radiology 150:305-309, 1984.)

from squamous cell carcinomas. In one study, however, esophageal adenocarcinomas were found to involve a longer vertical segment of the esophagus than squamous cell carcinomas.[102] Adenocarcinomas are also more likely to involve the distal esophagus,[101] so the presence of a long, infiltrating lesion in the distal esophagus should suggest the possibility of adenocarcinoma.

Less frequently, these tumors may appear as polypoid intraluminal masses (Fig. 27-19B) or as primary ulcerative lesions with a meniscoid ulcer surrounded by a thick rind of tumor (Fig. 27-19C).[101,102] Occasionally, these lesions may have a varicoid appearance due to submucosal spread of tumor (Fig. 27-19D).[101,102,143] Similar findings may be present in patients with squamous cell carcinoma. However, many patients with adenocarcinoma arising in Barrett's esophagus have associated hiatal hernias, gastroesophageal reflux, reflux esophagitis, or peptic strictures.[101,102] The possibility of adenocarcinoma should therefore be considered in any patient with esophageal cancer who has other clinical or radiologic signs of reflux disease.

When adenocarcinomas are located in the distal esophagus, they have a marked tendency to invade the gastric cardia or fundus.[101,102,139] Gastric involvement may be manifested on barium studies by a polypoid or ulcerated mass in the fundus. In other patients, these tumors may cause distortion

or obliteration of the normal anatomic landmarks at the cardia and irregular areas of ulceration without a discrete mass (Fig. 27-20).[101] The findings may be quite subtle, so that optimal double-contrast views of the gastric cardia and fundus are required to demonstrate these lesions. In general, esophageal adenocarcinoma invading the gastric cardia or fundus cannot be distinguished radiographically from carcinoma of the cardia or fundus invading the distal esophagus. However, esophageal adenocarcinomas usually have a greater degree of esophageal involvement in relation to that of the stomach, whereas gastric cardiac carcinomas have a greater degree of fundal involvement.

DIFFERENTIAL DIAGNOSIS

Early Esophageal Cancer

Early squamous cell carcinomas and adenocarcinomas usually appear on double-contrast esophagograms as plaquelike lesions or as flat, sessile polyps. However, squamous papillomas may also appear as small, sessile, slightly lobulated polyps that are indistinguishable from early esophageal cancers (see Chapter 26).[144] *Candida* esophagitis and glycogenic acanthosis usually produce multiple plaquelike defects in the esophagus, but a single large plaque can be mistaken for a plaquelike

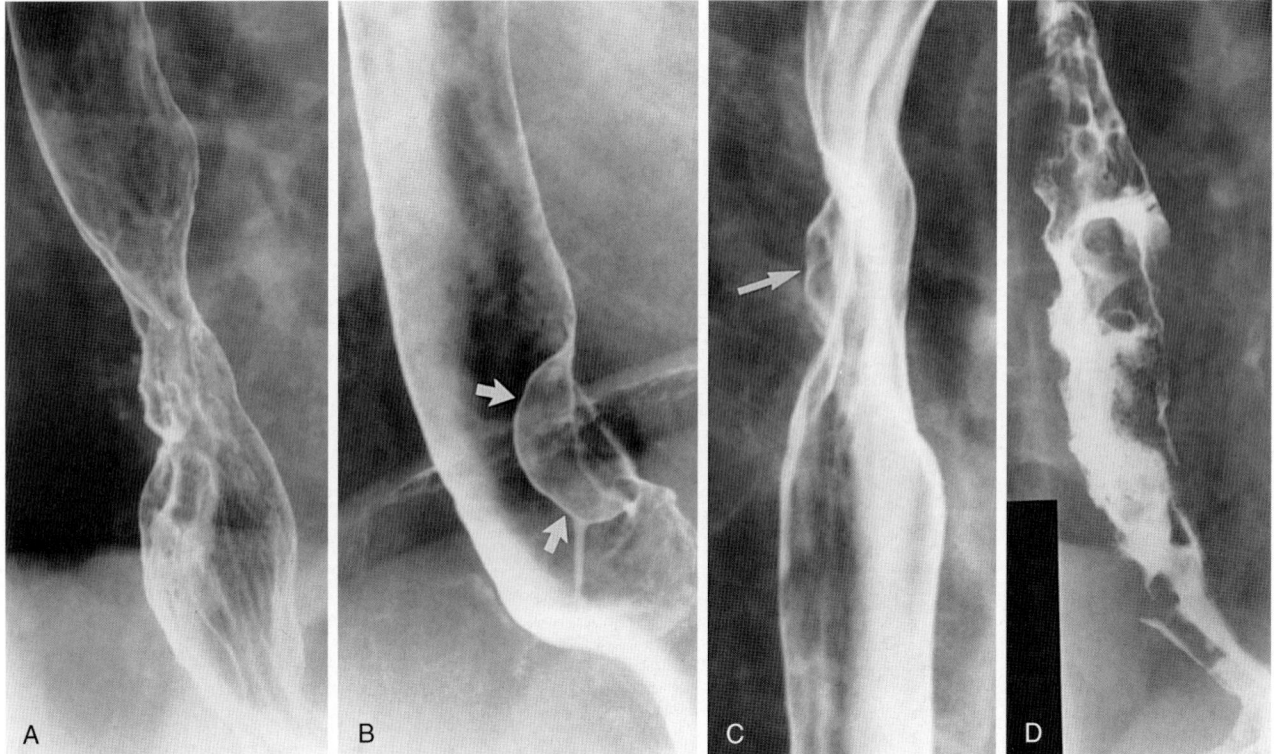

Figure 27-19. Advanced adenocarcinoma in Barrett's esophagus: patterns of tumor. A. Infiltrating lesion. **B.** Polypoid lesion (*arrows*). **C.** Ulcerative lesion (*arrow*). **D.** Varicoid lesion. (**B** from Levine MS: Radiology of the Esophagus. Philadelphia, WB Saunders, 1989; **C** and **D** from Levine MS, Caroline D, Thompson JJ, et al: Adenocarcinoma of the esophagus: Relationship to Barrett mucosa. Radiology 150:305-309, 1984.)

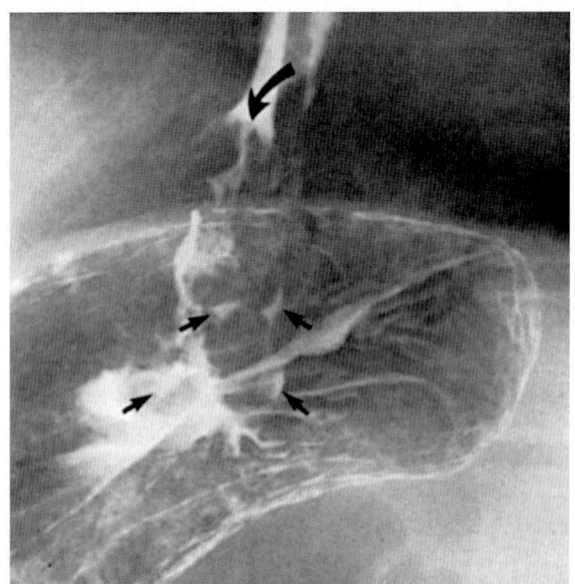

Figure 27-20. Adenocarcinoma in Barrett's esophagus invading the stomach. Double-contrast view of the gastric fundus shows obliteration of the normal anatomic landmarks at the cardia with irregular areas of ulceration (*straight arrows*). Also note tumor involving the distal esophagus (*curved arrow*). At surgery, this patient had a primary adenocarcinoma arising in Barrett's mucosa with secondary gastric involvement. (From Levine MS, Caroline D, Thompson JJ, et al: Adenocarcinoma of the esophagus: Relationship to Barrett mucosa. Radiology 150:305-309, 1984.)

carcinoma. Occasionally, inflammatory exudates or pseudomembranes associated with severe reflux esophagitis may also appear radiographically as plaquelike defects indistinguishable from early adenocarcinomas (Fig. 27-21).[145] However, pseudomembrane formation may be suggested by the presence of other discrete satellite lesions or by a change in the size and appearance of the lesions during the radiologic examination. When the radiographic findings are equivocal, endoscopy and biopsy are required for a definitive diagnosis.

Because superficial spreading carcinomas are manifested on double-contrast esophagograms by tiny nodules or plaques, a localized area of *Candida* esophagitis could conceivably produce a similar appearance (Fig. 27-22).[146] However, the plaquelike defects of candidiasis tend to be discrete lesions with well-defined borders and normal intervening mucosa, whereas the nodules or plaques of superficial spreading carcinoma tend to coalesce, producing a continuous area of disease. Superficial spreading carcinomas that are more extensive should be differentiated from other benign conditions causing a diffusely nodular mucosa, such as *Candida* esophagitis, glycogenic acanthosis, or, rarely, leukoplakia, acanthosis nigricans, and squamous papillomatosis.[146-150] However, the latter conditions also tend to produce discrete lesions rather than a continuous area of disease. Finally, superficial spreading carcinoma may produce a reticulonodular appearance that closely resembles the reticular pattern of Barrett's mucosa.[151] However, this last finding is usually associated with a midesophageal stricture, with the reticular pattern extending distally a variable distance from the stricture (see Chapter 23).

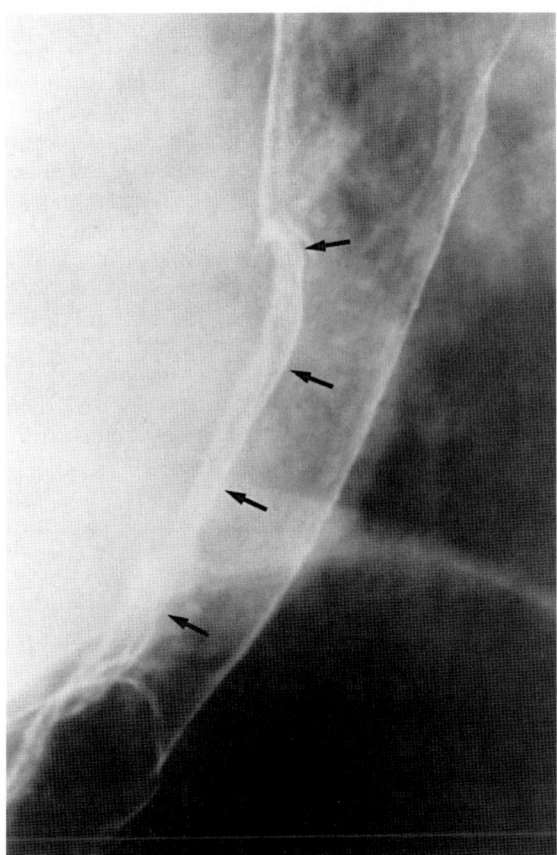

Figure 27-21. Reflux esophagitis with a large pseudomembrane, mimicking a plaquelike adenocarcinoma. There is a longitudinally oriented, plaquelike lesion (*arrows*) on the anterolateral wall of the distal esophagus. The radiographic findings are worrisome for a plaquelike carcinoma, but endoscopy revealed pseudomembranes due to severe reflux esophagitis without evidence of tumor. (From Levine MS, Cajade AG, Herlinger H, et al: Pseudomembranes in reflux esophagitis. Radiology 159:43-45, 1986.)

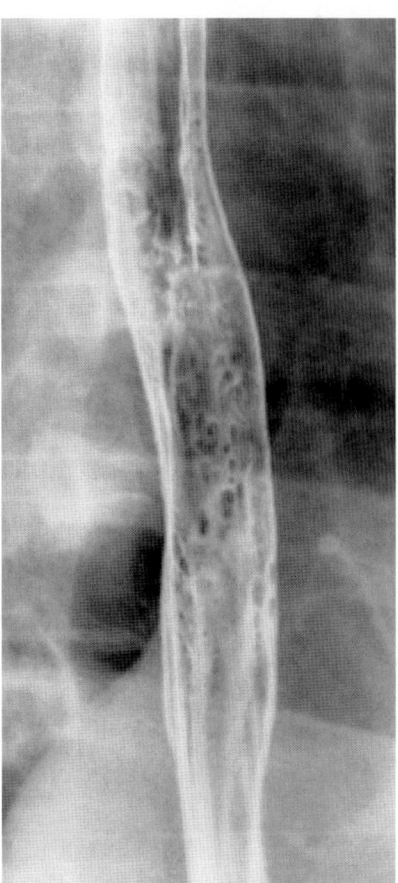

Figure 27-22. Localized area of *Candida* esophagitis. This appearance could be mistaken for a superficial spreading carcinoma. However, note how the plaques have discrete borders and are separated by short segments of normal mucosa. (From Levine MS: Radiology of the Esophagus. Philadelphia, WB Saunders, 1989.)

Advanced Carcinoma

Infiltrating esophageal carcinomas usually have an obvious malignant appearance. Occasionally, however, these lesions may resemble benign strictures, with concentric narrowing and relatively smooth, tapered borders (see Fig. 27-8B).[84,152] In such cases, an abrupt change in caliber or focal irregularity, nodularity, or stiffening of one wall of the stricture should suggest the possibility of malignant tumor, particularly an adenocarcinoma in Barrett's esophagus.[101,102] Fluoroscopic observation may also help differentiate benign and malignant strictures, because the wall of the esophagus is immobile when infiltrated by tumor, whereas normal peristalsis is usually observed in a benign stricture. Rarely, esophageal cancer may cause beaklike narrowing of the distal esophagus, mimicking the appearance of primary achalasia.[102] However, asymmetry, nodularity, or ulceration of the narrowed segment should suggest a malignant lesion.

When infiltrating cancers are detected in the esophagus, it may be difficult or impossible to differentiate a squamous cell carcinoma from an adenocarcinoma arising in Barrett's mucosa. However, adenocarcinomas tend to be located more distally in the esophagus and often invade the gastric cardia

or fundus, whereas squamous cell carcinomas rarely extend subdiaphragmatically to involve the stomach.[101,102,139] Other clinical or radiographic signs of reflux esophagitis should also favor adenocarcinoma. However, endoscopy and biopsy are required for a definitive diagnosis.

Although squamous cell carcinomas and adenocarcinomas sometimes appear as polypoid masses in the esophagus, the presence of a bulky intraluminal mass (especially one that expands the esophagus without causing obstruction) should suggest the possibility of other rare malignant tumors such as spindle cell carcinoma and primary malignant melanoma of the esophagus (see Chapter 28).[153,154] Rarely, benign tumors such as fibrovascular polyps may be manifested by polypoid lesions, but these tumors tend to appear as smooth, expansile, sausage-shaped masses in the upper thoracic esophagus (see Chapter 26).[155] Finally, impacted food in the esophagus may be confused radiographically with polypoid carcinomas. However, the presence of a stricture directly below the polypoid defect should suggest the possibility of a food impaction. Impacted debris may also obstruct the esophagus, whereas polypoid carcinomas rarely cause esophageal obstruction. Obviously, a history of sudden onset of dysphagia while eating meat or other bulky food products should suggest this complication.

Primary ulcerative carcinomas usually appear as distinctive meniscoid ulcers surrounded by a thick rim of malignant tissue. However, the adjacent tumor mass may be relatively subtle, so these lesions can occasionally be mistaken for benign ulcers. Conversely, some patients with esophagitis may have large, flat ulcers with a surrounding mound of edema, erroneously suggesting an ulcerated carcinoma. Ulcers associated with potassium chloride or quinidine ingestion or nasogastric intubation may have a particularly ominous appearance (see Chapter 25). Endoscopy and biopsy may therefore be required to exclude a malignant lesion.

Although varicoid carcinoma can mimic the appearance of esophageal varices on a single radiograph, these entities can usually be differentiated at fluoroscopy.[88-90,143] True varices tend to change in size and shape with peristalsis, respiration, and Valsalva maneuvers, whereas varicoid tumors have a rigid, fixed configuration, with an abrupt demarcation between the involved segment and the adjacent normal mucosa. Most varicoid carcinomas are squamous cell carcinomas or adenocarcinomas, but other malignant tumors such as lymphoma may occasionally produce similar findings.[156]

Rarely, localized submucosal extension of a squamous cell carcinoma or adenocarcinoma may produce a smooth submucosal mass, mimicking the appearance of a benign leiomyoma (Fig. 27-23).[157] However, a malignant lesion should be suspected if there is lobulation or ulceration of the mass.

STAGING

Although CT has been the mainstay for staging esophageal carcinoma, the increasing use of endoscopic ultrasound (EUS) and positron emission tomography (PET) has altered the staging algorithm for patients with newly diagnosed esophageal cancer. In the past, CT of the chest and upper abdomen was often the only preoperative staging test for esophageal cancer. Currently, however, a combination of CT, EUS, and PET is advocated to determine which patients should be treated with surgery, chemotherapy, or combined chemotherapy and radiation therapy. As with any cancer, staging criteria for esophageal carcinoma include detection of local invasion, regional lymph node involvement, and distant metastases. The different imaging modalities have different strengths and weaknesses for each of these parameters.

Computed Tomography

Technique

When CT is performed for esophageal cancer staging, the scan should include the upper abdomen as well as the thorax because of the high incidence of upper abdominal lymph node metastases at the time of diagnosis.[158] Distal esophageal cancers are more likely to be associated with upper abdominal lymph node involvement (Fig. 27-24); the frequency of

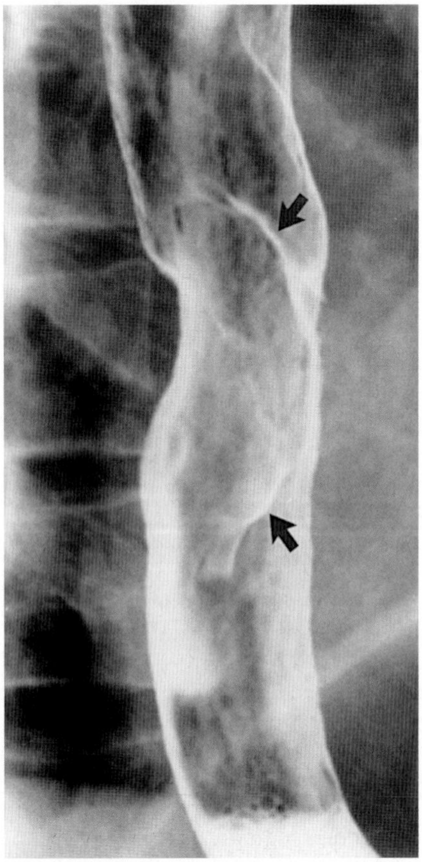

Figure 27-23. Esophageal carcinoma resembling a benign submucosal mass. However, this lesion (*arrows*) is larger and has a more irregular contour than most leiomyomas. (From Levine MS: Radiology of the Esophagus. Philadelphia, WB Saunders, 1989.)

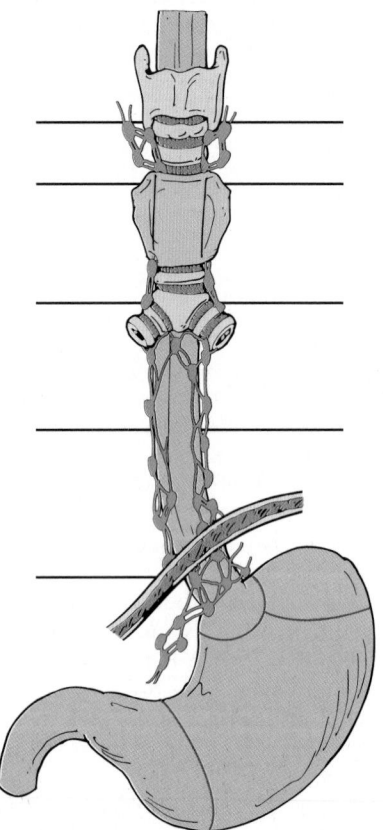

Figure 27-24. Longitudinal lymphatics of esophagus. Artist's drawing shows how the lymphatic channels surrounding the distal esophagus drain into paracardiac and lesser curvature lymph nodes in the upper abdomen, accounting for the high frequency of abdominal lymph node metastases in patients with distal esophageal cancers.

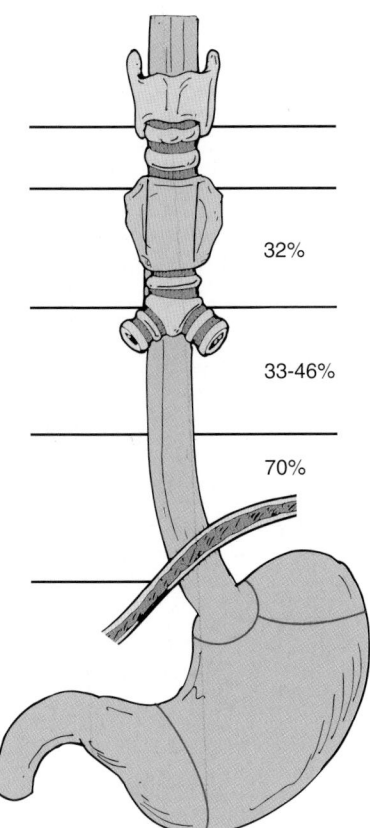

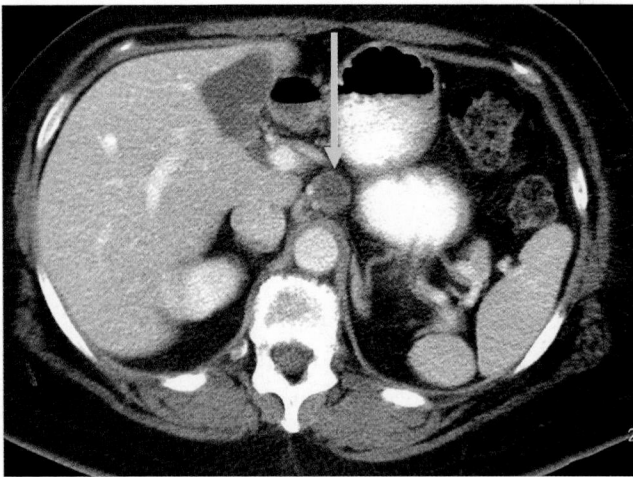

Figure 27-26. Enlarged subdiaphragmatic lymph node (*arrow*) due to lymphatic metastasis from esophageal carcinoma. Lymphatic metastases may occur at a considerable distance from the primary tumor because of the rich network of longitudinally oriented periesophageal lymphatics.

Figure 27-25. Relationship between frequency of subdiaphragmatic lymph node metastases and location of esophageal cancer. Artist's drawing shows how distal esophageal cancers have a substantially higher frequency of subdiaphragmatic lymph node metastases than cancer located more proximally in the esophagus.

abdominal lymph node metastases is about 30% for thoracic esophageal cancers above the level of the carina but increases to 70% for cancers below the carina (Fig. 27-25).[159] Because the lymphatic drainage of the esophagus is longitudinal rather than circumferential (as in the remainder of the gastrointestinal tract), lymph node metastases tend to occur above and below the site of the primary tumor, rather than immediately adjacent to the tumor (Fig. 27-26). Intravenous contrast material is administered whenever possible to increase detectability of hepatic metastases and better differentiate lymph nodes from vascular structures in the mediastinum. Currently, it is controversial whether staging CT should also include the neck to look for cervical lymph node metastases.

Staging Criteria

The major CT criteria for staging esophageal cancer include detection of (1) local invasion of the mediastinum; (2) regional lymph node involvement; and (3) distant metastases. CT is better at detecting local invasion of the mediastinum by esophageal cancer than it is at detecting local invasion by other gastrointestinal cancers, presumably because the mediastinum is a contained space. As a result, direct invasion can be predicted by mass effect criteria that are not useful elsewhere in the gastrointestinal tract.

The CT criteria for local invasion include (1) loss of the fat plane between the tumor and adjacent structures in the

mediastinum and (2) displacement or indentation of other mediastinal structures. The CT findings of displacement of the trachea or bronchus or indentation of the posterior wall of the trachea or bronchus by the tumor mass have been found to be highly accurate for predicting tracheal or bronchial invasion (Figs. 27-27 and 27-28).[160-165] The combined results from six studies with surgical confirmation revealed that CT had a sensitivity of 93%, a specificity of 98%, and an accuracy of 97% for predicting tracheobronchial invasion by esophageal cancer.[166]

Mass effect criteria can also be used to predict pericardial invasion. If the tumor extends to the posterior surface of the heart with no intervening fat plane and if the tumor bulges into the lumen of the left atrium on CT or MRI, pericardial invasion can be predicted with a high level of confidence (Fig. 27-29). The combined results of those same six studies revealed that CT had a sensitivity, specificity, and accuracy of 94% for predicting pericardial invasion.[166]

It is more difficult to predict aortic invasion because the esophagus normally contacts the aorta with no intervening fat plane (Fig. 27-30). Investigators have circumvented this problem by recognizing that the fat plane surrounding the aorta normally has a circumference of 360 degrees (similar to that of a compass). If an esophageal cancer obliterates the fat plane between the esophagus and aorta by more than one fourth of the circumference (greater than 90 degrees), tumor is considered to be invading the aorta (Fig. 27-31). If the tumor obliterates less than 45 degrees of the circumference, the aorta is not considered to be invaded by tumor (Fig. 27-32). Finally, if the tumor obliterates 45 to 90 degrees of the circumference, the CT findings are considered to be indeterminate for aortic invasion (Fig. 27-33). By using this criterion, the combined results of those same six studies revealed that CT had a sensitivity of 88%, a specificity of 96%, and an accuracy of 94% for predicting aortic invasion.[166]

Because lymph node enlargement is the CT criterion used to predict mediastinal or upper abdominal lymph node metastases, CT is limited by the fact that it cannot detect tumor in normal-sized lymph nodes. CT therefore fails to detect

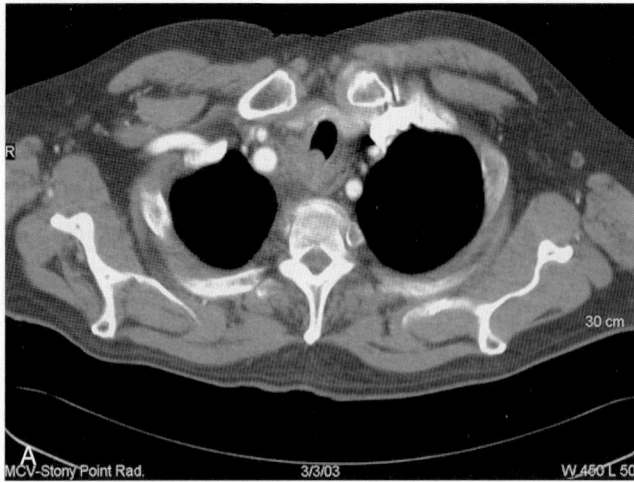

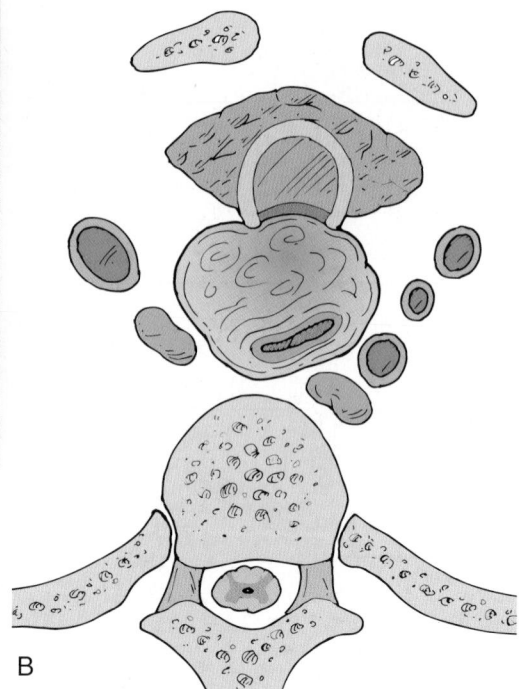

Figure 27-27. Tracheal invasion by esophageal carcinoma. A. CT shows esophageal tumor indenting posterior wall of trachea. This finding is diagnostic of tracheal invasion. **B.** Artist's drawing of tracheal invasion by esophageal tumor.

B

nodes that are involved by tumor in the absence of nodal enlargement. Enlarged lymph nodes adjacent to an esophageal cancer also may not be visualized because they are inseparable from the primary lesion. When enlarged mediastinal lymph nodes are detected, CT also cannot differentiate benign causes of lymph node enlargement from metastatic tumor. In one study, benign enlargement of lymph nodes occurred more frequently when the primary esophageal cancer was large and necrotic.[167] In general, CT has been found to be more accu-

rate for predicting upper abdominal lymph node metastases than mediastinal lymph node metastases.[168]

CT of the chest and upper abdomen can also detect distant metastases to the lungs, bones, liver, or other structures. These findings are useful for predicting long-term survival in patients with esophageal cancer. In one study, patients with CT findings of mediastinal or subdiaphragmatic invasion by tumor had a significantly shorter survival compared with patients without these findings.[168]

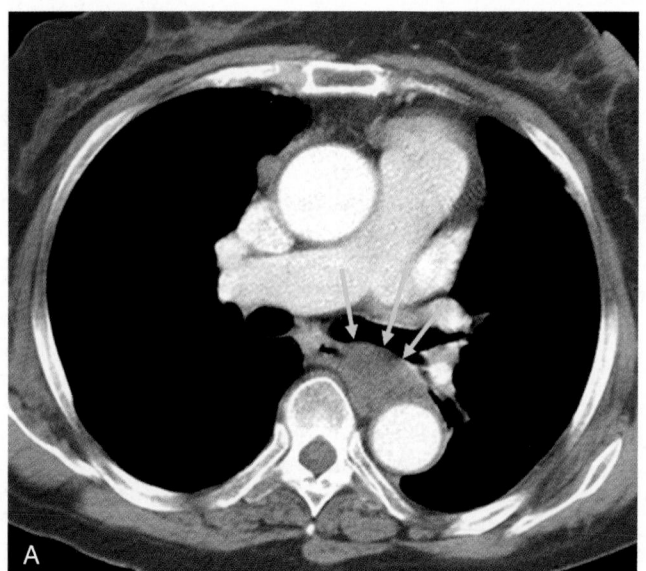

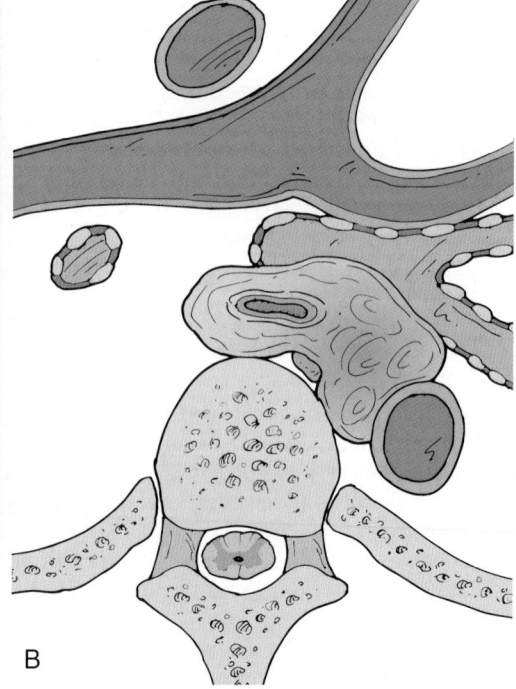

Figure 27-28. Bronchial invasion by esophageal carcinoma. A. CT shows esophageal tumor bowing and displacing posterior wall (*arrows*) of left main bronchus. This finding is diagnostic of bronchial invasion. **B.** Artist's drawing of bronchial invasion by tumor.

B

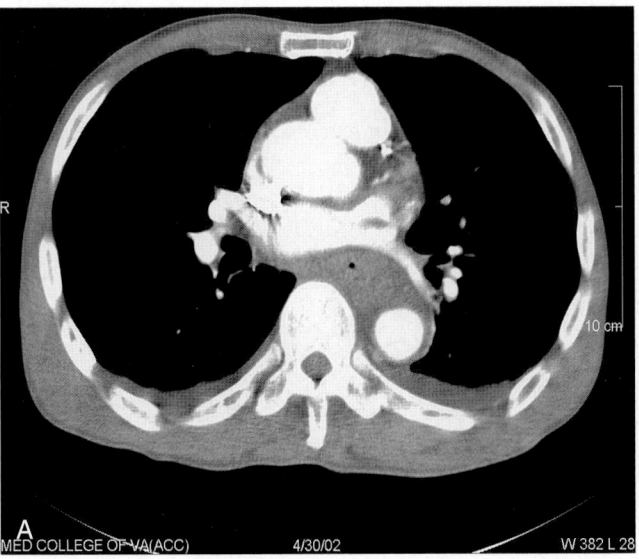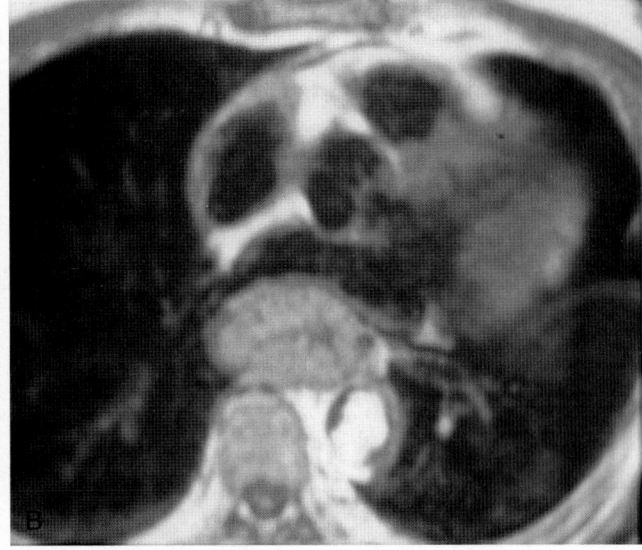

Figure 27-29. Pericardial invasion by esophageal carcinoma. A. CT shows esophageal tumor indenting posterior wall of left atrium. This finding is indicative of pericardial invasion. **B.** MRI also shows tumor indenting posterior wall of left atrium.

Endoscopic Ultrasound

Technique

The ultrasound probe is built into the tip of a fiberoptic endoscope designed specifically for EUS. The tip of the probe is covered by a distensible rubber balloon that can be filled with water to provide an acoustic interface between the transducer

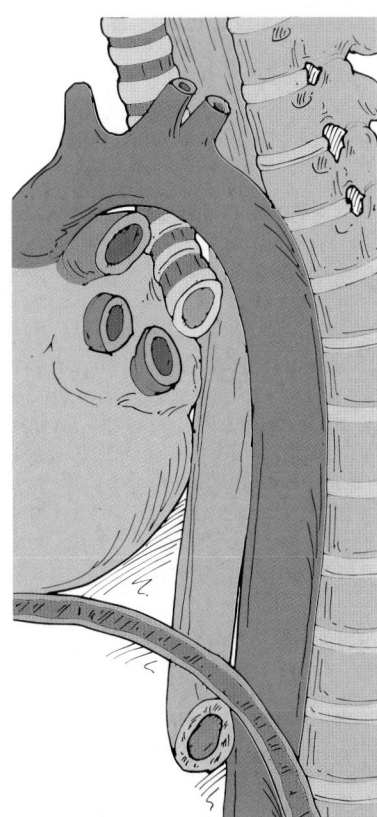

Figure 27-30. Normal contact between esophagus and descending thoracic aorta. Artist's drawing shows how there is direct contact between the esophagus and adjacent descending thoracic aorta.

and the esophageal wall. These ultrasound units are stand-alone devices separate from the upper gastrointestinal endoscope. The probes are similar in size to standard endoscopes, so that they cannot pass through areas of marked luminal narrowing caused by advanced esophageal cancers, preventing adequate staging of these tumors. Reported rates of non-traversability of the tumor at EUS have ranged from 20% to 45%.[169,170] More recently, a tiny probe has been developed that can pass through the biopsy channel of a standard upper gastrointestinal endoscope.[171,172] These probes have the advantage of being able to traverse a greater percentage of esophageal cancers because of the smaller probe caliber. At the same time, these smaller probes utilize very high frequency transducers, so that they have a more limited field of view.

Staging Criteria

EUS provides excellent visualization of the five layers of the esophageal wall. These layers are recognized on EUS as alternating layers of increased and decreased echogenicity, producing five rings (Fig. 27-34). The inner echogenic line represents the mucosal interface with the transducer, the central echogenic line represents submucosal fat (fat is echogenic on ultrasound), and the outer echogenic line represents serosal fat. Tumors are usually manifested by hypoechogenic masses causing disruption or widening of these esophageal rings (Fig. 27-35). EUS is excellent for detecting esophageal tumors and can often identify lesions that have spread beyond the wall, allowing differentiation of T2 tumors (which are confined to the esophageal wall) from T3 tumors (which extend beyond the esophageal wall into the periesophageal fat). The ability of EUS to detect T4 tumors (which are invading adjacent structures in the mediastinum) is limited by the inability to differentiate invasive tumors from those that extend to adjacent structures without actual invasion.

A meta-analysis of 13 studies evaluating the accuracy of EUS for esophageal cancer staging found that EUS had an overall accuracy of 89% for predicting the depth of tumor invasion in the esophageal wall and an accuracy of 79% for

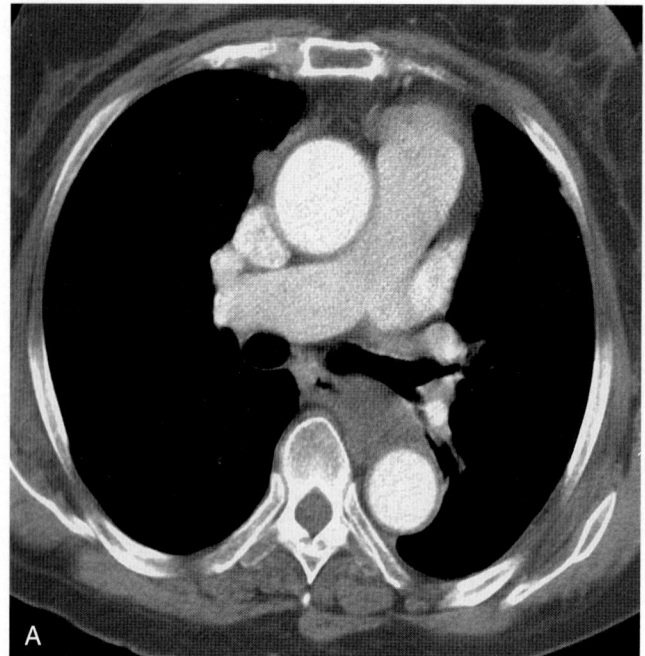

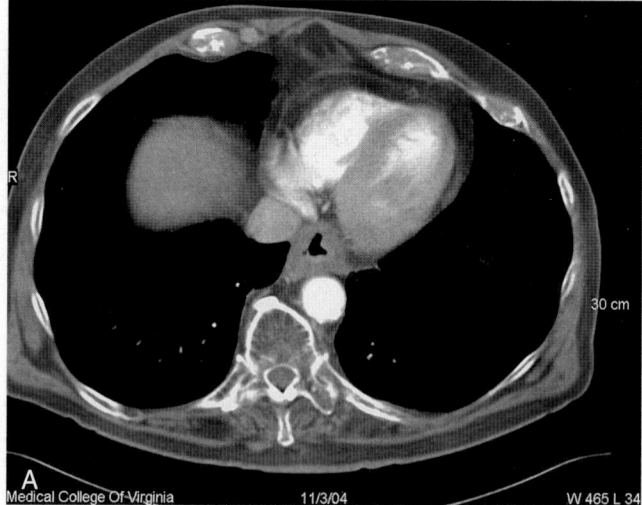

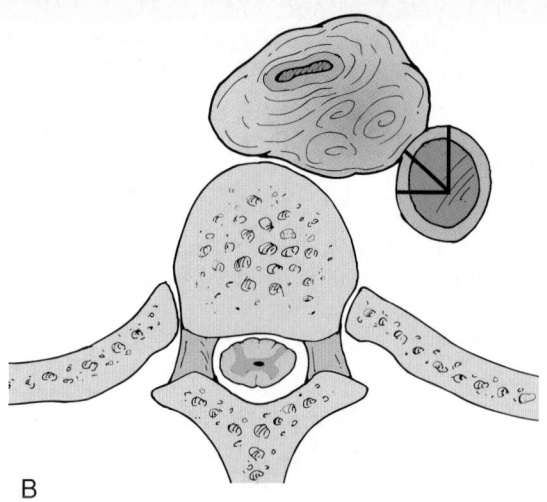

Figure 27-32. Esophageal carcinoma without evidence of aortic invasion. A. CT shows how there is less than 45 degrees of contact between the esophageal tumor and aorta. This finding indicates that the aorta is not invaded by tumor. **B.** Artist's drawing also shows how there is less than 45 degrees of contact between the esophageal tumor and aorta.

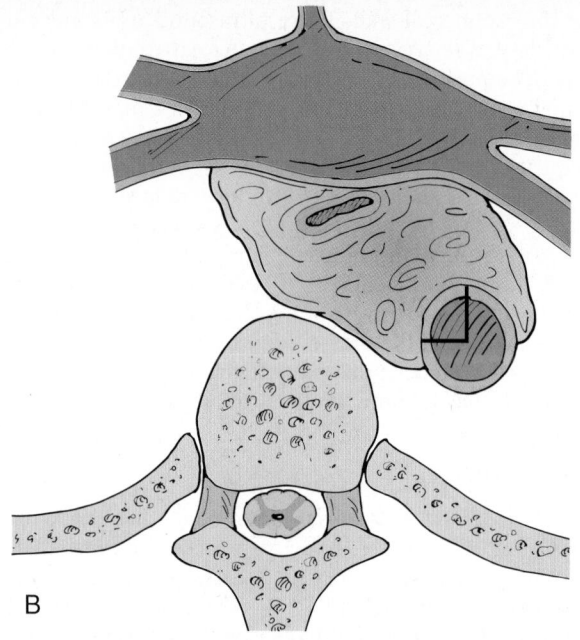

Figure 27-31. Aortic invasion by esophageal carcinoma. A. CT shows how there is greater than 90 degrees of contact between the esophageal tumor and aorta without intervening fat planes. This is a useful CT criterion for predicting aortic invasion. **B.** Artist's drawing also shows how there is greater than 90 degrees of contact between the tumor and aorta.

predicting mediastinal lymph node metastases (Fig. 27-36).[173] Many authors therefore believe that EUS should be complementary to helical CT for staging esophageal cancer. EUS is superior to CT for detecting the depth of invasion of the esophageal wall and mediastinal lymph node metastases, but CT is superior to EUS for detecting distant metastases. The ability of EUS to differentiate T2 from T3 tumors is particularly helpful for guiding treatment, because patients with T2 tumors usually undergo primary surgical resection whereas chemoradiation therapy is usually given to patients with T3

tumors. At institutions in which surgery is performed for both T2 and T3 tumors, however, this benefit of EUS is lost.

The accuracy of EUS for nodal staging can be increased by transesophageal EUS-guided fine-needle aspiration cytology of peritumoral lymph nodes in the mediastinum.[174] In one study, routine fine-needle aspiration of lymph nodes at EUS was found to have an accuracy of 93% for nodal staging versus an accuracy of 70% for EUS alone.[175] EUS with fine-needle aspiration can therefore improve local staging of esophageal cancer.

Positron Emission Tomography

PET using fluorodeoxyglucose (FDG) is another useful test for staging esophageal cancer. Because these tumors and their metastases to the liver, lungs, cervical lymph nodes, and other sites are relatively FDG avid (Figs. 27-37 and 27-38), PET or PET-CT can detect metastases that are not recognized on CT.[176] In one study, PET revealed metastases not visible on CT of the chest and upper abdomen in 17% of patients with

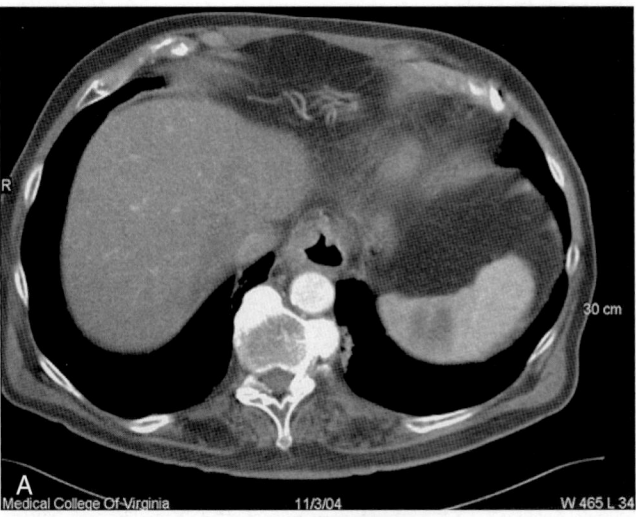

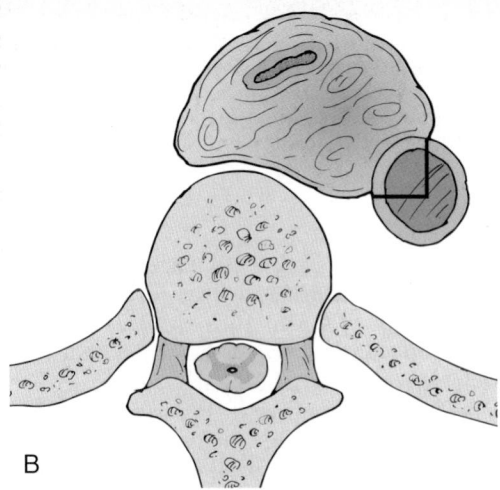

Figure 27-33. Indeterminate CT for aortic invasion by esophageal cancer. A. CT shows how there is between 45 and 90 degrees of contact between the esophageal tumor and aorta. This finding is indeterminate for aortic invasion. **B.** Artist's drawing also shows how there is between 45 and 90 degrees of contact between the esophageal tumor and aorta.

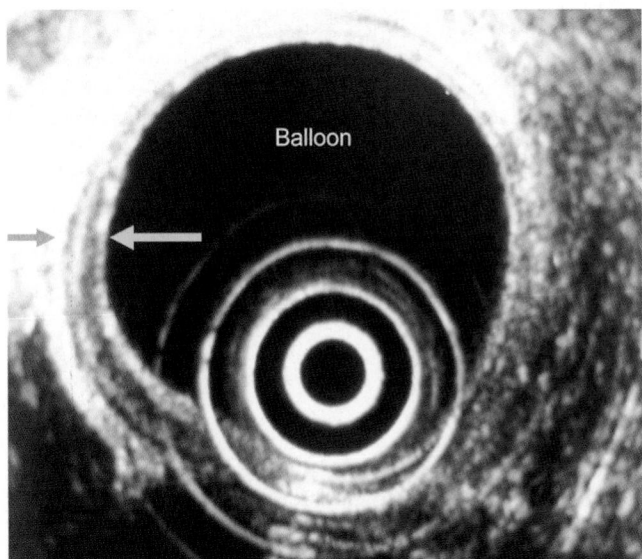

Figure 27-34. Normal endoscopic ultrasound showing all five layers (*arrows*) **of esophageal wall.**

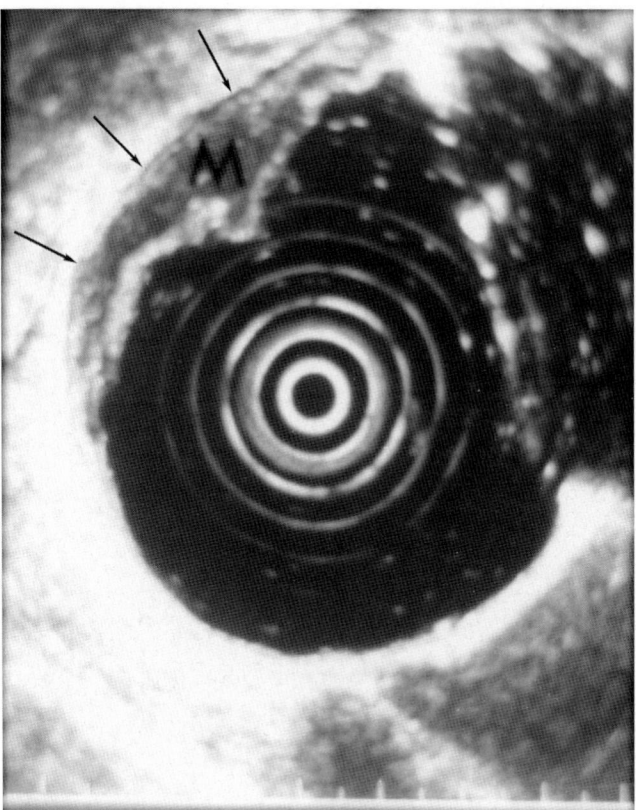

Figure 27-35. Endoscopic ultrasound of esophageal cancer. Endoscopic ultrasound shows a hypoechoic mass (M) causing focal widening of the esophageal wall. The thin black line peripherally (*arrows*) indicates that the tumor has not yet invaded the serosal fat.

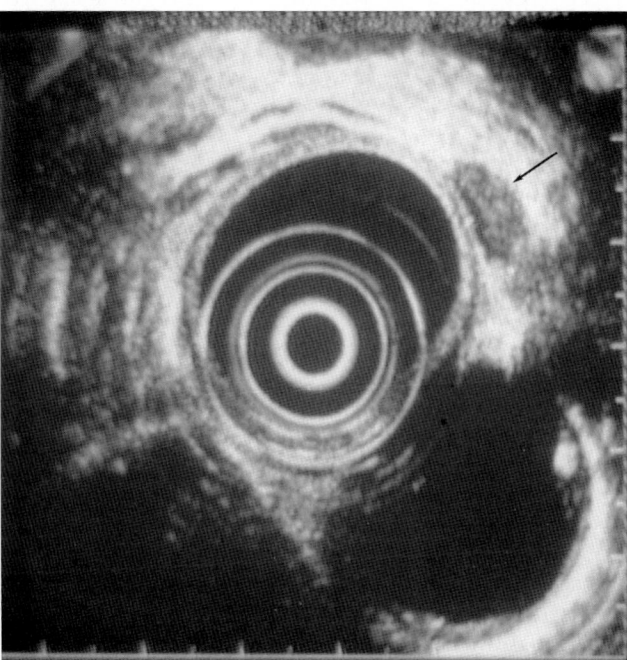

Figure 27-36. Endoscopic ultrasound of lymph node metastasis from esophageal carcinoma. The enlarged node is manifested by a hypoechoic focus (*arrow*).

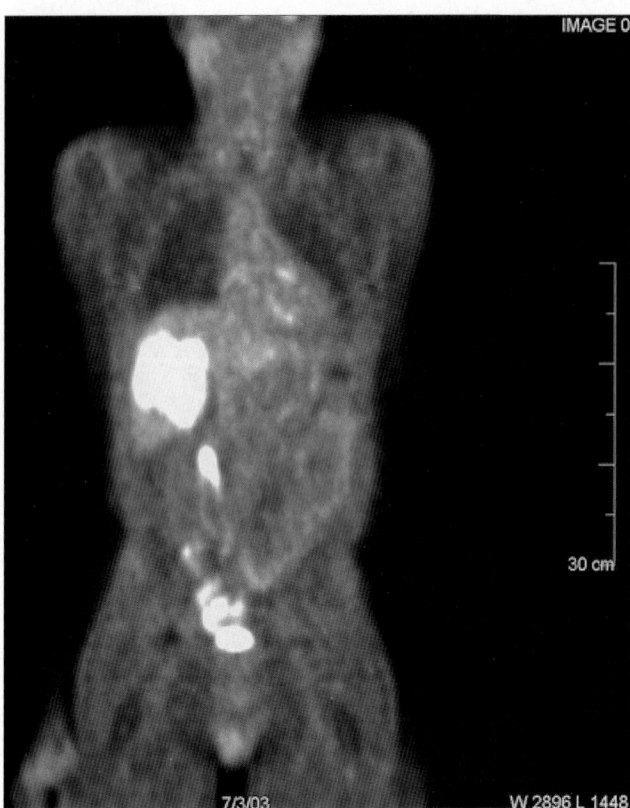

Figure 27-37. Liver metastasis from esophageal carcinoma on PET. Coronal PET image shows marked uptake of radionuclide in liver due to avidity of hepatic metastasis.

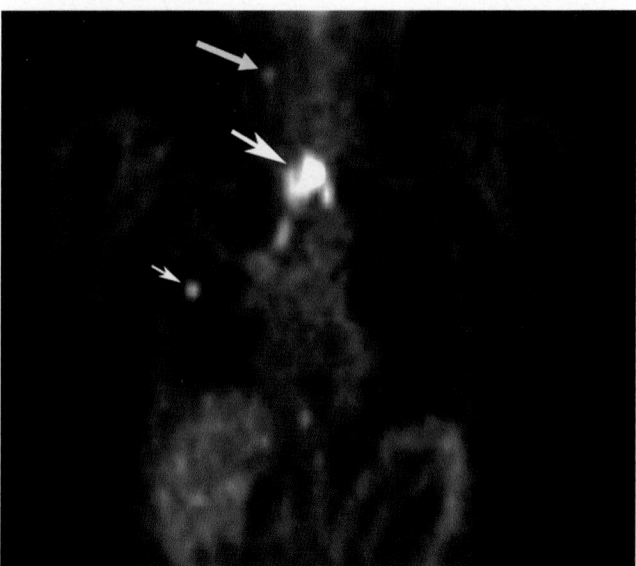

Figure 27-38. Cervical lymph node and pulmonary metastases from esophageal carcinoma on PET. Coronal PET image shows marked uptake of radionuclide (*large white arrow*) in bulky esophageal tumor in upper mediastinum. Also note uptake in metastases to right cervical lymph node (*yellow arrow*) and right lung (*small white arrow*).

esophageal cancer, including 38% of cervical lymph node metastases, 23% of bone metastases, and 15% of hepatic metastases.[177] PET is therefore particularly helpful when CT reveals no evidence of local invasion or distant metastases (Fig. 27-39). In another study, PET contributed important additional information for cancer staging in 14% of patients with esophageal cancer who underwent CT.[178]

Ultrasonography of the Neck

Cervical lymph nodes appear to be of greater importance for esophageal cancer staging than has previously been recognized. In one study, one third of patients who underwent esophagectomy for "curable" cancers of the thoracic esophagus were found to have cervical lymph node metastases when a lymph node dissection of the neck was performed at the time of esophagectomy.[179] In fact, lymph node metastases were found to be as common in the neck as in the mediastinum. The frequency of cervical lymph nodes metastases directly correlates with the location of the tumor in the esophagus; 80% of patients with tumors in the cervical esophagus have cervical lymph node metastases versus 52% with tumors in the proximal thoracic esophagus, 29% with tumors in the mid-thoracic esophagus, and 9% with tumors in the distal thoracic esophagus.[180]

Because of the high frequency of cervical lymph node metastases from esophageal cancer, Asian and European authors have advocated ultrasonography of the neck with fine-needle aspiration of suspicious lymph nodes as an alter-

native imaging test for staging esophageal cancer.[181,182] Neck ultrasonography is performed with a high-frequency transducer in the range of 7.5 to 10 MHz. This examination is relatively easy to perform because the lymph nodes of interest in the neck are within 3 cm of the skin surface. Lymph nodes are considered to be abnormal if they have a diameter larger than 5 mm or a short-to-long ratio of greater than 50%.[183] In one study, ultrasonography of the neck with fine-needle aspiration of suspicious nodes had a sensitivity of 88%, a specificity of 59%, and an accuracy of 78% for detecting cervical lymph node metastases from esophageal cancer.[184]

Staging Algorithm

CT is usually recommended as the initial test for esophageal cancer staging. If CT reveals local invasion or distant metastases, no further imaging is warranted. If, however, CT is negative or indeterminate for local invasion or distant metastases, the patient can be referred for EUS. If the tumor still appears to be resectable on EUS, then PET or PET-CT can be performed to detect local invasion or distant metastases not recognized on CT or EUS. Further investigation is needed to determine whether ultrasonography or CT of the neck should be performed routinely to assess for cervical lymph node metastases in these patients.

TREATMENT

Depending on the stage of the tumor at the time of diagnosis, esophageal cancer may be treated by curative or palliative measures. Curative therapy includes surgery, irradiation, and surgery combined with preoperative or postoperative radiation therapy or chemotherapy. Palliative therapy includes surgery, irradiation, chemotherapy, placement of an indwelling esophageal prosthesis, and laser treatment.

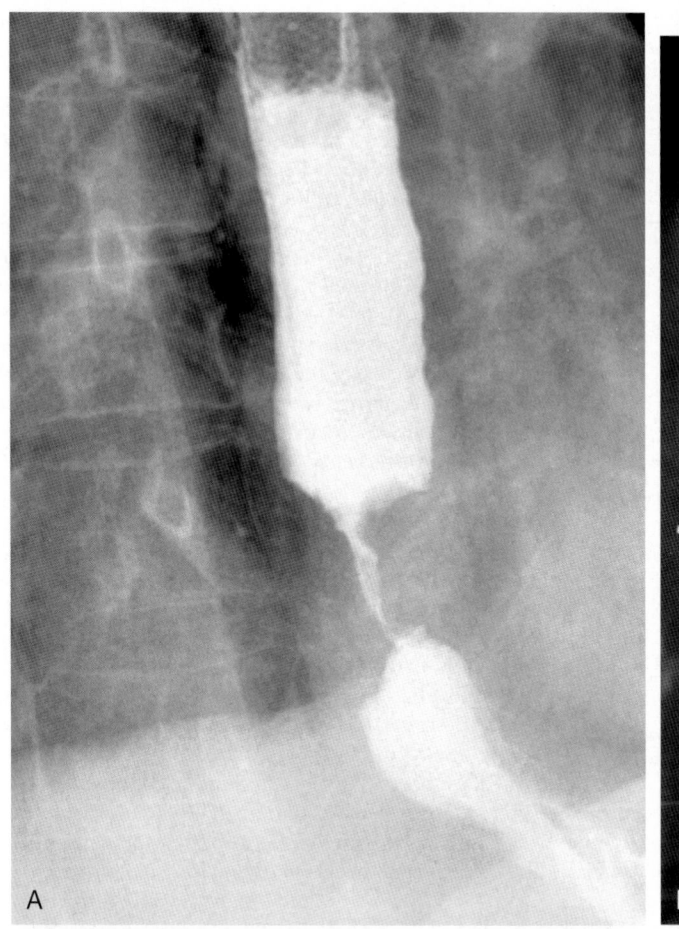

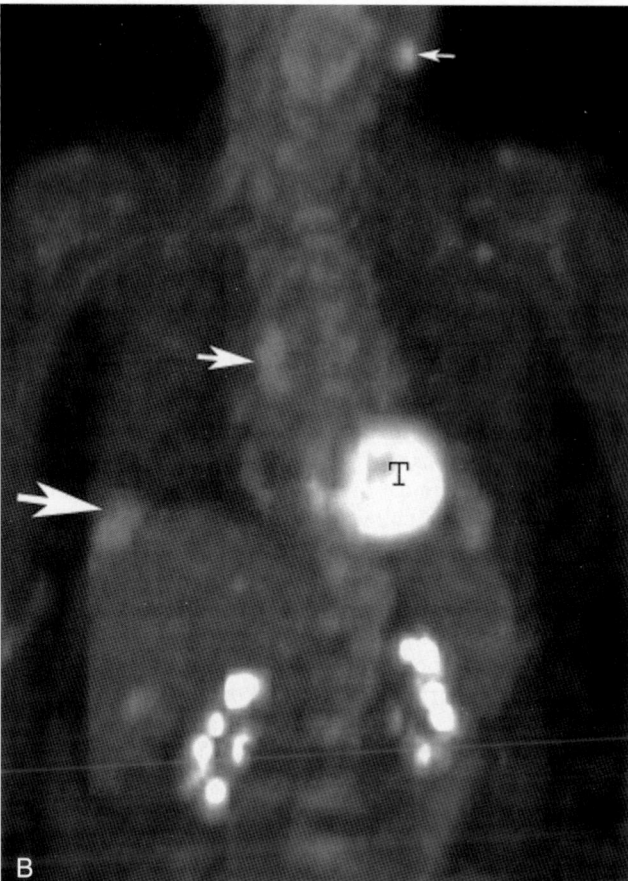

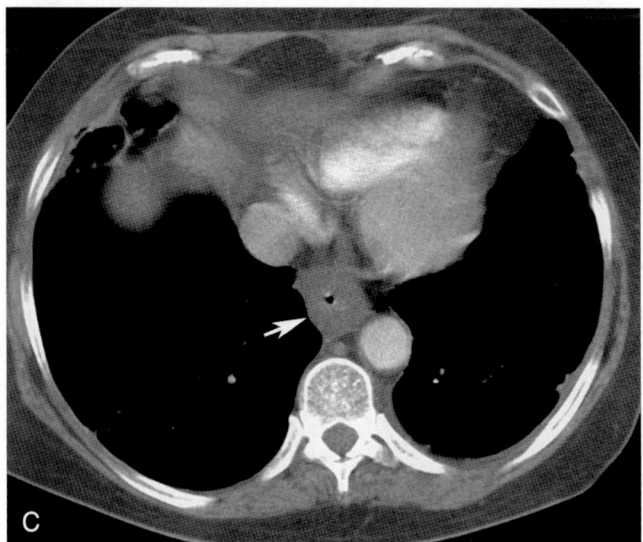

Figure 27-39. Value of PET for showing metastases not detected on CT.
A. Barium study shows a circumferentially infiltrating carcinoma of the distal esophagus. **B.** Coronal PET image shows marked uptake of radionuclide in distal esophageal tumor (T). However, there is also uptake in metastases to the liver (*large arrow*), mediastinum (*medium arrow*), and a left cervical lymph node (*small arrow*). The PET scan has therefore dramatically altered the staging of this patient's disease. **C.** CT shows marked esophageal wall thickening by tumor (*arrow*). However, this lesion is potentially resectable without CT findings of local or distant metastases. (Note how there is less than 45 degrees of contact between the tumor and adjacent aorta.)

Surgery

Curative resection of a carcinoma in the distal two thirds of the esophagus usually requires an esophagogastrectomy and gastric pull-through. Resection of a more proximal lesion may require a free jejunal graft for reconstruction of the pharyngoesophagus. Palliative surgery in patients with advanced esophageal cancer usually consists of an esophageal bypass procedure to control symptoms of obstruction or fistula formation. The most common bypass procedures include colonic interposition and creation of a gastric tube. Palliation may also be achieved by passage of an esophageal prosthesis (usually an expandable metallic stent) to bypass an obstruction or fistula. The normal and abnormal appearances after surgery or other palliative procedures for esophageal cancer are discussed in Chapter 31.

Radiation Therapy

Radiation therapy may be used for either palliative or definitive treatment of esophageal cancer. Squamous cell carcinomas tend to be more radiosensitive than adenocarcinomas.[185] Tumors in the cervical or upper thoracic esophagus also tend to be more radiosensitive than those located in the middle or distal thoracic esophagus.[185] Partial or total regression of tumor occurs in most patients who undergo this form of treatment.[186-188] Although these patients may have significant relief from dysphagia in the initial months after therapy, the lesions subsequently recur locally in 30% to 85% of cases.[185,188-190] Even when the tumor is eradicated from the esophagus, these patients often die as a result of widespread metastases to the liver, lungs, or mediastinum.[185,188,191] Increased morbidity or mortality may also be attributed directly to complications of radiation therapy, such as esophageal ulceration, perforation, and fistula formation.[190,192] As a result, the prognosis after radiation therapy is comparable with or slightly worse than that after surgery, with an average survival of only 9 to 10 months.

Partial regression of tumor after radiation therapy may be recognized on serial barium studies by a decrease in the size and bulk of the lesion. With total regression of tumor, esophagography may reveal a normal esophagus or a benign-appearing stricture at the site of the original lesion (Fig. 27-40).[188,189,193,194] In most cases, these strictures appear as smooth, tapered areas of narrowing without evidence of nodularity, mass effect, or ulceration to suggest residual tumor. Even when there is total regression of tumor, however, these patients often die as a result of distant metastases, presumably because of unrecognized lymphatic involvement at the time of therapy.[188] Thus, disappearance of the cancer on radiologic or endoscopic studies does not necessarily indicate a cure.

Although most patients have an initial clinical response to radiation therapy, recurrent dysphagia often occurs within 3 to 9 months after treatment because of local recurrence of tumor.[185,188,189] Recurrent carcinoma may be recognized on barium studies by the development of a polypoid, ulcerative, or infiltrating lesion within or just beyond the margins of the original radiation portal.[188] However, an exacerbation of symptoms in these patients may be caused not only by recurrent tumor but also by benign radiation strictures, fistula formation, perforation, or opportunistic esophageal infections such as *Candida* and herpes esophagitis.[188] Thus, radiologic studies may differentiate recurrent carcinoma from other complications in these patients.

Chemoradiation Therapy

Initial reports suggested that combined chemotherapy and radiation therapy of patients with esophageal carcinoma produced an immediate and dramatic response but that the long-term benefits of this approach were questionable. Preoperative chemoradiation therapy has also been advocated as an adjunct to surgery for patients with locally advanced tumors or regional lymphadenopathy.[2] Unfortunately, conflicting data have been reported about the value of multimodality therapy. In a study of patients with adenocarcinoma of the esophagus, preoperative chemoradiation therapy was found to be superior to surgery alone, with median survivals

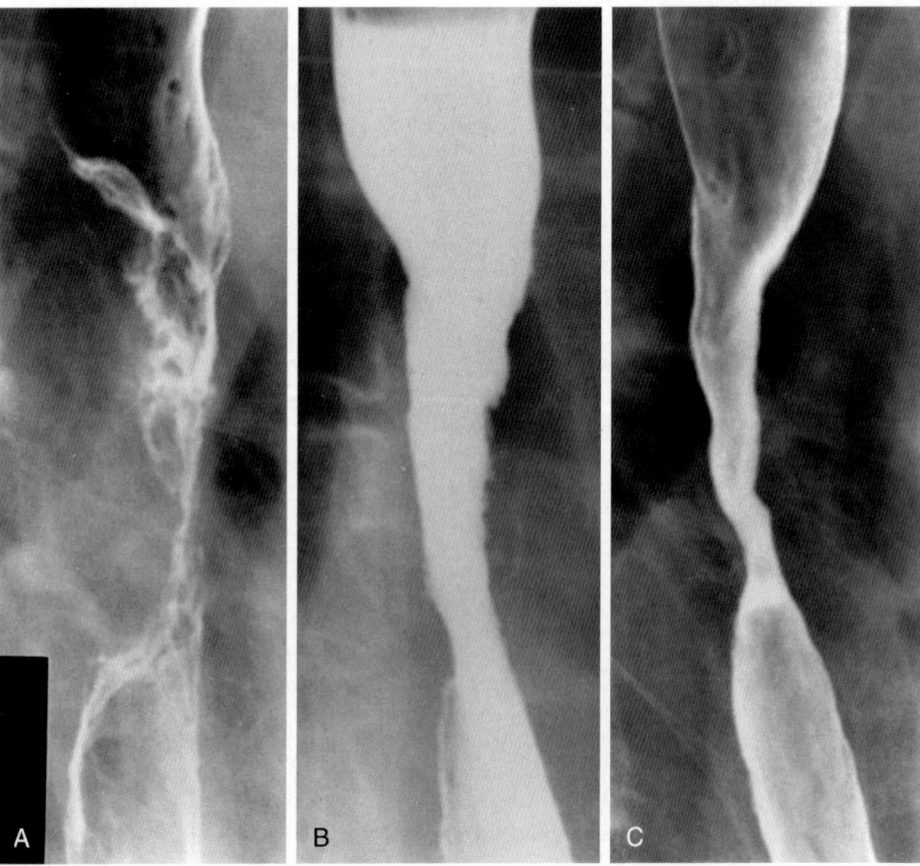

A   B   C

Figure 27-40. Total regression of esophageal carcinoma after radiation therapy with a benign residual stricture. A. Initial esophagogram shows an advanced, infiltrating carcinoma in the midesophagus. **B.** Second study 4 months after radiation therapy shows partial regression of the tumor with residual areas of shallow ulceration. **C.** Third study 2 months later shows total regression of the lesion with a smooth, tapered, benign-appearing radiation stricture in this location. (From Levine MS: Radiology of the Esophagus. Philadelphia, WB Saunders, 1989.)

of 15 months and 11 months, respectively.[195] In another study of patients with squamous cell carcinoma of the esophagus, however, preoperative chemoradiation therapy did not improve overall survival of these patients.[196] Nevertheless, combined chemoradiation therapy is a viable alternative to surgery in patients with advanced disease or medical conditions that preclude surgery.

References

1. Livstone EM, Skinner DB: Tumors of the esophagus. In Berk JE (ed): Gastroenterology. Philadelphia, WB Saunders, 1985, pp 818-850.
2. Wang KK, Wongkeesong M, Buttar NS: American Gastroenterological Association technical review on the role of the gastroenterologist in the management of esophageal carcinoma. Gastroenterology 128: 1471-1505, 2005.
3. Pottern LM, Morris LE, Blot WJ, et al: Esophageal cancer among black men in Washington, DC: Alcohol, tobacco, and other risk factors. J Natl Cancer Inst 67:777-783, 1981.
4. Engel LS, Chow WH, Vaughan TL, et al: Population attributable risks of esophageal and gastric cancers. J Natl Cancer Inst 95:1404-1413, 2003.
5. Fielding JE: Smoking: Health effects and control. N Engl J Med 313: 491-498, 1985.
6. Caygill CP, Johnston DA, Lopez M, et al: Lifestyle factors and Barrett's esophagus. Am J Gastroenterol 97:1328-1331, 2002.
7. Ribeiro U, Posner MC, Safatle-Ribeiro AV, et al: Risk factors for squamous cell carcinoma of the esophagus. Br J Surg 83:1174-1185, 1996.
8. Yang CS: Research on esophageal cancer in China: A review. Cancer Res 40:2633-2644, 1980.
9. Burrell RJW, Roach WA, Shadwell A: Esophageal cancer in the Bantu of the Transkei associated with mineral deficiency in garden plants. J Natl Cancer Inst 36:201-214, 1966.
10. Warwick GP, Harington JS: Some aspects of the epidemiology and etiology of esophageal cancer with particular emphasis on the Transkei, South Africa. Adv Cancer Res 17:81-229, 1973.
11. Amer MH, El-Yazigi A, Hannan MA, et al: Water contamination and esophageal cancer at Gassim Region, Saudi Arabia. Gastroenterology 98:1141-1147, 1990.
12. Stephen SJ, Uragoda CG: Some observations on oesophageal carcinoma in Ceylon, including its relationship to betel chewing. Br J Cancer 24:11-15, 1970.
13. Correa P: Precursors of gastric and esophageal cancer. Cancer 50: 2554-2565, 1982.
14. Craighead JE, Mossman BT: The pathogenesis of asbestos-associated diseases. N Engl J Med 306:1446-1455, 1982.
15. Chang F, Shen Q, Zhou J, et al: Detection of human papillomavirus DNA in cytologic specimens derived from esophageal precancer lesions and cancer. Scand J Gastroenterol 25:383-388, 1990.
16. Chang F, Syrjanen S, Shen Q, et al: Screening for human papillomavirus infections in esophageal squamous cell carcinomas by in situ hybridization. Cancer 72:2525-2530, 1993.
17. Just-Viera JO, Haight C: Achalasia and carcinoma of the esophagus. Surg Gynecol Obstet 128:1081-1093, 1969.
18. Seliger G, Lee T, Schwartz S: Carcinoma of the proximal esophagus: A complication of long-standing achalasia. Am J Gastroenterol 57:20-25, 1972.
19. Carter R, Brewer LA: Achalasia and esophageal carcinoma. Am J Surg 130:114-118, 1975.
20. Wychulis AR, Woolam GL, Andersen HA, et al: Achalasia and carcinoma of the esophagus. JAMA 215:1638-1641, 1971.
21. Hankins JR, McLaughlin JS: The association of carcinoma of the esophagus with achalasia. J Thorac Cardiovasc Surg 69:355-360, 1975.
22. Chuong JJH, DuBovik S, McCallum RW: Achalasia as a risk factor for esophageal carcinoma: A reappraisal. Dig Dis Sci 29:1105-1108, 1984.
23. Bigger IA, Vinson PP: Carcinoma secondary to burn of the esophagus from ingestion of lye. Surgery 28:887-889, 1950.
24. Imre J, Kopp M: Arguments against long-term conservative treatment of oesophageal strictures due to corrosive burns. Thorax 27:594-598, 1972.
25. Appleqvist P, Salmo M: Lye corrosion carcinoma of the esophagus: A review of 63 cases. Cancer 45:2655-2658, 1980.
26. Hopkins RA, Postlethwait RW: Caustic burns and carcinoma of the esophagus. Ann Surg 194:146-148, 1981.
27. Weaver A, Fleming SM, Knechtges TC, et al: Triple endoscopy: A neglected essential in head and neck cancer. Surgery 86:493-496, 1979.
28. Atkinson D, Fleming S, Weaver A: Triple endoscopy: A valuable procedure in head and neck surgery. Am J Surg 144:416-419, 1982.
29. McGuirt WF: Panendoscopy as a screening examination for simultaneous primary tumors in head and neck cancer: A prospective sequential study and review of the literature. Laryngoscope 92:569-576, 1982.
30. Wynder EL, Mushinski MH, Spivak JC: Tobacco and alcohol consumption in relation to the development of multiple primary cancers. Cancer 40:1872-1878, 1977.
31. Harris OD, Cooke WT, Thompson H, et al: Malignancy in adult coeliac disease and idiopathic steatorrhea. Am J Med 42:899-912, 1967.
32. Collins SM, Hamilton JD, Lewis TD, et al: Small bowel malabsorption and gastrointestinal malignancy. Radiology 126:603-609, 1978.
33. Chisholm M: The association between webs, iron and postcricoid carcinoma. Postgrad Med J 50:215-219, 1974.
34. Wynder EL, Hultberg S, Jacobsson F, et al: Environmental factors in cancer of the upper alimentary tract: A Swedish study with special reference to Plummer-Vinson (Paterson-Kelly) syndrome. Cancer 10: 470-487, 1957.
35. Chudecki B: Radiation cancer of the thoracic oesophagus. Br J Radiol 45:303-304, 1972.
36. O'Connell EW, Seaman WB, Ghahremani GG: Radiation-induced esophageal carcinoma. Gastrointest Radiol 9:287-291, 1984.
37. Ahsan H, Neugut AI: Radiation therapy for breast cancer and increased risk of esophageal carcinoma. Ann Intern Med 128:114-117, 1998.
38. Shine I, Allison PR: Carcinoma of the oesophagus with tylosis. Lancet 1:951-953, 1966.
39. Harper PS, Harper RMJ, Howel-Evans AW: Carcinoma of the oesophagus with tylosis. Q J Med 39:317-333, 1970.
40. Munyer TP, Margulis AR: Tylosis. AJR 136:1026-1027, 1981.
41. Blot W, Devesa S, Fraumeni J: Continued climb in rates of esophageal adenocarcinoma: An update. JAMA 270:1320, 1993.
42. Froelicher P, Miller G: The European experience with esophageal cancer limited to the mucosa and submucosa. Gastrointest Endosc 32:88-90, 1986.
43. Bonavina L: Early oesophageal cancer: Results of a European multicentre survey. Group European pour l'Etude des Maladies de l'Oesophage. Br J Surg 82:9-101, 1995.
44. Japanese Society for Esophageal Diseases: Guidelines for the clinical and pathologic studies on carcinoma of the esophagus. Jpn J Surg 6:69-78, 1976.
45. Roth MJ, Liu SF, Dawsey SM, et al: Cytologic detection of esophageal squamous cell carcinoma and precursor lesions using balloon and sponge samplers in asymptomatic adults in Linxian, China. Cancer 80:2047-2059, 1997.
46. Moss AA, Koehler RE, Margulis AR: Initial accuracy of esophagograms in detection of small esophageal carcinoma. AJR 127:909-913, 1976.
47. Zornoza J, Lindell MM: Radiologic evaluation of small esophageal carcinoma. Gastrointest Radiol 5:107-111, 1980.
48. Mannell A: Carcinoma of the esophagus. Curr Probl Surg 19:553-647, 1982.
49. Yamada A: Radiologic assessment of resectability and prognosis in esophageal carcinoma. Gastrointest Radiol 4:213-218, 1979.
50. Postlethwait RW: Carcinoma of the esophagus. Curr Probl Cancer 2:1-44, 1978.
51. Fitzgerald RH, Bartles DM, Parker EF: Tracheoesophageal fistulas secondary to carcinoma of the esophagus. J Thorac Cardiovasc Surg 82:194-197, 1981.
52. Little AG, Ferguson MK, DeMeester TR, et al: Esophageal carcinoma with respiratory tract fistula. Cancer 53:1322-1328, 1984.
53. Bottiglieri NG, Palmer ED, Briggs GW, et al: Aortoesophageal fistula complicating carcinoma of the esophagus. Am J Dig Dis 8:837-844, 1963.
54. Vennos AD, Templeton PA: Pneumopericardium secondary to esophageal carcinoma. Radiology 182:131-132, 1992.
55. Mandard AM, Chasle J, Marnay J, et al: Autopsy findings in 111 cases of esophageal cancer. Cancer 48:329-335, 1981.
56. Sannohe Y, Hiratsuka R, Doki K: Lymph node metastases in cancer of the thoracic esophagus. Am J Surg 141:216-218, 1981.
57. Rosengren JE, Goldstein HM: Radiologic demonstration of multiple foci of malignancy in the esophagus. Gastrointest Radiol 3:11-13, 1978.
58. Davis M, Gogel H, McIntire C, et al: Esophageal carcinoma multiplex with gastric metastasis. Gastrointest Radiol 14:6-8, 1989.
59. Glick SN, Teplick SK, Levine MS, et al: Gastric cardia metastasis in esophageal carcinoma. Radiology 160:627-630, 1986.

60. Glick SN, Teplick SK, Levine MS: Squamous cell metastases to the gastric cardia. Gastrointest Radiol 10:339-344, 1985.
61. Koehler RE, Moss AA, Margulis AR: Early radiographic manifestations of carcinoma of the esophagus. Radiology 119:1-5, 1976.
62. Skinner DB: Surgical treatment for esophageal carcinoma. Semin Oncol 11:136-143, 1984.
63. Levine MS, Dillon EC, Saul SH, et al: Early esophageal cancer. AJR 146:507-512, 1986.
64. Carey LC, Darin JC, Worman LW, et al: Upper gastrointestinal hemorrhage from carcinoma of esophagus. Arch Surg 90:460-464, 1965.
65. Barrie JR, Goodner JT: Hematemesis from cancer of the esophagus. J Thorac Cardiovasc Surg 56:289-292, 1968.
66. Ghosh BC, Choudhry KU, Beattie EJ: Massive bleeding from esophageal cancer. J Thorac Cardiovasc Surg 63:977-979, 1972.
67. Alrenga DP: Fatal hemorrhage complicating carcinoma of the esophagus: Report of four cases. Am J Gastroenterol 65:422-426, 1976.
68. Graham DY, Schwartz JT, Cain GD, et al: Prospective evaluation of biopsy number in the diagnosis of esophageal and gastric carcinoma. Gastroenterology 82:228-231, 1982.
69. Lal N, Bhasin DK, Malik AK, et al: Optimal number of biopsy specimens in the diagnosis of carcinoma of the oesophagus. Gut 33:724-726, 1992.
70. Suzuki H, Kobayashi S, Endo M, et al: Diagnosis of early esophageal cancer. Surgery 71:99-103, 1971.
71. Yamada A, Kobayashi S, Kawai B, et al: Study on x-ray findings of early oesophageal cancer. Australas Radiol 16:238-246, 1972.
72. Itai Y, Kogure T, Okuyama Y, et al: Superficial esophageal carcinoma: Radiological findings in double-contrast studies. Radiology 126:597-601, 1978.
73. Sato T, Sakai Y, Kajita A, et al: Radiographic microstructures of early esophageal carcinoma: Correlation of specimen radiography with pathologic findings and clinical radiography. Gastrointest Radiol 11:12-19, 1986.
74. Lee SS, Ha HK, Byun JH, et al: Superficial esophageal cancer: Esophagographic findings correlated with histopathologic findings. Radiology 236:535-544, 2005.
75. Itai Y, Kogure T, Okuyama Y, et al: Diffuse finely nodular lesions of the esophagus. AJR 128:563-566, 1977.
76. Schmidt LW, Dean PJ, Wilson RT: Superficially invasive squamous cell carcinoma of the esophagus. Gastroenterology 91:1456-1461, 1986.
77. Lindell MM, Hill CA, Libshitz HI: Esophageal cancer: Radiographic chest findings and their prognostic significance. AJR 133:461-465, 1979.
78. Putman CE, Curtis A, Westfried M, et al: Thickening of the posterior tracheal stripe: A sign of squamous cell carcinoma of the esophagus. Radiology 121:533-536, 1976.
79. Daffner RH, Postlethwait RW, Putman CE: Retrotracheal abnormalities in esophageal carcinoma: Prognostic implications. AJR 130:719-723, 1978.
80. Levine MS, Chu P, Furth EE, et al: Carcinoma of the esophagus and esophagogastric junction: Sensitivity of radiographic diagnosis. AJR 168:1423-1426, 1997.
81. DiPalma JA, Prechter GC, Brady CE: X-ray-negative dysphagia: Is endoscopy necessary? J Clin Gastroenterol 6:409-411, 1984.
82. Halpert RD, Feczko PJ, Spickler EM, et al: Radiologic assessment of dysphagia with endoscopy. Radiology 157:599-602, 1985.
83. Wiot JW, Felson B: Radiographic differential diagnosis of esophageal cancer. JAMA 226:1548-1552, 1973.
84. Goldstein HM, Zornoza J, Hopens T: Intrinsic diseases of the adult esophagus: Benign and malignant tumors. Semin Roentgenol 16:183-197, 1981.
85. Levine MSL: Esophageal cancer: Radiologic diagnosis. Radiol Clin North Am 35:265-279, 1997.
86. Iyer RB, Silverman PM, Tamm EP, et al: Diagnosis, staging, and follow-up of esophageal cancer. AJR 181:785-793, 2003.
87. Gloyna RE, Zornoza J, Goldstein HM: Primary ulcerative carcinoma of the esophagus. AJR 129:599-600, 1977.
88. Lawson TL, Dodds WJ, Sheft DJ: Carcinoma of the esophagus simulating varices. AJR 107:83-85, 1969.
89. Yates CW, LeVine MA, Jensen KM: Varicoid carcinoma of the esophagus. Radiology 122:605-608, 1977.
90. Sabedotti G, Dreweck MO, Sabedotti V, et al: Carcinoma of the esophagus: Varicoid pattern. RadioGraphics 26:271-274, 2006.
91. Cho SR, Schneider V, Beachley MC, et al: Carcinoma of the esophagus: Assessment of submucosal extent. J Can Assoc Radiol 33:154-157, 1982.
92. Steiner H, Lammer J, Hackl A: Lymphatic metastases to the esophagus. Gastrointest Radiol 9:1-4, 1984.
93. Allen HA, Bush JE: Midesophageal carcinoma metastatic to the stomach: Its unusual appearance on an upper gastrointestinal series. South Med J 76:1049-1051, 1983.
94. Raphael HA, Ellis FH, Dockerty MB: Primary adenocarcinoma of the esophagus: 18 year review and review of literature. Ann Surg 164:785-796, 1966.
95. Turnbull ADM, Goodner JT: Primary adenocarcinoma of the esophagus. Cancer 22:915-918, 1968.
96. Bosch A, Frias Z, Caldwell WL: Adenocarcinoma of the esophagus. Cancer 43:1557-1561, 1979.
97. Daly JM, Karnell LH, Menck HR: National Cancer Data Base report on esophageal carcinoma. Cancer 78:1820-1828, 1996.
98. Devesa SS, Blot WJ, Fraumeni JF: Changing patterns in the incidence of esophageal and gastric carcinoma in the United States. Cancer 83:2049-2053, 1998.
99. Bytzer P, Christensen PB, Damkier P, et al: Adenocarcinoma of the esophagus and Barrett's esophagus: A population-based study. Am J Gastroenterol 94:86-91, 1999.
100. Haggitt RC, Tryzelaar J, Ellis FH, et al: Adenocarcinoma complicating columnar epithelium-lined (Barrett's) esophagus. Am J Clin Pathol 70:1-5, 1978.
101. Levine MS, Caroline D, Thompson JJ, et al: Adenocarcinoma of the esophagus: Relationship to Barrett mucosa. Radiology 150:305-309, 1984.
102. Agha FP: Barrett carcinoma of the esophagus: Clinical and radiographic analysis of 34 cases. AJR 145:41-46, 1985.
103. Bozymski EM, Herlihy KJ, Orlando RC: Barrett's esophagus. Ann Intern Med 97:103-107, 1982.
104. Sjogren RW, Johnson LF: Barrett's esophagus: A review. Am J Med 74:313-321, 1983.
105. Spechler SJ, Goyal RK: Barrett's esophagus. N Engl J Med 315:362-371, 1986.
106. Levine MS, Herman JB, Furth EE: Barrett's esophagus and esophageal adenocarcinoma: The scope of the problem. Abdom Imaging 20:291-298, 1995.
107. Sarr MG, Hamilton SR, Marrone GC, et al: Barrett's esophagus: Its prevalence and association with adenocarcinoma in patients with symptoms of gastroesophageal reflux. Am J Surg 149:187-192, 1985.
108. Winters C, Spurling TJ, Chobanian SJ, et al: Barrett's esophagus: A prevalent, occult complication of gastroesophageal reflux disease. Gastroenterology 92:118-124, 1987.
109. Corder AP, Jones RH, Sadler GH, et al: Heartburn, oesophagitis and Barrett's oesophagus in self-medicating patients in general practice. Br J Clin Pract 50:245-248, 1996.
110. Csendes A, Smok G, Burdiles P, et al: Prevalence of Barrett's esophagus by endoscopy and histologic studies: A prospective evaluation of 306 control subjects and 376 patients with symptoms of gastroesophageal reflux disease. Dis Esophagus 13:5-11, 2000.
111. Paull A, Trier JS, Dalton MD, et al: The histologic spectrum of Barrett's esophagus. N Engl J Med 295:476-480, 1976.
112. Thompson JJ, Zinsser KR, Enterline HT: Barrett's metaplasia and adenocarcinoma of the esophagus and gastroesophageal junction. Hum Pathol 14:42-61, 1983.
113. Weinstein WM, Ippoliti AF: The diagnosis of Barrett's esophagus: Goblets, goblets, goblets. Gastrointest Endosc 44:91-95, 1996.
114. Hirota WK, Loughney TM, Lazas DJ, et al: Specialized intestinal metaplasia, dysplasia, and cancer of the esophagus and esophagogastric junction: Prevalence and clinical data. Gastroenterology 116:277-285, 1999.
115. Sharma P, Morales TG, Sampliner RE: Short segment Barrett's esophagus—the need for standardization of the definition and of endoscopic criteria. Am J Gastroenterol 93:1033-1036, 1998.
116. Skinner DB, Walther BC, Riddell RH, et al: Barrett's esophagus: Comparison of benign and malignant cases. Ann Surg 198:554-565, 1983.
117. Reid BJ: Barrett's esophagus and esophageal adenocarcinoma. Gastroenterol Clin North Am 20:817-834, 1991.
118. Spechler SJ, Robbins AH, Rubins HB, et al: Adenocarcinoma and Barrett's esophagus: An overrated risk? Gastroenterology 87:927-933, 1984.
119. Cameron AJ, Ott BJ, Payne WS: The incidence of adenocarcinoma in the columnar-lined (Barrett's) esophagus. N Engl J Med 313:857-859, 1985.
120. Shaheen NJ, Crosby MA, Bozymski EM, et al: Is there publication bias in the reporting of cancer risk for esophageal adenocarcinoma. Gastroenterology 119:333-338, 2000.
121. Berenson MM, Riddell RH, Skinner DB, et al: Malignant transformation of esophageal columnar epithelium. Cancer 41:554-561, 1978.

122. Hamilton SR, Smith RRL: The relationship between columnar epithelial dysplasia and invasive adenocarcinoma arising in Barrett's esophagus. Am J Clin Pathol 87:301-312, 1987.

123. Reid BJ, Weinstein WM, Lewin KJ, et al: Endoscopic biopsy can detect high-grade dysplasia or early adenocarcinoma in Barrett's esophagus without grossly recognizable neoplastic lesions. Gastroenterology 94:81-90, 1988.

124. Hameeteman W, Tytgat GNJ, Houthoff HJ, et al: Barrett's esophagus: Development of dysplasia and adenocarcinoma. Gastroenterology 96:1249-1256, 1989.

125. Sharma P, Morales TH, Bhattacharyya A, et al: Dysplasia in short-segment Barrett's esophagus: A prospective 3-year follow-up. Am J Gastroenterol 92:2012-2016, 1997.

126. Weston AP, Krmpotich PT, Cherian R, et al: Prospective long-term endoscopic and histological follow-up of short-segment Barrett's esophagus: Comparison with traditional long-segment Barrett's esophagus. Am J Gastroenterol 92:407-413, 1997.

127. Schnell TG, Sontag SJ, Chejfec G: Adenocarcinoma arising in tongues or short-segments of Barrett's esophagus. Dig Dis Sci 37:137-143, 1992.

128. Nishimaki T, Watanabe K, Suzuki T, et al: Early esophageal adenocarcinoma arising in a short-segment of Barrett's mucosa after total gastrectomy. Am J Gastroenterol 91:1856-1857, 1996.

129. Gossner L, Stolte M, Sroka R, et al: Photodynamic ablation of high-grade dysplasia and early cancer in Barrett's esophagus by means of 5-aminolevulinic acid. Gastroenterology 114:448-455, 1998.

130. Ell C, May A, Gossner L, et al: Endoscopic mucosal resection of early cancer and high-grade dysplasia in Barrett's esophagus. Gastroenterology 118:670-677, 2000.

131. Provenzale D, Kemp JA, Arora S, et al: A guide for surveillance of patients with Barrett's esophagus. Am J Gastroenterol 89:670-680, 1994.

132. Sharma P, McQuaid K, Dent J, et al: A critical review of the diagnosis and management of Barrett's esophagus: The AGA Chicago workshop. Gastroenterology 127:310-330, 2004.

133. Reid BJ, Blount PL, Rubin CE, et al: Flow-cytometric and histological progression to malignancy in Barrett's esophagus: Prospective endoscopic surveillance of a cohort. Gastroenterology 102:1212-1219, 1992.

134. Robaszkiewicz M, Reid BJ, Volant A, et al: Flow-cytometric DNA content analysis of esophageal squamous cell carcinomas. Gastroenterology 101:1588-1593, 1991.

135. McDonald GB, Brand DL, Thorning DR: Multiple adenomatous neoplasms arising in columnar-lined (Barrett's) esophagus. Gastroenterology 72:1317-1321, 1977.

136. Keeffe EB, Hiskin EC, Schubert F: Adenomatous polyp arising in Barrett's esophagus. J Clin Gastroenterol 8:271-274, 1986.

137. Recht MP, Levine MS, Katzka DA, et al: Barrett's esophagus in scleroderma: Increased prevalence and radiographic findings. Gastrointest Radiol 13:1-5, 1988.

138. Halpert RD, Laufer I, Thompson JJ, et al: Adenocarcinoma of the esophagus in patients with scleroderma. AJR 140:927-930, 1983.

139. Keen SJ, Dodd GD, Smith JL: Adenocarcinoma arising in Barrett's esophagus: Pathologic and radiologic features. Mt Sinai J Med 51:442-450, 1984.

140. Kalish RJ, Clancy PE, Orringer MB, et al: Clinical, epidemiologic, and morphologic comparison between adenocarcinomas arising in Barrett's esophageal mucosa and in the gastric cardia. Gastroenterology 86:461-467, 1984.

141. Dupas JL, Caproy JP, Lorriaux A: Endoscopic diagnosis of early primary adenocarcinoma in Barrett's columnar-lined esophagus. Endoscopy 7:98-101, 1975.

142. Wong A, Fitzgerald RC: Epidemiologic risk factors for Barrett's esophagus and associated adenocarcinoma. Clin Gastroenterol Hepatol 3:1-10, 2005.

143. Odes HS, Maor E, Barki Y, et al: Varicoid carcinoma of the esophagus: Report of a patient with adenocarcinoma and review of the literature. Am J Gastroenterol 73:141-145, 1980.

144. Montesi A, Alessandro P, Graziani L, et al: Small benign tumors of the esophagus: Radiological diagnosis with double contrast examination. Gastrointest Radiol 8:207-212, 1983.

145. Levine MS, Cajade AG, Herlinger H, et al: Pseudomembranes in reflux esophagitis. Radiology 159:43-45, 1986.

146. Levine MS, Macones AJ, Laufer I: *Candida* esophagitis: Accuracy of radiographic diagnosis. Radiology 154:581-587, 1985.

147. Glick SN, Teplick SK, Goldstein J, et al: Glycogenic acanthosis of the esophagus. AJR 139:683-688, 1982.

148. Itai Y, Kogure T, Okuyama Y, et al: Diffuse finely nodular lesions of the esophagus. AJR 128:563-566, 1977.

149. Itai Y, Kogure T, Okuyama Y, et al: Radiological manifestations of oesophageal involvement in acanthosis nigricans. Br J Radiol 49:592-593, 1976.

150. Nuwayhid NS, Ballard ET, Cotton R: Esophageal papillomatosis. Ann Otol Rhinol Laryngol 86:623-625, 1977.

151. Levine MS, Kressel HY, Caroline D, et al: Barrett esophagus: Reticular pattern of the mucosa. Radiology 147:663-667, 1983.

152. Agha FP, Whitehouse WM: Carcinoma of the esophagus: Its varied radiologic features. Mt Sinai J Med 51:430-441, 1984.

153. Agha FP, Keren DF: Spindle-cell squamous carcinoma of the esophagus: A tumor with biphasic morphology. AJR 145:541-545, 1985.

154. Yoo CC, Levine MS, McLarney JK, et al: Primary malignant melanoma of the esophagus: Radiographic findings in seven patients. Radiology 209:455-459, 1998.

155. Levine MS, Buck JL, Pantongrag-Brown L, et al: Fibrovascular polyps of the esophagus: Clinical, radiographic, and pathologic findings in 16 patients. AJR 166:781-787, 1996.

156. Caruso RD, Berk RN: Lymphoma of the esophagus. Radiology 95:381-382, 1970.

157. Engelman RM, Scialla AV: Carcinoma of the esophagus presenting radiologically as a benign lesion. Dis Chest 53:652-655, 1968.

158. Halvorsen RA, Thompson WM: CT of esophageal neoplasms. Radiol Clin North Am 27:667-685, 1989.

159. Akiyama H, Tsurumaru M, Kawamura T, et al: Principles of surgical treatment for carcinoma of the esophagus: Analysis of lymph node involvement. Ann Surg 194:438-445, 1981.

160. Thompson WM, Halvorsen RA, Foster WL, et al: Computed tomography for staging esophageal and gastroesophageal cancer: Re-evaluation. AJR 141:951-958, 1983.

161. Coulomb M, Leas JF, Sarrazin R, et al: Computed tomography and esophageal carcinoma. J Radiol 62:475-487, 1981.

162. Gayet B, Frija J, Cahuzac J, et al: The usefulness of computed tomography in esophageal carcinoma: A prospective and "blind" study. Gastroenterol Clin Biol 12:23-28, 1988.

163. Grosser G, Wimmer B, Ruf G: Computed tomography for carcinoma of the esophagus: A prospective study. Fortschr Geb Rontgenstr Nuklearmed Erganzungsband 143:288-293, 1985.

164. Muhling T, Kuklinski ME, Hubsch T, et al: Computed tomography of oesophageal carcinoma: A correlation of computed tomographic and post-operative findings. Fortschr Geb Rontgenstr Nuklearmed Erganzungsband 143:189-193, 1985.

165. Picus D, Balfe DM, Koehler RE, et al: Computed tomography in the staging of esophageal carcinoma. Radiology 146:433-438, 1983.

166. Halvorsen RA, Thompson WM: CT of esophageal neoplasms. Radiol Clin North Am 27:667-685, 1989.

167. Lackner K, Weiand G, Koster O, et al: Computed tomography for tumors of the esophagus and stomach. Fortschr Geb Rontgenstr Nuklearmed Erganzungsband 134:364-370, 1981.

168. Halvorsen RA, Magruder-Habib K, Foster W, et al: Esophageal cancer: Long-term follow-up of staging by computed tomography. Radiology 161:147-151, 1986.

169. Heidemann J, Schilling MK, Schmassmann A, et al: Accuracy of endoscopic ultrasonography in preoperative staging of esophageal carcinoma. Dig Surg 17:219-224, 2000.

170. Kelly S, Harris KM, Berry E, et al: A systematic review of the staging performance of endoscopic ultrasound in gastroesophageal carcinoma. Gut 49:534-539, 2001.

171. Koch J, Halvorsen RA, Thompson WM: Therapy hinges on staging in upper GI tract cancer. Diagn Imaging 15:74-81, 1993.

172. Menzel J, Domschke W: Gastrointestinal miniprobe sonography: The current status. Am J Gastroenterol 95:605-616, 2000.

173. Lightdale CJ, Kulkarni KG: Role of endoscopic ultrasonography in the staging and follow-up of esophageal cancer. J Clin Oncol 23:4483-4489, 2005.

174. Savides TJ: EUS FNA staging of esophageal cancer [editorial]. Gastroenterology 125:1883-1886, 2003.

175. Vasquez-Sequeiros E, Norton ID, Clain JE, et al: Impact of EUS-guided fine-needle aspiration on lymph node staging in patients with esophageal carcinoma. Gastrointest Endosc 53:751-757, 2001.

176. Kato H, Kuwano H, Nakajima M, et al: Comparison between positron emission tomography and computer tomography in the assessment of esophageal carcinoma. Cancer 94:921-928, 2002.

177. Imdahl A, Hentschel M, Kleimaier M, et al: Impact of FDG-PET for

staging of oesophageal cancer. Langenbecks Arch Surg 389:283-288, 2004.

178. Kato H, Miyazaki T, Nakajima M, et al: The incremental effect of positron emission tomography on diagnostic accuracy on the initial staging of esophageal cancer. Cancer 103:148-156, 2005.

179. Altorki NK, Skinnner DB: Occult cervical nodal metastasis in esophageal cancer: Preliminary results of three-field lymphadenectomy. J Thorac Cardiovasc Surg 113:540-544, 1997.

180. Griffith JF, Chanc ACW, Ahuja AT, et al: Neck ultrasound in staging squamous oesophageal carcinoma—a high yield technique. Clin Radiol 55:696-701, 2000.

181. Tachimori Y, Kato H, Watanabe H, et al: Neck ultrasonography for thoracic esophageal carcinoma. Ann Thorac Surg 57:1180-1183, 1994.

182. Van Overhagen H, Lameris JS, Berger MY, et al: Supraclavicular lymph node metastases in carcinoma of the esophagus and gastroesophageal junction: Assessment with CT, US, and US-guided fine-needle aspiration biopsy. Radiology 179:155-158, 1991.

183. Doldi SB, Lattuada E, Zappa MA, et al: Ultrasonographic evaluation of the cervical lymph nodes in preoperative staging of esophageal neoplasms. Abdom Imaging 23:275-277, 1998.

184. Natsugoe S, Yoshinaka H, Shimada M, et al: Assessment of cervical lymph node metastasis in esophageal carcinoma using ultrasonography. Ann Surg 229:62-66, 1999.

185. Beatty JD, DeBoer G, Rider WD: Carcinoma of the esophagus: Pretreatment assessment, correlation of radiation treatment parameters with survival, and identification and management of radiation treatment failure. Cancer 43:2254-2267, 1979.

186. Parker EF, Gregorie HB: Carcinoma of the esophagus: Long-term results. JAMA 235:1018-1020, 1976.

187. Rosenberg JS, Franklin B, Steiger Z: Esophageal cancer: An interdisciplinary approach. Curr Probl Cancer 11:1-52, 1981.

188. Levine MS, Langer J, Laufer I, et al: Radiation therapy of esophageal carcinoma: Correlation of clinical and radiographic findings. Gastrointest Radiol 12:99-105, 1987.

189. Pearson JG: The value of radiotherapy in the management of esophageal cancer. AJR 105:500-513, 1969.

190. Drucker MH, Mansour KA, Hatcher CR, et al: Esophageal carcinoma: An aggressive approach. Ann Thorac Surg 28:133-137, 1979.

191. Fraser RW, Wara WM, Thomas AN, et al: Combined treatment methods for carcinoma of the esophagus. Radiology 128:461-465, 1978.

192. Elkon D, Lee MS, Hendrickson FR: Carcinoma of the esophagus: Sites of recurrence and palliative benefits after definitive radiotherapy. Int J Radiat Oncol Biol Phys 4:615-620, 1978.

193. Leborgne R, Leborgne F, Barlocci L: Cancer of the oesophagus: Results of radiotherapy. Br J Radiol 36:806-811, 1963.

194. Wara WM, Mauch PM, Thomas AN, et al: Palliation for carcinoma of the esophagus. Radiology 121:717-720, 1976.

195. Walsh TN, Noonan N, Hollywood D, et al: A comparison of multimodal therapy and surgery for esophageal adenocarcinoma. N Engl J Med 335:462-467, 1996.

196. Bosset JF, Gignoux M, Triboulet JP, et al: Chemoradiotherapy followed by surgery compared with surgery alone in squamous-cell cancer of the esophagus. N Engl J Med 337:161-167, 1997.

Other Malignant Tumors of the Esophagus

Marc S. Levine, MD

METASTASES

Esophageal metastases are found at autopsy in less than 5% of patients dying of carcinoma. Most cases result from direct invasion by primary malignant tumors of the stomach, lung, and neck or from contiguous involvement by tumor-containing lymph nodes in the mediastinum. These various forms of esophageal involvement by metastatic tumor produce characteristic radiographic findings that are discussed separately in later sections.

Sites of Origin

Carcinoma of the stomach accounts for about 50% of all esophageal metastases.[1] Tumors involving the gastric cardia or fundus may invade the distal esophagus by contiguous spread through the diaphragmatic hiatus. Carcinomas of the lung

and breast are other less common causes of esophageal metastases.[2-4] Most cases result from direct extension of tumor to the esophagus or from contiguous esophageal involvement by lymphadenopathy in the posterior mediastinum. The esophagus may also be involved by contiguous spread of malignant tumors in the neck, such as laryngeal, pharyngeal, and thyroid carcinoma. Rarely, the esophagus may be involved by hematogenous metastases from tumors arising in distant locations such as the kidney, liver, rectum, prostate, cervix, and skin.[5-9] Thus, most malignant tumors are capable of metastasizing to the esophagus.

Clinical Findings

Patients with esophageal metastases may present with dysphagia as a result of esophageal compression by enlarged mediastinal lymph nodes or actual invasion of the esophagus by tumor. Although the presence of esophageal metastases usually indicates a poor prognosis, some patients (particularly those with breast or lung cancer) may present with dysphagia as the initial manifestation of their disease.[2,10] Also, patients with breast cancer often have late-onset metastases to the esophagus, with an average interval of approximately 8 years from the time of diagnosis to the development of dysphagia.[4,11] When dysphagia occurs, these patients usually have widespread metastatic disease.[3,11]

Radiographic Findings

Direct Invasion

Direct invasion of the cervical or thoracic esophagus by carcinoma of the larynx, pharynx, thyroid, or lung produces characteristic findings on barium studies. Early invasion may be manifested by a smooth or slightly irregular contour defect in the esophagus with gently sloping, obtuse borders and a contiguous soft tissue mass in the adjacent neck or mediastinum. The area of involvement may have a more serrated, scalloped, or nodular appearance as the esophageal wall is further infiltrated by tumor (Fig. 28-1). Eventually, there may be circumferential narrowing of the esophagus with mass effect, nodularity, ulceration, or even obstruction (Fig. 28-2).

Rarely, thyroid cancer invading the esophagus may be manifested by an expansile intraluminal mass, mimicking the appearance of a spindle cell carcinoma (see later section).[12]

Secondary esophageal involvement by carcinoma of the gastric cardia or fundus may be manifested radiographically by a polypoid mass extending from the fundus into the distal esophagus (Fig. 28-3) or by irregular narrowing of the distal esophagus without a discrete mass.[13,14] Esophageal involvement is usually confined to a short segment of the distal esophagus but may extend as far proximally as the aortic arch.[13] Occasionally, these tumors may cause smooth, tapered narrowing of the distal esophagus at or near the gastroesophageal junction, mimicking the appearance of achalasia (see next section on Secondary Achalasia).

When the distal esophagus appears to be involved by tumor on barium studies, the gastric cardia and fundus should also be evaluated radiographically to determine whether there is associated gastric involvement. In some cases, barium studies may demonstrate an obvious malignant tumor in the stomach (see Fig. 28-3). In others, however, the presence of tumor in the gastric fundus may be recognized only by distortion or obliteration of the normal anatomic landmarks at the cardia associated with relatively subtle areas of nodularity, mass effect, or ulceration (Fig. 28-4).[14,15] Thus, a meticulous double-contrast examination of the fundus is essential to rule out an underlying carcinoma of the cardia in these patients.

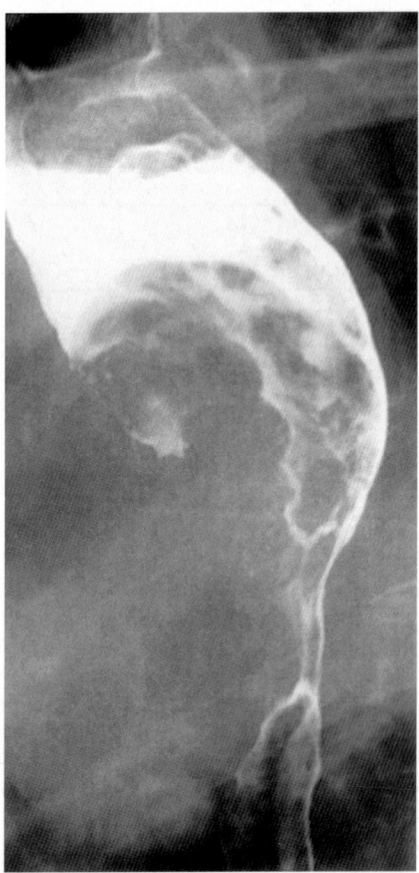

Figure 28-1. Direct esophageal invasion by carcinoma of the lung. Eccentric mass effect and narrowing of the esophagus by tumor in the adjacent mediastinum are noted. The scalloped contour of the esophagus in this region indicates direct invasion by tumor. (From Levine MS: Radiology of the Esophagus. Philadelphia, WB Saunders, 1989.)

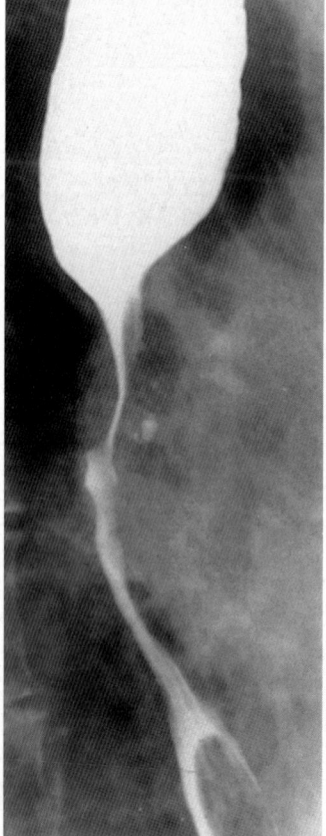

Figure 28-2. Direct esophageal invasion by carcinoma of the lung. This patient has a long segment of irregular narrowing in the midesophagus due to circumferential involvement by metastatic tumor in the mediastinum. (Courtesy of Robert A. Goren, MD, Philadelphia, PA.)

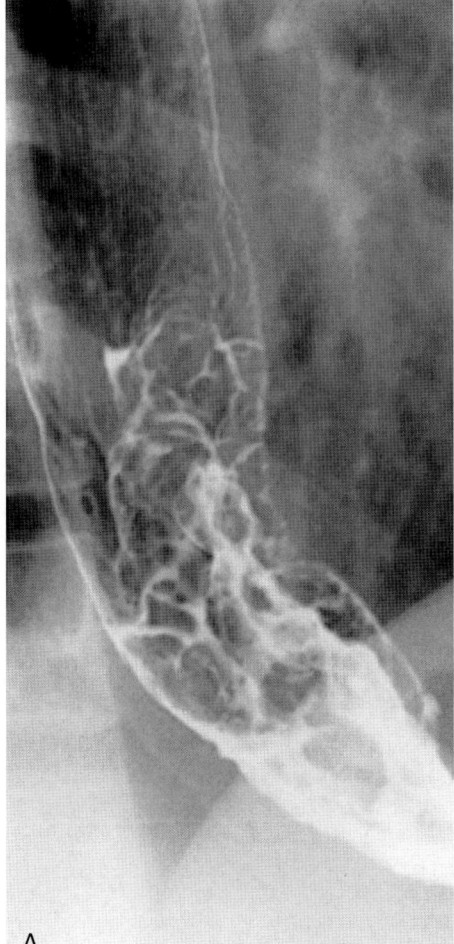

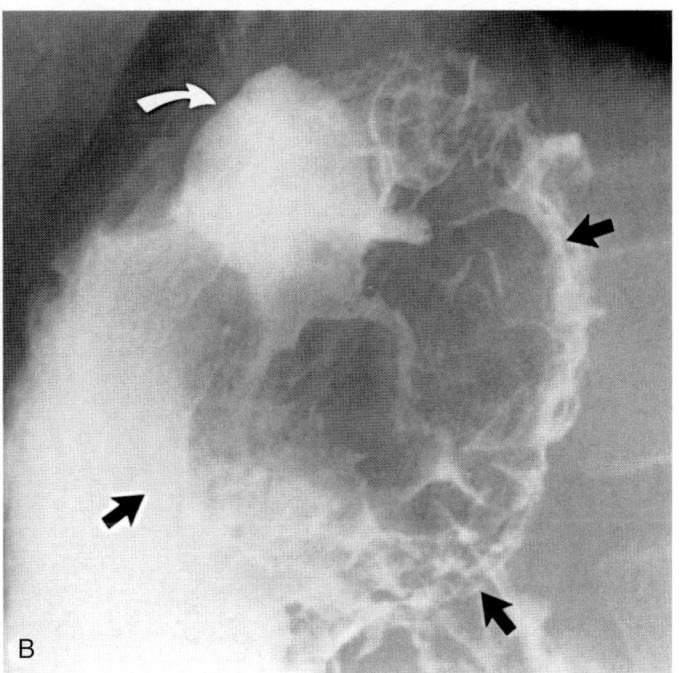

Figure 28-3. Direct esophageal invasion by gastric carcinoma. A. Double-contrast esophagogram shows a polypoid lesion in the distal esophagus that extends inferiorly to the gastroesophageal junction. **B.** Lateral view of the gastric fundus shows a large fundal mass (*black arrows*) containing an eccentric area of ulceration (*white arrow*). This patient had a primary gastric carcinoma invading the distal esophagus. (From Levine MS: Radiology of the Esophagus. Philadelphia, WB Saunders, 1989.)

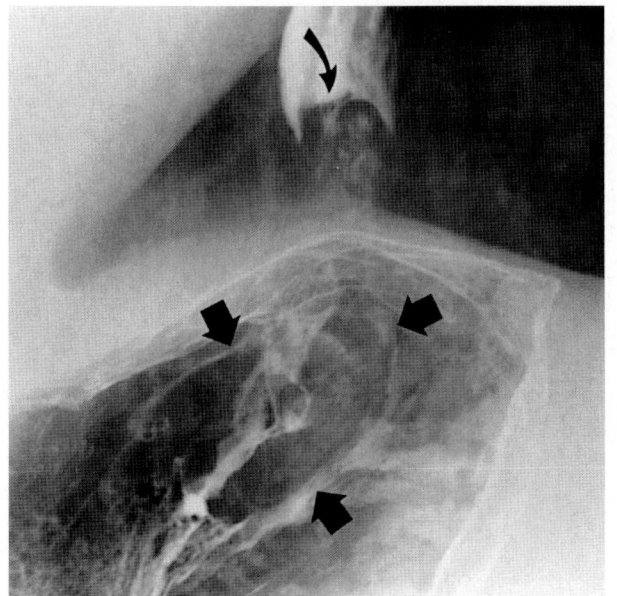

Figure 28-4. Direct esophageal invasion by carcinoma of the gastric cardia. Double-contrast view of the fundus shows obliteration of the normal anatomic landmarks at the cardia with a centrally ulcerated polypoid lesion (*straight arrows*) extending into the distal esophagus (*curved arrow*). (From Levine MS, Laufer I, Thompson JJ: Carcinoma of the gastric cardia in young people. AJR 140:69-72, 1983, © by American Roentgen Ray Society.)

Contiguous Involvement by Mediastinal Lymph Nodes

Although any neoplasm that metastasizes to mediastinal lymph nodes may secondarily involve the esophagus, carcinomas of the breast and lung are the most common underlying malignancies in these patients.[11] Because of the proximity of the midesophagus to subcarinal lymph nodes, esophageal involvement by mediastinal lymphadenopathy occurs most frequently at this level.[10,16] Barium studies typically reveal a smooth or slightly lobulated extrinsic indentation on the esophagus at or just below the carina (Fig. 28-5A).[10,16] When tumor directly invades the esophagus, it may have a more irregular contour, often with areas of ulceration (Fig. 28-6).[1,4,6] Eventually, the wall of the esophagus may be circumferentially infiltrated by tumor, producing an area of concentric narrowing with a surrounding soft tissue mass (Fig. 28-7).[2,4,6] When esophageal involvement by mediastinal tumor is suspected on barium studies, CT may be performed to show the extent and location of adenopathy in the mediastinum (Fig. 28-5B).

Hematogenous Metastases

True blood-borne or hematogenous metastases to the esophagus are extremely uncommon. Most cases are caused by carcinoma of the breast, but other distant tumors may also metastasize hematogenously to the esophagus. Surprisingly,

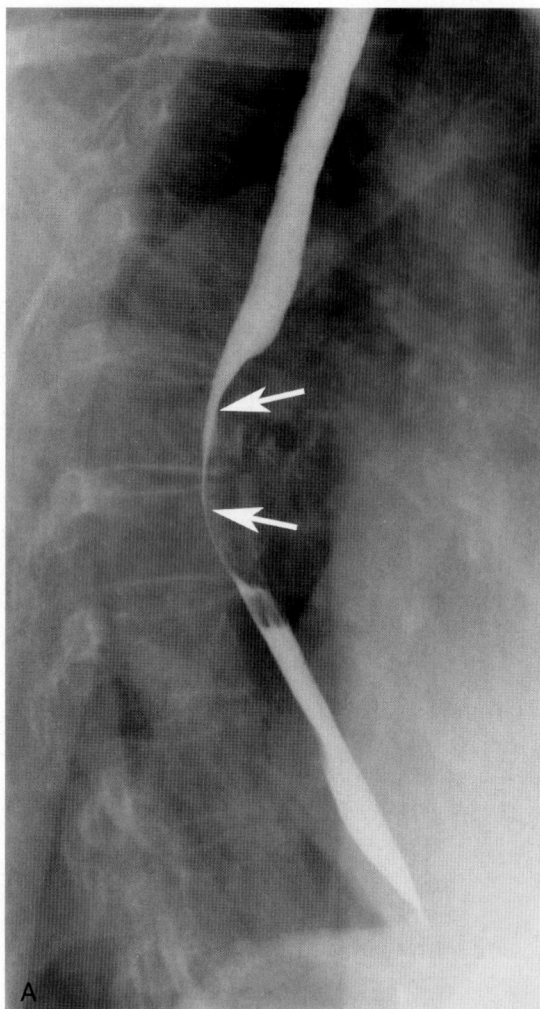

A

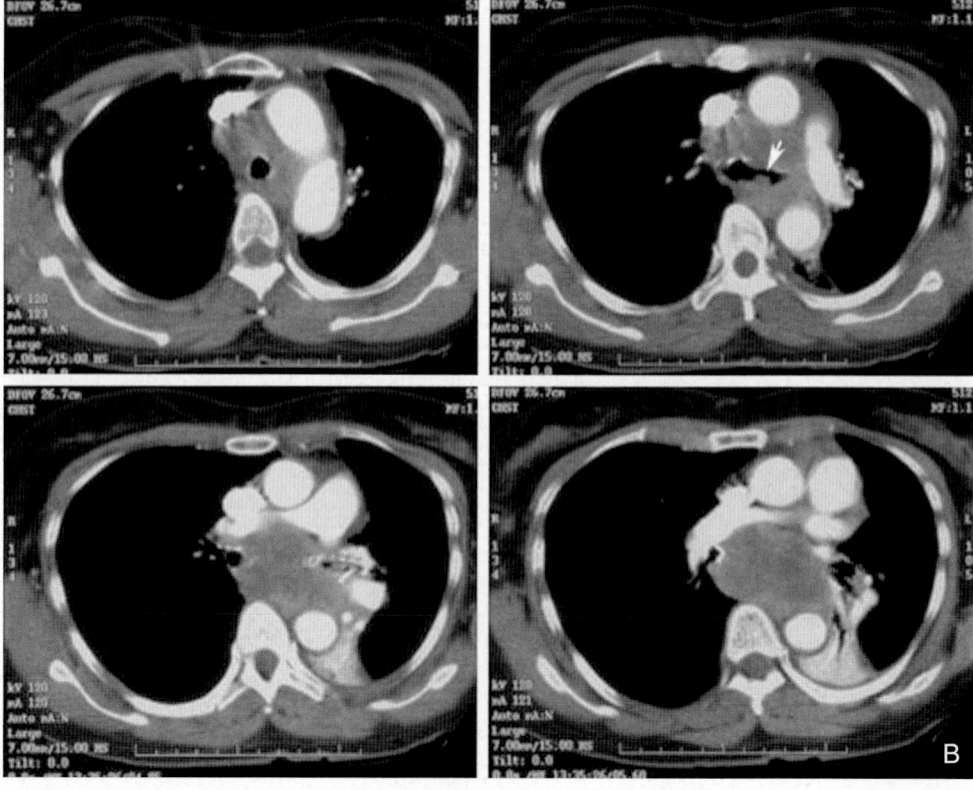

B

Figure 28-5. Esophageal compression by mediastinal lymphadenopathy from carcinoma of the lung. A. Barium study shows a large extrinsic indentation (*arrows*) on the anterolateral wall of the midesophagus just below the carina. **B.** CT shows bulky mediastinal and subcarinal adenopathy as the cause of this finding. An endobronchial lesion (*arrow*) is also seen in the left main bronchus near the carina. This patient was found to have a small cell carcinoma of the lung. (Courtesy of Vincent Low, MD, Perth, Australia.)

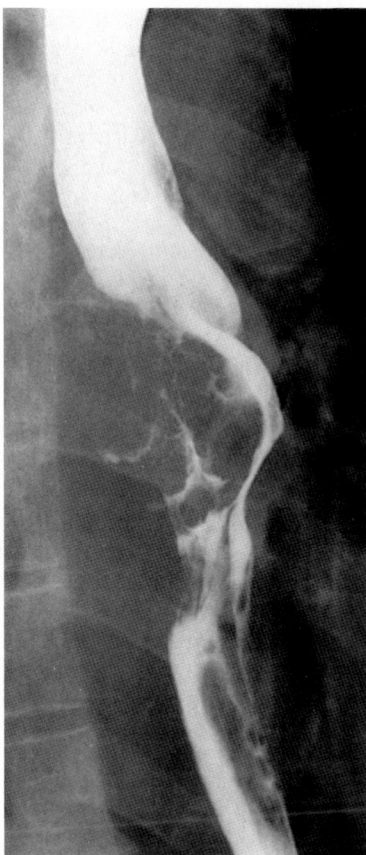

Figure 28-6. Esophageal involvement by mediastinal lymphadenopathy from carcinoma of the cervix. There is eccentric mass effect on the midesophagus with an irregular contour and areas of ulceration due to esophageal invasion by tumor in adjacent subcarinal nodes. (From Levine MS: Radiology of the Esophagus. Philadelphia, WB Saunders, 1989.)

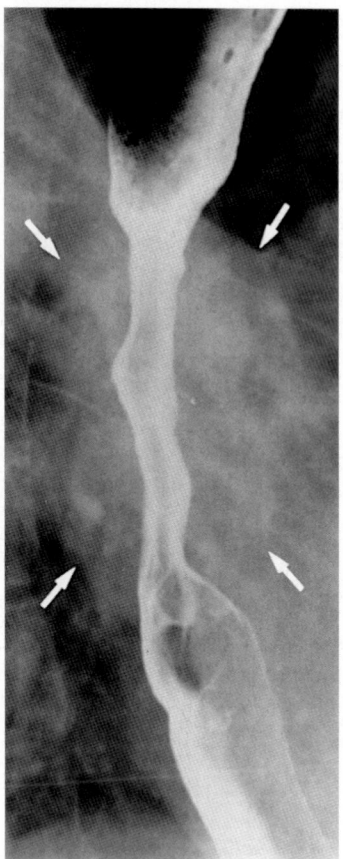

Figure 28-7. Circumferential esophageal involvement by metastatic breast cancer in the mediastinum. A relatively smooth, tapered area of narrowing is seen in the midesophagus. However, a surrounding soft tissue mass (*arrows*) in the mediastinum suggests esophageal involvement by lymphadenopathy. (From Levine MS: Radiology of the Esophagus. Philadelphia, WB Saunders, 1989.)

however, malignant melanoma (which has the highest percentage of blood-borne metastases to the gastrointestinal tract) rarely involves the esophagus.[5,9] Whatever the origin, blood-borne metastases to the esophagus usually appear on barium studies as short, eccentric strictures (most frequently in the middle third of the esophagus) with intact overlying mucosa and smooth, tapered margins (Fig. 28-8).[1,4,6,17] Although blood-borne metastases to the esophagus tend to be infiltrating lesions, they may occasionally be manifested by one or more discrete submucosal masses or centrally ulcerated "bull's-eye" lesions.[17]

Differential Diagnosis

A smooth or slightly lobulated indentation on the esophagus may be caused by a variety of extrinsic mass lesions, such as benign tumors and cysts in the mediastinum, aberrant vessels, and an ectatic aorta or aortic aneurysm compressing the esophagus. In contrast, esophageal invasion by metastatic tumor should be suspected when the area of mass effect has an irregular, serrated, or nodular contour associated with angulated, tethered folds or ulceration. As a result, malignant invasion of the esophagus usually can be distinguished radiographically from benign lesions in the mediastinum that are extrinsically compressing but not invading the esophagus.

The differential diagnosis for upper esophageal or midesophageal strictures caused by metastatic tumor includes Barrett's esophagus and scarring from mediastinal irradiation, caustic ingestion, eosinophilic esophagitis, or oral medications such as potassium chloride and quinidine. When these patients are known to have a previously irradiated malignant tumor in the thorax, however, the major diagnostic considerations include a benign radiation stricture and recurrent tumor. In such cases, CT may be used to differentiate recurrent tumor from a radiation stricture by showing a mediastinal mass or lymphadenopathy in the region of the stricture.

SECONDARY ACHALASIA

The terms *secondary achalasia* and *pseudoachalasia* are used interchangeably to describe an entity in which the clinical, radiographic, endoscopic, and manometric features may be indistinguishable from those of primary, or idiopathic, achalasia. Malignancy-induced secondary achalasia is an uncommon condition, accounting for only 2% to 4% of patients with findings of achalasia at manometry.[18] Nearly 75% of cases are caused by carcinoma of the gastric cardia or fundus directly invading the gastroesophageal junction or distal esophagus.[19-21] Less frequently, hematogenous metastases from other malignant tumors, including breast, lung, pancreatic, uterine, and

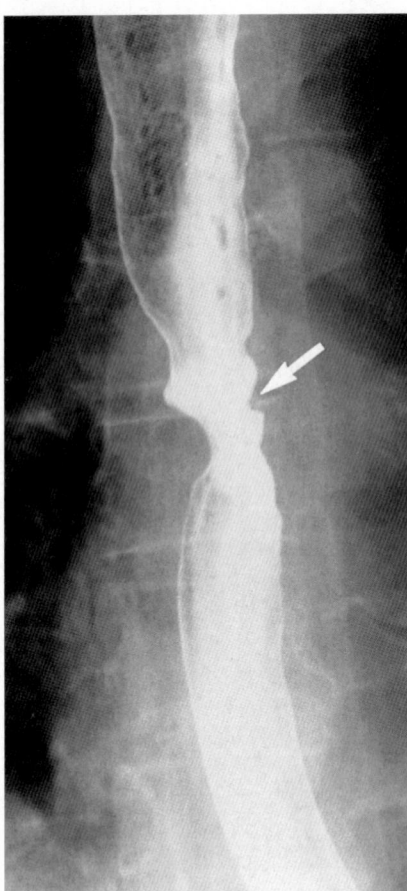

Figure 28-8. Hematogenous metastasis to the esophagus from carcinoma of the breast. The lesion is manifested by a short, benign-appearing stricture (*arrow*) in the midesophagus. (From Levine MS: Radiology of the Esophagus. Philadelphia, WB Saunders, 1989.)

prostate cancer may produce identical findings.[8,19,22,23] Occasionally, lymphoma or benign conditions such as Chagas' disease and amyloidosis may also produce an achalasia-like syndrome.[24-26] It is important to differentiate the two forms of achalasia, because primary achalasia may be treated by pneumatic dilatation, whereas secondary achalasia often necessitates exploratory laparotomy or other treatment for widespread metastatic disease.

Pathogenesis

Both primary achalasia and secondary achalasia are characterized by absent esophageal peristalsis and a hypertensive lower esophageal sphincter that fails to relax normally in response to deglutition. In patients with primary achalasia, the motor disorder is thought to be caused by degeneration and loss of the ganglion cells of Auerbach's plexus in the esophagus. However, the precise mechanism by which metastases to the gastroesophageal junction produce this motor disorder is uncertain. Some patients have tumor directly invading the distal esophagus with actual destruction of myenteric ganglia.[27] However, others have tumor confined to the gastroesophageal junction without involvement of the neural plexus in the esophagus.[28] In such cases, the motor disorder may be caused by extraesophageal metastases to the vagus nerve or dorsal

motor nucleus of the vagus nerve in the brain stem.[20,28] Secondary achalasia may also occur as a paraneoplastic phenomenon caused by circulating tumor products that alter esophageal motor function.[8] Studies have found that malignant neuroendocrine tumors (particularly small cell carcinoma of the lung) may express a variety of neural antigens that initiate an autoimmune response, with circulating antibodies (known as anti-Hu antibodies) that cause neural degeneration and subsequent findings of secondary achalasia.[29,30]

Clinical Findings

Although dysphagia occurs in both the primary and secondary forms of achalasia, other clinical features are often helpful in distinguishing these entities. Most patients with primary achalasia are between 20 and 50 years of age, and they have dysphagia for an average of 4 to 6 years before they seek medical attention.[18,31] In contrast, most patients with secondary achalasia are older than 50 years and the duration of symptoms is usually less than 6 months.[18,31] Secondary achalasia also is more likely to be associated with substantial weight loss.[32] An underlying malignant tumor should therefore be suspected whenever achalasia is diagnosed on radiographic, endoscopic, or manometric studies in elderly patients with recent onset of dysphagia and weight loss.[18,31,32] Nevertheless, some patients with primary achalasia may be older than 60 years and others may have a relatively short duration of symptoms.[31,33,34] Thus, it is not always possible to differentiate these conditions by clinical criteria.

Radiographic Findings

Secondary achalasia is classically manifested on barium studies by absent peristalsis in the body of the esophagus and smooth, tapered narrowing of the distal esophagus, producing a "birdbeak" configuration at or just above the gastroesophageal junction (Fig. 28-9).[8,19,31,35] Although the radiographic appearance may closely resemble that of primary achalasia, infiltration of the distal esophagus by tumor in secondary achalasia sometimes causes asymmetric or eccentric narrowing, abrupt transitions, rigidity, and mucosal nodularity or ulceration.[31,35] Another important sign of malignancy is the length of the narrowed segment, which may extend 3.5 cm or more above the gastroesophageal junction in secondary achalasia but rarely extends this far proximally in patients with primary achalasia (Fig. 28-10).[31] Finally, the degree of esophageal dilatation is usually less in patients with secondary achalasia because of the rapid onset of disease.[31] When findings of achalasia are present on barium studies, a narrowed distal esophageal segment longer than 3.5 cm with little or no proximal dilatation in a patient with recent onset of dysphagia should therefore be highly suggestive of secondary achalasia, even in the absence of other suspicious radiographic findings.[31]

Because secondary achalasia is usually caused by carcinoma of the gastric cardia or fundus invading the distal esophagus, careful radiologic examination of the fundus is essential in these patients. Not infrequently, an obvious polypoid, ulcerated, or infiltrating malignancy may be demonstrated in the fundus (see Fig. 28-9B). With less advanced lesions, no gross abnormalities may be identified in the gastric fundus on conventional single-contrast barium studies. However, double-

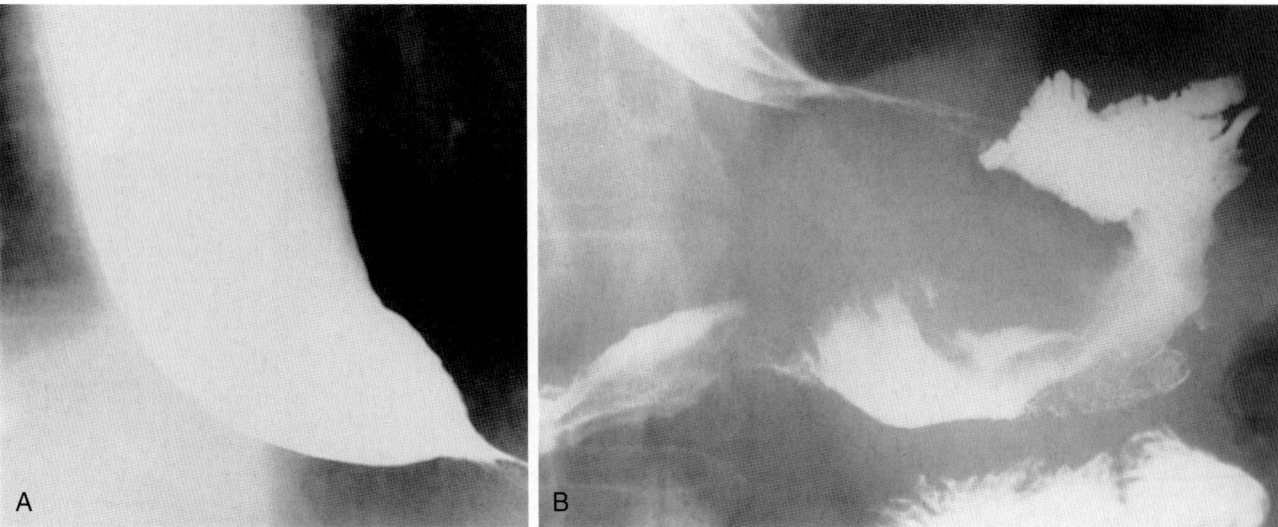

Figure 28-9. Secondary achalasia caused by gastric carcinoma. A. There is smooth, tapered narrowing of the distal esophagus, producing the characteristic "bird-beak" appearance of primary achalasia. **B.** However, a view of the stomach reveals a diffusely infiltrating carcinoma of the gastric body and fundus that has invaded the distal esophagus.

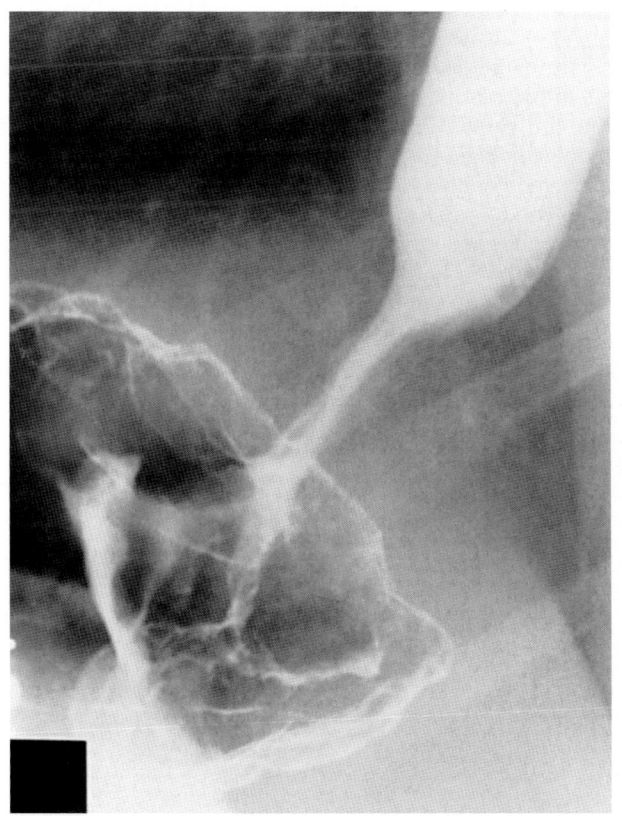

Figure 28-10. Secondary achalasia caused by carcinoma of the gastric cardia. There is smooth, tapered narrowing of the distal esophagus, but the narrowed segment extends a considerable distance from the gastroesophageal junction (a finding not often seen in patients with primary achalasia). Also note how the tumor causes marked nodularity of the gastric fundus with obliteration of the normal anatomic landmarks at the cardia. (From Levine MS: Radiology of the Esophagus. Philadelphia, WB Saunders, 1989.)

contrast studies of the fundus may demonstrate subtle evidence of tumor distorting or obliterating the normal anatomical landmarks at the cardia (see Fig. 28-10).[14,15] In contrast, the esophageal "rosette" that demarcates the gastric cardia on double-contrast studies should be normal in patients with primary achalasia.

CT is also helpful for evaluating patients with suspected achalasia. In primary achalasia, CT typically reveals little or no esophageal wall thickening and no evidence of mediastinal adenopathy or a mass at the cardia (Fig. 28-11).[36,37] In some cases, however, CT may reveal a pseudomass at the cardia because of inadequate distention of this region.[38] In contrast, CT may show asymmetric esophageal wall thickening, a soft tissue mass at the cardia, or mediastinal adenopathy in patients with secondary achalasia (Fig. 28-12).[39] CT may also be helpful for identifying the site of the primary tumor in patients with secondary achalasia caused by remote tumors.

LYMPHOMA

The esophagus is the least common site of gastrointestinal involvement by lymphoma, accounting for only about 1% of cases.[40] Both non-Hodgkin's and, less commonly, Hodgkin's lymphoma may involve the esophagus. These patients almost always have generalized lymphoma with direct invasion of the esophagus by lymphomatous nodes in the mediastinum, contiguous spread of lymphoma from the gastric fundus, or synchronous development of lymphoma in the wall of the esophagus.[41-45] Rarely, primary esophageal lymphoma (usually Hodgkin's disease) may occur without extraesophageal disease.[46-51] Cases of AIDS-related primary esophageal lymphoma have also been reported.[52,53] When esophageal lymphoma is suspected, endoscopy should be performed with deep esophageal biopsy specimens to confirm the diagnosis. However, false-negative biopsy specimens have been reported in 25% to 35% of cases because of the patchy nature of the disease and sampling error.[51] Thus, some patients may require surgery for a definitive diagnosis.

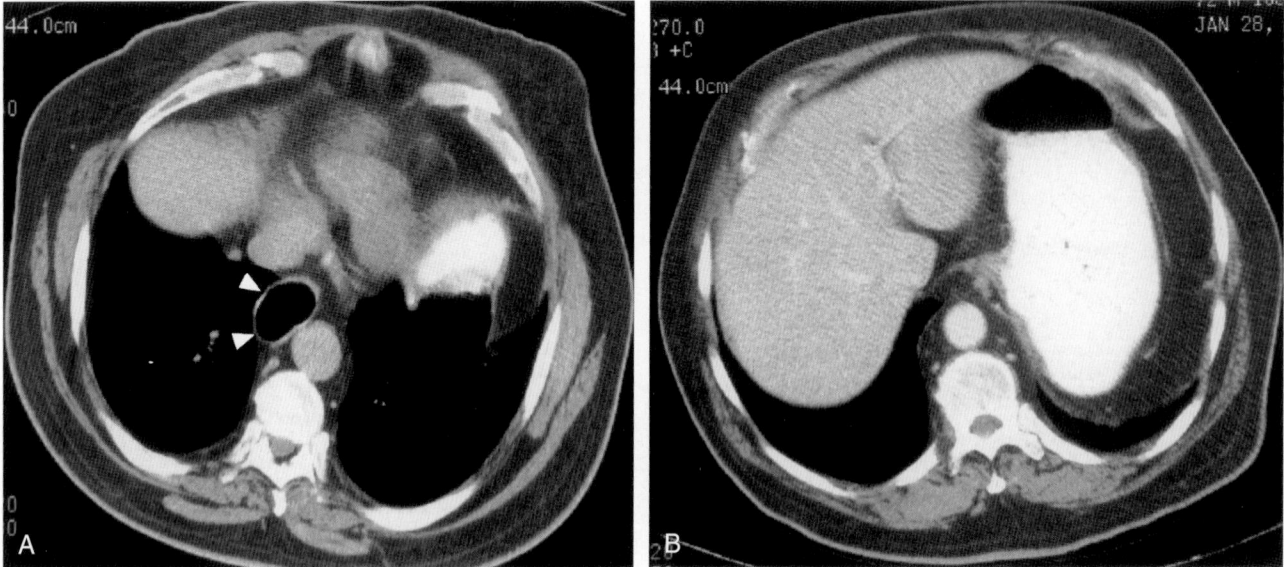

Figure 28-11. Primary achalasia on CT. A. CT scan shows a dilated esophagus (*arrowheads*) without esophageal wall thickening or mediastinal adenopathy. **B.** Another scan more caudally shows no evidence of a soft tissue mass at the gastroesophageal junction. (Note barium in the gastric fundus.) This patient had long-standing primary achalasia.

Clinical Findings

Most patients with esophageal lymphoma have no esophageal symptoms, so that the diagnosis is usually made at autopsy in patients with widespread disease.[40,41] However, some patients may develop dysphagia as a result of esophageal narrowing or obstruction by tumor.[42-44] Rarely, they may present with dysphagia as the initial manifestation of their disease.[54] Because many patients with lymphoma are treated by irradiation or chemotherapy, opportunistic esophagitis may be suspected as a more likely cause of dysphagia in these individuals.

Radiographic Findings

Secondary involvement of the esophagus by gastric lymphoma may be manifested on barium studies by irregular narrowing of the distal esophagus due to contiguous spread of tumor from the gastric fundus (Fig. 28-13).[42-45,55] In such cases, careful radiologic examination of the gastric cardia and fundus may demonstrate a polypoid, ulcerated, or infiltrating lesion in the fundus due to associated gastric lymphoma. Trans-cardiac extension of gastric lymphoma is thought to occur in about 10% of patients.[55] However, these lesions cannot be

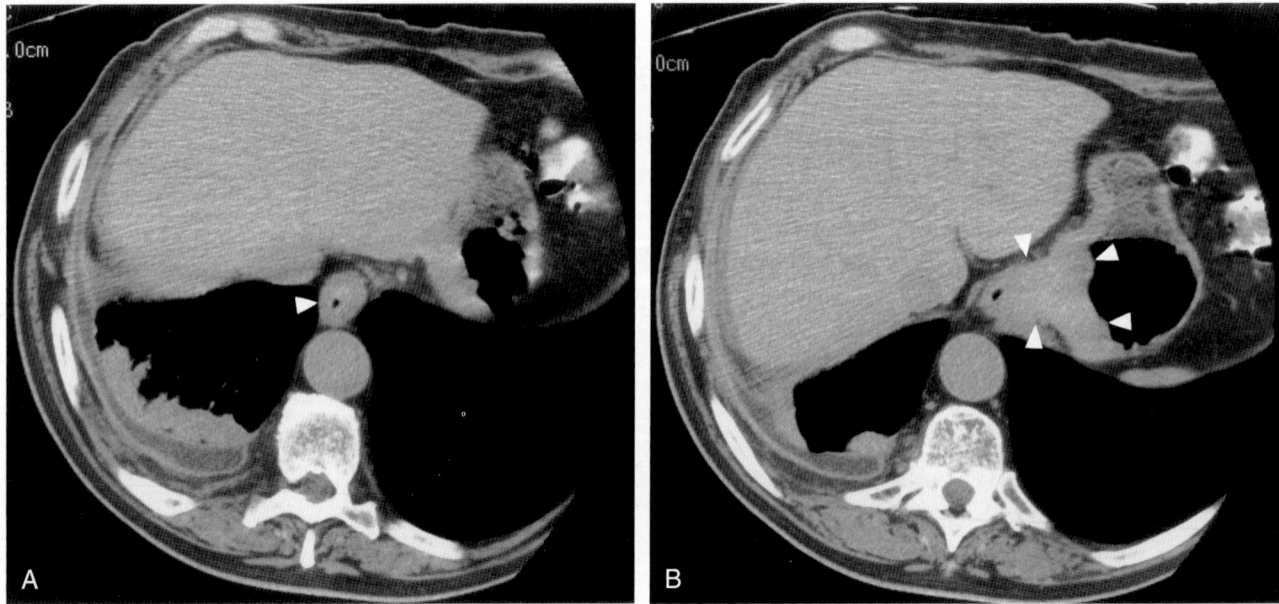

Figure 28-12. Secondary achalasia on CT. A. CT scan shows marked thickening of the esophageal wall (*arrowhead*) in the distal esophagus at the level of beaklike narrowing seen on a prior barium study (not shown). **B.** Another scan more caudally shows an asymmetric soft tissue mass (*arrowheads*) at the gastroesophageal junction protruding into the gas-filled fundus. This patient had a carcinoma of the cardia causing secondary achalasia.

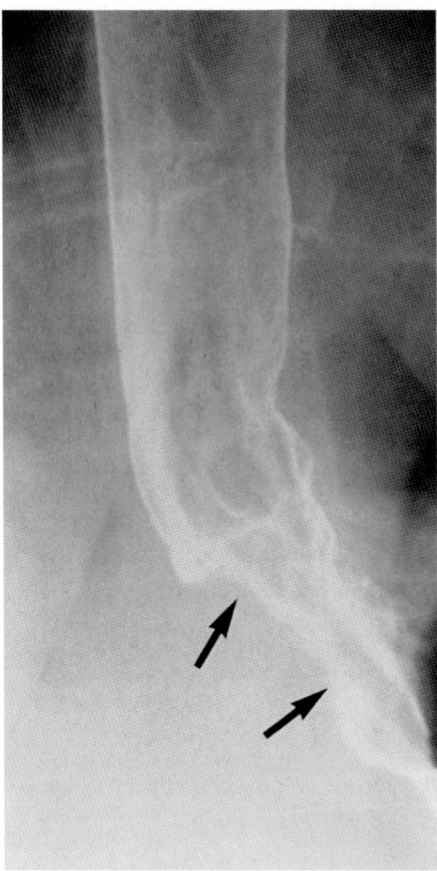

Figure 28-13. Esophageal involvement by gastric lymphoma. There is irregular narrowing (*arrows*) of the distal esophagus due to contiguous spread of lymphoma from the gastric fundus. Carcinoma of the gastric cardia invading the distal esophagus could produce identical findings. (From Levine MS: Radiology of the Esophagus. Philadelphia, WB Saunders, 1989.)

distinguished radiographically from carcinoma of the gastric fundus invading the distal esophagus.

Mediastinal lymphoma may cause extrinsic compression of the esophagus, resulting in a smooth indentation with obtuse, gently sloping borders.[41] Further esophageal involvement may be manifested by a more irregular or serrated contour abnormality due to invasion of the wall by tumor. Eventually, mediastinal lymphoma may cause diffuse esophageal narrowing (Fig. 28-14A). CT is particularly useful for determining the extent of disease in the mediastinum (Fig. 28-14B). Other patients may develop esophageal airway fistulas, usually as a complication of radiation therapy.[56,57]

Depending on the pattern of growth, intrinsic esophageal lymphoma may be manifested by a spectrum of abnormalities, including submucosal nodules, enlarged folds, polypoid masses, or strictures. The most common finding is a polypoid or ulcerated mass or an infiltrating stricture indistinguishable from esophageal carcinoma (Fig. 28-15).[42-45,48-52] Less frequently, lymphomatous infiltration of the submucosa may result in enlarged, tortuous longitudinal folds, mimicking the appearance of varices.[41-45] Occasionally, discrete submucosal masses may be found in the middle or distal third of the esophagus, suggesting multiple leiomyomas.[42,43] Other patients may have innumerable small submucosal nodules throughout the esophagus (Fig. 28-16).[58,59] Leukemic infiltrates, hematogenous metastases, Kaposi's sarcoma, multiple leiomyomas,

and esophageal retention cysts have also been described as rare causes of submucosal nodules, but the lesions tend to be larger and less numerous in these cases. Rarely, esophageal lymphoma may cause aneurysmal dilatation similar to that found in the small intestine.[51]

SPINDLE CELL CARCINOMA

Malignant polypoid epithelial tumors of the esophagus containing both carcinomatous and sarcomatous elements are exceedingly uncommon, accounting for only 0.5% to 1.5% of all esophageal neoplasms.[60] Terms formerly used to describe these lesions include carcinosarcoma, pseudosarcoma, polypoid carcinoma, and spindle cell variant of squamous cell carcinoma. However, many investigators believe that these lesions represent various expressions of a single malignant tumor, which has been designated *spindle cell squamous carcinoma*, or simply, *spindle cell carcinoma*.[61-63]

Pathology

In the past, classic carcinosarcomas of the esophagus were thought to contain a true mixture of carcinomatous and sarcomatous elements in which either element metastasized to regional lymph nodes or distant structures.[64,65] In contrast, pseudosarcomas were thought to be composed primarily of sarcoma-like spindle cells with adjacent areas of squamous cell carcinoma.[66-68] Because the sarcomatous portion of the tumor rarely metastasized to other structures, pseudosarcomas were thought to be less aggressive lesions and to have a better prognosis than carcinosarcomas.[65] In subsequent studies, however, it was shown that local or distant metastases occurred from the sarcomatous portion of so-called pseudosarcomas and that these lesions behaved as aggressively as carcinosarcomas.[61,69] Thus, carcinosarcoma and pseudosarcoma appear to be the same pathologic entity, with varying degrees of anaplastic spindle cell metaplasia of the carcinomatous portion of the tumor.[61,63,70]

Clinical Findings

Because spindle cell carcinomas are polypoid intraluminal tumors, affected individuals almost always present clinically with dysphagia and weight loss.[71] Most patients are elderly men, who often have a history of cigarette smoking or alcohol consumption.[68,71] The clinical presentation is therefore indistinguishable from that of squamous cell carcinoma.

It has previously been suggested that spindle cell carcinomas have a better prognosis than squamous cell carcinomas because they tend to remain superficial, with local invasion and regional or distant metastases occurring late in the course of the disease.[64,72] However, other investigators have found that as many as 50% of patients with spindle cell carcinoma have metastatic disease at the time of diagnosis, and the overall 5-year survival rate is only 2% to 8%.[65,71] Thus, the prognosis of this tumor is probably comparable with that of squamous cell carcinoma.

Radiographic Findings

Spindle cell carcinomas usually appear on barium studies as large polypoid intraluminal masses that expand or dilate the

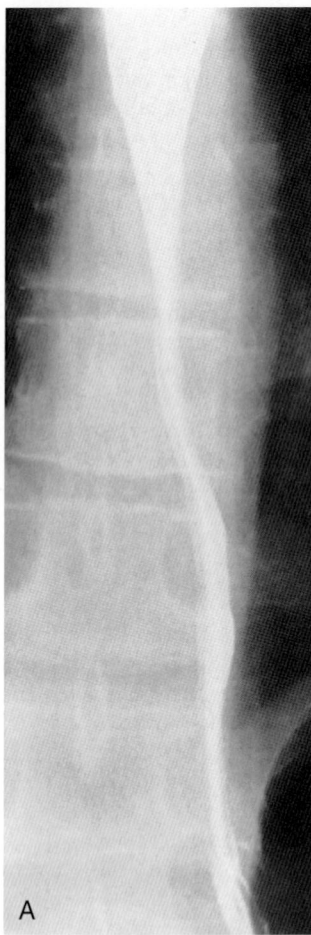

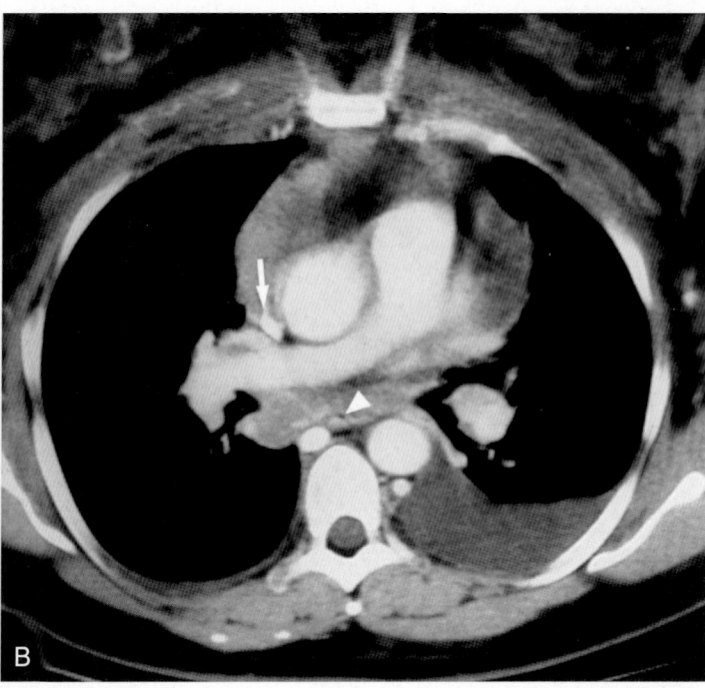

Figure 28-14. Esophageal involvement by mediastinal lymphoma. A. Barium study shows a long segment of smooth narrowing in the distal third of the esophagus due to circumferential involvement by mediastinal lymphoma. **B.** CT scan in another patient with large cell lymphoma of the mediastinum shows extensive mediastinal adenopathy compressing the esophagus (*arrowhead*) and superior vena cava (*arrow*). (**A** courtesy of Kyunghee C. Cho, MD, Newark, NJ; **B** courtesy of Richard M. Gore, MD, Evanston, IL.)

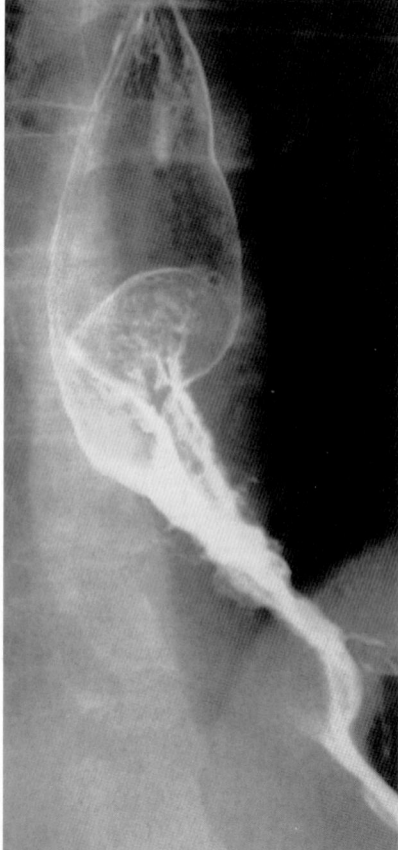

Figure 28-15. Primary AIDS-related non-Hodgkin's lymphoma of the esophagus. There is an irregular, ulcerated area of narrowing with a shelflike proximal border in the distal thoracic esophagus. This lesion is indistinguishable from an advanced esophageal carcinoma. (Courtesy of Jackie Brown, MD, Vancouver, British Columbia, Canada.)

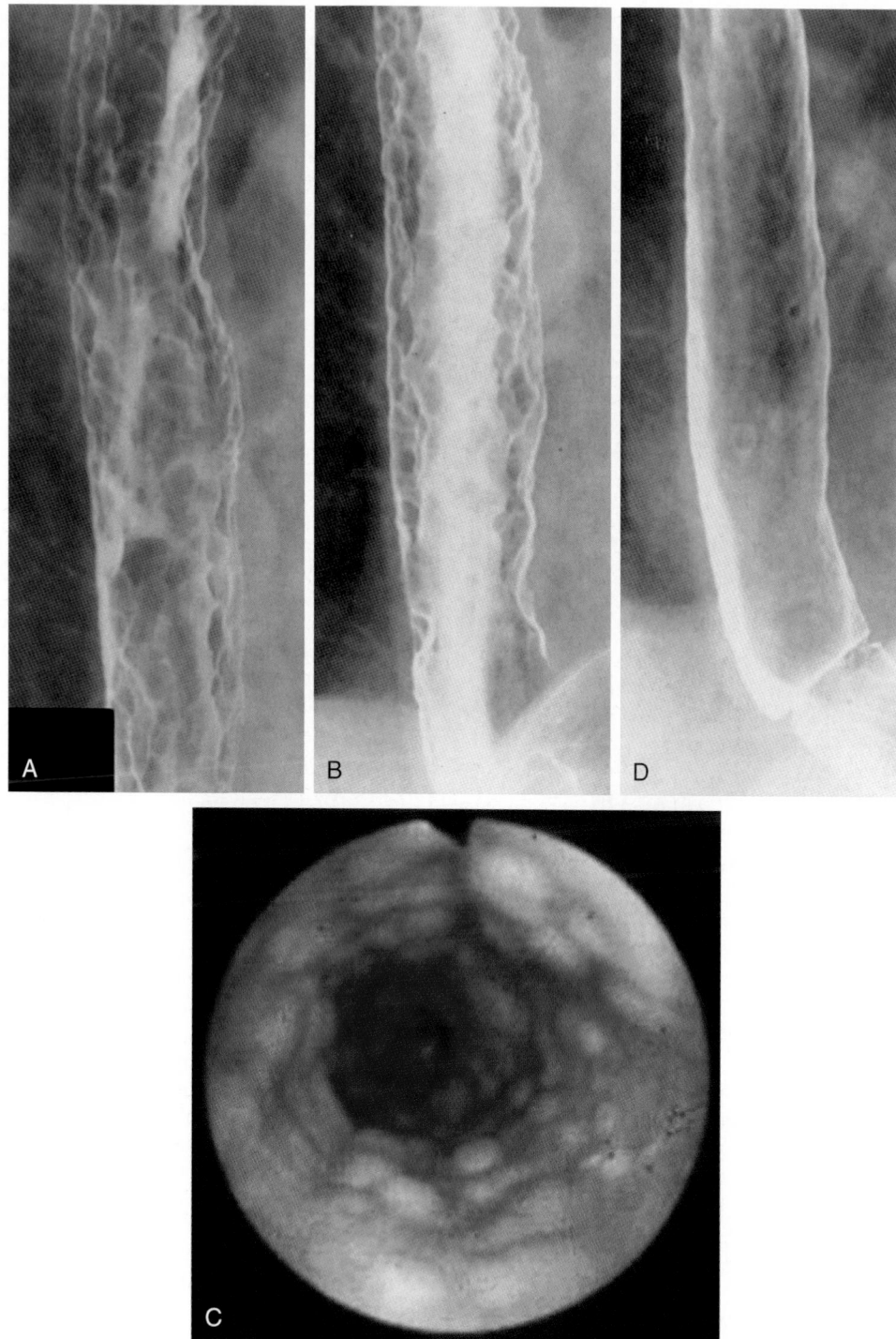

Figure 28-16. Generalized non-Hodgkin's lymphoma involving the esophagus. Double-contrast images of the middle (**A**) and distal (**B**) thoracic esophagus reveal innumerable 3- to 10-mm submucosal nodules extending from the thoracic inlet to the gastroesophageal junction. This appearance might initially be mistaken for that of varices, but the diffuse distribution and discrete margins of the lesions allow them to be differentiated from varices. **C.** Endoscopic photograph reveals multiple, discrete submucosal nodules that had a whitish-yellow appearance on visual examination. **D.** Repeat esophagogram obtained 2 months after chemotherapy reveals virtually complete healing of the submucosal nodules seen on the earlier study. (From Levine MS, Sunshine AG, Reynolds JC, et al: Diffuse nodularity in esophageal lymphoma. AJR 145:1218-1220, 1985, © by American Roentgen Ray Society.)

esophagus without causing obstruction (Fig. 28-17).[62,63,65,69,72] Similarly, CT may demonstrate a bulky soft tissue mass expanding the lumen of the esophagus. These tumors tend to be located in the middle or distal third of the esophagus.[63,68,71] In some cases, barium may form a dome over the intraluminal portion of the tumor, producing a "cupola" effect.[62,63,65] Occa-

sionally, a broad-based or narrow pedicle may be observed radiographically.[62,63,68,69] Rarely, torsion of the pedicle results in spontaneous sloughing of the tumor.[68] Most spindle cell carcinomas are polypoid lesions, but some can be infiltrating or annular lesions indistinguishable from squamous cell carcinomas.[65,71]

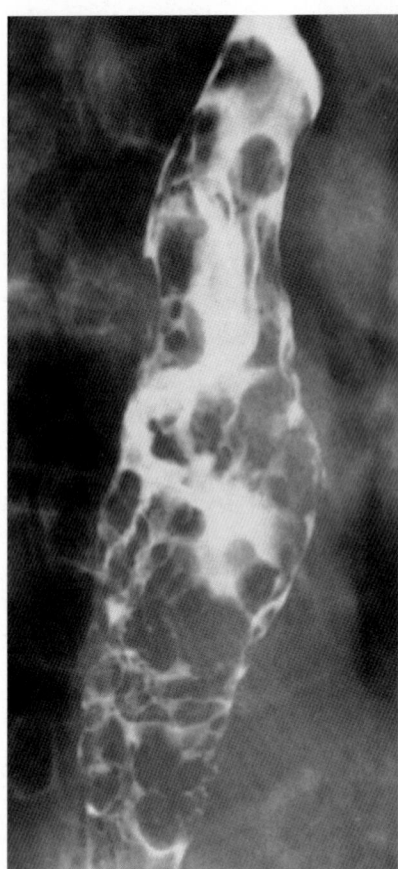

Figure 28-17. Spindle cell carcinoma of the esophagus. There is a long polypoid intraluminal mass in the midesophagus that expands the lumen without causing obstruction. This appearance is typical of spindle cell carcinoma but can also be seen with primary malignant melanoma of the esophagus (see Fig. 28-19). (From Laufer I, Levine MS [eds]: Double Contrast Gastrointestinal Radiology, 2nd ed. Philadelphia, WB Saunders, 1992.)

Differential Diagnosis

The differential diagnosis for a bulky, polypoid intraluminal mass includes other benign and malignant polypoid tumors of the esophagus. Benign lesions such as giant fibrovascular polyps, lipomas, or leiomyomas occasionally may produce similar findings, but these lesions tend to have a smoother contour and are less lobulated.[73] Squamous cell carcinomas and adenocarcinomas arising in Barrett's mucosa may be polypoid lesions, but as these tumors become more advanced, they tend to infiltrate and narrow the lumen rather than to expand it.[74] Other rare tumors of the esophagus such as leiomyosarcoma, lymphoma, Kaposi's sarcoma, and primary malignant melanoma of the esophagus may also be manifested by polypoid intraluminal masses. Thus, a definitive diagnosis of spindle cell carcinoma can be made only on histologic grounds.

LEIOMYOSARCOMA

Leiomyosarcomas of the esophagus are rare low-grade malignant tumors characterized by slow growth and late metastases.[75,76] These tumors are almost always thought to arise de novo rather than from preexisting leiomyomas.[77,78] They are usually located in the distal two thirds of the esophagus because this is the portion of the esophagus that is lined by smooth muscle.[79,80] The lesions may eventually spread by direct extension to the pleura, pericardium, diaphragms, and stomach, or they may metastasize hematogenously to the liver, lungs, and bones.[76,78,79] Because of their relatively slow growth rates, esophageal leiomyosarcomas have a better prognosis than squamous cell carcinomas, with 5-year survival rates approaching 35%.[79,81] Nevertheless, rapid progression of esophageal leiomyosarcomas has occasionally been documented.[81]

Clinical Findings

Esophageal leiomyosarcomas are usually found in middle-aged or elderly patients[76,82] and are slightly more common in men than in women.[79,82] Dysphagia is the most common presenting clinical complaint, but dysphagia can be minimal or absent if the tumor has a predominantly exophytic pattern of growth with little encroachment on the lumen.[83] When dysphagia does occur, it is often present for a longer interval (6 to 12 months) than in patients with esophageal carcinoma because of the slow growth of these tumors.[79] Although rare, gastrointestinal bleeding can occur if the lesion is ulcerated.[77]

An esophagectomy or esophagogastrectomy is the treatment of choice for esophageal leiomyosarcomas.[76,79,80,82] Even when metastases are present, resection of the primary tumor may lead to prolonged survival of these patients. Because leiomyosarcomas are radiosensitive, bulky lesions can also be palliated by radiation therapy in nonsurgical candidates.[76,79,80]

Radiographic Findings

Esophageal leiomyosarcomas sometimes contain large exophytic components that can be recognized on chest radiographs as mediastinal masses.[76,83,84] Rarely, chest radiographs may reveal dense calcification within the tumor.[85] Leiomyosarcomas may appear on barium studies as large, lobulated intramural masses containing areas of ulceration or tracking (Fig. 28-18A).[83] These tumors therefore have the same radiographic features as malignant gastrointestinal stromal tumors in the stomach and small bowel. Less commonly, they may appear as polypoid, expansile intraluminal masses in the esophagus[75,78,83,84,86] or even as infiltrative lesions with irregular luminal narrowing.[78,84]

Esophageal leiomyosarcomas are characterized on CT by heterogeneous masses containing large exophytic components, central areas of low density, and extraluminal gas or contrast material within the tumor (presumably because of necrosis and cavitation) (Fig. 28-18B).[78,80,81,83] Similar CT findings have been reported with malignant gastrointestinal stromal tumors elsewhere in the gastrointestinal tract, indicating that these tumors have the same gross pathologic features regardless of their location.

Esophageal leiomyosarcomas may be manifested on MRI by esophageal masses that are isointense with skeletal muscle on T1-weighted images (Fig. 28-18C) and hyperintense on T2-weighted images (Fig. 28-18D).[83,87] MRI may also reveal a central signal void caused by extraluminal gas within the tumor.[83] Esophageal leiomyosarcomas are characterized on endoscopic sonography by well-defined hyperechoic masses arising from the muscular layer of the esophageal wall.[81] These tumors can also be recognized on angiography as hyper-

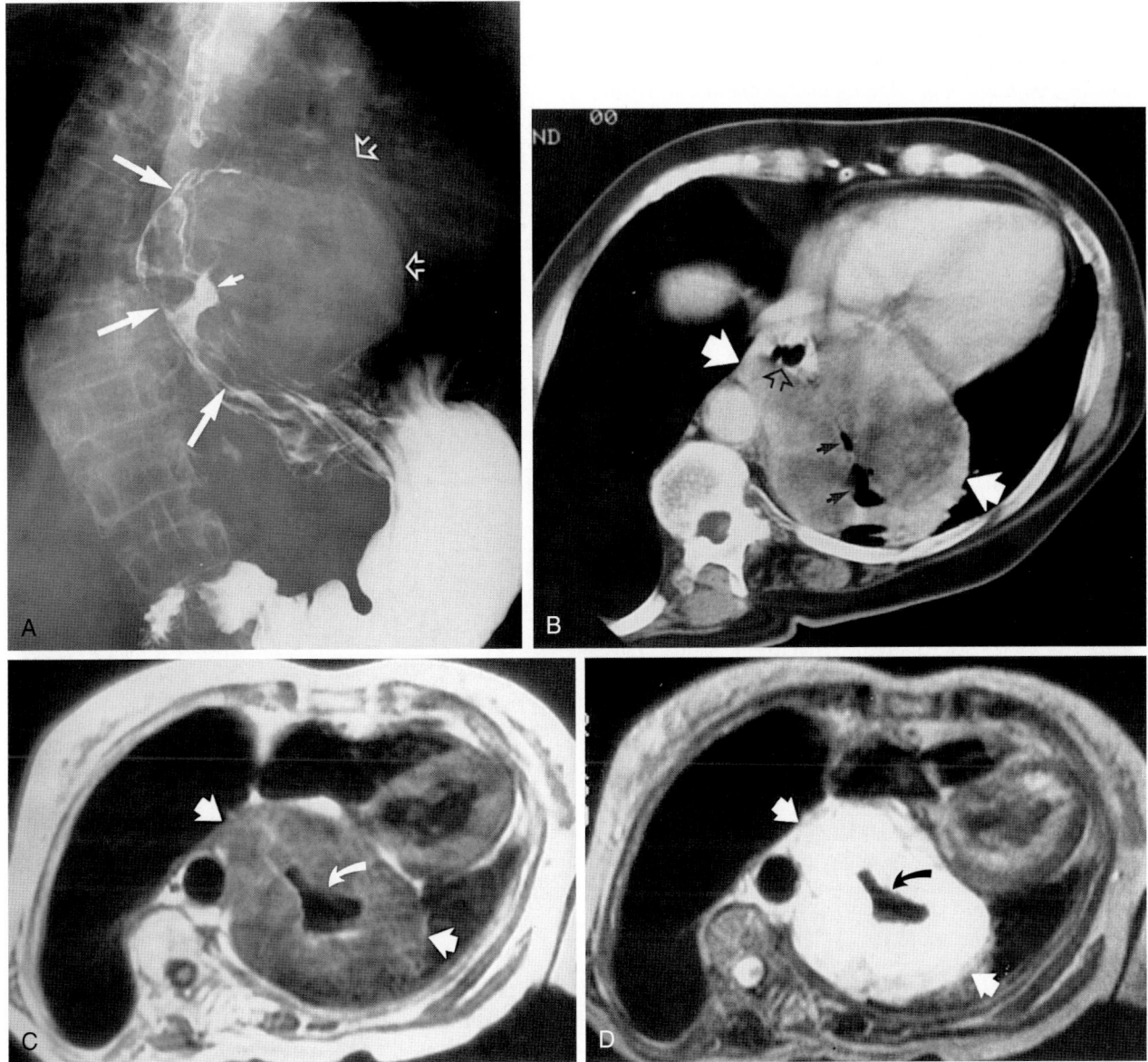

Figure 28-18. Esophageal leiomyosarcoma. A. Barium study shows a giant intramural mass (*large arrows*) with a bulky exophytic component in the mediastinum (*open arrows*). Note the relatively small central ulcer (*small arrow*) within the lesion. **B.** CT scan shows a heterogeneous mass (*white arrows*) in the left side of the mediastinum with central areas of low density. Note the extraluminal collections of gas (*solid black arrows*) within the lesion that are separate from the esophageal lumen (*open black arrow*). **C.** T1-weighted (TR/TE, 674/12) MR image also shows a mass (*straight arrows*) in the left side of the mediastinum. Note how the mass is isointense with skeletal muscle. **D.** T2-weighted (2697/80) MR image shows how the lesion (*straight arrows*) is markedly hyperintense relative to skeletal muscle. In both **C** and **D**, there is a focal area of signal void (*curved arrows*) caused by extraluminal gas within the tumor. (From Levine MS, Buck JL, Pantongrag-Brown L, et al: Leiomyosarcoma of the esophagus: Radiographic findings in 10 patients. AJR 167:27-32, 1996, © by American Roentgen Ray Society.)

vascular masses with tumor vessels, dilated vascular channels or venous lakes, and early venous drainage.[78]

Differential Diagnosis

Esophageal leiomyosarcomas that appear on barium studies as intramural masses must be differentiated from leiomyomas and other benign mesenchymal tumors in the esophagus. However, these benign intramural lesions tend to be smaller and less lobulated and rarely if ever contain areas of ulceration or tracking. Leiomyosarcomas that appear as polypoid masses must be differentiated from spindle cell sarcoma, lymphoma, Kaposi's sarcoma, and even primary malignant

melanoma of the esophagus. Giant fibrovascular polyps may also appear as expansile intraluminal masses, but these benign tumors usually have a much smoother contour and almost always arise in the cervical esophagus from the region of the cricopharyngeus.[73] Finally, leiomyosarcomas that appear as infiltrative lesions must be differentiated from squamous cell carcinomas or adenocarcinomas arising in Barrett's mucosa.[74]

MALIGNANT MELANOMA

Primary malignant melanoma of the esophagus is a rare but aggressive tumor that accounts for less than 1% of all malignant esophageal neoplasms.[88] In the past, these lesions were thought to represent metastases from occult melanomas of the eye, skin, or anus. However, esophageal metastases are rarely found in patients with documented melanomas elsewhere.[5,9] The seeming paradox of developing melanoma in a structure such as the esophagus is explained by the fact that small numbers of melanocytes are present in the esophageal mucosa in 2% to 8% of patients.[89-91] As in the skin, esophageal melanoma presumably develops because of malignant degeneration of these preexisting melanocytes. A review of the literature suggests that primary malignant melanoma is at least 10 times more common than metastatic melanoma involving the esophagus.[88]

Clinical Findings

Primary esophageal melanoma is an extremely aggressive tumor that is usually diagnosed in the elderly. Most patients present with dysphagia and weight loss,[88] but the diagnosis is rarely suggested on clinical grounds. These tumors can sometimes be recognized at endoscopy as darkly pigmented masses, but pigmentation is not always apparent on visual inspection.[88] The treatment of primary esophageal melanoma is surgical; an extensive esophageal resection is usually performed. However, these tumors tend to be advanced lesions at the time of diagnosis. As a result, affected individuals have a dismal prognosis, with 5-year survival rates of less than 5% and an average overall survival of only 10 to 13 months from the time of diagnosis.[88,92]

Radiographic Findings

Esophageal melanomas have strikingly similar findings on barium studies, appearing as bulky, polypoid intraluminal masses that expand the esophagus without causing obstruction (Fig. 26-19).[93-96] CT may also reveal large soft tissue masses expanding the esophagus.[95,96] These findings occur because melanoma tends to grow intraluminally along the longitudinal axis of the esophagus, producing a polypoid mass that widens the lumen as it enlarges.[95] Most esophageal melanomas are located in the lower half of the esophagus,[88] probably because of the greater concentration of melanocytes in this region.[89-91]

Differential Diagnosis

The major consideration in the differential diagnosis of a large polypoid intraluminal mass in the esophagus is spindle cell carcinoma.[62,63,65] Other rare tumors involving the esophagus that may produce similar findings include leiomyosarcoma, lymphoma, and Kaposi's sarcoma. In contrast, squamous cell carcinoma and adenocarcinoma of the esophagus rarely appear as expansile esophageal masses because these tumors tend to infiltrate and narrow the lumen rather than to expand it.

KAPOSI'S SARCOMA

Kaposi's sarcoma is a multifocal neoplasm of the reticuloendothelial system that is classically manifested by slow-growing cutaneous lesions on the lower extremities. However, a much more aggressive form of Kaposi's sarcoma has been recognized with increased frequency in patients with AIDS.

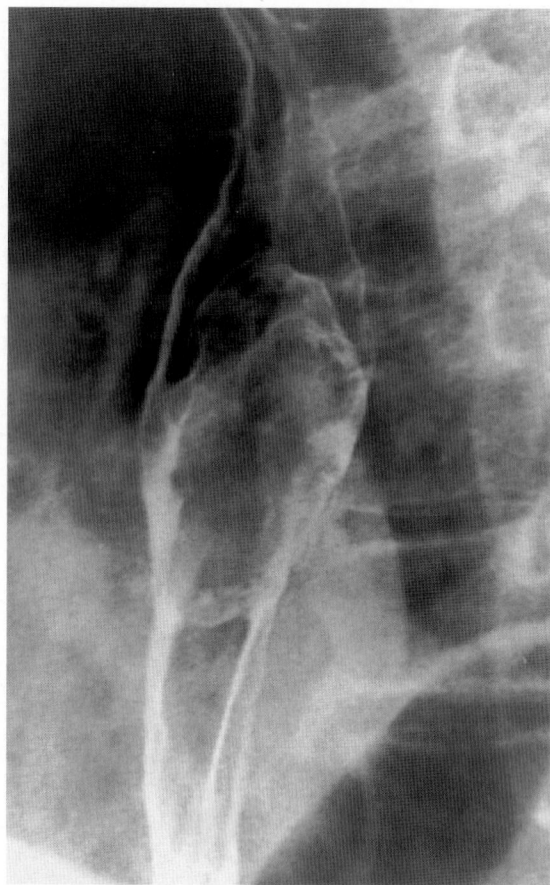

Figure 28-19. Primary malignant melanoma of the esophagus. There is a polypoid mass expanding the lumen of the distal esophagus. This lesion cannot be distinguished from spindle cell carcinoma (see Fig. 28-17) or other rare malignant tumors of the esophagus. (From Yoo CC, Levine MS, McLarney JK, et al: Primary malignant melanoma of the esophagus: Radiographic findings in seven patients. Radiology 209:455-459, 1998.)

More than 30% of AIDS patients in the United States have Kaposi's sarcoma,[97] and approximately 50% of patients with Kaposi's sarcoma have gastrointestinal involvement, manifested by submucosal nodules, polypoid lesions, or thickened folds in the stomach, duodenum, small bowel, or colon.[98,99] Rarely, esophageal involvement has also been reported.[98,100]

Radiographic Findings

Esophageal involvement by Kaposi's sarcoma may be manifested on barium studies by a single polypoid mass in the esophagus or by multiple submucosal lesions (Fig. 28-20).[98,100] When multiple submucosal lesions are present, the differential diagnosis includes lymphoma, leukemia, multiple leiomyomas, and, rarely, metastases from malignant melanoma. However, Kaposi's sarcoma should be suspected when one or more discrete esophageal lesions are found in patients with AIDS who have associated lesions on the skin.

SMALL CELL CARCINOMA

Primary small cell (or oat cell) carcinoma of the esophagus is a rare but aggressive malignant tumor characterized by

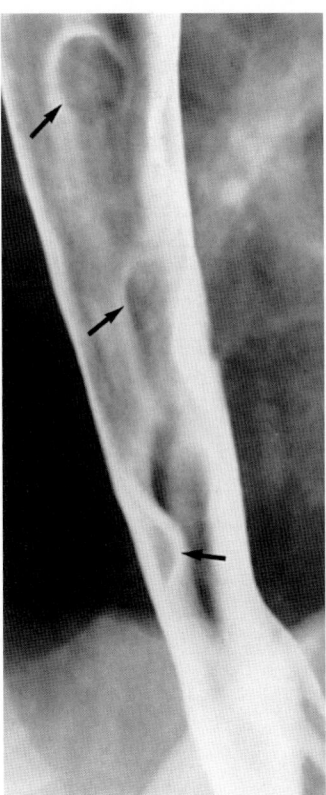

Figure 28-20. Kaposi's sarcoma involving the esophagus. Multiple submucosal masses (*arrows*) are seen in the esophagus. This patient had additional submucosal lesions elsewhere in the gastrointestinal tract. (Courtesy of Robert A. Goren, MD, Philadelphia, PA.)

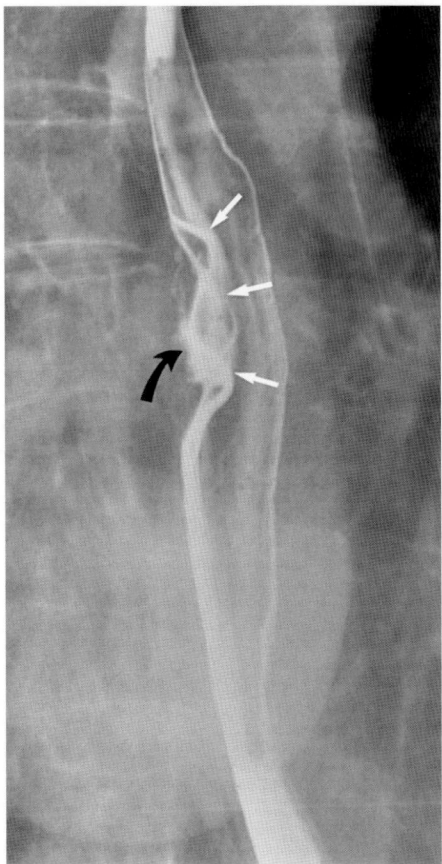

Figure 28-21. Small cell carcinoma of the esophagus. There is a smoothly marginated, sessile mass (*white arrows*) containing a relatively flat central area of ulceration (*black arrow*) on the right posterolateral wall of the midesophagus below the level of the carina. (From Levine MS, Pantongrag-Brown L, Buck JL, et al: Small-cell carcinoma of the esophagus: Radiographic findings. Radiology 199:703-705, 1996.)

early metastases and a rapidly fatal course. The tumor may be derived from argyrophilic cells or Kulchitsky cells of neuro-ectodermal origin.[90,101] Affected individuals typically present with rapidly progressive dysphagia and weight loss.[102,103] These patients have a dismal prognosis, with an average survival of 6 months or less from the time of diagnosis.[101-103] Because of the likelihood of distant metastases, surgery has been recommended primarily for palliation, whereas a multimodality approach with combination chemotherapy and radiation therapy has been advocated to improve patient survival.[101,103,104]

Radiographic Findings

Advanced small cell carcinomas of the esophagus may appear on barium studies as bulky polypoid or fungating masses, sometimes containing areas of ulceration or cavitation.[62,105,106] Less advanced lesions may be characterized by strikingly similar radiographic findings, appearing as smoothly marginated, sessile, centrally ulcerated masses, most commonly in the midesophagus near the level of the carina (Fig. 28-21).[107,108] Although this appearance is more likely to be caused by squamous cell carcinoma, it is important to obtain endoscopic biopsy specimens, because a preoperative histologic diagnosis of small cell carcinoma may dramatically alter the management of these patients. Rarely, regression of small cell carcinoma may be documented on follow-up barium studies after combination chemotherapy and radiation therapy.[107]

LEUKEMIA

Although rarely diagnosed before death, esophageal involvement by leukemia has been reported at autopsy in 2% to 13% of patients.[109,110] These leukemic deposits may appear on barium studies as one or more discrete nodular elevations (Fig. 28-22).[103,105] Coalescent intramural lesions may also be manifested by irregular areas of narrowing in the middle or distal third of the esophagus on barium studies (Fig. 28-23A) with esophageal wall thickening on CT (Fig. 28-23B).[111] Rarely, bulky leukemic deposits may appear as polypoid lesions in the esophagus.[112] These leukemic deposits may undergo marked regression after radiation therapy.[111] Esophageal symptoms may therefore be palliated by mediastinal irradiation, but the overall prognosis for this disease is unchanged.

MISCELLANEOUS TUMORS

Other rare malignant tumors that have been reported in the esophagus include adenoid cystic carcinoma,[113,114] chondrosarcoma,[115] synovial sarcoma,[116] and malignant carcinoid tumor.[117] In general, sarcomas tend to be more polypoid than carcinomas, which are more infiltrating lesions. Nevertheless, a definitive diagnosis can be made only on histologic criteria.

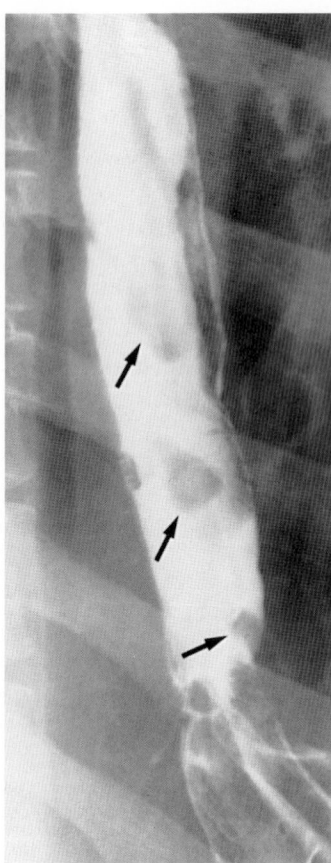

Figure 28-22. Leukemic infiltration of the esophagus. This patient has multiple submucosal masses (*arrows*) in the esophagus due to leukemic deposits. (Courtesy of Sadi R. Antonmattei, MD, Arecibo, Puerto Rico.)

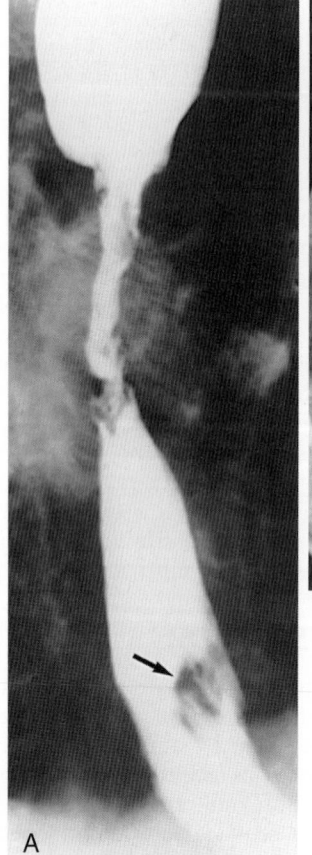

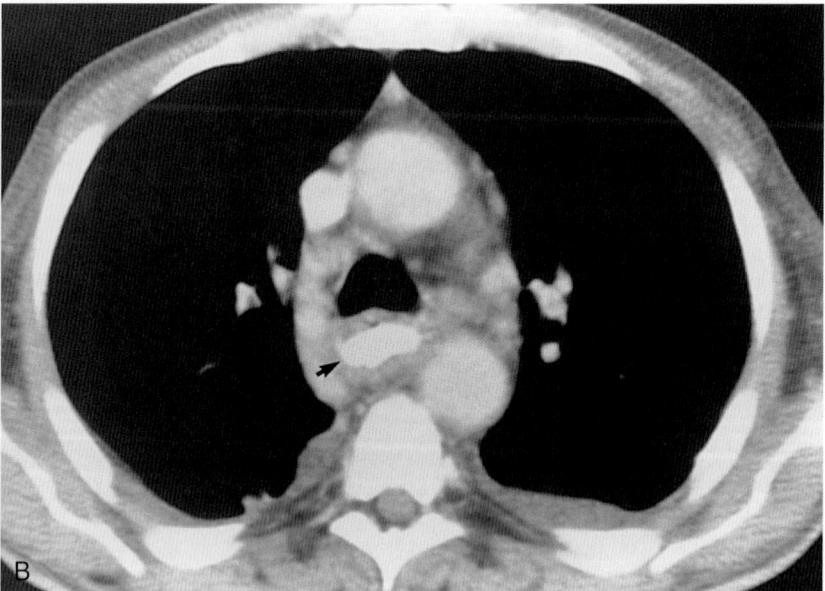

Figure 28-23. Leukemic infiltration of the esophagus. A. Esophagogram shows irregular narrowing of the midesophagus due to leukemic infiltration of the wall. Note a discrete leukemic deposit (*arrow*) in the distal esophagus. **B.** CT scan just above the level of the stricture shows contrast medium in a dilated lumen (*arrow*) with infiltration of the surrounding wall. (Courtesy of Duane G. Mezwa, MD, Royal Oak, MI.)

References

1. Agha FP: Secondary neoplasms of the esophagus. Gastrointest Radiol 12:187-193, 1987.
2. Polk HC, Camp FA, Walker AW: Dysphagia and esophageal stenosis: Manifestation of metastatic mammary cancer. Cancer 20:2002-2007, 1967.
3. Holyoke ED, Nemoto T, Dao TL: Esophageal metastases and dysphagia in patients with carcinoma of the breast. J Surg Oncol 1:97-107, 1969.
4. Anderson MF, Harell GS: Secondary esophageal tumors. AJR 135:1243-1246, 1980.
5. Wood CB, Wood RAB: Metastatic malignant melanoma of the esophagus. Am J Dig Dis 20:786-789, 1975.
6. Fisher MS: Metastasis to the esophagus. Gastrointest Radiol 1:249-251, 1976.
7. Gore RM, Sparberg M: Metastatic carcinoma of the prostate to the esophagus. Am J Gastroenterol 77:358-359, 1982.
8. Feczko PJ, Halpert RD: Achalasia secondary to nongastrointestinal malignancies. Gastrointest Radiol 10:273-276, 1985.
9. Schneider A, Martini N, Burt ME: Malignant melanoma metastatic to the esophagus. Ann Thorac Surg 55:516-517, 1993.
10. Stankey RM, Roshe J, Sogocio RM: Carcinoma of the lung and dysphagia. Dis Chest 55:13-17, 1969.
11. Varanasi RV, Saltzman JR, Krims P, et al: Breast carcinoma metastatic to the esophagus: Clinicopathological and management features of four cases, and literature review. Am J Gastroenterol 90:1495-1499, 1995.
12. Cooney BS, Levine MS, Schnall MD: Metastatic thyroid carcinoma presenting as an expansile intraluminal esophageal mass. Abdom Imaging 20:20-22, 1995.
13. Balthazar EJ, Goldfine S, Davidian NM: Carcinoma of the esophagogastric junction. Am J Gastroenterol 74:237-243, 1980.
14. Freeny PC, Marks WM: Adenocarcinoma of the gastroesophageal junction: Barium and CT examination. AJR 138:1077-1084, 1982.
15. Levine MS, Laufer I, Thompson JJ: Carcinoma of the gastric cardia in young people. AJR 140:69-72, 1983.
16. Fleischner FG, Sachsse E: Retrotracheal lymphadenopathy in bronchial carcinoma, revealed by the barium-filled esophagus. AJR 90:792-798, 1963.
17. Libshitz HI, Lindell MM, Dodd GD: Metastases to the hollow viscera. Radiol Clin North Am 20:487-499, 1982.
18. Parkman HP, Cohen S: Malignancy-induced secondary achalasia. Dysphagia 8:292-296, 1993.
19. Lawson TL, Dodds WJ: Infiltrating carcinoma simulating achalasia. Gastrointest Radiol 1:245-248, 1976.
20. McCallum RW: Esophageal achalasia secondary to gastric carcinoma: Report of a case and review of the literature. Am J Gastroenterol 71:24-29, 1979.
21. Kahrilas PJ, Kishk SM, Helm JF, et al: Comparison of pseudoachalasia and achalasia. Am J Med 82:439-446, 1987.
22. Joffe N: Right-angled narrowing of the distal oesophagus secondary to carcinoma of the tail of the pancreas. Clin Radiol 30:33-37, 1979.
23. Eaves R, Lambert J, Rees J, et al: Achalasia secondary to carcinoma of the prostate. Dig Dis Sci 28:278-284, 1983.
24. Davis JA, Kantrowitz PA, Chandler HL, et al: Reversible achalasia due to reticulum-cell sarcoma. N Engl J Med 293:130-132, 1975.
25. Ferreira-Santos R: Aperistalsis of the esophagus and colon (megaesophagus and megacolon) etiologically related to Chagas' disease. Am J Dig Dis 6:700-726, 1961.
26. Costigan DJ, Clouse RE: Achalasia-like esophagus from amyloidosis. Dig Dis Sci 28:763-765, 1983.
27. Simeone J, Burrell M, Toffler R: Esophageal aperistalsis secondary to metastatic invasion of the myenteric plexus. AJR 127:862-864, 1976.
28. Shulze KS, Goresky CA, Jabbari M, et al: Esophageal achalasia associated with gastric carcinoma: Lack of evidence for widespread plexus destruction. Can Med Assoc J 112:857-864, 1975.
29. Lee HR, Lennon VA, Camilleri M, et al: Paraneoplastic gastrointestinal motor dysfunction: Clinical and laboratory characteristics. Am J Gastroenterol 96:373-379, 2001.
30. Giorgio RD, Bovara M, Barbara G, et al: Anti-HuD-induced neuronal apoptosis underlying paraneoplastic gut dysmotility. Gastroenterology 125:70-79, 2003.
31. Woodfield CA, Levine MS, Rubesin SE, et al: Diagnosis of primary versus secondary achalasia: Reassessment of clinical and radiographic criteria. AJR 175:727-731, 2000.
32. Tucker HJ, Snape WJ, Cohen SC: Achalasia secondary to carcinoma: Manometric and clinical features. Ann Intern Med 89:315-318, 1978.
33. Sandler RS, Bozymski EM, Orlando RC: Failure of clinical criteria to distinguish between primary achalasia and achalasia secondary to tumor. Dig Dis Sci 27:209-213, 1982.
34. Tracey JP, Traube M: Difficulties in the diagnosis of pseudoachalasia. Am J Gastroenterol 89:2014-2018, 1994.
35. Seaman WB, Wells J, Flood CA: Diagnostic problems of esophageal cancer: Relationship to achalasia and hiatus hernia. AJR 90:778-791, 1963.
36. Rabushka LS, Fishman EK, Kuhlman JE: CT evaluation of achalasia. J Comput Assist Tomogr 15:434-439, 1991.
37. Tishler JM, Shin MS, Stanley RJ, et al: CT of the thorax in patients with achalasia. Dig Dis Sci 28:692-697, 1983.
38. Marks WM, Callen PW, Moss AA: Gastroesophageal region: Source of confusion on CT. AJR 136:359-362, 1981.
39. Carter M, Deckmann RC, Smith RC, et al: Differentiation of achalasia from pseudoachalasia by computed tomography. Am J Gastroenterol 92:624-628, 1997.
40. Rosenberg SA, Diamond HD, Jaslowitz B, et al: Lymphosarcoma: A review of 1,269 cases. Medicine (Baltimore) 40:31-84, 1961.
41. Caruso RD, Berk RN: Lymphoma of the esophagus. Radiology 95:381-382, 1970.
42. Carnovale RL, Goldstein HM, Zornoza J, et al: Radiologic manifestations of esophageal lymphoma. AJR 128:751-754, 1977.
43. Zornoza J, Dodd GD: Lymphoma of the gastrointestinal tract. Semin Roentgenol 15:272-287, 1980.
44. Agha FP, Schnitzer B: Esophageal involvement in lymphoma. Am J Gastroenterol 80:412-416, 1985.
45. Levine MS, Rubesin SE, Pantongrag-Brown L, et al: Non-Hodgkin's lymphoma of the gastrointestinal tract: Radiographic findings. AJR 168:165-172, 1997.
46. Stein HA, Murray D, Warner HA: Primary Hodgkin's disease of the esophagus. Dig Dis Sci 26:457-461, 1981.
47. Doki T, Hamada S, Murayama H, et al: Primary malignant lymphoma of the esophagus. Endoscopy 16:189-192, 1984.
48. Taal BG, Van Heerde P, Somers R: Isolated primary oesophageal involvement by lymphoma: A rare cause of dysphagia: Two case histories and a review of other published data. Gut 34:994-998, 1993.
49. Oguzkurt L, Karabulut N, Cakmakci E, et al: Primary non-Hodgkin's lymphoma of the esophagus. Abdom Imaging 22:8-10, 1997.
50. Gaskin CM, Low VHS, Ho LM: Isolated primary non-Hodgkin's lymphoma of the esophagus. AJR 176:551-552, 2001.
51. Coppens E, Nakadi IE, Nagy N, et al: Primary Hodgkin's lymphoma of the esophagus. AJR 180:1135-1337, 2003.
52. Radin DR: Primary esophageal lymphoma in AIDS. Abdom Imaging 18:223-224, 1993.
53. Sabate JM, Franquet T, Palmer J, et al: AIDS-related primary esophageal lymphoma. Abdom Imaging 22:11-13, 1997.
54. Traube M, Waldron JA, McCallum RW: Systemic lymphoma initially presenting as an esophageal mass. Am J Gastroenterol 77:835-837, 1982.
55. Hricak H, Thoeni RF, Margulis AR, et al: Extension of gastric lymphoma into the esophagus and duodenum. Radiology 135:309-312, 1980.
56. Lambert A: Malignant tracheoesophageal fistula secondary to Hodgkin's disease. J Thorac Cardiovasc Surg 69:820-826, 1975.
57. Kirsch HL, Cronin DW, Stein GN, et al: Esophageal perforation: An unusual presentation of esophageal lymphoma. Dig Dis Sci 28:371-374, 1983.
58. Levine MS, Sunshine AG, Reynolds JC, et al: Diffuse nodularity in esophageal lymphoma. AJR 145:1218-1220, 1985.
59. Gedgaudas-McClees RK, Maglinte DDT: Lymphomatous esophageal nodules: The difficulty in radiological differential diagnosis. Am J Gastroenterol 80:529-530, 1985.
60. Xu L, Sun C, Wu L, et al: Clinical and pathological characteristics of carcinosarcoma of the esophagus: report of four cases. Ann Thorac Surg 37:197-203, 1984.
61. Martin MR, Kahn LB: So-called pseudosarcoma of the esophagus: Nodal metastases of the spindle cell element. Arch Pathol Lab Med 101:604-609, 1977.
62. Olmsted WW, Lichtenstein JE, Hyams VJ: Polypoid epithelial malignancies of the esophagus. AJR 140:921-925, 1983.
63. Agha FP, Keren DF: Spindle-cell squamous carcinoma of the esophagus: A tumor with biphasic morphology. AJR 145:541-545, 1985.
64. Talbert JL, Cantrell JR: Clinical and pathological characteristics of carcinosarcoma of the esophagus. J Thorac Cardiovasc Surg 45:1-12, 1963.
65. McCort JJ: Esophageal carcinosarcoma and pseudosarcoma. Radiology 102:519-524, 1972.

66. Razzuk MA, Urschel HC, Race GJ, et al: Pseudosarcoma of the esophagus. J Thorac Cardiovasc Surg 61:650-653, 1971.

67. Postlethwait RW, Wechsler AS, Shelburne JD: Pseudosarcoma of the esophagus. Ann Thorac Surg 19:198-205, 1975.

68. Nichols T, Yokoo H, Craig RM, et al: Pseudosarcoma of the esophagus. Am J Gastroenterol 72:615-622, 1979.

69. Halvorsen RA, Foster WL, Williford ME, et al: Pseudosarcoma of the esophagus: Barium swallow and CT findings. J Can Assoc Radiol 34:278-281, 1983.

70. Osamura RY, Shimamora K, Hata J: Polypoid carcinoma of the esophagus: A unifying term for carcinosarcoma and pseudosarcoma. Am J Surg Pathol 2:201-208, 1978.

71. Hinderleider CD, Aguam AS, Wilder JR: Carcinosarcoma of the esophagus: A case report and review of the literature. Int Surg 64:13-19, 1979.

72. Kenneweg DJ, Cimmino CV: Carcinosarcoma of the esophagus. AJR 101:482-484, 1967.

73. Levine MS, Buck JL, Pantongrag-Brown L, et al: Fibrovascular polyps of the esophagus: Clinical, radiographic, and pathologic findings in 16 patients. AJR 166:781-787, 1996.

74. Levine MS: Esophageal cancer: Radiologic diagnosis. Radiol Clin North Am 35:265-279, 1997

75. Wolfel DA: Leiomyosarcoma of the esophagus. AJR 89:127-131, 1963.

76. Franklin GO, Antler AS, Thelmo WL, et al: Esophageal leiomyosarcoma. N Y State J Med 82:1100-1103, 1982.

77. Glanz I, Grunebaum M: The radiological approach to leiomyoma of the oesophagus with a long-term follow-up. Clin Radiol 28:197-200, 1977.

78. Balthazar EJ: Gastrointestinal leiomyosarcoma—unusual sites: Esophagus, colon, and porta hepatis. Gastrointest Radiol 6:295-301, 1981.

79. Weinstein EC, Kim YS, Young GJ, et al: Leiomyosarcoma of the esophagus. Milit Med 4:206-209, 1968.

80. Patel SR, Anandarao N: Leiomyosarcoma of the esophagus. N Y State J Med 90:371-372, 1990.

81. Koga H, Iida M, Suekane H, et al: Rapidly growing esophageal leiomyosarcoma: Case report and review of the literature. Abdom Imaging 20:15-19, 1995.

82. Choh JH, Khazei AH, Ihm HJ: Leiomyosarcoma of the esophagus: Report of a case and review of the literature. J Surg Oncol 32:223-226, 1986.

83. Levine MS, Buck JL, Pantongrag-Brown L, et al: Leiomyosarcoma of the esophagus: Radiographic findings in 10 patients. AJR 167:27-32, 1996.

84. Berk RN, Scher GS, Bode DF: Unusual tumors of the gastrointestinal tract. AJR 113:159-169, 1971.

85. Itai Y, Shimazu H: Leiomyosarcoma of the oesophagus with dense calcification. Br J Radiol 51:469-471, 1978.

86. Athanasoulis CA, Aral IM: Leiomyosarcoma of the esophagus. Gastroenterology 54:271-274, 1968.

87. Ohnishi T, Yoshioka H, Ishida O: MR imaging of gastrointestinal leiomyosarcoma. Radiat Med 9:114-117, 1991.

88. Sabanathan S, Eng J, Pradhan GN: Primary malignant melanoma of the esophagus. Am J Gastroenterol 84:1475-1481, 1989.

89. De la Pava S, Nigogosyan G, Pickren JW, et al: Melanosis of the esophagus. Cancer 16:48-50, 1963.

90. Tateishi R, Taniguchi H, Wada A, et al: Argyrophil cells and melanocytes in esophageal mucosa. Arch Pathol 98:87-89, 1974.

91. Sharma SS, Venkateswaran A, Chacko A, et al: Melanosis of the esophagus: An endoscopic, histochemical, and ultrastructural study. Gastroenterology 100:13-16, 1991.

92. Chalkiadakis G, Wihlm JM, Morand G, et al: Primary malignant melanoma of the esophagus. Ann Thorac Surg 39:472-475, 1985.

93. Isaacs JL, Quirke P: Two cases of primary malignant melanoma of the oesophagus. Clin Radiol 39:455-457, 1988.

94. Brown JH, Chew FS: Primary esophageal melanoma. AJR 157:318, 1991.

95. Yoo CC, Levine MS, McLarney JK, et al: Primary malignant melanoma of the esophagus: Radiographic findings in seven patients. Radiology 209:455-459, 1998.

96. Gollub MJ, Prowda JC: Primary melanoma of the esophagus: Radiologic and clinical findings in six patients. Radiology 213:97-100, 1999.

97. Friedman SL, Wright TL, Altman DF: Gastrointestinal Kaposi's sarcoma in patients with acquired immunodeficiency syndrome: Endoscopic and autopsy findings. Gastroenterology 89:102-108, 1985.

98. Rose HS, Balthazar EJ, Megibow AJ, et al: Alimentary tract involvement in Kaposi sarcoma: Radiographic and endoscopic findings in 25 homosexual men. AJR 139:661-666, 1982.

99. Wall SD, Friedman SL, Margulis AR: Gastrointestinal Kaposi's sarcoma in AIDS: radiographic manifestations. J Clin Gastroenterol 6:165-171, 1984.

100. Umerah BC: Kaposi sarcoma of the oesophagus. Br J Radiol 53:807-808, 1980.

101. Law SYK, Fok M, Lam KY, et al: Small cell carcinoma of the esophagus. Cancer 73:2894-2899, 1994.

102. Attar BM, Levendoglu HA, Rhee H: Small cell carcinoma of the esophagus. Dig Dis Sci 35:145-152, 1990.

103. Beyer KI, Marshall JB, Diaz-Arias AA, et al: Primary small-cell carcinoma of the esophagus: Report of 11 cases and review of the literature. J Clin Gastroenterol 13:135-141, 1995.

104. Hussein Am, Feun LG, Sridhar KS, et al: Combination chemotherapy and radiation therapy for small-cell carcinoma of the esophagus. Am J Clin Oncol 13:369-373, 1990.

105. Ignacio AG, Chintapalli K, Choi H: Primary oat cell carcinoma of the esophagus. Am J Gastroenterol 82:78-81, 1987.

106. Mulder LD, Gardiner GA, Weeks DA: Primary small cell carcinoma of the esophagus: Case presentation and review of the literature. Gastrointest Radiol 16:5-10, 1991.

107. Hirsch JA, Levine MS, Silberg DG, et al: Small-cell carcinoma of the esophagus with regression after combination chemotherapy and radiation therapy. Can Assoc Radiol J 46:45-47, 1995.

108. Levine MS, Pantongrag-Brown L, Buck JL, et al: Small-cell carcinoma of the esophagus: Radiographic findings. Radiology 199:703-705, 1996.

109. Prolla JC, Kirsner JB: The gastrointestinal lesions and complications of the leukemias. Ann Intern Med 61:1084-1103, 1964.

110. Givler RL: Esophageal lesions in leukemia and lymphoma. Am J Dig Dis 15:31-36, 1970.

111. Thompson BC, Feczko PJ, Mezwa DG: Dysphagia caused by acute leukemic infiltration of the esophagus [letter]. AJR 155:654, 1990.

112. Gildenhorn HL, Fahey JL, Solomon RD: Functional esophageal obstruction due to leukemic infiltration. AJR 88:736-740, 1962.

113. O'Sullivan JP, Cockburn JS, Drew CE: Adenoid cystic carcinoma of the esophagus. Thorax 30:476-480, 1975.

114. Kabuto T, Taniguchi K, Iwanaga T, et al: Primary adenoid cystic carcinoma of the esophagus. Cancer 43:2452-2456, 1979.

115. Yaghmai I, Ghahremani GG: Chondrosarcoma of the esophagus. AJR 126:1175-1177, 1976.

116. Block MJ, Iozzo RV, Edmunds LH, et al: Polypoid synovial sarcoma of the esophagus. Gastroenterology 92:229-233, 1987.

117. Brenner S, Heimlich H, Widman M: Carcinoid of esophagus. N Y State J Med 69:1337-1339, 1969.

Miscellaneous Abnormalities of the Esophagus

Marc S. Levine, MD

MALLORY-WEISS TEAR

Pathogenesis

Mallory-Weiss tear is recognized as a relatively common injury in which a sudden, rapid increase in intraesophageal pressure produces a linear mucosal laceration at or near the gastric cardia. These tears are usually caused by violent retching or vomiting after an alcoholic binge or by protracted vomiting for any reason.[1-3] Less commonly, Mallory-Weiss tears may be caused by prolonged hiccuping or coughing, seizures, straining at stool, childbirth, or blunt abdominal trauma.[4] Similar injuries may also result from direct laceration of the mucosa by an advancing endoscope or by a sharp foreign body in the esophagus, such as a piece of taco.[5-7]

Clinical Findings

Mallory-Weiss tears account for 5% to 10% of all cases of acute upper gastrointestinal bleeding.[8,9] Some patients may have massive hematemesis, but most tears heal spontaneously within 48 to 72 hours, so that bleeding is usually self-limited.[1,4,9] These patients therefore have an excellent prognosis, with an overall mortality rate of only about 3%.[2,4] Although most patients can be managed conservatively, selective intra-arterial infusion of vasopressin, transcatheter embolization, endoscopic electrocoagulation, or surgical repair of the tear may occasionally be required to control bleeding.[10-13]

Radiographic Findings

About 95% of Mallory-Weiss tears are diagnosed by endoscopy.[3] Nevertheless, these mucosal lacerations may occasionally be recognized on double-contrast esophagograms as shallow, longitudinally oriented, linear 1- to 4-cm collections of barium in the distal esophagus at or slightly above the gastroesophageal junction (Fig. 29-1). The radiographic appearance may be indistinguishable from that of a linear ulcer in the distal esophagus caused by reflux esophagitis. However, a history of recent vomiting or hematemesis (particularly in an alcoholic) should suggest the correct diagnosis.

ESOPHAGEAL HEMATOMA

Pathogenesis

Most esophageal hematomas are caused by a mucosal laceration or tear in the distal esophagus. If the tear is partially or completely occluded by edema or blood clot, continued hemorrhage may lead to progressive submucosal dissection of blood, producing an intramural hematoma.[14] As with Mallory-Weiss tears, the underlying laceration is usually caused by a

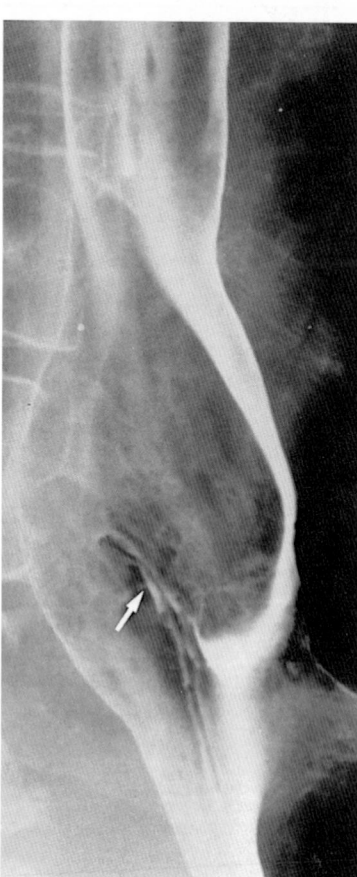

Figure 29-1. Mallory-Weiss tear. A linear collection of barium (*arrow*) is visible in the distal esophagus just above the gastroesophageal junction. Although a linear ulcer from reflux esophagitis could produce a similar appearance, the correct diagnosis was suggested by the clinical history. (Courtesy of Harvey M. Goldstein, MD, San Antonio, TX.)

sudden increase in intraesophageal pressure resulting from one or more episodes of violent retching or vomiting.[14,15] Esophageal hematomas may also be caused by esophageal instrumentation or, rarely, by blunt trauma to the chest or abdomen.[16-18] Occasionally, spontaneous hematomas may develop in patients who have impaired hemostasis because of thrombocytopenia, bleeding disorders, or anticoagulation.[19,20] In contrast to traumatic hematomas, which almost always occur as solitary lesions in the distal esophagus, spontaneous hematomas tend to spare the distal esophagus and occur at multiple sites.[15]

Clinical Findings

Patients with esophageal hematomas usually present with sudden onset of severe retrosternal chest pain, dysphagia, or hematemesis.[14,20,21] Despite the dramatic clinical findings, most esophageal hematomas resolve spontaneously within 1 to 2 weeks on conservative treatment with nasogastric suction, antibiotics, and intravenous fluids.[14,17,20,21] These lesions should therefore be considered self-limited because they almost never progress to complete transmural perforation.

Radiographic Findings

Esophageal hematomas usually appear on esophagography as solitary, ovoid, or elongated submucosal masses in the distal esophagus (Fig. 29-2).[14,17-19,22] As a result, they may be indistinguishable from leiomyomas or other benign intramural lesions. When a mucosal laceration is present, contrast medium may dissect beneath the mucosa into the hematoma. This intramural dissection produces a characteristic "double-barreled" appearance resulting from parallel collections of contrast medium in both true and false lumens separated by a thin, radiolucent stripe (Fig. 29-3).[16,23-25] Rarely, a double-barreled appearance may also be caused by intramural tracking of contrast medium as a result of Crohn's disease, *Candida* esophagitis, or tuberculous esophagitis.

Esophageal hematomas may be recognized on CT by the presence of an eccentric, well-defined intramural mass, which sometimes has a tubular appearance, extending a considerable distance along the long axis of the esophagus.[23,26,27] If the hematoma is acute or subacute, hyperdense areas may be present within the lesion.[26]

ESOPHAGEAL PERFORATION

Esophageal perforation is the most serious and rapidly fatal type of perforation in the gastrointestinal tract. Untreated thoracic esophageal perforations have a mortality rate of nearly 100% because of the fulminant mediastinitis that occurs after esophageal rupture.[28] Perforation of the cervical esophagus is a more common but less devastating injury. Early diagnosis of esophageal perforation is important because of the need for prompt surgical intervention in most cases.

Pathogenesis

Instrumentation

Endoscopic procedures are responsible for up to 75% of all esophageal perforations.[29,30] This complication occurs in

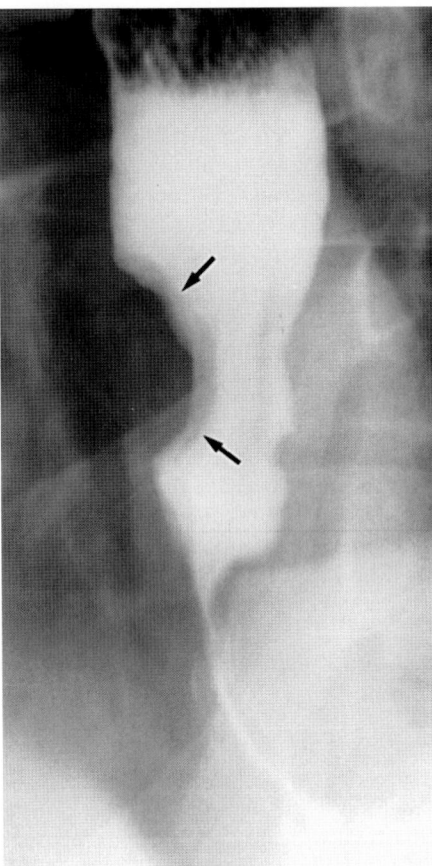

Figure 29-2. Esophageal hematoma. There is a smooth submucosal mass (*arrows*) in the distal esophagus. The hematoma was caused by a pneumatic dilatation procedure for achalasia. The esophagus is narrowed below the hematoma because of the patient's underlying achalasia. (From Levine MS: Radiology of the Esophagus. Philadelphia, WB Saunders, 1989.)

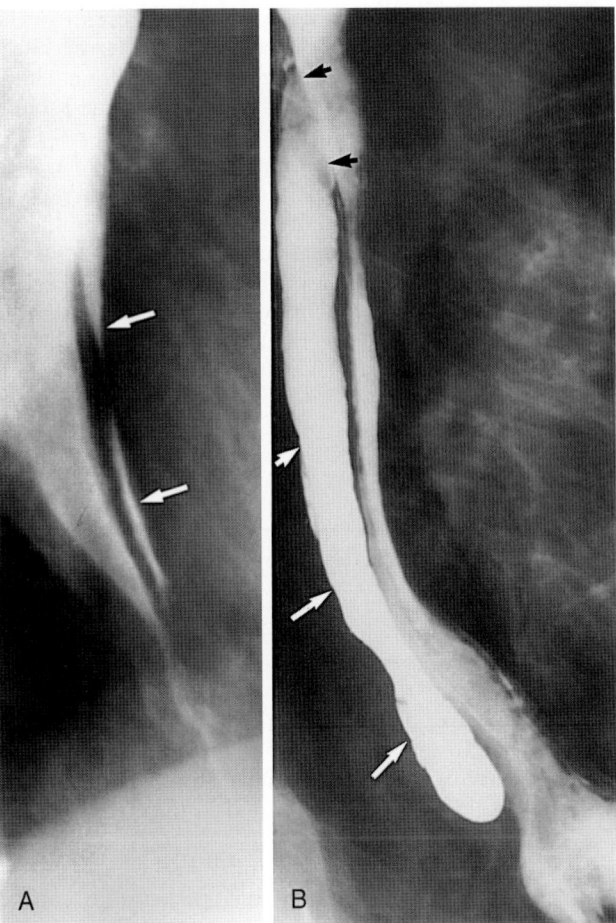

Figure 29-3. Two examples of intramural dissections with a double-barreled esophagus. A and **B.** The longitudinal intramural tracks (*white arrows*) are separated from the esophageal lumen by a radiolucent mucosal stripe. Both patients had traumatic dissections that occurred during esophageal instrumentation. The site of the laceration (*black arrows*) is well seen in **B**. (**A** courtesy of Sang Y. Han, MD, Birmingham, AL; **B** courtesy of Frank H. Miller, MD, Chicago, IL.)

about 1 in 3000 patients who undergo endoscopic examinations with modern fiberoptic instruments.[30] Most endoscopic perforations involve the piriform sinus or the posterior wall of the hypopharynx or cervical esophagus (at or just above the cricopharyngeus), where it is compressed against the cervical spine by the advancing endoscope.[29,31] The presence of cervical osteophytes or a pharyngeal diverticulum increases the risk of perforation.[30] In contrast to cervical esophageal perforations, which often occur in the absence of underlying disease, thoracic esophageal perforations usually result from endoscopic injury at or above esophageal strictures (benign or malignant) or from therapeutic maneuvers, such as variceal sclerotherapy, balloon dilatation, bougienage, placement of stents or nasogastric tubes, or foreign body removal.[30,32,33] Perforation may also occur after esophageal surgery, most frequently at the site of a ruptured anastomosis (see Chapter 31).

Foreign Bodies

Most foreign body perforations in adults are caused by impacted animal or fish bones in the hypopharynx that erode through the piriform sinus or cervical esophagus at or near the level of the cricopharyngeus. Rarely, foreign body obstructions in the thoracic esophagus also lead to perforation as a result of transmural inflammation and pressure necrosis at the site of impaction (see later section on Foreign Body Impaction). Esophageal perforation may also be caused by accidental or intentional ingestion of caustic agents (see Chapter 25).

Trauma

Penetrating injuries to the esophagus are most frequently caused by knife or bullet wounds. Because the neck lacks the bony protection afforded by the thorax, these injuries usually involve the cervical esophagus.[29] Rarely, blunt trauma to the neck, chest, or abdomen may also lead to pharyngeal or esophageal rupture or transection (see next section).[34]

Spontaneous Esophageal Perforation (Boerhaave's Syndrome)

In spontaneous esophageal perforation, a sudden, rapid increase in intraluminal esophageal pressure causes a full-thickness perforation of normal underlying esophageal tissue, with ensuing mediastinitis, sepsis, and shock. Most cases result from violent retching or vomiting, usually after an alcoholic binge.[35,36] Occasionally, however, spontaneous rupture of the esophagus may result from other causes of increased intra-esophageal pressure, such as coughing, weightlifting, childbirth, defecation, seizures, status asthmaticus, and blunt trauma to the chest or abdomen.[36]

Spontaneous esophageal perforations usually occur as 1- to 4-cm, vertically oriented, linear tears on the left lateral wall of the distal esophagus just above the gastroesophageal junction.[35,36] The distal esophagus is most vulnerable because of the lack of supporting mediastinal structures in this region. These perforations tend to be located on the left side of the distal esophagus because the right side is protected by the descending thoracic aorta.[29,36] Rarely, spontaneous perforation of the upper thoracic esophagus or even the cervical esophagus has been reported.[37,38]

Clinical Findings

Cervical Esophageal Perforation

Most cervical esophageal perforations occur as direct complications of endoscopy, but the endoscopist may be unaware that a perforation has occurred at the time of the examination. Subsequently, these patients may develop neck pain, dysphagia, or fever. Physical examination often reveals subcutaneous emphysema in the neck as a result of gas escaping from the pharynx into the adjacent soft tissues. If untreated, these patients may develop a retropharyngeal abscess with subsequent sepsis and shock.

Cervical esophageal perforations often heal with conservative medical treatment, so that small perforations can be treated nonoperatively. Larger perforations usually require a cervical mediastinotomy and open drainage to prevent abscess formation. With an overall mortality rate of less than 15%,[30] these injuries have a much better prognosis than thoracic esophageal perforations.

Thoracic Esophageal Perforation

Patients with thoracic esophageal perforation may present with the classic triad of vomiting, severe substernal chest pain, and subcutaneous emphysema of the chest wall and neck.[35,39] Some patients have atypical chest pain referred to the left shoulder or back,[35] whereas others have epigastric pain, particularly if the perforation involves the intra-abdominal segment of the esophagus below the diaphragmatic hiatus.[40] Furthermore, subcutaneous emphysema is not always present on physical examination. As a result, thoracic esophageal perforation can be mistaken for a variety of acute abdominal or cardiothoracic conditions, including perforated peptic ulcer, myocardial infarction, spontaneous pneumothorax, pulmonary infarct, acute pancreatitis, dissecting aortic aneurysm, or mesenteric infarction.[35,36,39] Occasionally, signs or symptoms of esophageal perforation can also be masked by treatment with corticosteroids.[41] Clinical confusion often leads to delayed diagnosis and treatment of a life-threatening condition. After 24 hours, the mortality rate for thoracic esophageal perforation is 70%.[35] Thus, early diagnosis is essential for improving survival of these patients.

In contrast to cervical esophageal perforations, which can often be treated conservatively, thoracic esophageal perforations usually require immediate thoracotomy (with surgical closure of the perforation and mediastinal drainage) to prevent the development of mediastinitis, sepsis, and death.[42] Rarely, thoracic esophageal perforations associated with Boerhaave's syndrome may heal spontaneously without surgical intervention.[43] Other small, self-contained perforations can sometimes be managed nonoperatively with broad-spectrum antibiotics and parenteral alimentation.[30] The overall mortality rate for all patients with thoracic esophageal perforation is about 25%.

Radiographic Findings

Plain Radiographs

Cervical Esophageal Perforation

Subcutaneous emphysema or retropharyngeal gas may be visible on anteroposterior or lateral radiographs of the neck within 1 hour after a pharyngeal or cervical esophageal perforation (Fig. 29-4A).[29] Subsequently, air may dissect along fascial planes from the neck into the chest, producing pneumomediastinum (see Fig. 29-4A).[29] Lateral radiographs of the neck may also demonstrate widening of the prevertebral space, anterior deviation of the trachea, and, eventually, a retropharyngeal abscess containing mottled gas or a single air-fluid level.

Thoracic Esophageal Perforation

About 90% of patients with thoracic esophageal perforations have abnormal chest radiographs.[44,45] The earliest findings include mediastinal widening and pneumomediastinum; the latter finding is usually recognized by the presence of radiolucent streaks of gas along the left lateral border of the aortic arch and descending thoracic aorta or along the right lateral border of the ascending aorta and heart (Fig. 29-5A).[29,35,36,45] Subsequently, gas in the mediastinum may dissect along fascial planes superiorly to the supraclavicular area, producing subcutaneous emphysema in the neck within several hours of the perforation.[36]

Seventy-five to 90 percent of thoracic esophageal perforations are associated with a pleural effusion or hydropneumothorax.[46] Distal esophageal perforations often result in a sympathetic left pleural effusion or atelectasis in the basilar segments of the left lung because of irritation of the adjacent mediastinal parietal pleura and pulmonary parenchyma (see Fig. 29-5A). Pleural effusions may be present within 12 hours of the perforation and are occasionally detected before the development of mediastinal or cervical emphysema. If the mediastinal pleura ruptures, gas and fluid may enter the pleural space directly from the mediastinum, producing a hydropneumothorax. Because the distal esophagus directly abuts the mediastinal parietal pleura on the left, 75% of hydropneumothoraces occur on the left side, whereas 5% occur on the right and 20% are bilateral.[35]

Rarely, abdominal radiographs may reveal extraluminal collections of gas in the lesser sac or retroperitoneum when the intra-abdominal segment of the distal esophagus is perforated below the diaphragmatic hiatus.[40,47] Such patients may have vague abdominal discomfort without chest pain or other classic signs of esophageal perforation, so that the diagnosis is often delayed. On the other hand, intra-abdominal esophageal perforations can have a more benign clinical course, because some of these perforations heal spontaneously with conservative treatment.[40,47]

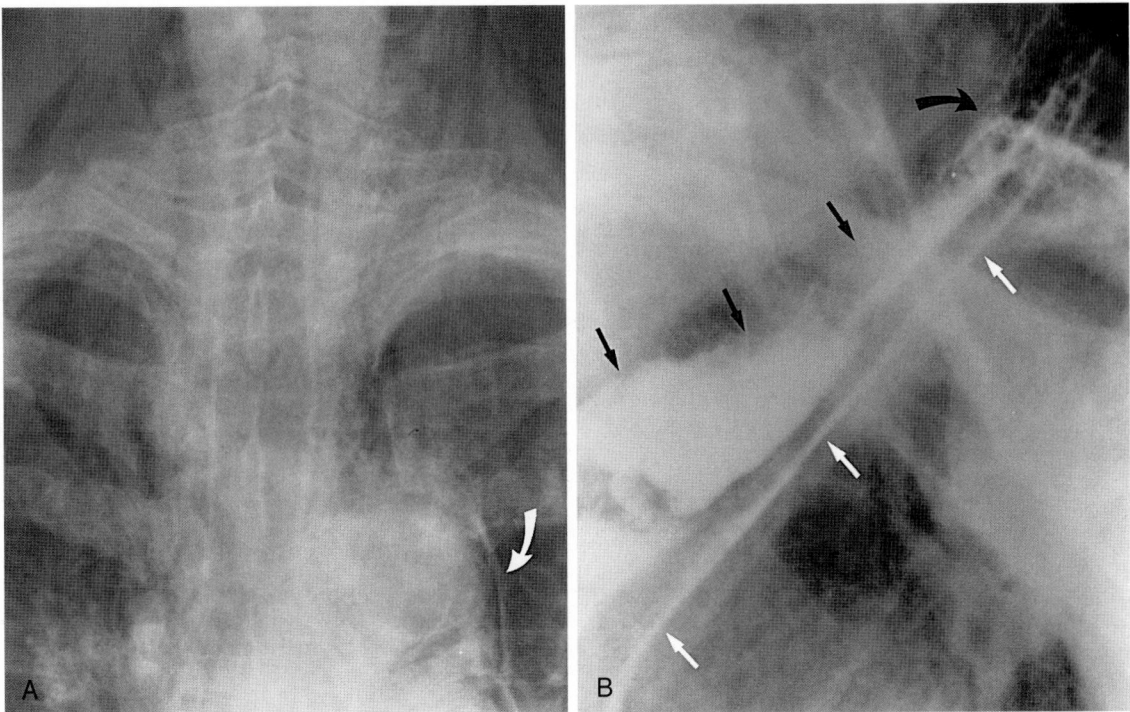

Figure 29-4. Cervical esophageal perforation by traumatic endoscopy. A. Close-up view from a posteroanterior chest radiograph obtained several hours after the procedure shows extensive subcutaneous emphysema in the neck and associated pneumomediastinum (*arrow*). **B.** Study using water-soluble contrast medium in a steep oblique projection reveals a cervical esophageal perforation (*curved black arrow*) with contrast medium extending inferiorly in the mediastinum (*straight black arrows*) behind the esophagus (*white arrows*). (From Levine MS: Radiology of the Esophagus. Philadelphia, WB Saunders, 1989.)

Contrast Studies

Fluoroscopic esophagography is the study of choice for suspected esophageal perforation. The ideal contrast agent for this examination provides diagnostic information about the site and extent of perforation without posing a risk to the patient. It has been shown experimentally that barium is capable of inciting an inflammatory reaction in the mediastinum with subsequent granuloma formation and fibrosis, whereas water-soluble contrast agents, such as diatrizoate meglumine and diatrizoate sodium (Gastroview), do not

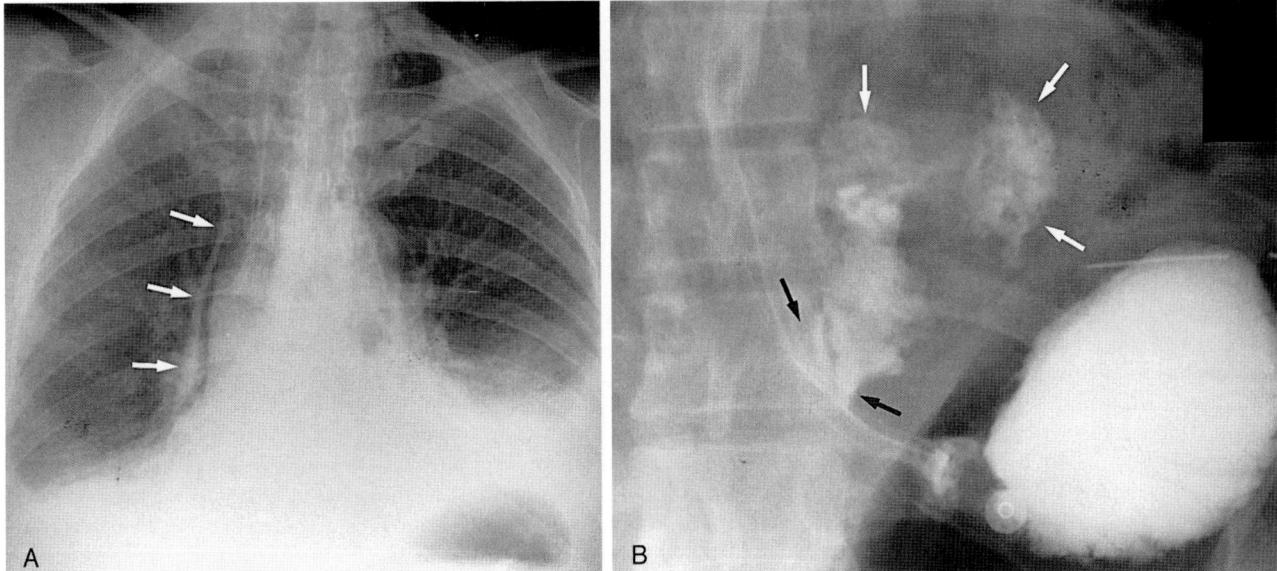

Figure 29-5. Spontaneous esophageal perforation or Boerhaave's syndrome. A. Posteroanterior chest radiograph shows a right-sided pneumomediastinum (*arrows*) and a left pleural effusion. These findings are highly suggestive of spontaneous esophageal perforation in a patient (particularly an alcoholic) with severe retching or vomiting. **B.** Subsequent study using water-soluble contrast medium confirms the presence of a localized perforation of the left lateral wall of the distal esophagus (*black arrows*), with extension of the leak laterally and superiorly in the mediastinum (*white arrows*). (Courtesy of Seth N. Glick, MD, Philadelphia, PA.)

produce a significant histologic response and have no known deleterious effects on the neck, mediastinum, and pleural or peritoneal cavities.[48,49] These water-soluble contrast agents also are rapidly absorbed from the mediastinum, so that follow-up studies to assess healing are not compromised by residual contrast medium in the mediastinum. The initial radiologic examination should therefore be performed with water-soluble contrast media. On the other hand, water-soluble contrast media are extremely hypertonic contrast agents that may cause severe pulmonary edema if aspirated into the lungs.[50] Some authors therefore advocate the use of low-osmolality, water-soluble contrast agents, such as metrizamide (Amipaque) and iohexol (Omnipaque), to avoid this risk.[51] Others have advocated the use of barium as the initial contrast agent for patients with suspected esophageal perforation if there is major clinical concern about aspiration.[52]

Water-soluble contrast agents have another disadvantage because they are less radiopaque than barium and less adherent to sites of leakage, limiting their ability to depict perforations, particularly if the perforations are subtle.[53] In various series, 50% of cervical esophageal perforations and 14% to 25% of thoracic esophageal perforations were missed on studies performed only with water-soluble contrast agents.[54-56] For this reason, when the initial study with water-soluble contrast medium fails to show a leak, the examination should immediately be repeated with barium to detect subtle leaks that are more likely to be visualized with a higher-density contrast agent (Fig. 29-6).[48,49,53,57-59] In such cases, the deleterious effects of barium in the mediastinum are more than offset by the earlier diagnosis and treatment of a potentially life-threatening condition.

In two studies, 38% and 22% of leaks missed on esophagograms with water-soluble contrast agents were visualized on esophagograms with 60% and 100% w/v barium suspensions, presumably because of the greater density of these bariums and greater adherence to sites of extraluminal leakage.[60,61] In another study, a 250% w/v barium suspension (i.e., the high-density barium used for double-contrast upper gastrointestinal examinations) detected 50% of pharyngeal or esophageal perforations that were not visualized with a water-soluble contrast agent.[62] Leaks detected only with high-density barium were more likely to be characterized by small, blind-ending tracks or tiny extraluminal collections than those visualized with a water-soluble contrast agent. Nevertheless, patient management was affected in the majority of cases.[62] High-density barium should therefore be used to optimize detection of esophageal perforation on radiographic studies when no leaks are detected with a water-soluble contrast agent.

Esophageal perforations are recognized on esophagography by extravasation of contrast medium from the esophagus into the neck or mediastinum. In patients with spontaneous perforation (Boerhaave's syndrome), contrast medium is usually seen extravasating from the left lateral wall of the distal esophagus into the adjacent mediastinum (Fig. 29-5B).[53] Rarely, spontaneous perforation of the upper thoracic or even the cervical esophagus may also be demonstrated (Fig. 29-7).[38] Regardless of the site of perforation, a sealed-off leak may be manifested by a self-contained extraluminal collection that communicates with the adjacent lumen (see Figs. 29-6B and 29-7A). In contrast, larger perforations may result in free extravasation of contrast medium into the mediastinum, with

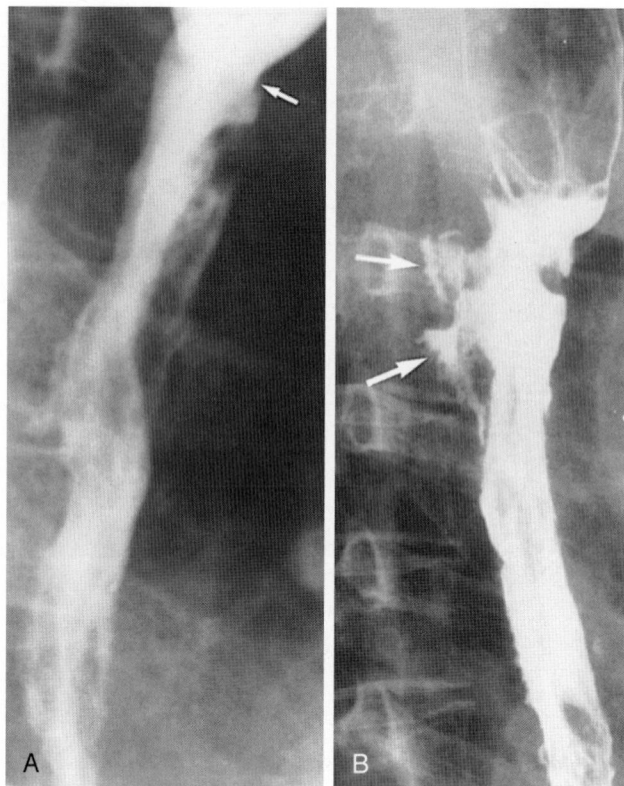

Figure 29-6. The importance of using barium for the diagnosis of subtle perforations. A. Initial study using water-soluble contrast medium after an esophagogastrectomy shows an irregular contour below the esophagogastric anastomosis (*arrow*), but no definite site of perforation is seen. **B.** Repeat examination performed moments later with barium sulfate shows a sealed-off anastomotic perforation (*arrows*) that was not visible with the water-soluble contrast medium. This case dramatically illustrates how barium should be given to all patients with suspected perforation if the initial study using water-soluble contrast medium fails to demonstrate a leak.

extension along fascial planes superiorly or inferiorly from the site of perforation (see Figs. 29-4B and 29-5B).

Computed Tomography

Computed tomography may also be performed on patients in whom esophageal perforation is suspected on clinical grounds. In such cases, the finding of extraluminal gas in the mediastinum should be highly suggestive of esophageal perforation.[63,64] Mediastinal, pleural, and pericardial fluid collections are other, less specific findings.[64] When a perforation is present, CT also is useful for determining the extent of extraluminal gas and fluid in the mediastinum and for monitoring patients who are treated nonoperatively.[64] A limitation of CT, however, is its frequent inability to locate the exact site of perforation. Helical CT esophagography with dilute low-osmolar contrast medium has been advocated as a better technique than conventional CT for showing the site of perforation in these patients.[65]

FOREIGN BODY IMPACTION

Nearly 80% of all pharyngeal or esophageal foreign body impactions occur in children who accidentally or intentionally

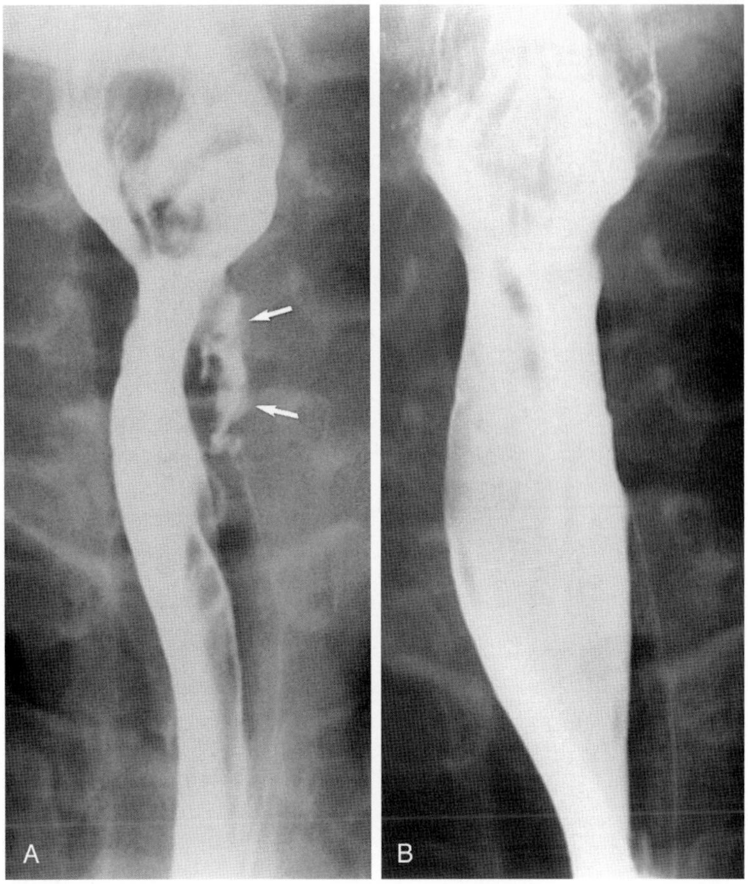

Figure 29-7. Spontaneous perforation of the cervical esophagus after an alcoholic binge. A. There is a small, sealed-off perforation (*arrows*) of the lower cervical esophagus. **B.** Follow-up esophagogram 6 weeks later shows complete healing of the perforation without evidence of a residual leak. (**A** and **B** from Isserow JA, Levine MS, Rubesin SE: Spontaneous perforation of the cervical esophagus after an alcoholic binge: Case report. Can Assoc Radiol J 49:241-243, 1998.)

ingest coins, toys, or other foreign objects.[66] Foreign body impactions in adults are usually caused by animal or fish bones or unchewed boluses of meat.[66,67] Bones tend to lodge in the pharynx near the level of the cricopharyngeus, whereas meat usually lodges in the distal esophagus near the gastroesophageal junction.[68] In contrast to impactions resulting from sharp foreign bodies, meat impactions are often caused by underlying esophageal rings or strictures. Although 80% to 90% of foreign bodies in the esophagus pass spontaneously, the remaining 10% to 20% require some form of therapeutic intervention.[66,69]

Clinical Findings

Animal or fish bones tend to lodge in the pharynx, often near the level of the cricopharyngeus.[68] The patient may complain of pharyngeal dysphagia or of a sensation of a foreign body in the throat. In contrast, meat bolus impactions tend to occur in the distal esophagus and are manifested by the sudden onset of substernal chest pain, odynophagia, or dysphagia.[68] Some patients with distal foreign body impactions may have dysphagia that is referred to the pharynx, however, so that the subjective site of obstruction is unreliable in determining the level of impaction.

Esophageal perforation occurs in less than 1% of all patients with foreign body impactions.[67] However, the risk of perforation increases substantially if the impaction persists more than 24 hours.[67,70] Perforation results from transmural esophageal inflammation and subsequent pressure necrosis at the

site of impaction. The development of mediastinitis may lead to sudden, rapid clinical deterioration, manifested by chest pain, sepsis, and shock.[70] Rarely, an impacted foreign body can erode through the wall of the esophagus, producing an aortoesophageal, esophagobronchial, or esophagopericardial fistula (see later section on Fistulas).

Radiographic Findings

Plain Radiographs

Anteroposterior and lateral radiographs of the neck and chest may occasionally demonstrate bones or other radiopaque foreign bodies in the pharynx or esophagus. Lateral radiographs of the neck are usually more helpful than anteroposterior radiographs in identifying animal or fish bones lodged in the pharynx or cervical esophagus (Fig. 29-8) because these bones are easily obscured by the overlying cervical spine on anteroposterior radiographs. Nevertheless, considerable difficulty may be encountered in differentiating small bone fragments from calcified thyroid or cricoid cartilage.

Contrast Studies

When a foreign body impaction in the pharynx or esophagus is suspected, an early barium swallow may be performed to determine whether a foreign body is present and whether it is causing obstruction. If the barium study confirms the presence of a foreign body in the esophagus, the radiologist may

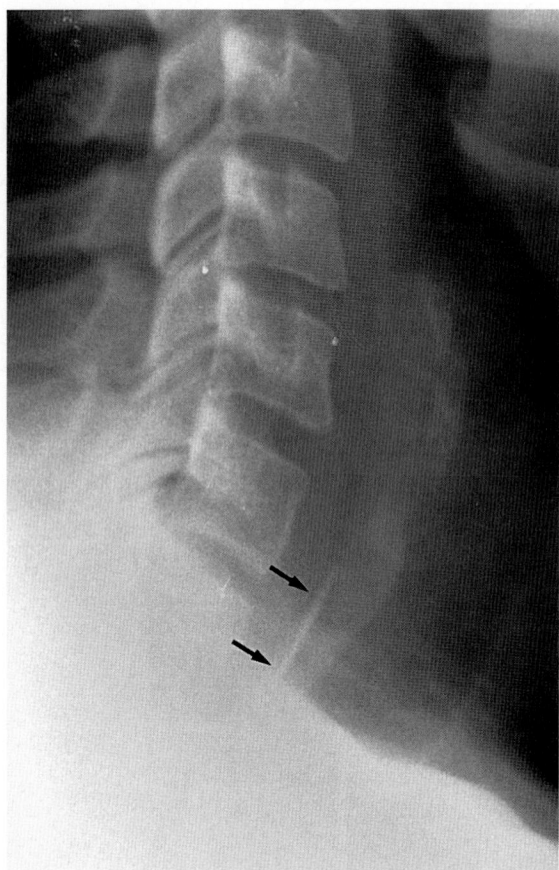

Figure 29-8. Swallowed pork bone in the neck near the pharyngoesophageal junction. Note the faintly calcified density (*arrows*) in the region of the cricopharyngeus on a lateral view of the neck. (From Levine MS: Radiology of the Esophagus. Philadelphia, WB Saunders, 1989.)

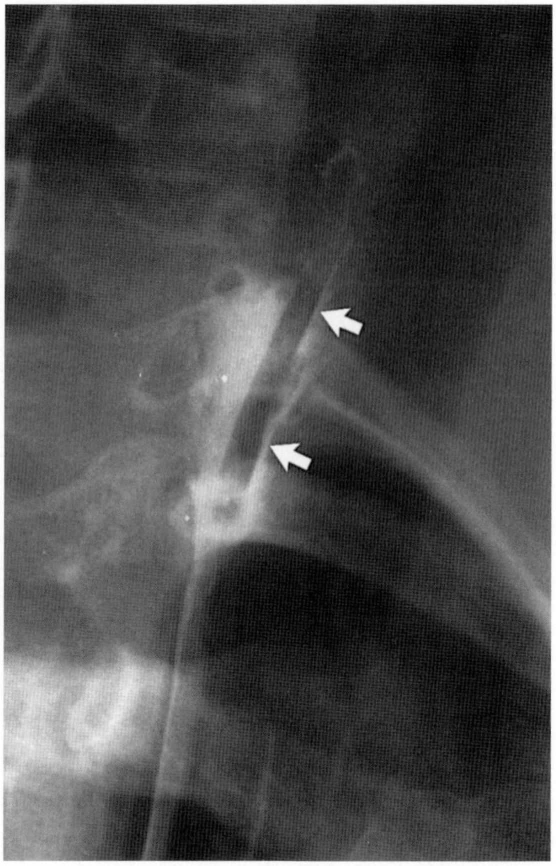

Figure 29-9. Turkey bone in the cervical esophagus. Barium swallow reveals a linear filling defect (*arrows*) resulting from a bone lodged in the cervical esophagus just below the cricopharyngeus. (From Levine MS: Radiology of the Esophagus. Philadelphia, WB Saunders, 1989.)

attempt to relieve the impaction by performing various therapeutic maneuvers under fluoroscopic guidance (see section on Treatment).

Animal or fish bones in the pharynx or cervical esophagus are easily obscured by barium, so that they may be difficult to detect on contrast examinations. These foreign bodies, however, can sometimes be recognized as linear filling defects in the vallecula, piriform sinus, or cricopharyngeal region (Fig. 29-9). In some cases, cotton balls or marshmallows soaked in barium may also be helpful for demonstrating small foreign bodies in the pharynx or esophagus.

Foreign body impactions in the thoracic esophagus usually result from a large bolus of unchewed meat that lodges above the gastroesophageal junction or above a pathologic area of narrowing, most commonly a Schatzki ring or peptic stricture.[66-68] When an impacted meat bolus causes esophageal obstruction, barium studies typically reveal a polypoid filling defect in the esophagus, with an irregular meniscus resulting from barium outlining the superior border of the impacted bolus (Figs. 29-10A and 29-11A). Although the radiographic appearance could be mistaken for a polypoid carcinoma obstructing the esophagus, the correct diagnosis is almost always apparent from the clinical history. In some cases, a small amount of barium may trickle around the impacted meat bolus into the distal esophagus, erroneously suggesting a stricture (see Fig. 29-11A). Thus, it may be ex-

tremely difficult to ascertain whether the underlying esophagus is normal or abnormal at the time of impaction because the impacted bolus prevents adequate visualization of the esophagus below this level.

When it occurs, esophageal perforation almost always develops more than 24 hours after the onset of impaction.[67] Rarely, however, perforation may occur within 6 hours.[71] When a perforation is present, esophagography may demonstrate not only the site of impaction but also extravasation of contrast medium into the mediastinum (Fig. 29-12). This extravasation raises concern about the appropriate choice of contrast agents because patients with food impactions also are at high risk for aspiration. When the disadvantages of barium in the mediastinum are weighed against the disadvantages of water-soluble contrast medium in the airway, it may be prudent to use barium as the initial contrast agent, giving the patient only a few small sips of barium to exclude a perforation before continuing the examination.[71] Alternately, patients with suspected food impaction could be given low-osmolality, water-soluble contrast agents such as iohexol to avoid the risk of pulmonary edema if aspiration occurs.[51]

After the food impaction has been relieved, a follow-up esophagogram should be performed to rule out a Schatzki ring or peptic stricture as the cause of the impaction (Fig. 29-10B).[66-68] Rarely, food impactions may be caused by malignant strictures or even by giant thoracic osteophytes

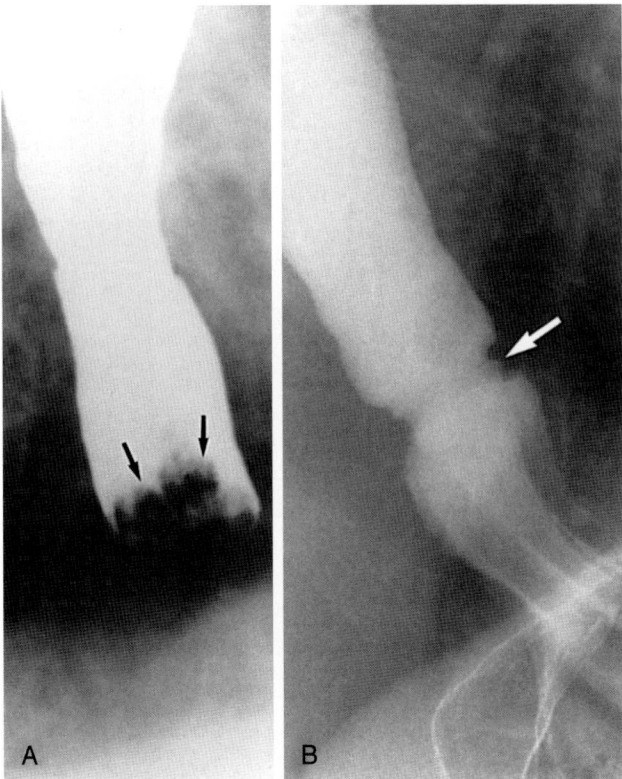

Figure 29-10. Distal foreign body obstruction due to an underlying Schatzki ring. A. Initial esophagram shows barium outlining the superior border of an impacted bolus of meat (*arrows*) in the distal esophagus, with complete obstruction at this level. **B.** Second esophagogram after endoscopic removal of the foreign body shows an underlying Schatzki ring (*arrow*) as the cause of this impaction.

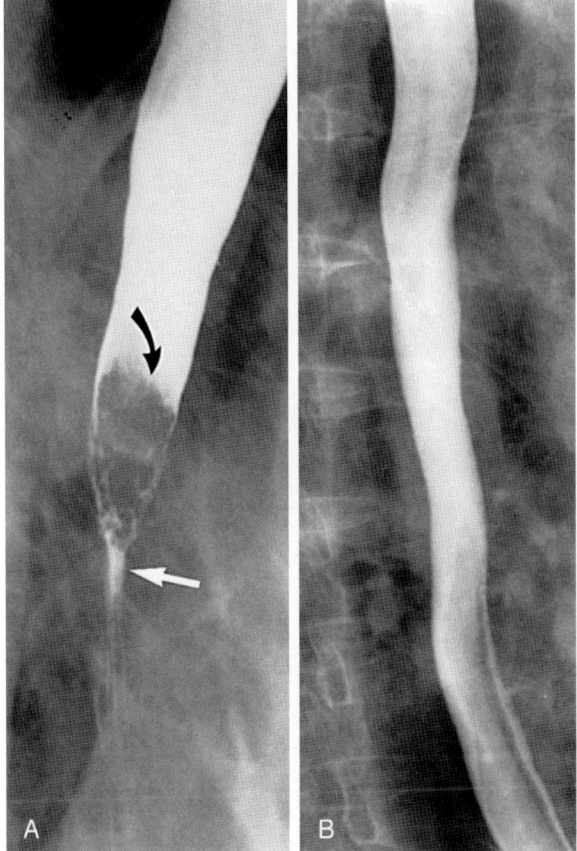

Figure 29-11. Foreign body obstruction in a normal esophagus. A. An impacted meat bolus in the midesophagus appears as a polypoid filling defect (*black arrow*). The incompletely distended esophagus below the impaction (*white arrow*) could be mistaken for a pathologic area of narrowing. **B.** Repeat esophagogram after removal of the foreign body shows a normal underlying esophagus. (From Levine MS: Radiology of the Esophagus. Philadelphia, WB Saunders, 1989.)

or other structures impinging on the esophagus.[66,72] In other patients, follow-up esophagography may reveal a normal underlying esophagus (Fig. 29-11B).

Treatment

When swallowed foreign bodies fail to pass spontaneously, some form of therapeutic intervention is required for their removal. Impacted foreign bodies in the pharynx or esophagus may be removed by endoscopy or by the use of a wire basket or a Foley catheter balloon under fluoroscopic guidance.[66-69,73-75] These techniques appear to be safe and effective for extracting blunt foreign bodies from the esophagus.

Radiologists may also attempt to relieve esophageal food impactions by various noninvasive maneuvers. A single dose of 1 mg of intravenous glucagon may facilitate passage of impacted food in the distal esophagus by relaxing the lower esophageal sphincter.[76,77] Glucagon is unlikely to be effective, however, if the impaction is located in the upper or middle third of the esophagus because glucagon does not affect motor activity in the body of the esophagus.[78] Administration of gas-forming agents (e.g., E-Z-Gas, E-Z-EM Company, Westbury, NY) has also been advocated to distend the esophagus above an obstructing food bolus and facilitate passage of the bolus into the stomach.[79] Combination therapy with glucagon, an effervescent agent, and water appears to be a particularly effective technique for relieving esophageal food impactions, with a success rate of 70%.[80-82] Rarely, however, abrupt dis-

tention of the obstructed esophagus by a gas-forming agent may cause esophageal perforation,[80] particularly if the obstructing bolus has been present long enough to produce ischemia or pressure necrosis at the site of impaction. For this reason, gas-forming agents should probably not be used if the obstruction has been present longer than 24 hours.

FISTULAS

Esophageal-Airway Fistula

Most esophageal-airway fistulas result from direct invasion of the tracheobronchial tree by advanced esophageal carcinomas. Tracheoesophageal or esophagobronchial fistulas (usually involving the left main bronchus) have been reported in 5% to 10% of patients with esophageal cancer.[83,84] The fistulas tend to occur after radiation therapy, presumably because radiation-induced tumor necrosis accelerates fistula formation. Other esophageal-airway fistulas may be caused by esophageal instrumentation, endobronchial stents that erode into the esophagus, foreign bodies, blunt or penetrating injuries to the chest, or, rarely, perforation of an esophageal diverticulum.[32,85] Esophagobronchial fistulas may also be caused by tuberculosis, histoplasmosis, or other granulomatous diseases

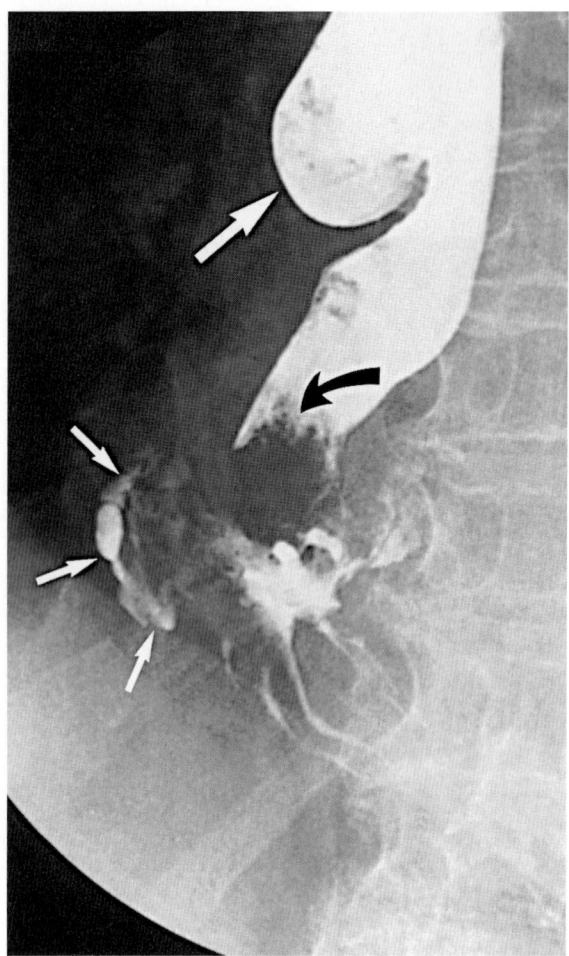

Figure 29-12. Foreign body obstruction with associated perforation. A polypoid defect (*black arrow*) is present in the distal esophagus as a result of an esophageal food impaction. In addition, there is extravasation of contrast medium into a focal collection (*small white arrows*) in the mediastinum, indicating perforation. Also note the large diverticulum (*large white arrow*) in the midesophagus. This perforation occurred within 6 hours of the onset of impaction. (From Gougoutas C, Levine MS, Laufer I: Esophageal food impaction with early perforation, AJR 171:427-428, 1998, © by American Roentgen Ray Society.)

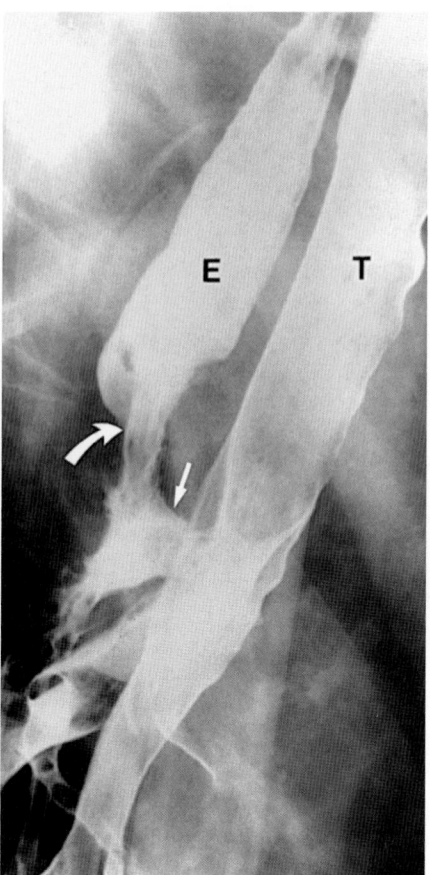

Figure 29-13. Esophagobronchial fistula. This fistula (*straight arrow*) was caused by an advanced, infiltrating esophageal carcinoma (*curved arrow*). E, esophagus; T, trachea. (From Levine MS: Radiology of the Esophagus. Philadelphia, WB Saunders, 1989.)

in which necrotic, caseating mediastinal lymph nodes erode into the esophagus and tracheobronchial tree.[86] Rarely, esophagobronchial fistulas may be congenital.[87]

Patients with esophageal-airway fistulas often present with paroxysmal coughing after ingestion of liquids. Some patients may have recurrent pneumonitis, hemoptysis, or a productive cough with particles of food in the sputum. These fistulas may be difficult to differentiate on clinical grounds from recurrent tracheobronchial aspiration.

When an esophageal-airway fistula is suspected, the radiologic examination should be performed with barium rather than water-soluble contrast agents because the latter agents are hypotonic and may draw fluid into the lungs, causing severe, potentially fatal pulmonary edema.[50] Most of these fistulas are readily demonstrated on barium studies and are found to arise within an advanced, infiltrating esophageal carcinomas (Fig. 29-13). Once barium has entered the trachea or bronchi, however, it can be coughed up into the proximal trachea or larynx, so that delayed overhead radiographs may erroneously suggest tracheobronchial aspiration. The initial

swallow should therefore be performed in a lateral projection (with a videorecording of the hypopharynx) to differentiate a fistula from aspiration.

Esophagopleural Fistula

Esophagopleural fistulas are usually caused by previous surgery, esophageal instrumentation, radiation, or advanced esophageal carcinoma directly invading the pleural space.[88] In contrast to patients with esophageal-airway fistulas, these individuals may have nonspecific clinical findings such as chest pain, fever, dysphagia, dyspnea, or foul-smelling regurgitations.[88,89] When an esophagopleural fistula is suspected, the diagnosis can be confirmed by recovery of ingested methylene blue in fluid aspirated during thoracentesis. Nonoperative management of esophagopleural fistulas is associated with mortality rates approaching 100%, where surgical repair is associated with mortality rates of about 50%.[90] Early diagnosis and surgical repair of these fistulas is therefore essential.

Chest radiographs may reveal a pleural effusion, pneumothorax, or hydropneumothorax on the side of the fistula (Fig. 29-14A).[88] Pneumomediastinum or mediastinal widening is usually not present on chest radiographs because the mediastinum tends not to be directly involved by the fistula. When an esophagopleural fistula is suspected because of the clinical or plain film findings, a study using water-soluble

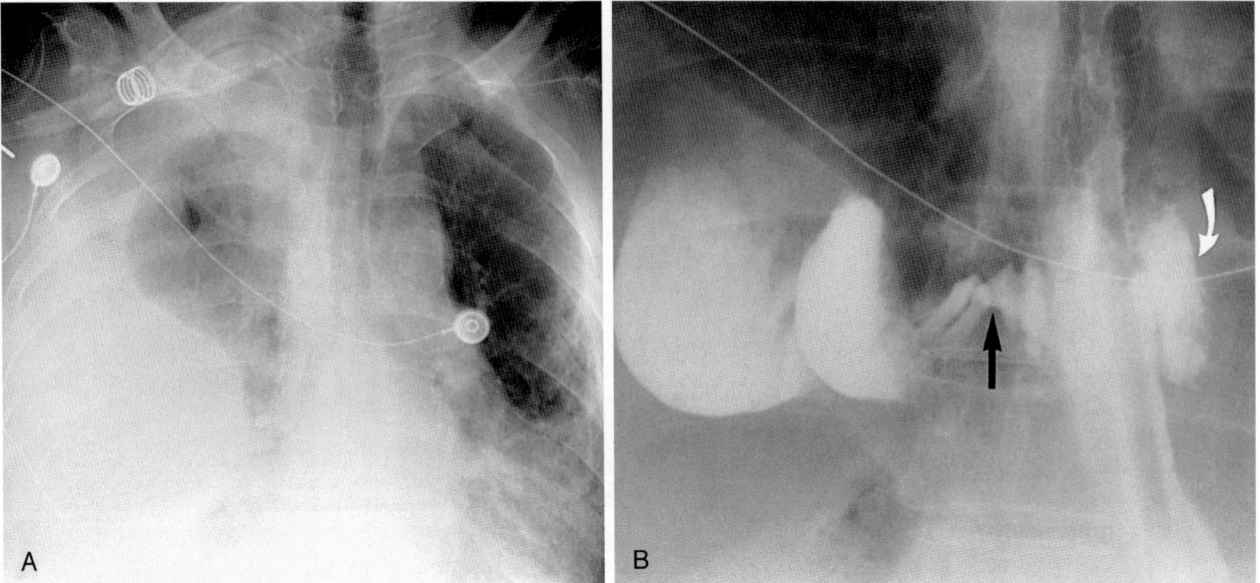

Figure 29-14. Esophagopleural fistula caused by endoscopic sclerotherapy of esophageal varices. A. Posteroanterior chest radiograph shows a large right pleural effusion. **B.** Study using water-soluble contrast medium reveals an esophagopleural fistula (*black arrow*) with contrast medium extending laterally in the right pleural space. There also is extravasated contrast medium in the mediastinum (*white arrow*). (From Levine MS: Radiology of the Esophagus. Philadelphia, WB Saunders, 1989.)

contrast medium should be performed to confirm the presence of a fistula and to determine its precise location (Fig. 29-14B). CT may also be helpful for demonstrating small collections of contrast medium, gas, or fluid in the pleural space.[91]

Occasionally, surgical disruption of the muscularis propria during a myotomy for achalasia, resection of a leiomyoma, or dissection of malignant tumor adherent to the esophagus may cause eccentric ballooning and thinning of the esophageal wall, resulting in the development of an esophagopleural fistula.[92] In such cases, CT or esophagography with water-soluble contrast agents may reveal an esophagopleural fistula at the site of esophageal ballooning or thinning (Fig 29-15).[92]

Aortoesophageal Fistula

Aortoesophageal fistulas are rare but highly lethal fistulas usually caused by intraesophageal rupture of an atherosclerotic, syphilitic, or dissecting aneurysm of the descending thoracic aorta.[93-95] Aortoesophageal fistulas may also be caused by a swallowed foreign body, esophageal carcinoma, an infected aortic graft, or erosion of an endovascular stent into the esophagus.[95,96]

Affected patients may initially present with several small "sentinel" episodes of arterial hematemesis, followed by a symptom-free latent period of hours to weeks and a sudden, final episode of massive hematemesis, exsanguination, and death.[93-95] This latent period has been attributed to blood clot occluding the fistula, hypotension, and vasoconstriction in response to severe hypovolemia.[93] As a result, early diagnosis of an impending aortoesophageal fistula provides the opportunity for definitive, potentially lifesaving surgery with placement of an aortic graft.

Aortoesophageal fistulas should be suspected in patients with arterial hematemesis who have a large atherosclerotic aneurysm of the descending thoracic aorta on chest radio-

graphs.[95] In such cases, studies using water-soluble contrast agents may reveal extrinsic compression or displacement of the esophagus by the aneurysm but rarely show leakage of contrast medium into the aorta because of the flow dynamics of these structures (Fig. 29-16A).[93] When an infected aortic graft has eroded into the esophagus, extravasated contrast medium from the esophagus may occasionally outline the coiled springs of the graft (Fig. 29-16C).[93,96] The presence of an aortoesophageal fistula may be confirmed by demonstrating extravasation of contrast medium from the aorta into the esophagus by aortography. The origin of the fistulous track is often occluded by thrombus, however, so that aortography may also fail to delineate the actual fistula in these patients (Fig. 29-16B).[94]

Esophagopericardial Fistula

Esophagopericardial fistulas are rare fistulas caused by severe esophagitis, esophageal cancer, swallowed foreign bodies, or prior surgery.[97] These fistulas usually lead to the rapid development of severe pericarditis or cardiac tamponade resulting from leakage of esophageal contents into the pericardial space. Chest radiographs reveal pneumopericardium or hydropneumopericardium in 25% to 50% of cases.[97] The diagnosis may be confirmed by having the patient swallow a water-soluble contrast agent to demonstrate the fistulous track or gross filling of the pericardial sac with contrast medium (Fig. 29-17).

DIVERTICULA

Esophageal diverticula may be classified by their location or by their mechanism of formation. The most common locations include the pharyngoesophageal junction (i.e., Zenker's diverticulum) (see Chapter 20), the midesophagus, and the distal esophagus just above the gastroesophageal junction

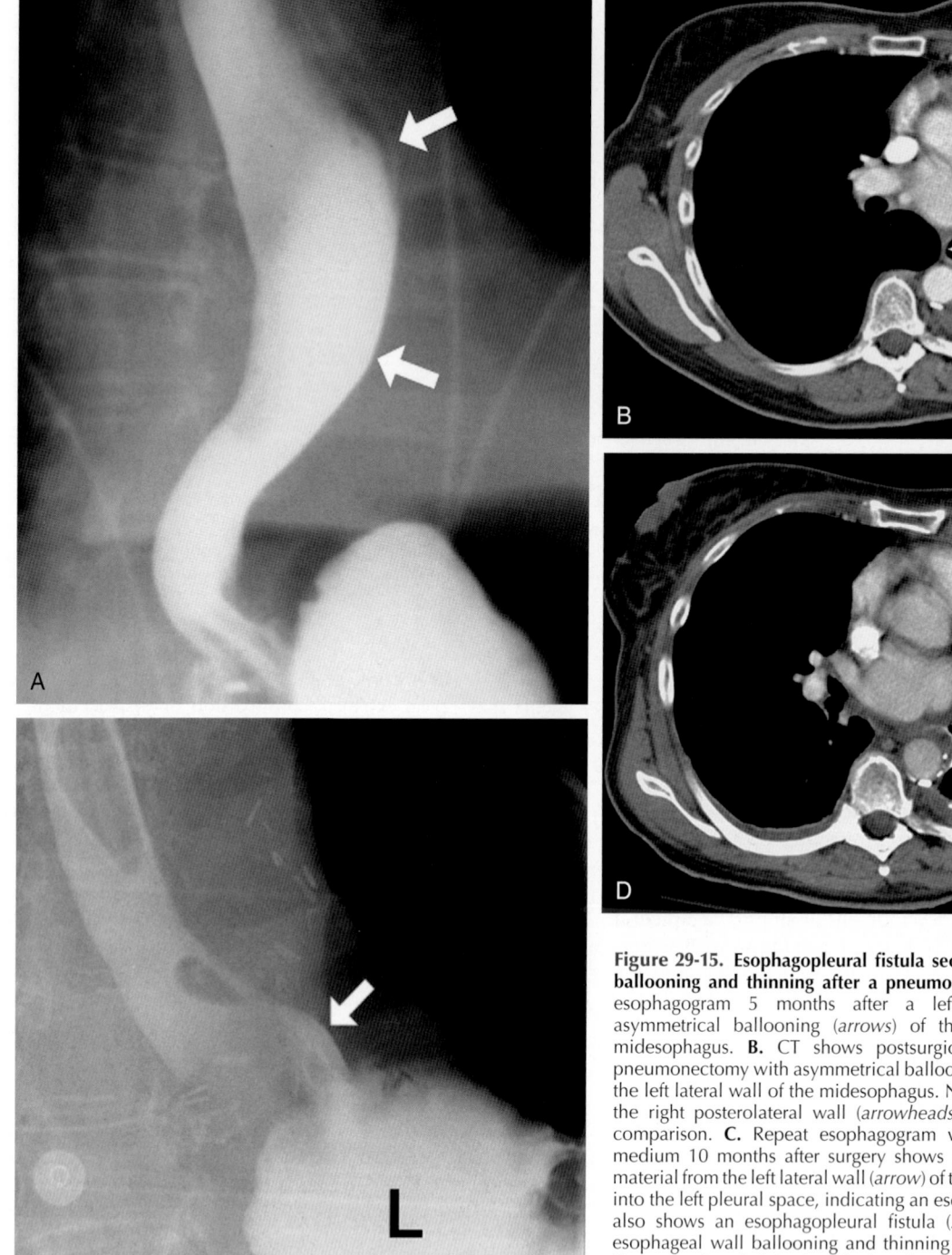

Figure 29-15. Esophagopleural fistula secondary to esophageal wall ballooning and thinning after a pneumonectomy. A. Single-contrast esophagogram 5 months after a left pneumonectomy shows asymmetrical ballooning (*arrows*) of the left lateral wall of the midesophagus. **B.** CT shows postsurgical changes from the left pneumonectomy with asymmetrical ballooning and thinning (*arrow*) of the left lateral wall of the midesophagus. Note the normal thickness of the right posterolateral wall (*arrowheads*) of the midesophagus for comparison. **C.** Repeat esophagogram with water-soluble contrast medium 10 months after surgery shows leakage (L) of oral contrast material from the left lateral wall (*arrow*) of the ballooned midesophagus into the left pleural space, indicating an esophagopleural fistula. **D.** CT also shows an esophagopleural fistula (*short arrow*) at the site of esophageal wall ballooning and thinning with oral contrast medium (*long arrow*) and air in the left pleural space. (From Liu PS, Levine MS, Torigian DA: Esophagopleural fistula secondary to esophageal wall ballooning and thinning after pneumonectomy: Findings on chest CT and esophagography. AJR 186:1627-1629, 2006. Reprinted with permission from the American Journal of Roentgenology.)

(i.e., epiphrenic diverticulum). Diverticula may be formed either by pulsion caused by increased intraluminal esophageal pressure associated with esophageal dysmotility (especially diffuse esophageal spasm) or by traction caused by fibrosis in adjacent periesophageal tissues. In the past, many midesopha-geal diverticula were thought to be traction diverticula caused by scarring from tuberculosis or histoplasmosis in perihilar or subcarinal lymph nodes. This type of diverticulum has decreased in frequency, however, so that most midesophageal diverticula are now thought to be of the pulsion variety.[98]

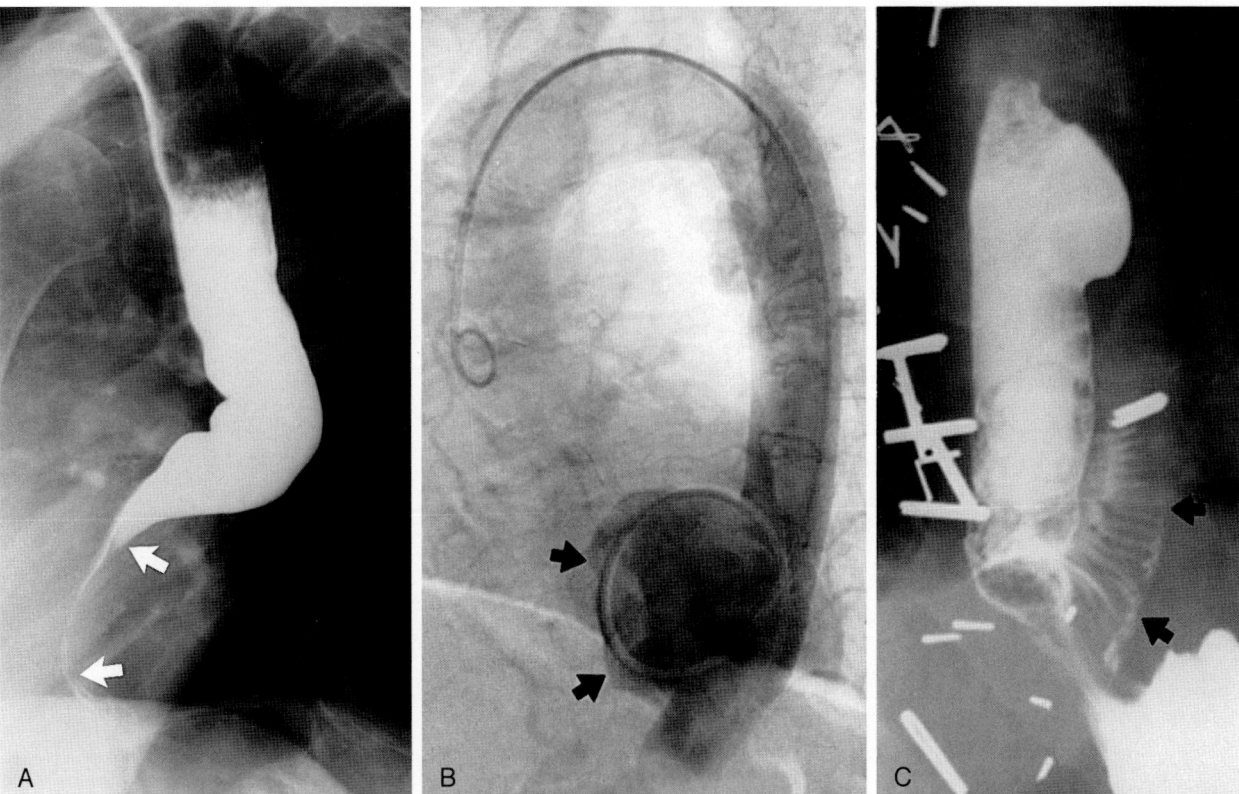

Figure 29-16. Aortoesophageal fistula caused by an aortic aneurysm. A. Initial esophagram shows anterior displacement and narrowing of the distal esophagus (*arrows*) by an aneurysm of the descending thoracic aorta. **B.** Subsequent aortogram reveals a saccular aneurysm with intraluminal thrombus (*arrows*) occluding the origin of the fistula. Although radiographic studies failed to demonstrate the fistula, an aortoesophageal fistula was found at surgery. **C.** Another esophagogram after placement of a Dacron aortic graft shows a recurrent aortoesophageal fistula with extravasated contrast medium from the esophagus outlining the aortic graft (*arrows*). This fistula was caused by infection of the graft. (From Baron RL, Koehler RE, Gutierrez FR, et al: Clinical and radiographic manifestations of aortoesophageal fistulas. Radiology 141:599-605, 1981.)

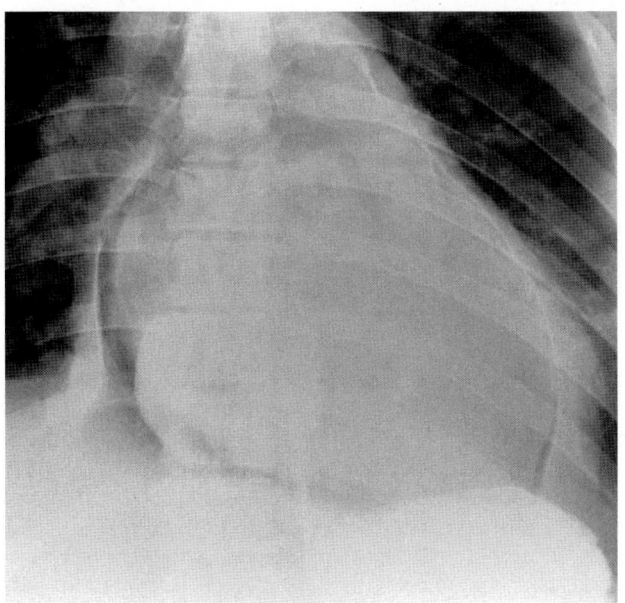

Figure 29-17. Esophagopericardial fistula caused by a perforated ulcer associated with severe reflux esophagitis. Posteroanterior chest radiograph after oral administration of water-soluble contrast medium reveals a pneumopericardium with free leakage of contrast medium into the pericardial space. Air and contrast medium outline the inner aspect of the pericardial sac. Also, contrast medium is seen faintly in a hiatal hernia. (From Cyrlak D, Cohen AJ, Dana ER: Esophagopericardial fistula: Causes and radiographic features. AJR 141:177-179, 1983, © by American Roentgen Ray Society.)

Pulsion and Traction Diverticula

Pulsion and traction diverticula are usually incidental findings in the esophagus without clinical significance. When symptoms are present in patients with one or more pulsion diverticula, they are typically related to the patient's underlying esophageal dysmotility,[99] but some diverticula that are extremely large may cause symptoms.

Radiographic Findings

Diverticula are readily detected on esophagograms as barium-filled outpouchings from the esophagus. They are best seen in profile, but they may be recognized en face as ring shadows on double-contrast studies. Once a diverticulum has been detected, it should be classified as either a pulsion diverticulum or a traction diverticulum. Pulsion diverticula are much more common, are usually located in the middle or distal thirds of the esophagus, and are often associated with other radiographic evidence of motor dysfunction. They usually have a rounded contour and a wide neck and are frequently multiple (Fig. 29-18). Because they contain no muscle in their wall, they tend to remain filled after the esophagus has emptied of barium (see Fig. 29-18B).

Traction diverticula are usually located in the midesophagus and have a tented or triangular configuration as a result of scarring and retraction from surgery, radiation, or granulomatous disease in the adjacent mediastinum (Fig. 29-19).

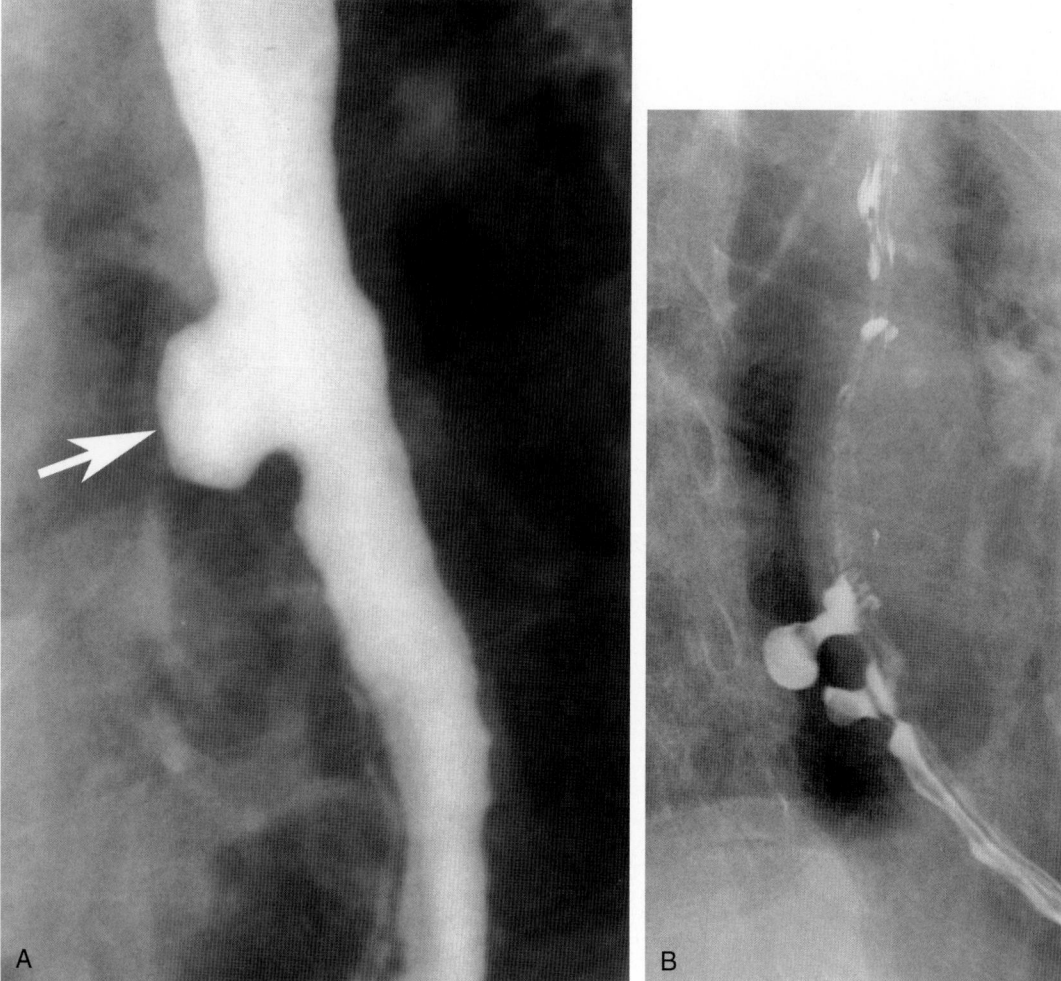

Figure 29-18. Pulsion diverticula. A. Note the smooth contour and wide neck of this pulsion diverticulum (*arrow*) in the midesophagus. There also is evidence of esophageal dysmotility with weak nonperistaltic contractions more distally. Pulsion diverticula are often associated with esophageal motor dysfunction, particularly diffuse esophageal spasm. **B.** In another patient, the pulsion diverticula remain filled after most of the barium has been emptied from the esophagus by peristalsis. Again note the rounded contour and wide necks of the diverticula. (**B** from Levine MS: Radiology of the Esophagus. Philadelphia, WB Saunders, 1989.)

Traction diverticula typically occur as solitary outpouchings containing all layers of the esophageal wall, including muscle, so that they tend to empty when the esophagus collapses. Thus, it is usually possible to distinguish pulsion and traction diverticula on radiologic grounds.

Epiphrenic Diverticulum

Epiphrenic diverticulum is an uncommon form of esophageal diverticulum that arises in the distal esophagus, usually within 10 cm from the gastroesophageal junction. It is generally believed to be a pulsion diverticulum caused by diffuse esophageal spasm with markedly increased intraluminal esophageal pressures.[99,100] In one study, however, diffuse esophageal spasm was found in less than 10% of patients with epiphrenic diverticula,[101] so other as yet undefined factors may also contribute to the development of these structures. Investigators have also found a significant correlation between the presence of symptoms and the size of the diverticulum (i.e., patients with epiphrenic diverticula greater than 5 cm in diameter are more likely to be symptomatic) and preferential filling on espha-

gography.[101] Thus, the development of symptoms appears to be related primarily to the morphologic features of the diverticulum rather than to underlying esophageal dysmotility in these patients.

When an epiphrenic diverticulum fills with food, it may compress the true lumen of the esophagus, causing dysphagia.[101,102] Food or fluid that accumulates within an epiphrenic diverticulum may also be regurgitated into the esophagus with subsequent reflux symptoms, chest pain, or aspiration.[101] Rarely, these diverticula may perforate into the mediastinum or form a fistula to the airway. When symptoms associated with an epiphrenic diverticulum are particularly severe or intractable, they may necessitate surgical intervention, most commonly a diverticulectomy and esophagomyotomy.[103,104]

Radiographic Findings

An epiphrenic diverticulum may occasionally be recognized on chest radiographs by the presence of a soft tissue mass (often containing an air-fluid level) that mimics a hiatal hernia (Fig. 29-20A and B). On barium studies, most patients have

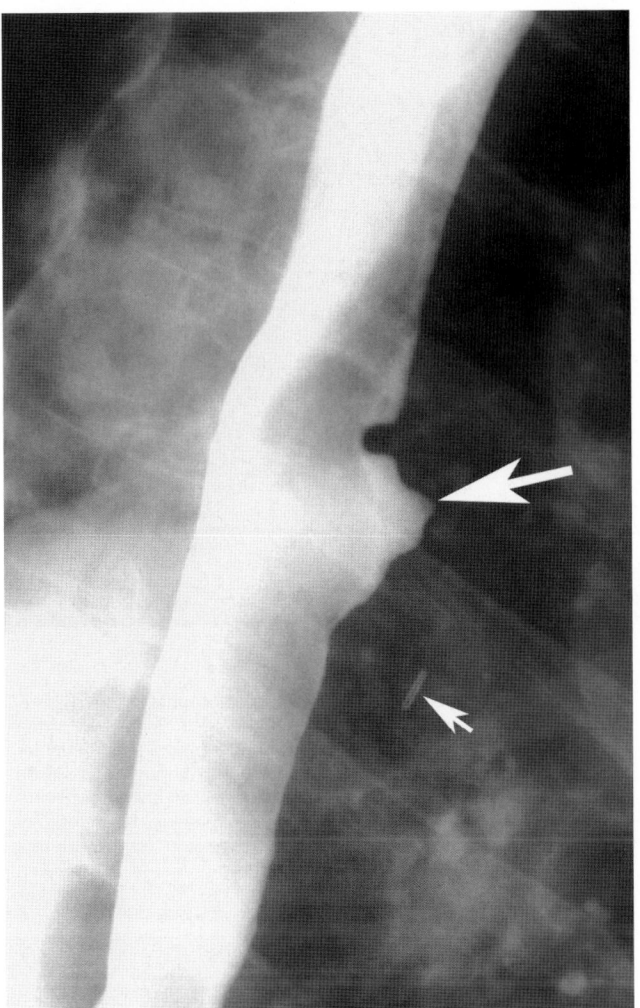

Figure 29-19. Traction diverticulum. The diverticulum has a pointed or triangular tip (*large arrow*) as a result of traction and volume loss in the adjacent mediastinum from prior surgery. A surgical clip (*small arrow*) is seen in the mediastinum. (From Levine MS: Radiology of the Esophagus. Philadelphia, WB Saunders, 1989.)

a solitary diverticulum arising from the right side of the distal esophagus (Fig. 29-20C), but the diverticula can occasionally be multiple or arise from the left side.[101] Epiphrenic diverticula vary markedly in size, ranging from 1 to 12 cm in largest diameter.[101] Barium studies may also reveal preferential filling or prolonged retention of barium within the diverticulum, regurgitation of barium or debris from the diverticulum, or compression of the adjacent esophagus.[101]

ECTOPIC GASTRIC MUCOSA

Ectopic gastric mucosa in the upper esophagus is a relatively common congenital anomaly, with a reported incidence of 4% to 10% at endoscopy.[105,106] In contrast to Barrett's mucosa, the ectopic gastric mucosa is thought to have no relationship to gastroesophageal reflux disease, and most patients with this finding are asymptomatic. Ectopic gastric mucosa is almost always located in the upper esophagus at or just above the thoracic inlet, hence the term *inlet patch*.[105]

Ectopic gastric mucosa in the esophagus can sometimes be recognized on double-contrast esophagography by a shallow depression with small indentations at its superior and inferior borders (Fig. 29-21).[107-109] These lesions are most commonly found on the right lateral wall of the upper thoracic esophagus at or near the thoracic inlet.[107-109] Although this depression could be mistaken on barium studies for ulceration or even an intramural dissection (see Fig. 29-21),[109] the appearance and location of ectopic gastric mucosa is so characteristic that endoscopy is probably not warranted in asymptomatic patients with this finding. Affected individuals may occasionally develop dysphagia because of associated webs or strictures in the upper esophagus.[110,111]

CONGENITAL ESOPHAGEAL STENOSIS

Congenital esophageal stenosis is a rare developmental anomaly caused by defective embryologic separation of the primitive foregut from the respiratory tract with sequestration of tracheobronchial precursor cells in the esophageal wall.[112,113]

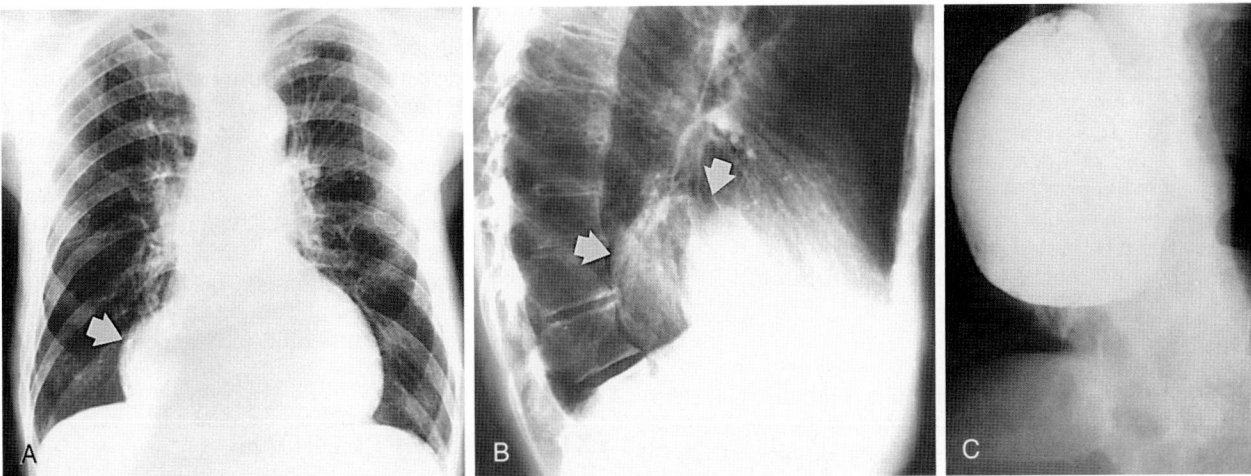

Figure 29-20. Large epiphrenic diverticulum. A. Posteroanterior chest radiograph shows a prominent bulge along the right border of the heart (*arrow*). **B.** Lateral chest radiograph shows a soft tissue mass (*arrows*) mimicking the appearance of a hiatal hernia. **C.** A barium study reveals a large epiphrenic diverticulum that remains filled with barium after the esophagus has emptied. (From Levine MS: Radiology of the Esophagus. Philadelphia, WB Saunders, 1989.)

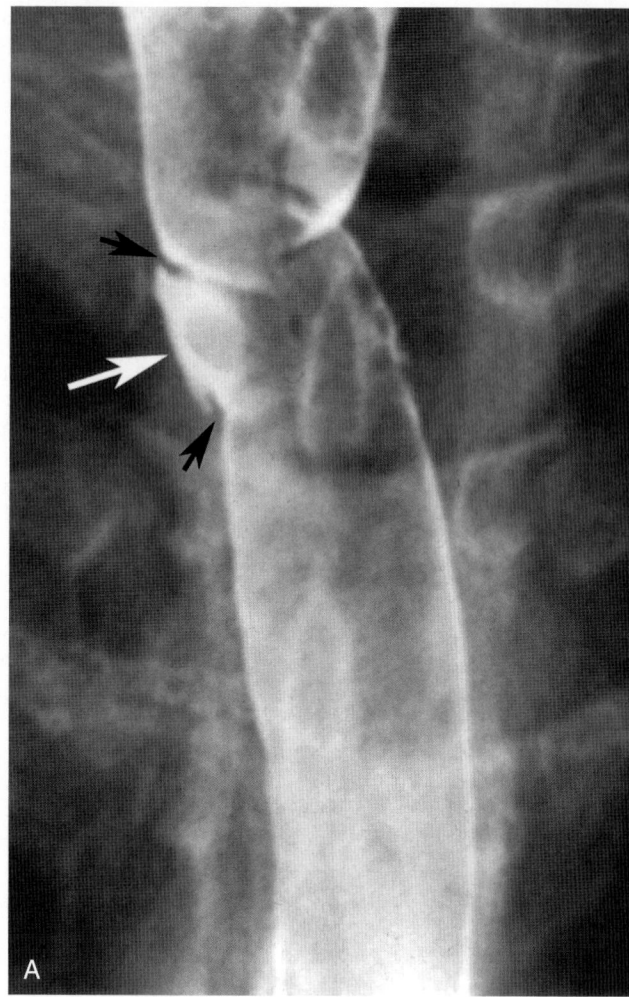

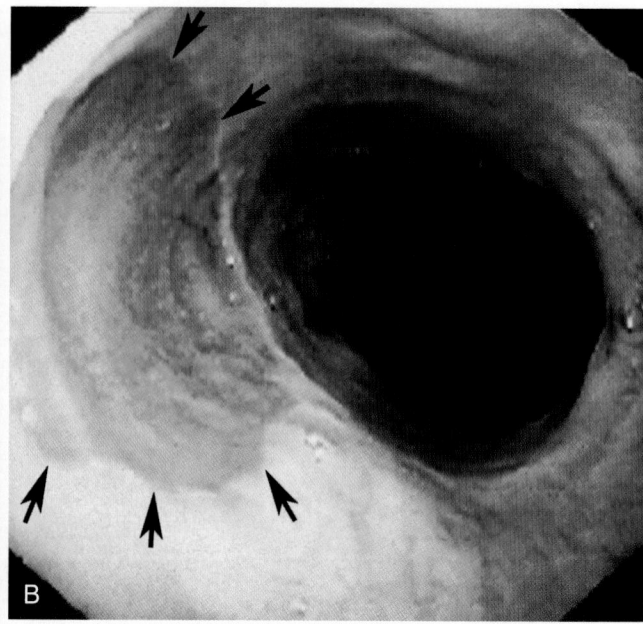

Figure 29-21. Ectopic gastric mucosa in the esophagus. A. There is a broad, flat depression (*white arrow*) on the right lateral wall of the upper esophagus near the thoracic inlet, with a pair of small indentations (*black arrows*) at both ends of the lesion. Although it could be mistaken for an ulcer, this lesion has the typical appearance and location of ectopic gastric mucosa in the esophagus. **B.** Endoscopy shows a reddish-brown epithelial-lined depression (*arrows*) in the upper esophagus characteristic of ectopic gastric mucosa. (From Lee J, Levine MS, Shultz CF: Ectopic gastric mucosa in the oesophagus mimicking ulceration. Eur J Radiol 31:97-200, 1997.)

Infants may have a severe form of congenital esophageal stenosis associated with esophageal atresia or tracheoesophageal fistulas,[114] but adults may have a mild form of the disease manifested by esophageal strictures.[115-117]

Clinical Findings

Patients with severe forms of congenital esophageal stenosis typically present during infancy with marked dysphagia and vomiting,[114,118] but patients with milder forms of stenosis may present during adolescence or early adulthood with a long-standing history of intermittent dysphagia, chest pain, and occasional food impactions.[115-117] For reasons that are unclear, almost all reported adults have been men.[115-117] Because symptoms are caused by underlying strictures, dysphagia is usually alleviated by endoscopic dilatation of the strictures.[114]

Radiographic Findings

Congenital esophageal stenosis in adults is usually characterized on esophagography by the presence of smooth, tapered strictures in the upper esophagus or midesophagus.[115,116,119,120] The strictures often contain multiple ringlike constrictions, producing a distinctive radiographic appearance on double-contrast esophagograms (Fig. 29-22).[120] The etiology of these ringlike constrictions is uncertain, but they may represent

cartilaginous rings similar to those found in the trachea.[120] Whatever the explanation, the presence of an esophageal stricture with distinctive ringlike constrictions should suggest congenital esophageal stenosis in the proper clinical setting.

Differential Diagnosis

Idiopathic eosinophilic esophagitis may also be manifested on esophagography by an esophageal stricture with distinctive ringlike indentations (see Fig. 25-13).[121] The correct diagnosis should be suggested, however, by the presence of an atopic history or peripheral eosinophilia. Ringlike indentations have also been described on double-contrast esophagograms in patients with fixed transverse folds, but these folds usually occur in the distal esophagus in patients with peptic strictures.[122] Fine transverse striations may also been seen in patients with a "feline" esophagus, but these transverse striations occur as a transient finding and are not associated with strictures.[123]

EXTRINSIC IMPRESSIONS

Normal Impressions

A variety of normal structures in the mediastinum, including the heart, aortic arch, and left main bronchus, may cause

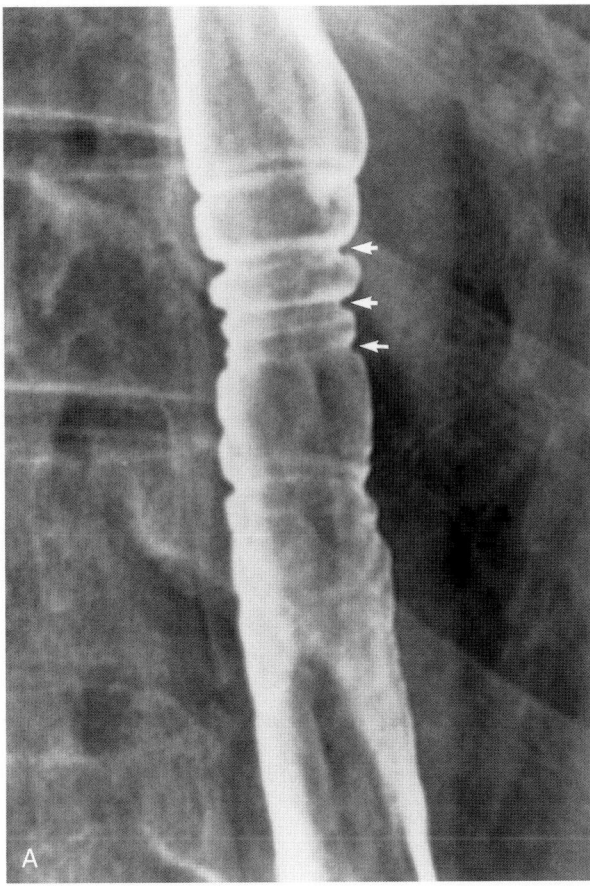

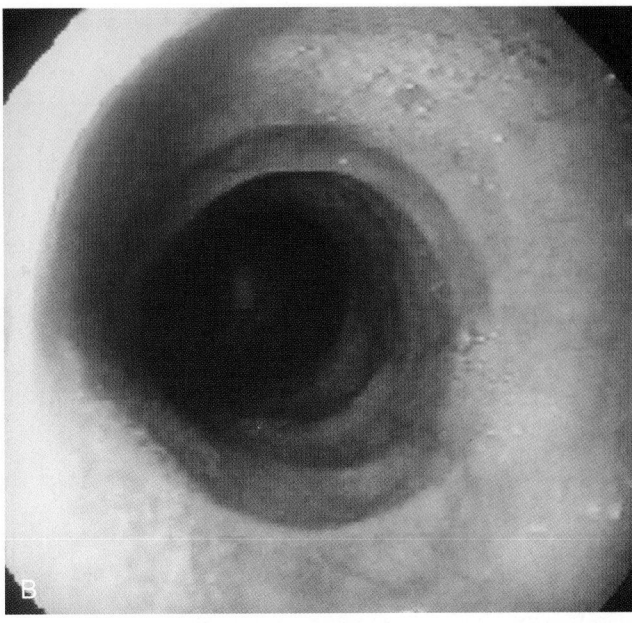

Figure 29-22. Congenital esophageal stenosis. A. There is a mild area of narrowing in the midesophagus with distinctive ringlike indentations (*arrows*) in the region of the stricture. **B.** Endoscopy also shows ringlike indentations that resemble tracheal rings. (**A** from Luedtke P, Levine MS, Rubesin SE, et al: Radiologic diagnosis of benign esophageal strictures: A pattern approach. RadioGraphics 23:897-909, 2003.)

extrinsic impressions on the esophagus (see Chapter 21). In about 10% of patients, a smooth, gently sloping indentation may also be seen on the right posterolateral wall of the upper thoracic esophagus between the thoracic inlet and the aortic arch (Fig. 29-23A).[124] Correlation with CT has shown that this impression is caused by an unusually prominent right inferior supra-azygous recess of the lung indenting the upper esophagus (Fig. 29-23B).[124] It is important to be aware of this finding, so that it is not mistaken for adenopathy or other masses in the mediastinum and unnecessary cross-sectional imaging of the chest can be avoided. A narrowed thoracic inlet (in the sagittal dimension) is another well-recognized anatomic variant that can result in extrinsic compression of the right side of the barium-filled esophagus, erroneously suggesting a mass lesion in this region.[125] In such patients, however, CT will reveal a narrowed thoracic inlet without evidence of a mass.[125]

Abnormal Impressions

Abnormal impressions are most commonly caused by the heart and great vessels. An enlarged left atrium or ventricle may produce a broad impression on the anterior wall of the distal esophagus. In contrast, a tortuous or ectatic descending thoracic aorta may cause a prominent impression on the posterior wall of the distal esophagus near the esophageal hiatus of the diaphragm (Fig. 29-24). In some patients, compression of the distal esophagus by the aorta may cause dysphagia (i.e., dysphagia aortica).[126] Similarly, congenital abnormalities of the great vessels, such as an aberrant sub-

clavian artery and double aortic arch, may compress the esophagus, causing dysphagia (i.e., dysphagia lusoria), as discussed in Chapter 117. The esophagus may also be compressed or displaced by masses in the mediastinum, including substernal thyroid goiters, mediastinal lymphadenopathy, and other benign or malignant neoplasms. In such cases, it is important to differentiate compression or displacement of the esophagus from actual invasion by an adjacent mediastinal mass (see Chapter 28).

Esophageal Retraction

Esophageal deviation may be caused by pulmonary, pleural, or mediastinal scarring, with retraction of the esophagus toward the diseased hemithorax (Fig. 29-25). It is usually possible to differentiate this retraction from esophageal displacement by a mediastinal mass, by using the radiologic sign illustrated in Figure 29-26.[127] When the esophagus is displaced or pushed by an extrinsic mass in the mediastinum, it tends to be narrower at this level than above or below the deviated segment (see Figs. 29-24 and 29-26A), whereas the esophagus tends to be wider at this level when it is retracted or pulled by pleuropulmonary scarring (see Figs. 29-25 and 29-26B).[127] When esophageal retraction is suggested by barium studies, chest radiographs should confirm the presence of tuberculosis, radiation damage, postsurgical changes, or other signs of scarring and volume loss in the affected hemithorax. It is important to determine whether the esophagus has been "pushed" or "pulled" from its normal midline position because esophageal retraction resulting from pleuropulmonary scarring

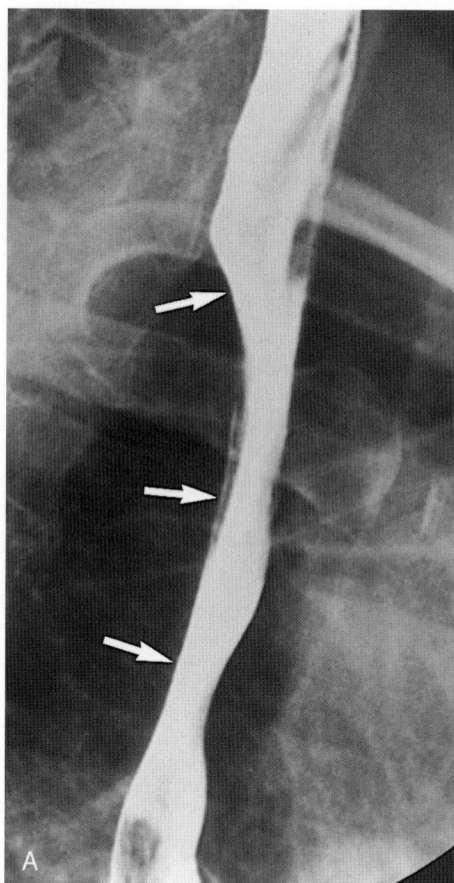

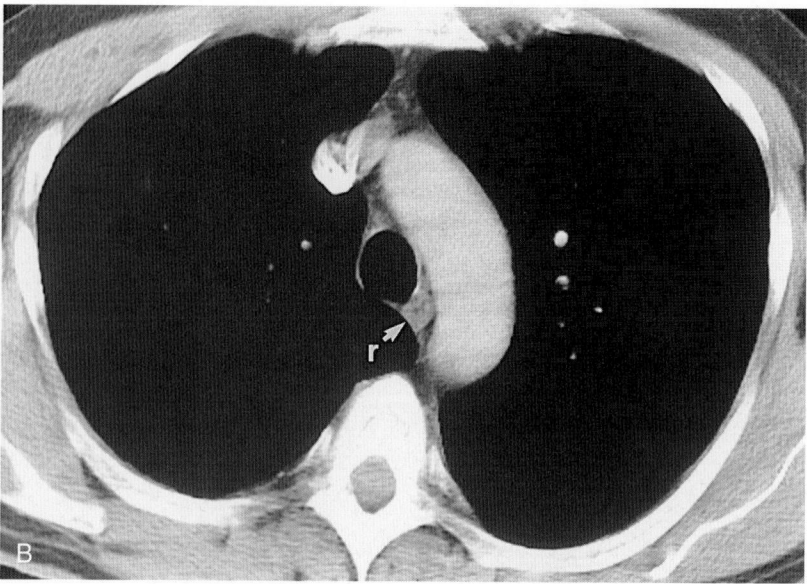

Figure 29-23. Extrinsic impression on the esophagus by a prominent right inferior supra-azygous recess. A. There is a smooth, gently sloping indentation (*arrows*) of the right posterolateral wall of the upper thoracic esophagus between the thoracic inlet and the aortic arch. **B.** In the same patient, CT of the chest shows a prominent right inferior supra-azygous recess (r) impinging on the right posterolateral wall of the upper esophagus (*arrow*). (From Sam JW, Levine MS, Miller WT: The right inferior supra-azygous recess: A cause of upper esophageal pseudomass on double-contrast esophagography. AJR 171:1583-1586, 1998, © by American Roentgen Ray Society.)

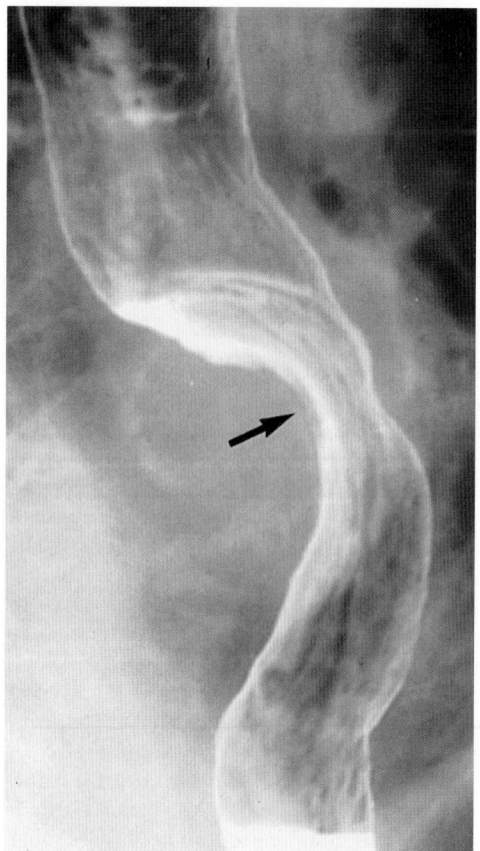

Figure 29-24. Esophageal impression (*arrow*) by an ectatic descending thoracic aorta. The esophagus is narrowed at the level of deviation. (From Levine MS, Gilchrist AM: Esophageal deviation: Pushed or pulled? AJR 149:513-514, 1987, © by American Roentgen Ray Society.)

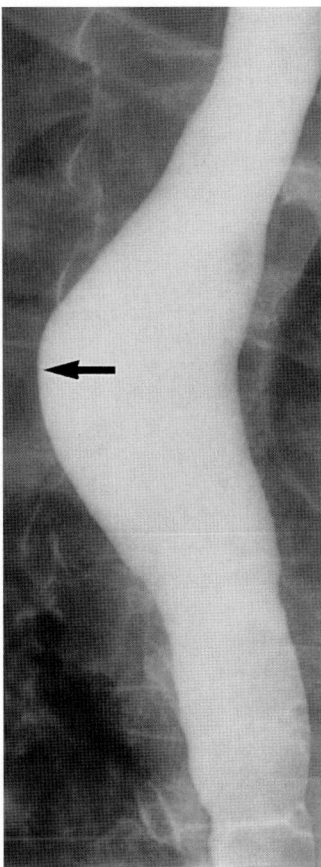

Figure 29-25. Esophageal retraction by pleuropulmonary scarring. The esophagus is deviated to the right (*arrow*) because of scarring and volume loss from right upper lobe tuberculosis. The esophagus is widened at the level of deviation. This characteristic widening indicates retraction of the esophagus toward the side of pleuropulmonary scarring rather than displacement by a mass on the opposite side.

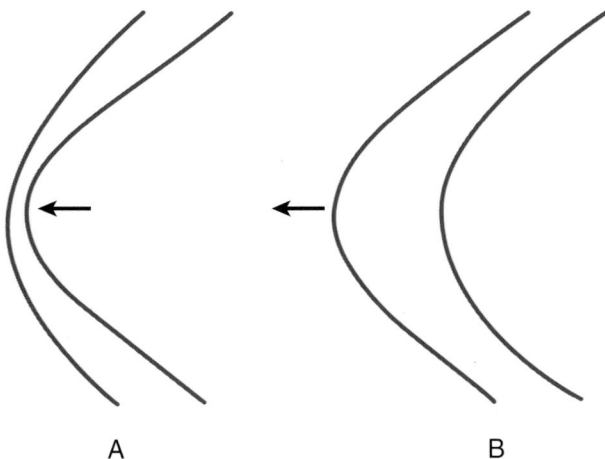

Figure 29-26. Pushed versus pulled esophagus. A. When the esophagus is displaced or pushed by an extrinsic mediastinal mass, it tends to be narrower at this level (*arrow*) than above or below the deviated segment. **B.** When the esophagus is retracted or pulled by pleuropulmonary scarring and volume loss, however, it tends to be wider at this level (*arrow*) than above or below the deviated segment. (From Levine MS, Gilchrist AM: Esophageal deviation: Pushed or pulled? AJR 149:513-514, 1987, © by American Roentgen Ray Society.)

usually represents an incidental finding, whereas esophageal displacement by a mediastinal mass may require further investigation with CT or MRI to determine the nature and extent of the mass.

VARICES

Uphill Varices

Pathophysiology

The development of uphill varices results from changes in the venous drainage of the esophagus caused by altered flow dynamics in patients with portal hypertension. Normally, the cervical esophagus and upper thoracic esophagus are drained by the supreme intercostal vein, bronchial veins, inferior thyroid vein, and other mediastinal collaterals; the midthoracic esophagus is drained by the azygos and hemiazygos veins; and the distal thoracic esophagus is drained by a periesophageal plexus of veins that communicate distally with the coronary vein. In turn, the coronary vein drains into the splenic vein near its junction with the portal vein or directly into the portal vein. In portal hypertension, however, increased portal venous pressure leads to reversal of venous flow through the coronary vein into a plexus of dilated esophageal and periesophageal veins that anastomose superiorly with collaterals from the azygos and hemiazygos venous systems. Because the azygos vein drains directly into the superior vena cava, portal venous blood returns to the right side of the heart via the superior vena cava rather than the inferior vena cava, thus bypassing the obstructed portal system.

Clinical Findings

Esophageal varices are important because of the potentially catastrophic consequences of variceal rupture and hemorrhage. Variceal bleeding occurs in 25% to 35% of patients with cirrhosis, and as many as 30% of these hemorrhages are fatal.[128,129] Although some patients have major variceal hemorrhage manifested by one or more episodes of massive hematemesis, others have intermittent, low-grade bleeding with melena, guaiac-positive stool, or iron-deficiency anemia. Surprisingly, however, the size and extent of varices correlate poorly with the degree of bleeding.

Radiographic Findings

Chest Radiographs

Esophageal varices may occasionally be manifested on chest radiographs by a retrocardiac posterior mediastinal mass. This finding is caused either by dilated esophageal or paraesophageal veins or, less commonly, by dilated azygos or hemiazygos veins.[130-132] The mass is usually more obvious on radiographs obtained with the patient in the recumbent position, as hydrostatic pressure tends to overcome portal pressure in the upright position, shifting blood flow to other, more dependent collateral vessels.

Barium Studies

Esophagography has not traditionally been considered a reliable technique for diagnosing esophageal varices. Some authors have advocated the use of anticholinergic agents such as propantheline bromide (Pro-Banthine) and hyoscine-N-butyl bromide (Buscopan) to improve visualization of varices by decreasing esophageal peristalsis.[133,134] However, anticholinergic agents such as Pro-Banthine may be contraindicated in patients with glaucoma, cardiac disease, or urinary retention. Although Buscopan has fewer side effects, it is not commercially available in the United States.

Whether or not pharmacologic agents are used, optimal demonstration of varices requires meticulous attention to radiographic technique, because varices can easily be obscured on overly distended or collapsed views of the esophagus (Fig. 29-27). The examination should be performed with the patient in a recumbent (usually prone right anterior oblique) position, using a high-density barium suspension or paste to increase adherence of barium to the esophageal mucosa. Mucosal relief views of the collapsed esophagus are particularly helpful for demonstrating varices (see Fig. 29-27D). However, peristalsis tends to squeeze blood from the thin-walled varices, rendering them invisible for as long as 15 to 30 seconds (see Fig. 29-27C). The fluoroscopist must therefore wait for the varices to refill before obtaining these mucosal relief views. If necessary, the patient should be asked to spit his or her saliva into a basin to avoid initiating a new peristaltic sequence and collapsing the varices again. With optimal technique, it has been shown that esophagography has an overall sensitivity of 89% and an overall accuracy of 87% in detecting esophageal varices.[135]

Because of the underlying venous anatomy, uphill varices tend to be most prominent in the distal third or half of the thoracic esophagus, fading gradually as they ascend to the level of entry of the azygos vein into the superior vena cava. As described previously, varices are usually best seen on mucosal relief views, appearing as tortuous or serpiginous longitudinal filling defects in the collapsed or partially collapsed esophagus (see Fig. 29-27D).[136] Varices may also be seen on double-contrast images when they are etched in white owing to trapping of barium between the edge of the lesions and the adjacent esophageal wall (see Fig. 29-27A). Because varices alternately distend and collapse with peristalsis, respiration, and varying degrees of esophageal distention, they may be observed as a transient finding, visible on only one or several spot images obtained during the radiologic examination.

Computed Tomography

Esophageal varices may be recognized on CT by a thickened, lobulated esophageal wall containing round, tubular, or serpentine structures that have homogeneous attenuation and enhance with contrast material to the same degree as adjacent vessels (Fig. 29-28).[137-139] CT may also reveal coronary, paraumbilical, perisplenic, retrogastric, paraesophageal, omental, mesenteric, and abdominal wall varices in patients with portal hypertension.[139] Occasionally, dilated azygos, hemiazygos, or paraesophageal veins can be mistaken for a posterior mediastinal mass on unenhanced CT.[132,140] However, the marked degree of enhancement that occurs within these dilated vascular structures after infusion of contrast should establish the correct diagnosis.[132,140]

Angiography

Arteriograms of the celiac artery, selective arteriograms of the superior mesenteric or splenic artery, or, less frequently,

portal venograms may be obtained to confirm the presence of uphill varices and to determine the nature and extent of underlying venous abnormalities. With portal hypertension, images obtained during the venous phase of the examination usually fail to demonstrate the portal vein because of reversal of blood flow through numerous collateral vessels to bypass the obstructed venous system. In almost all cases, the coronary vein acts to shunt portal blood through a periesophageal plexus of veins, producing uphill varices, which communicate with the azygos venous system and superior vena cava (Fig. 29-29). Delineation of the angiographic anatomy is important when a surgical shunt is contemplated to control variceal bleeding.

Differential Diagnosis

A confident diagnosis of esophageal varices can usually be made on the basis of radiologic criteria. Occasionally, however, submucosal edema and inflammation associated with esophagitis may be manifested by thickened, tortuous longitudinal folds, mimicking the appearance of varices.[141] Some esophageal carcinomas may also produce a varicoid appearance because of submucosal spread of tumor (Fig. 29-30).[142-144] However, varices tend to change in size and shape at fluoroscopy with respiration, peristalsis, and other maneuvers, whereas varicoid tumors have a more fixed, rigid appearance.[142-144] An abrupt demarcation between the involved segment and the adjacent normal esophagus should also favor tumor, because uphill varices tend to fade superiorly without an obvious demarcation. Finally, varicoid carcinomas may cause dysphagia, whereas this symptom rarely occurs in patients with varices. Thus, it is usually possible to differentiate these entities on clinical and radiologic grounds.

Treatment

The treatment of bleeding esophageal varices includes intravenous infusion of vasopressin or somatostatin analogues (e.g., octreotide), esophageal balloon tamponade, portosystemic shunt surgery, the Sugiura procedure, endoscopic sclerotherapy, endoscopic variceal ligation, and transjugular intrahepatic portosystemic shunt—the TIPS procedure (see Chapter 91).[128,145] The primary aims of therapy are to control active bleeding and to prevent rebleeding.

Endoscopic Sclerotherapy

Endoscopic sclerotherapy has emerged as a viable alternative to surgery for controlling variceal bleeding and decreasing the risk of recurrent bleeding with fewer complications than surgery.[146-148] Endoscopic sclerotherapy is performed by paravariceal injection or direct intraluminal injection of varices with a sclerosing solution via a fiberoptic endoscope. The sclerosing agent causes a severe inflammatory reaction and intramural fibrosis with mechanical obliteration of the varices. However, as many as 30% of patients who undergo sclerotherapy develop complications, including mild chemical esophagitis, ulceration, strictures, and esophageal perforation.[149-152]

Contrast studies performed immediately after sclerotherapy may reveal esophageal dysmotility, esophagitis, irregular luminal narrowing, or, rarely, intramural hematomas.[150,153,154] Mucosal sloughing at the injection sites may cause ulceration (Fig. 29-31A),[150,153] whereas transmural necrosis may

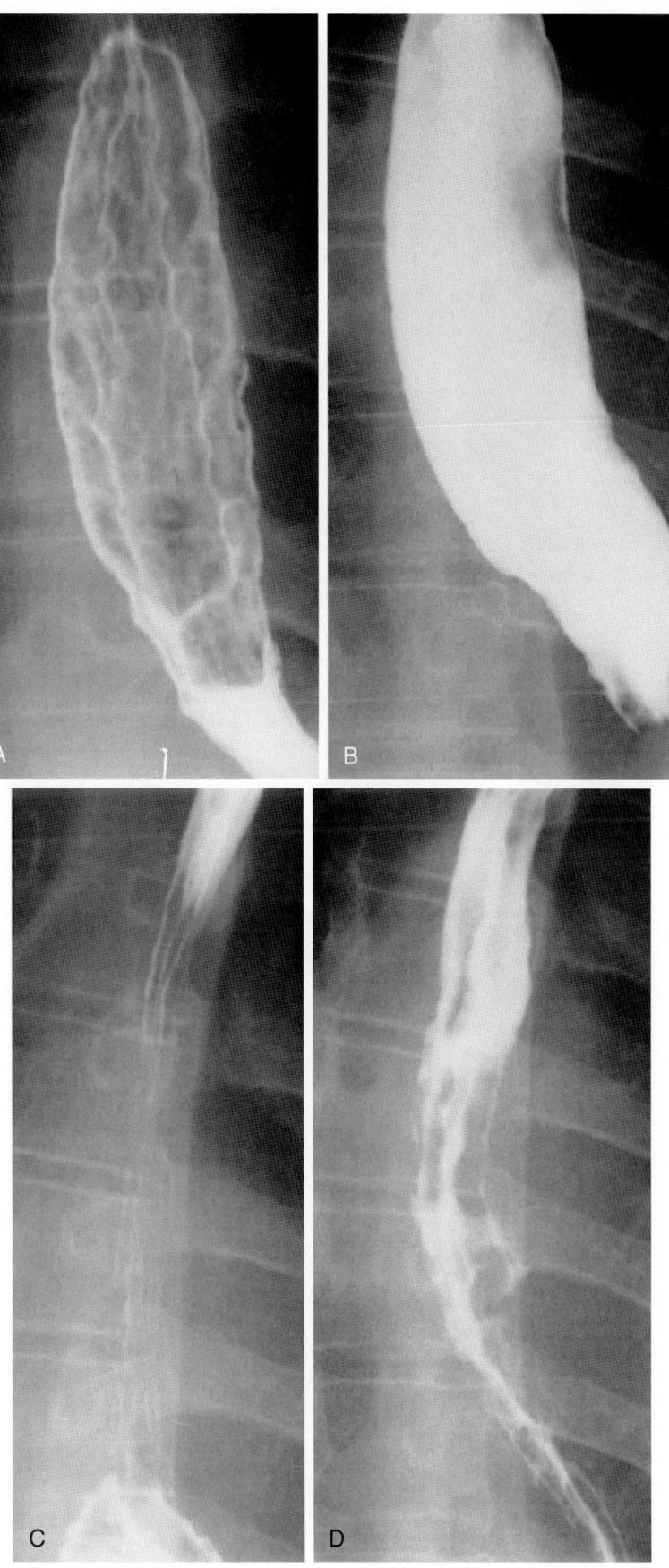

Figure 29-27. Uphill esophageal varices. A. Multiple varices are seen on a double-contrast esophagogram. Note how the varices are etched in white. **B.** The varices are obscured by intraluminal barium on a single-contrast image. **C.** The varices also are not visible on a mucosal relief view immediately after a peristaltic stripping wave that has squeezed blood from the dilated veins, causing them to collapse. **D.** However, the varices can be recognized as serpiginous filling defects on another view several seconds after passage of the peristaltic wave. (From Levine MS: Radiology of the Esophagus. Philadelphia, WB Saunders, 1989.)

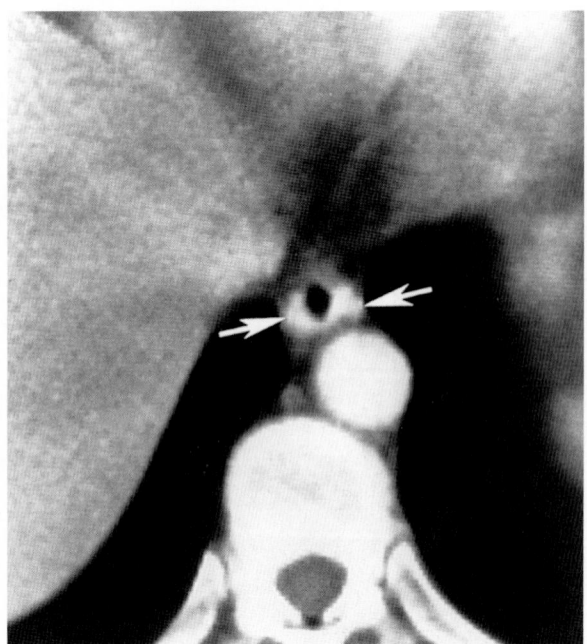

Figure 29-28. Esophageal varices: CT findings. CT during rapid infusion of intravenous contrast medium shows dense enhancement of the varices (*arrows*). (Courtesy of Robert A. Halvorsen, MD, San Francisco, CA.)

lead to the development of transverse or longitudinal intramural tracks (Fig. 29-31B), esophagopleural fistulas, or localized esophageal perforation (Fig. 29-31C).[153,155] Contrast studies performed 30 or more days after sclerotherapy may reveal esophageal strictures of varying length and caliber (Fig. 29-31D).[152]

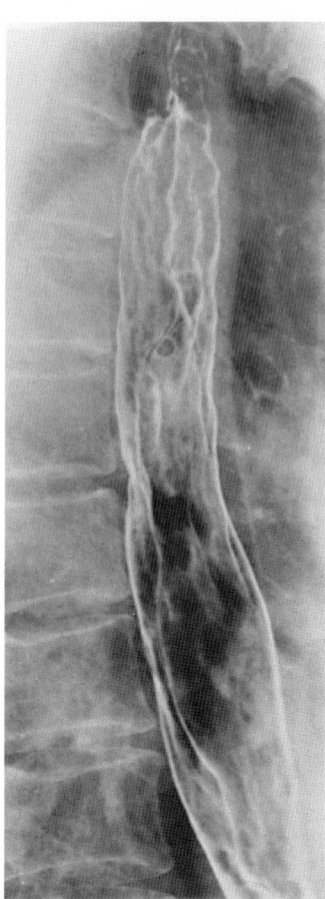

Figure 29-30. Varicoid carcinoma. Thickened, tortuous folds in the esophagus mimic the appearance of varices. This appearance is caused by submucosal spread of tumor. (Courtesy of Akiyoshi Yamada, MD, Tokyo, Japan.)

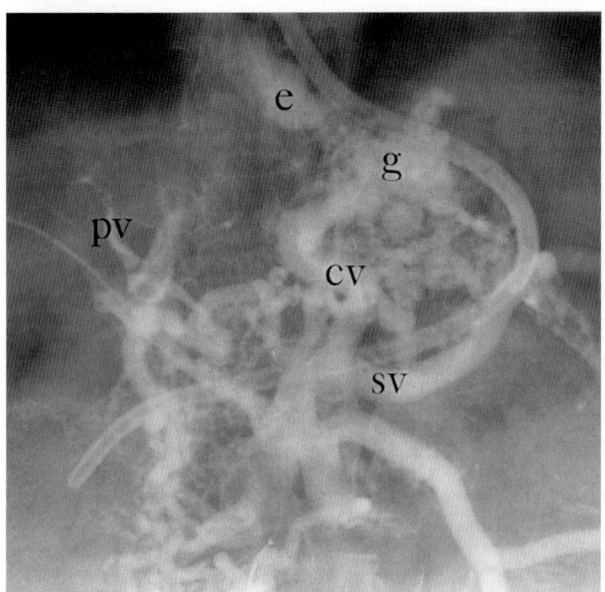

Figure 29-29. Angiographic demonstration of esophageal and gastric varices due to portal hypertension. This image from a portal venogram shows cavernous transformation of the portal vein (pv) with reversal of blood flow through the coronary vein (cv) and splenic vein (sv), producing gastric (g) and esophageal (e) varices. (Courtesy of Dana R. Burke, MD, Bethesda, MD.)

Sclerosed varices are usually manifested on CT by a thickened esophageal wall with outer high-attenuation and inner low-attenuation regions on contrast-enhanced scans, producing a characteristic laminated appearance.[156,157] This finding may result from a sclerosant-induced inflammatory reaction, edema, or hemorrhage within the esophageal wall, so that normal enhancement of varices no longer occurs. CT may also demonstrate a predominantly low-attenuation mediastinal effusion with obliteration of mediastinal fat planes caused by an acute paraesophageal reaction after sclerotherapy.[157] In contrast, a mediastinal abscess from esophageal perforation may be manifested on CT by a predominantly high-attenuation mediastinal effusion associated with mediastinal or pleural gas.[157] Thus, CT may be helpful in determining the nature and extent of postsclerotherapy complications in these patients.

Endoscopic Variceal Ligation

Endoscopic variceal ligation or banding is another technique for the treatment of bleeding esophageal varices in which the varices are ensnared and ligated with endoscopically placed rubber bands, causing strangulation, sloughing, fibrosis, and eventual obliteration of the varices.[158] It has been shown that variceal ligation is associated not only with lower rebleeding rates than endoscopic sclerotherapy but also with fewer complications.[159,160] Contrast studies may occasionally be

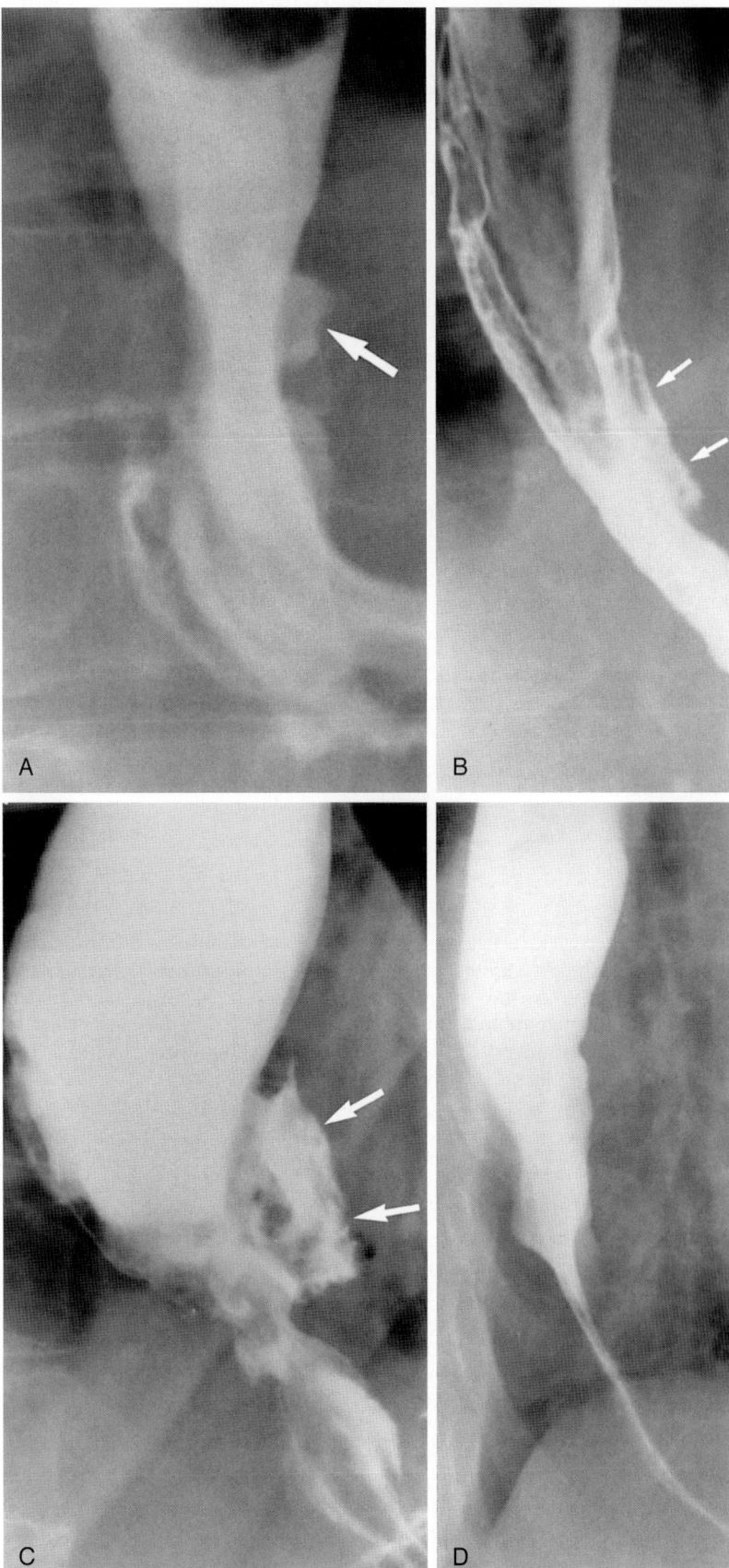

Figure 29-31. Complications of endoscopic sclerotherapy of varices. A. There is a relatively deep ulcer (*arrow*) with associated narrowing of the distal esophagus due to edema and spasm. **B.** This patient has a longitudinal intramural track (*arrows*) in the distal esophagus. **C.** Another patient has a focal, sealed-off perforation of the distal esophagus with contrast medium seen entering an extraluminal cavity (*arrows*). **D.** This patient has a long, tapered stricture in the distal esophagus several months after endoscopic sclerotherapy. (**A**, **B**, and **D** from Levine MS: Radiology of the Esophagus. Philadelphia, WB Saunders, 1989.)

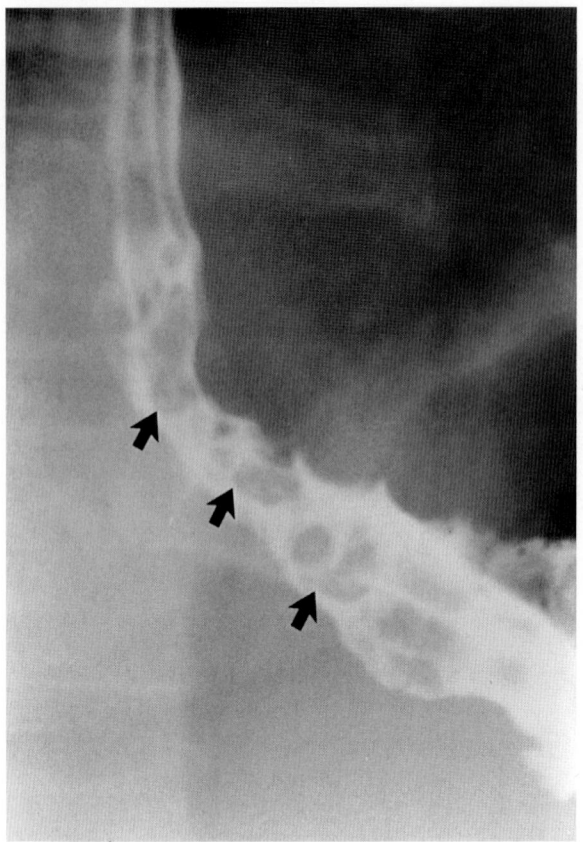

Figure 29-32. Appearance of ligated esophageal varices. A study with water-soluble contrast medium shows several smooth, rounded filling defects (*arrows*), which could be mistaken for neoplastic lesions in the distal esophagus. These represent banded varices 1 day after endoscopic variceal ligation.

performed after variceal ligation to rule out esophageal perforation. In such cases, the ligated varices may be recognized on esophagography as smooth, rounded filling defects in the distal esophagus that are indistinguishable from small polyps (Fig. 29-32).[161] However, the correct diagnosis should be apparent from the clinical history.

Downhill Varices

Pathophysiology

Because the venous structures draining the cervical and upper thoracic esophagus communicate with the supreme intercostal vein, bronchial veins, inferior thyroid vein, and other mediastinal collaterals, obstruction of the superior vena cava may lead to reversal of flow through those vessels into esophageal and paraesophageal veins to bypass the obstruction. Because blood flows downward in them, the dilated esophageal veins are called *downhill varices*.[162]

The location and extent of downhill varices depend pathophysiologically on whether the superior vena cava is obstructed above or below the site of entry of the azygos vein into the superior vena cava.[162,163] If the obstruction occurs above the entry of the azygos vein, downhill varices can return blood from the head and upper extremities via the azygos vein to the superior vena cava below the level of obstruction.

As a result, downhill varices are always confined to the upper or midthoracic esophagus in these cases. If, however, the obstruction occurs at or below the site of entry of the azygos vein into the superior vena cava, the azygos venous system can no longer be used to bypass the obstruction. In such cases, venous flow continues via downhill varices to the distal esophagus, where the coronary vein diverts blood to the portal vein and inferior vena cava, bypassing the obstructed superior vena cava. Thus, downhill varices of this type may involve the entire thoracic esophagus.

Downhill varices are often caused by bronchogenic carcinoma or, less frequently, by other metastatic tumors or lymphoma in the mediastinum.[162-164] When the superior vena cava is obstructed by malignant tumor, the patient rarely survives long enough for the varices to extend distally, so that they are almost always confined to the upper thoracic esophagus, regardless of whether the obstruction occurs above or below the entry of the azygos vein into the superior vena cava.[162] Occasionally, however, obstruction of the superior vena cava may be caused by benign lesions such as a substernal goiter or mediastinal fibrosis due to radiation or histoplasmosis (i.e., sclerosing mediastinitis).[165,166] In such cases, long-standing obstruction of the superior vena cava at or below the level of entry of the azygos vein may lead to the development of extensive downhill varices involving the entire thoracic esophagus.[162,166] With greater use of central venous catheters for hyperalimentation or chemotherapy, catheter-induced thrombosis has also been recognized as an increasingly common cause of superior vena cava obstruction.[167,168] Regardless of the cause of the obstruction, catheter-directed thrombolysis and/or endovascular stents have been shown to be safe and effective alternatives to surgical bypass for the treatment of these patients.[168,169]

Clinical Findings

Obstruction of the superior vena cava results in the superior vena cava syndrome, characterized by facial, periorbital, neck, and bilateral arm swelling and dilated superficial veins over the chest wall. Although most patients with downhill varices caused by the superior vena cava syndrome are asymptomatic, affected individuals may occasionally develop hematemesis or low-grade gastrointestinal bleeding with melena, guaiac-positive stool, or iron-deficiency anemia.[170] Downhill varices should therefore be suspected in any patient with superior vena cava obstruction who develops signs of upper gastrointestinal bleeding.

Radiographic Findings

Like uphill varices, downhill varices appear on barium studies as serpiginous longitudinal filling defects in the esophagus (Fig. 29-33).[164] However, they can be differentiated from uphill varices by their location, as they are almost always confined to the upper or middle third of the thoracic esophagus, whereas uphill varices are predominantly located in the distal third. As expected, downhill varices are best visualized on mucosal relief views of the collapsed or partially collapsed esophagus with the use of a high-density barium suspension.

When downhill varices are suspected on the basis of barium studies, the patient should be evaluated for other clinical or radiologic signs of superior vena cava obstruction.

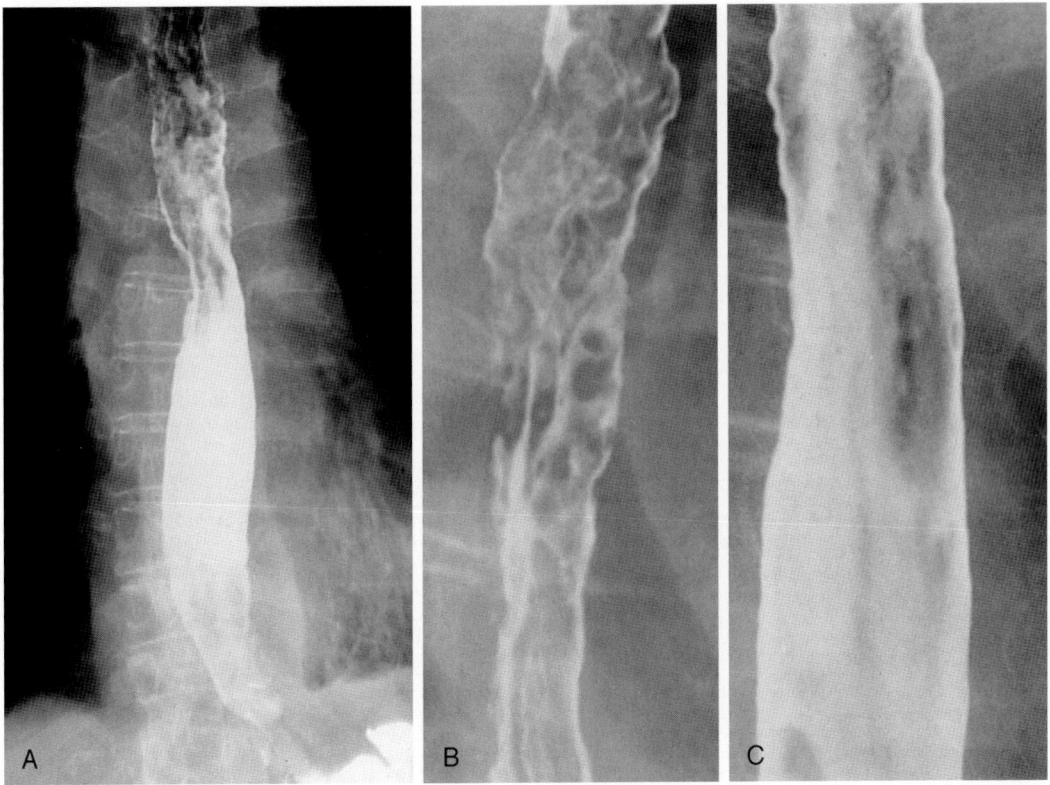

Figure 29-33. Downhill esophageal varices due to superior vena cava obstruction by bronchogenic carcinoma. A. Chest radiograph with barium in the esophagus shows thickened, nodular folds in the midesophagus with a normal-appearing esophagus below this level. Note how the superior mediastinum is widened because of adenopathy from metastatic lung cancer. **B.** Mucosal relief view of the esophagus shows prominent downhill varices. **C.** Another view moments later shows obliteration of the varices with greater esophageal distention. (From Levine MS: Radiology of the Esophagus. Philadelphia, WB Saunders, 1989.)

Chest radiography or CT may reveal obvious widening of the superior mediastinum due to mediastinal lymphadenopathy (see Fig. 29-33A), tumor, substernal thyroid goiter, or, less commonly, mediastinal fibrosis. Venography may be required to confirm the diagnosis and to determine the level and degree of stenosis or obstruction and extent of collateral circulation, particularly if a surgical shunt, catheter-directed thrombolysis, or endovascular stent is contemplated.

Differential Diagnosis

Downhill varices may be confused radiographically with varicoid carcinomas that produce thickened, tortuous folds in the upper esophagus or midesophagus as a result of submucosal spread of tumor (see Fig. 29-30).[142-144] However, downhill varices tend to change in size and shape at fluoroscopy whereas varicoid tumors have a more fixed appearance and more abrupt, well-defined borders.

Idiopathic Varices

Rarely, esophageal varices may occur in patients who have no other signs of hepatic cirrhosis, portal hypertension, or superior vena cava obstruction.[171,172] Because the mechanism of variceal formation is unknown, they have been called *idiopathic varices.* It has been postulated that these varices develop as a result of a congenital weakness in the venous channels of the esophagus.[171-173] Although idiopathic varices are extremely uncommon, they are important because of the risk of variceal bleeding.[171]

Radiographic Findings

Although uphill and downhill varices tend to occur as multiple lesions, an idiopathic varix usually occurs as a solitary lesion, appearing as a smooth, slightly lobulated submucosal mass in the esophagus (Fig. 29-34A).[174] As a result, the radiographic findings may erroneously suggest a submucosal tumor such as a leiomyoma. However, an idiopathic varix can usually be effaced or even obliterated by esophageal distention (Fig. 29-34B), so that images obtained with the patient in both upright and recumbent positions with variable esophageal distention should suggest the vascular origin of the lesion.[174] It is important for endoscopists to be aware of this entity, so that a varix is not inadvertently sampled without careful preliminary visual inspection.

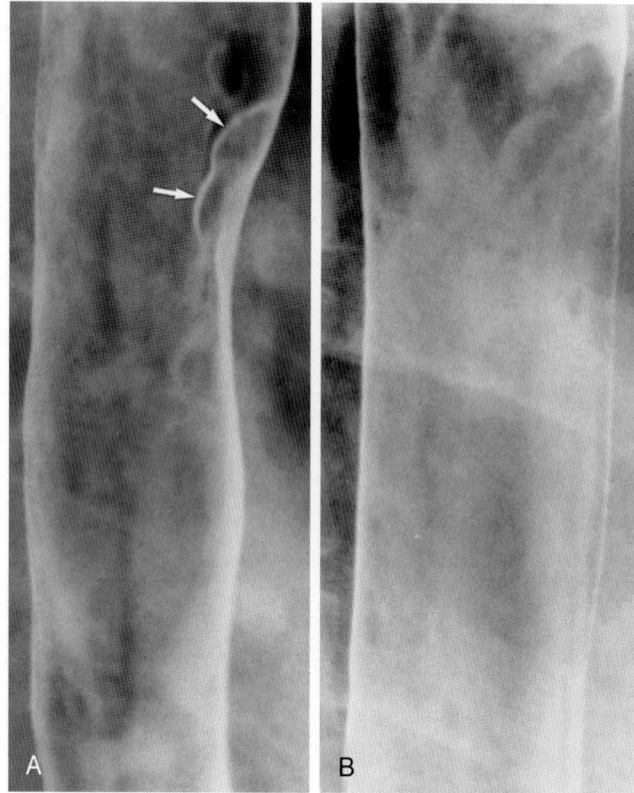

Figure 29-34. Idiopathic varix. A. There is a slightly lobulated, submucosal-appearing mass (*arrows*) that is indistinguishable from a leiomyoma or other submucosal tumor. **B.** Another view moments later shows obliteration of the varix with greater esophageal distention. (Courtesy of Seth N. Glick, MD, Philadelphia, PA.)

References

1. Ansari A: Mallory-Weiss syndrome: Revisited. Am J Gastroenterol 64:460-466, 1975.
2. Bubrick MP, Lundeen JW, Onstad GR, et al: Mallory-Weiss syndrome: Analysis of fifty-nine cases. Surgery 88:400-405, 1980.
3. Hastings PR, Peters KW, Cohn I: Mallory-Weiss syndrome: Review of 69 cases. Am J Surg 142:560-562, 1981.
4. Graham DV, Schwartz JT: The spectrum of the Mallory-Weiss tear. Medicine (Baltimore) 57:307-318, 1977.
5. Baker RW, Spiro AH, Trnka YM: Mallory-Weiss tear complicating upper endoscopy. Gastroenterology 82:140-142, 1982.
6. Hunter TB, Protell RL, Horsley WW: Food laceration of the esophagus: The taco tear. AJR 140:503-504, 1983.
7. Penston JG, Boyd EJ, Wormsley KG: Mallory-Weiss tears occurring during endoscopy: Report of four cases. Endoscopy 24:262-265, 1992.
8. Foster DN, Miloszewski K, Losowsky MS: Diagnosis of Mallory-Weiss lesions: A common cause of upper gastrointestinal bleeding. Lancet 2:483-485, 1976.
9. Knaver CM: Mallory-Weiss syndrome: Characterization of 75 Mallory-Weiss lacerations in 528 patients with upper gastrointestinal hemorrhage. Gastroenterology 71:5-8, 1976.
10. Clark RA: Intraarterial vasopressin infusion for treatment of Mallory-Weiss tears of the esophagogastric junction. AJR 133:449-451, 1979.
11. Carsen GM, Casarella WJ, Spiegel RM: Transcatheter embolization for treatment of Mallory-Weiss tears of the esophagogastric junction. Radiology 128:309-313, 1978.
12. Papp JP: Electrocoagulation of actively bleeding Mallory-Weiss tears. Gastrointest Endosc 2:128-130, 1980.
13. Harris JM, DiPalma JA: Clinical significance of Mallory-Weiss tears. Am J Gastroenterol 88:2056-2058, 1993.
14. Dallemand S, Amorosa JK, Morris DW, et al: Intramural hematomas of the esophagus. Gastrointest Radiol 8:7-9, 1983.
15. Shay SS, Berendson RA, Johnson LF: Esophageal hematoma: Four new cases, a review, and proposed etiology. Dig Dis Sci 26:1019-1024, 1981.
16. Bradley JL, Han SY: Intramural hematoma (incomplete perforation) of the esophagus associated with esophageal dilatation. Radiology 130:59-62, 1979.
17. Steenbergen WV, Fevery J, Broeckaert L, et al: Intramural hematoma of the esophagus: Unusual complication of variceal sclerotherapy. Gastrointest Radiol 9:293-295, 1984.
18. de Vries RA, Kremer-Schneider MME, Otten MH: Intramural hematoma of the esophagus caused by minor head injury 6 hours previously. Gastrointest Radiol 16:283-285, 1991.
19. Andress M: Submucosal haematoma of the oesophagus due to anticoagulant therapy. Acta Radiol Diagn 11:216-219, 1971.
20. Ashman FC, Hill MC, Saba GP, et al: Esophageal hematoma associated with thrombocytopenia. Gastrointest Radiol 3:115-118, 1978.
21. Meulman N, Evans J, Watson A: Spontaneous intramural haematoma of the oesophagus: A report of three cases and review of the literature. Aust N Z J Surg 64:190-193, 1994.
22. Chen P, Lebowitz R, Lewicki AM: Spontaneous hematoma of the esophagus. Radiology 100:281-282, 1971.
23. Lowman RM, Goldman R, Stern H: The roentgen aspects of intramural dissection of the esophagus. Radiology 93:1329-1331, 1969.
24. Joffe N, Millan VG: Postemetic dissecting intramural hematoma of the esophagus. Radiology 95:379-380, 1970.
25. Pellicano A, Watier A, Gentile J: Spontaneous double-barreled esophagus. J Clin Gastroenterol 9:149-154, 1987.
26. Demos TC, Okrent DH, Studlo JD, et al: Spontaneous esophageal hematoma diagnosed by computed tomography. J Comp Assist Tomogr 10:133-135, 1986.
27. Herbetko J, Delany D, Ogilvie BC, et al: Spontaneous intramural haematoma of the oesophagus: Appearance on computed tomography. Clin Radiol 44:327-328, 1991.
28. Campbell TC, Andrews JL, Neptune WB: Spontaneous rupture of the esophagus (Boerhaave's syndrome). JAMA 235:526-528, 1976.
29. Love L, Berkow AE: Trauma to the esophagus. Gastrointest Radiol 2:305-321, 1978.
30. Pasricha PJ, Fleischer DE, Kalloo AN: Endoscopic perforations of the upper digestive tract: A review of their pathogenesis, prevention, and management. Gastroenterology 106:787-802, 1994.
31. Meyers MA, Ghahremani GG: Complications of fiberoptic endoscopy: I. Esophagoscopy and gastroscopy. Radiology 115:293-300, 1975.
32. Baron TH: Expandable metal stents for the treatment of cancerous obstruction of the gastrointestinal tract. N Engl J Med 344:1681-1687, 2001.
33. Ghahremani GG, Turner MA, Port RB: Iatrogenic intubation injuries of the upper gastrointestinal tract in adults. Gastrointest Radiol 5:1-10, 1980.
34. Polsky S, Kerstein MD: Pharyngo-esophageal perforation due to blunt trauma. Am Surg 61:994-996, 1995.
35. O'Connell ND: Spontaneous rupture of the esophagus. AJR 99:186-203, 1967.
36. Rogers LF, Puig W, Dooley BN, et al: Diagnostic considerations in mediastinal emphysema: A pathophysiologic approach to Boerhaave's syndrome and spontaneous pneumomediastinum. AJR 115:495-511, 1972.
37. Bradham RR, deSaussure C, Lemel AL: Spontaneous perforation of the cervical esophagus. Arch Surg 111:284-285, 1976.
38. Isserow JA, Levine MS, Rubesin SE: Spontaneous perforation of the cervical esophagus after an alcoholic binge. Can Assoc Radiol J 49:241-243, 1998.
39. Janjua KJ: Boerhaave's syndrome. Postgrad Med J 73:265-270, 1997.
40. Han SY, Tishler JM: Perforation of the abdominal segment of the esophagus. AJR 143:751-754, 1984.
41. Klygis LM, Jutabha R, McCrohan MB, et al: Esophageal perforations masked by steroids. Abdom Imaging 18:10-12, 1993.
42. Berry BE, Ochsner JL: Perforation of the esophagus: A 30 year review. J Thorac Cardiovasc Surg 65:1-7, 1973.
43. Maglinte DDT, Edwards MC: Spontaneous closure of esophageal tear in Boerhaave's syndrome. Gastrointest Radiol 4:223-225, 1979.
44. Phillips LG, Cunningham J: Esophageal perforation. Radiol Clin North Am 22:607-613, 1984.
45. Han SY, McElvein RB, Aldrete JS, et al: Perforation of the esophagus: Correlation of site and cause with plain film findings. AJR 145:537-540, 1985.

46. Parkin GJS: The radiology of perforated esophagus. Clin Radiol 24: 324-332, 1973.

47. Healy ME, Mindelzun RE: Lesser sac pneumoperitoneum secondary to perforation of the intraabdominal esophagus. AJR 142:325-326, 1984.

48. James AE, Montali RJ, Chaffee V, et al: Barium or Gastrografin: Which contrast media for diagnosis of esophageal tears? Gastroenterology 68:1103-1113, 1975.

49. Vessal K, Montali RJ, Larson SM, et al: Evaluation of barium and Gastrografin as contrast media for the diagnosis of esophageal ruptures or complications. AJR 123:307-319, 1975.

50. Chiu CL, Gambach RR: Hypaque pulmonary edema: A case report. Radiology 111:91-92, 1974.

51. Brick SH, Caroline DF, Lev-Toaff AS, et al: Esophageal disruption: Evaluation with iohexol esophagography. Radiology 169:141-143, 1988.

52. Gollub MJ, Bains MS: Barium sulfate: A new (old) contrast agent for diagnosis of postoperative esophageal leaks. Radiology 202:360-362, 1997.

53. Rubesin SE, Levine MS: Radiologic diagnosis of gastrointestinal perforation. Radiol Clin North Am 41:1095-1115, 2003.

54. Foster JH, Jolly PC, Sawyers JL, et al: Esophageal perforation: Diagnosis and treatment. Ann Surg 161:701-709, 1965.

55. Berry BE, Ochsner JL: Perforation of the esophagus: A 30 year review. J Thorac Cardiovasc Surg 65:1-7, 1973.

56. Wychulis AR, Fontana RS, Payne WS: Instrumental perforations of the esophagus. Dis Chest 55:184-189, 1969.

57. Dodds WJ, Stewart ET, Vlymen WJ: Appropriate contrast media for evaluation of esophageal disruption. Radiology 144:439-441, 1982.

58. Foley MJ, Ghahremani GG, Rogers LF: Reappraisal of contrast media used to detect upper gastrointestinal perforations. Radiology 144:231-237, 1982.

59. Levine MS: What is the best oral contrast material to use for the fluoroscopic diagnosis of esophageal rupture? AJR 162:1243, 1994.

60. Tanomkiat W, Galassi W: Barium sulfate as contrast medium for evaluation of postoperative anastomotic leaks. Acta Radiol 41:482-485, 2000.

61. Buecker A, Wein BB, Neuerburg JM, et al: Esophageal perforation: Comparison of use of aqueous and barium-containing contrast media. Radiology 202:683-686, 1997.

62. Swanson JO, Levine MS, Redfern RO, et al: Usefulness of high-density barium for detection of leaks after esophagogastrectomy, total gastrectomy, and total laryngectomy. AJR 181:415-420, 2003.

63. Backer CL, LoCicero J, Hartz RS, et al: Computed tomography in patients with esophageal perforation. Chest 98:1078-1080, 1990.

64. White CS, Templeton PA, Attar S: Esophageal perforation: CT findings. AJR 160:767-770, 1993.

65. Fadoo F, Ruiz DE, Dawn SK, et al: Helical CT esophagography for the evaluation of suspected esophageal perforation or rupture. AJR 182:1177-1179, 2004.

66. Webb WA: Management of foreign bodies of the upper gastrointestinal tract. Gastroenterology 94:204-216, 1988.

67. Nandi P, Ong GB: Foreign bodies in the oesophagus: Review of 2,394 cases. Br J Surg 65:5-9, 1978.

68. Giordano A, Adams G, Boies L, et al: Current management of esophageal foreign bodies. Arch Otolaryngol 107:249-251, 1981.

69. Ginsberg GG: Management of ingested foreign objects and food bolus impactions. Gastrointest Endosc 41:33-38, 1995.

70. Barber GB, Peppercorn MA, Ehrlich C, et al: Esophageal foreign body perforation. Am J Gastroenterol 79:509-511, 1984.

71. Gougoutas C, Levine MS, Laufer I: Esophageal food impaction with early perforation. AJR 171:427-428, 1998.

72. Underberg-Davis S, Levine MS: Giant thoracic osteophyte causing esophageal food impaction. AJR 157:319-320, 1991.

73. Shaffer HA, Alford BA, de Lange EE, et al: Basket extraction of esophageal foreign bodies. AJR 147:1010-1013, 1986.

74. Macpherson RI, Hill JG, Othersen HB, et al: Esophageal foreign bodies in children: Diagnosis, treatment, and complications. AJR 166:919-924, 1996.

75. Harned RK, Strain JD, Hay TC, et al: Esophageal foreign bodies: Safety and efficacy of Foley catheter extraction of coins. AJR 168:443-446, 1997.

76. Ferrucci JT, Long JA: Radiologic treatment of esophageal food impaction using intravenous glucagon. Radiology 125:25-28, 1977.

77. Trenkner SW, Maglinte DDT, Lehman GA, et al: Esophageal food impaction: Treatment with glucagon. Radiology 149:401-403, 1983.

78. Hogan WJ, Dodds WJ, Hoke SE, et al: Effect of glucagon on esophageal motor function. Gastroenterology 69:160-165, 1975.

79. Rice BT, Spiegel PK, Dombrowski PJ: Acute esophageal food impaction treated by gas-forming agents. Radiology 146:299-301, 1983.

80. Smith JC, Janower ML, Geiger AH: Use of glucagon and gas-forming agents in acute esophageal food impaction. Radiology 159:567-568, 1986.

81. Kaszar-Seibert DJ, Korn WT, Bindman DJ, et al: Treatment of acute esophageal food impaction with a combination of glucagon, effervescent agent, and water. AJR 154:533-534, 1990.

82. Robbins MI, Shortsleeve MJ: Treatment of acute esophageal food impaction with glucagon, an effervescent agent, and water. AJR 162:325-328, 1994.

83. Fitzgerald RH, Bartles DM, Parker EF: Tracheoesophageal fistulas secondary to carcinoma of the esophagus. J Thorac Cardiovasc Surg 82:194-197, 1981.

84. Little AG, Ferguson MK, DeMeester TR, et al: Esophageal carcinoma with respiratory tract fistula. Cancer 53:1322-1328, 1984.

85. Spalding AR, Burney DP, Richie RE: Acquired benign bronchoesophageal fistulas in the adult. Ann Thorac Surg 28:378-383, 1979.

86. Vasquez RE, Landay M, Kilman WJ, et al: Benign esophagorespiratory fistulas in adults. Radiology 167:93-96, 1988.

87. Sheiner NM, LaChance C: Congenital esophagobronchial fistula in the adult. Can J Surg 23:489-491, 1980.

88. Weschler RJ, Steiner RM, Goodman LR, et al: Iatrogenic esophageal-pleural fistula: Subtlety of diagnosis in the absence of mediastinitis. Radiology 144:239-243, 1982.

89. Massard G, Wihlm JM: Early complications: Esophagopleural fistula. Chest Surg Clin North Am 9:617-631, 1999.

90. Massard G, Ducrocq X, Hentz JG, et al: Esophagopleural fistula: An early and long-term complication after pneumonectomy. Ann Thorac Surg 58:1437-1440, 1994.

91. Weschler RJ: CT of esophageal-pleural fistulae. AJR 147:907-909, 1986.

92. Liu PS, Levine MS, Torigian DA: Esophagopleural fistula secondary to esophageal wall ballooning and thinning after pneumonectomy: Findings on chest CT and esophagography. AJR 186:1627-1629, 2006.

93. Baron RL, Koehler RE, Gutierrez FR, et al: Clinical and radiographic manifestations of aortoesophageal fistulas. Radiology 141:599-605, 1981.

94. Khawaja FI, Varindani MK: Aortoesophageal fistula: Review of clinical, radiographic and endoscopic features. J Clin Gastroenterol 9:342-344, 1987.

95. Hollander JE, Quick G: Aortoesophageal fistula: A comprehensive review of the literature. Am J Med 91:279-287, 1991.

96. Seymour EQ: Aortoesophageal fistula as a complication of aortic prosthetic graft. AJR 131:160-161, 1978.

97. Cyrlak D, Cohen AJ, Dana ER: Esophagopericardial fistula: Causes and radiographic features. AJR 141:177-179, 1983.

98. Kaye MD: Oesophageal motor dysfunction in patients with diverticula of the mid-thoracic oesophagus. Thorax 29:666-672, 1974.

99. Debas HT, Payne WS, Cameron AJ, et al: Physiopathology of lower esophageal diverticulum and its implications for treatment. Surg Gynecol Obstet 151:593-600, 1980.

100. Dodds WJ, Stef JJ, Hogan WJ, et al: Radial distribution of peristaltic pressure in normal subjects and patients with esophageal diverticulum. Gastroenterology 69:584-590, 1975.

101. Fasano NC, Levine MS, Rubesin SE, et al: Epiphrenic diverticulum: Clinical and radiographic findings in 27 patients. Dysphagia 18:9-15, 2003.

102. Niv Y, Fraser G, Krugliak P: Gastroesophageal obstruction from food in an epiphrenic esophageal diverticulum. J Clin Gastroenterol 16:314-316, 1993.

103. Altorki NK, Sunagawa M, Skinner DB: Thoracic esophageal diverticula: Why is operation necessary? J Thorac Cardiovasc Surg 105:260-264, 1993.

104. Benacci JC, Deschamps C, Trastek VF, et al: Epiphrenic diverticulum: Results of surgical treatment. Ann Thorac Surg 55:1109-1114, 1993.

105. Jabbari M, Goresky CA, Lough J, et al: The inlet patch: Heterotopic gastric mucosa in the upper esophagus. Gastroenterology 89:352-356, 1985.

106. Borhan-Manesh F, Farnum JB: Incidence of heterotopic gastric mucosa in the upper oesophagus. Gut 32:968-972, 1991.

107. Ueno J, Davis SW, Tanakami A, et al: Ectopic gastric mucosa in the upper esophagus: Detection and radiographic findings. Radiology 191:751-753, 1994.

108. Takeji H, Ueno J, Nishitani H: Ectopic gastric mucosa in the upper esophagus: Prevalence and radiographic findings. AJR 164:901-904, 1995.
109. Lee J, Levine MS, Schultz CF: Ectopic gastric mucosa in the oesophagus mimicking ulceration. Eur J Radiol 31:197-200, 1997.
110. Buse PE, Zuckerman GR, Balfe DM: Cervical esophageal web associated with a patch of heterotopic gastric mucosa. Abdom Imaging 18:227-228, 1993.
111. Galan AR, Katzka DA, Castell DO: Acid secretion from an esophageal inlet patch demonstrated by ambulatory pH monitoring. Gastroenterology 115:1574-1576, 1998.
112. Anderson LS, Shackelford GD, Mancilla-Jimenez R, et al: Cartilaginous esophageal ring: A cause of esophageal stenosis in infants and children. Radiology 108:665-666, 1973.
113. Rose JS, Kassner EG, Jurgens KH, et al: Congenital esophageal strictures due to cartilaginous rings. Br J Radiol 48:16-18, 1975.
114. Yeung CK, Spitz L, Brereton RJ, et al: Congenital esophageal stenosis due to tracheobronchial remnants: A rare but important association with esophageal atresia. J Pediatr Surg 27:852-855, 1992.
115. McNally PR, Collier EH, Lopiano MC, et al: Congenital esophageal stenosis: A rare cause of food impaction in the adult. Dig Dis Sci 35:263-266, 1990.
116. McNally PR, Lemon JC, Goff JS, et al: Congenital esophageal stenosis presenting as noncardiac, esophageal chest pain. Dig Dis Sci 38:369-373, 1993.
117. Katzka DA, Levine MS, Ginsberg GG, et al: Congenital esophageal stenosis in adults. Am J Gastroenterol 95:32-36, 2000.
118. Murphy SG, Yazbeck S, Russo P: Isolated congenital esophageal stenosis. J Pediatr Surg 30:1238-1241, 1995.
119. Pokieser P, Schima W, Schober E, et al: Congenital esophageal stenosis in a 21-year-old man: Clinical and radiographic findings. AJR 170:147-148, 1998.
120. Oh CH, Levine MS, Katzka DA, et al: Congenital esophageal stenosis in adults: Clinical and radiographic findings in seven patients. AJR 176:1179-1182, 2001.
121. Zimmerman SL, Levine MS, Rubesin SE, et al: Idiopathic eosinophilic esophagitis in adults: The ringed esophagus. 236:159-165, 2005.
122. Levine MS, Goldstein HM: Fixed transverse folds in the esophagus: A sign of reflux esophagitis. AJR 143:275-278, 1984.
123. Gohel VK, Edell SL, Laufer I, et al: Transverse folds in the human esophagus. Radiology 128:303-308, 1978.
124. Sam JW, Levine MS, Miller WT: The right inferior supraazygous recess: A cause of upper esophageal pseudomass on double-contrast esophagography. AJR 171:1583-1586, 1998.
125. McClure MJ, Ellis PK, Kelly IMG, et al: Esophageal pseudomass: Extrinsic compression of the esophagus due to a narrow thoracic inlet. AJR 174:1003-1004, 2000.
126. Birholz JC, Ferrucci JT, Wyman SM: Roentgen features of dysphagia aortica. Radiology 111:93-96, 1974.
127. Levine MS, Gilchrist AM: Esophageal deviation: Pushed or pulled? AJR 149:513-514, 1987.
128. Sharara AI, Rockey DC: Gastroesophageal variceal hemorrhage. N Engl J Med 345:669-681, 2001.
129. Graham DY, Smith JL: The course of patients after variceal hemorrhage. Gastroenterology 80:800-809, 1981.
130. Jonsson K, Rian RL: Pseudotumoral esophageal varices associated with portal hypertension. Radiology 97:593-597, 1970.
131. Ishikawa T, Saeki M, Tsukune Y, et al: Detection of paraesophageal varices by plain films. AJR 144:701-704, 1985.
132. Lau KK, Phillips G, McKenzie A: Pseudotumoral paraesophageal varices. Gastrointest Radiol 17:193-194, 1992.
133. Ghahremani GG, Port RB, Winans CS, et al: Esophageal varices: Enhanced radiologic visualization by anticholinergic drugs. Am J Dig Dis 17:703-712, 1972.
134. Liu CI: Enhanced visualization of esophageal varices by Buscopan. AJR 121:232-235, 1974.
135. Farber E, Fischer D, Eliakim R, et al: Esophageal varices: Evaluation with esophagography with barium versus endoscopic gastroduodenoscopy in patients with compensated cirrhosis-blinded prospective study. Radiology 237:535-540, 2005.
136. Cockerill EM, Miller RE, Chernish SM, et al: Optimal visualization of esophageal varices. AJR 126:512-523, 1976.
137. Clark KE, Foley WD, Berland LL, et al: CT evaluation of esophageal and upper abdominal varices. J Comput Assist Tomogr 4:510-515, 1980.
138. Balthazar EJ, Naidich DP, Megibow AJ, et al: CT evaluation of esophageal varices. AJR 148:131-135, 1987.
139. Cho KC, Patel YD, Wachsberg RH, Seeff J: Varices in portal hypertension: Evaluation with CT. RadioGraphics 15:609-622, 1995.
140. Ishikawa T, Tsukune Y, Ohyama Y, et al: Venous abnormalities in portal hypertension demonstrated by CT. AJR 134:271-276, 1980.
141. Rabin M, Schmaman IB: Reflux esophagitis resembling varices. S Afr Med J 55:293-295, 1979.
142. Lawson TL, Dodds WJ, Sheft DJ: Carcinoma of the esophagus simulating varices. AJR 107:83-85, 1969.
143. Silver TM, Goldstein HM: Varicoid carcinoma of the esophagus. Dig Dis 19:56-58, 1974.
144. Yates CW, LeVine MA, Jensen KM: Varicoid carcinoma of the esophagus. Radiology 122:605-608, 1977.
145. Garcia-Tsao G: Current management of the complications of cirrhosis and portal hypertension: Variceal hemorrhage, ascites, and spontaneous bacterial peritonitis. Gastroenterology 120:726-748, 2001.
146. Macdougall BRD, Westaby D, Theodossi A, et al: Increased long-term survival in variceal haemorrhage using injection sclerotherapy: Results of a controlled trial. Lancet 1:124-127, 1982.
147. Hootegem PV, Van Besien K, Broeckaert L, et al: Endoscopic sclerotherapy of esophageal varices: Long-term follow-up, recurrence, and survival. J Clin Gastroenterol 10:368-372, 1988.
148. Infante-Rivard C, Esnaola S, Villeneuve JP: Role of endoscopic variceal sclerotherapy in the long-term management of variceal bleeding: A meta-analysis. Gastroenterology 96:1087-1092, 1989.
149. Barsoum MS, Abdel-Wahab MH, Bollous F, et al: The complications of injection sclerotherapy of bleeding oesophageal varices. Br J Surg 69:79-81, 1982.
150. Tihansky DP, Reilly JJ, Schade RR, et al: The esophagus after injection sclerotherapy of varices: Immediate postoperative changes. Radiology 153:43-47, 1984.
151. Korula J, Pandya K, Yamada S: Perforation of esophagus after endoscopic variceal sclerotherapy. Dig Dis Sci 34:324-329, 1989.
152. Guynn TP, Eckhauser FE, Knol JA, et al: Injection sclerotherapy-induced esophageal strictures: Risk factors and prognosis. Am Surg 57:567-571, 1991.
153. Agha FP: The esophagus after endoscopic injection sclerotherapy: Acute and chronic changes. Radiology 153:37-42, 1984.
154. Steenbergen WV, Fevery J, Broeckaert L, et al: Intramural hematoma of the esophagus: Unusual complication of variceal sclerotherapy. Gastrointest Radiol 9:293-295, 1984.
155. Wilbom SL, Rector WG, Schaefer JW: An esophagobronchial fistula after endoscopic variceal sclerotherapy. J Clin Gastroenterol 10:81-83, 1988.
156. Halden WJ, Harnsberger HR, Mancuso AA: Computed tomography of esophageal varices after sclerotherapy. AJR 140:1195-1196, 1983.
157. Mauro MA, Jaques PF, Swantkowski TM, et al: CT after uncomplicated esophageal sclerotherapy. AJR 147:57-60, 1986.
158. Stiegmann GV, Goff JS, Sun JH, et al: Endoscopic variceal ligation: An alternative to sclerotherapy. Gastrointest Endosc 35:431-434, 1989.
159. Stiegmann GV, Goff JS, Michaletz-Onody PA, et al: Endoscopic sclerotherapy as compared with endoscopic ligation for bleeding esophageal varices. N Engl J Med 326:1527-1532, 1992.
160. Laine L, el-Newihi HM, Migikovsky B, et al: Endoscopic ligation compared with sclerotherapy for the treatment of bleeding esophageal varices. Ann Intern Med 119:1-7, 1993.
161. Low VHS, Levine MS: Endoscopic banding of esophageal varices: Radiographic findings. AJR 172:941-942, 1999.
162. Felson B, Lessure AP: "Downhill" varices of the esophagus. Dis Chest 46:740-746, 1964.
163. Otto DL, Kurtzman RS: Esophageal varices in superior vena caval obstruction. AJR 92:1000-1012, 1964.
164. Mikkelsen WJ: Varices of the upper esophagus in superior vena caval obstruction. Radiology 81:945-948, 1963.
165. Salyer JM, Harrison HN, Winn DF, et al: Chronic fibrous mediastinitis and superior vena caval obstruction due to histoplasmosis. Dis Chest 35:364-377, 1959.
166. Sorokin JJ, Levine SM, Moss EG, et al: Downhill varices: Report of a case 29 years after resection of a substernal thyroid gland. Gastroenterology 73:345-348, 1977.
167. Chen JC, Bongard F, Klein SR: A contemporary perspective on superior vena cava syndrome. Am J Surg 160:207-211, 1990.
168. Kee ST, Kinoshita L, Razavi MK, et al: Superior vena cava syndrome: Treatment with catheter-directed thrombolysis and endovascular stent placement. Radiology 206:187-193, 1998.

169. Lanciego C, Chacon JL, Julian A, et al: Stenting as first option for endo-vascular treatment of malignant superior vena cava syndrome. AJR 177:585-593, 2001.

170. Fleig WE, Stange EF, Ditschuneit H: Upper gastrointestinal hemorrhage from downhill esophageal varices. Dig Dis Sci 27:23-27, 1982.

171. Schaefer J, Bramschreiber J, Mistilis S, et al: Gastroesophageal variceal bleeding in the absence of hepatic cirrhosis or portal hypertension. Gastroenterology 46:583-588, 1964.

172. Kelsen K, Burbige J: Idiopathic esophageal varices. Am J Gastroenterol 77:539-540, 1982.

173. Harinck E, Fernandes J, Vervat D: Congenital esophageal varices in identical twins without portal hypertension. J Pediatr Surg 6:488, 1971.

174. Trenkner SW, Levine MS, Laufer I, et al: Idiopathic esophageal varix. AJR 141:43-44, 1983.

Abnormalities of the Gastroesophageal Junction

Marc S. Levine, MD

The gastroesophageal junction has traditionally been a difficult area to evaluate on barium studies because the physiologic events associated with swallowing produce a dynamic, constantly changing appearance. The use of complicated, often contradictory terminology to describe both normal and abnormal findings at the cardia has also been a source of confusion. Evaluation of the cardia, perhaps more than of any other area in the upper gastrointestinal tract, requires meticulous attention to radiographic technique. Although rings, strictures, and hernias are best seen on conventional single-contrast barium studies, neoplastic lesions at the cardia are better delineated on double-contrast studies. Thus, radiologists must use different techniques during the fluoroscopic examination to optimally evaluate this area.

RADIOGRAPHIC TECHNIQUE

The gastric cardia is a notoriously difficult area to examine on single-contrast barium studies. Because of the overlying rib cage, the fundus is not accessible to manual palpation or compression. If the fundus is not fully distended, crowded gastric folds may obscure surface detail in this region. If larger volumes of barium are used to distend the fundus, however, it becomes relatively opaque, so that only contour abnormalities can be identified. Because of the inherent limitations of single-contrast barium studies in examining the cardia and fundus, double-contrast techniques have been used to improve radiographic visualization of this area.

The routine double-contrast esophagogram should include a double-contrast examination of the gastric cardia and fundus.[1,2] After upright double-contrast views of the esophagus have been obtained, the patient should be placed in the recumbent right lateral position (i.e., right side down) to directly visualize the gastric cardia en face. The cardia should be observed for several seconds, and, if it appears normal, a single spot image should be obtained. If the cardia appears abnormal, however, additional spot images should be taken as the patient is rotated farther, so that questionable lesions can be demonstrated both en face and in profile.

After the double-contrast portion of the study has been completed, the patient should be placed in the prone right anterior oblique position and instructed to rapidly gulp a thin, low-density barium suspension to achieve optimal distention of the distal esophagus. The single-contrast technique is particularly important for evaluating possible rings, strictures, or hernias in this region, because upright double-contrast views often fail to produce the degree of distention needed to optimally demonstrate these abnormalities.[3] If necessary, a bolster may be placed beneath the patient's upper abdomen to increase intra-abdominal pressure and improve esophageal distention. When a lower esophageal ring is detected, barium tablets or barium-impregnated marshmallows may also be used to help determine the caliber and obstructive potential of the ring and, if a marshmallow becomes impacted above the ring, to determine whether this impaction reproduces the patient's dysphagia.[4,5]

NORMAL RADIOGRAPHIC APPEARANCES

The esophagus is a relatively nondistensible tubular structure with a saccular distal segment that communicates with the stomach. The saccular segment has been called the *phrenic ampulla* or the *vestibule*, as it is the "entrance hall" to the stomach.[6] Manometric studies have shown that the esophageal vestibule corresponds to the location of the lower esophageal sphincter, a 2- to 4-cm high-pressure zone above the gastroesophageal junction that prevents reflux of peptic acid into the esophagus.[7,8] The vestibule extends inferiorly through the esophageal hiatus of the diaphragm before joining the stomach several centimeters below the hiatus. The short intra-abdominal segment of the esophagus terminates at the gastroesophageal junction or gastric cardia. The left lateral aspect of the cardia is demarcated anatomically by sling fibers that hook around a notch formed between the distal esophagus and the gastric fundus (i.e., the cardiac incisura). Important anatomic structures in this region that may be recognized on barium studies include the cardia, Z line, and lower esophageal mucosal and muscular rings. These structures are therefore discussed separately in the following sections.

Cardia

The gastric cardia is often not visualized on single-contrast barium studies because this region is obscured by barium in the fundus or by overlying gastric rugae. However, our ability to recognize the normal appearances of the cardia has improved dramatically with the use of double-contrast technique. In one study, the normal anatomic landmarks at the cardia were seen on more than 95% of double-contrast examinations but on only 20% of single-contrast examinations.[9] Thus, double-contrast technique is essential for evaluating this area.

The radiographic appearance of the cardia on double-contrast studies depends on how firmly it is anchored by the surrounding phrenoesophageal membrane to the esophageal hiatus of the diaphragm. When the cardia is well anchored, protrusion of the distal esophagus into the fundus produces a circular elevation containing four or five stellate folds that radiate to a central point at the gastroesophageal junction (i.e., the cardiac rosette) (Fig. 30-1A).[9,10] This elevation is demarcated from the adjacent fundus by a curved "hooding" fold that surrounds it laterally and superiorly. Several longitudinal folds are usually seen extending inferiorly from the cardiac rosette along the posterior wall of the lesser curvature. However, it should be recognized that the cardiac rosette reflects the closed, resting state of the lower esophageal sphincter, so that this landmark will be transiently obliterated by relaxation of the lower esophageal sphincter during deglutition.[10]

When the cardia is less firmly anchored to the surrounding phrenoesophageal membrane, the cardiac rosette may be visible without an associated protrusion or circular elevation (Fig. 30-1B).[10] With further ligamentous laxity, the rosette itself may vanish and the cardia may be characterized by only

a single undulant or crescentic line that crosses the area of the esophageal orifice (Fig. 30-1C).[10] Finally, severe ligamentous laxity may lead to the formation of a hiatal hernia, so that no cardiac structure is identified below the diaphragm. Instead, gastric folds may converge superiorly to a point several centimeters above the esophageal hiatus (Fig. 30-1D).[10] This finding should therefore suggest a sliding hiatal hernia, and a single-contrast esophagogram should be obtained with the patient in a prone position to confirm the presence of a hernia.

Radiologists should be familiar with the normal radiographic appearances of the cardia, because malignant lesions in this area may be recognized only by distortion, effacement, or obliteration of these landmarks (see later section on Carcinoma of the Cardia).

Z Line

The Z line is an irregular, serrated line that demarcates the squamocolumnar mucosal junction.[6,11] The Z line can sometimes be recognized on double-contrast esophagograms as a thin, radiolucent stripe in the distal esophagus with a characteristic zigzag appearance (Fig. 30-2). Occasionally, however, the Z line can be mistaken for superficial ulceration associated with reflux esophagitis, particularly if the esophagus is not completely distended. Because the Z line represents the histologic squamocolumnar junction, it is usually located at or near the gastroesophageal junction.

Mucosal Ring

A lower esophageal mucosal ring is the most common ringlike narrowing found in the distal esophagus. The ring consists of a membranous ridge that is covered by squamous epithelium superiorly and columnar epithelium inferiorly, so that it corresponds histologically to the squamocolumnar junction.[12,13] This lower esophageal mucosal ring, also known as a B ring, is manifested on barium studies by a thin, weblike area of narrowing at the gastroesophageal junction (Fig. 30-3).[11,13,14] The ring has smooth, symmetrical margins and a height of 2 to 4 mm.[11,13,14] Mucosal rings with a diameter greater than 20 mm rarely cause symptoms.[11] If the diameter of the ring is less than 20 mm, however, it may cause dysphagia and may therefore represent a pathologic finding (see later section on Schatzki Ring).

Lower esophageal mucosal rings are fixed, reproducible structures on barium studies, but the distal esophagus must be adequately distended to visualize these structures. Single-contrast technique with the patient in a prone right anterior oblique position is particularly well suited for demonstrating lower esophageal rings, because it is the best technique for achieving optimal distention of the distal esophagus. It has been shown that more than 50% of lower esophageal rings seen on prone single-contrast views of the esophagus are not visualized on the double-contrast phase of the examination.[3,15] Thus, biphasic studies are required to demonstrate these structures.

Muscular Ring

A muscular or contractile ring, also known as an A ring, is found much less frequently in the distal esophagus than a

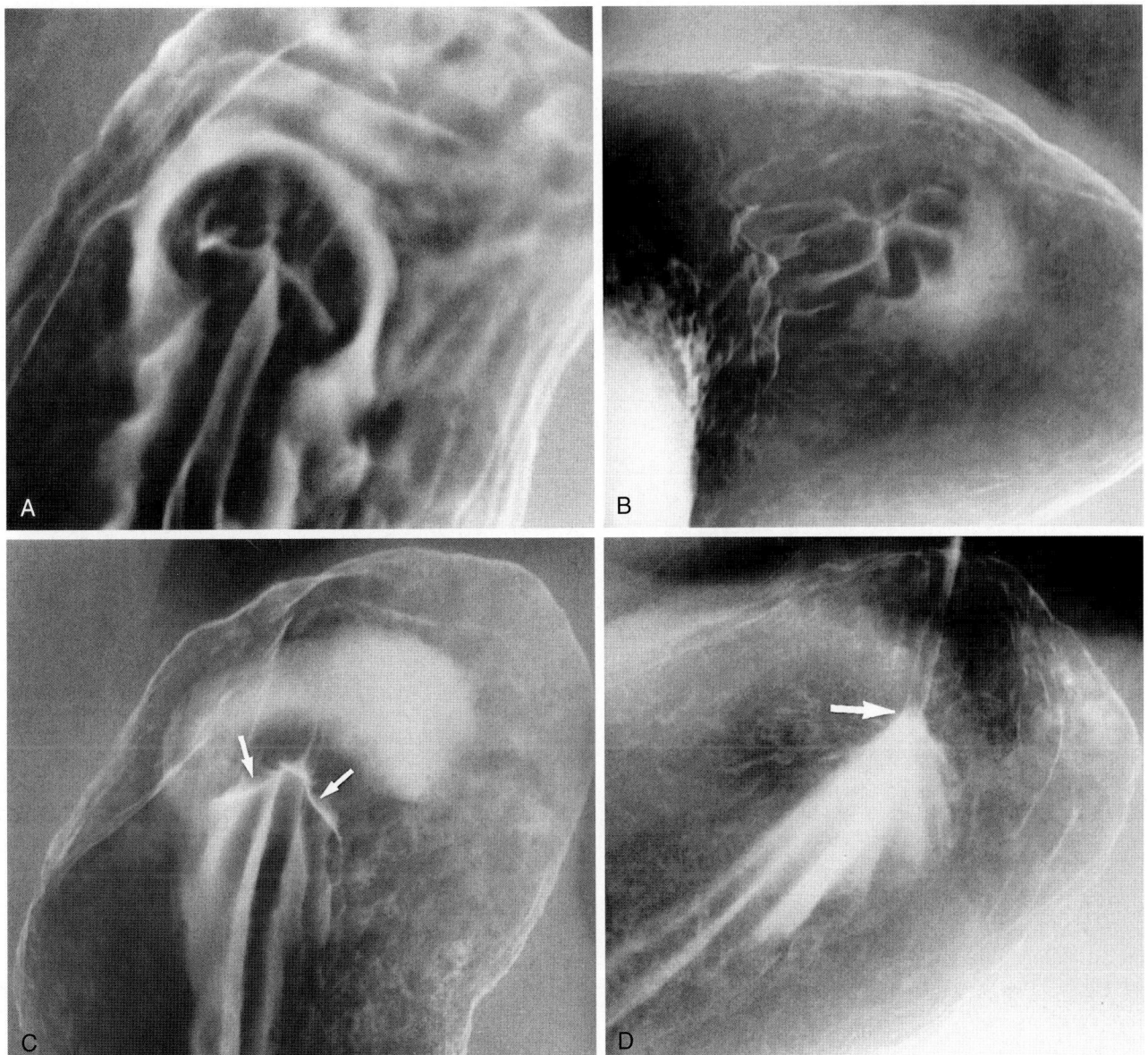

Figure 30-1. Normal appearances of the gastric cardia. A. This patient has a well-anchored cardia appearing as a circular protrusion with centrally radiating folds (i.e., the cardiac rosette). **B.** In another patient, there are stellate folds without a surrounding protrusion because of laxity of the ligaments surrounding the cardia. **C.** Further ligamentous laxity has resulted in obliteration of the cardiac rosette. Instead, this patient has a single crescentic line (*arrows*) at the cardia. **D.** In another patient with severe ligamentous laxity, gastric folds in a small hiatal hernia are seen converging superiorly toward a point (*arrow*) several centimeters above the esophageal hiatus of the diaphragm. (From Levine MS: Radiology of the Esophagus. Philadelphia: WB Saunders, 1989.)

mucosal ring. Muscular rings are located at the proximal end of the esophageal vestibule near the tubulovestibular junction and are completely covered by squamous epithelium.[8] Unlike a mucosal ring, which is a fixed anatomic structure, a muscular ring occurs as a transient physiologic phenomenon resulting from active muscular contraction in the distal esophagus.

A muscular ring usually appears on esophagography as a relatively broad, smooth area of narrowing that changes considerably in caliber and configuration during the fluoroscopic examination (see Fig. 30-3).[7,11,13] Because a muscular ring is caused by active muscular contraction, it may vanish completely with esophageal distention, so that it is observed as a transient finding at fluoroscopy.[7,11,13] Not infrequently, both

mucosal and muscular rings are visible during the same examination (see Fig. 30-3). In such cases, the fixed nature of the mucosal ring distinguishes it from the dynamic, changing appearance of the muscular ring above.

SCHATZKI RING

Although some investigators have used the terms *Schatzki ring* and *lower esophageal ring* interchangeably, Schatzki himself originally described this entity as a pathologically stenotic ring that caused dysphagia.[16] Because most lower esophageal rings do not cause symptoms, they probably should not be called Schatzki rings. Instead, the term should be reserved for

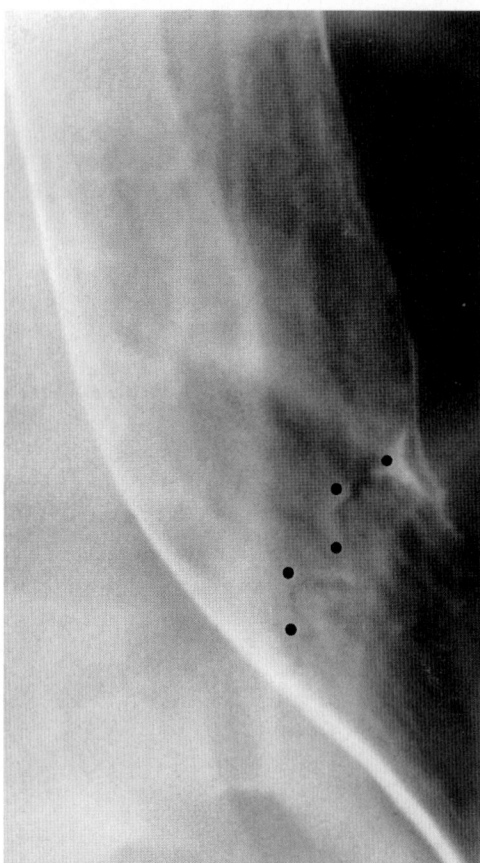

Figure 30-2. Z line. The normal Z line is seen as a thin, zigzagging, radiolucent stripe (*dots*) in the distal esophagus near the gastroesophageal junction. (From Levine MS: Radiology of the Esophagus. Philadelphia: WB Saunders, 1989.)

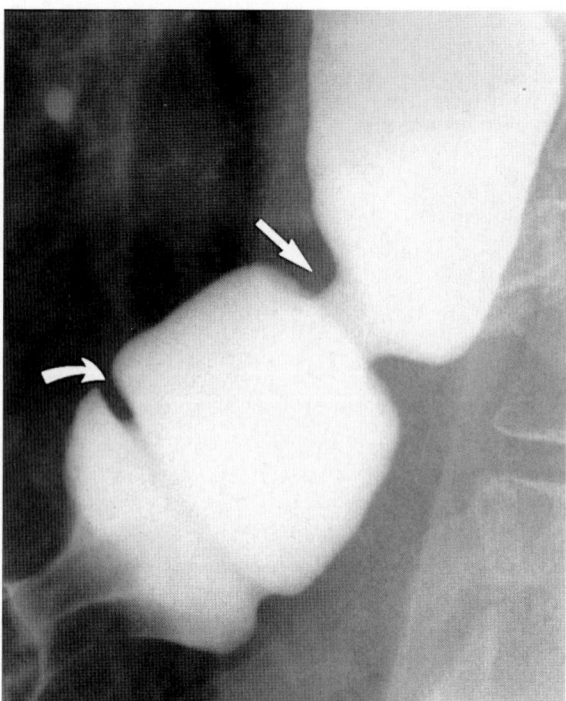

Figure 30-3. Lower esophageal rings. The mucosal ring appears on a prone single-contrast esophagogram as a thin, weblike constriction (*curved arrow*) at the gastroesophageal junction above a small hiatal hernia, whereas the muscular ring appears as a relatively broad area of narrowing (*straight arrow*) near the superior border of the esophageal vestibule. Unlike mucosal rings, muscular rings are often a transient finding at fluoroscopy. (From Levine MS: Radiology of the Esophagus. Philadelphia: WB Saunders, 1989.)

symptomatic patients with narrow-caliber rings at the gastroesophageal junction. Thus, the diagnosis of a Schatzki ring is made on the basis of clinical and radiographic criteria.

Pathogenesis

The pathogenesis of a Schatzki ring is uncertain. Some investigators have favored a congenital origin, but the rarity of symptoms before 50 years of age tends to refute this theory.[6] Other investigators believe that a Schatzki ring represents an annular, ringlike structure caused by scarring from reflux esophagitis.[6,13,17-19] This theory is supported by a study that showed that Schatzki rings progressed or underwent transformation into true peptic strictures on serial radiologic examinations.[18] Nevertheless, it is difficult to explain the frequent absence of reflux symptoms in these patients. The data are therefore inconclusive.

Clinical Findings

Schatzki rings are typically manifested by episodic dysphagia for solids.[15,16,20,21] In a study of 332 patients, Schatzki found that lower esophageal rings less than 13 mm in diameter almost always caused dysphagia, whereas rings greater than 20 mm in diameter almost never caused dysphagia.[20] A statistical analysis of Schatzki's original data 40 years later showed that a 1-mm decrease in ring diameter corresponded to a 46% increase in the likelihood that a patient has dysphagia.[22]

Patients with Schatzki rings may have minimal dysphagia or may be intermittently asymptomatic until a large bolus of food lodges above the ring. Because the most frequent offending agent is an inadequately chewed piece of meat, this condition has been described as the "steak house syndrome."[23] The impacted bolus in the distal esophagus may cause severe chest pain or an uncomfortable "sticking" sensation behind the lower sternum.[24] Resolution of symptoms almost always occurs when the impacted bolus is passed, regurgitated, or removed. Rarely, a prolonged bolus obstruction may lead to esophageal perforation.[13]

Relief from symptoms is often obtained by simply explaining the benign nature of the ring and advising these individuals to eat more slowly and chew their food more carefully. However, patients with recurrent dysphagia may require mechanical disruption of the ring by direct endoscopic rupture, bougienage, electrocautery incision, pneumatic dilatation, or, rarely, surgery.[21,25,26]

Radiographic Findings

A Schatzki ring usually appears on barium studies as a thin (2 to 4 mm in height), weblike constriction (less than 13 mm in diameter) at the gastroesophageal junction (Fig. 30-4).[11,13-16,20] A hiatal hernia is almost always observed below the level of the ring. Except for its smaller caliber, a Schatzki ring therefore has the same appearance and location as an asymptomatic mucosal ring. Almost all rings less than 13 mm in diameter cause dysphagia,[20] so that they may be classified as Schatzki rings on the basis of the radiographic findings. Occasionally,

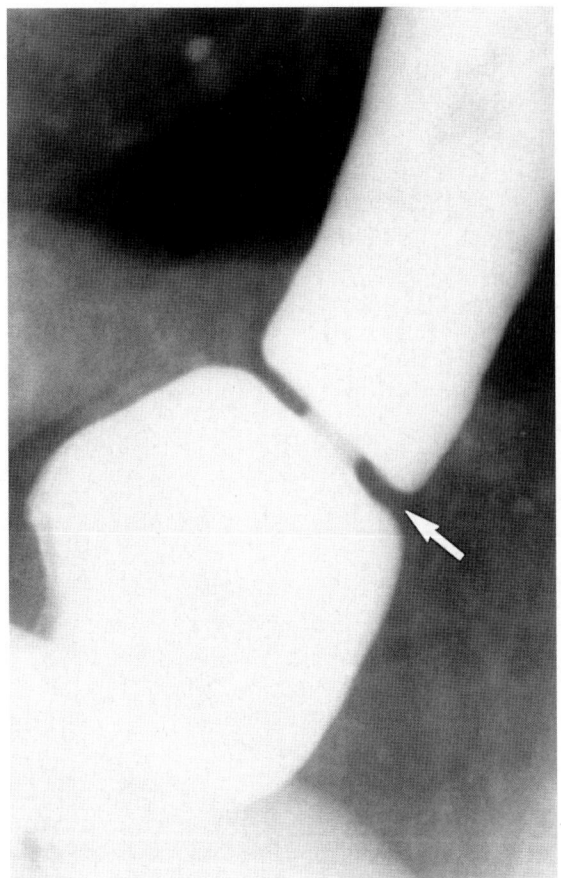

Figure 30-4. Schatzki ring. The ring appears on a prone single-contrast esophagogram as a thin, weblike (less than 13 mm in diameter) constriction (*arrow*) at the gastroesophageal junction above a hiatal hernia. Note that except for its smaller caliber, it has the same appearance and location as an asymptomatic mucosal ring. This patient presented with dysphagia.

however, rings between 13 and 20 mm may also cause symptoms, so that the diagnosis of a Schatzki ring in these patients requires some knowledge of the clinical history.

Like other rings in the lower esophagus, Schatzki rings are visualized on barium studies only if the lumen above and below the ring is distended beyond the caliber of the ring. As a result, single-contrast views of the distal esophagus with the patient prone may demonstrate Schatzki rings that are not visible, even in retrospect, on the double-contrast phase of the examination because of inadequate distention of this region (Fig. 30-5).[3,15] Conversely, overdistention of the hiatal hernia on prone views can result in overlap of the distal end of the esophagus and proximal end of the hernia, producing a double density of two superimposed, convex collections of barium that obscures the region of the gastroesophageal junction and prevents visualization even of high-grade Schatzki rings (Fig. 30-6A).[27] When this "overlap" phenomenon occurs, additional prone views of the distal esophagus should be obtained when the hiatal hernia is less distended to avoid overlap of the hernia and adjacent distal esophagus and allow visualization of these rings (Fig. 30-6B).[27] Carefully performed biphasic esophagography is thought to be even more sensitive than endoscopy for detecting Schatzki rings.[15]

Differential Diagnosis

A Schatzki ring has such a characteristic appearance that the radiographic findings are virtually diagnostic of this entity. Occasionally, however, other abnormalities may produce similar findings. Ringlike peptic strictures constitute as many as 40% of all peptic strictures in the distal esophagus.[28] These strictures often resemble Schatzki rings, but careful analysis may reveal that they have more tapered, asymmetric borders and a slightly greater length (4 to 10 mm) (see Fig. 23-18).[28]

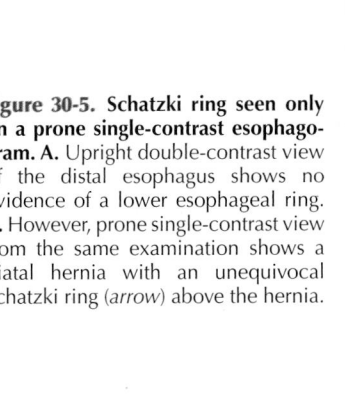

Figure 30-5. Schatzki ring seen only on a prone single-contrast esophagogram. A. Upright double-contrast view of the distal esophagus shows no evidence of a lower esophageal ring. **B.** However, prone single-contrast view from the same examination shows a hiatal hernia with an unequivocal Schatzki ring (*arrow*) above the hernia.

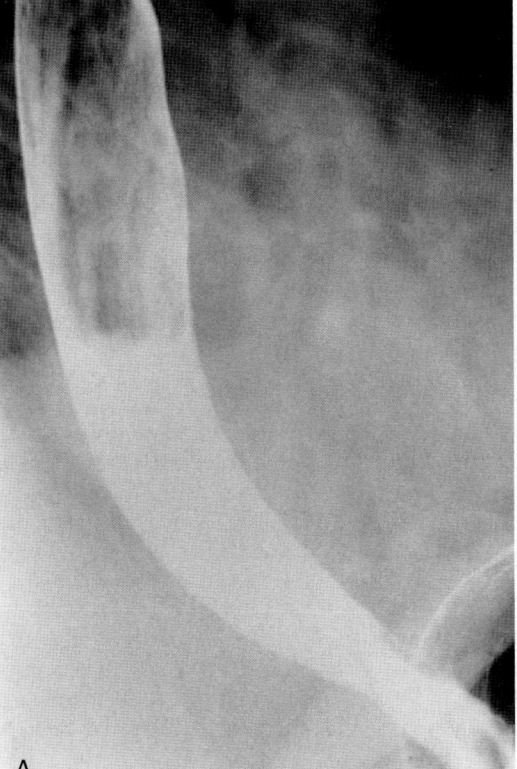

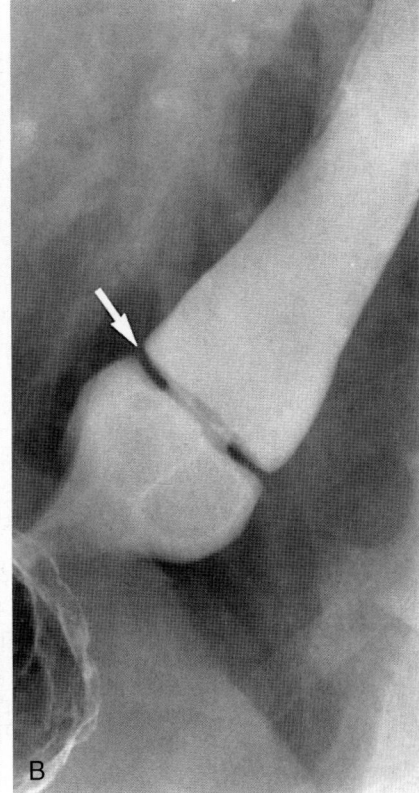

A

B

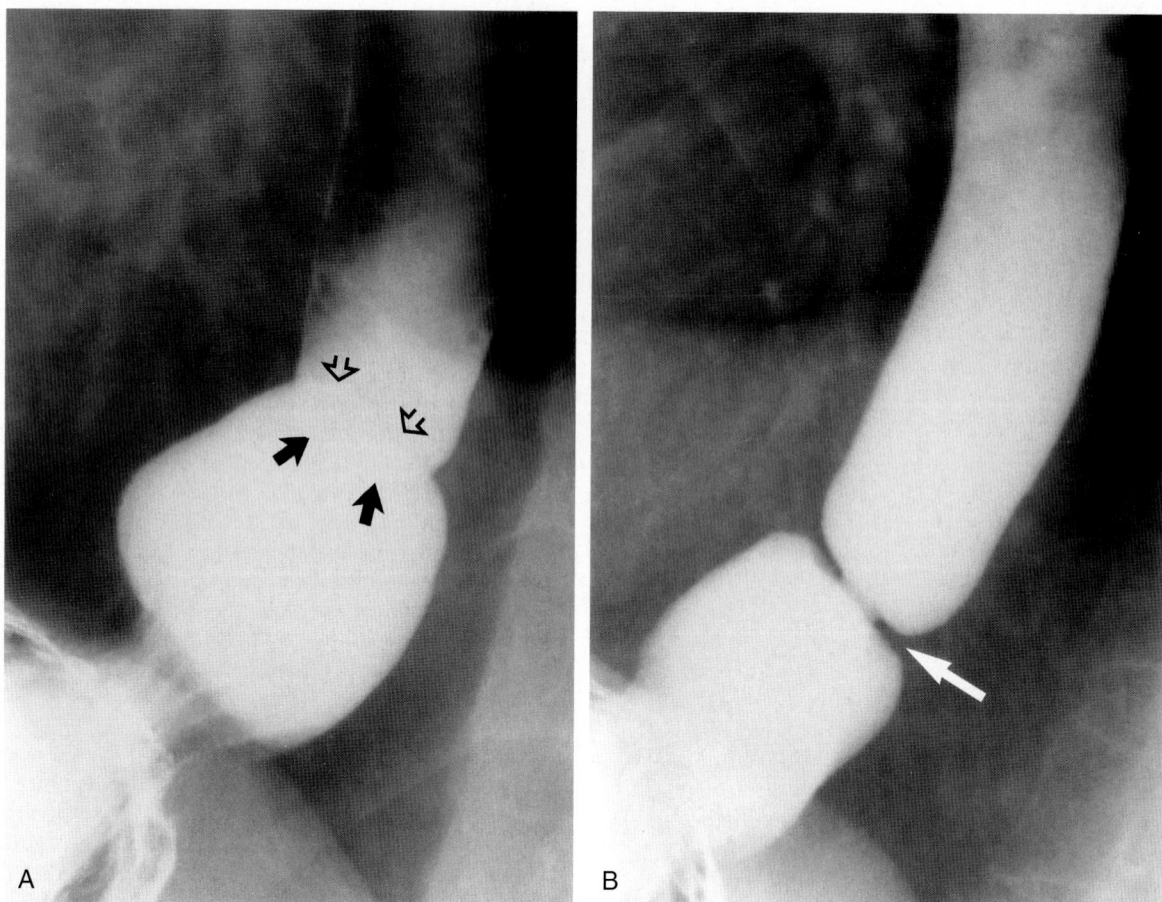

Figure 30-6. Overlap phenomenon obscuring Schatzki ring. A. Prone single-contrast view of the distal esophagus shows a hiatal hernia without evidence of a lower esophageal ring. However, there is a double density with two superimposed convex collections of barium, caused by overlap of the distal end of the esophagus (*solid arrows*) and the proximal end of the hernia (*open arrows*). **B.** Repeat view with less distention of the hernia shows a tight Schatzki ring (*arrow*) when the distal esophagus and adjacent hiatal hernia no longer overlap. (From Hsu WC, MS Levine, Rubesin SE, Overlap phenomenon: A potential pitfall in the radiographic detection of lower esophageal rings, AJR, 180, 745-747, 2003, © by American Roentgen Ray Society.)

Despite these subtle distinctions, there is probably overlap between ringlike peptic strictures and Schatzki rings detected on barium studies or endoscopy.

Esophageal webs may occasionally be found in the distal esophagus adjacent to the gastroesophageal junction.[29] These webs can be mistaken for Schatzki rings, but they tend to be located several centimeters or more above the gastroesophageal junction and are almost always associated with peptic strictures, so that they can usually be differentiated from lower esophageal rings on the basis of the radiographic findings.[29] Rarely, a focally infiltrating esophageal carcinoma can produce a localized constriction that superficially resembles a Schatzki ring. However, the presence of asymmetry, irregularity, and shelflike borders within the narrowed segment should indicate the need for early endoscopy to rule out a malignant lesion.

HIATAL HERNIA

Hiatal hernias are classified either as sliding or paraesophageal hernias, depending on the relationship of the cardia to the diaphragm and herniated portion of the stomach. About 99% of all hiatal hernias are sliding, and the remaining 1% are paraesophageal.[30] Despite its rarity, a paraesophageal hernia, unlike a sliding hernia, is considered to be a potentially life-threatening condition because of the risk of volvulus, incarceration, or strangulation of the herniated portion of the stomach.

Sliding Hiatal Hernia

Pathogenesis

The phrenoesophageal membrane is a firm, elastic structure surrounding the gastroesophageal junction that normally tethers the distal esophagus to the diaphragm and prevents the proximal portion of the stomach from herniating through the esophageal hiatus of the diaphragm into the chest. With aging, however, a lifetime of constant swallowing causes progressive wear and tear on the phrenoesophageal membrane, with eventual stretching or rupture of the membrane and axial herniation of the stomach into the chest.[7,8,30,31] Not surprisingly, the prevalence of hiatal hernias increases with age; 60% of elderly people in the United States are found to have a hiatal hernia on barium studies.[32]

Clinical Significance

Considerable controversy exists about the relationship between a sliding hiatal hernia and the subsequent development of gastroesophageal reflux and reflux esophagitis. Although some investigators believe that a hiatal hernia predisposes to gastroesophageal reflux disease, others believe that a hiatal hernia is of doubtful clinical significance when it occurs as an isolated finding without other clinical or radiologic signs of reflux disease.[33-35] This subject is discussed in greater detail in Chapter 23.

Radiographic Diagnosis

A sliding hiatal hernia may be recognized radiographically when the gastroesophageal junction is located above the esophageal hiatus of the diaphragm. Single-contrast barium studies with the patient prone are more likely to demonstrate a hiatal hernia than are double-contrast studies with the patient upright, because the hernia is frequently reduced into the abdomen in the upright position and because the hernia is more difficult to distend adequately when the patient is standing.[3] The patient should therefore be instructed to continuously drink a thin, low-density barium suspension in the prone right anterior oblique position for optimal demonstration of these structures.

Because a lower esophageal mucosal ring demarcates the anatomic location of the gastroesophageal junction, a sliding hiatal hernia may be diagnosed on barium studies obtained with the patient prone when a mucosal ring is observed 2 cm or more above the diaphragmatic hiatus (see Fig. 30-3).[11] Even in the absence of a definite mucosal ring, a hiatal hernia can often be recognized by the presence of gastric folds within the hernia (Fig. 30-7). These folds may continue inferiorly through the diaphragmatic hiatus into the abdominal portion of the stomach. Not infrequently, the hernia may be kinked or narrowed at the esophageal hiatus because of extrinsic compression by the surrounding diaphragm at this level. Occasionally, a prominent diagonal notch may also be seen on the left lateral and superior aspect of the hernia because of crossing gastric sling fibers at the cardiac incisura (Fig. 30-8).[30]

When a moderate-sized or large hiatal hernia is present, double-contrast views of the stomach obtained with the patient in an upright or right lateral recumbent position also permit assessment of the mucosa within the hernia for ulcers, neoplasms, or other abnormalities not easily seen on single-contrast images. Ulcers are particularly likely to develop at the hiatal orifice (so-called "riding" ulcers), where the gastric mucosa is repeatedly exposed to trauma on the ridge riding over the hiatus (Fig. 30-9).[36] Occasionally, gastric carcinomas that develop within hiatal hernias may be manifested on double-contrast studies by polypoid masses or infiltrative lesions with thickened, distorted folds in the hernia.[37]

When barium studies are performed on patients with large hiatal hernias (i.e., hernias containing 50% or more of the

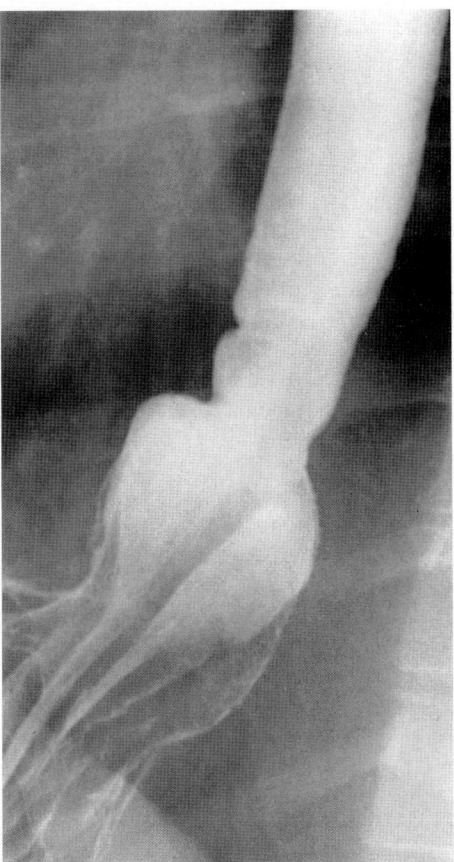

Figure 30-7. Sliding hiatal hernia. Gastric rugae are seen in the hernia on this prone, single-contrast view of the esophagus. (From Levine MS: Radiology of the Esophagus. Philadelphia: WB Saunders, 1989.)

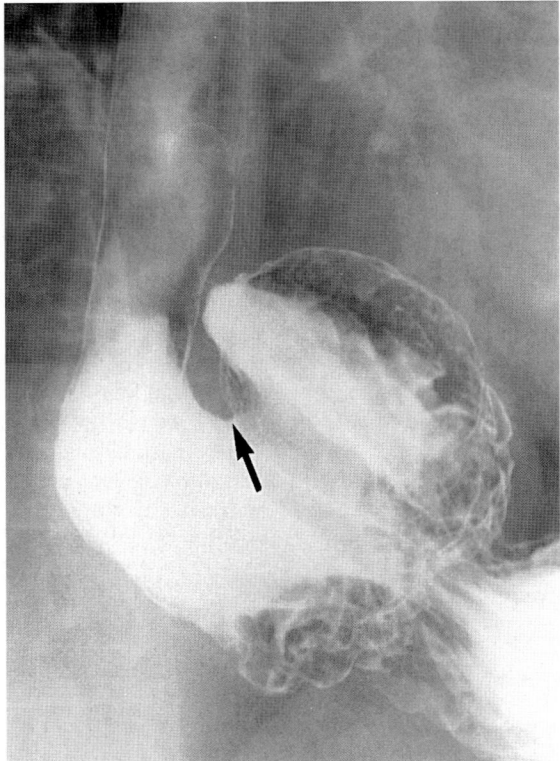

Figure 30-8. Large hiatal hernia. There is a prominent diagonal notch (*arrow*) on the superior aspect of the hernia due to crossing gastric sling fibers at the cardiac incisura. This appearance may erroneously suggest a mixed sliding-paraesophageal hernia. (From Levine MS: Radiology of the Esophagus. Philadelphia: WB Saunders, 1989.)

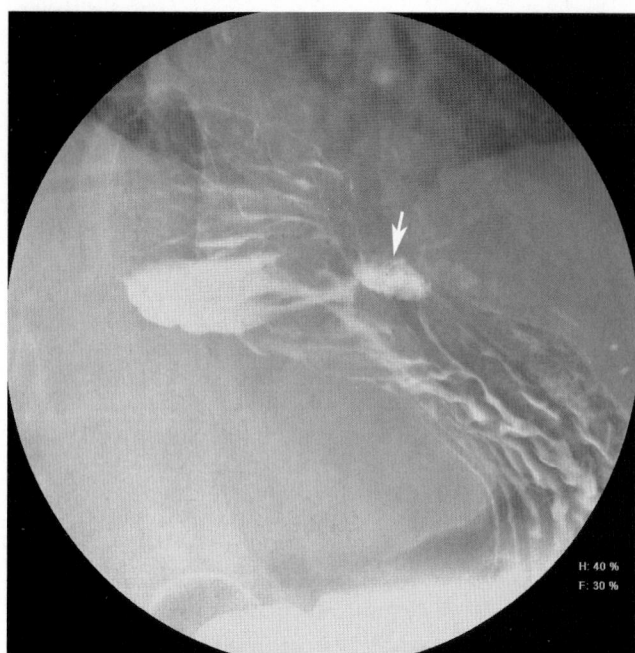

Figure 30-9. Hiatal hernia with a "riding" ulcer. There is a hiatal hernia with a large ulcer (*arrow*) in the proximal stomach where it traverses the esophageal hiatus of the diaphragm, probably because of repeated trauma to the gastric mucosa at the level of the hiatus.

stomach), the weight of the barium may cause the gastric fundus to droop inferiorly beneath the herniated gastric body (especially in the upright position), producing a distinctive radiographic appearance, also known as the "floppy" fundus (Fig. 30-10).[38] These patients may develop symptoms such as postprandial pain, early satiety, nausea, retching, and vomiting because of a mechanical effect of ingested food and liquids pooling in the floppy fundus or because of subsequent traction on the stomach that impedes emptying of the hernia.[38] Because symptoms result from distortion of the gastric anatomy, these symptoms usually resolve only after surgical repair of the hernia.[38]

A large hiatal hernia associated with a floppy fundus can be mistaken on barium studies for an organoaxial gastric volvulus, a potentially life-threatening condition because of the risk of incarceration, strangulation, and infarction of the involved stomach (see Chapter 38).[36,39,40] In organoaxial gastric volvulus, however, most or all of the stomach herniates above the diaphragm into the lower thorax, with the greater curvature of the stomach rotated above the lesser curvature, producing an upside-down intrathoracic stomach.[41,42] In contrast, normal anatomic relationships are preserved in patients with a floppy fundus.

Paraesophageal Hernia

Pathogenesis

In the rare paraesophageal hernia, a portion of the stomach herniates through the esophageal hiatus into the chest alongside the distal esophagus, while the cardia retains its normal position below the diaphragm. The hernia is thought to occur through a localized weakness or defect in the phrenoesophageal membrane.[36] These patients may eventually develop a

mixed sliding-paraesophageal hernia if the gastroesophageal junction also rises above the diaphragm.[43] Rarely, the entire stomach or a major portion of the stomach herniates through the esophageal hiatus, producing a gastric volvulus (see Chapter 38).

Clinical Significance

Many patients with paraesophageal hernias are asymptomatic, and the hernia is an incidental finding on barium studies performed for other reasons. Unlike sliding hiatal hernias, paraesophageal hernias are rarely associated with gastroesophageal reflux or reflux esophagitis. As the hernias enlarge, however, these patients can develop serious complications such as obstruction, incarceration, strangulation, and infarction.[43-47] Because of these potentially life-threatening complications, some authors believe that surgery is warranted in all patients with paraesophageal hernias (assuming they are surgical candidates), even if these patients are asymptomatic.[48,49] However, not all authors favor such an aggressive approach in elderly, often debilitated patients with paraesophageal hernias because of the high risk of surgery in this group. Laparoscopic repair of paraesophageal hernias has been advocated as a less invasive technique than traditional surgery.[50]

Radiographic Diagnosis

A paraesophageal hernia may be diagnosed on barium studies when the gastric fundus has herniated through the esophageal hiatus of the diaphragm alongside the distal esophagus while the cardia retains its normal position below the diaphragm (Fig. 30-11). In a mixed sliding-paraesophageal hernia, however, the cardia has also herniated above the diaphragm into the chest (Fig. 30-12). Occasionally, a sliding hiatal hernia can be mistaken radiographically for a mixed sliding-paraesophageal hernia because of a prominent notch on the superior aspect of the hernia that erroneously suggests a paraesophageal component (see Fig. 30-8).[30]

In patients with a gastric volvulus or upside-down, intrathoracic stomach, almost the entire stomach has herniated through the esophageal hiatus into the chest and has assumed an inverted or upside-down configuration (see Chapter 38). Rarely, traction or torsion of the stomach at or near the level of the hiatus may lead to obstruction, infarction, or perforation of the intrathoracic stomach.[41] These patients may undergo surgery on an emergent basis without preoperative barium studies because of their rapidly deteriorating clinical condition.

CARCINOMA OF THE CARDIA

The clinical and radiographic aspects of carcinoma of the cardia are discussed in detail in Chapter 36. On barium studies, advanced lesions at the cardia may appear as obvious exophytic or infiltrating lesions in the gastric fundus. However, other lesions at the cardia may be recognized only by relatively subtle nodularity, mass effect, or ulceration in this region with distortion, effacement, or obliteration of the normal anatomic landmarks at the cardia (Fig. 30-13).[9,10,51,52] Because these abnormalities at the cardia are extremely difficult to demonstrate on conventional single-contrast barium studies,

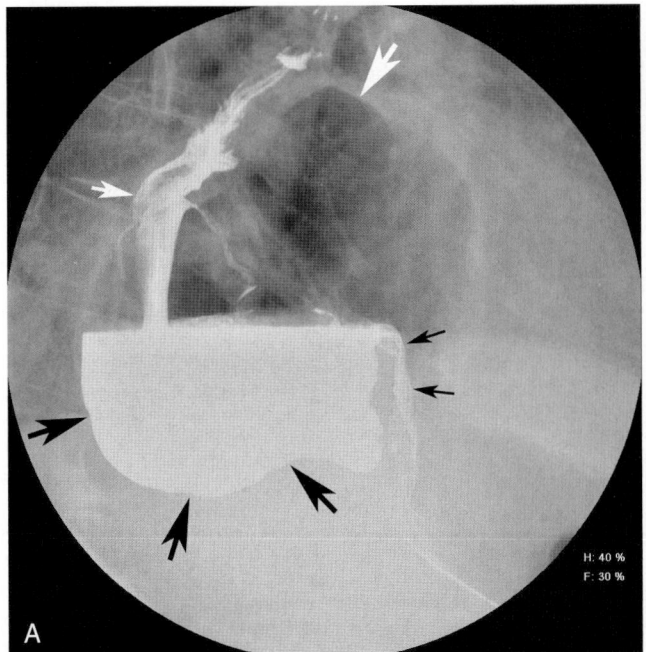

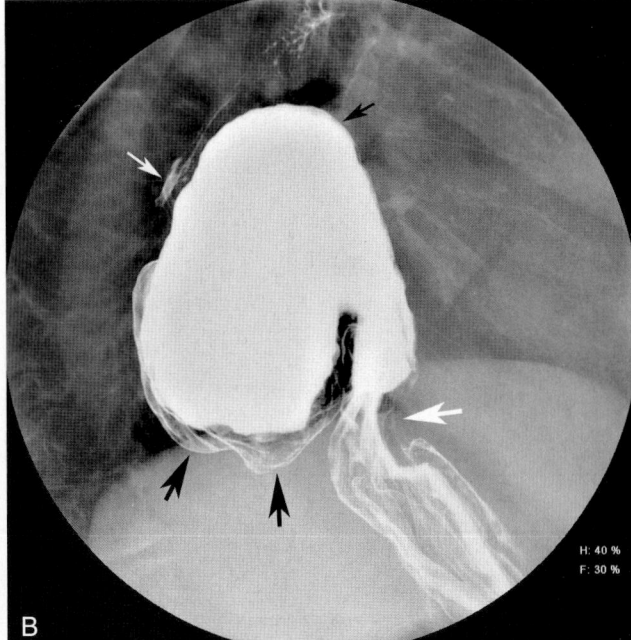

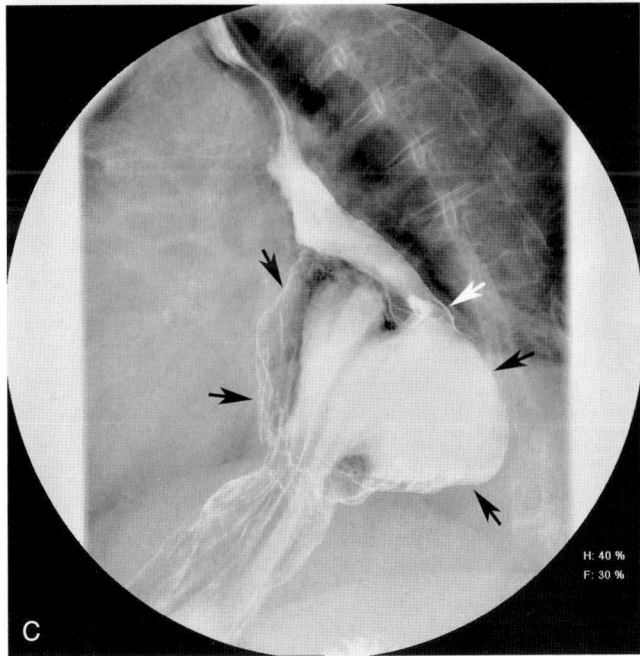

Figure 30-10. Large hiatal hernia with a "floppy" fundus. A. Upright double-contrast view shows a large hiatal hernia with the gastric fundus (*large black arrows*) flopping inferiorly beneath the most superior portion of the gas-filled gastric body (*large white arrow*). Note how there is pooling of barium in the floppy fundus, with a small amount of barium spilling over into the portion of the stomach (*small black arrows*) that traverses the diaphragm. **B.** Supine oblique view also shows a floppy fundus (*large black arrows*) inferior to the most superior portion of the gastric body (*small black arrow*). Again note how there is narrowing of the stomach (*large white arrow*) where it traverses the diaphragm. **C.** Prone oblique view now shows the gastric fundus (*black arrows*) in its expected location above the intrathoracic portion of the gastric body, so that the fundus is no longer flopped inferiorly. (In **A**, **B**, and **C**, the small white arrows denote the location of the gastroesophageal junction above the diaphragm.) (From Huang SY, Levine MS, Rubesin SE, et al: Large hiatal hernias with a floppy fundus. AJR 188:960-964, 2007, © by American Roentgen Ray Society.)

double-contrast technique is essential for detecting these lesions at the earliest possible stage.

PROLAPSED ESOPHAGOGASTRIC MUCOSA

Retrograde or antegrade prolapse of mucosa in the esophagogastric region may produce a polypoid filling defect in the distal esophagus or gastric fundus (Fig. 30-14A).[53,54] However, mucosal prolapse usually occurs as a transient phenomenon, so that the filling defect intermittently vanishes at fluoroscopy (Fig. 30-14B). The distal esophagus may also invaginate into a sliding hiatal hernia or a hiatal hernia may invaginate into the fundus, producing an apparent mass lesion (Fig. 30-15A).[55]

However, greater distention of the fundus with barium or gas usually displaces an invaginated hernia above the diaphragm and reduces the invaginated distal esophagus, so that this lesion is also observed as a transient finding during the radiologic examination (Fig. 30-15B). Thus, it is usually possible to differentiate prolapsed esophagogastric mucosa or invaginated hernias from true polypoid lesions at the cardia.

OTHER ABNORMALITIES

Other abnormalities occurring at or near the gastroesophageal junction include peptic strictures (see Chapter 23), inflammatory esophagogastric polyps (see Chapter 23), esophageal or gastric varices (see Chapters 29 and 38), primary or secondary

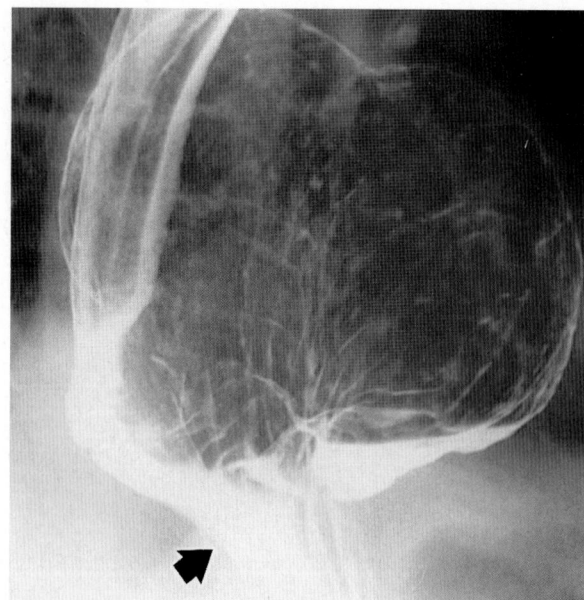

Figure 30-11. Paraesophageal hernia. The gastric fundus has herniated into the chest alongside the distal esophagus, but the gastric cardia (*arrow*) retains its normal position below the diaphragm. (From Levine MS: Radiology of the Esophagus. Philadelphia: WB Saunders, 1989.)

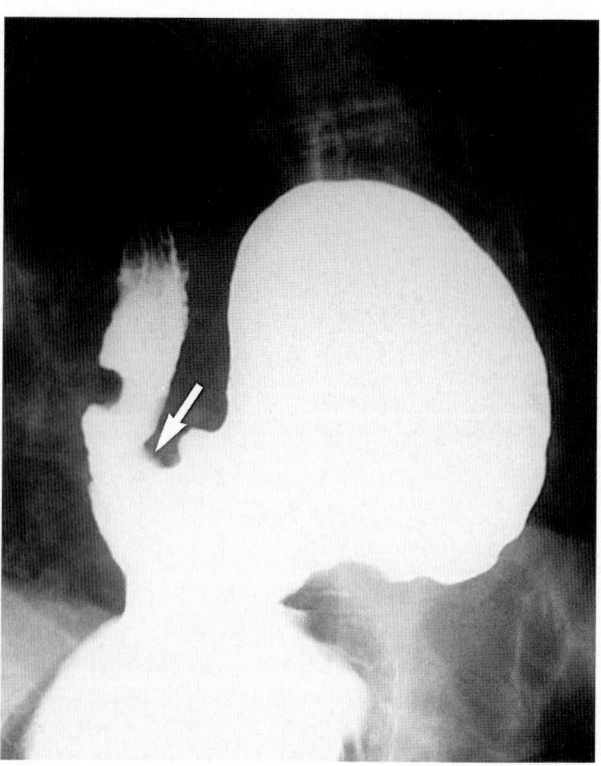

Figure 30-12. Mixed sliding-paraesophageal hernia. The gastric fundus has herniated into the chest alongside the distal esophagus. In this patient, however, the cardia (*arrow*) has also herniated above the diaphragm. These are features of a mixed hernia.

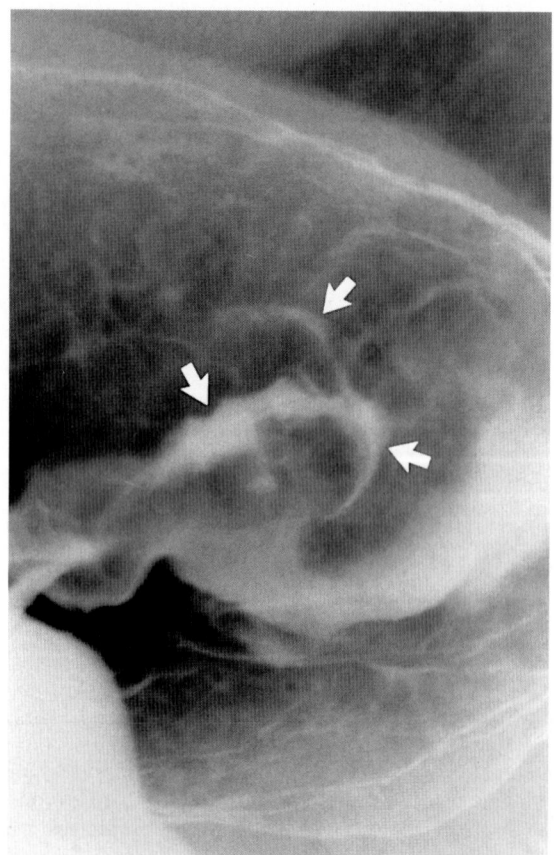

Figure 30-13. Carcinoma of the gastric cardia. The normal anatomic landmarks at the cardia have been obliterated and replaced by irregular areas of ulceration (*arrows*) due to tumor in this region. (From Levine MS: Radiology of the Esophagus. Philadelphia: WB Saunders, 1989.)

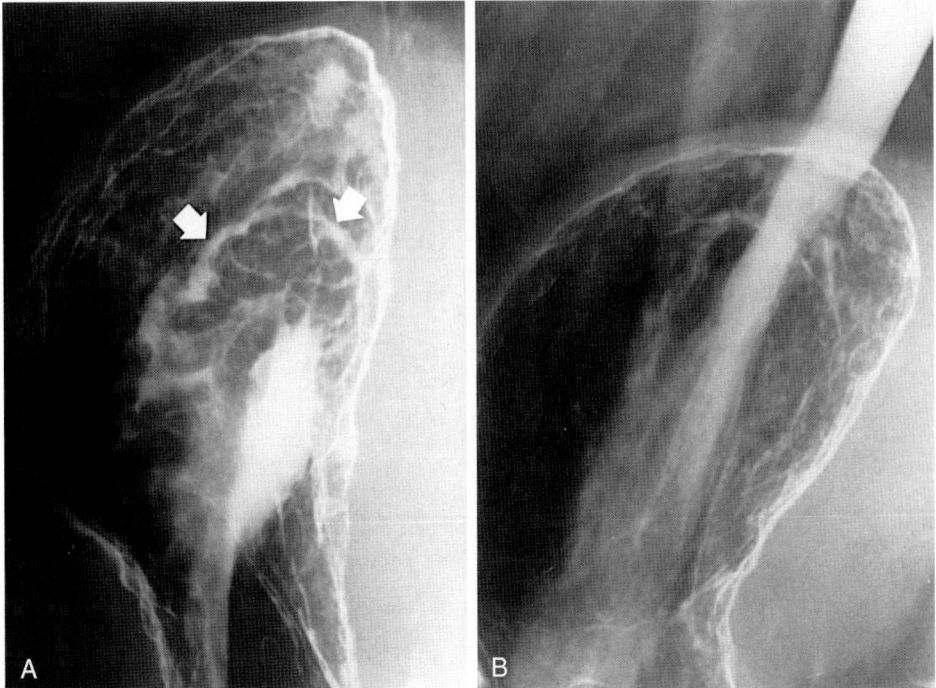

Figure 30-14. Pseudotumor in the gastric fundus due to retrograde prolapse of esophagogastric mucosa. A. Initial double-contrast view of the stomach shows an apparent polypoid mass (*arrows*) in the fundus at the expected location of the cardia. **B.** Repeat view as the patient swallows additional barium shows a normal fundus. This pseudotumor was caused by intermittent retrograde prolapse of mucosa in the esophagogastric region.

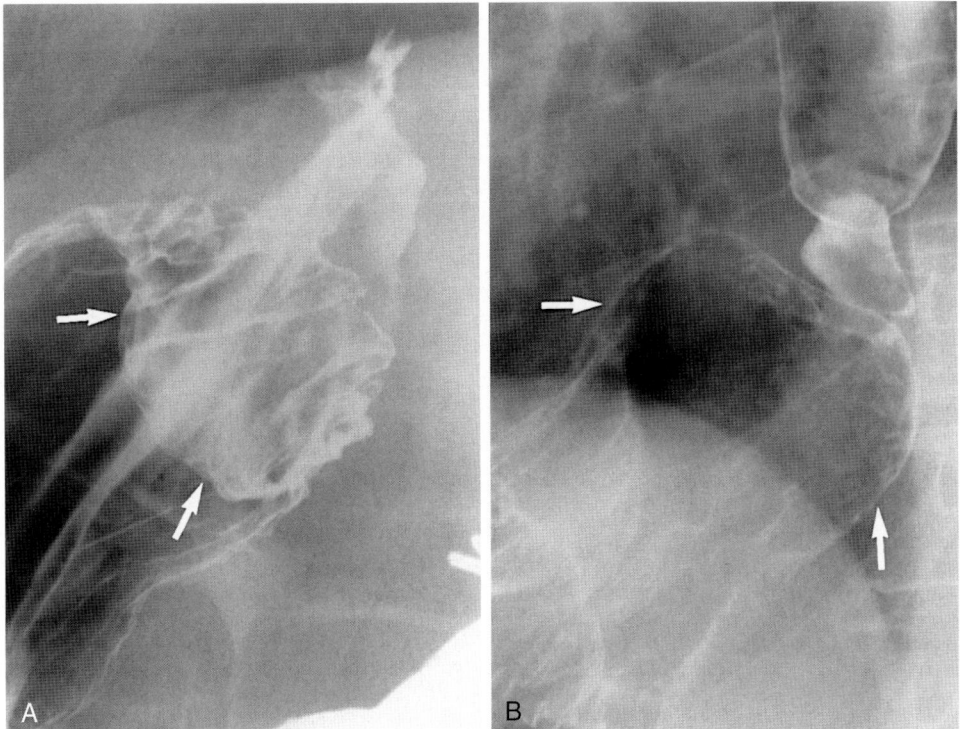

Figure 30-15. Pseudotumor in the gastric fundus due to an invaginated hiatal hernia. A. An apparent mass lesion (*arrows*) is seen in the fundus on a double-contrast radiograph. **B.** Moments later, the invaginated hernia (*arrows*) has risen above the diaphragm, and the pseudotumor is no longer seen.

achalasia (see Chapters 22 and 28), and squamous cell metastases to the cardia (see Chapter 27).

References

1. Levine MS, Rubesin SE, Herlinger H, et al: Double-contrast upper gastrointestinal examination: Technique and interpretation. Radiology 168:593-602, 1988.
2. Levine MS, Rubesin SE: Radiologic investigation of dysphagia. AJR 154:1157-1163, 1990.
3. Chen YM, Ott DJ, Gelfand DW, et al: Multiphasic examination of the esophagogastric region for strictures, rings, and hiatal hernia: Evaluation of the individual techniques. Gastrointest Radiol 10:311-316, 1985.
4. Wolf BS: Use of a half-inch barium tablet to detect minimal esophageal strictures. J Mt Sinai Hosp 28:80-95, 1961.
5. Ott DJ, Kelley TF, Chen YM, et al: Evaluation of the esophagus with a marshmallow bolus: Clarifying the cause of dysphagia. Gastrointest Radiol 16:1-4, 1991.
6. Friedland GW: Historical review of the changing concepts of lower esophageal anatomy: 430 B.C.-1977. AJR 131:373-388, 1978.
7. Wolf BS, Heitmann P, Cohen BR: The inferior esophageal sphincter, the manometric high pressure zone and hiatal incompetence. AJR 103:251-276, 1968.
8. Dodds WJ: Current concepts of esophageal motor function: Clinical implications for radiology. AJR 128:549-561, 1977.
9. Freeny PC: Double-contrast gastrography of the fundus and cardia: Normal landmarks and their pathologic changes. AJR 133:481-487, 1979.
10. Herlinger H, Grossman R, Laufer I, et al: The gastric cardia in double-contrast study: Its dynamic image. AJR 135:21-29, 1980.
11. Ott DJ, Gelfand DW, Wu WC, et al: Esophagogastric region and its rings. AJR 142:281-287, 1984.
12. Johnston JR, Griffin JC: Anatomic location of the lower esophageal ring. Surgery 61:528-534, 1967.
13. Goyal RK, Glancy JJ, Spiro HM: Lower esophageal ring. N Engl J Med 282:1298-1305, 1970.
14. Schatzki R, Gary JE: The lower esophageal ring. AJR 75:246-261, 1956.
15. Ott DJ, Chen YM, Wu WC, et al: Radiographic and endoscopic sensitivity in detecting lower esophageal mucosal ring. AJR 147:261-265, 1986.
16. Schatzki R, Gary JE: Dysphagia due to a diaphragm-like localized narrowing in the lower esophagus ("lower esophageal ring"). AJR 70:911-922, 1953.
17. Scharschmidt BF, Watts HD: The lower esophageal ring and esophageal reflux. Am J Gastroenterol 69:544-549, 1978.
18. Chen YM, Gelfand DW, Ott DJ, et al: Natural progression of the lower esophageal mucosal ring. Gastrointest Radiol 12:93-98, 1987.
19. Marshall JB, Kretschmar JM, Diaz-Arias AA: Gastroesophageal reflux as a pathogenic factor in the development of symptomatic lower esophageal rings. Arch Intern Med 150:1669-1672, 1990.
20. Schatzki R: The lower esophageal ring: Long term follow-up of symptomatic and asymptomatic rings. AJR 90:805-810, 1963.
21. DeVault KR: Lower esophageal (Schatzki's) ring: Pathogenesis, diagnosis and therapy. Dig Dis 14:323-329, 1996.
22. Pezzullo JC, Lewicki AM: Schatzki ring, statistically reexamined. Radiology 228:609-613, 2003.
23. Norton RA, King GD: "Steak house syndrome": The symptomatic lower esophageal ring. Lahey Clin Found Bull 13:55-59, 1963.
24. Desai DC, Rider JA, Puletti EJ, et al: Lower esophageal ring. Gastrointest Endosc 15:100-105, 1968.
25. Arvanitakis C: Lower esophageal ring: Endoscopic and therapeutic aspects. Gastrointest Endosc 24:17-18, 1977.
26. Burdick JS, Venu RP, Hogan WJ: Cutting the defiant lower esophageal ring. Gastrointest Endosc 39:616-619, 1993.
27. Hsu WC, Levine MS, Rubesin SE: Overlap phenomenon: A potential pitfall in the radiographic detection of lower esophageal rings. AJR 180:745-747, 2003.
28. Gupta S, Levine MS, Rubesin SE, et al: Usefulness of barium studies for differentiating benign and malignant strictures of the esophagus. AJR 180:737-744, 2003.
29. Weaver JW, Kaude JV, Hamlin DJ: Webs of the lower esophagus: A complication of gastroesophageal reflux? AJR 142:289-292, 1984.
30. Dodds WJ: Esophagus and esophagogastric region. In Margulis AR, Burhenne HJ (eds): Alimentary Tract Radiology, 3rd ed. St. Louis, CV Mosby, 1983, pp 529-603.
31. Wolf BS: Sliding hiatal hernia: The need for redefinition. AJR 117:231-247, 1973.
32. Ellis H: Diaphragmatic hernia—a diagnostic challenge. Postgrad Med J 62:325-327, 1986.
33. Cohen S, Harris LD: Does hiatus hernia affect competence of the gastroesophageal sphincter? N Engl J Med 284:1053-1056, 1971.
34. Behar J: Reflux esophagitis: Pathogenesis, diagnosis, and management. Arch Intern Med 136:560-566, 1976.
35. Wright RA, Hurwitz AL: Relationship of hiatal hernia to endoscopically proved reflux esophagitis. Dig Dis Sci 24:311-313, 1979.
36. Skinner DB: Hernias (hiatal, traumatic, and congenital). In Berk JE (ed): Bockus Gastroenterology, 4th ed. Philadelphia, WB Saunders, 1985, pp 705-716.
37. Maglinte DDT, Ghahremani GG, Gin FM, et al: Radiologic features of carcinomas arising in hiatal hernias. AJR 166:789-794, 1996.
38. Huang SY, Levine MS, Rubesin SE: Large hiatal hernias with a floppy fundus. AJR 188:960-964, 2007.
39. Babb RR, Peck OC, Jamplis RW: Gastric volvulus and obstruction in paraesophageal hiatus hernia: A surgical emergency. Am J Dig Dis 17:119-128, 1972.
40. McArthur KE: Hernias and volvulus of the gastrointestinal tract. In Feldman M, Scharschmidt BF, Sleisenger MH (eds): Sleisenger & Fordtran's Gastrointestinal and Liver Disease, 6th ed. Philadelphia, WB Saunders, 1998, pp 317-331.
41. Gerson DE, Lewicki AM: Intrathoracic stomach: When does it obstruct? Radiology 119:257-264, 1976.
42. Abbara S, Kalan MMH, Lewicki AM: Intrathoracic stomach revisited. AJR 181:403-414, 2003.
43. Wo JM, Branum GD, Hunter JG, et al: Clinical features of type III (mixed) paraesophageal hernia. Am J Gastroenterol 91:914-916, 1996.
44. Shocket E, Neber J, Drosg RE: The acutely obstructed, incarcerated paraesophageal hiatal hernia. Am J Surg 108:805-810, 1964.
45. Hill LD: Incarcerated paraesophageal hernia: A surgical emergency. Am J Surg 126:286-291, 1973.
46. Dunn DB, Quick G: Incarcerated paraesophageal hernia. Am J Emerg Med 8:36-39, 1990.
47. Landreneau RJ, Hazelrigg SR, Johnson JA, et al: The giant paraesophageal hernia: A particularly morbid condition of the esophageal hiatus. Mo Med 87:884-888, 1990.
48. Vitelli CE, Jaffe BM, Kahng KU: Paraesophageal hernia. N Y State J Med 89:654-657, 1989.
49. Landreneau RJ, Johnson JA, Marshall JB, et al: Clinical spectrum of paraesophageal herniation. Dig Dis Sci 37:537-544, 1992.
50. Oddsdottir M, Franco AL, Laycock WS, et al: Laparoscopic repair of paraesophageal hernia: New access, old technique. Surg Endosc 9:164-168, 1995.
51. Freeny PC, Marks WM: Adenocarcinoma of the gastroesophageal junction: Barium and CT examination. AJR 138:1077-1084, 1982.
52. Levine MS, Laufer I, Thompson JJ: Carcinoma of the gastric cardia in young people. AJR 140:69-72, 1983.
53. Kaye JJ, Stassa G: Mimicry and deception in the diagnosis of tumors of the gastric cardia. AJR 110:295-303, 1970.
54. Rudnick JP, Ferrucci JT, Eaton SB, et al: Esophageal pseudotumor: Retrograde prolapse of gastric mucosa into the esophagus. AJR 115:253-256, 1972.
55. Ghahremani GG, Collins PA: Esophago-gastric invagination in patients with sliding hiatus hernia. Gastrointest Radiol 1:253-261, 1976.

Postoperative Esophagus

Stephen E. Rubesin, MD • Noel N. Williams, MD

GENERAL PRINCIPLES

Radiologic evaluation of the postoperative esophagus requires an understanding of the operative procedures and of the normal postoperative radiologic appearances. The purpose of the radiologic examination is (1) to define the postoperative anatomy and establish a baseline; (2) to assess the efficacy of the procedure; and (3) to detect complications during the early (<4 weeks after surgery) or late (>4 weeks after surgery) postoperative periods.[1-5] During the early postoperative period, the most common complications include stasis resulting from adynamic ileus or vagotomy, obstruction resulting from anastomotic edema, and perforation resulting from anastomotic breakdown (Table 31-1).[1-5] During the late postoperative period, the most common complications include aspiration, gastroesophageal reflux, anastomotic strictures, and recurrent tumor (see Table 31-1).[1-5]

An anastomotic or staple line leak is the most common serious complication of esophageal surgery (Fig. 31-1). Sutures and staples hold less well in the esophagus than elsewhere in the gastrointestinal tract because the esophagus lacks a serosa, the esophageal muscle is stringy and soft, and the mucosa retracts from the cut esophageal margin because of mobility between the squamous mucosa, fatty submucosa, and muscularis propria.[2] A delay in the diagnosis of postoperative perforation leads to an increased morbidity and mortality resulting from mediastinitis, abscess formation, or sepsis.[4] Postoperative patients complaining of cervical, thoracic, or epigastric pain, fever, dysphagia, or respiratory distress may therefore require an emergent esophagogram. At our institution, esophagograms are routinely performed between

Table 31–1
Complications of Esophageal Surgery

Early Complications
Common
    Anastomotic or staple line leak
    Anastomotic narrowing
    Gastric or duodenal atony
    Aspiration
    Gastroesophageal reflux
    Delayed bypass emptying
        Anastomotic edema
        Anastomotic narrowing
        Gastric/duodenal atony
        Obstruction at diaphragm
            Pyloric channel obstruction or spasm
Uncommon
    Pneumothorax
    Pneumomediastinum
    Mediastinal hematoma
    Empyema
    Vocal cord paresis
    Chylothorax
    Ischemia of colonic or jejunal bypass
    Splenic injury
    Pancreatitis

Late Complications
Common
    Anastomotic stricture
    Aspiration
    Recurrent carcinoma
    Gastroesophageal reflux and its sequelae
Uncommon
    Delayed conduit emptying
    Tracheoesophageal fistula
    Anastomotic or staple line leak

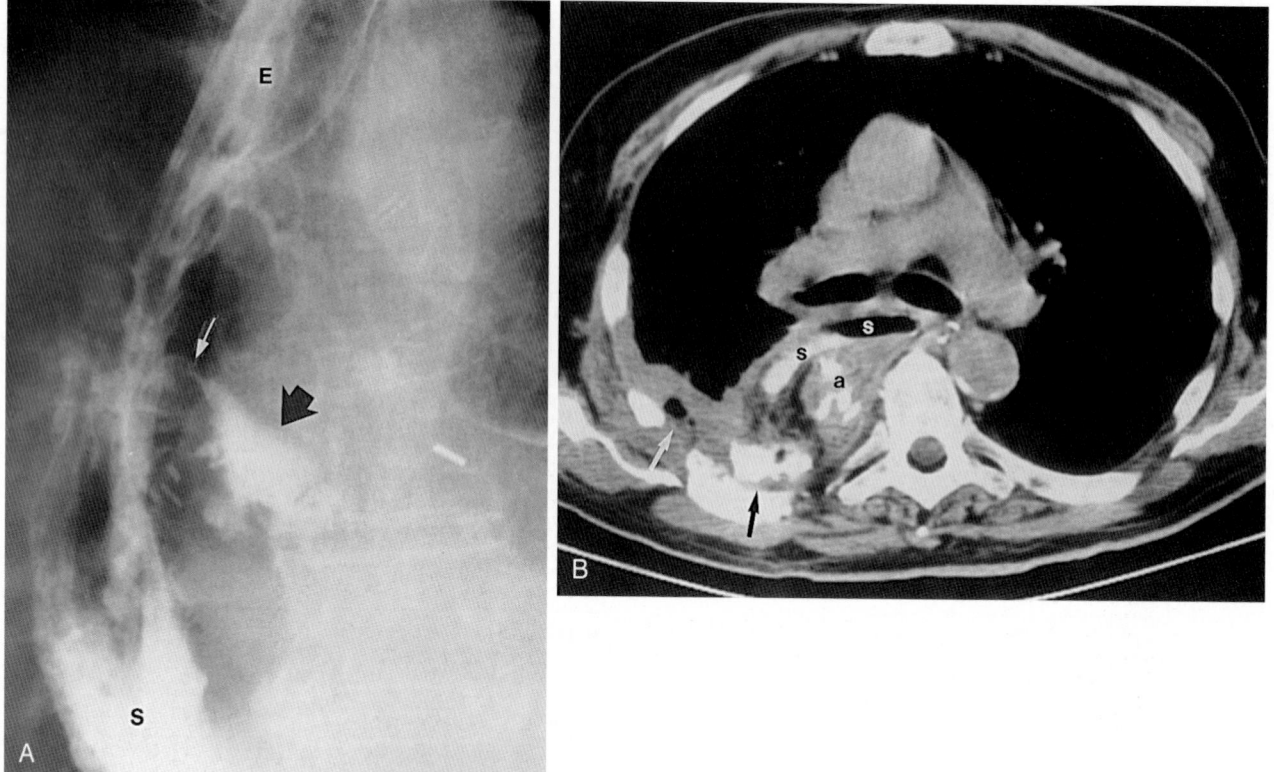

Figure 31-1. **Esophagogastrectomy with leak near esophagogastric anastomosis resulting in mediastinal abscess and empyema. A.** A collection filled with water-soluble contrast medium (*black arrow*) lies medial to the esophagogastric anastomosis. A thin track (*white arrow*) runs from the esophagogastric anastomosis to the collection. The esophagus (E) and stomach (S) are identified. **B.** CT at the level of the carina shows an extrinsic mass impression on the stomach (s) by a contrast-filled abscess (a) in the mediastinum. An empyema is manifested by contrast and gas collections (*arrows*) and associated soft tissue thickening in the pleural space. (Reproduced with permission from Rubesin SE, Beatty SM: The postoperative esophagus. Semin Roentgenol 39:401-410, 1994.)

the sixth and the eighth postoperative days, because some patients with esophageal perforation are asymptomatic and others have delayed leaks.[6] In contrast, gastric, small intestinal, or colonic anastomoses are not routinely evaluated in asymptomatic patients.

Edema, hemorrhage, and spasm at an anastomosis are the most common causes of obstruction in the early postoperative period. This obstruction usually resolves within 1 to 2 weeks after surgery. Obstruction may also occur where the viscus used as the esophageal substitute passes through the diaphragm (Fig. 31-2). In the late postoperative period, obstruction is usually caused by a benign stricture related to a healed anastomotic leak, ischemia at the anastomosis, or chronic gastroesophageal reflux. Other patients may have recurrent cancer or a tight diaphragmatic hiatus as the cause of this finding.

Esophageal dysmotility, delayed gastric emptying caused by pylorospasm or gastric atony, or diarrhea may be the result of manipulation, damage, or intentional surgical resection of the vagus nerve. Vocal cord paralysis or dysphagia with abnormal motility of the inferior constrictor muscles or proximal esophageal muscles may result from recurrent laryngeal injury.

Any form of esophageal surgery that disrupts the lower esophageal sphincter may result in gastroesophageal reflux. An antireflux procedure may be included as part of the esophagogastric anastomosis to prevent gastroesophageal reflux and

aspiration. The sequelae of postoperative gastroesophageal reflux include aspiration, reflux esophagitis, stricture formation, Barrett's esophagus, and adenocarcinoma arising in Barrett's esophagus.

The thoracic duct may also be damaged during surgery. The thoracic duct passes superiorly, anterior to the spine, between the aorta and the azygous vein. At the level of the T5 vertebral body, the thoracic duct crosses behind the esophagus and then continues cranially along the left side of the esophagus. Although uncommon, thoracic duct damage may result in chylothorax or chylous ascites.[2]

Early postoperative complications may be manifested by a variety of findings on chest and abdominal radiographs. A dilated viscus with air-fluid levels should suggest gastric outlet obstruction when the stomach is used to replace the esophagus. Pneumomediastinum, cervical or subcutaneous emphysema, a widened mediastinum, or a rapidly enlarging pleural effusion should suggest anastomotic breakdown and perforation.[7] Nevertheless, chest and abdominal radiographs may be normal in patients with perforation.

Laparoscopic surgery was introduced into routine surgical practice in the early 1990s and has been applied to several disorders of the esophagus.[4,5] Laparoscopic surgery is based on the principle of a minimally invasive approach to surgical problems that traditionally required open operations. Laparoscopic surgery is performed with the use of videoscopically guided instruments to allow dissection of anatomic structures

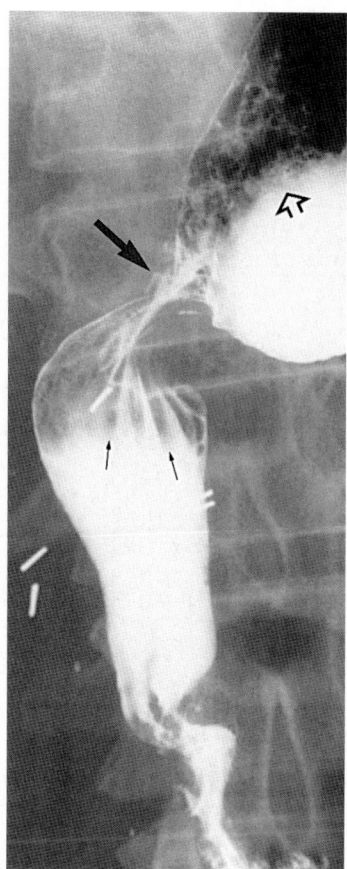

Figure 31-2. Postoperative obstruction after esophagogastrectomy. There is tapered narrowing of the stomach (*large arrow*) where it passes through the diaphragm. Below the diaphragm, twisting of the stomach is manifested radiographically by gastric folds (*small arrows*) radiating toward the area of narrowing. The stomach proximal to the obstruction shows dilatation, delayed emptying of barium, and retained debris (*open arrow*). (Reproduced with permission from Rubesin SE, Beatty SM: The postoperative esophagus. Semin Roentgenol 39:401-410, 1994.)

high-density barium should then be given for a more detailed examination.[1,19,20] Barium or low-osmolality, water-soluble contrast agents such as iohexol (Omnipaque) may be used as the primary contrast agent if aspiration or an esophageal-airway fistula is suspected. After the early postoperative period, the radiologic examination should be performed as a biphasic study that includes double-contrast views with high-density barium and single-contrast views with low-density barium.

GASTROESOPHAGEAL REFLUX AND HIATAL HERNIA

Patients with gastroesophageal reflux may undergo surgery because of intractable reflux esophagitis, peptic strictures, or Barrett's esophagus. With most of these surgical procedures, the crura are dissected, the esophagus is mobilized, the vagus nerves are preserved, the hiatal hernia is reduced, the diaphragm is repaired, and the intra-abdominal esophagus is restored. A variable portion of gastric fundus is usually wrapped around the proximal stomach.[4,21]

In a Nissen fundoplication, the gastric fundus is loosely wrapped 360 degrees around the intra-abdominal esophagus to create an antireflux valve.[22] A less than circumferential fundoplication wrap is used in patients with esophageal dysmotility and poor clearance of the bolus from the esophagus. In a Belsey Mark IV repair, the gastric fundus is sutured to the intra-abdominal esophagus, creating an acute esophagogastric junction angle (angle of His); a 270-degree fundoplication wrap around the left lateral aspect of the distal esophagus is then created.[23,24] In a Hill posterior gastropexy, the gastroesophageal junction is returned to an intra-abdominal location and anchored to the preaortic fascia (median arcuate ligament), thereby accentuating the esophagogastric junction angle and lengthening the segment of intra-abdominal esophagus.[25] However, a fundoplication is not performed. These procedures can be performed by a laparoscopic approach or open surgery. A Nissen fundoplication is usually performed laparoscopically via a transabdominal approach. A transthoracic approach is sometimes performed in complicated cases (e.g., patients with recurrent gastroesophageal reflux after an unsuccessful fundoplication, patients requiring concomitant esophageal myotomy for achalasia or diffuse esophageal spasm, or patients with a short, strictured esophagus). A Belsey Mark IV repair uses a left transthoracic approach, whereas a Hill posterior gastropexy uses a transabdominal approach.

Normal Postoperative Appearances

The Nissen fundoplication wrap normally appears as a large fundal mass with a smooth contour and surface (Fig. 31-3).[26,27] If the patient drinks barium in a recumbent, steep oblique or lateral position, the distal esophagus is shown to curve smoothly through the center of the fundoplication wrap.[28] The smooth, symmetrical wrap and its consistent relationship with the distal esophagus readily differentiate a fundoplication wrap from a true tumor in the fundus.

The gastric wrap of a Belsey Mark IV repair produces a smaller defect than a Nissen fundoplication.[29] The esophagus forms two distinct angles as it passes through the 270-degree fundoplication (Fig. 31-4).[30] The intra-abdominal esophagus has a shallow upper angle where the esophagus, fundus, and

in the abdominal cavity. The advantages of minimally invasive surgery include less wound pain because of smaller incisions, a better cosmetic result, shorter hospital stays, and less time away from the workplace. In the esophagus, laparoscopic surgery has been particularly successful for the treatment of patients with gastroesophageal reflux and achalasia. The operations performed are the same as those for open surgery and are therefore associated with the same complications. In addition, trocar injury to the small intestine may occur at the beginning of the procedure, causing postoperative peritonitis if this complication is not recognized at the time of surgery.

Depending on the nature of the surgery and the status of the patient, the postoperative radiologic examination should be tailored to demonstrate suspected complications. Barium and water-soluble contrast agents each have advantages and disadvantages in evaluating patients during the early postoperative period.[8-18] This subject is discussed in detail in Chapters 1 and 21. Briefly, water-soluble contrast agents should be used during the early postoperative period to rule out a perforation or anastomotic leak into the mediastinum or pleural space. If no water-soluble contrast medium is seen to extravasate from the esophagus on the initial spot images,

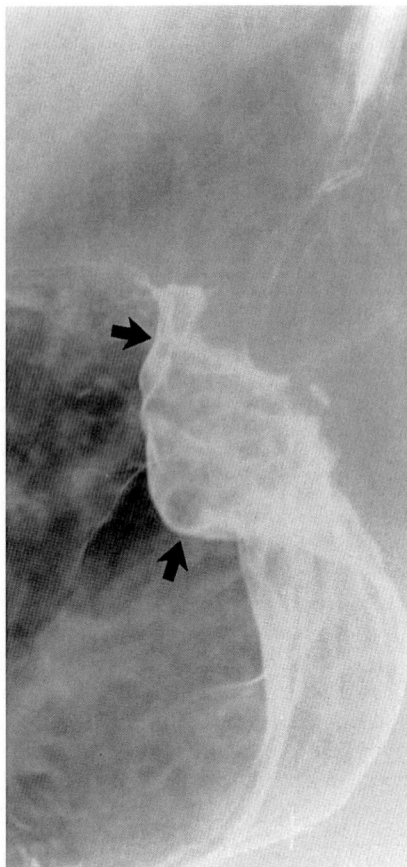

Figure 31-3. Normal Nissen fundoplication. The fundoplication wrap is seen as a smooth-surfaced, well-defined mass (*arrows*) in the gastric fundus. (From Rubesin SE, Levine MS: Postoperative esophagus. In Levine MS: Radiology of the Esophagus. Philadelphia, WB Saunders, 1989.)

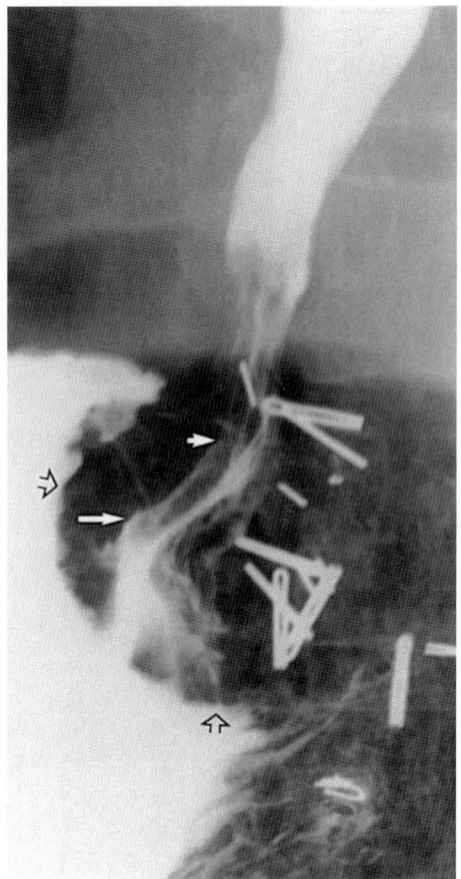

Figure 31-4. Normal Belsey Mark IV repair. The fundoplication wrap is seen as a well-circumscribed mass (*open arrows*) in the gastric fundus. As the esophagus passes through the fundoplication wrap, a shallow angle is formed where the esophagus, fundus, and diaphragm are sutured together (*short solid arrow*). A steeper angle (*long solid arrow*) is formed where the stomach is pulled upward toward the esophagus. (From Rubesin SE, Levine MS: Postoperative esophagus. In Levine MS: Radiology of the Esophagus. Philadelphia, WB Saunders, 1989.)

diaphragm are sutured together and a lower angle where the stomach is pulled upward toward the esophagus.[29]

In a Hill posterior gastropexy, the intra-abdominal esophagus is lengthened and the angle of His is accentuated.[30] Whatever antireflux operation is performed, neither gastroesophageal reflux nor a hiatal hernia should be observed after a successful repair.

Complications

Complications related directly to surgery include pneumothorax and pneumomediastinum. Acute hemorrhage usually arises from the short gastric vessels ligated at surgery or is related to operative injury of the spleen or liver. Instrumental perforation of the esophagus or stomach may be not detected during surgery and may lead to a left upper quadrant abscess. Late esophageal perforation may be caused by ischemia or diathermy injury.[2,4]

Obstruction

During the early postoperative period, edema of the fundoplication wrap may cause transient dysphagia. This complication may be manifested on esophagograms by a large, smooth fundal mass associated with smooth, tapered narrowing of the intra-abdominal esophagus and delayed emptying

of contrast material.[26] The edema usually subsides within 1 to 2 weeks, and a follow-up esophagogram demonstrates a much smaller defect in this region caused by the normal fundoplication wrap.

Some patients may have persistent narrowing of the esophagus, causing dysphagia or the "gas bloat" syndrome, with upper abdominal fullness and an inability to belch after meals.[21] Patients may also complain of inability to vomit and increased flatulence. In such cases, esophagograms may demonstrate fixed narrowing of the distal esophagus as a result of a tight fundoplication wrap (Fig. 31-5) or excessive closure of the esophageal hiatus of the diaphragm.[31,32]

Recurrent Hiatal Hernia and Gastroesophageal Reflux

Complete disruption of the fundoplication sutures is manifested radiographically by a recurrent hiatal hernia and gastroesophageal reflux without visualization of the fundoplication wrap (Fig. 31-6).[33,34] Partial disruption of the fundoplication sutures may be manifested by a partially intact wrap associated with one or more outpouchings from the gastric fundus (Fig. 31-7) or by an hourglass appearance of the stomach as the fundus slips through the fundoplication.[33,34] An hourglass

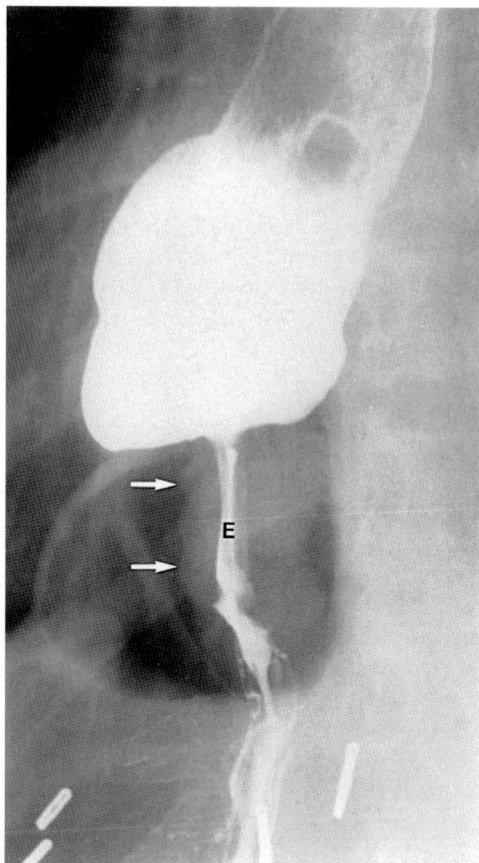

Figure 31-5. Persistent obstruction of the distal esophagus by a tight Nissen fundoplication wrap. The esophageal lumen (E) is narrowed by a tight fundoplication wrap (*arrows*). The proximal esophagus is dilated. There was delayed emptying of barium from the distal esophagus. (From Rubesin SE, Levine MS: Postoperative esophagus. In Levine MS: Radiology of the Esophagus. Philadelphia, WB Saunders, 1989.)

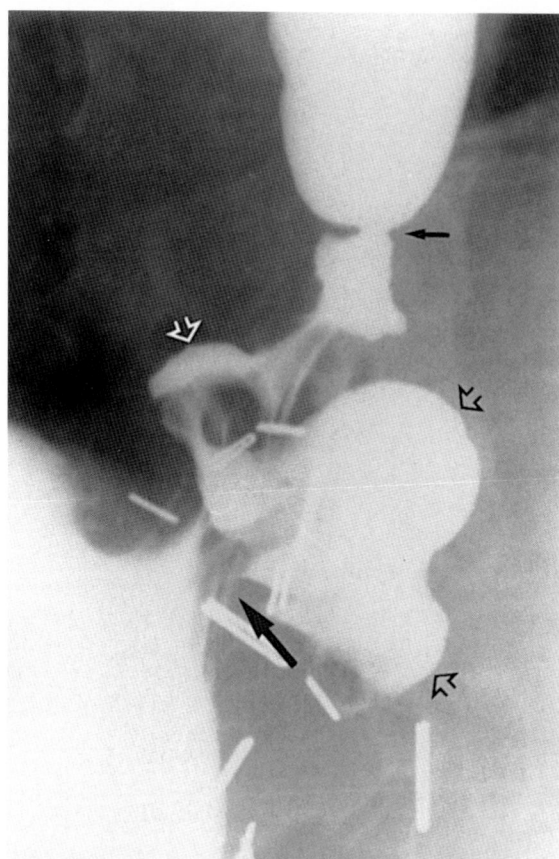

Figure 31-6. Breakdown of fundoplication wrap and recurrent hiatal hernia. Multiple gastric outpouchings (*open arrows*) are seen above the level of the diaphragm (*large black arrow*). The expected mass of the fundoplication wrap is not present in the gastric fundus. A focal peptic stricture is also seen at the gastroesophageal junction (*small black arrow*). (From Rubesin SE, Levine MS: Postoperative esophagus. In Levine MS: Radiology of the Esophagus. Philadelphia, WB Saunders, 1989.)

stomach may also be caused by inappropriate placement of the fundoplication around the gastric body. Finally, disruption of the diaphragmatic sutures (but not the fundoplication sutures) may result in a recurrent hiatal hernia with continued demonstration of an intact fundoplication wrap (Fig. 31-8).[33]

Other Considerations

In the past, the Angelchik antireflux prosthesis was used as a surgical alternative for the treatment of gastroesophageal reflux disease. A fundoplication wrap was created by placing a horseshoe-shaped silicon prosthesis around the intra-abdominal esophagus and gastric cardia.[35,36] Because of a high complication rate, this prosthesis is no longer used. Complications included migration of the prosthesis into the abdominal cavity or mediastinum, slippage of the prosthesis, and erosion of the prosthesis into the stomach.[36-42] Similar complications may result from laparoscopic placement of a gastric band for morbid obesity in which a prosthesis is placed around the gastric fundus.

BENIGN STRICTURES

Benign esophageal strictures may be treated by a variety of surgical and nonsurgical procedures, including esophageal

bougienage, fluoroscopically controlled balloon dilatation, and esophageal replacement with a gastric tube, jejunal graft, or colonic interposition. The site, extent, and cause of the stricture affect the therapeutic choice. Surgery is most frequently required for the treatment of lye strictures. Esophageal replacement surgery may also be performed on patients with intractable strictures caused by gastroesophageal reflux disease.

Peroral balloon or endoscopic dilatation of strictures under fluoroscopic guidance is an effective alternative to esophageal bougienage.[43,44] This procedure has a lower risk of perforation and a longer symptom-free interval than esophageal bougienage.[45-48]

CARCINOMA

Because they usually have advanced tumors at the time of diagnosis, patients with esophageal carcinoma continue to have 5-year survival rates of only 5% to 20%, despite advances in radiologic imaging, surgical technique, and treatment with radiation or chemotherapy.[49] Treatment for esophageal carcinoma is primarily palliative, focused on reversing starvation and cachexia by relieving dysphagia and restoring the ability to swallow. Palliation of advanced esophageal cancers

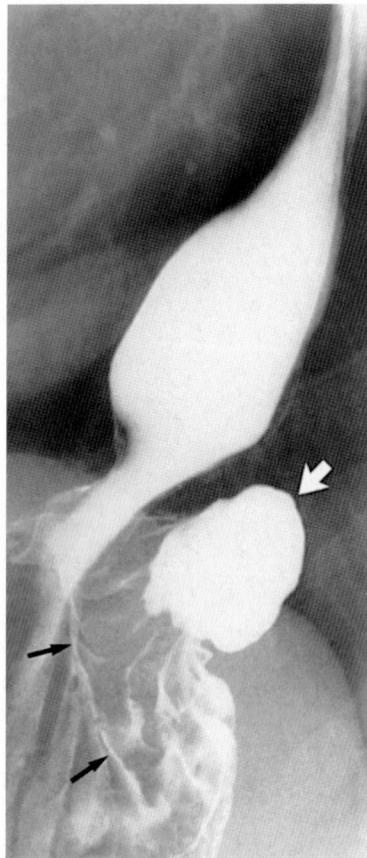

Figure 31-7. Partial breakdown of fundoplication wrap. The fundal wrap is partially intact (*small arrows*) but does not encircle the distal esophagus. A small fundal outpouching is present (*large arrow*). Barium is seen in the distal esophagus because of gastroesophageal reflux.

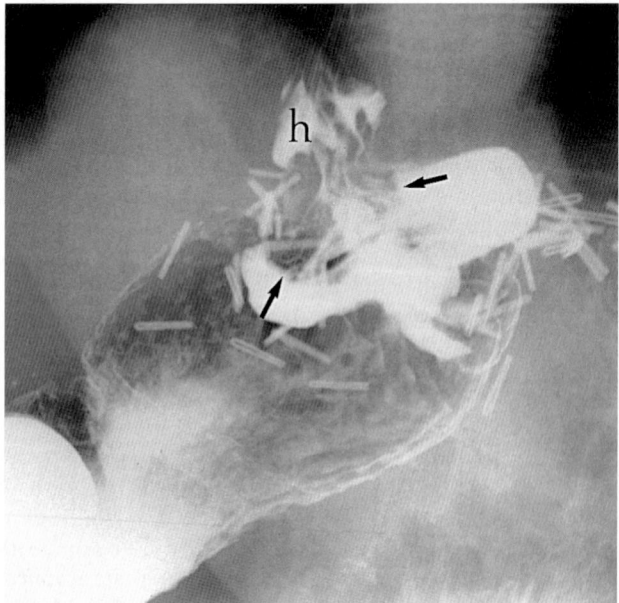

Figure 31-8. Recurrent hiatal hernia resulting from disruption of sutures closing the esophageal hiatus of the diaphragm. A small hiatal hernia (h) lies above the intact fundoplication wrap (*arrows*). (From Rubesin SE, Levine MS: Postoperative esophagus. In Levine MS: Radiology of the Esophagus. Philadelphia, WB Saunders, 1989.)

can be achieved not only by surgery but also by radiation therapy, esophageal stent placement, and endoscopic laser therapy.

Esophagogastrectomy

The esophagus can be removed by a transthoracic or a combined transhiatal/cervical approach. Distant metastases and aortic or tracheobronchial invasion by tumor are relative contraindications to surgery, but local extension of tumor and mediastinal adenopathy are not.[50]

Transthoracic Approach

A right-sided thoracotomy and abdominal incision (Ivor-Lewis operation) are performed on many patients with mid-thoracic esophageal cancers.[5,49] A left-sided thoracoabdominal incision is performed on patients with cancers involving the distal esophagus and cardia or lesions that have extensive nodal metastases near the celiac axis or lesser curvature of the stomach.[49] After resection of the diseased esophagus and cardia, the stomach is mobilized on its vascular pedicle and placed in the thorax with the lesser curvature facing the mediastinum (Fig. 31-9). A vertically oriented portion of the stomach may be removed, so that the stomach becomes tubular and functions as a conduit. An antireflux procedure may also be performed by invaginating the distal esophagus into the stomach. A gastric drainage procedure such as a pyloroplasty or pyloromyotomy is usually performed because the vagus nerves are sacrificed at surgery.

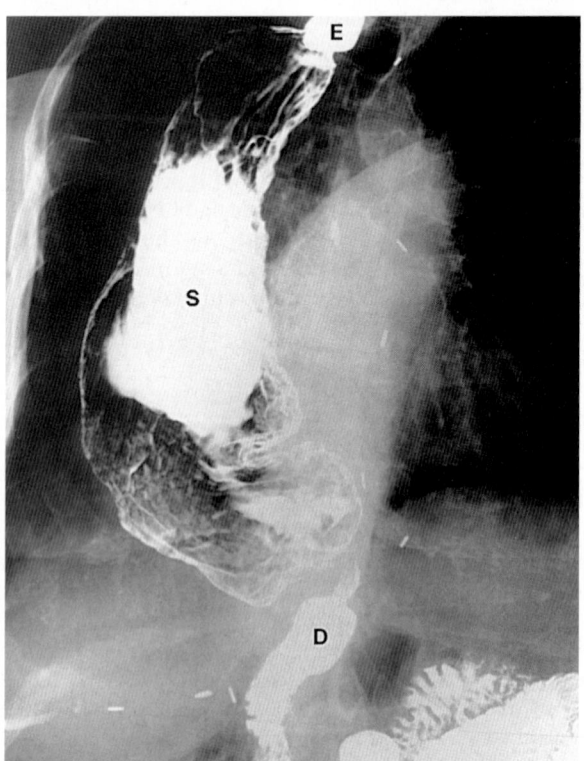

Figure 31-9. Normal right-sided esophagogastrectomy. The stomach (S) lies in the right hemithorax with the lesser curvature facing the mediastinum. The proximal duodenum (D) has been mobilized and stretched by a Kocher maneuver. Barium is seen in the distal esophagus (E) because of gastroesophageal reflux.

Transhiatal/Transcervical Approach

The stomach can also be used as a palliative bypass organ for advanced esophageal carcinoma without resorting to a thoracotomy.[51-53] In such cases, the stomach is brought superiorly through an anterior or posterior mediastinal tunnel (Fig. 31-10) into the neck via a combined transcervical/transhiatal approach. The fundus is then anastomosed to the cervical esophagus (and occasionally the pharynx) via a cervical approach. The diseased esophagus can be resected through the hiatal and cervical exposures, or it can be excluded. If the stomach has been placed substernally, the small opening of the thoracic inlet is widened by resecting the medial portion of the clavicle, sternoclavicular joint, and upper portion of the manubrium. A pyloromyotomy or pyloroplasty is performed to facilitate gastric emptying. A temporary feeding jejunostomy tube is usually inserted.

The transthoracic approach allows en bloc resection of the esophagus and local lymph nodes for complete staging and potential cure. Anastomotic or other staple line leaks in the middle mediastinum, however, are serious complications. The transhiatal approach allows removal of some, but not all cervical, intrathoracic, and intra-abdominal lymph nodes. A complete mediastinal lymph node exploration for staging or cure is not possible, but anastomotic leaks into the neck with the transhiatal approach are less serious than leaks into the mediastinum with the transthoracic approach. Nevertheless, the two techniques have about the same success rate for cure.[5]

Complications

The most common complications during the early postoperative period include anastomotic leaks, obstruction,

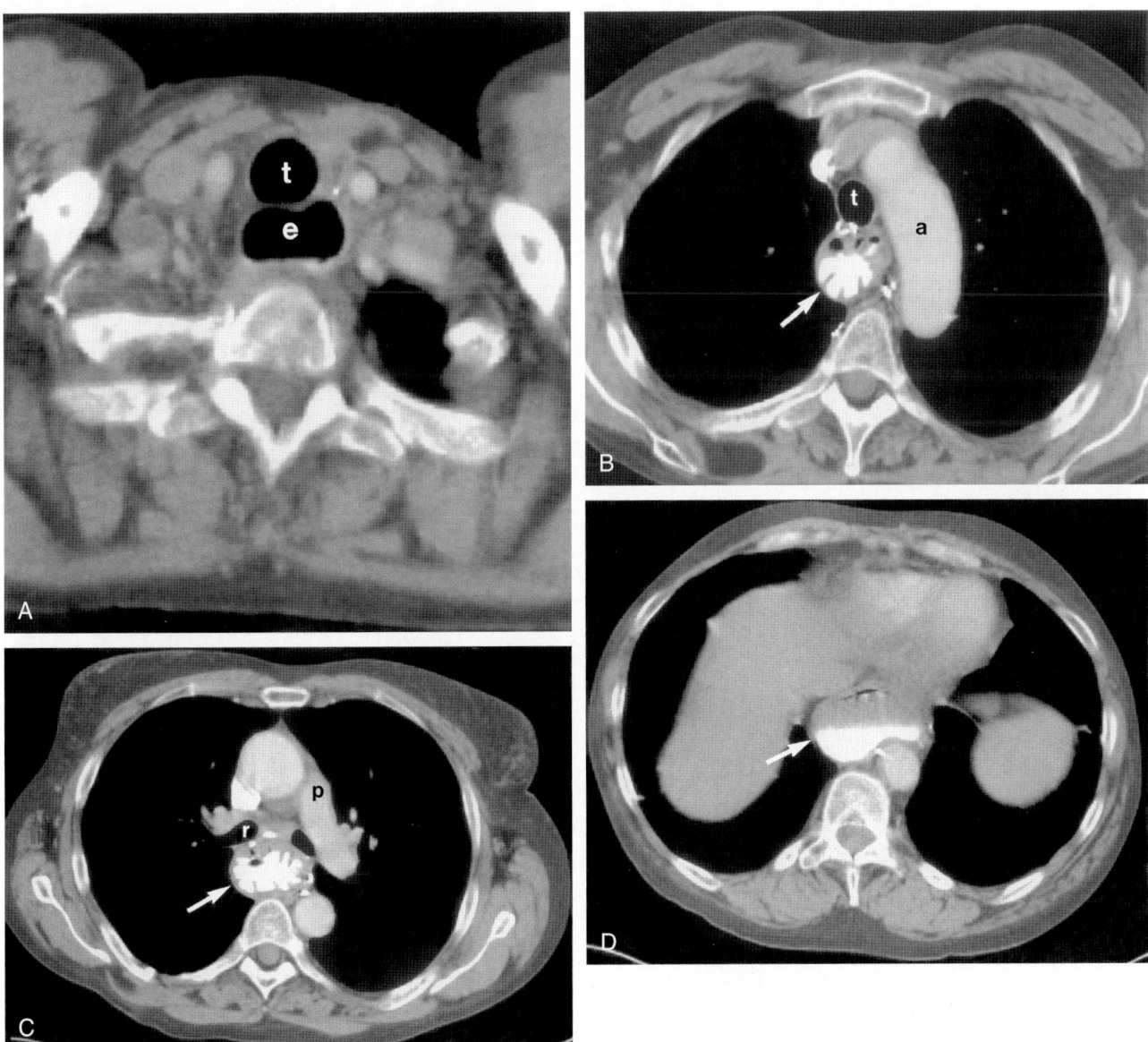

Figure 31-10. Normal transhiatal esophagogastrectomy on CT. A. Axial image of the neck shows the residual cervical esophagus (e) distended by air. The trachea (t) is seen anteriorly. **B.** Axial image at the level of the aortic arch (a) shows the intrathoracic stomach (*arrow*) lying posterior to the trachea (t), anterior to the spine, and abutting the aorta. Rugal folds are visible in the stomach. **C.** Axial image at the level of the main pulmonary artery (p) shows the intrathoracic stomach (*arrow*) posterior to the mainstem bronchi (right mainstem bronchus identified by r). **D.** Axial image at the level of the diaphragm shows the intrathoracic stomach (*arrow*). The rugal folds are not seen at this level because the stomach is more distended.

gastric atony and dilatation, and aspiration into the larynx. A study using water-soluble contrast medium (followed by high-density barium if there is no evidence of a leak[20]) is usually performed within 7 to 10 days after surgery to rule out a leak at the esophagogastric anastomosis, at the line of creation of the gastric tube, and at the pyloroplasty. Mechanical obstruction may occur at the esophagogastric anastomosis or pylorus (Fig. 31-11) because of edema, hemorrhage, or leak. Mechanical obstruction may also occur at the distal end of the intrathoracic portion of the stomach because of gastric volvulus or extrinsic compression by the diaphragm. Pancreatitis may rarely develop because the duodenum is freed from the pancreatic head to allow the stomach to be pulled superiorly into the chest.[2]

The most common complications during the late postoperative period include gastroesophageal reflux and its sequelae, anastomotic strictures, fistulas, and recurrent tumor.[50] Acute gastroesophageal reflux may result in aspiration pneumonia. Chronic gastroesophageal reflux may lead to reflux esophagitis (Fig. 31-12), peptic strictures (Fig. 31-13), Barrett's esophagus, and, eventually, esophageal adenocarcinoma (Fig. 31-14). Healing of anastomotic leaks may result in benign anastomotic strictures. Although recurrent tumor in the mediastinum is best demonstrated by CT or MRI, barium studies may reveal a smooth or spiculated area of extrinsic mass effect on the mediastinal border of the stomach (Fig. 31-15).[50,54] Recurrent esophageal carcinoma may also be demonstrated by

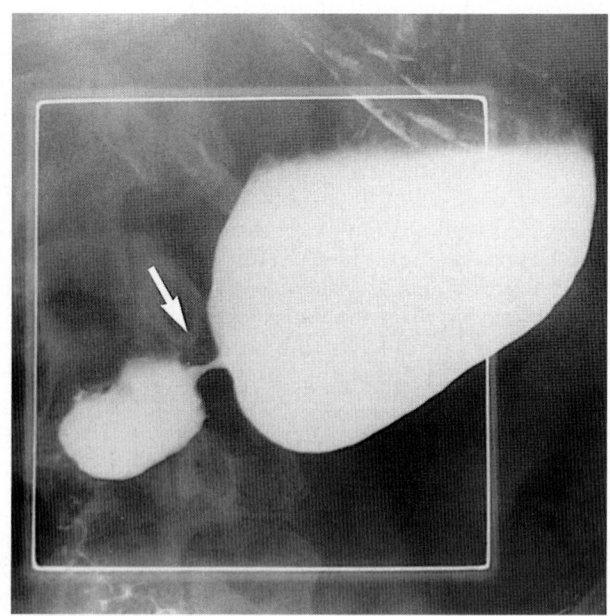

Figure 31-11. Obstruction at pylorus after pyloroplasty performed during esophagogastrectomy. There is smooth symmetrical narrowing of the pylorus (*arrow*). Obstruction was manifested fluoroscopically by delayed gastric emptying and radiographically by a barium-fluid-air level in the stomach, indicating retained fluid, rather than the normally expected barium-air level. (Reproduced with permission from Rubesin SE, Beatty SM: The postoperative esophagus. Semin Roentgenol 39: 401-410, 1994.)

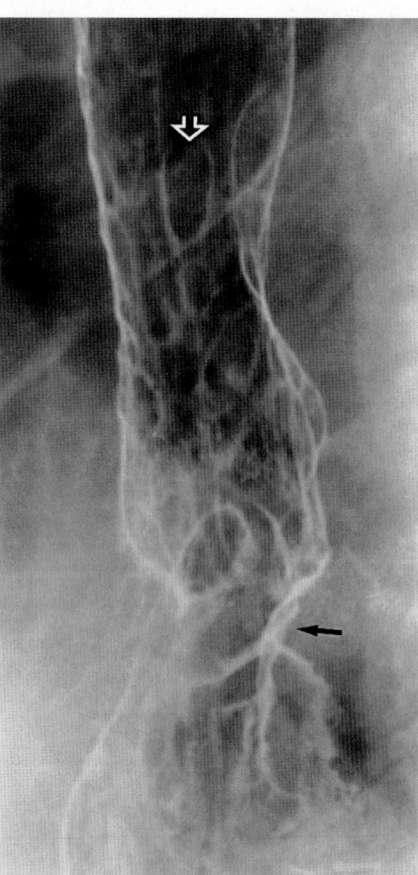

Figure 31-12. Esophagogastrectomy with reflux esophagitis. Numerous confluent plaques and pseudomembranes (*open arrow*) are seen on the esophageal mucosa above the esophagogastric junction (*solid arrow*). Free gastroesophageal reflux was seen at fluoroscopy.

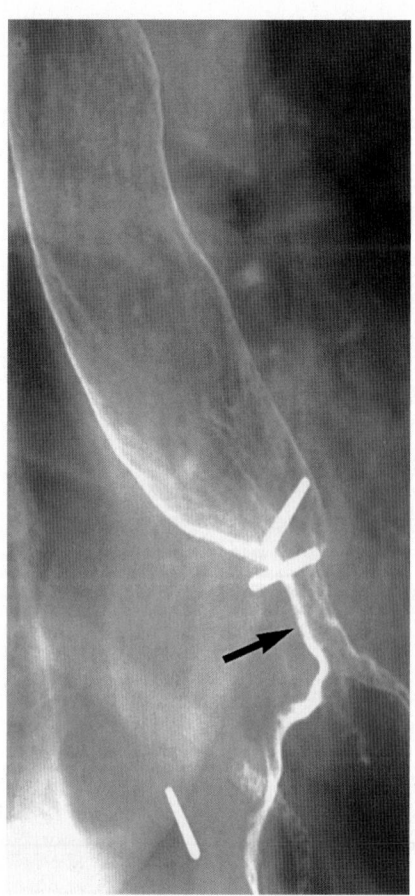

Figure 31-13. Esophagogastrectomy with peptic stricture. A smooth, tapered stricture (*arrow*) is seen above the esophagogastric anastomosis. (From Rubesin SE, Levine MS: Postoperative esophagus. In Levine MS: Radiology of the Esophagus. Philadelphia, WB Saunders, 1989.)

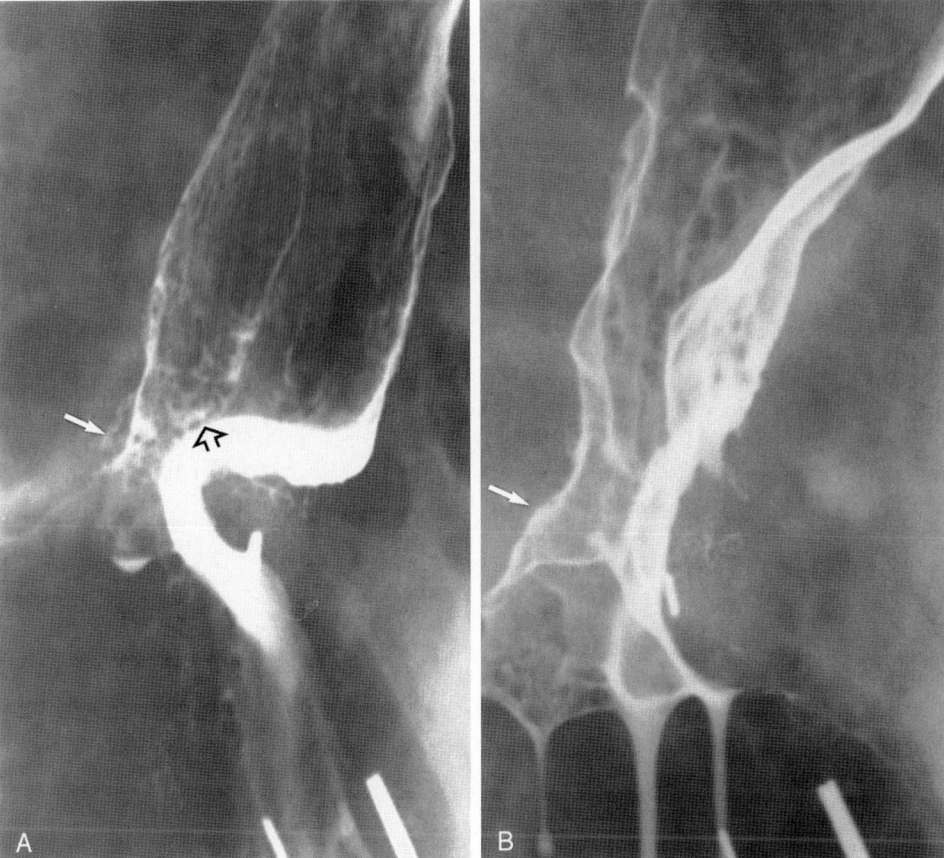

Figure 31-14. Esophagogastrectomy with a superimposed adenocarcinoma in Barrett's esophagus. A. Reflux esophagitis after esophagogastrectomy is manifested by a finely nodular mucosa (*open arrow*) just proximal to the esophagogastric anastomosis (*solid arrow*). **B.** Two years later, an irregular, infiltrating lesion with coarsely nodular mucosa is seen just above the esophagogastric anastomosis (*arrow*). Surgery revealed an adenocarcinoma arising in Barrett's mucosa. (From Rubesin SE, Levine MS: Postoperative esophagus. In Levine MS: Radiology of the Esophagus. Philadelphia, WB Saunders, 1989.)

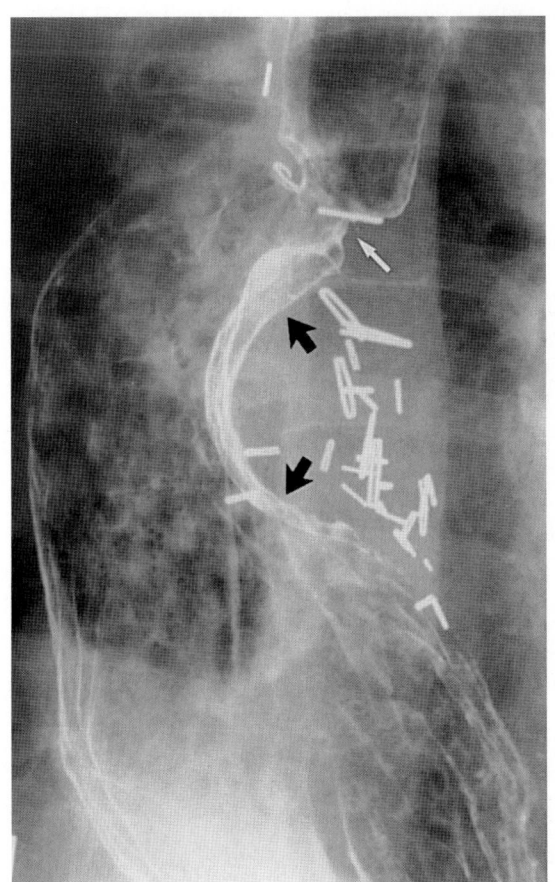

Figure 31-15. Esophagogastrectomy with recurrent mediastinal tumor. A smooth area of extrinsic mass effect (*black arrows*) is seen on the lesser curvature of the intrathoracic stomach below the esophagogastric anastomosis (*white arrow*). (From Rubesin SE, Levine MS: Postoperative esophagus. In Levine MS: Radiology of the Esophagus. Philadelphia, WB Saunders, 1989.)

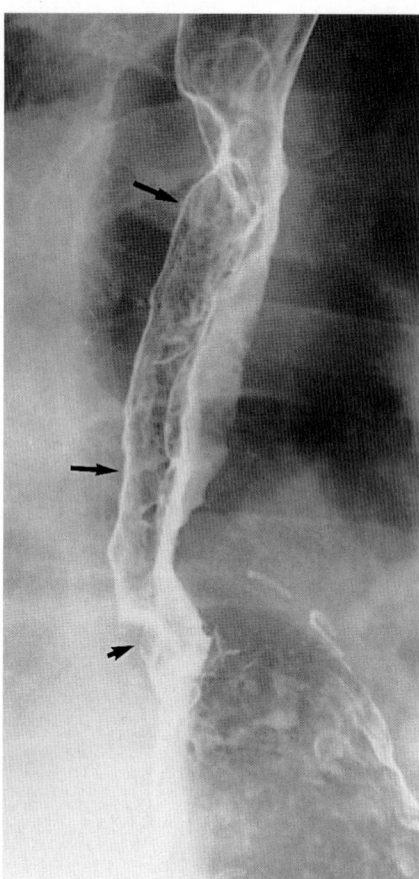

Figure 31-16. Esophagogastrectomy with recurrent esophageal carcinoma. The distal esophagus is diffusely narrowed and irregular (*long arrows*) and has a nodular surface pattern because of recurrent esophageal carcinoma. (The esophagogastric anastomosis is denoted by a *short arrow*.) (From Rubesin SE, Levine MS: Postoperative esophagus. In Levine MS: Radiology of the Esophagus. Philadelphia, WB Saunders, 1989.)

barium studies (Fig. 31-16). Any suspicious area should be further evaluated by endoscopy and biopsy. Delayed perforations may occasionally be caused by recurrent mediastinal tumor or mediastinal irradiation.

Several complications may be related to esophageal exclusion if the diseased esophagus has been bypassed but not resected. If the native esophagus is disrupted, a left subphrenic abscess may develop. The excluded esophagus may also form a posterior mediastinal mucocele (Fig. 31-17).[55] These mucoceles may become infected or compress the tracheobronchial tree. Symptoms may also be caused by gastroesophageal reflux into the excluded esophagus. Carcinoma may develop in an esophagus bypassed for a lye stricture.[55]

Colonic Interposition, Jejunal Interposition, and Free Jejunal Graft

Various segments of the colon and jejunum may be used to bypass severe peptic strictures, caustic strictures, or inoperable esophageal cancers. When colonic interposition is performed, the right or transverse colon is placed in an isoperistaltic direction (Fig. 31-18) whereas the left colon is placed in either an isoperistaltic or an antiperistaltic direction.[56] If the colon is placed in the anterior mediastinum, the cologastric anastomosis is usually located on the anterior wall of the stomach.[56] If the colon is placed in the posterior mediastinum, however, the cologastric anastomosis is located on the posterior wall of the upper stomach.[56] A vagotomy and pyloroplasty are also performed. A preoperative barium enema may be performed to rule out significant colonic disease before surgery. A preoperative angiogram may also be obtained to demonstrate the vascular anatomy of the colon and to rule out vascular disease, particularly in patients with suspected atherosclerosis.[57]

Colonic interposition is a procedure performed when the stomach cannot be used for esophageal replacement, for example, in patients with prior gastric surgery. Colonic

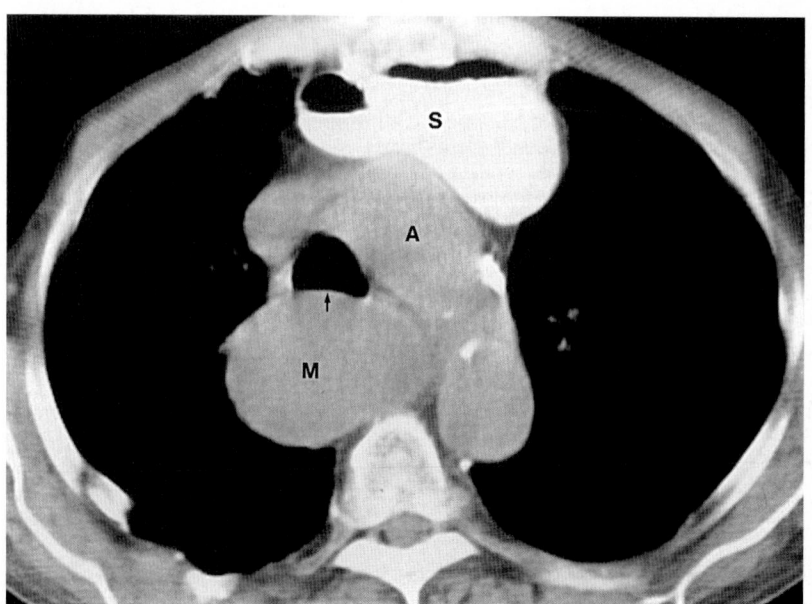

Figure 31-17. Mucocele arising in the excluded esophagus after esophageal bypass by stomach pulled through anterior mediastinal tunnel. CT at the level of the aortic arch (A) shows the substernal position of the stomach (S). A mucocele of the surgically isolated esophagus is manifested by a smooth-surfaced ovoid mass (M) in the right middle mediastinum. The mass indents the posterior tracheal wall (*arrow*). (Reproduced with permission from Rubesin SE, Beatty SM: The postoperative esophagus. Semin Roentgenol 39:401-410, 1994.)

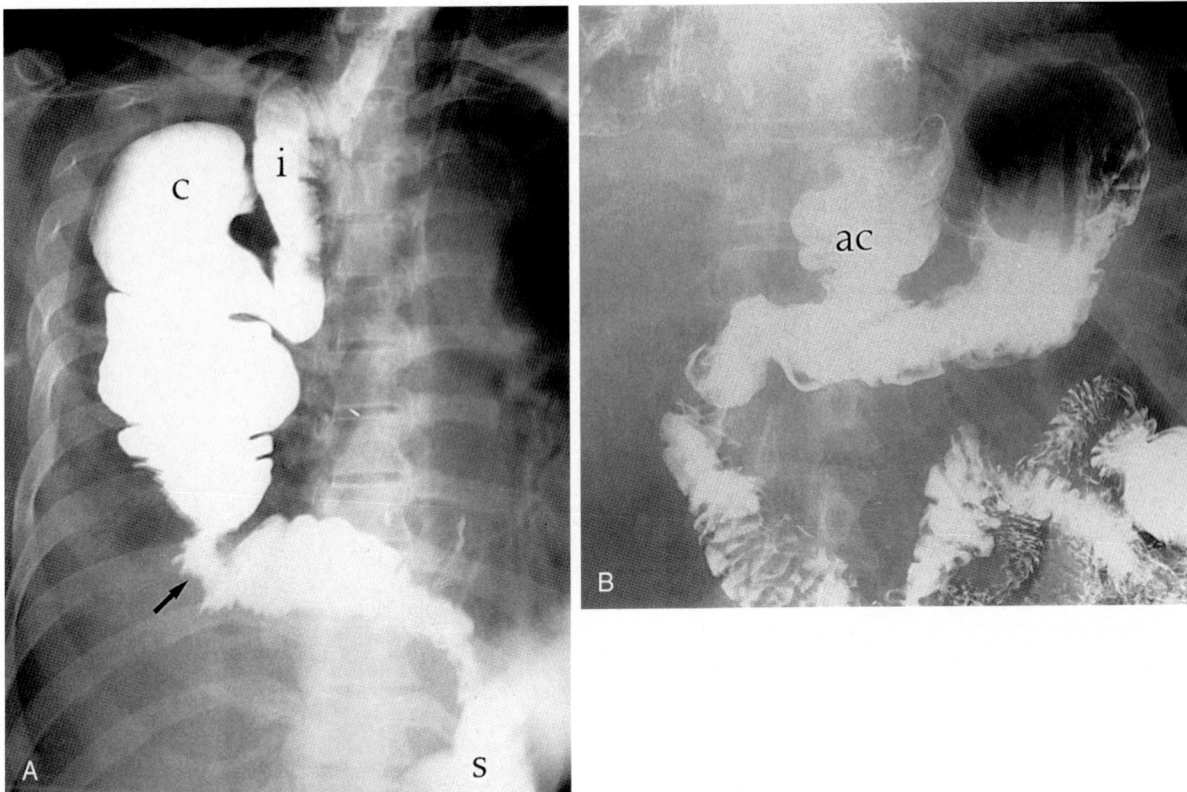

Figure 31-18. Normal colonic interposition. A. There is an isoperistaltic right colonic interposition with anastomosis of the terminal ileum (i) to the cervical esophagus. Mild narrowing of the colon is seen where it passes through the diaphragm (*arrow*). C, cecum; S, stomach. **B.** The ascending colon (ac) is anastomosed to the lesser curvature of the stomach. (From Rubesin SE, Levine MS: Postoperative esophagus. In Levine MS: Radiology of the Esophagus. Philadelphia, WB Saunders, 1989.)

interposition is associated with much higher morbidity and mortality rates than esophagogastrectomy. Anastomotic leaks occur in 25% to 40% of patients.[49,50] They are usually located at the proximal anastomosis, leading to abscess and stricture formation (Fig. 31-19).[57,58] Other postoperative complications include anastomotic edema and obstruction, chylothorax, mediastinal hematoma or abscess, empyema, and intra-abdominal abscess.[57] Ischemia of the transposed colon may be manifested radiographically by spasm, ulceration, loss of haustration, or a nodular mucosa.[58] Occasionally, during the early postoperative period, the mucosal folds in the interposed transverse colon may resemble jejunal folds, but this finding disappears after 1 to 3 months.[56]

Stricture formation at the proximal anastomosis is the most common late postoperative complication, occurring in 20% to 40% of patients (see Fig. 31-19).[56-58] The transposed colon may also become dilated and redundant, leading to the development of delayed graft emptying, with bloating, pain, and dysphagia. Other late complications include diverticulitis or carcinoma of the transposed colon, coloesophageal reflux, colobronchial fistulas, gastric outlet obstruction, and small bowel obstruction within the transverse mesocolon defect created at the time of surgery.[59]

Palliative Intubation

Palliative placement of an esophageal stent may be performed to allow oral feeding through advanced, obstructing esopha-

geal cancers or to obturate malignant tracheoesophageal fistulas. The use of expandable intraesophageal metallic stents (Fig. 30-20) has replaced the use of plastic tubes (e.g., Celestin tubes).[60-66] These metallic stents may be placed endoscopically, surgically, or fluoroscopically. A study using water-soluble contrast medium is performed after stent placement to evaluate stent position and patency and to rule out esophageal perforation. The stent should be fixed in position, with its upper tip proximal to the tumor and its lower tip distal to the tumor. Contrast medium should flow easily through the lumen of the stent.

Esophageal perforation is the most serious complication.[60,61,67] Obstruction of the stent may be caused by kinking of the stent or luminal obstruction resulting from mucosal prolapse, food impaction, or residual or recurrent tumor.[60,67-69] Reflux of gastric contents through the stent may lead to reflux esophagitis or aspiration pneumonia.[70,71] Reflux through a stent is such a common problem that stents with antireflux mechanisms have been designed.[72] Metallic stents may initially be malpositioned, or they can migrate.[55] Rarely, a stent may cause pressure necrosis of the esophageal wall, resulting in a mediastinal leak or aortoesophageal fistula. Ulceration of the esophagus or stomach may also occur.

Laser Therapy

Endoscopic laser therapy is a palliative procedure that provides transient relief from dysphagia in patients with unresectable

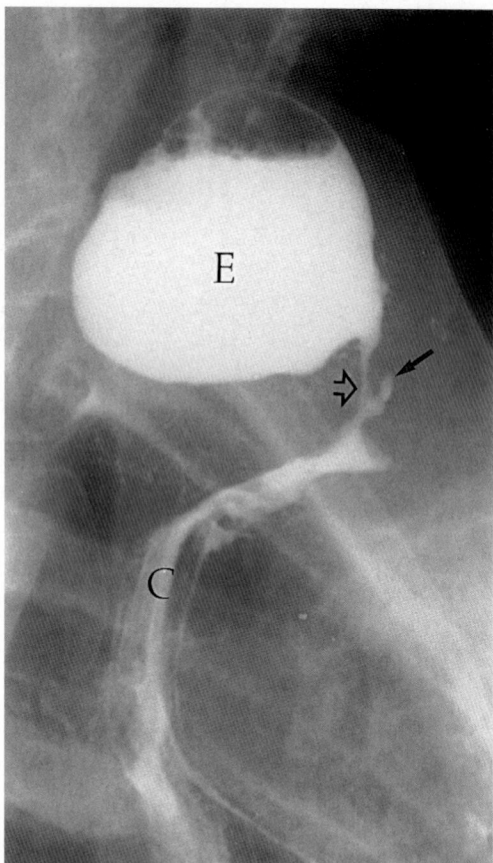

Figure 31-19. Colonic interposition with stricture formation after an anastomotic leak at the esophagocolonic anastomosis. A tight stricture (*open arrow*) is present at the anastomosis between the dilated esophagus (E) and the collapsed colon (C). A short, blind-ending track (*solid arrow*) is seen at the site of a prior anastomotic leak. (From Rubesin SE, Levine MS: Postoperative esophagus. In Levine MS: Radiology of the Esophagus. Philadelphia, WB Saunders, 1989.)

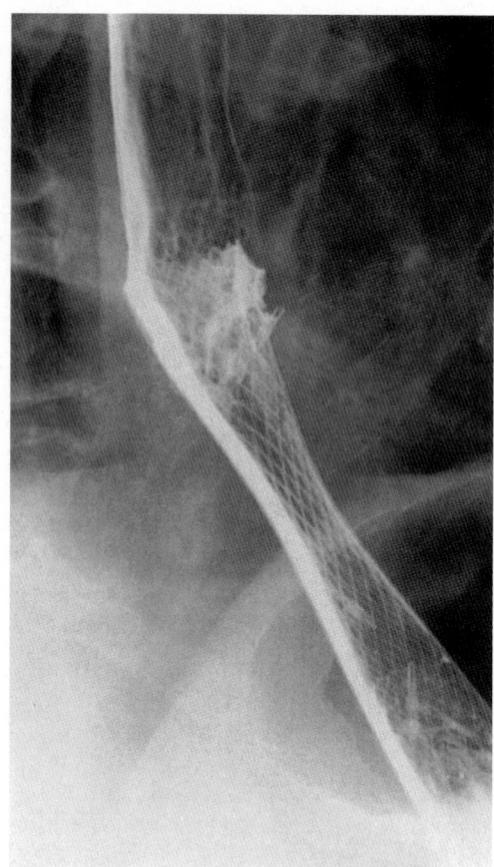

Figure 31-20. Esophageal stent. An endoscopically placed metallic stent is seen traversing an adenocarcinoma of the distal esophagus. Note how the distal end of the stent passes through the gastroesophageal junction into the gastric fundus.

or obstructing esophageal carcinomas.[73] The intraluminal portion of the tumor is coagulated and vaporized, resulting in a widened diameter of the esophageal lumen. A metallic stent may be placed after laser ablation of tumor. Photodynamic therapy may also be used, combining a chemical photosensitizer with laser treatment.[74,75] Laser therapy has a major advantage over radiation therapy because no damage occurs to adjacent organs.[76] Furthermore, patients may undergo multiple laser treatments whereas radiation therapy is limited by the total radiation dose to the mediastinum. Complications of laser therapy include esophageal perforation, tracheoesophageal fistulas, pneumopericardium, and pneumoperitoneum.[73,76]

ACHALASIA

Neither medical therapy nor surgery can correct the abnormal esophageal motility and lower esophageal sphincter dysfunction that occur in patients with achalasia. The two major forms of therapy, pneumatic dilatation and cardiomyotomy, are both aimed at improving esophageal emptying by disrupting the high-pressure lower esophageal sphincter. Intramuscular injection of botulinum toxin has also been used for the treatment of achalasia.[77]

Pneumatic Dilatation

The most serious complication of pneumatic dilatation is lower esophageal perforation, occurring in 1% to 4% of patients.[78] Although the presence of chest pain or fever after the procedure should suggest this complication, some patients may have clinically silent or delayed perforations.[79] A study using water-soluble contrast medium should therefore be performed after pneumatic dilatation to rule out a perforation, regardless of the patient's symptoms.[80,81] If no perforation is seen with water-soluble contrast medium, high-density barium should be given to demonstrate greater anatomic detail and subtle leaks. Perforations usually occur on the left posterolateral wall of the distal esophagus just above the diaphragm. Some patients may have small, sealed-off perforations that resemble intramural dissections, whereas others may have free perforations into the mediastinum or pleural space.[82,83] Increasing symptoms during the early postoperative period may necessitate a repeat esophagogram to demonstrate a delayed perforation or a perforation that was not initially visualized because of edema and spasm at the dilatation site. In addition, edema and spasm at the gastroesophageal junction may lead to delayed esophageal emptying despite adequate disruption of the lower esophageal sphincter fibers. Thus, the radiographic appearance immediately after dilatation is a poor predictor of the efficacy of the procedure.[81]

Cardiomyotomy

Cardiomyotomy, or Heller myotomy, is an effective form of therapy for patients with untreated achalasia or achalasia that is unresponsive to pneumatic dilatation. The procedure is performed using open or laparoscopic technique. During myotomy, the lower esophageal sphincter fibers are surgically divided, thereby disrupting the sphincter. Some surgeons perform a concomitant antireflux procedure. After cardiomyotomy, there should be free flow of contrast medium from the esophagus into the stomach with decreased esophageal dilatation and absence of the beaklike narrowing of the esophagogastric region associated with achalasia.[84] In about 50% of cases, there is eccentric ballooning of the esophagus at the site of Heller myotomy (Fig. 31-21).[85] The most common early postoperative complication is perforation of the distal esophagus.[86] Persistent dysphagia during the late postoperative period may indicate an incomplete myotomy or a tight fundoplication wrap. Conversely, postoperative gastroesophageal reflux, reflux esophagitis, and peptic strictures may indicate the need for an antireflux procedure.

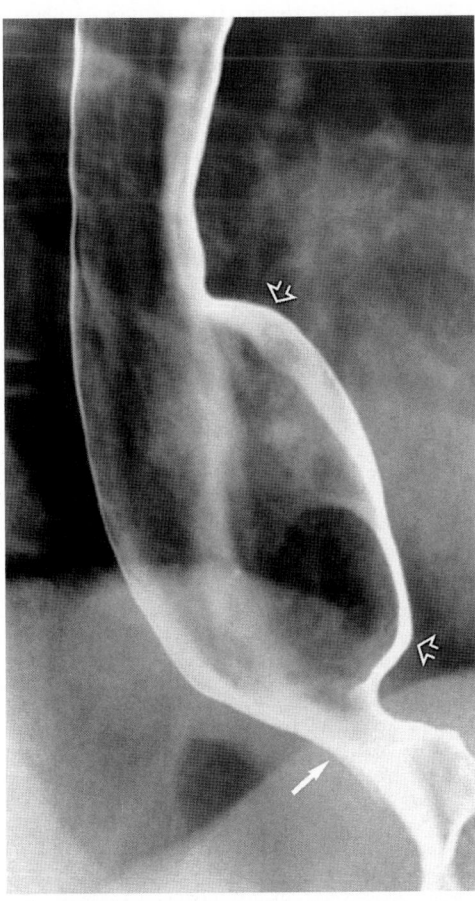

Figure 31-21. Ballooning of the distal esophagus after cardiomyotomy for achalasia. There is eccentric outpouching or ballooning of the distal esophageal wall at the cardiomyotomy site (*open arrows*). The gastroesophageal junction (*solid arrow*) is widely patent. (From Rubesin SE, Levine MS: Postoperative esophagus. In Levine MS: Radiology of the Esophagus. Philadelphia, WB Saunders, 1989.)

VARICES

Endoscopic sclerotherapy or variceal banding, transjugular intrahepatic portosystemic shunts, portosystemic shunt surgery, and esophageal devascularization procedures are the major forms of therapy for esophageal varices. Endoscopic sclerotherapy and variceal banding are discussed in Chapter 29.

Sugiura Procedure

The Sugiura procedure is a technique that was developed in Japan for surgical devascularization of esophageal varices.[87,88] Venous collaterals between paraesophageal varices and the wall of the esophagus are ligated from the level of the left inferior pulmonary vein to the esophageal hiatus. The esophagus is then transected at the level of the diaphragm and subsequently reanastomosed. Bridging veins between the abdominal esophagus and the proximal stomach as well as the stomach and the lesser curvature are also ligated. A splenectomy, selective vagotomy, and pyloroplasty are often performed. The Sugiura procedure does not alter hepatic function or cause hepatic encephalopathy.

A widely patent esophageal lumen should be demonstrated at the transection line after a Sugiura procedure.[89] Varices are found to decrease in size or disappear in more than 90% of patients within several months of surgery. The most common early postoperative complication is suture breakdown, leading to esophageal perforation and mediastinitis.[90] Other patients may develop hiatal hernias, gastroesophageal reflux, or anastomotic strictures after this procedure.

References

1. Rubesin SE, Levine MS: Postoperative esophagus. In Levine MS (ed): Radiology of the Esophagus. Philadelphia, WB Saunders, 1989, pp 267-290.
2. Orringer MB: Complications of esophageal surgery. In Zuidema GD (ed): Shackleford's Surgery of the Alimentary Tract, vol 1. Philadelphia, WB Saunders, 1991, pp 434-459.
3. Rubesin SE, Beatty SM: The postoperative esophagus. Semin Roentgenol 29:401-418, 1994.
4. Peters JH, DeMeester TR: Esophagus: Anatomy, physiology and gastroesophageal reflux disease. In Greenfield LJ, Mulholland MW, Oldham KT, et al (eds): Surgery: Scientific Principles and Practice. Philadelphia, Lippincott Williams & Wilkins, 2001, pp 659-692.
5. Orringer MB: Tumors, injuries, and miscellaneous conditions of the esophagus. In Greenfield LJ, Mulholland MW, Oldham KT, et al (eds): Surgery: Scientific Principles and Practice. Philadelphia, Lippincott Williams & Wilkins, 2001, pp 692-735.
6. Anbari M, Levine MS, Cohen R, et al: Delayed leaks and fistulas after esophagogastrectomy: Radiologic evaluation. AJR 160:1217-1220.
7. Dodds WJ, Stewart ET, Vlymen WJ: Appropriate contrast media for evaluation of esophageal disruption. Radiology 144:439-441, 1982.
8. Ott DJ, Gelfand DW: Gastrointestinal contrast agents: Indications, uses and risks. JAMA 249:2380-2384, 1984.
9. James AE, Montali RJ, Chaffee V, et al: Barium or Gastrografin: Which contrast media for diagnosis of esophageal tears. Gastroenterology 68:1103-1113, 1975.
10. Foley MJ, Ghahremani GG, Rogers LF: Reappraisal of contrast media used to detect upper gastrointestinal perforations. Radiology 144:231-237, 1982.
11. Dunbar JS, Skinner GB, Wortzman G, et al: An investigation of effects of opaque media on the lungs with comparison of barium, Lipiodol and Dionosil. AJR 82:902-926, 1959.
12. Reich SB: Production of pulmonary edema by aspiration of water-soluble nonabsorbable contrast media. Radiology 92:367-370, 1969.
13. Chiu CL, Gambach RR: Hypaque pulmonary edema: A case report. Radiology 111:91-92, 1974.

14. Ginai AZ, ten Kate FJW, ten Berg RGM, et al: Experimental evaluation of various contrast agents for use in the gastrointestinal tract in case of suspected leakage: Effects on the lungs. Br J Radiol 57:895-901, 1984.

15. Ginai AZ, ten Kate FJW, ten Berg RGM, et al: Experimental evaluation of various contrast agents for use in the gastrointestinal tract in case of suspected leakage: Effects on the mediastinum. Br J Radiol 58:585-592, 1985.

16. Ginai AZ: Clinical use of Hexabrix for radiological evaluation of leakage from the upper gastrointestinal tract based on experimental study. Br J Radiol 60:343-346, 1987.

17. Brick SH, Caroline DF, Lev-Toaff AS, et al: Esophageal disruption: Evaluation with iohexol esophagography. Radiology 169:141-143, 1988.

18. Gollub MJ, Bains MS: Barium sulfate: New (old) contrast agent for diagnosis of postoperative esophageal leaks. Radiology 202:360-362, 1997.

19. Reichle RL, Fishman EK, Nixon MS, et al: Evaluation of the postsurgical esophagus after partial esophagogastrectomy for esophageal cancer. Invest Radiol 28:247-257, 1993.

20. Swanson JO, Levine MS, Redfern RO, Rubesin SE: Usefulness of high-density barium for detection of leaks after esophagogastrectomy, total gastrectomy, and total laryngectomy. AJR 181:415-420, 2003.

21. Bredenburg CE: Gastrointestinal reflux and hiatus hernia. In Fromm D (ed): Gastrointestinal Surgery. New York, Churchill Livingstone, 1985, pp 163-205.

22. Nissen R: Gastropexy and "fundoplication" in surgical treatment of hiatal hernia. Am J Dig Dis 6:954-961, 1961.

23. Skinner DB, Belsey RHR: Surgical management of esophageal reflux and hiatus hernia: Long term results with 1030 patients. J Thorac Cardiovasc Surg 53:33-54, 1967.

24. Orringer MB, Skinner DB, Belsey RHR: Long term results of the Mark IV operation for hiatal hernia and analyses of recurrence and their treatment. J Thorac Cardiovasc Surg 63:25-33, 1972.

25. Hill LD: Management of recurrent hiatal hernia. Arch Surg 102:296-302, 1971.

26. Skucas J, Mangla JC, Adams JT, et al: An evaluation of the Nissen fundoplication. Radiology 118:539-543, 1976.

27. Thoeni RF, Moss AA: The radiographic appearance of complications following Nissen fundoplication. Radiology 131:17-21, 1979.

28. Cohen WN: The fundoplication repair of sliding esophageal hiatus hernia: The roentgenographic appearance. AJR 104:625-631, 1968.

29. Feigin DS, James AE, Stitik FP, et al: The radiological appearance of hiatal hernia repairs. Radiology 110:71-77, 1974.

30. Teixidor HS, Evans JA: Roentgenographic appearance of the distal esophagus and the stomach after hiatal hernia repair. AJR 119:245-258, 1973.

31. Demeester TR, Johnson LF, Kent AH: Evaluation of current operations for the prevention of gastroesophageal reflux. Ann Surg 180:511-525, 1974.

32. Polk HC: Fundoplication for reflux esophagitis: Misadventures with the operation of choice. Ann Surg 183:645-652, 1976.

33. Saik RP, Greenburg AG, Peskin GW: A study of fundoplication disruption and deformity. Am J Surg 134:19-24, 1977.

34. Hatfield M, Shapir J: The radiologic manifestations of failed antireflux procedures. AJR 144:1209-1214, 1985.

35. Angelchik JP, Cohen R: A new surgical procedure for the treatment of gastroesophageal reflux and hiatal hernia. Surg Gynecol Obstet 148:246-248, 1979.

36. Lewis RA, Angelchik JP, Cohen R: A new surgical prosthesis for hiatal hernia repair. Radiology 135:630, 1980.

37. Peloso OA: Intra-abdominal migration of an antireflux prosthesis. JAMA 248:351-353, 1982.

38. Starling JR, Reichelderfer MO, Pellett JR, et al: Treatment of symptomatic gastroesophageal reflux using Angelchik prosthesis. Ann Surg 195:686-691, 1982.

39. Haney PJ, Gunadi IK, Arnold J, et al: Spontaneous penetration of an antireflux prosthesis into the stomach. Gastrointest Radiol 8:303-305, 1983.

40. Lackey C, Potts J: Penetration into the stomach: A complication of the antireflux prosthesis. JAMA 248:350, 1982.

41. Burhenne LJW, Fratkins LB, Flak B, et al: Radiology of the Angelchik prosthesis for gastroesophageal reflux. AJR 142:507-511, 1984.

42. Curtis DJ, Benjamin SB, Kerr R, et al: Angelchik anti-reflux device: Radiographic appearance of complications. Radiology 151:311-313, 1984.

43. London RL, Trotman BW, DiMarino AJ, et al: Dilatation of severe esophageal strictures by inflatable balloon catheter. Gastroenterology 80:173-175, 1981.

44. Owman T, Lunderquist A: Balloon catheter dilatation of esophageal strictures—a preliminary report. Gastrointest Radiol 7:301-305, 1982.

45. Goldthorn JF, Ball WS, Wilkinson LG, et al: Esophageal strictures in children: Treatment by serial balloon catheter dilatation. Radiology 153:655-658, 1984.

46. Starck E, Paolucci V, Herzer M, et al: Esophageal stenosis: Treatment with balloon catheters. Radiology 153:637-640, 1984.

47. Dawson SL, Mueller PR, Ferrucci JT, et al: Severe esophageal strictures: Indications for balloon catheter dilatation. Radiology 153:631-635, 1984.

48. McLean GK, Cooper GS, Hartz WH, et al: Radiologically-guided balloon dilatation of gastrointestinal strictures: I. Technique and factors influencing procedural success. Radiology 165:35-40, 1987.

49. Meyer JA: Cancer of the esophagus. In Fromm D (ed): Gastrointestinal Surgery. New York, Churchill Livingstone, 1985, pp 207-232.

50. Owen JW, Balfe DM, Koehler RE, et al: Radiologic evaluation of complications after esophagogastrectomy. AJR 140:1163-1169, 1983.

51. Orringer MB, Sloan H: Substernal gastric bypass of the excluded esophagus for palliation of esophageal carcinoma. J Thorac Cardiovasc Surg 70:836-851, 1975.

52. Gandi SK, Naunheim, KS: Complications of transhiatal esophagectomy. Chest Surg Clin North Am 7:601-612, 1997.

53. Orringer MB, Marshall B, Stirling MC: Transhiatal esophagectomy: Clinical experience and refinements. Ann Surg 230:392-403:1999.

54. Agha FP, Orringer MB, Amendola MA: Gastric interposition following transhiatal esophagectomy: Radiographic evaluation. Gastrointest Radiol 10:17-24, 1985.

55. Glickstein M, Gefter WB, Low D, et al: Esophageal mucocele after surgical isolation of the esophagus. AJR 149:729-730, 1987.

56. Agha FP, Orringer MB: Colonic interposition: Radiographic evaluation. AJR 142:703-708, 1984.

57. Christensen LR, Shapir J: Radiology of colonic interposition and its associated complications. Gastrointest Radiol 11:233-240, 1986.

58. Larson TC, Shuman LS, Libshitz HI, et al: Complications of colonic interposition. Cancer 56:681-690, 1985.

59. Perlmutter DH, Tapper D, Teele RL, et al: Colobronchial fistula as a late complication of coloesophageal interposition. Gastroenterology 86:1570-1572, 1984.

60. Gollub MJ, Gerdes H, Bains MS: Radiographic appearances of esophageal stents. RadioGraphics 17:1169-1182, 1997.

61. Acunas B, Rozanes I, Akpinar S, et al: Palliation of malignant esophageal strictures with self-expanding nitinol stents: Drawbacks and complications. Radiology 199:648-652, 1996.

62. Han Y-M, Song H-Y, Lee J-M, et al: Esophagorespiratory fistulae due to esophageal carcinoma: Palliation with a covered Gianturco stent. Radiology 199:65-70, 1996.

63. Song H-Y, Park S-I, Do Y-S, et al: Expandable metallic stent placement in patients with benign esophageal strictures: Results of long-term follow-up. Radiology 203:131-136, 1997.

64. Nevitt AW, Kozarek RA, Kidd R: Expandable esophageal prostheses: Recognition, insertion techniques, and positioning. AJR 167:1009-1014, 1966.

65. Song H-Y, Park S-I, Jung H-Y, et al: Benign and malignant esophageal strictures: Treatment with polyurethane-covered retrievable expandable metallic stent. Radiology 203:747-752, 1999.

66. Therasse E, Oliva VL, Lafontaine E, et al: Balloon dilation and stent placement for esophageal lesions: Indications, methods and results. RadioGraphics 23:89-115, 2003.

67. Lipinski JK, Conway SS, Kottler RE, et al: The radiology of oesophageal tubes for malignant strictures. Clin Radiol 33:453-459, 1982.

68. Russell E, Shapiro R, Wilson GL: Radiologic aspects of Celestin tube intubation for incurable obstruction. Radiology 102:531-532, 1972.

69. Giarardet RE, Ransdell HT, Wheat MW: Palliative intubation in the management of esophageal carcinoma. Ann Thorac Surg 18:417-430, 1974.

70. Kairaluoma MI, Kalevi J, Karkola P, et al: Celestin tube palliation of unresectable esophageal carcinoma. J Thorac Cardiovasc Surg 73:783-786, 1977.

71. Haynes JW, Miller PR, Steiger Z, et al: Celestin tube use: Radiographic manifestations of associated complications. Radiology 150:41-44, 1984.

72. Hans-Ulrich L, Marriott A, Wilbraham L, et al: Effectiveness of open verus antireflux stents for palliation of distal esophageal carcinoma and prevention of symptomatic gastroesophageal reflux. Radiology 225:359-365, 2002.

73. Wolf EL, Frager J, Brandt LJ, et al: Radiographic appearance of the esophagus and stomach after laser treatment of obstructing carcinoma. AJR 146:519-522, 1986.

74. Lightdale CJ, Hier SK, Marcon NE, et al: Photodynamic therapy with porfimer sodium versus thermal ablation therapy with Nd:YAG laser for palliation of esophageal cancer: A multicenter randomized trial. Gastrointest Endosc 42:507-512, 1995.

75. McCaughan JS Jr, Ellison EC, Guy JY, et al: Photodynamic therapy for esophageal malignancy: A prospective twelve-year study. Ann Thorac Surg 62:1005-1110, 1996.

76. Fleischer D, Kessler F: Endoscopic Nd:YAG laser therapy for carcinoma of the esophagus: A new form of palliative treatment. Gastroenterology 85:600-606, 1985.

77. Pasricha PJ, Ravich WJ, Hendrix TR, et al: Treatment of achalasia with intrasphincteric injections of botulinum toxin—results of a pilot study. Gastroenterology 104:A168, 1993.

78. Okike N, Payne WS, Neufeld DM, et al: Esophagomyotomy versus forceful dilatation for achalasia of the esophagus: Results in 899 patients. Ann Thorac Surg 28:119-125, 1979.

79. Zegel HG, Kressel HY, Levine GM, et al: Delayed perforation after pneumatic dilatation for the treatment of achalasia. Gastrointest Radiol 4:219-221, 1979.

80. Stewart ET, Miller WN, Hogan WJ, et al: Desirability of roentgen esophageal examination immediately after pneumatic dilatation for achalasia. Radiology 130:589-591, 1979.

81. Ott DJ, Wu WC, Gelfand DW, et al: Radiographic evaluation of the achalasic esophagus immediately following pneumatic dilatation. Gastrointest Radiol 9:185-191, 1984.

82. Bradley JL, Han SY: Intramural hematoma (incomplete perforation) of the esophagus associated with esophageal dilatation. Radiology 130:59-62, 1979.

83. Agha FP, Lee HH: The esophagus after endoscopic pneumatic balloon dilatation for achalasia. AJR 146:25-29, 1986.

84. Meyer JA: Nonmalignant disease of the esophagus. In Fromm D (ed): Gastrointestinal Surgery. New York, Churchill Livingstone, 1985, pp 113-162.

85. Rubesin SE, Kennedy M, Levine MS, et al: Distal esophageal ballooning following Heller myotomy. Radiology 167:345-347, 1988.

86. Yoo C, Levine MS, Redfern RO, et al: Laparoscopic Heller myotomy and fundoplication: Findings and predictive value of early postoperative radiographic studies. Abdom Imaging 29:643-647, 2004.

87. Sugiura M, Futagawa S: A new technique for treating esophageal varices. J Thorac Cardiovasc Surg 66:677-685, 1973.

88. Sugiura M, Futagawa S: Further evaluation of the Sugiura procedure in the treatment of esophageal varices. Arch Surg 112:1317-1321, 1977.

89. Greenspan R, Kressel HY, Laufer I, et al: Radiographic findings in the esophagus following the Sugiura procedure. Radiology 144:245-247, 1982.

90. Koyama K, Takagi Y, Ouchi K, et al: Results of esophageal transection for esophageal varices: Experience in 100 cases. Am J Surg 139:204-209, 1980.

Esophagus: Differential Diagnosis

Marc S. Levine, MD

TABLE 32-1. ULCERATION	TABLE 32-5. THICKENED FOLDS
TABLE 32-2. MUCOSAL NODULARITY	TABLE 32-6. STRICTURES
TABLE 32-3. SOLITARY MASS LESIONS	
TABLE 32-4. MULTIPLE SUBMUCOSAL MASSES	

Table 32-1
Ulceration

Cause	Radiographic Findings	Distribution	Comments
Common			
Reflux esophagitis	Shallow, punctate, or linear ulcers; deep ulcers less common	Distal	Reflux symptoms, hiatal hernia, and/or gastroesophageal reflux
Candida esophagitis	Ulcers associated with diffuse plaque formation (i.e., "shaggy" esophagus)	Variable	Odynophagia in immunocompromised (usually AIDS) patients
Herpes esophagitis	Discrete, superficial ulcers	Middle or distal	Odynophagia in immunocompromised patients; occasionally in healthy patients
Drug-induced esophagitis	Discrete, superficial ulcers; occasionally giant, flat ulcers	Midesophagus near aortic arch or left main bronchus	Odynophagia in patients taking oral medications (e.g., doxycycline or tetracycline)
Uncommon			
Radiation esophagitis	Superficial or deep ulcers	Conform to radiation portal	History of radiation therapy
Caustic esophagitis	Superficial or deep ulcers	Variable	History of caustic ingestion
Tuberculous esophagitis	Superficial or deep ulcers	Variable	History of pulmonary tuberculosis or AIDS
Cytomegalovirus esophagitis	One or more giant, flat ulcers	Variable	AIDS patients
HIV esophagitis	One or more giant, flat ulcers	Variable	HIV-positive or AIDS patients with odynophagia
Crohn's disease	Aphthous ulcers	Variable	Advanced Crohn's disease in small bowel or colon
Nasogastric intubation	Shallow ulcers or giant, flat ulcers	Distal	History of intubation
Alkaline reflux esophagitis	Superficial or deep ulcers	Distal	Partial or total gastrectomy
Behçet's disease	Superficial ulcers	Variable	Oral and genital ulcers and ocular inflammation
Epidermolysis bullosa dystrophica	Superficial ulcers or bullae	Variable	Skin disease
Benign mucous membrane pemphigoid	Superficial ulcers or bullae	Variable	Skin disease

Table 32-2
Mucosal Nodularity

Cause	Radiographic Findings	Distribution	Comments
Common			
Reflux esophagitis	Nodular or granular mucosa (nodules poorly defined)	Distal one third or one half of thoracic esophagus	Reflux symptoms, hiatal hernia, and/or gastroesophageal reflux
Candida esophagitis	Discrete plaques	Localized or diffuse	Odynophagia in immunocompromised patients
Glycogenic acanthosis	Nodules or plaques	Localized or diffuse	Asymptomatic
Uncommon			
Barrett's esophagus	Reticular pattern	Localized	Often adjacent to distal aspect of midesophageal stricture
Radiation esophagitis	Granular mucosa and decreased distensibility	Conforms to radiation portal	Temporal relationship to radiation therapy
Superficial spreading carcinoma	Poorly defined, coalescent nodules or plaques	Localized or diffuse	May be asymptomatic
Esophageal papillomatosis	Multiple excrescences	Diffuse	Asymptomatic
Acanthosis nigricans	Tiny nodules	Diffuse	Skin disease
Cowden's disease	Tiny nodules (i.e., hamartomatous polyps)	Diffuse	Hereditary disorder with associated malignant tumors of skin, gastrointestinal tract, and thyroid
Leukoplakia	Tiny nodules	Localized or diffuse	Rare

Table 32-3
Solitary Mass Lesions

Cause	Radiographic Findings	Distribution	Comments
Mucosal Lesions			
Papilloma	Sessile or slightly lobulated polyp	Variable	Asymptomatic
Adenoma	Sessile or pedunculated polyp	Distal	Arises in Barrett's mucosa
Inflammatory esophagogastric polyp	Polypoid protuberance with contiguous fold arising near cardia	Distal	Associated reflux esophagitis
Adenocarcinoma or squamous cell carcinoma	Plaquelike, sessile, or polypoid lesion	Variable	Small lesions may be early esophageal cancers
Spindle cell carcinoma	Bulky polypoid mass	Variable	Expands lumen without causing obstruction
Primary malignant melanoma	Bulky polypoid mass	Variable	Expands lumen without causing obstruction
Submucosal Lesions			
Leiomyoma	Smooth submucosal mass	Variable	Usually asymptomatic; rarely ulcerated
Fibrovascular polyp	Large pedunculated mass with sausage-shaped appearance	Arises in cervical esophagus but extends distally	May be regurgitated into or occlude larynx, causing asphyxia and sudden death
Granular cell tumor	Smooth submucosal mass	Usually distal	Associated lesions on skin or tongue
Lipoma	Sessile or pedunculated lesion	Variable	Fat density on CT
Hemangioma	Smooth submucosal mass	Variable	Risk of exsanguination
Idiopathic varix	Smooth submucosal mass	Variable	Effaced or obliterated with esophageal distention (unless thrombosed)
Duplication cyst	Smooth submucosal mass	Right lateral wall of distal esophagus	Fluid density on CT

Table 32-4
Multiple Submucosal Masses

Cause	Distribution	Comments
Benign Lesions		
Leiomyomas	Middle or distal	May be asymptomatic
Granular cell tumors	Middle or distal	Associated lesions on skin or tongue
Hemangiomas	Diffuse	Osler-Weber-Rendu disease
Retention cysts (esophagitis cystica)	Distal	Asymptomatic
Malignant Lesions		
Hematogenous metastases	Middle or distal	Very rare in esophagus
Lymphoma	Diffuse	Usually non-Hodgkin's lymphoma
Leukemia	Diffuse	Usually asymptomatic
Kaposi's sarcoma	Diffuse	Patients with AIDS

Table 32-5
Thickened Folds

Cause	Radiographic Findings	Distribution	Comments
Varices	Tortuous or serpiginous folds	Uphill: distal Downhill: middle	Effaced or obliterated with esophageal distention; no dysphagia
Esophagitis	Smooth, nodular, or scalloped folds	Diffuse	Reflux symptoms or other findings of esophagitis
Varicoid carcinoma	Thickened, lobulated folds	Variable	Rigid, fixed appearance at fluoroscopy; dysphagia common
Lymphoma	Thickened, lobulated folds	Variable	Usually non-Hodgkin's lymphoma

Table 32-6
Strictures

Cause	Radiographic Findings	Comments
Distal Esophagus		
Peptic strictures	Symmetric or asymmetric; moderate length or ringlike	Associated hiatal hernia
Barrett's esophagus	Symmetric or asymmetric (i.e., peptic strictures)	Barrett's mucosa found in 40% of peptic strictures
Nasogastric intubation	Long area of narrowing	Rapidly progressive
Zollinger-Ellison syndrome	Long area of narrowing	May be initial manifestation of disease; hypergastrinemia
Crohn's disease	Short or long	Advanced Crohn's disease in small bowel or colon
Alkaline reflux strictures	Short or long	Rapidly progressive; seen after partial or total gastrectomy
Carcinoma (usually adenocarcinoma)	Irregular narrowing with nodularity or ulceration	Arises in Barrett's esophagus; often invades gastric cardia and fundus; recent dysphagia and weight loss
Midesophagus		
Barrett's esophagus	Tapered or ringlike	Hiatal hernia and/or gastroesophageal reflux; adjacent reticular pattern
Radiation	Usually tapered	History of radiation therapy (>50 Gy)
Eosinophilic esophagitis	Variable narrowing with concentric rings (ringed esophagus)	History of allergies and peripheral eosinophilia
Caustic ingestion	Single or multiple; long strictures common	History of caustic ingestion
Oral medications	Often near level of enlarged left atrium	Potassium chloride, quinidine, alendronate, nonsteroidal anti-inflammatory drugs
Opportunistic infection (usually candidiasis)	Short or long	History of *Candida* esophagitis
Epidermolysis bullosa dystrophica	High strictures or webs	Skin disease
Benign mucous membrane pemphigoid	High strictures or webs	Skin disease
Chronic graft-versus-host disease	Relatively long	History of marrow transplant
Glutaraldehyde-induced injury	Long and tapered	Rapidly progressive stricture within weeks of endoscopy
Congenital esophageal stenosis	Tapered narrowing with concentric rings	Long-standing dysphagia for solids; food impactions
Carcinoma (usually squamous cell carcinoma)	Irregular narrowing with nodularity or ulceration	History of smoking and/or alcohol consumption; recent dysphagia and weight loss
Metastatic tumor	Tapered or irregular narrowing	Usually lung or breast cancer

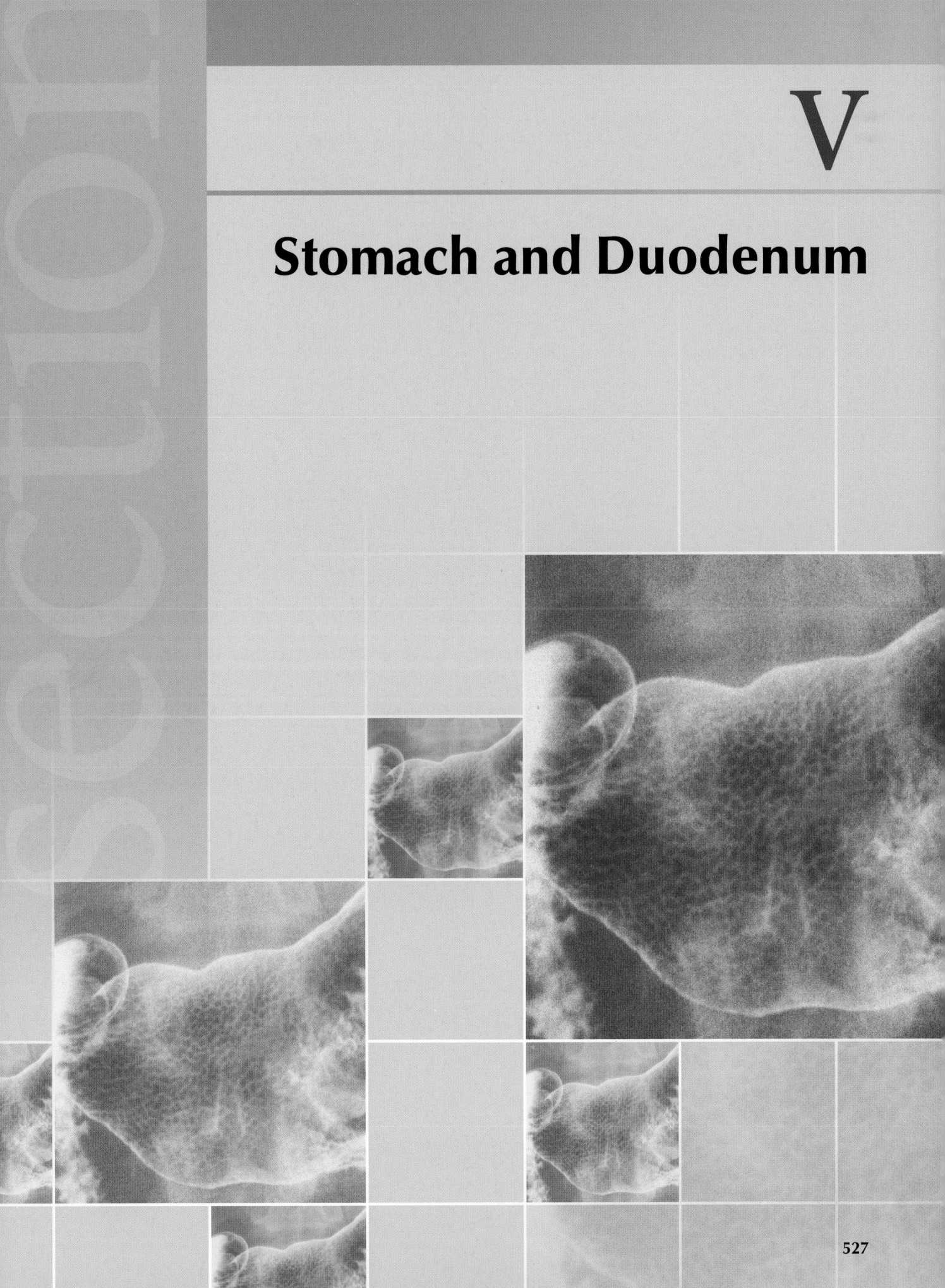

V

Stomach and Duodenum

Peptic Ulcers

Marc S. Levine, MD

Gastric or duodenal ulcers (i.e., peptic ulcers) are thought to occur in about 10% of the adult population in western countries.[1] Peptic ulcers are important not only because of the frequent occurrence of pain or other symptoms but also because of the morbidity and mortality associated with complications such as bleeding and perforation. It has been well established that *Helicobacter pylori* and nonsteroidal anti-inflammatory drugs (NSAIDs) have a major role in the development of ulcers. A better understanding of the pathophysiology has led to important breakthroughs in ulcer treatment. Although duodenal ulcers are virtually always benign, a small percentage of gastric ulcers are found to be malignant. Thus, gastric ulcers require careful evaluation and follow-up to differentiate benign and malignant lesions.

EPIDEMIOLOGY AND PATHOGENESIS

During the late 19th and early 20th centuries, gastric ulcers were much more common than duodenal ulcers.[2] Since that time there has been a dramatic reversal of this relationship, so that duodenal ulcers are now more common than gastric ulcers.[2] Although duodenal ulcers occur in adults of all ages, gastric ulcers are found predominantly in patients older than 40 years of age.[1,2] Regardless of the location of the ulcers,

the gender distribution is about equal.[3] Both gastric and duodenal ulcers are characterized by seasonal variations, with a higher frequency of ulcers in spring and autumn and a lower frequency in summer.[4]

A voluminous body of literature has shown convincingly that *H. pylori* or NSAIDs are responsible for most gastric ulcers and that *H. pylori* is the causative agent for almost all duodenal ulcers. Nevertheless, data indicate that the incidence of *H. pylori*–negative idiopathic ulcers is rising even in the absence of NSAID use.[5] Other possible causative agents include corticosteroids, tobacco, alcohol, coffee, stress, duodenogastric reflux of bile, and delayed gastric emptying. Hereditary factors have also been implicated. These subjects are discussed separately in the following sections.

Helicobacter pylori Gastritis

H. pylori (formerly known as *Campylobacter pylori*) is a gram-negative, spiral bacillus that was first isolated on endoscopic biopsy specimens from the stomach in 1983.[6] Since that time, *H. pylori* has been recognized as the major causative factor in the development of both gastric and duodenal ulcers (excluding those caused by NSAIDs or Zollinger-Ellison syndrome).[7-9] In various studies, the prevalence of *H. pylori* gastritis has ranged from 60% to 80% in patients with gastric ulcers and from 95% to 100% in patients with duodenal ulcers.[7,10,11]

The mechanism by which *H. pylori* predisposes to the development of ulcers remains uncertain. It has been shown, however, that patients with *H. pylori* gastritis have increased secretion of gastrin with high basal and peak acid outputs.[12] Gastrin-mediated increase in gastric acid secretion and inhibition of the normal physiologic mechanisms for controlling acid secretion appear to be key factors in the pathogenesis of peptic ulcers. Nevertheless, most people with *H. pylori* never develop ulcers. It has therefore been postulated that certain strains of *H. pylori* are more virulent and are more likely to be associated with ulcer formation.[12,13] A high prevalence and density of a particularly virulent *cagA*-positive strain of *H. pylori* in the duodenum has been associated with the development of duodenal ulcers.[14] Many patients with duodenal ulcers also have evidence of gastric metaplasia at the borders of the ulcers with infection of the metaplastic epithelium by *H. pylori*.[14,15] The infected mucosa may therefore be more susceptible to ulceration.

Nonsteroidal Anti-inflammatory Drugs

In various studies, the prevalence of gastric ulcers in patients receiving regular treatment with aspirin or other NSAIDs has ranged from 15% to 30%.[16-18] It has been shown that NSAIDs inhibit prostaglandin production by blocking the formation of cyclooxygenase (COX-1), a rate-limiting enzyme for the synthesis of prostaglandins.[18,19] This phenomenon occurs even with aspirin doses as low as 10 mg daily (compared with a dose of 81 mg daily for cardiovascular prophylaxis).[20] Because prostaglandins have cytoprotective properties in the stomach, inhibition of prostaglandin synthesis can lead to severe mucosal injury and ulceration.[18,19,21,22]

The ulcerogenic effects of NSAIDs are also related to a topical effect resulting from breakdown of the mucosal barrier.[19,22] It has been shown that aspirin disrupts the mucus gel layer of the stomach, allowing acid to damage the gastric mucosa even in the presence of normal or decreased acid secretion.[23] Altered mucosal resistance is therefore thought to be an important factor in ulcer pathogenesis. NSAID-induced ulcers are sometimes located on the greater curvature of the antrum, presumably because of localized mucosal injury as the ingested NSAID capsules collect by gravity in the most dependent portion of the stomach (see later section on Location). Nevertheless, the majority of NSAID-induced gastric ulcers occur in other portions of the stomach (away from the greater curvature). Studies have also shown that patients taking enteric-coated aspirin have the same risk of upper gastrointestinal bleeding as those taking non–enteric-coated aspirin.[24] Ulcers have also been induced in cats by intravenous infusion of aspirin.[25] Thus, the development of ulcers is ultimately mediated by a combination of the topical and systemic effects of NSAIDs.

Chronic NSAID use is associated not only with an increased frequency of ulcers but also with an increased frequency of complications such as perforation, obstruction, and bleeding.[26,27] Studies have shown that people taking NSAIDs have a twofold to sixfold higher incidence of clinically important upper gastrointestinal events than those not taking NSAIDs.[18] Clinical trials have also shown that such events occur annually in 3% to 4.5% of all arthritis patients taking

NSAIDs.[18] The risk increases even further in people older than 60 years of age.[21] A careful NSAID history should therefore be obtained in all *H. pylori*-negative patients with peptic ulcers because of the likelihood that these ulcers are NSAID related in the absence of *H. pylori*.

Corticosteroids

Some investigators believe that corticosteroids predispose to the development of peptic ulcers, particularly gastric ulcers. This concern often results in discontinuation of corticosteroid therapy in patients with ulcer symptoms or occult gastrointestinal bleeding. In a large double-blind study, however, patients receiving corticosteroids were found to have the same frequency of peptic ulcers as the general population.[28] It is therefore questionable whether corticosteroids have any role in ulcer pathogenesis. Nevertheless, corticosteroids can mask the clinical findings associated with peptic ulcers, so that a large ulcer or even a perforated ulcer may fail to produce symptoms in these patients.

Tobacco, Alcohol, and Coffee

Some investigators have found that cigarette smokers are more likely to have ulcers than nonsmokers[29,30] and that perforated ulcers are also more likely to occur in these individuals.[31] Others have found no significant correlation between smoking and peptic ulcers.[32] Although alcohol and coffee are thought to stimulate acid secretion, their role in ulcer pathogenesis remains uncertain.[29]

Stress

Some investigators believe that emotional stress contributes to the development of peptic ulcers by increasing secretion of peptic acid.[33,34] In one study, extreme emotional stress after a major earthquake in Japan resulted in an increased frequency of gastric ulcers, particularly bleeding ulcers.[35] Others have found that stressful life events are no more common in patients with ulcers than in the general population.[36] Thus, the role of stress in the development of peptic ulcers remains uncertain.

Gastroduodenal Reflux of Bile and Delayed Gastric Emptying

Some investigators have found that patients with gastric ulcers have an unusually high concentration of bile acids in the stomach.[37] As a result, duodenogastric reflux of bile has been implicated in ulcer pathogenesis. Others have found that gastric stasis resulting from any cause of gastric outlet obstruction or gastric atony may predispose to the development of gastric ulcers by prolonging exposure of the gastric mucosa to acid and pepsin in the stomach.[38] These stasis-induced gastric ulcers have come to be known as *Dragstedt's ulcers* based on the name of the investigator who described these lesions.[38]

Hereditary Factors

A small percentage of patients with peptic ulcers have a family history of ulcers.[39,40] This familial aggregation of ulcers is explained primarily by hereditary rather than environmental factors because studies of twins have found a much greater concordance of ulcers in monozygotic twins than in dizygotic twins.[39] Patients with blood type O also have a higher incidence of ulcers than those with other blood types.[39] Finally, peptic ulcers are more common in patients with genetic syndromes such as multiple endocrine neoplasia type 1, systemic mastocytosis, and tremor-nystagmus-ulcer syndrome.[39] Thus, hereditary factors have clearly been implicated in the development of peptic ulcers.

CLINICAL FINDINGS

Patients with peptic ulcers usually present with localized epigastric pain, consisting of a gnawing, aching, or burning discomfort between the xiphoid cartilage and the umbilicus.[41] Ulcer pain tends to have a rhythmic nature; gastric ulcer pain classically occurs less than 2 hours after meals, whereas duodenal ulcer pain occurs 2 to 4 hours after meals and is more likely to waken the patient at night.[41] Nevertheless, there is so much overlap in the timing and quality of the pain that it is difficult to differentiate gastric and duodenal ulcers on clinical grounds.

Other patients with peptic ulcers may have right upper quadrant, back, or chest pain or other symptoms such as bloating, belching, nausea, vomiting, anorexia, and weight loss.[41] Depending on the clinical presentation, the differential diagnosis includes reflux esophagitis, gastritis, duodenitis, cholecystitis, pancreatitis, gastroenteritis, irritable bowel syndrome, ischemic bowel disease, Crohn's disease, and gastric or pancreatic carcinoma.[41]

Still other patients with peptic ulcers may initially present with signs or symptoms caused by complications of their ulcers, such as perforation, obstruction, and bleeding. When ulcers on the posterior wall of the stomach or duodenum penetrate into the pancreas, the normally rhythmic epigastric pain associated with ulcers is replaced by a more constant pain that radiates to the back. In contrast, free perforation of a gastric or duodenal ulcer causes generalized peritonitis. The major factors contributing to mortality in patients with perforated peptic ulcers include age older than 60 years and a delay of more than 24 hours from the time of diagnosis to the time of surgery.[42]

Ulcers in the distal antrum, pyloric channel, or duodenum that are associated with edema, spasm, or scar formation may cause varying degrees of gastric outlet obstruction. Such patients may present with postprandial nausea and vomiting. Patients with pyloric channel ulcers sometimes develop a characteristic clinical syndrome (the pyloric channel syndrome) manifested by severe postprandial epigastric pain that is relieved by vomiting.[43,44]

Peptic ulcers are the most common cause of acute upper gastrointestinal bleeding, accounting for about 50% of cases.[45] Some patients have one or more episodes of massive hemorrhage, manifested by hematemesis, melena, or rectal bleeding, whereas others have chronic, low-grade hemorrhage, manifested by guaiac-positive stool or iron-deficiency anemia.[41] Gastric ulcers are more likely to bleed than duodenal ulcers, probably because of the greater size of the ulcer craters and older age of the patients.[41] When ulcers are present in the duodenum, however, postbulbar duodenal ulcers are more likely to be associated with upper gastrointestinal bleeding (particularly massive bleeding) than those in the duodenal bulb.[46] Bleeding from ulcers ceases spontaneously in about 80% of cases, but some form of medical, endoscopic, angiographic, or surgical therapy is required to control the bleeding in the remaining 20%.[45]

The diagnosis of peptic ulcer disease is complicated by the fact that 25% to 50% of patients with proven gastric or duodenal ulcers are asymptomatic.[41,47] Ulcers may be clinically silent until the development of an acute abdominal catastrophe caused by bleeding or perforation. Conversely, patients with classic ulcer symptoms are not always found to have ulcers on radiologic or endoscopic examinations.[48] Thus, peptic ulcer disease remains a challenging clinical diagnosis.

TREATMENT

The choice of treatment for peptic ulcer disease depends on the underlying cause. If *H. pylori* gastritis is confirmed either by endoscopy and biopsy or by noninvasive tests such as the urea breath test or serologic tests (see Chapter 34), there is considerable evidence that eradication of *H. pylori* leads to more rapid healing of both gastric and duodenal ulcers and to a much lower rate of ulcer recurrence.[49-51] On the basis of these findings, expert panels convened by the National Institutes of Health and the American Digestive Health Foundation concluded that all patients with gastric or duodenal ulcers who are infected by *H. pylori* should be treated with antimicrobial and antisecretory agents.[52,53] Various combinations of antibiotics (e.g., tetracycline, amoxicillin, clarithromycin, metronidazole, bismuth), H_2-receptor antagonists (e.g., cimetidine, ranitidine), and proton pump inhibitors (e.g., omeprazole) have been shown to be highly effective in eradicating *H. pylori*,[54-56] so that these patients can literally be "cured" of their ulcer disease.

In the absence of *H. pylori*, H_2-receptor antagonists such as cimetidine and ranitidine have proved to be highly effective in accelerating healing of both gastric and duodenal ulcers by suppressing acid secretion.[57] Proton pump inhibitors such as omeprazole are even more effective for suppressing acid secretion and accelerating ulcer healing by selectively inhibiting the gastric proton pump that controls the first step in the production of gastric acid.[58] Because patients with NSAID-related ulcers have decreased synthesis of prostaglandins (see earlier section on NSAIDs), misoprostol (a synthetic prostaglandin E analogue) has been used to accelerate ulcer healing.[59] Administration of prostaglandins and prostaglandin analogues to patients receiving NSAIDs also decreases the risk of developing gastric ulcers.[60] Sucralfate, colloidal bismuth, and carbenoxolone are other drugs that have been used with varying degrees of success for the treatment of ulcers.

Surgical intervention may ultimately be required for recurrent or intractable ulcers that fail to heal with medical therapy; for ulcer complications such as bleeding and perforation; and for ulcers that have equivocal or suspicious findings on radiologic studies or endoscopy. The most common operations include partial gastrectomy, vagotomy and pyloroplasty, and hyperselective vagotomy. These surgical procedures and their complications are discussed in Chapter 39. Because of better diagnosis and medical treatment of peptic ulcer disease, the need for surgery in these patients has decreased considerably since the late 1960s.[61,62] Advances in the treatment of peptic ulcers in *H. pylori*–positive patients may further decrease the need for surgery in the future.

RADIOGRAPHIC FINDINGS

Gastric Ulcers

Examination Technique

The double-contrast examination should be performed as a biphasic study that includes double-contrast views of the stomach with a high-density barium suspension and prone or upright compression views with a low-density barium suspension (see Chapter 21). Ulcer detection is facilitated by the routine administration of 0.1 mg of glucagon intravenously to induce gastric hypotonia. Ulcers located on the posterior wall or on the lesser or greater curvature of the stomach are usually well seen on double-contrast views obtained in supine or oblique projections. Flow technique can be used to better delineate shallow ulcers on the posterior wall or lesser curvature by slowly rotating the patient from side to side to manipulate a thin layer of high-density barium over the dependent surface of the stomach (Fig. 33-1).[63] Upright compression views are also helpful for evaluating ulcers on the lesser curvature. With the patient in an upright position, the weight of the barium tends to pull the antrum inferiorly and straighten the lesser curvature, so that these ulcers can be optimally demonstrated.[64]

It is important to be aware of the limitations of the double-contrast study in diagnosing ulcers on the anterior or nondependent wall of the stomach. Because of the effect of gravity, these ulcers may not be filled with barium on double-contrast views obtained in the usual supine or oblique projections (Fig. 33-2A). Prone compression views of the gastric antrum and body should therefore be obtained routinely to demonstrate ulcers on the anterior wall

(Fig. 33-2B). When ulcers or other lesions are suspected in this location, double-contrast views of the anterior wall can also be obtained by placing the patient in a prone Trendelenburg position.[65]

Shape

Gastric ulcers are classically seen as round or ovoid collections of barium (see Figs. 33-1B and 33-2B). Ulcer craters may have a variety of shapes and configurations, appearing as linear, rod-shaped, rectangular, serpiginous, or flame-shaped lesions (Fig. 33-3).[66-69] Linear ulcers constitute about 5% of all gastric ulcers diagnosed on double-contrast studies.[68] These linear ulcers probably represent a stage of ulcer healing in both the stomach and the duodenum.[68,69]

Size

The radiographic sensitivity in detecting gastric ulcers is related primarily to ulcer size; ulcers greater than 5 mm are more likely to be detected on barium studies.[70] A major advantage of double-contrast technique is its ability to distend the stomach and efface the normal mucosal folds, so that small ulcers can be demonstrated (Fig. 33-4). In fact, most gastric ulcers diagnosed on double-contrast studies are less than 1 cm.[69] The high prevalence of small ulcers may also be related to the aggressive medical treatment these patients often receive before they undergo radiologic investigations.

Large ulcers tend to be located more proximally in the stomach (Fig. 33-5).[71] These ulcers may occasionally be recognized on abdominal radiographs by the presence of gas in the ulcer crater. Giant gastric ulcers (i.e., ulcers > 3 cm) have a higher risk of complications such as bleeding and perforation.[72] However, most giant ulcers are found to be benign.[72] Thus, the size of the ulcer has no relationship to the presence of carcinoma.

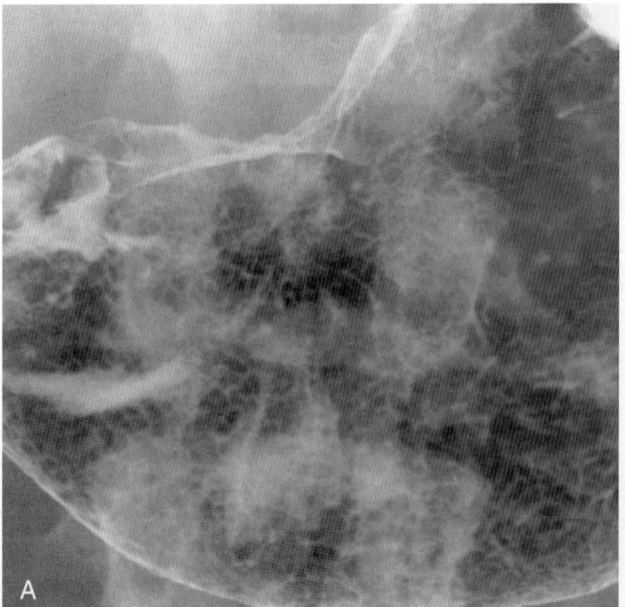
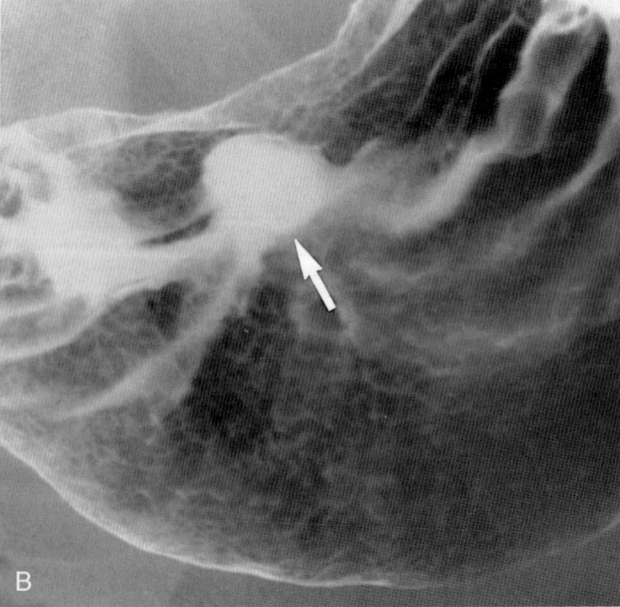

Figure 33-1. Importance of flow technique for posterior wall ulcers. A. Supine double-contrast view shows no evidence of an ulcer, even in retrospect. **B.** With flow technique, an ulcer (*arrow*) is seen on the posterior wall of the antrum. Note how folds radiate to the edge of the ulcer crater. (From Laufer I, Levine MS [eds]: Double Contrast Gastrointestinal Radiology, 2nd ed. Philadelphia, WB Saunders, 1992.)

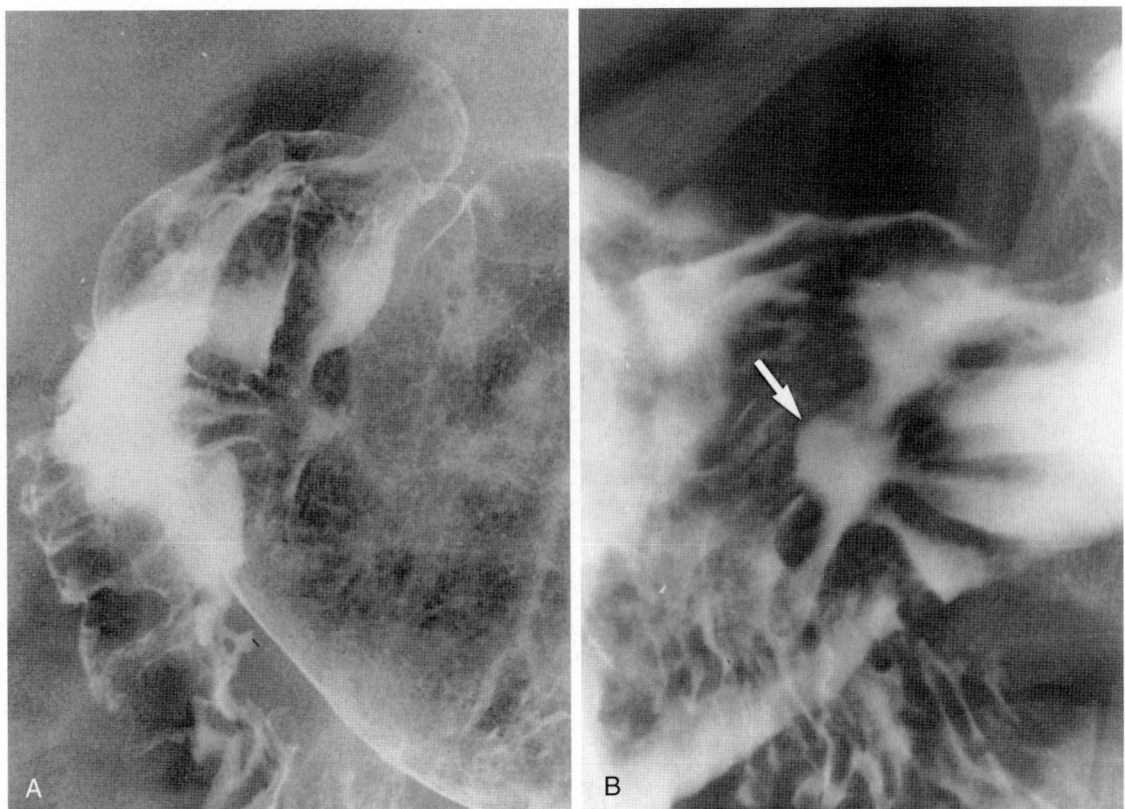

Figure 33-2. Importance of prone compression for anterior wall ulcers. A. Supine double-contrast view shows abnormal folds in the antrum without a definite ulcer. **B.** Prone compression view shows filling of an anterior wall ulcer (*arrow*). Note how folds radiate to the edge of the ulcer crater. (From Laufer I, Levine MS [eds]: Double Contrast Gastrointestinal Radiology, 2nd ed. Philadelphia, WB Saunders, 1992.)

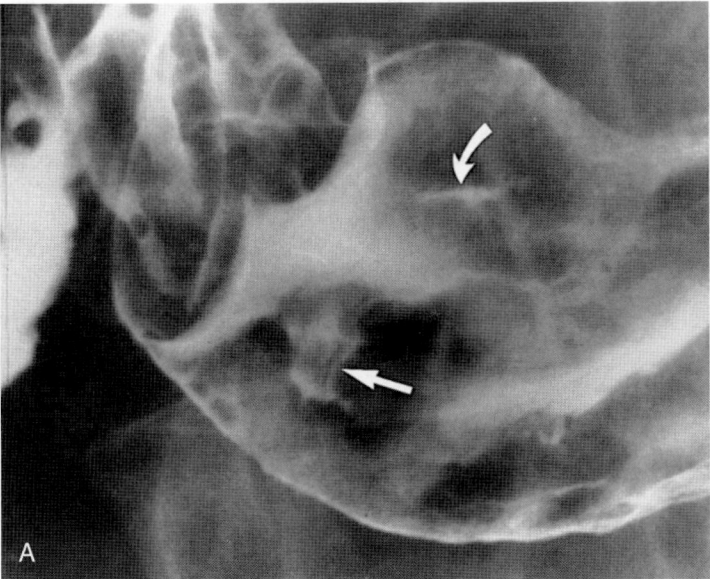

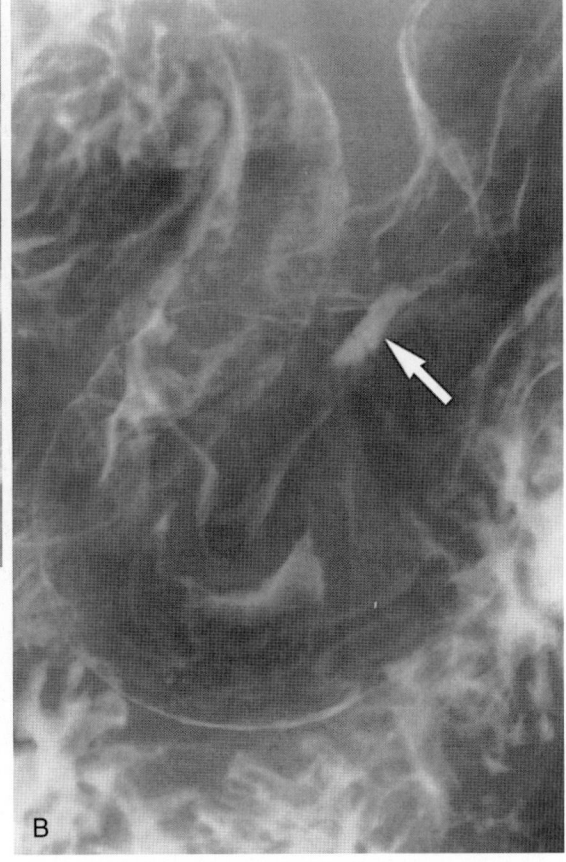

Figure 33-3. Gastric ulcers of different shapes. A. This patient has star-shaped (*straight arrow*) and linear (*curved arrow*) ulcers in the antrum. **B.** In another patient, a rod-shaped ulcer (*arrow*) is seen in the stomach.

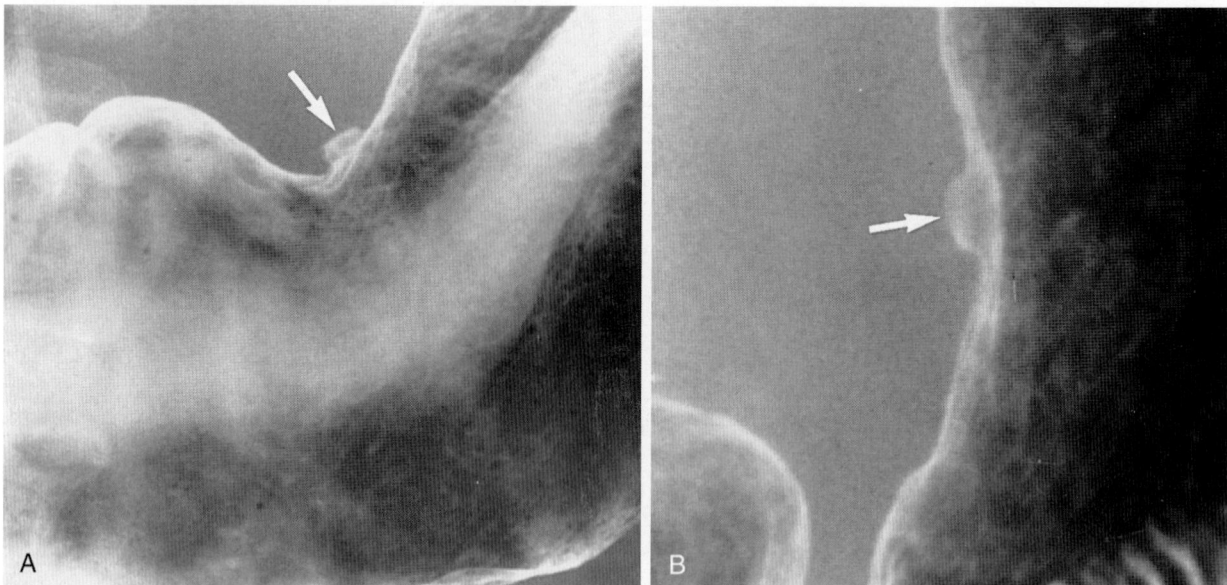

Figure 33-4. Small gastric ulcers. A and **B.** Despite their small size, these lesser curvature ulcers (*arrows*) are well seen on double-contrast radiographs.

Location

Most benign gastric ulcers are located on the lesser curvature or posterior wall of the antrum or body of the stomach.[69,71,73,74] In various studies, only 1% to 7% of benign ulcers are located on the anterior wall and 3% to 11% are on the greater curvature.[69,71,73,75] In younger people, ulcers tend to be located in the antrum, whereas in older people, they are more likely to be located in the upper body, particularly on the lesser curvature.[76,77] These high lesser curvature ulcers have been described as *geriatric ulcers.*[71]

Benign greater curvature ulcers are almost always located in the distal half of the stomach, and the vast majority are caused by ingestion of aspirin or other NSAIDs.[69,78] Because these ulcers rarely occur on the proximal half of the greater curvature, any ulcers in this location should be considered suggestive of malignant tumor until proved otherwise. Except for these ulcers high on the greater curvature, the location of the ulcer has no relationship to the presence of carcinoma.

Gastric ulcers are occasionally found in hiatal hernias.[79] They tend to occur on the lesser curvature aspect of the hernia, where the hernial sac is compressed by the esophageal hiatus of the diaphragm (see Fig. 30-9).[74] Because the hernia is inaccessible to palpation, double-contrast technique is particularly helpful for demonstrating these ulcers.

Morphologic Features

Ulcers on the lesser or greater curvature are readily visualized in profile on barium studies, permitting analysis of the size, shape, and depth of the ulcer crater as well as associated findings such as radiating folds, Hampton's line, or an ulcer mound or collar. Ulcers on the anterior or posterior wall may be difficult or impossible to visualize in profile, however, so that these lesions must be evaluated on the basis of their appearance en face. In such cases, double-contrast technique is particularly helpful in assessing the surrounding mucosa for signs of benign or malignant disease.

Lesser Curvature Ulcers

Ulcers on the lesser curvature typically appear as smooth, round or ovoid craters that project beyond the contour of the adjacent gastric wall (Fig. 33-6; see Fig. 33-4).[64,69,80,81] In

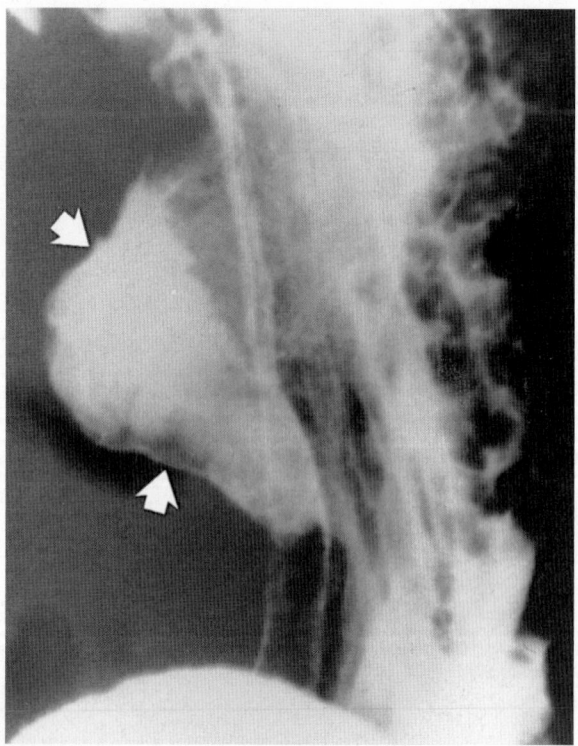

Figure 33-5. Giant gastric ulcer. A giant ulcer (*arrows*) is seen projecting from the lesser curvature of the upper gastric body. Large ulcers tend to be located more proximally in the stomach.

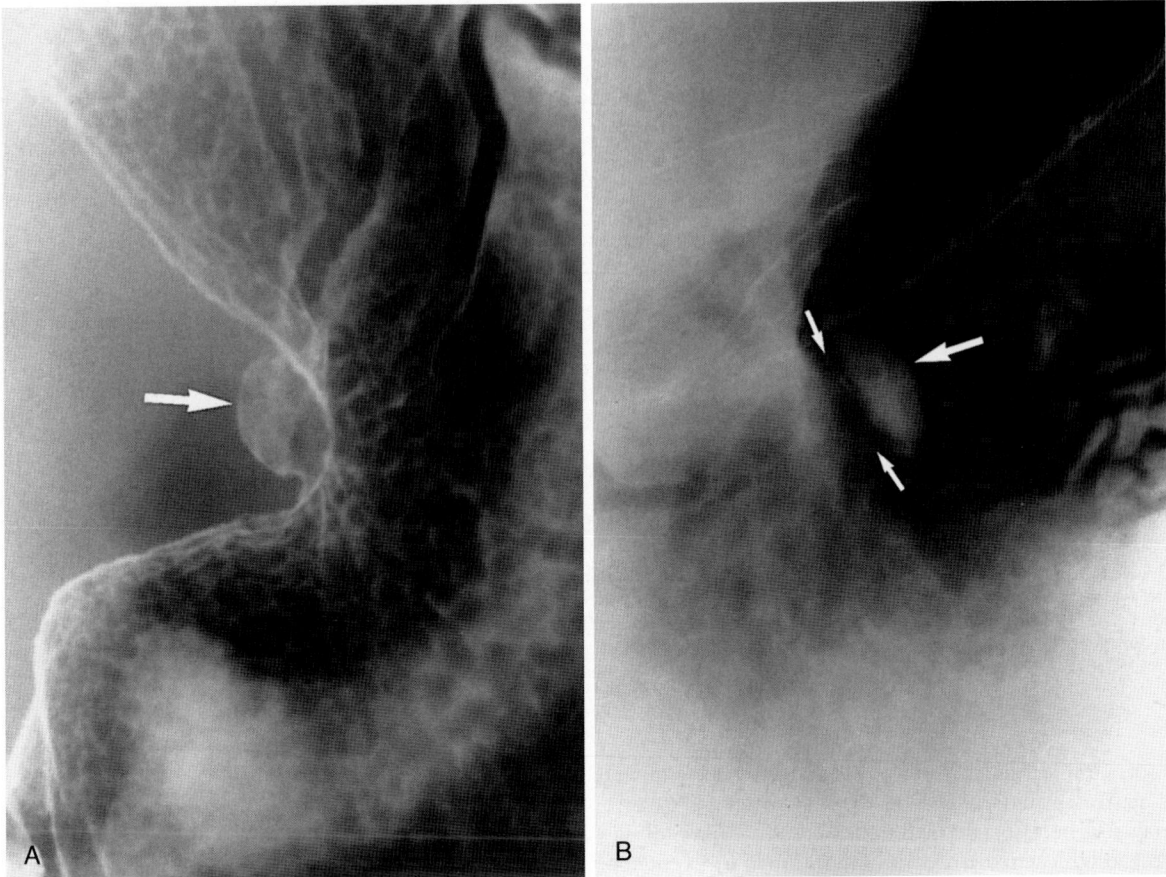

Figure 33-6. Lesser curvature ulcers. A. A smooth, round ulcer (*arrow*) is seen projecting beyond the lesser curvature. The radiating folds and enlarged areae gastricae in the adjacent mucosa are due to surrounding edema and inflammation. **B.** In another patient, a lesser curvature ulcer (*large arrow*) is demonstrated on a prone compression view. Note the radiolucent band of edema or ulcer collar (*small arrows*) adjacent to the ulcer. Both of these cases demonstrate classic features of benign gastric ulcers. (**A** from Levine MS, Creteur V, Kressel HY, et al: Benign gastric ulcers: Diagnosis and follow-up with double contrast radiography. Radiology 164:9-13, 1987.)

some patients with lesser curvature ulcers, upright compression views may reveal a thin, barely perceptible radiolucent line that separates barium in the ulcer crater from barium in the gastric lumen.[64,80] Also known as Hampton's line, this finding results from undermining of the mucosa surrounding the orifice of the ulcer crater.[64] In other patients, the rim of undermined mucosa may become more edematous, producing a wide, radiolucent band, or ulcer collar (see Fig. 33-6B).[64] Occasionally, edema and inflammation surrounding the ulcer produces an ulcer mound, seen in profile as a smooth, bilobed hemispheric mass projecting into the lumen on both sides of the ulcer.[64] Ulcer mounds usually have poorly defined outer borders that form obtuse, gently sloping angles with the adjacent gastric wall.[64] Hampton's lines, ulcer collars, and ulcer mounds are considered to be classic features of benign gastric ulcers, but these findings are present in only a small percentage of all patients with lesser curvature ulcers.

Retraction of the gastric wall adjacent to lesser curvature ulcers sometimes leads to the development of smooth, symmetric folds that radiate to the edge of the ulcer crater (see Fig. 33-6A).[69] Occasionally, these ulcers may be associated with retraction of the opposite wall, producing an incisura on the greater curvature. Other lesser curvature ulcers may be associated with focal enlargement of areae gastricae sur-

rounding the ulcer because of edema and inflammation of the adjacent mucosa (see Fig. 33-6A).[69]

Greater Curvature Ulcers

In the past, almost all ulcers on the greater curvature of the stomach were thought to be malignant.[82] It is now recognized that benign ulcers can occur on the distal half of the greater curvature in patients who are taking aspirin or other NSAIDs (Figs. 33-7 and 33-8).[69,78] The location of these ulcers on the greater curvature is presumably related to the effect of gravity because the dissolving aspirin tablets collect in the most dependent portion of the stomach, causing localized mucosal injury. Such lesions have been described as *sump ulcers* because of their typical location on the greater curvature.[78] A similar phenomenon may also account for the frequent finding of linear or serpiginous erosions in the body of the stomach, on or near the greater curvature in patients who are taking NSAIDs (see Chapter 34).[83] Because of their location, greater curvature ulcers have a tendency to penetrate inferiorly into the gastrocolic ligament, occasionally leading to the development of a gastrocolic fistula (see later section on Fistulas).

In contrast to ulcers on the lesser curvature, greater curvature ulcers may appear to have an intraluminal location

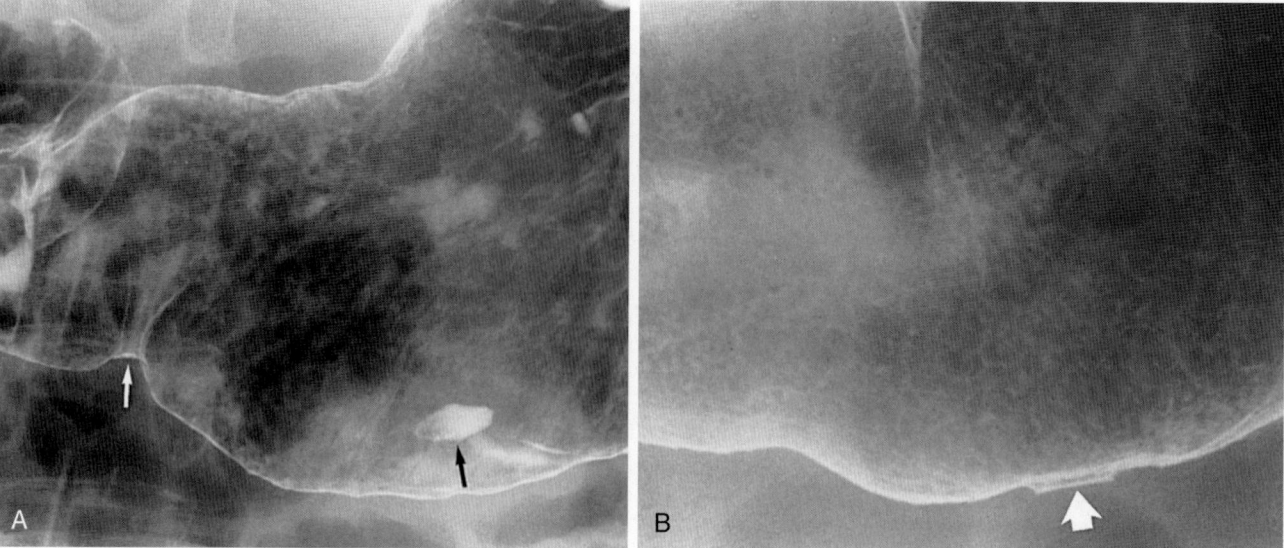

Figure 33-7. Greater curvature ulcers caused by aspirin and indomethacin. A. A small aspirin-induced ulcer (*black arrow*) is seen in the gastric body adjacent to the greater curvature. An area of scarring seen more distally on the greater curvature (*white arrow*) is due to a healed ulcer in this location. **B.** In another patient, an extremely shallow ulcer (*arrow*) is seen on the greater curvature as a result of ingestion of indomethacin. Radiating folds and other signs of ulcer disease are absent. This ulcer could easily be missed without optimal radiographic technique. (From Laufer I, Levine MS [eds]: Double Contrast Gastrointestinal Radiology, 2nd ed. Philadelphia, WB Saunders, 1992.)

because of circular muscle spasm and retraction of the adjacent gastric wall (see Fig. 33-8A).[84] Greater curvature ulcers may also be associated with considerable surrounding mass effect and thickened, irregular folds due to marked edema and inflammation (see Fig. 33-8).[69,84] Because of these morphologic features, benign greater curvature ulcers often have a suspicious radiographic appearance, so that the usual criteria for differentiating benign and malignant ulcers elsewhere in the stomach are unreliable for ulcers in this location.[69,84] Endoscopy and biopsy may therefore be required for some greater curvature ulcers despite a history of aspirin ingestion.

Posterior Wall Ulcers

Ulcers on the dependent or posterior wall of the gastric antrum or body may fill with barium, producing the conventional appearance of an ulcer crater (Fig. 33-9; see Fig. 33-1B). However, shallow ulcers on the posterior wall may appear as ring shadows on routine double-contrast views due to a thin layer of barium coating the rim of the unfilled crater (Fig. 33-10A). In such cases, flow technique can be used to manipulate the barium pool over the surface of the ulcer and demonstrate filling of the ulcer crater (Fig. 33-10B).[63] It is important not only to determine the size and shape of these posterior wall ulcers but also to assess the en face appear-

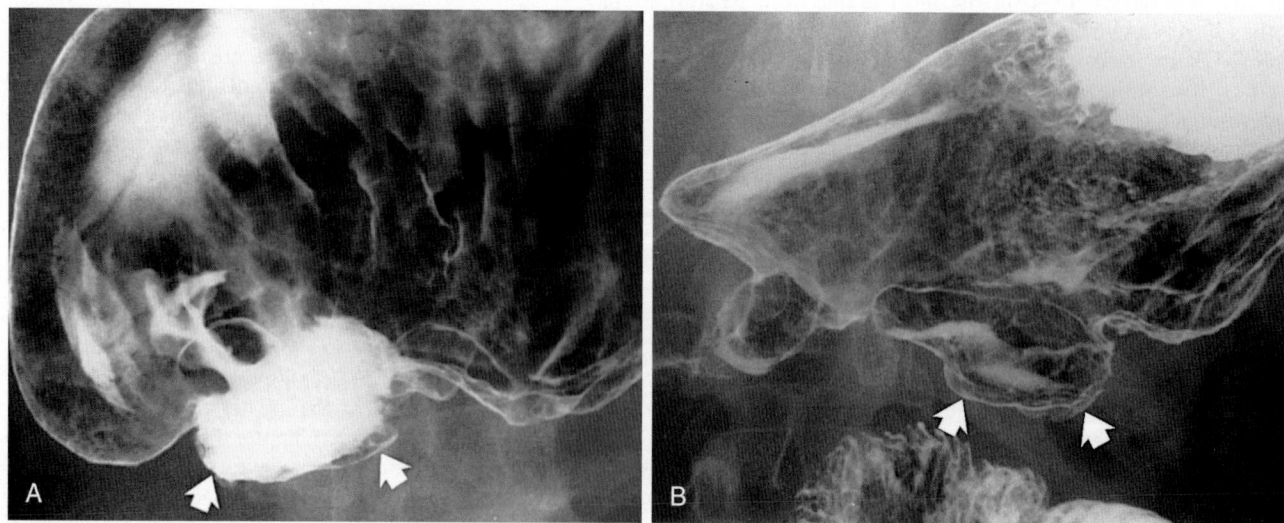

Figure 33-8. Giant greater curvature ulcers caused by aspirin. A. This large ulcer (*arrows*) on the greater curvature has an apparent intraluminal location and is associated with thickened, irregular folds and considerable mass effect from a surrounding mound of edema. **B.** In another patient, thickened, irregular folds are seen abutting a large greater curvature ulcer (*arrows*). In both cases, endoscopic biopsy specimens revealed no evidence of tumor, and follow-up studies after treatment with antisecretory agents showed complete healing of the ulcers. Both patients had taken high doses of aspirin. (**A** from Laufer I, Levine MS [eds]: Double Contrast Gastrointestinal Radiology, 2nd ed. Philadelphia, WB Saunders, 1992.)

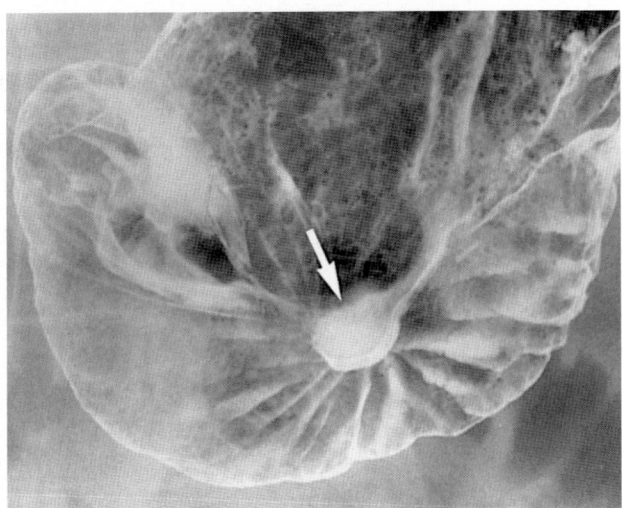

Figure 33-9. Posterior wall ulcer. A large ulcer (*arrow*) is present on the posterior wall of the stomach. Multiple folds are seen radiating to the edge of the ulcer crater. (From Laufer I, Levine MS [eds]: Double Contrast Gastrointestinal Radiology, 2nd ed. Philadelphia, WB Saunders, 1992.)

ance of the surrounding mucosa. Not infrequently, the areae gastricae are enlarged or distorted in the region of the ulcer because of edema and inflammation of the adjacent mucosa.[69] An ulcer collar or mound can sometimes be seen en face as a radiolucent halo of edematous tissue with poorly defined outer borders that fade peripherally into the adjacent mucosa.

Posterior wall ulcers may also be associated with a spectacular collection of folds that radiate to the edge of the ulcer crater or adjacent edematous mound.[69] Occasionally, the edema and spasm associated with antral ulcers may cause such severe narrowing and deformity of the distal stomach that it is difficult to evaluate these ulcers by the usual radiologic criteria (Fig. 33-11).

Anterior Wall Ulcers

Ulcers on the nondependent or anterior wall of the gastric antrum or body may also appear as ring shadows on routine double-contrast views because of barium coating the rim of the unfilled ulcer crater tangential to the central beam of the x-ray (Fig. 33-12A).[81,85] In such cases, the ulcer may be demonstrated by turning the patient 180 degrees to the prone position, so that the ulcer is located on the dependent wall and fills with barium (Fig. 33-12B). Prone compression views of the stomach with low-density barium should therefore be obtained routinely to demonstrate these anterior wall ulcers.

Multiplicity

With double-contrast technique, multiple ulcers have been detected in about 20% of patients with ulcers or ulcer scars,[86] a figure approximating the 20% to 30% prevalence of multiple ulcers at endoscopy, surgery, and autopsy.[87] It has sometimes been stated that the presence of multiple gastric ulcers favors benign disease. In one study, however, 20% of patients with multiple gastric ulcers had malignant lesions.[88] It is now recognized that patients may have coexisting benign

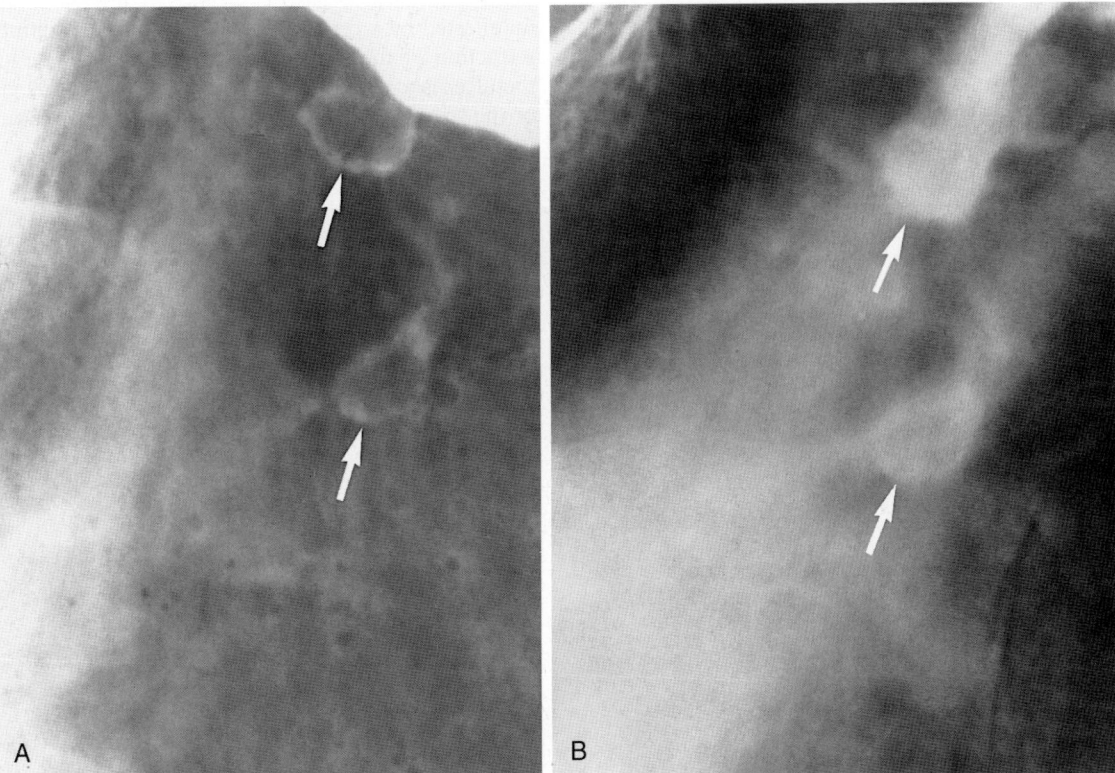

Figure 33-10. Ring shadows caused by shallow posterior wall ulcers. A. Supine double-contrast view shows two discrete ring shadows (*arrows*) in the upper body of the stomach where barium coats the rim of shallow, unfilled ulcers on the posterior wall. **B.** The use of flow technique to manipulate the barium pool over the surface of the ulcers results in filling of the ulcer craters (*arrows*).

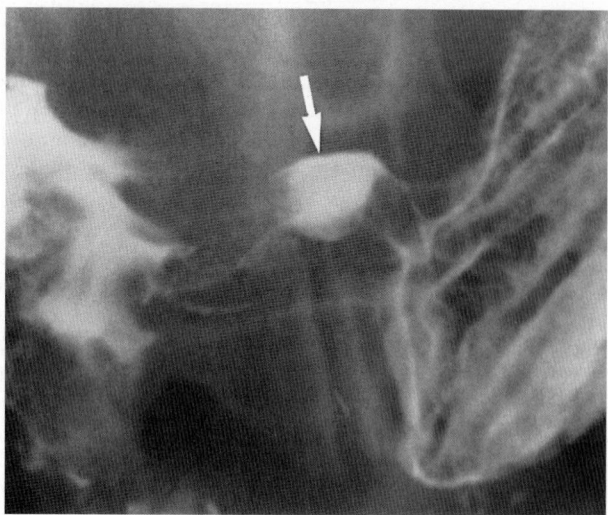

Figure 33-11. Antral ulcer associated with marked edema and spasm. A large ulcer (*arrow*) is seen in the gastric antrum. This ulcer is difficult to evaluate by the usual radiologic criteria because of antral narrowing and deformity due to edema and spasm accompanying the ulcer.

and malignant ulcers, so that each ulcer must be evaluated individually on barium studies.

When multiple gastric ulcers are present, they tend to be located in the gastric antrum or body (see Fig. 33-3A). Multiple gastric ulcers are more likely to occur in patients who are taking aspirin or other NSAIDs (see Fig. 33-7A). In one study, 80% of patients with multiple ulcers had a history of aspirin use.[87] A careful drug history should therefore be obtained from these patients.

Ulcer Healing and Scarring

The radiologic assessment of ulcer healing is important for evaluating the success or failure of medical therapy and for confirming the presence of benign ulcer disease (see next section on Benign Versus Malignant Ulcers). Ulcer healing may be manifested on barium studies not only by a decrease in the size of the ulcer crater but also by a change in its shape. Previously round or ovoid ulcers often have a linear appearance on follow-up studies, so that linear ulcers presumably represent a stage of ulcer healing (Fig. 33-13).[68,69] Other ulcers may undergo splitting, so that the original crater is replaced by two separate ulcer niches at the periphery of the original ulcer (Fig. 33-14).[69] This phenomenon probably occurs because healing and re-epithelialization are more rapid in the central portion of the ulcer than in the periphery.

Benign gastric ulcers usually respond dramatically to treatment with antisecretory agents. The average interval between the initial barium study showing the ulcer and the follow-up study showing complete healing is about 8 weeks.[69] Follow-up studies to demonstrate ulcer healing should therefore be performed after 6 to 8 weeks of medical treatment because studies performed sooner are unlikely to show complete healing.

In general, complete radiologic healing of a gastric ulcer has been considered a reliable sign that the ulcer is benign. Rarely, complete healing of malignant ulcers may occur with medical therapy.[89,90] However, nodularity of the ulcer scar or irregularity, clubbing, or amputation of radiating folds should suggest the possibility of an underlying malignant tumor. The surrounding gastric mucosa must therefore be evaluated carefully after ulcer healing has occurred. If suspicious findings are present, endoscopy and biopsy are still required to rule out a malignant lesion.

Ulcer healing may lead to the development of ulcer scars, which are visible on double-contrast studies in 90% of patients with healed gastric ulcers.[69] These scars are usually manifested by a central pit or depression, radiating folds, or retraction of the adjacent gastric wall.[69,91,92] The location of the ulcer is a major determinant of the morphologic features of the scar. Healing of ulcers on the lesser curvature is often

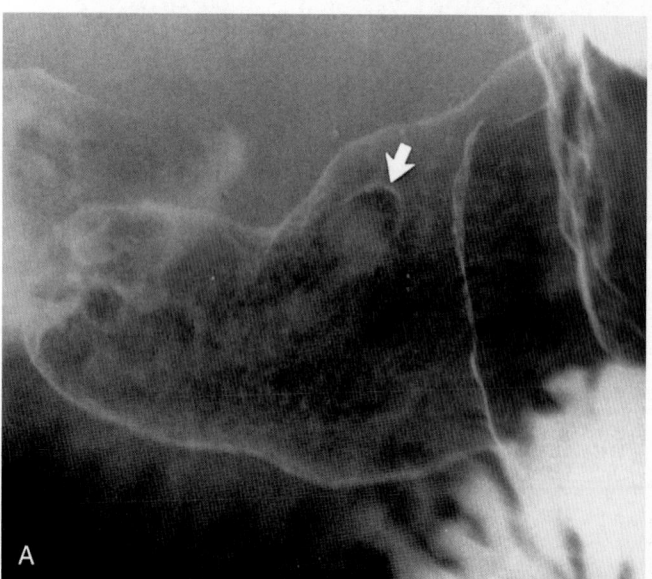

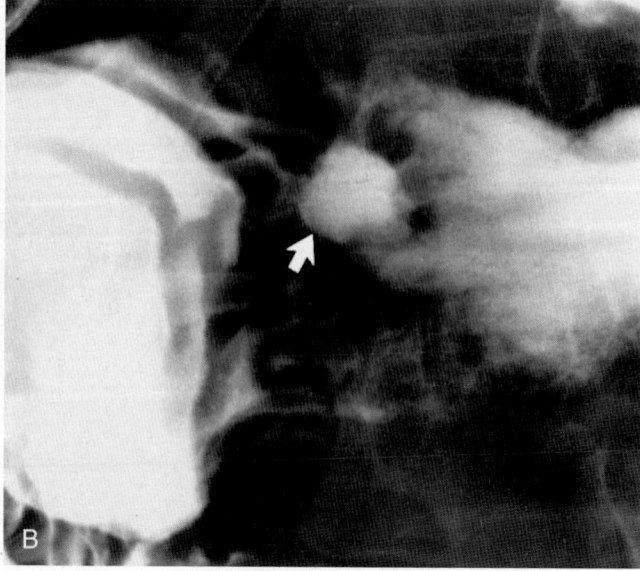

Figure 33-12. Partial ring shadow caused by an anterior wall ulcer. A. Supine double-contrast view shows a partial ring shadow (*arrow*) in the antrum. **B.** Prone compression view shows the anterior wall ulcer (*arrow*) filling with barium. (From Levine MS, Rubesin SE, Herlinger H, et al: Double contrast upper gastrointestinal examination: Technique and interpretation. Radiology 168:593-602, 1988.)

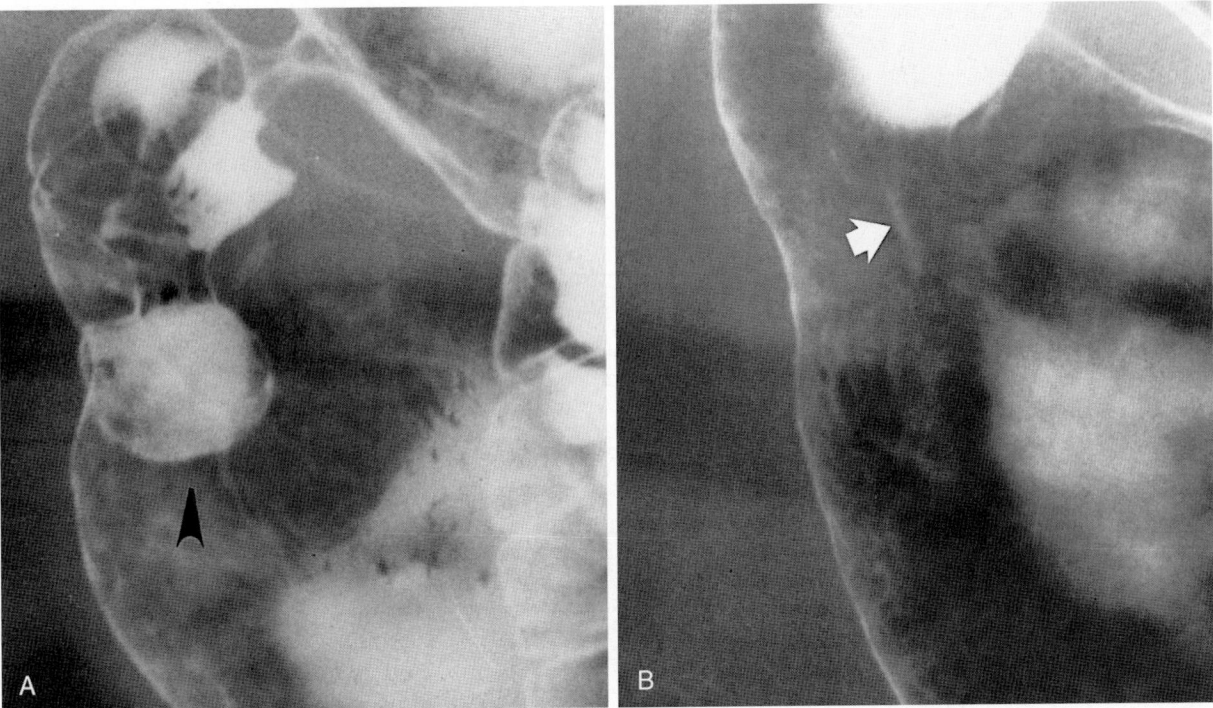

Figure 33-13.   Development of a linear ulcer during healing. A. A large, round ulcer (*arrowhead*) is seen on the posterior wall of the antrum. **B.** Follow-up study 8 weeks later shows substantial ulcer healing with a residual linear ulcer (*arrow*) in this location. (From Levine MS, Creteur V, Kressel HY, et al: Benign gastric ulcers: Diagnosis and follow-up with double-contrast radiography. Radiology 164:9-13, 1987.)

associated with the development of relatively innocuous scars, manifested by slight flattening or retraction of the adjacent gastric wall with or without radiating folds (Fig. 33-15).[69,91] In contrast, healing of ulcers on the greater curvature or posterior wall of the stomach is sometimes associated with the development of a spectacular collection of radiating folds

(Fig. 33-16).[69,81,91] The folds may converge to a central point or to a circular or linear pit or depression (Fig. 33-17).[69,91,92] This central depression can be mistaken radiographically for a shallow, residual ulcer crater. However, the central depression of an ulcer scar tends to have more gradually sloping margins than an ulcer crater and should remain unchanged

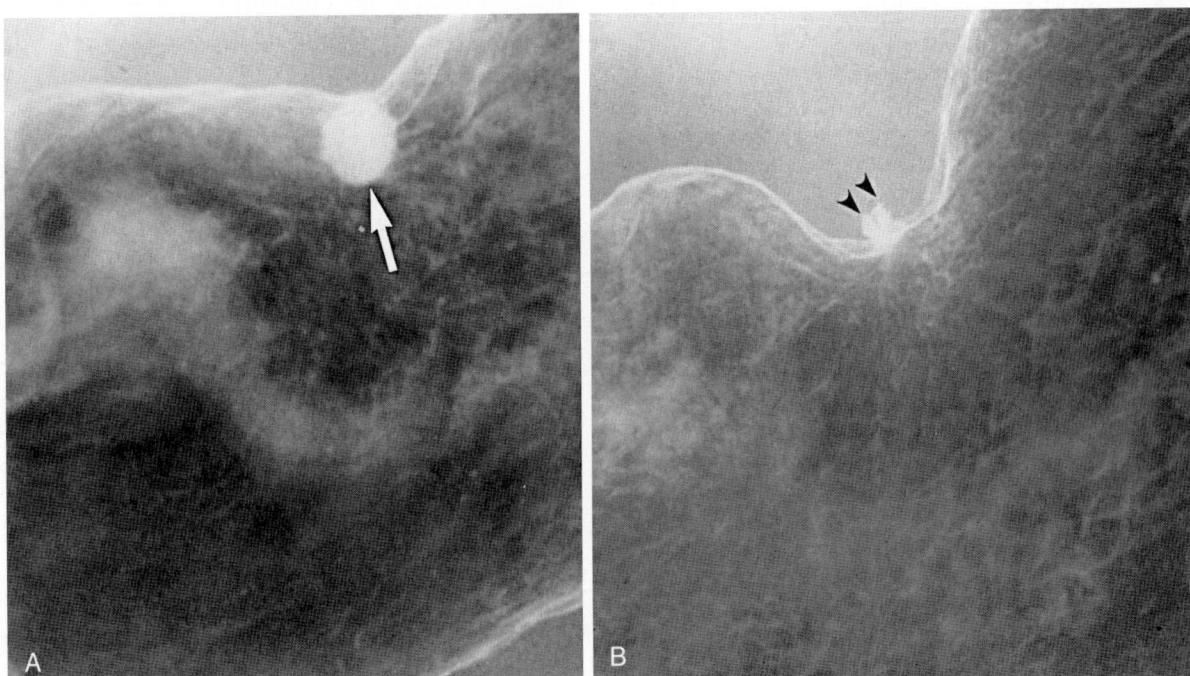

Figure 33-14.   Splitting of an ulcer during healing. A. A round ulcer (*arrow*) is seen adjacent to the lesser curvature. **B.** Follow-up study several weeks later shows splitting of the ulcer with two closely spaced niches (*arrowheads*) at the site of the original crater.

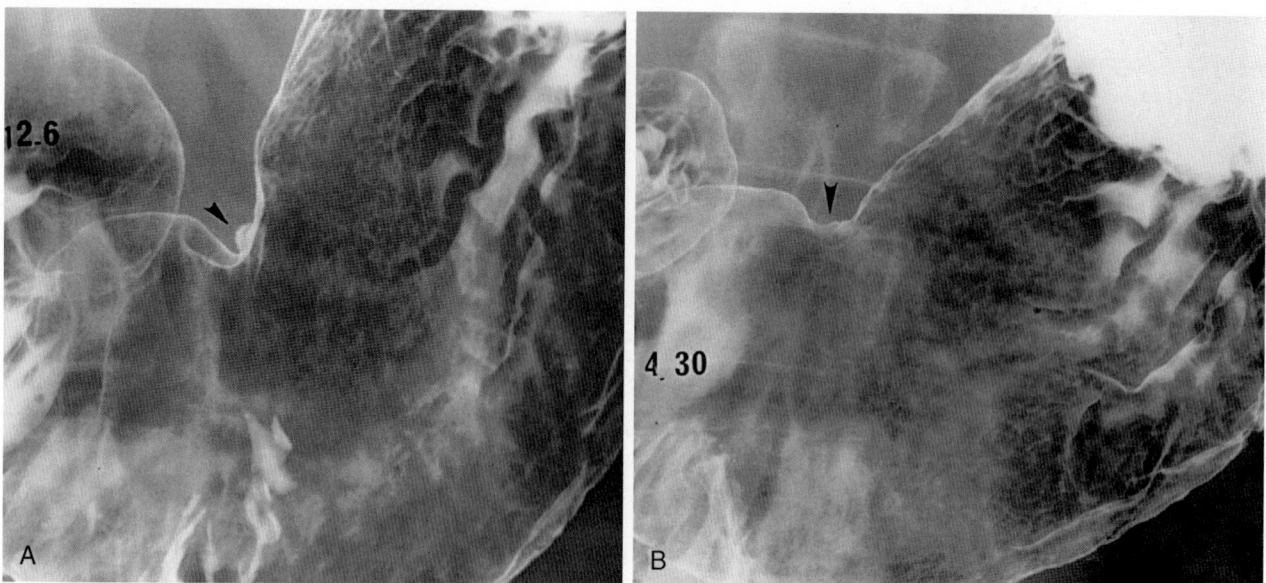

Figure 33-15. **Healing of a lesser curvature ulcer with scarring. A.** A small, benign-appearing ulcer (*arrowhead*) is seen on the lesser curvature. **B.** Follow-up study 5 months later shows complete healing of the ulcer with slight flattening and retraction of the adjacent gastric wall (*arrowhead*). (From Laufer I, Levine MS [eds]: Double Contrast Gastrointestinal Radiology, 2nd ed. Philadelphia, WB Saunders, 1992.)

on sequential follow-up studies. A re-epithelialized ulcer scar can also be differentiated from an active ulcer by the presence of normal areae gastricae within the central portion of the scar (Fig. 33-18).[69]

Healing of antral ulcers may also lead to the development of a prominent transverse fold that can be mistaken for an antral web or diaphragm.[91] In other patients, severe scar formation may be manifested by antral narrowing and deformity (Fig. 33-19A). The narrowed segment usually has a smooth, tapered appearance, but asymmetric scarring may result in flattening and shortening of the lesser or greater curvature, so that the pylorus has an eccentric location in relation to

the antrum and duodenal bulb (Fig. 33-19B). Occasionally, an ulcer scar may be associated with such irregular antral narrowing that it mimics the linitis plastica appearance of a primary scirrhous carcinoma of the stomach.[93] When antral scarring cannot be differentiated from a scirrhous carcinoma on radiologic criteria, endoscopy and biopsy are required for a more definitive diagnosis. Healing of ulcers on the lesser curvature of the gastric body may also lead to marked retraction and deformity of the opposite wall, producing a deep incisura on the greater curvature.[91,92] Rarely, scarring of the gastric body may result in the development of an "hourglass" stomach with marked narrowing of the gastric body (see Fig. 33-19C).

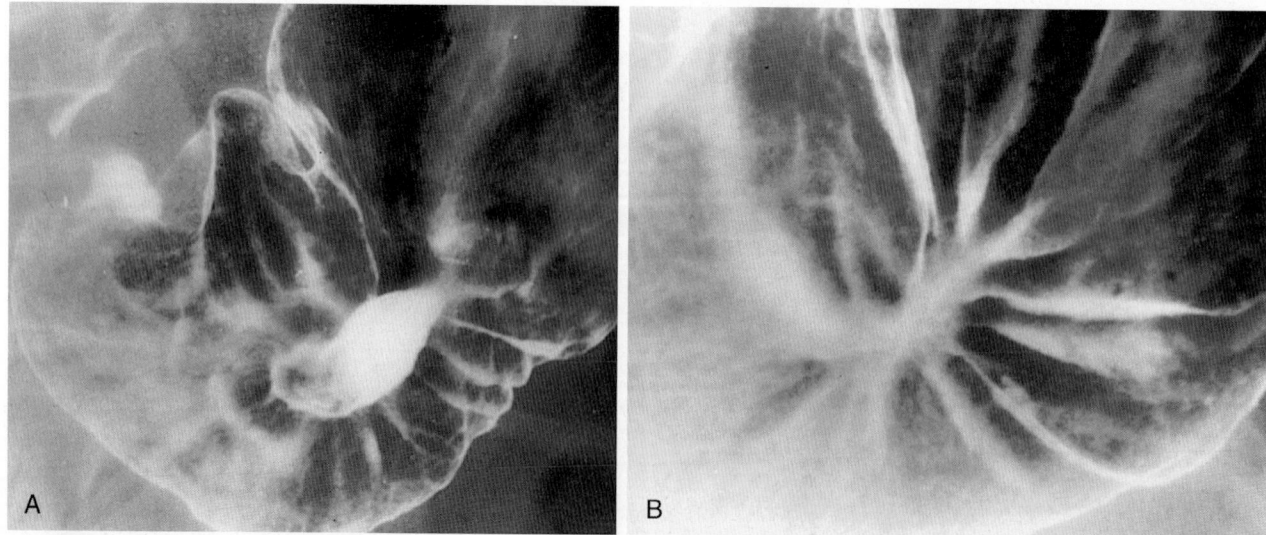

Figure 33-16. **Healing of a posterior wall ulcer with scarring. A.** There is a large posterior wall ulcer with multiple folds radiating to the edge of the ulcer crater. **B.** Follow-up study 8 weeks later shows complete healing of the ulcer with a spectacular collection of folds radiating to the site of the previous crater. (From Laufer I, Levine MS [eds]: Double Contrast Gastrointestinal Radiology, 2nd ed. Philadelphia, WB Saunders, 1992.)

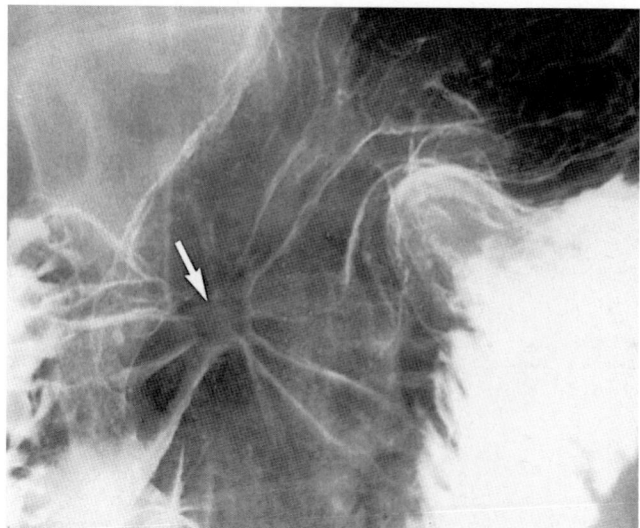

Figure 33-17. Ulcer scar with folds radiating to a central depression. Multiple folds are seen radiating to a central area (*arrow*) that could be mistaken for a shallow, residual ulcer crater. (From Levine MS, Creteur V, Kressel HY, et al: Benign gastric ulcers: Diagnosis and follow-up with double-contrast radiography. Radiology 164:9-13, 1987.)

Benign Versus Malignant Ulcers

More than 95% of gastric ulcers diagnosed in the United States are found to be benign.[64,94] Nevertheless, radiologic examinations are often thought to be unreliable in differentiating benign ulcers from ulcerated carcinomas. Previous reports indicate that 6% to 16% of gastric ulcers that appear benign on conventional single-contrast barium studies are malignant.[95-98] Although these studies were performed between 1955 and 1975, many gastroenterologists have used these data as the justification for performing endoscopy and biopsy on all patients with radiographically diagnosed gastric ulcers to rule out gastric carcinoma.

With double-contrast techniques, it is possible to obtain a much more detailed study of the mucosa surrounding the ulcer for signs of malignancy, such as irregular mass effect, nodularity, rigidity, or mucosal destruction. Several studies have found that virtually all gastric ulcers with an unequivocally benign appearance on double-contrast examinations are, in fact, benign lesions.[69,99] In those studies, about two thirds of all benign ulcers had a benign radiographic appearance, so that unnecessary endoscopy could be avoided in most patients with gastric ulcers diagnosed on double-contrast examinations. This finding has important implications for the evaluation of gastric ulcers in general because barium studies are safer and less expensive than endoscopy.

Unequivocally benign gastric ulcers are characterized en face by a round or ovoid ulcer crater surrounded by a smooth mound of edema or regular, symmetric mucosal folds that radiate to the edge of the crater (see Figs. 33-9, 33-13A, 33-14A, and 33-16A).[69,99] The areae gastricae adjacent to the ulcer may be enlarged as a result of inflammation and edema of the surrounding mucosa (see Fig. 33-6A).[69] When viewed in profile, benign gastric ulcers project outside the gastric lumen and are sometimes associated with a smooth, symmetric ulcer mound or collar or with smooth, straight mucosal folds that radiate to the edge of the ulcer crater (see Figs. 33-4, 33-6, and 33-15A).

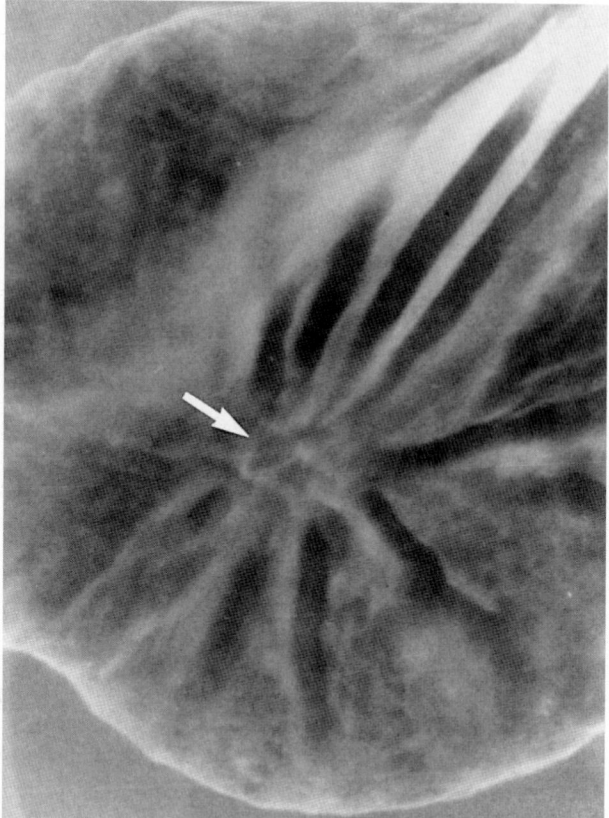

Figure 33-18. Re-epithelialized ulcer scar with centrally radiating folds. This scar can be differentiated from an active ulcer by the presence of normal areae gastricae within the central portion of the scar (*arrow*). (From Levine MS, Rubesin SE, Herlinger H, et al: Double contrast upper gastrointestinal examination: Technique and interpretation. Radiology 168:593-602, 1988.)

In contrast, malignant ulcers are characterized en face by an irregular ulcer crater eccentrically located within a discrete tumor mass.[69] There may be focal nodularity of the surrounding mucosa or distortion or even obliteration of adjacent areae gastricae as a result of tumor infiltrating this region.[69] Although radiating folds may be present, they are often nodular, clubbed, fused, or amputated because of infiltration of the folds by tumor (Fig. 33-20).[100] When viewed in profile, malignant ulcers do not project beyond the expected gastric contour, and there is often a discrete tumor mass that forms acute angles with the gastric wall rather than the obtuse, gently sloping angles expected for a benign mound of edema (Fig. 33-21).

Equivocal ulcers are those that have mixed features of benign and malignant disease, so that a confident diagnosis cannot be made on radiologic criteria. For example, edema and inflammation surrounding a benign ulcer may result in enlarged, distorted areae gastricae, mass effect, or thickened, irregular folds, producing an indeterminate radiographic appearance (Fig. 33-22). Similarly, NSAID-induced greater curvature ulcers that have an apparent intraluminal location or considerable associated mass effect and shouldered edges may result in equivocal radiographic findings (see Fig. 33-8). Most ulcers that have an equivocal appearance are ultimately found to be benign lesions. It seems prudent to err on the side of caution, however, by suggesting the possibility of

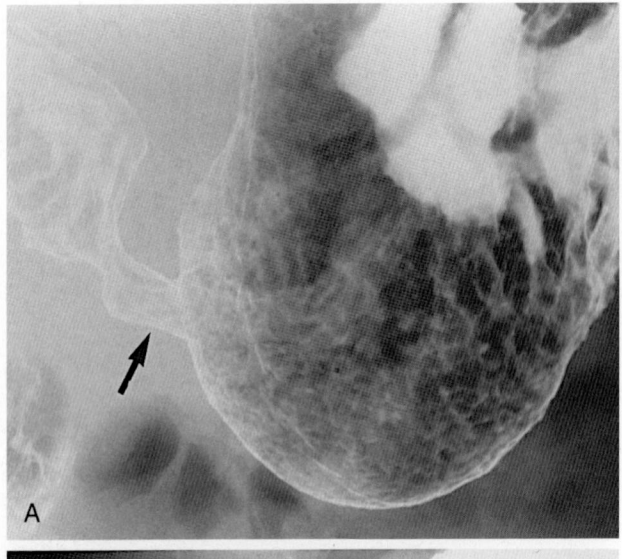

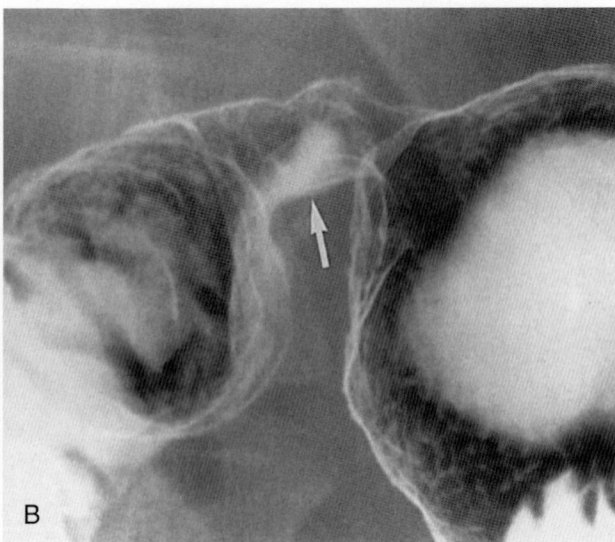

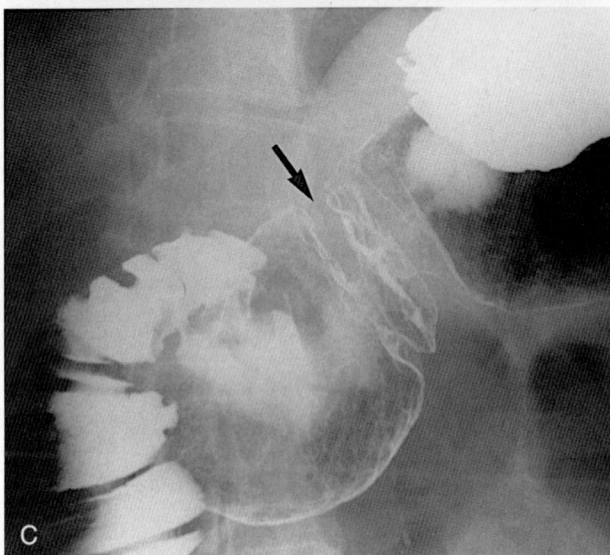

Figure 33-19. Various types of gastric scarring from ulcer disease. **A.** This patient has tapered narrowing and deformity of the antrum (*arrow*) caused by scarring from a previous antral ulcer. This degree of narrowing can lead to gastric outlet obstruction. **B.** Another patient has a widened, eccentric pylorus (*arrow*) caused by asymmetric scarring from peptic ulcer disease. **C.** A third patient has an hourglass stomach with focal narrowing of the gastric body (*arrow*) caused by severe ulcer scarring.

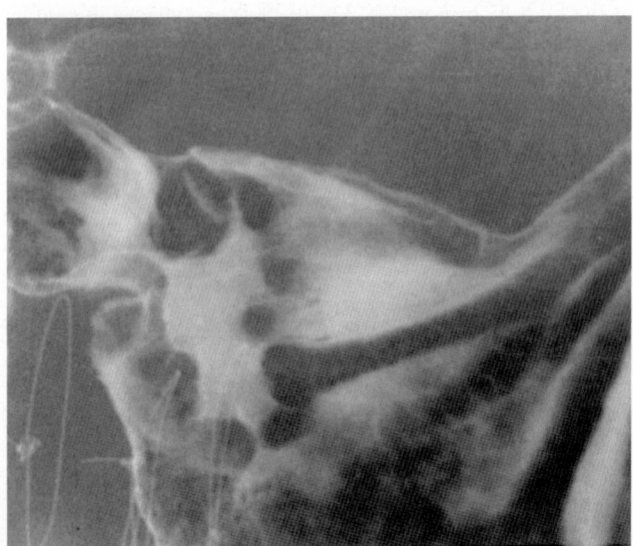

Figure 33-20. Malignant gastric ulcer. This patient has an irregular ulcer on the posterior wall of the antrum with scalloped borders and nodular, clubbed folds surrounding the ulcer. These are classic features of a malignant gastric ulcer. (From Levine MS, Creteur V, Kressel HY, et al: Benign gastric ulcers: Diagnosis and follow-up with double contrast radiography. Radiology 164:9-13, 1987.)

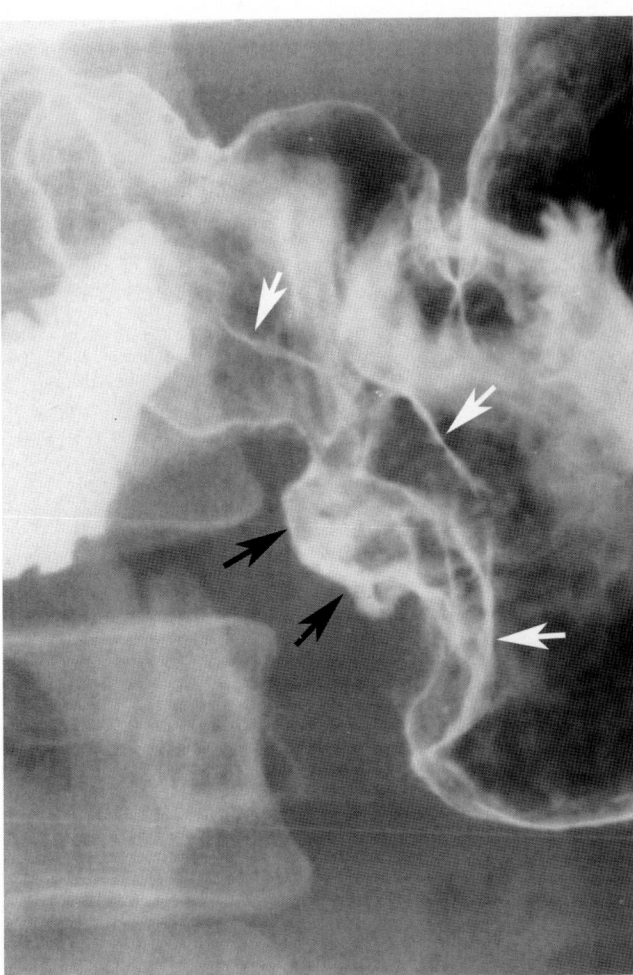

Figure 33-21. Malignant gastric ulcer. This patient has an ulcerated mass on the greater curvature of the antrum. Note how the ulcer (*black arrows*) projects inside the gastric lumen within a discrete tumor mass (etched in white) (*white arrows*) that forms acute angles with the adjacent gastric wall rather than the obtuse angles expected for a benign mound of edema. These are classic features of a malignant gastric ulcer.

malignant tumor in some benign lesions to avoid missing an early carcinoma.

Gastric ulcers that have an unequivocally benign appearance on double-contrast studies can be followed with serial double-contrast studies until complete healing without need for endoscopic evaluation.[69] However, ulcers that have an equivocal or suspicious appearance should be evaluated by endoscopy for a more definitive diagnosis. Although endoscopy is a sensitive technique for diagnosing gastric carcinoma, false-negative biopsy specimens and brushings have been reported in some patients with malignant lesions.[101] If the radiographic findings are suggestive of malignant tumor, negative histologic or cytologic findings should therefore not be taken as definitive evidence of a benign ulcer. Instead, follow-up barium studies should be performed at regular intervals until complete healing is demonstrated. If the ulcer fails to heal with adequate medical treatment or if it continues to have a suspicious radiographic appearance, repeat endoscopy and biopsy may be required. Even if endoscopic biopsy specimens and brushings remain negative, surgical resection should be considered for some patients with suspicious findings or intractable ulcers on serial barium studies.

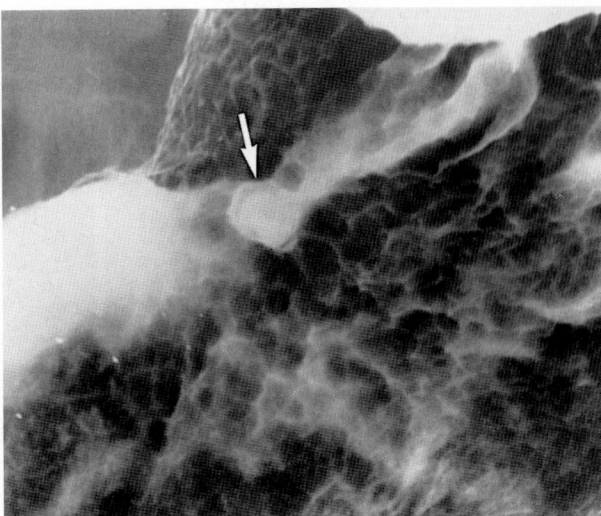

Figure 33-22. Benign gastric ulcer with an indeterminate radiographic appearance. A small ulcer (*arrow*) is seen near the lesser curvature with enlarged, nodular areae gastricae surrounding the ulcer because of edema and inflammation of the adjacent mucosa. Although the radiographic findings are equivocal, endoscopic biopsy specimens revealed no evidence of tumor, and a follow-up study after treatment showed complete healing of the ulcer.

Duodenal Ulcers

In contrast to gastric ulcers, duodenal ulcers are virtually always benign. When duodenal ulcers are detected on barium studies, these patients can therefore receive medical treatment without need for endoscopy. Unlike gastric ulcers, duodenal ulcers are often located on the anterior wall of the duodenal bulb, so that prone compression views of the duodenum should be obtained routinely to detect these lesions. Duodenal ulcers may also be obscured by edema, spasm, or scarring of the bulb. Conversely, barium trapped in the crevices of a deformed bulb can mimic ulcer craters. Radiologists should therefore be aware of the limitations of barium studies in diagnosing duodenal ulcers and of the need to perform a biphasic examination in these patients.

Examination Technique

Double-contrast views of the duodenum must be complemented by prone compression views to demonstrate ulcers on the anterior wall of the bulb.[102] These anterior wall ulcers may be hidden in the barium pool, however, unless adequate compression of the bulb is obtained with an inflatable balloon or other prone compression device (Fig. 33-23). Other duodenal ulcers are best seen on upright compression views. Thus, optimal radiologic evaluation of the duodenum requires a biphasic examination that includes double-contrast views of the duodenal bulb with high-density barium and prone or upright compression views with low-density barium.[103]

Shape

Most duodenal ulcers appear as round or ovoid collections of barium (Fig. 33-24). About 5% of duodenal ulcers diagnosed on double-contrast studies have a linear configuration (Fig. 33-25).[68,104] These linear ulcers tend to be located near the base of the duodenal bulb and often have a transverse

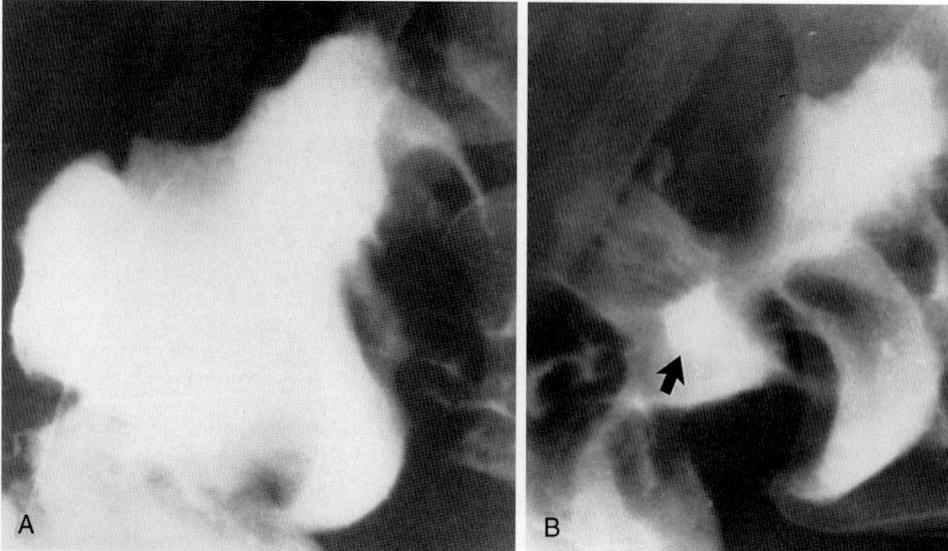

Figure 33-23. Importance of prone compression for anterior wall duodenal ulcers. A. Initial prone view shows no evidence of a duodenal ulcer. **B.** Prone compression of the bulb with an inflatable balloon clearly demonstrates an ulcer crater (*arrow*) on the anterior wall. This ulcer was hidden in the barium pool on the earlier radiograph.

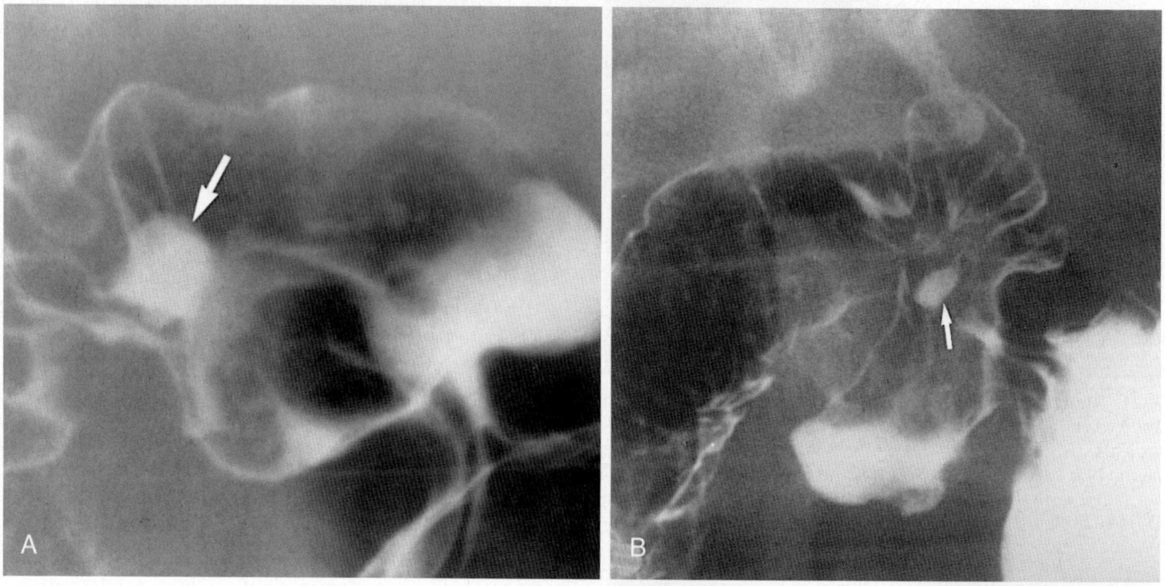

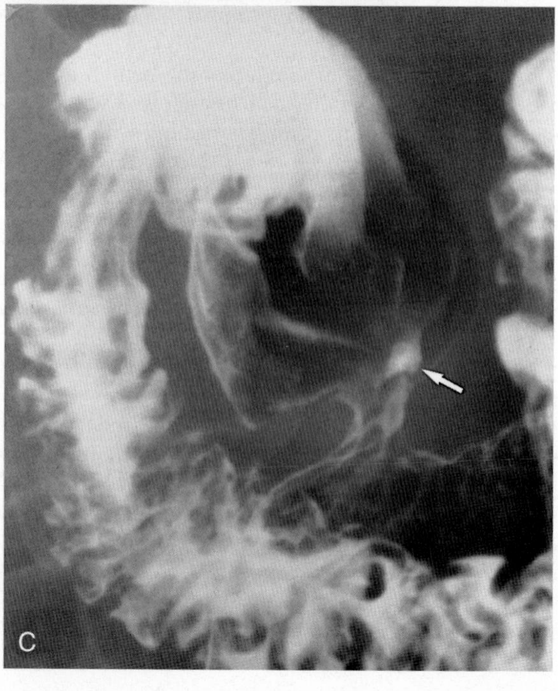

Figure 33-24. Duodenal ulcers in various locations. A. A large ulcer (*arrow*) is seen at the apex of the bulb. **B.** A small ulcer (*arrow*) is present in the central portion of the bulb. This ulcer is associated with radiating folds and bulbar deformity. **C.** A small ulcer (*arrow*) is seen at the base of the bulb, with folds radiating toward the ulcer crater. (**A** from Laufer I, Levine MS [eds]: Double Contrast Gastrointestinal Radiology, 2nd ed. Philadelphia, WB Saunders, 1992.)

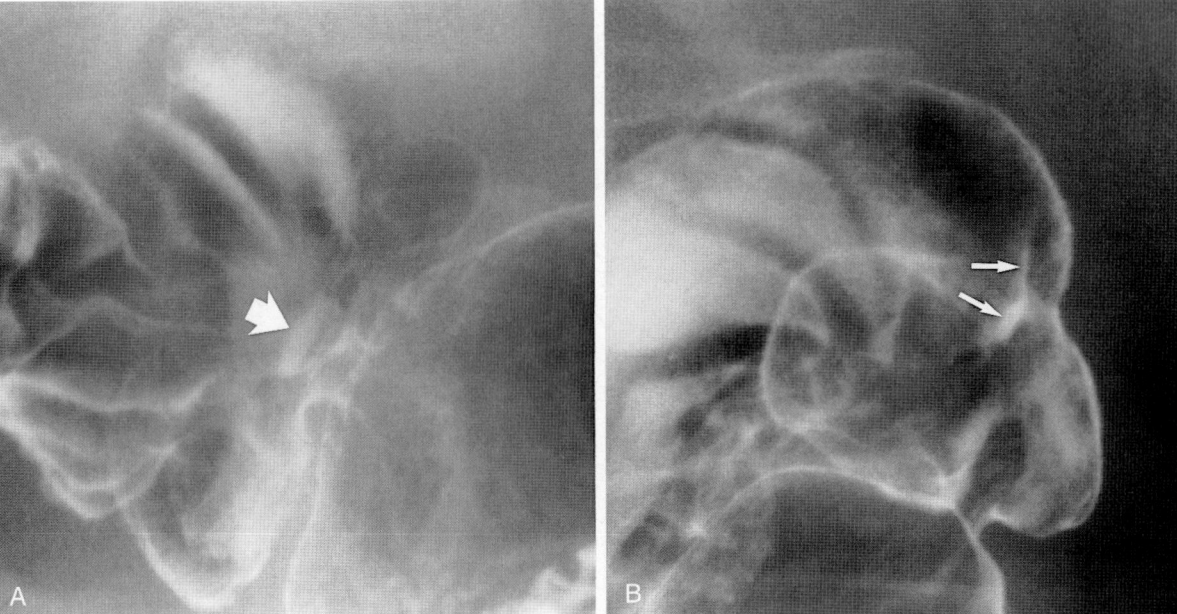

Figure 33-25. Linear duodenal ulcers. A. A linear ulcer (*arrow*) is seen at the base of the bulb. The ulcer has a transverse orientation in relation to the bulb. **B.** In another patient, a linear ulcer (*arrows*) is seen at the apex of the bulb. (From Laufer I, Levine MS [eds]: Double Contrast Gastrointestinal Radiology, 2nd ed. Philadelphia, WB Saunders, 1992.)

orientation in relation to the bulb (see Fig. 33-25A).[104] As in the stomach, linear ulcers are thought to represent a stage of healing.[66,104] In fact, they may be indistinguishable from linear ulcer scars.

Size

Most duodenal ulcers diagnosed on double-contrast studies are less than 1 cm. A major advantage of double-contrast technique is its ability to demonstrate small ulcers, frequently no more than several millimeters in diameter (see Fig. 33-24B and C). Nevertheless, giant ulcers are occasionally detected in the duodenum (see later section on Giant Duodenal Ulcers).

Location

About 90% of duodenal ulcers are located in the duodenal bulb and the remaining 10% are in the postbulbar duodenum.[46,105] Bulbar ulcers may involve the apex, central portion, or base of the bulb (see Fig. 33-24). Unlike gastric ulcers, which rarely develop on the anterior wall, as many as 50% of duodenal ulcers are located on the anterior wall of the bulb.[77,106] Postbulbar ulcers are usually located in the proximal descending duodenum above the papilla of Vater (see later section on Postbulbar Ulcers). Thus, the presence of one or more ulcers distal to the papilla should raise the possibility of Zollinger-Ellison syndrome (see later section on Zollinger-Ellison Syndrome).

Morphologic Features

Bulbar Ulcers

Ulcers in the duodenal bulb usually appear as discrete niches that can be visualized en face or in profile (see Fig. 33-24). The ulcers are often surrounded by a smooth, radiolucent mound

of edematous mucosa. Occasionally, the size of the ulcer mound may be quite striking in relation to the central crater (see Fig. 33-26B). Bulbar ulcers also tend to be associated with radiating folds that converge centrally at the edge of the crater (see Figs. 33-24B and C). In patients with shallow ulcers or small, healing ulcers, the ulcer crater may be visible only with optimal radiographic technique. Thus, the presence of radiating folds should prompt a careful search for an active ulcer at the site of fold convergence before attributing these folds to an ulcer scar.

As in the stomach, ulcers on the anterior wall of the duodenal bulb may be difficult to detect on routine double-contrast views. Other anterior wall ulcers may be manifested by a ring shadow caused by barium coating the rim of the unfilled ulcer crater (Fig. 33-26A).[85] These anterior wall ulcers can be demonstrated by obtaining prone or upright compression views of the bulb to fill the crater with barium (Fig. 33-26B).

Duodenal ulcers are often associated with significant deformity of the bulb caused by edema and spasm accompanying the ulcer or by scarring from a previous ulcer (see Fig. 33-24B).[102] This deformity may obscure small ulcers in the bulb, resulting in a substantial number of false-negative examinations. It is therefore important to recognize the limitations of the radiologic diagnosis of duodenal ulcers in the presence of a deformed bulb. Nevertheless, symptomatic patients with a deformed bulb on barium studies should probably be treated for an active duodenal ulcer because of the high risk of ulcer disease, whether or not an ulcer is demonstrated with certainty.

Postbulbar Ulcers

Postbulbar ulcers are usually located on the medial wall of the proximal descending duodenum above the papilla of Vater (Fig. 33-27).[46,105,107] These ulcers are notoriously difficult to demonstrate on barium studies, presumably because severe

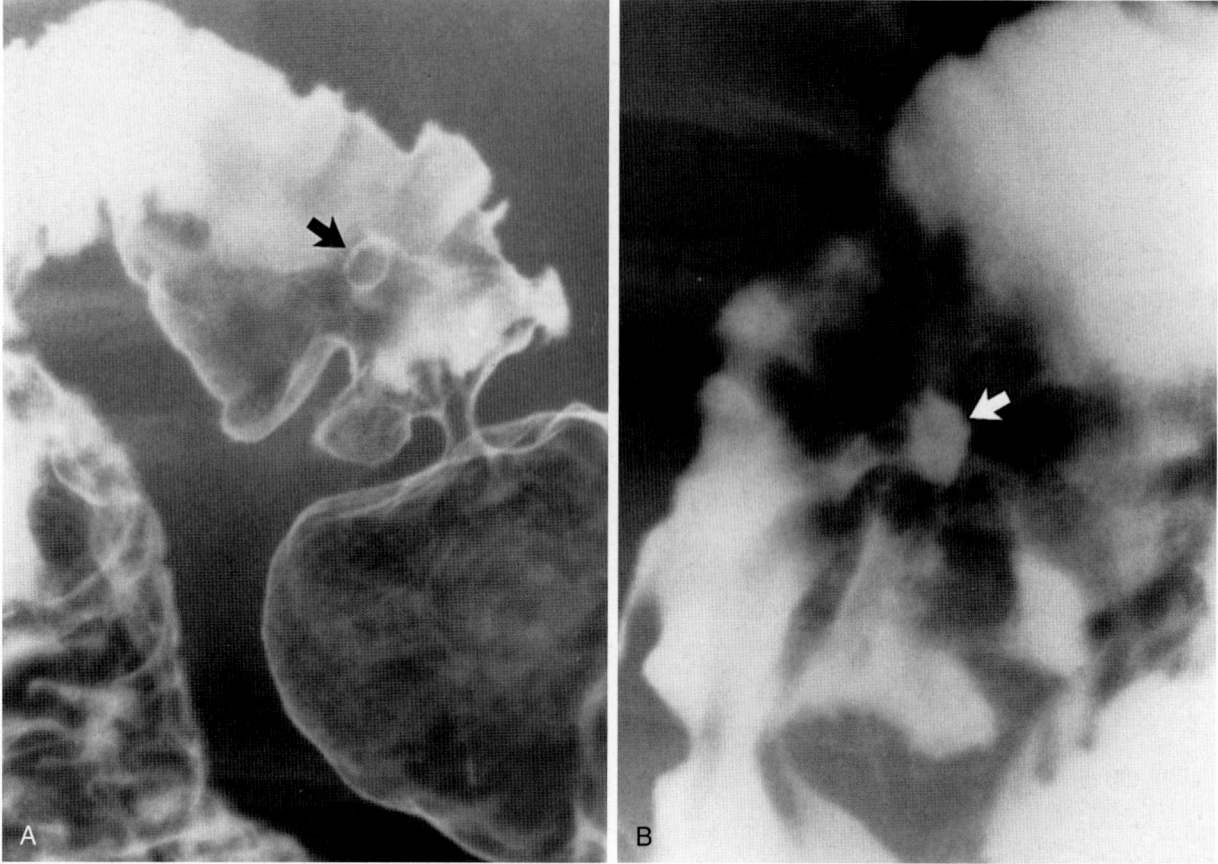

Figure 33-26. Ring shadow caused by an anterior wall duodenal ulcer. A. Supine oblique double-contrast view of the duodenum shows a ring shadow (*arrow*) in the bulb as a result of barium coating the rim of an unfilled ulcer on the nondependent surface. **B.** Prone compression view shows filling of the anterior wall ulcer (*arrow*). Note the large, radiolucent mound of edema surrounding the ulcer. (From Laufer I, Levine MS [eds]: Double Contrast Gastrointestinal Radiology, 2nd ed. Philadelphia, WB Saunders, 1992.)

edema and spasm accompanying the ulcer prevent visualization of the ulcer crater. The edema and spasm often result in circumferential narrowing of the adjacent lumen or eccentric narrowing with a smooth, rounded indentation on the lateral wall of the descending duodenum opposite the crater (see Fig. 33-27A).[107] If the ulcer crater itself is obscured by edema and spasm, this indentation may be the only radiologic sign of a postbulbar ulcer (Fig. 33-28).

Many postbulbar duodenal ulcers are greater than 1 cm, so that they tend to be larger than bulbar ulcers, which are usually less than 1 cm.[46] Large postbulbar ulcers may cause marked narrowing of the adjacent duodenum proximally and distally as a result of severe edema and spasm accompanying these ulcer craters (Fig. 33-29).[46] The larger size of the ulcers could help explain the higher prevalence of major upper gastrointestinal bleeding and the poorer response of postbulbar ulcers to medical therapy.[46] Healed postbulbar ulcers may occasionally be associated with focal scarring and fibrosis, resulting in the development of a "ring stricture" with eccentric narrowing of the postbulbar duodenum (Fig. 33-30).[108]

Giant Duodenal Ulcers

Giant duodenal ulcers are defined as duodenal ulcers greater than 2 cm.[109] These ulcers are important because of an increased risk of complications such as perforation, obstruc-

tion, and upper gastrointestinal bleeding.[110] Nevertheless, treatment with antisecretory agents may lead to dramatic ulcer healing, so that these patients can often be managed conservatively without need for surgery.[111] Giant duodenal ulcers are almost always located in the duodenal bulb and may be so large that they replace virtually the entire bulb (Figs. 33-31 and 33-32). Paradoxically, giant ulcers can be mistaken on barium studies for a scarred or even a normal bulb. However, the duodenal bulb would be expected to change in size and shape at fluoroscopy, whereas these giant ulcers will have a fixed, unchanging configuration (see Fig. 33-32).[109,111,112]

Giant duodenal ulcers may occasionally be recognized on ultrasound studies as discrete, hypoechoic cystic lesions anterolateral to the head of the pancreas.[113] The differential diagnosis for these lesions includes a duodenal diverticulum and pancreatic pseudocyst. In such cases, a barium study should be performed for a more certain diagnosis.

Multiplicity

About 15% of patients with duodenal ulcers have multiple ulcers.[114] Most of these ulcers are located in the duodenal bulb. The presence of multiple ulcers should raise the possibility of Zollinger-Ellison syndrome (see later section on Zollinger-Ellison syndrome).

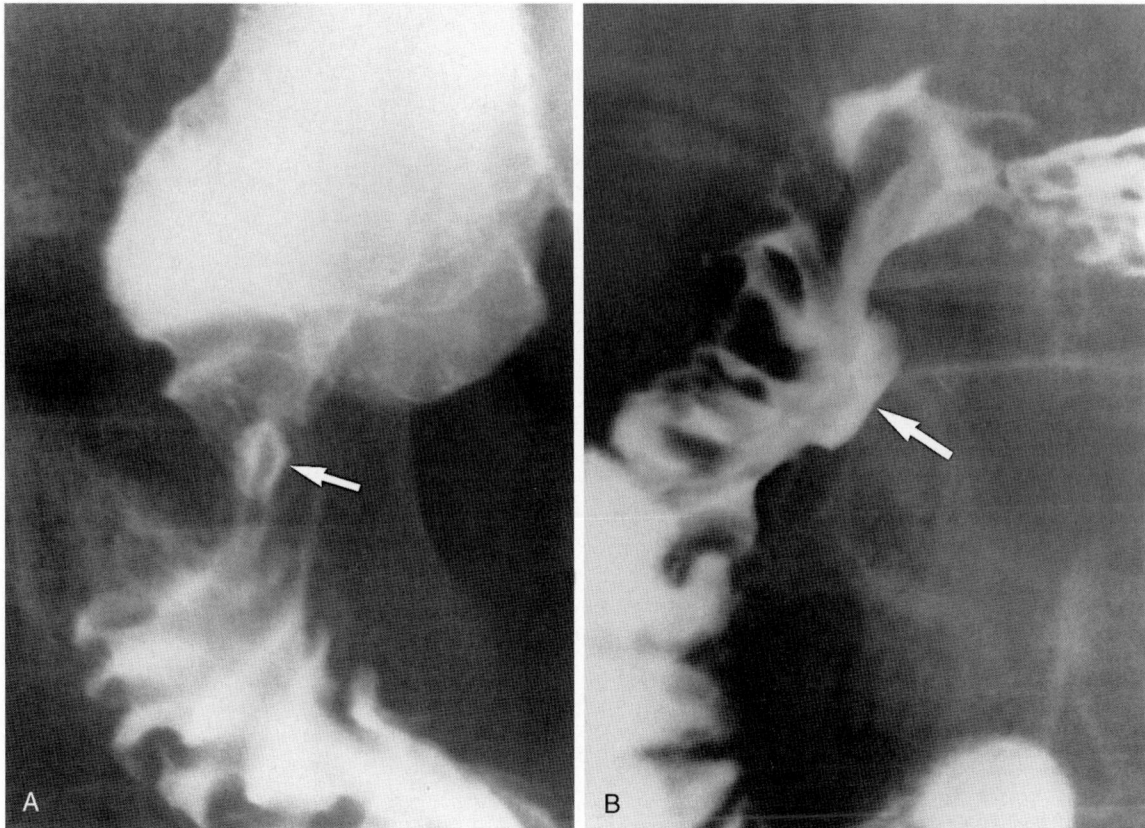

Figure 33-27. Postbulbar duodenal ulcers. A. An ulcer (*arrow*) is seen on the medial wall of the proximal descending duodenum. There is also a smooth, rounded indentation of the lateral wall as a result of associated edema and spasm. **B.** Another patient has a large, relatively flat ulcer (*arrow*) on the medial wall of the postbulbar duodenum above the papilla of Vater. The folds radiate toward the ulcer crater.

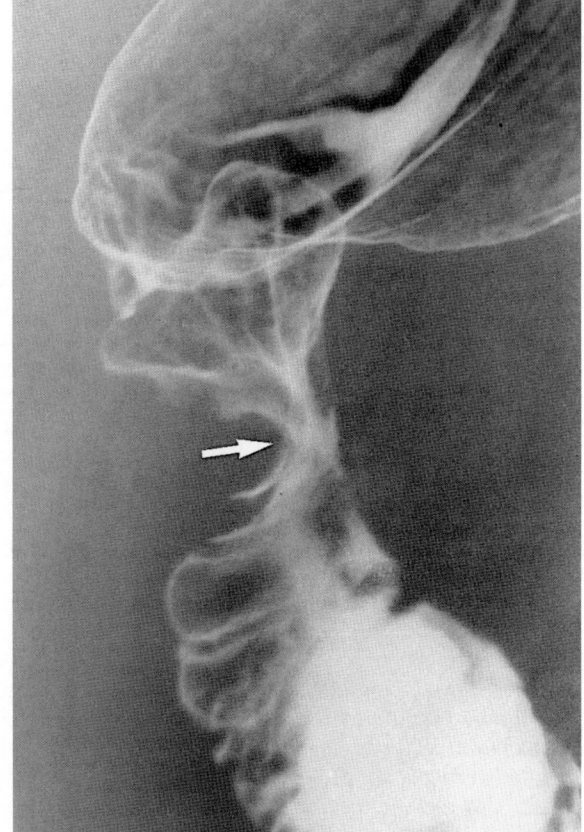

Figure 33-28. Postbulbar duodenal ulcer not visualized on barium study. A prominent indentation is seen on the lateral aspect of the proximal descending duodenum (*arrow*) as a result of edema and spasm accompanying a postbulbar ulcer that was not visualized on this study. The ulcer was seen at subsequent endoscopy.

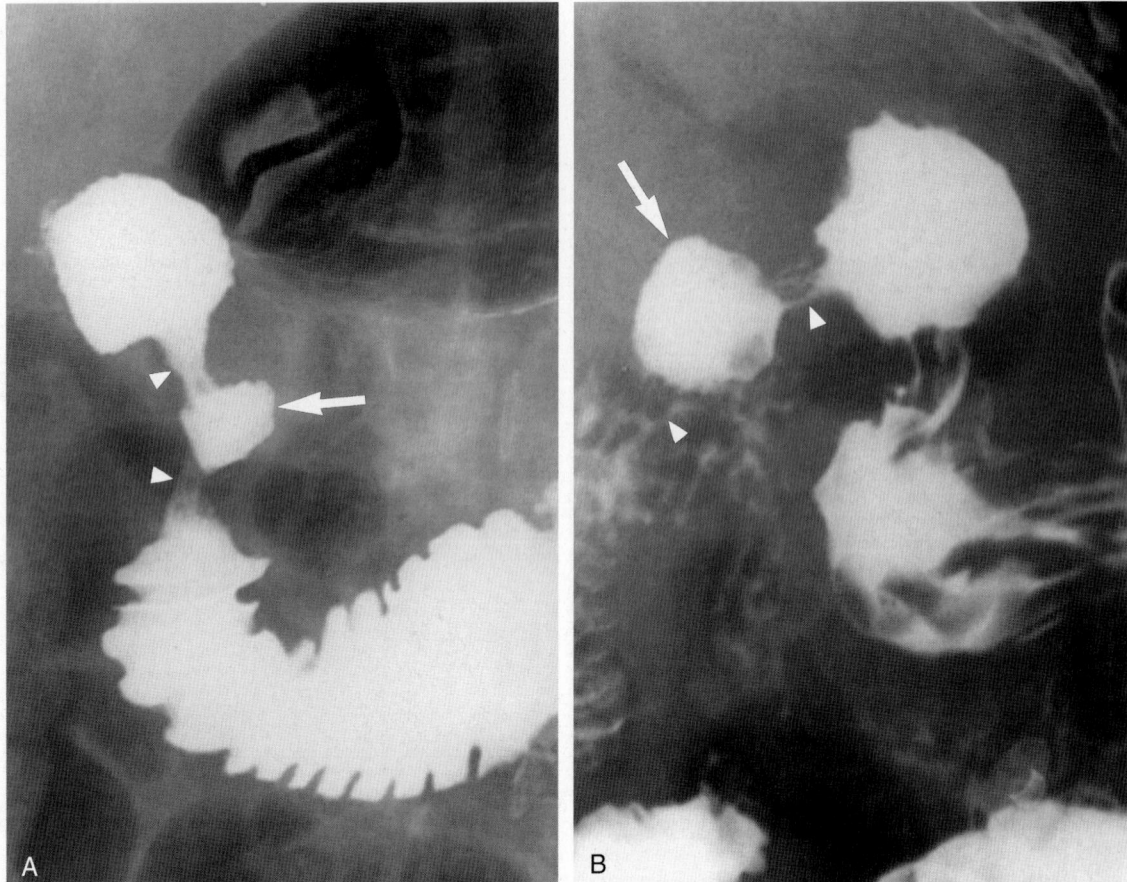

Figure 33-29. **Large postbulbar duodenal ulcers. A** and **B.** Two patients with large postbulbar ulcers (*arrows*) in the proximal descending duodenum. In both cases, note marked narrowing of the adjacent duodenum proximally and distally (*arrowheads*) as a result of severe edema and spasm accompanying these ulcer craters. (From Carucci LR, Levine MS, Rubesin SE, et al: Upper gastrointestinal tract barium examination of postbulbar duodenal ulcers. AJR 182:927-930, 2004; © by American Roentgen Ray Society.)

Ulcer Healing and Scarring

Duodenal ulcers usually heal rapidly during treatment with antisecretory agents. As the ulcers decrease in size, they often have a linear configuration.[66,104] Ulcer healing may lead to the development of an ulcer scar, manifested by radiating folds, bulbar deformity, or both. When radiating folds are present, they almost always converge at the site of the previous ulcer. In some patients, a residual depression in the central portion of the scar may simulate an active ulcer crater. As a result, it is often difficult to differentiate small, healing ulcers from ulcer scars. Nevertheless, follow-up barium studies to demonstrate ulcer healing are probably unnecessary for patients with uncomplicated duodenal ulcers who have an adequate clinical response to medical therapy because these ulcers are virtually always benign. Follow-up studies should therefore be reserved for patients with intractable ulcer symptoms or ulcer complications such as obstruction.

Bulbar deformity results from asymmetric scarring and retraction of the duodenal bulb during ulcer healing. Uninvolved segments of the bulb may balloon out between areas of fibrosis, producing one or more pseudodiverticula, which can usually be differentiated from ulcers by their tendency to change in size and shape at fluoroscopy. When multiple pseudodiverticula are present, the duodenal bulb may have a classic "cloverleaf" appearance (Fig. 33-33).

Pyloric Channel Ulcers

Pyloric channel ulcers should be treated as gastric ulcers rather than duodenal ulcers in terms of the need for aggressive evaluation and follow-up to differentiate these lesions from ulcerated carcinomas. Most pyloric channel ulcers are less than 1 cm, and they are usually located on the lesser curvature aspect of the pylorus. They also tend to be located on the anterior wall of the pylorus, so that they may appear as ring shadows on routine double-contrast views (Fig. 33-34A).[115] In such cases, the ulcers should fill with barium on prone or upright compression views (Fig. 33-34B). Some pyloric channel ulcers may cause marked edema and spasm of the pylorus and distal antrum, so that optimal radiologic evaluation of this area is not always possible.

Pyloric channel ulcers must be differentiated on barium studies from pseudodiverticula caused by scarring from previous ulcer disease or a surgical pyloroplasty. However, ulcers usually have a fixed configuration, whereas pseudodiverticula are more likely to change in size and shape at fluoroscopy. The presence of mucosal folds in the region of the outpouching should also suggest a pseudodiverticulum rather than an ulcer. Occasionally, adult hypertrophic pyloric stenosis may be manifested by a narrowed, elongated pyloric channel with diamond-shaped outpouchings or dimples extending superiorly or inferiorly from this region, but these patients

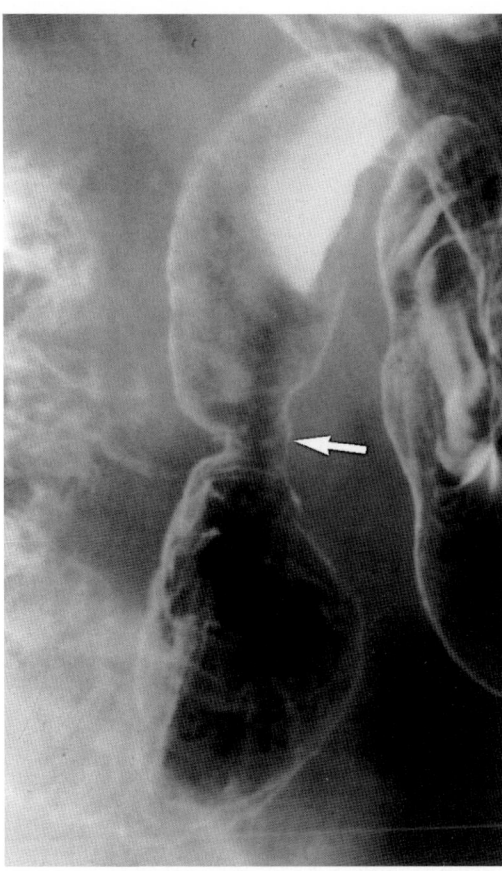

Figure 33-30. Postbulbar ring stricture. There is eccentric narrowing (*arrow*) of the postbulbar duodenum due to scarring and fibrosis from a previous ulcer in this location. (From Laufer I, Levine MS [eds]: Double Contrast Gastrointestinal Radiology, 2nd ed. Philadelphia, WB Saunders, 1992.)

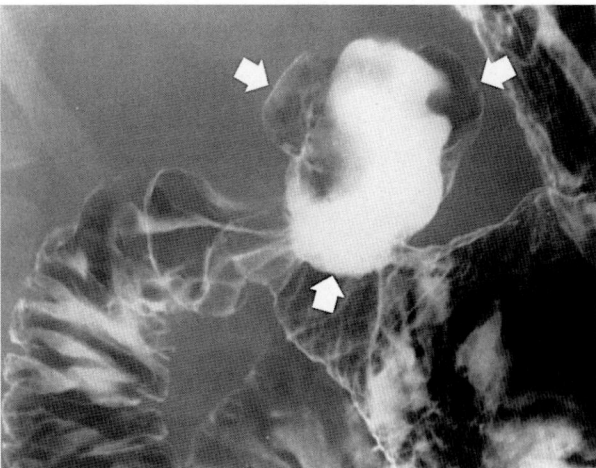

Figure 33-31. Giant duodenal ulcer. This giant ulcer (*arrows*) has replaced virtually the entire duodenal bulb. Paradoxically, such ulcers can be mistaken for a scarred or even a normal bulb.

usually have a long-standing history of obstructive symptoms. Healing of pyloric channel ulcers may lead to narrowing, elongation, or angulation of the pylorus, sometimes associated with gastric outlet obstruction.

DIFFERENTIAL DIAGNOSIS

Gastric or duodenal ulcers may occasionally be simulated by a variety of double-contrast artifacts, including barium precipitates, "stalactites," and see-through phenomena (see Chapter 4).[116] An inadequate or poorly prepared barium suspension may result in the development of barium precipitates that resemble tiny ulcers in the stomach or duodenum. However, these precipitates can be differentiated from ulcers by their failure to project beyond the contour of the stomach or duodenum in profile and by the absence of associated findings such as mucosal edema or radiating folds. Stalactites are hanging droplets of barium that are sometimes seen on the nondependent or anterior gastric wall.[117] Although a stalactite can be mistaken for a small ulcer on a single view, the transient nature of this finding at fluoroscopy differentiates a stalactite from a true ulcer. Finally, calcified densities (e.g., renal calculi or calcified splenic arteries) or contrast-containing structures (e.g., colonic diverticula) overlying the stomach or duodenum can be mistaken for ulcers on double-contrast

images. These artifacts are easily recognized by obtaining multiple images in different projections.

The most important consideration in the differential diagnosis of a benign gastric ulcer is an ulcerated gastric carcinoma (see earlier section on Benign Versus Malignant Ulcers). An ulcer that is surrounded by a discrete mound of edema can also be mistaken for an ulcerated submucosal mass such as a gastrointestinal stromal tumor.[118,119] However, the edematous mass surrounding an ulcer usually has poorly defined borders that form obtuse angles with the adjacent gastric wall whereas a submucosal mass has well-defined borders that form right angles with the adjacent gastric wall.[119] When gastric ulcers are associated with massive edema, there may be such narrowing and deformity that the radiographic findings erroneously suggest an infiltrating carcinoma. This problem is more likely to occur with prepyloric ulcers that cause gastric outlet obstruction, so that it is not possible to adequately assess the distal antrum. If a malignant lesion cannot be excluded on radiologic criteria, endoscopy and biopsy should be performed for a more definitive diagnosis.

Although multiple gastric or duodenal ulcers may be present in patients with uncomplicated peptic ulcer disease, this finding should raise the possibility of Zollinger-Ellison syndrome, cytomegalovirus infection, caustic ingestion, lymphoma, and other granulomatous conditions such as Crohn's disease, tuberculosis, sarcoidosis, and syphilis (see Chapters 34 and 37). In many cases, the correct diagnosis is suggested by the clinical history.

Gastric ulcer scars that are manifested by radiating folds must be differentiated from early gastric cancers, in which the folds tend to have a more lobulated, nodular, or irregular appearance.[100] If the radiographic findings are equivocal, endoscopy and biopsy should be performed for a more certain diagnosis. Benign-appearing ulcer scars may also result from healing of lymphomatous gastric lesions treated with chemotherapy (see Chapter 37).[120] Finally, ulcer scars may resemble surgical scars resulting from prior gastrostomy, cystogastrostomy (internal drainage of a pancreatic pseudocyst into the stomach), or wedge resection of the stomach.[92] However, ulcer scars can usually be differentiated from surgical scars on the basis of the clinical history.

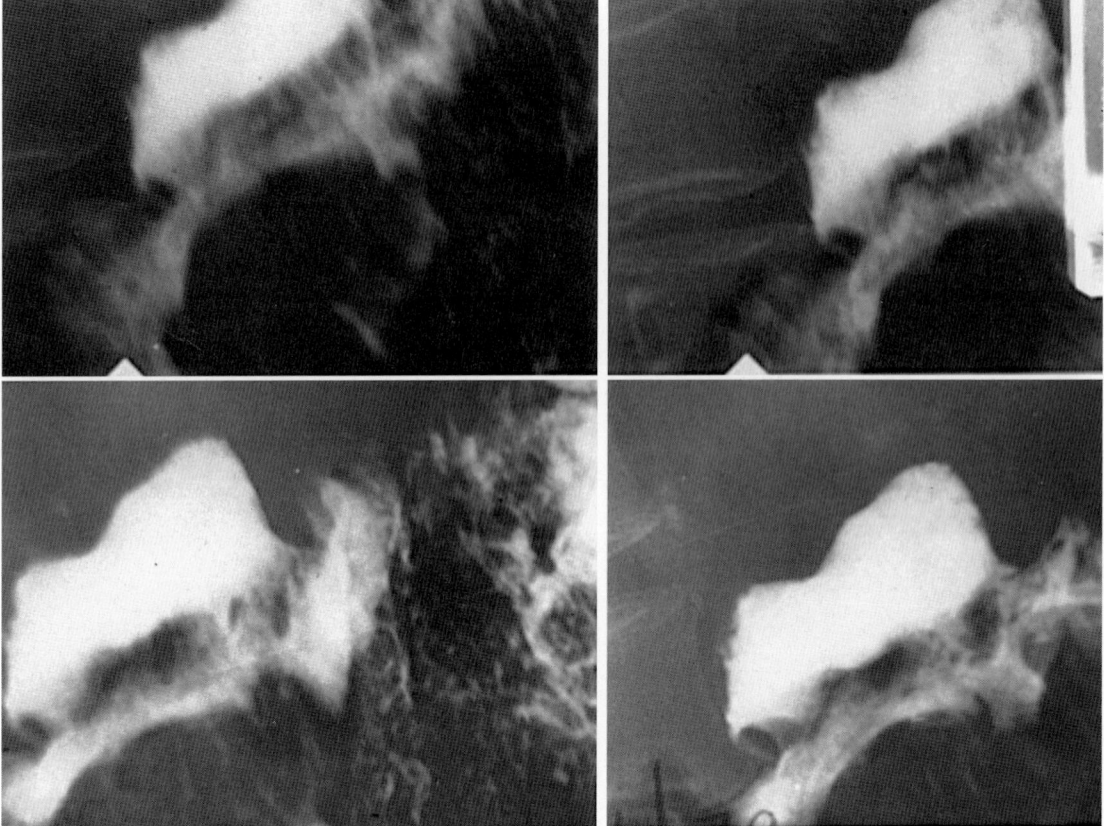

Figure 33-32.   Giant duodenal ulcer. Four spot images of the bulb show a giant ulcer that has a constant size and shape. In contrast, the duodenal bulb usually has a changing appearance at fluoroscopy. Also note the large radiolucent band of edema adjacent to the ulcer.

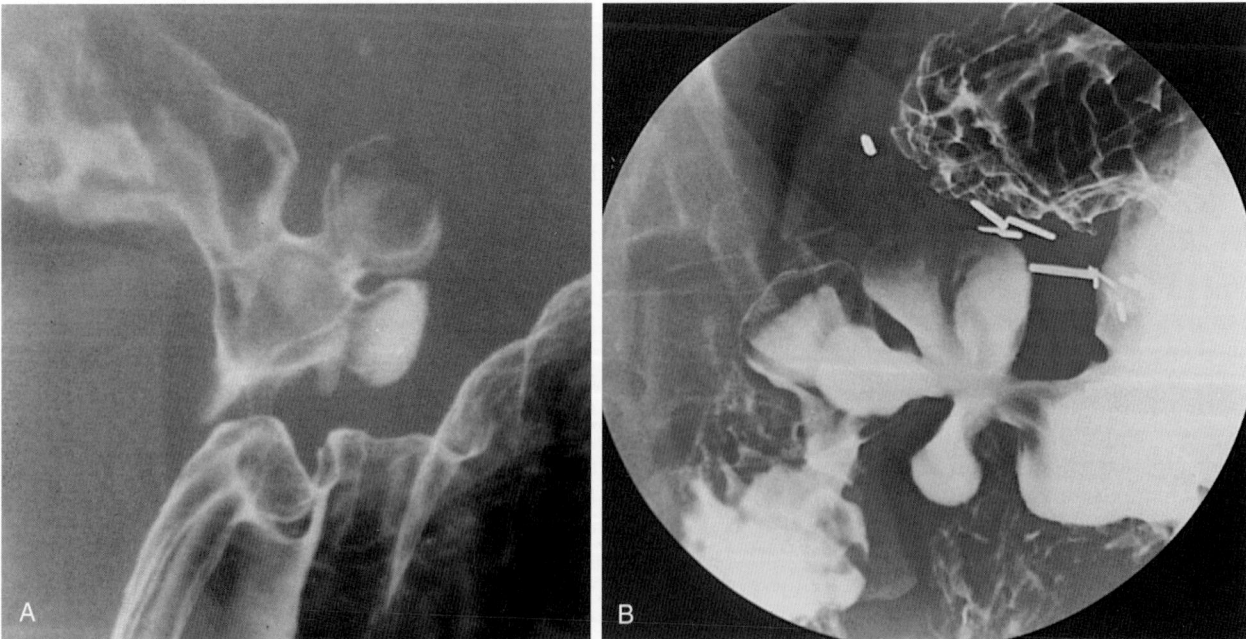

Figure 33-33.   Scarred duodenal bulb. A and **B.** Two examples of marked bulbar deformity with multiple pseudodiverticula, producing a cloverleaf appearance.

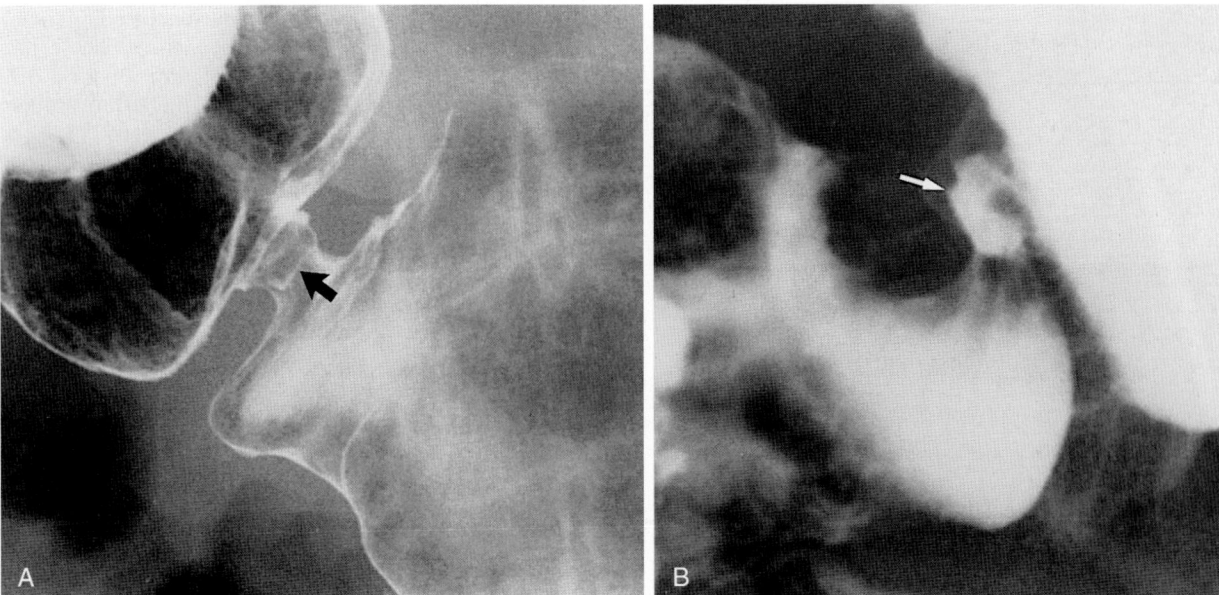

Figure 33-34. Pyloric channel ulcer. A. Initial double-contrast view with the patient in a supine position shows a partial ring shadow (*arrow*) in the region of the pylorus. **B.** Prone compression view shows barium filling an ulcer crater (*arrow*) on the anterior wall of the pyloric channel.

APPROACH TO ULCERS

In view of current recommendations that all *H. pylori*–positive patients with gastric or duodenal ulcers be treated with antimicrobial and antisecretory agents,[52,53] it is important to determine whether patients with ulcers are infected with *H. pylori*. Although endoscopy and biopsy may be performed to document the presence of *H. pylori* gastritis, highly accurate tests for *H. pylori* such as the urea breath test and serologic tests, are widely available (see Chapter 34). The combination of a double-contrast upper gastrointestinal examination and noninvasive testing for *H. pylori* could therefore replace endoscopy as a rational approach for evaluating patients with dyspepsia, epigastric pain, or other upper gastrointestinal symptoms.[8]

Here is one scenario. Patients with persistent upper gastrointestinal symptoms who fail to respond to an empirical trial of antisecretory agents could undergo a double-contrast barium study as the first diagnostic examination. If the barium study reveals a gastric or duodenal ulcer, a noninvasive test for *H. pylori* could be performed to determine whether the patient should receive antibiotics as well as conventional antisecretory agents. If the barium study reveals gastritis or duodenitis without an ulcer, however, there is not yet enough evidence to justify treatment with antibiotics even if these patients are infected with *H. pylori* (see Chapter 34). Thus, testing for *H. pylori* would not be required in most cases. Finally, if the barium study reveals a suspicious gastric ulcer or any abnormality that is equivocal or suspicious for malignant tumor, endoscopy should be performed for a more definitive diagnosis.

If randomized, controlled trials ultimately reveal that symptomatic patients with *H. pylori* gastritis should be treated with antimicrobial agents in the absence of ulcers, then noninvasive tests for *H. pylori* could be performed routinely at the time of the initial barium study. Clinical decisions regarding treatment with antisecretory agents or antibiotics

could then be made on the basis of the combined results of the barium study and noninvasive tests for *H. pylori*. Nevertheless, endoscopy would still be required for patients with equivocal or suspicious radiographic findings.

COMPLICATIONS

The major complications of peptic ulcers include upper gastrointestinal bleeding, obstruction, and perforation. These complications are often life-threatening, so that early treatment is essential for decreasing morbidity and mortality. Radiologists therefore have a major role in the recognition of these complications.

Upper Gastrointestinal Bleeding

Bleeding peptic ulcers may be manifested by sudden, massive upper gastrointestinal hemorrhage with hematemesis, melena, or rectal bleeding or by chronic, low-grade hemorrhage with guaiac-positive stool or iron-deficiency anemia. Endoscopy has a sensitivity of more than 90% in detecting the bleeding site in these patients.[121] Barium studies are less accurate because of the difficulty in obtaining adequate mucosal coating in the presence of bleeding and the inability to determine whether a radiographically diagnosed lesion is the actual source of bleeding. Nevertheless, double-contrast studies have a reported sensitivity of 70% to 80% in detecting the bleeding site in patients with acute upper gastrointestinal hemorrhage.[121,122]

The most frequent radiologic sign of bleeding in a gastric or duodenal ulcer is a blood clot at the base of the ulcer, typically seen as a smooth or irregular filling defect in the barium-filled ulcer crater (Fig. 33-35).[122] Granulation tissue or debris in the ulcer may produce similar findings. However, the defect is likely to represent an adherent blood clot in patients who have a history of recent upper gastrointestinal

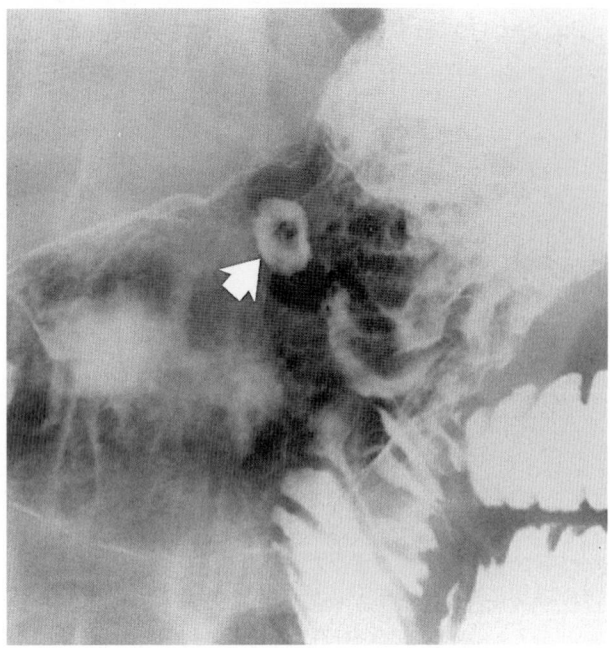

Figure 33-35. Ulcer with blood clot. A radiolucent filling defect is seen in the central portion of a barium-filled ulcer (*arrow*) on the posterior wall of the stomach. This patient presented with hematemesis 1 day earlier. (From Laufer I, Levine MS [eds]: Double Contrast Gastrointestinal Radiology, 2nd ed. Philadelphia, WB Saunders, 1992.)

bleeding. If the clot is dislodged, recurrent bleeding may occur with potentially catastrophic consequences. These patients should therefore be observed carefully for a period of 24 to 48 hours when a blood clot is detected on barium studies.

Obstruction

Although ulcers in the fundus, body, or proximal antrum of the stomach rarely cause gastric outlet obstruction, ulcers in the distal antrum, pyloric channel, or duodenum may cause obstruction resulting from edema and spasm associated with the ulcer crater or from scarring and fibrosis associated with ulcer healing. In patients with severe gastric outlet obstruction, abdominal radiographs may reveal a dilated stomach containing food and debris (Fig. 33-36A). This food or fluid in the stomach may dilute ingested barium, compromising the radiographic examination (Fig. 33-36B). The stomach should therefore be decompressed with a nasogastric tube before performing barium studies on these patients.

Severe scarring from ulcers in the distal antrum or pyloric channel may be manifested on barium studies by a relatively short segment of narrowing with delayed emptying of barium from the stomach (see Fig. 33-19A). It is sometimes difficult to differentiate these areas of scarring from localized scirrhous carcinomas involving the prepyloric region of the antrum.[123] Irregular narrowing and abrupt, shelflike proximal borders should favor a malignant lesion (see Chapter 36). If the findings are equivocal or suspicious for tumor, endoscopy and biopsy should be performed for a more certain diagnosis.

Although scarring from duodenal ulcers rarely causes obstruction, postbulbar ulcers may lead to the development of strictures in the proximal descending duodenum with

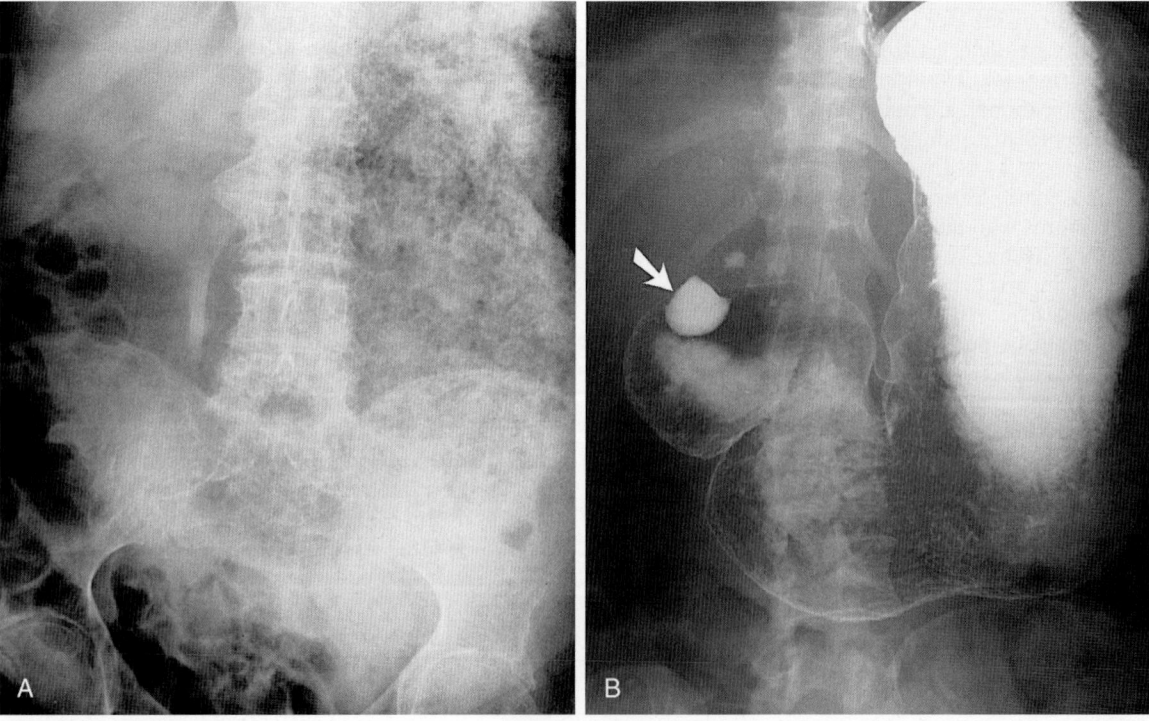

Figure 33-36. Gastric outlet obstruction caused by pyloric channel ulcers. A. Abdominal radiograph shows a markedly dilated stomach with retained food and debris resulting from gastric outlet obstruction. After the stomach was decompressed, endoscopy revealed a pyloric channel ulcer causing the obstruction. **B.** In another patient, an overhead radiograph from a barium study shows a dilated stomach with retained fluid diluting the barium and no emptying into the duodenum. A large pyloric channel ulcer (*arrow*) is also seen.

subsequent obstruction (see earlier section on Postbulbar Ulcers). Other causes of duodenal narrowing and obstruction include Crohn's disease, tuberculosis, tumors, hematomas, duplication cysts, and extrinsic compression of the duodenum by an annular pancreas, pancreatitis, pancreatic pseudocysts, or pancreatic carcinoma.

Perforation

Penetrating ulcers on the anterior wall of the stomach or duodenum may perforate directly into the peritoneal cavity, whereas penetrating ulcers on the posterior wall of the stomach or duodenum usually result in a walled-off or "confined" perforation. Some penetrating ulcers may also involve other hollow organs, producing a fistula. These various types of perforations are considered separately in the following sections.

Free Perforation

Ulcers on the anterior wall of the stomach or duodenum directly abut the peritoneal cavity, so that perforation of a penetrating ulcer in this location may result in acute peritonitis with free spillage of gastric and duodenal contents into the peritoneal cavity. Because duodenal ulcers are often located on the anterior wall of the bulb, perforated duodenal ulcer is the most common cause of peritonitis in the adult population. The volume of gas that escapes into the peritoneal cavity from a perforated peptic ulcer depends on how quickly the site of perforation seals off. In one study, free intraperitoneal air was detected on abdominal radiographs in only about two thirds of patients with perforated duodenal ulcers.[124] The presence of pneumoperitoneum in an acutely ill patient therefore strongly supports the diagnosis of a perforated ulcer, but the absence of pneumoperitoneum in no way excludes this diagnosis.

If abdominal radiographs reveal pneumoperitoneum in patients with clinical signs of peritonitis, immediate surgery is warranted. If there is no evidence of pneumoperitoneum, studies with water-soluble contrast agents or CT may be performed to determine whether a perforation has occurred. Only about 50% of patients with perforated duodenal ulcers are found to have extravasation of contrast medium from the duodenum, presumably because the perforation has sealed off by the time the examination is performed.[125] When extravasation of contrast medium does occur, about half the patients are found to have a generalized leak into the peritoneal cavity and half are found to have a walled-off leak (Fig. 33-37)[125] (see next section on Confined Perforation).

With an ulcer causing free perforation, studies with water-soluble contrast agents may show contrast medium leaking from the stomach or duodenum into the subhepatic space or elsewhere into the peritoneal cavity. CT may reveal inflammatory changes in the perigastroduodenal soft tissues, extraluminal fluid or contrast material, and varying amounts of free intraperitoneal air.[126] The site of perforation can sometimes be identified on CT by interruption of the enhanced gastroduodenal wall or by tiny extraluminal air bubbles in close proximity to the perforation.[127]

Less frequently, ulcers on the posterior wall of the stomach may perforate into the lesser peritoneal cavity or lesser sac, a potential space between the stomach and pancreas. An abscess

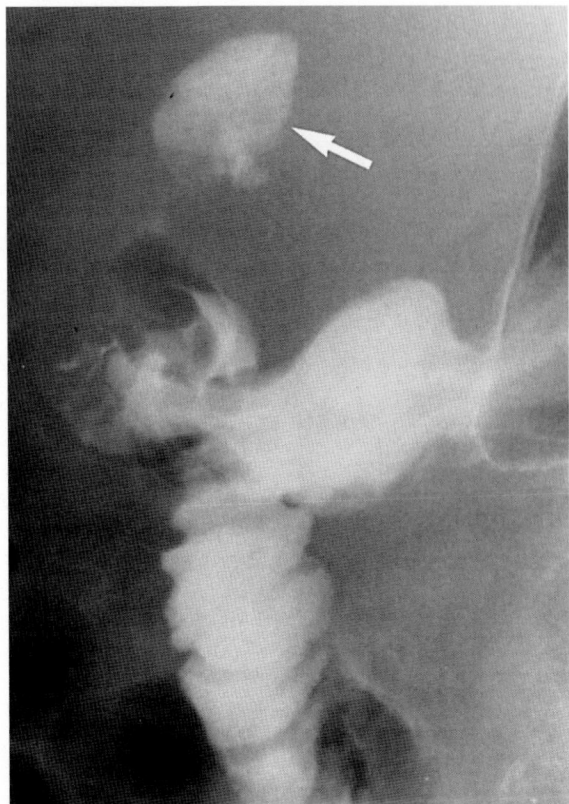

Figure 33-37. Perforated duodenal ulcer. Water-soluble contrast medium is seen tracking superiorly from the region of the duodenal bulb into a sealed-off collection (*arrow*). This patient presented with clinical signs of peritonitis.

in the lesser sac may be manifested by extraluminal gas collections in the left upper quadrant on abdominal radiographs (Fig. 33-38) or by extrinsic mass effect on the posterior wall of the stomach or actual leakage of contrast material into the lesser sac on studies with water-soluble contrast agents. CT is extremely useful for documenting these lesser sac collections or abscesses.[128]

Confined Perforation

Penetrating ulcers on the posterior wall of the stomach or duodenum are often associated with the development of a walled-off or confined perforation resulting from an inflammatory reaction and fibrous adhesions that seal off the perforation site as the ulcer enters adjacent structures. The pancreas is involved in the majority of patients with confined perforations. Other less common sites of involvement include the lesser omentum, transverse mesocolon, liver, spleen, biliary tract, and colon. If the affected structure is a hollow organ, such as the colon or biliary tract, this process may lead to the development of a fistula (see later section on Fistulas).

Less than 50% of patients with posterior penetrating ulcers and confined perforations have evidence of extraluminal gas or contrast medium collections on studies with water-soluble contrast agents. A posterior penetrating ulcer should be suspected, however, when an unusually deep ulcer crater is seen in profile on the posterior wall of the stomach or duodenum. In such cases, CT may be helpful for demonstrating signs

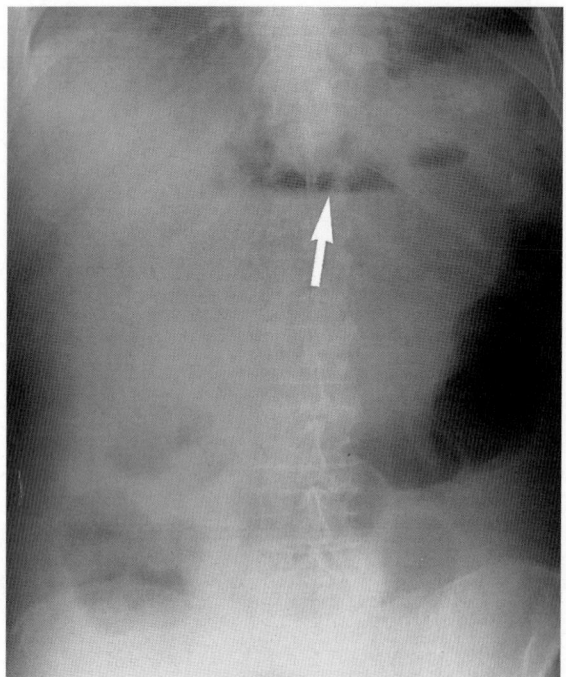

Figure 33-38. Lesser sac abscess caused by a perforated gastric ulcer. Upright abdominal radiograph shows an air-fluid level (*arrow*) in the lesser sac caused by a lesser sac abscess. Subsequent study with a water-soluble contrast agent revealed a perforated posterior wall gastric ulcer with leakage of the contrast agent directly into the lesser sac.

of pancreatic penetration, including loss of fascial planes and the presence of soft tissue bands or low-density sinus tracks between these structures.[129]

Penetrating ulcers on the lesser curvature of the stomach occasionally enter the adjacent hepatic parenchyma, resulting in the development of an abscess in the left lobe of the liver. This complication should be suspected when contrast studies demonstrate a deep ulcer on the lesser curvature associated with a large area of extrinsic mass effect on the adjacent gastric wall (Fig. 33-39A). In such cases, CT can be used to demonstrate the presence of a confined perforation involving the liver (Fig. 33-39B).

Splenic penetration by a gastric ulcer is extremely unusual because of the rarity of benign ulcers on the posterior wall or greater curvature of the gastric fundus. Although barium studies are usually nonspecific, transmural penetration by an ulcer high on the greater curvature or posterior wall of the stomach may be suspected if the ulcer extends well beyond the adjacent gastric contour.[130] In such cases, CT may demonstrate extension of the ulcer directly into the substance of the spleen.[131] If CT confirms splenic penetration by a benign gastric ulcer, early surgery is required because of the risk of massive, potentially life-threatening gastrointestinal bleeding if the ulcer ruptures into the spleen.[131]

Fistulas

Penetrating ulcers in the stomach or duodenum may occasionally erode through the wall of adjacent hollow organs, producing a variety of fistulas, including gastroduodenal, gastrocolic, duodenocolic, choledochoduodenal, duodeno-

renal, and gastropericardial fistulas. These fistulas are considered separately in the following sections.

Gastroduodenal Fistulas (Double-Channel Pylorus)

The double-channel pylorus is an acquired gastroduodenal fistula caused by a penetrating ulcer in the distal antrum that erodes directly into the base of the duodenal bulb.[132-134] These ulcers are usually located on the lesser curvature of the prepyloric antrum but are occasionally located on the greater curvature.[133,134] Paradoxically, the development of a double-channel pylorus may lead to improved ulcer symptoms, possibly because the fistula facilitates gastric emptying.[134]

Although the double-channel pylorus is difficult to visualize on endoscopy, it is readily detected on barium studies.[133,134] The double-channel pylorus is typically manifested by two discrete tracks extending from the distal antrum into the base of the duodenal bulb (Fig. 33-40). The track on the greater curvature side of the stomach usually represents the true pyloric channel, whereas the track on the lesser curvature side represents the fistula. The barium-filled tracks are often separated by a thin, radiolucent bridge or septum that is best seen on prone compression views. Sequential barium studies may show progression from a penetrating prepyloric ulcer to a double-channel pylorus.

Gastrocolic Fistulas

In the past, most gastrocolic fistulas were thought to be caused by primary carcinoma of the stomach or transverse colon invading the gastrocolic ligament.[135] With the increasing use of aspirin and other NSAIDs in today's pill-oriented society, however, benign NSAID-induced ulcers on the greater curvature of the stomach have become a more common cause of gastrocolic fistulas than carcinoma of the stomach or transverse colon.[78,136-138] Affected individuals typically have a history of taking high doses of aspirin or other NSAIDs. As the ulcers enlarge, they penetrate inferiorly into the gastrocolic ligament, eventually producing a gastrocolic fistula. These fistulas are classically manifested by the triad of feculent vomiting, foul-smelling eructations, and diarrhea,[135] but some patients may present with abdominal pain or other nonspecific clinical findings.[137] When a gastrocolic fistula is suspected on clinical grounds, endoscopy is contraindicated because of the risk of perforation and peritonitis.[136] In contrast to gastrocolic fistulas caused by malignant tumors, fistulas complicating NSAID-induced greater curvature ulcers sometimes heal on medical treatment without need for surgery.[137,139]

In patients with gastrocolic fistulas complicating NSAID-induced ulcers, barium studies may reveal giant ulcers on the greater curvature of the gastric antrum or body with early filling of the transverse colon via the fistula (Fig. 33-41).[136,137] Because of the greater pressures generated during a barium enema examination, this technique can sometimes demonstrate fistulas that are not visualized on upper gastrointestinal studies.[138] When fistulas are shown on barium studies, patients should be questioned about a possible history of NSAID use. Other causes of gastrocolic fistulas include gastric or colonic carcinoma, lymphoma, Crohn's disease, and tuberculosis.

Duodenocolic Fistulas

Duodenocolic fistulas are usually caused by carcinoma of the ascending colon or hepatic flexure invading the descending duodenum. Occasionally, these fistulas may result from pene-

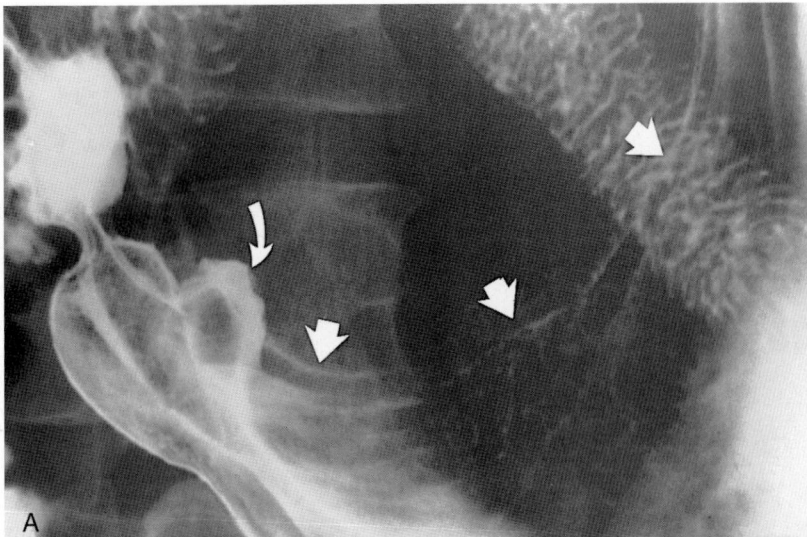

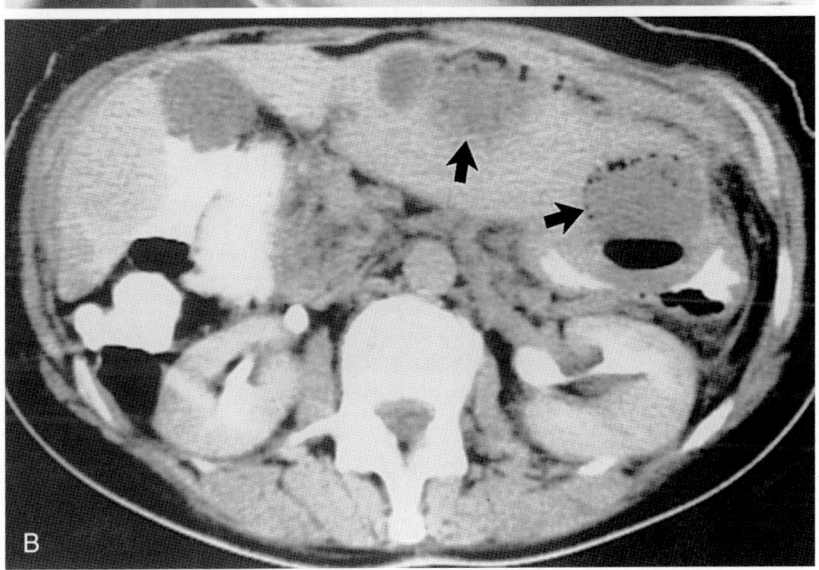

Figure 33-39. Penetrating lesser curvature ulcer with an associated hepatic abscess. A. Barium study shows a deep ulcer (*curved arrow*) on the lesser curvature of the distal antrum. Also note the large area of extrinsic mass effect (*straight arrows*) on the adjacent gastric wall. **B.** CT scan reveals several gas- and fluid-containing abscess cavities (*arrows*) in the left lobe of the liver. These abscesses were caused by penetration of the ulcer into the hepatic parenchyma.

trating ulcers in the duodenal bulb or postbulbar duodenum that have eroded into the hepatic flexure of the colon.[140,141] Affected individuals may present with abdominal pain, diarrhea, feculent vomiting, foul-smelling eructations, or undigested food in the stool. Although upper gastrointestinal studies may fail to demonstrate the fistula, barium enema examinations are often successful because of the greater pressures generated by this technique.[141]

Choledochoduodenal Fistulas

About 90% of enterobiliary fistulas occur as complications of stones in the biliary tract.[142] Only about 5% are caused by peptic ulcer disease.[142] Most of these patients have penetrating duodenal ulcers that rupture into the common bile duct, producing a choledochoduodenal fistula.[142] These patients usually have symptoms related to their underlying ulcers but occasionally present with abnormal liver function tests, jaundice, or ascending cholangitis.[143] Abdominal radiographs may reveal pneumobilia with gas in the gallbladder or bile ducts (Fig. 33-42), and barium studies may demonstrate a duodenal ulcer or duodenal scarring, sometimes associated with reflux of barium into the biliary tree.[143-145] Rarely, these

ulcers may lead to the development of cholecystoduodenal, cholecystogastric, or choledochogastric fistulas.[142]

Duodenorenal Fistulas

Penetrating postbulbar duodenal ulcers rarely may rupture posteriorly into the pyelocalyceal system of the right kidney, producing a duodenorenal fistula. These fistulas may be demonstrated on barium studies or retrograde pyelography. Other rare causes of duodenorenal fistulas include malignant tumors, infection, and trauma.

Gastropericardial Fistulas

Benign ulcers in the intrathoracic portion of the stomach (either a hiatal hernia or a gastric pull-through after esophagogastrectomy) rarely erode through the pericardium, producing a gastropericardial fistula.[146] This complication is catastrophic for the patient because it usually leads to the rapid development of purulent pericarditis, cardiac tamponade, and death. The sudden appearance of pneumopericardium on chest radiographs of an acutely ill patient with an intrathoracic stomach should therefore raise the possibility of a gastropericardial fistula. Upper gastrointestinal studies with

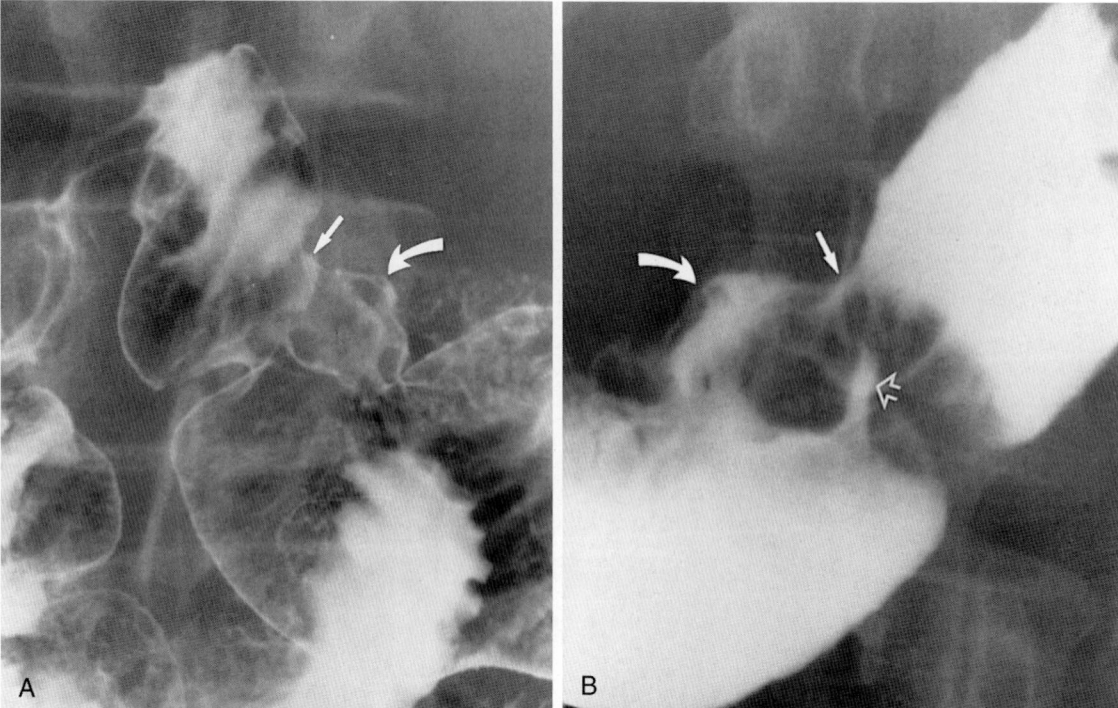

Figure 33-40. Double channel pylorus. A. Double-contrast view of the antrum shows a prepyloric lesser curvature ulcer (*curved arrow*) that communicates distally with the base of the duodenal bulb (*straight arrow*). **B.** Prone view of the antrum also delineates the lesser curvature ulcer (*curved arrow*) with a track (*straight arrow*) extending from the ulcer into the duodenum. Note the normal pyloric channel (*open arrow*) inferiorly.

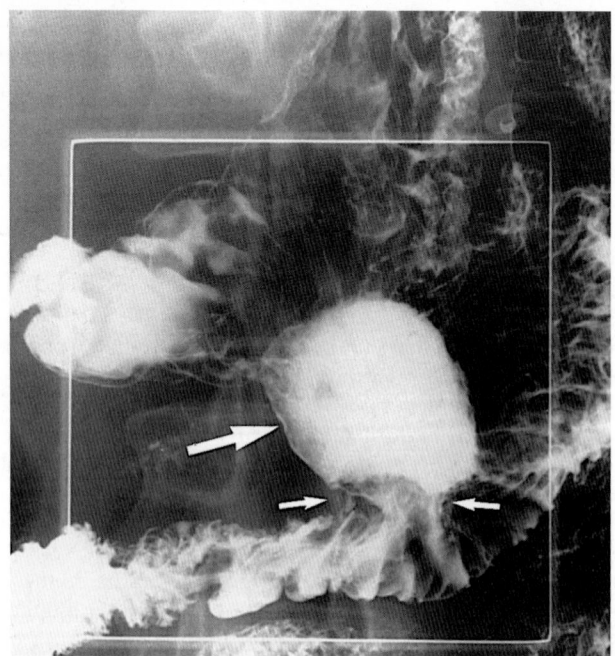

Figure 33-41. Gastrocolic fistula caused by an aspirin-induced greater curvature ulcer. Double-contrast upper gastrointestinal study reveals a giant ulcer (*large arrow*) on the greater curvature of the stomach with barium entering a wide fistulous track (*small arrows*) that communicates directly with the transverse colon. This patient had been taking high doses of aspirin. (From Levine MS, Kelly MR, Laufer I, et al: Gastrocolic fistulas: The increasing role of aspirin. Radiology 187:359-361, 1993.)

water-soluble contrast agents may document the presence of a fistula by showing extravasation of contrast medium into the pericardial sac.[147] Because of the high mortality associated with this complication, the best hope for survival is early surgery with drainage of the pericardium and closure of the fistula.[146]

ZOLLINGER-ELLISON SYNDROME

Since its original description by Zollinger and Ellison in 1955,[148] Zollinger-Ellison syndrome has been recognized as a life-threatening condition characterized by marked hypersecretion of gastric acid and a severe form of peptic ulcer disease resulting from high levels of gastrin in patients with underlying gastrinomas. These tumors not only may cause a devastating ulcer diathesis but may also behave as malignant lesions, metastasizing to the liver or other structures (see Chapter 99). The development of potent antisecretory agents for controlling acid secretion as well as sophisticated techniques for localizing these islet cell tumors have had a major impact on patient survival. Although barium studies may reveal typical features of peptic ulcer disease, it is sometimes possible to suggest the diagnosis of Zollinger-Ellison syndrome on the basis of the radiographic findings.

Pathology

Zollinger-Ellison syndrome is caused by the uncontrolled release of gastrin from autonomously functioning non–beta islet cell tumors known as *gastrinomas* (see Chapter 99). About 75% of these tumors are located in the pancreas, 15% in the duodenum, and 10% in other extraintestinal locations,

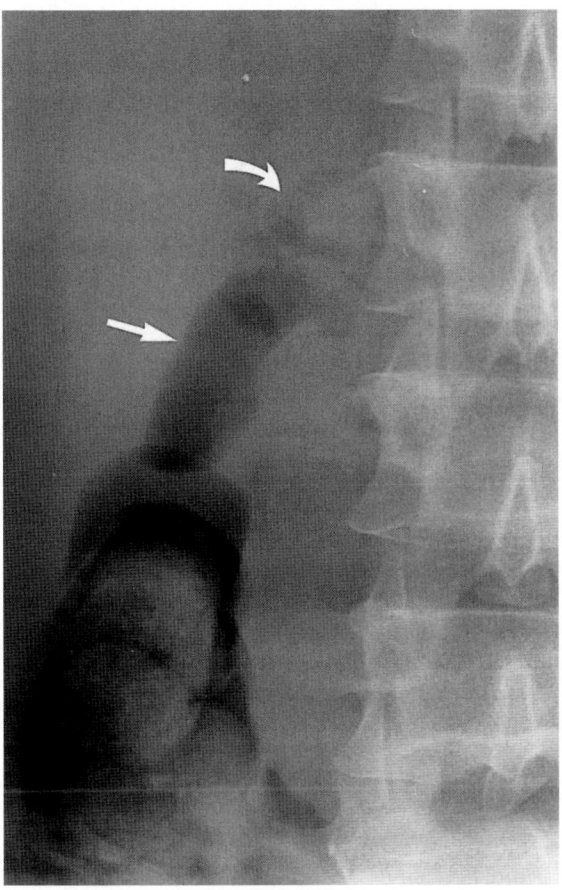

Figure 33-42. Pneumobilia caused by a choledochoduodenal fistula.
Close-up view from an abdominal radiograph shows gas in the gallbladder (*straight arrow*) and bile ducts (*curved arrow*) caused by a
choledochoduodenal fistula in a patient with a giant duodenal ulcer.

including the liver, ovaries, and lymph nodes.[149,150] Most
gastrinomas are thought to be malignant; multiple tumors
or metastases are found at the time of diagnosis in 30 to 50%
of patients.[150] The liver is the most frequent site of metastatic
disease.

Most gastrinomas occur as sporadic tumors. About 25%,
however, are genetically transmitted as part of the hereditary
syndrome multiple endocrine neoplasia type 1.[151] This syndrome is characterized not only by pancreatic tumors but also
by parathyroid, pituitary, and adrenal tumors.

Clinical Aspects

More than 90% of patients with Zollinger-Ellison syndrome
have upper gastrointestinal ulcers caused by hypersecretion
of gastric acid.[150] The presenting signs and symptoms may be
indistinguishable from those associated with ordinary peptic
ulcers. However, the possibility of Zollinger-Ellison syndrome
should be considered in patients who have multiple ulcers,
ulcers in unusual locations, ulcers that are resistant to medical
therapy, or postoperative recurrence of ulcers.[149,150]

The second most common clinical problem in Zollinger-
Ellison syndrome is diarrhea, which occurs in up to 50% of
patients and is the presenting symptom in 35%.[149,150] This
diarrhea is related primarily to the severe volume load caused
by the secretion of several liters of acid into the intestines

each day. The acidic pH of the small bowel may also damage
the intestinal mucosa, resulting in a spruelike state with villous
atrophy, malabsorption, and steatorrhea.[152] Other patients
may initially present with reflux symptoms or dysphagia
caused by the development of severe reflux esophagitis or
peptic strictures.[153]

The diagnosis of Zollinger-Ellison syndrome is established by the demonstration of hypergastrinemia and gastric
acid hypersecretion in a patient with peptic ulcers, diarrhea,
or other clinical features of a gastrinoma. In the appropriate
clinical setting, fasting serum gastrin levels greater than 1000
pg/mL should be virtually diagnostic of Zollinger-Ellison
syndrome.[150] However, not all patients have such high serum
gastrin levels. Furthermore, hypergastrinemia may occur in
patients with atrophic gastritis, gastric outlet obstruction,
and G-cell hyperplasia.

In the past, total gastrectomy was the treatment of choice
for preventing hypersecretion of acid and its complications
in patients with Zollinger-Ellison syndrome. However, H_2-
receptor antagonists (e.g., cimetidine and ranitidine) and,
more recently, proton pump inhibitors (e.g., omeprazole) have
proved to be extremely effective in suppressing acid secretion and promoting ulcer healing without need for surgery.[150,154,155] Total gastrectomy should therefore be reserved
for noncompliant patients.

As fewer patients succumb to the ulcer diathesis in
Zollinger-Ellison syndrome, malignant spread of gastrinomas
has become a major cause of long-term morbidity and mortality in these individuals. Greater attention has therefore been
focused on early detection and excision of the underlying gastrinomas before the development of hepatic metastases.[156,157]
Although the primary tumors are often difficult to detect on
preoperative imaging studies, successful localization of gastrinomas can be achieved by CT, angiography, or selective portal
venous sampling for gastrin or by whole-body imaging with
somatostatin scintigraphy.[158-161] The most important prognostic factor affecting survival is the extent of tumor at the
time of surgery. Patients with no tumor or lesions that are
resectable at laparotomy have 5-year survival rates greater
than 90%, whereas patients with liver metastases have 5-year
survival rates less than 20%.[150]

Radiographic Findings

Zollinger-Ellison syndrome may be manifested on barium
studies by a characteristic constellation of findings.[162-166]
Hypersecretion of acid often results in a large volume of
fluid in the stomach, duodenum, and proximal jejunum that
dilutes the barium and compromises mucosal coating. Many
patients have markedly thickened gastric folds, particularly
in the fundus and body of the stomach, not only because of
edema and inflammation but also because of gastrin-induced
parietal cell hyperplasia (Fig. 33-43A). Duodenal and jejunal
folds may also have a grossly thickened, edematous appearance
because of a severe inflammatory response to the enormous
amount of gastric secretions entering the proximal small
bowel. Although thickened folds may be caused by a variety
of conditions in the stomach and duodenum (see next section
on Differential Diagnosis), the combination of thickened folds
and excessive fluid in the stomach, duodenum, and proximal
jejunum should suggest the possibility of Zollinger-Ellison
syndrome.

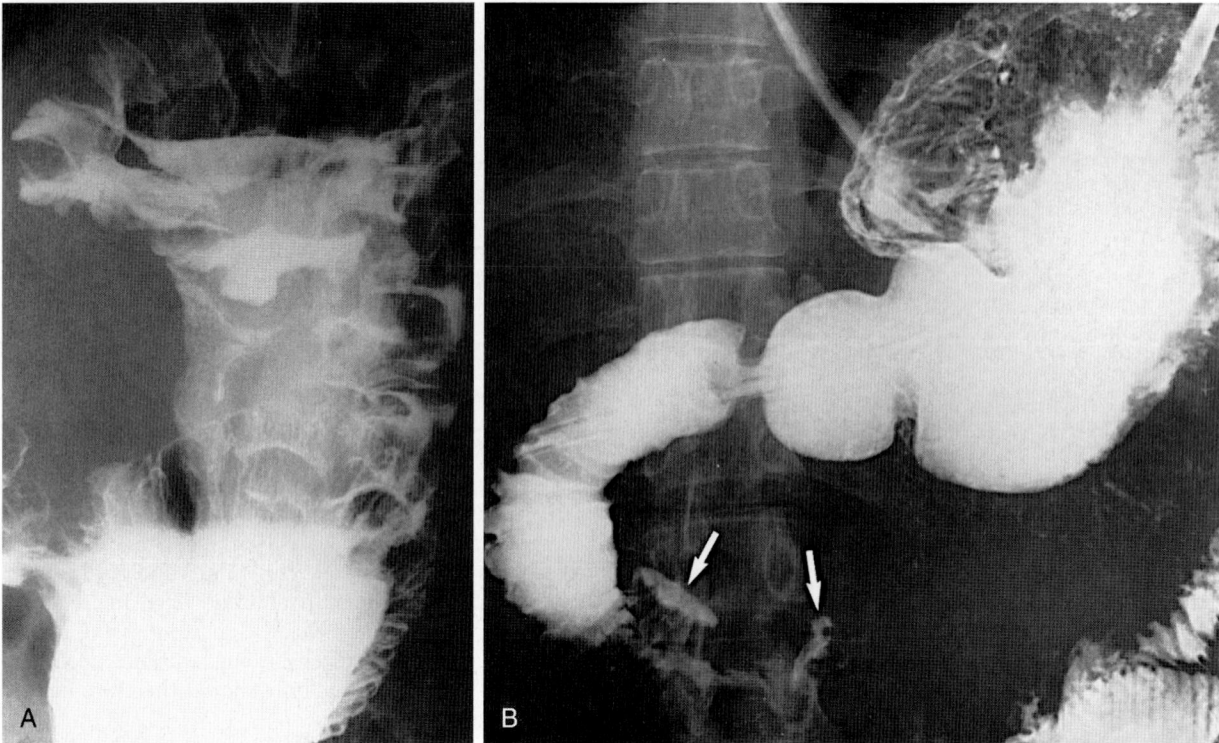

Figure 33-43. Zollinger-Ellison syndrome. A. There are markedly thickened folds in the gastric fundus and body. Also note how the barium is diluted by excessive fluid in the stomach. **B.** In another patient, two discrete ulcers (*arrows*) are seen in the third and fourth portions of the duodenum. Ordinary peptic ulcers rarely occur distal to the papilla of Vater, so that ulcers in this location should suggest the possibility of Zollinger-Ellison syndrome. (**B** courtesy of Stephen W. Trenkner, MD, Minneapolis, MN.)

Approximately 75% of the ulcers in Zollinger-Ellison syndrome are located in the stomach or duodenal bulb, so that they cannot be differentiated from ordinary peptic ulcers.[167] The remaining 25% are located in the postbulbar duodenum or proximal jejunum.[167] Because peptic ulcers rarely occur distal to the papilla of Vater, the presence of one or more ulcers in the third or fourth portion of the duodenum or in the proximal jejunum should be highly suggestive of Zollinger-Ellison syndrome (Fig. 33-43B). Patients with this syndrome are also more likely to have multiple ulcers than other patients with peptic ulcer disease.[167]

Differential Diagnosis

Markedly thickened gastric folds may be present in a variety of conditions, including *H. pylori* gastritis, hypertrophic gastritis, Ménétrier's disease, and lymphoma. Similarly, thickened duodenal or jejunal folds may be caused by a host of inflammatory or infectious processes. Although thickened folds are a nonspecific finding, the simultaneous presence of increased fluid in the upper gastrointestinal tract and one or more ulcers in unusual locations should strongly suggest Zollinger-Ellison syndrome. If this syndrome is suspected on the basis of the radiographic findings, a fasting serum gastrin level should be obtained for a more definitive diagnosis.

References

1. Boyd EJS, Wormsley KG: Etiology and pathogenesis of peptic ulcer. In Berk JE, Haubrich WS, Kalser MH, et al (eds): Bockus Gastroenterology, 4th ed. Philadelphia, WB Saunders, 1985, pp 1013-1059.
2. Bonnevie O: Changing demographics of peptic ulcer disease. Dig Dis Sci 30(Suppl 11):85-145, 1985.
3. Kurata JH, Haile BM, Elashoff JD: Sex differences in peptic ulcer disease. Gastroenterology 88:96-100, 1985.
4. Sonnenberg A, Wasserman IH, Jacobsen SJ: Monthly variation of hospital admission and mortality of peptic ulcer disease: A reappraisal of ulcer periodicity. Gastroenterology 103:1192-1198, 1992.
5. Hung LCT, Ching JYL, Sung JJY, et al: Long-term outcome of *Helicobacter pylori*-negative idiopathic bleeding ulcers: A prospective cohort study. Gastroenterology 128:1845-1850, 2005.
6. Warren JR, Marshall BJ: Unidentified curved bacilli on gastric epithelium in active chronic gastritis. Lancet 2:1273-1275, 1983.
7. Peterson WL: *Helicobacter pylori* and peptic ulcer disease. N Engl J Med 324:1043-1048, 1991.
8. Levine MS, Rubesin SE: The *Helicobacter pylori* revolution: Radiologic perspective. Radiology 195:593-596, 1995.
9. Pattison CP, Combs MK, Marshall BJ: *Helicobacter pylori* and peptic ulcer disease: Evolution to revolution to resolution. AJR 168:1415-1420, 1997.
10. Yardley JH, Paull G: *Campylobacter pylori*: A newly recognized infectious agent in the gastrointestinal tract. Am J Surg Pathol 12(Suppl):89-99, 1988.
11. Chamberlain CE, Peura DA: *Campylobacter (Helicobacter) pylori*: Is peptic disease a bacterial infection? Arch Intern Med 150:951-955, 1990.
12. Peek RM, Blaser MJ: Pathophysiology of *Helicobacter pylori*-induced gastritis and peptic ulcer disease. Am J Med 102:200-207, 1997.
13. Graham DU: *Helicobacter pylori* infection in the pathogenesis of duodenal ulcer and gastric cancer: A model. Gastroenterology 113:1983-1991, 1997.
14. Hamlet A, Thoreson AC, Nilsson O, et al: Duodenal *Helicobacter pylori* infection differs in *cagA* genotype between asymptomatic subjects and patients with duodenal ulcers. Gastroenterology 116:259-268, 1999.
15. Moss S, Calam J: *Helicobacter pylori* and peptic ulcers: The present position. Gut 33:289-292, 1992.
16. Larkai EN, Smith JL, Lidsky MD, et al: Gastroduodenal mucosa and dyspeptic symptoms in arthritic patients during chronic nonsteroidal anti-inflammatory drug use. Am J Gastroenterol 82:1153-1158, 1987.

17. Bellary SV, Isaacs PET, Lee FI: Upper gastrointestinal lesions in elderly patients presenting for endoscopy: Relevance of NSAID usage. Am J Gastroenterol 86:961-964, 1991.

18. Laine L: Approaches to nonsteroidal anti-inflammatory drug use in the high-risk patient. Gastroenterology 120:594-606, 2001.

19. Hawkey CJ: Nonsteroidal anti-inflammatory drug gastropathy. Gastroenterology 119:521-535, 2000.

20. Cryer B, Feldman M: Effects of very low dose daily, long-term aspirin therapy on gastric, duodenal, and rectal prostaglandin levels and on mucosal injury in healthy humans. Gastroenterology 117:17-25, 1999.

21. Lanza FL: NSAIDs and the gastrointestinal tract. Abdom Imaging 22:1-4, 1997.

22. Wallace JL: Nonsteroidal anti-inflammatory drugs and gastroenteropathy: The second hundred years. Gastroenterology 112:1000-1016, 1997.

23. Davenport HW: Salicylate damage to the gastric mucosal barrier. N Engl J Med 276:1307-1312, 1967.

24. Kelly JP, Kaufman DW, Jurgelon JM, et al: Risk of aspirin-associated major upper gastrointestinal bleeding with enteric-coated or buffered product. Lancet 348:1413-1416, 1996.

25. Bugat R, Thompson MR, Aures D, et al: Gastric mucosal lesions produced by intravenous infusion of aspirin in cats. Gastroenterology 7:754-759, 1976.

26. Lanas A, Serrano P, Bajador E, et al: Evidence of aspirin use in both upper and lower gastrointestinal perforation. Gastroenterology 112:683-689, 1997.

27. Wilcox CM, Alexander LN, Cotsonis GA, et al: Nonsteroidal anti-inflammatory drugs are associated with both upper and lower gastrointestinal bleeding. Dig Dis Sci 42:990-997, 1997.

28. Conn HO, Blitzer BL: Nonassociation of adrenocorticosteroid therapy and peptic ulcer. N Engl J Med 294:473-479, 1976.

29. Friedman GD, Siegelaub AB, Seltzer CC: Cigarettes, alcohol, coffee, and peptic ulcer. N Engl J Med 290:469-473, 1974.

30. Piper DW, Nasiry R, McIntosh J, et al: Smoking, alcohol, analgesics, and chronic duodenal ulcer. Scand J Gastroenterol 19:1015-1021, 1984.

31. Svanes C, Soreide JA, Skarstein A, et al: Smoking and ulcer perforation. Gut 41:177-180, 1997.

32. Wormsley KG: Smoking and duodenal ulcer. Gastroenterology 75:139-142, 1978.

33. Peters MN, Richardson CT: Stressful life events, acid hypersecretion, and ulcer disease. Gastroenterology 84:114-119, 1983.

34. Walker P, Luther J, Samloff IM, et al: Life events, stress and psychosocial factors in men with peptic ulcer disease. Gastroenterology 94:323-330, 1988.

35. Aoyama N, Kinoshita Y, Fujimoto S, et al: Peptic ulcers after the Hanshin-Awaji earthquake: Increased incidence of bleeding ulcers. Am J Gastroenterol 93:311-316, 1998.

36. Thomas J, Greig M, Piper DW: Chronic gastric ulcer and life events. Gastroenterology 78:905-911, 1980.

37. Rhodes J, Barnardo DE, Phillips SF, et al: Increased reflux of the bile into the stomach in patients with gastric ulcers. Gastroenterology 57:241-252, 1969.

38. Dragstedt LR: A concept of the etiology of gastric and duodenal ulcers. Gastroenterology 30:208-220, 1956.

39. Rotter JI: The genetics of peptic ulcers: More than one gene, more than one disease. Prog Med Genet 4:1-58, 1980.

40. Tarpila S, Samloff IM, Pikkarainen P, et al: Endoscopic and clinical findings in first-degree relatives of duodenal ulcer patients and control subjects. Scand J Gastroenterol 17:503-506, 1982.

41. Roth JLA, Stein GN, Morissey JR, et al: Diagnosis of peptic ulcer. In Berk JE, Haubrich WS, Kalser MH, et al (eds): Bockus Gastroenterology, 4th ed. Philadelphia, WB Saunders, 1985, pp 1060-1115.

42. Krippaehne WW, Fletcher WS, Dunphy JE: Acute perforation of duodenal and gastric ulcer: Factors affecting mortality. Arch Surg 88:874-882, 1964.

43. Burge H, Gill AM, Lewis RH: The pyloric-channel syndrome and gastric ulceration. Lancet 1:73-75, 1963.

44. Glickman MG, Szemes G, Loeb P, et al: Peptic ulcer of the pyloric region. AJR 113:147-158, 1971.

45. Laine L, Peterson WL: Bleeding peptic ulcer. N Engl J Med 331:717-727, 1994.

46. Carucci LR, Levine MS, Rubesin SE, et al: Upper gastrointestinal tract barium examination of postbulbar duodenal ulcers. AJR 182:927-930, 2004.

47. Dunn JP, Etter LE: Inadequacy of the medical history in the diagnosis of duodenal ulcer. N Engl J Med 266:68-72, 1962.

48. Sharma MP, Choudhari G: Nocturnal pain and duodenal ulcer. Br J Clin Pract 42:198-199, 1967.

49. Graham DY, Lew GM, Klein PD, et al: Effect of treatment of Helicobacter pylori infection on the long-term recurrence of gastric or duodenal ulcer. Ann Intern Med 116:705-708, 1992.

50. Hentschel E, Brandstatter G, Dragosics B, et al: Effect of ranitidine and amoxicillin plus metronidazole on the eradication of Helicobacter pylori and the recurrence of duodenal ulcer. N Engl J Med 328:308-312, 1993.

51. Van der Hulst RWM, Rauws EAJ, Koycu B, et al: Prevention of ulcer recurrence after eradication of Helicobacter pylori: A prospective long-term follow-up study. Gastroenterology 113:1082-1086, 1997.

52. NIH Consensus Development Panel on Helicobacter pylori in Peptic Ulcer Disease: Helicobacter pylori in peptic ulcer disease. JAMA 272:65-69, 1994.

53. International Update Conference on Helicobacter pylori: The Report of the Digestive Health Initiative International Update Conference on Helicobacter pylori. Gastroenterology 113:S4-S8, 1997.

54. Walsh JH, Peterson WL: The treatment of Helicobacter pylori infection in the management of peptic ulcer disease. N Engl J Med 333:984-991, 1995.

55. Bayerdorffer E, Miehlke S, Mannes GA, et al: Double-blind trial of omeprazole and amoxicillin to cure Helicobacter pylori infection in patients with duodenal ulcers. Gastroenterology 108:1412-1417, 1995.

56. Lazzaroni M, Bargiggia S, Porro GB: Triple therapy with ranitidine or lansoprazole in the treatment of Helicobacter pylori–associated duodenal ulcer. Am J Gastroenterol 92:649-652, 1997.

57. Isenberg JI, McQuaid KR, Laine L, et al: Acid-peptic disorders. In Yamada T (ed): Textbook of Gastroenterology. Philadelphia, JB Lippincott, 1991, pp 1241-1339.

58. McFarland RJ, Bateson MC, Green JRB, et al: Omeprazole provides quicker symptom relief and duodenal ulcer healing than ranitidine. Gastroenterology 98:278-283, 1990.

59. Agrawal NM, Saffouri B, Kruss DM, et al: Healing of benign gastric ulcers: A placebo-controlled comparison of two dosage regimens of Misoprostol, a synthetic analogue of prostaglandin E_1. Dig Dis Sci 30(Suppl 11):164S-170S, 1985.

60. Gilbert DA, Surawicz CM, Silverstein FE, et al: Prevention of acute, aspirin-induced gastric mucosal injury by 15-R-15 methyl prostaglandin E_2: An endoscopic study. Gastroenterology 86:339-345, 1984.

61. Penn I: The declining role of the surgeon in the treatment of acid-peptic disease. Arch Surg 115:134-135, 1980.

62. Gustavsson S, Kelly KA, Melton LJ, et al: Trends in peptic ulcer surgery: A population-based study in Rochester, Minnesota, 1956-1985. Gastroenterology 94:688-694, 1988.

63. Kikuchi Y, Levine MS, Laufer I, et al: Value of flow technique for double-contrast examination of the stomach. AJR 147:1183-1184, 1986.

64. Nelson SW: The discovery of gastric ulcers and the differential diagnosis between benignancy and malignancy. Radiol Clin North Am 7:5-25, 1969.

65. Goldsmith MR, Paul RE, Poplack WE, et al: Evaluation of routine double contrast views of the anterior wall of the stomach. AJR 126:1159-1163, 1976.

66. Poplack WE, Paul RE, Goldsmith MR, et al: Linear and rod-shaped peptic ulcers. Radiology 122:317-321, 1977.

67. Amaral NM: Radiographic diagnosis of shallow gastric ulcers: A comparative study of technique. Radiology 129:597-600, 1978.

68. Braver JM, Paul RE, Philipps E, et al: Roentgen diagnosis of linear ulcers. Radiology 132:29-32, 1979.

69. Levine MS, Creteur V, Kressel HY, et al: Benign gastric ulcers: Diagnosis and follow-up with double-contrast radiography. Radiology 164:9-13, 1987.

70. Ott DJ, Gelfand DW, Wu WC: Detection of gastric ulcer: Comparison of single- and double-contrast examination. AJR 139:93-97, 1982.

71. Gelfand DW, Dale WJ, Ott DJ: The location and size of gastric ulcers: Radiologic and endoscopic evaluation. AJR 143:755-758, 1984.

72. Barragry TP, Blatchford JW, Allen MO: Giant gastric ulcers: A review of 49 cases. Ann Surg 203:255-259, 1986.

73. Sun DCH, Stempien SJ: The Veterans Administration Cooperative Study on Gastric Ulcer: Site and size of the ulcer as determinants of outcome. Gastroenterology 61:576-584, 1971.

74. Thompson G, Stevenson GW, Somers S: Distribution of gastric ulcers by double-contrast barium meal with endoscopic correlation. J Can Assoc Radiol 34:296-297, 1983.

75. Findley JW: Ulcers on the greater curvature of the stomach. Gastroenterology 40:183-187, 1961.

76. Amberg JR, Zboralske FF: Gastric ulcers after 70. AJR 96:393-399, 1966.
77. Sheppard MC, Holmes GKT, Cockel R: Clinical picture of peptic ulceration diagnosed endoscopically. Gut 18:524-530, 1977.
78. Kottler RE, Tuft RJ: Benign greater curve gastric ulcer: the "sump-ulcer." Br J Radiol 54:651-654, 1981.
79. Hocking BV, Alp MH, Grant AK: Gastric ulceration within hiatus hernia. Med J Aust 2:207-208, 1976.
80. Wolf BS: Observations on roentgen features of benign and malignant ulcers. Semin Roentgenol 6:140-150, 1971.
81. Levine MS: Erosive gastritis and gastric ulcers. Radiol Clin North Am 32:1203-1214, 1994.
82. Pack GT: The relationship of gastric ulcer to gastric cancer. Cancer 3:515-522, 1950.
83. Levine MS, Verstandig A, Laufer I: Serpiginous gastric erosions caused by aspirin and other nonsteroidal antiinflammatory drugs. AJR 146:31-34, 1986.
84. Zboralske FF, Stargardter FL, Harell GS: Profile roentgenographic features of benign greater curvature ulcers. Radiology 127:63-67, 1978.
85. Linbert M, Krause GR: The "ring" shadow in the diagnosis of ulcer. AJR 90:767-773, 1963.
86. Bloom SM, Paul RE, Matsue H, et al: Improved radiologic detection of multiple gastric ulcers. AJR 128:949-952, 1977.
87. Dagradi AE, Falkner RE, Lee ER: Multiple benign gastric ulcers. Am J Gastroenterol 62:36-45, 1974.
88. Taxin RN, Livingston PA, Seamon WB: Multiple gastric ulcers: A radiographic sign of benignity? Radiology 114:23-27, 1975.
89. Sakita T, Ogura Y, Takasu S, et al: Observations on the healing of ulcerations in early gastric cancer. Gastroenterology 60:835-844, 1971.
90. Kagan RA, Steckel RJ: Gastric ulcer in a young man with apparent healing. AJR 128:831-834, 1977.
91. Keller RJ, Wolf BS, Khilnani MT: Roentgen features of healing and healed benign gastric ulcers. Radiology 97:353-359, 1970.
92. Gelfand DW, Ott DJ: Gastric ulcer scars. Radiology 140:37-43, 1981.
93. Levine MS, Kong V, Rubesin SE, et al: Scirrhous carcinoma of the stomach: Radiologic and endoscopic diagnosis. Radiology 175:151-154, 1990.
94. Wenger J, Brandborg LL, Spellman FA: Cancer: I. Clinical aspects. Gastroenterology 61:598-605, 1971.
95. Hayes MA: The gastric ulcer problem. Gastroenterology 29:609-620, 1955.
96. Kirsch IE: Benign and malignant gastric ulcers: Roentgen differentiation. Radiology 64:357-365, 1955.
97. Elliott GU, Wald SM, Benz RI: A roentgenologic study of ulcerating lesions of the stomach. AJR 77:612-622, 1957.
98. Schulman A, Simpkins KC: The accuracy of radiological diagnosis of benign, primarily and secondarily malignant gastric ulcers and their correlation with three simplified radiological types. Clin Radiol 26:317-325, 1975.
99. Thompson G, Somers S, Stevenson GW: Benign gastric ulcer: A reliable radiologic diagnosis? AJR 141:331-333, 1983.
100. Ichikawa H: Differential diagnosis between benign and malignant ulcers of the stomach. Clin Gastroenterol 2:329-332, 1973.
101. Segal AW, Healy MJR, Cox AG, et al: Diagnosis of gastric cancer. BMJ 2:669-672, 1975.
102. Stein GN, Martin RD, Roy RH, et al: Evaluation of conventional roentgenologic techniques for demonstration of duodenal ulcer craters. AJR 91:801-807, 1964.
103. Levine MS, Rubesin SE, Herlinger H, et al: Double contrast upper gastrointestinal examination: Technique and interpretation. Radiology 168:593-602, 1988.
104. de Roos A, Op den Orth JO: Linear niches in the duodenal bulb. AJR 140:941-944, 1983.
105. Rodriguez HP, Aston JK, Richardson CT: Ulcers in the descending duodenum: Postbulbar ulcers. AJR 119:316-322, 1973.
106. Classen M: Endoscopy in benign peptic ulcer. Clin Gastroenterol 2:315-318, 1973.
107. Ball RP, Segal AL, Golden R: Postbulbar ulcers of the duodenum. AJR 59:90-99, 1948.
108. Bilbao MK, Frische LH, Rosch J, et al: Postbulbar duodenal ulcer and ring-stricture. Radiology 100:27-35, 1971.
109. Mistilis SP, Wiot JF, Nedelman SH: Giant duodenal ulcer. Ann Intern Med 59:155-164, 1963.
110. Eisenberg RL, Margulis AR, Moss AA: Giant duodenal ulcers. Gastrointest Radiol 2:347-353, 1978.
111. Jaazewski R, Crane SA, Cid AA: Giant duodenal ulcers: Successful healing with medical therapy. Dig Dis Sci 28:486-489, 1983.
112. Kirsh IE, Brendel T: The importance of giant duodenal ulcer. Radiology 91:14-19, 1968.
113. Parulekar SG, Lubert M: Ultrasound demonstration of giant duodenal ulcer. Gastrointest Radiol 8:29-31, 1983.
114. Kawai K, Ida K, Misaki F, et al: Comparative study for duodenal ulcer by radiology and endoscopy. Endoscopy 5:7-13, 1973.
115. Wills JS: Pyloric channel ulcers and the air-contrast examination. Radiology 130:250-252, 1979.
116. Gobel VK, Kressel HY, Laufer I: Double contrast artifacts. Gastrointest Radiol 3:139-146, 1978.
117. Op den Orth JO, Ploem S: The stalactite phenomenon on double contrast studies of the stomach. Radiology 117:523-525, 1975.
118. Linsman JR: Gastric ulcers simulating intramural, extramucosal tumors. AJR 101:421-424, 1967.
119. Bonfield RE, Mantel W: The problem of differentiating benign antral ulcers from intramural tumors. Radiology 106:25-27, 1973.
120. Fox ER, Laufer I, Levine MS: Radiographic response of gastric lymphoma to chemotherapy. AJR 142:711-714, 1984.
121. Thoeni RF, Cello JP: A critical look at the accuracy of endoscopy and double-contrast radiography of the upper gastrointestinal (UGI) tract in patients with substantial UGI hemorrhage. Radiology 135:305-308, 1980.
122. Fraser GM: The double contrast barium meal in patients with acute upper gastrointestinal bleeding. Clin Radiol 29:625-634, 1978.
123. Balthazar EJ, Rosenberg H, Davidian MM: Scirrhous carcinoma of the pyloric channel and distal antrum. AJR 134:669-673, 1980.
124. Edwards RH, Foster JH: Pneumoperitoneum in perforated duodenal ulcer. Am J Surg 104:551-554, 1962.
125. Jacobson G, Berne CJ, Meyers HI, et al: The examination of patients with suspected perforated ulcer using a water-soluble contrast medium. AJR 86:37-49, 1961.
126. Fultz PJ, Skucas J, Weiss SL: CT in upper gastrointestinal tract perforations secondary to peptic ulcer disease. Gastrointest Radiol 17:5-8, 1992.
127. Ongolo-Zogo P, Borson O, Garcia P, et al: Acute gastroduodenal peptic ulcer perforation: Contrast-enhanced and thin-section spiral CT findings in 10 patients. Abdom Imaging 24:329-332, 1999.
128. Jeffrey RB, Federle MP, Wall S: Value of computed tomography in detecting occult gastrointestinal perforation. J Comput Assist Tomogr 7:825-827, 1983.
129. Madrazo BL, Halpert RD, Sandler MA, et al: Computed tomographic findings in penetrating peptic ulcer. Radiology 153:751-754, 1984.
130. Joffe N, Antonioli DA: Penetration into spleen by benign gastric ulcers. Clin Radiol 32:177-181, 1981.
131. Glick SN, Levine MS, Teplick SK, et al: Splenic penetration by benign gastric ulcer: Preoperative recognition with CT. Radiology 163:637-639, 1987.
132. Farack UM, Goresky CA, Jabbari M, et al: Double pylorus: A hypothesis concerning its pathogenesis. Gastroenterology 66:596-600, 1974.
133. Jamshidnejad J, Koehler RE, Narayan D: Double channel pylorus. AJR 130:1047-1050, 1978.
134. Hegedus V, Poulsen PE, Reichardt J: The natural history of the double pylorus. Radiology 126:29-34, 1978.
135. Smith DL, Dockerty MB, Black BM: Gastrocolic fistulas of malignant origin. Surg Gynecol Obstet 134:829-832, 1972.
136. Laufer I, Thornley GD, Stolberg H: Gastrocolic fistula as a complication of benign gastric ulcer. Radiology 119:7-11, 1976.
137. Levine MS, Kelly MR, Laufer I, et al: Gastrocolic fistulas: The increasing role of aspirin. Radiology 187:359-361, 1993.
138. Tavenor T, Smith S, Sullivan S: Gastrocolic fistula: A review of 15 cases and an update of the literature. J Clin Gastroenterol 16:189-191, 1993.
139. Thyssen EP, Weinstock LB, Balfe DM, et al: Medical treatment of benign gastrocolic fistula. Ann Intern Med 118:433-435, 1993.
140. Sasson L, Weiskopf S: Duodenocolic fistula as a complication of peptic ulcer. Am J Gastroenterol 29:51-58, 1958.
141. Starzl TE, Dorr TW, Meyer WH: Benign duodenocolic fistula. Arch Surg 78:611-619, 1959.
142. Berguer LH: Internal biliary fistulas. Am J Gastroenterol 43:11-22, 1965.
143. Constant E, Turcotte JG: Choledochoduodenal fistula: The natural history and management of an unusual complication of peptic ulcer disease. Ann Surg 167:221-228, 1968.
144. McEwan-Alvarada G, Dysart DN: Choledochoduodenal fistulas complicating duodenal ulcer. Am J Dig Dis 12:947-954, 1967.

145. Hoppenstein JM, Medoza CB, Watne AL: Choledochoduodenal fistula due to perforating duodenal ulcer disease. Ann Surg 173:145-147, 1971.

146. West AB, Nolan N, O'Brian DS: Benign peptic ulcers penetrating pericardium and heart: Clinicopathological features and factors favoring survival. Gastroenterology 94:1478-1487, 1988.

147. O'Driscoll J, Hourihane JB: Intrapericardial barium in a case of peptic ulceration. Br J Radiol 49:177-179, 1976.

148. Zollinger RM, Ellison EH: Primary peptic ulcerations of the jejunum associated with islet cell tumors of the pancreas. Ann Surg 142:709-728, 1955.

149. Wolfe MM, Jensen RT: Zollinger-Ellison syndrome: Current concepts in diagnosis and management. N Engl J Med 317:1200-1209, 1987.

150. Del Valle J, Yamada T: Zollinger-Ellison syndrome. In Yamada T (ed): Textbook of Gastroenterology. Philadelphia, JB Lippincott, 1991, pp 1340-1352.

151. Ballard HS, Frane B, Havtsock RJ: Familial multiple endocrine adenoma-peptic ulcer complex. Medicine (Baltimore) 43:481-516, 1964.

152. Mausbach CM II, Wilkins RM, Dobbins WO, et al: Intestinal mucosal function and structure in the steatorrhea of Zollinger-Ellison syndrome. Arch Intern Med 121:487-494, 1968.

153. Miller LS, Vinayek R, Frucht H, et al: Reflux esophagitis in patients with Zollinger-Ellison syndrome. Gastroenterology 98:341-346, 1990.

154. Maton PN, Vinayek R, Frucht H, et al: Long-term efficacy and safety of omeprazole in patients with Zollinger-Ellison syndrome: A prospective study. Gastroenterology 97:827-836, 1989.

155. Lew EA, Pisegna JR, Starr JA, et al: Intravenous pantoprazole rapidly controls gastric acid hypersecretion in patients with Zollinger-Ellison syndrome. Gastroenterology 118:696-704, 2000.

156. Fraker DL, Norton JA, Alexander HR, et al: Zollinger-Ellison syndrome: Surgery should still play an important role in its management. Ann Surg 220:320-330, 1994.

157. Norton JA, Fraker DL, Alexander HR, et al: Surgery to cure the Zollinger-Ellison syndrome. N Engl J Med 341:635-644, 1999.

158. Wank SA, Doppman JL, Miller DL, et al: Prospective study of the ability of computerized axial tomography to localize gastrinomas in patients with Zollinger-Ellison syndrome. Gastroenterology 92:905-912, 1987.

159. Maton PN, Miller DL, Doppman JL, et al: The role of selective angiography in the management of patients with Zollinger-Ellison syndrome. Gastroenterology 92:913-918, 1987.

160. Cherner JA, Doppman JL, Norton JA, et al: Selective venous sampling for gastrin to localize gastrinomas: A prospective assessment. Ann Intern Med 105:841-847, 1986.

161. Gibril F, Reynolds JC, Doppman JL, et al: Somatostatin receptor scintigraphy: Its sensitivity compared with that of other imaging methods in detecting primary and metastatic gastrinomas: A prospective study. Ann Intern Med 125:26-34, 1996.

162. Amberg JR, Ellison EH, Wilson SD, et al: Roentgenographic observations in the Zollinger-Ellison syndrome. JAMA 190:185-187, 1964.

163. Missakian MM, Carlson HC, Huzenga KA: Roentgenographic findings in Zollinger-Ellison syndrome. AJR 94:429-437, 1965.

164. Nelson SW, Christoforidis AJ: Roentgenologic features of the Zollinger-Ellison syndrome: Ulcerogenic tumor of the pancreas. Semin Roentgenol 3:254-266, 1968.

165. Zboralske FF, Amberg JR: Detection of the Zollinger-Ellison syndrome: The radiologist's responsibility. AJR 104:529-543, 1968.

166. Nelson SW, Lichtenstein JE: The Zollinger-Ellison syndrome. In Marshak RH (ed): Radiology of the Stomach. Philadelphia, WB Saunders, 1983, pp 334-381.

167. Ellison EH, Wilson SD: The Zollinger-Ellison syndrome: Reappraisal and evaluation of 260 registered cases. Ann Surg 160:514-530, 1964.

Inflammatory Conditions of the Stomach and Duodenum

Marc S. Levine, MD

EROSIVE GASTRITIS

Erosions are defined histologically as epithelial defects that do not penetrate beyond the muscularis mucosae. Although erosive gastritis is rarely diagnosed on conventional single-contrast barium studies, it has become a relatively frequent finding on double-contrast studies, with an overall prevalence of 0.5% to 20% reported in the radiologic literature.[1-6] However, not all patients with erosive gastritis are symptomatic. Thus, it is difficult to be certain of the clinical significance of gastric erosions demonstrated on radiologic or endoscopic examinations.

Pathogenesis

Aspirin or other nonsteroidal anti-inflammatory drugs (NSAIDs) are thought to be the most common cause of erosive gastritis, accounting for about 50% of cases.[7] Other causes include alcohol, stress, trauma, burns, Crohn's disease, viral or fungal infection, and endoscopic heater probe therapy or other iatrogenic trauma.[8-13] However, some patients with erosive gastritis have no apparent predisposing factors for this condition.[14] Such cases presumably occur as a variant of peptic ulcer disease.

Considerable attention has been focused on the role of aspirin and other NSAIDs in the development of erosive gastritis. Both clinical and laboratory investigations have shown that these agents are capable of disrupting the mucosal barrier in the stomach, causing erosive gastritis and gastric ulcers (see Chapter 33).[8,15-18] In one study, 40% of patients receiving aspirin for 3 months or longer had endoscopic evidence of erosive gastritis.[16] Other studies of healthy volunteers have shown that as few as two aspirin tablets may cause an acute erosive gastritis that is recognized endoscopically within 24 hours.[17,18] Maximal damage usually occurs by 1 to 3 days, and evidence of healing may be documented endoscopically by 1 week.[19] Thus, gastric erosions may form rapidly after ingestion of aspirin or other NSAIDs and may heal rapidly when these drugs are withdrawn.

Clinical Findings

Some patients with erosive gastritis present with dyspepsia, epigastric pain, or signs or symptoms of upper gastrointestinal bleeding.[20] However, other patients are asymptomatic. In fact, gastric erosions can persist for years in the absence of clinical symptoms.[21] Because erosions may be detected as an incidental finding on radiologic or endoscopic examinations, it is important to rule out other abnormalities in the stomach and duodenum before assuming that these erosions are the cause of the patient's symptoms.

Radiographic Findings

Two types of erosions may be identified on double-contrast studies. The most common type is the *complete*, or *varioliform*, erosion in which punctate or slitlike collections of barium representing the epithelial defects are surrounded by radiolucent halos of edematous, elevated mucosa (Fig. 34-1).[3,5,14] Varioliform erosions typically occur in the gastric antrum and are often aligned on the crests of the rugal folds.[3,5,20] Because they are shallow lesions, erosions on the dependent or posterior wall may be better delineated by the use of flow technique to manipulate a thin layer of barium over the mucosal surface.[22] Some of the surrounding mounds of edema may prevent filling of the central pits or depressions, so that these erosions appear as filling defects in the thin barium pool without central collections of barium. In other patients, erosive gastritis may be manifested only by scalloped antral folds (Fig. 34-2A). Depending on the quality of mucosal coating, erosions may be faintly seen on the crest of the folds (Fig. 34-2B). These scalloped antral folds often persist after the erosions have healed. Occasionally, residual epithelial nodules or polyps may be detected at the site of the healed erosions. These hyperplastic polyps are thought to represent the sequelae of chronic erosive gastritis.[20]

Incomplete or *"flat"* erosions are epithelial defects without elevation of the surrounding mucosa. They appear radi-

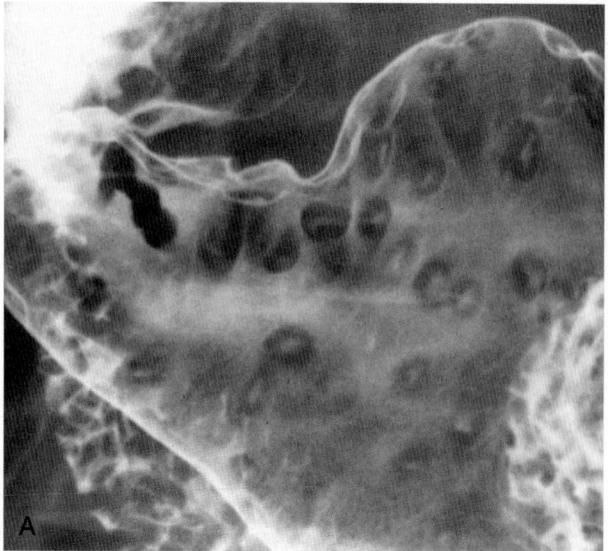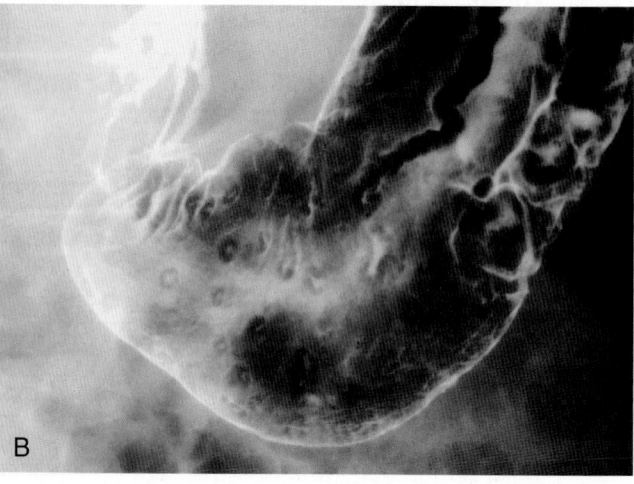

Figure 34-1. Erosive gastritis with varioliform erosions. A and **B.** In both patients, multiple varioliform erosions are seen in the antrum as tiny barium collections with surrounding halos of edematous mucosa. (**A** from Laufer I, Levine MS [eds]: Double Contrast Gastrointestinal Radiology, 2nd ed. Philadelphia, WB Saunders, 1992.)

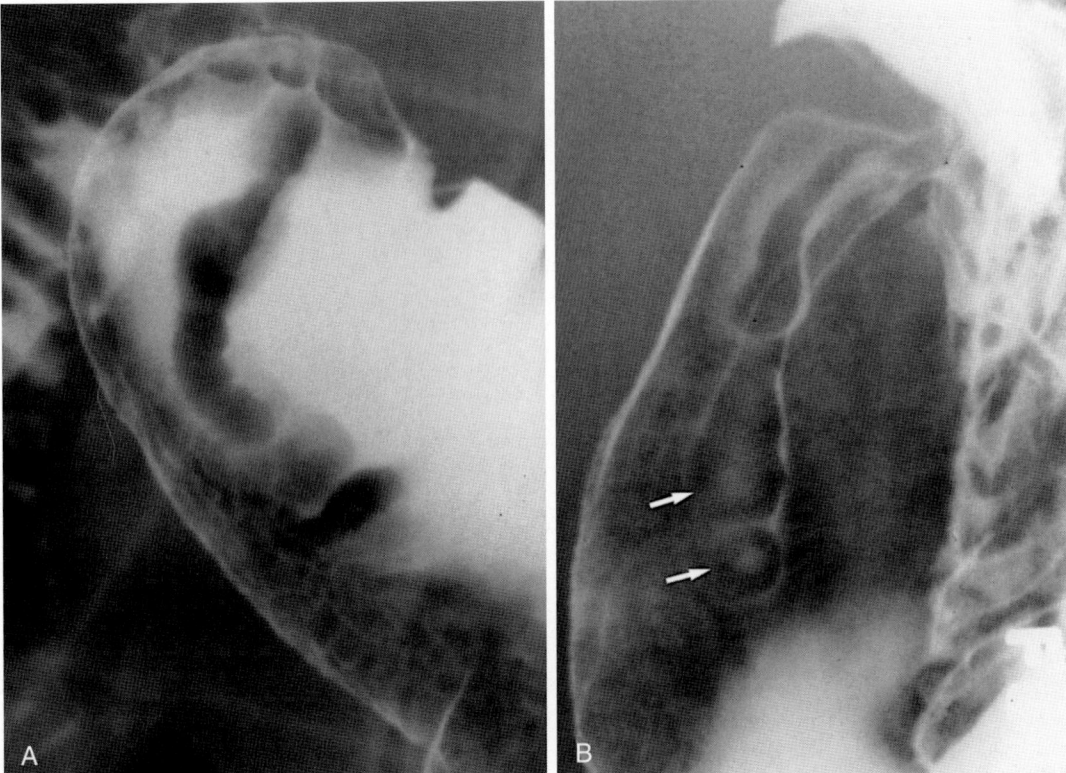

Figure 34-2. Erosive gastritis with scalloped antral folds. A. A thickened, lobulated fold is present in the gastric antrum. **B.** In another patient, several erosions (*arrows*) can be seen on the crest of a scalloped fold.

ographically as linear streaks or dots of barium (Fig. 34-3).[6,14] Because the surrounding mucosa is normal, incomplete erosions are much more difficult to detect than are varioliform erosions, accounting for only 5% to 19% of all erosions diagnosed on double-contrast studies.[6,7]

Although no causative significance is generally attributed to the shape or location of gastric erosions diagnosed on double-contrast studies, aspirin and other NSAIDs sometimes produce incomplete, linear or serpiginous erosions that tend to be clustered in the body of the stomach on or near the greater curvature (Fig. 34-4).[23] It has been postulated that these erosions result from localized mucosal injury that occurs as the dissolving tablets collect by gravity in the dependent portion of the stomach. Whatever the explanation, these distinctive linear or serpiginous erosions should be highly suggestive of recent aspirin or other NSAID use. Nevertheless, the majority of patients with NSAID-induced erosive gastritis have typical varioliform erosions in the gastric antrum.[7,23] Aspirin or other NSAIDs should therefore still be considered as the most likely cause of erosive gastritis, even when the erosions are confined to the antrum and have a varioliform appearance. Recurrent episodes of NSAID-induced erosion formation and healing may eventually lead to relatively subtle flattening and deformity of the greater curvature of the antrum, a radiologic sign of NSAID-related gastropathy (Fig. 34-5).[24,25] Detection of any of these findings should lead to careful questioning of the patient about a possible history of aspirin or other NSAID use. If recent ingestion of these drugs is confirmed in symptomatic patients, withdrawal of the offending agent usually produces a dramatic clinical response.[23]

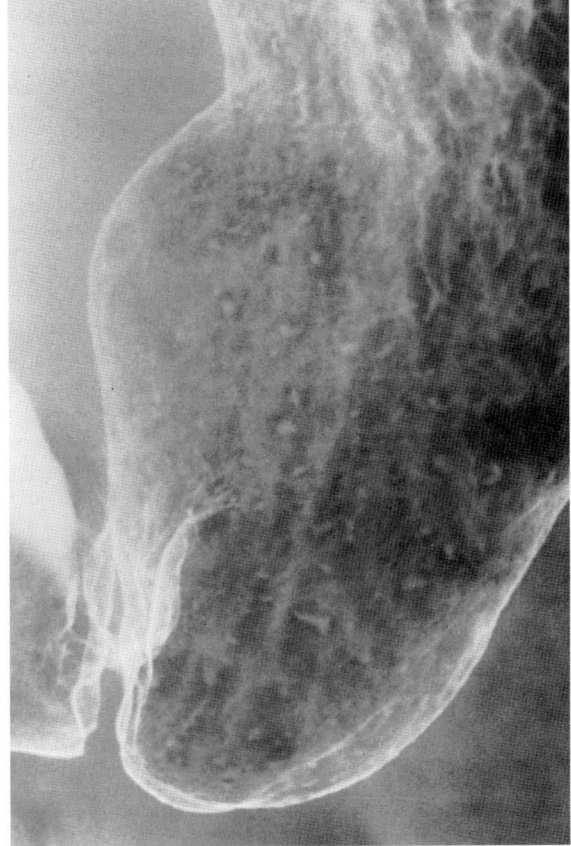

Figure 34-3. Erosive gastritis with incomplete erosions. Numerous linear and punctate erosions are seen in the gastric antrum and body. Many of the erosions are incomplete (i.e., they are not surrounded by mounds of edema).

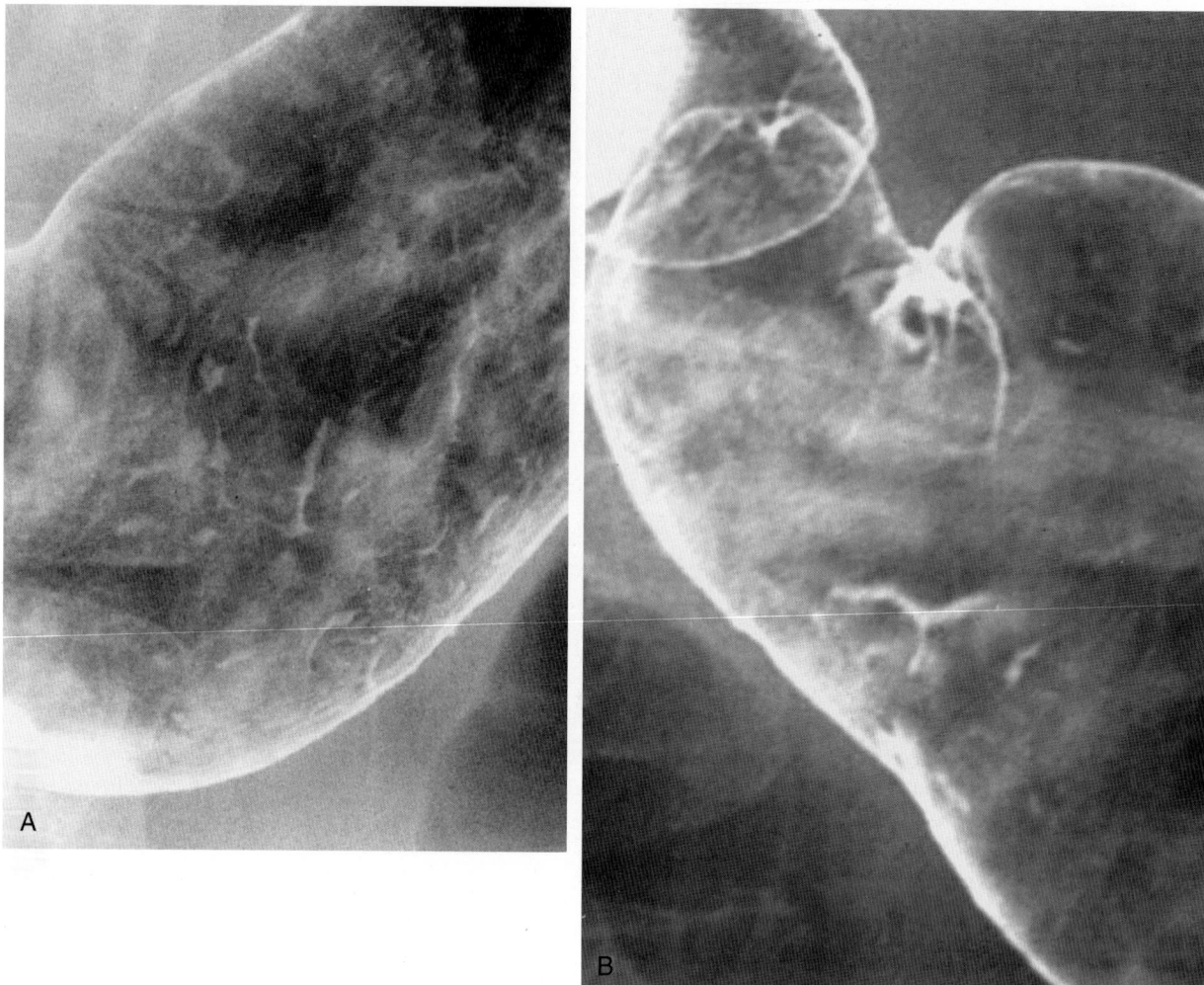

Figure 34-4. Erosive gastritis caused by nonsteroidal anti-inflammatory drugs (NSAIDs). A and **B.** Distinctive linear and serpiginous erosions are clustered in the body (**A**) and antrum (**B**) of the stomach near the greater curvature as a result of NSAID ingestion. The patient in **A** was taking naproxen, and the patient in **B** was taking ibuprofen. (**A** from Levine MS, Verstandig A, Laufer I: Serpiginous gastric erosions caused by aspirin and other nonsteroidal antiinflammatory drugs. AJR 146:31-34, 1986, © by American Roentgen Ray Society.)

Crohn's disease is another condition that may be manifested on double-contrast studies by multiple erosions or "aphthoid" ulcers in the stomach.[10,11] However, these patients almost always have associated Crohn's disease involving the small bowel or colon (see later section on Crohn's Disease). Shallow ulcers or erosions may also result from opportunistic infection by cytomegalovirus (CMV) in patients with AIDS (see later section on Cytomegalovirus),[26] or they may occur as a complication of endoscopic heater probe therapy or other iatrogenic trauma (Fig. 34-6).[13]

Differential Diagnosis

Gastric erosions can sometimes be mistaken on barium studies for ulcerated submucosal masses or "bull's-eye" lesions in the stomach. However, the central ulcer of a "bull's-eye" lesion is considerably larger than an erosion, and the surrounding mass tends to be larger than the radiolucent mound of edema surrounding an erosion (see Chapter 37). "Bull's-eye" lesions also tend to be less numerous than erosions and are not typically aligned on the crests of the folds. Thus, it is usually possible to distinguish these lesions by radiographic criteria.

ANTRAL GASTRITIS

Some patients have a form of gastritis that is confined to the gastric antrum, an entity also known as antral gastritis. Alcohol, tobacco, coffee, and, more recently, *Helicobacter pylori* have been implicated in the development of antral gastritis (see later section on *Helicobacter pylori* Gastritis). Some patients with this condition have increased secretion of peptic acid, but others have normal or even decreased acid secretion. Affected individuals may present with dyspepsia, epigastric pain, or other symptoms that are indistinguishable from those of peptic ulcer disease. Treatment is generally aimed at suppressing acid secretion in the stomach.

Radiographic Findings

Antral gastritis may be manifested on barium studies by thickened folds, antral erosions (see earlier section on Erosive Gastritis), crenulation of the lesser curvature, mucosal nodularity, transverse antral striae, a hypertrophied antral-pyloric fold, and antral narrowing.

Some patients have thickened, scalloped or lobulated folds that are oriented longitudinally in the antrum (Fig. 34-7A),

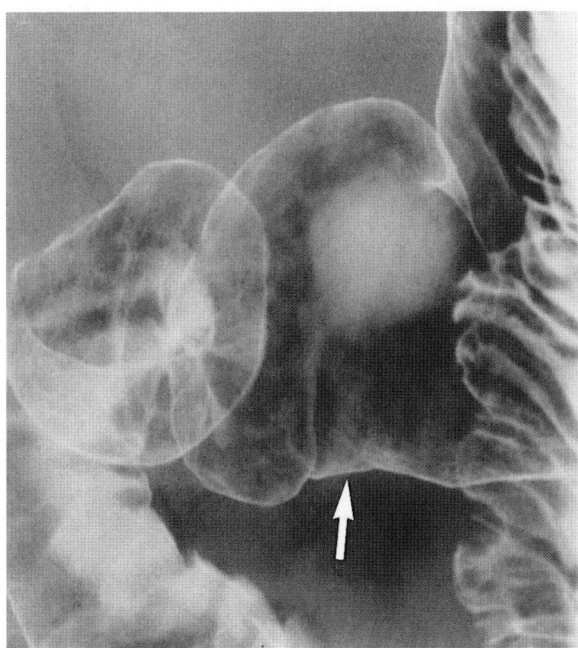

Figure 34-5. Antral flattening caused by NSAIDs. There is flattening and deformity of the greater curvature of the distal antrum (*arrow*) due to chronic aspirin therapy. This finding is characteristic of NSAID-related gastropathy.

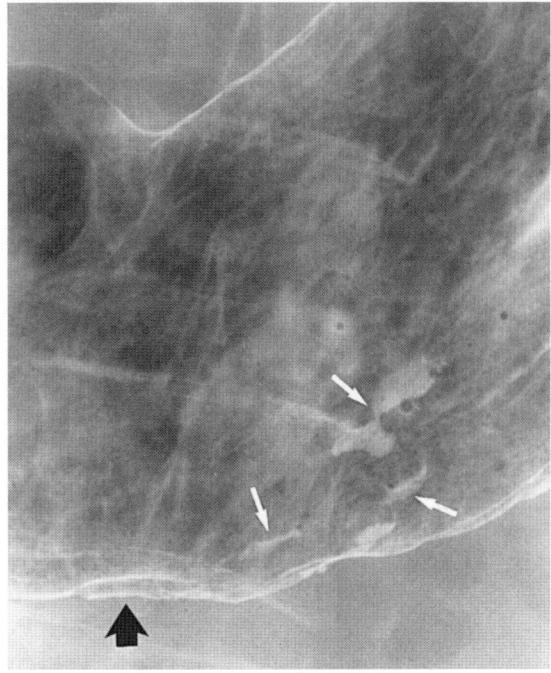

Figure 34-6. Heater-probe ulcers and erosions. Shallow, irregular ulcers and linear erosions are seen en face (*white arrows*) and in profile (*black arrow*) on the greater curvature of the stomach. These ulcerations occurred as a direct complication of endoscopic heater probe therapy. (From Rummerman J, Rubesin SE, Levine MS, et al: Gastric ulceration caused by heater probe coagulation. Gastrointest Radiol 13:200-202, 1988. With kind permission from Springer Science and Business Media.)

whereas others have thickened transverse antral folds (Fig. 34-7B). Thickened antral folds should be recognized as the single most common sign of antral gastritis on double-contrast barium studies; thickened folds are detected in about 75% of patients with radiographically diagnosed antral gastritis.[7] The vast majority of these patients are found to have *H. pylori* as the cause of their gastritis (see later section on *Helicobacter pylori* Gastritis).[7]

Crenulation or irregularity of the lesser curvature of the distal antrum may also be recognized as a transient or per-sistent finding at fluoroscopy (see Fig. 34-7B).[27] Other patients may have fine transverse striations or striae as a sign of chronic antral gastritis,[28] although this finding can also be seen as a normal variant.[29] Still other patients may have a single lobulated fold that arises on the lesser curvature of the prepyloric antrum and extends into the pylorus or base of the duodenal bulb (Fig. 34-8).[30,31] This hypertrophied

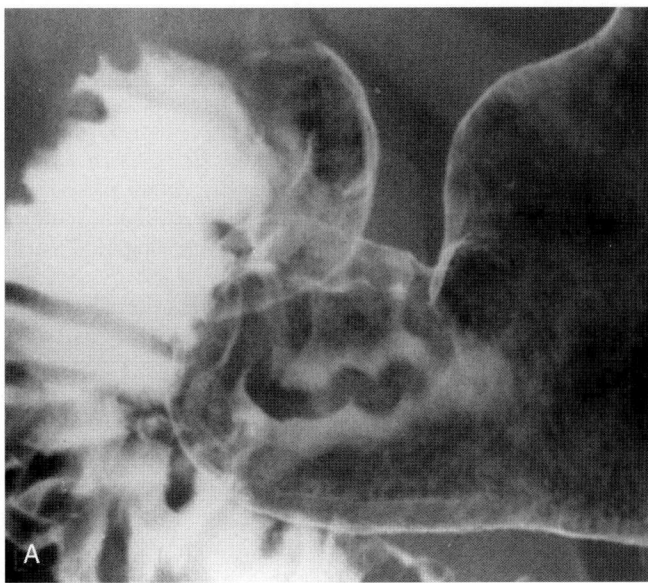
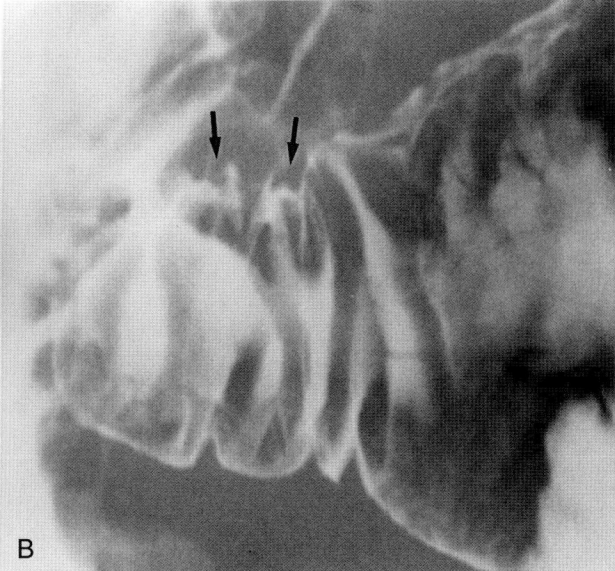

Figure 34-7. Antral gastritis. A. This patient has thickened, scalloped folds that are oriented longitudinally in the antrum. **B.** In another patient, there are thickened transverse folds in the antrum with fine nodularity and crenulation of the adjacent lesser curvature (*arrows*).

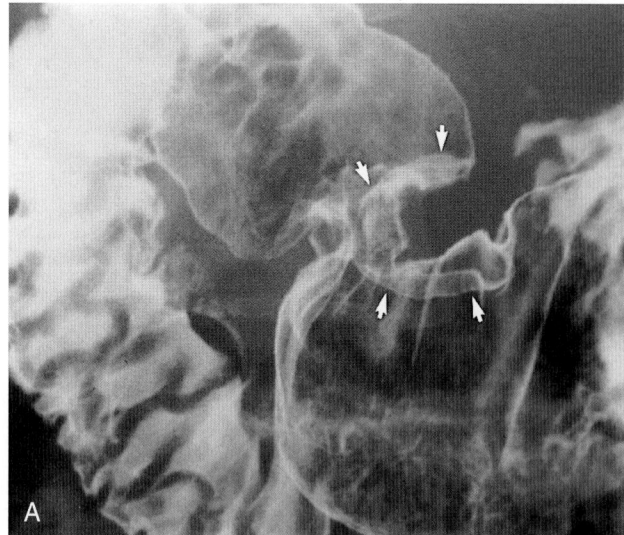

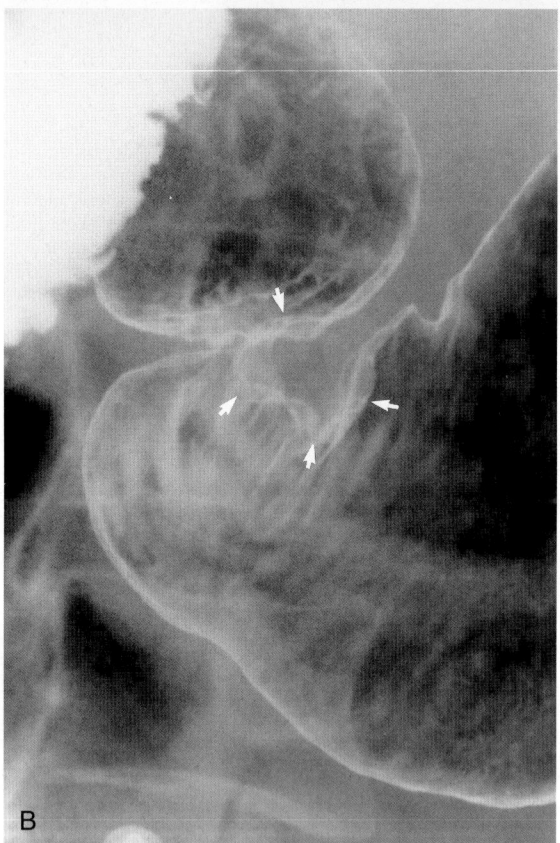

Figure 34-8. Hypertrophied antral-pyloric fold. A and **B.** In both patients, a single lobulated fold (*arrows*) on the lesser curvature of the distal antrum extends through the pylorus into the base of the duodenal bulb. The characteristic appearance and location of this fold should differentiate it from a polypoid or plaquelike antral carcinoma.

antral-pyloric fold is thought to be a sequela of chronic antral gastritis and is often associated with other radiographic signs of gastritis. Endoscopy is not warranted when a characteristic antral-pyloric fold is seen on barium studies.[31] If the fold cannot be distinguished from a polypoid or plaquelike carcinoma on the lesser curvature, however, endoscopy and biopsy should be performed to rule out malignant tumor.

Differential Diagnosis

Severe antral gastritis associated with antral narrowing must be differentiated from gastric carcinoma. With malignant tumors, however, the narrowed antrum tends to have a more abrupt transition with the adjacent stomach and a more fixed, rigid contour. Thus, it is usually possible to differentiate these conditions by radiographic criteria. When the folds are markedly thickened and lobulated, antral gastritis can also mimic the appearance of lymphoma or even a submucosally infiltrating carcinoma.[32] In such cases, endoscopy may be required for a more definitive diagnosis.

HELICOBACTER PYLORI GASTRITIS

H. pylori (formerly known as *Campylobacter pylori*) is a gram-negative bacillus that was first isolated from the stomach on endoscopic biopsy specimens in 1983.[33] Since that time, *H. pylori* has been recognized as the most common cause of chronic active gastritis.[34,35] The organism is usually found in clusters or clumps beneath the mucus layer on surface epithelial cells or, less commonly, superficial foveolar cells in the stomach.[36] *H. pylori* gastritis is characterized pathologically by an acute inflammatory reaction in the mucosa with accumulation of neutrophils, plasma cells, and, eventually, lymphoid nodules.[36] The gastric antrum has been the most common site of involvement, but the proximal half of the stomach or even the entire stomach may be involved by this disease.[35,37] *H. pylori* gastritis is important not only because it may cause upper gastrointestinal symptoms but also because it is associated with the development of gastric and duodenal ulcers (see Chapter 33), gastric carcinoma (see Chapter 36), and low-grade, B-cell, mucosa-associated lymphoid tissue (MALT) lymphoma (see Chapter 37).

Clinical Findings

H. pylori infection is acquired by oral ingestion of the bacterium and is mainly transmitted within families during early childhood.[38] *H. pylori* is a worldwide pathogen, being most common in developing countries. In developed countries, *H. pylori* is more common in lower socioeconomic populations.[35,38] The prevalence of *H. pylori* also increases with age; more than 50% of Americans older than 60 years of age are infected by this organism.[39] Some people with *H. pylori* may present with dyspepsia, epigastric pain, or other upper gastrointestinal symptoms.[35] However, most people with *H. pylori* are asymptomatic.[39] Even when symptoms are present, it is difficult to prove that the symptoms are caused by *H. pylori* because of the high prevalence of this infection in the population.

H. pylori gastritis can effectively be eradicated from the stomach by treatment with a combination of antimicrobial agents (e.g., amoxicillin, clarithromycin, metronidazole, tetracycline, or bismuth) and antisecretory agents (i.e., proton pump inhibitors).[40] In a consensus development panel sponsored by the National Institutes of Health in 1994 and a subsequent international update conference sponsored by the American Digestive Health Foundation in 1997, combination treatment with antimicrobial and antisecretory agents was recommended for all *H. pylori*-positive patients with gastric or duodenal ulcers to accelerate healing of ulcers and decrease the rate of ulcer recurrence.[41,42] There are conflicting

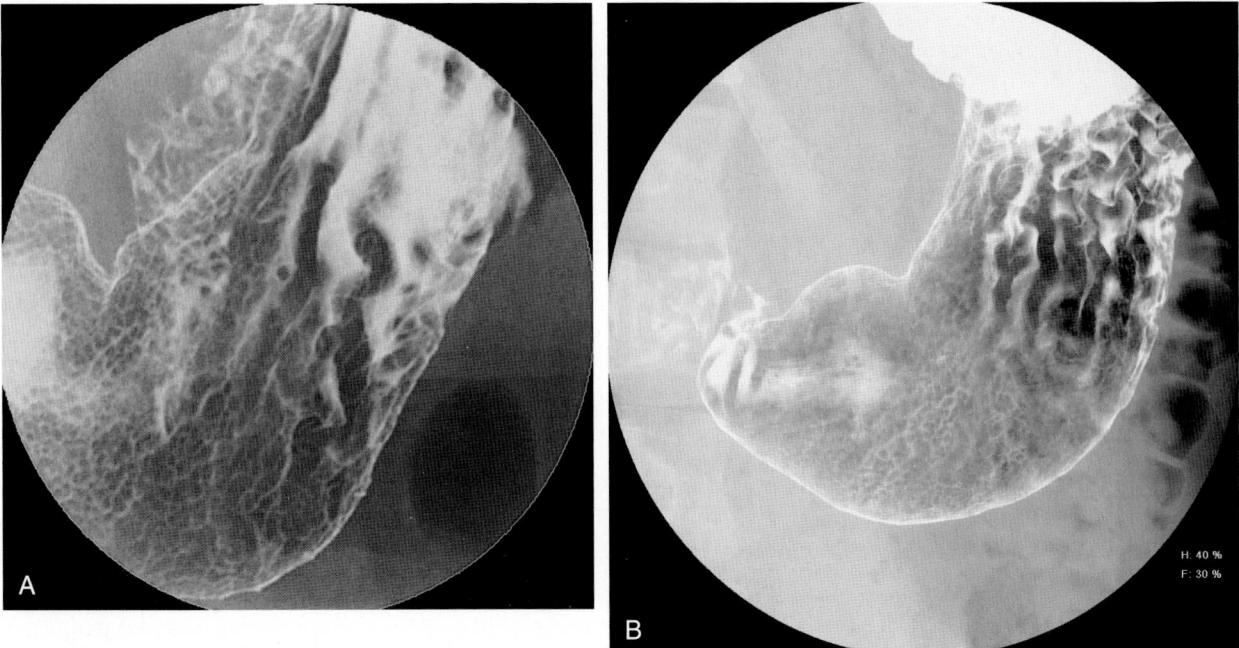

Figure 34-9. *H. pylori* **gastritis. A** and **B.** In both patients, thickened folds are seen in the body of the stomach and enlarged areae gastricae in the proximal antrum as a result of chronic infection by *H. pylori*. (**A** from Levine MS, Laufer I: The gastrointestinal tract: Dos and don'ts of digital imaging. Radiology 207:311-316, 1998.)

data, however, about the value of antimicrobial therapy for *H. pylori*–positive patients with nonulcer dyspepsia.[43-45] As a result, the panels did not recommend treatment for this subset of patients.[41,42] It therefore remains unclear whether antimicrobial agents should be reserved for patients with *H. pylori* who have gastric or duodenal ulcers or whether patients with *H. pylori* who have nonulcer dyspepsia would also benefit from treatment.

H. pylori gastritis can accurately be diagnosed at endoscopy on the basis of histologic specimens, cultures, and the rapid urease test.[46,47] However, noninvasive tests for *H. pylori*, such as the urea breath test (using orally administered ^{14}C-labeled or ^{13}C-labeled urea) and serologic tests, have reported sensiti-

vities and specificities of greater than 90%.[38,46,47] Highly accurate noninvasive tests are therefore available for detecting this infection.

Radiographic Findings

H. pylori gastritis is by far the most common cause of thickened folds in the gastric antrum or body on double-contrast barium studies (Fig. 34-9).[7,48-52] However, other patients may have diffusely thickened folds in the stomach or thickened folds that are confined to the fundus.[49] Still others with *H. pylori* gastritis may have markedly thickened, lobulated gastric folds (i.e., polypoid gastritis) in either a diffuse (Fig. 34-10) or

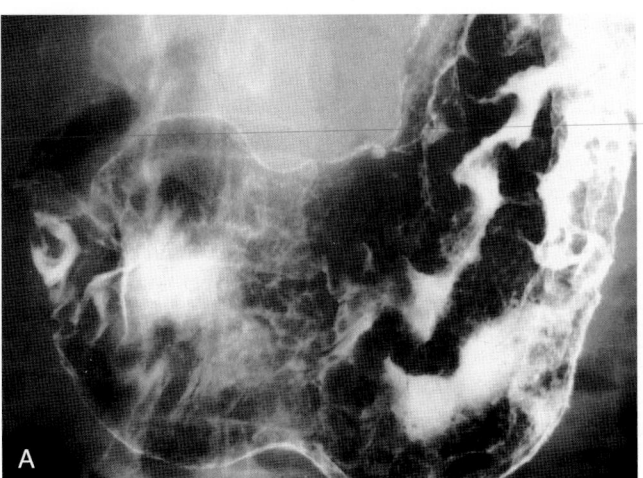
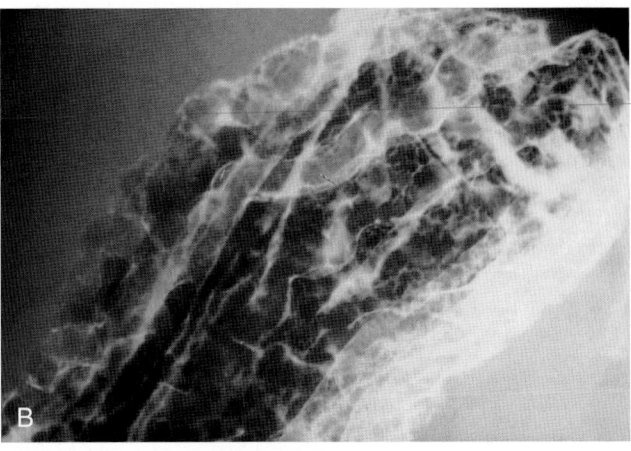

Figure 34-10. *H. pylori* **causing diffuse polypoid gastritis. A** and **B.** Markedly thickened, lobulated folds are seen in the gastric body (**A**) and fundus (**B**). This appearance could be mistaken for severe hypertrophic gastritis, Ménétrier's disease, or lymphoma, but endoscopic biopsy specimens revealed *H. pylori* gastritis without evidence of tumor. (From Sohn J, Levine MS, Furth EE, et al: *Helicobacter pylori* gastritis: Radiographic findings. Radiology 195:763-767, 1995.)

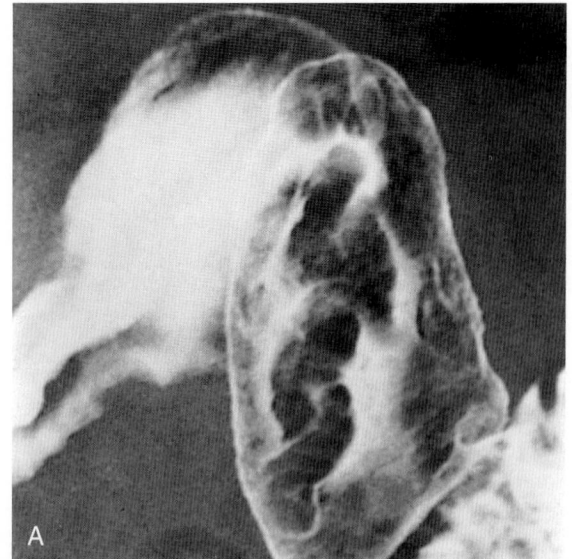

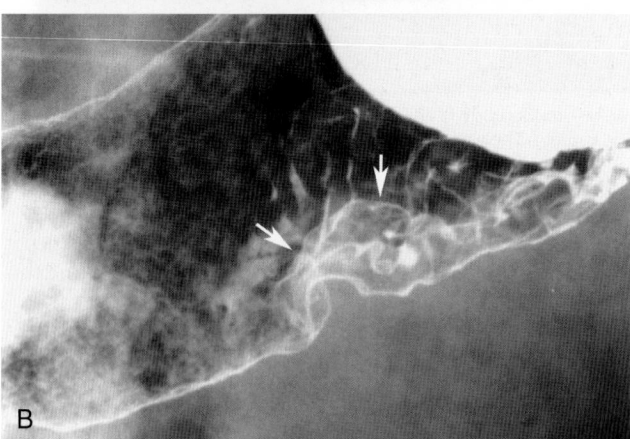

Figure 34-11. *H. pylori* **causing localized polypoid gastritis. A** and **B.** Focally thickened, lobulated folds are seen in the gastric antrum in **A** and in the gastric body (*arrows*) in **B**. These findings are worrisome for a localized lymphoma or submucosally infiltrating carcinoma. In both patients, however, endoscopic biopsy specimens revealed *H. pylori* gastritis without evidence of tumor.

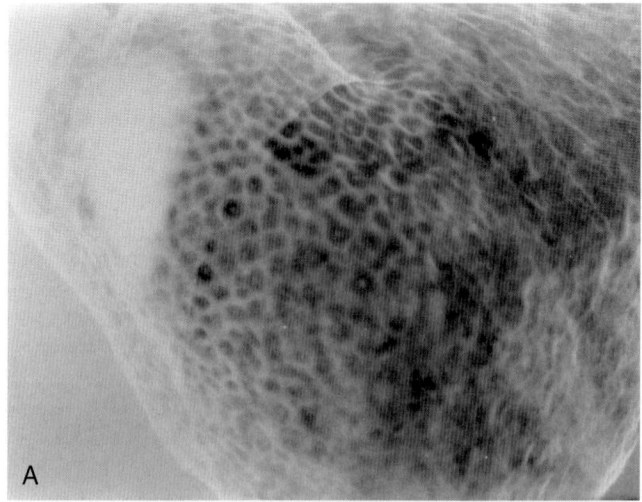

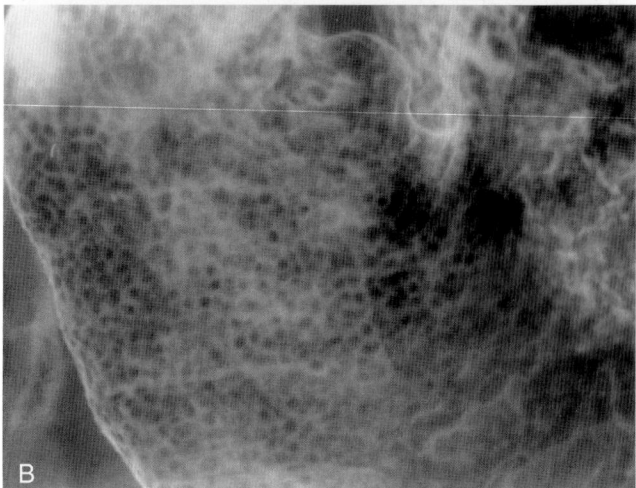

Figure 34-12. *H. pylori* **gastritis with lymphoid hyperplasia. A** and **B.** In both patients, enlarged lymphoid follicles are seen as innumerable tiny, round nodules that carpet the mucosa of the gastric antrum. In **A**, note how many of the nodules have central umbilications with punctate collections of barium seen en face in the lesions. (From Torigian DA, Levine MS, Gill NS, et al: Lymphoid hyperplasia of the stomach: Radiographic findings in five adult patients. AJR 177:71-75, 2001, © by American Roentgen Ray Society.)

localized (Fig. 34-11) distribution.[7,49] In such cases, it may be difficult or impossible to differentiate *H. pylori* gastritis from other infiltrative conditions or even malignant tumor involving the stomach (see next section on Differential Diagnosis).

H. pylori gastritis may also be manifested on double-contrast studies by enlarged areae gastricae (≥3 mm in diameter) in the stomach (see Fig. 34-9).[7,49] In the past, enlarged areae gastricae have been associated with hypersecretory states and duodenal ulcers.[53,54] In retrospect, however, this association is probably related to underlying *H. pylori* gastritis in many patients. The presence of enlarged areae gastricae should therefore suggest the possibility of *H. pylori*, particularly if associated with thickened gastric folds.[7,49]

Patients with chronic *H. pylori* gastritis may gradually acquire lymphoid tissue in the gastric mucosa, resulting in the development of intramucosal aggregates of lymphocytes or lymphoid follicles containing germinal centers.[55,56] This phenomenon is almost always thought to be mediated by a

specific immune response to *H. pylori*.[57] In one study, more than 90% of patients with lymphoid hyperplasia of the stomach were found to have *H. pylori* gastritis.[2] Lymphoid hyperplasia is therefore a potential marker for *H. pylori* gastritis even in the absence of other findings. These enlarged lymphoid follicles are manifested on double-contrast barium studies by innumerable tiny (1 to 3 mm in diameter), round, frequently umbilicated nodules that carpet the mucosa of the gastric antrum or antrum and body (Fig. 34-12).[58] The radiographic findings are therefore similar to those of lymphoid hyperplasia of the small bowel or colon.

Differential Diagnosis

The radiographic findings of *H. pylori* gastritis may be indistinguishable from those of hypertrophic gastritis, Ménétrier's disease, or lymphoma when the thickened, lobulated folds have a diffuse distribution,[59] and the findings may be indistinguishable from malignant tumors such as lymphoma or a submucosally infiltrating carcinoma when the enlarged, polypoid folds have a focal distribution.[7,49] In other patients with *H. pylori* gastritis, CT may reveal circumferential thickening of the antrum or focal thickening of the posterior gastric wall, occasionally simulating a gastric carcinoma.[60] Endoscopy and biopsy are required for a definitive diagnosis when malignant tumor is suspected on the basis of the radiographic findings. Nevertheless, it is important to be aware of the association between *H. pylori* and this polypoid form of gastritis, so that careful testing for the organism is performed at the time of endoscopy in these patients.

When *H. pylori* gastritis is associated with lymphoid hyperplasia of the stomach, the major consideration in the differential diagnosis is low-grade gastric MALT lymphoma (see Chapter 37). However, gastric MALT lymphoma is manifested on double-contrast studies by multiple round, variably sized, often confluent nodules with poorly defined borders (Fig. 34-13).[61] In contrast, the nodules of gastric lymphoid hyperplasia have more discrete borders, a more uniform size, and, not infrequently, central umbilications (see Fig. 34-12).[58] Lymphoid hyperplasia of the stomach should also be differentiated from enlarged areae gastricae, another finding associated with *H. pylori* gastritis.[7,46] However, enlarged areae gastricae have a more polygonal or angulated configuration, producing a sharply marginated reticular network (see Fig. 34-9), and they do not contain central umbilications. Other unusual neoplastic lesions such as leukemic infiltrates or even polyposis syndromes may also be manifested on double-contrast studies by multiple small nodules, but the nodules tend to have a more variable size and a more sporadic distribution. Thus, it is usually possible to differentiate lymphoid hyperplasia of the stomach from other conditions on radiographic criteria. If the findings are equivocal, however, endoscopic biopsy specimens should be obtained for a more definitive diagnosis.

HYPERTROPHIC GASTRITIS

Hypertrophic gastritis, also known as hypertrophic hypersecretory gastropathy, is characterized by marked glandular hyperplasia and increased secretion of acid in the stomach.[62,63] Gastric folds may be thickened not only because of glandular hyperplasia but also because of edema and inflammation. Although the pathogenesis of this condition is uncertain, glandular hyperplasia in the stomach may be caused by pituitary, hypothalamic, or vagal stimuli.[62] These patients may present with epigastric pain, nausea and vomiting, or, less frequently, signs or symptoms of upper gastrointestinal bleeding.[62,63] If the radiographic or endoscopic findings support the diagnosis of hypertrophic gastritis, treatment with antisecretory agents is usually recommended to suppress acid secretion in the stomach.

Radiographic Findings

Hypertrophic gastritis is manifested on barium studies by thickened folds, predominantly in the gastric fundus and body, because the acid-secreting portion of the stomach is most affected by this condition (Fig. 34-14). Several studies have shown a significant correlation between the degree of fold thickening and the amount of acid secretion in the stomach.[64,65] The presence of markedly thickened, lobulated folds in the stomach should therefore suggest the possibility of hypertrophic gastritis. In retrospect, however, many if not most cases of previously diagnosed hypertrophic gastritis probably resulted from infection by *H. pylori*, a much more common cause of thickened gastric folds (see previous section on *Helicobacter pylori* Gastritis).

Differential Diagnosis

H. pylori gastritis, Ménétrier's disease, and lymphoma are the major considerations in the differential diagnosis of thickened, lobulated gastric folds. *H. pylori* gastritis can usually be differentiated from hypertrophic gastritis by noninvasive tests for *H. pylori*, such as the urea breath test and serologic tests (see previous section on *Helicobacter pylori* Gastritis). Ménétrier's disease should be suspected in patients who have normal or decreased acid secretion and a protein-losing enteropathy (see next section on Ménétrier's Disease), whereas lymphoma should be suspected when associated findings such as ulcers, masses, or "bull's-eye" lesions are present in the stomach (see Chapter 37). Gastric carcinoma is a less common cause of thickened folds, and it is usually associated with loss of distensibility and decreased or absent peristalsis in the involved portion of the stomach.[66] If the radiographic findings are equivocal, endoscopy and biopsy may be required to rule out malignant tumor. Rarely, other conditions such as Zollinger-Ellison syndrome, eosinophilic gastritis, and varices may be manifested by thickened folds in the stomach, but the correct diagnosis can usually be suggested on the basis of the clinical history and presentation.

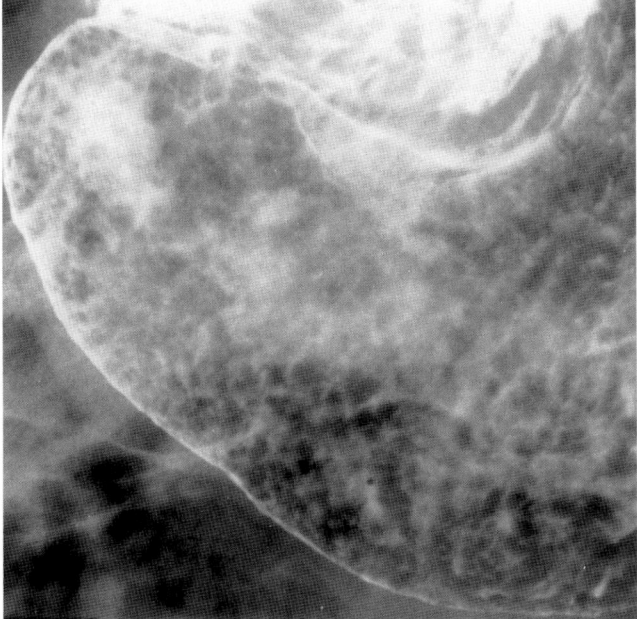

Figure 34-13. Low-grade gastric MALT lymphoma. There are multiple round, variably sized, confluent nodules with poorly defined borders in the gastric antrum. These are characteristic findings of gastric MALT lymphoma. In contrast, the nodules of lymphoid hyperplasia have more discrete borders and a more uniform size (see Fig. 34-12). (From Yoo CC, Levine MS, Furth EE, et al: Gastric mucosa-associated lymphoid tissue lymphoma: Radiographic findings in six patients. Radiology 208:239-243, 1998.)

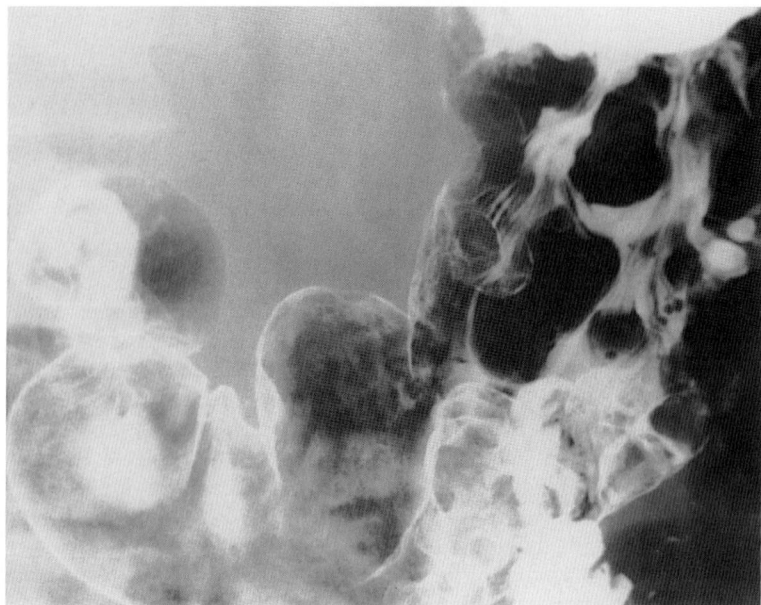

Figure 34-14. Hypertrophic gastritis. Markedly thickened, lobulated folds are seen in the body of the stomach. The antrum appears normal. (From Laufer I, Levine MS [eds]: Double Contrast Gastrointestinal Radiology. 2nd ed. Philadelphia, WB Saunders, 1992.)

MÉNÉTRIER'S DISEASE

Since its original description by Ménétrier in 1898, Ménétrier's disease has been recognized as a rare condition of unknown cause characterized by marked foveolar hyperplasia in the stomach, enlarged gastric rugae, hypochlorhydria, and hypoproteinemia. In the past, this condition has also been called cystic gastritis, giant hypertrophic gastritis, giant mucosal hypertrophy, and hyperplastic gastropathy. Ménétrier's disease may cause chronic, disabling symptoms, occasionally necessitating a gastric resection. Despite its rarity, this entity has received considerable attention in the radiologic literature because of its often dramatic appearance on barium studies.

Pathology

Ménétrier's disease is characterized histologically by thickening and hyperplasia of the mucosa as a result of cystic dilatation and elongation of gastric mucous glands associated with deepening of the foveolar pits.[67,68] Despite these findings, gastric acid output is decreased or absent in about 75% of cases.[69] Some patients have a protein-losing enteropathy resulting from loss of protein from the hyperplastic mucosa into the gastric lumen.[70] Others have varying degrees of gastritis in either a patchy or diffuse distribution.

Clinical Findings

Ménétrier's disease tends to occur in older patients and is more common in men than in women.[69] Affected individuals often present with epigastric pain, nausea and vomiting, diarrhea, anorexia, weight loss, or peripheral edema.[67,69,71] Laboratory studies may reveal hypoalbuminemia resulting from a protein-losing enteropathy, hypochlorhydria resulting from decreased acid secretion, or both.[67] Rarely, the development of gastric carcinoma has been described in patients with preexisting Ménétrier's disease.[72,73] It is unclear, however, whether Ménétrier's disease is a premalignant condition or whether this association is coincidental.

Some patients with Ménétrier's disease have spontaneous remission of symptoms, and others respond to treatment with antisecretory agents, vagotomy, or antibiotics. However, most patients have a prolonged illness with intractable symptoms.[71] A total gastrectomy may be required for patients who are unresponsive to medical therapy.

Radiographic Findings

Ménétrier's disease is classically manifested on barium studies by grossly thickened, lobulated folds in the gastric fundus and body with relative sparing of the antrum (Fig. 34-15A).[74] In one study, however, the antrum was involved in nearly 50% of patients,[75] so that diffuse thickening of gastric folds in no way precludes this diagnosis. The greatest degree of fold thickening usually occurs on or near the greater curvature.[74] When the disease is confined to one portion of the stomach, focally enlarged folds may erroneously suggest a polypoid carcinoma (Fig. 34-15B).[74] In other patients, excessive mucus in the stomach may dilute the barium and compromise mucosal coating.

Ménétrier's disease is characterized on CT by a markedly thickened gastric wall with masslike elevations representing giant, heaped-up folds protruding into the lumen (Fig. 34-15C). When Ménétrier's disease is suspected on barium studies or CT, full-thickness endoscopic biopsy specimens should be obtained to confirm the diagnosis.

Differential Diagnosis

Although a variety of conditions may be manifested by thickened gastric folds, these conditions rarely produce the degree of fold thickening seen in Ménétrier's disease. When *H. pylori* gastritis is associated with markedly thickened, lobulated folds, the radiographic findings may be indistinguishable from those of Ménétrier's disease.[46] Gastric lymphoma is sometimes associated with enlarged folds, but neoplastic infiltration should be suggested by the presence of polypoid masses,

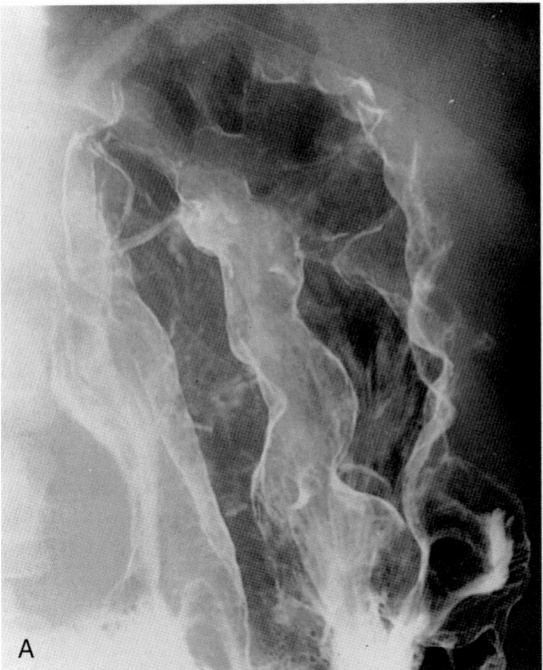

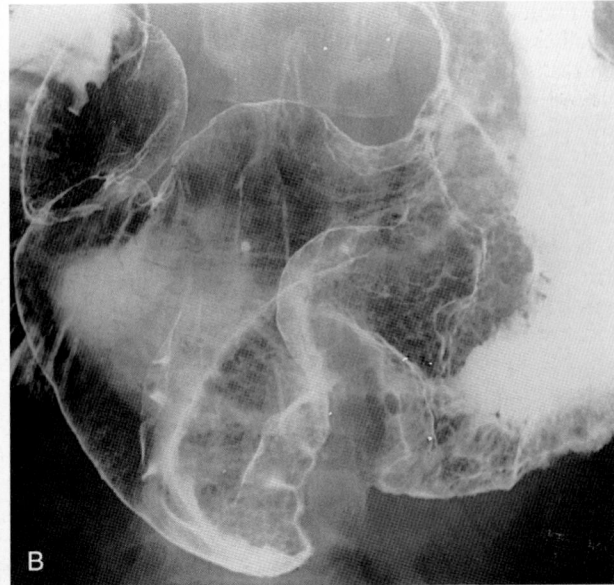

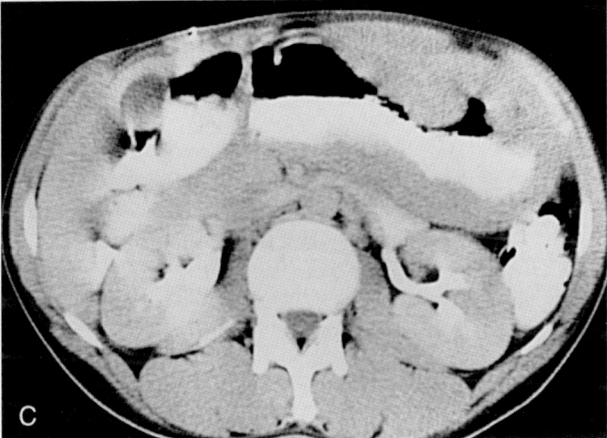

Figure 34-15. Ménétrier's disease. A. Grossly thickened folds are present in the gastric fundus. **B.** In another patient, masslike protrusions of the folds are seen on the greater curvature of the gastric body. This appearance could be mistaken for a polypoid gastric carcinoma. The distal antrum is relatively spared. **C.** In the patient shown in **B**, a CT scan shows massive thickening of the gastric wall with masslike protrusions into the lumen. Endoscopic biopsy specimens in this patient revealed typical pathologic findings of Ménétrier's disease without evidence of tumor. (**A** from Laufer I, Levine MS [eds]: Double Contrast Gastrointestinal Radiology, 2nd ed. Philadelphia, WB Saunders, 1992.)

ulcers, or "bull's-eye" lesions in these patients (see Chapter 37). Occasionally, gastric carcinoma may be manifested by thickened folds, but infiltrating cancers tend to narrow the lumen, whereas the stomach usually remains pliant and distensible in patients with Ménétrier's disease. Zollinger-Ellison syndrome may also be characterized by thickened folds, but the presence of increased secretions in the stomach or other associated abnormalities (e.g., ulcers and thickened folds) in the duodenum and proximal jejunum should suggest the correct diagnosis (see Chapter 33). Gastric varices should also be included in the differential diagnosis, but varices tend to have a more serpiginous appearance and are usually confined to the region of the gastric cardia or fundus (see Chapter 38). Other conditions involving the stomach, such as Crohn's disease, eosinophilic gastritis, sarcoidosis, tuberculosis, and syphilis, may also be manifested by thickened folds. In such cases, however, the correct diagnosis is usually suggested by the clinical history and presentation.

ATROPHIC GASTRITIS

Atrophic gastritis is important because of its association with pernicious anemia, a megaloblastic anemia caused by decreased synthesis of intrinsic factor and subsequent mal-

absorption of vitamin B_{12}. Pernicious anemia is a disease of the elderly; it accounts for 50 of every 100,000 hospital admissions in the United States.[76] Although the pathogenesis of this disease is uncertain, an autoimmune mechanism has been postulated because of the frequent finding of parietal cell or intrinsic factor antibodies in these individuals.[77]

More than 90% of patients with pernicious anemia have underlying atrophic gastritis, characterized pathologically by atrophy of mucosal glands, loss of parietal and chief cells, thinning of the mucosa, and, eventually, intestinal metaplasia.[78] The finding of intestinal metaplasia is particularly worrisome because it is widely believed to be the precursor lesion of the intestinal type of gastric cancer. The literature has also implicated chronic *H. pylori* infection as a major cause of atrophic gastritis, intestinal metaplasia, and gastric carcinoma (see Chapter 36).

Pathogenesis

Atrophic gastritis may be classified into two types (type A and type B), which have different histologic, immunologic, and secretory characteristics.[36,79,80] In type A gastritis, mucosal atrophy is confined to the gastric fundus and body with antral sparing. This type of atrophic gastritis is thought to result from immunologic injury (i.e., antiparietal cell antibodies) and is usually associated with pernicious anemia.[79]

In contrast, type B gastritis is characterized by predominant antral disease with limited involvement of the fundus and body. This form of atrophic gastritis is more common and usually results from mucosal injury by *H. pylori* or, less commonly, by other endogenous or exogenous agents such as bile acids or alcohol.[36,79,80] In patients with *H. pylori,* it has been postulated that the organism progressively damages the gastric mucus layer, causing chronic atrophic gastritis and gastric atrophy.[34,81] A particular strain of *H. pylori* known as *cagA* (cytotoxin-associated gene A) has been associated with an increased prevalence and degree of atrophic gastritis (predisposing these patients to the development of gastric carcinoma),[82] so that the risk of malignant degeneration may not be the same for all patients with this infection.

Clinical Findings

Although atrophic gastritis rarely causes symptoms, some patients with pernicious anemia may initially present with neurologic symptoms as a result of long-standing vitamin B_{12} deficiency. Early diagnosis of pernicious anemia is therefore important, so that vitamin B_{12} replacement therapy can be initiated before irreversible neurologic sequelae develop. Because the average adult has a 3- to 6-year body store of vitamin B_{12}, the gastric lesion in pernicious anemia may antedate the hematologic and neurologic abnormalities in this condition by several years. The diagnosis of atrophic gastritis on upper gastrointestinal studies might therefore permit these patients to be treated with vitamin B_{12} supplements before the full-blown clinical entity of pernicious anemia has developed.

Relationship to Gastric Carcinoma

Patients with atrophic gastritis and pernicious anemia are at increased risk for the development of gastric carcinoma. In one study, the risk of developing gastric cancer in these patients was found to be about three times greater than that in the general population.[83] Although some investigators advocate endoscopic or radiologic surveillance of patients with known pernicious anemia, others believe that the risk of cancer is not high enough to warrant routine screening.[84-86] Nevertheless, any patient with pernicious anemia who has occult gastrointestinal bleeding should be evaluated aggressively to rule out a superimposed gastric carcinoma.

The literature suggests that patients with *H. pylori*–associated atrophic gastritis have a substantially increased risk of developing gastric carcinoma (see Chapter 36). Evidence from several studies shows that the risk of gastric cancer in *H. pylori*–positive patients is about four times greater than that in patients without this infection.[87] Because of the high prevalence of *H. pylori* in the population, however, it remains unclear whether widespread eradication of *H. pylori* is justified from a societal perspective to prevent the development of cancer.

Radiographic Findings

The diagnosis of atrophic gastritis may be suggested on single-contrast studies by the presence of a narrowed, tubular stomach with decreased or absent mucosal folds, predominantly in the body and fundus (i.e., the "bald" fundus) (Fig. 34-16).[88] In one study, 80% of patients with atrophic gastritis and pernicious anemia had a fundal diameter of 8 cm or less, absent folds in the fundus and body, and small

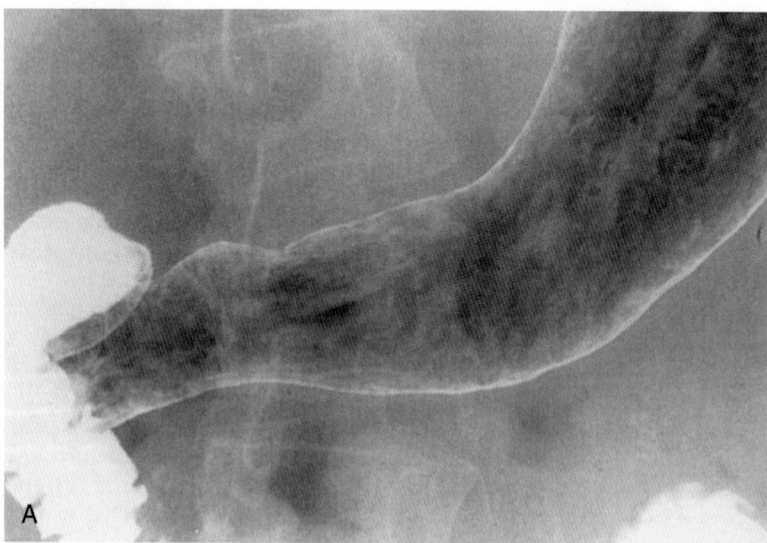

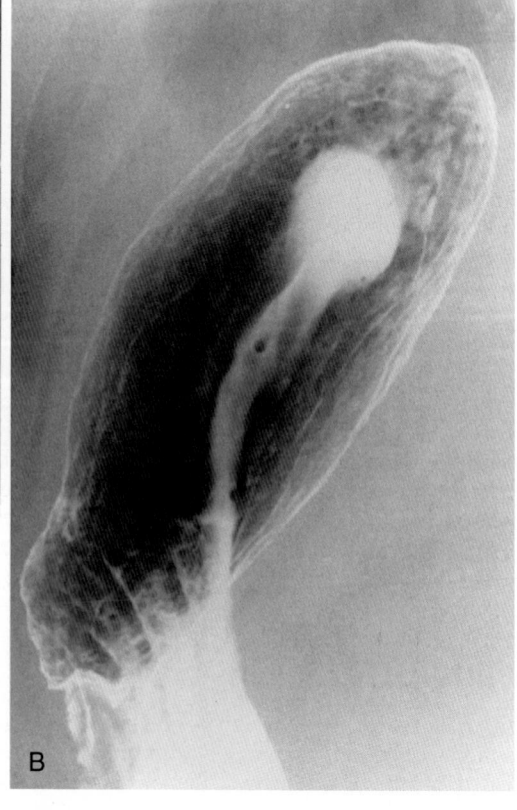

Figure 34-16. Atrophic gastritis. A and **B.** The stomach has a tubular configuration with decreased distensibility, a paucity of mucosal folds, and absence of discernible areae gastricae. These findings are characteristic of atrophic gastritis.

(1 to 2 mm in diameter) or absent areae gastricae in the stomach.[89] However, this combination of findings was also present in about 10% of age-matched controls.[89] The radiologic diagnosis of atrophic gastritis in patients with pernicious anemia has therefore been limited by a lack of criteria that are both sensitive and specific for this condition. When atrophic gastritis is suspected on double-contrast studies, serum vitamin B_{12} levels should be obtained to determine whether vitamin B_{12} replacement therapy is indicated.

Many questions remain about the appearance of the areae gastricae in patients with atrophic gastritis. It has previously been postulated that variations in the size of the areae gastricae depend on parietal cell mass.[90] Thus, the small size and frequent absence of areae gastricae in patients with atrophic gastritis may be explained by the loss of parietal cells in these individuals. In contrast, focal enlargement of the areae gastricae should raise the possibility of intestinal metaplasia or even a superficial spreading carcinoma, so that this finding should be evaluated by endoscopy and biopsy.

Differential Diagnosis

Scirrhous carcinoma of the stomach (i.e., linitis plastica) is the most important consideration in the differential diagnosis of atrophic gastritis. However, scirrhous tumors are usually characterized by a nodular, distorted mucosa and thickened, irregular folds,[91] whereas atrophic gastritis is characterized by a smooth, featureless mucosa and decreased or absent mucosal folds. Thus, scirrhous carcinomas can almost always be differentiated from atrophic gastritis by radiologic criteria. Scarring from peptic ulcer disease or other conditions may also be characterized by gastric narrowing, but the antrum and body tend to be involved rather than the fundus.

GRANULOMATOUS CONDITIONS

Crohn's Disease

Although Crohn's disease primarily affects the small bowel and colon, early signs of upper gastrointestinal involvement may be detected on double-contrast barium studies in more than 20% of patients with granulomatous ileocolitis.[92] Occasionally, the onset of upper gastrointestinal disease coincides with or even precedes the onset of ileal or colonic disease, so that these patients do not necessarily have known Crohn's disease when they seek medical attention. Endoscopic biopsy specimens from the stomach or duodenum may fail to reveal granulomas because of the superficial nature of the biopsy specimens and the patchy distribution of the disease.[93] Thus, the absence of definitive histologic findings should not discourage a diagnosis of gastroduodenal Crohn's disease if the clinical and radiographic findings suggest this condition.

Clinical Findings

Patients with early gastroduodenal involvement by Crohn's disease are often asymptomatic. Patients with more advanced disease may present with pain, vomiting, weight loss, or signs and symptoms of upper gastrointestinal bleeding.[94,95] Some patients may also have diarrhea because of associated ileocolic Crohn's disease. The development of a gastrocolic or duodenocolic fistula is classically manifested by feculent vomiting, diarrhea, and weight loss.[96] This triad of findings is present in only about 30% of patients, however, so that gastrocolic fistulas are not often suspected on clinical grounds.[97]

Asymptomatic patients with early gastroduodenal Crohn's disease require no specific treatment. In patients with more advanced disease, sulfasalazine (Azulfidine) or corticosteroids may effectively relieve epigastric pain or other upper gastrointestinal complaints.[94] In contrast, a surgical bypass procedure such as a gastrojejunostomy or duodenojejunostomy may be required to alleviate symptoms of gastric outlet obstruction.[94]

Radiographic Findings

As in the ileum or colon, gastroduodenal Crohn's disease is characterized by nonstenotic and stenotic phases of involvement. The initial nonstenotic phase is manifested by a spectrum of findings, including aphthoid ulcers, larger ulcers, thickened folds, and distorted, effaced, or, rarely, "cobblestoned" mucosa. Subsequent scarring and fibrosis may cause antral, pyloric, or duodenal narrowing with progressive gastric outlet obstruction. Thus, the radiologic features of gastroduodenal Crohn's disease are similar to those found in the small bowel and colon.

Gastric Involvement

Gastric Crohn's disease almost always involves the antrum or antrum and body of the stomach.[98] More proximal extension of Crohn's disease is unusual, and isolated fundal involvement rarely occurs.[99] When the stomach is affected by Crohn's disease, the duodenum also tends to be involved.[98,100,101] Most patients have associated granulomatous ileocolitis, but the diagnosis of Crohn's disease may not be known at the time of clinical presentation. When gastric involvement is suggested by upper gastrointestinal studies, a small bowel follow-through or barium enema should be performed to determine whether there is concomitant ileocolic disease.

Aphthoid ulcers, the earliest histologic lesions of Crohn's disease, are detected in the stomach on double-contrast studies in more than 20% of patients with granulomatous ileocolitis.[92] These aphthoid ulcers tend to be located in the antrum or antrum and body, appearing as punctate or slitlike collections of barium surrounded by radiolucent mounds of edema (Fig. 34-17).[11,92,102] As a result, these lesions may be indistinguishable from varioliform gastric erosions (see earlier section on Erosive Gastritis).

More advanced gastroduodenal Crohn's disease may be manifested by one or more larger ulcers, thickened folds (Fig. 34-18), or a nodular or cobblestoned mucosa in the gastric antrum or body.[98,100] Subsequent scarring may lead to the development of a narrowed, tubular, funnel-shaped antrum that has been likened to the sacramental ram's horn, or shofar, used to sound the advent of the Jewish New Year (Fig. 34-19).[103] In other patients, combined gastroduodenal scarring may produce a single, continuous tubular structure involving the antrum and duodenum with obliteration of the normal anatomic landmarks at the pylorus (Fig. 34-20).[94,100] Because of its resemblance to a postsurgical stomach after a Billroth I partial gastrectomy, this finding has been described as the *pseudo-Billroth I* sign of gastroduodenal Crohn's disease.[104] Rarely, filiform polyps may be found in the stomach as a sequela of severe granulomatous gastritis (Fig. 34-21).[105]

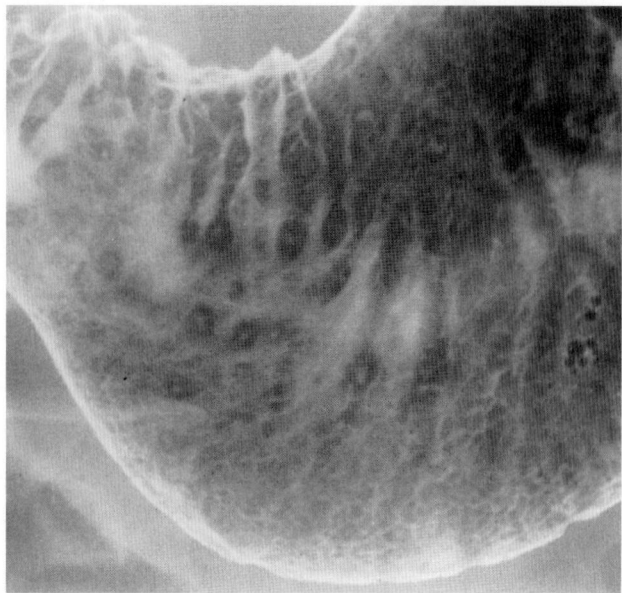

Figure 34-17. Early gastric Crohn's disease with aphthoid ulcers. These lesions are indistinguishable from varioliform erosions in the stomach. This patient had typical findings of Crohn's disease in the terminal ileum. (Courtesy of Robert A. Goren, MD, Philadelphia, PA.)

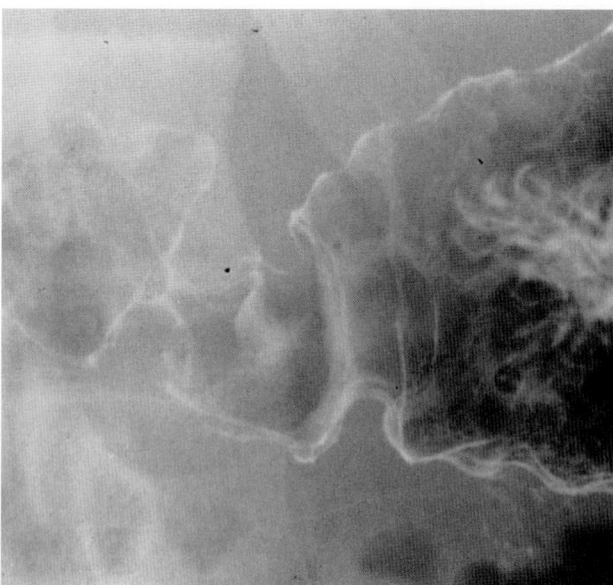

Figure 34-18. Gastric Crohn's disease. Thickened, nodular folds are seen in the antrum of the stomach. (From Levine MS: Crohn's disease of the upper gastrointestinal tract. Radiol Clin North Am 25:79-91, 1987.)

Patients with Crohn's disease may occasionally develop gastrocolic fistulas.[96,97,106] These individuals usually have underlying Crohn's disease of the transverse colon with extension of a fistula via the gastrocolic ligament to the greater curvature of the stomach. On barium studies, the greater curvature may have a nodular or spiculated appearance with thickened, distorted folds in the region of the fistula. These findings probably represent a nonspecific inflammatory response to the adjoining fistula rather than actual extension of Crohn's disease to the stomach. Gastrocolic fistulas are demonstrated on only about one third of upper gastrointestinal examinations, so that barium enemas are often required for diagnosis of these fistulas.[97]

Although patients with ileocolic Crohn's disease are thought to be at increased risk for developing carcinoma of the small bowel and colon, the relationship between gastric Crohn's disease and gastric carcinoma remains controversial. Anecdotal cases of gastric cancer have been reported in patients with long-standing gastric Crohn's disease,[107] but it is uncertain whether this association is coincidental.

Duodenal Involvement

Although duodenal involvement by Crohn's disease is usually associated with antral involvement, isolated duodenal Crohn's disease occurs more frequently than isolated Crohn's disease of the stomach.[100] As elsewhere in the gastrointestinal

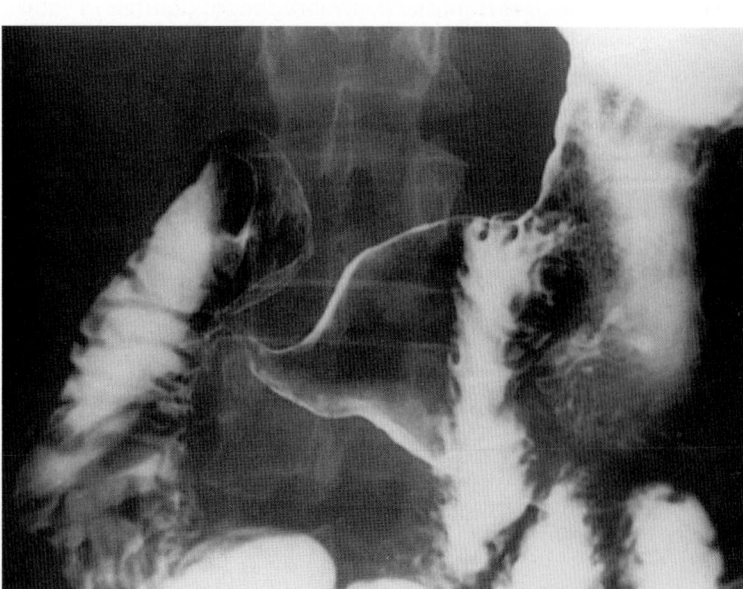

Figure 34-19. Gastric Crohn's disease with antral narrowing. There is smooth, funnel-shaped narrowing of the antrum, resulting in the classic "ram's horn" sign of gastric Crohn's disease. (From Levine MS: Crohn's disease of the upper gastrointestinal tract. Radiol Clin North Am 25:79-91, 1987.)

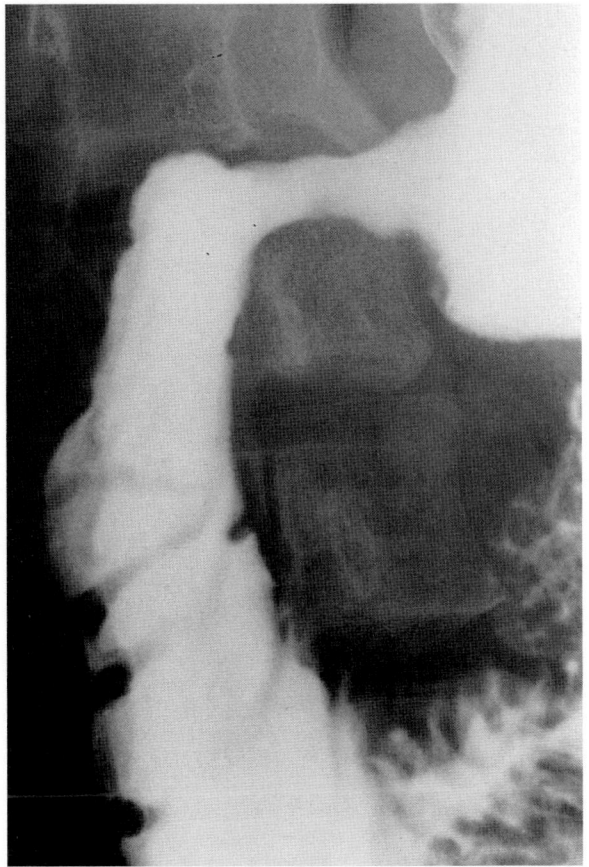

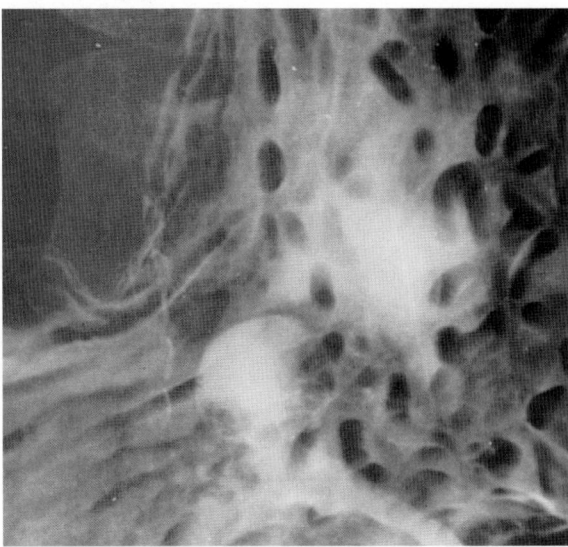

Figure 34-21. Gastric Crohn's disease with filiform polyps. Multiple linear and ovoid filling defects are seen in the stomach in a patient with long-standing Crohn's disease. (From Levine MS: Crohn's disease of the upper gastrointestinal tract. Radiol Clin North Am 25:79-91, 1987.)

Figure 34-20. Gastroduodenal Crohn's disease. There is contiguous narrowing of the antrum and duodenum, with obliteration of the normal anatomic landmarks at the pylorus. Because the antrum and duodenum merge together as a single tubular structure, this finding has been described as the pseudo-Billroth I sign of gastroduodenal Crohn's disease. (From Levine MS: Crohn's disease of the upper gastrointestinal tract. Radiol Clin North Am 25:79-91, 1987.)

tract, aphthoid ulcers represent the earliest morphologic abnormality on double-contrast studies of the duodenum (Fig. 34-22).[11,102] With progression, duodenal Crohn's disease may be manifested by thickened, nodular folds (Fig. 34-23), ulcers, or even a cobblestoned appearance because of intersecting linear ulcers similar to those found in advanced ileocolitis.[108]

Subsequent scarring may lead to the development of one or more areas of asymmetric duodenal narrowing with outward ballooning or sacculation of the duodenal wall between areas of fibrosis.[108] These strictures typically involve the postbulbar duodenum, appearing as smooth, tapered areas of narrowing that extend from the apical portion of the duodenal bulb into the descending duodenum (Fig. 34-24).[104,108]

Figure 34-22. Duodenal Crohn's disease with aphthoid ulcers. Several discrete aphthoid ulcers (*arrows*) are seen in the distal duodenum near the ligament of Treitz. Note the stellate configuration of the ulcers. (Courtesy of Louis Engelhom, MD, Brussels, Belgium.)

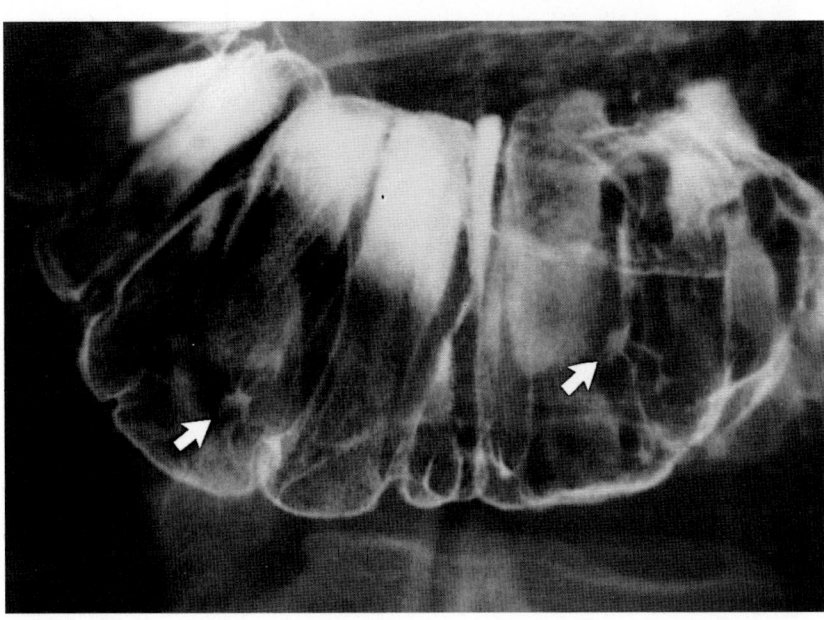

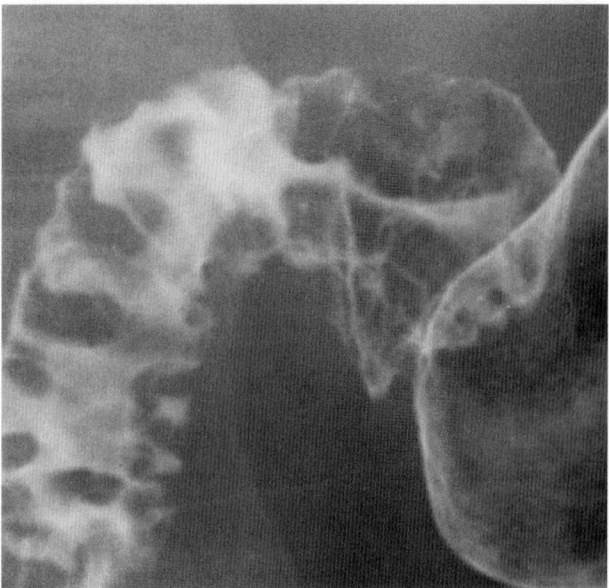

Figure 34-23. Duodenal Crohn's disease with thickened folds. The folds have a thickened, nodular appearance in the proximal duodenum. Peptic duodenitis could produce similar findings.

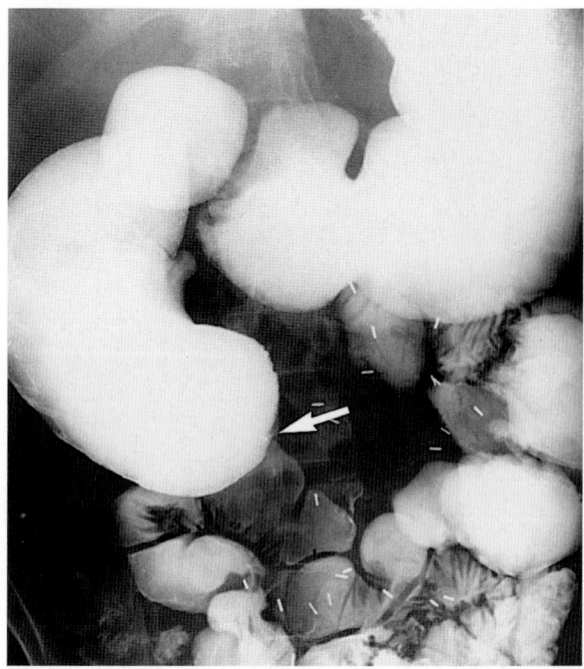

Figure 34-25. Duodenal Crohn's disease with a megaduodenum. There is high-grade obstruction (*arrow*) of the distal duodenum with marked duodenal dilatation above this level. (From Levine MS: Crohn's disease of the upper gastrointestinal tract. Radiol Clin North Am 25:79-91, 1987.)

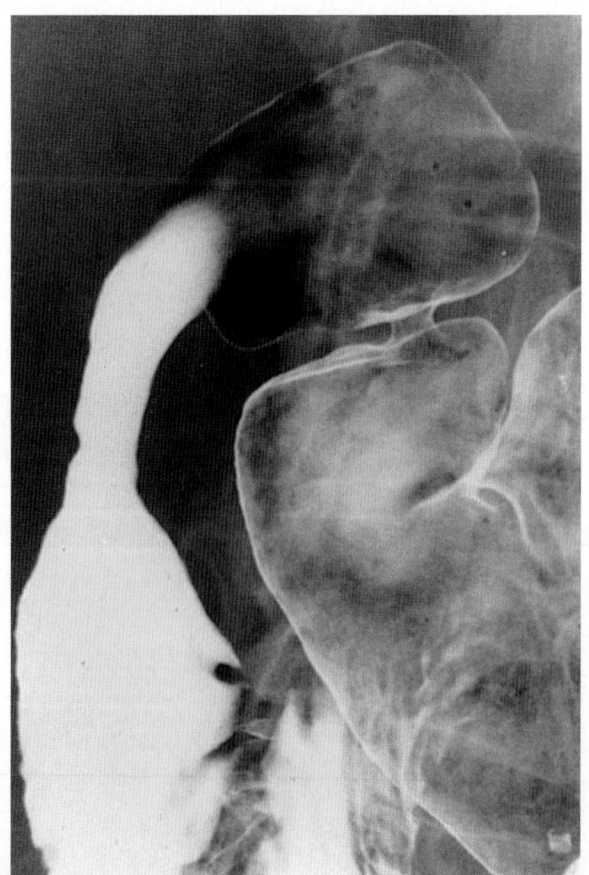

Figure 34-24. Duodenal Crohn's disease with stricture formation. There is smooth, tapered narrowing of the apical portion of the bulb and adjacent segment of the descending duodenum. This appearance is characteristic of Crohn's disease.

As a result, scarring from duodenal Crohn's disease can usually be differentiated on barium studies from the "cloverleaf" bulbar deformity associated with scarring from peptic ulcer disease.[104] Other patients may have one or more strictures in the second or third portions of the duodenum that cause marked obstruction and proximal dilatation, resulting in a so-called megaduodenum (Fig. 34-25).[108]

Primary duodenal Crohn's disease is rarely associated with the development of fistulas. However, duodenocolic fistulas may occasionally result from advanced Crohn's disease involving the transverse colon with subsequent fistulization to the third or fourth portions of the duodenum (Fig. 34-26).[104,109] Thickened, spiculated folds may be demonstrated in the affected duodenum, but the fistula itself is more likely to be visualized on barium enema than on upper gastrointestinal examination because of the higher pressures generated with this technique. Because these duodenal changes represent a nonspecific inflammatory response rather than actual involvement of the duodenum by Crohn's disease, follow-up barium studies after resection of the fistula may show a completely normal duodenum.[109]

Differential Diagnosis

Stomach

Aphthoid ulcers in the stomach may be indistinguishable on double-contrast studies from gastric erosions resulting from NSAIDs or other causes. Although gastric involvement by Crohn's disease is much less common than erosive gastritis, the possibility of Crohn's disease should be suspected when gastric erosions are present in patients with crampy abdominal pain and diarrhea, and a small bowel follow-through

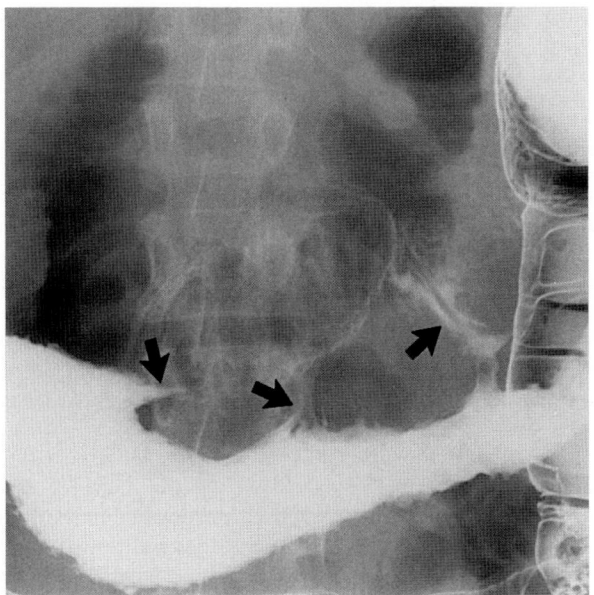

Figure 34-26. Crohn's disease with duodenocolic fistulas. Barium enema shows three separate fistulous tracks (*arrows*) extending from the superior border of the transverse colon to the third and fourth portions of the duodenum. The tubular, severely ulcerated appearance of the transverse colon is due to advanced granulomatous colitis. Duodenocolic fistulas almost always result from primary Crohn's disease of the colon with nonspecific inflammatory changes in the duodenum adjoining the fistula. (From Levine MS: Crohn's disease of the upper gastrointestinal tract. Radiol Clin North Am 25:79-91, 1987.)

should be performed to evaluate the terminal ileum in these individuals.

The funnel-shaped antral narrowing associated with more advanced gastroduodenal Crohn's disease must be differentiated from other conditions, particularly a scirrhous gastric carcinoma. In one study, about one third of patients with antral narrowing caused by Crohn's disease underwent surgery because the radiographic findings simulated a scirrhous carcinoma.[103] However, the narrowed antrum of Crohn's disease tends to have a smooth, tubular configuration, whereas scirrhous carcinoma produces a linitis plastica appearance with a distorted, more irregular mucosal contour.[91] Antral narrowing may also be caused by a variety of other conditions, including scarring from peptic ulcer disease, sarcoidosis, tuberculosis, syphilis, eosinophilic gastritis, caustic ingestion, and radiation. In such cases, the correct diagnosis is often suggested by the clinical history and presentation.

Gastrocolic fistulas may be caused not only by Crohn's disease but also by benign, penetrating ulcers on the greater curvature of the stomach in patients who are taking aspirin or other NSAIDs (see Chapter 33).[110] Occasionally, these fistulas may also be caused by carcinoma of the stomach or transverse colon invading the gastrocolic ligament.[106] When Crohn's disease is responsible for the fistula, a barium enema examination usually reveals findings of advanced granulomatous colitis in the transverse colon.

Duodenum

Aphthoid ulcers in the duodenum may be indistinguishable on double-contrast studies from varioliform duodenal erosions (see later section on Duodenitis). However, erosive duodenitis usually involves the duodenal bulb, whereas the aphthoid ulcers of Crohn's disease may be located anywhere in the duodenum from the bulb to the ligament of Treitz. The presence of one or more ulcers in the duodenal bulb or postbulbar duodenum should raise the possibility of Zollinger-Ellison syndrome, but these patients usually have markedly thickened folds and increased secretions in the stomach (see Chapter 33). Thickened, nodular folds in the descending duodenum may be caused not only by Crohn's disease but also by duodenitis, pancreatitis, or other conditions.

Although a smooth segment of tapered narrowing in the postbulbar duodenum is characteristic of the stenotic phase of Crohn's disease, scarring from uncomplicated postbulbar duodenal ulcers may produce a similar appearance.[111] In contrast, annular duodenal carcinomas can usually be differentiated from benign strictures by their shelflike, overhanging borders. When duodenal involvement by Crohn's disease is suspected on upper gastrointestinal examination, a small bowel follow-through or barium enema should be performed to search for associated Crohn's disease in the small bowel or colon.

Sarcoidosis

Sarcoidosis is a systemic granulomatous disease of unknown origin, characterized pathologically by the presence of non-caseating granulomas. Most patients have thoracic sarcoidosis with bilateral hilar lymphadenopathy or fibronodular pulmonary infiltrates on chest radiographs. About 40% of patients have extrathoracic disease involving the eye, skin, lymph nodes, liver, spleen, heart, and musculoskeletal or nervous system. Although sarcoidosis is rarely thought to affect the gastrointestinal tract, one investigator found noncaseating granulomas on mucosal biopsy specimens from the stomach in 10% of patients with known sarcoidosis.[112] Thus, gastrointestinal involvement by sarcoidosis may be more common than is generally recognized.

Clinical Findings

Sarcoidosis involves the stomach more frequently than any other portion of the gastrointestinal tract. Most patients with gastric sarcoidosis are asymptomatic,[112] but some may present with nausea, vomiting, bloating, or weight loss because of gastric outlet obstruction.[113] Others may present with epigastric pain or signs or symptoms of upper gastrointestinal bleeding resulting from ulceration of the overlying mucosa.[114] Treatment with corticosteroids produces a dramatic clinical response in about two thirds of symptomatic patients.[113] Surgical intervention may occasionally be required for patients who have persistent gastric outlet obstruction, massive bleeding, or radiographic or endoscopic findings that are suggestive of malignant tumor.

Radiographic Findings

Gastric sarcoidosis may be manifested by a spectrum of radiographic findings. In patients with superficial disease, double-contrast studies may reveal a localized area of mucosal nodularity or thickened, irregular folds (Fig. 34-27A).[115,116] Other patients may have benign-appearing or malignant-appearing ulcers in the stomach.[114,116] More advanced sarcoidosis may result in smooth, cone-shaped antral narrowing and

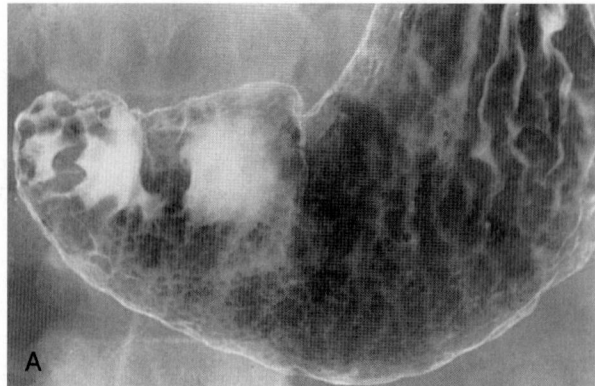
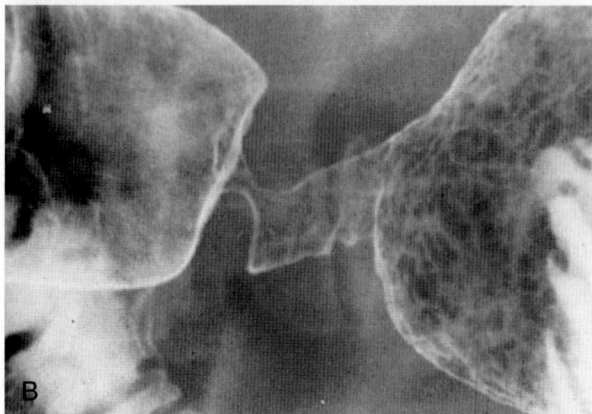

Figure 34-27. Gastric sarcoidosis. A. Double-contrast study shows considerable nodularity of the mucosa in the gastric antrum. This patient had pulmonary sarcoidosis, and endoscopic biopsy specimens revealed noncaseating granulomas in the stomach. **B.** In another patient, more advanced gastric sarcoidosis is manifested by marked antral narrowing and deformity. (**B** courtesy of Seth N. Glick, MD, Philadelphia, PA.)

deformity (Fig. 34-27B).[114] Similar findings may be caused by scarring from peptic ulcer disease, caustic ingestion, radiation, and a variety of other granulomatous conditions, including Crohn's disease, tuberculosis, and syphilis. Rarely, sarcoidosis may produce more irregular gastric narrowing, mimicking the linitis plastica appearance of an advanced scirrhous carcinoma of the stomach.[117] The possibility of gastric sarcoidosis should be suspected, however, when chest radiographs reveal characteristic findings of sarcoidosis in the thorax.

Tuberculosis

Gastroduodenal involvement occurs in less than 0.5% of all patients with tuberculosis.[118] The stomach and duodenum are rarely involved because of the paucity of lymphoid tissue in the upper gastrointestinal tract, the high acidity of peptic secretions, and the rapid passage of ingested organisms into the small bowel. Most patients with gastric or duodenal tuberculosis are found to have generalized tuberculosis. Gastroduodenal infection is presumably caused by ingestion of the bacillus or by hematogenous spread to lymphatics in the wall of the stomach or duodenum.[119] Although routine pasteurization of milk has dramatically decreased the incidence of gastrointestinal tuberculosis in the United States, some patients may travel to the United States from other countries such as South Africa or India, where tuberculosis is endemic.

Gastric and duodenal tuberculosis has been encountered with increased frequency in patients with AIDS, particularly those of Haitian origin.[120]

Clinical Findings

Patients with gastric or duodenal tuberculosis may present with epigastric pain or signs or symptoms of upper gastrointestinal bleeding.[121-123] Subsequently, they may develop nausea and vomiting because of progressive scarring and gastric outlet obstruction.[123] Although the clinical findings are nonspecific, the possibility of gastroduodenal tuberculosis should be considered in patients who have known pulmonary tuberculosis or who have migrated from areas where tuberculosis is endemic.

Stool cultures for tuberculosis are unreliable; some patients with pulmonary tuberculosis have positive culture results in the absence of gastrointestinal infection, whereas others have negative culture results despite gastrointestinal infection.[119] A definitive diagnosis of gastroduodenal tuberculosis can be made when endoscopic biopsy specimens reveal caseating granulomas in the stomach or duodenum, but these granulomas may not be demonstrated because of their submucosal location and the small size of the specimen samples.[123] Depending on the severity of disease, gastroduodenal tuberculosis may be treated by antituberculous drug therapy or, if necessary, gastric resection or bypass.

Radiographic Findings

Gastric tuberculosis may be manifested on barium studies by one or more areas of ulceration, most frequently on the lesser curvature of the antrum or in the region of the pylorus.[120,124] Subsequent scarring may cause marked antral narrowing, eventually leading to the development of gastric outlet obstruction.[124,125] Occasionally, the narrowed antrum may have an irregular contour, simulating the linitis plastica appearance of a primary scirrhous carcinoma of the stomach.[124] As in the ileocecal region, advanced gastric tuberculosis may be associated with the development of multiple tracks and fistulas.[124]

Duodenal tuberculosis may also be manifested on barium studies by ulcers, thickened folds, narrowing, or fistulas.[126-128] As in Crohn's disease, duodenal tuberculosis is often associated with contiguous involvement of the distal antrum. Enlarged tuberculous lymph nodes adjacent to the duodenum may cause widening, narrowing, or obstruction of the duodenal sweep.[128] Rarely, duodenorenal fistulas may result from spread of tuberculosis from the right kidney to the duodenum.[129]

Syphilis

Gastric syphilis is a rare disease, occurring in less than 1% of all patients with secondary or tertiary syphilis.[130] Nevertheless, gastric involvement should be suspected in young patients with untreated lues who develop epigastric pain, nausea, vomiting, or signs or symptoms of upper gastrointestinal bleeding.[131] The diagnosis of gastric syphilis can be confirmed by isolating *Treponema pallidum* on endoscopic biopsy specimens or by demonstrating the typical spirochetes on darkfield microscopy.[132] Affected individuals usually have a marked

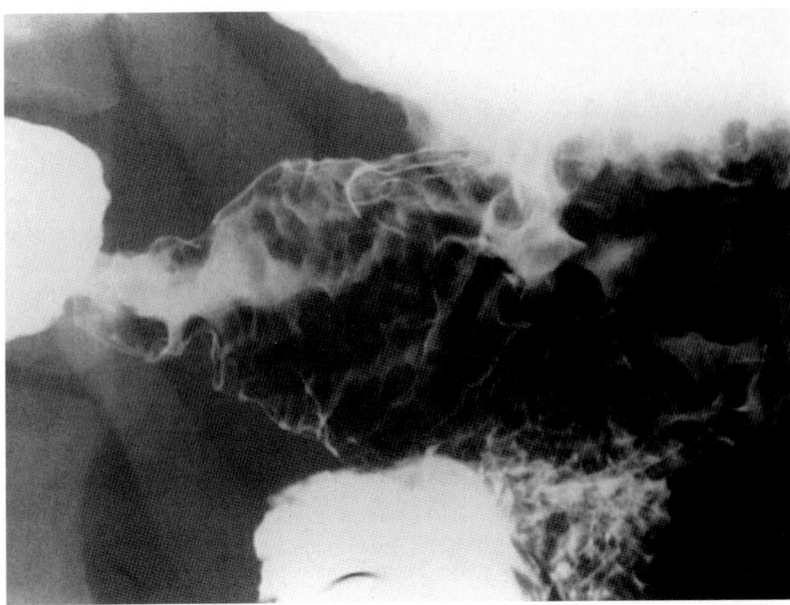

Figure 34-28. Gastric syphilis. Mucosal nodularity and thickened folds are seen in the antrum in this patient with proven gastric syphilis.

clinical response to antiluetic therapy if they are treated before substantial gastric scarring has occurred.

Radiographic Findings

Secondary syphilis involving the stomach is sometimes associated with a severe form of acute gastritis. In such cases, barium studies may reveal mucosal nodules, erosions, shallow or deep ulcers, and thickened folds, predominantly in the antrum (Fig. 34-28).[130,131,133] In contrast, tertiary syphilis involving the stomach is characterized by progressive scarring and fibrosis, eventually producing a tubular, funnel-shaped antrum.[130,133] This appearance may be indistinguishable from antral narrowing caused by Crohn's disease, caustic ingestion, radiation, or other granulomatous conditions such as tuberculosis and sarcoidosis. Other patients with tertiary syphilis may have focal narrowing of the gastric body, producing an hourglass- or dumbbell-shaped stomach.[133] Rarely, the narrowed stomach may have a more irregular contour, mimicking the linitis plastica appearance of a primary scirrhous carcinoma of the stomach.[134] When gastric syphilis is suspected on the basis of the clinical and radiographic findings, endoscopic biopsy specimens are required for a definitive diagnosis.

Fungal Diseases

A variety of fungal diseases may rarely involve the stomach. Gastric histoplasmosis may be manifested by thickened folds, ulceration, or narrowing of the stomach.[135] Gastric candidiasis may be associated with the development of large aphthoid ulcers or even centrally ulcerated "bull's-eye" lesions.[12,136] Other rare fungal infections of the stomach include actinomycosis and mucormycosis.[137,138]

OTHER INFECTIONS

Cytomegalovirus Infection

Cytomegalovirus (CMV), a member of the herpesvirus group, is the most common viral pathogen affecting the gastro-intestinal tract in patients with AIDS.[139] Although the esophagus and colon are more frequent sites of involvement (see Chapters 24 and 62), human immunodeficiency virus (HIV)-positive patients may occasionally develop CMV gastritis and duodenitis.[26,140-144] Affected individuals may present with severe abdominal pain or signs or symptoms of upper gastrointestinal bleeding.[143] The treatment of CMV gastritis or duodenitis includes relatively toxic antiviral agents such as ganciclovir (which is associated with bone marrow suppression).[145] Thus, endoscopic biopsy specimens, brushings, or cultures are required for a definitive diagnosis before treating these patients.

Radiographic Findings

CMV gastritis may be manifested on barium studies by mucosal nodularity, erosions, ulcers, thickened folds, and, in severe cases, irregular antral narrowing (Fig. 34-29).[26,140,141] Other opportunistic infections such as cryptosporidiosis and toxoplasmosis may occasionally produce similar findings in patients with AIDS (see later sections on Cryptosporidiosis and Toxoplasmosis). Rarely, deep ulcers can result in the development of fistulas to adjacent structures such as the colon.[142] When CMV gastritis is suspected, the diagnosis may be confirmed by demonstrating characteristic inclusion bodies on endoscopic biopsy specimens or brushings or by obtaining positive cultures for CMV.

CMV duodenitis may be manifested on barium studies by luminal narrowing with thickened or effaced folds in the proximal duodenum (Fig. 34-30).[143,144] The differential diagnosis includes other opportunistic infections in the duodenum in patients with AIDS, such as cryptosporidiosis, strongyloidiasis, and tuberculosis. Endoscopic biopsy specimens, brushings, or viral cultures for CMV are therefore required for a definitive diagnosis.

Cryptosporidiosis

Cryptosporidium, a protozoan, may infect the small bowel in patients with AIDS, causing a profuse secretory diarrhea

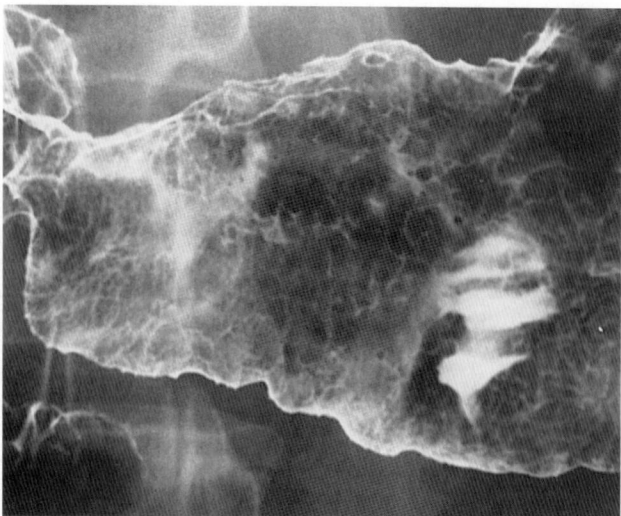

Figure 34-29. Cytomegalovirus gastritis. Mucosal nodularity and tiny ulcerations are seen in the gastric antrum. Note the irregular contour of the stomach. This patient had AIDS.

(see Chapter 46). Much less frequently, cryptosporidiosis may involve the stomach.[140,146,147] In such cases, barium studies may demonstrate antral narrowing and rigidity, occasionally associated with one or more deep ulcers.[140,146,147] CT may also reveal a narrowed antrum with marked thickening of the gastric wall.[148] CMV gastritis should be the major consideration in the differential diagnosis of antral narrowing and ulceration in patients with AIDS (see earlier section on Cytomegalovirus). When infectious gastritis is suspected on the basis of the radiographic findings, biopsy specimens,

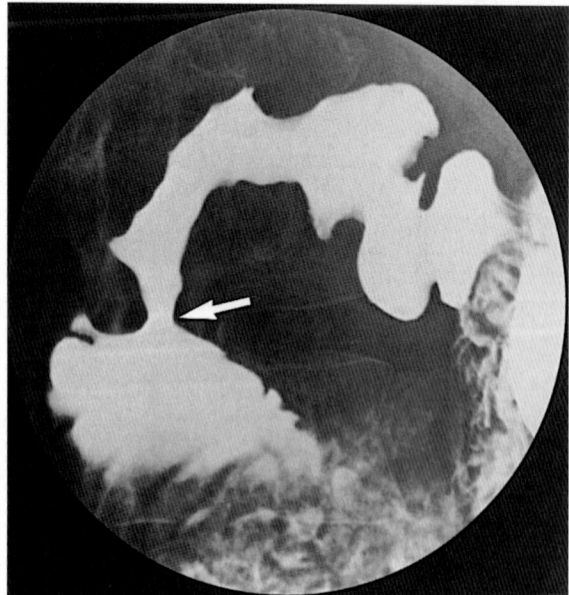

Figure 34-30. Cytomegalovirus duodenitis. There is marked narrowing and effacement of the proximal descending duodenum and a relatively abrupt transition (*arrow*) to normal-appearing duodenum more distally. This patient had AIDS. (From Mong A, Levine MS, Furth EE, et al: Cytomegalovirus duodenitis in an AIDS patient. AJR 172:939-940, 1999, © by American Roentgen Ray Society.)

brushings, or viral cultures should be obtained from the stomach for a more definitive diagnosis.

Toxoplasmosis

Opportunistic infection of the stomach by toxoplasmosis is a rare cause of antral narrowing on barium studies or of a thickened gastric wall on CT in patients with AIDS.[149,150] The diagnosis may be confirmed by demonstration of the teardrop-shaped trophozoites in histologic specimens from the stomach.[149,150] Toxoplasmosis should therefore be included in the differential diagnosis of gastric narrowing or wall thickening in HIV-positive patients.

Strongyloidiasis

Strongyloides stercoralis is a parasite of worldwide distribution that causes infection of the stomach, duodenum, and proximal small bowel.[151-153] Cases are occasionally encountered in metropolitan areas of the United States in patients who have emigrated from areas of endemic infection, such as Africa, Asia, and South America.[153] Strongyloidiasis also occurs as an opportunistic infection in patients with AIDS. Affected individuals may present with abdominal pain, nausea and vomiting, diarrhea, malabsorption, or hypoalbuminemia as a result of a protein-losing enteropathy.[152] A peripheral eosinophilia is present in 25% to 35% of cases.[152]

Radiographic Findings

Gastric involvement by strongyloidiasis may occasionally be manifested on barium studies by antral gastritis or narrowing.[151,153] However, the duodenum and proximal jejunum are more common sites of involvement. Barium studies may reveal thickened or effaced mucosal folds, ulceration, and narrowing or dilatation of the affected bowel (Fig. 34-31A).[151-153] As the disease progresses, there may be tubular narrowing of the lumen and obliteration of the normal fold pattern in the duodenum, producing a classic "lead pipe" appearance (Fig. 34-31B). Some patients may eventually develop a massively dilated duodenum, or megaduodenum (see Fig. 34-31B). Other conditions associated with a megaduodenum include Zollinger-Ellison syndrome, scleroderma, and celiac disease. Occasionally, scarring of the duodenal wall permits reflux of barium into the biliary tree via an incompetent sphincter of Oddi.[152,153] Although strongyloidiasis is rarely found in the United States, this diagnosis should be considered when barium studies reveal characteristic findings in patients with AIDS or in patients who have a recent history of travel to endemic areas.

EOSINOPHILIC GASTRITIS

Eosinophilic gastroenteritis is an unusual condition characterized by eosinophilic infiltration of the gastrointestinal tract, primarily the stomach and small bowel.[154,155] In some patients, the esophagus may be involved by this disease (see Chapter 25). Most patients with eosinophilic gastroenteritis have a peripheral eosinophilia ranging from 10% to 80%.[154,155] About half the patients have a history of allergic diseases.[155] The clinical symptoms are related to the site and extent of gastrointestinal involvement. Patients with eosinophilic gastritis

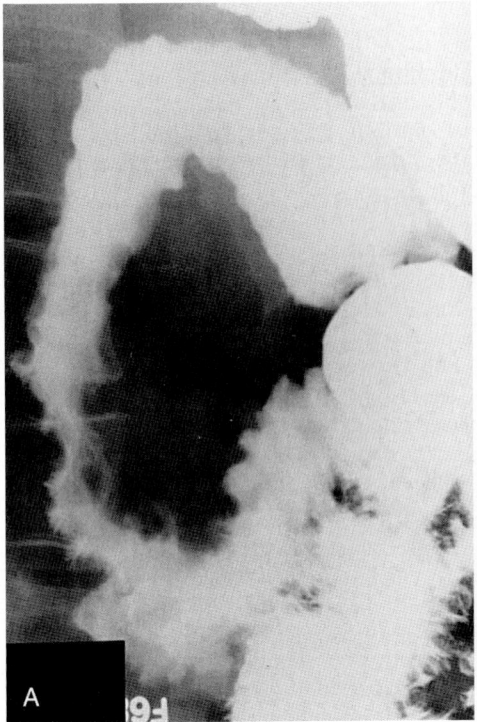 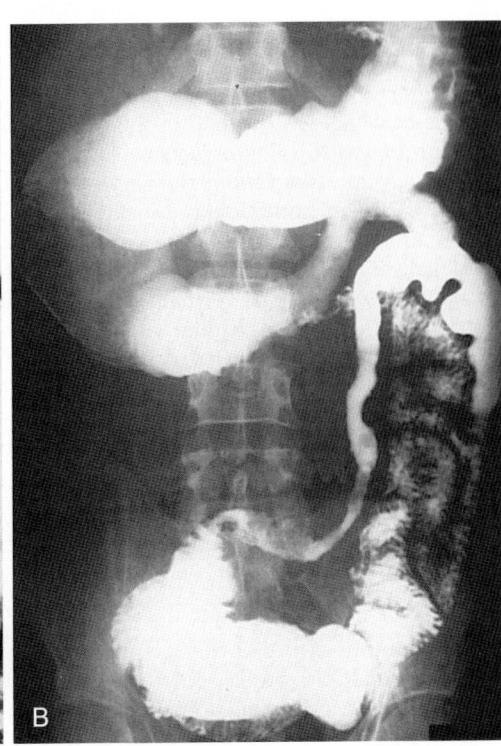

Figure 34-31. Duodenal strongyloidiasis. A. Markedly thickened, edematous folds are present in the duodenum. This patient had AIDS. **B.** In another patient with more advanced disease, there is a markedly dilated duodenum (i.e., a megaduodenum) with effaced mucosal folds. Also note the smooth, tubular appearance of the proximal jejunum, producing a lead pipe appearance. This patient had recently immigrated to the United States from an area where strongyloidiasis was endemic. (**B** courtesy of Murray K. Dalinka, MD, Philadelphia, PA.)

may present with epigastric pain, nausea and vomiting, or, less frequently, signs or symptoms of upper gastrointestinal bleeding.[154,155] In contrast, patients with eosinophilic enteritis may have diarrhea, malabsorption, or a protein-losing enteropathy.[154,155] Although treatment with corticosteroids often produces a dramatic clinical response, eosinophilic gastroenteritis is a chronic, relapsing disease with intermittent exacerbations sometimes occurring after long asymptomatic intervals.[154,155]

Radiographic Findings

Eosinophilic gastritis usually involves the antrum or antrum and body of the stomach.[154,156] Rarely, however, disease may be confined to the proximal portion of the stomach with antral sparing.[157] Barium studies may reveal mucosal nodularity, thickened folds, or narrowing and rigidity of the distal half of the stomach (Fig. 34-32).[154,158] Occasionally, severe antral narrowing may cause gastric outlet obstruction.[159] About 50% of patients with eosinophilic gastritis have concomitant involvement of the small bowel, manifested by diffuse thickening and nodularity of small bowel folds (see Chapter 47).[158]

Differential Diagnosis

When eosinophilic gastritis is manifested by thickened folds, the differential diagnosis includes antral gastritis, *H. pylori* gastritis, hypertrophic gastritis, Ménétrier's disease, Zollinger-Ellison syndrome, lymphoma, and other conditions associated with thickened folds. Despite its rarity, eosinophilic gastritis should be considered in patients who have a peripheral eosinophilia or history of allergic diseases. When eosinophilic gastritis causes antral narrowing, the differential diagnosis includes a primary scirrhous carcinoma of the

stomach, caustic ingestion, radiation, Crohn's disease, and other granulomatous conditions involving the stomach, such as sarcoidosis, tuberculosis, and syphilis. In such cases, the correct diagnosis may be suggested by the clinical history and presentation. When eosinophilic gastritis is suspected on the basis of the upper gastrointestinal examination, a small bowel follow-through should be performed to determine whether the small bowel is also involved by this disease.

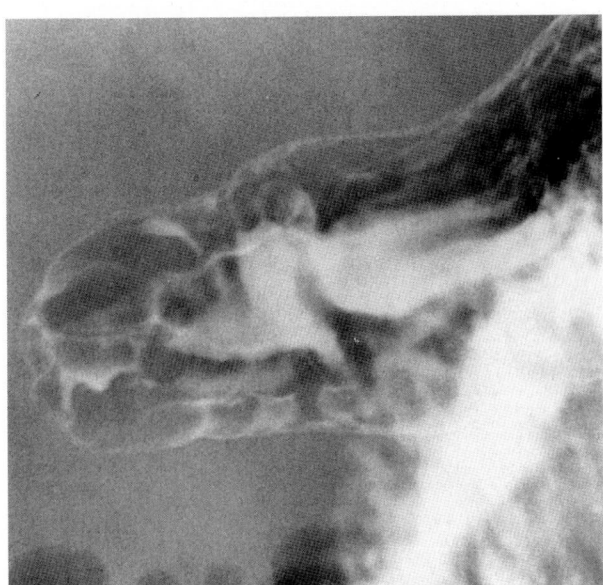

Figure 34-32. Eosinophilic gastritis. Thickened, nodular folds are seen in the gastric antrum. Other causes of antral gastritis could produce identical findings. (From Herlinger H, Maglinte D [eds]: Clinical Radiology of the Small Intestine. Philadelphia, WB Saunders, 1989.)

EMPHYSEMATOUS GASTRITIS

Emphysematous gastritis is a rare type of phlegmonous gastritis in which gas is found in the gastric wall because of infection by gas-forming organisms such as *Escherichia coli, Proteus vulgaris, Clostridium perfringens,* and *Staphylococcus aureus.*[160,161] This condition is usually caused by profound insults to the stomach, such as caustic ingestion, gastroduodenal surgery, or gastric volvulus.[160] Subsequent ischemia or necrosis permits gas-forming organisms to enter the gastric wall. Affected individuals may present with an acute, fulminating illness characterized by severe abdominal pain, hematemesis, tachycardia, fever, and shock.[160] Supportive therapy with parenteral fluids and antibiotics should be initiated, but a nasogastric tube should not be placed in the stomach because of the high risk of perforation. Despite intensive treatment, mortality rates as high as 60% have been reported.[160]

Radiographic Findings

Emphysematous gastritis is characterized on abdominal radiographs by multiple streaks, bubbles, or mottled collections of gas in the wall of the stomach, silhouetting the gastric shadow (Fig. 34-33).[160,161] These intramural gas collections have a constant relationship to the stomach with changes in the patient's position, so that they can be differentiated from residue or food, which shifts to the dependent portion of the stomach on upright or decubitus views.[160] Studies with

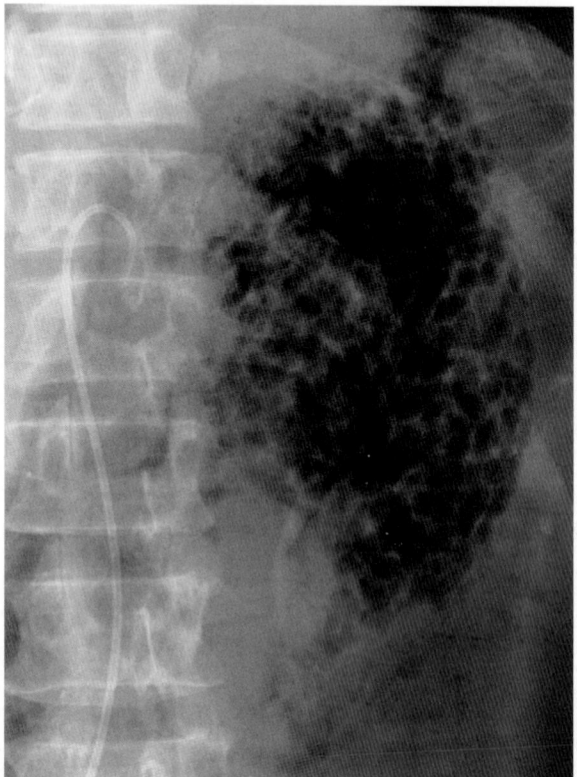

Figure 34-33. Emphysematous gastritis. Close-up view from an abdominal radiograph shows numerous mottled and bubbly collections of gas in the wall of the stomach. An attempted embolization of a gastric carcinoma led to gastric necrosis and subsequent infection by gas-forming organisms.

water-soluble contrast agents may be performed to confirm the extraluminal location of these gas collections. In other patients, intramural dissection or actual extravasation of contrast medium may be demonstrated. Occasionally, CT may reveal small collections of gas in the gastric wall that are not recognized on abdominal radiographs.[162]

Differential Diagnosis

Emphysematous gastritis must be differentiated from other rare conditions known as gastric emphysema and gastric pneumatosis. In contrast to emphysematous gastritis, gastric emphysema is characterized by long, linear collections of intramural gas that extend circumferentially around the stomach (see Chapter 38).[161,163] In gastric emphysema, gas is thought to enter the wall of the stomach via mucosal rents caused by increased intraluminal pressure associated with gastric outlet obstruction or by iatrogenic trauma resulting from endoscopy or other gastric instrumentation. Despite the dramatic radiographic findings, affected individuals are often asymptomatic. Thus, gastric emphysema can usually be differentiated from emphysematous gastritis by clinical and radiographic criteria.

Gastric pneumatosis is an extremely rare form of pneumatosis intestinalis in which multiple gas-filled cysts or blebs are found in the wall of the stomach.[161] This condition much more commonly involves the small bowel or colon (see Chapter 16). When present in the stomach, the gas-filled intramural cysts may be indistinguishable from the bubbly gas collections associated with emphysematous gastritis. However, patients with gastric pneumatosis are usually asymptomatic, whereas patients with emphysematous gastritis are acutely ill. Thus, these conditions can be differentiated on the basis of the clinical history and presentation.

CAUSTIC INGESTION

Accidental or intentional ingestion of caustic agents may lead to severe injury of the upper gastrointestinal tract. Although the esophagus is more commonly involved (see Chapter 25), gastroduodenal injury may also occur. The esophagus is classically damaged by strong alkaline agents such as liquid lye (i.e., concentrated sodium hydroxide), whereas the stomach and duodenum are more likely to be damaged by strong acids such as hydrochloric, sulfuric, acetic, oxalic, carbolic, and nitric acid. Nevertheless, esophageal injury often occurs in patients who ingest strong acids, and gastroduodenal injury occurs in 5% to 10% of patients who ingest strong alkali.[164] Pathologically, injury to the stomach and duodenum occurs in three phases, including (1) an acute necrotic phase 1 to 4 days after caustic ingestion; (2) an ulceration-granulation phase 5 to 28 days after caustic ingestion; and (3) a final phase of cicatrization and scarring beginning 3 to 4 weeks after caustic ingestion.[164,165]

Patients with gastroduodenal injury by caustic agents may present with severe abdominal pain, nausea, vomiting, hematemesis, fever, and shock.[165,166] Studies with water-soluble contrast agents are sometimes performed to assess the extent and severity of injury to the upper gastrointestinal tract. In patients who are stable and have no evidence of perforation, conservative treatment can be initiated with antibiotics, corticosteroids, and parenteral feedings.[166] After a latent period of 3 to 4 weeks, however, many patients develop rapidly progressive gastric outlet obstruction because of antral scarring and fibrosis.[166] As a result, a gastroenterostomy or partial gastrectomy is sometimes required in these individuals.[165]

Radiographic Findings

Ingested caustic agents tend to flow down the lesser curvature of the stomach into the antrum, causing severe pylorospasm that delays emptying into the duodenum.[167] As a result, the lesser curvature and distal antrum of the stomach sustain the greatest degree of damage, whereas the duodenum is relatively spared.[167] During the acute phase of injury, studies with water-soluble contrast agents may reveal thickened folds, ulceration, gastric atony, or mural defects resulting from edema and hemorrhage.[167] In fulminating cases, gastric necrosis may be manifested on abdominal radiographs or CT by streaky, bubbly, or mottled collections of intramural gas that are unaffected by changes in the patient's position.[168] These intramural collections may result either from mechanical disruption of the wall or from secondary infection by gas-forming organisms.[168] In such cases, studies with water-soluble contrast agents may reveal a confined perforation with intramural dissection of contrast medium or loculated perigastric collections (Fig. 34-34). Rarely, these studies may reveal free perforation into the peritoneal cavity. A case of delayed gastric perforation 2 days after ingestion of hydrochloric acid has been reported in which necrosis of the gastric wall was recognized on CT by absence of the normally enhancing mucosa and remaining gastric wall.[169]

If patients survive the acute illness, barium studies performed 4 weeks or more after caustic ingestion may reveal progressive narrowing and deformity of the antrum or antrum and body of the stomach.[167,170] In some patients the narrowed antrum may have a smooth, tubular configuration (Fig. 34-35A), whereas in others it may have a more irregular contour, mimicking the appearance of a primary scirrhous

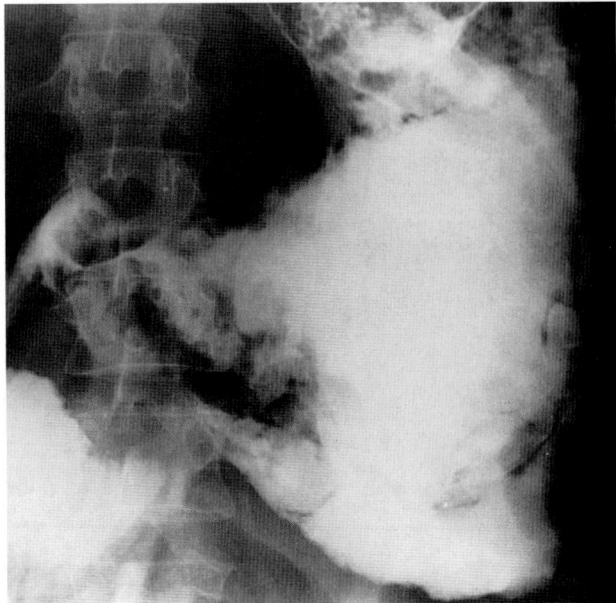

Figure 34-34. Severe gastric injury caused by caustic ingestion. Study with water-soluble contrast medium shows a grossly abnormal stomach with intramural dissection of contrast medium and numerous mural defects resulting from edema and hemorrhage after acid ingestion.

carcinoma of the stomach (Fig. 34-36).[167,171] Other conditions in the differential diagnosis of antral narrowing include Crohn's disease, sarcoidosis, tuberculosis, syphilis, radiation, and severe scarring from peptic ulcer disease. However, the diagnosis of caustic injury is usually apparent from the clinical history. About 20% of patients with antral scarring from caustic ingestion have associated esophageal scarring (Fig. 34-35B).[170]

Because caustic agents cause intense pylorospasm (which has a protective effect on the duodenum), the duodenal

Figure 34-35. Caustic scarring of the stomach and esophagus. A. Double-contrast study of the stomach shows marked antral narrowing and deformity as a result of scarring from previous lye ingestion. **B.** Esophagogram shows an associated stricture in the esophagus, extending distally from the carina (*arrows*) to the gastroesophageal junction. Aspirated barium is also present in both main bronchi. (From Levine MS: Radiology of the Esophagus. Philadelphia, WB Saunders, 1989.)

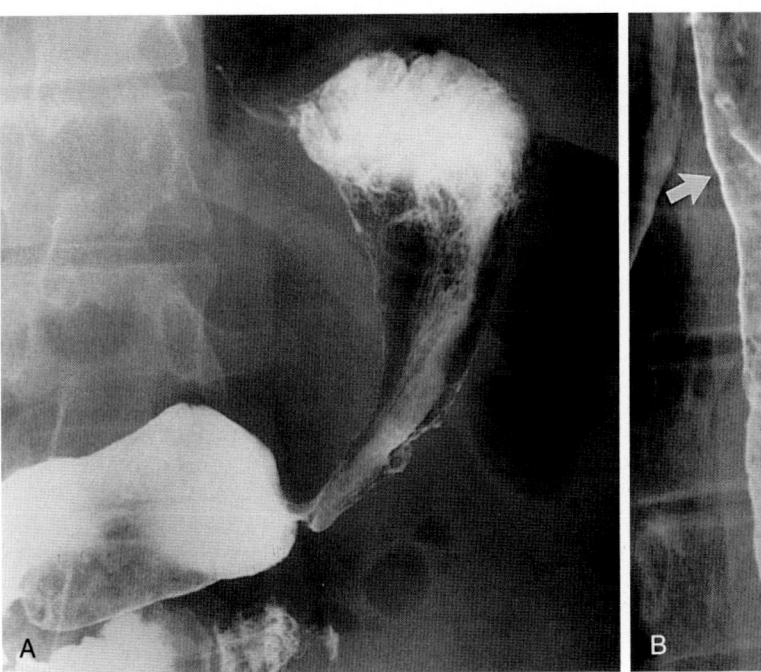
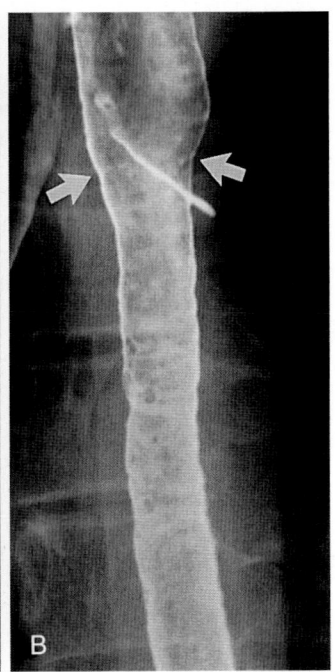

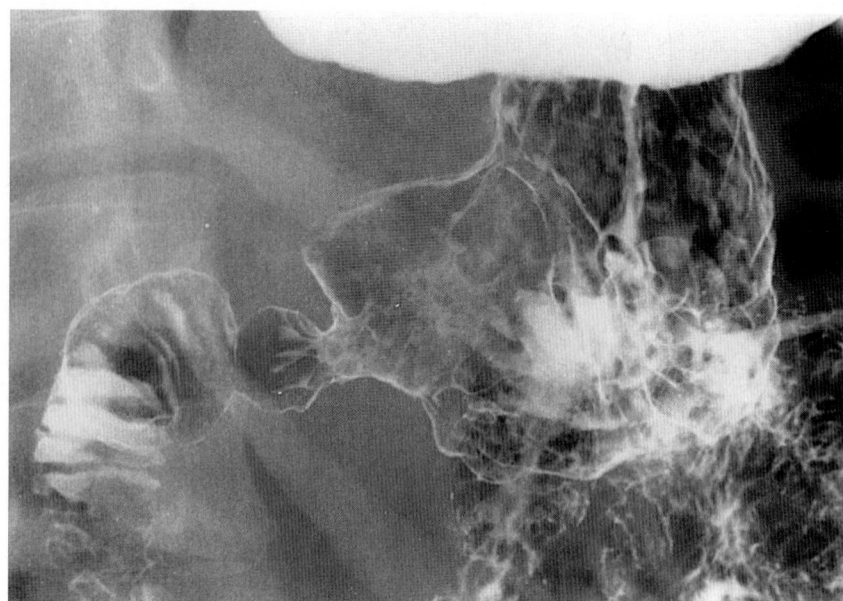

Figure 34-36. Caustic scarring of the stomach. Asymmetric narrowing and deformity of the distal antrum due to scarring are noted as a result of previous acid ingestion. This appearance could be mistaken for a scirrhous carcinoma of the antrum. The duodenum appears normal.

bulb and sweep may appear normal in patients with marked antral scarring (see Fig. 34-36). Occasionally, however, severe duodenal injury may be manifested on barium studies by thickened folds, spasm, atony, ulceration, and, eventually, strictures in the duodenum anywhere from the bulb to the ligament of Treitz.[167] These patients almost always have evidence of associated gastric injury.

RADIATION

Radiation doses of 50 Gy or more to the upper abdomen may cause significant injury to the stomach and duodenum when these structures are included in the radiation portal.[172-174] The distal antrum and pyloric region are most commonly affected, but the duodenal sweep may also be involved in patients who have received radiation to the right upper quadrant. Inflammatory changes in the stomach and duodenum typically occur 1 to 6 months after radiation therapy, whereas scarring and fibrosis occur 6 months or more after treatment.[172,173] Affected individuals may present with dyspepsia, epigastric pain, nausea, vomiting, or signs or symptoms of upper gastrointestinal bleeding.[172,173] Although the symptoms may suggest peptic ulcer disease, the possibility of radiation injury should be considered in any patient who has received radiation therapy to the upper abdomen during the previous 12 months.

Radiographic Findings

The acute phase of radiation injury to the stomach may be manifested radiographically by gastroparesis, spasm, thickened folds, or ulceration, predominantly involving the distal antrum and pyloric region and, occasionally, the duodenum.[172-174] Rarely, perforation of deep ulcers may result in acute peritonitis.[172] Subsequent scarring may lead to the development of antral or, less commonly, duodenal narrowing 6 months or more after completion of radiation therapy.[172,174] In such cases, CT may reveal luminal narrowing with non-specific gastric wall thickening and stranding in the perigastric fat.[174] Rarely, the narrowed antrum may have an irregular contour, simulating a scirrhous carcinoma of the stomach.[175]

FLOXURIDINE TOXICITY

Because floxuridine (5-FUDR) is extracted almost completely by the liver after infusion into the hepatic artery it is the agent of choice for hepatic artery infusion chemotherapy in patients with unresectable liver metastases. In the past, 5-FUDR was administered via catheters placed percutaneously into the hepatic artery, but surgically implantable infusion pumps have replaced external catheter systems at many hospitals as the primary means of delivering 5-FUDR into the liver in patients with liver metastases.[176] Although uncommon, gastroduodenal inflammation, ulceration, and bleeding may occur as a direct complication of this form of chemotherapy.

Pathogenesis

In patients who are receiving 5-FUDR via catheters placed percutaneously into the hepatic artery, gastroduodenal toxicity occurs because the drug is infused directly into vessels supplying the stomach and duodenum, such as the gastroduodenal and right gastric arteries. In patients who have hepatic artery infusion pumps, the gastroduodenal and right gastric arteries are surgically ligated at the time of pump placement to prevent overflow of the drug into these vessels. Despite such precautions, gastroduodenal toxicity has been reported as a complication of 5-FUDR therapy via a hepatic artery infusion pump,[177-179] presumably because of the development of small collateral channels between the hepatic artery and the gastroduodenal or right gastric arteries after these vessels have been ligated. Whatever the explanation, it is important to recognize that severe gastroduodenal toxicity may occur as a complication of hepatic artery infusion of 5-FUDR not only via an external catheter system but also via an implantable pump.

Clinical Findings

Gastroduodenal toxicity should be suspected when patients who are receiving hepatic artery infusion of 5-FUDR develop intractable nausea, vomiting, epigastric pain, or signs or symptoms of upper gastrointestinal bleeding.[179] Although the possibility of metastatic tumor may be considered in these patients, the temporal relationship between 5-FUDR therapy and the onset of symptoms should suggest the correct diagnosis. In most cases, cessation of chemotherapy produces rapid clinical improvement.

Radiographic Findings

Gastroduodenal toxicity resulting from 5-FUDR may be manifested on barium studies by gastroduodenal ulceration or by severe gastritis or duodenitis with markedly thickened, edematous folds in the stomach or duodenum (Fig. 34-37).[179-182] Ischemia, bleeding, vasculitis, or other inflammatory or infectious conditions may produce similar findings. However, the temporal relationship between 5-FUDR therapy and the onset of symptoms should suggest the correct diagnosis.

DUODENITIS

The pathophysiology of duodenitis is controversial. Because this condition is often associated with gastric hyperacidity, it has been postulated that duodenitis represents part of the spectrum of peptic ulcer disease.[183-185] However, some patients with duodenitis have normal or even decreased gastric acid secretion, so that it may be a distinct clinical entity unrelated to peptic ulcer disease.[186-188] Other data suggest that *H. pylori* may also have a role in the development of this condition.[189]

Whatever the pathophysiology, duodenitis is thought to be an important cause of upper gastrointestinal symptoms, including dyspepsia, epigastric pain, nausea, fatty food intolerance, and early satiety.[183,184,187,190] Less frequently, erosive duodenitis may be associated with signs or symptoms of upper gastrointestinal bleeding, such as hematemesis, melena, or guaiac-positive stool.[187]

Radiographic Findings

The diagnosis of duodenitis may be suggested on barium studies in patients who have a spastic, irritable duodenal bulb or thickened, nodular folds in the proximal duodenum (Fig. 34-38).[191] For reasons that are unclear, patients with chronic renal failure who are undergoing dialysis often have enlarged duodenal folds to a degree rarely encountered in other patients with duodenitis (Fig. 34-39).[192,193] However, thickened folds are sometimes present on barium studies in patients in whom there is no endoscopic or histologic evidence of inflammation, so that duodenitis has not generally been considered to be a reliable radiologic diagnosis.[194]

With double-contrast technique, it is possible to demonstrate more subtle signs of inflammatory disease in the duodenum. This inflammation may be manifested by mucosal nodules or nodular folds or by diffuse coarsening of the mucosal surface pattern of the bulb with lucent areas surrounded by barium-filled grooves that resemble the areae gastricae in the stomach.[194-196] With double-contrast technique, it is also possible to diagnose erosive duodenitis, a condition previously thought to be solely in the domain of the endoscopist.[6,194,196] These erosions may be found in the duodenal bulb or, less commonly, in the descending duodenum. As in the stomach, incomplete erosions appear as tiny flecks of barium in the duodenum, whereas complete or varioliform erosions appear as central barium collections surrounded by radiolucent halos of edematous mucosa (Fig. 34-40).[6,194,196] False-positive radiologic diagnoses may occasionally result from normal mucosal pits in the duodenum that are mistaken for incomplete erosions on double-contrast studies (Fig. 34-41).[197] Thus, a confident diagnosis of erosive duodenitis can be made only when true varioliform erosions are demonstrated.

Some patients with celiac disease (nontropical sprue) may have severe duodenitis with thickened folds, nodular

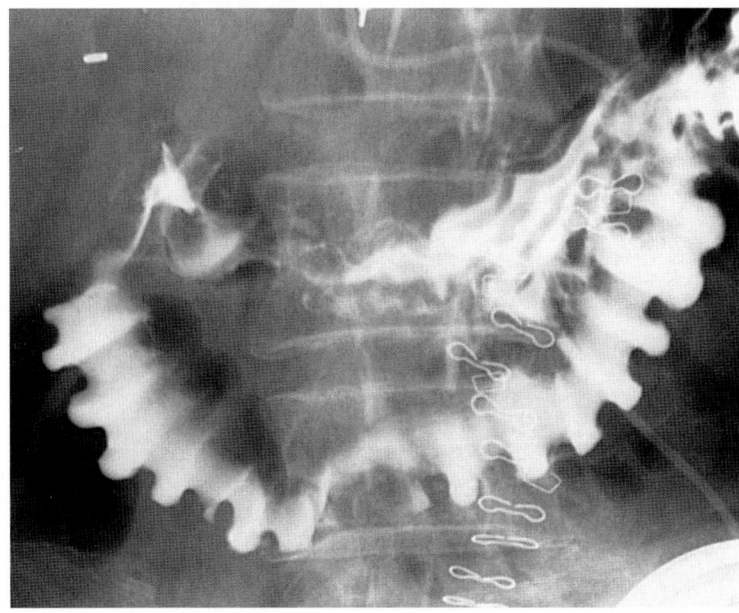

Figure 34-37. Severe duodenitis caused by 5-floxuridine (FUDR) toxicity. A barium study shows markedly thickened, edematous folds in the duodenum to the level of the ligament of Treitz. This patient was receiving 5-FUDR via a hepatic artery infusion pump. (Reprinted from, by permission of the publisher, Hiehle JF, Levine MS: Gastrointestinal toxicity of 5-FU and 5-FUDR: Radiographic findings. Can Assoc Radiol J 42:109-112, 1991.)

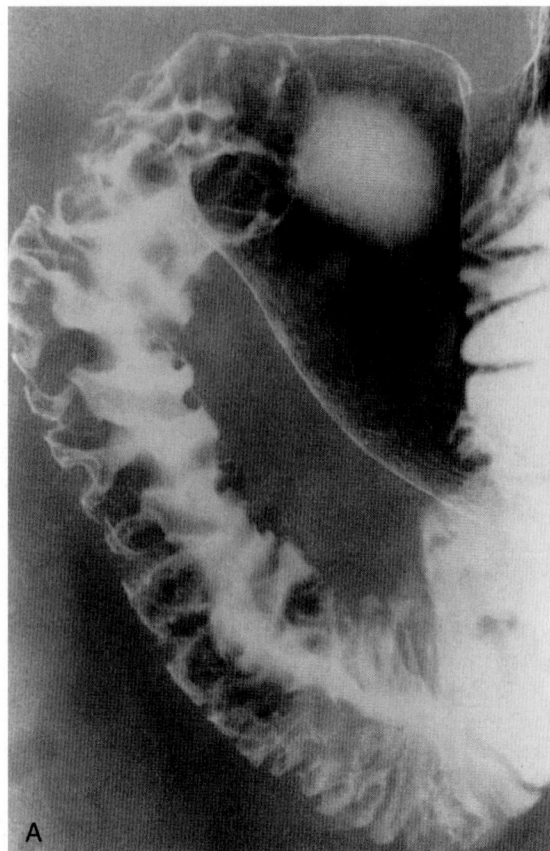

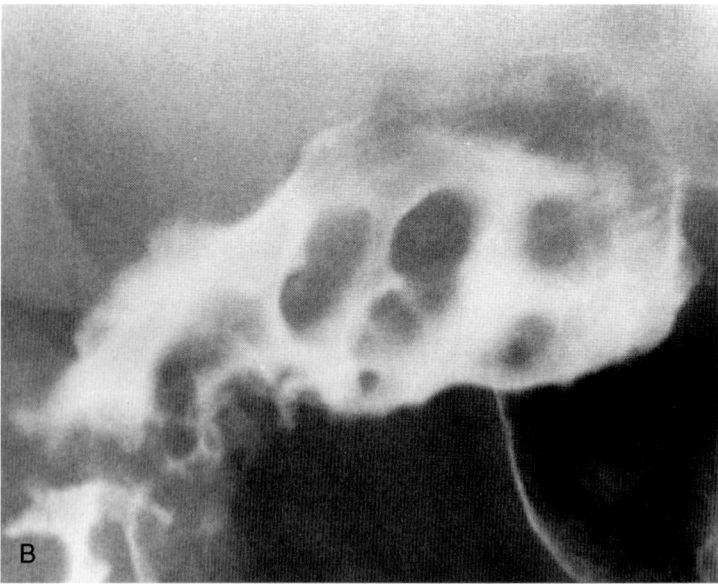

Figure 34-38. Duodenitis. A. Thickened, irregular folds are seen in the proximal duodenum. **B.** In another patient, thickened folds and mucosal nodularity are present in the duodenal bulb.

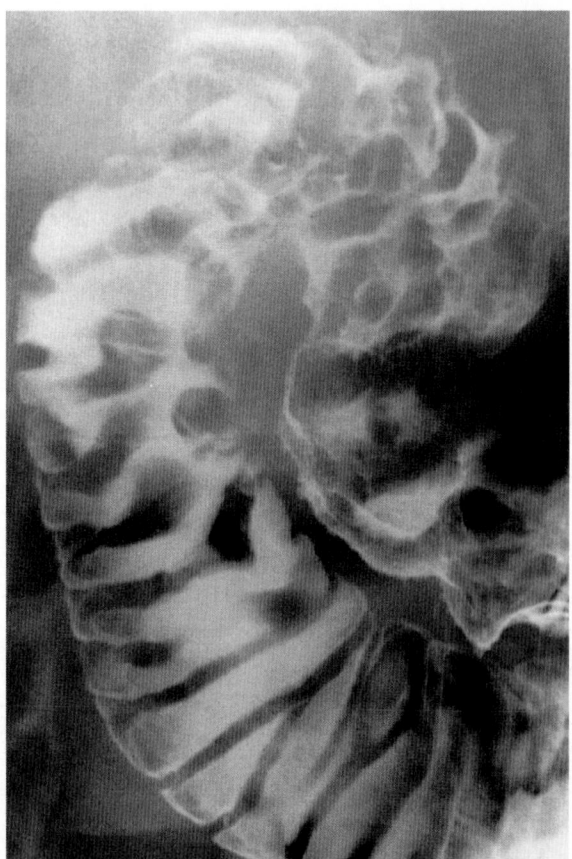

Figure 34-39. Severe duodenitis associated with chronic renal failure. Grossly thickened, polypoid folds are seen in the proximal duodenum. This patient was undergoing dialysis for chronic renal failure. (From Laufer I, Levine MS [eds]: Double Contrast Gastrointestinal Radiology, 2nd ed. Philadelphia, WB Saunders, 1992.)

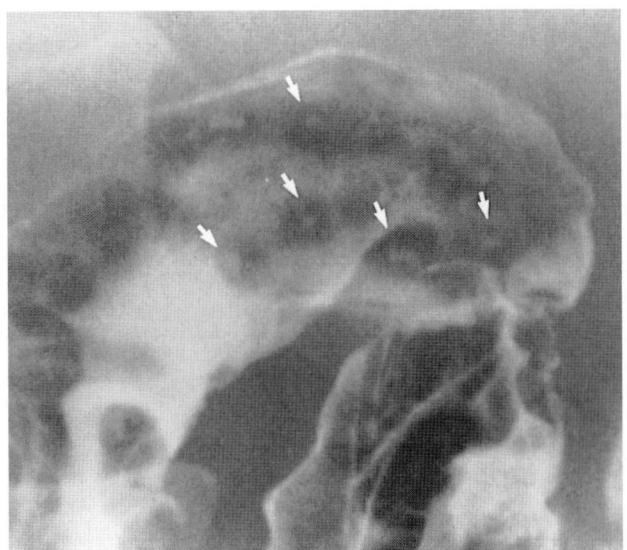

Figure 34-40. Erosive duodenitis. Varioliform erosions are seen in the duodenum as tiny flecks of barium surrounded by radiolucent mounds of edematous mucosa (*arrows*). (From Levine MS, Rubesin SE, Herlinger H, et al: Double-contrast upper gastrointestinal examination: technique and interpretation. Radiology 168:593-602, 1988.)

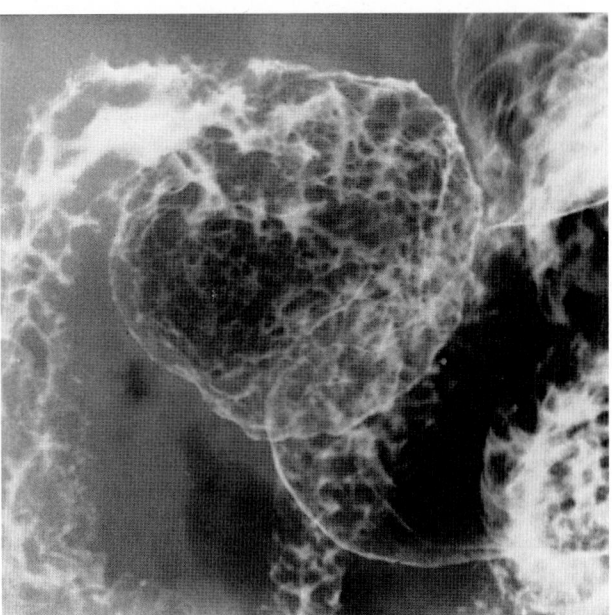

Figure 34-42. Celiac disease with a bubbly bulb. There are multiple hexagonal filling defects in the duodenal bulb and thickened, irregular folds in the descending duodenum as a result of associated duodenitis. (From Jones B, Bayless TM, Hamilton SR, et al: "Bubbly" duodenal bulb in celiac disease: Radiologic-pathologic correlation. AJR 142:119-122, 1984, © by American Roentgen Ray Society.)

mucosa, ulcers, or strictures in the descending duodenum.[198,199] Others may have small (1 to 4 mm), hexagonal filling defects in the duodenal bulb, producing a distinctive mosaic pattern or "bubbly" bulb (Fig. 33-42).[200] In contrast to heterotopic gastric mucosa, which predominantly involves the juxtapyloric region of the bulb (see Chapter 35), these nodules tend to be distributed more diffusely throughout the bulb. The presence of a bubbly bulb or thickened duodenal folds should therefore suggest the possibility of celiac disease in patients with

malabsorption. A small bowel enema or small bowel biopsy may be required for a definitive diagnosis (see Chapter 47).

Duodenitis may also be caused by Crohn's disease, caustic ingestion, radiation, 5-FUDR toxicity, and infectious processes such as tuberculosis and strongyloidiasis. These conditions and their radiographic findings are discussed elsewhere in this chapter. Finally, duodenitis may occur in patients with underlying pancreatitis involving the head of the pancreas. In such cases, the correct diagnosis is suggested by thickened, spiculated duodenal folds associated with widening of the duodenal sweep or compression of the medial aspect of the descending duodenum (see Chapter 38). When underlying pancreatitis is suspected as the cause of these findings, CT should be performed for a more definitive diagnosis.

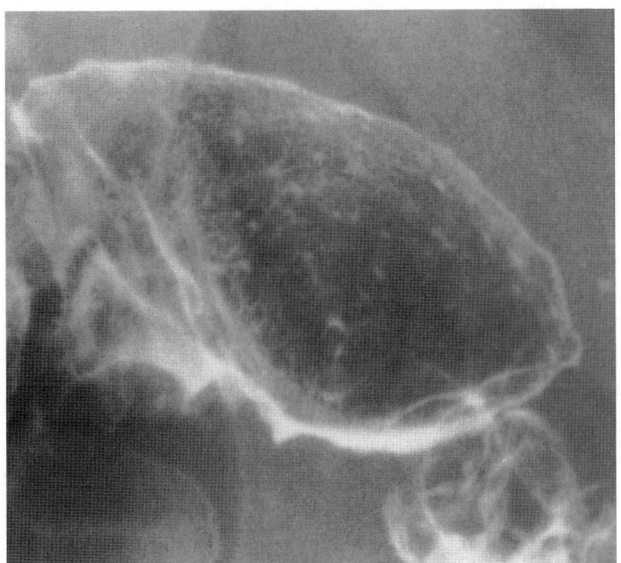

Figure 34-41. Mucosal pits simulating erosive duodenitis. Punctate collections of barium trapped in tiny, epithelialized pits can be mistaken for duodenal erosions. However, these collections are not surrounded by radiolucent mounds of edema. (From Bova JG, Kamath V, Tio FO, et al: The normal mucosal surface pattern of the duodenal bulb: Radiologic-histologic correlation. AJR 145:735-738, 1985, © by American Roentgen Ray Society.)

References

1. Poplack W, Paul RE, Goldsmith M, et al: Demonstration of erosive gastritis by the double-contrast technique. Radiology 117:519-521, 1975.
2. Laufer I: An assessment of the accuracy of double contrast gastroduodenal radiology. Gastroenterology 71:874-878, 1976.
3. Op den Orth JO, Dekker W: Gastric erosions: Radiological and endoscopic aspects. Radiol Clin (Belg) 45:88-89, 1976.
4. Op den Orth JO, Dekker W: Gastric polyps or erosions. AJR 129:357-358, 1977.
5. Tragardh B, Wehlin L, Ohashi K: Radiologic appearance of complete gastric erosions. Acta Radiol Diagn (Stockh) 19:634-642, 1978.
6. Catalano D, Pagliari U: Gastroduodenal erosions: Radiological findings. Gastrointest Radiol 7:235-240, 1982.
7. Dheer S, Levine MS, Redfern RO, et al: Radiographically diagnosed antral gastritis: Findings in patients with and without *Helicobacter pylori* infection. Br J Radiol 75:805-811, 2002.
8. Lanza F, Royer G, Nelson R: An endoscopic evaluation of the effects of non-steroidal anti-inflammatory drugs on the gastric mucosa. Gastrointest Endosc 21:103-105, 1975.
9. Roberts DM: Chronic gastritis, alcohol, and non-ulcer dyspepsia. Gut 13:768-774, 1972.

10. Laufer I, Trueman T: Multiple superficial gastric erosions due to Crohn's disease of the stomach: Radiologic and endoscopic diagnosis. Br J Radiol 49:726-728, 1976.

11. Ariyama J, Wehlin L, Lindstrom CG, et al: Gastroduodenal erosions in Crohn's disease. Gastrointest Radiol 5:121-125, 1980.

12. Cronan J, Burrell M, Trepeta R: Aphthoid ulcerations in gastric candidiasis. Radiology 134:607-611, 1980.

13. Rumerman J, Rubesin SE, Levine MS, et al: Gastric ulceration caused by heater probe coagulation. Gastrointest Radiol 13:200-202, 1988.

14. Laufer I, Hamilton J, Mullens JE: Demonstration of superficial gastric erosions by double contrast radiography. Gastroenterology 68:387-391, 1975.

15. MacDonald WC: Correlation of mucosal histology and aspirin intake in chronic gastric ulcer. Gastroenterology 65:381-389, 1973.

16. Silvoso GR, Ivey KJ, Butt JH, et al: Incidence of gastric lesions in patients with rheumatic disease on chronic aspirin therapy. Ann Intern Med 91:517-520, 1979.

17. O'Laughlin JC, Hoftiezer JW, Ivey KJ: Effect of aspirin on the human stomach in normals: Endoscopic comparison of damage produced one hour, 24 hours, and 2 weeks after administration. Scand J Gastroenterol 16:211-214, 1981.

18. Lanza FL, Nelson RS, Rack MF: A controlled endoscopic study comparing the toxic effects of sulindac, naproxen, aspirin, and placebo on the gastric mucosa of healthy volunteers. J Clin Pharmacol 24:89-95, 1984.

19. Graham DY, Smith JL, Dobbs SM: Gastric adaptation occurs with aspirin administration in man. Dig Dis Sci 28:1-6, 1983.

20. McLean AM, Paul RE, Philipps E, et al: Chronic erosive gastritis-clinical and radiological features. J Can Assoc Radiol 33:158-162, 1982.

21. McAdam WAF, Morgan AG, Jackson A, et al: Multiple persisting idiopathic gastric erosions. Gut 16:410, 1975.

22. Kikuchi Y, Levine MS, Laufer I, et al: Value of flow technique for double contrast examination of the stomach. AJR 147:1183-1184, 1986.

23. Levine MS, Verstandig A, Laufer I: Serpiginous gastric erosions caused by aspirin and other nonsteroidal anti-inflammatory drugs. AJR 146:31-34, 1986.

24. Laveran-Stiebar RL, Laufer I, Levine MS: Greater curvature antral flattening: A radiologic sign of NSAID-related gastropathy. Abdom Imaging 19:295-297, 1994.

25. Catalano O: Greater curvature antral flattening due to nonsteroidal antiinflammatory drugs. Fortschr Rontgenstr 167:122-124, 1997.

26. Balthazar EJ, Megibow AJ, Hulnick DH: Cytomegalovirus esophagitis and gastritis in AIDS. AJR 144:1201-1204, 1985.

27. Turner CJ, Lipitz LR, Pastore RA: Antral gastritis. Radiology 113:305-312, 1974.

28. Cho KC, Gold BM, Printz DA: Multiple transverse folds in the gastric antrum. Radiology 164:339-341, 1987.

29. Seymour EQ, Meredith HC: Antral and esophageal rimple: A normal variation. Gastrointest Radiol 3:147-149, 1978.

30. Glick SN, Cavanaugh B, Teplick SK: The hypertrophied antral-pyloric fold. AJR 145:547-549, 1985.

31. Arora R, Levine MS, Harvey RT, et al: Hypertrophied antral-pyloric fold: Reassessment of radiographic findings in 40 patients. Radiology 213:347-351, 1999.

32. Lewis TD, Laufer I, Goodacre RL: Arteriovenous malformation of the stomach: Radiologic and endoscopic features. Am J Dig Dis 23:467-470, 1978.

33. Warren JR, Marshall BJ: Unidentified curved bacilli on gastric epithelium in active chronic gastritis. Lancet 2:1273-1275, 1983.

34. Kuipers EJ, Uyterlinde AM, Pena AS, et al: Long-term sequelae of Helicobacter pylori gastritis. Lancet 345:1525-1528, 1995.

35. Pattison CP, Combs MJ, Marshall BJ: Helicobacter pylori and peptic ulcer disease: Evolution to revolution to resolution. AJR 168:1450-1420, 1997.

36. Appelman HD: Gastritis: Terminology, etiology, and clinicopathological correlations: another biased view. Hum Pathol 25:1006-1019, 1994.

37. Bayerdorffer E, Lehn N, Hatz R, et al: Difference in expression of Helicobacter pylori gastritis in antrum and body. Gastroenterology 102:1575-1582, 1992.

38. Suerbaum S, Michetti P: Helicobacter pylori infection. N Engl J Med 347:1175-1186, 2002.

39. Dooley CP, Cohen H, Fitzgibbons PL, et al: Prevalence of Helicobacter pylori infection and histologic gastritis in asymptomatic patients. N Engl J Med 321:1562-1566, 1989.

40. Hopkins RJ: Current FDA-approved treatments for Helicobacter pylori and the FDA approval process. Gastroenterology 113:S126-S130, 1997.

41. NIH Consensus Development Panel on Helicobacter pylori in peptic ulcer disease: Helicobacter pylori in peptic ulcer disease. JAMA 272:65-69, 1994.

42. International Update Conference on Helicobacter pylori: The Report of the Digestive Health Initiative International Update Conference on Helicobacter pylori. Gastroenterology 113:S4-S8, 1997.

43. McColl K, Murray L, El-Omar E, et al: Symptomatic benefit from eradicating Helicobacter pylori infection in patients with nonulcer dyspepsia. N Engl J Med 339:1869-1874, 1998.

44. Blum AL, Talley NJ, O'Morain C, et al: Lack of effect of treating Helicobacter pylori infection in patients with nonulcer dyspepsia. N Engl J Med 339:1875-1881, 1998.

45. Talley NJ, Vakil N, Ballard ED, et al: Absence of benefit of eradicating Helicobacter pylori in patients with nonulcer dyspepsia. N Engl J Med 341:1106-1111, 1999.

46. Cutler AF, Havstad S, Ma CK, et al: Accuracy of invasive and non-invasive tests to diagnose Helicobacter pylori infection. Gastroenterology 109:136-141, 1995.

47. Thijs JC, van Zwet AA, Thijs WJ, et al: Diagnostic tests for Helicobacter pylori: A prospective evaluation of their accuracy, without selecting a single test as the gold standard. Am J Gastroenterol 91:2125-2129, 1996.

48. Morrison S, Dahms BB, Hoffenberg E, et al: Enlarged gastric folds in association with Campylobacter pylori gastritis. Radiology 171:819-821, 1989.

49. Sohn J, Levine MS, Furth EE, et al: Helicobacter pylori gastritis: Radiographic findings. Radiology 195:763-767, 1995.

50. Mond DJ, Pochaczevsky R, Vernace F, et al: Can the radiologist recognize Helicobacter pylori gastritis? J Clin Gastroenterol 20:199-202, 1995.

51. Crocker JD, Bender GN: Antral nodularity, fold thickness, and narrowing: Signs on the upper gastrointestinal series that may indicate chronic active gastritis secondary to Helicobacter pylori. Invest Radiol 30:4 80-483, 1995.

52. Rubesin SE, Furth EE, Levine MS: Gastritis from NSAIDs to Helicobacter pylori. Abdom Imaging 30:142-159, 2005.

53. Rose C, Stevenson GW: Correlation between visualization and size of the areae gastricae and duodenal ulcer. Radiology 139:371-374, 1981.

54. Watanabe H, Magota S, Shiiba S, et al: Coarse areae gastricae in the proximal body and fundus: A sign of gastric hypersecretion. Radiology 146:303-306, 1983.

55. Genta RM, Hamner HW, Graham DY: Gastric lymphoid follicles in Helicobacter pylori infection: Frequency, distribution, and response to triple therapy. Hum Pathol 24:577-583, 1993.

56. Genta RM, Hamner HW: The significance of lymphoid follicles in the interpretation of gastric biopsy specimens. Arch Pathol Lab Med 118:740-743, 1994.

57. Wyatt JI, Rathbone BJ: Immune response of the gastric mucosa to Campylobacter pylori. Scand J Gastroenterol Suppl 142:44-49, 1988.

58. Torigian DA, Levine MS, Gill NS, et al: Lymphoid hyperplasia of the stomach: Radiographic findings in five adult patients. AJR 177:71-75, 2001.

59. Chaloupka JC, Gay BB, Caplan D: Campylobacter gastritis simulating Ménétrier's disease by upper gastrointestinal radiography. Pediatr Radiol 20:200-201, 1990.

60. Urban BA, Fishman EK, Hruban RH: Helicobacter pylori gastritis mimicking gastric carcinoma at CT evaluation. Radiology 179:689-691, 1991.

61. Yoo CC, Levine MS, Furth EE, et al: Gastric mucosa-associated lymphoid tissue lymphoma: Radiographic findings in six patients. Radiology 208:239-243, 1998.

62. Stempien SJ, Dagradi AE, Reingold IM, et al: Hypertrophic hypersecretory gastropathy. Am J Dig Dis 9:471-493, 1964.

63. Tan DTD, Stempien SJ, Dagradi AE: The clinical spectrum of hypertrophic hypersecretory gastropathy. Gastrointest Endosc 18:69-73, 1971.

64. Moghadam M, Gluckmann R, Eyler WR: The radiological assessment of gastric acid output. Radiology 89:888-895, 1967.

65. Press AJ: Practical significance of gastric rugal folds. AJR 125:172-183, 1975.

66. Balthazar EJ, Davidian MM: Hyperrugosity in gastric carcinoma: Radiographic, endoscopic, and pathologic features. AJR 136:531-535, 1981.

67. Fieber SS, Rickert RR: Hyperplastic gastropathy. Am J Gastroenterol 76:321-329, 1981.

68. Wolfsen HC, Carpenter HA, Talley NJ: Ménétrier's disease: A form of hypertrophic gastropathy or gastritis? Gastroenterology 104:1310-1319, 1993.

69. Scharschmidt BF: The natural history of hypertrophic gastropathy (Ménétrier's disease). Am J Med 63:644-652, 1977.

70. Jarnum S, Jensen KB: Plasma protein turnover (albumin, transferrin, IgG, IgM) in Ménétrier's disease (giant hypertrophic gastritis): Evidence of non-selective protein loss. Gut 13:128-137, 1972.

71. Searcy RM, Malagelada JR: Ménétrier's disease and idiopathic hypertrophic gastropathy. Ann Intern Med 100:560-565, 1984.

72. Rubin RG, Fink H: Giant hypertrophy of the gastric mucosa associated with carcinoma of the stomach. Am J Gastroenterol 47:379-388, 1967.

73. Williams SM, Harned RK, Settles RH: Adenocarcinoma of the stomach in association with Ménétrier's disease. Gastrointest Radiol 3:387-390, 1978.

74. Reese DF, Hodgson JR, Dockerty MB: Giant hypertrophy of the gastric mucosa (Ménétrier's disease): A correlation of the roentgenographic, pathologic, and clinical findings. AJR 88:619-626, 1962.

75. Olmsted WW, Cooper PH, Madewell JE: Involvement of the gastric antrum in Ménétrier's disease. AJR 126:524-529, 1976.

76. Maxfield DL, Boyd WC: Pernicious anemia: A review, an update, and an illustrative case. J Am Osteopath Assoc 8:133-142, 1983.

77. Jeffries GH, Sleisenger MH: Studies of parietal cell antibody in pernicious anemia. J Clin Invest 44:2021-2038, 1965.

78. Joske RA, Finckh ES, Wood IJ: Gastric biopsy: A study of 1,000 consecutive successful gastric biopsies. Q J Med 24:269-294, 1955.

79. Strickland RG, Mackay IR: A reappraisal of the nature and significance of chronic atrophic gastritis. Am J Dig Dis 18:426-440, 1973.

80. Furth EE, Rubesin SE, Levine MS: Pathologic primer on gastritis: An illustrated sum and substance. Radiology 197:693-698, 1995.

81. Kuipers EJ, Klinkenberg-Knol EC, Vandenbroucke-Grauls JE, et al: Role of *Helicobacter pylori* in the pathogenesis of atrophic gastritis. Scand J Gastroenterol 32(Suppl):28-34, 1997.

82. Sozzi M, Valentini M, Figura N, et al: Atrophic gastritis and intestinal metaplasia in *Helicobacter pylori* infection: The role of CagA status. Am J Gastroenterol 93:375-379, 1998.

83. Elsborg L, Mosbech J: Pernicious anaemia as a risk factor in gastric cancer. Acta Med Scand 206:315-318, 1979.

84. Cheli R, Santi L, Ciancamerla G, et al: A clinical and statistical follow-up study of atrophic gastritis. Am J Dig Dis 18:1061-1066, 1973.

85. Siurala M, Lehtola J, Ihamaki T: Atrophic gastritis and its sequelae: Results of 19-23 years follow-up examinations. Scand J Gastroenterol 9:441-446, 1974.

86. Borch K: Epidemiologic, clinicopathologic, and economic aspects of gastroscopic screening of patients with pernicious anemia. Scand J Gastroenterol 21:21-30, 1986.

87. Asaka M, Takeda H, Sugiyama T, et al: What role does *Helicobacter pylori* play in gastric cancer? Gastroenterology 113:S56-S60, 1997.

88. Laws JW, Pitman RG: The radiological features of pernicious anaemia. Br J Radiol 33:229-237, 1960.

89. Levine MS, Palman CL, Rubesin SE, et al: Atrophic gastritis in pernicious anemia: Diagnosis by double-contrast radiography. Gastrointest Radiol 14:215-219, 1989.

90. Mackintosh CE, Kreel L: Anatomy and radiology of the areae gastricae. Gut 18:855-864, 1977.

91. Levine MS, Kong V, Rubesin SE, et al: Scirrhous carcinoma of the stomach: Radiologic and endoscopic diagnosis. Radiology 175:151-154, 1990.

92. Levine MS: Crohn's disease of the upper gastrointestinal tract. Radiol Clin North Am 25:79-91, 1987.

93. Danzi JT, Farmer RG, Sullivan BH, et al: Endoscopic features of gastroduodenal Crohn's disease. Gastroenterology 70:9-13, 1976.

94. Nugent FW, Richmond M, Park SK: Crohn's disease of the duodenum. Gut 18:115-120, 1977.

95. Wagtmans MJ, Verspaget HW, Lamers CB, et al: Clinical aspects of Crohn's disease of the upper gastrointestinal tract: A comparison with distal Crohn's disease. Am J Gastroenterol 92:1467-1470, 1997.

96. Metzger WH, Ranganath KA: Crohn's disease presenting as a gastrocolic fistula. Am J Gastroenterol 65:258-261, 1976.

97. Kokal W, Pickleman J, Steinberg JJ: Gastrocolic fistula in Crohn's disease. Surg Gynecol Obstet 146:701-704, 1978.

98. Marshak RH, Maklansky D, Kurzban JD, et al: Crohn's disease of the stomach and duodenum. Am J Gastroenterol 77:340-343, 1982.

99. Gray RR, Grosman H: Crohn's disease involving the proximal stomach. Gastrointest Radiol 10:43-45, 1985.

100. Legge DA, Carlson HC, Judd ES: Roentgenologic features of regional enteritis of the upper gastrointestinal tract. AJR 110:355-360, 1970.

101. Beaudin D, DaCosta LR, Prentice RSA, et al: Crohn's disease of the stomach. Am J Dig Dis 18:623-629, 1973.

102. Kelvin FM, Gedgaudas RK: Radiologic diagnosis of Crohn's disease (with emphasis on its early manifestations). Crit Rev Diagn Imaging 16:43-91, 1981.

103. Farman J, Faegenburg D, Dallemand S, et al: Crohn's disease of the stomach: the "ram's horn" sign. AJR 123:242-251, 1975.

104. Nelson SW: Some interesting and unusual manifestations of Crohn's disease ("regional enteritis") of the stomach, duodenum, and small intestine. AJR 107:86-101, 1969.

105. Zegel HG, Laufer I: Filiform polyposis. Radiology 127:615-619, 1978.

106. Laufer I, Joffe N, Stolberg H: Unusual causes of gastrocolic fistula. Gastrointest Radiol 2:21-25, 1977.

107. Patel M, Banerjee B, Block JG, et al: Gastric Crohn's disease complicated by adenocarcinoma of the stomach: Case report and review of the literature. Am J Gastroenterol 92:1368-1371, 1997.

108. Thompson WM, Cockrill H, Rice RP: Regional enteritis of the duodenum. AJR 123:252-261, 1975.

109. Herlinger H, O'Riordan D, Saul S, et al: Nonspecific involvement of bowel adjoining Crohn's disease. Radiology 159:47-51, 1986.

110. Laufer I, Thornley GD, Stolberg H: Gastrocolic fistula as a complication of benign gastric ulcer. Radiology 119:7-11, 1976.

111. Bilbao MK, Frische LH, Rosch J, et al: Postbulbar duodenal ulcer and ring-stricture. Radiology 100:27-35, 1971.

112. Palmer ED: Note on silent sarcoidosis of the gastric mucosa. J Lab Clin Med 52:231-234, 1958.

113. Chinitz MA, Brandt LJ, Frank MS, et al: Symptomatic sarcoidosis of the stomach. Dig Dis Sci 30:682-688, 1985.

114. Dunbar RD: Sarcoidosis and its radiologic manifestations. Crit Rev Diagn Imaging 28:185-220, 1978.

115. Levine MS, Ekberg O, Rubesin SE, et al: Gastrointestinal sarcoidosis: Radiographic findings. AJR 153:293-295, 1989.

116. Farman J, Ramirez G, Rybak B, et al: Gastric sarcoidosis. Abdom Imaging 22:248-252, 1997.

117. Bellan L, Semelka R, Warren CPW: Sarcoidosis as a cause of linitis plastica. J Can Assoc Radiol 39:72-74, 1988.

118. Chazan BI, Aitchison JD: Gastric tuberculosis. BMJ 2:1288-1290, 1960.

119. Thoeni RF, Margulis AR: Gastrointestinal tuberculosis. Semin Roentgenol 14:283-294, 1979.

120. Brody JM, Miller DK, Zeman RK, et al: Gastric tuberculosis: A manifestation of acquired immunodeficiency syndrome. Radiology 159:342-348, 1986.

121. Subei I, Attar B, Schmitt G, et al: Primary gastric tuberculosis. Am J Gastroenterol 82:769-772, 1987.

122. Misra D, Rai RR, Nundy S, et al: Duodenal tuberculosis presenting as bleeding peptic ulcer. Am J Gastroenterol 83:203-204, 1988.

123. Nair KV, Pai CG, Rajogopal KP, et al: Unusual presentations of duodenal tuberculosis. Am J Gastroenterol 86:756-760, 1991.

124. Pinto RS, Zausner J, Beranbaum ER: Gastric tuberculosis. AJR 110:808-812, 1970.

125. Jadvar H, Mindelzun RE, Olcott EW, et al: Still the great mimicker: Abdominal tuberculosis. AJR 168:1455-1460, 1997.

126. Black GA, Carsky EW: Duodenal tuberculosis. AJR 131:329-330, 1978.

127. Tishler JMA: Duodenal tuberculosis. Radiology 130:593-595, 1979.

128. Gupta SK, Jain AK, Gupta JP, et al: Duodenal tuberculosis. Clin Radiol 39:159-161, 1988.

129. Schwartz DT, Garnes HA, Lattimer JK, et al: Pyeloduodenal fistula due to tuberculosis. J Urol 104:373-375, 1970.

130. Cooley RN, Childers JH: Acquired syphilis of the stomach. Gastroenterology 39:201-207, 1960.

131. Reisman TN, Leverett FL, Hudson JR, et al: Syphilitic gastropathy. Am J Dig Dis 20:588-593, 1975.

132. Sachar DB, Klein RS, Swerdlow F, et al: Erosive syphilitic gastritis: Dark-field and immunofluorescent diagnosis from biopsy specimen. Ann Intern Med 80:512-515, 1974.

133. Jones BV, Lichtenstein JE: Gastric syphilis: Radiologic findings. AJR 160:59-61, 1993.

134. Anai H, Okada Y, Okubo K, et al: Gastric syphilis simulating linitis plastica type of gastric cancer. Gastrointest Endosc 36:624-626, 1990.

135. Fisher JR, Sanowski RA: Disseminated histoplasmosis producing hypertrophic gastric folds. Am J Dig Dis 23:282-285, 1978.

136. Nelson RS, Bruni HC, Goldstein HM: Primary gastric candidiasis in uncompromised subjects. Gastrointest Endosc 22:92-94, 1975.

137. Van Olmen G, Larmuseau MF, Geboes K, et al: Primary gastric actinomycosis. Am J Gastroenterol 79:512-516, 1984.

138. Lawson H, Schmaman A: Gastric phycomycosis. Br J Surg 61:743-746, 1974.

139. Rotterdam H, Tsang P: Gastrointestinal disease in the immuno-compromised patient. Hum Pathol 25:1123-1140, 1994.

140. Falcone S, Murphy BJ, Weinfeld A: Gastric manifestations of AIDS: Radiographic findings on upper gastrointestinal examination. Gastrointest Radiol 16:95-98, 1991.

141. Farman J, Lerner ME, Ng C, et al: Cytomegalovirus gastritis: Protean radiologic manifestations. Gastrointest Radiol 17:202-206, 1992.

142. Agel NM, Tanner P, Drury A, et al: Cytomegalovirus gastritis with perforation and gastrocolic fistula formation. Histopathology 18:165-168, 1991.

143. Wilcox CM, Schwartz DA: Symptomatic CMV duodenitis. J Clin Gastroenterol 14:293-297, 1992.

144. Mong A, Levine MS, Furth EE, et al: Cytomegalovirus duodenitis in an AIDS patient. AJR 172:939-940, 1999.

145. Buhles WC, Mastre BJ, Tinker AJ, et al: Ganciclovir treatment of life- or sight-threatening cytomegalovirus infection: Experience in 314 immunocompromised patients. Rev Infect Dis 10(Suppl 3):S495-S506.

146. Berk RN, Wall SD, McArdle CB, et al: Cryptosporidiosis of the stomach and small intestine in patients with AIDS. AJR 143:549-554, 1984.

147. Ventura G, Cauda R, Larocca LM, et al: Gastric cryptosporidiosis complicating HIV infection: Case report and review of the literature. Eur J Gastroenterol Hepatol 9:307-310, 1997.

148. Soulen MC, Fishman EK, Scatarige JC, et al: Cryptosporidiosis of the gastric antrum: Detection using CT. Radiology 159:705-706, 1986.

149. Smart PE, Weinfeld A, Thompson NE, et al: Toxoplasmosis of the stomach: A cause of antral narrowing. Radiology 174:369-370, 1990.

150. Alpert L, Miller M, Alpert E, et al: Gastric toxoplasmosis in acquired immunodeficiency syndrome: Antemortem diagnosis with histopathologic characterization. Gastroenterology 110:258-264, 1996.

151. Louisy CL, Barton CJ: The radiological diagnosis of *Strongyloides stercoralis* enteritis. Radiology 98:535-541, 1971.

152. Berkman YM, Rabinowitz J: Gastrointestinal manifestations of strongyloidiasis. AJR 115:306-311, 1972.

153. Dallemand S, Waxman M, Farman J: Radiological manifestations of *Strongyloides stercoralis*. Gastrointest Radiol 8:45-51, 1983.

154. Goldberg HI, O'Kieffe D, Jenis EH, et al: Diffuse eosinophilic gastroenteritis. AJR 119:342-351, 1973.

155. Vitellas KM, Bennett WF, Bova JG, et al: Radiographic manifestations of eosinophilic gastroenteritis. Abdom Imaging 20:406-413, 1995.

156. Burhenne HJ, Carbone JV: Eosinophilic (allergic) gastroenteritis. AJR 96:332-338, 1966.

157. Balfe DM: Eosinophilic gastritis. AJR 152:1322, 1989.

158. Wehunt WD, Olmsted WW, Neiman HL, et al: Eosinophilic gastritis. Radiology 120:85-89, 1976.

159. Freundlich IM, Schaupp R, Lehman JS: Eosinophilic gastroenteritis: A case report with extensive jejunal involvement. Radiology 86:493-495, 1966.

160. Meyers HJ, Parker JJ: Emphysematous gastritis. Radiology 89:426-431, 1967.

161. Nelson SW: Extraluminal gas collections due to diseases of the gastrointestinal tract. AJR 115:225-248, 1972.

162. Monteferrante M, Shimkin P: CT diagnosis of emphysematous gastritis. AJR 153:191-192, 1989.

163. Schorr S, Marcus M: Intramural gastric emphysema. Br J Radiol 35:641-644, 1962.

164. Franken EA: Caustic damage of the gastrointestinal tract: Roentgen features. AJR 118:77-85, 1973.

165. Citron BP, Pincus IJ, Geokas MC, et al: Chemical trauma of the esophagus and stomach. Surg Clin North Am 48:1303-1311, 1968.

166. Goldman LP, Weigert JM: Corrosive substance ingestion: A review. Am J Gastroenterol 79:85-90, 1984.

167. Muhletaler CA, Gerlock AJ, de Soto L, et al: Gastroduodenal lesions of ingested acids: Radiographic findings. AJR 135:1247-1252, 1980.

168. Levitt R, Stanley RJ, Wise L: Gastric bullae: An early roentgen finding in corrosive gastritis following alkali ingestion. Radiology 115:597-598, 1975.

169. Kanne JP, Gunn M, Blackmore CC: Delayed gastric perforation resulting from hydrochloric acid ingestion. AJR 185:682-683, 2005.

170. Poteshman NL: Corrosive gastritis due to hydrochloric acid ingestion. AJR 99:182-185, 1967.

171. Kleinhaus U, Rosenberger A, Adler O: Early and late radiological features of damage to the stomach caused by acid ingestion. Radiol Clin (Belg) 46:26-37, 1977.

172. Roswit B, Malsky SJ, Reid CB: Severe radiation injuries of the stomach, small intestine, colon, and rectum. AJR 114:460-475, 1972.

173. Goldstein HM, Rogers LF, Fletcher GH, et al: Radiological manifestations of radiation-induced injury to the normal upper gastrointestinal tract. Radiology 117:135-140, 1975.

174. Capps GW, Fulcer AS, Szucs RA, et al: Imaging features of radiation-induced changes in the abdomen. RadioGraphics 17:1455-1473, 1997.

175. Lane D: Irradiation gastritis simulating carcinoma. Med J Aust 2:576-577, 1970.

176. Williams NN, Daly JM: Infusional versus systemic chemotherapy for liver metastases from colorectal cancer. Surg Clin North Am 69:401-410, 1989.

177. Wells JJ, Nostrant TT, Wilson JAP, et al: Gastroduodenal ulcerations in patients receiving selective hepatic artery infusion chemotherapy. Am J Gastroenterol 80:425-429, 1985.

178. Shike M, Gillin JS, Kemeny N, et al: Severe gastroduodenal ulcerations complicating hepatic artery infusion chemotherapy for metastatic colon cancer. Am J Gastroenterol 81:176-179, 1986.

179. Hiehle JF, Levine MS: Gastrointestinal toxicity of 5-FU and 5-FUDR: Radiographic findings. J Can Assoc Radiol 42:109-112, 1991.

180. Hall DA, Clouse ME, Gramm HF: Gastroduodenal ulceration after hepatic arterial infusion chemotherapy. AJR 136:1216-1218, 1981.

181. Chuang VP, Wallace S, Stroehlein J, et al: Hepatic artery infusion chemotherapy: Gastroduodenal complications. AJR 137:347-350, 1981.

182. Mann FA, Kubal WS, Ruzicka FF: Radiographic manifestations of gastrointestinal toxicity associated with intraarterial 5-fluorouracil infusion. RadioGraphics 2:329-339, 1982.

183. Thomson WO, Robertson AG, Imrie CW, et al: Is duodenitis a dyspeptic myth? Lancet 1:1197-1198, 1977.

184. Greenlaw R, Sheehan DG, DeLuca V, et al: Gastroduodenitis: A broader concept of peptic ulcer disease. Dig Dis Sci 25:660-662, 1980.

185. Sircus W: Duodenitis: A clinical, endoscopic, and histopathologic study. Q J Med 56:593-600, 1985.

186. Gelzayd EA, Gelfand DW, Rinaldo JA: Nonspecific duodenitis: A distinct clinical entity? Gastrointest Endosc 19:131-133, 1973.

187. Gelzayd EA, Biederman MA, Gelfand DW: Changing concepts of duodenitis. Am J Gastroenterol 64:213-216, 1975.

188. Collen MJ, Loebenberg MJ: Basal gastric acid secretion in nonulcer dyspepsia with or without duodenitis. Dig Dis Sci 34:246-250, 1989.

189. Wyatt JI, Rathbone BJ, Dixon MF, et al: *Campylobacter pyloridis* and acid induced gastric metaplasia in the pathogenesis of duodenitis. J Clin Pathol 40:841-848, 1987.

190. Cheli R: Symptoms in chronic non-specific duodenitis. Scand J Gastroenterol 17(Suppl):84-86, 1982.

191. Fraser GM, Pitman RG, Lawrie JH, et al: The significance of the radiological finding of coarse mucosal folds in the duodenum. Lancet 2:979-982, 1964.

192. Wiener SN, Vertes V, Shapiro H: The upper gastrointestinal tract in patients undergoing chronic dialysis. Radiology 92:110-114, 1969.

193. Zukerman GR, Mills BA, Koehler RE, et al: Nodular duodenitis: Pathologic and clinical characteristics in patients with end-stage renal disease. Dig Dis Sci 11:1018-1024, 1983.

194. Levine MS, Turner D, Ekberg O, et al: Duodenitis: A reliable radiologic diagnosis? Gastrointest Radiol 16:99-103, 1991.

195. Glick SN, Gohel VK, Laufer I: Mucosal surface patterns of the duodenal bulb. Radiology 150:317-322, 1984.

196. Gelfand DW, Dale WJ, Ott DJ, et al: Duodenitis: Endoscopic-radiologic correlation in 272 patients. Radiology 157:577-581, 1985.

197. Bova JG, Kamath V, Tio FO, et al: The normal mucosal surface pattern of the duodenal bulb: radiologic-histologic correlation. AJR 145:735-738, 1985.

198. Marn CS, Gore RM, Ghahremani GG: Duodenal manifestations of nontropical sprue. Gastrointest Radiol 11:30-35, 1986.

199. Schweiger GD, Murray JA: Postbulbar duodenal ulceration and stenosis associated with celiac disease. Abdom Imaging 23:347-349, 1998.

200. Jones B, Bayless TM, Hamilton SR, et al: "Bubbly" duodenal bulb in celiac disease: Radiologic-pathologic correlation. AJR 142:119-122, 1984.

Benign Tumors of the Stomach and Duodenum

Marc S. Levine, MD

Between 85% and 90% of all neoplasms in the stomach and duodenum are benign.[1] About half are mucosal lesions and half are submucosal. Most of these benign neoplasms are discovered fortuitously on radiologic or endoscopic studies performed for other reasons. Tumors that are large or ulcerated, however, may cause abdominal pain or upper gastrointestinal bleeding. Depending on their histologic features, some benign tumors are also important because of an associated risk of malignancy. Although gastric and duodenal polyps are rarely diagnosed on single-contrast barium studies, the use of double-contrast technique has led to greater detection of these lesions.

MUCOSAL LESIONS

Gastric polyps comprise about 50% of all benign neoplasms in the stomach.[2] Polyps are much less common in the duodenum. In the past, gastric polyps were rarely detected on single-contrast barium studies, with a reported incidence of only 0.01% to 0.05%.[3] However, the routine use of double-contrast technique has dramatically improved our ability to detect gastric polyps, with a reported incidence of 1% to 2% on double-contrast studies.[4,5] Most are small, innocuous hyperplastic polyps, but some larger lesions are adenomatous polyps that are capable of undergoing malignant degeneration

via an adenoma-carcinoma sequence similar to that in the colon. The need for endoscopic biopsy and removal of these polyps is directly related to their size and appearance. Radiologists, therefore, have an important role in the detection of gastric polyps and in subsequent decisions about patient management.

Hyperplastic Polyp

Hyperplastic polyps are by far the most common benign epithelial neoplasms in the stomach, comprising 75% to 90% of all gastric polyps.[6] Because hyperplastic polyps are not premalignant, they must be differentiated from adenomatous polyps, which have a known risk of malignant degeneration. Although histologic specimens are required for a definitive diagnosis, hyperplastic polyps have such a characteristic appearance on double-contrast barium studies that they can usually be differentiated from adenomatous polyps without need for endoscopy.

Pathology

Hyperplastic polyps consist histologically of elongated, branching, cystically dilated glandular structures.[7,8] They usually appear grossly as one or more small, sessile nodules with a smooth, dome-shaped contour. Because these polyps have a self-limited growth pattern, most are less than 1 cm.[4,8] Hyperplastic polyps rarely undergo malignant degeneration.[8,9] Nevertheless, patients with hyperplastic polyps are at increased risk for harboring separate, coexisting gastric carcinomas. In various series, 8% to 28% of patients with hyperplastic polyps in the stomach have been found to have synchronous gastric carcinomas.[7,9] This association is probably related to the presence of underlying atrophic gastritis, which predisposes to the development of both polyps and cancer.[8] Hyperplastic polyps are therefore important because of the increased risk of gastric carcinoma in these patients.

Fundic gland polyps appear to be a variant of hyperplastic polyps arising within fundic gland mucosa in the fundus and body of the stomach.[10] They consist histologically of cystically dilated, hyperplastic fundic glands that have no malignant potential.[11] Because affected individuals almost always have multiple (up to 50) gastric polyps, this entity has been called *fundic gland polyposis*.[11] Affected individuals are typically middle-aged women.[12] Fundic gland polyposis can occur as an isolated condition in the stomach but also develops in about 40% of patients with familial adenomatous polyposis syndrome (FAPS) (see Chapter 65).[13] Thus, colonoscopy is often recommended in patients with fundic gland polyposis to determine whether they have FAPS and whether colonic surveillance is warranted.

Clinical Findings

Most hyperplastic polyps are small (<1 cm), innocuous lesions that are detected as incidental findings on radiologic or endoscopic examinations.[4] Rarely, polyps that have a friable or ulcerated surface may cause low-grade upper gastrointestinal bleeding and pedunculated polyps in the gastric antrum may prolapse through the pylorus, causing intermittent symptoms of gastric outlet obstruction.[14]

Radiographic Findings

Most hyperplastic polyps in the stomach appear on double-contrast studies as smooth, sessile, round or ovoid nodules, ranging from 5 to 10 mm.[4,8] They tend to occur as multiple lesions in the gastric fundus or body (Fig. 35-1).[4] When multiple polyps are present, they also tend to be similar in size.[8]

Hyperplastic polyps on the dependent surface of the stomach (i.e., the posterior wall) typically appear on double-contrast studies as smooth, round filling defects in the barium pool, whereas polyps on the nondependent surface (i.e., the

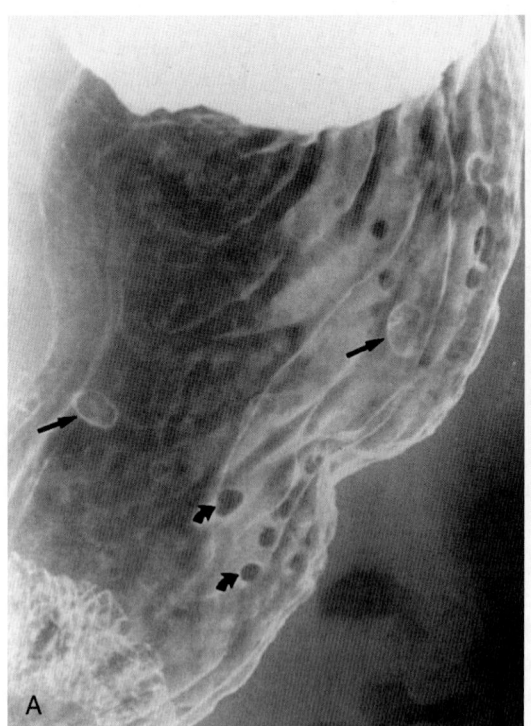
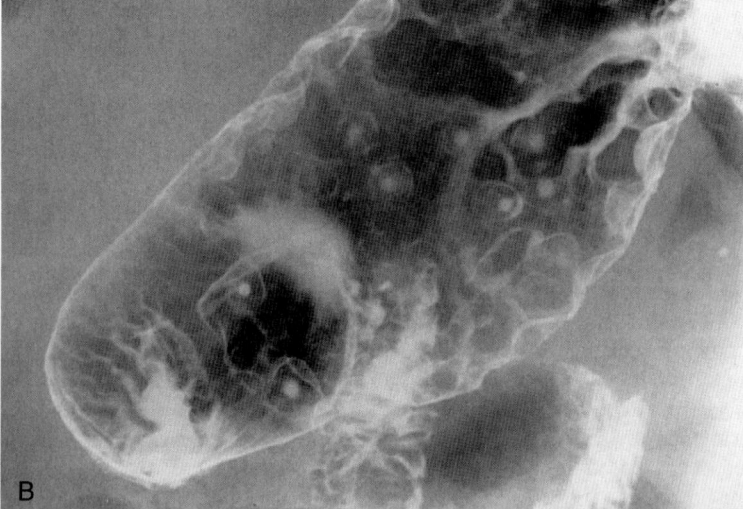
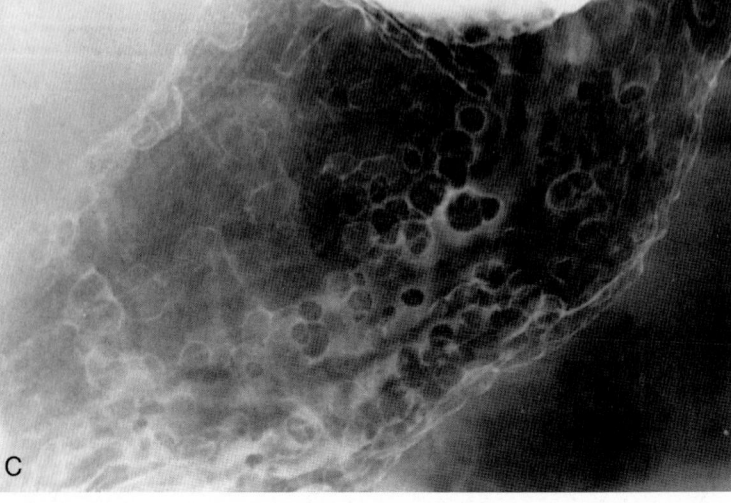

Figure 35-1. Multiple hyperplastic polyps. A. Polyps on the dependent surface or posterior wall appear as filling defects in the barium pool (*curved arrows*), whereas polyps on the nondependent surface or anterior wall are etched in white (*straight arrows*). **B.** This patient has multiple anterior wall polyps containing hanging droplets of barium, or stalactites, that could be mistaken for central areas of ulceration. **C.** Innumerable hyperplastic polyps are present in the gastric body. (**B** from Laufer I, Levine MS [eds]: Double Contrast Gastrointestinal Radiology, 2nd ed. Philadelphia, WB Saunders, 1992.)

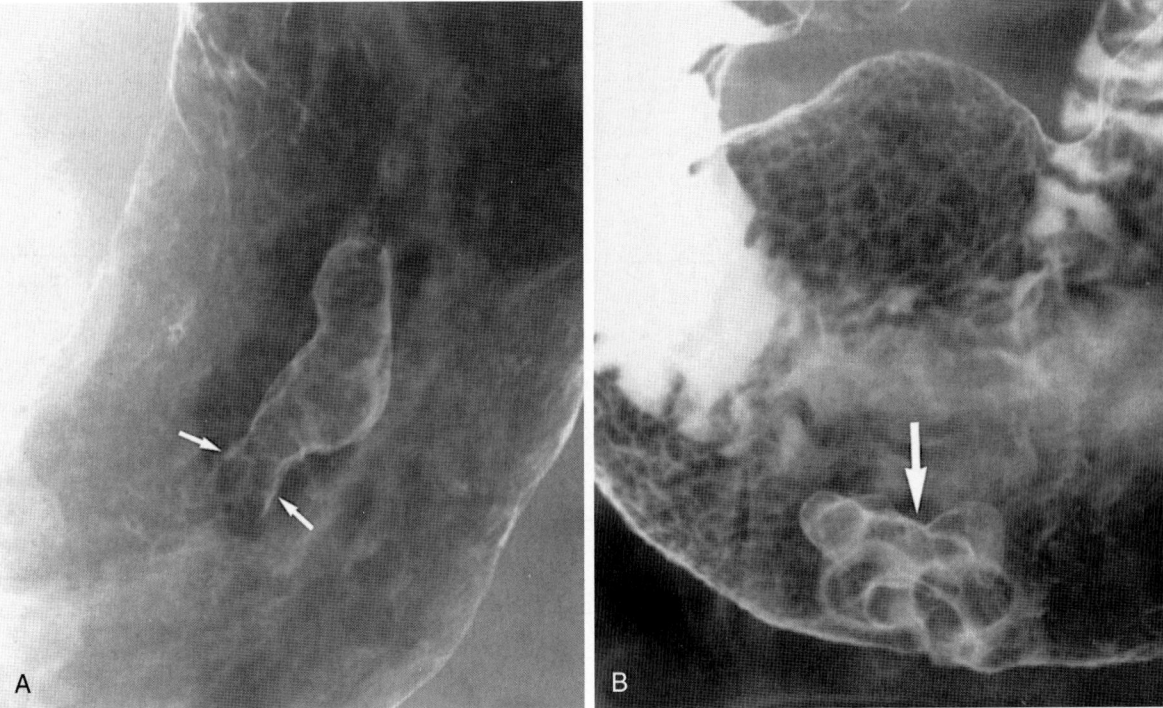

Figure 35-2. Atypical hyperplastic polyps. A. A long, pedunculated polyp is present in the gastric body. The polyp has a discrete stalk (*arrows*). This patient had pernicious anemia. **B.** A conglomerate mass of hyperplastic polyps (*arrow*) is seen in the antrum in another patient. This lesion is quite lobulated and could be mistaken for a polypoid carcinoma.

anterior wall) appear as ring shadows that are etched in white because of trapping of barium between the edge of the polyp and the adjacent mucosa (see Fig. 35-1A). A small hanging droplet of barium, or "stalactite," on a nondependent or anterior wall polyp can be mistaken en face for a central area of ulceration (see Fig. 35-1B),[15] but this droplet of barium is seen as a transient finding at fluoroscopy. Occasionally, one or more stalactites may be present as the only sign of hyperplastic polyps on the anterior wall.[16] In such cases, careful examination of the area with prone compression views should demonstrate the underlying polyps responsible for this phenomenon.

Although most hyperplastic polyps are less than 1 cm, some can be as large as 2 to 6 cm, appearing as lobulated or pedunculated lesions (Fig. 35-2).[14,17] A giant hyperplastic polyp or conglomerate mass of hyperplastic polyps can occasionally be mistaken for a polypoid gastric carcinoma (see Fig. 35-2B).[14,17] Rarely, pedunculated hyperplastic polyps in the antrum may prolapse through the pylorus into the duodenum, causing gastric outlet obstruction (Fig. 35-3).[14]

Fundic gland polyps appear on double-contrast examinations as multiple small (<1 cm), rounded nodules in the gastric fundus or body that are indistinguishable from typical hyperplastic polyps (Fig. 35-4).[11,12,18] In some patients, spontaneous regression of fundic gland polyps has been reported.[12,13,18]

Differential Diagnosis

Hyperplastic polyps that appear as ring shadows on double-contrast studies must be differentiated from shallow ulcers on the dependent or posterior gastric wall and from unfilled ulcers on the nondependent or anterior wall. With flow technique, however, ulcer craters on the dependent wall should fill with barium, producing a discrete niche or collection.[19] In

contrast, ulcers on the nondependent wall should fill with barium on prone compression views of the stomach. Thus, it is usually possible to differentiate these lesions by performing a biphasic examination that includes flow technique and prone compression.

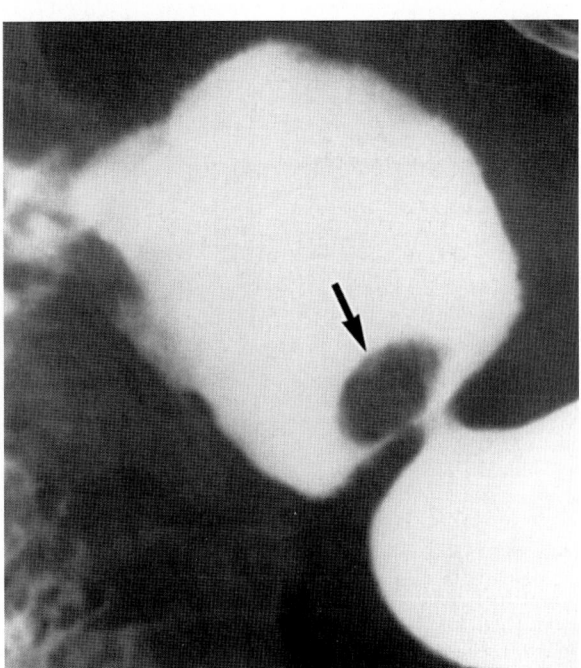

Figure 35-3. Prolapsed hyperplastic polyp. This patient has a pedunculated polyp (*arrow*) that has prolapsed from the antrum into the base of the duodenal bulb.

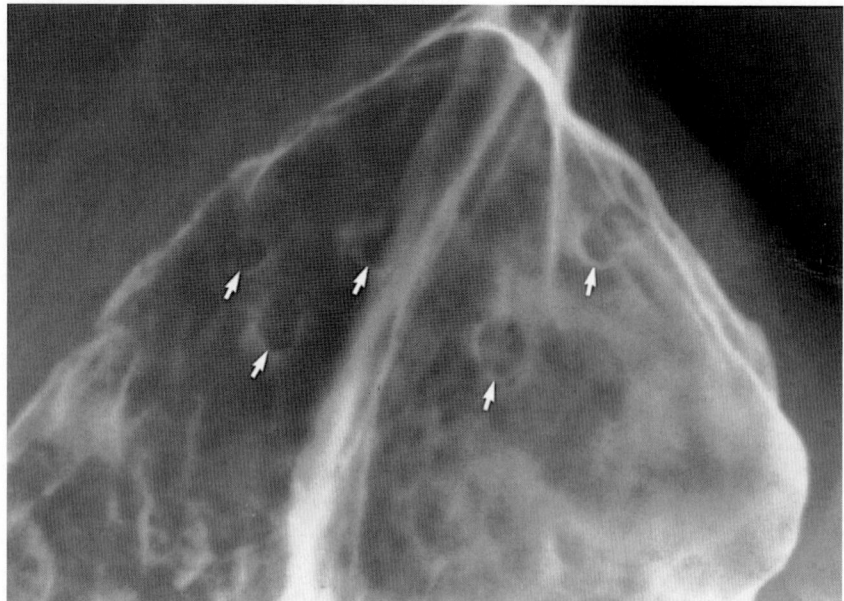

Figure 35-4. Fundic gland polyposis. Multiple tiny polyps (*arrows*) are present in the gastric fundus. These lesions have no malignant potential and are indistinguishable radiographically from hyperplastic polyps.

Polyps that appear as ring shadows must also be distinguished from "see-through" artifacts caused by overlying structures that are calcified (e.g., phleboliths) or partially filled with contrast material (e.g., barium-containing colonic diverticula). Such structures can mimic the appearance of anterior wall polyps on a single view (Fig. 35-5A), but their location outside the stomach is readily apparent on images obtained in other projections (Fig. 35-5B).

Hyperplastic polyps that have a lobulated appearance or are larger than 1 cm cannot be distinguished from adenomatous polyps on radiographic criteria. Rarely, giant hyperplastic polyps or a conglomerate mass of hyperplastic polyps can mimic the appearance of a polypoid gastric carcinoma (see Fig. 35-2B).[14,17] Thus, polyps that are unusually large or lobulated should be evaluated by endoscopy and biopsy or, if necessary, resected for a definitive diagnosis.

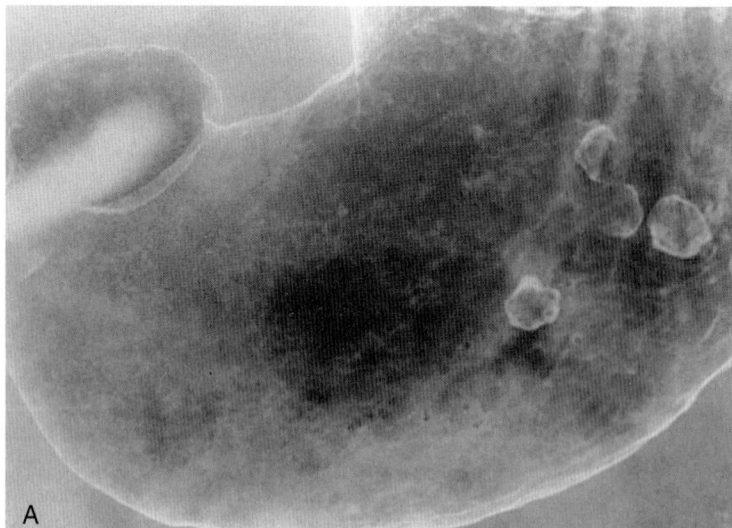

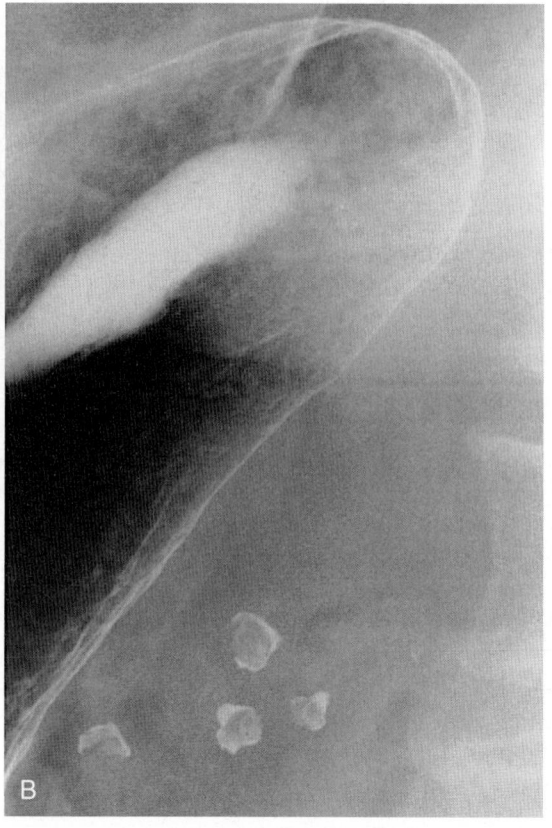

Figure 35-5. See-through artifacts mimicking hyperplastic polyps in the stomach. A. Multiple ring shadows are seen in the gastric body. These could represent hyperplastic polyps on the anterior wall that are etched in white. **B.** Lateral view shows multiple barium-filled colonic diverticula posterior to the stomach. (From Laufer I, Levine MS [eds]: Double Contrast Gastrointestinal Radiology, 2nd ed. Philadelphia, WB Saunders, 1992.)

The differential diagnosis of multiple hyperplastic polyps in the stomach includes multiple adenomatous polyps and gastric involvement by a polyposis syndrome. However, adenomatous polyps tend to be larger and less numerous and are more lobulated than most hyperplastic polyps. Both types of polyps can occur simultaneously in some patients,[14] but an adenomatous polyp should be suspected if one lesion is disproportionately larger than the others.[4] A generalized polyposis syndrome should be suspected if multiple polyps are also present in the small bowel or colon (see Chapter 65).

Management

Almost all smooth, sessile polyps less than 1 cm are hyperplastic polyps with no malignant potential. Small, round or ovoid gastric polyps detected on double-contrast studies should therefore be considered innocuous lesions without need for further investigation or treatment. Endoscopic biopsy or polypectomy should be performed, however, if the polyp is lobulated or pedunculated, if it is larger than 1 cm, or if it enlarges on follow-up radiologic studies.

Adenomatous Polyp

Adenomatous polyps constitute less than 20% of all gastric polyps.[4,5,9] Nevertheless, these polyps are important because they are capable of undergoing malignant degeneration. As a result, they must be treated more aggressively than hyperplastic polyps in the stomach.

Pathology

Adenomatous polyps are composed of dysplastic epithelium. Depending on the predominant glandular architecture, they may be classified as tubular, villous, or tubulovillous adenomas; the vast majority are tubular or mixed tubulovillous adenomas.[7] Malignant degeneration of these lesions occurs via an adenoma-carcinoma sequence similar to that in the colon. Foci of carcinoma in situ or invasive carcinoma are present in nearly 50% of resected adenomatous polyps larger than 2 cm, but malignant changes are rarely found in smaller lesions.[7,20] As in the colon, the risk of malignancy therefore depends primarily on polyp size. Nevertheless, adenocarcinoma is 30 times more common than adenomatous polyps in the stomach, so that most gastric cancers are thought to originate de novo and not from preexisting polyps.[8,9]

Adenomatous polyps are often found in the stomach in patients with chronic atrophic gastritis.[21,22] Because of the association between atrophic gastritis and gastric carcinoma (see Chapter 36), the risk of developing a separate gastric cancer may be greater than the risk of malignant degeneration in an adenomatous polyp.[8] As many as 30% to 40% of patients with adenomatous polyps in the stomach have been found to have gastric carcinomas.[8,9] Thus, detection of an adenomatous polyp in the stomach should lead to a careful search for other lesions.

Clinical Findings

Because of their greater size, adenomatous polyps in the stomach produce symptoms more frequently than hyperplastic polyps. These patients may present with epigastric pain,

bloating, upper gastrointestinal bleeding, or, rarely, symptoms of gastric outlet obstruction.[23,24]

Radiographic Findings

Most adenomatous polyps diagnosed in the stomach on barium studies are larger than 1 cm.[5,9,22] They usually occur as solitary lesions (most frequently in the antrum) (Fig. 35-6),[8,20] but multiple adenomatous polyps are sometimes found (Fig. 35-7). The polyps may be sessile or pedunculated, and they tend to be more lobulated than hyperplastic polyps (see Figs. 35-6 and 35-7). When the lesions are pedunculated, the stalk may be seen en face as an inner ring shadow overlying the head of the polyp, producing the "Mexican hat" sign that is classically found with pedunculated polyps in the colon (see Fig. 35-6B). Rarely, pedunculated antral polyps may prolapse through the pylorus, causing intermittent gastric outlet obstruction.[3]

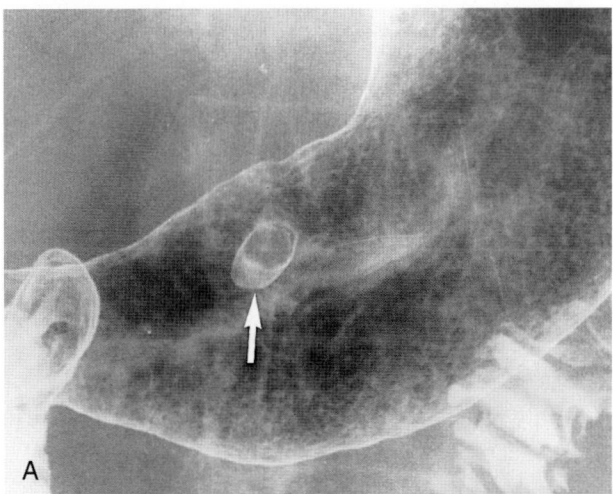

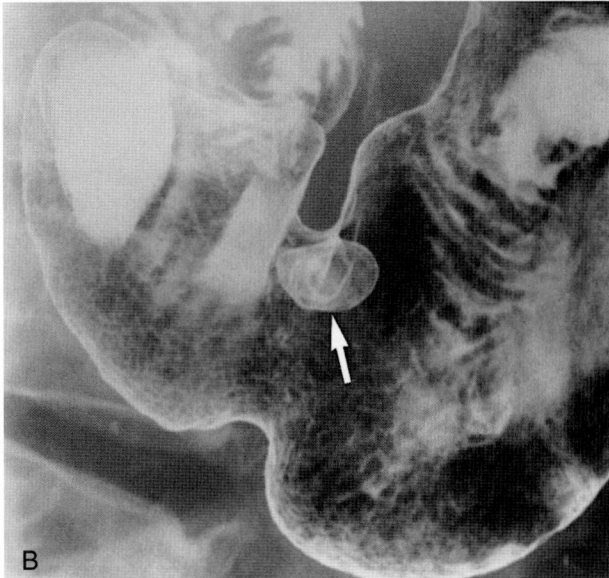

Figure 35-6. Adenomatous polyps. A. A sessile polyp (*arrow*) is present in the antrum. **B.** A pedunculated antral polyp (*arrow*) is seen in another patient. The stalk appears as an inner ring shadow overlying the head of the polyp, producing the "Mexican hat" sign. (**B** courtesy of Dean D. T. Maglinte, MD, Indianapolis, IN.)

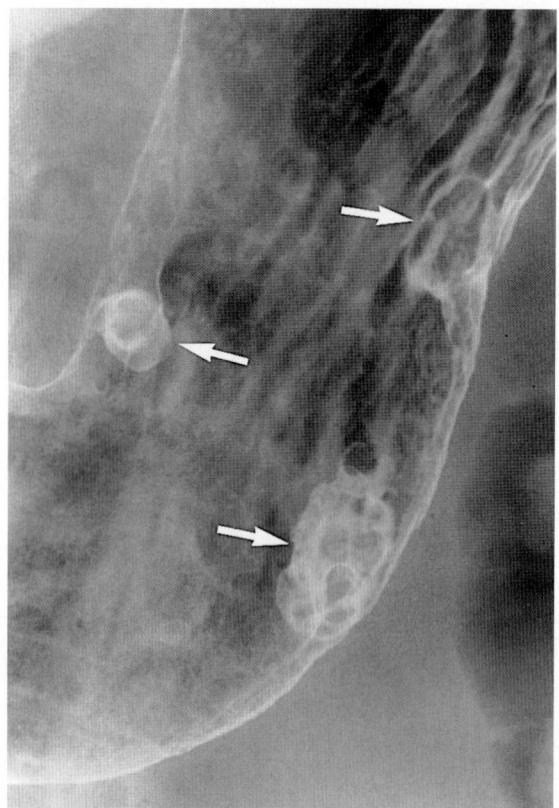

Figure 35-7. Multiple adenomatous polyps. The polyps (*arrows*) are larger and more lobulated than most hyperplastic polyps in the stomach. The most distal lesion on the greater curvature is indistinguishable from a polypoid carcinoma. (From Laufer I, Levine MS [eds]: Double Contrast Gastrointestinal Radiology, 2nd ed. Philadelphia, WB Saunders, 1992.)

As with hyperplastic polyps, lesions on the nondependent or anterior wall may be etched in white on double-contrast views. Occasionally, a hanging droplet of barium, or stalactite, on these nondependent lesions can mimic the appearance of ulceration.[15] However, adenomatous polyps are rarely ulcerated.

Differential Diagnosis

Adenomatous polyps in the stomach that appear as smooth, sessile lesions may be difficult to distinguish on barium studies from hyperplastic polyps. However, most adenomatous polyps are greater than 1 cm and they usually occur as solitary lesions whereas hyperplastic polyps are almost always smaller than 1 cm and are often multiple.[4] Adenomatous polyps that are sessile and have a smooth contour can also be mistaken for benign gastrointestinal stromal tumors (GISTs) or other submucosal lesions. Finally, adenomatous polyps that are larger and more lobulated may be indistinguishable from polypoid gastric carcinomas (see Fig. 35-7). In fact, adenomatous polyps often harbor one or more foci of carcinoma in situ or invasive carcinoma, so that aggressive management of these lesions is required.

Management

When a gastric polyp is detected on barium studies, endoscopic biopsy specimens should be obtained if the lesion has features of an adenomatous polyp (i.e., it is larger than 1 cm, is lobulated or pedunculated, or enlarges on follow-up barium studies). If biopsy specimens confirm the presence of an adenomatous polyp, it should be resected because of the risk of malignant degeneration.[25] Regardless of the endoscopic findings, polyps larger than 2 cm should always be resected because of the even greater likelihood that they are adenomatous and the high risk of malignant tumor in adenomatous polyps of this size.[3,5,9] If invasive carcinoma is present in the resected specimen, a wedge resection of the stomach or partial gastrectomy may be required.[26] As in the colon, a much more aggressive approach is therefore warranted in the management of adenomatous polyps than hyperplastic polyps because of the increased cancer risk in these patients.

Duodenal Polyp

Duodenal polyps are much less common than gastric polyps. Hyperplastic polyps (which constitute most gastric polyps) are rarely found in the duodenum. Instead, most duodenal polyps are adenomatous.[27] Because these polyps rarely cause symptoms, they are usually detected as incidental findings on radiologic or endoscopic examinations. Occasionally, however, duodenal polyps may cause low-grade upper gastrointestinal bleeding or obstructive jaundice.[28]

Radiographic Findings

Duodenal polyps usually appear on barium studies as smooth, sessile lesions in the first or second portion of the duodenum (Fig. 35-8). They tend to be less than 2 cm, but giant duodenal polyps have occasionally been described.[29] Most duodenal polyps occur as solitary lesions, but multiple adenomatous, hamartomatous, or inflammatory polyps may be found in the duodenum as part of a diffuse polyposis syndrome (see Chapter 65).

Differential Diagnosis

Sessile polyps in the duodenum may be difficult to distinguish on barium studies from benign GISTs, Brunner gland hamartomas, or other submucosal masses, so that endoscopy may be required for a definitive diagnosis. Occasionally, antral mucosa or even pedunculated antral polyps that prolapse through the pylorus can be mistaken for polypoid lesions in the duodenum (Fig. 35-9; see also Fig. 35-3). However, prolapsed antral mucosa is usually manifested by a characteristic mushroom-shaped defect at the base of the bulb. In other patients, apparent polypoid lesions may result from heaped-up areas of redundant mucosa on the inner aspect of the superior duodenal flexure between the first and second portions of the duodenum (Fig. 35-10). However, these "flexural pseudolesions" can usually be differentiated from true polyps by their characteristic location and changeable appearance at fluoroscopy.[30,31]

Villous Tumor

Adenomatous polyps in the stomach and duodenum that contain predominantly villous elements have been called villous adenomas, papillary adenomas, papillomas, or adenomatous papillomas.[32] Because of their high malignant potential,

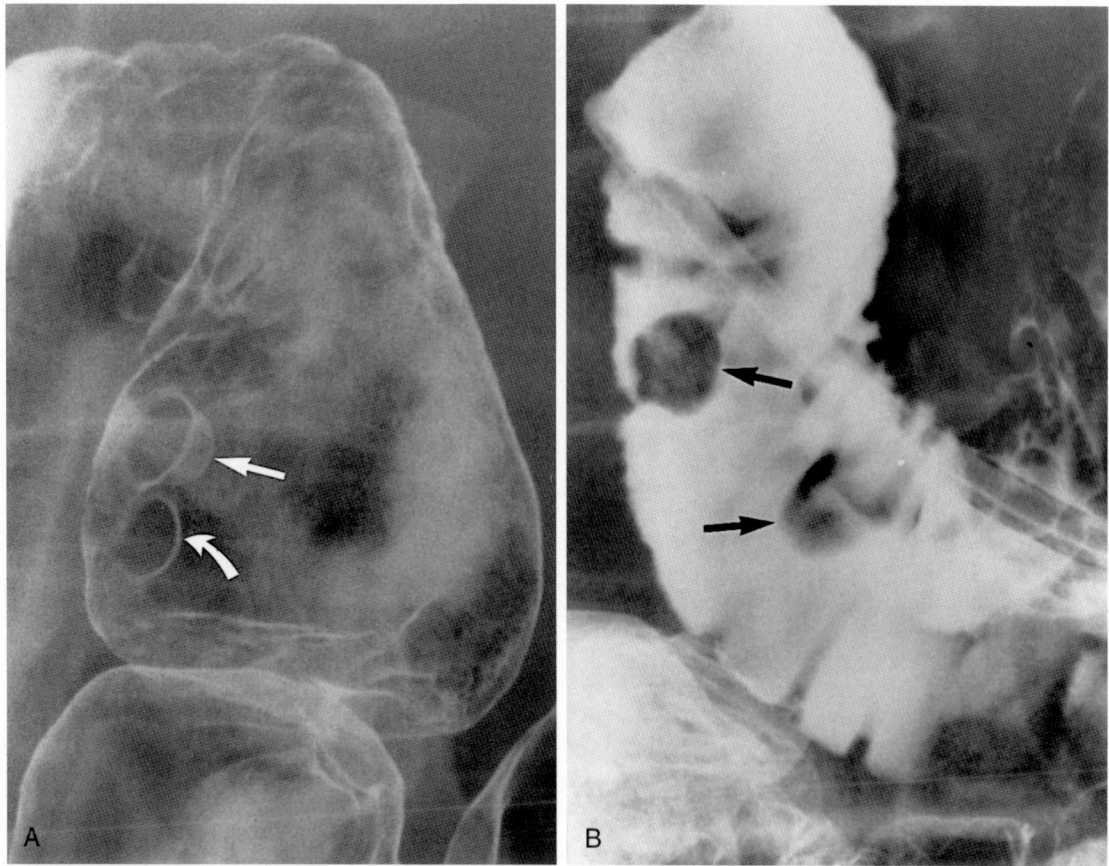

Figure 35-8. Duodenal polyps. A. Two polyps are present in the duodenal bulb. The lower polyp is seen as a ring shadow (*curved arrow*) and the higher polyp as a bowler hat (*straight arrow*). **B.** Several adenomatous polyps (*arrows*) are seen in the descending duodenum in another patient. This study was performed by injecting barium through a tube in the proximal duodenum. (**A** from Laufer I, Levine MS [eds]: Double Contrast Gastrointestinal Radiology, 2nd ed. Philadelphia, WB Saunders, 1992.)

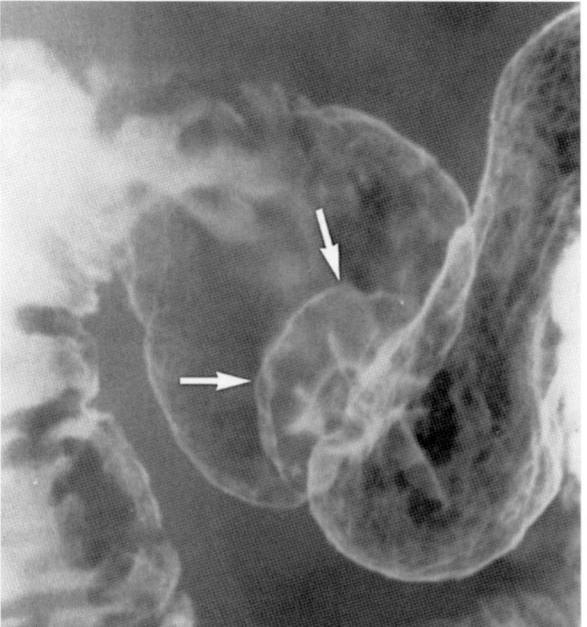

Figure 35-9. Prolapsed antral mucosa. The prolapsed mucosa produces a mushroom-shaped defect (*arrows*) at the base of the duodenal bulb. The characteristic appearance and location of the prolapsed antral mucosa should differentiate this finding from a true polypoid lesion. (From Laufer I, Levine MS [eds]: Double Contrast Gastrointestinal Radiology, 2nd ed. Philadelphia, WB Saunders, 1992.)

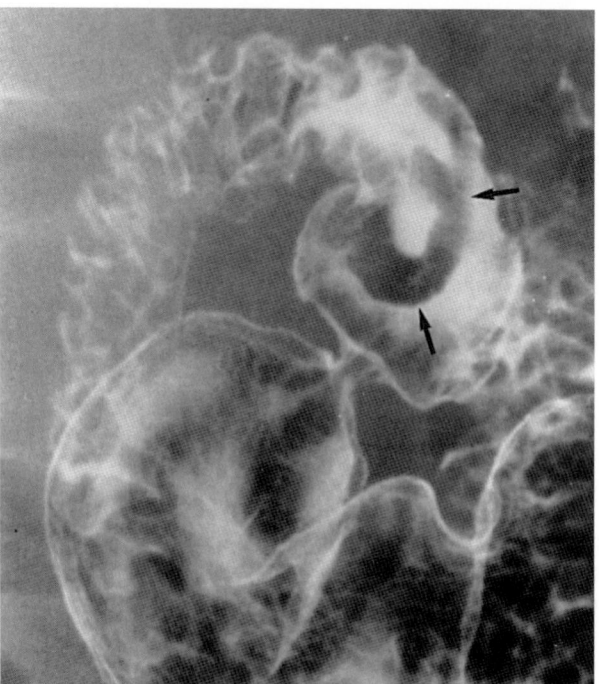

Figure 35-10. Duodenal pseudolesion. Redundant mucosa at the superior duodenal flexure simulates an ulcerated mass (*arrows*) at the apex of the duodenal bulb. However, the characteristic appearance and location of this finding should suggest a flexural pseudolesion.

however, the term *villous tumors* is probably best because it avoids the erroneous impression that these lesions are always benign.[33,34]

Pathology

Villous tumors in the stomach and duodenum closely resemble those in the colon, appearing grossly as polypoid masses with numerous frondlike projections. They usually occur as solitary lesions, ranging from 3 to 9 cm, but giant villous tumors as large as 15 cm have been reported.[34,35] Villous tumors rarely cause gastric outlet obstruction because of the soft consistency of these lesions. They are equally distributed in the stomach, but duodenal lesions tend to be located in the descending duodenum near the papilla of Vater.[33-35]

Villous tumors in the stomach and duodenum are associated with an even higher risk of malignant change than villous tumors in the colon. The risk of malignancy is directly related to the size of the lesion. In the stomach, malignant changes are found in 50% of lesions 2 to 4 cm in size and in 80% of lesions larger than 4 cm. Similarly, malignant changes are found in 30% to 60% of villous tumors in the duodenum, with the highest cancer risk in lesions larger than 4 cm.[32,33] Although villous tumors in the stomach and duodenum have been classified as benign neoplasms in this chapter, for all practical purposes they should be treated as malignant lesions.

Clinical Findings

Most patients with villous tumors in the stomach and duodenum are older than 50 year of age. They may present with signs or symptoms of upper gastrointestinal bleeding, such as melena, guaiac-positive stool, and iron-deficiency anemia.[33,34] Because villous tumors in the duodenum are often located near the papilla of Vater, some patients may develop obstructive jaundice.[33,34] In contrast to villous tumors in the colon, however, villous tumors in the stomach and duodenum rarely cause diarrhea or electrolyte depletion.[33,34] Although gastric and duodenal lesions have the same secretory capabilities as those in the colon, reabsorption of fluid and electrolytes in the small and large bowel apparently prevents the development of a diarrheal syndrome.

Villous tumors in the stomach and duodenum should be resected because of the high risk of malignant degeneration. Some benign lesions can be removed by endoscopy, but those harboring invasive carcinoma require surgery.[32,33,35]

Radiographic Findings

Villous tumors in the stomach and duodenum usually appear on barium studies as polypoid masses, ranging from 2 to 9 cm.[34-36] The lesions often have a reticular or "soap bubble" appearance with serrated, feathery margins because of trapping of barium in multiple clefts between the frondlike projections of the tumor (Figs. 35-11 and 35-12).[30,36,37] Thus, villous tumors in the stomach and duodenum have the same radiographic features as those in the colon.

Villous tumors in the duodenum tend to be located near the papilla of Vater (see Fig. 35-12)[33-35] but occasionally are found as far proximally as the duodenal bulb.[38] Because these lesions are easily obscured by superimposed mucosal folds,

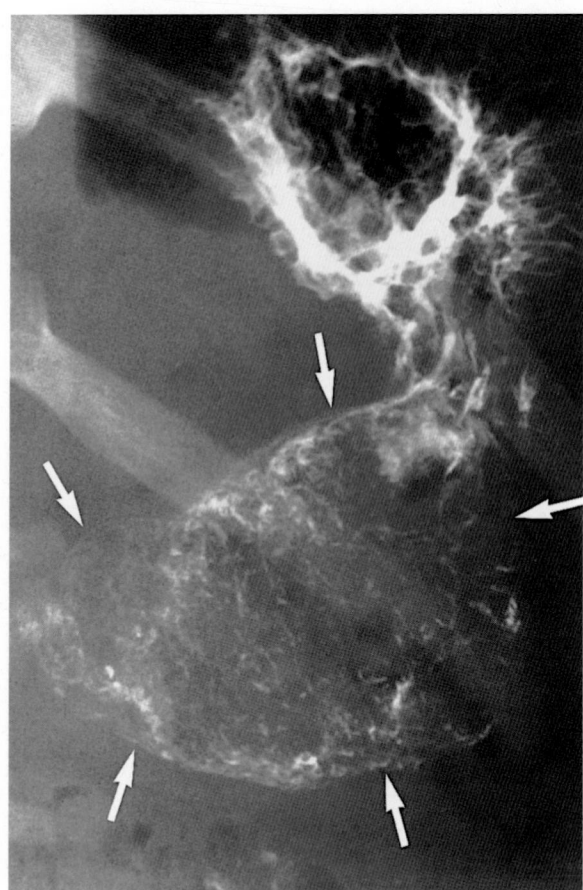

Figure 35-11. Villous tumor in the stomach. A giant villous tumor (*arrows*) in the gastric antrum has a characteristic soap bubble appearance because of trapping of barium between the frondlike projections of the tumor. This lesion could be mistaken for a bezoar, but, in contrast to bezoars, it did not move with changes in the patient's position. (Courtesy of Abraham Ghiatis, MD, San Antonio, TX.)

they are best visualized on double-contrast studies with optimal distention of the duodenum. Hypotonic duodenography (after intravenous administration of 1 mg of glucagon) is a particularly effective technique for effacing the overlying folds, so that subtle lesions in the periampullary duodenum are better seen (see Fig. 35-12B).[35,37]

Differential Diagnosis

A large gastric bezoar may occasionally produce a soap bubble appearance mimicking that of a villous tumor in the stomach as a result of barium trapped in the interstices of the bezoar. However, the freely mobile nature of the bezoar with changes in the patient's position should suggest the correct diagnosis. Carcinoma or lymphoma of the stomach or duodenum may also be manifested by a bulky intraluminal mass, but these lesions rarely produce a soap bubble appearance.

Polyposis Syndromes

With the widespread use of double-contrast radiography and endoscopy, gastroduodenal involvement by the polyposis syndromes has proved to be far more common than was previously recognized (see Chapter 65). In patients with FAPS, detection of adenomatous polyps in the stomach or duodenum

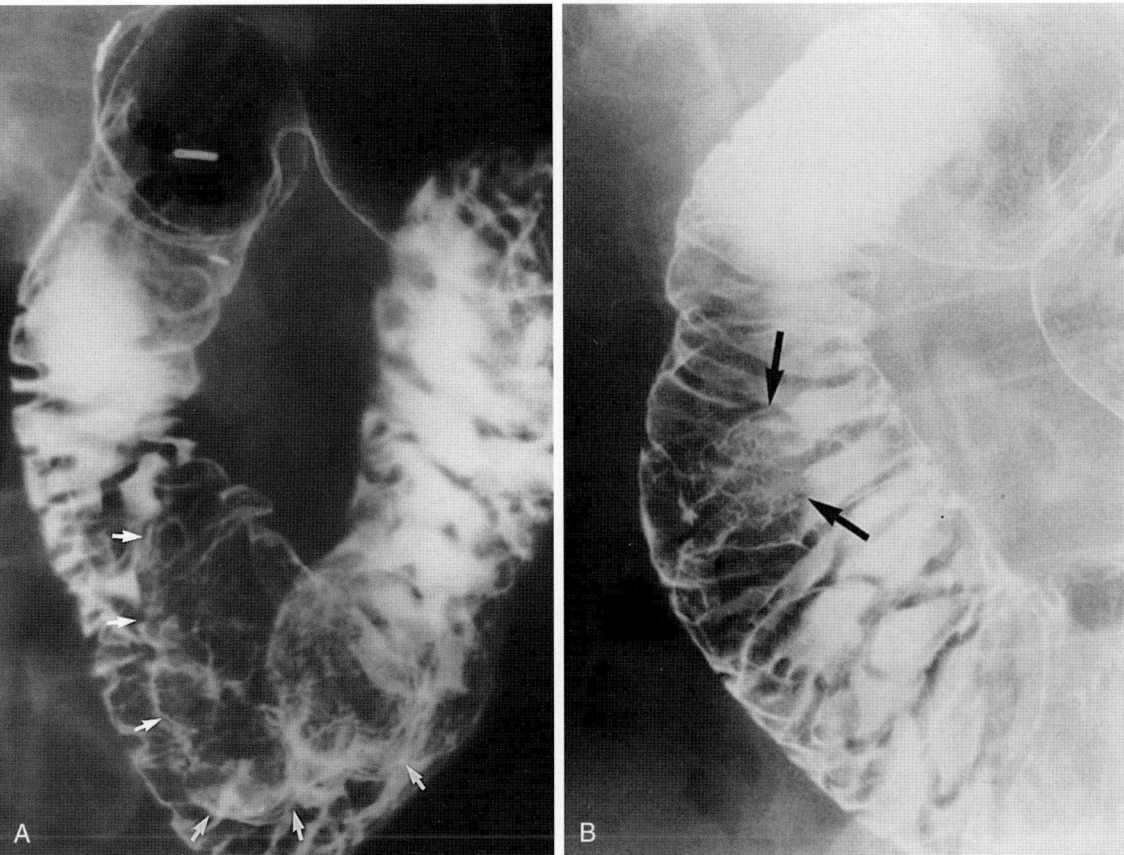

Figure 35-12. Villous tumors in the duodenum. A. This villous tumor appears as a polypoid mass (*arrows*) just below the level of the papilla. Note the characteristic reticular surface of the lesion. **B.** In another patient, a more subtle villous tumor (*arrows*) is seen with optimal distention of the descending duodenum. Again, note the reticular surface of the lesion. (**A** from Laufer I, Levine MS [eds]: Double Contrast Gastrointestinal Radiology, 2nd ed. Philadelphia, WB Saunders, 1992.)

is particularly important because of the malignant potential of these lesions and the increased risk of gastric or duodenal carcinoma. Some investigators therefore believe that periodic surveillance of the upper gastrointestinal tract should be performed on all patients with FAPS. Other polyposis syndromes involving the stomach and duodenum include Peutz-Jeghers syndrome, Cronkhite-Canada syndrome, juvenile polyposis, and Cowden's disease (see Chapter 65). In patients with Cronkhite-Canada syndrome, barium studies may reveal distinctive "whiskering" along the margins of the stomach because of trapping of barium between tiny mucosal excrescences (Fig. 35-13).[39] When accompanied by characteristic ectodermal findings, this appearance should be highly suggestive of Cronkhite-Canada syndrome.

Figure 35-13. Cronkhite-Canada syndrome involving the stomach. A single-contrast view shows whiskering (*arrows*) of the greater curvature because of trapping of barium between tiny mucosal excrescences. This finding is characteristic of gastric involvement by Cronkhite-Canada syndrome.

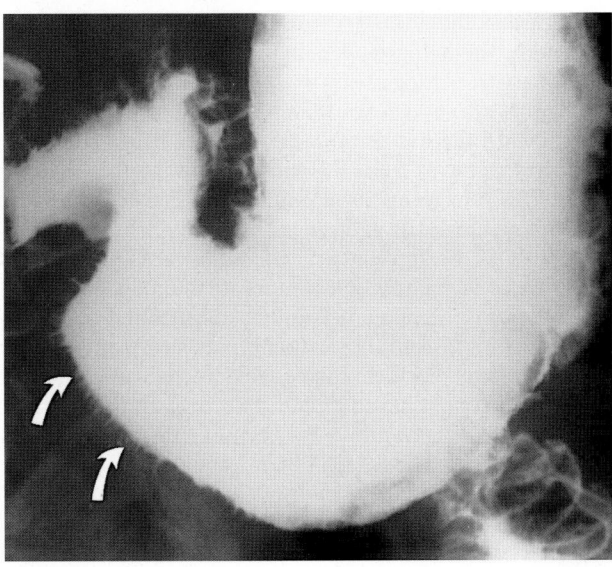

SUBMUCOSAL LESIONS

The terms *submucosal* and *intramural* are used interchangeably in this chapter. It should nevertheless be recognized that all submucosal lesions are intramural but not all intramural lesions are submucosal, because they can also arise from the muscularis propria or even the subserosa. These mesenchymal lesions constitute about half of all benign gastroduodenal neoplasms.[2] Nearly 90% are GISTs.[40] Other less common submucosal lesions include leiomyoblastomas, lipomas, hemangiomas, lymphangiomas, glomus tumors, neural tumors, granular cell tumors, inflammatory fibroid polyps, ectopic pancreatic rests, Brunner gland hamartomas, and duplication cysts. Most benign submucosal tumors are discovered as incidental findings at surgery or autopsy. However, lesions that are large or ulcerated may cause abdominal pain or upper gastrointestinal bleeding. Other mesenchymal tumors are important because of an associated risk of malignancy. Submucosal masses may be difficult to visualize at endoscopy because the overlying mucosa appears normal. As a result, barium studies are particularly helpful for detecting these lesions.

Benign Gastrointestinal Stromal Tumor

Although GISTs were once thought to represent smooth muscle tumors (leiomyomas and leiomyosarcomas), they are now believed to arise from the interstitial cells of Cajal and can be identified using immunohistochemistry for expression of CD-117, also known as c-kit protein (a cell membrane receptor with tyrosine kinase activity).[41] In one study, almost all submucosal masses previously classified as smooth muscle tumors were found to be GISTs, with the exception of submucosal masses in the esophagus, where true leiomyomas were far more common.[42] GISTs constitute about 90% of mesenchymal tumors and 40% of all benign tumors in the stomach and duodenum.[1,40,43] These lesions are important not only because they may cause symptoms but also because a small percentage are found to be malignant.

Pathology

Benign GISTs consist histologically of intersecting bundles of spindle-shaped cells in a characteristic whorling pattern that distinguishes these tumors from normal smooth muscle.[40,44] Depending on their growth pattern, GISTs may appear grossly as endogastric, exogastric, or "dumbbell"-shaped lesions.[1] About 80% are endogastric lesions that remain intramural but grow toward the lumen. Another 15% are exogastric lesions that grow outward from the stomach toward the peritoneal cavity. The remaining 5% are dumbbell-shaped lesions that have both endogastric and exogastric components.

Almost all benign gastric and duodenal GISTs occur as solitary lesions, but multiple tumors are found in 1% to 2% of patients.[1] Most benign GISTs in the stomach and duodenum are less than 3 cm, but some patients may have giant lesions as large as 25 cm.[44] As these tumors enlarge, they often outgrow their blood supply, causing central necrosis and ulceration.[45] In various series, ulceration has been documented in 50% to 70% of all gastric GISTs larger than 2 cm.[1,45]

About 90% of GISTs in the stomach are found to be benign lesions.[1] However, it is often difficult to differentiate benign from malignant GISTs by histopathologic criteria.[46,47]

The most commonly accepted microscopic index of malignancy is the degree of mitotic activity in the tumor.[44] Nevertheless, mitotic activity may be increased in only a portion of a malignant GIST, so that random biopsy specimens or frozen sections may erroneously suggest a benign lesion. Thus, a definitive diagnosis of malignancy ultimately depends on the tumor's biologic behavior and the demonstration of invasive growth beyond the stomach via direct extension, lymphatic spread, or hematogenous metastases (see Chapter 37).[43]

Clinical Findings

Benign gastric and duodenal GISTs occur with about equal frequency in men and women. Affected individuals are usually older than 50 years of age.[44] Most patients with lesions smaller than 3 cm are asymptomatic. As these tumors enlarge, ulceration of the lesion may cause epigastric pain or upper gastrointestinal bleeding, manifested by hematemesis, melena, guaiac-positive stool, or iron-deficiency anemia.[43,44] Occasionally, pedunculated leiomyomas in the gastric antrum may cause nausea and vomiting as a result of intermittent gastric outlet obstruction.[48,49]

Radiographic Findings

Most benign GISTs are not diagnosed on abdominal radiographs, but a large tumor in the stomach can occasionally be recognized as a soft tissue mass indenting the gastric air shadow.[2] Rarely, benign GISTs in the stomach contain irregular streaks or clumps of mottled calcification that are visible on abdominal radiographs, barium studies, or CT (Fig. 35-14).[50,51] Mucinous adenocarcinomas of the stomach may also calcify, but the calcification in these lesions tends to have a punctate, granular, or finely stippled appearance (see Chapter 36).[52] The differential diagnosis for left upper quadrant calcification also includes calcified adrenal, renal, or splenic lesions.

Benign GISTs typically appear on barium studies as discrete submucosal masses (Figs. 35-15 through 35-17). These tumors have the same radiographic features as intramural, extramucosal lesions elsewhere in the gastrointestinal tract. When viewed in profile, the lesions have a smooth surface that is etched in white on double-contrast images, and their borders form right angles or slightly obtuse angles with the adjacent gastric or duodenal wall (see Fig. 35-15A). When viewed en face, the intraluminal surface of these tumors has abrupt, well-defined borders (see Fig. 35-15B). Because the overlying mucosa is usually intact, a normal areae gastricae pattern can sometimes be seen overlying these lesions.

Gastric GISTs vary in size from tiny lesions of several millimeters to enormous masses that encroach substantially on the lumen (see Fig. 35-16).[44] Tumors larger than 2 cm frequently contain areas of ulceration, manifested by a central barium-filled crater within the surrounding submucosal mass (see Fig. 35-17A). Because of their characteristic appearance, centrally ulcerated GISTs have been described as "bull's-eye" or "target" lesions. Occasionally, a hanging droplet of barium (i.e., stalactite) on an anterior wall GIST can mimic the appearance of ulceration (see Fig. 35-15B), but the stalactite can usually be recognized as a transient finding at fluoroscopy.[15]

Because ulcerated GISTs may cause major upper gastrointestinal bleeding, ulceration is generally considered an

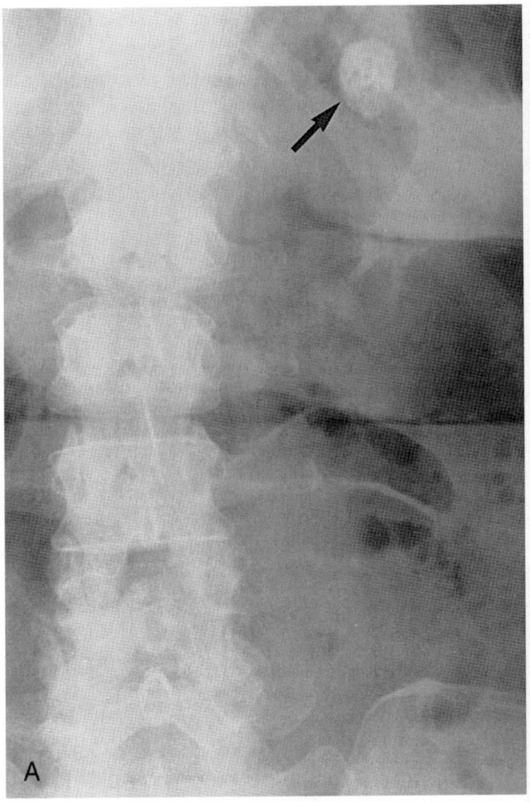

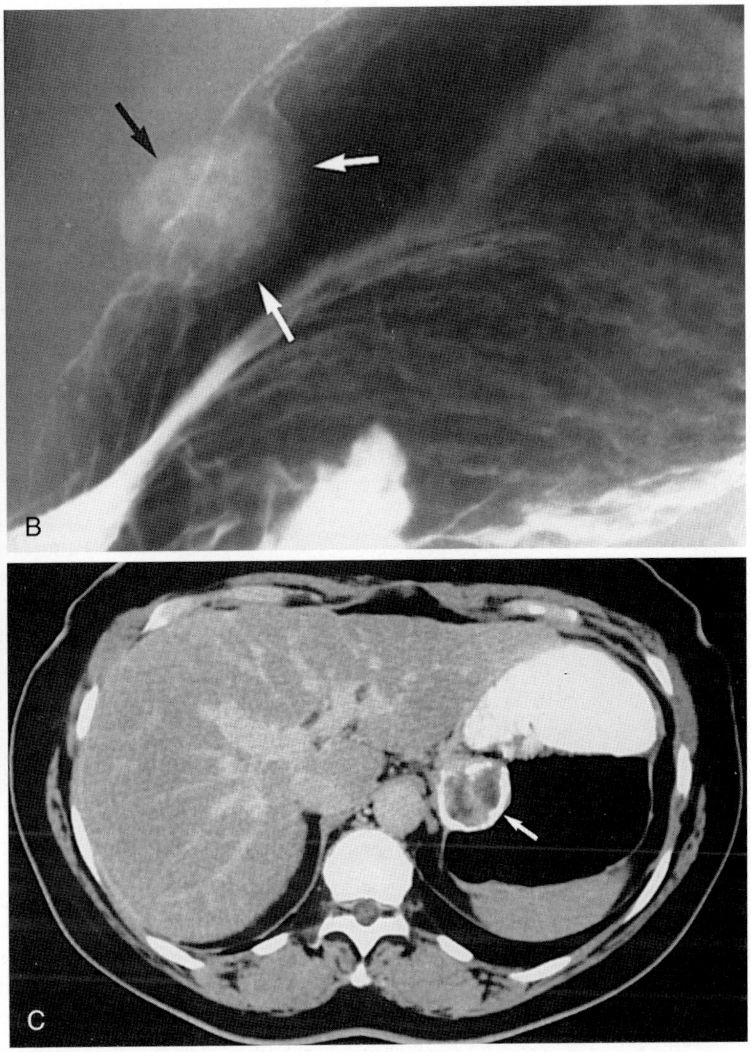

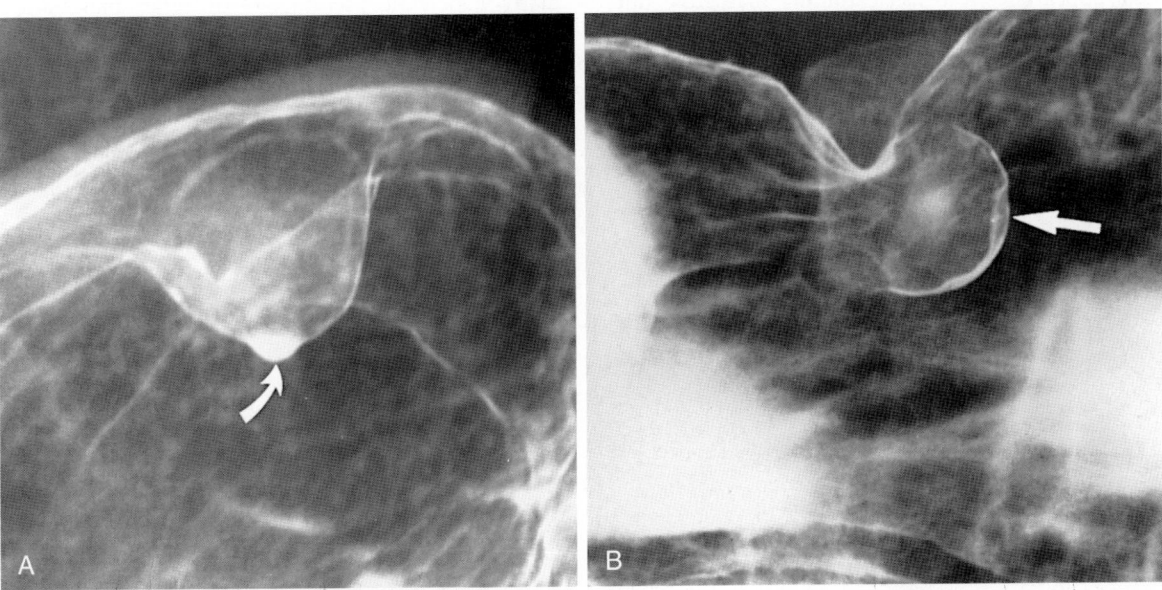

Figure 35-14. Benign GISTs with calcification. A. Close-up view of an abdominal radiograph reveals a dense clump of calcification (*arrow*) in the left upper quadrant. **B.** Barium study shows that this calcification (*black arrow*) is located within a discrete submucosal mass (*white arrows*) in the stomach. At surgery, the lesion was found to be a benign GIST. **C.** In another patient, a peripherally calcified benign GIST (*arrow*) is shown on a CT scan. (**C** courtesy of Alec J. Megibow, MD, New York, NY.)

Figure 35-15. Benign GISTs. A. A submucosal mass is seen in profile in the gastric fundus. The lesion has smooth borders that form slightly obtuse angles with the adjacent gastric wall. This view was taken with the patient upright, and a barium stalactite (*arrow*) is seen hanging down from the inferior surface of the lesion. **B.** In another patient, a small GIST is seen en face (*arrow*) in the gastric body. This lesion also has typical features of a submucosal mass with smooth, well-defined borders. A hanging droplet of barium or stalactite is visible on the surface of this anterior wall lesion. (From Laufer I, Levine MS [eds]: Double Contrast Gastrointestinal Radiology, 2nd ed. Philadelphia, WB Saunders, 1992.)

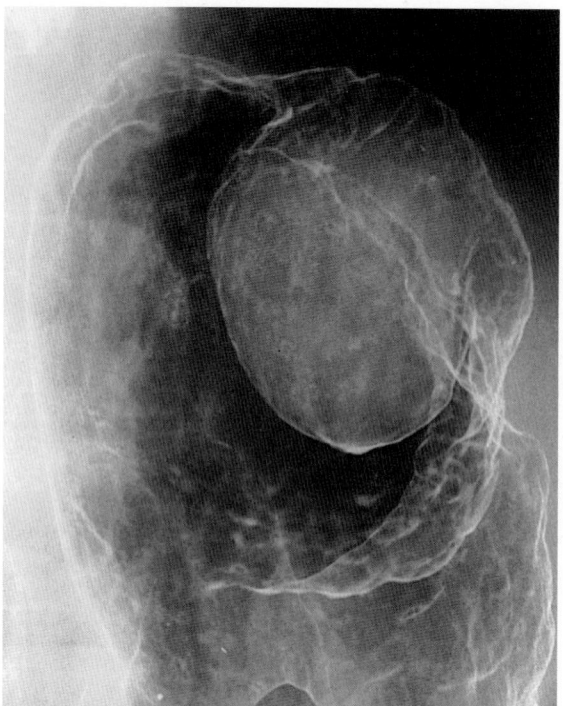

Figure 35-16. Giant benign GIST. This lesion in the gastric fundus encroaches considerably on the lumen. (From Laufer I, Levine MS [eds]: Double Contrast Gastrointestinal Radiology, 2nd ed. Philadelphia, WB Saunders, 1992.)

indication for surgery. Rarely, however, complete healing of ulceration in benign gastric GISTs can occur in patients treated with antisecretory agents (see Fig. 35-17), so that medical therapy may lead to cessation of bleeding when surgery is contraindicated.[53] If necessary, bleeding can be controlled angiographically by selective embolization of feeding vessels.[54]

Although most benign GISTs in the stomach have a typical submucosal appearance, exogastric tumors that grow outward from the stomach may be difficult to differentiate from extrinsic mass lesions. The presence of a central dimple or spicule at the apex of the mass should suggest an intramural

rather than an extrinsic lesion.[55] This area of tenting probably results from traction on the gastric wall by the base or pedicle of the mass as it enlarges. Other GISTs that grow intraluminally may develop pseudopedicles. Rarely, pedunculated antral GISTs may prolapse into the duodenum or act as the lead point for a gastrogastric or gastroduodenal intussusception.[48,49]

Differential Diagnosis

GISTs are by far the most common benign submucosal tumors in the stomach and duodenum. However, other intramural lesions such as lipomas, neurofibromas, hemangiomas, and ectopic pancreatic rests may also be manifested by discrete submucosal masses. Occasionally, lipomas can be recognized by their tendency to change in size and shape at fluoroscopy (see later section on Lipoma). Ectopic pancreatic rests may be suggested by their characteristic location on the greater curvature of the distal antrum (see later section on Ectopic Pancreatic Rest). In most cases, however, these submucosal lesions cannot be differentiated by radiologic criteria.

Centrally ulcerated GISTs appear as typical bull's-eye or target lesions. Although a solitary bull's-eye lesion in the stomach or duodenum is most likely to represent an ulcerated GIST on empirical grounds, other benign mesenchymal tumors that are ulcerated can produce identical findings. In contrast, the presence of multiple bull's-eye lesions should suggest a malignant tumor such as metastatic disease, lymphoma, or Kaposi's sarcoma, because GISTs are rarely multiple.[1]

An antral or duodenal ulcer surrounded by a radiolucent mound of edema may also simulate an ulcerated GIST. Conversely, an ulcerated GIST may erroneously suggest an ulcer in the stomach or duodenum.[56] However, a benign GIST usually has discrete borders, whereas the edematous mound surrounding a gastric or duodenal ulcer tends to have a more gradual transition.

Exogastric GISTs are often difficult to distinguish on barium studies from extrinsic masses involving the stomach, particularly pancreatic pseudocysts or other pancreatic lesions. Gastric compression by an enlarged liver, spleen, kidney, or other abdominal mass may produce similar findings. As indicated earlier, however, the presence of a central dimple or

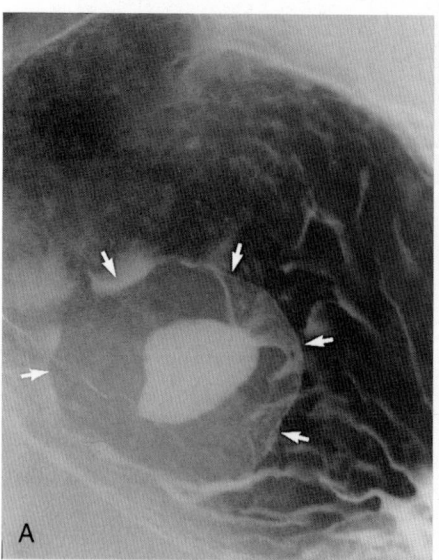

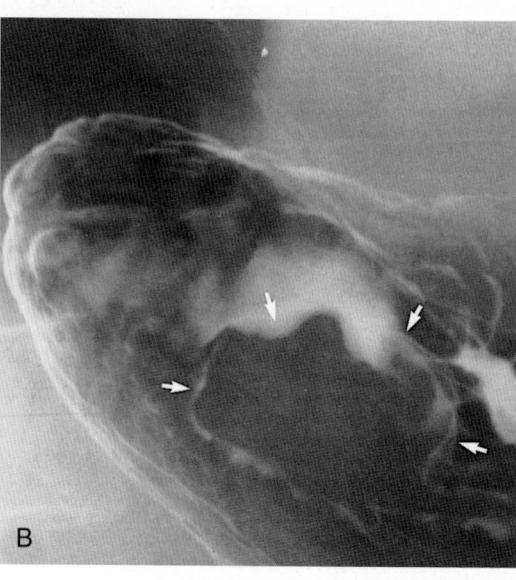

Figure 35-17. Ulcerated GIST with complete healing of the ulcer. A. Initial study reveals a relatively large benign GIST (*arrows*) in the fundus with a central area of ulceration, producing a bull's-eye lesion. **B.** Follow-up study 3 years later shows complete healing of the ulcer within the tumor (*arrows*). (From O'Riordan D, Levine MS, Yeager BA: Complete healing of ulceration within a gastric leiomyoma. Gastrointest Radiol 10: 47-49, 1985. With kind permission from Springer Science and Business Media.)

spicule at the apex of the mass should suggest an exogastric, intramural lesion such as a GIST.[55] When extrinsic mass lesions are suspected, ultrasound, CT, and MRI may be helpful for establishing the correct diagnosis.

Management

Small, asymptomatic submucosal masses that are detected in the stomach or duodenum on barium studies can probably be followed conservatively without need for endoscopic or surgical intervention because most of these lesions are found to be benign stromal tumors. In such cases, follow-up barium studies or endoscopy may be performed at yearly intervals to be certain that the tumor is not enlarging. However, ulcerated lesions or lesions larger than 2 cm should probably be resected because of the risk of malignancy and the difficulty in distinguishing benign and malignant stromal tumors by histopathologic criteria.[1,41,43] Depending on the size of the lesion, it can be enucleated, locally excised, or, if necessary, removed by partial gastrectomy or duodenectomy.[43,44]

Leiomyoblastoma

Leiomyoblastomas are unusual smooth muscle tumors that occur predominantly in the stomach. However, these tumors have also been reported in the small bowel, retroperitoneum, and uterus.[57] Leiomyoblastomas differ histologically from GISTs, but the gross morphologic findings are virtually identical.[44] As with other gastrointestinal stromal tumors, leiomyoblastomas are important because of the risk of malignancy in these lesions.

Pathology

Leiomyoblastomas consist histologically of round, polygonal, or epithelioid cells with eccentric nuclei, perinuclear vacuolization, and a clear or acidophilic cytoplasm.[57-59] Because of the histologic findings, these tumors have also been called *epithelioid leiomyomas*.[58,59] Most leiomyoblastomas are benign lesions, but metastases to the liver or other structures occur in about 10% of patients.[60] As with other GISTs, malignant lesions usually have increased mitotic activity on microscopic examination.[58] Size is also an important factor in predicting biologic behavior because metastases rarely occur with lesions smaller than 6 cm.[58] Nevertheless, many authors believe that all leiomyoblastomas should be resected because of the difficulty in distinguishing benign and malignant lesions by histopathologic criteria.[57,59]

Gastric leiomyoblastomas tend to occur as solitary lesions, most frequently in the antrum, but multiple tumors have been reported.[58,61] As with leiomyomas, most lesions appear as submucosal masses, often with central necrosis and ulceration.[60,61] Occasionally, they may have an exogastric pattern of growth.[61]

Clinical Findings

In contrast to leiomyomas, leiomyoblastomas are more common in men than in women.[60,61] These patients may be asymptomatic, or they may present with pain, vomiting, upper gastrointestinal bleeding, or a palpable abdominal mass.[57,60,61] Occasionally, giant exogastric leiomyoblastomas may rupture suddenly into the peritoneal cavity, causing catastrophic intraperitoneal bleeding.[62]

Radiographic Findings

Gastric leiomyoblastomas are indistinguishable on barium studies from other GISTs (see earlier section on Benign Gastrointestinal Stromal Tumor). Most appear as smooth submucosal masses, often containing central areas of ulceration (Fig. 35-18).[61] Some endogastric lesions can become pedunculated, whereas exogastric lesions can be mistaken for extrinsic masses involving the stomach (Fig. 35-19A).[61] Cystic degeneration of these exogastric leiomyoblastomas is occasionally manifested on CT by a cystic mass abutting the stomach (Fig. 35-19B).[63,64] Rarely, CT may show areas of calcification within the tumor.[64] The differential diagnosis for these lesions is discussed in detail in the previous section on Benign Gastrointestinal Stromal Tumor.

Lipoma

Gastric lipomas are rare tumors, accounting for only about 5% of gastrointestinal tract lipomas and fewer than 1% of all gastric neoplasms.[65] Duodenal lipomas are even rarer. Most of these lesions are detected as incidental findings on barium study, endoscopy, or autopsy. Thus far, no cases of malignant degeneration of gastrointestinal lipomas have been reported. Occasionally, however, lesions that are large or ulcerated may cause obstruction or bleeding. Although lipomas are difficult to differentiate on barium studies from other submucosal masses in the stomach or duodenum, CT has proved to be a valuable technique for diagnosing these lesions.

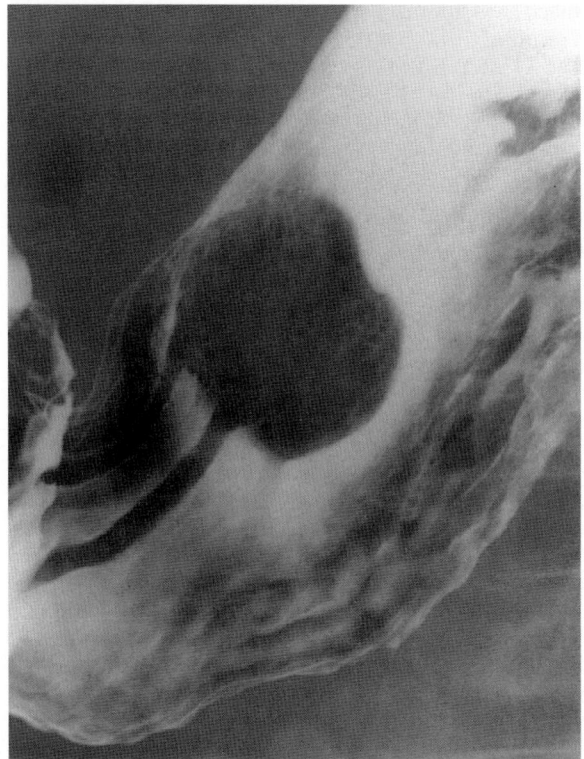

Figure 35-18. Gastric leiomyoblastoma. A large submucosal mass is present in the gastric body. This lesion is indistinguishable from a benign GIST.

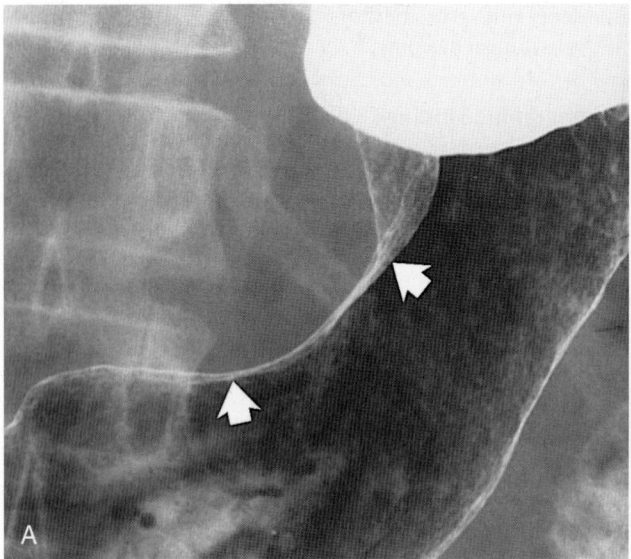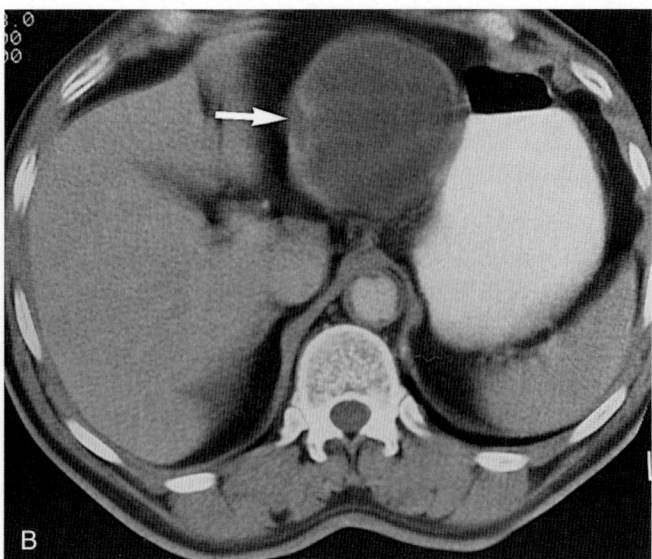

Figure 35-19. Exogastric leiomyoblastoma. A. Barium study shows a smooth extrinsic impression (*arrows*) on the lesser curvature of the gastric body. **B.** CT scan shows a smooth, well-defined cystic mass (*arrow*) abutting the stomach. At surgery, this patient was found to have an exogastric leiomyoblastoma with cystic degeneration of the tumor. (Courtesy of Kyunghee C. Cho, MD, Newark, NJ.)

Pathology

Lipomas are composed of mature fat cells surrounded by a fibrous capsule. They tend to occur as solitary lesions, most frequently in the gastric antrum.[66-68] About 95% are endo-gastric lesions that arise in the submucosa and grow toward the lumen, whereas the remaining 5% are exogastric lesions that arise in the subserosa and grow outward from the stomach.[66] As lipomas enlarge, they may develop central ulcers as a result of pressure necrosis of the overlying mucosa.[67]

Clinical Findings

Small lipomas usually cause no symptoms, but larger lesions may undergo ulceration, causing abdominal pain or upper gastrointestinal bleeding.[66,67,69] Rarely, pedunculated antral lipomas that prolapse through the pylorus may cause inter-mittent gastric outlet obstruction with recurrent nausea and vomiting.[66] Small lipomas in asymptomatic patients can be followed without need for surgery. However, larger lesions that cause symptoms should be resected.[67]

Radiographic Findings

Large gastric and duodenal lipomas containing a sufficient amount of fat may occasionally appear as radiolucent shadows on abdominal radiographs. Barium studies typically reveal a smooth submucosal mass or centrally ulcerated bull's-eye lesion indistinguishable from a benign GIST or other mesen-chymal tumor (Fig. 35-20A).[68] Most lipomas occur as iso-lated antral lesions,[66-68] but multiple lipomas are occasionally present in the stomach or duodenum.[70] Because lipomas have a soft consistency, the correct diagnosis can be suggested if the lesions change in size and shape with peristalsis or palpa-tion at fluoroscopy (Fig. 35-20B).[70] Rarely, pedunculated antral lipomas may prolapse into the duodenum or act as the lead point for a gastroduodenal intussusception.[68]

CT has proved to be of considerable value for diagnosing gastrointestinal lipomas.[71-75] These lesions typically appear on CT as well-circumscribed lesions of uniform fatty den-sity with an attenuation of −70 to −120 Hounsfield units (Fig. 35-20C).[71,74] Occasionally, CT may reveal linear strands of soft-tissue density or ulceration within the tumor.[68,74] It should therefore be recognized that these findings occur in a benign lipoma and are not signs of a liposarcoma, which is extremely rare in the gastrointestinal tract. Thus, a gastric or duodenal lipoma can be definitively diagnosed by CT and unnecessary endoscopy or surgery can be avoided.

Hemangioma

Hemangiomas constitute less than 2% of all benign tumors in the stomach. They are even rarer in the duodenum. The lesions may be classified as capillary hemangiomas composed of numerous tiny vascular structures or, less commonly, as cavernous hemangiomas composed of large blood spaces or sinusoids lined by endothelial tissue. It is uncertain whether these lesions are congenital malformations or true neoplasms capable of autonomous growth. They tend to occur as soli-tary lesions, but multiple hemangiomas may be present in the stomach, small bowel, and colon. Occasionally, gastrointestinal hemangiomas are associated with telangiectasia of the skin.[76]

Although sarcomatous changes are rarely found in gastro-intestinal hemangiomas, these highly vascular lesions are dangerous because of the risk of massive upper gastro-intestinal bleeding. Endoscopy typically reveals a bluish black submucosal lesion. Surgical resection is usually curative.

Radiographic Findings

Hemangiomas in the stomach typically appear on barium studies as smooth submucosal masses that are indistinguish-able from GISTs or other mesenchymal tumors.[76] However,

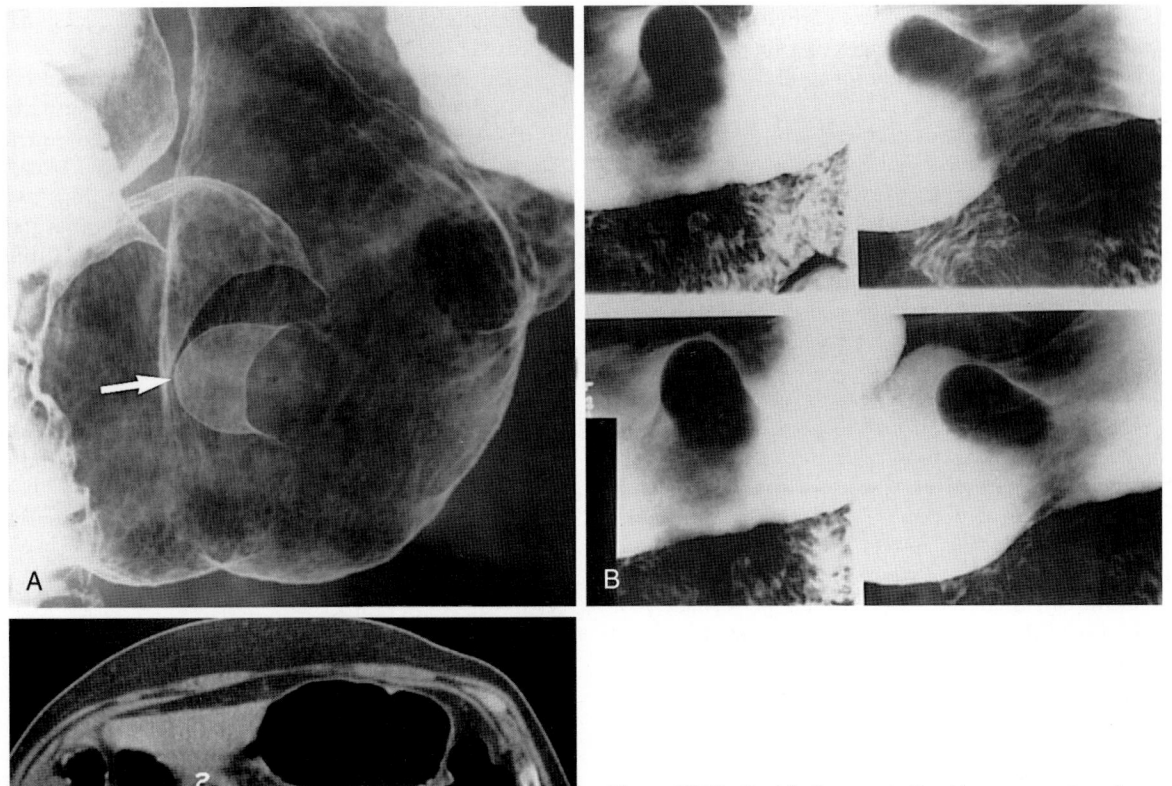

Figure 35-20. Gastric lipoma. A. Double-contrast view shows a smooth submucosal mass (*arrow*) in the antrum. **B.** Prone single-contrast views show how the lesion changes in size and shape with varying degrees of compression. This changing appearance should be highly suggestive of a lipoma. **C.** CT scan shows how the lesion in the antrum (*cursor 2*) has the same density as perirenal fat (*cursor 1*), confirming the presence of a lipoma. (From Laufer I, Levine MS [eds]: Double Contrast Gastrointestinal Radiology, 2nd ed. Philadelphia, WB Saunders, 1992.)

the presence of phleboliths within the lesion should be virtually pathognomonic of a hemangioma.[77] Such phleboliths are occasionally visible on abdominal radiographs, and their intimate relationship to the stomach may be confirmed on barium studies or CT.[77] The presence of additional hemangiomas on the skin should also suggest the correct diagnosis.

Lymphangioma

Lymphangiomas are rare benign tumors of the stomach and duodenum.[78] These lesions consist histologically of irregularly dilated lymphatic channels lined by benign-appearing endothelial cells. Lymphangiomas are thought to be developmental malformations arising from sequestered lymphatic tissue.[78] These lesions often have a cystic appearance because of progressive accumulation of fluid.

Although they may occur anywhere in the body, lymphangiomas rarely affect the gastrointestinal tract. These lesions are usually detected as incidental findings in asymptomatic patients. Occasionally, however, they are large enough to cause obstruction or intussusception.[78] Gastric and duodenal lymphangiomas that cause symptoms should be resected.

Radiographic Findings

Lymphangiomas may appear on barium studies as smooth intramural masses that are indistinguishable from benign GISTs or other mesenchymal tumors in the stomach and duodenum.[78] Because of their cystic nature, these lesions may be pliable at fluoroscopy and are occasionally seen to change in shape with manual compression.[78] However, gastric and duodenal lipomas may produce identical findings.

Glomus Tumor

Glomus tumors are derived from glomus bodies, specialized arteriovenous communications that regulate temperature in the skin.[79] Because glomus bodies are particularly abundant in the nail beds and pads of the finger tips and toes, glomus tumors are classically subungual in location. Rarely, glomus tumors are found in the stomach.[79-81]

Most patients with glomus tumors in the stomach are asymptomatic. However, ulcerated tumors may cause upper gastrointestinal bleeding.[79,81] Local excision is usually curative, but these highly cellular lesions can appear malignant on frozen sections at the time of surgery, so that an unnecessarily extensive resection is sometimes performed.[79,80]

Radiographic Findings

Glomus tumors in the stomach usually occur as solitary lesions in the antrum, ranging from 1 to 4 cm.[80] These tumors appear on barium studies as smooth submucosal masses (with or without ulceration) and are therefore indistinguishable from benign GISTs or other more common mesenchymal tumors in the stomach (Fig. 35-21).[82] Occasionally, glomus tumors contain tiny flecks of calcification.[79] These tumors also have a soft consistency, so that they can be mistaken for lipomas because of their tendency to change in size and shape at fluoroscopy.[82]

Neural Tumor

Neural tumors constitute 5% to 10% of benign gastric tumors.[1] Most are nerve sheath tumors (neurilemomas, schwannomas, or neuromas). The tumors are composed histologically of Schwann cells with elongated nuclei in a palisade arrangement. As they outgrow their blood supply, these lesions may undergo central necrosis and ulceration with subsequent upper gastrointestinal bleeding. Most nerve sheath tumors are benign, but sarcomatous changes have occasionally been reported.[1]

Neurofibromas are other less common neural tumors in the stomach. These tumors arise from sympathetic nerves of the Auerbach myenteric plexus or, less frequently, the Meissner plexus.[83] Gastric neurofibromas are usually small lesions that are detected as incidental findings at surgery or autopsy. Occasionally, however, these tumors may cause epigastric pain, nausea, vomiting, or upper gastrointestinal bleeding.[83] They tend to be isolated lesions, but multiple neurofibromas may be present in the stomach and duodenum in patients with generalized neurofibromatosis or von Recklinghausen's disease.[84,85] This condition is characterized by cutaneous, intracranial, or intraspinal neurofibromas, skin pigmentation, bone abnormalities, and other congenital malformations. About 10% of neurofibromas in the stomach eventually undergo malignant degeneration.[83] The risk of malignancy seems to be greatest in lesions associated with generalized neurofibromatosis.

Radiographic Findings

Neural tumors in the stomach usually appear on barium studies as discrete submucosal masses (with or without ulceration) that are indistinguishable from benign GISTs or other mesenchymal tumors (Fig. 35-22). However, some exogastric lesions may grow outward from the stomach, projecting as lobulated masses into the peritoneal cavity.[83] Others may have an hourglass or dumbbell configuration.[83] Although they are rare lesions, gastric and duodenal neurofibromas should be suspected when multiple submucosal masses are found in the stomach and duodenum in patients with cutaneous neurofibromas or other stigmata of neurofibromatosis (Fig. 35-23).

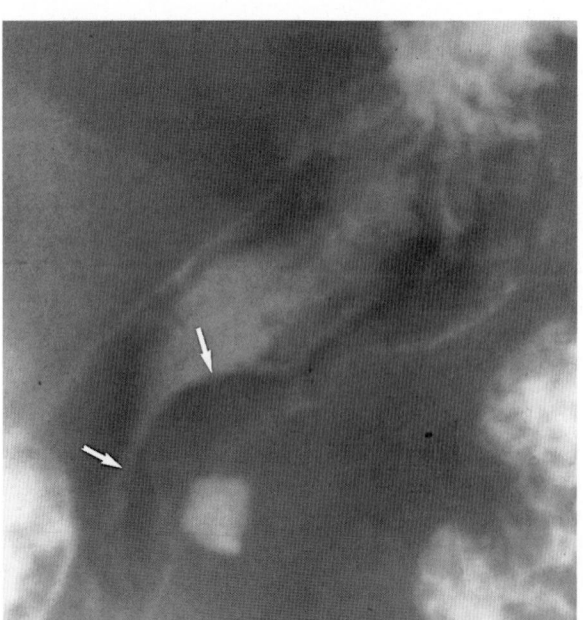

Figure 35-21. Glomus tumor. An ulcerated submucosal mass (*arrows*) is seen on the greater curvature of the antrum. This lesion cannot be distinguished from other, more common mesenchymal tumors in the stomach. (Courtesy of Bruce Knox, MD, Norfolk, VA.)

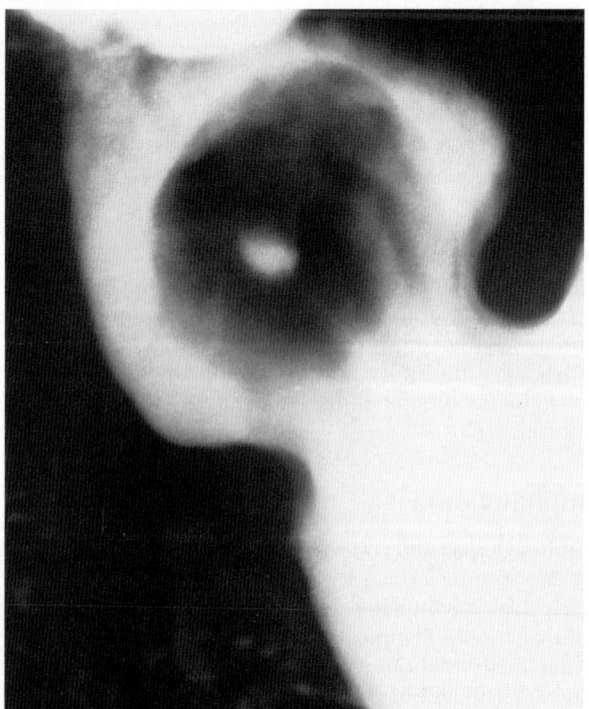

Figure 35-22. Gastric neurofibroma. An ulcerated submucosal mass is seen en face in the antrum. This lesion cannot be distinguished from an ulcerated GIST. (Courtesy of Sat Somers, MD, Ontario, Canada.)

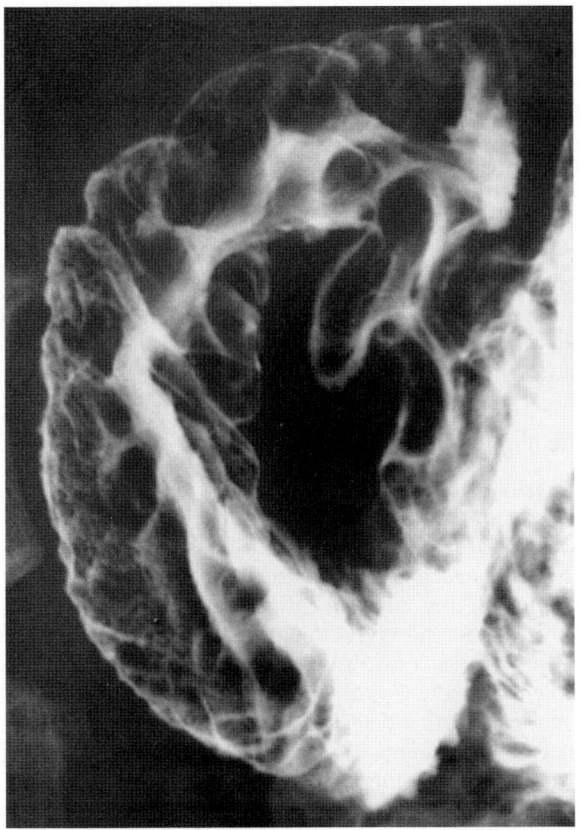

Figure 35-23. Duodenal neurofibromas in a patient with neurofibromatosis. Multiple submucosal masses are present in the first and second portions of the duodenum. This patient also had cutaneous neurofibromas and other stigmata of neurofibromatosis. (Courtesy of Seth N. Glick, MD, Philadelphia, PA.)

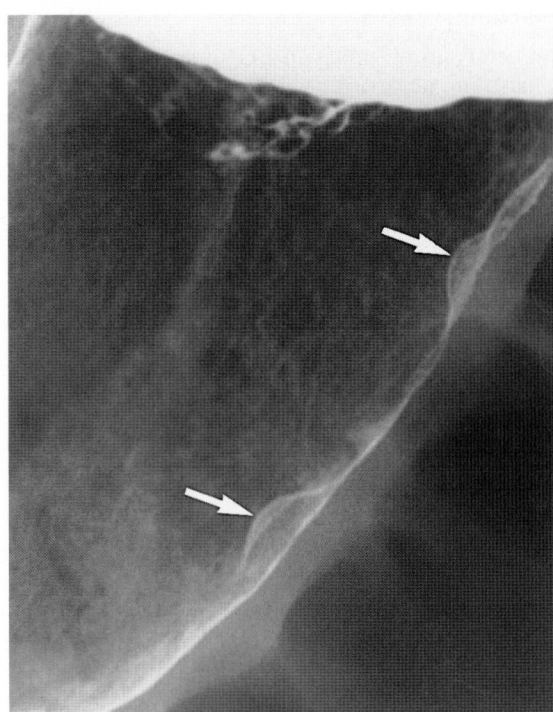

Figure 35-24. Granular cell tumors. Several small submucosal masses (*arrows*) are present on the greater curvature of the stomach. This patient had additional granular cell tumors on the tongue.

Granular Cell Tumor

Granular cell tumors are rare benign tumors that occur predominantly in the skin, tongue, breast, and subcutaneous tissues.[86] These tumors originally were called granular cell myoblastomas, but more recent histochemical and electron microscopic data suggest that they have a neural derivation, arising from Schwann cells.[87] The lesions consist histologically of sheets of polygonal tumor cells containing an eosinophilic-staining, granular cytoplasm.[87] About 7% of granular cell tumors are located in the gastrointestinal tract, including the esophagus, stomach, colon, appendix, and biliary tree.[88] Granular cell tumors in the stomach are usually found unexpectedly at surgery or autopsy.[89] Occasionally, however, ulcerated lesions may cause epigastric pain or upper gastrointestinal bleeding.[89] Surgical resection is almost always curative.

Radiographic Findings

Granular cell tumors in the stomach usually appear on barium studies as discrete submucosal masses, ranging from 0.5 to 2.5 cm.[89] Occasionally, multiple granular cell tumors are present in the stomach (Fig. 35-24).[90] Despite their rarity, granular cell tumors should be suspected when submucosal lesions are found in the stomach in patients who have additional lesions involving the skin, tongue, or breast.

Inflammatory Fibroid Polyp

Inflammatory fibroid polyps are uncommon submucosal lesions characterized histologically by whorls of fibrous tissue and blood vessels associated with an inflammatory infiltrate containing a high percentage of eosinophils.[91] These lesions tend to occur in the stomach but are also found in the small bowel and colon. Because of the histologic findings, inflammatory fibroid polyps have also been called eosinophilic granulomas and fibromas with eosinophilic infiltration.[92] However, inflammatory fibroid polyps are unrelated to eosinophilic granulomas of the lung or bone, which are composed primarily of histiocytes rather than fibroblasts. These lesions are not associated with a peripheral eosinophilia as is eosinophilic gastroenteritis, a separate and more diffuse condition.

Although the pathogenesis is uncertain, it has been postulated that inflammatory fibroid polyps have an allergic or inflammatory origin and are therefore not true neoplasms. One theory is that a localized break in the mucosa incites an inflammatory response in the adjacent submucosa, with connective tissue proliferation in the form of a polypoid mass. Whatever their origin, inflammatory fibroid polyps are benign lesions without any known risk of malignant degeneration.

Clinical Findings

Most patients with inflammatory fibroid polyps are asymptomatic, but some may present with epigastric pain or upper gastrointestinal bleeding because of superficial ulceration of the lesions.[91] Rarely, pedunculated polyps in the distal antrum may cause intermittent symptoms of gastric outlet obstruction.[91]

Radiographic Findings

Inflammatory fibroid polyps in the stomach are usually located in the antrum, occurring as solitary lesions that range from 1 to 5 cm.[93,94] The lesions may appear on barium studies as sessile or, less frequently, pedunculated polyps with a smooth or slightly lobulated contour (Fig. 35-25).[93,94] As a result, they may be indistinguishable from adenomatous polyps in the stomach. Other inflammatory fibroid polyps that have a submucosal appearance may be indistinguishable from benign GISTs.[94] When these lesions are pedunculated, they may occasionally prolapse through the pylorus, causing gastric outlet obstruction. Rarely, inflammatory fibroid polyps are larger or more lobulated, mimicking the appearance of polypoid gastric carcinomas.[91]

Ectopic Pancreatic Rest

Although they are not true neoplasms, ectopic pancreatic rests are included in this chapter because they are submucosal lesions that are difficult to distinguish from GISTs or other mesenchymal tumors in the stomach and duodenum. Most ectopic pancreatic rests are discovered as incidental findings in patients seeking medical attention for other reasons. It may be necessary to resect these lesions, however, if they cause symptoms or if a neoplastic condition cannot be excluded on radiologic or endoscopic examinations.

Pathology

Ectopic pancreatic rests consist histologically of all pancreatic elements, including acini, ducts, and islet cells, but ductal structures tend to be arranged more haphazardly in these lesions than in normal pancreatic tissue. Ectopic pancreatic rests are thought to result from abnormal embryologic development in which fragments of the ventral or dorsal pancreatic anlage are implanted in the intestinal wall.[95] These primitive epithelial buds may undergo varying degrees of differentiation toward

mature glandular tissue. The term *adenomyosis* has been used to encompass a histologic spectrum of lesions, ranging from undifferentiated glandular epithelium to well-differentiated pancreatic tissue.[96] Lesions consisting of poorly differentiated acinar and ductal structures have been called adenomyomas, whereas well-differentiated nodules of pancreatic tissue have been called ectopic, heterotopic, or aberrant pancreatic rests.[96,97]

Ectopic pancreatic rests occur throughout the gastrointestinal tract, but about 80% are located in the stomach, duodenum, or proximal jejunum.[98] Occasionally, this anomaly is found in the gallbladder, biliary tree, liver, spleen, omentum, mesentery, appendix, mediastinum, or even Meckel's diverticulum.[99]

Clinical Findings

Most patients with ectopic pancreatic rests in the stomach or duodenum are asymptomatic, but some may present with epigastric pain or upper gastrointestinal bleeding.[100,101] It has been postulated that complications result from irritation or ulceration of the adjacent gastric or duodenal mucosa by pancreatic secretions.[95] Occasionally, lesions arising near the pylorus may cause gastric outlet obstruction.[102] Rarely, ectopic pancreatic rests develop the same diseases that affect normal pancreatic tissue, including pancreatitis, pseudocysts, and benign or malignant pancreatic tumors.[103] Because upper gastrointestinal symptoms are more likely to be caused by peptic ulcer disease or other unrelated disorders, this anomaly should not be accepted as the source of the patient's symptoms without careful radiographic or endoscopic evaluation of the entire stomach and duodenum. Ectopic pancreatic rests should be resected only if the patient is symptomatic or if a significant neoplasm cannot be excluded nonoperatively.

Radiographic Findings

Ectopic pancreatic rests in the stomach and duodenum usually appear on barium studies as smooth, broad-based submucosal masses, closely resembling benign GISTs or other mesenchymal tumors (Fig. 35-26).[95,98,104,105] They almost always occur as solitary lesions, ranging from 1 to 3 cm.[106] Ectopic pancreatic rests in the stomach tend to be located on the greater curvature of the distal antrum 1 to 6 cm from the pylorus (see Fig. 35-26),[104,105] whereas duodenal lesions are most frequently found in the proximal duodenum between the duodenal bulb and the papilla of Vater.

Ectopic pancreatic rests in the stomach and duodenum often contain a central umbilication or dimple, representing the orifice of a primitive ductal system.[104,105] In about 50% of patients, this orifice is manifested by a central collection of barium, ranging from 1 to 5 mm in diameter and 5 to 10 mm in depth.[104] When viewed en face, these umbilicated lesions have the typical bull's-eye appearance of ulcerated GISTs or other mesenchymal tumors. Rarely, barium may reflux into rudimentary ductal structures that terminate in tiny club-shaped pouches, a finding that is virtually pathognomonic of ectopic pancreatic rests.[95]

Differential Diagnosis

The presence of a centrally umbilicated submucosal mass on the greater curvature of the gastric antrum 1 to 6 cm from the

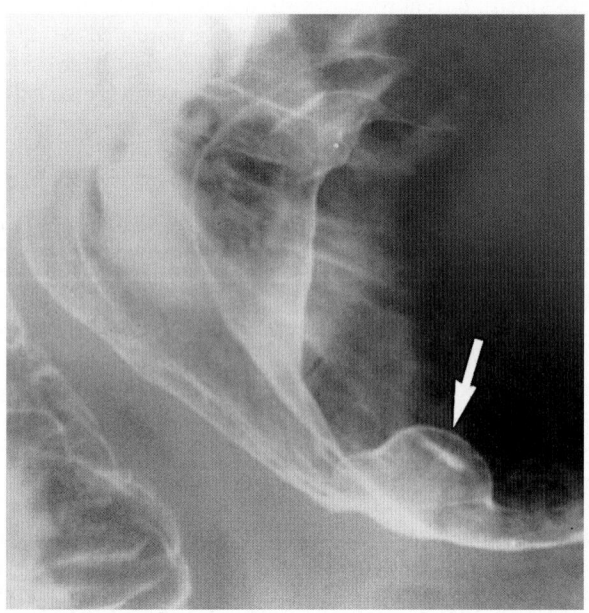

Figure 35-25. Inflammatory fibroid polyp. A sessile, slightly lobulated polyp (*arrow*) is seen on the greater curvature of the gastric antrum. This lesion is indistinguishable from an adenomatous polyp in the stomach.

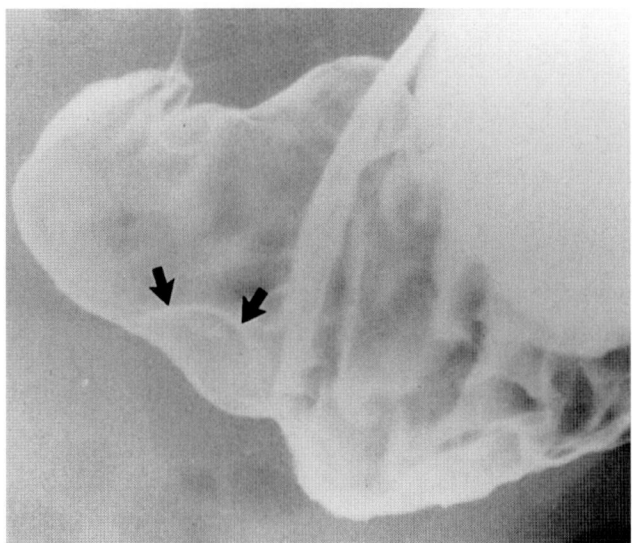

Figure 35-26. Ectopic pancreatic rest. The lesion appears as a discrete submucosal mass (*arrows*) on the greater curvature of the distal antrum. This is a characteristic location for ectopic pancreatic rests. (From Laufer I, Levine MS [eds]: Double Contrast Gastrointestinal Radiology, 2nd ed. Philadelphia, WB Saunders, 1992.)

pylorus should be highly suggestive of an ectopic pancreatic rest. Benign GISTs on the greater curvature may produce similar findings, but these lesions often contain areas of ulceration, and their location in the stomach is more variable. Other conditions such as metastatic disease, lymphoma, and Kaposi's sarcoma may also be manifested by bull's-eye lesions, but these patients usually have multiple lesions in the stomach and duodenum, whereas ectopic pancreatic rests almost always occur as solitary lesions. If the radiographic findings are equivocal, endoscopy and biopsy should be performed for a more definitive diagnosis.

Brunner Gland Hyperplasia (Brunner Gland Hamartoma)

Brunner glands in the duodenum normally secrete an alkaline mucus that protects the mucosa from the damaging effects of acidic gastric juices entering the duodenum. Brunner gland hyperplasia is therefore thought to occur as a response to hypersecretion of acid in the stomach.[106] However, hyperchlorhydria has been documented by gastric analysis in less than 50% of patients with this condition[107] so that a causal relationship between gastric hyperacidity and Brunner gland hyperplasia has not been proved.

Pathology

Hyperplastic Brunner glands may be manifested grossly by diffuse enlargement of Brunner glands throughout the proximal duodenum or by massive enlargement of a single gland. In the past, solitary lesions have been called Brunner gland adenomas.[108,109] However, pathologic examination of these lesions has revealed an intimate admixture of ducts, acini, smooth muscle, and adipose tissue without evidence of cellular atypia, so that many investigators now believe that these lesions should be classified as hamartomas rather than true

neoplasms.[110,111] Their hamartomatous origin is supported by the absence of malignant degeneration in these enlarged glands. Nevertheless, Brunner gland hamartomas are important because they can be mistaken for neoplastic lesions on radiologic or endoscopic examinations and because they may occasionally cause symptoms.

Clinical Findings

Except for its association with duodenal ulcers and gastric hypersecretory states,[106] the diffuse form of Brunner gland hyperplasia has no clinical significance. In contrast, solitary Brunner gland hamartomas may occasionally cause obstructive symptoms, epigastric pain, or upper gastrointestinal bleeding because of ulceration of the overlying mucosa.[108,111,112] Although the diffuse form of Brunner gland hyperplasia requires no specific treatment, solitary lesions should be resected if they cause symptoms or if the pathologic diagnosis is in doubt.[111] An endoscopic polypectomy may be feasible if the lesion is small or pedunculated, but surgery may be required for larger lesions.[111,112]

Radiographic Findings

The diffuse form of Brunner gland hyperplasia is manifested on barium studies by multiple small, rounded nodules in the proximal duodenum, producing a characteristic "cobblestone" or "Swiss cheese" appearance (Fig. 35-27A).[113,114] The nodules tend to be most abundant in the duodenal bulb with fewer nodules in the descending duodenum, so that the lesions correspond to the normal anatomic distribution of Brunner glands.[113] Occasionally, central flecks of barium may be identified in the nodules. As a result, it has been postulated that these lesions represent chronic duodenal erosions in various stages of re-epithelialization.[115]

Brunner gland hamartomas may appear as one or more submucosal or sessile lesions, ranging from several millimeters to several centimeters (Fig. 35-27B).[109,111,113,114,116,117] Some patients with giant Brunner gland hamartomas may have large polypoid defects in the duodenum (Fig. 35-27C).[118] Other patients with enlarged Brunner glands may have markedly thickened, irregular folds in the proximal duodenum because of concomitant duodenitis (Fig. 35-27D).[117] Rarely, large intramural masses may cause mechanical obstruction of the duodenum or act as the lead point for a duodenojejunal intussusception.[111,116,119]

Differential Diagnosis

The differential diagnosis for the diffuse form of Brunner gland hyperplasia includes the various polyposis syndromes, benign lymphoid hyperplasia, heterotopic gastric mucosa, and nodular duodenitis. Although the polyposis syndromes may be manifested by multiple rounded nodules in the duodenum, these individuals almost always have a generalized intestinal polyposis, whereas Brunner gland hyperplasia is confined to the duodenum. Similarly, benign lymphoid hyperplasia is characterized by multiple small nodules in the duodenal bulb and proximal duodenum (Fig. 35-28).[120] However, these patients often have generalized lymphoid hyperplasia of the small bowel or colon. Heterotopic gastric mucosa in the duodenum is characterized by angulated or polygonal 1- to

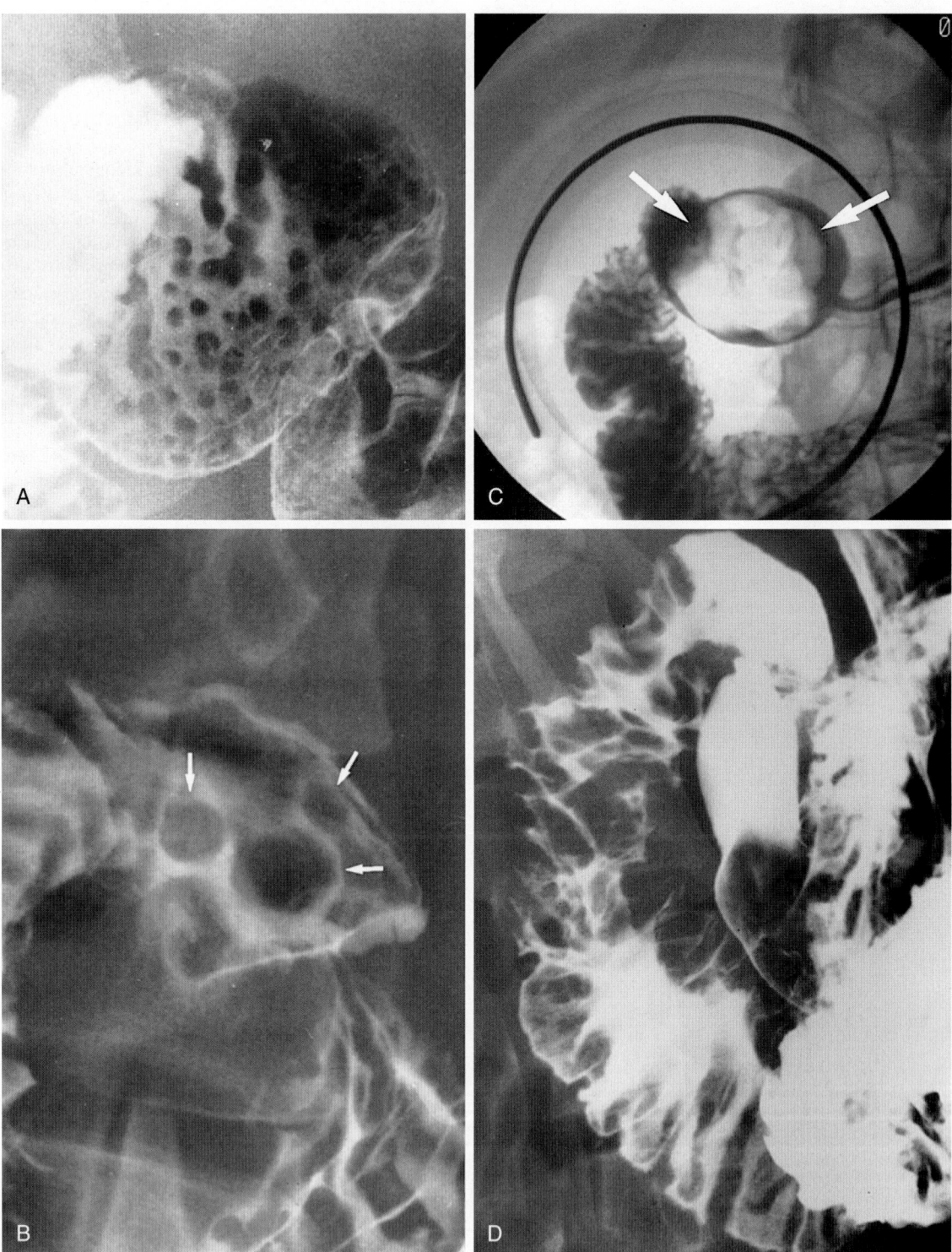

Figure 35-27. Brunner gland hyperplasia: spectrum of findings. A. Multiple tiny, rounded nodules are present in the duodenal bulb in a patient with diffuse Brunner gland hyperplasia. **B.** This patient has several Brunner gland hamartomas in the duodenum, manifested by submucosal masses (*arrows*) in the bulb. **C.** A large polypoid defect (*arrows*) is seen in the duodenal bulb in another patient with a giant Brunner gland hamartoma. **D.** A fourth patient with enlarged Brunner glands has markedly thickened, disorganized folds in the descending duodenum because of concomitant duodenitis. (**A** from Laufer I, Levine MS [eds]: Double Contrast Gastrointestinal Radiology, 2nd ed. Philadelphia, WB Saunders, 1992; **C** courtesy of Jackie Brown, MD, Vancouver, Canada; **D** courtesy of Dean D. T. Maglinte, MD, Indianapolis, IN.)

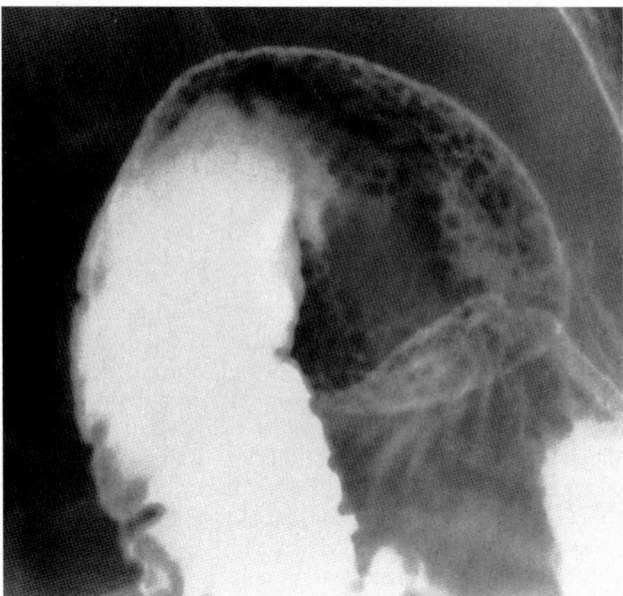

Figure 35-28. Benign lymphoid hyperplasia. Innumerable tiny nodules are present in the duodenal bulb. This patient had hypogammaglobulinemia. (From Laufer I, Levine MS [eds]: Double Contrast Gastrointestinal Radiology, 2nd ed. Philadelphia, WB Saunders, 1992.)

5-mm nodules or plaques that, in contrast to Brunner glands, tend to be clustered near the base of the duodenal bulb (Fig. 35-29).[121,122] Finally, nodular duodenitis may be manifested by thickened, nodular folds that can resemble hyperplastic Brunner glands. However, the nodular folds tend to coalesce in the inflamed duodenum whereas enlarged Brunner glands have more discrete borders.

Solitary Brunner gland hamartomas are difficult to distinguish from other polypoid lesions in the duodenum. Depend-

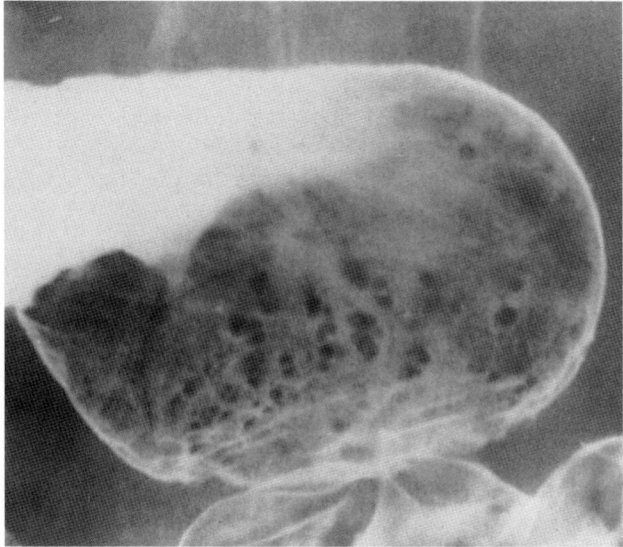

Figure 35-29. Heterotopic gastric mucosa in the duodenum. There are discrete, angulated filling defects near the base of the duodenal bulb. This appearance is so characteristic of heterotopic gastric mucosa that a confident diagnosis can be made on the basis of double-contrast studies without need for endoscopy. (From Laufer I, Levine MS [eds]: Double Contrast Gastrointestinal Radiology, 2nd ed. Philadelphia, WB Saunders, 1992.)

ing on their appearance, they can resemble mucosal lesions such as adenomatous polyps or submucosal lesions such as benign GISTs. Occasionally, prolapsed gastric mucosa in the duodenal bulb may produce a similar appearance. However, prolapsed mucosa is usually recognized as a mushroom-shaped defect at the base of the bulb that occurs as a transient finding at fluoroscopy (see Fig. 35-9). Rarely, a pedunculated polyp in the gastric antrum that has prolapsed into the duodenum can also be mistaken for a duodenal lesion such as a Brunner gland hamartoma.[3]

Duplication Cyst

Duplication cysts are hollow, epithelium-lined, spherical or tubular structures that are directly attached to some portion of the gastrointestinal tract, most frequently the distal ileum.[123,124] They tend to occur on the mesenteric border of the bowel, often sharing a common blood supply and muscular coat with the adjacent bowel wall. Most duplication cysts are spherical duplications that have no direct communication with the normal gastrointestinal tract.[124,125] However, the rare tubular form of duplication cyst may communicate with the gastrointestinal lumen at its proximal or distal end.[124,125]

Duplication cysts of the stomach and duodenum are uncommon lesions, comprising only 4% to 5% of all intestinal duplications.[125,126] However, they may be associated with a variety of complications such as bleeding, obstruction, or perforation. These lesions should therefore be surgically repaired or removed whenever feasible.

Pathology

Gastrointestinal duplication cysts are congenital malformations, probably resulting from faulty embryologic budding or defective recanalization of the alimentary tube during early fetal life.[124,127,128] Histologically, they are fluid-filled cysts containing a well-developed smooth muscle layer and mucous membrane lining. This mucous membrane is usually identical to that of the parent bowel, but duplication cysts may occasionally contain gastric, intestinal, pancreatic, or even respiratory epithelium.[124,129] When ectopic gastric mucosa is present in the cyst, secretion of peptic acid may cause ulceration or bleeding.[129] Depending on the volume of secretions within the cysts, they may vary from 1 to 25 cm.[129] Duplication cysts of the stomach usually arise from the greater curvature of the antrum or body,[123,126] whereas duplication cysts of the duodenum usually arise from the medial aspect of the first or second portion of the duodenum.[125,127,129]

Duplication cysts of the stomach and duodenum may be associated with a variety of other congenital anomalies, including intestinal or biliary atresia, malrotation, imperforate anus, double gallbladder, and double uterus. These patients also tend to have duplication cysts elsewhere in the gastrointestinal tract.[130] In contrast to mediastinal duplication cysts, duplication cysts of the stomach and duodenum are rarely associated with hemivertebrae or other vertebral anomalies.[126,129]

Clinical Findings

Gastric duplication cysts are twice as common in women as in men,[130] whereas duodenal duplication cysts have an approximately equal sex distribution.[127] Because most gastric duplication cysts cause symptoms during the first year of life, they are almost always diagnosed during early childhood.[126,130] In contrast, 35% to 40% of duodenal duplication cysts are discovered in patients older than age 20.[129,131]

Children or adults with duplication cysts of the stomach or duodenum most commonly present with a palpable abdominal mass and vomiting as the enlarging cyst encroaches on the adjacent stomach or duodenum.[126,127,129,130] In infants with gastric duplication cysts, nonbilious vomiting may erroneously suggest hypertrophic pyloric stenosis.[132] In contrast, duodenal duplication cysts tend to be associated with bilious vomiting.[125] Less frequently, older children or adults may present with abdominal pain, weight loss, fever, or upper gastrointestinal bleeding.[125-127,129,130] Abdominal pain probably results from progressive distention of the cyst by its own secretions. Fever occurs if the cyst becomes infected. Upper gastrointestinal bleeding is caused by localized pressure necrosis of the adjacent gastric or duodenal wall or by ulceration of a cyst that communicates directly with the stomach or duodenum.[125,127] Duodenal duplication cysts may occasionally compress the ampulla of Vater or the pancreatic or common bile ducts, causing acute pancreatitis or obstructive jaundice.[127,129] Rarely, duplication cysts may present as surgical emergencies because of torsion or perforation of the cyst with associated peritonitis.[129,133]

Because of these complications, duplication cysts of the stomach and duodenum should be treated surgically. Gastric duplication cysts can often be excised without difficulty from their attachment to the greater curvature of the stomach.[130] Because of their proximity to the ampulla of Vater, how-ever, duodenal duplication cysts frequently cannot be resected without performing a pancreaticoduodenectomy and reconstructive biliary surgery. Alternatively, some surgeons prefer to create a window between the cyst and the duodenum by excising a portion of the common wall between these structures to permit internal drainage and decompression of the cyst.[125,129]

Radiographic Findings

Duplication cysts of the stomach and duodenum may occasionally be recognized on abdominal radiographs by the presence of a soft tissue mass indenting the gastric or duodenal air shadows. The transverse colon may also be displaced inferiorly by gastric duplication cysts. Rarely, curvilinear calcification may be identified in the cyst wall.[134,135] However, calcification is more commonly seen in mesenteric, renal, or adrenal cysts.

Gastric duplication cysts typically appear on barium studies as intramural or extrinsic mass lesions involving the greater curvature or, less commonly, the posterior wall or lesser curvature of the gastric antrum (Fig. 35-30A).[123,136] Similarly, duodenal duplication cysts may be recognized as smooth intramural or extrinsic masses involving the medial wall of the descending duodenum (Fig. 35-31).[125,129,131] As gastric and duodenal duplication cysts enlarge, they may encroach considerably on the lumen of the stomach and duodenum, causing progressive obstruction. Rarely, communicating duplication cysts can be recognized as ovoid or tubular, barium-filled structures adjacent to the stomach or duodenum because of opacification of the cyst lumen (Fig. 35-32).[137,138]

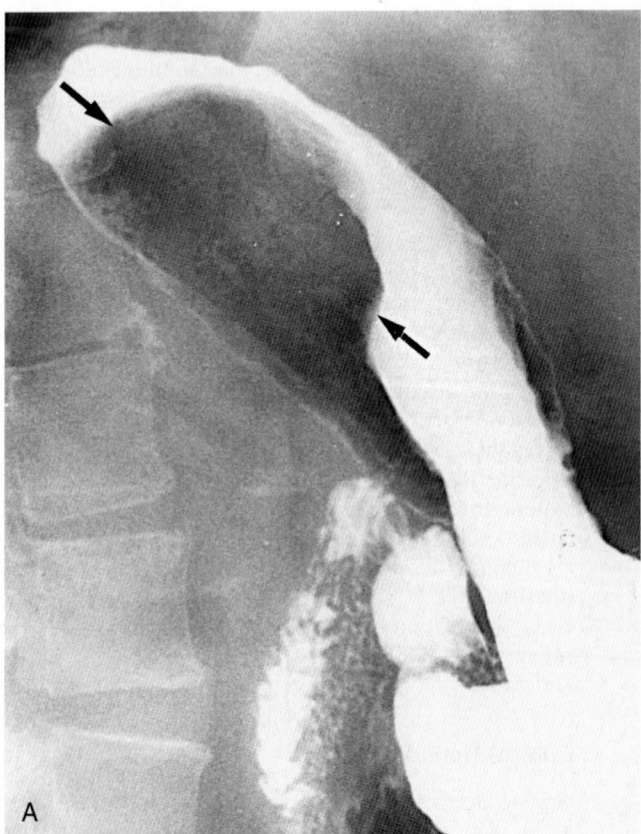

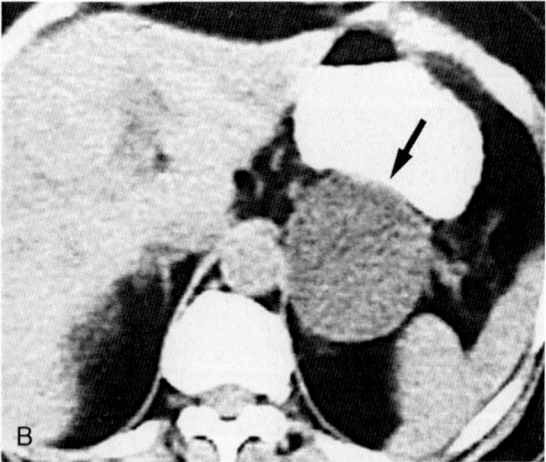

Figure 35-30. Gastric duplication cyst. A. Barium study shows a smooth mass (*arrows*) indenting the posterior wall of the gastric fundus. **B.** CT scan shows a thin-walled, fluid-filled mass (*arrow*) abutting the stomach. (From Thornhill BA, Cho KC, Morehouse HT: Gastric duplication associated with pulmonary sequestration: CT manifestations. AJR 138:1168-1171, 1982, © by American Roentgen Ray Society.)

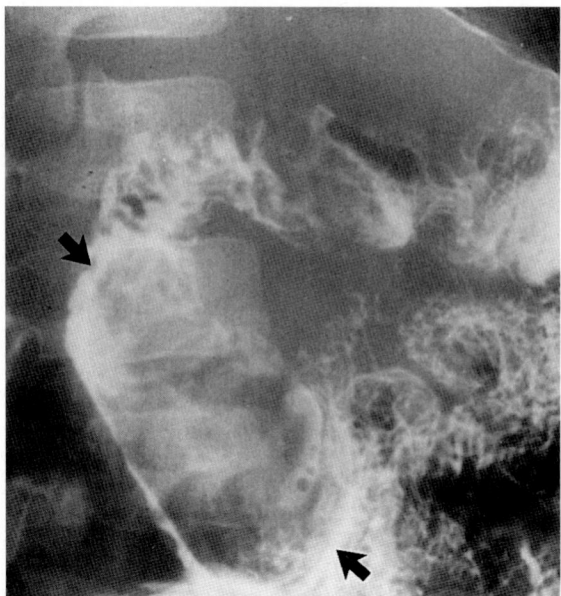

Figure 35-31. Duodenal duplication cyst. There is a large intramural mass (*arrows*) in the descending duodenum. Note the smooth contour of the lesion. An intramural hematoma or choledochal cyst could produce similar findings.

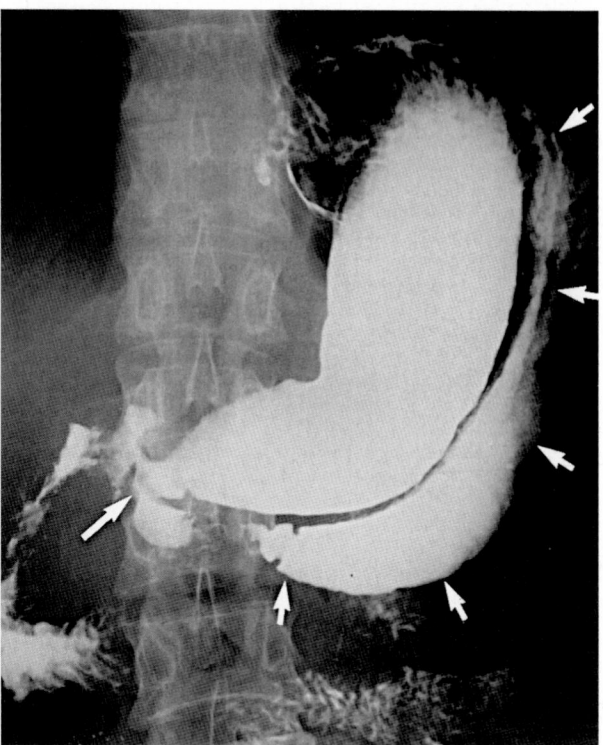

Figure 35-32. Communicating gastric duplication. Barium has entered a long, tubular duplication cyst (*short arrows*) on the greater curvature of the stomach. The duplication extends from the fundus to the pylorus, where it communicates with the lumen (*long arrow*). This form of duplication is extremely uncommon. (From Marshak RH, Lindner AE, Maklansky D [eds]: Radiology of the Stomach. Philadelphia, WB Saunders, 1983.)

Both ultrasonography and CT may be helpful in confirming the cystic nature of gastric and duodenal duplications that are visualized indirectly on barium studies. These structures usually appear on ultrasound examination as sonolucent masses with strong posterior wall echoes and through-transmission.[138,139] In some patients, the mucosal lining of the cyst is manifested by an echogenic inner ring surrounded by a relatively hypoechoic muscle layer.[138,139] Echogenic internal components may occasionally be seen in cysts that are infected or hemorrhagic.[139] These duplication cysts can also be recognized on CT as thin-walled, fluid-filled structures abutting the greater curvature of the stomach or medial wall of the descending duodenum (Fig. 35-30B).[135,137,140] Rarely, CT may demonstrate cyst wall calcification or enteroliths within the cyst.[140]

Differential Diagnosis

The finding on barium studies of a smooth intramural lesion on the greater curvature of the gastric antrum or medial wall of the descending duodenum should suggest the possibility of a duplication cyst, particularly in children. Other intramural lesions (i.e., benign GISTs, lipomas, or hematomas) or extrinsic lesions (i.e., pancreatic tumors or pseudocysts or choledochal cysts) involving the stomach or duodenum may produce similar findings. When duplication cysts are suspected on barium studies, ultrasonography or CT may be helpful for documenting the cystic nature of these structures. Other cystic lesions in the upper abdomen, such as choledochal cysts, mesenteric cysts, omental cysts, and pancreatic pseudocysts, may resemble duplication cysts on ultrasound or CT studies.[139,140] Nevertheless, the finding of a cystic mass that is contiguous with the greater curvature of the stomach or medial wall of the duodenum but separable from the gallbladder, extrahepatic biliary tree, and pancreas should be highly suggestive of a duplication cyst.

References

1. Good CA: Benign tumors of the stomach and duodenal bulb. J Can Assoc Radiol 16:92-104, 1965.
2. Ochsner SF, Janetos GP: Benign tumors of the stomach. JAMA 191:881-887, 1965.
3. Marshak RH, Feldman F: Gastric polyps. Am J Dig Dis 10:909-935, 1965.
4. Gordon R, Laufer I, Kressel HY: Gastric polyps found on routine double-contrast examination of the stomach. Radiology 134:27-30, 1980.
5. Feczko PJ, Halpert RD, Ackerman LV: Gastric polyps: Radiological evaluation and clinical significance. Radiology 155:581-584, 1985.
6. Ming S-C: The classification and significance of gastric polyps. In Yardly JH, Morson BC, Abell M (eds): The Gastrointestinal Tract. International Academy of Pathology Monograph. Baltimore, Williams & Wilkins, 1977, pp 149-175.
7. Tomosulo J: Gastric polyps: Histologic types and their relationship to gastric carcinoma. Cancer 27:1346-1355, 1971.
8. Ming S-C: The adenoma-carcinoma sequence in the stomach and colon: II. Malignant potential of gastric polyps. Gastrointest Radiol 1:121-125, 1976.
9. Ming S-C, Goldman H: Gastric polyps: A histogenetic classification and its relation to carcinoma. Cancer 18:721-726, 1965.
10. Burt RW: Gastric fundic gland polyps. Gastroenterology 125:1462-1469, 2003.
11. Iida M, Yao T, Watanabe H, et al: Fundi gland polyposis in patients without familial adenomatosis coli: Its incidence and clinical features. Gastroenterology 86:1437-1442, 1984.
12. Tsuchigame T, Saito R, Ogata Y, et al: Clinical evaluation of gastric fundic gland polyps without familial polyposis coli. Abdom Imaging 20:101-105, 1995.
13. Iida M, Yao T, Itoh H, et al: Natural history of fundic gland polyposis in patients with familial adenomatosis coli/Gardner's syndrome. Gastroenterology 89:1021-1025, 1985.

14. Joffe N, Antonioli DA: Atypical appearances of benign hyperplastic polyps. AJR 131:147-152, 1978.
15. Op den Orth JO, Ploem S: The stalactite phenomenon on double contrast studies of the stomach. Radiology 117:523-525, 1975.
16. Aronchick J, Laufer I, Glick SN: Barium stalactites: Observations on their nature and significance. Radiology 149:588-591, 1983.
17. Smith HJ, Lee EL: Large hyperplastic polyps of the stomach. Gastroint Radiol 8:19-23, 1983.
18. Hizawa K, Iida M, Matsumoto T, et al: Natural history of fundic gland polyposis without familial adenomatosis coli: Follow-up observations in 31 patients. Radiology 189:429-432, 1993.
19. Kikuchi Y, Levine MS, Laufer I, et al: Value of flow technique for double-contrast examination of the stomach. AJR 147:1183-1184, 1986.
20. Op den Orth JO, Dekker W: Gastric adenomas. Radiology 141:289-293, 1981.
21. Laxen F: Gastric carcinoma and pernicious anaemia in long-term endoscopic follow-up of subjects with gastric polyps. Scand J Gastroenterol 19:535-540, 1984.
22. Borch K: Epidemiologic, clinicopathologic, and economic aspects of gastroscopic screening of patients with pernicious anaemia. Scand J Gastroenterol 21:21-30, 1986.
23. Bone GE, McClelland RN: Management of gastric polyps. Surg Gynecol Obstet 142:933-938, 1976.
24. Kumar A, Quick CRG, Carr-Locke DL: Prolapsing gastric polyp, an unusual cause of gastric outlet obstruction: A review of the pathology and management of gastric polyps. Endoscopy 28:452-455, 1996.
25. Lanza FL, Graham DY, Nelson RS, et al: Endoscopic upper gastrointestinal polypectomy: Report of 73 polypectomies in 63 patients. Am J Gastroenterol 75:345-348, 1981.
26. ReMine SG, Hughes RW Jr, Weiland LH: Endoscopic gastric polypectomies. Mayo Clin Proc 56:371-375, 1981.
27. Hancock RJ: An 11-year review of primary tumours of the small bowel including the duodenum. Can Med Assoc J 103:1177-1179, 1970.
28. Griffen WO, Schaefer JW, Schindler S, et al: Ampullary obstruction by benign duodenal polyps. Arch Surg 97:444-449, 1968.
29. Deutschberger O, Tchertkoff V, Daino J, et al: Benign duodenal polyp: Review of the literature and report of a giant adenomatous polyp of the duodenal bulb. Am J Gastroenterol 38:75-84, 1962.
30. Nelson JA, Sheft DJ, Minagi H, et al: Duodenal pseudopolyp: The flexural fallacy. AJR 123:262-267, 1975.
31. Burrell M, Toffler R: Flexural pseudolesions of the duodenum. Radiology 120:313-315, 1976.
32. Schulten MF, Dyasu R, Beal JM: Villous adenoma of the duodenum: A case report and review of the literature. Am J Surg 132:90-96, 1976.
33. Mir-Madjlessi S-H, Farmer RG, Hawk WA: Villous tumors of the duodenum and jejunum: Report of four cases and review of the literature. Am J Dig Dis 18:467-476, 1973.
34. Miller JH, Gisvold JJ, Weiland LH, et al: Upper gastrointestinal tract: Villous tumors. AJR 134:933-936, 1980.
35. Kutim ND, Ranson JHC, Gouge TH, et al: Villous tumors of the duodenum. Ann Surg 181:164-168, 1975.
36. Gaitini O, Kleinhaus U, Munichor M, et al: Villous tumors of the stomach. Gastrointest Radiol 13:105-108, 1988.
37. Ring EJ, Ferucci JT, Eaton SB, et al: Villous adenoma of the duodenum. Radiology 104:45-48, 1972.
38. Boyer CW: Adenoma of the duodenal bulb: A case report. AJR 90:753-755, 1963.
39. Kilcheski T, Kressel HY, Laufer I, et al: The radiographic appearance of the stomach in Cronkhite-Canada syndrome. Radiology 141:57-60, 1981.
40. Salmela H: Smooth muscle tumors of the stomach. Acta Chir Scand 134:384-391, 1968.
41. Hwang JH, Kimmey MB: The incidental upper gastrointestinal subepithelial mass. Gastroenterology 126:301-307, 2004.
42. Miettinen M, Sobin LH, Sarlomo-Rikala M: Immunohistochemical spectrum of GISTs at different sites and their differential diagnosis with a reference to CD117 (KIT). Mod Pathol 13:1134-1142, 2000.
43. Delikaris P, Golematis B, Missitzis G, et al: Smooth muscle neoplasms of the stomach. South Med J 76:440-442, 1983.
44. Morrissey K, Cho ES, Gray GF, et al: Muscular tumors of the stomach: Clinical and pathological study of 113 cases. Ann Surg 178:148-155, 1973.
45. Tayiem AK: Recurrent massive gastrointestinal bleeding due to gastric leiomyoma. J Kans Med Soc 81:460-461, 1980.
46. Suster S: Gastrointestinal stromal tumors. Semin Diagn Pathol 13:297-313, 1996.
47. Sanders L, Silverman M, Rossi R, et al: Gastric smooth muscle tumors: Diagnostic dilemmas and factors affecting outcome. World J Surg 20:992-995, 1996.
48. Short WF, Young BR: Roentgen demonstration of prolapse of benign polypoid gastric tumors into the duodenum, including a dumbbell-shaped leiomyoma. AJR 103:317-320, 1968.
49. Grundy A, Rayter Z, Shorthouse AJ: Gastrogastric intussuscepting leiomyomas. Gastrointest Radiol 9:319-321, 1984.
50. Crummy AB, Juhl JH: Calcified gastric leiomyoma. AJR 87:727-728, 1962.
51. Graham JC, Blanchard IT, Scatliff JH: Calcified gastric leiomyoma presenting as a mediastinal mass. AJR 114:529-531, 1972.
52. McGinnis GO: Adenocarcinoma of the stomach with calcification: A case report. Gastroenterology 39:90-93, 1960.
53. O'Riordan D, Levine MS, Yeager BA: Complete healing of ulceration within a gastric leiomyoma. Gastrointest Radiol 10:47-49, 1985.
54. Cho KJ, Reuter SR: Angiography of duodenal leiomyomas and leiomyosarcomas. AJR 135:31-35, 1980.
55. Herlinger H: The recognition of exogastric tumours: Report of six cases. Br J Radiol 39:25-36, 1966.
56. Stassa G, Klingensmith WC: Primary tumors of the duodenal bulb. AJR 107:105-110, 1969.
57. Lavin P, Hajdu SI, Foote FW: Gastric and extragastric leiomyoblastomas: Clinicopathologic study of 44 cases. Cancer 29:305-311, 1972.
58. Appelman HD, Helwig EB: Gastric epithelioid leiomyoma and leiomyosarcoma (leiomyoblastoma). Cancer 38:708-728, 1976.
59. Dalaker K, Harket R: Leiomyoblastoma (epithelioid leiomyoma) of the stomach. Acta Chir Scand 146:141-144, 1980.
60. van Steenbergen W, Kojima T, Geboes K, et al: Gastric leiomyoblastoma with metastases to the liver: A 36-year follow-up study. Gastroenterology 89:875-881, 1985.
61. Faegenburg D, Farman J, Dallemand S: Leiomyoblastoma of the stomach. Radiology 117:297-300, 1975.
62. Kelsey JR: Leiomyoblastoma of the stomach presenting as acute intraperitoneal hemorrhage. Gastroenterology 51:539-541, 1966.
63. Choi BI, Ok ID, Im JG, et al: Exogastric cystic leiomyoblastoma with unusual CT appearance. Gastrointest Radiol 13:109-111, 1988.
64. Lerner ME, Farman J, Cho K, et al: Leiomyoblastoma: Varied CT appearance. Clin Imaging 16:194-197, 1992.
65. Fernandez MJ, Davis RP, Nora PF: Gastrointestinal lipomas. Arch Surg 118:1081-1083, 1983.
66. Turkington RW: Gastric lipoma: Report of a case and review of the literature. Am J Dig Dis 10:719-726, 1965.
67. Maderal F, Hunter F, Fuselier G, et al: Gastric lipomas: An update of clinical presentation, diagnosis, and treatment. Am J Gastroenterol 79:964-967, 1984.
68. Taylor AJ, Stewart ET, Dodds WJ: Gastrointestinal lipomas: A radiologic and pathologic review. AJR 155:1205-1210, 1990.
69. Chu AG, Clifton JA: Gastric lipoma presenting as peptic ulcer: Case report and review of the literature. Am J Gastroenterol 78:615-618, 1983.
70. Deeths TM, Madden PN, Dodds WJ: Multiple lipomas of the stomach and duodenum. Dig Dis 20:771-774, 1975.
71. Megibow AJ, Redmond PE, Bosniak MA, et al: Diagnosis of gastrointestinal lipomas by CT. AJR 133:743-745, 1979.
72. Heiken JP, Forde KA, Gold RP: Computed tomography as a definitive method for diagnosing gastrointestinal lipomas. Radiology 142:409-414, 1982.
73. Imoto T, Nobe T, Koga M, et al: Computed tomography of gastric lipomas. Gastrointest Radiol 8:129-131, 1983.
74. Thompson WM, Kende AI, Levy AD: Imaging characteristics of gastric lipomas in 16 adult and pediatric patients. AJR 181:981-985, 2003.
75. Mendez-Uriburu L, Ahualli J, Mendez-Uriburu J, et al: CT appearances of intraabdominal and intrapelvic fatty lesions. AJR 183:933-943, 2004.
76. Kerekes ES: Gastric hemangioma. Radiology 82:468-469, 1964.
77. Simms SM: Gastric hemangioma associated with phleboliths. Gastrointest Radiol 10:51-53, 1985.
78. Davis M, Fenoglio-Preiser C, Haque AK: Cavernous lymphangioma of the duodenum. Gastrointest Radiol 12:10-12, 1987.
79. Harig BM, Rosen Y, Dallemand S, et al: Glomus tumor of the stomach. Am J Gastroenterol 63:423-428, 1975.
80. Appelman HD, Helwig EB: Glomus tumors of the stomach. Cancer 23:203-213, 1969.
81. Weitzner S: Glomus tumor of the stomach: Report of a case and review of the literature. Am J Gastroenterol 51:322-328, 1969.
82. Schneider HJ: Glomus tumor of the stomach. AJR 92:1026-1028, 1964.

83. Banks BM: Neurofibroma of the stomach. Gastroenterology 41:158-167, 1950.
84. Perea VD, Gregory LJ: Neurofibromatosis of the stomach: Report of a case associated with von Recklinghausen's disease and review of the literature. JAMA 182:259-263, 1962.
85. Hoare AM, Elkington SG: Gastric lesions in generalized neurofibromatosis. Br J Surg 63:449-451, 1976.
86. Lack EE, Worsham GF, Callihan MD, et al: Granular cell tumor: A clinicopathologic study of 110 patients. J Surg Oncol 13:301-306, 1980.
87. Fisher ER, Wechsler H: Granular cell myoblastoma—a misnomer: Electron microscopic and histochemical evidence concerning its Schwann cell derivation and nature (granular cell schwannoma). Cancer 15:936-954, 1962.
88. Johnston J, Helwig EB: Granular cell tumors of the gastrointestinal tract and perianal region: A study of 74 cases. Dig Dis Sci 26:807-816, 1981.
89. Naidech HJ, Axelrod RS, Seliger G: Granular cell tumor (myoblastoma) of the stomach. AJR 113:245-247, 1971.
90. Schwartz DT, Gaetz HP: Multiple granular cell myoblastomas of the stomach. Am J Clin Pathol 44:453-457, 1965.
91. Carlson E, Ward JG: Inflammatory gastric polyps (eosinophilic granulomas of the stomach). Am J Surg 99:352-357, 1960.
92. Salm R: Gastric fibroma with eosinophilic infiltration. Gut 6:85-91, 1965.
93. Allman RN, Cavanagh RC, Helwig EB, et al: Inflammatory fibroid polyp. Radiology 127:69-73, 1978.
94. Harned RK, Buck JL, Shekitka KM: Inflammatory fibroid polyps of the gastrointestinal tract: Radiologic evaluation. Radiology 182:863-866, 1992.
95. Besemann EF, Auerbach SH, Wolfe WW: The importance of roentgenologic diagnosis of aberrant pancreatic tissue in the gastrointestinal tract. AJR 107:71-76, 1969.
96. Bush WH, Hall DG, Ward BH: Adenomyosis of the gastric antrum in children. Radiology 111:179-181, 1974.
97. Goldberg HI, Margulis AR: Adenomyoma of the stomach. AJR 96:382-386, 1966.
98. Copleman B: Aberrant pancreas in the gastric wall. Radiology 81:107-111, 1963.
99. Martinez LO, Gregg M: Aberrant pancreas in the gallbladder. J Can Assoc Radiol 24:234-235, 1973.
100. Tonkin RD, Field TE, Wykes PR: Pancreatic heterotopia as a cause of dyspepsia. Gut 3:135-139, 1962.
101. Clark RE, Teplick SK: Ectopic pancreas causing massive gastrointestinal hemorrhage: Report of a case diagnosed angiographically. Gastroenterology 69:1331-1333, 1975.
102. Matsumoto Y, Kawai Y, Kimura K: Aberrant pancreas causing pyloric obstruction. Surgery 76:827-829, 1974.
103. Green PHR, Barratt PJ, Percy JP, et al: Acute pancreatitis occurring in gastric aberrant pancreatic tissue. Am J Dig Dis 22:734-740, 1977.
104. Kilman WJ, Berk RN: The spectrum of radiographic features of aberrant pancreatic rests involving the stomach. Radiology 123:291-296, 1977.
105. Thoeni RF, Gedgaudas RK: Ectopic pancreas: Usual and unusual features. Gastrointest Radiol 5:37-42, 1980.
106. Franzin G, Musola R, Ghidini O, et al: Nodular hyperplasia of Brunner's glands. Gastrointest Endosc 31:374-378, 1985.
107. Kaplan EL, Dyson WL, Fitts WT: The relationship of gastric hyperacidity to hyperplasia of Brunner's glands. Arch Surg 98:636-639, 1969.
108. Nelson OF, Whitaker EG, Roberts FM: Adenoma of Brunner's glands. Am J Surg 110:977-980, 1965.
109. Osborne R, Toffler R, Lowman RM: Brunner's gland adenoma of the duodenum. Am J Dig Dis 18:689-694, 1973.
110. ReMine WH, Brown PW, Gomes MMR, et al: Polypoid hamartomas of Brunner's glands. Arch Surg 100:313-316, 1970.
111. Strutynsky N, Posniak R, Mori K: Obstructing hamartoma of Brunner's glands of the duodenum. Dig Dis Sci 27:279-282, 1982.
112. Ponka JL, Shaalan AK: Massive gastrointestinal hemorrhage secondary to tumors of Brunner's glands. Am J Surg 108:51-56, 1964.
113. Dodd GD, Fishler JS, Park OK: Hyperplasia of Brunner's glands: Report of two cases with review of the literature. Radiology 60:814-823, 1953.
114. Weinberg PE, Levin B: Hyperplasia of Brunner's glands. Radiology 84:259-262, 1965.
115. Walk L: Nodular hyperplasia of duodenal Brunner's glands—does it exist? Endoscopy 14:162-165, 1982.
116. Maglinte DDT, Mayes SL, Ng AC, et al: Brunner's gland adenoma: Diagnostic considerations. J Clin Gastroenterol 4:127-131, 1982.
117. Merine D, Jones B, Ghahremani GG, et al: Hyperplasia of Brunner glands: The spectrum of its radiographic manifestations. Gastrointest Radiol 16:104-108, 1991.
118. van Rooij WJJ, ven der Horst JJ, Stuifbergen WNHM, et al: Extreme diffuse adenomatous hyperplasia of Brunner's glands: Case report. Gastrointest Radiol 15:285-287, 1990.
119. Lempke RE: Intussusception of the duodenum: Report of a case due to Brunner's gland hyperplasia. Ann Surg 150:160-166, 1959.
120. Govoni AF: Benign lymphoid hyperplasia of the duodenal bulb. Gastrointest Radiol 1:267-269, 1976.
121. Langkemper R, Hoek AC, Dekker W, et al: Elevated lesions in the duodenal bulb caused by heterotopic gastric mucosa. Radiology 137:621-624, 1980.
122. Agha FP, Ghahremani GG, Tsang TK, et al: Heterotopic gastric mucosa in the duodenum: Radiographic findings. AJR 150:291-294, 1988.
123. Kremer RM, Lepoff RB, Izant RJ: Duplication of the stomach. J Pediatr Surg 5:360-364, 1970.
124. Taft DA, Hairston JT: Duplication of the alimentary tract. Am Surg 42:455-462, 1976.
125. Soper RT, Selke AC: Duplication cyst of the duodenum: Case report and discussion. Surgery 68:562-566, 1970.
126. Pruksapong C, Donovan RJ, Pinit A, et al: Gastric duplication. J Pediatr Surg 14:83-85, 1979.
127. Inouye WY, Farrell C, Fitts WT, et al: Duodenal duplication: Case report and literature review. Ann Surg 162:910-916, 1965.
128. Agha FP, Gabriele OF, Abdulla FH: Complete gastric duplication. AJR 137:406-407, 1981.
129. Thompson NW, Labow SS: Duplication of the duodenum in the adult. Arch Surg 94:301-306, 1967.
130. Bartels RJ: Duplication of the stomach. Am Surg 33:747-752, 1967.
131. Faegenburg D, Bosniak M: Duodenal anomalies in the adult. AJR 88:642-657, 1962.
132. Kammerer M: Duplication of the stomach resembling hypertrophic pyloric stenosis. JAMA 207:2101-2102, 1969.
133. Kleinhaus S, Boley SJ, Winslow P: Occult bleeding from a perforated gastric duplication in an infant. Arch Surg 116:122, 1981.
134. Alford BA, Armstron P, Franken EA, et al: Calcification associated with duodenal duplications in children. Radiology 134:647-648, 1980.
135. Omojola MF, Hood IC, Stevenson GW: Calcified gastric duplication. Gastrointest Radiol 5:235, 1980.
136. Bower RJ, Sieber WK, Kiesewetter WB: Alimentary tract duplications in children. Ann Surg 188:669-674, 1978.
137. McAlister WH, Siegel MJ: Duodenal duplication. AJR 152:1328-1329, 1989.
138. Hulnick DH, Balthazar EJ: Gastric duplication cyst: GI series and CT correlation. Gastrointest Radiol 12:106-108, 1987.
139. Kangarloo H, Sample WF, Hansen G, et al: Ultrasonic evaluation of abdominal gastrointestinal tract duplication in children. Radiology 131:191-194, 1979.
140. Bar-Ziv J, Katz R, Nobel M, et al: Duodenal duplication cyst with enteroliths: Computed tomography and ultrasound diagnosis. Gastrointest Radiol 14:220-222, 1989.

Carcinoma of the Stomach and Duodenum

Marc S. Levine, MD • Alec J. Megibow, MD • Michael L. Kochman, MD

GASTRIC CARCINOMA

There has been a dramatic decline in the incidence of gastric carcinoma since the late 1940s.[1-4] Nevertheless, it remains a deadly disease, with overall 5-year survival rates of less than 20%.[4-8] Since the 1980s, attention has been focused on the role of double-contrast barium studies and endoscopy for the early diagnosis of gastric cancer. The Japanese have had tremendous success in detecting early gastric cancer by mass screening of the adult population with these techniques. However, it is difficult to justify such screening programs outside Japan because of the lower incidence of this malignancy. Thus, the prognosis for gastric carcinoma remains dismal in most parts of the world.

Epidemiology

Gastric carcinoma has striking geographic variations, with the highest incidences reported in Japan, Chile, Finland, Poland, and Iceland.[3,8] However, Japanese immigrants and their offspring living in the United States have a significantly lower incidence of gastric cancer than those living in Japan.[8,9] Such epidemiologic data suggest that environmental factors have a major role in the development of gastric carcinoma. Dietary habits may be particularly important in explaining the observed geographic differences in cancer risk. *Helicobacter pylori* infection of the stomach has also increasingly been implicated as a major risk factor in the development of gastric carcinoma in various parts of the world. Other predisposing conditions include atrophic gastritis, pernicious anemia,

gastric polyps, partial gastrectomy, Ménétrier's disease, and hereditary factors. These various risk factors for gastric cancer are discussed separately in the following sections.

Dietary Factors

Studies have shown that diets rich in salted, smoked, or poorly preserved foods are associated with an increased risk of gastric cancer[4,10,11] whereas diets rich in fruits and vegetables are associated with a decreased risk.[4,12] Foods containing nitrates or nitrites have also been implicated in the development of gastric cancer.[4, 9] These compounds are converted by bacteria to nitrosamines, which are thought to have a carcinogenic effect on the stomach.[13] Thus, populations with a higher average intake of nitrates and nitrites probably have a higher gastric cancer risk. Conversely, vitamin C (ascorbic acid) appears to have a protective effect by reducing nitrites to nitric oxide and preventing the formation of nitrosamine compounds.[14] This could explain why consumption of fruit and vegetables is associated with a decreased risk of gastric cancer. A recent study also found that high intake of cereal fiber is associated with a significantly lower risk of gastric cardiac cancer,[15] possibly because of the nitrite-scavenging properties of cereal fiber.

Helicobacter pylori Gastritis

H. pylori has increasingly been implicated as a major risk factor in the pathogenesis of gastric carcinoma. Various studies have found that people with *H. pylori* gastritis have a two to six times greater risk of developing gastric cancer than those without this infection.[16-18] It has been well documented that people with long-standing *H. pylori* gastritis are more likely to develop atrophic gastritis.[19-21] Over a period of years, chronic atrophic gastritis may progress to gastric atrophy, intestinal metaplasia, dysplasia, and, eventually, gastric carcinoma.[4, 22-24] Other studies have found that people with *H. pylori* gastritis are more likely to develop the intestinal type of gastric carcinoma than people without this infection (see later section on Pathology of Gastric Carcinoma).[25,26] It has also been shown that certain strains of *H. pylori*, which produce a vacuolating cytotoxin (*cagA*), are associated with a higher prevalence of atrophic gastritis and gastric carcinoma.[27,28] A meta-analysis of 16 studies from the literature found that infection with *cagA*-positive strains of *H. pylori* substantially increases the risk of gastric cancer over the risk associated with *H. pylori* infection irrespective of *cagA* status.[29]

Nevertheless, gastric cancer develops in only a tiny percentage of all people with *H. pylori* gastritis, so other environmental or genetic factors presumably have a role in cancer pathogenesis. In a cost-effectiveness model, Parsonnet and colleagues found that widespread screening and treatment of adults for *H. pylori* is a potentially cost-effective strategy for the prevention of gastric cancer, particularly in high-risk populations.[30] However, further investigation is needed to determine whether such an approach is justified.

Atrophic Gastritis

Atrophic gastritis has been classified into two types, which have different histologic, immunologic, and secretory characteristics. Type A gastritis is usually associated with pernicious anemia (see next section). In contrast, type B gastritis (which is more common) predominantly involves the antrum and usually results from mucosal injury by *H. pylori* or, less commonly, by other toxic agents[31] (see Chapter 34). Long-term studies indicate that about 10% of patients with type B gastritis develop gastric carcinoma within 10 to 20 years.[32,33] It has been postulated that chronic atrophic gastritis leads to the development of intestinal metaplasia, dysplasia, and, eventually, adenocarcinoma.[4,22,23] This pathologic sequence of events is supported by the frequent association of gastric carcinoma and intestinal metaplasia on surgical specimens.[22,23] Thus, chronic atrophic gastritis and intestinal metaplasia are thought to be important precursor conditions for the development of gastric carcinoma.

Pernicious Anemia

Type A gastritis predominantly involves the gastric fundus and body and is usually thought to result from immunologic injury by antiparietal cell antibodies in patients with pernicious anemia.[31] This type of gastritis may also be associated with an increased risk of gastric cancer. In various studies, the incidence of gastric cancer in patients with pernicious anemia has been two to three times greater than that expected for the general population.[34,35] Most such tumors involve the gastric fundus or body. Although some investigators advocate radiologic or endoscopic surveillance of patients with known pernicious anemia, others believe that the cancer risk is not high enough to warrant routine surveillance.[36] Nevertheless, any patient with pernicious anemia who has guaiac-positive stool or other upper gastrointestinal complaints should be aggressively evaluated for possible gastric carcinoma.

Gastric Polyps

Adenomatous polyps account for less than 20% of all gastric polyps.[37] Despite their rarity, these polyps are premalignant lesions that are capable of undergoing malignant degeneration via an adenoma-carcinoma sequence similar to that found in the colon.[38] Nearly 50% of gastric adenomas larger than 2 cm are found to harbor carcinomatous foci.[39,40] All adenomatous polyps should therefore be resected because of the risk of malignant transformation. Nevertheless, adenocarcinoma is about 30 times more common than adenomatous polyps in the stomach, so most gastric cancers are thought to originate de novo and not from preexisting polyps.[38]

Partial Gastrectomy

Patients who undergo partial gastrectomy may be at increased risk for the development of gastric carcinoma. A *gastric stump cancer* is defined as a primary carcinoma of the gastric remnant occurring a minimum of 5 years after partial gastrectomy for gastric ulcers or other benign disease.[41] Affected individuals have usually undergone a Billroth II rather than a Billroth I procedure.[42,43] These tumors tend to be located in the distal portion of the gastric remnant near the gastrojejunal anastomosis. It has been postulated that recurrent bile reflux above the anastomosis causes chronic gastritis, intestinal metaplasia, and, eventually, gastric carcinoma. In various studies, the mortality from gastric cancer 15 or more years after partial gastrectomy has been three to seven times greater than that expected for the general population.[43-45] Some authors therefore advocate routine endoscopic surveillance of the gastric remnant starting 15 years after surgery.[45] However, other investigators have found no greater incidence of gastric carcinoma than that expected for the general population as long as 25 years after surgery.[46] Thus, the need for surveillance in these patients remains controversial.

Gastric carcinoma has also been reported as a late complication of gastrojejunostomy for benign disease in the absence of partial gastrectomy.[47,48] As in patients who have undergone a Billroth II procedure, bile reflux gastritis and intestinal metaplasia are thought to be predisposing factors. Whatever the explanation, the risk of developing gastric carcinoma also appears to be increased in patients who undergo a gastrojejunostomy without a gastric resection.

Ménétrier's Disease

Ménétrier's disease is a rare disorder of unknown etiology characterized by a hypertrophic gastropathy associated with decreased gastric acid secretion and protein-losing enteropathy (see Chapter 34). Anecdotal cases of gastric carcinoma have been described in patients with Ménétrier's disease.[49] However, it is unclear whether this association is coincidental or whether Ménétrier's disease is a premalignant condition.

Hereditary Factors

Hereditary factors have also been implicated in the development of gastric cancer, because a positive family history has been associated with an increased risk of this malignancy.[50] In one study, the prevalence of *H. pylori* gastritis was significantly higher in subjects who had parents with gastric cancer than among other subjects.[51] Such findings suggest that familial aggregation of gastric cancer may be explained at least partly by familial clustering of *H. pylori* gastritis. Patients with gastric cancer also have been found to have a higher frequency of blood type A and a lower frequency of blood type O than the general population.[52]

Pathology

Gross Features

Most gastric carcinomas are polypoid or ulcerated lesions.[53-55] Polypoid carcinomas have a plaquelike, lobulated, or fungating appearance. Ulcerated carcinomas may contain deep, irregular or broad, shallow areas of ulceration due to necrosis and excavation of the tumor.[53] The ulcer may be surrounded by a thin rind of malignant tissue or by an obvious mass lesion, so that many polypoid tumors have ulcerated components. Less commonly, gastric carcinomas may be diffusely infiltrative lesions that spread along the gastric wall with relatively little intraluminal growth.[53] These "scirrhous" tumors may produce a classic *linitis plastica* appearance due to submucosal thickening and fibrosis incited by the tumor. Other gastric carcinomas may be superficial spreading lesions that are confined to the mucosa or submucosa without invading the deep muscle layers of the gastric wall.[53]

Rarely, patients with gastric carcinoma have multiple primary lesions separated by normal intervening mucosa. In various series, two or more synchronous tumors have been found in 2% to 8% of all patients with gastric cancer.[56,57] In such cases, individual lesions may have different morphologic features.

Histologic Features

More than 95% of malignant neoplasms in the stomach are adenocarcinomas.[3] The remaining lesions consist of lymphoma, gastrointestinal stromal tumor, Kaposi's sarcoma, carcinoid, and other rare malignant tumors (see Chapter 37). Gastric adenocarcinomas may be subdivided into two categories: (1) an intestinal type characterized by well-formed glandular structures that tend to grow in a fungating manner and (2) a diffuse type characterized by poorly cohesive cells that tend to infiltrate and thicken the gastric wall without producing a discrete mass.[58] Intestinal-type lesions are more likely to involve the distal stomach and to occur in patients with underlying atrophic gastritis. In contrast, diffuse-type lesions are more likely to involve the entire stomach (especially the cardia) and are associated with a worse prognosis.[59]

Gastric carcinomas have been further classified by the World Health Organization into the following subtypes: papillary, tubular, mucinous, and signet-ring cell.[60] Most tumors that are capable of forming glandular structures secrete mucinous substances.[53] Occasionally, excessive mucin accumulates extracellularly in colloid or mucinous adenocarcinomas.[53] Other adenocarcinomas are composed of distinctive signet-ring cells, containing large amounts of intracytoplasmic mucin and compressed, eccentric nuclei.[53] As they infiltrate the gastric wall, these signet-ring cells often incite a marked desmoplastic response in the submucosa and muscularis propria, producing the classic pathologic features of a primary

scirrhous carcinoma. In various series, scirrhous tumors have been found to account for 5% to 15% of all gastric cancers.[5,7]

Most adenocarcinomas of the stomach are diagnosed at an advanced stage. By definition, *advanced gastric cancers* have already invaded the muscularis propria. These tumors are usually associated with metastases to regional lymph nodes or other local or distant structures. In contrast, *early gastric cancers* are defined histologically as cancers in which malignant invasion is limited to the mucosa or submucosa, regardless of the presence or absence of lymph node metastases.[61,62] The largest number of early gastric cancers has been reported in Japan as a result of mass screening of the adult population. Unlike advanced carcinomas, which have a dismal prognosis, early gastric cancers are curable lesions with 5-year survival rates of greater than 90% (see later section on Treatment and Prognosis).

Distribution

At one time, most gastric carcinomas were located in the antrum.[63] Since the late 1940s, however, there has been a gradual shift in the distribution of gastric cancer from the antrum proximally to the body and fundus.[1,63,64] This changing distribution has been attributed primarily to an increasing incidence of carcinoma of the gastric cardia, which has increased at a rate exceeding that of any other cancer.[4,65-67] As a result, these lesions now have a relatively even distribution in the stomach, with about 30% located in the antrum, 30% in the body, and 40% in the fundus or cardiac region.[1,6,7,64] This changing pattern of disease has important implications for cancer detection, because the gastric cardia and fundus must be carefully evaluated for signs of malignancy in all patients who undergo barium studies or endoscopy to rule out gastric carcinoma.

Routes of Spread

Gastric carcinoma may invade local, regional, or distant structures by four pathways: direct extension, lymphatic spread, intraperitoneal seeding, and hematogenous metastases. The various pathways of spread are discussed separately in the following sections.

Direct Extension

Gastric carcinoma has a tendency to involve contiguous structures such as the liver, pancreas, and spleen.[55,68] Longitudinal spread of tumor along the gastrointestinal tract is also relatively common. The distal esophagus is directly involved by carcinoma of the cardia in about 60% of patients,[69] whereas the duodenum is involved by carcinoma of the antrum in 5% to 25% of patients.[70-72] Tumor involving the greater curvature of the stomach may spread inferiorly via the gastrocolic ligament to the transverse colon, occasionally resulting in the development of a gastrocolic fistula.[73]

Lymphatic Spread

Because of the abundant lymphatics in the stomach, lymph node metastases are found in 74% to 88% of patients with gastric carcinoma.[53] These patients may initially have involvement of local (perigastric) nodes and, subsequently, regional (celiac, hepatic, left gastric, and splenic) or distant (left supraclavicular and left axillary) nodes.[8] The frequency of lymphatic metastases is related to the size and depth of penetration of the tumor. Nevertheless, lesions are still classified histologically as early gastric cancers, regardless of the presence of lymph node metastases, if malignant invasion is confined to the mucosa or submucosa.[61]

Intraperitoneal Seeding

Patients with advanced gastric carcinoma may have intraperitoneal-seeded or omental metastases.[68] Diffuse carcinomatosis may be associated with small bowel obstruction and ascites. Some patients with signet-ring cell adenocarcinomas have bilateral "drop" metastases to the ovaries, known as *Krukenberg tumors.*[74] Although other malignant tumors can metastasize to the ovaries, gastric carcinoma is responsible for the majority of cases.[74] In fact, some patients with gastric carcinoma may present with bilateral ovarian masses as the initial manifestation of their disease.

Hematogenous Metastases

Because the stomach is drained by the portal vein, the liver is the most common site of hematogenous (i.e., blood-borne) metastases from gastric carcinoma.[55] Other less common sites of hematogenous spread include the lungs, adrenals, kidneys, bones, and brain.

Clinical Findings

Gastric carcinoma is usually considered a disease of middle and late life, with a peak incidence between 50 and 70 years of age.[8,54,75] However, 3% to 5% of patients with gastric cancer are younger than 35 years of age and 1% are younger than 30 years.[76-78] Furthermore, the percentage of young patients with gastric cancer has more than doubled since 1970.[77] These patients tend to have more aggressive lesions, so they have a worse prognosis than most patients with gastric carcinoma.[77,78]

Gastric carcinoma is twice as common in men as in women.[2,8,11] However, carcinoma of the cardia has a much greater predilection for men (7:1) than carcinoma elsewhere in the stomach.[79,80] The explanation for this discrepancy is unclear.

Most patients with gastric carcinoma are symptomatic only when they have advanced tumors with local or distant metastases.[8,9] The most common presenting findings include epigastric pain, bloating, early satiety, nausea, vomiting, dysphagia, anorexia, weight loss, and signs or symptoms of upper gastrointestinal bleeding, such as hematemesis, melena, guaiac-positive stool, and iron-deficiency anemia.[8,9,54] However, similar findings may be caused by ulcers, gastritis, or other benign conditions. As a result, there is often a considerable lag between the onset of symptoms and the diagnosis of gastric cancer.

The clinical presentation is also affected by the location and morphologic features of the tumor. For example, nausea and vomiting are common findings in patients with obstructing lesions involving the distal antrum or pyloric region.[4] In contrast, patients with scirrhous carcinomas may develop early satiety because of the decreased compliance of a stomach that is diffusely infiltrated by tumor.[81] Paradoxically, gastric emptying may be more rapid than normal in these individ-

uals. Other patients with carcinoma of the cardia may present with recent onset of dysphagia caused by tumor obstructing the cardia.[82,83] Some patients complain of food sticking behind the lower sternum, whereas others have a sensation of blockage referred to the thoracic inlet or pharynx. The gastric cardia and fundus should therefore be carefully evaluated in all patients with dysphagia, regardless of the subjective site of obstruction, to rule out a carcinoma of the cardia masquerading as a pharyngeal or esophageal disorder.

Other patients with advanced gastric cancer may initially present with signs or symptoms of metastatic disease, such as anorexia, weight loss, abdominal masses, hepatic enlargement, jaundice, ascites, back pain, or neurologic findings. Patients with ovarian metastases may have bilateral pelvic masses (Krukenberg tumors), and patients with drop metastases to the rectosigmoid colon may have a Blumer shelf found on rectal examination.

Endoscopic Findings

When biopsy specimens and brushings are obtained, endoscopy has a reported overall sensitivity of 94% to 98% in the diagnosis of gastric carcinoma.[84-87] However, multiple biopsy specimens should be taken from suspicious lesions to decrease the risk of sampling error. It should also be recognized that endoscopy is a much less reliable technique for diagnosing scirrhous tumors. In various series, the sensitivity of endoscopy in detecting these lesions has ranged from only 33% to 70%.[88-90] False-negative endoscopic biopsy specimens or brushings may occur not only because scirrhous tumors are located predominantly in the submucosa but also because the tumor cells are often separated by large areas of fibrosis. In some cases, three or more endoscopic examinations may be required for a definitive histologic diagnosis.[90] Thus, excessive reliance on negative endoscopic findings may cause inordinate delays in the treatment of these patients. It is also important to be aware of the limitations of endoscopy in detecting scirrhous tumors based on the gross endoscopic appearance; the overlying mucosa often appears normal, so the presence and extent of tumor is easily underestimated at endoscopy.[91]

Radiographic Findings

Early Gastric Cancer

The double-contrast upper gastrointestinal examination has been widely recognized as the best radiologic technique for the diagnosis of early gastric cancer.[92-95] The Japanese Endoscopic Society has divided these lesions into three basic types.[96] Type I lesions are elevated lesions that protrude more than 5 mm into the lumen. Type II lesions are superficial lesions that are further subdivided into three groups—types IIa, IIb, and IIc—depending on their morphologic features. Type IIa lesions are elevated but protrude less than 5 mm into the lumen. Type IIb lesions are essentially flat. Type IIc lesions are slightly depressed but do not penetrate beyond the muscularis mucosae. Type III lesions are true mucosal ulcerations, with the ulcer penetrating the muscularis mucosae but not the muscularis propria. When early gastric cancers exhibit more than one of these morphologic features, they may have a dual classification, with the most predominant pattern listed first (e.g., type III + IIc).

Type I early gastric cancers typically appear as small, elevated lesions in the stomach.[93,94] Because adenomatous polyps may undergo malignant degeneration (see earlier section on Gastric Polyps), the possibility of early gastric cancer should be suspected for any sessile or pedunculated polyps larger than 1 cm. Other type I lesions may protrude considerably into the lumen and still be classified histologically as early gastric cancers (Fig. 36-1A).[94] Thus, polypoid carcinomas cannot be diagnosed definitively as early or advanced lesions on the basis of the radiographic findings.

Type II early gastric cancers are superficial lesions with elevated (IIa), flat (IIb), or depressed (IIc) components. These lesions may be manifested by plaquelike elevations, mucosal nodularity, shallow areas of ulceration, or some combination of these findings (Fig. 36-1B and C).[92-95] Occasionally, type II lesions may be quite extensive and involve a considerable surface area of the stomach.

Type III early gastric cancers are characterized by shallow, irregular ulcer craters with nodularity of the adjacent mucosa and clubbing, fusion, or amputation of radiating folds (Fig. 36-1D).[93,94] Careful analysis of the radiographic findings

usually allows these lesions to be distinguished from benign gastric ulcers, which have different radiographic features (see Chapter 33). Although some lesions with an equivocal or suspicious appearance are found to be benign ulcers, endoscopy and biopsy should be performed for all lesions with suspicious radiographic findings to avoid missing early cancers.

About 70% of the ulcers in type IIc or III early gastric cancers are reported to undergo significant healing on medical treatment.[97] It has been postulated that these cancers are characterized by a cycle of ulceration, healing, and recurrent ulceration. Rarely, complete healing of malignant ulcers has also been described.[97] However, malignant tumors may still be suspected on follow-up barium studies if mucosal nodularity or other abnormalities are detected at the site of the previous ulcer.

Japanese researchers have reported an incidence of early gastric cancer (i.e., the percentage of all gastric cancers that are detected as early lesions) of 25% to 46%[98-101] compared with an incidence of only 5% to 24% in Western countries.[93-95,102-108] This discrepancy can be attributed to mass screening of the adult population in Japan because of the

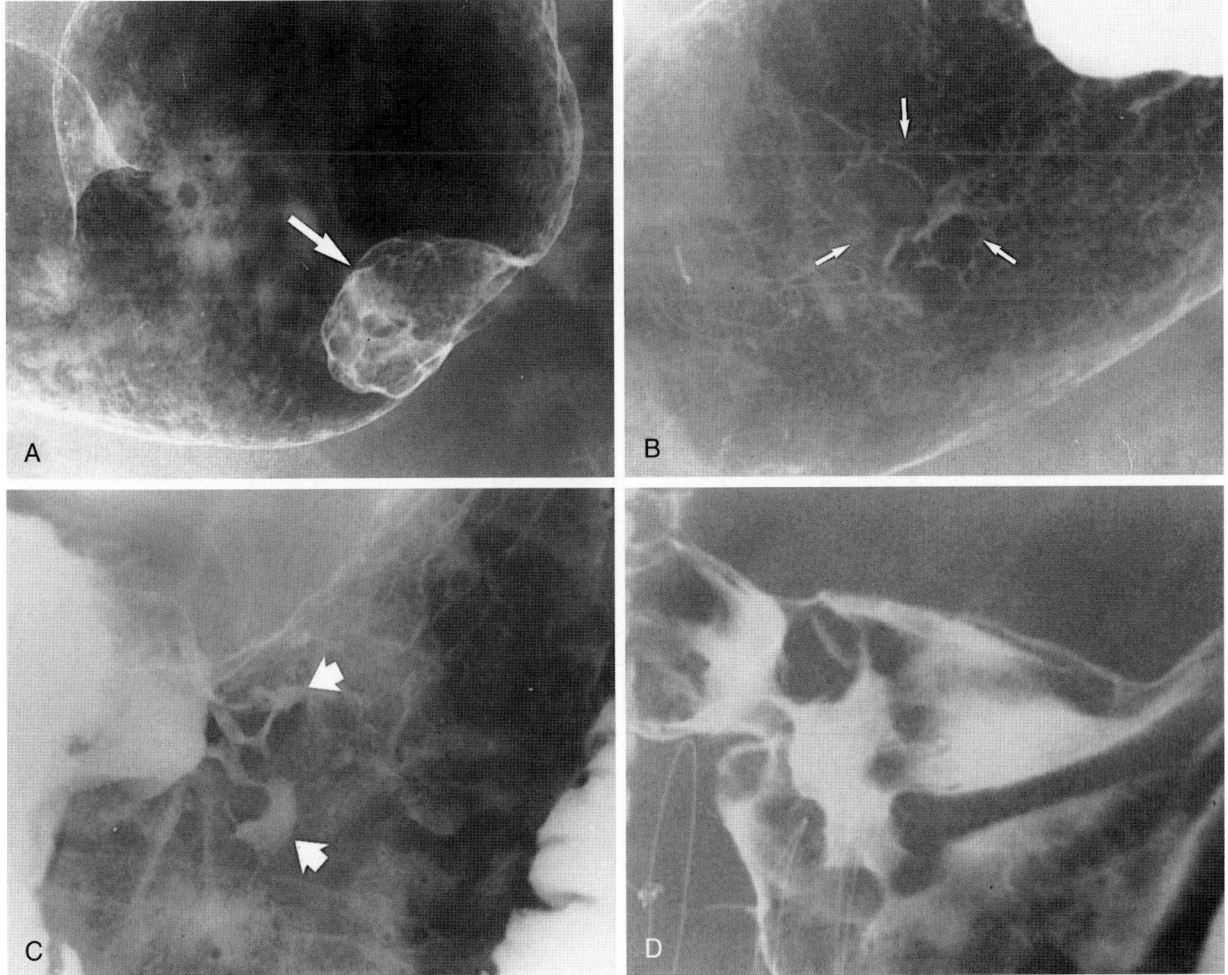

Figure 36-1. Early gastric cancers. A. A type I lesion is seen as a polypoid mass (*arrow*) on the greater curvature of the gastric body. Despite its size, this lesion was found to be an early cancer. **B.** A type IIa lesion is manifested by a focal cluster of shallow elevations and nodules (*arrows*) in the gastric body. **C.** A type IIc lesion is manifested by shallow, irregular areas of ulceration and nodularity (*arrows*) in the gastric antrum. **D.** A type III lesion is seen as a scalloped, irregular antral ulcer with nodular, clubbed folds surrounding the ulcer crater. (**A** courtesy of Kyunghee C. Cho, MD, Newark, NJ; **B** from Laufer I, Levine MS [eds]: Double Contrast Gastrointestinal Radiology, 2nd ed. Philadelphia, WB Saunders, 1992; **D** from Levine MS, Creteur V, Kressel HY, et al: Benign gastric ulcers: diagnosis and follow-up with double-contrast radiography. Radiology 164:9-13, 1987.)

unusually high prevalence of gastric carcinoma in that country. Occasionally, early gastric cancers may be detected in symptomatic patients with epigastric pain, upper gastrointestinal bleeding, or other complaints.[95] Early gastric cancers may also be discovered fortuitously in patients who undergo radiologic or endoscopic examinations for other reasons. Nevertheless, radiologists and endoscopists in the West are unlikely to detect a substantial number of early gastric cancers as long as these examinations are performed predominantly on symptomatic patients.[95]

Advanced Carcinoma

Abdominal Radiographs

Polyarchy gastric carcinomas are occasionally recognized on abdominal radiographs by the presence of a soft tissue mass indenting the gastric air shadow (Fig. 36-2A). Primary scirrhous carcinomas may also be recognized by a narrowed, tubular configuration of the gas-filled stomach (Fig. 36-2B). Rarely, mucin-producing scirrhous carcinomas contain gross areas of calcification that have a stippled, punctate, or sandlike appearance (Fig. 36-3A).[109-111] When abdominal radiographs raise suspicion of gastric carcinoma, barium studies should be performed for a more definitive diagnosis (Fig. 36-3B). CT is a particularly sensitive technique for demonstrating calcification in these tumors (Fig. 36-3C).

Barium Studies

Accurate diagnosis of gastric cancer has always been an important goal of barium studies of the upper gastrointestinal tract. Unfortunately, single-contrast examinations have an overall sensitivity of only 75% in diagnosing these tumors.[112] In one study of 80 patients with gastric carcinoma, however, the lesion was detected on double-contrast examinations in 99% of cases, and malignant tumor was diagnosed or suspected on the basis of the radiographic findings in 96%.[112] In the same study, it was found that endoscopy had been recommended because of radiographic findings that were equivocal

or suggestive of tumor in only 4% of all patients who underwent double-contrast examinations during this period. Thus, a high sensitivity can be achieved in the diagnosis of gastric carcinoma on double-contrast studies without exposing an inordinate number of patients to unnecessary endoscopy. In another study, missed gastric cancers most often resulted from perceptual errors related to subtle depressed lesions overlooked in the thin barium pool with compression or flow technique.[113]

Advanced gastric carcinomas may appear as polypoid, ulcerative, or infiltrating lesions. However, many lesions have mixed morphologic features, so there is considerable overlap in the classification of these tumors. Because scirrhous carcinoma and carcinoma of the cardia produce distinctive radiographic findings, these lesions are considered separately in later sections.

Polypoid carcinomas are lobulated or fungating masses that protrude into the lumen (Figs. 36-4 and 36-5). On double-contrast studies, lesions on the dependent or posterior wall are seen as filling defects in the barium pool, whereas lesions on the nondependent or anterior wall are etched in white by a thin layer of barium trapped between the edge of the mass and the adjacent mucosa. These tumors often contain one or more irregular areas of ulceration. Occasionally, polypoid antral carcinomas may prolapse through the pylorus into the duodenum, appearing as mass lesions at the base of the bulb (Fig. 36-6). Rarely, two or more synchronous carcinomas may be present in the stomach (see Fig. 36-5).[56,57,114]

Ulcerated carcinomas are those in which the bulk of the tumor mass has been replaced by ulceration (Figs. 36-7 and 36-8). Although these lesions are often called malignant ulcers, the term is a misnomer because it is not the ulcer but the surrounding tumor that is malignant. In general, malignant ulcers are characterized en face by an irregular ulcer crater eccentrically located in a rind of malignant tissue.[115,116] The ulcers may have scalloped, angular, or stellate borders. Discrete tumor nodules are often seen in the adjacent mucosa. Folds converging to the edge of the ulcer may be blunted, nodular, clubbed, or fused as a result of tumor infiltration.[115,116] On

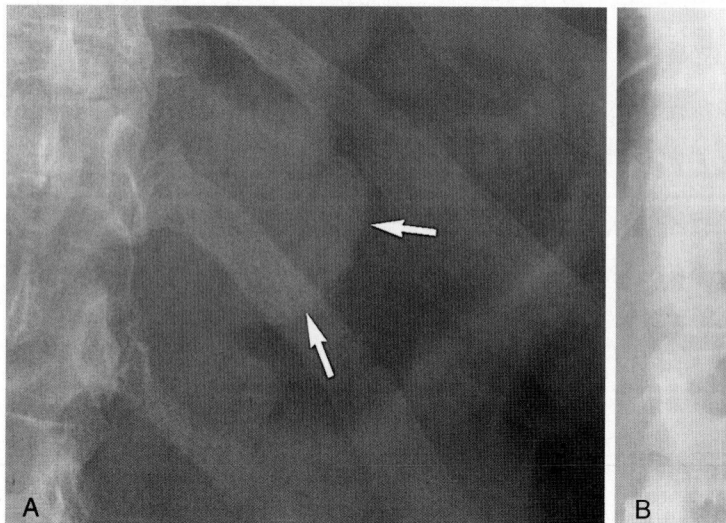
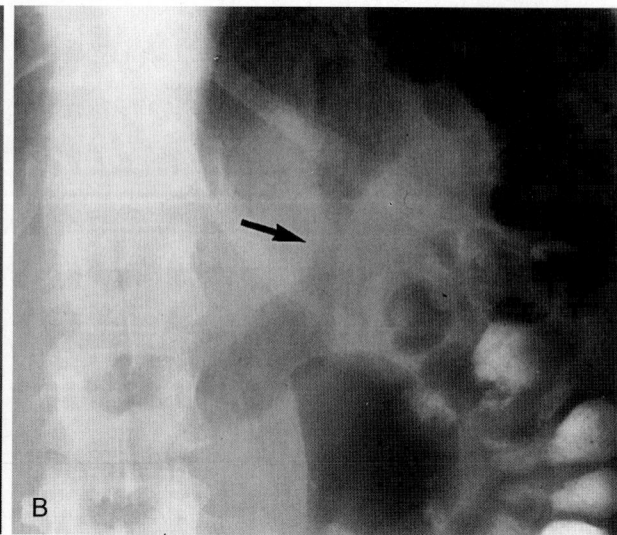

Figure 36-2. Plain abdominal radiographic findings of gastric carcinoma. A. Close-up view from an abdominal radiograph shows a soft tissue mass (*arrows*) indenting the lesser curvature of the gas-filled stomach. This was a polypoid gastric carcinoma. **B.** In another patient, the gas-filled stomach has a narrowed, tubular appearance (*arrow*) due to a scirrhous carcinoma (linitis plastica).

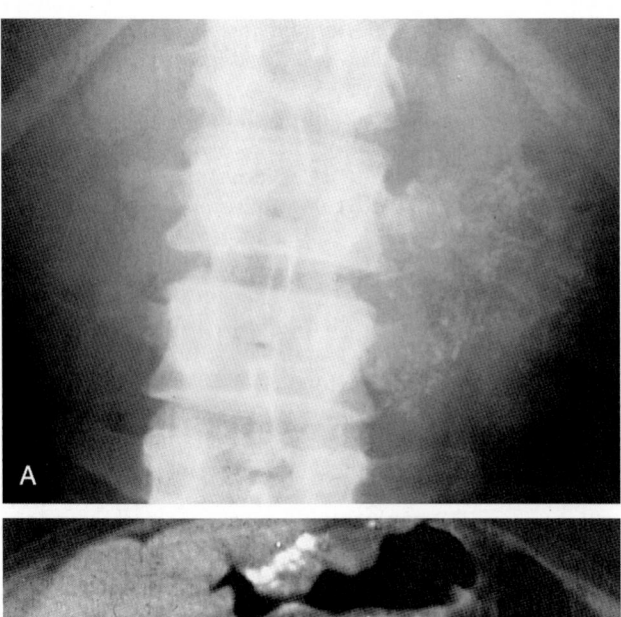

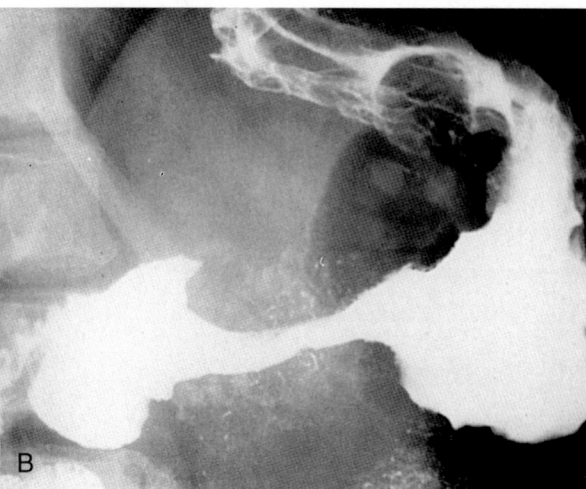

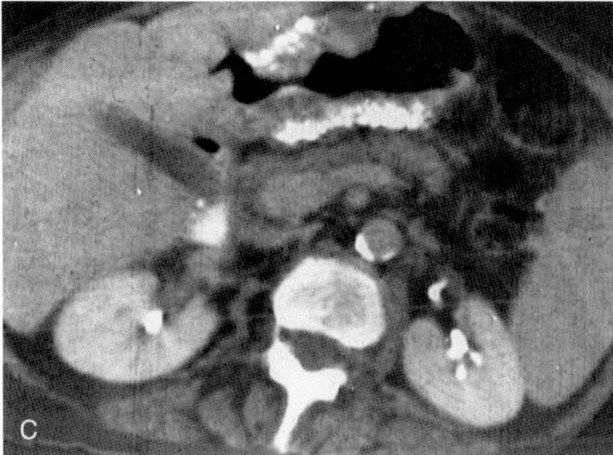

Figure 36-3. Calcified scirrhous carcinoma. A. Close-up view from an abdominal radiograph shows a large cluster of punctate or sandlike calcifications in the region of the stomach. **B.** Barium study in the same patient reveals marked antral narrowing caused by a scirrhous carcinoma of the stomach. Again, note multiple calcifications in this mucin-producing tumor. **C.** CT scan shows lobulated thickening of the gastric wall with extensive calcification in another patient with a scirrhous carcinoma. (**C** courtesy of Eugene Libson, MD, Jerusalem, Israel.)

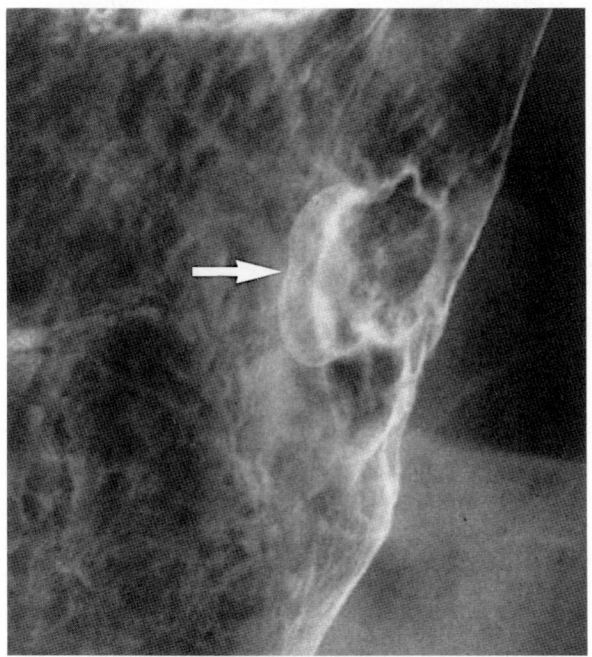

Figure 36-4. Polypoid gastric carcinoma. A polypoid mass (*arrow*) is seen on the greater curvature of the stomach.

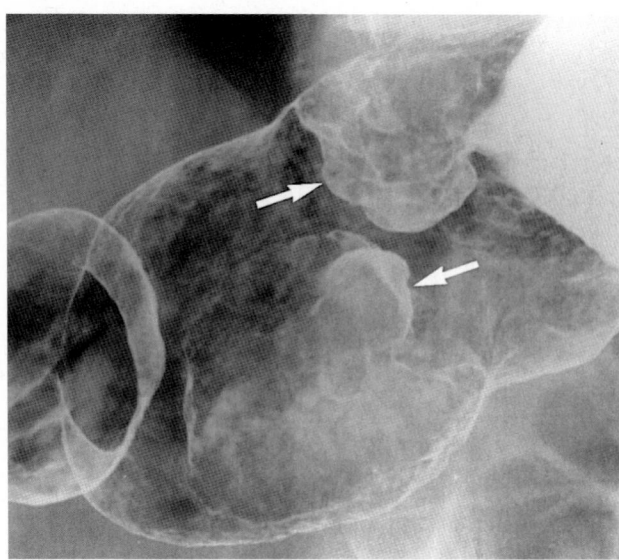

Figure 36-5. Synchronous gastric carcinomas. Two discrete polypoid masses (*arrows*) are seen in the stomach due to separate primary gastric carcinomas.

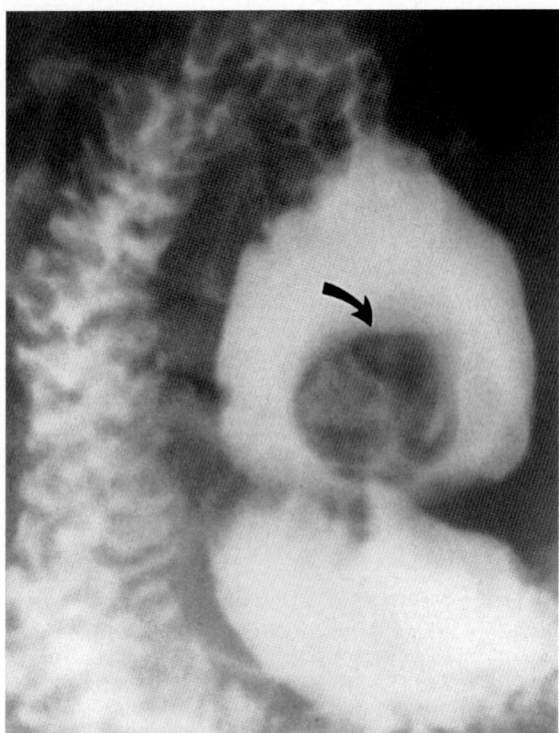

Figure 36-6. Prolapsed antral carcinoma. A polypoid mass (*arrow*) is seen at the base of the duodenal bulb. This patient had an antral carcinoma that had prolapsed into the duodenum.

double-contrast studies, malignant ulcers on the nondependent or anterior wall may be etched in white, so a double-ring shadow is observed in the stomach, with the outer ring representing the edge of the tumor and the inner ring representing the edge of the ulcer (see Fig. 36-7A). In such cases, prone compression views should demonstrate filling of the ulcer crater within a discrete tumor mass on the anterior wall (see Fig. 36-7B). A biphasic examination is therefore essential for detecting these lesions.

When viewed in profile, malignant ulcers usually have an intraluminal location, often within a discrete tumor mass (see Figs. 36-8B and C) whereas benign ulcers project beyond the adjacent contour of the stomach.[115,116] However, this criterion can be used only for ulcers on or near the lesser or greater curvature. The tumor mass surrounding malignant ulcers usually forms acute angles with the adjacent gastric wall rather than the obtuse, gently sloping angles expected for a benign mound of edema.[115,116] Clubbed or nodular folds may also be seen radiating to the edge of the ulcer crater or to the edge of the surrounding mass as a result of tumor infiltrating the folds (see Fig. 36-8B).

No sign in gastrointestinal radiology has generated more confusion than the meniscus sign of a malignant ulcer, which was originally described by Carman in 1921[117] and refined by Kirkland in 1934.[118] The Carman-Kirkland meniscus complex is caused by a cancer straddling the lesser curvature of the gastric antrum or body in which the tumor is a broad, flat lesion with central ulceration and elevated margins. Careful

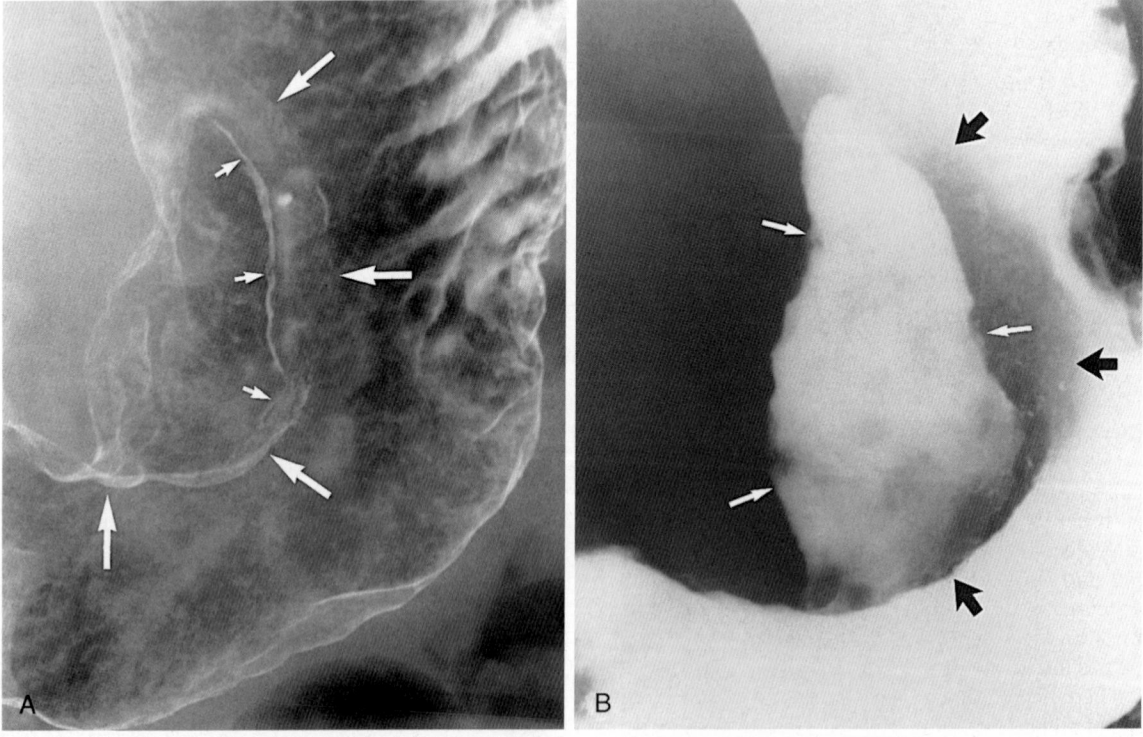

Figure 36-7. Ulcerated gastric carcinoma. A. Double-contrast view of the stomach shows a relatively large mass that is etched in white (*large arrows*) near the lesser curvature of the gastric body. Also note a second curvilinear density (*small arrows*) due to barium coating the rim of an unfilled central ulcer. **B.** Prone compression view shows the mass as a radiolucent filling defect (*black arrows*) on the anterior wall of the stomach. Note how the central ulcer (*white arrows*) fills with barium when the patient is in the prone position. The ulcer has a convex inner border and an intraluminal location, demonstrating the features of a Carman-Kirkland meniscus complex. (From Laufer I, Levine MS [eds]: Double Contrast Gastrointestinal Radiology, 2nd ed. Philadelphia, WB Saunders, 1992.)

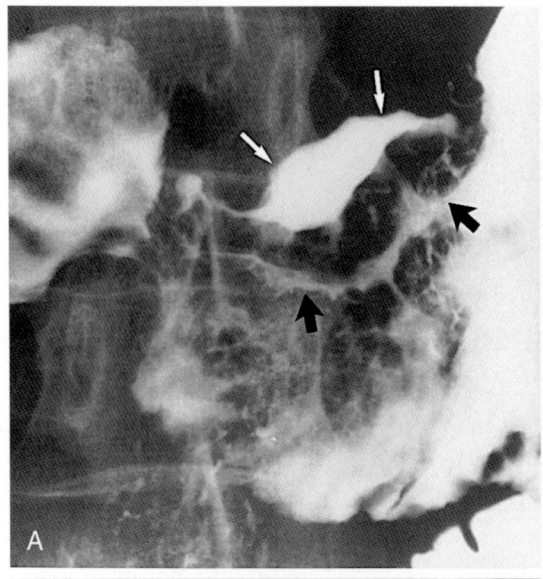
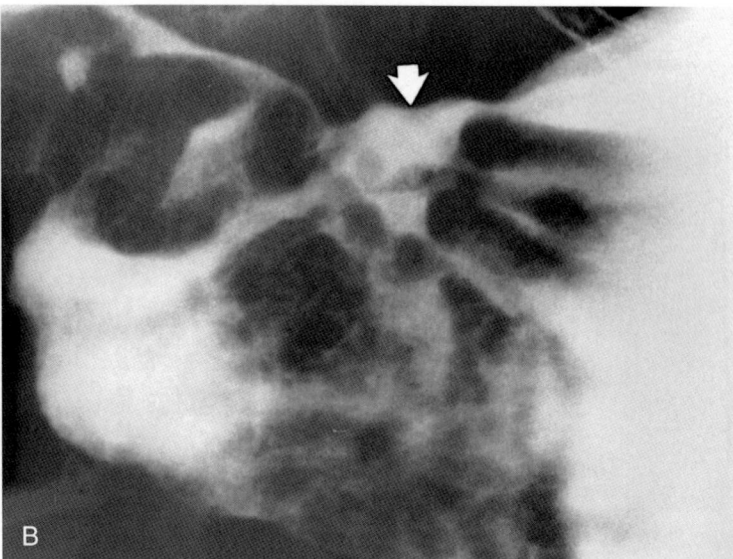
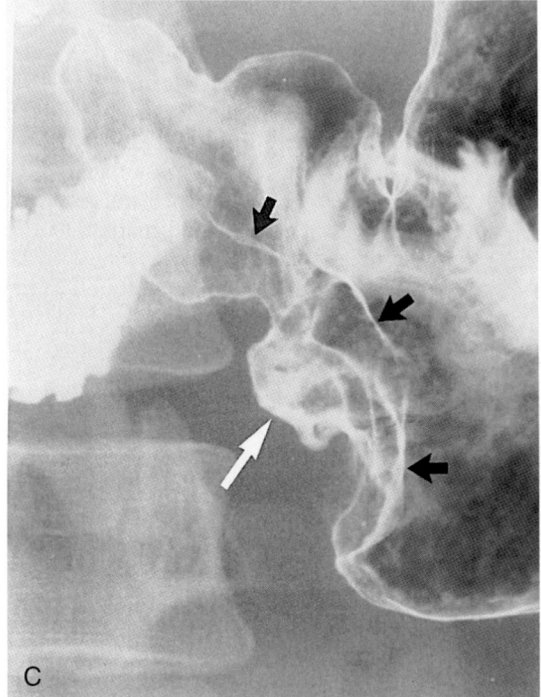

Figure 36-8. Malignant gastric ulcers. A. A meniscoid ulcer (*white arrows*) is seen on the lesser curvature of the antrum. Note the rind of malignant tumor (*black arrows*) surrounding the ulcer. **B.** Another malignant ulcer (*arrow*) is seen on the lesser curvature of the antrum. This ulcer has an intraluminal location. Also note how the folds converging to the ulcer have a nodular, clubbed appearance due to infiltration by tumor. **C.** A third patient has an ulcerated mass on the greater curvature of the antrum. Again note how the ulcer (*white arrow*) has an intraluminal location. Also note how the mass itself is etched in white (*black arrows*).

compression of the lesion may reveal a meniscoid ulcer with a convex inner border and a concave outer border that does not project beyond the expected gastric contour (see Figs. 36-7B and 36-8A).[115,116] A radiolucent halo may be seen abutting the meniscus due to apposition of the elevated edges of the tumor on the anterior and posterior walls. Although the Carman-Kirkland meniscus complex is a reliable radiologic sign of malignancy, it can be demonstrated in only a small percentage of all patients with malignant ulcers.

Infiltrating carcinomas are manifested by irregular narrowing of the stomach with nodularity and spiculation of the mucosa (Fig. 36-9). Some infiltrating lesions may have polypoid or ulcerated components. In advanced cases, these lesions may cause gastric outlet obstruction.

Transpyloric spread of antral carcinoma into the duodenum can be demonstrated on barium studies in 5% to 25% of patients.[70-72] Duodenal involvement is manifested by mass effect, nodularity, ulceration, or irregular narrowing of the proximal duodenum. Although transpyloric spread of tumor occurs in a higher percentage of patients with gastric lymphoma, gastric carcinoma is more likely to produce this finding because of its higher incidence.[72]

Rarely, advanced gastric carcinomas on the greater curvature of the stomach may spread inferiorly via the gastrocolic ligament to the superior border of the transverse colon, resulting in the development of a gastrocolic fistula.[73] Although these fistulas may occasionally be shown by an upper gastrointestinal study, they are more likely to be demonstrated by

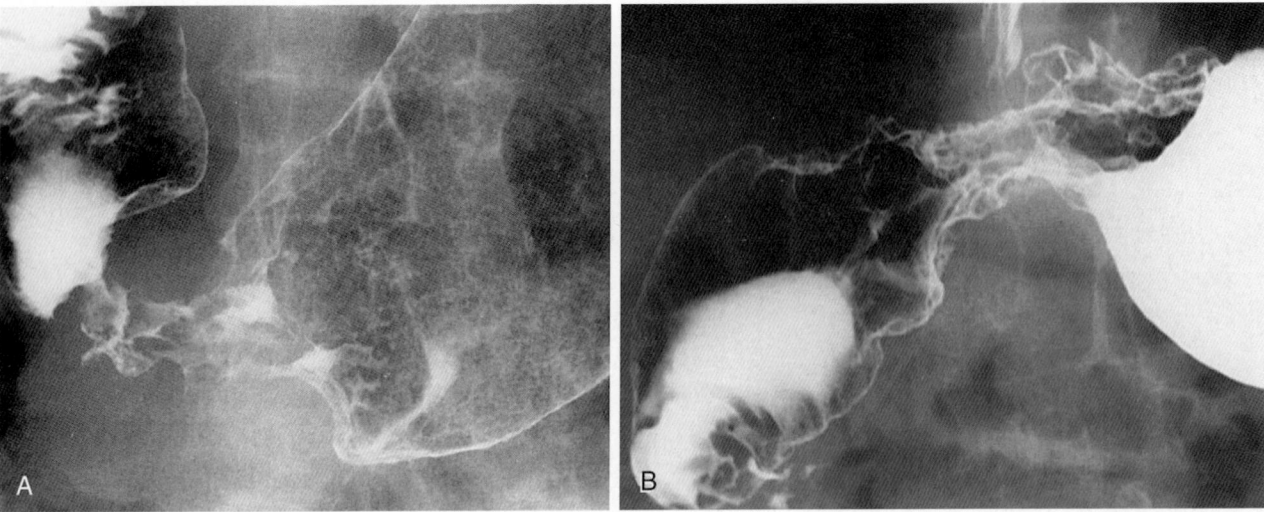

Figure 36-9. Infiltrating gastric carcinomas. A. Irregular narrowing and ulceration are seen in the antrum due to an advanced, infiltrating carcinoma. **B.** In another patient, an infiltrating carcinoma of the proximal stomach causes marked narrowing and spiculation of the upper gastric body.

a barium enema because of the higher pressures generated during this examination.

Scirrhous Carcinoma

Scirrhous gastric carcinomas are traditionally thought to involve the distal half of the stomach, arising near the pylorus and gradually extending upward from the antrum into the body and fundus.[81,119] These tumors are classically manifested on barium studies by irregular narrowing and rigidity of the

stomach, producing a *linitis plastica* or "leather bottle" appearance (Fig. 36-10).[81,119] In advanced cases, the stomach may be diffusely infiltrated by tumor (see Fig. 36-10B). Other patients may have localized scirrhous tumors that are confined to the prepyloric region of the antrum, appearing as short, annular lesions with shelflike proximal borders (Fig. 36-11).[120] With double-contrast technique, however, 20% to 40% of patients with scirrhous tumors are found to have localized lesions involving the gastric fundus or body with sparing of the antrum (Figs. 36-12 and 36-13).[90,91] Detection

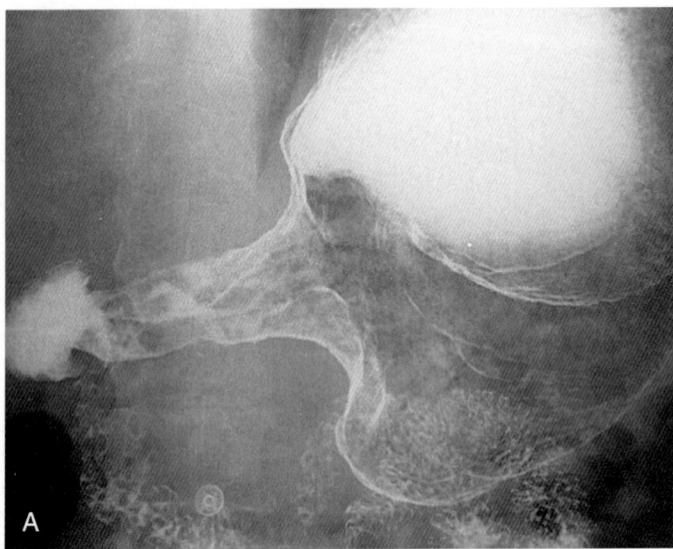

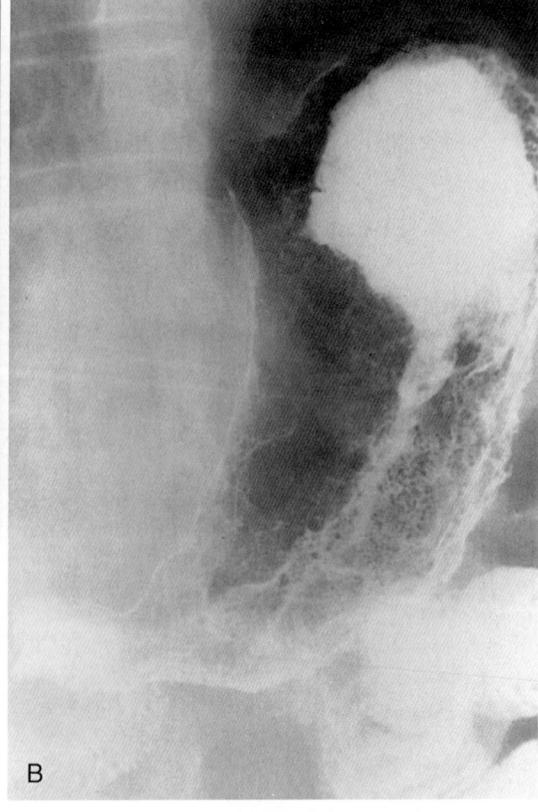

Figure 36-10. Scirrhous carcinomas of the stomach. A. There is marked narrowing of the antrum due to infiltration of the wall by tumor. **B.** In another patient there is encasement of the entire stomach by a scirrhous tumor, producing a diffuse linitis plastica appearance.

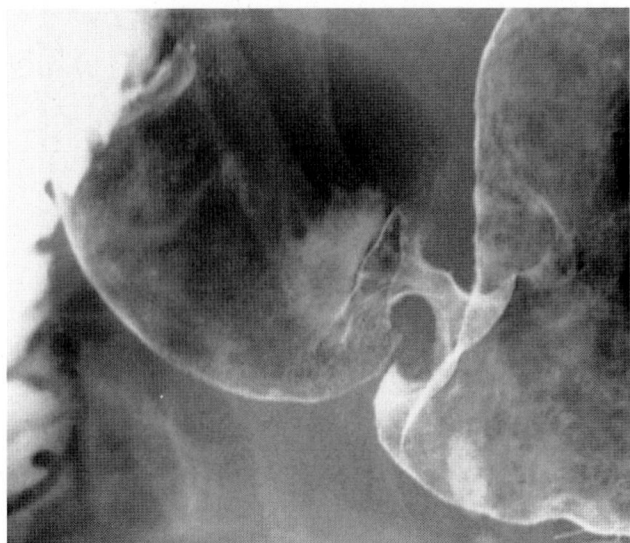

Figure 36-11. Localized scirrhous carcinoma of the distal antrum. A short, annular lesion is seen in the prepyloric region of the antrum. Note how the lesion has an abrupt, shelflike proximal border. (From Laufer I, Levine MS [eds]: Double Contrast Gastrointestinal Radiology, 2nd ed. Philadelphia, WB Saunders, 1992.)

of these lesions is presumably improved because of better gaseous distention of the proximal stomach on double-contrast studies. Whatever the explanation, radiologists should be aware that a significant percentage of patients with scirrhous tumors have localized lesions involving the gastric fundus or body rather than the classic form of linitis plastica involving the distal stomach.

Although scirrhous carcinomas are classically manifested by gastric narrowing and rigidity, some tumors may cause only mild loss of distensibility. Instead, these lesions may be recognized on double-contrast studies primarily by distortion of the normal surface pattern of the stomach with mucosal

nodularity, spiculation, ulceration, or thickened, irregular folds (see Fig. 36-13).[90] Thus, some lesions are likely to be missed if the radiologist relies too heavily on gastric narrowing as the major criterion for diagnosing these tumors.

Carcinoma of the Cardia

Tumors arising at the cardia are notoriously difficult to detect on conventional single-contrast barium studies. Because the overlying rib cage precludes manual palpation or compression of the fundus, even large lesions at the cardia may be obscured by crowded folds or relatively opaque barium that prevents adequate visualization of this region. With double-contrast technique, however, it is possible to evaluate the normal anatomic landmarks at the cardia and surrounding gastric mucosa for signs of malignancy. As a result, double-contrast barium studies may detect lesions at the cardia that are missed on conventional single-contrast examinations.[121-125]

When viewed en face, the normal cardia often appears on double-contrast studies as a circular elevation containing four or five stellate folds that radiate to a central button at the gastroesophageal junction (the cardiac "rosette") (see Chapter 30).[122,123] Some lesions at the cardia may be recognized only by relatively subtle nodularity, mass effect, or ulceration in this region with distortion, effacement, or obliteration of this rosette (Fig. 36-14).[122-125] Enlargement or lobulation of the surrounding elevation should also suggest a neoplastic lesion. Finally, an abnormal protrusion at the cardia should persist when additional barium is swallowed, whereas an apparent abnormality at the cardia must be an artifact if it vanishes as the lower esophageal sphincter relaxes and the cardia opens.[123]

Advanced carcinomas of the gastric cardia or fundus may be polypoid or infiltrating lesions. Polypoid tumors usually appear as lobulated intraluminal masses in the gastric fundus, often containing irregular areas of ulceration.[125,126] In contrast, infiltrating lesions are manifested by thickened, nodular

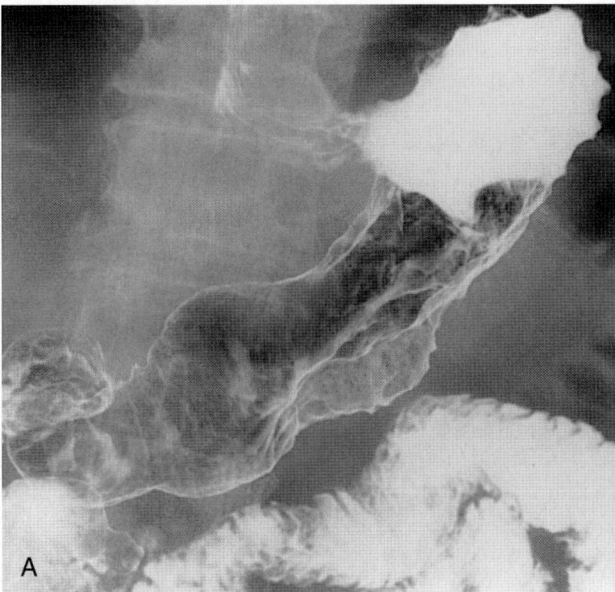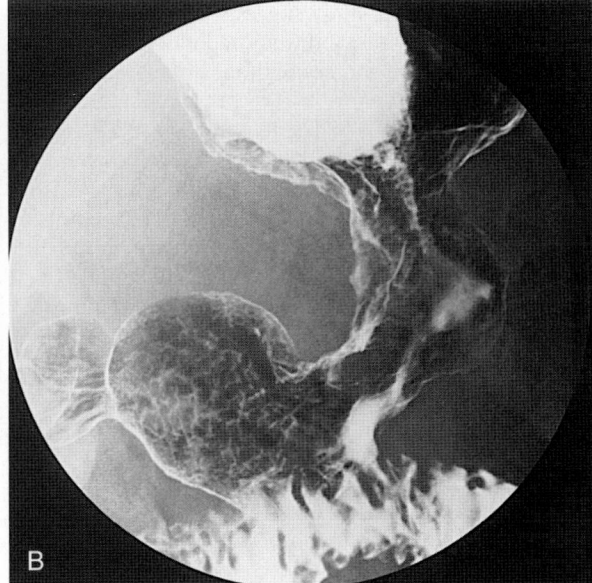

Figure 36-12. Localized scirrhous carcinomas of the proximal stomach. A. Irregular narrowing is seen in the gastric fundus and body with sparing of the antrum. **B.** Another patient has a scirrhous carcinoma of the gastric body with sparing of the fundus and antrum. (**A** from Laufer I, Levine MS [eds]: Double Contrast Gastrointestinal Radiology, 2nd ed. Philadelphia, WB Saunders, 1992.)

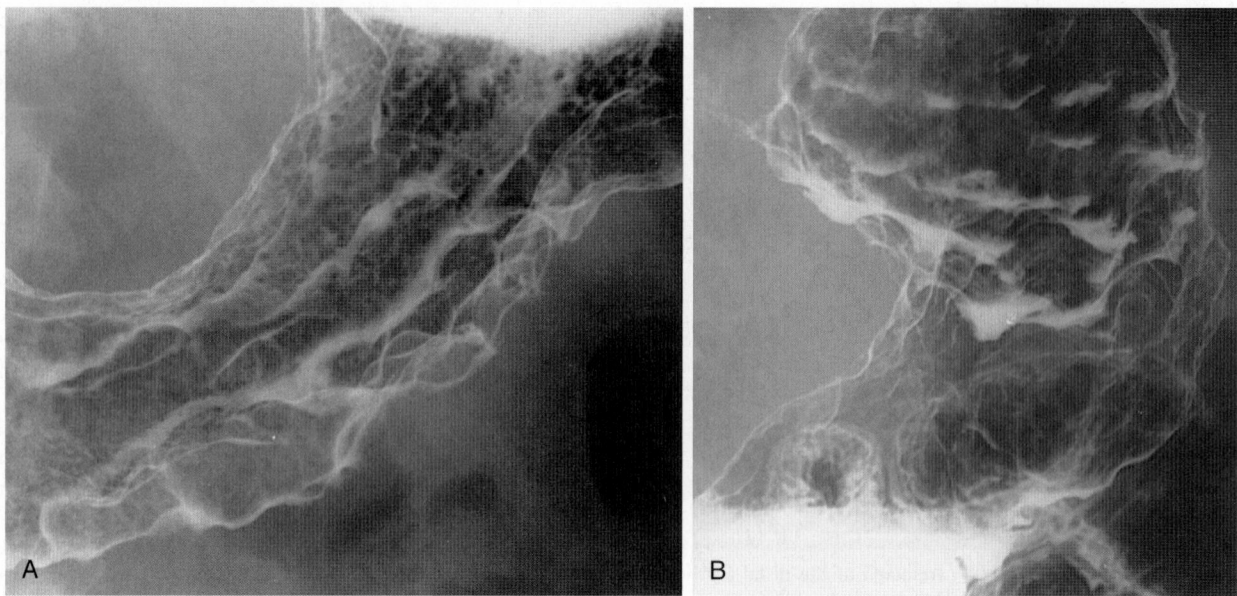

Figure 36-13. Scirrhous carcinomas of the proximal stomach with thickened folds. A. This patient has a localized scirrhous carcinoma of the gastric body. The tumor has caused only mild loss of distensibility. However, there is distortion of the normal surface pattern of the stomach with thickened, irregular folds and mucosal nodularity. **B.** In another patient, a scirrhous carcinoma of the fundus and body is manifested by thickened, lobulated folds without significant narrowing. (**A** from Levine MS, Kong V, Rubesin SE, et al: Scirrhous carcinoma of the stomach: Radiologic and endoscopic diagnosis. Radiology 175:151-154, 1990.)

folds and decreased distensibility of the fundus.[125,126] Advanced tumors may completely encase the fundus, producing a linitis plastica appearance (Fig. 36-15).

When an equivocal or suspicious lesion is detected in the region of the gastric cardia or fundus, endoscopy should be performed for a more definitive diagnosis. Nevertheless, radiographically demonstrated lesions at the cardia may occasionally be missed at endoscopy.[127] The barium study should therefore be repeated despite a negative endoscopic examination if the initial barium study suggests a malignant lesion. Rarely, some patients with continuing radiologic evidence of malignancy may require surgery without preoperative histologic confirmation.

Secondary esophageal involvement by advanced lesions may be manifested on barium studies by a polypoid or fungating mass that extends from the fundus into the distal esophagus or by thickened folds or irregular narrowing of the distal esophagus without a discrete lesion (see Fig. 36-14B and C).[125,126] Esophageal involvement is usually confined to a 4- to 5-cm segment above the gastroesophageal junction but may extend as far proximally as the aortic arch.[126] Submucosal spread of tumor may also result in secondary achalasia with tapered, beaklike narrowing of the distal esophagus at or just above the gastroesophageal junction (see Fig. 36-15A) (see Chapter 28).[126,128] However, certain morphologic features such as asymmetry, abrupt transitions, and mucosal nodularity or ulceration should suggest an underlying malignancy.[128] Secondary achalasia should also be suspected when the narrowed segment extends proximally a discrete distance from the gastroesophageal junction.[129] In such cases, careful radiologic evaluation of the fundus is essential to rule out a carcinoma of the cardia as the cause of these findings.

Computed Tomographic Findings

The widespread availability of multidetector CT (MDCT) scanners has improved the diagnosis of gastric carcinoma on CT because of the ability to create high-quality images in any conceivable view plane (Fig. 36-16). Detection of these lesions requires optimal gastric distention to efface the overlying rugal folds and accentuate areas of asymmetry along the contour of the gastric wall. Some authors recommend oral administration of a neutral (water-attenuation) contrast agent,[130-133] whereas others recommend the use of an oral effervescent agent (as is used for double-contrast barium studies of the stomach) to optimize gastric distention.[134,135]

Gastric carcinoma may be manifested on MDCT by polypoid, fungating, ulcerated, or infiltrating lesions (Fig. 36-17).[136] In one study, focal wall thickening (>1 cm) had a sensitivity of 100% for the detection of gastric carcinoma but a specificity of less than 50%.[137] Localized wall thickening is a particularly frequent finding at the gastroesophageal junction and in the gastric antrum,[138] leading to false-positive diagnoses. When a mass is suspected at the gastroesophageal junction, repeat scanning with oral effervescent agent in the prone or left-side down decubitus position may efface the wall and accentuate the presence of tumor in this region.[139] When there is a high index of suspicion, endoscopic ultrasonography (EUS) is recommended to confirm the diagnosis. When there is a lower index of suspicion, a double-contrast barium study may be performed as a cost-effective test to confirm that the stomach is normal. Similarly, smooth antral wall thickening (up to 12 mm) with or without submucosal low attenuation is frequently seen as a normal finding.[138] The symmetry of gastric wall thickening and uniformity of contrast enhancement are also features that distinguish benign from malignant causes

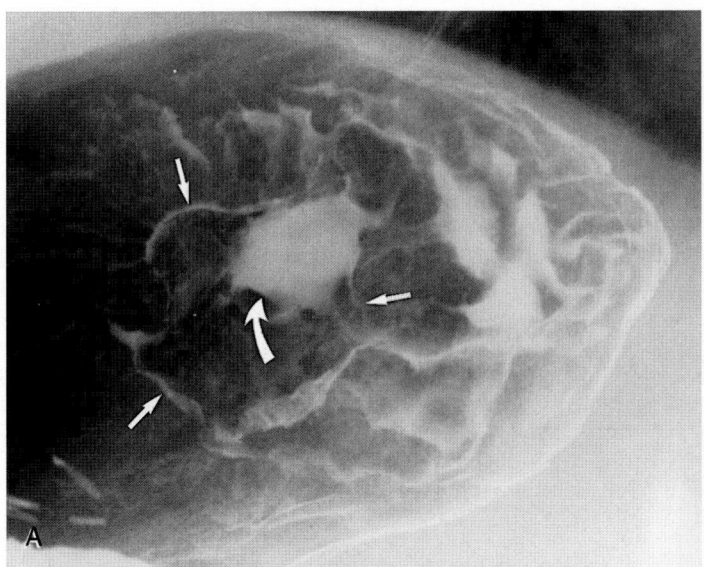

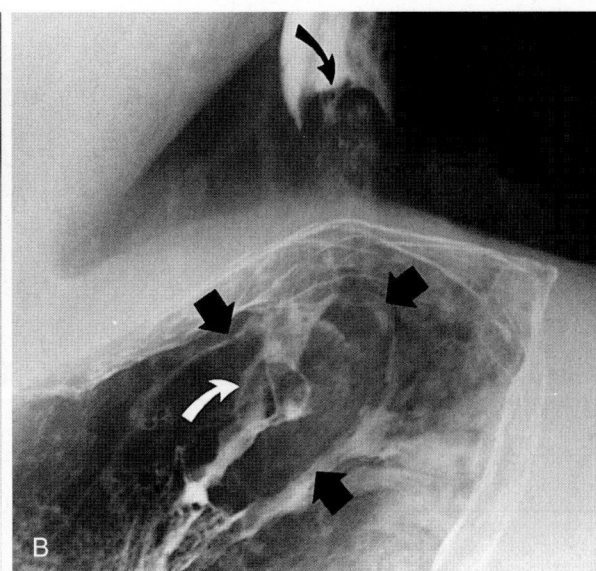

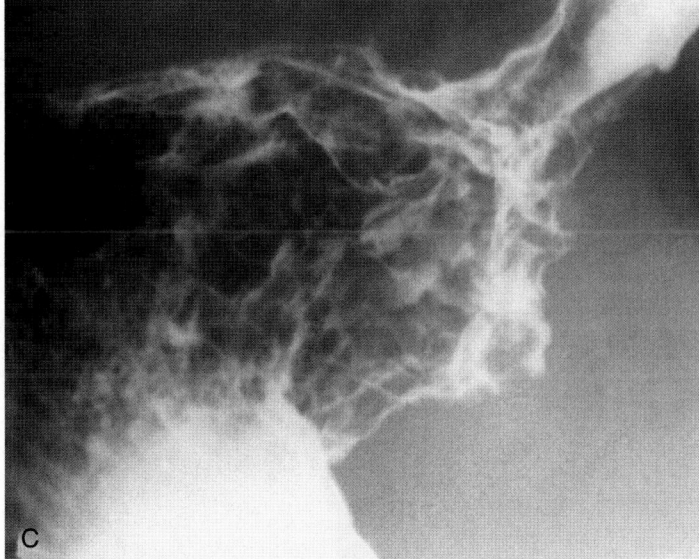

Figure 36-14. Carcinoma of the cardia. A. The normal anatomic landmarks at the cardia have been obliterated and replaced by a plaquelike lesion (*straight arrows*) containing a shallow area of ulceration (*curved arrow*). **B.** In another patient, the cardiac rosette has been replaced by a relatively flat mass (*straight black arrows*) with a central ulcer (*white arrow*). The tumor extends into the distal esophagus (*curved black arrow*). **C.** In a third patient, there is diffuse nodularity in the fundus with obliteration of the normal cardiac landmarks. Also note involvement of the distal esophagus. (**B** from Levine MS, Laufer I, Thompson JJ: Carcinoma of the gastric cardia in young people. AJR 140:69-72, 1983, © by American Roentgen Ray Society.)

Figure 36-15. Secondary achalasia caused by gastric carcinoma. A. There is smooth, tapered narrowing of the distal esophagus, producing the classic beaklike appearance of achalasia. **B.** A radiograph of the stomach, however, reveals an advanced, scirrhous carcinoma of the gastric fundus that has invaded the distal esophagus. (From Levine MS: Radiology of the Esophagus. Philadelphia, WB Saunders, 1989.)

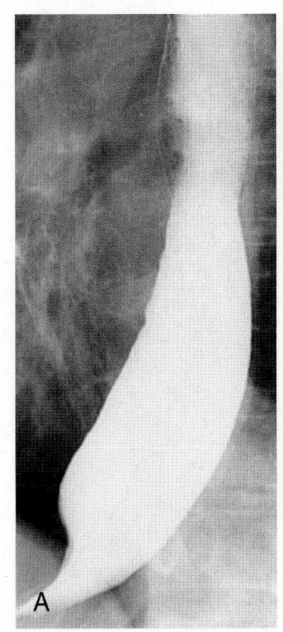

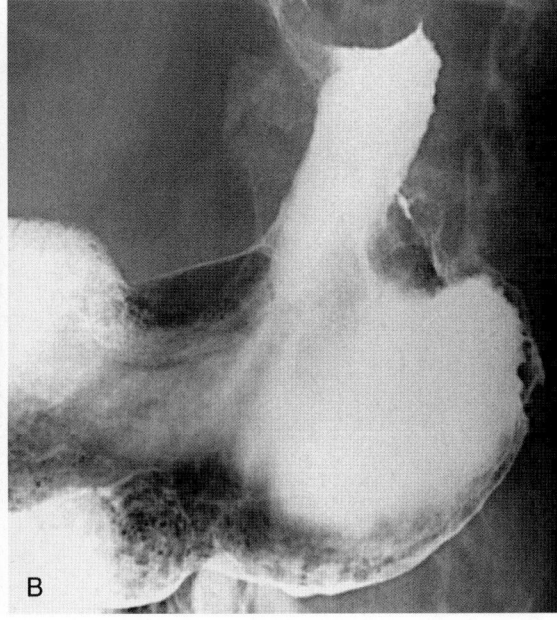

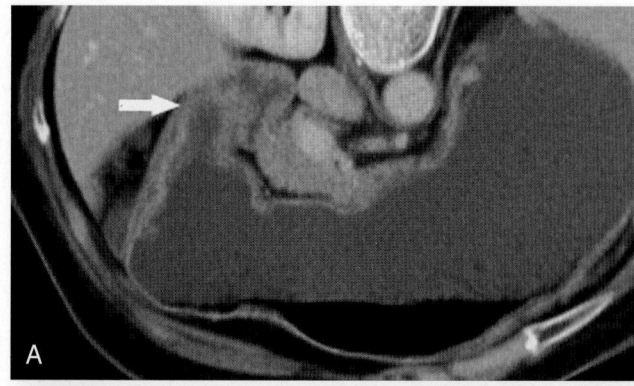

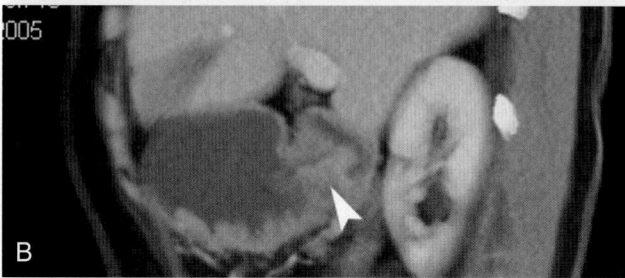

Figure 36-16. MDCT evaluation of gastric carcinoma. Three-dimensional volume-rendered CT in a patient with gastric carcinoma manifested by localized wall thickening in the antropyloric region of the stomach. **A.** This image shows the lesion (*arrow*) in a rendering that simulates a "left posterior oblique" view from an upper gastrointestinal series. **B.** Another image shows the lesion (*arrowhead*) in an orientation that simulates a "right anterior oblique" view from an upper gastrointestinal series. Note the importance of obtaining adequate gastric distention for optimal visualization of this tumor.

of wall thickening. In general, CT cannot be used to predict tumor histology but calcification or low attenuation within a thickened gastric wall should suggest the presence of a mucinous adenocarcinoma (Fig. 36-18).[140]

After intravenous administration of contrast material (delivered at rates of $3 \geq$ mL/s), gastric carcinomas may display a stratified enhancement pattern characterized by brightly enhancing mucosal and serosal layers with less enhancement of the submucosal and muscular layers of the gastric wall (Fig. 36-19).[131,141] Radiopathologic correlation has shown that the degree of enhancement relates to differences in proliferation of cancer cells; more tightly aggregated cancer cells enhance more brightly, whereas more scattered cancer cells result in regions of lower attenuation (Fig. 36-20).[142] Data from intravenous-enhanced MDCT can also be used to produce high-quality CT angiograms that serve as roadmaps for laparoscopic surgery.[143]

Differential Diagnosis

Early Gastric Cancer

Early gastric cancers may appear on barium studies as depressed (i.e., ulcerated), elevated (i.e., polypoid), or superficial lesions. Ulcerated cancers must be distinguished from benign gastric ulcers (see earlier section on Early Gastric Cancer). Occasionally, early gastric lymphomas may also appear as ulcerated lesions (see Chapter 37). Polypoid cancers must be distinguished from adenomatous or hyperplastic polyps or other benign or malignant tumors in the stomach. Finally, superficial cancers must be distinguished from a focal area of gastritis or intestinal metaplasia. When early gastric cancer is suspected on barium studies, endoscopy and biopsy are required for a definitive diagnosis.

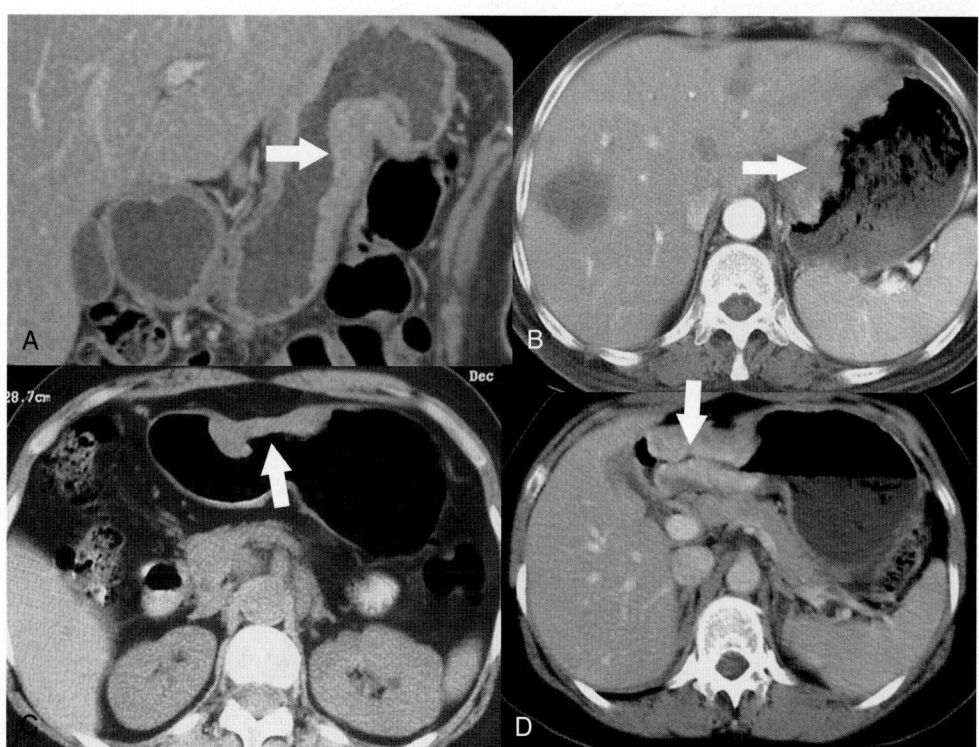

Figure 36-17. MDCT of gastric carcinoma. CT images from four different patients show the various CT appearances of gastric carcinoma (*arrows*). **A.** Polypoid carcinoma. **B.** Fungating carcinoma. Also note the presence of multiple hepatic metastases in this patient. **C.** Ulcerated carcinoma. **D.** Infiltrating carcinoma.

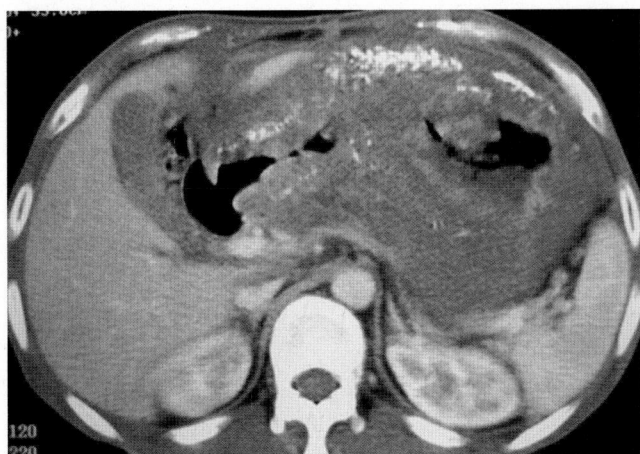

Figure 36-18. Mucinous adenocarcinoma of the stomach. CT image shows massive thickening of the gastric wall and marked luminal narrowing by an advanced infiltrating carcinoma. Also note extensive calcification within the tumor. This type of calcification is characteristic of mucinous adenocarcinomas of the stomach.

Advanced Carcinoma

The major consideration in the differential diagnosis of an ulcerated gastric carcinoma is a benign gastric ulcer with a surrounding mound of edema (see Chapter 33). Polypoid or ulcerated carcinomas must also be distinguished from other polypoid or ulcerated malignant tumors such as lymphoma and malignant gastrointestinal stromal tumors (see Chapter 37). Although the presence of a large, lobulated submucosal mass should favor the diagnosis of lymphoma or a malignant

stromal tumor, histologic specimens are ultimately required to differentiate these lesions.

Most cases of linitis plastica are caused by gastric carcinoma, but metastatic breast cancer, omental metastases, and non-Hodgkin's lymphoma involving the stomach may produce similar radiographic findings (Fig. 36-21) (see Chapter 37).[90,144-147] Cone-shaped antral narrowing and deformity may also be caused by scarring from peptic ulcer disease, caustic ingestion, radiation, or a variety of granulomatous diseases, including Crohn's disease, tuberculosis, sarcoidosis, and syphilis (see Chapter 34).[148] Antral narrowing may also occur in elderly patients with a "senile" antrum due to gastric atrophy.[149] In general, a smooth antral contour and lack of nodularity, spiculation, or ulceration should suggest benign disease. Rarely, however, these conditions may produce more irregular gastric narrowing, mimicking the appearance of malignant linitis plastica.

Carcinoma of the cardia invading the distal esophagus may be indistinguishable from a primary adenocarcinoma in Barrett's esophagus invading the stomach (see Chapter 27).[150] However, carcinoma of the cardia tends to have a greater degree of gastric involvement in relation to that of the esophagus. Squamous cell carcinoma of the esophagus may also spread distally via submucosal esophageal lymphatics to the gastric cardia or fundus, producing a polypoid lesion in the fundus (see Chapter 27).[151,152] Occasionally, a conglomerate mass of varices in the fundus may be manifested by a single lobulated lesion that closely resembles a polypoid fundal or cardiac carcinoma (see Chapter 38).[153,154] Inadequate gaseous distention of the fundus can also mimic the appearance of an infiltrating fundal tumor on double-contrast studies (Fig. 36-22A). However, additional views of the stomach after

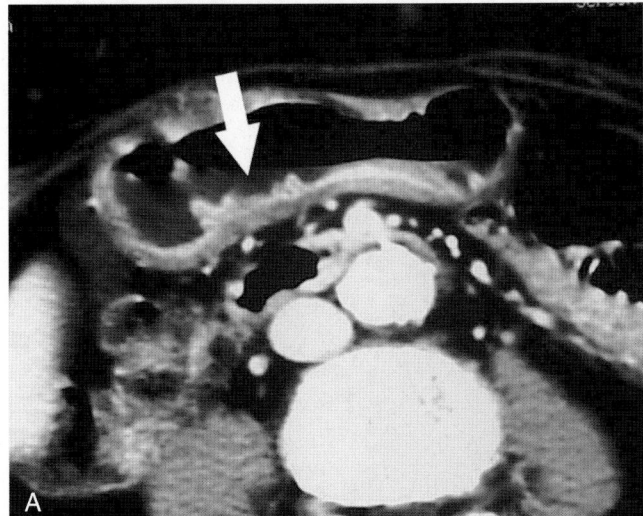

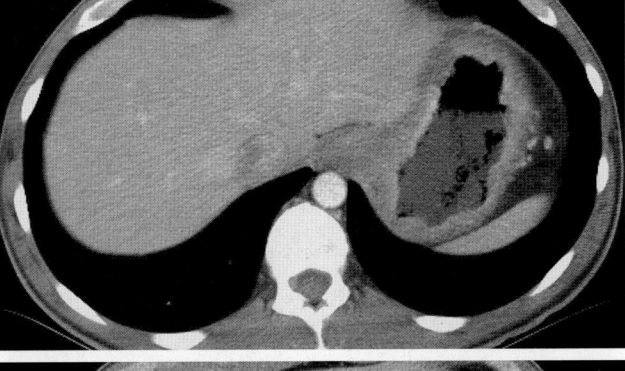

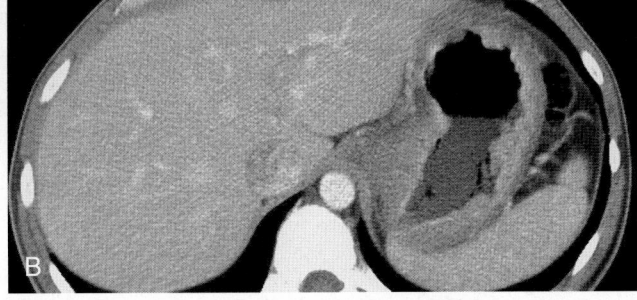

Figure 36-19. Gastric carcinoma with stratified enhancement patterns on CT. A. Contrast-enhanced CT image shows a malignant posterior wall ulcer (*arrow*) with irregular margins. Note decreased enhancement of the adjacent mucosa and a relatively hypodense submucosa. **B.** Contrast-enhanced CT images through the proximal stomach in 35-year-old man show an irregularly thickened gastric wall extending to the gastroesophageal junction due to a primary scirrhous carcinoma producing a linitis plastica. Note variable enhancement of the mucosa, prominent hyperdensity interspersed throughout the submucosa, and poor margination at the serosa.

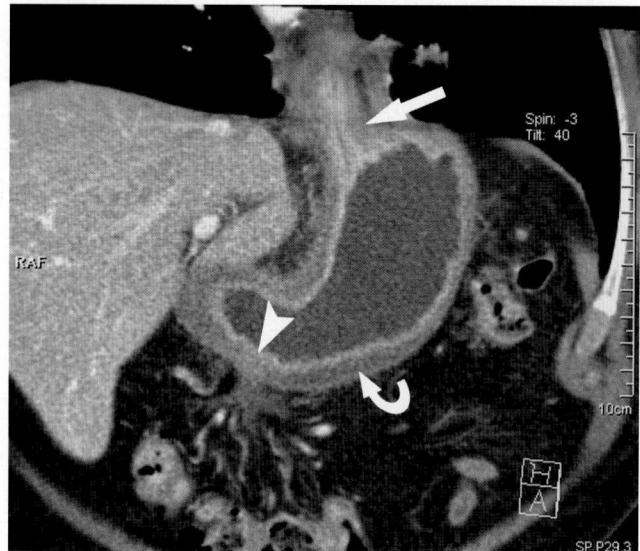

Figure 36-20. Gastric carcinoma with differential wall enhancement on CT. Three-dimensional MDCT image shows mural thickening and hyperdense attenuation in the distal esophagus and region of the gastroesophageal junction (*straight arrow*). The entire gastric wall appears infiltrated by tumor. Note how the mucosal layer is thin and enhances uniformly. In contrast, the submucosal layer is thickened and hypodense (*curved arrow*), possibly as a result of edema. A focal area of increased density is seen within the submucosa (*arrowhead*) along the greater curvature of the distal antrum. Soft tissue density extends into the adjacent perigastric fat, suggesting extension of tumor in this region.

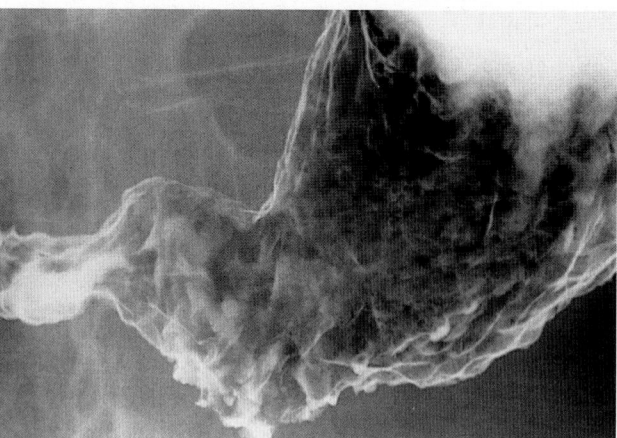

Figure 36-21. Metastatic breast cancer involving the stomach. There is antral narrowing with distortion of the normal surface pattern and a nodular, irregular mucosa in this region. A primary scirrhous carcinoma of the stomach could produce identical findings. (From Levine MS, Kong V, Rubesin SE, et al: Scirrhous carcinoma of the stomach: Radiologic and endoscopic diagnosis. Radiology 175:151-154, 1990.)

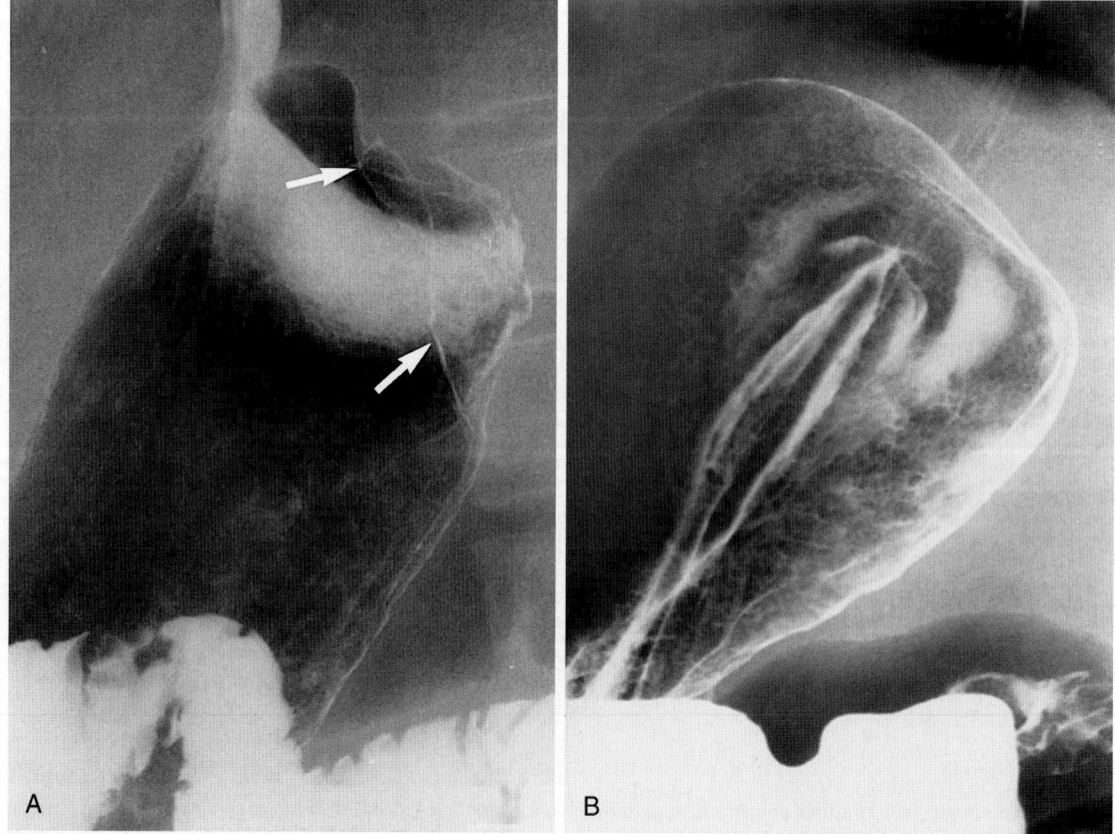

Figure 36-22. Inadequate gaseous distention mimicking a fundal tumor. A. Double-contrast radiograph of the stomach shows a possible infiltrating lesion (*arrows*) on the posterior wall of the fundus. **B.** After administration of additional effervescent agent, there is better distention of the fundus, eliminating the possibility of tumor. Note how the normal cardiac rosette is now visible.

administration of a second dose of effervescent agent should show that the fundus is normal in these patients (Fig. 36-22B).

Staging

Both CT and EUS have important roles in the evaluation and staging of patients with gastric carcinoma. These techniques are therefore discussed separately in the following sections.

Computed Tomography

The widespread availability of MDCT scanners and the ability to create high-quality images in multiple planes has rekindled interest in the value of CT for staging patients with gastric carcinoma. MDCT provides a rapid, global assessment of the stomach, surrounding fat, supporting structures, adjacent organs, and entire abdominal cavity. This global assessment allows for identification of local, regional, and distant spread of tumor.

Technique

Gastric carcinoma is most commonly characterized by wall thickening on MDCT. Detection of these lesions requires optimal gastric distention to efface the overlying rugal folds and accentuate areas of asymmetry along the contour of the stomach. Some authors recommend oral administration of neutral (water-attenuation) contrast agents,[130-133] whereas others recommend the use of oral effervescent agents (as used for double-contrast barium studies of the stomach) to optimize gastric distention.[134,135]

Imaging data should be collected with the thinnest possible detector configuration (0.625 to 1 mm, depending on the manufacturer). Overlapping reconstructions enable creation of 3D datasets with near isotropic voxels. Display images are created at 3 to 4 mm and are transmitted directly to the picture archiving communications system (PACS) or to hard copy images. Simultaneously, the thin-slice imaging data are transmitted to a workstation, allowing for construction of 3D images. Clinically useful 3D images displaying the gastric tumor and extragastric extension of tumor can be created, and selected images can be sent to the patient's imaging data record. All of the thin section data do not have to be permanently archived, but any 3D renderings created from these sections can be archived.

Administration of intravenous contrast material is critical for local staging and detection of distant metastases. The CT scans should include the pelvis as well as the abdomen because of the tendency for gastric cancers to disseminate within the peritoneal cavity, producing so-called "drop metastases" in the pelvis.

Results

Multidetector CT has substantially improved radiologic staging of gastric carcinoma. In a study of 106 patients with endoscopically proven gastric cancer, accurate staging by T classification increased from 77% on axial CT imaging to 84% on volumetric CT imaging.[155] This accuracy is also improved by analyzing the pattern of wall enhancement. In another study of 65 patients with gastric carcinoma, MDCT had an accuracy of 96% for detecting advanced gastric cancer and 41% for early gastric cancer, with an overall T classification accuracy of 85%.[142] Despite the low detection rate of early cancers, detection of these lesions was twice as high as that using 5-mm axial images alone. In another study of 41 patients, MDCT had an accuracy of 93% for detecting serosal invasion.[156] Not surprisingly, in all of these studies, as T classification increased, so did the accuracy of MDCT staging.

The gastric wall contains an abundant network of communicating lymphatic channels, providing collateral pathways that facilitate spread of tumor to lymph nodes at both local and distant sites (Fig. 36-23). The CT accuracy of staging based on N classification is less than that for T classification

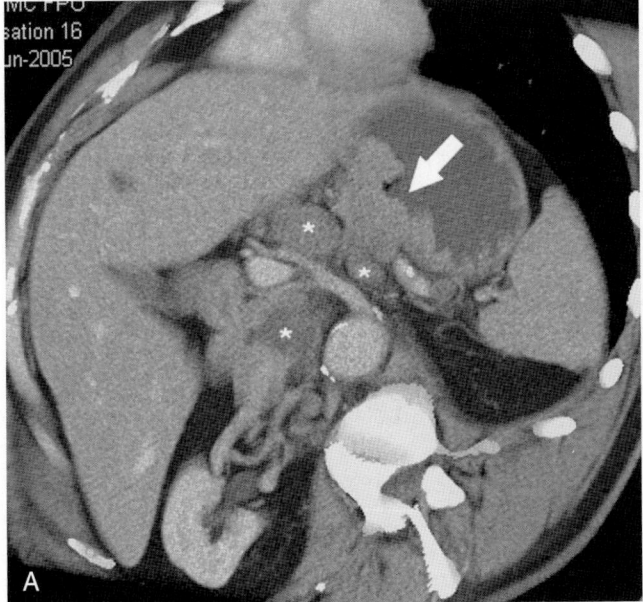
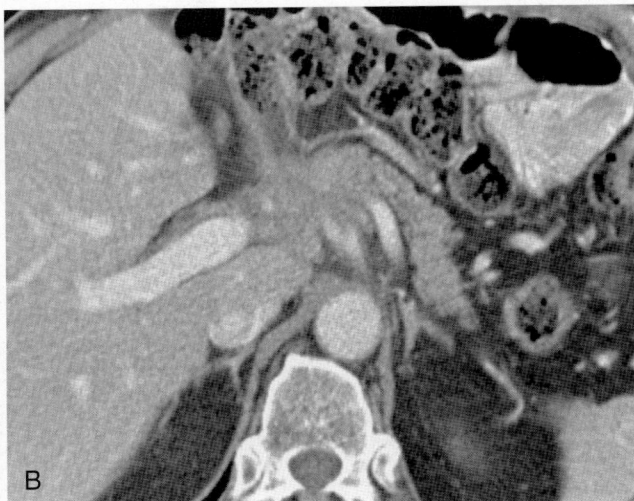

Figure 36-23. Perigastric lymph node metastases from gastric carcinoma. A. 3D MDCT image shows an ulcerated carcinoma of the gastroesophageal junction manifested by an irregular mass with central ulceration (*arrow*). Enlarged perigastric lymph nodes (*asterisks*) are present in a periceliac distribution due to lymphatic metastases. **B.** In another patient who underwent a previous gastrectomy for gastric carcinoma, an MDCT image shows peripancreatic lymphadenopathy simulating a carcinoma of the head of the pancreas.

despite technologic advances in CT. The overall N classification accuracy of MDCT in studies reported after 2000 has ranged from 60% to 80%. In two studies in which N classification accuracy was compared with EUS, both modalities had accuracies of 70% to 75% without statistically significant differences.[157,158] Nevertheless, most authors agree that EUS is more accurate in detecting local lymph node metastases adjacent to the primary tumor. Although this is important prognostic information, detection of distant nodal metastases is more important for determining surgical therapy and decreasing regional therapeutic failures.

Gastric carcinoma can metastasize by a variety of routes, including (1) direct extension across supporting ligamentous structures; (2) intraperitoneal dissemination; (3) lymphatic extension; and (4) hematogenous spread. Each of these modes of spread can be detected on MDCT imaging. Carcinoma of the cardia tends to extend into the gastrohepatic ligament and may invade the liver. In contrast, carcinoma of the gastric body or antrum may spread via the gastrocolic ligament to encase portions of the transverse colon (Fig. 36-24). Intraperitoneal dissemination of tumor may be manifested on CT by characteristic findings of peritoneal carcinomatosis, including the development of nodules in peritoneal reflections, retraction of the mesenteric root, omental caking, and loculated ascites. Once tumor has entered the peritoneal cavity, malignant cells tend to gravitate to its most dependent portions. As a result, the ovaries are frequently seeded in these patients (Fig. 26-25).[159] Kruckenberg tumors are classically defined as solid ovarian metastases from signet-ring cell adenocarcinomas, but the term is currently applied to any metastases to the ovaries, regardless of the site of the primary

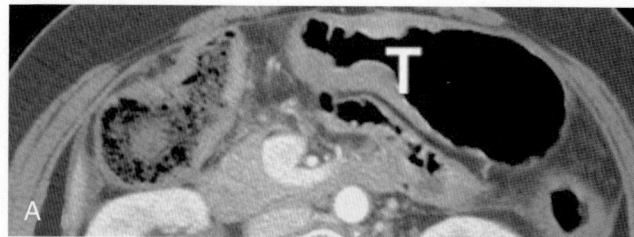
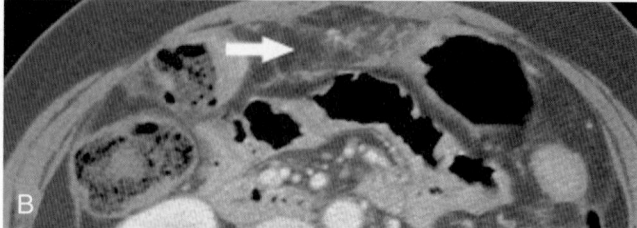
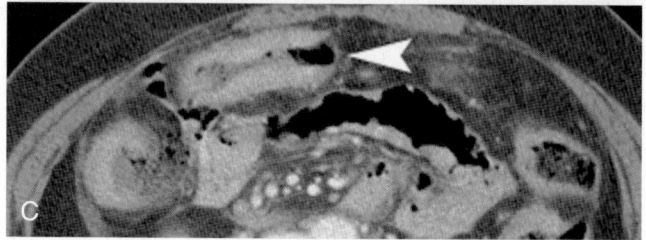

Figure 36-24. Gastric carcinoma invading the transverse colon via the gastrocolic ligament on sequential axial CT images. A. The gastric tumor (T) is manifested by localized wall thickening in the midportion of the stomach. **B.** Nodular densities are identified in the gastrocolic ligament (*arrow*) due to extension of tumor from the stomach. **C.** Another segment of localized wall thickening (*arrowhead*) is seen in the transverse colon due to direct invasion by tumor.

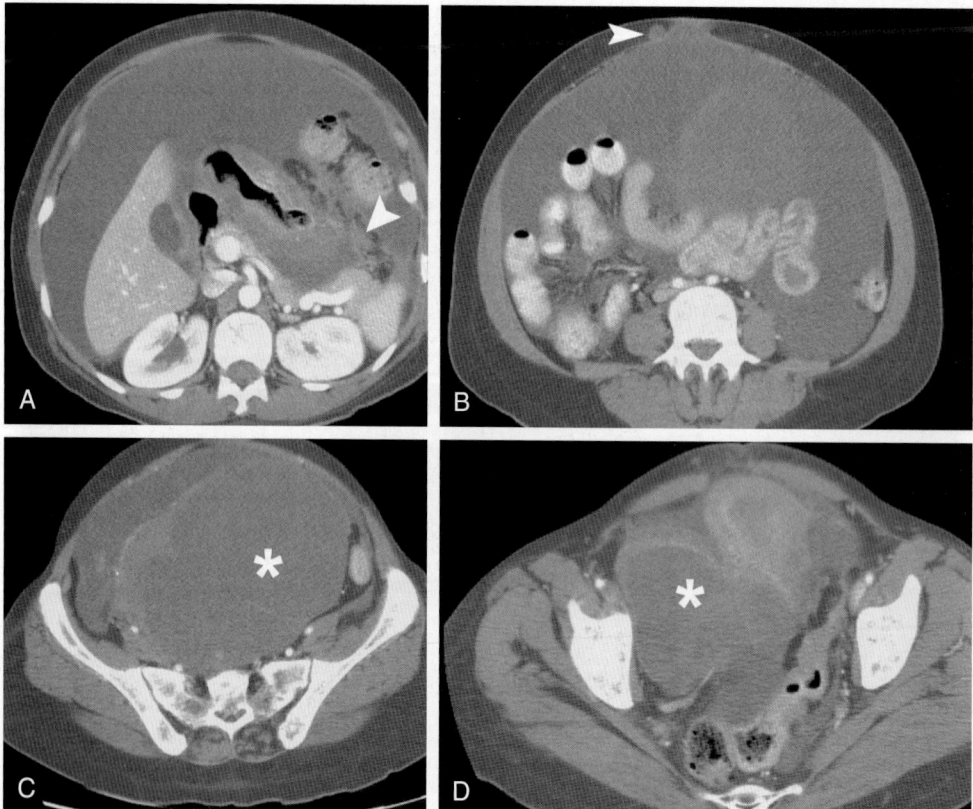

Figure 36-25. Gastric carcinoma with peritoneal and ovarian metastases. A. MDCT image shows a linitis plastica type neoplasm infiltrating the gastric wall. Multiple nodules are seen in the gastrocolic ligament (*arrowhead*) associated with large volume ascites. **B.** A "Sister Mary Joseph" nodule is seen to the right of the umbilicus (*arrowhead*). **C** and **D.** Left and right adnexal masses (*asterisks*) are present. The morphology is similar to that of epithelial ovarian neoplasms. Although the term *Kruckenberg tumor* classically applies only to solid ovarian masses arising from signet-ring cell carcinomas of the stomach, it is generally used for any ovarian metastases from any primary source.

tumor. Tumor can also extend through regional lymphatics in a sheetlike fashion, invading the retroperitoneum with resulting ureteral obstruction. Hematogenous metastases are most frequently found in the liver, but metastatic gastric carcinoma has been reported in a wide variety of sites.

Endoscopic Ultrasonography

The introduction and dissemination of EUS has substantially improved the accuracy of local staging of gastric carcinoma.[160] A major advantage of EUS is its ability to visualize the layers of the gastric wall, perigastric lymph nodes, and the relationship of the tumor to the surrounding tissues, allowing determination of the depth of wall invasion and the extent of regional lymph node involvement by tumor. Nevertheless, EUS is best performed as a complementary test to cross-sectional imaging studies such as CT for local tumor staging.

Technique

EUS employs high-frequency transducers, typically in the frequency range of 5 to 12 MHz, yielding an effective usable clinical resolution of 200 μm. There are two basic types of endosonographic equipment available for clinical use—a dedicated EUS endoscope with maneuvering and biopsy capabilities and a standard endoscope in which the EUS equipment is fitted on catheters and passed through the endoscope. The vast majority of published literature in the United States is based on data obtained with dedicated EUS endoscopes.

EUS requires a trained examiner and is therefore operator dependent.[161] The examination is usually performed under conscious sedation in an outpatient setting. Dedicated echoendoscopes have a suction capability, so that air can be removed from the stomach and deaerated water instilled to allow for acoustic coupling. An inflatable balloon surrounds the transducer and is filled with deaerated water to increase the surface contact area and improve the imaging window.

With standard technique, EUS typically visualizes the stomach as a five-layered structure, with each layer corresponding to histologically defined layers of the gastric wall

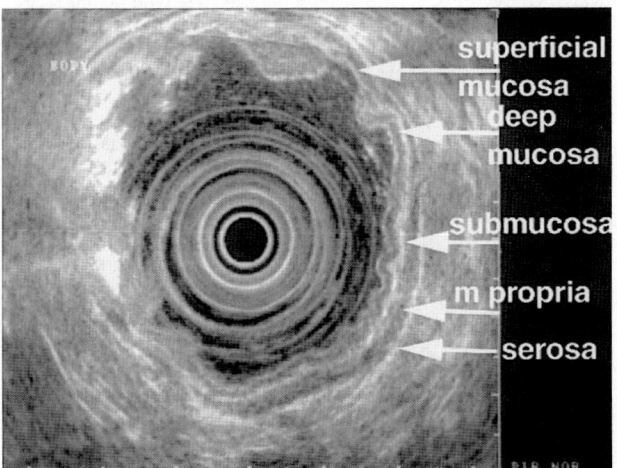

Figure 36-26. Endoscopic ultrasound appearance of the normal gastric wall. Note the typical five-layer wall pattern with a total wall thickness of only several millimeters. (*Arrows* denote the corresponding wall layers.)

(Fig. 36-26).[162] The first hyperechoic layer represents the balloon-mucosal interface, the second hypoechoic layer represents the deep mucosa, the third hyperechoic layer represents the submucosa, the fourth hypoechoic layer represents the muscularis propria, and the fifth hyperechoic layer represents the subserosa and serosa. With proper sonographic technique, EUS may visualize these gastric wall layers and surrounding tissues without air-induced artifacts or interference from gastric contents.

EUS is performed from the transgastric position, allowing visualization of the gastric wall, adjacent lymph nodes, and nearby organs, including the pancreas, spleen, left kidney, and, to a limited degree, the liver. However, EUS is limited by its inability to assess for distant metastases in the right lobe of the liver or elsewhere secondary to a limited depth of penetration and imaging window.

If the diagnosis of gastric cancer has not been established before EUS, the examination can be combined with a standard upper endoscopy, so that biopsy specimens of the primary tumor can be obtained.[163] As on CT, it may be difficult on EUS to differentiate neoplastic involvement of the stomach from inflammatory processes or fibrosis. EUS also cannot differentiate an early gastric cancer from an adenoma based on echogenicity alone, but evidence of disruption of the normal layers of the gastric wall, local invasion, or suspicious lymph nodes should be highly suggestive of malignant tumor.

Results

EUS has been shown to be a highly accurate technique for assessing the depth of tumor invasion and the presence or absence of regional lymph node involvement in patients with gastric carcinoma.[164-166] In most studies, the overall accuracy of EUS for T-staging has ranged from 85% to 88%.[167-169] Nevertheless, EUS does have limitations in staging by T classification of gastric cancer, because differentiation of subserosal (T2) from serosal (T3) invasion can be extremely difficult. EUS may also overestimate the depth of tumor invasion because of peritumoral inflammation and fibrosis or may underestimate the extent of tumor because of microscopic tumor infiltration of deeper layers of the gastric wall or microscopic nodal metastases.[170]

The finding of a thickened muscularis propria is virtually pathognomonic of a malignant gastric tumor, most often gastric adenocarcinoma and, less frequently, lymphoma (Fig. 36-27).[171,172] EUS is also the most sensitivity image technique for detecting perigastric lymph nodes. Unlike CT, in which the detection of abnormal lymph nodes depends entirely on size, the EUS criteria for involved lymph nodes include roundness and hypoechogenecity.[173,174] Malignant lymph nodes can be detected on EUS with a specificity of nearly 90%, but the sensitivity is lower, ranging from 55% to 80%.[164,168,175,176]

The overall diagnostic accuracy of EUS for determining nodal status (N classification) has ranged from 70% to 90%. A major limitation of EUS is its inability to detect nonenlarged nodes more than 3 cm from the gastric wall. Thus, unless the nodes are markedly enlarged and within range of the transducer, EUS may have limited value in planning the extent of lymphadenectomy. The development of real-time guided fine-needle aspiration technique increases the accuracy of lymph node assessment, because individual lymph nodes may be sampled for tumor.[177] Nevertheless, the role of this

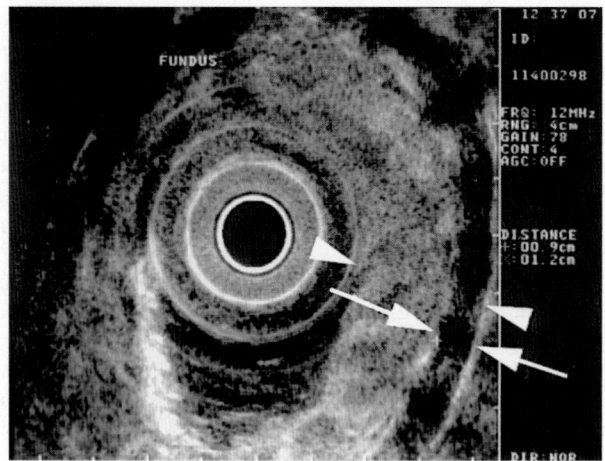

Figure 36-27. Endoscopic ultrasound appearance of linitis plastica. There is marked thickening of the entire gastric wall (*arrowheads*) with associated thickening of the muscularis propria (*arrows*).

technique in the routine staging of gastric cancer remains to be determined.

Summary

The approach to the preoperative staging of patients with gastric carcinoma remains controversial and depends to a major degree on the available imaging, oncologic, and surgical expertise.[163] After the histologic diagnosis of gastric cancer has been made, a cross-sectional imaging study (usually MDCT) is performed to exclude liver metastases or direct extension of tumor into adjacent organs. In patients without metastases or disseminated tumor, EUS can then be performed for local staging of tumor. In such cases, EUS may help select patients with advanced carcinoma in whom neoadjuvant radiation or chemotherapy should be administered before surgery. Patients with T1 to T3 tumors will most likely undergo attempts for curative resection and possibly multimodality therapy, whereas patients with T4 tumors may undergo a palliative bypass procedure or endoscopic palliation. Rare patients with T1 N0 M0 lesions may also undergo endoscopic therapy for attempts at cure if they are not reasonable candidates for surgery.[178] Thus, MDCT and EUS should be considered complementary tests for preoperative evaluation of patients with gastric carcinoma and selection of optimal treatment regimens.[179]

Treatment and Prognosis

Surgery is the only curative form of therapy in patients with gastric carcinoma. Depending on the location of the tumor, a subtotal or total gastrectomy or an esophagogastrectomy may be performed. Unfortunately, about 60% of patients who undergo surgery are found to have unresectable tumors.[8] Nevertheless, a palliative resection or bypass procedure may still be performed on these patients to prevent complications such as bleeding or obstruction. Radiation therapy has also been advocated for palliation of inoperable lesions. Adjuvant chemotherapy has been used in some patients, but the benefits of this treatment remain uncertain. Laser therapy and intraluminal stents have sometimes been used for treatment of patients with obstructing tumors. A detailed discussion

of the various operations and postoperative complications is presented in Chapter 39.

Patients with advanced gastric carcinoma have a dismal prognosis, with 5-year survival rates of only 3% to 21%.[4-7] In contrast, patients with early gastric cancer have 5-year survival rates of 85% to 100%.[99,100,107,108,180] Early detection of these lesions is therefore essential for improving patient survival. Thus far, most early gastric cancers have been detected in Japan as a result of mass screening of the adult population in that country. However, some symptomatic patients with gastric cancer in the West are also found to have early lesions. Because it is frequently not possible to distinguish early gastric cancer from advanced carcinoma on preoperative studies, an aggressive surgical approach is justified for all patients with resectable lesions.

DUODENAL CARCINOMA

Duodenal carcinoma is a rare malignant tumor, accounting for less than 1% of all gastrointestinal neoplasms.[181] Almost all of these lesions are located in the second, third, or fourth portions of the duodenum at or distal to the ampulla of Vater.[182,183] Patients with advanced duodenal cancer usually present with nausea, vomiting, abdominal pain, weight loss, or signs or symptoms of upper gastrointestinal bleeding. Rarely, however, early duodenal cancer may be detected on double-contrast barium studies or endoscopy in symptomatic patients.[184] An increased incidence of duodenal carcinoma has been reported in patients with Gardner's syndrome (see Chapter 65) and celiac disease (see Chapter 47), so that some form of radiologic or endoscopic surveillance may be warranted for these patients.[185,186] Duodenal carcinoma has also been associated with Crohn's disease and neuro-fibromatosis.[187-189]

Duodenal carcinomas usually appear on barium studies as polypoid, ulcerated, or annular lesions at or, more commonly, distal to the ampulla of Vater (Fig. 36-28). Some polypoid carcinomas may arise in preexisting villous tumors (see Chapter 35). Occasionally, duodenal carcinomas have a

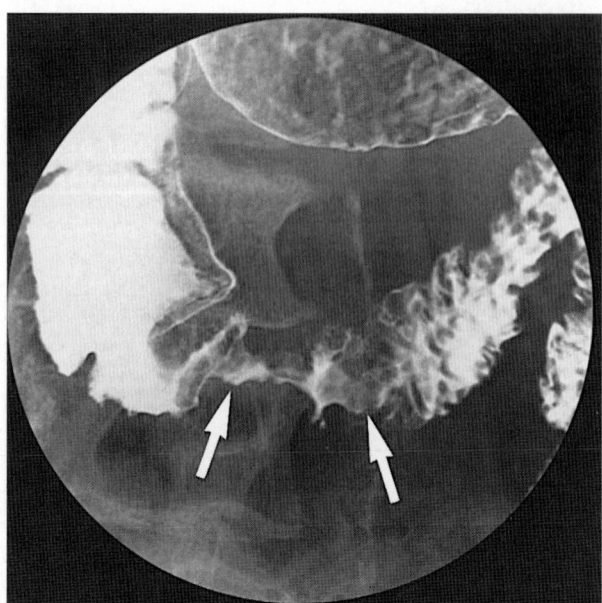

Figure 36-28. Duodenal carcinoma. An annular, ulcerated lesion (*arrows*) is seen in the third portion of the duodenum.

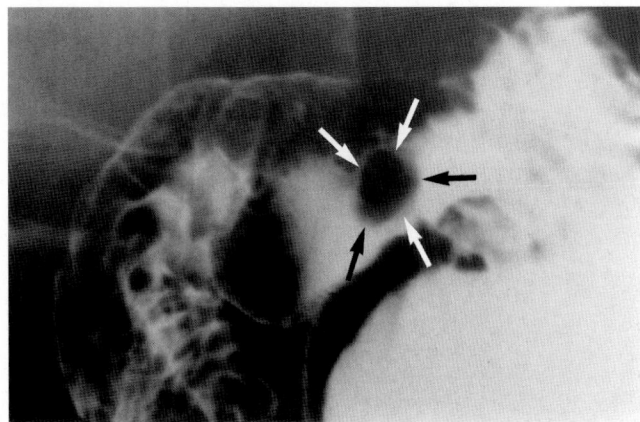

Figure 36-29. Early duodenal cancer. Double-contrast spot image of the duodenum shows a sessile, slightly lobulated, 1.3-cm polypoid lesion (*arrows*) in the duodenal bulb. This was an early cancer that was confined to the mucosa. (From Bradford D, Levine MS, Hoang D, et al: Early duodenal cancer: Detection on double-contrast upper gastrointestinal radiography. AJR 174:1564-1566, 2000. Reprinted with permission from the American Journal of Roentgenology.)

more proximal location, appearing as ulcerated masses in the proximal descending duodenum or even the duodenal bulb.[190] Nevertheless, the vast majority of duodenal ulcers are benign, so endoscopy should be considered only for lesions that have suspicious radiographic features. Rarely, early duodenal cancers may appear on double-contrast barium studies as small (<2 cm), sessile, polypoid or ulcerated lesions in the duodenum (Fig. 36-29).[184]

Duodenal carcinoma is usually manifested on CT by a localized area of wall thickening, producing a soft tissue mass (Fig. 36-30). Features such as tumor necrosis and ulceration are readily identified.[191] When CT reveals an exophytic or intramural mass containing central necrosis and ulceration, this combination of findings is reported to have a sensitivity of 100% and an accuracy of 86% for the detection of malignant tumor.[192]

CT is also useful for differentiating primary duodenal carcinoma from extrinsic tumors involving the duodenum, most frequently from the pancreas.[193] Recent literature has shown that 3D MDCT is particularly helpful for localizing neoplasms to the duodenum and for accurately defining tumor extent (Fig. 36-31).[194] The differential diagnosis of duodenal wall thickening on CT includes lymphoma, Crohn's disease, hematomas, and duodenitis from a wide variety of causes. It is usually possible to suggest the correct diagnosis, however, on

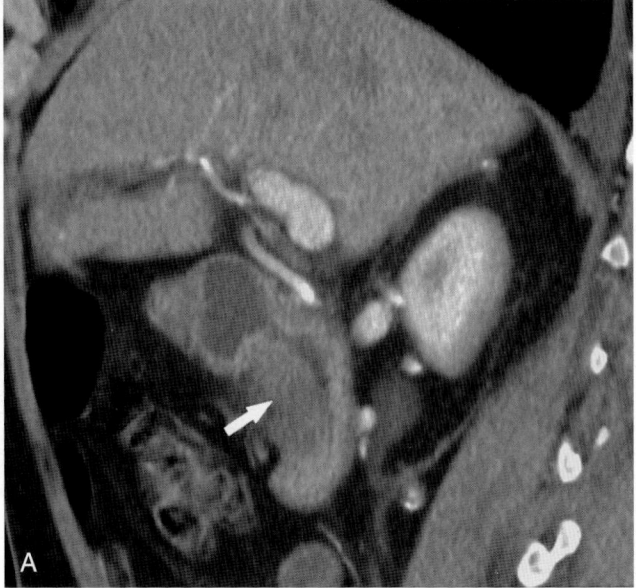

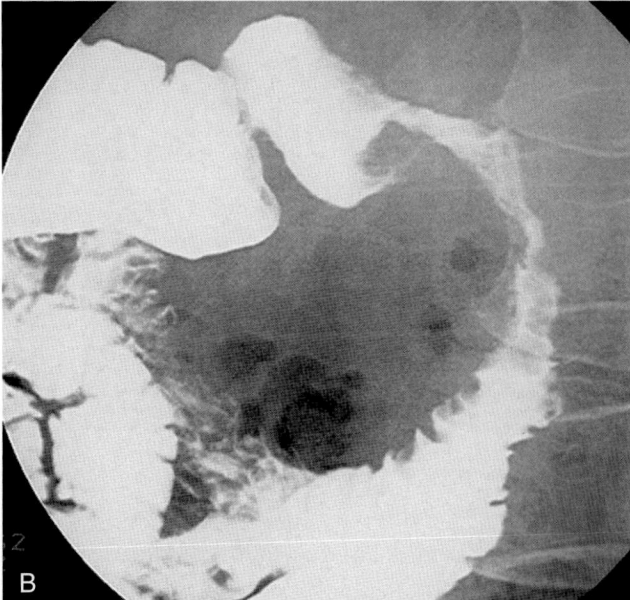

Figure 36-30. Duodenal carcinoma. A. Three-dimensional volume-rendered MDCT shows narrowing of the postbulbar duodenum by an eccentric soft tissue mass arising in the wall (*arrow*). **B.** Barium study from the same patient shows an advanced infiltrating carcinoma of the descending duodenum.

Figure 36-31. Periampullary duodenal carcinoma. Volume-rendered MDCT image shows a lobulated mass (*arrowhead*) in the duodenum, obstructing the common bile duct. MDCT is particularly helpful for determining the etiology of periampullary biliary obstruction.

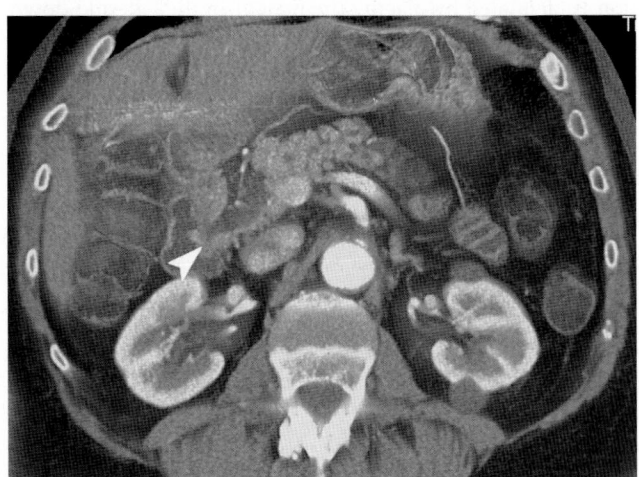

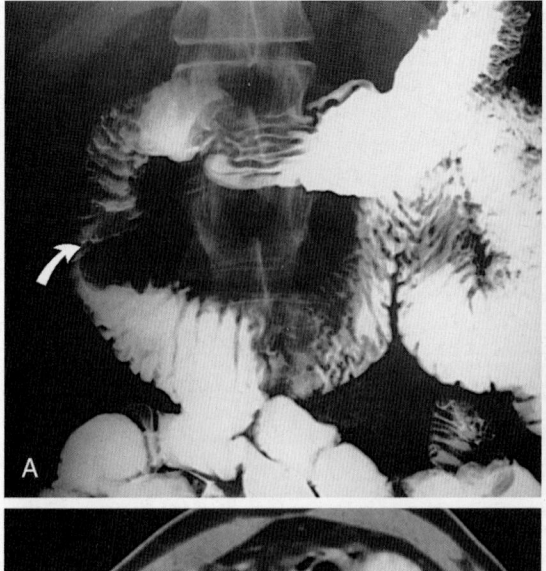
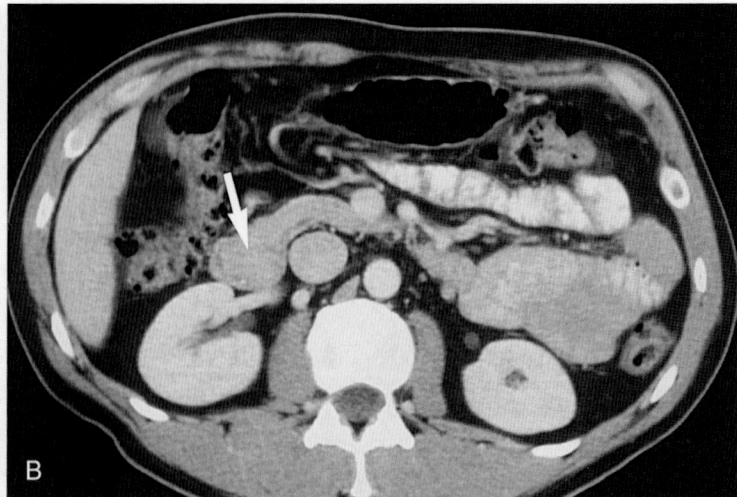
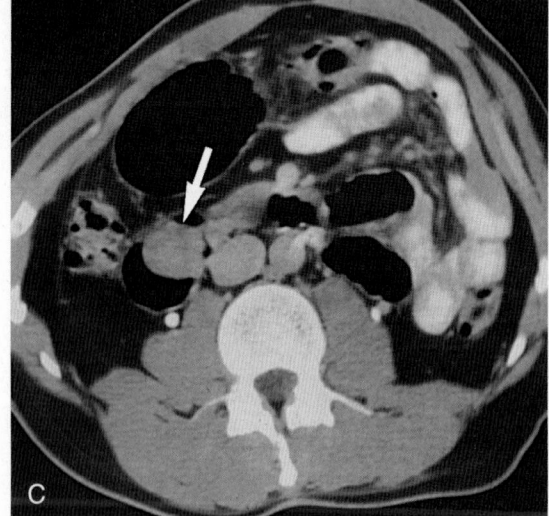

Figure 36-32. Ampullary carcinoma. A. Barium study shows a mass (*arrow*) on the medial aspect of the descending duodenum at the level of the papilla. **B.** CT scan also shows a soft tissue mass (*arrow*) in this region. **C.** After administration of additional effervescent agent and 1.0 mg of intravenous glucagon, a subsequent scan with the patient in the left-side-down decubitus position clearly delineates this intraluminal mass (*arrow*) in the descending duodenum.

the basis of the clinical history and the findings on barium studies and CT.

Although ampullary and periampullary carcinomas may be confused with primary pancreatic carcinomas, it is important to distinguish these lesions because ampullary tumors have a much better prognosis. Hypotonic CT duodenography may be useful for differentiating these tumors. The examination is facilitated by placing the patient in the left-side-down decubitus position after administration of an effervescent agent and 1.0 mg of intravenous glucagon to obtain scans of the gas-filled duodenal sweep. Both ampullary and periampullary lesions may be well demonstrated with this technique (Fig. 36-32).[195]

References

1. Cady B, Ramsden DA, Stein A, et al: Gastric cancer: Contemporary aspects. Am J Surg 133:423-429, 1977.
2. Devesa SS, Silverman DT: Cancer incidence and mortality trends in the United States: 1935-74. J Natl Cancer Inst 60:545-571, 1978.
3. Howson CP, Hiyama T, Wynder EL: The decline in gastric cancer: Epidemiology of an unplanned triumph. Epidemiol Rev 8:1-27, 1986.
4. Fuchs CS, Mayer RJ: Gastric carcinoma. N Engl J Med 333:32-41, 1995.
5. Moore JR: Gastric carcinoma: 30-year review. Can J Surg 29:25-28, 1986.
6. McBride CM, Boddie AW: Adenocarcinoma of the stomach: Are we making any progress? South Med J 80:283-286, 1987.
7. Cady B, Rossi RL, Silverman ML, et al: Gastric adenocarcinoma: A disease in transition. Arch Surg 124:303-308, 1989.
8. Boland CR, Scheiman JM: Tumors of the stomach. In Yamada T (ed): Textbook of Gastroenterology. Philadelphia, JB Lippincott, 1991, pp 1353-1379.
9. Kurtz RC, Sherlock P: Carcinoma of the stomach. In Berk JE (ed): Bockus Gastroenterology. Philadelphia, WB Saunders, 1985, pp 1278-1304.
10. Oiso T: Incidence of stomach cancer and its relation to dietary habits and nutrition in Japan between 1900 and 1975. Cancer Res 35: 3254-3258, 1975.
11. Neugut AI, Hayek M, Howe G: Epidemiology of gastric cancer. Semin Oncol 23:281-291, 1996.
12. Harrison LE, Zhang ZF, Karpeh MS, et al: The role of dietary factors in the intestinal and diffuse histologic subtypes of gastric adenocarcinoma. Cancer 80:1021-1028, 1997.
13. Mirvish SS: The etiology of gastric cancer: Intragastric nitrosamide formation and other theories. J Natl Cancer Inst 71:629-647, 1983.
14. Mirvish SS: Effects of vitamins C and E on *N*-nitroso compound formation, carcinogenesis, and cancer. Cancer 58:1842-1850, 1986.
15. Terry P, Lagergren J, Ye W, et al: Inverse association between intake of cereal fiber and risk of gastric cardia cancer. Gastroenterology 120:387-391, 2001.
16. Parsonnet J, Friedman GD, Vandersteen DP, et al: *Helicobacter pylori* infection and the risk of gastric carcinoma. N Engl J Med 325: 1127-1131, 1991.
17. Forman D, Newell DG, Fullerton F, et al: Association between infection

with *Helicobacter pylori* and risk of gastric cancer: Evidence from a prospective investigation. BMJ 302:1302-1305, 1991.

18. Nomura A, Stemmermann GN, Chyou PH, et al: *Helicobacter pylori* infection and gastric carcinoma among Japanese Americans in Hawaii. N Engl J Med 325:1132-1136, 1991.

19. Asaka M, Takeda H, Sugiyama T, et al: What role does *Helicobacter pylori* play in gastric cancer? Gastroenterology 113(Suppl):S56-S60, 1997.

20. Kuipers EJ, Klinkenberg-Knol EC, Vandenbroucke-Grauls JE, et al: Role of *Helicobacter pylori* in the pathogenesis of atrophic gastritis. Scand J Gastroenterol 32(Suppl 223):28-34, 1997.

21. McFarlane GA, Munro A: *Helicobacter pylori* and gastric cancer. Br J Surg 84:1190-1199, 1997.

22. Morson BC: Carcinoma arising from areas of intestinal metaplasia in the gastric mucosa. Br J Cancer 9:377-385, 1955.

23. Correa P, Haenszel W, Cuello C, et al: Gastric precancerous process in a high risk population: Cross sectional studies. Cancer Res 50:4731-4736, 1990.

24. Craanen ME, Dekker W, Blok P, et al: Intestinal metaplasia and *Helicobacter pylori:* An endoscopic bioptic study of the gastric antrum. Gut 33:16-20, 1992.

25. Hansson LE, Engstrand L, Nyren O, et al: Prevalence of *Helicobacter pylori* infection in subtypes of gastric cancer. Gastroenterology 109: 885-888, 1995.

26. Martin-de-Argila C, Boixeda D, Redondo C, et al: Relation between histologic subtypes and location of gastric cancer and *Helicobacter pylori.* Scand J Gastroenterol 32:303-307, 1997.

27. Sozzi M, Valentini M, Figura N, et al: Atrophic gastritis and intestinal metaplasia in *Helicobacter pylori* infection: The role of CagA status. Am J Gastroenterol 93:375-379, 1998.

28. Blaser MJ, Perez-Perez GI, Kleanthous H, et al: Infection with *Helicobacter pylori* strains possessing cagA is associated with an increased risk of developing adenocarcinoma of the stomach. Cancer Res 55:2111-2115, 1995.

29. Huang JQ, Zheng GF, Sumanac K, et al: Meta-analysis of the relationship between *cagA* seropositivity and gastric cancer. Gastroenterology 125:1636-1644, 2003.

30. Parsonnet J, Harris RA, Hack HM, et al: Modelling cost-effectiveness of *Helicobacter pylori* screening to prevent gastric cancer: A mandate for clinical trials. Lancet 348:150-154, 1996.

31. Strickland RG, Mackay IR: A reappraisal of the nature and significance of chronic atrophic gastritis. Am J Dig Dis 18:426-440, 1973.

32. Walker IR, Strickland RG, Ungar B, et al: Simple atrophic gastritis and gastric carcinoma. Gut 12:906-911, 1971.

33. Cheli R, Santi L, Ciancamerla G, et al: A clinical and statistical follow-up study of atrophic gastritis. Am J Dig Dis 18:1061-1066, 1973.

34. Elsborg L, Mosbech J: Pernicious anaemia as a risk factor in gastric cancer. Acta Med Scand 206:315-318, 1979.

35. Brinton L, Gridley G, Hrubec Z, et al: Cancer risk following pernicious anaemia. Br J Cancer 59:810-813, 1989.

36. Schafer LW, Larson DE, Metton LJ, et al: Risk of development of gastric carcinoma in patients with pernicious anemia: A population-based study in Rochester, Minnesota. Mayo Clin Proc 60:444-448, 1985.

37. Ming S-C: The classification and significance of gastric polyps. In Yardley JH, Morson BC, Abell M (eds): The Gastrointestinal Tract. Interna-tional Academy of Pathology Monograph. Baltimore, Williams & Wilkins, 1977, pp 149-175.

38. Ming S-C: The adenoma-carcinoma sequence in the stomach and colon: II. Malignant potential of gastric polyps. Gastrointest Radiol 1:121-125, 1976.

39. Tomosulo J: Gastric polyps. Histologic types and their relationship to gastric carcinoma. Cancer 27:1346-1355, 1971.

40. Op den Orth JO, Dekker W: Gastric adenomas. Radiology 141:289-293, 1981.

41. Feldman F, Seaman WB: Primary gastric stump carcinoma. AJR 115: 257-267, 1972.

42. Morgenstein L, Yamakawa T, Seltzer D: Carcinoma of the gastric stump. Am J Surg 125:29-38, 1973.

43. Caygill CPJ, Hill MJ, Kirkham JS, et al: Mortality from gastric cancer following gastric surgery for peptic ulcer. Lancet 1:929-931, 1986.

44. Offerhaus GJA, Tersmette AC, Huibregtse K: Mortality caused by stomach cancer after remote partial gastrectomy for benign conditions: 40 years of follow up of an Amsterdam cohort of 2633 postgastrectomy patients. Gut 29:1588-1590, 1980.

45. Viste A, Opheim P, Thunold J, et al: Risk of carcinoma following gastric operations for benign disease. Lancet 2:502-504, 1986.

46. Schafer LW, Larson DE, Melton LJ, et al: The risk of gastric carcinoma after surgical treatment for benign ulcer disease: A population-based study in Olmsted County, Minnesota. N Engl J Med 309:1210-1213, 1983.

47. Dougherty SH, Foster CA, Eisenberg MM: Stomach cancer following gastric surgery for benign disease. Arch Surg 117:294-297, 1982.

48. Goodman P, Levine MS, Gohil MN: Gastric carcinoma after gastro-jejunostomy for benign disease: Radiographic findings. Gastrointest Radiol 17:211-213, 1992.

49. Williams SM, Harned RK, Settles RH: Adenocarcinoma of the stomach in association with Menetrier's disease. Gastrointest Radiol 3:387-390, 1978.

50. La Vecchia C, Negri E, Franceschi S, et al: Family history and the risk of stomach and colorectal cancer. Cancer 70:50-55, 1992.

51. Brenner H, Bode G, Boeing H: *Helicobacter pylori* infection among offspring of patients with stomach cancer. Gastroenterology 118:31-35, 2000.

52. Bentall HH, Aird I: A relationship between cancer of stomach and the ABO blood groups. BMJ 1:799-801, 1953.

53. Ming S-C: Atlas of Tumor Pathology, Fascicle 7, Tumors of the Esophagus and Stomach. Washington, DC, Armed Forces Institute of Pathology, 1973, pp 144-205.

54. Olearchyk AS: Gastric carcinoma: A critical review of 243 cases. Am J Gastroenterol 70:25-45, 1978.

55. Wanke M, Schwan H: Pathology of gastric cancer. World J Surg 3: 675-684, 1979.

56. Moertel CG, Bargen JA, Soule EH: Multiple gastric cancers. Gastro-enterology 32:1095-1103, 1957.

57. Mitsudomi T, Watanabe A, Matsusake T, et al: A clinicopathological study of synchronous multiple gastric cancers. Br J Surg 76:237-240, 1989.

58. Lauren P: The two histological main types of gastric carcinoma: Diffuse and so-called intestinal-type carcinoma. Acta Pathol Microbiol Scand 64:31-49, 1965.

59. Lauren PA, Nevalainen JT: Epidemiology of intestinal and diffuse types of gastric carcinoma: A time-trend study in Finland with comparison between studies from high- and low-risk areas. Cancer 71:2926-2933, 1993.

60. Watanabe H, Jass JR, Sobin LH: Histologic Typing of Oesophageal and Gastric Tumors, 2nd ed. Berlin, Springer-Verlag, 1990.

61. Shirakabe H, Nishizawa M, Maruyama M, et al: Atlas of X-ray Diagnosis of Early Gastric Cancer. New York, Igaku-Shoin, 1982, pp 1-18.

62. Antonioli DA: Precursors of gastric carcinoma: A critical review with a brief description of early (curable) gastric cancer. Hum Pathol 25: 994-1005, 1994.

63. Meyers WC, Damiano RJ, Rotolo FS, et al: Adenocarcinoma of the stomach: Changing patterns over the last 4 decades. Ann Surg 205:1-8, 1987.

64. Antonioli DA, Goldman H: Changes in the location and type of gastric adenocarcinoma. Cancer 50:775-781, 1982.

65. Powell J, McConkey CC: Increasing incidence of adenocarcinoma of the gastric cardia and adjacent sites. Br J Cancer 62:440-443, 1990.

66. Blot WJ, Devesa SS, Kneller RW, et al: Rising incidence of adeno-carcinoma of the esophagus and gastric cardia. JAMA 265:1287-1289, 1991.

67. Pera M, Cameron AJ, Trastek VF, et al: Increasing incidence of adenocarcinoma of the esophagus and esophagogastric junction. Gastroenterology 104:510-513, 1993.

68. Fenoglio-Preiser CM, Noffsinger AE, Belli J, et al: Pathologic and pheno-typic features of gastric cancer. Semin Oncol 23:292-306, 1996.

69. Dodge OG: The surgical pathway of gastro-oesophageal carcinoma. Br J Surg 49:121-125, 1961.

70. Koehler RE, Hanelin LG, Laing FC, et al: Invasion of the duodenum by carcinoma of the stomach. 128:201-205, 1977.

71. Menuck L: Transpyloric extension of gastric carcinoma. Am J Dig Dis 23:269-274, 1978.

72. Cho KC, Baker SR, Alterman DD, et al: Transpyloric spread of gastric tumors: Comparison of adenocarcinoma and lymphoma. AJR 167: 467-469, 1996.

73. Smith DL, Dockerty MB, Black BM: Gastrocolic fistulas of malignant origin. Surg Gynecol Obstet 134:829-834, 1972.

74. Holtz F, Hart WR: Krukenberg tumors of the ovary: A clinicopathologic analysis of 27 cases. Cancer 50:2438-2447, 1982.

75. Hansen RM, Hanson GA: Gastric carcinoma. Am J Gastroenterol 74:497-503, 1980.

76. Bloss RS, Miller TA, Copeland EM: Carcinoma of the stomach in the young adult. Surg Gynecol Obstet 150:883-886, 1980.

77. Holburt E, Freedman SI: Gastric carcinoma in patients younger than 36 years. Cancer 60:1395-1399, 1987.
78. Grabiec J, Owen DA: Carcinoma of the stomach in young persons. Cancer 56:388-396, 1985.
79. MacDonald WC: Clinical and pathologic features of adenocarcinoma of the gastric cardia. Cancer 29:724-731, 1972.
80. Morales TG: Adenocarcinoma of the gastric cardia. Dig Dis 15:346-356, 1997.
81. Raskin MM: Some specific radiological findings and consideration of linitis plastica of the gastrointestinal tract. Crit Rev Diagn Imaging 8:87-105, 1976.
82. Fierst SM: Carcinoma of the cardia and fundus of the stomach. Am J Gastroenterol 57:403-409, 1972.
83. Webb JN, Busuttil A: Adenocarcinoma of the oesophagus and of the oesophagogastric junction. Br J Surg 65:475-479, 1978.
84. Qizilbash AH, Castelli M, Kowalski MA, et al: Endoscopic brush cytology and biopsy in the diagnosis of cancer of the upper gastrointestinal tract. Acta Cytol 24:313-318, 1980.
85. Llanos O, Guzman S, Duarte I: Accuracy of the first endoscopic procedure in the differential diagnosis of gastric lesions. Ann Surg 195:224-226, 1982.
86. Graham DY, Schwartz JT, Cain GD, et al: Prospective evaluation of biopsy number in the diagnosis of esophageal and gastric cancer. Gastroenterology 82:228-231, 1982.
87. Tatsuta M, Iishi H, Okuda S, et al: Prospective evaluation of diagnostic accuracy of gastrofibroscopic biopsy in diagnosis of gastric cancer. Cancer 63:1415-1420, 1989.
88. Winawer SJ, Posner G, Lightdale CJ, et al: Endoscopic diagnosis of advanced gastric cancer: Factors influencing yield. Gastroenterology 69:1183-1187, 1975.
89. Evans E, Harris O, Dickey D, et al: Difficulties in the endoscopic diagnosis of gastric and oesophageal cancer. Aust N Z J Surg 55:541-544, 1985.
90. Levine MS, Kong V, Rubesin SE, et al: Scirrhous carcinoma of the stomach: Radiologic and endoscopic diagnosis. Radiology 175:151-154, 1990.
91. Park MS, Ha HK, Choi BS, et al: Scirrhous gastric carcinoma: Endoscopy versus upper gastrointestinal radiography. Radiology 231:421-426, 2004.
92. Koga M, Nakata H, Kiyonari H, et al: Roentgen features of the superficial depressed type of early gastric carcinoma. Radiology 15:289-292, 1975.
93. Montesi A, Graziani L, Pesaresi A, et al: Radiologic diagnosis of early gastric cancer by routine double-contrast examination. Gastrointest Radiol 7:205-215, 1982.
94. Gold RP, Green PH, O'Toole KM, et al: Early gastric cancer: Radiographic experience. Radiology 152:283-290, 1984.
95. White RM, Levine MS, Enterline HT, et al: Early gastric cancer: Recent experience. Radiology 155:25-27, 1985.
96. Murakami T: Pathomorphological diagnosis. In Murakami T (ed): Early Gastric Cancer. Tokyo, University of Tokyo Press, 1971, pp 53-55.
97. Sakita T, Ogura Y, Takasu S, et al: Observations on the healing of ulcerations in early gastric cancer: The life cycle of the malignant ulcer. Gastroenterology 60:835-844, 1971.
98. Kawai K: Diagnosis of early gastric cancer. Endoscopy 1:23-28, 1971.
99. Kaneko E, Nakamura T, Umeda N, et al: Outcome of gastric carcinoma detected by gastric mass survey in Japan. Gut 18:626-630, 1977.
100. Okui K, Tejima H: Evaluation of gastric mass survey. Acta Chir Scand 146:185-187, 1980.
101. Kaibara N, Kawaguchi H, Nishidoi H, et al: Significance of mass survey for gastric cancer from the standpoint of surgery. Am J Surg 142:543-545, 1981.
102. Evans DMD, Craven JL, Murphy F, et al: Comparison of early gastric cancer in Britain and Japan. Gut 19:1-9, 1978.
103. Seifert E, Butke H, Gail K, et al: Diagnosis of early gastric cancer. Am J Gastroenterol 71:563-567, 1979.
104. Ohman U, Emas S, Rubio C: Relation between early and advanced gastric cancer. Am J Surg 140:351-355, 1980.
105. Green PH, O'Toole KM, Weinberg LM, et al: Early gastric cancer. Gastroenterology 81:247-256, 1981.
106. Busuttil A, Webb JN: Early carcinoma of the stomach: A ten-year survey. J R Coll Surg Edinb 26:322-327, 1981.
107. Carter KJ, Schaffer HA, Ritchie WP: Early gastric cancer. Ann Surg 199:604-609, 1984.
108. Green PHR, O'Toole KM, Slonim D, et al: Increasing incidence and excellent survival of patients with early gastric cancer: Experience in a United States medical center. Am J Med 85:658-661, 1988.
109. Thomas RL, Rice RP: Calcifying mucinous adenocarcinoma of the stomach. Radiology 88:1002-1003, 1967.
110. Balthazar E, Rosenthal N: Calcifying mucin-producing adenocarcinoma of stomach. N Y State J Med 73:2704-2706, 1973.
111. Lwin TOM, Soodeen TH: A case report of calcified mucinous adenocarcinoma of the stomach. J Can Assoc Radiol 24:370-373, 1973.
112. Low VHS, Levine MS, Rubesin SE, et al: Diagnosis of gastric carcinoma: Sensitivity of double-contrast barium studies. AJR 162:329-334, 1994.
113. Shindoh N, Nakagawa T, Ozaki Y, et al: Overlooked gastric carcinoma: Pitfalls in upper gastrointestinal radiology. Radiology 217:409-414, 2000.
114. Brandt D, Muramatsu Y, Ushio K, et al: Synchronous early gastric cancer. Radiology 173:649-652, 1989.
115. Nelson SW: The discovery of gastric ulcers and the differential diagnosis between benignancy and malignancy. Radiol Clin North Am 7:5-25, 1969.
116. Wolf BS: Observations on roentgen features of benign and malignant gastric ulcers. Semin Roentgenol 6:140-150, 1971.
117. Carman RD: A new roentgen-ray sign of ulcerating gastric cancer. JAMA 77:990-992, 1921.
118. Kirklin BR: The value of the meniscus sign in the roentgenologic diagnosis of ulcerating gastric carcinoma. Radiology 22:131-135, 1934.
119. Marshak RH, Lindner AE, Maklansky D: Carcinoma of the stomach. In Marshak RH, Lindner AE, Maklansky D (eds): Radiology of the Stomach. Philadelphia, WB Saunders, 1983, pp 108-146.
120. Balthazar EJ, Rosenberg H, Davidian MM: Scirrhous carcinoma of the pyloric channel and distal antrum. AJR 134:669-673, 1980.
121. Kobayashi S, Yamada A, Kawai B, et al: Study on early cancer of the cardiac region: X-ray findings of the surrounding area of the oesophagogastric junction. Australas Radiol 16:258-270, 1972.
122. Freeny PC: Double-contrast gastrography of the fundus and cardia: Normal landmarks and their pathologic changes. AJR 133:481-487, 1979.
123. Herlinger H, Grossman R, Laufer I, et al: The gastric cardia in double-contrast study: Its dynamic image. AJR 135:21-29, 1980.
124. Levine MS, Laufer I, Thompson JJ: Carcinoma of the gastric cardia in young people. AJR 140:69-72, 1983.
125. Freeny PC, Marks WM: Adenocarcinoma of the gastroesophageal junction: Barium and CT examination. AJR 138:1077-1084, 1982.
126. Balthazar EJ, Goldfine S, Davidian NM: Carcinoma of the esophagogastric junction. Am J Gastroenterol 74:237-243, 1980.
127. Milnes JP, Hine KR, Holmes GKT, et al: Limitations of endoscopy in the diagnosis of carcinoma of the cardia of the stomach. Br J Radiol 55:593-595, 1982.
128. Lawson TL, Dodds WJ: Infiltrating carcinoma simulating achalasia. Gastrointest Radiol 1:245-248, 1976.
129. Woodfield CA, Levine MS, Rubesin SE, et al: Diagnosis of primary versus secondary achalasia: Reassessment of clinical and radiographic criteria. AJR 175:727-731, 2000.
130. Ba-Ssalamah A, Prokop M, Uffmann M, et al: Dedicated multidetector CT of the stomach: Spectrum of diseases. RadioGraphics 23:625-644, 2003.
131. Wei WZ, Yu JP, Li J, et al: Evaluation of contrast-enhanced helical hydro-CT in staging gastric cancer. World J Gastroenterol 11:4592-4595, 2005.
132. Vorbeck F, Osterreicher C, Puspok A, et al: Comparison of spiral-computed tomography with water-filling of the stomach and endosonography for gastric lymphoma of mucosa-associated lymphoid tissue-type. Digestion 65:196-199, 2002.
133. Mani NB, Suri S, Gupta S, et al: Two-phase dynamic contrast-enhanced computed tomography with water-filling method for staging of gastric carcinoma. Clin Imaging 25:38-43, 2001.
134. Kim JH, Park SH, Hong HS, et al: CT gastrography. Abdom Imaging 30:509-517, 2005.
135. Inamoto K, Kouzai K, Ueeda T, et al: CT virtual endoscopy of the stomach: Comparison study with gastric fiberoscopy. Abdom Imaging 30:473-479, 2005.
136. Kim JP, Lee JH, Kim SJ, et al: Clinicopathologic characteristics and prognostic factors in 10783 patients with gastric cancer. Gastric Cancer 1:125-133, 1998.
137. Insko EK, Levine MS, Birnbaum BA, et al: Benign and malignant lesions of the stomach: Evaluation of CT criteria for differentiation. Radiology 228:166-171, 2003.
138. Pickhardt PJ, Asher DB: Wall thickening of the gastric antrum as a normal finding: Multidetector CT with cadaveric comparison. AJR 181:973-979, 2003.

139. Thompson WM, Halvorsen RA, Foster W, et al: Computed tomography of the gastroesophageal junction: Value of the left lateral decubitus view. J Comput Assist Tomogr 8:346-349, 1984.

140. Park MS, Yu JS, Kim MJ, et al: Mucinous versus nonmucinous gastric carcinoma: Differentiation with helical CT. Radiology 223:540-546, 2002.

141. Lee DH, Seo TS, Ko YT: Spiral CT of gastric carcinoma: Staging and enhancement pattern. Clin Imaging 25:32-37, 2001.

142. Shimizu K, Ito K, Matsunaga N, et al: Diagnosis of gastric cancer with MDCT using the water-filling method and multiplanar reconstruction: CT-histologic correlation. AJR 185:1152-1158, 2005.

143. Usui S, Hiranuma S, Ichikawa T, et al: Preoperative imaging of surrounding arteries by three-dimensional CT: Is it useful for laparoscopic gastrectomy? Surg Laparosc Endosc Percutan Tech 15:61-65, 2005.

144. Joffe N: Metastatic involvement of the stomach secondary to breast carcinoma. AJR 123:512-521, 1975.

145. Cormier WJ, Gaffey TA, Welch JM, et al: Linitis plastica caused by metastatic lobular carcinoma of the breast. Mayo Clin Proc 55:747-753, 1980.

146. Rubesin SE, Levine MS, Glick SN: Gastric involvement by omental cakes. Gastrointest Radiol 11:223-228, 1986.

147. Levine MS, Pantongrag-Brown L, Aguilera NS, et al: Non-Hodgkin lymphoma of the stomach: A cause of linitis plastica. Radiology 201:375-378, 1996.

148. Eisenberg RL: Gastrointestinal Radiology: A Pattern Approach, 2nd ed. Philadelphia, JB Lippincott, 1990, pp 205-222.

149. Bryk D, Elguezabal A: Roentgen problems in evaluating the atrophic stomach of the elderly. AJR 123:236-241, 1975.

150. Levine MS, Caroline D, Thompson JJ, et al: Adenocarcinoma of the esophagus: Relationship to Barrett mucosa. Radiology 150:305-309, 1984.

151. Allen HA, Bush JE: Midesophageal carcinoma metastatic to the stomach: Its unusual appearance on an upper gastrointestinal series. South Med J 76:1049-1051, 1983.

152. Glick SN, Teplick SK, Levine MS, et al: Gastric cardia metastasis in esophageal carcinoma. Radiology 160:627-630, 1986.

153. Anderson MF, Dunnick NR: Pseudotumor caused by gastric varices. Am J Dig Dis 22:929-932, 1977.

154. Carucci LR, Levine MS, Rubesin SE, et al: Tumorous gastric varices: Radiographic findings in 10 patients. Radiology 212:861-865, 1999.

155. Kim HJ, Kim AY, Oh ST, et al: Gastric cancer staging at multi-detector row CT gastrography: Comparison of transverse and volumetric CT scanning. Radiology 236:879-885, 2005.

156. Kumano S, Murakami T, Kim T, et al: T staging of gastric cancer: Role of multi-detector row CT. Radiology 237:961-966, 2005.

157. Polkowski M, Palucki J, Wronska E, et al: Endosonography versus helical computed tomography for locoregional staging of gastric cancer. Endoscopy 36:617-623, 2004.

158. Habermann CR, Weiss F, Riecken R, et al: Preoperative staging of gastric adenocarcinoma: Comparison of helical CT and endoscopic US. Radiology 230:465-471, 2004.

159. Kim SH, Kim WH, Park KJ, et al: CT and MR findings of Krukenberg tumors: Comparison with primary ovarian tumors. J Comput Assist Tomogr 20:393-398, 1996.

160. Rosch T: Endoscopic ultrasonography. Endoscopy 26:148-168, 1994.

161. Kochman ML, Scheiman JM: Endosonography—is it sound for the masses? J Clin Gastroenterol 19:2-5, 1994.

162. Kimmey MB, Martin RW, Haggitt RC, et al: Histological correlates of gastrointestinal endoscopic ultrasound images. Gastroenterology 96:433-441, 1989.

163. Kadish S, Kochman ML: Applications of gastrointestinal endoscopy in oncology. Oncology 9:967-980, 1995.

164. Botet JF, Lightdale CJ, Zauber AG: Preoperative staging of gastric cancer: Comparison of endoscopic US and dynamic CT. Radiology 181:426-432, 1991.

165. Abe S, Lightdale CJ, Brennan MF: The Japanese experience with endoscopic ultrasonography in the staging of gastric cancer. Gastrointest Endosc 39:586-591, 1993.

166. Rosch T: Endosonographic staging of gastric cancer: A review of literature results. Gastrointest Endosc Clin North Am 5:549-557, 1995.

167. Murata Y, Suzuki S, Hashimoto H: Endoscopic ultrasonography of the upper gastrointestinal tract. Surg Endosc 2:180-183, 1988.

168. Dittler JH, Siewert JR: Role of endoscopic ultrasonography in gastric carcinoma. Endoscopy 25:162-166, 1993.

169. Colin Jones DG, Rosch T, Dittler HL: Staging of gastric cancer by endoscopy. Endoscopy 25:34-38, 1993.

170. Tio TL, Coene PPLO, Schouwink MH, et al: Esophagogastric carcinoma. Preoperative TNM classification with endosonography. Radiology 173:411-417, 1989.

171. Andriulli A, Recchia S, De Angelis C, et al: Endoscopic ultrasonographic evaluation of patients with biopsy negative gastric linitis plastica. Gastrointest Endosc 36:611-615, 1990.

172. Mendis RE, Gerdes H, Lightdale CJ, et al: Large gastric folds: A diagnostic approach using endoscopic ultrasonography. Gastrointest Endosc 40:437-441, 1994.

173. Hildebrandt U, Feifel G: Endosonography in the diagnosis of lymph nodes. Endoscopy 25:243-245, 1993.

174. Faigel DO, Ginsberg GG, Furth EE, et al: Endosonography for malignant lymphadenopathy: Caveats and pitfalls. Gastrointest Endosc 43:294, 1996.

175. Akahoshi K, Misawa T, Fujishima H, et al: Regional lymph node metastasis in gastric cancer: Evaluation with endoscopic US. Radiology 182:559-564, 1992.

176. Tio TL, Kallimanis GE: Endoscopic ultrasonography of perigastrointestinal lymph nodes. Endoscopy 26:776-779, 1994.

177. Wiersema MJ, Kochman ML, Cramer HM, et al: Endosonography-guided real-time fine-needle aspiration biopsy. Gastrointest Endosc 40:700-707, 1994.

178. Akahoshi K, Chijiiwa Y, Hamada S, et al: Endoscopic ultrasonography: A promising method for assessing the prospects of endoscopic mucosal resection in early gastric cancer. Endoscopy 29:614-619, 1997.

179. Gore RM: Upper gastrointestinal tract tumours: Diagnosis and staging strategies. Cancer Imaging 5:95-98, 2005.

180. Everett SM, Axon ATR: Early gastric cancer in Europe. Gut 41:142-150, 1997.

181. Spira IH, Ghazi A, Wolff WI: Primary adenocarcinoma of the duodenum. Cancer 39:1721-1726, 1977.

182. Cortese AF, Cornell GN: Carcinoma of the duodenum. Cancer 29:1010-1015, 1972.

183. Joesting DR, Beart RW Jr, van Heerden JA, et al: Improving survival in adenocarcinoma of the duodenum. Am J Surg 141:228-231, 1981.

184. Bradford D, Levine MS, Hoang D, et al: Early duodenal cancer: Detection on double-contrast upper gastrointestinal radiography. AJR 174:1564-1566, 2000.

185. Itoh H, Iida M, Kuroiwa S, et al: Gardner's syndrome associated with carcinoma of the duodenal bulb: Report of a case. Am J Gastroenterol 80:248-250, 1985.

186. Levine ML, Dorf BS, Bank S: Adenocarcinoma of the duodenum in a patient with nontropical sprue. Am J Gastroenterol 81:800-802, 1986.

187. Meiselman MS, Ghahremani GG, Kaufman MW: Crohn's disease of the duodenum complicated by adenocarcinoma. Gastrointest Radiol 12:333-336, 1987.

188. Slezak P, Rubio C, Blomqvist L, et al: Duodenal adenocarcinoma in Crohn's disease of the small bowel: A case report. Gastrointest Radiol 16:15-17, 1991.

189. McGlinchey JJ, Santer GJ, Haggani MT: Primary adenocarcinoma of the duodenum associated with cutaneous neurofibromatosis. Postgrad Med J 58:115-116, 1982.

190. Barloon TJ, Lu CH, Honda H, et al: Primary adenocarcinoma of the duodenal bulb: Radiographic and pathologic findings in two cases. Gastrointest Radiol 14:223-225, 1989.

191. Farah MC, Jafri SZ, Schwab RE, et al: Duodenal neoplasms: Role of CT. Radiology 162:839-843, 1987.

192. Kazerooni EA, Quint LE, Francis IR: Duodenal neoplasms: Predictive value of CT for determining malignancy and tumor resectability. AJR 159:303-309, 1992.

193. Jayaraman MV, Mayo-Smith WW, Movson JS, et al: CT of the duodenum: An overlooked segment gets its due. RadioGraphics 21:S147-S160, 2001.

194. House MG, Yeo CJ, Cameron JL, et al: Predicting resectability of periampullary cancer with three-dimensional computed tomography. J Gastrointest Surg 8:280-288, 2004.

195. Bree RL, Megibow AJ: Hypotonic CT duodenography in the evaluation of periampullary neoplasms. Radiology 177:251, 1990.

Other Malignant Tumors of the Stomach and Duodenum

Marc S. Levine, MD • Alec J. Megibow, MD

METASTASES

Gastric metastases are found at autopsy in less than 2% of patients who die of carcinoma.[1] Duodenal metastases are even rarer. Nevertheless, metastases to the stomach and duodenum have been encountered more frequently as combined treatment with surgery, radiation therapy, or chemotherapy has led to prolonged survival of patients with widespread metastatic disease. Most lesions are hematogenous metastases from malignant melanoma or carcinoma of the breast or lung. Less frequently, the stomach or duodenum may be involved by lymphatic spread of tumor or by direct extension of tumor from neighboring structures or mesenteric reflections such as the gastrocolic ligament, transverse mesocolon, and greater omentum. These various forms of spread produce characteristic radiographic findings that are considered separately in the following sections.

Clinical Findings

Most gastroduodenal metastases are discovered unexpectedly at surgery or autopsy.[2] However, some patients with ulcerated metastases may develop signs or symptoms of upper gastrointestinal bleeding, such as hematemesis, melena, and guaiac-positive stool.[3,4] Others may present with epigastric pain, nausea, vomiting, early satiety, anorexia, or weight loss. One or more of these findings are sometimes caused by systemic chemotherapy or the hypercalcemia associated with widespread metastatic disease.[5] As a result, gastroduodenal metastases may not be suspected even if symptoms are present.

Most patients with gastroduodenal metastases have a known underlying malignancy. Occasionally, however, metastases to the stomach or duodenum may occur as the initial manifestation of an occult primary tumor.[4] Certain malignancies such as carcinoma of the breast and kidney can also metastasize to the stomach or duodenum many years after treatment of the original lesion.[5,6] It is therefore important to obtain a detailed clinical history in these patients.

Radiographic Findings

Hematogenous Metastases

True hematogenous or blood-borne metastases to the stomach or duodenum may be caused by a variety of malignant tumors. Although malignant melanoma has the highest percentage of hematogenous metastases,[7] breast cancer is such a common disease that it rivals melanoma as the most common cause of metastases to the bowel.[5] Much less frequently, the stomach or duodenum may be involved by hematogenous metastases from thyroid or testicular carcinoma or from other remote tumors.[1]

Hematogenous metastases usually appear on barium studies as one or more discrete submucosal masses in the stomach, duodenum, or small intestine (Fig. 37-1).[5,8-11] When multiple lesions are present, they tend to be of varying sizes because of periodic showers of tumor emboli into the arterial supply of the bowel.[8,12] As these submucosal masses outgrow their blood supply, they may undergo central necrosis and ulceration, resulting in the development of classic "bull's-eye" or "target" lesions (Fig. 37-2).[8,10-13] In general, bull's-eye lesions have large central ulcers in relation to the size of the surrounding mass.[8,12] Superficial fissures may occasionally radiate toward the central ulcer crater, producing a characteristic spokewheel pattern (see Fig. 37-2B).[8]

Hematogenous metastases to the stomach or duodenum are sometimes manifested by larger, more lobulated masses that can be mistaken radiographically for malignant gastrointestinal stromal tumors (GISTs) or even polypoid carcinomas (Fig. 37-3).[13] Other metastases, particularly those from malignant melanoma, may become necrotic, resulting in the development of giant, cavitated lesions. These cavitated metastases can be recognized on barium studies as amorphous collections of barium (usually 5 to 15 cm in size) that communicate with the lumen (Fig. 37-4).[11,14] CT is particularly well suited for demonstrating these giant, cavitated lesions.[15]

Hematogenous metastases to the stomach from the infiltrating lobular form of breast carcinoma may produce a linitis plastica or "leather bottle" appearance indistinguishable from that of a primary scirrhous carcinoma of the stomach (Fig. 37-5).[5,8,9,11] This linitis plastica appearance is caused not by fibrosis (as in patients with scirrhous carcinoma) but rather by highly cellular infiltrates of metastatic tumor in the gastric wall.[8] Although some cases may be manifested by only mild loss of distensibility, these lesions can still be recognized on double contrast studies by distortion of the normal surface pattern of the stomach, with mucosal nodularity, spiculation, ulceration, or thickened, irregular folds (see Fig. 37-5).[16] Some of these lesions may involve the proximal portion of the stomach with antral sparing (see Fig. 37-5B).[16] The possibility of metastatic disease should therefore be considered in any patient with linitis plastica who has a history of breast carcinoma.

CT is frequently performed on patients with metastatic disease involving the stomach. In two studies, metastases to the stomach were detected on CT in 5% to 27% of patients

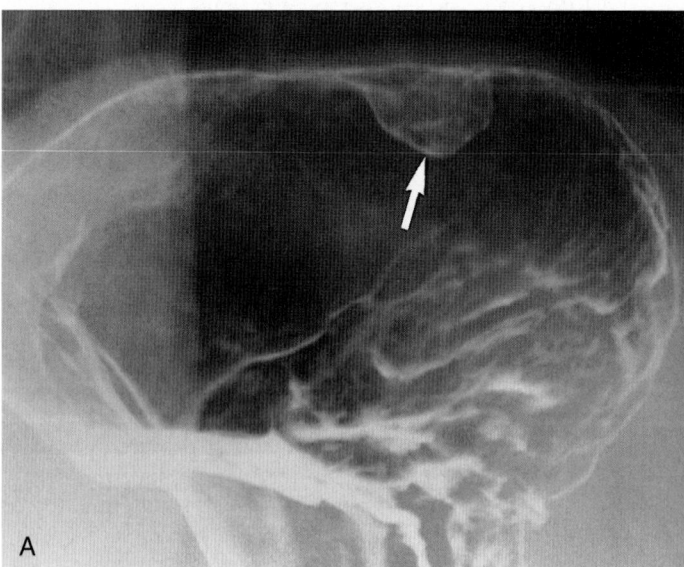

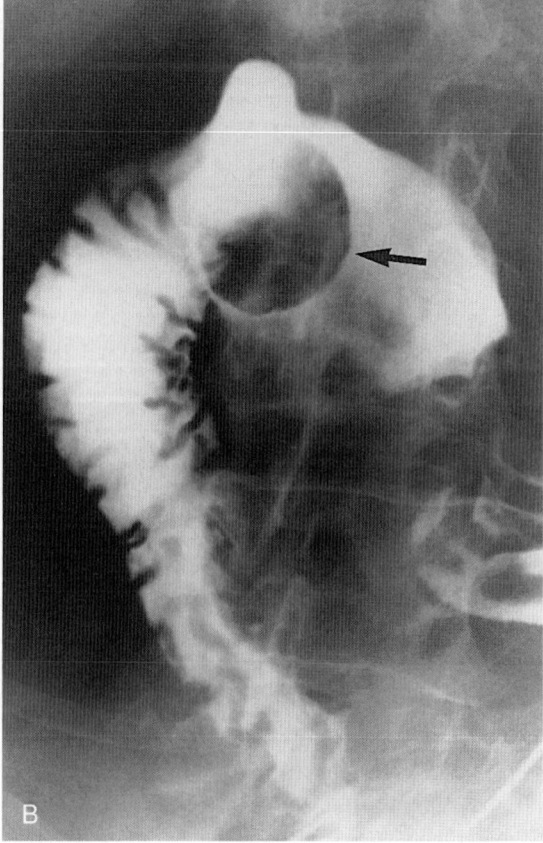

Figure 37-1. Gastric metastases from malignant melanoma. A. A discrete submucosal mass (*arrow*) is seen in the gastric fundus. **B.** In another patient, a large submucosal mass (*arrow*) is present in the duodenal bulb.

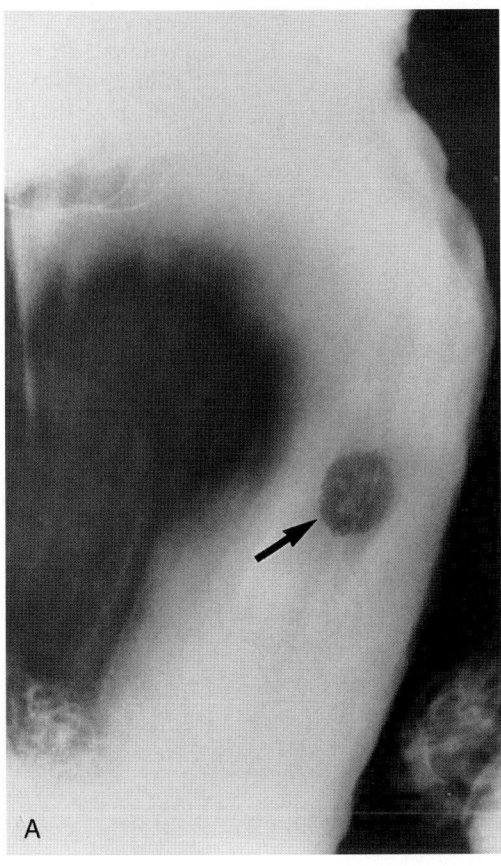

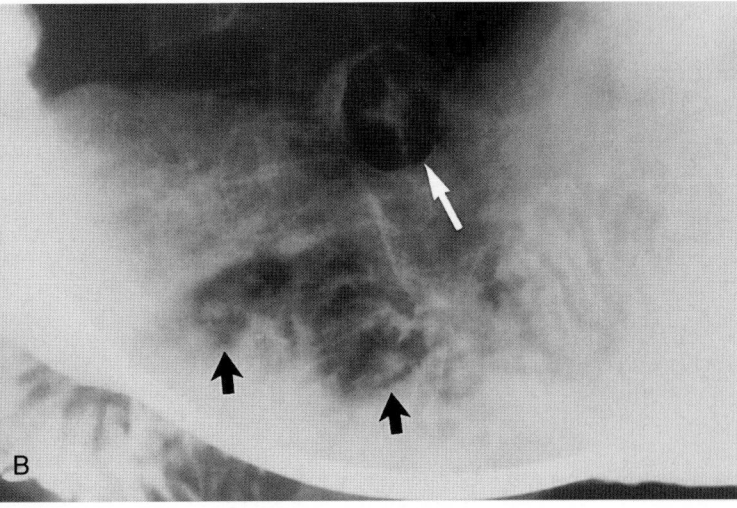

Figure 37-2. Ulcerated gastric metastases from malignant melanoma. A. A centrally ulcerated submucosal mass or bull's-eye lesion (*arrow*) is seen in the gastric body. **B.** In another patient, a prone compression view reveals multiple bull's-eye lesions (*black arrows*) in the stomach. Superficial fissures are seen radiating from the central ulcer of a metastasis on the lesser curvature, producing a spoke-wheel pattern (*white arrow*).

with breast carcinoma.[17,18] CT may reveal marked thickening of the gastric wall (sometimes associated with increased attenuation of the wall after intravenous contrast enhancement), producing a linitis plastica appearance that simulates a primary scirrhous carcinoma of the stomach (Fig. 37-6). In other patients with metastatic breast cancer, CT may reveal more focal wall thickening (Fig. 37-7). Because these tumors often reside deeply within the gastric wall, it may be difficult to obtain a definitive pathologic diagnosis from endoscopic

biopsy specimens. Nevertheless, the CT findings should be highly suggestive of metastatic breast cancer involving the stomach in the proper clinical setting.[19]

Hematogenous metastases to the stomach from malignant melanoma, bronchogenic carcinoma, and Kaposi's sarcoma may also be detected on CT.

Lymphatic Spread

Gastric metastases are found at autopsy in 2% to 15% of patients who die of squamous cell carcinoma of the esophagus.[20] These metastases are thought to be caused by tumor emboli that seed the gastric cardia or fundus via submucosal esophageal lymphatics extending subdiaphragmatically to paracardiac, lesser curvature, and celiac nodes. Squamous cell metastases to the gastric fundus may appear on barium studies as giant submucosal masses, often containing central areas of ulceration (Fig. 37-8).[20,21] As a result, these lesions can be mistaken for benign or malignant GISTs or even adenocarcinomas.[22] Squamous cell metastases to paracardiac or other lymph nodes in the upper abdomen are sometimes recognized on CT scans as multiple low-attenuation masses relative to skeletal muscle (Fig. 37-9).

The duodenum is occasionally involved by peripancreatic lymphadenopathy from pancreatic carcinoma, lymphoma, or other malignant tumors. In such cases, barium studies may reveal nodular indentations on the medial border of the descending duodenum or widening of the duodenal sweep. Pancreatic carcinoma, pancreatic pseudocysts, and pancreatitis, however, can produce identical radiographic findings. CT is extremely helpful for determining the cause of a widened

Figure 37-3. Gastric metastasis from malignant melanoma. There is a large, lobulated mass (*arrows*) on the greater curvature of the stomach. This lesion could be mistaken for a malignant gastrointestinal stromal tumor or even an adenocarcinoma.

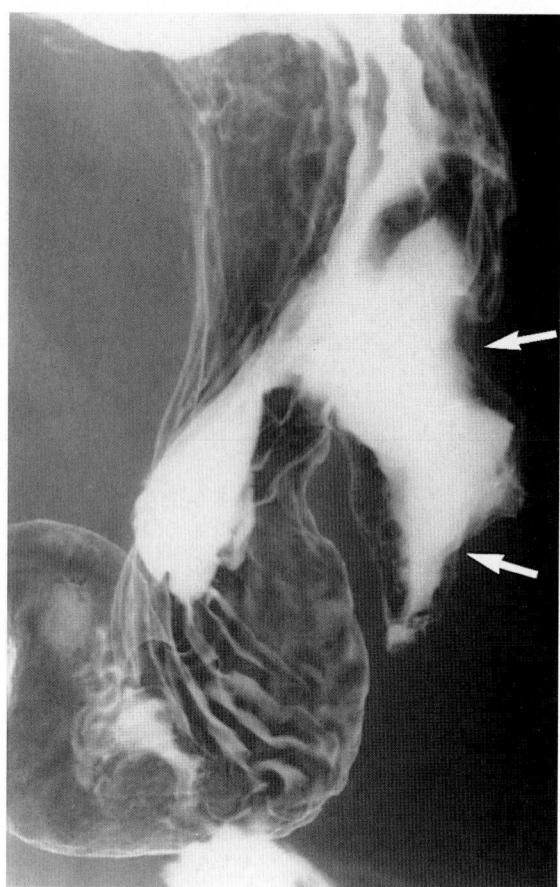

Figure 37-4. Cavitated metastasis from malignant melanoma. A giant, cavitated lesion (*arrows*) is seen on the greater curvature of the stomach. A malignant gastrointestinal stromal tumor or lymphoma could produce similar findings. (From Laufer I, Levine MS [eds]: Double Contrast Gastrointestinal Radiology, 2nd ed. Philadelphia, WB Saunders, 1992.)

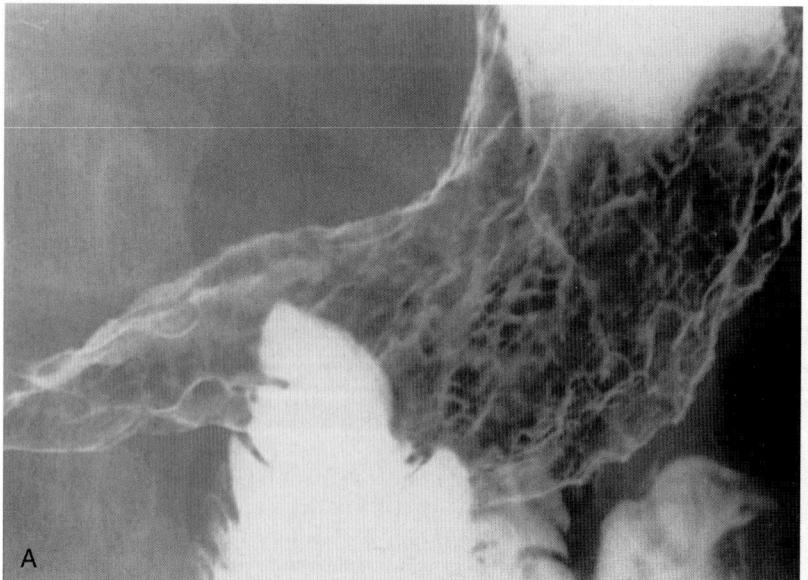

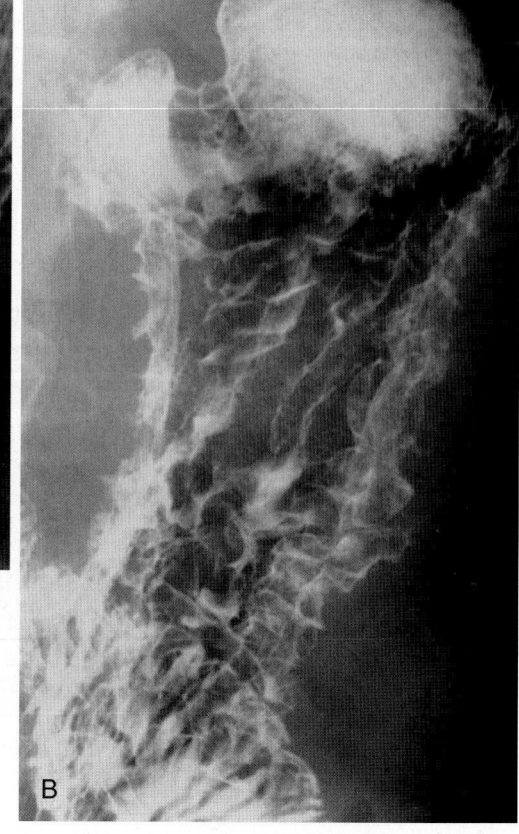

Figure 37-5. Metastatic breast cancer involving the stomach with a linitis plastica appearance. A. There is only mild loss of distensibility of the gastric antrum and body, but the mucosa has a nodular, irregular appearance because of infiltration by metastatic tumor. **B.** In another patient, the area of involvement is confined to the proximal half of the stomach. The fundus and body have an irregular contour with thickened, spiculated folds. (From Levine MS, Kong V, Rubesin SE, et al: Scirrhous carcinoma of the stomach: Radiologic and endoscopic diagnosis. Radiology 175:151-154, 1990.)

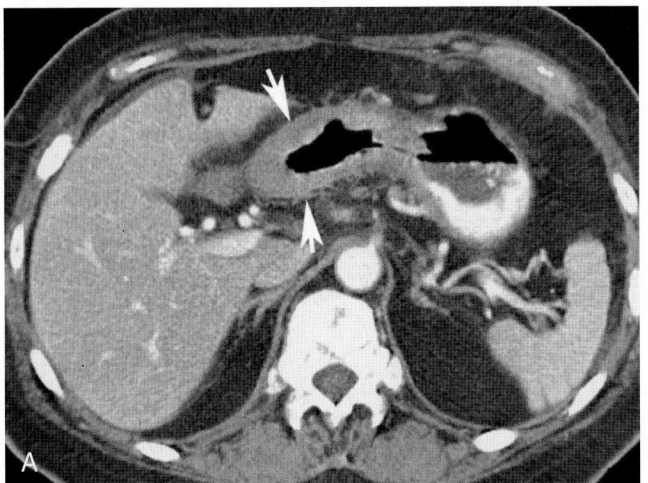

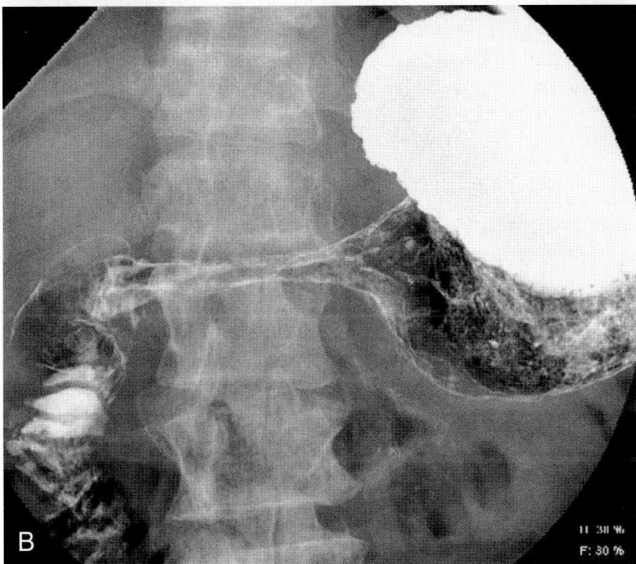

Figure 37-6. Metastatic breast cancer to the stomach with a linitis plastica appearance on CT. A. MDCT image in an elderly woman with metastatic breast carcinoma and early satiety shows marked thickening of the wall of the gastric antrum (*arrows*). The radiographic findings are indistinguishable from those of a primary scirrhous carcinoma of the stomach. **B.** Barium study in the same patient shows marked narrowing of the antrum, producing a classic linitis plastica appearance.

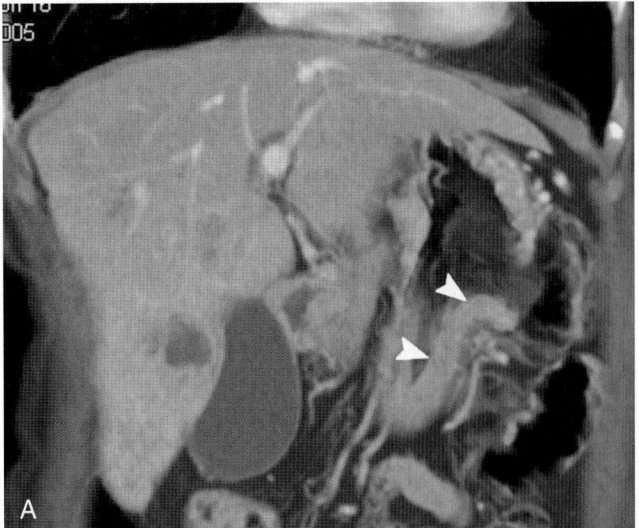

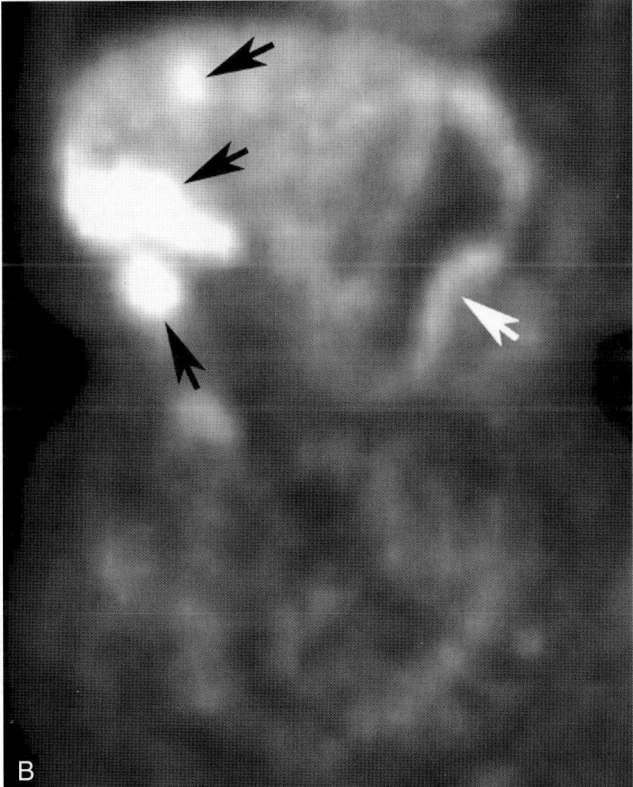

Figure 37-7. Metastatic breast cancer to the gastric wall on CT. A. MDCT image in a middle-aged woman with metastatic breast carcinoma shows localized thickening of the greater curvature of the stomach (*arrowheads*). **B.** FDG PET image in the same patient shows increased activity in the gastric wall (*white arrow*) and in the liver (*black arrows*).

duodenal sweep and for differentiating a pancreatic mass from adjacent lymphadenopathy.

Malignant tumors that metastasize to retroperitoneal lymph nodes near the superior mesenteric root may be manifested on barium studies by extrinsic mass effect, nodular indentations, ulceration, or, in advanced cases, obstruction of the distal duodenum near the ligament of Treitz (Fig. 37-10A).[23] CT is ideally suited for demonstrating retroperitoneal adenopathy as the cause of these abnormalities (Fig. 37-10B). Occasionally, retroperitoneal tumor involving the duodenum may cause delayed gastric emptying and massive gastric dilatation out of proportion to the degree of duodenal dilatation (Fig. 37-11).[24] This disproportionate gastric dilatation is probably related to vagal destruction by retroperitoneal tumor, which decreases gastric peristalsis and exacerbates gastric distention.

Direct Invasion

The stomach and duodenum may be directly invaded by malignant tumors arising in neighboring structures such as the esophagus, pancreas, and kidney. The stomach and duodenum may also be involved by direct extension of colonic carcinoma along mesenteric reflections (including the gastrocolic ligament and transverse mesocolon) or by contiguous spread of tumor from the greater omentum. Because the radiographic findings depend on the pathways of spread, the

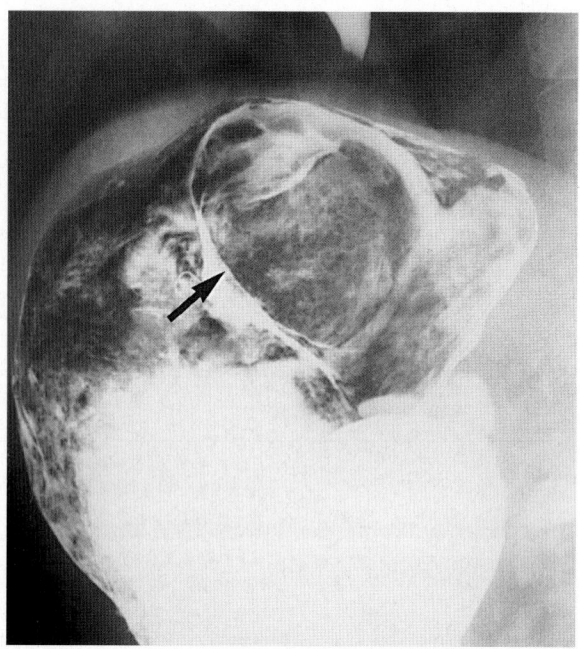

Figure 37-8. Squamous cell metastasis to the gastric cardia. A giant submucosal mass (*arrow*) in the fundus could be mistaken for a benign or malignant gastrointestinal stromal tumor. (From Glick SN, Teplick SK, Levine MS: Squamous cell metastases to the gastric cardia. Gastrointest Radiol 10:339-344, 1985. With kind permission from Springer Science and Business Media.)

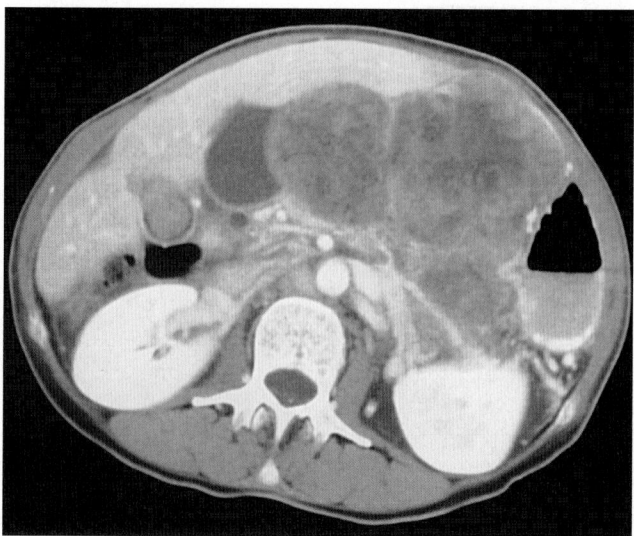

Figure 37-9. Metastatic adenopathy from squamous cell carcinoma of the esophagus. A bulky mass of adenopathy is seen in the region of the lesser sac. The low attenuation of the enlarged nodes is characteristic of squamous cell metastases.

various primary malignant tumors are discussed separately in the following sections.

Esophageal Carcinoma

In contrast to squamous cell carcinomas of the esophagus, adenocarcinomas arising in Barrett's mucosa have a marked

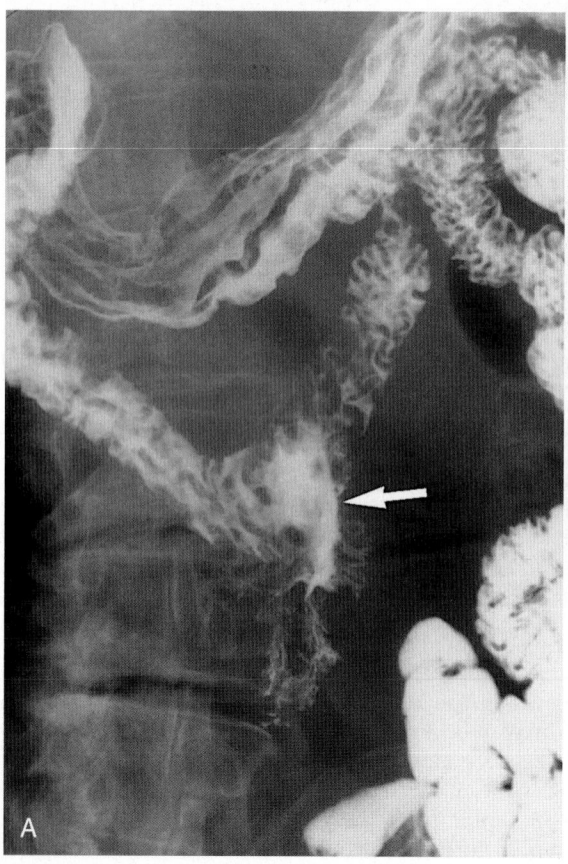

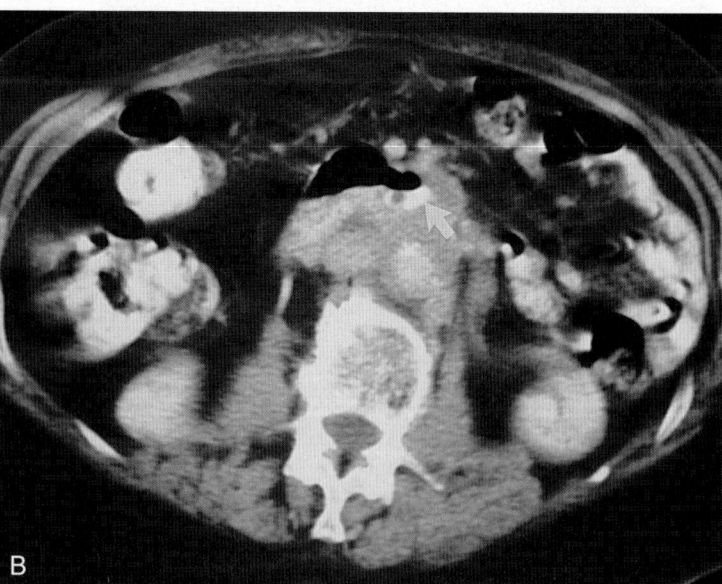

Figure 37-10. Duodenal invasion by retroperitoneal adenopathy. A. Barium study shows an ulcerated lesion (*arrow*) at the junction of the third and fourth portions of the duodenum. **B.** CT scan reveals a conglomerate mass of para-aortic adenopathy encasing the distal duodenum with associated ulceration (*arrow*).

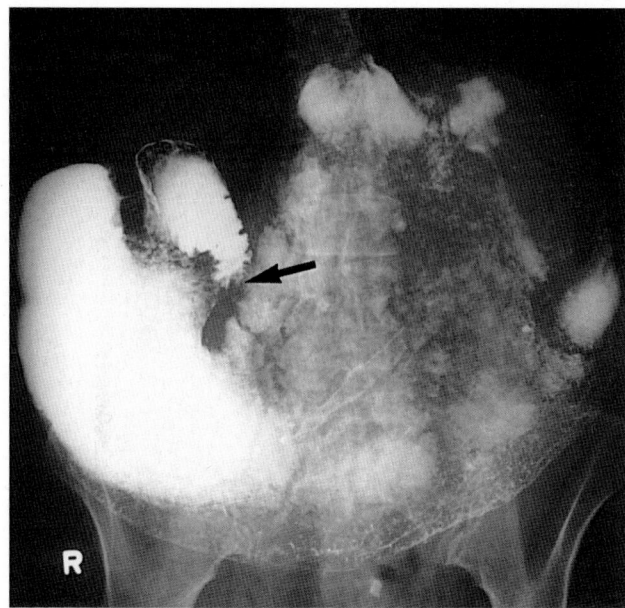

Figure 37-11. Duodenal obstruction by retroperitoneal metastases. Delayed overhead radiograph from an upper gastrointestinal study shows abrupt narrowing of the descending duodenum (*arrow*) with massive gastric dilatation out of proportion to the degree of duodenal dilatation. The dilated stomach extends inferiorly into the pelvis. (From Shammash JB, Rubesin SE, Levine MS: Massive gastric distention due to duodenal involvement by retroperitoneal tumors. Gastrointest Radiol 17:214-216, 1992. With kind permission from Springer Science and Business Media.)

tendency to invade the gastric cardia or fundus.[25,26] Gastric involvement may be manifested on barium studies by a large polypoid or ulcerated mass in the gastric fundus. In other cases, however, double-contrast views of the fundus may reveal more subtle findings, with distortion or obliteration of the normal anatomic landmarks at the cardia (i.e., the cardiac rosette) and irregular areas of ulceration or nodularity (see Chapter 27).[25] It is sometimes difficult to determine whether these tumors at the gastroesophageal junction have arisen in the esophagus or in the stomach. In general, however, esophageal adenocarcinomas have a disproportionate degree of esophageal involvement in relation to that of the stomach, whereas gastric or cardiac carcinomas have a greater degree of fundal involvement.

Pancreatic Carcinoma

The radiographic manifestations of gastroduodenal involvement by pancreatic carcinoma depend on whether the underlying tumor is located in the head, body, or tail of the pancreas. Carcinoma of the pancreatic head may cause widening of the duodenal loop or extrinsic compression of the medial border of the descending duodenum or greater curvature of the gastric antrum, whereas carcinoma of the pancreatic body or tail may cause extrinsic compression of the posterior wall of the gastric fundus and body or the superior border of the distal duodenum near the ligament of Treitz.[27] Actual invasion of the stomach or duodenum may be manifested on barium studies by spiculated mucosal folds, nodularity, mass effect, ulceration, obstruction, or, rarely, fistula formation (Figs. 37-12 to 37-14).[27]

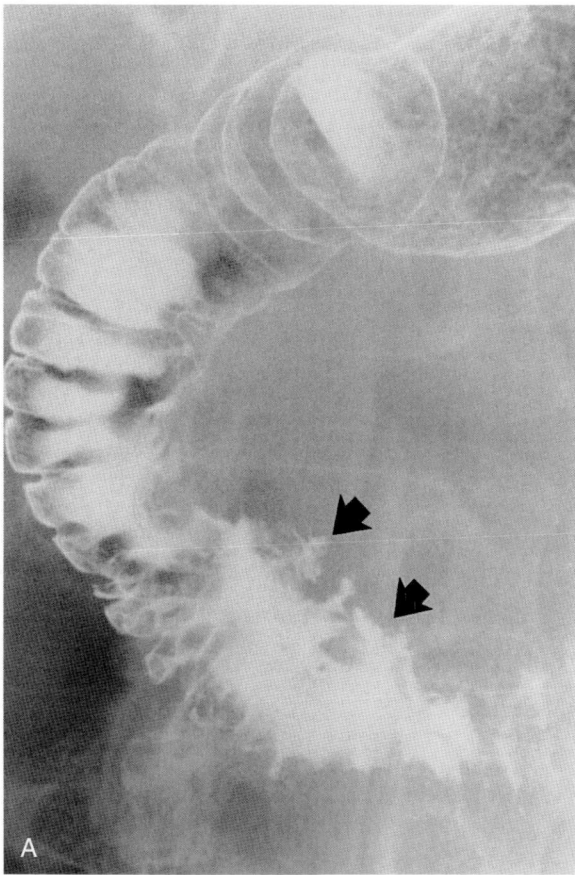

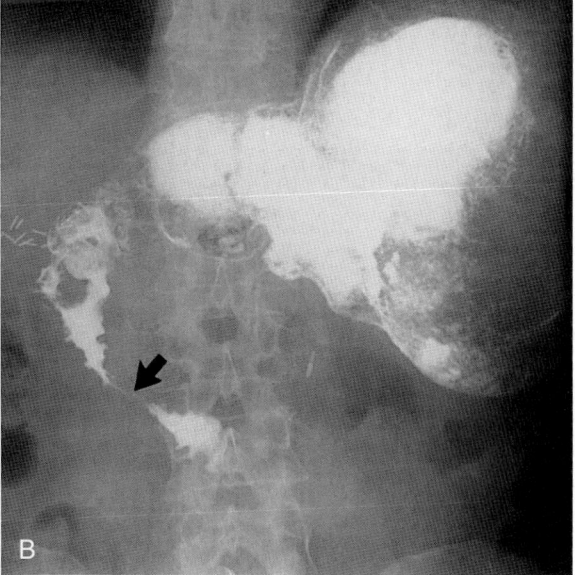

Figure 37-12. Duodenal invasion by pancreatic carcinoma. **A.** Irregular ulceration (*arrows*) is seen on the medial border of the descending duodenum as a result of invasion by pancreatic carcinoma. **B.** In another patient, there is narrowing and obstruction of the descending duodenum (*arrow*) by an advanced pancreatic carcinoma. This patient has gastric outlet obstruction with a dilated, fluid-filled stomach. (**A** from Laufer I, Levine MS [eds]: Double Contrast Gastrointestinal Radiology, 2nd ed. Philadelphia, WB Saunders, 1992.)

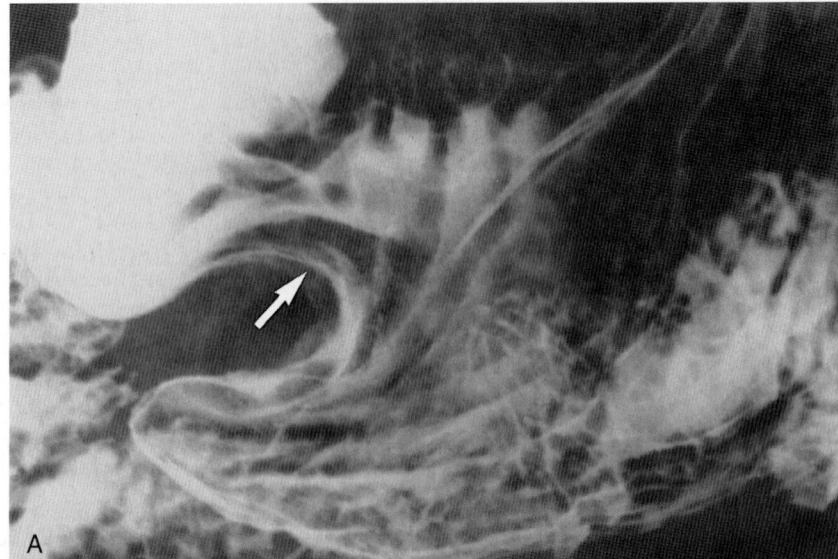

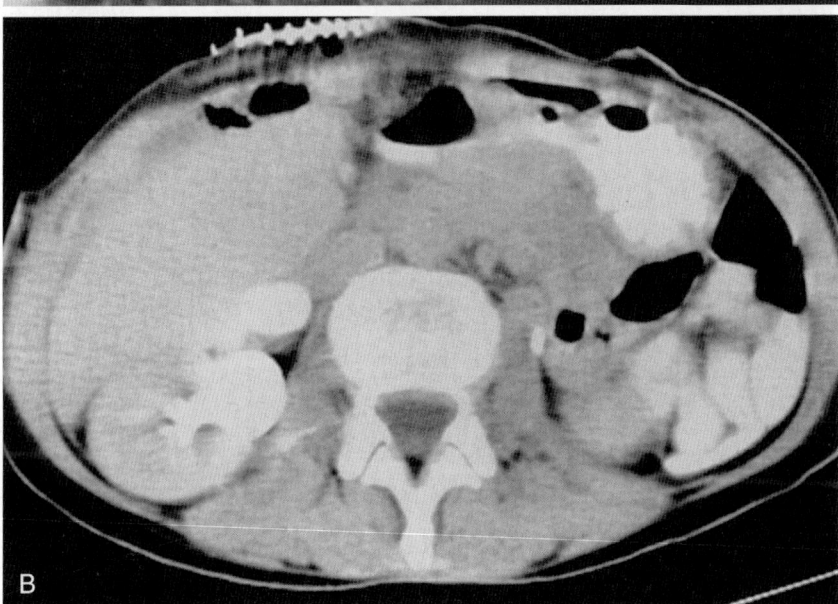

Figure 37-13. Gastric invasion by pancreatic carcinoma. A. Barium study shows a focal area of mass effect (*arrow*) on the greater curvature of the stomach. **B.** CT scan reveals an advanced pancreatic carcinoma invading the stomach.

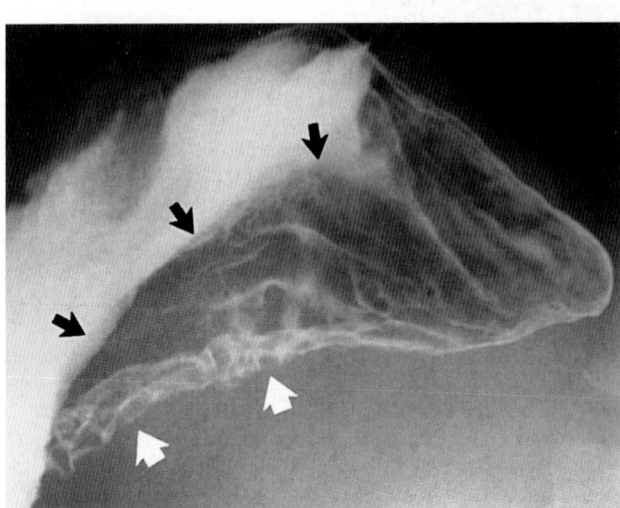

Figure 37-14. Gastric invasion by pancreatic carcinoma. There is extrinsic mass effect (*black arrows*) on the posterior wall of the gastric fundus due to an adjacent carcinoma of the pancreatic tail. The spiculated gastric contour (*white arrows*) indicates gastric invasion by tumor. (From Laufer I, Levine MS [eds]: Double Contrast Gastrointestinal Radiology, 2nd ed. Philadelphia, WB Saunders, 1992.)

Many patients with suspected pancreatic neoplasms undergo CT as the initial diagnostic examination. Although CT is of limited value in predicting minimal duodenal invasion by pancreatic carcinoma, distention of the duodenum with gas or water can facilitate detection of subtle findings of invasion. CT is of greater value in determining the cause of an abnormal retrogastric impression because it can differentiate pancreatic carcinoma from pancreatic pseudocysts (Fig. 37-15), retrogastric varices, or other abnormalities in the retroperitoneum.[28,29]

Renal Cell Carcinoma

Direct invasion of the duodenum by right-sided renal cell carcinoma may be manifested on barium studies by mass effect, nodularity, or ulceration of the posterolateral border of the descending duodenum. However, renal cell carcinoma tends not to elicit a desmoplastic response in the wall of the bowel, so that duodenal involvement is sometimes manifested by a polypoid intraluminal mass, mimicking the appearance of a primary duodenal carcinoma.[6,8] In patients with advanced renal cell carcinoma, CT is useful for determining the extent of tumor and its proximity to the duodenum. When a contiguous lesion is identified, however, CT is not reliable for determining whether tumor is invading the duodenum.

Colonic Carcinoma

Colonic carcinoma may involve the stomach or duodenum by direct extension along mesenteric reflections such as the gastrocolic ligament or transverse mesocolon. The gastrocolic ligament is the proximal portion of the greater omentum that extends superiorly from the anterosuperior border of the transverse colon to the greater curvature of the stomach (Fig. 37-16). Because of this anatomic relationship, carcinoma of the transverse colon may invade the stomach via the gastrocolic ligament, producing mass effect, nodularity, and spiculated, tethered mucosal folds on the greater curvature of the gastric antrum or body.[8] In other patients, carcinoma of the ascending colon or hepatic flexure may invade the

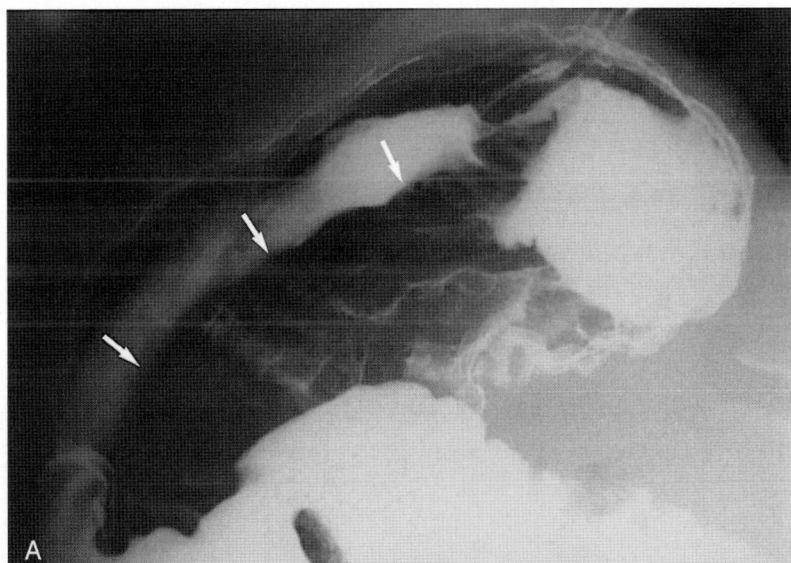

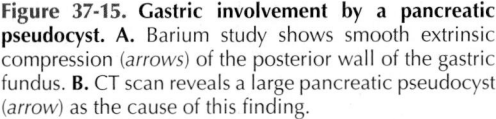

Figure 37-15. Gastric involvement by a pancreatic pseudocyst. A. Barium study shows smooth extrinsic compression (*arrows*) of the posterior wall of the gastric fundus. **B.** CT scan reveals a large pancreatic pseudocyst (*arrow*) as the cause of this finding.

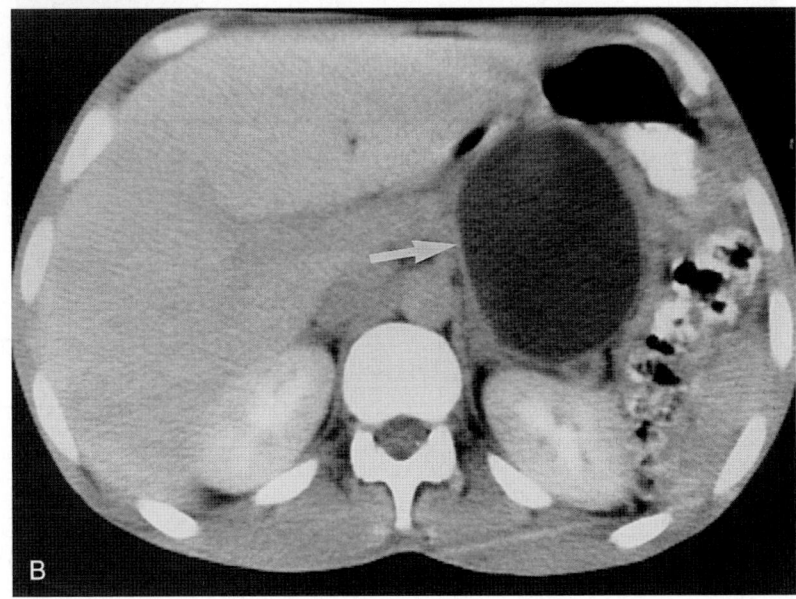

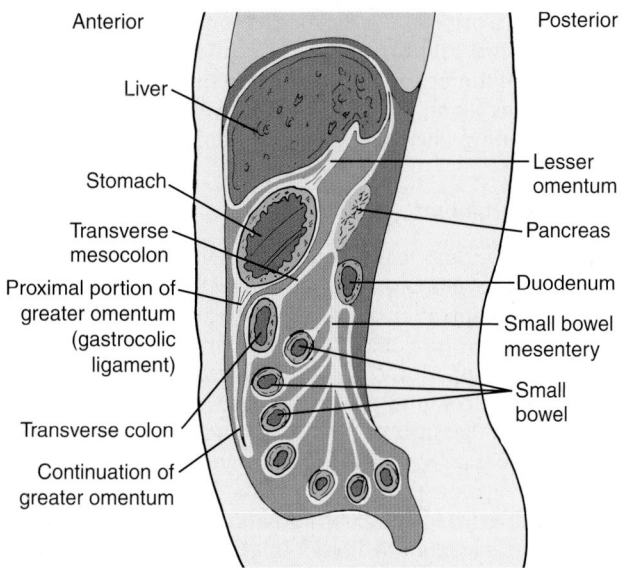

Figure 37-16. Sagittal diagram shows the mesenteric attachments of the stomach, small bowel, and colon. Because the proximal portion of the greater omentum (i.e., the gastrocolic ligament) inserts along the greater curvature of the stomach, contiguous spread of tumor from the transverse colon or greater omentum primarily affects this region. (From Rubesin SE, Levine MS: Omental cakes: colonic involvement by omental metastases. Radiology 154:593-596, 1985.)

duodenum via the lateral reflection of the transverse mesocolon, producing mass effect, nodularity, ulceration, or spiculated mucosal folds on the lateral border of the descending duodenum (Fig. 37-17A).[30,31] In such cases, a barium enema examination may show the underlying colonic neoplasm

responsible for these findings, and CT may show the mode of spread to the stomach or duodenum (Fig. 37-17B).

Carcinoma of the transverse colon invading the stomach or carcinoma of the hepatic flexure invading the duodenum may occasionally lead to the development of a gastrocolic or duodenocolic fistula (see Chapter 38).[32] In today's pill-oriented society, however, most such fistulas are caused by benign, aspirin-induced greater curvature gastric ulcers that penetrate via the gastrocolic ligament into the transverse colon (see Chapter 33).

Gallbladder Carcinoma

Advanced carcinoma of the gallbladder may directly invade adjacent structures such as the liver, duodenum, and hepatic flexure of the colon. Duodenal involvement by tumor has been reported in about 20% of patients.[33] CT is particularly useful for showing gastric and duodenal invasion by tumor (Fig. 37-18).

Omental Metastases

Bulky metastatic deposits in the greater omentum, or so-called omental "cakes," usually result from widespread intraperitoneal dissemination of ovarian carcinoma or, less frequently, cervical, uterine, bladder, gastric, colonic, pancreatic, or breast carcinoma.[34] These omental deposits may spread superiorly to the stomach via the proximal portion of the greater omentum, also known as the gastrocolic ligament (see Fig. 37-16). Gastric involvement by omental metastases is characterized on barium studies by mass effect, nodularity, flattening, or spiculated, tethered mucosal folds on the greater curvature of the gastric antrum or body (Fig. 37-19A).[35] These

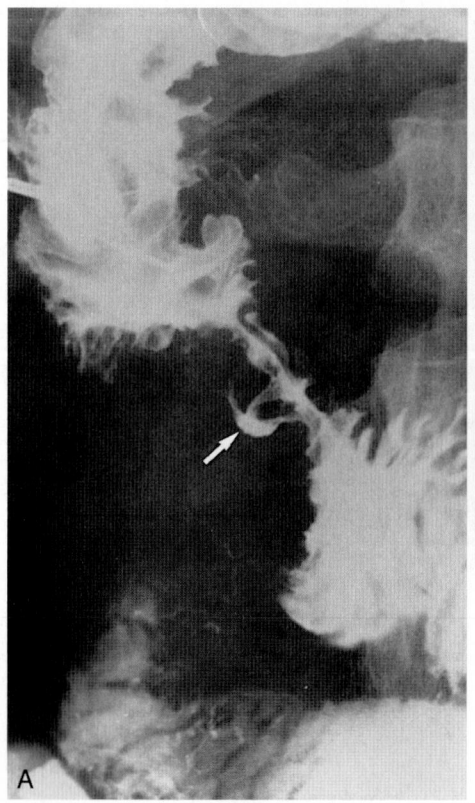

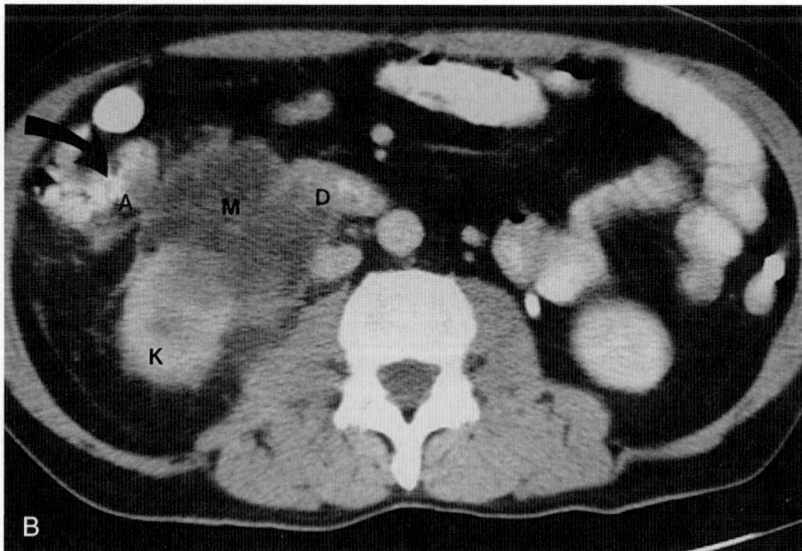

Figure 37-17. Duodenal invasion by colonic carcinoma. A. A large area of mass effect is seen on the lateral border of the descending duodenum with associated ulceration (*arrow*). This finding was caused by carcinoma of the hepatic flexure invading the duodenum. **B.** In another patient, CT scan shows invasion of the duodenum by recurrent carcinoma arising from the region of an ileotransverse colonic anastomosis (A). A heterogeneous mass (M) is seen invading the duodenum (D) and right kidney (K). Contrast medium is present in the bowel (*arrow*) adjacent to the anastomosis.

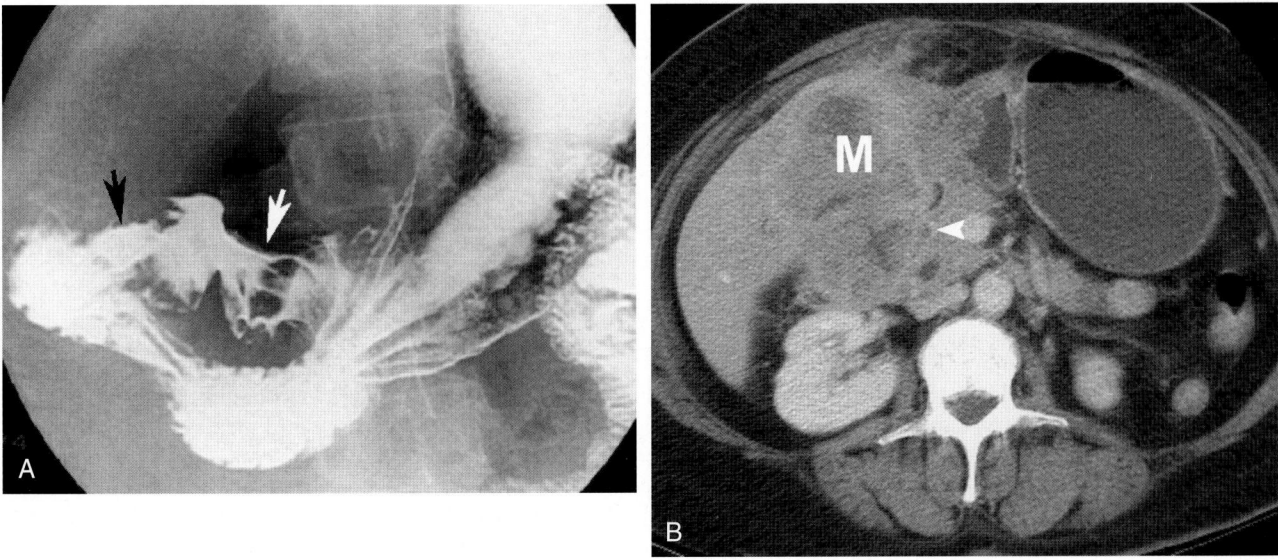

Figure 37-18. Gallbladder carcinoma invading the stomach and duodenum. A. Barium study shows narrowing and ulceration of the postbulbar duodenum (*black arrow*) and distortion of the duodenal sweep by tumor. Also note narrowing and deformity of the distal gastric antrum (*white arrow*) due to invasion by tumor. **B.** CT scan in the same patient shows an advanced carcinoma of the gallbladder (M) directly encasing and narrowing the descending duodenum (*arrowhead*). Also note tumor invading the distal stomach and infiltrating the peritoneal cavity.

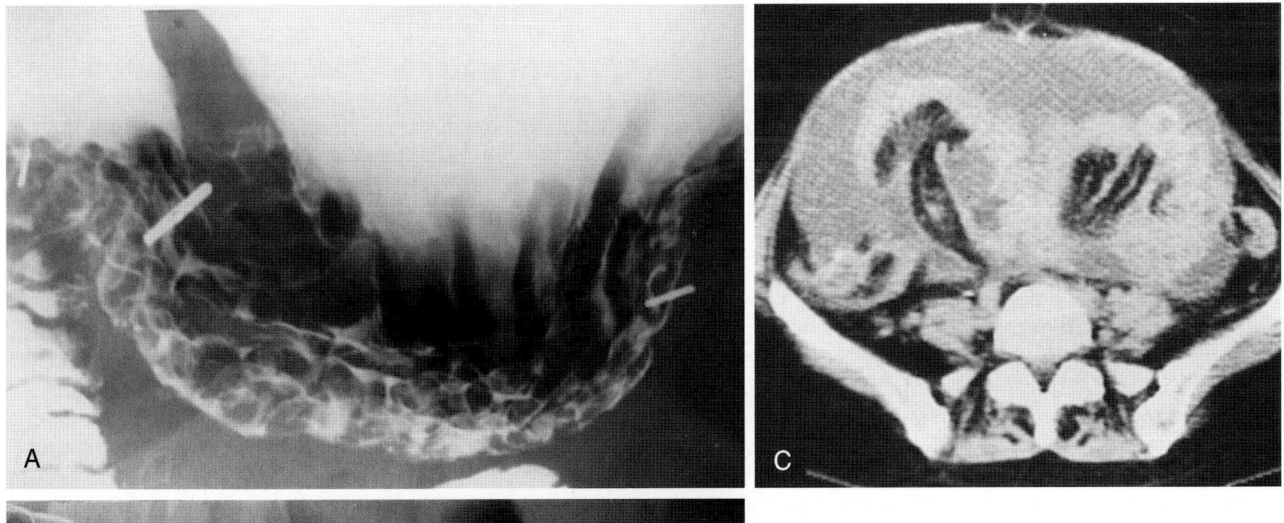

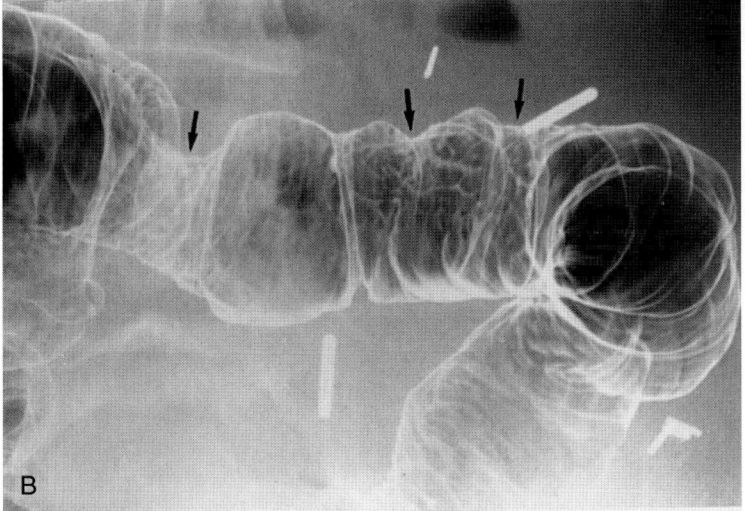

Figure 37-19. Gastric and colonic involvement by omental metastases from ovarian carcinoma. A. Upper gastrointestinal study shows spiculated folds and nodularity on the greater curvature of the gastric antrum and body as a result of direct extension of tumor from the greater omentum. **B.** Barium enema shows spiculation and tethering of the superior border of the transverse colon (*arrows*) as a result of simultaneous colonic involvement by omental tumor. **C.** In another patient, CT scan reveals ascites with a bulky omental cake separating the small bowel from the anterior abdominal wall. (**C** from Laufer I, Levine MS [eds]: Double Contrast Gastrointestinal Radiology, 2nd ed. Philadelphia, WB Saunders, 1992.)

changes reflect serosal involvement by tumor as well as a desmoplastic response that occurs along the insertion of the gastrocolic ligament on the greater curvature. In advanced cases, there may be circumferential narrowing of the gastric antrum resulting from encasement by metastatic tumor.[35]

Carcinoma of the transverse colon invading the stomach via the gastrocolic ligament may produce identical radiographic findings (see earlier section on Colonic Carcinoma).[8] In such cases, however, a barium enema examination should demonstrate the primary colonic carcinoma responsible for these findings. In contrast, patients with omental metastases involving the stomach almost always have associated colonic involvement by omental tumor, with mass effect, nodularity, and spiculated mucosal folds on the superior border of the transverse colon or, in advanced cases, circumferential narrowing of the bowel (Fig. 37-19B).[36] In our experience, gastric involvement by omental metastases is much more common than gastric invasion by colonic carcinoma via the gastrocolic ligament.

When gastric involvement by omental metastases is suspected on barium studies, CT is extremely helpful in delineating the extent of metastatic tumor. Although conventional barium studies provide indirect evidence of omental disease, CT can reveal omental masses as small as 1 cm in diameter.[37] More extensive omental metastases may be manifested on CT by a spectrum of findings, ranging from a lacy reticular appearance to bulky masses.[37] Non-neoplastic processes involving the omentum (notably tuberculous peritonitis) can simulate omental tumor. When the greater omentum is diffusely infiltrated by tumor, an omental cake may displace the colon or small bowel from the anterior abdominal wall (Fig. 37-19C).[34,38] Unless the lumen of the bowel is distended with contrast medium or gas, however, it is difficult to determine whether tumor is invading the stomach or transverse colon.

Differential Diagnosis

Hematogenous metastases that appear as small, nodular lesions in the stomach or duodenum may be difficult to differentiate on barium studies from multiple hyperplastic or adenomatous polyps. Metastases that have a more typical submucosal appearance can be mistaken for benign intramural lesions such as GISTs, lipomas, or ectopic pancreatic rests. However, these benign mesenchymal tumors tend to occur as solitary lesions, whereas metastases are usually multiple. Centrally ulcerated bull's-eye lesions may be caused not only by hematogenous metastases but also by lymphoma, Kaposi's sarcoma, or carcinoid tumors. Occasionally, varioliform erosions surrounded by unusually prominent mounds of edema can be mistaken for bull's-eye lesions. However, varioliform erosions are rarely greater than 1 cm, and the central barium collections are considerably smaller than those seen in ulcerated submucosal masses.

Giant, cavitated lesions in the stomach and duodenum may be caused not only by metastatic disease (particularly malignant melanoma) but also by lymphoma or malignant GISTs. However, malignant GISTs tend to occur as solitary lesions, so that the presence of multiple cavitated masses in the stomach, duodenum, or small bowel should favor a diagnosis of metastatic disease or lymphoma.

The linitis plastica appearance caused by metastatic breast cancer may be indistinguishable on barium studies from that of a primary scirrhous carcinoma of the stomach. Circumferential gastric involvement by pancreatitis, pancreatic carcinoma, colonic carcinoma, omental metastases, lymphoma, or Crohn's disease and scarring from various types of severe gastritis may produce similar findings. Nevertheless, the possibility of metastatic disease should be considered when a linitis plastica appearance is detected in patients who have previously been treated for breast carcinoma.

Direct invasion of the stomach and duodenum by metastatic tumor may be simulated by various benign and malignant conditions in the upper abdomen. Compression or displacement of the greater curvature or posterior wall of the stomach or of the medial border of the descending duodenum may be caused not only by pancreatic carcinoma but also by pancreatitis, pancreatic pseudocysts (see Fig. 37-15), peripancreatic lymphadenopathy, abdominal aortic aneurysms, or other retroperitoneal processes. Various signs of bowel wall invasion (i.e., mass effect nodularity and spiculated, tethered mucosal folds) may also result from a nonspecific desmoplastic response to inflammatory conditions involving the stomach. Thus, pancreatitis may produce changes on the greater curvature that are impossible to distinguish radiographically from pancreatic or colonic carcinoma or omental metastases involving the stomach. Other imaging techniques such as CT are usually helpful for differentiating these conditions.

LYMPHOMA

Lymphoma involves the stomach more frequently than any other portion of the gastrointestinal tract. Gastric lymphoma accounts for 50% of all gastrointestinal lymphomas, 25% of all extranodal lymphomas, and 3% to 5% of all malignant tumors in the stomach.[39-41] More than 50% of patients with gastric lymphoma have localized disease that is confined to the stomach and regional lymph nodes (i.e., primary gastric lymphoma); the remainder have generalized lymphoma with associated gastric involvement (i.e., secondary gastric lymphoma).[41] When it occurs, duodenal lymphoma usually results from contiguous transpyloric spread of lymphoma from the stomach. Because of its rarity, duodenal lymphoma is considered separately in a later section.

The vast majority of gastric lymphomas are non-Hodgkin's lymphomas of B-cell origin.[42] There is considerable evidence that these lymphomas arise from mucosa-associated lymphoid tissue (MALT) occurring in patients with chronic *Helicobacter pylori* gastritis.[43] It has therefore been postulated that most primary non-Hodgkin's gastric lymphomas originate as low-grade MALT lymphomas, which, if untreated, eventually progress to more high-grade lymphomas. In the past, low-grade proliferation of lymphoid tissue in the stomach has sometimes been called *pseudolymphoma*.[44] However, these pseudolymphomas are currently thought to represent monoclonal B-cell proliferations or true B-cell MALT lymphomas.[45,46] As a result, the term *pseudolymphoma* has largely been abandoned.

Because the gross pathologic findings are nonspecific, gastric lymphoma is often difficult to differentiate from gastric carcinoma on radiologic or endoscopic examinations. However, gastric lymphoma has a much better prognosis than gastric carcinoma, with overall 5-year survival rates of 50% to 60%.[47-49] Thus, failure to obtain biopsy specimens from an advanced lesion that is assumed to be inoperable gastric cancer may deprive the patient of the opportunity for cure or long-term palliation. Proper staging of the tumor is also important, so that a rational decision can be made about treatment options such as surgery, radiation therapy, and chemotherapy.

Pathology

The vast majority of gastric lymphomas are non-Hodgkin's lymphomas. Only rarely are these patients found to have Hodgkin's disease. Because of confusion with prior classification systems, pathologists at the National Cancer Institute developed a working formulation that recognizes three prognostic categories of non-Hodgkin's lymphoma: low grade, intermediate grade, and high grade.[50] Advanced lesions are usually classified as high-grade lymphomas of the large cell or immunoblastic type.[51]

The literature suggests that most primary non-Hodgkin's gastric lymphomas are low-grade B-cell lymphomas that arise from MALT.[52,53] These lesions have been classified as marginal zone B-cell MALT lymphomas by the International Lymphoma Study Group.[54] Paradoxically, these low-grade MALT lymphomas often occur in the stomach, which normally contains no organized lymphoid tissue.[52,53] However, it has been well documented that chronic *H. pylori* gastritis leads to the acquisition of lymphoid follicles and aggregates in the lamina propria (i.e., MALT)[55-57] and the subsequent development of low-grade B-cell MALT lymphomas.[52,53,58] Data also suggest that almost all patients with low-grade MALT lymphomas have particular strains of *H. pylori* containing cytotoxin-associated antigen (*cagA*),[59] so that these strains may have an important role in the pathogenesis of gastric MALT lymphoma.

Gastric MALT lymphomas are manifested pathologically by infiltration of the epithelium with small centrocyte-like cells, giving rise to the lymphoepithelial lesions that are characteristic of these tumors.[54] In various series, MALT lymphomas have been found to constitute as many as 50% to 72% of all primary gastric lymphomas,[60,61] so that this is a much more common tumor than has previously been recognized.

It has been shown that regions of low-grade MALT lymphoma are present on histopathologic examination in approximately 30% of patients with high-grade gastric lymphoma.[60,62] The findings from these studies support the concept that most non-Hodgkin's gastric lymphomas originate as low-grade gastric MALT lymphomas, which subsequently undergo transformation to intermediate or high-grade lymphomas. These low-grade MALT lymphomas could therefore be considered to be a form of early gastric lymphoma (defined as lymphoma limited to the mucosa or submucosa of the gastric wall, regardless of the presence or absence of lymph node metastases).[46]

Primary gastric lymphoma is usually confined to the stomach or regional lymph nodes at the time of diagnosis. In the Ann Arbor staging system,[41] stage I_E lesions involve the gastric wall; stage II_E lesions involve regional lymph nodes in the abdomen; stage III lesions involve lymph nodes above and below the diaphragm; and stage IV lesions are widely dis-seminated lymphomas that involve extra-abdominal lymph nodes as well as the omentum, mesentery, peritoneum, liver, spleen, lungs, or brain. The major factors affecting survival of patients with primary gastric lymphoma are the depth of invasion of the gastric wall and the presence or absence of nodal disease.

Clinical Findings

Gastric lymphoma occurs more frequently in men than in women, and the average age at the time of diagnosis is 55 to 60 years.[63] Patients with advanced lesions may present with abdominal pain, nausea, vomiting, anorexia, weight loss, a palpable epigastric mass, or signs or symptoms of upper gastrointestinal bleeding.[63] Occasionally, these patients may develop an acute abdomen because of spontaneous perforation of an ulcerated gastric lymphoma or perforation complicating systemic chemotherapy.[64] Patients with generalized lymphoma may also present with a fever or other signs of systemic disease. Whether or not affected individuals have primary gastric lymphoma or generalized lymphoma with gastric involvement, these lesions are often quite extensive in relation to the clinical presentation. Gastric lymphoma should therefore be suspected when a relatively advanced lesion in the stomach is associated with a paucity of clinical complaints.

In contrast to patients with early gastric cancer, who are usually asymptomatic (see Chapter 36), patients with early gastric lymphoma (particularly those with low-grade B-cell MALT lymphoma) may present with epigastric pain, dyspepsia, bloating, nausea, or vomiting.[65-67] The symptoms at presentation are therefore indistinguishable from those caused by gastric or duodenal ulcers, gastritis, or duodenitis. In fact, some patients may have underlying *H. pylori* gastritis as the cause of their symptoms. Whatever the explanation, the development of symptoms provides an opportunity to diagnose these low-grade gastric MALT lymphomas before they progress to more advanced lesions.

Endoscopic Findings

Low-grade gastric MALT lymphomas may be manifested at endoscopy by shallow ulcers, polypoid lesions, or erythematous, nodular mucosa.[65,67] In contrast, high-grade lymphomas may be manifested by enlarged rugal folds, infiltrative masses, or nodular, polypoid, or ulcerated lesions in the stomach.[68,69] Occasionally, endoscopy may reveal a characteristic "volcano crater" with a discrete ulcer surrounded by a narrow ridge of tumor.[69] Depending on the endoscopic findings, gastric lymphomas may be difficult to differentiate from carcinomas, benign GISTs, metastatic disease, Ménétrier's disease, hypertrophic gastritis, or even benign gastric ulcers. Endoscopic biopsy specimens are therefore required for a definitive diagnosis. Superficial biopsy specimens may be nondiagnostic because lymphomas often infiltrate the gastric wall beneath an intact mucosa. Whenever possible, multiple brushings and biopsy specimens should therefore be obtained from ulcerated or polypoid areas where tumor is more likely to be present. Deep biopsy specimens should also be obtained when the overlying mucosa appears normal. With adequate cytologic and biopsy specimens, endoscopy has a reported sensitivity of 85% to 95% in diagnosing gastric lymphoma.[70-72]

Treatment and Prognosis

When the diagnosis of gastric lymphoma has been established, proper staging of the tumor is needed to determine the appropriate treatment and assess prognosis. Additional diagnostic examinations include chest radiography, chest and abdominal CT scans, and fluorodeoxyglucose (FDG)-labeled CT/PET imaging. When both CT and FDG CT/PET scans are normal, routine staging laparotomy is probably unnecessary.[73]

Many investigators believe that the best treatment for early or localized gastric lymphoma with or without regional lymph node involvement (i.e., stage I_E or stage II_E lesions) is a subtotal gastrectomy with postoperative radiation or chemotherapy.[41,49,63,72,74,75] Although the role of systemic chemotherapy for localized gastric lymphoma remains controversial, advanced gastric lymphoma (i.e., stage III or stage IV lesions) is sometimes treated by radiation therapy, chemotherapy, or both without a gastric resection.[63] Massive upper gastrointestinal bleeding or even gastric perforation may occur as a complication of systemic chemotherapy, resulting in treatment failures.[64]

In contrast to high-grade gastric lymphomas, low-grade MALT lymphomas can often be treated successfully with antibiotics. In various studies, complete or partial regression of tumor has been reported in 60% to 80% of patients after eradication of *H. pylori* from the stomach.[66,76] One theory is that *H. pylori* evokes an immunologic response that stimulates growth of the tumor. Whatever the explanation, eradication of *H. pylori* from the stomach with antibiotics appears to be a viable alternative to surgery, chemotherapy, or radiation therapy as first-line treatment for low-grade gastric MALT lymphomas.

Long-term survival depends primarily on the stage of the tumor at the time of diagnosis. In various studies, reported 5-year survival rates have ranged from 62% to 90% for stage I_E lesions and from 29% to 50% for stage II_E lesions, but substantially lower rates are reported for stage III and stage IV lesions.[47,49,72,77] Patients with low-grade gastric MALT lymphomas have a much better prognosis than patients with high-grade lymphomas; low-grade lymphomas are associated with 5-year survival rates of 75% to 91%,[60,67] whereas high-grade MALT lymphomas are associated with 5-year survival rates of less than 60%.[67]

After treatment, some patients may develop recurrent gastric lymphoma whereas others are found to have recurrent tumor in distal nodal groups without evidence of gastric disease. Patients with recurrent lymphoma almost always become symptomatic within 2 years of treatment, so that the prognosis is excellent for patients who remain asymptomatic for more than 5 years.[78] Gastric lymphoma has a better prognosis than gastric carcinoma because of its inherent growth characteristics and its tendency to remain in the gastric wall for prolonged periods.

Radiographic Findings

Low-Grade MALT Lymphoma

Low-grade gastric MALT lymphomas may be manifested on double-contrast studies by variably sized, rounded, often confluent nodules involving a focal or, less frequently, diffuse segment of the stomach (Fig. 37-20).[79-82] Other MALT lymphomas may appear as small polypoid or ulcerated lesions;

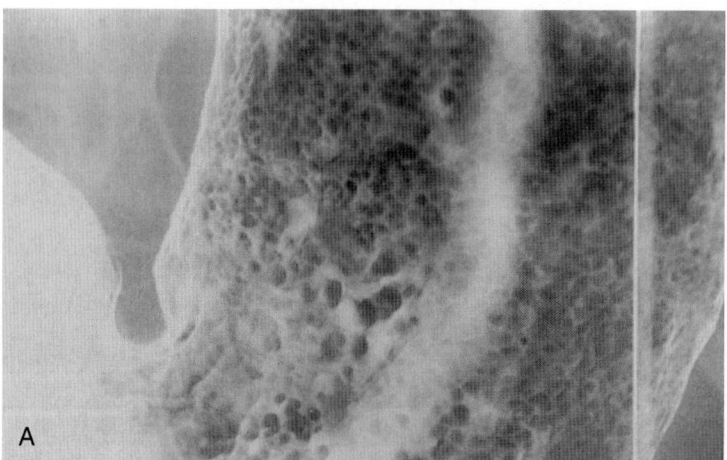
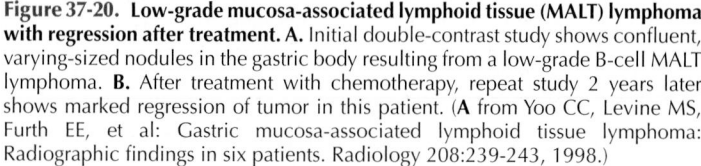
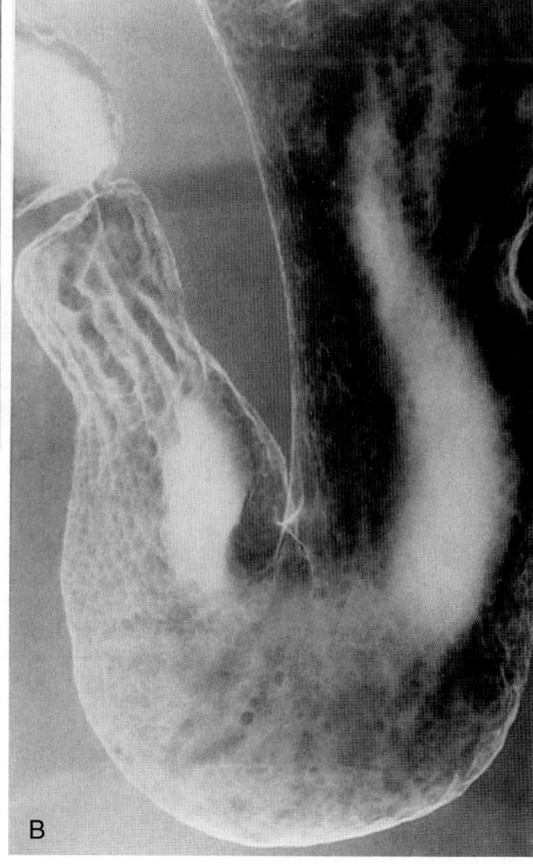

Figure 37-20.   Low-grade mucosa-associated lymphoid tissue (MALT) lymphoma with regression after treatment. A. Initial double-contrast study shows confluent, varying-sized nodules in the gastric body resulting from a low-grade B-cell MALT lymphoma. **B.** After treatment with chemotherapy, repeat study 2 years later shows marked regression of tumor in this patient. (**A** from Yoo CC, Levine MS, Furth EE, et al: Gastric mucosa-associated lymphoid tissue lymphoma: Radiographic findings in six patients. Radiology 208:239-243, 1998.)

shallow, irregular ulcers with nodular surrounding mucosa; or focally distorted, enlarged rugal folds.[80-82] These early lymphomas may be indistinguishable radiographically from early gastric cancer.

Endoscopic biopsy specimens should be obtained for a definitive diagnosis when low-grade MALT lymphomas are suspected on the basis of the radiographic findings. Although some patients may be found to have other conditions such as *H. pylori* gastritis without evidence of tumor (see Differential Diagnosis), it seems reasonable to accept a certain percentage of false-positive diagnoses because of the importance of detecting gastric MALT lymphomas at an early, curable stage.

Advanced Gastric Lymphoma

Advanced gastric lymphomas have an average diameter of 10 cm or more at the time of diagnosis.[40] Although the entire stomach may be infiltrated by tumor, most cases involve the antrum and body.[83] Depending on the gross pathologic features, gastric lymphomas may be classified radiographically as infiltrative, ulcerative, polypoid, or nodular lesions.[40,83-86] There is considerable overlap between these types, however, with many lesions having combined radiographic features.

Infiltrative gastric lymphomas are characterized by focal or diffuse enlargement of rugal folds resulting from submucosal spread of tumor (Fig. 37-21A).[40,83-86] The folds can be massively enlarged and often have a distorted, nodular contour, so that they can be mistaken for polypoid masses. Even with extensive lymphomatous infiltration, the stomach classically remains pliable and distensible because of the absence of associated fibrosis.[40,83] However, some non-Hodgkin's lymphomas may produce a linitis plastica appearance indistinguishable from that of a primary scirrhous carcinoma of the stomach.[87] These lesions are characterized by varying degrees of narrowing of the gastric antrum, body, or fundus, with nodularity, ulceration, and thickened or effaced mucosal folds (Fig. 37-21B). This linitis plastica appearance is caused by dense infiltrates of lymphomatous tissue in the gastric wall without associated fibrosis.[87] The histopathologic findings are therefore similar to those of metastatic breast cancer, in which gastric narrowing is caused by highly cellular deposits of metastatic tumor.[88] Conversely, Hodgkin's disease involving the stomach produces a linitis plastica appearance by inciting a marked desmoplastic response similar to that of a primary scirrhous carcinoma.[89]

Ulcerative lymphomas are characterized by one or more ulcerated lesions in the stomach (Fig. 37-21C).[40,83-86] Occasionally, the ulcers may be surrounded by a smooth mound of tumor or symmetric, radiating folds, mimicking the appearance of benign gastric ulcers.[84] More frequently, however, these ulcers have an irregular configuration associated with nodular surrounding mucosa or thickened, irregular folds resulting from lymphomatous infiltration of the gastric wall (see Fig. 37-21C).[40,84-86] Other gastric lymphomas may appear as giant, cavitated lesions as a result of necrosis and excavation of the tumor.[84,86]

Polypoid gastric lymphomas are characterized by one or more lobulated intraluminal masses indistinguishable from polypoid carcinomas (Fig. 37-21D).[40,83,84] Finally, the nodular form of gastric lymphoma is characterized by multiple submucosal nodules or masses, ranging from several millimeters to several centimeters.[84,85] These submucosal masses

often ulcerate, producing typical bull's-eye or target lesions (Fig. 37-21E).[90] In such cases, the central barium collections tend to be relatively large in relation to the surrounding elevations. Other patients may have multiple polyps indistinguishable from those associated with the various polyposis syndromes.

About 10% of patients with gastric lymphoma have contiguous transcardiac spread of tumor from the gastric fundus into the distal esophagus.[91] Esophageal involvement is usually manifested by thickened, irregular folds, luminal narrowing, or, less frequently, a polypoid mass in the distal esophagus.[91] Because adenocarcinoma is a much more common malignant tumor in the stomach, these findings are more likely to result from distal esophageal involvement by a fundal or cardiac carcinoma.

Gastric lymphoma may also extend into the duodenum by contiguous transpyloric spread. In various series, 30% to 40% of patients with gastric lymphoma had associated duodenal involvement on barium studies (see later section on Duodenal Lymphoma).[91,92] Because gastric carcinoma invades the duodenum in only 5% to 25% of patients,[92,93] it has been suggested that concomitant involvement of the stomach and duodenum by tumor should favor a diagnosis of lymphoma. However, adenocarcinoma is so much more common than lymphoma that it is still the most likely diagnosis on empirical grounds.[92]

Patients with advanced gastric lymphoma are sometimes treated exclusively with radiation therapy or chemotherapy. Follow-up barium studies or CT scans are useful in these patients for documenting the response to treatment and for evaluating gastrointestinal bleeding or other symptoms that develop after the initiation of radiation therapy or chemotherapy (Figs. 37-22 and 37-23).[94,95] Follow-up studies may show dramatic regression or resolution of the lymphomatous lesions, often with narrowing and deformity of the stomach as a result of residual scarring and fibrosis.[95] In other patients, chemotherapy may lead to marked regression of ulcerated mass lesions with the development of benign-appearing ulcers or ulcer scars at the site of the previous lesions (see Fig. 37-22C).[94] Chemotherapy may also lead to further ulceration, a confined perforation, or, rarely, free perforation of these lymphomatous lesions, with the development of massive upper gastrointestinal bleeding or peritonitis (see Figs. 37-22B and 37-23B).[94]

Computed Tomography

CT is the primary imaging modality for the pretreatment evaluation of abdominal lymphoma. It is important to recognize gastric involvement at the time of the initial study. Gastric lymphoma may be characterized on CT by polypoid, infiltrating, or hypertrophic lesions.[96,97] The most common CT finding is marked thickening of the gastric wall due to infiltration by tumor (Fig. 37-24). The degree of wall thickening is usually greater than that in patients with gastric carcinoma. The gastric wall also tends to display a more uniform enhancement pattern than in patients with gastric cancer (unless areas of ulceration or cavitation are present) (see Fig. 37-24). The rugal folds may be substantially thickened. Although the gastric contour is usually preserved, the mural stratification seen in the normal stomach and accentuated in hypertrophic gastritis is lost.[96,97] Any portion of the

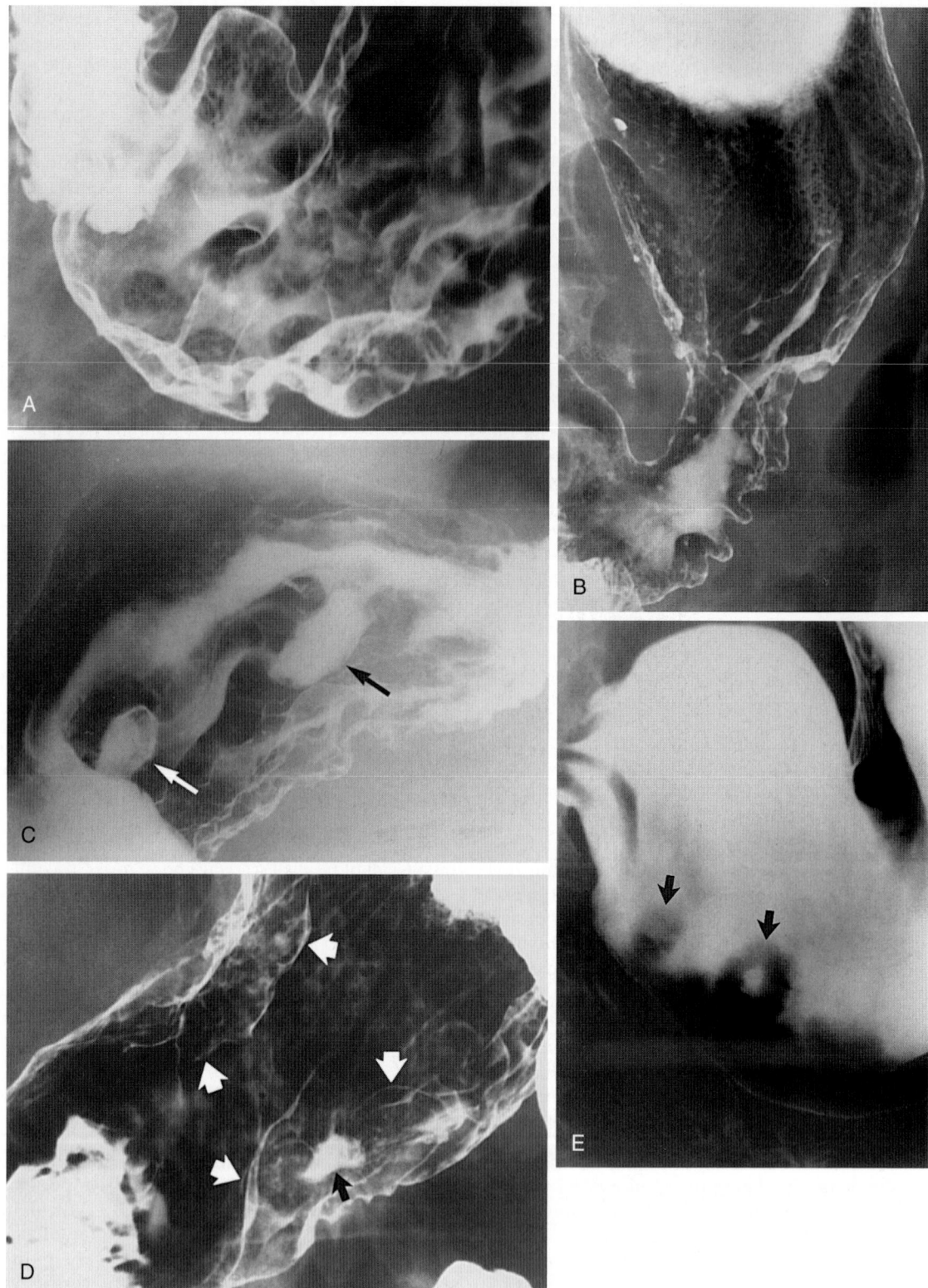

Figure 37-21. Various forms of gastric lymphoma. A. Diffusely thickened, irregular folds are present in the stomach due to lymphomatous infiltration of the gastric wall. **B.** This patient has linitis plastica, manifested by focal narrowing of the gastric body with nodularity and sacculation of the adjacent greater curvature. **C.** Several discrete ulcers (*arrows*) and thickened, lobulated folds are seen in the fundus. **D.** Two separate polypoid masses (*white arrows*) are seen on the lesser and greater curvature of the stomach. The greater curvature mass is ulcerated (*black arrow*). **E.** Two centrally ulcerated submucosal masses or bull's-eye lesions (*arrows*) are present in the gastric antrum. (**A** and **E** from Laufer I, Levine MS [eds]: Double Contrast Gastrointestinal Radiology, 2nd ed. Philadelphia, WB Saunders, 1992; **B** from Levine MS, Pantongrag-Brown L, Aguilera NS, et al: Non-Hodgkin lymphoma of the stomach: A cause of linitis plastica. Radiology 201:375-378, 1996; **D** courtesy of Duane G. Mezwa, MD, Royal Oak, MI.)

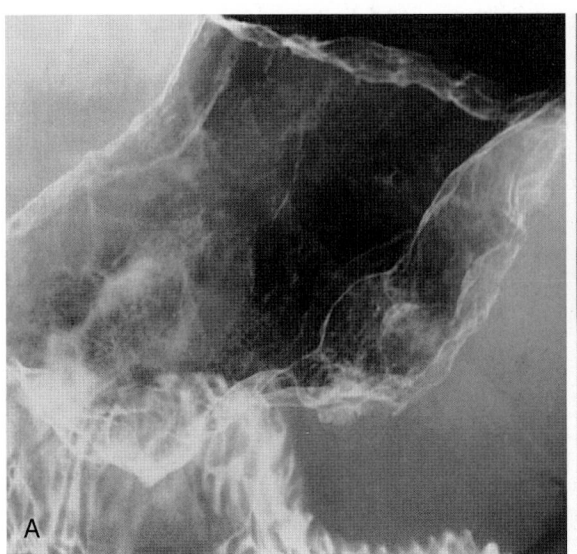

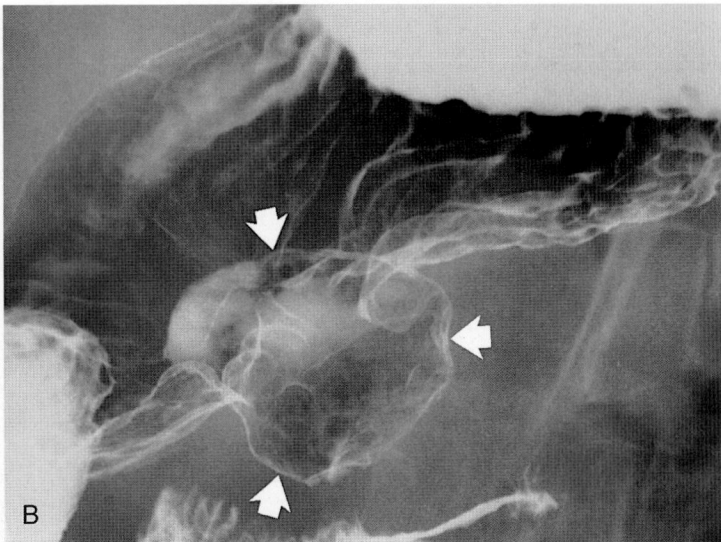

Figure 37-22. Response of gastric lymphoma to chemotherapy. A. Initial barium study shows thickened, irregular folds on the greater curvature of the gastric body due to lymphoma. **B.** After treatment with chemotherapy, follow-up study 6 months later shows regression of the lymphoma with a large area of cavitation (*arrows*) adjacent to the posterior wall of the stomach. **C.** Another follow-up study 1 year later shows further regression of the lymphoma with radiating folds and a tiny, benign-appearing residual ulcer (*arrow*) at the site of the previous excavation. (From Laufer I, Levine MS [eds]: Double Contrast Gastrointestinal Radiology, 2nd ed. Philadelphia, WB Saunders, 1992.)

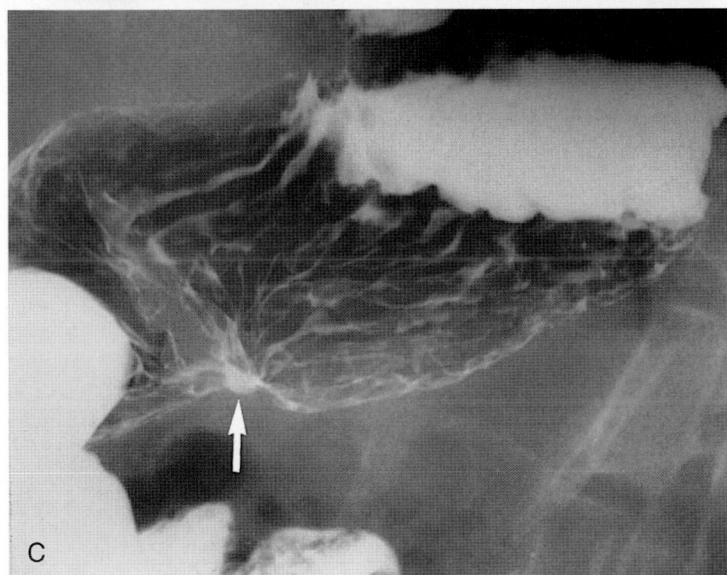

stomach may be involved by tumor, and transpyloric spread of lymphoma into the duodenum is commonly detected on CT (Fig. 37-25). The presence of lymphadenopathy beyond the expected drainage pathways of primary gastric carcinoma should also suggest a diagnosis of gastric lymphoma. When gastric lymphoma is suspected on CT, histologic confirmation should be obtained before treating these patients.

CT is a less sensitive technique for detecting low-grade gastric MALT lymphomas. In one study, CT revealed abnormalities in the stomach in about 50% of patients with these tumors.[98] The major findings on CT included segmental or diffuse gastric wall thickening or a polypoid or ulcerated mass lesion.[98] In such cases, endoscopy and biopsy are required for a definitive diagnosis.

Endoscopic Ultrasonography

Endoscopic ultrasonography (EUS) has been shown to be a valuable technique for staging patients with non-Hodgkin's gastric lymphoma, with an overall accuracy of approximately 90%.[99,100] The findings on EUS may be highly suggestive of lymphoma, but histologic specimens are required for a definitive diagnosis. Non-Hodgkin's gastric lymphoma may be manifested on EUS by a spectrum of findings, ranging from a hypoechoic mass that disrupts the normal wall layer pattern to selective thickening of the second and third echogenic layers or diffuse thickening of all five wall layers.[100] In patients who are treated nonoperatively, EUS is also useful for documenting the response to therapy.

Differential Diagnosis

Gastric MALT lymphomas that appear as small polypoid or ulcerated lesions in the stomach may be indistinguishable on barium studies from early gastric cancer. When MALT lymphomas are manifested by multiple, confluent, rounded nodules in the stomach, the differential diagnosis includes severe gastritis, lymphoid hyperplasia, or even a polyposis syndrome involving the stomach. In some cases, this mucosal nodularity may be difficult to differentiate from enlarged areae gastricae, a finding often associated with *H. pylori* gastritis.[101] However, areae gastricae tend to be more uniform

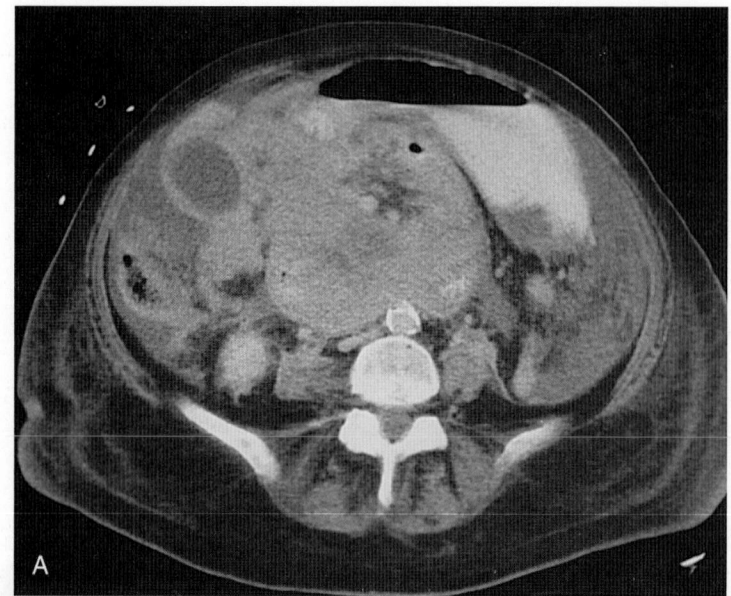

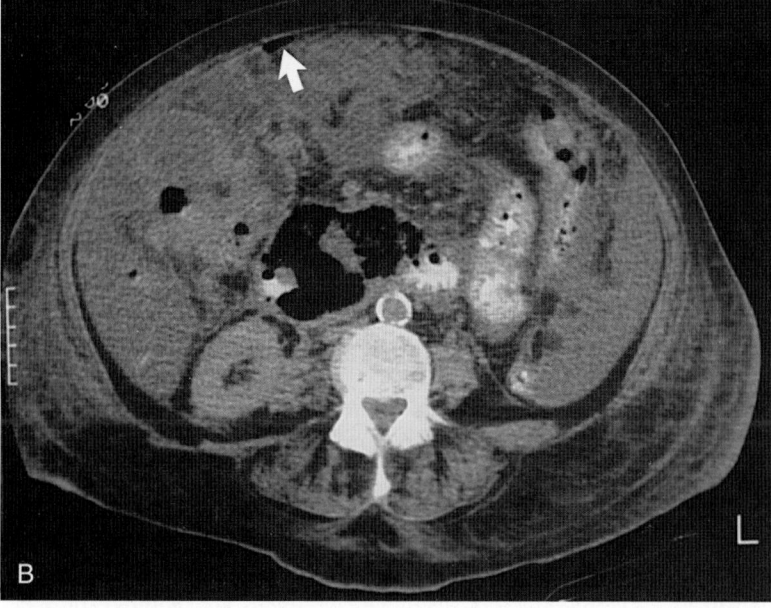

Figure 37-23. Response of duodenal lymphoma to chemotherapy. A. A conglomerate mass of adenopathy surrounds the mesenteric vessels. The duodenum is engulfed by this mass. **B.** Repeat CT scan after two cycles of chemotherapy shows multiple tiny collections of gas in the duodenal wall as a result of rapid tumor lysis and mural necrosis. A tiny amount of free air (*arrow*) is seen in the peritoneal cavity. This patient had developed clinical signs of peritonitis.

in size, producing a sharply marginated reticular network. Lymphoid hyperplasia associated with chronic *H. pylori* gastritis may also be manifested by innumerable nodules in the stomach (see Chapter 34).[102] However, the nodules of lymphoid hyperplasia appear as innumerable, tiny, rounded lesions carpeting the antrum or antrum and body of the stomach. Unlike the poorly defined, confluent nodules in low-grade MALT lymphoma, the nodules of lymphoid hyperplasia also tend to have more discrete borders, a more uniform size, and, not infrequently, central umbilications.[102]

Advanced infiltrative gastric lymphomas may be difficult to distinguish radiographically from other causes of thickened gastric folds, such as *H. pylori* gastritis, hypertrophic gastritis, Ménétrier's disease, and gastric carcinoma. Other infiltrative lymphomas may produce a linitis plastica appearance indistinguishable from that of a primary scirrhous carcinoma.[16] Deep endoscopic biopsy specimens are therefore required for a definitive diagnosis.

Ulcerated gastric lymphomas may be impossible to distinguish radiographically from ulcerated carcinomas. Much less frequently, ulcerated lymphomas that have a relatively innocuous appearance can be mistaken for benign gastric ulcers.[84] When lymphoma is characterized by multiple areas of ulceration, the differential diagnosis includes various inflammatory or infectious conditions involving the stomach, such as Zollinger-Ellison syndrome, Crohn's disease, tuberculosis, syphilis, and cytomegalovirus (see Chapters 33 and 34). However, the correct diagnosis is often suggested by the clinical history.

Polypoid gastric lymphomas may be indistinguishable from polypoid carcinomas. Other lymphomas that appear as submucosal masses can be mistaken for malignant GISTs. Although uncommon, giant, cavitated lymphomas may be impossible to differentiate from cavitated GISTs or cavitated metastases. However, malignant GISTs tend to occur as solitary lesions in the stomach, whereas lymphoma and metas-

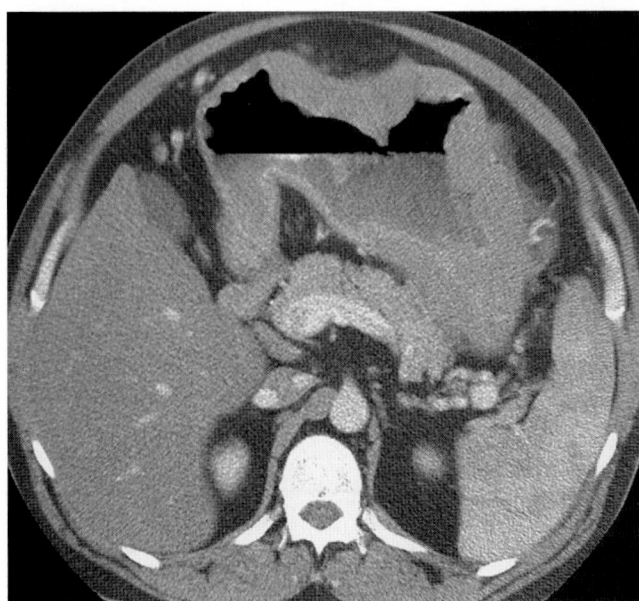

Figure 37-24. Gastric lymphoma on CT. CT scan shows marked thickening of the gastric wall with homogeneous enhancement due to the infiltrative form of gastric lymphoma. Small perigastric lymph nodes are present in the adjacent fat.

tatic disease are usually manifested by multiple lesions in the stomach, duodenum, and small bowel. In patients with gastric lymphoma, exophytic masses typically demonstrate homogeneous attenuation on CT,[96,97] whereas malignant GISTs often have a heterogeneous appearance because of areas of liquefactive necrosis (see later section on malignant GISTs).

Bull's-eye lesions in the stomach may be caused not only by lymphoma but also by Kaposi's sarcoma, carcinoid tumors, or metastases (particularly those from malignant melanoma). However, lymphomatous lesions tend to be of relatively uniform size, whereas metastases are often of variable size as a result of periodic showers of tumor emboli into the bowel.[8,12] Benign GISTs that are ulcerated may also have a bull's-eye appearance, but they usually occur as solitary lesions in the stomach or duodenum.

Duodenal Lymphoma

Duodenal involvement by lymphoma usually results from contiguous spread of tumor from the distal stomach or proximal jejunum (see Fig. 37-25) or from encasement of the duodenum by a conglomerate mass of lymphomatous nodes in the retroperitoneum (see Fig. 37-23A).[103] Because of the paucity of lymphoid tissue in the duodenum, primary duodenal lymphomas are rare lesions, constituting less than 5% of all small bowel lymphomas.[104] As in the stomach, duodenal lymphoma is characterized radiographically by infiltrative, ulcerative, polypoid, and nodular forms.

Duodenal lymphoma may be manifested by a variety of appearances on CT, including marked soft tissue thickening of the duodenal wall (Fig. 37-26), an ulcerated mass (Fig. 37-27), or exaggerated folds in the duodenum (Fig. 37-28).

Occasionally, duodenal or small bowel lymphoma may occur as a complication of long-standing celiac disease.[105,106] Treatment with a gluten-free diet has not been effective in preventing this complication. Thus, periodic radiologic surveillance of the duodenum and small bowel has been advocated to detect developing lymphomas at the earliest possible stage.[106]

MALIGNANT GASTROINTESTINAL STROMAL TUMOR

Malignant gastrointestinal stromal tumors (GISTs) are uncommon tumors that constitute only 1% to 3% of all malignant neoplasms in the stomach.[63,107,108] These tumors are often confined to the wall of the stomach for prolonged periods

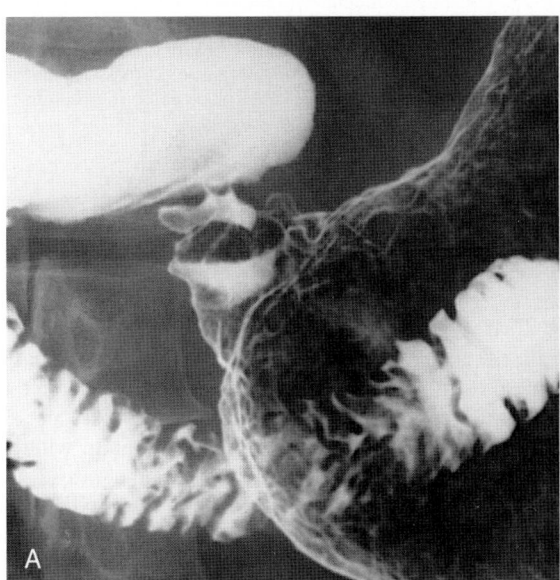
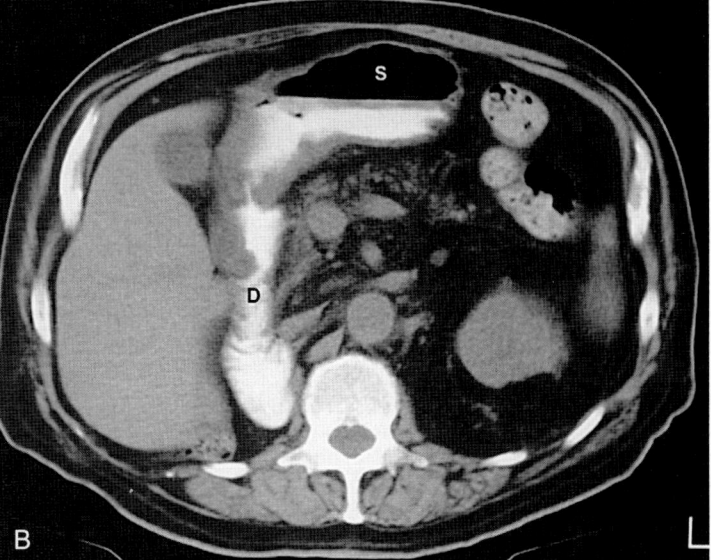

Figure 37-25. Transpyloric spread of lymphoma into the duodenum. A. Barium study shows nodularity and deformity of the distal antrum and pyloric region due to gastric lymphoma. The duodenal bulb appears normal. **B.** CT scan reveals a lymphomatous mass extending from the distal antrum into the proximal duodenum. Even in retrospect, duodenal involvement is not seen on the barium study. S, stomach; D, duodenum. (Courtesy of Edward Lubat, MD, Ridgewood, NJ.)

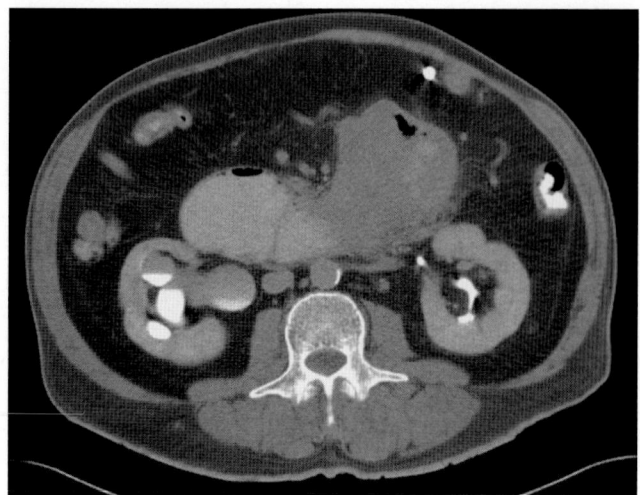

Figure 37-26. Duodenal lymphoma on CT. CT scan in an HIV-positive patient shows a large soft tissue mass encasing the third and fourth portions of the duodenum.

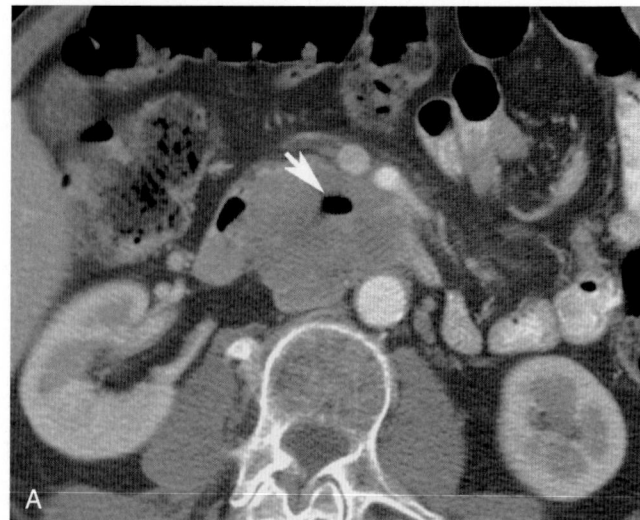

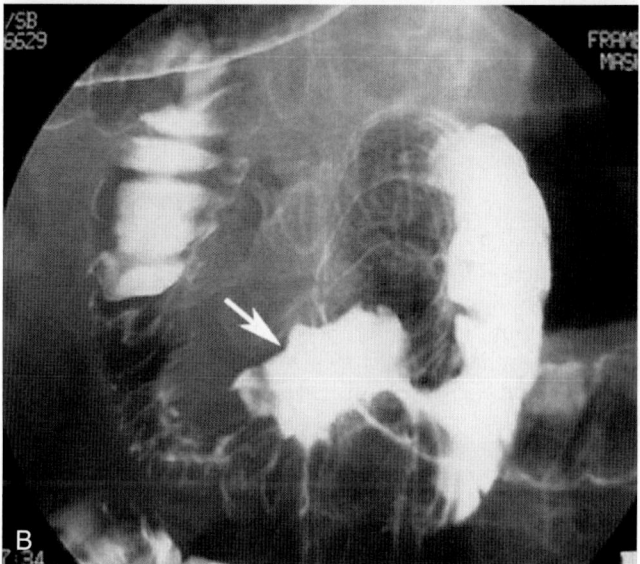

Figure 37-27. Ulcerated duodenal lymphoma on CT. A. CT scan from a 6-year-old boy shows a soft tissue mass in the duodenum with an air-filled central ulcer crater (*arrow*). Endoscopic biopsy specimens revealed non-Hodgkin's lymphoma. **B.** Barium study shows a mass lesion with thickened, irregular folds and a large area of ulceration (*arrow*) in the third portion of the duodenum.

before invading adjacent structures, so that they have a better prognosis than gastric adenocarcinomas. Because of their rarity, malignant GISTs in the duodenum are considered separately in a later section.

Pathology

GISTs are the most common mesenchymal tumors in the gastrointestinal tract. Most of these tumors are incompletely differentiated or undifferentiated and do not fulfill modern pathologic criteria for classification as leiomyomas or leiomyosarcomas. As a result, the generic designation of "gastrointestinal stromal tumors" has been widely adopted.[109] GISTs are characterized by positive immunoreactivity for KIT (CD 117), a tyrosine kinase growth factor receptor, allowing differentiation from true leiomyomas or leiomyosarcomas.[110] Pharmacologic targeting of these receptors with KIT/tyrosine kinase inhibitors has been shown to be of clinical utility in treating patients with GISTs.

GISTs usually consist histologically of interlacing whorls of spindle-shaped cells with eosinophilic cytoplasm and elongated nuclei.[111] Occasionally, these tumors contain distinctive epithelioid cells with eccentric nuclei and perinuclear vacuolization. In the past, GISTs with an epithelioid morphology were called *epithelioid leiomyosarcomas* or *leiomyoblastomas*.[112]

Malignant GISTs most commonly arise in the stomach. About 90% involve the fundus and body, and the remaining 10% involve the antrum.[107] These tumors are mesenchymal lesions, usually originating from the outer layer of the muscularis propria. Malignant stromal tumors involving the stomach tend to be large lesions with an average diameter of 10 cm at the time of diagnosis.[107] They often contain large cystic cavities or ulcers because of hemorrhage or necrosis within the tumor.[111]

Malignant GISTs of the stomach may have endogastric or exogastric patterns of growth, but because of their origin in the outer muscular layer they have a propensity for exogastric growth into the abdominal cavity.[111] As they enlarge, exogastric lesions may invade adjacent structures such as the

pancreas, colon, or diaphragm. Patients with advanced lesions often have widespread intraperitoneal seeding or hematogenous metastases to the liver.[113] Unlike gastric carcinomas, however, malignant GISTs rarely metastasize to regional lymph nodes.[113]

The most commonly accepted index of malignancy is the degree of mitotic activity in the tumor; gastric GISTs that are less than 5 cm and with five or fewer mitoses per 50 consecutive high-power fields are probably benign, whereas GISTs larger than 10 cm and with more than five mitoses per 50 high-power fields are considered malignant, and GISTs that fall between these categories are considered indeterminate lesions with uncertain malignant potential.[114] Finally, GISTs with more than 50 mitoses per 50 high-power fields are considered high-grade malignancies with an extremely aggressive malignant behavior.[114] However, the degree of mitotic activity, cellular atypia, and nuclear pleomorphism may vary

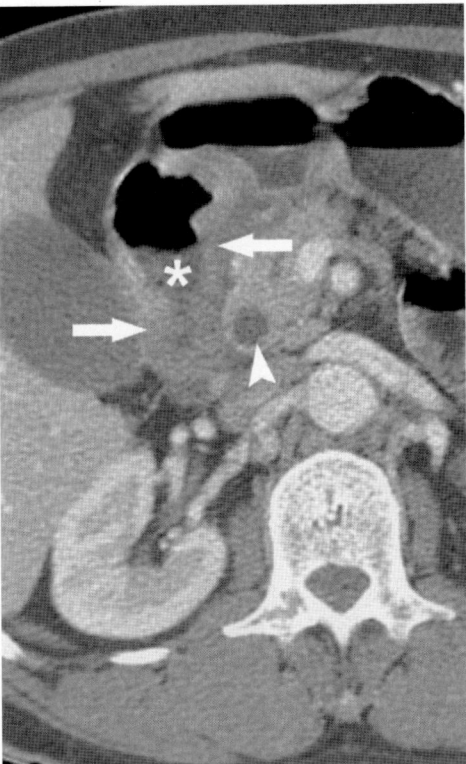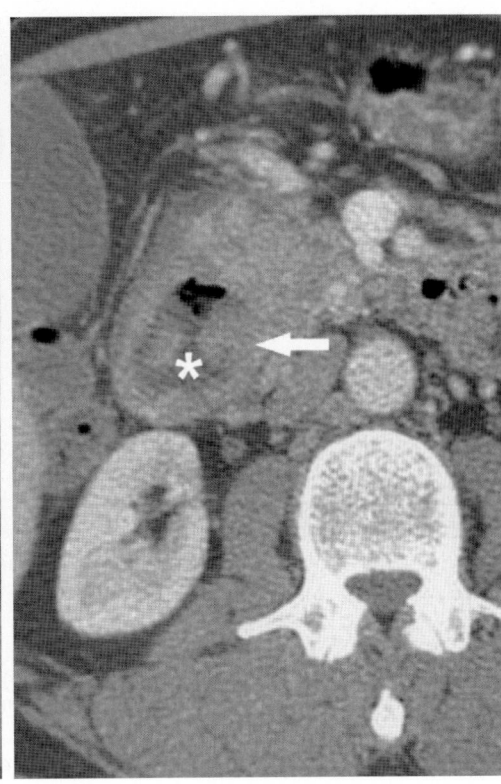

Figure 37-28. Duodenal lymphoma with exaggerated duodenal folds on CT. Sequential CT images in a patient with jaundice show deformity of the descending duodenum with a homogeneously thickened wall and exaggerated folds (*arrows*) due to biopsy-proven non-Hodgkin's lymphoma. The duodenal lumen contains both air and fluid (*asterisks*). Also note dilatation of the common bile duct (*arrowhead*).

markedly within an individual lesion, so that histopathologic criteria are not always reliable for differentiating benign and malignant GISTs.

Clinical Findings

Malignant GISTs of the stomach are more common in men.[115] These individuals are usually older than 50 years of age.[116] The average duration of symptoms at the time of diagnosis is 4 to 6 months.[107] Because malignant GISTS frequently ulcerate, affected individuals most commonly present with signs or symptoms of upper gastrointestinal bleeding, including hematemesis, melena, guaiac-positive stool, and iron-deficiency anemia.[109,111] Other presenting findings include nausea, vomiting, abdominal pain, weight loss, and a palpable abdominal mass.[111] However, some patients with exogastric tumors may remain asymptomatic until the lesions have reached enormous sizes.

It is important to be aware of the limitations of endoscopy in diagnosing malignant GISTs because positive endoscopic biopsy specimens may not be obtained unless the overlying mucosa is ulcerated. CT may also be performed to determine the relationship of suspicious lesions to the gastric wall and to guide needle aspiration biopsies of endoscopically inaccessible lesions.

Patients with malignant GISTs of the stomach generally have a better prognosis than patients with gastric carcinomas; reported 5-year survival rates range from 20% to 55%.[107,117] Tumors smaller than 5 cm have the best possibility for cure, although it is questionable whether these lesions are all malignant. In contrast, tumors greater than 8 cm are often found to be advanced, unresectable lesions at the time of diagnosis.[118] Surgery is the only curative form of therapy. Depending on

the extent of tumor, a wedge resection or a subtotal or total gastrectomy may be required. However, malignant GISTs rarely metastasize to regional lymph nodes, so that a lymph node dissection is of little therapeutic benefit to these patients. Although the role of radiation or chemotherapy is uncertain, some authors advocate chemotherapy when hepatic metastases are present.[108]

Radiographic Findings

Abdominal radiographs generally have limited value for diagnosing malignant GISTs involving the stomach. Occasionally, however, these tumors may be recognized by the presence of a soft tissue mass indenting the gastric bubble.[119] One or more extraluminal gas collections may also be seen in the left upper quadrant as a result of necrosis and cavitation of the tumor.[120] Rarely, abdominal radiographs may reveal mottled areas of calcification (see Fig. 37-31), but CT is a more sensitive technique for demonstrating this finding.[121]

More than 90% of patients with malignant GISTs of the stomach have abnormal barium studies,[108] but the correct diagnosis is suggested in only about half the cases because of difficulty in distinguishing these lesions from benign GISTs or other benign or malignant lesions in the stomach. Intramural lesions typically appear as large, lobulated submucosal masses in the gastric fundus or body (Fig. 37-29).[108] Malignant GISTs may contain one or more ulcers or, not infrequently, large areas of cavitation (Fig. 37-30).[108] Exogastric lesions may be manifested by giant soft tissue masses that cause extrinsic compression of the adjacent gastric wall (Figs. 37-31 and 37-32).[108,122] An important clue to the diagnosis of an exogastric tumor is the presence of a central dimple or spicule at the site of attachment or pedicle of the mass (see Fig. 37-32A).[123]

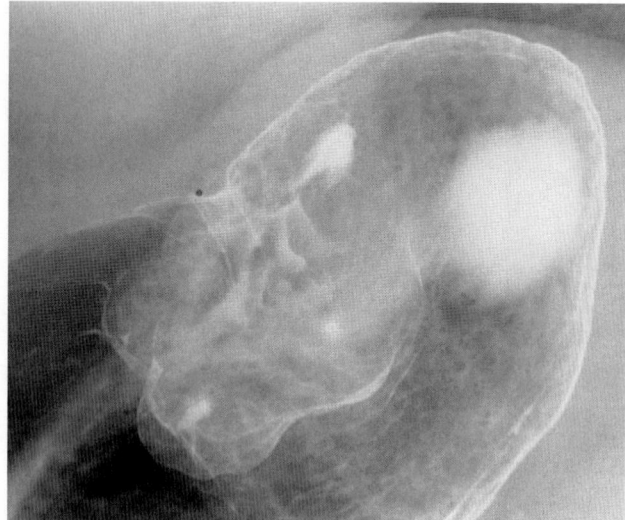

Figure 37-29. Malignant gastrointestinal stromal tumor. A large, lobulated submucosal mass is seen in the gastric fundus.

Rarely, endogastric tumors may appear as polypoid intraluminal masses indistinguishable from primary gastric carcinomas.[111]

The diagnosis of a malignant GIST should be suggested on CT by the presence of a large exogastric, heterogeneously enhancing mass (Fig. 37-33).[111,124-126] Peripheral enhancement corresponds to peripheral areas of viable tumor, whereas central areas of low attenuation correspond to areas of hemorrhage or necrosis.[111] These lesions are substantially larger than benign GISTS, usually greater than 5 cm in diameter; size has been shown to be the single most accurate predictive feature of malignancy.[126] Ulceration or cavitation within malignant GISTs is easily recognized on CT (see Fig. 37-33A). CT is also helpful for demonstrating the extent of the mass and invasion of adjacent structures (Fig. 37-34).[127-129] Rarely,

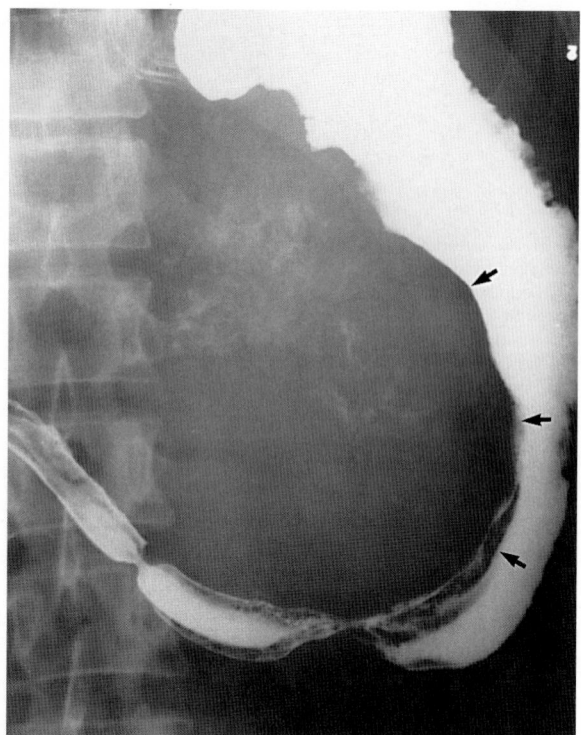

Figure 37-31. Exogastric malignant gastrointestinal stromal tumor with calcification. A giant exogastric mass causes displacement and compression (*arrows*) of the lesser curvature of the stomach. Mottled areas of calcification are seen in the tumor.

malignant GISTs may be so necrotic that they appear as water-density lesions (Fig. 37-35).

Malignant GISTs of the stomach most commonly metastasize to the liver and peritoneal cavity. Metastatic lesions are usually large and heterogeneous. Like the primary lesions, metastases may be multilocular lesions containing fluid-fluid

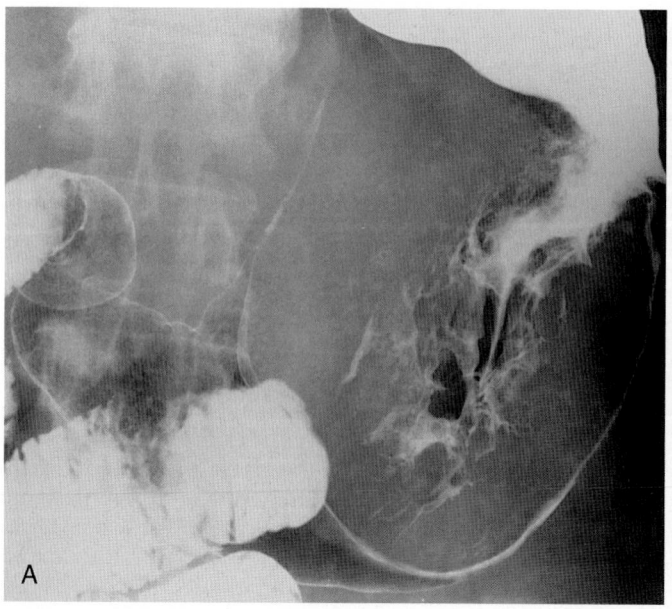
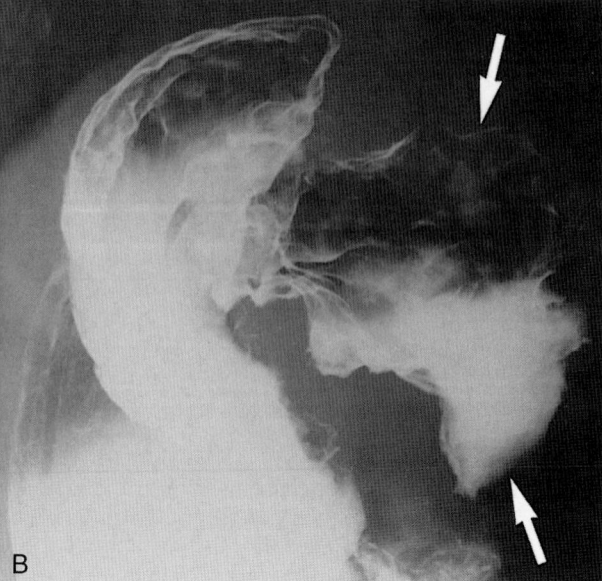

Figure 37-30. Malignant gastrointestinal stromal tumor with cavitation. A. A giant mass is present in the stomach. Barium is trapped within irregular cavities in the mass. **B.** Another cavitated lesion is manifested by a giant extraluminal collection of barium (*arrows*). (**A** courtesy of Hans Herlinger, MD, Philadelphia, PA.)

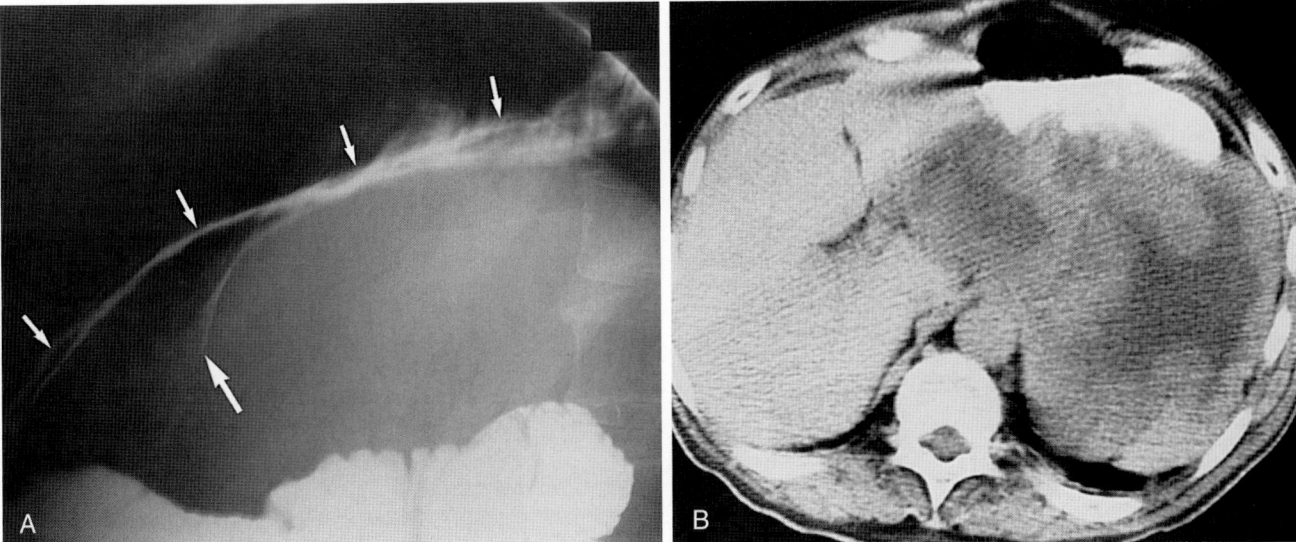

Figure 37-32. Exogastric malignant gastrointestinal stromal tumor. A. Lateral radiograph of the stomach shows a giant exogastric mass compressing the posterior wall of the gastric fundus (*small arrows*). A central dimple or spicule (*large arrow*) is seen at the site of attachment of the mass. This finding should suggest the possibility of an exogastric GIST. **B.** CT scan reveals a giant heterogeneous mass with multiple low-density areas due to necrosis of tumor. This heterogeneous appearance is characteristic of malignant GISTs on CT. (Courtesy of Hans Herlinger, MD, Philadelphia, PA.)

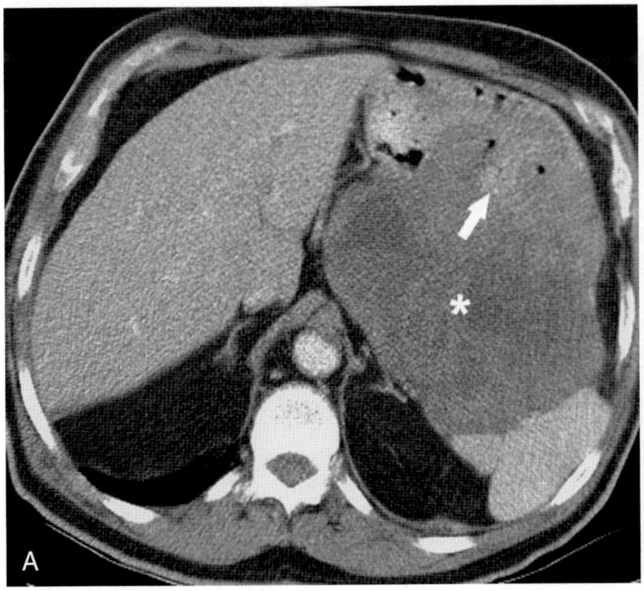

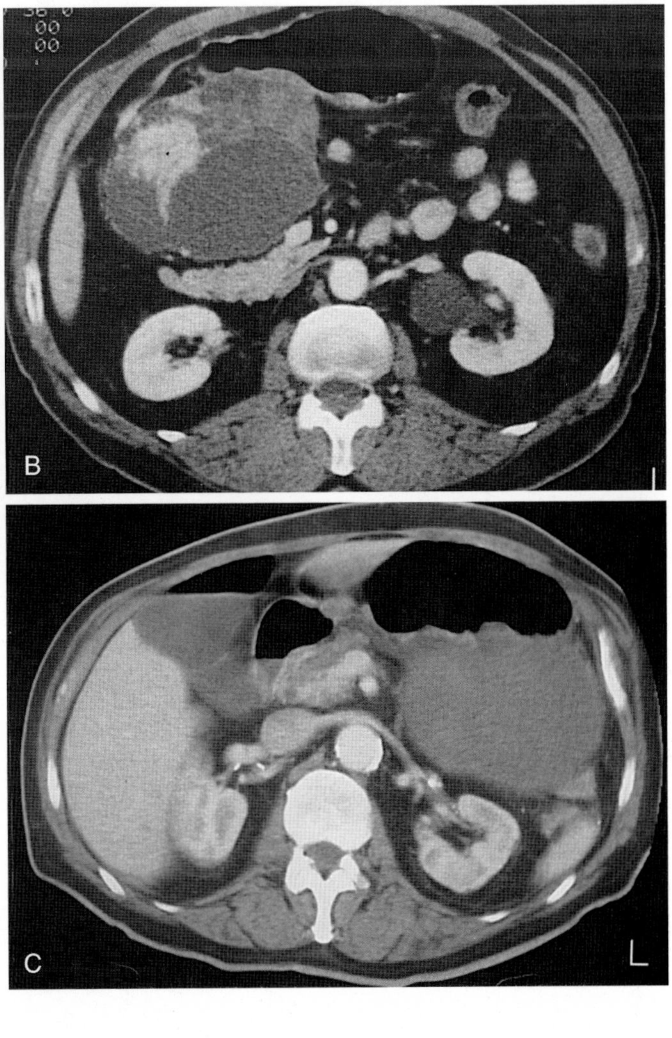

Figure 37-33. Malignant gastrointestinal stromal tumors on CT. A. A large, heterogeneous exogastric mass (*asterisk*) is seen arising from the posterior wall of the stomach. An ulcer crater (*arrow*) on the posterior wall of the stomach identifies the gastric wall as the origin of this mass. The heterogeneous enhancement and large size of the lesion strongly correlate with malignant histology. **B.** In another patient, a heterogeneous exogastric mass is seen insinuating between the stomach and pancreas. **C.** In a third patient, a gas- and fluid-filled mass projects posteriorly from the stomach. Although uncommon, this degree of necrosis can occur with malignant GISTs.

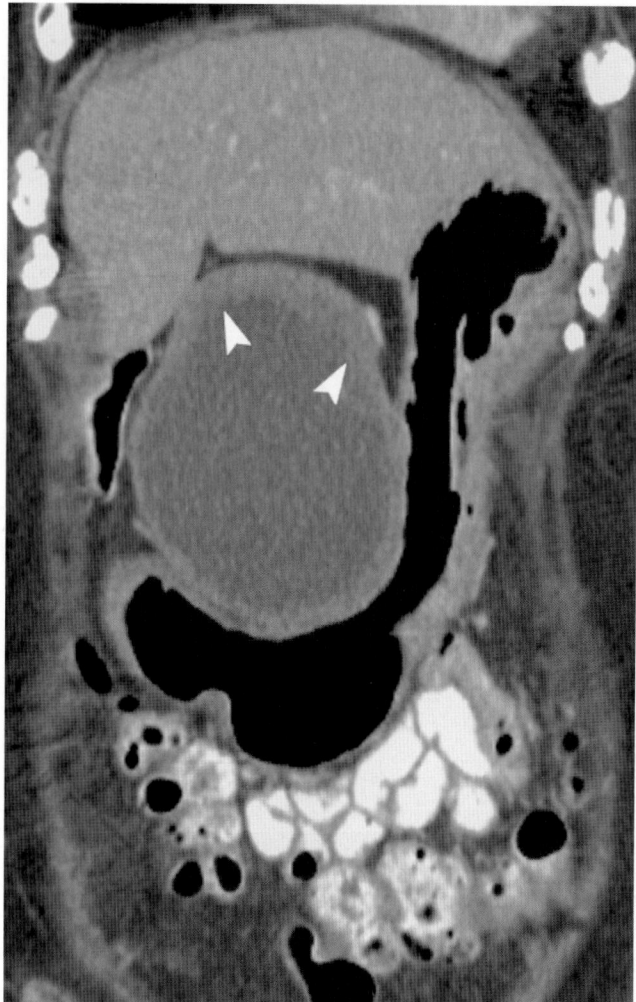

Figure 37-34. Malignant gastrointestinal stromal tumor on CT. Off-axis coronal volume-rendered MDCT image shows a large mass arising from the lesser curvature of the stomach. The wall of the lesion (*arrowheads*) is irregularly thickened.

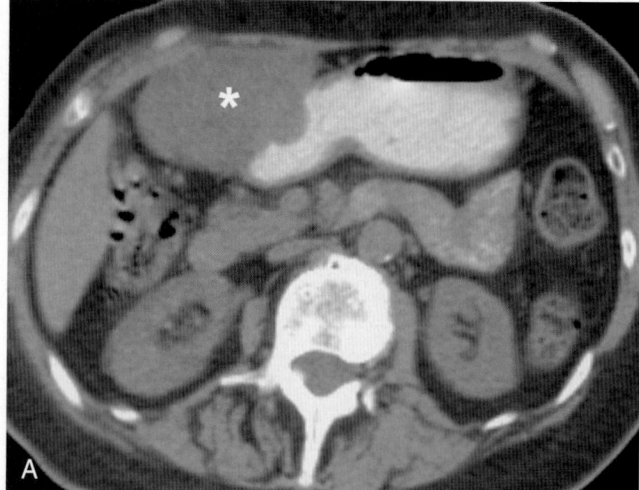

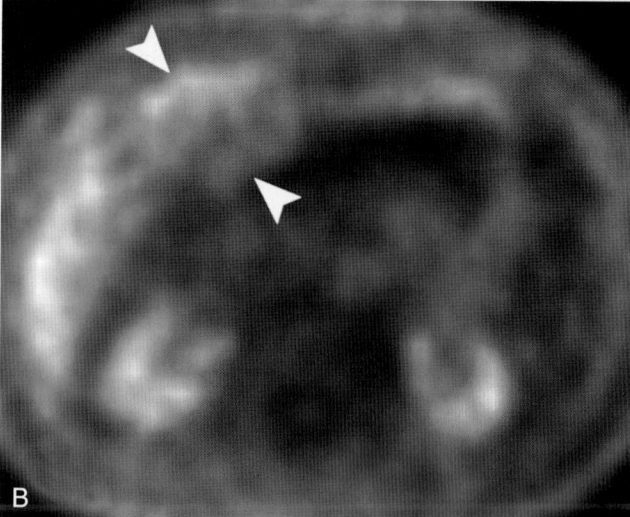

Figure 37-35. Malignant gastrointestinal stromal tumor with necrosis on CT. A. Non–contrast-enhanced CT scan shows a water-attenuation mass (*asterisk*) arising from the anterolateral wall of the stomach. **B.** FDG PET image shows increased activity (*arrowheads*) in the periphery of the mass. Viable tissue is typically located in the periphery of malignant GISTs that are highly necrotic.

levels and are usually positive on PET (Fig. 37-36). Peritoneal involvement by tumor is indistinguishable on CT from other intraperitoneal-seeded metastases.[130]

Malignant GISTs of the stomach are characterized on angiography by relatively well-circumscribed, hypervascular masses with huge feeding arteries and draining veins and intense tumor staining.[131] It is not possible, however, to differentiate benign and malignant stromal tumors by angiographic criteria. Angiography also is not able to distinguish malignant GISTs from other hypervascular lesions such as carcinoids, neurogenic tumors, or vascular metastases.

Differential Diagnosis

Because some malignant GISTs may be as small as 2 cm, it is not always possible to distinguish benign and malignant stromal tumors by radiographic criteria.[108] In general, however, submucosal masses that are larger and more lobulated or contain areas of necrosis or ulceration are more likely to be malignant. The major considerations in the differential diagnosis include lymphoma and other benign or malignant

tumors of mesenchymal origin. Cavitated GISTs may be impossible to distinguish radiographically from lymphoma or metastases from malignant melanoma or other tumors. However, patients with lymphoma or metastatic melanoma often have multiple lesions in the stomach and small bowel, whereas cavitary GISTs almost always occur as solitary lesions.

Malignant GISTs that have an exogastric growth pattern can mimic the appearance of extrinsic mass lesions arising in the liver, pancreas, kidney, or mesentery. In such cases, the typical CT finding of a bulky, heterogeneous mass involving the gastric wall should suggest the correct diagnosis (see Figs. 37-32B and 37-33). Exophytic adenocarcinomas have also been reported, but these lesions are extremely rare.[132] Occasionally, water-density GISTs may be difficult to distinguish from cystic pancreatic neoplasms or pancreatic pseudocysts. Angiography may be helpful in determining the origin of the mass in these patients. Duplication cysts may also appear on CT as water-density lesions involving the greater curvature of the stomach. Duplication cysts tend to be smaller,

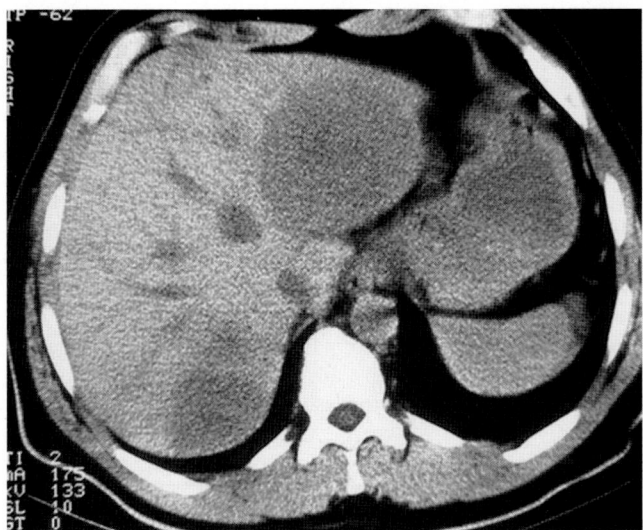

Figure 37-36. Metastases to the liver from a malignant gastrointestinal stromal tumor. CT scan shows multiple large, low-attenuation masses in the liver. The size and attenuation of these lesions are characteristic of hepatic metastases from malignant GISTs.

however, and may occasionally communicate with the gastric lumen.[133,134]

Malignant Duodenal Gastrointestinal Stromal Tumors

Malignant GISTs constitute only 10% of all malignant tumors in the duodenum.[135] The sex distribution is approximately

equal, in contrast to that in malignant GISTs of the stomach.[135,136] These patients may present with signs or symptoms of upper gastrointestinal bleeding, weight loss, abdominal pain, a palpable mass, or obstructive jaundice.[135,137] Many patients remain asymptomatic until they have advanced lesions. Aggressive surgical treatment (i.e., duodenectomy or pancreaticoduodenectomy) is often advocated.[135,137] Because malignant duodenal GISTs often invade adjacent structures or metastasize to the liver, these patients have a relatively poor prognosis.[137]

About 80% of malignant duodenal GISTs are located in the second or third portion of the duodenum.[135] Intramural lesions may appear on barium studies as submucosal masses, often containing areas of ulceration or cavitation (Fig. 37-37A).[135,137] Despite their large size, they rarely cause duodenal obstruction. Other tumors that have an exoenteric growth pattern may be indistinguishable on barium studies from pancreatic neoplasms, pancreatic pseudocysts, or other extrinsic mass lesions involving the duodenum. Malignant duodenal GISTs usually appear on CT as bulky exophytic masses with a heterogeneously enhancing soft tissue rim surrounding a low-density center, often containing gas, fluid, and/or contrast material due to a variable degree of necrosis, ulceration, or cavitation (Fig. 37-37B).[138] A central scar is sometimes seen on both CT and MRI.

KAPOSI'S SARCOMA

The classic form of Kaposi's sarcoma occurs primarily in elderly men and is manifested by slow-growing violaceous or hemorrhagic lesions on the lower extremities. Since the 1980s, however, patients with AIDS have developed a much

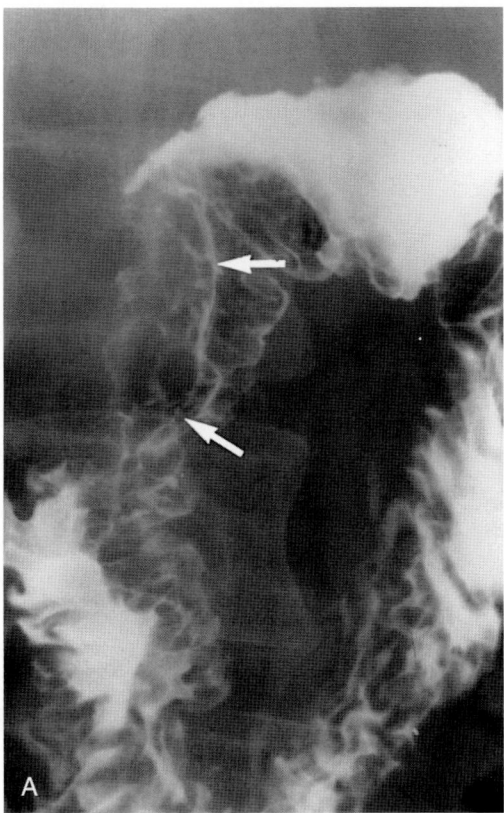

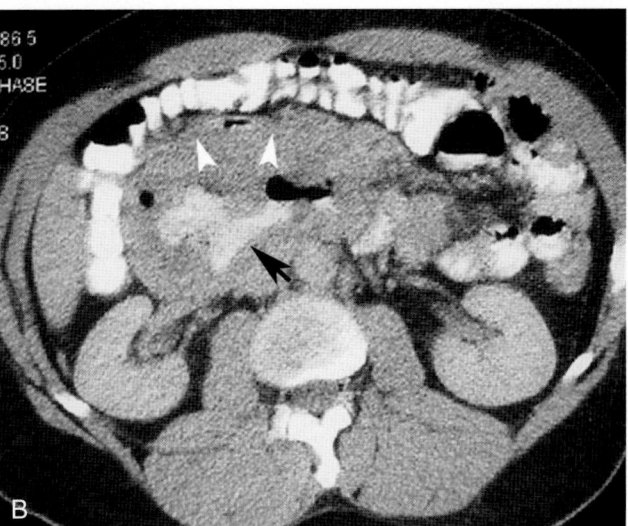

Figure 37-37. Malignant gastrointestinal stromal tumor of the duodenum. A. Barium study shows a large intramural mass (*arrows*) on the lateral border of the descending duodenum. **B.** In another patient, CT scan shows a bulky mass with a large area of central ulceration (*arrow*) in the second and third portions of the duodenum. Note how the duodenal lumen is displaced anteriorly (*arrowheads*) over the mass.

more aggressive form of Kaposi's sarcoma characterized by widespread visceral lesions, particularly in the gastrointestinal tract. In various series, about 35% of patients with AIDS have Kaposi's sarcoma,[139-142] and about 50% with Kaposi's sarcoma have gastrointestinal involvement.[140,143-145] The stomach, duodenum, and small bowel are the most common sites of involvement.[143,146] The colon is affected less frequently, and the esophagus is rarely involved by Kaposi's sarcoma.[143,146] Demonstration of these lesions has important prognostic implications, so that optimal radiographic technique is required whenever barium studies are performed on human immunodeficiency virus (HIV)-positive patients.

Clinical Findings

For reasons that are unclear, most AIDS patients with Kaposi's sarcoma are homosexuals rather than intravenous drug abusers or transfusion recipients.[142,147,148] Gastrointestinal involvement by Kaposi's sarcoma is almost always associated with cutaneous disease, but occasional cases have been reported in the absence of skin lesions.[145,148] Although some patients may present with abdominal pain or upper gastrointestinal bleeding, Kaposi's sarcoma involving the stomach or duodenum rarely causes symptoms, even if multiple lesions are present.[148] Instead, gastrointestinal symptoms usually result from recurrent opportunistic infection in these patients. In fact, patients with Kaposi's sarcoma have a worse prognosis than other patients with AIDS because they are even more likely to develop severe opportunistic infections.[141,142,148] In general, gastrointestinal involvement by Kaposi's sarcoma requires treatment only if it causes symptoms because these enteric lesions rarely affect the progression of AIDS or contribute directly to the patient's death.[148] Radiation therapy or chemotherapy are occasionally used to treat gastrointestinal Kaposi's sarcoma, but these forms of therapy pose substantial risks in patients who are already immunocompromised.[148]

Pathologic and Endoscopic Findings

Kaposi's sarcoma is probably a lesion of vascular origin, consisting histologically of whorled bundles of spindle-shaped cells in a matrix of vascular clefts containing red blood cells and hemosiderin.[146,149] Gastroduodenal involvement by Kaposi's sarcoma may be manifested on endoscopy by a variety of findings, including flat, hemorrhagic patches or macular discolorations; raised, reddish purple nodules, often containing central areas of ulceration (i.e., volcano lesions); and coalescent plaques or masses.[143,144,146,148] Although the gross appearance at endoscopy is characteristic, false-negative mucosal biopsy specimens are often obtained because of the submucosal origin of the lesions.[140,141,143,144,148]

Radiographic Findings

Small macular discolorations of the mucosa cannot be shown on barium studies, so that endoscopy is a much more sensitive technique for detecting the earliest gastrointestinal lesions of Kaposi's sarcoma.[143,144,146] However, elevated lesions can be shown on barium studies, particularly if double-contrast technique is used.[140] Gastroduodenal involvement may be manifested on barium studies by one or more submucosal defects, ranging from 0.5 to 3.0 cm (Fig. 37-38).[140,146,150,151] As these nodules enlarge, they often ulcerate, producing one or more bull's-eye or target lesions (Fig. 37-39).[143,146,151] Other patients may have thickened, nodular folds or polypoid masses in the stomach or duodenum (Fig. 37-40).[140,146] Rarely, an infiltrating form of Kaposi's sarcoma involving the stomach may produce a linitis plastica appearance indistinguishable from that of a primary scirrhous carcinoma (Fig. 37-41).[152] When suspicious lesions are detected in the stomach or duodenum, a small bowel follow-through may be performed to determine whether additional lesions are present in the small bowel.

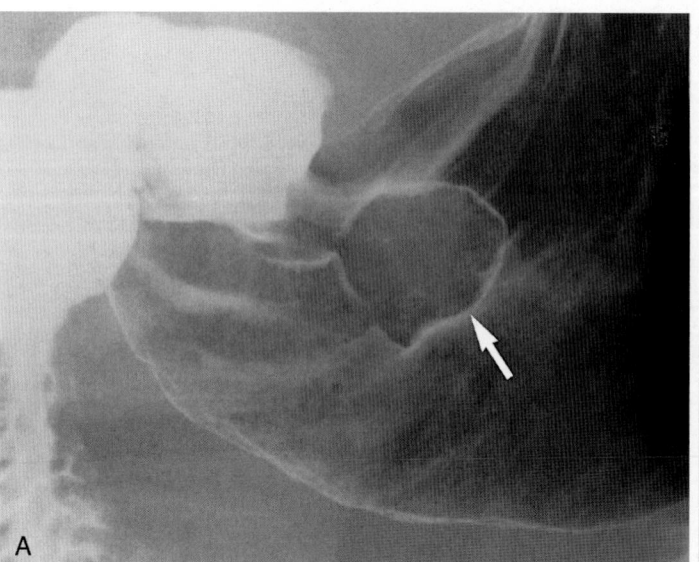 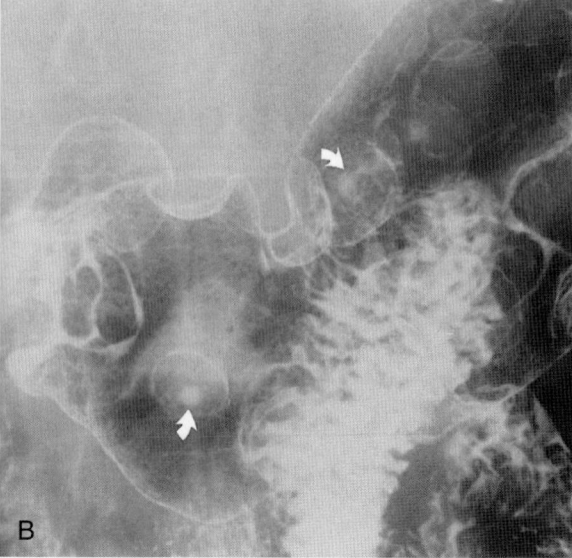

Figure 37-38. Kaposi's sarcoma with submucosal masses in AIDS patients. A. A solitary submucosal mass (*arrow*) is seen in the gastric antrum. **B.** In another patient, multiple submucosal masses are present in the stomach. The tiny collections of barium (*arrows*) seen overlying several anterior wall lesions represent hanging droplets of barium, or "stalactites," rather than ulcers.

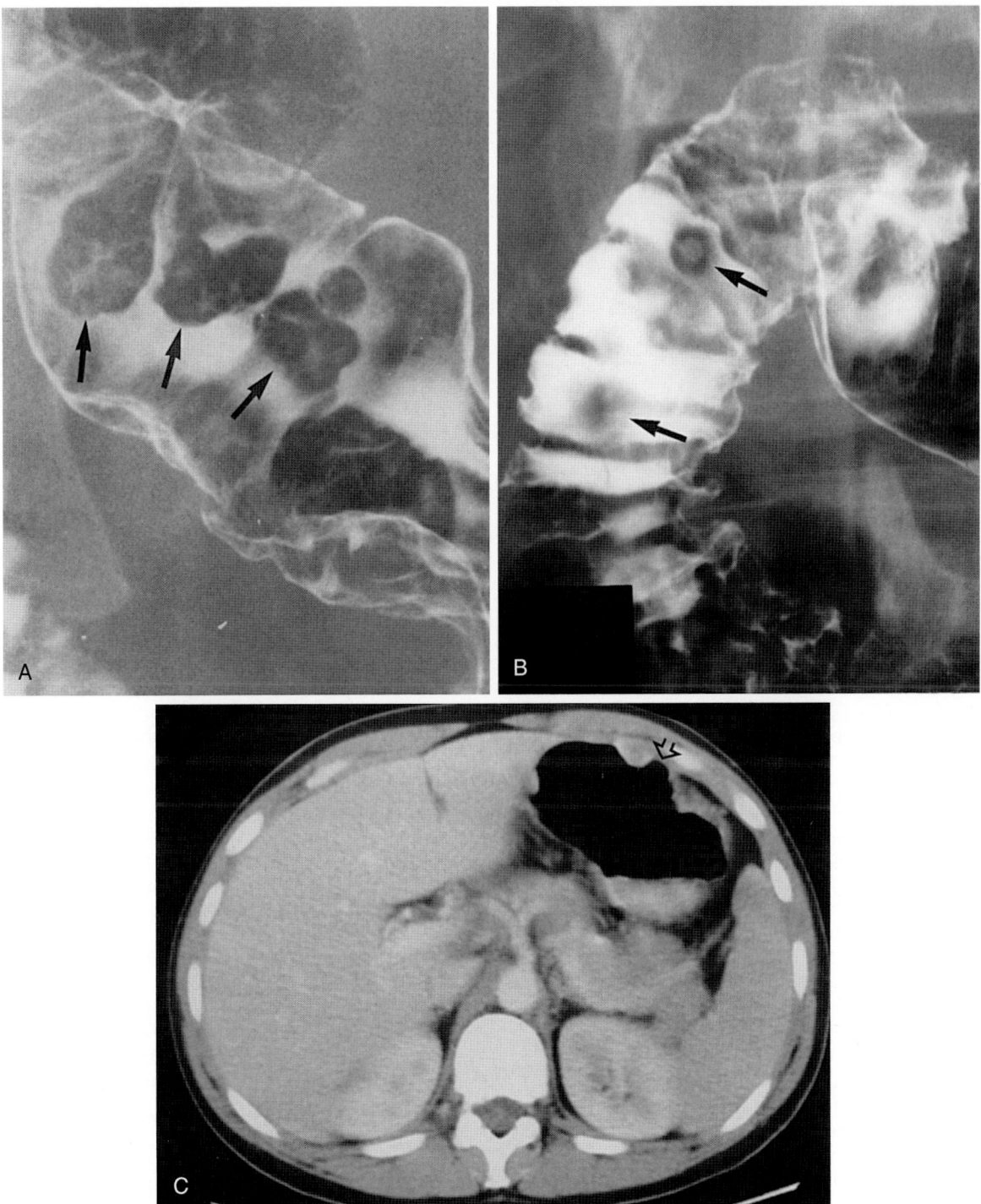

Figure 37-39. Kaposi's sarcoma with bull's-eye lesions in AIDS patients. A. Multiple bull's-eye lesions or centrally ulcerated submucosal masses (*arrows*) are present in the gastric antrum. **B.** In another patient, several bull's-eye lesions (*arrows*) are seen in the descending duodenum. **C.** In a third patient, CT scan shows an ulcerated submucosal mass on the anterior wall of the stomach. Gas outlines the ulcer (*arrow*). (**B** courtesy of Robert Goren, MD, Philadelphia, PA.)

CT may occasionally demonstrate tumor nodules in the stomach or duodenum resulting from Kaposi's sarcoma in AIDS patients who are being evaluated for opportunistic infection (see Fig. 37-39C).[153,154] CT can also be used to determine whether retroperitoneal adenopathy, splenomegaly, or other evidence of Kaposi's sarcoma is present in the abdomen.[155,156]

Differential Diagnosis

Kaposi's sarcoma and non-Hodgkin's lymphoma are the major considerations in the differential diagnosis of multiple, small nodular elevations in the stomach or duodenum in patients with AIDS.[140,146] Metastases, leukemic infiltrates, or multiple polyps (i.e., a polyposis syndrome) may produce similar findings, but the correct diagnosis can usually be suggested

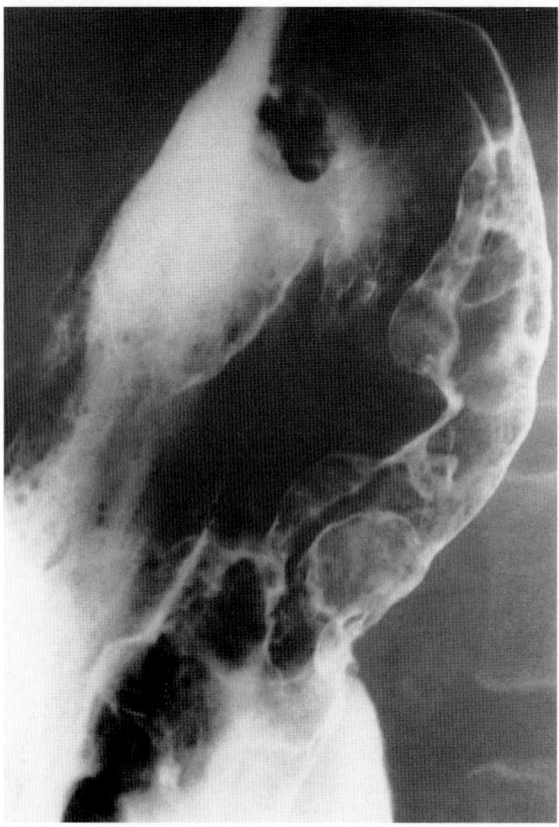

Figure 37-40. Kaposi's sarcoma in an AIDS patient. Multiple polypoid masses are seen on the posterior wall of the fundus.

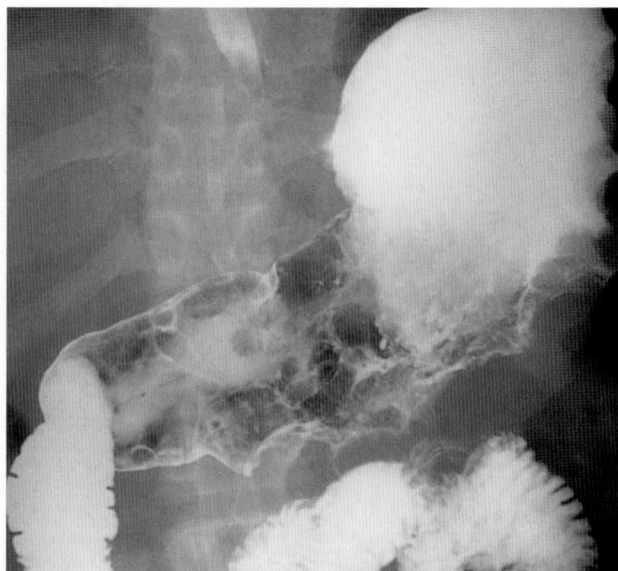

Figure 37-41. Kaposi's sarcoma with a linitis plastica appearance in an AIDS patient. The stomach has a markedly narrowed, irregular appearance caused by the infiltrating form of Kaposi's sarcoma.

on the basis of the clinical history. Kaposi's sarcoma and lymphoma are also the major considerations for multiple bull's-eye lesions in patients with AIDS.[140,146] When ulceration, narrowing, or thickened folds are demonstrated in the stomach, the possibility of opportunistic infections such as cryptosporidiosis, cytomegalovirus infection, and tuberculosis should also be considered.[151] Endoscopic biopsy specimens, brushings, and cultures are therefore required to differentiate Kaposi's sarcoma or other infiltrative lesions from the various opportunistic infections that occur in these patients.

CARCINOID TUMORS

Carcinoids are endocrine tumors that are capable of producing a variety of vasoactive substances. Only 2% to 3% of all gastrointestinal carcinoids are located in the stomach or duodenum.[157,158] Nevertheless, these lesions are important because they are slow-growing tumors with a well-recognized malignant potential.

Pathology

Carcinoid tumors of the stomach usually originate from enterochromaffin-like cells (Kulchitsky cells) arising in the gastric mucosa.[159,160] These tumors are argyrophilic but argentaffin-negative and lack the enzyme required for synthesis of 5-hydroxytryptamine (serotonin), so that they rarely show evidence of endocrine function.[161] As a result, patients with gastric carcinoids almost never exhibit symptoms of the carcinoid syndrome.

Gastric carcinoids have been found with increased frequency in patients with Zollinger-Ellison syndrome (usually associated with multiple endocrine neoplasia type 1) or chronic atrophic gastritis (with or without pernicious anemia).[159,160,162-164] It has been shown that hypergastrinemia in these patients causes proliferation of enterochromaffin-like cells with the subsequent development of gastric carcinoids. The carcinoids associated with hypergastrinemia usually appear as multiple small polyps in the gastric fundus with little, if any malignant potential, so that these patients have an excellent prognosis.[159,162] In contrast, sporadic gastric carcinoids (i.e., those not associated with hypergastrinemia) usually occur as solitary lesions that are more likely to exhibit invasive growth, metastasize to distant sites, or both.[159,162]

Duodenal carcinoids rarely arise from enterochromaffin cells or produce detectable serotonin levels, so that these lesions almost never result in the development of the carcinoid syndrome.[165] Duodenal carcinoids may be associated with Zollinger-Ellison syndrome or neurofibromatosis type 1.[165]

Clinical Findings

Gastric carcinoids have an equal sex distribution and usually occur in patients older than 40 years of age.[161] Many patients are asymptomatic, but some may present with abdominal pain, nausea, vomiting, weight loss, anorexia, or signs or symptoms of upper gastrointestinal bleeding.[161,165-168] Although larger lesions are more likely to bleed, massive bleeding of ulcerated carcinoids as small as 1 cm has been described.[169] Gastric carcinoids may be associated with primary hypergastrinemia in patients with Zollinger-Ellison syndrome or with secondary hypergastrinemia in patients with chronic atrophic gastritis.[159,162,163]

Gastric carcinoids are low-grade malignant tumors that can eventually metastasize to the liver or other structures. Metastases are found in 20% to 30% of patients with gastric carcinoids at the time of diagnosis,[158] but long-term survival

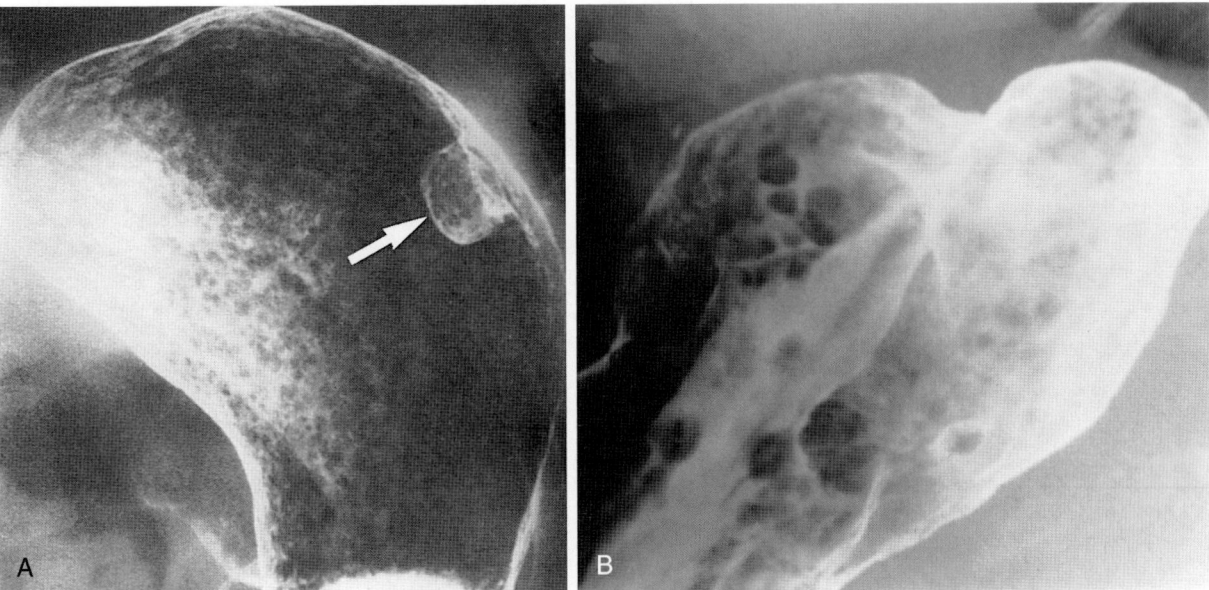

Figure 37-42. Gastric carcinoid tumors. A. A solitary submucosal mass (*arrow*) is seen in the gastric fundus. **B.** In another patient, multiple submucosal nodules are present in the fundus.

has been reported even when regional or hepatic metastases are present. Overall 5-year survival rates for patients with localized gastric carcinoids approach 95% versus 5-year survival rates of approximately 50% for gastric carcinoids of all stages.[160] These patients therefore have a much better prognosis than those with gastric carcinoma.

Radiographic Findings

Gastric carcinoid tumors associated with hypergastrinemia usually appear on barium studies as multiple small polyps in the gastric fundus or body.[163] In contrast, sporadic carcinoids may be manifested by one or more submucosal masses in the stomach (Figs. 37-42 and 37-43).[161] Some of these masses

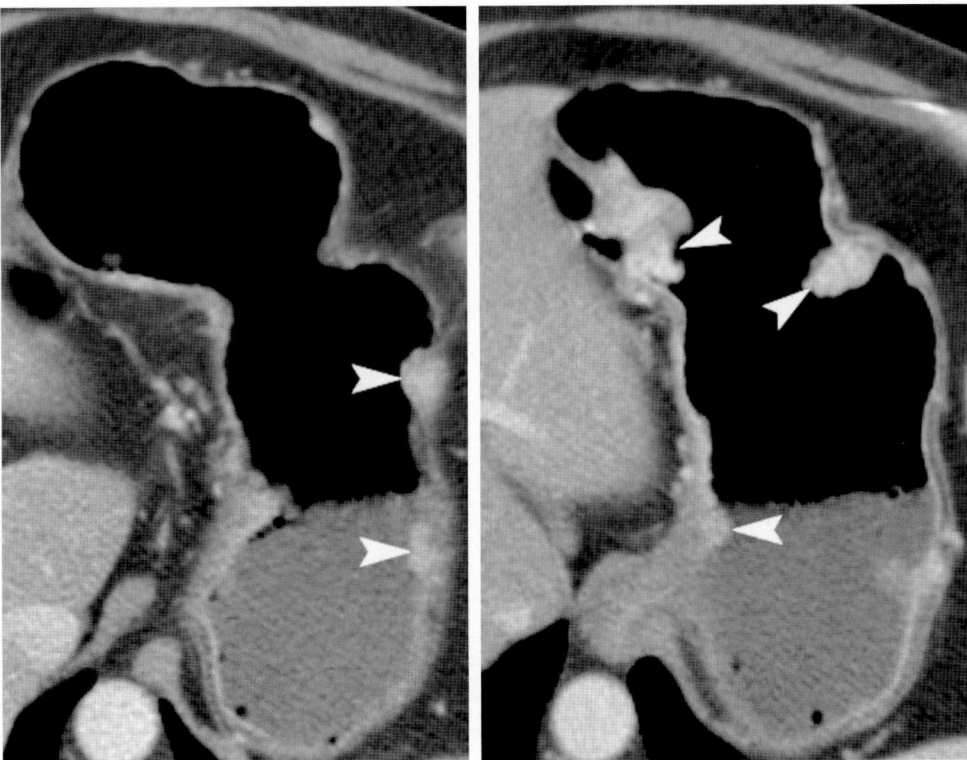

Figure 37-43. Gastric carcinoid tumors on CT. Sequential CT scans show multiple carcinoid tumors in the proximal stomach as enhancing polypoid masses (*arrowheads*).

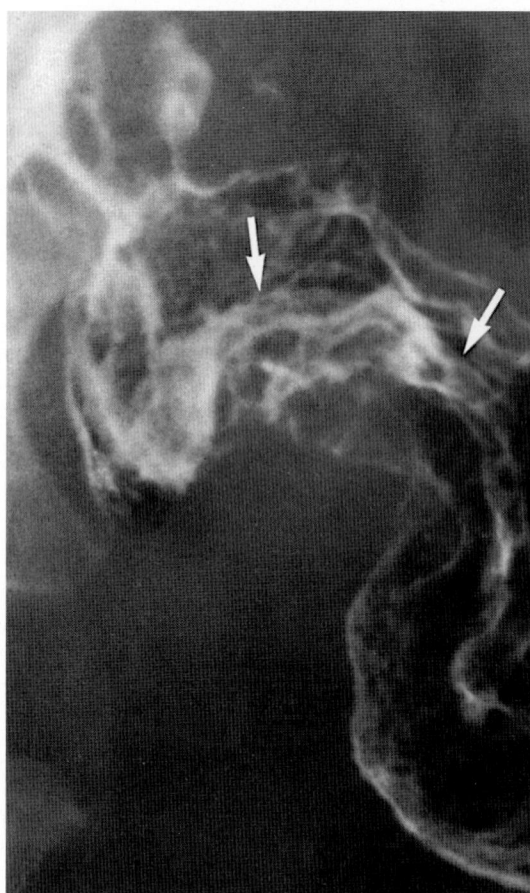

Figure 37-44. Gastric carcinoid tumor. A polypoid mass (*arrows*) is present on the greater curvature of the gastric antrum. This lesion is indistinguishable from other polypoid tumors in the stomach.

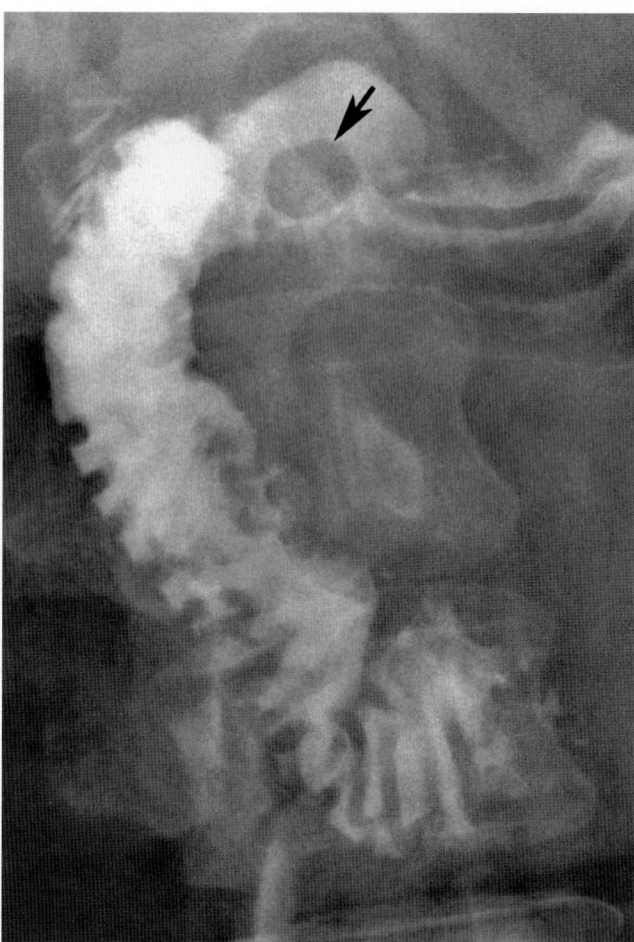

Figure 37-45. Duodenal carcinoid. Barium study shows a smooth, round submucosal mass (*arrow*) in the duodenal bulb. At surgery, this patient was found to have a malignant duodenal carcinoid tumor involving periduodenal lymph nodes.

may ulcerate, producing typical bull's-eye lesions.[161] The differential diagnosis for solitary submucosal-appearing gastric carcinoids includes benign GISTs, ectopic pancreatic rests, or other mesenchymal tumors, whereas the differential diagnosis for multiple gastric carcinoids includes metastases, lymphoma, Kaposi's sarcoma, or gastric involvement by one of the polyposis syndromes. Other patients may have sessile or pedunculated lesions that are indistinguishable from hyperplastic or adenomatous polyps.[170,171] Still other patients may have benign-appearing or malignant-appearing gastric ulcers.[163] Occasionally, advanced carcinoid tumors may appear as large polypoid masses that are indistinguishable from polypoid carcinomas (Fig. 37-44).[161,172]

Duodenal carcinoids may be manifested as one or more polypoid defects in the duodenal bulb or proximal descending duodenum.[165,173-175] These tumors may appear as discrete submucosal masses or intraluminal polyps (Fig. 37-45) or, less frequently, as polypoid or ulcerated lesions on barium studies or CT (Fig. 37-46).[165,173-175] When gastric or duodenal carcinoids are detected radiographically, endoscopic biopsy specimens are required for a definitive diagnosis.

MISCELLANEOUS TUMORS

Other rare malignant tumors that may occur in the stomach or duodenum include liposarcomas, fibrosarcomas, neurofibrosarcomas, plasmacytomas, hemangioendotheliomas,

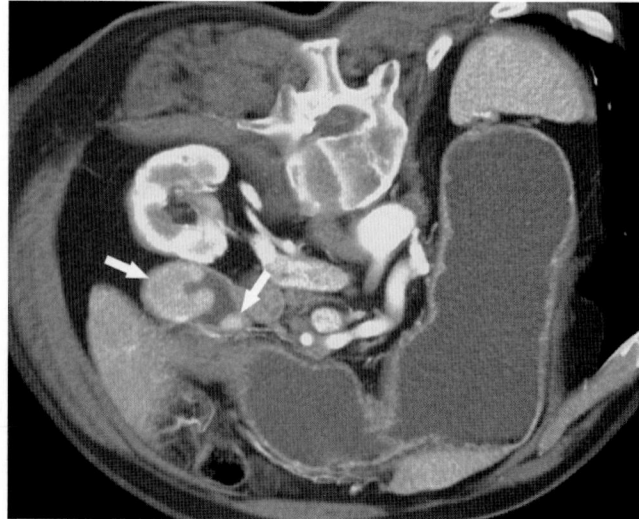

Figure 37-46. Duodenal carcinoids on CT. Arterial phase 3D volume-rendered MDCT image shows two hyperdense masses (*arrows*) in the duodenal bulb. The larger mass contains a central area of ulceration. Endoscopic biopsy specimens revealed duodenal carcinoid tumors.

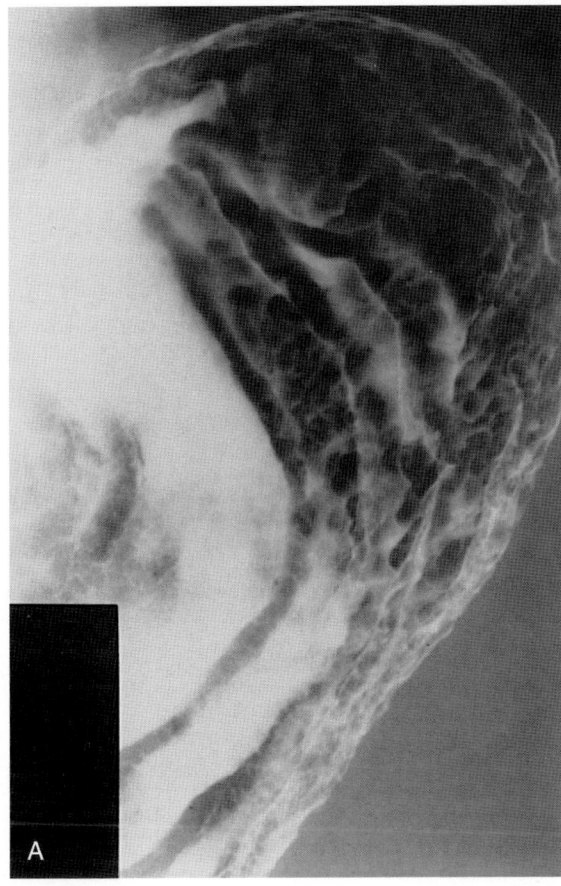

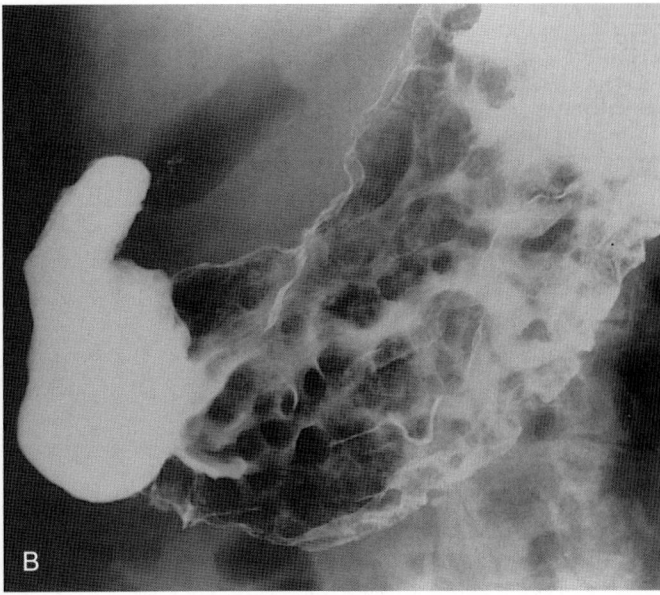

Figure 37-47. Other malignant tumors involving the stomach. A. Innumerable tiny nodules are seen in the gastric fundus as a result of chronic lymphocytic leukemia. **B.** In another patient, multiple submucosal masses are seen in the stomach as a result of multiple myeloma.

hemangiopericytomas, choriocarcinomas, and malignant autonomic nerve tumors.[176-181] Rarely, the stomach may be involved by leukemia or multiple myeloma (Fig. 36-47).[182,183] Squamous cell carcinomas and mixed adenosquamous carcinomas have also been described as rare malignant tumors in the stomach, arising from congenital rests of squamous epithelium or from preexisting areas of squamous meta-plasia.[184,185]

References

1. Menuck LS, Amberg JR: Metastatic disease involving the stomach. Am J Dig Dis 20:903-913, 1975.
2. Asch MJ, Wiedel PD, Habif DV: Gastrointestinal metastases from carcinoma of the breast: Autopsy study and 18 cases requiring operative intervention. Arch Surg 96:840-843, 1968.
3. Klein MS, Sherlock P: Gastric and colonic metastases from breast carcinoma. Am J Dig Dis 17:881-886, 1972.
4. Hsu CC, Chen JJ, Changchien CS: Endoscopic features of metastatic tumors in the upper gastrointestinal tract. Endoscopy 28:249-253, 1996.
5. Chang SF, Burrell MI, Brand MH, et al: The protean gastrointestinal manifestations of metastatic breast carcinoma. Radiology 126:611-617, 1978.
6. Khilnani MT, Wolf BS: Late involvement of the alimentary tract by carcinoma of the kidney. Am J Dig Dis 5:529-540, 1960.
7. Das Gupta TK, Brasfield RD: Metastatic melanoma of the gastrointestinal tract. Arch Surg 88:969-973, 1964.
8. Meyers MA, McSweeney J: Secondary neoplasms of the bowel. Radiology 105:1-11, 1972.
9. Joffe N: Metastatic involvement of the stomach secondary to breast carcinoma. AJR 123:512-521, 1975.
10. Goldstein HM, Beydonn MT, Dodd GD: Radiologic spectrum of metas-tatic melanoma to the gastrointestinal tract. AJR 129:605-612, 1977.
11. Lipshutz HI, Lindell MM, Dodd GD: Metastases to the hollow viscera. Radiol Clin North Am 20:487-499, 1982.
12. Felson B: "Bull's eye" lesions: Solitary or multiple nodules in the gastro-intestinal tract with large central ulceration. JAMA 229:825-826, 1974.
13. McDermott VG, Low VHS, Keogan MT, et al: Malignant melanoma metastatic to the gastrointestinal tract. AJR 166:809-813, 1996.
14. Zornoza J, Goldstein HM: Cavitating metastases of the small intestine. AJR 129:613-615, 1977.
15. Radin DR, Halls JM: Cavitating metastases of the stomach and duo-denum. J Comput Assist Tomogr 11:283-287, 1987.
16. Levine MS, Kong V, Rubesin SE, et al: Scirrhous carcinoma of the stomach: Radiologic and endoscopic diagnosis. Radiology 175:151-154, 1990.
17. Caskey CI, Scatarige JC, Fishman EK: Distribution of metastases in breast carcinoma: CT evaluation of the abdomen. Clin Imaging 15:166-171, 1991.
18. Taal BG, Peterse H, Boot H: Clinical presentation, endoscopic features, and treatment of gastric metastases from breast carcinoma. Cancer 89:2214-2221, 2000.
19. Winston CB, Hadar O, Teitcher JB, et al: Metastatic lobular carcinoma of the breast: Patterns of spread in the chest, abdomen, and pelvis on CT. AJR 175:795-800, 2000.
20. Glick SN, Teplick SK, Levine MS, et al: Gastric cardia metastasis in esophageal carcinoma. Radiology 160:622-630, 1986.
21. Glick SN, Teplick SK, Levine MS: Squamous cell metastases to the gastric cardia. Gastrointest Radiol 10:339-344, 1985.
22. Allen HA, Bush JE: Midesophageal carcinoma metastatic to the stomach: Its unusual appearance on an upper gastrointestinal series. South Med J 76:1049-1051, 1983.
23. Smith SJ, Carlson HC, Gisvold JJ: Secondary neoplasms of the small bowel. Radiology 125:29-33, 1977.
24. Shammash JB, Rubesin SE, Levine MS: Massive gastric distention due to duodenal involvement by retroperitoneal tumors. Gastrointest Radiol 17:214-216, 1992.
25. Levine MS, Caroline D, Thompson JJ, et al: Adenocarcinoma of the esophagus: Relationship to Barrett mucosa. Radiology 150:305-309, 1984.

26. Keen SJ, Dodd GD, Smith JL: Adenocarcinoma arising in Barrett's esophagus: Pathologic and radiologic features. Mt Sinai J Med 51:442-450, 1984.

27. Mani JR, Zboralske F, Margulis AR: Carcinoma of the body and tail of the pancreas. AJR 96:429-446, 1966.

28. Balthazar EJ, Megibow AJ, Naidich DP, et al: Computed tomographic recognition of gastric varices. AJR 142:1121-1125, 1984.

29. Marn CS, Glazer GM, Williams DM, et al: CT-angiographic correlation of collateral venous pathways in isolated splenic vein occlusion: New observations. Radiology 175:375-380, 1990.

30. Treitel H, Meyers MA, Maza V: Changes in the duodenal loop secondary to carcinoma of the hepatic flexure of the colon. Br J Radiol 43:209-213, 1970.

31. Meyers MA, Whalen JP: Roentgen significance of the duodenocolic relationships: An anatomic approach. AJR 117:263-274, 1973.

32. Vieta JO, Blanco R, Valentine GR: Malignant duodenocolic fistula: Report of two cases with one or more synchronous gastrointestinal cancers. Dis Colon Rectum 19:542-552, 1976.

33. Yamaguchi K, Enjoji M: Carcinoma of the gallbladder: A clinicopathology of 103 patients and a newly proposed staging. Cancer 62:1425-1432, 1988.

34. Levitt RG, Koehler RE, Sagel SS, et al: Metastatic disease of the mesentery and omentum. Radiol Clin North Am 20:501-510, 1982.

35. Rubesin SE, Levine MS, Glick SN: Gastric involvement by omental cakes: Radiologic findings. Gastrointest Radiol 11:223-228, 1986.

36. Rubesin SE, Levine MS: Omental cakes: Colonic involvement by omental metastases. Radiology 154:593-596, 1985.

37. Walkey MM, Friedman AC, Radecki PD: Computed tomography of peritoneal carcinomatosis. Radiology 171:152-170, 1989.

38. Levitt RG, Sagel SS, Stanley RJ: Detection of neoplastic involvement of the mesentery and omentum by computed tomography. AJR 131:835-838, 1978.

39. Freeman C, Berg JW, Cutler SJ: Occurrence and prognosis of extranodal lymphomas. Cancer 29:252-260, 1972.

40. Menuck LS: Gastric lymphoma: A radiologic diagnosis. Gastrointest Radiol 1:157-161, 1976.

41. Brady LW: Malignant lymphoma of the gastrointestinal tract. Radiology 137:291-298, 1980.

42. Papadimitriou CS, Papacharalampous NX, Kittas C: Primary gastrointestinal lymphoma: A morphologic and immunohistochemical study. Cancer 55:870-879, 1985.

43. Farinha P, Gascoyne RD: *Helicobacter pylori* and MALT lymphoma. Gastroenterology 128:1579-1605, 2005.

44. Orr RK, Lininger JR, Lawrence W: Gastric pseudolymphoma: A challenging clinical problem. Ann Surg 200:185-194, 1984.

45. Harris NL: Extranodal lymphoid infiltrates and mucosa-associated lymphoid tissue (MALT): A unifying concept. Am J Surg Pathol 15:879-884, 1991.

46. Kitamura K, Yamaguchi T, Okamoto K, et al: Early gastric lymphoma. Cancer 77:850-857, 1996.

47. Dworkin B, Lightdale CJ, Weingrad DN, et al: Primary gastric lymphoma: A review of 50 cases. Dig Dis Sci 27:986-992, 1982.

48. Brooks JJ, Enterline HT: Primary gastric lymphomas: A clinicopathologic study of 58 cases with long-term follow-up and literature review. Cancer 51:701-711, 1983.

49. Brands F, Monig SP, Raab M: Treatment and prognosis of gastric lymphoma. Eur J Surg 163:803-813, 1997.

50. National Cancer Institute: The non-Hodgkin's lymphoma pathologic classification project (summary and description of a working classification for clinical usage). Cancer 48:2112-2135, 1982.

51. Lewin KJ, Ranchod M, Dorfman RF: Lymphomas of the gastrointestinal tract. Cancer 42:693-707, 1978.

52. Wotherspoon AC, Ortiz-Hidalgo C, Falzon MR, et al: *Helicobacter pylori*–associated gastritis and primary B-cell gastric lymphoma. Lancet 338:1175-1176, 1991.

53. Eidt S, Stolte M, Fischer R: *Helicobacter pylori* gastritis and primary gastric non-Hodgkin's lymphomas. J Clin Pathol 47:436-439, 1994.

54. Harris NL, Jaffe ES, Stern H, et al: A revised European-American classification of lymphoid neoplasms: A proposal from the International Lymphoma Study Group. Blood 84:1361-1392, 1994.

55. Stolte M, Eidt S: Lymphoid follicles in antral mucosa: Immune response to *Campylobacter pylori*? J Clin Pathol 42:1269-1271, 1989.

56. Eidt S, Stolte M: Prevalence of lymphoid follicles and aggregates in *Helicobacter pylori* gastritis in antral and body mucosa. J Clin Pathol 46:832-835, 1993.

57. Genta RM, Hamner HW, Graham DY: Gastric lymphoid follicles in *Helicobacter pylori* infection: Frequency, distribution, and response to triple therapy. Hum Pathol 24:577-583, 1993.

58. Isaacson P, Wright DH: Extranodal malignant lymphoma arising from mucosa-associated lymphoid tissue. Cancer 53:2515-2524, 1984.

59. Eck M, Schmauber B, Haas R, et al: MALT-type lymphoma of the stomach is associated with *Helicobacter pylori* strains expressing the CagA protein. Gastroenterology 112:1482-1486, 1997.

60. Cogliatti SB, Schmid U, Schumacher U, et al: Primary B-cell gastric lymphoma: A clinicopathological study of 145 patients. Gastroenterology 101:1159-1170, 1991.

61. Akaza K, Motoori T, Nakamura S, et al: Clinicopathologic study of primary gastric lymphoma of B cell phenotype with special reference to low-grade B cell lymphoma of mucosa-associated lymphoid tissue among the Japanese. Pathol Int 45:832-845, 1995.

62. Chan JKC, Ng CS, Isaacson PG: Relationship between high-grade lymphoma and low-grade B-cell mucosa–associated lymphoid tissue lymphoma (MALToma) of the stomach. Am J Pathol 136:1153-1164, 1990.

63. Nelson RS, Lanza FL: Malignant tumors of the stomach. In Berk JE, Haubrich WS, Kalser MH, et al (eds): Bockus Gastroenterology, 4th ed. Philadelphia, WB Saunders, 1985, pp 1267-1277.

64. Sandler RS: Primary gastric lymphoma. Am J Gastroenterol 79:21-25, 1984.

65. Seifert E, Schulte F, Weismuller J, et al: Endoscopic and bioptic diagnosis of malignant non-Hodgkin's lymphoma of the stomach. Endoscopy 25:497-501, 1993.

66. Roggero E, Zucca E, Pinotti G, et al: Eradication of *Helicobacter pylori* infection in primary low-grade gastric lymphoma of mucosa-associated lymphoid tissue. Ann Intern Med 122:767-769, 1995.

67. Taal BG, Boot H, van Heerde P, et al: Primary non-Hodgkin lymphoma of the stomach: Endoscopic pattern and prognosis in low versus high grade malignancy in relation to the MALT concept. Gut 39:556-561, 1996.

68. Grossman E, Winawer SJ: Diffuse gastrointestinal lymphosarcoma: Gastroscopic and proctoscopic observations. Gastrointest Endosc 16:202-204, 1970.

69. Nelson RS, Lanza FL: The endoscopic diagnosis of gastric lymphoma: Gross characteristics and histology. Gastrointest Endosc 20:183-184, 1974.

70. Cabre-Fiol V, Vilardell F: Progress in the cytological diagnosis of the gastric lymphoma. Cancer 41:1456-1461, 1978.

71. Spinelli P, Gullo CL, Pizzetti P: Endoscopic diagnosis of gastric lymphomas. Endoscopy 12:211-214, 1980.

72. Shin MH, Karas M, Nisce L, et al: Management of primary gastric lymphoma. Ann Surg 195:196-202, 1982.

73. Shen YY, Kao A, Yen FR: Comparison of ^{18}F-fluoro-2-deoxyglucose positron emission tomography and gallium-67 citrate scintigraphy for detecting malignant lymphoma. Oncol Rep 9:321-325, 2002.

74. Mittal B, Wasserman TH, Griffith RC: Non-Hodgkin's lymphoma of the stomach. Am J Gastroenterol 78:780-787, 1983.

75. Amer MH, El-Akkad S: Gastrointestinal lymphoma in adults: Clinical features and management of 300 cases. Gastroenterology 106:846-858, 1994.

76. Bayerdorffer E, Neubauer A, Rudolph B, et al: Regression of primary gastric lymphoma of mucosa-associated lymphoid tissue after cure of *Helicobacter pylori* infection. Lancet 345:1591-1594, 1995.

77. Lim FE, Hartman AS, Tan EGC, et al: Factors in the prognosis of gastric lymphoma. Cancer 39:1715-1720, 1977.

78. Loehr WJ, Mujahed Z, Zahn RD, et al: Primary lymphoma of the gastrointestinal tract: A review of 100 cases. Ann Surg 170:232-238, 1969.

79. Levine MS, Elmas N, Furth EE, et al: *Helicobacter pylori* and gastric MALT lymphoma. AJR 166:85-86, 1996.

80. Yoo CC, Levine MS, Furth EE, et al: Gastric mucosa-associated lymphoid tissue lymphoma: Radiographic findings in six patients. Radiology 208:239-243, 1998.

81. Kim YH, Lim HK, Han JK, et al: Low-grade gastric mucosa-associated lymphoid tissue lymphoma: Correlation of radiographic and pathologic findings. Radiology 212:241-248, 1999.

82. Park MS, Kim KW, Yu JS, et al: Radiographic findings of primary B-cell lymphoma of the stomach: Low-grade versus high-grade malignancy in relation to the mucosa-associated lymphoid tissue concept. AJR 179:1297-1304, 2002.

83. Sherrick DW, Hodgson JR, Dockerty MB: The roentgenologic diagnosis of primary gastric lymphoma. Radiology 84:925-932, 1965.

84. Zornoza J, Dodd GD: Lymphoma of the gastrointestinal tract. Semin Roentgenol 15:272-287, 1980.
85. Fork FT, Ekberg O, Haglund U: Radiology in primary gastric lymphoma. Acta Radiol Diagn 25:481-488, 1984.
86. Levine MS, Rubesin SE, Pantongrag-Brown L, et al: Non-Hodgkin's lymphoma of the gastrointestinal tract: Radiographic findings. AJR 168:165-172, 1997.
87. Levine MS, Pantongrag-Brown L, Aguilera NS, et al: Non-Hodgkin lymphoma of the stomach: A cause of linitis plastica. Radiology 201:375-378, 1996.
88. Joffe N: Metastatic involvement of the stomach secondary to breast carcinoma. AJR 123:512-521, 1975.
89. Bloch C: Roentgen features of Hodgkin's disease of the stomach. AJR 99:175-181, 1967.
90. Ounnick NR, Harell GS, Parker BR: Multiple "bull's-eye" lesions in gastric lymphoma. AJR 126:965-969, 1976.
91. Hricak H, Thoeni RJ, Margulis AR, et al: Extension of gastric lymphoma into the esophagus and duodenum. Radiology 135:309-312, 1980.
92. Cho KC, Baker SR, Alterman DD, et al: Transpyloric spread of gastric tumors: Comparison of adenocarcinoma and lymphoma. AJR 167:467-469, 1996.
93. Koehler RE, Hanelin LG, Laing FC, et al: Invasion of the duodenum by carcinoma of the stomach. AJR 128:201-205, 1977.
94. Fox ER, Laufer I, Levine MS: Response of gastric lymphoma to chemotherapy: Radiographic appearance. AJR 142:711-714, 1984.
95. Libshitz HI, Lindell MM, Maor MH, et al: Appearance of the intact lymphomatous stomach following radiotherapy and chemotherapy. Gastrointest Radiol 10:25-29, 1985.
96. Buy JN, Moss AA: Computed tomography of gastric lymphoma. AJR 138:859-865, 1982.
97. Megibow AJ, Balthazar EJ, Naidich DP, et al: Computed tomography of gastrointestinal lymphoma. AJR 141:541-547, 1983.
98. Choi D, Lim HK, Lee SJ, et al: Gastric mucosa-associated lymphoid tissue lymphoma: Helical CT findings and pathologic correlation. AJR 178:1117-1122, 2002.
99. Tio TL, den Hartog-Jager FC, Tytgat GN: Endoscopic ultrasonography of non-Hodgkin lymphoma of the stomach. Gastroenterology 91:401-408, 1986.
100. Caletti G, Ferrari A, Brocchi E, et al: Accuracy of endoscopic ultra-sonography in the diagnosis and staging of gastric cancer and lymphoma. Surgery 113:14-27, 1993.
101. Van Dam J: The role of endoscopic ultrasonography in monitoring treatment: Response to chemotherapy in lymphoma. Endoscopy 26:772-773, 1994.
102. Torigian DA, Levine MS, Gill NS, et al: Lymphoid hyperplasia of the stomach: Radiographic findings in five adult patients. AJR 177:71-75, 2001.
103. Meyers MA, Katzen B, Alonso DR: Transpyloric extension to duodenal bulb in gastric lymphoma. Radiology 115:575-580, 1975.
104. Balikian JP, Nassar NT, Shamma'a MH, et al: Primary lymphomas of the small intestine including the duodenum: A Roentgen analysis of twenty-nine cases. AJR 107:131-141, 1969.
105. Holmes GKT, Stokes PL, Sorahan TM, et al: Coeliac disease, gluten-free diet, and malignancy. Gut 17:612-619, 1976.
106. Collins SM, Hamilton JD, Lewis TD, et al: Small-bowel malabsorption and gastrointestinal malignancy. Radiology 126:603-609, 1978.
107. Bedikian AY, Khankhanian N, Vadivieso M, et al: Sarcoma of the stomach: Clinicopathologic study of 43 cases. J Surg Oncol 13:121-127, 1980.
108. Nauert TC, Zornoza J, Ordonez N: Gastric leiomyosarcomas. AJR 139:291-297, 1982.
109. Suster S: Gastrointestinal stromal tumors. Semin Diagn Pathol 13:297-313, 1996.
110. Sarlomo-Rikala M, Kovatich AJ, Barusevicius A, et al: CD117: A sensitive marker for gastrointestinal stromal tumors that is more specific than CD34. Mod Pathol 11:728-734, 1998.
111. Levy AD, Remotti HE, Thompson WM, et al: Gastrointestinal stromal tumors: Radiologic features with pathologic correlation. RadioGraphics 23:283-304, 2003.
112. Appelman HD, Helwig EB: Gastric epithelioid leiomyoma and leiomyosarcoma (leiomyoblastoma). Cancer 38:708-728, 1976.
113. Burkill GJC, Badran M, Al-Muderis O, et al: Malignant gastrointestinal stromal tumor: Distribution, imaging features, and pattern of metastatic spread. Radiology 226:527-532, 2003.
114. Franquemont DW: Differentiation and risk assessment of gastrointestinal stromal tumors. Am J Clin Pathol 103:41-47, 1995.
115. Miettinen M, Sarlomo-Rikala M, Lasota J: Gastrointestinal stromal tumors: Recent advances in understanding of their biology. Hum Pathol 30:1213-1220, 1999.
116. Ludwig DJ, Traverso LW: Gut stromal tumors and their clinical behavior. Am J Surg 173:390-394, 1997.
117. Ranchod M, Kempson RL: Smooth muscle tumors of the gastrointestinal tract and retroperitoneum. Cancer 39:255-262, 1977.
118. Bedikian AY, Khankhanian N, Heilbrun LK, et al: Primary lymphomas and sarcomas of the stomach. South Med J 73:21-24, 1980.
119. Stauber SL, Messer J, Berger HW: Gastric leiomyosarcoma diagnosed on chest roentgenogram: Importance of the stomach bubble. Mt Sinai J Med 50:514-516, 1983.
120. Phillips JC, Lindsay JW, Kendall JA: Gastric leiomyosarcoma: Roentgenologic and clinical findings. Am J Dig Dis 15:239-246, 1970.
121. Scatarige JC, Fishman EK, Jones B, et al: Gastric leiomyosarcoma; CT observations. J Comput Assist Tomogr 9:320-327, 1985.
122. Train JS, Hertz I, Keller RJ: Exogastric smooth muscle tumors. Am J Gastroenterol 76:544-550, 1981.
123. Herlinger H: The recognition of exogastric tumours: Report of six cases. Br J Radiol 39:25-34, 1966.
124. Sharp RM, Ansel HJ, Keel SB: Best cases from the AFIP: Gastrointestinal stromal tumor. RadioGraphics 21:1557-1560, 2001.
125. Horton KM, Juluru K, Montgomery E, et al: Computed tomography imaging of gastrointestinal stromal tumors with pathologic correlation. J Comput Assist Tomogr 28:811-817, 2004.
126. Kim HC, Lee JM, Kim KW, et al: Gastrointestinal stromal tumors of the stomach: CT findings and prediction of malignancy. AJR 183:893-898, 2004.
127. McLeod AJ, Zornoza J, Shirkhoda A: Leiomyosarcoma: Computed tomographic findings. Radiology 52:133-136, 1984.
128. Megibow AJ, Balthazar EJ, Hulnick DH, et al: CT evaluation of gastrointestinal leiomyomas and leiomyosarcomas. AJR 144:727-733, 1985.
129. Disler DG, Chew FS: Gastric leiomyosarcoma. AJR 159:58, 1992.
130. Villanueva A, Perez C, Sabate JM, et al: CT manifestations of peritoneal leiomyosarcomatosis. Eur J Radiol 17:166-169, 1993.
131. Granmayeh M, Jonsson K, McFarland W, et al: Angiography of abdominal leiomyosarcoma. AJR 130:725-730, 1978.
132. Lee DH, Choi BI, Lee MG, et al: Exophytic adenocarcinoma of the stomach: CT findings. AJR 163:77-80, 1994.
133. Lo J, Sage MR, Paterson HS, et al: Gastric duplication in an adult. J Comput Assist Tomogr 7:328-330, 1983.
134. Hulnick DH, Balthazar EJ: Gastric duplication cyst: GI series and CT correlation. Gastrointest Radiol 12:106-108, 1987.
135. Pujari BD, Deadhare SG: Leiomyosarcoma of the duodenum. Int Surg 61:237-238, 1976.
136. McBrien MP, Garrett PEM: Leiomyosarcoma of the duodenum. Br J Surg 58:685-689, 1971.
137. Kanematsu M, Imaeda T, Iianuma G, et al: Leiomyosarcoma of the duodenum. Gastrointest Radiol 16:109-112, 1991.
138. Kim HC, Lee JM, Son KR, et al: Gastrointestinal stromal tumors of the duodenum: CT and barium study findings. AJR 183:415-419, 2004.
139. Hill CA, Harle TS, Mansell PWA: The prodrome, Kaposi sarcoma, and infections associated with acquired immunodeficiency syndrome: Radiologic findings in 39 patients. Radiology 149:393-399, 1983.
140. Wall SD, Friendman SL, Margulis AR: Gastrointestinal Kaposi's sarcoma in AIDS: Radiographic manifestations. J Clin Gastroenterol 6:165-171, 1984.
141. Friedman SL, Wright TL, Altman DF: Gastroenterology Kaposi's sarcoma with acquired immunodeficiency syndrome. Gastroenterology 89:102-108, 1985.
142. Henderson RG, Rahmatulla TD: An epidemic tumour. Br J Radiol 60:511-512, 1987.
143. Saltz RK, Kurtz RC, Lightdale CJ, et al: Kaposi's sarcoma: Gastrointestinal involvement correlation with skin findings and immunologic function. Dig Dis Sci 29:817-823, 1984.
144. Ell C, Matek W, Gramatzki M, et al: Endoscopic findings in a case of Kaposi's sarcoma with involvement of the large and small bowel. Endoscopy 17:161-164, 1985.
145. Lustbader I, Sherman A: Primary gastrointestinal Kaposi's sarcoma in a patient with acquired immune deficiency syndrome. Am J Gastroenterol 82:894-895, 1987.
146. Rose HS, Balthazar EJ, Megibow AJ, et al: Alimentary tract involvement in Kaposi sarcoma: Radiographic and endoscopic findings in 25 homosexual men. AJR 139:661-666, 1982.

147. Jaffe HW, Bregman DJ, Selik RM: Acquired immune deficiency syndrome in the United States: The first 1,000 cases. J Infect Dis 148:339-345, 1983.

148. Friedman SL: Gastrointestinal and hepatobiliary neoplasms in AIDS. Gastroenterol Clin North Am 17:465-486, 1988.

149. Balthazar EJ, Richman A: Kaposi's sarcoma of the stomach. Am J Gastroenterol 67:375-379, 1977.

150. Frager DH, Frager JD, Brandt LJ, et al: Gastrointestinal complications of AIDS: Radiologic features. Radiology 158:597-603, 1986.

151. Falcone S, Murphy BJ, Weinfeld A: Gastric manifestations of AIDS: Radiographic findings on upper gastrointestinal examination. Gastrointest Radiol 16:95-98, 1991.

152. Hadjiyane C, Lee YH, Stein L, et al: Kaposi's sarcoma presenting as linitis plastica. Am J Gastroenterol 86:1823-1825, 1991.

153. Leibman AJ, Gold BM: Gastric manifestations of autoimmune deficiency syndrome-related Kaposi's sarcoma on computed tomography. J Comput Tomogr 10:85-88, 1986.

154. Jeffrey RB Jr, Goodman PC, Olsen WL, et al: Radiologic imaging of AIDS. Curr Probl Diagn Radiol 17:73-117, 1988.

155. Jeffrey RB, Nyberg DA, Bottles K, et al: Abdominal CT in acquired immunodeficiency syndrome. AJR 146:7-13, 1986.

156. Herts BR, Megibow AJ, Birnbaum BA, et al: High attenuation lymphadenopathy in AIDS patients: Significance of findings on CT. Radiology 185:777-781, 1992.

157. Godwin JD: Carcinoid tumors: An analysis of 2837 cases. Cancer 36:560-569, 1975.

158. Balthazar EJ: Carcinoid tumors of the alimentary tract. Gastrointest Radiol 3:47-56, 1978.

159. Modlin IM, Tang LH: The gastric enterochromaffin-like cell: An enigmatic cellular link. Gastroenterology 111:783-810, 1996.

160. Modlin IM, Sandor A, Tang LH, et al: A 40-year analysis of 265 gastric carcinoids. Am J Gastroenterol 92:633-638, 1997.

161. Balthazar EJ, Megibow A, Bryk D: Gastric carcinoid tumors: Radiographic features in eight cases. AJR 139:1123-1127, 1982.

162. Rindi G, Luinetti O, Cornaggia M, et al: Three subtypes of gastric argyrophil carcinoid and the gastric neuroendocrine carcinoma: A clinicopathologic study. Gastroenterology 104:994-1006, 1993.

163. Berger MW, Stephens DH: Gastric carcinoid tumors associated with chronic hypergastrinemia in a patient with Zollinger-Ellison syndrome. Radiology 201:371-373, 1996.

164. Sculco D, Bilgrami S: Pernicious anemia and gastric carcinoid tumor: Case report and review. Am J Gastroenterol 92:1378-1380, 1997.

165. Levy AD, Taylor LD, Abbott RM, et al: Duodenal carcinoids: Imaging features with clinical-pathologic comparison. Radiology 237:967-972, 2005.

166. DeLuca RF, Ferrer JP, Gambescia RA, et al: Gastric carcinoid endoscopically simulating leiomyoma. Am J Gastroenterol 70:163-166, 1978.

167. Wengrower D, Fich A: Primary duodenal carcinoid. Am J Gastroenterol 82:1069-1070, 1987.

168. Abrams JS: Multiple malignant carcinoids of the stomach. Arch Surg 115:1219-1221, 1980.

169. Honig LJ, Weingarten G: A gastric carcinoid tumor with massive bleeding. Am J Gastroenterol 61:40-44, 1974.

170. Gueller R, Haddad JK: Gastric carcinoids simulating benign polyps. Gastrointest Endosc 21:153-155, 1975.

171. Syre-Smith G: Polypoid carcinoid tumor of the stomach. J Can Assoc Radiol 28:217-218, 1977.

172. Okeon MM, Bieber WP: Carcinoid tumor of the stomach resembling carcinoma. AJR 103:314-316, 1968.

173. Seymour EQ, Griffin CN, Kurtz SM: Carcinoid tumors of the duodenal cap presenting as multiple polypoid defects. Gastrointest Radiol 7:19-21, 1982.

174. Clements JL, Roche RR: Carcinoid of the duodenum: A report of six cases. Gastrointest Radiol 9:17-21, 1984.

175. Eschelman DJ, Duva-Frissora AD, Martin LC, et al: Metastatic carcinoid presenting as a duodenal mass. AJR 156:1301-1302, 1991.

176. Lopez-Negrete L, Luyando L, Sala J, et al: Liposarcoma of the stomach. Abdom Imaging 22:373-375, 1997.

177. Godard JE, Fox JE, Levinson MJ: Primary gastric plasmacytoma. Am J Dig Dis 18:508-512, 1973.

178. Yoon SE, Ha HK, Lee YS, et al: Upper gastrointestinal series and CT findings of primary gastric plasmacytoma: Report of two cases. AJR 173:1266-1268, 1999.

179. Pentimone F, Camici M, Cini G, et al: Duodenal plasmacytoma: A rare extramedullary location simulating a carcinoma. Acta Haematol 61:155-160, 1979.

180. Jindrak K, Bochetto JF, Alpert LI: Primary gastric choriocarcinoma. Hum Pathol 7:595-604, 1976.

181. Jain KA, Gerscovich EO, Goodnight JJ: Malignant autonomic nerve tumor of the duodenum. AJR 168:1461-1463, 1997.

182. Feingold ML, Goldstein MJ, Lieberman PH: Multiple myeloma involving the stomach: Report of a case with gastroscopic observations. Gastrointest Endosc 16:107-110, 1969.

183. Kwak HS, Jin GY, Lee JM: Radiologic findings of multiple myeloma with gastric involvement: A case report. Korean J Radiol 3:133-135, 2002.

184. Won OH, Farman J, Krishnan MN, et al: Squamous cell carcinoma of the stomach. Am J Gastroenterol 69:594-598, 1978.

185. Straus R, Heschel S, Fortmann DJ: Primary adenosquamous carcinoma of the stomach. Cancer 24:985-995, 1969.

Miscellaneous Abnormalities of the Stomach and Duodenum

Ronald L. Eisenberg, MD • Marc S. Levine, MD

VARICES

Gastric Varices

Pathophysiology

Portal Hypertension

The gastric fundus contains a venous plexus that is normally drained by numerous short gastric veins anastomosing distally with the splenic vein and proximally with branches of the coronary vein as well as venous channels surrounding the distal esophagus. Blood in the short gastric veins normally empties via the splenic vein into the portal venous system. In patients with portal hypertension, however, increased pressure in the portal and splenic veins leads to reversal of blood flow through the short gastric veins into the fundal venous plexus, producing fundal varices. As a result, gastric varices develop in

20% of patients with portal hypertension.[1] Because elevated portal pressure also causes reversal of flow through the coronary vein (producing uphill esophageal varices), some patients with portal hypertension have combined gastric and esophageal varices. However, others with portal hypertension have isolated gastric varices and an even greater number have isolated esophageal varices (see Chapter 29).

One explanation for the frequent failure to visualize gastric varices in patients with portal hypertension is that the venous channels in the gastric fundus have thicker, better connective tissue support than the thin-walled, loosely supported veins in the distal esophagus. As a result, varices may be more likely to form in the esophagus than in the stomach, despite comparable elevations in pressure. Even when gastric varices are present, they may be obscured on barium studies or endoscopy by overlying gastric rugae.

Splenic Vein Obstruction

In patients with splenic vein obstruction, increased pressure in the splenic vein beyond the obstruction leads to reversal of flow through the short gastric veins to the fundal plexus of veins, producing gastric varices. Because these patients have normal portal pressure, however, venous blood from the dilated fundal plexus can enter the portal venous system via the coronary vein without producing uphill esophageal varices. Unlike portal hypertension, splenic vein obstruction is therefore characterized by isolated varices in the gastric fundus without associated varices in the esophagus.

Splenic vein obstruction may result from intrinsic thrombosis or, more commonly, from extrinsic compression of the splenic vein by a variety of benign or malignant conditions, including pancreatitis, pancreatic pseudocysts, pancreatic carcinoma, metastatic disease, lymphoma, and retroperitoneal fibrosis or bleeding.[2-5] Intrinsic thrombosis of the splenic vein may be idiopathic or may result from polycythemia or other myeloproliferative disorders (see Chapter 92).[3]

Clinical Findings

Gastric varices are important because of the risk of gastrointestinal bleeding, which can range from low-grade, intermittent bleeding to massive hematemesis.[6,7] Gastric varices are less likely to bleed than esophageal varices because of their subserosal location and the greater thickness of overlying gastric tissue.[8] When gastric variceal bleeding occurs, however, it tends to be more severe than esophageal variceal bleeding and is associated with a higher mortality rate.[1] When gastric varices are associated with esophageal varices, affected individuals usually have the stigmata of portal hypertension. In contrast, patients with isolated gastric varices caused by splenic vein obstruction may present with abdominal pain and weight loss from underlying pancreatitis or pancreatic carcinoma.[3] Splenomegaly is also a frequent finding in splenic vein obstruction, but a normal-sized spleen does not exclude this condition.[9]

Radiographic Findings

Abdominal Radiographs

Large gastric varices may occasionally be recognized on chest or abdominal radiographs as one or more lobulated soft tissue densities in the gas-filled fundus. Depending on the cause of the varices (portal hypertension or splenic vein obstruction), abdominal radiographs may also reveal splenomegaly, ascites, or pancreatic calcification. When gastric varices are suspected on the basis of abdominal radiographs, barium studies or endoscopy should be performed for a more definitive diagnosis.

Barium Studies

Conventional single-contrast barium studies are thought to be unreliable for diagnosing gastric varices. Double-contrast technique has therefore been advocated to improve visualization of these structures.[5,10] Gastric varices may be recognized by the presence of thickened, tortuous folds or discrete, round submucosal filling defects in the gastric fundus, resembling the appearance of a bunch of grapes (Fig. 38-1).[3,5] Less frequently, a conglomerate mass of fundal varices, also known as tumorous gastric varices, may be manifested by a large polypoid mass that can be mistaken on barium studies for a polypoid carcinoma or even a malignant gastrointestinal stromal tumor (Figs. 38-2 and 38-3).[3,10-13] Tumorous varices have characteristic features, however, appearing in profile as smooth submucosal masses with an undulating contour and discrete borders on the posteromedial wall of the gastric fundus (see Figs. 38-2 and 38-3) and en face as thickened, tortuous folds that fade peripherally into the adjacent mucosa.[13] These radiographic features should allow differentiation from polypoid gastric neoplasms in most cases. Rarely, dilated gastroepiploic veins may be manifested by varices in the antrum or body of the stomach (Fig. 38-4).[14]

When gastric varices are detected on barium studies, it is important to determine whether uphill esophageal varices are also present in these patients. The presence of combined esophageal and gastric varices almost always indicates portal hypertension as the underlying cause. In contrast, the presence

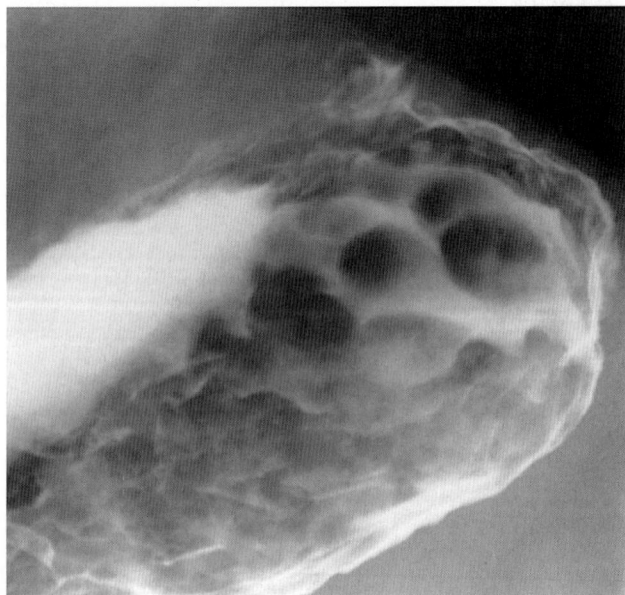

Figure 38-1. Gastric varices. Tortuous folds and submucosal filling defects are seen in the gastric fundus, resembling the appearance of a bunch of grapes. (From Levine MS, Kieu K, Rubesin SE, et al: Isolated gastric varices: Splenic vein obstruction or portal hypertension? Gastrointest Radiol 15:188-192, 1990. With kind permission from Springer Science and Business Media.)

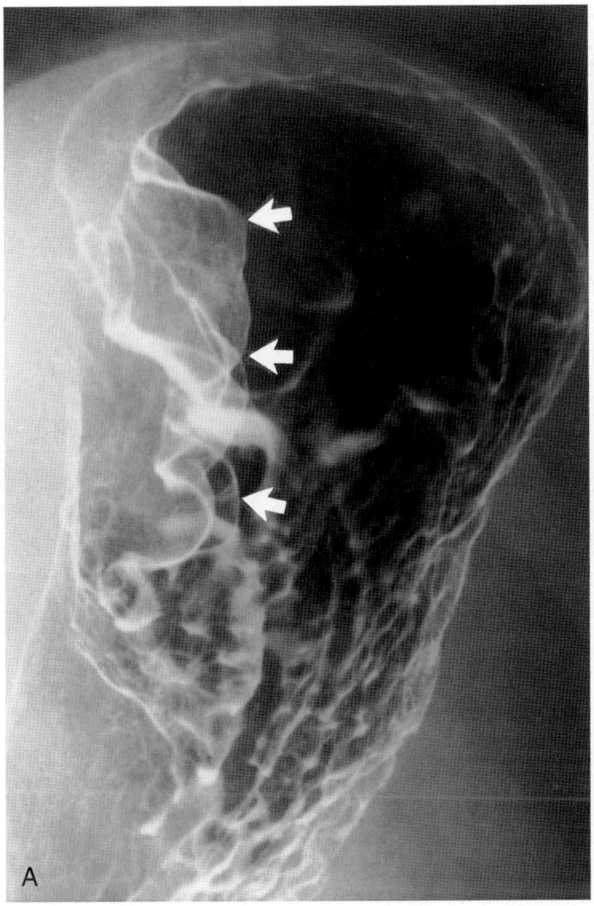

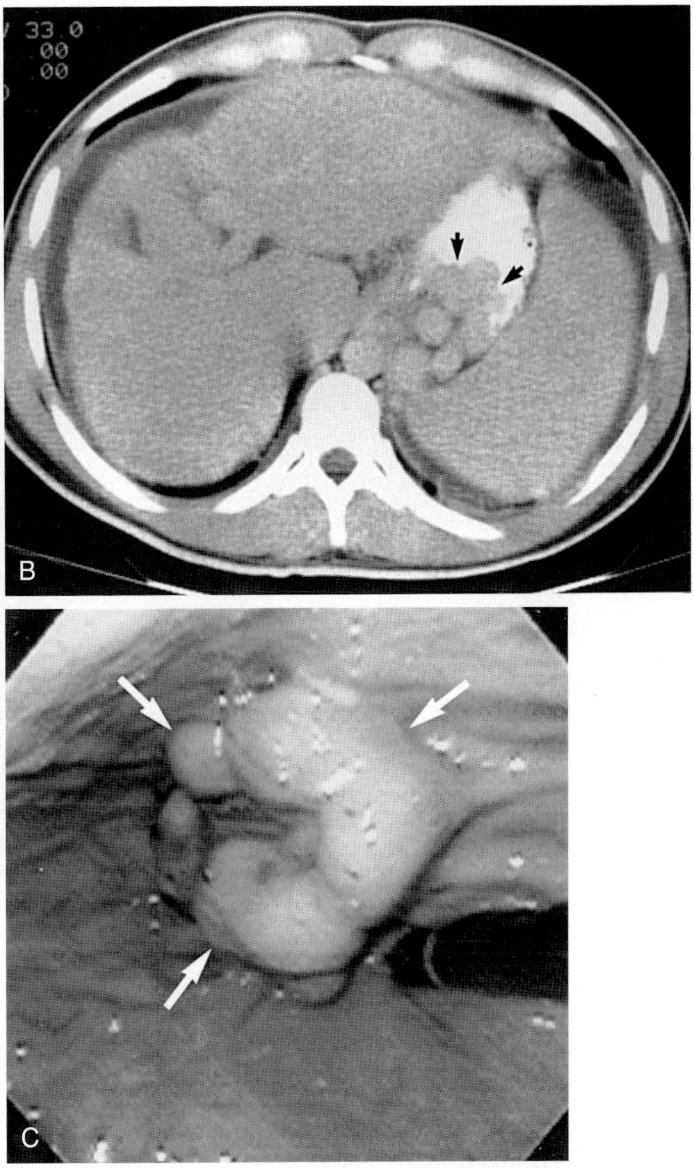

Figure 38-2. Conglomerate mass of gastric varices (also known as tumorous varices). A. Barium study shows a large, lobulated submucosal mass (*arrows*) on the medial aspect of the gastric fundus. Although this lesion could be mistaken for a malignant gastrointestinal stromal tumor or even a polypoid carcinoma, note its smooth, undulating contour. **B.** Unenhanced CT scan shows a lobulated soft tissue mass (*arrows*) on the posteromedial wall of the fundus. **C.** Endoscopic photograph shows a conglomerate mass of varices (*arrows*) in the gastric fundus adjacent to the cardia. This patient had underlying portal hypertension. (**B** and **C** from Levine MS, Kieu K, Rubesin SE, et al: Isolated gastric varices: Splenic vein obstruction or portal hypertension? Gastrointest Radiol 15:188-192, 1990. With kind permission from Springer Science and Business Media.)

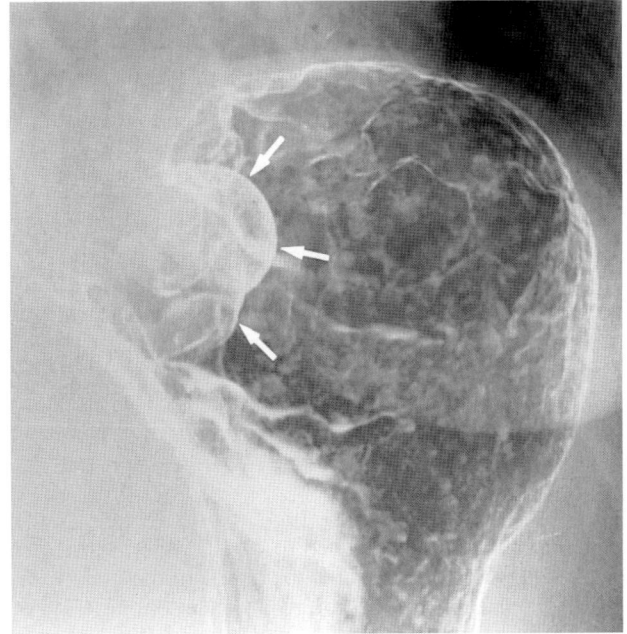

Figure 38-3. Conglomerate mass of isolated gastric varices due to splenic vein obstruction. A smooth, undulating mass (*arrows*) is seen on the posteromedial wall of the gastric fundus. Note the resemblance to the gastric varices in Figure 38-2. This patient had underlying pancreatitis causing splenic vein obstruction. (Courtesy of William M. Thompson, MD, Minneapolis, MN.)

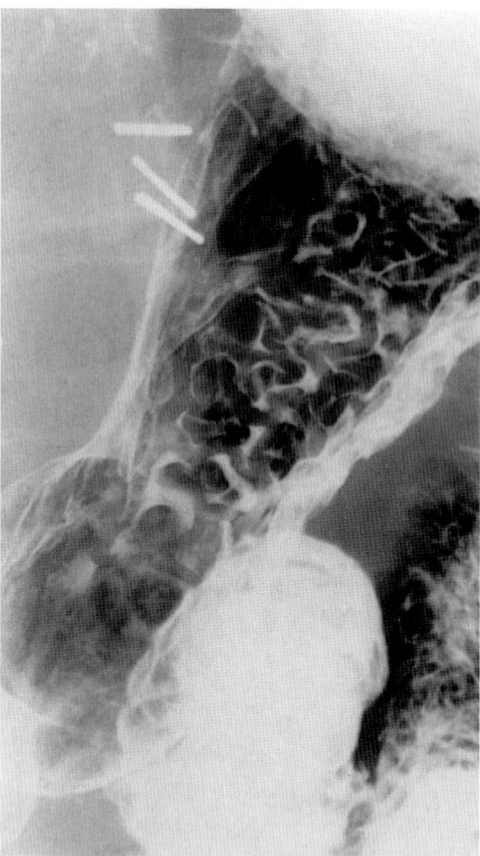

Figure 38-4. Nonfundal gastric varices. Thickened, tortuous folds are seen in the body of the stomach due to markedly dilated gastroepiploic veins. This patient had severe portal hypertension. (From Levine MS: Radiology of the Esophagus. Philadelphia, WB Saunders, 1989.)

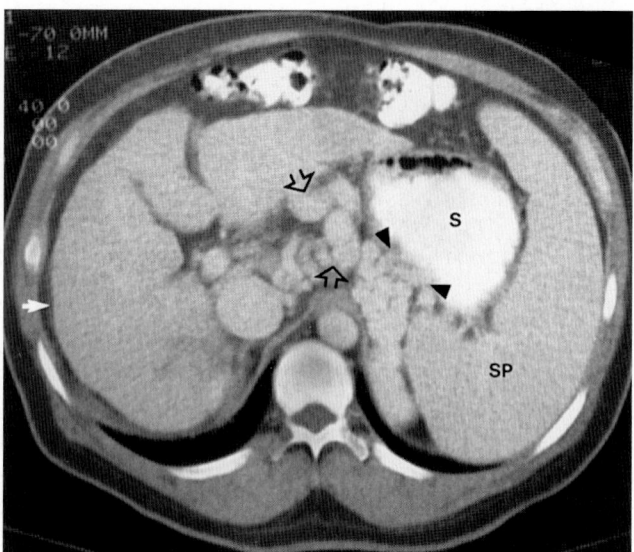

Figure 38-5. Gastric varices on CT. Enhancing collaterals are seen in the gastric wall (*arrowheads*), gastrohepatic ligament (*open arrows*), and left retroperitoneal space. This patient also has cirrhosis with splenomegaly and minimal ascites (*solid arrow*) due to portal hypertension. S, stomach; SP, spleen. (Courtesy of Richard M. Gore, MD, Evanston, IL.)

of isolated gastric varices should raise the possibility of splenic vein obstruction with a patent portal vein (see Fig. 38-3).[3,5] Nevertheless, portal hypertension is so much more common than splenic vein obstruction that most patients with gastric varices, even in the absence of esophageal varices, are found to have portal hypertension as the underlying cause (see Fig. 38-2).[15] If necessary, CT or angiography may be performed to document the presence of varices and elucidate their pathophysiology.

Computed Tomography

Gastric varices are usually recognized on CT as enhancing, well-defined, round or tubular densities on the posterior or posteromedial wall of the gastric fundus (Fig. 38-5).[16] CT is more sensitive than conventional radiologic examinations in detecting these lesions, because barium studies can only demonstrate varices that protrude into the lumen, whereas CT can delineate deeper intramural and perigastric varices.[16] CT may also reveal cirrhotic liver disease, splenomegaly, or ascites in patients with portal hypertension (see Fig. 38-5) and splenomegaly or pancreatic disease in patients with splenic vein obstruction.

Angiography

Angiography may be performed to confirm the presence of gastric varices and to determine the nature of the underlying venous abnormality. With portal hypertension, reversal of

flow through the coronary and short gastric veins leads to the formation of esophageal and gastric varices, with absent visualization of the portal and splenic veins. With splenic vein obstruction, however, delayed images reveal normal filling of a patent portal vein without evidence of esophageal varices, as blood is diverted from the fundal plexus of veins via the coronary vein to the portal venous system, bypassing the obstructed splenic vein (Fig. 38-6). Thus, portal hypertension can usually be differentiated from splenic vein obstruction by angiography, so that appropriate therapy can be instituted in these patients.

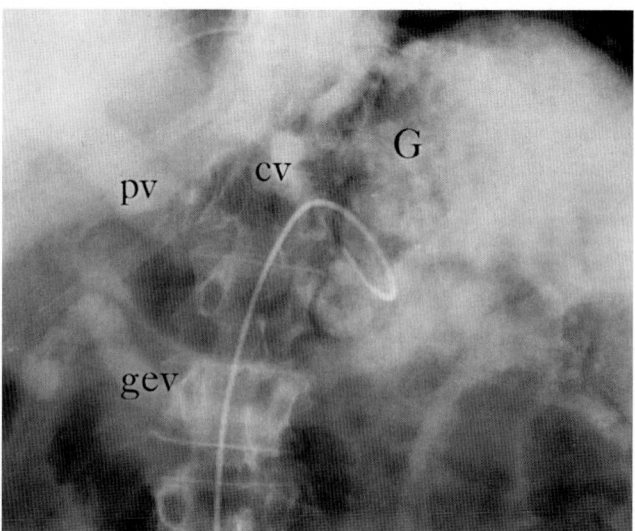

Figure 38-6. Angiographic demonstration of gastric varices due to splenic vein obstruction. Image from the venous phase of a splenic arteriogram shows a densely opacified spleen with absent visualization of the splenic vein, extensive gastric varices (G), and a dilated coronary vein (cv) diverting blood from the fundal plexus of veins to the portal vein (pv). Note the presence of a dilated gastroepiploic vein (gev). (Courtesy of Dana R. Burke, MD, Bethesda, MD.)

Differential Diagnosis

When gastric varices are manifested on barium studies by thickened, nodular folds in the fundus, the differential diagnosis includes *Helicobacter pylori* gastritis, Ménétrier's disease, Zollinger-Ellison syndrome, pancreatitis, and lymphoma.[17] However, varices tend to be more tortuous or lobulated, and they are often associated with esophageal varices. Less frequently, a conglomerate mass of fundal varices may resemble a polypoid carcinoma or even a malignant gastrointestinal stromal tumor (see Figs. 38-2 and 38-3).[3,10-13] However, the vascular origin of these lesions is suggested by their smooth, undulating contour and typical location on the posteromedial wall of the gastric fundus. CT or angiography may be required for a definitive diagnosis. It is particularly important to differentiate gastric varices from other lesions before performing endoscopic biopsy or surgery, because inadvertent perforation of a varix may lead to catastrophic gastrointestinal bleeding.

Treatment

Emergent treatment for bleeding gastric varices is rarely necessary. When major bleeding does occur in patients with splenic vein obstruction, the patients are almost always cured by simple splenectomy, because portal venous pressure is normal in these individuals.[18] In contrast, some form of portosystemic shunt may be required for gastric varices caused by portal hypertension because splenectomy alone has no effect on portal venous pressure in these patients. Thus, the choice of treatment for gastric varices depends on the underlying cause.

Duodenal Varices

Duodenal varices typically appear on barium studies as thickened, serpiginous folds in the proximal duodenum (Fig. 38-7). They are almost always associated with esophageal varices and may be complicated by gastrointestinal bleeding. Occasionally, an isolated duodenal varix can present as a solitary filling defect.[19]

PORTAL HYPERTENSIVE GASTROPATHY

Portal hypertensive gastropathy is a distinct pathologic entity caused by chronic portal hypertension.[20] Chronic venous congestion in the stomach results in mucosal hyperemia, capillary ectasia, and increased numbers of submucosal arteriovenous communications, with dilated arterioles, capillaries, and veins in the gastric wall.[21] For reasons that are unclear, portal hypertensive gastropathy occurs more frequently in patients with cirrhosis than in other patients with portal hypertension. This condition has important clinical implications because it is a cause of both acute and chronic upper gastrointestinal bleeding even in the absence of esophageal or gastric varices. It has been estimated that nonvariceal bleeding from portal hypertensive gastropathy is responsible for up to 30% of all cases of upper gastrointestinal bleeding in patients with portal hypertension.[22]

Radiographic Findings

Portal hypertensive gastropathy predominantly involves the gastric fundus and is manifested on barium studies by thickened, nodular folds with undulating contours and indistinct borders (Fig. 38-8).[23] Although the pathophysiologic basis for this fold thickening is uncertain, it could result from a

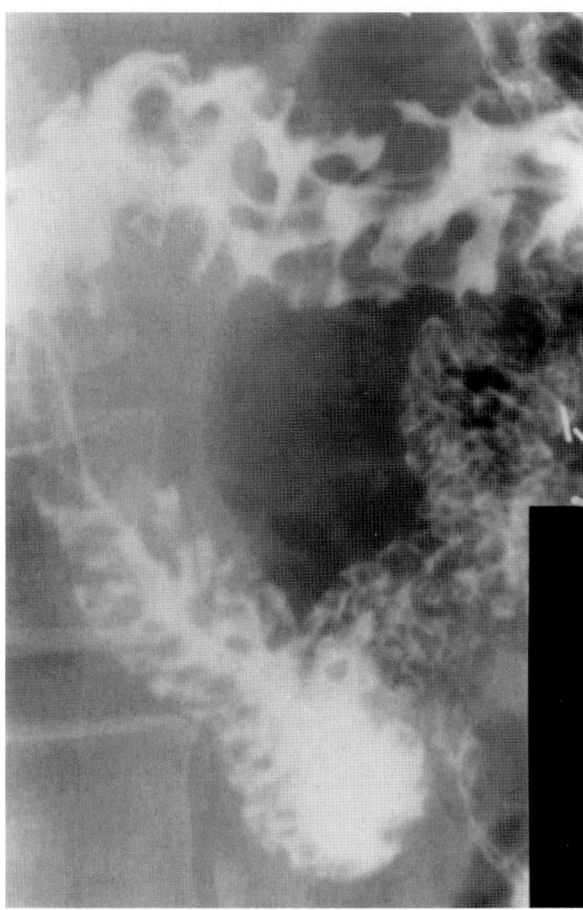

Figure 38-7. Duodenal varices. Thickened, serpiginous folds are seen in the proximal descending duodenum.

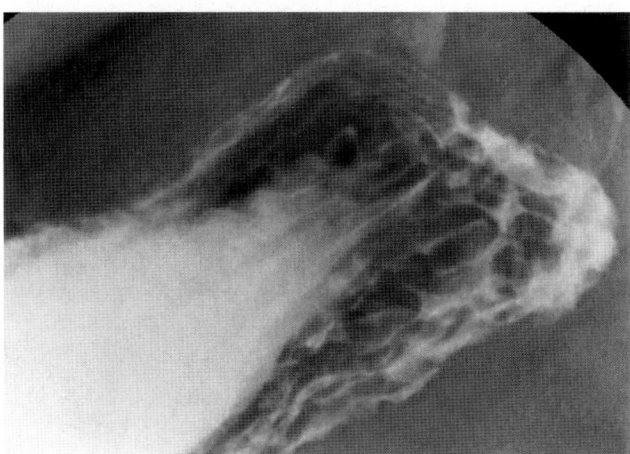

Figure 38-8. Portal hypertensive gastropathy. Thickened, nodular folds are seen in the gastric fundus. Note how the folds have an undulating contour and indistinct borders. Although gastric varices could produce a similar appearance, they tend to have a more serpentine configuration and are often associated with discrete submucosal masses (see Fig. 38-1). (From Chang D, Levine MS, Ginsberg GG, et al: Portal hypertensive gastropathy: Radiographic findings in eight patients. AJR 175:1609-1612, 2000, © by American Roentgen Ray Society.)

combination of mucosal hyperemia and dilated submucosal vessels. Gastric varices may also appear as thickened folds on barium studies, but the folds tend to have a more serpentine configuration and are often associated with discrete submucosal masses (see Fig. 38-1). The differential diagnosis also includes various forms of gastritis (especially *H. pylori* gastritis), lymphoma, and, rarely, Ménétrier's disease.

DIVERTICULA

Gastric Diverticula

Gastric diverticula almost always arise from the posterior wall of the fundus and usually cause no symptoms. A large gastric diverticulum that fails to fill with gas or barium can mimic a smooth-bordered submucosal mass. On further examination, barium is usually seen to enter the diverticulum, establishing the correct diagnosis (Fig. 38-9). A collection of barium may sometimes pool within a gastric diverticulum, mimicking an area of ulceration (see Fig. 38-9).

Intramural or partial gastric diverticulum is a rare anomaly of no clinical significance that is characterized by focal invagination of the mucosa into the muscular layer of the gastric wall.[24] These structures are almost always located on the greater curvature of the distal antrum. The diverticulum may be manifested on barium studies by a tiny collection of barium extending outside the contour of the adjacent gastric wall (Fig. 38-10). Although these structures can be mistaken for ulcers or even ectopic pancreatic rests on the greater curvature, they tend to have a changeable configuration at fluoroscopy, whereas true ulcers will have a fixed appearance.

Duodenal Diverticula

True Diverticula

Duodenal diverticula are detected as incidental findings on barium studies of the upper gastrointestinal tract in up to 15%

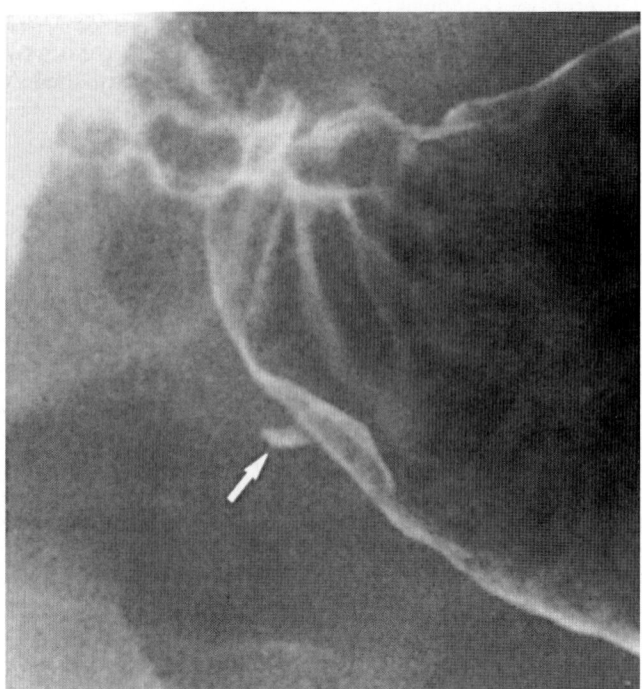

Figure 38-10. Intramural or partial gastric diverticulum. A tiny, barium-filled outpouching (*arrow*) is seen on the greater curvature of the distal antrum. There is a heaped-up area overlying the diverticulum that could be mistaken for an ectopic pancreatic rest.

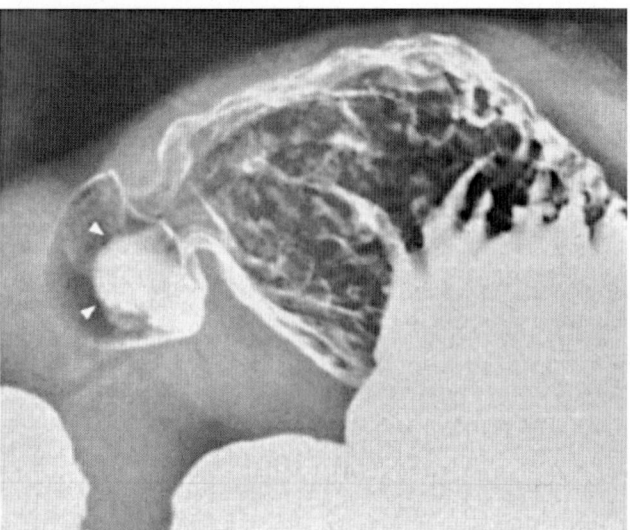

Figure 38-9. Gastric diverticulum. A large diverticulum is seen arising from the posterior wall of the fundus. Pooling of barium (*arrowheads*) in the diverticulum could be mistaken for an area of ulceration. (From Eisenberg RL: Gastrointestinal Radiology: A Pattern Approach, 3rd ed. Philadelphia, JB Lippincott, 1996.)

of patients. The diverticula are acquired lesions, consisting of a sac of mucosal and submucosal layers herniating through a muscular defect. These diverticula often fill and empty by gravity as a result of pressure generated by duodenal peristalsis. Most duodenal diverticula are located on the medial border of the descending duodenum in the periampullary region (Fig. 38-11), but they not infrequently are found in the third or fourth portion of the duodenum and can even occur on the lateral border of the descending duodenum (Fig. 38-12).

Duodenal diverticula typically appear on barium studies as smooth, round or ovoid outpouchings arising on a discrete neck from the medial border of the descending duodenum (see Fig. 38-11). They are often multiple and may change configuration during the course of the study. The lack of inflammatory reaction (i.e., spasm or edema) allows a duodenal diverticulum to be differentiated from a postbulbar ulcer. Bizarre, multilobulated or giant diverticula are occasionally seen.[25] Filling defects representing inspissated food particles or blood clots can sometimes be found within the diverticulum (Fig. 38-13).

When duodenal diverticula contain gas or a combination of fluid and gas, they are readily visible on CT. However, a diverticulum that is predominantly fluid filled can occasionally mimic the CT findings of a cystic neoplasm in the head of the pancreas (Fig. 38-14A).[26] The correct diagnosis can still be established, however, if intradiverticular gas is identified (Fig. 38-14B).[26]

More than 90% of patients with duodenal diverticula are asymptomatic.[27] Occasionally, however, these patients may develop serious complications such as duodenal diverticulitis, upper gastrointestinal bleeding, gastric outlet obstruction, and pancreaticobiliary disease. Duodenal diverticulitis can mimic

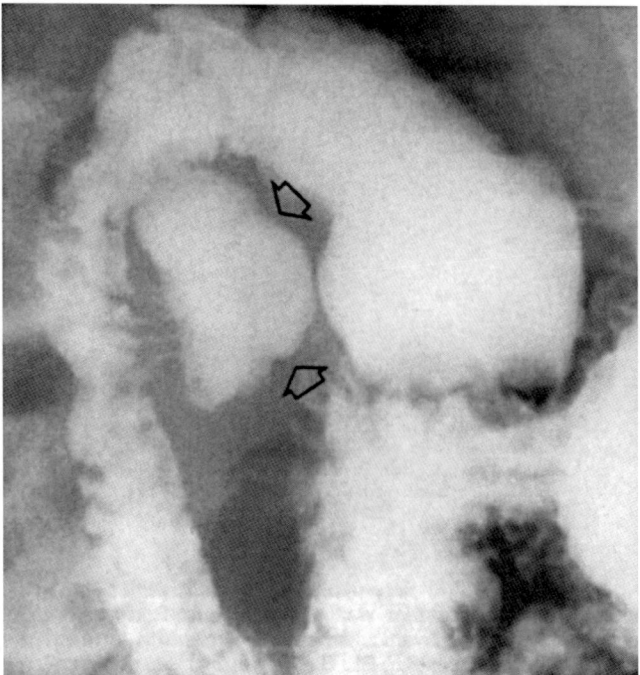

Figure 38-11. Duodenal diverticulum. A typical diverticulum (*arrows*) is seen arising from the medial border of the descending duodenum. (From Eisenberg RL: Gastrointestinal Radiology: A Pattern Approach, 3rd ed. Philadelphia, JB Lippincott, 1996.)

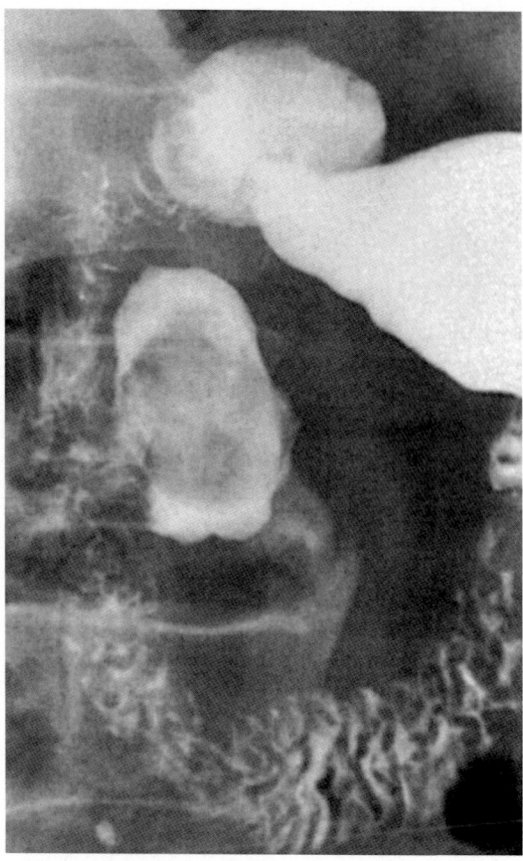

Figure 38-13. Duodenal diverticulum with a blood clot. This diverticulum contains a large, irregular filling defect representing a blood clot in a patient with recent upper gastrointestinal bleeding. (From Eisenberg RL: Gastrointestinal Radiology: A Pattern Approach, 3rd ed. Philadelphia, JB Lippincott, 1996.)

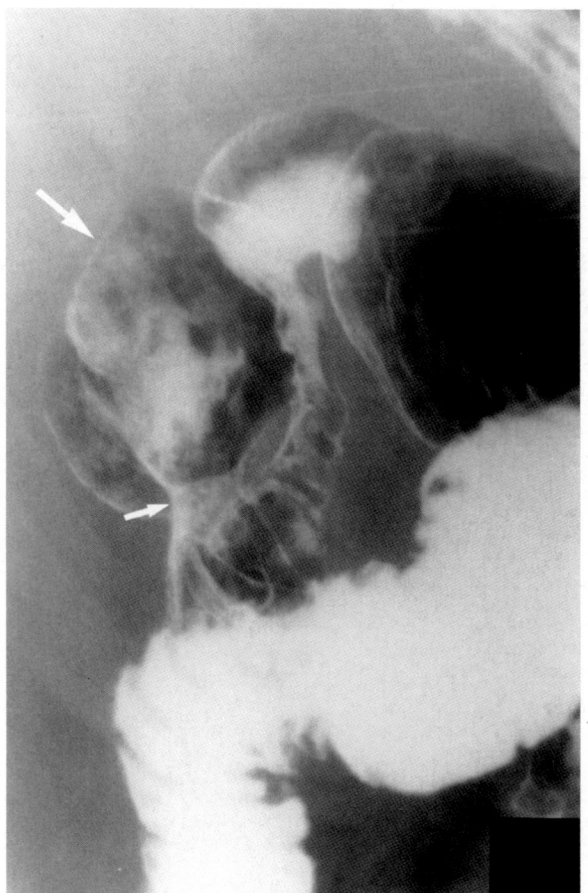

Figure 38-12. Lateral duodenal diverticulum. A diverticulum (*large arrow*) is seen arising from the lateral border of the descending duodenum. Note how the diverticulum has a discrete neck (*small arrow*). Also note how the diverticulum is compressing the adjacent duodenum.

other acute abdominal conditions such as cholecystitis, peptic ulcer disease, and pancreatitis; it is therefore a diagnosis of exclusion. Because duodenal diverticula are retroperitoneal structures, perforation can occur without clinical signs of peritonitis or radiographic signs of free intraperitoneal air. Instead, abdominal radiographs may reveal localized retroperitoneal gas adjacent to the duodenum and the upper pole of the right kidney.[28] Studies with barium or water-soluble contrast agents may demonstrate extravasation of contrast material from the perforated diverticulum or a deformed diverticulum representing the site of a sealed-off perforation.[29] CT is particularly helpful for showing a contained perforation or inflammatory changes involving adjacent structures.[30]

Rarely, duodenal diverticula may cause massive upper gastrointestinal bleeding.[31] In such cases, scanning with technetium Tc 99m–labeled red blood cells or angiography may be required to localize the site of bleeding.[31] Duodenal diverticula have also been described as a rare cause of duodenal or even biliary obstruction. Anomalous insertion of the common bile duct and pancreatic duct into a duodenal diverticulum can be demonstrated in about 3% of carefully performed T-tube cholangiograms.[32] This anatomic arrangement appears to interfere with the normal emptying mechanisms of the ductal systems, predisposing these patients to biliary obstruction, bile duct stones, and pancreatitis.

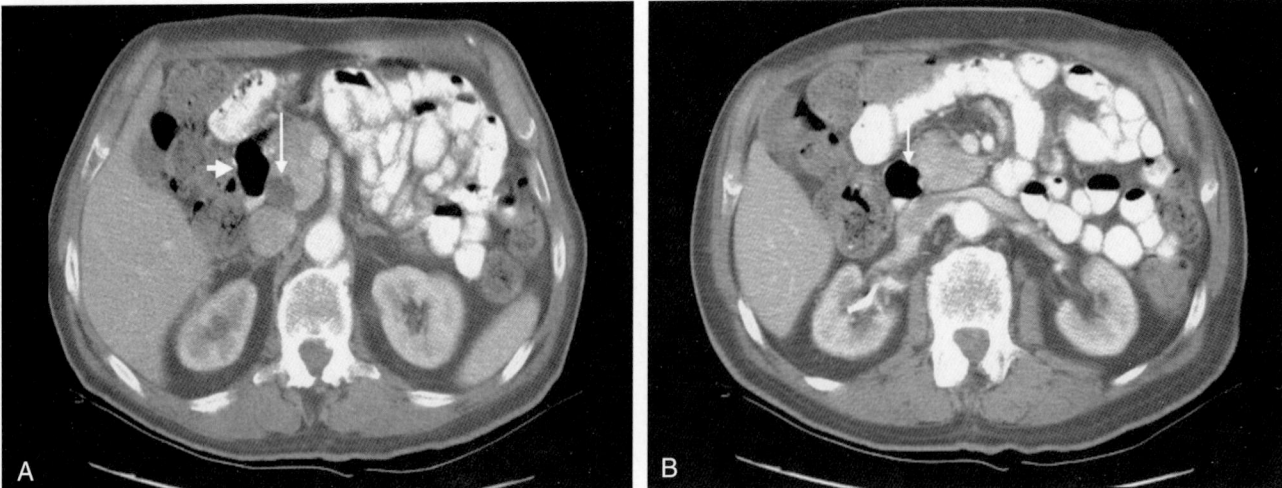

Figure 38-14. Duodenal diverticulum mimicking a cystic pancreatic neoplasm on CT. A. CT scan with oral and intravenous contrast material at the level of the pancreatic head shows a fluid-filled cystic lesion (*long arrow*) that was initially thought to represent a cystic pancreatic tumor. Note air and contrast material in the duodenum (*short arrow*). **B.** A follow-up CT scan at a similar level 6 months later shows filling of the diverticulum with gas (*arrow*), confirming the diagnosis of a duodenal diverticulum. (From Macari M, Lazarus D, Israel G, et al: Duodenal diverticula mimicking cystic neoplasms of the pancreas: CT and MR imaging findings in seven patients. AJR 180:195-199, 2003, © by American Roentgen Ray Society.)

Pseudodiverticula

Pseudodiverticula are exaggerated outpouchings or sacculations of the inferior and superior recesses of the duodenal bulb related to acute or chronic duodenal ulcer disease (Fig. 38-15). The sacculations may be caused by edema and spasm associated with an active ulcer or by asymmetric fibrosis and retraction associated with scarring from a healed ulcer. The degree of deformity, however, is not directly related to ulcer size; small ulcers may produce large sacculations, whereas large ulcers may produce little or no alteration in the contour of the bulb.

Intraluminal Diverticula

An intraluminal duodenal diverticulum is a sac of duodenal mucosa originating in the second portion of the duodenum near the papilla of Vater. The diverticulum forms from a congenital duodenal web or diaphragm that gradually elongates intraluminally over time as a result of mechanical factors such as forward pressure by food and duodenal peristalsis.[33] When filled with barium, an intraluminal duodenal diverticulum appears on barium studies as a finger-like sac separated from barium in the adjacent duodenal lumen by a radiolucent band representing the wall of the diverticulum (the "halo" sign) (Fig. 38-16).[33] CT may also be useful for showing these blind-ending saccular structures.[34]

Both intraluminal duodenal diverticula and congenital duodenal diaphragms can be associated with other anomalies, including annular pancreas, midgut volvulus, situs inversus, choledochocele, congenital heart disease, Down syndrome, imperforate anus, Hirschsprung's disease, omphalocele, hypoplastic kidneys, and exstrophy of the bladder.

Patients with intraluminal duodenal diverticula may sometimes develop nausea and vomiting from associated duodenal obstruction.[33] The usual treatment is surgery, but some patients have benefited from endoscopic incision of these structures.[33]

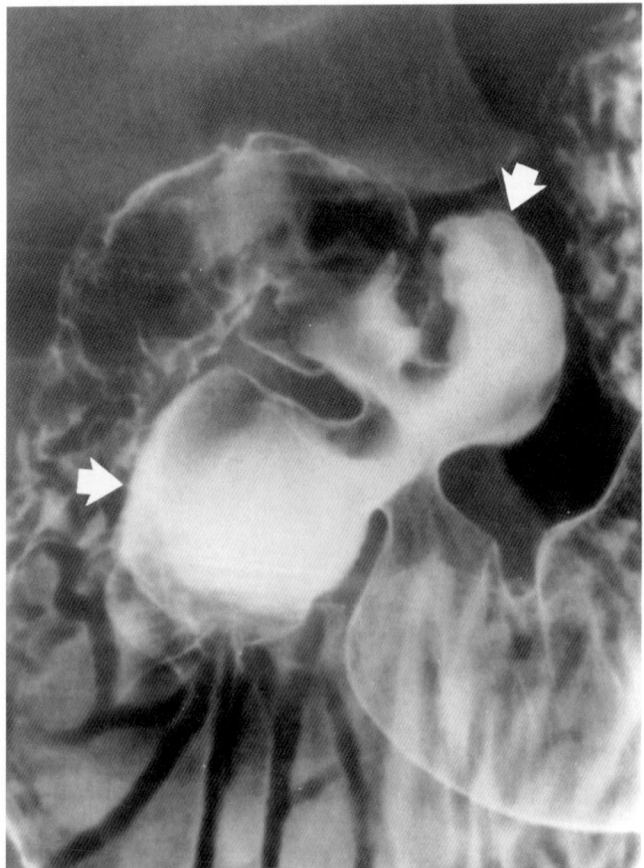

Figure 38-15. Duodenal pseudodiverticula. Two exaggerated outpouchings or pseudodiverticula (*arrows*) are seen at the base of the bulb due to scarring from previous peptic ulcer disease.

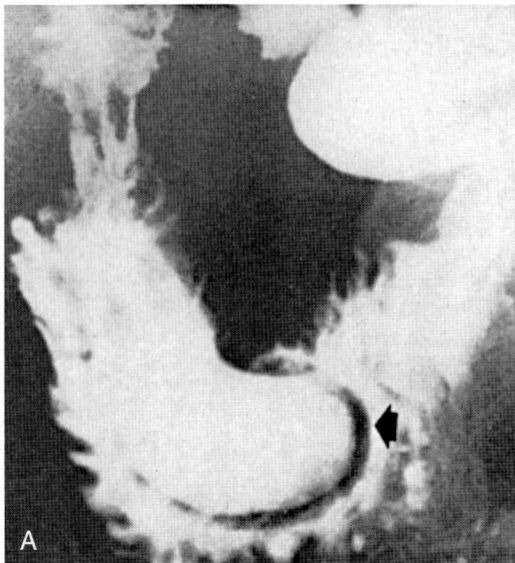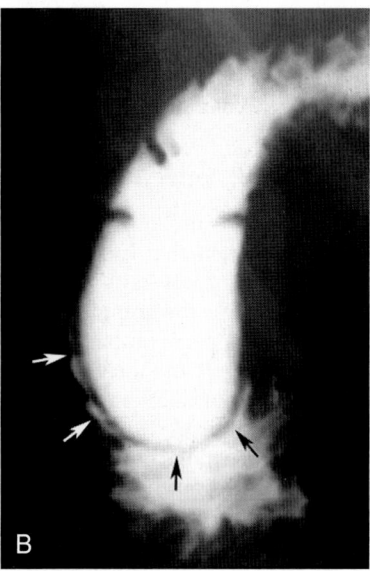

Figure 38-16. Intraluminal duodenal diverticulum. A and **B.** In both patients, the intraluminal finger-like sacs are separated from barium in the adjacent duodenal lumen by a radiolucent band (*arrows*) representing the wall of the diverticulum. (**A** from Laudan JCH, Norton GI: Intraluminal duodenal diverticulum. AJR 90:756-760, 1963, © by American Roentgen Ray Society.)

WEBS AND DIAPHRAGMS

Antral Webs and Diaphragms

Antral webs and diaphragms are thin, membranous septa that are usually located within 3 cm of the pyloric canal and are oriented perpendicular to the long axis of the stomach.[35] Clinical symptoms of partial gastric outlet obstruction (epigastric pain, fullness, and vomiting, particularly after a heavy meal) correlate with the size of the central aperture of the web or diaphragm. Symptoms of obstruction do not occur if the diameter of the aperture is greater than 1 cm. Even with minute central orifices as small as 2 mm, these diaphragms may not cause obstructive symptoms until adult life.

Nonobstructive antral webs and diaphragms appear on barium studies as persistent, sharply defined, 2- to 3-cm-wide bandlike defects in the barium column occurring at right angles to the gastric wall (Fig. 38-17).[35] A similar appearance may be produced by a prominent transverse antral fold, but transverse folds do not generally extend across the gastric lumen, and they are not perfectly straight. Antral webs and diaphragms are best visualized when the antrum is adequately distended proximal and distal to this structure. Occasionally, the antrum distal to the web can be mistaken radiographically for the duodenal bulb (Fig. 38-18). The distal antrum can also be mistaken for a gastric diverticulum or ulcer. On close inspection, however, it clearly lies within the

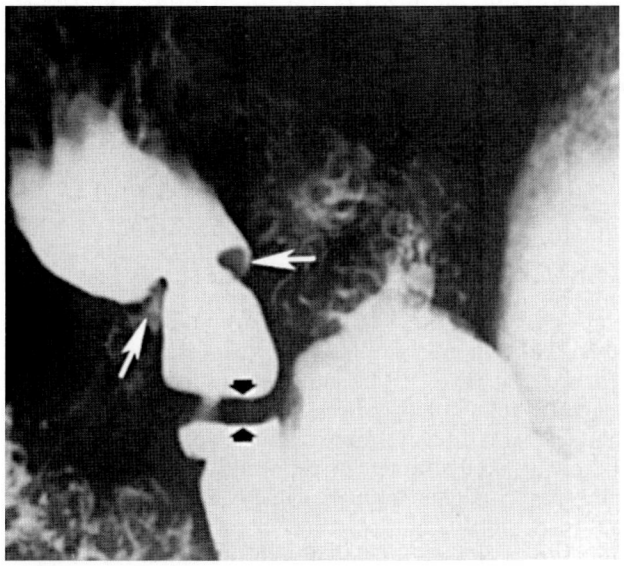

Figure 38-17. Antral mucosal diaphragm. A bandlike defect (*black arrows*) is seen arising at right angles to the gastric wall. The web is approximately 5 mm in thickness. The pyloric channel is denoted by *white arrows*. (From Bjorgvinsson E, Rudzki C, Lewicki AM: Antral web. Am J Gastroenterol 79:663-665, 1984, © by The American College of Gastroenterology.)

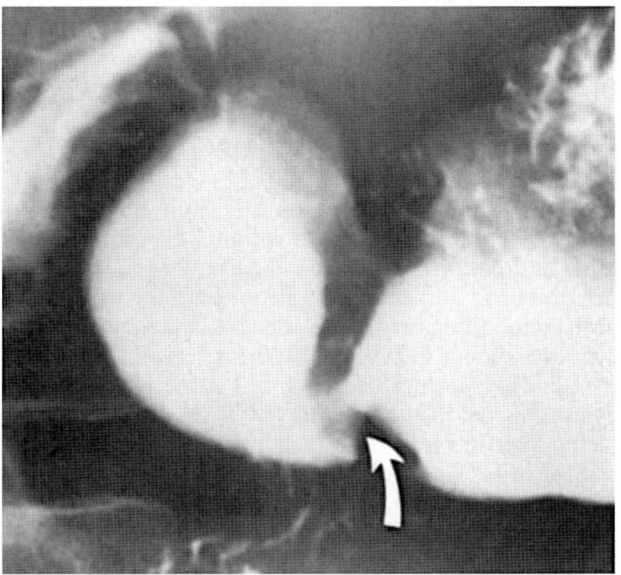

Figure 38-18. Antral mucosal diaphragm. The lumen is so narrowed by the diaphragm (*arrow*) that the antrum distal to the diaphragm could be mistaken for the duodenal bulb. (From Eisenberg RL: Gastrointestinal Radiology: A Pattern Approach, 3rd ed. Philadelphia, JB Lippincott, 1996.)

expected contour of the stomach and changes in size and shape at fluoroscopy.[35] With severe obstruction, gastric emptying is greatly delayed, and barium can be seen to pass in a thin stream (jet phenomenon) through the center of the orifice.[36]

Duodenal Webs and Diaphragms

Duodenal webs and diaphragms are weblike projections in the duodenal lumen that cause varying degrees of obstruction. Most reported cases have involved the second portion of the duodenum near the ampulla of Vater. A congenital duodenal web usually appears on barium studies as a thin, radiolucent line extending across the lumen, often associated with proximal duodenal dilatation (Fig. 38-19). Because the obstruction is incomplete, small amounts of gas may be present in more distal portions of the bowel.[37] Rarely, a web may balloon distally, forming an intraluminal duodenal diverticulum (see earlier section on Intraluminal Diverticula). Although the vast majority of duodenal webs and diaphragms are thought to be congenital, acquired duodenal diaphragms similar to those in the small bowel have been described as a rare complication of long-term use of nonsteroidal antiinflammatory drugs.[38]

ADULT HYPERTROPHIC PYLORIC STENOSIS

The histologic, anatomic, and radiographic abnormalities in adult hypertrophic pyloric stenosis are indistinguishable from those in the infantile form.[39] In fact, the disease in adults may represent a milder form of the same entity observed in infants and children. Most cases of adult hypertrophic pyloric stenosis go unrecognized because these individuals are asymptomatic. However, some patients complain of nausea and vomiting, epigastric pain, weight loss, or anorexia. Approximately 50%

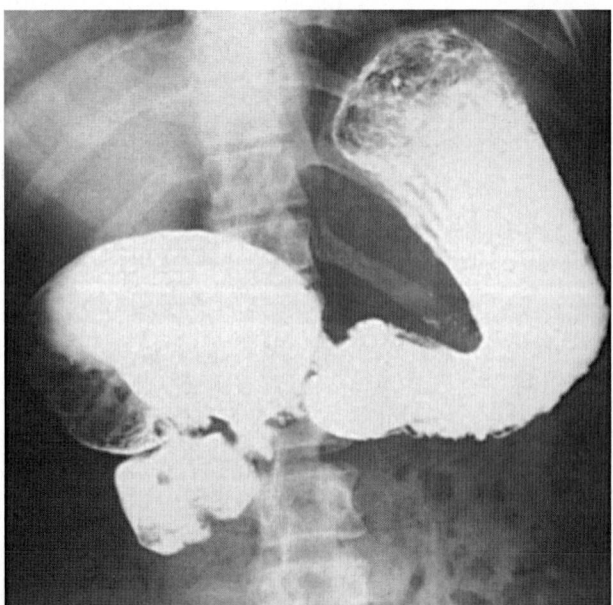

Figure 38-19. Duodenal web. There is high-grade stenosis of the second portion of the duodenum. The presence of gas in the bowel distal to the web indicates that the obstruction is incomplete. (From Eisenberg RL: Gastrointestinal Radiology: A Pattern Approach, 3rd ed. Philadelphia, JB Lippincott, 1996.)

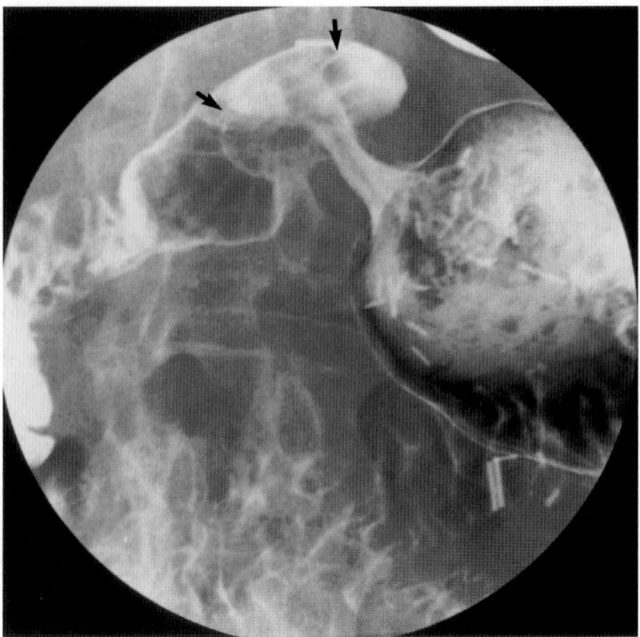

Figure 38-20. Adult hypertrophic pyloric stenosis. The pyloric canal is narrowed and elongated with a characteristic concave indentation (*arrows*) on the base of the duodenal bulb due to bulging of the pyloric muscle mass into the duodenum.

of patients with adult hypertrophic pyloric stenosis have associated gastric ulcers. These ulcers probably develop as a result of delayed gastric emptying with increased gastrin production and hyperacidity. In contrast to children, adults with this condition rarely develop high-grade gastric outlet obstruction.

Adult hypertrophic pyloric stenosis is typically manifested on barium studies by elongation and narrowing of the pyloric canal (Fig. 38-20).[39] The pylorus can measure 2 to 4 cm in length (the normal length is less than 1 cm in adults). The pylorus is also narrowed as a result of hypertrophy of the musculature. The proximal end of the narrowed pylorus merges gradually with the adjacent antrum, producing a smooth, tapered juncture without the shoulders expected for a malignant neoplasm. In contrast, the distal end of the hypertrophied pyloric muscle may bulge into the duodenum, producing a distinctive concave indentation on the base of the duodenal bulb (see Fig. 38-20).[39]

GASTRIC OUTLET OBSTRUCTION

Peptic ulcer disease is by far the most common cause of gastric outlet obstruction in adults, accounting for about two thirds of cases (Fig. 38-21). The ulcers are usually located in the duodenal bulb, but they may also be located in the pyloric channel or gastric antrum or, rarely, in the gastric body. Narrowing of the lumen in peptic ulcer disease can result from spasm, acute inflammation and edema, muscular hypertrophy, or fibrosis and scarring. In many cases, more than one of these factors contribute to the development of gastric outlet obstruction. Most patients with peptic ulcer disease causing pyloric obstruction have a long-standing history of ulcer symptoms. A gastric carcinoma should therefore be suspected when gastric outlet obstruction develops in previously asymptomatic patients.

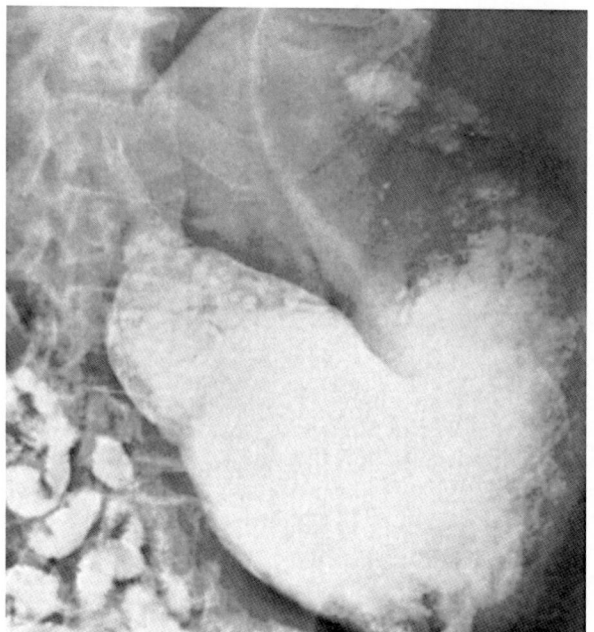

Figure 38-21. Gastric outlet obstruction caused by peptic ulcer disease. Note gastric distention and dilution of the barium by retained fluid in the stomach. (From Eisenberg RL: Gastrointestinal Radiology: A Pattern Approach, 3rd ed. Philadelphia, JB Lippincott, 1996.)

An annular carcinoma of the distal antrum or pylorus is the second most common cause of gastric outlet obstruction, accounting for nearly one third of cases (Fig. 38-22). Occasionally, metastases to the stomach or other malignant tumors also produce obstructive symptoms. In contrast to patients with peptic ulcer disease, patients with gastric outlet obstruction caused by malignant tumors may have recent onset of abdominal pain and weight loss.[40]

Abdominal radiographs in patients with gastric outlet obstruction often demonstrate the outline of the dilated, gas-filled stomach. Barium studies may reveal a mottled density of nonopaque material representing retained food and debris in the stomach. Depending on the degree of obstruction, there may be a marked delay in gastric emptying, with barium sometimes retained in the stomach for 24 hours or longer. Over time, the stomach may become enormously dilated, extending inferiorly into the lower abdomen or even the pelvis. In patients with gastric outlet obstruction, the radiologist must always attempt to differentiate a benign lesion (e.g., peptic ulcer disease) from a malignant lesion (e.g., gastric carcinoma) as the cause of obstruction on barium studies. The presence of a persistent collection of barium within the duodenal bulb, the pyloric channel, or the prepyloric gastric antrum should suggest peptic ulcer disease as the likely cause of obstruction. Distortion and scarring of the bulb with associated pseudodiverticula should also suggest ulcer disease as the likely cause of obstruction. Conversely, the presence of a discrete mass, nodularity, or irregularity in the adjacent antrum should suggest a malignant tumor. Nevertheless, it is not always possible to differentiate benign and malignant cases of gastric outlet obstruction on radiographic criteria. When gastric carcinoma cannot be excluded, endoscopy or even surgical exploration may be required for a definitive diagnosis.

Gastric outlet obstruction may occasionally be caused by other conditions involving the stomach and duodenum. Granulomatous diseases such as Crohn's disease, sarcoidosis, syphilis, and tuberculosis may cause marked antral narrowing and obstruction (Fig. 38-23). Severe pancreatitis or cholecystitis may cause intense spasm and edema of the adjacent duodenum with associated gastric outlet obstruction.[41] Antral narrowing and obstruction may also be caused by other rare conditions such as amyloidosis (see later section on Amyloidosis) and scarring from previous ingestion of corrosive substances.

Prolapse of a benign antral polyp into the duodenum may occasionally produce intermittent gastric outlet obstruction,

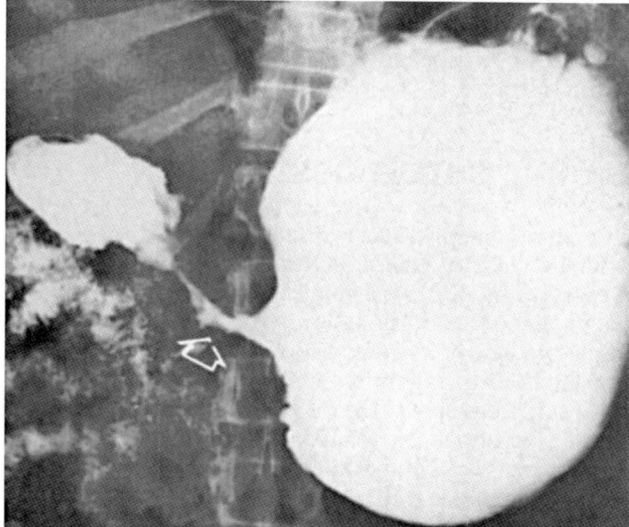

Figure 38-22. Gastric outlet obstruction caused by an annular carcinoma of the antrum. There is irregular narrowing of the distal antrum (*arrow*) with proximal dilatation of the stomach. (From Eisenberg RL: Gastrointestinal Radiology: A Pattern Approach, 3rd ed. Philadelphia, JB Lippincott, 1996.)

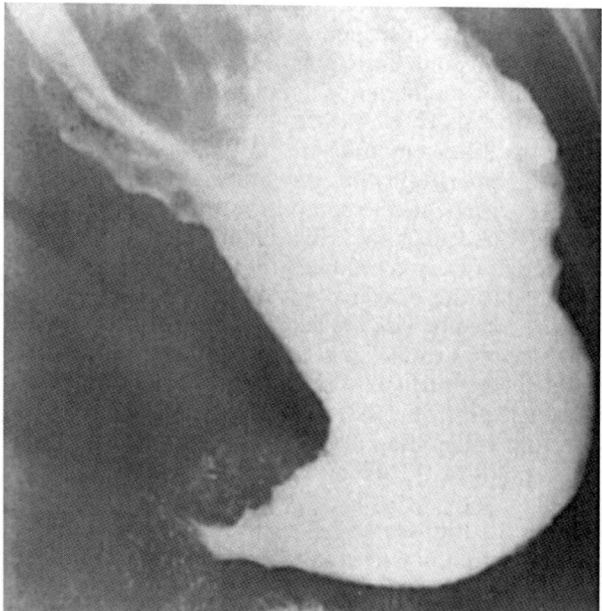

Figure 38-23. Gastric outlet obstruction caused by Crohn's disease. There is tapered narrowing of the distal antrum due to Crohn's disease involving the stomach. (From Eisenberg RL: Gastrointestinal Radiology: A Pattern Approach, 3rd ed. Philadelphia, JB Lippincott, 1996.)

with an intraluminal filling defect seen at the base of the duodenal bulb. Other conditions causing gastric outlet obstruction include antral mucosal webs and diaphragms, adult hypertrophic pyloric stenosis, and gastric volvulus (these conditions are discussed elsewhere in the chapter).

DUODENAL OBSTRUCTION

A variety of congenital anomalies, inflammatory disorders, and malignant tumors may cause duodenal obstruction. Many of these conditions are discussed elsewhere in the text.

Superior Mesenteric Root Syndrome

The transverse portion of the duodenum has a fixed position in the retroperitoneum. As a result, this portion of the duodenum is in a closed compartment bounded anteriorly by the root of the mesentery, which carries the superior mesenteric vessel sheath (artery, vein, and nerve), and posteriorly by the aorta and lumbar spine (at the L2-3 level, where the lumbar lordosis is most pronounced). Even in asymptomatic people, there is often a transient delay of barium where the transverse duodenum crosses the spine. This delay can be associated with mild, inconstant dilatation of the proximal duodenum (Fig. 38-24).

Any process that tends to close the nutcracker-like jaws of the aorticomesenteric angle results in some degree of compression of the transverse portion of the duodenum. This phenomenon is most likely to occur in asthenic persons, particularly those who rapidly lose weight and retroperitoneal fat because of debilitating illness; the increased dragging effect of the mesenteric root in these patients narrows the aorticomesenteric angle. Prolonged bed rest or immobilization in the supine position (e.g., patients with body casts or whole-body burns or patients who are fixed in a position of hyper-

extension after spinal injury or surgery) also causes the mesenteric root to compress the anterior aspect of the transverse duodenum, resulting in relative duodenal obstruction.[42,43]

In patients with scleroderma or other causes of decreased duodenal peristalsis, the combination of the lumbar spine, aorta, and mesenteric root may constitute enough of a barrier to cause significant obstruction of the transverse duodenum. As a result, the superior mesenteric root syndrome sometimes occurs in patients with scleroderma, who have a dilated, atonic duodenum proximal to the level of the superior mesenteric root (Fig. 38-25). Other collagen diseases such as dermatomyositis and systemic lupus erythematosus may produce similar radiographic findings. In Chagas' disease, inflammatory destruction of intramural autonomic plexuses by *Trypanosoma cruzi* can lead to generalized gastrointestinal aperistalsis and dilatation that most frequently involve the esophagus and colon but can also affect the duodenum. Disordered duodenal motility and dilatation can also occur as a result of neuropathies associated with diabetes, porphyria, and thiamine deficiency or as a result of surgical vagotomy for peptic ulcer disease or chemical vagotomy caused by ingestion of drugs such as atropine, morphine, and diphenoxylate (Lomotil).

Any space-occupying process within the aorticomesenteric angle can also compress the transverse duodenum, causing the superior mesenteric root syndrome. As a result, inflammatory thickening of the bowel wall or mesenteric root by pancreatitis, Crohn's disease, and peptic ulcer disease or neoplastic thickening of the mesenteric root by metastases to the mesentery or mesenteric lymph nodes can lead to relative duodenal obstruction.[44] Occasionally, metastatic tumor involving the duodenum may cause delayed gastric emptying and massive gastric dilatation out of proportion to the degree of duodenal obstruction, possibly because of injury to the vagal nerve by retroperitoneal tumor.[45]

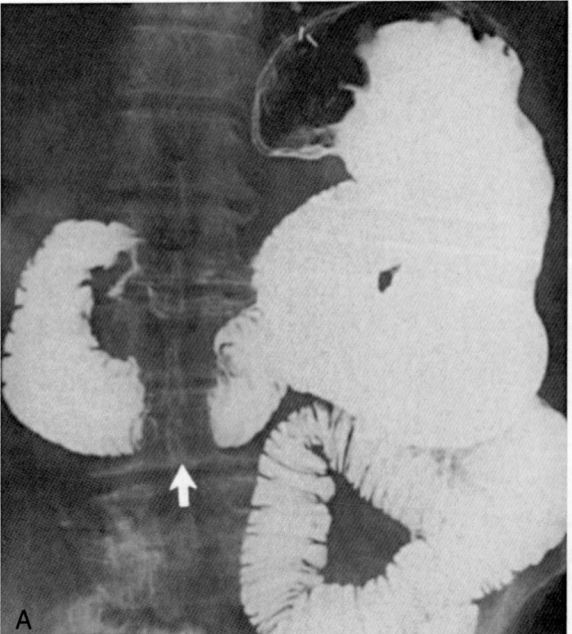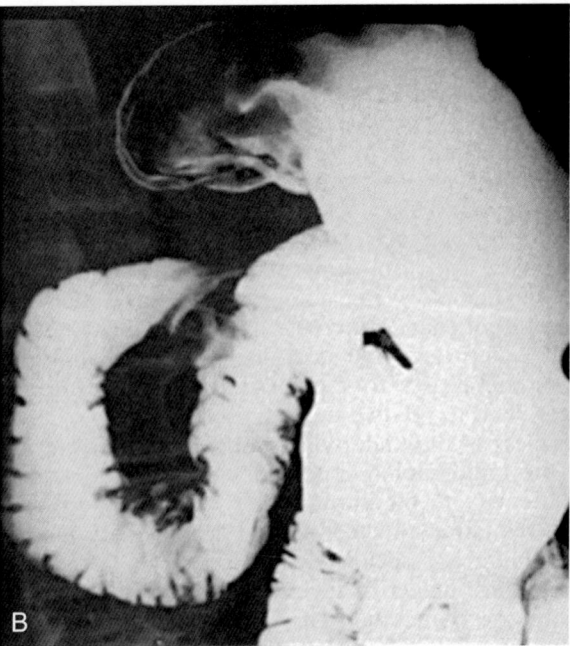

Figure 38-24. Asymptomatic patient with findings mimicking those in superior mesenteric root syndrome. A. Frontal view shows an extrinsic, vertically oriented, bandlike defect (*arrow*) and apparent obstruction of the third portion of the duodenum by the superior mesenteric root. **B.** Prone right anterior oblique view obtained moments later shows a normal duodenal sweep without evidence of obstruction.

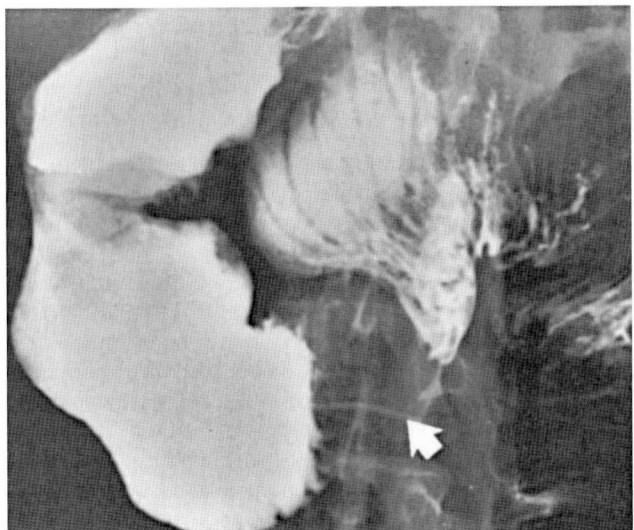

Figure 38-25. Superior mesenteric root syndrome caused by sclero-derma. The duodenum is markedly dilated and atonic proximal to an extrinsic, vertically oriented, bandlike defect (*arrow*) at the aortico-mesenteric angle. (From Eisenberg RL: Gastrointestinal Radiology: A Pattern Approach, 3rd ed. Philadelphia, JB Lippincott, 1996.)

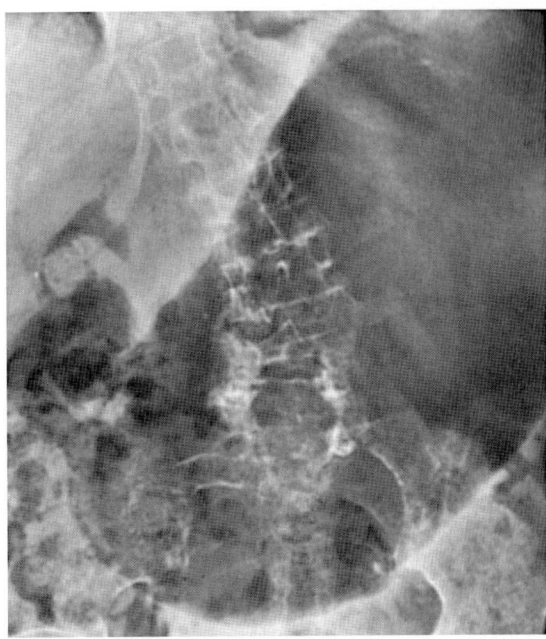

Figure 38-26. Massive gastric dilatation. Abdominal radiograph shows an enormous amount of gas filling a markedly dilated stomach that extends inferiorly into the pelvis. (From Eisenberg RL: Gastrointestinal Radiology: A Pattern Approach, 3rd ed. Philadelphia, JB Lippincott, 1996.)

Regardless of the underlying pathophysiologic mechanism, the superior mesenteric root syndrome is associated with characteristic radiographic findings. Barium studies usually reveal marked dilatation of the first and second portions of the duodenum associated with an extrinsic, vertically oriented, bandlike defect in the transverse portion of the duodenum overlying the spine (see Fig. 38-25). In some cases, the obstruction may be partially relieved by placing the patient in the prone position. CT may demonstrate beaklike compression of the third portion of the duodenum between the superior mesenteric vessels and aorta, thereby confirming the diagnosis of the superior mesenteric root syndrome.[46]

Other Causes

Intramural hematoma, intraluminal duodenal diverticulum, and aortoduodenal fistula (all discussed elsewhere in this chapter) are other causes of duodenal obstruction. Ulceration with stricture formation can also be a complication of radiation therapy to the upper abdomen.[47] A rare cause of duodenal obstruction is the preduodenal portal vein, which crosses in front of the duodenum rather than behind it. This anomaly is associated with other malformations such as duodenal bands and annular pancreas, which are more likely to be the cause of obstruction than the anomalous crossing vessel. In fact, the major reason to be aware of the preduodenal portal vein is so that it is not injured at the time of surgery for these other malformations.[48]

GASTRIC DILATATION WITHOUT GASTRIC OUTLET OBSTRUCTION

Acute or chronic dilatation of the stomach with prolonged retention of food and barium can occur without any organic gastric outlet obstruction. *Gastric retention* is defined as vomiting of food eaten more than 6 hours earlier or the presence of food in the stomach at the time of an upper gastro-

intestinal series (assuming that the patient has not eaten for 8 to 10 hours). However, gastric retention is not synonymous with gastric outlet obstruction, and "corrective" surgery is not always indicated in these patients.[49]

The appearance of nonobstructive gastric dilatation is indistinguishable from that of organic gastric outlet obstruction on abdominal radiographs. Large quantities of air and fluid may fill a massively enlarged stomach that can extend even to the floor of the pelvis (Fig. 38-26). Administration of barium usually reveals a large amount of solid gastric residue. Peristalsis is irregular, sluggish, and ineffectual. When barium studies show retained food and debris in the stomach without evidence of gastric outlet obstruction, the various nonobstructive causes of gastric retention must be excluded before accusing the patient of disregarding instructions and eating before the examination.

Acute Gastric Dilatation

Acute gastric dilatation is characterized by sudden and severe distention of the stomach by gas and fluid, usually accompanied by vomiting, dehydration, and peripheral vascular collapse. Within minutes to hours, a normal stomach can expand into a hyperemic, cyanotic, atonic sac that fills the abdomen. Most cases of acute gastric dilatation occur during the first several days after abdominal surgery (Fig. 38-27). This postoperative complication has decreased dramatically in incidence as a result of improved operative and postoperative care, including meticulous handling of tissues at surgery, better anesthetics, nasogastric suction, and careful monitoring of acid-base and electrolyte balances. Acute gastric dilatation can also occur as a complication of other medical or surgical conditions, including abdominal trauma and peritoneal inflammatory processes.

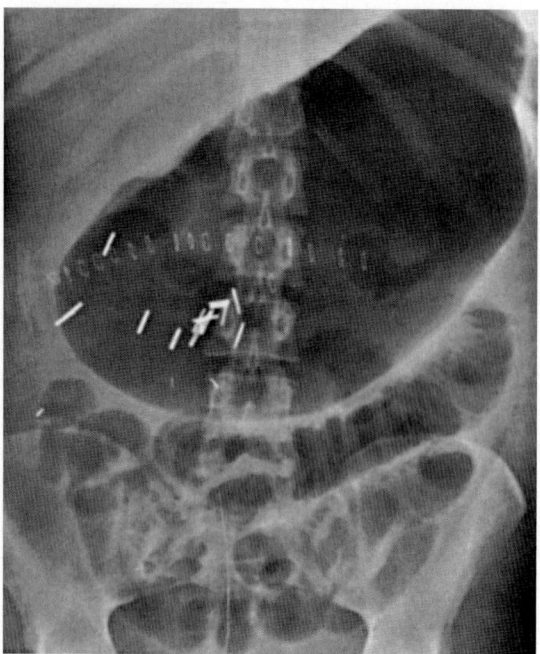

Figure 38-27. Acute gastric dilatation resulting from recent abdominal surgery. (From Eisenberg RL: Gastrointestinal Radiology: A Pattern Approach, 3rd ed. Philadelphia, JB Lippincott, 1996.)

vomiting, aspiration, fluid and electrolyte disturbances, dehydration, perforation, peritonitis, and shock.[50]

Chronic Gastric Dilatation and Gastroparesis

The two most common causes of chronic gastric dilatation and gastroparesis are diabetes and narcotics. Some patients are asymptomatic, but others develop chronic nausea, vomiting, and postprandial abdominal fullness.[51-53] About 40% of patients with diabetes have a dilated stomach with decreased or absent gastric peristalsis (i.e., diabetic gastroparesis) and delayed gastric emptying.[52] Most of these patients have long-standing, poorly controlled diabetes associated with a peripheral neuropathy or other complications.[51,53] Narcotic medications may also cause marked gastroparesis that gradually resolves after withdrawal of the offending agents. Other patients with neurologic abnormalities (e.g., brain tumors, bulbar poliomyelitis, and tabes dorsalis) may develop chronic gastric retention, although in these conditions, decreased peristalsis and dilatation more commonly involve the esophagus. Marked gastric dilatation may also develop in patients with scleroderma, polymyositis, dermatomyositis, and myotonic muscular dystrophy.[54,55] Other causes include electrolyte and acid-base imbalances, lead poisoning, and porphyria (Fig. 38-28).

ABNORMAL EXTRINSIC MASSES

Stomach

Extrinsic impressions on the stomach may be caused by a prominent left lobe of the liver, aberrant position of the spleen or left kidney, or pathologic enlargement of any of these structures (Fig. 38-29). CT can aid in differentiating these extrinsic defects from true intragastric lesions.

Appropriate therapy usually produces a rapid clinical response but, if untreated, acute gastric dilatation may be a life-threatening condition. Pain is seldom severe until these patients have marked gastric dilatation. Distention may also progress rapidly because of aerophagia (air swallowing). In fulminant cases, acute gastric dilatation may cause severe

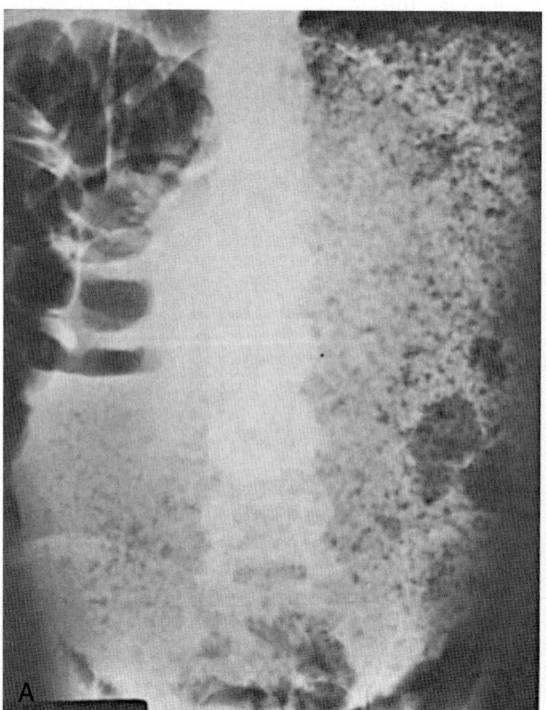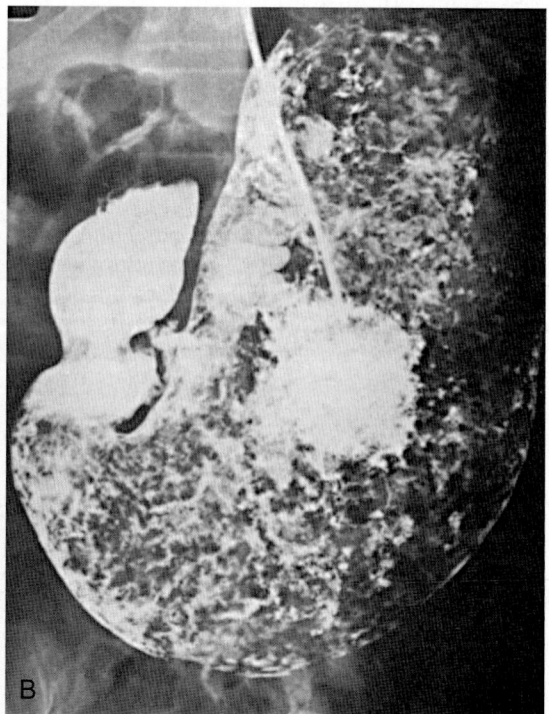

Figure 38-28. Chronic gastric dilatation caused by severe electrolyte and acid-base imbalance. A. Abdominal radiograph shows a marked amount of particulate material in a dilated stomach. **B.** Contrast study confirms the presence of marked gastric dilatation.

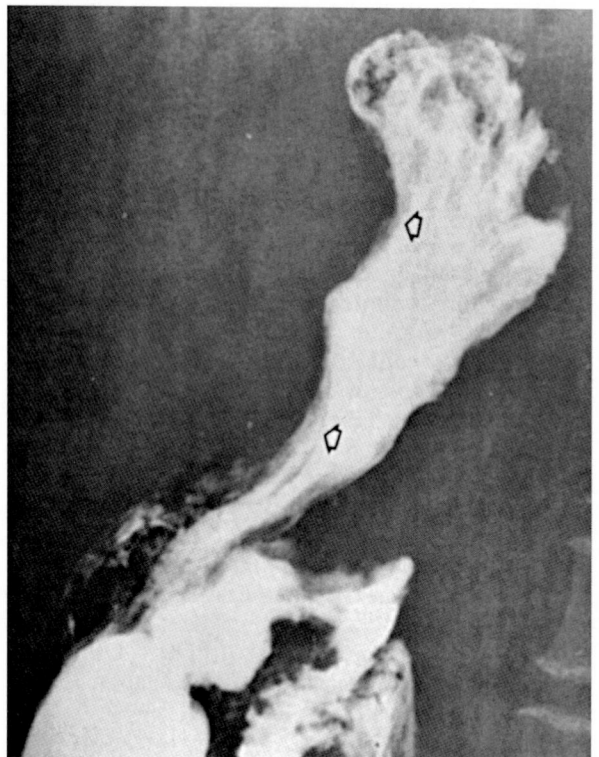

Figure 38-29. Gastric impressions by a polycystic liver. Two large extrinsic impressions (*arrows*) on the anterior aspect of the stomach could be mistaken for intramural lesions. (From Eisenberg RL: Gastrointestinal Radiology: A Pattern Approach, 3rd ed. Philadelphia, JB Lippincott, 1996.)

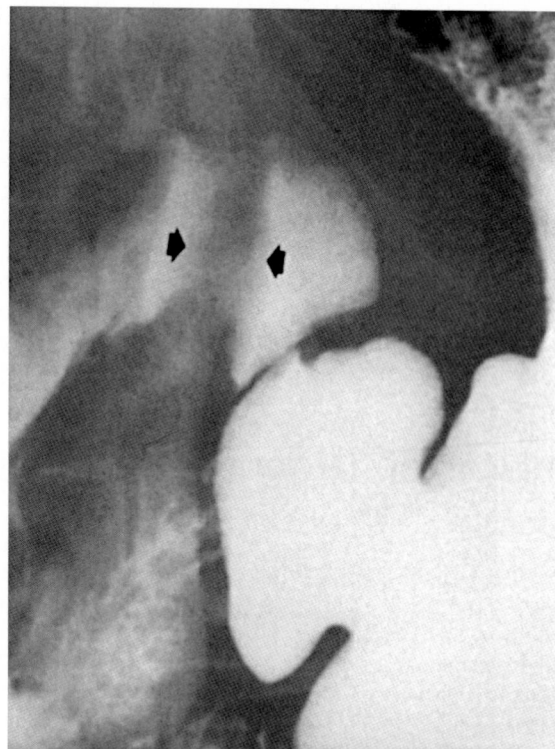

Figure 38-30. Duodenal impression by a dilated common bile duct. The dilated duct produces a characteristic tubular impression (*arrows*) on the duodenum near the apex of the bulb. (From Eisenberg RL: Gastrointestinal Radiology: A Pattern Approach, 3rd ed. Philadelphia, JB Lippincott, 1996.)

Duodenum

A variety of abnormalities involving organs in the right upper quadrant may cause displacement of or extrinsic pressure on the duodenal bulb and sweep. Even when normal, the common bile duct may produce a linear or small, rounded impression on the duodenal bulb. A dilated common bile duct typically produces a large tubular defect in the duodenal bulb that has an oblique orientation (Fig. 38-30). Extrinsic compression of the duodenum may also result from any cause of enlargement of the gallbladder (e.g., hydrops, carcinoma, and pericholecystic abscess).

Hepatomegaly or anomalous lobes of the liver may cause leftward displacement of the duodenal bulb and sweep.[56] Duodenal displacement may be particularly marked when there is hypertrophy of the caudate lobe. Hepatic cysts and tumors as well as metastatic lymphadenopathy in the periportal region may also produce one or more extrinsic impressions on the duodenal bulb and sweep.

Masses in the right kidney or adrenal gland can impress the posterolateral aspect of the duodenal sweep.[57] Generalized renal enlargement (secondary to a bifid collecting system or hydronephrosis), multiple cysts, polycystic disease, or renal cell carcinoma may also compress and displace the duodenum (Fig. 38-31). In other patients, anterior displacement of the duodenum may be caused by an enlarged right adrenal gland as a result of Addison's disease or adrenal carcinoma.

The midportion of the descending duodenum is crossed anteriorly by the transverse colon. In approximately 3% of patients there is an abnormally close positional relationship

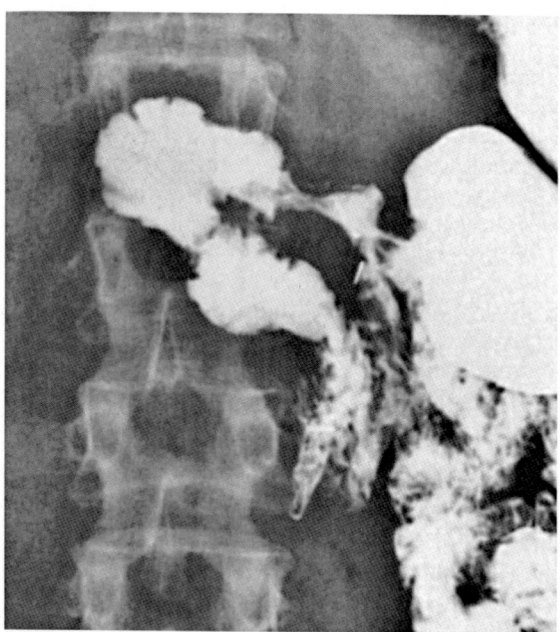

Figure 38-31. Duodenal impression by a polycystic right kidney. The duodenum is displaced to the left of the spine by the polycystic kidney. (From Eisenberg RL: Gastrointestinal Radiology: A Pattern Approach, 3rd ed. Philadelphia, JB Lippincott, 1996.)

between these two structures, resulting in a mutual indentation.[58] Carcinoma of the right side of the colon, especially the hepatic flexure, can result in an extrinsic impression on the outer border of the descending duodenum.[59] This finding may be caused by adjacent adenopathy or by direct extension of tumor across the short fascial plane of the lateral reflection of the transverse mesocolon, which attaches the hepatic flexure of the colon to the lower portion of the descending duodenum.

Dilated vessels can also produce one or more impressions on the outer wall of the duodenal bulb and sweep. These impressions may be caused by duodenal varices associated with portal hypertension or by dilated arterial collateral pathways resulting from occlusion of the celiac axis or superior mesenteric artery.[60]

WIDENING OF THE DUODENAL SWEEP

Although widening of the duodenal sweep on barium studies is often considered to be synonymous with an enlarged head of the pancreas, this finding is not always caused by pancreatic disease, so it must be interpreted with caution. There is great variation in the configuration of the duodenal sweep among normal patients, and slight degrees of widening are difficult to recognize with confidence. In heavy patients, the combination of a high transverse stomach and a long vertical course of the descending duodenum can also create the erroneous impression of a widened sweep.

True widening of the duodenal sweep may be caused by pancreatic neoplasms or by benign pancreatic disease (pancreatitis or pancreatic pseudocysts) (Figs. 38-32 and 38-33) (see next section). Although there are numerous radiographic criteria for distinguishing benign and malignant pancreatic disease involving the duodenum, this differentiation is often difficult on the basis of barium studies. When pancreatic abnormalities are suspected, CT or other cross-sectional imaging studies should therefore be obtained for a more definitive diagnosis.

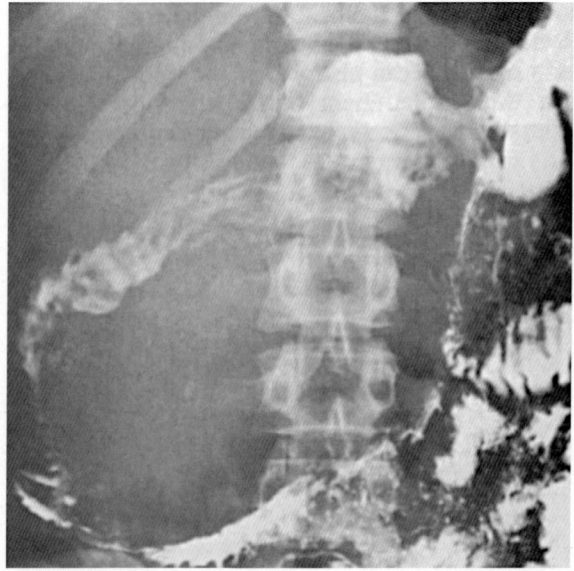

Figure 38-33. Widening of the duodenal sweep by a pancreatic pseudocyst. Pancreatitis or pancreatic carcinoma could produce similar findings (see Fig. 38-32). (From Eisenberg RL: Gastrointestinal Radiology: A Pattern Approach, 3rd ed. Philadelphia, JB Lippincott, 1996.)

Lymphoma, metastases, or inflammatory conditions involving pancreaticoduodenal or subpyloric lymph nodes may cause enlargement of these peripancreatic nodes and associated widening of the duodenal sweep (Fig. 38-34).[61] Depending on their location, mesenteric cysts or tumors may

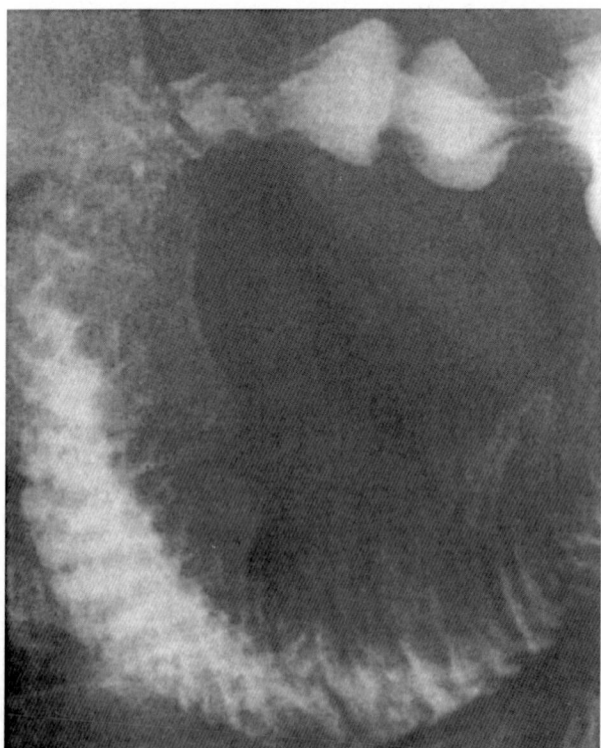

Figure 38-34. Widening of the duodenal sweep by peripancreatic lymphoma. Enlarged peripancreatic lymph nodes have produced a double contour on the medial border of the duodenum with associated spiculation. Pancreatitis or pancreatic carcinoma could produce similar findings (see Fig. 38-36). (From Eisenberg RL: Gastrointestinal Radiology: A Pattern Approach, 3rd ed. Philadelphia, JB Lippincott, 1996.)

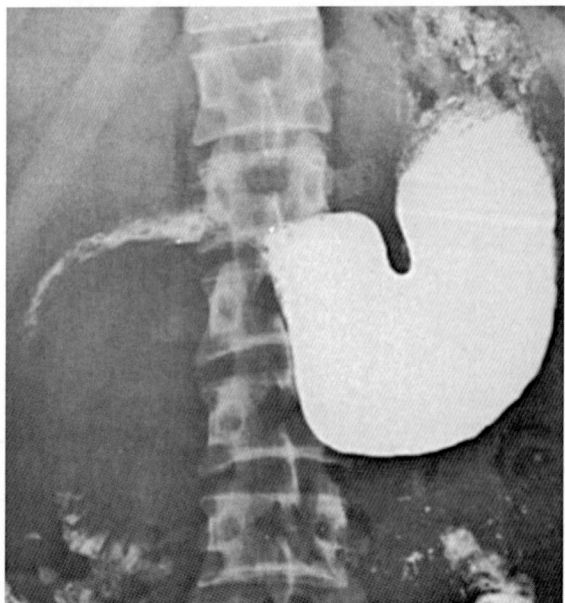

Figure 38-32. Widening of the duodenal sweep caused by acute pancreatitis. (From Eisenberg RL: Gastrointestinal Radiology: A Pattern Approach, 3rd ed. Philadelphia, JB Lippincott, 1996.)

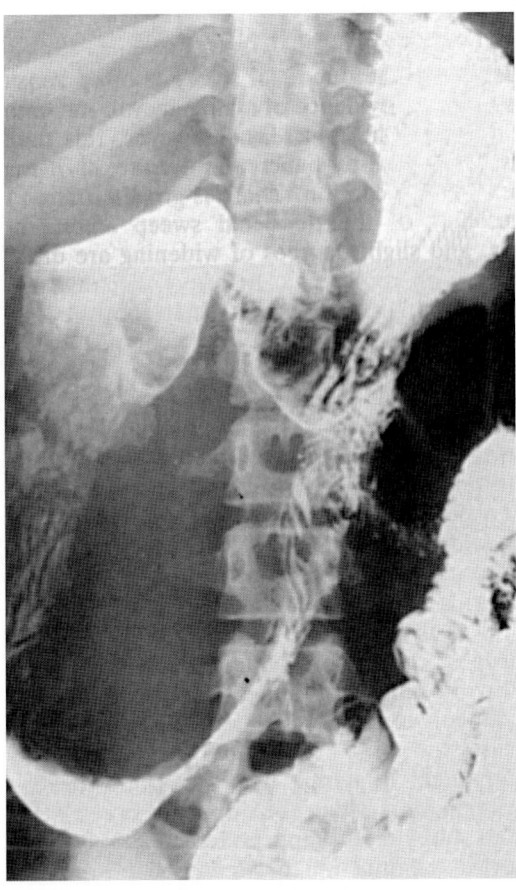

Figure 38-35. Widening of the duodenal sweep by a choledochal cyst. (From Eisenberg RL: Gastrointestinal Radiology: A Pattern Approach, 3rd ed. Philadelphia, JB Lippincott, 1996.)

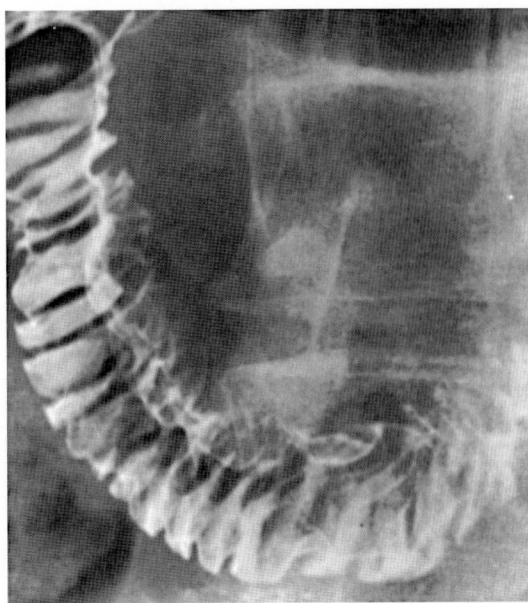

Figure 38-36. Duodenal involvement by pancreatic carcinoma. An enlarged pancreatic head produces a double contour on the medial border of the duodenal sweep. (From Eisenberg RL: Gastrointestinal Radiology: A Pattern Approach, 3rd ed. Philadelphia, JB Lippincott, 1996.)

produce similar findings. Rarely, dilated pancreaticoduodenal collateral vessels in patients with an occluded celiac axis or superior mesenteric artery can produce a smooth, concave impression on the medial aspect of the descending duodenum that simulates a mass in the head of the pancreas.

Retroperitoneal masses (primary or metastatic neoplasms or cysts) can also widen the duodenal sweep.[62] Downward displacement of the third portion of the duodenum by an aortic aneurysm can produce a similar radiographic appearance. A choledochal cyst (localized dilatation of the common bile duct) near the ampulla of Vater can result in generalized widening of the duodenal sweep (Fig. 38-35) or a localized impression near the papilla.

PANCREATIC DISEASES AFFECTING THE STOMACH AND DUODENUM

Before the advent of ultrasound, CT, and MR, alterations in the configuration and mucosal pattern of the antrum and duodenal sweep were carefully evaluated on barium studies as indirect signs of inflammatory or neoplastic disease involving the head of the pancreas. Although primarily of historical interest, radiographic changes on upper gastrointestinal series may occasionally suggest otherwise unexpected pancreatic disease.

Enlargement of the head of the pancreas can produce a mass impression on the inner aspect of the duodenal sweep that creates a double contour effect (Fig. 38-36). This appearance results from differential filling of the duodenum, with the interfold spaces along the inner aspect of the sweep containing less barium than the corresponding spaces along the outer aspect. Another nonspecific sign, originally attributed to malignant disease but probably more common in inflammatory disorders, is the "inverted-3" sign of Frostberg (Fig. 38-37). The central limb of the 3 represents the point of fixation of the duodenal wall, where the pancreatic and common bile ducts insert into the papilla. The impressions above and below this point reflect tumor mass, edema of the major and minor papillae, or smooth muscle spasm and edema in the duodenal wall.

Fine or coarse sharpening and elongation of barium-filled crevices between duodenal folds (i.e., spiculation) may be caused by mucosal edema or irritation (Fig. 38-38). This appearance can be seen in patients with pancreatitis or pancreatic carcinoma. Displacement or frank splaying of the spikes suggests tumor infiltration of the wall with traction and fixation of folds.

In advanced disease, duodenal involvement by pancreatitis, pancreatic pseudocysts, or pancreatic carcinoma may be manifested by the development of ulcers, cavities, or even pancreaticoduodenal fistulas. Pancreatitis, pseudocysts, or neoplasms involving the head of the pancreas may also produce a smooth area of extrinsic mass effect on the greater curvature of the gastric antrum (i.e., the "antral pad" sign).[63] Further infiltration of the stomach by the inflammatory process or tumor may result in an irregular gastric contour with spiculated, tethered mucosal folds on the greater curvature (Fig. 38-39). Similarly, disease involving the body or tail of the pancreas may be manifested by extrinsic compression, flattening, or spiculation of the posterior wall of the gastric fundus or body (Fig. 38-40A and B). When gastric involvement by pancreatic disease is suspected on the basis of barium

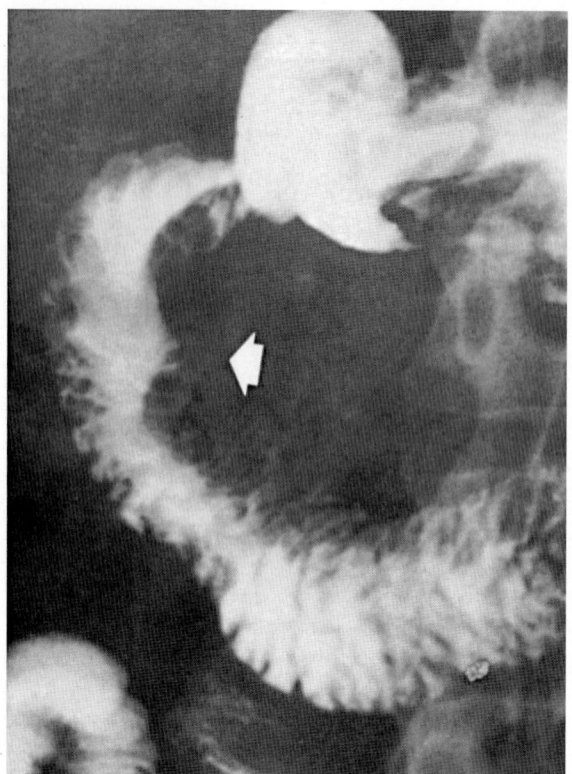

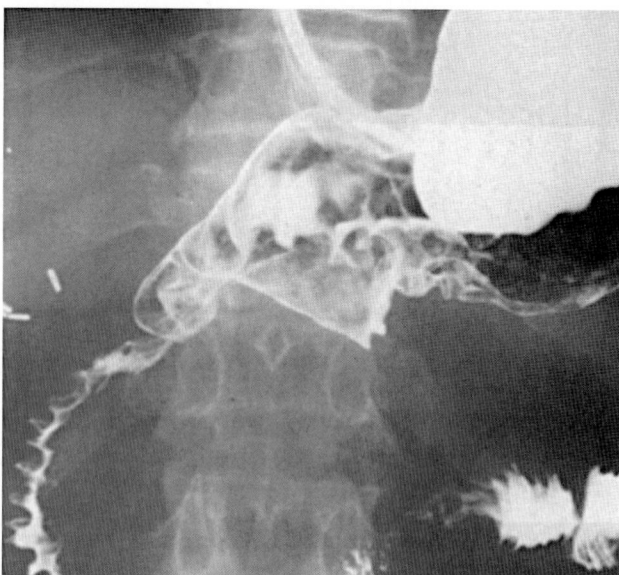

Figure 38-39. Gastric involvement by pancreatitis. There is flattening, irregularity, and spiculation of the greater curvature of the antrum due to extension of the inflammatory process to the stomach. Also note involvement of the proximal descending duodenum.

Figure 38-37. The inverted-3 sign of Frostberg. There is a widened duodenal sweep with fixation of the duodenal wall at the papilla (*arrow*), producing the inverted-3 sign. This patient had acute pancreatitis, so that the inverted-3 sign is not specific for pancreatic carcinoma.

studies, CT, MR, or ultrasonography should be performed for a more definitive diagnosis (Fig. 38-40C).

UNUSUAL FILLING DEFECTS

Bezoars

A bezoar is an intragastric mass consisting of accumulated ingested material. *Phytobezoars* (composed of undigested vegetable matter) have classically been associated with the eating of unripe persimmons, a fruit containing substances that coagulate on contact with gastric acid to produce a sticky gelatinous material, which then traps seeds, skin, and other foodstuffs. *Trichobezoars* (composed of hair) occur predominantly in women, especially those with schizophrenia or other mental illnesses. The accumulated, matted mass of hair can enlarge to occupy the entire lumen of the stomach, often assuming the shape of the organ. A small percentage of bezoars are composed of both hair and vegetable matter and are called *trichophytobezoars*.

Symptoms of gastric bezoars result from the mechanical effects of the foreign body in the stomach, including crampy epigastric pain and a sense of fullness or heaviness in the upper abdomen. There is a high prevalence of associated peptic ulcers, especially with the more abrasive phytobezoars. Large bezoars may also cause symptoms of gastric outlet obstruction.

A bezoar is sometimes visible on abdominal radiographs as a soft tissue mass floating in the stomach at the air-fluid interface (Fig. 38-41). Barium studies may show a conglomerate mass of debris with barium trapped in the interstices of the bezoar, producing a characteristic mottled appearance (Fig. 38-42). With changes in patient position, most bezoars are freely movable within the gastric lumen. A bezoar can also form in the gastric remnant after a partial gastrectomy

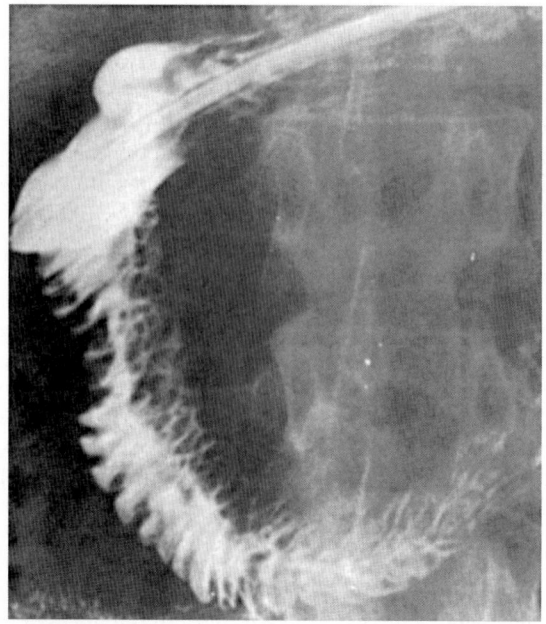

Figure 38-38. Duodenal involvement by pancreatitis. There is an extrinsic impression on the medial border of the descending duodenum with spiculated mucosal folds. (From Eisenberg RL: Gastrointestinal Radiology: A Pattern Approach, 3rd ed. Philadelphia, JB Lippincott, 1996.)

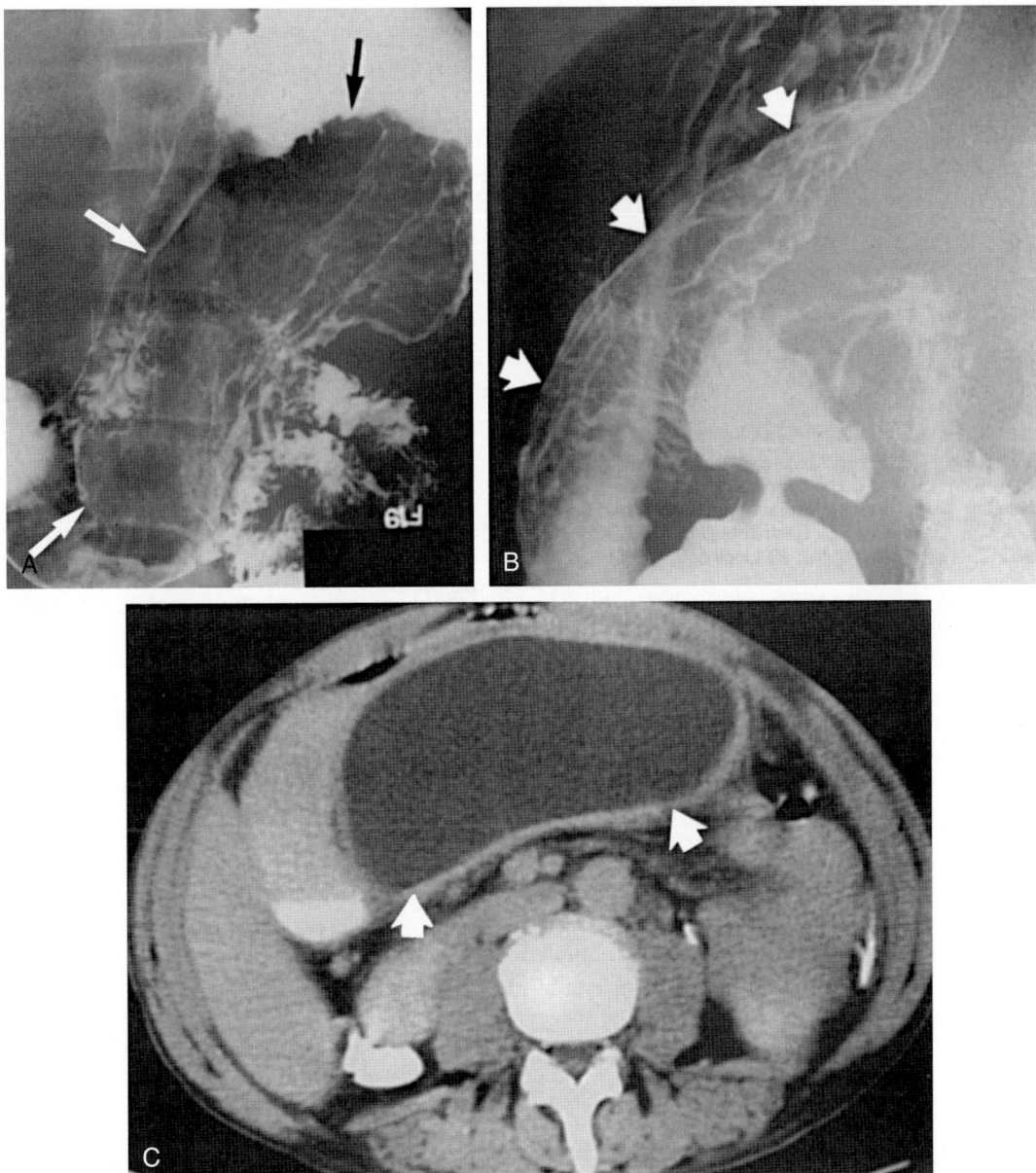

Figure 38-40. Gastric involvement by a pancreatic pseudocyst. A. Supine view of the stomach shows a large area of extrinsic mass effect (*arrows*) on the gastric fundus and body. **B.** Lateral view shows the retrogastric mass (*arrows*) in profile. **C.** CT scan reveals a large pancreatic pseudocyst (*arrows*) compressing and displacing the stomach. (From Laufer I, Levine MS [eds]: Double Contrast Gastrointestinal Radiology, 2nd ed. Philadelphia, WB Saunders, 1992.)

(Billroth I or II) when strictures develop at the gastroduodenal or gastrojejunal anastomosis, delaying emptying of ingested food. Occasionally, the bezoar may be unusually smooth, simulating an enormous gas bubble (Fig. 38-43). A bezoar is characterized on CT by an inhomogeneous intraluminal mass with a mottled gas pattern, often seen to be floating at the air-fluid interface (Fig. 38-44).[64]

Foreign Bodies

Foreign bodies may appear as radiolucent filling defects in the barium-filled stomach or duodenum. This appearance is produced by a variety of ingested substances, including food, pills, and nondigestible material.

Hematomas

In patients with upper gastrointestinal bleeding, blood clots may appear as one or more filling defects in the stomach or duodenum. Hemorrhage into the wall of the stomach secondary to a bleeding diathesis, anticoagulant therapy, or trauma can lead to the development of a large intramural gastric mass, most commonly involving the fundus.

Intramural duodenal hematoma is a recognized complication of blunt trauma to the abdomen. More than 80% of reported cases have occurred in children or young adults; child abuse is a major cause in infants and young children.[65] It is believed that the hematoma results from the bowel being crushed between the anterior abdominal wall and the

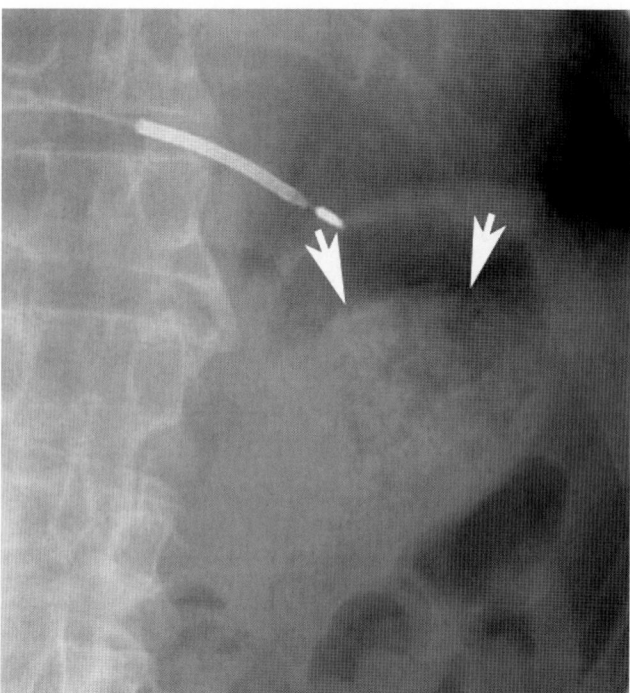

Figure 38-41. Gastric bezoar. Supine abdominal radiograph shows a gastric bezoar as a mottled soft tissue mass (*arrows*) floating in the stomach at the air-fluid interface.

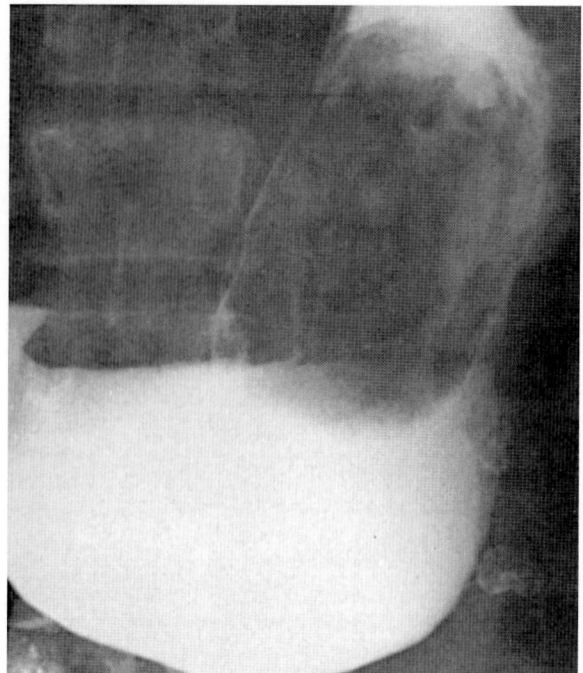

Figure 38-43. Gastric bezoar. The bezoar appears as a smooth filling defect in the stomach that could be mistaken for an enormous gas bubble. This patient was a model airplane builder who had been ingesting glue. (From Eisenberg RL: Gastrointestinal Radiology: A Pattern Approach, 3rd ed. Philadelphia, JB Lippincott, 1996.)

vertebral column. Because the second and third portions of the duodenum are fixed in a retroperitoneal position, they are prone to this type of injury if enough force is applied to the anterior abdominal wall. When the mucosa is separated from the loose submucosa, blood may dissect along submucosal compartments. Intramural duodenal hematomas may also be caused by a bleeding diathesis, anticoagulation, or endoscopic trauma.[66]

Intramural duodenal hematomas may appear on barium studies as well-circumscribed intramural masses with discrete margins. Some degree of stenosis and obstruction is usually present (Fig. 38-45A). CT may reveal marked thickening of the duodenal wall in these patients.[67] CT is also helpful for differentiating duodenal perforation from a hematoma without perforation. The presence of perforation is indicated by extraluminal gas or extravasated contrast material in the

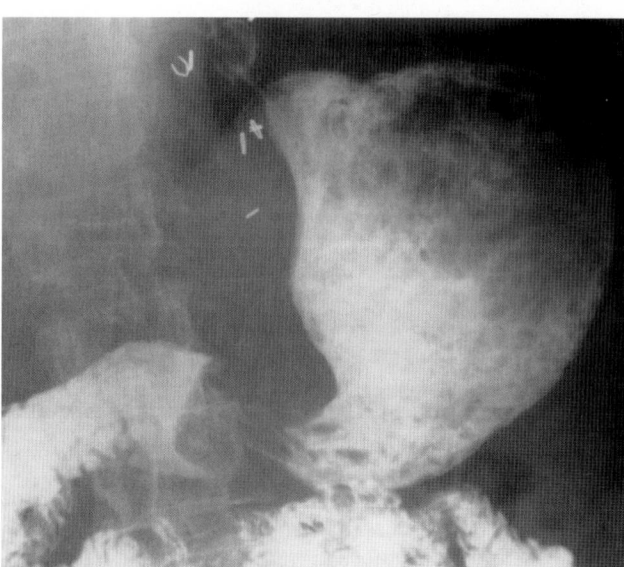

Figure 38-42. Gastric bezoar. The bezoar is manifested by a conglomerate mass of debris with barium trapped in its interstices, producing a characteristic mottled appearance.

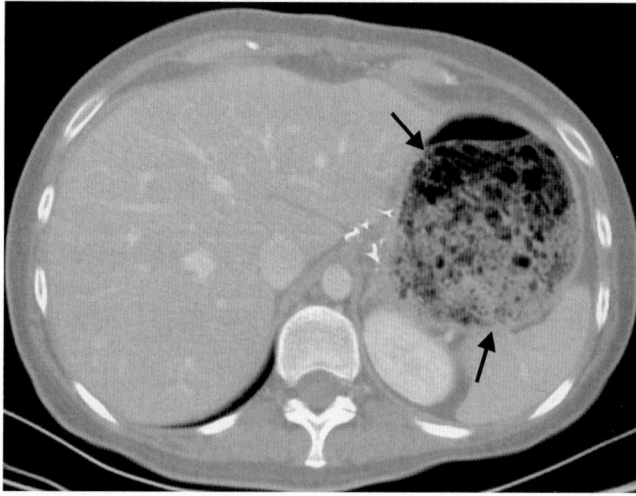

Figure 38-44. Gastric bezoar on CT. The bezoar is characterized on CT by an inhomogeneous intraluminal mass with a mottled gas pattern (*arrows*). This patient had undergone a partial gastrectomy with a bezoar in the gastric remnant because of a stricture at the gastrojejunal anastomosis (not visualized on this image). (From Woodfield CA, Levine MS: The postoperative stomach. Eur J Radiol 53:341-352, 2005.)

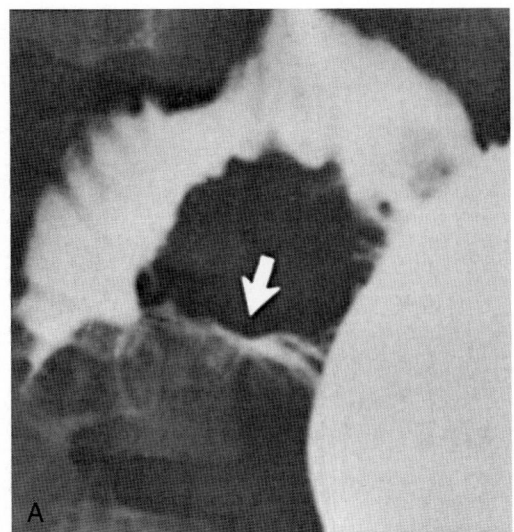

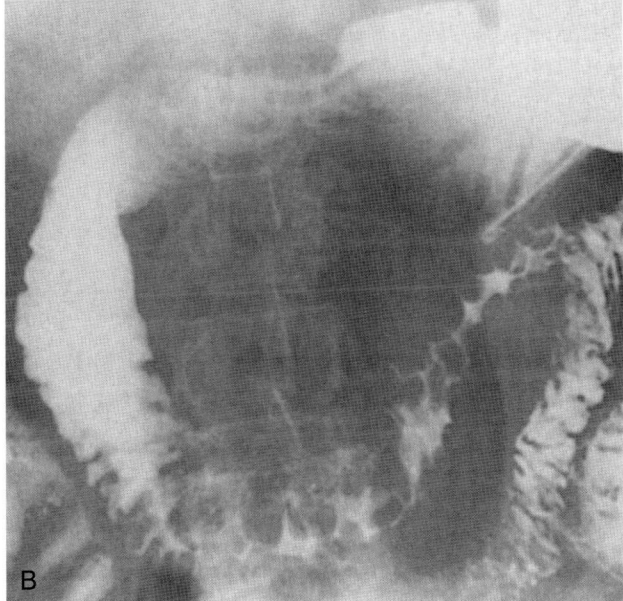

Figure 38-45. Intramural duodenal bleeding. A. There is marked narrowing of the distal descending duodenum (*arrow*) due to a large hematoma in a young child who had been kicked in the abdomen by his father. **B.** In another patient who had been undergoing anticoagulant therapy for a prosthetic heart valve there is thumbprinting of the distal duodenum due to extensive intramural hemorrhage. (**A** from Eisenberg RL: Gastrointestinal Radiology: A Pattern Approach. 3rd ed. Philadelphia, JB Lippincott, 1996; **B** courtesy of Richard L. Baron, MD, Pittsburgh, PA.)

right anterior pararenal space.[67] The right psoas margin may be obliterated because of associated retroperitoneal bleeding. A "coil spring" appearance has been described, and, rarely, delayed rupture into the peritoneal or retroperitoneal space may occur. Although some patients have discrete hematomas, others have diffuse hemorrhage in the duodenal wall, manifested by thickened, spiculated folds or thumbprinting (Fig. 38-45B).

Intragastric and Intraduodenal Gallstones

An intragastric gallstone is an extremely rare cause of a filling defect in the stomach. Gallstones may enter the stomach or

duodenum in patients with cholecystogastric or cholecystoduodenal fistulas. Similar to other foreign bodies in the stomach, intragastric gallstones may cause mucosal irritation, ulceration, bleeding, perforation, and even obstruction. Erosion of a gallstone into the duodenal bulb may also cause gastric outlet obstruction (Bouveret's syndrome), a rare but life-threatening condition.[68,69]

GASTRIC VOLVULUS

Gastric volvulus is an uncommon acquired twist of the stomach on itself that can lead to obstruction or strangulation with potentially life-threatening gastric infarction. It is usually associated with a large defect in the diaphragm that allows all or part of the stomach to herniate into the thorax. Free upward movement of the stomach into the chest is normally limited by various ligaments that anchor the stomach within the abdomen. The most rigid point of attachment is the site at which the second portion of the duodenum assumes a retroperitoneal position, thus becoming fixed to the posterior abdominal wall. The gastrocolic and gastrolienal ligaments also contribute to fixation of the stomach. Because of these points of anatomic fixation, torsion of the stomach may occur with significant degrees of gastric herniation. Less frequently, gastric volvulus may be associated with eventration or paralysis of the diaphragm without a true hernia. Cases of idiopathic gastric volvulus without apparent cause have also been reported.

With small herniations, the proximal portion of the stomach enters the hernial sac first. Obstruction or strangulation almost never occurs at this stage. As herniation progresses, the body and a variable portion of the antrum come to lie above the diaphragm, so that the stomach can become an entirely intrathoracic organ that is prone to a volvulus. *Organoaxial volvulus* refers to rotation of the stomach upward around its long axis (a line connecting the cardia with the pylorus). In this condition, the antrum moves from an inferior to a superior position, with the intrathoracic stomach predominantly in the right hemithorax. In mesenteroaxial volvulus, the stomach rotates from right to left or left to right about the long axis of the gastrohepatic omentum (a line connecting the middle of the lesser curvature with the middle of the greater curvature), with the intrathoracic stomach predominantly in the left hemithorax.[70]

Patients with gastric volvulus may be asymptomatic if there is no gastric outlet obstruction or vascular compromise. Other patients may develop postprandial pain or vomiting if there is partial gastric outlet obstruction.[71] In contrast, an acute gastric volvulus may present as a surgical emergency if the vascular supply to the stomach is compromised. An acute volvulus should be suggested by the classic triad of violent retching with production of little vomitus, constant severe epigastric pain, and an inability to advance a nasogastric tube beyond the distal esophagus. Vascular occlusion causes gastric necrosis, perforation, and shock, with a mortality rate of approximately 30%.

The radiographic signs of gastric volvulus are characteristic. Chest radiographs may reveal an intrathoracic stomach with a double air-fluid level in the chest when the patient is upright. Barium studies may reveal inversion of the intrathoracic stomach with the greater curvature above the level of the lesser curvature, the cardia and pylorus positioned in

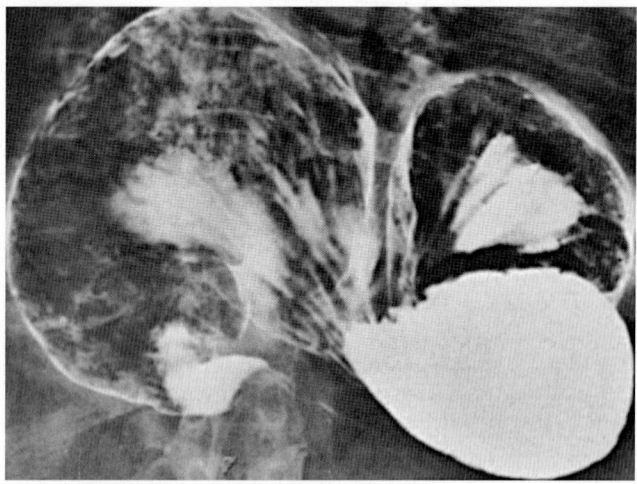

Figure 38-46. Gastric volvulus. This patient has an organoaxial volvulus of the stomach causing gastric outlet obstruction. The stomach is located above the diaphragm with inversion of the greater curvature above the lesser curvature and downward pointing of the pylorus. (From Eisenberg RL: Gastrointestinal Radiology: A Pattern Approach, 3rd ed. Philadelphia, JB Lippincott, 1996.)

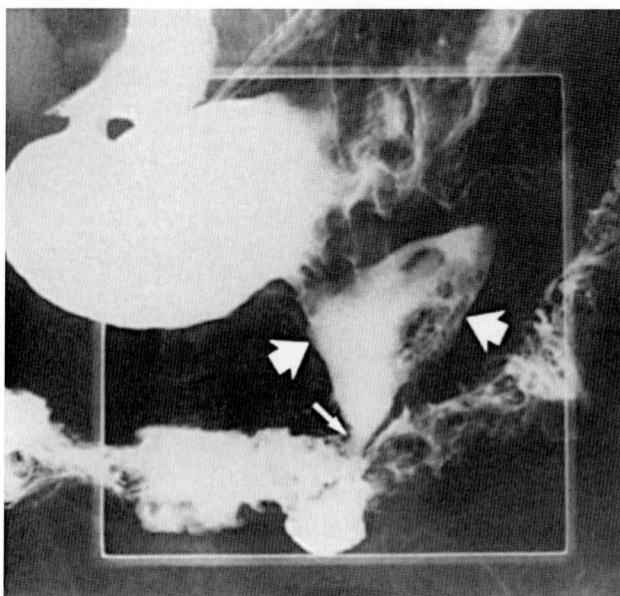

Figure 38-47. Gastrocolic fistula caused by a benign greater curvature ulcer. Upper gastrointestinal study shows a giant ulcer (*large arrows*) on the greater curvature of the stomach with barium entering a fistula (*small arrow*) that communicates with the superior border of the transverse colon. (From Levine MS, Kelly MR, Laufer I, et al: Gastrocolic fistulas: The increasing role of aspirin. Radiology 187:359-361, 1993.)

close proximity, and downward pointing of the pylorus and duodenum (also described as an upside-down intrathoracic stomach (Fig. 38-46).[72] Gastric volvulus may also be recognized on CT by the presence of an enlarged, twisted stomach in the thorax with identification of one or more sites of torsion.[73] Barium studies are useful for showing gastric outlet obstruction, whereas CT is useful for showing signs of ischemia.

GASTRODUODENAL AND DUODENOJEJUNAL INTUSSUSCEPTIONS

Gastroduodenal and duodenojejunal intussusceptions are rare entities, usually associated with gastric or duodenal tumors that serve as the lead point for the intussusception. In gastroduodenal intussusception, characteristic radiographic signs include foreshortening and narrowing of the gastric antrum, converging or telescoping mucosal folds in the antrum or duodenum, prepyloric collar-shaped outpouchings, widening of the pyloric channel, a coil spring appearance of duodenal mucosal folds, and widening of the duodenum with an associated intraluminal mass.[74,75] Similarly, duodenojejunal intussusception produces an intraluminal mass associated with a characteristic coil spring pattern.[76]

FISTULAS

Gastrocolic and Duodenocolic Fistulas

Fistulous communications between the stomach and duodenum and other abdominal organs may occur as a complication of benign or malignant disease. In the past, gastrocolic fistulas most commonly resulted from primary carcinomas of the colon or stomach.[77] In today's pill-oriented society, however, benign greater curvature gastric ulcers caused by aspirin or other nonsteroidal anti-inflammatory drugs have become a more common cause of gastrocolic fistulas than malignant tumors.[78] Occasionally, these greater curvature

ulcers may penetrate inferiorly via the gastrocolic ligament to the superior border of the transverse colon, which is almost always the site of the colonic end of the fistula (Fig. 38-47).

Malignant tumors causing gastrocolic (Fig. 38-48) or duodenocolic (Fig. 38-49) fistulas tend to be bulky, infiltrating lesions associated with a marked inflammatory reaction. These tumors apparently extend from the serosa of one viscus into the wall of another, followed by lumen-to-lumen necrosis. The presence of a fibrous stroma within the wall of a malignant fistula accounts for the length of these tracks and the relative separation of bowel loops.[77]

Malignant gastrocolic fistulas are frequently demonstrated on barium enema examinations but are rarely detected on upper gastrointestinal series. Increased intraluminal pressure in the colon at the time of a barium enema examination may overcome the resistance of a rigid, nondistensible fistula, allowing passage of barium into the stomach. In contrast, intraluminal pressure in the stomach at the time of an upper gastrointestinal examination may not be sufficient to overcome this resistance.[79]

A fistulous communication between the stomach, the jejunum, and the colon (gastrojejunocolic fistula) or directly between the stomach and the colon represents a serious complication of marginal ulceration after gastric surgery for peptic ulcer disease (Fig. 38-50).[80] Most patients with this condition have diarrhea and weight loss; pain, vomiting, and bleeding occur in one third to one half of cases. These patients have a high mortality rate, especially if diagnosis of the fistulas is delayed.

Cholecystoduodenal Fistulas

Fistulas between the gallbladder and duodenum may be caused by acute cholecystitis (90%) or severe peptic ulcer disease

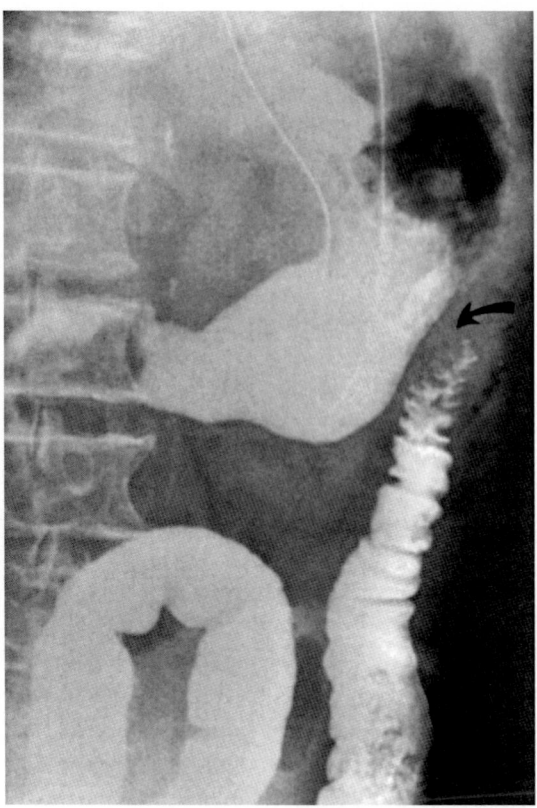

Figure 38-48. Gastrocolic fistula caused by carcinoma of the splenic flexure. Barium enema shows an annular carcinoma of the splenic flexure with barium entering the stomach via a gastrocolic fistula (*arrow*). (From Eisenberg RL: Gastrointestinal Radiology: A Pattern Approach. 3rd ed. Philadelphia, JB Lippincott, 1996.)

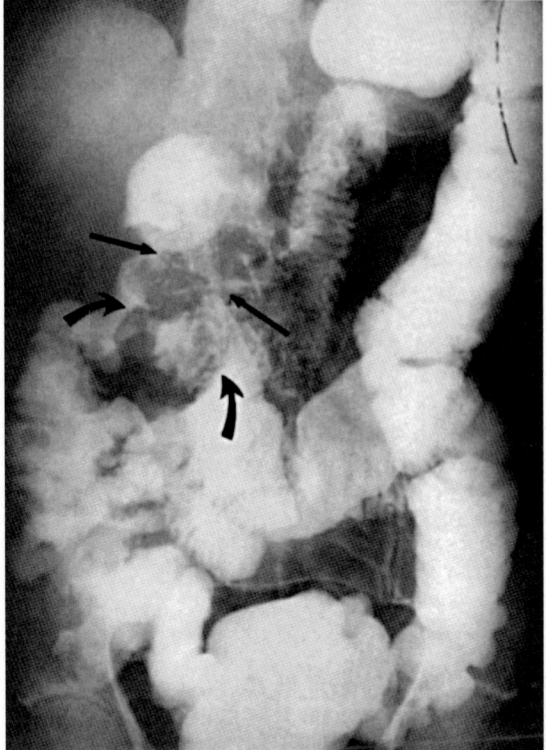

Figure 38-49. Duodenocolic fistula caused by carcinoma of the proximal transverse colon. Barium enema shows an annular carcinoma (*curved arrows*) of the proximal transverse colon, with barium entering the duodenum via a duodenocolic fistula (*straight arrows*). (From JO Vieta, R Blanco, GR Valentini: Malignant duodenocolic fistula: Report of two cases, each with one or more synchronous gastrointestinal cancers. Dis Colon Rectum 19:542-552, 1976, © by American Society of Colon and Rectal Surgeons, Inc.)

(6%). The remaining cases are caused by trauma or tumor. Acute cholecystitis most commonly results in the development of a cholecystoduodenal fistula, but the inflamed gallbladder can also perforate into the stomach, jejunum, or hepatic flexure of the colon. In patients with severe peptic ulcer disease, a penetrating duodenal or gastric ulcer can perforate into the gallbladder or bile duct.[81] Regardless of the cause, abdominal radiographs often show gas in the biliary tree. On upper gastrointestinal studies, barium may fill the cholecystoduodenal fistula (Fig. 38-51).

Other Fistulas

Aortoduodenal fistulas can occur as a complication of abdominal aortic aneurysms or of prosthetic vascular grafts. Pressure necrosis of the third portion of the duodenum, which is fixed and apposed to the anterior wall of an aortic aneurysm, can lead to digestion of the aortic wall by enteric secretions with the development of an aortoduodenal fistula. Secondary fistulas result from pseudoaneurysm formation with erosion into the adherent duodenum or dehiscence of the suture line associated with leakage of intestinal contents through the duodenum, whose blood supply has been compromised at surgery. Aortoduodenal fistula is often a fatal condition, characterized by abdominal pain, gastrointestinal bleeding, and a palpable, pulsatile mass. Barium studies may demonstrate compression or displacement of the third portion of the duodenum by an extrinsic mass (Fig. 38-52A). Rarely, in patients with aortic

grafts, the wall of the abdominal aorta may be outlined by extraluminal contrast medium tracking along the graft into the paraprosthetic space (Fig. 38-52B).[82]

Fistulas between the duodenum and right kidney may occasionally develop as a complication of pyelonephritis, particularly tuberculous pyelonephritis. The pathologic mechanism is usually rupture of a perirenal abscess into the duodenum, which is best demonstrated on retrograde pyelography. Rarely, a duodenal ulcer may penetrate into the right kidney, producing a duodenorenal fistula.

GASTRIC AND DUODENAL PERFORATION

The most frequent cause of pneumoperitoneum in patients with peritonitis is a perforated peptic ulcer, either a gastric ulcer or, more commonly, a duodenal ulcer (Fig. 38-53A). In approximately 30% of patients with perforated ulcers, however, there is no evidence of free intraperitoneal air on abdominal radiographs. The failure to demonstrate pneumoperitoneum is therefore of little value in excluding the possibility of a perforated ulcer. In general, the absence of gas in the stomach and presence of gas in small and large bowel should suggest a gastric perforation as the cause of pneumoperitoneum. Conversely, the absence of colonic gas and presence of a gastric air-fluid level and small bowel distention make a colonic perforation more likely. The findings on abdominal radiographs can be misleading, however, so that a firm diagnosis of the

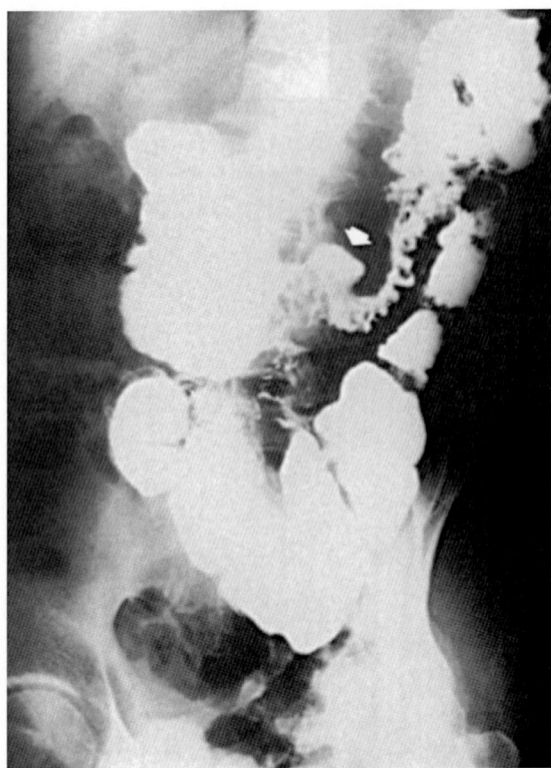

Figure 38-50. Gastrojejunocolic fistula. This patient had undergone a partial gastrectomy and gastrojejunostomy. There is a large anastomotic ulcer (*arrow*) at the gastrojejunostomy with filling of the jejunum and transverse colon via a gastrojejunocolic fistula. (From Thoeni RH, Hodgson JR, Scudamore HH: The roentgenologic diagnosis of gastrocolic and gastrojejunocolic fistulas. AJR 83:876-881, 1960 © by American Roentgen Ray Society.)

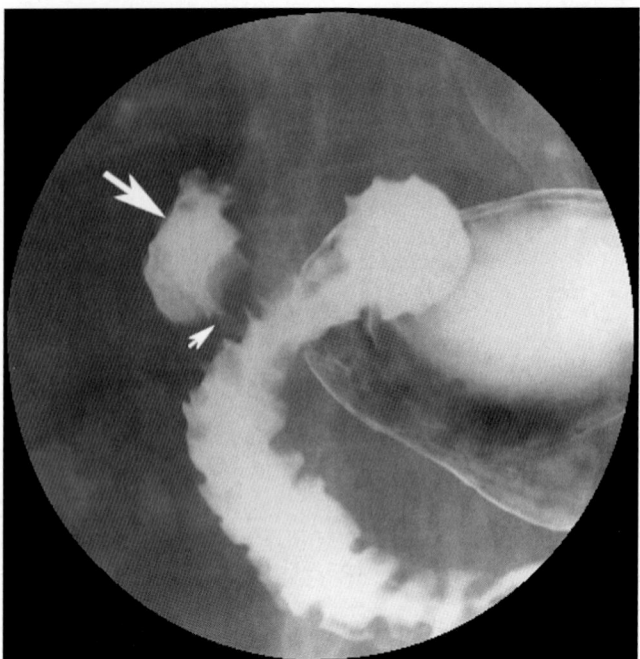

Figure 38-51. Cholecystoduodenal fistula. Barium study shows barium filling the gallbladder (*large arrow*) via a fistula (*small arrow*) from the descending duodenum. Also note thickened folds and decreased distensibility of the duodenum in this patient with a long-standing history of ulcer disease. The fistula presumably developed as a complication of a penetrating postbulbar duodenal ulcer.

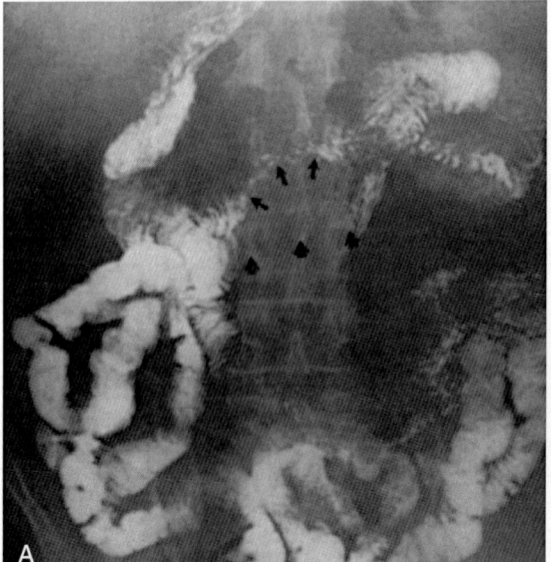
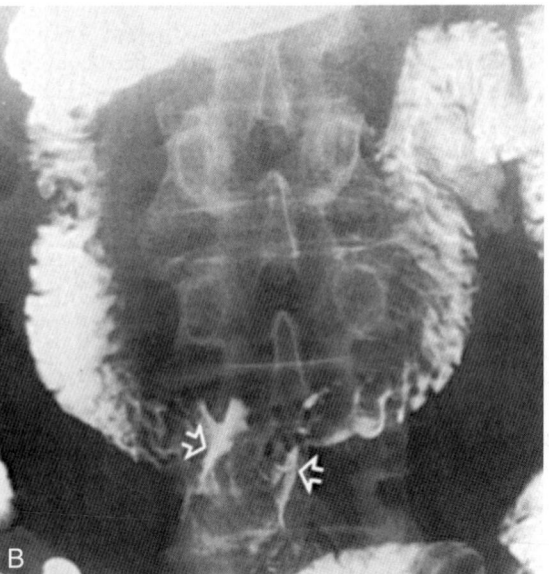

Figure 38-52. Aortoduodenal fistulas. A. The fistula causes extrinsic compression of the third portion of the duodenum (*thin arrows*) and displacement of an adjacent loop of jejunum (*thick arrows*). No contrast medium is seen entering the fistula. **B.** In another patient with an aortic graft, extravasated contrast medium from the distal duodenum is seen tracking between the graft and the aorta (*arrows*). (**A** from Wyatt GM, Rauchway MI, Spitz HB: Roentgen findings in aorto-enteric fistulae. AJR 126:714-722, 1976, © by American Roentgen Ray Society.)

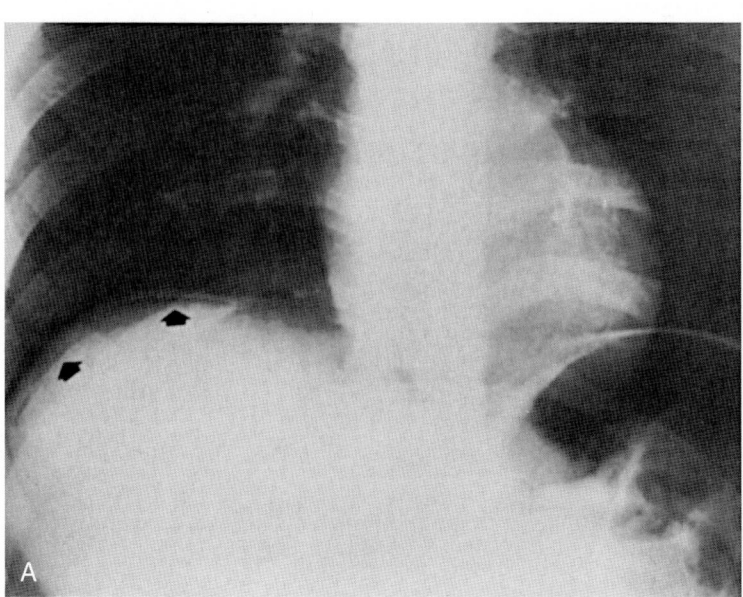
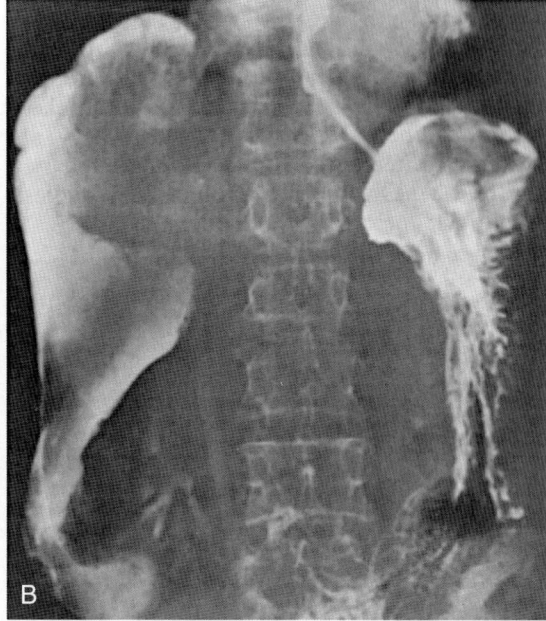

Figure 38-53. Pneumoperitoneum caused by a perforated duodenal ulcer. A. Free intraperitoneal air is seen beneath the right hemidiaphragm (*arrows*). **B.** Study using a water-soluble contrast agent shows free extravasation of the contrast agent from the duodenum into the right side of the peritoneal cavity. (From Eisenberg RL: Gastrointestinal Radiology: A Pattern Approach, 3rd ed. Philadelphia, JB Lippincott, 1996.)

site of perforation requires study with a water-soluble contrast agent (Fig. 38-53B).[83]

BENIGN GASTRIC EMPHYSEMA

Gas in the wall of the stomach is usually a sign of infection, ischemia, increased intraluminal pressure, or severe vomiting, but benign gastric emphysema may occasionally be demonstrated in the absence of underlying disease.[84] Although pneumatosis cystoides intestinalis can affect the wall of the stomach, it more commonly involves the small bowel or colon (see Chapter 16). Gastric emphysema may also be caused by spontaneous or traumatic rupture of a pulmonary bulla into the areolar tissue surrounding the esophagus. Changes in intrapulmonary pressure may force this gas into the upper portion of the esophagus, creating a valvelike mechanism with gradual downward extension of gas into the submucosal or subserosal layers of the gastric wall. When gas is seen on abdominal radiographs in the wall of the stomach in patients who are asymptomatic, gastric pneumatosis, traumatic emphysema of the stomach secondary to endoscopic perforation, and rupture of a pulmonary bulla into the esophageal wall are the most likely diagnostic possibilities (Fig. 38-54).

AMYLOIDOSIS

Deposition of an amorphous, eosinophilic, extracellular protein-polysaccharide complex of amyloid in the stomach can produce a broad spectrum of radiographic findings. Amyloid infiltration is sometimes associated with marked narrowing and rigidity of the wall of the stomach (especially the antrum), producing a linitis plastica appearance.[85] Generalized thickening of gastric folds can also occur (Fig. 38-55).

CYSTIC FIBROSIS

Cystic fibrosis is sometimes manifested on barium studies by a thickened, coarse fold pattern in the duodenum (Fig. 38-56). Associated findings include nodular indentations on the duodenal wall; smudging or poor definition of the mucosal fold pattern; and redundancy, distortion, and kinking of the duodenal contour.[86,87] These changes are usually confined to the first and second portions of the duodenum but occasionally extend into the proximal jejunum. The cause of duodenal fold

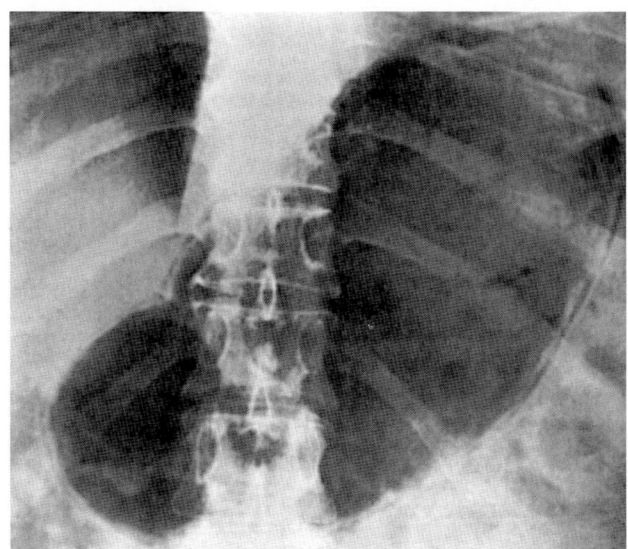

Figure 38-54. Benign gastric emphysema. Linear collections of gas are seen in the gastric wall as a complication of endoscopy. (From Eisenberg RL: Gastrointestinal Radiology: A Pattern Approach, 3rd ed. Philadelphia, JB Lippincott, 1996.)

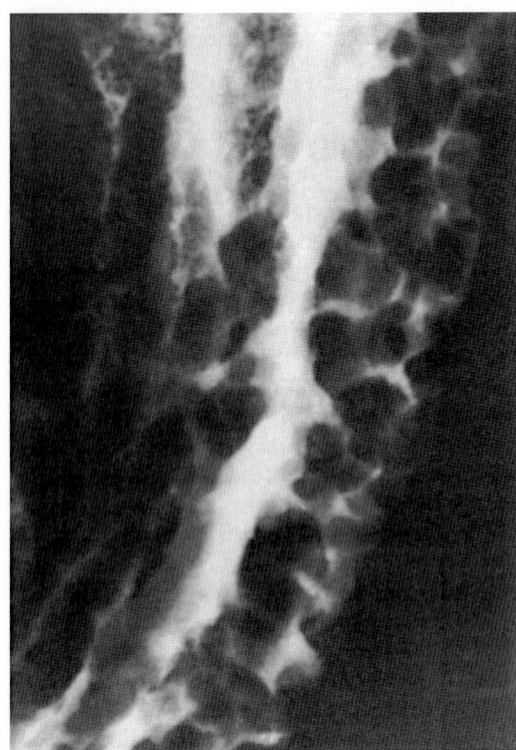

Figure 38-55. Gastric involvement by amyloidosis. There are thickened, nodular folds in the stomach due to infiltration of the gastric wall by amyloidosis. (From Eisenberg RL: Gastrointestinal Radiology: A Pattern Approach, 3rd ed. Philadelphia, JB Lippincott, 1996.)

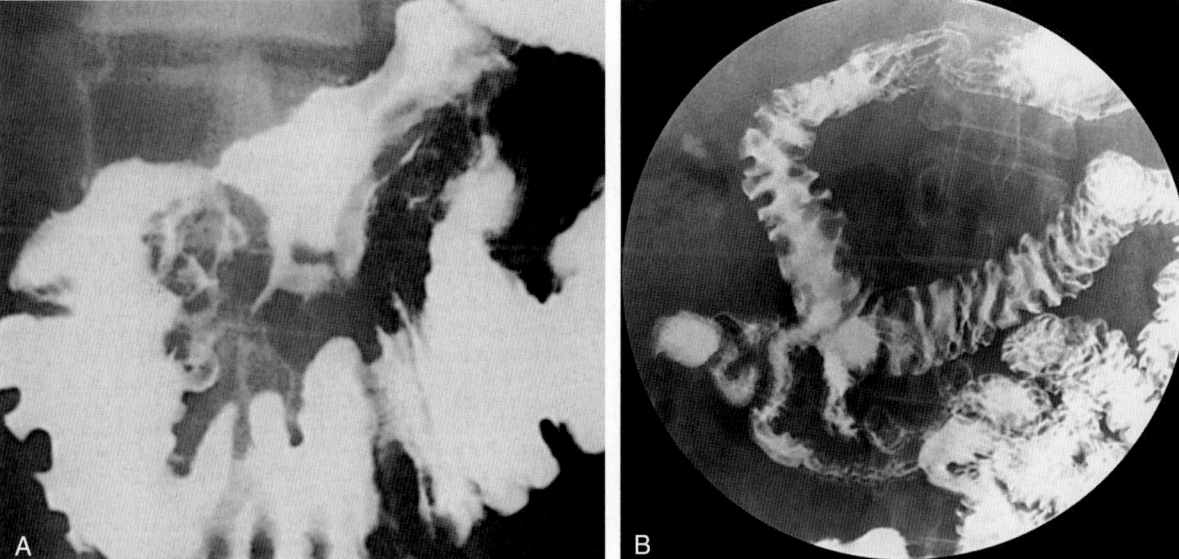

Figure 38-56. Duodenal involvement by cystic fibrosis. A and **B.** In both cases, a thickened, coarse fold pattern is seen in the duodenum. (**A** from Eisenberg RL: Gastrointestinal Radiology: A Pattern Approach, 3rd ed. Philadelphia, JB Lippincott, 1996.)

thickening in cystic fibrosis is uncertain. It has been postulated that a lack of secretion of pancreatic bicarbonate results in inadequate buffering of gastric acid, causing irritation and inflammation of the duodenum in these patients.[87]

References

1. Ryan BM, Stockbrugger RW, Ryan JM: A pathophysiologic, gastro-enterologic, and radiologic approach to the management of gastric varices. Gastroenterology 126:1175-1189, 2004.
2. Sutton JP, Yarborough DY, Richards JT: Isolated splenic vein occlusion. Arch Surg 100:623-626, 1970.
3. Muhletaler C, Gerlock J, Goncharenko V, et al: Gastric varices secondary to splenic vein occlusion: Radiographic diagnosis and clinical significance. Radiology 132:593-598, 1979.
4. Lavender S, Lloyd-Davies RW, Thomas ML: Retroperitoneal fibrosis causing localized portal hypertension. BMJ 3:627-628, 1970.
5. Cho KJ, Martel W: Recognition of splenic vein occlusion. AJR 131: 439-443, 1978.
6. Hershfield NB, Morrow I: Gastric bleeding due to splenic vein thrombosis. Can Med Assoc J 98:649-652, 1968.

7. Goldstein GB: Splenic vein thrombosis causing gastric varices and bleeding. Am J Gastroenterol 58:319-325, 1972.

8. Okuda K, Yasumoto M, Goto A, et al: Endoscopic observations of gastric varices. Am J Gastroenterol 60:357-365, 1973.

9. Itzchak Y, Glickman MG: Splenic vein thrombosis in patients with a normal size spleen. Invest Radiol 12:158-163, 1977.

10. Rice RP, Thompson WM, Kelvin FM, et al: Gastric varices without esophageal varices: An important pre-endoscopic diagnosis. JAMA 237:1976-1979, 1977.

11. Belgrad R, Carlson HC, Payne WS, et al: Pseudotumoral gastric varices. AJR 91:751-756, 1964.

12. Kaye JJ, Stassa G: Mimicry and deception in the diagnosis of tumors of the gastric cardia. AJR 110:295-303, 1970.

13. Carucci LR, Levine MS, Rubesin SE, et al: Tumorous gastric varices: Radiographic findings in 10 patients. Radiology 212:861-865, 1999.

14. Sos T, Meyers MA, Baltaxe HA: Nonfundic gastric varices. Radiology 105:579-580, 1972.

15. Levine MS, Kieu K, Rubesin SE, et al: Isolated gastric varices: Splenic vein obstruction or portal hypertension? Gastrointest Radiol 15:188-192, 1990.

16. Balthazar EJ, Megibow A, Naidich D, et al: Computed tomographic recognition of gastric varices. AJR 142:1121-1125, 1984.

17. Marshall JP, Smith PD, Hoyumpa AM: Gastric varices: Problems in diagnosis. Am J Dig Dis 22:947-955, 1977.

18. Babb RR: Splenic vein obstruction: A curable cause of variceal bleeding. Am J Dig Dis 21:512-513, 1976.

19. Bateson EM: Duodenal and antral varices. Br J Radiol 42:744-747, 1969.

20. Smart HL, Triger DR: Clinical features, pathophysiology, and relevance of portal hypertensive gastropathy. Endoscopy 23:224-228, 1991.

21. Panes J, Bordas JM, Pique JM, et al: Increased gastric mucosal perfusion in cirrhotic patients with portal hypertensive gastropathy. Gastroenterology 103:1875-1882, 1992.

22. Balan KK, Grime JS, Sutton R, et al: Do alterations in the rate of gastric emptying after injection sclerotherapy for esophageal varices play any role in the development of portal hypertensive gastropathy? HPB Surg 11:141-148, 1999.

23. Chang D, Levine MS, Ginsberg GG, et al: Portal hypertensive gastropathy: Radiographic findings in eight patients. AJR 175:1609-1612, 2000.

24. Treichel J, Gerstenberg E, Palme G, et al: Diagnosis of partial gastric diverticula. Radiology 119:13-18, 1976.

25. Millard JR, Ziter FMH, Slover WP: Giant duodenal diverticula. AJR 121:334-337, 1974.

26. Macari M, Lazarus D, Israel G, et al: Duodenal diverticula mimicking cystic neoplasms of the pancreas: CT and MR imaging findings in seven patients. AJR 180:195-199, 2003.

27. Afridi SA, Fichtenbaum CJ, Taubin H: Review of duodenal diverticula. Am J Gastroenterol 86:935-938, 1991.

28. Wolfe RD, Pearl MJ: Acute perforation of duodenal diverticulum with roentgenographic demonstration of localized retroperitoneal emphysema. Radiology 104:301-302, 1972.

29. Pugash RA, O'Brien SE, Stevenson GW: Perforating duodenal diverticulitis. Gastrointest Radiol 15:156-158, 1990.

30. Gore RM, Ghahremani GG, Kirsch MD, et al: Diverticulitis of the duodenum: Clinical and radiological manifestations of seven cases. Am J Gastroenterol 86:981-985, 1991.

31. Rioux L, Des Groseilliers S, Fortin M, et al: Massive upper gastrointestinal bleeding originating from a fourth-stage duodenal diverticulum. Can J Surg 39:510-512, 1996.

32. Nelson JA, Burhenne HJ: Anomalous biliary and pancreatic duct insertion into duodenal diverticula. Radiology 120:49-52, 1976.

33. Materne R: The duodenal wind sock sign. Radiology 218:749-750, 2001.

34. Johnston P, Desser TS: MDCT of intraluminal "windsock" duodenal diverticulum with surgical correlation and multiplanar reconstruction. AJR 183:249-250, 2004.

35. Clements JL, Jinkins JR, Torres WE, et al: Antral mucosal diaphragms in adults. AJR 133:1105-1111, 1979.

36. Bjorgvinsson E, Rudzki C, Lewicki AM: Antral web. Am J Gastroenterol 79:663-665, 1984.

37. Pratt AD: Current concepts of the obstructing duodenal diaphragm. Radiology 100:637-643, 1971.

38. Rha SE, Lee JH, Lee SY, et al: Duodenal diaphragm associated with long-term use of nonsteroidal antiinflammatory drugs: A rare cause of duodenal obstruction in an adult. AJR 175:920-921, 2000.

39. Balthazar EJ: Hypertrophic pyloric stenosis in adults: Radiographic features. Am J Gastroenterol 78:449-453, 1983.

40. Balthazar EJ, Rosenberg H, Davidian MM: Scirrhous carcinoma of the pyloric channel and distal antrum. AJR 134:669-674, 1980.

41. Aranha GV, Prinz RA, Greenlee HB, et al: Gastric outlet and duodenal obstruction from inflammatory pancreatic disease. Arch Surg 119:833-835, 1984.

42. Berk RN, Coulson DB: The body cast syndrome. Radiology 94:303-305, 1970.

43. Wallace RG, Howard WB: Acute superior mesenteric artery syndrome in the severely burned patient. Radiology 94:307-310, 1970.

44. Simon M, Lerner MA: Duodenal compression by the mesenteric root in acute pancreatitis and in inflammatory conditions of the bowel. Radiology 79:75-81, 1962.

45. Shammash JB, Rubesin SE, Levine MS: Massive gastric distention due to duodenal involvement by retroperitoneal tumors. Gastrointest Radiol 17:214-216, 1992.

46. Ooi GC, Chan KL, Ko KF, et al: Computed tomography of the superior mesenteric artery syndrome. Clin Imaging 21:210-212, 1997.

47. Rogers LF, Goldstein HM: Roentgen manifestations of radiation injury to the gastrointestinal tract. Gastrointest Radiol 2:281-291, 1977.

48. Braun P, Collins PP, Ducharme JC: Preduodenal portal vein: A significant entity? Report of two cases and a review of the literature. Can J Surg 17:316-322, 1974.

49. Rimer DG: Gastric retention without mechanical obstruction. Arch Intern Med 117:287-299, 1966.

50. Horowitz M, Fraser RJL: Gastroparesis: Diagnosis and management. Scand J Gastroenterol 30(Suppl 213):7-16, 1995.

51. Gramm HF, Reuter K, Costello P: The radiologic manifestations of diabetic gastric neuropathy and its differential diagnosis. Gastrointest Radiol 3:151-155, 1978.

52. Parkman HP, Hasler WL, Fisher RS: American Gastroenterological Association medical position statement: Diagnosis and treatment of gastroparesis. Gastroenterology 127:1589-1591, 2004.

53. Friedenberg FK, Parkman HP: Management of delayed gastric emptying. Clin Gastroenterol Hepatol 3:642-646, 2005.

54. Horowitz M, McNeil JD, Maddern GJ, et al: Abnormalities of gastric and esophageal emptying in polymyositis and dermatomyositis. Gastroenterology 90:434-439, 1986.

55. Nowak TV, Ionasescu V, Anuras S: Gastrointestinal manifestations of the muscular dystrophies. Gastroenterology 82:800-810, 1982.

56. Chon H, Arger PH, Miller WT: Displacement of duodenum by an enlarged liver. AJR 119:85-88, 1973.

57. Bluth I, Vitale P: Right renal enlargement causing alterations in the descending duodenum: A radiographic demonstration. Radiology 76:777-784, 1961.

58. Poppel MH: Duodenocolic apposition. AJR 83:851-856, 1960.

59. Treitel H, Meyers MA, Maza V: Changes in the duodenal loop secondary to carcinoma of the hepatic flexure of the colon. Br J Radiol 43:209-213, 1970.

60. Shimkin PM, Pearson KD: Unusual arterial impressions upon the duodenum. Radiology 103:295-297, 1972.

61. Zeman RK, Schiebler M, Clark LR, et al: The clinical and imaging spectrum of pancreaticoduodenal lymph node enlargement. AJR 144:1223-1227, 1985.

62. Leonidas JC, Kopel FB, Danese CA: Mesenteric cysts associated with protein loss in the gastrointestinal tract. AJR 112:150-154, 1971.

63. Asrani AV: The antral pad sign. Radiology 229:421-422, 2003.

64. Ripolles T, Garcia-Aguayo G, Martinez MJ, et al: Gastrointestinal bezoars: Sonographic and CT characteristics. AJR 177:65-69, 2001.

65. Kleinman PK, Brill PW, Winchester P: Resolving duodenal-jejunal hematoma in abused children. Radiology 160:747-750, 1986.

66. Ghishan FK, Werner M, Vieira P, et al: Intramural duodenal hematoma: An unusual complication of endoscopic small bowel biopsy. Am J Gastroenterol 82:368-370, 1987.

67. Kunin JR, Korobkin M, Ellis JH, et al: Duodenal injuries caused by blunt abdominal trauma: Value of CT in differentiating perforation from hematoma. AJR 160:221-223, 1993.

68. Singh AK, Shirkhoda A, Lal N, et al: Bouveret's syndrome: Appearance on CT and upper gastrointestinal radiography before and after stone obturation. AJR 181:828-830, 2003.

69. Brennan GB, Rosenberg RD, Arora S: Bouveret syndrome. RadioGraphics 24:1171-1175, 2004.

70. Gerson DE, Lewicki AM: Intrathoracic stomach: When does it obstruct? Radiology 119:257-264, 1976.

71. Allen MS, Trastek VF, Deschamps C, et al: Intrathoracic stomach: Presentation and results of operation. J Thorac Cardiovasc Surg 105:253-258, 1993.

72. Scott RL, Felker R, Winer-Muram H, et al: The differential retrocardiac air-fluid level: A sign of intrathoracic gastric volvulus. J Can Assoc Radiol 37:119-121, 1986.

73. Chiechi MV, Hamrick-Turner J, Abbitt PL: Gastric herniation and volvulus: CT and MR appearance. Gastrointest Radiol 17:99-101, 1992.

74. Meyers MA: Gastroduodenal intussusception. Am J Med Sci 254:347-355, 1967.

75. Choi SH, Han JK, Kim SH, et al: Intussusception in adults: From stomach to rectum. AJR 183:691-698, 2004.

76. Van Beers B, Trigau JP, Pringot J: Duodenojejunal intussusception secondary to duodenal tumors. Gastrointest Radiol 13:24-26, 1988.

77. Smith DL, Dockerty MD, Black BM: Gastrocolic fistulas of malignant origin. Surg Gynecol Obstet 134:829-832, 1972.

78. Levine MS, Kelly MR, Laufer I, et al: Gastrocolic fistulas: The increasing role of aspirin. Radiology 187:359-361, 1993.

79. Martinez LO, Manheimer LH, Casal GL, et al: Malignant fistulae of the gastrointestinal tract. AJR 131:215-218, 1978.

80. Swartz MJ, Paustian FF, Chleborad WJ: Recurrent gastric ulcer with spontaneous gastrojejunal and gastrocolic fistulas. Gastroenterology 44:527-531, 1963.

81. Haff RC, Wise L, Ballinger WF: Biliary-enteric fistulas. Surg Gynecol Obstet 133:84-88, 1971.

82. Wyatt GM, Rauchway MI, Spitz HB: Roentgen findings in aortoenteric fistulae. AJR 126:714-722, 1976.

83. Miller RE: The radiological evaluation of intraperitoneal gas (pneumoperitoneum). Crit Rev Diagn Imaging 4:61-85, 1973.

84. Lee S, Rutledge JN: Gastric emphysema. Am J Gastroenterol 79:899-904, 1984.

85. Carlson HC, Breen JF: Amyloidosis and plasma cell dyscrasias: Gastrointestinal involvement. Semin Roentgenol 21:128-138, 1986.

86. Phelan MS, Fine DR, Zentler-Munro L, et al: Radiographic abnormalities of the duodenum in cystic fibrosis. Clin Radiol 34:573-577, 1983.

87. Agrons GA, Corse WR, Markowitz RI, et al: Gastrointestinal manifestations of cystic fibrosis: Radiologic-pathologic correlation. RadioGraphics 16:871-893, 1996.

Postoperative Stomach and Duodenum

Richard M. Gore, MD • Claire H. Smith, MD

Radiologic evaluation of patients who have undergone gastric and duodenal surgery requires an understanding of the operative procedures and an appreciation of the normal postoperative appearance of the gut. The radiologist is frequently asked to define the postsurgical anatomy, to assess the efficacy of the procedures, to establish a postoperative baseline appearance, and to detect early and late postoperative complications. In this chapter we describe the more common operations performed on the stomach and duodenum, detail the rationale for surgery, provide a basic approach to contrast agent examinations in these patients, and discuss the normal postoperative appearance and common complications.

Gastric and duodenal operations are performed to control obesity, resect malignant or benign masses, and treat peptic ulcer disease and its complications, such as bleeding, perforation, and obstruction. Fifteen to 20 percent of postsurgical patients present with new or recurrent symptoms related to physiologic, metabolic, or anatomic factors (Table 39-1).[1,2] A multispecialty team approach is often needed to diagnose and treat these patients.

TERMINOLOGY

Guidelines describing postoperative changes of the stomach and duodenum have been well established. Radiologic evaluation should include the extent of bowel resection; the type, location, and diameter of the anastomosis; and the speed, direction, and completeness of gastric emptying.[3-5]

Several common eponyms deserve further explanation. The Billroth I procedure (Fig. 39-1) entails partial gastric re-

section (antrectomy) with gastroduodenostomy. The Billroth II procedure involves gastric resection with gastrojejunostomy and either Roux-en-Y or loop-type gastroenteric anastomosis. With the Roux-en-Y anastomosis, the jejunum is divided, the proximal end or side of the small bowel is attached to the stomach, and the distal end of the loop is anastomosed to the side of the distal jejunum (Fig. 39-2). With a loop-type gastroenterostomy, the stomach is joined to the side of the small bowel. A variable length of duodenum and jejunum forms a proximal or afferent loop, which carries pancreaticobiliary secretions toward the stomach, and a distal or efferent loop, which flows in a downstream direction. The gastroenterostomy may be anterior to the transverse colon (antecolic), or the small bowel may be brought up through an opening made in the transverse mesocolon to lie along the posterior wall of the stomach in a retrocolic location. The anastomosis is placed at the dependent portion of the stomach to facilitate gastric emptying.[3-5]

Further definition of the loop-type configuration describes how the afferent loop is related to the curvatures of the stomach. In a right-to-left (isoperistaltic) anastomosis (Fig. 39-3), the proximal loop of small bowel is first attached to the right or lesser curvature portion of the stomach with the distal loop of small bowel on the left or greater curvature area. A left-to-right (antiperistaltic) anastomosis defines the opposite configuration (Fig. 39-4). Choice of configuration depends on the surgeon's preference and the patient's body habitus.

Different terms are used for gastric operations performed for weight control.[6] For gastric stapling operations without

Table 39-1
Complications of Gastric and Duodenal Surgery

Esophageal dysmotility
   Tissue damage at operation
   After vagotomy
Esophagitis
   Gastroesophageal reflux
   Alkaline reflux
   Alimentary tube use
Gastric-emptying problems
   Gastric stasis
   Secondary gastric effects from impaired small bowel motility
   Dumping syndrome
   Generalized bowel ileus
   Bezoar formation
Gastritis and gastric remnant ulcerations
   Technical factors
      Indication for original operation
      Type of operation
      Experience of surgeon
      Adequacy of surgery
      Presence of unabsorbable sutures
   Presence of hypersecretory states
      Incomplete vagotomy
      Gastrinoma with Zollinger-Ellison syndrome
      Antral G-cell hyperplasia
      Retained antrum syndrome
      Hyperparathyroidism
   Ulcerogenic substance use
      Cigarette and tobacco products
      Ulcerogenic drugs
   Alkaline reflux
Neoplasm
   Recurrent tumor
   Gastric remnant cancer
Anastomotic leak or bowel perforation
   Abscess
   Fistula
Bowel obstruction
   Narrow anastomotic or channel diameter
      Edema
      Marginal ulcer
      Stricture after ulcer healing
      Prolapse and intussusception
   Bezoar formation
Gastrojejunocolic fistula
Jejunitis
Metabolic effects
   Malabsorption
      Steatorrhea with decreased vitamin D absorption
      Shortened intestinal transit time
      Inadequate mixture of pancreatic juices, bile salts, and food
   Iron-deficiency anemia
      Inadequate diet
      Impaired resorption of dietary iron
      Chronic blood loss
   Vitamin B_{12} anemia
      Decrease of gastric intrinsic factor
      Bacterial overgrowth (rare)
   Weight loss and malnutrition
      Insufficient caloric intake
      Incomplete digestion of food
      Inadvertent gastroileostomy
      Diarrhea
Psychologic effects
   Phantom ulcer syndrome
Nutritional support problems
   Intraperitoneal leakage of gastric contents
   Tube malposition, dislodgment, or blockage
   Gastroesophageal reflux and aspiration

Adapted from Smith C, Gardiner R: Postoperative stomach and recurrent abdominal pain. In Thompson WM (ed): Common Problems in Gastrointestinal Radiology. Chicago, Year Book Medical, 1989, pp 202-211.

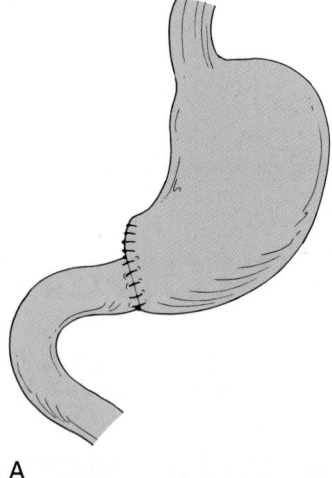

A

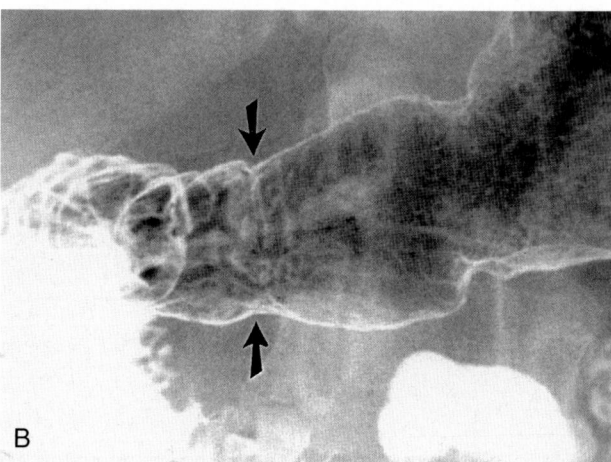

B

Figure 39-1. Billroth I gastroduodenostomy. Several modifications have been devised, but the basic operation ensures that the duodenal passage remains intact. **A.** Diagram of gastroduodenostomy. **B.** Upper gastrointestinal series shows minimal indentation (*arrows*) at the widely patent anastomosis. (**A** from Smith C, Deziel DJ: Radiology of the postoperative stomach. In Taveras JM, Ferrucci JT [eds]: Radiology: Diagnosis, Imaging, Intervention. Philadelphia, Lippincott-Raven, 1995, pp 1-16.)

bowel anastomosis, a small proximal gastric pouch and a narrow channel lead to the distal stomach. Gastric bypass operations create a restricted proximal gastric pouch and a narrow anastomosis or channel to the small bowel via the standard loop or Roux-en-Y configuration. The stomach is not resected, but there may or may not be gastric transection between the staple lines.

DIAGNOSTIC TESTING FOR POSTOPERATIVE COMPLICATIONS

The diagnostic approach to patients with suspected postsurgical complications depends on the patient's condition, the length of time since surgery, and the presenting complaint.[7,8]

Contrast Agent Studies

Water-soluble contrast agents are generally used in the immediate postoperative period when anastomotic leaks, staple line dehiscences, bowel perforations, fistulas, or abscesses are suspected. Plain radiographs should be obtained before all

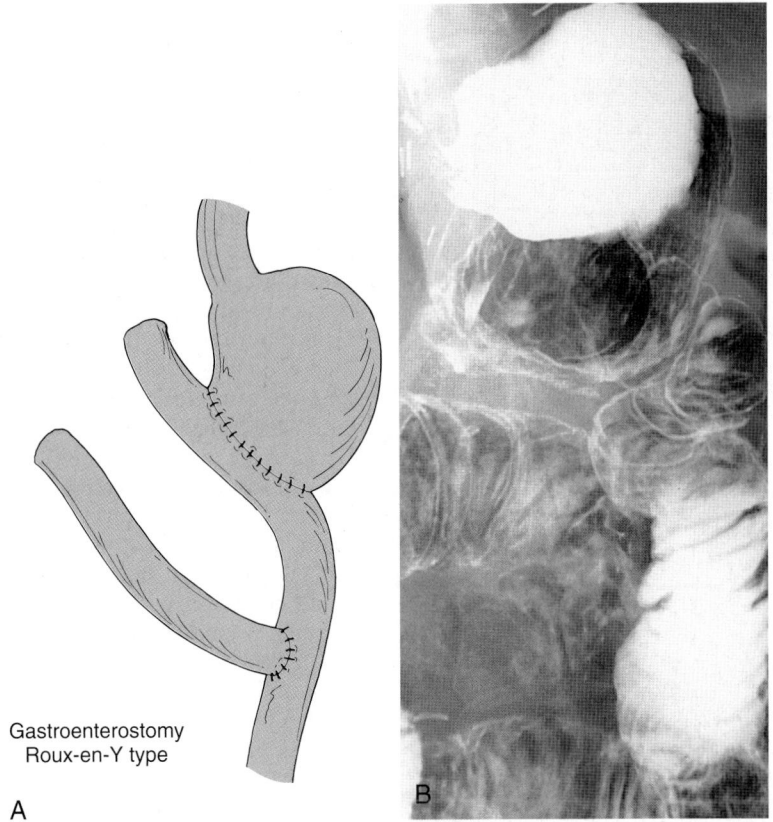

Figure 39-2. Partial gastrectomy with Roux-en-Y gastrojejunostomy. A. Diagram depicts the end-to-side gastrojejunostomy and enteroenterostomy. **B.** Barium study shows that the Roux-en-Y loop does not readily fill with contrast material and the distal enteroenterostomy may not be readily localized. Surgical clips are present at the gastroesophageal junctions from prior vagotomy. (**A** and **B** from Smith C, Deziel DJ, Kubicka RA: Evaluation of the postoperative stomach and duodenum. RadioGraphics 14:67-86, 1994.)

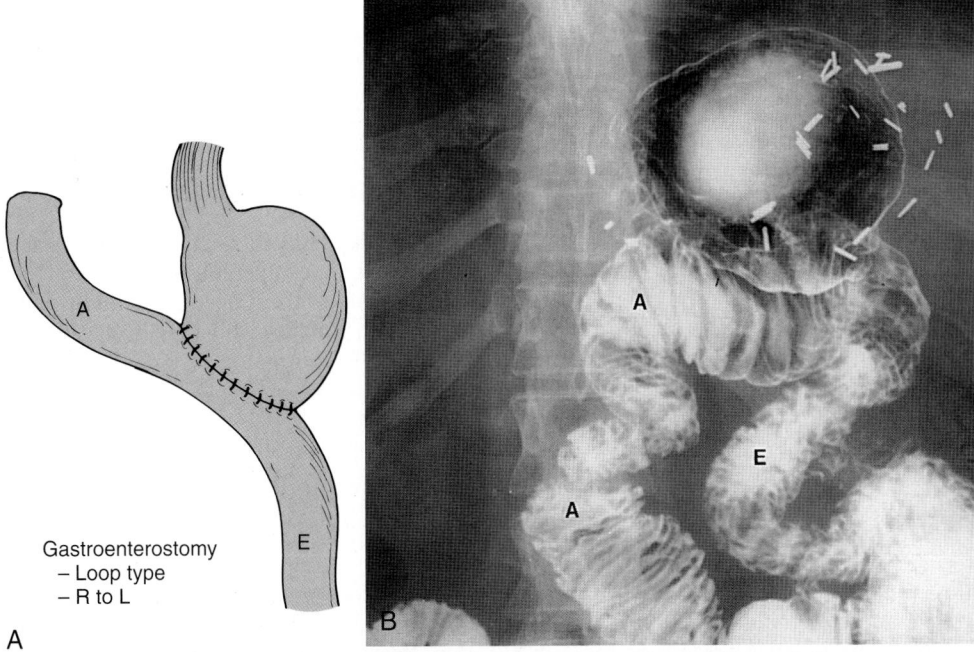

Figure 39-3. Billroth II gastrojejunostomy: isoperistaltic configuration. Diagram (**A**) and barium study (**B**) show loop-type, right-to-left configuration after gastric resection. In this modification, the afferent loop (A) swings to the left, and the anastomosis is carried from the greater curvature or left side of the stomach to the lesser curvature or right side. E, efferent limb. (**A** and **B** from Smith C, Deziel DJ, Kubicka RA: Evaluation of the postoperative stomach and duodenum. RadioGraphics 14:67-86, 1994.)

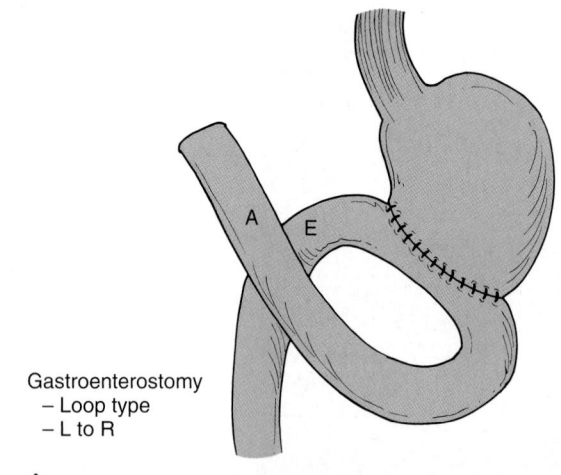

Gastroenterostomy
– Loop type
– L to R

A

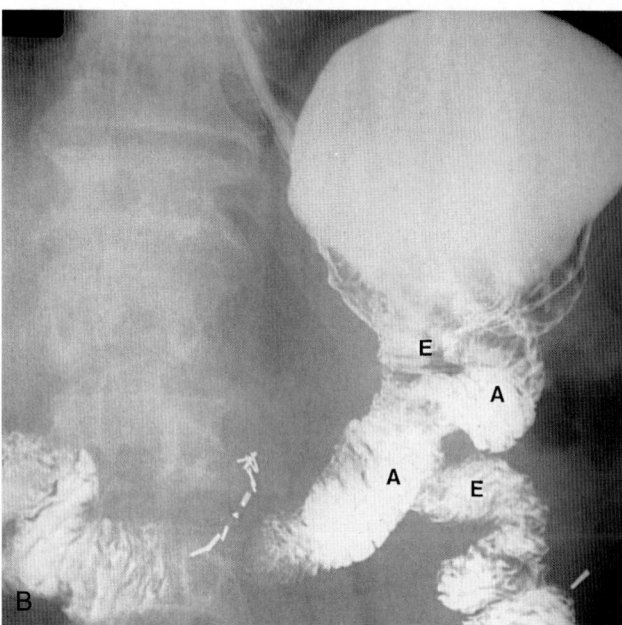

Figure 39-4. Billroth II gastrojejunostomy: antiperistaltic configuration. Diagram (**A**) and barium study (**B**) show the loop-type, left-to-right configuration after gastric resection. The small bowel is first anastomosed to the right side of the stomach and is then carried to the left. The length of the afferent (A) loop varies; the efferent loop (E) carries contents away from the stomach. (**A** and **B** from Smith C, Deziel DJ, Kubicka RA: Appearances of the postoperative alimentary tract. Radiol Clin North Am 31:1235-1253, 1993.)

contrast agent studies because the configuration of surgical staples, clips, and drains provides clues to the type of operation that has been performed. Foreign bodies or abnormal gas collections may also be found.[5] In morbidly obese patients, fluoroscopic evaluation may be limited or impossible and bowel perforation may be recognized only by seeing surgical drains outlined with contrast material on later films when compared with radiographs obtained before contrast agent enhancement.[6]

Positive contrast studies provide a reliable overview of surgically created anatomic alterations, and the choice of single- or double-contrast techniques depends on the clinical circumstances.[7] Single-contrast examinations are helpful for detecting fistulas, evaluating the rate and direction of liquid

flow, and examining debilitated patients who are unable to rapidly change position.[8] Essentials of single-contrast techniques are careful fluoroscopic tracking of contrast material, palpation, and mucosal relief films.

Double-contrast techniques depict exquisite mucosal detail, but patient cooperation is more critical for these studies. The fluoroscopist must maintain a careful balance between mucosal coating and egress of barium and gas through the anastomosis. This is facilitated by use of glucagon, initial administration of only small amounts of barium, prompt positioning of the patient, and timely elevation and lowering of the fluoroscopy table. Esophageal motility can be evaluated and compression films of the anastomosis obtained by using the same low-density contrast agents as employed in routine biphasic upper gastrointestinal studies.[2,8-12]

For obese patients whose gastric restrictive procedures have not resulted in weight loss, examination methods must also be altered.[13-38] Because fluoroscopic evaluation is limited, the first swallow of contrast material must be promptly filmed with the patient in the proper position.[13] Contrast material should be administered slowly to prevent overdistention of the small proximal gastric pouch and vomiting. In patients with gastric bypass procedures, the channel and small bowel loops can be examined reliably but the distal stomach is more difficult to evaluate. Fluoroscopically guided percutaneous injection of contrast material directly into the distal stomach has been used.[14,15] Endoscopy of the distal stomach using a pediatric colonoscope is the preferred route, particularly in perioperative patients. It is successful in at least 70% of patients after gastric bypass.[16]

Limitations of contrast agent studies in patients with prior gastric or duodenal surgery include apparent masses caused by postsurgical plication defects, contrast material trapped within deformed perianastomotic folds simulating recurrent ulcers, and edema or suture granulomas mimicking gastric neoplasm.[8] Alternatively, ulcers or masses may be falsely attributed to postsurgical deformities. Also, early mucosal changes of metaplasia associated with alkaline reflux usually escape radiologic detection.[9,17] Lastly, some anatomic configurations preclude adequate contrast agent examination despite meticulous fluoroscopic technique.

Computed Tomography

Oral, rectal, and intravenous contrast agents are needed to evaluate the postoperative patient on CT.[18] If patients are too ill to drink, contrast agents should be injected via alimentary tubes. In patients who have had gastric bypass procedures for weight control or in patients with long Roux-en-Y or afferent loops, CT may be helpful in evaluating these portions of the gut.[19]

Nuclear Medicine

Scintigraphic emptying studies are useful for patients with suspected postgastrectomy stasis syndromes, afferent loop dysfunction, motility problems of dumping and diarrhea, and postoperative symptoms of unclear cause.[20,21] The tests are easily performed with radiolabeled solids and liquids and can detect and quantitate subtle abnormalities of gastric emptying (see Chapter 14).[22]

Endoscopy

Endoscopy is useful in the detection of immediate postoperative problems and the diagnosis and treatment of some chronic complications. Although long Roux-en-Y loops or gastric bypass procedures may make endoscopy difficult, significant unexpected pathologic alterations can be detected.[23] In patients with less complicated postoperative anastomoses, experienced endoscopists can differentiate significant perianastomotic disease from normal postoperative deformities.[24]

Endoscopy is required to detect the early mucosal changes of alkaline reflux gastritis, the most common cause of postoperative dyspepsia. Because alkaline reflux gastritis may require surgical revision, accurate detection is crucial and barium examinations do not reliably diagnose this disorder in its early stages.[24-26]

Disadvantages of endoscopy include the risk of bowel perforation, cost, and technical factors related to altered anatomy and the expertise of the endoscopist.

DISEASES AND THEIR OPERATIONS

Surgery for Weight Control

Over the past decade, the number of surgical procedures for morbid obesity has dramatically increased.[13-38] In 2006, medical claims related to bariatric surgery exceeded $5 billion.[28] This impressive growth can be attributed to a number of factors, including the increasing prevalence of morbid obesity, the incorporation of laparoscopy into bariatric procedures, and the popularization of surgical treatment by the media and public. In the United States more than 30% of adults are obese and 2% to 3% of men and 6% to 7% of women are morbidly obese—some 12 million Americans.[14,15] Indeed, given the current epidemic, obesity and physical inactivity have become two of the most urgent public health issues in the United States. An estimated $50 billion is spent annually treating diseases associated with obesity, with total cost to society estimated at $150 billion.[14,15] Annual health care costs are 44% higher for patients who have a body mass index (BMI) greater than 35 than in patients who have a BMI of 20 to 24. Direct and indirect costs of obesity are estimated to be 7% of total national health care expenditures in the United States and between 1% and 5% in Europe.[25,28]

Obesity is defined by a BMI of 30 kg/m^2 or more; morbid obesity as a BMI of 40 kg/m^2 or 35 kg/m^2 with comorbidities; and super obesity as a BMI of 50 kg/m^2. Comorbidities associated with obesity include coronary artery disease, hyperlipidemia, type II diabetes, gallstones, hypertension, osteoarthritis, hypoventilation syndrome, and sleep apnea. There is also a significant positive association between obesity and high death rates for cancer of the esophagus, colorectum, liver, gallbladder, pancreas, stomach, kidney, prostate, breast, uterus, cervix, and ovary. A prospective cancer prevention cohort study estimated that overweight and obesity account for 14% of cancer deaths in men and 20% of those in women. This study estimated that over 90,000 cancer deaths per year in the United States could be avoided if the adult population all maintained a normal weight (BMI < 25).

In patients in whom other weight loss options have failed, bariatric surgery is the most reliable method of weight reduction that provides significant weight loss, extended weight maintenance, and control or reversal of obesity-related health problems. Morbid obesity is associated with excess mortality, and a number of therapeutic measures have been developed.[27] Although dietary and behavioral therapy and gastric balloons and bubbles are available, present-day operations are more effective in reducing excess body weight in the morbidly obese patient.[28]

Bariatric surgery began in 1953 with the jejunoileal bypass procedure but was associated with a high incidence of malnutrition, hepatic failure, nephrolithiasis, and arthritis. This led to the development of a number of other procedures, including the loop gastric bypass, the vertical banded gastroplasty, and Roux-en-Y gastric bypass (RYGB). Currently, RYGB, biliary-pancreatic diversion/duodenal switch (BPD/DS), and gastric banding procedures are the major surgical approaches employed. Laparoscopic Roux-en-Y gastric bypass (LRYGB) has become the gold standard for bariatric surgery in the United States, although laparoscopic adjustable gastric banding (LAGB) is becoming increasingly popular. Duodenal switch and biliopancreatic diversions are associated with protein-calorie malnutrition problems.[25]

Bariatric procedures fall into one of two categories: bypass and restrictive procedures (or a combination of both). Restrictive procedures involve placing a foreign body such as an adjustable silicone band around the gastric outlet to produce a feeling of early satiety. This technique is effective in reducing the volume of solid food intake, but liquid and semisolid foods can pass through the banded outlet without creating a sense of satiety. Accordingly, it is ineffective in a morbidly obese eater of sweet foods.[25]

Bypass procedures attempt to create a "controlled" state of malabsorption. The duodenal switch and biliopancreatic diversion produce malabsorption by reducing contact of digested food with small bowel, pancreatic and biliary secretions, or both.

Laparoscopic Roux-En-Y Gastric Bypass

The LRYGB (Fig. 39-5) has elements of both restriction and malabsorption by creating a small gastric pouch to lead to early satiety and bypassing 100 to 200 cm of small bowel. This does create malabsorption of important micronutrients such as calcium, iron, and vitamin B_{12}, which must be supplemented in the patient's diet.

In this procedure, a gastric pouch measuring 10 to 30 mL is created by surgical separation from the remainder of the stomach—the excluded gastric remnant. A mobilized loop of jejunum is anastomosed end-to-side to the gastric pouch. A side-to-side anastomosis is made between this Roux limb (the efferent loop) to the proximal jejunum to permit digestion with biliary and pancreatic secretions. The Roux limb can be brought to the pouch either dorsally, through the transverse mesocolon (retrocolic), or anterior to the transverse colon (antecolic). In this procedure 95% of the stomach, all of the duodenum, and a portion of the proximal jejunum of variable length are excluded from the digestive tract. In morbidly obese patients 30 cm of jejunum is excluded, and in super obese patients some 150 cm of jejunum is excluded. There are two afferent loops in this procedure: the duodenum and a small loop at the gastrojejunal anastomosis.[25]

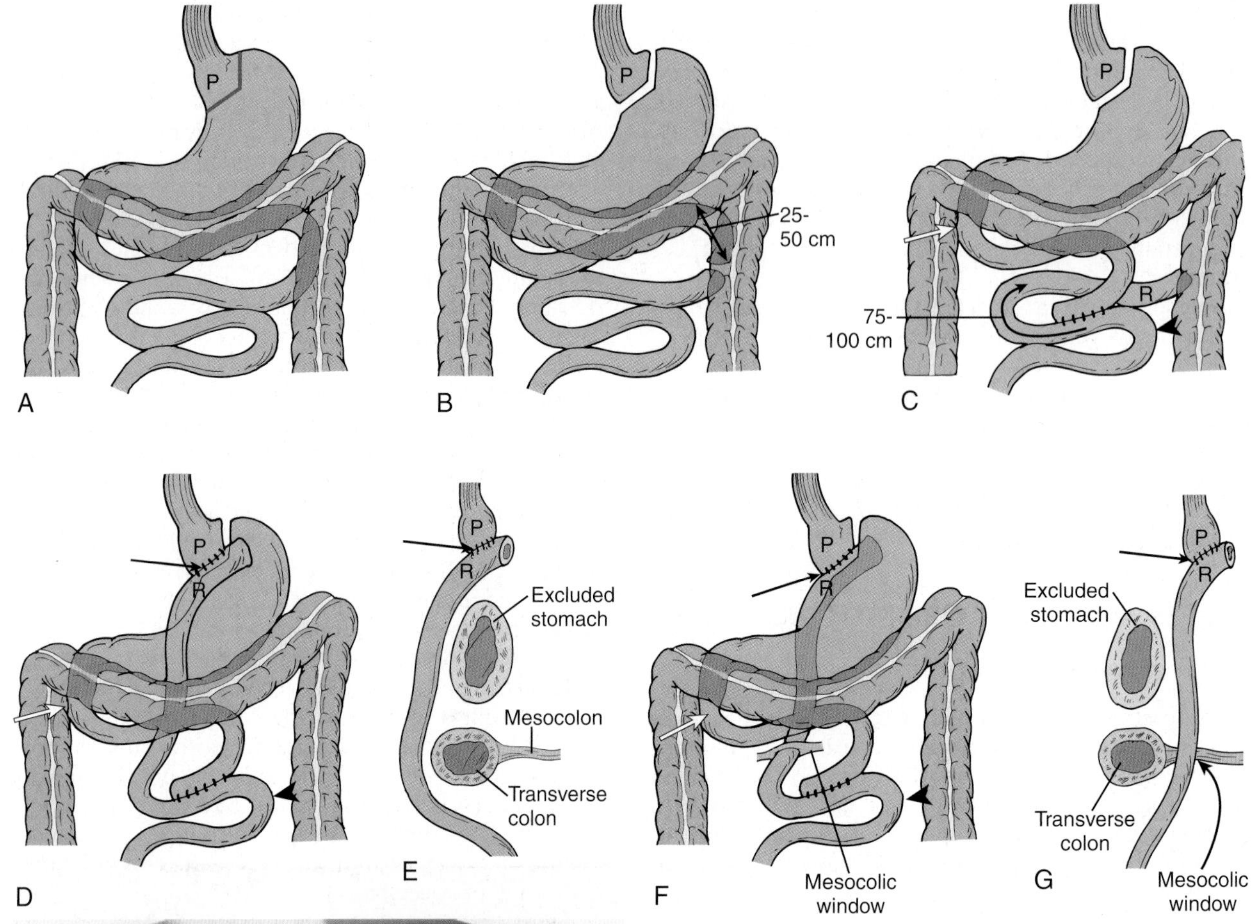

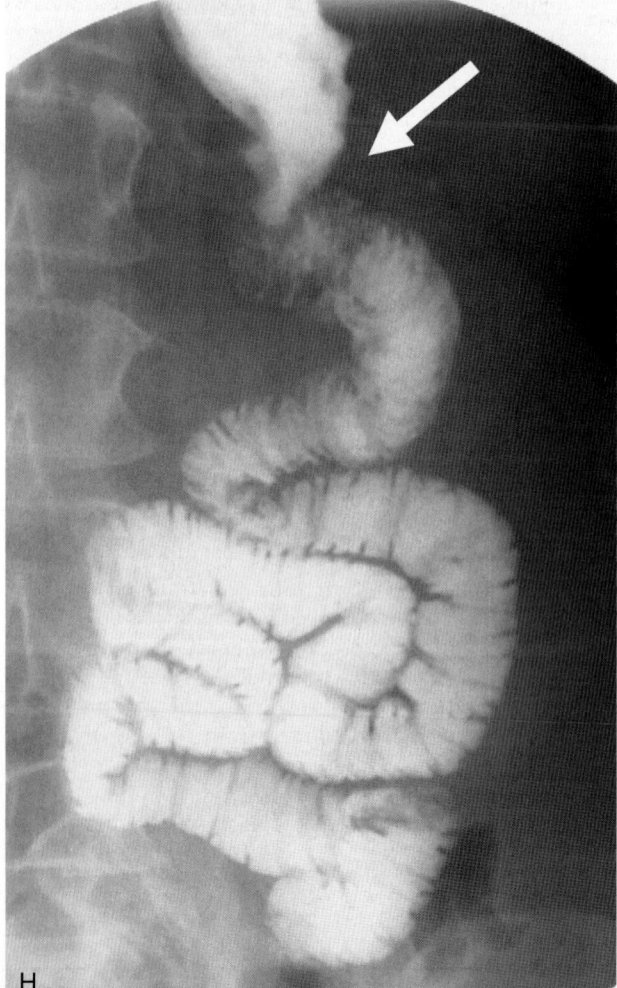

Figure 39-5. Laparoscopic creation of a Roux-en-Y gastric bypass.
A. A gastric pouch (P) is created by dividing the stomach primarily along the lesser curvature. **B.** The jejunum is divided 25 to 50 cm distal to the ligament of Treitz. The biliopancreatic limb (*arrow*) is temporarily excluded from the remainder of the small bowel. P, gastric pouch. **C.** The Roux limb (R) is measured to 75 to 100 cm and attached to the biliopancreatic limb (*arrow*) with a side-to-side anastomosis. There are now three distinct portions of small bowel: the biliopancreatic limb, the Roux limb, and the common channel (*arrowhead*) distal to the anastomosis. P, gastric pouch. Frontal (**D**) and lateral (**E**) views show antecolic-antegastric placement of the Roux limb (R), which is brought anterior to the transverse colon and stomach. P, pouch; *black arrow,* gastrojejunal anastomosis; *white arrow* in **D,** biliopancreatic limb; *arrowhead* in **D,** common channel. Frontal (**F**) and lateral (**G**) views show retrocolic-retrogastric placement of the Roux limb (R), which is tunneled posteriorly through a surgically created defect in the transverse mesocolon. P, pouch; *black arrow,* gastrojejunal anastomosis; *white arrow* in **F,** biliopancreatic limb; *arrowhead* in **F,** common channel. **H.** Contrast study showing normal postoperative appearance of gastric bypass. *Arrow,* gastrojejunostomy. (**A-G** from Scheiry CD, Scholz FJ, Shah PC, et al: Radiology of the laparoscopic Roux-en-Y gastric bypass procedure: Conceptualization and precise interpretation of results. RadioGraphics 26:1355-1371, 2006.)

Patients who undergo LRYGB show sustained weight reduction with a mean weight loss of the one third of body weight. Most comorbidities, especially diabetes, improve or completely resolve in the majority of patients within 1 year of LRYGB.

The mortality rate for this procedure ranges up to 3%. The most common causes of death include pulmonary embolism, anastomotic leak, respiratory failure, sepsis, cardiac arrhythmia, Roux limb necrosis, and upper gastrointestinal hemorrhage.[19]

Laparoscopic Adjustable Laparoscopic Banding Procedure

This procedure consists of looping a non-radiopaque silicon band around the fundus of the stomach approximately 3 cm beneath the gastroesophageal junction (Fig. 39-6). This creates a small proximal gastric pouch with a stoma to the remainder of the stomach. Seroserosal stitching of the band to the stomach is performed anteriorly to anchor it to the gastric wall. The size of the stoma between the small proximal pouch and the remainder of the stomach is adjustable because

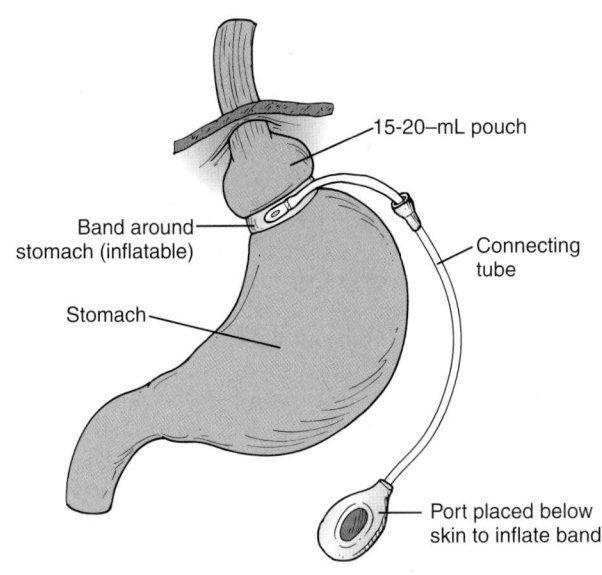

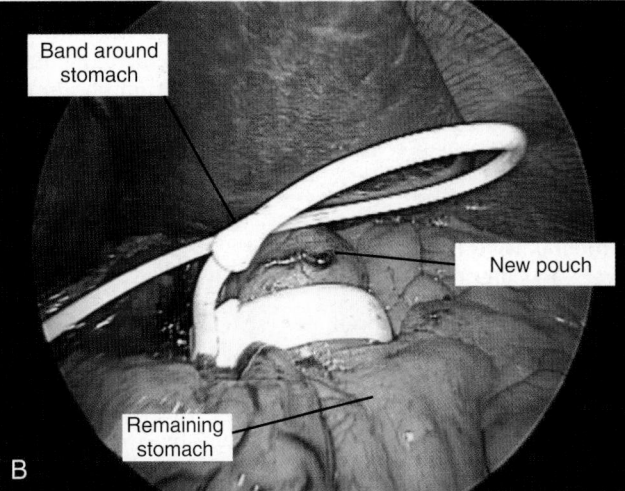

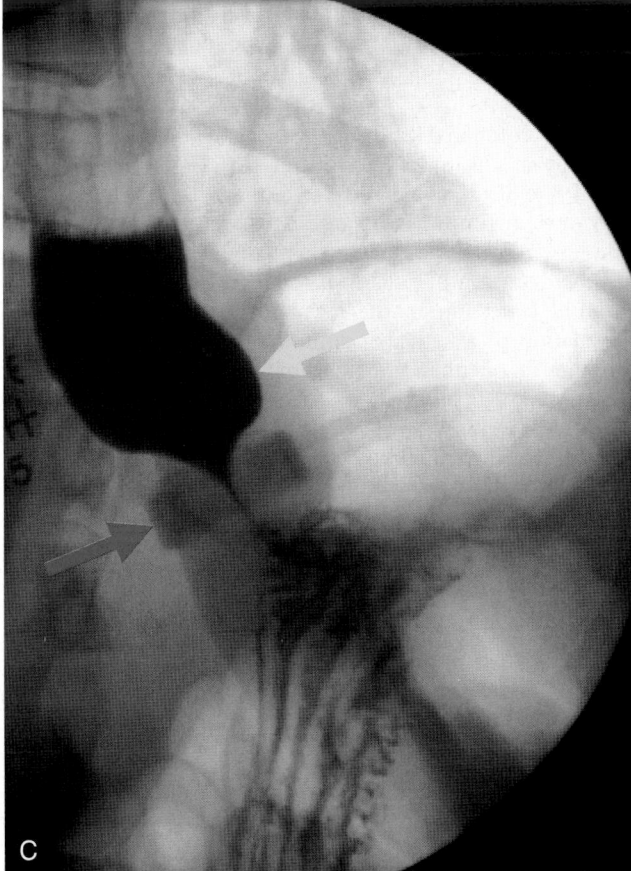

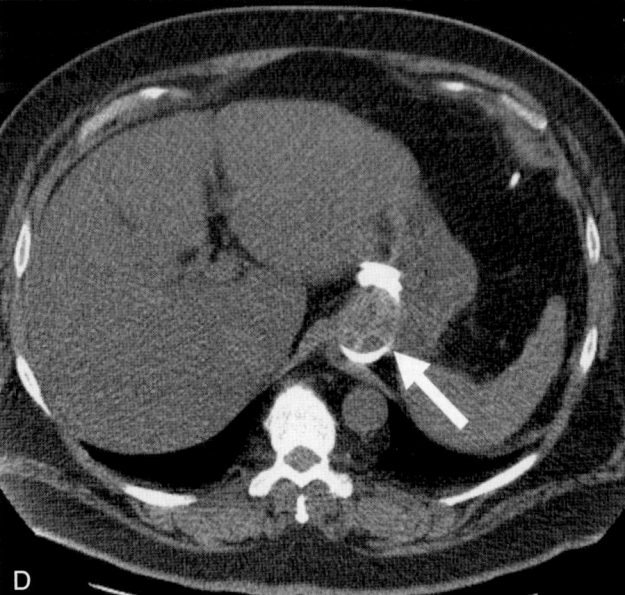

Figure 39-6. Adjustable laparoscopic banding procedure. A. Diagram illustrating the principles behind the gastric banding procedure. **B.** Intraoperative image showing the gastric band creating a new pouch. **C.** Upper gastrointestinal series shows the band (*red arrow*) and the gastric pouch (*yellow arrow*). **D.** CT scan shows the gastric band (*arrow*) encircling the proximal stomach.

the inner surface of the band is inflatable and connected by a thin silicone tube to a radiopaque access port with a self-sealing membrane. This access port is sutured in the anterior rectus sheath, typically bellow the caudal margin of the left rib cage during this laparoscopic procedure.[25]

Up to 8 mL of fluid can be injected into the band. It is usually left empty at the time of surgery because stomal edema in the early postoperative period will reduce the size of the stoma. The patient then returns in 3 to 4 weeks, and 4 to 5 mL of contrast agent is injected through the skin into the port under fluoroscopic guidance. The patient may then return additional times to optimize stoma size. The advantages of this technique include neither the stomach nor small bowel is opened and the stoma size can be tailored to the individual patient by a minimally invasive approach. Complications include band slippage with enlargement of the upper gastric pouch, pouch prolapse, band erosion, and band and port infection.[16]

Duodenal Switch/Biliary-Pancreatic Diversion Operation

The DS/BPD procedure combines restrictive and malabsorptive elements to achieve weight loss in the most morbidly obese patients (Fig. 39-7). The restrictive component of this procedure includes a partial gastrectomy, which reduces the stomach along the *greater curvature*, effectively restricting its capacity while maintaining its normal functionality. The

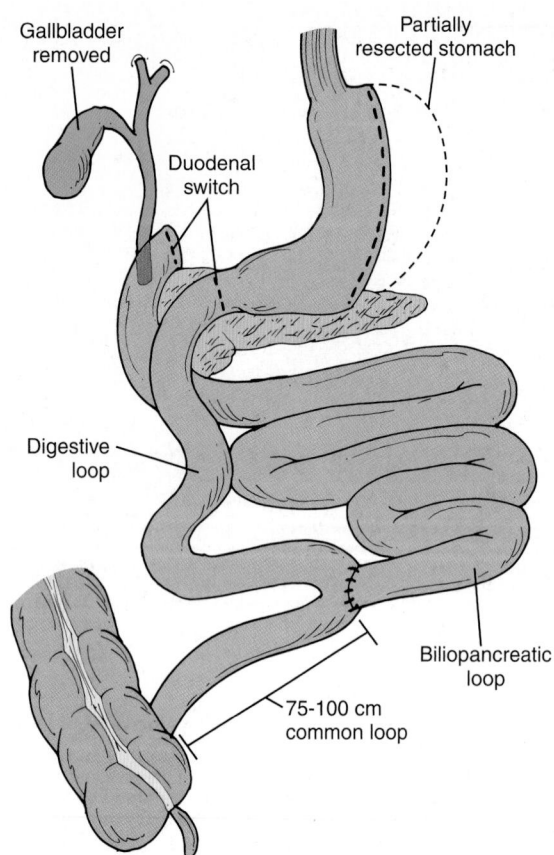

Figure 39-7. Duodenal switch/biliopancreatic diversion operation. This procedure consists of a 75% longitudinal gastrectomy, with creation of an alimentary limb that is approximately 50% of total small bowel length and a common channel length of 100 cm.

DS procedure keeps the pyloric valve intact, which potentially eliminates the complications of the dumping syndrome, marginal ulcers, stoma closures, and blockages. The DS procedure keeps a portion of the duodenum in the food stream. The preservation of the pylorus/duodenum pathway means that food is digested normally (to an optimally absorbable consistency) in the stomach before being excreted by the pylorus into the small intestine.[17,18]

The malabsorptive component of the DS/BPD procedure rearranges the small intestine to separate the flow of food from the flow of bile and pancreatic juices. This inhibits the absorption of calories and some nutrients. The divided intestinal paths are rejoined some 75 to 80 cm proximal to the ileocecal valve.

Complications of Operations for Weight Control

Complications (Figs. 39-8 to 39-13; see Table 39-1) are reported in 20% to 25% of patients undergoing RYGB, with 2% to 5% requiring reoperation. Complications include anastomotic leaks, gastrogastric fistulas, small bowel obstruction, deep venous thrombosis, fascial dehiscence, internal hernia formation, stenosis at the mesocolon, wound infection, inadequate weight control (due to too wide a gastrojejunostomy), strictures, marginal ulcerations, pancreatitis, esophagitis, cholelithiasis, and nutritional deficiencies that may cause a peripheral neuropathy secondary to vitamin B_{12} deficiency. LRYGB has a reported mortality rate less than 1%, usually due to pulmonary embolism or overwhelming peritonitis. The radiologist is often the first person to recognize these complications because diagnostic physical examination is frequently difficult to perform on these patients.

Anastomotic leaks (see Fig. 39-8) occur in 1% to 6% of patients after RYGB and more commonly occur at the site of the gastrojejunal anastomosis than at the site of the jejunojejunostomy. This complication is more common in laparoscopic compared with open bypass surgery. Leaks may develop at any time, from immediately after the operation until 7 to 10 days later. To detect these leaks, it is routine to perform an upper gastrointestinal study on the day after surgery. CT is more sensitive than upper gastrointestinal series in the detection of small leaks. On CT, leaks may present as a fluid collection in the left upper quadrant or with the formation of a fistula or sinus tract. These collections may show a rim of enhancement even if they are not infected. Most collections are subclinical and do not require intervention. These collections can be drained percutaneously under CT guidance if there is clinical suspicion of infection.

Gastrogastric fistulas are seen in approximately 3% of RYGB procedures and are usually due to staple gun failure. It is manifested radiologically by the presence of dense contrast material in the excluded stomach. In the absence of leak or peritonitis, these fistulas do not usually require surgical intervention but there is an increased risk of marginal ulceration and the efficacy of the procedure may be reduced. Enterocutaneous fistula may develop secondary to an anastomotic leak, and it is often better seen on CT than on upper gastrointestinal studies.

Anastomotic edema is a common finding in the initial postoperative period. This may lead to delayed gastric emptying, but this is usually self limited and resolves spontaneously on follow-up examination.

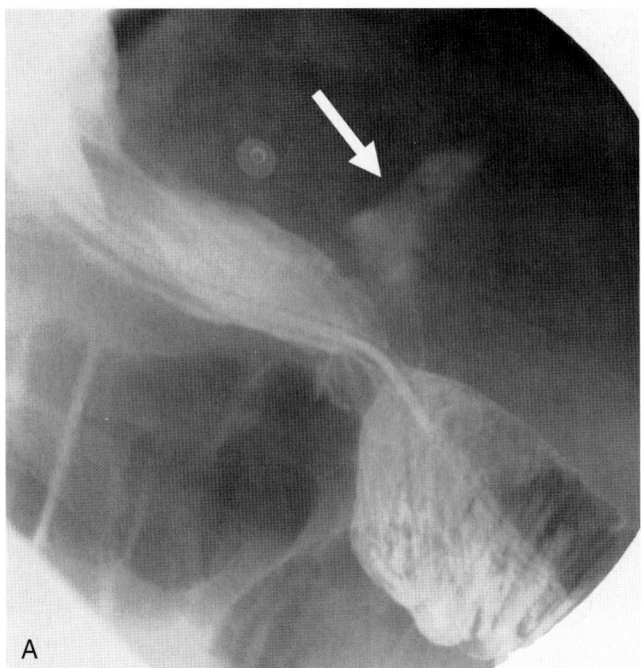

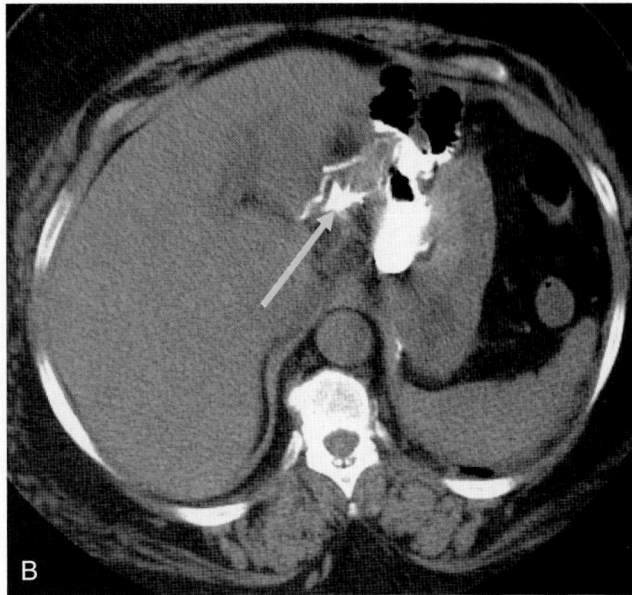

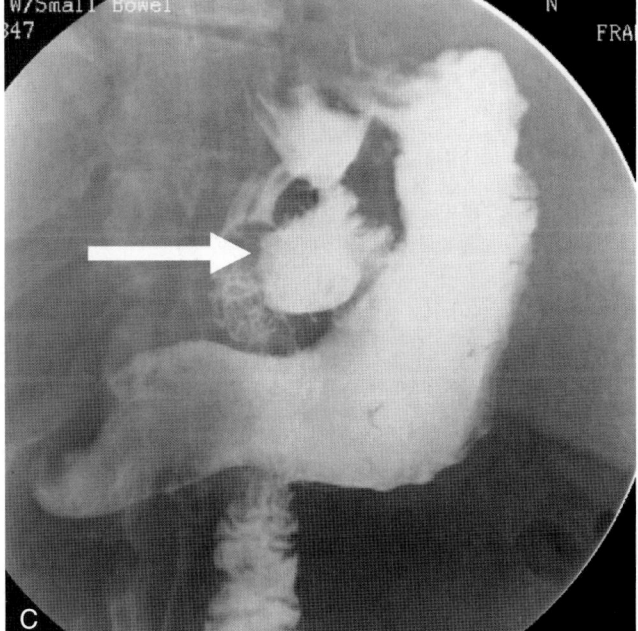

Figure 39-8. Complications of Roux-en-Y gastric bypass: anastomotic leaks, fistula. A. Extravasation of contrast medium is identified along the lateral aspect (*arrow*) of the gastrojejunostomy. **B.** CT scan shows contrast medium extravasation (*arrow*) in the region of the gastrohepatic ligament in a different patient. **C.** This upper gastrointestinal series demonstrates a fistula from the gastric pouch to the excluded stomach (*arrow*).

Gastric and small bowel obstruction develop in 3% to 5% of patients, and this usually is due to internal hernias, anastomotic strictures, adhesions, mesocolic tunnel stenosis, and, less commonly, intussusception or obstruction due to bezoar formation. With the introduction of laparoscopic technique, the number of obstructions due to adhesions has diminished while that of those due to internal hernias and anastomotic strictures has increased.

Adhesions can be seen after any abdominal operation. These adhesions can be low grade, which causes mild, chronic morbidity, or high grade, with closed loop, strangulating obstruction that requires emergency surgery. Most patients can be treated with bowel rest and do not require reoperation.

The transmesocolic type (see Fig. 39-11) is the most common internal hernia after LRYGB. It occurs through a defect in the transverse mesocolon through which the Roux limb is

brought to anastomose with the gastric pouch. The Roux limb itself and a variable amount of additional small bowel is typically herniated. The herniated gut is at risk for strangulation. Multidetector row CT findings include distended bowel loops anterior to the pancreas and above the transverse colon; crowding, engorgement, and deviation of mesenteric vessels; abrupt change in gut caliber proximal to the jejunojejunostomy; and inferior displacement of the transverse colon. Multiplanar reformatted views in the coronal and sagittal plane are very helpful in establishing the diagnosis.

The small bowel can easily pass between the Roux limb and the transverse mesocolon, a space known as Peterson's defect. This hernia does not have a defining sac or characteristic location and is difficult to diagnose.

It is often difficult to differentiate transmesenteric hernia from mesocolic tunnel stenosis. This later disorder, seen in

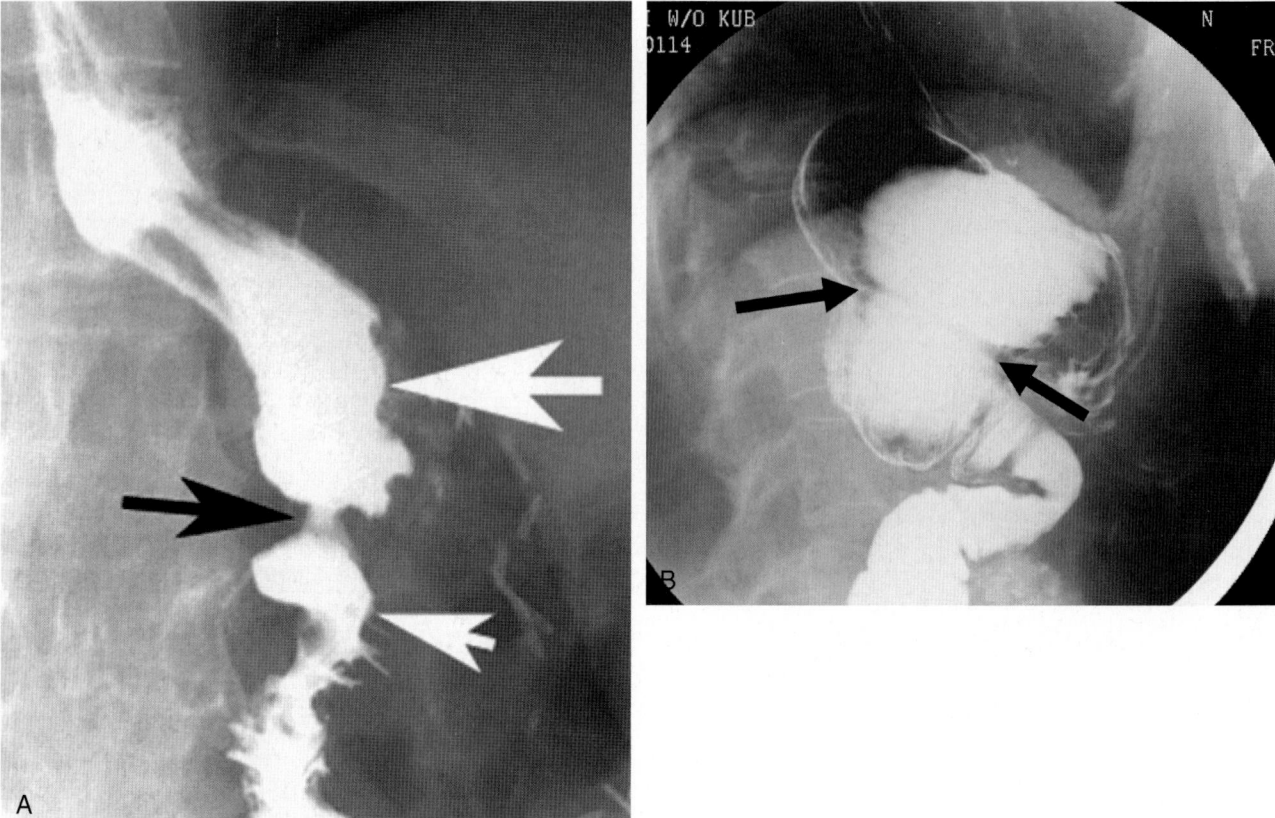

Figure 39-9. Complications of Roux-en-Y gastric bypass: gastrojejunostomy dysfunction. A. A 29-year-old woman presented with epigastric pain after gastric bypass surgery. Frontal view from single-contrast upper gastrointestinal study shows inferiorly located anastomotic stricture in profile (*black arrow*). Because anastomosis is located on inferior wall of gastric pouch (*large white arrow*), this stricture is clearly visible on frontal image. *Small white arrow,* proximal jejunum. **B.** A 36-year-old women complained of regaining weight after successful weight loss. The gastrojejunostomy is patulous (*arrows*), compromising the restrictive effect of the operation. (**A** from Jha S, Levine MS, Rubesin SE, et al: Detection of strictures on upper gastrointestinal tract radiographic examinations after laparoscopic Roux-en-Y gastric bypass surgery: Importance of projection. AJR 186:1090-1093, 2006. Reprinted with permission from the American Journal of Roentgenology.)

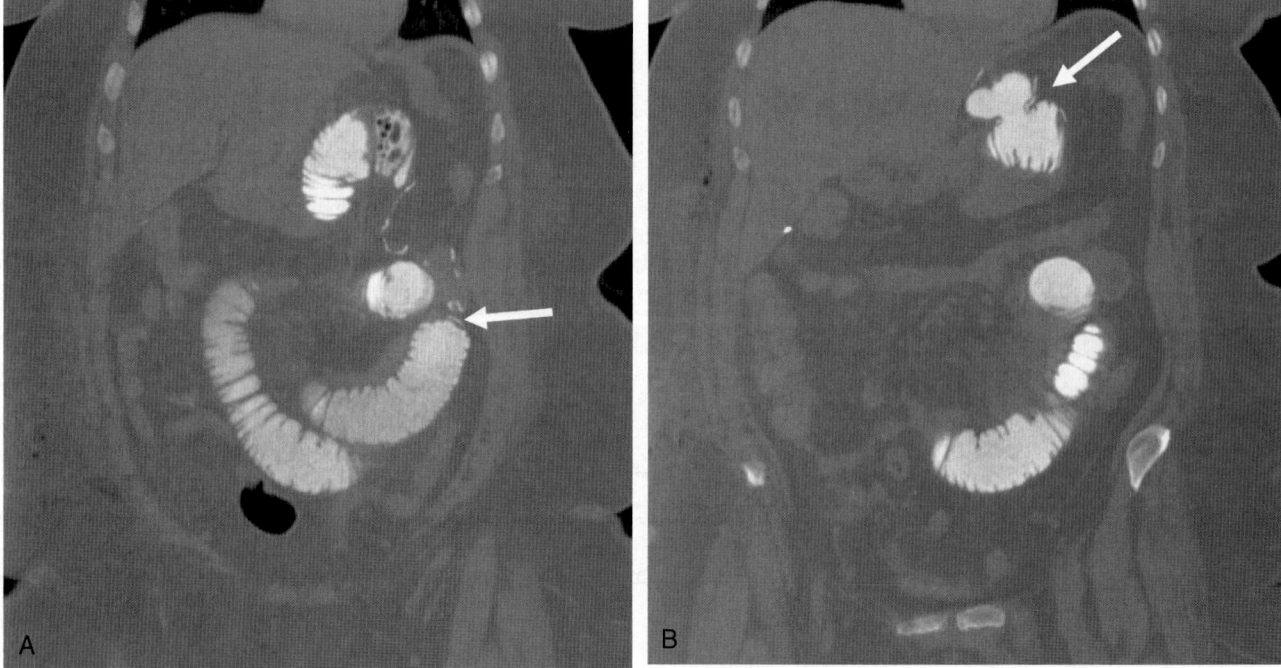

Figure 39-10. Complications of Roux-en-Y gastric bypass: obstruction. A. Coronal reformatted image shows obstruction of the Roux limb at the jejunal-jejunal anastomosis (*arrow*). **B.** Coronal reformatted image shows a normal appearing gastrojejunostomy (*arrow*).

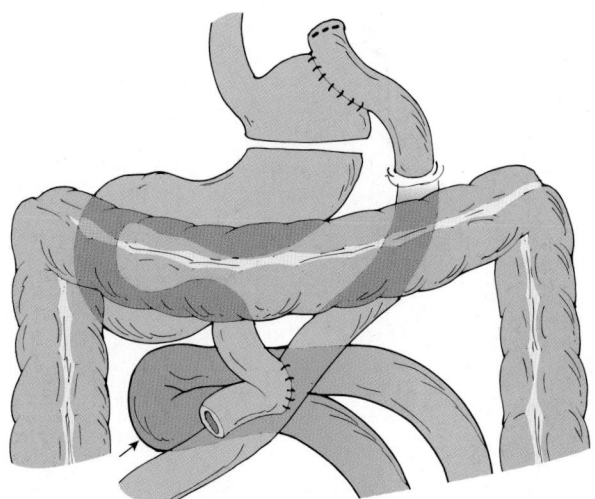

Figure 39-11. Diagram shows retrocolic Roux-en-Y gastric bypass procedure. *Arrow* indicates loop of small bowel protruding posterior to enteroenterostomy, in keeping with a retroanastomotic internal hernia. Illustration shows retrocolic Roux-en-Y procedure. (From Martin LC, Merkle EM, Thompson WM: Review of internal hernias: Radiographic and clinical findings. AJR 186:703-717, 2006. Reprinted with permission from the American Journal of Roentgenology.)

1% to 2% of retrocolic RYGB procedures, is caused by narrowing of the rent made in the transverse mesocolon to bring the jejunum to the stomach.[33-36] This tunnel stenosis obviously does not occur in patients who have undergone antecolic placement of the Roux loop, although this later technique does have a higher incidence of gastrojejunostomy stricture. Stenosis at the jejunojejunostomy can simulate mesocolic tunnel stenosis. In the later disorder, the duodenal-biliary-pancreatic loop is not distended. In the former, the efferent Roux limb is dilated down to a transition point, which is proximal to the sutures of the jejunojejunostomy site.

Incisional trocar hernias occur in 10% to 20%[33-36] of gastric bypass wounds (see Fig. 39-13). Trocar site hernias may cause small bowel obstruction and should be suspected when there is a short transition zone on the anterior abdominal wall with stranding of the subcutaneous fat.

Stenosis of the gastric pouch outlet develops in 3% to 27% of patients.[33-36] Dysphagia, vomiting, dehydration, and excessive weight loss are the typical presenting symptoms. On upper gastrointestinal studies, the gastric pouch has a spherical shape, with delayed emptying. Endoscopy with balloon dilation is often successful in treating these strictures. Jejunojejunostomy strictures are uncommon and may require surgery if symptomatic.

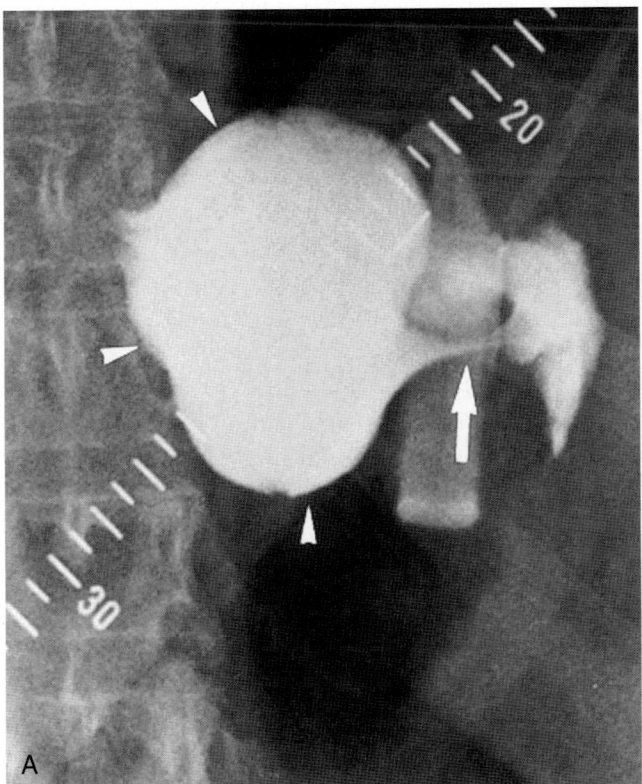

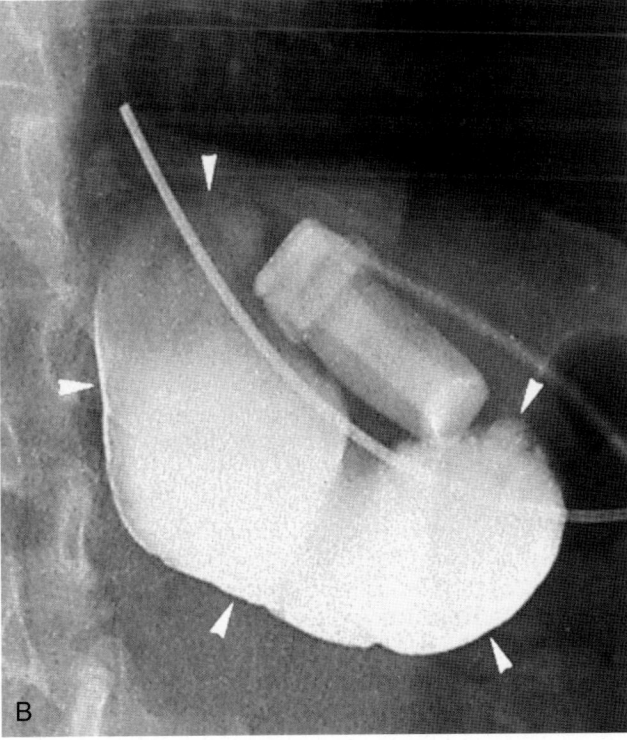

Figure 39-12. Complications of gastric bands. A. Fluoroscopic anteroposterior view shows acute concentric pouch dilatation (*arrowheads*) secondary to a too narrow stoma (*arrow*) after overinflation of the band by the radiologist. Notice the normal position of the band. Scale is in centimeters. **B.** Fluoroscopic view demonstrates partial gastric volvulus after posterior band slippage and extensive eccentric pouch dilatation (*arrowheads*). (From Wiesner W, Schöb O, Renward S, et al: Adjustable laparoscopic gastric banding in patients with morbid obesity: Radiographic management, results, and postoperative complications. Radiology 216:389-394, 2000.)

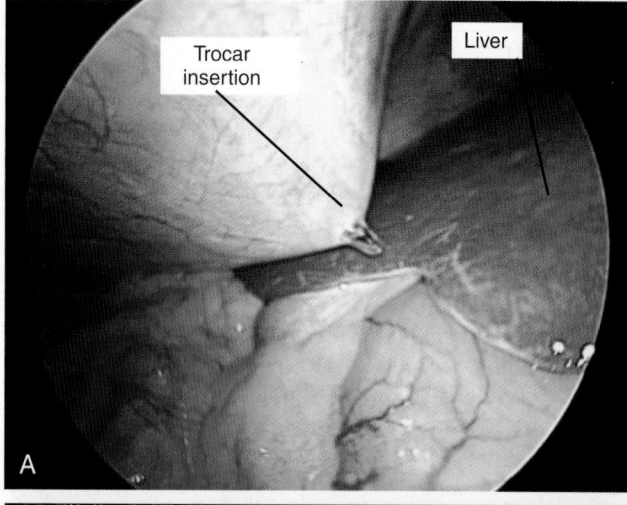

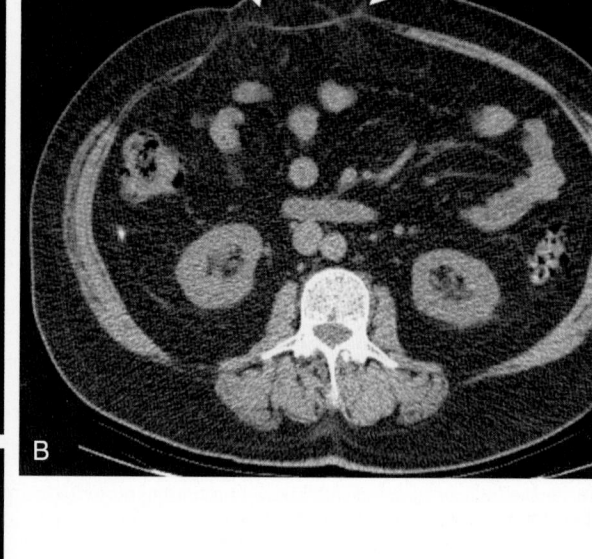

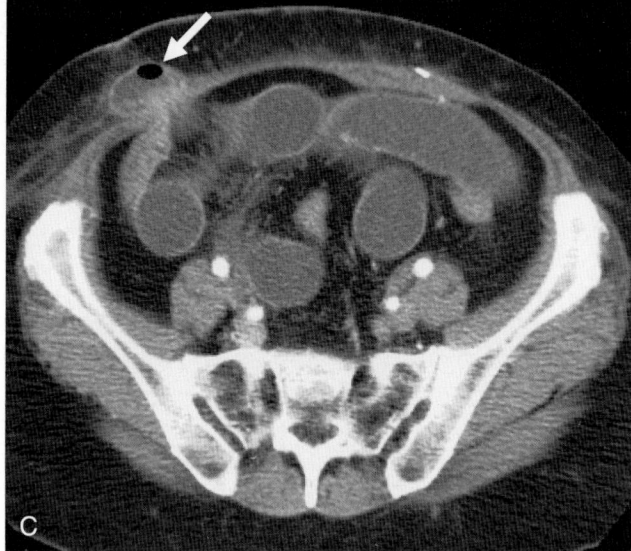

Figure 39-13. Complications of laparoscopic surgery: trocar hernias. A. Intraoperative image shows the stab wound being created. **B.** The defect (*arrows*) created weakens the abdominal wall and may lead to hernia formation. **C.** Trocar hernia in another patient. The loop of herniated ileum (*arrow*) is causing small bowel obstruction.

Marginal ulcerations develop in 3% to 10% of cases, and typically the ulcer is on the jejunal side of the gastrojejunostomy.[29-32] These lesions, which may result from anastomotic ischemia or excessive acid bathing of the jejunal limb, manifest as pain or bleeding. Marginal ulcerations occur more commonly in patients with fistulas to the gastric remnant. Medical therapy is usually successful in these patients, but surgery may be needed if it is not.

Bezoars can form in patients after surgery, and the most common site of obstruction is the proximal jejunum. Phytobezoars due to ingested fruit with seeds may simulate feces as a mottled soft tissue mass containing gas bubbles.

Other postsurgical complications include hepatic and splenic infarction, abscesses unrelated to an anastomotic leak, hematoma, and free intraperitoneal fluid in 10% of patients.

Specific complications of the LAGB procedure (see Fig. 39-12) include too tight or too patulous stoma between the pouch and the remainder of the stomach (which is easily corrected); pouch dilatation; prosthesis migration; prosthesis erosion into the stomach; and access port complications.

Specific complications of the DS/BPD procedure include gastric leaks at the angle of His, gastroparesis, duodenal-ileal anastomosis leaks and strictures, stenosis of the gastric sleeve, and gastroparesis.

Twenty-five to 30 percent of patients undergoing bariatric surgery have inadequate weight loss.[21] Weight loss is most dramatic for the first 3 postoperative months and is slower from months 3 through 12 until a plateau is reached. Often, patients will express concern that the operation is no longer working. An upper gastrointestinal examination is indicated to ensure the structural integrity of the gastric reconstruction.

Outlet Obstruction

Gastric outlet obstruction is not uncommon in the early postoperative period.[30] Vomiting must be controlled because regurgitation can stress the staple lines and cause dehiscence or gastric perforation. Early outlet problems are usually due to edema at the anastomosis in suture line, and symptoms resolve with supportive measures.

When the channel lumen is less than 6 to 8 mm wide, chronic problems appear. The stenosis usually occurs more than 6 weeks after surgery. Because weight loss is dramatic, patients often do not seek prompt follow-up. Patients return because of symptoms resulting from gastroesophageal reflux or because of accumulation of debris in the proximal gastric pouch. Techniques of balloon dilatation of channel stenoses now provide effective alternatives to reoperation.[31]

Surgery for Gastric Cancer and Gastric Masses

A variety of procedures are used to treat gastric carcinomas.[38] In patients undergoing operation for potential cure, the location of the primary tumor dictates the choice of resection.[39] Tumors located within 5 cm of the gastroesophageal junction undergo proximal gastric resection, esophagogastric anastomosis, and pyloroplasty. With a loop-type gastro-jejunostomy, the stomach and jejunum are anastomosed in one contiguous segment.[40] An alternative approach is total gastrectomy with or without splenectomy, but this approach is associated with greater postoperative morbidity as a result of complications of the reconstruction. For lesions located along the greater curvature, subtotal gastric resection for a distance of 5 to 6 cm around the lesion with omentectomy and splenectomy is performed followed by creation of a gastroenterostomy or gastroduodenostomy. Antral cancers are removed by subtotal gastric resection with wide proximal margins. Some cancers require total gastrectomy, and the distal esophagus is sutured to jejunum (Fig. 39-14) that has been brought up to the anastomosis as part of a Roux-en-Y procedure.[40]

Postoperative Complications

Perioperative and postoperative morbidity is common after surgery for gastric cancer because resections are extensive

and the patients are generally debilitated. The consequences of dumping, diarrhea, weight loss, and malnutrition increase postoperative difficulties.

Physiologic and Metabolic Problems

Subtotal gastric resection, removal of the pylorus, and extensive denervation of the stomach can alter gastric and intestinal motility, absorption, and biliary kinetics and cause a variety of physiologic problems.[41] Gastric emptying is often impaired when the normal pyloric channel is altered or when a previously unrecognized motility disorder becomes accentuated postoperatively.[38,42-45]

Anemia

Extensive gastric resection may lead to anemia because of malabsorption, inadequate oral intake, or chronic blood loss. Iron-deficiency anemia after gastric surgery may be related to rapid food passage in the duodenum and proximal jejunum. where iron is absorbed. and to decreased levels of acid and pepsin, which help convert organic iron to inorganic iron, which the gut can absorb.[46,47]

Vitamin B_{12} deficiency is caused by loss of intrinsic factor rather than bacterial overgrowth, as previously thought.

These metabolic deficiencies are accentuated in patients with total gastrectomy. Chronic nutritional problems far outweigh mechanical postgastrectomy syndromes or the rapid weight loss seen in the early postoperative course.[48]

Recurrent Carcinoma

Patients who have had a partial gastrectomy for localized gastric cancer are at considerable risk for developing recurrent tumor.[47-49] Recurrent tumor can appear infiltrating (Fig. 39-15), polypoid, or ulcerating on barium studies. Because surgically created plication defects can produce a mass effect simulating a malignancy, it is important to obtain a baseline postoperative examination in these patients.

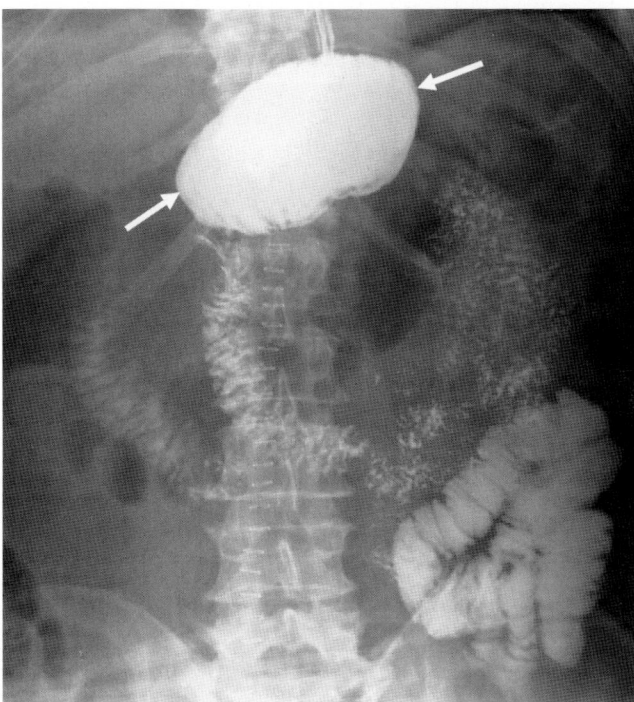

Figure 39-14. Esophagojejunostomy. Diffuse gastric neoplasms often necessitate complete gastric resection. A reservoir (*arrows*) constructed of jejunum is demonstrated on this upper gastrointestinal series. The reservoir is dilated due to edema at the entero-enterostomy.

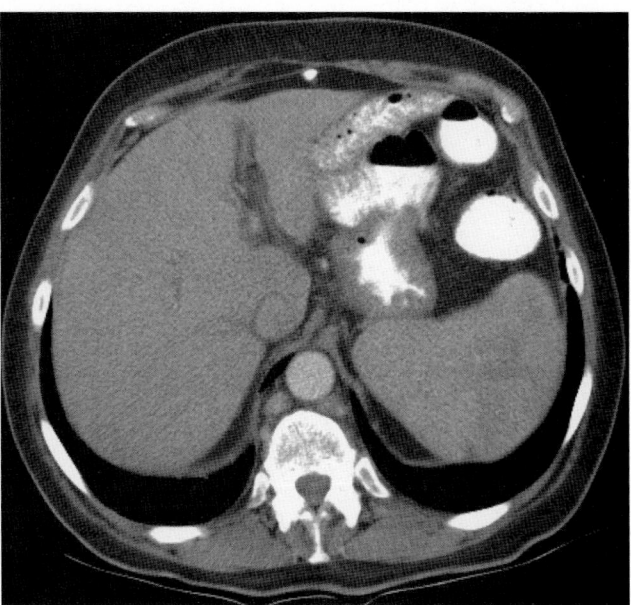

Figure 39-15. Recurrent gastric neoplasm. CT scan shows recurrent neoplasm near the contrast medium-filled proximal bowel.

Surgery for Peptic Ulcer Disease

The number of operations for peptic ulcer disease has declined significantly over the past 3 decades. This trend can be attributed to the development of histamine-2 blockers, proton pump inhibitors, agents that protect the gastric mucosa (e.g., sucralfate, prostaglandin analogs), and an understanding of the role of *Helicobacter pylori* and nonsteroidal anti-inflammatory agents in the origin of gastritis.

Duodenal Ulcers

With the advent of proton pump inhibitors, H_2 blockers, and other antiulcer regimens, surgery for gastric and duodenal ulcers has become far less frequent. Vagotomy and pyloroplasty (Fig. 39-16) are central to all surgical procedures for duodenal ulcer diathesis.[43] Acid secretion and parietal cell response to gastrin and other stimulants decrease after vagotomy.

Because vagotomy also causes gastric stasis, a pyloroplasty must be performed. Ulcers recur in 4% to 27% of patients who have had truncal vagotomy and pyloroplasty.[50-55] Antral resection is usually performed in conjunction with vagotomy to further reduce acid production by removing the antral source of gastrin and to prevent gastric stasis. Although ulcer recurrence after antrectomy is less than 1%, the side effects of diarrhea, dumping, and weight loss are increased.[56,57]

Highly selective vagotomy (parietal cell vagotomy) is a procedure in which branches of the vagus nerves that supply the fundic portion of the stomach are sectioned but hepatic, celiac, and motor branches are preserved so that an emptying procedure need not be performed. The operation is less traumatic, does not require anastomosis or creation of a suture line, does not alter gastric emptying, and has no physiologic or metabolic side effects. Ulcer recurrence rates range between 4% and 11%.[56,58]

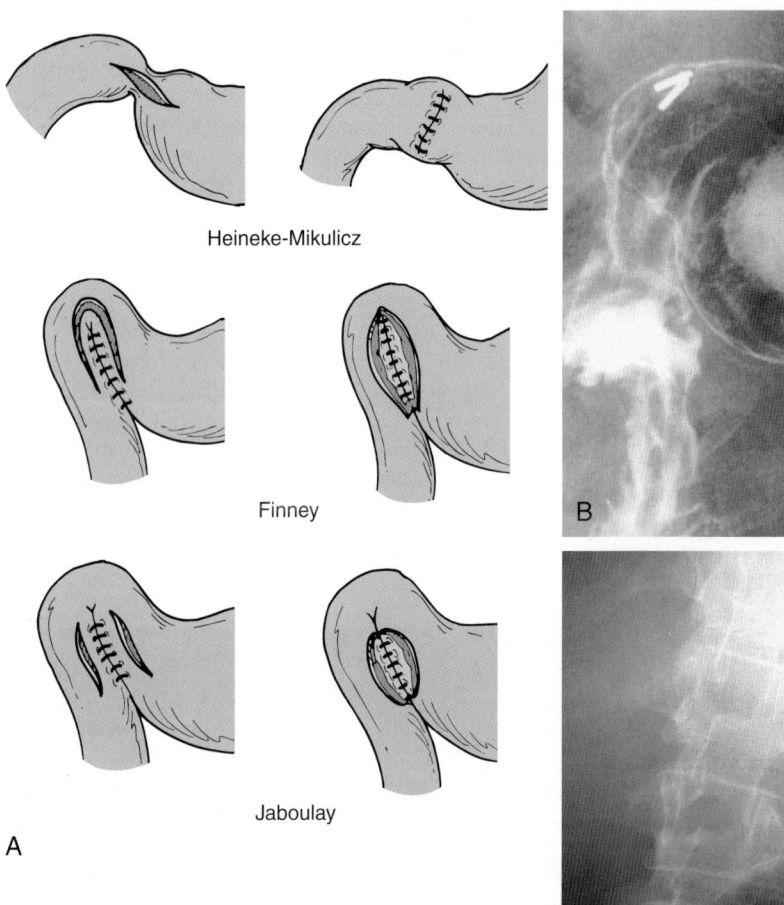

Heineke-Mikulicz

Finney

Jaboulay

A

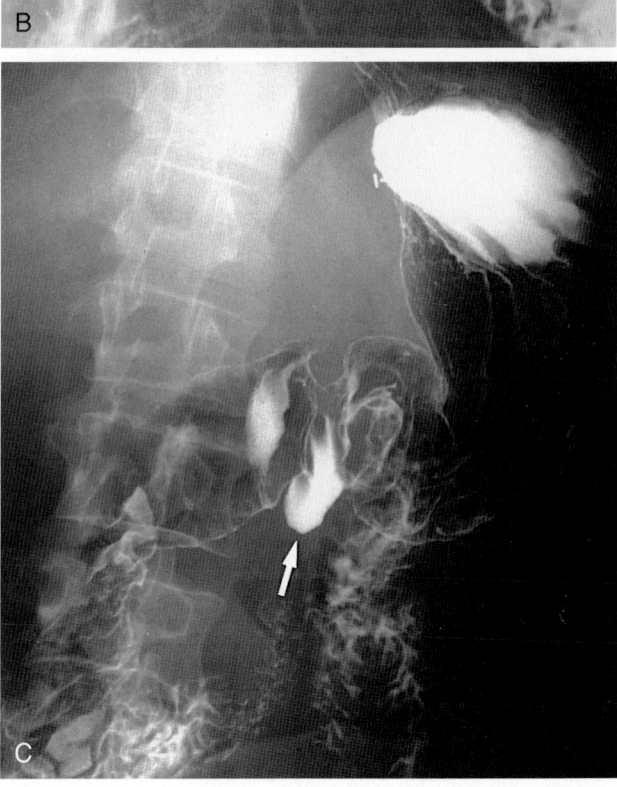

Figure 39-16. Vagotomy and pyloroplasty. A. Diagrams depict the three major types of pyloroplasties. The pyloroplasty may appear as a widened pylorus (**B**) or cause a pseudodiverticulum (**C**) (*arrow*) on barium studies. (**A** from Chung RS: Peptic ulcer surgery and its complications. In Achkar E, Farmer RG, Fleshler B [eds]: Clinical Gastroenterology. Philadelphia, Lea & Febiger, 1992, pp 261-273.)

Gastric Ulcers

Indications for Operation: Complications of Ulcers

The primary indications for surgery in patients with peptic ulcer disease are perforation, ulcer intractability, hemorrhage, and obstruction.[49,57,58] Patients with ulcers that fail to heal despite 12 to 15 weeks of intensive medical therapy and patients who have recurrent ulceration despite adequate medical care are also surgical candidates.

PERFORATION

In patients with acute perforation, the surgeon must decide whether to oversew the ulcer or perform definitive therapy.[59,60] In young patients without scarring, simple closure of duodenal ulcers involves a less than 20% chance of recurrence. In older patients, a simple patch is often insufficient.[60] Perforated gastric ulcers are usually treated with partial gastrectomy with or without vagotomy. Parietal cell vagotomy without drainage is an alternative approach.[57]

ULCER INTRACTABILITY

Ulcer intractability is a major indication for surgical resection. In 10% to 15% of patients, duodenal ulcers do not heal after 6 weeks of high-dose H_2-blockers and proton pump inhibitors; and in 15% to 30% of patients who do heal initially, relapse occurs eventually.[49,61,62] A high degree of safety and a low postoperative recurrence are noted when surgery is performed electively.

HEMORRHAGE

Approximately 70% of major bleeding from ulcers stops spontaneously.[60] Surgery is needed when shock occurs and when bleeding continues despite adequate medical, endoscopic, and transcatheter therapy. The optimal operation for duodenal ulcer bleeding is controversial; vagotomy plus pyloroplasty and vagotomy plus antrectomy are acceptable approaches.[49]

OBSTRUCTION FROM EDEMA OR FIBROSIS

Duodenal obstruction occurs in less than 10% of patients with peptic ulcer disease. Acutely, the patient is decompressed with a nasogastric tube and supported parenterally.[49] Vagotomy with gastric resection or drainage is the standard approach. If scarring is marked, a gastrojejunostomy may be needed.

Postoperative Complications

GASTRIC STASIS

Gastric stasis causes postprandial bloating, vomiting, pain, and weight loss in the absence of mechanical obstruction (Fig. 39-17A). Symptoms develop in 1% to 25% of patients, depending on the type of bowel reconstruction.[43] Although the exact pathophysiology of gastric stasis is unknown, ineffective gastric emptying, impaired bowel motility, and alkaline reflux gastritis have been implicated.[43,44] When severe, gastric stasis may require surgery to fashion the anastomosis into a different configuration or even total gastrectomy.

Nuclear medicine emptying studies are required to quantitate the rate of gastric emptying when the anastomotic diameter is normal.[20,21]

BEZOAR FORMATION

Bezoar formation (Fig. 39-17B) is a complication of subtotal gastrectomy, particularly when combined with vagotomy in an edentulous patient. Diminished peristalsis and absence of gastric acid allow poorly chewed fibrous material to be retained and form a matted mass. This complication should be suspected radiologically whenever a large, discrete mass

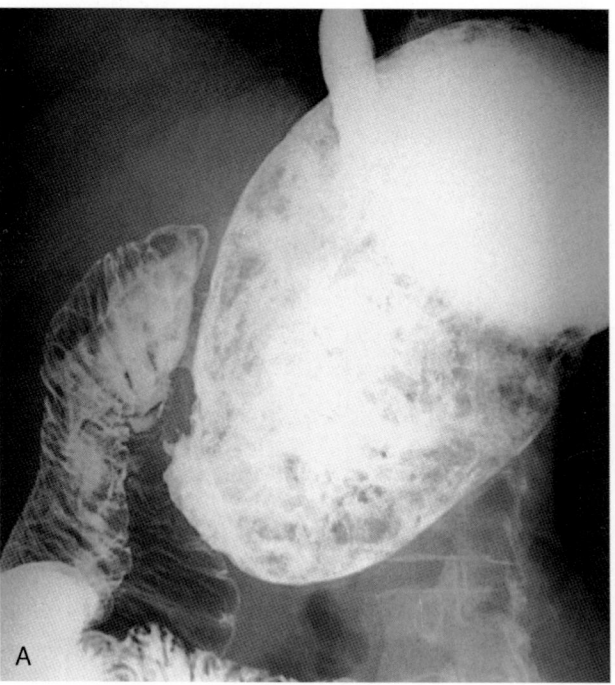 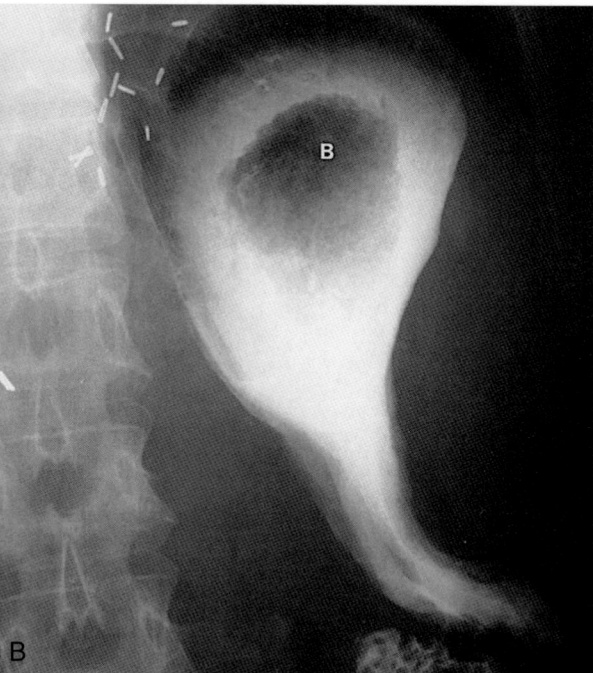

Figure 39-17. Functional complications of Billroth II gastrojejunostomy. A. Abundant retained secretions and food are present within the gastric remnant. The anastomosis was patent, and scintigraphic emptying studies showed significant gastric stasis. **B.** Bezoar (B) formation is a common complication of Billroth II surgery.

of food is encountered in a partially resected stomach in a fasting patient. Semisolid food will exit the stomach with the barium flow, whereas a bezoar remains in the stomach.

DUMPING SYNDROME

Patients with the dumping syndrome present with vasomotor and cardiovascular symptoms: weakness, dizziness, sweating, nausea, colic, diarrhea, and an urgent desire to lie down after eating.[44,45] Dumping has been reported to occur in 5% to 50% of patients, depending on the type of operation.[45] Most patients improve with dietary changes. Surgical reconstruction is usually unrewarding.[42,45]

ANASTOMOTIC LEAKS

Breakdown of a suture line and surgical anastomosis can occur at any anastomosis between the stomach and the small bowel, any enteroenteric anastomosis associated with gastric surgery, as well as the oversewn proximal end of the duodenum after a Billroth II procedure.[36] These complications are identified radiographically by contrast material exiting the gut lumen, filling an abscess cavity, a fistula, or the peritoneal cavity. CT may be needed to fully define the abscess cavity and to direct percutaneous drainage.[7]

STOMAL ULCERATION

Recurrent ulceration after Billroth I and II procedures for peptic ulcer disease commonly occurs on the duodenal or jejunal side of the anastomosis, respectively.[61,62] These marginal or postanastomotic ulcers develop in the following situations: inadequate gastric resection, retained antral remnant, gastrinoma, and excessively long afferent loop.[63] These ulcers are difficult to identify radiologically because the overlapping fold pattern and plication defects produced by surgery may obscure their detection.[64] When large, a frank ulcer crater may be identified (Fig. 39-18). Secondary signs include stiffness at the anastomosis, an edematous-appearing mass, or unusually thickened folds.

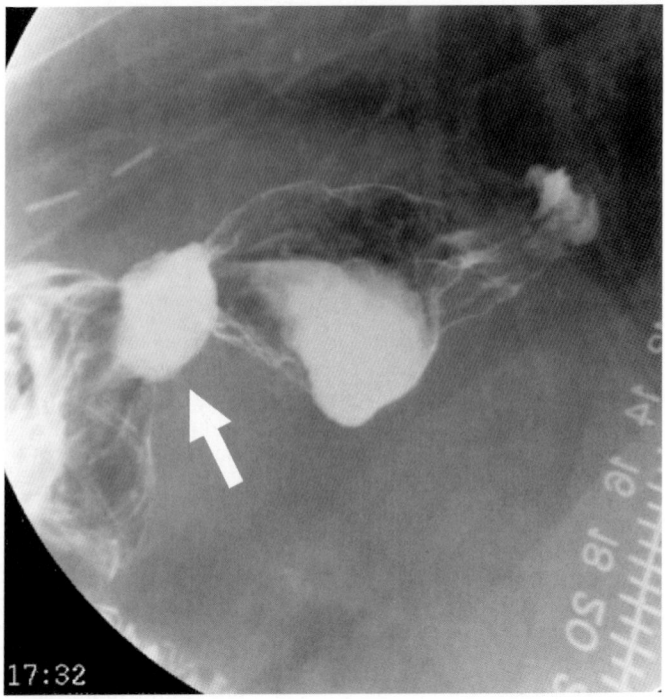

Figure 39-18. Marginal ulcer. A large marginal ulcer (*arrow*) is identified at the gastrojejunostomy.

JEJUNOGASTRIC INTUSSUSCEPTION

This rare complication of Billroth II gastric surgery can occur as an acute or a chronic process.[65] Retrograde prolapse of the small bowel adjacent to the gastroenterostomy into the stomach can cause partial or complete obstruction and can occasionally cause vascular compromise. Radiologically, there is a large intraremnant filling defect (Fig. 39-19), often suggestive of intussusception in its configuration.

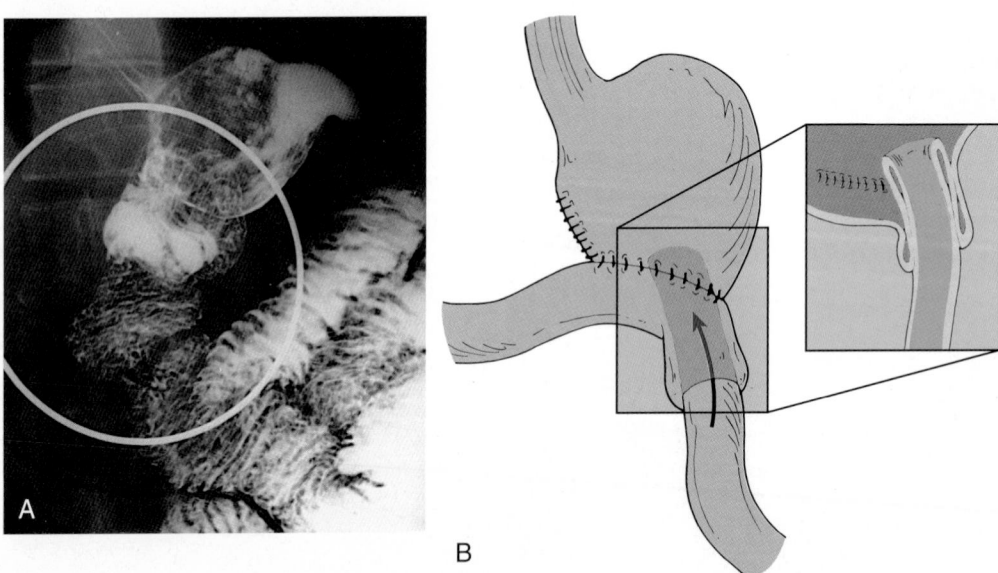

Figure 39-19. Jejunogastric intussusception. Intussusception of the efferent limb is present on the gastrointestinal study (**A**) and illustrated in the diagram (**B**). (**B** from Chung RS: Peptic ulcer surgery and its complications. In Achkar E, Farmer RG, Fleshler B [eds]: Clinical Gastroenterology. Philadelphia, Lea & Febiger, 1992, pp 261-273.)

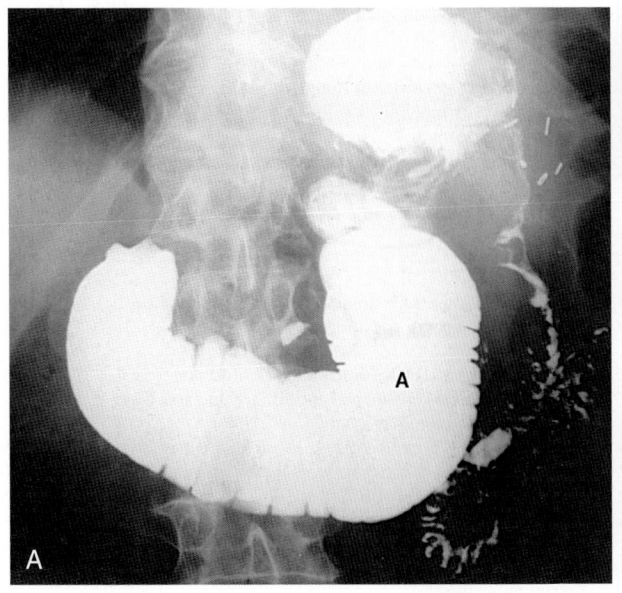

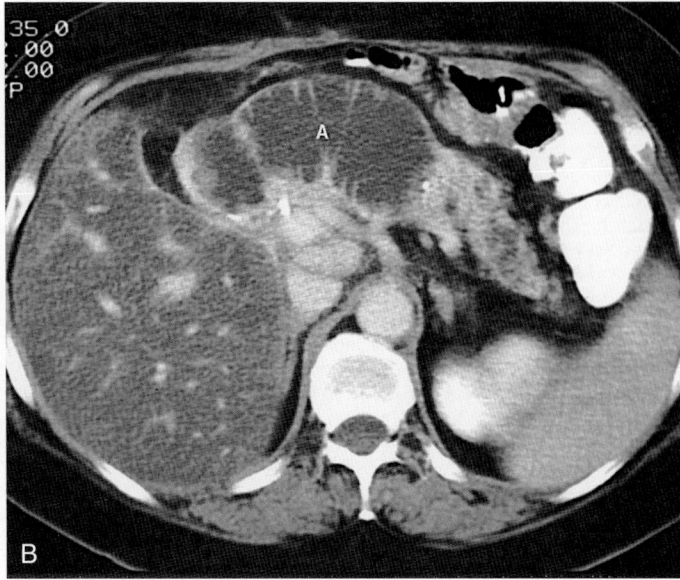

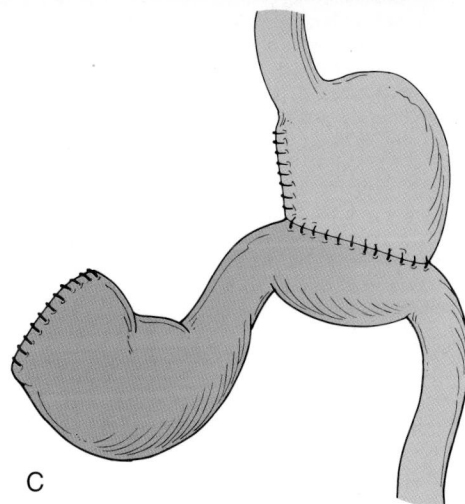

Figure 39-20. Afferent loop syndrome. A. Dilatation of a poorly emptying afferent loop (A) is demonstrated on a gastrointestinal study. **B.** CT scan performed on a different patient shows a dilated segment of jejunum (A) in the right upper quadrant. **C.** Schematic depiction of afferent loop syndrome. (**C** from Chung RS: Peptic ulcer surgery and its complications. In Achkar E, Farmer RG, Fleshler B [eds]: Clinical Gastroenterology. Philadelphia, Lea & Febiger, 1992, pp 261-273.)

AFFERENT LOOP SYNDROME

The afferent loop can become dilated (Fig. 39-20) in patients after Billroth II surgery for several reasons and can cause considerable epigastric distress, nausea, vomiting, postprandial fullness, and, rarely, obstructive jaundice. Causes of the afferent loop syndrome include internal hernia, kinking of the anastomosis, volvulus, adhesions, and stomal stenosis. First, there may be partial obstruction of the afferent loop at the gastrojejunostomy, leading to accumulation of pancreatic, biliary, and duodenal secretions and lumen dilatation. In this syndrome, CT and ultrasonography show a dilated, fluid-filled afferent loop and hepatobiliary scintigraphy reveals isotope retention in a dilated proximal segment; these are the main methods of establishing the diagnosis. Second, the gastrojejunostomy may be constructed so that food and fluid flow preferentially from the esophagus into the afferent loop, causing its dilatation.

NEOPLASM AFTER SURGERY FOR ULCER DISEASE

Partial gastrectomy for benign disorders, particularly peptic ulcer disease, is associated with an increased risk of gastric stump cancer.[66] There is a 15- to 20-year latent period after

which the relative risk increases threefold to sixfold. This delay probably reflects the time required for a gradual progression of normal mucosa to intestinal metaplasia to dysplasia and cancer as a result of prolonged achlorhydria and enterogastric reflux after enterostomy.[67] Truncal vagotomy, used to reduce gastric acid, may potentiate this transition.[68]

CHRONIC REMNANT GASTRITIS

One of the most common complications after gastric surgery is chronic gastritis. Without an intervening pylorus, chronic reflux of bile and pancreatic secretions produces inflammatory change in the gastric remnant. This manifests radiologically as enlarged gastric rugal folds.[66-69]

SUMMARY

The evaluation of patients with gastric and duodenal operations is challenging. A thorough understanding of the complex anatomic and physiologic alterations that occur after surgery and the close communication between physician and health care colleagues are essential to ensure accurate diagnosis and effective management strategies.[70]

References

1. Gore RM, Smith C: Postoperative findings. In Margulis AR (ed): Advances in Radiology of the Alimentary Tube. Heidelberg, Springer-Verlag, 1998, pp 305-334.
2. Steffes C, Fromm D: Postgastrectomy syndromes. In Zuidema GD (ed): Shackelford's Surgery of the Alimentary Tract, 4th ed. Philadelphia, WB Saunders, 1996, pp 166-184.
3. Smith C, Gardiner R: Postoperative stomach and recurrent abdominal pain. In Thompson WM (ed): Common Problems in Gastrointestinal Radiology. Chicago, Year Book Medical, 1989, pp 202-211.
4. Burhenne HJ: Roentgen anatomy and terminology of gastric surgery. AJR 91:731-743, 1964.
5. Burhenne HJ: The post-operative stomach. In Taveras JM, Ferruci JT (eds): Radiology: Diagnosis, Imaging, Intervention. Philadelphia, JB Lippincott, 1986, pp 1-11.
6. Smith C, Gardiner R, Kubicka RA, et al: Radiology of gastric restrictive surgery. RadioGraphics 5:193-216, 1985.
7. Derby CD, Minasi JS: Postgastrectomy and postvagotomy syndromes. In Brandt LJ (ed): Clinical Practice of Gastroenterology. New York, Churchill Livingstone, 1999, pp 404-414.
8. Laufer I: Barium studies. In Gore RM, Levine MS, Laufer I (eds): Textbook of Gastrointestinal Radiology. Philadelphia, WB Saunders, 1994, pp 292-303.
9. Ominsky SH, Moss AA: The postoperative stomach: Comparative study of double-contrast barium examinations and endoscopy. Gastrointest Radiol 4:17-21, 1979.
10. Gold RP, Seaman WB: The primary double-contrast examination of the postoperative stomach. Radiology 124:297-305, 1977.
11. Gohel VK, Laufer I: Double-contrast examination of the postoperative stomach. Radiology 129:601-607, 1978.
12. Odo Op Den Orth J: The postoperative stomach. In Laufer I, Levine MS (eds): Double Contrast Gastrointestinal Radiology, 2nd ed. Philadelphia, WB Saunders, 1992, pp 287-320.
13. Smith C, Gardiner R, Kubicka RA, et al: Gastric restrictive surgery for obesity: Early radiologic evaluation. Radiology 153:321-327, 1984.
14. Li Z, Bowerman S, Heber D: Health care ramifications of the obesity epidemic. Surg Clin North Am 85:681-702, 2005.
15. DeMaria EJ, Jamal MK: Laparoscopic adjustable gastric banding: Evolving clinical experience. Surg Clin North Am 85:773-788, 2005.
16. Provost DA: Laparoscopic adjustable gastric banding: an attractive alternative. Surg Clin North Am 85:789-806, 2005.
17. Anthone GJ: The duodenal switch operation for morbid obesity. Surg Clin North Am 85:819-834, 2005.
18. Brolin RE: Long limb Roux en Y gastric bypass revisited. Surg Clin North Am 85:807-818, 2005.
19. Livingston EH: Complications of bariatric surgery. Surg Clin North Am 85:853-868, 2005.
20. Jha S, Levine MS, Rubesin SE, et al: Detection of strictures on upper gastrointestinal tract radiographic examinations after laparoscopic Roux-en-Y gastric bypass surgery: Importance of projection. AJR 186:1090-1093, 2006.
21. Sandrasegaran K, Rajesh A, Lall C, et al: Gastrointestinal complications of bariatric Roux-en-Y gastric bypass surgery. Eur Radiol 15:254-262, 2005.
22. Blachar A, Federle MP, Paler KM, et al: Gastrointestinal complications of laparoscopic Roux-en-Y gastric bypass surgery: Clinical and imaging findings. Radiology 223:625-632, 2002.
23. Yu J, Turner MA, Cho SR, et al: Normal anatomy and complications after gastric bypass surgery: Helical CT findings. Radiology 231:753-760, 2004.
24. Srikanth MS, Keskey T, Fox SR, et al: Computed tomography patterns in small bowel obstruction after open distal gastric bypass. Obes Surg 14:811-822, 2004.
25. McNatt SS, Longhi JJ, Goldman CD, et al: Surgery for obesity: A review of the current state of the art and future directions. J Gastrointest Surg 11:377-397, 2007.
26. Carucci LF, Turner MA, Conklin RC, et al: Roux-en-Y gastric bypass surgery for morbid obesity: Evaluation of postoperative extraluminal leaks with upper gastrointestinal series. Radiology 238:119-127, 2006.
27. Hainaux B, Agneessens E, Rubesova E, et al: Intragastric band erosion after laparoscopic adjustable gastric banding for morbid obesity: Imaging characteristics of an underreported complication. AJR 184:109-112, 2005.
28. Kendrick ML, Dakin GF: Surgical approaches to obesity. Mayo Clin Proc 81(10 Suppl):S18-S24, 2006.
29. Scheirey CD, Scholz FJ, Shah PC, et al: Radiology of the laparoscopic Roux-en-Y gastric bypass procedure: Conceptualization and precise interpretation of results. RadioGraphics 26:1355-1371, 2006.
30. Mitchell MT, Pizzitola VJ, Knuttinen MG, et al: Atypical complications of gastric bypass surgery. Eur J Radiol 53:366-373, 2005.
31. Esmailzadeh H, Powell W, Lourie D, et al: Use of computed tomography in diagnosis of major postoperative gastrointestinal complications of laparoscopic Roux-en-Y gastric bypass surgery. Am Surg 70:964-966, 2004.
32. Lyass S, Khalili TM, Cunneen S, et al: Radiological studies after laparoscopic Roux-en-Y gastric bypass: Routine or selective? Am Surg 70:918-921, 2004.
33. Carucci LR, Turner MA: Radiologic evaluation following Roux-en-Y gastric bypass surgery for morbid obesity. Eur J Radiol 53:353-365, 2005.
34. Merkle EM, Hallowell PT, Crouse C, et al: Roux-en-Y gastric bypass for clinically severe obesity: Normal appearance and spectrum of complications at imaging. Radiology 234:674-683, 2005.
35. Cho M, Pinto D, Carrodeguas L, et al: Frequency and management of internal hernias after laparoscopic antecolic antegastric Roux-en-Y gastric bypass without division of the small bowel mesentery or closure of mesenteric defects: Review of 1400 consecutive cases. Surg Obes Relat Dis 2:87-91, 2006.
36. Singh R, Fisher BL: Sensitivity and specificity of postoperative upper GI series following gastric bypass. Obes Surg 13:73-75, 2003.
37. Nosher JL, Bodner LJ, Girgis WS, et al: Percutaneous gastrostomy for treating dilatation of the bypassed stomach after bariatric surgery for morbid obesity. AJR 183:1431-1435, 2004.
38. Kim KW, Choi BI, Han JK, et al: Postoperative anatomic and pathologic findings at ct following gastrectomy. RadioGraphics 22:323-338, 2002.
39. Fuchs CS, Mayer RJ: Gastric carcinoma. N Engl J Med 333:32-41, 1995.
40. Yoo SY, Kim KW, Han JK, et al: Helical CT of postoperative patients with gastric carcinoma: Value in evaluating surgical complications and tumor recurrence. Abdom Imaging 28:617-623, 2003.
41. Katai H: Function-preserving surgery for gastric cancer. Int J Clin Oncol 11:357-366, 2006.
42. Zissin R, Hertz M, Paran H, et al: Computed tomographic features of afferent loop syndrome: Pictorial essay. Can Assoc Radiol J 56:72-78, 2005.
43. Fich A, Neri M, Camilleri M, et al: Stasis syndromes following gastric surgery: Clinical and motility features of 60 symptomatic patients. J Clin Gastroenterol 12:505-512, 1990.
44. Woodward ER, Hocking MP: Postgastrectomy syndromes. Surg Clin North Am 67:509-520, 1987.
45. Alexander-Williams J, Hoare AM: The stomach: II. Partial gastric resection. Clin Gastroenterol 8:321-353, 1979.
46. Bradley EL III: The stomach: III. Total gastrectomy. Clin Gastroenterol 8:354-371, 1979.
47. Schrock TR, Way LW: Total gastrectomy. Am J Surg 135:348-355, 1978.
48. Tovey FI, Godfrey JE, Lewis MR: A gastrectomy population: 25-30 years on. Postgrad Med J 66:450-456, 1990.
49. Mulholland MW, Debas HT: Chronic duodenal and gastric ulcer. Surg Clin North Am 67:489-507, 1987.
50. McConnell DB, Baba GC, Deveney CW: Changes in surgical treatment of peptic ulcer disease within a veterans hospital in the 1970s and the 1980s. Arch Surg 124:1164-1167, 1989.
51. Elashoff JD, Grossman MI: Trends in hospital admissions and death rates for peptic ulcer disease in the United States from 1970 to 1978. Gastroenterology 78:280-285, 1980.
52. Kurata JH, Honda GD, Frankl H: Hospitalization and mortality rates for peptic ulcers: A comparison of a large health maintenance organization and United States data. Gastroenterology 83:1008-1016, 1982.
53. Bardhan KD, Cust G, Hinchliffe RFC, et al: Changing pattern of admissions and operations for duodenal ulcer. Br J Surg 76:230-236, 1989.
54. Sheaff CM, Nyhus LM: Recurrent ulcer. In Nyhus LM, Wastell C (eds): Surgery of the Stomach and Duodenum. Boston, Little, Brown, 1986, pp 516-534.
55. Stabile BE, Passaro E Jr: Recurrent peptic ulcer. Gastroenterology 76:124-135, 1976.
56. Jordan PH Jr, Thornby J: Should it be parietal cell vagotomy or selective vagotomy-antrectomy for treatment of duodenal ulcer? A progress report. Ann Surg 205:572-590, 1986.
57. Kocer B, Surmeli S, Solak C, et al: Factors affecting mortality and morbidity in patients with peptic ulcer perforation. J Gastroenterol Hepatol 22:565-570, 2007.
58. Soll AH: Peptic ulcer and its complications. In Feldman M, Scharchmidt

BF, Sleisenger MH (eds): Sleisenger and Fordtran's Gastrointestinal and Liver Disease, 6th ed. Philadelphia, WB Saunders, 1998, pp 620-678.

59. Steinberg SM, Lambiase L: Postoperative stomach. In DiMarino AJ, Benjamin SB (eds): Gastrointestinal Disease: An Endoscopic Approach. Malden, MA, Blackwell Science, 1997, pp 397-408.

60. Jordan PH Jr, Morros C: Perforated peptic ulcer. Surg Clin North Am 68:315-329, 1988.

61. Boyd EJS, Johnston DA, Penston JG, et al: Does maintenance therapy keep duodenal ulcers healed? Lancet 1:1324-1327, 1988.

62. Schirmer BD, Meyers WC, Hanks JB, et al: Marginal ulcer: A difficult surgical problem. Ann Surg 195:653-661, 1982.

63. Metz DC: Peptic ulcer disease: Diagnosis and management. In DiMarino AJ, Benjamin SB (eds): Gastrointestinal Disease: An Endoscopic Approach. Malden, MA: Blackwell Science, 1997, pp 285-304.

64. Chung RS: Peptic ulcer surgery and its complications. In Achkar E, Farmer RG, Fleshler B (eds): Clinical Gastroenterology. Philadelphia, Lea & Febiger, 1992, pp 261-273.

65. Poppel MH: Gastric intussusceptions. Radiology 78:602-608, 1962.

66. Goodman PC, Levine MS, Gohil MN: Gastric carcinoma after gastro-jejunostomy for benign disease: Radiographic findings. Gastrointest Radiol 17:211-213, 1992.

67. Kodera Y, Yamamura Y, Torii A, et al: Gastric remnant carcinoma after partial gastrectomy for benign and malignant gastric lesions. J Am Coll Surg 182:1-6, 1996.

68. Kim H-C, Han JK, Kim KW, et al: Afferent loop obstruction after gastric surgery: Helical CT findings. Abdom Imaging 28:624-630, 2003.

69. Kodera Y, Yamamura Y, Yokoyama I, et al: Early gastric cancer after gastrojejunostomy: Clinical pathologic aspects. Am J Gastroenterol 90:2213-2216, 1996.

70. Woodfield CA, Levine MS: The postoperative stomach. Eur J Radiol 53:341-352, 2005.

Stomach and Duodenum: Differential Diagnosis

Marc S. Levine, MD

Table 40-1
Gastric Ulcers (No Mass)

Cause	Location	Comments
Erosions		
Idiopathic	Antrum or body; often aligned on rugal folds	Varioliform erosions
Aspirin or other nonsteroidal anti-inflammatory drugs	Antrum or body; may be on or near greater curvature	Varioliform, linear, or serpiginous erosions
Crohn's disease	Antrum or body	Associated Crohn's disease in small bowel or colon
Ulcers		
Helicobacter pylori	Usually on lesser curvature or posterior wall of antrum or body	Accounts for 60%-80% of gastric ulcers
Aspirin or other nonsteroidal anti-inflammatory drugs	Distal half of greater curvature	May simulate malignant ulcer
Gastritis	Variable	Hypertrophic gastritis, granulomatous conditions, radiation, caustic ingestion, infections
Zollinger-Ellison syndrome	Variable	Associated ulcers in atypical locations; hypergastrinemia
Early gastric cancer	Variable	Nodular or deformed folds surrounding ulcer

Table 40-2
Gastric Mass Lesions

Cause	Radiographic Findings	Comments
Benign Mucosal Lesions		
Hyperplastic polyps	Round, sessile polyps in fundus or body; usually multiple	Not premalignant
Adenomatous polyps	Lobulated or pedunculated polyps in antrum; often solitary	Premalignant
Polyposis syndromes	Multiple polyps in stomach (also in small bowel or colon)	Familial adenomatosis polyposis, Peutz-Jeghers syndrome, Cronkhite-Canada syndrome, juvenile polyposis, Cowden's disease
Villous tumor	Giant mass with "soap bubble" appearance	Premalignant; rare in stomach
Bezoar	Giant masslike filling defect; freely movable	Unusual eating habits; gastroparesis or gastric outlet obstruction

Continued

Table 40-2
Gastric Mass Lesions—*cont'd*

Cause	Radiographic Findings	Comments
Malignant Mucosal Lesions		
Carcinoma	Polypoid mass; ulceration common	Usually advanced gastric cancer but may occasionally be early cancer
Benign Submucosal Lesions		
Benign gastrointestinal stromal tumor	Smooth submucosal mass; ulceration common; rarely multiple	May be difficult to differentiate from malignant gastrointestinal stromal tumor
Leiomyoblastoma	Smooth submucosal mass; ulceration common	Risk of malignancy
Lipoma	Submucosal mass with changeable shape at fluoroscopy; fat density on CT	Usually asymptomatic
Hemangioma	Submucosal mass with phleboliths	Risk of massive gastrointestinal bleeding
Lymphangioma	Submucosal mass	Rare
Glomus tumor	Submucosal mass	Usually asymptomatic
Neurofibroma	Solitary or multiple submucosal masses	Von Recklinghausen's disease
Granular cell tumor	Solitary or multiple submucosal masses	Associated lesions on skin or tongue
Inflammatory fibroid polyp	Sessile or pedunculated polyp in antrum; usually solitary	Usually asymptomatic
Ectopic pancreatic rest	Submucosal mass with central umbilication; usually on greater curvature of distal antrum	Usually asymptomatic
Duplication cyst	Submucosal mass on greater curvature of antrum or body; rarely communicates with lumen	Usually symptomatic during first year of life
Varices	Multiple submucosal masses in fundus (likened to bunch of grapes)	Portal hypertension or splenic vein obstruction
Malignant Submucosal Lesions		
Malignant gastrointestinal stromal tumor	Solitary, lobulated submucosal mass; ulceration or cavitation common	Better prognosis than carcinoma
Metastases	One or more submucosal masses; ulceration or cavitation common; bull's-eye lesions of varying sizes	Most commonly malignant melanoma or metastatic breast cancer
Lymphoma	One or more submucosal masses; ulceration or cavitation common; bull's-eye lesions of similar sizes	Usually non-Hodgkin's lymphoma
Kaposi's sarcoma	Multiple submucosal masses or bull's-eye lesions	Homosexuals with AIDS; usually have Kaposi's sarcoma on skin
Carcinoid	Multiple submucosal masses or bull's-eye lesions	Carcinoid syndrome uncommon
Leukemia	Multiple submucosal masses or polyps	Rare
Multiple myeloma	Multiple submucosa masses	Rare

Table 40-3
Thickened Gastric Folds

Cause	Distribution	Comments
Benign Conditions		
Antral gastritis	Antrum	Epigastric pain or dyspepsia
Helicobacter pylori gastritis	Usually antrum or antrum and body; sometimes diffuse	Associated with peptic ulcer disease
Hypertrophic gastritis	Fundus and body	Increased acid secretion; frequent duodenal ulcers
Ménétrier's disease	Fundus and body (massive folds)	Hypochlorhydria and hypoproteinemia
Zollinger-Ellison syndrome	Fundus and body (increased secretions; ulcers common)	Hypergastrinemia resulting from non-beta islet cell tumors
Varices	Fundus and cardia (serpentine folds)	Portal hypertension or splenic vein obstruction
Eosinophilic gastritis	Antrum	Peripheral eosinophilia; history of allergic diseases
Crohn's disease	Antrum and body	Associated Crohn's disease in small bowel or colon
Sarcoidosis	Antrum	Pulmonary sarcoidosis
Tuberculosis	Antrum	History of AIDS or travel to endemic areas
Caustic ingestion	Antrum	History of caustic ingestion
Radiation	Antrum	History of radiation therapy (>50 Gy)
Floxuridine toxicity	Antrum and body	Hepatic artery infusion chemotherapy
Amyloidosis	Antrum	Systemic amyloidosis
Malignant Conditions		
Lymphoma	Localized or diffuse	May have generalized lymphoma
Carcinoma	Localized or diffuse	Associated narrowing and rigidity of stomach

Table 40-4
Gastric Narrowing

Cause	Radiographic Findings	Comments
Benign Conditions		
Scarring from peptic ulcer disease	Smooth or asymmetric antral narrowing	History of ulcers
Atrophic gastritis	Diffusely narrowed, tubular stomach with decreased or absent folds	Pernicious anemia
Eosinophilic gastritis	Antral narrowing	Peripheral eosinophilia; history of allergic diseases
Crohn's disease	Funnel-shaped antral narrowing ("ram's horn" or "shofar" sign)	Associated Crohn's disease in small bowel or colon
Sarcoidosis	Cone-shaped antral narrowing	Pulmonary sarcoidosis
Tuberculosis	Antral narrowing; fistulas common	History of AIDS or travel to endemic areas
Syphilis	Funnel-shaped antral narrowing	Occurs in < 1% of patients with syphilis
Caustic ingestion	Narrowing of antrum or antrum and body	History of caustic ingestion; esophageal scarring in 20%
Radiation	Antral narrowing	History of radiation therapy (>50 Gy)
Cytomegalovirus infection	Antral narrowing and ulceration	History of AIDS
Amyloidosis	Antral narrowing	Systemic amyloidosis
Antral diaphragm or web	Transverse, weblike area of antral narrowing	May be asymptomatic
Malignant Conditions		
Scirrhous carcinoma	Linitis plastica	Antral narrowing classic, but isolated involvement of proximal stomach in 40%
Metastatic breast cancer	Linitis plastica	Recent or remote history of breast cancer
Omental cake	Mass effect and spiculated folds on greater curvature; occasionally circumferential	Omental metastases from ovarian carcinoma or other malignant neoplasms
Non-Hodgkin's lymphoma	Linitis plastica	May have generalized lymphoma
Hodgkin's disease	Linitis plastica	May have generalized Hodgkin's disease
Kaposi's sarcoma	Linitis plastica	Homosexuals with AIDS; usually have Kaposi's sarcoma on skin

Table 40-5
Gastric Outlet Obstruction

Cause	Radiographic Findings	Comments
Peptic ulcer disease	Antral, pyloric, or duodenal ulcer with spasm, edema, or scarring	Difficult to differentiate from tumor if high-grade obstruction
Antral scarring	Antral narrowing	Crohn's disease, sarcoidosis, tuberculosis, syphilis, caustic ingestion, radiation
Carcinoma	Infiltrating antral or pyloric channel tumor	Usually advanced lesions
Other malignant tumors	Irregular narrowing or extrinsic compression of antrum or duodenum	Pancreatic carcinoma, lymphoma, retroperitoneal metastases
Hypertrophic pyloric stenosis	Elongated, narrowed pylorus	Uncommon cause of obstruction in adults
Antral diaphragm or web	Transverse, weblike area of antral narrowing	Degree of obstruction depends on size of central aperture of web
Gastric volvulus	Dilated, upside-down, intrathoracic stomach	Surgical emergency if incarcerated or strangulated
Gastroparesis	Flaccid stomach with decreased or absent peristalsis but no gastric outlet obstruction	History of diabetes, narcotic use, or other conditions associated with gastroparesis

Table 40-6
Duodenal Filling Defects

Cause	Radiographic Findings	Comments
Non-neoplastic Conditions		
Prolapsed antral mucosa	Mushroom-shaped defect at base of bulb	Usually asymptomatic
Flexural pseudotumor	Filling defect at superior duodenal flexure resulting from redundant mucosa	May simulate mass
Heterotopic gastric mucosa	Tiny, polygonal or angulated nodules at base of bulb	No clinical significance
Brunner gland hyperplasia	Multiple rounded nodules in proximal duodenum ("Swiss cheese" appearance)	Associated with duodenitis
Benign lymphoid hyperplasia	Multiple tiny, rounded nodules in proximal duodenum	Associated with immunologic disorders
Choledochocele	Submucosal mass in region of ampulla	Congenital anomaly
Duplication cyst	Submucosal mass on medial wall of descending duodenum	Congenital anomaly
Intramural hematoma	Submucosal mass on medial wall of duodenum	Bleeding diathesis, anticoagulation, or trauma
Benign Tumors		
Polyps	Smooth, sessile elevations; usually solitary	Hyperplastic or adenomatous
Polyposis syndromes	Multiple polypoid lesions	Familial adenomatous polyposis, Peutz-Jeghers syndrome, Cronkhite-Canada syndrome, juvenile polyposis
Villous adenoma	Polypoid mass with frondlike projections; usually near ampulla	High malignant potential
Mesenchymal lesions	Submucosal mass, often with central ulceration or umbilication	Leiomyoma, lipoma, neurogenic tumor, Brunner gland hamartoma, ectopic pancreatic rest
Malignant Tumors		
Duodenal carcinoma	Polypoid mass at or distal to papilla of Vater	Gastrointestinal bleeding or obstruction
Ampullary carcinoma	Polypoid mass in region of ampulla	Jaundice common
Malignant gastrointestinal stromal tumor	Lobulated submucosal mass; ulceration or cavitation common	Better prognosis than carcinoma
Metastases	Multiple submucosal masses or bull's-eye lesions	Most commonly malignant melanoma or metastatic breast cancer
Lymphoma	Multiple submucosal masses or bull's-eye lesions	Usually non-Hodgkin's lymphoma
Kaposi's sarcoma	Multiple submucosal masses or bull's-eye lesions	Homosexuals with AIDS; usually have Kaposi's sarcoma on skin
Carcinoid	Multiple submucosal masses or bull's-eye lesions	Carcinoid syndrome uncommon

Table 40-7
Thickened Duodenal Folds

Cause	Radiographic Findings	Comments
Duodenitis	Thickened, nodular folds in proximal duodenum; occasionally associated with erosions	Not a reliable diagnosis unless folds grossly thickened
Brunner gland hyperplasia	Thickened, nodular folds in proximal duodenum	Usually associated with duodenitis
Chronic renal failure	Markedly thickened, nodular folds, particularly in bulb	Usually on dialysis
Pancreatitis	Thickened folds associated with medial compression or widening of duodenal sweep	Elevated serum amylase level; CT, MRI, or ultrasound for confirmation
Zollinger-Ellison syndrome	Thickened folds in stomach, duodenum, and proximal jejunum	Ulcers in atypical locations
Crohn's disease	Thickened folds, ulceration, or strictures	Associated Crohn's disease in small bowel or colon
Parasitic infection (giardiasis and strongyloidiasis)	Thickened or effaced folds, irritability, and spasm in duodenum and proximal jejunum	Stool cultures or small bowel brushings and biopsy specimens for diagnosis
Cryptosporidiosis	Thickened folds in duodenum and small bowel	History of AIDS; profuse secretory diarrhea
Celiac disease	Thickened folds in proximal duodenum	Often associated with "bubbly" bulb
Intramural hemorrhage	Thickened, spiculated folds or thumbprinting	History of bleeding diathesis, anticoagulation, or trauma
Varices	Serpentine folds in proximal duodenum	Portal hypertension
Lymphoma	Thickened folds or thumbprinting	Usually non-Hodgkin's lymphoma

Table 40-8
Dilated Duodenum (Megaduodenum)

Cause	Associated Radiographic Findings	Comments
Scleroderma	Dilated small bowel with hide-bound appearance	Systemic signs of scleroderma
Celiac disease	Dilated small bowel with decreased number of folds in jejunum	Malabsorption
Zollinger-Ellison syndrome	Thickened folds and increased secretions in stomach and duodenum; one or more ulcers	Hypergastrinemia
Strongyloidiasis	Thickened or effaced folds, ulceration, or "lead pipe" appearance in duodenum and jejunum	History of AIDS or travel to endemic areas
Superior mesenteric root syndrome	Broad, linear crossing defect on distal duodenum by mesenteric root	Thin or bedridden patients
Vagotomy	Dilated small bowel	Appropriate surgical history
Obstruction	Benign or malignant narrowing or extrinsic compression of duodenum	Postbulbar ulcer, Crohn's disease, pancreatitis, metastatic disease
Ileus	Dilated duodenum without mechanical obstruction	Postoperative ileus, metabolic imbalance, pancreatitis

Table 40-9
Extrinsic Impressions on the Duodenum

Cause	Location	Radiographic Findings	Comments
Pancreatic disease	Medial	Widened duodenal sweep	Pancreatitis, pancreatic pseudocyst, or pancreatic carcinoma
Peripancreatic adenopathy	Medial	Widened duodenal sweep	Peripancreatic metastases or lymphoma
Aortic aneurysm	Medial	Widened duodenal sweep	Aortoduodenal fistula is a rare complication
Gallbladder disease	Superior	Extrinsic compression of bulb or proximal duodenum	Acute or chronic cholecystitis or hydrops of the gallbladder
Liver disease	Superior	Extrinsic compression of bulb or proximal duodenum	Hepatomegaly of any cause
Renal disease	Posterolateral	Extrinsic compression of descending duodenum	Polycystic kidney, renal cell carcinoma
Colonic disease	Anterolateral	Extrinsic compression of descending duodenum	Carcinoma of the hepatic flexure

VI

Small Bowel

STEPHEN E. RUBESIN
Section Editor

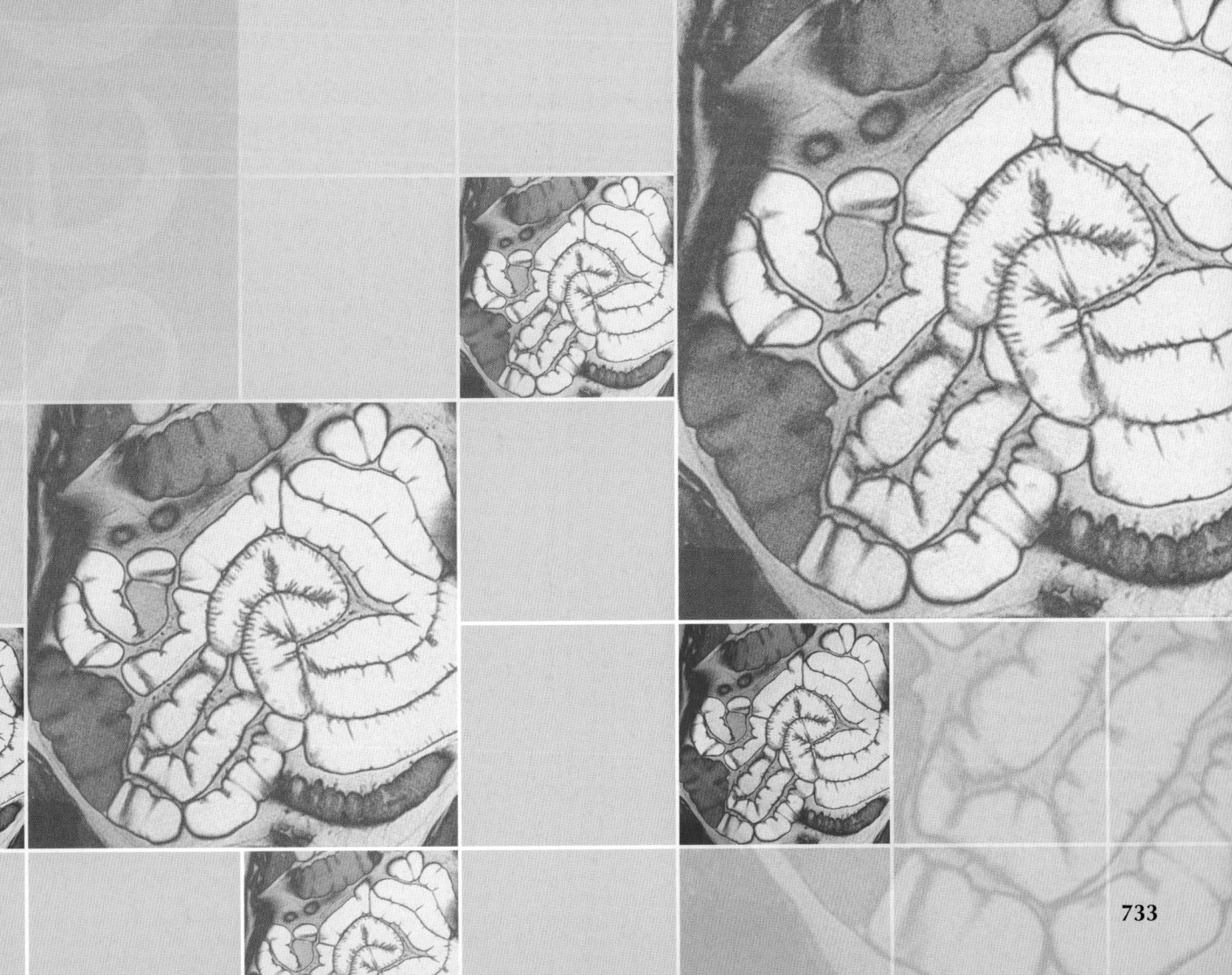

Barium Examinations of the Small Intestine

Stephen E. Rubesin, MD

The focus of this chapter is on barium examinations of the mesenteric small intestine. Normal anatomy pertinent to understanding barium examinations is presented. The variety of contrast examinations for studying the small intestine is then described. Finally, a symptom-based approach to contrast imaging of the small intestine is presented.

NORMAL SMALL INTESTINE

The small intestine is extremely tortuous, beginning at the pylorus and extending about 11 feet in the living human from the pylorus to the ileocecal valve. Intestinal length is extremely variable, depending on neuromuscular tone and vascular flow. For example, the denervated, bloodless intestine stretched at autopsy varies from 10 to 30 feet.[1] A patient with a small bowel obstruction will have a tortuous, long and wide small intestine in which the jejunum may fall deep into the pelvis.

The mesenteric portion of the small intestine is suspended from the retroperitoneum by the relatively short root of the small bowel mesentery, extending about 15 cm from the duodenojejunal junction to the right iliac fossa.[2] The mesenteric small intestine is divided into the jejunum and ileum. The jejunum arbitrarily comprises the proximal 40% of the mesenteric small intestine and the ileum makes up the distal 60% (Fig. 41-1). The jejunum typically occupies the left upper quadrant, and the ileum occupies the pelvis and right lower quadrant. The location of the jejunum and ileum is often variable, however, given the mobility of the intestine on the root of the mesentery. Not infrequently, the jejunum flops into the right upper quadrant or changes position during fluoroscopic examination of the small bowel.

The small intestine has a smooth, curvilinear contour, as readily seen on abdominal radiographs or cross-sectional imaging studies in patients with free intraperitoneal air. The

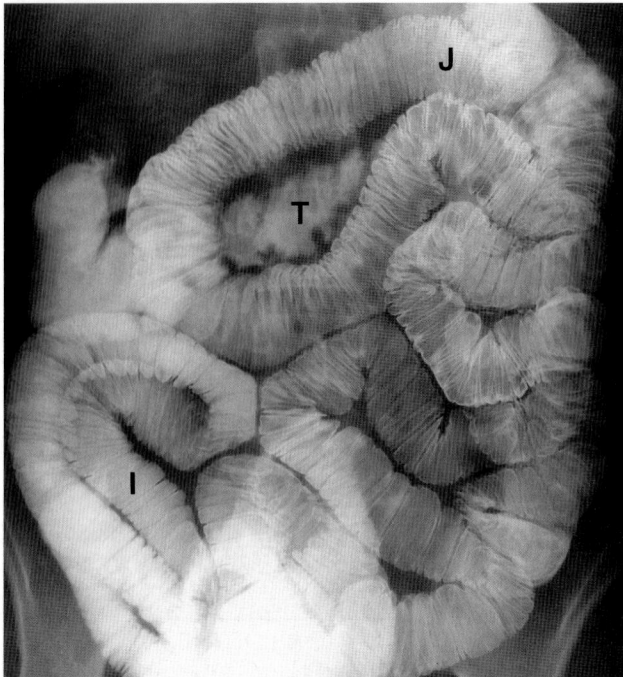

Figure 41-1. Normal small intestine. Overhead radiograph from enteroclysis (small bowel enema) shows the jejunum (J) in the left upper quadrant and the ileum (I) in the right lower quadrant. The transverse colon is also seen (T). The folds are more numerous, taller, and slightly thicker in the jejunum than in the ileum. The jejunum can be up to 4 cm in diameter and the ileum up to 3 cm in diameter.

inner contour of the intestine is characterized by folds that encircle the lumen, known as the folds of Kerckring, valvulae conniventes, or plicae circulares (Fig. 41-2). These folds are composed of mucosa and submucosa (Fig. 41-3) and increase the surface area of the small intestine by 300%.[1] The small

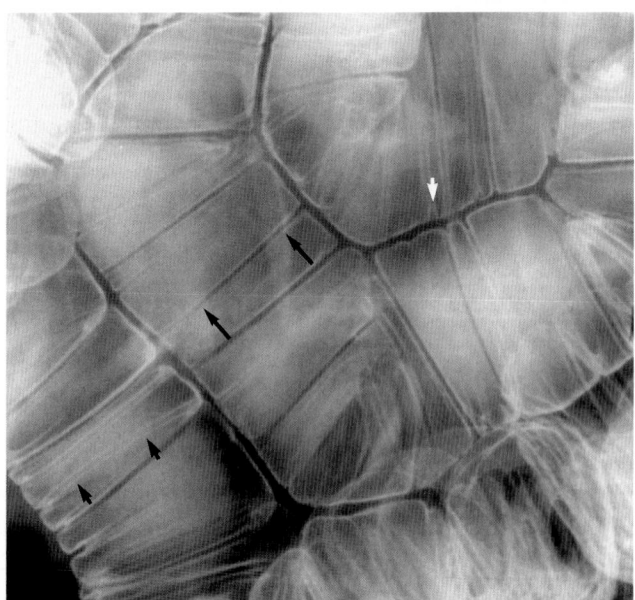

Figure 41-2. Normal small bowel folds. Spot image of the mid small intestine from enteroclysis shows the folds as linear radiolucent filling defects (*long black arrows*) in the shallow barium pool. In contrast, nondependent folds are etched in white (*short black arrows*). The height of the folds (*white arrow*) indicates that this image was obtained from the distal jejunum/proximal ileum. The mucosal surface is smooth.

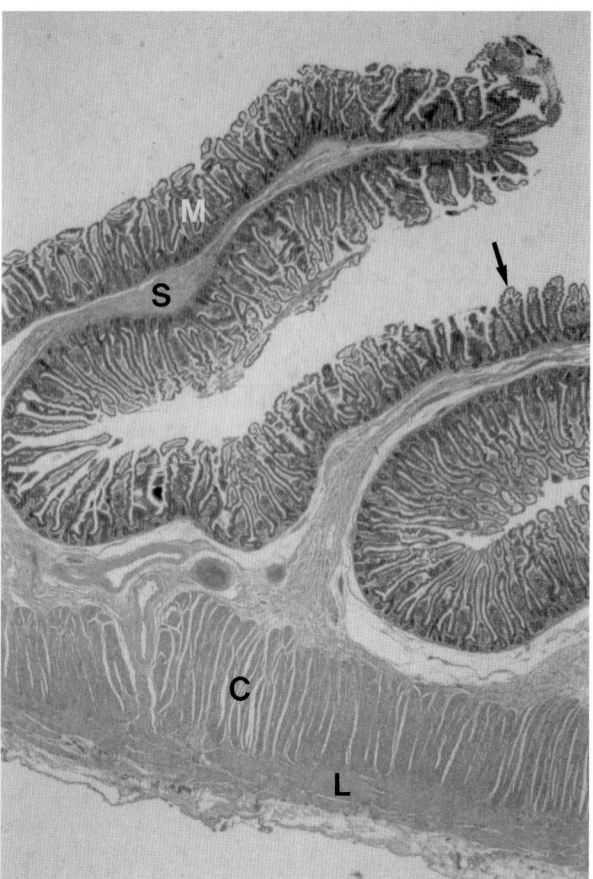

Figure 41-3. Normal small bowel folds. Portions of two small bowel folds are present on this histologic photomicrograph. Each fold (plica) is composed of a mucosal layer (M) (epithelium, lamina propria, and muscularis mucosae) covering a submucosal core (S). Each villus (*arrow*) is composed of a single layer of epithelial cells covering a core of lamina propria. The muscularis propria is composed of an inner circular muscle layer (C) and an outer longitudinal muscle layer (L).

bowel folds lie perpendicular to the longitudinal axis of the intestine and are thicker, taller, and more numerous in the jejunum than in the ileum (Table 41-1).[2,3] Villi are leaf- or finger-shaped protrusions of epithelium and lamina propria (see Fig. 41-3) that stud the surface of the folds. Each villus

Table 41-1
Normal Parameters for Enteroclysis and Small Bowel Follow-Through

	Enteroclysis	Small Bowel Follow-Through
Number Folds per Inch		
Jejunum	4-7	Difficult to count
Ileum	2-4 (or less)	Difficult to count
Fold Thickness		
Jejunum	1-2 mm	2-3 mm
Ileum	1-1.5 mm	1-2 mm
Fold Height		
Jejunum	3-7 mm	Difficult to asses
Ileum	1-3 mm	Difficult to assess
Lumen Width		
Jejunum	<4 cm	<3 cm
Ileum	<3 cm	<2 cm

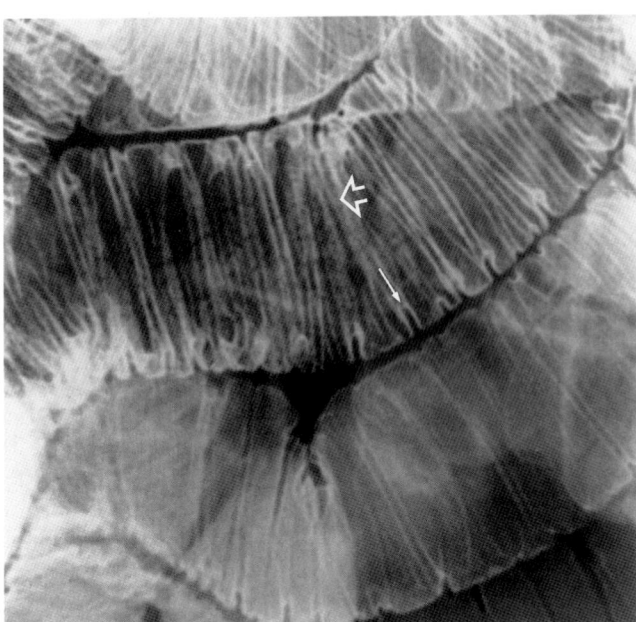

Figure 41-4. Normal villi demonstrated by enteroclysis. Spot image of the jejunum shows villi in one loop as tiny, submillimeter, round radiolucent filling defects (*open arrow*). This loop can be identified as jejunum by the relatively tall height of the folds (*thin arrow*).

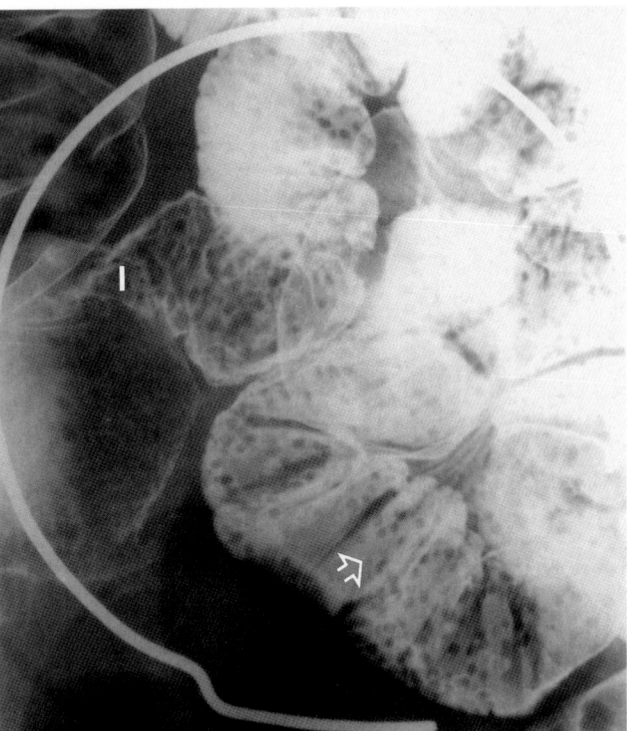

Figure 41-5. Lymphoid hyperplasia of the distal ileum due to common variable immunodeficiency. Spot image of the distal ileum shows numerous 1- to 2-mm round/ovoid radiolucent filling defects (*arrow*) in the shallow barium pool. These lymphoid follicles are more numerous and extend more proximally than usual. The ileal side of the ileocecal valve is identified (I).

has a core of lamina propria containing a cellular stroma, capillaries, a lacteal, and nerves. Villi are tall and thin in the jejunum and shorter and broader in the ileum.[1] Duodenal villi are more variable and can be short and broad, leaf-shaped, or branched.[1] The villi are about 1 mm in cross-section and are just at the limits of fluoroscopic resolution (Fig. 41-4). In contrast, the microvillous brush border of the small intestine is invisible on all radiographic examinations.

The small intestine is one of the largest immunologic organs of the body and a major site of interaction with foreign food antigens, pathogens, and toxins.[4] The host defenses begin at the epithelial surface with a mucus layer containing immunoglobulins (especially secretory IgA) and enzymes. This mucus prevents microbes from adhering to the epithelium and acts as a buffer and lubricant.[1] A variety of other defenses also protect the host from these food antigens, including intraluminal gastric acid, bile salts, and pancreatic enzymes, and small bowel peristalsis.

The small bowel epithelium is composed of a single layer of cells bound by tight junctions impermeable to large molecules and pathogens. Intramucosal phagocytes include granulocytes, macrophages, and Paneth cells. Three distinct lymphocyte populations are present in the intestine within the epithelium, lamina propria, and Peyer's patches. Intraepithelial lymphocytes are located in the basal portion of the epithelium and compose up to 30% of the cell population in the mucosa. Immunocytes in the lamina propria are composed mainly of IgA-secreting plasma cells and lymphocytes. T lymphocytes of both helper-inducer and suppressor-cytotoxic types are present. Lymphoid aggregates span the muscularis mucosae, with portions of these aggregates in the lamina propria and submucosa. These lymphoid aggregates increase in size and number in the distal ileum (Fig. 41-5), forming confluent Peyer's patches in the lower ileum. A specialized epithelium

that is one cell layer in thickness separates these lymphoid aggregates from the lumen, facilitating antigen processing. The lymphoid aggregates do not have a capsule, defined borders, a medulla, or afferent lymphatics that are present in lymph nodes.[1] The follicular areas are composed of B cells, and the parafollicular regions, of T cells.

PRINCIPLES FOR PERFORMING AND INTERPRETING SMALL BOWEL EXAMINATIONS

The small intestine is a difficult structure to image. The intraluminal environment is hostile to barium preparations. A large amount of fluid (approximately 9 L) enters the small intestine each day, with only 1.5 to 1.9 L entering the colon.[5] Bile acids, gastric acids, pancreatic secretions, and the epithelial mucus layer interact with barium in the small intestine. Fortunately, most modern barium suspensions no longer suffer from flocculation and clumping, as often occurred in the past.

Because of the inherent length and motility of the small intestine, imaging of this structure can take a long time. Intestinal loops overlap and change in size, shape, and position with peristalsis. Normal small bowel transit ranges from 30 to 120 minutes. Transit time can be lengthened dramatically in patients with obstruction or adynamic ileus from a variety of causes.

The radiologist evaluates the overall location, course, and size of various portions of the small intestine.[6] For example,

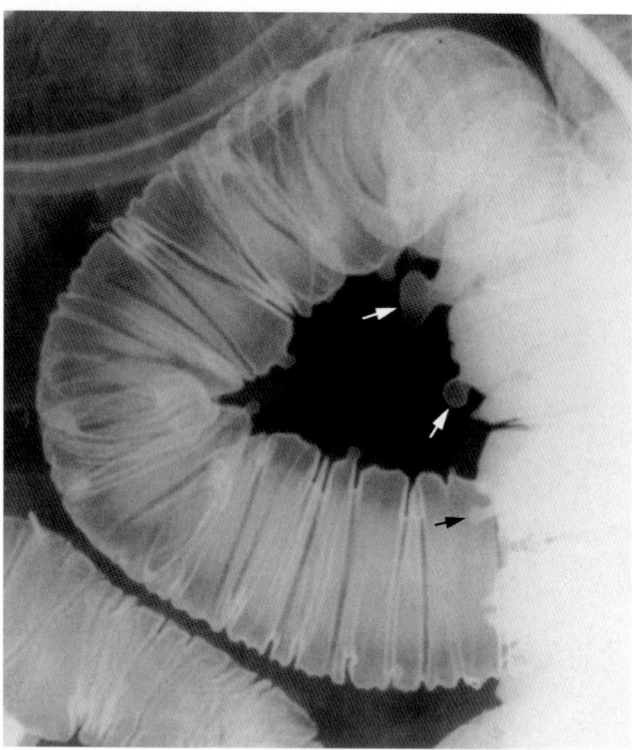

Figure 41-6. Jejunal diverticula. Spot image from enteroclysis shows at least 10 small diverticula extending from the mesenteric border of a jejunal loop. Some diverticula are etched in white by barium (*white arrows*), and others (*black arrow*) are filled with barium.

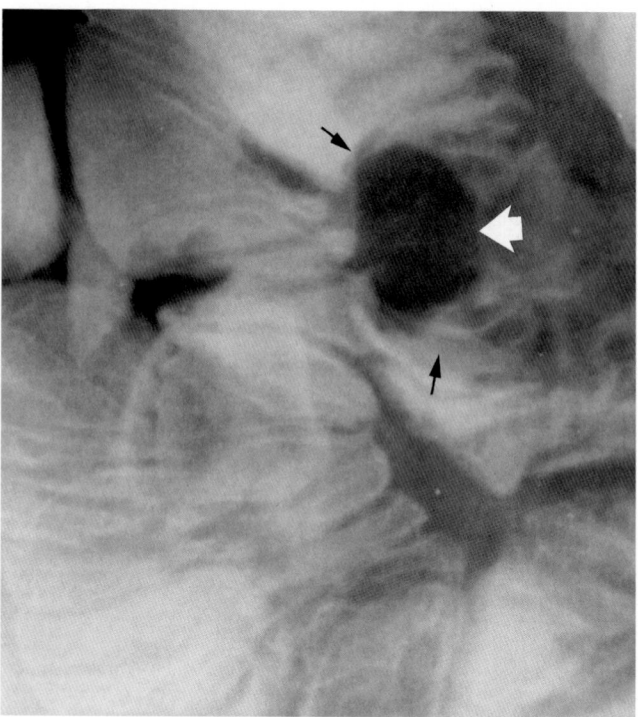

Figure 41-7. Carcinoid tumor in the ileum. Spot image of the distal ileum shows a 1.5-cm ovoid radiolucent filling defect (*white arrow*) protruding into the barium column. Note how the folds (*black arrows*) are pulled toward the tumor by a desmoplastic reaction at the base of the lesion. The adjacent ileal loop is also pulled toward the tumor. This desmoplastic reaction is typical of carcinoid tumors or intraperitoneal metastases.

the radiologist determines the location of the duodenojejunal junction and the location of the first loops of jejunum. The radiologist also evaluates the luminal contour and searches for abnormalities that extend beyond the small intestine (e.g., diverticula [Fig. 41-6], sacculations, ulcers, and exoenteric masses) or lesions that protrude into the lumen (e.g., polyps [Fig. 41-7] and abnormal folds). The small bowel folds are best evaluated when the lumen is fully distended and the folds lie perpendicular to the longitudinal axis of the bowel. Fold width also depends on the degree of luminal distention; the greater the distention, the thinner the folds appear (Fig. 41-8). The folds are best shown after mucus has been washed off the luminal surface by the barium column. If folds are evaluated long after the barium column has passed, intestinal secretions can lift barium away from the mucosal surface, so that the folds may erroneously appear thickened. En face mucosal detail is seen during compression of the barium column or with double-contrast technique. Visualization of this mucosal detail is necessary for detecting mucosal granularity or nodularity or small ulcers such as aphthoid ulcers (Fig. 41-9).

Fluoroscopy is a key component of any small bowel examination. The radiologist examines the head of the barium column to understand the course of the small intestine and to detect contour abnormalities or filling defects in the barium column. The radiologist also assesses bowel motility, distensibility, and pliability during the fluoroscopic examination. Fixation of intestinal loops can also be recognized by manual palpation of the bowel.

SMALL BOWEL FOLLOW-THROUGH

There are many ways to perform a small bowel follow-through examination. In this chapter I discuss the technique that I use. A small bowel follow-through is a single contrast examination of the esophagus, stomach, and small intestine that employs barium most appropriate for the small bowel. For this examination, the patient drinks a large volume (500 to 1000 mL) of low-density (30 to 50% w/v) barium specifically designed for evaluating the small intestine.

The patient should not eat or drink after 9 to 11 PM the day before the examination. If a peroral pneumocolon is to be performed, the patient should receive a barium enema preparation to cleanse the terminal ileum and right side of the colon.

A single-contrast upper gastrointestinal series is often performed (using 1 to 2 cups of low-density barium) as a prelude to examining the small bowel. The purpose of the upper gastrointestinal series is to show gross upper gastrointestinal involvement by diseases that affect the small bowel, such as Crohn's disease and scleroderma. Esophageal or gastric abnormalities may also be detected as incidental findings, given the high frequency of upper gastrointestinal disorders such as gastroesophageal reflux disease. However, a double-contrast upper gastrointestinal examination using high-density barium is not performed, because this barium is not designed for evaluating the small intestine, and, if used, high-density barium often prevents adequate visualization of pelvic small bowel loops. The radiologist therefore sacrifices

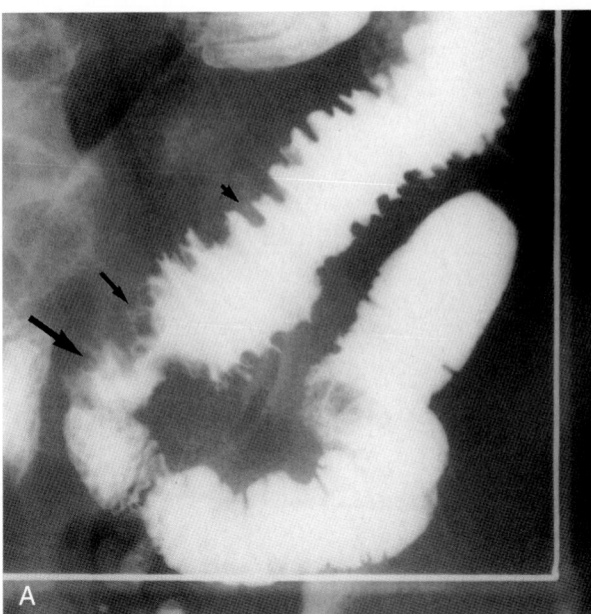 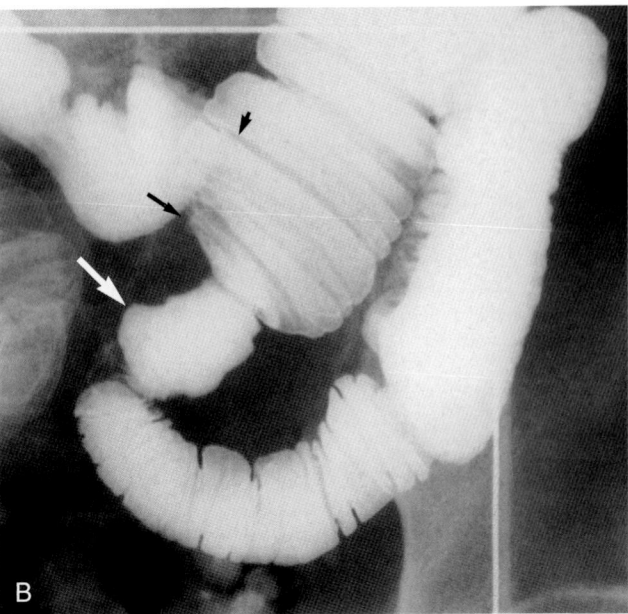

Figure 41-8. Variation in the width of small bowel folds with luminal distention. A. Spot image obtained during early single-contrast phase of enteroclysis shows a focal area of tapered narrowing (*medium-sized black arrow*) containing an irregular collection of barium (*long black arrow*). Note apparent widening of the small bowel folds (*short black arrow*) when the lumen is incompletely distended. **B.** Spot image obtained during early phase of methylcellulose filling (the loop is still visualized mainly in single contrast before a transradiant methylcellulose effect has been achieved) shows how the narrowed segment has a more abrupt proximal margin (*long black arrow*). An amorphous collection of barium (*white arrow*) disrupts the normal luminal contour and fold pattern. This was an ulcerated adenocarcinoma of the distal jejunum causing low-grade small bowel obstruction. Note the normal width of the small bowel folds (*short black arrow*) in the distended jejunum proximal to the tumor.

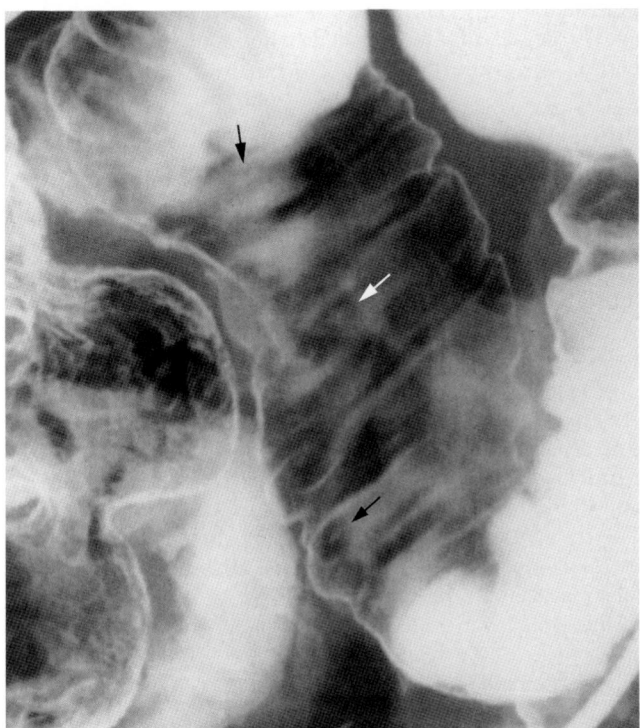

Figure 41-9. Aphthoid ulcers in Crohn's disease. Spot image of the terminal ileum from a peroral pneumocolon shows aphthoid ulcers (*arrows*) as punctate barium collections surrounded by radiolucent halos of edema.

double-contrast evaluation of the upper gastrointestinal tract to ensure a more optimal examination of the small intestine. After the esophagus, stomach, and duodenum are evaluated, the patient leaves the fluoroscopic suite and slowly sips an additional 1 to 2 cups of low-density barium.

In some practices, a technologist obtains overhead radiographs and a radiologist evaluates the overheads views, only fluoroscoping and palpating the small bowel when an abnormality is suspected or when barium has reached the terminal ileum. Such an approach is strongly discouraged. A small bowel follow-through relies on fluoroscopic detection and spot image documentation of all abnormalities. Each loop of small bowel is palpated when it is optimally distended by low-density barium (Fig. 41-10). The radiologist should therefore evaluate the patient at least several times: about 15 to 30 minutes after the single contrast upper gastrointestinal series is performed and then at 15- to 45-minute intervals, depending on how fast the barium column is progressing through the small intestine. The patient is turned into various positions, and manual palpation (including supine, lateral, and prone compression views) is used to "splay out" individual small bowel loops. In my practice, I no longer obtain overhead radiographs. If the "big picture" is required, a digital spot radiograph obtained at the lowest magnification is usually adequate for this purpose.

The length of the examination can be shortened by administering a standard dose of 20 mg of metoclopramide (Reglan) orally 20 to 30 minutes before the study or 10 mg intravenously at the beginning of the examination.[7-9] Metoclopramide accelerates gastric emptying and small bowel transit. Unfortunately, metoclopramide also increases resting muscle

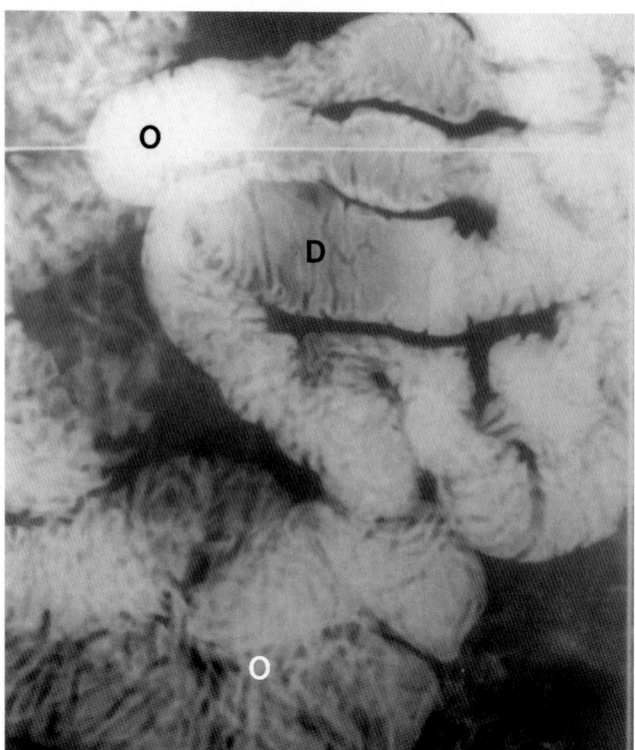

Figure 41-10. Normal small bowel follow-through. Spot radiograph with compression shows the distal jejunum. When the loops are well distended (D) and separated from each other, an image from a small bowel follow-through is comparable to that from enteroclysis. When loops are overlapping (black O), however, the density of the barium may obscure anatomic detail. When loops are overlapping and partially collapsed, the overlapping folds may form a "feathery" pattern (white O).

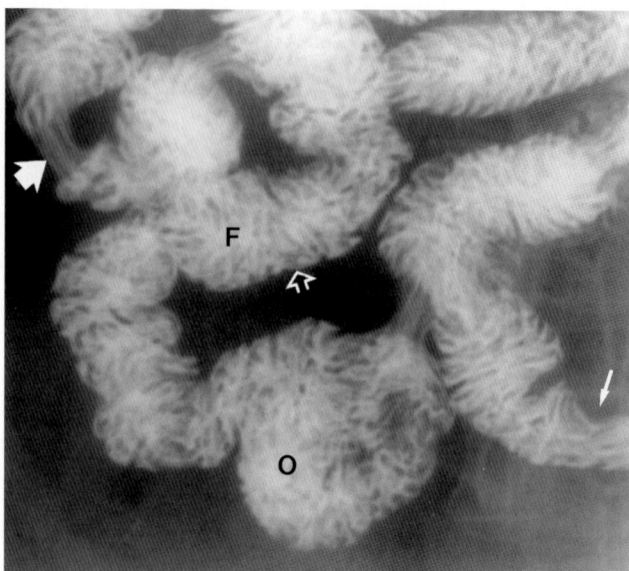

Figure 41-11. Partially distended small bowel during small bowel follow-through. Folds (F) in a partly distended proximal ileal loop have a feathery pattern. The contour is well visualized (*open arrow*) when a loop is isolated. When loops are contracting (*thin arrow*), a smooth impression is seen on the mesenteric border, mimicking an extrinsic lesion indenting the small bowel. When a loop is collapsed or contracting, folds lie parallel to the longitudinal axis of the small bowel (*thick arrow*). Dense areas of barium may result from overlapping loops (black O) that can be separated by compression.

tone, resulting in incomplete small bowel distention.[10] The result is a faster but less optimal examination.

Some radiologists administer two to three doses of effervescent agent (600 to 900 mL of CO_2) when the barium column reaches pelvic loops of ileum or the terminal ileum. This technique shortens the examination and demonstrates small bowel loops on an air-contrast study. Nevertheless, administration of an effervescent agent can be uncomfortable, because large volumes of gas can incite intestinal cramping. It also results in decreased luminal distention in comparison to enteroclysis, and only one third to one half of the small bowel is shown on the air-contrast study.[11]

Some radiologists employ a premade mixture of 24% w/v barium suspended in methylcellulose. This barium suspension produces greater luminal distention than a routine small bowel follow-through as well as a transradiant effect that mimics enteroclysis.[12] However, the barium is not as dense as that used for a routine small bowel follow-through, so that it can be more difficult to detect filling defects in the barium column. Luminal distention also is less than that in enteroclysis, because it is limited by the rate of gastric emptying at the pylorus.

The small bowel follow-through has two important limitations. Even with the use of metoclopramide, the pylorus delays emptying of barium from the stomach, so that the small bowel may be incompletely distended. As a result, it can be difficult to evaluate luminal contour (Fig. 41-11) or to detect filling defects in the barium column. Because normal transit time for the small bowel is 30 to 120 minutes, it also is not feasible for the radiologist to remain in the fluoroscopy suite for the entire examination. As a result, the small bowel can only be evaluated intermittently and lesions can be missed, depending on the degree of filling and distention of individual small bowel loops at the time of fluoroscopy.

Peroral Pneumocolon

A peroral pneumocolon may be performed in conjunction with a small bowel follow-through.[13-16] This is a double-contrast examination, primarily used to evaluate patients with suspected Crohn's disease in the terminal ileum or to evaluate the right side of the colon in patients in whom a barium enema or colonoscopy failed to adequately visualize this portion of the bowel.

The patient undergoes a barium enema preparation to clear feces from the terminal ileum and right side of the colon. After a routine small bowel follow-through has been performed, 1 mg of glucagon is administered intravenously and air is insufflated into the rectum via a Foley catheter. The colon is slowly distended with air as the patient is turned into various positions to manipulate air into the cecum and terminal ileum. Air can be refluxed successfully into the terminal ileum in 85% to 90% of patients. Double-contrast spot images of the pelvic ileum, terminal ileum, and right side of the colon are then obtained (Fig. 41-12).

ENTEROCLYSIS

The small intestine has been examined via intubation techniques since the 1920s.[17-20] All of these techniques entail positioning a tube beyond the pylorus, overdistending the small

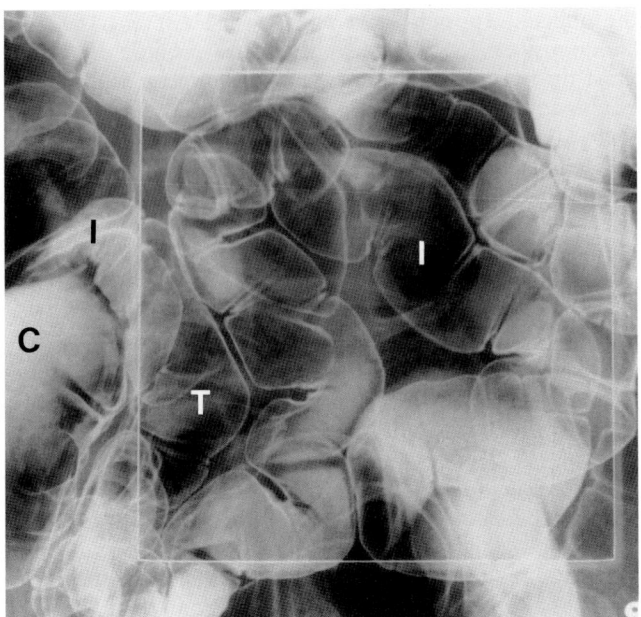

Figure 41-12. Normal distal ileum demonstrated during peroral pneumocolon. Spot radiograph shows the terminal ileum (T) and distal ileum (white I) in air-contrast study. The mucosa is smooth and featureless. The cecum (C) and ileal side of the ileocecal valve (black I) are also identified.

bowel with various contrast agents, and detecting abnormalities at fluoroscopy. The multiplicity of techniques for performing enteroclysis reflects the imperfections of each individual technique. Lack of universal acceptance of this procedure by the radiologic community is related to the relatively high level of expertise needed to perform enteroclysis and to patient discomfort during the intubation procedure.

Preparation

An unprepped patient often has feces in the terminal ileum and right side of the colon. This fecal matter obscures mucosal detail, mimics polyps, and impedes passage of contrast material through the distal ileum.[21] A preparation is therefore given to clear feces from the terminal ileum and right colon before the examination. This can be a full barium-enema type preparation, including osmotic cathartics such as magnesium citrate and colonic stimulants such as bisacodyl. At my institution, I have achieved successful cleansing of the right side of the colon with a clear liquid diet the day before the examination combined with four 5-mg tablets of bisacodyl the evening before the examination. The patient does not eat or drink after midnight. On the day of the examination, the patient should temporarily discontinue medications such as narcotics that decrease small bowel peristalsis.

Metoclopramide

Metoclopramide is administered orally or intravenously before the examination.[21,22] Metoclopramide begins to take effect 1 to 3 minutes after intravenous injection of a 10-mg dose or 30 to 60 minutes after ingestion of two 10-mg tablets.[23] This drug facilitates passage of the enteroclysis catheter by relaxing the pyloric sphincter and duodenal bulb and by increasing

gastric antral contractions.[24,25] Passage of barium through the small bowel is accelerated because metoclopramide increases peristalsis in the duodenum and jejunum. Metoclopramide may also improve visualization of strictures in Crohn's disease (Fig. 41-13). However, its use is contraindicated in patients with known pheochromocytomas, because it may stimulate catecholamine release from these lesions, precipitating a hypertensive crisis.[26] Metoclopramide is also contraindicated in patients with epilepsy or and in patients receiving drugs that may cause extrapyramidal reactions, because it increases the frequency and severity of seizures associated with these reactions.

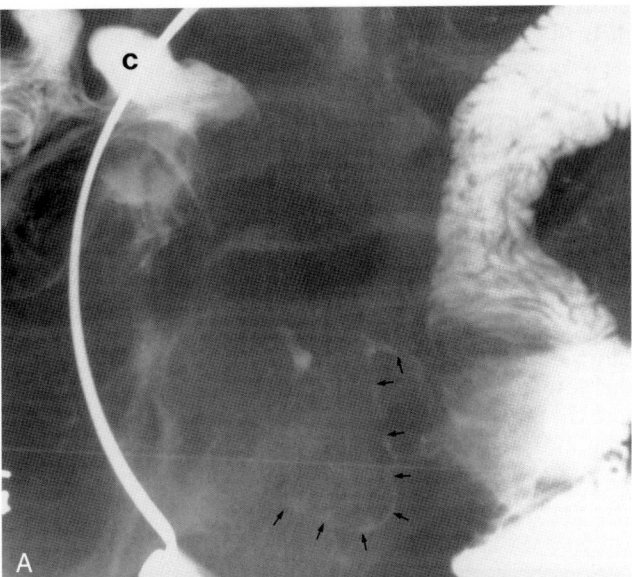

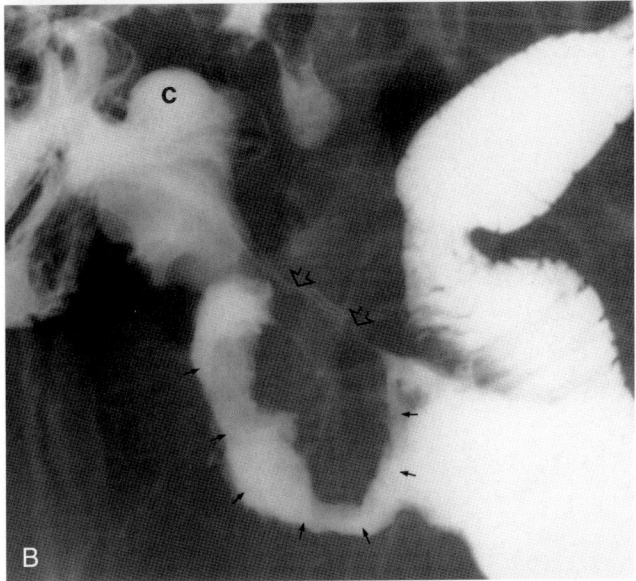

Figure 41-13. Value of metoclopramide for evaluating narrowing of the terminal ileum in a patient with Crohn's disease. A. Spot radiograph from a small bowel follow-through shows a stringlike segment of narrowing (*arrows*) in the terminal ileum inferior to the cecum (C). **B.** After metoclopramide has been administered, the narrowed segment (*short arrows*) distends considerably but is still abnormal with effaced folds and nodular mucosa due to Crohn's disease. An ileoileal fistula (*open arrows*) is also visualized. These images show how narrowing in Crohn's disease may be caused by a combination of spasm, edema, inflammatory change, and fibrosis.

Anesthesia

The major complaint patients have about enteroclysis is intubation. Patients can be made more comfortable by the use of conscious sedation.[27] One protocol for conscious sedation includes a combination of fentanyl or diazepam for analgesia and midazolam for an amnesic effect.[21] Oral diazepam alone can be used as an alternative.[24]

Intubation

A variety of enteroclysis catheters are available from several manufacturers.[28-30] The catheters have a diameter of 8 to 13 French, an end hole or side holes, and a balloon attached to their tips. One manufacturer has a multiple-lumen catheter capable of both a diagnostic study and therapeutic decompression.[31]

We suggest having the patient ingest a small amount (15 to 30 mL) of enteroclysis barium orally before intubation. This barium coats the antrum, pylorus, and duodenal bulb, which are important landmarks that guide the radiologist in passing the enteroclysis catheter.

A complete description of intubation techniques is beyond the scope of this chapter but is described in several references.[6,21,22,24] The enteroclysis catheter can be passed into the oropharynx via an oral or nasal route. The oral route has the advantage of allowing visualization of catheter passage into the throat but the disadvantage of causing more gagging. Oral intubation is made easier by the use of a topical anesthetic spray. In contrast, the nasal route causes less gagging, because there is less contact of the catheter with the base of the tongue and posterior pharyngeal wall. However, nasal intubation may cause nasal bleeding and may result in prolonged nasal discomfort as the catheter is manipulated during the examination. Nasal intubation is made easier with the use of topical lidocaine jelly in the intubated naris.

The major purpose of the catheter guidewire is to torque or guide the tip of the catheter along the longitudinal axis of the bowel. The guidewire is sometimes placed at the tip of the catheter, with appropriate torquing to guide the catheter in the proper direction. At other times, the guidewire is retracted, allowing the soft tip of the catheter to pass through sensitive regions such as the pylorus or to curve around tight bends such as the apex of the duodenal bulb (Fig. 41-14). Passage of the catheter into the duodenum is also facilitated by changing the configuration of the bowel with manual compression (Fig. 41-15) or by turning the patient on the fluoroscopic table. The tip of the catheter can be left in the second portion of the duodenum for single-contrast or air-contrast enteroclysis. When methylcellulose is used, however, the tip of the catheter should ideally be placed in the first loop of jejunum to limit reflux of methylcellulose into the stomach. Inflation of the balloon on the catheter also helps prevent methylcellulose from refluxing into the stomach. If the patient complains of discomfort during inflation of the balloon, it should immediately be deflated until the discomfort subsides. Duodenal perforation has been reported in one patient during intubation for enteroclysis.[32]

Successful intubation during enteroclysis depends on the skill and experience of the examining radiologist (whether or not sedation is used) and the patient's anatomy. Intubation is more difficult in patients with a prominent cricopharyngeus,

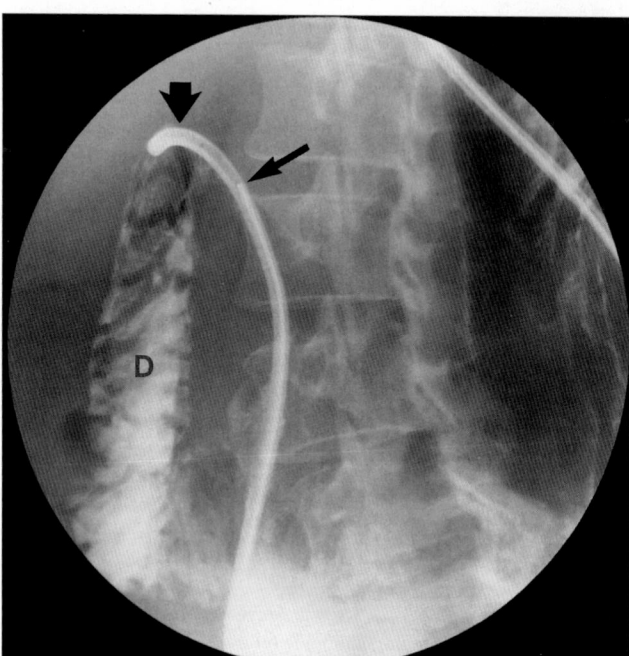

Figure 41-14. Enteroclysis catheter directed around the apex of the duodenal bulb. The soft tip of the enteroclysis catheter is bending around the 180-degree turn (*thick arrow*) between the duodenal bulb and proximal descending duodenum. The wire (*thin arrow*) has been retracted, allowing the catheter tip to be more pliable, so that it can bend around this curve. Contrast in the duodenum (D) is the residue of 30 mL of barium swallowed at the outset of the study to outline the anatomy of the pyloric region and facilitate passage of the catheter.

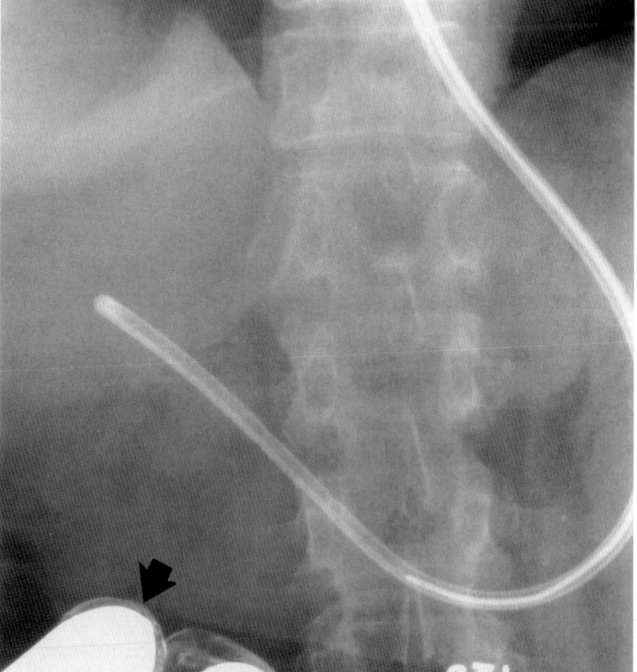

Figure 41-15. Compression by examiner to guide the enteroclysis catheter. The hand of the examiner covered by a lead glove (*arrow*) pushes on the greater curvature of the stomach. This directs the enteroclysis catheter toward the pylorus. Note how the guidewire is retracted from the tip of the catheter.

hiatal hernia, and transversely oriented stomach. Intubation is also potentially more difficult in patients with a dilated, atonic stomach due to diabetes or other causes.

Contrast material can be infused through the enteroclysis catheter with syringes or a variety of pumps. The use of an electric pump (e.g., a mini dialysis pump, RS-7800; Renal Systems, Minneapolis, MN) enables the radiologist to accurately control the infusion rate, which can be adjusted during the examination.[33] If the infusion rate is too fast, overdistention of the jejunum may cause hypotonia of the bowel. If the infusion rate is too slow, however, the lumen may be suboptimally distended, prolonging the examination time. Flow rates are generally between 50 and 150 mL/min.

The following descriptions of the various types of enteroclysis reflect my own experience and feelings about these techniques. Each radiologist should carefully evaluate the advantages and disadvantages of each before choosing a particular method for performing enteroclysis.

Single-Contrast Enteroclysis

A low-density (20% to 40% w/v) barium is the usual contrast agent for single-contrast enteroclysis.[25,34] In rare cases of suspected perforation, water-soluble contrast agents (e.g., meglumine diatrizoate/diatrizoate sodium) can be used. The enteroclysis catheter is passed into the proximal duodenum. Contrast is instilled via a syringe, pump, or gravity-feed bag. Between 600 and 1200 mL of barium are injected at an initial rate of about 75 mL/min. After administering a large volume of barium, water may be instilled into the catheter to push barium into the distal ileum and obtain a moderate double-contrast effect.

Single-contrast studies are simpler to perform than other types of enteroclysis, because only one contrast agent is employed. Reflux of barium into the stomach rarely induces vomiting, as sometimes occurs with methylcellulose. With air- or methylcellulose-contrast techniques, the mucosal surface of the small bowel is readily demonstrated en face. With single-contrast technique, however, evaluation of mucosal detail en face depends on compression and analysis of fold morphology. Although single-contrast technique is inferior to double-contrast techniques for visualizing mucosal detail, the diagnosis of many small bowel abnormalities (e.g., adhesions, tumors, and hernias) does not require subtle demonstration of surface detail. In patients with known or suspected malabsorption, however, double-contrast enteroclysis techniques are recommended.

Air-Contrast Enteroclysis

Air contrast is the standard form of enteroclysis in Japan and has become a favorite technique of Dean Maglinte, MD, one of the leading proponents of enteroclysis.[21,35-37] I have used the technique at one of my institutions, where an electric pump is not available for methylcellulose infusion. After intubation of the proximal duodenum, between 300 and 600 mL of barium varying from 50% to 80% w/v is instilled by gravity, syringe, or pump. The infusion rate of barium is altered to preserve peristalsis and for uniform distention of the proximal and mid small bowel. Room air or carbon dioxide is administered when barium reaches the pelvic small bowel[21] or terminal ileum.[37] Small bowel hypotonia may be induced by intravenous injec-

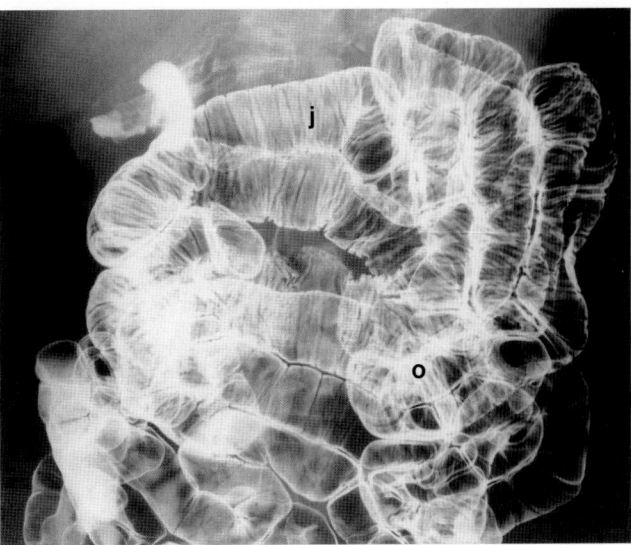

Figure 41-16. Jejunum during air-contrast enteroclysis. Coned-down view from an overhead radiograph demonstrates the small intestine in an air-contrast study. The jejunum (j) is well shown where loops are seen without overlap. When loops overlap (o), however, the small bowel is not optimally visualized.

tion of 1 mg of glucagon after barium has reached the right side of the colon.[6]

Air-contrast enteroclysis produces spectacular mucosal detail in loops coated by barium and distended by gas (Fig. 41-16). However, I have found it difficult to titrate the amount of barium necessary to coat the bowel without having too much barium in the lumen. Unlike double-contrast studies of the stomach and colon, it is more difficult to manipulate the barium pool, so that some loops are visualized only with dense barium, despite using various patient positions and compression (Fig. 41-17). Overlap of barium-filled loops with air-filled loops also results in radiographic overexposure of the loops demonstrated in air contrast. Distention of pelvic loops with air is sometimes incomplete.

Another disadvantage of air-contrast enteroclysis is that injection of large volumes of air into the small intestine may cause considerable discomfort. Sedation of these patients is therefore strongly recommended by some authors.[21]

In summary, I have achieved beautiful demonstration of the jejunum but suboptimal demonstration of pelvic ileal loops with air-contrast enteroclysis. Air-contrast techniques are more likely to be of value for patients with intestinal disease involving long segments of small bowel (e.g., malabsorptive states or Crohn's disease). Methylcellulose-contrast enteroclysis is more effective, however, for patients with adhesions or other lesions involving shorter segments of bowel.

Methylcellulose-Contrast Enteroclysis

During methylcellulose-contrast enteroclysis, a small volume of barium is propelled through the small intestine by a large volume of radiolucent liquid (the methylcellulose) (Fig. 41-18).[22,38] Medium-density (50% to 80% w/v) barium coats the intestinal mucosa, and methylcellulose distends the lumen. This is a biphasic examination. The radiologist follows the column of barium, looking for obstructing lesions (see Fig. 41-8) or lesions in the barium pool (Fig. 41-19). The small

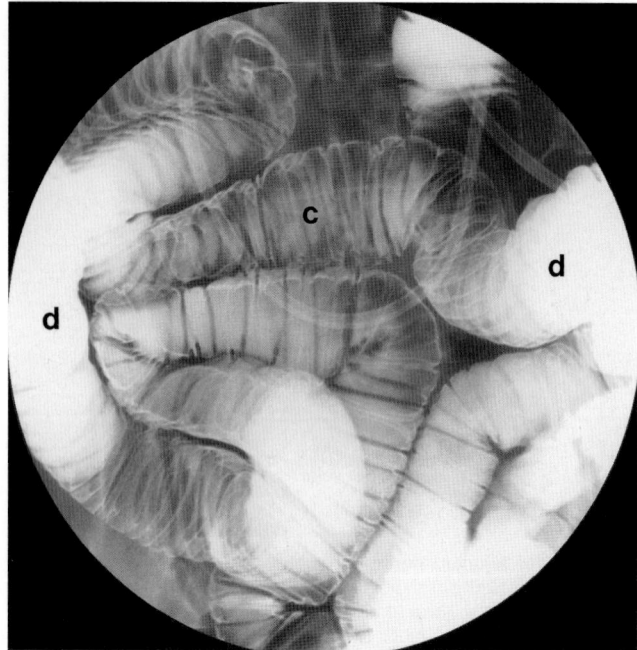

Figure 41-17. Too much barium on air-contrast enteroclysis. Mid small bowel loops are well visualized (c) in some areas. In other areas, however, dense barium (d) obscures folds and mucosal detail. It is sometimes difficult to titrate the appropriate volume of barium for air-contrast enteroclysis.

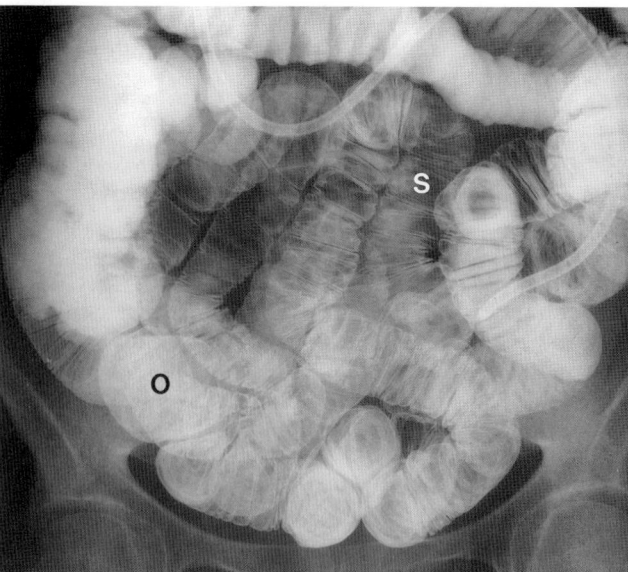

Figure 41-18. Methylcellulose-contrast enteroclysis. Overhead radiograph obtained at the end of the enteroclysis examination shows exquisite anatomic detail in nonoverlapping loops (S). Anatomic detail may be difficult to visualize, however, when loops overlap (O), even though the methylcellulose allows partial visualization of these overlapping loops, termed a *transradiant effect*.

bowel folds and en face mucosal detail are then evaluated when the lumen is distended by methylcellulose. Full luminal distention by methylcellulose straightens the valvulae conniventes, better delineates en face mucosal detail, and over-distends the lumen, increasing conspicuity of low-grade obstructing lesions.

Varying amounts and densities of barium have been employed for methylcellulose-contrast enteroclysis. I routinely use 220 to 300 mL of 80% w/v barium, infusing barium at 60 to 80 mL/min via a syringe until about one half of the expected intestinal loops are visualized. Herlinger and associates use 180 to 220 mL of 80% w/v barium.[24] Maglinte and

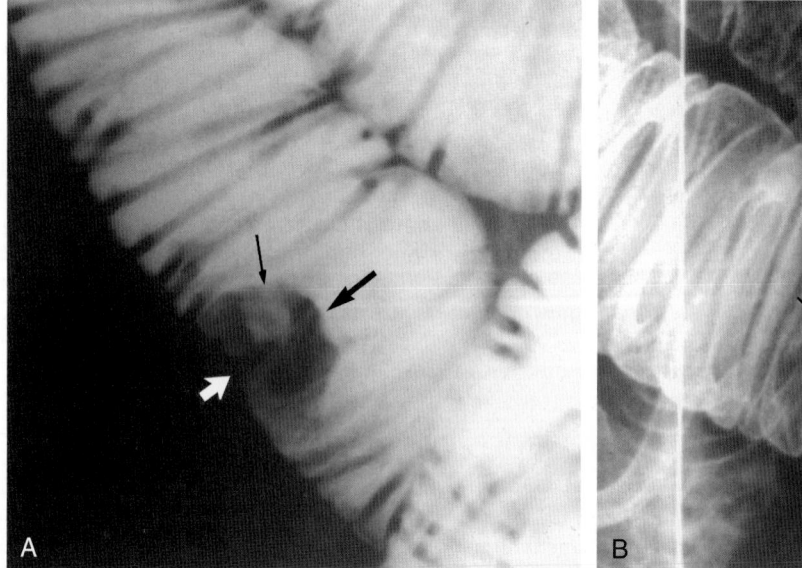
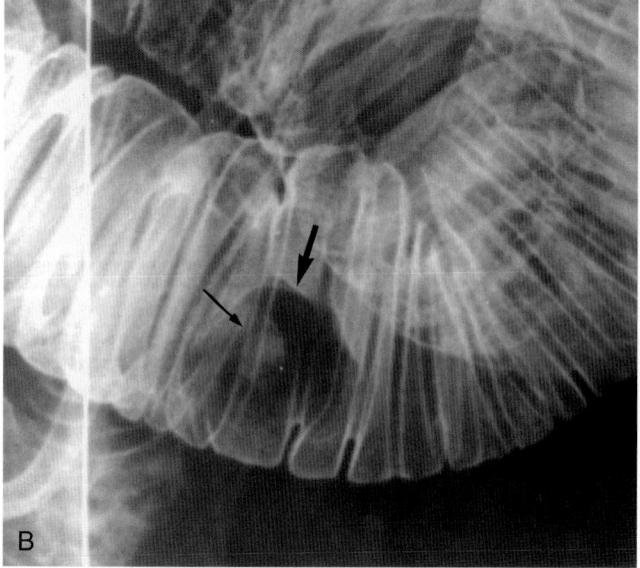

Figure 41-19. Metastatic melanoma demonstrated during enteroclysis. A. Spot image obtained during the single-contrast phase of enteroclysis shows a polypoid mass as a lobulated radiolucent filling defect (*thick black arrow*) in the barium column. The normal luminal contour is disrupted (*white arrow*). A central barium collection is seen (*thin black arrow*). **B.** Spot radiograph obtained during the methylcellulose phase again shows a slightly lobulated radiolucent filling defect (*thick arrow*) with a central barium collection (*thin arrow*), representing an ulcer. Apart from the ulceration, the surface of the polyp is smooth, indicating the submucosal origin of the lesion.

colleagues recommend infusing 300 to 600 mL of 50% w/v barium until pelvic loops of ileum are filled.[39] The amount of barium infused for this examination ultimately depends on the perceived length and diameter of the small intestine and on the presence or absence of obstruction or increased intraluminal fluid.

The use of methylcellulose enables the radiologist to see through overlapping small bowel loops to a greater degree than that allowed with single-contrast or air-contrast enteroclysis. However, methylcellulose-contrast enteroclysis also has several disadvantages. Methylcellulose is a thick, sticky substance that may require dilution in the "barium kitchen." Bubbles will form if methylcellulose is shaken, not stirred. Unless an electric pump is used, methylcellulose is messy and difficult to instill. The enteroclysis catheter tip should be placed in the jejunum, because reflux of methylcellulose into the stomach may induce projectile vomiting. If the radiologist needs to visualize the duodenum, the catheter should therefore be retracted to the proximal duodenum at the end of the examination and additional barium infused (Fig. 41-20). Once methylcellulose has reached the colon, uncontrollable diarrhea may ensue, requiring placement of an enema tip in

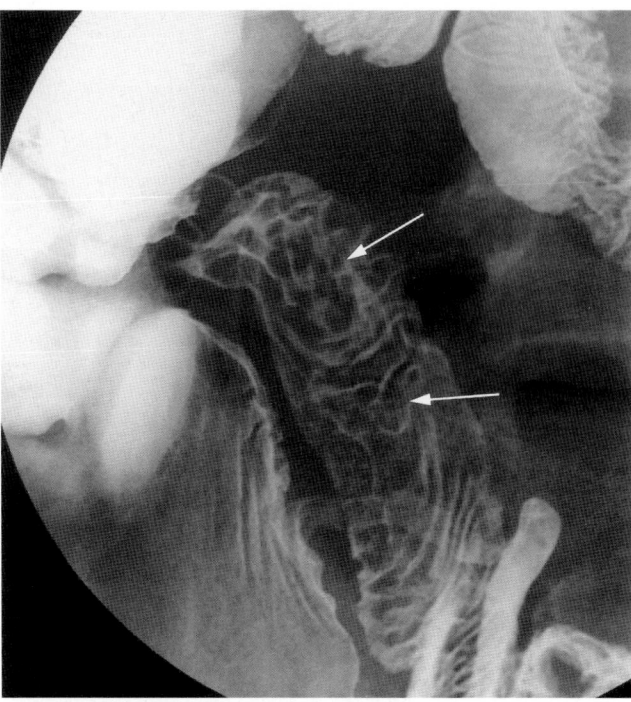

Figure 41-21. Crohn's disease demonstrated by enteroclysis. Spot image shows thickened, nodular folds (*arrows*) in the terminal ileum.

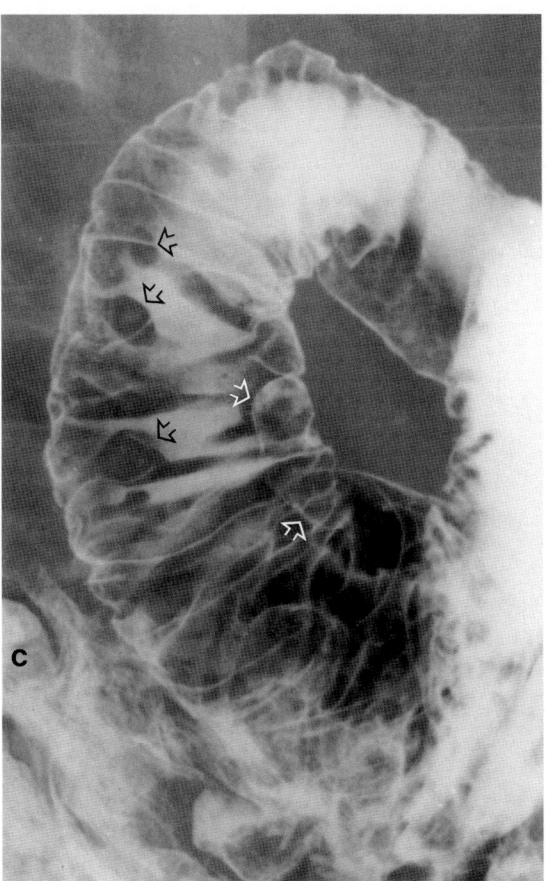

Figure 41-20. Air-contrast examination of duodenum after enteroclysis. Spot radiograph shows multiple small polyps (several identified by *black arrows*) as radiolucent filling defects in the shallow barium pool on the posterior wall of the descending duodenum. The papilla of Vater is enlarged (*white arrows*). Contrast in the colon (c) partly obscures the third portion of the duodenum. This patient had familial adenomatous polyposis syndrome. The polyps were tubular adenomas; the enlarged papilla of Vater resulted from an adenocarcinoma arising in a tubulovillous adenoma.

the rectum to allow rectal drainage and alleviate patient discomfort and embarrassment.

Methylcellulose-contrast enteroclysis almost always results in excellent double contrast in the jejunum. With infusion of enough methylcellulose, a double-contrast examination of the terminal ileum may also be achieved (Fig. 41-21). However, barium diffusion into the methylcellulose may result in a poor double-contrast effect in the ileum, resulting in only a single-contrast examination of the distal ileum (Fig. 41-22). To prevent diffusion of barium into the methylcellulose, the radiologist limits compression, especially in pelvic loops of ileum. Thus, the double-contrast barium enema and peroral pneumocolon are more reliable techniques if a detailed double-contrast examination of the terminal ileum is required.

Hypotonic Duodenogram

A hypotonic duodenogram is a detailed examination of the duodenum and, in some patients, the first two loops of jejunum.[6] This examination is used to elucidate confusing radiographic, CT, or endoscopic findings in the duodenum and first loop of jejunum. High-density barium is administered via an enteroclysis catheter placed in the proximal descending duodenum. After high-density barium has entered the duodenum and first jejunal loop, the patient is rotated on the fluoroscopic table to coat the mucosa. A standard dose of 1 mg of glucagon is administered intravenously to induce intestinal hypotonia. Air is then injected into the catheter to distend the duodenal lumen, and spot images are obtained (Fig. 41-23).

A similar examination can be performed in a less invasive way by having the patient swallow an effervescent agent and high-density barium. The patient is then placed with his or her right side down. When the duodenum has adequately filled

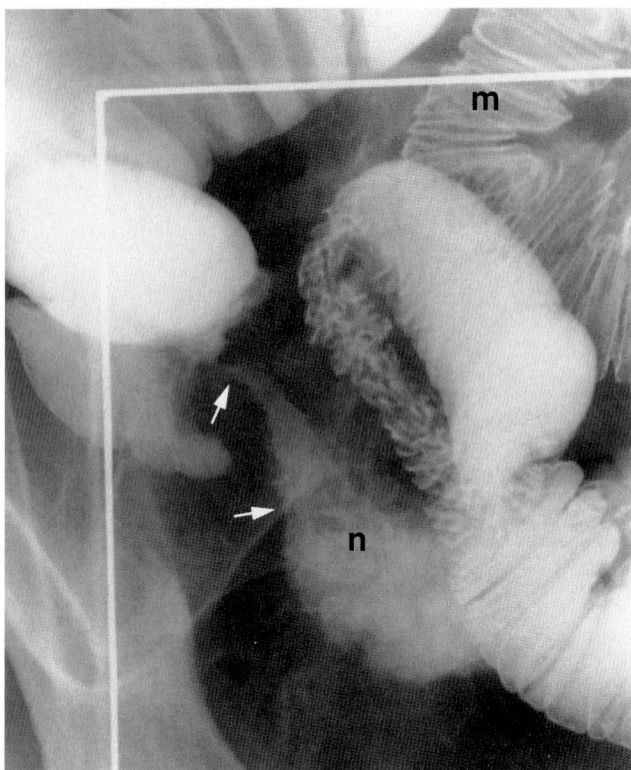

Figure 41-22. Diffusion of barium into methylcellulose column in neo-terminal ileum in Crohn's disease. Spot image shows tapered narrowing of the neoterminal ileum (*arrows*) with minimal nodularity of the mucosa (n). The neoterminal ileum is seen only in single contrast, whereas a double contrast effect (m) is seen more proximally. This patient underwent prior resection of the terminal ileum, cecum, and proximal ascending colon for Crohn's disease. This image shows recurrent Crohn's disease in the neoterminal ileum.

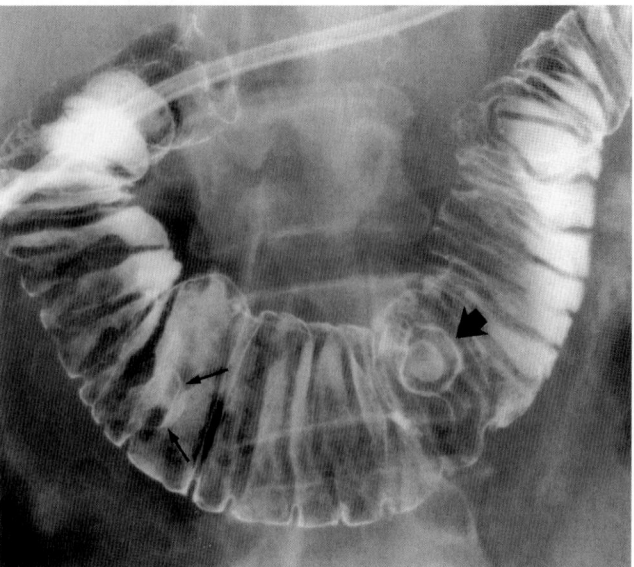

Figure 41-23. Hypotonic duodenogram. Upper endoscopy revealed a polypoid lesion in the duodenum. A radiographic study was requested for clarification. Spot image of the distal duodenum in air-contrast study shows a 1.8-cm polypoid lesion (*thin arrows*) etched in white in the second portion of the duodenum. A 2-cm polypoid lesion (*thick arrow*) is also seen at the junction of the third and fourth portions of the duodenum. Repeat endoscopy with biopsy and subsequent surgery revealed an adenocarcinoma of the second portion of the duodenum and a hemangioma of the fourth portion.

with barium, 1 mg of glucagon is injected intravenously to induce intestinal hypotonia. The patient is then rotated on the table to coat the mucosa, and spot images are obtained. This technique is limited, however, because there is less control over the volume of barium and air in the duodenum with the oral route than with the intubation technique.

SMALL BOWEL STUDIES USING WATER-SOLUBLE CONTRAST AGENTS

The small intestine is a hostile environment for imaging with water-soluble contrast agents. These hyperosmolar agents draw fluid into the intestinal lumen and are further diluted by excess fluid in the lumen in patients with hypotonia or obstruction. As a result, the radiographic density of water-soluble contrast agents is generally inadequate for diagnostic purposes in patients with small bowel obstruction. These contrast agents are therefore not indicated for examining the small bowel, except in patients with suspected leaks.

In general, leaks arising in the duodenum or first several loops of jejunum can be demonstrated by water-soluble contrast studies. Leaks in the mid or distal small bowel, however, are often missed because of dilution of the water-soluble contrast agent with fluid. When a leak is suspected in the distal small bowel (particularly at an ileocolic anastomosis), it may

therefore be preferable to perform a water-soluble contrast enema with reflux of contrast medium into the distal ileum.

Suspected leaks in the mid small bowel initially may be evaluated by CT. If the small bowel is not dilated, enteroclysis using water-soluble contrast may then be performed (Fig. 41-24).[6]

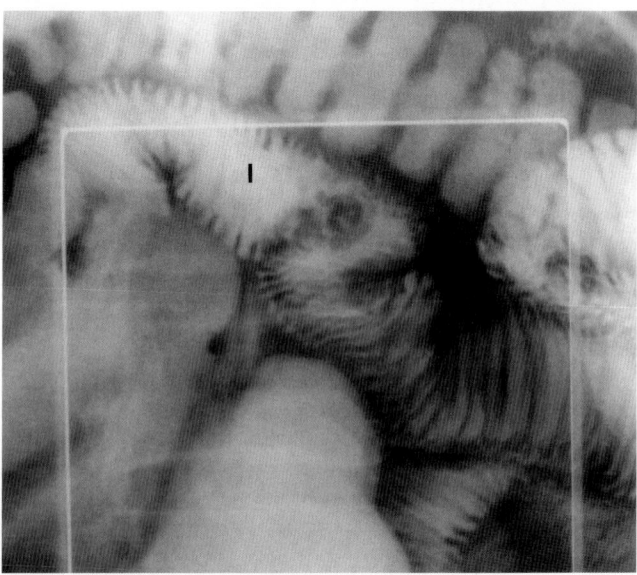

Figure 41-24. Enteroclysis using water-soluble contrast. Spot image from water-soluble contrast enteroclysis shows a normal proximal fold pattern (I). When the small bowel is not distended, a study using water-soluble contrast can demonstrate anatomic detail. When the small bowel is hypomotile or distended, however, intraluminal fluid dilutes the water-soluble contrast, limiting visualization of the bowel.

RETROGRADE EXAMINATIONS OF THE SMALL INTESTINE

Barium Enema

The barium enema is an underutilized but powerful examination for imaging the terminal ileum and distal small bowel.[40] If plain abdominal radiographs or CT cannot differentiate a distal small bowel obstruction from an adynamic ileus, a single-contrast barium enema may be extremely helpful in these patients. The study can be used not only to rule out an obstructing lesion in the colon as a cause of dilated small bowel but also to evaluate the distal ileum by refluxing barium through the ileocecal valve. Reflux of barium into a dilated terminal ileum indicates the presence of an adynamic ileus, whereas reflux of barium into a narrowed terminal ileum (with dilated, gas-filled ileal loops more proximally) indicates the presence of a small bowel obstruction. In many cases, barium can be refluxed in a retrograde fashion to the site of transition, enabling the radiologist to determine the site and cause of obstruction (see Chapter 50). In patients with high-grade small bowel obstruction, a barium enema is faster and easier on the patient than an enteroclysis examination or small bowel follow-through.

A single contrast or double-contrast barium enema may be performed in patients with suspected Crohn's disease. Double-contrast studies have the advantage of being able to diagnose early inflammatory lesions of Crohn's disease, such as aphthoid ulcers (Fig. 41-25). In contrast, single-contrast studies are more reliable for refluxing large volumes of barium into the distal small bowel when it is important to assess the terminal ileum and distal ileum for radiographic signs of Crohn's disease.

In patients who are not obstructed, a standard barium enema preparation may be helpful. In patients with high-grade small bowel obstruction, however, an oral preparation is contraindicated. Such studies should be performed without any preparation or after gentle cleansing enemas.

A standard dose of 1 mg of glucagon is administered intravenously to relax the colon and ileocecal valve. Up to 2.5 L of 20% to 30% w/v barium is instilled via an enema bag/tip. Reflux of barium through the ileocecal valve is possible in about 85% of patients. If a distal small bowel obstruction is present, an attempt should be made to reflux barium directly to the site of obstruction. In some cases, water can be added to the enema bag to propel the barium retrograde through the distal ileum.

Ileostomy Enema

The small bowel proximal to an ileostomy can easily be evaluated by a retrograde examination through the ileostomy stoma. If there is clinical suspicion of a leak or obstruction, no preparation is used. If there is clinical suspicion of recurrent Crohn's disease, however, an oral preparation (e.g., magnesium citrate or Phospho-Soda) may be helpful for eliminating debris from the small bowel before performing the examination. The patient is also instructed not to eat solids the day before the procedure.

A soft catheter (e.g., a Foley catheter) is inserted into the ileostomy. If disease is suggested at the ileostomy or near the peritoneal reflection (e.g., Crohn's disease or a stricture or leak), the balloon of the catheter should not be inflated. If injection of barium shows no evidence of disease in the distal ileum at or near the peritoneal reflection, the catheter balloon may be inflated with 3 to 5 mL of air or saline and the catheter is retracted to the peritoneal reflection. If there is doubt about disease at the ileostomy, the opening can be explored with a small finger. If inflation of the balloon is contraindicated, and barium leaks out from the ileostomy stoma, the radiologist can withdraw the catheter, distend the balloon outside the ostomy, and push the distended balloon against the outside of the ileostomy to seal the ileostomy opening.

A wide variety of contrast agents can be injected via the catheter. If a leak from the distal small bowel is suspected, water-soluble contrast agents may be employed. If a distal small bowel obstruction is suspected, a single-contrast ileostomy enema can be performed with 30% to 50% w/v barium. Thin barium is injected via a syringe until the site of obstruction is reached and characterized. If Crohn's disease or tumor is suspected, a double-contrast ileostomy enema can be performed, first injecting 50% to 80% w/v barium into the proximal ileum, followed by air or methylcellulose to visualize mucosal detail (Fig. 41-26). As with all small bowel studies, fluoroscopy and spot images are the mainstays of diagnosis. The ileostomy and small bowel adjacent to the anterior abdominal wall are best visualized with the patient in a lateral position. The ileostomy is best filled after the catheter is removed, the ostomy bag is replaced, and the patient is turned to an orthogonal position (usually a steep oblique or lateral position).

CHOICE OF FLUOROSCOPIC EXAMINATION

Zealots of enteroclysis, small bowel follow-through, CT, CT enteroclysis, MR enteroclysis, and capsule enteroscopy abound. This section attempts to provide a rational approach to fluoroscopic imaging of the small bowel.

The unifying feature of all forms of barium diagnosis is palpation of each loop of small intestine when the loop is

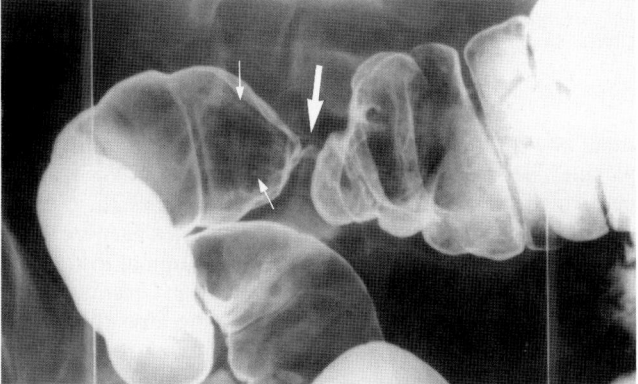

Figure 41-25. Barium enema demonstrating recurrent Crohn's disease. On previous endoscopy, it was not possible to pass the endoscope through the ileocolic anastomosis into the neoterminal ileum in a patient who had prior surgery for Crohn's disease. A double-contrast barium enema shows a short stricture (*large arrow*) at the ileocolic anastomosis. Aphthoid ulcers (*small arrows*) are also seen in the adjacent neoterminal ileum.

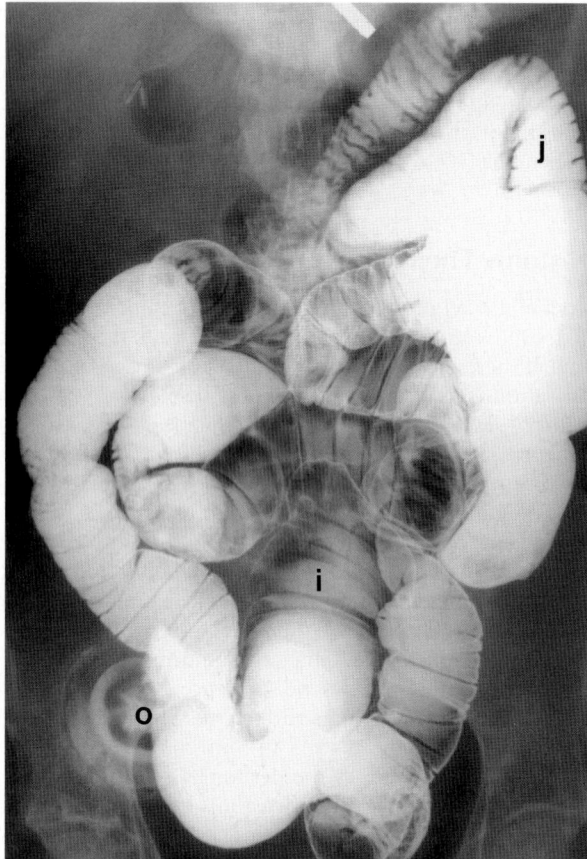

Figure 41-26. Ileostomy enema. This patient complained of abdominal pain and distention. A total colectomy had previously been performed. CT revealed dilated small bowel. An overhead radiograph obtained at the end of a retrograde ileostomy enema shows diffuse dilatation of small bowel to the level of the proximal jejunum (j). No site of narrowing or obstruction is identified in this patient with an intestinal ileus. Air-contrast effect in the ileum (i) results from air present in the small bowel before barium was instilled via the ostomy (o).

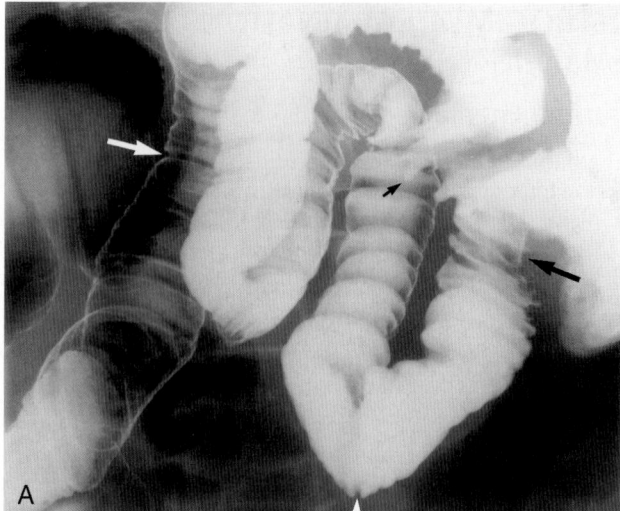

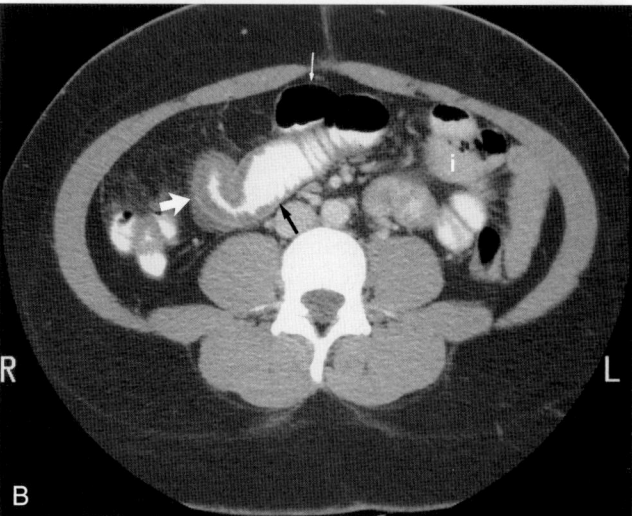

Figure 41-27. Long segment of radiation enteropathy demonstrated by small bowel follow-through. A. Spot image shows abnormal loops of ileum (*between long arrows*). The folds are thickened but retain their normal orientation perpendicular to the longitudinal axis of the small bowel. Two areas of angulation (*short arrows*) are identified as a result of radiation serositis. No obstruction was seen. **B.** CT shows marked wall thickening (*thick white arrow*) in a loop of ileum. Mild fold thickening is seen more proximally (*black arrow*). Note the normal wall thickness (*thin white arrow*) in small bowel proximal to the diseased segment. Little anatomic detail is available in some loops (i).

optimally distended. This necessitates that the radiologist remain with the patient during enteroclysis or return to the fluoroscopic suite at 15- to 30-minute intervals for small bowel follow-through studies, depending on the rate of progression of barium through the small intestine. Because of emphasis on fluoroscopic and spot image diagnosis, enteroclysis is associated with only a slightly higher radiation dose to the patient than the small bowel follow-through.[41] A single-contrast examination evaluates the luminal contour and filling defects in the barium column. A double-contrast examination evaluates the luminal contour, filling defects in the barium column or pool, and mucosal detail en face. The small bowel folds are well evaluated by either technique only when the lumen is fully distended.

The major advantage of the small bowel follow-through over enteroclysis is that it is easier on the patient and avoids the need for intubation of the small intestine (so that sedation is unnecessary). Long segments of abnormal bowel are easy to visualize (Fig. 41-27) as long as frequent fluoroscopy is performed. As a result, diseases involving long segments of small bowel, such as Crohn's disease, ischemia, and radiation change, are readily detected on a small bowel follow-through. However, enteroclysis has a number of important advantages over the

small bowel follow-through. Because the radiologist is at the patient's side for the entire examination, fluoroscopy can be performed whenever needed. During enteroclysis, the pylorus also is bypassed, so that radiographic contrast agents can be instilled at an optimal rate for obtaining luminal distention. Short lesions such as tumors or skip lesions in Crohn's disease are better demonstrated by enteroclysis because the lumen is overdistended, making subtle areas of focal narrowing more conspicuous (see Fig. 41-7). The small bowel folds are also better evaluated by enteroclysis because the lumen is distended and the folds are straightened.[42] Major mucosal abnormalities such as cobblestoning can be demonstrated on single-contrast small bowel follow-throughs with compression, but demonstration of subtle mucosal abnormalities requires double-contrast technique (Fig. 41-28).

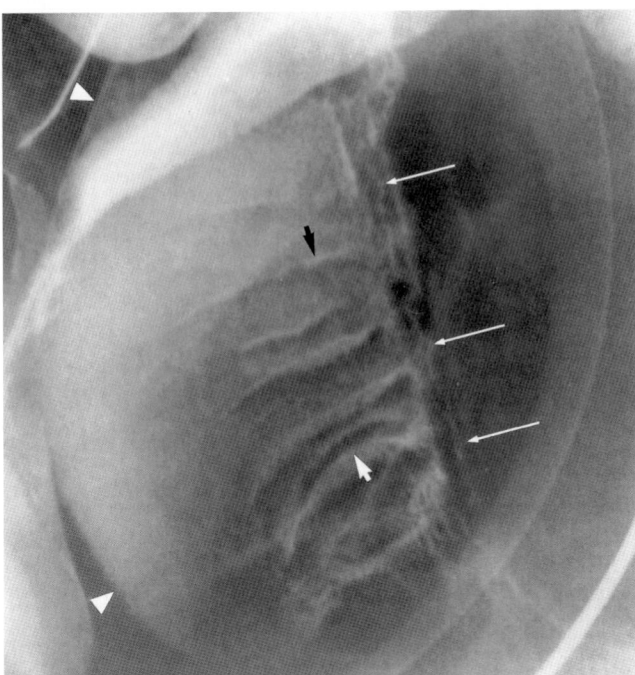

Figure 41-28. Mesenteric border ulcer demonstrated on enteroclysis in a patient with Crohn's disease. Spot image shows a thin, linear collection of barium (*long arrows*) along the mesenteric border of the distal ileum. Folds (*short arrow*) are pulled toward the site of ulceration, leading to sacculation (*arrowheads*) of the relatively uninvolved antimesenteric border.

The choice of which radiographic study to perform (small bowel follow-through versus enteroclysis) depends primarily on the indication for the examination. Various clinical settings for evaluating the small bowel are discussed in the following sections.

Chronic Diarrhea

Small bowel follow-through is an adequate examination for the diagnosis of Crohn's disease or other inflammatory diseases involving long segments of bowel.[24] In general, a small bowel follow-through can demonstrate cobblestoning, mesenteric border ulcers, fissures, fistulas (Fig. 41-29), and long segments of narrowing. However, the small bowel follow-through can miss short skip lesions in Crohn's disease as well as the aphthoid ulcers of early Crohn's disease. If a surgeon desires a full evaluation of disease extent and possible skip lesions before surgery in a patient with known Crohn's disease, enteroclysis is a better preoperative examination. If a patient has a normal-appearing terminal ileum during a small bowel follow-through but there is a strong clinical suspicion of Crohn's disease, a peroral pneumocolon can be obtained for air-contrast views of the terminal ileum. Ideally, this study should be performed after the patient has received a barium enema preparation to eliminate debris from the distal ileum and right side of the colon. A peroral pneumocolon or double-contrast barium enema with reflux of barium into the terminal ileum enables much better detection of mucosal nodularity and aphthoid ulcers (Fig. 41-30) than a conventional small bowel follow-through.

Enteroclysis may not visualize the terminal ileum any better than a small bowel follow-through (see Fig. 41-22). Over-

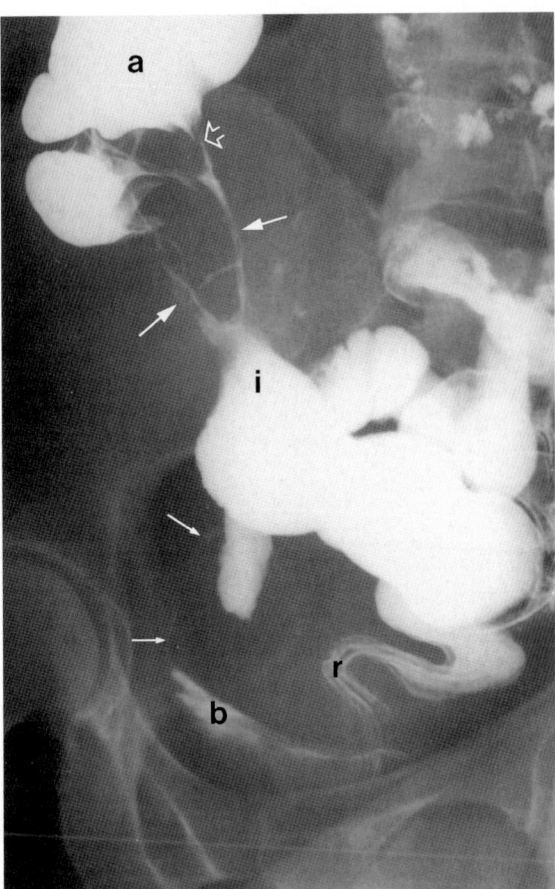

Figure 41-29. Multiple fistulas demonstrated on small bowel follow-through in a patient with Crohn's disease. An overhead radiograph obtained after barium reached the colon (r, rectum) shows several tracks (*thick arrows*) coursing from the dilated distal ileum (i) to the ascending colon (a); one of these is a diseased terminal ileum and the other is an ileocolic fistula. Another fistula (*open arrow*) enters the medial wall of the ascending colon above the ileocecal valve. A thin, barium-etched fistula (*thin arrows*) courses from the ileum to the barium-filled urinary bladder (b).

distention of ileal loops in the pelvis during enteroclysis may cause so much overlap of loops that it is difficult to demonstrate the terminal ileum in isolation. The double-contrast effect of enteroclysis using methylcellulose is often lost before barium has reached the terminal ileum because of progressive mixing of barium and methylcellulose. An air-contrast enteroclysis may be performed, but a peroral pneumocolon or double-contrast barium enema are easier on the patient and will enable air-contrast images of the terminal ileum to be obtained in the 85% of patients in whom air or barium can be refluxed into the terminal ileum.

Small Bowel Obstruction

As described in Chapter 50, the sun never sets on patients with suspected small bowel obstruction without these patients undergoing abdominal CT (unless they go directly to surgery). CT has a major advantage over barium studies in that it does not rely on barium reaching the site of obstruction but rather uses intraluminal fluid to outline the transition zone. CT also is a considerably shorter procedure than an antegrade barium study in patients with high-grade obstruction. A

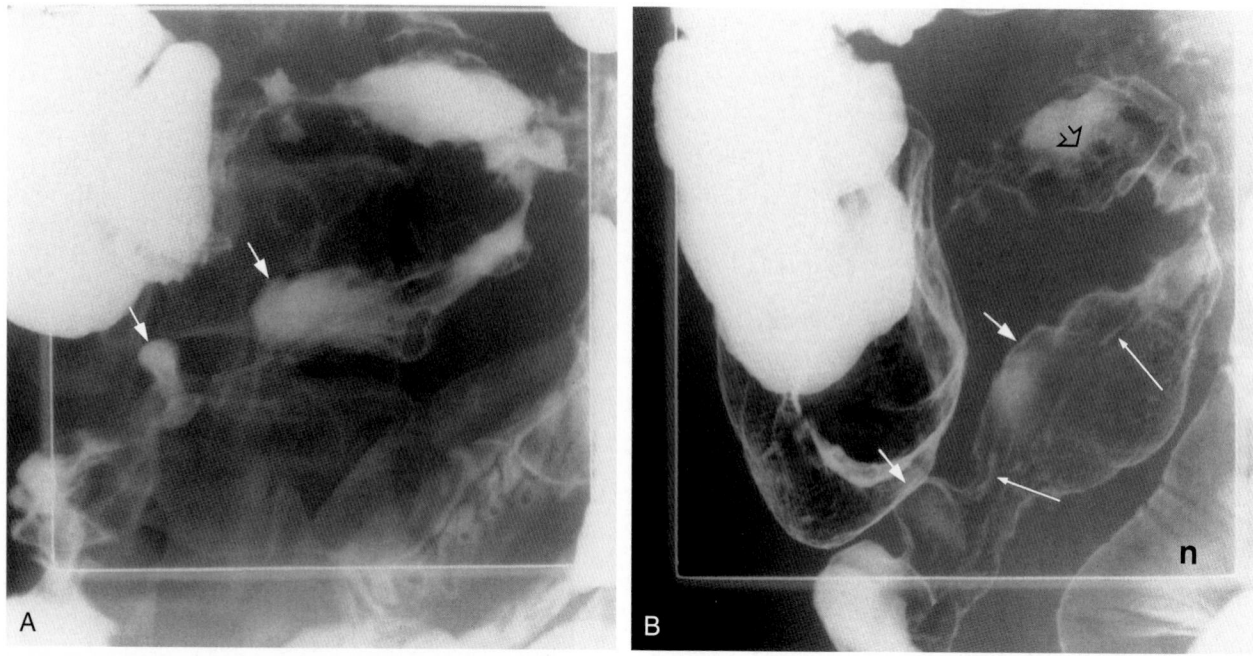

Figure 41-30. Peroral pneumocolon in a patient with suspected Crohn's disease. A. Spot radiograph from small bowel follow-through shows an abnormal terminal ileum, manifested by sacculations (*arrows*) alternating with areas of narrowing. **B.** Spot image from peroral pneumocolon shows that most of the areas of narrowing are more distensible than shown in **A**. Several mesenteric border ulcers (*long arrows*) and sacculations (*short arrows*) characteristic of Crohn's disease are now visualized. The mucosa is focally nodular (*open arrow*). Compare and contrast the appearance of the mucosa in the terminal ileum with that in an adjacent loop of normal ileum (n).

small bowel follow-through and enteroclysis are therefore discouraged in patients with high-grade small bowel obstruction shown by plain abdominal radiographs or CT. Retrograde examination of the small bowel by barium enema (Fig. 41-31) or colostomy enema is the preferred examination in the setting of high-grade distal small bowel obstruction or if there is a question of whether the patient has an adynamic ileus, proximal colonic lesion, or distal small bowel obstruction. An antegrade study can be performed after decompression by a nasogastric tube or long tube (Kantor or Miller-Abbott tube) (Fig. 41-32) or through a combination enteroclysis/decompression catheter.

Vomiting is more a symptom of gastroduodenal or proximal small bowel disease than of distal small bowel disease. In patients with vomiting and no evidence of plain radiographic or CT findings of distal small bowel obstruction, a single- or double-contrast upper gastrointestinal series with evaluation of the proximal small bowel may be performed. Alternatively, if an upper endoscopy has cleared the stomach and proximal duodenum, enteroclysis or a hypotonic duodenogram extending into the first several small bowel loops may be considered.

Abdominal Pain

Unexplained abdominal pain can be evaluated by a small bowel follow-through or enteroclysis. The small bowel follow-through is superior to enteroclysis for evaluation of small bowel transit time and the motility component of motor disorders. In contrast, enteroclysis is superior for showing the structural components of motor disorders (e.g., diverticula in jejunoileal diverticulosis and sacculations or an increased number of small bowel folds in scleroderma). Enteroclysis

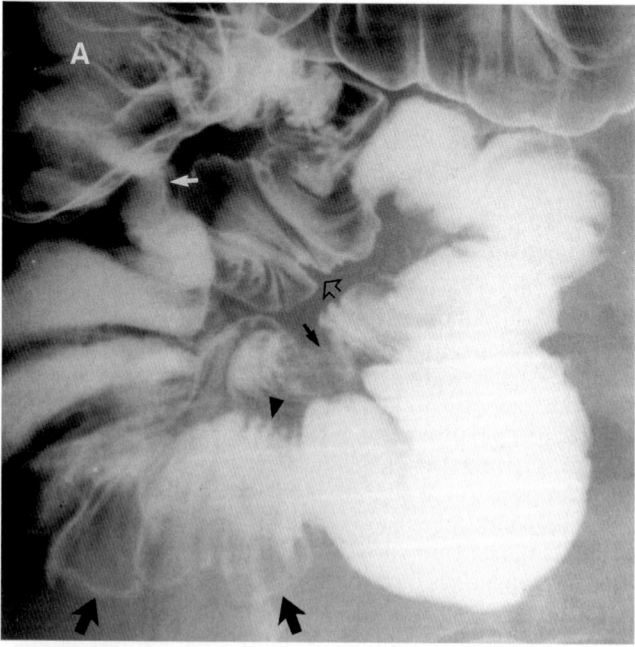

Figure 41-31. Recurrent carcinoid tumor with small bowel obstruction on barium enema. The distal ileum is dilated, and small bowel folds are tethered (*open arrow*). In one loop, folds are bunched together (*arrowhead*) by the mesenteric desmoplastic process, and the opposite walls are sacculated (*large arrows*). Several short segments of narrowing (*short arrows*) are also seen. The ascending colon is identified (A).

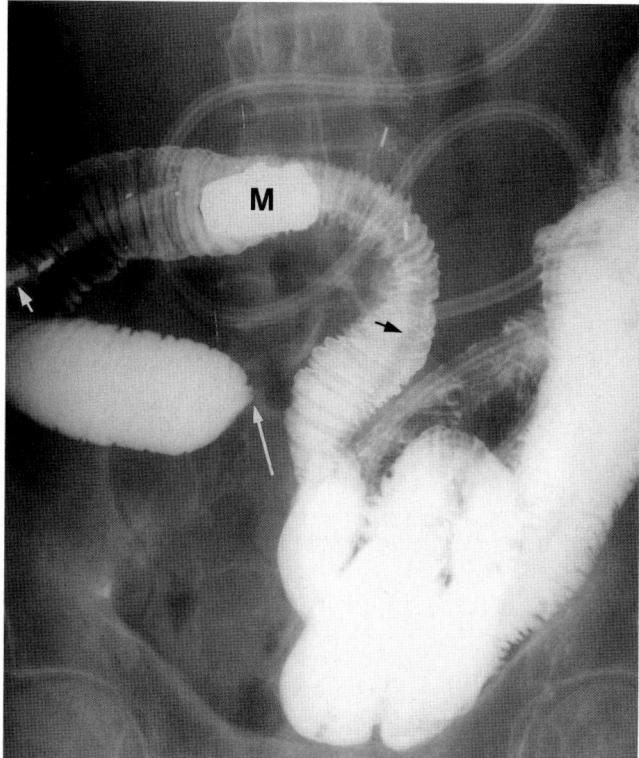

Figure 41-32. Complete small bowel obstruction demonstrated on enteroclysis after decompression of the small bowel by a Miller-Abbott tube. There is an abrupt, beaklike cutoff in the ileum (*long white arrow*) with complete small bowel obstruction caused by an adhesion. The proximal small intestine has been decompressed by a Miller-Abbott tube (the tip of the tube is denoted by a *short white arrow*) and is only mildly dilated. The mercury-filled bag (M) has flipped in a retrograde fashion. Note how the tube is seen as a filling defect (*black arrow*) in the barium column.

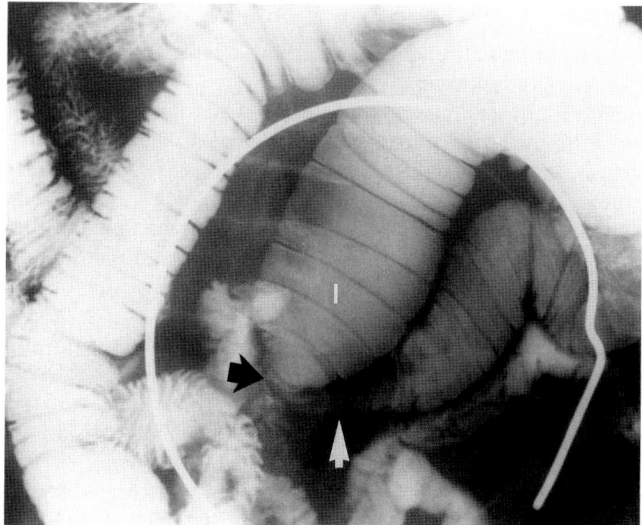

Figure 41-33. Adhesions and low-grade small bowel obstruction demonstrated on enteroclysis. This patient had intermittent abdominal pain and distention and a history of prior abdominal surgery. There is abrupt angulation (*black arrow*) of the ileum, with narrowing (*white arrow*) distal to the site of angulation. The folds in the transition zone are preserved, and the mucosa is smooth. The ileum (I) proximal to the adhesion is mildly dilated.

is also superior for showing short lesions such as isolated adhesions (Fig. 41-33) or tumors that may account for abdominal pain.

Transient intussusceptions usually occur as normal variants or are associated with motor disorders. When a transient intussusception shown on CT is associated with signs of obstruction or tumor, the radiologist should perform enteroclysis, because this technique is superior for excluding short lesions such as tumors and adhesions that may cause intussusception. However, most transient intussusceptions are not associated with signs of obstruction or tumor. In this scenario, it is unclear whether a small bowel follow-through is sufficient for excluding a structural abnormality. Clearly, enteroclysis will provide a more confident diagnosis of normality for ruling out tumor or an adhesion in this setting.

Suspected Perforation

As described previously, suspected perforation of the duodenum and proximal jejunum can be adequately evaluated with a water-soluble small bowel follow-through. Diagnosis of perforation in the presence of dilated small intestine from obstruction or ileus is difficult, however, because water-soluble contrast agents provide inadequate density when diluted by intraluminal fluid. Water-soluble contrast agents are further diluted because of their hyperosmolar nature, which causes more fluid to be drawn into the small bowel lumen. In the presence of dilated distal small intestine, retrograde examination of the small bowel with water-soluble contrast agents is therefore preferable for excluding a distal small bowel leak (particularly a leak at an ileocolic anastomosis). Water-soluble enteroclysis (see Fig. 41-24) should be performed after intestinal decompression in patients with suspected perforation of the mid or distal small bowel.

Malabsorption

A classification and discussion of malabsorption is presented in Chapter 47. A small bowel follow-through is adequate for detecting large structural lesions that cause bacterial overgrowth (e.g., jejunoileal diverticulosis or Crohn's disease with obstruction). However, enteroclysis is the procedure of choice for showing malabsorptive disorders involving the mucosa and submucosa of the bowel (e.g., celiac disease [Fig. 41-34], Whipple's disease, and amyloidosis). A strong argument can therefore be made for air-contrast enteroclysis in the setting of malabsorption, because the mucosal surface of the jejunum, the most common site of disorders causing malabsorption, can be exquisitely shown. CT is also a helpful adjunct for diagnosing disorders primarily or secondarily involving lymph nodes.

Unexplained Gastrointestinal Bleeding

A small bowel follow-through is quite limited for detecting causes of small intestinal bleeding.[39,43-46] Small tumors are easily missed.[45] In one study comparing expertly performed enteroclysis with non–expertly performed small bowel follow-through procedures, enteroclysis detected 90% of tumors diagnosed at surgery, whereas small bowel follow-through detected only 33%.[45] It is therefore difficult to establish a

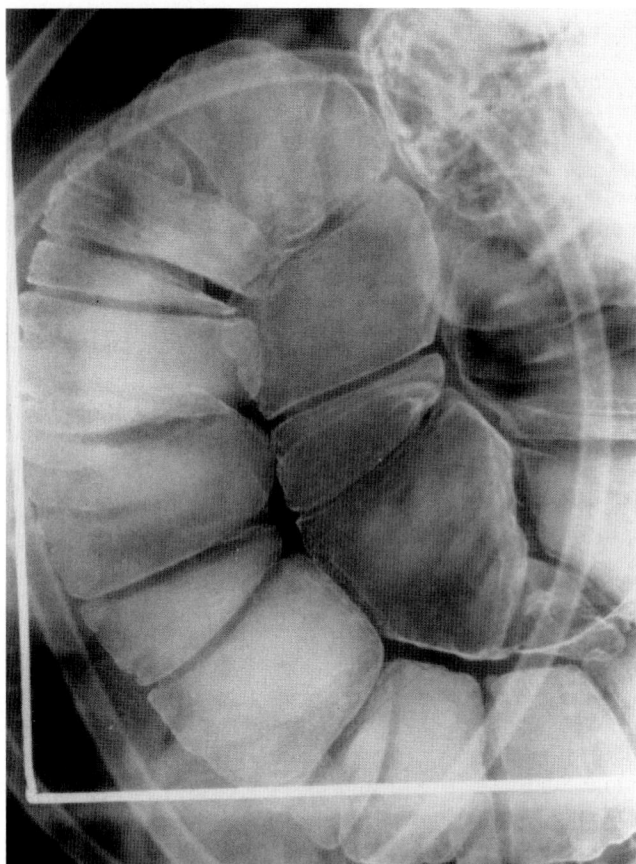

Figure 41-34. Celiac disease demonstrated on enteroclysis. Spot image shows a decreased number of folds per inch in the jejunum.

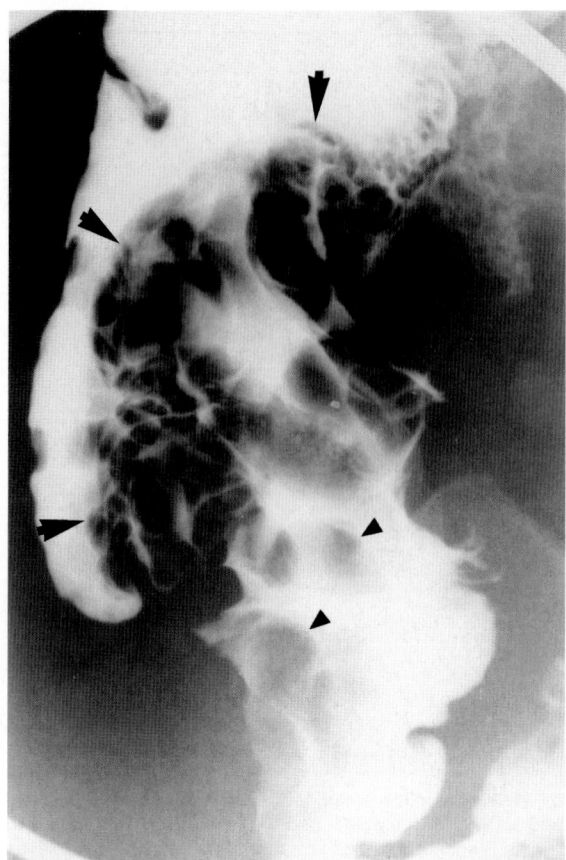

Figure 41-35. Ileocecal lymphoma demonstrated on small bowel follow-through. Spot image of the ileocecal region shows marked lobulation and enlargement of the ileocecal valve (*arrows*) with spread of tumor into the medial wall of the cecum and ascending colon. The folds of the distal ileum also are marked enlargement and lobulated (*arrowheads*). This patient with mantle cell lymphoma presented with gastrointestinal bleeding.

confident diagnosis of normalcy on a small bowel follow-through. A combination of a small bowel follow-through (to exclude obstruction/stricture) and capsule endoscopy may be an acceptable alternative for evaluating patients with gastrointestinal bleeding. However, capsule endoscopy also has its limitations. Because normal small bowel transit varies from 30 to 120 minutes, the gastroenterologist or physician's assistant will spend an inordinate amount of time at a computer workstation evaluating the images. Capsule endoscopy also has limited ability to localize lesions. Finally, capsule endoscopy is not infallible, because a considerable portion of the intestine is not examined by the video capsule.

Methylcellulose-contrast enteroclysis is adequate for demonstration of most small bowel tumors (see Fig. 41-7). However, it usually will not detect varices, arteriovenous malformations, or nonsteroidal anti-inflammatory drug–induced erosions or potassium chloride–induced erosions as well as capsule endoscopy. Air-contrast enteroclysis may allow diagnosis of subtle ulcerative lesions in the proximal small intestine with greater sensitivity than methylcellulose-contrast enteroclysis. Although I have not had great success with air-contrast enteroclysis in the pelvic ileum, this is the standard enteroclysis technique performed in Japan.

In summary, a small bowel follow-through is indicated only when assessing for large structural causes of gastrointestinal bleeding (Fig. 41-35). This test is probably indicated only if there is low suspicion of an abnormality, if a large lesion such as lymphoma, gastrointestinal stromal tumor (Fig. 41-36), is-

chemia, or hematoma is suspected, or if capsule endoscopy is planned as a follow-up.

Air-contrast enteroclysis is indicated when looking for subtle erosions in patients taking nonsteroidal anti-inflammatory drugs. Methylcellulose-contrast enteroclysis and air-contrast enteroclysis are satisfactory when searching for subtle lesions or small tumors. In patients with known malignant tumors, enteroclysis will permit a more confident diagnosis of normalcy or of metastatic disease than will a small bowel follow-through.

The role of CT or MR angiography for bleeding tumors has yet to be established. CT and MR enterography are inferior to enteroclysis because they do not assess en face mucosal detail and they have lower resolution than enteroclysis. As a result, barium enteroclysis should be superior to CT or MR enteroclysis for the diagnosis of Crohn's disease, diseases causing malabsorption, or primary tumors. I believe that if a patient is to undergo intubation, a barium enteroclysis study should be performed (rather than CT or MR enteroclysis), except perhaps when searching for a cause of gastrointestinal bleeding.

A summary of the choice of examinations for evaluating the small bowel in various clinical settings is presented in Table 41-2.

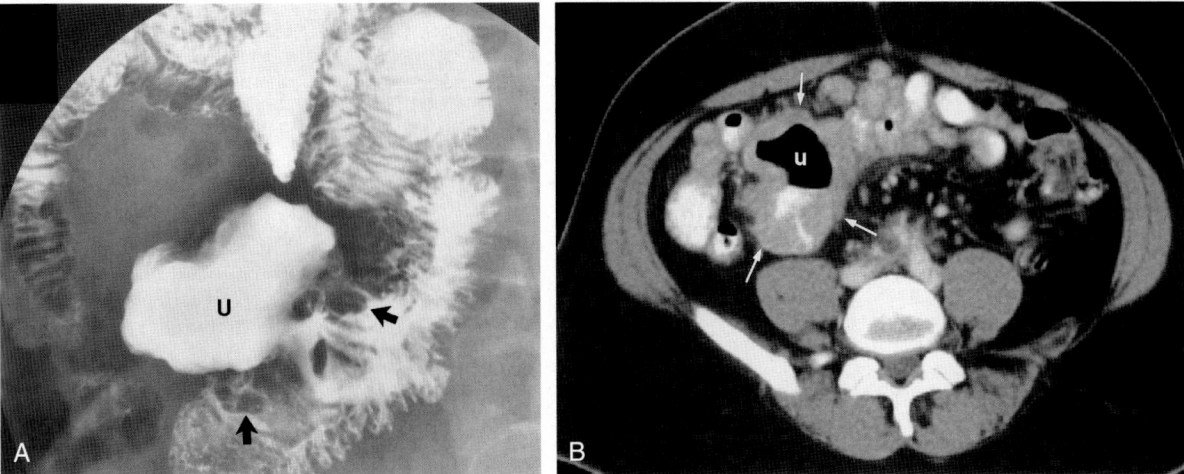

Figure 41-36. Gastrointestinal stromal tumor demonstrated on small bowel follow-through. A. Spot image shows a large, irregular barium-filled cavity (U) on the mesenteric border of the mid small bowel. Coarse, lobulated tumor nodules (*arrows*) are present adjacent to the cavity. **B.** Axial CT shows the bulk of the tumor (*arrows*) surrounding the cavity (u). The mucosal changes are not apparent. This patient presented with gastrointestinal bleeding.

Table 41-2
Choice of Barium Studies for Evaluating Small Bowel in Various Clinical Settings

Clinical Scenario	Initial Study
Chronic diarrhea (excluding Crohn's disease)	Small bowel follow-through
Known Crohn's disease	
Acute abdominal pain	CT to exclude abscess
Anastomotic recurrence	Barium enema
Exclude skip lesion before surgery	Enteroclysis
Acute abdominal pain	CT (ultrasound if gynecologic disease suspected)
Chronic abdominal pain	Small bowel follow-through followed by enteroclysis if still suspicion of small bowel disease
Small bowel obstruction	CT followed by barium enema as problem-solving tools for high-grade distal small bowel or proximal colonic obstruction
Low-grade obstruction	Small bowel follow-through or enteroclysis
Vomiting	Upper gastrointestinal series with evaluation of proximal small bowel
Malabsorption	Enteroclysis (consider air-contrast)
Unexplained gastrointestinal bleeding	Small bowel follow-through/capsule endoscopy
	Methylcellulose enteroclysis
	Air-contrast enteroclysis if NSAID erosions must be excluded
	CT angiography: role to be determined
Suspected hematogenous metastases	Enteroclysis
Suspected perforation	CT can suggest presence of perforation; suboptimal for evaluating site and cause of perforation
Upper gastrointestinal tract	Water-soluble contrast upper gastrointestinal series
Bypassed duodenum	HIDA scan or injection of water-soluble contrast agent into indwelling duodenal/biliary tube
Proximal jejunum	Small bowel follow-through with water-soluble contrast
Mid small bowel	Water-soluble contrast enema or water-soluble contrast enteroclysis
Distal small bowel/ileocolic anastomosis	Water-soluble contrast enema

NSAID, nonsteroidal anti-inflammatory drug; HIDA, hepatoiminodiacetic acid.

References

1. Fenolgio-Preiser CM, Hoffsinger AE, Stemmermann GN, et al: Normal anatomy of the small intestine. In Fenolgio-Preiser CM, Hoffsinger AE, Stemmermann GN, et al (eds): Gastrointestinal Pathology: An Atlas and Text, 2nd ed. Philadelphia, Lippincott-Raven, 1999, pp 275-309.
2. Herlinger H: Anatomy of the small intestine. In Herlinger H, Maglinte DDT, Birnbaum BA (eds): Clinical Imaging of the Small Intestine, 2nd ed. New York, Springer-Verlag, 1999, pp 3-12.
3. Rubesin SE, Furth EE: Differential diagnosis of small intestinal abnormalities with radiologic-pathologic correlation. In Herlinger H, Maglinte DDT, Birnbaum BA (eds): Clinical Imaging of the Small Intestine, 2nd ed. New York, Springer, 1999, pp 527-566.
4. Tlaskalova-Hogenova H, Farre-Castany MA, Stapankova R, et al: The gut as a lymphoepithelial organ: The role of intestinal epithelial cells in mucosal immunity. Fol Microbiol 40:385-391, 1995.
5. Montrose MH, Keely SJ, Barrett KE: Electrolyte secretion and absorption: Small intestine and colon. In Yamada T, Alpers DH, Kaplowitz N, et al (eds):Textbook of Gastroenterology, 4th ed. Philadelphia, Lippincott Williams & Wilkins, 2003, pp 308-340.
6. Rubesin SE, Levine MS: Principles of Performing a Small Bowel Examination. Westbury, NY, E-Z-EM, 2005.
7. Grivaux M, Cornet A, Wattez E: Le metoclopramide en radiologie digestive. Semin Hosp Paris 44:2338-2345, 1964.

8. Howarth FH, Cockel R, Roper BW, et al: The effect of metoclopramide upon gastric motility and its value in barium progress meals. Clin Radiol 20:294-300, 1969.

9. Kreel L: The use of oral metoclopramide in the barium meal and follow-through examination. Br J Radiol 43:31-35, 1970.

10. Grumbach K, Herlinger H, Laufer I, et al: Metoclopramide-ceruletide–assisted small bowel examination. ROFO 149:47-51, 1988.

11. Fraser GM, Preston PG: The small bowel follow-through enhanced with an oral effervescent agent. Clin Radiol 34:673-679, 1983.

12. Fitch D: The small-bowel see-through: An improved method of radiographic small-bowel visualization. Can J Med Radiat Tech 26:167-171, 1995.

13. Kressel HY, Evers KA, Glick SN, et al: The peroral pneumocolon examination: Technique and indications. Radiology 144:414-416, 1982.

14. Kellett MJ, Zboralske FF, Margulis AR: Peroral pneumocolon examination of the ileocecal region. Gastrointest Radiol 1:361-365, 1977.

15. Kelvin FM, Gedgaudas RK, Thompson WM, et al: The peroral pneumocolon examination: Its role in evaluating the terminal ileum. AJR 139:115-121, 1982.

16. Fitzgerald EJ, Thompson GT, Somers SS, at al: Pneumocolon as an aid to small bowel studies. Clin Radiol 36:633-637, 1985.

17. Einhorn M: The Duodenal Tube and Its Possibilities, 2nd ed. Philadelphia, FA Davis, 1926.

18. Pesquera GS: Method for direct visualization of lesions in the small intestine. AJR 22:254-257, 1929.

19. Gershon-Cohen J, Shay H: Barium enteroclysis method for direct immediate examination of the small intestine by single and double contrast technique. AJR 42:456-458, 1939.

20. Schatzki R: Small bowel enema. AJR 50:743-751, 1943.

21. Maglinte DDT, Lappas JC, Heitkamp DE, et al: Technical refinements in enteroclysis. Radiol Clin North Am 41:213-229, 2003.

22. Herlinger H: A modified technique for the double contrast small bowel enema. Gastrointest Radiol 3:201-207, 1978.

23. Schulze-Delrieu K: Metoclopramide drug therapy. N Engl J Med 305:28-33, 1981.

24. Herlinger H, Maglinte DDT, Tsuneyosi Y: Enteroclysis: Technique and variations. In Herlinger H, Maglinte DDT, Birnbaum BA (eds): Clinical Imaging of the Small Intestine, 2nd ed. New York, Springer-Verlag, 1999, pp 95-124.

25. Nolan DJ, Cadman PJ: The small bowel enema made easy. Clin Radiol 38:295-301, 1987.

26. Plovin PF, Mennard J, Corrol P: Hypertensive crisis in patients with pheochromocytoma given metoclopramide. Lancet 2:1357-1358, 1976.

27. Maglinte DDT, Lappas JC, Chernish SM, et al: Improved tolerance of enteroclysis by use of sedation. AJR 151:951-952, 1988.

28. Maglinte DDT: Balloon enteroclysis catheter. AJR 143:761-762, 1984.

29. Taverner DS, Odurny A: Enteroclysis—the influence of tube design. Clin Radiol 49:176-178, 1994.

30. Traill ZC, Nolan DL: Technical report: Intubation fluoroscopy times using new enteroclysis tube. Clin Radiol 50:339-340, 1994.

31. Maglinte DDT, Stevens LH, Hall RC, et al: Dual purpose tube for enteroclysis and nasogastric-nasoenteric decompression. Radiology 185:281-282,1992.

32. Diner WC: Duodenal perforation during intubation for small bowel enema study. Radiology 168:39-41, 1988.

33. Maglinte DDT, Miller RE: A comparison of pumps used for enteroclysis. Radiology 152:815, 1984.

34. Sellink JL, Miller RE: Radiology of the Small Bowel: Modern Enteroclysis Technique and Atlas. The Hague, Martinus Nijhoff, 1982.

35. Kobayashi S, Nishizawa M, Mizuno K, et al: X-ray examination of the small intestine: I. Double contrast method as a routine examination [in Japanese]. Jpn J Clin Radiol 19:619-625, 1974.

36. Kobayashi S, Nishizawa M: X-ray examination of small intestine-double contrast method by duodenal intubation. Stomach Intest 11:157-165, 1976.

37. Shirakabe H, Kobayashi S: Air double contrast barium study of the small bowel. In Herlinger H, Maglinte D (eds): Clinical Radiology of the Small Intestine. Philadelphia, WB Saunders, 1989, pp 139-145.

38. Trickey SE, Halls J, Hodson CJ: A further development of the small bowel enema. J R Soc Med 56:1070-1073, 1963.

39. Maglinte DDT, Lappas JC, Kelvin FM, et al: Small bowel radiography: How, when and why? Radiology 163:297-305, 1987.

40. Miller RE: Complete reflux examination of the small bowel. Radiology 84:457-462, 1986.

41. Salomonowitz E: Radiation dose of double contrast and single contrast examinations. In Herlinger H, Maglinte D (eds): Clinical Radiology of the Small Intestine. Philadelphia, WB Saunders, 1989, pp 147-150.

42. Taverne PP, van der Jagt EJ: Small bowel radiography: A prospective comparative study of three techniques in 200 patients. ROFO 143:293-297, 1985.

43. Maglinte DDT, Elmore MF, Eisenberg M, et al: Meckel diverticulum: Radiologic demonstration by enteroclysis. AJR 134:925-932, 1980.

44. Maglinte DDT, Burney BT, Miller RE: Lesions missed on small bowel follow-through: Analysis and recommendations. Radiology 144:737-739, 1982.

45. Bessette JR, Maglinte DDT, Kelvin FM, et al: Primary malignant tumors in the small bowel: A comparison of the small-bowel enema and conventional follow-through examination. AJR 153:741-744, 1989.

46. Hara AK, Leighton JA, Sharma UK, Fleischer DE: Small bowel: Preliminary comparison of capsule endoscopy with barium study and CT. Radiology 230:260-65, 2004.

Computed Tomographic Enteroclysis

Dean D. T. Maglinte, MD • John C. Lappas, MD • Kumaresan Sandrasegaran, MD

TECHNICAL MODIFICATIONS

Used with Neutral Enteral and IV Contrast

Used with Positive Enteral Contrast

CLINICAL INDICATIONS

Small Bowel Obstruction

Crohn's Disease

Small Bowel Tumors

Unexplained Gastrointestinal Bleeding

Miscellaneous Applications

ROLE IN THE ERA OF VIDEO CAPSULE ENDOSCOPY

Before Capsule Endoscopy

After Capsule Endoscopy

DISADVANTAGES

SUMMARY

Barium enteroclysis overcomes most of the inherent limitations of the small bowel follow-through and has proven to be the most reliable of the conventional contrast methods of radiographic examination.[1,2] Computed tomography has shown that barium small bowel radiography fails to demonstrate important extraintestinal manifestations of small bowel disease.[3-5] A comparison of barium enteroclysis and abdominal CT in small bowel Crohn's disease has shown that the advantages of CT are its ability to depict mural and extraintestinal complications of the disease. The advantages of enteroclysis are the demonstration of low-grade obstruction, small sinus tracts, fistulas, and ulcerations that are often missed on CT. This higher sensitivity is principally due to the volume challenge presented to the small bowel wall by the controlled infusion.[6] Computed tomographic enteroclysis (CTE) was introduced to overcome the individual deficiencies of CT and barium enteroclysis and to combine the advantages of both examinations into one technique (Table 42-1). Kloppel and coworkers showed CTE to be highly accurate in depicting mucosal abnormalities, bowel thickening, fistulas, and extraintestinal complications of Crohn's disease.[7] The first North American study focused on patients with partial small bowel obstruction[8] and concluded that CTE overcame the poor sensitivity of conventional CT for the diagnosis of low-grade small bowel obstruction.

The introduction of multidetector CT (MDCT) technology allowed faster scanning and thinner collimation. It is now possible on 40- and 64-channel scanners to routinely acquire isotropic resolution voxels of the abdomen and pelvis within 15 seconds, which permits creation of high-quality multiplanar reformat (MPR) views.[9-12] In this chapter we review the modifications of CTE that have evolved since its original

Table 42-1

Conventional CT and Enteroclysis in Demonstrating Features of Small Bowel Crohn's Disease

Feature	Conventional CT		Enteroclysis	
	No. of Patients	%	No. of Patients	%
Ulcerations	7	19	29	78 †
Mural edema	15	41	17	46
Obstruction	6	16	17	46 †
Stricture	4	11	14	38 †
Sinus tract	2	5	10	27 †
Fistula	3	8	9	24 †
Abscess	10	27*	7	19
Extraintestinal disease	3	0	0	0
Total No. of lesions	47		54	

*and † demonstrate the added value of CT enteroclysis over conventional CT and fluoroscopic enteroclysis.
From Maglinte DD, Hallet R, Rex D: Imaging of small bowel Crohn's disease: Can abdominal CT replace barium radiography? Emerg Radiol 8:127-133, 2001.

description, present an overview of its clinical applications, and analyze its role in the era of video capsule endoscopy (VCE).

TECHNICAL MODIFICATIONS

Since the original reports that used dilute positive enteral contrast, CTE has evolved into two distinct modifications, one using neutral enteral contrast with intravenous (IV) contrast enhancement and the other employing positive (water-soluble) enteral contrast without IV contrast.[13-16] Each modification has technical differences that are described separately. For both techniques bowel preparation includes a low-residue diet, ample fluids, a laxative on the day before the examination, and nothing orally on the day of the examination. As with barium enteroclysis, when using a 13-F enteroclysis catheter (Cook Inc., Bloomington, IN) patients are given an option of conscious sedation.[13]

Used with Neutral Enteral and IV Contrast

Enteral contrast media used with this method are water (Fig. 42-1), 0.5% methylcellulose, and dilute barium (VoLumen, EZEM, Westbury, NY). These agents have been used successfully, and the choice mainly depends on individual preference. Methylcellulose was used initially because of its perceived slower absorption compared with water.[17] Water is the neutral enteral contrast of our choice because it is inexpensive, has lower attenuation, and has reduced tendency to cause vomiting and diarrhea. The lower attenuation of water, compared with methylcellulose and VoLumen (which contains 0.1% barium sulfate), allows better contrast between the bowel lumen and IV contrast–enhanced mucosa. Given the speed of MDCT there is insufficient time for significant water absorption; thus, using water does not usually result in nondistended loops. However, if it known that there will be a long delay between the enteral infusion and CT, an alternative contrast such as VoLumen may be considered. This agent has additives to give flavor and to decrease bowel absorption. It is also the ideal agent for oral hyperhydration during CT enterography. The amount and rate of administration of IV contrast used in CTE will depend on the radiologist's individual preference. We prefer CT acquisition during the late arterial/early portal venous phase when maximum intestinal mucosal enhancement occurs.[18]

Due to the low viscosity of neutral enteral agents, a small balloon catheter (9-F MCTE catheter, EZEM, Westbury, NY) can be used without the need for conscious sedation. The catheter tip is ideally positioned left of midline, and the balloon is inflated with 30 to 40 mL of air before infusion. Sixty milliliters of air is injected into the infusion lumen to ensure that the tip is not in a diverticulum. Our technique of performing CTE with neutral enteral and IV contrast is summarized in Box 42-1. The rate of enteral infusion starts at 60 mL/min and is gradually increased. The rate is reduced if the patient experiences symptoms such as pain or nausea or if the force of infusion retropulses the balloon into the second portion of the duodenum. The rate of infusion is increased by 20 mL/min when the patient is on the CT scanner table. If the patient rectally evacuates the enteral agent a further 1500 mL of the agent is given while on the CT table, before IV contrast agent administration.

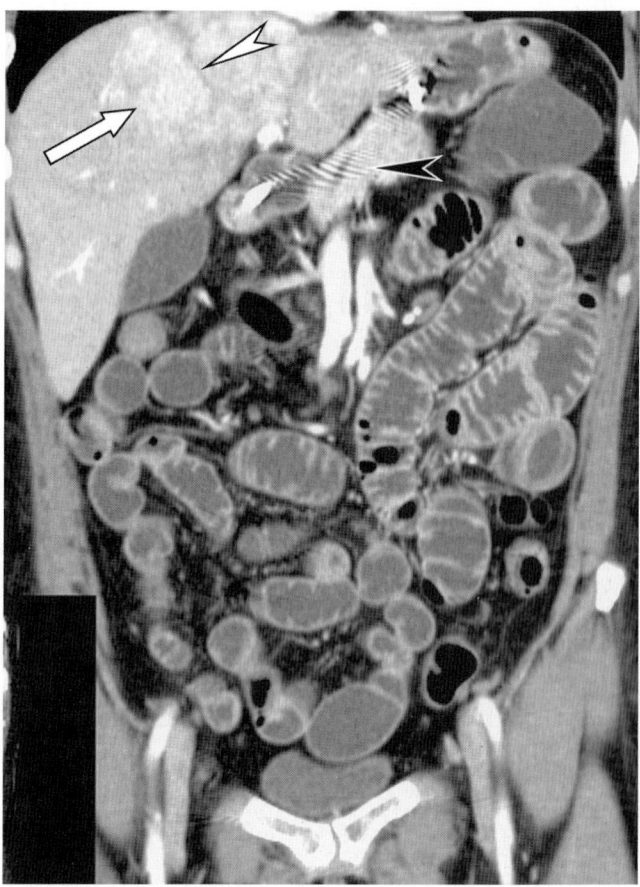

Figure 42-1. Neutral enteral contrast CTE in a 47-year-old woman with Crohn's disease and abdominal pain. Coronal reformat of isotropic resolution acquisition shows no small bowel abnormality. Incidental hypervascular liver mass (*arrow*) with scar (*white arrowhead*) was demonstrated and later proven to be focal nodular hyperplasia. Note dark and bright stripes (*black arrowhead*) adjacent to the nasoduodenal tube. This (Feldkamp) artifact is due to the off-center modulation of pixel noise in the z position when dealing with a wide cone beam (40-channel CT used in this study). The artifact is most obvious on coronal or sagittal reformats at sites where x-ray attenuation changes rapidly along the z direction.

Used with Positive Enteral Contrast

Positive enteral contrast ranges from a 4% to 15% water-soluble contrast solution to a dilute 6% barium solution (Fig. 42-2).[13] Because the infusion of enteral contrast is done under fluoroscopic control, the balloon and catheter tip can

BOX 42-1	**Computed Tomographic Enteroclysis with Neutral Enteral and IV Contrast**

Fluoroscopic Phase
1. Position balloon to the left of the spine.
2. Give 0.3 mg glucagon IV.
3. Infuse 2 L of water at 60-120 mL/min. Transfer to CT table.

CT Phase
4. Give 0.3 mg glucagon IV.
5. Infuse 1 L of water at 100-150 mL/min.
6. IV contrast: 4 mL/s; total 150 mL. CT acquired at 50-s delay.
7. Deflate balloon, aspirate refluxed water in stomach, withdraw catheter.

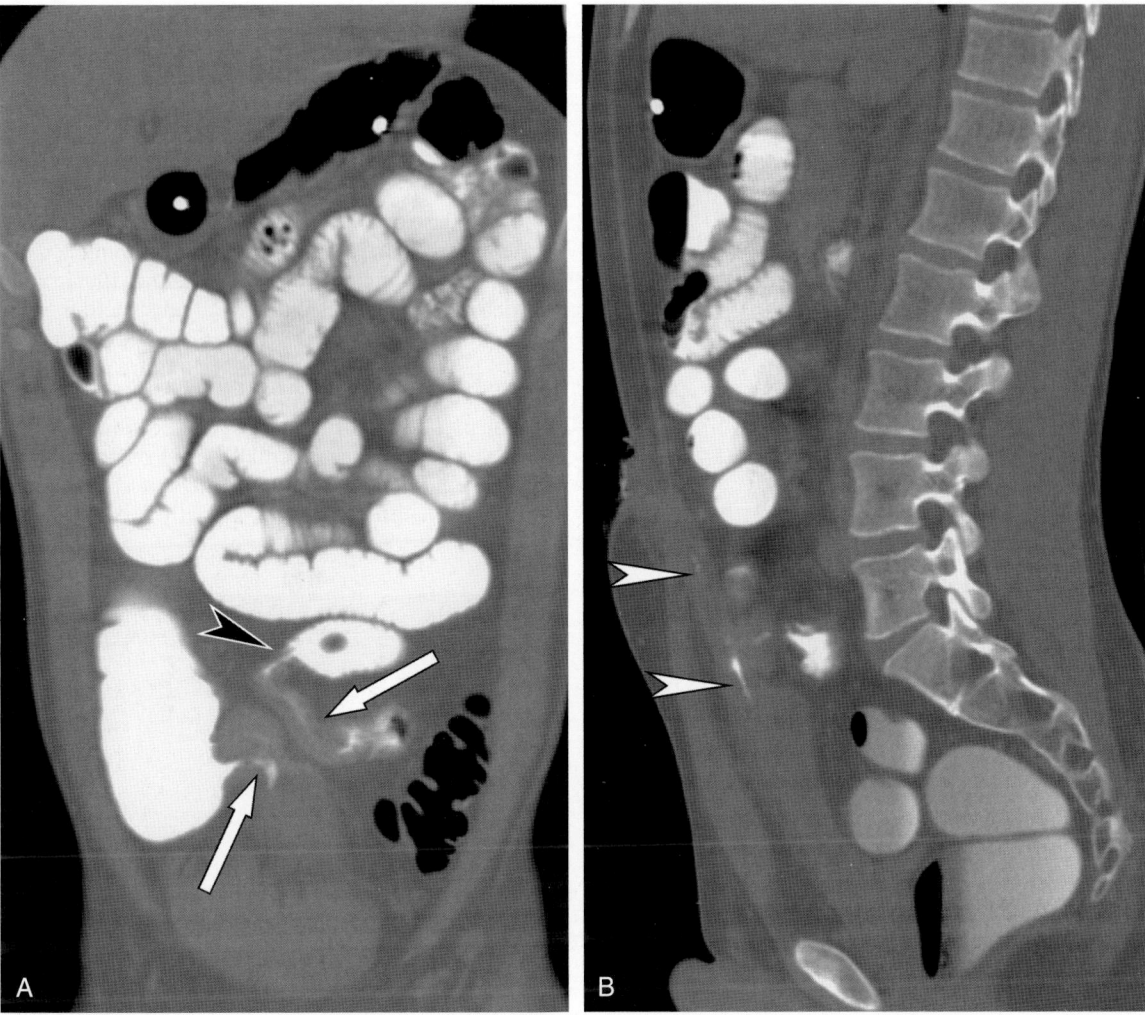

Figure 42-2. Positive-contrast CTE in 29-year-old man with Crohn's disease. A. Coronal reformat shows low-grade small bowel obstruction with sharp transition point (*black arrowhead*). The cause of obstruction was a long segment of fibrostenosis (*arrows*). **B.** Sagittal reformat shows enteric fistula (*white arrowheads*). Because of fibrostenosis, patient was not treated with infliximab (inhibitor of tumor necrosis factor-α).

be positioned in the descending duodenum. Because of the viscosity of the contrast material used, a 13-F diagnostic enteroclysis or a 13.5-F decompression/enteroclysis catheter is used. Box 42-2 shows our CTE protocol with positive enteral contrast.

BOX 42-2 | **Computed Tomographic Enteroclysis with Positive Enteral Contrast (No IV Contrast)**

Fluoroscopic Phase
1. Position balloon catheter tip in descending duodenum.
2. Infuse 12% water-soluble contrast: 2 L plus. Infusion rate is 55-150 mL/min (adjusted for optimal enteral volume challenge).
3. Limit fluoroscopy until contrast is in cecum.

CT Phase
4. Infuse 500-1000 mL on CT table before and during scanning. Increase infusion rate by 10 mL/min from rate of infusion during fluoroscopy.
5. Withdraw enteroclysis catheter to stomach, suction contrast, and withdraw catheter.

Determination of optimal infusion rate during the fluoroscopic phase is important because this is the main factor that keeps the small intestine distended during the CT acquisition. Newer digital fluoroscopic units allow diagnostic single-contrast examinations when using 12% solution of meglumine diatrizoate. In some instances subtle gradients of low-grade partial obstruction may be observed during the fluoroscopic phase and not on the CT images. The etiology of the obstruction, however, is usually not evident on fluoroscopy. When combined with the CT images, fluoroscopic observations recorded on the spot radiographs add confidence to the diagnosis.

Box 42-3 lists our CT parameters using 4-, 16-, 40-, and 64-channel scanners. A window width of 360 Hounsfield units (HU) and a level of 40 HU are used with neutral enteral and IV contrast. Small bowel windows (width of 1200 HU, level of 200 HU) are used for viewing positive enteral contrast CT.

Strategies are required for handling the large number of source images produced by isotropic imaging to reduce the number of images to be reviewed by the radiologists. Interpretation is done on a separate workstation using interactive 2D viewing of thicker axial, coronal, and sagittal reformats with cross-referencing of abnormal or questionable findings.

BOX 42-3 **Computed Tomographic Parameters**

These parameters apply to scanners from Phillips Medical Systems; similar parameters could be used on other scanners.
- 4-channel: 3.2-mm section (slice) width at 1.3-mm reconstruction interval
- 16-channel: 2.0 mm at 1.0-mm reconstruction interval
- 40- or 64-channel: detector configuration: 40 (or 64) × 0.625 mm
  Original axial source images (isotropic resolution): 0.9 mm at 0.45 mm (kept on scanner and not sent to PACS)
  Reformats: axial, coronal, and sagittal 4 mm at 3 mm (made on the scanner and sent to PACS)

Selected images are sent to a picture archiving and communications system (PACS) and are of value in case conferences and planning surgery.

CLINICAL INDICATIONS

The clinical applications of the two modifications of CTE overlap. In our early experience, we used CTE with positive enteral contrast for most small bowel investigations. Since the introduction of MDCT, CTE with neutral enteral and IV contrast is our primary method of investigation when the small bowel is not distended on abdominal radiography or conventional CT and there is no contraindication to the use of iodinated contrast. This technique is faster, is reproducible, and allows a more global detailed evaluation, not only of the small intestine but the entire abdomen. It is well tolerated when simple technical guidelines are observed and uses less radiation than CTE with positive enteral contrast. Box 42-4

BOX 42-4 **Indications for Neutral Enteral and IV Contrast Computed Tomographic Enteroclysis**

1. Unexplained gastrointestinal bleeding or anemia, especially in children or young adults
2. Staging of known Crohn's disease
3. Small bowel obstruction—no significant small bowel distention on plain radiograph
4. Alternative examination:
   Before or after wireless capsule endoscopy
   When double-contrast carbon dioxide/barium enteroclysis is not technically possible

BOX 42-5 **Indications for Positive Enteral Contrast Computed Tomographic Enteroclysis**

1. Suspected recurrent small bowel obstruction or unexplained abdominal pain with negative conventional exams and IV contrast contraindicated
2. Suspected small bowel disease (unexplained lower gastrointestinal bleeding, anemia, diarrhea, and history of NSAID intake) where IV contrast is contraindicated or carbon dioxide/barium enteroclysis not technically possible
3. Patients with small bowel obstruction in whom general surgeons prefer conservative management (see text)

summarizes the current clinical indications of CTE with neutral enteral and IV contrast. Box 42-5 summarizes the current clinical indications of CTE with positive enteral contrast.

Small Bowel Obstruction

The initial North American reports on CTE focused on patients with partial small bowel obstruction.[8,19,20] The sensitivity and specificity of CTE (89% and 100%, respectively) in detecting partial small bowel obstruction were higher than those of conventional CT (50% and 94%, respectively) (Fig. 42-3). This difference was even more marked in patients with known or suspected abdominal malignancy.[19]

The precise localization and classification of adhesions, the most common cause of small bowel obstruction, is readily made on CTE with interactive 2D interpretation. This has management implications especially when a laparoscopic

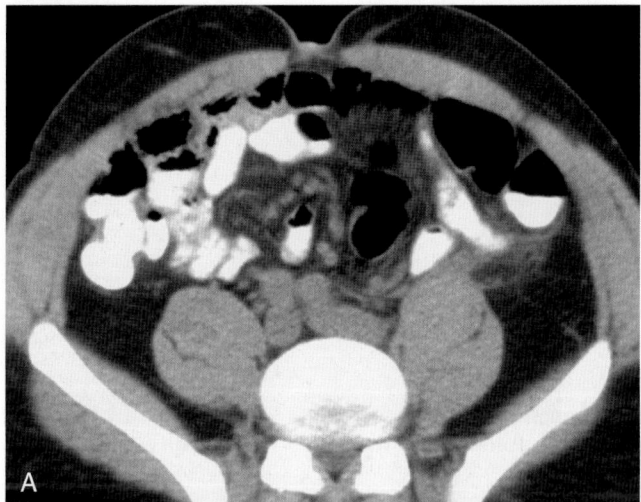

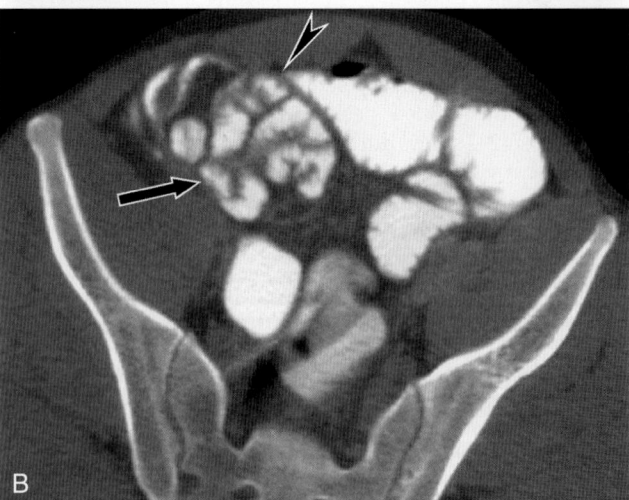

Figure 42-3. A 38-year-old man with a prior appendicectomy presented with intermittent abdominal pain. A. Conventional CT scan shows no evidence of distended small bowel. **B.** CTE with positive enteral contrast, performed 3 days later, demonstrates distended proximal bowel loop with abrupt tapering of caliber (*arrowhead*) adjacent to anterior parietal peritoneum. Distal small bowel contains enteral contrast but is non-distended (*arrow*). Low-grade obstruction was diagnosed and surgically proven as being due to adhesions.

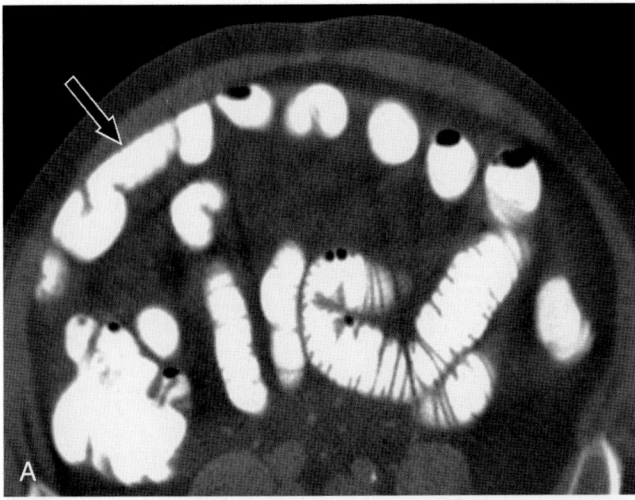

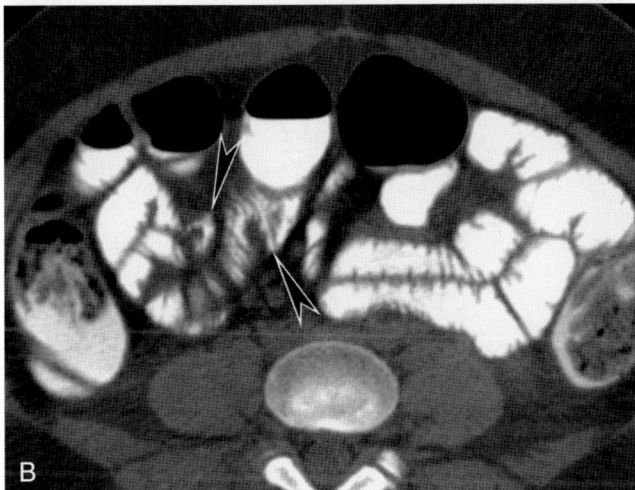

Figure 42-4. Parietal and visceral adhesions shown by positive contrast CTE. A. A 64-year-old man with prior hernia repair showed a long loop of nondistended small bowel (*arrow*) closely applied to anterior parietal peritoneum, consistent with parietal adhesions. **B.** A 34-year-old woman with abdominal pain and history of appendicectomy, right oophorectomy, and hysterectomy. Multiple loops of nondistended small bowel in midabdomen showed kinks (*arrowheads*) and mild fold thickening. This appearance suggested visceral adhesions.

surgical approach is used.[21] Interactive 2D interpretation allows categorization of small bowel adhesions into parietal and visceral adhesions (Fig. 42-4).[11] Single and multiple points of obstruction are readily demonstrated as in barium enteroclysis, but their precise location is made easier by CTE. A volume-rendered surgical perspective can be added to 2D imaging and may simplify the understanding of the obstructive process as well as assist in surgical planning.[22]

There is a subset of patients with small bowel obstruction in whom surgeons prefer conservative management: early postoperative obstruction (within 2 weeks of surgery), Crohn's disease, carcinomatosis, and prior radiation or multiple surgeries.[23] In this group the multipurpose enteroclysis tube (13.5-F MDEC tube, Cook Inc., Bloomington, IN) is used to decompress the small bowel to a much greater degree than is achievable with a standard nasogastric tube.[24] After overnight decompression of the distended small bowel a slow infusion (typically 40 to 75 mL/min) is used to deliver sufficient contrast to the point of obstruction to determine if the obstruc-

tion is partial or complete. If initial infusion shows hypotonic fluid-filled small bowel with little or no flow of enteral contrast, the authors perform CT without further infusion after a 3-hour delay. A further delayed scan (12 hours after start of infusion) is done if there is no evidence of enterally infused contrast in the collapsed distal small bowel loops or colon. In complete obstruction, water-soluble contrast does not pass the point of obstruction after a delay of 12 hours or more. After the examination, the balloon of the catheter is deflated and continuous or intermittent suction is given depending on the severity of small bowel obstruction.[25] The differentiation of early postoperative mechanical small bowel obstruction from severe ileus is made more conclusively by CTE.[11]

Crohn's Disease

An early report[7] showed CTE to be highly accurate in depicting mural abnormalities, stenosis, fistulas, and extraintestinal manifestations. The main groups of Crohn's disease are active inflammatory, fibrostenosing, chronic smoldering, and fistulous types.[14,26,27] Differentiation is important in deciding therapy with immunosuppressant, anticytokine drugs and surgery. For instance, inhibitors of the cytokine tumor necrosis factor-α have been shown to useful in healing fistulous disease[28] but have no known beneficial effect on, or may exacerbate, fibrostenotic segments. These drugs are expensive, and careful patient selection is required.

In determining the severity and extent of known active Crohn's disease neutral enteral contrast with IV iodinated contrast is the optimal technique. Mucosal hyperenhancement, submucosal edema, wall thickening, and mesenteric hypervascularity ("comb sign") are well demonstrated by this technique (Fig. 42-5). Enteric fistula, fibrostenotic segments, and abscess are also diagnosed by this technique (Fig. 42-6). We use positive enteral contrast when there is a contraindication to use of IV contrast or when plain radiography shows distended small bowel. Aphthoid lesions of suspected early Crohn's disease, increasingly diagnosed by WCE, are usually not visible on CTE (Fig. 42-7).[29] If radiologic investigation is required in such cases, we use barium and air double-contrast fluoroscopic enteroclysis. In all cases of CTE, the routine use of MPR views and 2D interactive interpretation is valuable for precise diagnosis and planning surgery.[26]

Small Bowel Tumors

Recent reports have confirmed the efficacy of CTE in the diagnosis of small bowel tumors.[17,30] In one report, CTE was superior to capsule endoscopy in the diagnosis of small bowel tumors.[30] In our experience, WCE may miss small submucosal tumors, which may be mistaken for folds in the bowel wall. Thus, it is useful to perform CTE in patients with negative or equivocal WCE (Fig. 42-8).

In carcinoid tumors the site and number of primary tumors (30% have multiple primary sites) are best diagnosed with CTE.[8,20] Because of its ability to evaluate the small bowel wall and the presence of liver metastases, CTE with neutral enteral and IV contrast is the preferred technique. The distention of small bowel that is achievable by CTE can help differentiate malignant from benign strictures (Fig. 42-9).

Staging of ovarian carcinoma involves determination of local extension to bowel. Serosal attachment to the small

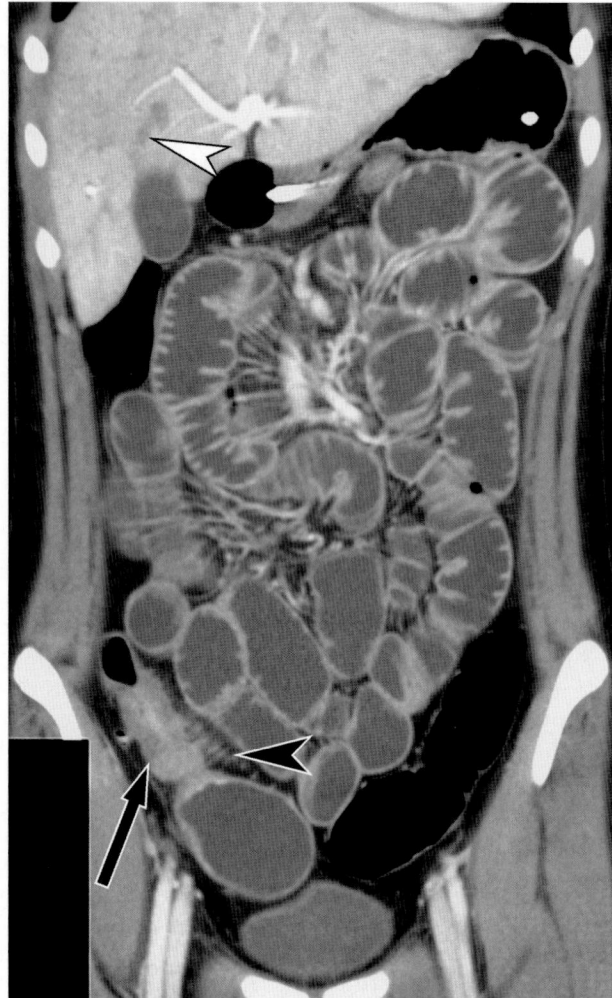

Figure 42-5. Neutral enteral contrast CTE in 59-year-old woman with active Crohn's disease. Note thick-walled distal ileum (*arrow*) with mucosal enhancement and mesenteric hypervascularity (*black arrowhead*), the "comb sign." Note mild, irregular bile duct dilation (*white arrowhead*) indicating sclerosing cholangitis.

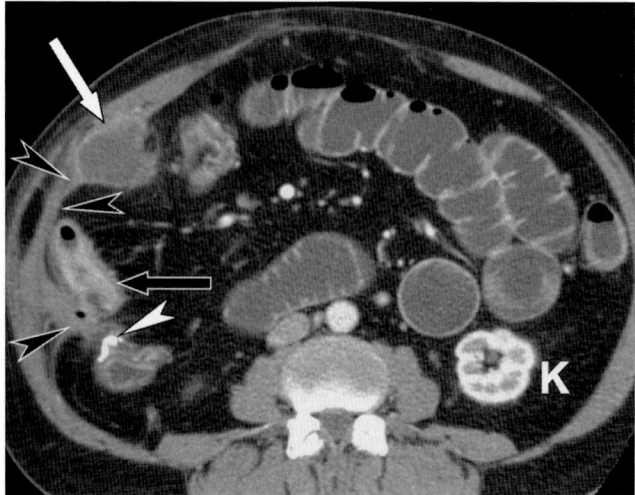

Figure 42-6. Crohn's disease fistula. Axial image of neutral enteral contrast CTE in a 62-year-old woman with Crohn's disease shows a long fistulous track (*black arrowheads*) extending from inflamed cecum (*black arrow*) to an abscess (*white arrow*). Evidence of prior terminal ileal resection shown by surgical clips (*white arrowhead*). Note the late arterial phase of IV contrast bolus, indicated by enhancement of left renal cortex (K).

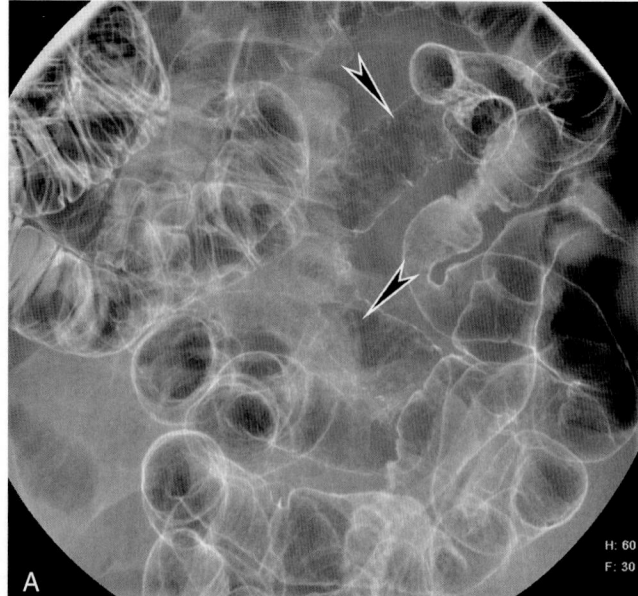

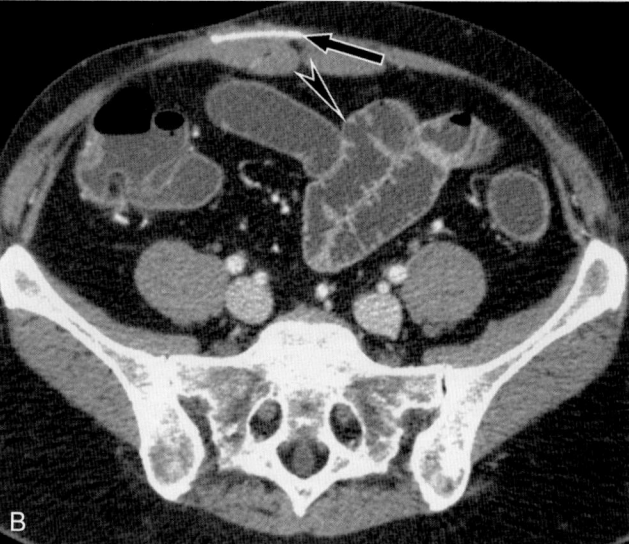

Figure 42-7. Crohn's disease. Double-contrast carbon dioxide/barium small bowel fluoroscopic enteroclysis (**A**) and neutral enteral contrast CTE (**B**) performed within 2 weeks of each other in a 54-year-old woman with suspected Crohn's disease. Fluoroscopic study showed minute aphthous ulcers in small bowel loops (**A**, *arrowheads*), whereas CTE of same loop (**B**, *arrowhead*) showed no abnormality. Note incidental abdominal wall mesh (**B**, *arrow*).

bowel changes the stage and requires the presence of gastrointestinal surgeon and gynecologist at surgery. Maximum distention of small bowel loops at CTE allows serosal metastases to be identified more confidently (Fig. 42-10).[11]

Unexplained Gastrointestinal Bleeding

Thirty-eight to 66 percent of patients with gastrointestinal bleeding have identifiable vascular malformations. Barium examination has a low yield examination in this population, with reported sensitivity of less than 10%.[31] Vascular malformations have been diagnosed on helical CT with IV contrast, and two cases have been demonstrated by CTE with neutral enteral and IV contrast.[20] There are, however, no reports on

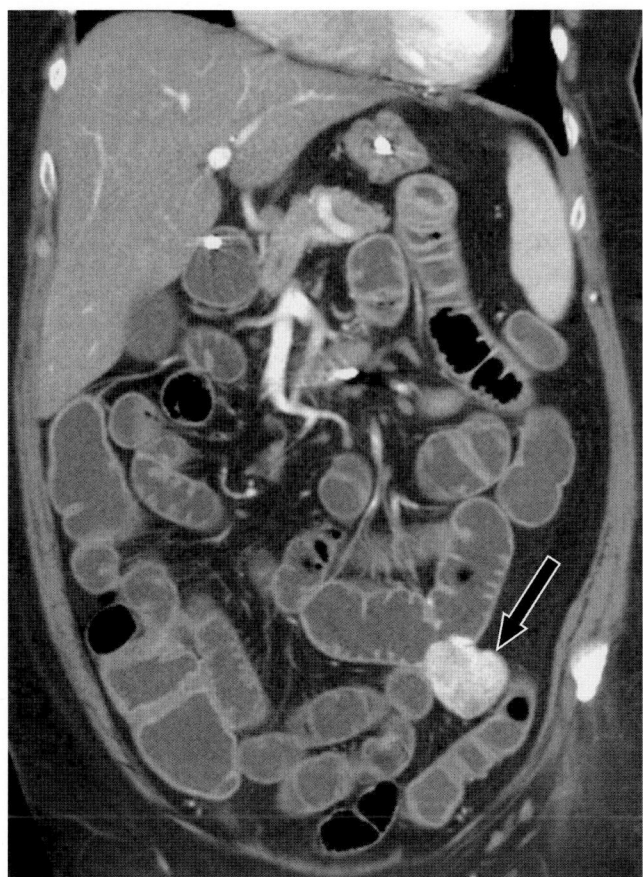

Figure 42-8. Neutral enteral contrast CTE in a 63-year-old woman with unexplained gastrointestinal bleeding. Wireless capsule endoscopy shows jejunal angioectasia (not shown). CTE showed 3-cm hypervascular submucosal mass (*arrow*) arising from mid small bowel, which proved at surgery to be a gastrointestinal stromal tumor.

the efficacy of CTE in this group of patients. In our experience, angioectasia, commonly diagnosed by WCE, is not diagnosable by CTE even with arterial and venous phase post-contrast acquisitions.

Four to 15 percent of patients with occult or recurrent gastrointestinal bleeding of the small bowel have tumors.[32] These are diagnosed accurately with CT enteroclysis.[17,30] Vasculitis may present as unexplained anemia. Diffuse small bowel mucosal enhancement is easily appreciated on neutral enteral and IV contrast CTE (Fig. 42-11).

Miscellaneous Applications

Computed tomographic enteroclysis has been of value in resolving the false-positive and false-negative interpretations of other imaging studies. Diagnostic errors may arise with conventional CT as a result of poor distention or peristalsis simulating small bowel wall thickening. Mixing artifacts from use of positive oral contrast may be mistaken for filling defects.[11] Conventional CT may also fail to diagnose proximal (within the first two loops of jejunum) small bowel obstruction. CTE with the catheter tip in the descending duodenum allows more precise diagnosis (Fig. 42-12).

CTE may indirectly help with diagnosis of functional bowel disorders. The high infusion rate used with CTE may result in abdominal pain and nausea in patients with irritable bowel

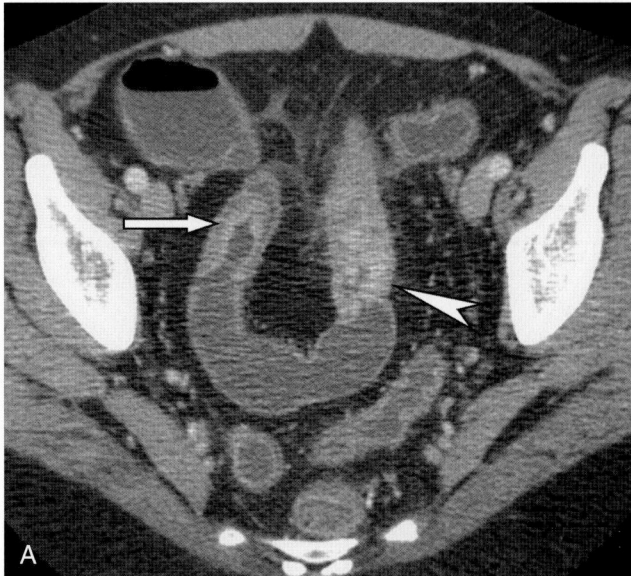

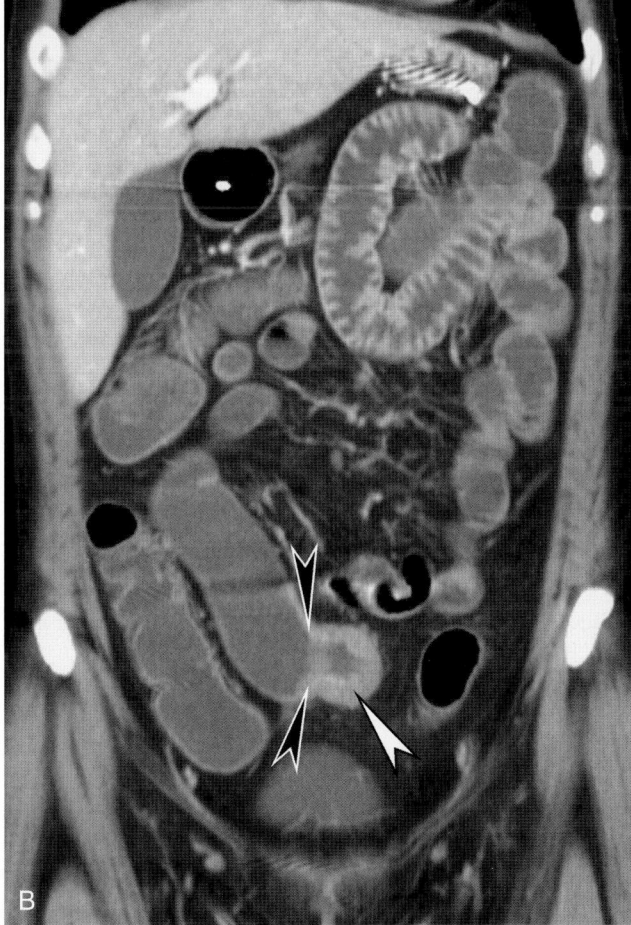

Figure 42-9. Refractory Crohn's disease in a 41-year-old woman. Axial image (**A**) and coronal reformat (**B**) of CTE with neutral enteral and IV contrast demonstrates mild wall thickening of terminal ileum (**A**, *arrow*). Note mural heterogeneity with enhancement of mucosa and edema in submucosa. More proximally an 8-cm segment of significant wall thickening with homogeneous enhancement was seen (**A** and **B**, *white arrowhead*). There appeared to be proximal shouldering (**B**, *black arrowheads*). At surgery, the distal ileal lesion was Crohn's disease; the more proximal abnormality was adenocarcinoma. Good bowel distention during CTE allowed the differentiation of inflammatory and neoplastic strictures.

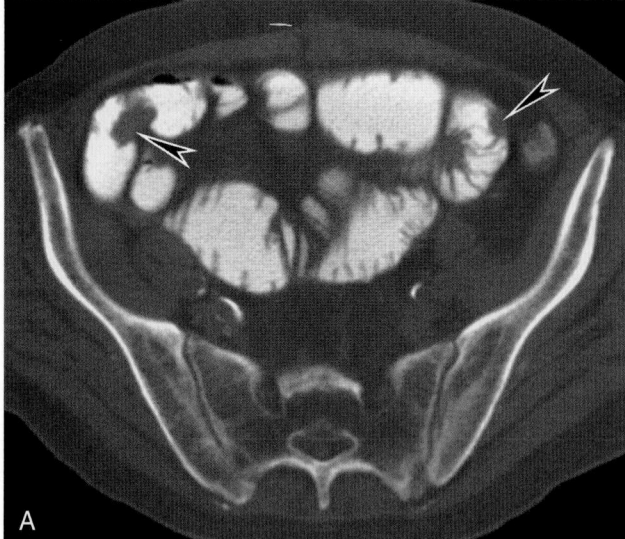

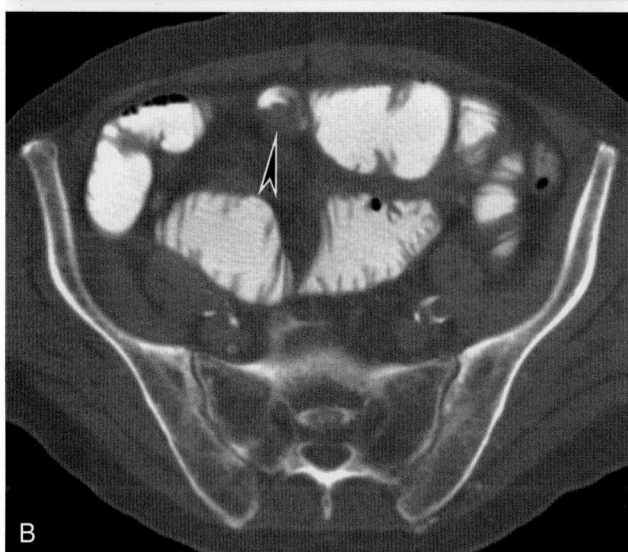

Figure 42-10. Serosal metastases. A and **B.** Axial images of positive contrast CTE in an 80-year-old man with a history of colon cancer showed multiple masses in small bowel (*arrowheads*) consistent with serosal metastases, proven at surgery to be a cause of small bowel obstruction. Prior conventional CT (not shown) did not reveal metastases and suggested adhesions as cause of the obstruction.

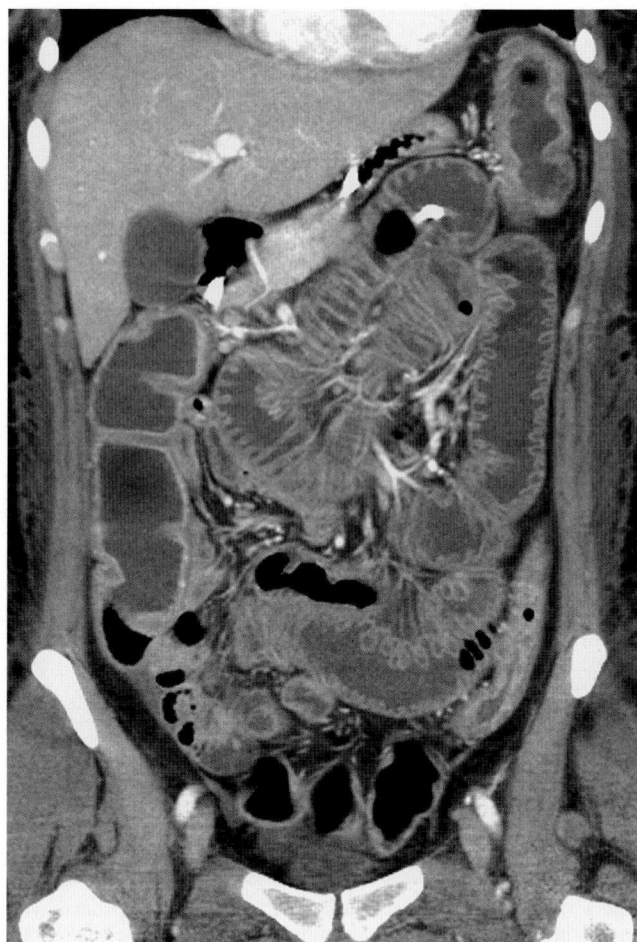

Figure 42-11. Neutral contrast CTE in a 27-year-old woman with chronic diarrhea and anemia. Prior history included systemic lupus erythematosus. Coronal reformat reveals diffuse smooth small bowel wall and fold thickening. Small bowel biopsy showed vasculitis.

syndrome, similar to the symptoms usually experienced by the patient.[11]

ROLE IN THE ERA OF VIDEO CAPSULE ENDOSCOPY

Before Capsule Endoscopy

Conventional CT is likely to remain the primary diagnostic test for assessment of small bowel disease in the acute setting. With the advent of VCE the role of imaging is likely to be curtailed in the elective work-up of patients with suspected small bowel disease. This group includes patients with unexplained abdominal pain, diarrhea, or gastrointestinal bleeding. In patients without clinical evidence for a potentially obstructing small bowel lesion, radiology may have a limited

role. CTE should be considered before capsule endoscopy when there is a risk of an obstructing lesion, to avoid the risk of entrapment of the capsule by such a lesion (see Fig. 42-12). As stated earlier, when the indication raises the possibility of early Crohn's or nonsteroidal anti-inflammatory drug (NSAID) enteropathy, air double-contrast enteroclysis is a reliable method of imaging.

After Capsule Endoscopy

The clinical significance of the small arteriovenous malformations without evidence of bleeding or superficial mucosal "scratches" shown by VCE is increasingly questioned. Therefore, although VCE may have a high sensitivity it may not be specific (see Chapter 44). We have seen many situations in which findings seen on VCE may not be the source of patients' symptoms. For instance, VCE showed proximal vascular malformations in a patient with unexplained anemia but missed the gastrointestinal stromal tumor that was shown on subsequent CTE (see Fig. 42-8). In another instance, VCE, interpreted by experienced gastroenterologists, suggested Crohn's disease but subsequent enteroclysis showed diaphragm disease and superficial ulcers of NSAID enteropathy.

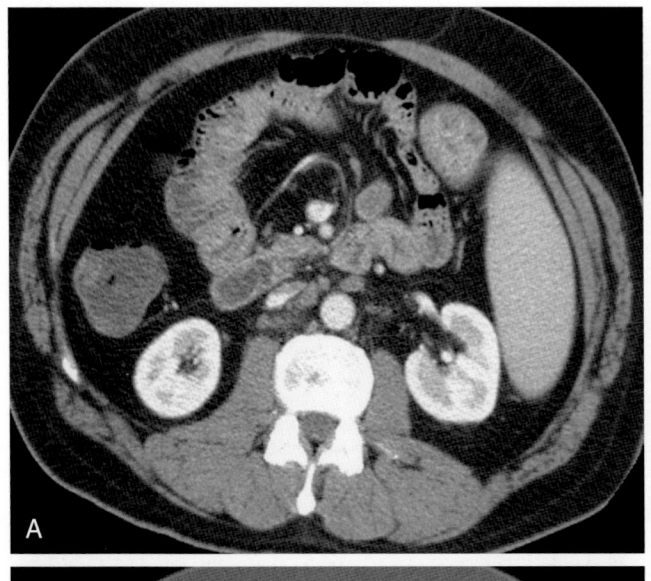
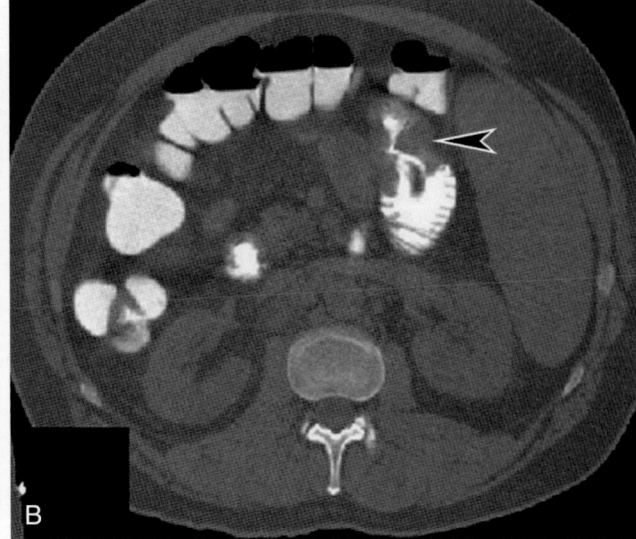
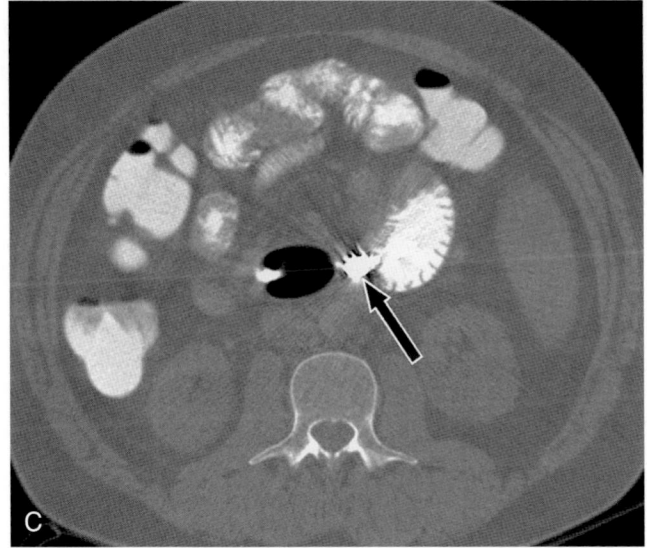

Figure 42-12. Jejunal adenocarcinoma. Axial CT (**A**) and positive contrast CTE (**B** and **C**) in a 48-year-old man presenting with vomiting and weight loss. CT showed no obstruction or mass. Wireless capsule enteroscopy performed after CT was unsuccessful because the capsule was trapped in proximal small bowel. CTE shows annular mass (**B**, arrowhead) in proximal jejunum proven to be adenocarcinoma and capsule trapped in distal duodenum (**C**, arrow).

VCE may miss Meckel's diverticulum. It is therefore useful to consider CTE or double-contrast air-barium enteroclysis in patients with negative or equivocal VCE.

DISADVANTAGES

The necessity of nasoenteric tube placement for infusion and its associated discomfort is alleviated by the use of conscious sedation and the use of smaller tubes. Conscious sedation requires dedicated personnel and makes the procedure longer and more expensive. In smaller institutions this may not be practical. The logistics of performing CT when the fluoroscopic suite is physically separated from the CT scanners is a deterrent. The addition of CT to enteroclysis increases the cost of the procedure and exposure of radiation to patients and radiologic personnel.

Radiation doses remain an issue with CTE. This factor has been one of the arguments favoring MR enteroclysis over CTE. However, a recent prospective comparison of MR enteroclysis and CTE has shown that the latter has diagnostic superiority and better interobserver agreement in the detection of small

bowel lesions.[33] The use of higher multichannel CT (16-, 40- and 64-channels) has reduced radiation by 10% to 66%.[34] This reduction has been achieved by wider cone beams (reducing the wasted penumbra radiation) and automatic tube current modulation.

SUMMARY

Computed tomographic enteroclysis combines the advantages of CT and barium enteroclysis in the investigation of small bowel disease. The use of multichannel technology and 2D reformatting has made organs that are longer than wide, such as the small bowel, easier to examine with CTE. As more experience with VCE and the patency capsule is reported, the role of radiologic investigations in the elective clinical investigation of small bowel disease will need to be reevaluated. In a market-driven health care environment, radiologic tests with low sensitivity and poor negative predictive values may not be justified. CTE will continue to be used in specific clinical situations where it has a high degree of accuracy or where other tests such as conventional CT or VCE are inconclusive.[36-40]

References

1. Maglinte DD: Small bowel imaging—a rapidly changing field and a challenge to radiology. Eur Radiol 16:967-971, 2006.
2. Maglinte DD, Kelvin FM, O'Connor K, et al: Current status of small bowel radiography. Abdom Imaging 21:247-257, 1996.
3. Kala Z, Valek V, Kysela P, et al: A shift in the diagnostics of the small intestine tumors. Eur J Radiol Mar 5, 2007 [E pub ahead of print].
4. Fishman EK, Wolf EJ, Jones B, et al: CT evaluation of Crohn's disease: Effect on patient management. AJR 148:537-540, 1987.
5. Merine D, Fishman EK, Jones B: CT of the small bowel and mesentery. Radiol Clin North Am 27:707-715, 1989.
6. Maglinte DD, Hallet R, Rex D: Imaging of small bowel Crohn's disease: Can abdominal CT replace barium radiography? Emerg Radiol 8:127-133, 2001.
7. Koppel R, Thiele J, Bosse J: The Sellink CT method [in German]. Rofo Fortschr Geb Rontgenstr Neuen Bildgeb Verfahr 156:91-92, 1992.
8. Bender GN, Timmons JH, Williard WC, Carter J: Computed tomographic enteroclysis: One methodology. Invest Radiol 31:43-49, 1996.
9. Caoili EM, Paulson EK: CT of small-bowel obstruction: Another perspective using multiplanar reformations. AJR 174:993-998, 2000.
10. Horton KM, Fishman EK: The current status of multidetector row CT and three-dimensional imaging of the small bowel. Radiol Clin North Am 41:199-212, 2003.
11. Maglinte DD, Bender GN, Heitkamp DE, et al: Multidetector-row helical CT enteroclysis. Radiol Clin North Am 41:249-262, 2003.
12. Ros PR, Ji H: Special focus session: Multisection (multidetector) CT: Applications in the abdomen. RadioGraphics 22:697-700, 2002.
13. Maglinte DD, Lappas JC, Heitkamp DE, et al: Technical refinements in enteroclysis. Radiol Clin North Am 41:213-229, 2003.
14. Rollandi GA, Curone PF, Biscaldi E, et al: Spiral CT of the abdomen after distention of small bowel loops with transparent enema in patients with Crohn's disease. Abdom Imaging 24:544-549, 1999.
15. Schober E, Turetschek K, Schima W: Methylcellulose enteroclysis spiral CT in the preoperative assessment of Crohn's disease: Radiologic pathologic correlation [abstract]. Radiology 205:717, 1997.
16. Schoepf UJ, Holzknecht N, Matz C: New developments in imaging the small bowel with multislice computed tomography and negative contrast medium. In Reiser MF (ed): Multislice CT. Heidelberg, Springer, 2005, pp 49-60.
17. Romano S, De LE, Rollandi GA, et al: Multidetector computed tomography enteroclysis (MDCT-E) with neutral enteral and IV contrast enhancement in tumor detection. Eur Radiol 15:1178-1183, 2005.
18. Horton KM, Eng J, Fishman EK: Normal enhancement of the small bowel: Evaluation with spiral CT. J Comput Assist Tomogr 24:67-71, 2000.
19. Walsh D, Bender GN, Timmons JH: Comparison of computed tomography-enteroclysis and traditional computed tomography in the setting of suspected partial small bowel obstruction. Emerg Radiol 5:29-37, 1998.
20. Bender GN, Maglinte DD, Kloppel VR, Timmons JH: CT enteroclysis: A superfluous diagnostic procedure or valuable when investigating small-bowel disease? AJR 172:373-378, 1999.
21. Maglinte DD, Gage SN, Harmon BH, et al: Obstruction of the small intestine: Accuracy and role of CT in diagnosis. Radiology 188:61-64, 1993.
22. Gollub MJ: Multidetector computed tomography enteroclysis of patients with small bowel obstruction: A volume-rendered "surgical perspective." J Comput Assist Tomogr 29:401-407, 2005.
23. Bass KN, Jones B, Bulkley GB: Current management of small-bowel obstruction. Adv Surg 31:1-34, 1997.
24. Suter M, Zermatten P, Halkic N, et al: Laparoscopic management of mechanical small bowel obstruction: Are there predictors of success or failure? Surg Endosc 14:478-483, 2000.
25. Maglinte DD, Balthazar EJ, Kelvin FM, Megibow AJ: The role of radiology in the diagnosis of small-bowel obstruction. AJR 168:1171-1180, 1997.
26. Maglinte DD, Gourtsoyiannis N, Rex D, et al: Classification of small bowel Crohn's subtypes based on multimodality imaging. Radiol Clin North Am 41:285-303, 2003.
27. Furukawa A, Saotome T, Yamasaki M, et al: Cross-sectional imaging in Crohn disease. Radiographics 24:689-702, 2004.
28. Holtmann MH, Neurath MF: Anti-TNF strategies in stenosing and fistulizing Crohn's disease. Int J Colorectal Dis 20:1-8, 2005.
29. Maglinte DD: Invited commentary. RadioGraphics 25:711-718, 2005.
30. Boudiaf M, Jaff A, Soyer P, et al: Small-bowel diseases: Prospective evaluation of multi-detector row helical CT enteroclysis in 107 consecutive patients. Radiology 233:338-344, 2004.
31. Rex DK, Lappas JC, Maglinte DD, et al: Enteroclysis in the evaluation of suspected small intestinal bleeding. Gastroenterology 97:58-60, 1989.
32. Maglinte DD, O'Connor K, Bessette J, et al: The role of the physician in the late diagnosis of primary malignant tumors of the small intestine. Am J Gastroenterol 86:304-308, 1991.
33. Schmidt S, Lepori D, Meuwly JY, et al: Prospective comparison of MR enteroclysis with multidetector spiral-CT enteroclysis: Interobserver agreement and sensitivity by means of "sign-by-sign" correlation. Eur Radiol 13:1303-1311, 2003.
34. Kalra MK, Rizzo SM, Novelline RA: Technologic innovations in computer tomography dose reduction: Implications in emergency settings. Emerg Radiol 11:127-128, 2005.
35. Minordi LM, Vecchioli A, Guidi L, et al: Multidetector CT enteroclysis versus barium enteroclysis with methylcellulose in patients with suspected small bowel disease. Eur Radiol 16:1527-1536, 2006.
36. Di Mizio R, Rollandi GA, Bellomi M, et al: Multidetector-row helical CT enteroclysis. Radiol Med (Torino) 111:1-10, 2006.
37. Romano S, De Lutio E, Rollandi GA, et al: Multidetector computed tomography enteroclysis (MDCT-E) with neutral enteral and IV contrast enhancement in tumor detection. Eur Radiol 15:1178-1183, 2005.
38. Parrish FJ: Small bowel CT-enteroclysis: Technique, pitfalls and pictorial review. Australas Radiol 50:289-297, 2006.
39. Pilleul F, Penigaud M, Milot L, et al: Possible small-bowel neoplasms: Contrast-enhanced and water-enhanced multidetector CT enteroclysis. Radiology 241:796-801, 2006.
40. Johanssen S, Boivin M, Lochs H, Voderholzer W: The yield of wireless capsule endoscopy in the detection of neuroendocrine tumors in comparison with CT enteroclysis. Gastrointest Endosc 63:660-665, 2006.
41. Triester SL, Leighton JA, Leontiadis GI, et al: A meta-analysis of the yield of capsule endoscopy compared to other diagnostic modalities in patients with non-stricturing small bowel Crohn's disease. Am J Gastroenterol 101:954-964, 2006.

Magnetic Resonance Enteroclysis of the Small Bowel

Nicholas C. Gourtsoyiannis, MD • Nickolas Papanikolaou, PhD

Magnetic resonance imaging of the gastrointestinal tract is gaining increasing clinical acceptance. Recent advances in MRI hardware and software allow for rapid acquisition of high-resolution images of the gastrointestinal tract, and a number of clinical indications have evolved.[1-3] MRI of the small bowel appears to be a most challenging application, despite the presence of a number of other sensitive, direct or indirect, techniques available. MR enteroclysis is an emerging technique for imaging of the small bowel, combining the advantages of conventional enteroclysis with those of cross-sectional imaging.[4,5] This technique has the potential to provide anatomic and functional information. The technical aspects, clinical applications, and limitations of MR enteroclysis are reviewed in this chapter.

TECHNICAL CONSIDERATIONS

Contrast Agents

Various contrast agents have been proposed for MR enteroclysis of the small bowel.[1,4,6-20] The most important characteristics for gastrointestinal intraluminal contrast agents include uniform and homogeneous opacification with adequate distention throughout the entire small bowel lumen, high-contrast resolution between the lumen and bowel wall, no significant adverse effects, and low cost. In addition, minimal mucosal absorption and absence of artifact formation are desirable. Gastrointestinal contrast agents can be classified according to their effect on the MR signal intensity of the bowel lumen as positive, negative, and biphasic. Positive contrast agents such as ferrous ammonium citrates,[6] iron phytate,[7] or manganese chloride,[8] produce increased intraluminal signal intensity, whereas negative contrast agents such as barium sulfate,[11] superparamagnetic iron oxide (SPIO), oral magnetic particles (OMP), AMI-121,[12] kaolin,[13] and perflubron[14] result in decreased signal intensity of the bowel lumen. On T2-weighted images, the uniform distribution of the negative contrast within the small and large bowel allows easier visualization of the dark bowel loops within the hyperintense mesenteric fat tissue, thus improving overall image quality. Moreover, the drop of the intraluminal signal intensity (SI) on T2-weighted images facilitates the discrimination between normal bowel wall and hyperintense pathologic processes.[21] The combination of negative intraluminal contrast agents and postgadolinium T1-weighted images produces high contrast between the bowel wall and the lumen. Biphasic contrast agents, such as methylcellulose, mannitol, sorbitol, or polyethylene glycol (PEG) water solutions,[4] behave as positive or negative, depending on the applied pulse sequence (Fig. 43-1).

Route of Contrast Administration

Two different approaches have been developed for MRI of the small bowel. These include MR enterography and MR enteroclysis. MR enterography is based on the oral ingestion of an adequate amount of contrast agent (600 to 1000 mL) and

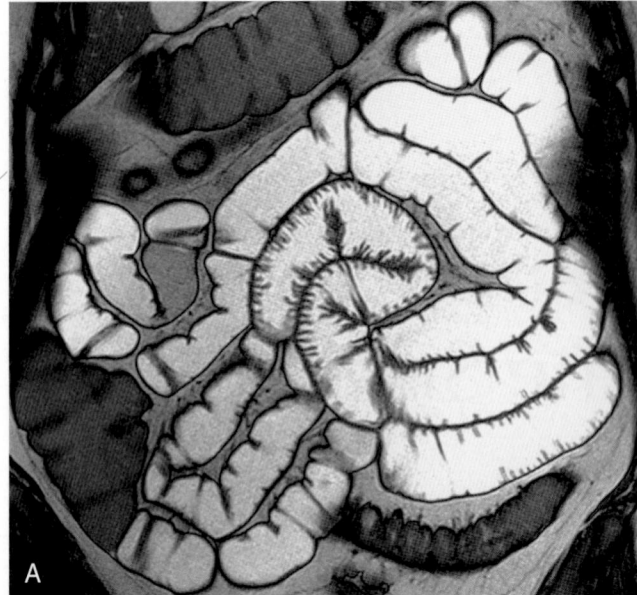

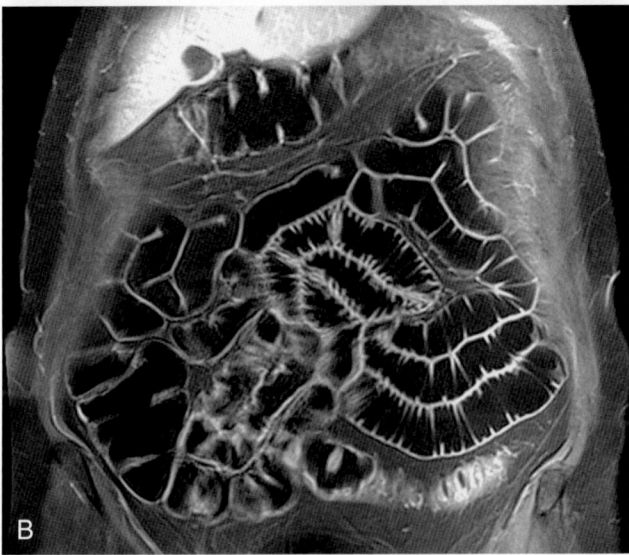

Figure 43-1. Normal MR enteroclysis study. Coronal true FISP image (**A**), and 2D fast low-angle shot (FLASH) image (**B**) with fat saturation acquired 75 seconds after intravenous injection of gadolinium. Iso-osmotic water solution renders the lumen with high signal intensity on **A** due to increased T2/T1 value and low signal intensity on **B**, while normal intestinal wall presents with high signal intensity due to increased gadolinium uptake.

and the contrast agent is administrated in two phases. At first, a flow rate of 80 to 120 mL/min is utilized until the contrast agent reaches the terminal ileum. In the second phase, the flow rate is increased up to 300 mL/min to create reflex atony.

Pulse Sequences

The small bowel is optimally imaged with fast and ultrafast pulse sequences. The spatial resolution of these sequences should be high enough to allow the demonstration of small lesions, such as superficial ulceration or mucosal nodularity. These sequences have inherently poor signal-to-noise ratio (SNR), so they must be optimized to achieve clinically acceptable image quality. All these requirements can be fulfilled by using high-end MR scanners, with field strength of at least 1.5 Tesla, that can provide higher SNR. Short repetition and echo times, which are of great importance in ultrafast imaging, can be only achieved when using advanced gradient systems. Dedicated abdominal phased-array radiofrequency (RF) coils should be utilized to further increase the limited SNR of the ultrafast pulse sequences.

MRI examination protocols of the small bowel should include T1- and T2-weighted sequences in the axial and coronal planes. Both T1- and T2-weighted sequences should be fast enough to allow comfortable breath-hold acquisition times and reduce motion-related artifacts. For T1-weighted images, most authors use spoiled gradient-echo (SGRE) sequences in 2D and 3D acquisition modes with or without fat-saturation prepulses.[22] T2-weighted images are obtained using turbo spin-echo (TSE) and half-Fourier acquisition single-shot turbo spin-echo (HASTE) sequences.[21,23] More recently, the true fast imaging with steady-state precession (FISP) sequence has been shown to provide high-resolution images of the bowel wall (see Fig. 43-1A) and mesentery.[4] Fat-suppressed TSE or short tau inversion recovery (STIR) sequences have also been employed to assess the activity in Crohn's disease.[21]

CLINICAL APPLICATIONS

Crohn's Disease

Modern imaging is assuming an increasingly important role in the classification of Crohn's disease subtypes (see Chapter 45). MR enteroclysis has shown to be highly sensitive in demonstrating superficial, mural, and extramural lesions in patients with Crohn's disease. Subtle lesions such as mucosal nodularity, superficial ulcerations, and thickening of the folds (Fig. 43-2) may be depicted by MR enteroclysis, although with a lower sensitivity as compared with conventional enteroclysis, owing to its lower spatial resolution.[24] Using true FISP images, MR enteroclysis can demonstrate the characteristic discrete ulceration of Crohn's disease[23-26]; linear ulcers appear as thin lines of high signal intensity, longitudinally or transversely (fissure ulcers) oriented within the thickened bowel wall (Fig. 43-3). Cobblestoning can also be appreciated as sharply demarcated, patchy areas of moderate signal intensity, corresponding to remaining islands of thickened mucosa, surrounded by longitudinal and transverse ulcers of high signal intensity (Fig. 43-4).

True FISP MR images are superior to HASTE images in demonstrating linear ulcers, cobblestoning, and intramural tracts, whereas T1-weighted SGRE images are less sensitive. Wall thickening is clearly shown by all MR enteroclysis

acquisition of consecutive sequences. Early acquisitions are utilized for the study of jejunal loops, whereas late images, acquired with a delay of 25 to 30 minutes, are used for distal ileal loops and the ileocecal valve evaluation.[19] Recently, a modified technique comprising oral administration of 1000 to 1500 mL of hyperosmotic water solutions (mannitol and locust bean gum) and intravenous administration of erythromycin in healthy volunteers resulted in considerable luminal distention.[20]

However, luminal distention can only reliably be achieved with MR enteroclysis.[4,5] In this technique, patients are examined in the prone position, utilizing a phased-array coil. A total amount of 1500 to 2000 mL of an iso-osmotic water solution (PEG) is administered through a nasojejunal catheter, using an MR compatible pump. Controlled infusion is employed

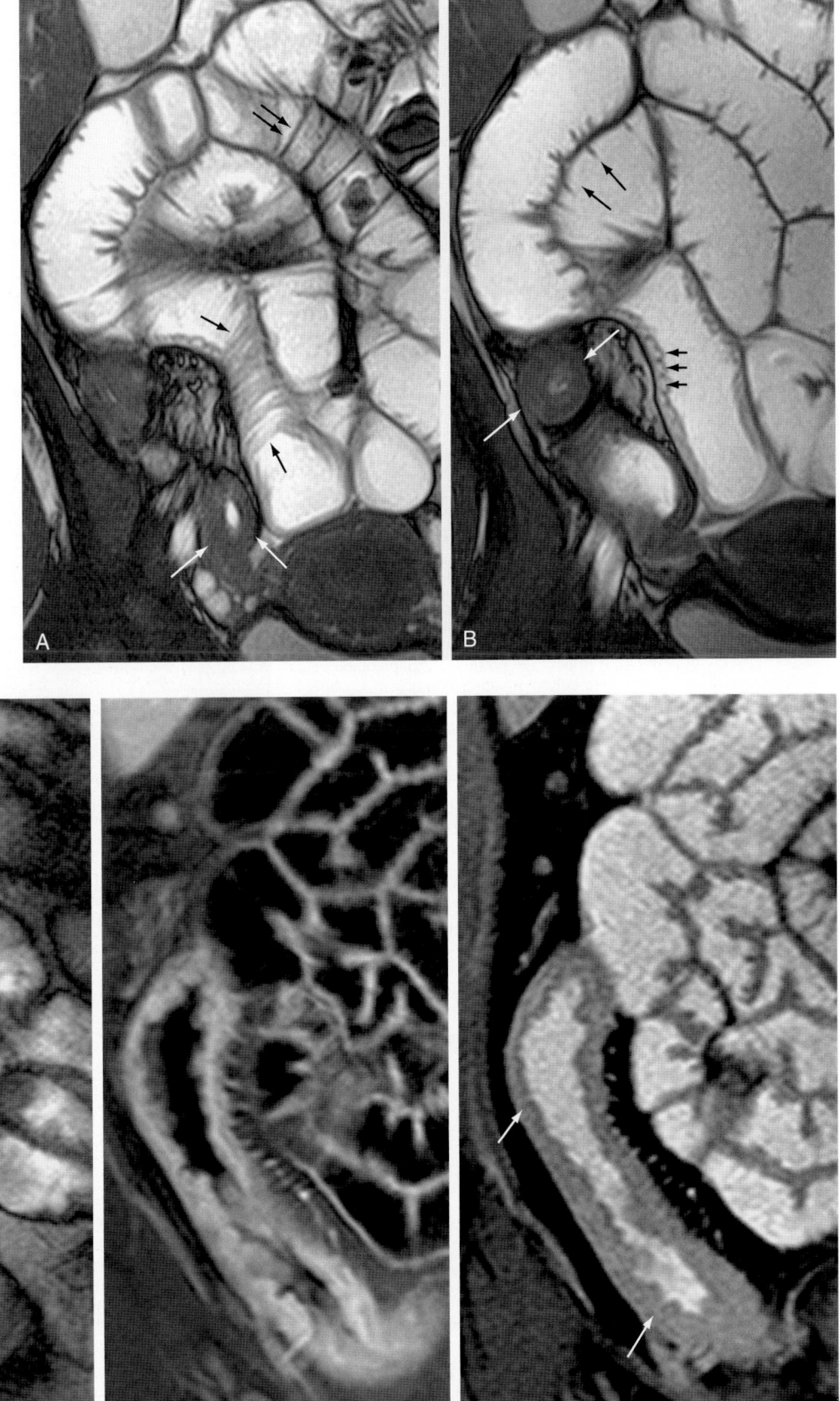

Figure 43-2. Crohn's disease: mural thickening. A 46-year-old woman presented with Crohn's disease diagnosed 10 years ago (Crohn's Disease Activity Index [CDAI] = 120). Tangential (**A**) and perpendicular (**B**) appearances of segmental fold thickening are demonstrated on coronal spot views of the distal ileum, using a true FISP sequence. High signal intensity of the thickened folds indicates edema (*short black arrows*). Note that normal folds are presented with low signal intensity (*long black arrows*). Concentric and symmetric wall thickening is also demonstrated in the terminal ileum (*white arrows*). (Used with permission from Gourtsoyiannis N, Papanikolaou N, Grammatikakis J, et al: Assessment of Crohn's disease activity in the small bowel with MR and conventional enteroclysis: Preliminary results. Eur Radiol 14:1017-1024, 2004.)

Figure 43-3. Crohn's disease: ulcerations. A. Coronal true FISP image demonstrates an abnormal ileal segment with wall thickening, moderate signal intensity of the wall, and multiple ulceration. **B.** Postgadolinium 2D SGRE reveals an inhomogeneous moderate enhancement pattern. **C.** Postgadolinium true FISP image with 2-mm thick slices shows the mucosa as a thin black line. The diagnosis of ulceration can be easily made on the basis of the discontinuity of this black line as shown in the areas marked with *arrows*.

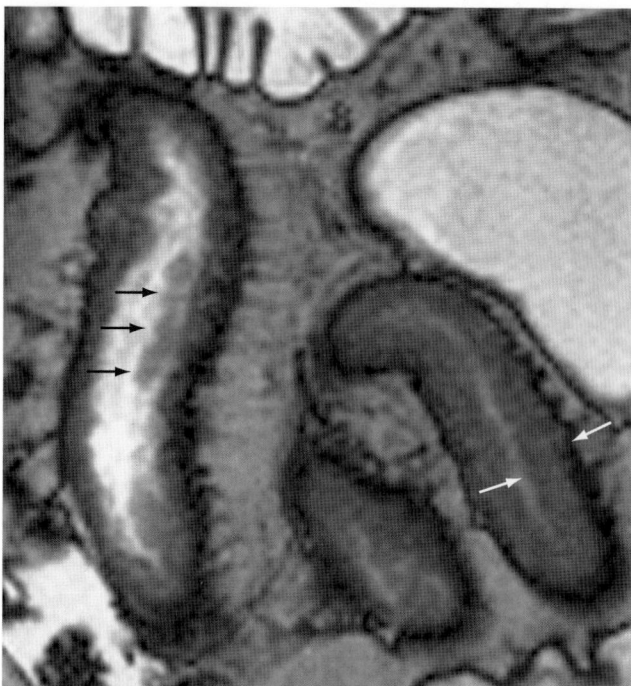

Figure 43-4. Crohn's disease: cobblestone mucosa. Coronal true FISP spot view demonstrates significant mural thickening (*white arrows*) in an ileal loop. Cobblestoning is depicted as sharply demarcated patchy areas of moderate signal intensity in an adjacent affected segment (*arrows*). (Used with permission from Prassopoulos P, Papanikolaou N, Grammatikakis J, et al: MR enteroclysis imaging findings in Crohn's disease. RadioGraphics 21:S161-S172, 2001.)

sequences, provided that the bowel lumen is adequately distended (Fig. 43-5).[23-26] In the absence of extensive edema, thickened small bowel wall exhibits low to moderate signal intensity on true FISP and HASTE images.

Accurate measurements of bowel wall thickening and estimation of the length of disease involvement can be obtained on MR enteroclysis images. Luminal narrowing and associated prestenotic small bowel dilatation are easily recognized with all sequences (Figs. 43-6 and 43-7).

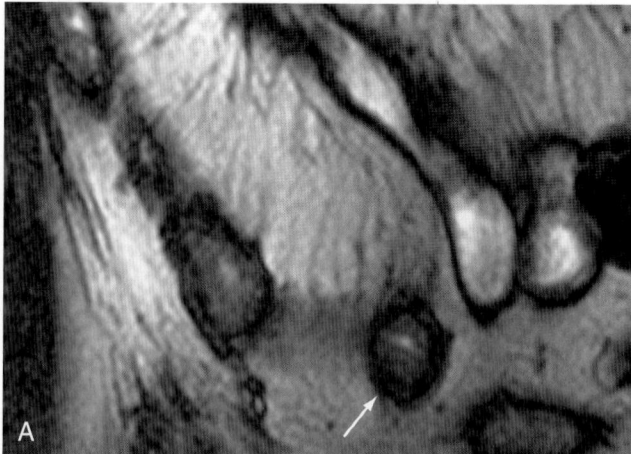

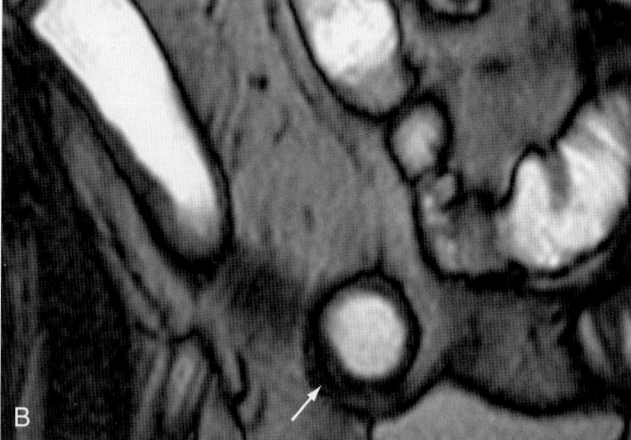

Figure 43-5. The importance of luminal distention. A. Suboptimal luminal distention in a patient with Crohn's disease may result in over-estimation of wall thickness measurements (*arrow*). **B.** Sufficient luminal distention on the same patient can guarantee accurate wall thickness measurements (*arrow*). (Used with permission from Gourtsoyiannis N, Papanikolaou N, Karantanas A: Tratto gastrointestinale. In Bartolozzi C, Lencioni R [eds]: Risonanza Magnetica dell'Addome Superiore Inferiore. 2 volumi Piza, UTET, 2005, pp 271-284.)

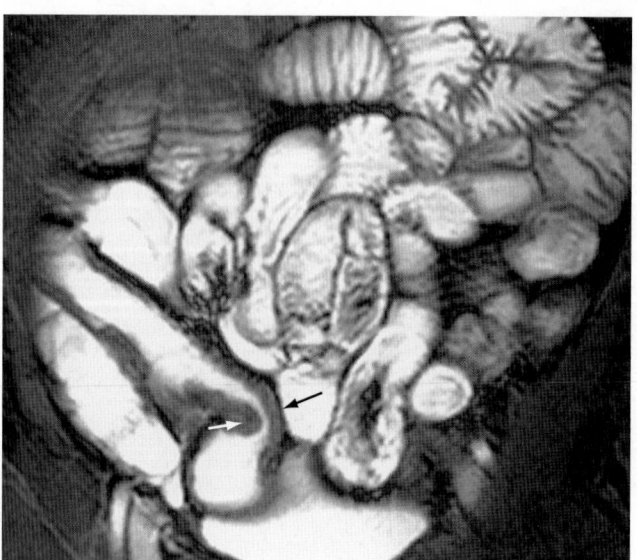

Figure 43-6. Crohn's disease: stricture with prestenotic dilatation. Coronal true FISP image in a patient who presented with obstructive symptoms shows a tight stricture (*arrows*), with prestenotic dilatation. (Used with permission from Gourtsoyiannis N, Papanikolaou N, Karantanas A: Tratto gastrointestinale. In Bartolozzi C, Lencioni R [eds]: Risonanza Magnetica dell'Addome Superiore Inferiore. 2 volumi Piza, UTET, 2005, pp 271-284.)

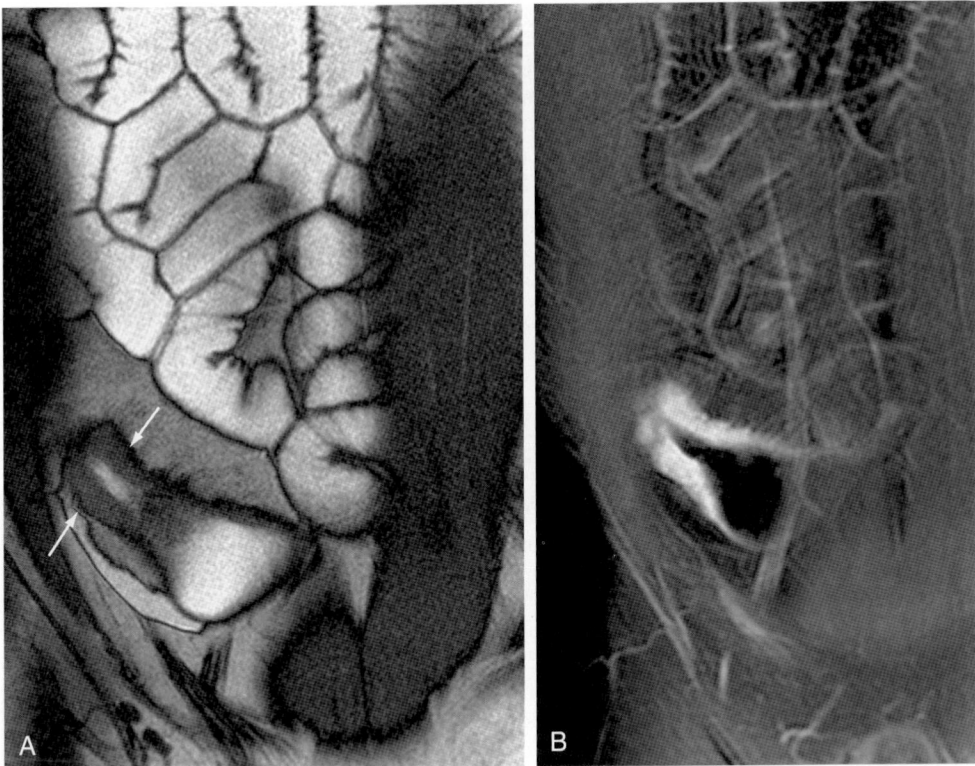

Figure 43-7. Crohn's disease: mural thickening, lumen narrowing, and fibrofatty proliferation of the mesentery. Mural thickening of the terminal ileum demonstrated on both coronal true FISP (*arrows*, **A**) and postgadolinium 2D FLASH (**B**) images. Luminal narrowing and associated prestenotic dilatation can be seen on true FISP image and diffused, marked enhancement on postgadolinium 2D FLASH images. Fibrofatty proliferation of the mesentery is accompanying the involved segment.

In a recent study,[24] MR enteroclysis was found to be equivalent to conventional enteroclysis in detecting, localizing, and estimating the length of disease involvement and in assessing mural thickening, luminal narrowing, and high-grade stenoses. MR enteroclysis has a clear advantage over conventional enteroclysis in the demonstration of extraluminal manifestations or complications of Crohn's disease.[23-26] The extent of creeping fat of the mesentery (fibrofatty proliferation) and its fatty or fibrotic composition can be directly assessed on true FISP images, while it can be inferred on conventional enteroclysis. Fibrofatty proliferation may present as mass effect, separating and/or displacing small bowel loops (Fig. 43-8). The involved mesentery may contain small (< 8 mm) lymph nodes that are easily identified on true FISP images by their low signal intensity against the bright mesenteric fat (Fig. 43-9). These lymph nodes often are not clearly demonstrated on HASTE images owing to k-space filtering effects or on T1-weighted SGRE images owing to saturation of mesenteric fat signal. Sinus tracts and fistulas are demonstrated by the high signal intensity of their fluid content on true FISP (Fig. 43-10A) and HASTE images and by the low signal intensity with a peripheral high signal intensity halo due to inflammation on postgadolinium T1-weighted SGRE images (Fig. 43-10B). Abscesses can be recognized by their fluid content and wall enhancement.

Recent reports have shown that MRI using oral ingestion of a solution containing locust bean gum and mannitol as intraluminal contrast agent is feasible.[27] Simultaneous visualization of both the small and large bowel can be achieved by rectal administration of water.[27] With this technique, inflammatory lesions in the colon and terminal ileum, as well as lesions located in the proximal small bowel, not reachable by endoscopic procedures, can be depicted.

The most appealing application of MR enterography using oral administration of PEG is in children with Crohn's disease. This approach can provide diagnostic information regarding

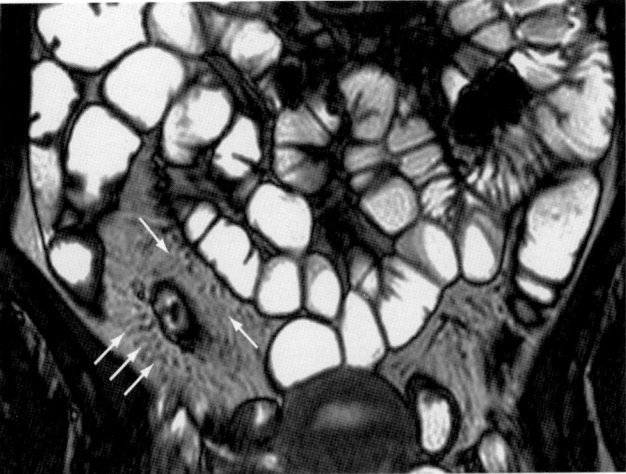

Figure 43-8. Crohn's disease: fibrofatty proliferation of the mesentery. Extensive fibrofatty proliferation of the mesentery (*arrows*), associated with diseased ileum is demonstrated on a coronal true FISP image. (Used with permission from Gourtsoyiannis N, Papanikolaou N, Rieber A, et al: Evaluation of the small intestine by MR imaging. In Gourtsoyiannis N [ed]: Radiological Imaging of the Small Intestine. New York, Springer, 2002, pp 157-170.)

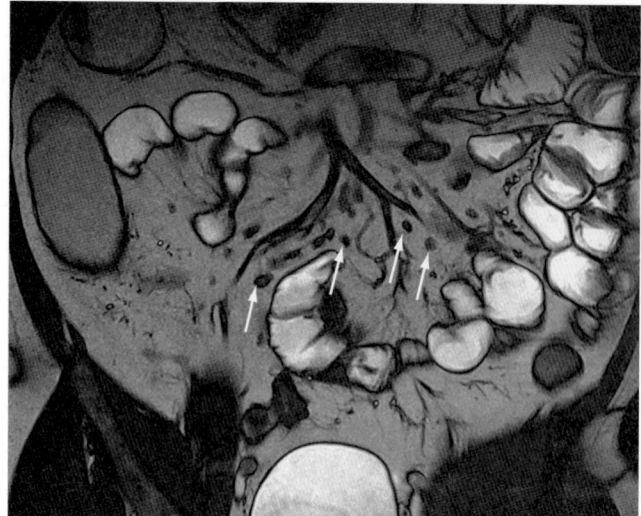

Figure 43-9. Mesenteric lymph nodes. Multiple, small mesenteric lymph nodes can be easily recognized (*arrows*) on true FISP images as low signal intensity round or oval structures against the bright mesenteric fat.

the extent and severity of intramural and extramural abnormalities. It can also demonstrate colonic cobblestoning and stenosis in most patients. The overall concordance between MR enterography and endoscopy approaches 90%.[28] The only drawback is its inability to demonstrate superficial ulceration.[28]

Disease Activity

Assessment of Crohn's disease activity is crucial in optimizing patient management. This is currently accomplished by clinical and/or laboratory parameters. No single test has been established as the gold standard. The most widely used method is the Crohn's Disease Activity Index (CDAI). Several MRI features[21,29-34] are reported to reflect or measure disease activity, including mucosal hyperemia, intramural edema, transmural ulceration, wall thickening and enhancement (Fig. 43-11), and mesenteric involvement, due either to vascular engorgement or to the presence of enhancing mesenteric lymph nodes (Fig. 43-12).

The severity of disease process can be ranked using measurements of wall thickening, the length of the involved segment, and gadolinium uptake in comparison to renal cortex enhancement.[32] Measurements of bowel wall thickness might be influenced by the degree of luminal distention in normal or involved bowel loops, with no extensive fibrosis present. A reproducible threshold for bowel wall thickening measurements corresponding to active disease requires optimal luminal distention, achieved either by duodenal intubation or an appropriate oral contrast agent resulting in adequate distention.

Active disease may also manifest as high signal intensity of intestinal wall on T2-weighted images,[21] due to the long T2 relaxation time of edema. Fat-suppressed T2-weighted images may be more sensitive in demonstrating submucosal edema due to scaling effects that are responsible for gray-scale rearrangement during the image reconstruction process. The presence of submucosal edema results in the so-called multilayered enhancement pattern on postgadolinium T1-weighted SGRE images (see Fig. 43-11).

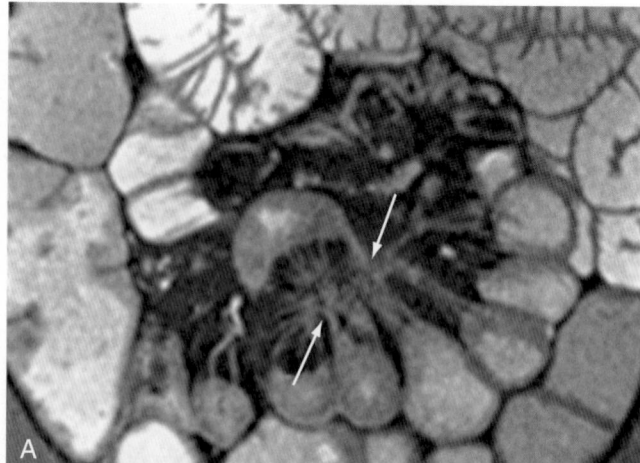

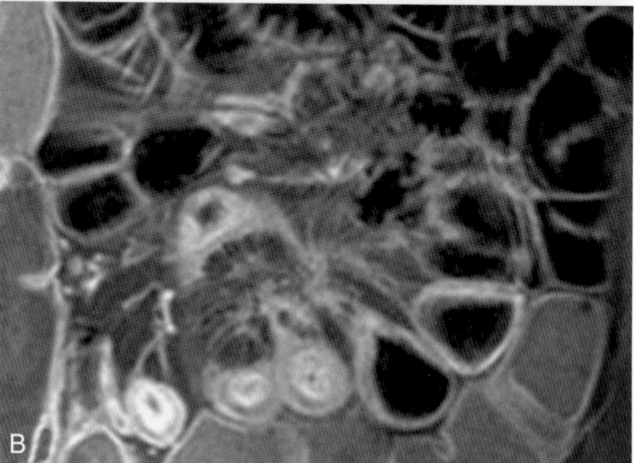

Figure 43-10. Enteroenteric fistulas. Multiple enteroenteric fistulas resulting in the so-called star sign (*arrows*) on a coronal true FISP image with fat saturation (**A**) and on a postgadolinium 2D FLASH image with fat saturation (**B**).

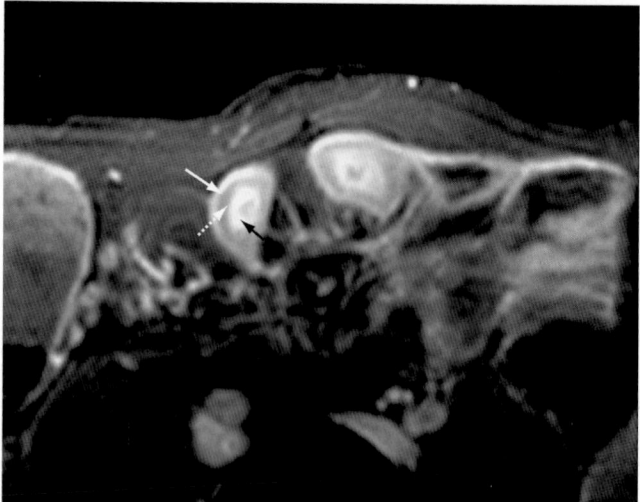

Figure 43-11. Crohn's disease: mural hyperemia and stratification. Patient with active Crohn disease (CDAI = 276). Axial postgadolinium FLASH image shows a multilayered contrast enhancement pattern in the affected small bowel segments. Hyperemic mucosal layer exhibits high signal intensity, owing to increased gadolinium uptake (*black arrow*), as opposed to submucosal edema showing no enhancement (*dotted white arrow*). The outer layer of muscularis and serosa have high gadolinium uptake (*white arrow*).

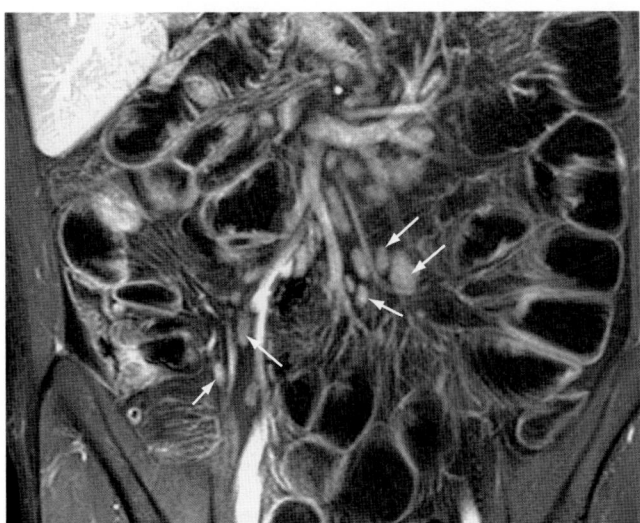

Figure 43-12. Crohn's disease: enhancing mesenteric lymph nodes. Coronal 2D FLASH image reveals a number of enhancing mesenteric lymph nodes (*arrows*) along the superior mesenteric artery and its main branches after gadolinium administration.

Mural enhancement is considered one of the most important indicators of disease activity,[21,29] and it can be appreciated on T1-weighted SGRE images. This enhancement can be quantified by determining the signal intensity of the affected intestinal wall before and after the intravenous administration of gadolinium on T1-weighted SGRE images.[29,33,34] There is good statistical correlation between biologic activity and MRI parameters of wall enhancement, wall T2 hyperintensity, and T2 hyperintensity of fibrofatty proliferation on fat-suppressed images.[21]

The presence of deep ulceration, severe wall thickening, and mesenteric lymph nodes that enhance strongly after paramagnetic contrast administration showed an excellent correlation with the CDAI.[30] Identification of deep ulcers was the most sensitive MRI criterion for disease activity, because more than one deep ulcer was invariably present in active Crohn's disease. Adequate luminal distention and high-resolution dedicated pulse sequences are the key requirements for the demonstration of these lesions.

Enhancing mesenteric lymph nodes are highly suggestive of active Crohn's disease (see Fig. 43-12). A few small non-enhancing mesenteric lymph nodes may occasionally be seen close to nonactive bowel segments, whereas strong nodal enhancement typically is seen adjacent to segments with active inflammation.[30] The amount of contrast enhancement can be quantified by means of region of interest measurements on the corresponding lymph node and a nearby vessel taking the ratio between them as a quantitative index.

The so-called comb sign, corresponding to increased mesenteric vascularity, is nicely depicted on true FISP images close to the mesenteric border of an involved small bowel segment. These engorged vessels manifest as short, parallel, low-signal intensity linear structures perpendicular to the long axis of the diseased small bowel loop.[26] The comb sign can be demonstrated on T1-weighted SGRE images as high signal intensity linear structures due to vascular enhancement (Fig. 43-13). On CT,[35] vascular engorgement has been reported to express acute exacerbation of Crohn's disease. This has not yet been confirmed on MRI.[30] Mesenteric hypervascularity is not considered as specific feature of active Crohn's disease because it has been found in cases of lupus mesenteric vasculitis, other vasculitides, as well as ulcerative colitis.

Neoplasms

Magnetic resonance enteroclysis incorporates the advantages of MRI with those of volume challenge and has been found to be sensitive in the detection of small bowel tumors. The

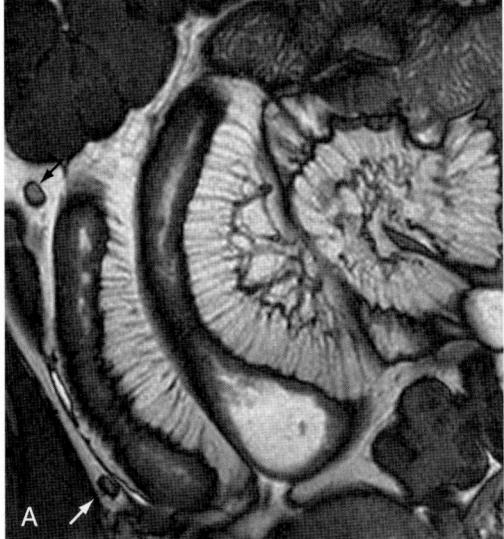
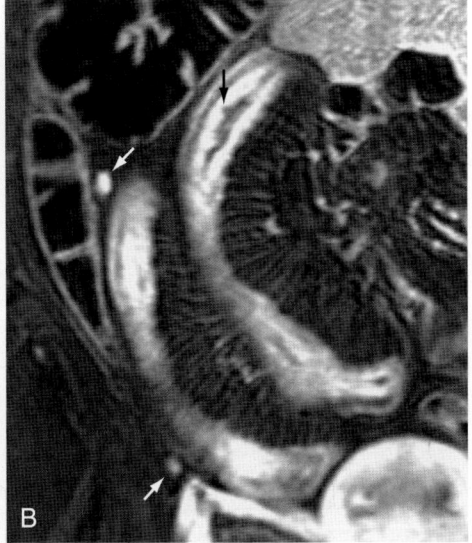

Figure 43-13. Crohn's disease: comb sign. A 32-year-old woman presented with active Crohn's disease (CDAI = 257). Extensive ileal involvement with mural thickening and lumen narrowing is demonstrated on a coronal true FISP (**A**) spot view. Two small mesenteric lymph nodes with moderate signal intensity (*arrows*) are also seen. (**B**) Postgadolinium T1-weighted SGRE image demonstrates mural stratification of both involved segments, marked enhancement of the mesenteric lymph nodes (*white arrows*), and a discrete ulcer (*black arrow*). Increased mesenteric vascularity ("comb" sign) is depicted on both (**A**) and (**B**) images. (Used with permission from Gourtsoyiannis N, Papanikolaou N, Grammatikakis J, et al: Assessment of Crohn's disease activity in the small bowel with MR and conventional enteroclysis: Preliminary results. Eur Radiol 14:1017-1024, 2004.)

high signal intensity of the intraluminal fluid and mesenteric fat on true FISP images allows for the depiction of tumors exhibiting intermediate signal intensity. Small bowel neoplasms are mildly hypointense to isointense in comparison with the intestinal wall on precontrast non–fat-suppressed T1-weighted SGE images and present various enhancement patterns (Fig. 43-14).[36] High contrast between the tumor and surrounding bright fat enables MRI to accurately demonstrate the local extension of the lesions.

Small bowel stromal tumors, adenocarcinoma, carcinoid tumor, and lymphoma exhibit contrast enhancement that is better appreciated on fat-suppressed T1-weighted SGRE images. Marked contrast enhancement can be seen with carcinoid tumors and benign or malignant stromal tumors. Lymphomas present with increased signal intensity on diffusion-weighted images (Fig. 43-15). This behavior is due to tumor hypercellularity that is causing restricted diffusion of the water molecules.

Lipomatous tumors and tumor hemorrhage can be detected on nonenhanced, non–fat-suppressed T1-weighted SGRE images, which should be acquired in addition to the MR enteroclysis comprehensive imaging protocol. Small bowel loop distortion and neoplastic invasion are depicted by all MR enteroclysis sequences. Lymphadenopathy is best demonstrated on true FISP and T1-weighted SGRE images.

Small Bowel Obstruction

Magnetic resonance enteroclysis can provide anatomic and functional information identical to that provided by conventional enteroclysis in cases of small bowel obstruction.[5] In addition, extraluminal causes are better illustrated using MR enteroclysis. MR fluoroscopy, utilizing dynamic projectional steady-state turbo spin-echo (SSTSE) sequences, is extremely helpful in diagnosing low-grade stenosis and in determining the level of obstruction. True FISP and postgadolinium enhanced T1-weighted SGRE images can disclose the level

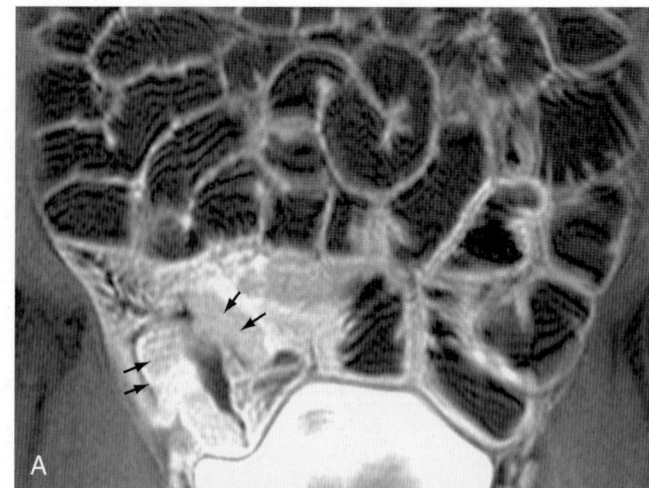
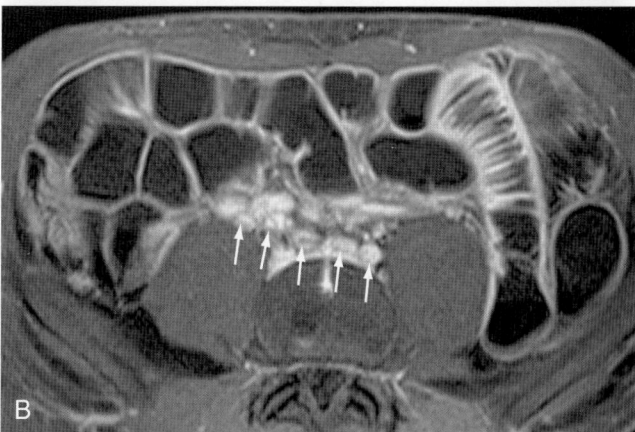

Figure 43-14. Lymphoma of the terminal ileum. Coronal (**A**) and axial (**B**) postgadolinium 2D FLASH images demonstrate homogeneous moderate enhancement of the tumor (*black arrows*) and luminal distension locally. Multiple, large, enhancing lymph nodes (*white arrows,* **B**) are also seen.

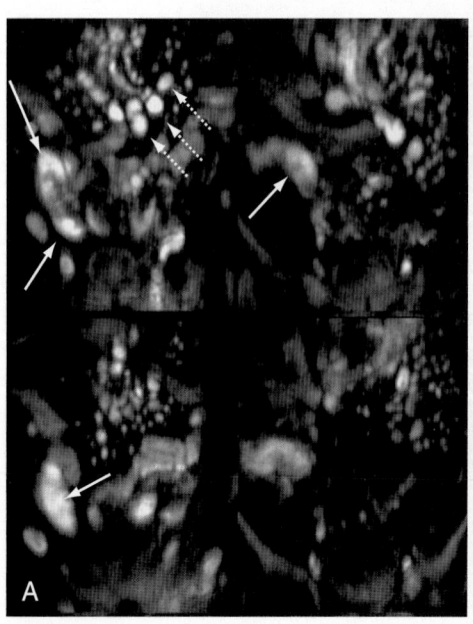
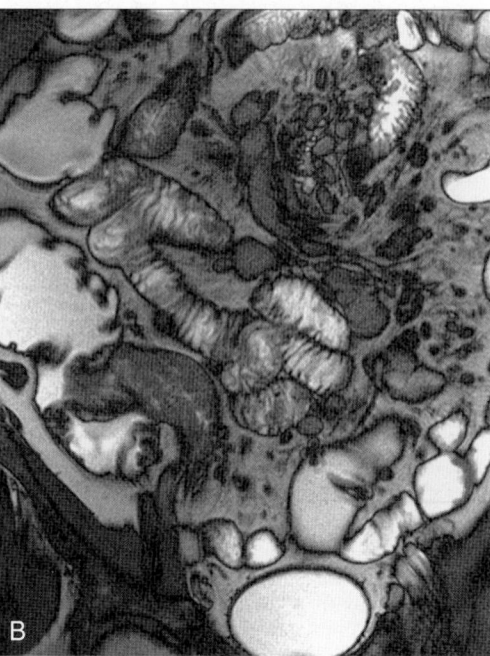

Figure 43-15. Small bowel lymphoma. A. Four coronal consecutive diffusion weighted images (b = 3000) demonstrating high signal intensity due to hypercellularity on the terminal ileum (*arrows*) and several small and large, in size, mesenteric lymph nodes (*dotted arrows*). **B.** The true FISP coronal spot view confirms the presence of an involved terminal ileum and multiple mesenteric lymph nodes.

and the cause of obstruction. In a recent study of 27 patients with postsurgical adhesions, cine MRI using the true FISP technique resulted in a sensitivity of 87.5% and a specificity of 92.5%.[37]

In patients with malignancy who have symptoms of bowel obstruction, gadolinium-enhanced MRI can distinguish benign from malignant causes of bowel obstruction with an accuracy of 92%.[38] Features indicating the malignant cause of the obstruction include the presence of a mass, localized segmental mural thickening, and moderate or marked peritoneal thickening and enhancement. Benign intestinal obstruction is indicated by the absence of a true mass and more generalized mural thickening.[38]

Malabsorption

Malabsorption, especially celiac disease, is another indication for MRI of the small bowel.[39] The role of diagnostic imaging in celiac disease is usually limited, because the final diagnosis is obtained by jejunal biopsy. However, MRI might be useful both for diagnosis and follow-up, because it can provide, noninvasively, morphologic information such as bowel dilatation, ileal jejunization, jejunoileal reversal pattern, and, at the same time, extraintestinal findings, such as mesenteric vascular congestion, lymphadenopathy, hyposplenism, or the presence of intussusception.[39]

Cystic Fibrosis

Magnetic resonance imaging is able to provide information on the extension of the intestinal involvement and in differentiating acute edematous from chronic inflammatory patterns of cystic fibrosis.[40] Recognition of such patterns is clinically important to assess prognosis and treatment, because fibrosis indicates irreversibility of the disease process. The severity of inflammation seems to parallel the degree of gadolinium uptake on T1-weighted images and the hyperintensity on T2-weighted images of the bowel wall.[12]

Ischemia—Bleeding

The role of MRI in small bowel ischemia has not yet been established. Limited experience indicates that bowel wall changes, vascular engorgement, and mesenteric edema can be appreciated on MRI.[41] Superior mesenteric artery blood flow changes in chronic mesenteric ischemia can also be studied with phase-contrast cine-MRI.[42] In addition, there are indications from animal studies that gastrointestinal bleeding can be diagnosed by dynamic post–contrast-enhanced 3D MR angiography, using a blood pool agent.[43]

SUMMARY

Magnetic resonance enteroclysis is an important tool in the diagnostic assessment of small intestinal disease. The most important advantages of MR enteroclysis include superb soft tissue contrast; the ability to obtain functional information; direct multiplanar imaging; and lack of ionizing radiation. Adequate bowel distention, homogeneous lumen opacification, fast sequences with breath-hold acquisition times, both T1- and T2-weighted imaging, and contrast enhancement are need to optimize the MR enteroclysis examination.[44,45]

We recommend the following comprehensive MR enteroclysis protocol for the small intestine: SSTSE, true FISP, HASTE, and fat-suppressed T1-weighted SGRE sequences. SSTSE is utilized for monitoring the infusion process and performing MR fluoroscopy, whereas true FISP and HASTE are mainly used for anatomic demonstration and detection of the pathology. T1-weighted SGRE sequences after intravenous gadolinium injection assist tissue characterization. Inflammatory or neoplastic diseases, including intestinal wall abnormalities, exoenteric disease manifestations and complications, disease activity, and, to a lesser extent, mucosal abnormalities can be appreciated on MR enteroclysis. Furthermore, accurate individual lesion detection, provided by MR enteroclysis, may successfully address clinical questions related to classification of Crohn's disease subtypes.

References

1. Low RN, Francis IR: MR Imaging of gastrointestinal tract with IV gadolinium and diluted barium oral contrast media compared with unenhanced MR imaging and CT. AJR 169:1051-1059, 1997.
2. Luboldt W, Steiner P, Bauerfeind P, et al: Detection of mass lesions with MR colonography: Preliminary report. Radiology 207:59-65, 1998.
3. Marciani L, Gowland PA, Spiller RC, et al: Effect of meal viscosity and nutrients on satiety, intragastric dilution, and emptying assessed by MRI. Am J Physiol Gastrointest Liver Physiol 280:G1227-G1233, 2001.
4. Gourtsoyiannis N, Papanikolaou N, Grammatikakis J, et al: Magnetic resonance imaging of the small bowel using a true-FISP sequence after enteroclysis with water solution. Invest Radiol 35:707-711, 2000.
5. Umschaden HW, Szolar D, Gasser J, et al: Small-bowel disease: Comparison of MR enteroclysis images with conventional enteroclysis and surgical findings. Radiology 215:717-725, 2000.
6. Kivelitz D, Gehl HB, Heuck A, et al: Ferric ammonium citrate as a positive bowel contrast agent for MR imaging of the upper abdomen: Safety and diagnostic efficacy. Acta Radiol 40:429-435, 1999.
7. Hahn PF: Advances in contrast enhanced MR imaging: Gastrointestinal contrast agents. AJR 156:252-254, 1991.
8. Small WC, DeSimone-Macchi D, Parker JR, et al: A multisite phase III study of the safety and efficacy of a new manganese choride–based gastrointestinal contrast agent for MRI of the abdomen and pelvis. JMRI 10:15-24, 1999.
9. Mirowitz SA, Susman N: Use of a nutritional support formula as a gastrointestinal contrast agent for MRI. J Comput Assist Tomogr 16:908-915, 1992.
10. Karantanas AH, Papanikolaou N, Kalef-Ezra J, et al: Blueberry juice used per os in upper abdominal MR imaging: Composition and initial clinical data. Eur Radiol 10:909-913, 2000.
11. Rubin DL, Muller HH, Young SW: Formulation of radiographically detectable gastrointestinal contrast agents for magnetic resonance imaging: Effects of barium sulfate additive on MR contrast agent effectiveness. Magn Reson Med 23:154-165, 1992.
12. Faber SC, Stehling MK, Holzknecht N, et al: Pathologic conditions in the small bowel: Findings at fat-suppressed gadolinium-enhanced MR imaging with an optimized suspension of oral magnetic particles. Radiology 205:278-282, 1997.
13. Mitchell DG, Vinitski S, Mohamed FB, et al: Comparison of Kaopectate with barium for negative and positive enteric contrast at MR imaging. Radiology 181:475-480, 1991.
14. Mattrey RF, Trambert MA, Brown JJ, et al: Perflubron as an oral contrast agent for MR Imaging: Results of a phase III clinical trial. Radiology 191:841-848, 1994.
15. Weinreb JC, Maravilla KR, Redman HC, Nunnally R: Improved MR imaging of the upper abdomen with glucagon and gas. J Comput Assist Tomogr 8:835-838, 1984.
16. Rieber A, Aschoff A, Nussle K, et al: MRI in the diagnosis of small bowel disease: Use of positive and negative oral contrast media in combination with enteroclysis. Eur Radiol 10:1377-1382, 2000.
17. Papanikolaou N, Prassopoulos P, Grammatikakis J, et al: Optimization of a contrast medium suitable for conventional enteroclysis, MR enteroclysis, and virtual MR enteroscopy. Abd Imaging 27:517-522, 2002.
18. Giovagnoni A, Fabbri A, Maccioni F: Oral contrast agents in MRI of the gastrointestinal tract. Abdom Imaging 27:367-375, 2002.

19. Laghi A, Paolantonio P, Iafrate F, et al: Oral contrast agent for MRI of the bowel. Topics in MRI 13:389-396, 2002.
20. Ajaj W, Goyen M, Schneemann H, et al: Oral contrast agents for small bowel MRI: Comparison of different additives to optimize bowel distension. Eur Radiol 14:458-464, 2004.
21. Maccioni F, Viscido A, Broglia L, et al: Evaluation of Crohn's disease activity with magnetic resonance imaging. Abdom Imaging 25:219-228, 2000.
22. Gourtsoyiannis N, Papanikolaou N, Grammatikakis J, et al: MR enteroclysis protocol optimization: Comparison between 3D FLASH with fat saturation after intravenous gadolinium injection and true FISP sequences. Eur Radiol 11:908-913, 2001.
23. Prassopoulos P, Papanikolaou N, Grammatikakis J, et al: MR enteroclysis imaging findings in Crohn's disease. RadioGraphics 21:S161-S172, 2001.
24. Gourtsoyiannis NC, Grammatikakis J, Papamastorakis G, et al: Imaging of small intestinal Crohn's disease: Comparison between MR enteroclysis and conventional enteroclysis. Eur Radiol 16:1915-1925, 2006.
25. Gourtsoyiannis N, Papanikolaou N, Grammatikakis J, Prassopoulos P: MR Enteroclysis: Technical considerations and clinical applications. Eur Radiol 12:2651-2658, 2002.
26. Gourtsoyiannis N, Papanikolaou N, Rieber A, et al: Evaluation of the small intestine by MR imaging. In Gourtsoyiannis N (ed): Radiological Imaging of the Small Intestine. Berlin, Springer, 2002, pp 157-170.
27. Narin B, Ajaj W, Gohde S, et al: Combined small and large bowel MR imaging in patients with Crohn's disease: A feasibility study. Eur Radiol 14:1535-1542, 2004.
28. Magnano G, Granata C, Barabino A, et al: Polyethylene glycol and contrast-enhanced MRI of Crohn's disease in children: Preliminary experience. Pediatr Radiol 33:385-391, 2003.
29. Masselli G, Vecchioli A, Gualdi GF: Crohn disease of the small bowel: MR enteroclysis versus conventional enteroclysis. Abdom Imaging 31:400-409, 2006.
30. Gourtsoyiannis N, Papanikolaou N, Grammatikakis J, et al: Assessment of Crohn's disease activity in the small bowel with MR and conventional enteroclysis: Preliminary results. Eur Radiol 14:1017-1024, 2004.
31. Masselli G, Casciani E, Polettini E, et al: Assessment of Crohn's disease in the small bowel: Prospective comparison of magnetic resonance enteroclysis with conventional enteroclysis. Eur Radiol 16:2817-2827, 2006.
32. Wiarda BM, Kuipers EJ, Heitbrink MA, et al: MR enteroclysis of inflammatory small-bowel diseases. AJR Am J Roentgenol 187:522-531, 2006.
33. Sempere GA, Sanjuan V, Chulia E, et al: MRI evaluation of inflammatory activity in Crohn's disease. AJR 184:1829-1235, 2005.
34. Florie J, Wasser MN, Arts-Cieslik K, et al: Dynamic contrast-enhanced MRI of the bowel wall for assessment of disease activity in Crohn's disease. AJR 186:1384-1392, 2006.
35. Lee SS, Ha HK, Yang SK, et al: CT of prominent pericolic or perienteric vasculature in patients with Crohn's disease: Correlation with clinical disease activity and findings on barium studies. AJR 179:1029-1036, 2002
36. Semelka RC, John G, Kelekis N, et al: Small bowel neoplastic disease: Demonstration by MRI. JMRI 6:855-860, 1996.
37. Lienemann A, Sprenger D, Steitz HO, et al: Detection and mapping of intraabdominal adhesions by using functional cine MR imaging: Preliminary results. Radiology 217:421-425, 2000.
38. Low RN, Chen SC, Barone R: Distinguishing benign from malignant bowel obstruction in patients with malignancy: Findings at MR imaging. Radiology 228:157-165, 2003.
39. Laghi A, Paolantonio P, Catalano C, et al: MR imaging of the small bowel using polyethylene glycol solution as an oral contrast agent in adults and children with celiac disease: Preliminary observations. AJR 180:191-194, 2003.
40. Almberger M, Iannicelli E, Antonelli M, et al: The role of MRI in the intestinal complications in cystic fibrosis. Clin Imaging 25:344-348, 2001.
41. Ha HK, Lee EH, Lim CH, et al: Application of MRI for small intestinal diseases. JMRI 8:375-383, 1998.
42. Li KC, Whitney WS, McDonnell CH, et al: Chronic mesenteric ischemia: Evaluation with phase-contrast cine MR imaging. Radiology 190:175-179, 1994.
43. Hilfiker PR, Weishaupt D, Kacl GM, et al: Comparison of three dimensional magnetic resonance imaging in conjunction with a blood pool contrast agent and nuclear scintigraphy for the detection of experimentally induced gastrointestinal bleeding. Gut 45:581-587, 1999.
44. Gourtsoyiannis NC, Papanikolaou N: Magnetic resonance enteroclysis. Semin Ultrasound CT MR. 26:237-246, 2005.
45. Maglinte DD: Small bowel imaging—a rapidly changing field and a challenge to radiology. Eur Radiol 16:967-971, 2006.

Video Capsule Endoscopy

Frans-Thomas Fork, MD, PhD • Samuel Nathan Adler, MD

In 2001 a commercially available video capsule was introduced that was disposable, ingestible, and dedicated to the examination of the whole small bowel mucosa.[1-6] Since that time, video capsule endoscopy (VCE) has revolutionized small bowel imaging and is now accepted as the most sensitive means of evaluating the mucosa of the small bowel.[7]

TECHNICAL DESCRIPTION

The capsule measures 11 × 23 mm and contains a complementary metal-oxide semiconductor chip camera, a transmitter, two silver oxide batteries, and light-emitting diodes inside a clear, transparent dome with no light absorption. Sharp images are obtained from very short distances with good feel for depth of space. The capsule has a panoramic, 130-degree view of the interior of the small bowel with a magnification factor of eight. It continuously transmits images at two frames per second during its peristalsis-propelled passage through the intestines. The capsule also harbors an antenna for radio transmission of the images to an aerial system of electrodes attached to the surface of the abdomen. A video recorder, carried in a waist belt together with batteries then records the signals during an 8- to 10-hour examination period. This recorder is later connected to a computer workstation that processes the images. The study is viewed in a video mode at various speeds, with facilities for pausing and rewinding. An ordinary VCE study comprises two images per second, approximately 50,000 images in total. In general, the reading time ranges from 45 minutes to 1 hour.

PROCEDURE

The patient fasts for the 12 hours before the VCE; however, water is permitted. Many physicians do not require any bowel preparations and do not restrict the patient's ordinary daily activities during the video recording. However, others prefer to add a purgative the evening before the procedure.[8]

Sometimes the VCE is incomplete, most often owing to gastric retention and slow bowel transit and sometimes owing to residual small bowel content, which obscures mucosal visualization.[9] Research aimed at promoting the passage of the capsule and cleansing the small bowel is underway. Tegaserod, a selective serotonin type 4 receptor partial agonist, has been approved for treatment of patients with irritable bowel syndrome, and preliminary results on shortening capsule transit time are promising.

The localization of a VCE screen-depicted lesion is inaccurate. Areas that have a fixed location in the abdominal cavity, such as the retroperitoneally located duodenal sweep or the ileocecal valve, are more easily located. The overall transit time, as well as transit time per sector of the gastrointestinal tract, can be calculated accurately. For this reason, position of the capsule in the small bowel may be estimated from the amount of time that has passed from the entrance of the capsule into the duodenum until it reached a specific location while relating this to total small bowel transit time. The time bar is complemented by the locator system, which essentially represents an electronic small bowel follow-through tracing.

Currently, the capsule designed for diagnosing the small bowel disease is the only one with extensive clinical documentation. An esophageal capsule is marketed for the diagnosis of gastroesophageal reflux and Barrett's esophagus.[10] Other capsules for visualization of the stomach and colon are being developed.

INDICATIONS

Video capsule endoscopy is indicated to rule out mucosal disease of the small bowel. Until recently, most patients who underwent VCE had prior panendoscopy and small bowel enterography. An antecedent small bowel follow-through is performed to exclude a small bowel stricture that might cause capsule impaction.

The most frequent indications for VCE are gastrointestinal bleeding (obscure, occult, or macroscopic); Crohn's disease; NSAID-induced enteropathy; neoplastic lesions of the small bowel; and malabsorption. VCE has a low diagnostic yield in patients with chronic pain or with symptoms similar to irritable bowel syndrome.

VCE has proven so successful that there is now debate as to whether capsule enteroscopy should be used as a first-line investigation of the small bowel instead of being the last one. This is based on the observation that detailed examination of the small bowel mucosa and the detection of stenotic lesions with radiologic means is difficult. In fact, the clinically proven low risk for capsule retention and the ineffectiveness of small bowel series to predict capsule retention have led to updated policies that neither endoscopy nor any other procedure needs to precede a VCE.[11,12]

Exclusion Criteria

Patients with severe dysphagia and gastric outlet problems should not swallow the capsule but rather have it deposited in the duodenum via gastroscopic intubation. Patients with a known or suspected stricture of the gut, and those who have had extensive abdominal surgery, should be tested with a radiopaque sham capsule intended to verify the functional patency of the gastrointestinal tract. This "patency capsule" has the same outer dimensions as the video capsule and harbors a small radiofrequency identification tag. Free passage is proven when the capsule is passed intact within 40 hours or not detected by fluoroscopy or an external scanner after 36 hours. A retained patency capsule may indicate stenosis, and a planned VCE may have to be reconsidered. Because the patency capsule disintegrates within 40 to 100 hours, the risk for impaction is eliminated.

Until further experience has been gained, VCE might be performed after careful consideration in pregnant women. It is still contraindicated in patients with cardiac pacemakers and other implanted electrical medical devices. VCE is effective in diagnosing suspected Crohn's disease in pediatric patients.[13,14]

ENDOSCOPIC FINDINGS

The eightfold magnified images (Figs. 44-1 to 44-8) provided by VCE depict the small bowel mucosa in great detail, down to an individual villous structure. VCE has great potential to unveil and identify lesions of the small bowel mucosa that cause loss of villi; change in color; surface structure; and lumen caliber. Lesions include mucosal breaks, erosions, tiny and superficial ulcers (elongated, dendritic and round ones), angiodysplasia, hemangioma, varices, anastomotic strictures, and benign, early, and advanced malignant tumors.[15]

VCE cannot distinguish a true submucosal small bowel wall lesion, such as a gastrointestinal stromal tumor from an extra-intestinal one. A discrete, dark bluish color is identified when the small bowel loop abuts on a solid organ or a tumor mass.

Recent technical improvement of VCE facilitates the identification of blood in the small bowel by marks shown on the time column displayed on the screen. A further improvement includes the coloration of the time bar, which helps identify the transition from small bowel to colon and from stomach to small bowel.

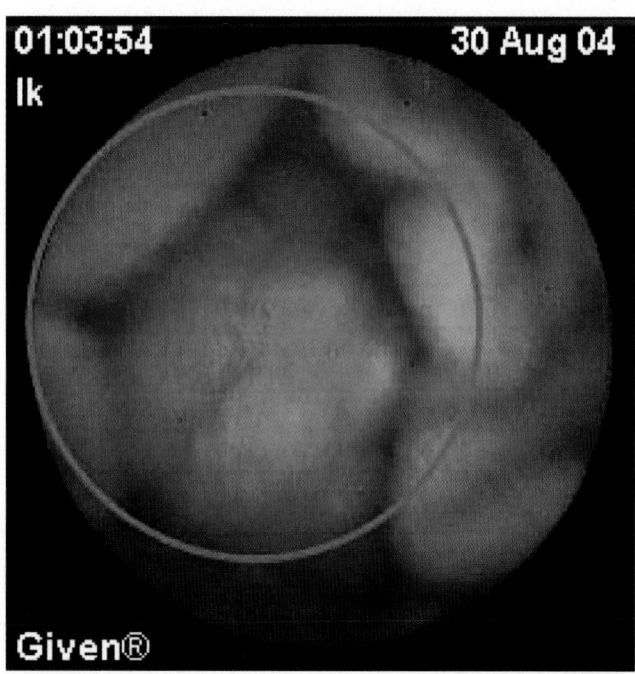

Figure 44-1. Benign hamartoma. This 3-cm polyp was surgically removed.

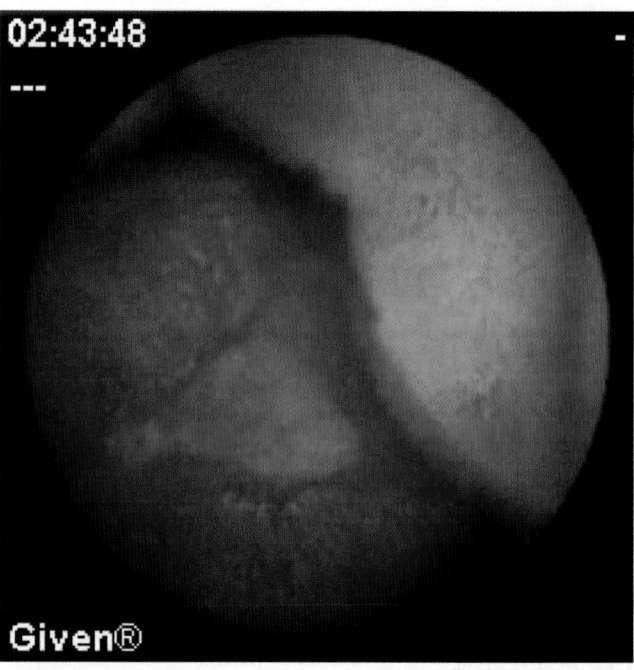

Figure 44-2. Ulcerated small bowel tumor. MALT lymphoma of the small bowel.

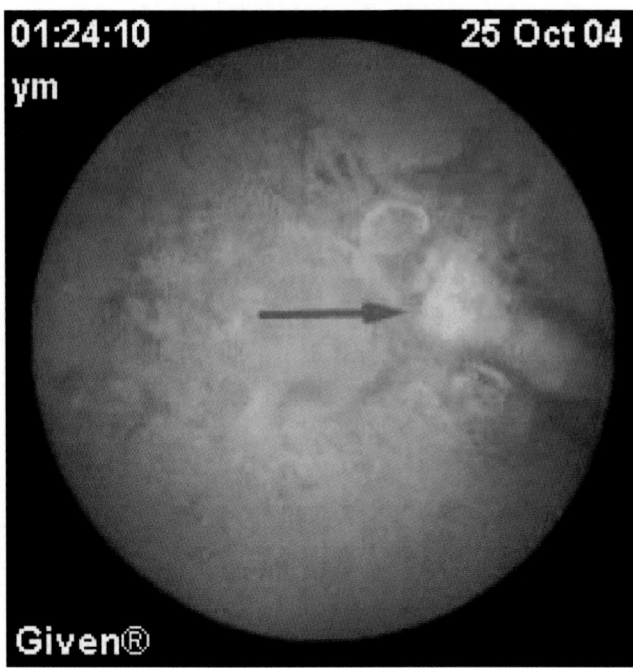

Figure 44-3. Crohn's disease. Small bowel ulcer with inflamed surrounding tissue and mucosal hemorrhages.

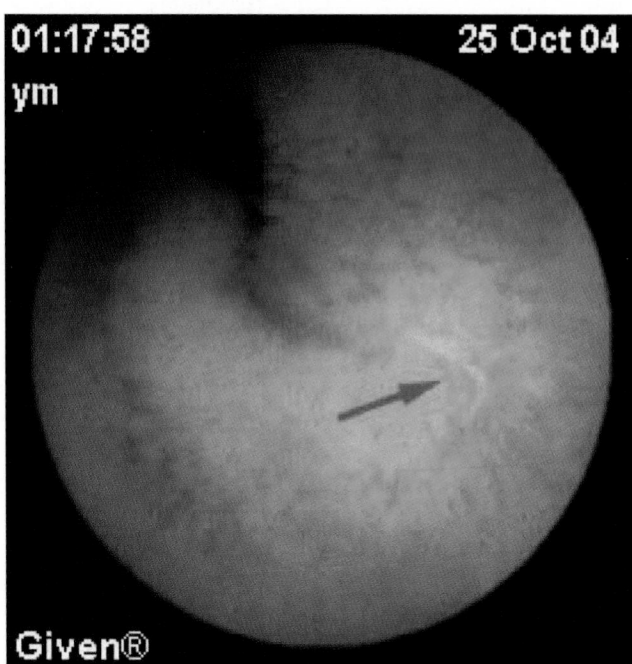

Figure 44-4. Crohn's disease. Linear superficial ulceration/erosion.

RADIOLOGIC FINDINGS

Small Bowel Bleeding

The diagnostic work-up of patients with unexplained iron-deficiency anemia should always include upper and lower endoscopies of the gastrointestinal tract. In the precapsule era, standard radiology of the small bowel was routinely performed, most often as a tube enteroclysis or as dedicated single-contrast enterography. These studies typically had a diagnostic yield in the range of 10% to 20%.[16] Since its introduction in 2001, the capsule has gained a well-established role in the investigation of patients with recurrent occult gastrointestinal bleeding in whom small bowel barium enema studies, gastroscopy, and colonoscopy fail to reveal the source.[17,18]

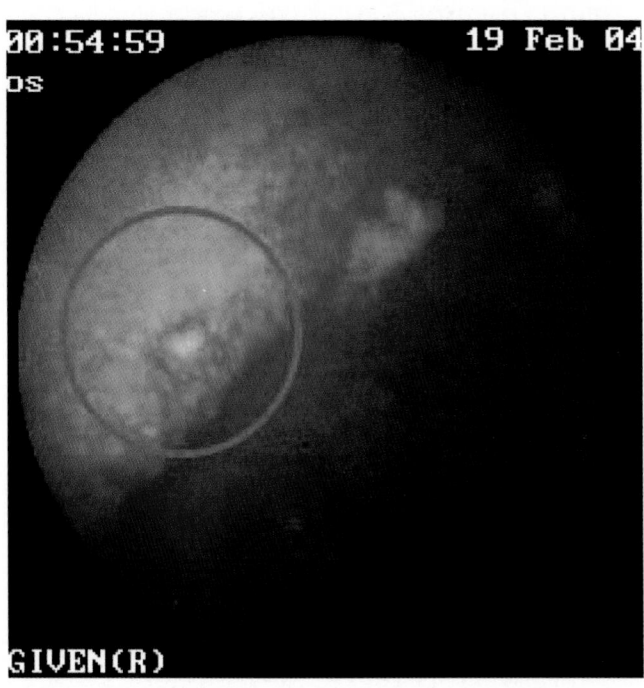

Figure 44-5. Aphthous lesion in a patient with Crohn's disease.

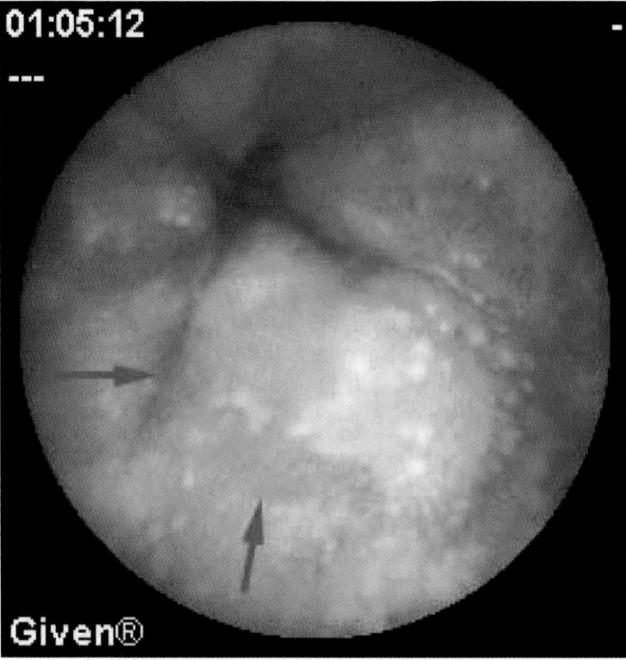

Figure 44-6. Radiation enteritis with loss of villi. The whitish dots represent dilated lymphatics.

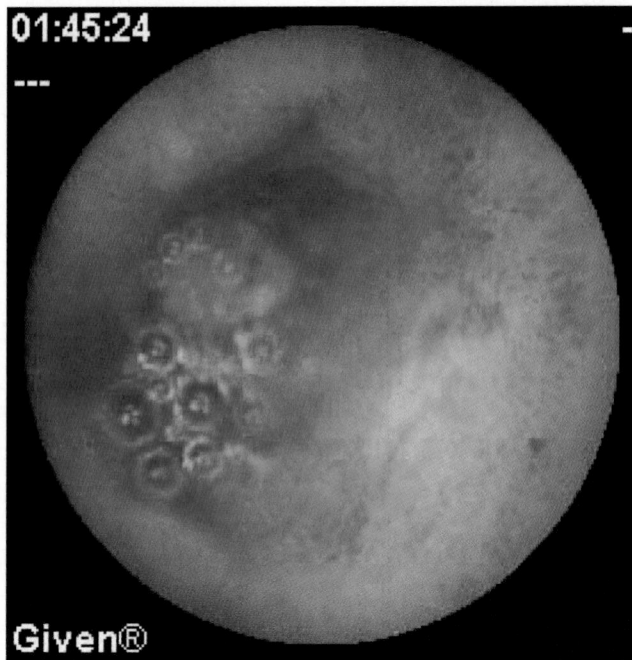

Figure 44-7. Radiation enteritis and spontaneous bleeding after pressure contact with the video capsule.

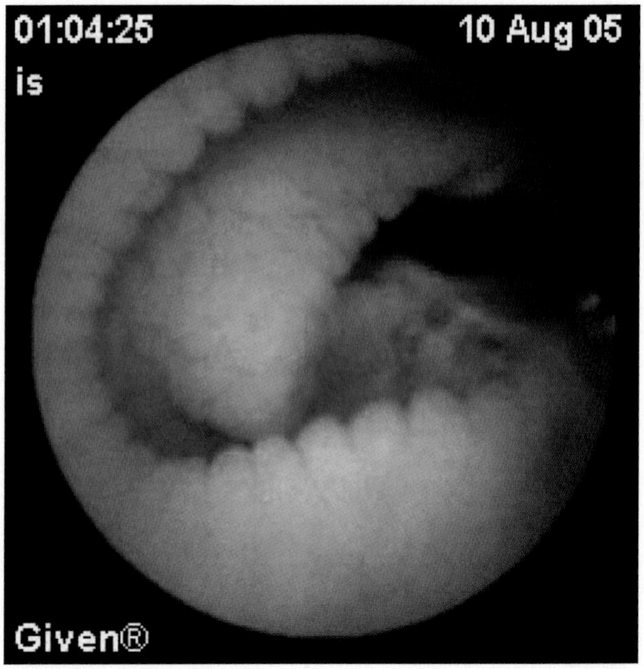

Figure 44-8. Extensive scalloping of the valvulae conniventes in a patient with celiac disease.

VCE depicts lesions that are not detected by other means: superficial, small, and shallow lesions; angiodysplasia; and erosions and ulcers.[9,19] In a series of 32 patients with small bowel bleeding, VCE findings were positive in 21 (66%), whereas selective angiography of the celiac and mesenteric arteries was positive in 4 of 26 and scintigraphy was negative in all 13 patients examined. The diagnostic sensitivities of enteroclysis, angiography, scintigraphy, and conventional enteroscopy in patients with obscure bleeding range from only 10% to 20%.[20,21] A single study group reported an exceptional 60% diagnostic sensitivity for radiology.[22] Positive findings on enteroclysis include sporadic cases with motility disorder and mucosal abnormalities but mainly adhesions, filling defects and masses, strictures, and small bowel diverticulosis. Patients with risk for capsule retention should undergo a patency capsule examination or an enterography as a fallback technique before VCE.[12]

The highest yield of positive small bowel studies is probably found in patients with symptoms related to the gut and unequivocally normal evaluations of the upper gastrointestinal tract and colon. No other clinical parameter has been shown to be associated with a positive or negative small bowel study.[19]

Inflammation

The small bowel has a limited number of ways to react to a variety of inflammation agents: edema and swelling of the mucosa, loss of villi, and formation of erosions and ulcers of various depth and extension. Shallow erosions, limited to the inner mucosal layer, usually heal without scars, whereas penetrating ulcers may heal with scar formation and strictures. These complications occur in patients with Crohn's

disease and in those on certain medications, such as NSAIDs and potassium chloride supplements.[23]

VCE is useful in assessing the severity and extent of sprue. Scalloping of the mucosa and villous atrophy (see Fig. 44-8) are observed.[24] VCE is also used to evaluate patients with refractory sprue, ulcerative jejunitis, adenocarcinoma, or lymphoma of the small bowel.

Crohn's Disease

Signs of Crohn's disease evident with VCE include villous denudation, aphthoid ulcerations, or erosions distributed from the pylorus to the distal ileum. These lesions are far more reliably seen on VCE when compared with radiographic methods including CT enteroclysis.[25,26] Crohn's disease of the terminal ileum and the ileocecal valve is better assessed, however, by ileocolonoscopy.[27]

Endoscopy with biopsy plays an integral role in the initial diagnosis of Crohn's disease. Conventional diagnostic modalities may be normal, even in patients with significant symptoms. "New" lesions, compatible with Crohn's disease, may be revealed in 40% to 65% of VCE examinations.[28] In patients with known Crohn's disease, additional lesions not detected by other modalities may be disclosed by VCE in 47% of cases and lesions detected by other modalities may be ruled out in 16% of cases.[29] Strictures are present in as many as 25% of patients with Crohn's disease. VCE is contraindicated in these individuals. Abscess, phlegmon, creeping fat of the mesentery, fistulas, sinus tracts, and mural thickening are better depicted on MRI and multidetector CT than with VCE. VCE and CT/MRI are complementary tools for diagnosing small bowel Crohn's disease, with the former capable of detecting mucosal lesions and the latter, transmural and extraintestinal ones.[30,31]

COST-EFFECTIVENESS

Crohn's disease causes a life-long burden of remissions punctuated by recurrences. The inability of traditional diagnostic methods to image the entire small bowel and the low diagnostic yield of these tests add health care costs, especially when the tests have to be repeated. Published results for work-up of Crohn's disease show unanimously that VCE, when appropriate, has a higher average diagnostic yield, as compared with small bowel radiology and colonoscopy. VCE as a first-line diagnostic procedure has therefore been suggested not only from a payer perspective but also for the benefit of the patient. The idea that disclosure of minute lesions also translates into early disease seems to justify VCE. Earlier diagnosis may also have a significant therapeutic impact through earlier treatment.[32] The detailed exploration of the mucosa by VCE may widen the indications to include documentation of early or failed response to medical treatment.

FUTURE INDICATIONS

Video capsule endoscopy has the potential to significantly impact on the clinical management of patients with Crohn's disease and occult gastrointestinal bleeding.[33-35]

Although conventional endoscopic examinations (i.e., push-enteroscopy, and ileocolonoscopy) are less sensitive for revealing obscure small bowel lesions, these procedures will remain first-line techniques owing to their general availability and means for simultaneous treatment.[35] Sonde enteroscopy as a method for examining the entire small bowel is being replaced by the VCE, whereas virtual enteroscopies based on CT and MRI techniques are still experimental. The hardware and software needed for VCE are undergoing rapid technical improvements that may relegate push-enteroscopy and intraoperative enteroscopy to those cases in which biopsies or therapy are required. At the same time, enteroscopes for total enteroscopy are also being improved and may become more widely available, allowing biopsies and therapy in all segments of the small intestine, without the need for operative intervention.[36] Capsule technique for real-time diagnosis of the small bowel mucosa is soon to be launched. Furthermore, capsules that provide cytologic and chemical sampling of the small bowel are being developed.

SUMMARY

Video capsule endoscopy is a patient-friendly means of reliably detecting gastrointestinal disorders, including occult bleeding, Crohn's disease, and nonsteroidal anti-inflammatory drug–induced enteropathy. Its ability to depict small and early mucosal lesions is unrivalled by any present radiographic technique.[37-41]

References

1. Lewis BS: The history of enteroscopy. Gastrointest Endosc Clin North Am 9:1-11, 1999.
2. Meron G: The development of the swallowable video-capsule (M2A). Gastrointest Endosc 52:817-819, 2000.
3. Swain CP, Gong F, Mills TN: Wireless transmission of a colour television moving image from the stomach using a miniature CCD camera, light source and microwave transmitter. Gut 39:A26, 1996.
4. Swain CP, Gong F, Mills TN: Wireless transmission of a colour television moving image from the stomach using a miniature CCD camera, light source and microwave transmitter. Gastrointest Endosc 45:AB40, 1997.
5. Mosse CA, Swain CP: Technical advances and experimental devices for enteroscopy. Gastrointest Endosc Clin North Am 9:145-161, 1999.
6. Iddan G, Meron G, Glukhovsky A, Swain P: Wireless capsule endoscopy: Brief communications. Nature 405:417, 2000.
7. Swain P: Wireless capsule endoscopy and Crohn's disease. Gut 54:323-326, 2005.
8. de Franchis R, Avgerinos A, Barkin J, et al: ICCE consensus for bowel preparation and prokinetics. Endoscopy 37:1040-1045, 2005.
9. De Leusse A, Landi B, Edery J, et al: Video capsule endoscopy for investigation of obscure gastrointestinal bleeding: Feasibility, results, and interobserver agreement. Endoscopy 37:617-621, 2005.
10. Eliakim R, Sharma VK, Yassin K, et al: A prospective study of the diagnostic accuracy of PillCam ESO esophageal capsule endoscopy versus conventional upper endoscopy in patients with chronic gastroesophageal reflux diseases. J Clin Gastroenterol 39:572-578, 2005.
11. Fireman Z, Eliakim R, Adler S, Scapa E: Capsule endoscopy in real life: A four-centre experience of 160 consecutive patients in Israel. Eur J Gastroenterol Hepatol 16:927-931, 2004.
12. Ell C, Remke S, May A, et al: The first prospective controlled trial comparing wireless capsule endoscopy with push enteroscopy in chronic gastrointestinal bleeding. Endoscopy 34:685-689, 2002.
13. Guilhon de Araujo Sant'Anna AM, Dubois J, Miron MC, Seidman EG: Wireless capsule endoscopy for obscure small-bowel disorders: Final results of the first pediatric controlled trial. Clin Gastroenterol Hepatol 3:264-270, 2005.
14. Arguelles-Arias F, Caunedo A, Romero J, et al: The value of capsule endoscopy in pediatric patients with a suspicion of Crohn's disease. Endoscopy 36:869-873, 2004.
15. Sturniolo GC, Di Leo V, Vettorato MG, D'Inca R: Clinical relevance of small-bowel findings detected by wireless capsule endoscopy. Scand J Gastroenterol 40:725-733, 2005.
16. Bouhnik Y, Bitoun A, Coffin B, et al: Two way push videoenteroscopy in investigation of small bowel disease. Gut 43:280-284, 1998.
17. Mylonaki M, Fritscher-Ravens A, Swain P: Wireless capsule endoscopy: A comparison with push enteroscopy in patients with gastroscopy and colonoscopy negative gastrointestinal bleeding. Gut 52:1122-1126, 2003.
18. Schulmann K, Hollerbach S, Kraus K, et al: Feasibility and diagnostic utility of video capsule endoscopy for the detection of small bowel polyps in patients with hereditary polyposis syndromes. Am J Gastroenterol 100:27-37, 2005.
19. Rex DK, Lappas JC, Maglinte DD, et al: Enteroclysis in the evaluation of suspected small bowel bleeding. Gastroenterology 97:58-60, 1989.
20. Lingenfelser T, Ell C: Lower gastrointestinal bleeding. Best Pract Res Clin Gastroenterol 15:135-153, 2001.
21. Van Gossum A: Obscure digestive bleeding. Best Pract Res Clin Gastroenterol 15:155-174, 2001.
22. Zuckerman GR, Prakash C, Askin MP, Lewis BS: AGA technical review on the evaluation and management of occult and obscure gastrointestinal bleeding. Gastroenterology 119:1431-1438, 2000.
23. Goldstein JL, Eisen GM, Lewis B, et al: Video capsule endoscopy to prospectively assess small bowel injury with celecoxib, naproxen plus omeprazole, and placebo. Clin Gastroenterol Hepatol 3:133-141, 2005.
24. Joyce AM, Burns DL, Marcello PW, et al: Capsule endoscopy findings in celiac disease associated enteropathy–type intestinal T-cell lymphoma. Endoscopy 37:594-596, 2005.
25. Adler SN, Jacob H: Occult inflammatory small-bowel disease: Not so occult anymore. Scand J Gastroenterol 40:360-364, 2005.
26. Eliakim R, Adler SN: Capsule video endoscopy in Crohn's disease—the European experience. Gastrointest Endosc Clin North Am 14:129-137, 2004.
27. Voderholzer WA, Beinhoelzl J, Rogalla P, et al: Small bowel involvement in Crohn's disease: A prospective comparison of wireless capsule endoscopy and computed tomography enteroclysis. Gut 54:369-373, 2005.
28. Ge ZZ, Hu YB, Xiao SD: Capsule endoscopy in diagnosis of small bowel Crohn's disease. World J Gastroenterol 10:1349-1352, 2004.
29. Eliakim R, Fischer D, Suissa A, et al: Wireless capsule video endoscopy is a superior diagnostic tool in comparison to barium follow-through and computerized tomography in patients with suspected Crohn's disease. Eur J Gastroenterol Hepatol 15:363-367, 2003.
30. Albert JG, Martiny F, Krummenerl A, et al: Diagnosis of small bowel Crohn's disease: A prospective comparison of capsule endoscopy with magnetic resonance imaging and fluoroscopic enteroclysis. Gut, Epub July 14, 2005.

31. Eliakim R, Suissa A, Yassin K, et al: Wireless capsule video endoscopy compared to barium follow-through and computerised tomography in patients with suspected Crohn's disease—final report. Dig Liver Dis 36:519-522, 2004.

32. Goldfarb NI, Pizzi LT, Fuhr JP Jr, et al: Diagnosing Crohn's disease: An economic analysis comparing wireless capsule endoscopy with traditional diagnostic procedures. Dis Manag 7:292-304, 2004.

33. Malik A, Lukaszewski K, Caroline D, et al: A retrospective review of enteroclysis in patients with obscure gastrointestinal bleeding and chronic abdominal pain of undetermined etiology. Dig Dis Sci 50:649-655, 2005.

34. Adler DG, Knipschield M, Gostout C: A prospective comparison of capsule endoscopy and push enteroscopy in patients with GI bleeding of obscure origin. Gastrointest Endosc 59:492-498, 2004.

35. Rossini FP, Pennazio M: Small-bowel endoscopy. Endoscopy 32:138-145, 2000.

36. Lee SD, Cohen RD: Endoscopy of the small bowel in inflammatory bowel disease. Gastrointest Endosc Clin North Am 12:485-493, 2002.

37. Eliakim R: Wireless capsule video endoscopy: Three years of experience. World J Gastroenterol 10:1238-1239, 2004.

38. Hara AK, Leighton JA, Sharma VK, et al: Imaging of small bowel disease: Comparison of capsule endoscopy, standard endoscopy, barium examination, and CT. RadioGraphics 25:697-711, 2005.

39. Hara AK, Leighton JA, Heigh RI, et al: Crohn disease of the small bowel: Preliminary comparison among CT enterography, capsule endoscopy, small-bowel follow-through, and ileoscopy. Radiology 238:128-134, 2006.

40. Carey EJ, Leighton JA, Heigh RI, et al: A single-center experience of 260 consecutive patients undergoing capsule endoscopy for obscure gastrointestinal bleeding. Am J Gastroenterol 102:89-95, 2007.

41. Eliakim R: The impact of capsule endoscopy on Crohn's disease. Dig Liver Dis 39:1545-1546, 2007.

Crohn's Disease of the Small Bowel

Richard M. Gore, MD • Gabriele Masselli, MD • Dina F. Caroline, MD, PhD

Crohn's disease is an idiopathic inflammatory disease that can affect any part of the gastrointestinal tract from the mouth to the anus. The small bowel is the major site of involvement. With the exception of malignant neoplasms, Crohn's disease can be the most devastating disease to involve the gastrointestinal tract. It has a worldwide distribution but is most common in northern Europe, North America, and Japan. Prevalence has increased, mostly in younger age groups, with a peak age between 15 and 25 years.[1-3] What was formerly believed to be a second incidence peak in older patients is now thought to have been caused primarily by ischemic colitis. Both genders are equally affected. A familial tendency has frequently been described.[1-3]

The small bowel is involved by Crohn's disease in 80% of patients, with the terminal ileum by far the most common location. Disease is confined to the small bowel in 30% of patients and affects the colon together with the small bowel in 50% of patients. Isolated involvement of the colon occurs in 15% to 20%, and isolated perianal disease occurs in 2% to 3%.[4] Upper gastrointestinal tract involvement is recognized

with increasing frequency but almost invariably occurs with small bowel or colonic disease. The gastric and duodenal manifestations of Crohn's disease are discussed in Chapter 34, and the colonic features of this disease are discussed in Chapter 61.

CLINICAL CONSIDERATIONS

Although the focus of this chapter is on Crohn's disease of the small bowel, differences in presentation from colonic disease must be mentioned. Patients with colonic Crohn's disease are more likely to present with blood loss, perianal disease, toxic megacolon, and extraintestinal complications. Crohn's disease in the small bowel has a slightly better prognosis, although there are more likely to be complications such as abscesses, fistulas, and obstruction. Abdominal pain, mild diarrhea, weight loss, and pyrexia are common clinical findings. Other patients may present with a right lower quadrant mass, representing the diseased ileum or cecum. Delays of 3 to 4 years have been reported between the onset of often subtle symptoms and the diagnosis of Crohn's disease in the small bowel.[4]

Many factors contribute to the development of diarrhea in patients with Crohn's disease. An inflamed bowel mucosa causes increased secretion of fluid and electrolytes. Extensive terminal ileal disease or resection impairs bile salt reabsorption, leading to malabsorption of fat and fat-soluble vitamins. Bacterial overgrowth secondary to strictures, fistulas to colon, adhesions, aneurysmal dilation, or bypassed loops can also cause diarrhea. The combination of decreased food absorption and intermittent obstruction may lead to significant weight loss in these patients.[4,5]

DIAGNOSTIC TOOLS

There are a large number of examinations available for diagnosing, staging, and following Crohn's disease of the small bowel. These include ileocolonoscopy with direct inspection of the terminal ileum, video capsule endoscopy, conventional small bowel follow-through, conventional enteroclysis, multidetector-row CT (MDCT), MDCT enteroclysis, MDCT enterography, ultrasonography, MRI, and MR enteroclysis. These studies are used:

- To demonstrate the early changes of Crohn's disease.
- To depict the full extent of involvement and the possible presence of skip lesions if surgery is contemplated.
- To determine the cause of any clinical deterioration in previously stable patients with Crohn's disease.
- To distinguish between spasm, active stenotic disease, and a fibrous stricture.
- To investigate postoperative complications of Crohn's disease.
- To definitively rule out the presence of Crohn's disease in the small bowel.

CLASSIFICATION AND THERAPY

Crohn's disease is a chronic relapsing disease, usually characterized by periods of symptom exacerbation alternating with periods of clinical remission. Its variable behavior has led to the following classification system[6]: active inflammatory; fibrostenotic; fistulizing/perforating; or reparative/regenerative (Table 45-1). Each of these subtypes has different therapeutic and prognostic implications. Also, different phases of the disease may be present within different segments of small bowel in the same patient.

Medications useful in the active inflammatory subtype of Crohn's disease include 5-aminosalicylate-based drugs, corticosteroid based drugs, and antibiotics (e.g., metronidazole, ciprofloxacin). Second-line medications are immunosuppressive agents such as azathioprine, 6-mercaptopurine, and methotrexate.[7,8] Recently, targeted monoclonal antibodies such as infliximab, which targets human tumor necrosis factor-β, and natalizumab, which targets β_4 integrin, a leukocyte adhesion molecule, have become available.[8] These drugs are very expensive and have complications. This arsenal of medications has prompted the need for noninvasive, reproducible, and objective measurements of Crohn's disease activity.

The fistulizing/perforating type requires antibiotics to treat the active infection, and the monoclonal antibodies have proven effective in patients with refractory fistulas and sinus tracts. Percutaneous abscess drainage is a suitable means of treating Crohn's disease–related abscesses. The fibrostenotic

Table 45-1

Radiologic Classification of Crohn's Disease of the Small Bowel

Active Inflammatory Subtype
Minimal changes
Superficial ulcerations (aphthae)
Minimal fold thickening or distortion (edema)
Severe changes
Deep ulcers, cobblestone mucosa
Marked wall thickening due to transmural inflammation (mural stratification and target sign)
Obstruction secondary to spasm
Comb sign

Fibrostenotic Subtype
Minimal stenosis
Minimal decrease in luminal diameter, mild prestenotic dilatation
Minimal wall thickening, no bowel wall edema
Severe stenosis
Marked decrease in luminal diameter with obvious prestenotic dilatation
Marked wall thickening with loss of mural stratification

Fistulizing/Perforating Subtype
Deep fissuring ulcers, sinus tracts
Fistulas to adjacent organs, bowel, skin
Associated inflammatory mass

Reparative/Regenerative Subtype
Mucosal atrophy
Regenerative polyps
Minimal decrease in lumen diameter—no mural edema

From Maglinte DDT, Gourtsoyiannis N, Rex D, et al: Classification of small bowel Crohn's subtypes based on multimodality imaging. Radiol Clin North Am 41:285-303, 2003.

subtype of Crohn's disease may need strictureplasty or bowel resection because small bowel obstruction is the major clinical manifestation of this type. The reparative type of Crohn's disease requires maintenance medication.[9]

ILEOCOLONOSCOPY AND VIDEO CAPSULE ENDOSCOPY

Ileocolonoscopy (Figs. 45-1 and 45-2) allows accurate diagnosis of Crohn's disease of the colon and terminal ileum. It provides assessment of disease activity and consequences of inflammation, including strictures, mass lesions, bleeding, and the development of dysplasia or malignancy.

Video capsule endoscopy is a new means of directly inspecting the entire length of the small bowel. It employs an ingested sealed capsule that measures 27 mm in length and 11 mm in width. The camera within the capsule, which also contains a light source, takes two photographs at eight times magnification every second and runs on electricity supplied by onboard batteries. During the typical small bowel examination, an average of about 55,000 photographs are taken. The capsule is propelled through the gastrointestinal tract by peristalsis. The images are transmitted in radiofrequency signals to, and stored on, a recorder device placed in a belt worn by the patient throughout the day of the procedure. The capsule is disposable and is not recovered after the test. At the end of the study, the recorder device is retrieved and the images obtained are downloaded onto a computer. The computer

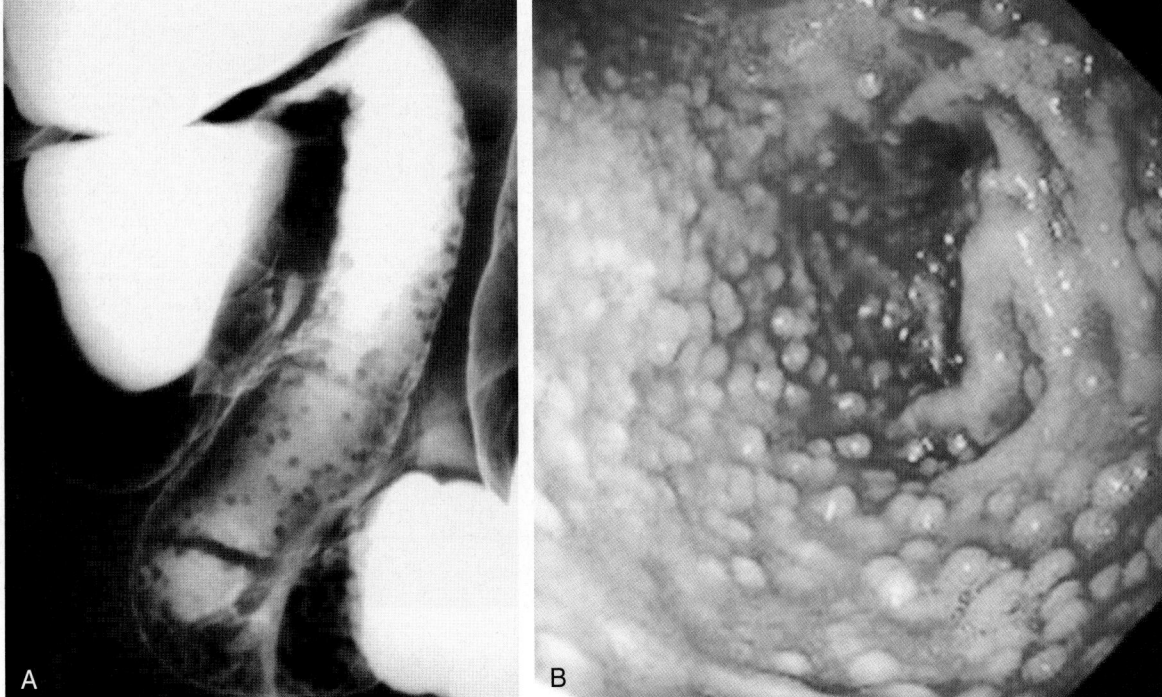

Figure 45-1. Early active inflammatory Crohn's diseases: enlarged lymphoid follicles. A. Double-contrast barium enema examination with reflux into the terminal ileum shows prominent lymphoid follicles. This is a nonspecific finding that can be found in a variety of infectious, inflammatory, immunologic, and neoplastic disease. **B.** Image from an ileocolonoscopy study shows multiple lymphoid follicles in this patient with early Crohn's disease.

generates a video that is then reviewed for relevant pathology.[10] This technique is discussed in greater detail in Chapter 44.

Early studies have shown video capsule endoscopy (see Fig. 45-2B) to be the most sensitive means of diagnosing non-stricturing Crohn's disease.[11-16] The presence of stricture is a contraindication to this procedure.

BARIUM CONTRAST EXAMINATIONS

Active Inflammatory Disease

Early Active Inflammatory Disease

The pathologic and radiologic findings correlate well in early Crohn's disease.[17-23] The earliest histologic changes consist of hyperplasia of lymphoid tissue (see Fig. 45-1A) and obstructive lymphedema in the submucosa. Because the submucosa extends into the core of mucosal folds, the folds may thicken at this stage in a smooth, symmetric manner.

Hyperplasia of lymphoid follicles (see Fig. 45-1) in the lamina propria can be associated with shallow, 1- to 3-mm mucosal erosions surrounded by a small halo of edema, also known as *aphthoid ulcers* (see Fig. 45-2).[24-27]

Intermediate Active Inflammatory Disease

As the disease gradually extends transmurally, further changes take place in the mucosa and submucosa. Progressive submucosal edema may cause the base of the folds to widen until some folds are partially or completely obliterated. This process is similar to the thumbprinting that occurs in patients

with bowel ischemia. In patients with ischemia, however, the fold abnormalities change over a period of days to weeks, whereas in patients with Crohn's disease, the fold abnormalities persist and are usually associated with changes of more advanced Crohn's disease elsewhere in the small bowel. The mucosal inflammatory infiltrate tends to vary focally in intensity. This infiltrate, together with patchy submucosal fibrosis, leads to distortion and interruption of folds.[24-28]

Some aphthoid ulcers may enlarge and deepen, producing a stellate or rose thorn appearance. Other aphthoid ulcers may fuse with adjacent ulcers, producing crescentic or linear shapes. A typical finding is that of a long, linear ulcer on the mesenteric border, which may be accentuated by a parallel radiolucency caused by fusion of thickened transaxially oriented folds. The mesenteric border ulcer is associated with thickening, sclerosis, and retraction of the adjacent mesentery and of the straightened mesenteric border of the involved bowel. At the same time, the unaffected, redundant antimesenteric border becomes pleated or sacculated.

An inflammatory cellular infiltrate with focally pronounced edema and granulation tissue can give rise to localized mucosal elevations or inflammatory polyps. These lesions are common in the colon but infrequent in the small bowel. Inflammatory polyps usually occur in small numbers in an area of mucosa that is denuded of folds. Occasionally, a bowel segment contains many inflammatory polyps (up to 1 cm in diameter), separated from one another by curving lines of barium occupying the crevices between the elevations. When seen in profile, the polyps appear as notches demarcated by protrusions of barium. The diameter of such bowel segments is not reduced. This is called the *nodular pattern* of Crohn's disease to

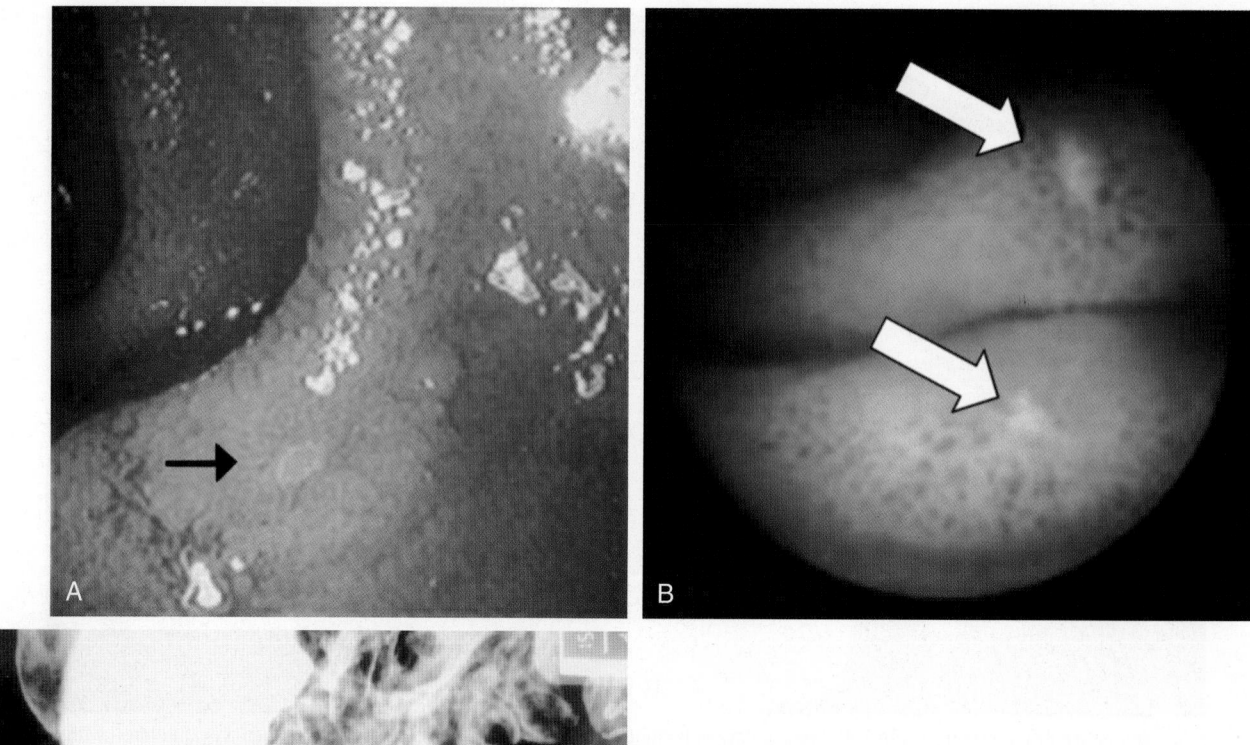

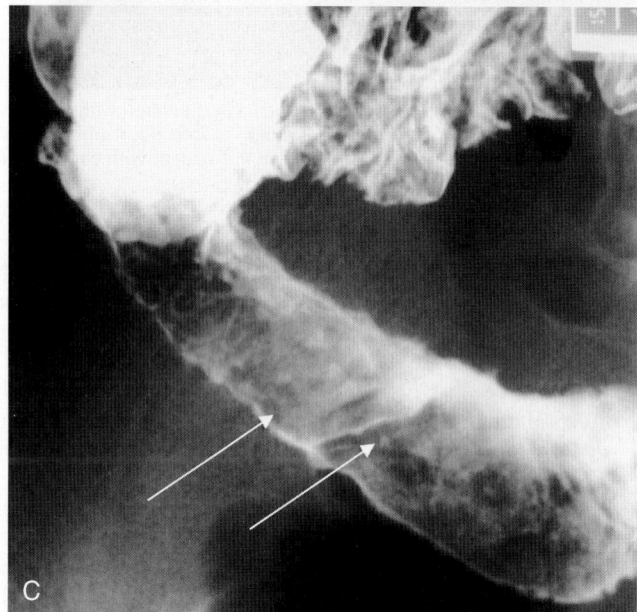

Figure 45-2. Early active inflammatory Crohn's disease: aphthoid ulcerations. A. Image of the terminal ileum obtained during ileocolonoscopy demonstrates an aphthoid ulcer (*arrow*). **B.** Small bowel video capsule study shows two aphthoid ulcerations (*arrows*) in the distal ileum. **C.** Double-contrast image of the terminal ileum shows multiple aphthoid ulcerations (*arrows*).

underscore its essential difference from the ulceronodular or "cobblestone" pattern (Fig. 45-3) of advanced, fissuring, ulcer-related Crohn's disease.[24-28]

Advanced Active Inflammatory Disease

In advanced Crohn's disease, the process has extended transmurally to the serosa and beyond. Deep linear clefts of ulceration, or fissures, are typical of this stage of the disease (Fig. 45-4). Islands of surviving mucosa surrounded by extensive ulceration give the appearance of elevations above the ulcerated background. These islands of mucosa are therefore known as *pseudopolyps.* The deep fissures characteristic of this advanced stage may be manifested by a combination of axial and transaxial fissuring, which separates the pseudopolyps

from one another. This finding is always associated with lumen reduction and is referred to as the *ulceronodular* or *cobblestone* pattern of advanced Crohn's disease (see Fig. 45-3).[24-28] This pattern should not be confused with the nodular pattern of less advanced Crohn's disease.

Changes associated with linear mesenteric ulceration advance in a caudad direction as the disease progresses. Antimesenteric redundancy of the opposite bowel wall gradually disappears as it is incorporated in the transaxial extension of ulcerated Crohn's disease (Fig. 45-5). The bowel wall is now thickened by a combination of fibrosis and inflammatory infiltrate. Another feature of transmural disease is the so-called fat wrapping that occurs as hypertrophied subperitoneum is tethered toward the bowel wall by mesenteric perivascular fibrosis.[28]

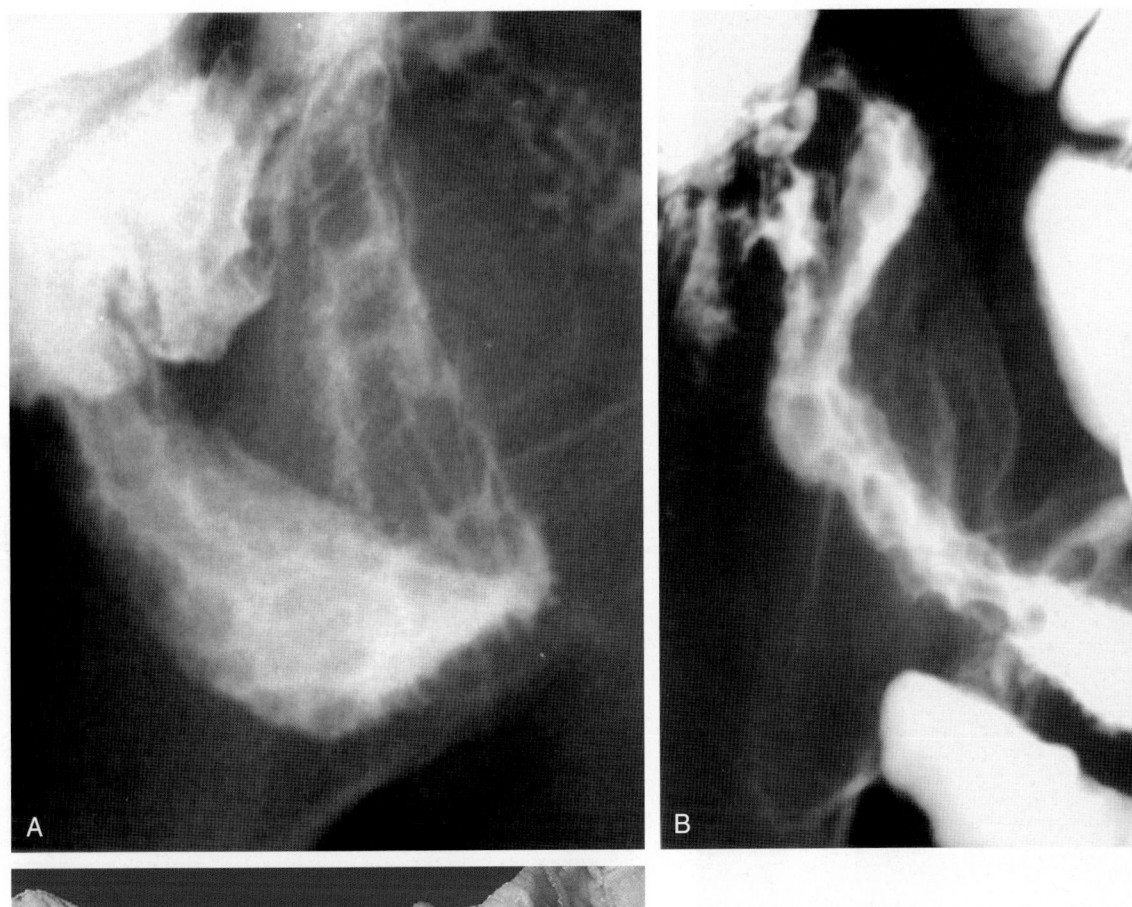

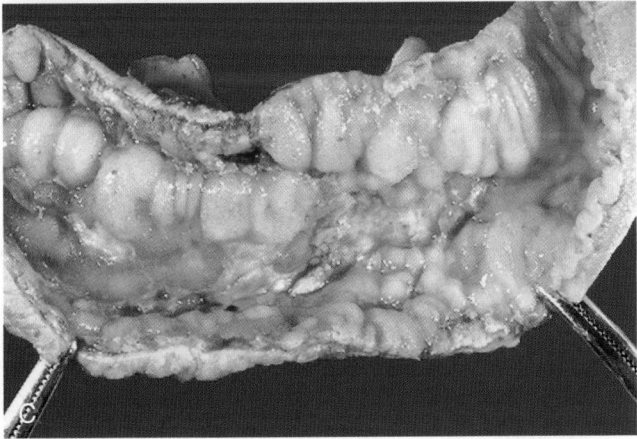

Figure 45-3. Active inflammatory Crohn's disease: cobblestone mucosa. A and **B.** Multiple transverse and longitudinal ulcerations of the terminal ileum are identified on conventional small bowel examinations performed in these two different patients with Crohn's disease. **C.** Specimen showing cobblestone mucosa.

Fibrostenotic Disease

The strictures (Figs. 45-6 and 45-7) of small bowel Crohn's disease are caused by collagen deposition, predominantly in the submucosa. These strictures are an important cause of small bowel obstruction, often necessitating surgery. Strictures or stricture-like findings are reported in 21% of patients with small bowel Crohn's disease.[4,27] MDCT, MRI, CT enterography, CT enteroclysis, and MR enteroclysis are valuable techniques for differentiating fibrotic strictures from lumen narrowing by spasm or active ulcerated stenotic disease. Obstruction by a fibrous stricture may require surgery, whenever possible consisting of strictureplasty to avoid bowel resection.[28] Some patients with Crohn's disease may develop high-

grade small bowel obstruction; this complication is reliably documented by MDCT and MR.

Other patients with Crohn's disease may have multiple strictures, representing advanced skip lesions. Stasis related to strictures can be associated with bacterial overgrowth. This is especially true in patients who develop aneurysmal dilation of the small bowel (see Fig. 45-7), usually between two strictures. Strictures are generally well shown by barium study.

Resection of bowel in patients with Crohn's disease is followed by a high frequency (85%) of disease recurrence. Indeed, recurrent inflammation has been detected within 8 days of surgery, provided that exposure to the fecal stream had been reestablished. Multiple resections have made Crohn's

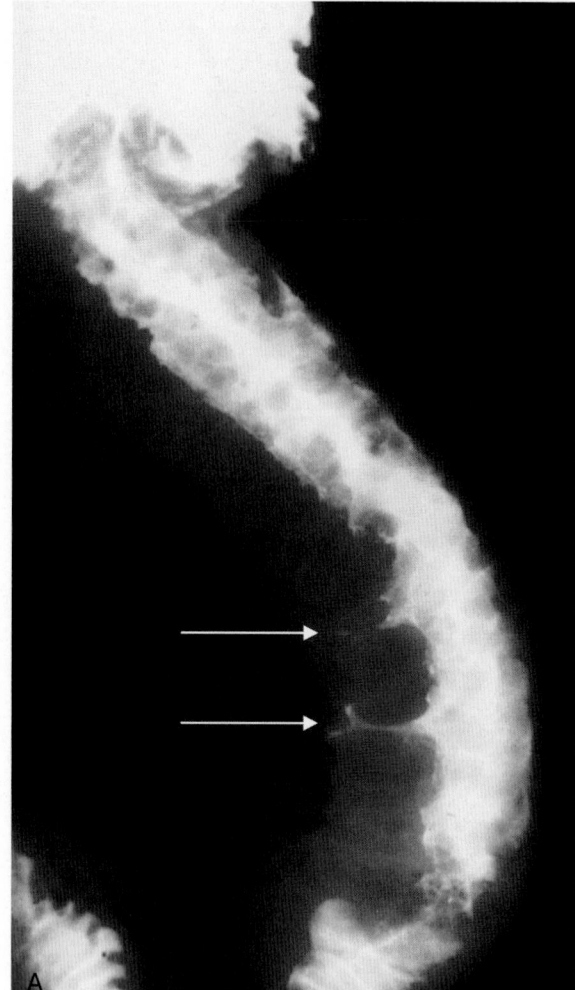

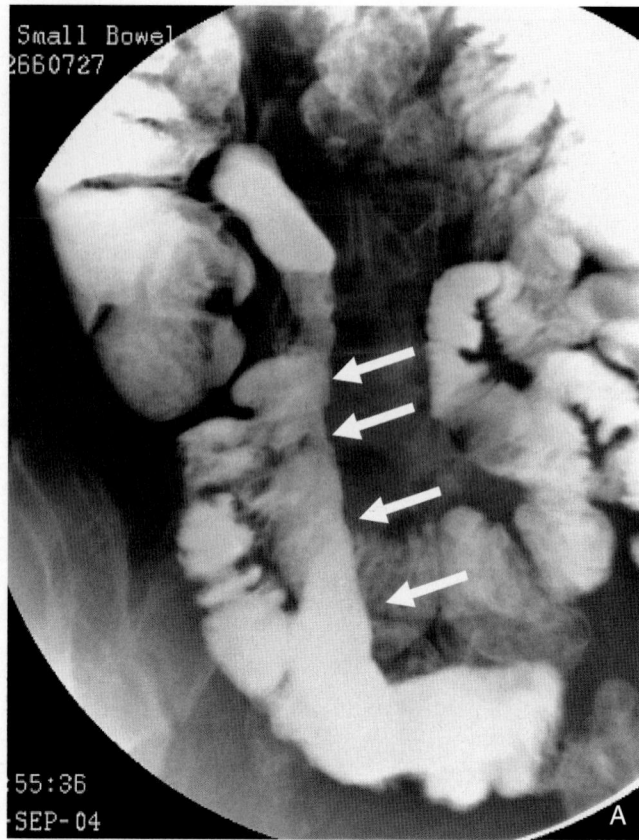

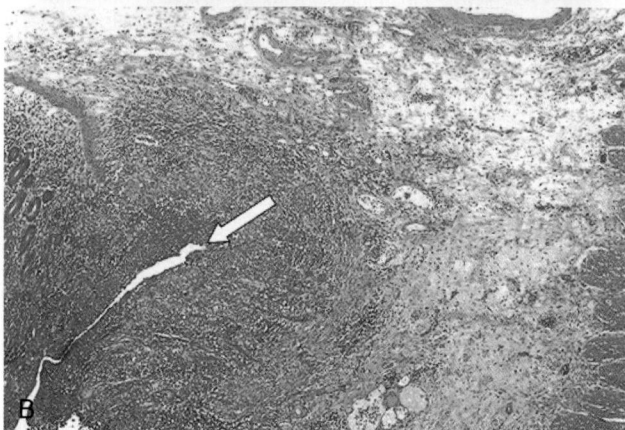

Figure 45-4. Deep ulcerations of fistulizing/perforating Crohn's disease. A. Specimen radiograph shows two deep ulcerations (*arrows*) penetrating into the fat of the small bowel mesentery. **B.** A fissuring ulcer (*arrow*) is identified on this pathologic image.

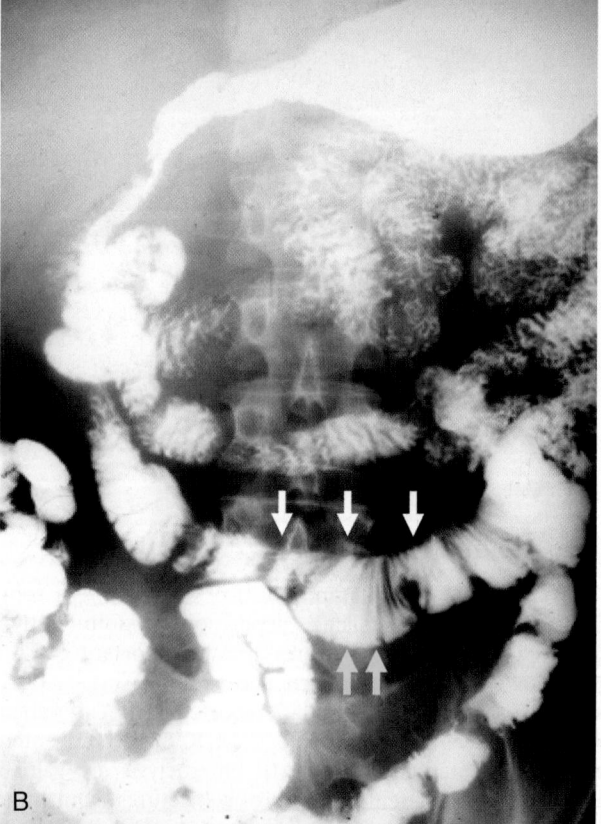

Figure 45-5. Sacculations in Crohn's disease. A. There is straightening of the mesenteric border (*arrows*) of the terminal ileum due to fibrofatty proliferation of the mesentery. **B.** Multiple segments of small bowel show straightening and shortening of the mesenteric border (*white arrows*) with a redundant antimesenteric border forming sacculations (*yellow arrows*).

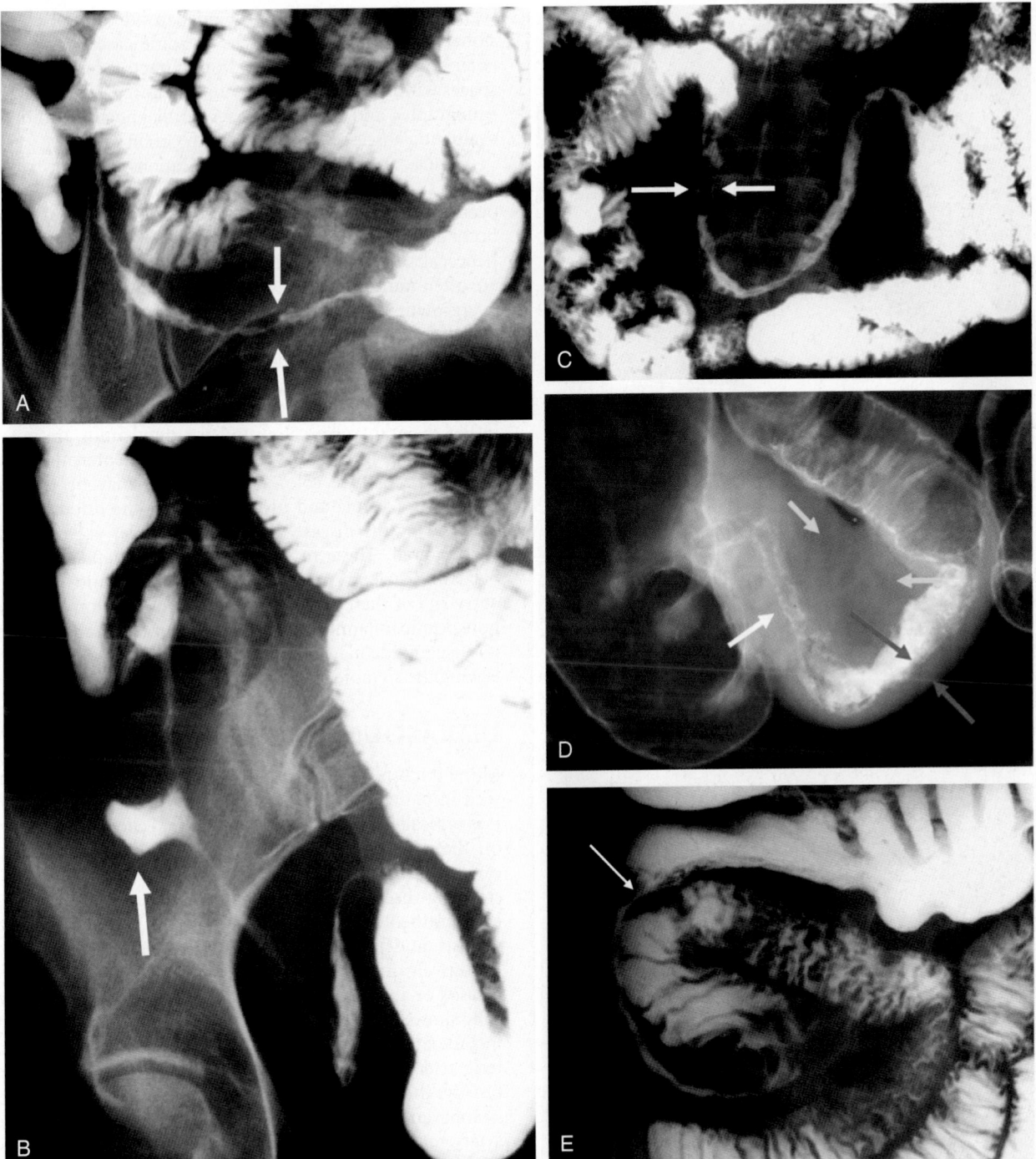

Figure 45-6. Fibrostenotic Crohn's disease. These four patients demonstrate the "string sign" of Crohn's disease with narrowing and rigidity of the involved segments due to cicatrizing Crohn's disease. **A.** The terminal ileum is narrowed (*arrows*) and there is minimal proximal dilation. **B.** There is a sacculation (*arrow*) identified along the antimesenteric border of this very narrowed ileum. **C.** A segment of marked luminal narrowing (*arrows*) is identified in the distal jejunum. **D.** Specimen radiograph shows narrowing of the lumen of the terminal ileum (*white arrow*) associated with mural thickening (*red arrows*). Note the "creeping fat" (*yellow arrows*) on the mesenteric size of the distal ileum. **E.** Recurrent, stricturing Crohn's disease is evident on both sides of the ileocolic anastomosis (*arrow*).

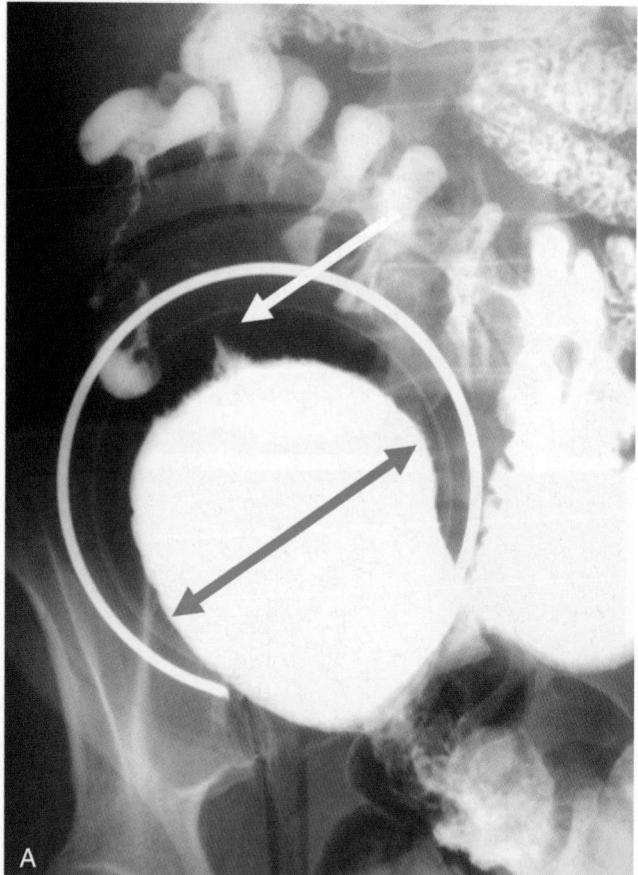

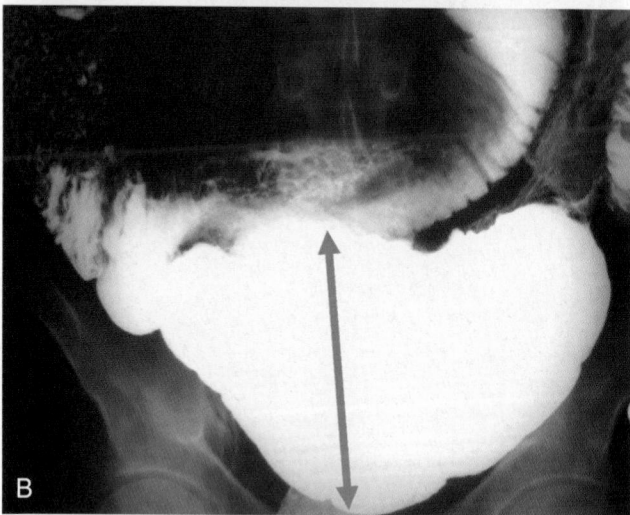

Figure 45-7. Aneurysmal dilation of fibrostenotic small bowel in Crohn's disease. A. There is segmental marked dilation (*red arrow*) of a segment of the terminal ileum due to a distal stricture (*white arrow*). **B.** There is a long segment of aneurysmal dilation (*red arrow*) of distal ileum located between two strictures.

disease of the small bowel a major cause of the short bowel syndrome.[4,27]

Fistulizing/Perforating Disease

Abscesses develop in some 20% of patients with Crohn's disease, and most can be treated with percutaneous drainage.[4] Inflammatory lesions may remain closely related to a diseased segment of bowel or may extend beyond the bowel, occasionally into the psoas muscle. In some cases, barium may enter an abscess cavity, a collection of tracts, or multiple small spaces within an inflammatory mass. However, MDCT, ultrasonography, and MRI are preferred diagnostic methods for evaluating abscesses in patients with Crohn's disease.

Fistulas are abnormal communications between two epithelial surfaces or an epithelial surface and the skin, which occur in 6% to 33% of patients with Crohn's disease.[4] Fistulas occur as a result of transmural extension of disease (Fig. 45-8). Ileocecal and enteroenteric fistulas are the most common and are often multiple. An enterocolic fistula may lead to bacterial overgrowth and is one of the causes of malabsorption associated with Crohn's disease. Enterocutaneous fistulas can be well shown by barium studies, MDCT, and MRI.

Because the attachment of the transverse mesocolon crosses the mid-descending duodenum, Crohn's-related fistulas between the transverse colon and the duodenum are not unusual. Recurrent Crohn's disease in the neoterminal ileum after ileotransverse colonic anastomosis may be associated with such a fistula and invariably leaves the duodenum uninvolved by the disease. Ileosigmoid fistulas are more often encountered. These fistulas may serve a useful purpose by bypassing strictures in the ileocecal area. In most cases, the entry site of these fistulas into the sigmoid colon shows only nonspecific inflammatory changes. If surgery is contemplated, it is usually adequate to resect the diseased ileum and stricture, leaving the sigmoid colon intact.[4]

ULTRASOUND EXAMINATIONS

Mural thickening (Fig. 45-9) is the most common abnormality seen in patients with Crohn's disease of the small bowel.[29-47] It is typically concentric, and the mural echogenicity depends on the degree of inflammatory infiltration and fibrosis. In early acute disease, mural stratification is retained. With long-standing disease, a target or pseudokidney appearance may be identified. In patients with "burned out," long-standing disease, fat deposition in the submucosa may be present.

Actively inflamed gut appears rigid and fixed with decreased or absent peristalsis.[29-47] Color Doppler imaging typically shows hyperemia. Findings on spectral Doppler analysis include increased superior mesenteric and/or inferior mesenteric artery blood flow, increased pulsatility index, decreased resistive index, and increased portal vein velocity.[29-47] Increased systolic and diastolic flow through the superior mesenteric artery may also be seen attesting to disease activity. Creeping fat of the mesentery manifests as a uniform echogenic halo around the mesenteric border of the encased gut. As on barium study, MDCT, and MRI, this abnormal fat causes separation of bowel loops.

Prominent lymph nodes are seen in most patients with the active inflammatory phase of Crohn's disease. These perienteric lymph nodes, which are located in the subperitoneal space of the small bowel mesentery, present as focal hypoechoic masses that are spherical and have lost their normal echogenic streak emanating from the nodal hilum. These nodes are typically hyperemic, moderate in size, and tender. Abnormal lymph nodes are not commonly seen in quiescent Crohn's disease.[29-47]

Crohn's disease strictures show mural thickening of the gut with the luminal surfaces of the involved segments in

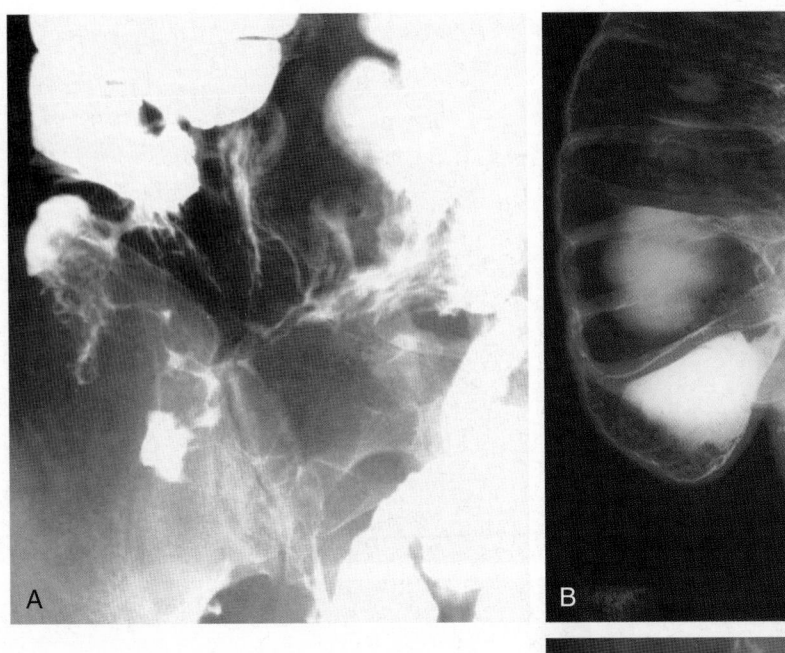
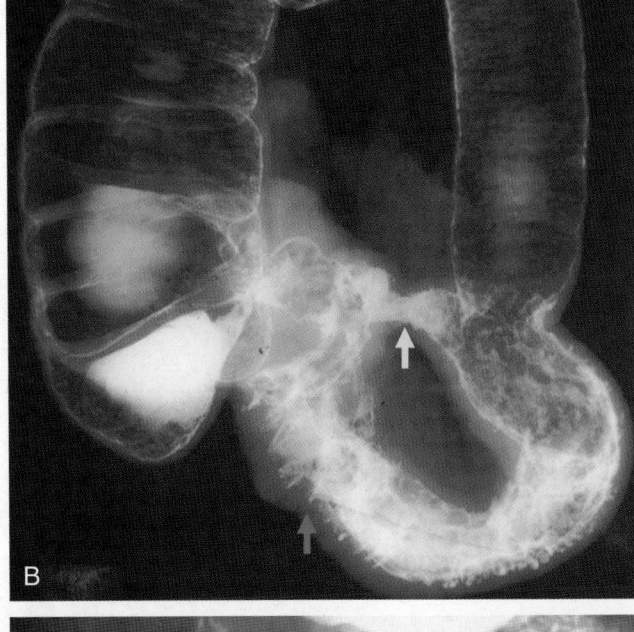
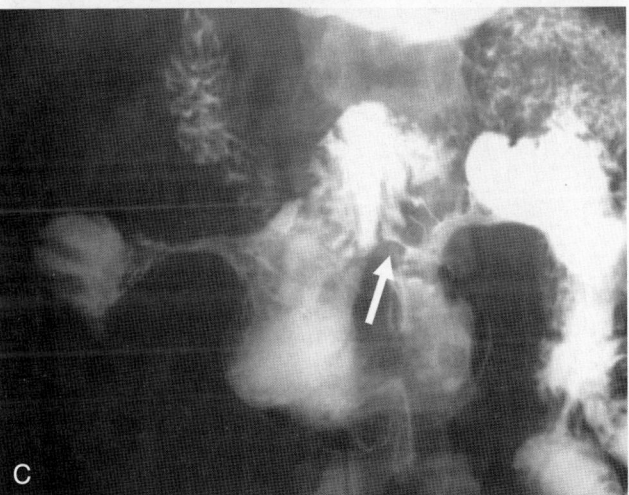

Figure 45-8. Fistulizing/perforating Crohn's disease.
A. Multiple ileocolic and ileoileal fistula are shown on this small bowel series. **B.** Specimen radiograph shows an ileoileal fistula (*arrow*). Note the cobblestone mucosa and deep ulcerations (*red arrow*) associated with mural thickening. **C.** Fistula between the proximal small bowel and colon (*arrow*) are demonstrated on this radiograph.

apposition (Fig. 45-10). The lumen may appear as a narrow linear echogenic central region within the thickened segment of small bowel. Dilated, hyperperistaltic segments can be seen proximal to the strictured segments. Aneurysmal dilatation and sacculation may be seen proximal to the involved segments.

Fistula appear as linear bands of varying echogenicity (Fig. 45-11) extending from the gut to the bladder, other segment of bowel, or bladder. Gas within the fistula will appear echogenic and may show the "ring-down" artifact. An empty or partially closed tract will appear as a hypoechoic segment of bowel, or bladder. Abscesses on ultrasound manifest as a fluid-filled or complex mass that may contain gas.[29-47]

MAGNETIC RESONANCE IMAGING

Magnetic resonance imaging has become a well-established technique in evaluating patients with known or suspected Crohn's disease by virtue of its ability to help confirm the diagnosis; localize lesions; assess their severity, extent, and inflammatory activity; and identify extraintestinal complica-

tions that may require surgical intervention.[48-65] MR enteroclysis is an emerging diagnostic tool that combines the advantages of conventional enteroclysis and MRI.

Technique

Adequate distention of the bowel lumen is very important in MRI because collapsed bowel loops can hide lesions or mimic pathology. Different methods have been used to achieve adequate distention. MR enteroclysis provides distention of the entire small bowel, visualizes mucosal abnormalities, and obtains functional information about small bowel mobility.[48-65]

T2-weighted half-Fourier rapid acquisition with relaxation enhancement (RARE) or half-Fourier acquisition single-shot turbo spin-echo (HASTE) and T1-weighted gadolinium-enhanced spoiled gradient-echo (SGE) are important sequences in evaluating the location, extent, and severity of Crohn's disease.[48-65]

Gadolinium-enhanced SGE sequences are very effective at demonstrating severity of inflammatory changes and length of diseased bowel. The lack of magnetic susceptibility and

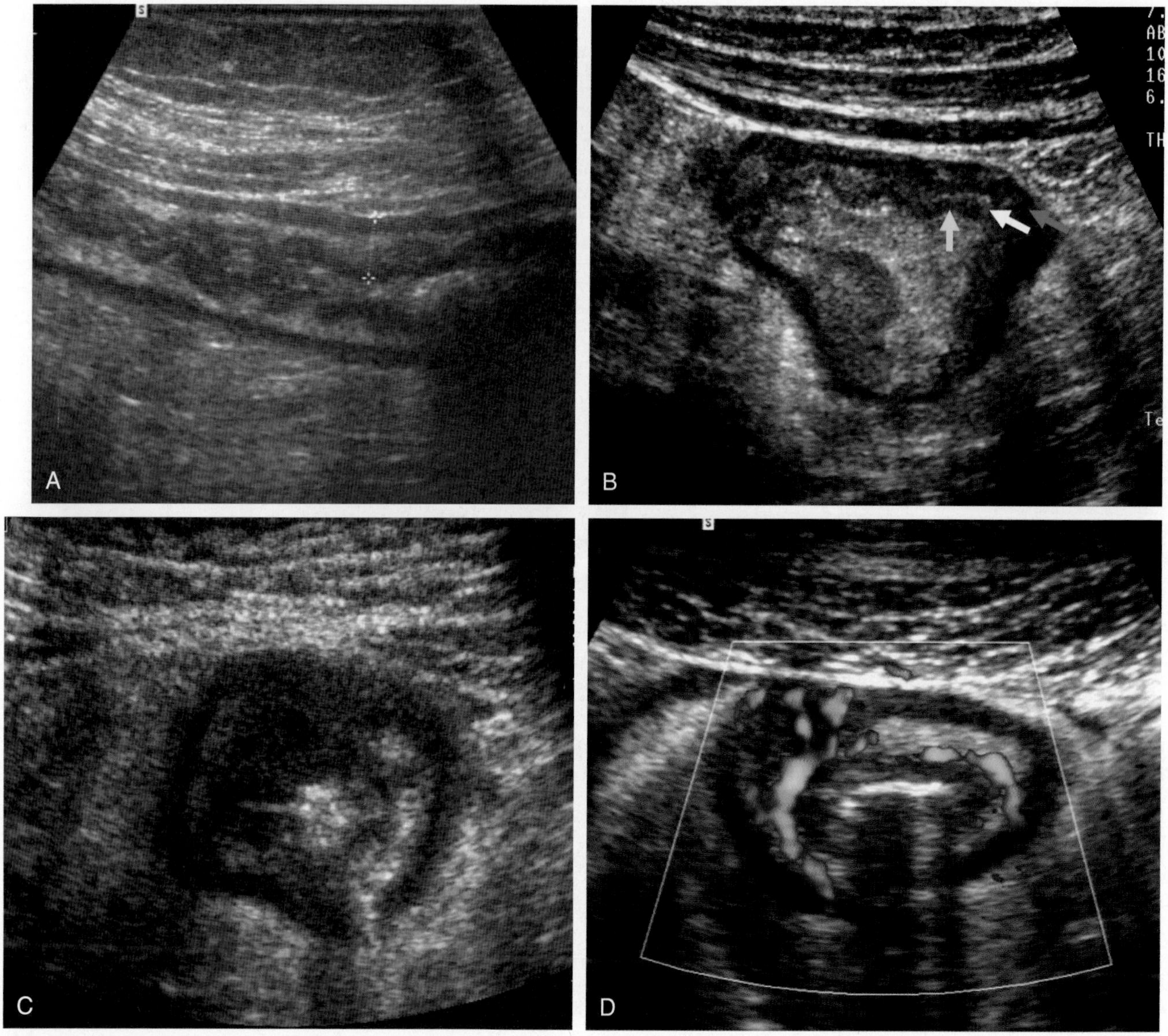

Figure 45-9. Crohn's disease: sonographic features. A. Mural thickening is the sonographic hallmark of Crohn's disease. **B.** In acute disease, mural stratification is maintained. Yellow arrow, mucosa-muscularis mucosae; white arrow, submucosa; red arrow, muscularis mucosae. **C.** In chronic Crohn's disease, mural stratification is lost. **D.** The density of vessels seen on color flow Doppler ultrasound correlates with the degree of disease activity. (Courtesy of Dr. Pierre-Jean Valette, Lyons, France.)

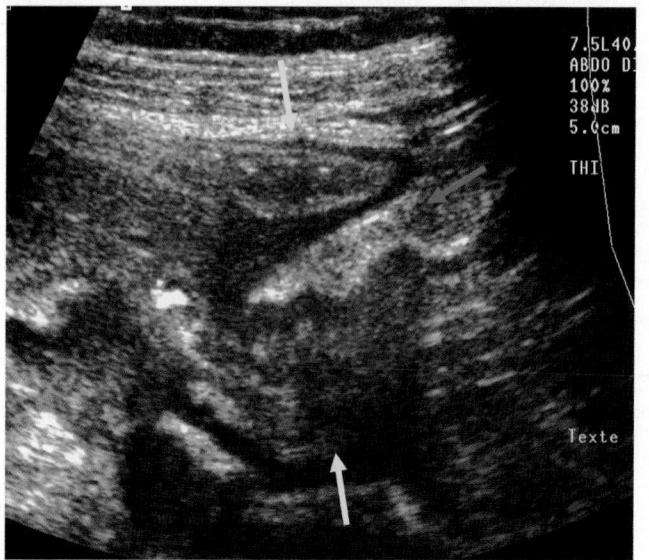

Figure 45-10. Fibrostenosing Crohn's disease: sonographic features. Marked thickening of a segment of ileum (*yellow arrows*) is identified causing dilation of the proximal small bowel (*red arrow*). (Courtesy of Dr. Pierre-Jean Valette, Lyons, France.)

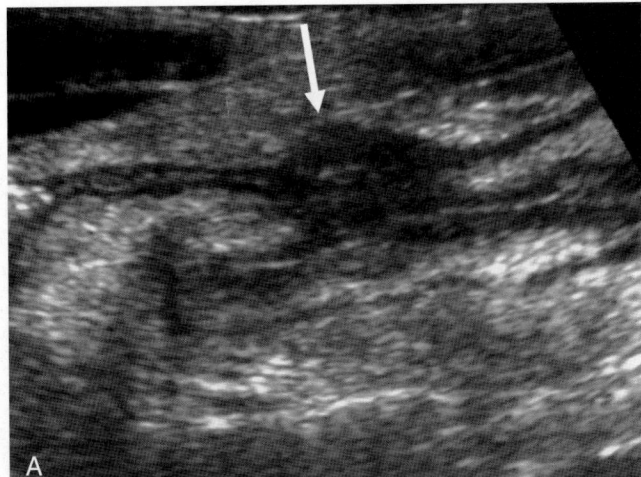

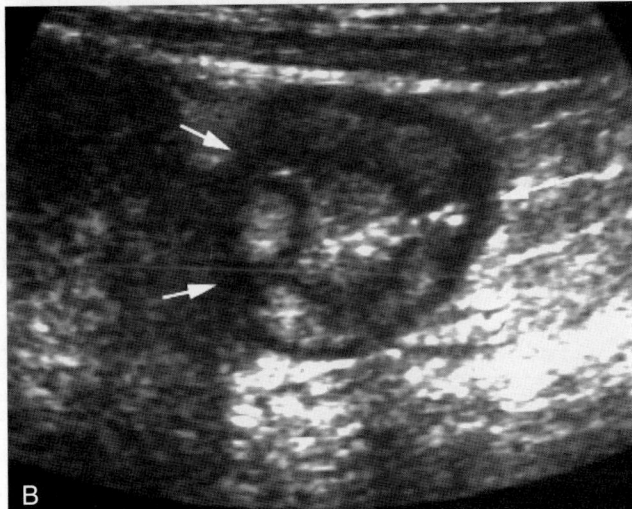

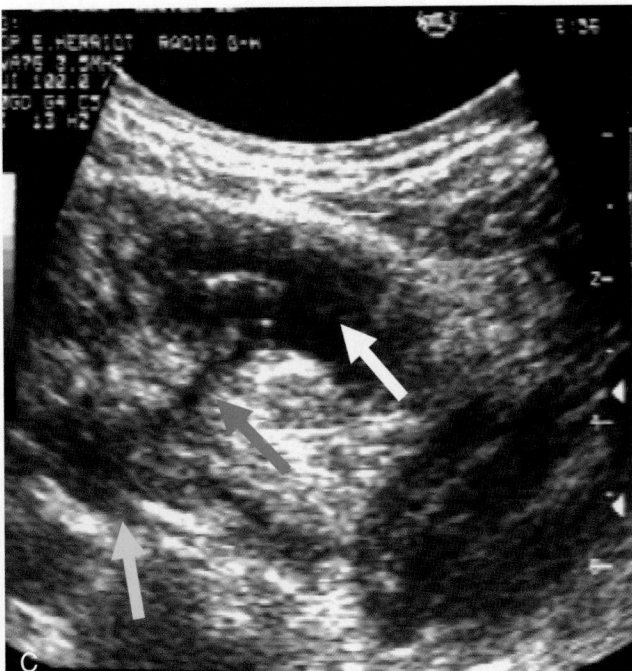

Figure 45-11. Fistulizing/perforating subtype Crohn's disease: deep ulcerations. An affected segment scanned longitudinally (**A**) and axially (**B**) shows mural thickening with deep ulcerations (*arrows*) and lumen stenosis. **C.** A fistula (*red arrow*) is seen extending from a diseased segment of ileum (*white arrow*) to a small abscess cavity (*yellow*). (Courtesy of Dr. Pierre-Jean Valette, Lyons, France.)

bowel artifacts theoretically make the HASTE sequence ideal for imaging bowel.[48-65]

The true-FISP (fast imaging with steady-state precision) sequence is particularly good for obtaining information about mural and extraintestinal complications; mural ulcers and mesenteries are very well visualized and lymph nodes are very conspicuous with this technique. The black boundary artifact encountered with the true-FISP sequence at fat/water interfaces may hamper the perception of subtle thickening of the bowel wall.[48-65]

Mucosal Abnormalities

Images achieved with MR enteroclysis provide sufficient resolution to detect early lesions of Crohn's disease, such as blunting, flattening, thickening, distortion of small bowel folds, mucosal nodularity, and aphthous-type ulcers (Fig. 45-12). MR enteroclysis is less sensitive than conventional enteroclysis in the detection of early mucosal abnormalities owing to low spatial resolution and lack of compression techniques.

Aphthoid ulcerations may enlarge and coalesce to form deeper, usually linear ulcerations, which frequently assume a longitudinal and transverse orientation. On T2-weighted images, they appear as thin lines of high signal intensity within the thickened bowel wall (Fig. 45-13).

Cobblestoning manifests on MR images as patchy, sharply demarcated areas of high signal intensity along affected small bowel segments (Fig. 45-14). This mucosal pattern reflects severe edema between longitudinal and transverse ulcerations, which results in the cobblestone appearance. Mucosal nodularity, ulcerations, and cobblestoning are best seen on true FISP images (see Fig. 45-14).[48-65]

Mucosal hyperemia and mild submucosal edema are best seen with gadolinium-enhanced T1-weighted sequences with fat saturation. The abnormal gut appears as an inner ring of mucosal enhancement highlighted against a low-intensity ring resulting from submucosal edema. This abnormal mural enhancement is sensitive in revealing early inflammatory changes, even in absence of bowel wall thickening (Fig. 45-15).

Transmural Abnormalities

Bowel wall thickening, usually ranging from 1 to 2 cm, is the most consistent feature of Crohn's disease on MRI (Figs. 45-16 to 45-18). It is important that the bowel be distended when assessing bowel wall thickening. On T1-weighted images there is low signal intensity in the center from the fluid in the lumen surrounded by a thin enhancing inner layer followed by a thicker intermediate layer with low enhancement and a thin outer layer with strong enhancement (see Fig. 45-18).

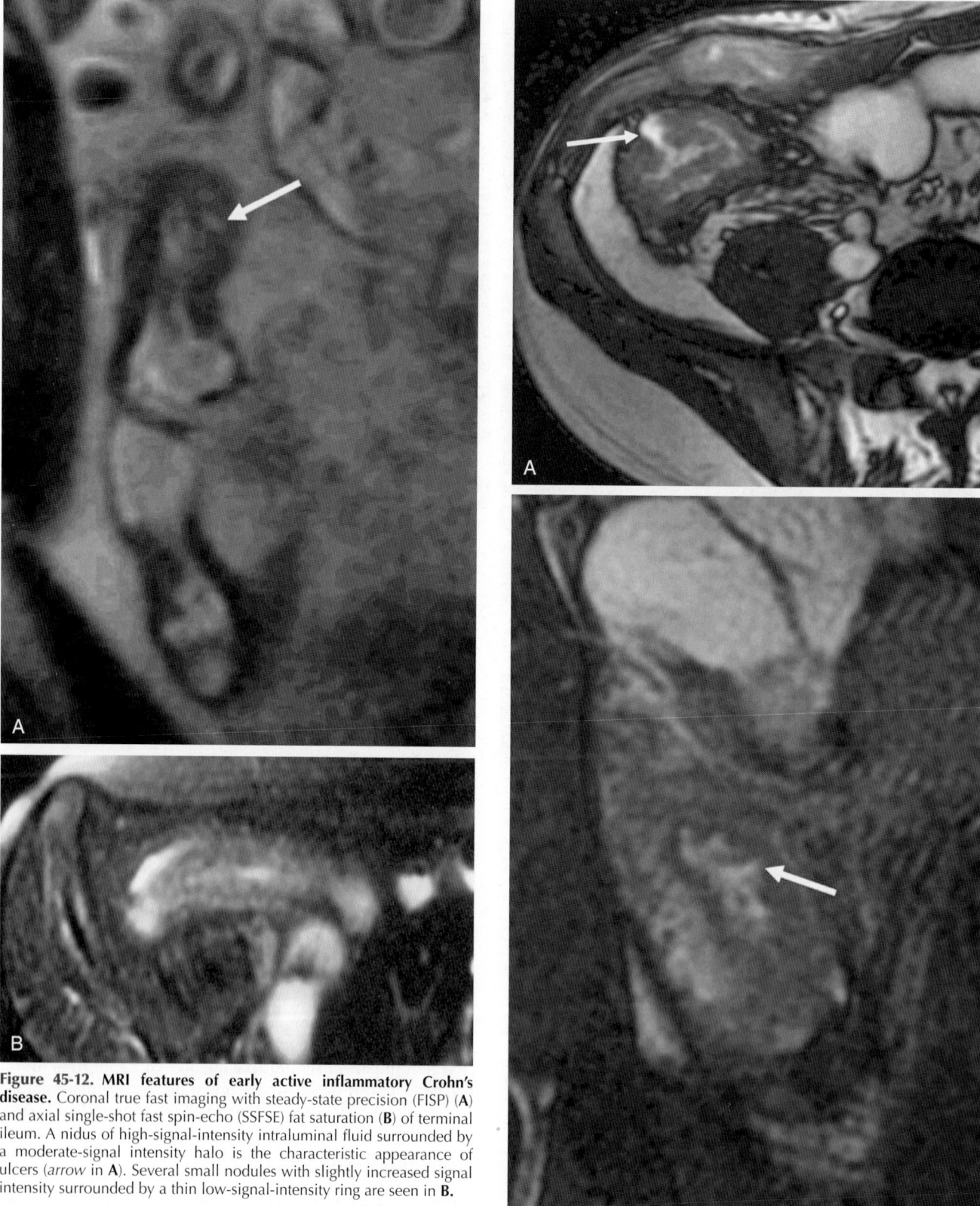

Figure 45-12. MRI features of early active inflammatory Crohn's disease. Coronal true fast imaging with steady-state precision (FISP) (**A**) and axial single-shot fast spin-echo (SSFSE) fat saturation (**B**) of terminal ileum. A nidus of high-signal-intensity intraluminal fluid surrounded by a moderate-signal intensity halo is the characteristic appearance of ulcers (*arrow* in **A**). Several small nodules with slightly increased signal intensity surrounded by a thin low-signal-intensity ring are seen in **B**.

Figure 45-13. Deeper ulcerations in active inflammatory Crohn's disease: MRI features. Axial (**A**) and coronal (**B**) true FISP MR images of terminal ileum. Ulcers are visualized as thin lines of high signal intensity, longitudinally or transversely (fissure ulcers) (*arrows*) oriented within the thickened bowel wall.

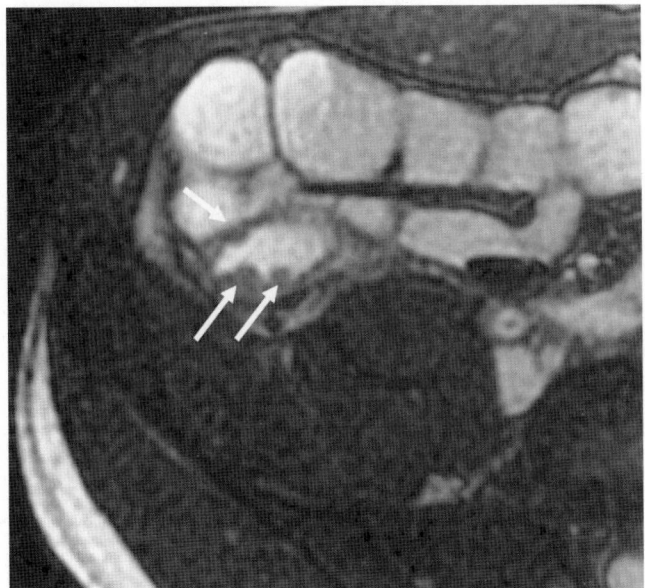

Figure 45-14. Active inflammatory Crohn's disease with inflammatory pseudopolyps: MRI features. Axial true FISP scan of distal ileum shows pseudopolyps as small nodular defects protruding through the thickened bowel wall (*arrows*).

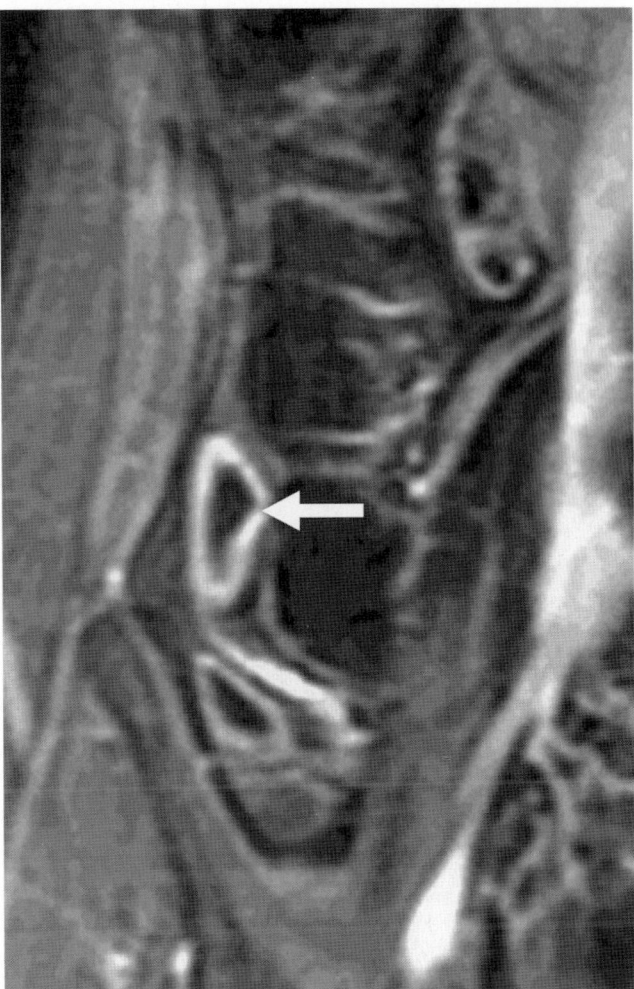

Figure 45-15. MR image of Crohn's disease: abnormal mural enhancement. Contrast-enhanced coronal fat-saturated T1-weighted image of terminal ileum shows intense wall enhancement (*arrow*) in a segment that shows normal thickness, a finding that indicates early inflammatory changes.

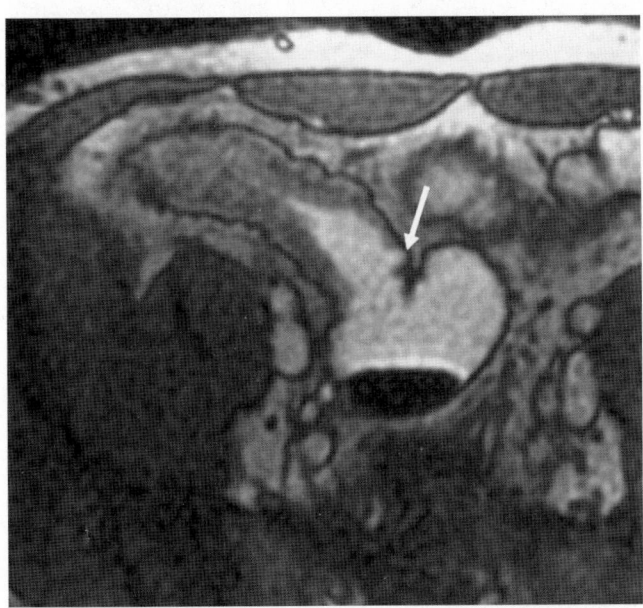

Figure 45-16. MR image of Crohn's disease: mural thickening. Axial true FISP image of distal ileum shows wall thickening with marked narrowing of the lumen. Note small ulcer in thickened wall (*arrow*).

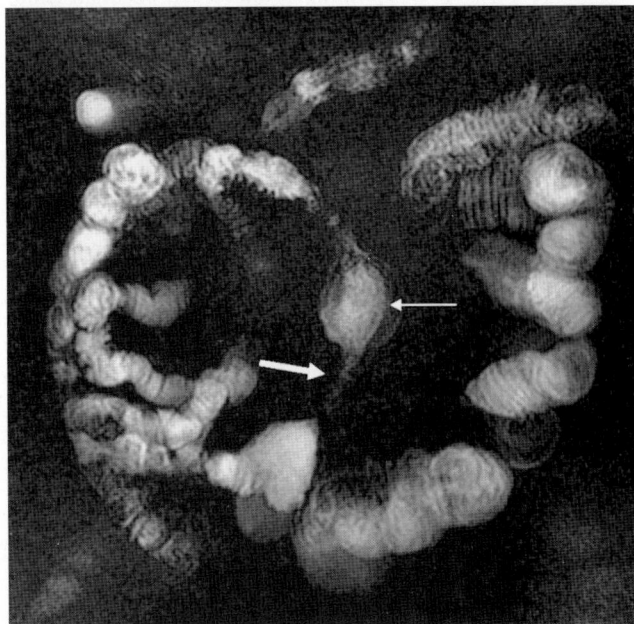

Figure 45-17. Fibrostenotic Crohn's disease: MRI features. MR fluoroscopic image shows high-grade stenosis of distal ileum (*arrow*) with prestenotic dilatation (*thin arrow*).

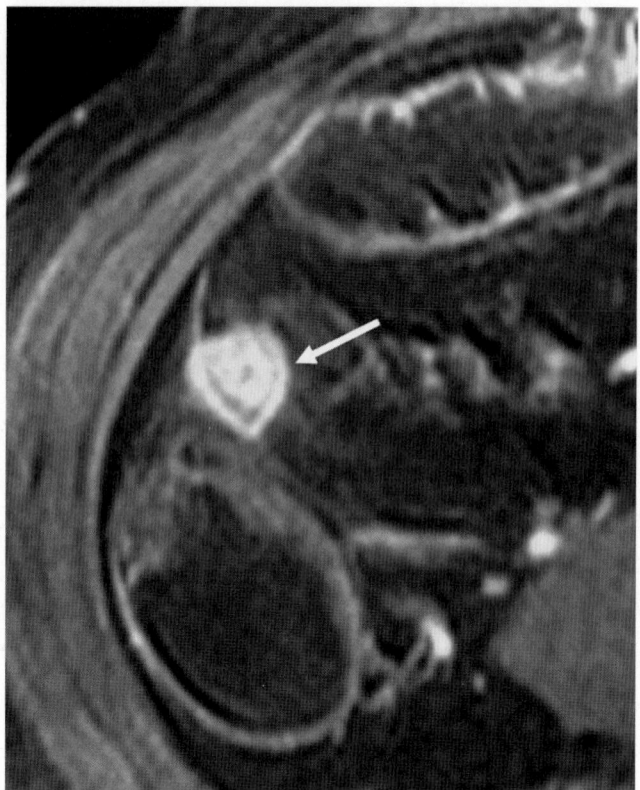

Figure 45-18. Crohn's disease: mural stratification on MRI. Axial fat-saturated T1-weighted image of terminal ileum shows a target pattern consisting of low signal intensity in the center (from the fluid in the lumen), surrounded by a thin enhancing mucosal layer, followed by a thicker intermediate layer with low enhancement, and a thin serosal layer with strong enhancement.

A target pattern is often observed on gadolinium-enhanced T1-weighted images in patients with acute Crohn's disease, but this is a nonspecific finding and also can occur in acute infectious and ischemic disease. Although the target pattern on enhanced T1-weighted images is nonspecific, it is unusual to observe a target pattern in small bowel tumors, and this can be helpful in differentiating tumors from other small bowel lesions.[48-65]

The differentiation between a high-grade and a low-grade partial small bowel obstruction frequently often cannot be appreciated by static cross-sectional sequences, but MR fluoroscopy is particular useful in this distinction (see Fig. 45-17). MR fluoroscopic images can be reviewed in a cine loop format to obtain functional information concerning bowel obstruction.

The ability of MR fluoroscopy to demonstrate the enteric agent makes it ideal for assessment of the severity of small-bowel obstruction and of the presence of prestenotic dilatation, a question frequently posed by physicians who treat patients with mechanical obstruction of the small bowel.

Extramural Manifestations and Complications

On MRI, sinus tracts and fistulas are demonstrated by the high signal intensity of their fluid content on true FISP and HASTE images (Fig. 45-19). On contrast-enhanced, fat-

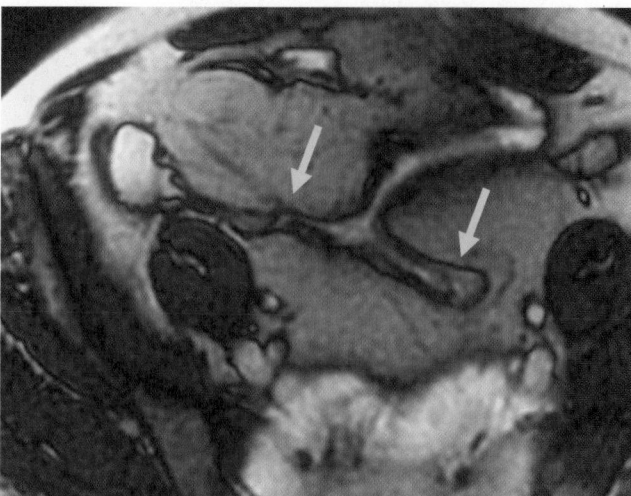

Figure 45-19. Fistulizing/perforating Crohn's disease: MRI finding. Axial true FISP image shows multiple ileoileal fistulas that contain high-signal-intensity fluid (*arrows*).

suppressed T1-weighted, 3D gradient-recalled-echo images, the central cavity has low signal intensity and is surrounded by a brightly enhancing rim (Fig. 45-20).

However, because these findings are of clinical importance and can be observed (using cross-sectional imaging techniques) in up to 50% of patients (fibrofatty proliferation) and 35% of patients (abscesses), respectively,[26] these are important to diagnose, and abscesses need to be drained.

Fibrofatty proliferation of the mesentery develops in nearly 50% of patient's with Crohn's disease and is the most common cause of bowel loop separation. The fibrofatty prolifera-

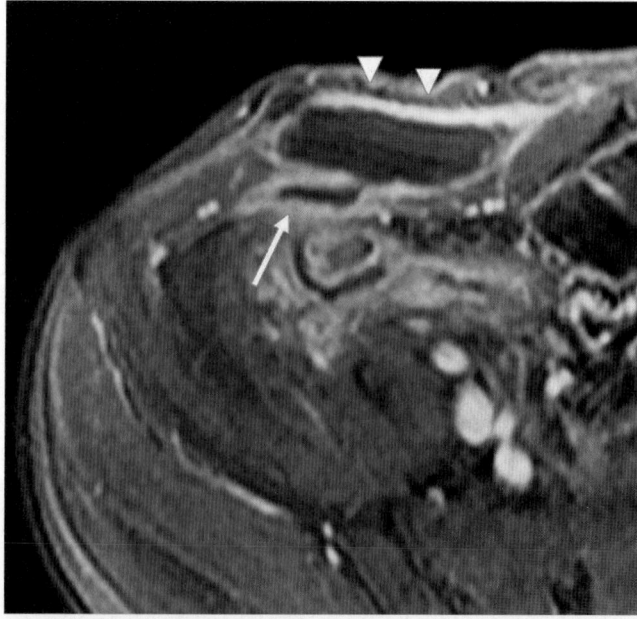

Figure 45-20. Fistulizing/perforating Crohn's disease: MRI features. Axial T1-weighted fat saturation image of the terminal ileum shows a sinus tract (*arrow*) communicating between terminal ileum and fluid containing abscess collection into abdominal wall (*arrowheads*).

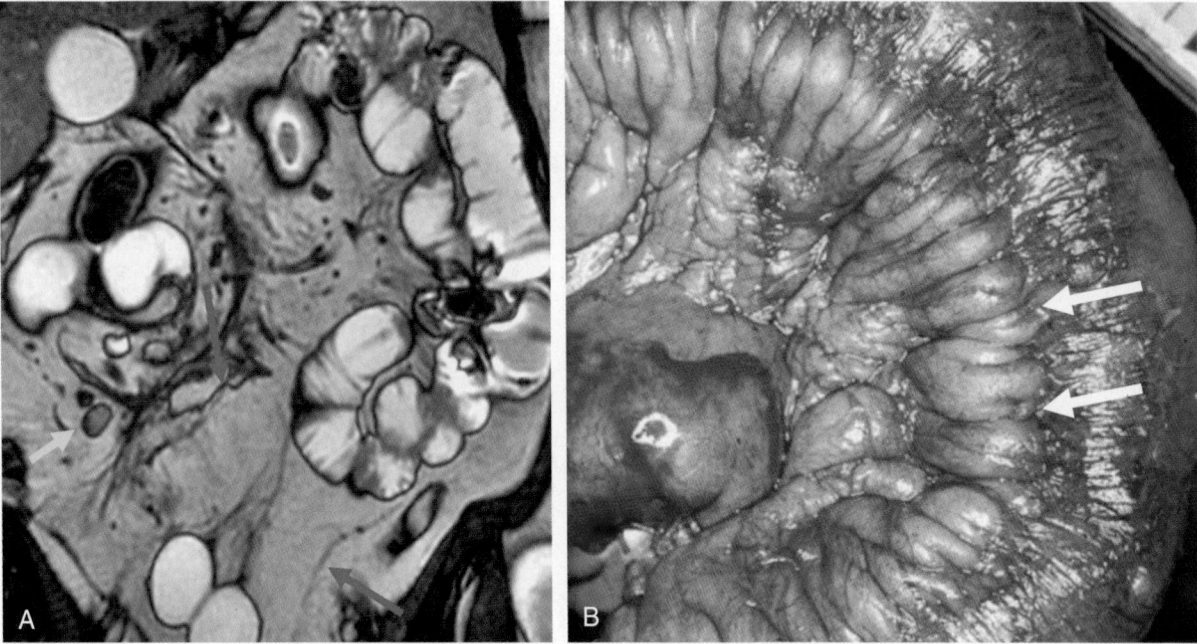

Figure 45-21.   Creeping fat of the mesentery: MRI and pathologic features. A. Coronal true FISP image shows fibrofatty proliferation of the mesentery appearing as linear low-signal-intensity structures separating bowel loops (*red arrows*); small mesenteric nodes are demonstrated by their low signal intensity within the bright mesenteric fat (*yellow arrow*). **B.** Surgical specimen shows abnormal fat on the mesenteric side of the small bowel, "creeping" (*arrows*) toward the antimesenteric side.

tion is the result of perivascular inflammation. FISP sequences are preferred in imaging the mesenteric fat (Fig. 45-21).

The "comb sign" seen on MDCT can also be depicted with MR as short, parallel, low-signal-intensity linear structures perpendicular to the intestinal long axis of the diseased bowel.[48-65] They are best demonstrated on contrast-enhanced T1-weighted images as high-signal-intensity linear structures due to vascular enhancement (Fig. 45-22).

Small mesenteric lymph nodes are easily detected by their low signal intensity scattered within the bright mesenteric fat on true FISP sequence (see Fig. 45-21). Gadolinium uptake on 3D gradient-recalled-echo images allows the identification of small inflammatory nodes. Moreover, extraluminal findings are useful in differential diagnosis: fibrofatty proliferation is a hallmark of Crohn's disease and can aid in the diagnosis if other signs of disease are less obvious and do not permit distinction between ulcerative colitis and Crohn's disease. The comb sign and the presence of enhancing mesenteric nodes may be useful in the differential diagnosis of lymphoma and metastases, which are usually hypovascular lesions.[1]

The most remarkable feature of postoperative recurrence in patients with Crohn's disease is its striking predilection for the new terminal ileum, either on the proximal side of the ileocolonic anastomosis or immediately proximal to the ileostomy. The spectrum of MR appearances is similar to that seen in unoperated patients (Figs. 45-22 and 23).

Assessment of Disease Activity

Magnetic resonance imaging has the potential to make the classification system of subtypes of Crohn's disease more objective and reproducible and can help the clinician plan appropriate therapy. Indeed, differentiation between fibrotic and edematous stenosis based on MR properties is useful for selecting patients for medical (edematous) versus surgical (fibrotic) treatment.

Active Inflammatory Disease

The active inflammatory subtype of Crohn's disease is characterized by focal inflammation, superficial and deep ulcers, and an often-transmural inflammatory reaction with lymphoid aggregates and granuloma formation. As with MDCT, mural stratification with low-signal-intensity intraluminal fluid, surrounded by a thin, enhancing mucosal layer, which in turn is surrounded by a thicker intermediate layer with low enhancement and a thin serosal layer with strong enhancement, is highly specific for active inflammation (see Fig. 45-18).[48-65]

Enhancing mesenteric lymph nodes are highly suggestive of active Crohn's disease (see Fig. 45-22). Increased mesenteric vascularity, the so-called comb sign, is an indicator of disease activity. Hypervascularity at the level of the vasa recta may be associated with perivascular fibrotic tissue.[48-65]

MRI also may have a role in the evaluation of acute exacerbations of Crohn's disease. Specifically, in patients with long-standing disease, marked enhancement of the mucosa with a thickened and minimally enhancing outer layer is suggestive of acute-on-chronic involvement.[49-65]

Stricturing Disease

Small bowel obstruction is the predominant clinical manifestation of this disease subtype. MRI demonstrates a fixed narrowing of the involved bowel with associated wall thickening. There is marked prestenotic dilatation (Fig. 45-24).

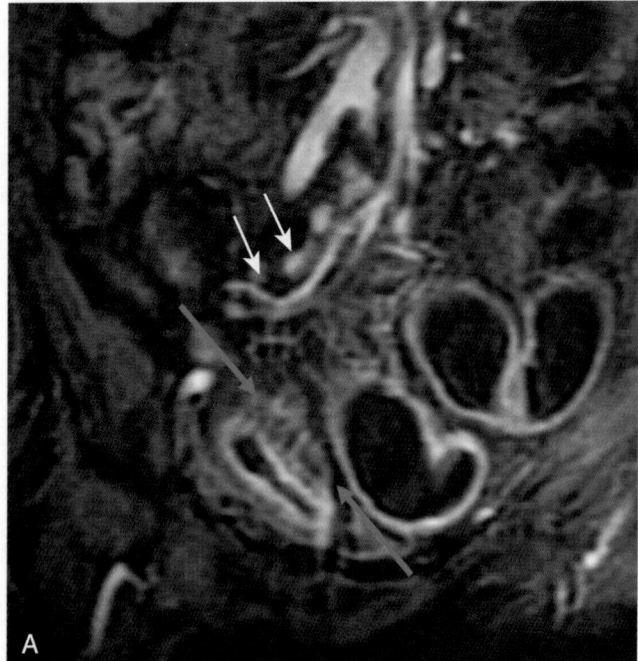

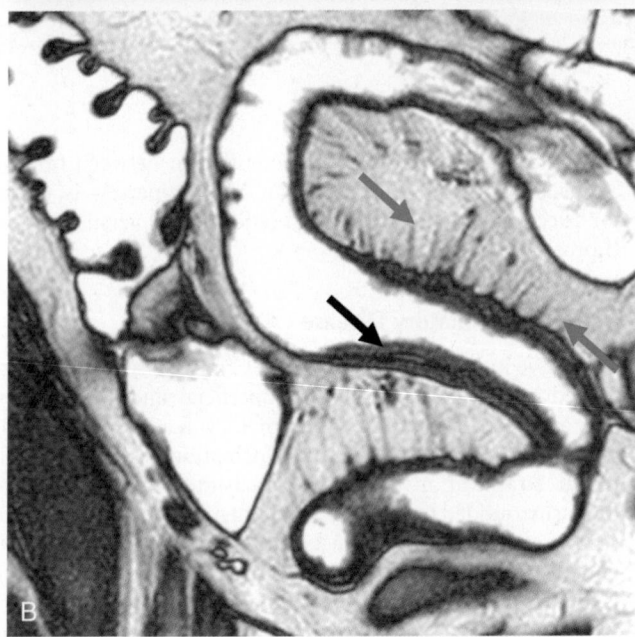

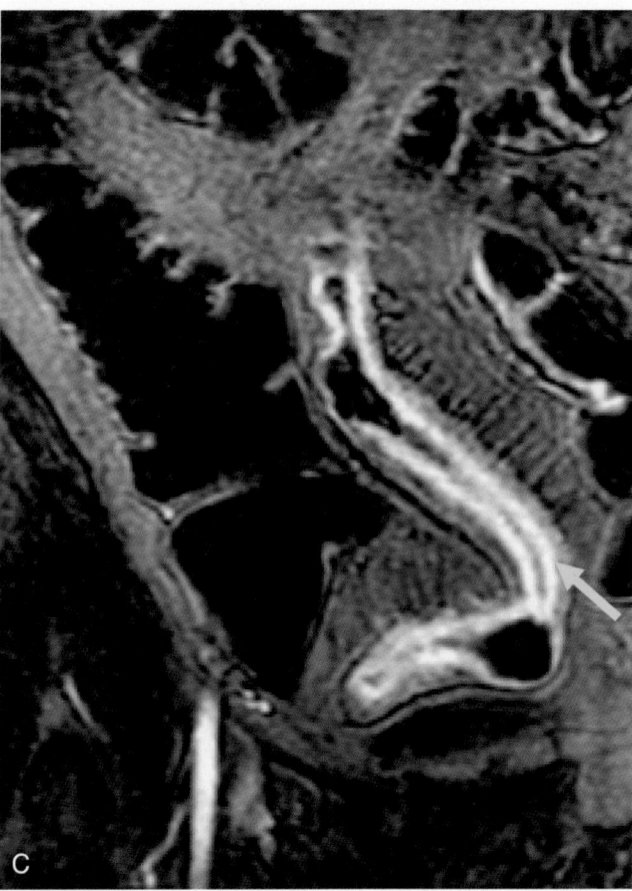

Figure 45-22. Comb sign of active Crohn's disease: MRI findings.
A. T1-weighted coronal MR image shows high signal of mucosal and serosal surfaces with low signal intensity in muscularis and submucosa (preserved mural stratification pattern). Note increased vascularity in the adjacent small-bowel mesentery, the so-called comb sign (*red arrows*) and enhancing mesenteric lymph nodes (*white arrows*). These findings are suggestive of active Crohn's disease. **B.** MR enteroclysis, coronal scan, shows mural thickening (*black arrow*) of the terminal ileum with engorged vasa rectae in the ileocolic mesentery (*red arrows*). **C.** Contrast-enhanced MR image in a different patient shows marked mucosal enhancement (*arrow*) of an inflamed segment of distal ileum. (**B** and **C** courtesy of Dr. Georg DeBatin, Essen, Germany.)

Additionally, mural enhancement is reduced and mural stratification is lost. This indicates that transmural fibrosis has supervened (Fig. 45-25).

Fistulizing/Penetrating Disease

This Crohn's subtype is characterized by transmural extension of the inflammatory process with resultant fistula formation or perforation. Deep ulcers precede sinus and fistula formation to adjacent organs and the development of abscesses (Fig. 45-26).

Sinus tracts and fistulas are demonstrated by the high signal intensity of their fluid content on true FISP and HASTE images. The multiplanar imaging capabilities of MR are particularly useful in depicting complex fistulas and sinus tracts.

MULTIDETECTOR COMPUTED TOMOGRAPHY

There are three major MDCT techniques employed in the evaluation of Crohn's disease of the small bowel: conventional positive intraluminal contrast studies, CT enterography, and CT enteroclysis.[66-78]

Computed Tomographic Enterography

CT enterography employs MDCT with narrow section thickness and reconstruction interval, intravenous contrast material, and large volumes of neutral contrast agent to distend the lumen in an effort to improve the detection of small bowel inflammation and extracolonic complications. MDCT can be

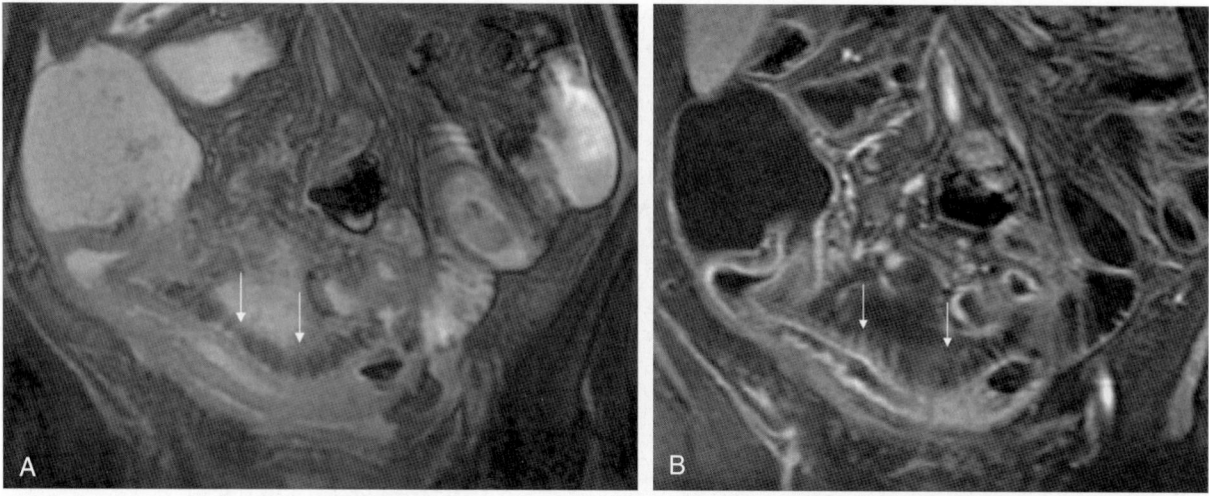

Figure 45-23. Recurrent Crohn's disease: MRI findings. Coronal true FISP fat saturation (**A**) and coronal gadolinium enhanced fat-suppressed T1-weighted (**B**) images show thickening of new terminal ileum with layered enhancement pattern: the comb sign (*arrows*).

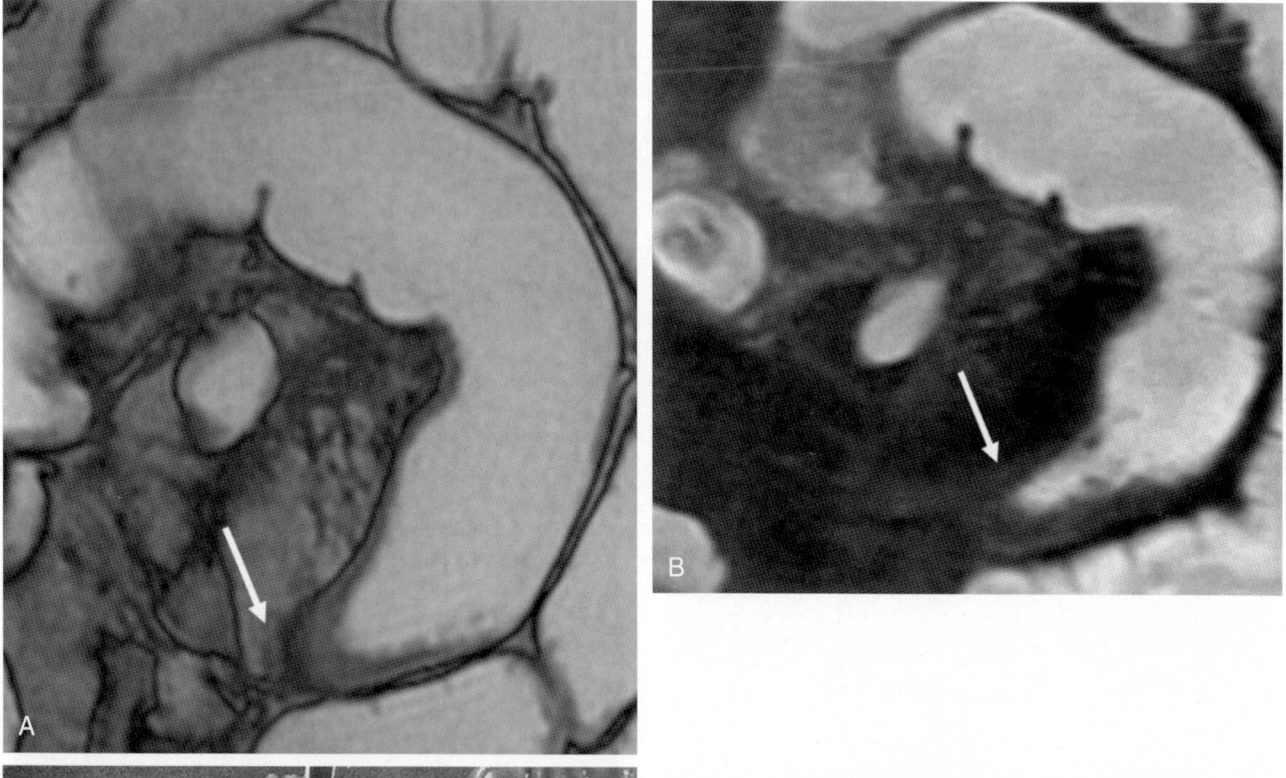

Figure 45-24. Stenosing Crohn's disease: MRI and pathologic features. Coronal true FISP (**A**) and coronal SSFSE fat saturation (**B**) MR images show marked narrowing of the distal ileum (*arrow*) with prestenotic dilatation. **C.** Surgical specimen shows a region of stenosis and prestenotic dilatation.

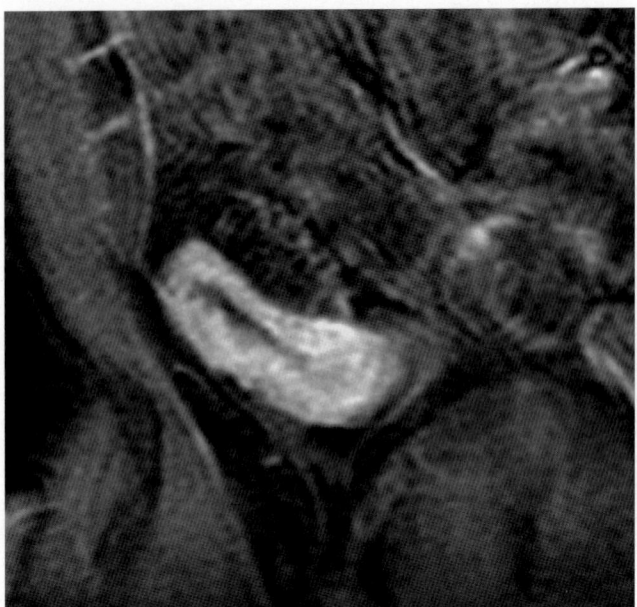

Figure 45-25. Coronal gadolinium-enhanced T1-weighted 3D gradient-recalled-echo MR image shows thickened wall with uniform enhancement.

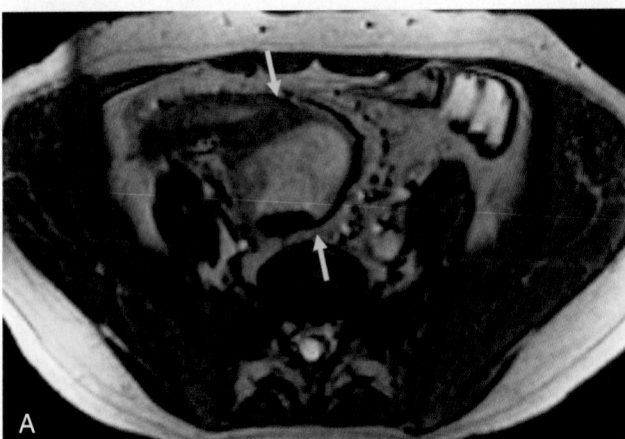

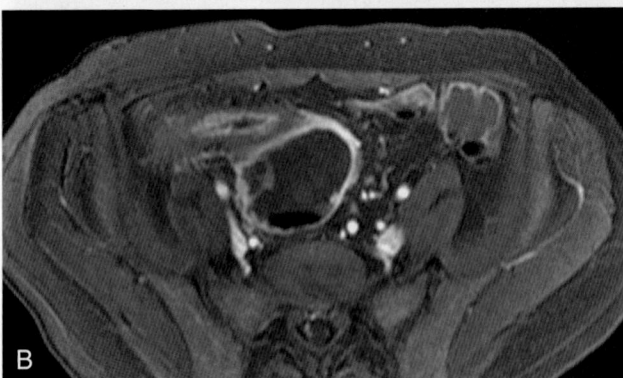

Figure 45-26. Abscess secondary to fistulizing/perforating Crohn's disease. **A.** Axial true FISP image obtained in the prone position show high-signal-intensity fluid and dark gas within the abscess (*arrows*). Image was taken with the patient in the prone position. **B.** Axial T1-weighted 3D gradient-recalled-echo (B) image shows enhancement of the abscess wall after the intravenous administration of gadolinium. Image was taken with the patient in the prone position.

performed during the enteric phase (45 seconds after injection) and the portal venous phase (70 seconds after injection). Jejunal attenuation is greater than ileal attenuation, and collapsed bowel loops demonstrate greater attenuation than distended bowel loops. Mural hyperenhancement and increased mural thickness are the most sensitive CT findings of active Crohn's disease.[66,67]

Computed Tomographic Enteroclysis

Computed tomographic enteroclysis employs contrast material infused through a nasojejunal tube. Both positive (dilute barium) and neutral contrast (water, methylcellulose, Enterovu) may be administered. The technique of CT enteroclysis is discussed in Chapter 42.

Active Inflammatory Disease

Enlarged lymphoid follicles, small ulcers, and aphthae are not demonstrated on MDCT. Mucosal hyperemia and submucosal edema can be appreciated when a bolus of intravenous contrast is administered (Fig. 45-27)

Cobblestone mucosa can be appreciated as deep longitudinal and transverse ulcers with thickened, edematous mucosa interposed. With more severe disease, deep ulcerations manifest as protrusions of intraluminal fluid or contrast agent into the edematous wall.

Mural stratification of the wall in patients with Crohn's disease indicates the presence of edema from active inflammation (Figs. 45-28 and 45-29). This target appearance is composed of an inner ring of mucosal enhancement, an outer ring of enhancement of the muscularis propria and serosa, and an intermediate low-density ring reflecting submucosal edema. The degree of enhancement of these various layers reflects the underlying disease activity, and changes in the degree of enhancement can be used to direct clinical decisions. Indeed, quantitative measurements of mural enhancement and wall thickening at CT enterography correlate highly with ileoscopic and histologic findings of active inflammatory Crohn's disease.[66,67]

The assessment of mural enhancement is hindered by the presence of positive intraluminal contrast because this contrast isoattenuates the inner ring of mucosal enhancement to some degree. In patients with chronic disease, fat rather then fluid (edema) is identified in the submucosa of the affected segments.[70,71]

Patients with active Crohn's disease also show engorgement of the vasa rectae, the so-called comb sign. This indicates perienteric hyperemia.[72,73] Creeping fat of the mesentery is also well depicted on MDCT (Fig. 45-30).

Fistulizing/Perforating Disease

In this more advanced form of disease, there is transmural extension of disease with fistula formation (Fig. 45-31) and perforation. Deep ulcerations progress into sinus tracts and fistulas to adjacent organs. Abscesses (Fig. 45-32) also result from this process. MDCT has become the primary means of diagnosing and treating Crohn's disease–related abscesses (Fig. 45-33).[79]

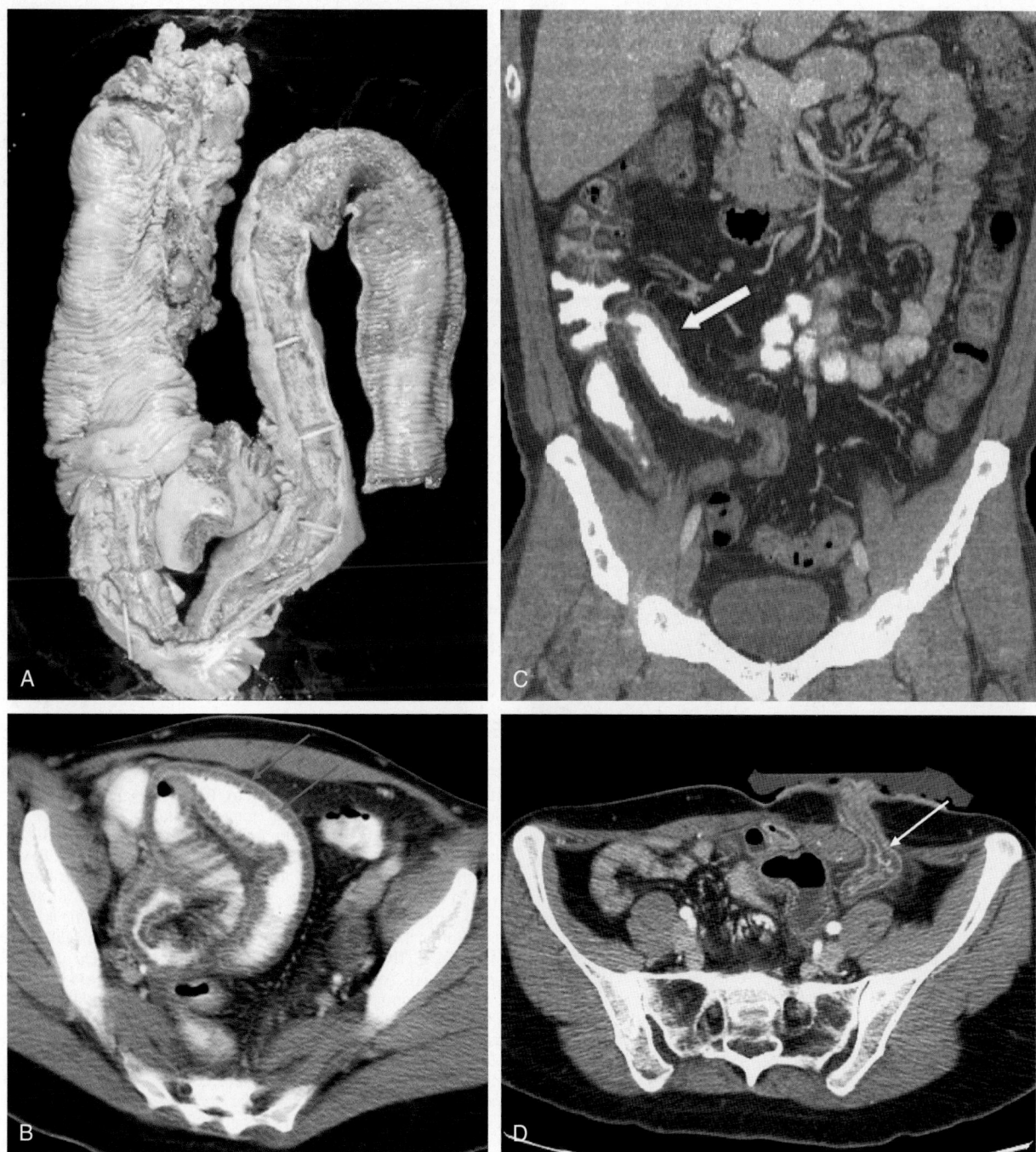

Figure 45-27. Mural thickening in Crohn's disease: CT and pathologic findings. A. Surgical specimen shows thickening and rigidity of the distal ileum, the so-called garden hose appearance. **B.** Axial image shows submucosal edema with ulcerations (*arrows*) involving a thickened segment of distal ileum. **C.** Coronal reformatted image also shows the abnormal mural thickening and submucosal edema (*arrow*). **D.** Recurrent Crohn's disease in a patient with an ileostomy. Note the mural stratification, submucosal edema, and mucosal enhancement in the segment of ileum (*arrow*) proximal to the stoma.

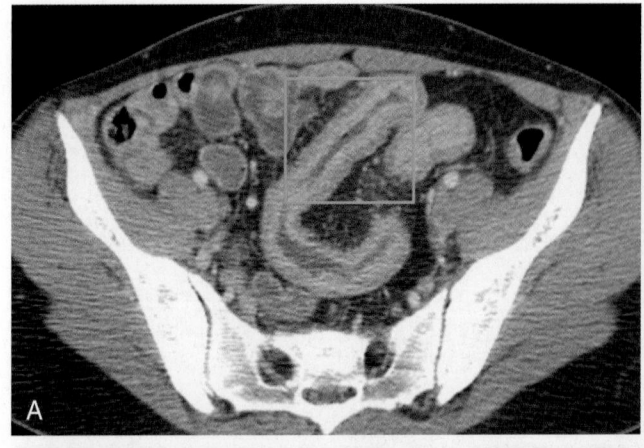

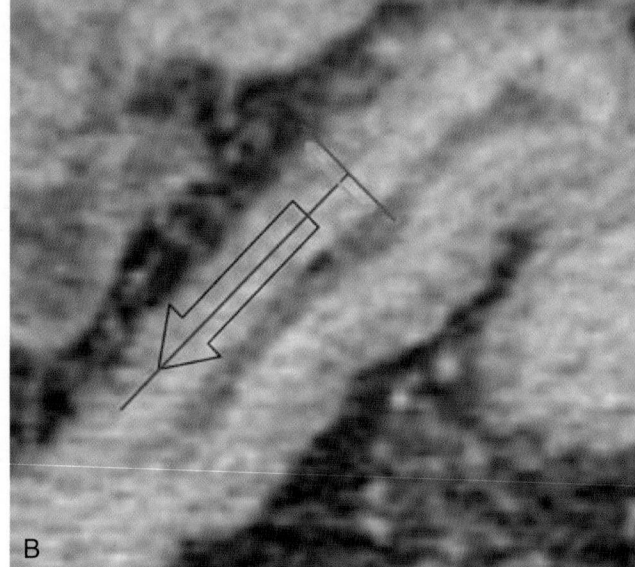

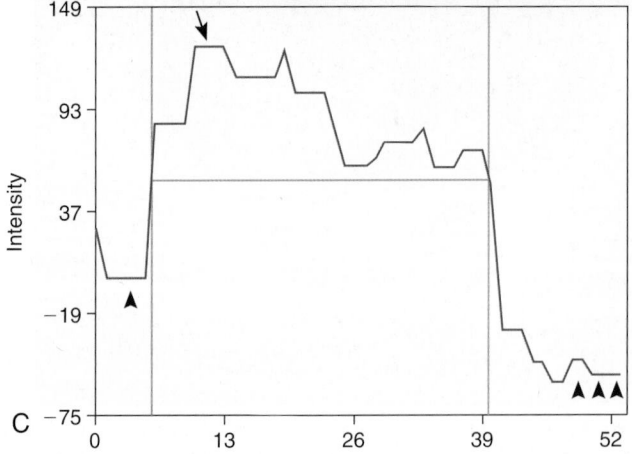

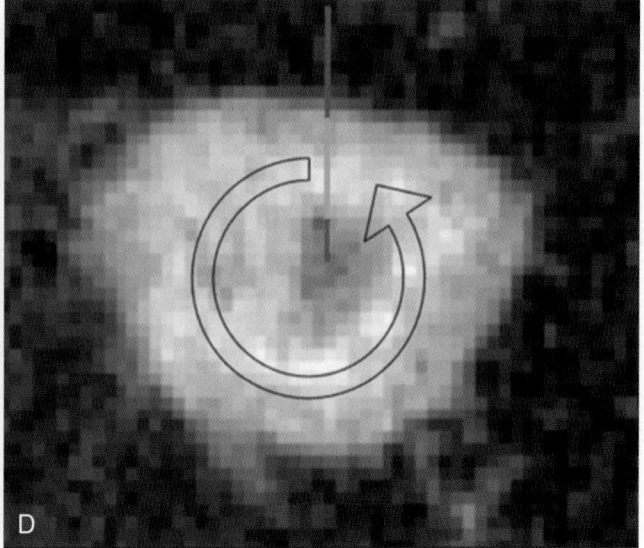

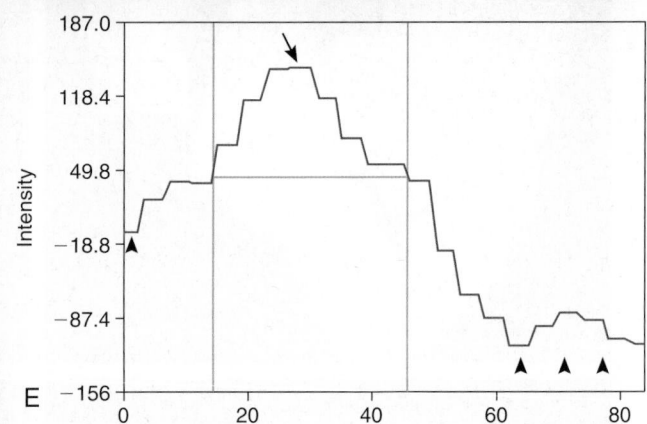

Figure 45-28. Semiautomated measurement of terminal ileal attenuation assess disease activity. (A) Transverse CT image of inflamed ileal loop shows that the gut lumen is transected parallel to the transverse cut plane. The *green box* indicates the portion of the image that is cropped to isolate the bowel segment to be analyzed. **B.** Within the cropped image, the line tool (*red line*) was placed over the bowel wall to obtain measurements of mural attenuation and wall thickness every 1 mm along a 3.0-cm bowel segment (along the *blue line,* in the direction of the *open arrow*). **C.** Graph corresponding to ileal measurements in **B.** The numbers on the y-axis are Hounsfield units; those on the x-axis represent distance in millimeters. The *red curve* plots CT attenuation versus distance, with values corresponding to the *red line* traversing the bowel wall in **B.** Graph shows maximum mural attenuation (*arrow*), with the automated mural thickness measurement obtained by using a full width at half-maximum technique (*H-shaped measurement*) and attenuation values corresponding to luminal fluid (*large arrowhead*) and perienteric fat (*small arrowheads*). **D.** Transverse CT image demonstrates analysis of another ileal segment in which the gut lumen is transected perpendicular to the transverse cut plane, with the line tool (*green and red line*) placed in the center of the bowel lumen to obtain measurements of mural attenuation and wall thickness at 15-degree increments rotating around the central axis of the bowel. **E.** Graph corresponding to ileum in **D** shows maximum mural attenuation (*arrow*), the automated mural thickness measurement obtained by using a full width at half-maximum technique (*H-shaped measurement*) and attenuation values corresponding to luminal fluid (*large arrowhead*) and perienteric fat (*small arrowheads*). (From Bodily KD, Fletcher JG, Solem CA, et al: Crohn disease: Mural attenuation and thickness at contrast-enhanced CT enterography—correlation with endoscopic and histologic findings. Radiology 238:505-516, 2006.)

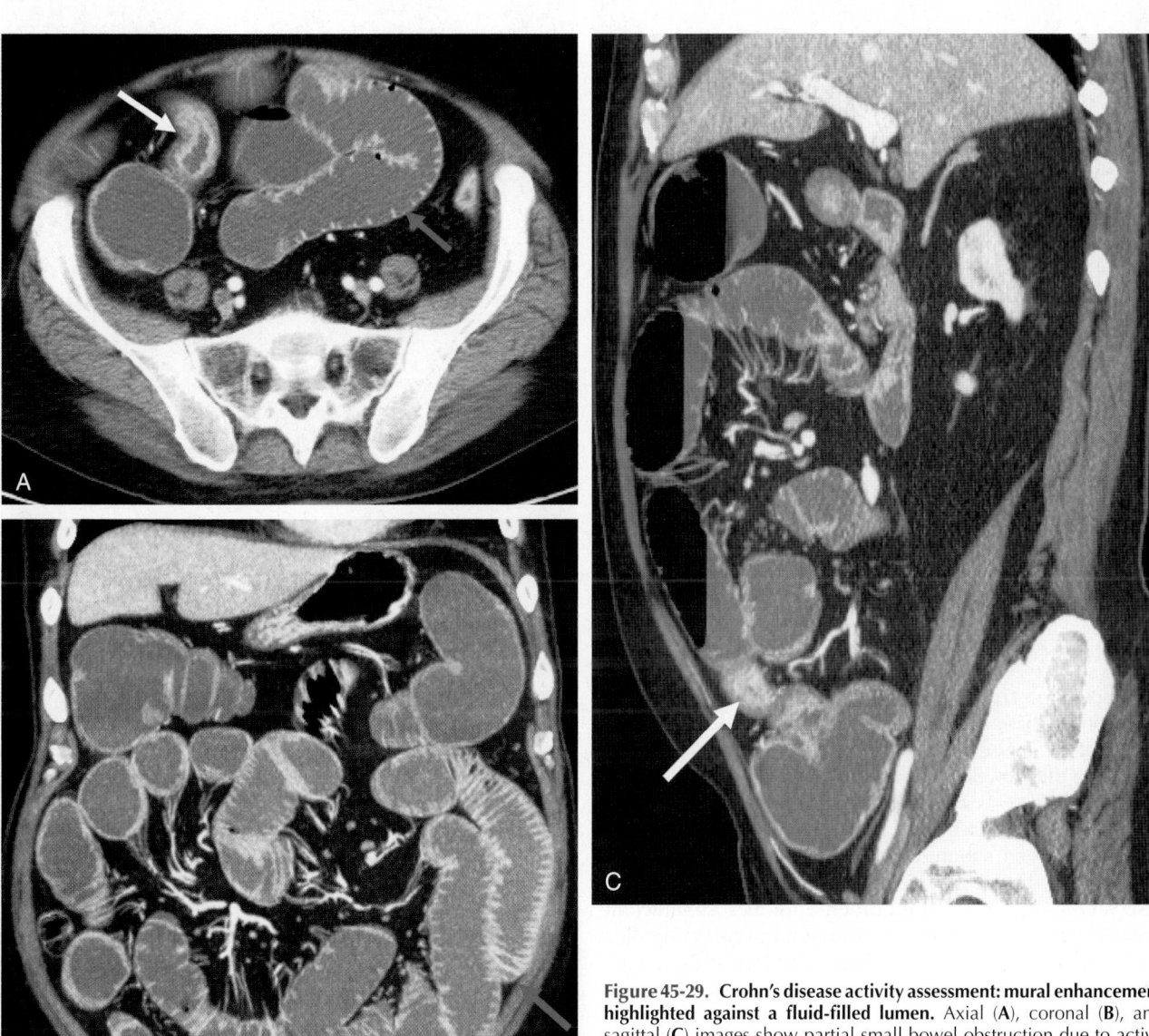

Figure 45-29. Crohn's disease activity assessment: mural enhancement highlighted against a fluid-filled lumen. Axial (**A**), coronal (**B**), and sagittal (**C**) images show partial small bowel obstruction due to active Crohn's disease with submucosal edema. The narrowed segments (*white arrows*) show mural thickening, mural stratification, and robust mucosal enhancement. Red arrows, dilated, fluid-filled small bowel proximal to the distal partial obstruction.

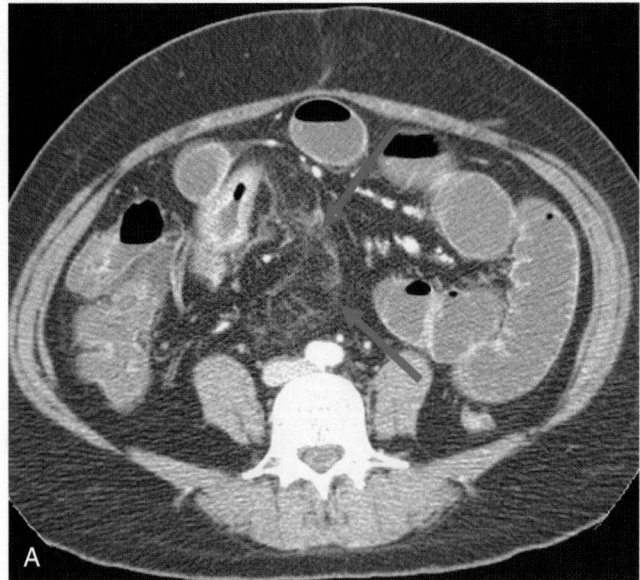

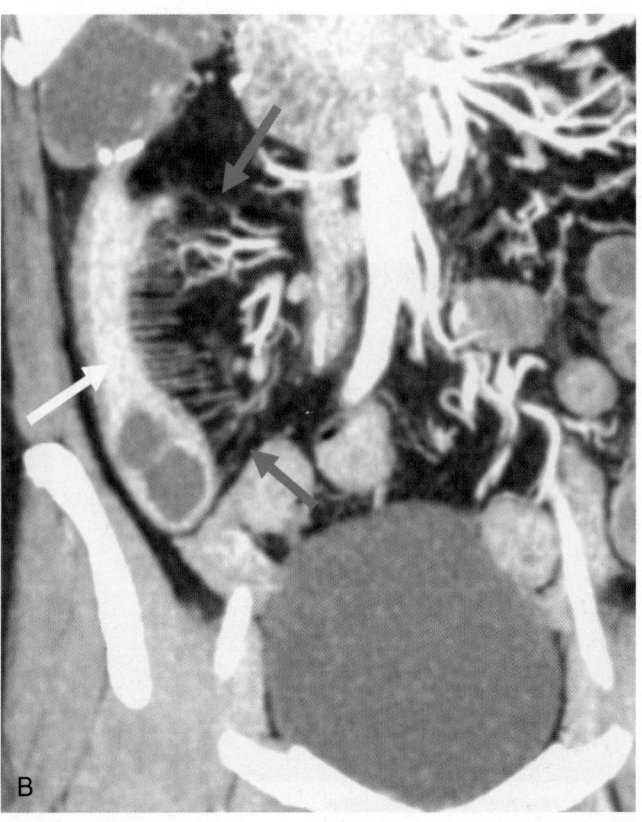

Figure 45-30. Creeping fat of the mesentery: CT features. A. Abnormal attenuation is identified in the ileocolic mesentery (*arrows*). There is a paucity of bowel loops in this region. **B.** The comb sign (*red arrows*) within abnormal fat is demonstrated along the mesenteric border of this abnormal segment of ileum. Note the mural hyperenhancement (*white arrow*).

Fibrostenotic Phase

Small bowel obstruction is the major manifestation of the fibrostenotic phase of Crohn's disease. MDCT demonstrates a fixed narrowing of the involved bowel with mural thickening. Here, the bowel uniformly enhances with soft tissue attenuation; there is no submucosal edema. This type of disease must be differentiated from small bowel obstruction due to spasm and submucosal edema resulting from active inflammatory disease in which the target sign is visible. The preservation of mural stratification indicates submucosal edema and active disease that may respond to corticosteroids and other immunosuppressive agents. The loss of this stratification often indicates transmural fibrosis that may require surgical intervention.

Reparative/Regenerative Phase

Inactive Crohn's disease can be associated with other phases of Crohn's disease in other portions of the gut. There may be a decrease in the lumen diameter but not active inflammation as identified in the "burned out" segment.

CROHN'S JEJUNOILEITIS

Diffuse jejunoileitis forms a subset of Crohn's enteritis in which the distal ileum may be spared and disease progression may be craniad. It affects less than 10% of patients with

Crohn's disease of the small bowel.[4] Jejunoileitis affects younger patients, has a more acute onset, and requires more extensive bowel resections than distal Crohn's disease. In some cases, craniad progression with involvement of the duodenum has been noted.

CROHN'S CARCINOMA

An increased prevalence of small bowel carcinoma has been reported in patients with Crohn's disease involving the small bowel. Most investigators agree that Crohn's cancers exhibit special features: younger persons are more likely to be affected; the distal ileum is the usual site of involvement; and areas of long-standing disease are more likely to undergo malignant change, rendering a radiologic diagnosis more difficult. Surgically bypassed bowel is another site more likely to be involved by tumor when radiologic diagnosis is extremely difficult, but this form of surgery is no longer performed. Carcinoma may also arise at the site of fistulas, so that any bleeding from such fistulas should be viewed with suspicion. A preoperative radiologic diagnosis is almost always impossible because of the absence of characteristic features; this is also usually the case at laparotomy. It is not surprising that patients with Crohn's carcinoma have a dismal prognosis, with an overall survival from the time of diagnosis measured in months.[79-81]

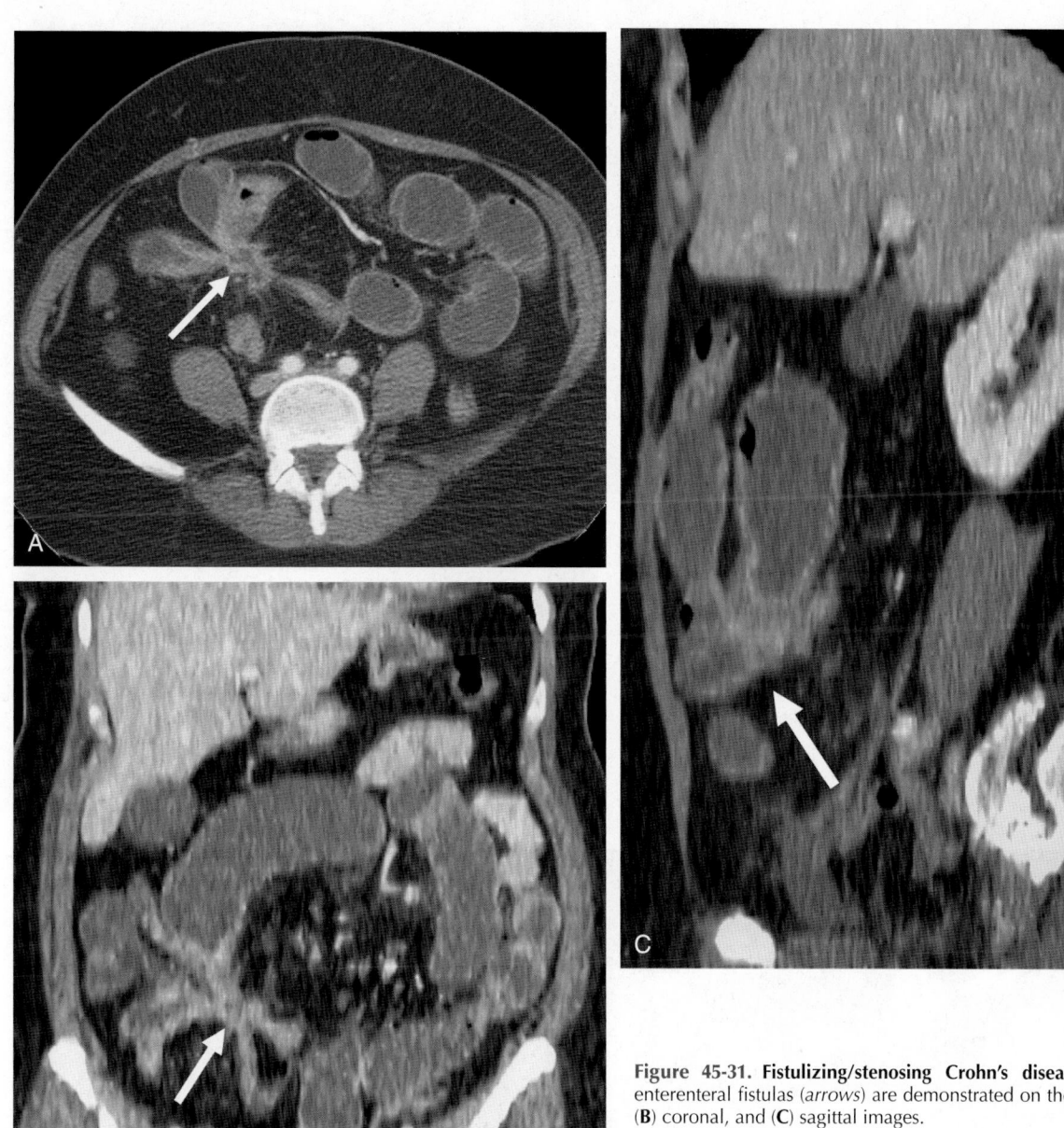

Figure 45-31. Fistulizing/stenosing Crohn's disease. Multiple enterenteral fistulas (*arrows*) are demonstrated on these (**A**) axial, (**B**) coronal, and (**C**) sagittal images.

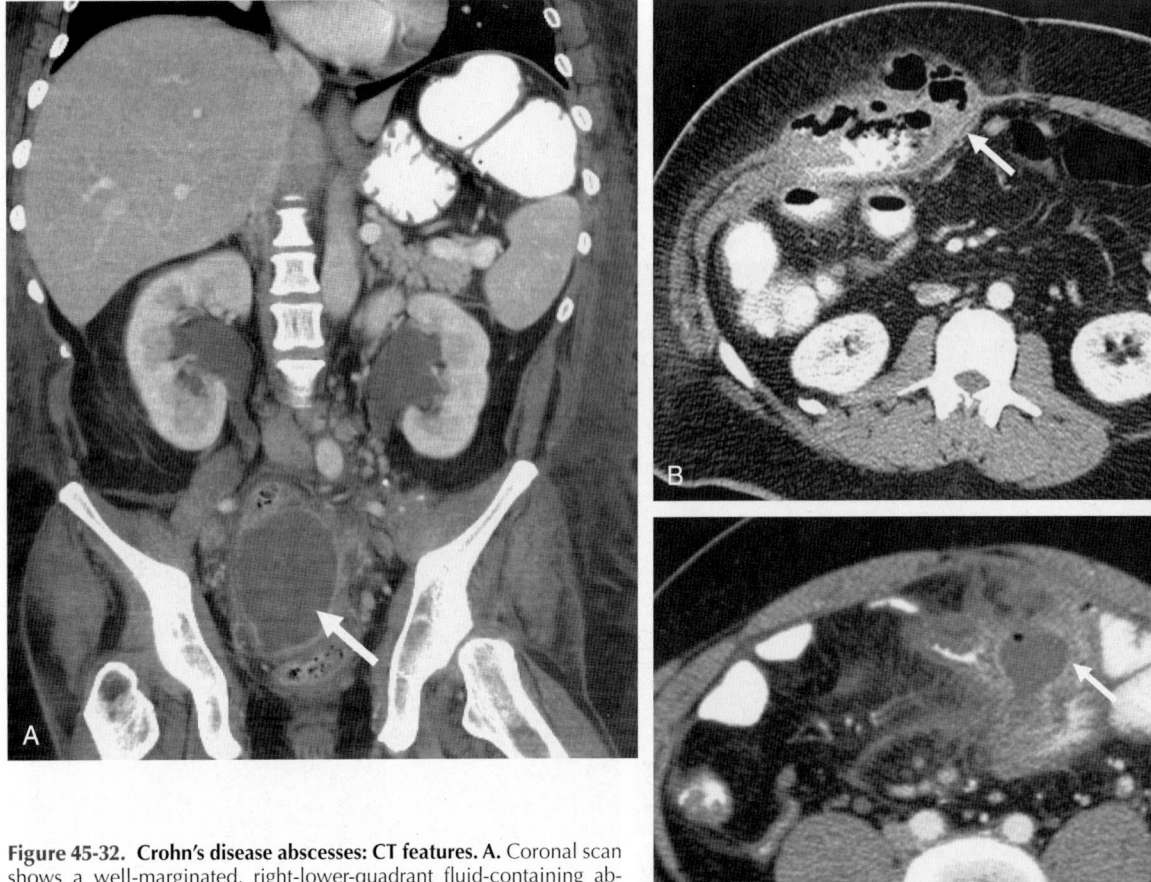

Figure 45-32. Crohn's disease abscesses: CT features. A. Coronal scan shows a well-marginated, right-lower-quadrant fluid-containing abscess cavity (*arrow*) secondary to ileal Crohn's disease. There is bilateral hydronephrosis. **B.** Axial image in a different patient shows an abscess cavity (*arrow*) containing gas and contrast secondary to fistulizing ileal Crohn's disease. **C.** An interloop gas-containing abscess (*arrow*) is seen in the small bowel mesentery due to distal jejunal Crohn's disease.

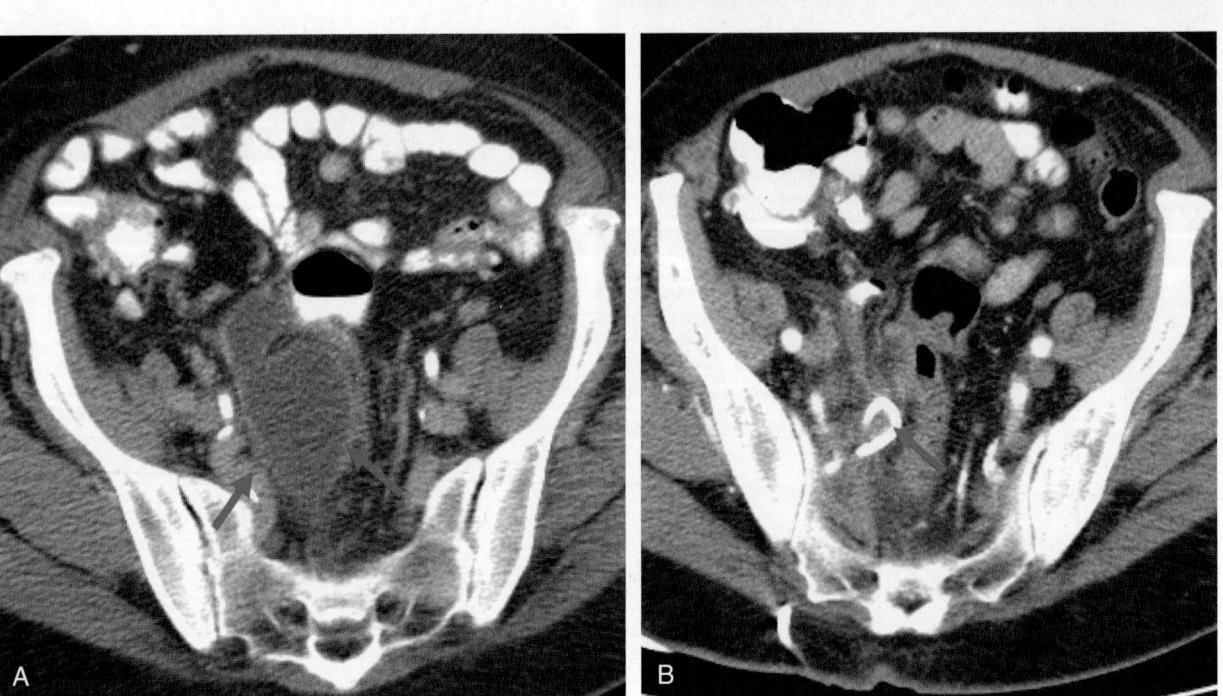

Figure 45-33. Crohn's disease abscess drainage. A. An abscess is present in the right lower quadrant (*arrows*). **B.** This abscess was percutaneously drained (*arrow*) via a right transgluteal approach.

References

1. Barreiro-de Acosta M, Dominguez-Munoz JE, Nunez-Pardo de Vera MC, et al: Relationship between clinical features of Crohn's disease and the risk of developing extraintestinal manifestations. Eur J Gastroenterol Hepatol 19:73-78, 2007.

2. Bernstein CN, Wajda A, Svenson LW, et al: The epidemiology of inflammatory bowel disease in Canada: A population-based study. Am J Gastroenterol 101:1559-1568, 2006.

3. Bernstein CN, Rawsthorne P, Cheang M, et al: A population-based case control study of potential risk factors for IBD. Am J Gastroenterol 101:993-1002, 2006.

4. Munkholm P, Binder V: Clinical features and natural history of Crohn's disease. In Sartor RB, Sandborn WJ (eds): Kirsner's Inflammatory Bowel Diseases, 6th ed. Edinburgh, Saunders, 2004, pp 289-300.

5. Riddell RH: Pathology of idiopathic inflammatory bowel disease. In Sartor RB, Sandborn WJ (eds): Kirsner's Inflammatory Bowel Diseases, 6th ed. Edinburgh, Saunders, 2004, pp 399-424.

6. Maglinte DDT, Gourtsoyiannis N, Rex D, et al: Classification of small bowel Crohn's subtypes based on multimodality imaging. Radiol Clin North Am 41:285-303, 2003.

7. van Assche G: Emerging drugs to treat Crohn's disease. Expert Opin Emerg Drugs 12:49-59, 2007.

8. Creed TJ, Probert CS: Review article: Steroid resistance in inflammatory bowel disease—mechanisms and therapeutic strategies. Aliment Pharmacol Ther 25:111-122, 2007.

9. Teitelbaum JE, Saeed S, Triantafyllopoulou M, et al: Infliximab in pediatric Crohn disease patients with enterovesicular fistulas. J Pediatr Gastroenterol Nutr 44:279-282, 2007.

10. Valle J, Alcantara M, Perez-Grueso MJ, et al: Clinical features of patients with negative results from traditional diagnostic work-up and Crohn's disease findings from capsule endoscopy. J Clin Gastroenterol 40:692-696, 2006.

11. Marmo R, Rotondano G, Piscopo R, et al: Capsule endoscopy versus enteroclysis in the detection of small-bowel involvement in Crohn's disease: A prospective trial. Clin Gastroenterol Hepatol 3:772-776, 2005.

12. Triester SL, Leighton JA, Leontiadis GI, et al: A meta-analysis of the yield of capsule endoscopy compared to other diagnostic modalities in patients with non-stricturing small bowel Crohn's disease. Am J Gastroenterol 101:954-964, 2006.

13. Bruining DH, Loftus EV: Evolving diagnostic strategies for inflammatory bowel disease. Curr Gastroenterol Rep 8:478-485, 2006.

14. Hara AK, Leighton JA, Sharma VK, et al: Imaging of small bowel disease: Comparison of capsule endoscopy, standard endoscopy, barium examination, and CT. RadioGraphics 25:697-711, 2005.

15. Hara AK, Leighton JA, Heigh RI, et al: Crohn disease of the small bowel: Preliminary comparison among CT enterography, capsule endoscopy, small-bowel follow-through, and ileoscopy. Radiology 238:128-134, 2006.

16. Hara AK, Leighton JA, Sharma VK, et al: Small bowel: Preliminary comparison of capsule endoscopy with barium study and CT. Radiology 230:260-265, 2004.

17. Goldberg HI, Caruthers SB, Nelson JA, et al: Radiographic findings of the National Cooperative Crohn's Disease Study. Gastroenterology 77:925-937, 1979.

18. Maglinte DDT, Chernish SM, Kelvin FM, et al: Crohn disease of the small intestine: Accuracy and relevance of enteroclysis. Radiology 184:1-6, 1992.

19. Glick SN: Crohn's disease of the small intestine. Radiol Clin North Am 25:25-45, 1987.

20. Rubesin SE, Bronner M: Radiologic-pathologic concepts in Crohn's disease. Adv Gastrointest Radiol 1:27-55, 1991.

21. Ekberg O, Lindstrom C: Superficial lesions in Crohn's disease of the small bowel. Gastrointest Radiol 4:389-393, 1979.

22. Jones B, Hamilton SR, Rubesin SE, et al: Granular small bowel mucosa: A reflection of villous abnormality. Gastrointest Radiol 12:219-225, 1987.

23. Nolan DJ, Gourtsoyiannis NC: Crohn's disease of the small intestine: A review of the radiological appearances in 100 consecutive patients examined by a barium infusion technique. Gastrointest Radiol 31:597-603, 1980.

24. Marshak RH, Wolf BS: Roentgen findings in regional enteritis. AJR 74:1000-1014, 1955.

25. Herlinger H, Rubesin SE, Furth EE: Mesenteric border linear ulcer in Crohn's disease: Historical, radiologic and pathologic perspectives. Abdom Imaging 23:122-126, 1998.

26. Buck JL, Dachman AH, Sobin LH: Polypoid and pseudopolypoid manifestations of inflammatory bowel disease. RadioGraphics 11:293-304, 1991.

27. Nolan DJ, Piris J: Crohn's disease of the small intestine: A comparative study of the radiological and pathological appearances. Clin Radiol 31:591-596, 1980.

28. Herlinger H, Furth EE, Rubesin SE: Fibrofatty proliferation of the mesentery in Crohn's disease: The query corner. Abdom Imaging 23:001-003, 1998.

29. Tarjan Z, Toth G, Gyorke T, et al: Ultrasound in Crohn's disease of the small bowel. Eur J Radiol 35:176-182, 2000.

30. Maconi G, Sampietro GM, Parente F, et al: Contrast radiology, computed tomography and ultrasonography in detecting internal fistulas and intra-abdominal abscesses in Crohn's disease: A prospective comparative study. Am J Gastroenterol 98:1545-1555, 2003.

31. Parente F, Maconi G, Bollani S, et al: Bowel ultrasound in assessment of Crohn's disease and detection of related small bowel strictures: A prospective comparative study versus x ray and intraoperative findings. Gut 50:490-495, 2002.

32. Bru C, Sans M, Defelitto MM, et al: Hydrocolonic sonography for evaluating inflammatory bowel disease. AJR 177:99-105, 2001.

33. Byrne MF, Farrell MA, Abass S, et al: Assessment of Crohn's disease activity by Doppler sonography of the superior mesenteric artery, clinical evaluation and the Crohn's disease activity index: A prospective study. Clin Radiol 56:973-978, 2001.

34. Maconi G, Radice E, Greco S, et al: Bowel ultrasound in Crohn's disease. Best Pract Res Clin Gastroenterol 20:93-112, 2006.

35. Fraquelli M, Colli A, Casazza C, et al: Role of US in detection of Crohn disease: Meta-analysis. Radiology 236:95-101, 2005.

36. Spalinger J, Patriquin H, Miron M-C, et al: Doppler US in patients with Crohn disease: Vessel density in the diseased bowel reflects disease activity. Radiology 217:787-793, 2000.

37. De Pascale A, Garofalo G, Perna M, et al: Contrast-enhanced ultrasonography in Crohn's disease. Radiol Med (Torino) 111:539-550, 2006.

38. Calabrese E, La Seta F, Buccellato A, et al: Crohn's disease: A comparative prospective study of transabdominal ultrasonography, small intestine contrast ultrasonography, and small bowel enema. Inflamm Bowel Dis 11:139-145, 2005.

39. Yekeler E, Danalioglu A, Movasseghi B, et al: Crohn disease activity evaluated by Doppler ultrasonography of the superior mesenteric artery and the affected small-bowel segments. J Ultrasound Med 24:59-65, 2005.

40. Parente F, Greco S, Molteni M, et al: Modern imaging of Crohn's disease using bowel ultrasound. Inflamm Bowel Dis 10:452-461, 2004.

41. Miao YM, Koh DM, Amin Z, et al: Ultrasound and magnetic resonance imaging assessment of active bowel segments in Crohn's disease. Clin Radiol 57:913-918, 2002.

42. Potthast S, Rieber A, Von Tirpitz C, et al: Ultrasound and magnetic resonance imaging in Crohn's disease: A comparison. Eur Radiol 12:1416-1422, 2002.

43. Rispo A, Imbriaco M, Celentano L, et al: Noninvasive diagnosis of small bowel Crohn's disease: Combined use of bowel sonography and Tc-99m-HMPAO leukocyte scintigraphy. Inflamm Bowel Dis 11:376-382, 2005.

44. Ruess L, Blask ARN, Bulas DI, et al: Inflammatory bowel disease in children and young adults: Correlation of sonographic and clinical parameters during treatment. AJR 175:79-84, 2000.

45. Maconi G, Di Sabatino A, Ardizzone S, et al: Prevalence and clinical significance of sonographic detection of enlarged regional lymph nodes in Crohn's disease. Scand J Gastroenterol 40:1328-1333, 2005.

46. Bremner AR, Pridgeon J, Fairhurst J, et al: Ultrasound scanning may reduce the need for barium radiology in the assessment of small-bowel Crohn's disease. Acta Paediatr 93:479-481, 2004.

47. Valette PJ, Rioux M, Pilleul F, et al: Ultrasonography of chronic inflammatory bowel diseases. Eur Radiol 11:1859-1866, 2001.

48. Wiarda BM, Kuipers EJ, Heitbrink MA, et al: MR Enteroclysis of inflammatory small-bowel diseases. AJR 187:522-531, 2006.

49. Masselli G, Casciani E, Polettini E, et al: Assessment of Crohn's disease in the small bowel: Prospective comparison of magnetic resonance enteroclysis with conventional enteroclysis. Eur Radiol 16:2817-2724, 2006.

50. Pauls S, Gabelmann A, Schmidt SA, et al: Evaluating bowel wall vascularity in Crohn's disease: A comparison of dynamic MRI and wideband harmonic imaging contrast-enhanced low MI ultrasound. Eur Radiol 16:2410-2417, 2006.

51. Gourtsoyiannis NC, Grammatikakis J, Papamastorakis G, et al: Imaging of small intestinal Crohn's disease: comparison between MR enteroclysis and conventional enteroclysis. Eur Radiol 16:1915-1925, 2006.

52. Rottgen R, Herzog H, Lopez-Haninnen E, et al: Bowel wall enhancement in magnetic resonance colonography for assessing activity in Crohn's disease. Clin Imaging 30:27-31, 2006.

53. Maccioni F, Bruni A, Viscido A, et al: MR imaging in patients with Crohn disease: Value of T2- versus T1-weighted gadolinium-enhanced MR sequences with use of an oral superparamagnetic contrast agent. Radiology 238:517-530, 2006.

54. Koh M, Miao Y, Chinn RJS, et al: MR imaging evaluation of the activity of Crohn's disease. AJR 177:1325-1332, 2001.

55. Gourtsoyiannis NC, Papanikolaou N: Magnetic resonance enteroclysis. Semin Ultrasound CT MRI 26:237-246, 2005.

56. Wiarda BM, Kuipers EJ, Houdijk LP, et al: MR enteroclysis: Imaging technique of choice in diagnosis of small bowel diseases. Dig Dis Sci 50:1036-1040, 2005.

57. Horsthuis K, Lavini Mphil C, Stoker J: MRI in Crohn's disease. J Magn Reson Imaging 22:1-12, 2005.

58. Laghi A, Paolantonio P, Passariello R: Small bowel. Magn Reson Imaging Clin North Am 13:331-348, 2005.

59. Zalis M, Singh AK: Imaging of inflammatory bowel disease: CT and MR. Dig Dis 22:56-62, 2004.

60. Narin B, Ajaj W, Gohde S, et al: Combined small and large bowel MR imaging in patients with Crohn's disease: A feasibility study. Eur Radiol 14:1535-1542, 2004.

61. Gourtsoyiannis N, Papanikolaou N, Grammatikakis J, et al: Assessment of Crohn's disease activity in the small bowel with MR and conventional enteroclysis: Preliminary results. Eur Radiol 14:1017-1024, 2004.

62. Low RN, Sebrechts CP, Politoske DA, et al: Crohn disease with endoscopic correlation: Single-shot fast spin-echo and gadolinium-enhanced fat-suppressed spoiled gradient-echo MR imaging. Radiology 222:652-660, 2002.

63. Sempere GAJ, Sanjuan VM, Chulia EM, et al: MRI evaluation of inflammatory activity in Crohn's disease. AJR 184:1829-1835, 2005.

64. Schunk K: Small bowel magnetic resonance imaging for inflammatory bowel disease. Top Magn Reson Imaging 13:409-425, 2002.

65. Maccioni F, Bruni A, Viscido A, et al: MR imaging in patients with Crohn disease: Value of T2- versus T1-weighted gadolinium-enhanced MR sequences with use of an oral superparamagnetic contrast agent. Radiology 238:517-530, 2006.

66. Booya F, Fletcher JG, Huprich JE, et al: Active Crohn disease: CT findings and interobserver agreement for enteric phase CT enterography. Radiology 241:787-795, 2006.

67. Bodily KD, Fletcher JG, Solem CA, et al: Crohn disease: Mural attenuation and thickness at contrast-enhanced CT enterography—correlation with endoscopic and histologic findings of inflammation. Radiology 238:505-516, 2006.

68. Colombel JF, Solem CA, Sandborn WJ, et al: Quantitative measurement and visual assessment of ileal Crohn's disease activity by computed tomography enterography: Correlation with endoscopic severity and C reactive protein. Gut 55:1561-1567, 2006.

69. Wold PB, Fletcher JG, Johnson CD, et al: Assessment of small bowel Crohn disease: Noninvasive peroral CT enterography compared with other imaging methods and endoscopy-feasibility study. Radiology 229:275-281, 2003.

70. Maglinte DD: Science to practice: Do mural attenuation and thickness at contrast-enhanced CT enterography correlate with endoscopic and histologic findings of inflammation in Crohn disease? Radiology 238:381-382, 2006.

71. Sailer S, Peloschek P, Schobe E, et al: Diagnostic value of CT enteroclysis compared with conventional enteroclysis in patients with Crohn's disease. AJR 185:1575-1581, 2005.

72. Hara AK, Leighton JA, Heigh RI, et al: Crohn disease of the small bowel: Preliminary comparison among CT enterography, capsule endoscopy, small-bowel follow-through, and ileoscopy. Radiology 238:128-134, 2006.

73. Paulsen SR, Huprich JE, Fletcher JG, et al: CT enterography as a diagnostic tool in evaluating small bowel disorders: Review of clinical experience with over 700 cases. RadioGraphics 26:641-657, 2006.

74. Liu YB, Liang CH, Zhang ZL, et al: Crohn disease of small bowel: Multidetector row CT with CT enteroclysis, dynamic contrast enhancement, CT angiography, and 3D imaging. Abdom Imaging, September 12, 2006 (Epub ahead of print).

75. Zissin R, Hertz M, Paran H, et al: Small bowel obstruction secondary to Crohn disease: CT findings. Abdom Imaging 29:320-325, 2004.

76. Lee SS, Ha HK, Yang S-K, et al: CT of prominent pericolic or perienteric vasculature in patients with Crohn's disease: Correlation with clinical disease activity and findings on barium studies. AJR 179:1029-1036, 2002.

77. Choi D, Jin Lee S, Ah Cho Y, et al: Bowel wall thickening in patients with Crohn's disease: CT patterns and correlation with inflammatory activity. Clin Radiol 58:68-74, 2001.

78. Furukawa A, Saotome T, Yamasaki M, et al: Cross-sectional imaging in Crohn disease. RadioGraphics 24:689-702, 2004.

79. Rypens F, Dubois J, Garel L, et al: Percutaneous drainage of abdominal abscesses in pediatric Crohn's disease. AJR 188:579-585, 2007.

80. Friedman S: Cancer in Crohn's disease. Gastroenterol Clin North Am 35:621-639, 2006.

81. Sands BE: Inflammatory bowel disease: Past, present, and future. J Gastroenterol 42:16-25, 2007.

Inflammatory Disorders of the Small Bowel Other Than Crohn's Disease

Stephen E. Rubesin, MD

A variety of inflammatory diseases of the small bowel are typically associated with diarrhea. Inflammatory disorders that cause malabsorption are discussed in Chapter 47, and Crohn's disease is given special treatment in Chapter 45.

More textbook pages are devoted to Crohn's disease than all other inflammatory conditions of the small bowel combined. This reflects several factors, including the frequent evaluation of acute infections involving the small bowel by stool cultures, toxin titers, and endoscopic biopsies rather than by imaging studies. In addition, most chronic infections of the small bowel that are the scourges of underdeveloped countries are unusual in the United States or other countries that have modern water and sewage treatment systems. Finally, radiologic imaging has a vital role in the diagnosis of Crohn's disease and its complications.

Despite these considerations, radiologists in the United States and other developed countries need to be familiar with inflammatory diseases of the small intestine other than Crohn's disease. With immigration, tourism, and globalization of the economy, infectious conditions of the small bowel are more likely to be encountered. Some of these patients with acute infectious diseases may undergo imaging studies for symptoms such as diarrhea or right lower quadrant pain (Figs. 46-1 and 46-2). In this chapter a review is presented of the wide spectrum of inflammatory and infectious disorders involving the small bowel other than Crohn's disease.

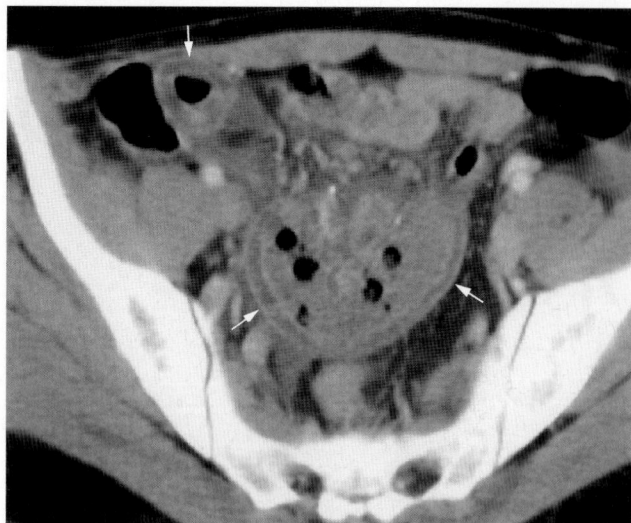

Figure 46-1. An oncologist presented with 7 days of diarrhea and right lower quadrant pain after returning from a conference in the Caribbean. CT through the pelvis shows a thickened bowel wall (*arrows*) in the distal ileum with a mural stratification pattern of enhancing mucosa, thickened but low-attenuation submucosa, and enhancing muscularis propria. The patient's symptoms resolved within 3 weeks. A follow-up CT was normal. Although stool cultures were negative, the presumptive diagnosis was acute infectious enteritis.

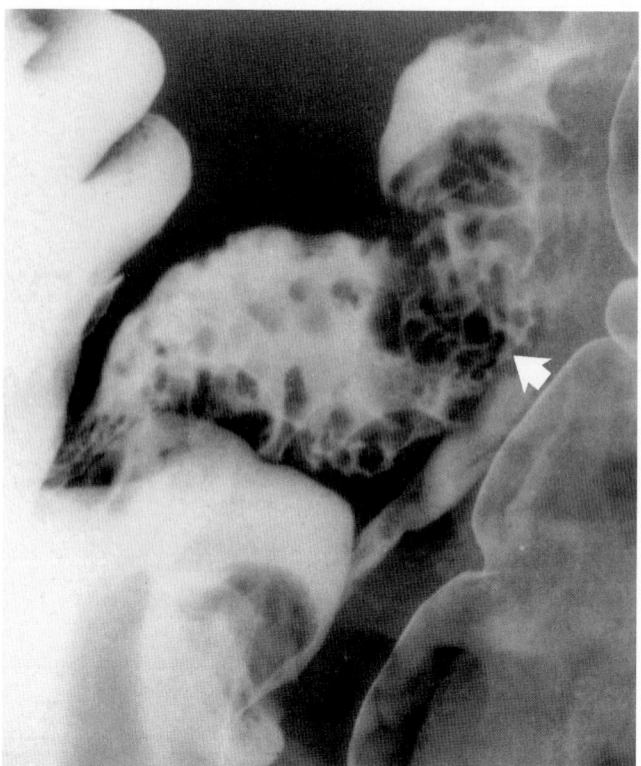

Figure 46-2. A young man presented with 2 weeks of right lower quadrant pain and mild diarrhea. Spot image from a peroral pneumocolon shows numerous smooth, ovoid, 3- to 5-mm nodules in the terminal ileum. Endoscopic follow-up was recommended because of the degree of nodularity and the confluent appearance of the nodules (*arrow*). Endoscopic biopsy specimens obtained several days later showed acute inflammatory changes in the terminal ileum. A follow-up barium study was normal. Although no stool cultures were obtained, the presumptive diagnosis was acute infectious ileitis.

THE SMALL INTESTINE AS AN IMMUNOLOGIC ORGAN

The microflora of the upper gastrointestinal tract originates from swallowed food and from the oral cavity. Small amounts of bacteria and yeasts are present in the esophagus, stomach, and duodenum—about 10^6 bacteria/mL compared with 10^{11} to 10^{12} bacteria/mL in the distal small bowel and colon.[1]

A variety of mechanisms prevent bacterial colonization of the small intestine. Secretion of water, electrolytes, and mucus by epithelial cells is an important component of host protection. Mucous secretions help prevent adherence of infectious agents to epithelial cells or penetration of toxins into these cells. Intestinal motility and fluid flow also impede bacterial colonization of the small bowel. Diarrhea due to increased secretion of fluid and electrolytes also facilitates passage of infectious agents from the small intestine. Nevertheless, bacterial colonization may occur if there is small bowel stasis due to a motor disorder, diverticulosis, or strictures.

The small intestine is one of the largest immunologic organs in the body, because it has an enormous surface area that is constantly exposed to foreign antigens. In healthy individuals, the small intestine is in a chronic state of low-grade inflammation and immune activity.[2] In most people, however, foreign antigens are eliminated without producing clinical symptoms. The small intestine can exclude foreign antigens without inducing autoimmune intestinal disease due to cross-reactivity of foreign and host antigens.

The immune system includes intraepithelial lymphocytes, lymphoid tissue in Peyer's patches in the lamina propria, neutrophils, macrophages, and mast cells. Peyer's patches are unencapsulated lymphoid clusters spanning the lamina propria.[2] A specialized epithelium overlies the Peyer's patches; M cells in this specialized epithelium transport antigens to the underlying lymphoid tissue.

B cells in the lamina propria synthesize immunoglobulin A (IgA) and, to a lesser degree, IgM, IgG, and IgE. Intraluminal secretion of IgA inhibits bacterial adherence to the epithelium, preventing bacterial colonization. IgA also neutralizes bacterial toxins, minimizing any deleterious effects on epithelial cell function. IgA also blocks absorption of intraluminal antigens. IgA helps neutralize intracellular pathogens but does not cause their destruction.

Intraepithelial lymphocytes are primarily T cells. These cells lie in the basal epithelium, secrete cytokines, and are involved with antigen recognition and tolerance to oral antigens. These cells also perform immunosurveillance against abnormal epithelial cells. T cells are markedly increased in number in graft-versus-host disease, celiac disease, and protozoal infections.

Polymorphonuclear neutrophils differentiate in the bone marrow, leave the peripheral circulation, enter the lamina propria, and traverse the epithelium to enter the intestinal lumen. Neutrophils recognize and phagocytize antibody-coated bacteria. Macrophages in the lamina propria are derived from monocytes produced in the bone marrow. These cells also pass through the epithelium into the lumen. Macrophages are important in bacterial phagocytosis and killing. Mast cells are found in all layers of the bowel wall. These cells contain granules with preformed mediators of inflammation such as histamine and 5-hydroxytryptamine. Mast cells are important in the defense against intestinal parasites and food antigens.

PARASITIC INFESTATIONS

Worms and protozoa infect more than one fourth of the world's population. Helminths (worms) are divided into roundworms (nematodes), tapeworms (cestodes), and flukes (trematodes). Nematodes are round and unsegmented. They have a body cavity and are divided into separate sexes.[2] Cestodes are tape-like and segmented and are hermaphrodites. Trematodes are leaf shaped and unsegmented and are also hermaphrodites.

Ascariasis

Ascaris lumbricoides is the most common intestinal worm, infecting about one fourth of the world's population, most frequently people living in the tropics and subtropics.[3] Ascariasis is acquired by ingesting mature eggs from contaminated soil, food, or water. Two to 3 weeks after ingestion of eggs, larvae develop in the small intestine. The larvae penetrate the mucosa, enter vessels in the bowel wall to reach the portal venous system, and migrate through the liver and heart to the lungs. The larvae then penetrate the alveoli, enter the tracheobronchial tree, and are swallowed. Development is completed in the small intestine, where the worms attach to the mucosal surface of the midjejunum. Worms may grow up to 40 cm in length.

Symptoms include abdominal pain and malabsorption. If the worms are present in large numbers, ascariasis can cause small bowel obstruction due to luminal obturation or intussusception.[4,5] Mature worms that migrate into the bile or pancreatic ducts may cause cholangitis or pancreatitis.

Ascaris can be identified on plain abdominal radiographs, barium studies, and CT. Long tubular filling defects are seen in the intestinal lumen on barium studies (Fig. 46-3) or CT.[6]

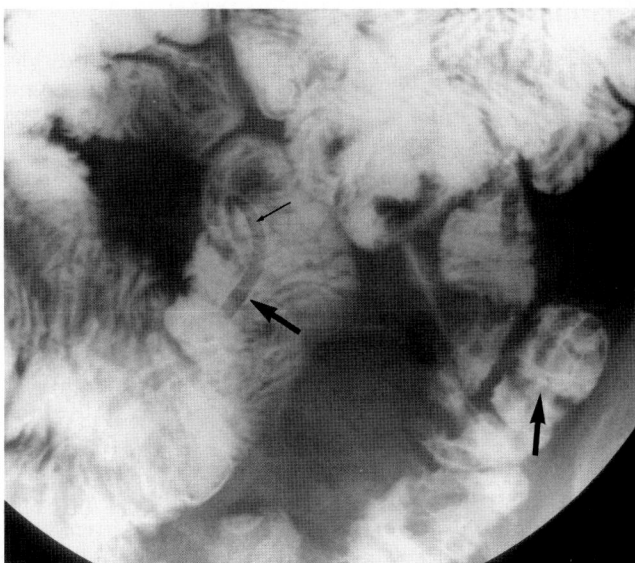

Figure 46-3. Ascariasis: a young man presented with crampy abdominal pain and mild diarrhea 1 month after returning from a vacation in Central America. Spot image of the ileum from a small bowel follow-through shows numerous smooth, tubular filling defects in the barium column (representative ascarids identified by *thick arrows*). Barium faintly stains the body cavity of one worm (*thin arrow*). (From Forbes A, Misiewicz JJ, Compton CC, et al: Atlas of Clinical Gastroenterology, 3rd ed. Edinburgh, Elsevier-Mosby, 2005.)

If barium enters the worm's intestinal tract, a long, thin line of barium will be present within the tubular radiolucent filling defect caused by the worm (see Fig. 46-3). Small bowel folds are usually of normal size but may be enlarged. Small nodules reflect submucosal cysts surrounded by fibrotic tissue. The radiographic diagnosis can be confirmed by detection of ova in stool specimens.

Hookworm Infestation (Ancylostomiasis)

Hookworms are small (8 to 10 mm) nematodes that infect almost 1 billion people worldwide.[2] Near adult-stage larvae and adult worms attach to the small intestinal mucosa. Ova are secreted into the feces. Infection results primarily from filarial invasion of the feet (in people who walk barefoot) or hands. *Ancylostoma duodenale* is found in southern Europe, the Mediterranean region, and the western coast of South America. *Necator americanus* causes hookworm infestation in the southern United States, the Caribbean, and South America. Both species are found in India and southeast Asia.[7] The incidence of hookworm disease has decreased markedly in the southern United States with improved sanitation.

Although hookworm infestation can cause abdominal pain, diarrhea, or acute gastrointestinal bleeding, iron-deficiency anemia is the most common clinical presentation. Peripheral eosinophilia is present in most patients.

The jejunal mucosa is edematous and hemorrhagic at sites of intestinal attachment. Hookworms have not been demonstrated on barium studies. Jejunal fold thickening and irritability may be present.[8] Ileal strictures have also been reported.[2] Regional lymphadenopathy may be present. A definitive diagnosis requires demonstration of ova in stool specimens or worms in jejunal aspirates or biopsy specimens.

Strongyloidiasis

Strongyloides stercoralis is a nematode most commonly found in the tropics and subtropics and in areas of poor sanitation or areas where human waste is used as fertilizer. In the United States, strongyloidiasis is found in people living in Appalachia,[9] military personnel returning from endemic regions, and patients who are immunocompromised due to malnutrition, steroid use, AIDS, or other causes.

Filariform larvae about 0.5 mm long penetrate the skin, migrate through the venous system to the lungs, penetrate the alveoli, enter the tracheobronchial tree, and are swallowed. The larvae are transformed into adult worms in the small intestine. The females penetrate the mucosa of the duodenum and proximal jejunum and live in the superficial layers of the proximal small bowel. Male worms are expelled. Female worms are about 2 mm in length.

Strongyloidiasis differs from other nematode diseases because autoinfection may occur; these infections may be life threatening in immunocompromised hosts. Eggs released into the intestinal lumen form rhabditiform larvae that develop into infective filariform larvae in the intestinal lumen or in the soil. The filariform larvae may reinvade intestinal mucosa or perianal skin. Most larvae die in lymphatics in the wall of the small bowel or in the mesentery.

Strongyloidiasis may cause a wide variety of clinical symptoms, including abdominal pain, diarrhea, weight loss, and malabsorption.

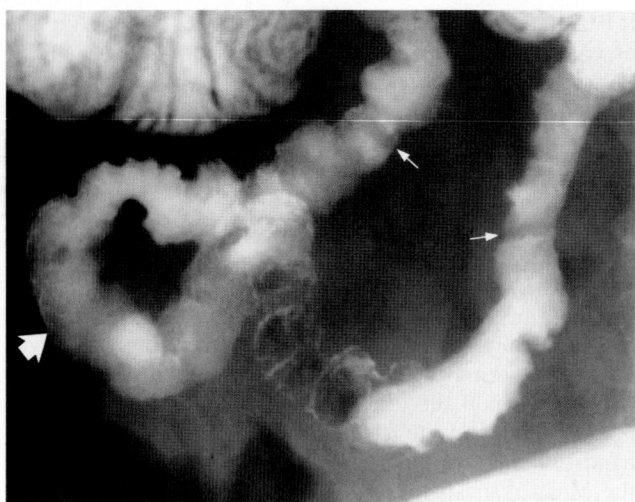

Figure 46-4. Strongyloidiasis. Coned-down view of overhead radiograph from a small bowel follow-through shows markedly thickened folds (*thin arrows*) in several loops of jejunum. In some areas, the inflammatory process is so severe that the folds are effaced or lost (*thick arrow*). (Courtesy of Jack Farman, MD, New York; from the teaching files of Hans Herlinger, MD.)

Mild infestation by strongyloidiasis cannot be detected on imaging studies. With chronic infection, thickened folds are seen in the duodenum and jejunum on barium studies.[10] With severe infection, the small bowel folds are effaced or obliterated and the jejunum can assume a narrowed, tubular configuration (Fig. 46-4).[11,12] Strongyloidiasis is also a cause of papillary stenosis and small intestinal dilatation. A definitive diagnosis can be made by duodenal aspiration or biopsy.[13]

Anisakiasis

Members of the Anisakidae family are nematode parasites of marine mammals. *Anisakis* larvae are found in intermediate hosts such as squid and fish (including salmon, cod, anchovy, tuna, mackerel, Pacific pollock, Pacific red snapper, and herring).[14] Human infection is acquired by eating raw, inadequately cooked, or pickled fish. Anisakiasis is most common in areas where raw fish such as sushi or sashimi is frequently eaten. Ingested larvae most frequently attach and invade the stomach, but small or large bowel involvement may occur. Edema and inflammation develop at the site of attempted larval penetration. Ulceration and perforation with formation of inflammatory masses have been reported. Symptoms of small bowel involvement can mimic those of acute appendicitis, Crohn's disease, or small bowel obstruction.

Anisakis larvae have been detected on barium studies of the stomach and colon but not of the small intestine.[15] Focal, irregular fold thickening may be seen in the small bowel. Strictures and short, ulcerated lesions have also been described.[8] Perforation with mesenteric abscess formation may lead to a mesenteric mass/abscess detected on cross-sectional imaging studies.[16]

Tapeworm (Cestode) Infestation

Cestodes live as adults in the gastrointestinal tract of definitive hosts and as cysticerci in the tissue of intermediate hosts. Humans are the definitive hosts for *Taenia saginata*

(beef tapeworm), *Taenia solium* (pork tapeworm), *Hymenolepis nana* (dwarf tapeworm), and *Diphyllobothrium latum* (fish tapeworm). In contrast, humans are intermediate hosts for *Echinococcus granulosus, Echinococcus multilocularis,* and *Taenia solium.* These ribbon-like worms may vary in length from several millimeters to several meters. They attach to the intestinal mucosa by a scolex. A connecting region is followed by the strobila and a chain of developing segments (the proglottids). The number of proglottids varies from 3 to 4000, and the length of the cestode varies from several millimeters to several meters.[17]

Humans are infected by eating inadequately cooked beef, pork, or fish (including pike, salmon, trout, whitefish, and turbot). After infected flesh is ingested, the cysticercus breaks down, releasing a scolex that attaches in the upper jejunum. The adult worm develops, and proglottids and ova are released into the lumen. Tapeworm infection usually causes no symptoms. Because of its long length (up to 4 to 6 meters), *T. saginata* may cause obstructive symptoms. In contrast, *D. latum* may cause vitamin B_{12} deficiency and macrocytic anemia.

Trematode (Flukes) Infestation

A variety of flukes may involve the liver, biliary tract, and intestines. The genus *Schistosoma* infects more than 150 million people worldwide.[2] *S. mansoni* is endemic in Africa, the Middle East, and Latin America; *S. japonicum* is endemic primarily in Asia; and *S. haematobium* is endemic in the Middle East and Africa. *S. haematobium* mainly causes genitourinary disease but is occasionally found in the appendix. Because colonic infection by schistosomiasis is more common than small bowel infection, this disease is discussed in Chapter 62.

Giardiasis

Giardiasis is the most common parasitic disease worldwide. In the United States,[18,19] giardiasis is most frequently found in the Rocky Mountain states. Surface water contaminated by feces from wild animals is the principal source of infection. Cysts remain viable in cold water for 1 to 3 months.[2] Cysts can also survive the chlorine levels of many municipal water systems. Giardiasis is also transmitted by homosexual behavior and by fecal-oral transmission from contaminated food and pets. The risk of infection is greater in patients with immunodeficiency states and hypochlorhydria.

After cyst ingestion, trophozoites emerge in the duodenum and proximal jejunum. The trophozoites remain in the intestinal lumen or penetrate the mucus gel layer of the proximal intestine to attach to the glycocalyx of the enterocytes. The trophozoites do not invade the epithelium. Mature cysts are excreted in the stool.

The infection varies from the asymptomatic carrier state, to self-limited diarrhea or chronic, watery diarrhea. Because the infection is patchy, biopsy specimens may be normal in infected patients. Some patients may have villous atrophy with crypt hyperplasia and variable inflammation, and others may have lymphoid hyperplasia.

The small intestine frequently appears normal on small bowel follow-through studies. In about one half of patients there is increased intraluminal fluid and rapid small bowel

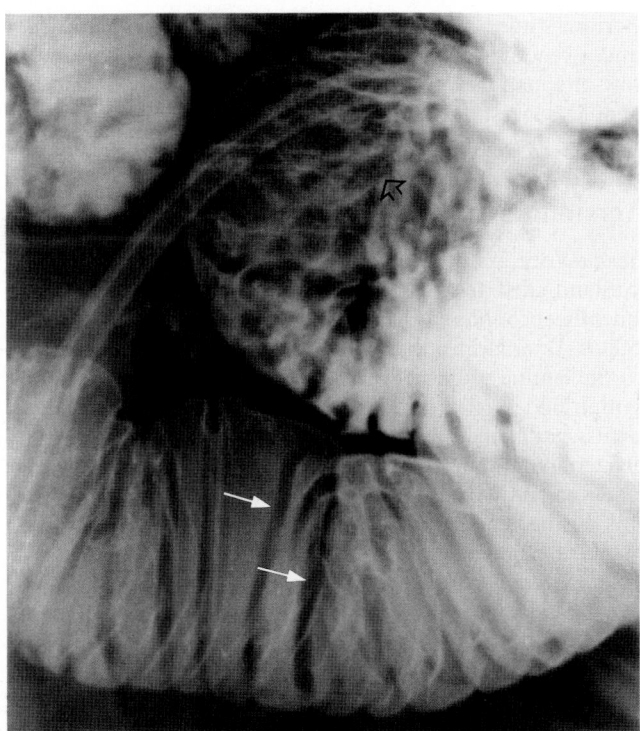

Figure 46-5. Giardiasis. Spot image of the jejunum from an enteroclysis examination shows mildly thickened folds (*arrows*). Tiny mucosal nodules (*open arrow*) reflect enlargement of villi. (From the teaching files of Hans Herlinger, MD.)

transit. Some reports have described thickened folds and irritability in the duodenum and jejunum (Fig. 46-5).[20,21] Because barium studies are abnormal in fewer than one half of infected patients and the radiographic findings are nonspecific, the diagnosis depends on detection of cysts and trophozoites on stool examinations, detection of trophozoites on duodenal biopsies or aspirates, or a positive fluorescent antibody test.[22]

Trypanosomiasis

Chagas' disease is caused by the protozoan *Trypanosoma cruzi*, spread by the bite of the reduviid bug. Chagas' disease is endemic in central Brazil, northern Argentina, and Venezuela but has also been reported in southern areas of the United States. It is estimated that 350,000 people in the United States are seropositive for this infection.[23] *T. cruzi* produces a neurotoxin that attacks autonomic ganglion cells throughout the body, including those in the heart, gastrointestinal tract, urinary tract, and respiratory tract.[24] The esophagus, duodenum, and colon are the gastrointestinal organs most commonly affected, resulting in secondary achalasia, megaduodenum, and megacolon. Involvement of the mesenteric small bowel leads to dilatation of the small bowel with delayed transit.

BACTERIAL INFECTIONS

Traveler's diarrhea and foodborne diseases are common problems related to tainted water supplies and improperly prepared or stored food. Bacteria are the organisms usually responsible for traveler's diarrhea, which explains why prophylactic use of antibiotics decreases the incidence of traveler's

diarrhea.[25] Chemicals, viruses, and parasites are less frequent causes of traveler's diarrhea. Any microbial pathogen that causes diarrhea may be responsible. Enterotoxigenic *E. coli* is the most common cause of traveler's diarrhea. Enteroadherent and enteropathogenic *E. coli* are less frequent causes. *Shigella* and *Campylobacter jejuni* are the next most common pathogens, but these bacteria usually involve the colon. This infection is rarely diagnosed on imaging studies, because acute, watery diarrhea develops during or shortly after a period of travel.

Tuberculosis

Tuberculosis is endemic in Asia. Intestinal tuberculosis, however, is uncommon in western countries, usually occurring in the homeless, alcoholics, inmates, farm workers, immigrants, or people infected with human immunodeficiency virus (HIV). With the rise of AIDS and immigration, intestinal tuberculosis is becoming more common in developed countries. In one hospital in London with an extensive population of Asian immigrants, new diagnoses of tuberculosis were almost as common as new diagnoses of Crohn's disease.[26,27] The proposed mechanisms of infection of the gastrointestinal tract include (1) ingestion of infected sputum or milk and (2) hematogenous spread to submucosal lymphatics.[28] Intestinal tuberculosis frequently occurs without radiographic evidence of pulmonary disease.[26-28]

Intestinal tuberculosis primarily occurs in the ileocecal region. The distribution of tuberculosis parallels the distribution of the lymphatics. In one autopsy series of over 1000 cases, 90% of patients had ileal disease and 75% had cecal disease. Other sites were not infrequently involved, however, including the ascending colon in 51%, the transverse colon in 33%, the descending colon in 23%, and the appendix in 33%.[29] Skip lesions may be present.

The three classic forms of gastrointestinal tuberculosis are the ulcerative, hypertrophic, and ulcerohypertrophic forms.[30] Sloughing of mucosa overlying submucosal tubercles results in ulceration. These ulcers usually appear as short (3 to 6 mm in length) collections perpendicular to the longitudinal axis of the bowel. The ulcers may be stellate or longitudinal. Extensive inflammation and fibrosis of the bowel wall results in the hypertrophic form of tuberculosis associated with extensive mesenteric lymphadenopathy and adhesions. Bacilli are found primarily in necrotic mesenteric lymph nodes rather than the intestinal wall. Endoscopic biopsy specimens and tissue cultures are frequently negative.[31,32] In one study, acid-fast bacilli and caseating necrosis were found in only 32% and 50% of patients with gastrointestinal tuberculosis, respectively.[33] In some cases, laparoscopic diagnosis with cultures and histologic examination of ascitic fluid may be helpful. Not infrequently, however, the diagnosis of tuberculosis is made only by pathologic examination of resected surgical specimens.

Complications of small bowel tuberculosis include strictures and obstruction, fistulas, enteroliths, and chronic appendicitis.

Barium studies may reveal perpendicular, stellate, or longitudinal ulcers of varying size with heaped-up margins in the colon or ileum (usually the terminal ileum).[34] Short or long strictures may be associated with nodular mucosa. A narrow, contracted cecum associated with a gaping ileocecal valve and disproportionate inflammation of the ascending colon are

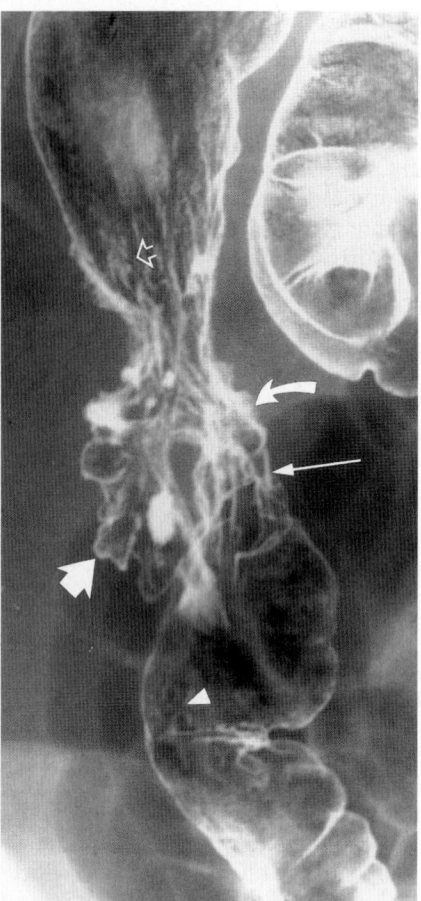

Figure 46-6. Ileocecal tuberculosis. Spot image of the ascending colon from a double-contrast barium enema shows disproportionately severe disease in the cecum versus the terminal ileum. The cecum is contracted and sacculated (*large arrow*). Granular and nodular mucosa (*open arrow*) is present in the cecum and ascending colon. The ileocecal valve is gaping (*curved arrow*). Only the distal 2 cm of the terminal ileum is narrowed (*thin arrow*). The remainder of the terminal ileum has a finely nodular mucosa (*arrowhead*). (From Rubesin SE, Bartram CI, Laufer I: Inflammatory bowel disease. In Levine MS, Rubesin SE, Laufer I [eds]: Double Contrast Gastrointestinal Radiology, 3rd ed. Philadelphia, WB Saunders, 2000, pp 417-470.)

findings that help to distinguish ileocecal tuberculosis from Crohn's disease (Fig. 46-6).[35] However, longitudinal ulceration, sinus tracts, and fistulas in the terminal ileum may be indistinguishable from those in Crohn's disease on barium studies.

CT often reveals thickening of the ileocecal valve. The medial wall of the cecum is disproportionately thickened and often associated with a soft tissue mass that engulfs the terminal ileum.[36] Wall thickening may be uniform or heterogeneous. Lymphadenopathy predominates in the pericecal region but may extend into the mesentery.

Historically, radiologic differentiation of tuberculosis from Crohn's disease was facilitated by predominance of the tuberculous inflammatory process in the cecum and ascending colon with a patulous ileocecal valve lumen and thickened ileocecal valve lips in patients with tuberculosis. However, tuberculosis and Crohn's disease may have a similar lymphatic distribution and overlapping radiographic findings. The clinical history and patient demographics should therefore be considered before suggesting the diagnosis of Crohn's disease.

Barium studies showing disease predominantly in the cecum and ascending colon with cecal contraction and CT showing low-attenuation lymph nodes indicative of caseous necrosis should suggest tuberculosis rather than Crohn's disease as the diagnosis in these patients.[37]

Yersiniosis

Yersinia are gram-negative cocci acquired after ingestion of contaminated food or water. *Y. enterocolitica* is more frequently encountered than *Y. pseudotuberculosis* in the United States. *Yersinia* invades epithelial cells, enters Peyer's patches in the lamina propria/submucosa, and spreads to mesenteric lymph nodes.[38] Ileitis, colitis, mesenteric adenitis, periappendicitis, and hemolytic-uremic syndrome have been reported.[39] Bacterial multiplication in Peyer's patches and regional lymph nodes can result in distant infections, including chronic hepatis, ankylosing spondylitis, and lung and kidney infections.[40]

Yersinia infection leads to the development of aphthoid ulcers overlying hyperplastic lymph follicles in the bowel. Hyperplasia of follicular and interfollicular regions results in massive lymphadenopathy.[41] Acute vasculitis may cause ischemia.

The radiographic appearance in *Yersinia* enterocolitis depends on the course of infection. Early in the disease, aphthoid ulcers and thickened folds may be the predominant findings in the terminal ileum.[42] Later in the disease, the ulcers disappear but thickened, undulating folds persist (Fig. 46-7).

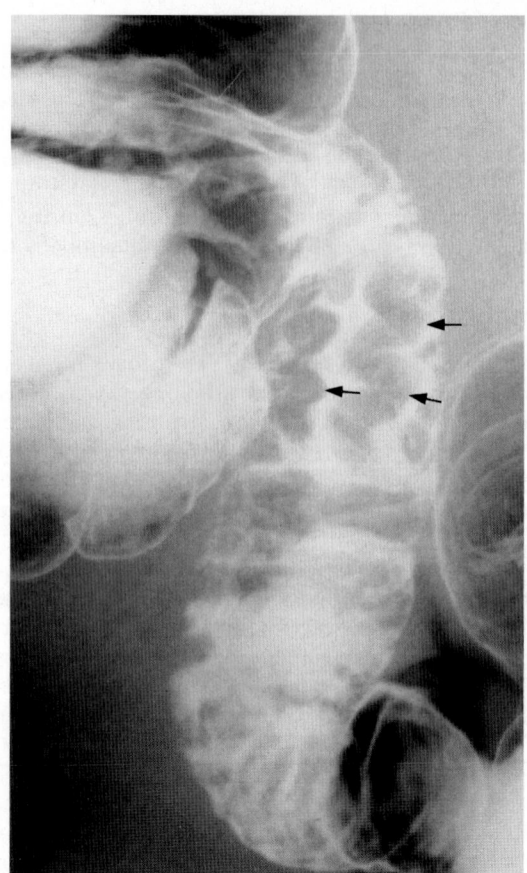

Figure 46-7. *Yersinia* ileitis. Spot image of the terminal ileum from a double-contrast barium enema shows thickened, undulating folds (*arrows*) in the terminal ileum. No ileal narrowing is seen.

The inflammatory process is distinguished from Crohn's disease by the absence of luminal narrowing, fissures, or fistulas. The inflammatory process usually resolves in 4 to 6 weeks.

Salmonellosis

Salmonella is a species of infection that is classified into subgroups.[1] In humans, most *Salmonella* pathogens belong to subgroup A. Gastrointestinal *Salmonella* infections may have distinct clinical forms, including typhoid fever, gastroenteritis, and an asymptomatic carrier state.

Foodborne outbreaks resulting in diarrhea are usually due to *S. enteritidis* and *S. typhimurium*, found in a wide variety of sources, including eggs, poultry, and livestock. Diarrheal outbreaks due to fecal-oral spread from human reservoirs are less common.[1] *Salmonella* enter and multiply in M cells and enterocytes and then disseminate to lymphoid tissue and macrophages in the submucosa and mesenteric lymph nodes. The diarrheal form of salmonellosis varies from a few loose stools to a severe watery diarrheal state. The diarrhea usually lasts from 3 to 7 days. Bacteremia is uncommon, occurring in 6% to 8% of patients.[1]

Typhoid fever is most commonly caused by *S. typhi* and *S. paratyphi*. Humans are the reservoir for *S. typhi*. The organism is transmitted by the fecal-oral route, so that this disease is usually found in regions with contaminated water and poor waste treatment. In most patients, a brief episode of diarrhea precedes the febrile illness. A systemic, acute febrile illness then lasts for 3 to 5 weeks, accompanied by nonspecific symptoms such as headaches, malaise, abdominal discomfort, and arthralgias. Complications of *Salmonella* include gastrointestinal bleeding and perforation related to a lymphoid reaction in the ileocecal region. Bacteremia can lead to other infections, including meningitis, pericarditis, orchitis, and splenic or liver abscesses. Hepatosplenomegaly may be present. Perforation or peritonitis may cause an adynamic ileus.

Salmonella may be manifested on barium studies by longitudinally oriented ulcers in the distal ileum overlying Peyer's patches.[2] Prominent lymphoid hyperplasia may be present, and vascular thrombosis may be seen. The disease is sometimes detected on CT performed to evaluate hepatosplenomegaly, right lower quadrant pain, and fever. CT may reveal circumferential thickening of the terminal ileum.[43] Barium studies may demonstrate nonspecific fold thickening in the terminal ileum.

Campylobacteriosis

Campylobacter comprises a group of gram-negative rods, including *C. jejuni, C. fetus,* and *C. coli.* These organisms may cause an acute enteritis or colitis, or affected individuals may remain in an asymptomatic carrier state. Colonic infections may be severe, resulting in fulminant colitis with gastrointestinal bleeding or toxic megacolon.[44] Systemic manifestations (including arthritis, endocarditis, genital infections, and urinary infections) may occur. Cross-reactivity of *C. jejuni* and neural antigens may result in Guillain-Barré syndrome.[2]

When the small intestine is involved, multiple superficial ulcers may develop in the distal ileum and region of the ileocecal valve. Barium studies may reveal thickened folds and aphthoid ulcers in the distal ileum and terminal ileum.[45,46]

The radiographic findings are indistinguishable from those of yersiniosis or early Crohn's disease.

FUNGAL INFECTIONS

Histoplasmosis

Histoplasma capsulatum is a dimorphic fungus commonly found in the Mississippi and Ohio River valleys. This fungus occurs in a mycelial form at ambient temperature and in a yeast form at body temperature.[47] The fungus usually infects elderly patients or immunocompromised hosts. Small bowel infection is common in patients with disseminated disease, but clinical symptoms are usually minimal. Ileocecal disease is characterized by ulceration, mucosal nodularity, strictures, and lymphadenopathy.[47] Intestinal perforation and peritonitis may also be seen.[48,49]

VIRAL INFECTIONS

Numerous viruses may infect the small intestine, resulting in an acute diarrheal state. Radiologic studies are rarely performed in this clinical setting. The diagnosis can be made by viral cultures or by enzyme-linked immunosorbent assay or electron microscopy of stool specimens. Cytomegalovirus involving the small bowel is described in a later section on immunocompromised patients.

DRUG-INDUCED DISORDERS

Drugs may cause a variety of abnormalities in the small intestine. Ischemia can result from systemic hypotension and hypovolemia, mesenteric arterial vasoconstriction, and slow mesenteric flow with venous thrombosis (Table 46-1).[50] Ischemia is discussed in Chapter 51. Anticoagulants may cause gastrointestinal bleeding. Small bowel hypomotility can result from narcotics and other drugs with anticholinergic properties or neurotoxic side effects (Table 46-2). Drugs may cause

Table 46-1
Drugs Causing Small Bowel Ischemia

Antihypertensive drugs/diuretics
Norepinephrine
Dopamine
Vasopressin
Digoxin
Cocaine
Ergotamines
  Ergotamine
  Methysergide
Oral contraceptives

Table 46-2
Drugs Associated with Small Bowel Hypomotility

Anticholinergic drugs
Phenothiazines
Tricyclic antidepressants
Verapamil
Clonidine
Vincristine
Narcotics

Table 46-3
Drugs Associated with Various Forms of Malabsorption

Tetracycline
Cholestyramine
Colchicine
Neomycin
Methotrexate
Methyldopa
Allopurinol
Thiazide diuretics
Clofazimine

malabsorption by a number of mechanisms, including interference with fat digestion and absorption; decreased gastric, pancreatic, and biliary secretions; increased intestinal transit, and small bowel mucosal injury (Table 46-3). Alcohol may also cause malabsorption by damage to intestinal crypts and villi. Metals such as aluminum, lead, gold, cadmium, mercury, zirconium, and iron may also damage small bowel epithelium.

Ulcers and Stenoses Related to NSAIDs

The small bowel is probably the most frequent site of gastrointestinal blood loss caused by nonsteroidal anti-inflammatory drug (NSAID) use. NSAID-related lesions are being detected with increased frequency by capsule endoscopy, enteroscopy, and enteroclysis. Small bowel ulcers are found at autopsy in approximately 8% of people who take NSAIDs.[51,52] The mechanism of injury is unknown.

NSAID-related injury is found primarily in the ileum. Punctate, linear, or circumferential ulcers secondary to NSAIDS may cause gastrointestinal bleeding or perforation. Chronic inflammation and scarring leads to the formation of charac-

teristic weblike diaphragms and ringlike strictures in the small bowel.[53-55] The mucosal diaphragms vary from slightly enlarged valvulae conniventes to thick, rigid, ringlike areas of narrowing. Pathologically, thick layers of hyalinized collagen are found to interdigitate with the muscularis mucosae.[2,56]

NSAID-induced ulcers may be detected on air contrast enteroclysis. Any form of enteroclysis can detect small bowel strictures, but thin webs may be difficult to differentiate from prominent small bowel folds. Thicker webs may be seen as 2- to 5-mm thick rings encircling the bowel associated with a tapered contour (see Chapter 50).[54]

Fluorinated Antipyrimidines

Cells in the small bowel crypts have a high turnover rate and are particularly susceptible to chemotherapeutic drugs that inhibit cell proliferation. Mucosal damage occurs within the first 3 days of chemotherapy. Mucosal regeneration occurs within several weeks after cessation of chemotherapy.[50] Enteritis may be caused by chemotherapeutic agents such as dactinomycin, bleomycin, cytarabine, doxorubicin, methotrexate, 5-fluorouracil, and vincristine.[50]

Enteritis related to chemotherapy can sometimes be detected on CT performed in patients with known metastatic disease who have abdominal pain and diarrhea.

Two antipyrimidines, 5-fluorouracil (5-FU) and floxuridine (5-FUDR), are used for the treatment of colonic carcinoma metastatic to the liver. Direct infusion of these agents into the hepatic artery may cause severe gastroduodenal inflammation and ulceration.[57] Intravenous infusion may also produce a severe form of gastroduodenitis and associated enteropathy, manifested by nausea, vomiting, and diarrhea. CT (usually performed for follow-up of liver metastases) may reveal marked wall thickening in the distal ileum (Fig. 46-8).[58] Barium studies may show smooth, thickened or effaced ileal folds (Fig. 46-9).[59] The diagnosis is suggested based on the

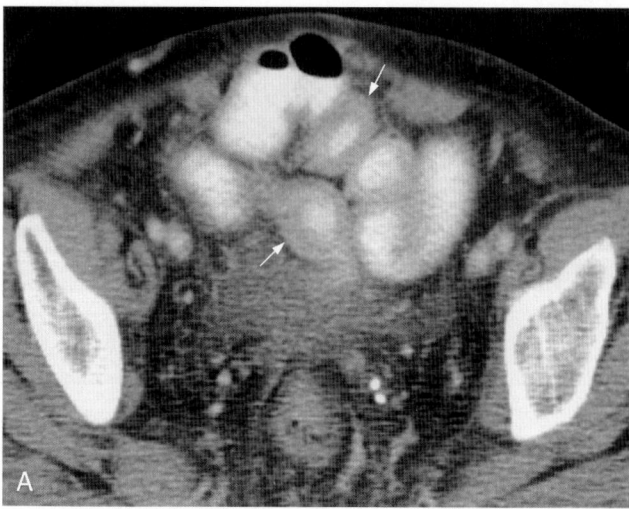
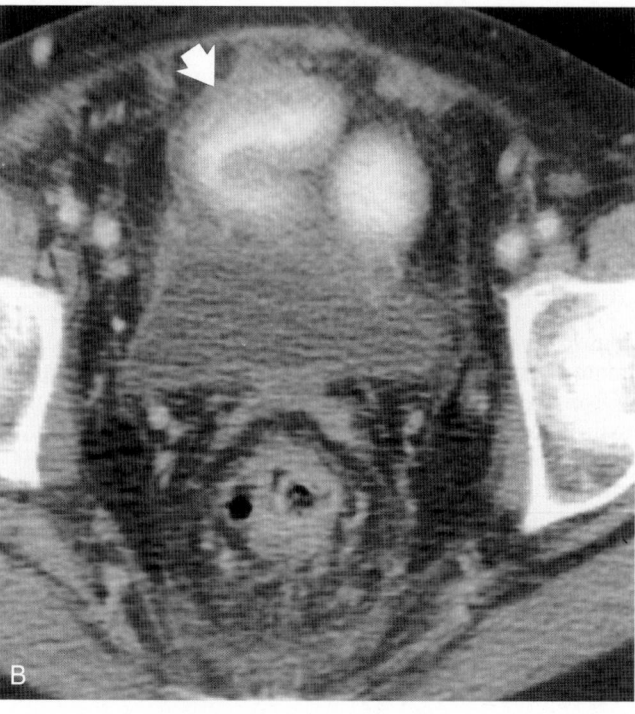

Figure 46-8. 5-FUDR chemotoxicity. A. CT through the upper pelvis shows thickening of the wall of several small bowel loops (*arrows*). **B.** CT at the level of the acetabula shows wall thickening of an ileal loop in profile (*arrow*).

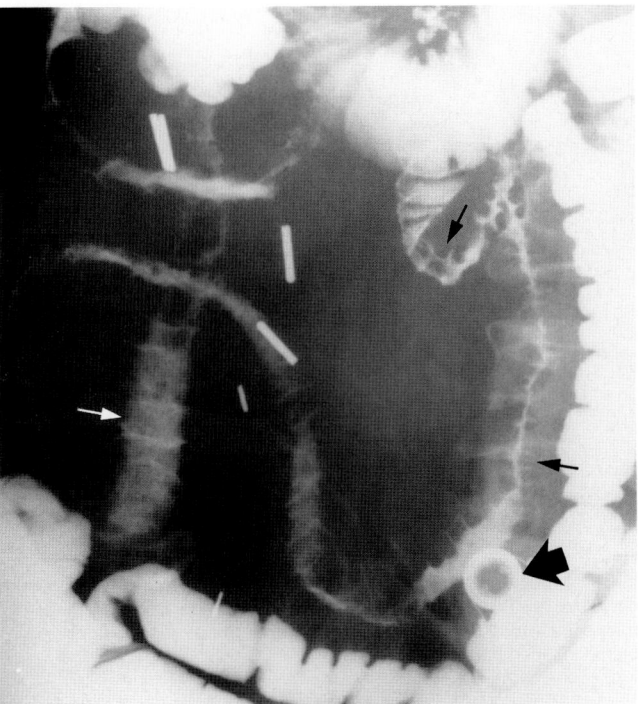

Figure 46-9. 5-FUDR chemotoxicity. Spot image of the right lower quadrant shows three loops of neoterminal ileum with markedly thickened, relatively smooth folds (*thin arrows*) perpendicular to the longitudinal axis of the bowel. A portion of the infusion pump is identified (*thick arrow*). The ascending colon and cecum are surgically absent after a right hemicolectomy for colonic cancer.

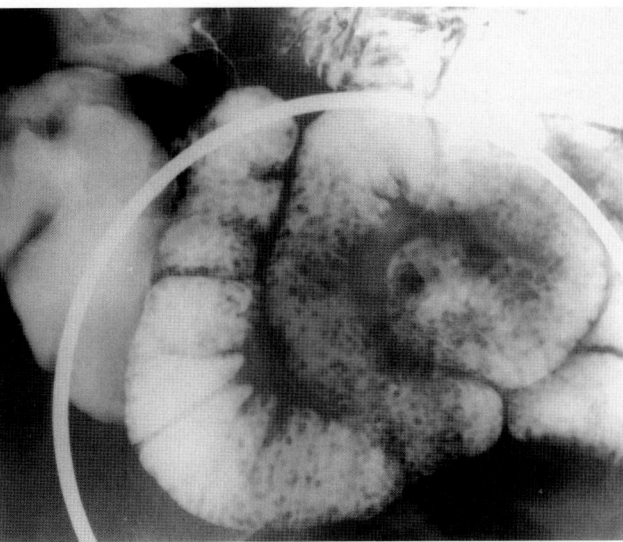

Figure 46-10. Marked lymphoid hyperplasia in a patient with common variable immunodeficiency. Spot image from a small bowel follow-through shows innumerable 1- to 2-mm, round nodules in the distal ileum and terminal ileum. These lymphoid follicles are increased in number and extent in comparison to the usual lymphoid pattern confined primarily to the terminal ileum. The lymphoid follicles are not enlarged or confluent.

clinical history of recent chemotherapy with 5-FU or 5-FUDR. The diagnosis is confirmed if there is improvement or resolution of clinical symptoms after cessation of chemotherapy and regression of radiologic abnormalities on follow-up imaging studies.

INFLAMMATORY DISEASE IN IMMUNODEFICIENCY

Selective Immunoglobulin A and Common Variable Immunodeficiency

Selective immunoglobulin A and common variable immunodeficiency are the most common primary immune deficiency states in adults.[60] In selective IgA deficiency there are a decreased number of IgA-producing plasma cells in the lamina propria and submucosa.[2] Gastrointestinal tract infections are uncommon, however, because there is a compensatory increase in IgM-producing plasma cells. Bacterial and viral infections of the sinonasal regions cause the majority of clinical complaints. There is a questionable increase in giardial infections. On barium studies, nodular lymphoid hyperplasia of the ileum is often present.

Common variable immunodeficiency is a heterogeneous group of varying B- and T-cell abnormalities that result in decreased production of IgG, IgM, and IgA, with an abnormal response to antigens and increased susceptibility to gastrointestinal and respiratory infections. This heterogeneous disorder is associated with autoimmune diseases such as autoimmune hepatitis and sclerosing cholangitis. About one third of patients have the autoimmune form of atrophic gastritis with pernicious anemia and its increased risk of gastric carcinoma. Splenomegaly is frequently found. There may also be an increased risk of small bowel lymphoma in these patients.[61,62]

Polyclonal B-cell lymphoid hyperplasia is present in the small intestine.[2] Lymphoid aggregates of T cells are present in the epithelium and lamina propria. A varying amount of villous atrophy is seen. Unlike gluten-sensitive enteropathy, however, a paucity of inflammatory cells is present in the lamina propria. A granulomatous reaction may also be present.

Barium studies may reveal extensive nodular lymphoid hyperplasia in the ileum (Fig. 46-10).[63,64] The nodules are slightly larger and are more numerous and more widely distributed than the usual lymphoid follicles seen in the terminal ileum in children and young adults.

Giardiasis is common in patients with common variable immunodeficiency. Unlike disease in immunocompetent individuals, giardiasis in common variable immunodeficiency may cause severe mucosal damage and malabsorption. There is also an increased risk of colonic infections (such as salmonellosis) that can mimic ulcerative colitis.[60]

Graft-versus-Host Disease

Gastrointestinal epithelium is damaged during the induction protocols for bone marrow transplantation. Anorexia, cramping, abdominal pain, and watery diarrhea occur immediately after induction by chemotherapy or radiation. Within 3 weeks, the enterocyte population is restored and symptoms subside. However, acute graft-versus-host disease (GVHD) develops in 30% to 50% of patients 3 to 11 weeks after allogeneic bone marrow transplantation. This condition is manifested clinically by diarrhea, anorexia, vomiting, abdominal pain, gastrointestinal bleeding and protein loss, and secondary infections.[2,60]

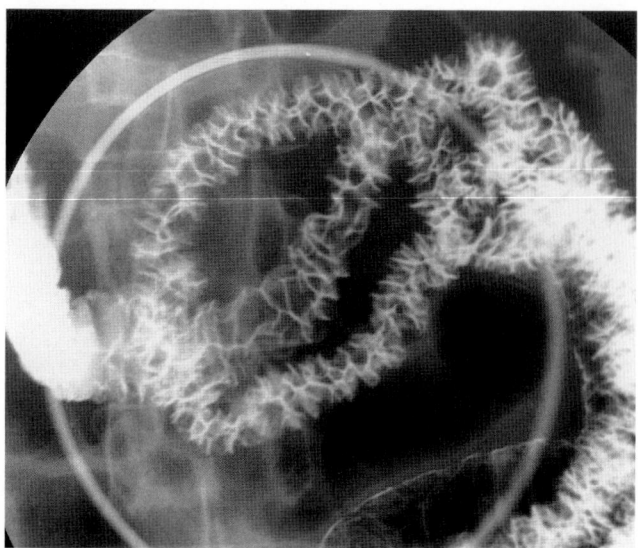

Figure 46-11. Graft-versus-host disease. Spot image from a small bowel follow-through shows diffuse fold thickening in the jejunum.

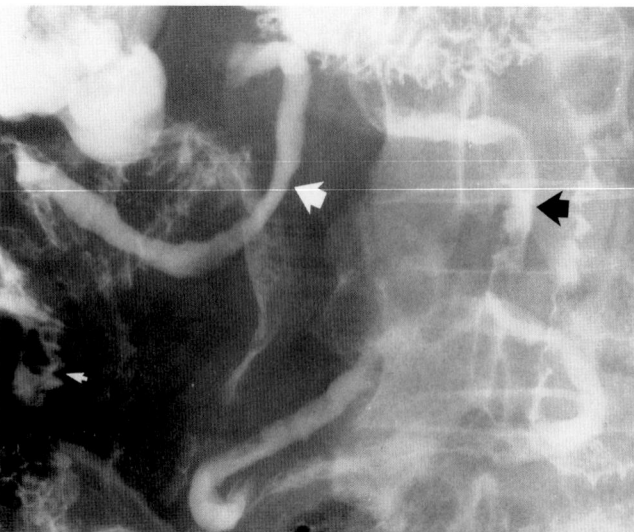

Figure 46-12. Graft-versus-host disease. Spot image from a small bowel follow-through shows that the jejunum and upper ileum have a diffusely narrowed, tubular appearance. In some loops the folds are markedly thickened (*small arrow*), whereas in other loops the folds are completely effaced (*large arrows*).

In patients with this disease, CD4[+] T lymphocytes from the donor graft recognize host histocompatibility antigens as foreign, leading to a T-cell–mediated attack on various tissues of the host. Tissue damage is most clinically evident in the skin, liver, mucous membranes, eyes, and gastrointestinal tract. A maculopapular rash may be present on the palms, soles, and trunk. Acute watery diarrhea results from denudation of the intestinal epithelium. Biopsy findings vary from individual crypt cell death to total necrosis of the epithelium. Submucosal edema is present. Acute GVHD is often complicated by cytomegalovirus, astrovirus, adenovirus, and *Clostridium difficile* infections.[65,66] Cholestasis and mild hepatocellular necrosis are reflected by abnormal results of liver function tests.

Chronic GVHD develops 3 to 13 months after transplantation and occurs without prior acute GVHD in one fourth of patients. Esophageal changes are seen in 15% of patients, as described in Chapter 25.[67] Unlike acute GVHD, which is characterized by enterocyte necrosis, chronic GVHD is characterized by patchy fibrosis of the lamina propria and submucosa with bacterial overgrowth.

Barium studies may confirm the diagnosis of acute or chronic GVHD and show the extent of disease. Thickened folds and nodular mucosa may be seen (Fig. 46-11). A tubular ("ribbon-like" or "toothpaste") bowel may result from sloughing of the epithelium or such rapid transit that barium fails to coat the surface of the small bowel (Fig. 46-12).[68-70] Barium may also adhere to the necrotic bowel surface, so that it is sometimes detected on abdominal radiographs or CT performed after the initial barium study.[71,72] CT may reveal a diffusely thickened small bowel wall (Fig. 46-13) with extensive submucosal edema (i.e., a target sign) or pneumatosis.[73] The mesentery may also be engorged, and ascites may be present.

Typhlitis

Neutropenic enterocolitis primarily affects the cecum and, to a lesser degree, the terminal ileum and appendix. Neutropenic enterocolitis is sometimes detected on CT scans to evaluate abdominal pain or fever in patients with various forms of

leukemia (Fig. 46-14). This entity is discussed in detail in Chapter 62.

Gastrointestinal Infections in AIDS

About one half of patients infected with HIV have chronic diarrhea.[74,75] This can be related to AIDS enteropathy, infectious enteritis or colitis, motility disturbances, or drug-induced side effects of antiretroviral and antimicrobial agents.[76] A wide variety of viruses, bacteria, protozoa, and fungi can infect the small bowel in patients with AIDS. Some pathogens such as *Mycobacterium avium-intracellulare* are unique to AIDS. Other pathogens such as *Salmonella* have an increased incidence in patients with AIDS in comparison to immunocompetent patients. Patients with AIDS often have several concurrent infections, resulting in chronic diarrhea, malabsorption, protein-calorie malnutrition, and weight loss.

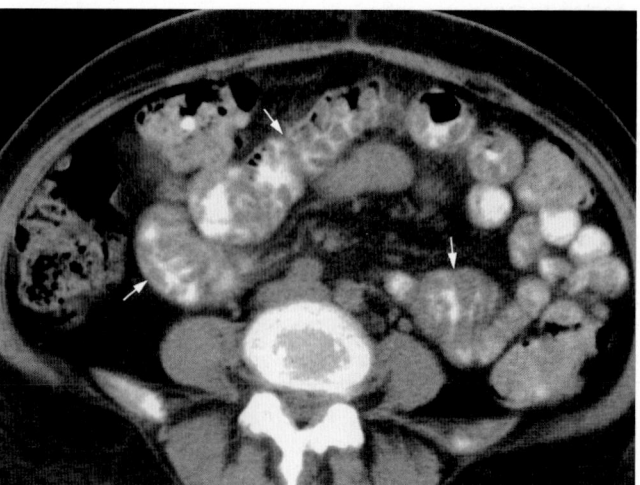

Figure 46-13. Graft-versus-host disease. CT through the top of the iliac crest shows extensive fold thickening (*arrows*) in mid small bowel loops.

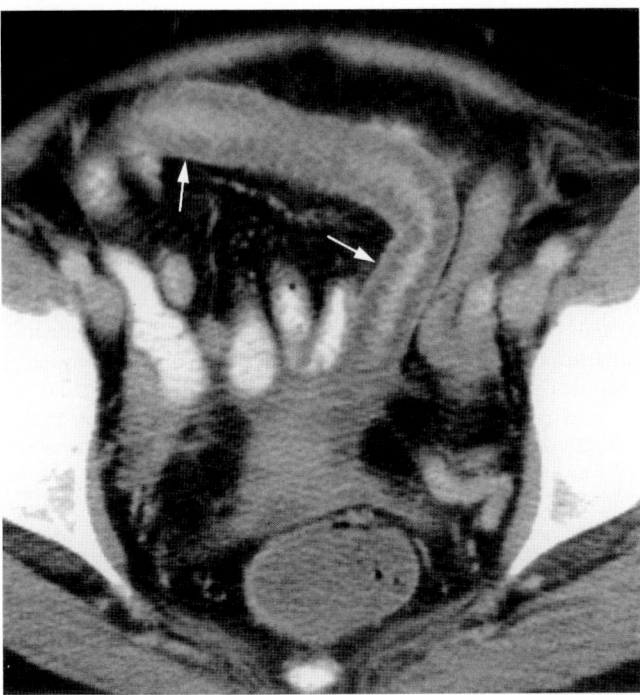

Figure 46-14. Neutropenic enteritis. CT through the pelvis shows marked thickening of an ileal loop (*arrows*) with a mural stratification pattern due to low-attenuation submucosal edema and inflammation. Other images revealed marked cecal inflammation compatible with typhlitis.

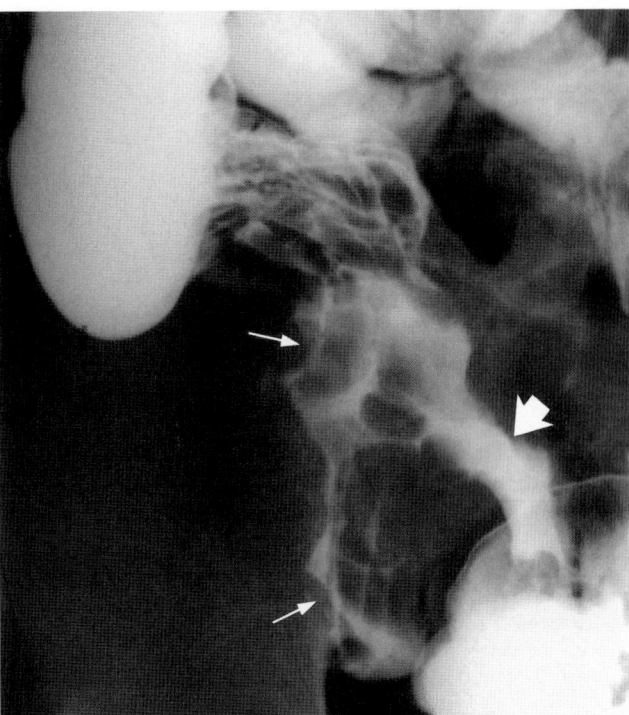

Figure 46-15. Cytomegalovirus infection in a patient with AIDS. Spot image of the terminal ileum from a small bowel follow-through shows large, lobulated folds (*thin arrows*) and barium-filled grooves due to ulceration. Localized perforation is manifested by a barium-filled track (*thick arrow*) extending into the mesentery. (Courtesy of Emil J. Balthazar, MD, New York; from the teaching files of Hans Herlinger, MD.)

Human Immunodeficiency Virus Enteritis

The gastrointestinal tract can be a portal of entry for the HIV virus through tears in the rectal mucosa or even intact intestinal epithelium. HIV adheres to M cells in the intestinal epithelium.[77] The virus is subsequently delivered to intraepithelial lymphocytes, to lymphocytes in lymphoid follicles, and to macrophages in the lamina propria.[78] HIV infection results in near-complete destruction of CD4+ intraepithelial lymphocytes, leading to abnormal differentiation of IgA-secreting B cells and decreased numbers of mucosal IgA plasma cells. HIV also alters enterocyte differentiation.[79] As a result, HIV infection causes villous atrophy, crypt hyperplasia, edema, and chronic inflammation.[80] Nutrient absorption is impaired because of the loss of mature enterocytes.

An acute self-limited diarrhea lasting 1 to 3 weeks occurs in approximately one third of patients with acute HIV infection. The radiologist is not usually involved at this stage. AIDS enteropathy is defined as osmotic diarrhea and malabsorption occurring without evidence of other enteric infections. The radiologist may be asked to perform imaging studies on patients with chronic diarrhea, however, because endoscopy can establish the diagnosis in only about 40% of patients with suspected small bowel infection and stool analysis can establish the diagnosis in only about 60% of patients.[81-83] Imaging studies are used to show the presence of small bowel disease and can sometimes aid in the differential diagnosis of these conditions.

Cytomegalovirus Infection

Cytomegalovirus is a double-stranded DNA virus in the herpesvirus group. A self-limited diarrheal infection can be seen in immunocompetent individuals.[84] After the initial infection, the virus enters a latent phase in circulating mononuclear cells throughout the gastrointestinal tract.[85] The virus is most frequently reactivated when the host becomes immunocompromised. CMV accumulates in nuclear and cytoplasmic inclusions in epithelial cells, mononuclear cells, endothelial cells, fibroblasts, histiocytes, and smooth muscle cells of the gastrointestinal tract. The infection results in varying degrees of inflammation and necrosis. Endothelial cell damage causes submucosal ischemia with secondary epithelial ulceration. Ulceration leads to pseudomembrane formation and perforation.

In the small intestine, discrete erosions and penetrating ulcers are separated by normal mucosa.[86] Barium studies and CT usually show ulceration in the distal small bowel and terminal ileum (Figs. 46-15 and 46-16) and in the cecum and ascending colon.[86,87] However, some patients primarily have duodenal or jejunal disease or even diffuse small bowel disease.[88-90] Intestinal perforation and ileocolic intussusceptions associated with lymphoid hyperplasia have also been described.[91]

Cryptosporidiosis

Cryptosporidium parvum is a unicellular, spore-forming coccidial protozoan that causes an acute self-limited diarrhea in immunocompetent patients. In patients with CD4+ counts less than 200 cells/mm³, however, *C. parvum* may cause a diffuse mucosal enteropathy, resulting in chronic, voluminous, watery diarrhea and malabsorption.[92] This parasite is transmitted by

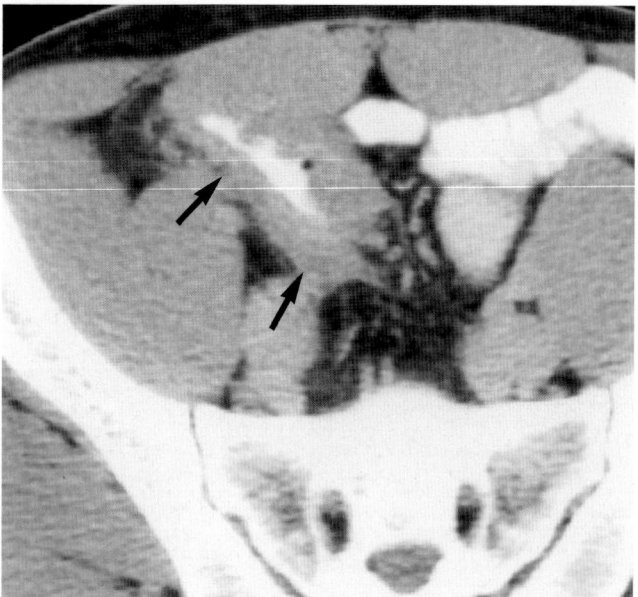

Figure 46-16. Cytomegalovirus infection in a patient with AIDS. CT through the pelvis shows marked wall thickening of the distal ileum (*arrows*). There also is irregularity of the mucosal surface due to ulceration. (Courtesy of Emil J. Balthazar, MD, New York; from the teaching files of Hans Herlinger, MD.)

the fecal/oral route via contaminated water or by person to person or pet to person contact.[93] Cryptosporidia are present in vacuoles beneath the membrane of epithelial cells at the villous tips but outside the epithelial cell cytoplasm. Infection results in a spectrum of findings, ranging from a normal histologic appearance to villous atrophy with severe inflammation.

Barium studies may reveal a variable degree of fold thickening in the duodenum and mesenteric small bowel (Fig. 46-17).[94,95] One series reported proximal small bowel predominance with cryptosporidial enteritis.[96]

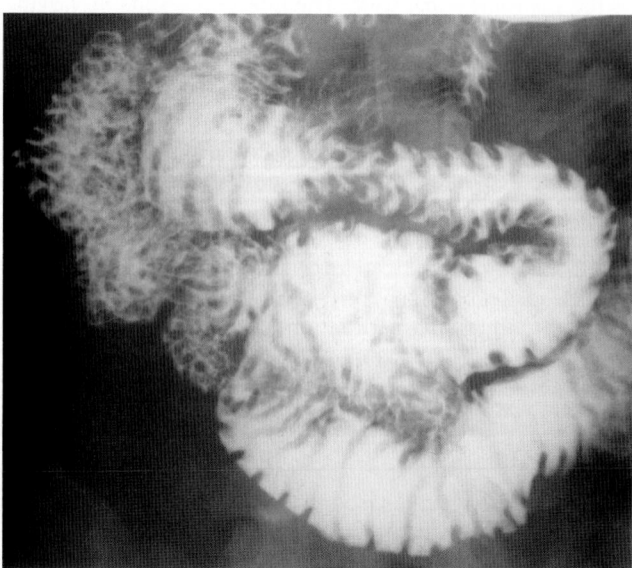

Figure 46-17. Cryptosporidiosis. Spot image of the mid small bowel shows mild, diffuse thickening of the folds. (From the teaching files of Hans Herlinger, MD.)

Isosporiasis and Other Intracellular Protozoans

Isospora belli is an obligate intracellular protozoan acquired by ingestion of contaminated food or water or by homosexual transmission.[97] Invasion of villous enterocytes results in villous atrophy and inflammation, often associated with extensive eosinophilic infiltration of the small bowel wall. Profuse watery diarrhea and malabsorption may ensue. Barium studies may reveal thickened small bowel folds, primarily in the duodenum and proximal small intestine.[98]

Cyclospora cayetanensis is an obligate intracellular protozoan that also causes villous atrophy and acute and chronic inflammation in normal or immunocompromised people. A chronic or relapsing watery diarrhea is usually present.

Microsporidia are a group of spore-forming obligate intracellular protozoans that infect the small intestine or disseminate to other organs, depending on the species.[99,100] A chronic watery diarrhea is usually present.

Enterocytozoon bieneusi infects 10% to 34% of patients with HIV infection and CD4+ counts of less than 50 cells/mm^3. This protozoan infects enterocytes in the jejunum, resulting in villous atrophy and inflammation.[101]

Mycobacterium avium-intracellulare Complex

Two acid-fast obligate intracellular mycobacteria, *M. avium* and *M. intracellulare*, form the *Mycobacterium avium-intracellulare* (MAI) complex. These organisms are ubiquitous in the environment and are not enteric pathogens in immunocompetent patients. However, immunosuppressed patients exposed to aerosols, soil, or food containing MAI may develop disseminated infection. Genetic analysis of MAI isolated from AIDS patients has shown that most of these infections are caused by *M. avium*, so that the term *M. avium* complex (MAC) is currently favored.[102] HIV-infected patients with CD4+ counts less than 100 cell/mm^3 may have disseminated MAC infection involving the liver, spleen, bone marrow, lymph nodes, and gastrointestinal tract. Gastrointestinal involvement may cause chronic diarrhea, abdominal pain, malabsorption, weight loss, hepatosplenomegaly, and lymphadenopathy (Fig. 46-18).

The small intestine is the most severely infected portion of the gastrointestinal tract. Both jejunal and ileal predominance

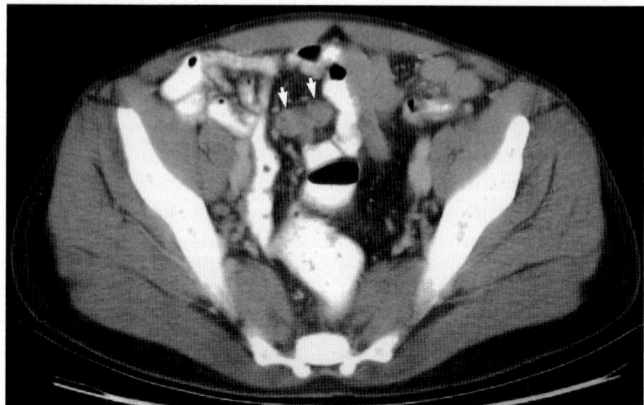

Figure 46-18. Mesenteric lymphadenopathy in a patient with *Mycobacterium avium* complex enteritis. CT through the pelvis shows enlarged lymph nodes (*arrows*) in the small bowel mesentery. The ileal wall is questionably thickened.

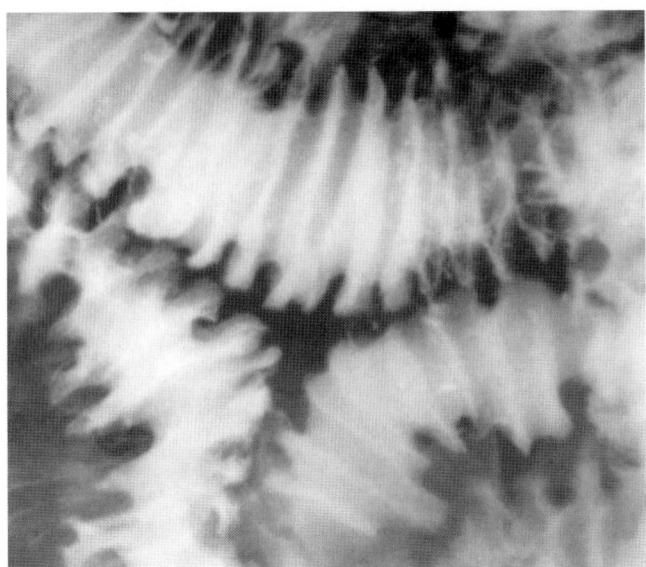

Figure 46-19. *Mycobacterium avium* **complex enteritis.** Spot image from a small bowel follow-through shows moderately thickened, smooth folds in the affected small bowel.

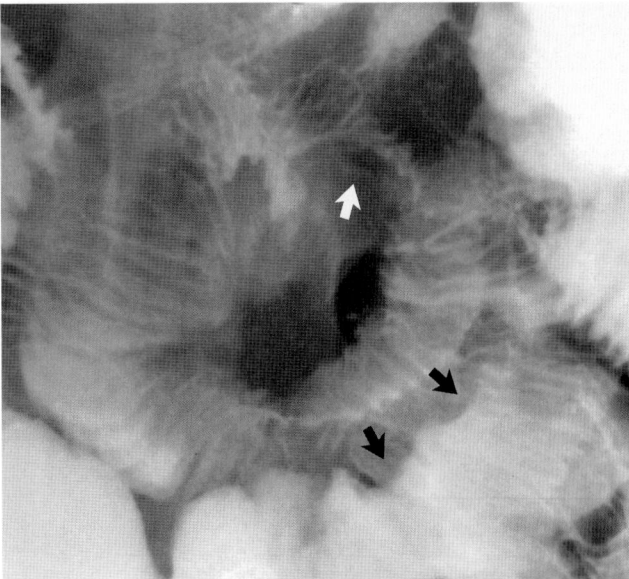

Figure 46-21. Tuberculous peritonitis in a patient with AIDS. Spot image from an enteroclysis examination shows extrinsic mass impressions (*arrows*) on the mesenteric border of midjejunal loops. Small bowel folds are also mildly enlarged.

have been described.[85,103,104] Barium studies may reveal thickened small bowel folds due to infiltration of the lamina propria and submucosa by macrophages packed with acid-fast organisms (Fig. 46-19). Fine mucosal nodularity may also be seen as a result of villous blunting from diffuse infiltration of the lamina propria. Aphthoid ulcers have also been described.[105] CT may reveal mesenteric lymphadenopathy, which is often more prominent than the retroperitoneal lymphadenopathy in these patients. Enlarged lymph nodes may have normal or low attenuation (Fig. 46-20). Hepatomegaly, splenomegaly, and ascites may also be detected in patients with disseminated infection.[106]

Small bowel infection by *M. tuberculosis* in patients with AIDS produces radiographic findings similar to those in immunocompetent patients with *M. tuberculosis*.[107] However, disseminated tuberculosis involving the peritoneum (Fig. 46-21), liver, spleen, and pancreas is more common in patients with

AIDS.[108] The findings of tuberculous peritonitis include high-attenuation ascites, peritoneal and omental nodules, and low-attenuation lymphadenopathy (see Chapter 112).

Actinomycosis

Actinomyces israelii is a filamentous bacterium that is part of the normal oral flora. Gastrointestinal actinomycosis most frequently involves the terminal ileum (Fig. 46-22) and appendix. A transmural infection mimicking Crohn's disease may be seen.[109] Fistulas are often present.

Candidiasis

Fungal spores or hyphae of *Candida* may be found as a result of noninvasive colonization of blind loops or necrotic tissue. In contrast, invasive candidiasis may occur in the small intestine in patients with disseminated candidal infections, including patients with AIDS.[110,111] Mucosal invasion causes ulceration and even perforation. Barium studies may reveal thickened small bowel folds.

DIFFERENTIAL DIAGNOSIS

The radiologist most frequently encounters infectious disease of the small intestine during the work-up of patients with acute right lower quadrant pain or during the work-up of patients with chronic diarrhea, malabsorption, and weight loss.[112] Acute enteritis that causes abdominal pain rather than diarrhea can mimic appendicitis on clinical grounds. If CT to rule out acute appendicitis shows thickened ileal folds (Fig. 46-23) or regional mesenteric lymphadenopathy, various infectious pathogens (such as *Yersinia*) must be considered. However, a CT diagnosis of "mesenteric adenitis" is not indicative of a specific etiology. A definitive diagnosis therefore requires stool cultures and biopsy specimens. Unfortunately,

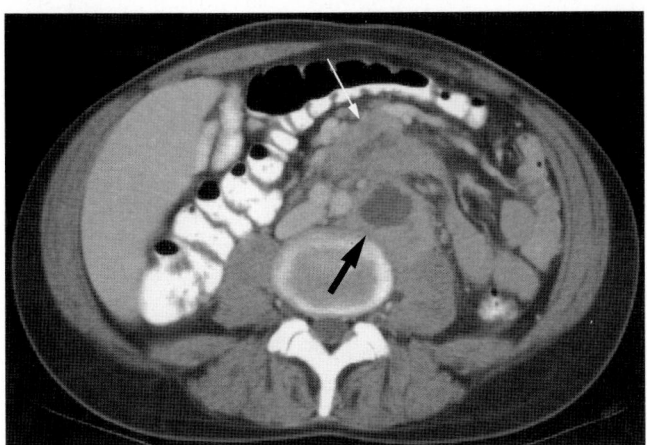

Figure 46-20. Mesenteric and retroperitoneal lymphadenopathy in a patient with *Mycobacterium avium* complex enteritis. CT through the tip of the liver shows a large left para-aortic nodal mass with a low-attenuation center (*black arrow*). Masslike infiltration of the small bowel mesentery (*white arrow*) is also present.

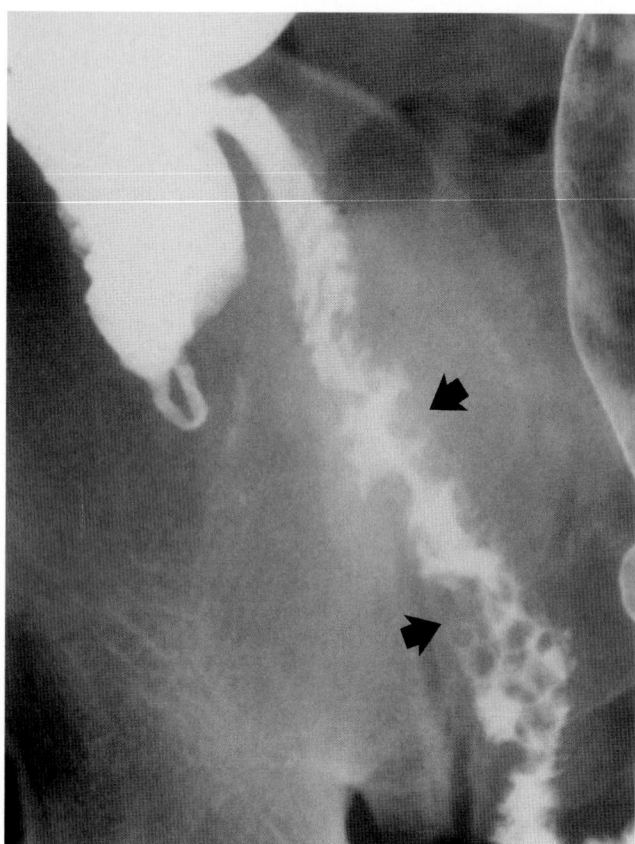

Figure 46-22. Actinomycosis in a patient with AIDS. Spot image from a double-contrast barium enema shows mucosal nodularity (*arrows*) and irregular fold thickening in the terminal ileum.

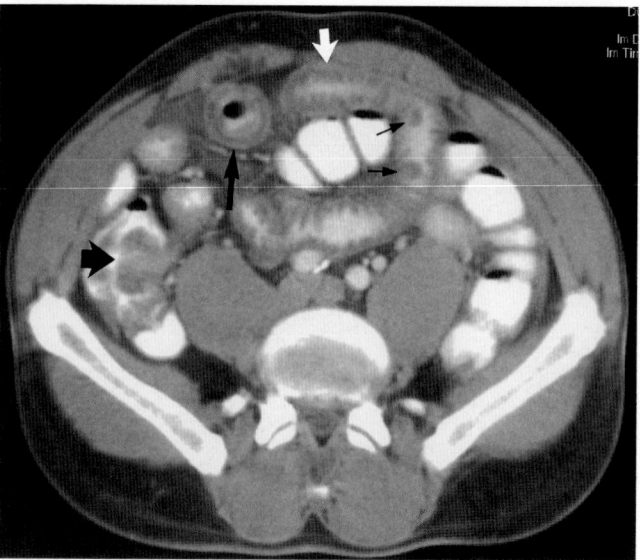

Figure 46-23. Acute enteritis in a patient presenting with acute right lower quadrant pain. CT shows thickened folds (*white arrow*) and nodules (*short, thin black arrows*) in a loop of ileum. A mural stratification pattern is present in a loop seen in cross section (*long black arrow*). The ileocecal valve is enlarged (*short, thick black arrow*).

Fig. 46-7), tuberculosis (see Fig. 46-6), and lymphoma. In patients with acute diarrhea, aphthoid ulcers are not specific for Crohn's disease, because they reflect nonspecific inflammation of lymphoid tissue with erosion of the overlying mucosa. Any acute infection or inflammatory process can therefore lead to the development of aphthoid ulcers or thickened folds in the terminal ileum. In fact, an acute infection such as yersiniosis should be favored in patients with these radiographic findings who have acute diarrhea or abdominal

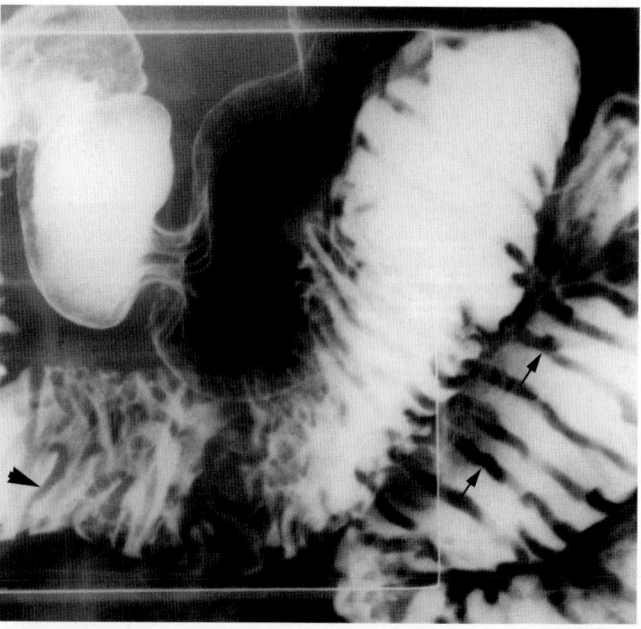

Figure 46-24. Proximal small bowel fold thickening in a patient with AIDS. Spot image from a small bowel follow-through shows mildly thickened undulating folds (*thin arrows*) in a proximal loop of jejunum. Compare these jejunal folds with folds in the third portion of the duodenum (*thick arrow*). Normal duodenal folds should be slightly thicker than jejunal folds. Enteroscopic biopsy specimens revealed cryptosporidiosis.

these cultures and biopsies are often negative or nonspecific in patients with acute infections. In such cases, follow-up CT or endoscopy may be needed to rule out small bowel lymphoma.

CT or barium studies may be performed in patients with chronic diarrhea or abdominal pain. Because the small bowel folds are composed of mucosa and submucosa, thickened folds on CT or barium studies indicate disease involving the mucosa and submucosa (Fig. 46-24; see also Fig. 46-23). Enlargement of the villous pattern (with fine nodularity) reflects abnormal villi. The inflammatory response to a variety of damaging agents such as chemical toxins, radiation, and infection is often similar. As a result, the radiographic findings of thickened folds or villous enlargement are often nonspecific in patients with chronic diarrhea. When small bowel folds are thickened, the radiologist should therefore consider the age, travel history, and immune status of the patient. Proximal or diffuse small bowel fold thickening in patients with AIDS is caused by a variety of infections, including MAC, cryptosporidiosis (see Fig. 46-24), and isosporiasis. Patients receiving 5-FU or 5-FUDR may have intestinal chemotoxicity (see Figs. 46-8 and 46-9). Patients who have received allogeneic bone marrow transplants may have GVHD (see Figs. 46-11 to 46-13) or cytomegalovirus infection. Patients with proximal or diffuse small bowel fold thickening and a clinical history of malabsorption may have other types of disorders that are discussed in Chapter 47.

Disease involving the distal ileum usually indicates a disorder that has an affinity for lymphatic tissue in the small intestine, including Crohn's disease, *Yersinia* enterocolitis (see pain. Unfortunately, it may be difficult to obtain a definitive diagnosis in these patients, because cultures and biopsy specimens are often negative for a specific pathogen.

Aphthoid ulcers, mesenteric border ulcers, cobblestoning, strictures, and fistulas should be highly suggestive of Crohn's disease in patients with chronic diarrhea (see Chapter 45). However, these findings are not always specific for Crohn's disease. If, for example, there is a clinical history of an immune deficiency state or if the patient has lived in a region of the world where tuberculosis in endemic, then tuberculosis (see Fig. 46-6), actinomycosis (see Fig. 46-22), Behçet's disease, and cytomegalovirus (see Figs. 46-15 and 46-16) should be considered (depending on the clinical history). The CT findings of bowel wall thickening, mesenteric lymphadenopathy, and mesenteric infiltration or abscess formation also are not specific for Crohn's disease, so that further work-up is required.

Florid lymphoid reactions in the terminal ileum may result from prior enteric infection, immune deficiency states (in particular, common variable immunodeficiency), and lymphoma. Small (1 to 2 mm), round, uniform nodules separated by normal mucosa are indicative of lymphoid hyperplasia (Fig. 46-25), which can probably be followed without further diagnostic testing. However, lymphoid nodules that are larger (>2 mm), more confluent, and not round, smooth, and uniform should be investigated for lymphoma (Fig. 46-26).

Bowel wall thickening on CT also is not a specific finding. In the small intestine, however, a mural stratification pattern with a low-attenuation submucosa may be caused by a vascular or inflammatory process (see Fig. 46-1) but not malignant tumor. Lack of contrast enhancement should suggest necrosis

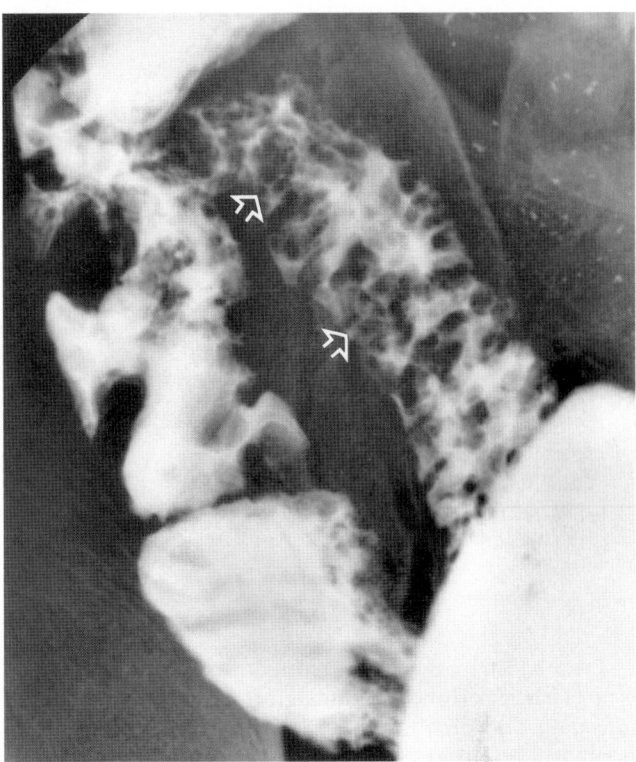

Figure 46-26. Mantle cell lymphoma in the terminal ileum. Spot image from a small bowel follow-through shows small, round, ovoid or polygonal nodules ranging from 1 to 4 mm. The nodules are confluent in some areas (*arrows*). This type of mucosal nodularity requires endoscopic biopsies to rule out lymphoma. The nodularity does not resemble cobblestoning, because transversely and longitudinally oriented barium-filled clefts are not seen.

and a possible vascular component to the disease. Fat deposition in the small bowel submucosa should suggest Crohn's disease. Ileal wall thickening in patients with AIDS may be caused by inflammatory conditions or AIDS-related lymphoma (Fig. 46-27).

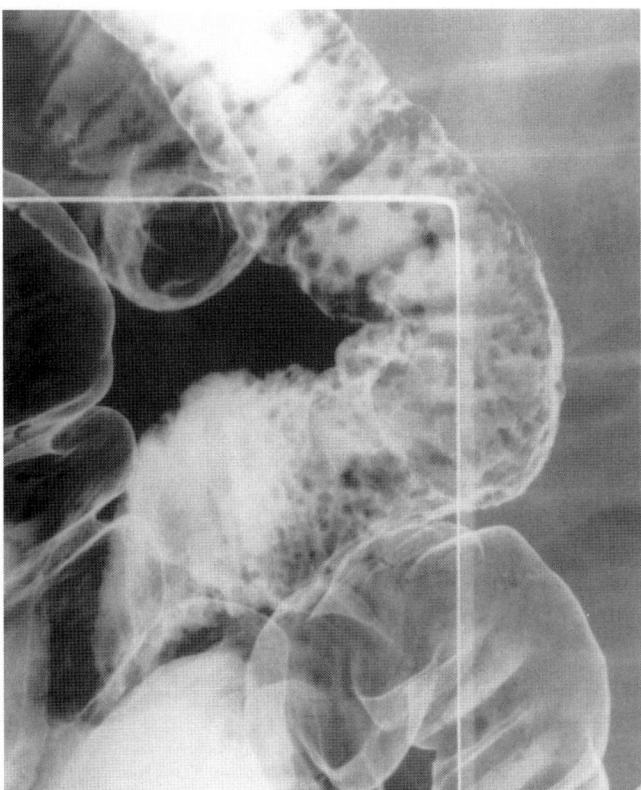

Figure 46-25. Lymphoid hyperplasia in the terminal ileum. Spot image from a double-contrast barium enema shows discrete, round, uniform-sized, one to two radiolucent filling defects in the terminal ileum separated by normal mucosa.

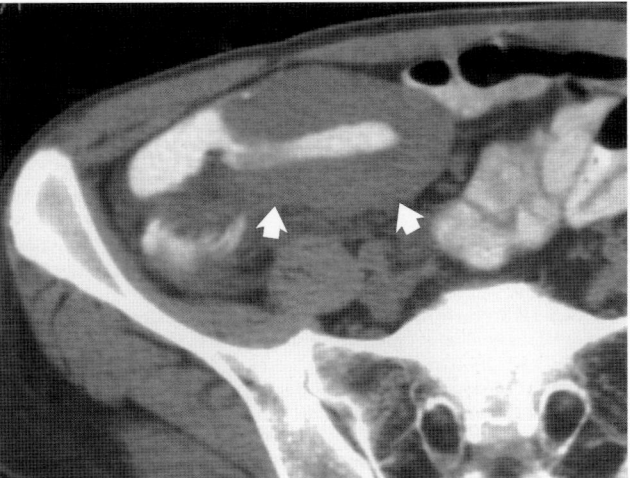

Figure 46-27. Ileal wall thickening in a patient with AIDS. CT through the pelvis shows marked (1.5 to 2 cm) wall thickening (*arrows*) of uniform attenuation in the terminal ileum. The medial wall of the cecum is also thickened. Biopsy specimens revealed lymphoma. Marked wall thickening of uniform attenuation should be considered highly worrisome for small bowel lymphoma.

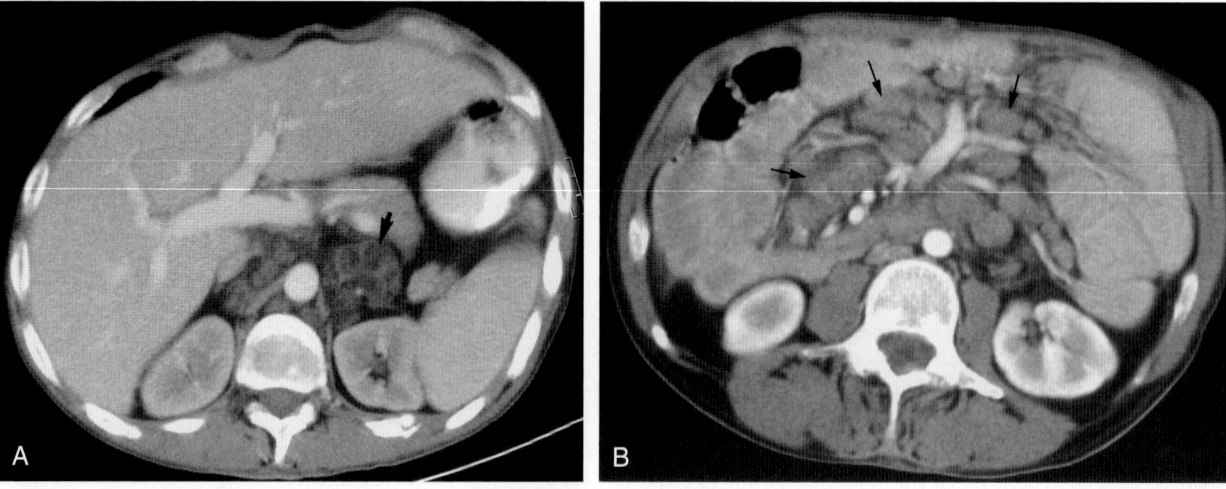

Figure 46-28. Lymphadenopathy in Whipple's disease. A. CT through the liver shows low-attenuation lymphadenopathy in the retrocaval, retrocrural and left para-aortic (*arrow*) regions. **B.** An image caudal to **A** shows marked mesenteric lymphadenopathy (*arrows*) of more uniform and higher attenuation.

Lymphadenopathy adjacent to abnormal small bowel loops is not a particularly helpful finding, because it can be seen with infectious disorders, Crohn's disease, carcinoid tumor, intraperitoneal metastases, and lymphoma. Extensive mesenteric lymphadenopathy in patients with chronic diarrhea or malabsorption is typically seen in patients with gluten-sensitive enteropathy, Whipple's disease (Fig. 46-28), and MAI infections. Lymphadenopathy in celiac disease is usually reactive, but lymphoma cannot be excluded.

References

1. Greenberg HB, Matsui SM, Holodniy M: Small intestine: Infections with common bacterial and viral pathogens. In Yamada T, Alpers DH, Kaplowitz N, et al (eds): Textbook of Gastroenterology, 4th ed. Philadelphia, Lippincott Williams & Wilkins, 2003, pp 1530-1560.
2. Fenoglio-Preiser CM, Noffsinger AE, Stemmermann GN, et al: Non-neoplastic lesions of the small intestine. In Gastrointestinal Pathology: An Atlas and Text, 2nd ed. Philadelphia, Lippincott-Raven, 1999, pp 309-358.
3. Pawloski ZS: Ascariasis: Host-pathogen biology. Rev Infect Dis 4: 806-814, 1982.
4. Wynne JM, Ellman BAH: Bolus obstruction by *Ascaris lumbricoides*. S Afr Med J 63:644-646, 1983.
5. Blumenthal DS, Schultz MG: Incidence of intestinal obstruction in children infected with *Ascaris lumbricoides*. Am J Trop Med Hyg 24: 801-804, 1975.
6. Hommeyer SC, Hamill GS, Johnson JA: CT diagnosis of intestinal ascariasis. Abdom Imaging 20:315-316, 1995.
7. Markell EK, Voge M: Medical Parasitology, 4th ed. Philadelphia, WB Saunders, 1976.
8. Herlinger H: Parasitic and bacterial inflammatory diseases. In Herlinger H, Maglinte DDT, Birnbaum BA (eds): Clinical Imaging of the Small Intestine, 2nd ed. New York, Springer, 1999, pp 291-309.
9. Berk SL, Verghese A, Alvarez S, et al: Clinical and epidemiologic features of strongyloidiasis: A prospective study in rural Tennessee. Arch Intern Med 147:1257-1264, 1987.
10. Drasin GF, Moss JPO, Cheng SH: *Strongyloides stercoralis* colitis: Findings in four cases. Radiology 126:619-621, 1978.
11. Medina LS, Heiken JP, Gold RP: Pipestem appearance of small bowel in strongyloidiasis is not pathognomonic of fibrosis and irreversibility. AJR 159:543-544, 1992.
12. Dallemand S, Waxman M, Farman J: Radiological manifestations of *Strongyloides stercoralis*. Gastrointest Radiol 8:45-51, 1983.
13. Hizawa K, Iida M, Aoyagi K, et al: Early detection of strongyloidiasis using endoscopic duodenal biopsy: Report of a case. J Clin Gastroenterol 22:157-159, 1996.
14. Muraoka A, Suehiro I, Fuigii M, et al: Acute gastric anisakiasis: 28 cases during the last 10 years. Dig Dis Sci 41:2362-2365, 1996.
15. Matsui T, Iida M, Murakami M, et al: Intestinal anisakiasis: Clinical and radiologic features. Radiology 157:299-302, 1985.
16. Cespedes M, Saez A, Rodriguez I, et al: Chronic anisakiasis presenting as a mesenteric mass. Abdom Imaging 25:548-550, 2000.
17. Pearson RD: Parasitic diseases: Helminths. In Yamada T, Alpers DH, Kaplowitz N, et al (eds): Textbook of Gastroenterology, 4th ed. Philadelphia, Lippincott Williams & Wilkins, 2003, pp 2608-2625.
18. Kapus KD, Lundgren RG Jr, Juranek DD, et al: Intestinal parasitism in the United States: Update on a continuing problems. Am J Trop Med Hyg 50:705, 1994.
19. Katelaris PH, Farthing MJG: Diarrhea and malabsorption in giardiasis: A multifactorial process? Gut 33:295-297, 1992.
20. Farthing MJ: Giardiasis. Gastroenterol Clin North Am 25:493-515, 1996.
21. Brandon J, Glick SN, Teplick SK: Intestinal giardiasis: Importance of serial filming. AJR 144:581-584, 1985.
22. Li E, Stanley SL: Parasitic diseases: Protozoa. In Yamada T, Alpers DH, Kaplowitz N, et al (eds): Textbook of Gastroenterology, 4th ed. Philadelphia, Lippincott Williams & Wilkins, 2003, pp 2588-2607.
23. Holbert RD, Margiros E, Hirsch CP, Nunenmacher SJ: Chagas disease: A case in south Mississippi. J Miss State Med Assoc 36:1-5, 1995.
24. Smith B: The myenteric plexus in Chagas disease. J Pathol Bacteriol 94:462-463, 1967.
25. Olsen SJ, MacKinnon LC, Goudling JS, et al: Surveillance for foodborne-disease outbreaks—United States, 1993-1997. MMWR Morb Mortal Wkly Rep 49(SS-1):1-62, 2000.
26. Palmer KR, Patil DH, Basran GS, et al: Abdominal tuberculosis in urban Britain—a common disease. Gut 26:1296-1305, 1985.
27. Ahmed FB: Tuberculous enteritis: A serious possibility in some patients. Grand Rounds-Hammersmith Hospital. BMJ 31:215-217, 1996.
28. Carreera GF, Young S, Lewicki AM: Intestinal tuberculosis. Gastrointest Radiol 1:147-155, 1976.
29. Cullen JH: Intestinal tuberculosis: Clinical pathological study. Q Bull Sea View Hosp 5:143-160, 1940.
30. Thoeni RF, Margulis AR: Gastrointestinal tuberculosis. Semin Roentgenol 14:283-294, 1979.
31. Ferentzi CV, Sieck JO, Ali MA: Colonoscopic diagnosis and medical treatment of ten patients with colonic tuberculosis. Endoscopy 20:62-65, 1988.
32. Hoshino M, Shibata M, Goto N, et al: A clinical study of tuberculous colitis. Gastroenterol Jpn 14:299-305, 1979.
33. Kim KM, Lee A, Choi KY: Intestinal tuberculosis: Clinicopathologic analysis and diagnosis by endoscopic biopsy. Am J Gastroenterol 93:606-609, 1998.
34. Nakano H, Jaramillo E, Watanabe M, et al: Intestinal tuberculosis: Findings on double-contrast barium enema. Gastrointest Radiol 17:108-114, 1992.

35. Brombart M, Massion J, et al: Radiologic differences between ileocecal tuberculosis and Crohn's disease. Am J Dig Dis 6:589-612, 1961.
36. Balthazar EJ, Gordon R, Hulnick D: Ileocecal tuberculosis: CT and radiologic evaluation. AJR 154:499-503, 1990.
37. Park SJ, Han JK, Kim TK, et al: Tuberculous colitis: Radiologic-colonoscopic correlation. AJR 175:121-128, 2000.
38. Hanski C, Autschka U, Schmoranzer HP, et al: Immunohistochemical and electron microscopic study of interaction of *Yersinia enterocolitica* serotype 08 with intestinal mucosa during experimental enteritis. Infect Immun 57:673-678, 1989.
39. VanTrappen G, Agg HO, Ponette E, et al: *Yersinia* enteritis and enterocolitis: Gastroenterological aspects. Gastroenterology 72:220-227, 1977.
40. Saebo A, Lasser J: *Yersinia* enterocolitica, an inducer of chronic inflammations. Int J Tissue React 16:51-57, 1994.
41. Compton CC: Case 28-1990. In Scully E (ed): Case records of the Massachusetts General Hospital. N Engl J Med 323:121-123, 1990.
42. Ekberg O, Sjostrom B, Brahme F: Radiological findings in *Yersinia* ileitis. Radiology 123:15-19, 1977.
43. Balthazar EJ, Charles HW, Megibow AJ: *Salmonella* and *Shigella*-induced ileitis. CT findings in four patients. J Comput Assist Tomogr 20:375-378, 1996.
44. McKinley MJ, Taylor M, Sangree MH: Toxic megacolon with *Campylobacter* colitis. Conn Med 44:496-497, 1980.
45. Brodey PA, Fertig S, Aron JM: *Campylobacter* enterocolitis: Radiographic feature. AJR 139:1199-1201, 1982.
46. Herlinger H: Parasitic and bacterial inflammatory diseases. In Herlinger H, Maglinte DDT, Birnbaum BA (eds): Clinical Imaging of the Small Intestine, 2nd ed. New York, Springer, 1999, pp 291-308.
47. Fantry GT, Fantry LE, James SP: Chronic infections of the small intestine. In Yamada T, Alpers DH, Kaplowitz N, et al: (eds): Textbook of Gastroenterology, 4th ed. Philadelphia, Lippincott Williams & Wilkins, 2003, pp 1561-1579.
48. Alterman DD, Cho KC: Histoplasmosis involving the omentum in an AIFS patient: CT demonstration. J Comput Assist Tomogr 12:664-665, 1988.
49. Heneghan SJ, Li J, Petrossian E, Bizer LS: Intestinal perforation from gastrointestinal histoplasmosis in acquired immunodeficiency syndrome: Case report and review of the literature. Arch Surg 128:464-466, 1993.
50. Levin MS: Miscellaneous diseases of the small intestine. In Yamada T, Alpers DH, Kaplowitz N, et al: (eds): Textbook of Gastroenterology, 4th ed. Philadelphia, Lippincott Williams & Wilkins, 2003, pp 1663-1684.
51. Allison MC, Howatson AG, Torrance CJ, et al: Gastrointestinal damage associated with the use of nonsteroidal antiinflammatory drugs. N Engl J Med 327:749-754, 1992.
52. Morris AJ, Madhok R, Sturrock RD, et al: Enteroscopic diagnosis of small bowel ulceration in patients receiving non-steroidal antiinflammatory drugs. Lancet 337:520, 1991.
53. Bjarnason I, Price AB, Zanelli G, et al: Clinicopathological features of nonsteroidal antiinflammatory drug-induced small intestinal strictures. Gastroenterology 94:1070-1074, 1988.
54. Levi S, deLacey G, Price AB, et al: "Diaphragm-like" strictures of the small bowel in patients treated with non-steroidal antiinflammatory drugs. Br J Radiol 63:186-189, 1990.
55. Wilson IH, Cooley NV, Luibel FJ: Nonspecific stenosing small bowel ulcers. Am J Gastroenterol 50:449-455, 1968.
56. Lang J, Price AB, Levi AJ, et al: Diaphragm disease: Pathology of disease of the small intestine induced by non-steroidal anti-inflammatory drugs. J Clin Pathol 41:516-526, 1988.
57. Hiehle JF, Levine MS: Gastrointestinal toxicity of 5-FU and 5-FUDR: Radiographic findings. Can Assoc Rad J 42:109-112, 1991.
58. Carucci LR, Rubesin SE, Pretorius ES, et al: Toxic effects of fluorouracil on the small bowel. RSNA Gastrointestinal cases of the day [serial online]. RSNA Link Web, July 2002.
59. Kelvin FM, Gramm HF, Gluck WL, et al: Radiologic manifestations of small bowel toxicity due to floxuridine therapy. AJR 146:39-43, 1977.
60. Shanahan F: Gastrointestinal manifestations of immunologic disorders. In Yamada T, Alpers DH, Kaplowitz N, et al (eds): Textbook of Gastroenterology, 4th ed. Philadelphia, Lippincott Williams & Wilkins, 2003, pp 2705-2722.
61. Sander CA, Medeiros LJ, Weiss LM, et al: Lymphoproliferative lesions in patients with common variable immunodeficiency syndrome. Am J Surg Pathol 16:1170-1183, 1992.
62. Chiaramonte C, Glick SN: Nodular lymphoid hyperplasia of the small bowel complicated by jejunal lymphoma in a patient with common variable immunodeficiency syndrome. AJR 163:1118-1119, 1994.
63. Crooks DJM, Brown WR: The distribution of intestinal nodular lymphoid hyperplasia in immunoglobulin deficiency. Clin Radiol 31:701-706, 1980.
64. Herlinger H: Immune deficiency diseases. In Herlinger H, Maglinte DDT, Birnbaum BA (eds): Clinical Imaging of the Small Intestine, 2nd ed. New York, Springer, 1999, pp. 309-330.
65. Cox G, Matsui S, Lo R, et al: Etiology and outcome of diarrhea after marrow transplantation: A prospective study. Gastroenterology 107:1398-1407, 1994.
66. Jones B, Kramer SS, Saral R, et al: Gastrointestinal inflammation after bone marrow transplantation: Graft-versus host disease or opportunistic infection. AJR 150:277-281, 1988.
67. McDonald GB, Sullivan KM, Plumley TF: Radiographic features of esophageal involvement in chronic graft-versus-host disease in humans. AJR 142:501-506, 1984.
68. Fisk JD, Shulman HM, Greening RR, et al: Gastrointestinal radiographic features of human graft-versus-host-disease. AJR 136:329-336, 1981.
69. Rosenberg HK, Serota FT, Koch, et al: Radiographic features of gastrointestinal graft-versus-host disease. Radiology 38:371-374, 1981.
70. Gramm HF, Vincent ME, Braver JM: Differential diagnosis of tubular small bowel. Curr Imaging 2:62-70, 1990.
71. Ma LD, Jones B, Lazenby AJ, et al: Persistent oral contrast lining the intestine in severe mucosal disease: Elucidation of radiographic appearance. Radiology 191:747-749, 1981.
72. Jones B, Fishman EK, Kramer S, et al: Computed tomography of gastrointestinal inflammation after bone marrow transplantation. AJR 146:691-695, 1986.
73. Navari RM, Sharma P, Deeg HJ, et al: Pneumatosis cystoides intestinalis following allogeneic marrow transplantation. Transplant Proc 15:1720-1724, 1983.
74. Smith PD, Janoff EN: Gastrointestinal complications of the acquired immunodeficiency syndrome. In Yamada T, Alpers DH, Kaplowitz N, et al (eds): Textbook of Gastroenterology, 4th ed. Philadelphia, Lippincott Williams & Wilkins, 2003, pp 2567-2589.
75. Dworkin B, Wormser GP, Rosenthal WS, et al: Gastrointestinal manifestations of the acquired immunodeficiency syndrome: A review of 22 cases. Am J Gastroenterol 80:774-778, 1985.
76. Poles M, Fuerst M, McGowan I, et al: HIV-related diarrhea is multifactorial and fat malabsorption is commonly present, independent of HAART. Am J Gastroenterol 96:1831-1837, 2001.
77. Fenoglio-Prieser CM, Noffsinger AE, Stemmermann GN, et al: AIDS-related diseases. In Gastrointestinal Pathology: An Atlas and Text, 2nd ed. Philadelphia, Lippincott-Raven, 1999, pp 563-595.
78. Amerongen HM, Weltzin R, Farnet CM, et al: Transepithelial transport of HIV-1 by intestinal M cells: A mechanism for transmission of AIDS. J AIDS 4:760-765, 1991.
79. Heise C. Dandekar S, Kumar P, et al: Human immunodeficiency virus infection of enterocytes and mononuclear cells in human jejunal mucosa. Gastroenterology 100:1521-1527, 1991.
80. Kotler DP, Reka S, Clayton F: Intestinal mucosal inflammation associated with human immunodeficiency virus infection. Dig Dis Sci 38:1119-1126, 1993.
81. Greenson JK, Belitsos PC, Yardley JH, et al: AIDS enteropathy: Occult enteric infections and duodenal mucosal alterations in chronic diarrhea. Ann Intern Med 114:366-372, 1991.
82. Wilcox CM, Schwartz DA, Cotsonis G, Thompson SE: Chronic unexplained diarrhea in human immunodeficiency virus infection: Determination of the best diagnostic approach. Gastroenterology 110:30-37, 1996.
83. Rene E, Marche C, Regnier B, et al: Intestinal infections in patients with acquired immunodeficiency syndrome: A prospective study in 132 patients. Dig Dis Sci 34:773-780, 1989.
84. Surawicz C, Myerson D: Self-limited cytomegalovirus colitis in immunocompetent individuals. Gastroenterology 94:194-199, 1988.
85. Pantongrag-Brown L, Nelson AM, Brown AE, et al: Gastrointestinal manifestations of acquired immunodeficiency syndrome: Radiologic-pathologic correlation. RadioGraphics 15:1155-1178, 1995.
86. Balthazar EJ, Martino JM: Giant ulcers of the ileum and colon caused by cytomegalovirus in patients with AIDS. AJR 166:1275-1276, 1996.
87. Balthazar EJ, Megibow AJ, Fazzini E, et al: Cytomegalovirus virus colitis in AIDS: Radiographic findings in 11 patients. Radiology 155:585-589, 1985.
88. Teixidor HS, Honig CL, Norsoph E, et al: Cytomegalovirus infection of the alimentary canal: Radiologic findings with pathologic correlation. Radiology 163:317-323, 1987.

89. DeRiso A, Kemeny MM, Torres RA, Oliver JML: Multiple jejunal perforations second to cytomegalvirus in a patient with acquired immune deficiency syndrome. Dig Dis Sci 34:623-629, 1989.
90. Williams CM, Schwartz DA: Symptomatic CMV duodenitis: An important clinical problem in AIDS. J Clin Gastroenterol 14:293-297, 1992.
91. Kram HB, Shoemaker WC: Intestinal perforation due to cytomegalovirus infection. Dis Colon Rectum 33:1037-1040, 1990.
92. Phillips AD, Thomas AG, Walker-Smith JA: *Cryptosporidium,* chronic diarrhea and the proximal small intestinal mucosa. Gut 33:1057-1061, 1992.
93. DuPont HL, Chappell, CL, Sterling CR, et al: The infectivity of cryptosporidium parvum in healthy volunteers. N Engl J Med 332:855-859, 1995.
94. Wall S, Ominsky S, Altman DF, et al: Multifocal abnormalities of the gastrointestinal tract in AIDS. AJR 146:1-5, 1986.
95. Megibow AJ, Balthazar EJ, Hulnick DH: Radiology of non-neoplastic gastrointestinal disorders in acquired immune deficiency syndrome. Semin Roentgenol 22:31-41, 1987.
96. Berk RN, Wall SD, McCardle CB, et al: Cryptosporidiosis of the stomach and small intestine in patients with the acquired immunodeficiency syndrome. AJR 143:549-554, 1984.
97. DeHovitz JA, Pape JW, Boncy M, Johnson WD: Clinical manifestations and therapy of *Isospora belli* infections in patients with acquired immunodeficiency syndrome. N Engl J Med 315:87-90, 1986.
98. Shein R, Gleb A: *Isospora belli* in a patient with acquired immunodeficiency syndrome. J Clin Gastroenterol 6:525-528, 1984.
99. Leder K, Ryan N, Spelman D, Crowe SM: Microsporidial disease in HIV-infected patients: A report of 42 patients and review of the literature. Scand J Infect Dis 30:331-338, 1998.
100. Case 51-1993. Case Records of the Massachusetts General Hospital (Microsporidiosis). 329:1946-1954, 1993.
101. Kotler DP, Francisco A, Clayton F, et al: Small intestinal injury and parasitic diseases in AIDS. Ann Intern Med 113:444-449, 1991.
102. Yakrus MA, Good RCL: Geographic distribution, frequency, and specimen source of *Mycobacterium avium* complex serotypes isolated from patients with acquired immunodeficiency syndrome. J Clin Microbiol 28:926-929, 1990.
103. Vincent ME, Robbins AR: *Mycobacterium avium-intracellulare complex* enteritis: Pseudo-Whipple's disease in acquired immunodeficiency. AJR 144:921-922, 1985.
104. Schneedbaum GW, Novick DM, Chabon AB, et al: Terminal ileitis associated with *Mycobacterium avium-intracellulare* infection in a homosexual man with acquired immune deficiency syndrome. Gastroenterology 92:1127-1132, 1987.
105. Frager DH, Frager JD, Brandt LJ, et al: Gastrointestinal complications of AIDS: Radiologic features. Radiology 158:597-605, 1986.
106. Nyberg DA, Federle MP, Jeffrey RB, et al: Abdominal CT findings of disseminated *Mycobacterium avium-intracellulare* in AIDS. AJR 145:297-299, 1985.
107. Jadvar H, Mindelzun RE, Olcott EW, Levitt DB: Still the great mimicker: Abdominal tuberculosis. AJR 168:1455-1460, 1997.
108. Radin DR: Intraabdominal *Mycobacterium tuberculosis* vs. *Mycobacterium avium-intracellulare* infections in patients with AIDS: Distinction based on CT findings. AJR 156:487-491, 1991.
109. Litt HI, Levine MS, Maki DD, et al: Ileal actinomycosis in a patient with AIDS. AJR 172:1297-1299, 1999.
110. Joshi SN, Garvin PJ, Sunwoo YC: Candidiasis of the duodenum and jejunum. Gastroenterology 80:829-833, 1981.
111. Radin DR, Fong T, Halls JM, Pontrelli GN: Monilial enteritis in acquired immunodeficiency syndrome. AJR 141:1289-1290, 1983.
112. Rubesin SE, Furth EE: Differential diagnosis of small intestinal abnormalities with radiologic-pathologic explanation. In Herlinger H, Maglinte DDT, Birnbaum BA (eds): Clinical Imaging of the Small Intestine, 2nd ed. New York, Springer, 1999, pp 527-566.

Malabsorption

Stephen E. Rubesin, MD

Malabsorption is caused by a variety of diseases originating in the liver and biliary tree, pancreas, and small intestine.[1-3] A discussion of normal digestion and absorption and a description of diseases of the small intestine that result in malabsorption are presented in this chapter.

DIGESTION AND ABSORPTION

The components of most foods (carbohydrates, proteins, and fats) cannot be utilized in their natural states. Foods must first be digested and then absorbed by the gastrointestinal tract. Proper functioning of the liver and biliary tree, pancreas, and small bowel, and, to a lesser degree, salivary glands, stomach, and colon is required for normal digestion and absorption of food.

Carbohydrate Digestion and Absorption

Carbohydrates account for 40% to 50% of daily caloric intake.[4] Ingested carbohydrates are derived from plants, except for lactose, which originates in dairy products. *Simple sugars* include the monosaccharides, fructose and glucose, and the disaccharides, sucrose and lactose. *Starches* are soluble polymers of glucose found in the cell walls of plants. The starches are α-amylose, a linear polymer of glucose and amylopectin, a branched form of glucose. *Dietary fibers* are nondigestible carbohydrates (i.e., nonstarch polysaccharides) that are structural components of plant cell walls.

The gastrointestinal tract is adapted for digesting carbohydrates to a monosaccharide form that can be transported across the epithelium of the small intestine. Luminal digestion of starches is accomplished by α-amylase secreted by the parotid gland and pancreas. Salivary amylase is of minor importance because this enzyme is deactivated in the acidic environment of the stomach. Amylase digestion of starches is so efficient that starch digestion is more dependent on the form of the starch than on the availability of luminal amylase.[4] Amylase deficiency is present only in cases of severe pancreatic insufficiency.

Enzymes on the apical membrane of the enterocytes are responsible for further digestion of the products of luminal digestion and breakdown of disaccharides. For example, sucrase-isomaltase is an enzyme that cleaves sucrose into glucose and fructose. Brush border lactase cleaves lactose into glucose and galactose. This enzyme is critical for mammalian survival, because early nutrition is provided by the mother's milk.[4] The monosaccharides are then brought across the epithelium by passive diffusion, facilitative transport of proteins, or a sodium-coupled active transport.

Colonic bacteria digest dietary fiber that reaches the colon, producing a variety of products, including short-chain fatty acids, methane, and hydrogen. Short-chain fatty acids are rapidly absorbed in the colon, providing energy for colonic epithelial cells.

Digestion of lactose, sucrose, and starches is incomplete, because digestion depends on the type of food and contact time with the brush border. Between 2% and 20% of starch is not digested.[4] Most small bowel diseases result in global dysfunction of intestinal mucosa leading to carbohydrate malabsorption, with subsequent diarrhea, flatulence, and weight loss. Specific disaccharidase deficiencies result in similar symptoms. For example, trehalose is a disaccharide of glucose found in insects, yeasts, and mushrooms. As a result, people who are trehalase deficient have severe diarrhea after ingestion of mushrooms.

Protein Digestion and Absorption

Proteins in the lumen of the gastrointestinal tract derive from the diet (70 to 100 g/day); from salivary, gastric, pancreatic, and biliary secretions (30 g/day); and from sloughed epithelial cells (30 g/day).[5] Protein digestion begins in the stomach. Inactive precursors (pepsinogens) are secreted from chief cells and are activated to pepsins in the acidic environment of the stomach. Proteins in the gastric lumen are digested to a mixture of large polypeptides, smaller oligopeptides, and free amino acids.

The exocrine pancreas secretes five inactive precursor zymogens into the duodenal lumen. Enteropeptidase (enterokinase) on the brush border of the duodenal enterocytes converts trypsinogen into trypsin. Trypsin then activates the remainder of the pancreatic zymogens (chymotrypsinogen, proelastase, and procarboxypeptidases A and B).[5] These pancreatic enzymes break proteins into oligopeptides (60% to 70%) and free amino acids (30% to 40%).[5] Peptidases on the brush border of the enterocytes further degrade the intraluminal oligopeptides, resulting in a mixture of tripeptides, dipeptides, and free amino acids. Distinct transport systems separately transport free amino acids and peptides of two to three amino acids into the epithelial cells. Various peptidases within the enterocytes further digest the small polypeptides. Amino acids leave the enterocytes via transport mechanisms across the basal membrane, passing into the portal circulation.

Fat Digestion and Absorption

The sources of fat include diet (120 to 150 g), biliary secretions (40 to 50 g), and sloughed intestinal cells and bacteria.[6] Most dietary fat is composed of neutral fats—long chain triglycerides. Phospholipids and sterols (including cholesterol) comprise only a small percentage of dietary fat.[6]

Lipid digestion begins in the stomach with hydrolysis of triglycerides by gastric and salivary lipase. Twenty to 30% of intraluminal fat digestion occurs in the stomach. The grinding action of the antrum helps reduce triglycerides into smaller particles. The fat globules are dispersed in a stable form with a large surface area, termed *emulsification*. Gastric lipid digestion has an increased role in patients with cystic fibrosis or partial gastrectomy.[6]

After chyme reaches the small intestine, bile salts and lecithin secreted by the liver solubilize the fat, allowing the fat to be broken into smaller droplets by the agitating action of the small bowel. Lipolytic enzymes secreted by the pancreas break triglycerides, phospholipids, and sterol esters into their component monoglycerides and free fatty acids. Bile salts combine with the monoglycerides and free fatty acids to form micelles. The micelles deliver the breakdown products of fat to the microvilli of the epithelial cell brush border.

After brush border uptake, long-chain fatty acids and monoglycerides are delivered to smooth endoplasmic reticulum in the cytoplasm for resynthesis into complex lipids.[6] Phospholipids, an important component of cell membranes, are synthesized in the rough endoplasmic reticulum. Triglycerides resynthesized in the endoplasmic reticulum of enterocytes are secreted by enterocytes as lipoproteins. These lipoproteins are multimolecular aggregates of lipid and protein with a configuration that allows transport through aqueous intracellular fluid or plasma. Lecithin is the primary phospholipid in lipoproteins and is derived primarily from bile salts (10 to 20 g/day) or diet (5 to 10 g/day). Cholesterol is primarily derived from biliary secretions (1 to 2 g/day) with a minor component (0.2 to 0.5 g/day) from the diet.

Most dietary fat enters the lymphatic circulation through lacteals located in each villus and is then passed via mesenteric lymphatics to the thoracic duct and superior vena cava. About 25% of triglycerides are transported to the liver bound to albumin.

Digestion of fat is very efficient. Almost all dietary triglyceride is absorbed by enterocytes. No ingested triglyceride is found in the colon. The small amount of fecal fat (less than 7 g/day) is derived from phospholipids in sloughed intestinal membranes or intestinal bacteria. After micelle delivery, bile salts return to the small bowel lumen to solubilize more free fatty acids and monoglycerides. Eventually, conjugated bile salts (95%) are resorbed in the ileum as an active sodium-coupled process. Some bile salts are passively absorbed in the proximal small intestine. Fecal loss of bile salts is balanced by synthesis of bile in the liver.

Fluids and Electrolytes

Diarrhea and malabsorption are not synonymous. Malabsorption may occur in some diarrheal states. A large volume of fluid (8 to 10 L) enters the gastrointestinal lumen each day, but only 100 mL of fluid is normally excreted in the feces.[7] The daily fluid load includes about 2 L of oral intake, 0.5 to 1.5 L of saliva, 2.5 L of gastric juice, 0.5 L of bile, 1.5 L of pancreatic secretion, and 1 L of intestinal secretions. The small bowel absorbs about 7 L of fluid daily, with 1.5 to 1.9 L of fluid reaching the colon. The colon is capable of resorbing up to 4 L of fluid on a daily basis. Diarrhea therefore occurs if more than 4 L of fluid reaches the colon or if abnormally functioning colonic mucosa cannot resorb the 1.9 L of fluid that normally enters the colon each day.

ANATOMIC CLASSIFICATION OF MALABSORPTION

From the above discussion of digestion and absorption, it is clear that carbohydrate digestion requires a functioning pancreas and small bowel brush border enzymes. Normal protein digestion requires adequate gastric and pancreatic function and small bowel brush border enzymes. Fat digestion requires normal hepatic, biliary, exocrine pancreatic, and small bowel function. As a result, malabsorption may be caused by abnormalities of the liver, biliary tree, stomach, and small intestine (Table 47-1).[3]

Hepatobiliary and Pancreatic Disorders

Bile salt insufficiency due to biliary obstruction or decreased hepatic synthesis leads to mild malabsorption. Any disease that destroys pancreatic exocrine tissue decreases bicarbonate and pancreatic enzyme secretion. Maldigestion does not occur until 90% of the pancreatic exocrine tissue has been destroyed.[4] The most common cause of pancreas-related maldigestion is alcohol-related pancreatitis. Patients with cystic fibrosis have malabsorption, but this is less common.

Gastric Disorders

Diseases of the stomach may cause mild malabsorptive states. Patients with pernicious anemia have decreased production of intrinsic factor, leading to vitamin B_{12} deficiency. In patients with Zollinger-Ellison syndrome, inflammation and ulceration in the duodenum and first several loops of jejunum causes diarrhea, not malabsorption. About one third of patients with Zollinger-Ellison syndrome have diarrhea related to gastric hypersecretion and intestinal mucosal damage. Mild malabsorption results from excess acid entering the duodenum that inactivates pancreatic enzymes.

Small Bowel Disorders

Malabsorption can result from a wide variety of mechanisms associated with diseases of the small intestine (see Table 47-1).

Bacterial Overgrowth

Any disease that causes stasis in the lumen of the small intestine can lead to bacterial overgrowth and small bowel dysfunction (Table 47-2).[3] Disorders that cause chronic small bowel obstruction (e.g., Crohn's disease and adhesions) may result in stagnation and bacterial overgrowth. Diseases with intrinsic small bowel hypomotility (e.g., diabetes, scleroderma, and jejunal diverticulosis) can also lead to stasis and bacterial overgrowth. Stasis in surgical blind loops or the afferent loop of a gastrojejunostomy can also result in bacterial overgrowth.

In patients with bacterial overgrowth, malabsorption is related to several mechanisms, including intraluminal bacterial deconjugation of bile salts and fermentation of carbohydrates. Concomitant epithelial cell dysfunction may be present.

Table 47-1
Anatomically Oriented Classification of Malabsorption

Organ	Disease or Condition	Pathophysiology
Stomach	Zollinger-Ellison syndrome	Pancreatic enzyme inactivation by acid
	Post gastrectomy	Rapid transit of nutrients, dilution pancreatic enzymes
	Pernicious anemia	Intrinsic factor deficiency (vitamin B_{12} malabsorption)
Pancreas	Chronic pancreatitis, cystic fibrosis, pancreatic cancer	Decreased pancreatic enzyme and bicarbonate secretion
Liver, biliary tree	Severe parenchymal liver disease	Decreased bile salt formation
	Cholestatic liver disease (primary biliary cirrhosis, drug-induced cholestasis), bile duct obstruction (bile duct carcinoma, pancreatic cancer, gallstones, sclerosing cholangitis)	Decreased bile salt delivery to duodenum
Small intestine	Jejunal diverticulosis, scleroderma, small intestinal fistulas, stricture in Crohn's disease, diabetes, pseudo-obstruction	Stasis with bacterial overgrowth, bile salt deconjugation
	Crohn's disease, small intestinal resection, cholecystocolonic fistula	Increased bile salt loss
	Lactase deficiency, Crohn's disease	Disaccharidase deficiency
	Celiac disease, tropical sprue, Whipple's disease, eosinophilic gastroenteritis, radiation enteropathy, Crohn's disease, intestinal ischemia, ileal resection	Loss of normal epithelial cells
	Abetalipoproteinemia	Nonformation chylomicrons
	Lymphangiectasia, lymphoma, tuberculosis, carcinoid	Lymphatic obstruction
	Diabetes mellitus, giardiasis, adrenal insufficiency, hyperthyroidism, hypogammaglobulinemia, amyloidosis, AIDS	Multiple causes

Reproduced with permission from Rubesin SE, Rubin RA, Herlinger H: Small bowel malabsorption: Clinical and radiological perspectives. Radiology 184:297-305, 1992.

Table 47-2

Diseases Causing Small Bowel Hypomotility and Malabsorption*

Genetic disorders
Familial visceral neuropathies
Familial visceral myopathies
Muscular dystrophy

Collagen-Vascular Disorders
Progressive systemic sclerosis
Dermatomyositis/polymyositis
Periarteritis nodosa
Systemic lupus erythematosus

Endocrine Disorders
Diabetes mellitus
Hypothyroidism
Hyperthyroidism (hypermotility)†
Hypoparathyroidism

Neurologic Diseases
Parkinson's disease
Multiple sclerosis
Chagas' disease
Spinal cord injury

Drugs
Narcotics
Phenothiazines
Antiparkinson's medications
Ganglionic blockers
Tricyclic antidepressants

Other
Celiac disease
Radiation enteritis
Jejunal diverticulosis
Amyloidosis
Lead poisoning

*Disorders typically having a malabsorptive state are highlighted in bold.
†In hyperthyroidism, small bowel transit time is rapid, not slow.
Reproduced with permission from Rubesin SE: Diseases of the small bowel causing malabsorption. In Taveras JM, Ferrucci JT (eds): Radiology: Diagnosis, Imaging, Intervention. Philadelphia, JB Lippincott, 1993, pp 1-17.

Bacterial digestion of malabsorbed fat forms compounds that can stimulate small bowel or colonic secretion. Solutes of malabsorbed carbohydrates and deconjugated bile salts are also osmotically active, resulting in water and electrolyte loss.

Brush Border Disease

Brush border enzyme deficiencies or transport mechanism deficiencies may cause osmotic diarrhea, malabsorption, or both. The most common example of osmotic diarrhea due to brush border disaccharidase deficiency is lactase "deficiency" (lactose-phlorizin hydrolase deficiency) with lactose intolerance.[4] The norm for most human populations is for brush border lactose-phlorizin hydrolase levels to decline to 5% to 10% of childhood levels in older children and adolescents. As a result, ingestion of dairy products can lead to diarrhea, flatulence, and cramps in most adult populations and is the true norm. Preservation of lactose-phlorizin hydrolase is an autosomally recessive trait, found typically in northern Europeans. Intermediate activity of this enzyme is found in heterozygotes.

Mucosal Damage

Damage to surface epithelial cells causes malabsorption of electrolytes and nutrients. Inflammation of crypt cells and immature villus cells causes secretory diarrhea. Blood, pus, and mucus in the intestinal lumen leads to osmotic diarrhea. Widespread epithelial damage is therefore characterized by a combination of osmotic and secretory diarrhea and nutrient malabsorption. Diseases that destroy proximal small bowel epithelium cause generalized malabsorption of fats, proteins, carbohydrates, iron, and folate, whereas diseases that damage distal ileal mucosa primarily cause malabsorption of fat due to bile salt loss and vitamin B_{12} deficiency. Mucosal diseases causing malabsorption involve relatively long segments of small bowel. These diseases are relatively uncommon, however, and include celiac disease, tropical sprue, Whipple's disease, and eosinophilic enteritis.

Postmucosal Disease

Any disorder that obstructs lacteals in the villi or lymphatics in the small bowel mesentery may cause fat malabsorption. In primary lymphangiectasia, for example, abnormal formation of lymphatics results in impaired absorption of chylomicrons and fat-soluble vitamins and loss of lymph into the intestinal lumen from lymphoenteric fistulas.

Diseases with Multifactorial Causes

Malabsorption is caused by several mechanisms in many diseases. In amyloidosis, for example, malabsorption can be attributed to stasis with bacterial overgrowth, mucosal destruction due to ischemia, and disruption of nutrient absorption by amyloid deposition in the lamina propria. Fat malabsorption in hyperthyroidism is attributed to rapid small bowel transit.

DIAGNOSIS OF MALABSORPTION: CLINICAL PERSPECTIVE

Malabsorption is characterized by diarrhea, steatorrhea, excessive gas, abdominal pain, and weight loss. Diarrhea is caused by decreased intestinal absorption, colonic secretion of fluid induced by hydroxy fatty acids, and osmotic overload of bile salts and fatty acids. *Steatorrhea* is the term used for the bulky, foul-smelling, greasy stools caused by malabsorption of fat. Excessive gas production related to fermentation of carbohydrates by intestinal bacteria results in borborygmi, flatulence, and abdominal distention. Abdominal pain is due to a variety of causes, including pancreatic inflammation, biliary disease, small bowel obstruction, and ischemia.

The clinician has a broad array of laboratory tests and biopsies to make a diagnosis of malabsorption. The reader is referred to textbooks of gastroenterology for further description of these tests. Radiologic imaging in patients with a clinical diagnosis of malabsorption is performed as an adjunct to help identify diseases (e.g., jejunoileal diverticulosis) that cause malabsorption. Radiologic imaging is also used to detect complications of diseases that cause malabsorption (e.g., T-cell lymphoma arising in celiac disease).

Unfortunately, adults with malabsorption often have an insidious presentation. Steatorrhea may be so mild that it is unrecognized by the patient. Mild steatorrhea is typical of low-grade bile duct obstruction, chronic hepatic disease, mild to moderate pancreatic insufficiency, and even mild celiac disease. Many patients with malabsorption present with symptoms related to specific vitamin or nutrient deficiencies. For example, vitamin A deficiency may cause night blindness; vitamin K deficiency results in easy bruisability, petechiae, or hematuria; vitamin D or calcium malabsorption results in paresthesias, tetany or bone pain; and decreased absorption of folate, vitamin B, or iron may cause pallor, glossitis, stomatitis, and cheilosis.

BACTERIAL OVERGROWTH

A wide variety of disorders may cause small bowel hypomotility with resulting stasis and bacterial overgrowth (see Table 47-2) or intestinal pseudo-obstruction.

Jejunoileal Diverticulosis

Small bowel diverticula are acquired protrusions of mucosa and submucosa on the mesenteric border of the small bowel, where the vasa recta pierce the muscularis propria. The diverticula are larger and more numerous in the jejunum, decreasing in size and number as they progress into the ileum.[8,9] Jejunoileal diverticula develop in a heterogeneous group of disorders associated with abnormalities of smooth muscle or the myenteric plexus. Small bowel dysmotility is frequent. Some cases of jejunoileal diverticulosis may be a manifestation of systemic sclerosis or a forme fruste of isolated scleroderma.[10]

Jejunoileal diverticulosis is not uncommon, occurring in about 2% of the population,[8] but most people with jejunal diverticulosis are asymptomatic. In patients with numerous diverticula, stasis with bacterial overgrowth and malabsorptive symptoms may occur. Complications of jejunal diverticula, including gastrointestinal obstruction or perforation, may cause abdominal symptoms.

Diverticula are readily identified on barium studies as 1- to 7-cm round, barium-filled sacs on the mesenteric border of the small bowel (Fig. 47-1). The mouths of the diverticula are broad based and the necks are variable in length. Air-fluid levels may be present on upright or cross-table lateral radiographs. If there are numerous diverticula, the course of the small bowel may be obscured by the numerous sacs (Fig. 47-2). The motor disorder seen in jejunoileal diverticulosis is manifested by decreased peristalsis, increased intraluminal fluid and gas, luminal dilatation, and prolonged transit time.

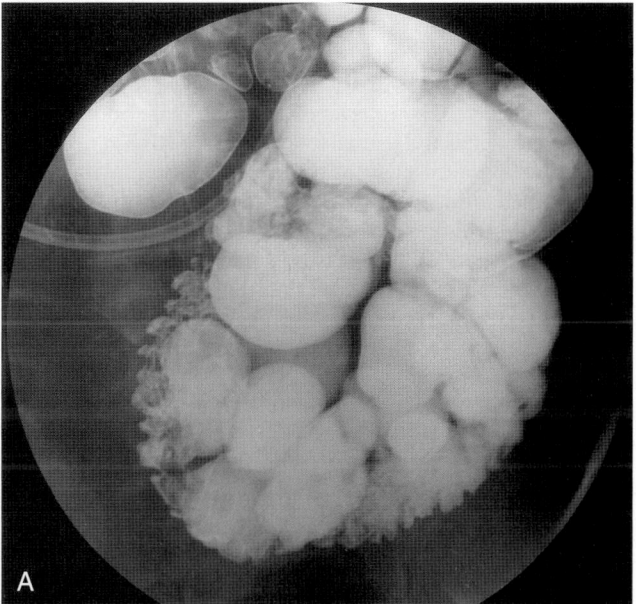

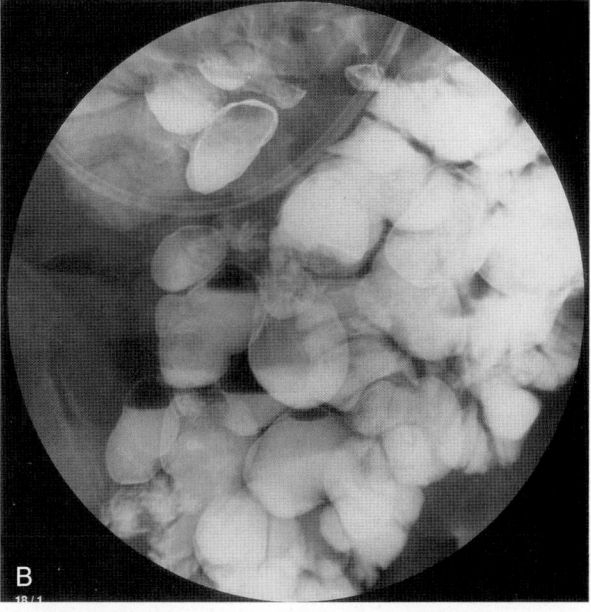

Figure 47-2. Jejunoileal diverticulosis causing malabsorption. A. Spot image from enteroclysis shows innumerable barium-filled diverticula obscuring the underlying small bowel loops from which they arise. **B.** Upright spot image shows multiple air-fluid levels and air-barium levels in the diverticula.

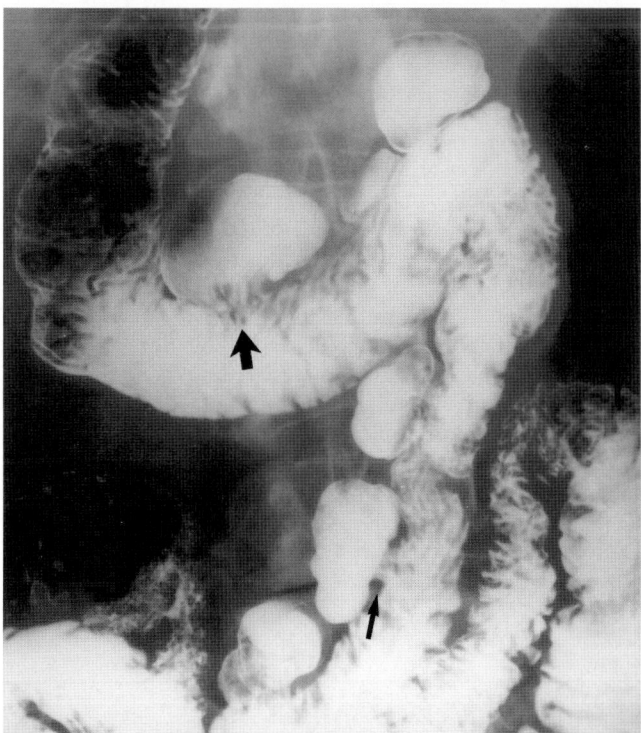

Figure 47-1. Jejunal diverticulosis. Coned-down view of overhead radiograph from small bowel follow-through shows multiple large diverticula on the mesenteric border of the distal duodenum and proximal jejunum. The sacs are smooth, but many have a lobulated contour. The mouth (*small arrow*) of one diverticulum is visualized in profile. Folds are seen radiating (*large arrow*) into another diverticulum. This degree of diverticulosis does not usually cause malabsorption.

Although other small bowel disorders may be associated with sacculations or diverticula, jejunoileal diverticulosis is easily differentiated from the sacculations in Crohn's disease, scleroderma, or prior surgery; a solitary Meckel diverticulum; or diverticula confined to the terminal ileum.[1,10]

Jejunoileal diverticulosis may be complicated by pneumatosis cystoides intestinalis or free intraperitoneal air due to perforation or benign pneumatosis.[10,11] Rarely, diverticulitis may cause small bowel perforation. Jejunal diverticulitis can also result in abdominal pain, obstruction, or gastrointestinal bleeding.[12-16] Mechanical obstruction may result from volvulus, enterolith impaction, or diverticulitis. Heterotopic tissue or neoplasms are rare complications.

Progressive Systemic Sclerosis, Visceral Neuropathies, and Myopathies

The small intestine is involved in about 40% of patients with progressive systemic sclerosis (scleroderma).[17] The smooth muscle, especially that of the circular muscle layer, degenerates and is replaced by collagen.[18] The muscular abnormalities result in duodenal and jejunal dilatation (Fig. 47-3) and hypomotility, with prolonged small bowel transit time and increased intraluminal fluid. Patchy and predominant fibrosis of the circular muscle layer leads to bunching of small bowel folds, producing the so-called *hidebound bowel* (see Fig. 47-3).[19] Despite luminal dilatation, an increased number of small bowel folds per inch is usually seen. Asymmetric scarring leads to wide-mouthed sacculations, most frequently on the mesenteric border of the small bowel (Fig. 47-4).[20,21] As with any small bowel disorder characterized by hypomotility, transient

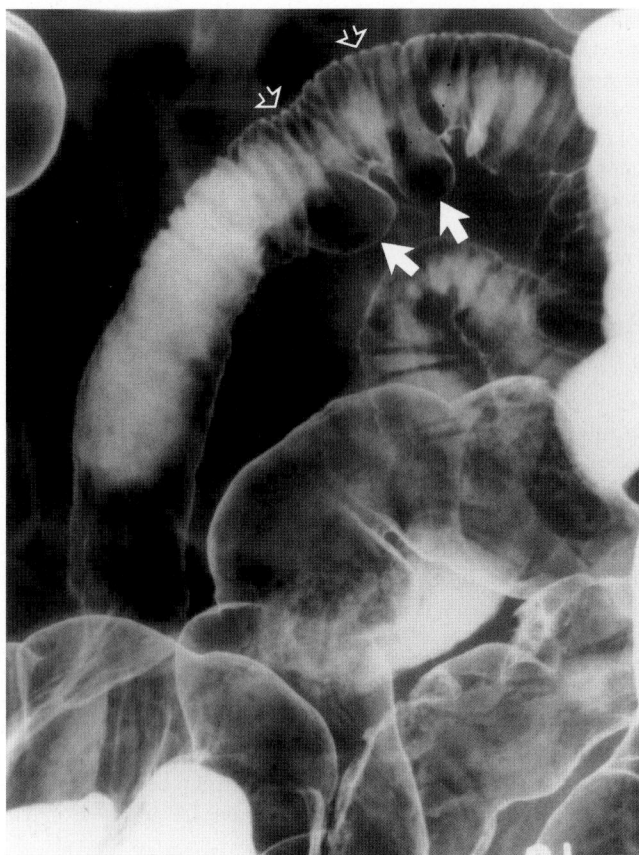

Figure 47-4. Scleroderma. Spot image from double-contrast barium enema shows sacculation of the mesenteric border (*closed arrows*) of the terminal ileum with bunching of folds (*open arrows*) on the antimesenteric border due to fibrosis in the muscular layers.

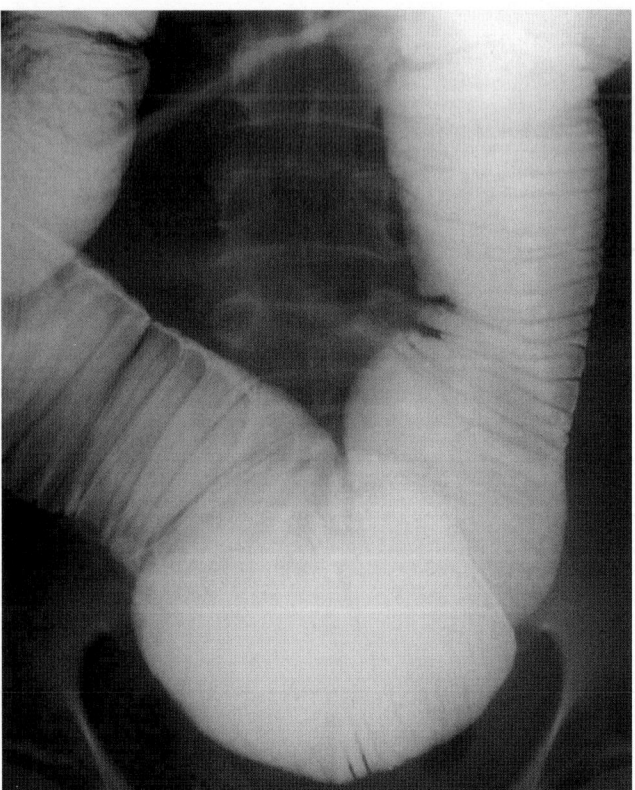

Figure 47-3. Scleroderma. Spot radiograph from enteroclysis shows massively dilated small bowel. (Compare the diameter of the lumen with the size of a lumbar vertebral body.) There is also an increased number of folds per inch, producing the *hidebound sign*.

intussusceptions and pneumatosis intestinalis may occur with or without pneumoperitoneum.

Several forms of visceral myopathies and neuropathies may present as malabsorption or intestinal pseudo-obstruction. These include autosomal dominant and recessive conditions or isolated cases.[22] The visceral myopathies are characterized histologically by degeneration and fibrosis of both the inner circular and outer longitudinal smooth muscle layers.[23] Congenital neuropathies are characterized by degeneration of the myenteric plexus of the bowel. Decreased or absent peristalsis is seen in visceral myopathies and scleroderma, but large amplitude nonpropulsive contractions are seen only in visceral neuropathies.[23] Marked duodenal enlargement typically occurs in visceral myopathies, whereas small bowel dilatation may be present in both visceral myopathies and neuropathies. The increased number of folds and sacculations typical of scleroderma are not found. The colon demonstrates hypercontractility in visceral neuropathy and dilatation and lack of haustration in visceral myopathy.[23]

EPITHELIAL CELL DAMAGE

Celiac Disease

Celiac disease (gluten-sensitive enteropathy or celiac sprue) is a chronic disease in which the gliadin fraction of wheat gluten causes damage to the small bowel mucosa. Removal of wheat products from the diet reverses this mucosal damage.

Although the mechanism of celiac is not completely understood, it is postulated that there is a suspension of the normal immune tolerance to foreign food antigens.[24] The gliadin fraction of ingested wheat products stimulates an immune response in the epithelium of the small intestine, leading to mucosal inflammation and destruction. Lymphocytic infiltration may also occur in the stomach (as lymphocytic gastritis) or in the colon.[25]

Celiac disease is uncommon and is most frequently encountered in whites, particularly northern Europeans and people from Ireland.[26] Children may present with diarrhea, abdominal distention, weight loss, and failure to thrive. Young adults may present with diarrhea, steatorrhea, or infertility. Older adults may present with steatorrhea, anemia, weight loss, or other symptoms. Patients who develop symptoms in adulthood or who develop celiac disease de novo in adulthood may present with symptoms related to malabsorption of specific nutrients such as vitamin A or B$_{12}$. Bleeding or purpura related to vitamin K deficiency may be present. Aphthous stomatitis, cheilosis, and glossitis are not infrequent. In adults, symptoms in celiac disease may be precipitated by pregnancy, respiratory therapy, and gastric surgery.[27] Gluten-sensitive enteropathy is seen in patients with dermatitis herpetiformis.[28] Celiac disease has also been associated with other skin diseases such as psoriasis, eczema, cutaneous amyloid, and mycosis fungoides.[24]

Recent research advances have shown that celiac disease is much more common than previously thought, occurring in about 1 in 200 whites.[24] Most people with celiac disease ignore minor symptoms or are asymptomatic. The diagnosis of celiac disease can be made when physicians test for serum antibodies associated with celiac disease in patients with minimal gastrointestinal complaints or indicators of malabsorption, such as vitamin deficiencies. IgA and IgG antibodies to gliadin are elevated in 75% to 85% of patients with celiac disease.[29] These antibodies may also be elevated in some patients with inflammatory bowel disease or liver disease.[24] Endomysial antibody is also elevated in a large percentage of patients with celiac disease.[30,31] The antigen for antiendomysial antibody is tissue transglutaminase (tTG). An enzyme-linked immunoadsorbent assay (ELISA) test for IgA anti-tTG is reported to have a sensitivity of 90% to 95% in the diagnosis of celiac disease. Other studies have shown less favorable results for antiendomysial antibody.[31] Some patients with celiac disease have IgA deficiency, so this test will have false-negative results in these patients. Small bowel biopsies and follow-up biopsies after gluten withdrawal are usually required for a definitive diagnosis.[32]

Biopsy specimens in celiac disease classically reveal loss of intestinal villi associated with crypt hyperplasia and infiltration of the lamina propria by plasma cells and lymphocytes (Fig. 47-5).[33] Lesser degrees of villous atrophy may be present, however, ranging from mild flattening to partial villous atrophy or a flat mucosa. Because other diseases may cause loss of intestinal villi, biopsy-proven reversal of mucosal changes after gluten withdrawal is essential for confirming this diagnosis. Nevertheless, some patients may develop disease that is refractory to gluten withdrawal.

Radiographic Findings

Although endoscopic or capsular biopsy is required for a definitive diagnosis of celiac disease, enteroclysis may also be

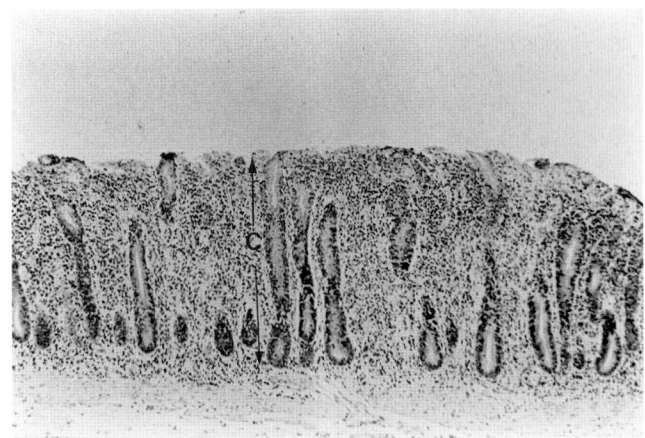

Figure 47-5. Complete villous atrophy in celiac disease. Medium-power photomicrograph shows complete absence of villi. The crypts (representative crypt identified by C) extend to the surface of the epithelium. The height of the mucosa is somewhat preserved by crypt hyperplasia with edema and inflammation of the lamina propria (hematoxylin and eosin). (From Rubesin SE, Herlinger H, Saul SH, et al: Adult celiac disease and its complications. RadioGraphics 9:1045-1066, 1989.)

performed to establish the diagnosis in patients with atypical symptoms.[34] Enteroclysis is particularly of value for detecting complications in patients with known celiac disease and a poor response to medical therapy or in patients with recurrent symptoms despite gluten withdrawal.[34-36]

The small bowel findings in celiac disease reflect the underlying villous atrophy. With extensive villous atrophy, there is loss of the surface area of the mucosa. This loss of mucosa in celiac disease is manifested by a decreased number of folds in the proximal jejunum (Fig. 47-6), the portion of the small

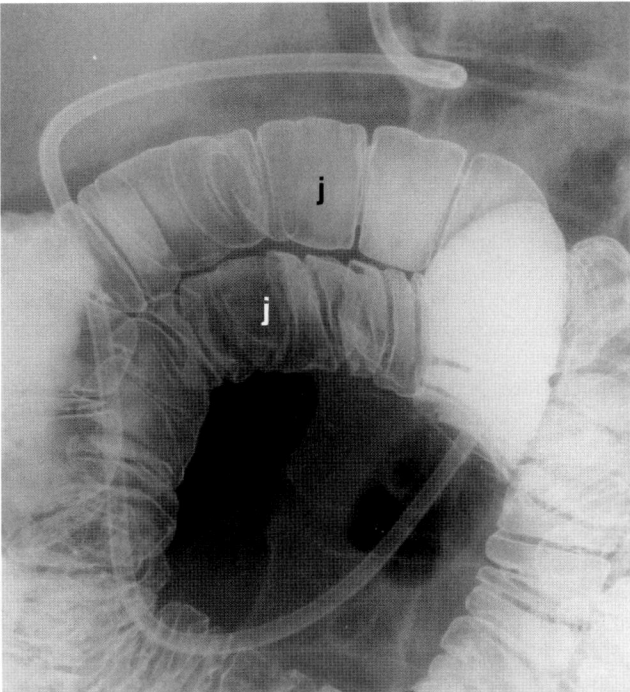

Figure 47-6. Celiac disease. Spot radiograph from enteroclysis shows a paucity of folds (two to three folds per inch) in two loops of jejunum (j). However, the folds are of normal thickness.

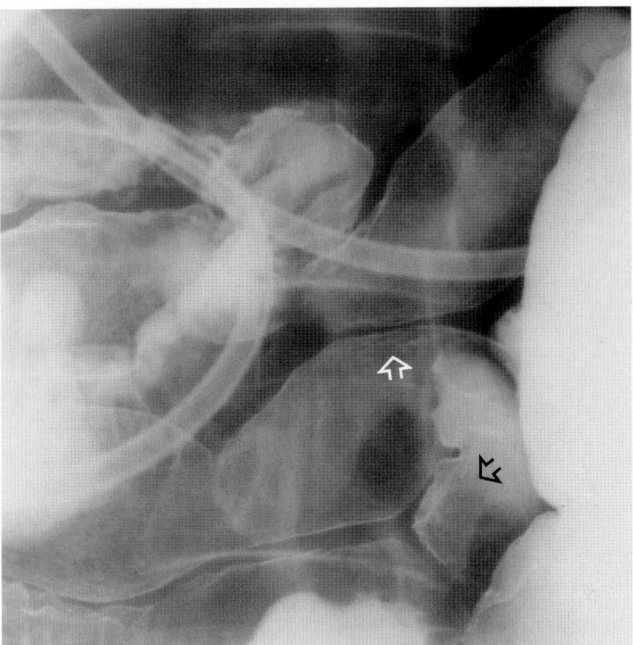

Figure 47-7. Mosaic pattern in celiac disease. Spot radiograph of the jejunum from enteroclysis shows a tubular configuration with near complete absence of folds. A subtle, finely nodular surface pattern is seen in some regions (*arrows*), reflecting the mosaic pattern of atrophic mucosa. (From Rubesin SE, Herlinger H, Saul SH, et al. Adult celiac disease and its complications. RadioGraphics 9:1045-1066, 1989, expanded view of Fig. 7.)

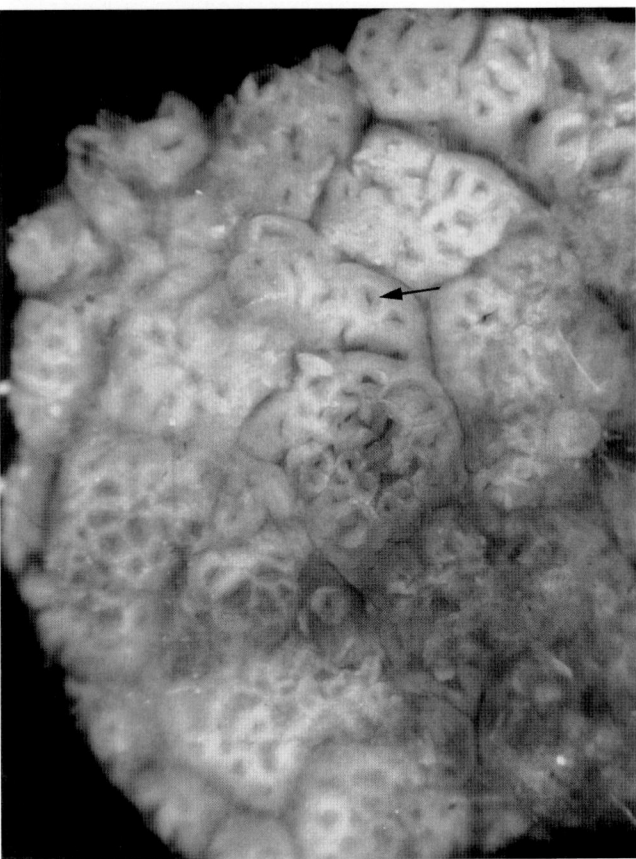

Figure 47-8. Mosaic pattern in celiac disease. Dissecting photomicrograph of the jejunum shows islands of mucosa surrounded by deep grooves. Crypt openings (*arrow*) are visible on the surface of each mucosal island. (Courtesy of M. S. Losowsky, MD, Leeds, England; from Rubesin SE, Herlinger H, Saul SH, et al: Adult celiac disease and its complications. RadioGraphics 9:1045-1066, 1989.)

bowel that is most severely involved by this disease. Three or fewer folds per inch are present in 75% of adult patients with known or suspected celiac disease.[34] Four folds per inch in the proximal jejunum is indeterminate for celiac disease, because the proximal jejunum normally has four to seven folds per inch. The mucosal surface pattern may appear finely reticular in uncomplicated celiac disease with polygonal radiolucent islands of mucosa surrounded by barium-filled grooves (Fig. 47-7).[34,35] This radiographic pattern reflects the "mosaic" pattern visualized when celiac mucosa is examined under a dissecting microscope (Fig. 47-8).[37] Villous atrophy reveals the underlying groove pattern of the mucosa and the crypt openings (see Fig. 47-8).

In contrast, ileal folds may be increased in number and thicker than normal in celiac disease, an adaptive response to increase the mucosal surface area of the small bowel.[38] This phenomenon has been termed *jejunization* of the ileum. If jejunal or proximal ileal folds are enlarged or nodular, complications such as ulcerative jejunoileitis, lymphoma, or edema related to hypoproteinemia (Fig. 47-9) should be suspected.[35] Nevertheless, thickened, nodular folds and discrete mucosal nodules can be seen in the duodenum in patients with uncomplicated celiac disease. Abnormalities of the duodenal folds reflect the effect of gastric acid on duodenal mucosa damaged by celiac disease, with some combination of inflammation, Brunner's gland hyperplasia, and gastric metaplasia.[39-41]

Enteroclysis is much more accurate than small bowel follow-through studies for evaluating fold patterns and establishing the diagnosis of celiac disease or one of its complications. However, transient intussusceptions occur in 25% of patients with celiac disease, and these intussusceptions are better shown on small bowel follow-throughs (Fig. 47-10).[42,43]

Diffuse hypomotility in celiac disease may also be better shown on small bowel follow-through studies.

Complications

The major complications of celiac disease include malabsorption refractory to gluten withdrawal, hyposplenism, neuropathy, intestinal ulceration and pneumatosis, lymphadenopathy, the cavitary mesenteric lymph node syndrome, and malignancy.[35,37,44,45] In patients with known celiac disease, complications are frequently heralded by the development of fever, acute abdominal pain, abdominal distention, weight loss, or steatorrhea despite adherence to a gluten-free diet. CT and enteroclysis are complementary radiologic tests for the diagnosis of these complications.[46]

Splenic atrophy occurs in one third to one half of patients with celiac disease.[47-49] Decreased splenic size correlates with decreased splenic function.[49] A small spleen may be shown on any radiologic test capable of visualizing the spleen.

Mesenteric and retroperitoneal lymphadenopathy is not uncommon in celiac disease and usually is caused by reactive lymphoid hyperplasia.[50,51] Mesenteric or retroperitoneal lymphadenopathy can be of low attenuation (Fig. 47-11), reflecting fat deposition in lymph nodes, or of normal attenuation. The cavitary mesenteric lymph node syndrome is a rare, usually

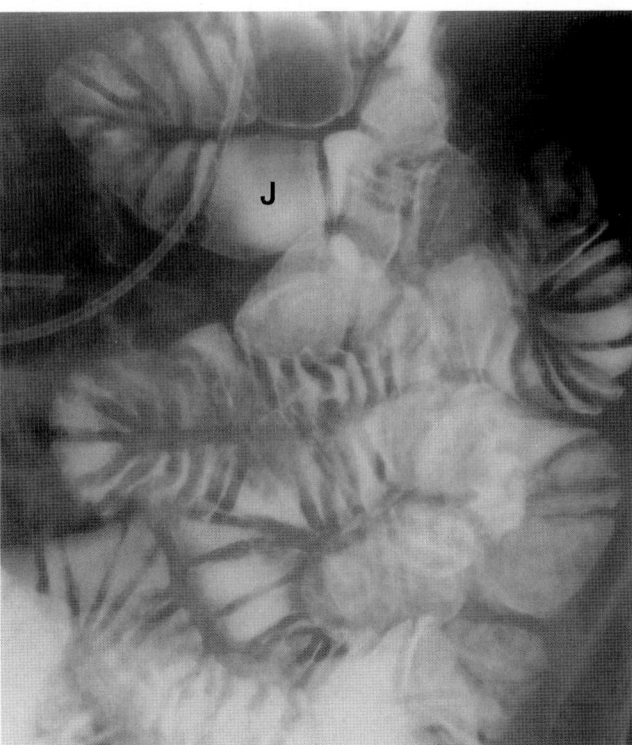

Figure 47-9. Small bowel edema due to hypoproteinemia in celiac disease. Spot radiograph from enteroclysis shows a decreased number of folds per inch in the jejunum (J). The folds are also thickened due to a protein-losing enteropathy with a low serum albumin. (From the teaching files of Hans Herlinger, MD.)

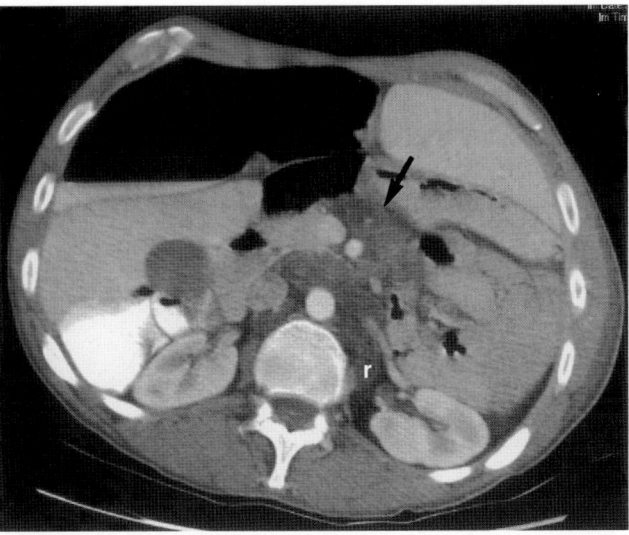

Figure 47-11. Lymphadenopathy in celiac disease. CT shows numerous low-attenuation lymph nodes (*arrow*) in the root of the small bowel mesentery and in the retroperitoneum (r).

fatal disorder, typically occurring in patients with celiac disease or in patients with small bowel villous atrophy refractory to a gluten-free diet.[52-54] This condition is characterized by markedly enlarged, cavitary lymph nodes filled with lipid-rich hyaline material. CT may reveal mesenteric or retroperitoneal masses of low attenuation with or without fat-fluid levels (Fig. 47-12).[35]

Although numerous malignant tumors have been described in patients with celiac disease, there is definitely an increased incidence of squamous cell carcinoma of the pharynx and esophagus and adenocarcinoma and lymphoma of the small bowel in these patients.[24,55-62] In fact, malignant tumors are the most common cause of death in adults with celiac disease.[59-63]

Small bowel lymphomas are T-cell lymphomas in patients with celiac disease. These tumors have a 300-fold higher incidence in celiac disease than in the general population and are the most common malignant tumors complicating celiac disease.[24,57,58] Lymphomas in celiac disease are distinct

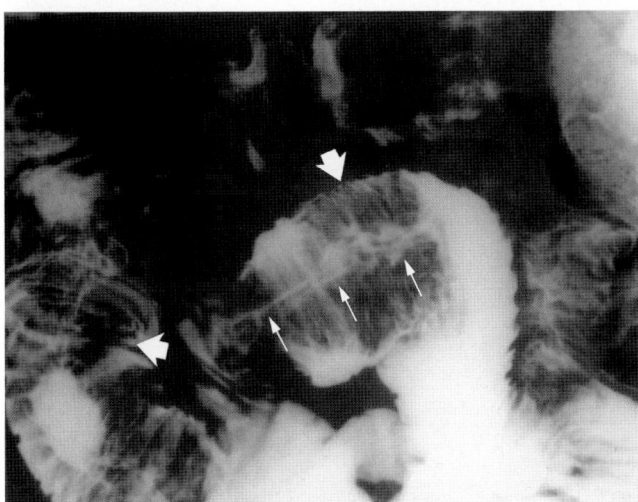

Figure 47-10. Transient intussusceptions in celiac disease. Spot radiograph from small bowel follow-through shows two transient intussusceptions (*large arrows*). An intraluminal filling defect (the intussusceptum) is surrounded by barium coursing between the wall of the intussusceptum and the mucosa of the intussuscipiens. The collapsed lumen of the intussusceptum (*small arrows*) is filled with barium. (From Rubesin SE, Herlinger H, Saul SH, et al: Adult celiac disease and its complications. RadioGraphics 9:1045-1066, 1989.)

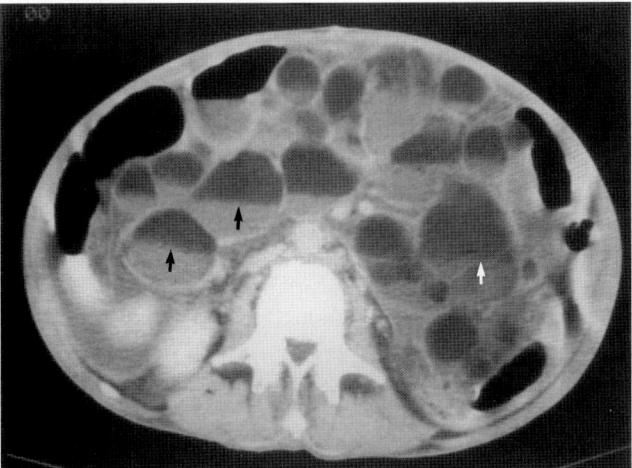

Figure 47-12. Cavitary mesenteric lymph node syndrome. CT shows numerous ovoid masses in the abdomen. The masses have fat/debris levels (*arrows*). These represent enlarged, cavitary lymph nodes that could be mistaken for loops of small bowel with air-fluid levels. However, the fat and fluid attenuation of the nodes and the lack of opacification by positive oral contrast should suggest the correct diagnosis. (From Rubesin SE, Herlinger H, Saul SH, et al: Adult celiac disease and its complications. RadioGraphics 9:1045-1066, 1989.)

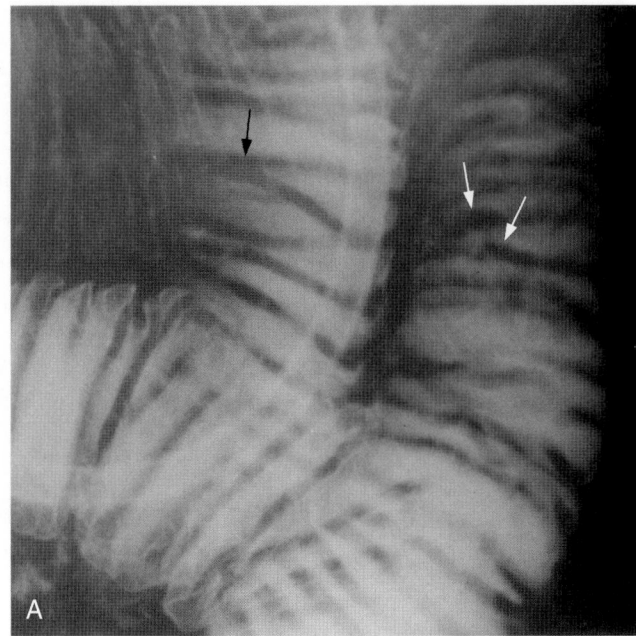

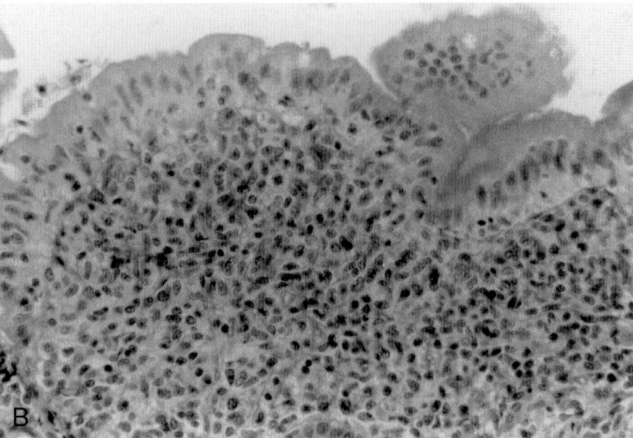

Figure 47-13. T-cell lymphoma complicating celiac disease. A. Spot radiograph from enteroclysis shows mildly thickened, undulating, slightly nodular folds (*arrows*) in the proximal jejunum. **B.** Biopsy specimen from the jejunum shows a monomorphic lymphomatous infiltrate expanding the lamina propria due to T-cell lymphoma (hematoxylin and eosin). (From Rubesin SE, Herlinger H, Saul SH, et al: Adult celiac disease and its complications. RadioGraphics 9:1045-1066, 1989.)

from typical B-cell small bowel lymphomas, involving long segments of bowel or having a multifocal distribution. Unlike most small bowel lymphomas, these tumors tend to be located in the jejunum rather than in the ileum.[35] T-cell lymphomas are usually manifested on barium studies by thickened, nodular folds in long segments of jejunum (Fig. 47-13).[35] In some patients, however, radiographic studies may reveal a cavitary or annular lesion (Fig. 47-14).

Radiologic differentiation of T-cell lymphoma from ulcerative jejunoileitis is not possible. Ulcerative jejunoileitis is an entity in which multiple ulcers develop in the small bowel during the fifth or sixth decades of life.[64,65] About 75% of these patients have celiac disease or villous atrophy unresponsive to gluten withdrawal.[46] They usually present as fever, abdominal pain, weight loss, or abdominal distention. This entity is complicated by gastrointestinal bleeding, perforation, or obstruction. Ulceration is most prominent in the jejunum but is also seen in the ileum or colon. Thickened, nodular folds may be present in the jejunum, mimicking the radiographic appearance of lymphoma (Fig. 47-15). Some cases of ulcerative jejunoileitis may progress to stricture formation (Fig. 47-16).

Small bowel adenocarcinomas are usually annular, infiltrating lesions involving the duodenum or jejunum.[35] These tumors have a threefold higher incidence in celiac disease than in the general population. They are usually advanced tumors at the time of diagnosis.[53]

Tropical Sprue

Tropical sprue is a disease that occurs in residents of endemic tropical or subtropical areas such as the Caribbean, southeast Asia, and India. Visitors to endemic areas usually develop tropical sprue only after prolonged visits. The disease is uncommon in children. Patients initially suffer a watery diarrheal illness that may remit or progress to chronic malabsorption. Although unproven, it has been postulated that colonization of the small intestine by toxigenic strains of coliform bacteria

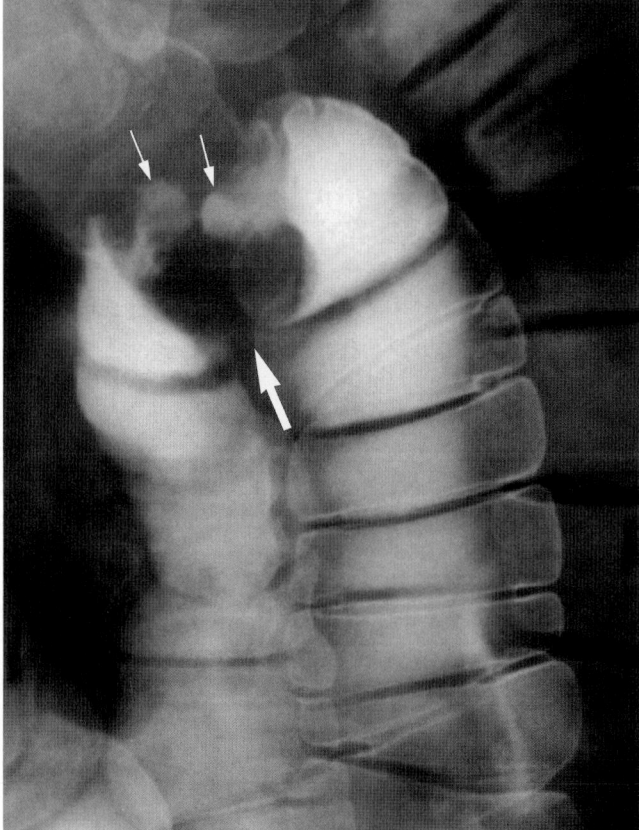

Figure 47-14. T-cell lymphoma complicating celiac disease. Spot radiograph from enteroclysis shows a short, annular lesion (*large arrow*) with central ulceration (*small arrows*) in the jejunum. Note the decreased number of jejunal folds proximal to the lesion due to underlying celiac disease.

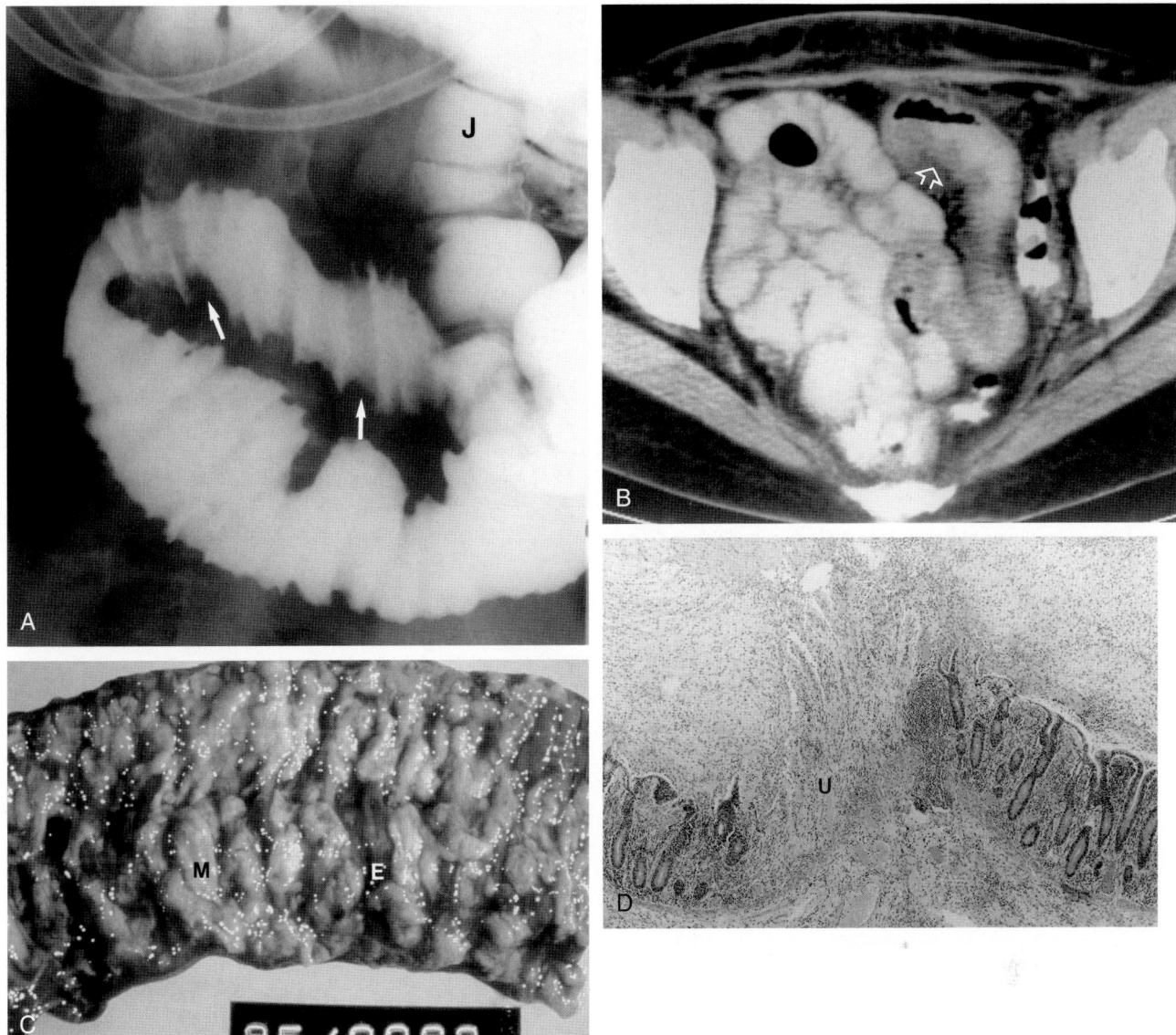

Figure 47-15. Ulcerative jejunoileitis complicating celiac disease. A. Spot radiograph during early phase of enteroclysis shows a loop of jejunum with moderately thickened, irregular folds (*arrows*) due to ulcerative jejunoileitis. Also note a decreased number of normal-sized folds more proximally in the jejunum (J) due to underlying celiac disease. **B.** CT shows irregular thickening of the wall of a loop of small bowel, predominantly on its mesenteric border. **C.** Specimen photograph shows white pseudomembranes (M) covering ulcerated epithelium (E). **D.** Low-power photomicrograph shows a focal area of ulceration (U). The mucosal surface is covered with inflammatory cells, fibrin, and sloughed epithelial cells. Also note villous atrophy due to celiac disease. (**A** to **C** from Rubesin SE, Herlinger H, Saul SH, et al: Adult celiac disease and its complications. RadioGraphics 9:1045-1066, 1989.)

causes tropical sprue.[66] Combined folate and vitamin B_{12} deficiency in tropical sprue can lead to megaloblastic anemia. In contrast to celiac disease, villous atrophy is partial and crypt hyperplasia is not severe. This disease responds to antibiotic and folate therapy.[24]

Tropical sprue is radiographically distinct from celiac disease. Thickened folds are seen in the jejunum (Fig. 47-17) and even the ileum, in contrast to the normal-sized folds (though decreased in number) in uncomplicated celiac disease.

Giardiasis

The protozoan *Giardia lamblia* is a frequent cause of endemic and epidemic diarrhea worldwide. Outbreaks of diarrhea are less frequent in the United States. Rarely, however, giardiasis is heralded by malabsorptive symptoms.[67] Barium studies in patients with giardiasis usually show no abnormalities. The protozoan attaches to the mucosal surface of the intestine, causing little damage to the underlying small bowel.[33] In severe cases, thickened folds may be seen in the distal duodenum and proximal jejunum (Fig. 47-18).[68,69] There also may be rapid transit of barium and spasm in the proximal small bowel.[70,71] Other causes of malabsorption associated with intestinal hypermotility include Zollinger-Ellison syndrome and diabetes.

Whipple's Disease

Tropheryma whippelii is a gram-positive bacillus with a thick wall and a trilaminar membrane.[72] This recently cultured

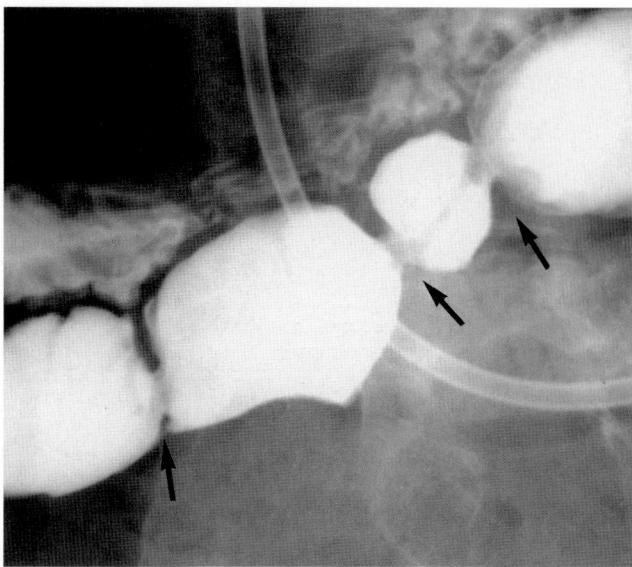

Figure 47-16. Strictures in ulcerative jejunoileitis complicating celiac disease. Spot radiograph from enteroclysis shows three short segments of ringlike narrowing (*arrows*) in the jejunum. (From Rubesin SE, Herlinger H, Saul SH, et al: Adult celiac disease and its complications. RadioGraphics 9:1045-1066, 1989.)

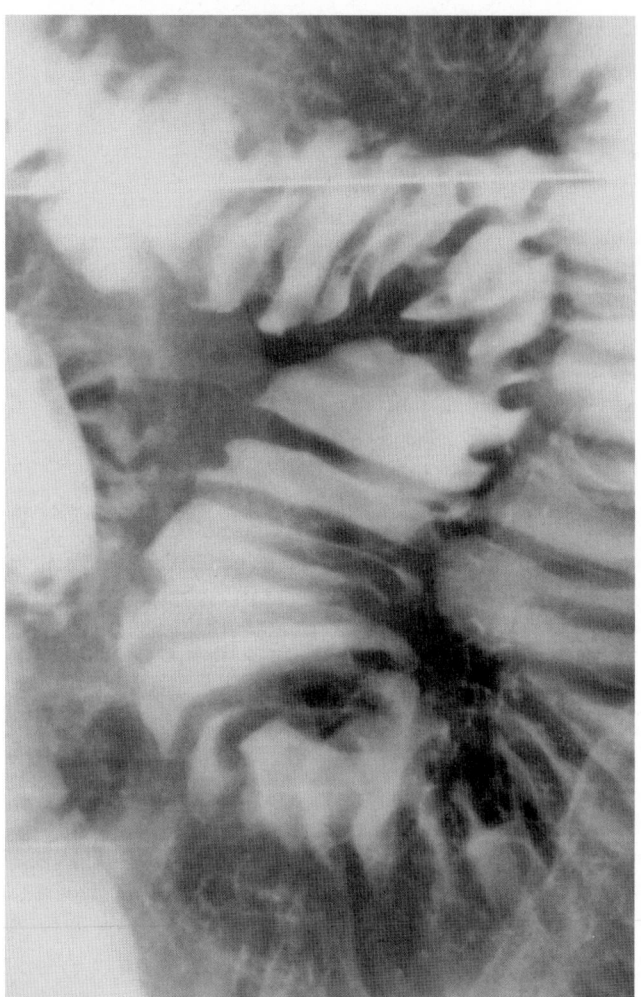

Figure 47-17. Tropical sprue. Spot radiograph from small bowel follow-through shows moderately thickened, slightly undulating folds in the jejunum. Unlike celiac disease, the number of folds per inch in the jejunum is normal.

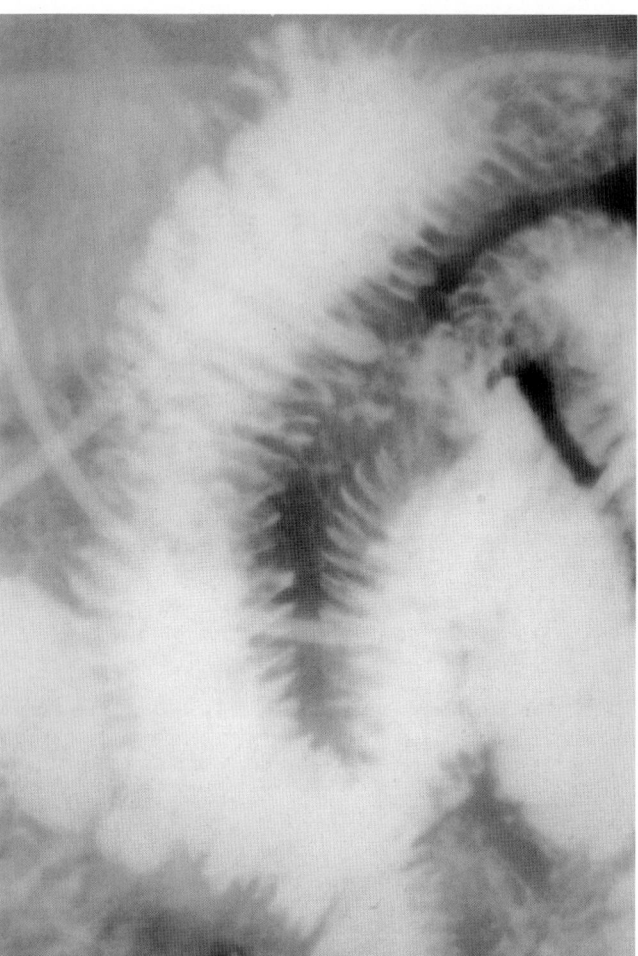

Figure 47-18. Giardiasis. Spot radiograph from enteroclysis shows mildly thickened, straight folds in the proximal jejunum. (From Rubesin SE: Diseases of small bowel causing malabsorption. In Taveras JM, Ferrucci JT [eds]: Radiology: Diagnosis, Imaging, Intervention. Philadelphia, JB Lippincott, 1993, pp 1-17.)

bacterium is responsible for the rare systemic bacterial disease first described by George Whipple in 1907.[73] It has been postulated that a defect in monocyte/macrophage function prevents affected individuals from eliminating the Whipple's bacillus.

Whipple's disease usually occurs in whites, particularly men, with a male predominance of 6 to 1.[74] Gastrointestinal symptoms include bloating, weight loss, and steatorrhea. Extraintestinal manifestations include arthritis, arthralgias, cardiac disease, fever, and multiple central nervous findings (including dementia and myoclonus). Arthritis is the most common extraintestinal manifestation. These patients typically have a migratory arthritis involving large and small joints. Cardiac involvement is characterized by pericarditis, valvular defects, and congestive heart failure. Peripheral lymphadenopathy is not uncommon.

Whipple's disease is typically manifested on barium studies by thickened, nodular folds, primarily in the distal duodenum and jejunum (Fig. 47-19).[75] Fine mucosal nodularity is sometimes demonstrated (Fig. 47-20) as a result of villous blunting due to expansion of the lamina propria by lacteals distended with fat and by innumerable macrophages containing digested bacilli (Fig. 47-21).[33]

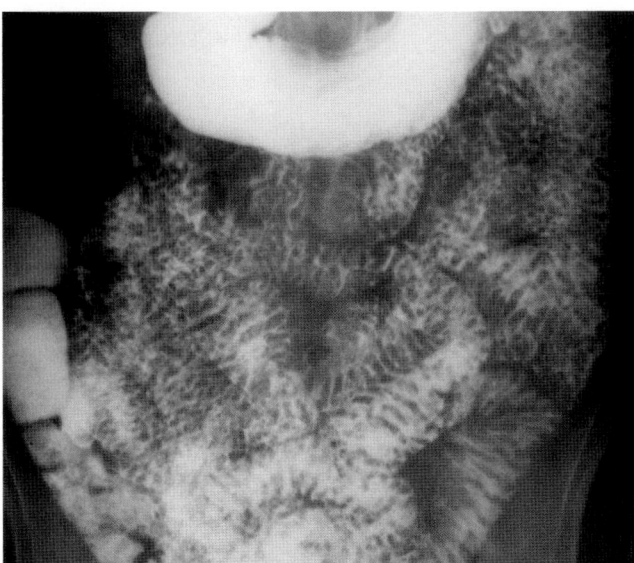

Figure 47-19. Whipple's disease. Overhead radiograph from small bowel follow-through shows thickened, nodular folds in the proximal and mid small bowel.

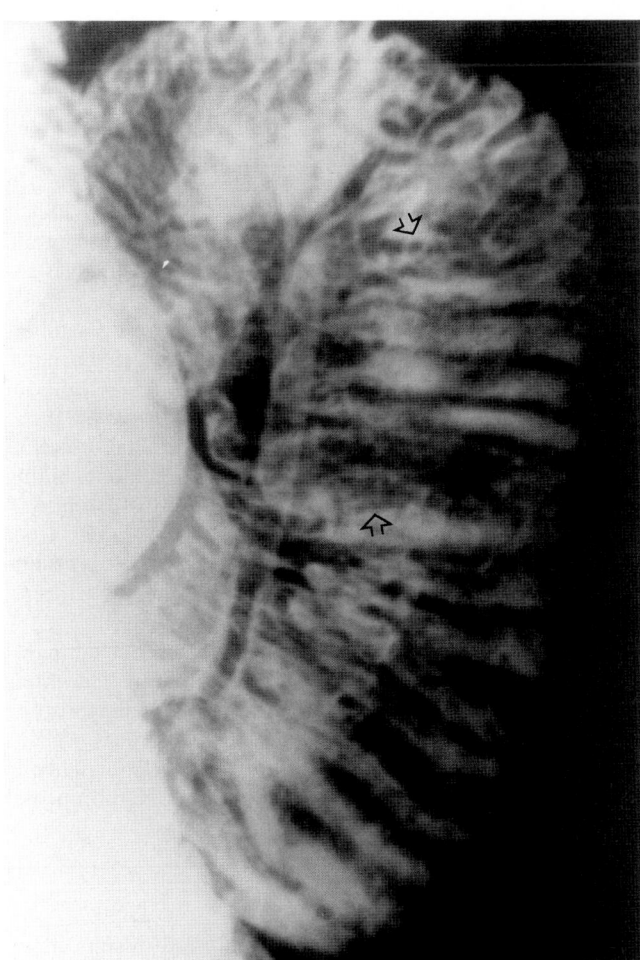

Figure 47-20. Whipple's disease. Spot radiograph from enteroclysis show mildly thickened folds in the proximal jejunum. Also note nodularity of the mucosa (*arrows*) due to villous enlargement. (Courtesy of Dr. Salomonowicz, Vienna, Austria.)

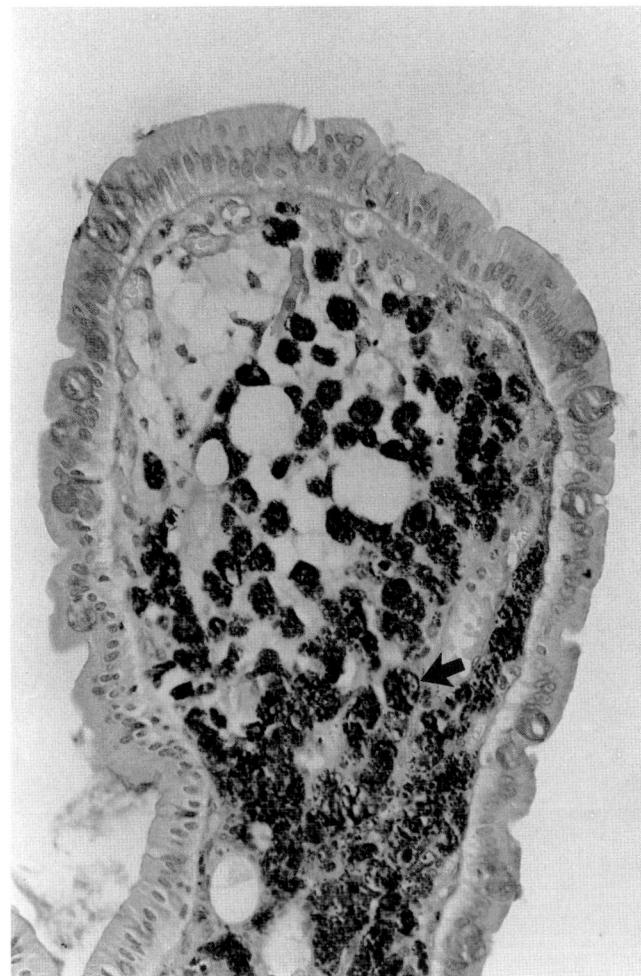

Figure 47-21. Whipple's disease. Photomicrograph of a villus in a patient with Whipple's disease shows how this structure is enlarged and bulbous. The lamina propria is expanded by macrophages (*arrow*) packed with periodic acid–Schiff-positive material derived from the capsules of *Tropheryma whippelii* (PAS, original magnification ×400). (From Rubesin SE, Furth EE: Differential diagnosis of small intestinal abnormalities with radiologic-pathologic correlation. In Herlinger H, Maglinte DDT, Birnbaum BA [eds]: Clinical Imaging of the Small Intestine, 2nd ed. New York, Springer, 1999, pp 527-566.)

CT may reveal enlarged, low-attenuation lymph nodes in the mesentery and retroperitoneum (Fig. 47-22).[76] Fat accumulation in obstructed lymph nodes accounts for this low-attenuation lymphadenopathy. Other causes of low-attenuation mesenteric and retroperitoneal lymphadenopathy include *Mycobacterium avium-intracellulare* infection in patients with AIDS, celiac disease, and metastatic testicular carcinoma.[35,78,79]

The diagnosis of Whipple's disease is confirmed on biopsy specimens showing a lamina propria packed with periodic acid–Schiff (PAS)-positive macrophages containing gram-positive, acid-fast negative bacilli.[33] Electron micrography may be performed to verify the diagnosis.

Eosinophilic Gastroenteritis

Eosinophilic enteritis is a rare, heterogeneous group of disorders characterized by an eosinophilic infiltrate in various

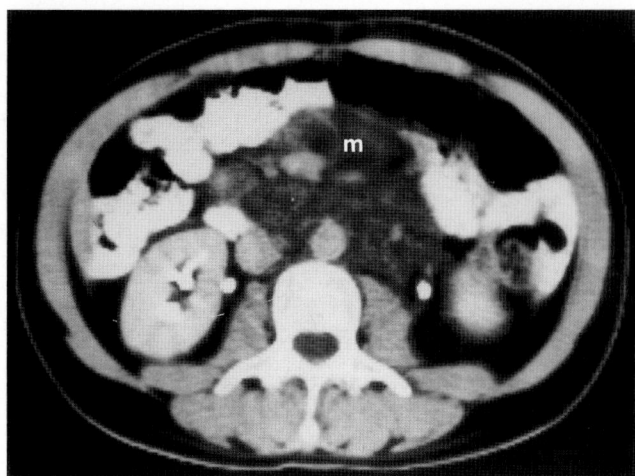

Figure 47-22. Whipple's disease. CT shows expansion of the root of the small bowel mesentery (m) as well as the aortocaval and left para-aortic regions, with separation of vessels, lateral displacement of small bowel loops, and focally decreased attenuation of expanded "mesenteric fat." At surgery, there was marked lymphadenopathy due to lymphatic infiltration by Whipple's disease rather than abnormal mesenteric fat. (From Rubesin SE, Rubin RA, Herlinger H: Small bowel malabsorption: Clinical and radiologic perspectives. Radiology 184:297-305, 1992.)

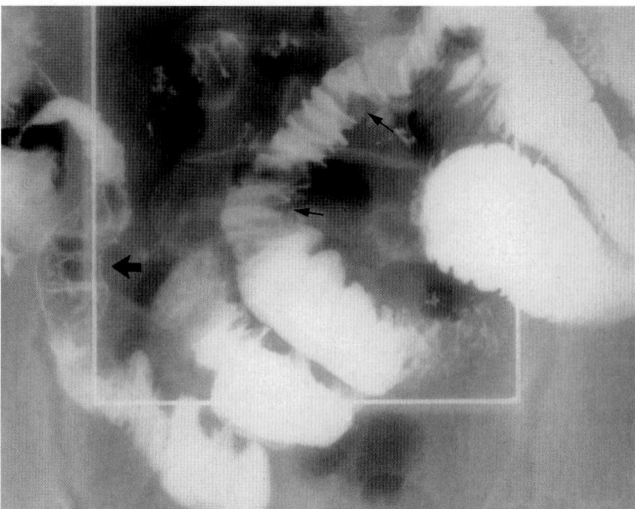

Figure 47-23. Eosinophilic enteritis. Spot radiograph from small bowel follow-through shows thickened, straight folds (*small arrows*) in several loops of distal small bowel and an abnormal surface pattern (*large arrow*) in the terminal ileum.

organs and various layers of the gastrointestinal tract. Symptoms depend on the distribution and location of the eosinophilic infiltrate. If the small bowel mucosa and submucosa are infiltrated by eosinophils, mild steatorrhea, protein loss, weight loss, and iron deficiency may occur. Eosinophilic infiltration of the muscularis propria results in gastric outlet obstruction or small bowel obstruction.[79] Eosinophilic infiltration involving primarily the serosa of the small bowel is rare but can result in eosinophilic ascites.[80] Eosinophilic enteritis usually develops during the third to sixth decades of life. About 50% of patients have a peripheral eosinophilia or an allergic history (including asthma, hay fever, drug sensitivity, or urticaria). The diagnosis of eosinophilic enteritis requires biopsy confirmation of eosinophilic infiltration of the small bowel wall in the absence of extraintestinal disease or parasitic infection.

Eosinophilic infiltration of the small bowel can involve the jejunum or the entire small bowel, is typically patchy, and can be unifocal or multifocal. With the mucosal form of eosinophilic enteritis, barium studies may reveal smooth or nodular, thickened folds perpendicular to the longitudinal axis of the small bowel (Fig. 47-23).[81,82] Spasm is a frequent finding. Eosinophilic enteritis can mimic the radiographic findings of other diseases causing submucosal bleeding (e.g., ischemia) in the small bowel. Concomitant gastric disease is found in about 50% of patients. In such cases, barium studies may reveal antral polyps or thickened, nodular antral folds. Thus, clues to the diagnosis of eosinophilic enteritis include simultaneous involvement of the gastric antrum and small bowel, a peripheral eosinophilia, and a history of allergic diseases.

Amyloidosis

Amyloidosis is a group of diseases characterized by extracellular deposition of insoluble fibrillar proteins with specific histologic staining and characteristic features on electron microscopy. In primary amyloidosis and amyloidosis associated with multiple myeloma, a variable portion of an immunoglobulin light chain is deposited predominantly in the muscular layers of the small bowel. This results in small bowel hypomotility. Primary amyloidosis also affects the tongue, heart, kidneys, blood vessels, nerves, and muscles. In secondary and hereditary forms of amyloidosis, amyloid is primarily deposited in the mucosa, resulting in malabsorption. Secondary amyloidosis is associated with chronic gastrointestinal diseases such as Crohn's disease and schistosomiasis and chronic systemic inflammatory diseases such as tuberculosis, rheumatoid arthritis, leprosy, chronic osteomyelitis, and familial Mediterranean fever. Ischemia and infarction can result from amyloid deposition in blood vessels.

Barium studies reveal abnormalities in the small bowel in about 40% of patients with primary amyloidosis, including decreased small bowel motility, transient intussusceptions, thickened, nodular folds, focal ulceration, and, rarely, acute perforation.[83-85] Small bowel enemas may reveal a finely granular mucosal surface pattern, reflecting blunting of villi and deposition of amyloid in the lamina propria (Fig. 47-24).[85,86] Large amyloid deposits in the lamina propria may be manifest by 4- to 10-mm, smooth-surfaced nodular elevations (Fig. 47-25).[85] Chronic ischemia and infarction may also be manifested by numerous 3- to 4-mm nodules as well as erosions and thickened mucosal folds.[85] Although ischemic changes are reversible, the fine granularity and submucosal nodules do not respond to therapy.[85]

Short-Gut Syndrome

Resection of large lengths of small intestine results in an acute diarrheal illness and a long-term malabsorptive state.[87] Disease states that lead to extensive small bowel resections include vascular damage from volvulus, superior mesenteric artery embolus, superior mesenteric vein thrombosis, and

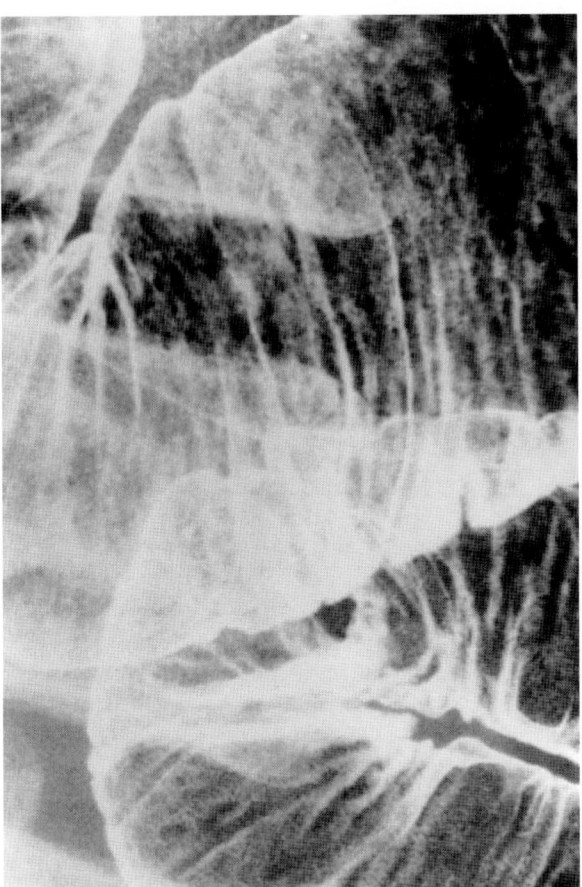

Figure 47-24. Amyloidosis involving the small bowel. Air-contrast enteroclysis shows fine granularity of the mucosa. Histologic examination revealed wide, blunted villi expanded by amyloid deposits in the lamina propria. (A courtesy of Tada S, et al: Amyloidosis of the small intestine: Findings on double-contrast radiographs. AJR 156:741-744, 1991.)

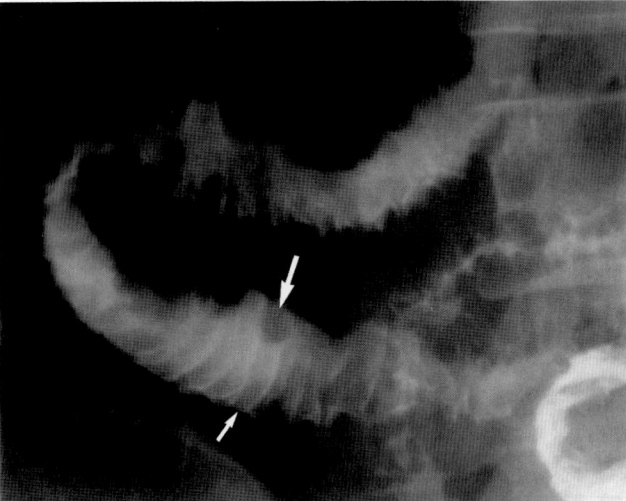

Figure 47-25. Amyloidosis involving the small bowel. Spot radiograph from small bowel follow-through shows smooth, thickened folds (*small arrow*) due to edema from low-grade ischemia as well as focal nodularity (*large arrow*) due to amyloid deposits in the submucosa.

esters are secreted from cells in association with the large hydrophobic protein apo-B. MTTP is an enzyme found in the endoplasmic reticulum that is necessary for assembly of apo-B–containing lipoproteins.[24] Without functioning MTTP, apo-B cannot form a protein capable of transporting fats from the basal membrane of enterocytes. This results in accumulation of absorbed fats and fat-soluble vitamins within enterocytes. Triglycerides also accumulate in hepatocytes.

Symptoms and age at onset vary, depending on the specific defect in apo-B–lipoprotein synthesis. Clinically apparent malabsorption may develop at any time from infancy to early adulthood. Vitamin E deficiency results in spinocerebellar

strangulated hernia; Crohn's disease; radiation enteropathy; and abdominal trauma.[87] Barium studies are of value for documenting the amount of small intestine remaining (Fig. 47-26) and the presence of residual or recurrent small bowel disease (usually the same disease that necessitated small bowel resection). Barium studies may also reveal postsurgical complications such as adhesions and anastomotic strictures. Other complications include gastric hypersecretion with ulcer formation and renal calculi due to hyperoxaluria after ileal resection. Ileal resection can also leads to cholelithiasis.

In some patients, portions of the remaining small intestine compensate for the loss of bowel by increasing the thickness and number of folds to increase the absorptive capability of the small bowel.[88] As a result, barium studies may reveal an increased number of ileal folds as well as an increase in their height and thickness.

NONFORMATION OF CHYLOMICRONS

Abetalipoproteinemia

Abetalipoproteinemia is a rare, autosomally transmitted disorder that is heterogeneous at the molecular level.[24,89] This disorder is linked to a defect in the microsomal triglyceride transport protein (MTTP).[24,89] Triglycerides and cholesterol

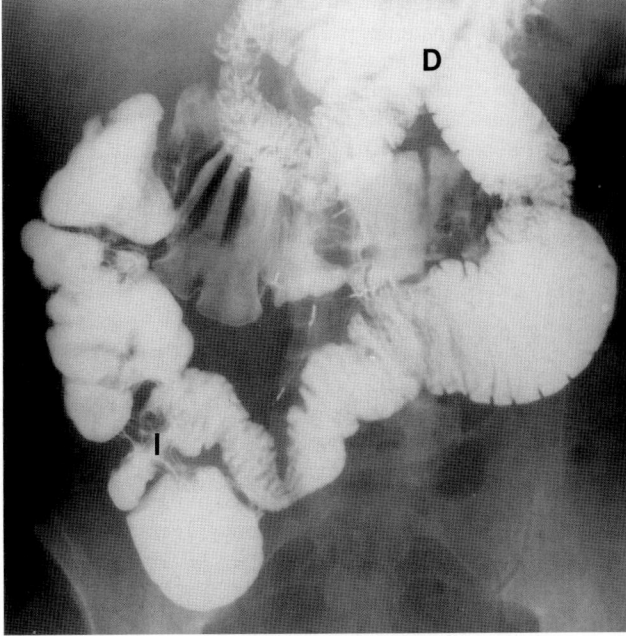

Figure 47-26. Short-gut syndrome. Overhead radiograph shows a total of only three loops of small bowel from the duodenojejunal junction (D) to the ileocecal valve (I). The small bowel is dilated but not obstructed.

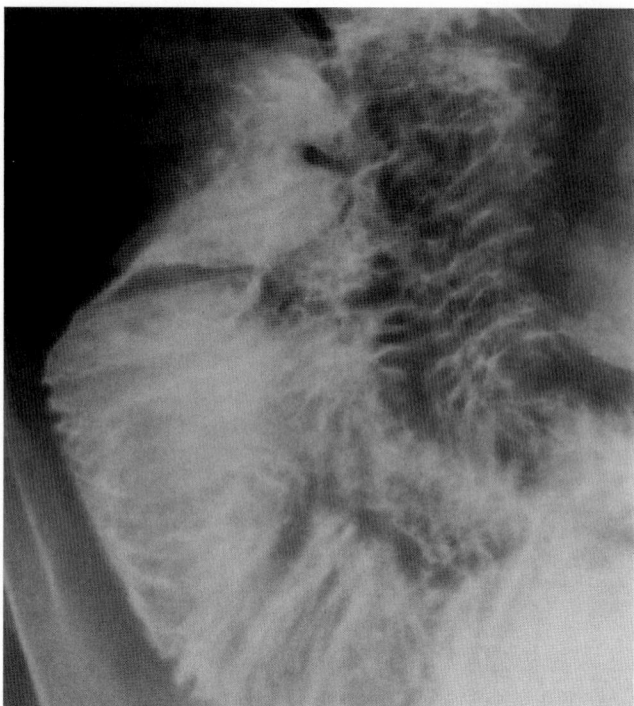

Figure 47-27. Abetalipoproteinemia. Spot radiograph of small bowel shows mildly thickened, irregular folds, possibly because of intestinal secretions that prevent barium from adequately coating the mucosal surface, as the microscopic pathology does not explain the apparent fold thickening in this condition. (From the teaching files of Hans Herlinger, MD.)

degeneration and acanthocytosis. Vitamin A deficiency results in retinitis pigmentosa, which typically develops during the second decade of life. Mental retardation may also be present.

Barium studies may reveal moderately thickened, nodular folds in the duodenum and proximal jejunum (Fig. 47-27).[26,90] It is difficult to explain the radiographic findings on the basis of the underlying pathology. There is no villous distortion or infiltration of the submucosa in abetalipoproteinemia, only accumulation of fat in enterocytes near the tips of the villi. No fat droplets are seen in the intercellular spaces or lymphatics. It has therefore been postulated that these "thickened folds" on barium studies are an artifact of malabsorption, in which increased secretions prevent barium from adequately coating the mucosa.[91]

LYMPHATIC OBSTRUCTION/ LYMPHANGIECTASIA

Intestinal lymphangiectasia results from a congenital abnormality of lymphatic development or from lymphatic obstruction in the small bowel wall and mesentery. Lymphatic obstruction results in abnormal absorption of chylomicrons and fat-soluble vitamins, excessive leakage of lymph into the intestinal lumen, and impaired circulation of enteric lymphocytes. Chylous ascites results from serosal and mesenteric lymphatic obstruction. Blockage of the thoracic duct causes chylous pleural effusions.

In patients with primary lymphangiectasia, symptoms usually develop in older children and young adults. Diarrhea is present in 80% of patients. Steatorrhea is less common,

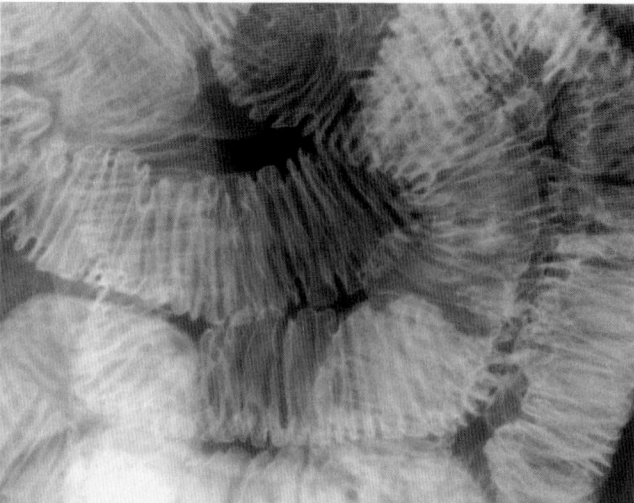

Figure 47-28. Lymphangiectasia. Spot radiograph of jejunum from enteroclysis shows smooth, mildly thickened, slightly undulating folds.

occurring in 20% of patients.[92] Edema of the extremities and chylous pleural effusions are common. Patients may develop hypogammaglobulinemia, lymphocytopenia (particularly of T lymphocytes), and hypoproteinemia.

Lymphatic obstruction in secondary lymphangiectasia is caused by cardiac failure, retroperitoneal fibrosis, radiation therapy, or mesenteric lymph node involvement by Whipple's disease, tuberculosis, sarcoidosis, lymphoma, or carcinoid tumor.

Barium studies typically reveal thickened, straight, parallel, relatively smooth folds in the jejunum and ileum (Fig. 47-28).[92] Disproportionate involvement of the duodenum and jejunum occurs in some patients.[93] Dilated lymphatic lacteals may cause villous distention and blunting (Fig. 47-29), manifested radiographically by sharply defined 1-mm nodular radiolucencies in the small bowel (Fig. 47-30). Luminal distention is uncommon. CT may reveal a thickened small bowel wall (Fig. 47-31). In patients with secondary lymphangiectasia, CT may also reveal lymphadenopathy of normal or low attenuation.

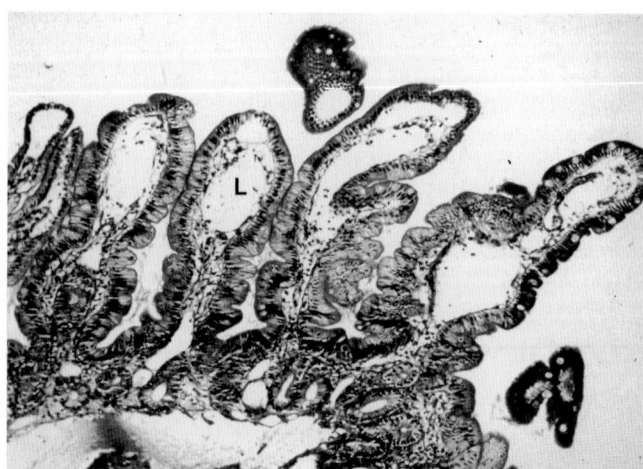

Figure 47-29. Lymphangiectasia. Medium-power photomicrograph shows dilated lacteals (representative lacteal identified by L) distending villi.

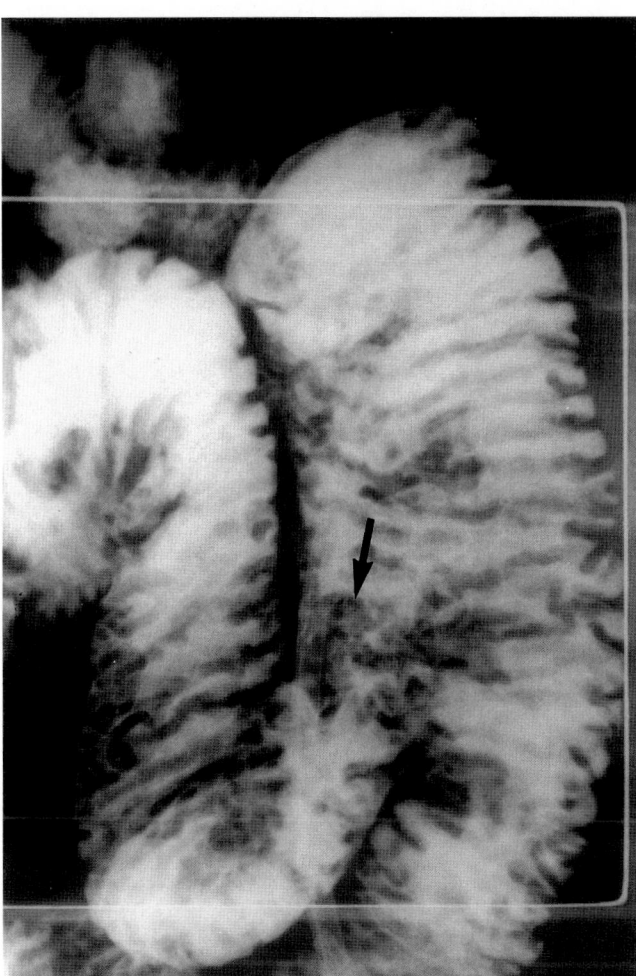

Figure 47-30. Lymphangiectasia. Spot radiograph from enteroclysis shows mildly thickened, irregular folds. Tiny mucosal nodules (*arrow*) are seen in one region due to enlarged, bulbous villi.

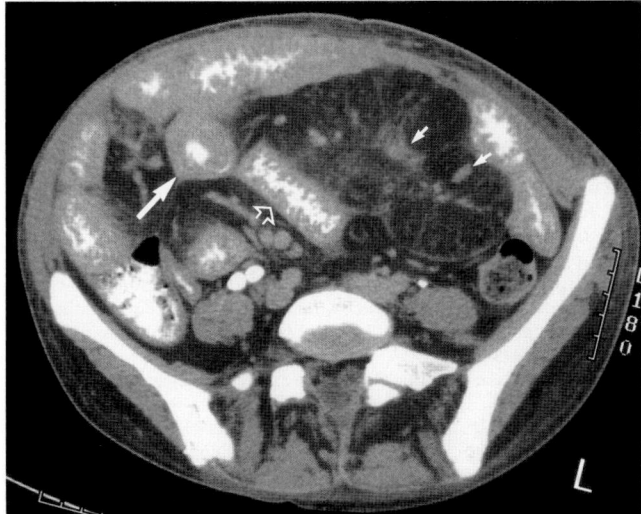

Figure 47-31. Lymphangiectasia. CT through upper pelvis shows diffuse thickening of the small bowel wall both in profile (*open arrow*) and en face (*large arrow*). Stranding of the small bowel mesentery reflects dilated lymphatics and mild mesenteric lymph node enlargement (*small arrows*).

MULTIFACTORIAL DISEASES

Diabetes Mellitus

Between 10% and 20% of patients with severe diabetes mellitus have diarrhea without malabsorption.[94] Steatorrhea, if present, is usually mild. Steatorrhea in patients with diabetes mellitus has a variety of causes, including hypomotility with bacterial overgrowth, pancreatic exocrine insufficiency, malabsorption of bile salts, and abnormal small bowel absorption or secretion. The pathogenesis of diabetic malabsorption is uncertain. The proximal vagus nerves and sympathetic nerves of the small bowel show varying demyelination, but the myenteric and submucosal plexi are histologically normal.[95] As a result, diabetics with symptoms related to the small bowel usually have a severe neuropathy and often also have a nephropathy and retinopathy. Barium studies may reveal small bowel transit that is normal, slow, or rapid. Some patients may have accompanying gastroparesis.

Cystic Fibrosis

Cystic fibrosis is an autosomal recessive disorder caused by a variety of defects in the cystic fibrosis transmembrane conductance regulator gene *(CFTR)* on chromosome 7q32.[96] At least 1000 mutations have been discovered in this gene, accounting for the wide variation in the severity and presentation of cystic fibrosis. The epithelial cells of the small intestine express the *CFTR* gene, resulting in abnormal duodenal bicarbonate secretion,[97] abnormal activity of peptide hydrolases, and abnormal chloride secretion. Loss of pancreatic enzyme secretion and subsequent maldigestion further compounds small bowel problems. Malabsorption, if present, is related to bile acid and pancreatic exocrine abnormalities.[96,98]

Although cystic fibrosis does not cause a small bowel–related malabsorptive syndrome, it does lead to a meconium ileus equivalent, often leading to distal small bowel obstruction or even intussusception of the distal ileum.[99,100] The proximal colon and distal small bowel are filled with thick, viscous fecal material. Cystic fibrosis is included in this discussion because folds in the duodenum and mesenteric small bowel may appear thickened in patients with this condition (Fig. 47-32).[101] The cause of these thickened folds is uncertain. It has been postulated that thick secretions coating the mucosa prevent barium from approaching the epithelial layer, leading to the erroneous impression of thickened folds. Whatever the explanation, the possibility of ischemia or other malabsorptive states may be considered because of this finding.

DIFFERENTIAL DIAGNOSIS OF FOLD ENLARGEMENT IN MALABSORPTION

Small bowel folds are composed of mucosa and submucosa. Small bowel folds are therefore enlarged by diseases involving the mucosa and submucosa.[91] Smooth enlargement of folds usually indicates edema, hemorrhage, or inflammation in the lamina propria and submucosa. In contrast, tiny (0.5 to 2 mm) nodules usually indicate villous enlargement by mucosal inflammation, amyloid infiltration, or lacteal obstruction. Finally, gross nodularity of folds usually indicates focal deposition of inflammatory cells, amyloid, or tumor.

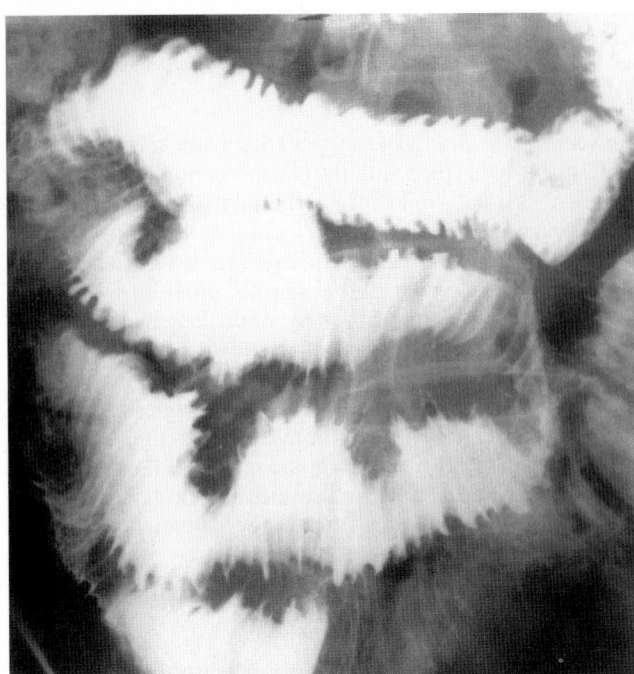

Figure 47-32. Cystic fibrosis. Spot radiograph from small bowel follow-through shows luminal dilatation and moderately thickened, straight folds.

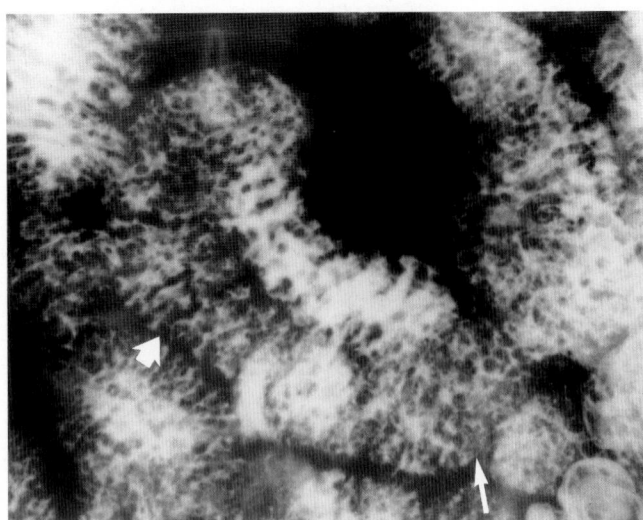

Figure 47-33. Lymphoma as a cause of diffuse nodular fold thickening. Spot radiograph from small bowel follow-through shows moderately thickened, nodular small bowel folds (*short arrow*). Tiny nodules reflect villous enlargement (*long arrow*). This radiographic appearance is unusual for non-Hodgkin's lymphoma involving the small bowel but can be seen in T-cell lymphoma complicating celiac disease, Mediterranean lymphoma associated with immunoproliferative small intestinal disease, and lymphoma in patients with AIDS. (Courtesy of K. Cho, MD, Scarsdale, NY.)

Malabsorptive diseases that are manifested by thickened, smooth folds include giardiasis, lymphangiectasia, tropical sprue, and celiac disease complicated by severe hypoproteinemia. Fold changes in giardiasis and celiac disease occur in the proximal jejunum, whereas lymphangiectasia is more evenly distributed throughout the small bowel. Giardiasis is further characterized by rapid small bowel transit and spasm. Celiac disease is usually associated with a decreased number of folds per inch.

Malabsorptive diseases that are manifested by thickened, nodular folds include celiac disease complicated by lymphoma or ulcerative jejunoileitis, Whipple's disease, amyloidosis, eosinophilic enteritis, abetalipoproteinemia, and mastocytosis. Thickened, nodular folds in celiac-related lymphoma or ulcerative jejunoileitis are usually focal and are located in the jejunum. There also is a decreased number of folds per inch in 75% of patients with celiac disease. In Whipple's disease and abetalipoproteinemia, the folds are more diffusely abnormal, although jejunal predominance occurs in some patients. Whipple's disease is typically a disease of middle-aged white men, whereas abetalipoproteinemia is associated with retinitis pigmentosa and spinocerebellar degeneration that develop during the second and third decades of life. Eosinophilic gastroenteritis typically has a multifocal distribution, often associated with ileal predominance and skip areas. About 50% of patients with eosinophilic enteritis have a peripheral eosinophilia or allergic history. Amyloidosis is more diffusely distributed throughout the small bowel. Coarse mucosal deposits (nodules larger than 5 mm) of amyloid may be present. Fine mucosal nodules (enlarged villi due to dilated lacteals) may also be seen in patients with lymphangiectasia if optimal radiographic technique is employed.

Other diseases of the small bowel may produce thickened, finely nodular folds, but malabsorption is not present. About 50% of patients with mastocytosis have flushing, tachycardia, headaches, and urticaria pigmentosa. Mucosal nodularity is usually multifocal. However, malabsorption is rare in patients with mastocytosis. Some patients with diffuse lymphoma have diffusely thickened, nodular folds in large segments of the small intestine (Fig. 47-33). This radiographic pattern is present in patients with mantle cell lymphoma and Mediterranean lymphoma associated with immunoproliferative small intestinal disease (IPSID).

References

1. Rubesin SE: Diseases of small bowel causing malabsorption. In Taveras JM, Ferrucci JT (eds): Radiology: Diagnosis, Imaging, Intervention. Philadelphia, JB Lippincott, 1993, pp 1-17.
2. Powel DW: Approach to the patient with diarrhea. In Yamada T, Alpers DH, Kaplowitz N, et al (eds): Textbook of Gastroenterology, 4th ed. Philadelphia, Lippincott Williams & Wilkins, 2003, pp 844-894.
3. Rubesin SE, Rubin RA, Herlinger H: Small bowel malabsorption: Clinical perspectives. Radiology 184:297-305, 1992.
4. Traber P: Carbohydrate assimilation. In Yamada T, Alpers DH, Kaplowitz N, et al (eds): Textbook of Gastroenterology, 4th ed. Philadelphia, Lippincott Williams & Wilkins, 2003, pp 389-413.
5. Ganapathy V, Ganapathy ME, Leibach FH: Protein digestion and assimilation. In Yamada T, Alpers DH, Kaplowitz N, et al (eds): Textbook of Gastroenterology, 4th ed. Philadelphia, Lippincott Williams & Wilkins, 2003, pp 438-449.
6. Davidson NO: Intestinal lipid absorption. In Yamada T, Alpers DH, Kaplowitz N, et al (eds): Textbook of Gastroenterology, 4th ed. Philadelphia, Lippincott Williams & Wilkins, 2003, pp 413-437.
7. Devroede GJ, Philips SF: Conservation of sodium, chloride and water by the human colon. Gastroenterology 56:125-142, 1969.
8. Maglinte DDT, Chernish SM, D'Weese R, et al: Acquired jejunoileal diverticular disease: Subject review. Radiology 158:577-580, 1986.
9. Salmonowitz E, Wittich G, Hajek P, et al: Detection of intestinal diverticula by double contrast small bowel enema: Differentiation from other intestinal diverticula. Gastrointest Radiol 8:271-278, 1983.
10. Krishnamurthy S, Kelly MM, Rohrman CA, et al: Jejunal diverticulosis: A heterogeneous disorder caused by a variety of abnormalities of

smooth muscle and myenteric plexus. Gastroenterology 85:538-547, 1983.

11. Dunn V, Nelson JA: Jejunal diverticulosis and chronic pneumoperitoneum. Gastrointest Radiol 4:165-168, 1979.

12. Chow DC, Babaian M, Taubin HL: Jejunoileal diverticula. Gastroenterologist 5:78-84, 1997.

13. Ross CB, Richards WO, Sharp KW, et al: Diverticular disease of the jejunum and its complications. Am Surg 56:319-324, 1990.

14. Benya EC, Ghahremani GG, Brosnan JJ: Diverticulitis of the jejunum: Clinical and radiological features. Gastrointest Radiol 16:24-28, 1991.

15. Greenstein S, Jones B, Fishman EK, et al: Small bowel diverticulitis: CT findings. AJR 147:271-174, 1986.

16. Baskin RH, Mayo CW: Jejunal diverticulosis: A clinical study of 87 cases. Surg Clin North Am 32:1185-1196, 1952.

17. Schuffler MD: Neuromuscular abnormalities of the small and large intestine. In White R (ed): Gastrointestinal and Oesophageal Pathology. Edinburgh, Churchill-Livingstone, 1995, pp 407-430.

18. D'Angelo WA, Fries JF, Msai AST et al: Pathologic observations in systemic sclerosis (scleroderma): A study of fifty-eight matched controls. Am J Med 46:428-440, 1969.

19. Horowitz AL, Meyers MA: The "hide-bound" small bowel of scleroderma: Characteristic mucosal fold pattern. AJR 119:332-334, 1973.

20. Queloz JM, Woloshin HJ: Sacculation of the small intestine in scleroderma. Radiology 105:513-515, 1972.

21. Olmsted WW, Madewell JE: The esophageal and small bowel manifestations of progressive systemic sclerosis. Gastrointest Radiol 1:33-36, 1976.

22. Camilleri M: Dysmotility of the small intestine. In Yamada T, Alpers DH, Kaplowitz N, et al (eds): Textbook of Gastroenterology, 4th ed. Philadelphia, Lippincott Williams & Wilkins, 2003, pp 1486-1529.

23. Rohrmann CA, Ricci MT, Krishnamurthy S, et al: Radiologic and histologic differentiation of neuromuscular disorders of the gastrointestinal tract: Visceral myopathies, visceral neuropathies, and progressive systemic sclerosis. AJR 143:933-941, 1981.

24. Ciclitira PJ, Ellis HJ: Celiac disease. In Yamada T, Alpers DH, Kaplowitz N, et al (eds): Textbook of Gastroenterology, 4th ed. Philadelphia, Lippincott Williams & Wilkins, 2003, pp 1580-1599.

25. Feely KM, Heneghan MA, Stevens FM, et al: Lymphocytic gastritis and coeliac disease: Evidence of a positive association. J Clin Pathol 51:207-210, 1998.

26. Herlinger H, Metz DC: Malabsorption states. In Herlinger H, Maglinte DDT, Birnbaum BA (eds): Clinical Imaging of the Small Intestine, 2nd ed. New York, Springer, 1999, pp 331-376.

27. Bai J, Moran C, Martinez C, et al: Celiac sprue after surgery of the upper gastrointestinal tract. J Clin Gastroenterol 13:521-524, 1991.

28. Brow JR, Parker F, Weinstein WM, et al: The small intestinal mucosa in dermatitis herpetiformis: I. Severity and distribution of the small intestinal lesions and associated malabsorption. Gastroenterology 60:355-361, 1971.

29. Stern M: Comparative evaluation of serological tests for celiac disease: A European initiative towards standardization. Working Group on Serological Screening for Celiac Disease. J Pediatr Gastroenterol Nutr 31:513-519, 2000.

30. McMillan SA, Haughton DJ, Biggart JD, et al: Predictive value for celiac disease of antibodies to gliadin, endomysium and jejunum in patients attending for jejunal biopsy. BMJ 303:1163-1166, 1991.

31. Rostami K, Kerckhaert J, Tiemessen R, et al: Sensitivity of antiendomysium and antigliadin antibodies in untreated celiac disease: Disappointing in clinical practice. Am J Gastroenterol 94:888-894, 1999.

32. Saverymuttu SH, Sabbat J, Burke M, et al: Impact of endoscopic duodenal biopsy on the detection of small intestinal villous atrophy. Postgrad Med J 67:47-49, 1991.

33. Fenoglio-Preiser CM, Noffsinger AE, Stemmermann GN, et al (eds): Gastrointestinal Pathology, 2nd ed: An Atlas and Text. Philadelphia, Lippincott-Raven, 1999, pp 459-512.

34. Herlinger H, Maglinte DDT: Jejunal fold separation in adult celiac disease: Relevance of enteroclysis. Radiology 158:605-611, 1986.

35. Rubesin SE, Herlinger H, Saul SH, et al: Adult celiac disease and its complications. RadioGraphics 9:1045-1065, 1989.

36. La Seta F, Salerno G, Brucellato A, et al: Radiologic indicants of adult coeliac disease assessed by double contrast enteroclysis. Eur J Radiol 15:157-162, 1992.

37. Cooke WT, Holmes GKT: Coeliac Disease. Edinburgh, Churchill Livingstone, 1984.

38. Bova JG, Friedman AC, Weser E, et al: Adaptation of the ileum in non-

39. Knauer CM, Monroe LS: The roentgenographic abnormalities of the duodenum in celiac sprue. Digestion 101:129-136, 1964.

40. Jones B, Bayless TM, Hamilton SR, et al: "Bubbly" duodenal bulb in celiac disease: Radiologic-pathologic correlation. AJR 142:119-122, 1984.

41. Marm CS, Gore RM, Ghahremani GG: Duodenal manifestations of nontropical sprue. Gastrointest Radiol 1:30-35, 1986.

42. Ruoff M, Lindner AE, Marshak RH: Intussusception in sprue. AJR 104:525-528, 1968.

43. Cohen MD, Lintott DJ: Transient small bowel intussusceptions in adult coeliac disease. Clin Radiol 29:529-534, 1978.

44. Trier JS: Celiac sprue. N Engl J Med 325:1709-1719, 1991.

45. Trier JS: Case records of the Massachusetts General Hospital, case 15, 1990. N Engl J Med 322:1067-1075, 1990.

46. Baer AN, Bayless TM, Yardley JH: Intestinal ulceration and malabsorption syndromes. Gastroenterology 79:754-765, 1980.

47. Robertson DAF, Swinson CN, Hall R, et al: Coeliac disease, splenic function and malignancy. Gut 23:666-669, 1982.

48. O'Grady JG, Stevens FM, Harding B, et al: Hyposplenism and gluten-sensitive enteropathy. Gastroenterology 87:1326-1331, 1984.

49. Robinson PJ, Bullen AW, Hall R, et al: Splenic size and function in adult coeliac disease. Br J Radiol 53:532-537, 1980.

50. Simmonds JP, Rosenthal FD: Lymphadenopathy in coeliac disease. Gut 22:756-758, 1981.

51. Jones B, Bayless STM, Fishman EK, et al: Lymphadenopathy in celiac disease: Computed tomographic observations. AJR 142:1127-1132, 1984.

52. Matuchansky C, Colin R, Hemet J: Cavitation of mesenteric lymph nodes, splenic atrophy and a flat small intestinal mucosa: Report of 6 cases. Gastroenterology 87:606-614, 1984.

53. Holmes GKT: Mesenteric lymph node cavitation in coeliac disease. Gut 27:728-733, 1986.

54. Howat AJ, McPhie JL, Smith DA, et al: Cavitation of mesenteric lymph nodes: A rare complication of coeliac disease associated with poor outcome. Histopathology 27:349-354, 1995.

55. Brunton FJ, Guyer PB: Malignant histiocytosis and ulcerative jejunitis of the small intestine. Clin Radiol 34:291-295, 1983.

56. Wright BH, Jones DB, Clark H, et al: Is adult-onset coeliac disease due to a low-grade lymphoma of intraepithelial lymphocytes? Lancet 337:1373-1374, 1991.

57. Isaacson PG, Spencer J, Conolly CE, et al: Malignant histiocytosis of the intestine: A T-cell lymphoma. Lancet 2:699-691, 1985.

58. Swinson CM, Salvin G, Coles EC, et al: Coeliac disease and malignancy. Lancet 1(8316):111-115, 1983.

59. Holmes GKT, Dunn GI, Cockel R, et al: Adenocarcinoma of the upper small bowel complicating coeliac disease. Gut 21:1010-1016, 1980.

60. O'Brien CJ, Saverymuttu S, Hodgson HJF, et al: Coeliac disease, adenocarcinoma of jejunum and in situ squamous carcinoma of oesophagus. J Clin Pathol 36:62-67, 1983.

61. Straker RJ, Gunasekaren S, Brady PG: Adenocarcinoma of the jejunum in association with celiac sprue. J Clin Gastroenterol 11:320-323, 1989.

62. Dannenberg A, Godwin T, Raybourn J, et al: Multifocal adenocarcinoma of the small intestine in a patient with celiac sprue. J Clin Gastroenterol 11:73-76, 1989.

63. Logan RFA, Rifkind EA, Turner ID, et al: Mortality in celiac disease. Gastroenterology 97:265-271, 1989.

64. Lamont CM, Adams FG, Mills PR: Radiology in idiopathic chronic ulcerative enteritis. Clin Radiol 3:283-287, 1982.

65. Zaplosky JH, Janower ML: Idiopathic chronic ulcerative enteritis: A report of two cases. Radiology 155:39-40, 1985.

66. Fantry GT, Fantry LE, James SP: Chronic infections of the small intestine. In Yamada T, Alpers DH, Kaplowitz N, et al (eds): Textbook of Gastroenterology, 4th ed. Philadelphia, Lippincott Williams & Wilkins, 2003, pp 1561-1579.

67. Yardley JH, Bayless TM: Giardiasis. Gastroenterology 52:301-304, 1967.

68. Peterson GM: Intestinal changes in *Giardia lamblia* infestation. AJR 77:670-677, 1957.

69. Marshak RH, Ruoff M, Lindner AE: Roentgen manifestations of giardiasis. AJR 104:557-560, 1968.

70. Fisher CH, Oh KS, Bayless TM, et al: Current perspectives on giardiasis. AJR 125:207-217, 1975.

71. Brandon J, Glick SN, Teplick SK: Intestinal giardiasis: The importance of serial filming. AJR 144:581-584, 1985.

72. Relman DA, Schmidt TM , MacDermott RP, et al: Identification of the uncultured bacillus of Whipple's disease. N Engl J Med 327:293-301, 1993.

73. Whipple GH: A hitherto undescribed disease characterized anatomically by deposits of fat and fatty acids in the intestinal and mesenteric lymphatic tissues. Bull Johns Hopkins Hosp 18:382, 1907.

74. Durand DV, Lecomte C, Cathebras P, et al: Whipple disease: Clinical review of 52 cases. The SNFMI Research Group on Whipple Disease. Société Nationale Française de Médecine Interne. Medicine 76:170-184, 1997.

75. Philips RL, Carson HC: The roentgenographic and clinical findings in Whipple's disease: A review of 8 patients. AJR 123:268-273, 1975.

76. Davis SJ, Patel A: Case report: Distinctive echogenic lymphadenopathy in Whipple's disease. Clin Radiol 42:60-62, 1990.

77. Jeffrey RBJR, Nyberg DA, Bottles K, et al: Abdominal CT in acquired immunodeficiency syndrome. AJR 146:7-13, 1986.

78. Radin DR: Intraabdominal mycobacterium tuberculosis vs. *Mycobacterium avium intracellulare* infections in patients with AIDS: Distinction based on CT findings. AJR 156:487-491, 1991.

79. Marshak RH, Linder A, Maklansky D, et al: Eosinophilic gastroenteritis. JAMA 245:1677-1680, 1981.

80. Smith TR, Schmiedeberg P, Flax H, et al: Nonmucosal predominantly serosal eosinophilic enteritis: A case report. Clin Imaging 14:235-238, 1990.

81. MacCarty RL, Talley NJ: Barium studies in diffuse eosinophilic gastroenteritis. Gastrointest Radiol 15:183-187, 1990.

82. Schulman A, Morton PCG, Dietrich BE: Eosinophilic gastroenteritis. Clin Radiol 31:101-104, 1980.

83. Legge DA, Wollaeger AE, Carlson HC: Intestinal pseudo-obstruction in systemic amyloidosis. Gut 11:764-767, 1970.

84. Yamada M, Hatakeyama S, Tsukagoshhi H: Gastrointestinal amyloid deposition in AL (primary or myeloma associated) and AA (secondary) amyloidosis: Diagnostic value of gastric biopsy. Hum Pathol 16: 1206-1211, 1985.

85. Tada S, Iida M, Matsui T, et al: Amyloidosis of the small intestine: Findings on double-contrast radiographs. AJR 156:741-744, 1991.

86. Smith TR, Cho KC: Small intestine amyloidosis producing a stippled punctate mucosal pattern: Radiological-pathological correlation. Am J Gastroenterol 81:477-479, 1986.

87. Thompson JS: Surgical aspects of the short-bowel syndrome. Am J Surg 170:532-536, 1995.

88. Gouttebel MC, Saint Aubert B, Colette C, et al: Intestinal adaptation in patients with short bowel syndrome. Dig Dis Sci 34:709-715, 1989.

89. Sharp D, Binderman L, Combs KA, et al: Cloning and gene defects in microsomal triglyceride transfer protein associated with abetalipoproteinemia. Nature 365:65, 1993.

90. Weinstein MA, Pearson KD, Agus SG: Abetalipoproteinemia. Radiology 108:269-273, 1973.

91. Rubesin SE, Furth EE: Differential diagnosis of small intestinal abnormalities with radiologic-pathologic explanation. In Herlinger H, Maglinte DDT, Birnbaum BA (eds): Clinical Imaging of the Small Intestine, 2nd ed. New York, Springer, 1999, pp 527-566.

92. Shimkin P, Waldman T, Krugman R: Intestinal lymphangiectasia. AJR 110:827-841, 1970.

93. Kingham JGC, Moriarty KJ, Furness M, et al: Lymphangiectasia of the colon and small intestine. Br J Radiol 55:774-777, 1982.

94. Valdovinos MA, Camilleri M, Zimmerman BR: Chronic diarrhea in diabetes mellitus: Mechanisms and an approach to diagnosis and treatment. Mayo Clin Proc 68:691, 1993.

95. Yoshida MM, Schuffler MD, Sumi SM: There are no morphologic abnormalities of the gastric wall or abdominal vagus in patients with diabetic gastroparesis. Gastroenterology 94:907-914, 1988.

96. Whitcomb DC: Hereditary diseases of the pancreas. In Yamada T, Alpers DH, Kaplowitz N, et al (eds): Textbook of Gastroenterology, 4th ed. Philadelphia, Lippincott Williams & Wilkins, 2003, pp 2147-2165.

97. Robinson PJ, Smith AL, Sly PD: Duodenal pH in cystic fibrosis and its relationship to fat malabsorption. Dig Dis Sci 35:1299-1304, 1990.

98. Gaskin KJ, Waters DLM, Howman-Giles R, et al: Liver disease and common bile duct stenosis in cystic fibrosis. N Engl J Med 318:340-346, 1988.

99. Park RW, Grand RJ: Gastrointestinal manifestations of cystic fibrosis: A review. Gastroenterology 81:1143-1161, 1981.

100. Matsehe J, Go V, Di Magno E: Meconium ileus equivalent complicating cystic fibrosis in postneonatal children and young adults. Gastroenterology 72:732-736, 1977.

101. Taussig L, Saldino R, di Sent'Agnese P: Radiographic abnormalities of the duodenum and small bowel in cystic fibrosis of the pancreas (mucoviscidosis). Radiology 106:369-376, 1973.

Benign Tumors of the Small Bowel

John C. Lappas, MD • Dean D. T. Maglinte, MD •
Kumaresan Sandrasegaran, MD

CLINICAL CONSIDERATIONS

Primary neoplasms of the small bowel are uncommon, and although about 40 different histologic types of benign and malignant tumors have been identified, these lesions constitute only 1% to 5% of all gastrointestinal neoplasms.[1,2] Nearly 75% of small bowel tumors found at autopsy are benign, whereas most of the symptomatic tumors and tumors detected at surgery are malignant.[2] Regardless of the relative incidence of benign and malignant small bowel tumors, the low susceptibility of the small bowel to neoplastic transformation is remarkable when one considers its length, total mucosal surface area, and diversity of structural elements.

Benign small bowel tumors are usually discovered in people between 50 and 80 years of age and occur with equal frequency in men and women. Symptomatic patients may present with abdominal pain and other clinical features of partial or intermittent intestinal obstruction.[3] Small bowel obstruction may be caused by intussuscepting neoplasms, and benign tumors are involved in the majority of adult patients. Bleeding from benign tumors occurs in 40% to 50% of symptomatic patients.[3-5] Anemia, occult bleeding, or intermittent gastrointestinal hemorrhage may be caused by ulceration of an epithelial adenoma or of the mucosa overlying an intramural tumor. In clinical investigations in which enteroclysis was used to evaluate gastrointestinal bleeding, small bowel neoplasms accounted for 50% of the cases, with nearly equal detection of benign and malignant tumors.[6,7] Constitutional symptoms such as malaise, anorexia, and weight loss are uncommon in patients with benign small bowel neoplasms.

IMAGING CONSIDERATIONS

Although it has been difficult for any one institution to have wide experience in the management of benign small bowel neoplasms, sufficient cumulative experience from different centers indicates that delayed or inaccurate diagnosis of small bowel tumors is common.[1-5] This diagnostic dilemma is related not only to the infrequent occurrence of such neoplasms but also to the vagueness and paucity of symptoms and the difficulty in detecting these lesions on conventional small bowel follow-through barium studies. For all these reasons, more sophisticated diagnostic methods of intestinal evaluation have been advocated for patients with suspected small bowel neoplasms.[8]

Barium-based methods of enteroclysis have been shown to be a reliable technique for the demonstration of small bowel tumors and for the evaluation of occult gastrointestinal bleeding and intestinal obstruction.[8-10] Enteroclysis may also allow for accurate differentiation of benign small bowel tumors.[9-11] Because CT has increasingly been utilized for the evaluation of patients with nonspecific abdominal symptoms, it may provide the initial opportunity to detect and characterize tumors of the small bowel. Certain CT findings can differentiate benign and malignant small bowel tumors, and for some benign tumors such as lipomas and leiomyomas CT may allow for a specific diagnosis.[11-13] CT enteroclysis represents a newer modification of these radiologic methods of investigation that combines the techniques of small bowel infusion enteroclysis with the imaging advantages inherent in multidetector CT scanners.[14,15]

Whether performed with positive enteral contrast media (e.g., iodinated water-soluble contrast agents) or preferably with neutral enteral contrast media (e.g., water) with intravenous contrast enhancement, CT enteroclysis has been shown to be an accurate method for the diagnosis of small bowel neoplasms.[16,17] CT enterography (an enteric CT study without intubated intestinal infusion) and MR enteroclysis are also emerging as improved imaging methods for the investigation of small bowel neoplasms.[18,19] Although small bowel capsule endoscopy is a sensitive technique for detection of mucosal disease (including intestinal polyposis), this technique has a number of limitations in the diagnosis of small bowel tumors.[17,20,21]

SPECIFIC TUMORS

Although numerous benign tumors can be found in the small bowel, approximately 90% are adenomas, leiomyomas, lipomas, or hemangiomas. Reports of benign tumors arising from virtually all mesenchymal cell types have appeared sporadically in the literature.[22] Benign small bowel tumors often display similar morphologic features on imaging studies. Although a specific histologic diagnosis may be difficult, useful diagnostic observations can be made based on the number and location of tumors and on certain radiologic features that help to differentiate these lesions.

Adenoma

Small bowel adenomas are benign glandular epithelial neoplasms that have the same classifications as colonic adenomas and may exhibit a malignant predisposition. Approximately 40% are villous adenomas, whereas the remainder have a tubular or tubulovillous histologic architecture. As with colonic adenomas, the finding of cellular atypia, a villous component, or larger size increases the risk for malignancy. Most patients with adenomas are asymptomatic, but these individuals may occasionally present with gastrointestinal bleeding or intestinal obstruction resulting from small bowel intussusception.

Typical adenomas are small (1 to 2 cm), smooth or slightly lobulated lesions. They may appear on barium studies as sessile or pedunculated intraluminal polyps or as small mural nodules on enteroclysis (Fig. 48-1). Radiologic differentiation from other polypoid lesions such as a polypoid carcinoma, hamartomatous or inflammatory polyps, or other small submucosal neoplasms is difficult.

Although small bowel adenomas usually occur as solitary lesions, they may occasionally be multiple, especially in patients with hereditary multiple polyposis syndromes (e.g., familial adenomatous polyposis syndrome or Gardner's syndrome).[2] Villous adenomas are larger than most adenomatous polyps, are sessile and lobulated, have a strong predilection for the duodenum, and have a high risk of malignant degeneration.[23]

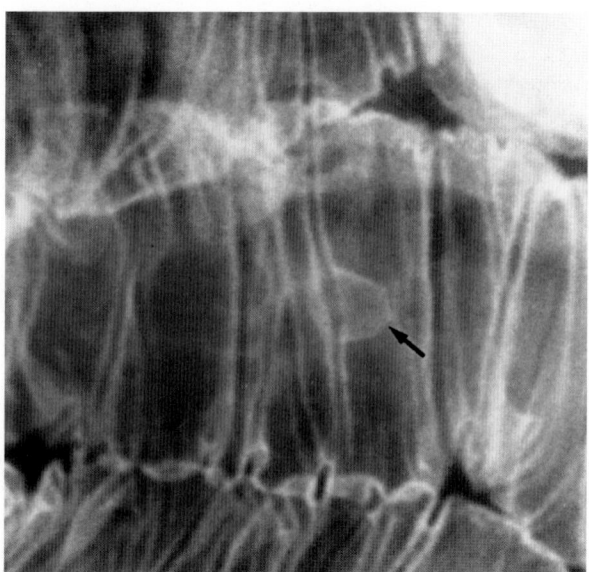

Figure 48-1. Adenoma. Enteroclysis shows a small (8-mm) jejunal adenoma with a smooth, sessile mucosal nodule (*arrow*).

Gastrointestinal Stromal Tumor

Gastrointestinal stromal tumors (GISTs) constitute the major subset of gastrointestinal mesenchymal neoplasms, encompassing most tumors previously classified as smooth muscle tumors. GISTs display spindle cell or epithelioid morphology and certain immunohistochemical markers with KIT (CD117) protein, a tyrosine kinase growth factor receptor, being most specific for GISTs and expression of α-smooth muscle actin being frequent in GISTs of the small bowel (gastrointestinal leiomyogenic tumor [GILT]).[24] Accordingly, true benign leiomyomas (also leiomyosarcomas and schwannomas) are not derived from GIST precursor cells and are different from GISTs in biological behavior and immunology.[24,25]

GISTs are common benign small bowel tumors arising from the muscularis propria and consisting of well-differentiated smooth muscle. These tumors are typically single, firm, well-circumscribed neoplasms that demonstrate a slight predilection for the jejunum.[1-3] Different growth patterns are observed; GISTs may develop as discrete masses that protrude in an inward (submucosal or endoenteric), outward (subserosal or exoenteric), or bidirectional fashion relative to the intestinal wall and lumen. Gastrointestinal bleeding is the most frequent clinical presentation because these tumors are highly vascular and may ulcerate. Obstruction from intussusception or from intraluminal growth and compression by tumor is also a common clinical manifestation.

In patients with small bowel tumors, features on barium enteroclysis allowed for the accurate preoperative diagnosis of GISTs in 83% to 100% of cases.[9,26] Submucosal tumors appear as smooth, round, or semilunar mural defects that are demarcated by sharp angles to the intestinal wall (Fig. 48-2). Small tumors show subtle findings of focal stretching or flattening of the overlying mucosal folds and minimal intraluminal protrusion. Subserosal tumors produce mass effect on adjacent bowel loops or can result in displacement of intestinal loop segments. Actual tumor size may be underestimated on fluoroscopic barium studies, whereas cross-sectional imaging studies are ideal for showing the extraluminal component

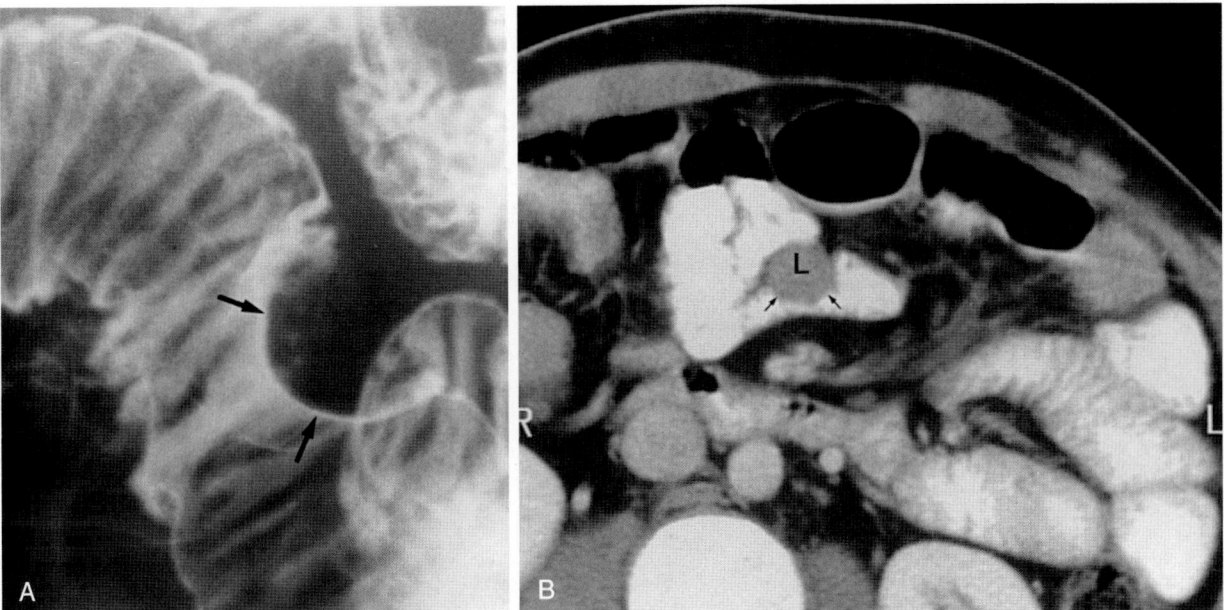

Figure 48-2. Benign Gastrointestinal stromal tumor. A. The submucosal nature of the tumor is recognized on barium study, with an area of semi-circular mass effect within the lumen (*arrows*). The smooth surface results from stretching of the overlying normal mucosa. **B.** CT of the GIST (L) shows a smooth submucosal mass of homogeneous soft tissue (muscle) attenuation compressing the lumen (*arrows*).

of these lesions (Fig. 48-3). Finally, tumors with bidirectional growth may demonstrate both luminal protrusion and displacement of adjacent bowel loops.

CT is particularly useful in depicting the nature and extent of small bowel GISTs.[27,28] The tumors may appear on CT as sharply defined spherical masses that display a homogeneous soft tissue density and uniform contrast enhancement (see Fig. 48-3). Although it is difficult to predict the malignant potential of these tumors, experience with CT suggests that malignant GISTs are larger than benign tumors and less

uniform in shape and have a more heterogeneous tissue attenuation.[28] Tumor size is the single most predictive factor of metastatic potential; tumors smaller than 2 cm are usually benign, whereas those larger than 5 cm are usually malignant.

Lipoma

Lipomas of the small bowel account for 20% to 25% of all gastrointestinal lipomas, and the small bowel represents the second most common site of gastrointestinal involvement by

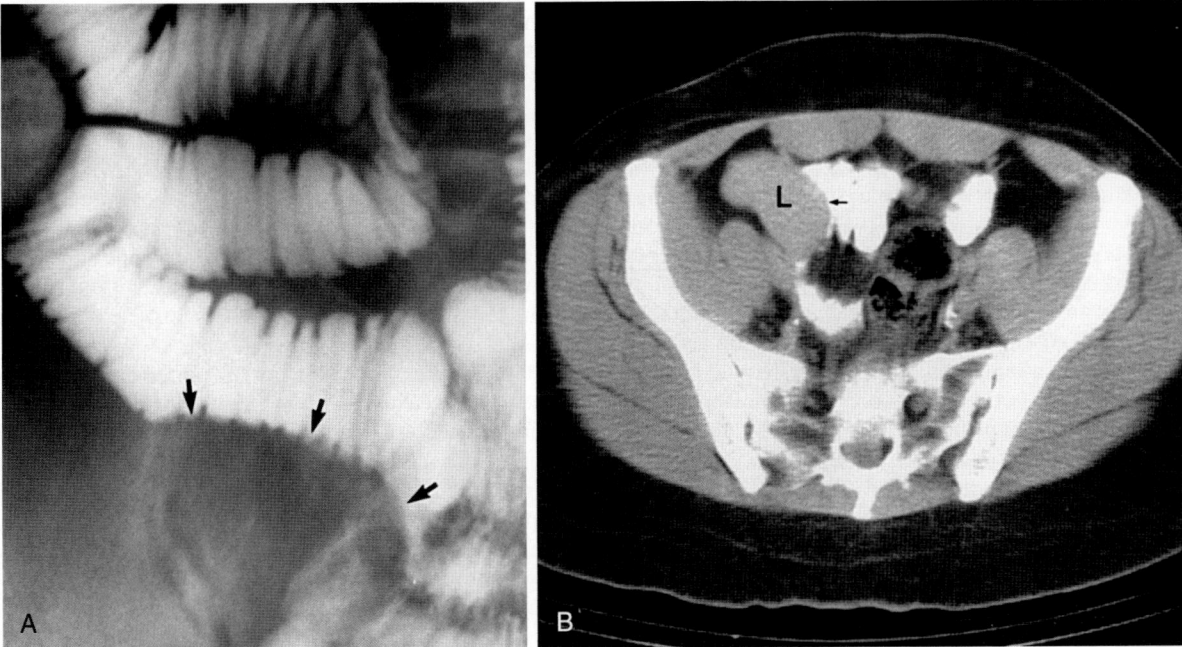

Figure 48-3. Benign gastrointestinal stromal tumor in a patient with a palpable abdominal mass. A. Barium study shows a mild area of mass effect (*arrows*) on the bowel. **B.** CT shows a soft tissue mass representing an exoenteric GIST (L) arising from the small bowel (*arrow*).

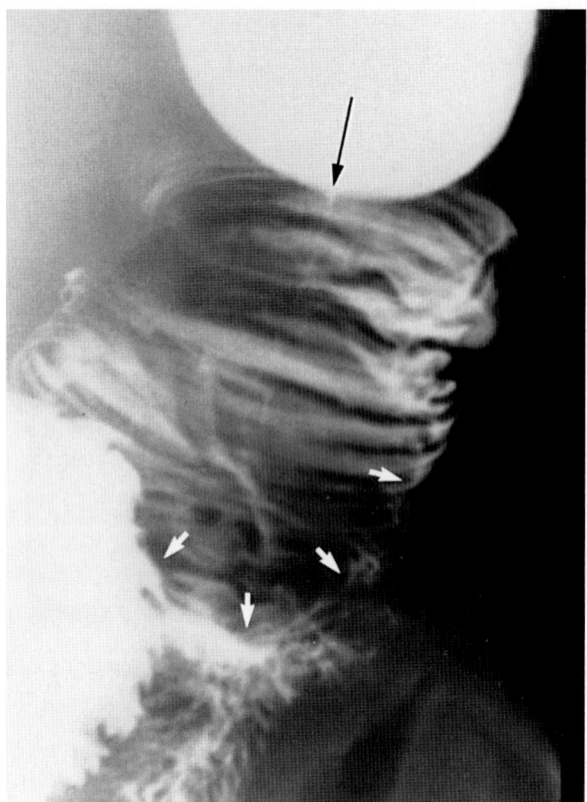

Figure 48-4. Lipoma with intussusception. A dilated small bowel loop shows an abrupt narrowing of its lumen at the entry into the intussusception (*black arrow*). Also note the stretched "coiled spring" pattern of folds typical of intussusception. The contour of the lipoma is visible at the apex of the intussusception (*white arrows*).

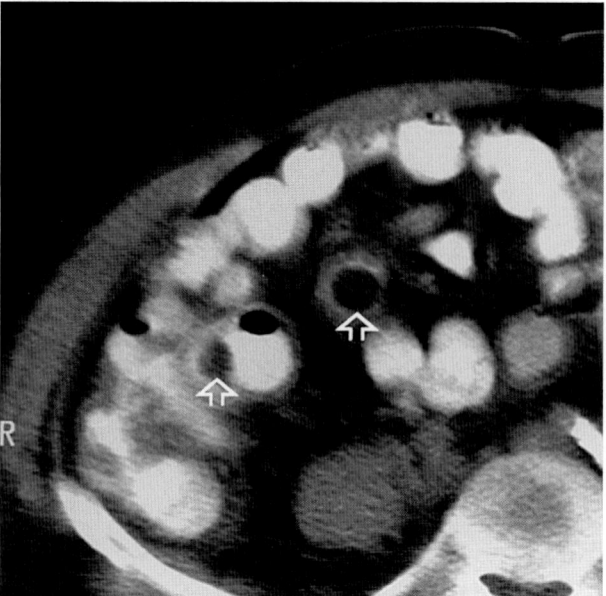

Figure 48-5. Lipoma. CT shows two lipomas protruding into the bowel lumen (*arrows*). A well-circumscribed, intraluminal homogeneous mass with negative attenuation consistent with fat is characteristic of an enteric lipoma on CT.

these tumors.[29] Lipomas arise as well-circumscribed submucosal proliferations of fat that usually grow intraluminally; outward extension of these tumors tends to be impeded by the firmness of the muscularis propria. Small bowel lipomas are usually solitary, relatively avascular lesions of variable size (1 to 6 cm). Most of these tumors occur in the ileum. Although most patients with lipomas are asymptomatic, some may present with intermittent intestinal obstruction, usually resulting from small bowel intussusception (Fig. 48-4).

Barium studies may reveal a sharply demarcated, often pedunculated tumor that tends to conform to the contour of the small bowel lumen.[29,30] Because of the soft consistency of lipomas, their configuration may change at fluoroscopy with compression or peristalsis of the small bowel. CT can establish the diagnosis of a small bowel lipoma by showing that the lesion has attenuation values consistent with fat.[30] A homogeneous mass between −80 and −120 Hounsfield units is considered to be diagnostic of a lipoma (Fig. 48-5). The presence of soft tissue stranding within an otherwise uniform lipoma on CT has been attributed to fibrovascular changes associated with ulceration of the tumor.[30,31]

Hemangioma

Benign angiomatous tumors are hamartomatous vascular growths that are most likely congenital. Two principal forms have been described: the papillary (capillary) hemangioma and the cavernous hemangioma. Cavernous hemangiomas predominate in the small bowel, occurring either as simple polypoid tumors or, rarely, as diffusely expansile lesions.[32] Microscopically, these submucosal neoplasms consist of enlarged vascular channels or sinuses, lined by endothelium and surrounded by minimal stromal tissue. Hemangiomas may be single or multiple. Although most hemangiomas are only millimeters in size, some may enlarge and protrude into the lumen. Direct invasion of the mucosa or penetration beyond the serosa is uncommon.

In contrast to other small bowel tumors, which are less likely to cause symptoms, 80% of patients with hemangiomas are symptomatic. Most patients present with gastrointestinal bleeding that is often acute, severe, and intermittent. Anemia and occult fecal blood loss are other common clinical findings.

Hemangiomas must be of sufficient size to produce an intraluminal or intramural nodular defect on barium studies (Fig. 48-6). Although a rare occurrence, the finding of calcified phleboliths on abdominal radiographs can suggest the diagnosis. When discovered in patients with vascular cutaneous lesions or with tuberous sclerosis, Turner's syndrome, or Osler-Weber-Rendu disease, such radiographic findings should increase the suspicion for intestinal hemangiomas. Mesenteric arteriography may be performed to demonstrate an intestinal vascular abnormality, but differentiation between small vascular tumors and other vascular malformations is difficult. In one reported case, CT demonstrated a large jejunal hemangioma that appeared as a heterogeneous mass with prominent mesenteric vasculature.[33] CT enteroclysis and CT enterography performed with neutral enteral and intravenous contrast media have the potential to demonstrate vascular hemangiomas, providing that the tumor is of sufficient size and that the intestinal lumen is adequately distended for optimal visualization of the bowel wall.[15]

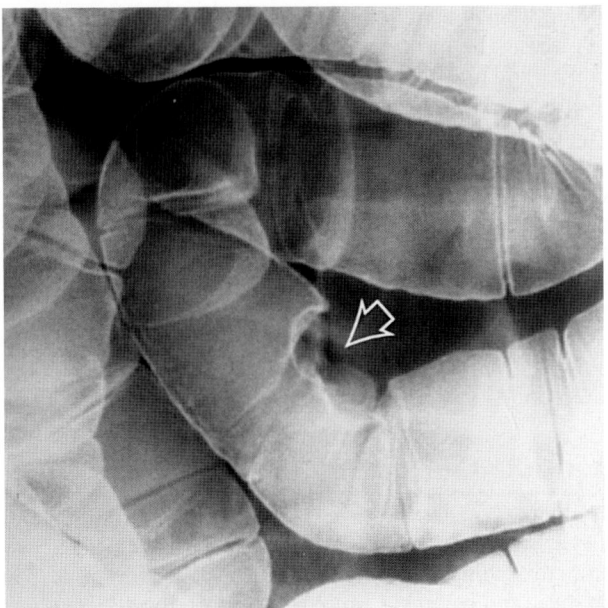

Figure 48-6. Hemangioma. Double-contrast enteroclysis shows a 1.5-cm, slightly lobulated mural nodule (*arrow*) in a patient with occult gastrointestinal bleeding. A hemangioma was confirmed at surgery. (From Maglinte DDT, Lappas JC, Kelvin FM, et al: Small bowel radiography: How, when, and why? Radiology 163:297-305, 1987.)

Uncommon Tumors

Neurogenic tumors arise from the intramural neural plexus of the small bowel. Neurofibromas are the nerve tumors encountered most frequently and are composed of nerve sheath elements, notably Schwann cells and fibroblasts. Neurofibromas may occur as solitary lesions or, more commonly, as multiple lesions with or without systemic neurofibromatosis type 1. Although rare in the general population, neural tumors of the small bowel are reported in 10% to 25% of patients with neurofibromatosis.[34] Neurofibromas in neurofibromatosis type 1 that cause symptoms are most common in the jejunum. The clinical manifestations vary depending on tumor extent; mucosal involvement may lead to gastrointestinal bleeding or obstruction from intussusception or volvulus. Neurofibromas may originate within the intestinal wall, appearing as solitary or multifocal intraluminal or intramural masses. Diffusely elongated tumors may be manifested by mural thickening on CT, whereas barium studies may reveal scalloping of the intestinal wall from the intramural and intraluminal components of these tumors.[34] Neurofibromas of mesenteric origin may encroach on adjacent small bowel loops, producing mass effect on the serosal surface, or may directly infiltrate the intestinal wall, producing focal or diffuse mural thickening and rigidity, or submucosal or mucosal masses. *Ganglioneuromas* arising from sympathetic ganglia may appear as focal polypoid lesions, multifocal polyps (ganglioneuromatous polyposis), or diffusely infiltrating lesions (ganglioneuromatosis). Imaging characteristics of these tumors are similar to those seen with other neurofibromas.[34]

Inflammatory fibroid polyps, also referred to as inflammatory pseudotumors, are encountered almost exclusively in the ileum. They are usually solitary and are composed of a vascular fibrous stroma with a diffuse inflammatory infiltrate. Their specific etiology remains uncertain, but these lesions most likely develop as a result of an exuberant response to local intestinal injury.[9,35] Barium studies may reveal a nonspecific smooth, rounded mass in the distal small bowel. Affected individuals may occasionally present with obstructive symptoms resulting from intussusception of the polyps.[35]

Myoepithelial hamartoma is a rare developmental tumor consisting of varying amounts of pancreatic tissue, smooth muscle, and epithelial structures. The term *ectopic pancreatic rest* is used to describe these lesions when there is a predominance of pancreatic acinar tissue. Most myoepithelial hamartomas occur in the gastric antrum or duodenum, but some have been reported in the mesenteric small bowel.[22] Myoepithelial hamartomas are solitary, small lesions that appear on barium studies as smooth, mural masses with occasional umbilication.

Heterotopic gastric mucosa may occur as an isolated lesion in the mesenteric small bowel, or it may be associated with malformations such as Meckel's diverticulum or an enteric duplication. Occasionally, barium studies may reveal a sessile or pedunculated polyp.

POLYPOSIS SYNDROMES

Familial Adenomatous Polyposis Syndrome

Familial adenomatous polyposis syndrome (FAPS) and its variant syndromes (Gardner's syndrome and Turcot's syndrome) are different manifestations of a hereditary disorder caused by a germline mutation of the adenomatous polyposis coli gene.[36] Adenomatous polyps in FAPS typically involve the colon, but to a lesser degree the small bowel may also be involved; such patients may have multiple duodenal and jejunoileal adenomas and ileal lymphoid polyps. Small bowel adenomas have also been reported to develop in the ileum after restorative proctocolectomy for FAPS.[37] About 75% of patients with duodenal adenomas are found to have adenomas in the proximal jejunum on endoscopy, and about 25% of patients have additional distal jejunal and ileal polyps on capsule endoscopy.[38] Isolated adenomas of the distal jejunum or ileum are rare, occurring in only 3% of FAPS patients.[38] Because small bowel polyps in FAPS occur more frequently in those patients with "sentinel" duodenal adenomas, enteroclysis and capsule endoscopy may have an important role for the diagnosis and surveillance of small bowel disease in patients with duodenal polyps.[20,21,38]

FAPS can also be associated with the development of desmoid tumors, which are rare, benign proliferations of musculoaponeurotic fibrous tissue that are locally aggressive and tend to recur without distant metastases. Desmoid tumors are reported in 10% of patients with FAPS, with 50% of the tumors being intra-abdominal and 85% to 100% localized to the mesentery.[39] CT is an ideal imaging test for the detection of desmoids because it can show the extent of tumor invasion within the mesentery and affected small bowel.[40,41]

Peutz-Jeghers Syndrome

Peutz-Jeghers syndrome (PJS) is an unusual autosomal-dominant disorder with variable penetrance; about 50% of cases are familial and 50% are new mutations. PJS is characterized by gastrointestinal hamartomatous polyps, mucocutaneous melanotic pigmentation, and a substantial risk of

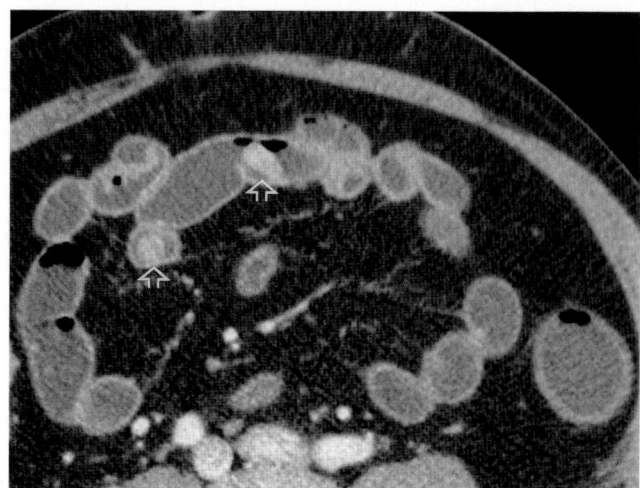

Figure 48-7. Peutz-Jeghers syndrome. CT enteroclysis performed with enteral water infusion and intravenous contrast enhancement shows multiple intraluminal polyps within the jejunum (*arrows*). The fluid density of the neutral enteral contrast medium is juxtaposed to the enhancing bowel wall, increasing conspicuity of the tumor.

developing a variety of malignant tumors.[42,43] Affected individuals present in early life with pigmented macules on the lips, buccal mucosa, and volar surfaces of the hands and feet. Cutaneous lesions often predate the formation of gastrointestinal polyps but typically fade during adolescence, with only the buccal lesions persisting into adulthood. Signs of gastrointestinal polyps may be evident during the second or third decades of life, with gastrointestinal bleeding or abdominal pain caused by transient small bowel intussusceptions.

Histologically, the polyps in PJS are benign hamartomas containing a proliferative smooth muscle core and are lined by normal intestinal epithelium. PJS polyps are more commonly found in the jejunum than in the ileum but may also occur in the stomach or colon. Patients with PJS are at increased risk for the development of intestinal and extraintestinal malignancies, including esophageal, gastric, small bowel, colorectal, breast, ovarian, and pancreatic cancers.[42,43] Most of the reported gastrointestinal cancers in PJS patients appear to develop from coexisting adenomas rather than from hamartomas, but a hamartoma-adenoma-carcinoma sequence is suspected in some cases.[43]

Barium studies may demonstrate luminal polyps of variable size in the small bowel. Larger polyps (2 to 3 cm) typically have a lobulated contour and pedunculated lesions with broad-based attachments may also be found.[44,45] Diffuse proliferation of intestinal polyps is atypical for PJS, because uninvolved small bowel segments usually alternate with other segments containing sporadic hamartomas. PJS polyps may be detected on CT as soft tissue masses within the contrast medium–filled intestinal loops and are exquisitely displayed on CT enteroclysis (Fig. 48-7).[46]

Cowden's Disease

Cowden's disease, or multiple hamartoma-neoplasia syndrome, is an inherited condition characterized by hamartomas and other abnormalities of the skin, breast, thyroid gland, and intestinal tract.[42] Eighty percent of patients present with benign dermatologic manifestations that serve as markers of the disease, the most common being facial trichilemmomas, lipomas, and mucocutaneous keratoses. Patients with Cowden's syndrome are at particularly high risk for developing breast and thyroid cancers.[42] Gastrointestinal polyposis is reported in 30% to 60% of patients and includes hamartomas indistinguishable from the polyps seen in JPS or from lipomatous or inflammatory polyps.[42,44] One or more portions of the gastrointestinal tract (especially the colon) or the entire gastrointestinal tract may be involved. In one review of Cowden's disease, the small bowel was involved in 14 of 32 patients.[47] Enteroclysis may reveal multiple polyps, producing a nodular mucosal surface pattern in patients with diffuse small bowel disease.[47]

Cronkhite-Canada Syndrome

Cronkhite-Canada syndrome is a nonfamilial condition characterized by diffuse gastrointestinal polyposis associated with distinctive clinical findings. Symptoms of abdominal pain, diarrhea, and anorexia precede or occur together with the development of ectodermal changes, including alopecia, hyperpigmentation, and dystrophy of nails. Disease onset is usually gradual, and older adults are primarily affected. Intestinal malabsorption and protein loss can be severe, and affected individuals often have a downhill clinical course with eventual death. Polyps occur in the stomach and colon in virtually all patients, with the small bowel involved in more than 50% of cases. Cronkhite-Canada polyps are inflammatory and consist of dilated cystic interstitial glands, closely resembling the hamartomas in PJS. Certain patterns of gastrointestinal involvement have been described on barium studies: (1) diffuse involvement with innumerable small polyps (most common); (2) scattered polyps of various sizes; and (3) sparse involvement with few small polyps.[48] Barium studies may also reveal thickened folds and increased luminal secretions in the small bowel due to hypoproteinemia and malabsorption.

References

1. O'Riordan BG, Vilor M, Herrera L: Small bowel tumors: An overview. Dig Dis Sci 14:245-257, 1996.
2. Gill SS, Heuman DM, Mihas AA: Small intestinal neoplasms. J Clin Gastroenterol 33:267-282, 2001.
3. Rangiah DS, Cox M, Richardson M, et al: Small bowel tumours: A 10 year experience in four Sydney teaching hospitals. Aust NZ J Surg 74:788-792, 2004.
4. Minardi AJ Jr, Zibari GB, Aultman DF, et al: Small-bowel tumors. J Am Coll Surg 186:664-668, 1998.
5. Ciresi DL, Scholten DJ: The continuing dilemma of primary tumors of the small intestine: Am Surg 61: 698-702, 1995.
6. Rex DK, Lappas JC, Maglinte DDT, et al: Enteroclysis in the evaluation of suspected small intestinal bleeding. Gastroenterology 97:58-60, 1989.
7. Moch A, Herlinger H, Kochman ML, et al: Enteroclysis in the evaluation of obscure gastrointestinal bleeding. AJR 163:1381-1384, 1994.
8. Lappas JC, Maglinte DDT: Radiological approach to investigation of the small intestine. In Gourtsoyiannis N (ed): Radiological Imaging of the Small Intestine. New York, Springer-Verlag, 2002, pp 447-463.
9. Nagi B, Verma V, Vaiphei K, et al: Primary small bowel tumors: A radiologic-pathologic correlation. Abdom Imaging 26:474-480, 2001.
10. Gourtsoyiannis NC, Bays D, Papaioannou N, et al: Benign tumors of the small intestine: Preoperation evaluation with a barium infusion technique. Eur J Radiol 16:115-125, 1993.
11. Gourtsoyiannis NC, Mako E: Imaging of primary small intestinal tumors by enteroclysis and CT with pathological correlation. Eur Radiol 7: 625-642, 1997.
12. Laurent F, Raynaud M, Biset JM, et al: Diagnosis and categorization

of small bowel neoplasms: Role of computed tomography. Gastrointest Radiol 16:115-119, 1991.

13. Buckley JA, Fishman EK: CT evaluation of small bowel neoplasms: Spectrum of disease. RadioGraphics 18:379-392, 1998.

14. Maglinte DDT, Lappas JC, Heitkamp DE, et al: Technical refinements in enteroclysis. Radiol Clin North Am 41:213-229, 2003.

15. Maglinte DDT, Bender GN, Heitkamp DE, et al: Multidetector-row helical CT enteroclysis. Radiol Clin North Am 41:249-262, 2003.

16. Romano S, De LE, Rollandi GA, et al: Multidetector computed tomography enteroclysis (MDCT-E) with neutral enteral and IV contrast enhancement in tumor detection. Eur Radiol 15:1178-1183, 2005.

17. Boudiaf M, Jaff A, Soyer P, et al: Small-bowel diseases: Prospective evaluation of multi-detector row helical CT enteroclysis in 107 consecutive patients. Radiology 233:338-344, 2004.

18. Horton KM, Fishman EK: The current status of multidetector row CT and three-dimensional imaging of the small bowel. Radiol Clin North Am 41:199-211, 2003.

19. Umschaden HW, Gasser J: MR enteroclysis. Radiol Clin North Am 41:231-248, 2003.

20. Hara AK, Leighton JA, Virender K, et al: Imaging of small bowel disease: Comparison of capsule endoscopy, standard endoscopy, barium examination, and CT. RadioGraphics 25:697-718, 2005.

21. Maglinte DDT: Capsule imaging and the role of radiology in the investigation of diseases of the small bowel. Radiology 236:763-767, 2005.

22. Olmsted WW, Ros PR, Hjermstad BM, et al: Tumors of the small intestine with little or no malignant predisposition: A review of the literature and report of 56 cases. Gastrointest Radiol 12:231-239, 1987.

23. Witteman BJM, Janssens AR, Griffioen G, et al: Villous tumors of the duodenum: An analysis of the literature with emphasis on malignant transformation. Neth J Med 42:5-11, 1993.

24. Miettinen M, Lasota J: Gastrointestinal stromal tumors: Definition, clinical, histological, immunohistochemical, and molecular genetic features and differential diagnosis. Virchows Arch 438:1-12, 2001.

25. Pidhorecky I, Cheney RT, Kraybill WG, Gibbs JF: Gastrointestinal stromal tumors: Current diagnosis, biologic behavior, and management. Ann Surg Oncol 7:705-712, 2000.

26. Gourtsoyiannis NC, Bays D, Malames M, et al: Radiological appearances of small intestinal leiomyomas. Clin Radiol 45:94-103, 1992.

27. Megibow AJ, Balthazar EJ, Hulnick DH, et al: CT evaluation of gastrointestinal leiomyomas and leiomyosarcomas. AJR 144:727-731, 1985.

28. Sandrasegaran K, Rajesh A, Rydberg J, et al: Gastrointestinal stromal tumors: Clinical, radiologic, and pathologic features. AJR 184:803-811, 2005.

29. Taylor AJ, Stewart ET, Dodds WJ: Gastrointestinal lipomas: A radiologic and pathologic review. AJR 155:1205-1210, 1990.

30. Thompson WM: Imaging and findings of lipomas of the gastrointestinal tract. AJR 184:1163-1171, 2005.

31. Kakitsubata Y, Kakitsubata S, Nagatomo H, et al: CT manifestations of lipomas of the small intestine and colon. Clin Imaging 17:179-184, 1993.

32. Lightdale CJ, Hornsby-Lewis L: Tumors of the small intestine. In Haughbrich WS, Schaffner F (eds): Bockus Gastroenterology, 5th ed. Philadelphia, WB Saunders, 1995, pp 1274-1290.

33. Varma JD, Hill MC, Harvey LAC: Hemangioma of the small intestine manifesting as gastrointestinal bleeding. RadioGraphics 18:1029-1033, 1998.

34. Levy AD, Patel N, Dow N, et al: From the archives of the AFIP: Abdominal neoplasms in patients with neurofibromatosis type 1: Radiologic-pathologic correlation. RadioGraphics 25:455-480, 2005.

35. Harned RK, Buck JL, Shekitka KM: Inflammatory fibroid polyps of the gastrointestinal tract: Radiological evaluation. Radiology 182:863-866, 1992.

36. Bronner MP: Gastrointestinal inherited polyposis syndromes. Mod Pathol 16:359-365, 2003.

37. Wu JS, McGannon EA, Church JM: Incidence of neoplastic polyps in the ileal pouch of patients with familial adenomatous polyposis after restorative proctocolectomy. Dis Colon Rectum 41:552-556, 1998.

38. Schulmann K Hollerbch S, Kraus K, et al: Feasibility and diagnostic utility of video capsule endoscopy for the detection of small bowel polyps in patients with hereditary polyposis syndromes. Am J Gastroenterol 100: 27-37, 2005.

39. Knudsen AL, Bulow S: Desmoid tumour in familial adenomatous polyposis: A review of literature. Fam Cancer 1:111-119, 2001.

40. Casillas J, Sais GJ, Greve JL, et al: Imaging of intra- and extraabdominal desmoid tumors. RadioGraphics 11:959-968, 1991.

41. Einstein DM, Tagliabue JR, Desai RK: Abdominal desmoids: CT findings in 25 patients. AJR 157:275-279, 1991.

42. Schreibman RI, Baker M, Amos C, McGarrity TJ: The hamartomatous polyposis syndromes: A clinical and molecular review. Am J Gastroenterol 100:476-490, 2005.

43. McGarrity TJ, Kulin HE, Zaino RJ: Peutz-Jeghers syndrome. Am J Gastroenterol 95:596-604, 2000.

44. Cho GJ, Bergquist K, Schwartz AM: Peutz-Jeghers syndrome and the hamartomatous polyposis syndromes: Radiologic-pathologic correlation. RadioGraphics 17:785-791, 1997.

45. Buck JL, Harned RK, Lichtenstein JE, Sobin LH: Peutz-Jeghers syndrome. RadioGraphics 12:365-378, 1992.

46. Sener RN, Kumcuoglu Z, Elmas N, et al: Peutz-Jeghers syndrome: CT and US demonstration of small bowel polyps. Gastrointest Radiol 16:21-23, 1991.

47. Chen YM, Ott DJ, Wu WC, et al: Cowden's disease: A case report and literature review. Gastrointest Radiol 12:325-329, 1987.

48. Dachman AH, Buck JL, Burke AP, et al: Cronkhite-Canada syndrome: Radiologic features. Gastrointest Radiol 14:285-290, 1989.

Malignant Tumors of the Small Bowel

Dean D. T. Maglinte, MD • John C. Lappas, MD •
Kumaresan Sandrasegaran, MD

GENERAL CONSIDERATIONS

Incidence

Although the small intestine represents 75% of the length and
90% of the mucosal surface of the alimentary tract, primary
malignant tumors of the small bowel constitute less than 2%
of all gastrointestinal neoplasms.[1,2] Adenocarcinoma, carcinoid, gastrointestinal stromal tumor (GIST), and lymphoma
account for about 45%, 30%, 13%, and 12% of these primary
malignant small bowel tumors, respectively.[2,3]

Delays in Diagnosis: Contributions of Clinician and Radiologist

Despite substantial improvements in diagnostic techniques
and operative mortality, the survival of patients with primary
malignant tumors of the small intestine has not changed in
the past 40 years.[4] Unfortunately, many patients have advanced
tumors at the time of surgery because of delayed diagnosis.
These delays may occur for a variety of reasons, including
failure of patients to report symptoms, failure of physicians to
order appropriate diagnostic tests, and failure of radiologists

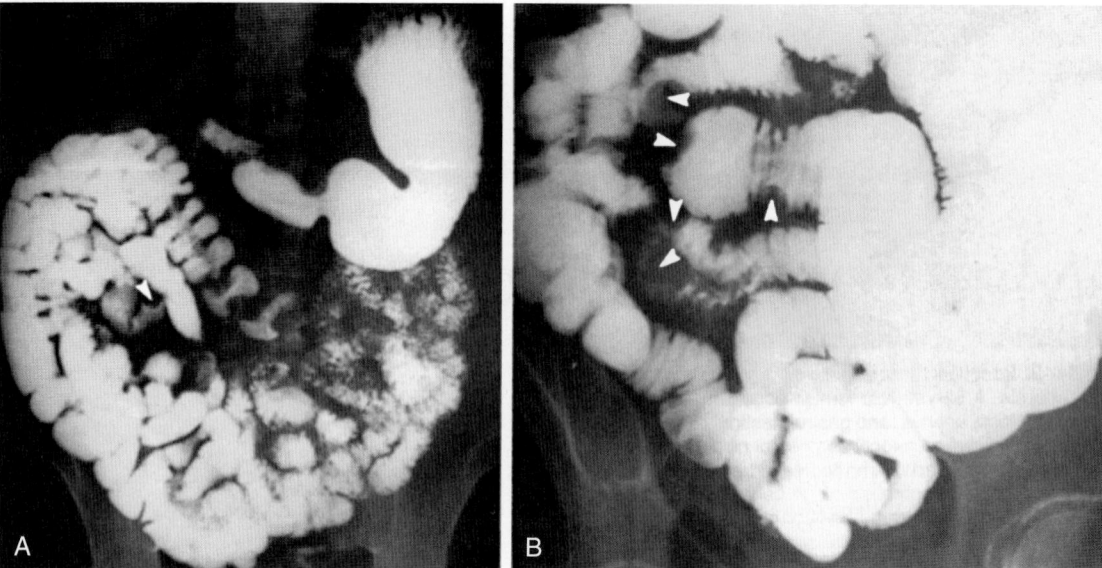

Figure 49-1. Delayed diagnosis of malignant tumor in a 78-year-old woman with recurrent abdominal pain and anemia. A. Prone overhead radiograph from a small bowel follow-through at another institution was interpreted as normal. In retrospect, there is a suggestion of a polypoid defect (*arrowhead*) in a loop of ileum in the right abdomen. **B.** Enteroclysis performed 6 months later shows multiple intramural defects (*arrowheads*) with partial obstruction by the largest lesion. Surgery revealed a multifocal carcinoid with extension to mesenteric nodes.

to arrive at a correct diagnosis. Most of these delays occur after patients seek medical attention. Although radiologists are responsible for only a minority of physician errors, these errors may cause the longest delays in diagnosis (Fig. 49-1). Greater awareness of the small intestine as a potential source of unexplained abdominal symptoms is needed, so that appropriate radiologic tests may be performed for early diagnosis and treatment of malignant small bowel tumors. The low prevalence of small bowel tumors and the nonspecificity of clinical symptoms underscore the need for imaging methods with a high negative predictive value and sensitivity.

IMAGING CONSIDERATIONS

Barium Studies

Conventional barium studies are relatively inaccurate tests for the diagnosis of malignant small bowel tumors. In various series, abnormalities were present on small bowel follow-through studies in 53% to 83% of patients with primary malignant small bowel tumors, but direct evidence of tumor was found in only 30% to 44% of cases.[5] A study comparing enteroclysis and small bowel follow-through showed sensitivities of 95% for enteroclysis versus 61% for small bowel follow-through.[6] Nevertheless, a major limitation of enteroclysis is the lack of demonstration of extraintestinal abnormalities.

Newer Imaging Techniques

Computed tomography (CT) can be used for tumor staging, showing such features as transmural extension, mesenteric involvement, and distant spread. Several modifications in CT techniques have been increasingly utilized in recent years. In the past, positive oral contrast media (usually dilute iodinated contrast media) were widely used. These contrast media were safe and allowed good opacification of the small bowel.

However, the current approach favors neutral oral contrast media combined with intravenous contrast media when there is a suspicion of small bowel tumor. Advantages of this technique include fewer artifacts due to uneven mixing with enteric contents, better visualization of enhancing small bowel tumors (Fig. 49-2), and easier processing of CT angiograms and 3D techniques. One disadvantage of oral neutral contrast media is reduced distention of the distal small bowel secondary to peristalsis. This disadvantage can be overcome either by infusion of enteral contrast media under hydrostatic pressure

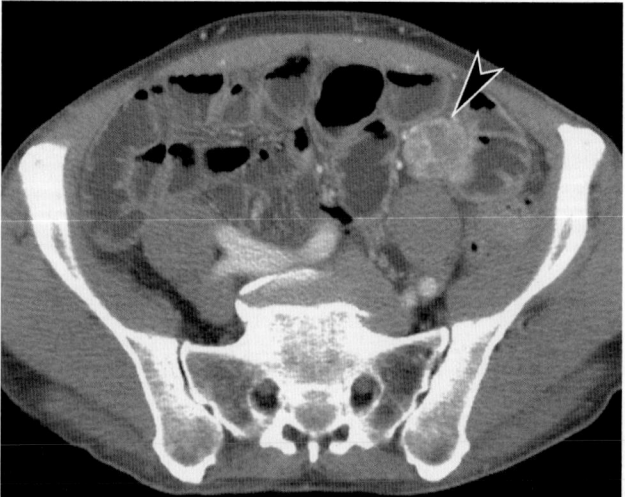

Figure 49-2. Value of neutral enteral contrast medium in a 58-year-old man with unexplained anemia. CT enteroclysis with neutral enteral and intravenous contrast media shows a partially enhancing mass (*arrowhead*) closely adherent to a loop of mid jejunum. The mass proved to be a gastrointestinal stromal tumor. This lesion was not seen on a routine CT performed at an outside institution with positive oral contrast media (*not shown*).

using a nasoenteric tube (CT enteroclysis) or by having patients ingest large volumes of contrast material, usually 1.5 to 2 L, in predetermined aliquots over a period of time (CT enterography). Details of CT enteroclysis are provided in Chapter 42. Water is the most commonly used neutral enteral contrast agent; other proprietary preparations include VoLumen (EZ-EM, Westbury, NY), which contains agents to reduce absorption and add flavor. Multiplanar reformats are helpful in unraveling loops of small bowel and planning surgery.

Ultrasonography is used extensively in Europe to investigate the small bowel. However the negative predictive value of ultrasound is low. MRI of the small bowel is still evolving; gadolinium-enhanced, fat-suppressed spin-echo images can produce a high-quality examination.[7] Of the newer methods of small bowel imaging, CT enteroclysis using neutral enteral and intravenous contrast media appears to be the most accurate.[8,9] Conventional angiography has been largely replaced by CT angiography, which provides excellent delineation of superior mesenteric artery branches to the vasa recta.

Nuclear medicine techniques, particularly positron emission tomography (PET), have value in selected patients for staging small bowel tumors and assessing the response to therapy. It seems likely that the sensitivity of this technique will be increased by newer-generation PET/CT scanners that also allow an optimal contrast-enhanced CT examination to be performed. At this time, however, there are no published data on the use of PET/CT for diagnosing small bowel tumors.

The role of capsule endoscopy for patients with suspected small bowel neoplasms has not been established. This tool is likely to complement rather than replace existing imaging techniques for diagnosing small bowel tumors.

ADENOCARCINOMA

Epidemiology

The incidence of colorectal cancer is 50 times greater than that of small bowel cancer. Possible explanations for the relative resistance of small bowel mucosa to carcinogenesis include rapid transit (reducing the time of mucosal exposure to carcinogens), a high volume of fluid diluting intraluminal carcinogens, the absence of bacterial degradation of bile salts, a high proliferation rate of mucosal cells competitively inhibiting the growth of malignant cells, and immunomodulation by the high levels of immunoglobulin A produced by abundant ileal lymphoid tissue.[10] Despite its lower prevalence, small bowel carcinoma has a number of features in common with colorectal carcinoma, including its frequent development via an adenoma-carcinoma sequence and the presence of mutations in key regulatory genes such as ki-*RAS* and *TP53*. The presence of gene mutations may explain the high incidence of associated extraintestinal malignant tumors in patients with small bowel cancer.

Pathology

Adenocarcinoma is more common in the jejunum than in the ileum, occurring predominantly in its first 30 cm.[11] These tumors are usually well differentiated, even when metastases are present. A mucin-producing columnar epithelium is frequently identified.

Associated Conditions

Patients with celiac disease have a higher than expected incidence of non-Hodgkin's lymphoma of the small bowel as well as carcinoma of the small bowel and esophagus.[12] Clinical deterioration of a patient with celiac disease on a gluten-free diet should therefore raise the possibility of a complicating malignancy.

There is an increased incidence of carcinoma in patients with Crohn's disease, particularly those with long-standing disease (>10 years), enteric fistulas, or surgically created nonfunctional bowel loops.[13,14] Carcinoma complicating Crohn's disease (i.e., Crohn's carcinoma) differs from de novo cancer of the small bowel in that younger male patients are more likely to be affected, and the ileum is a more common site of involvement. These tumors may be difficult to differentiate from Crohn's disease both preoperatively and at surgery, so that the diagnosis of carcinoma is often made only on frozen sections (Fig. 49-3). Because of difficulties in diagnosis, the mean survival of patients with Crohn's carcinoma is less than 12 months.[13]

There is a significantly increased risk of developing gastric, jejunal, and colonic cancers in patients with Peutz-Jeghers syndrome. Compared with the general population, relative risk ratios of 100 to 250 have been reported.[15,16] There is continuing debate as to whether the hamartomatous polyps in Peutz-Jeghers syndrome harbor adenomatous components or directly transform into cancer.[15,16] Other hereditary gastrointestinal cancer syndromes such as familial adenomatous polyposis syndrome and hereditary nonpolyposis colorectal cancer syndrome are also associated with a higher risk of small bowel cancer.

Imaging Findings

Enteroclysis is superior to small bowel follow-through for the diagnosis of small bowel carcinoma, with reported sensitivities of 95% and 61%, respectively.[6] Because of the usual location of small bowel carcinomas within 25 cm of the duodenojejunal junction, a patient referred for an upper gastrointestinal examination because of pain, vomiting, or anemia should have a barium study not only of the duodenum but also of the proximal jejunum. Suspicion should also be raised when the dilated distal duodenum or proximal jejunum contains excess fluid.

Due to delays in diagnosis, 60% of small bowel cancers present as "apple core" lesions. These annular tumors are typically manifested by short segments of circumferential narrowing with mucosal irregularity and overhanging edges (Fig. 49-4). The malignant strictures usually have a fixed, unchanging appearance during compression. However, an annular lesion of the distal ileum is more likely to be caused by a metastasis from colon cancer than by a primary small bowel carcinoma.[17] Other less common radiographic features of small bowel carcinoma include a polypoid mass with or without ulceration (Fig. 49-5) or multiple lobulated filling defects. These findings are more commonly seen in the duodenum than in the mesenteric small bowel.

Carcinoma of the small bowel is typically manifested on CT by a solitary soft tissue mass in the proximal jejunum causing concentric or asymmetric luminal narrowing and obstruction (Fig. 49-6). These lesions may have a heterogeneous

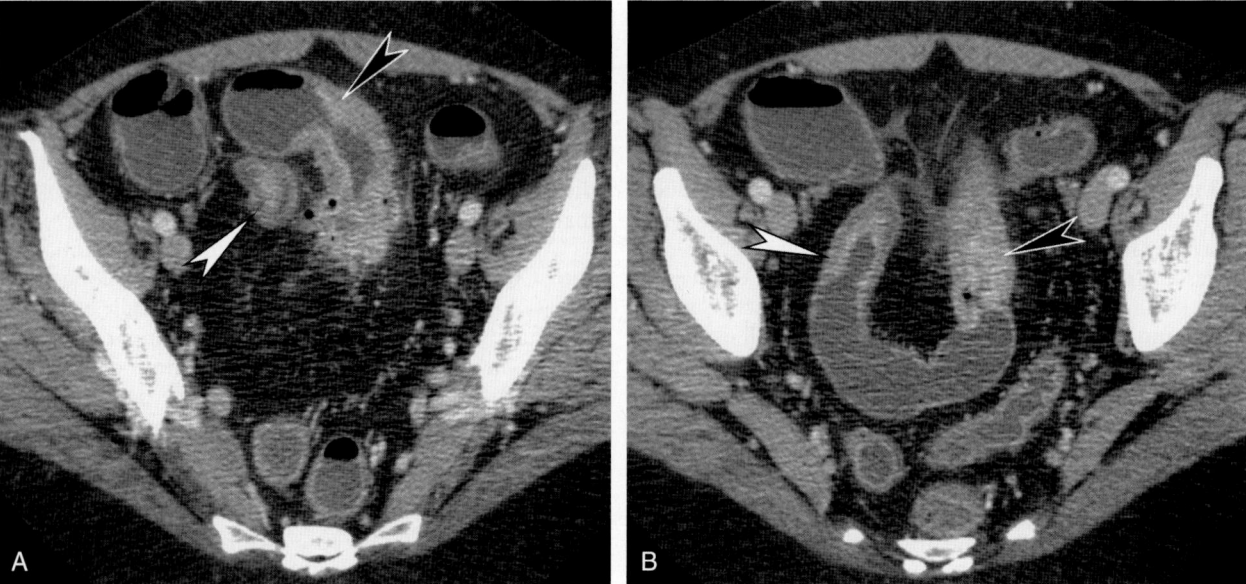

Figure 49-3. Refractory Crohn's disease in a 41-year-old woman. A and **B.** Axial images from CT enteroclysis with neutral enteral and intravenous contrast media show mild wall thickening (*white arrowheads*) in the terminal ileum. Note mural heterogeneity with enhancement of the mucosa and edema in the submucosa. More proximally, there is an 8-cm segment of marked wall thickening with homogeneous enhancement (*black arrowheads*) and proximal shouldering (*best seen in* **A**). At surgery, the wall thickening in the distal ileum was caused by Crohn's disease, and the more proximal lesion was caused by adenocarcinoma. Optimal bowel distention during CT enteroclysis allowed differentiation of these inflammatory and neoplastic strictures.

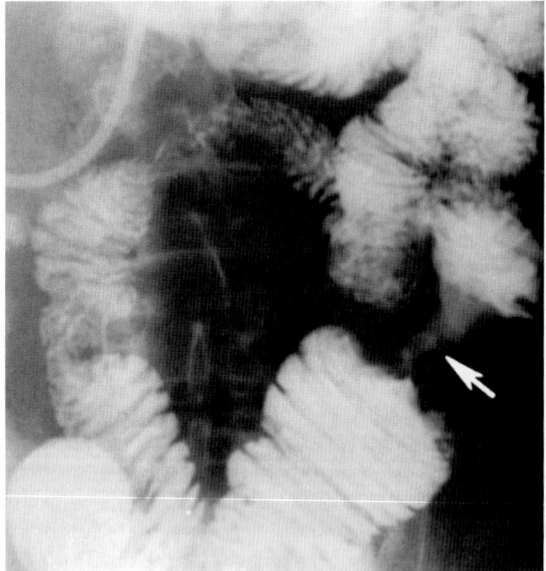

Figure 49-4. Enteroclysis for diagnosing jejunal adenocarcinoma in a 69-year-old man with vomiting. Enteroclysis shows a short segment of circumferential narrowing in the proximal jejunum with mucosal destruction and overhanging edges (*arrow*). These are the typical findings of an "apple core" lesion in a patient with jejunal adenocarcinoma. A small bowel follow-through 3 weeks earlier failed to demonstrate the lesion (*not shown*). (From Maglinte DDT, O'Connor K, Bessette J, et al: The role of the physician in the late diagnosis of primary malignant tumors of the small intestine. Am J Gastroenterol 86:304-308, 1991, © by The American College of Gastroenterology.)

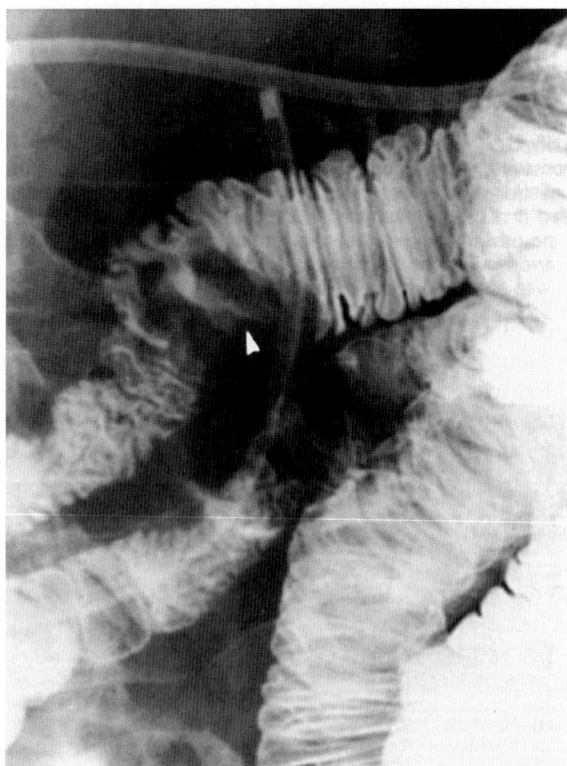

Figure 49-5. Atypical jejunal adenocarcinoma in a 63-year-old man with abdominal pain. Enteroclysis shows an eccentric, ulcerated mass (*arrowhead*) in the proximal jejunum. The radiographic findings are more suggestive of lymphoma, but the location is typical of adenocarcinoma, which was found at surgery.

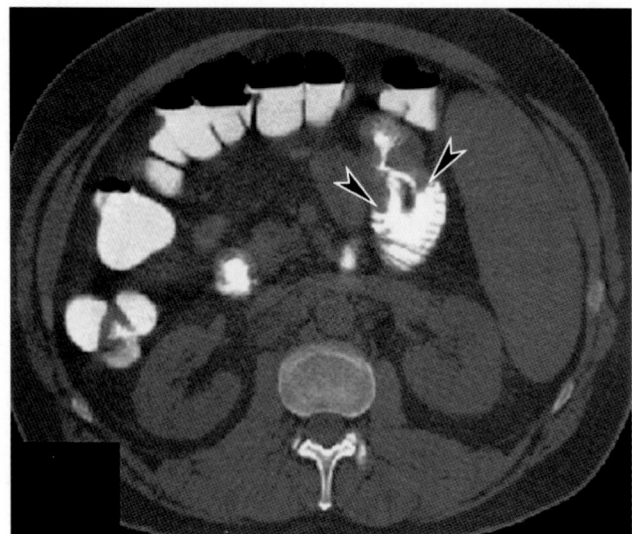

Figure 49-6. Jejunal adenocarcinoma in a 47-year-old man with abdominal pain and bloating. Capsule endoscopy was unsuccessful as the capsule became lodged in the proximal small bowel. CT enteroclysis shows an ulcerated, annular lesion (*arrowheads*) in the proximal jejunum. This proved to be a jejunal adenocarcinoma.

attenuation and moderate enhancement after administration of intravenous contrast material. The liver, peritoneal surfaces, local lymph nodes, and ovaries may be secondarily involved. Small bowel carcinomas infrequently cause intussusception. It may not be possible on imaging studies to differentiate small bowel carcinomas from other malignant neoplasms such as lymphoma or inflammatory processes such as Crohn's disease.

Treatment and Prognosis

The only curative therapy for small bowel cancer is radical surgery. The proximity of invaded nodes to major vessels often prevents an adequate radical resection. Radiation therapy and chemotherapy are usually not helpful. A 5-year survival rate of 46% has been reported for carcinoma of the jejunum versus 20% for carcinoma of the ileum.[18] In comparison, patients with small bowel carcinoid tumors have 5-year survival rates of more than 50%.[19,20]

CARCINOID TUMORS

Carcinoid tumors originate from the ectodermal cells of the neural crest. These tumors may occur at any site in which such cells are located, including the gastrointestinal, pancreatic, biliary, respiratory, and genitourinary tracts as well as the thymus. Carcinoids represent a heterogeneous group of tumors with different forms of biologic behavior. An imprecise classification differentiates carcinoid tumors into foregut, midgut, and hindgut lesions based on their embryonic origin. In the future, carcinoid tumors may be categorized using molecular genetics.[19]

The small bowel is the most common site of malignant carcinoid tumors, and the distal 50 cm of the ileum is the common site of small bowel involvement. Thirty to 50 percent of patients with small bowel carcinoid tumors develop a second primary malignancy.[19,20]

All carcinoid tumors are potentially malignant. Invasiveness is a function of time, anatomic location, and size. There are no clear histologic differences between benign and malignant carcinoid tumors. The malignant nature of these tumors can be confirmed only if local invasion or distant metastases are observed. About 95% of carcinoid tumors larger than 2 cm metastasize versus only 50% of tumors smaller than 1 cm.[20] Extension beyond the bowel wall is found in 30% to 67% of ileal lesions at the time of diagnosis.[2]

Pathophysiology

Hormonally active substances secreted by ileal carcinoid tumors include serotonin (5-hydroxytryptophan) and bradykinin. Deamination by the liver converts serotonin to 5-hydroxyindoleacetic acid (5-HIAA), which is excreted in the urine.

When the tumor has invaded the muscle layer of the bowel wall, the local action of several polypeptide growth factors, such as connective tissue growth factor and platelet-derived growth factor, provokes an intense fibroblastic reaction.[19] The resulting mesenteric fibrosis causes indrawing, kinking, and, occasionally, obstruction of small bowel loops. Vasoactive amines such as serotonin are no longer thought to be the primary cause of this mesenteric fibrosis.[19] Occlusion of mesenteric vessels may also cause bowel ischemia. Mesenteric metastases often exceed the primary tumor in size and endocrine activity. Advanced ileal carcinoid tumors can metastasize widely to the omentum, peritoneal surfaces, lymph nodes, liver, and lungs.

Clinical Aspects

Ileal carcinoids may cause no symptoms and may be detected as incidental findings on imaging studies. Many patients have nonspecific gastrointestinal symptoms for several years before these tumors are discovered. The carcinoid syndrome is characterized by periodic cutaneous flushing, diarrhea, and, less frequently, bronchospasm. This syndrome occurs in about 10% of patients with ileal carcinoids. Significantly elevated blood levels of serotonin and urine levels of 5-HIAA are usually detected. Extensive hepatic metastases are present in 95% of patients with the carcinoid syndrome; almost all of these patients are found to have primary ileal carcinoid tumors. Occasionally, however, the carcinoid syndrome may occur in the absence of hepatic disease,[21,22] for example, when the primary carcinoid tumor or its mesenteric metastases communicate with the systemic circulation via retroperitoneal veins. Subendothelial fibrosis in the heart may cause right-sided valvular stenosis or irregular septal contractions. In contrast, the left side of the heart is protected because of the ability of the lungs to deaminate serotonin.

Survival rates in patients with malignant carcinoid tumors vary from less than 20% if metastatic disease is found at the time of presentation to 75% if complete resection of the tumor is possible.[23]

Imaging Findings

Carcinoid tumor should be the leading consideration when a small tumor is detected in the distal ileum on enteroclysis (Fig. 49-7). Other diagnostic considerations include leiomyomas

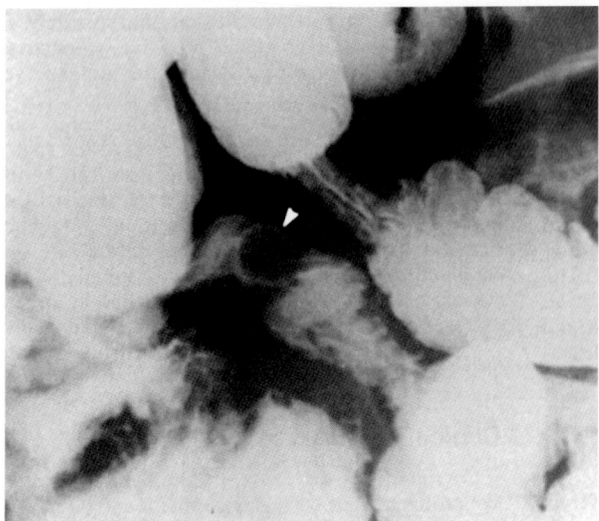

Figure 49-7. Carcinoid tumor in a 69-year-old man with lower gastro-intestinal bleeding. Enteroclysis shows a small, rounded submucosal mass (*arrowhead*) in the terminal ileum. This was a proven ileal carcinoid. Adjacent lymph nodes were negative for metastases. Prior radionuclide scintigraphy, angiography, and CT (*not shown*) failed to reveal the lesion.

and adenomas. The presence of multiple distal small bowel nodules increases the likelihood of a carcinoid (see Fig. 49-1),[24] but multiple nodules can also be seen with lymphoma or metastases from breast cancer or malignant melanoma. Unlike mesenteric lesions, the primary carcinoid tumor usually has a smooth, rounded configuration. On multislice CT performed with neutral oral and intravenous contrast media, the primary tumor may be manifested by an enhancing polypoid mass in the wall of the bowel (Fig. 49-8). In most cases, however, CT fails to reveal the primary tumor.

With tumor growth into the mesentery, the typical CT appearance is that of a spiculated mesenteric mass with curvilinear stranding and indrawing of adjacent bowel loops (Fig. 49-9). Calcification of mesenteric lesions is common (70%).[25] Invasion or constriction of mesenteric blood vessels may cause small bowel ischemia, manifested by nonspecific thickening of the bowel wall (Fig. 49-10). Occasionally, desmoid tumors and sclerosing mesenteritis may produce similar findings in the mesentery on CT. The latter disease is an idiopathic fibrotic condition similar histologically to primary retroperitoneal fibrosis. Isotropic imaging with maximum intensity projections and multiplanar reformats may help in planning surgery for carcinoid tumors.[26]

Liver lesions are best demonstrated on dual-phase CT with imaging in the late arterial and venous phases. On the

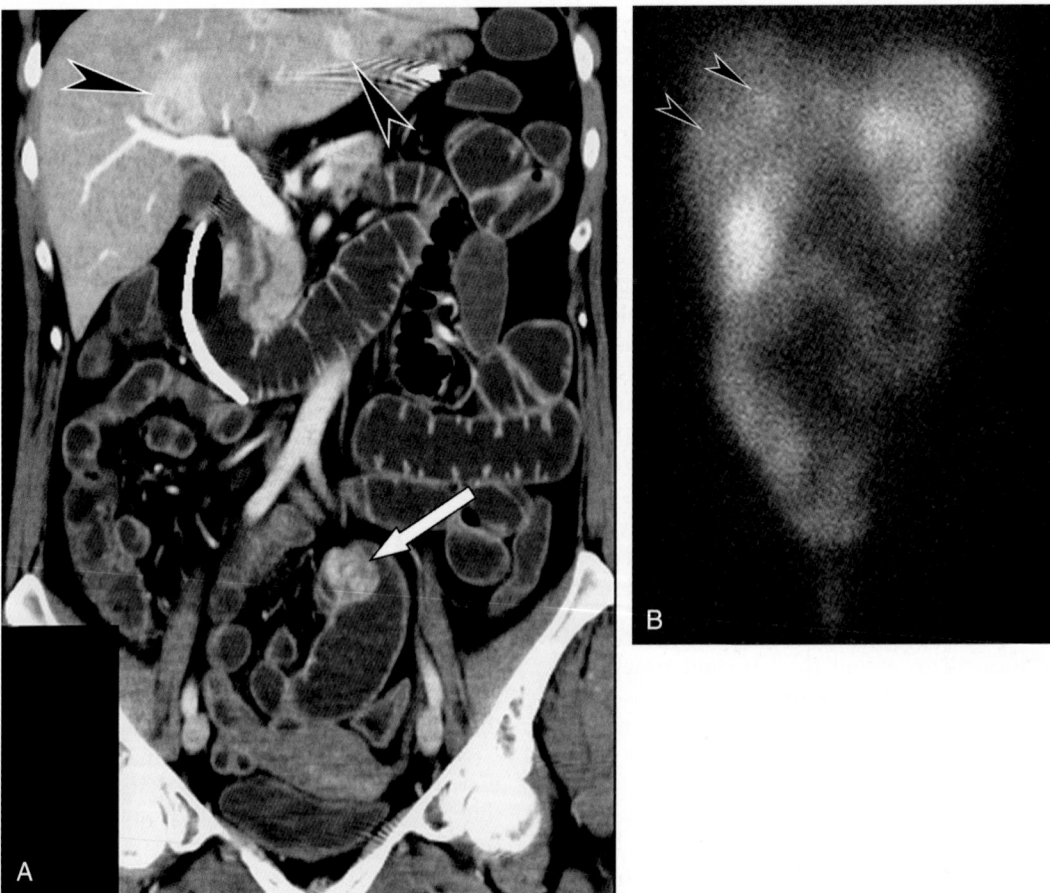

Figure 49-8. Metastatic carcinoid tumor in a 59-year-old woman with diarrhea and wheezing. A. Coronal reformat from isotropic resolution CT enteroclysis performed with neutral enteral contrast media shows a 3-cm hypervascular mass (*arrow*) in the distal ileum. There also are multiple hypervascular liver metastases (*arrowheads*). **B.** Indium-111 octreotide scan shows the liver metastases as foci of slightly increased uptake (*arrowheads*). The primary tumor was not seen on this scan.

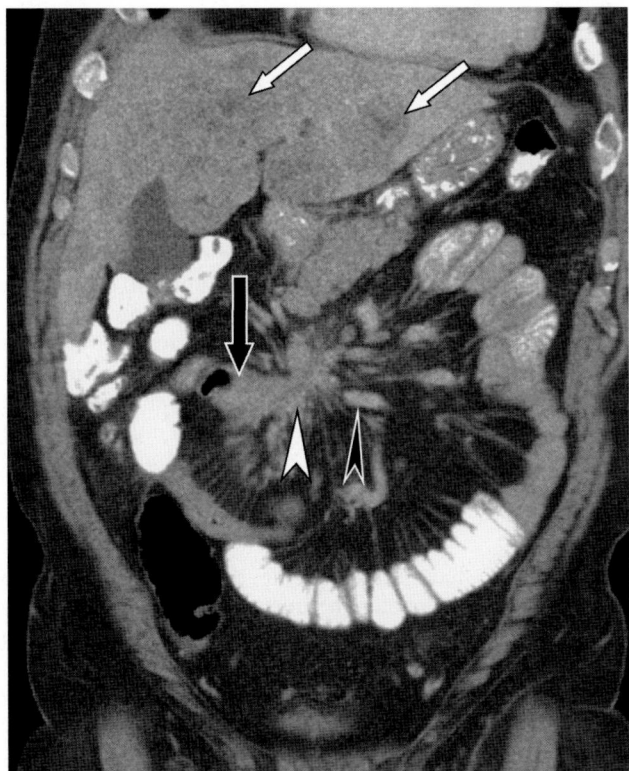

Figure 49-9. Carcinoid syndrome in a 58-year-old man. Coronal reformat from CT without intravenous contrast media shows a spiculated mesenteric mass (*white arrowhead*). A loop of small bowel (*black arrow*) is adherent to this mass. Adjacent mesenteric vessels are mildly dilated (*black arrowhead*). Also note the presence of liver metastases (*white arrows*).

arterial phase, smaller metastases are usually hypervascular (see Fig. 49-8A). Larger lesions are often heterogeneous with peripheral hyperdensity. On the hepatic venous phase, liver metastases may become isoattenuating and 10% of these metastases are undetectable. Cystic changes, necrosis, or gas formation may also be seen after embolic therapy.

On MRI, the primary tumors are usually hypointense and hyperintense on precontrast T1- and T2-weighted images, respectively, and show intense enhancement with gadolinium.[27] Liver metastases are hypointense on T1-weighted images and enhance during the arterial phase of gadolinium injection. They are hyperintense to a variable degree on T2-weighted sequences.[28,29]

Iodine-123 (^{123}I)–labeled metaiodobenzylguanidine (MIBG) has been used for locating the site of the primary tumor and sites of metastatic disease, but this imaging technique has a low sensitivity (55%-70%).[19] Nevertheless, MIBG imaging may be used if other techniques have failed to localize the tumor or if therapy with iodine-131 (^{131}I)-MIBG is being considered.[30] Indium-111 (^{111}In)- or ^{123}I-labeled diethylenetriaminepentaacetic acid (DTPA) octreotide, a long-acting analog of somatostatin, has been shown to have a sensitivity of 80% to 100% in diagnosing carcinoid tumors (see Fig. 49-8B).[30] Anatomic localization is improved with the use of single photon emission CT (SPECT). Somatostatin receptor scanning has been claimed to be more cost effective than conventional imaging for detecting these tumors.[31] Fluorine-18 (^{18}F)-fluorodeoxyglucose (FDG) PET may be used for detection of poorly differentiated primary tumors that are not seen with other techniques (Fig. 49-11). For most small bowel carcinoid tumors, which have slow proliferation, FDG-PET is of limited value.[30] In small studies, PET scanning with ^{18}F-dopa, gallium-68 (^{68}Ga)–labeled octreotide, or carbon-11 (^{11}C)–labeled tryptophan has been shown to be very sensitive in

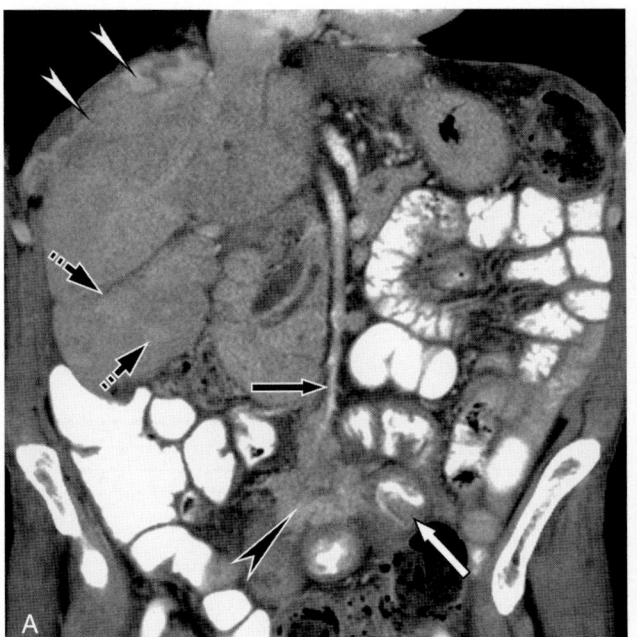
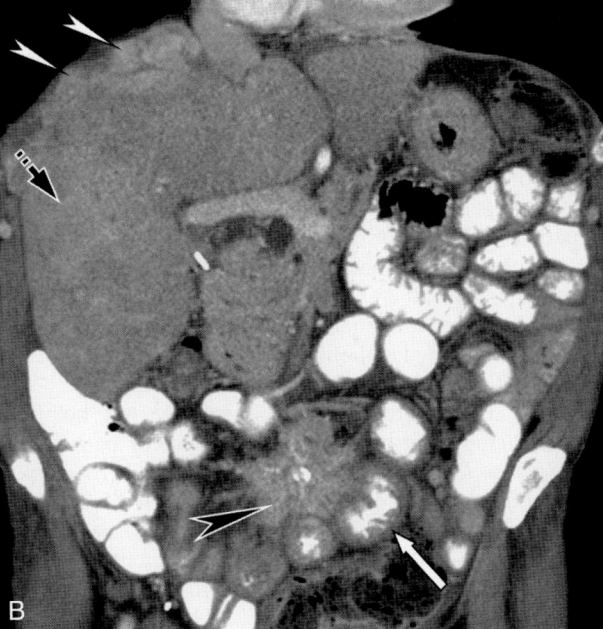

Figure 49-10. Carcinoid syndrome in a 69-year-old man. A and **B.** Coronal CT reformats show a spiculated mass (*black arrowheads*) in the mesentery with calcification. The superior mesenteric artery (*black arrow in* **A**) is encased by this mass. There is associated wall thickening (*white arrows*) of an adjacent small bowel loop due to proven ischemia. Also note liver parenchymal (*dashed arrows*) and surface (*white arrowheads*) metastases.

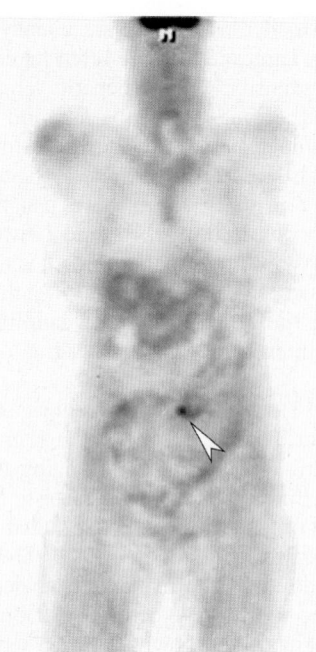

Figure 49-11. Carcinoid syndrome in a 59-year-old woman. CT and octreotide scans (*not shown*) failed to reveal the primary tumor or evidence of metastases. Fluoro-18-deoxyglucose PET scan shows intense uptake (*arrowhead*) in the mid small bowel corresponding to the primary carcinoid tumor. This patient presumably had the carcinoid syndrome because the venous drainage of the tumor communicated with the systemic circulation via retroperitoneal veins.

localizing tumor extent,[19,30,32] but these agents have limited availability.

Treatment

All small bowel carcinoids are potentially malignant and should be resected with a clear margin together with radical resection of regional lymph nodes. Surgical debulking of liver metastases or liver transplantation are options in selected patients with metastatic disease. Radiofrequency or cryoprobe ablation are associated with good symptomatic relief and reduction of urinary markers in the first year, but significant recurrence rates have been reported by 2 years.[19]

Hepatic arterial embolization with a mixture of cytotoxic agents, gelatin sponges, and polyvinyl alcohol particles can produce a biochemical and clinical response in up to 60% of patients.[19] However, the median response time is about 7 months,[19] and repeated embolization of alternating liver lobes or subsequent systemic chemotherapy may be necessary.[33]

Systemic chemotherapy per se is usually not helpful. Radiation therapy can be used for palliation of pain from bone metastases. Radionuclides such as ^{131}I-MIBG and ^{111}In-octreotide achieve tumor stability in 40% to 80% of patients but induce remission in less than 10% of patients.[30] Better tumor regression (up to 40%) is achieved with yttrium-90 1,4,7,10-tetraazacyclododecane-1,4,7,10-tetraacetic acid (DOTA)-octreotide or lutetium-177 DOTA octreotate. Interferon-alfa increases the radiosensitivity of these tumors by upregulating somatostatin type 2 receptors, so this agent may be combined with peptide receptor radionuclides for a better patient response.

GASTROINTESTINAL STROMAL TUMORS

Gastrointestinal stromal tumors are the most common mesenchymal tumors arising in the gastrointestinal tract. These tumors are characterized by expression of a tyrosine kinase growth factor receptor, also called KIT receptor or CD117.[34] This allows unchecked growth of tumor and resistance to apoptosis. These tumors differ immunohistologically and in their behavior from other mesenchymal tumors such as leiomyosarcomas, which do not express KIT antigen. In the past, GISTs were misdiagnosed as smooth muscle tumors because these tumors share many features on light microscopy. Unlike breast, lung, and colon cancers, in which the development of tumor requires multiple mutations of different genes, most GISTs occur due to a single gain-of-function mutation of the *KIT* gene.

Pathology

GISTs tend to have an exophytic growth pattern. These tumors commonly involve the muscularis propria and show mucosal ulceration in 50% of cases.[35] GISTs are thought to originate from stem cells (which normally expresses CD117) rather than from smooth muscle cells. The histologic classification is based on the predominant cell type, either spindle cell or epithelioid.[36] Twenty to 30 percent of GISTs are found to be malignant at the time of presentation.[36,37] Features associated with a worse prognosis include a distal small bowel location, tumor size, and high mitotic activity.[38] Tumor size is the best factor for predicting metastatic potential.[39,40] Tumors less than 2 cm usually do not metastasize, whereas those larger than 5 cm are usually malignant.[41] Nevertheless, many pathologists believe that all GISTs will eventually become malignant and that smaller tumors should be classified as at low risk for malignancy rather than as benign.[42]

Mesenchymal tumors are classified not only on their appearance at light microscopy but also on their immunochemical findings. Table 49-1 shows a simplified version of the current classification.[34] Specific markers for glial tumors include S-100 and glial fibrillary acidic protein; markers for smooth muscle tumors include α-smooth muscle antigen and desmin; and markers for fibrous tumors include vimentin. In the future, molecular genetics may help determine which GISTs will become malignant. In general, certain mutations, such as a gain-of-function mutation in exon 11 of the c-kit

Table 49-1

Immunohistochemical Properties of Gastrointestinal Mesenchymal Tumors

	CD117	S-100	Alpha SMA	Vimentin
GIST	Positive	May be positive	Usually negative	Negative
GIGT	Negative	Positive	Negative	Negative
GILT	Negative	Negative	Positive	Negative
GIFT	Negative	Negative	Negative	Positive

GIST, gastrointestinal stromal tumor; GIGT, gastrointestinal glial tumor; GILT, gastrointestinal leiomyogenic tumor (includes leiomyosarcoma); GIFT, gastrointestinal fibrous tumor; CD117, c-*kit* antigen; Alpha SMA, smooth muscle antigen.
From Sandrasegaran K, Rajesh A, Rydberg J, et al: Gastrointestinal stromal tumors: Clinical, radiologic, and pathologic features. AJR 184: 803-811, 2005.

antigen, and increased numbers of mutations are associated with a higher malignant potential.[38,43] At the same time, 5% of GISTs are weak or negative for c-kit antigen expression but instead are highly positive for platelet-derived growth factor-α. This subset of predominantly gastric GISTs (95% are of gastric origin) may be associated with different growth patterns, because these tumors are less likely to metastasize but also have less of a response to different forms of chemotherapy (see later).[44]

Clinical Aspects

The clinical presentation of patients with GISTs is often non-specific. Abdominal pain or distention is the most common presenting finding.[45] Gastrointestinal bleeding and unexplained anemia are also frequent findings. Despite the large size of these tumors, intestinal obstruction is rare. Patients with small bowel GISTs have a worse prognosis than those with gastric GISTs, most likely because these individuals have more advanced tumors at the time of presentation.

Imaging Findings

Most small bowel GISTs are large tumors at the time of diagnosis, usually greater than 5 cm. The predominant CT appearance is a heterogeneously enhancing exophytic mass (Fig. 49-12).[46,47] Homogeneous, intense enhancement may sometimes be seen with tumors less than 5 cm (Fig. 49-13). Despite their tendency for exophytic growth, most GISTs also have an intraluminal component on CT. Like lymphoma, GISTs may cause marked expansion of the lumen with aneurismal dilatation of the affected bowel. This finding may be partly related to the cavitary nature of these fast-growing tumors with apparent enlargement of the lumen. GISTs may also damage the myenteric plexus, causing the lumen to dilate. Calcification is uncommon at presentation but may be detected in metastatic lesions after chemotherapy.

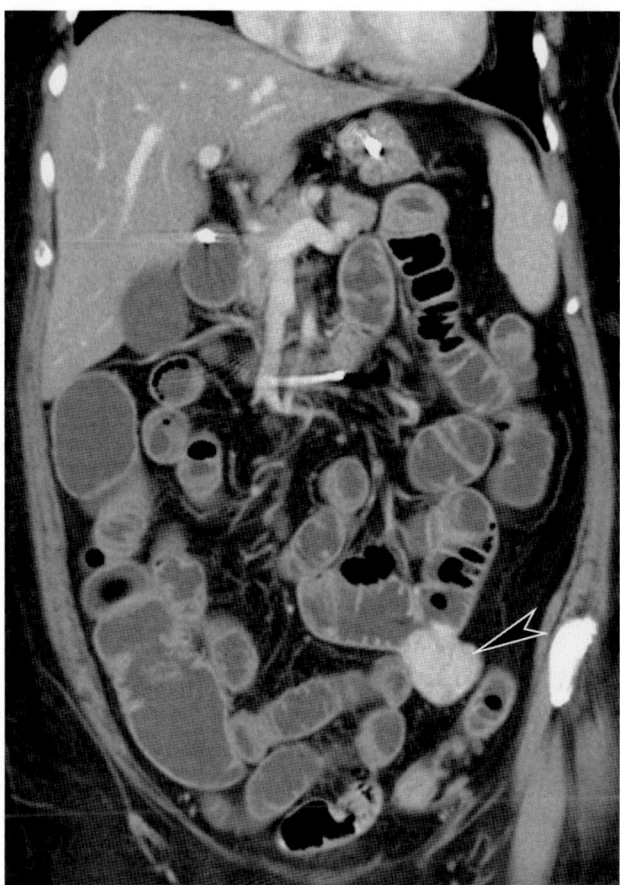

Figure 49-13. Gastrointestinal stromal tumor in a 63-year-old woman with unexplained gastrointestinal bleeding. CT enteroclysis shows a 3-cm hypervascular submucosal mass (*arrow*) arising from the mid small bowel. This was a proven GIST at surgery. Prior capsule endoscopy showed jejunal angioectasia (*not shown*) but not the small bowel tumor.

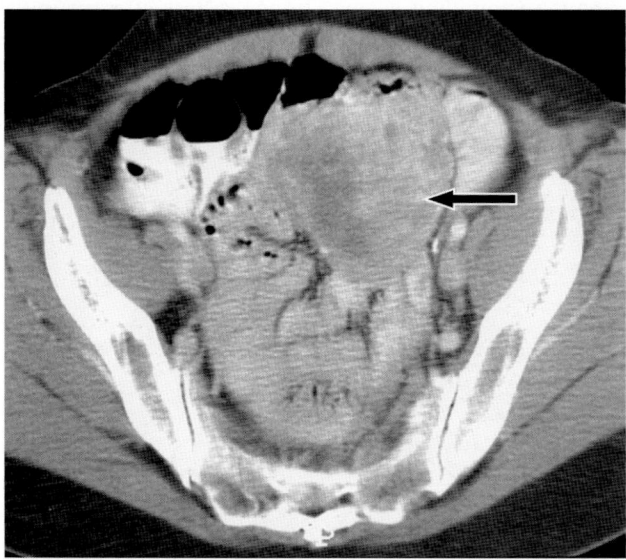

Figure 49-12. Gastrointestinal stromal tumor in a 50-year-old woman with chronic abdominal pain. CT of the pelvis shows a heterogeneously enhancing exophytic mass (*arrow*) adherent to small bowel loops. This was a proven GIST.

Unlike adenocarcinoma and lymphoma, lymphatic spread does not usually occur in patients with GISTs.[46,47] The presence of substantial adenopathy should therefore raise the possibility of an alternative diagnosis. Mesenteric masses are usually smooth surfaced and do not show spiculation or indrawing of the mesentery (Fig. 49-14). Many mesenteric masses have low-density centers, even when the primary tumor is hypervascular. Mesenteric metastases are common at relapse. Large mesenteric masses may grow around mesenteric vessels but do not usually cause distal venous thrombosis. CT is better at detecting mesenteric metastases than MRI.

Omental disease is seen less frequently than mesenteric disease. Omental masses are usually small (<2 cm) and homogeneously enhancing. Omental caking is sometimes present on CT. Because of the mobility of the omentum, some masses may be in different locations on subsequent CT scans. Despite a high risk of solid metastases to the mesentery, ascites is uncommon and is more likely to result from chemotherapy.[48]

Small liver metastases are usually hypervascular on CT and MRI before chemotherapy.[46,47] Dual-phase CT or MRI with gadolinium may show bright homogeneous enhancement in the late arterial (portal venous inflow) phase and almost complete washout on the hepatic venous phase. As a result, untreated liver metastases may be missed on a single venous phase CT study. However, not all metastases have

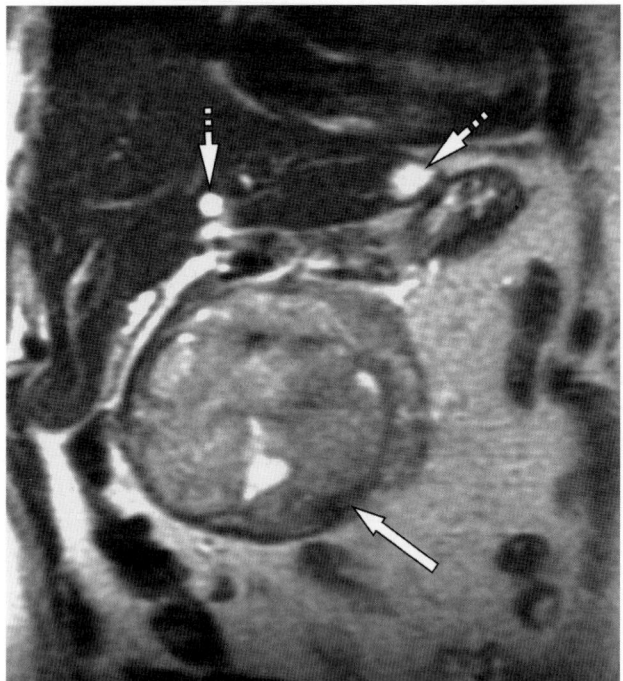

Figure 49-14. A 75-year-old woman receiving treatment with imatinib for a known gastrointestinal stromal tumor. T2-weighted coronal fast spin-echo MRI sequence shows a 10-cm mildly hyperintense abdominal mass (*solid arrow*) caused by mesenteric metastases from her known GIST. Note how the mass has a smooth surface. Hyperintense liver metastases (*dashed arrows*) are also seen.

similar vascularity. In the same liver, there may be hypovascular and hypervascular masses, possibly representing different generations of metastases. On MRI, metastases usually have low- or intermediate-signal intensity on precontrast T1-weighted sequences and marginally bright signal intensity on T2- weighted sequences (see Fig. 49-14). Necrosis is common in larger masses. Lung metastases are extremely rare in GISTs, even in the presence of extensive liver and peritoneal metastases. This is a major difference in the pattern of metastatic spread between GISTs and leiomyosarcomas.

Metastases to the mesentery and liver may become hypovascular and often completely cystic on CT as little as 1 month after targeted chemotherapy (Fig. 49-15).[49] These metastases may therefore be mistaken for simple cysts. MRI is superior to single-phase CT in assessing the viability of metastases.[47] Changes in T2-weighted signal intensity on MRI and cystic changes on CT are predictive of a successful tumor response. Tumor size measurements are less accurate in charting tumor response.[47,50] One of the first signs of relapse may be a new enhancing focus within a stable cystic metastasis.[51]

Uptake of ^{18}F-FDG by metastatic GISTs is variable, so that PET is not as sensitive as CT in detecting metastases.[52] In tumors that take up ^{18}F-FDG, however, PET may determine the response of metastatic GISTs to imatinib earlier than CT.[53]

Treatment

In the absence of metastatic disease, complete surgical excision of GISTs should be undertaken and offers the best hope for cure.[54,55] Unlike small bowel carcinomas, resection of GISTs does not require a wide bowel excision.[43] Lymphadenectomy also is usually unnecessary, because these tumors generally do not metastasize to lymph nodes.[41,43] Despite an apparently complete resection with clear margins, however, the recurrence rate is high; hepatic or mesenteric recurrences occur in 40% to 90% of patients after surgery.[39,40] This high recurrence rate may be partly related to the development of mesenteric implants if the tumor is disrupted at surgery; hence the importance of meticulous surgical technique.[41] For this reason, percutaneous biopsies are best avoided.[45] Radiation therapy and standard chemotherapy have not been found to be successful in treating this disease.[39,56,57]

Since 2000, the standard chemotherapy for metastatic or large (>10 cm) GISTs has been imatinib mesylate (Gleevec, Novartis, East Hanover, NJ). At least initially, this agent is effective in 80% of patients with GISTs.[58] Imatinib blocks tyrosine kinase receptors and accelerates apoptosis of GISTs. Apoptosis and the absence of necrosis may explain why treated GIST metastases often appear cystic on CT and MRI without surrounding edema. Tumor relapse after an initial response is sometimes seen after the first year of therapy due to secondary mutations of tyrosine kinase domain.[59]

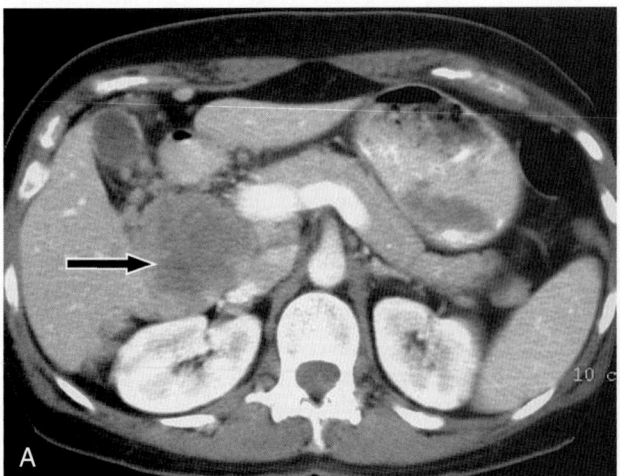
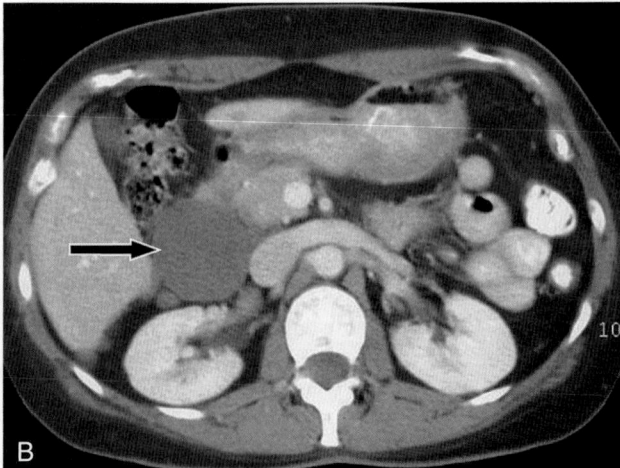

Figure 49-15. A 49-year-old woman with a history of a "leiomyosarcoma" and recurrent abdominal pain. A. Pretreatment CT shows a solid mesenteric metastasis (*arrow*). A gastrointestinal stromal tumor was diagnosed on immunohistochemical studies. **B.** After 3 months of imatinib therapy, the mass (*arrow*) has decreased in size; there is also a substantial decrease in the density of the lesion, which now resembles a benign cyst.

NON-HODGKIN'S LYMPHOMA

Gastrointestinal lymphoma may be primary or secondary. A diagnosis of primary gastrointestinal lymphoma can be made when the following criteria are met: (1) lymphadenopathy is confined to the area of bowel abnormality; (2) peripheral white cell counts and bone marrow aspirates are normal; and (3) there is no evidence of disease in the liver or spleen. Secondary gastrointestinal lymphoma usually affects multiple sites. Gross or microscopic evidence of gastrointestinal involvement has been found at autopsy in about 50% of cases of disseminated lymphoma. In primary gastrointestinal lymphoma, the stomach is most commonly involved (40% to 75%), followed by the small intestine (20% to 40%), ileocecal region (10% to 20%), colon (10% to 15%), and esophagus (less than 1%).[60,61]

The overall prognosis of primary small bowel lymphoma is only fair, with expected 5-year survival rates of 25% to 30%.[60] Predictors of poor prognosis include a stage greater than IIE2; tumor size larger than 10 cm; immunoblastic histology; T-cell type; and an acute abdomen at the time of clinical presentation.[62,63]

Classification and Staging

Non-Hodgkin's lymphomas are classified on the basis of their histologic composition. Immunohistochemical methods have increasingly been utilized in combination with the histologic findings to classify these tumors. Unlike in the stomach, most small bowel lymphomas have high-grade histology. They usually are non-Hodgkin's lymphomas with B-cell immunophenotype. Histologically, most of these lymphomas are the diffuse large cell variety.[60,61,63]

Staging refers to the distribution and extent of lymphoma within the body. The Ann Arbor staging system for Hodgkin's disease has been modified for staging of non-Hodgkin's lymphoma. The subscript E is used to designate disease in extranodal sites. Stage I_E means disease is confined to a single extranodal site (the small bowel). Stage II_{E1} indicates associated involvement of a group of regional lymph nodes. More

extensive subdiaphragmatic nodal involvement is identified as stage II_{E2}. Stage III_E refers to small bowel lymphoma with lymphadenopathy on both sides of the diaphragm. Stage IV implies widespread organ dissemination. It is generally agreed that staging of non-Hodgkin's lymphoma is more relevant for selecting treatment options than the histologic classification of the tumor. Cases of stage I_E small bowel lymphoma are rare; nearly half of small bowel lymphomas are stage II_E. Patients in both groups should have surgery before additional treatment is instituted. Complete excision of the tumor improves survival.

Clinical Aspects

Patients with small bowel lymphoma typically present with abdominal pain, often associated with nausea or vomiting, anemia, weight loss, and pyrexia. A palpable abdominal mass or small bowel obstruction may be present. Malabsorption and diarrhea are rare presenting features in the western form of lymphoma. This presentation is more likely to occur in Mediterranean (B-cell) lymphoma and enteropathy-associated (T-cell) lymphoma.

Imaging Findings

The diverse radiographic appearances of small bowel lymphoma on barium studies reflect the gross morphology of the disease. From a radiologic perspective, gastrointestinal lymphomas may be classified as infiltrating, cavitary, aneurysmal (or saccular), nodular, and mesenteric nodal forms.[64] In one study, the infiltrating form was the most frequent, followed by the cavitary form.[65]

Circumferentially infiltrating non-Hodgkin's lymphoma involves a variable length of small intestine with thickening and subsequent effacement of folds (Fig. 49-16A). A desmoplastic reaction is not usually seen. The lumen is more often widened than narrowed. CT with intravenous contrast media may show one or more segments of circumferential wall thickening with mild or moderate homogeneous enhancement (Fig. 49-16B).

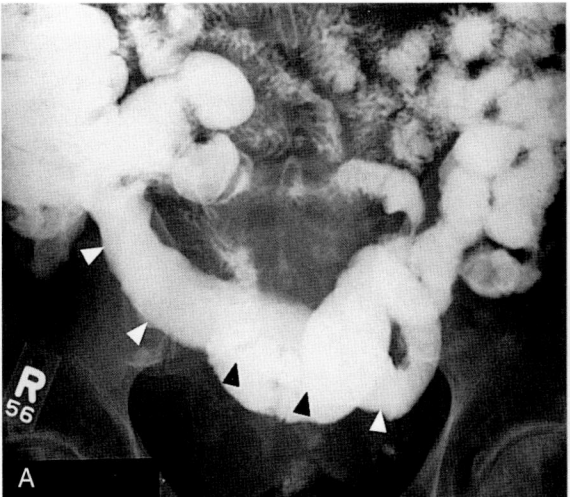 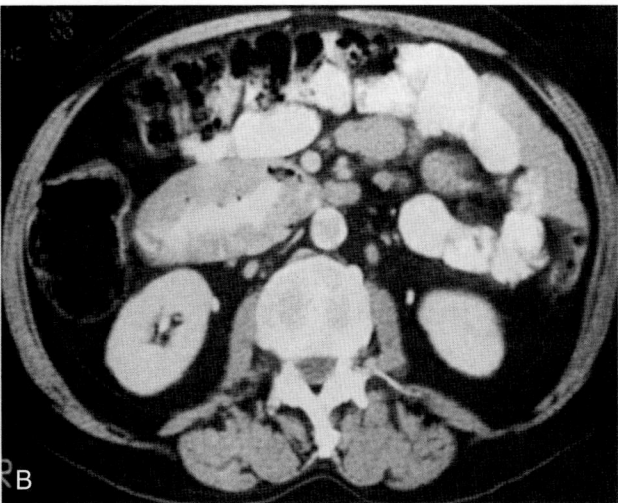

Figure 49-16. Infiltrating non-Hodgkin's lymphoma in a 62-year-old woman with abdominal pain and weight loss. A. Enteroclysis shows a slightly widened segment of terminal ileum (*arrowheads*) with effacement of folds. **B.** Axial CT shows sausage-shaped thickening of the affected bowel wall with homogeneous enhancement.

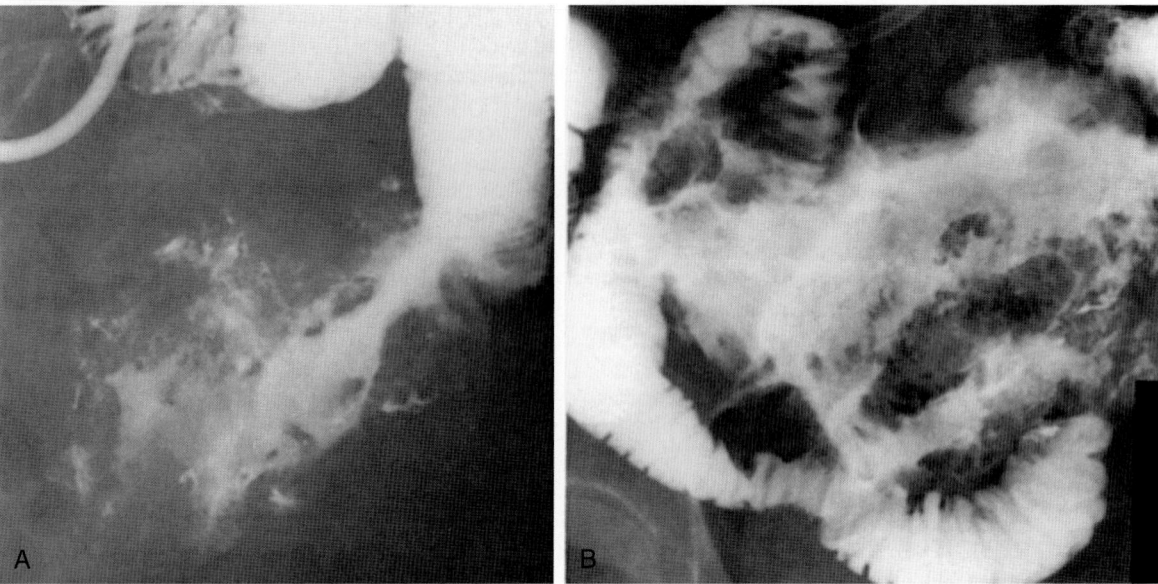

Figure 49-17. Cavitary non-Hodgkin's lymphoma in an elderly woman with abdominal pain and weight loss for 5 months. A. Enteroclysis shows barium extravasating into an exoenteric space. **B.** Later image from the same examination shows a large barium-, air-, and debris-filled cavity occupying the mesenteric border of several small bowel loops. (From Fishman EK, Kuhlman JE, Jones RC: CT of lymphoma: Spectrum of disease. RadioGraphics 11:647-669, 1991.)

Transmural infiltration by lymphoma may cause a localized perforation, resulting in a sealed-off mesenteric cavity (Fig. 49-17). There is usually bowel wall and fold thickening. This cavitary form of lymphoma requires extensive bowel resection.

Aneurysmal bowel dilatation may occur as a result of destruction of the autonomic nerve plexus. These lesions appear as focally ballooned segments of bowel showing reduced peristalsis and no proximal obstruction (Fig. 49-18). With aneurysmal dilatation, the air- and debris-containing space is bounded entirely by the bowel wall (unlike the cavitary form). The bowel contour may revert to normal after treatment; however, perforation is a life-threatening complication. For this reason, complete resection of the tumor should be attempted whenever possible before initiating chemotherapy.[66]

The nodular form of small bowel lymphoma is less common and is primarily seen in patients with disseminated lymphoma involving the gastrointestinal tract. The nodular form is characterized on barium studies by multiple small (0.5-2.0 cm) submucosal nodules in the small bowel (Fig. 49-19), often containing central areas of umbilication or ulceration. The nodules may protrude into the lumen or, rarely, they may act as the lead point for a small bowel intussusception. Multiple lymphomatous polyposis is a rare type of primary gastrointestinal lymphoma, usually associated with mantle cell histology.[67,68] This form of lymphoma is usually manifested by innumerable sessile polyps of varying sizes in the ileocecal region. The prognosis is extremely poor.

Mesenteric nodal lymphoma may secondarily involve contiguous loops of small bowel. Barium studies may reveal

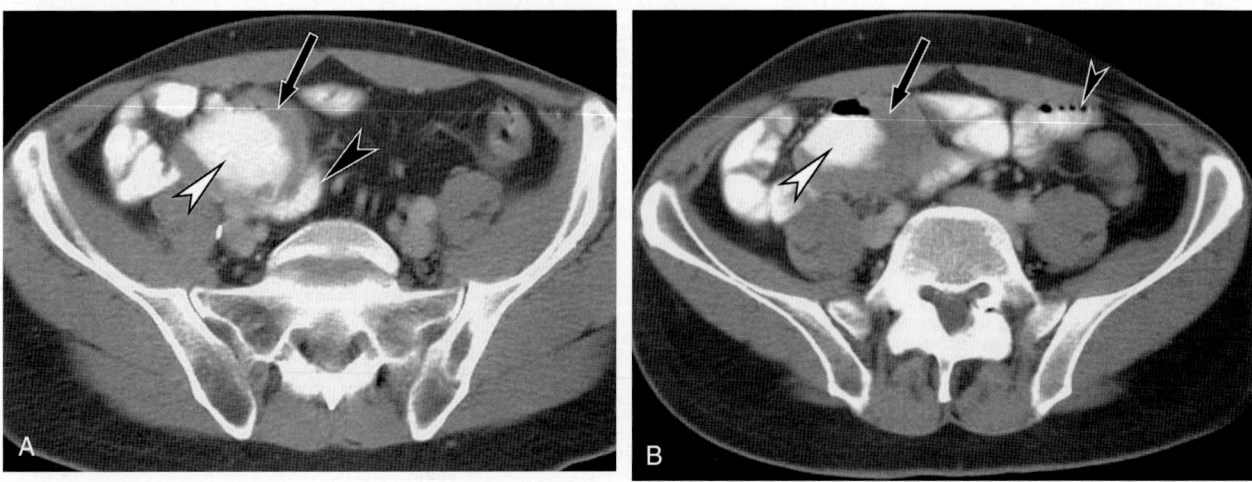

Figure 49-18. Non-Hodgkin's lymphoma causing aneurysmal dilatation in a 64-year-old man with night sweats and weight loss. A and **B.** CT shows a small bowel mass (*arrow*) with a markedly dilated lumen (*white arrowhead*). The bowel serosa or lymphomatous mass itself surrounds the distended lumen, differentiating this from the cavitary form of lymphoma. Note nondilated small bowel (*black arrowhead*) more proximally.

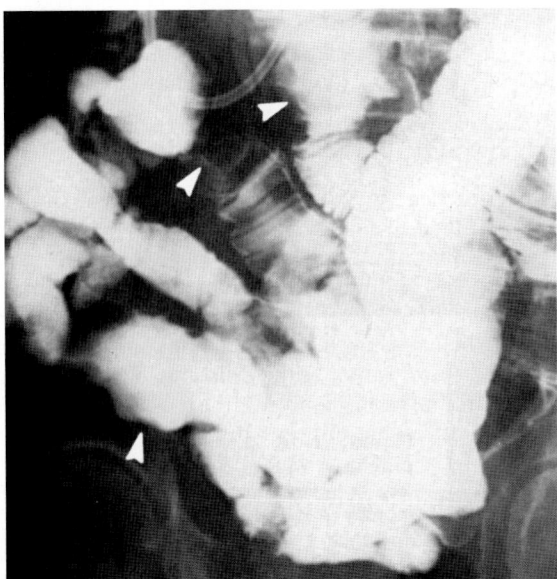

Figure 49-19. Nodular form of non-Hodgkin's lymphoma in a 62-year-old woman with abdominal pain and weight loss. Small bowel follow-through shows multiple small polypoid lesions and short ulcerated segments (*arrowheads*).

a positive FDG-PET scan after the completion of chemotherapy in patients with small bowel lymphoma is a strong predictor of relapse. PET is reported to have a higher accuracy than CT in the detection of residual disease after therapy.[72]

Other Forms of Lymphoma

The uncommon American form of Burkitt's lymphoma predominantly affects children and mainly involves the ileocecal area. This form of lymphoma has one of the most rapid doubling times of any tumor. Like the more common Burkitt lymphoma endemic in Africa, it is associated with the Epstein-Barr virus. Barium studies may show irregular fold thickening, luminal narrowing, and ulceration of the diseased bowel (Fig. 49-21). Lymph nodes are rarely affected.

Mediterranean lymphoma is at the malignant end of a spectrum of a group of pathologic processes termed *immunoproliferative small intestinal disease*.[73,74] At the benign end of this spectrum there is polyclonal infiltration of the bowel mucosa by plasma cells and pleomorphic lymphocytes, presumably in response to yet unidentified microbes. Monoclonal proliferation of all layers of the bowel wall by atypical B lymphocytes typifies the more malignant forms of immunoproliferative small intestinal disease. The pathogenesis of this disease is similar to that of low-grade gastric lymphoma, which develops as a chronic immune response to *Helicobacter pylori*. If diagnosed at an early stage, immunoproliferative small intestinal disease may regress after treatment with antibiotics and corticosteroids.[73,75] Mediterranean lymphoma mainly affects socioeconomically poor, young adults of Arab, Jewish, and Mediterranean origin. The most common presentation is intractable diarrhea and malabsorption. This entity is also found in other populations, including South African blacks and Mexican Americans. Barium studies may reveal thickened folds and multiple nodular filling defects.

Enteropathy-associated T-cell lymphoma is discussed in Chapter 47. Lymphoma complicating immunodeficiency states is discussed in Chapter 53.

displacement and compression of these loops by an adjacent mesenteric mass (Fig. 49-20A). These masses are usually best visualized by CT (Fig. 49-20B). Some lobulated mesenteric masses may encase adjacent small bowel loops, producing a classic "sandwich" appearance (see Fig. 49-20B).[69]

The sonographic and MRI appearances of gastrointestinal lymphoma have been described,[70,71] but these techniques have not gained widespread acceptance in the diagnosis or staging of non-Hodgkin's lymphoma. In general, these tumors have homogeneous low-signal and heterogeneous high-signal intensity on T1- and T2-weighted MR sequences, respectively. Despite mild physiologic uptake in the gastrointestinal tract,

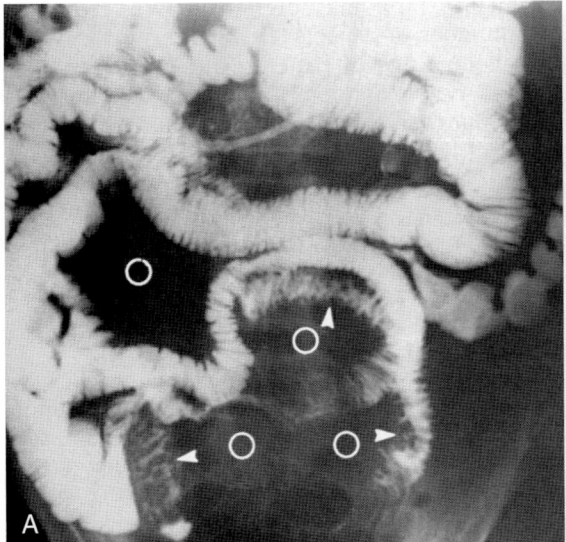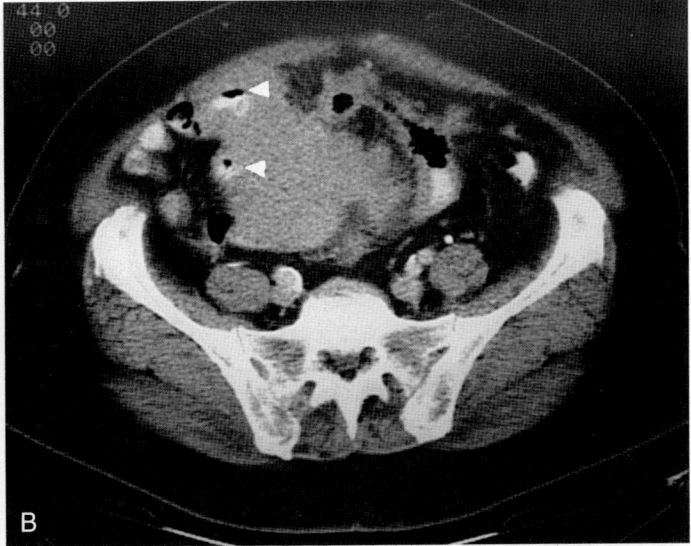

Figure 49-20. Mesenteric nodal form of non-Hodgkin's lymphoma in a 71-year-old man. A. Multiple loops of small bowel are displaced by mesenteric masses (*open circles*). Involved folds are thickened and nodular (*arrowheads*). There is no evidence of obstruction. **B.** CT shows a large mesenteric mass displacing and compressing loops of ileum. Two segments of small bowel (*arrowheads*) are surrounded by the nodal mass, producing a typical "sandwich" appearance.

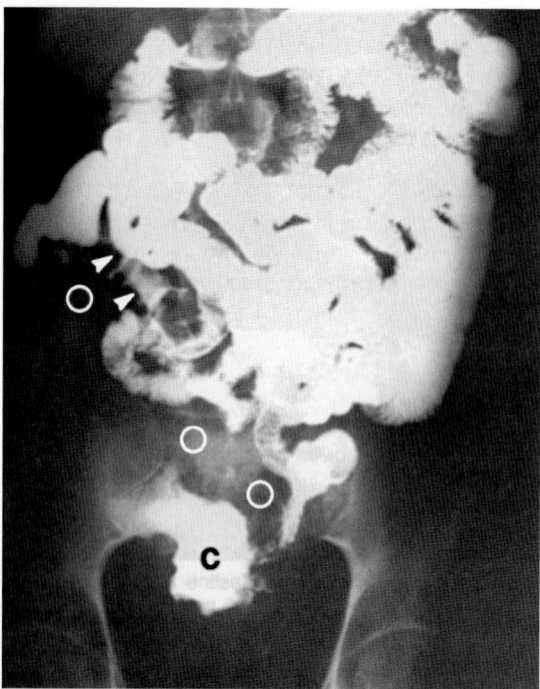

Figure 49-21. Burkitt's lymphoma in a 14-year-old boy with a right lower quadrant abdominal mass. Small bowel follow-through shows a large tumor (*open circles*) infiltrating the distal small bowel and cecum (C). Note how involved small bowel loops have flattened, nodular folds (*arrowheads*). This patient had Burkitt's lymphoma.

Hodgkin's Disease

Involvement of the gastrointestinal tract by Hodgkin's disease is extremely rare. Radiologic findings of gastrointestinal lymphoma in a patient with Hodgkin's disease warrant a review of the original histologic findings. The development of non-Hodgkin's lymphoma has been documented after treatment of Hodgkin's disease.[76] Hodgkin's disease has been reported to cause fibrosis of the bowel wall with tapered, eccentric narrowing of the involved segment but not the overhanging edges seen in carcinoma. There may be displacement of uninvolved small bowel loops by nodal masses.

METASTASES

The small intestine may be the only site of metastases from an extraintestinal malignant tumor. More frequently, metastatic involvement of the small bowel is discovered in patients with widespread abdominal carcinomatosis. Tumor may involve the small bowel via several pathways: (1) intraperitoneal spread; (2) hematogenous dissemination; and (3) extension from an adjacent tumor either directly or via lymphatic channels.[77] Intraperitoneal spread is the most frequent pathway for spread of malignant tumor to the small bowel.[2]

Intraperitoneal Spread

Dependent areas in the abdomen and pelvis in which ascitic fluid accumulates before overflowing to an adjacent space are preferred sites for malignant cell deposition. These sites include the posterior pelvic cul-de-sac, small bowel mesentery near the ileocecal valve, sigmoid mesocolon, and right paracolic gutter.

CT is the most common technique for detecting intraperitoneal-seeded metastases. The sensitivity of this technique is improved by optimizing distention of the bowel lumen (such as with CT enteroclysis) (Fig. 49-22). The etiology of small bowel obstruction after therapy for abdominal malignancy includes adhesions, metastases, or radiation enteropathy. The findings on CT enteroclysis enable differentiation of these conditions in more than two thirds of cases. Adhesions usually have a sharp zone of transition, often adjacent to the anterior parietal peritoneum. The presence of rounded, nodular defects or focal enhancement of the bowel wall favors metastases. Irregular wall thickening of pelvic small bowel loops with normal thickness of abdominal bowel loops favors radiation therapy. These conditions may coexist.

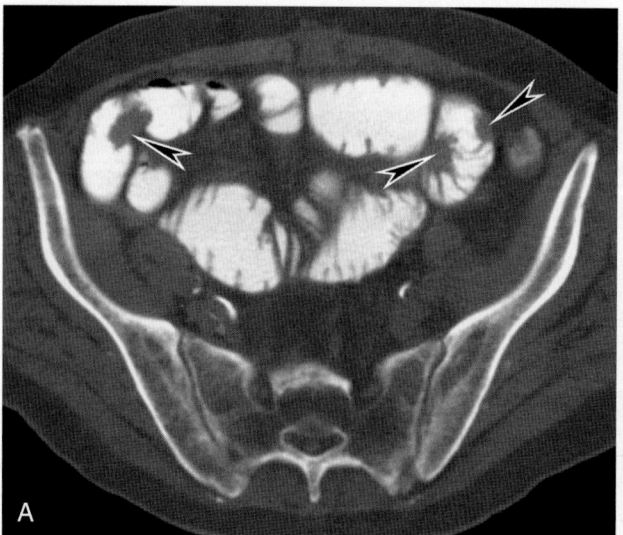
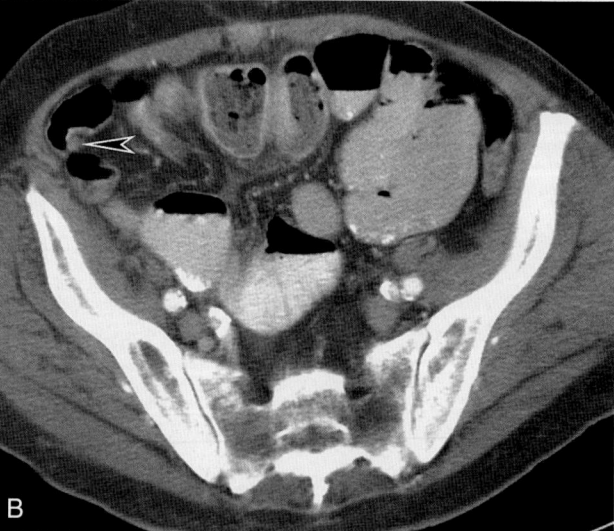

Figure 49-22. Small bowel obstruction in an 80-year-old man with a history of colon cancer. A. Axial image from positive contrast CT enteroclysis shows multiple masses (*arrowheads*) in the small bowel wall compatible with serosal metastases as the cause of this patient's small bowel obstruction. **B.** These lesions were not reported on a prior CT with oral and intravenous contrast media. In retrospect, one of the serosal metastases (*arrowhead*) is visible.

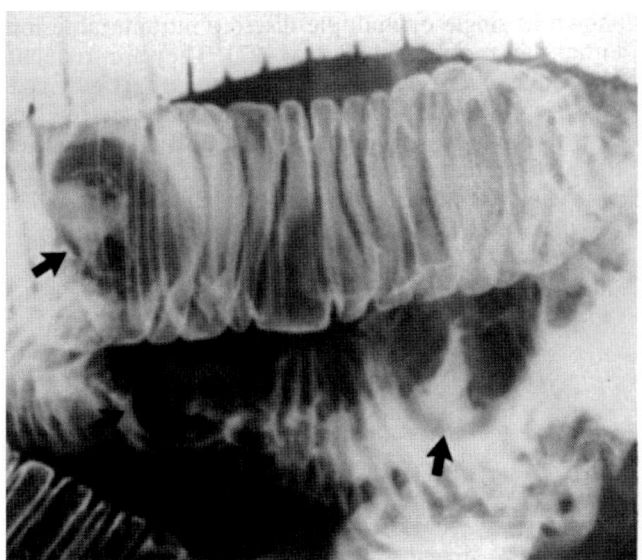 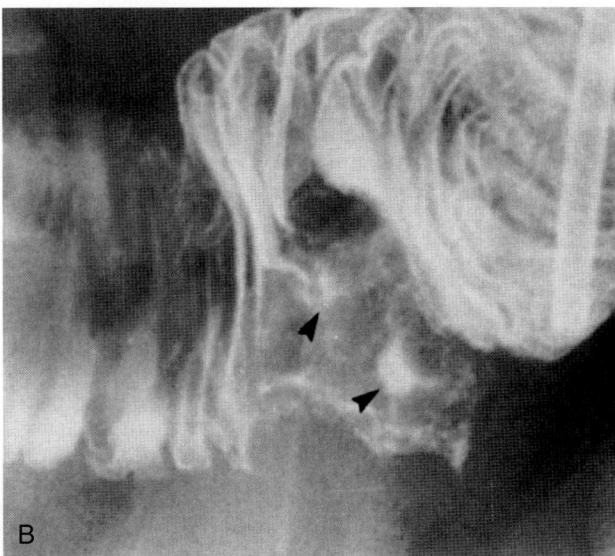

Figure 49-23. A 65-year-old man with a history of malignant melanoma. A. At least two bull's-eye lesions (*arrows*) are present in the jejunum. Note the large size of the ulcers. **B.** A larger polypoid metastasis with radiating linear ulcerations (*arrowheads*) produces the typical spokewheel pattern of metastases from malignant melanoma. Note how there is no evidence of small bowel obstruction. (From Herlinger H, Maglinte D [eds]: Clinical Radiology of the Small Intestine. Philadelphia, WB Saunders, 1989.)

Hematogenous Spread

Hematogenous metastases to the small intestine are most commonly from malignant melanoma, breast cancer, and lung cancer. In some patients, metastases from breast cancer or melanoma may come to clinical attention many years after diagnosis and treatment of the original tumor. With carcinoma of the lung, however, there is no lag time and the clinical features of the primary tumor usually overshadow symptoms caused by the metastases. Patients with hematogenous metastases to the small bowel usually present with gastrointestinal bleeding and generalized deterioration rather than intestinal obstruction.

In patients with malignant melanoma and breast cancer, metastases usually appear as smoothly rounded polypoid lesions of different sizes on the antimesenteric border of the bowel. "Target" or "bull's-eye" lesions (i.e., nodules with central ulcers) occur less often in the mesenteric small intestine than in the stomach and may show a spokewheel pattern of fissuring extending from the edge of the central ulcer to the periphery of the mass (Fig. 49-23). Intestinal obstruction is rare unless there is associated intussusception. Large melanoma deposits may grow through the small bowel wall and cavitate, simulating aneurysmal dilatation. Desmoplasia with bowel obstruction is more often seen with metastases from lung cancer. The discrepancy between the autopsy findings and the premortem findings of metastatic melanoma to the small bowel suggests that currently used imaging techniques (small bowel follow-through and CT) are not sensitive in identifying the number and location of these metastases.[78]

Other Metastatic Pathways

Lymph node metastases from a left-sided colon carcinoma can invade the proximal jejunum near the ligament of Treitz via lymphatic vessels that course adjacent to the ascending left colic branch of the inferior mesenteric artery. Residual tumor after resection of a cecal carcinoma or of a gynecologic malignancy can involve the distal ileum by direct extension through the subperitoneal space.[77] Blockage of a proximal lymph node by tumor may lead to retrograde flow of lymph and tumor emboli with involvement of adjacent segments of bowel. This mechanism may be responsible for spread of tumor to small bowel adjacent to the anastomotic site after resection of colonic carcinoma.

SUMMARY

The prognosis for many malignant tumors of the small bowel has not improved substantially in the past few decades, primarily because these patients already have advanced disease at the time of clinical presentation. Radiologists could help reduce the lag time before diagnosis by performing state-of-the-art CT. The optimal CT technique for these examinations includes the use of neutral oral and intravenous contrast media, isotropic imaging (possible with 16-channel and higher scanners) with high-quality nonaxial reformats, and adequate distention of the small intestine by oral hyperhydration (CT enterography) or enteric infusion under hydrostatic pressure (CT enteroclysis).

Capsule endoscopy is clearly superior to other imaging techniques for diagnosing Crohn's disease and vascular malformations in the small intestine. This is not the case with small bowel tumors, however, particularly small submucosal neoplasms. Imaging will also be required to assess tumor extent and the response to therapy. In the future, PET/CT may also have a substantial role in the management of these patients.

References

1. Neugut AI, Marvin MR, Rella VA, Chabot JA: An overview of adenocarcinoma of the small intestine. Oncology (Williston Park) 11:529-536, 1997.

2. Maglinte DDT, Herlinger H: Small bowel neoplasms. In Herlinger H, Maglinte DDT, Birnbaum BA (eds): Clinical Imaging of the Small Intestine. New York, Springer-Verlag, 1999, pp 377-438.

3. North JH, Pack MS: Malignant tumors of the small intestine: A review of 144 cases. Am Surg 66: 46-51, 2000.

4. Maglinte DD, O'Connor K, Bessette J, et al: The role of the physician in the late diagnosis of primary malignant tumors of the small intestine. Am J Gastroenterol 86:304-308, 1991.

5. Zollinger RM Jr: Primary neoplasms of the small intestine. Am J Surg 151:654-658, 1986.

6. Bessette JR, Maglinte DD, Kelvin FM, Chernish SM: Primary malignant tumors in the small bowel: A comparison of the small-bowel enema and conventional follow-through examination. AJR 153:741-744, 1989.

7. Kettritz U, Shoenut JP, Semelka RC: MR imaging of the gastrointestinal tract. Magn Reson Imaging Clin North Am 3:87-98, 1995.

8. Boudiaf M, Jaff A, Soyer P, et al: Small-bowel diseases: Prospective evaluation of multi-detector row helical CT enteroclysis in 107 consecutive patients. Radiology 233:338-344, 2004.

9. Romano S, De LE, Rollandi GA, et al: Multidetector computed tomography enteroclysis (MDCT-E) with neutral enteral and IV contrast enhancement in tumor detection. Eur Radiol 15:1178-1183, 2005.

10. Delaunoit T, Neczyporenko F, Limburg PJ, Erlichman C: Pathogenesis and risk factors of small bowel adenocarcinoma: A colorectal cancer sibling? Am J Gastroenterol 100:703-710, 2005.

11. Frost DB, Mercado PD, Tyrell JS: Small bowel cancer: A 30-year review. Ann Surg Oncol 1:290-295, 1994.

12. Green PH, Fleischauer AT, Bhagat G, et al: Risk of malignancy in patients with celiac disease. Am J Med 115:191-195, 2003.

13. Bernstein D, Rogers A: Malignancy in Crohn's disease. Am J Gastroenterol 91:434-440, 1996.

14. Palascak-Juif V, Bouvier AM, Cosnes J, et al: Small bowel adenocarcinoma in patients with Crohn's disease compared with small bowel adenocarcinoma de novo. Inflamm Bowel Dis 11:828-832, 2005.

15. McGarrity TJ, Kulin HE, Zaino RJ: Peutz-Jeghers syndrome. Am J Gastroenterol 95:596-604, 2000.

16. Schreibman IR, Baker M, Amos C, McGarrity TJ: The hamartomatous polyposis syndromes: A clinical and molecular review. Am J Gastroenterol 100:476-490, 2005.

17. Levine MS, Drooz AT, Herlinger H: Annular malignancies of the small bowel. Gastrointest Radiol 12:53-58, 1987.

18. Johnson AM, Harman PK, Hanks JB: Primary small bowel malignancies. Am Surg 51:31-36, 1985.

19. Modlin IM, Kidd M, Latich I, et al: Current status of gastrointestinal carcinoids. Gastroenterology 128:1717-1751, 2005.

20. Gore RM, Berlin JW, Mehta UK, et al: GI carcinoid tumours: Appearance of the primary and detecting metastases. Best Pract Res Clin Endocrinol Metab 19:245-263, 2005.

21. Lightdale C, Hornsby-Lewis L: Tumors of the small intestine. In Berk JE (ed): Bockus Gastroenterology. Philadelphia, WB Saunders, 1995, pp 1274-1290.

22. Hossain J, al-Mofleh I, Tandon R, Dhahada NM: Carcinoid syndrome without liver metastasis. Postgrad Med J 65:597-599, 1989.

23. Gore RM: Small bowel cancer: Clinical and pathologic features. Radiol Clin North Am 35:351-360, 1997.

24. Jeffree MA, Nolan DJ: Multiple ileal carcinoid tumours. Br J Radiol 60:402-403, 1987.

25. Sugimoto E, Lorelius LE, Eriksson B, Oberg K: Midgut carcinoid tumours: CT appearance. Acta Radiol 36:367-371, 1995.

26. Horton KM, Kamel I, Hofmann L, Fishman EK: Carcinoid tumors of the small bowel: A multitechnique imaging approach. AJR Am J Roentgenol 182:559-567, 2004.

27. Kim KW, Ha HK: MRI for small bowel diseases. Semin Ultrasound CT MR 24:387-402, 2003.

28. Bader TR, Semelka RC, Chiu VC, et al: MRI of carcinoid tumors: Spectrum of appearances in the gastrointestinal tract and liver. J Magn Reson Imaging 14:261-269, 2001.

29. Dromain C, de BT, Baudin E, et al: MR imaging of hepatic metastases caused by neuroendocrine tumors: Comparing four techniques. AJR 180:121-128, 2003.

30. Oberg K, Eriksson B: Nuclear medicine in the detection, staging and treatment of gastrointestinal carcinoid tumours. Best Pract Res Clin Endocrinol Metab 19:265-276, 2005.

31. Debas HT, Mulvihill SJ: Neuroendocrine gut neoplasms: Important lessons from uncommon tumors. Arch Surg 129:965-971, 1994.

32. Orlefors H, Sundin A, Garske U, et al: Whole-body (11)C-5-hydroxy-tryptophan positron emission tomography as a universal imaging technique for neuroendocrine tumors: Comparison with somatostatin receptor scintigraphy and computed tomography. J Clin Endocrinol Metab 90:3392-3400, 2005.

33. Moertel CG, Johnson CM, McKusick MA, et al: The management of patients with advanced carcinoid tumors and islet cell carcinomas. Ann Intern Med 120:302-309, 1994.

34. Sandrasegaran K, Rajesh A, Rydberg J, et al: Gastrointestinal stromal tumors: Clinical, radiologic, and pathologic features. AJR 184:803-811, 2005.

35. Suster S: Gastrointestinal stromal tumors. Semin Diagn Pathol 13:297-313, 1996.

36. Miettinen M, Lasota J: Gastrointestinal stromal tumors—definition, clinical, histological, immunohistochemical, and molecular genetic features and differential diagnosis. Virchows Arch 438:1-12, 2001.

37. Joensuu H, Fletcher C, Dimitrijevic S, et al: Management of malignant gastrointestinal stromal tumours. Lancet Oncol 3:655-664, 2002.

38. Rudolph P, Chiaravalli AM, Pauser U, et al: Gastrointestinal mesenchymal tumours—immunophenotypic classification and survival analysis. Virchows Arch 441:238-248, 2002.

39. Dematteo RP, Lewis JJ, Leung D, et al: Two hundred gastrointestinal stromal tumors: Recurrence patterns and prognostic factors for survival. Ann Surg 231:51-58, 2000.

40. Ng EH, Pollock RE, Munsell MF, et al: Prognostic factors influencing survival in gastrointestinal leiomyosarcomas: Implications for surgical management and staging. Ann Surg 215:68-77, 1992.

41. Dematteo RP: The GIST of targeted cancer therapy: A tumor (gastrointestinal stromal tumor), a mutated gene (c-kit), and a molecular inhibitor (STI571). Ann Surg Oncol 9:831-839, 2002.

42. Joensuu H, Fletcher C, Dimitrijevic S, et al: Management of malignant gastrointestinal stromal tumours. Lancet Oncol 3:655-664, 2002.

43. Berman J, O'Leary TJ: Gastrointestinal stromal tumor workshop. Hum Pathol 32:578-582, 2001.

44. Corless CL, Schroeder A, Griffith D, et al: PDGFRA mutations in gastrointestinal stromal tumors: Frequency, spectrum and in vitro sensitivity to imatinib. J Clin Oncol 23:5357-5364, 2005.

45. Pidhorecky I, Cheney RT, Kraybill WG, Gibbs JF: Gastrointestinal stromal tumors: Current diagnosis, biologic behavior, and management. Ann Surg Oncol 7:705-712, 2000.

46. Burkill GJ, Badran M, Al-Muderis O, et al: Malignant gastrointestinal stromal tumor: Distribution, imaging features, and pattern of metastatic spread. Radiology 226:527-532, 2003.

47. Sandrasegaran K, Rajesh A, Rushing DA, et al: Gastrointestinal stromal tumors: CT and MRI findings. Eur Radiol 15:1407-1414, 2005.

48. Dagher R, Cohen M, Williams G, et al: Approval summary: Imatinib mesylate in the treatment of metastatic and/or unresectable malignant gastrointestinal stromal tumors. Clin Cancer Res 8:3034-3038, 2002.

49. Chen MY, Bechtold RE, Savage PD: Cystic changes in hepatic metastases from gastrointestinal stromal tumors (GISTs) treated with Gleevec (imatinib mesylate). AJR 179:1059-1062, 2002.

50. Choi H, Charnsangavej C, de Castro FS, et al: CT evaluation of the response of gastrointestinal stromal tumors after imatinib mesylate treatment: A quantitative analysis correlated with FDG PET findings. AJR 183:1619-1628, 2004.

51. Shankar S, van Sonnenberg E, Desai J, et al: Gastrointestinal stromal tumor: New nodule-within-a-mass pattern of recurrence after partial response to imatinib mesylate. Radiology 235:892-898, 2005.

52. Goerres GW, Stupp R, Barghouth G, et al: The value of PET, CT and in-line PET/CT in patients with gastrointestinal stromal tumours: Long-term outcome of treatment with imatinib mesylate. Eur J Nucl Med Mol Imaging 32:153-162, 2005.

53. Gayed I, Vu T, Iyer R, et al: The role of ^{18}F-FDG PET in staging and early prediction of response to therapy of recurrent gastrointestinal stromal tumors. J Nucl Med 45:17-21, 2004.

54. Crosby JA, Catton CN, Davis A, et al: Malignant gastrointestinal stromal tumors of the small intestine: A review of 50 cases from a prospective database. Ann Surg Oncol 8:50-59, 2001.

55. Ludwig DJ, Traverso LW: Gut stromal tumors and their clinical behavior. Am J Surg 173:390-394, 1997.

56. Plaat BE, Hollema H, Molenaar WM, et al: Soft tissue leiomyosarcomas and malignant gastrointestinal stromal tumors: Differences in clinical outcome and expression of multidrug resistance proteins. J Clin Oncol 18:3211-3220, 2000.

57. Conlon KC, Casper ES, Brennan MF: Primary gastrointestinal sarcomas: Analysis of prognostic variables. Ann Surg Oncol 2:26-31, 1995.

58. van der Zwan SM, Dematteo RP: Gastrointestinal stromal tumor: 5 years later. Cancer 104:1781-1788, 2005.

59. Chen LL, Sabripour M, Andtbacka RH, et al: Imatinib resistance in gastrointestinal stromal tumors. Curr Oncol Rep 7:293-299, 2005.

60. Liang R, Todd D, Chan TK, et al: Prognostic factors for primary gastrointestinal lymphoma. Hematol Oncol 13:153-163, 1995.

61. d'Amore F, Brincker H, Gronbaek K, et al: Non-Hodgkin's lymphoma of the gastrointestinal tract: A population-based analysis of incidence, geographic distribution, clinicopathologic presentation features, and prognosis. Danish Lymphoma Study Group. J Clin Oncol 12:1673-1684, 1994.

62. Gill SS, Heuman DM, Mihas AA: Small intestinal neoplasms. J Clin Gastroenterol 33:267-282, 2001.

63. Domizio P, Owen RA, Shepherd NA, et al: Primary lymphoma of the small intestine: A clinicopathological study of 119 cases. Am J Surg Pathol 17:429-442, 1993.

64. Marshak RH, Lindner AE, Maklansky D: Lymphoreticular disorders of the gastrointestinal tract: Roentgenographic features. Gastrointest Radiol 4:103-120, 1979.

65. Rubesin SE, Gilchrist AM, Bronner M, et al: Non-Hodgkin lymphoma of the small intestine. RadioGraphics 10:985-998, 1990.

66. Baildam AD, Williams GT, Schofield PF: Abdominal lymphoma—the place for surgery. J R Soc Med 82:657-660, 1989.

67. Moynihan MJ, Bast MA, Chan WC, et al: Lymphomatous polyposis: A neoplasm of either follicular mantle or germinal center cell origin. Am J Surg Pathol 20:442-452, 1996.

68. Vignote ML, Chicano M, Rodriguez FJ, et al: Multiple lymphomatous polyposis of the GI tract: Report of a case and review. Gastrointest Endosc 56:579-582, 2002.

69. Fishman EK, Kuhlman JE, Jones RJ: CT of lymphoma: Spectrum of disease. RadioGraphics 11:647-669, 1991.

70. Chou CK, Chen LT, Sheu RS, et al: MRI manifestations of gastrointestinal lymphoma. Abdom Imaging 19:495-500, 1994.

71. Goerg C, Schwerk WB, Goerg K: Gastrointestinal lymphoma: Sonographic findings in 54 patients. AJR 155:795-798, 1990.

72. Kumar R, Xiu Y, Potenta S, et al: ^{18}F-FDG PET for evaluation of the treatment response in patients with gastrointestinal tract lymphomas. J Nucl Med 45:1796-1803, 2004.

73. Fine KD, Stone MJ: Alpha-heavy chain disease, Mediterranean lymphoma, and immunoproliferative small intestinal disease: A review of clinicopathological features, pathogenesis, and differential diagnosis. Am J Gastroenterol 94:1139-1152, 1999.

74. Witzig TE, Wahner-Roedler DL: Heavy chain disease. Curr Treat Options Oncol 3:247-254, 2002.

75. O'Keefe SJ, Winter TA, Newton KA, et al: Severe malnutrition associated with alpha-heavy chain disease: Response to tetracycline and intensive nutritional support. Am J Gastroenterol 83:995-1001, 1988.

76. Castellino RA, Blank N, Hoppe RT, Cho C: Hodgkin disease: Contributions of chest CT in the initial staging evaluation. Radiology 160:603-605, 1986.

77. Oliphant M, Berne AS, Meyers MA: Imaging the direct bidirectional spread of disease between the abdomen and the female pelvis via the subperitoneal space. Gastrointest Radiol 13:285-298, 1988.

78. Bender GN, Maglinte DD, McLarney JH, et al: Malignant melanoma: Patterns of metastasis to the small bowel, reliability of imaging studies, and clinical relevance. Am J Gastroenterol 96:2392-2400, 2001.

Small Bowel Obstruction

Stephen E. Rubesin, MD • Richard M. Gore, MD

Many of the diseases causing small bowel obstruction are described and illustrated in detail in other chapters. The purpose of this chapter is to provide a working classification for patients with small bowel obstruction. This chapter not only describes the causes of small bowel obstruction (Table 50-1) but also presents an overall radiologic approach for the diagnostic work-up of patients with suspected small bowel obstruction. Specific imaging studies used to evaluate these patients are described in detail in Chapters 41 to 44.

DEFINITIONS

Small bowel obstruction is a condition not a disease. The term *small bowel obstruction* does not indicate the cause or degree of obstruction. The term *ileus* comes from the Greek, variably meaning "to twist up," "to wrap," or "to roll up,"[1] implying that a patient is "rolled up" in discomfort. The term *ileus* also means that the bowel lumen is dilated, but it must have a qualifier before it implies either neuromuscular-based dilatation or mechanical obstruction. *Functional ileus, paralytic ileus, functional obstruction,* and *adynamic ileus* are equivalent terms implying that the bowel is dilated because there is abnormal intestinal motility that prevents succus entericus from progressing along the gastrointestinal tract. Common causes of adynamic ileus include drugs that alter bowel motility (e.g., narcotics), recent abdominal surgery, intestinal ischemia, peritonitis, neuromuscular disorders (e.g., scleroderma), and endocrine disturbances (e.g., diabetes or hypothyroidism). If succus entericus cannot progress through the small bowel because the lumen is mechanically obstructed, the terms *small bowel obstruction, mechanical ileus,* or *mechanical obstruction* can be used. To avoid confusion, we prefer to use two distinct terms, *adynamic ileus* and *small bowel obstruction,* for describing these conditions.

Simple obstruction implies that the lumen is partially or completely occluded but that blood flow is preserved. *Strangulation* or *strangulated obstruction* means that blood flow is compromised, leading to bowel wall edema, intestinal ischemia, and, eventually, necrosis and perforation. A simple obstruction can be *complete* (i.e., no fluid or gas passes beyond the site of obstruction) or *incomplete* (i.e., some fluid or gas does pass beyond the site of obstruction). In *open-loop obstruction,* intestinal flow is blocked distally but proximal loops are open and can be decompressed by vomiting or nasogastric intubation. In *closed-loop obstruction,* flow into and out of the closed loop is blocked, resulting in progressive accumulation of fluid and gas within this loop.

PATHOPHYSIOLOGY

After food has been digested in the stomach and duodenum, most of the contents entering the jejunum are in a fluid state. If the neuromuscular function of the bowel is preserved, a large degree of luminal narrowing is needed to produce obstruction. Narrowing may be caused by abrupt angulation, kinking, or compression of the lumen by extrinsic disease; circumferential compromise of the lumen by intrinsic disease; intussusception; and obturation by intraluminal contents.

A series of physiologic factors leads to progressive accumulation of fluid in obstructed small bowel loops. Elevated intraluminal pressures stimulate secretion of water and electrolytes into the lumen.[2] Release of hormones such as vasoactive intestinal polypeptide (VIP) and various prostaglandins stimulates epithelial secretion and inhibits fluid resorption.[3,4]

Table 50-1
Small Bowel Obstruction In Adults

Extrinsic Lesions
Adhesions
Hernias
  External
    Inguinal
    Femoral
    Obturator
    Sciatic
    Perineal
    Supravesical
    Spigelian
    Lumbar
    Incisional
    Umbilical
  Internal
    Paraduodenal
    Epiploic foramen
    Diaphragmatic (traumatic)
    Transomental
    Transmesenteric
    Iliac fossa
Extrinsic tumors in mesentery
    Lymphoma
    Peritoneal metastases
    Carcinoid
    Desmoid
Abscess
    Diverticulitis
    Pelvic inflammatory disease
    Crohn's disease
Aneurysm
Hematoma
Endometriosis
Congenital
    Annular pancreas
    Ladd's bands

Intramural Lesions
Tumors infiltrating small bowel wall
    Adenocarcinoma
    Carcinoid tumor
    Lymphoma (rare)
    Gastrointestinal stromal tumors (rare)
Inflammatory conditions
    Crohn's disease
    Tuberculosis
    Potassium chloride or nonsteroidal anti-inflammatory
        drug-induced stricture
    Eosinophilic gastroenteritis
Vascular
    Radiation enteropathy
    Ischemia
Hematoma
    Post-traumatic hematoma
    Thrombocytopenia
    Anticoagulants
    Henoch-Schönlein purpura
Congenital
    Atresia, stricture, stenosis
    Duplication
    Meckel's diverticulum

Intraluminal Causes
Obturation
Gallstone
Bezoar
Foreign body
Ascaris
Meconium (cystic fibrosis)
Intussuscepting tumor
Inverted Meckel's diverticulum

Enzymatic breakdown of intraluminal contents increases the osmolality of intraluminal contents, also drawing more fluid into the lumen.

Intraluminal pressures are higher with closed-loop obstruction than with open-loop obstruction.[2] This leads to even further secretion of fluid into the closed loop. High intraluminal pressures eventually exceed venous pressures and even capillary pressures. Loss of blood flow leads to the potential cascade of small bowel ischemia, necrosis, and perforation. Stasis in closed-loop obstruction also leads to bacterial overgrowth. Subsequent bacterial invasion of the bowel leads to further edema and inflammation, and release of bacterial toxins into the circulation leads to shock.[2]

In open-loop obstruction involving the proximal small intestine, vomiting or intubation leads to loss of gastric, pancreatic, and biliary secretions. Loss of electrolytes in these secretions results in dehydration, metabolic alkalosis, hypochloremia, hypokalemia, and hyponatremia. Only minor changes in fluids and electrolytes are seen with open-loop obstruction involving the distal small bowel because less fluid is lost.

CLINICAL PRESENTATION

Open-loop obstruction of the proximal small bowel is characterized by frequent, large volume, often bilious vomiting.[2] Abdominal pain is intense but is often relieved by further vomiting. Abdominal distention and tenderness are minimal because the small bowel is decompressed by vomiting.

In open-loop obstruction of the distal small bowel, fluid fills distensible small bowel loops. As a result, vomiting is less frequent and of lower volume. Abdominal distention is moderate to marked.

In closed-loop obstruction, reflex vomiting may be present, even if the obstruction is distal. Abdominal distention is often absent. Abdominal pain is progressive and may worsen rapidly if intestinal ischemia progresses to infarction and perforation.

CLASSIFICATION

Extrinsic Lesions

Adhesions

Adhesions are the most common cause of small bowel obstruction, accounting for about two thirds of cases.[5,6] Most adhesions form after abdominal surgery. Ten percent to 15% of adhesions are attributed to prior or concurrent inflammation.[6] A small fraction of adhesions are thought to be congenital. Although adhesions form in more than 90% of patients who have undergone laparotomy, only 5% of these patients develop an adhesive obstruction.[5,7]

Less than 1% of patients develop small bowel obstruction during the immediate postoperative period. About 90% of these early postoperative obstructions are caused by adhesions, 7% by hernias, and the remainder by abscesses or intussusception.[8,9]

The most important radiographic finding in the diagnosis of small bowel obstruction is an abrupt transition from dilated to nondilated small intestine at the site of obstruction. On barium studies, a sharp, straight, or curved edge is seen where the adhesive band crosses the bowel lumen (Fig. 50-1). The

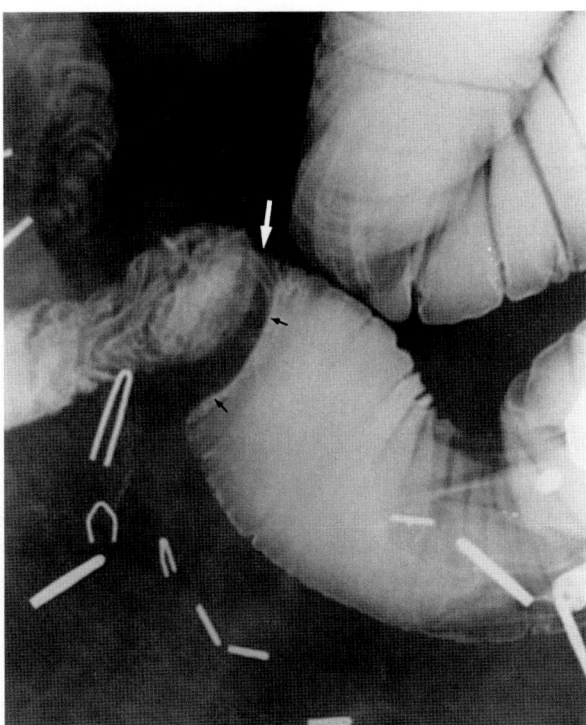

Figure 50-1. Partial small bowel obstruction by an adhesive band. Spot radiograph from enteroclysis shows a long, linear lucency (*black arrows*) representing an adhesive band crossing the ileum. The ileum is focally narrowed (*white arrow*) by the band. Note preservation of small bowel folds (*white arrow*) in the area of narrowing with dilated bowel proximally and collapsed bowel distally.

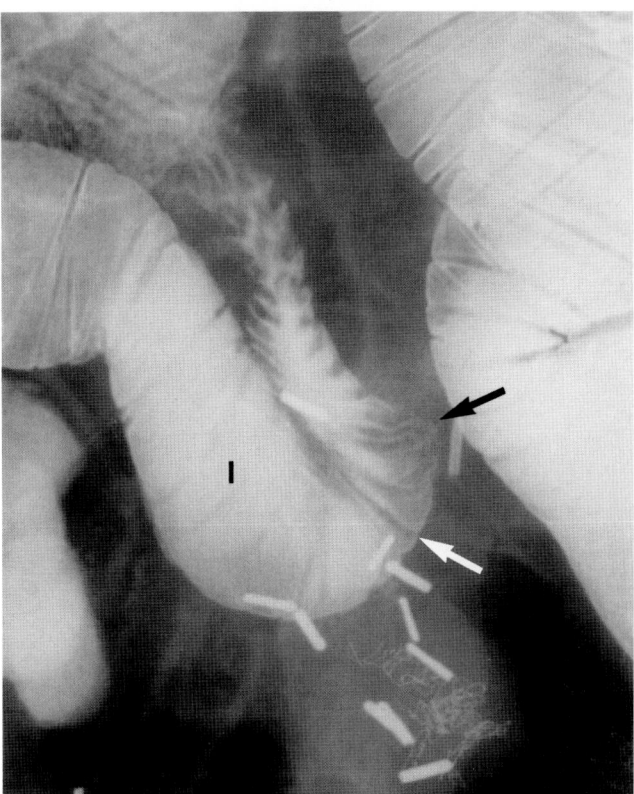

Figure 50-2. Partial small bowel obstruction by an adhesive band. Spot radiograph from enteroclysis shows a thin radiolucent band (*white arrow*) crossing the lumen of the ileum. The folds are tethered by the adhesive process (*black arrow*). The ileum (I) proximal to the band is dilated.

adhesion itself may be manifested by a narrow, bandlike radiolucency crossing the lumen between dilated proximal and collapsed distal small bowel loops (see Fig. 50-1). The bowel may be angulated toward the adhesion (Fig. 50-2), and smooth, thin folds may be tethered toward the extraluminal adhesive process. The bowel may be completely cut off with a rounded, beaklike or sharp edge (Figs. 50-3 and 50-4). Small

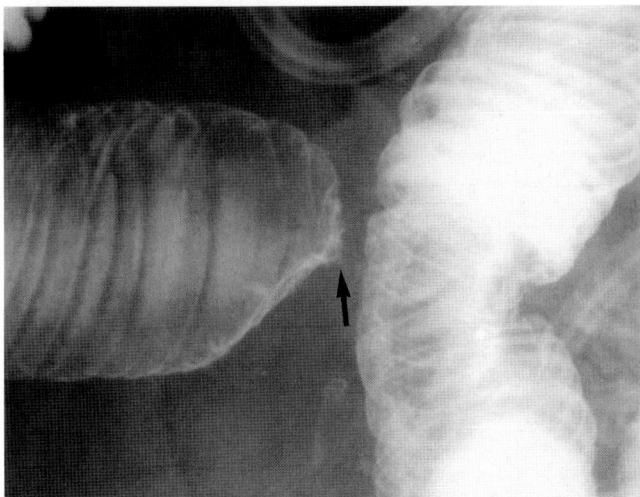

Figure 50-3. Adhesion causing complete small bowel obstruction. Abrupt beaklike narrowing (*arrow*) represents the site of an adhesion completely obstructing the mid small bowel. (From the teaching files of Hans Herlinger, MD.)

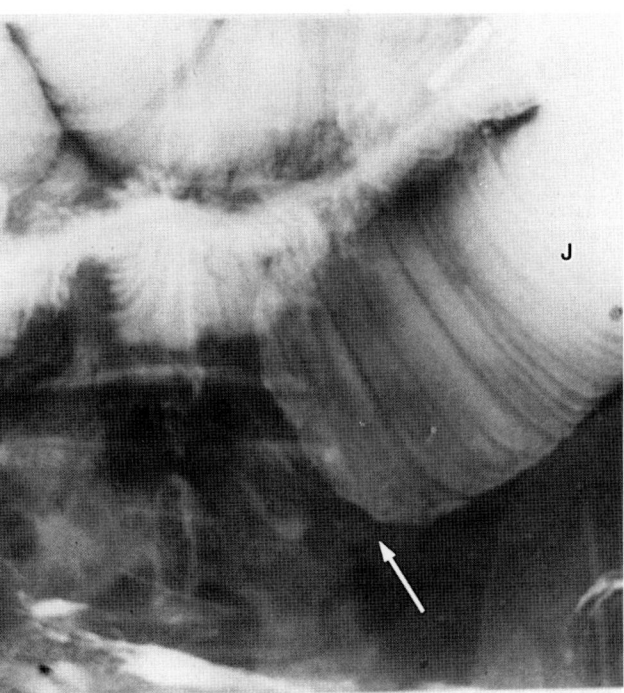

Figure 50-4. Adhesion causing near-complete small bowel obstruction. The lumen of the small bowel is abruptly cut off (*arrow*). Folds are preserved in the jejunum (J) proximal to the adhesion.

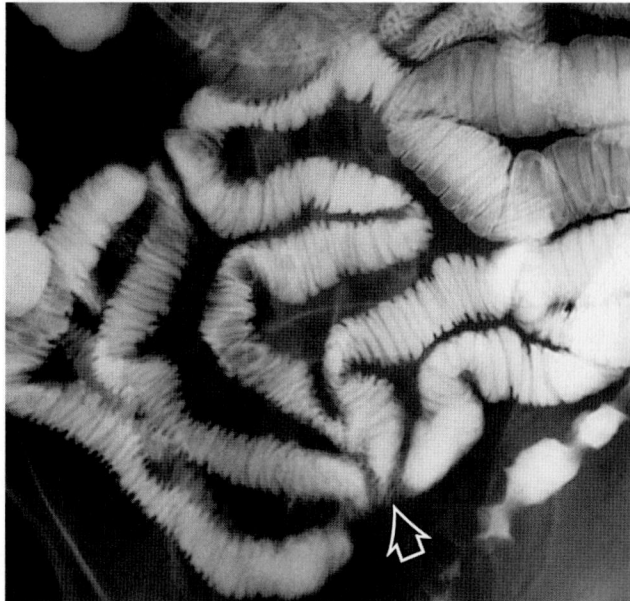

Figure 50-5. Fixation of loops at adhesive site. Spot radiograph from enteroclysis shows three loops of intestine pulled toward the site of an adhesion (*arrow*). The loops could not be separated by manual palpation at fluoroscopy.

bowel folds are preserved, and no mucosal nodularity or mass is present. Several loops may be pulled toward the site of the adhesions (Fig. 50-5). Multiple bands (Fig. 50-6) or extensive adhesions may be present. Multiple bands are often associated with scar formation along the anterior abdominal wall at prior incision sites. Extensive adhesions are often caused by previous intra-abdominal inflammatory processes

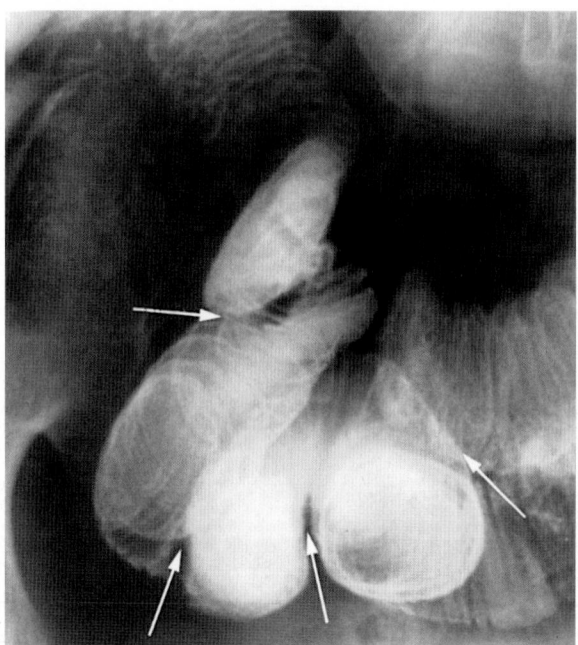

Figure 50-6. Multiple adhesive bands causing low-grade small bowel obstruction. Spot radiograph from enteroclysis shows four linear radiolucent bands (*arrows*) crossing two loops of ileum. The normal shape of the loops is disrupted. A lateral view (not shown) showed adhesions extending from the anterior abdominal wall.

such as traumatic perforation, peritonitis, and postoperative abscesses.

Adhesions are not usually seen on CT. As a result, there is an abrupt transition from dilated to collapsed small intestine without an apparent cause (Fig. 50-7).[10] The transition zone may appear rounded or beaklike (Fig. 50-8).[11,12] Thus, adhesive obstruction is a diagnosis of exclusion on CT; an adhesion is thought to be present when no other cause for small bowel obstruction can be identified. The cause of the transition zone also may not be apparent on CT in patients with small primary tumors (e.g., carcinoid tumors) or intraperitoneal metastases and in patients with short inflammatory, ischemic, or drug-related strictures.[10] However, the diagnosis of adhesive

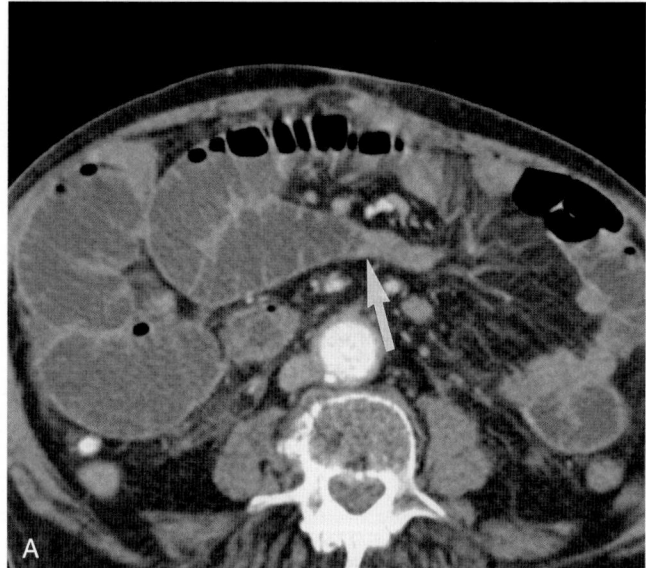

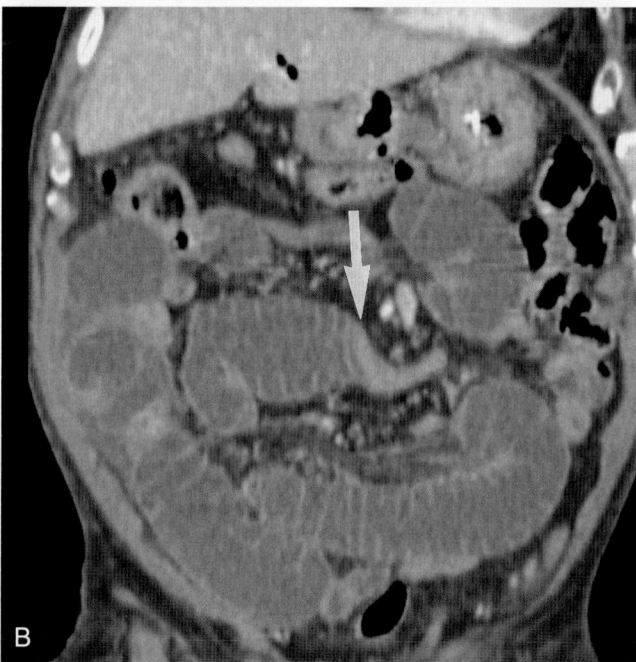

Figure 50-7. CT of small bowel obstruction due to adhesions. Axial (**A**) and coronal multiplanar reconstruction (**B**) images show dilated, fluid-filled small bowel to the level of an adhesion in the distal jejunum. Note the abrupt transition (*arrow*) between dilated small bowel proximal to the site of obstruction and collapsed small bowel distally. (Courtesy of Jay P. Heiken, MD, St. Louis, MO.)

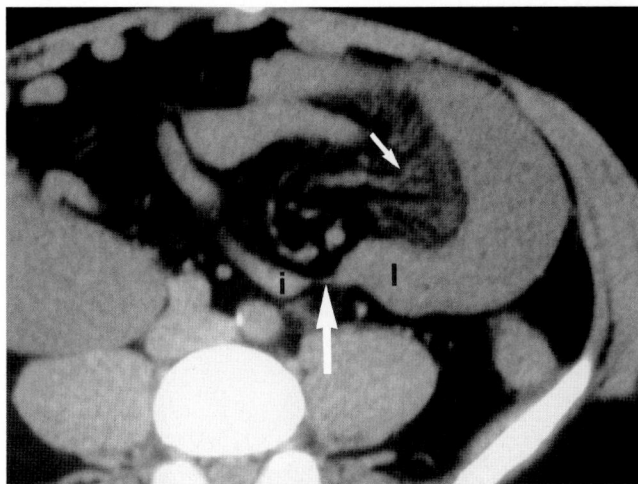

Figure 50-8. CT of small bowel obstruction due to an adhesion. Axial image shows tapered, beaklike narrowing (*large arrow*) at the transition zone between dilated ileum (I) proximally and collapsed ileum (i) distally. Vessels in the small bowel mesentery are engorged (*small arrow*). (Courtesy of Jay P. Heiken, MD, St. Louis, MO.)

obstruction on CT is supported by a history of prior laparotomy in the absence of known tumor with a predilection for intraperitoneal spread (e.g., ovarian carcinoma) or a known history of inflammatory bowel disease. The CT diagnosis of adhesions has been found to be accurate in 70% to 95% of patients.[12-18]

Closed-Loop Obstruction and Strangulation

The most common causes of closed-loop obstruction are single adhesive bands, internal or external hernias, and rents in the mesentery.[19] The trapped small bowel loop or loops become progressively dilated and fluid filled. The vessels feeding the trapped intestine may be compressed by the band or hernia opening or occluded by twisting of the mesentery; either process can lead to strangulation of the bowel. The risk of strangulation of the trapped loops depends on the duration and degree of compression or twisting.

The radiographic findings of a strangulated obstruction depend on the level of trapping and twisting (Fig. 50-9). Initially, the closed loop may not be dilated on CT. In the usual patient, however, the closed loop is considerably dilated and fluid filled and contains little or no intraluminal gas. If the closed loop or loops are parallel to the plane of reconstruction on CT, they may have a C-shaped or U-shaped configuration (Fig. 50-10).[20,21] If the loops are perpendicular to the plane of reconstruction they have a radial configuration, with the trapped mesentery pointing toward the band or hernial opening. The loops that enter and exit the closed loop lie side by side and are narrowed or tapered at the level of the band or mesenteric rent.[22] The entry and exit site may have a beaklike appearance when imaged in cross section. Small bowel proximal to the closed loop may also be dilated and fluid filled, whereas small bowel distal to the closed loop is collapsed. Mesenteric vessels are often seen radiating to the site of obstruction.

With a strangulated obstruction, there is a continuum from bowel wall edema to mild to moderate ischemia, transmural infarction, and, eventually, intestinal perforation. CT has a sensitivity of approximately 80% in the diagnosis of strangulation in closed-loop obstruction.[20] CT may reveal circumferential bowel wall thickening of low, normal, or high attenuation, indicating strangulation (Fig. 50-11). With the use of intravenous contrast material, wall thickening may show early enhancement, delayed enhancement,[23] or no enhancement.[24] On unenhanced CT scans, high-attenuation bowel wall thickening implies hemorrhage with ischemia. The absence of contrast enhancement is clear evidence of vascular obstruction.[24] A mural stratification pattern or *target sign* (with low attenuation of the submucosa reflecting submucosal edema) may indicate a spectrum of pathology ranging from bowel wall edema to full-thickness infarction (see Fig. 50-11). Pneumatosis in the wall of the closed loop indicates a rent in the mucosa associated with strangulation. Sloughed mucosa or debris in the lumen may have the appearance of feces. In general, CT cannot accurately predict viability of bowel (even if pneumatosis is present).[24] Air in the mesenteric veins or portal venous system, however, should be highly suggestive of nonviable bowel.

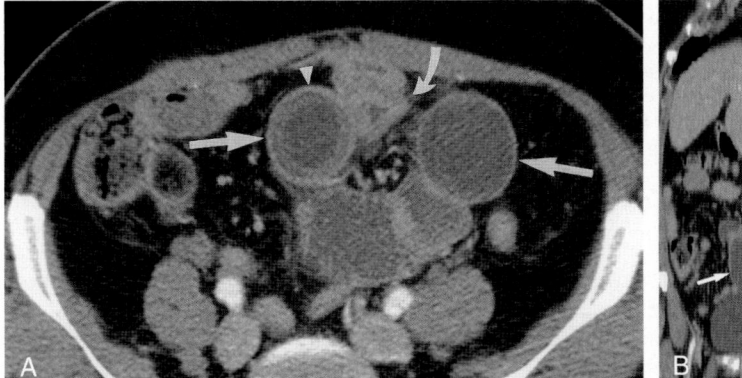
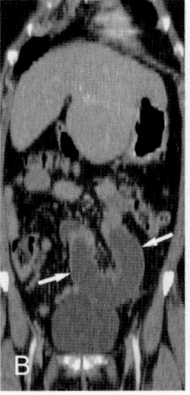
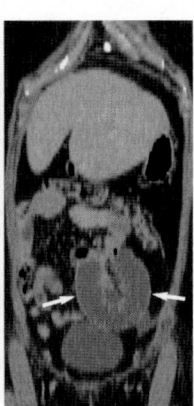

Figure 50-9. CT of closed-loop obstruction due to an internal hernia. A. Axial CT scan shows dilated, fluid-filled ileum (*straight arrows*) within the closed loop. Note the collapsed segments of bowel (*curved arrow*) where they enter the hernia sac. One loop has a thickened wall with a mural stratification pattern (*arrowhead*), indicating bowel wall edema/ischemia. **B.** Coronal images show the U shape of the obstructed closed loop (*arrows*).

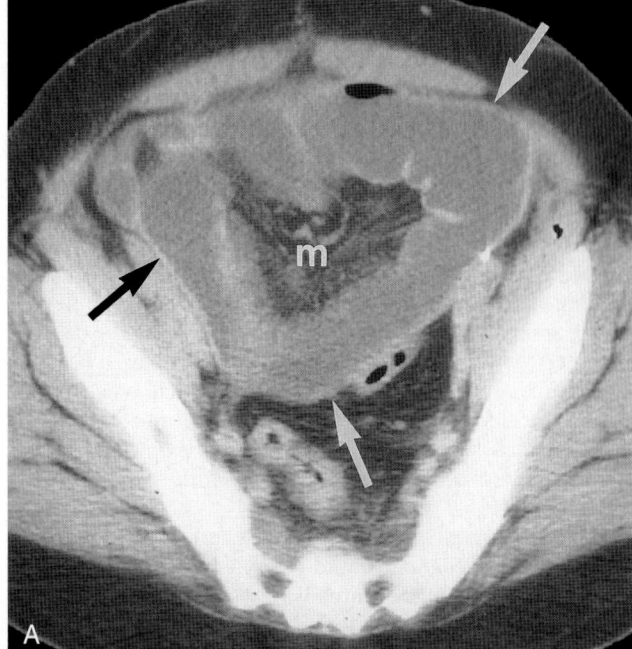

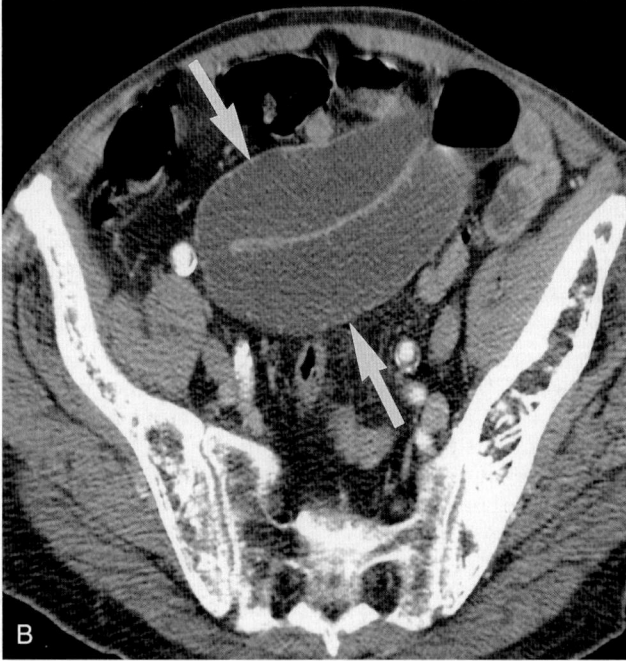

Figure 50-10. Closed-loop obstructions. A. U-shaped closed-loop obstruction (*arrows*). The small bowel mesentery (m) is engorged, but the wall of the involved bowel is not thickened or abnormally enhancing. **B.** C-shaped closed-loop obstruction (*arrows*). Focally dilated small bowel loops in a U-shaped (**A**) or C-shaped (**B**) configuration provide a clue that a closed-loop obstruction is present.

If the closed loop is twisted, its mesentery appears twisted or whirled.[25,26] Fluid in the leaves of the small bowel mesentery is not specific for ischemia, because intraperitoneal fluid is commonly seen in simple small bowel obstructions. However, strangulation is implied by haziness of the mesenteric fat and large mesenteric vessels, findings reflecting mesenteric edema and venous engorgement related to compression or twisting of mesenteric vessels.

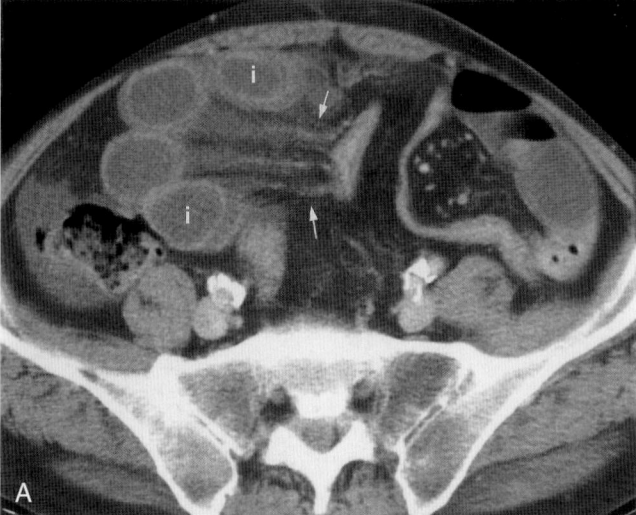

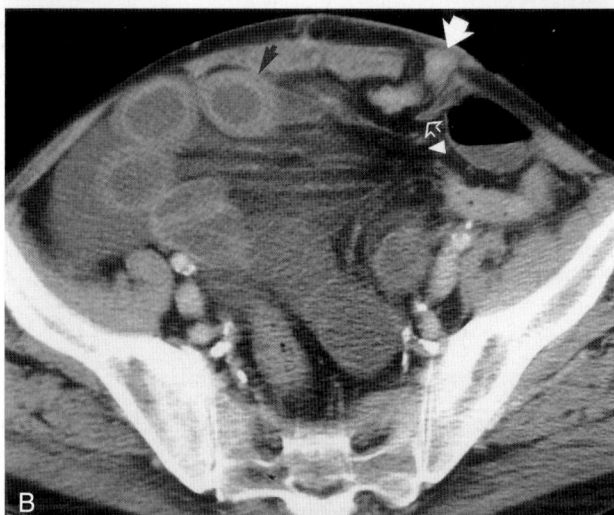

Figure 50-11. CT of Spigelian hernia resulting in a closed-loop obstruction with strangulation. A. Axial image through pelvis shows four loops of small bowel (between i and i) with their mesentery radiating toward the midline (*arrows*). Haziness of the small bowel mesentery results from vascular engorgement. **B.** Axial image just caudad to **A** shows the mesentery radiating toward the left anterior abdominal wall (*arrowhead*). The radially arranged bowel loops have a thickened wall with a mural stratification pattern (*black arrow*) indicative of submucosal edema due to ischemia. A loop of small bowel is trapped in a spigelian hernia (*closed arrow*) with twisting and angulation of the loop (*open arrow*) exiting the hernia, producing a small bowel volvulus with a closed-loop obstruction. At surgery, a twist of the loop exiting the Spigelian hernia was found to have caused irreversible small bowel ischemia.

Enteroclysis and small bowel follow-through studies should not be performed in patients with high-grade small bowel obstruction and suspected closed-loop obstruction. However, low-grade, partial closed-loop obstructions may occasionally be found on barium studies in less symptomatic patients (Fig. 50-12).[27,28] In such cases there is compression of the inflow and outflow limbs of small bowel, as the trapped loops course beneath the responsible band (see Fig. 50-12) or through the responsible hernia.[27,28] Volvulus is implied by twisting of folds at the site of obstruction. Smooth, thickened small bowel folds in a partially closed loop indicate bowel wall edema with possible ischemia.

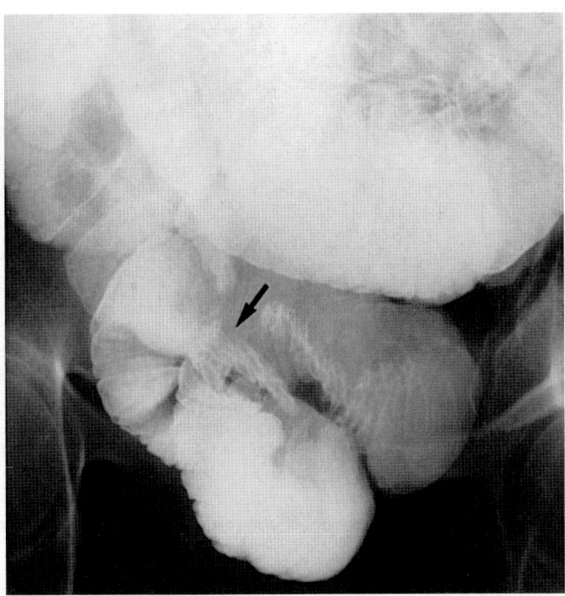

Figure 50-12. Partial closed-loop obstruction on enteroclysis. Two loops of small bowel are focally angulated and narrowed (*arrow*) where they pass beneath an adhesive band.

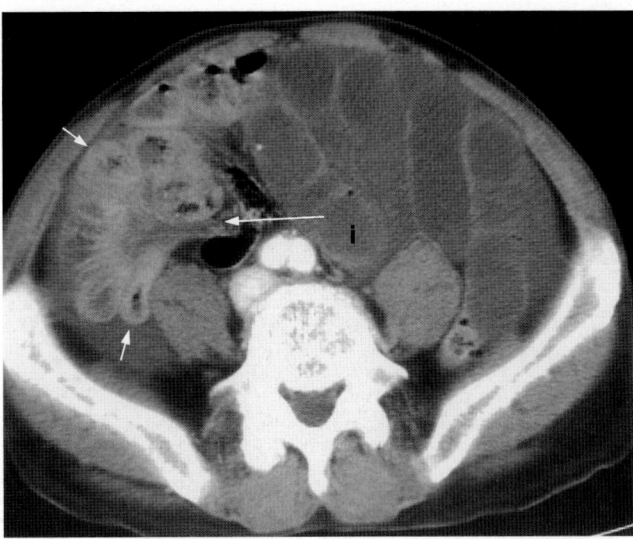

Figure 50-13. CT of internal hernia beneath an adhesive band. Several loops of small bowel are radially arranged (*short arrows*) toward the site of an adhesive band (*long arrow*). The herniated loops are collapsed and show intense enhancement. The ileum (i) proximal to the band is dilated. At surgery, irreversible ischemia of the herniated small bowel was found.

Hernias

Prior to the era of laparotomy, hernias were the most common cause of small bowel obstruction. There is a 5% to 10% lifetime risk of developing an anterior abdominal wall hernia.[2] These hernias are described in detail in Chapter 114.

The only skeletal support of the abdomen is the lowermost ribs, lumbar spine, sacrum, and pelvis. The viscera are held in the abdomen by muscles, aponeuroses, fascial layers, and peritoneum. The paired rectus abdominis muscles form the anterior muscular anchor of the abdomen, coursing from the xiphoid process and midline rib cage to the symphysis pubis. The external oblique muscles run in a posterosuperior to anteroinferior direction. Conversely, the internal oblique muscles run in a posteroinferior to anterosuperior direction at a near 90-degree angle to the external oblique muscles. The fibers of the transverses abdominis muscles course transversely. The joined aponeuroses of the external and internal oblique muscles and transversus abdominis muscles surround the rectus muscles and form the linea alba in the midline. Hernias occur at predictable sites of weakness in the abdominal wall, where there is only fascia and peritoneum between the viscera and skin. A wide variety of internal hernias occur at sites of mesenteric and omental weakness, at normal openings of the peritoneal surface, and beneath congenital or adhesive bands (Fig. 50-13).[29-32]

Complications of hernias include incarceration, obstruction, and strangulation. *Incarcerated hernias* are not reducible, usually because of adhesions in the hernia sac. Urgent treatment is not required, because incarceration is not equivalent to obstruction or strangulation. Incarceration is not a radiologic diagnosis, unless the fluoroscopist manually reduces the hernia (indicating that it is not incarcerated) or the hernia retracts with changes in the patient's position. When incarcerated hernias cause small bowel obstruction, the obstruction tends to be high grade or complete.[2] Strangulation is a serious, often life-threatening complication. Strangulated hernias are tense and irreducible.

Inguinal hernias comprise about 80% of anterior abdominal wall hernias, and femoral hernias comprise only about 5%.[2] Inguinal hernias are more common in men than in women (7:1), whereas femoral hernias are more common in women than in men (1.8:1).[33] Most patients with inguinal hernias have a patent processus vaginalis as the cause of the hernias. These hernias usually result from elevated abdominal pressures related to pregnancy, coughing, constipation, obesity, prostatism, or physical exertion. Inguinal hernias may also be caused by weakening of the muscular aponeurosis and fascia due to age, cigarette smoking, or collagen deficiency (e.g., Marfan's, Ehlers-Danlos, and Hunter-Hurler syndromes).[33]

Direct inguinal hernias occur at Hesselbach's triangle, bounded anterosuperiorly by the inguinal ligament, medially by the rectus abdominis muscle, and laterally by the inferior epigastric vessels that form the lateral umbilical fold. Herniations occur inferiorly, where this region is covered only by peritoneum and the transversalis fascia. *Indirect inguinal hernias* occur in the deep inguinal ring in a fossa bounded medially by the inferior epigastric vessels (Fig. 50-14). Because of this anatomy, indirect inguinal hernias occur lateral and direct inguinal hernias medial to the inferior epigastric vessels. Congenital indirect inguinal hernias enter a patent tunica vaginalis. The risk of a major complication in a patient with an inguinal hernia is low.

Weakness in the linea alba at the umbilicus leads to *umbilical/paraumbilical hernias* (Fig. 50-15). Most pediatric umbilical hernias close spontaneously, but persistent umbilical hernias require surgery.[2]

Epigastric hernias also occur in defects in the linea alba. These hernias are more frequent in men than in women. Multiple hernias are seen in 20% of patients. Epigastric hernias usually contain incarcerated preperitoneal fat but not a peritoneal sac. Gastric herniation is uncommon.

Complications in *parastomal hernias* are uncommon. However, peritoneal herniation develops in more than 50% of patients who have had a colostomy for 5 years or longer.

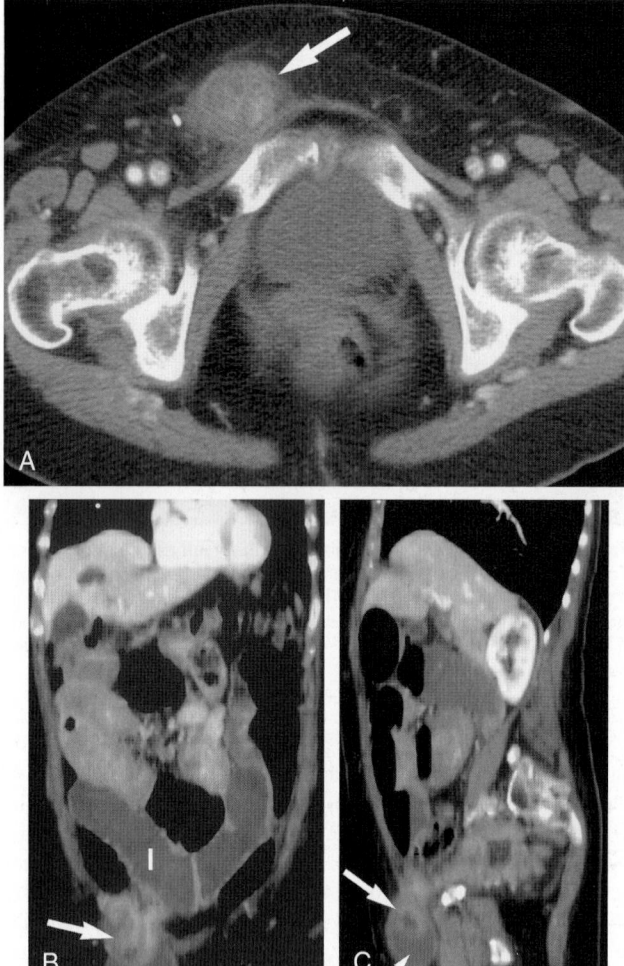

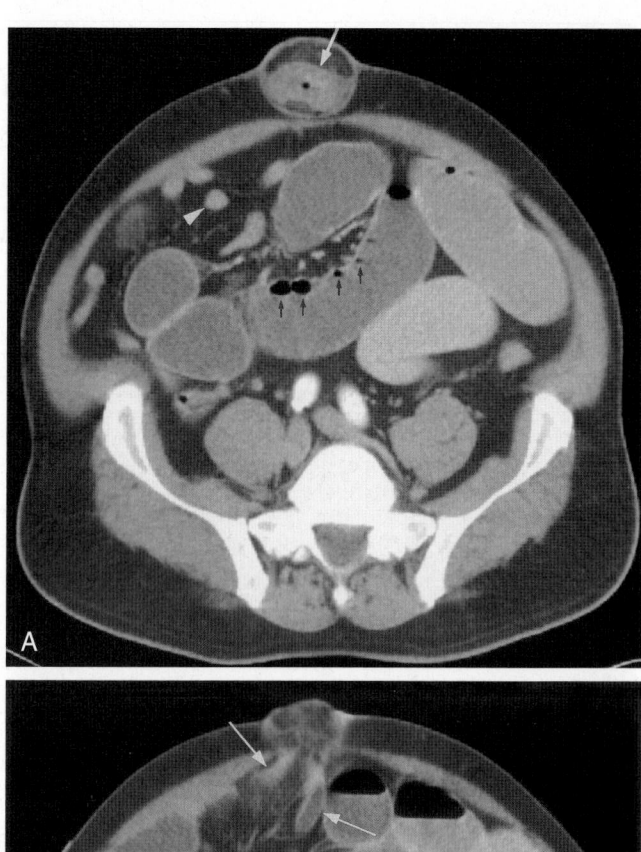

Figure 50-14. CT of inguinal hernia. A. Axial image through the level of the urinary bladder shows a right inguinal hernia (*arrow*). Coronal (**B**) and sagittal (**C**) multiplanar reconstructions show dilated, fluid-filled ileum (I) to the level of the hernia. Collapsed, hyperemic ileum (*long arrows*, **B** and **C**) enters the hernia sac. Also note fluid in the hernia sac (*short arrow*, **C**).

Spigelian hernias occur below the level of the semilunar line (line of Spigel). The aponeurosis of each internal oblique muscle splits above the semilunar line to surround the rectus abdominis muscle, with its posterior half joining the aponeurosis of the transversus abdominis muscle posterior to the ipsilateral rectus abdominis muscle. Below the line of Spigel, the aponeuroses of the external and internal oblique muscles and the transversus abdominis muscle pass anterior to the rectus abdominis muscle. Spigelian hernias occur below this transition point. These hernias are usually small (1 to 2 cm) and intraparietal, rarely penetrating the fascia of the external oblique muscles (Fig. 50-16). Spigelian hernias may contain omentum, small bowel, or colon. Incarceration and strangulation are common complications (see Fig. 50-11).

Richter's hernias are any hernias in which only one wall of a loop of bowel enters the hernia. The involved bowel wall may be ischemic or gangrenous.

The obturator foramen is covered by the obturator internus and externus muscles. A small superolateral corner of the obturator fossa is weakened at the site of penetration by the

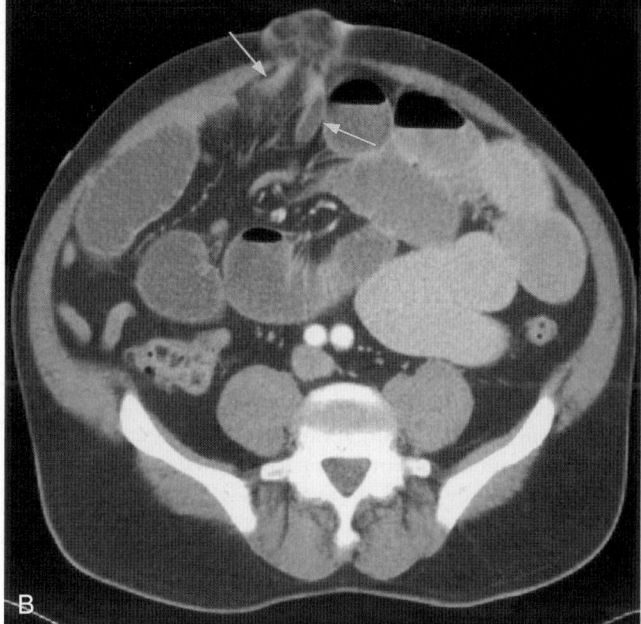

Figure 50-15. CT of umbilical hernia resulting in small bowel obstruction and strangulation. A. The umbilical hernia contains a loop of small bowel with a thickened wall (*white arrow*). The proximal small bowel is dilated and fluid filled. The CT equivalent of a *string of pearls* sign is present (*black arrows*) due to bubbles of gas trapping along the nondependent surface of a fluid-filled loop. Small bowel distal to the obstruction is collapsed (*arrowhead*). **B.** Axial image just caudal to **A** shows collapsed loops (*arrows*) entering and exiting the hernia. The fat in the umbilical hernia is engorged. At surgery, the ileum within the hernia sac showed irreversible ischemia.

obturator nerve and vessel. *Obturator hernias* can occur at this superolateral site (Fig. 50-17).

CT and barium studies may reveal smooth, tapered compression of the bowel loops entering and exiting the hernia, with the degree of narrowing determined by the width of the luminal opening.[33,34] Dilatation of small bowel proximal to the hernia indicates obstruction at the entry site due to com-

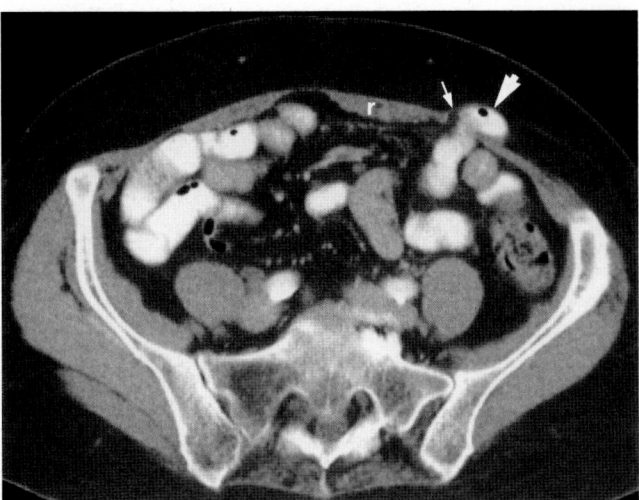

Figure 50-16. Intraparietal Spigelian hernia on CT. Axial CT shows a loop of ileum (*large arrow*) protruding just lateral to the left rectus sheath (r). The hernia is intraparietal, as it is covered by the fascia of the external oblique muscle *(small arrow)*.

pression, twisting, and/or narrowing of the bowel. Dilatation of loops with the hernia itself suggests obstruction at the outflow loop. The radiographic findings of strangulation are similar to those of adhesive obstruction. The sigmoid colon is usually found in a left inguinal hernia, and the distal ileum is in a right inguinal hernia (Fig. 50-18), although the cecum and appendix can also be drawn into a right inguinal hernia (see Fig. 50-18). Lateral or steep oblique views are extremely helpful for showing midline (Figs. 50-19 and 50-20) or obturator hernias on barium studies. Upright views or views obtained during a Valsalva maneuver are also helpful for showing pelvic hernias at fluoroscopy. Similarly, lateral views while the patient performs a Valsalva maneuver enable visualization of anterior abdominal wall hernias on CT.[35]

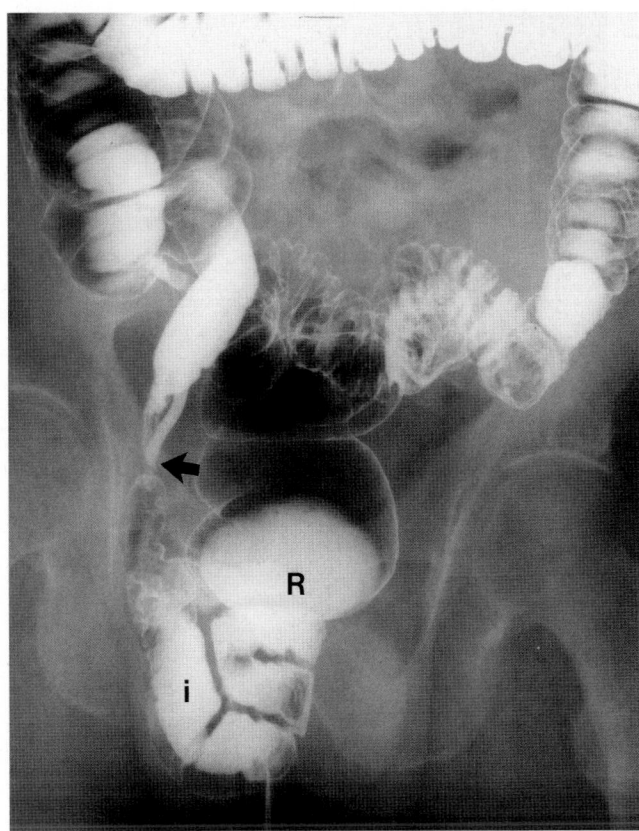

Figure 50-18. Right inguinal hernia containing ileum and appendix. Overhead radiograph from double-contrast barium enema shows loops of ileum (i) below and to the right of the rectal ampulla (R). The tip of the appendix (*arrow*) also enters the right inguinal canal. (From Forbes A, Misiewicz JJ, Compton CC, et al: Atlas of Clinical Gastroenterology, 3rd ed. Edinburgh, Elsevier Mosby, 2005.)

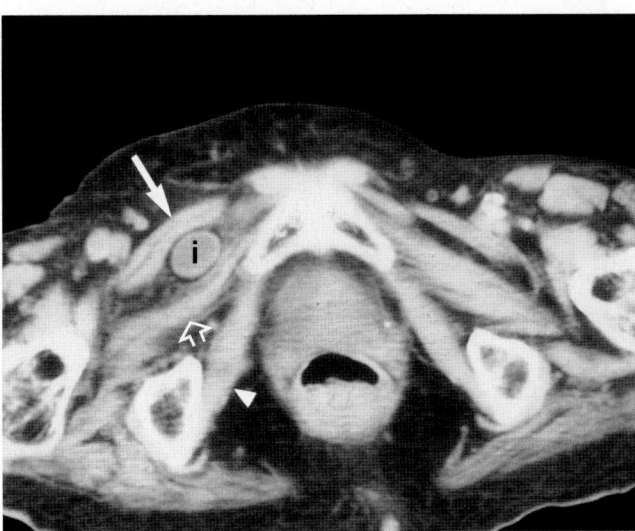

Figure 50-17. Obturator hernia on CT. Axial CT through pelvis shows a loop of ileum (i) between the pectineus muscle (*large arrow*) and the external obturator muscle (*open arrow*). The internal obturator muscle is identified by the *arrowhead*.

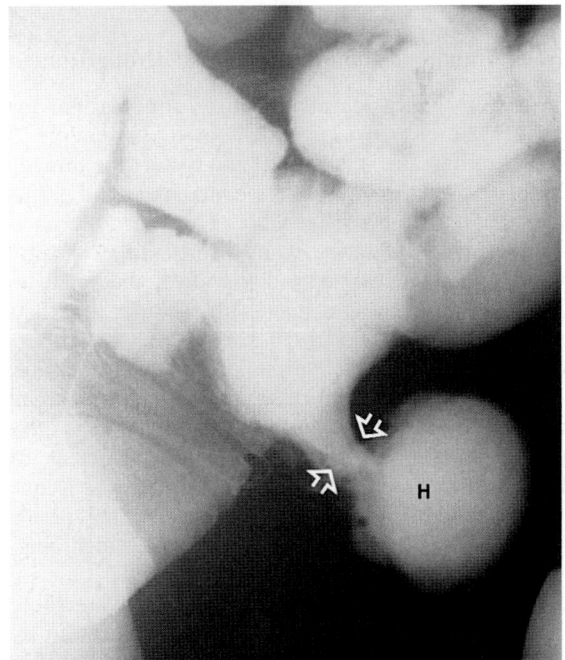

Figure 50-19. Anterior abdominal wall hernia causing high-grade small bowel obstruction. Steep left posterior oblique view from enteroclysis shows a loop small bowel (H) protruding beyond the contour of the anterior abdominal wall. The small bowel loops entering and exiting the hernia (*arrows*) are narrowed. This was a clinically unsuspected incisional hernia.

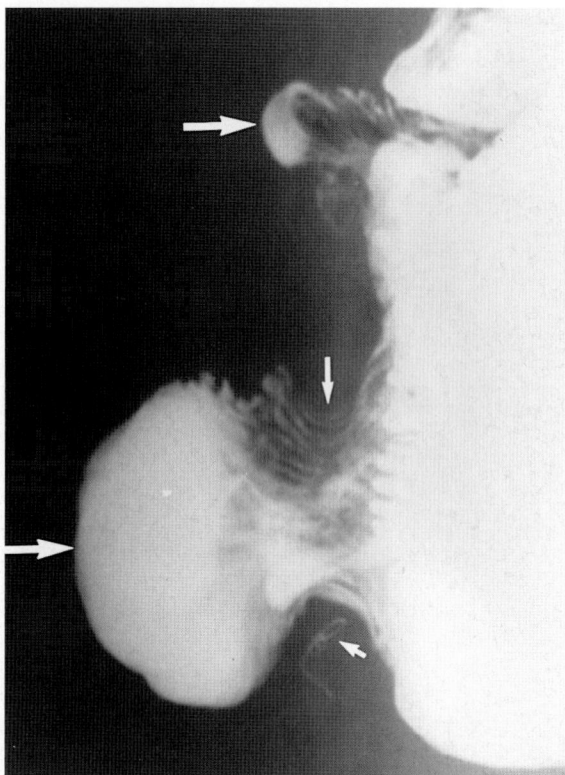

Figure 50-20. Incisional hernias detected on lateral view from small bowel follow-through. Spot radiograph from small bowel follow-through with the patient in a lateral position shows intestinal loops (*large arrows*) protruding beyond the expected contour of the anterior abdominal wall (identified by wire sutures—*small arrow*). Mild, smooth compression of the lower loop with preservation of normal folds (*mid-sized arrow*) is present at the neck of the lower hernia sac.

Extrinsic Tumors in the Mesentery or Retroperitoneum

A variety of neoplastic, inflammatory, and vascular masses extrinsic to bowel may cause small bowel obstruction. These masses compress the small bowel and distort the lumen by a desmoplastic reaction involving the mesentery and peritoneal surfaces of the bowel.

Spread of inflammation from diverticulitis (usually sigmoid diverticulitis) can secondarily affect the small bowel. The inflammatory process may cause an adynamic ileus or small bowel obstruction (Fig. 50-21).

Carcinomatosis involving the small bowel mesentery is most frequently caused by disseminated ovarian carcinoma in women and by carcinomas arising from organs adjacent to the peritoneum (including the stomach, pancreas, colon, and liver) in men and women. Carcinomatosis is frequently multifocal, occurring at dependent sites in the peritoneal cavity in which ascitic fluid accumulates (including the mesenteric border of the distal ileum, medial base of the cecum, sigmoid mesentery, pararectal fossae, and rectouterine or rectovesical space).[36] Carcinomatosis produces an extensive desmoplastic reaction, manifested by extrinsic mass effect (Fig. 50-22), angulation of small bowel loops (Fig. 50-23), luminal narrowing, and tethering of folds (Fig. 50-24) both on CT and barium studies.[37,38] CT may reveal underlying ascites, often with peritoneal implants on the surface of the liver, peritoneum, omentum, or mesentery. CT may also reveal

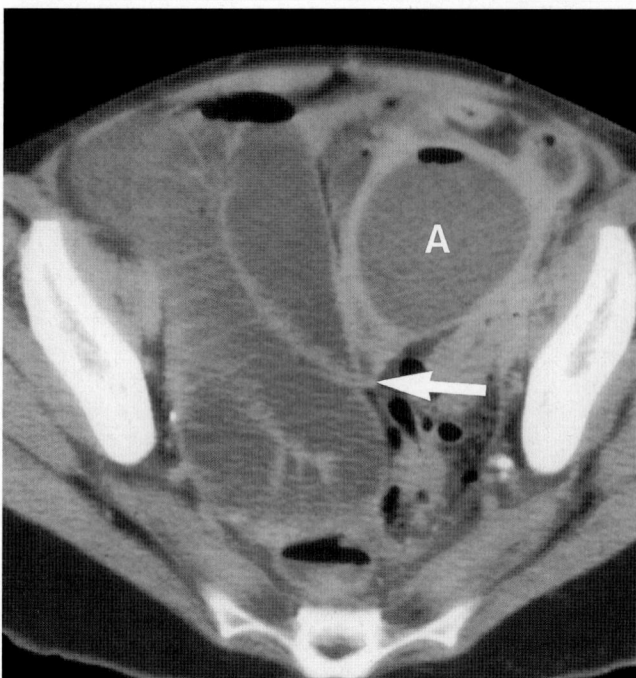

Figure 50-21. Diverticulitis causing small bowel obstruction. Axial CT through the pelvis shows a large, thick-walled abscess (A) containing fluid and an air bubble. The abscess was related to diverticulitis (not depicted on this image). There is dilatation of the pelvic ileum with beak-like narrowing (*arrow*) of an ileal loop at the site of obstruction.

the underlying malignant tumor responsible for the ascites. Carcinoid tumors, mycobacterial infection, and desmoid tumors can mimic intraperitoneal metastases. Metastases or lymphoma in retroperitoneal lymph nodes may secondarily extend into the root of the mesentery, causing small bowel obstruction. Retroperitoneal nodal invasion may also resemble

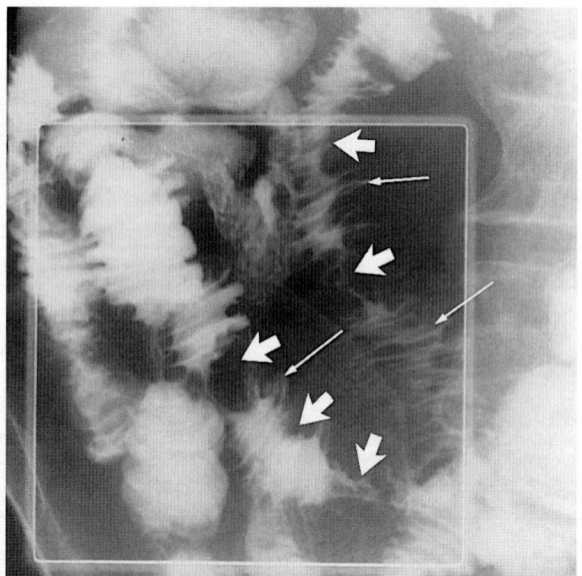

Figure 50-22. Intraperitoneal metastases from ovarian carcinoma. Multiple smooth-surfaced extrinsic masses indent the mesenteric border of the distal ileum (*short arrows*). Ileal folds (*long arrows*) are retracted toward the root of the small bowel mesentery.

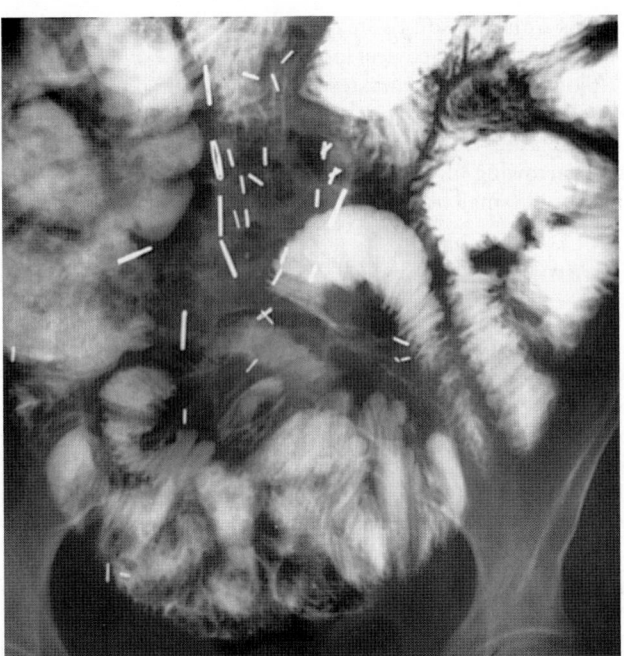

Figure 50-23. Intraperitoneal metastases from ovarian carcinoma. The entire pelvic ileum shows numerous kinked and angulated loops with extrinsic mass impressions and normal-sized folds tethered toward the mesentery. Identical radiographic findings may be caused by severe radiation damage, metastatic carcinoid tumor, and mesenteric fibrosis.

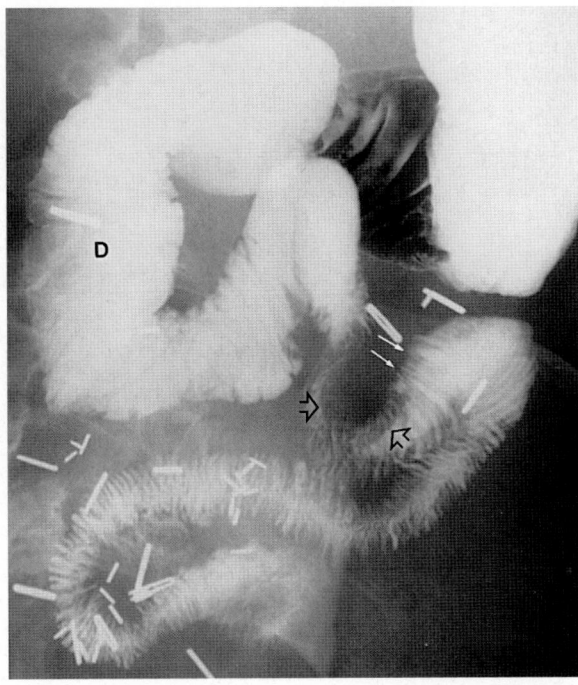

Figure 50-25. Retroperitoneal metastases from bladder cancer secondarily obstructing the jejunum. Overhead radiograph from small bowel follow-through shows an extrinsic mass impression (*open arrows*) and tethering of mucosal folds (*closed arrows*) just beyond the ligament of Trietz. Partial obstruction is manifested by duodenal dilatation (D). Retroperitoneal lymphadenopathy from transitional cell carcinoma of the bladder typically spreads through the root of the small bowel mesentery, causing obstruction of the proximal jejunum at or near the ligament of Treitz.

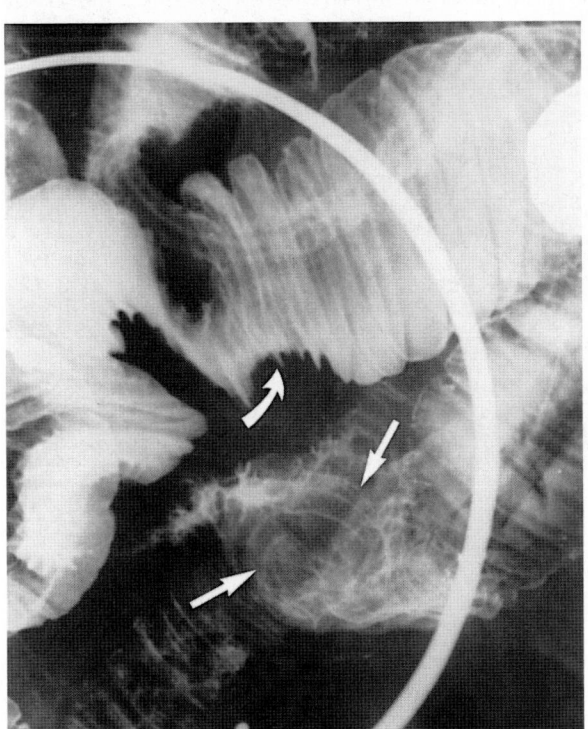

Figure 50-24. Intraperitoneal metastases from ovarian carcinoma. Spot radiograph from enteroclysis shows focal extrinsic mass effect and spiculation of the bowel contour (*curved arrow*) at the site of intraperitoneal implants. The adjacent small bowel is kinked and angulated. Tethered folds are seen en face (*straight arrows*) in a circular arrangement indicative of twisting at the site of the implants.

intraperitoneal metastases, with mass effect and desmoplastic tethering of the adjacent bowel (Fig. 50-25).

Small carcinoid tumors typically appear as smooth-surfaced submucosal masses of 1 to 2 cm in diameter.[37] Once carcinoid tumors have infiltrated the deep layers of the small bowel wall or the adjacent mesentery, however, they may be indistinguishable from intraperitoneal metastases on imaging studies. An intense desmoplastic reaction causes focal or multifocal angulation of the bowel wall, luminal narrowing, and tethering of mucosal folds toward the side of mass effect.[39] Invasive carcinoid tumors cannot be differentiated on barium studies from intraperitoneal metastases, because both diseases are located in the distal ileum and can be multifocal. However, CT demonstration of a large central mesenteric nodal metastasis (with calcification in 50%) is virtually diagnostic of a malignant carcinoid tumor (Fig. 50-26).[40]

Primary non-Hodgkin's lymphoma of the small bowel does not usually cause obstruction because it is a soft tumor that causes only mild luminal narrowing.[41] However, non-Hodgkin's lymphomas arising in mesenteric lymph nodes or extending from the retroperitoneum into the small bowel mesentery may cause small bowel obstruction due to tumor infiltration and luminal narrowing (Fig. 50-27).[41]

Enteric duplication cysts may compress the adjacent small bowel, causing obstruction. Duplication cysts are typically located on the mesenteric border of the distal ileum. As a result, barium studies may reveal an extrinsic mass impression on the adjacent ileum's mesenteric border. Communication with the lumen of the small bowel is uncommon. CT typically

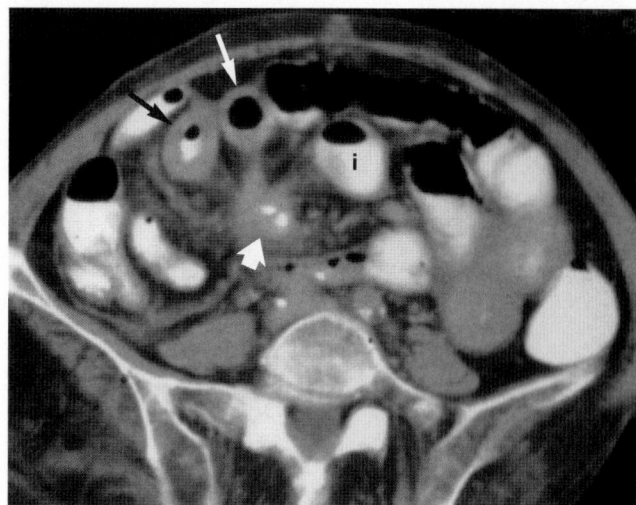

Figure 50-26. Carcinoid tumor causing partial obstruction and small bowel ischemia. Axial CT through pelvis shows dilated ileum (i) with contrast material in the colon, indicating partial small bowel obstruction. A centrally calcified mass (*short thick arrow*) is seen at the root of the small bowel mesentery. Thick strands of tumor radiate from the mass towards the ileum. Two ileal loops (*thin black and white arrows*) have uniformly thickened walls. These findings are characteristic of a carcinoid tumor involving the mesentery. At surgery, the carcinoid tumor had spread to the root of the small bowel mesentery, causing ischemic changes in adjacent ileal loops. (From Rubesin SE: Small bowel tumors. Contemp Diagn Radiol 27:1-6, 2004.)

reveals a mass of soft tissue or fluid density on the mesenteric border of the affected ileal loop.

Slowly leaking aneurysms of the abdominal aorta or iliac vessels or surgery for such aneurysms may also cause a severe desmoplastic reaction that can lead to marked distortion and narrowing of small bowel loops, causing partial or even high-grade small bowel obstruction.

Intramural Lesions

Intrinsic tumors or inflammatory processes that infiltrate the submucosa and muscularis propria may cause obstruction by narrowing the lumen of the affected small bowel. Marked circumferential luminal narrowing is necessary to obstruct the bowel because of the liquid contents of the small intestine. Such lesions include primary small bowel carcinoma, Crohn's disease, and radiation enteropathy. Polypoid lesions of the small bowel may also cause obstruction by intussusception.

Primary Tumors

Adenocarcinoma of the small bowel has a predilection for the second to fourth portions of the duodenum and proximal jejunum. When patients with small bowel carcinoma present with clinical signs of obstruction, these tumors are almost always at an advanced stage. Barium studies may reveal a short, annular segment of narrowing with abrupt, shelflike

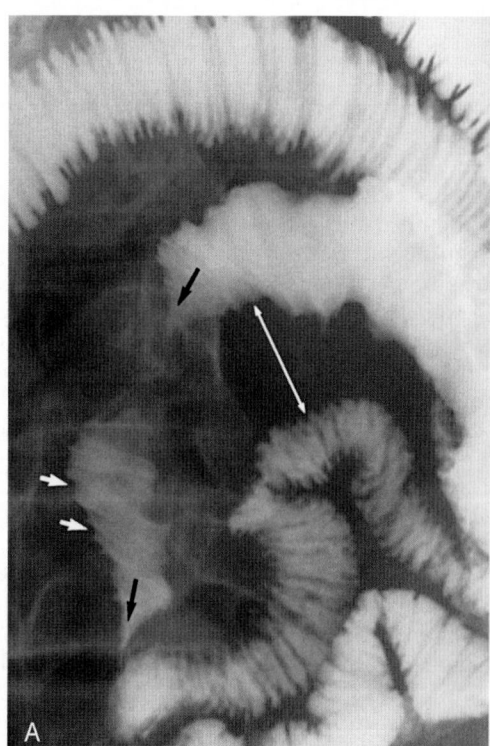
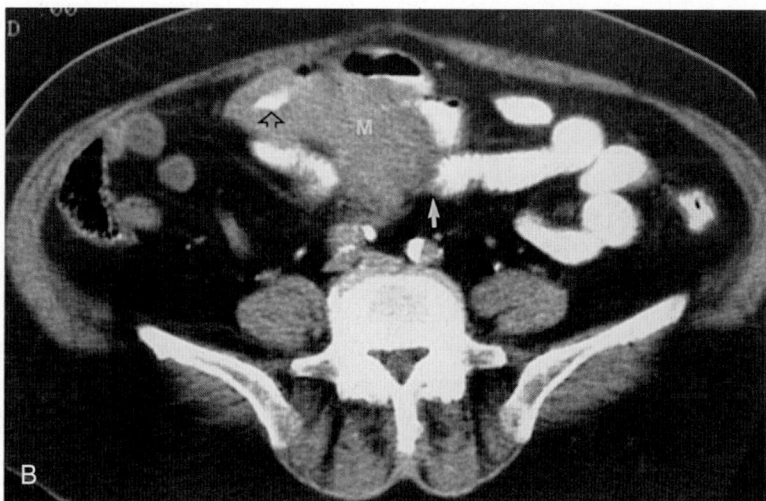

Figure 50-27. Non-Hodgkin's lymphoma in mesenteric lymph nodes causing partial small bowel obstruction. A. Overhead radiograph from enteroclysis shows that pelvic ileal loops are separated (*double arrow*) by a presumed mass in the small bowel mesentery. The small bowel is narrowed, tapered, and partially obstructed at several sites (*black arrows*). Thickened small bowel folds (*white arrows*) could be secondary to ischemia from venous/lymphatic obstruction in the mesentery or direct tumor invasion. **B.** Axial CT image shows how small bowel loops are separated by a large, homogeneous mesenteric mass (M). A loop of small bowel is tapered and partially obstructed (*closed arrow*). Tumor circumferentially infiltrates another small bowel loop (*open arrow*), accounting for the thickened folds seen on enteroclysis. (**A** from Rubesin SE, Gilchrist AM, Bronner M, et al: Non-Hodgkin lymphoma of the small intestine. RadioGraphics 10:985-998, 1990.)

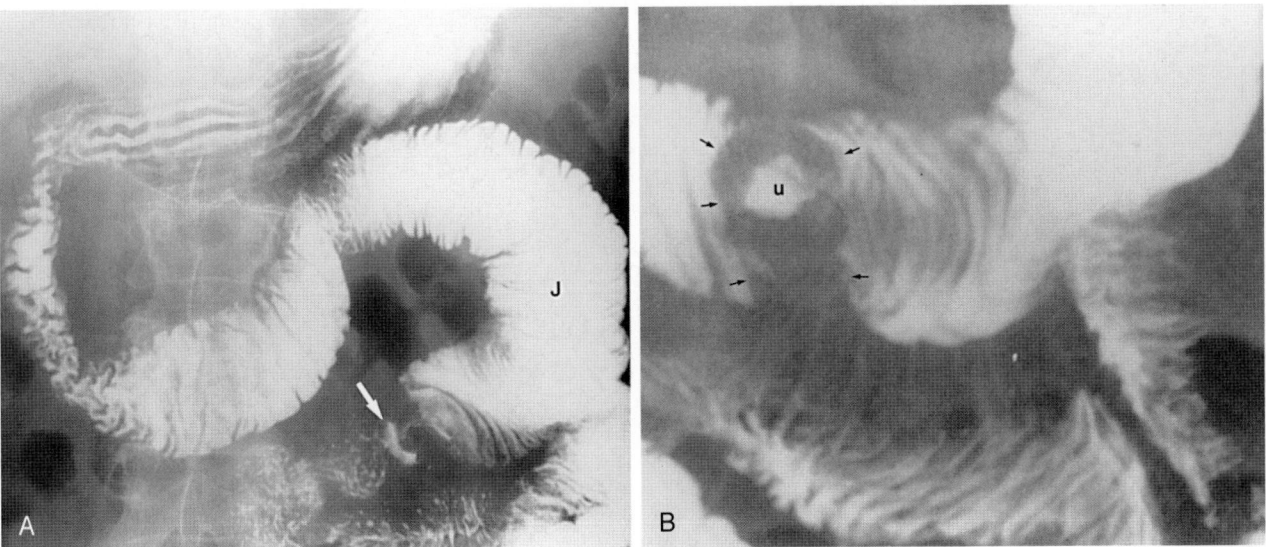

Figure 50-28. Adenocarcinoma of the jejunum causing partial small bowel obstruction. A. Overhead radiograph from an upper gastrointestinal series shows dilated distal duodenum and jejunum (J) proximal to a focally ulcerated lesion (*arrow*). **B.** Spot radiograph shows a circumferential mass (*arrows*) with central ulceration (u). This case illustrates the importance of converting an upper gastrointestinal series to a small bowel study when the distal duodenum is dilated.

margins (Fig. 50-28).[37] Nodularity or ulceration may be seen at the center of the lesion. The tumor is rigid and does not change in shape with manual compression or peristalsis. A primary small bowel tumor may sometimes be confused with an annular intraperitoneal metastasis (Fig. 50-29) or an adhesive band. However, intraperitoneal metastases tend to involve the distal small bowel, the bowel wall is angulated, and the folds are spiculated and tethered (Fig. 50-30).[42] An adhesive band may circumferentially narrow the lumen, but the mucosa is smooth, and the folds are tethered rather than nodular (Fig. 50-31).[43]

Primary lymphoma of the small bowel rarely causes obstruction, because this is a soft, infiltrative tumor that destroys the muscular wall, usually resulting in dilatation or cavitation.[41] Even when primary lymphomas are circumferential and narrow the lumen, high-grade small bowel obstruction is

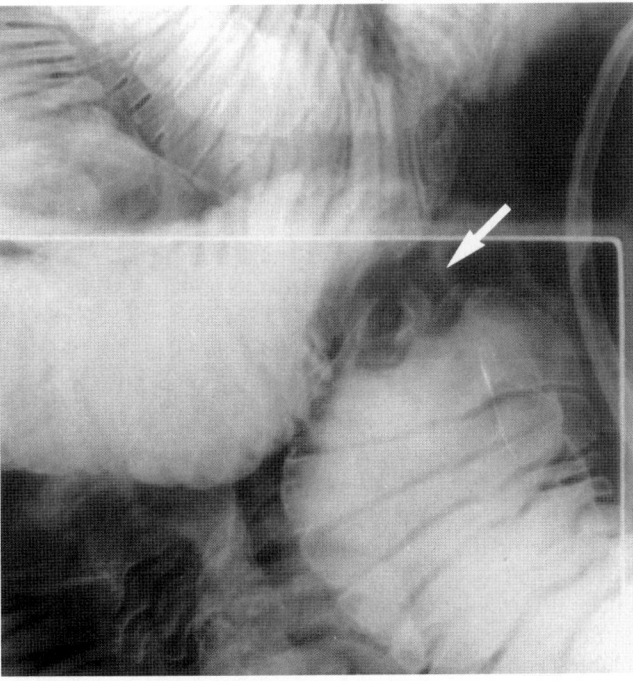

Figure 50-29. Annular intraperitoneal metastasis from colonic carcinoma. Spot radiograph from enteroclysis shows a short, annular lesion (*arrow*) in the small bowel. The margins of the lesion are shelflike but smooth, and the mucosa is probably preserved. It is difficult to determine with certainty whether this is an annular intraperitoneal metastasis or a primary malignant small bowel tumor. (From the teaching files of Hans Herlinger, MD.)

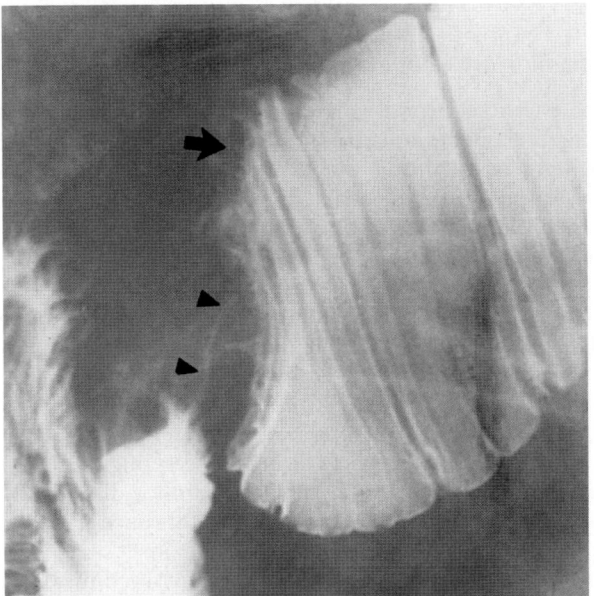

Figure 50-30. Annular metastasis from colonic carcinoma. Spot radiograph from enteroclysis shows a short, annular lesion with a markedly angulated, pencil-thin lumen (*arrowheads*). Although the proximal margin is abrupt, the folds are preserved and tethered (*arrow*).

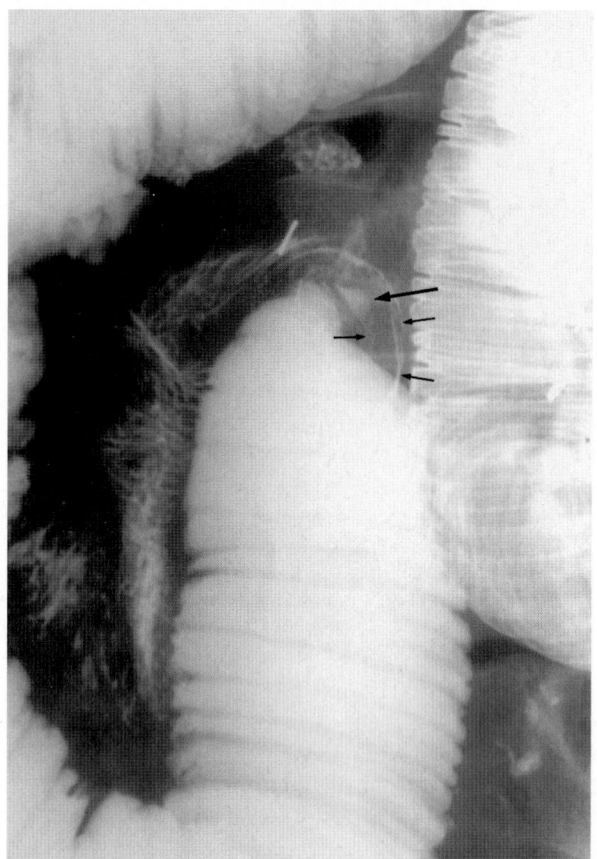

Figure 50-31. Circumferential adhesive band. Spot radiograph from enteroclysis shows abrupt angulation (*long arrow*) at the site of obstruction. The small bowel just distal to the angulation is markedly narrowed (*short arrows*), but folds are preserved throughout this region. (From the teaching files of Hans Herlinger, MD.)

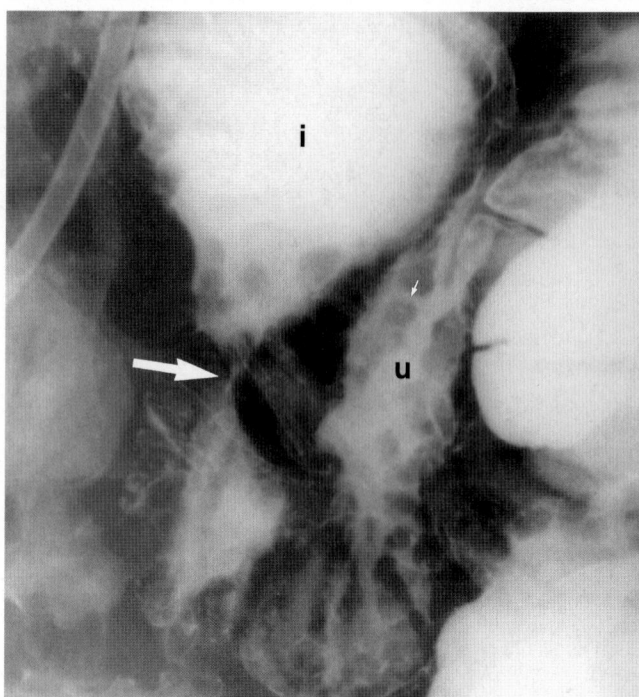

Figure 50-32. Crohn's disease causing partial small bowel obstruction. Spot radiograph from enteroclysis shows dilated ileum (i) proximal to a short, very tight stricture (*large arrow*). An ulceronodular pattern (cobblestoning) (u) is seen in the ileum distal to the stricture, manifested by transverse and longitudinal barium-filled, knifelike clefts/ulcers (*small arrow*) separating polygonal islands of relatively spared mucosa. (From the teaching files of Hans Herlinger, MD.)

extremely unusual because of the soft cellular nature of these lesions.

Inflammatory Conditions

The advanced stenotic phase of Crohn's disease may cause recurrent episodes of partial small bowel obstruction. Although high-grade obstructions are uncommon, small bowel obstruction is the most frequent indication for surgery in patients with Crohn's disease.[44] When luminal narrowing is seen on barium studies (Fig. 50-32) or CT (Fig. 50-33), the narrowing may be caused by edema, spasm, inflammation, fibrosis, or, rarely, a superimposed carcinoma.[45] The diameter of the stricture may change during the course of the examination or on delayed images. Severe narrowing may produce the classic "string" sign. In such cases, the use of metoclopramide or high-volume administration of contrast material at enteroclysis may distend the lumen to varying degrees, often associated with an ulceronodular pattern. Obstruction is diagnosed on barium studies or CT by delayed passage of contrast medium through the diseased segment with proximal small bowel dilatation.[46-48] Bowel wall thickening or localized mesenteric disease does not aid in the CT diagnosis of obstruction. Stenoses that resist the pressure of enteroclysis may require surgery.

Other inflammatory causes of small bowel obstruction are rare. Acute infections such as yersiniosis rarely cause small bowel obstruction because the acute inflammatory process heals without fibrosis. Tuberculosis is unusual in Western countries but may be seen in returning visitors or immigrants from Asia.[49] Tuberculosis may produce radiographic findings identical to those of Crohn's disease, but the cecum and ascending colon tend to be more severely involved than the terminal ileum. Patients with tuberculosis may also have a patulous ileocecal valve rather than the narrowed ileocecal valve typically seen in Crohn's disease. A definitive diagnosis of ileocecal tuberculosis requires culture and biopsy specimens.

Vascular Diseases

Radiation Enteropathy

Radiation enteropathy may cause mild to moderate small bowel obstruction due to a combination of serositis, adhesions, bowel wall fibrosis, and dysmotility. The changes occur within a preexisting radiation portal, usually in pelvic loops of ileum. Barium studies may reveal submucosal edema and fibrosis, manifested by smooth, straight, parallel, thickened folds that traverse the small bowel lumen (Fig. 50-34).[37] Barium filling compressed interstices between the folds may produce *interspace spikes*. The lumen of the affected bowel may also be narrowed as a result of submucosal fibrosis. Radiation-induced serositis and adhesions result in fixation and angulation of

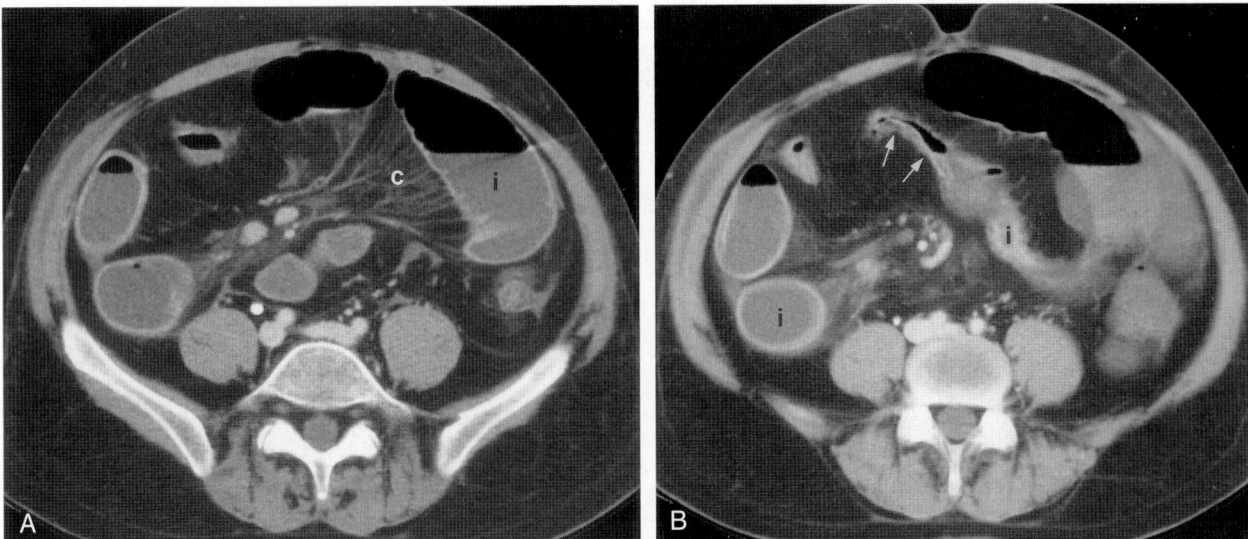

Figure 50-33. Crohn's disease causing partial small bowel obstruction. A. Axial CT through pelvis shows dilated ileum (i). Inflammation tracking up lymphatics and veins produces prominent mesenteric vessels, the so-called comb sign (c). **B.** Axial image cranial to **A** shows a segment of tapered narrowing, with wall thickening along the mesenteric border (*arrows*) of the bowel. Dilated right lower quadrant ileal loops (i) have mildly thickened walls. Inflammatory changes are also present in the mesentery. (From Forbes A, Misiewicz JJ, Compton CC, et al: Atlas of Clinical Gastroenterology, 3rd ed. Edinburgh, Elsevier Mosby, 2005.)

small bowel loops and tethering of folds similar to any extensive adhesive process (Fig. 50-35).[50] CT may also reveal thickening of the bowel wall and small bowel folds, with an associated target sign due to submucosal edema (Fig. 50-36).[51] Small bowel obstruction is suggested by dilatation of proximal small bowel loops with angulation of the diseased ileal loops in the pelvis (see Fig. 50-36B). Adhesive bands may form where small bowel enters the radiation portal. Smooth, tapered strictures may develop 6 months or more after radiation therapy (Fig. 50-37). Surgery in patients with radiation

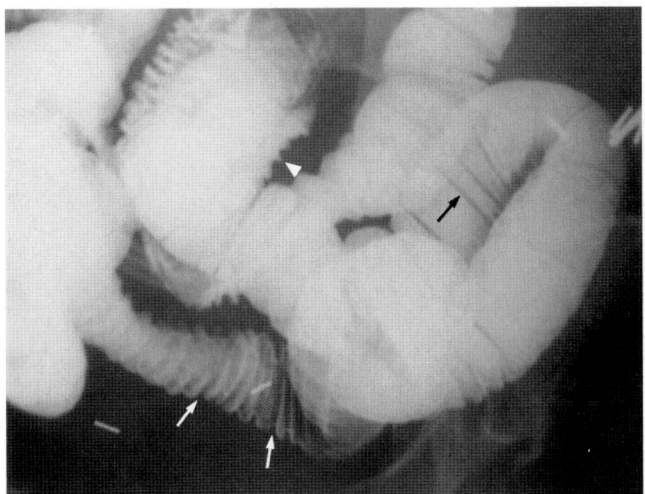

Figure 50-34. Radiation enteropathy causing low-grade small bowel obstruction. Spot radiograph from enteroclysis shows smooth, thickened folds (*white arrows*) in several pelvic loops of ileum. The folds are slightly angulated, indicating radiation serositis. In profile, the spaces between the thickened folds have a spikelike appearance (*arrowhead*), also known as *interspace spikes*. A nearby loop has normal-sized folds (*black arrow*) for comparison.

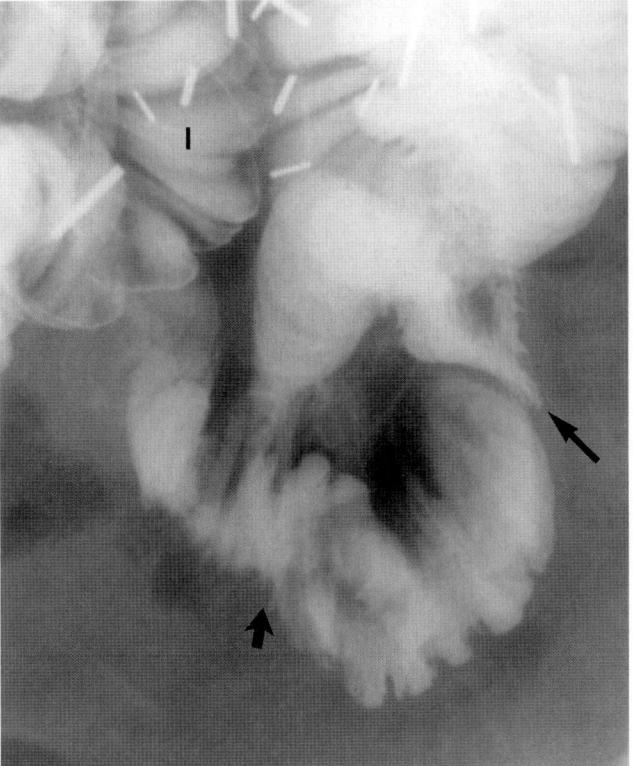

Figure 50-35. Radiation enteropathy causing low-grade small bowel obstruction. Smooth, thickened folds (*short arrow*) are seen in several loops of pelvic ileum. Extensive radiation serositis also causes angulation and narrowing of these loops (*long arrow*). Mild scarring produces a scalloped contour in a left-sided ileal loop (I). Intraperitoneal implants could produce similar radiographic findings.

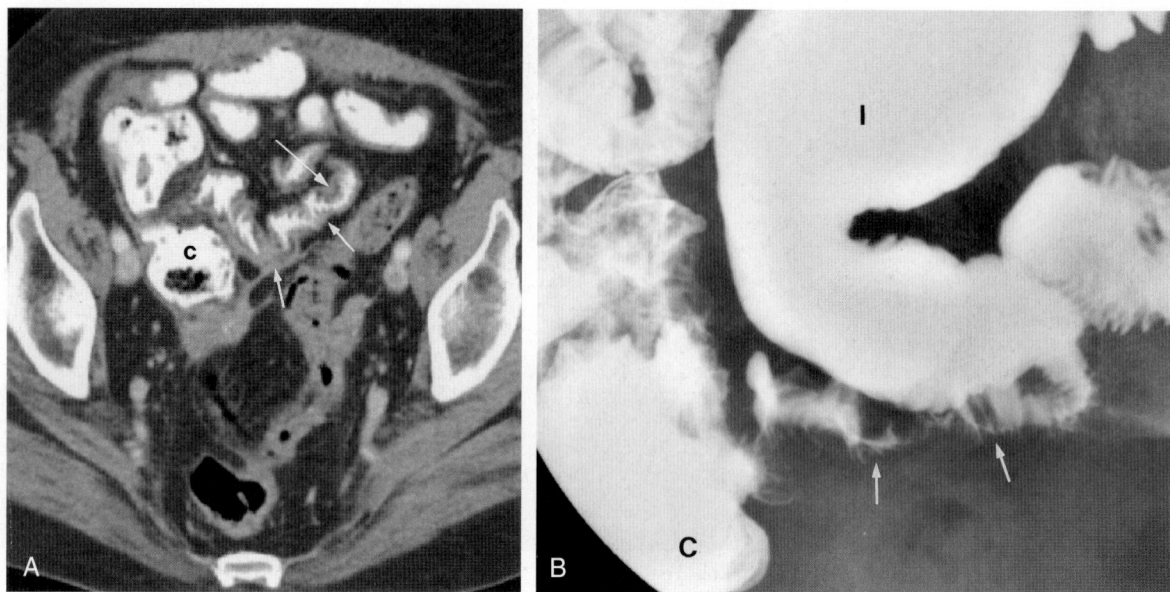

Figure 50-36. Radiation enteropathy causing low-grade small bowel obstruction. A. Axial CT through pelvis shows angulation and wall thickening (*short arrows*) in the terminal ileum. There also is a mural stratification pattern (*long arrow*) due to submucosal edema. c, cecum. **B.** Spot radiograph from a small bowel follow-through shows angulation and smooth, thickened folds (*arrows*) in the terminal ileum. The ileum (I) proximal to this segment of radiation change is dilated. C, cecum.

enteropathy is not without risk, because these patients may develop postoperative fistulas and interloop abscesses.[2]

Other Vascular Causes

Blunt abdominal trauma (often a seat-belt injury) may result in stricture formation due to small bowel ischemia or healing

of bowel wall hematomas. However, most hematomas resolve without sequelae on conservative treatment.[52] Strictures developing at enteroenterostomy sites (Fig. 50-38) may be the sequelae of ischemia, prior leaks with subsequent scarring, or surgical technique.

Acute inflammation, ischemia, and ulceration related to nonsteroidal anti-inflammatory drugs (NSAIDs) or potassium chloride tablets may also result in stricture formation.[53] In such cases, barium studies may reveal ringlike strictures (Fig. 50-39) with tiny central openings.

Figure 50-37. Radiation stricture. A short, smooth segment of narrowing (*open arrows*) is present at the edge of the radiation portal. Smooth, straight, thickened folds perpendicular to the longitudinal axis of the bowel (*closed arrows*) are typical of radiation change due to submucosal edema or fibrosis.

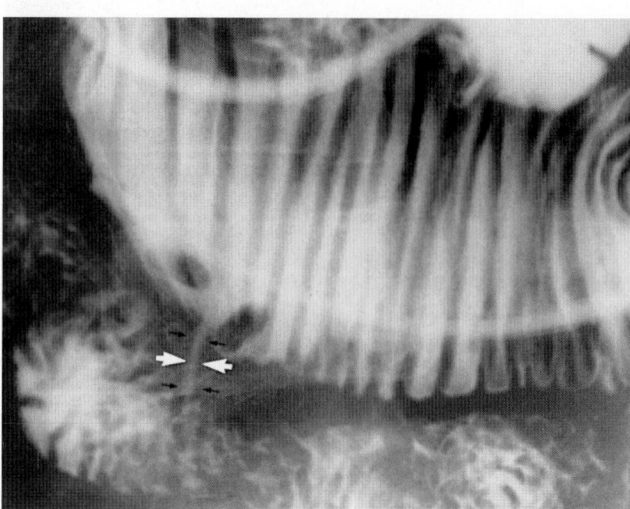

Figure 50-38. High-grade obstruction due to a stricture at the site of an enteroenterostomy. A 1- to 2-mm in width, barium-filled side-to-side enteroenterostomy (*arrows*) is present. The jejunum proximal to the obstruction is markedly dilated.

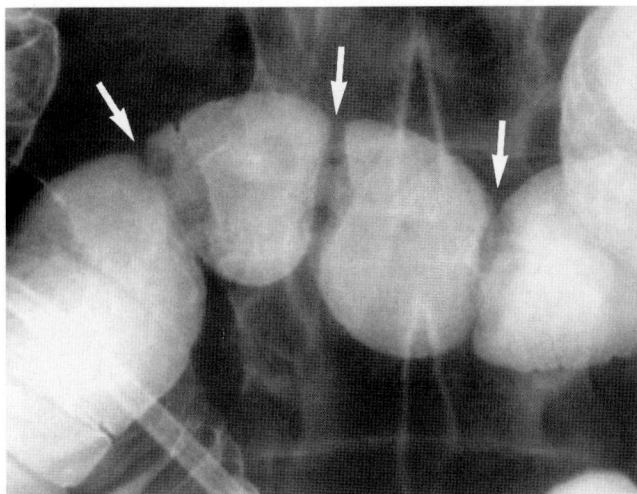

Figure 50-39. Ringlike strictures due to nonsteroidal anti-inflammatory drug use. Spot radiograph from enteroclysis shows three ringlike areas of narrowing (*arrows*) in the jejunum. (Courtesy of Arunas Gasparitis, MD.)

Intraluminal Causes

Gallstones, bezoars, foreign bodies, meconium, and tangles of *Ascaris* worms may obturate the small bowel lumen, causing obstruction.

Gallstone-induced small bowel obstruction (also known as *gallstone ileus*) usually occurs in elderly patients, especially women. With acute cholecystitis, a gallstone can erode through a distended gallbladder into the duodenum or colon, producing a biliary-enteric fistula. Most such fistulas extend from the gallbladder fossa to the duodenum. These intraluminal gallstones may pass through the small bowel until they become lodged in its narrowest segment (typically the terminal ileum at or near the ileocecal valve), causing small bowel obstruction. Calcified, ectopic gallstones are visible on plain abdominal radiographs in only about 15% of patients (Fig. 50-40). CT is superior for demonstration of calcified gallstones (Fig. 50-41) as the cause of small bowel or colonic obstruction in these patients.[54] The classic triad of a calcified gallstone, gas in a shrunken gallbladder or biliary tree, and small bowel obstruction is found in only a minority of patients on plain abdominal radiographs[55] but is better detected on CT. In some patients, a gallstone may be detected on small bowel follow-through studies as a calcified or noncalcified radiolucent filling defect at the site of transition between dilated and nondilated small bowel (Fig. 50-42).

Foreign body impactions in the small bowel (Fig. 50-43) are much less common than foreign body impactions in the pharynx and esophagus.[56] Small bowel obstruction by foreign bodies usually occurs in psychiatric or mentally challenged patients or in drug smugglers. Some people who eat indigestible food substances such as persimmons can develop small bowel bezoars.[57] These patients often have undergone a partial gastrectomy or gastroenterostomy and may have an underlying small bowel obstruction.

In adults with cystic fibrosis, inspissation of bowel contents may cause small bowel obstruction (meconium ileus equivalent). These patients may have a history of decreased intake of pancreatic enzyme supplements or narcotic use.

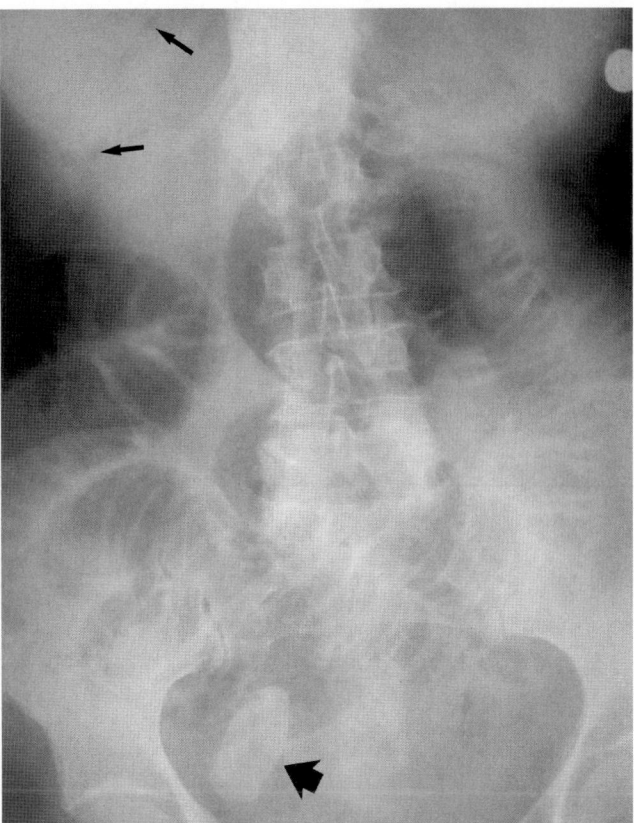

Figure 50-40. Gallstone causing distal small bowel obstruction ("gallstone ileus"). A large, ovoid calcification is seen in the right lower quadrant (*thick arrow*). The small bowel proximal to the gallstone is diffusely dilated. Air is also present in the biliary tree (*thin arrows*). This triad of findings is characteristic of gallstone ileus. (From the teaching files of Hans Herlinger, MD.)

Intussusception

Various extrinsic, intrinsic, and intraluminal processes result in small bowel intussusception. A loop of small intestine with part of its mesentery invaginates into the lumen of an

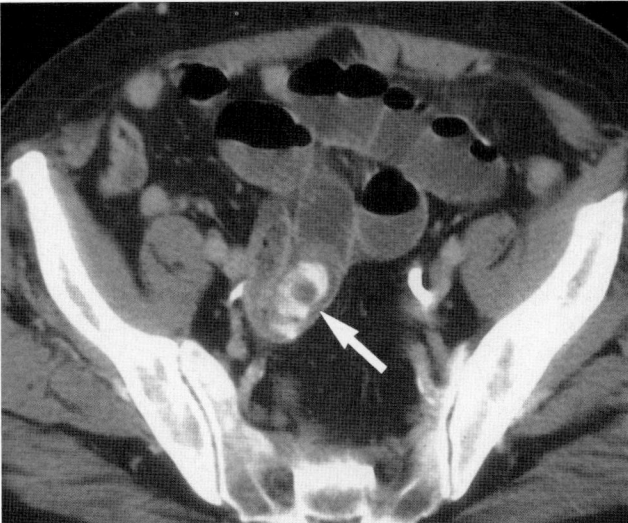

Figure 50-41. Gallstone causing small bowel obstruction. Axial CT image shows a calcified gallstone (*arrow*) in the distal ileum. The small bowel proximal to the gallstone is dilated and partially fluid filled.

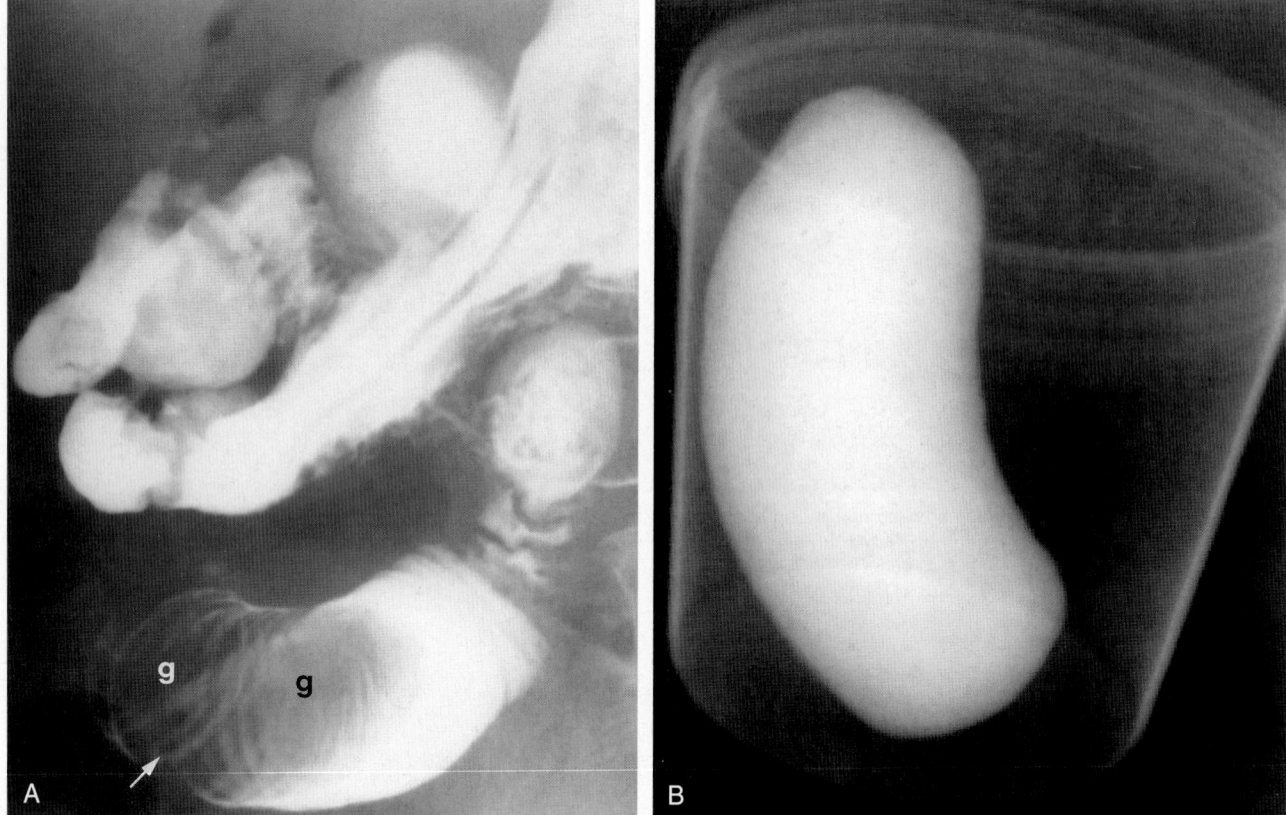

Figure 50-42. Gallstone causing proximal small bowel obstruction. A. A 10-cm radiolucent filling defect (g) is present in a dilated jejunal loop. Barium outlining jejunal folds gives the false impression of an intussusception. **B.** Specimen radiograph demonstrates this giant gallstone in a cup. (Courtesy of Vincent Low, MD.)

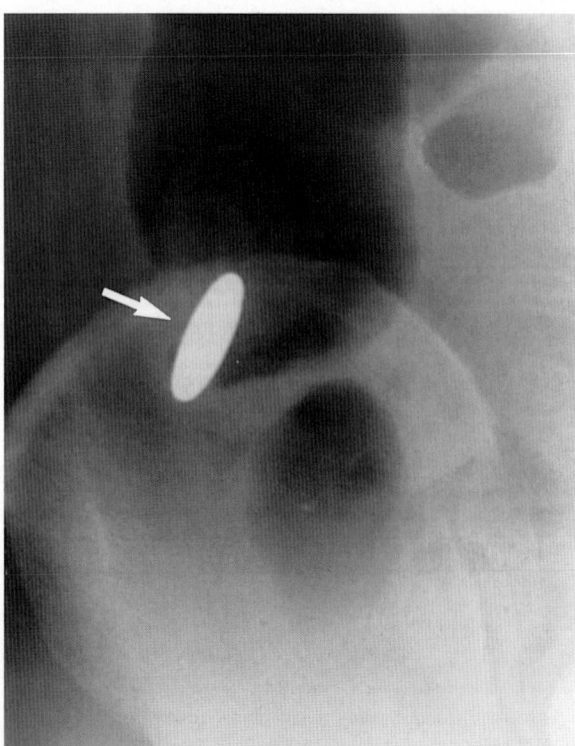

Figure 50-43. Coin impacted in the small intestine. Coned-down view from an abdominal radiograph shows a coin (*arrow*) in the right lower quadrant. The ileum is dilated in the region of the coin. According to this patient, the coin had been present in his abdomen for more than 20 years. Subsequent enteroclysis (not shown) revealed a focal small bowel stricture at the site of the coin.

adjacent small bowel segment distally. The inner, advancing segment is termed the *intussusceptum* and the outer, receiving segment the *intussuscipiens*. Most intussusceptions are nonobstructive, transient intussusceptions without a lead point that are detected on abdominal CT performed for other reasons.[58,59] Nonobstructive, transient intussusceptions are also seen in small bowel disorders associated with dysmotility, such as scleroderma and celiac disease. Benign or malignant polypoid tumors are the most common causes of small bowel intussusception in adults presenting with small bowel obstruction.[60] In postoperative patients, intussusceptions may be related to suture lines, adhesions, or intestinal tubes.[61]

Barium studies typically reveal a narrowed, tapered, barium-filled channel outlining the mucosa of the intussusceptum (Fig. 50-44).[37] If barium refluxes between the outer wall of the intussusceptum and the mucosal surface of the intussuscipiens, the mucosal folds of the intussuscipiens will be seen as parallel folds perpendicular to the longitudinal axis of the bowel, producing a *coil-spring* appearance (see Fig. 50-44). Coil-spring folds that appear thicker than normal small bowel folds indicate that there is associated edema due to lymphatic or venous congestion. If the intussusception is caused by an underlying tumor, a polypoid lead point may be identified. Barium filling the interstices of the lead point suggests that the tumor is a mucosal lesion such as an adenoma or hamartoma. In contrast, a round, smooth-surfaced polypoid lead point suggests a submucosal lesion such as a lipoma or metastatic melanoma (Fig. 50-45).

Small bowel intussusception may be manifested on CT by a pair of concentric soft tissue rings with an eccentrically

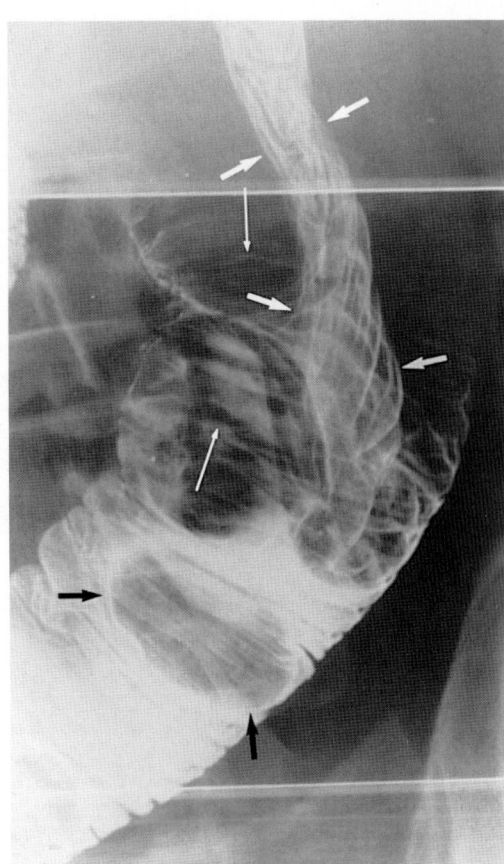

Figure 50-45. Metastatic melanoma causing intussusception and partial small bowel obstruction. Spot radiograph from enteroclysis shows the lumen of the intussusceptum as a narrowed, tubular structure lined by twisted mucosal folds (*short white arrows*). Retrograde flow of barium outlines the folds of the intussuscipiens (*long white arrows*). The folds of the intussuscipiens are thickened by edema. A large, smooth-surfaced polypoid lesion (*black arrows*) is the cause of the intussusception.

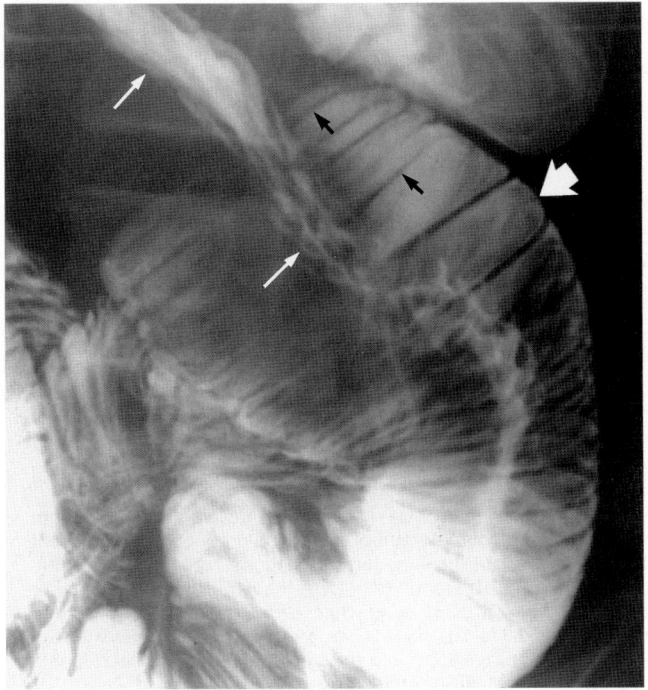

Figure 50-44. Jejunal intussusception due to an adhesion. The lumen of the intussusceptum is narrowed and outlined by barium (*thin white arrows*). Barium refluxes in a retrograde fashion between the serosal surface of the intussusceptum and the mucosal surface of the intussuscipiens (*thick white arrow*). Barium coating the mucosal surface of the intussuscipiens reveals mucosal folds (*short black arrows*), the so-called coil-spring sign. At surgery, the intussusception was found to occur at a site of adhesions.

located area of fat attenuation inside the outer ring.[62-64] The outer ring of soft tissue represents the intussuscipiens, whereas the inner ring represents the wall of the intussusceptum, and the eccentrically located fat represents the mesentery of the intussusceptum (Figs. 50-46 and 50-47). Vessels in the invaginating mesentery may be visible as punctate dots or thin, undulating strands of soft tissue or intravenous contrast attenuation. If the wall of the intussuscipiens is thickened, the possibility of bowel wall edema and ischemia should be considered.[63] Obstruction is suggested by dilatation of small bowel proximal to the intussusception with collapsed small bowel distally.

The clinical history is extremely helpful for evaluating patients with small bowel intussusception. Most patients with metastatic melanoma as the lead point have a history of prior surgical removal of malignant melanoma from the skin. Occasionally, however, these patients may present with an intussusception caused by metastatic melanoma as the initial manifestation of their disease.[65] Most patients with Peutz-Jeghers syndrome, an autosomal dominant disorder, have a family history of this syndrome. However, 45% of cases of Peutz-Jeghers syndrome occur as spontaneous mutations, so that these patients may initially present with small bowel symptoms related to intussuscepting hamartomas. Most patients

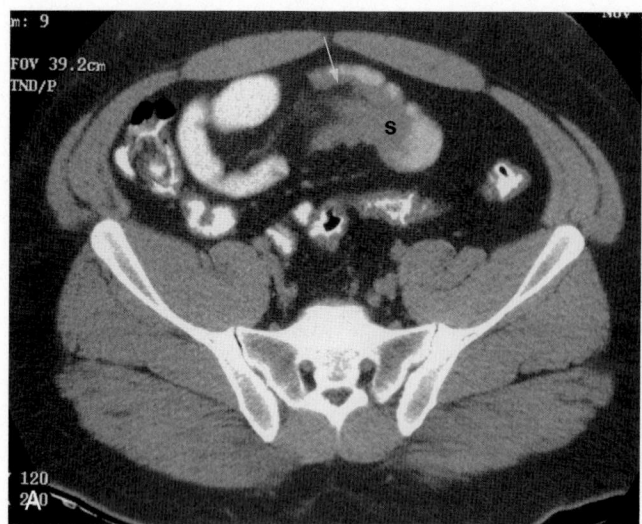

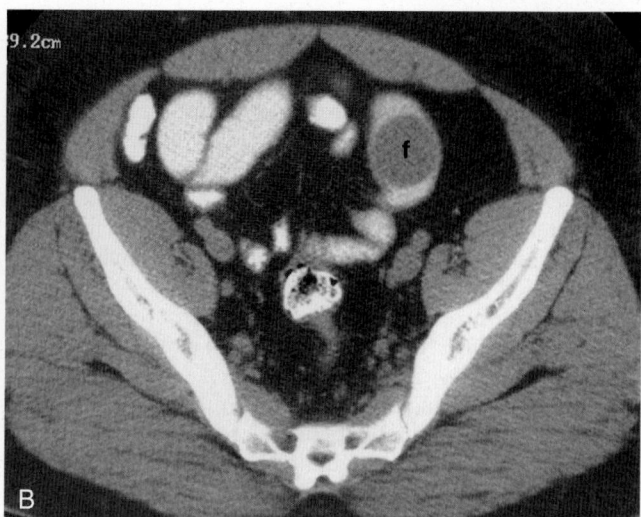

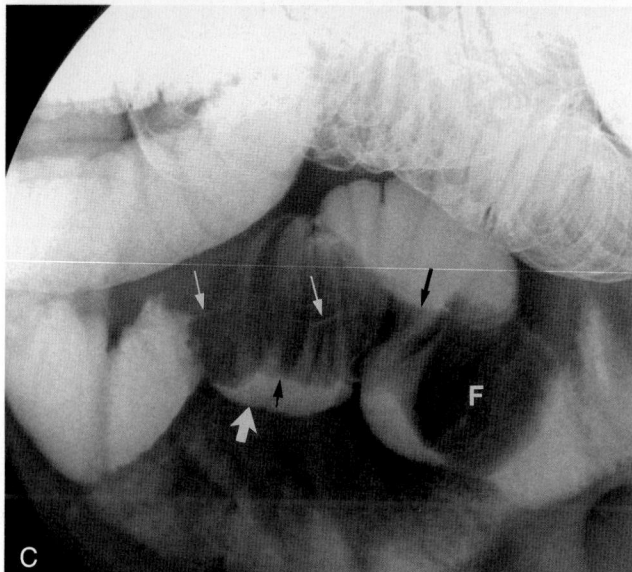

Figure 50-46. Inflammatory fibroid polyp causing intussusception.
A. Axial CT through pelvis shows the stalk of a polyp (S) within the lumen of the ileum. The mesentery (*white arrow*) is being drawn into the lumen. **B.** Image just caudad to **A** shows a round, soft tissue attenuation intraluminal mass (f). **C.** Spot radiograph from enteroclysis shows the head of the polyp (F), the stalk of the polyp (*long black arrow*), the lumen of the intussusceptum (*thin white arrows*), the serosal surface of the intussusceptum (*short black arrow*) and retrograde flow of barium into the intussuscipiens (*thick white arrow*). (From Rubesin SE: Small bowel tumors. Contemp Diagn Radiol 27:1-6, 2004.)

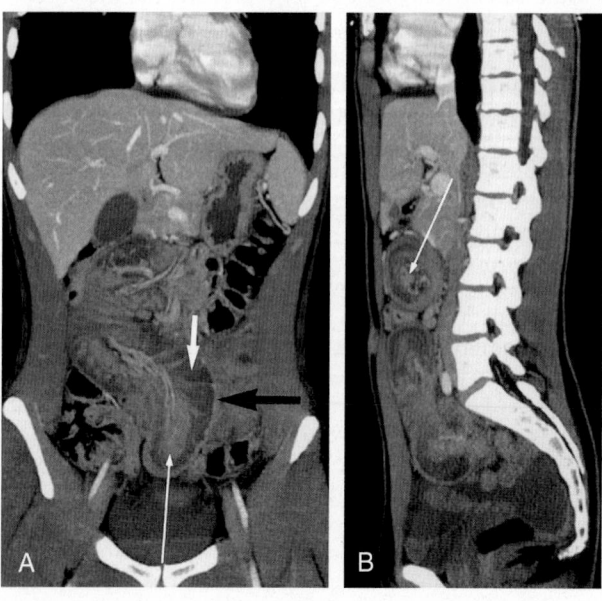

Figure 50-47. Mesenteric fat invaginating during intussusception.
Coronal (**A**) and sagittal (**B**) multiplanar CT reconstructions in a patient with a jejunal lipoma show the intussusception as a pair of concentric rings: the outer ring (*black arrow*) represents the wall of the intussuscipiens; the inner ring of soft tissue (*long white arrows*) is the intussusceptum. Eccentrically located fat (*short white arrow*) is the mesentery of the intussusceptum invaginating into the intussuscipiens. An ileal lipoma (not shown) was the cause of the intussusception.

with Peutz-Jeghers syndrome also have pigmented lesions on the lips, oral mucosa, face, or extremities.[66] However, pigmented lesions may be overlooked in patients of African or Asian origin; these patients may initially present with gastrointestinal bleeding or abdominal pain caused by an intussuscepting hamartoma.

The location of the intussusception is of little value in distinguishing polyps of different histologic types. Peutz-Jeghers polyps and adenomas are most frequently located in the proximal jejunum, whereas stromal tumors, metastatic melanoma, and lipomas have a relatively uniform distribution in the small bowel.

When small bowel intussusception occurs, barium filling the interstices of an intussusception should suggest that the lead point is a tumor of mucosal origin, such as a Peutz-Jeghers polyp or adenoma. Intussuscepting lesions that are centrally umbilicated or ulcerated are usually submucosal tumors such as stromal tumors or metastatic melanoma (see Fig. 50-45). In fact, melanoma metastases are central umbilicated or ulcerated in more than 50% of cases.[67] Intussusception by soft melanoma metastases may be intermittent and may not cause obstruction. Multiple polypoid tumors in the jejunum or mid small intestine should suggest a diagnosis of Peutz-Jeghers syndrome or metastases, especially from malignant melanoma. Lipomas are smooth, pliable, often pedunculated lesions that have fat attenuation on CT (Fig. 50-48), so they must be distinguished from the invaginating mesentery of an intussuscepting polyp. Inflammatory fibroid polyps are typically located in the distal ileum (see Fig. 50-46). Pedunculated polyps with long stalks that intussuscept are usually inflammatory fibroid polyps (see Fig. 50-46), lipomas, or an inverted Meckel diverticulum (Fig. 50-49).[68,69] Other causes of intussusception include Henoch-Schönlein purpura, lymphoma, hematomas, and mesenteric lymphadenopathy. Causes of intussusception in patients with AIDS include B-cell lymphoma, Kaposi's sarcoma, mesenteric lymphadenopathy, lymphoid hyperplasia, and intestinal dysmotility.[70]

RADIOLOGIC IMAGING

The role of radiologic imaging in the diagnosis of small bowel obstruction is (1) to confirm the diagnosis of obstruction;

(2) to locate the site or sites and degree of obstruction; and (3) to diagnose the cause of obstruction.[71] A particular imaging technique is helpful if it can distinguish partial from complete obstruction and open- from closed-loop obstruction and if it can detect strangulation. Radiologic imaging modalities such as CT have been described in detail in other chapters. The focus of this discussion is on the role of a variety of imaging modalities in patients with small bowel obstruction.

Plain Abdominal Radiographs

The plain abdominal radiograph has traditionally been used as the first radiologic study in the work-up of acute abdominal pain and suspected small bowel obstruction.[72,73] Many adults admitted with a clinical suspicion of acute small bowel obstruction undergo surgery on the basis of the clinical, physical, and laboratory findings in conjunction with the findings on plain abdominal radiographs. The diagnosis of small bowel obstruction on abdominal radiographs requires demonstration of dilated loops of small bowel, identified by their smooth luminal contour, valvulae conniventes, and central location in the abdomen (Fig. 50-50A). Air-fluid levels may traverse the entire lumen of the bowel (Fig. 50-50B) or may be trapped as bubbles between folds at the top of a fluid-filled bowel loop, resulting in a "string of pearls" sign (Fig. 50-50B). Fluid-filled loops may not be seen on supine abdominal radiographs but may be recognized on upright or cross-table lateral decubitus radiographs (Fig. 50-51).

Plain abdominal radiographs have only moderately accuracy for the diagnosis of small bowel obstruction. In one series, abdominal radiographs had a sensitivity of 86% for the diagnosis of high-grade obstruction but a sensitivity of only 56% for the diagnosis of low-grade obstruction.[14] In another series, abdominal radiographs revealed small bowel obstruction in 78% of patients with this condition.[74] Obstructions can be missed on abdominal radiographs if vomiting or nasogastric intubation leads to decompression of dilated small bowel loops. Fluid-filled loops also may not be visible, leading to a false-negative diagnosis or erroneous interpretation of the level of obstruction (Fig. 50-52). Occasionally, abdominal radiographs may be obtained too early in the course of the obstruction for fluid and air to be present in dilated small

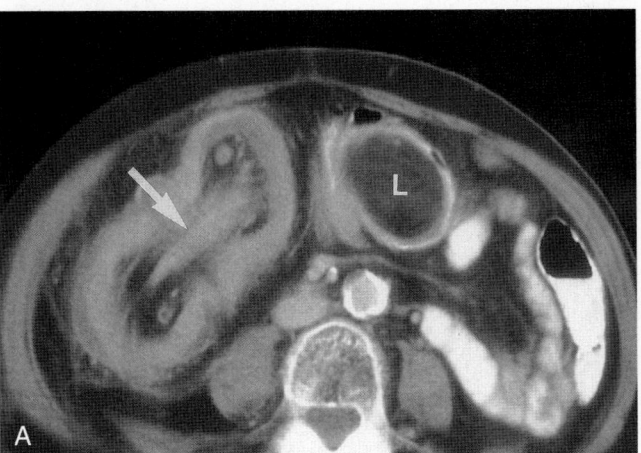
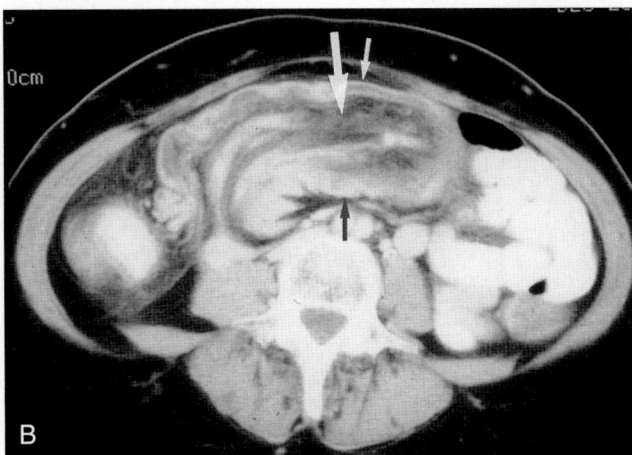

Figure 50-48. Ileal lipoma causing ileocolic intussusception. A. Axial CT shows an ileocolic intussusception with a lipoma (L) serving as the lead point of the intussusceptum (*arrow*) and its surrounding mesentery. **B.** Axial image caudad to **A** shows the dilated colon (intussuscipiens) (*small arrows*) containing the intussuscepted distal ileum and proximal colon (*large arrow*).

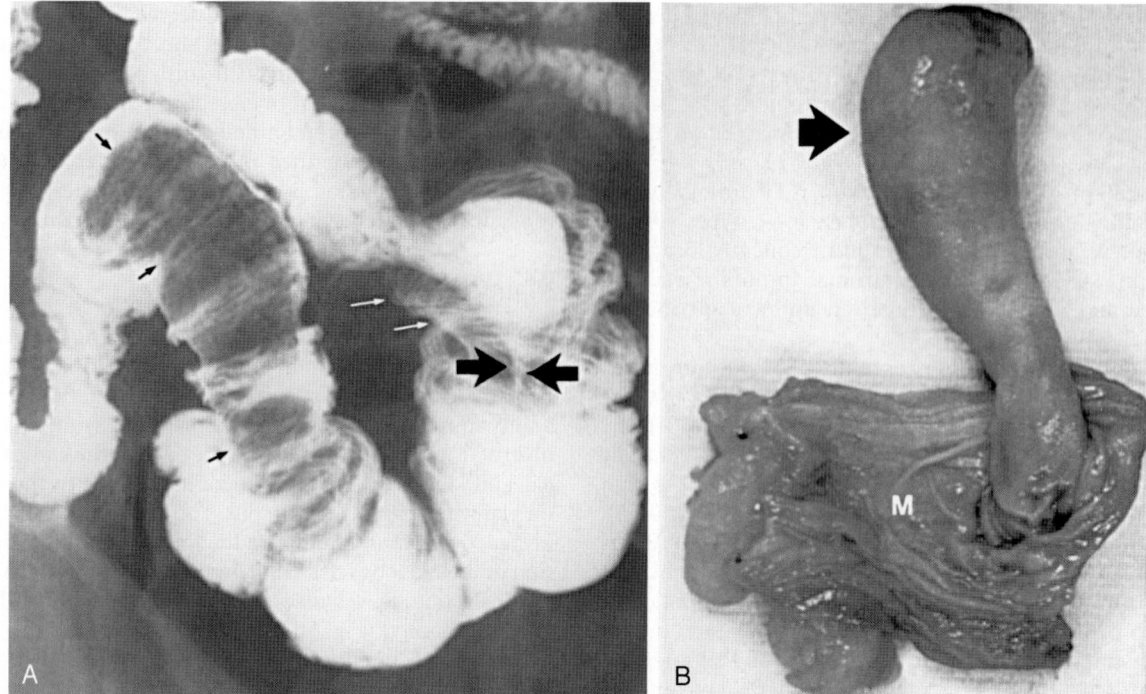

Figure 50-49. Inverted Meckel's diverticulum causing intussusception. A. Spot radiograph from small bowel follow-through shows tapered narrowing of the ileum (*large black arrows*) at the narrowest point of the intussusceptum. The mucosa of the intussuscipiens is outlined by refluxed barium (*white arrows*). A long polypoid intraluminal filling defect (*small black arrows*) is the invaginated Meckel diverticulum. **B.** The surgically resected specimen shows the invaginated Meckel diverticulum as a long polypoid projection (*arrow*) from the mucosal surface (M) of the bowel. (From Rubesin SE, Herlinger H, DeGaeta L: Interlude: Test your skills. Radiology 176:636 and 644, 1990.)

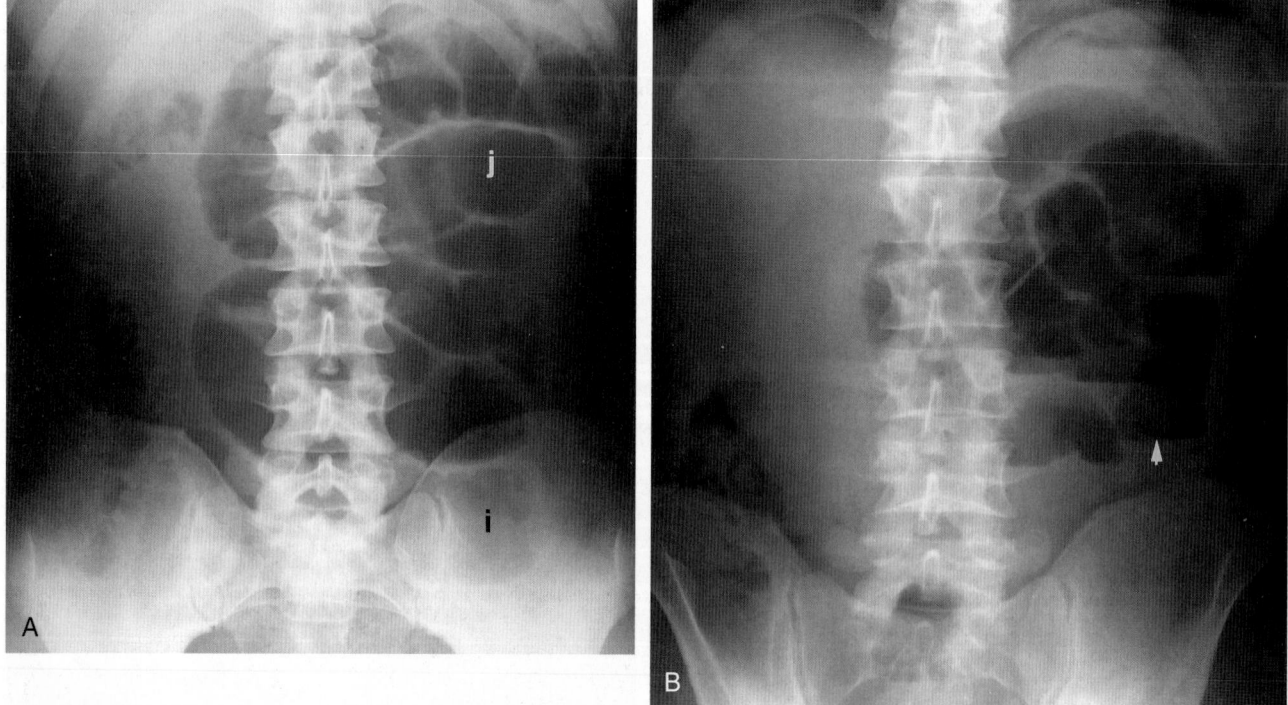

Figure 50-50. Plain abdominal radiographs showing small bowel obstruction. A. Supine abdominal radiograph shows diffuse dilatation of jejunum (j) and proximal ileum (i). **B.** Upright abdominal radiograph shows numerous air-fluid levels (*arrow*) in dilated small bowel.

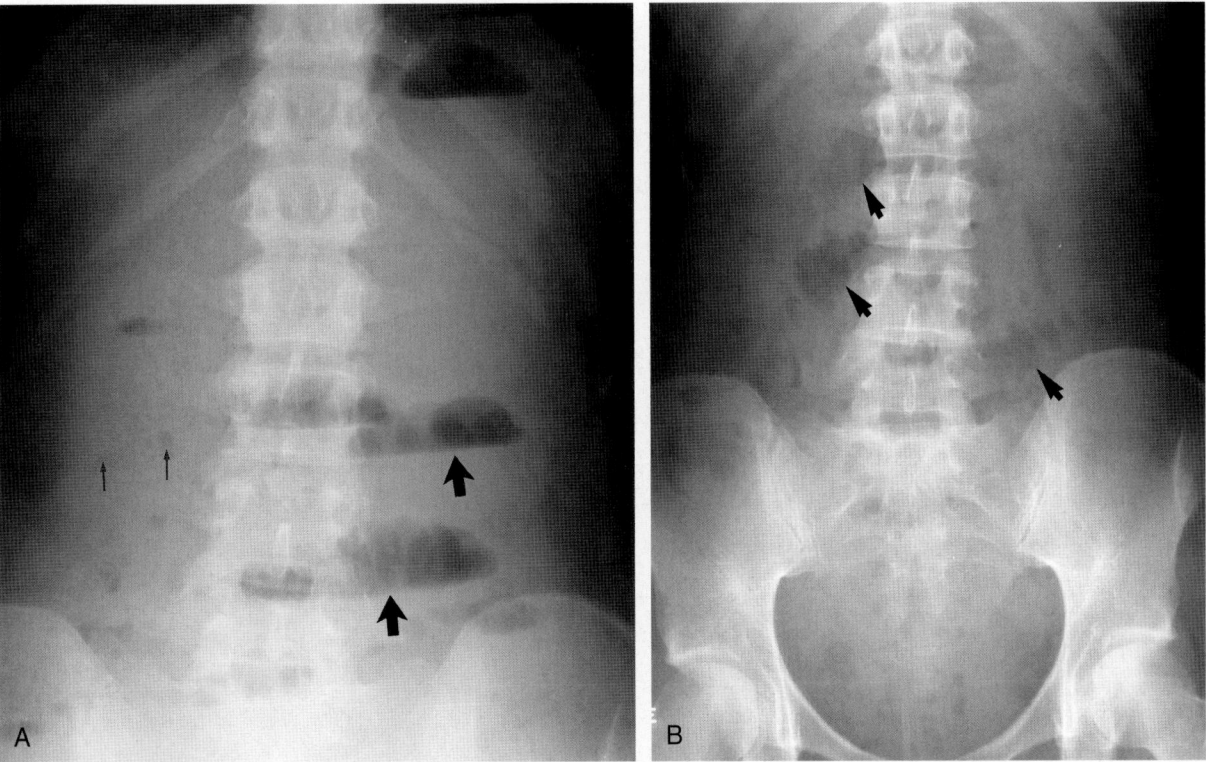

Figure 50-51. Supine abdominal radiograph not indicating extent of small bowel obstruction. A. Supine abdominal radiograph shows only minimal distention of several gas-filled small bowel loops (*arrows*). **B.** Upright abdominal radiograph shows several long air-fluid levels (*large arrows*). Tiny collections of gas are also seen as contiguous bubbles (*small arrows*) between small bowel folds ("string of pearls" sign).

bowel. A false-positive diagnosis of obstruction also occurs in up to 44% of patients, often resulting from an adynamic ileus or aerophagia that is mistaken for obstruction. The level of obstruction can be accurately predicted in about 75% of patients.[74]

Unfortunately, plain abdominal radiographs have little value in suggesting the diagnosis of strangulation.[75,76] In patients with strangulating obstruction, the underlying small bowel obstruction can be diagnosed on abdominal radiographs in only about 50% of patients.[75,76] Strangulation is suggested on abdominal radiographs by demonstration of smooth, thickened folds in dilated small bowel loops. Portal venous gas or linear pneumatosis paralleling the wall of the small bowel should strongly suggest superimposed ischemia and infarction. Closed-loop obstructions are often not visible because they are fluid filled. However, a disproportionately dilated, fluid-filled loop that has a fixed appearance on serial abdominal radiographs should suggest a closed-loop obstruction.

Computed Tomography

Given the limitations of plain abdominal radiographs, CT has become an important technique (if not the modality of choice) for the diagnosis of small bowel obstruction. Some radiologists even believe that CT should replace abdominal radiographs as the first imaging test for the diagnosis of small bowel obstruction and its complications, although this subject remains controversial.[72,77] CT has a vital role in these patients because it is readily available, fast, and noninvasive. In comparison to barium studies, CT does not require contrast material to reach the site of obstruction but instead uses

intestinal fluid proximal to the obstruction to outline the transition zone (Fig. 50-53).[78] As a result, CT has become the procedure of choice for diagnosing a variety of abdominal conditions, including (1) adynamic ileus; (2) acute or prolonged, high-grade small bowel obstruction; (3) suspected strangulation (see Fig. 50-11) or perforation; and (4) acute inflammatory processes such as appendicitis, Crohn's disease (see Fig. 50-33), and diverticulitis causing small bowel obstruction. CT is also the best examination for evaluating patients with to suspected metastatic disease causing small bowel obstruction (Fig. 50-54).

CT has an accuracy of about 80% for the diagnosis of high-grade small bowel obstruction versus an accuracy of only 50% for low-grade obstruction.[14] CT can accurately predict the cause of obstruction in 70% to 95% of patients[12,15,18,78] and can often suggest superimposed intestinal ischemia, infarction, and perforation. The entire abdomen is evaluated by CT, providing a vast array of important information not available on plain abdominal radiographs. For example, CT can identify a variety of causes of small bowel obstruction, including carcinoid tumor, intraperitoneal or hematogenous metastasis, Crohn's disease, appendicitis, and diverticulitis.[79]

CT does have limitations, however, in the evaluation of patients with suspected small bowel obstruction. The degree of small bowel dilatation does not always correlate with the presence or degree of obstruction. It may also be difficult to distinguish an adynamic small bowel ileus from a distal small bowel obstruction if a transition zone is not identified.[79] It can also be difficult to determine the location of the transition zone along the course of the dilated small bowel, even with the ability to "scroll" through a scan on a picture archiving and

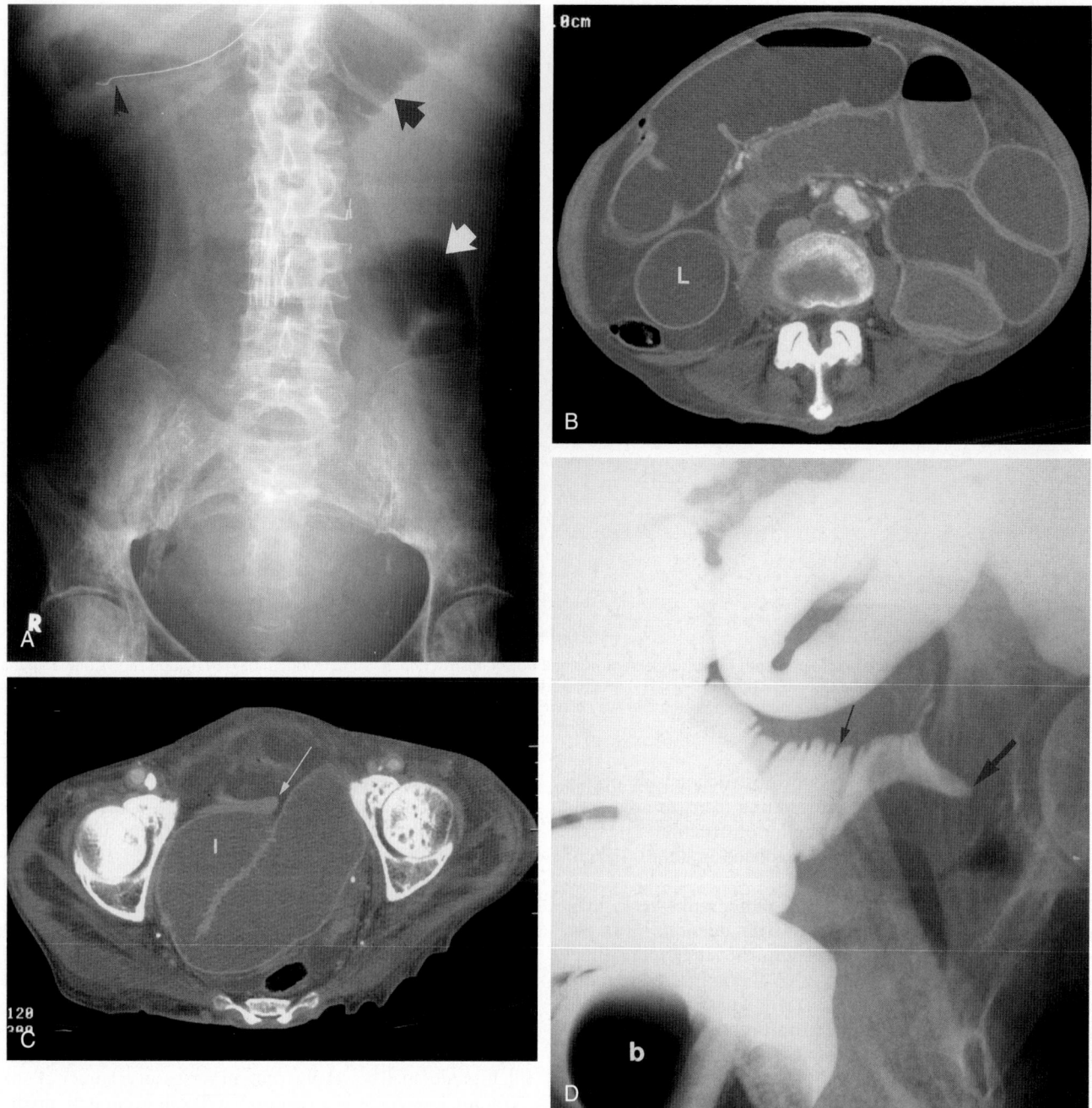

Figure 50-52. Plain abdominal radiograph that is misleading about the level of obstruction. A. Abdominal radiograph shows a markedly dilated loop of small intestine in the left upper quadrant (*thick black arrow*). A dilated loop of bowel (*white arrow*) is also present in the left midabdomen. Is this small bowel or colon? The gastric antrum and tip of the nasogastric tube (*arrowhead*) are deviated to the right. **B.** Axial CT through abdomen shows marked small bowel dilatation. Many loops are gasless and only filled with fluid (L), explaining why they were not visualized on the abdominal radiograph. Ascites is also present. **C.** Axial image through pelvis shows the transition zone (*arrow*) between dilated ileum (I) proximal to the site of obstruction and collapsed ileum distally. No soft tissue mass is identified at the site of transition (*arrow*), so the obstruction is presumed to be caused by an adhesion. **D.** Single-contrast barium enema with reflux of barium into the ileum (*small arrow*) shows smooth, tapered narrowing (*large arrow*) at the site of obstruction compatible with an adhesion. The balloon (b) of the enema tip is identified. The diagnosis of adhesions was confirmed at surgery. (From Forbes A, Misiewicz JJ, Compton CC, et al: Atlas of Clinical Gastroenterology, 3rd ed. Edinburgh, Elsevier Mosby, 2005.)

communications system workstation or to reconstruct 3D images. Unfortunately, the location of the transition zone to one abdominal quadrant is not accurate in diagnosing the site of obstruction, because markedly dilated jejunum may fall into the pelvis and obstructed distal ileum may rotate into the left upper quadrant. Finally, CT is an excellent technique for suggesting strangulation, but it cannot be used to predict

whether a small bowel loop has reversible or irreversible ischemia and whether the affected bowel will be viable at surgery.[80,81] Abnormal bowel wall thickening or mesenteric engorgement also cannot be used to predict surgical viability of bowel. In the setting of ischemia, CT finding of pneumatosis indicates breakdown in the mucosal integrity of the bowel wall and is strongly suggestive of ischemia. However, even the CT

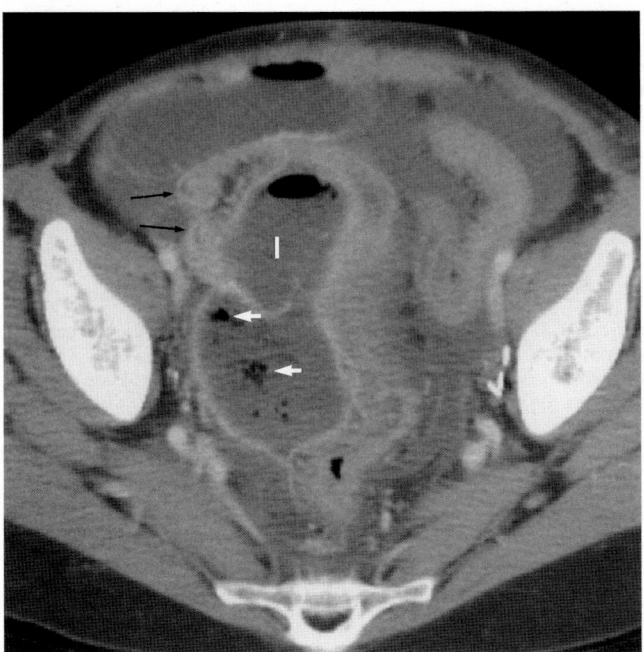

Figure 50-53. Small bowel obstruction on CT without evidence of a mass at the transition zone. Axial image through pelvis shows dilated, fluid-filled ileum (I). Note air bubbles (*white arrows*) trapped in debris. There is no evidence of a mass at the site of transition. A collapsed loop of ileum (*black arrows*) seen in cross section near the site of transition was found at surgery to be a loop of small bowel trapped beneath an adhesion.

finding of pneumatosis does not predict irreversible ischemia at surgery. In contrast, the CT findings of free intraperitoneal gas and portomesenteric gas indicate a much greater likelihood of irreversible transmural necrosis than pneumatosis alone. Despite these limitations, CT is currently the modality of choice in acutely ill patients with suspected high-grade or complete small bowel obstruction, suspected strangulation, or suspicion of an inflammatory process such as appendicitis or Crohn's disease or a hernia as the cause of obstruction.[82-84]

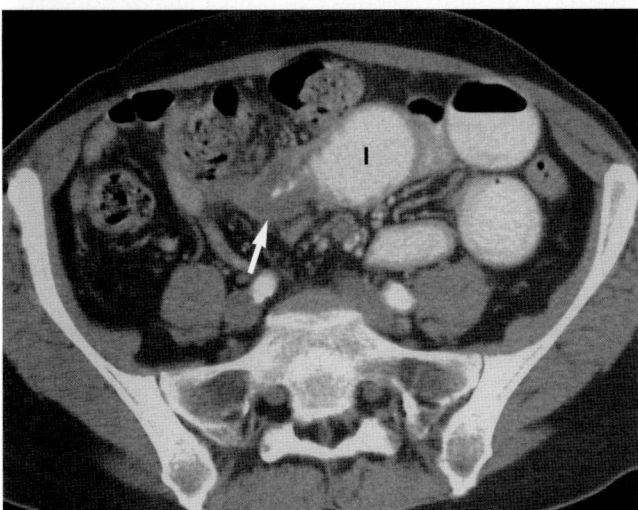

Figure 50-54. Small bowel obstruction on CT with evidence of a mass at the transition zone. Axial CT image through pelvis shows dilated ileum (I). There is uniform, circumferential thickening (*white arrow*) of the bowel wall at the site of transition. A metastasis from lung carcinoma was found at surgery.

Barium Studies

A variety of barium studies may be performed on patients with suspected small bowel obstruction, including small bowel follow-through, enteroclysis (i.e., small bowel enema), barium enema, and studies performed via indwelling nasogastric, nasojejunal, or jejunostomy tubes. These studies are described in detail in Chapter 41.

The use of barium is safe in patients with suspected small bowel obstruction, because barium does not form concretions in the small bowel lumen proximal to an obstructing lesion. In such patients, residual fluid in dilated small bowel loops prevents barium from dehydrating and agglomerating. Barium also does not form concretions in the proximal ascending colon. However, concretions may form in the remainder of the colon as water is resorbed from the barium sulfate suspension. As a result, barium should not be administered orally or via a proximal bowel tube in a patient with an obstructing lesion distal to the hepatic flexure of the colon, because dense barium concretions can form in these patients, with the possibility of stercoral ulceration and perforation. If there is any doubt about the location of bowel obstruction, CT or barium enema should be performed before barium is administered proximal to the site of a distal colonic obstruction.

The presence of barium proximal to a small bowel obstruction makes surgery more hazardous, because barium spilling into the peritoneal cavity can incite a granulomatous form of peritonitis. Some surgeons therefore request that small bowel studies be performed using water-soluble contrast material rather than barium in this clinical setting. Small bowel follow-throughs with water-soluble contrast material have been advocated as a therapeutic technique to improve small bowel obstructions.[85] The use of water-soluble contrast material in patients with small bowel obstruction, however, does not make sense on radiographic or surgical grounds. Because water-soluble contrast agents are markedly hyperosmolar, they draw fluid into the bowel lumen, whereas the aim of therapy is to decompress the small bowel. Dilution of water-soluble contrast material by retained fluid in the dilated small bowel also results in poor radiographic detail (Fig. 50-55), compromising the ability to diagnose small bowel obstruction and determine its site and cause on these studies. Therefore, the only valid indication for using water-soluble contrast material for an antegrade small bowel study is the suspicion of a leak, primarily when small bowel obstruction is proximal or the small bowel is not dilated. If perforation is suspected in patients with distal small bowel obstruction, CT or retrograde water-soluble contrast enemas are better choices. Rarely, enteroclysis can be performed with water-soluble contrast material to exclude a small bowel leak.

Small bowel follow-through and enteroclysis studies are poor examinations for evaluating patients with high-grade distal small bowel obstruction. Because of small bowel dilatation and decreased small bowel peristalsis, it may take an inordinate period of time for barium to reach the site of obstruction. Not infrequently, 24-hour follow-up images are required to visualize the site of high-grade distal small bowel obstruction. By this time, the barium suspension is diluted and there is poor anatomic visualization of the transition zone (Fig. 50-56), which can even be obscured by superimposed barium-filled loops of dilated small bowel.

If a study must be performed from above in a patient with a high-grade small bowel obstruction, prior passage of

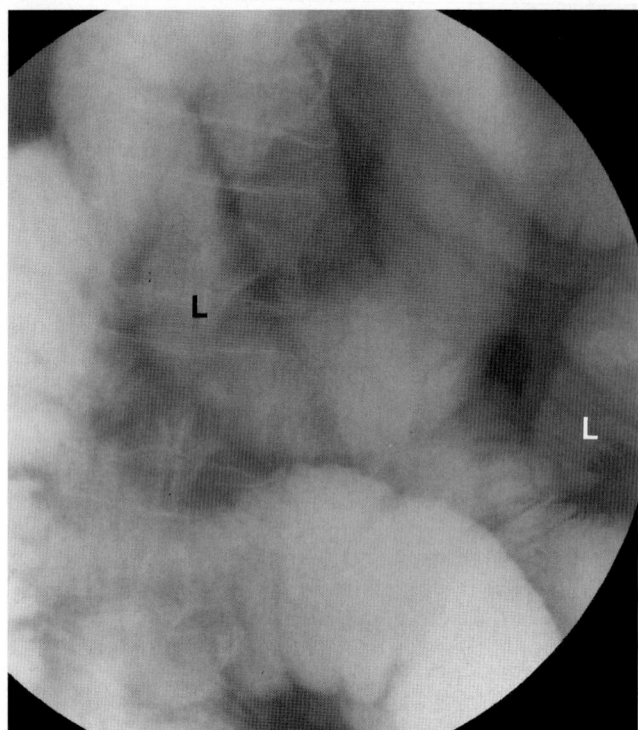

Figure 50-55. Small bowel follow-through with water-soluble contrast material shows little anatomic detail. Mid small bowel loops are dilated without demonstration of small bowel folds (black L). The folds are seen only when the small bowel is less distended (white L).

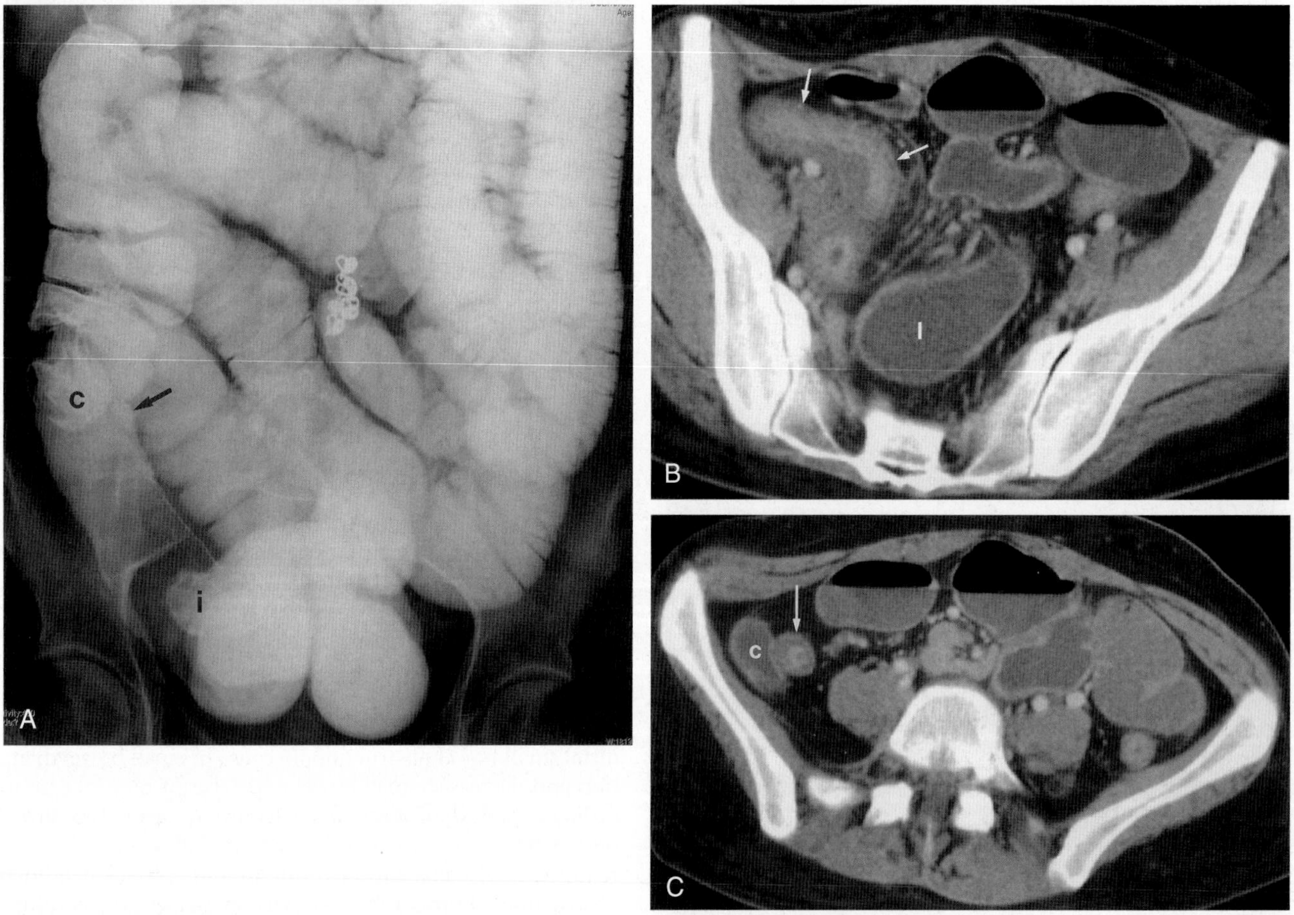

Figure 50-56. Small bowel obstruction with poor demonstration of site of transition on small bowel follow-through. A young woman presented with acute abdominal pain and distention. **A.** Barium had not reached the colon after 10 hours. An overhead radiograph obtained 24 hours after ingestion of barium shows diffuse small bowel dilatation. There are a relatively collapsed cecum (c) and terminal ileum (*arrow*) with dilated ileum (i) proximal to the terminal ileum but poor delineation of the site of transition. **B.** Axial CT through pelvis shows dilated ileum (I) with a thick-walled distal ileum (*arrows*). **C.** Axial CT craniad to **B** shows thickened terminal ileum with a mural stratification pattern (*arrow*). c, cecum. At surgery, this patient was found to have Crohn's disease as the cause of high-grade small bowel obstruction.

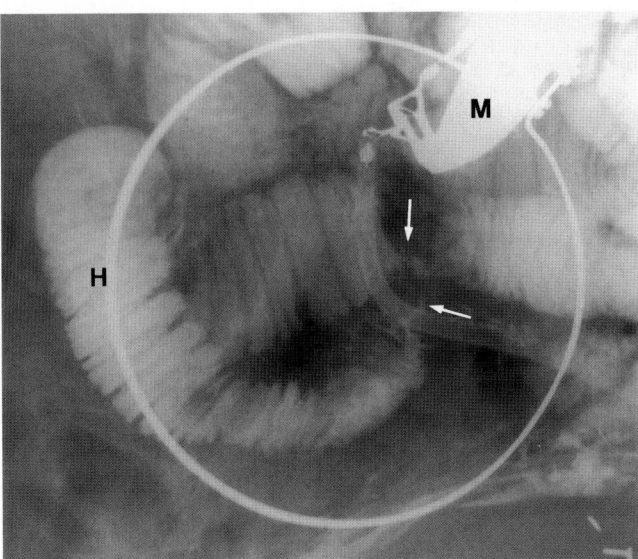

Figure 50-57. Small bowel enema performed after long-tube decompression. Spot radiograph shows the mercury-filled bag (M) of a long decompression tube (a Kantor tube). A loop of small bowel (H) has herniated underneath an adhesion. The adhesion compresses the entry and exit sites (*arrows*) of the loop. This patient had a partial closed-loop obstruction. (From the teaching files of Hans Herlinger, MD.)

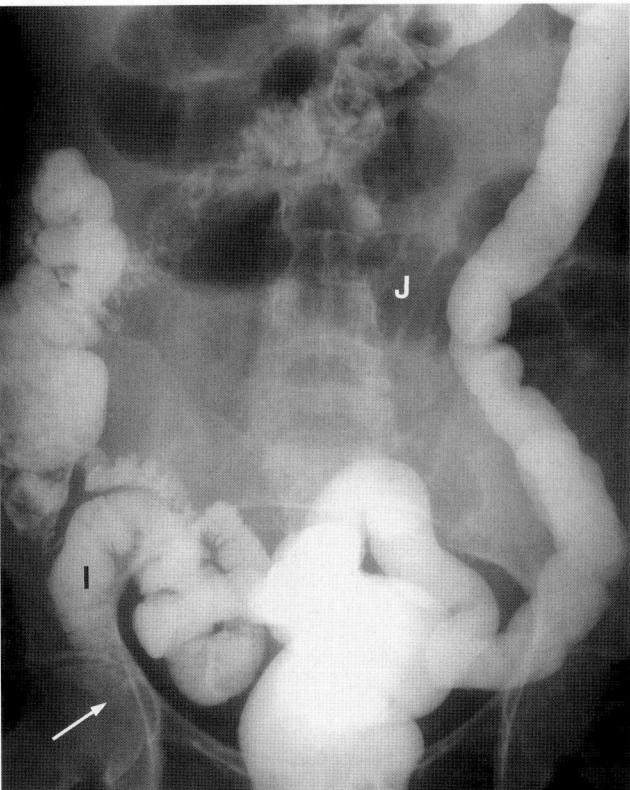

Figure 50-58. Barium enema demonstrating high-grade small bowel obstruction from an incarcerated inguinal hernia. An overhead radiograph from a single-contrast barium enema shows dilated, gas-filled loops of jejunum (J) in the upper abdomen. Barium has refluxed from the colon into the distal ileum (I), where it stops at the internal ring of the right inguinal canal (*arrow*).

a Miller-Abbott tube, Kantor tube (Fig. 50-57), or enteroclysis catheter with a built-in suction port is helpful.[86,87] The small bowel is decompressed, and an antegrade barium study is performed.

If more information is needed after CT, a single-contrast barium enema with reflux of barium into the distal small bowel to the site of obstruction is often better than an antegrade study in patients with high-grade distal small bowel obstruction (Fig. 50-58; see Fig. 50-52D). After administration of 1 mg of intravenous glucagon to relax the ileocecal valve, barium can be refluxed into the distal ileum in 85% of patients. Barium is then propelled in a retrograde fashion by addition of water to the enema bag. This is an excellent technique that can easily visualize pelvic loops of ileum and even the proximal ileum and jejunum. The barium enema is also an excellent examination in patients with an ileocecal anastomosis. A long length of small intestine can be visualized by retrograde flow of barium, with demonstration of the transition zone in patients with small bowel obstruction.

In patients with an ileostomy or colostomy, a retrograde ileostomy or colostomy enema can also be performed to evaluate for distal small bowel obstruction.

Enteroclysis and small bowel follow-through studies are reserved for patients with known or suspected low-grade small bowel obstruction. Enteroclysis should not be performed in patients with high-grade small bowel obstruction, suspected strangulation or perforation, or adynamic ileus. Enteroclysis is superior to small bowel follow-through studies in demonstration of short lesions such as strictures or tumors. By overdistending the small intestine, enteroclysis can demonstrate even subtle adhesions (see Fig. 50-2). Obstruction is suggested by distention of the jejunal diameter to greater than 4 cm and the ileal diameter to greater than 3 cm. A high-grade obstruction is implied by delayed passage of contrast to the site of the transition zone, dilution of contrast material, and

minimal passage of contrast material through the transition zone. A low-grade obstruction is diagnosed if there is delayed passage of contrast material at the transition zone itself. Small bowel follow-through studies are more physiologic, however, with inherent small bowel motility propelling the barium along the gastrointestinal tract, allowing a more accurate estimate of transit time. Small bowel follow-through examinations are also much easier on both the patient and examiner, but only in the setting of low-grade or absent small bowel obstruction. Long lesions such as Crohn's disease and ischemia (Fig. 50-59) can be easily be demonstrated on small bowel follow-throughs in patients with low-grade obstruction. Small bowel follow through examinations (especially with a peroral pneumocolon) are probably superior in demonstration of the terminal ileum in comparison to enteroclysis.

Other Examinations

CT and MR enteroclysis are intubation techniques discussed in earlier chapters.[88] The authors of the chapter believe these techniques combine the worst of both modalities: the difficulty and discomfort of intubation and the lower resolution and lack of en face mucosal detail in CT and MR. Like enteroclysis, these techniques have little or no role in patients with suspected high-grade small bowel obstruction. Blinded studies are needed to determine if these modalities add to multidetector-row CT or enteroclysis in the diagnosis of

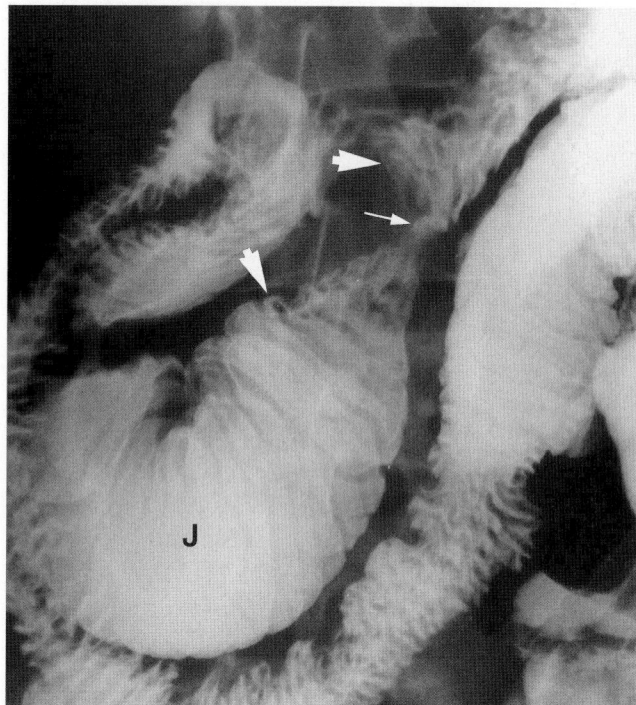

Figure 50-59. Small bowel follow-through demonstrating low-grade obstruction by an ischemic stricture. A spot radiograph shows a segment of tapered small bowel narrowing (*thick arrows*) with a small central ulcer (*thin arrow*) and preserved folds. The jejunum (J) is dilated proximal to the stricture. (From Rubesin SE, Furth EE: Differential diagnosis of small intestinal abnormalities with radiologic-pathologic explanation. In Herlinger H, Maglinte DDT, Birnbaum BA [eds]: Clinical Imaging of the Small Intestine, 2nd ed. New York, Springer, 1999, pp 527-566.)

suspected low-grade small bowel obstruction. Perhaps these techniques will be of value in patients with carcinoid tumor, radiation therapy, and peritoneal metastasis. Ultrasonography is a modality that should also be considered for evaluating small bowel obstruction in adults if CT or contrast studies are unavailable.[89-92]

References

1. Haubrich WS: Medical Meanings: A Glossary of Word Origins, 2nd ed. Philadelphia, College of Physicians, 2003.
2. Soybel DI: Ileus and bowel obstruction. In Greenfield LJ, Mulholland MW, Oldham DT, et al (eds): Surgery: Scientific Principles and Practice. Philadelphia, Lippincott Williams & Wilkins, 2001, pp 798-812.
3. Basson M, Fielding LP, Bilchik A, et al: Does vasoactive intestinal polypeptide mediate the pathophysiology of bowel obstruction? Am J Surg 157:109, 1989.
4. Ohman U: Studies on small intestinal obstruction: I. Intraluminal pressure in experiment low obstruction in the cat. Acta Chir Scand 141:413, 1975.
5. Ellis H, Moran BJ, Thompson JN, et al: Adhesion-related hospital readmissions after abdominal and pelvic surgery: A retrospective cohort study. Lancet 353:1476-1480, 1999.
6. Markogiannakis H, Messaris E, Dardamanis D, et al: Acute mechanical bowel obstruction: Clinical presentation, etiology, management and outcome. World J Gastroenterol 13:432-437, 2007.
7. Petrovic B, Nikolaidis P, Hammond NA, et al: Identification of adhesions on CT in small-bowel obstruction. Emerg Radiol 12:88-93, 2006.
8. Coletti L, Bossart PA: Intestinal obstruction in the early postoperative period. Arch Surg 55:385, 1989.
9. Foster NM, McGory ML, Zingmond DS, et al: Small bowel obstruction: A population-based appraisal. J Am Coll Surg 203:170-176, 2006.
10. Birnbaum BA, Maglinte DDT: Small bowel obstruction. In Herlinger H,
Maglinte DDT, Birnbaum BA (eds): Clinical Imaging of the Small Intestine. New York, Springer, 1999, pp 467-506.
11. Megibow AJ, Balthazar EJ, Cho KC, et al: Bowel obstruction: Evaluation with CT. Radiology 180:313-318, 1991.
12. Fukuya T, Hawes DR, Lu CC, et al: CT diagnosis of small bowel obstruction: Efficacy in 60 patients. AJR 158:765-769, 1992.
13. Thompson WM, Kilani RK, Smith BB, et al: Accuracy of abdominal radiography in acute small-bowel obstruction: Does reviewer experience matter? AJR Am J Roentgenol 188:W233-238, 2007.
14. Yaghmai V, Nikolaidis P, Hammond NA, et al: Multidetector-row computed tomography diagnosis of small bowel obstruction: Can coronal reformations replace axial images? Emerg Radiol 13:69-72, 2006.
15. Gazelle GS, Goldberg MA, Wittenberg J, et al: Efficacy of CT in distinguishing small-bowel obstruction from other causes of small bowel dilatation. AJR 162:43-47, 1994.
16. Maglinte DDT, Nolan DJ, Herlinger H: Preoperative diagnosis by enteroclysis of unsuspected closed-loop obstruction in medically managed patients. J Clin Gastroenterol 13:308-312, 1991.
17. Balthazar EJ: CT of small-bowel obstruction. AJR 162:255-261, 1994.
18. Taourel PG, Fabre JM, Pradel JA, et al: Value of CT in diagnosis and management of patients with suspected acute small-bowel obstruction. AJR 165:1187-192, 1995.
19. Maglinte DDT, Herliner H, Nolan DJ: Radiologic features of closed loop obstruction: Analysis of 25 confirmed cases. Radiology 179:383-387, 1991.
20. Balthazar EJ, Birnbaum BA, Megibow AJ et al: Closed-loop and strangulating intestinal obstruction: CT signs. Radiology 185:769-775, 1992.
21. Cho KC, Hoffman-Tretin JC, Alterman DD: Closed-loop obstruction of the small bowel: CT and sonographic appearance. J Comput Assist Tomogr 13:256-257, 1989.
22. Frager D, Baer JW, Medwid SW, et al: Detection of intestinal ischemia in patients with acute small-bowel obstruction due to adhesions or hernia: Efficacy of CT. AJR 166:67-71, 1996.
23. Zaleman M, van Gansbeke D, Lalmand B, et al: Delayed enhancement of the bowel wall: A new CT sign of small bowel strangulation. J Comput Assist Tomogr 20:379-381, 1996.
24. Sheedy SP, Earnest F 4th, Fletcher JG, et al: CT of small-bowel ischemia associated with obstruction in emergency department patients: Diagnostic performance evaluation. Radiology 241:729-736, 2006.
25. Goodman P, Raval B: CT diagnosis of acquired small bowel volvulus. Am Surg 56:628-631, 1990.
26. Shaff MI, Himmelfarb E, Sacks GA, et al: The whirl sign: A CT finding in volvulus of the large bowel. J Comput Assist Tomogr 9:410, 1985.
27. Price J, Nolan DJ: Closed-loop obstruction: Diagnosis by enteroclysis. Gastrointest Radiol 14:251-254, 1989.
28. Maglinte DDT, Herlinger H, Nolan DJ: Radiologic features of closed loop obstruction: Analysis of 25 confirmed cases. Radiology 179:383-387, 1991.
29. Mathieu D, Luciani A: Internal abdominal herniations. AJR 183:397-404, 2004.
30. Yu C-Y, Lin C-C, Yu J-C, et al: Strangulated transmesosigmoid hernia: CT diagnosis. Abdom Imaging 29:158-160, 2004.
31. Haku T, Daidougi K, Kawamura H, Matsuzaki M: Internal herniation through a defect of the broad ligament of the uterus. Abdom Imaging 29:161-163, 2004.
32. Catqalano OA, Bencivenga A, Abbate M, et al: Internal hernia with volvulus and intussusception: Case report. Abdom Imaging 29:164-165, 2004.
33. Ihedioha U, Alani A, Modak P, et al: Hernias are the most common cause of strangulation in patients presenting with small bowel obstruction. Hernia 10:338-340, 2006.
34. Aguirre DDA, Casola G, Sirlin C: Abdominal wall hernias: MDCT findings. AJR 183:681-690, 2004.
35. Emby DJ, Aoun G: CT technique for suspected anterior abdominal wall hernia. AJR 181:431-433, 2003.
36. Meyers MA: Intraperitoneal spread of malignancies. In Meyers MA (ed): Dynamic Radiology of the Abdomen, 5th ed. New York, Springer, 2000, pp 131-255.
37. Rubesin SE, Furth EE: Differential diagnosis of small intestinal abnormalities with radiologic-pathologic explanation. In Herlinger H, Maglinte DDT, Birnbaum BA (eds): Clinical Imaging of the Small Intestine, 2nd ed. New York, Springer-Verlag, 1999, pp 527-566.
38. Zboralske FF, Bessolo RJ: Metastatic carcinoma to the mesentery and gut. Radiology 88:302-310, 1967.
39. Moertel CJ, Sauer WG, Dockerty MB, et al: Life history of the carcinoid tumor of the small intestine. Cancer 14:901-912, 1961.

40. Horton KM, Kamel I, Hofmann L, Fishman EK: Carcinoid tumors of the small bowel: A multi-technique imaging approach. AJR 182:559-567, 2004.

41. Rubesin SE, Gilchrist AM, Bronner M, et al: Non-Hodgkin lymphoma of the small intestine. RadioGraphics 10:985-998, 1990.

42. Levine MS, Drooz AT, Herlinger H: Annular malignancies of the small bowel. Gastrointest Radiol 12:53-58, 1987.

43. Caroline DF, Herlinger H, Laufer I, et al: Small-bowel enema in the diagnosis of adhesive obstruction. AJR 142:1133-1139, 1984.

44. Mekhijian HS, Switz DM, Watts HD, et al: National cooperative Crohn's disease study: Factors determining recurrence of Crohn's disease after surgery. Gastroenterology 77:907, 1979.

45. Graham MF, Diegelmann RF, Elson CO, et al: Collagen contents and types in the intestinal stricture of Crohn's disease. Gastroenterology 84:257-265, 1988.

46. Zissin R, Hertz M, Paran H, et al: Small bowel obstruction secondary to Crohn disease: CT findings. Abdom Imaging 29:320-325, 2003.

47. Gore RM, Balthazar EJ, Ghahremani GG, Miller FH: CT features of ulcerative colitis and Crohn's disease. AJR 167:3-15, 1996.

48. Greenstein-Orel S, Rubesin SE, Jones B, et al: Computed tomography vs barium studies in the acutely symptomatic patient with Crohn's disease. J Comput Assist Tomogr 11:1009-1016, 1987.

49. Palmer KR, Patil DH, Basran GS, et al: Abdominal tuberculosis in urban Britain—a common disease. Gut 26:1296-1305, 1985.

50. Mendelsohn RM, Nolan DJ: The radiological features of radiation enteritis. Clin Radiol 36:141-148, 1985.

51. Fishman EK, Zinreich JS, Jones B, et al: Computed tomographic diagnosis of radiation ileitis. Gastrointest Radiol 9:149-152, 1984.

52. Czyrko C, Weltz CR, Markowitz RI, et al: Blunt abdominal trauma resulting in intestinal obstruction: when to operate? J Trauma 30:1567-1571, 1990.

53. Bjarnason I, Price AB, Zanelli G, et al: Clinicopathological features of nonsteroid antiinflammatory drug-induced small intestinal strictures. Gastroenterology 94:1070-1074, 1988.

54. Grumbach K, Levine MS, Wexler JA: Gallstone ileus diagnosed by computed tomography. J Comput Assist Tomogr 10:146-148, 1986.

55. Balthazar EJ, Schechter LS: Gallstone ileus: The importance of contrast examinations in the roentgenographic diagnosis. AJR 125:374-378, 1975.

56. Bloom RR, Nakano PH, Gray SW, et al: Foreign bodies of the gastrointestinal tract. Am J Surg 52:618-621, 1986.

57. Price JE, Michael SL, Morgenstein L: Fruit pit obstruction: The propitious pit. Arch Surg 111:773-775, 1976.

58. Sandrasegaran K, Kopecky KK, Rajesh A, Lappas J: Proximal small bowel intussusceptions in adults: CT appearance and clinical significance. Abdom Imaging 29:653-657, 2004.

59. Lvoff N, Breiman RS, Coakley, et al: Distinguishing features of self-limiting adult small bowel intussusception identified at CT. Radiology 227:68-72, 2003.

60. Warshauer DM, Lee JK: Adult intussusception detected at CT or MR imaging: Clinical imaging correlation. Radiology 212:853-860, 1999.

61. Sarr MG, Nagorney, DM, McIlrath DC: Post-operative intussusception in the adult. Arch Surg 116:144, 1981.

62. Curcio CM, Feinstein RS, Humphrey RL, et al: Computed tomography of enteroenteric intussusception. J Comput Assist Tomogr 6:969-974, 1982.

63. Balik AA, Ozturk G, Aydinli B, et al: Intussusception in adults. Acta Chir Belg 106:409-412, 2006.

64. Balthazar EJ: CT of the gastrointestinal tract: Principles and interpretation. AJR 156:23-32, 1991.

65. Das Gupta T, Brasfield R: Metastatic melanoma-clinicopathological study. Cancer 17:1323-1339, 1969.

66. Dormandy TL: Gastrointestinal polyposis with mucocutaneous pigmentation (Peutz-Jeghers syndrome). N Engl J Med 256:1093-1103, 1957.

67. Goldstein HM, Beydoon MT, Dodd GD: Radiologic spectrum of melanoma metastatic to the gastrointestinal tract. AJR 129:605-612, 1977.

68. Rubesin SE, Herlinger H, DeGaeta L: Interlude: Test your skills. Inverted Meckel's diverticulum. Radiology 178:636-644, 1990.

69. Ghahremani GG: Radiology of Meckel's diverticulum. Crit Rev Diagn Imaging 26:1-43, 1986.

70. Wood GJ, Kumar, PN, Cooper C, et al: AIDS-associated intussusception in young adults. J Clin Gastroenterol 21:158-162, 1995.

71. Rubesin SE, Herlinger H: CT evaluation of bowel obstruction: A landmark article. [editorial]. Radiology 180:307-308, 1991.

72. Baker SR: Unenhanced helical CT versus plain abdominal radiography: A dissenting opinion. Radiology 205:45-47, 1997.

73. Mucha P Jr: Small intestinal obstruction. Surg Clin North Am 67:597-620, 1987.

74. Shrake PD, Rex DK, Lappas JC, et al: Radiographic evaluation of suspected small bowel obstruction. Am J Gastroenterol 86:175-178, 1991.

75. Sarr MG, Bulkley GB, Zuidema GD: Preoperative recognition of intestinal strangulation obstruction: Prospective evaluation of diagnostic capability. Am J Surg 145:176-182, 1983.

76. Otamiri T, Sjoedahl R, Ihse I: Intestinal obstruction with strangulation of the small bowel. Acta Chir Scand 153:307-310, 1987.

77. Mindelzun RE, Jeffrey RB: Unenhanced helical CT for evaluating acute abdominal pain: A little more cost, a lot more information. Radiology 205:43-45, 1997.

78. Maglinte DDT, Balthazar EJ, Kelvin FM, Megibow AJ: The role of radiology in the diagnosis of small bowel obstruction. AJR 168:1171-1180, 1997.

79. Balthazar EJ. CT of the gastrointestinal tract: Principles and interpretation. AJR 156:23-32, 1991.

80. Balthazar EJ, Liebeskind ME, Macari M: Intestinal ischemia in patients in whom small bowel obstruction is suspected: Evaluation of accuracy, limitation and clinical implications of CT in diagnosis. Radiology 205:510-522, 1997.

81. Kernagis LY, Levine MS, Jacobs JE: Pneumatosis intestinalis in patients with ischemia. Correlation of CT findings with viability of the bowel. AJR 180:733-736, 2003.

82. Macari M, Megibow A: Imaging of suspected acute small bowel obstruction. Semin Roentgenol 36:108-117, 2001.

83. Furukawa A, Yamasaki M, Takahashi M, et al: CT diagnosis of small bowel obstruction: Scanning technique, interpretation and role in the diagnosis. Semin Ultrasound CT MRI 24:336-352, 2003.

84. Obuz F, Terzi C, Sokmen S, et al: The efficacy of helical CT in the diagnosis of small bowel obstruction. Eur J Radiol 48:299-304, 2003.

85. Assalia A, Shein M, Kopelman D, et al: Therapeutic effect of oral Gastrografin in adhesive, partial small bowel obstruction: A prospective randomized trial. Surgery 115:433-437, 1994.

86. Maglinte DDT, Steven LH, Hall RC, et al: Dual purpose tube for enteroclysis and nasogastric/nasoenteric decompression. Radiology 185:281-282, 1992.

87. Maglinte DDT, Kelvin FM, Milcon LT, et al: Nasointestinal tube for decompression or enteroclysis: Experience with 150 patients. Abdom Imaging 19:108-112, 1994.

88. Bender GN, Maglinte DDT, von Kloeppel R, et al: CT enteroclysis: A superfluous diagnostic procedure or valuable when investigating small-bowel disease [review]? AJR 172:373-378, 1999.

89. Noone TC, Semelka RC, Chaney DM, et al: Abdominal imaging studies: Comparison of diagnostic accuracies resulting from ultrasound, computed tomography, and magnetic resonance imaging in the same individual. Magn Reson Imaging 22:19-24, 2004.

90. O'Malley ME, Wilson SR: US of gastrointestinal tract abnormalities with CT correlation. RadioGraphics 23:59-72, 2003.

91. Maglinte DD: Small bowel imaging—a rapidly changing field and a challenge to radiology. Eur Radiol 16:967-971, 2006.

92. Hong SS, Kim AY, Byun JH, et al: MDCT of small-bowel disease: Value of 3D imaging. AJR Am J Roentgenol 187:1212-1221, 2006.

93. Jaffe TA, Martin LC, Thomas J, et al: Small-bowel obstruction: Coronal reformations from isotropic voxels at 16-section multi-detector row CT. Radiology 238:135-142, 2006.

Vascular Disorders of the Small Intestine

Karen M. Horton, MD • Elliot K. Fishman, MD

Small bowel pathology continues to be a diagnostic challenge for both clinicians and radiologists. Clinicians struggle to diagnose many small bowel diseases because patients typically present with very nonspecific complaints, such as abdominal pain, weight loss, or anemia. Therefore, in most cases, the diagnosis of small bowel pathology relies on the radiologist. Traditional barium studies of the small intestine are still helpful in diagnosing many small bowel diseases. However, they are inherently limited because they only image the lumen of the bowel and give very little information about extramural disease. Since its introduction in the late 1970s, computed tomography has been used to image the small intestine and is now routinely employed to evaluate small bowel obstruction and Crohn's disease. With the advent of the multidetector scanner, CT has taken on a larger diagnostic role in small bowel disease, including diagnosis of vascular disorders of the small intestine.

Vascular disorders of the small intestine encompass a variety of conditions that primarily affect the mesenteric vasculature. These conditions are typically very difficult to diagnose both clinically and radiographically; often angiography or surgery is ultimately relied on to establish the diagnosis. With the introduction of multidetector CT (MDCT), which allows faster scanning and thinner collimation along with the development of sophisticated 3D imaging tools, it is now possible to image the small bowel vasculature as well as the small intestine in a single examination. This offers a comprehensive evaluation of patients with a wide variety of suspected small bowel vascular disorders.

In this chapter we review the current status of imaging of a variety of vascular disorders of the small intestine, including mesenteric ischemia and infarction, vasculitis, hemangiomas, aneurysms, and radiation enteritis. Although a variety of imaging modalities are discussed, the focus is on the use of MDCT and 3D imaging for the diagnosis of these conditions.

COMPUTED TOMOGRAPHIC IMAGING

Computed tomographic imaging of the gastrointestinal tract has undergone considerable improvement over the past several years. The introduction of 64-slice MDCT now allows submillimeter imaging and the creation of isotropic datasets. This, along with significant advancements in 3D imaging software, now makes it possible to obtain high-resolution images of the small intestine as well as of the mesenteric arteries and veins. In the past, patients with suspected vascular disorders of the small intestine required conventional angiography. CT can now be used initially as a primary imaging modality in these patients.

If a vascular disorder of the small intestine is suspected clinically, a dedicated examination of the small bowel and mesentery should be obtained. Because vascular disorders can affect both the mesenteric arteries as well as veins, it is necessary to obtain dual-phase imaging through the entire abdomen and pelvis. At our institution, approximately 120 mL of nonionic contrast is injected at a rapid rate (3 to 5 mL/s) through a large-caliber peripheral catheter. Arterial phase images are obtained approximately 30 seconds after the start of the injection, and venous phase images are obtained approximately 50 seconds after the start of the injection. This dual-phase imaging allows excellent visualization of the mesenteric arteries and the mesenteric veins.

Thin collimation is essential to maintain high resolution in all imaging planes. At this point we use our 64-slice scanner and the 0.6-mm collimator setting. This allows creation of 0.75-mm slices, which are reconstructed every 0.5 mm for 3D imaging. Because of the complexity of the mesenteric vasculature, multiplanar reformat (MPR) views and preferably volume-rendered 3D imaging are necessary to completely visualize all of the branches. The choice of the 3D rendering algorithm is crucial in this clinical setting. There are currently three main rendering algorithms available: shaded surface (SS), volume rendering (VR), and maximum intensity projection (MIP). Shaded surface rendering is the most basic of the three but of limited value for evaluating the mesenteric arteries and bowel. Therefore, it is usually a combination of volume rendering and MIP that is most valuable for this clinical indication.

Anatomy of the small bowel and the mesenteric vasculature is complicated so it is usually necessary to use a variety of

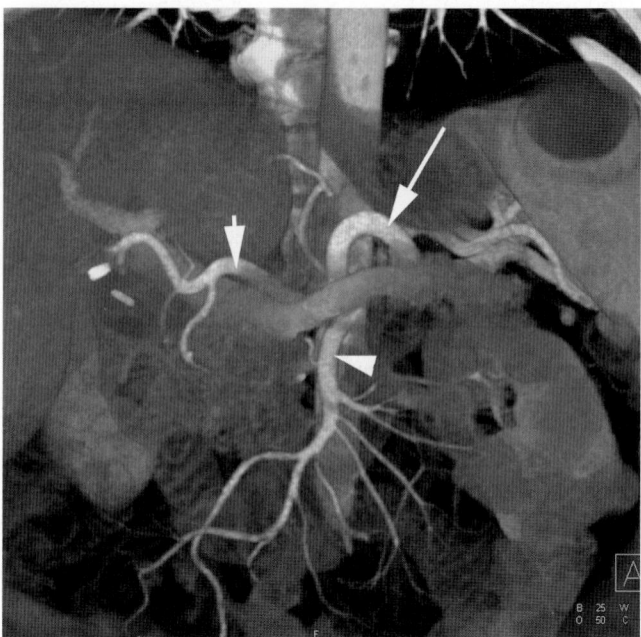

Figure 51-2. Normal celiac and superior mesenteric artery coronal anatomy. Coronal volume-rendered 3D CT angiogram shows normal anatomy of the celiac axis (splenic artery [*long arrow*], common hepatic artery [*short arrow*]) and SMA (*arrowhead*). The coronal projection allows easy identification of the branches of the SMA.

imaging planes. For visualization of the proximal portion of the celiac axis, the superior mesenteric artery (SMA), and the inferior mesenteric artery (IMA), a sagittal projection is most helpful (Fig. 51-1). However, to adequately visualize the complicated vascular branching of the vessels, coronal or coronal oblique planes are usually needed (Fig. 51-2). Similarly, the mesenteric veins are best seen in a coronal projection (Fig. 51-3). This can be performed easily in real time using new advanced 3D imaging software. After adequate evaluation of the vessels it is also important to comprehensively image the bowel (Fig. 51-4). This typically relies on using cut planes to remove overlapping bowel loops. Usually coronal and/or sagittal or axial oblique imaging planes are most helpful.

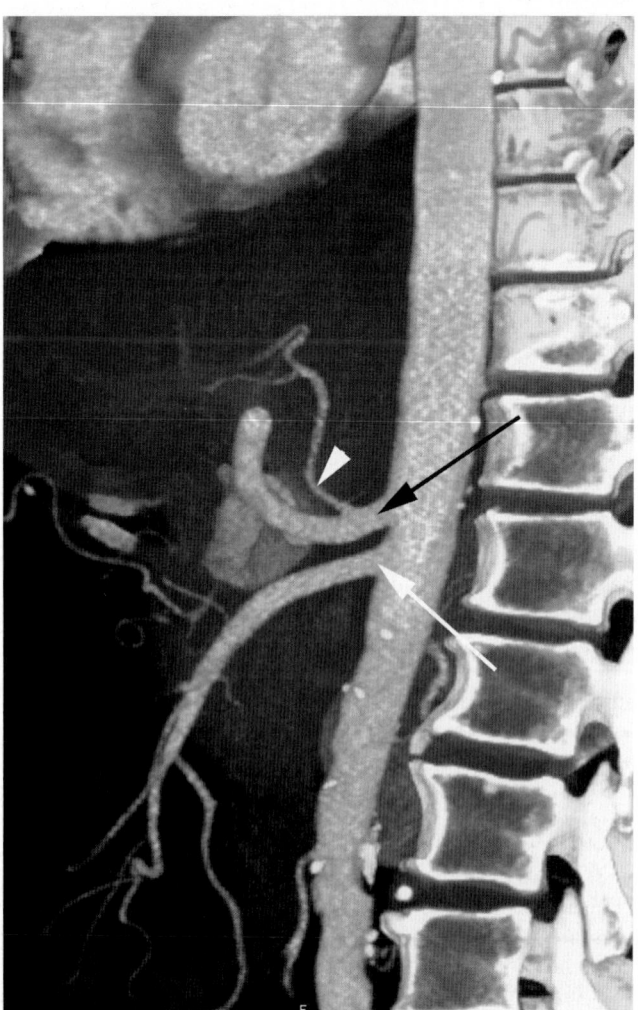

Figure 51-1. Normal celiac and superior mesenteric artery sagittal anatomy. Sagittal volume-rendered 3D CT angiogram shows normal anatomy of the celiac axis (*black arrow*) and SMA (*white arrow*). The left gastric artery (*arrowhead*) can also be seen arising from the celiac artery.

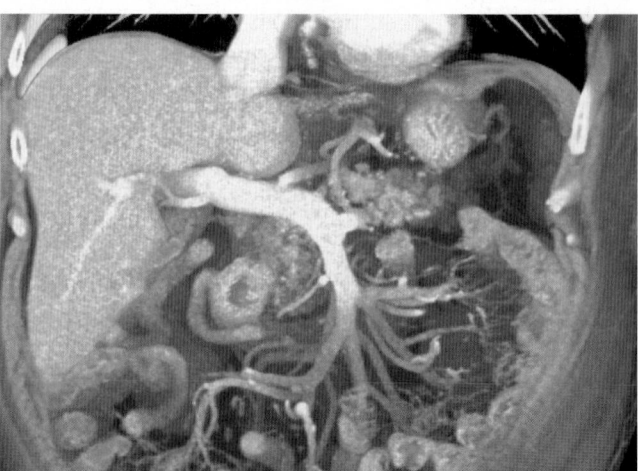

Figure 51-3. Normal mesenteric veins. Coronal volume-rendered 3D CT demonstrates the normal appearance of the mesenteric veins as they join the splenic vein and portal vein at the confluence.

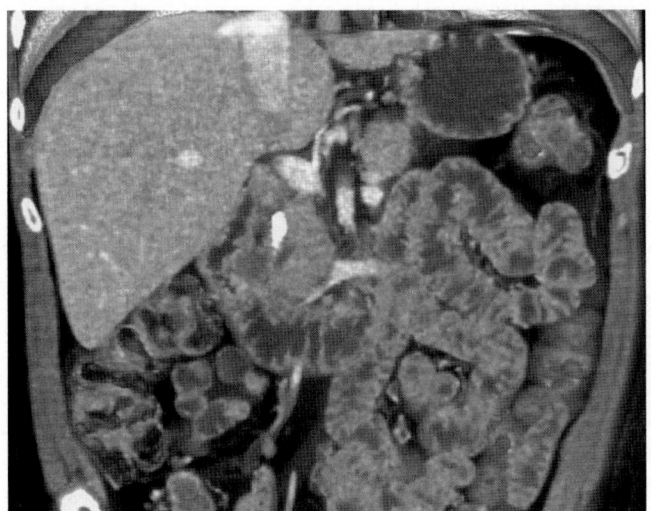

Figure 51-4. Normal small bowel: coronal volume-rendered image.

MESENTERIC ISCHEMIA

Mesenteric ischemia is a complicated disorder that is increasing in incidence as the population ages, accounting for approximately 1% of all cases of the acute abdomen[1,2] and 0.1% of all hospital admissions.[3] Despite its frequency as well as heightened clinical awareness of the condition, morbidity and mortality rates for mesenteric ischemia have remained high, largely related to delay in diagnosis.[4,5] Delay in diagnosis and treatment is due to the lack of accurate and safe imaging tools. Angiography is considered to be the gold standard for the radiographic diagnosis of ischemia and in some cases not only can make the diagnosis but also can provide transcatheter therapy.[6] Early implementation of angiography has been the main factor in improved mortality rates over the past 30 years.[7] However, angiography is expensive, invasive, and sometimes risky to perform in the population in which intestinal ischemia most commonly occurs. Therefore, CT is often used as the first-line imaging modality to confirm the diagnosis or to suggest alternative conditions, which may explain the patient's symptoms.

Mesenteric ischemia occurs when there is compromised blood flow to the small intestine. It can result in a broad spectrum of disorders, depending on etiology, onset, and duration of the injury. The variability in these factors influences the clinical presentation as well as the radiographic findings and often dictates the appropriate treatment and ultimate prognosis. Mesenteric ischemia is typically classified into two categories: acute mesenteric ischemia and chronic mesenteric ischemia.

Acute Mesenteric Ischemia

Acute mesenteric ischemia is one of the most serious and life-threatening abdominal conditions and has an estimated mortality of 60% to 80%.[3,6]

Acute ischemia results from a significant and usually rapid reduction of blood flow to the intestines. The major causes of acute mesenteric ischemia include arterial or venous occlusion or nonocclusive reduction of intestinal blood flow. Acute thrombosis or embolization to the SMA accounts for 60% to 70% of cases, whereas mesenteric vein thrombosis repre-

sents 5% to 10% of cases. Nonocclusive ischemia resulting from low flow states accounts for up to 30% of cases. Therefore, comprehensive radiographic examination of patients with suspected mesenteric ischemia requires high-resolution evaluation of the mesenteric vessels (arteries and veins) as well as the small bowel and colon.

Emboli to the superior mesenteric artery typically are associated with cardiac arrhythmias such as atrial fibrillation but can also occur in valvular disease, recent myocardial infarction or mycotic aneurysms of the thoracic aorta.[8] The wide-caliber lumen and narrow-angle takeoff of the SMA make it especially susceptible to emboli.[9] A large embolus can lodge in the proximal portion of the SMA, resulting in extensive involvement of the entire mesenteric small bowel and right colon. The embolus most often lodges in the proximal SMA, 3 to 10 cm from the origin (Figs. 51-5 and 51-6).[9] Smaller emboli will lodge more distally and may affect only small segments of bowel, owing to the availability of collateral flow.

Thrombi originating in the SMA are less common than emboli but can occur in patients with hypercoagulable conditions, such as protein C or S antithrombin III deficiency. Thrombus can also form in areas of severe atherosclerotic narrowing, typically occurring at the origin of the SMA and/or celiac axis (Fig. 51-7).[4]

Acute arterial ischemia can also occur in the absence of thrombus in patients with vasculitis and in patients with complicated bowel obstruction or be due to mesenteric vessel encasement by tumors (Fig. 51-8). Any condition that results in an abrupt decreased in arterial perfusion to the intestines can result in acute ischemia.

Acute ischemia can result from thrombosis of the mesenteric veins (Figs. 51-9 and 51-10). SMV thrombosis can occur in patients with hypercoagulable states, polycythemia rubra vera, carcinomatosis, portal hypertension, or patients taking oral contraceptives. Mesenteric vein thrombosis can also occur in patients with infectious disorders such as diverticulitis or appendicitis. Historically, no identifiable cause is be found in 20% to 30% of cases.[10]

The third major category of acute mesenteric ischemia is the nonocclusive type. This accounts for approximately 30% of all cases and is associated with a 70% mortality rate.[11] Nonocclusive mesenteric ischemia occurs when there is a decrease in blood pressure, typically associated with cardiac failure, trauma (Fig. 51-11), or widespread sepsis in patients with underlying significant atherosclerotic disease. Certain drugs such as digitalis can decrease the mesenteric blood flow and result in ischemia. In younger patients, nonocclusive mesenteric ischemia has been reported with cocaine use (Fig. 51-12), which results in splanchnic vasoconstriction to preserve blood flow to the heart and brain.[12]

Computed Tomographic Findings

The sensitivity of CT for the diagnosis of acute ischemia has increased significantly over the years, from a low of 39% to a recent high of 82%, which is comparable to catheter angiography.[13-15] The typical CT features of acute mesenteric ischemia include the following:

1. *Dilatation.* Small bowel dilatation is a common, nonspecific finding (see Fig. 51-5), reported in 8 of 9 patients in one series.[16] Bowel dilatation is more commonly found in mural infarction than in reversible

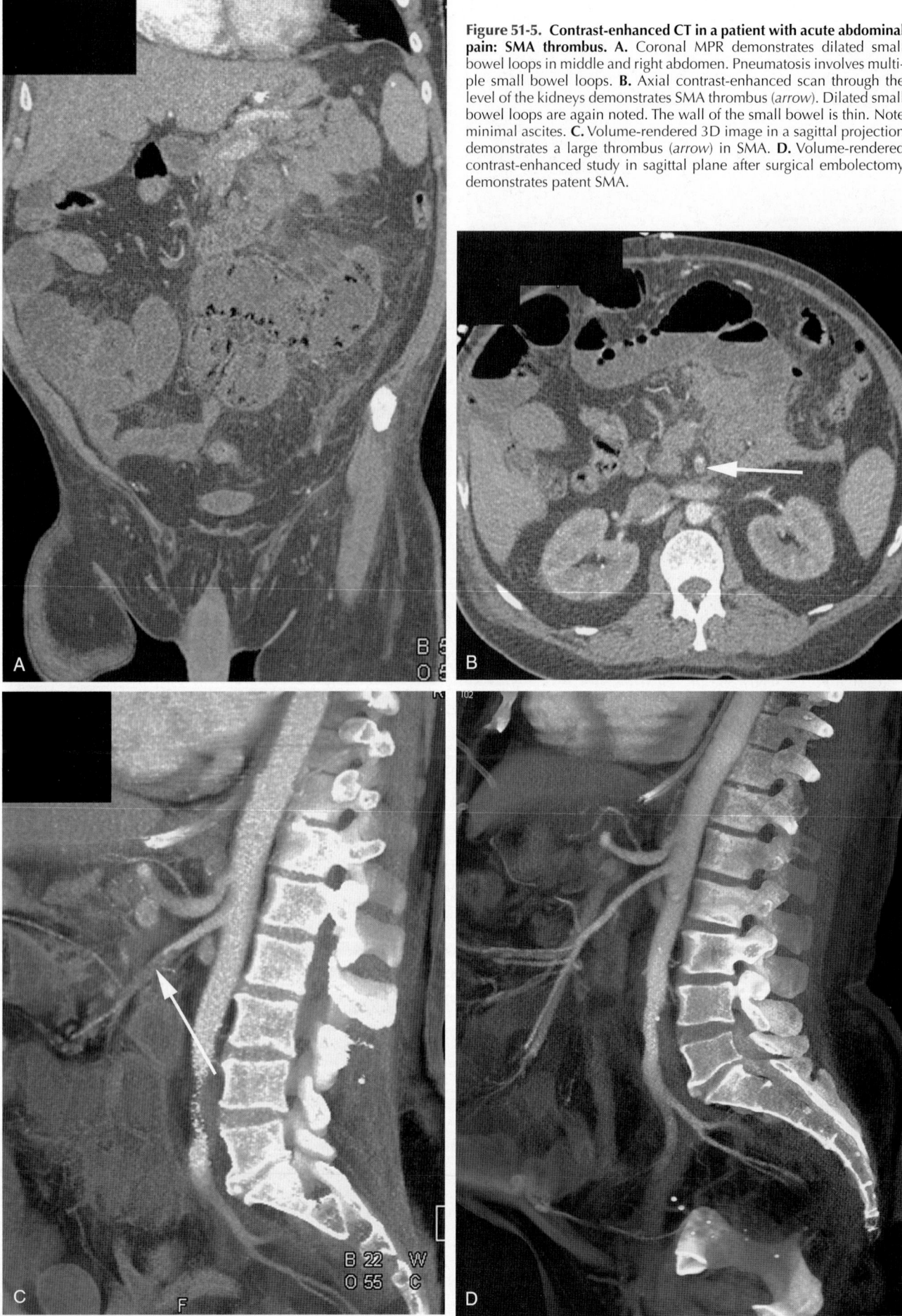

Figure 51-5. Contrast-enhanced CT in a patient with acute abdominal pain: SMA thrombus. A. Coronal MPR demonstrates dilated small bowel loops in middle and right abdomen. Pneumatosis involves multiple small bowel loops. **B.** Axial contrast-enhanced scan through the level of the kidneys demonstrates SMA thrombus (*arrow*). Dilated small bowel loops are again noted. The wall of the small bowel is thin. Note minimal ascites. **C.** Volume-rendered 3D image in a sagittal projection demonstrates a large thrombus (*arrow*) in SMA. **D.** Volume-rendered contrast-enhanced study in sagittal plane after surgical embolectomy demonstrates patent SMA.

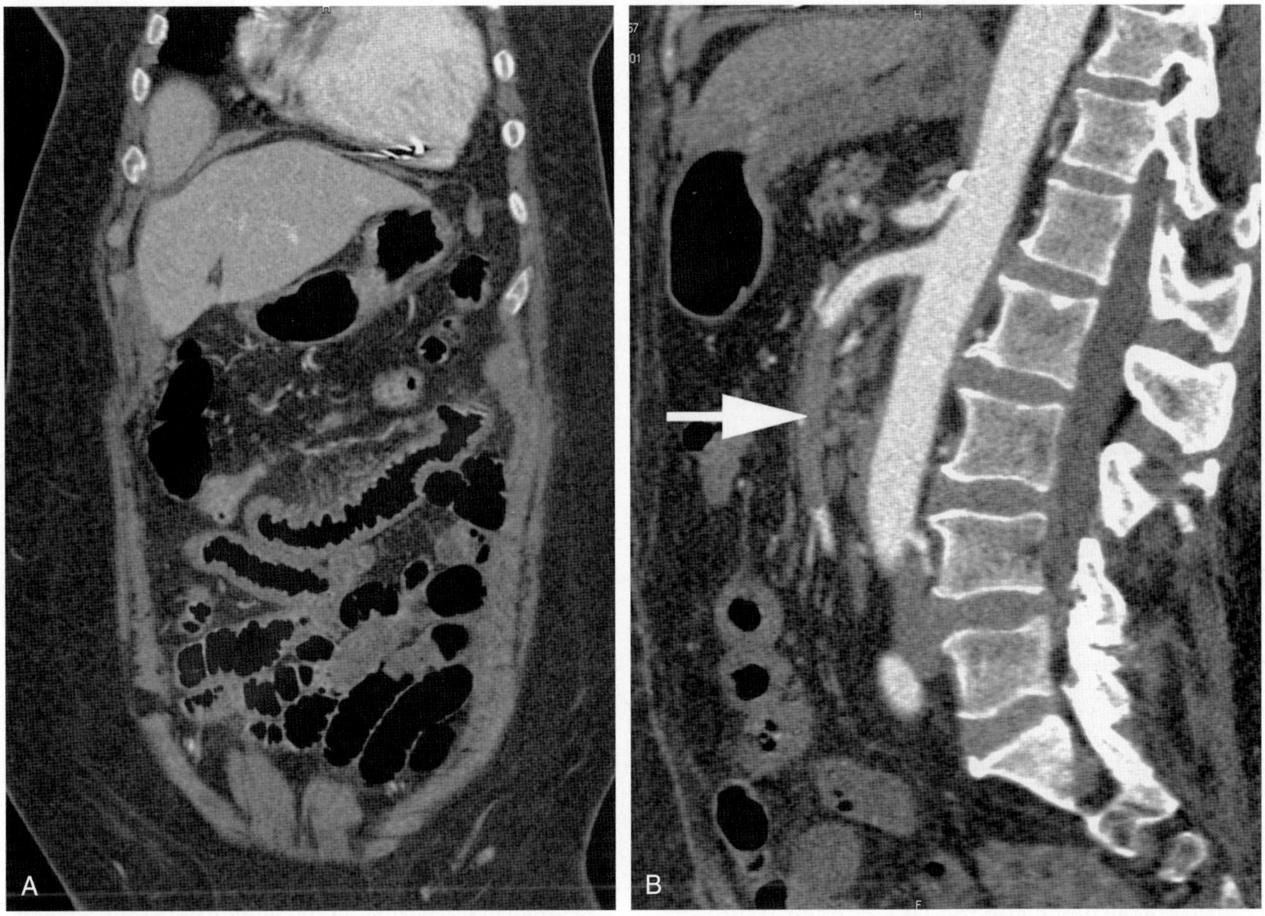

Figure 51-6. Patient with acute abdominal pain: SMA thrombus. A. Coronal MPR demonstrates minimal-to-moderate thickening of multiple small bowel loops in the midabdomen. The wall appears homogeneous in density. **B.** Sagittal MPR demonstrates moderate thrombus (*arrow*) in the SMA. There is also calcification and narrowing of the origin of the celiac artery, which is probably related to chronic atherosclerotic disease.

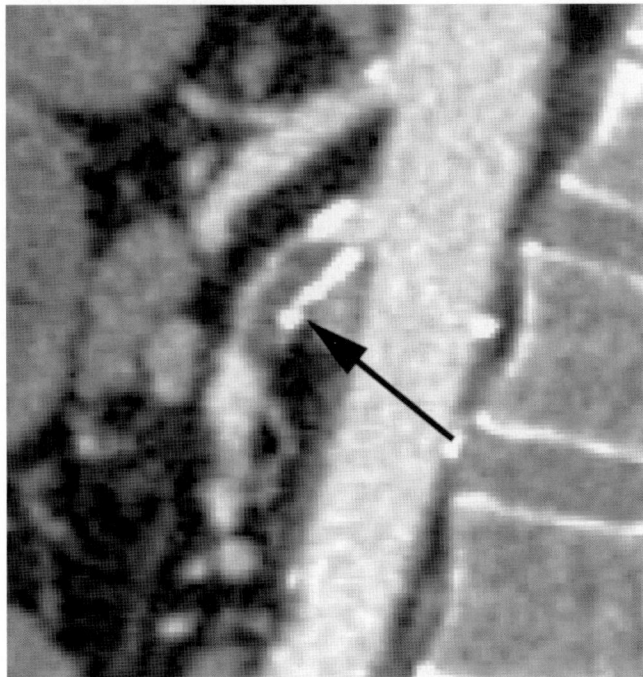

Figure 51-7. Superior mesenteric artery thrombus. Sagittal volume-rendered 3D CT scan demonstrates thrombus (*arrow*) formation at the origin of the SMA in a region of calcified atherosclerotic plaque.

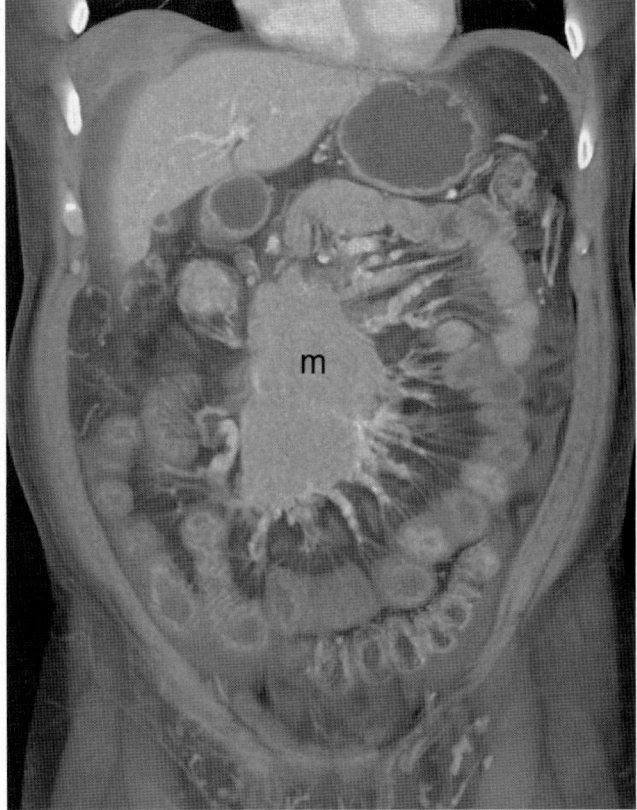

Figure 51-8. Mesenteric carcinoid. Coronal volume-rendered 3D CT scans demonstrate a large mesenteric carcinoid tumor (m) encasing the mesenteric vessels resulting in small bowel wall thickening related to ischemia.

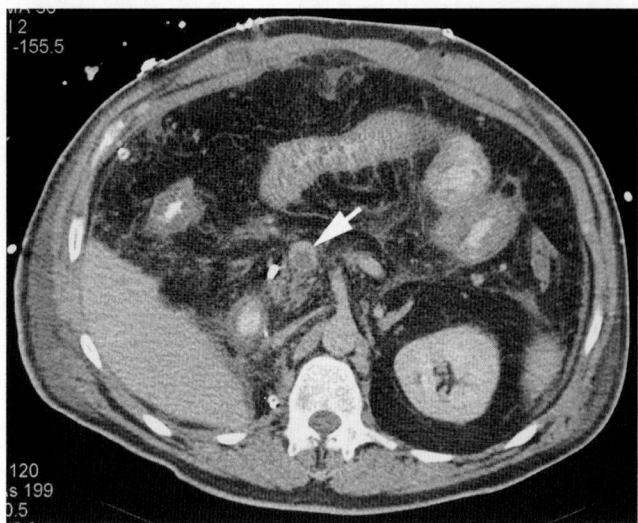

Figure 51-9. Superior mesenteric vein thrombus. Contrast-enhanced CT in a patient with acute abdominal pain demonstrates SMV thrombus (*arrow*). Note the moderate small bowel and right colon thickening.

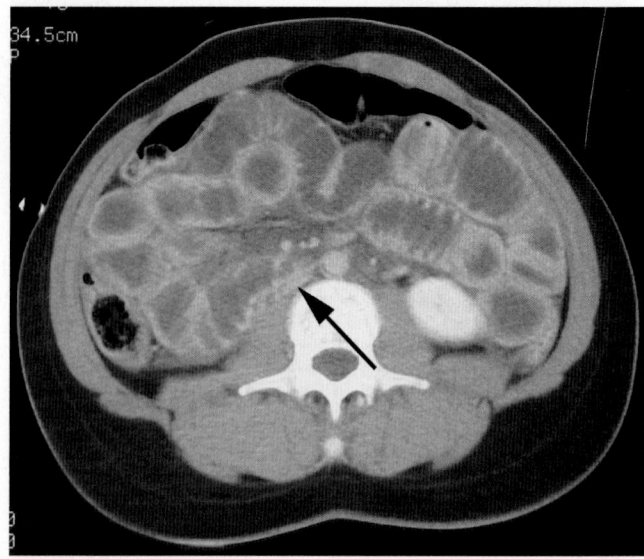

Figure 51-11. Evaluation of a 23-year-old woman in shock after motor vehicle accident. Contrast-enhanced CT demonstrates pneumoperitoneum. The inferior vena cava is flat (*arrow*), compatible with hypovolemia. The bowel is thickened with increased enhancement, compatible with shock bowel.

disease, presumably owing to disruption of normal peristalsis.[17,18]

2. *Bowel wall thickening.* Mural thickening is a very common finding in patients with ischemia. It is usually more prominent in patients with venous thrombosis than arterial thrombosis (see Figs. 51-9 and 51-10).[19] In one series, bowel wall thickening up to 1.5 cm was noted in patients with mesenteric vein thrombosis.[16] Significant bowel wall thickening is also more common in patients with reversible disease, whereas transmural infarction is more likely to result in dilated loops with a paper thin wall, owing to the destruction of intestinal musculature and intramural nerves.[14,15,17,20] Although small bowel wall thickening is a common finding, the presence and degree of bowel wall thickening does not usually correlate with the severity of the ischemic damage.[20]

3. *Abnormal bowel wall attenuation.* The appearance of the bowel wall varies. Typically, the bowel has a target

appearance due to low-density submucosal edema.[21] Intramural hemorrhage can also occur, resulting in high density, either in the submucosa or throughout the bowel wall.[22]

4. *Abnormal mural enhancement.* Small bowel ischemia can result in hyperemia of the affected segments, which can result in increased enhancement after intravenous contrast administration. This increased enhancement can be homogenous and diffuse or can be limited to the mucosa, causing a target appearance (Fig. 51-13).[21] Hyperemia and hyperperfusion of the bowel have been reported to have a sensitivity of 33% and a specificity of 71% for acute mesenteric ischemia.[15] Increased enhancement actually is a positive prognostic sign, because it indicates viable bowel. Absence of enhancement is an uncommon finding but is highly specific for ischemia/infarction.[15] In some patients with ischemia, delayed enhancement of the affected loops can be seen, resulting from delayed delivery of contrast. Similarly, there may be prolonged contrast enhancement in the ischemic segment, owing to delayed washout.

5. *Pneumatosis/portomesenteric venous air.* Pneumatosis and portomesenteric venous gas are uncommon but relatively specific signs that indicate mucosal breakdown and transmural ischemia (Fig. 51-14). Pneumatosis is present in 6% to 28% of cases, and portomesenteric gas occurs in 3% to 14%.[14,15,17,23] The specificity of pneumatosis and portomesenteric venous gas approaches 100%, but these features can also be seen in nonischemic conditions such as infectious and inflammatory enteritis and iatrogenic mucosal injuries.[20]

6. *Stranding and ascites.* Ascites and mesenteric stranding are nonspecific findings in patients with bowel ischemia (see Figs. 51-5 and 51-8). Their presence

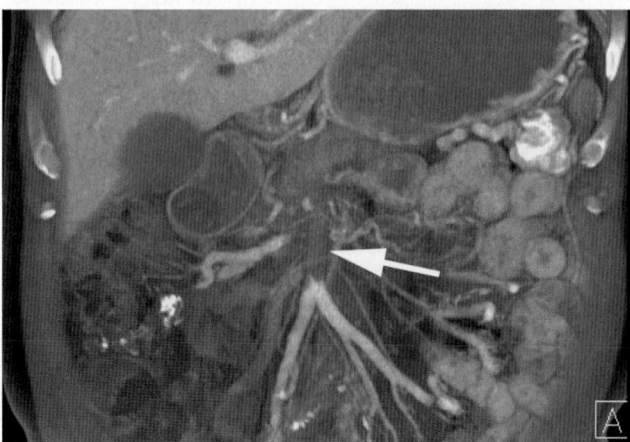

Figure 51-10. Superior mesenteric vein thrombus. Coronal volume-rendered 3D CT shows moderate thickening of the small bowel. A large thrombus (*arrow*) is seen in the SMV.

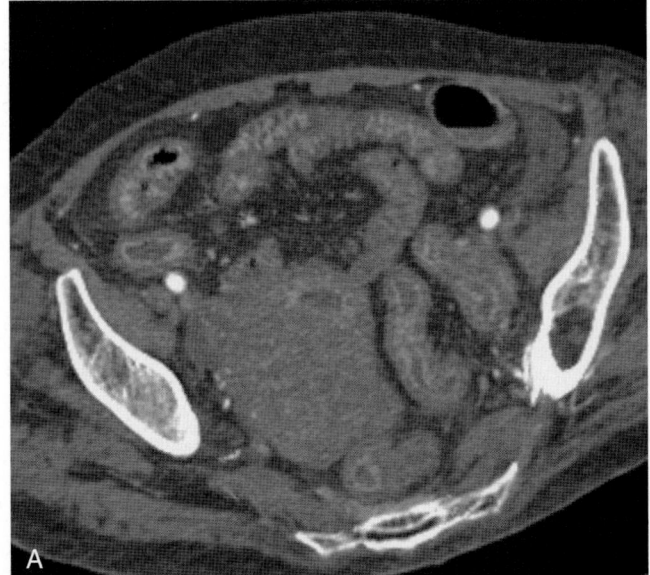
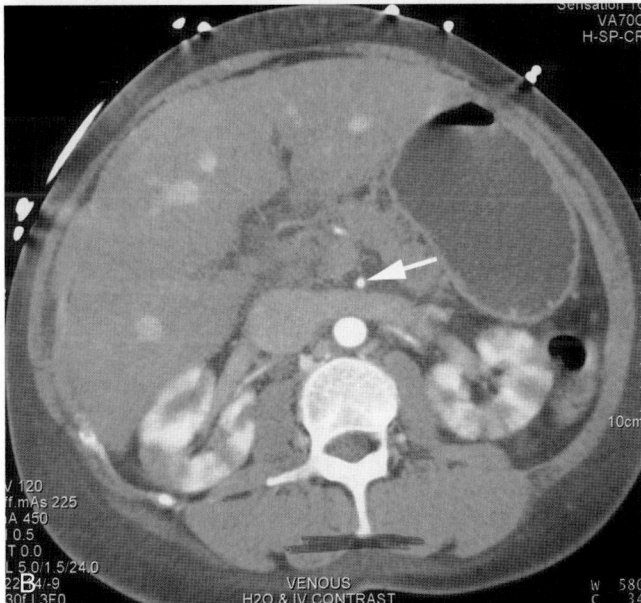
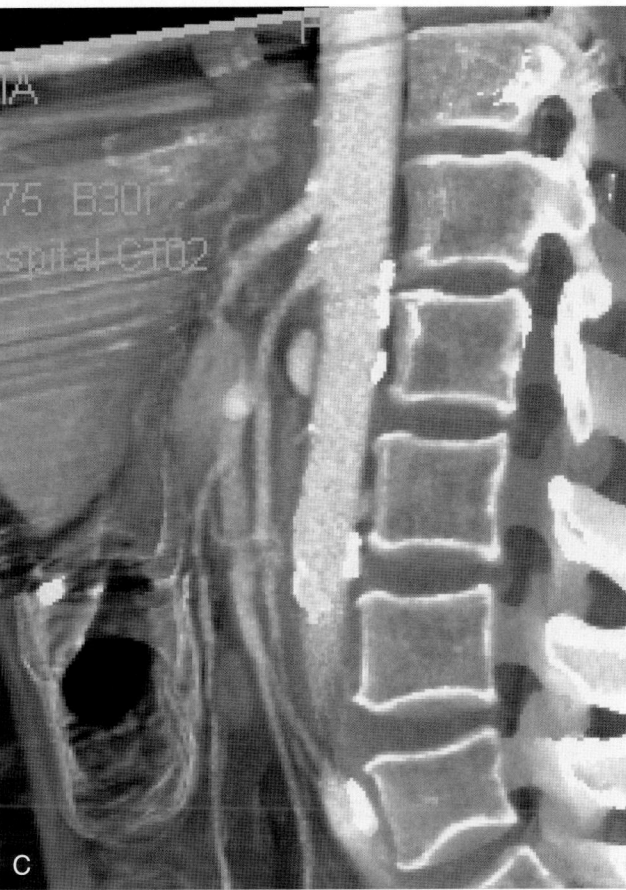

Figure 51-12. **An intravenous drug abuser presented complaining of pain after recent cocaine use. A.** Axial image through the pelvis demonstrates moderate small bowel and right colon thickening. The small bowel demonstrates mucosal hyperemia and low density in the submucosa. **B.** Contrast-enhanced CT through the level of the kidneys demonstrates multiple bilateral renal infarcts. The caliber of the SMA is small (*arrow*). **C.** Sagittal MPR demonstrates narrowing of the SMA compatible with a vasculitis.

depends on the pathogenesis, duration, and severity as well as on the site of involvement.[20] For example, mesenteric fat stranding, fluid, and ascites, respectively, have sensitivities of 8%, 88%, and 75% and specificities of 79%, 90%, and 76%, respectively, for the diagnosis of ischemia in patients with complicated bowel obstruction.[24]

Chronic Mesenteric Ischemia

Chronic mesenteric ischemia (CMI) is less common than acute mesenteric ischemia and typically has a more indolent presentation. CMI is most common in elderly patients with widespread atherosclerotic disease.[25] Patients usually complain of abdominal pain, which is often associated with meals, as well as weight loss. Because these are very nonspecific complaints, it is usually necessary to eliminate a variety of other conditions before considering the diagnosis of CMI. The diag-

nosis requires a careful clinical history because there are currently no sensitive or specific tests for a functional diagnosis of CMI.[26]

Atherosclerotic disease of the mesenteric vessels is the main cause of CMI. Usually there is disease of at least two of the three major mesenteric arteries (celiac axis, superior mesenteric artery, and inferior mesenteric artery) (Fig. 51-15). In the majority of cases, atheromas involve the proximal segments of the mesenteric arteries. Fatty infiltration of the wall of the arteries may lead to stenosis or occlusion.[26] However, the mere presence of atherosclerotic disease in the mesenteric arteries does not necessarily mean that CMI is present. For example, ultrasound and autopsy studies have consistently shown that severe atherosclerotic disease can be present in multiple mesenteric arteries in patients without symptoms of ischemia.[27-29] The key to the diagnosis is the demonstration of not only the atherosclerotic stenosis or occlusion but also the collateral pathways.

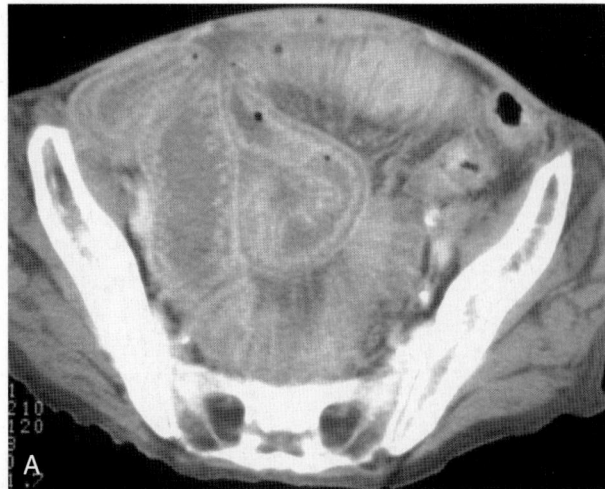

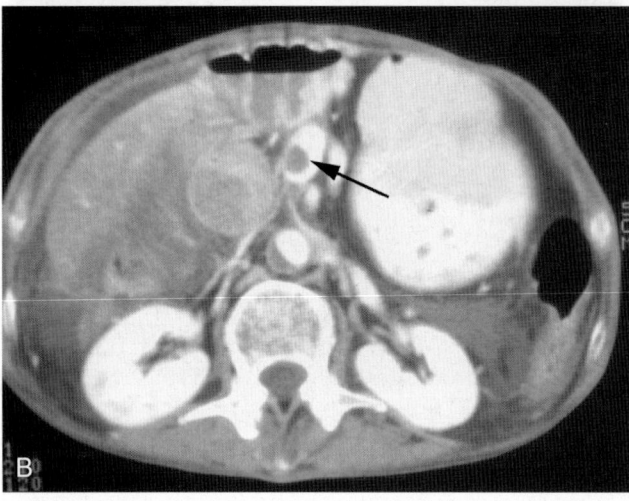

Figure 51-13. Superior mesenteric vein thrombus. A. Contrast-enhanced CT demonstrates thickening of the small bowel and right colon with the so-called target appearance due to submucosal edema. **B.** Thrombus (*arrow*) is seen in the SMV.

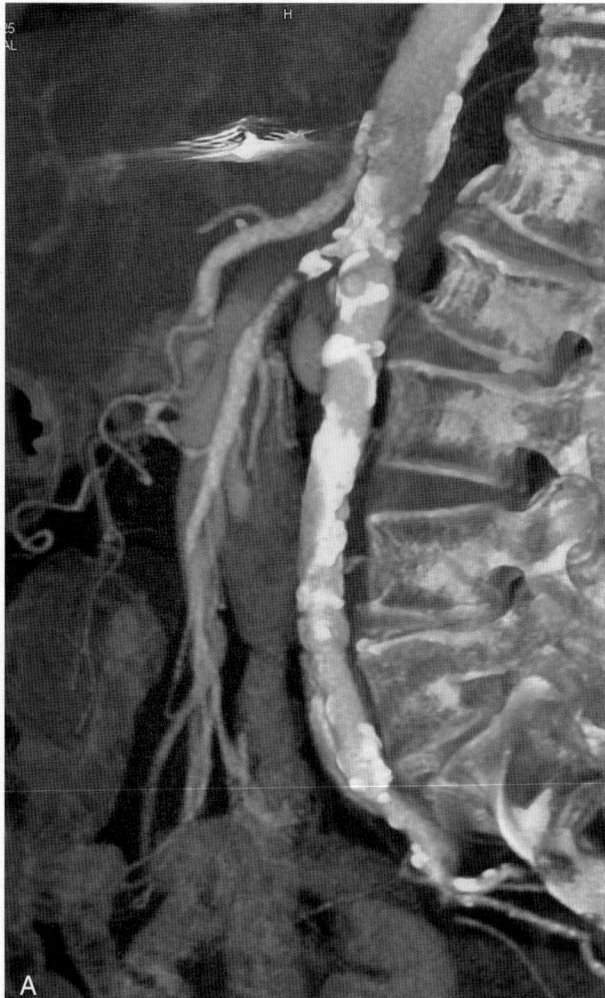

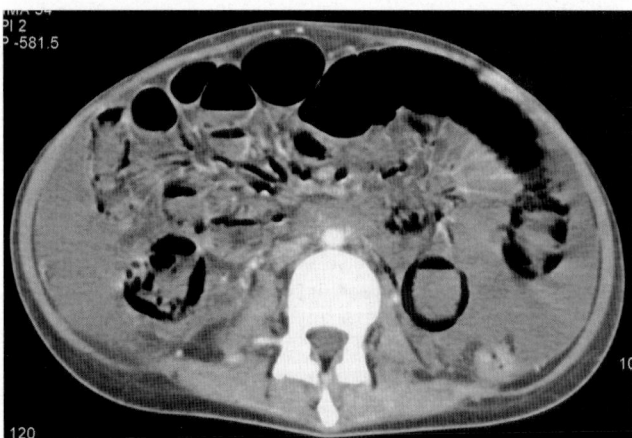

Figure 51-14. Mesenteric ischemia and infarction. Contrast-enhanced CT scan in a patient with mesenteric ischemia and infarcted bowel shows ascites, extensive pneumatosis, and air within mesenteric veins. Despite emergent surgery, the patient died.

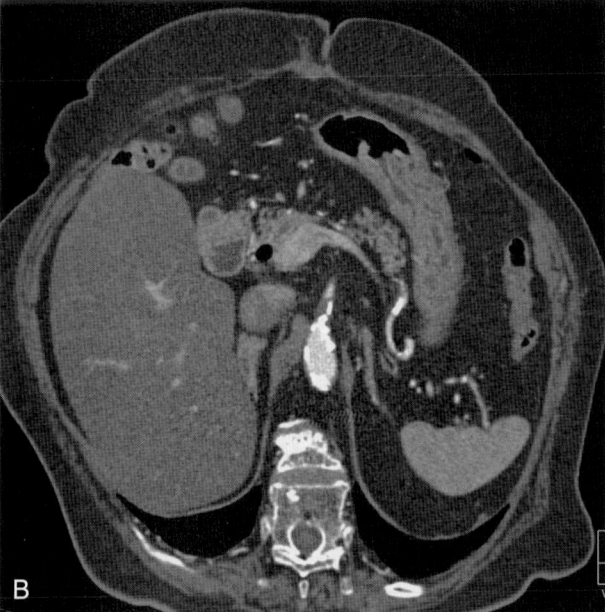

Figure 51-15. Chronic mesenteric ischemia. A. Sagittal CT angiogram demonstrates calcified atherosclerotic plaque at the origins of the celiac artery and SMA. **B.** Axial oblique MPR demonstrates both calcified and soft plaque at the SMA origin.

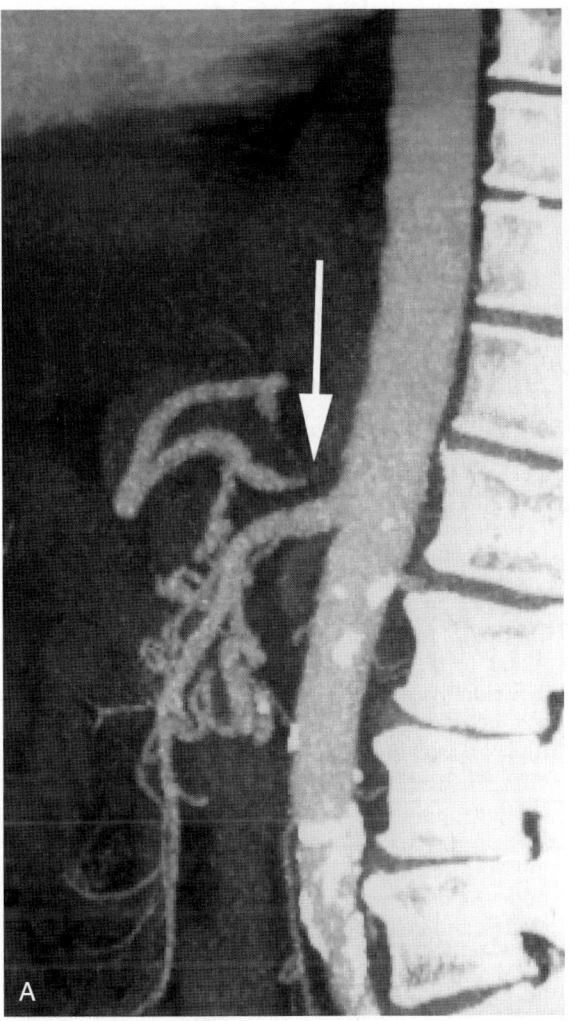

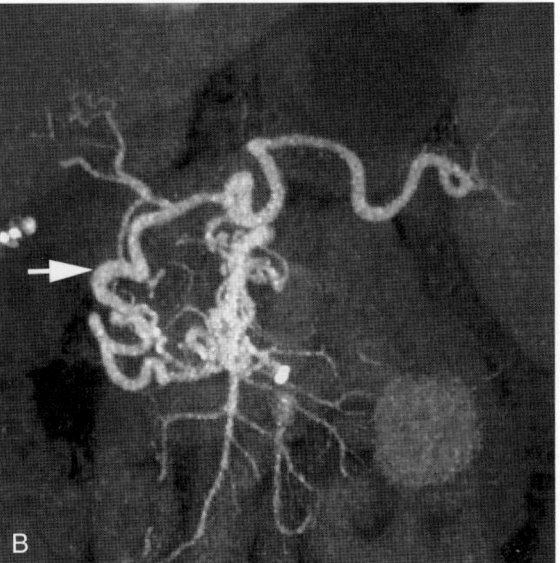

Figure 51-16. CT angiogram in a patient with celiac stenosis. A. Sagittal volume rendering shows marked narrowing (*arrow*) at the SMA origin. **B.** Coronal image shows the pancreaticoduodenal collateral pathways (*arrow*), which have developed between the SMA and celiac axis.

Two major collateral pathways are common. The pancreaticoduodenal arteries connect the celiac axis and SMA and can flow in either direction, depending on the site of occlusion (Fig. 51-16).[26] The Riolan arch and the marginal artery of Drummond (Fig. 51-17) allow communication between the SMA and IMA.[26] In severe cases when the celiac artery, SMA, and IMA are compromised, then pelvic, lumbar, or phrenic collateral vessels develop.[26]

In the past, patients with suspected CMI underwent conventional angiography. Cross-sectional imaging studies are now being utilized with greater frequency to screen for this disease. Duplex ultrasound has proven to be an accurate screening test for the proximal arteries.[30-32] Magnetic resonance angiography has also been shown to correlate accurately with conventional angiography and has the advantage of being safe in patients with renal insufficiency.[33,34] Given the widespread availability of MDCT scanners and sophisticated 3D imaging software, CT is usually the initial imaging modality performed in patients suspected of having CMI. CT can also determine whether the patient will benefit from catheter angiography and percutaneous interventions or a surgical bypass procedure.

Nonatheromatous disease can also affect the mesenteric vessels, resulting in CMI. This includes vasculitis, median arcuate ligament syndrome, and radiation injury (see later for a discussion of these disorders).

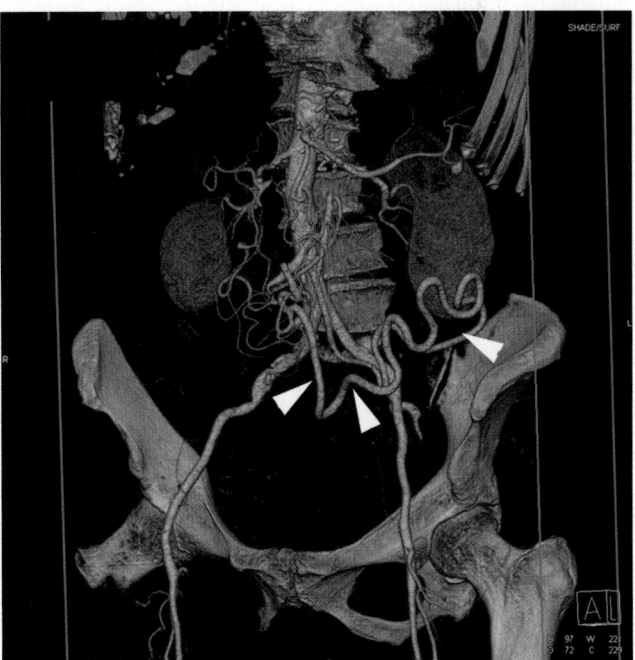

Figure 51-17. Collateral vessels. Marginal artery of Drummond (*arrowheads*) in a patient with SMA stenosis demonstrates the collateral pathways between the IMA and SMA (*arrowhead*).

Computed Tomographic Findings

In most patients with CMI, CT demonstrates relatively normal mural thickness and enhancement of the small intestine because collateral vessels have developed and maintain adequate blood flow to the bowel. Only when flow is critically compromised will changes in small bowel enhancement and mural thickening occur. Atherosclerotic plaque, lumen occlusion, and pattern of collaterals are easily identified and can help dictate patient treatment.[35-38]

VASCULITIS

Vasculitis is a general term for a group of diseases that result in inflammation and necrosis of blood vessels. It is often classified according to the size of the affected blood vessels. Large vessel vasculitis affects the aorta and its major branches, medium vessel vasculitis involves the visceral arteries and their branches, and small vessel vasculitis affects arterioles, venules and capillaries.[39]

Large vessel vasculitis includes giant cell arteritis and Takayasu's arteritis. Medium vessel vasculitis includes polyarteritis nodosa and Kawasaki disease. Small vessel vasculitis includes Wegener's granulomatosis, Churg-Strauss syndrome, microscopic polyangiitis, Henoch-Schönlein syndrome, systemic lupus erythematosus, rheumatoid vasculitis, and Behçet's syndrome.

Large Vessel Vasculitis

Of the large vessel vasculitides, Takayasu's arteritis is the most likely to involve the mesenteric vessels. Takayasu's arteritis is a chronic inflammatory disease of large arteries; usually the aorta and its main branches are affected.[39] Women are affected 10 times more often than men. Takayasu's arteritis classically involves the aortic arch but can also affect the abdominal aorta mesenteric branches, resulting in abdominal pain, acute or chronic ischemia, hemorrhage, or stricture.[39]

The radiographic diagnosis of mesenteric involvement by Takayasu's arteritis is typically made using conventional angiography. However, these findings can also be appreciated on detailed CT imaging of the mesenteric vessels using thin-collimation MDCT and 3D imaging software. The walls of the superior mesenteric artery appear thickened, similar in appearance to atherosclerotic disease, although the vascular involvement is more regular and more extensive. Significant stenosis of the SMA can occur along with poststenotic dilation, aneurysms, and, in severe cases, occlusion with collateral vessel formation. Unlike conventional angiography, CT also has the advantage of being able to directly visualize mural changes, including increased or decreased enhancement, wall thickening, mesenteric stranding, ascites, or, in cases of infarction, pneumatosis or mesenteric venous gas.

Medium Vessel Vasculitis

Of the medium-sized vessel vasculitides, polyarteritis nodosa is the most likely one to affect the mesenteric arteries. It is a necrotizing vasculitis that weakens the arterial wall (Fig. 51-18), leading to the formation of aneurysms, typically at branch points. The kidneys and renal arteries are affected in up to 80% to 90% of patients. Small intestine and mesenteric vessels are involved in over 50% of cases, and this carries a poor prognosis.[40] Abdominal pain is reported in up to half of patients with this disorder, and it usually results from ischemia.[41] In a series of 24 patients with polyarteritis nodosa and gastrointestinal tract involvement, 54% developed a surgical abdomen, 3 of whom died.[40]

Radiologic diagnosis can be made on conventional or CT angiography by the demonstration of the aneurysms involving the renal and mesenteric, hepatic, splenic, and/or peripancreatic arteries.[42]

Small Vessel Vasculitis

Of the small vessel vasculitides, the most likely to involve the small intestine are Henoch-Schönlein purpura, systemic lupus erythematosus, and Behçet's disease.

Henoch-Schönlein Purpura (HSP)

HSP is a small vessel vasculitis that most commonly affects children.[43] It is characterized by the deposition of IgA complexes in the skin, joints, kidneys, and gastrointestinal tract. The skin disease is typically the first manifestation, appearing as a petechial rash with purpura, often on the lower extremities.[43] Gastrointestinal tract involvement can occur in up to 60% of adults, resulting in abdominal pain related to ischemia and, in some cases, hemorrhage.[44] The CT features of HSP (Fig. 51-19) include wall thickening, luminal narrowing, fold thickening, and ulceration.[45,46] Enlarged mesenteric nodes, small bowel dilatation, engorged mesenteric vasculature, ascites, and mesenteric stranding have also been reported.[46]

Systemic Lupus Erythematosus

Systemic lupus erythematosus (SLE) is a complex autoimmune disease with multisystem involvement. It can affect any portion of the gastrointestinal tract, which is especially susceptible to small vessel vasculitis.[39,47] In addition, 27% to 42% of patients with SLE have a antiphospholipid syndrome that places them at risk for the development of mesenteric arterial or venous thrombosis.[48,49] The end result of the vasculitis or thrombus formation is bowel ischemia. CT will demonstrate the typical findings of small bowel ischemia (Fig. 51-20), including bowel thickening, edema, intramural hemorrhage, altered enhancement, or, in more advanced cases, pneumatosis or mesenteric venous gas.[47] 3D imaging of the mesenteric vessels can also be useful to detect the presence of thrombus in the mesenteric vasculature. In cases of vasculitis induced ischemia, beading or pruning of the mesenteric artery branches may be apparent.

Behçet's Disease

Behçet's disease usually affects young males aged 11 to 30 and is characterized by oral and genital ulcers and ocular inflammation. It is an uncommon inflammatory condition of unknown etiology that may involve multiple organs, including the gastrointestinal tract, in up to 50% of cases. Diagnosis is typically made by biopsy of the mucosal ulcers. Corticosteroids are the usual treatment.

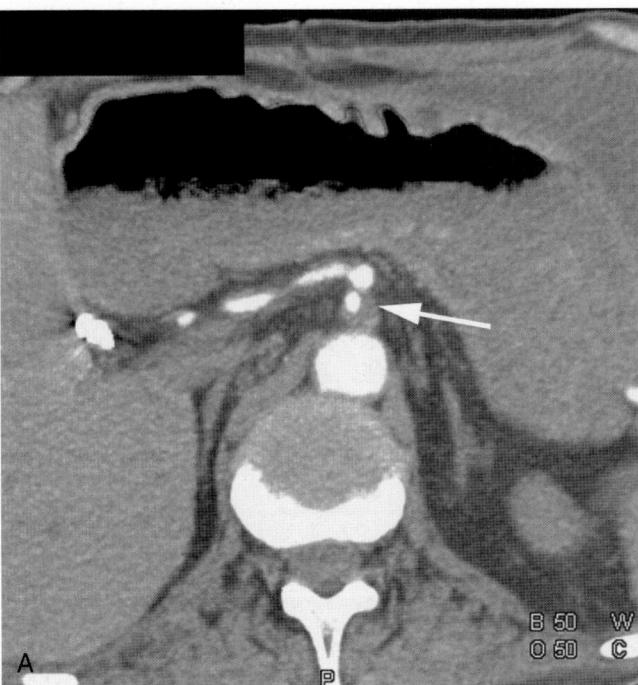

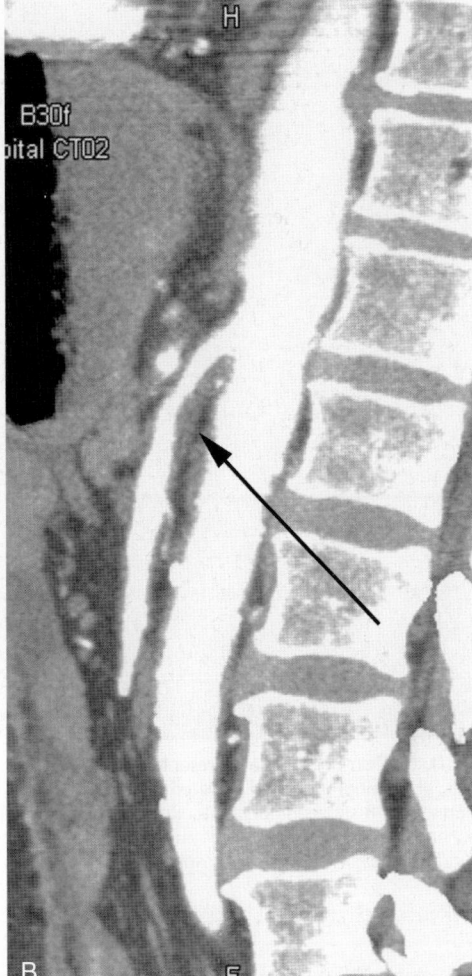

Figure 51-18. Patient with abdominal pain and polyarteritis nodosa. **A.** Axial contrast-enhanced CT demonstrates mural thickening of the SMA (*arrow*). **B.** Sagittal MPR demonstrates mural thickening (*arrow*) of the proximal portion of the SMA, a classic finding in polyarteritis nodosa.

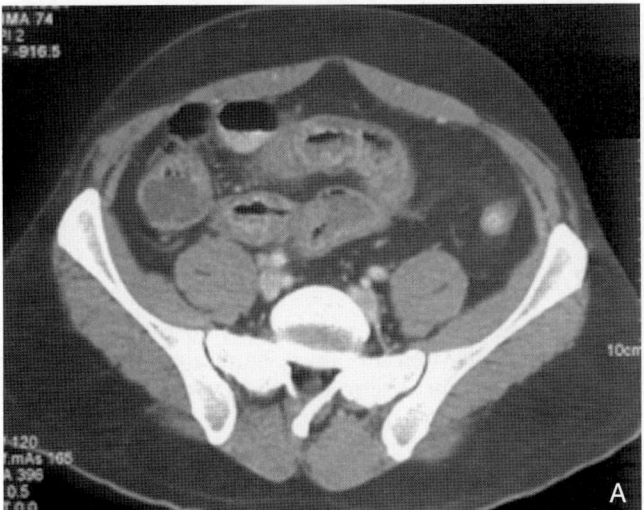

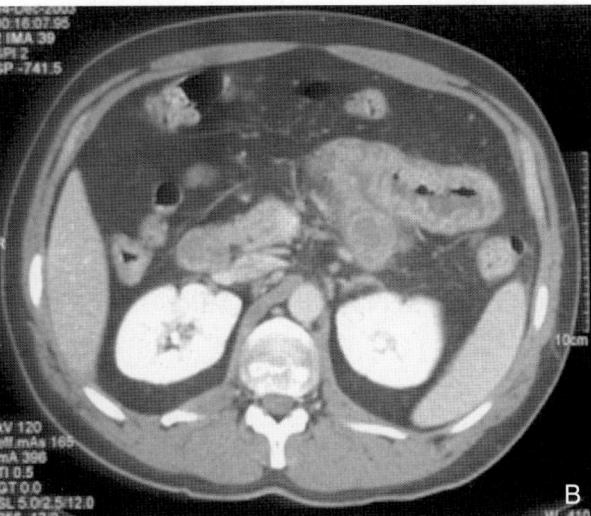

Figure 51-19. Henoch-Schönlein purpura. Contrast-enhanced CT demonstrates moderate small bowel thickening with submucosal edema producing the so-called target appearance. This is pathologically proven Henoch-Schönlein purpura.

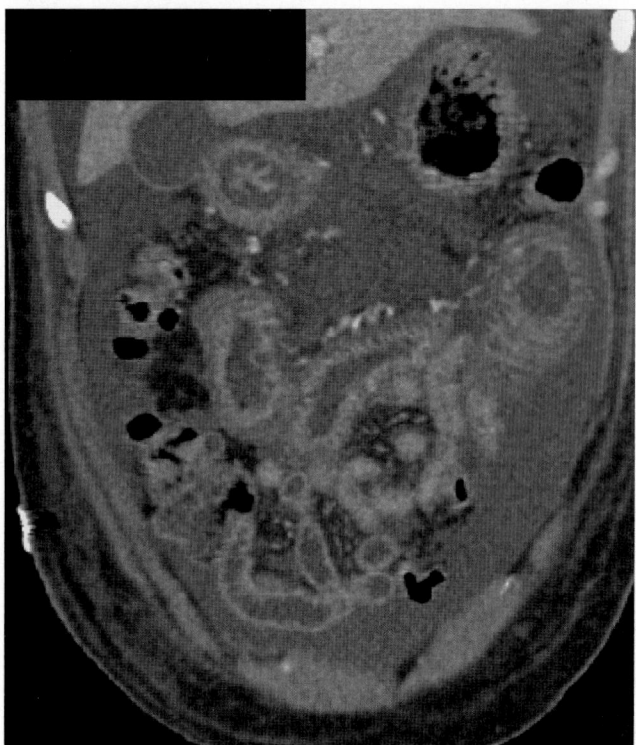

Figure 51-20. A 32-year-old woman presented with systemic lupus erythematosus, abdominal pain, and elevated lactic acid level. Coronal contrast-enhanced MPR shows moderate ascites. The small bowel in the midabdomen and left upper quadrant is thickened. There is mucosal hyperemia, and low density is seen in the submucosa.

Intestinal Behçet's disease mimics Crohn's disease on barium studies and CT, with inflammatory change most pronounced in the ileum. Focal and masslike small bowel fold thickening is often present, simulating small bowel lymphoma or neoplasm. Discrete ulcers may be present and in the proper clinical setting often suggest the correct diagnosis. In one series of 28 patients with intestinal Behçet's disease, with and without complications, small bowel thickening and/or polypoid lesions were reported.[50] Polypoid lesions were more common in patients without complications, whereas bowel thickening was more common in patients with complications.[50] Severe mesenteric infiltration/infiltration was also more common in patients with complications such as peritonitis or perforation.

SUPERIOR MESENTERIC ARTERY DISSECTION

Aortic dissection can involve the SMA (Figs. 51-21 and 51-22). The dissection flap can extend into the proximal portion of the vessel or can occlude the origin. In either case, blood flow to the small intestine can become compromised, resulting in ischemia. In rare cases, spontaneous isolated SMA dissection can occur without an associated aortic dissection. This is most likely a result of cystic medial necrosis and fibromuscular dysplasia.[51] Patients typically present with clinical symptoms related to either intestinal ischemia or hemorrhage. The dissection flap can easily be visualized on CT angiography and typically is located a few centimeters distal to the SMA origin, often resulting in narrowing of the lumen.[52]

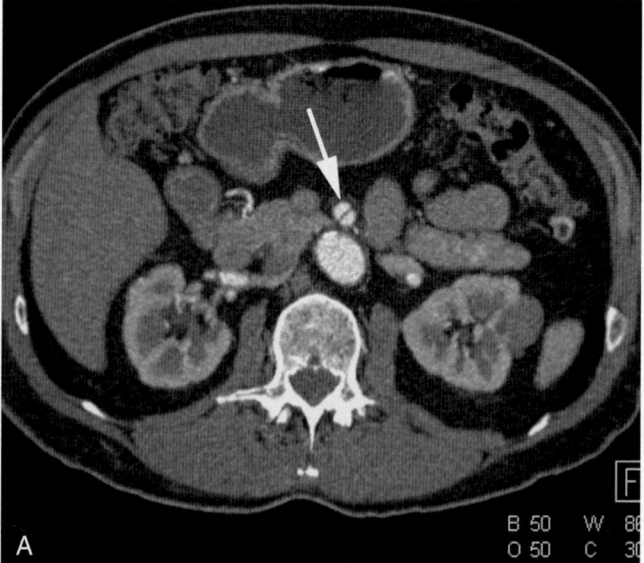

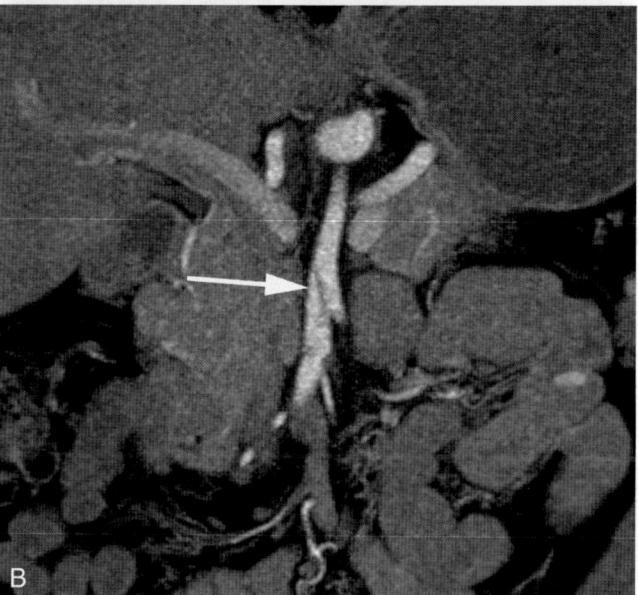

Figure 51-21. Superior mesenteric artery dissection. A. Axial contrast-enhanced CT through the level of the kidneys shows an SMA dissection. **B.** Coronal MPR shows the dissection flap (*arrow*).

TRAUMA

Bowel and mesenteric injury is found in 5% of patients undergoing laparotomy after significant blunt abdominal trauma.[52] The mesenteric side of the small intestine is more vulnerable to vascular tears and results in mesenteric hematoma.[53] The antimesenteric border on the other hand is more likely to perforate.[53] Mesenteric injuries are notoriously difficult to detect, and any fluid or increased density in the mesentery must be viewed with suspicion even when there is no pneumoperitoneum.

RADIATION ENTERITIS

The small intestine is the most common site of injury in patients undergoing radiation therapy, particularly patients

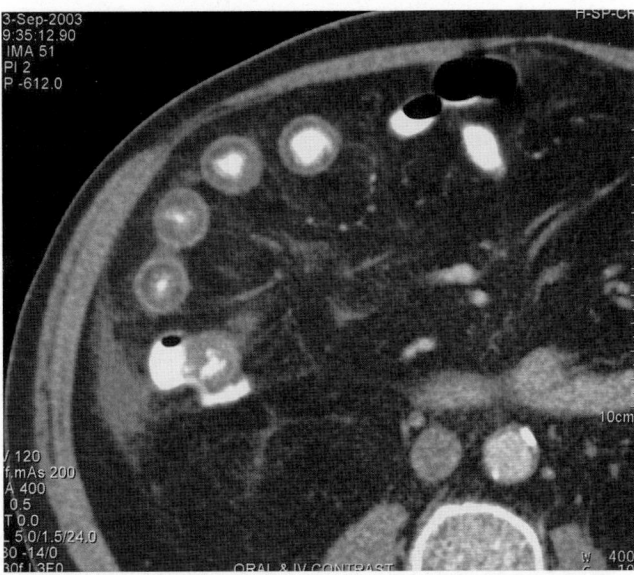

Figure 51-23. Radiation enteritis. Axial contrast-enhanced CT in a patient after radiation therapy for lymphoma shows moderate thickening of several small bowel loops in the right abdomen, compatible with radiation enteritis. There is minimal mesenteric stranding and ascites.

receiving high doses of radiation over a relatively short period of time, Patients with a history of previous intra-abdominal surgery or peritonitis are especially susceptible, owing to immobility of the intestine caused by adhesions. Patients with diabetes or atherosclerotic disease are also at increased risk, because the radiation results in an endarteritis and, ultimately, fibrosis. Patients can present with signs and symptoms of radiation enteritis (pain, diarrhea, bleeding) acutely during the radiation therapy. The features of chronic radiation injury (pain, obstruction, malabsorption) can develop as late as 25 years after therapy.

The diagnosis of radiation enteritis is usually made clinically. Small bowel series and CT can help confirm the diagnosis and determine the severity and extent of involvement. In patients with acute radiation enteritis, CT and small bowel series typically demonstrate thickening of the small bowel folds and wall as well as mucosal ulceration (Fig. 51-23). Intramural hemorrhage and/or edema will often be present. Over time, patients with chronic radiation injury will demonstrate stenosis, adhesions, and/or fistulas. In some cases, the small bowel mucosa is destroyed, resulting in a featureless appearance referred to as "ribbon" or "toothpaste" bowel.

SPLANCHNIC ARTERY ANEURYSM

Splanchic artery aneurysms are rare, with an incidence of 0.01% to 0.25% in routine autopsy series.[54] Most patients with splanchnic artery aneurysms are asymptomatic, and the diagnosis is usually made incidentally.[55] These aneurysms can rupture, causing abdominal pain and bleeding. The splenic artery is most commonly involved (60%), followed by the hepatic artery (20%), SMA (5.5%), celiac artery (4%), pancreatic arteries (2%), and gastroduodenal artery (1.5%).[56,57] Diagnosis can be made on CT, MRI, ultrasound, or angiography.

The most common location for an SMA aneurysm is within the first 5 cm of its origin.[55] The most common causes are endocarditis, atherosclerosis, and pancreatitis.[58] Complications

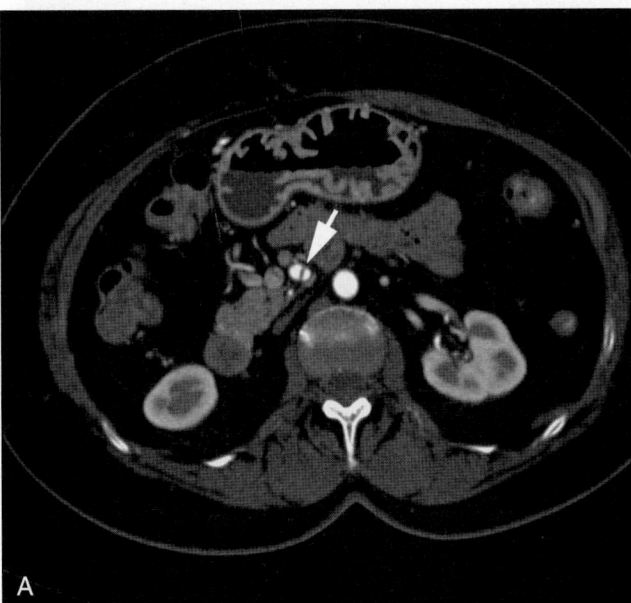

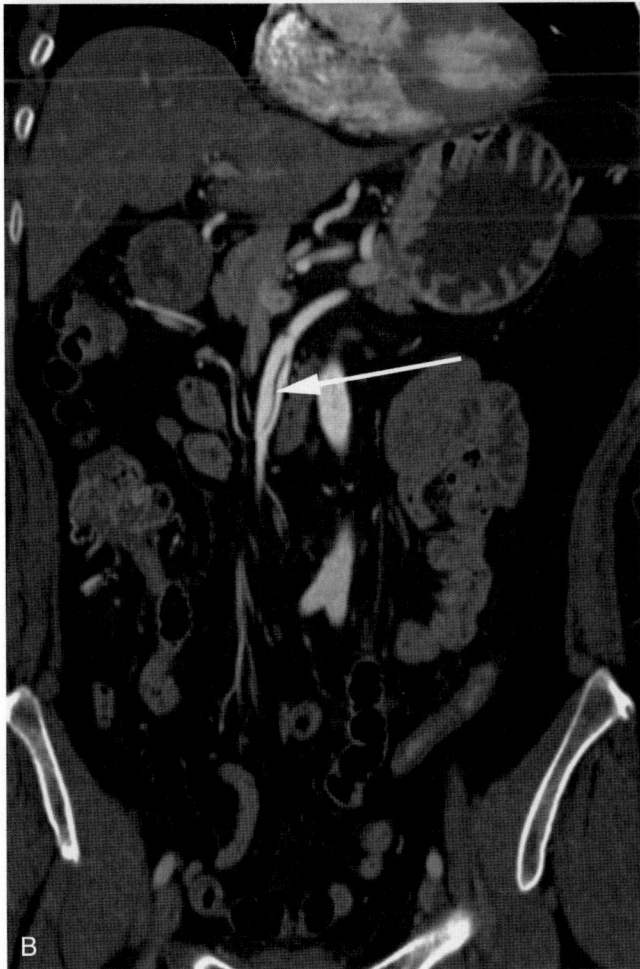

Figure 51-22. Superior mesenteric artery dissection. A. Contrast-enhanced CT through the level of the kidneys shows a dissection flap in the SMA. **B.** Coronal MPR shows the dissection flap (*arrow*) in the midmesenteric artery.

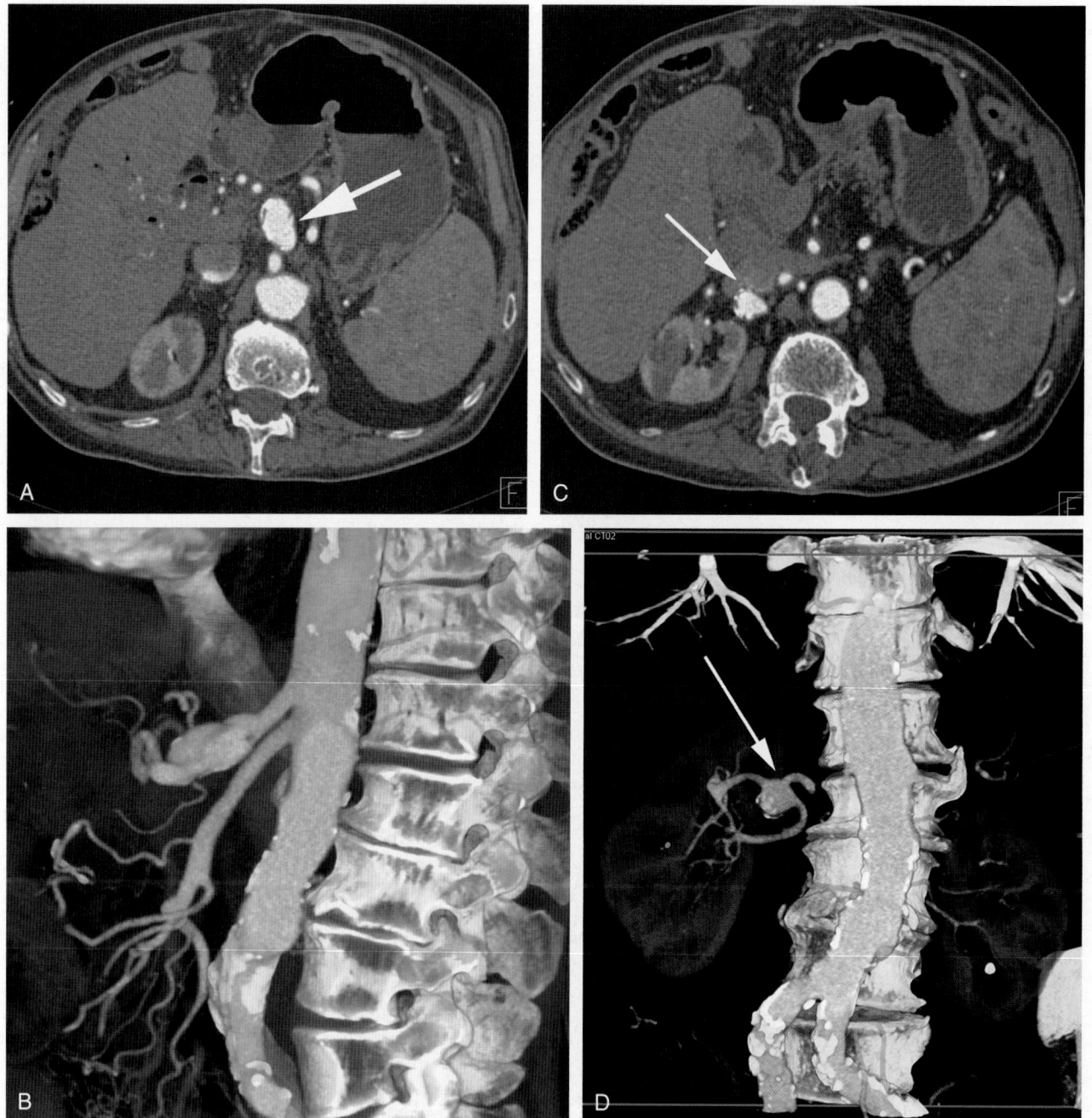

Figure 51-24. Celiac axis aneurysm. A. Axial contrast-enhanced CT in the arterial phase shows an aneurysm (*arrow*) of the celiac axis. **B.** Volume-rendered CT angiogram nicely demonstrates the complex shape of the celiac axis aneurysm, which begins approximately 1.5 cm distal to the origin. **C.** Contrast-enhanced CT through the level of the kidneys demonstrates an aneurysm of the right renal artery (*arrow*). **D.** Volume-rendered CT angiogram of the right renal artery shows a right renal artery aneurysm (*arrow*).

include thrombosis, ischemia, and rupture and carry a high mortality rate.

Celiac artery aneurysms occur more often in men, and 75% will have symptoms, typically pain (Figs. 51-24 and 51-25).[57] The risk of rupture is 13%, with a 100% mortality rate when rupture occurs.[58] The most common cause is atherosclerosis, and most aneurysms develop at or near the vessel origin.

MEDIAN ARCUATE LIGAMENT SYNDROME

The median arcuate ligament is a fibrous arch that unites the crura on either side of the aortic hiatus. In most people,

the ligament crosses above the celiac origin and anterior to the aorta. However, in 10% to 24% of people, the ligament has a low insertion across the origin of the celiac axis.[59] The compression can be hemodynamically significant, resulting in collateral flow to the celiac artery from the SMA (Fig. 51-26). A small subset of people with this low insertion will be symptomatic, presenting with symptoms similar to those of CMI. The cause of pain in patients with median arcuate ligament syndrome is controversial. Some authorities believe the pain is a result of compromised blood flow and requires percutaneous transluminal angioplasty or stent placement. Others believe the pain is a result of compression of the celiac plexus.[26,60-62]

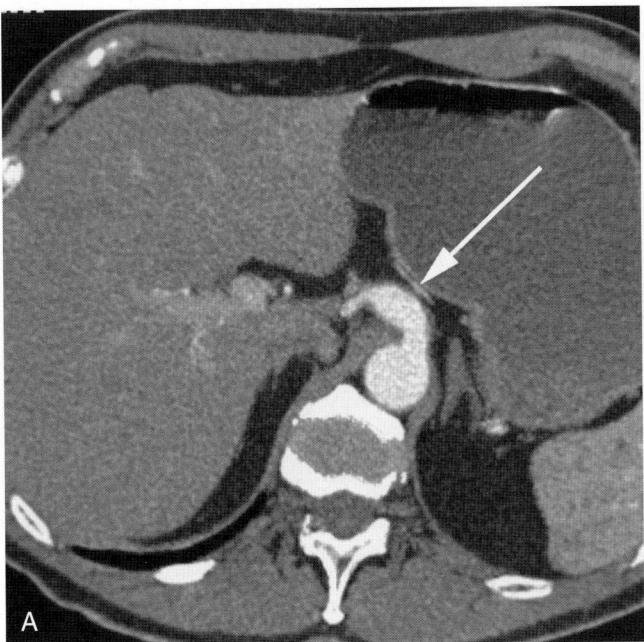

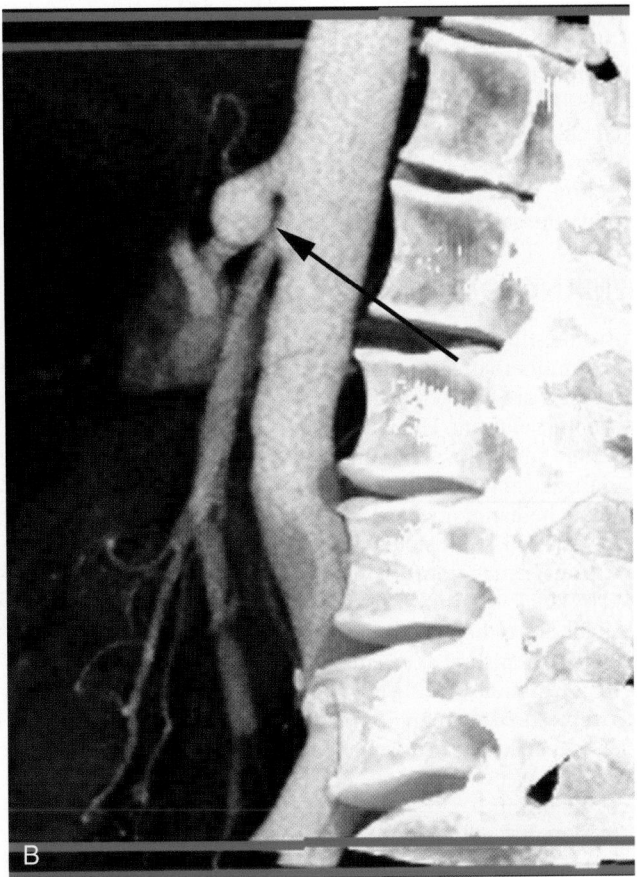

Figure 51-25. Celiac artery aneurysm. Aneurysmal dilatation of the celiac axis (*arrow*) is identified on axial (**A**) and sagittal (**B**) images.

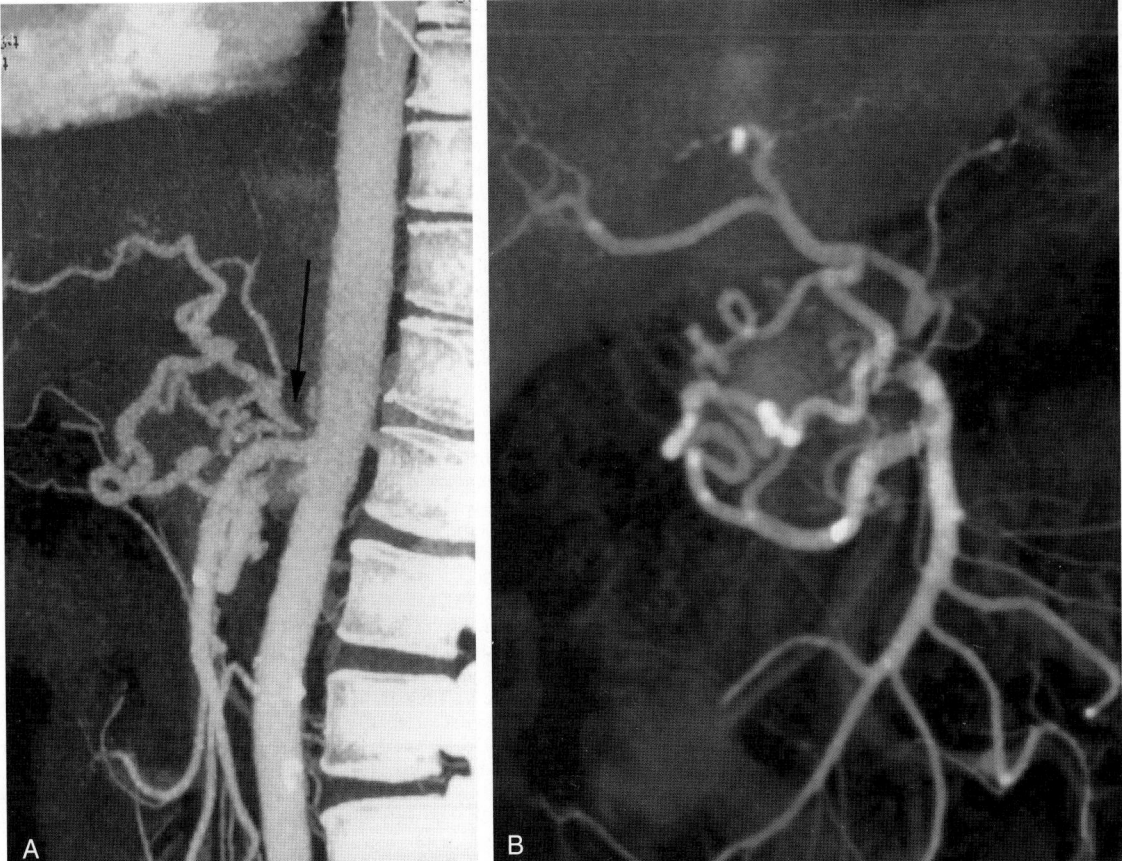

Figure 51-26. Median arcuate ligament syndrome. A. Sagittal contrast-enhanced MPR shows "hook-like" appearance of the proximal celiac axis, which is narrowed. **B.** Coronal 3D CT angiogram shows enlarged and dilated collateral supplying the celiac artery from the SMA.

The diagnosis was typically made with catheter angiography but has also been reported with ultrasonography and CT. On CT angiography, the low insertion of the median arcuate ligament results in a characteristic impression on the proximal celiac axis, causing a "hooked" appearance. When the compression is hemodynamically significant, poststenotic dilatation is seen as well as collateral flow from the SMA through the gastroduodenal and peripancreatic arteries.[63]

HEMANGIOMAS

Gastrointestinal hemangiomas are relatively rare benign vascular tumors that can occur anywhere in the gastrointestinal tract. They are most frequently located in the small intestine, usually the jejunum. Hemangiomas account for 7% to 10% of all benign small bowel tumors.[64] Histologically, hemangiomas are classified and named according to their major components. Capillary hemangiomas are composed of small capillaries with thin walls and blood-filled spaces lined by endothelial cells. Cavernous hemangiomas consist of larger blood-filled sinuses lined by single or multiple layers of endothelial cells.

Small bowel hemangiomas can be single or multiple and in some patients are associated with hemangiomas or vascular malformations in other organs such as the liver and skin. Gastrointestinal hemangiomas have been associated with Osler-Weber-Rendu syndrome, Maffucci's syndrome, Klippel-Trenaunay-Weber syndrome, and congenital blue rubber bleb nevus syndrome.

Patients usually present with gastrointestinal bleeding. However, large lesions can cause abdominal pain or bowel obstruction.

Small bowel hemangiomas are difficult to diagnose radiographically. In a review of the Japanese literature by Akamatsu and coworkers, a preoperative diagnosis was possible in 24% of patients using small bowel series, angiography, or scintigraphy.[65] Occasionally, plain films of the abdomen may demonstrate small vascular calcifications. Small bowel series can occasionally demonstrate a polypoid mass, which changes shape or collapses on compression. Angiography or scintigraphy can also be helpful. In the past, CT was only able to identify larger lesions. However, with the introduction of MDCT scanners and 3D imaging software, smaller hemangiomas can now be diagnosed (Fig. 51-27).

Gastrointestinal hemangiomatosis is a vascular malformation that presents in infancy and childhood with gastrointestinal bleeding. This is manifested by diffuse infiltration of the gut and mesentery with hemangiomas. Radiographically, calcifications and phleboliths are identified throughout the gastrointestinal tract. CT can demonstrate marked vascular enhancement of the bowel after rapid administration of intravenous contrast.

The recently introduced capsule endoscopy may also aid in detecting small bowel hemangiomas in patients with unexplained gastrointestinal blood loss.

SUMMARY

Recent advances in CT technology and software have lead to a proliferation of new CT applications in the gut. CT can now be used as a first-line imaging study in patients with suspected vascular disorders of the small intestines. CT can accurately image the small bowel and mesenteric vasculature

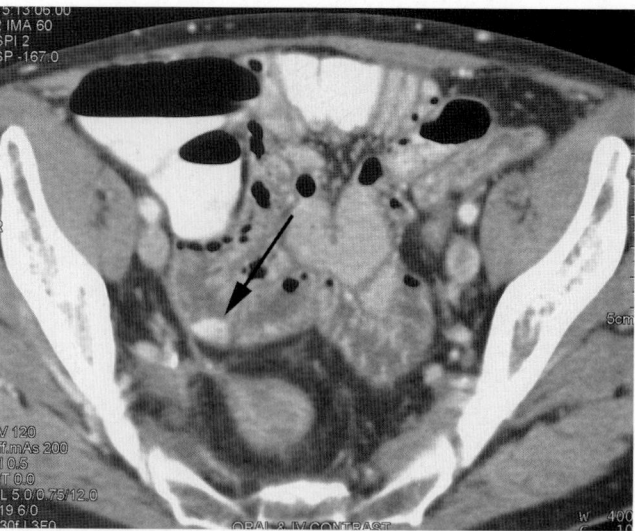

Figure 51-27. Small bowel hemangioma. Contrast-enhanced axial CT demonstrates a 9-mm enhancing distal small bowel (*arrow*) hemangioma.

and identify a wide range of pathology, and it can therefore be used to confirm or exclude the suspected diagnosis and triage patients to appropriate treatment.[66-68]

References

1. Sreenarasimhaiah J: Chronic mesenteric ischemia. Curr Treat Options Gastroenterol 10:3-9, 2007.
2. Ruotolo R, Evans S: Mesenteric ischemia in the elderly. Gastroenterology 15:527-557, 1999.
3. Greenwald D, Brandt L, Reinus J: Ischemic bowel disease in the elderly. Gastroenterol Clin North Am 30:445-465, 2004.
4. McKinsey J, Gerwertz B: Acute mesenteric ischemia. Surg Clin North Am 77:307-318, 1997.
5. Heys S, Brittenden J, Crofts T: Acute mesenteric ischemia: the continuing difficulty in early diagnosis. Postgrad Med 69:48-51, 1993.
6. Freeman A, Graham J: Damage control surgery and angiography in cases of acute mesenteric ischemia. Aust NZ J Surg 75:308-317, 2005.
7. Bolen S, Brandt L, Sammartano R: History of mesenteric ischemia: The evolution of a diagnosis and management. Surg Clin North Am 77:275-288, 1997.
8. Batellier J, Kierny R: Superior mesenteric artery embolism: Eighty-two cases. Ann Vasc Surg 4:112-116, 1990.
9. Tendler D: Acute intestinal ischemia and infarction. Semin Gastroenterol Dis 11:66-76, 2003.
10. Rhee R, Gloviczki P, Mendonea C, et al: Mesenteric venous thrombosis: Still a lethal disease in the 1990s. J Vasc Surg 20:688-697, 1994.
11. Bassiouny H: Nonocclusive mesenteric ischemia. Surg Clin North Am 77:319-326, 1997.
12. Suhaker C, Al-Hakeem M, MacAurthur J, et al: Mesenteric ischemia secondary to cocaine abuse: Case reports and literature review. Am J Gasterenterol 92:1053-1054, 1997.
13. Smerud M, Johnson C, Stephens D: Diagnosis of bowel infarction: A comparison of plain films and CT scans in 23 patients. AJR 154:99-103, 1990.
14. Klein H, Lensing R, Klosterhalfen B, et al: Diagnostic imaging of mesenteric infarction. Radiology 197:79-82, 1995.
15. Taourel P, Deneuville M, Pradel J, et al: Acute mesenteric ischemia: Diagnosis with contrast enhanced CT. Radiology 199:632-636, 1996.
16. Lee R, Tung H, Tung, PHM, et al: CT in acute mesenteric ischemia. Clin Radiol 58:279-287, 2002.
17. Alpen M, Glazer G, Francis I: Ischemia of infarcted bowel's findings. Radiology 166:149-152, 1988.
18. Sheedy SP, Earnest F 4th, Fletcher JG, et al: CT of small-bowel ischemia associated with obstruction in emergency department patients: Diagnostic performance evaluation. Radiology 241:729-736, 2006.
19. Kim J, Ha H, Byun J: Intestinal infarction secondary to mesenteric venous thrombosis. J Comput Assist Tomogr 17:382-385, 1993.

20. Wiesner W, Khurana B, Hoon J, Ros P: CT of acute bowel ischemia. Radiology 226:635-650, 2003.
21. Bartnicke B, Balfe D: CT appearance of intestinal ischemia and intramural hemorrhage. Radiol Clin North Am 32:845-860, 1994.
22. Horton K, Corl F, Fishman E: CT of nonneoplastic diseases of the small bowel: Spectrum of disease. J Comput Assist Tomogr 23:417-428, 1999.
23. Salzano A, De Rosa A, Carbone M, et al: Computerized tomography features of intestinal infarction: 56 surgically treated patients of which 5 with reversible mesenteric ischemia. Radiol Med (Torino) 97:246-250, 1999.
24. Fujimoto T, Fukuda T, Uetani M, et al: Helical CT signs in the diagnosis of intestinal ischemia in small bowel obstruction. AJR 176:1167-1171, 2000.
25. Moawad J, Gewertz B: Chronic mesenteric ischemia. Surg Clin North Am 77:357-369, 1997.
26. Cognet F, Salem D, Dranssart M, et al: Chronic mesenteric ischemia; imaging and percutaneous treatment. RadioGraphics 22:863-879, 2002.
27. Jarvinen O, Laurikka J, Sisto T, et al: Atherosclerosis of visceral arteries. Vasa 24:9-14, 1995.
28. Biebl M, Oldenburg WA, Paz-Fumagalli R, et al: Surgical and interventional visceral revascularization for the treatment of chronic mesenteric ischemia—when to prefer which? World J Surg 31:562-568, 2007.
29. Roobottom C, Dubbins P: Significant disease of the celiac and superior mesenteric arteries in asymptomatic patients, predictive value of Doppler sonography. AJR 161:985-988, 1993.
30. Moneta G, Lee RW, Yeager R, et al: Mesenteric duplex scanning: A blinding prospective study. J Vasc Surg 17:79-84, 1993.
31. Perko M: Duplex ultrasound for assessment of superior mesenteric artery blood flow. Eur J Vasc Endovasc Surg 21:106-117, 2001.
32. Zwolak R, Fillinger M, Walsh D, et al: Mesenteric and celiac duplex scanning: A validation study. J Vasc Surg 27:1078-1087, 1998.
33. Shih MC, Angle JF, Leung DA, et al: CTA and MRA in mesenteric ischemia: Part 2, Normal findings and complications after surgical and endovascular treatment. AJR Am J Roentgenol 188:462-471, 2007.
34. Ernst O, Asnar V, Sergent G, et al: Comparing contrast-enhanced breath hold MR angiography and conventional angiography in the evaluation of the mesenteric circulation. AJR 174:433-439, 2000.
35. Horton K, Fishman E: 3D CT angiography of the celiac and superior mesenteric arteries with multidetector CT data sets: Preliminary observations. Abdom Imaging 25:523-525, 2000.
36. Horton K, Fishman E: Multidetector row and 3D CT of the mesenteric vasculature: Normal anatomy and pathology. Semin Ultrasound CT MR 24:353-363, 2003.
37. Horton K, Fishman E: Volume -rendered 3D CT of the mesenteric vasculature: Normal anatomy, anatomic variants, and pathologic conditions. RadioGraphics 22:161-172, 2002.
38. Horton K, Fishman E: Multi-detector row CT of mesenteric ischemia: Can it be done? RadioGraphics 21:1463-1473, 2001.
39. Ha H, Lee S, Rha S, et al: Radiologic features of vasculitis involving the gastrointestinal tract. RadioGraphics 20:779-794, 2000.
40. Levine S, Hellman D, Stone J: Gastrointestinal involvement in polyarteritis nodosa (1986-2000): Presentation and outcomes in 24 patients. Am J Med 112:386-391, 2002.
41. Bassel K, Harford W: Gastrointestinal manifestation of collagen vascular disease. Semin Gastrointest Dis 6:228-240, 1995.
42. Kato T, Fujii K, Ishii E, et al: A case of polyarteritis nodosa with lesions of the superior mesenteric artery illustrating the diagnostic usefulness of three-dimensional computed tomographic angiography. Clin Rheumatol 24:628-631, 2005.
43. Mills J, Michel B, Bloch D, et al: The American College of Rheumatology 1990 criteria for the classification of Henoch-Schönlein purpura. Arth Rheum 33:1114-1121, 1990.
44. Jeong Y, Ha H, Yoon C, et al: Gastrointestinal involvement in Henoch-Schönlein syndrome. AJR 168:965-968, 1997.
45. Siskind B, Burrell M, Pun H, et al: CT demonstration of gastrointestinal involvement in Henoch-Schönlein syndrome. Gastrointest Radiol 10:352-354, 1985.
46. Jeong Y, Ha H, Yoon C, et al: Gastrointestinal involvement in Henoch-Schönlein syndrome: CT findings. AJR 168:965-968, 1997.
47. Lalani T, Kanne J, Hatfield G, Chen P: Imaging findings in systemic lupus erythematosus. RadioGraphics 24:1069-1086, 2004.
48. Espinosa G, Cervera R, Font J, Shoenfeld Y: Antiphospholipid syndrome: Pathogenic mechanisms. Autoimmune Rev 2:677-696, 2003.
49. Andrews P, Frampton G, Cameron J: Antiphospholipid syndrome and systemic lupus erythematosus. Lancet 342:988-989, 1993.
50. Ha H, Lee H, Yang S, et al: Intestinal Behçet syndrome: CT features of patients with and without complications. Radiology 209:449-454, 1998.
51. Okino Y, Kiyosue H, Mori H, et al: Root of the small-bowel mesentery: Correlative anatomy and CT features of pathologic conditions. RadioGraphics 21:1475-1490, 2001.
52. Corbetti F, Vigo M, Bulzacchi A, et al: CT diagnosis of spontaneous dissection of the superior mesenteric artery. J Comput Assist Tomogr 13:965-967, 1989.
53. Nghiem H, Jeffrey R, Mindelzun R: CT of blunt trauma to the bowel and mesentery. AJR 160:53-58, 1993.
54. Stanley J, Thompson N, Fry W: Splanchnic artery aneurysms. Arch Surg 101:689-697, 1970.
55. Pilleul F, Beuf O: Diagnosis of splanchnic artery aneurysms and pseudo-aneurysms, with special reference to contrast enhanced 3D magnetic angiography: A review. Acta Radiol 45:702-708, 2004.
56. Rokke O, Sondenaa K, Amundsen S, et al: The diagnosis and management of splanchnic artery aneurysms. Scand J Gastroenterol 1:737-743, 1996.
57. Messina L, Shanley C: Visceral artery aneurysms. Surg Clin North Am 77:425-442, 1997.
58. Shanley C, Shah N: Uncommon splanchnic artery aneurysms: Splenic, hepatic and celiac. Ann Vasc Surg 10:506-515, 1996.
59. Linder H, Kemprud E: A clinicoanatomic study of the arcuate ligament of the diaphragm. Arch Surg 103:600-605, 1971.
60. Nyman O, Ivancev K, Lindle M, Uher P: Endovascular treatment of chronic mesenteric ischemia: Report of five cases. Cardiovasc Intervent Radiol 31:305-313, 1998.
61. Matsumoto A, Tegtmeyer C, Fitzcharles E, et al: Percutaneous transluminal angioplasty of visceral arterial stenosis: Results and long term clinical follow-up. J Vasc Interv Radiol 6:165-174, 1995.
62. Roayaie S, Jossart G, Gitlitz D, et al: Laparoscopic release of celiac artery compression syndrome facilitated by laparoscopic ultrasound scanning to confirm restoration of blood flow. J Vasc Surg 32:814-817, 2000.
63. Horton K, Talamini M, Fishman E: Median arcuate ligament syndrome: Evaluation with CT angiography. RadioGraphics 25:1177-1182. 2005.
64. Sorbi D, Conio M, Gostout C: Vascular disorders of the small bowel. Gastrointest Endosc Clin North Am 9:71-92, 1999.
65. Ramanujam P, Venkatesh K, Bettinger L, et al: Hemangioma of the small intestine: Case report and literature review. Am J Gasterenterol 90:2063-2064, 1995.
66. Hong SS, Kim AY, Byun JH, et al: MDCT of small-bowel disease: Value of 3D imaging. AJR Am J Roentgenol 187:1212-1221, 2006.
67. Romano S, Lassandro F, Scaglione M, et al: Ischemia and infarction of the small bowel and colon: spectrum of imaging findings. Abdom Imaging 31:277-292, 2006.
68. Maglinte DD: Small bowel imaging—a rapidly changing field and a challenge to radiology. Eur Radiol 16:967-971, 2006.

Postoperative Small Bowel

John C. Lappas, MD • Kumaresan Sandrasegaran, MD •
Dean D. T. Maglinte, MD

Surgical treatment of diseases of the small bowel requires the use of relatively few operative techniques, and most of these surgical interventions are applicable to any segment of the jejunum and ileum. Such interventions include enterotomy for removal of polyps or foreign bodies; enteroplasty for treatment of strictures; enterectomy for resection of obstructed, traumatized, neoplastic, or necrotic segments; plication to prevent intestinal obstruction; and creation of ostomies or mucous fistulas for feeding or drainage purposes.[1] The small bowel is also used for surgical construction of reservoirs after gastrectomy and proctocolectomy and for the reconstitution of biliary and pancreatic flow into the gastrointestinal tract. Small bowel transplantation has also become a surgical option for treatment of selected patients with short bowel syndrome and intestinal failure.

Radiographic studies are seldom performed as routine follow-up for small bowel surgery but rather to assess the integrity of the postoperative small bowel or to investigate postoperative complications. In patients with a history of small bowel surgery who present with gastrointestinal symptoms, the postoperative anatomy and site of anastomoses should be carefully evaluated by radiographic studies (Figs. 52-1 and 52-2). Small bowel enteroclysis techniques combined with fluoroscopic observation of luminal infusion can readily demonstrate the anatomic detail of the surgically altered intestine.[2,3] CT enteroclysis techniques are well suited for the evaluation of postoperative small bowel obstruction or small bowel dysmotility after various surgical procedures.[4] Recognition of enteric suture material on abdominal CT alerts the radiologist to the presence of surgically altered bowel and prompts a search for possible postoperative abnormalities or complications. Appreciation of the postoperative anatomy

and associated intestinal alterations can be especially important, because the pertinent surgical history may be incomplete or even unknown at the time of diagnostic imaging.

SMALL BOWEL AFTER GASTRIC SURGERY

Important alterations in small intestinal physiology or anatomy may occur after various forms of surgery on the stomach. In the postgastrectomy syndrome, pathophysiologic disorders

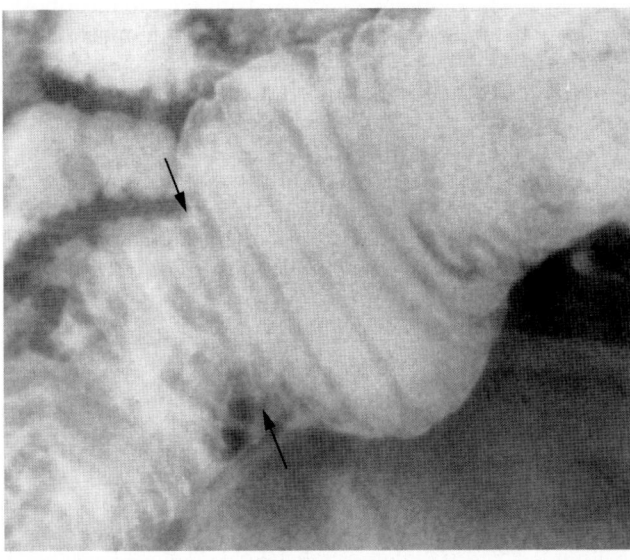

Figure 52-1. Jejunal end-to-end anastomosis. Luminal distention achieved by enteroclysis infusion facilitates accurate delineation of a normal anastomosis (*arrows*).

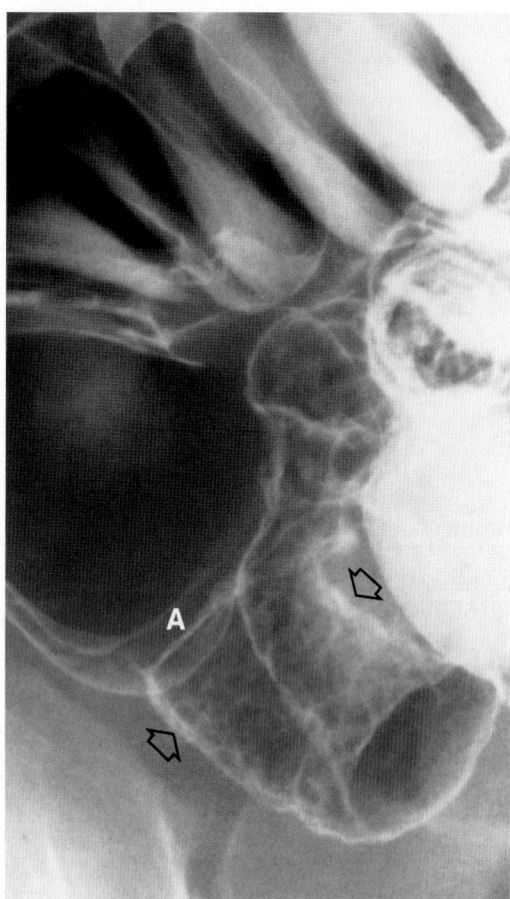

Figure 52-2. Ileocolic anastomosis. Peroral pneumocolon technique (performed with retrograde air insufflation and glucagon-induced hypotonia) optimizes distention of the anastomotic region. The ileocolic anastomosis (A) is patent, but nodularity and narrowing of the neoterminal ileum (*arrows*) indicate recurrent Crohn's disease.

can result from interruption of the pyloric sphincter mechanism or as the sequelae of vagotomy. Rapid influx of hyperosmotic gastric contents into the small bowel may be manifested clinically by the dumping syndrome with symptoms of postprandial cramping and urgent diarrhea. Mild luminal dilatation and hypermotility of the efferent jejunum can sometimes be observed on small bowel studies. Serotonin, enteroglucagon, and vasoactive intestinal polypeptide are also released systemically by the small intestine in response to luminal distention and are partly responsible for the vasomotor component of the dumping syndrome.[5] Small bowel dysmotility (with bacterial overgrowth and intestinal malabsorption) and impaired pancreatic and biliary function may also contribute to postvagotomy diarrhea.[6]

Afferent Loop Obstruction

An afferent loop may be created with an esophago-, gastro-, or enteroenterostomy performed in conjunction with various gastric or pancreaticogastric operations. In Billroth II gastrojejunostomy, the duodenum is the afferent loop; in Whipple's procedure, the Roux jejunal limb is the afferent loop; and in Roux-en-Y gastric bypass, the duodenum and proximal jejunum compose the afferent loop. Afferent loop obstruction (also referred to as biliopancreatic limb obstruction) is an

uncommon complication of these surgical procedures that occurs with variable clinical severity and acuteness or chronicity.[7] Afferent loop syndrome refers to chronic partial obstruction of the afferent loop. Major causes of this syndrome include stenosis of the anastomosis, postsurgical adhesions, retrograde intussusception, volvulus, internal hernia, recurrent neoplasm, and inflammatory disease.[7,8] The clinical diagnosis of afferent loop obstruction can be difficult, because some patients have vague symptoms rather than the classic finding of abdominal pain relieved by bilious vomiting. Acute obstruction can result in pancreatitis, whereas chronic afferent loop syndrome can result in malabsorption, gastrointestinal bleeding, or perforation.[9]

Abdominal radiographs are often normal because the obstructed afferent loop is fluid filled, owing to ongoing accumulation of biliary, pancreatic, and intestinal secretions. Barium studies may suggest the diagnosis if there is nonfilling of the afferent loop or preferential filling of a dilated afferent loop associated with stasis (Fig. 52-3). However, the efficacy of barium studies is questionable because the afferent loop fails to opacify in 20% of normal postoperative patients.[10]

CT and ultrasound permit direct visualization of the obstructed afferent loop and are the preferred methods for diagnostic imaging.[10-12] CT may demonstrate thinly marginated, round or tubular cystic structures in the periportal or peripancreatic region, forming a characteristic U-shaped afferent

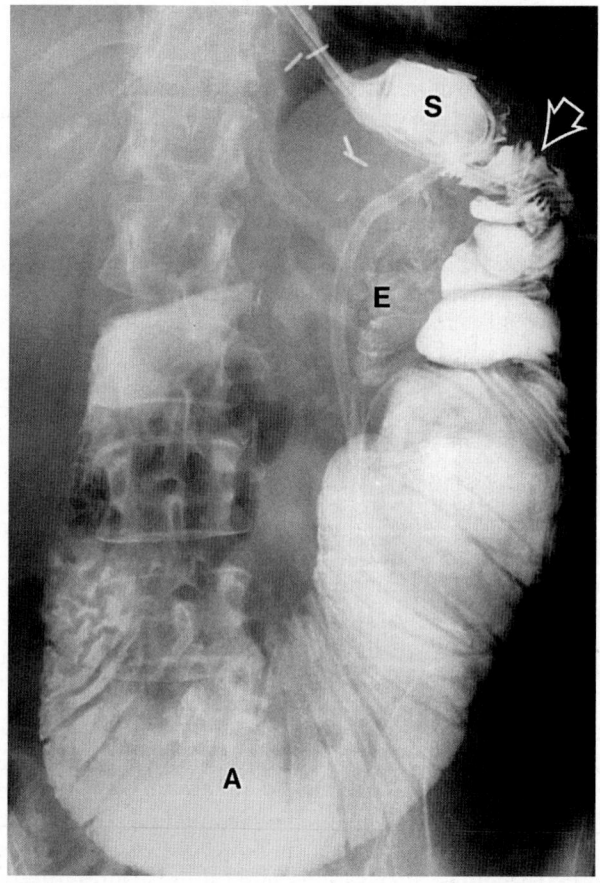

Figure 52-3. Afferent loop obstruction. Injection of barium into a small gastric remnant (S) results in preferential filling of a dilated afferent loop (A). Only minimal contrast material enters the efferent (E) small intestine. Distorted bowel margins are due to kinking and tethering from adhesions (*arrow*).

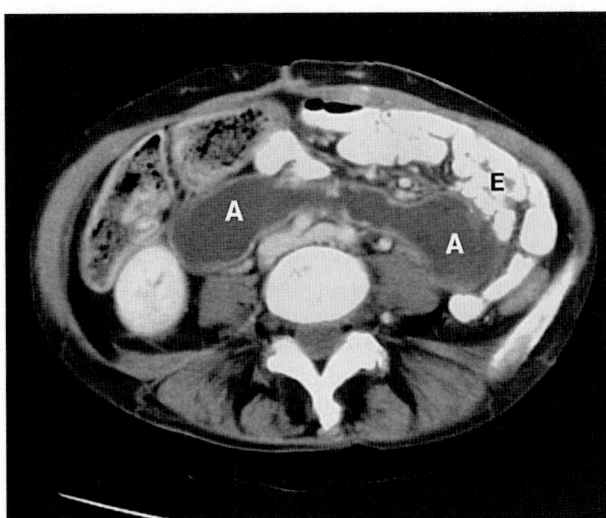

Figure 52-4. CT of afferent loop obstruction. Oral contrast medium opacifies the normal efferent small bowel loops (E), while the uniformly dilated afferent loop (A) remains nonopacified.

loop that traverses the midline on sequential axial images (Fig. 52-4). Nonopacification of the afferent loop is common after oral administration of contrast material. Transmitted pressure from the obstruction may be sufficient to distend the gallbladder and bile ducts, creating additional cystic structures.[11,12] Coronal CT images aid in identifying the course of the obstructed loop and in differentiating the dilated afferent loop from other fluid collections (Fig. 52-5).[7] The uniform size of the obstructed afferent loop and anterior displacement of the superior mesenteric artery may be additional diagnostic

clues. Ultrasound may also demonstrate the dilated afferent loop as a cystic or tubular structure in continuity with the gastric anastomosis and biliary system.[12,13]

Inadvertent Gastroileostomy

Gastroileostomy represents a surgical misadventure in which an anastomosis is inadvertently created between the stomach and ileum instead of the jejunum. This error usually occurs during a difficult operation complicated by the presence of dense adhesions and is the result of improper identification of the ligament of Treitz. Intestinal malrotation and obesity may also be contributing factors. Gastroileostomy usually leads to the development of severe diarrhea and weight loss shortly after surgery. Affected individuals may also present with malabsorption, anemia, and electrolyte imbalances due to short-circuiting of the small bowel. The signs and symptoms of gastroileostomy can mimic those associated with postgastrectomy diarrhea, gastrojejunocolic fistulas, or short bowel syndrome.

The essential diagnostic feature for the diagnosis of gastroileostomy is recognition of a distal efferent loop that crosses from the left upper quadrant of the abdomen directly into the right lower quadrant, resulting in unexpectedly rapid opacification of the cecum with contrast medium (Fig. 52-6).[14]

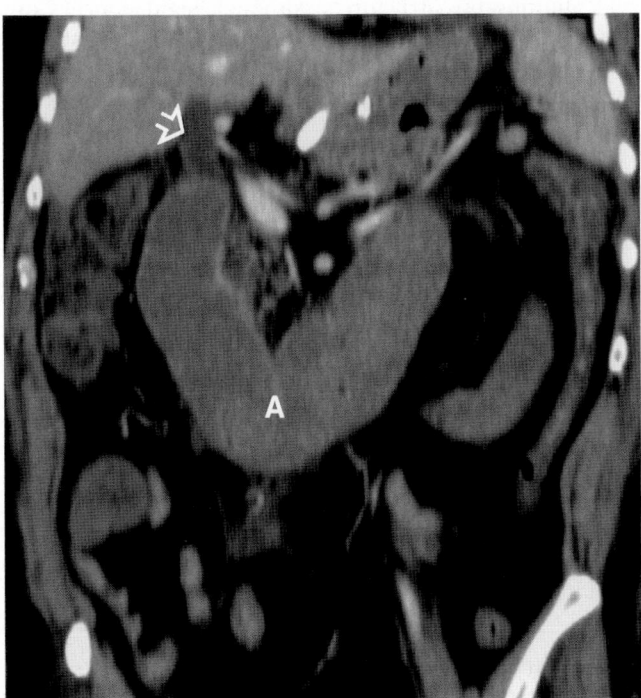

Figure 52-5. CT of afferent loop obstruction after Roux-en-Y esophagojejunostomy. Coronal CT shows distention of the afferent biliopancreatic limb (A) and common bile duct (*arrow*). The scan was performed with intravenous but not oral contrast media.

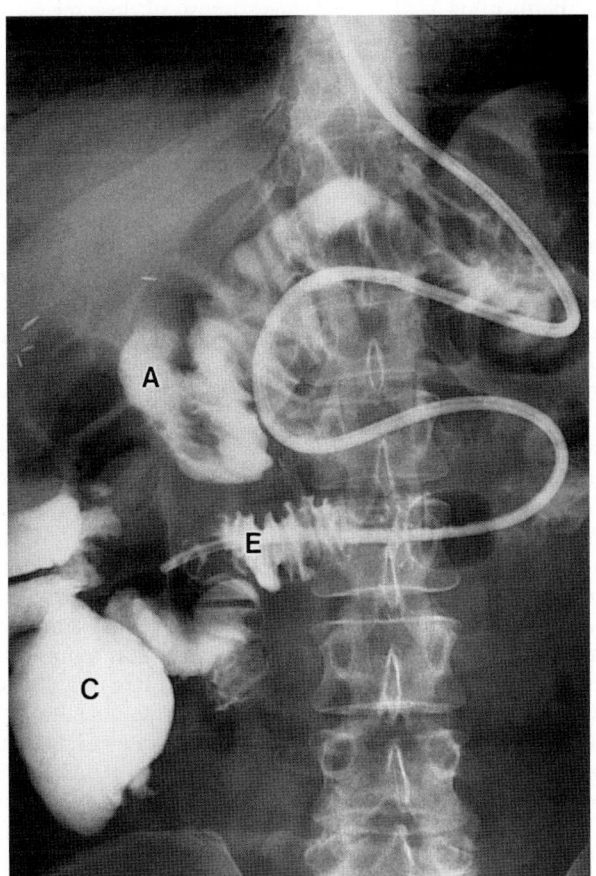

Figure 52-6. Inadvertent gastroileostomy after subtotal gastric resection and planned Billroth II gastroenterostomy. An enteroclysis catheter passes through the gastric remnant into the shortened efferent loop (E). Contrast infusion results in abnormally rapid filling of the cecum (C) and reflux of barium into the proximal afferent loop (A).

ENTERECTOMY AND ANASTOMOSIS

Enterectomy refers to surgical excision of the intestine and its corresponding mesentery for a wide variety of clinical conditions. Segmental resection of the small bowel is usually accompanied by a primary enteroenteric anastomosis, but in some cases an external ostomy is created in conjunction with a distal mucous fistula or a blind-ending distal pouch.

Anastomosis of the small bowel is one of the most commonly performed gastrointestinal surgical procedures, because it is required for reconstituting continuity of the intestine after resection, for bypassing an obstructed intestinal segment, and for creation of an enteric reservoir. Mechanical sutures and staples or manual suturing techniques may be employed for all types of intestinal operations.[15] An ideal anastomosis should be watertight and well vascularized, with an adequate stoma and a suture line free from tension. Anastomoses created under conditions of contamination, marked edema, or excessive tissue friability are associated with a high rate of breakdown.

Intestinal anastomoses can be constructed end to end (see Fig. 52-1), functionally end to end (anatomic side to side), end to side, or side to side (Fig. 52-7). An end-to-end anastomosis is the preferred technique for reestablishing continuity of the small bowel, as long as there is minimal disparity in luminal size between the anastomosed loops. An end-to-end anastomosis is also best for avoiding small bowel stasis syndromes. Closing the two ends of an excised bowel segment and performing a side-to-side anastomosis in close proximity to the closed ends is another technique for producing a functional end-to-end anastomosis that provides an increased anastomotic surface and decreases the risk of anastomotic strictures. An end-to-side anastomosis is used to compensate for disproportionate proximal and distal luminal sizes, and a side-to-side anastomosis is used to bypass an intestinal obstruction, as in patients with extensive neoplastic disease of the small bowel. When an end-to-side anastomosis is performed, the end of the proximal intestinal lumen is anastomosed to the side of the distal lumen. This arrangement ensures that peristalsis within the blind (distal) segment is directed antegrade toward and beyond the anastomotic opening, thereby preventing or minimizing stasis (Fig. 52-8).[1]

Given the high frequency of surgical enteroenteric anastomoses, intestinal obstruction related to the development of strictures or kinking at the anastomotic site is uncommon. Despite careful preoperative patient preparation and meticulous surgical technique, dehiscence of small bowel anastomoses can occur. Apart from technical considerations, several factors may adversely affect the success of an anastomosis, including sepsis, tissue hypoxia, malignancy, and advanced patient age. Intestinal perforation from an anastomotic dehiscence may be detected by the presence of free intraperitoneal air on abdominal radiographs. Water-soluble contrast studies or CT may be performed to demonstrate anastomotic leaks, but CT can also be used to localize contaminated peritoneal fluid and visualize associated abscess collections. Extra-intestinal fluid collections, which may progressively increase in volume during the postoperative period, should be suggestive of anastomotic disruption on CT, and extravasation of enteric contrast is diagnostic of this complication (Fig. 52-9). Suture dehiscence with a small or contained intestinal leak can also incite a localized perianastomotic inflammatory process or phlegmon, causing partial small bowel obstruction (Fig. 52-10).

Postoperative Blind Pouch and Loop

Although anatomic end-to-end and functional end-to-end surgical anastomoses have largely replaced side-to-side anastomoses for restoring bowel continuity, the latter procedure is occasionally performed, and this type of anastomosis can lead to the development of postoperative blind pouches. When a side-to-side anastomosis is created, division of the circular muscle can result in local dysmotility with stasis, progressive dilatation of the proximal anastomotic segment, and formation of a blind intestinal pouch. An incorrectly performed end-to-side anastomosis (side of the proximal segment of intestine sutured to the end of the distal segment) creates a similar anatomic abnormality. Occasionally, blind pouches may develop in patients with previously functional end-to-end (anatomic side-to-side) surgical anastomoses due to abnormal peristalsis and stasis. Dilatation of anastomotic intestinal segments usually develops 5 to 15 years after surgery.

In addition to intestinal stasis (with the potential for bacterial overgrowth), a postoperative blind pouch can be associated with inflammation, ulceration, and gastrointestinal bleeding.[14] Abdominal pain and distention, episodic diarrhea, and a history of previous intestinal anastomosis should suggest the clinical syndrome of a postoperative blind pouch, but a definitive diagnosis requires radiologic imaging. Segmental resection of the pouch and a restorative end-to-end anastomosis are corrective and eliminate the associated complications.

Abdominal radiographs may suggest the presence of a blind pouch if they reveal a fluid-filled soft tissue mass or gas-filled structure of variable size and shape. Small bowel contrast studies, particularly enteroclysis and CT enteroclysis, should demonstrate the pouch and its anastomotic relationships (Fig. 52-11). A blind intestinal pouch may be recognized on CT as a distinct saccular enteric structure with surgical clips abutting this structure.[16] Although blind pouches can range from 4 to 10 cm in size, obstruction of the small intestine related to the pouch and the anastomotic site is unusual.[16]

Although the blind loop syndrome has some clinical features in common with the blind pouch syndrome, the anatomic abnormalities associated with the blind loop syndrome are different. In blind loop syndrome, a segment of small intestine has been completely bypassed from the enteric stream by an enteroenteric anastomosis. Stasis of small bowel contents within the blind loop leads to bacterial overgrowth, which can approximate the composition of normal colonic flora in the most severely affected patients. Bacterial overgrowth in the small intestine may result in profound disturbances of absorptive function with marked malabsorption of lipids and vitamin B_{12}.[17] As a result, clinical signs and symptoms of this syndrome include diarrhea, steatorrhea, anemia, and nutritional deficiencies. As in the diagnosis of blind pouch, dedicated small bowel contrast studies can accurately demonstrate the postoperative anatomic abnormality. The clinical syndromes of malabsorption associated with blind pouch and blind loop are discussed in further detail in Chapter 47.

Short Bowel Syndrome

The short bowel syndrome is characterized by malnutrition, steatorrhea, and acidic diarrhea resulting from extensive surgical resection of the small intestine. Conditions requiring such major small bowel resections include mesenteric ischemia

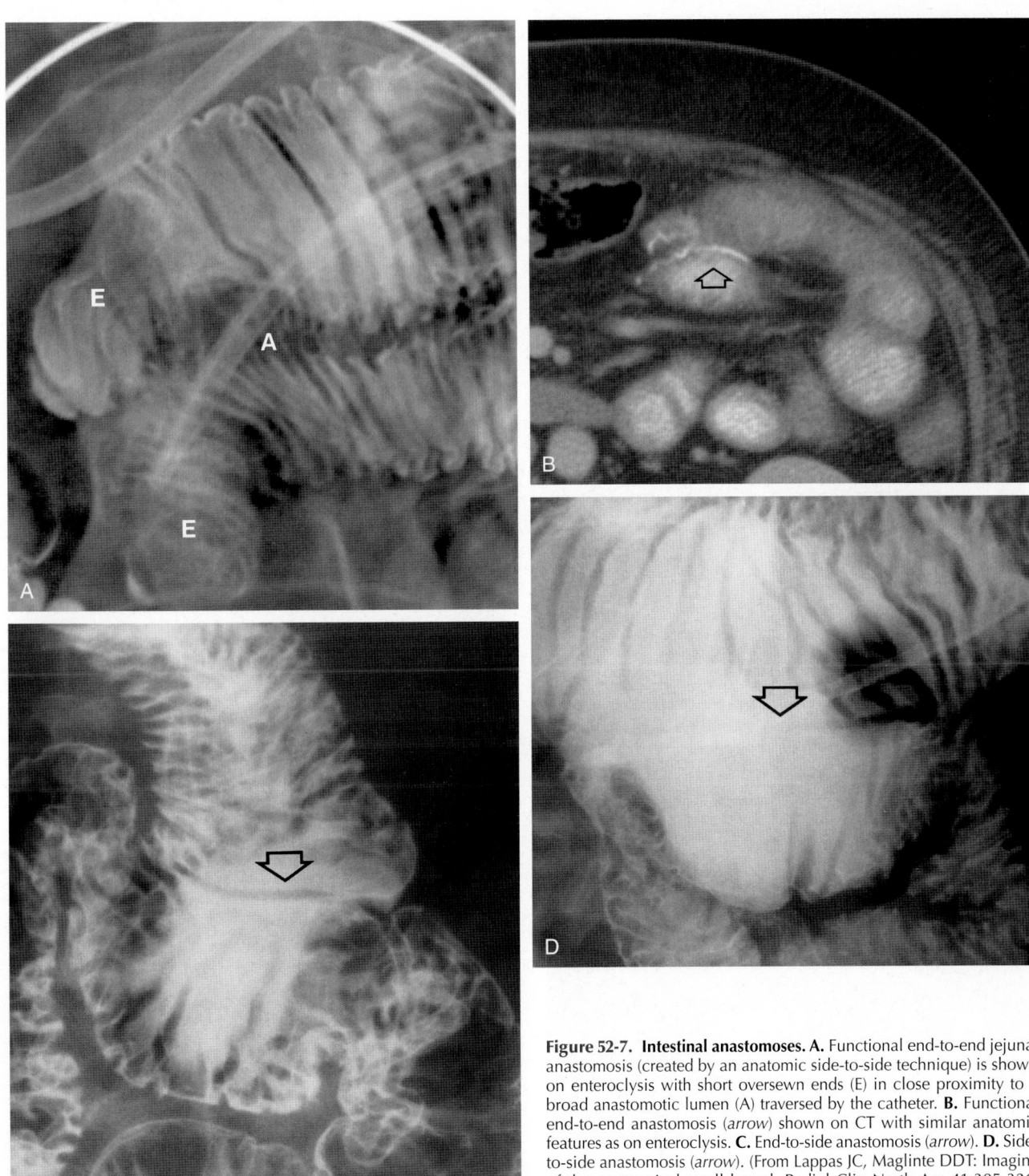

Figure 52-7. Intestinal anastomoses. A. Functional end-to-end jejunal anastomosis (created by an anatomic side-to-side technique) is shown on enteroclysis with short oversewn ends (E) in close proximity to a broad anastomotic lumen (A) traversed by the catheter. **B.** Functional end-to-end anastomosis (*arrow*) shown on CT with similar anatomic features as on enteroclysis. **C.** End-to-side anastomosis (*arrow*). **D.** Side-to-side anastomosis (*arrow*). (From Lappas JC, Maglinte DDT: Imaging of the postsurgical small bowel. Radiol Clin North Am 41:305-326, 2003.)

with infarction, strangulated internal hernias, volvulus, Crohn's disease, and intestinal trauma in adults and gastroschisis, necrotizing enterocolitis, and intestinal atresia in children. The degree of malabsorption and fluid loss depends on the length and location of the resected small bowel, the amount of residual colon, and the nature of the underlying disease

process. A jejunal length of less than 200 cm (especially if no colon remains) may necessitate nutritional supplements.[18] An adaptive response of villous hypertrophy and mucosal cellular hyperplasia in the ileum may compensate to varying degrees for resection of a large part of the jejunum. However, the unique ability of the terminal ileum to selectively transport

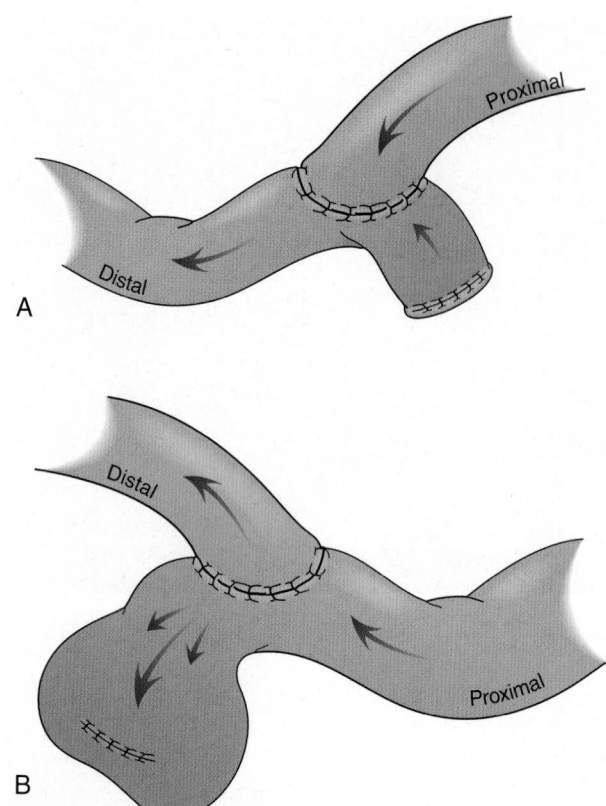

Figure 52-8. End-to-side anastomosis. A. With proper surgical technique, the end of the proximal small bowel segment is anastomosed to the side of the distal small bowel segment, allowing intestinal contents to flow in a normal peristaltic direction (*arrows*) through a patent bowel lumen. **B.** An improper anastomosis, with the side of the proximal small bowel segment sutured to the end of the distal small bowel segment, allows intestinal peristalsis (*arrows*) to be directed into the blind segment, leading to luminal dilatation (pouch formation) and intestinal stasis.

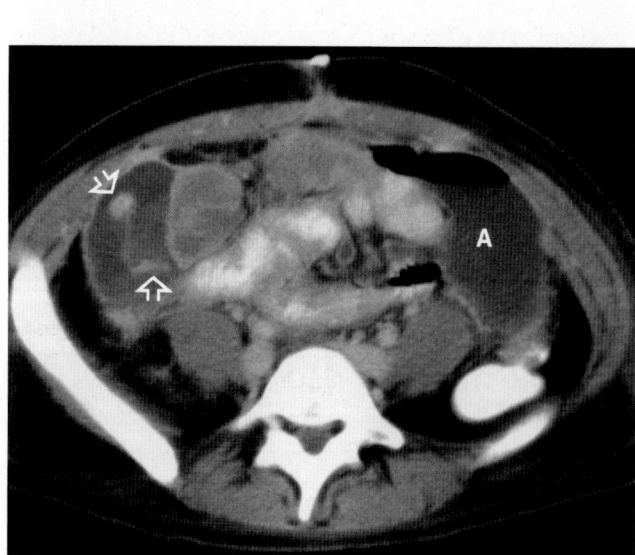

Figure 52-9. Dehiscence of small bowel anastomosis with abscess formation. CT shows an intraperitoneal abscess (A) containing extraluminal gas, fluid, and extravasated enteric contrast medium (*arrows*). These findings indicate breakdown of an enteric anastomosis. (From Lappas JC, Maglinte DDT: Imaging of the postsurgical small bowel. Radiol Clin North Am 41:305-326, 2003.)

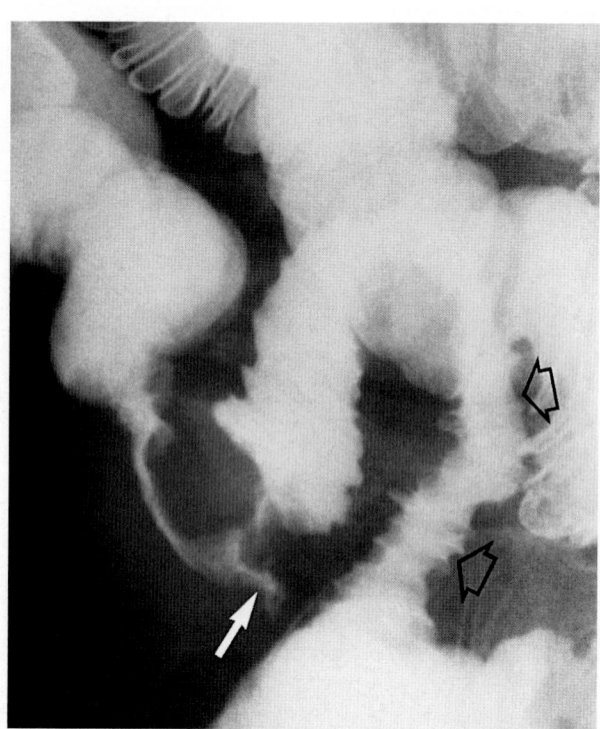

Figure 52-10. Perianastomotic phlegmon with intestinal narrowing. Symptoms of obstruction developed in this patient shortly after a segmental ileal resection with an end-to-end anastomosis had been performed for benign disease. Enteroclysis shows a short segment of luminal narrowing with a tiny leak (*closed arrow*) and thickened folds (*open arrows*) in the adjacent ileal loop. At surgery, ischemic dehiscence of the anastomosis was associated with a localized inflammatory reaction and mural edema of the proximal small bowel segment.

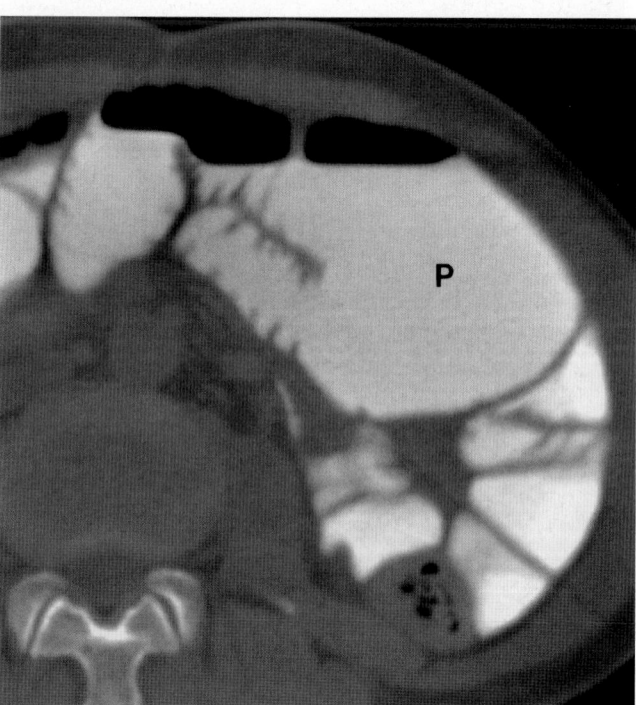

Figure 52-11. Blind pouch. CT enteroclysis shows formation of a blind, saccular pouch (P) associated with a side-to-side jejunal anastomosis.

intrinsic factor/vitamin B$_{12}$ complex and bile salts cannot be effectively restored after a resection of more than 100 cm (approximately 50%) of the distal ileum. Recognition of the metabolic consequences of substantial intestinal resection and aggressive correction of fluid and electrolyte deficits has decreased the mortality of these patients during the early postoperative period.[18]

Assessment of the length of residual small bowel is important in planning nutritional therapy and affects surgical decisions should further resection be necessary. Radiographic measurements of shortened small bowel (<200 cm) based on the findings of barium studies are comparable to those obtained at surgery and are sufficiently accurate to influence management decisions.[19] Barium studies also indicate the degree of ileal adaptation, as shown by an increased number of thickened folds and an increased luminal diameter. Recurrent or progressive small bowel disease (for which the small bowel resection was originally performed) can also be assessed.

ENTEROSTOMY

An enterostomy refers to an intestinal opening that is surgically designed to communicate with the skin and can function on either a temporary or permanent basis. To prevent intraabdominal leaks from the intestinal lumen, an enterostomy is made in those small bowel segments that are sufficiently mobile to be brought in contact with the anterior abdominal wall.

Jejunostomy

A jejunostomy is an ideal route for administering nutritional support.[1] Advantages of a feeding jejunostomy over a feeding gastrostomy include reduced nausea and vomiting and a lower risk of pulmonary aspiration from gastroesophageal reflux. Surgical feeding jejunostomies are performed in malnourished patients with a lengthy anticipated postoperative course; in patients with upper gastrointestinal pathology, including gastroparesis, malignant tumors, and fistulas or anastomotic leaks proximal to the potential jejunostomy site; and in patients who are not candidates for endoscopic, fluoroscopic, or laparoscopic insertion of feeding jejunostomies or who have failed these approaches. Direct intubated jejunostomies satisfy temporary nutritional requirements, but longterm jejunal feeding is best accomplished by a Roux-en-Y type jejunostomy. Surgical placement of the jejunostomy at least 70 cm distal to the duodenojejunal junction and fixation of the jejunal loop to the peritoneum are common techniques employed during jejunostomy construction. Some surgeons prefer to have the jejunostomy catheter routinely injected with water-soluble contrast media before initiating enteric feeding to ascertain proper catheter position and prevent misdirected infusions.

Various complications can be associated with any of the surgical jejunostomy techniques.[1,20] In a series of patients with jejunostomy tubes, radiographic studies demonstrated complications related to catheter placement in 14% of cases and various mechanical problems were attributed to the location or function of the catheter in 19% of cases.[21] Abnormalities include enterogastric reflux of the alimentation fluid, malpositioning of the catheter, dislodgment with intra-abdominal

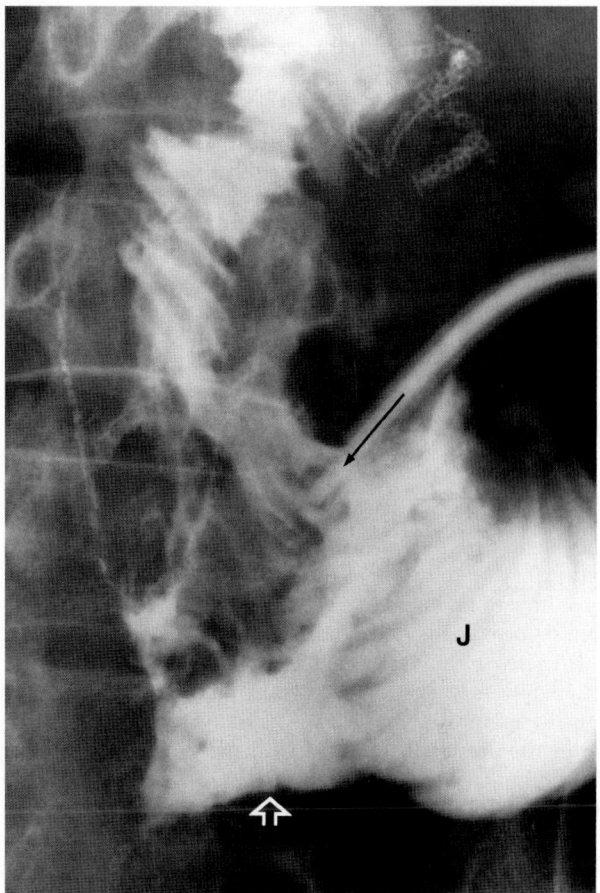

Figure 52-12. Jejunostomy catheter malpositioning. Injection of watersoluble contrast medium (*closed arrow*) shows incomplete purchase of the catheter within the jejunal lumen (J), resulting in tracking of contrast medium into a focal extraluminal collection (*open arrow*). Proper positioning of the catheter may be achieved by manipulating the catheter under fluoroscopic guidance.

leakage (Fig. 52-12), and small bowel obstruction at or near the jejunostomy site.[21]

Ileostomy

A distal enterostomy or ileostomy is primarily used for evacuation of intestinal contents in patients with diseases such as ulcerative colitis or familial adenomatous polyposis syndrome that necessitate a total colectomy. Conventional (end) ileostomy with total proctocolectomy provides a relatively simple and often curative surgical approach that mitigates the future risk of malignancy or recurrent inflammation with these diseases. However, loss of fecal continence and its attendant physical and psychological effects are major drawbacks of this surgery. Since the development of ileoanal reservoir procedures, the use of conventional end-ileostomy is usually restricted to the elderly or to patients with extensive Crohn's proctocolitis, anal sphincter dysfunction, or reservoir failure.[22] Another form of distal enterostomy, the loop (doublebarrel) ileostomy, is sometimes performed for temporary intestinal diversion in patients with acute intestinal obstruction or Crohn's disease complicated by extensive fistulas or abscesses or as an adjunct to complex operations requiring protection of a distal enteric anastomosis to promote healing.

Creation of a conventional Brooke or everting end-ileostomy involves transection of the ileum with mobilization of a 5-cm ileal segment through an abdominal wall defect and a specific suturing technique to allow for ileostomy maturation.[22] Malfunction of an ileostomy may result from adhesions, prestomal narrowing of the ileal lumen, paraileostomy hernias, and recurrent disease. These abnormalities can present early or late after end-ileostomy and usually occur at or near the ileostomy site, producing symptoms of diarrhea or intestinal obstruction.

Evaluation of patients with an ileostomy and suspected ileostomy dysfunction or other complications can be safely performed by retrograde contrast media examinations, including enteroclysis. Specific techniques are described for adapting enteroclysis catheters, small Foley catheters, and externally applied ostomy cones for ileostomy intubation.[23] Although retrograde ileostomy infusion allows better visualization of the distal small bowel and is preferred for most ileostomy examinations, good diagnostic results have also been reported with antegrade small bowel enteroclysis.[24]

In cases of partial small bowel obstruction, antegrade enteroclysis may accurately demonstrate the presence of functionally significant adhesions.[23] Fascial scarring with narrowing of the prestomal segment of ileum as it passes through the abdominal wall may also be a cause of intestinal obstruction and resulting ileostomy dysfunction.[25] In patients with parastomal hernias, contrast studies can demonstrate the herniated bowel and any associated obstruction, provided that lateral radiographs are obtained (Fig. 52-13). CT has demonstrated a higher incidence of parastomal ileostomy hernias than clinical examination in patients with conventional ileostomies (36% vs. 10%, respectively).[26] The hernias are usually lateral to the stoma and are often associated with large (>3 cm) defects in the anterior abdominal wall at the stomal site (Fig. 52-14).[26] Because CT accurately detects parastomal ileostomy hernias, it is the recommended study for the evaluation of ileostomy patients with unexplained stoma-related abdominal symptoms.

ILEAL RESERVOIRS

Ileal reservoirs are continence-preserving surgical procedures that offer patients the advantage of an improved body image and active lifestyle. Many surgeons consider the presence of Crohn's disease a contraindication for this procedure because of the high risk of recurrent inflammatory bowel disease and the potential need for additional small bowel resections in these patients.[27]

Continent Ileostomy Reservoir

Kock introduced the concept of an internal reservoir associated with a postcolectomy ileostomy in 1969 and demonstrated that the terminal ileum could function as a low-pressure, highly compliant reservoir.[28] The complexity of Kock pouch construction and function now limits the application of the procedure to selected patients with prior colectomy and conventional ileostomy or failed or contraindicated ileoanal pouch surgery.[27,29]

Creation of a continent ileostomy involves the use of the distal 45 cm of ileum, with the most proximal ileal segment fashioned into a spherical reservoir by complex suturing techniques. By design, opposing directions of peristalsis prevent propulsive activity from emptying the pouch. Continence is further maintained by intussusception of the efferent ileal segment into the pouch to form a valve mechanism, whereas the end of the ileum creates the abdominal wall stoma. Suturing of the pouch to the anterior abdominal wall provides stability and prevents volvulus of the pouch and peripouch herniation. Successful construction of a Kock pouch eliminates the need for an external ileostomy appliance, because the contents of the ileal reservoir are evacuated by stomal intubation.

Complications of the Kock pouch usually occur months after surgery and include various forms of valve dysfunction, nonspecific inflammation of the reservoir or the afferent ileal segment (pouch ileitis), and fistulas. Although the Koch pouch achieves reasonable functional results with long-term continence, surgical revision of the continent ileostomy is often required.[30]

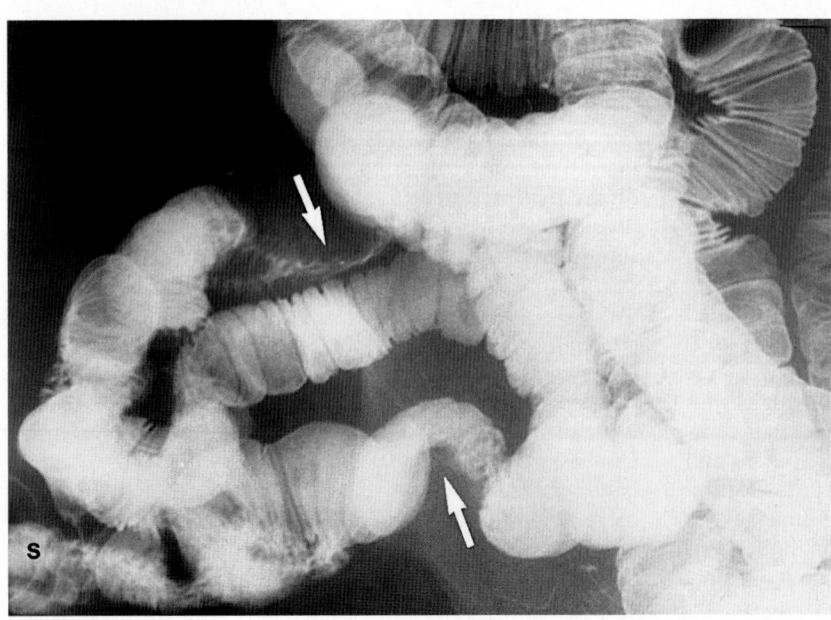

Figure 52-13. Parastomal ileostomy hernia. Lateral view during enteroclysis shows small bowel loops herniating through the anterior abdominal wall, with mild luminal compression (*arrows*) at the site of the abdominal wall defect. Antegrade infusion more accurately depicts the functional degree of obstruction in patients with an ileostomy. S, ileostomy stoma.

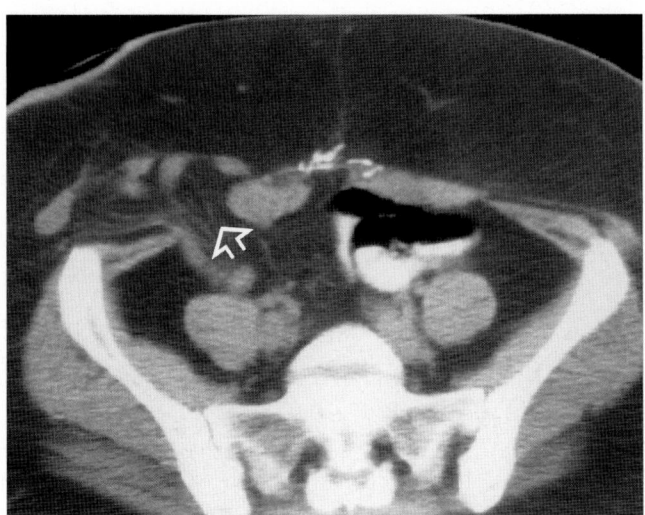

Figure 52-14. CT of parastomal ileostomy hernia. CT shows a large anterior abdominal wall defect (*arrow*) with herniation of small bowel loops and the adjacent mesentery. This diagnosis requires careful review of several scan slices, because the herniated loops and ileostomy stoma are often in different axial scan planes.

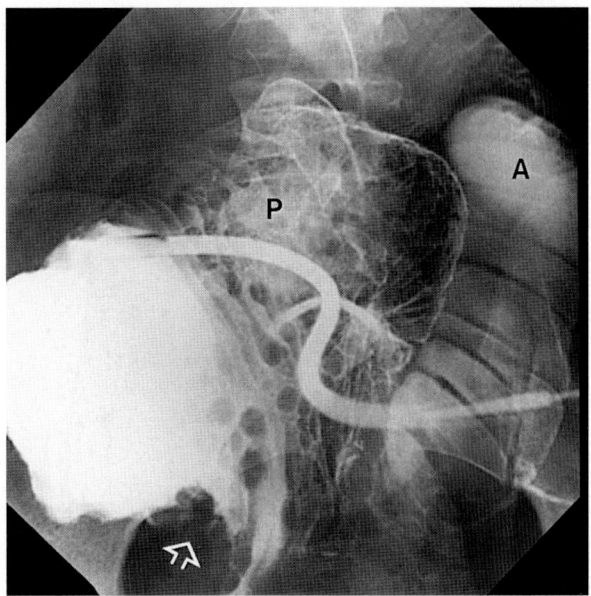

Figure 52-15. Kock pouch in a patient with familial adenomatous polyposis syndrome. Contrast medium injection of the pouch (P) after catheterization of the efferent limb shows multiple round mucosal defects representing recurrent adenomas. An irregular mass (*arrow*) suggests malignant tumor. A, afferent limb.

Retrograde double-contrast barium examination after cleansing irrigation of the reservoir is the recommended technique for evaluation of the Kock pouch.[31] Radiography in an oblique or lateral view is required to adequately visualize the efferent ileal segment and ileostomy stoma. If there is a clinical suspicion of suture dehiscence in the immediate postoperative period or of pouch perforation after intubation, the pouch should be evaluated using water-soluble contrast media rather than barium.

Barium studies of the normal reservoir show typical small bowel fold patterns interrupted by a linear mucosal ridge representing the suture line between the two anastomosed ileal segments.[31] Surface granularity is seen with mild pouchitis, whereas ulceration and mucosal fold distortion occur with more severe inflammation of the pouch.[32] The intact continence valve appears as a tubular or round, lobular structure invaginating within the reservoir, often associated with an array of stabilizing surgical clips. Sliding and eversion of the valve from the pouch results in valve shortening with progressive lengthening and tortuosity of the efferent ileal segment abutting the stoma.[32] Difficulty in pouch intubation, chronic outflow obstruction, and incontinence ensue. Adenomas may develop in the continent ileostomy, and surveillance of the reservoir is required in patients who underwent surgery for any of the polyposis syndromes (Fig. 52-15).

Ileoanal Pouches

Creation of an ileal reservoir with ileoanal anastomosis after colectomy and rectal mucosectomy has become an important surgical alternative for patients requiring total proctocolectomy. In patients with primary colonic mucosal disease, including chronic ulcerative colitis and familial adenomatous polyposis syndrome, this innovative operation removes potential disease-bearing mucosa while preserving anal continence and the normal defecatory pathway.

Several types of ileoanal pouches have been described, but the J-pouch configuration is preferred because of the simplicity of its construction, an adequate reservoir capacity, ease of emptying, and the absence of a potentially obstructing efferent limb.[27,33] An ileoanal J pouch is constructed from the distal 25 cm of ileum, fashioned into a J shape, and secured by side-to-side anastomosis of two adjacent loops (Fig. 52-16A). After anorectal mucosectomy and a rectal transection that maintains the integrity of the anal sphincter, the constructed ileal pouch is anastomosed to the dentate line of the rectal cuff. A proximal diverting ileostomy is often performed, and the extensive anastomoses in the ileoanal pouch are allowed to heal for a period of 8 to 12 weeks before closure of the protective ileostomy.

Although excellent functional results are often achieved in patients with an ileoanal reservoir, the procedure can be associated with major complications.[34,35] Common problems include pouchitis, small bowel obstruction, anastomotic dehiscence or strictures, fistulas, and pelvic abscesses. Most complications are adequately managed, but ileoanal pouch failure occurs in about 10% of patients.[34] Radiologic evaluation of the ileoanal reservoir is required to assess its function and to exclude anastomotic leaks from the reservoir or other postoperative complications.[36-39] In centers performing restorative proctocolectomy as a single-stage operation, postoperative imaging of the ileoanal pouch and anastomosis is not routinely performed but is reserved for investigation of clinically suspected complications.[40]

Contrast ileography or pouchograms can be performed antegrade through the ileostomy stoma or, preferably, retrograde through a soft rectal catheter inserted via the anus to visualize the ileal pouch and ileoanal anastomosis. Water-soluble contrast media are used for early postoperative examinations or if there is a clinical suspicion of a pouch leak, whereas barium is used for routine evaluation of the pouch. The normal J pouch is depicted on contrast studies as an ovoid structure with distinctive vertical raphes corresponding

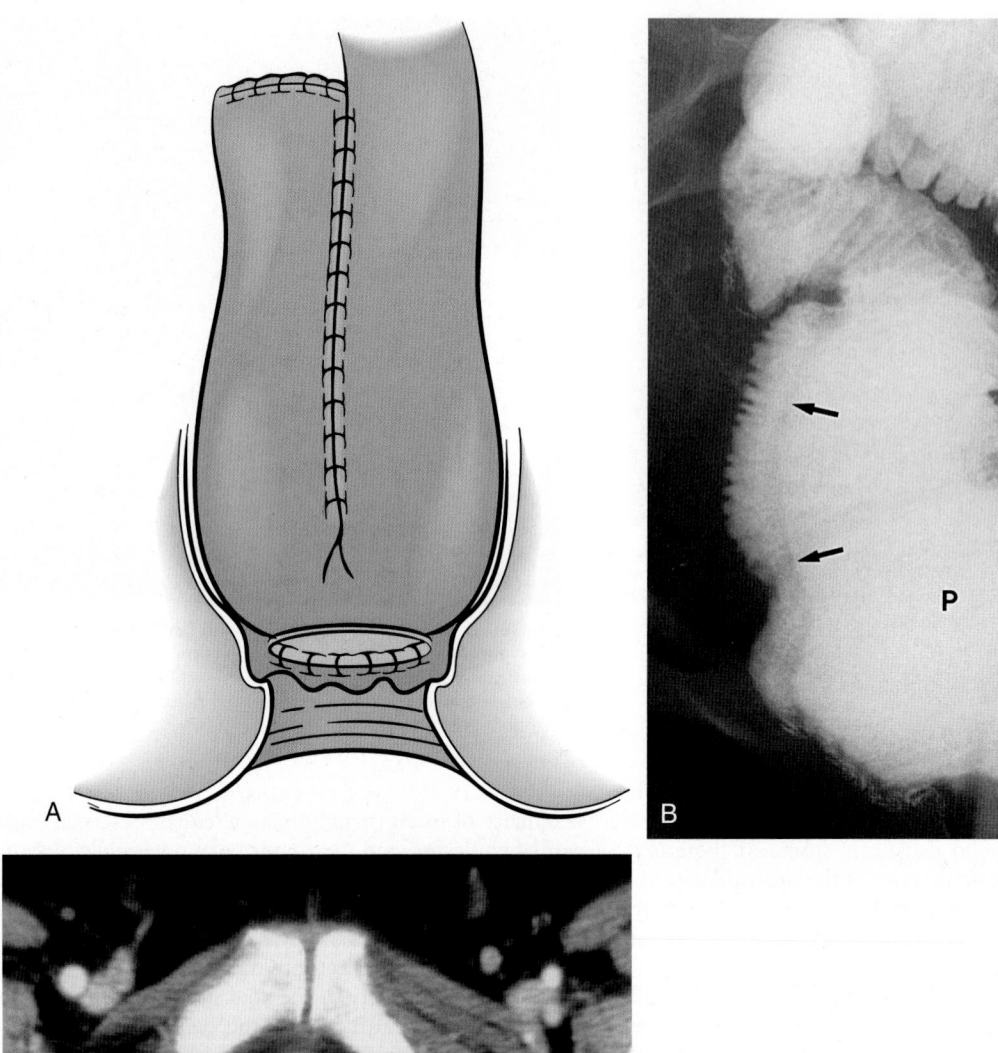

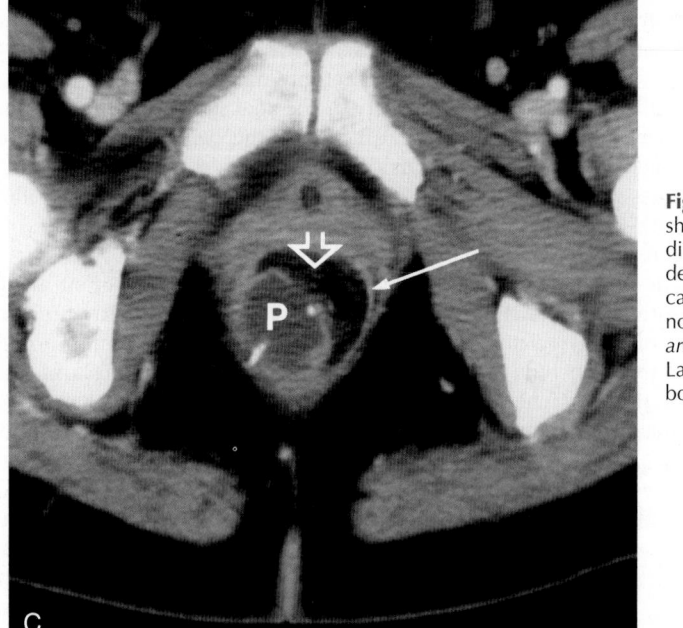

Figure 52-16. Ileoanal-J pouch. A. Schematic representation shows side-to-side anastomosis of adjacent ileal loops and direct anastomosis of the inferior apex of the reservoir to the dentate line. **B.** Normal pouchogram shows characteristic vertical raphe (*arrows*) created by the anastomotic line. **C.** CT of normal pouch (P) with surrounding ileal mesentery (*open arrow*) and thin muscular anorectal wall (*closed arrow*). (From Lappas JC, Maglinte DDT: Imaging of the postsurgical small bowel. Radiol Clin North Am 41:305-326, 2003.)

to the lines of anastomosis (Fig. 52-16B). CT may reveal a thin, surgically stapled pouch wall with normal adjacent fat (Fig. 52-16C).[36,37]

Pouchitis (mucosal inflammation of the ileoanal pouch) occurs in nearly 50% of patients who undergo this procedure. Affected individuals often present with a clinical syndrome of fever, abdominal cramping, and diarrhea. Contrast poucho-

grams are nonspecific but may demonstrate spasm and thickened ileal pouch folds. In patients with anastomotic dehiscence and pelvis sepsis, pouchograms with water-soluble contrast media may reveal extravasation of contrast material; extraluminal gas; thickened, spiculated pouch folds; or extrinsic mass effect on the pouch by an adjacent inflammatory mass or abscess (Fig. 52-17A). Clinically silent leaks from the ileal

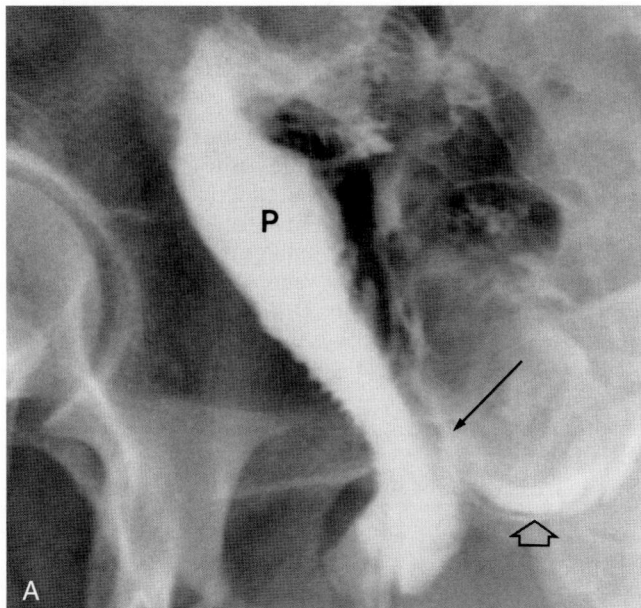

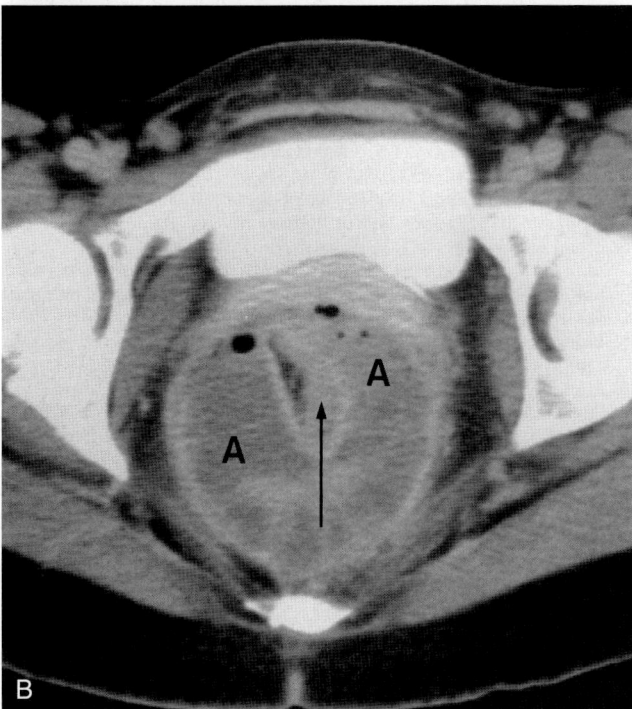

Figure 52-17. Peripouch abscess. A. J-pouch ileogram shows breakdown (*closed arrow*) of the ileoanal anastomosis with extravasation of water-soluble contrast medium (*open arrow*) into the pelvis. Adjacent pelvic inflammation results in narrowing and irregularity of the pouch (P). **B.** CT shows a large multilocular abscess (A) encircling the collapsed pouch and its fat-density mesentery (*arrow*). Note how the inflammatory process causes rectal wall thickening and stranding of the perirectal fat. (From Lappas JC, Maglinte DDT: Imaging of the postsurgical small bowel. Radiol Clin North Am 41:305-326, 2003.)

pouch may also be demonstrated on water-soluble contrast studies.[39] Patients with postoperative pelvic infections may have an abnormal pouch and inflammatory infiltration of the peripouch and perirectal fat on CT. Abscesses typically occur in the peripouch region between the ileal mesenteric fat and the adjacent rectal muscularis (Fig. 52-17B). In patients with

infectious complications after ileoanal pouch surgery, the findings on ileography are often nonspecific, whereas CT more accurately delineates the inflammatory process and can also direct therapeutic intervention.[37,38] Signs and symptoms of intestinal obstruction may become apparent after closure of the ileostomy and commonly involve the closure site or the distal small bowel. Adhesions, volvulus, and anastomotic strictures may also develop as a result of the extensive surgical resection and bowel manipulations.[33,34] Diagnostic studies such as barium enteroclysis or CT enteroclysis are effective in delineating the site and degree of small bowel obstruction in these patients.

SMALL BOWEL TRANSPLANTATION

Intestinal transplantation has emerged as a treatment for patients with short bowel syndrome and intestinal failure who can no longer tolerate total parenteral nutrition (TPN). Although intestinal transplantation has developed more slowly than other organ transplantation, the introduction of the potent immunosuppressant agent tacrolimus (in conjunction with other agents) has made transplantation feasible. As of 2003, nearly 1000 transplantations had been performed in over 60 surgical programs worldwide, with 1-year graft and patient survival rates approaching the results of liver transplantation.[41] More than 80% of all current survivors have stopped parenteral nutrition and resumed normal daily activities.

Intestinal failure may result from surgical or anatomic loss of intestine (short bowel syndrome) or from a significant functional abnormality. Other conditions treated by small bowel transplantation include volvulus, necrotizing enterocolitis, and intestinal atresia in children, and vascular disorders, Crohn's disease, and intestinal trauma in adults. TPN, the primary treatment for most patients with intestinal failure, can also lead to life-threatening hepatic failure. These factors can influence the decision for intestinal transplantation and the specific transplant procedure utilized.[42]

Three types of transplant operations are performed.[42,43] Isolated intestinal transplantation is performed in patients who maintain good hepatic function (Fig. 52-18), whereas combined intestinal and liver transplantation is performed in those patients with TPN-related or inborn hepatic dysfunction, and abdominal multivisceral grafts (intestine, liver, stomach, duodenum, and pancreas) are reserved for patients with extensive gastrointestinal tract abnormalities caused by vascular, absorptive, or motility disorders. In small bowel transplantation, the donor intestine is anastomosed to the recipient colon with creation of a diverting ileostomy that can be closed several months after transplantation if the patient's condition has stabilized and there is no evidence of graft rejection or infection. Current surgical practice usually excludes the colon from intestinal allografts.

Before transplantation, gastrointestinal contrast examinations may be performed to assess the nature and extent of bowel abnormalities and, in patients with short bowel syndrome, to map the amount of remaining intestine. If liver transplantation is planned, CT may also be performed to assess the hepatic parenchyma and vasculature.[44] After transplantation, contrast studies may be useful for evaluating anastomoses, gastric emptying, intestinal transit, and small bowel mucosal patterns. The normal postsurgical anatomy includes and normal patency of the critical vasculature.[45] Varying degrees of intra-abdominal fluid are common during the early postoperative period and consist of interloop ascites or loculated fluid collections with or without infection. CT may reveal a variety of abnormalities after intestinal transplantation, including intestinal dilatation associated with ileus or obstruction and nonspecific bowel wall thickening caused by preservation injury, graft rejection, infection, or ischemia. CT may also reveal a spectrum of findings related to anastomotic leaks, thrombosis of arterial or venous grafts, post-transplant lymphoproliferative disorders (PTLD), and complications specific to liver transplantation.[44,45] PTLD is more common after intestinal transplants than after other organ transplants because of the greater degree of immunosuppression. This condition may be manifested on CT by abdominal lymphadenopathy and the development of masses in the gastrointestinal tract or solid organs.

References

1. Lui KIM, Walker FW: Surgical procedures on the small intestine. In Zuidema GD (ed): Surgery of the Alimentary Tract, 4th ed. Philadelphia, WB Saunders, 1996, pp 267-288.
2. Lappas JC, Maglinte DDT: Radiological approach to investigation of the small intestine. In Gourtsoyiannis N (ed): Medical Radiology—Diagnostic Imaging; Radiological Imaging of the Small Intestine. New York, Springer-Verlag, 2002, pp 447-463.
3. Maglinte DDT, Lappas JC, Heitkamp DE, et al: Technical refinements in enteroclysis. Radiol Clin North Am 41:213-229, 2003.
4. Maglinte DDT, Bender GN, Heitkamp DE, et al: Multidetector-row helical CT enteroclysis. Radiol Clin North Am 41:249-262, 2003.
5. Abumrad NN, Sawyers JL, Richards WO: Dumping syndrome and other early postgastrectomy sequelae. In Scott HJ, Sawyers JL (eds): Surgery of the Stomach, Duodenum, and Small Intestine, 2nd ed. Boston, Blackwell Scientific Publications, 1992, pp 620-631.
6. Eagon JC, Miedema BW, Kelly KA: Postgastrectomy syndromes. Surg Clin North Am 72:445-465, 1992.
7. Sandrasegaran K, Maglinte DDT, Rajesh A, et al: CT of acute biliopancreatic limb obstruction. AJR 186:104-109, 2006.
8. Jones KB: Biliopancreatic limb obstruction in gastric bypass at or proximal to the jejunojejunostomy: A potentially deadly, catastrophic event. Obes Surg 6:485-493, 1996.
9. Conter RL, Converse JO, McGarrity TJ, Koch KL: Afferent loop obstruction presenting as acute pancreatitis and pseudocyst: Case reports and review of the literature. Surgery 108:22-27, 1990.
10. Wise SW: Case 24: Afferent loop syndrome. Radiology 216:142-145, 2000.
11. Gayer G, Barsuk D, Hertz M, et al: CT diagnosis of afferent loop syndrome. Clin Radiol 57:835-839, 2002.
12. Hasuda K, Makino Y, Arata T, Yamada T: Afferent loop obstruction diagnosed by sonography and computed tomography. Br J Radiol 64:1156-1158, 1991.
13. Lee DH, Lim JH, Ko YT: Afferent loop syndrome: Sonographic findings in seven cases. AJR 157:41-43, 1991.
14. Lappas JC, Maglinte DDT: Imaging of the postsurgical small bowel. Radiol Clin N Am 41:305-326, 2003.
15. Steichen FM, Galibert LA, Wolsch RA, et al: Stapling techniques in operations on the gastrointestinal tract. In Baker RJ, Fischer JE (eds): Mastery of Surgery, 4th ed. Philadelphia, Lippincott Williams & Wilkins, 2001, pp 201-225.
16. Sandrasegaran K, Maglinte DDT, Rajesh A, et al: CT findings of postsurgical blind pouch of small bowel. AJR 186:110-113, 2006.
17. Keusch GT, Gorbach SL: Enteric microbial ecology and infection. In Haubrich WS, Schaffner F (eds). Bockus-Gastroenterology, 5th ed. Philadelphia, WB Saunders, 1995, pp 1115-1145.
18. Loeff DS, Imbembo AL, Bohrer S: Small-intestinal insufficiency and the short-bowel syndrome. In Zuidema GD (ed): Surgery of the Alimentary Tract, 4th ed. Philadelphia, WB Saunders, 1996, pp 333-374.
19. Nightingale JMD, Bartram CI, Lennard-Jones JE: Length of residual small bowel after partial resection: Correlation between radiographic and surgical measurements. Gastrointest Radiol 16:305-306, 1991.

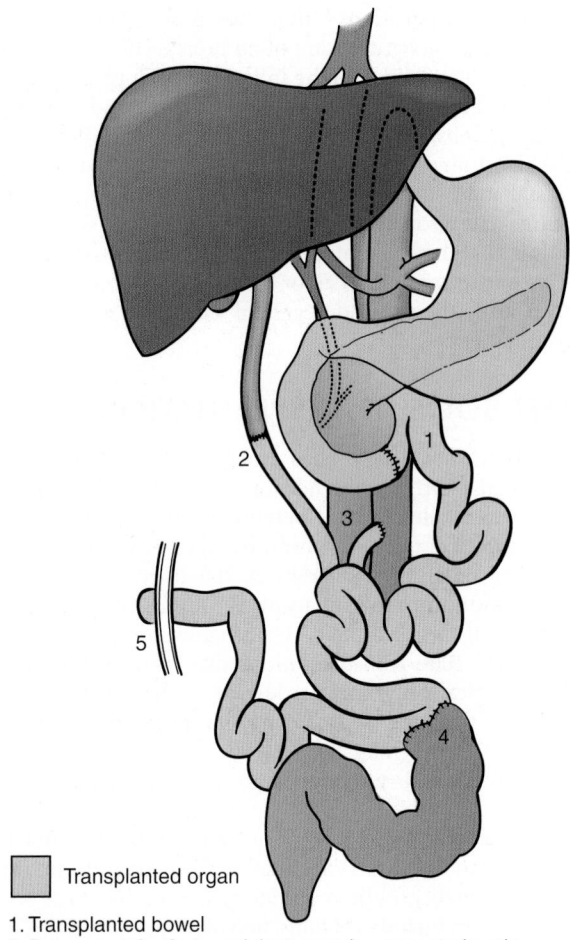

Transplanted organ

1. Transplanted bowel
2. Donor portal vein to recipient superior mesenteric vein
3. Donor superior mesenteric artery to recipient aorta
4. Recipient colon to transplanted bowel
5. Ileostomy

Figure 52-18. Schematic representation of isolated small bowel transplantation (*donor small intestine shaded gray*). After critical donor-recipient arterial and venous anastomoses are established, the intestinal graft is anastomosed to the recipient colon with a temporary ileostomy.

a native-to-donor jejunojejunal, duodenojejunal, or gastrogastric anastomosis and a donor-to-native ileocolic anastomosis with an end-ileostomy. Healthy allografts show normal bowel caliber and mucosal patterns, active peristalsis, and normal transit times.

Abnormalities on early postoperative gastrointestinal contrast studies include gastric atony and slow small bowel transit with varying degrees of luminal dilatation.[44] Thickened, edematous folds may be present in the graft during the early postoperative period due to harvesting injury. In contrast, fold thickening during the later postoperative period should raise concern about infection, rejection, or ischemia of the transplanted intestine.[44] Loss of the normal fold pattern, resulting in a tubular appearance of the intestinal graft, may be caused by both acute and chronic rejection and by infection with cytomegalovirus. However, radiographic studies are insensitive for detection of acute graft rejection or infection, which are more accurately diagnosed by frequent surveillance ileoscopy with mucosal biopsies and zoom video endoscopy.[43]

Uncomplicated small bowel grafts may be manifested on CT by nondilated intestinal loops with normal wall thickness

20. McGonigal MD, Lucas CE, Ledgerwood AM: Feeding jejunostomy in patients who are critically ill. Surg Gynecol Obstet 168:275-277, 1989.
21. Carucci LR, Levine MS, Rubesin SE, et al: Evaluation of patients with jejunostomy tubes: Imaging findings. Radiology 223:241-247, 2002.
22. Becker JM: Surgical therapy for ulcerative colitis and Crohn's disease. Gastroenterol Clin North Am 28:371-390, 1999.
23. Lappas JC, Maglinte DDT. Advances in enteroclysis. In Margulis AR (ed): Modern Imaging of the Alimentary Tube. Berlin, Springer-Verlag, 1997, pp 129-142.
24. Kay VJ, Nolan DJ: The small bowel enema in the patient with an ileostomy. Clin Radiol 39:418-422, 1988.
25. Zagoria RJ, Gelfand DW, Ott DJ: Retrograde examination of the small bowel in patients with an ileostomy. Gastrointest Radiol 11:97-101, 1986.
26. Etherington RJ, Williams JG, Hayward MWJ, et al: Demonstration of para-ileostomy herniation using computed tomography. Clin Radiol 41:333-336, 1990.
27. Becker JM: Surgical therapy for ulcerative colitis and Crohn's disease. Gastroenterol Clin North Am 28:371-390, 1999.
28. Kock NG: Continent ileostomy. Prog Surg 12:180-201, 1973.
29. Peiser JG, Cohen Z, McLeod RS: Surgical treatment of ulcerative colitis—continent ileostomy. In Allan RN, Rhodes JM, Hanauer SB, et al (eds): Inflammatory Bowel Diseases. New York, Churchill Livingstone, 1997, p 753.
30. Castillo E, Thomassie LM, Whitlow CB, et al: Continent ileostomy: Current experience. Dis Colon Rectum 48:1263-1268, 2005.
31. Lycke KG, Gothlin JH, Jensen JK, et al: Radiology of the continent ileostomy reservoir: Method of examination and normal findings. Abdom Imaging 19:116-123, 1994.
32. Lycke KG, Gothlin JH, Jensen JK, et al: Radiology of the continent ileostomy reservoir: Findings in patients with late complications. Abdom Imaging 19:124-131, 1994.
33. Cima RR, Young-Fadok T, Pemberton JH: Procedures for ulcerative colitis. In Souba WW, Fink MP, Jurkovich GJ, et al (eds): ACS Surgery, Principles and Practice. New York, Web MD Inc., 2005, pp 674-684.
34. Marcello PW, Roberts PL, Schoetz DJ Jr, et al: Long-term results of the ileoanal pouch procedure. Arch Surg 128:500-504, 1993.
35. Meagher AP, Farouk R, Dozios RR, et al: J ileal pouch-anal anastomosis for chronic ulcerative colitis: Complications and long term outcome in 1310 patients. Br J Surg 85:800-803, 1998.
36. Alfisher MM, Scholz FJ, Roberts PL, Counihan T: Radiology of the ileal pouch-anal anastomosis: Normal findings, examination pitfalls, and complications. RadioGraphics 17:81-98, 1997.
37. Brown JJ, Balfe DM, Heiken JP, et al: Ileal J pouch: Radiologic evaluation in patients with and without postoperative infectious complications. Radiology 174:115-120, 1990.
38. Thoeni RF, Fell SC, Engelstad B, et al: Ileoanal pouches: Comparison of CT, scintigraphy, and contrast enemas for diagnosing postsurgical complications. AJR 154:73-78, 1990.
39. Hrung JM, Levine MS, Rombeau JL, et al: Total proctocolectomy and ileoanal pouch: The role of contrast studies for evaluating postoperative leaks. Abdom Imaging 23:375-379, 1998.
40. Mowschenson PM, Critshlow JF: Outcome of early surgical complications following ileoanal pouch operation without diverting ileostomy. Am J Surg 169:1143-1145, 1995.
41. Grant D, Abu-Elmagd K, Reyes J, et al: 2003 Report of the intestine transplant registry: A new era has dawned. Ann Surg 241:607-613, 2005.
42. Abu-Elmagd K, Reyes J, Fung JJ: Clinical intestinal transplantation: Recent advances and future considerations. In Norman DJ, Turka LA (eds): Primer on Transplantation, 2nd ed. Mt. Laurel, NJ, American Society of Transplantation, 2001, pp 610-625.
43. Abu-Elmagd K, Bond G: Gut failure and abdominal visceral transplantation. Proc Nutr Soc 62:727-737, 2003.
44. Campbell WL, Abu-Elmagd K, Furukawa H, et al: Intestinal and multi-visceral transplantation. Radiol Clin North Am 33:595-614, 1995.
45. Bach DB, Levin MF, Vellet AD, et al: CT findings in patients with small-bowel transplants. AJR 159:311-315, 1992.

chapter

53

Miscellaneous Abnormalities of the Small Bowel

Stephen E. Rubesin, MD

ABNORMALITIES OF SMALL BOWEL DEVELOPMENT IN ADULTS

Meckel's Diverticulum

Midgut Duplications

Heterotopic Tissue

Segmental Dilatation

Intestinal Malrotation

Paraduodenal (Mesocolic) Hernias

ENDOMETRIOSIS

PNEUMATOSIS INTESTINALIS

INTESTINAL EDEMA

ENTEROLITHS AND BEZOARS

ABNORMALITIES OF SMALL BOWEL DEVELOPMENT IN ADULTS

Meckel's Diverticulum

The yolk sac provides nutrition to the fetus before the placenta develops. The yolk sac is connected to the midgut by the omphalomesenteric duct (vitellointestinal duct). This duct is obliterated during the seventh to eighth weeks of embryogenesis, as the placenta assumes the nutritional feeding of the fetus.[1] Persistence of various portions of the omphalomesenteric duct leads to a variety of anomalies. Failure of the entire omphalomesenteric duct to atrophy leads to an entero-umbilical fistula. Failure of one portion of the duct to atrophy may result in a fusiform area of dilatation, termed an *omphalomesenteric cyst*. Persistence of the vitellointestinal duct as a fibrous cord can lead to volvulus or compressive obstruction.

Meckel's diverticulum results from persistence of the omphalomesenteric duct at its attachment to the ileum. It is the most common congenital abnormality of the gastrointestinal tract; the prevalence of Meckel's diverticulum at autopsy is 1% to 4%.[2,3] However, the majority of people with this congenital anomaly never develop symptoms.

Meckel's diverticulum arises from the antimesenteric border of the ileum, usually within 100 cm of the ileocecal valve. It may be connected to the umbilicus by a fibrous band or to other intestinal loops by congenital bands or adhesions. The diverticulum usually varies from 2 to 15 cm in length and is about 2 cm in width.[1] Meckel's diverticulum contains all layers of the intestinal wall. The cyst is lined by small bowel epithelium and often contains heterotopic gastric or pancreatic tissue or Brunner's glands.[1]

Infants (younger than 2 years of age) with Meckel's diverticulum may present with gastrointestinal bleeding due to secretion of acid by ectopic gastric mucosa and subsequent ulceration. Adults may present with gastrointestinal bleeding, obstruction, or perforation.[4-7] Diverticulitis results from ulceration and focal perforation of the diverticulum due to ectopic gastric mucosa or an enterolith or foreign body impaction.[8] Obstruction results from a variety of mechanisms, including intussusception, volvulus around a persistent fibrous or adhesive band, or ileal narrowing related to ulceration. The diverticulum may become incarcerated in an inguinal, femoral, or umbilical hernia, also known as a hernia of Littré.[9] A variety of tumors may arise in Meckel's diverticulum, including carcinoid tumors, adenocarcinomas, and benign or malignant mesenchymal tumors.[10]

Technetium pertechnetate scintigraphy can detect ectopic gastric mucosa in more than 85% of infants, children, and adults with Meckel's diverticulum who have acute or chronic gastrointestinal bleeding.[5,11-13] However, most adults are asymptomatic or develop symptoms related to obstruction. All imaging modalities (except enteroclysis) have a poor sensitivity for detection of Meckel's diverticulum. In a small percentage of cases, plain abdominal radiographs may reveal radiopaque enteroliths in a Meckel diverticulum[14,15] or a dilated, gas-filled diverticulum in the right lower quadrant.

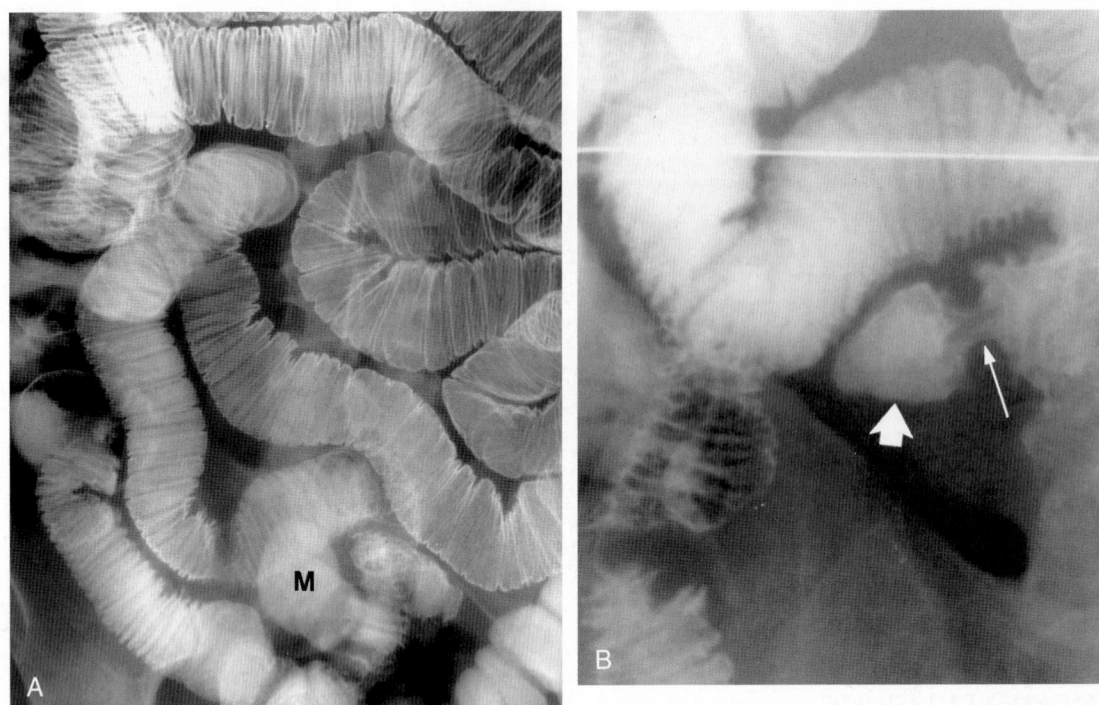

Figure 53-1. Meckel's diverticulum. A. Overhead radiograph from enteroclysis shows a saccular structure (M) in a pelvic loop of ileum. Note how this portion of the bowel is blind ending and does not contain normal folds. **B.** A spot image when the diverticulum was incompletely distended shows a triangular sac (*thick arrow*) arising from the distal ileum. Smooth folds (*thin arrow*) radiate to the origin of the diverticulum. Note how this Meckel's diverticulum appears to arise from the concave border of the bowel. This image demonstrates how the concave border of a small bowel loop is not always its true mesenteric border, as Meckel's diverticulum arises from the antimesenteric border of the ileum.

Meckel's diverticulum is rarely diagnosed on small bowel follow-throughs, except in patients with excessive mesenteric fat related to obesity or Crohn's disease.[16,17] CT or ultrasound may demonstrate a cystic or tubular structure attached to bowel in the right lower quadrant.

In adults without gastrointestinal bleeding, enteroclysis is by far the best radiologic test for Meckel's diverticulum. Enteroclysis has been shown to detect Meckel's diverticulum in 2% to 3% of patients, approaching the incidence at autopsy.[18-20] A blind-ending tubular or cystic sac is usually seen to communicate with the antimesenteric border of the distal ileum (Fig. 53-1).[21] One clue to the presence of the diverticulum is a triradiate fold pattern at the junction of the sac with the intestinal lumen (Fig. 53-2). Folds in the diverticulum will be perpendicular to folds in the adjacent ileum. The surface of the diverticulum may be abnormal, containing a granular mucosa (Fig. 53-3), focal ulceration, or a focal polypoid mound of ectopic gastric mucosa or tumor. In other patients, an inverted Meckel diverticulum may appear as a polypoid intraluminal lesion (Fig. 53-4), which sometimes acts a lead point for a small bowel intussusception.[21-24]

Midgut Duplications

Most midgut duplications involve the ileum, particularly the region of the ileocecal valve, and also the duodenum. These are usually elongated lesions attached to the muscular layer of the adjacent small bowel. If secretions accumulate, the duplication may become a cystic mass protruding into the small bowel mesentery. Multiple duplications are found in about 5% of patients.[25,26] About 20% of these duplications commu-

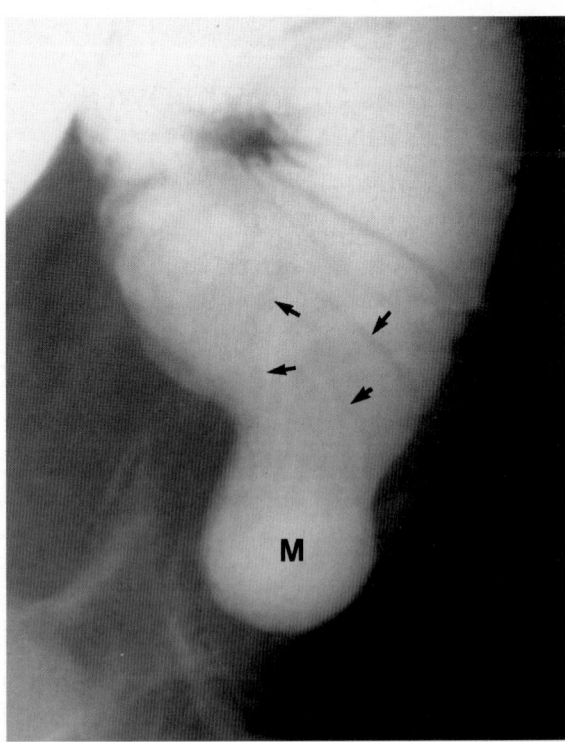

Figure 53-2. Meckel's diverticulum. Steep oblique spot image shows a blind-ending saccular structure (M) arising from the antimesenteric border of the ileum. Note how folds (*arrows*) radiate to the edges of the diverticulum and to its opening. (From Herlinger H, Jones B, Jacobs JE: Miscellaneous abnormalities of the small bowel. In Gore RM, Levine MS [eds]: Textbook of Gastrointestinal Radiology. Philadelphia, WB Saunders, 2000, pp 865-883.)

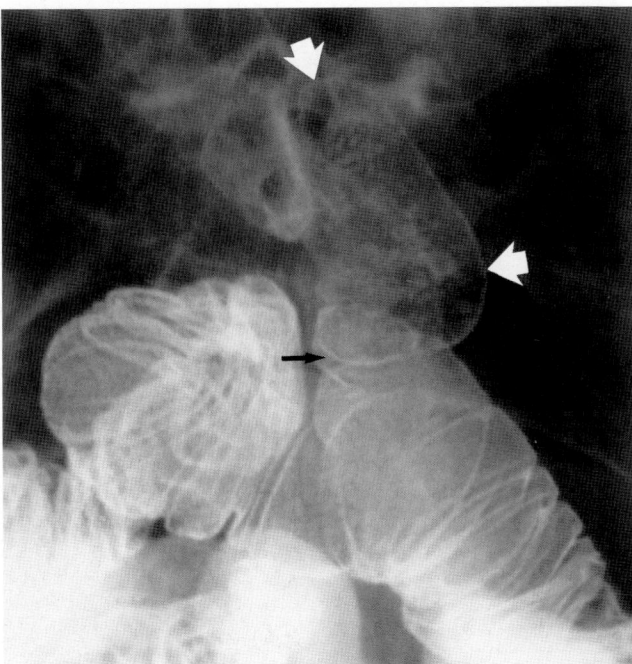

Figure 53-3. Meckel's diverticulum. A blind-ending sac (*white arrows*) arises from the distal ileum. The surface of the diverticulum has a granular appearance. At pathology, the mucosal surface of the diverticulum showed chronic inflammation but no ectopic gastric epithelium was found. Note the fold pattern at the entrance of the diverticulum (*black arrow*).

nicate with the bowel lumen at the proximal or distal end of the cyst or at both ends.[27] Midgut duplication cysts contain all layers of the bowel wall, including a mucosa, submucosa, and inner circular muscle layer with its associated myenteric plexus.[1] Duplication cysts may also contain gastric mucosa, pancreatic tissue, thyroid stroma, ciliated bronchial epithelium, lung, and cartilage.[1] The mucosal lining of these cysts is usually intestinal.

Ectopic gastric epithelium lining a duplication cyst may cause peptic ulceration with subsequent gastrointestinal bleeding or perforation.[28] Obstruction may result from volvulus, intussusception, or compression of the adjacent bowel by the cyst. Rarely, duplication cysts are complicated by tumor.

Duplication cysts may be manifested on barium studies by an extrinsic mass indenting and compressing the mesenteric border of the adjacent bowel.[29] Barium enters the cyst in only a small percentage of cases (Fig. 53-5). CT or ultrasound may show a cystic mass embedded in the small bowel wall.[29,30] If there is concern about gastrointestinal ulceration or bleeding, a ^{99m}Tc pertechnetate scan usually reveals heterotopic gastric mucosa in the cyst.

Heterotopic Tissue

Ectopic gastric mucosa is present in a wide variety of locations in the gastrointestinal tract, including the esophagus, duodenum, and mesenteric small intestine as well as in congenital abnormalities such as duplication cysts and Meckel's diverticulum. Congenital ectopic mucosa contains an orderly arrangement of superficial foveolar epithelium and underlying fundic glands partially lined by parietal and chief cells.[31] Ectopic mucosa should be distinguished from the more common

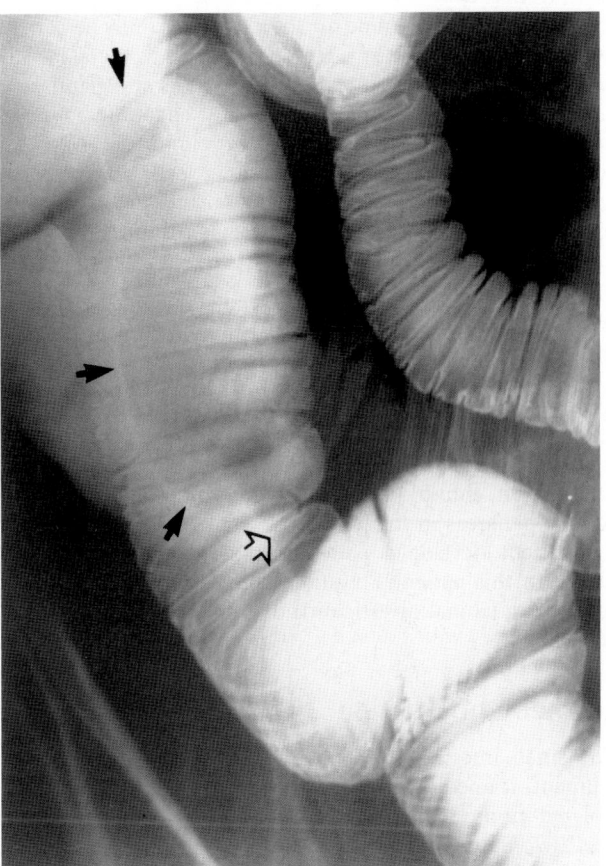

Figure 53-4. Inverted Meckel's diverticulum. Enteroclysis shows a long, smooth-surfaced, polypoid intraluminal filling defect (*closed arrows*) in the distal ileum. A tubular radiolucent filling defect (*open arrow*) resembles a stalk. This inverted Meckel's diverticulum could be mistaken for a pedunculated ileal polyp such as a lipoma or inflammatory fibroid polyp. (Reprinted with permission from Rubesin SE, Herlinger H, DeGaeta L: Interlude: Test Your Skills. Inverted Meckel's diverticulum. Radiology 176:636 and 644, 1990.)

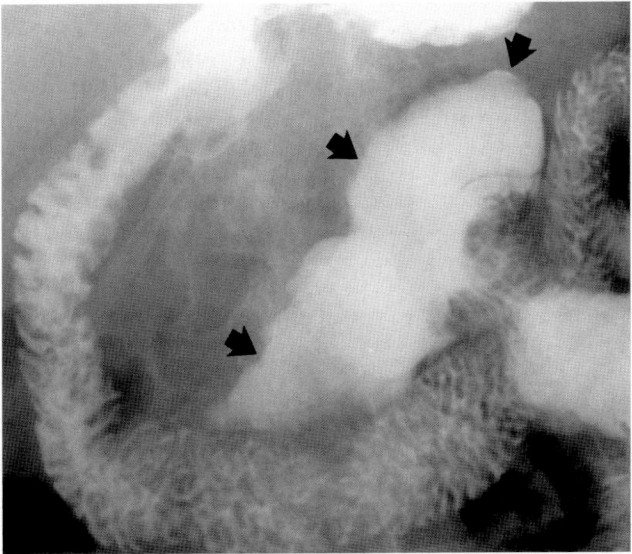

Figure 53-5. Duodenal duplication. Barium fills a 10-cm cavitary lesion that parallels the inner border of the third and fourth portions of the duodenum. The adjacent duodenum has normal folds. It is difficult to distinguish this duplication from an exophytic cavitary mass such as a gastrointestinal stromal tumor. (From the teaching files of Hans Herlinger, MD.)

foveolar metaplasia found in the duodenal bulb in patients with peptic duodenitis.[32] However, foveolar metaplasia in peptic duodenitis lacks organized gastric pits and glands.[1]

Ectopic pancreas is most frequently encountered in the duodenum (28%), stomach (26%), or jejunum (16%).[33] The ectopic tissue may arise from various levels of the bowel wall, including the mucosa, submucosa, and serosa.[31] Ectopic pancreatic tissue is composed of varying numbers of acini, ducts, and islet cells. Ectopic pancreas has also been reported in jejunal and ileal diverticula and Meckel's diverticulum as well as in the gallbladder, bile ducts, umbilicus, and fallopian tubes.

Ectopic pancreas in the mesenteric small bowel is usually discovered incidentally as a nodule or mass of lobulated solid or cystic tissue abutting the bowel in patients operated on for other causes. Although microscopic pancreatitis is not uncommon, clinical pancreatitis is very unusual. One case of ectopic pancreas in the jejunum has been reported in which the patient developed pancreatitis and pseudocyst formation.[34] In this patient, a cystic lesion abutted a jejunal loop, mimicking jejunal diverticulitis or a small, perforated tumor (Fig. 53-6).

Segmental Dilatation

The small intestine may have a focally dilated, aperistaltic segment, termed *segmental dilatation.*[35,36] In most cases, the isolated atonic loop is in the ileum, giving rise to the term *ileal dysgenesis.* The etiology of this condition is uncertain, but it has been postulated that it results from congenital neuromuscular dysfunction. In children, ileal dysgenesis is associated with Meckel's diverticulum and omphaloceles.[37,38] Ectopic mucosa (especially gastric mucosa) may be found in the dilated segment and may cause ulceration.

Segmental dilatation may be manifested on barium studies by a focally dilated, spherical or tubular segment of ileum (Figs. 53-7 and 53-8) in direct contiguity with the adjacent inflow and outflow loops of ileum.[39] The aperistaltic segment functions as a barrier to intestinal flow, resulting in partial small bowel obstruction. Ulcerated mucosa may be present in some patients. This condition can be distinguished from Meckel's diverticulum by its direct continuity with adjacent ileal loops. Ileal dysgenesis can also be distinguished from primary small bowel lymphoma with aneurysmal dilatation by the normal mucosal surface of the dilated ileal loop.

Intestinal Malrotation

Symptomatic patients with intestinal malrotation are usually infants and children with high-grade obstruction due to midgut volvulus or Ladd's bands. The embryologic, clinical, and radiographic aspects of intestinal malrotation in infants and children are described in detail in Chapters 115 and 119. Adults with intestinal malrotation are usually asymptomatic or have vague abdominal complaints.[40-42]

Intestinal malrotation encompasses a number of variations based on the degree of rotation of the midgut when it returns to the coelomic cavity. During the eighth fetal week, the midgut loop rotates 90 degrees counterclockwise while it is within the umbilical cord, so that the cecum lies on the left side of the fetus and the jejunum on the right.[1] If the midgut returns to the abdomen without further rotation, it maintains this orientation. Although this variation represents a

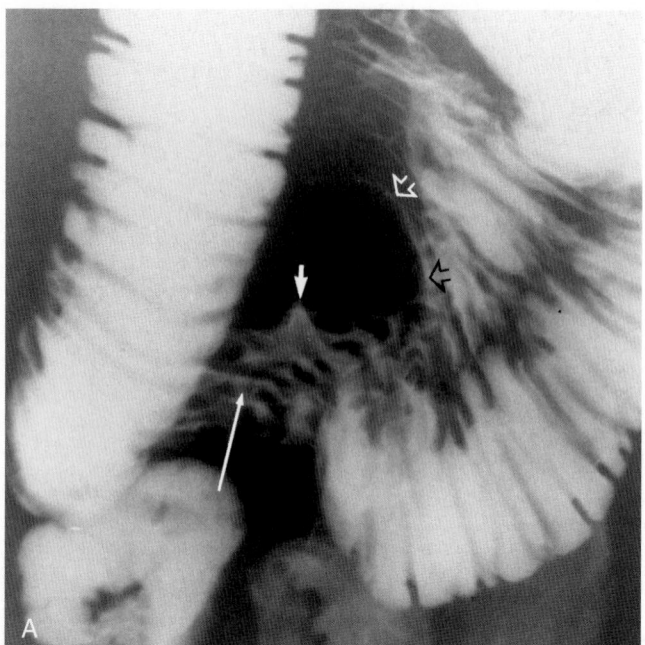

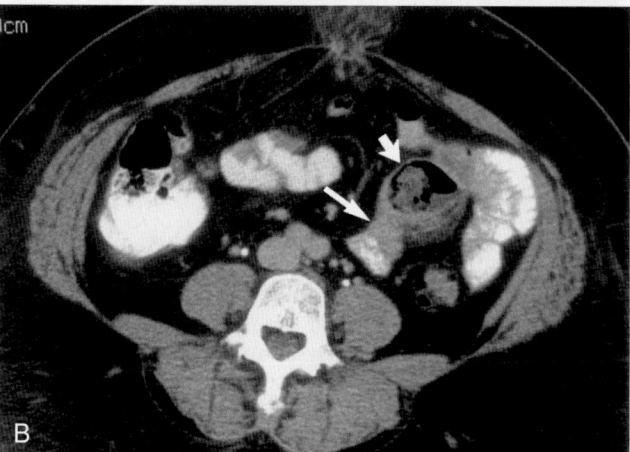

Figure 53-6. Ectopic pancreas in the jejunum complicated by pancreatitis and pseudocyst formation. A. Enteroclysis shows a tiny barium collection (*short arrow*) in the jejunum. Small bowel folds in this region are mildly thickened and undulating (*long arrow*) and are parallel to the longitudinal axis of the bowel rather than straight and perpendicular to the bowel, as seen in normal adjacent jejunum. Mass effect (*open arrows*) is also seen at the edge of the lesion. **B.** CT shows a soft tissue mass (*long arrow*) replacing the contrast-filled lumen of the bowel. A central cavity (*short arrow*) contains air and soft tissue. At pathology, the soft tissue mass was ectopic pancreatic tissue with associated pancreatitis, and the cavity was a pseudocyst that communicated with the lumen. This lesion could easily be confused with jejunal diverticulitis or a cavitary mass such as lymphoma.

90-degree rotation, it has been confusingly termed *nonrotation* because the small bowel is not rotating within the coelomic cavity. *Nonrotation* therefore actually represents small bowel rotation that stopped at 90 degrees of counterclockwise rotation. The third and fourth portions of the duodenum and duodenojejunal flexure are absent. Instead, the jejunum is a direct continuation of the second portion of the duodenum (Fig. 53-9). The jejunum and ileum lie in the right side of the abdomen, whereas the colon lies on the left side. The cecum is in the midline, with the terminal ileum entering the cecum from its right side. The appendix originates from a midline position, often low in the midline of the abdomen.[43]

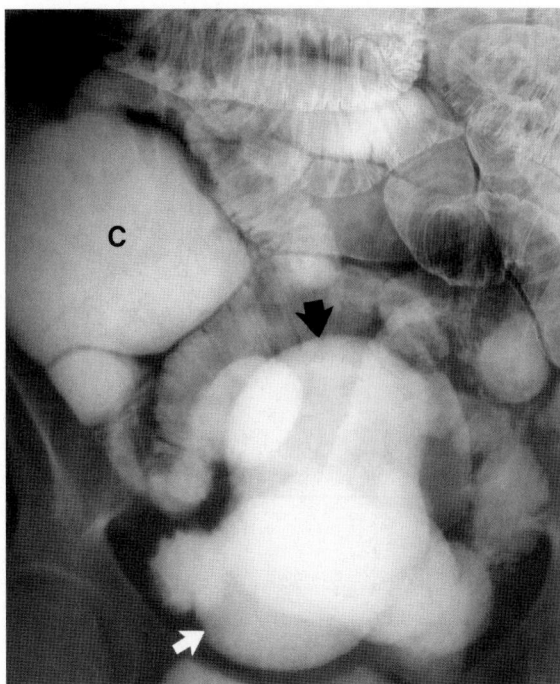

Figure 53-7. Ileal dysgenesis. Overhead radiograph from enteroclysis shows several round, focal, markedly dilated segments of pelvic ileum (*arrows*). The cecum (C) is identified. Normal-sized ileal loops were seen entering and exiting the dilated ileum at fluoroscopy.

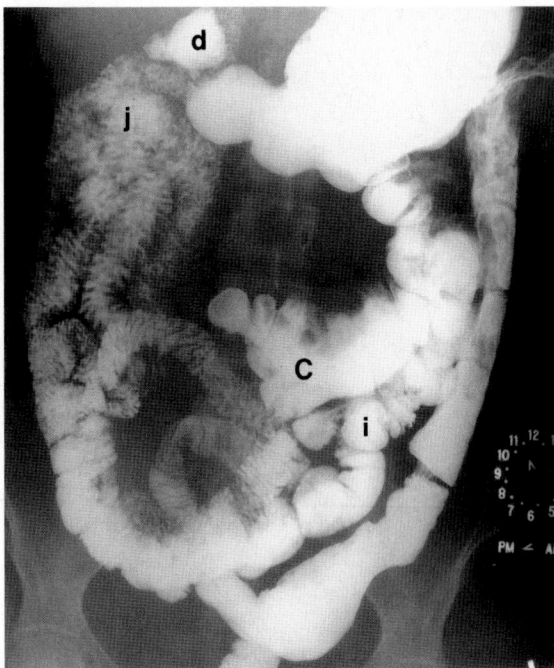

Figure 53-9. Intestinal nonrotation. Overhead radiograph from small bowel follow-through shows the duodenal bulb (d) in a normal location, with lack of the third and fourth portions of the duodenum and lack of a duodenojejunal junction to the left of the spine. The jejunum (j) is in the right upper quadrant, and most of the ileum is also in the right abdomen, with the distal ileum (i) crossing to the left to join a midline cecum (C). The colon lies in the left abdomen.

During the 10th fetal week, the midgut normally rotates another 90 degrees counterclockwise within the umbilical cord, so that the cecum lies superiorly on the right and the jejunum inferiorly on the left.[43] The jejunum is then the first midgut loop to enter the coelomic cavity, passing behind the superior mesenteric artery. During this part of rotation, the jejunum comes to lie between the posterior duodenum and anteriorly positioned colon. During the 11th week, the cecum

rotates still another 90 degrees into the right lower quadrant, completing a 270-degree counterclockwise rotation.

Intestinal malrotation occurs when the midgut fails to complete its 180-degree counterclockwise rotation. The duodenojejunal junction is not fixed in its normal location to the left of the spine but instead lies inferiorly and to the right of the spine. The small bowel lies predominantly in the right or mid abdomen. Mesenteric bands from the liver and posterior abdominal wall cross the second portion of the duodenum and extend to the cecum (Ladd's bands).

Intestinal hyperrotation occurs when the small intestine has rotated more than the usual 180 degrees, resulting in a long ascending colon with the cecum located in the left upper quadrant. In a *reversed rotation*, the bowel enters the abdomen with a clockwise rotation, so that the transverse colon lies posterior to the duodenum in the right upper quadrant.

The location of the duodenojejunal junction should be ascertained in any adult with vomiting or abdominal pain. The normal duodenojejunal junction lies to the left of the spine at about the level of the duodenal bulb. When the ligament of Treitz is in its normal position, the jejunum may cross to the right of the spine as a normal variant (as long as the jejunum is not entering a right paraduodenal hernia). On the other hand, the duodenojejunal junction not infrequently has an abnormal location. An abnormally positioned duodenojejunal junction is important because it may cause twisting and obstruction of the proximal small bowel, manifested by duodenal dilatation and slow transit of contrast material on barium studies. However, the typical "corkscrew" sign of intestinal malrotation and midgut volvulus in infants (see Chapter 115) is rarely found in adults.[44] Intestinal malrotation in adults is often recognized on CT, MRI, or ultrasound by an

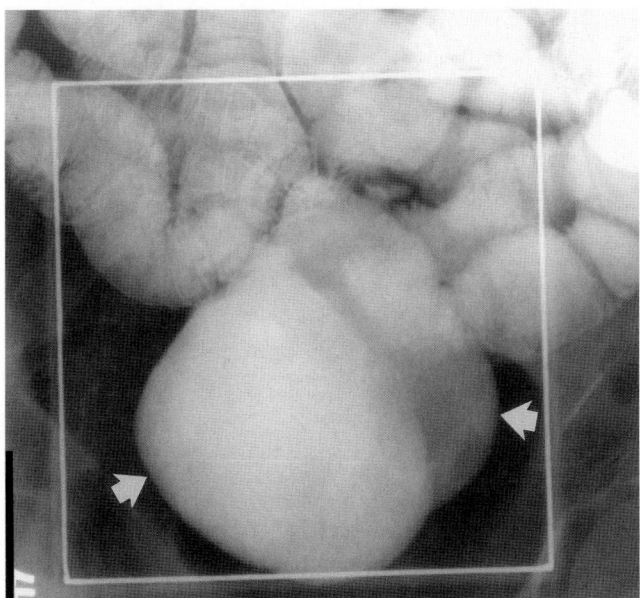

Figure 53-8. Ileal dysgenesis. Enteroclysis shows a large bilobed ileal segment (*arrows*). Normal entry and exit loops of pelvic ileum were seen on other views.

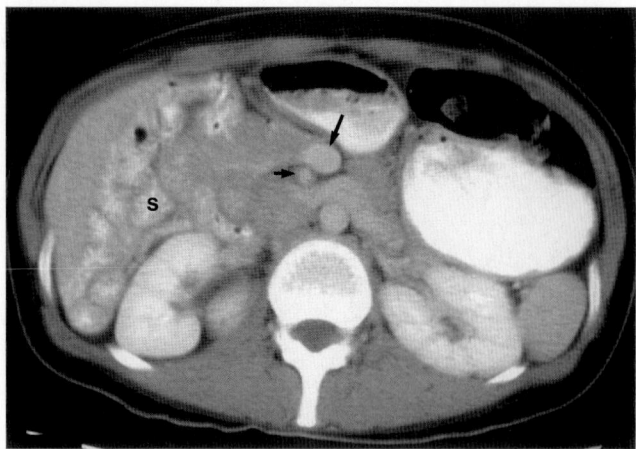

Figure 53-10. Intestinal malrotation. Axial CT through the tip of the liver shows that the superior mesenteric vein (*long arrow*) lies anterior and to the left of the superior mesenteric artery (*short arrow*). The jejunum (s) lies in the right upper quadrant.

abnormal relationship between the superior mesenteric artery and superior mesenteric vein, so that the vein lies anterior and to the left of the artery (Fig. 53-10).

Paraduodenal (Mesocolic) Hernias

Paraduodenal hernias are the most common internal abdominal hernias, accounting for about one half of all such hernias. Although abdominal hernias are discussed in detail in Chapter 113, paraduodenal hernias are discussed here, because these hernias relate to abnormal rotation and fixation of the colonic mesentery to the retroperitoneum.[45,46]

A left paraduodenal hernia represents a hernia into the mesentery of the descending colon. The opening of a left paraduodenal hernia is just lateral to the fourth portion of the duodenum at the fossa of Landzert, an anatomic fossa found at autopsy in 2% of patients.[47] This fossa is present when the inferior mesenteric vein and ascending left colon artery are incompletely fixed to the retroperitoneum. Loops of jejunum can herniate beneath the left colonic mesentery, potentially causing small bowel obstruction or ischemia.

A left paraduodenal hernia may be manifested on barium studies by a variable number of jejunal loops clumped together in the left upper quadrant lateral to the fourth portion of the duodenum (Fig. 53-11). The inlet and outlet loops may be focally narrowed where they are compressed at the hernia orifice (see Fig. 53-11). The loops do not change position with time or palpation, because they are fixed within the hernia sac. Barium may be retained in these loops on delayed images due to obstruction. Abdominal CT may reveal a cluster of small bowel loops lateral to the duodenum between the adrenal gland and the transverse or descending colon.[48]

A right paraduodenal hernia occurs at the mesentericoparietal fossa (the fossa of Waldeyer), which is found in about 1% of autopsies.[47] This fossa lies in the upper portion of the jejunal mesentery behind the superior mesenteric artery and inferior to the third portion of the duodenum. The orifice of the hernia is bounded superiorly by the superior mesenteric artery and vein (small bowel mesentery). Once the proximal jejunum enters the orifice, it herniates to the right beneath the mesenteries of the transverse or ascending colon. Thus, a

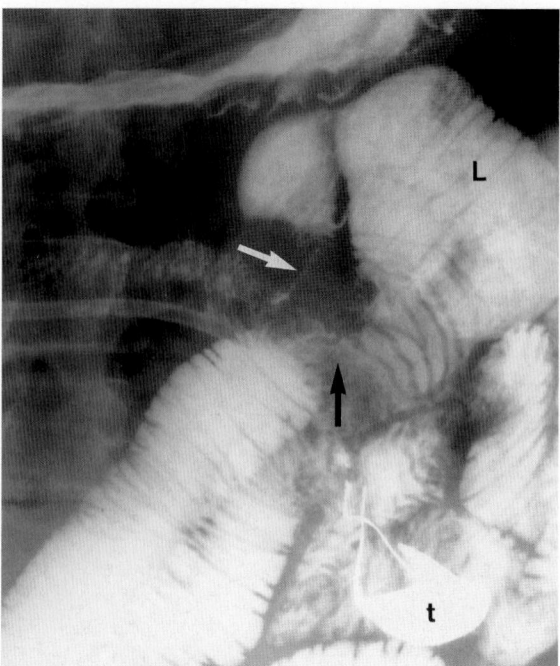

Figure 53-11. Left paraduodenal hernia. Coned-down image from overhead radiograph on enteroclysis performed via a Kantor tube (t) shows a cluster of jejunal loops (L) in the left upper quadrant. These loops are extrinsically compressed (*arrows*) at the entry site to the fossa of Lanzert. (From the teaching files of Hans Herlinger, MD.)

right paraduodenal hernia is best thought of as a hernia into the mesentery of the ascending colon.[45]

A right paraduodenal hernia may be manifested on barium studies by a variable number of jejunal loops clumped together in the right abdomen inferior to the third portion of the duodenum (Fig. 53-12). The herniated loops may be

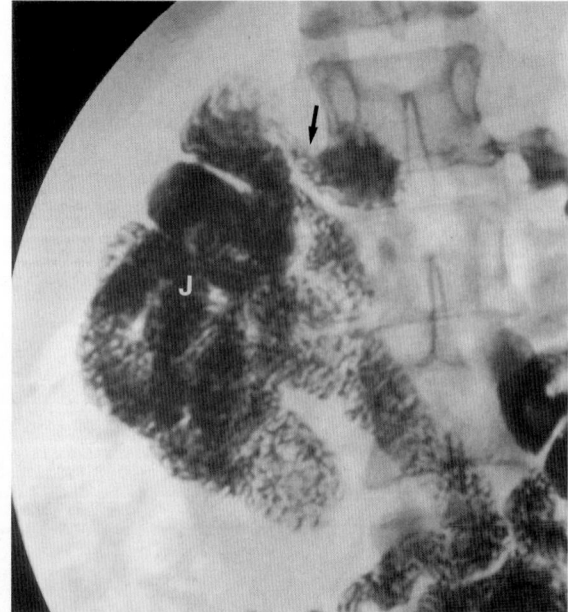

Figure 53-12. Right paraduodenal hernia. Low-power spot image from a small bowel follow-through shows a large cluster of jejunal loops (J) clumped together in the right upper quadrant. Note how there is compression of one loop (*arrow*) at the inlet to the fossa of Waldeyer.

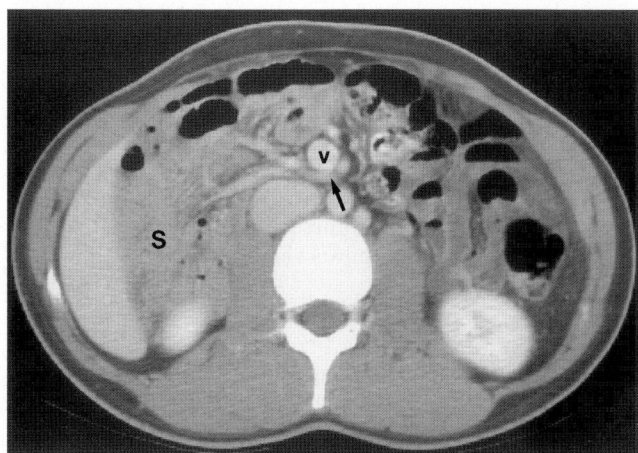

Figure 53-13. Right paraduodenal hernia. Axial CT through the tip of the liver shows collapsed bowel (S) in the right upper quadrant. A tributary (*arrow*) of the superior mesenteric vein is looping behind this vein (V). (Reprinted with permission from Herlinger H, Jones B, Jacobs JE: Miscellaneous abnormalities of the small bowel. In Gore RM, Levine MS [eds]: Textbook of Gastrointestinal Radiology. Philadelphia, WB Saunders, 2000, pp 865-883.)

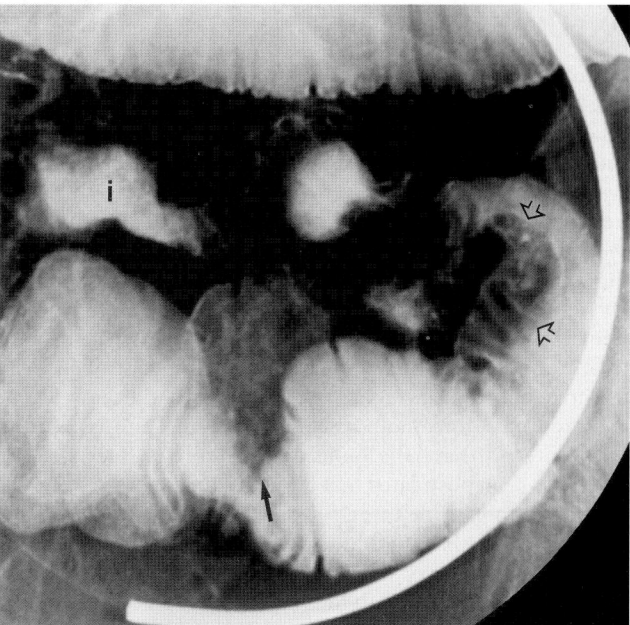

Figure 53-14. Ileal endometriosis. Spot image obtained during enteroclysis shows a focal, smooth, extrinsic mass impression (*open arrows*) on the mesenteric border of a pelvic loop of ileum. At a second site, there is another focal extrinsic mass impression (*arrow*) and tethering of folds toward the mesenteric border. The ileal mucosa is preserved. The distal ileum (i) is collapsed. These endometriosis implants in the ileum are indistinguishable from intraperitoneal metastases to the small bowel.

dilated and may show delayed emptying of barium. The inlet and outlet loops are closely apposed and narrowed due to extrinsic compression at the hernia orifice. CT or MRI may also reveal a focal cluster of jejunal loops in the right side of the abdomen inferior to the duodenum.[49] The branches of the superior mesenteric artery and vein are whirled posteriorly and to the right behind these vessels (Fig. 53-13), extending toward the right-sided jejunal loops.

ENDOMETRIOSIS

Endometrial tissue found outside the uterus is termed *endometriosis*. This ectopic endometrial tissue primarily involves the peritoneal surfaces of the pelvis and pelvic organs, including the ovaries, fallopian tubes, and pouch of Douglas. Colonic involvement is found in 15% to 37% of women who undergo surgery for endometriosis.[50,51] Ileal involvement is much less frequent, found in only 1% to 7% of surgical cases.[52,53] Ectopic endometrial tissue usually has a serosal or subserosal location, but endometrial tissue may burrow into the muscularis propria, the submucosa, or even the mucosa. The endometrial tissue goes through the proliferative and secretory phases of the menstrual cycle, with sloughing and bleeding, leading to regeneration of endometrial tissue and fibrosis.[1] Bowel involvement is primarily characterized by extensive subserosal fibrosis and serosal puckering. Endometrial tissue burrowing into the muscularis propria may result in increased muscle thickness. Small bowel involvement results in crampy abdominal or pelvic pain or symptoms of intestinal obstruction.[54-57] Cyclic pain associated with menses is found in a minority (14% to 40%) of patients.[57,58]

Endometriosis may be manifested radiographically by findings similar to those found with intraperitoneal spread of malignant tumor or inflammatory diseases. Barium studies may reveal focal or multifocal areas of extrinsic mass effect on ileal loops associated with spiculation of the bowel contour and tethering of mucosal folds (Fig. 53-14).[59,60] Circumferential narrowing may be present, but mucosal folds are preserved. The radiographic or CT findings can mimic those of intraperitoneal metastases to the bowel (Fig. 53-15) or of a carcinoid tumor with intraperitoneal spread. Rarely, a solitary deposit of ileal endometriosis can mimic a primary carcinoid tumor or appendicitis secondarily involving the adjacent ileum.[60]

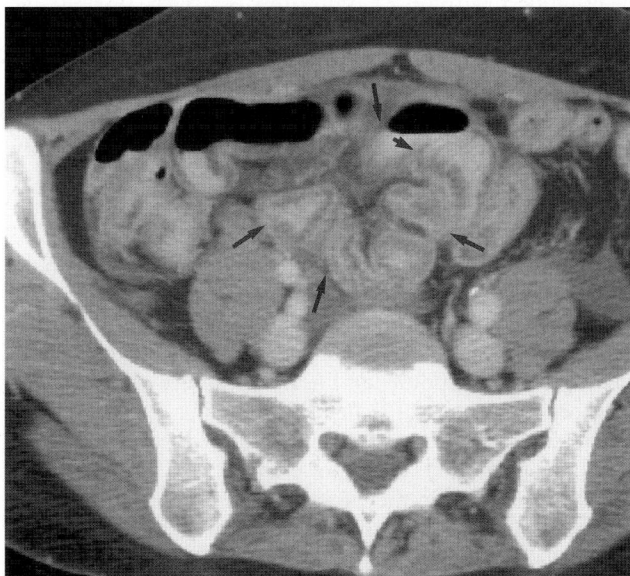

Figure 53-15. Ileal endometriosis. Axial CT through the pelvis shows ileal loops (*long arrows*) pulled toward the mesentery with associated tethering of folds (*small arrow*). The submucosa has slightly low attenuation.

PNEUMATOSIS INTESTINALIS

Pneumatosis means gas in the bowel wall. This entity is discussed in detail and illustrated in Chapters 16 and 51. This discussion will focus on pneumatosis as it pertains to the small intestine. In *pneumatosis intestinalis*, multiple gas-filled cysts are present in any layer of the small bowel wall, most frequently the subserosa,[61] but also the submucosa and even the mucosa.[1] However, pneumatosis intestinalis rarely involves the muscularis propria. The gas-filled spaces may vary from several millimeters to several centimeters. The cysts have an unorganized lining of flat cells and giant cells, often associated with a mild surrounding inflammatory infiltrate. The cysts do not communicate macroscopically with the bowel wall and are found to contain gas but not fluid. The gas in these cysts does not have the same composition as intestinal air, and it has been postulated that the gas may arise from bacterial fermentation in some cases.

Pneumatosis has traditionally been divided into two categories based on the clinical history and the appearance of the gas collections on plain abdominal radiographs. *Pneumatosis cystoides* was thought to be a relatively benign condition characterized by cystic, bubbly gas-filled blebs in the wall of the bowel due to a host of underlying causes. In contrast, *linear pneumatosis* was thought to be an ominous sign of intestinal necrosis due to ischemia and infarction of bowel. However, further review and correlation with abdominal CT has led to revision of this traditional classification of pneumatosis.[61-64]

Pneumatosis is currently thought to be a nonspecific finding associated with a wide variety of conditions. Some patients with pneumatosis have increased intraluminal pressures due to small bowel obstruction or hyperperistalsis associated with diarrheal states. In other patients, pneumatosis is probably related to bacterial invasion through rents in the mucosa.[61] This theory explains the association of pneumatosis with iatrogenic trauma caused by feeding tubes and endoscopic biopsies and by surgical trauma. Other conditions associated with pneumatosis include nonsteroidal anti-inflammatory drug-induced erosions, Crohn's disease, celiac disease, and ischemia bowel disease with or without infarction.[61-65] Bacterial invasion associated with luminal stasis may explain pneumatosis associated with motility disorders such as scleroderma and jejunal diverticulosis. Bacterial invasion is also postulated in immunocompromised patients with AIDS and bone marrow transplants[66] and in patients receiving chemotherapy, radiation therapy, or corticosteroids. The etiology of pneumatosis in patients with chronic obstructive pulmonary disease, asthma, cystic fibrosis, and barotrauma remains uncertain.

Pneumatosis is manifested on plain abdominal radiographs by round, ovoid, or linear collections of gas along the margins of the bowel wall (see Chapter 16). Intramural gas collections that have a finely mottled or linear appearance are thought to be more worrisome for ischemia bowel disease. CT is a more sensitive technique for showing these linear or cystic collections in various layers of the bowel wall.[67-70] Neither the extent of pneumatosis nor the presence of intraperitoneal gas is an accurate predictor of the severity of disease. Evaluation of bowel wall thickness, lack of bowel wall enhancement with intravenous contrast medium, vascular engorgement or fluid in the adjacent mesentery, and the presence of mesenteric or portal venous gas are much more important parameters on CT for the assessment of ischemia or infarction (see Chapter

51). Gas in the portomesenteric venous system is a particularly ominous sign on plain abdominal radiographs in patients with ischemia,[71] because abdominal radiographs can detect only large amounts of gas in the peripheral portal veins or branches of the portomesenteric venous system, findings generally indicative of nonviable bowel. Because CT can identify much smaller amounts of gas in the portal venous system, however, detection of portomesenteric venous gas by CT is not a reliable predictor of bowel viability at surgery.[72,73]

INTESTINAL EDEMA

The small bowel has a limited number of ways to react to various insults. Bowel wall edema is one component of this reaction to a wider variety of inflammatory or ischemic conditions. The current discussion focuses on bowel wall edema as the predominant component of this reaction.

Edema of the small intestine occurs primarily in the lamina propria and submucosa. This process is characterized by dilatation of mucosal and submucosal lymphatics and increased interstitial fluid. Isolated bowel wall edema is most frequently associated with diseases that cause hypoalbuminemia (with a serum albumen less than 2 g/dL).[74,75] The two most common causes of small bowel edema are cirrhosis and the nephrotic syndrome. However, any intestinal disease associated with hypoalbuminemia related to malabsorption can cause bowel wall edema. For example, patients with gluten-sensitive enteropathy and hypoalbuminemia can have diffuse fold enlargement due to small bowel edema. Any intestinal disease that causes intraluminal protein loss can also result in hypoalbuminemia, including the enteropathy associated with congestive heart failure, constrictive pericarditis, and burns; Ménétrier's disease; lymphangiectasia; and Crohn's disease.[74,76]

Several factors account for small bowel edema in patients with cirrhosis. Oncotic pressure is low as a result of hypoalbuminemia and hypovolemia. Small intestinal capillary pressure may also be elevated because of portal hypertension, congestive heart failure, and water and salt retention due to

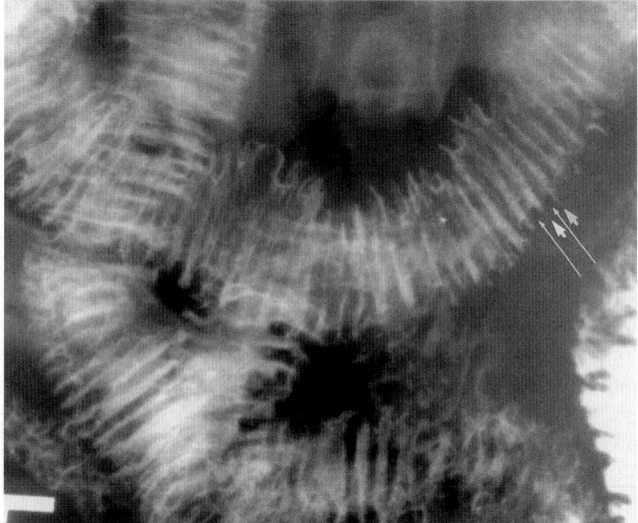

Figure 53-16. Small bowel edema in a patient with cirrhosis and hypoalbuminemia. Spot image from a small bowel follow-through shows diffusely thickened, smooth, straight folds (*long arrows*) that are perpendicular to the longitudinal axis of the bowel. Barium trapped between the folds forms the so-called interspace spikes (*short arrows*).

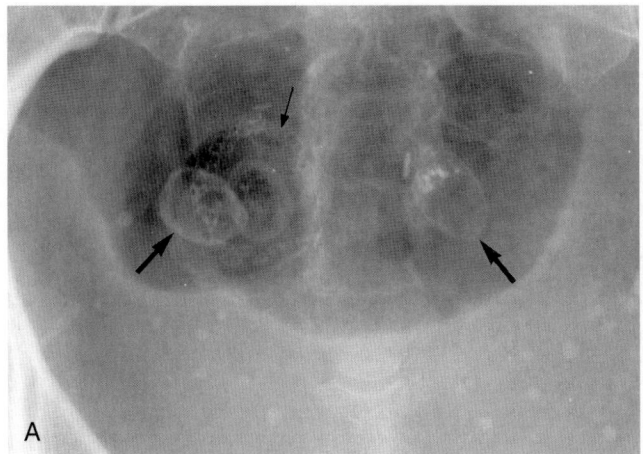

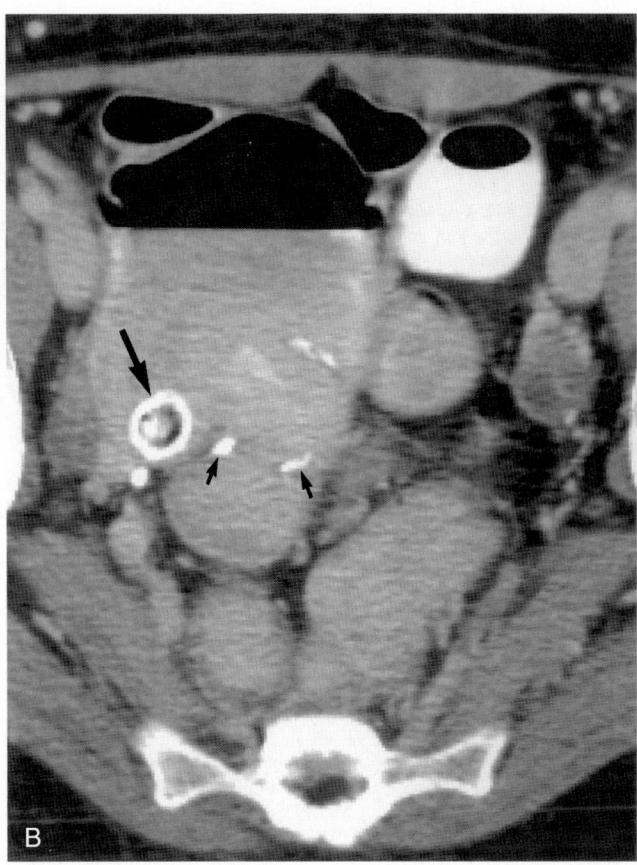

Figure 53-17. Enteroliths proximal to a stricture at the ileorectal anastomosis. A. Coned-down view from plain abdominal radiograph shows three peripherally calcified ovoid structures (*large arrows*) near an anastomotic staple line (*small arrow*). **B.** Axial CT image through the pelvis shows one of the enteroliths as a peripherally calcified structure (*large arrow*) containing central bubbles of air and soft tissue attenuation. Part of the staple line (*small arrows*) is identified.

decreased aldosterone catabolism and associated renal dysfunction.[74-76] In cirrhotics, congestive changes in the jejunum are similar to portal hypertensive gastropathy in the stomach, with an increased size and number of capillaries and venules in the lamina propria and submucosa.[1,77]

Barium studies of the small bowel in patients with hypoalbuminemia may show smooth, straight or slightly undulating, mildly thickened folds that are diffusely distributed throughout the small intestine (Fig. 53-16) although generally best visualized in the jejunum.[76] The luminal diameter of the jejunum is slightly increased.[75] CT can also show edema of the small bowel mesentery in 86% of patients. Omental and retroperitoneal edema is seen less frequently (56%).[78]

ENTEROLITHS AND BEZOARS

Bezoar derives from the Persian root *Padzahr,* meaning antidote.[79] A bezoar was a calculus found in the stomach or gallbladder of wild goats that lived in northeastern Persia. Bezoars were believed to have a variety of medicinal properties, especially as antidotes for poisoning. In humans, most bezoars are found in the stomach and are composed of indigestible organic substances such as hair (trichobezoars) or fruit (phytobezoars). Any vegetable or fruit with high fiber content can result in bezoar formation.

Bezoars and enteroliths are uncommon in the small intestine.[80] Bezoars form in areas of stasis such as jejunal diverticula, Meckel's diverticulum, and bypassed small bowel loops after surgery for Crohn's disease. Bezoars also form proximal to strictures related to Crohn's disease, tuberculosis, or other causes. Small intestinal bezoars are composed of hair, un-

digested food, or medications such as nonabsorbable antacids. In areas of the world where persimmons are eaten, most phytobezoars are related to ingestion of unripe persimmons.[81,82]

Small intestinal bezoars or enteroliths are intraluminal masses of mixed density/attenuation on CT (Fig. 53-17). These intraluminal masses may contain air, soft tissue, or calcium (see Fig. 53-17).[83,84] Peripheral or laminated calcification may be present (see Fig. 53-17). Small intestinal bezoars are typically found in the distal ileum (the narrowest portion of the small bowel) or just proximal to pathologic areas of narrowing, such as strictures, anastomoses, or tumors. Bezoars can be confused with intraluminal gallstones associated with gallstone ileus. However, no air is identified in the biliary tree in patients with bezoars.

References

1. Fenoglio-Preiser CM, Noffsinger AE, Stemmermann GN, et al: (eds): Nonneoplastic lesions of the small intestine. In Gastrointestinal Pathology, an Atlas and Text, 2nd ed. Philadelphia, Lippincott-Raven, 1999, pp 309-458.
2. Mackey WC, Dineen P: A fifty-year experience with Meckel's diverticulum. Surg Gynecol Obstet 156:56-64, 1983.
3. Levy A, Hobbs CM: Meckel diverticulum: Radiologic features with pathologic correlation. RadioGraphics 24:565-587, 2004.
4. Yamaguchi M, Takeuchi S, Awazu S: Meckel's diverticulum: Investigation of 600 patients in the Japanese literature. Am J Surg 136:247-249, 1978.
5. Maglinte DDT, Jordan LG, Van Hove ED, et al: Chronic gastrointestinal bleeding from Meckel's diverticulum: Radiologic considerations. J Clin Gastroenterol 3:47-52, 1981.
6. Leijonmarck CE, Bonman-Sandelin K, Frisell J, et al: Meckel's diverticulum in the adult. Br J Surg 73:146-149, 1986.
7. Arnold H, Pellicane JV: Meckel's diverticulum: A 10-year experience. Am Surg 63:354-355, 1997.

8. Bennet GL, Birnbaum BA, Balthazar EJ: CT of Meckel diverticulitis in 11 patients. AJR 182:625-629, 2004.

9. Perlman JA, Hoover HC, Safer PK: Femoral hernia with strangulated Meckel's diverticulum (Littre's hernia). Am J Surg 139:286-289, 1980.

10. Dixon AY, McAnaw M, McGregor DH, et al: Dual carcinoid tumors of Meckel's diverticulum presenting as metastasis in an inguinal hernia sac: Case report with literature review. Am J Gastroenterol 83:1283-1288, 1988.

11. Sfakianakis GN, Conway JJ: Detection of ectopic gastric mucosa in Meckel's diverticulum and in other aberrations by scintigraphy: Indications and methods—a 10 year experience. J Nucl Med 22:647-654 (part I), 732-738 (part II), 1981.

12. Fries M, Mortensen W, Robertson B: Technetium pertechnetate scintigraphy to detect ectopic gastric mucosa in Meckel's diverticulum. Acta Radiol Diagn 25:417-422, 1984.

13. Dixon PM, Nolan DJ: The diagnosis of Meckel's diverticulum: A continuing challenge. Clin Radiol 38:615-619, 1987.

14. Benahmou G: Small intestinal obstruction by an enterolith from a Meckel's diverticulum. Int Surg 64:43-45, 1979.

15. Pantongrag-Brown J, Levine MS, Buetow PC, et al: Meckel's enteroliths: Clinical, radiologic and pathologic findings. AJR 167:1447-1150, 1996.

16. Ekman CN: Regional enteritis associated with Meckel's diverticulum: A report of five cases. Gastroenterology 13:130-134, 1958.

17. Glick SN, Maglinte DDT, Herlinger H: Association of Meckel's diverticulum and Crohn's disease. Gastrointest Radiol 13:67-71, 1988.

18. Maglinte DDT, Elmore MF, Isenberg M, et al: Meckel diverticulum: Radiologic demonstration by enteroclysis. AJR 134:925-932, 1980.

19. Maglinte DDT, Burney BT, Miller RE: Lesions missed on small bowel follow-through: Analysis and recommendations. Radiology 144:737-739, 1982.

20. Salomonowitz E, Wittich G, Hajek P, et al: Detection of intestinal diverticula by double contrast small bowel enema: Differentiation from other intestinal diverticula. Gastrointest Radiol 8:271-278, 1983.

21. Ghahremani GG: Radiology of Meckel's diverticulum. Crit Rev Diagn Imaging 26:1-43, 1986.

22. Freeny PC, Walker JH: Inverted diverticula of the gastrointestinal tract. Gastrointest Radiol 4:57-59, 1979.

23. Rubesin SE, Herlinger H: Test your skills: Inverted Meckel's diverticulum. Radiology 176:636 and 644, 1990.

24. Hamada T, Ishida O, Yasutomi M: Inverted Meckel diverticulum with intussusception. CT findings. J Comput Assist Tomogr 19:808-810, 1995.

25. Bower RJ, Sieber WK, Kiesewetter WB: Alimentary duplications in children. Ann Surg 188:669-674, 1978.

26. Buras RR, Guzetta PC, Majd M: Multiple duplications of the small intestine. J Pediatr Surg 21:957-959, 1986.

27. Scully RE, Galldabini JJ, McNeely BV: Case records of the Massachusetts General Hospital. N Engl J Med 17:958-962, 1980.

28. Gilchrist AM, Sloan JM, Logan CJH, Mils JOM: Case report: Gastrointestinal bleeding due to multiple ileal duplications diagnosed by scintigraphy and barium studies. Clin Radiol 41:134-136, 1990.

29. Ros PR, Olmsted WW, Moser RP Jr, et al: Mesenteric and omental cysts: Histologic classification with imaging correlation. Radiology 164:327-332, 1987.

30. Kelly RB, Mahoney PD, Johnson JF: CT demonstration of an unusual enteric duplication cyst. J Comput Assist Tomogr 10:506-507, 1986.

31. Fenoglio-Preisser CM, Pascal RR, Perzin KH: Tumors of the Intestines, Atlas of Tumor Pathology, 2nd series, fascicle 27. Washington, DC, Armed Forces Institute of Pathology, 1980, pp 405-411.

32. Rubesin SE, Furth EE, Herlinger H: "Bubbly" duodenal bulb in clinically unsuspected or refractory adult celiac disease. Abdom Imaging 23:449-452, 1988.

33. Lai EC, Tompkins RK: Heterotopic pancreas: Review of a 26-year experience. Am J Surg 151:697-700, 1985.

34. Rubesin SE, Furth EE, Birnbaum BA, et al: Ectopic pancreas complicated by pancreatitis and pseudocyst formation mimicking jejunal diverticulitis. Br J Radiol 70:311-313, 1997.

35. Musselman JA, Ghahremai GG, Bordin GM, et al: Idiopathic localized dilatation of the ileum in adults. Gastrointest Radiol 6:267-268, 1981.

36. Ratcliffe J, Tait J, Lisle D, et al: Segmental dilatation of the small bowel: Report of three cases and literature review. Radiology 171:827-830, 1989.

37. Bell BR, Ternberg JL, Bower RJ: Ileal dysgenesis in infants and children. J Pediatr Surg 17:395-399, 1982.

38. Morewood DJ, Cunningham ME: Case report: Segmental dilatation of the ileum presenting with anemia. Clin Radiol 36:267-268, 1985.

39. Javors BR, Gold RP, Ghahremani GG, et al: Idiopathic localized dilatation of the ileum in adults: Findings on barium studies. AJR 164:87-90, 1994.

40. Balthazar EJ: Intestinal malrotation in adults: Roentgenographic assessment with emphasis on isolated complete and partial nonrotations. AJR 126:358-367, 1976.

41. Berardi RS: Anomalies of midgut rotation in the adult. Surg Gynecol Obstet 151:113-124, 1980.

42. Kern IB, Curie BG: The presentation of malrotation of the intestine in adults. Ann R Coll Surg Engl 72:239-242, 1990.

43. Houston CS, Wittenborg MH: Roentgen evaluation of anomalies of rotation and fixation of the bowel in children. Radiology 84:1-17, 1965.

44. Fukuya T, Brown BP, Lu CC: Midgut volvulus as a complication of intestinal malrotation in adults. Dig Dis Sci 38:438-444, 1993.

45. Meyers MA: Internal abdominal hernias. In Meyers MA (ed): Dynamic Radiology of the Abdomen, 5th ed. New York, Springer, 2000, pp 712-728.

46. Suchato C, Pekanan P, Panjapiyakul C: CT findings in symptomatic left paraduodenal hernia. Abdom Imaging 21:148-149, 1996.

47. Parsons PB: Paradudodenal hernia. AJR 69:563-589, 1953.

48. Olazabal A, Guasch I, Casas D: Case Report: CT diagnosis of nonobstructive left paraduodenal hernia. Clin Radiol 46:288-289, 1992.

49. Warshauer DM, Mauro MA: CT diagnosis of paraduodenal hernia. Gastrointest Radiol 17:13-15, 1992.

50. Aronchick CA, Brooks FP, Dyson WL, et al: Ileocecal endometriosis presenting with abdominal pain and gastrointestinal bleeding. Dig Dis Sci 28:566-572, 1983.

51. Brosens JA: Endometriosis: Current issues in diagnosis and medical management. J Reprod Med 43:281-286, 1998.

52. McAfee CH, Greer HL: Intestinal endometriosis: A report of 29 cases with a review of the literature. J Obstet Gynecol 67:539-555, 1960.

53. Martinbeau PW, Pratt JH, Gaffy TA: Small bowel obstruction secondary to endometriosis. Mayo Clin Proc 50:239-243, 1975.

54. LiVolsi VA, Perzin KH: Endometriosis of the small intestine producing intestinal obstruction or simulating neoplasm. Am J Dig Dis 19:100-107, 1974.

55. Croom RD, Donovan ML, Schweisinger WH: Intestinal endometriosis. Am J Surg 148:660-667, 1984.

56. Gindoff PR, Jewelewicz R: Ileal resection in the operative treatment of endometriosis. Obstet Gynecol 69:511-513, 1987.

57. Minocha A, Davis MS, Wright RA: Small bowel endometriosis masquerading as regional enteritis. Dig Dis Sci 39:1126-1133, 1994.

58. Badawy SZY, Freedman L, Numann P, et al: Diagnosis and management of intestinal endometriosis: A report of five cases. J Reprod Med 33:851-855, 1988.

59. Nitsch B, Ho C-S, Cullen J: Barium study of small bowel endometriosis. Gastrointest Radiol 13:361-363, 1988.

60. Scarmato V, Levine MS, Herlinger HH, et al: Ileal endometriosis: Radiographic findings in five cases. Radiology 214:509-512, 2000.

61. Feczko PJ, Mezwa DG, Farah MC, et al: Clinical significance of pneumatosis of the bowel wall. RadioGraphics 12:1069-1078, 1992.

62. Scheidler J, Stabler A, Kleber G, et al: Computed tomography in pneumatosis intestinalis: Differential diagnosis and therapeutic consequences. Abdom Imaging 20:523-528, 1995.

63. Heng Y, Schuffler MD, Haggitt RC, et al: Pneumatosis intestinalis: A review. Am J Gastroenterol 90:1747-1758, 1995.

64. Pear BL: Pneumatosis intestinalis: A review. Radiology 207:13-19, 1998.

65. Galandiuk S, Fazio VW: Pneumatosis cystoides intestinalis: A review of the literature. Dis Colon Rectum 29:358-363, 1986.

66. Navari RM, Sharma P, Deeg HJ, et al: Pneumatosis cystoides intestinalis following allogeneic marrow transplantation. Transplant Proc 15:1720-1724, 1983.

67. Kelvin FM, Korobkin M, Rauch RF, et al: Computed tomography of pneumatosis intestinalis. J Comput Assist Tomogr 8:276-280, 1984.

68. Clark RA: Computed tomography of bowel infarction. J Comput Assist Tomogr 11:757-762, 1987.

69. Perez C, Llauger L, Puig J, Palmer J: Computed tomographic findings in bowel ischemia. Gastrointest Radiol 14:241-245, 1989.

70. Smerud MJ, Johnson CD, Stephens DH: Diagnosis of bowel infarction: A comparison of plain films and CT scans in 23 cases. AJR 154:99-103, 1990.

71. Dodds WJ, Stewart ET, Goldberg HI: Pneumatosis intestinalis associated with hepatic portal venous gas. Am J Dig Dis 21:992-995, 1976.

72. Weisner W, Mortele KJK, Glickman JN, et al: Pneumatosis intestinalis and portomesenteric venous gas in intestinal ischemia: Correlation CT findings with severity of ischemia and clinical outcome. AJR 177:1319-1323, 2001.

73. Kernagis LY, Levine MS, Jacobs JE: Pneumatosis intestinalis in patients with ischemia: Correlation of CT findings with viability of the bowel. AJR 180:733-736, 2003.

74. Marshak RH, Khilnani M, Eliasoph J, Wolf BS: Intestinal edema. AJR 101:379-387, 1967.
75. Farthing MJG, Madewell JE, Bartram CI, et al: Radiologic features of the jejunum in hypoalbuminemia. AJR 136:883-886, 1981.
76. Balthazar EJ, Gade MF: Gastrointestinal edema in cirrhotics: Radiographic manifestations with emphasis on colonic involvement. Gastrointest Radiol 1:215-223, 1976.
77. Nagral AS, Joshi AS, Bhatia P, et al: Congestive jejunopathy in portal hypertension. Gut 34:694-697, 1993.
78. Chopra S, Dodd GD, Chintapalli KN, et al: Mesenteric, omental and retroperitoneal edema in cirrhosis: Frequency and spectrum of CT findings. Radiology 211:737-742, 1999.
79. Elgood C (trans): A treatise on the bezoar stone. By the late Mahmud bin Masud the imad-ul-din the physician of Ispahan. Ann Med History 7:73-80, 1935.
80. Javors BR, Bryk D: Enterolithiasis: Report of four cases. Gastrointest Radiol 8:359-362, 1983.
81. Kaplan O, Klausner JM, Lelcuk S, et al: Persimmon bezoars as a cause of intestinal obstruction: Pitfalls in their surgical management. Br J Surg 72:242-243, 1985.
82. Verstandig AG, Klin B, Bloom RA, et al: Small bowel phytobezoars: Detection with radiography. Radiology 172:705-707, 1989.
83. Ripolles T, Garcia-Aguayo J, Marinez M-J, Gil P: Gastrointestinal bezoars: Sonographic and CT characteristics 177:65-69, 2001.
84. Quirogoga S, Alvarez-Castells AA, Sebastia MC, et al: Small bowel obstruction secondary to bezoar: CT diagnosis. Abdom Imaging 22:315-317, 1997.

Small Intestine: Differential Diagnosis

Stephen E. Rubesin, MD

Complex insight into differential diagnosis requires more than the memorization of gamuts. The tables in this chapter concerning the differential diagnosis of small bowel diseases are not meant to be exhaustive. The lists of differential diagnoses presented here cannot possibly include all of the information found in the chapters on the small bowel in this textbook or in other texts. Instead, the tables present an approach for classifying the most common causes of various radiographic abnormalities in the small bowel in relation to the size, location, distribution, and radiographic characteristics of these abnormalities. A list of references is included for further reading.[1-50]

Table 54-1
Normal Small Bowel Parameters

	Jejunum	Ileum
Normal Parameters for Enteroclysis		
Folds per inch length	4-7	2-4
Thickness of folds	1-2 mm	1.0-1.5 mm
Diameter of lumen	up to 4 cm	up to 3 cm
Wall thickness	1.0-1.5 mm	1.0-1.5 mm
Normal Parameters for Small Bowel Follow-Through		
Thickness of folds	2-3 mm	1-2 mm
Diameter of lumen	up to 3 cm	up to 2 cm

Data from references 1 and 2.

Table 54-2
Small Bowel Lumen Dilated, Normal Fold Thickness

	Cause	Comments
Diffuse Small Bowel Dilatation	Mechanical obstruction, small bowel or colon	Air-fluid levels on abdominal radiographs (CT if high grade, ultrasound if CT unavailable); barium studies for partial or intermittent obstruction
		Common causes: adhesions, hernias, metastases, radiation enteropathy, colonic carcinoma with back-up into dilated small bowel
	Adynamic ileus	Air-fluid levels, but aperistaltic; CT shows absence of obstruction
		Common causes: postoperative, medications, ischemia, vagotomy
		Less common causes: systemic sclerosis (dilated duodenum, hidebound small bowel), amyloidosis, peritonitis, electrolyte imbalances (hypokalemia, uremia), blunt trauma, diabetes, hypothyroidism
Focal Small Bowel Dilatation	Proximal obstruction	Fluid levels in few small bowel loops in upper abdomen: primary adenocarcinoma, postoperative strictures, adhesions
	Focal adynamic ileus	Pancreatitis, postoperative manipulation or leak, pelvic irradiation
	Closed-loop obstruction	Group of air-fluid levels unchanging in position
		CT for possible strangulation
	Internal hernia	Focal region of dilated loops with air-fluid levels
		CT and barium for diagnosis
	Celiac disease	Jejunal dilatation; history can be atypical
		Enteroclysis: wide separation of jejunal folds

Data from references 1 to 6.

SMALL BOWEL FOLDS AND MUCOSAL CHANGES

Small bowel villi are formed by a single-cell epithelial surface covering a lamina propria filled with fat, vessels, inflammatory cells, and a central lacteal. Fine nodularity of the mucosal surface (also termed *micronodularity* or a *sandlike pattern*) therefore reflects enlargement of villi, usually by an abnormality in the lamina propria, such as edema, inflammation, or infiltration by amyloid or other substances. Small bowel folds are composed of mucosa and submucosa. Enlarged or effaced small bowel folds therefore reflect edema, hemorrhage, inflammation, or infiltration of the lamina propria and submucosa.

A large variety of diseases cause abnormal villi and abnormal small bowel folds. Tables 54-3 through 54-7 are only a guide to stratify these diseases by their location in the small bowel and whether the folds are smoothly enlarged or are enlarged and nodular. Many diseases have both abnormal villi and enlarged folds, because the pathologic process involves both the lamina propria and submucosa. Smooth fold thickening usually implies edema related to hypoalbuminemia or edema/hemorrhage related to vascular causes. Nodular fold thickening implies inflammation or infiltration by tumor, amyloid, or other substances. In reality, it is often difficult to distinguish smooth fold enlargement from mildly nodular folds. The radiographic findings of diseases associated with edema or hemorrhage can therefore overlap with those of inflammatory/infiltrative diseases.

Table 54-3
Smooth, Straight, Thickened Folds

	Cause	Comments
Diffusely Distributed	Edema	Hypoalbuminemia: cirrhosis, nephrotic syndrome
		Protein-losing enteropathy
		Congestive heart failure
		Portal hypertension
	Eosinophilic enteritis	Mucosal type with fold thickening extensive or multisegmental
		Antral nodularity
		Asthma, peripheral eosinophilia in 50%
Focal Smooth Fold Thickening	Intramural hemorrhage	Segmental stack of coins appearance; interspace spikes; thumbprinting on mesenteric border
	Ischemia	
	Anticoagulants	Most patients return to normal within 2 to 3 weeks
	Coagulopathies	
	Superior mesenteric vein thrombosis	
	Vasculitides	Ischemic changes, hemorrhage, ulceration/necrosis with small vessel disease (lupus, Henoch-Schönlein purpura)
	Blunt trauma	CT: look for possible perforation—mesenteric haziness/fluid, thickened bowel wall, lack of bowel contrast enhancement, focal pneumatosis, free air
	Radiation enteropathy	Clinical history
		Thickened folds, narrow interfold spaces (interspace spikes); barium changes resemble picket fence
		Changes confined to radiation portal

Data from references 1, 7 to 12, and 49.

Table 54-4
Micronodularity* (1- to 2-mm Mucosal Nodules)

Cause	Comments
Whipple's disease	White males with arthralgias, cardiovascular and neurologic symptoms
	CT: low-attenuation mesenteric lymph node mass
Mycobacterium avium-intracellulare (MAI) complex enteritis	AIDS
	MAI-laden macrophages in lamina propria
	CT shows necrosis in enlarged lymph nodes
Abetalipoproteinemia	Adolescent with retinitis pigmentosa, acanthocytosis, spinocerebellar degeneration
	Retained fat globules in villous enterocytes
Histoplasmosis	*Histoplasma*-laden macrophages in lamina propria
Lymphangiectasia	Villi enlarged by dilated lacteals in primary form
	Edema in submucosa
	Mesenteric adenopathy causes secondary form
Macroglobulinemia	IgM macroglobulin in lamina propria
	Lymphoma may occur
Radiation therapy	Associated with smooth, thickened, straight folds
Crohn's disease	Distal/terminal ileum
	Aphthoid ulcers/mesenteric border ulcers; cobblestoning; strictures, fissures, fistulas

*Micronodularity implies villous enlargement due to infiltrative process in lamina propria. This table lists diseases that often involve the mucosa and submucosa and also produce abnormal folds.
Data from references 1 to 11 and 13 to 18.

Table 54-5
Irregular Fold Thickening, Diffuse

Cause	Comments
Lymphangiectasia, primary	Submucosal edema plus micronodularity
	Congenital hypoplasia of lymphatics
Lymphangiectasia, secondary	Small bowel changes as above
	Obstruction of lymph drainage by retroperitoneal fibrosis, radiation, mesenteric lymphadenopathy (Whipple's, lymphoma)
Amyloidosis, AA and AL	Fold thickening if deposits in vessels cause ischemia.
	Micronodularity in secondary amyloidosis reflects amyloid deposits in lamina propria
	Four- to 10-mm nodules in submucosa (AL)
Mastocytosis	Histamine release-associated headaches, flushing, diarrhea; urticaria pigmentosa (50%), bone lesions (20%)
	Stomach/duodenum: ulcers
	Small bowel: multiple urticaria-like nodules
	Thickened folds are often segmental
Immunoproliferative small intestinal disease (IPSID)	Relates to multiple parasitic/bacterial infections
	Patient from Mediterranean region
	Extensive lymphoid hyperplasia
	Responds to treatment
Mediterranean lymphoma	Young patient with progression of IPSID to monoclonal lymphomatous infiltrate
	Lymphoid nodules enlarged, nonuniform, confluent
	Lymph node masses
	Associated with α heavy-chain disease
AIDS	Large variety of infections cause diffuse thickened folds.
Graft-versus-host disease	Often with CMV infection (see Table 54-8)

Data from references 1 and 17 to 20.

Table 54-6
Irregular Fold Thickening, Proximal Small Bowel

Cause	Comments
T-cell lymphoma complicating celiac disease	Diarrhea recurs despite gluten-free diet
	Nodular fold thickening in long segments
	May have annular lesions
Ulcerative jejunoileitis	Complicates celiac disease
	Before inflammatory infiltrate changes to monoclonal lymphoma
	Radiographically indistinguishable from T-cell lymphoma
Tropical sprue	History of sojourn in tropics
	Unlike celiac disease, folds are thickened and separation of jejunal folds does not occur
Zollinger-Ellison syndrome	Gastric and duodenal ulcers
	Increased intraluminal fluid
Strongyloidiasis	Effaced folds, tubular bowel contour with severe disease
AIDS-related infections	MAI, isosporiasis, cryptosporidiosis
Gastrojejunostomy	Thick folds in efferent loop just distal to gastrojejunal anastomosis

Data from references 1, 2, 5, and 21.

Table 54-7
Irregular Fold Thickening, Distal Ileum

	Cause	Comments
With Minimal Luminal Narrowing	Crohn's disease, early	Coarse villous pattern, aphthous ulcers
		Uncommon pattern if no associated colonic disease
		Not an unusual pattern in neoterminal ileum
	Yersinia enterocolitis	Early: thickened, nodular folds, ulcers
		5-8 weeks: lymphoid hyperplasia
		8-12 weeks: normal terminal ileum
	Salmonellosis, campylobacteriosis	Similar to *Yersinia* but more ulceration
	Mantle cell lymphoma	Part of systemic disease
		Multiple nodules, mesenteric masses
		Prognosis poor
	Cecal carcinoma	Cecal mass associated with retrograde extension of tumor via lymphatics into terminal ileum
		Thickened, nodular folds
		Only superficial resemblance to Crohn's disease
With Moderate to Marked Luminal Narrowing	Crohn's disease	Narrowing may change in diameter if due to spasm, edema, or inflammation rather than fibrosis
		Mild: mesenteric border ulceration and antimesenteric sacculation
		Moderate: transmural extension with luminal narrowing and ulceronodular pattern
		Severe: strictures, fissures, fistulas
		CT best to determine presence of mesenteric abscesses
	Tuberculosis	Patient from endemic area or immunodeficient
		More pronounced in cecum/right colon
		Ulcers, transverse folds, patulous ileocecal valve, retracted cecum
		May be indistinguishable from Crohn's disease
	Behçet's disease	Associated with uveitis, genital ulcers, arthritis
		Penetrating ulcers, especially in colon
	AIDS-related infections	Cytomegalovirus, actinomycosis

Data from references 1 and 22 to 27.

Table 54-8
Tubular Bowel with Luminal Narrowing

Cause	Comments
Graft-versus-host disease	Often complicated by cytomegalovirus infection
	Diffuse small bowel involvement
	"Toothpaste" appearance is a function of rapid transit
	Prolonged adherence of barium
Chronic ischemic changes	Radiation or amyloidosis
	Involved bowel hypoperistaltic or aperistaltic
Burnt-out Crohn's disease	Distal ileum
	Active disease may be present nearby
Strongyloidiasis	Jejunum
	Severe disease, but reversible

Data from references 1, 8, 12, 19, 20, 27, and 28.

Table 54-9
Tubular Bowel Without Luminal Narrowing

Cause	Comments
Primary lymphoma	Segmental infiltrate effaces fold pattern
	Five to 15 cm in length.
Celiac disease, long standing	Near absence of folds in proximal jejunum
	Associated with a mosaic pattern

Data from references 1, 2, 3, 5, and 21.

Table 54-10
Solitary Polyp

Cause	Comments
Carcinoid, early	80% of carcinoid tumors in distal ileum
	Polyp in ileum: exclude carcinoid
	30% multiple
	Early form of tumor (0.5-2.0 cm) before invasion and desmoplastic effect
Lipoma	Elongated lesions with pseudopedicle
	May ulcerate; change in shape
	CT: fat attenuation
Adenoma	85% of adenomas in duodenum
	10% of adenomas in jejunum
Brunner gland polyp	First or second portions of duodenum
Hemangioma	Sessile polyp or carpet lesion
	May contain phleboliths
Gastrointestinal stromal tumor	Sessile polyp or target lesion
	Cavitary mass when large
Neurofibroma	Association with neurofibromatosis
Gangliocytic paraganglionoma	Near papilla of Vater
Inverted Meckel's diverticulum	Elongated intraluminal "polyp" in distal ileum
	Associated with intussusception
Inflammatory fibroid polyp	Usually in ileum
	Elongated polyp composed of granulation tissue with eosinophils

Data from references 1 and 29 to 35.

Table 54-11
Multiple Polyps and Polyposis Syndromes

	Cause	Comments
Multiple Polyps	Hematogenous metastases	Most commonly metastatic melanoma
		Submucosal mass
	Kaposi's sarcoma	Known AIDS
		Plaque, submucosal mass, or target lesion
	Carcinoid tumor	Multiple in 30% (see Table 54-10)
	Disseminated lymphoma	Multiple submucosal masses or target lesions
	Mantle cell lymphoma	Lymphomatous polyposis
	Multiple myeloma	Rare
Polyposis Syndromes	Peutz-Jeghers syndrome	Autosomal dominant, but 40% are spontaneous mutations
		Sessile or pedunculated polyp with lobulated or villous surface
		Jejunum
		Young patients with bleeding or pain; pigmented lesions on mouth, lips, palms
	Cowden's disease	Autosomal dominant
		Polyps of varying histologies but hamartomatous polyps more often in colon than in small bowel
		Facial papillomas
		Associated thyroid disease (66%) and breast carcinoma (33%-50%)
	Cronkhite-Canada syndrome	Nonhereditary; mean age of 60 years
		Diarrhea, ectodermal changes, protein loss
		Inflammatory polyps more frequent in stomach and in colon than in duodenum or small bowel
	Familial adenomatous polyposis syndrome	Autosomal dominant; 10%-30% are spontaneous mutations
		Mutations in various portions of *APC* gene produce the various clinical syndromes (e.g., Gardner's, Turcot's)
		Small bowel adenomas primarily in duodenum
		12% develop periampullary carcinomas
		Desmoid tumors in root of small bowel mesentery
	Neurofibromatosis	Known clinical diagnosis

Data from references 1 and 36.

Table 54-12
Multiple Target Lesions

Cause	Comments
Melanoma metastases	Hematogenous spread
	Submucosal lesions, often on antimesenteric border
	Large ulcer with "spokewheel" radiating folds
Other hematogenous metastases	Breast and lung cancer
Lymphoma, disseminated	Involves stomach more frequently than small bowel
Kaposi's sarcoma	Involves stomach and duodenum more frequently than small bowel
	Plaquelike lesion or thickened folds more common morphologic forms
	Homosexuals with AIDS

Data from references 1, 11, and 15.

Table 54-13
Annular Lesion with Shelflike Margins

Cause	Comments
Small bowel obstruction by adhesive band	Transition zone with sharply demarcated band compressing against distended proximal and collapsed distal small bowel
	Shelflike or beaklike narrowing
	Adjacent folds are normal; no mucosal nodularity
Adenocarcinoma, primary	Proximal jejunum
	Short lesion with shouldering
	Central ulceration; folds destroyed or nodular
	Obstruction not severe, unless late diagnosis
Metastases	Colon cancer most frequent primary tumor
	Mid to distal small bowel
	Desmoplasia with angulation causing obstruction
	Folds relatively preserved but may be tethered
Primary small bowel lymphoma	Long lesion without obstruction
	Nodular folds and effaced mucosa
	Center bulges aneurysmally
	Multiple in up to 25% of patients
Carcinoid	Misleading en face appearance of "saddle" lesion (polypoid lesion spreading circumferentially)
Anastomotic stricture	Clinical history; staple line
NSAID stricture	Multiple, ringlike thickened webs causing low-grade obstruction

Data from references 1, 11, 21, 32, and 37-43.

Table 54-14
Annular Lesion with Tapered Edges

Cause	Comments
Adhesion	Beaklike tapering with smooth folds
Crohn's disease	Stricture due to primary disease or skip lesion
	Associated cobblestoning or mesenteric border ulcers
Radiation enteropathy	Strictures within area of severe damage or at entry site into radiation field
	Bowel loops often angulated; folds tethered due to serositis/fibrosis
Ischemia	Usually low-grade obstruction
	May be related to trauma

Data from references 1, 12, 26, and 27.

Table 54-15
Exoenteric Cavitary Lesions

	Comments
Common Causes	
Primary non-Hodgkin's lymphoma	Transmural ulceration with perforation into mesentery or cavitation of tumor that has invaded mesentery
Metastatic melanoma	Large, deeply ulcerated metastases
Malignant gastrointestinal stromal tumor	Cavity due to central necrosis in tumor that subsequently communicates with bowel lumen or to ischemic necrosis of epithelium overlying tumor with secondary ulceration
Uncommon Causes	
Adenocarcinoma	Deeply ulcerated tumor perforates
Jejunal diverticulitis with abscess cavity	
Ectopic pancreas with pancreatitis and pseudocyst formation	
Hematogenous metastasis from pulmonary carcinoma	
Crohn's disease	Fistula or perforation forms abscess cavity
	Other findings of Crohn's disease

Data from references 1, 11, 21, 41, and 45 to 47.

Table 54-16
Separation of Bowel Loops without Tethering

Cause	Comments
Prominent fat within small bowel mesentery	Most common of cause of separated loops
	More pronounced in ileum
	Loops retain normal pliability and mobility
Ascites	Small bowel loops centrally located
	CT for etiology
Mesenteric masses	Lymphoma of mesenteric nodal origin: enlarges and displaces bowel; may surround it without obstruction (sandwich sign); later infiltrates intestinal wall causing obstruction
	Desmoid tumor related to familial adenomatous polyposis syndrome
Crohn's disease	CT for diagnosis:
	Fibrovascular extension of Crohn's disease causing prominent mesenteric fat
	Abscess

Data from references 1, 21, and 36.

Table 54-17
Mass Effect with Tethering of Mucosal Folds

Causes	Comments
Intraperitoneal metastases	Right lower quadrant, pelvis
	Multiple hemispheric masses on mesenteric border of distal ileum with crowded, tethered folds
Carcinoid tumor, early	Hemispheric sessile polyp with adjacent desmoplastic crowding of folds
	Multiple in 30%
Carcinoid tumor, advanced	Intense desmoplastic effect on adjacent bowel loops
	Mesenteric metastases grow larger than primary tumor
	CT: central mesenteric mass (calcified in 50%), mesenteric stranding
	Associated with ascites, small bowel ischemia
Interloop or omental abscess	Extrinsic mass with mildly edematous folds radiating toward abscess
Retractile mesenteritis	Intestinal loops separated and pulled toward mesentery
	CT shows soft tissue mesenteric masses
Endometriosis	Sharply demarcated plaques invade serosa causing pleating of underlying mucosa
	Infrequent in terminal ileum; more often involves rectosigmoid colon
Pancreatitis	Desmoplastic changes in left upper quadrant: jejunum and splenic flexure
Root of mesentery nodal metastasis	At or left of duodenojejunal junction: left-sided colon cancer, transitional cell carcinoma of bladder
	Near second portion or duodenum: right-sided colon cancer
Cecal/appendiceal process involving terminal ileum	Cecal lymphoma, carcinoma
	Appendicitis
	Appendiceal tumors
Crohn's disease	Abscess/inflammatory process in mesentery
	Other findings of Crohn's disease

Data from references 1, 32, 46, and 47.

Table 54-18
Site Predilection of Diseases

Proximal Jejunum
Adenocarcinoma
Jejunal diverticulosis
Infections: giardiasis, Whipple's disease, cryptosporidiosis, isosporiasis
Celiac disease
Zollinger-Ellison related pathology
Polyps in Peutz-Jeghers syndrome

Distal Ileum
Crohn's disease
Carcinoid tumors
Ileitis caused by *Yersinia, Campylobacter*, cytomegalovirus, Behçet's disease
Intraperitoneal metastases
Secondary involvement by inflammatory or neoplastic disease of cecum or appendix
Radiation enteropathy
Tuberculosis (right-sided colonic predominance)

Antimesenteric Border
Meckel's diverticulum
Hematogenous metastases
Sacculation in Crohn's disease

Mesenteric Border
Linear ulcers in Crohn's disease
Peritoneally seeded metastases
Jejunal diverticula
Thumbprinting due to intramural bleeding
Mesenteric hematoma
Intestinal duplication
Cavitation in primary intestinal lymphoma

Data from references 1 to 6, 10, 12, 13, 15, 21, 24 to 27, 36, 38, and 46 to 49.

Table 54-19
Association with Gastroduodenal Changes

Disease	Comments
Crohn's disease	Aphthoid ulcers in stomach Proximal duodenal ulceration/cobblestoning/strictures Gastrocolic fistula via gastrocolic ligament or duodenocolic fistula via transverse mesocolon
Zollinger-Ellison syndrome	Peptic ulcers more frequent in stomach and duodenum than in jejunum High acid output causes fold edema/ulceration
Eosinophilic enteritis	Patchy elevations in gastric antrum
Systemic mastocytosis	Histamine-related peptic ulceration Nodules in duodenum and jejunum
Cystic fibrosis in adult	Irregular fold thickening in duodenum and ileum Irregular meshlike pattern in small bowel Changes reflect adherent mucus

Data from references 1, 9, 25, 48, and 49.

References

1. Herlinger H, Maglinte DDT, Birnbaum BB: Clinical Radiology of the Small Intestine. New York, Springer-Verlag, 1999.
2. Herlinger H, Maglinte DDT: Jejunal fold separation in adult celiac disease: Relevance of enteroclysis. Radiology 158:605-611, 1986.
3. Rubesin SE, Rubin RA, Herlinger H: Small bowel malabsorption: Clinical and radiologic perspectives. How we see it. Radiology 184:297-305, 1992.
4. Horowitz AL, Meyers MA: The "hide-bound" small bowel of scleroderma: Characteristic mucosal fold pattern. AJR 119:332-334, 1973.
5. Rubesin SE, Grumbach K, Herlinger H, et al: Adult celiac disease and its complications. RadioGraphics 9:1045-1066, 1989.
6. Bova JG, Friedman AC, Weser E, et al: Adaptation of the ileum in nontropical sprue: Reversal of the jejunal fold pattern. AJR 144:299-302, 1985.
7. Marshak RH, Ruoff M, Lindner AE: Roentgen manifestations of giardiasis. AJR 104:557-560, 1968.
8. Dallemand S, Waxman M, Farman J: Radiologic manifestations of *Strongyloides stercoralis*. Gastrointest Radiol 8:45-51, 1983.
9. Schulman A, Morton PCG, Dietrich BE: Eosinophilic gastroenteritis. Clin Radiol 31:101-104, 1980.
10. Khilnani MT, Marshak RH, Eliasoph J, et al: Intramural intestinal hemorrhage. AJR 92:1061-1071, 1964.
11. Rubesin SE, Laufer I: Pictorial glossary of double contrast radiology. In Gore RM, Levine MS (eds): Textbook of Gastrointestinal Radiology. Philadelphia, WB Saunders, 2000, pp 44-66.
12. Mendelson RM, Nolan DJ: The radiological features of radiation enteritis. Clin Radiol 36:141-148, 1985.
13. Philips RL, Carlson HC: The roentgenographic and clinical findings in Whipple's disease: A review of 8 patients. AJR 123:268-273, 1975.
14. Vincent ME, Robbins AH: *Mycobacterium avium-intracellulare* complex enteritis: Pseudo-Whipple's disease in AIDS. AJR 144:921-922, 1985.
15. Berk RN, Wall SD, McArdle CT, et al: Cryptosporidiosis of the stomach and small intestine in patients with AIDS. AJR 143:549-554, 1984.
16. Jones B, Hamilton SR, Rubesin SE, et al: Granular small bowel mucosa: A reflection of villous abnormality. Gastrointest Radiol 12:319-225, 1987.
17. Olmsted WW, Madewell JE: Lymphangiectasia of the small intestine. Gastrointest Radiol 1:241-243, 1976.
18. Kingham JGC, Moriarty KJ, Furness M, et al: Lymphangiectasia of the colon and small intestine. Br J Radiol 55:774-777, 1982.
19. Legge DA, Carlson HC, Wollaeger EE: Roentgenologic appearance of systemic amyloidosis involving the gastrointestinal tract. AJR 110:/'406-410, 1970.
20. Tada S, Iida M, Matsui T, et al: Amyloidosis of the small intestine: Findings on double contrast radiographs. AJR 156:741-744, 1991.
21. Rubesin SE, Gilchrist AM, Bronner M, et al: Non-Hodgkin lymphoma of the small intestine. RadioGraphics 10:985-998, 1990.
22. Glick SN, Teplick SK: Crohn's disease of the small intestine: Diffuse mucosal granularity. Radiology 154:313-317, 1985.
23. Ekberg O, Lindstom C: Superficial lesions in Crohn's disease of the small bowel. Gastrointest Radiol 4:389-393, 1979.
24. Ekberg O, Sjostrom B, Brahme F: Radiological findings in *Yersinia* ileitis. Radiology 123:15-19, 1977.
25. Goldberg HI, Caruthers SB, Nelson JA, et al: Radiographic findings of the National Cooperative Crohn's disease study. Gastroenterology 77:925-937, 1979.
26. Herlinger H, Rubesin SE, Furth EE: Mesenteric border ulcers in Crohn's disease: Historical, radiologic and pathologic perspectives. Abdom Imaging 23:122-126, 1998.
27. Rubesin SE, Bronner M: Radiologic-pathologic concepts in Crohn's disease. Adv Gastrointest Radiol 1:27-55, 1991.
28. Jones B, Kramer S, Saral R, et al: Gastrointestinal inflammation after bone marrow transplantation: Graft-versus-host disease or opportunistic infection? AJR 150:277-281, 1988.
29. Fenoglio-Preiser CM, Pascal RR, Perzin KH: Tumors of the intestines. Atlas of Tumor Pathology, second series, fascicle 27. Washington, DC, Armed Forces Institute of Pathology, 1990.
30. Hoffman JW, Fox PS, Wilson SD: Duodenal wall tumors and the Zollinger-Ellison syndrome. Arch Surg 107:334-339, 1973.
31. Perzin KH, Bridge MF: Adenomas of the small intestine: A clinicopathologic review of 51 cases and a study of their relationship to carcinoma. Cancer 48:799-819, 1981.
32. Moertel CG, Saver WG, Dockerty MB, et al: Life history of the carcinoid tumor of the small intestine. Cancer 14:901-912, 1961.
33. Hansen PS: Hemangioma of the small intestine with special reference to intussusception: Review of the literature and report of 3 new cases. Am J Clin Pathol 18:414-42, 1948.
34. Shimer GR, Helwig EB: Inflammatory fibroid polyps of the intestine. Am J Clin Pathol 81:708-714, 1984.
35. Lee SM, Mosental WT, Weissman RE: Tumorous heterotopic gastric mucosa in the small intestine. Arch Surg 100:619-622, 1970.

36. Franzin G, Zamboni G, Scarpa A: Polyposis syndromes. In Whitehead R (ed): Gastrointestinal and Oesophageal Pathology. Edinburgh, Churchill Livingstone, 1995, pp 892-905.

37. Collier PE, Turowski P, Diamond DL: Small intestinal adenocarcinoma complicating regional enteritis. Cancer 55:516-521, 1985.

38. Bridge MF, Perzin KH: Primary adenocarcinoma of the jejunum and ileum: A clinicopathologic study. Cancer 36:1876-1887, 1975.

39. Levine MS, Drooz AT, Herlinger H: Annular malignancies of the small bowel. Gastrointest Radiol 12:53-58, 1987.

40. Issacson P: B cell lymphomas of the gastrointestinal tract: Am J Surg Pathol 9:117-128, 1985.

41. Ranchod M, Kempson RL: Smooth muscle tumors of the gastrointestinal tract and retroperitoneum. Cancer 39:255-262, 1977.

42. Wilson IH, Cooley NV, Luibel FJ: Nonspecific stenosing small bowel ulcers. Am J Gastroenterol 50:449-455, 1968.

43. Lang J, Price AB, Levi AJ, et al: Diaphragm disease: Pathology of disease of the small intestine induced by non-steroidal anti-inflammatory drugs. J Clin Pathol 41:516-526, 1988.

44. Greenstein S, Jones B, Fishman EK, et al: Small bowel diverticulitis: CT findings. AJR 147:271-274, 1986.

45. Rubesin SE, Furth EE, Birnbaum BA, et al: Ectopic pancreas complicated by pancreatitis and pseudocyst formation mimicking jejunal diverticulitis. Br J Radiol 70:311-313, 1997.

46. Meyers MM: Clinical involvement of mesenteric and antimesenteric borders of small bowel loops. Gastrointest Radiol 1:41-47, 1976.

47. Meyers MM: Clinical involvement of mesenteric and antimesenteric borders of small bowel loops: II. Radiologic interpretation of pathologic alterations. Gastrointest Radiol 1:49-58, 1976.

48. Vaidya MG, Sodhi JS: Gastrointestinal tract tuberculosis: A study of 102 cases including 55 hemicolectomies. Clin Radiol 29:189-195, 1978.

49. Rubesin SE, Furth EE: Differential diagnosis of small intestinal abnormalities with radiologic-pathologic explanation. In Herlinger H, Maglinte DDT, Birnbaum BA (eds): Clinical Imaging of the Small Intestine, 2nd ed. New York, Springer, 1999, pp 527-566.

50. Rubesin SE: The simplified approach to differential diagnosis of small bowel abnormalities. Radiol Clin North Am 41:343-364, 2003.

Colon

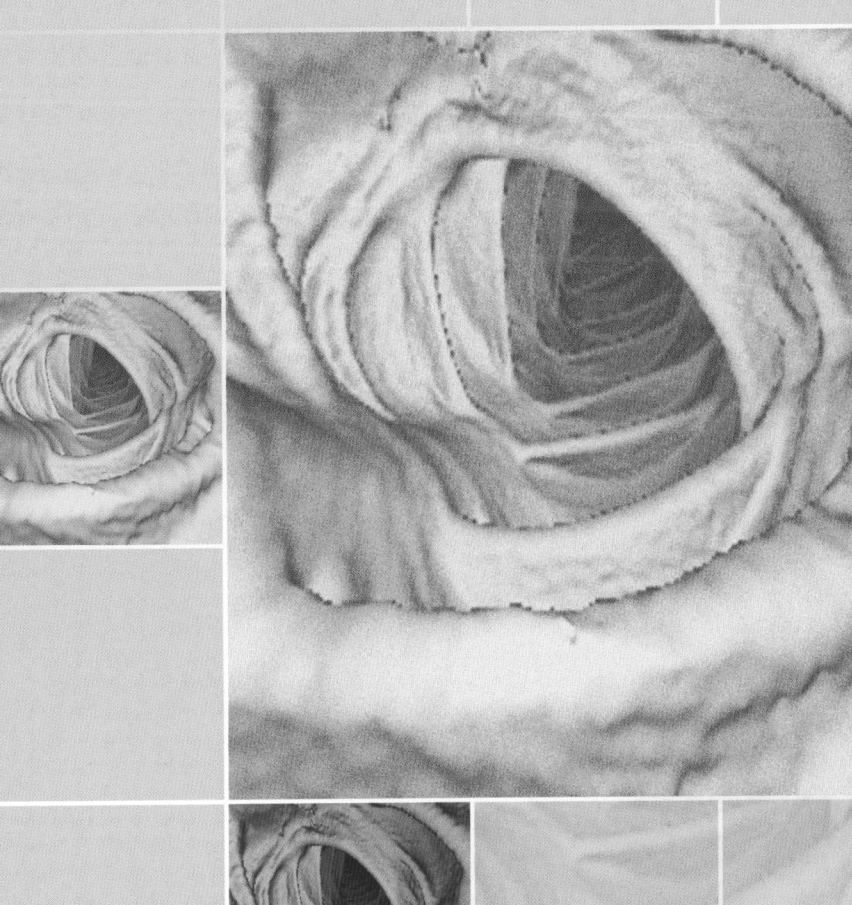

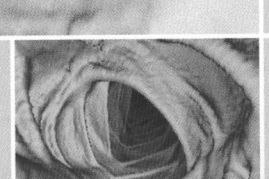

Barium Studies of the Colon

Igor Laufer, MD • Marc S. Levine, MD

Barium examination of the colon is designed primarily for the detection of mucosal lesions. In this regard, it competes directly with colonoscopy. Although colonoscopy has an advantage in the ability to detect changes in color and the ability to obtain biopsy specimens, a properly performed barium study should be fully competitive in the detection of gross as well as subtle colonic lesions.

Barium studies are also suitable for the detection of intramural lesions in the colon. For this purpose, the barium examination is clearly superior to endoscopy. Cross-sectional imaging studies such as CT, MRI, and endoscopic ultrasonography can then be performed for further evaluation of the lesion's morphology.

Extrinsic lesions affecting the colon can also be clearly demonstrated on barium studies. However, the extramural component of the lesion is much better demonstrated by CT, MRI, or endoscopic ultrasonography.

SINGLE- VERSUS DOUBLE-CONTRAST TECHNIQUE

It is generally agreed that double-contrast technique is superior to single-contrast technique for the detection of small polypoid lesions and the early changes of inflammatory bowel disease. Double-contrast technique is also acknowledged to be superior for examination of the rectum. In addition, there are specific signs (e.g., mucosal spiculation in endometriosis

or metastatic disease) that are much more clearly demonstrated on double-contrast studies (see Chapter 5).

Single-contrast technique is preferred for particular indications, including mechanical problems (e.g., obstruction or fistulas) and in cases in which control of the barium column is required, as in suspected diverticulitis or intussusception. In cases of suspected ischemic colitis, single-contrast technique is also preferred because double-contrast studies may efface the thumbprinting that is characteristic of ischemia.[1] The details for performing and interpreting single-contrast barium studies are discussed in Chapter 3. The remainder of this chapter deals more specifically with the double-contrast barium enema.

DOUBLE-CONTRAST BARIUM ENEMA

Preparation of the Patient

Although a variety of preparation regimens are used,[2] most entail the following basic components:
- A clear liquid diet is followed for 24 hours.
- One or preferably two sets of laxatives are taken on the afternoon and evening before the examination.
- A suppository is taken on the morning of the examination.

This basic preparation is effective in most patients when it is followed, but noncompliance with the prescribed preparation is often a problem. Patients should be asked when they arrive in the department whether they have taken the preparation and whether it has been effective in producing clear, watery bowel movements. If there is any doubt about the adequacy of the preparation, a preliminary abdominal radiograph should be obtained. If this radiograph shows indisputable evidence of fecal residue in the colon, the examination is rescheduled after an additional 24 hours of preparation.

Cleansing enemas improve the cleanliness of the colon but are difficult to perform on outpatients from a logistic viewpoint. These enemas also tend to result in significant residual fluid within the colon, which deteriorates the quality of mucosal coating. The same may be said of oral lavage regimens using solutions such as GoLYTELY.[3]

Materials

The choice of barium suspension is critical. We prefer a suspension of medium viscosity at approximately 100% w/v (liquid Polibar, E-Z-EM Company, Westbury, NY). The barium suspension must coat the mucosal surface well and for a prolonged period, so that artifacts do not develop as the examination proceeds.

The Miller air enema tip is ideal for double-contrast studies because it allows for barium infusion and air insufflation via the enema tip.[4] Although a retention balloon is attached to the end of the tip, it is not routinely inflated. Instead, the balloon is inflated only if the patient is unable to retain the barium or air. When required, the retention balloon should be inflated under direct fluoroscopic control with no more than 100 mL of air. The balloon need not fill the lumen of the rectum. It should be retracted distally against the anal verge to act as a plug and minimize leakage of barium around the balloon. A hypotonic agent such as glucagon (1 mg) should be administered intravenously on a routine basis to improve the quality of the examination and decrease patient discomfort.

As with double-contrast upper gastrointestinal studies, radiographs are exposed on a 400 speed system at 105 kV(p).

Table 55-1
Routine Double-Contrast Enema

Position	Views
Spot Radiographs	
Prone	Rectum
Left posterior oblique	Sigmoid colon
Left lateral	Rectum
Supine	Cecum
Upright	Hepatic and splenic flexures
Supine	All remaining colonic segments
Overhead Radiographs	
Vertical beam	Posteroanterior
Angled (prone)	Rectosigmoid
Horizontal beam	Left and right lateral decubitus views; cross-table lateral view of rectum

We rely primarily on fluoroscopy and spot images for diagnostic purposes, but these are supplemented by a series of routine overhead radiographs, as outlined in Table 55-1. The overheads include a series of horizontal beam radiographs that are particularly valuable in patients whose preparation is less than perfect (Fig. 55-1). The quality of these radiographs can be improved by the use of a wedge filter, which evens out the density over the entire image.[5] Fluoroscopy and radiography can now be performed more easily using digital fluoroscopic equipment.[6]

ROUTINE EXAMINATION

A routine sequence of spot radiographs is summarized in Table 55-1, and selected views are illustrated in Figure 55-2. Several key points are worth noting. The fluoroscopist should start with the patient in the prone or left lateral position, so that the sigmoid colon and descending colon are in the dependent position and are easier to fill. It is important to

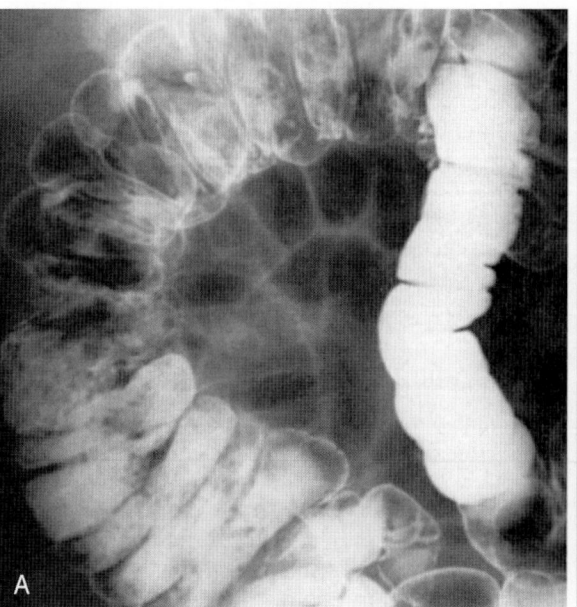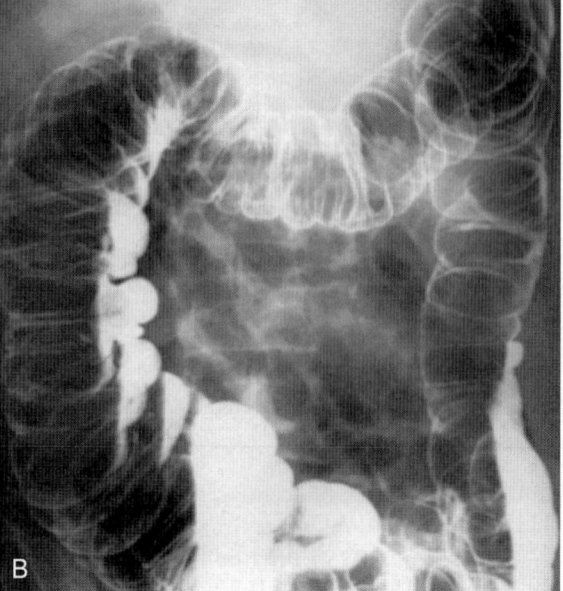

Figure 55-1. Importance of the decubitus view with imperfect bowel preparation. A. Oblique radiograph shows considerable fecal residue in the right colon. **B.** Left lateral decubitus radiograph shows fecal debris layering out in the barium, enabling a clear view of most of the right colon.

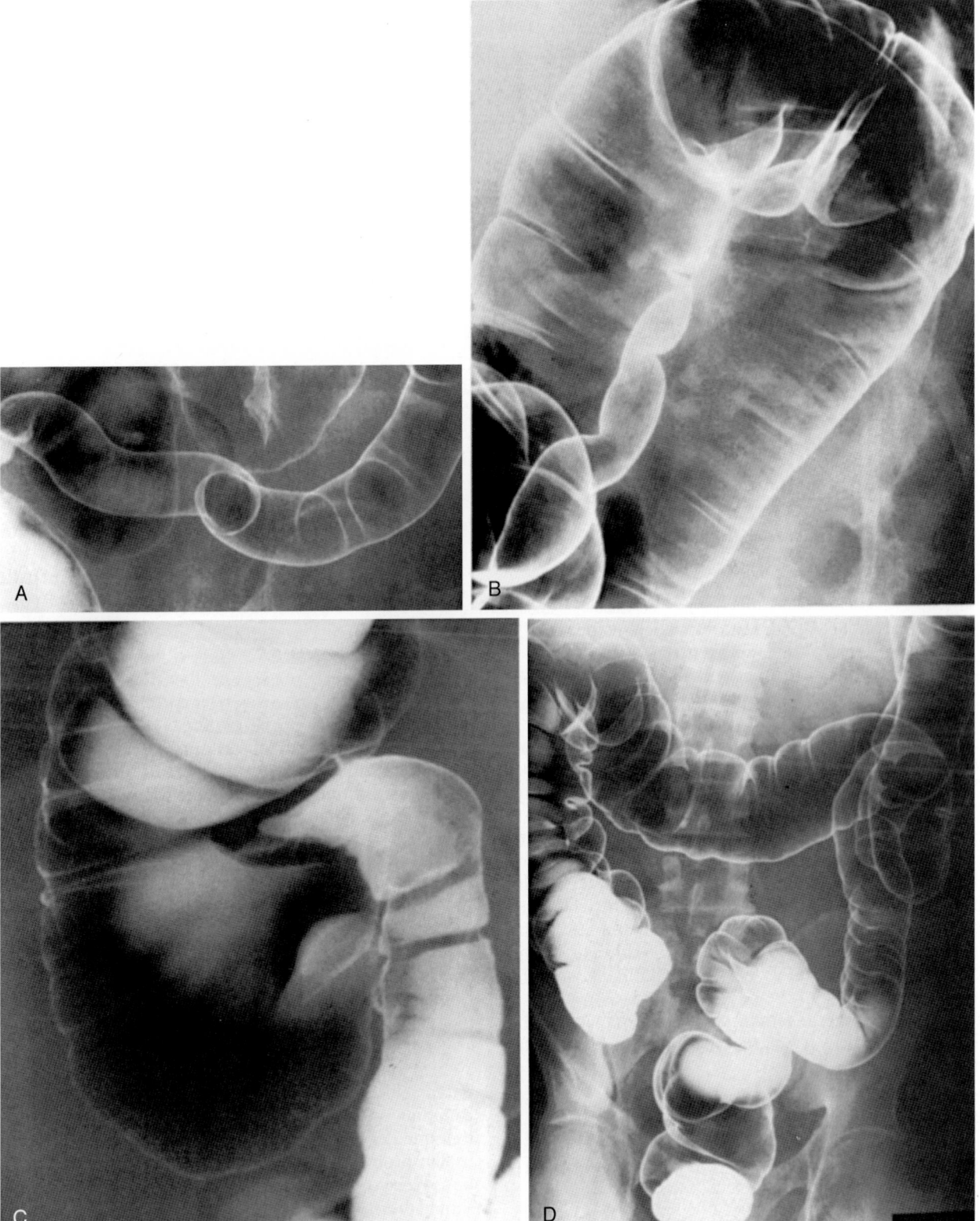

Figure 55-2. Selected radiographs from normal examinations. A. Spot radiograph of the sigmoid colon in the left posterior oblique position.
B. Upright spot radiograph of the splenic flexure in the right posterior oblique position. **C.** Spot radiograph of the cecum and terminal ileum in the supine position. **D.** Overhead radiograph in the prone position.

Continued

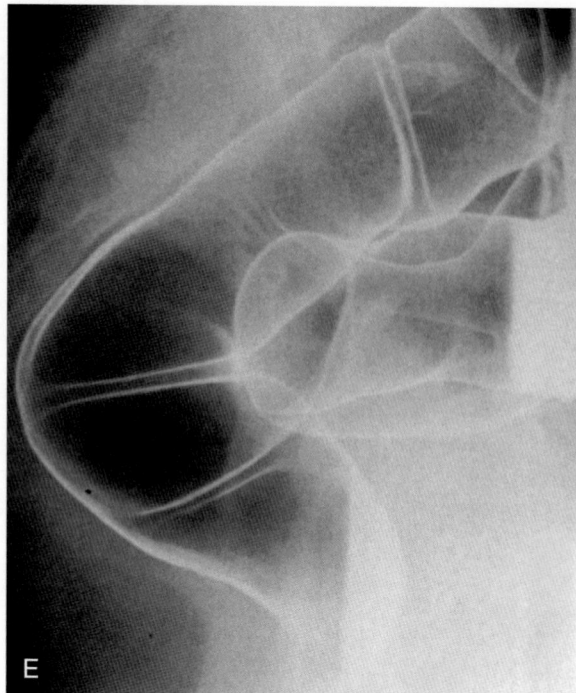
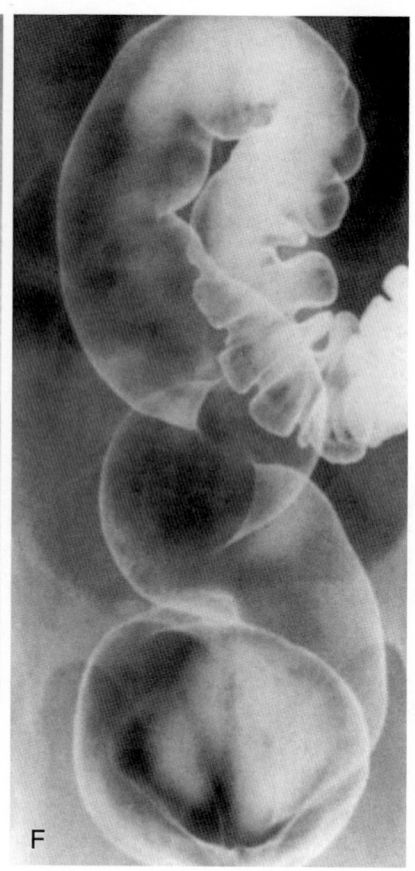

Figure 55-2, cont'd. E. Prone, cross-table lateral view of the rectum. **F.** Prone, angled view of the rectosigmoid colon. (**B** and **D** from Laufer I, Levine MS [eds]: Double Contrast Gastrointestinal Radiology, 2nd ed. Philadelphia, WB Saunders, 1992.)

be certain that barium has passed around the splenic flexure before insufflation of air is begun. The air is used to propel the barium across the transverse colon and into the ascending colon. At several points during the procedure, barium is drained from the rectum by dropping the enema bag onto the floor. As the patient turns, it is useful to watch the flow of barium across the mucosal surface because this "flow technique" may be valuable for demonstrating superficial lesions. The upright position ensures that barium drops into the cecum and provides the best views of the hepatic and splenic flexures and upper half of the colon. With digital techniques, postprocessing of the images should be considered a routine aspect of interpretation.[6] Subtle mucosal alterations and differences in density may become apparent only after the image has been altered.[7]

NORMAL APPEARANCES

Surface Pattern

The mucosal surface of the colon usually has a smooth, featureless appearance (Fig. 55-3A). In some patients, the mucosal surface may harbor a fine network of lines, also known as the innominate grooves or areae colonicae (Fig. 55-3B).[8] These patterns may be visualized en face with double-contrast technique or in profile in the barium-filled colon that is partially collapsed (Fig. 55-3C).[9] Occasionally, double-contrast studies may reveal innominate pits rather than grooves (Fig. 55-3D).[10] This is a normal appearance that should not be mistaken for superficial ulceration. This fine network

pattern is seen more frequently in countries such as Japan, where a barium suspension of lower density and lower viscosity is routinely used. In other patients, fine, transverse striations are seen as a transient phenomenon, probably secondary to contraction of the muscularis mucosae (Fig. 55-3E).

Lymphoid Follicles

In some patients, a pattern of fine 1- to 3-mm nodules is seen on the mucosal surface. These represent lymphoid follicles (Fig. 55-4A). They are regularly identified in children[11] but may also be seen in older individuals.[12] As long as the follicles are less than 2 to 3 mm in diameter, they can be considered a normal phenomenon. However, enlargement of these lymphoid follicles may be associated with a variety of diseases, including inflammation, Crohn's disease, lymphoma, and immune deficiency states.[13] It also has been shown that unusually prominent lymphoid follicles in older individuals may be associated with colonic tumors (Fig. 55-4B).[14] This finding should therefore promote a vigorous search for the presence of underlying colonic neoplasms.

Terminal Ileum

Lymphoid follicles are typically seen in the terminal ileum, particularly in younger patients (Fig. 55-4C). This is a normal appearance, but these lymphoid follicles may become enlarged and are particularly prominent in patients with conditions such as *Yersinia* enteritis or lymphoma.

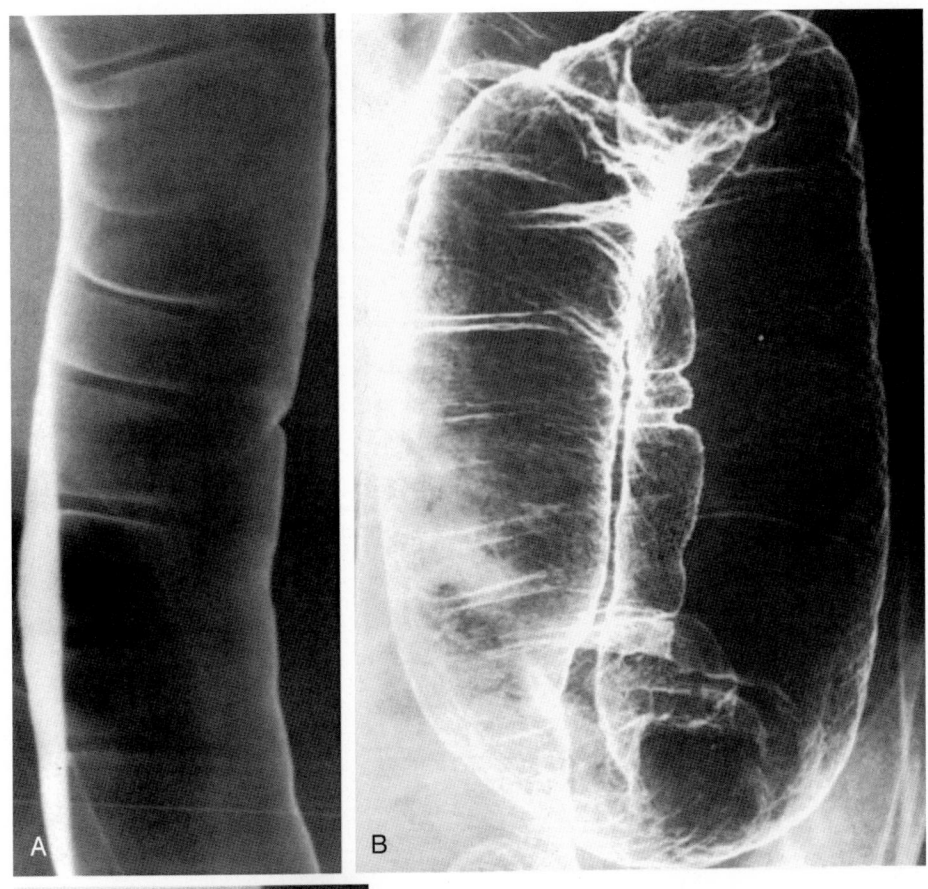

Figure 55-3. Normal mucosal surface. A. The smooth, featureless surface of the colon usually seen on double-contrast studies. **B.** Innominate grooves on the surface of the colon. **C.** Single-contrast view shows the profile appearance of the innominate lines. These lines should not be mistaken for ulcers.

Continued

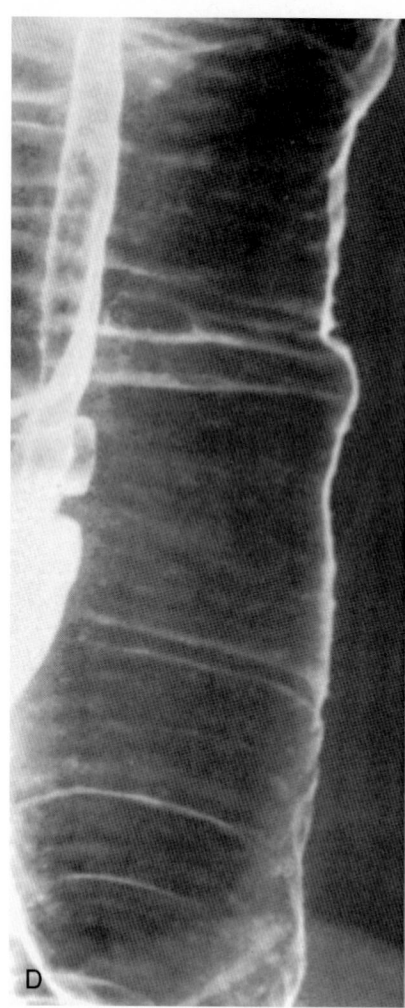

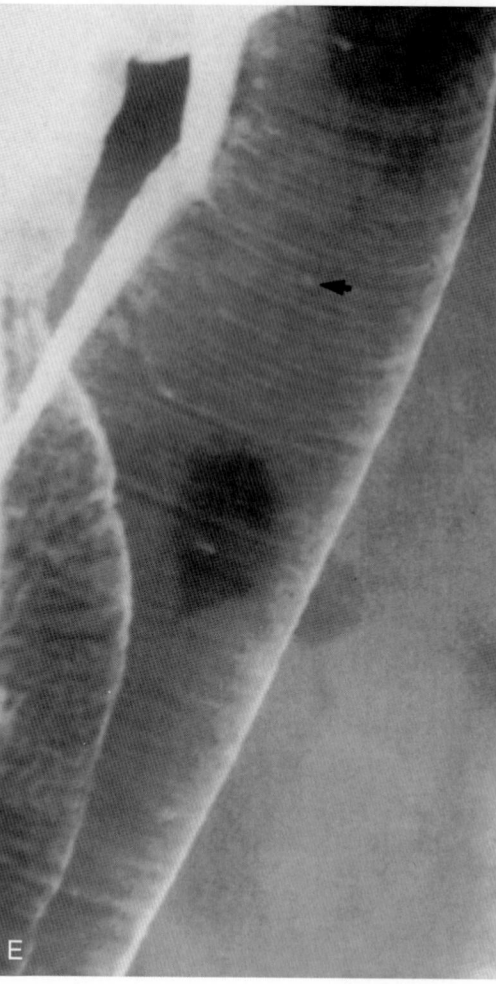

Figure 55-3, cont'd D. Surface pattern in a normal adult showing pinpoint barium collections (innominate pits) both en face and in profile. **E.** Transient striations in the transverse colon due to contraction of the muscularis mucosae. There are also punctate barium collections representing tiny diverticula (*arrow*). (**B** from Laufer I: Double Contrast Gastrointestinal Radiology with Endoscopic Correlation. Philadelphia, WB Saunders, 1979; **C** and **D** from Laufer I, Levine MS [eds]: Double Contrast Gastrointestinal Radiology, 2nd ed. Philadelphia, WB Saunders, 1992.)

TECHNICAL PROBLEMS

Poor Preparation

Poor colonic preparation remains a major obstacle to the performance of diagnostic double-contrast barium enemas. Poor preparation can simulate pathologic conditions such as inflammatory bowel disease (Fig. 55-5). Nevertheless, with the use of horizontal beam radiography (upright and lateral decubitus views), relatively small lesions can still be detected in the presence of fecal debris. In this regard, it is important to keep in mind the distinction between protrusions on the dependent and nondependent surfaces; fecal residue is invariably found only on the dependent surface, whereas, with appropriate manipulation, true polypoid lesions can be seen "etched in white" on the nondependent surface (Fig. 55-6) (see Chapter 4).

Diverticulosis

The presence of marked sigmoid diverticulosis poses a diagnostic dilemma because it may be difficult to detect polypoid lesions in the presence of multiple air-filled diverticula. In such cases, it may be necessary to reexamine the sigmoid colon by single-contrast technique (Fig. 55-7)[15] or to recommend flexible sigmoidoscopy to further evaluate the sigmoid colon.

Incontinence

Patient incontinence may be a limiting factor in the performance of single- or double-contrast barium enema examinations. An intravenous injection of glucagon helps to relieve spasm, and inflation of the retention balloon (as described previously) under direct visualization may also overcome this problem.

Nonfilling of the Right Colon

For various reasons, it may be difficult or impossible to fill the right colon. In some cases, if the patient is asked to evacuate the barium, barium and air are also propelled retrograde into the right colon, enabling adequate visualization of the cecum and ascending colon on postevacuation radiographs. If this fails, however, it may be necessary to convert the examination to a single-contrast barium enema to obtain adequate filling of the right colon.[16]

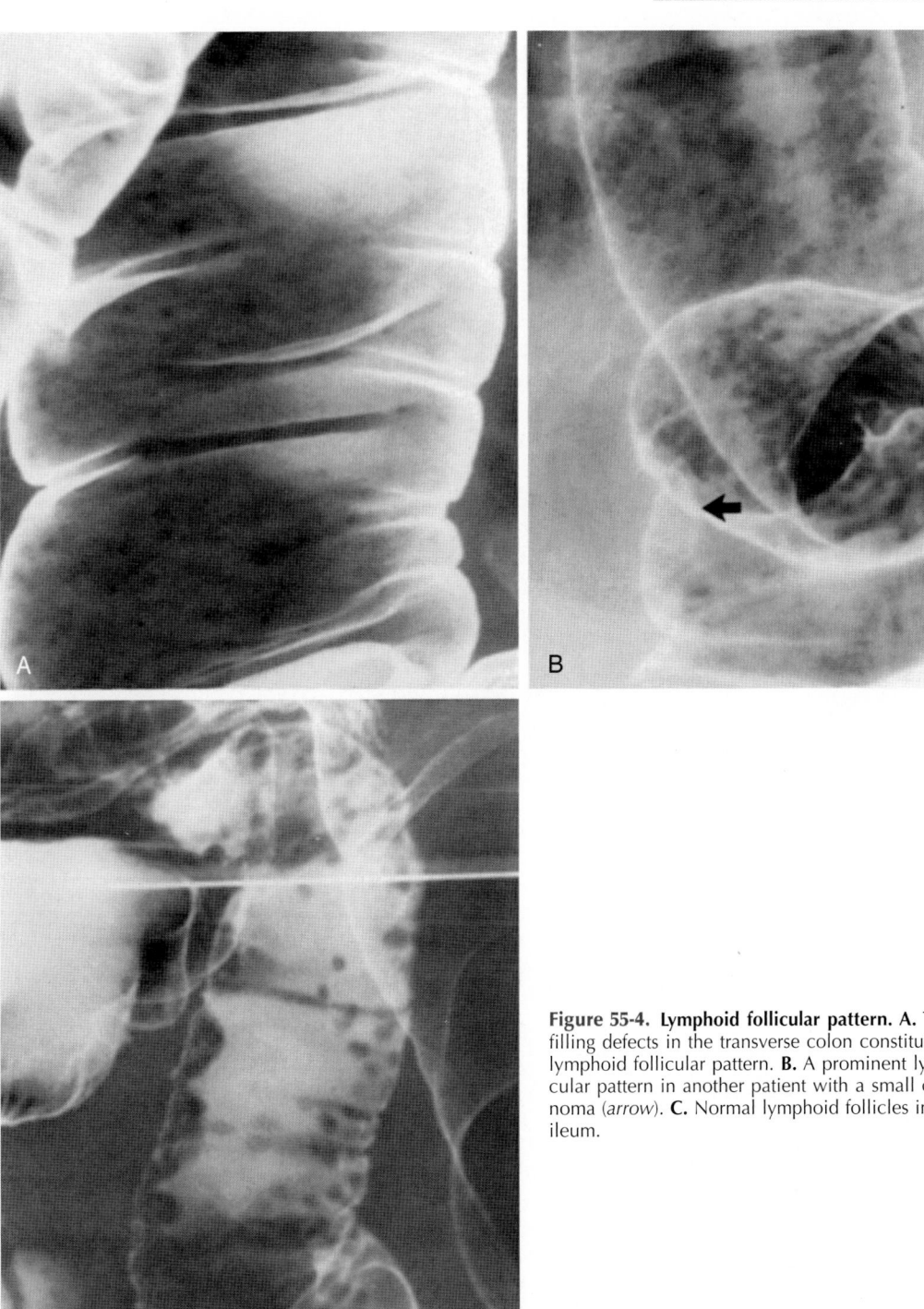

Figure 55-4. Lymphoid follicular pattern. A. Tiny, rounded filling defects in the transverse colon constitute the normal lymphoid follicular pattern. **B.** A prominent lymphoid follicular pattern in another patient with a small colonic carcinoma (*arrow*). **C.** Normal lymphoid follicles in the terminal ileum.

COMPLICATIONS

Many patients experience gas pains during and after the procedure.[17] These can be minimized by using carbon dioxide instead of air for gaseous distention.[18] The most serious complication is perforation of the bowel.[19] In most cases, the perforation occurs in the rectum and is usually related to inflation of a retention balloon in a diseased rectum. A follow-up contrast study with water-soluble contrast medium may show the contrast medium dissecting into the wall of the rectum and even extending into the retroperitoneum (Fig. 55-8A).

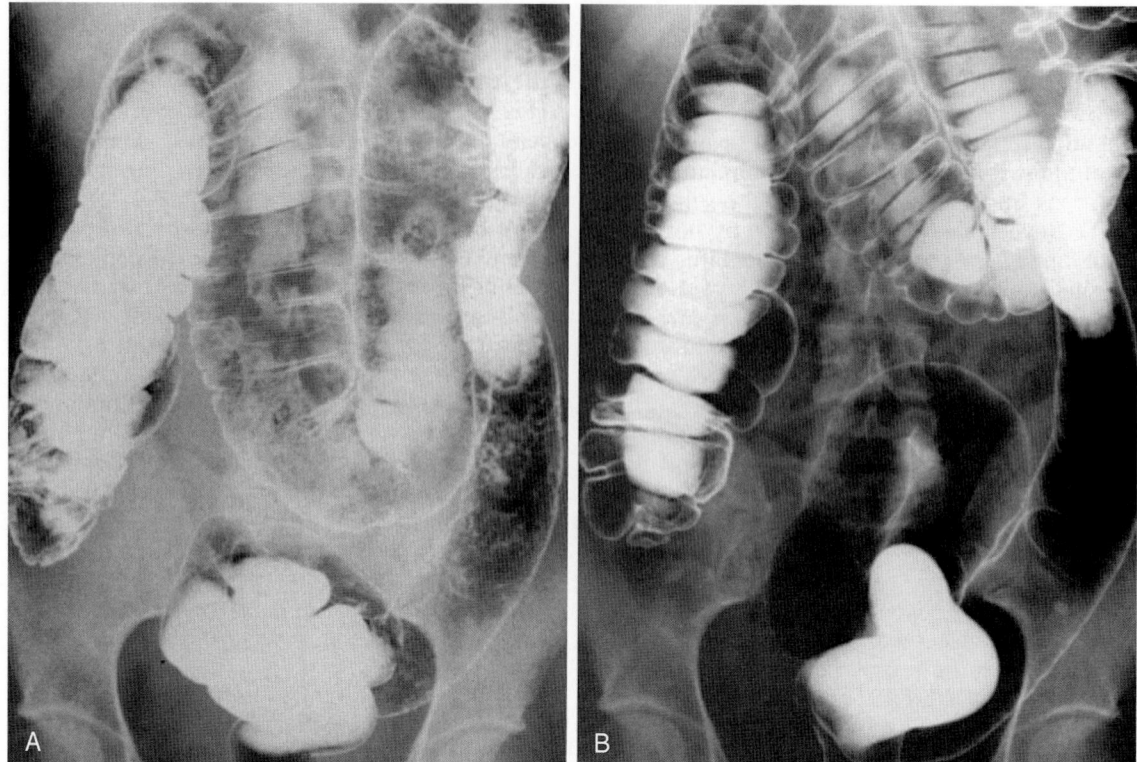

Figure 55-5. Poor preparation simulating inflammatory bowel disease. A. Initial study suggests that the mucosa is abnormal throughout the colon. **B.** Another examination with adequate preparation shows that the mucosal surface is normal.

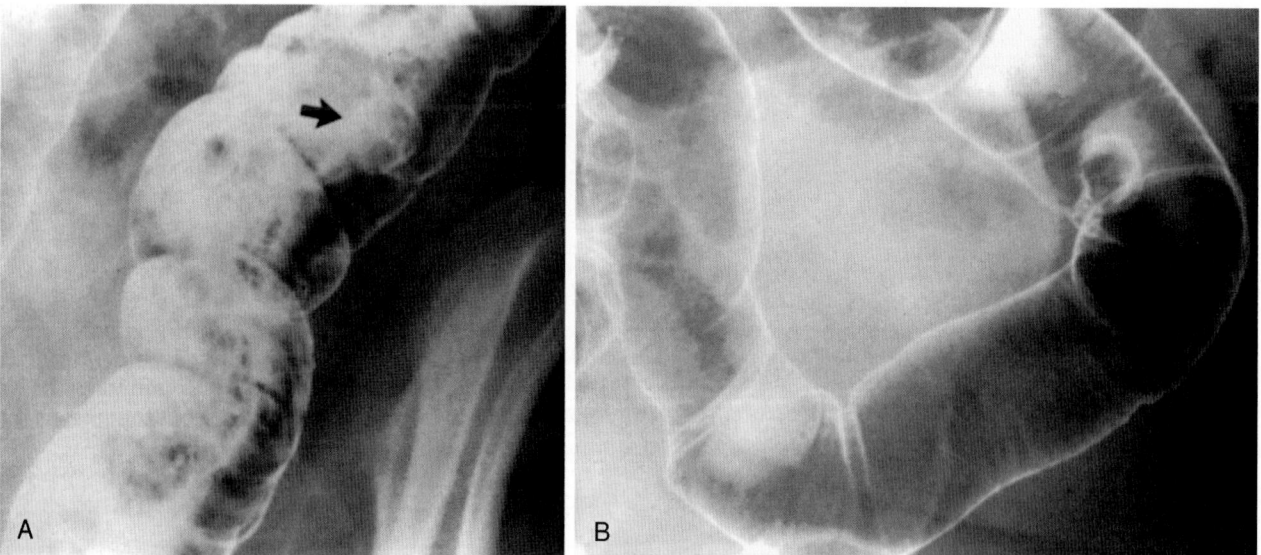

Figure 55-6. Detection of a polyp despite fecal debris. A. There is considerable fecal debris in the left side of the colon. Nevertheless, a polyp can be recognized as a lesion that is etched in white (*arrow*). **B.** After the fecal material has been cleared away, a repeat spot radiograph shows the pedunculated polyp.

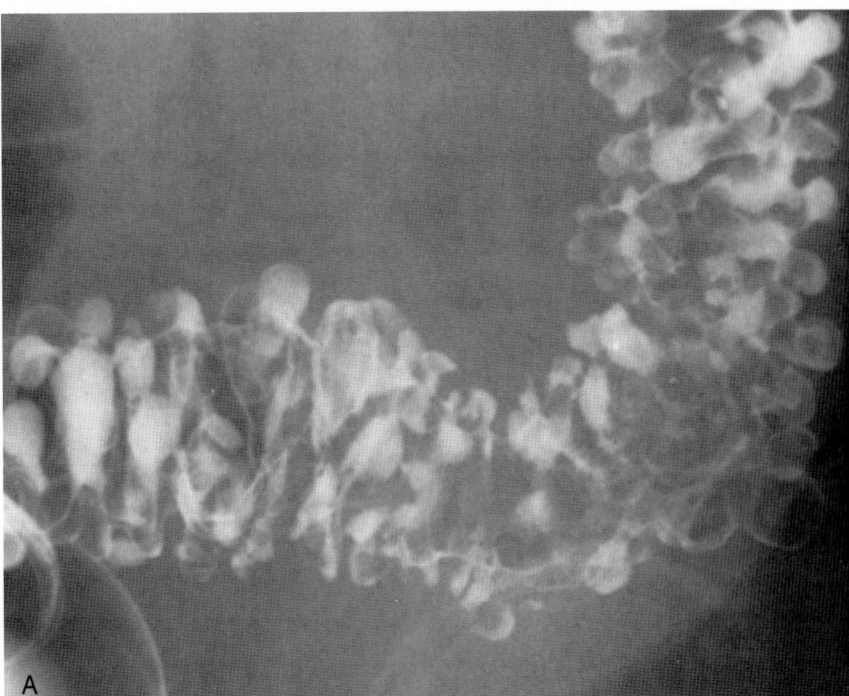

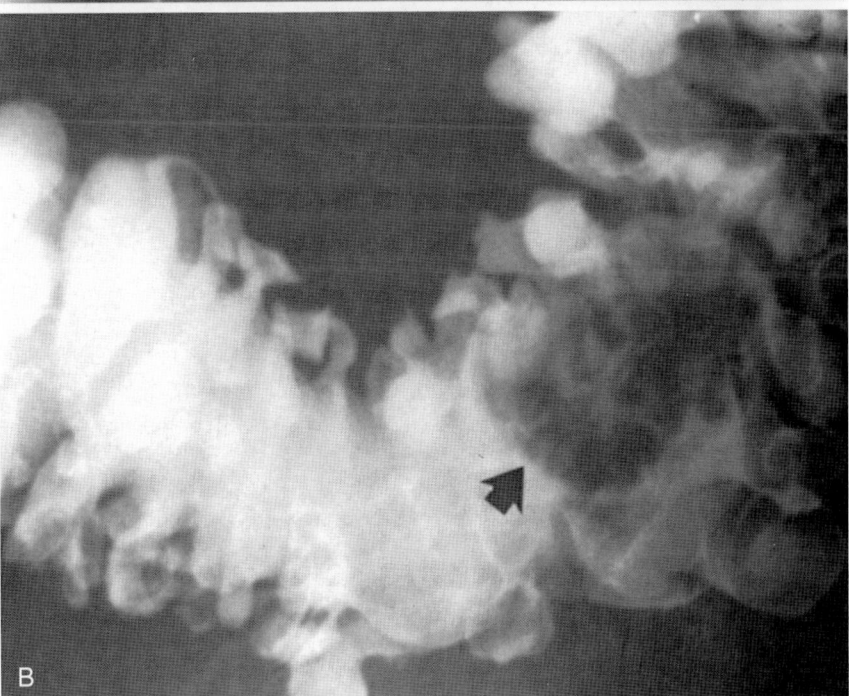

Figure 55-7. Diverticulosis with sigmoid flush. A. The diverticula are obvious on the double-contrast study, but a polypoid cancer cannot be identified. **B.** After refilling the colon with single-contrast barium, the polypoid cancer (*arrow*) is seen. (From Laufer I, Levine MS [eds]: Double Contrast Gastrointestinal Radiology, 2nd ed. Philadelphia, WB Saunders, 1992.)

Less frequently, there is a perforation of the intraperitoneal portion of the colon, almost always at the site of diseased bowel (Fig. 55-8B). In patients with diverticulosis, air alone may extravasate during the double-contrast barium enema and can be recognized as retroperitoneal or intraperitoneal air on spot radiographs (Fig. 55-8C).

A barium enema examination should never be performed immediately after endoscopic biopsy of normal or inflamed rectal mucosa with large biopsy forceps. This sequence is a major cause of rectal perforation.[20,21] If a deep rectal biopsy has been obtained, the barium enema study should therefore be postponed for at least 5 days. Biopsies of tumors or biopsies performed with a small forceps through flexible endoscopes need not force such long postponements.

Allergic complications are rare but have become more prominent in the past few years.[22] These may represent reactions to the barium, the glucagon, or even the latex in the rectal catheters. In fact, the latex in the retention balloons has been replaced by silicone because it was thought to be responsible for several severe allergic reactions.[23,24]

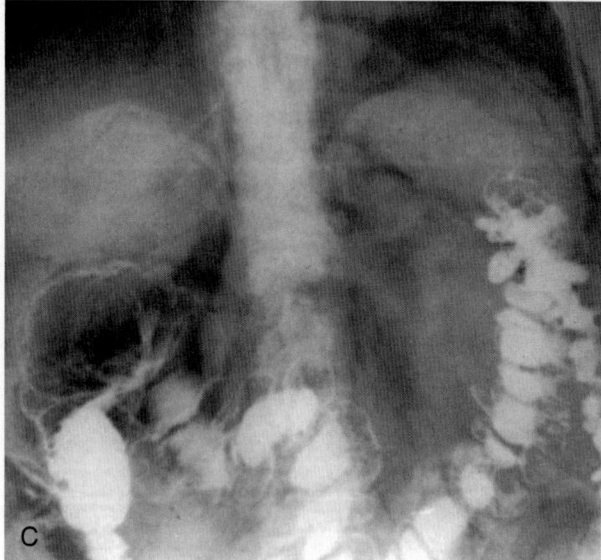

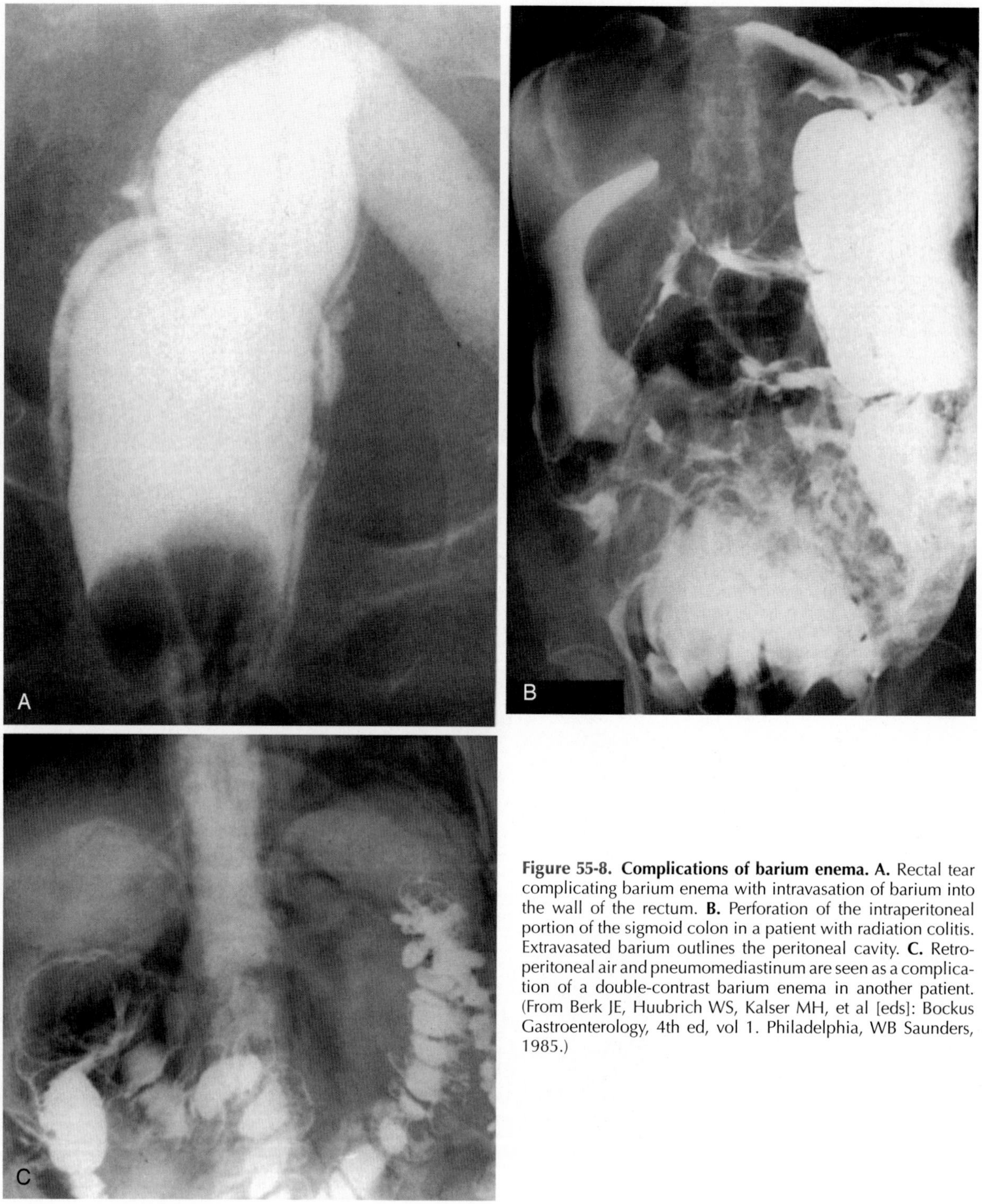

Figure 55-8. Complications of barium enema. A. Rectal tear complicating barium enema with intravasation of barium into the wall of the rectum. **B.** Perforation of the intraperitoneal portion of the sigmoid colon in a patient with radiation colitis. Extravasated barium outlines the peritoneal cavity. **C.** Retroperitoneal air and pneumomediastinum are seen as a complication of a double-contrast barium enema in another patient. (From Berk JE, Huubrich WS, Kalser MH, et al [eds]: Bockus Gastroenterology, 4th ed, vol 1. Philadelphia, WB Saunders, 1985.)

Transient bacteremia has been reported in some studies after barium enema, although clinical problems have not been reported.[25] Nevertheless, in patients with high-risk cardiac lesions, such as artificial heart valves, it may be prudent to use antibiotic prophylaxis, as recommended by the American Heart Association.[26] This prophylaxis consists of amoxicillin, 3 g, by mouth 1 hour before the study and 1.5 g at 6 hours afterward.

In patients with severe ulcerative disease of the bowel, air and contrast medium may enter the perirectal veins and gas may even be seen in the portal vein.[27] This may occur as a fatal event.

VARIATIONS IN TECHNIQUE

Suspected Perforation

When colonic perforation is suspected, the barium enema study should be performed with a water-soluble contrast

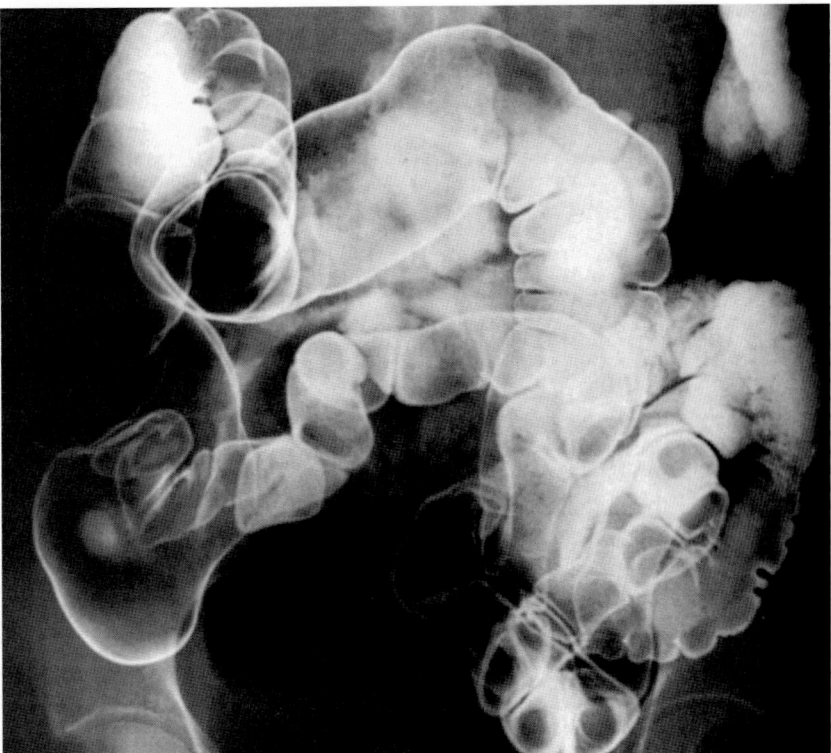

Figure 55-9. Peroral pneumocolon. Excellent visualization of the right colon and distal small bowel is obtained. (From Laufer I, Levine MS [eds]: Double Contrast Gastrointestinal Radiology, 2nd ed. Philadelphia, WB Saunders, 1992.)

agent such as diatrizoate meglumine and diatrizoate sodium (Gastroview; Mallinckrodt, St. Louis, MO). If extravasation is not demonstrated, it may be prudent to repeat the examination with barium for better definition and detail. In patients with cystic fibrosis, a water-soluble enema can be administered for diagnostic and therapeutic purposes.[28] In such patients, the hyperosmolar agent can draw fluid into the bowel and liquefy the viscous stool, sometimes with therapeutic results.

Peroral Pneumocolon

When the primary diagnostic interest is in the terminal ileum and cecum, an excellent examination can be achieved by use of the peroral pneumocolon.[29] The patient should undergo preparation of the colon as for a barium enema. After orally administered barium has reached the right colon, 1 mg of glucagon is administered intravenously and air is insufflated through the rectum. This provides excellent double-contrast views of the cecum and terminal ileum (Fig. 55-9) (see also Chapter 41).

Colostomy Enema

Double-contrast examinations of excellent quality can be performed through a colostomy. This is particularly important in patients who are being observed after resection of a previous rectal carcinoma because they have a significant risk of developing a metachronous primary colon cancer at a later point in time. Although a variety of devices have been described, we prefer the technique in which a Foley catheter is inserted through a nipple that is held against the colostomy (Fig. 55-10).[30]

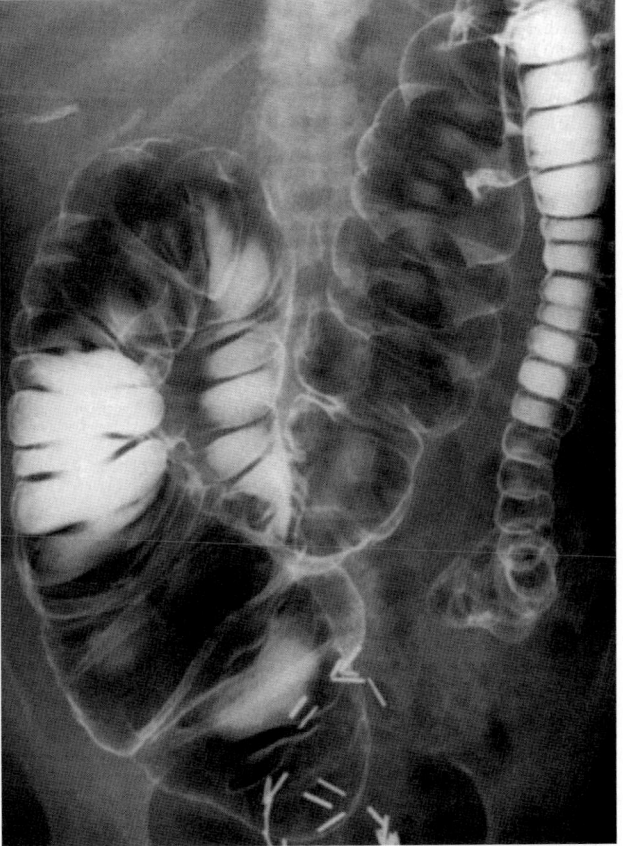

Figure 55-10. Colostomy enema. Excellent visualization of the residual colon is obtained after a colostomy. (From Laufer I, Levine MS [eds]: Double Contrast Gastrointestinal Radiology, 2nd ed. Philadelphia, WB Saunders, 1992.)

References

1. Bartram CI: Obliteration of thumbprinting with double contrast enemas in acute ischemic colitis. Gastrointest Radiol 4:85-88, 1979.
2. Fork ET, Ekberg O, Nilsson G, et al: Colon cleansing regimens. Gastrointest Radiol 7:383-389, 1982.
3. Bakran A, Bradley JA, Breshnihan E, et al: Whole gut irrigation: An inadequate preparation for double contrast barium enema examination. Gastroenterology 73:28-30, 1977.
4. Miller RE: A new enema tip. Radiology 92:1492, 1969.
5. De Lacey G, Wignall B, Ambrose J, et al: The double contrast barium enema: Improvements to lateral decubitus views including the use of a wedge filter. Clin Radiol 29:197-199, 1978.
6. Levine MS, Laufer I: The gastrointestinal tract: Dos and don'ts of digital imaging (state of the art). Radiology 207:311-316, 1998.
7. Kaiser JS, Levine MS, Laufer I, et al: Value of digital fluoroscopy for the diagnosis of pneumatosis coli. Eur J Radiol 29:21-24, 1998.
8. Matsuura K, Nakata H, Takeda N, et al: Innominate lines of the colon. Radiology 123:581-584, 1977.
9. Williams I: Innominate grooves in the surface of the mucosa. Radiology 84:877-880, 1965.
10. Frank DF, Berk RN, Goldstein HM: Pseudoulcerations of the colon on barium enema examination. Gastrointest Radiol 2:129-131, 1977.
11. Laufer I, deSa D: The lymphoid follicular pattern: A normal feature of the pediatric colon. AJR 130:51-55, 1978.
12. Kelvin FM, Max RJ, Norton GA, et al: Lymphoid follicular pattern of the colon in adults. AJR 133:821-825, 1979.
13. Glick SN, Teplick SK, Goren RA: Small colonic nodularity and the double contrast barium enema. RadioGraphics 1:73-86, 1981.
14. Bronen RA, Glick SN, Teplick SK: Diffuse lymphoid follicles of the colon associated with colonic carcinoma. AJR 142:105-109, 1984.
15. Lappas JC, Maglinte DDT, Kopecky KK, et al: Diverticular disease: Imaging with post-double-contrast sigmoid flush. Radiology 168:35-37, 1988.
16. Levine MS, Gasparaitis AE: Barium filling for glucagon-resistant spasm on double-contrast barium enema examinations. Radiology 160:264-265, 1986.
17. Gelfand DW: Complications of gastrointestinal radiologic procedures: I. Complications of routine fluoroscopic studies. Gastrointest Radiol 5:293-315, 1980.
18. Bessette JR, Maglinte DDT: Double-contrast barium enema study: Simple conversion to CO_2. Radiology 162:274-275, 1987.
19. Gelfand DW, Ott DJ, Ramquist NA: Pneumoperitoneum occurring during double-contrast enema. Gastrointest Radiol 4:307-308, 1979.
20. Maglinte DDT, Strong RC, Strate RW, et al: Barium enema after colorectal biopsies: Experimental data. AJR 139:693-697, 1982.
21. Harned RK, Consigny PM, Cooper NB: Barium enema examination following biopsy of the rectum or colon. Radiology 145:11-16, 1982.
22. Schwartz EE, Glick SN, Foggs MB, et al: Hypersensitivity reactions after barium enema examination. AJR 143:103-104, 1984.
23. Smith HJ: Performance of barium examination after acute myocardial infarction: Report of a survey. AJR 149:63-65, 1987.
24. Gelfand DW: Barium enemas, latex balloons and anaphylactic reactions. AJR 156:1-2, 1991.
25. Butt J, Hentges D, Pelican G, et al: Bacteremia during barium enema study. AJR 130:715-718, 1978.
26. Dajani AS, Bisno AL, Kyung J, et al: Prevention of bacterial endocarditis: Recommendations by the American Heart Association. JAMA 264:2919-2922, 1990.
27. Stein MG, Crues JV III, Hamlin JA: Portal venous air associated with barium enema. AJR 140:1171-1172, 1983.
28. Glick SN, Kressel HY, Laufer I, et al: Meconium ileus equivalent: Treatment with Hypaque enema. Diagn Imaging 49:149-152, 1980.
29. Kressel HY, Evers KA, Glick SN, et al: The peroral pneumocolon examination: Technique and indication. Radiology 144:414-416, 1982.
30. Goldstein HM, Miller RH: Air contrast colon examination in patients with colostomies. AJR 127:607-610, 1976.

Dynamic Evaluation of the Anorectum

Sat Somers, MBChB • Clive Bartram, MD • Julia R. Fielding, MD • Kang Hoon Lee, MD • Richard M. Gore, MD

The pelvic floor is a complex system of muscles, ligaments, nerves, and fascial planes that support the pelvic organs, maintain rectal and urinary continence, and coordinate relaxation during urination and defecation. It must endure a lifetime of straining at defecation, laughing, lifting, sneezing, coughing, increasing body weight, and, in the case of women, the trauma of childbirth. It is not surprising that pelvic floor weakness is a common clinical problem, particularly in multiparous women older than 50 years of age, and is a major health issue impacting on the quality of life. One half of women with pelvic floor weakness have some degree of pelvic prolapse. Ten to 20 percent of this group present with a variety of clinical problems, including pain, pressure, urinary and fecal incontinence, prolapse, and defecatory dysfunction. These conditions are worsened by obesity, multiparity, menopause, and chronic obstructive pulmonary disease.

The management of pelvic floor dysfunction is becoming increasingly dependent on imaging. The chances of successful medical and surgical treatment are enhanced when a complete understanding of the global nature of the pathology has been elucidated by imaging.

At the present time, there are three major methods of evaluating the anorectum radiographically: fluoroscopic evacua-tion proctography, ultrasonography, and MRI. The virtues and limitations of each of these modalities are considered in this chapter.

Traditionally, the pelvic floor is divided into an anterior, middle, and posterior compartment. The peritoneal cavity and its pelvic contents can be considered a fourth compartment. This classification is somewhat artificial because the structures of the pelvic floor are so intimately related that patients with abnormalities in one compartment often have disorders in others (Fig. 56-1).

ANATOMY OF THE ANORECTUM

Ligaments and Fasciae

The fasciae and ligaments of the pelvic floor provide passive support, while the muscles, primarily the levator ani, provide active support of the pelvis. The fasciae form condensations (ligaments) that are attached to the bony ring of the pelvis. The pelvic floor has three layers from superior to inferior: the pelvic fascia, pelvic diaphragm, and urogenital diaphragm, with their associated supportive structures, which are intimately

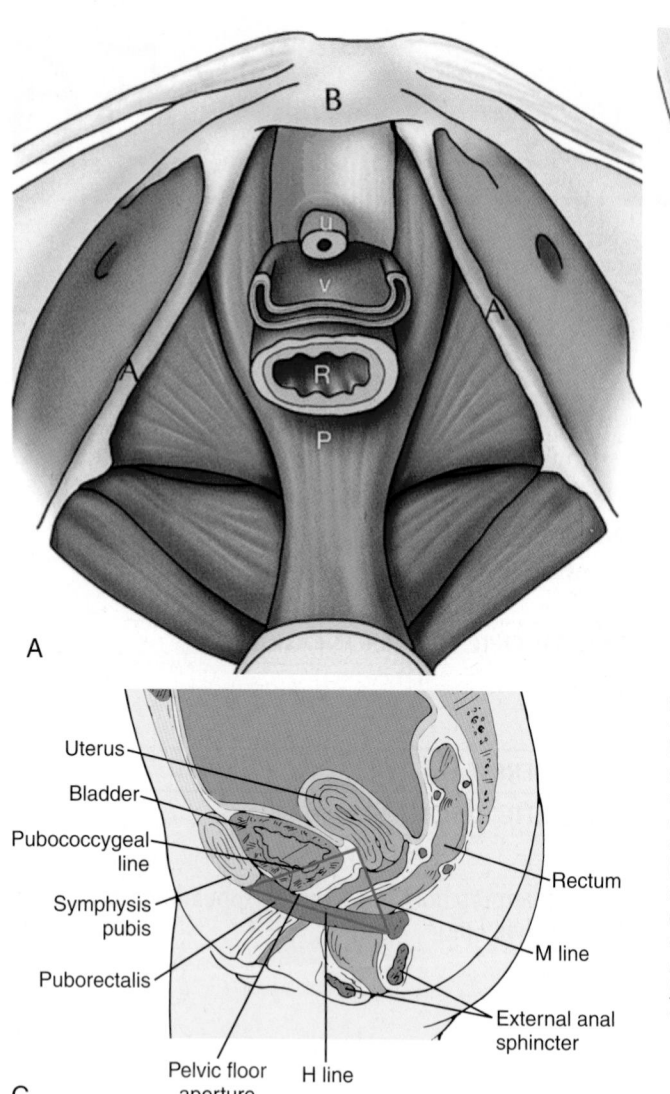

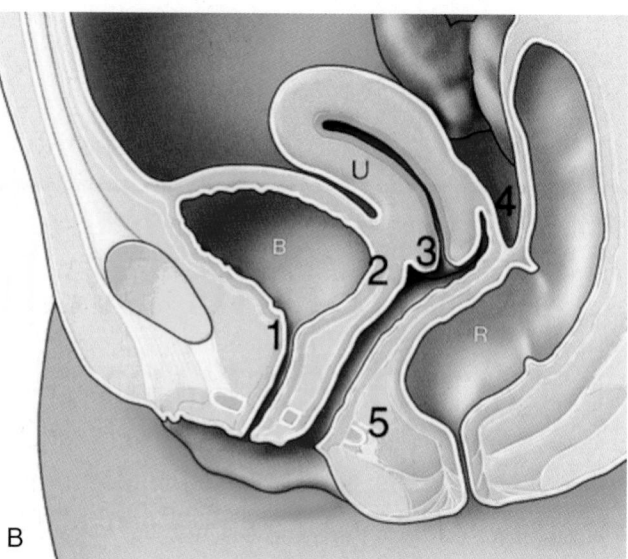

Figure 56-1. Schematic depiction of normal pelvic anatomy. A. Axial schematic diagram shows the anatomic structures that provide pelvic floor support. A, arcus tendineus fascia pelvis ("white line"); B, pubic bone; P, puborectalis sling; R, rectum; U, urethra, V, vagina. **B.** Sagittal schematic of the pelvis demonstrates various sites of prolapse, including the bladder neck and urethra (1), bladder base (2), cervicovaginal vault (3), cul-de-sac (4), and rectum (5). B, bladder, R, rectum, U, uterus. **C.** Drawing of the sagittal midline view of the female pelvis shows bony landmarks and the puborectal muscle, also called the levator sling. The pubococcygeal, H, and M lines and the levator plate are delineated in red. (**A** and **B** from Pannu HK, Kaufman HS, Cundiff GW, et al: Dynamic MR imaging of pelvic organ prolapse: Spectrum of abnormalities. RadioGraphics 20:1567-1582, 2000; **C** from Fielding JR: Practical MR imaging of female pelvic floor weakness. Radio-Graphics 22:295-304, 2002.)

related to the urogenital region, urethra, anal sphincter, and vagina in women.

Anorectal Musculature

The levator ani plate consists of three muscles that form the posterior pelvic diaphragm. The iliococcygeus muscle origi-nates from the ischial spine and obturator fascia and passes caudally, posteriorly, and medially to insert on the sacrum at S4 and S5 and the anococcygeal raphe. The pubococcygeus muscle originates from the obturator fascia and pubis and passes posteriorly, caudally, and medially to decussate with fibers from the contralateral side. The fibers from the medial part of the pubococcygeus fuse with the perineal body, pros-tate, and vagina and form part of the longitudinal muscle bundle as it travels in the intersphincteric plane.

The puborectalis muscle arises with the pubococcygeus from the pubis and urogenital diaphragm and proceeds poste-riorly alongside the anorectal junction. Fibers from one side join with fibers from the other to form a sling behind the rectum at the anorectal ring. This ring is an important land-mark, and its dysfunction leads to a variety of clinical disorders. The puborectalis muscle receives innervation from S3 and S4.

The rectococcygeus muscle arises from the coccyx and passes forward and downward to blend with the longitudinal muscle fibers of the rectum and pelvic fascia. These muscles tether the rectum to the coccyx. The coccygeus muscle supports the rectum and brings the coccyx forward during squeezing.

The internal anal sphincter (IAS) forms the innermost muscular layer of the anal canal and is a continuation of the circular muscle of the rectum and ends with a pronounced rounded edge 1 to 1.5 cm caudal to the dentate line and slightly cranial to the terminus of the external anal sphincter (EAS). The IAS is 2.5 to 4 cm in length and 0.5 cm thick and is the terminal condensation of the circular rectal smooth muscle. The IAS is smooth muscle that has autonomous innervation from sympathetic presacral nerves. The longitudinal anal muscle is the continuation of the longitudinal muscle of the rectal wall and pubococcygeus muscle. Inferiorly, fibers course through the IAS and EAS, with some gaining attachment to the perianal skin. These dermal terminations are called the corrugator cutis ani.

The EAS is the outermost muscle of the distal anal canal and is slightly longer (1 cm) than the IAS and occupies a posi-tion outside the IAS, enveloping it throughout its length. The EAS is an elliptical cylinder of muscle that is continuous with the puborectalis muscle superiorly. Caudally, it becomes subcutaneous and lies laterally and more inferiorly than the IAS. The EAS is divided into deep and superficial compartments. Dorsally, the EAS is attached to the skin superficially and the sacrococcygeal raphe and coccyx more deeply. The EAS is continuous with the puborectalis muscle at the level of the anorectal ring. Ventrally, the EAS is attached to the skin superficially, to the transverse peroneus muscle slightly more deeply, and proceeds most deeply with the puborectalis muscle toward the pubis at the level of the anorectal ring. The EAS is under voluntary control and is innervated by the pudendal nerves (S2 through S4).

INDICATIONS FOR EXAMINATION

Patients with pelvic floor abnormalities present with a variety of sign, symptoms, and physical findings.

Constipation

Constipation is a very subjective description of inadequate bowel function. Patients may present with difficulty in initiating defecation, with incomplete defecation, or with the need for considerable straining with defecation. Some patients may also complain of constipation if stool is of inadequate size, weight, or water content. These symptoms may be accompanied by a variety of complaints, including bloating and abdominal pain. Clinically, mechanical abnormalities such as intussusception and prolapse are often suspected in patients with incomplete defecation. Some of these patients may need to resort to digital or positional maneuvers to assist defecation.

The clinical presentation of incontinence ranges from constant soiling of clothes as a result of slow intermittent leakage to the inability to retain any stool.

Disorders of defecation affects the female population more than males. In the average practice, usually 80% of patients are women. Painful defecation, perineal pain, dyspareunia, rectal bleeding, and the solitary rectal ulcer syndrome are other chief complaints.

EVACUATION PROCTOGRAPHY

The dynamic assessment of defecation was first described by Burhenne in 1964, and now most investigators use a modification of the examination described by Mahieu and colleagues.[1-9] This modification consists of opacifying the rectum and having the patient sit on a commode and go through a series of maneuvers, including defecation. In women, the vagina is also opacified. The technique may be further modified by opacifying the small bowel, introducing intraperitoneal contrast material, and opacifying the bladder; these modifications facilitate the diagnosis of enteroceles and sigmoidoceles.[9-15] Preparation of the bowel with laxatives or enemas is not necessary; however, some authors believe that a limited bowel preparation will be more comfortable for the patient and will also provide a more standardized examination.[16] The entire procedure is recorded on spot films and videotape. The examination is usually completed in about 15 minutes.

In patients who are incontinent and have great difficulty in retaining the rectal contrast, the examination may be done in the left lateral decubitus position.

The entire procedure should be explained to the patient to help ensure that the patient understands all the instructions during the actual examination. Often, it is useful to ask the patient to practice the maneuvers, such as squeezing the buttocks to demonstrate lift, while the patient is sitting on the side of a stretcher before instillation of contrast medium.

Technique

Small Bowel Opacification

The small bowel is opacified with the same barium used for examination of the small intestine. The volume used is 400 to 600 mL; it is given 45 to 60 minutes before the fluoroscopic study. Some authors suggest a waiting time of up to 3 hours.

Bladder Opacification

Bladder opacification can be achieved with any contrast agent used for cystography. The volume of contrast that is introduced should be sufficient to opacify the bladder without distending it to the point that it becomes uncomfortable for the patient. Two hundred milliliters is usually adequate. Overdistention of the bladder may also mask enteroceles.

Positive Contrast Peritoneography

Enteroceles, sigmoidoceles, and prolapse of other pelvic structures such as rectum, bladder, and uterus can be detected by opacifying the pouch of Douglas. Peritoneography can be performed by instilling 20 to 60 mL of nonionic contrast material into the peritoneal cavity while the patient, with an empty bladder, is lying supine on the fluoroscopy table.[11-13] The puncture site can be in the midline 2 cm below the umbilicus,[11] 3 cm below the umbilicus and 4 cm to the left,[13] or any other suitable point on the anterior abdominal wall that avoids intra-abdominal structures.

Ultrasonography may be used to avoid injury to the bowel and bladder when the puncture needle is being placed. With sterile technique, contrast material is injected into the peritoneal cavity with a 22-gauge needle. Intermittent fluoroscopy ensures correct placement of the needle by observing free flow of contrast material into the peritoneal cavity. The needle is then withdrawn, and the table is tilted approximately 30 degrees upward to allow flow of the contrast material into the pouch of Douglas. The remainder of the examination is performed in the usual way.

Vaginal Opacification

In women, the vagina is opacified after the small bowel loops in the pelvis have filled with contrast material or have been outlined by peritoneography. The agent used for opacification varies.[18] A vaginal tampon soaked with a water-soluble contrast agent used to be the standard vaginal marker, but the tampon can act as a pelvic strut, obscuring diagnostic information.[14] Instead, a radiopaque gel is a preferred vaginal marker (Fig. 56-2). The gel can be made with equal parts of Ortho Gynol II Gel, a contraceptive gel (Johnson and Johnson, Inc., Montreal, Canada), and a high-density water-soluble contrast medium. A combination of 14 mL of Ortho Gynol II Gel and 14 mL of iodixanol (Visipaque 320—Amersham Health,

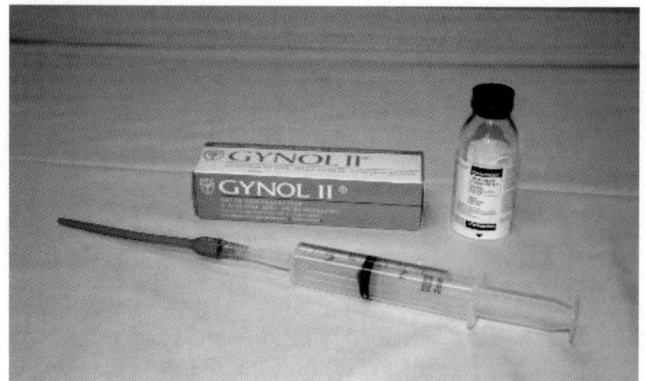

Figure 56-2. Materials useful for vaginal catheterization and opacification for the defecography procedure.

Montreal, Canada) or iohexol (Omnipaque) is instilled into the vagina with a bladder irrigation syringe connected to a pediatric enema tip (see Fig. 56-2). Barium paste works equally well. The patient is placed in the lithotomy or left lateral decubitus position, the tip of the enema tube is inserted into the vaginal vault, and the contrast medium is injected as the tip is withdrawn.

Rectal Opacification

The next step is opacification of the rectum. A barium paste with a consistency similar to that of stool is preferred. Liquid barium is not physiologic and stresses even a normal continence mechanism. It may also result in abnormal contraction of the pelvic floor and anal muscles at rest, preventing recognition of abnormal muscular resting tone.[6]

A barium paste prepared with barium and potato starch has the appropriate consistency.[4] Commercial preparations such as Anatrast (Lafayette Pharmaceuticals, Lafayette, IN, 47904) are also accurate, although these preparations are slightly less viscous. A disadvantage of the barium and potato starch mixture is that it does not coat the walls of the lumen well. This problem can be overcome by instilling 30 to 50 mL of high-density liquid barium (e.g., Polibar Plus, E-Z-EM Company) before introducing the barium-starch mixture. The barium-starch mixture is also difficult to instill into the rectum with a regular caulking gun. An orthopedic glue gun, although more expensive, is much easier to use because it is geared and lasts for years. If an orthopedic glue gun is used, a 50-cm half-inch tube that is filled with high-density liquid barium and is attached to the glue gun at one end and to a wide-bore enema tip at the other is ideal for the introduction of both rectal contrast agents.

Contrast medium is introduced until the patient reports the sensation of rectal fullness and the desire to evacuate. The position of the anal orifice is marked with a radiopaque paste. The paste is made with 50 g of petrolatum mixed with 50 g of Ultra-R barium sulfate (E-Z-EM Company). The marker facilitates measurement of the anal canal. The patient is then led to the commode for the dynamic portion of the study.

Commode

The defecography commode needs to fulfill the following requirements: it must be sturdy so that the patient is not afraid to sit on it; it must be radiolucent; and it must be designed to allow filming in both lateral and frontal projections. It should also have an anchoring mechanism to attach it safely to a fluoroscopic table. Attachment to the fluoroscopic table allows movement of the commode with the table movement control buttons. Commodes can be built with a personal design or a published design, or they may be purchased from commercially available sources.[20] We use a commode designed by Bernier and associates (Fig. 56-3).[20] It has a centimeter ruler in the midline for direct measurement of midline sagittal structures on the films (Fig. 56-4).

Documentation

The radiation dose needed to record this examination should be as low as possible. Many investigators therefore perform the study with only videofluoroscopy. However, the resolution is not sufficient to detect subtle radiographic changes, so spot films are recommended. In general, videofluoroscopy should be performed during the entire examination, with spot filming of key events. If stimulatable phosphors or digital radiography is used for the spot films, the radiation dose can be reduced.

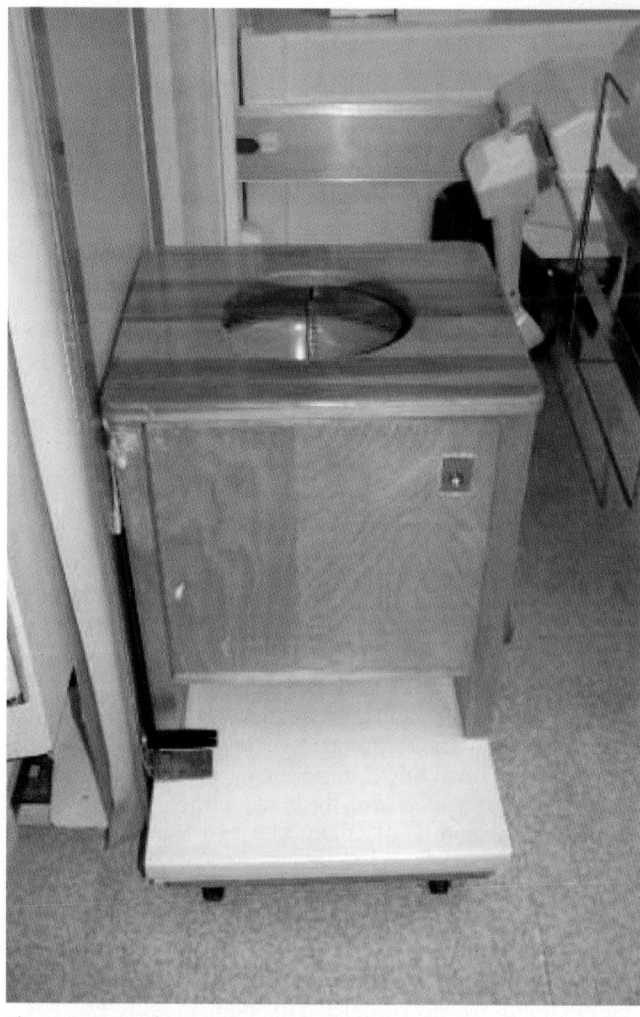

Figure 56-3. Defecography commode. The commode is shown attached to a remote-control fluoroscopic table. The midline centimeter ruler can be seen. The ruler permits direct measurements of midline sagittal structures.

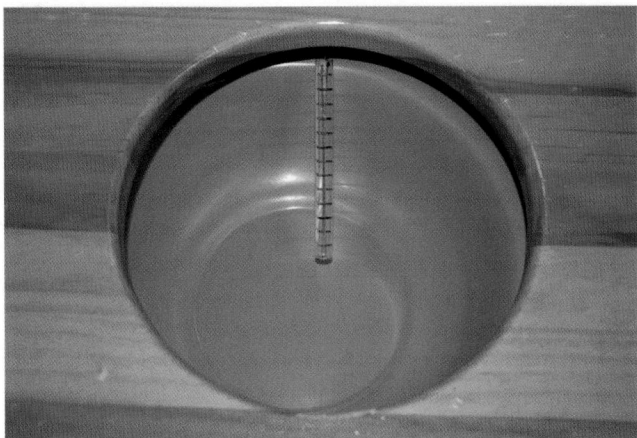

Figure 56-4. Close-up of the dish in the defecography commode. Note the ruler.

To enable the patient to feel more comfortable during the procedure, it is preferable to use a remote-control fluoroscopy room that has subdued lighting and is cleared of all personnel. The comfort of the patient is extremely important if an accurate assessment of the defecation process is to be obtained.

Spot radiographs are obtained in the lateral position with the patient responding to requests to rest (Fig. 56-5), lift (Fig. 56-6) (or squeeze), cough (Fig. 56-7), strain, defecate, and strain after defecation.

At rest, there is no conscious contraction of the pelvic musculature (see Fig. 56-5). During lifting, the patient maxi-

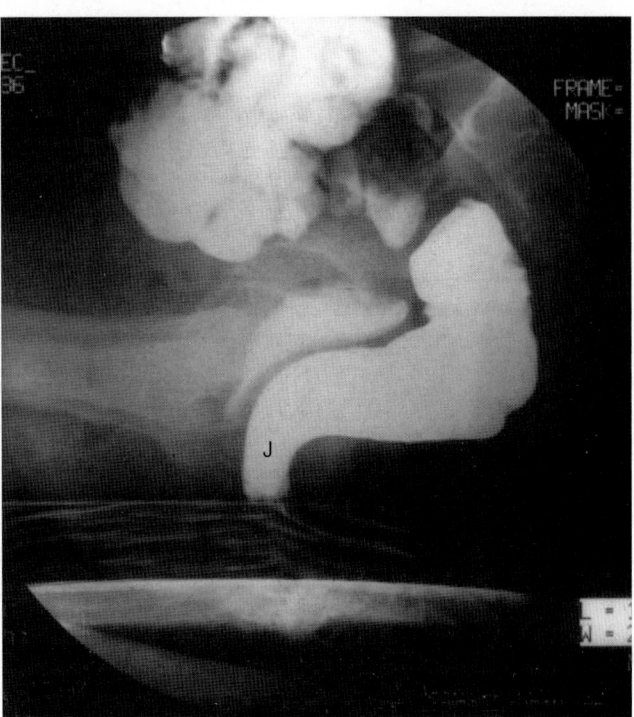

Figure 56-6. Normal appearance of the proctogram during lift. There is good contraction of the puborectalis and the levator ani. The anorectal junction (J) level is raised well above the level of the ischial tuberosities.

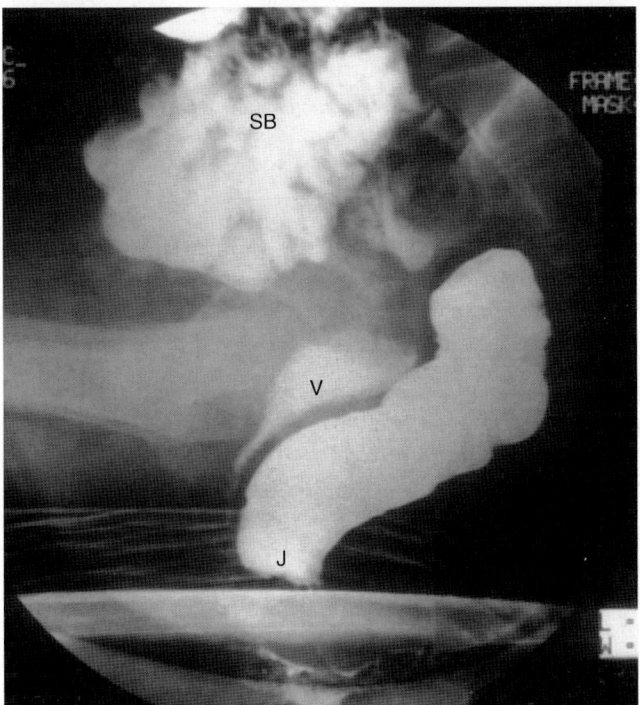

Figure 56-5. Normal appearance of the proctogram during rest. Note the opacified vagina (V) and its close relationship to the anterior rectal wall, as well as the level of the anorectal junction (J). The opacified small bowel (SB) is also seen.

mally contracts the pelvic floor musculature and elevates the entire pelvic floor (see Fig. 56-6).[21] The muscles involved are the puborectalis and levator ani. As a result, the anorectal angle becomes acute and the anal canal lengthens. These changes can be measured and are indicators of the continence mechanism. When asked to cough, the patient should produce a powerful cough in the rest position. This action simultaneously increases intra-abdominal pressure and contraction of the anal and pelvic floor muscles. In normal individuals, there is minimal or no descent of the pelvic floor and total continence. When asked to strain, the patient should strain downward maximally without evacuating. This maneuver stresses the continence mechanism and gives a measure of pelvic floor descent. The anal canal shortens during straining in most women (mean change, 2 mm).[21] Nearly all patients demonstrate some perineal descent, but this is the least reliable portion of the examination because some patients paradoxically contract the pelvic floor muscles, perhaps for fear of incontinence.

Finally, spot radiographs are obtained during defecation and postdefecation straining (Figs. 56-7 and 56-8). These films give a measurement of pelvic floor descent and an estimate of the completeness of emptying. Morphologic abnormalities such as intussusception and rectoceles are often visualized at this time, and the changes contributing to difficulty in defecation can be analyzed. Rectoceles are outpouchings of the rectum beyond the expected contour of the rectal wall (Fig. 56-9). They are often normal and are more common in women.[21] If a rectocele does not empty completely during defecation, it may produce a feeling of incomplete evacuation of the rectum.

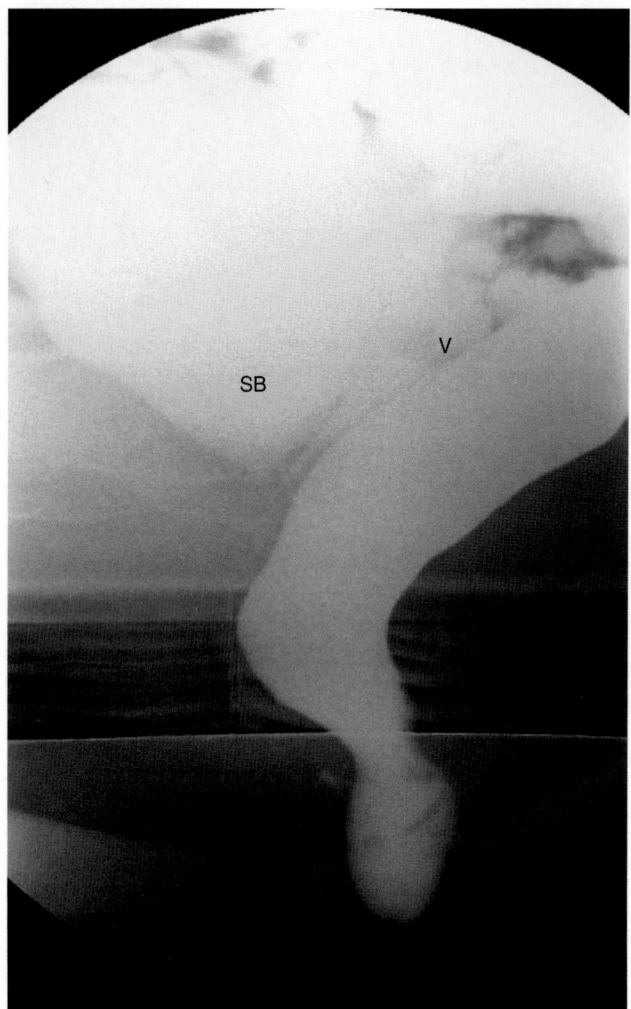

Figure 56-7. Normal appearance of the proctogram during defecation. The anorectal angle has increased considerably in comparison with the resting position, and the anal canal is open with evacuation in progress. The vagina (V) and small bowel (SB) maintain their position in relation to the rectum.

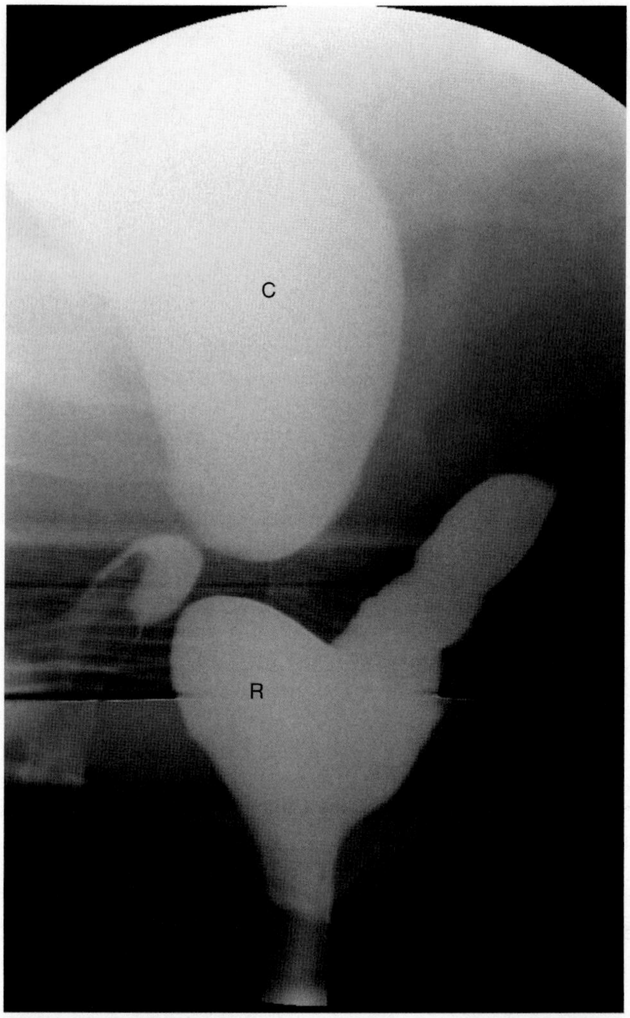

Figure 56-8. Normal appearance of the proctogram during end of defecation straining. The rectum is almost empty, and an anterior rectocele (R) and a transient cystocele (C) are seen during straining. The rectocele and cystocele retract with relaxation, and the anatomy returns to normal.

Measurements

Measurements taken from spot radiographs include the anorectal angle, anal canal length, level of the anorectal junction, and descent and elevation of the anorectal junction.

Anorectal Angle

The anorectal angle (Fig. 56-10) is measured between the axis of the anal canal and the tangent to the posterior wall of the rectum. It can be difficult to measure because the posterior wall of the rectum is often not clearly delineated and the angle becomes highly subjective.[22] Caution should therefore be exercised in assessing its significance. At rest, this angle is usually no greater than 120 degrees in control subjects. However, the angle has a normal range of 70 to 134 degrees, with a mean of about 95 degrees.[21] When the patient squeezes or lifts the buttocks, the anorectal angle decreases to a mean of 19 degrees (range, 6 to 26 degrees) in women and a mean of 28 degrees (range, 12 to 45 degrees) in men.[21] This angle increases during straining and defecation. The mean anorectal angle during straining in normal young women is 103 degrees, with a range of 75 to 108 degrees. In men, the mean angle is slightly lower at 98 degrees, with a range of 67 to 123 degrees.[21]

Anal Canal Length

Anal canal length is the distance traversed by the parallel borders of the anal canal before they form the diverging walls of the distal rectum. At rest, the mean length of the anal canal is 16 mm (range, 6 to 26 mm) in women and 22 mm (range, 10 to 38 mm) in men. During lifting (squeezing), the anal canal lengthens to a mean of 19 mm (range, 9 to 26 mm) in women and 28 mm (range, 12 to 45 mm) in men. During straining, the canal shortens slightly and has a mean length of 14 mm (range, 6 to 20 mm) in young women and 17 mm (range, 9 to 27 mm) in young men.[21]

Level of Anorectal Junction

The anorectal junction is the uppermost point of the anal canal. Its position is measured from an easily visualized fixed point, the ischial tuberosity. A positive value indicates a

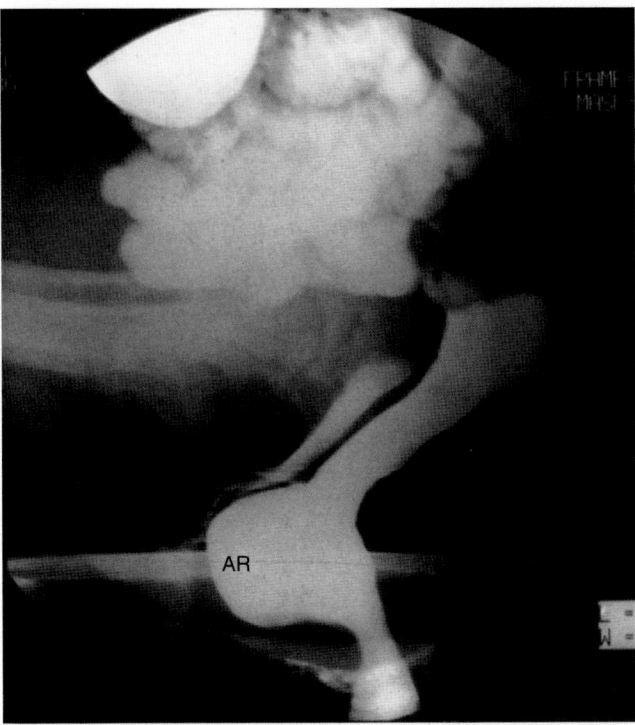

Figure 56-9. Anterior rectocele. An outpouching is seen at the anterior wall of the rectum. Anterior rectoceles (AR) of moderate size are normal during evacuation in young women.

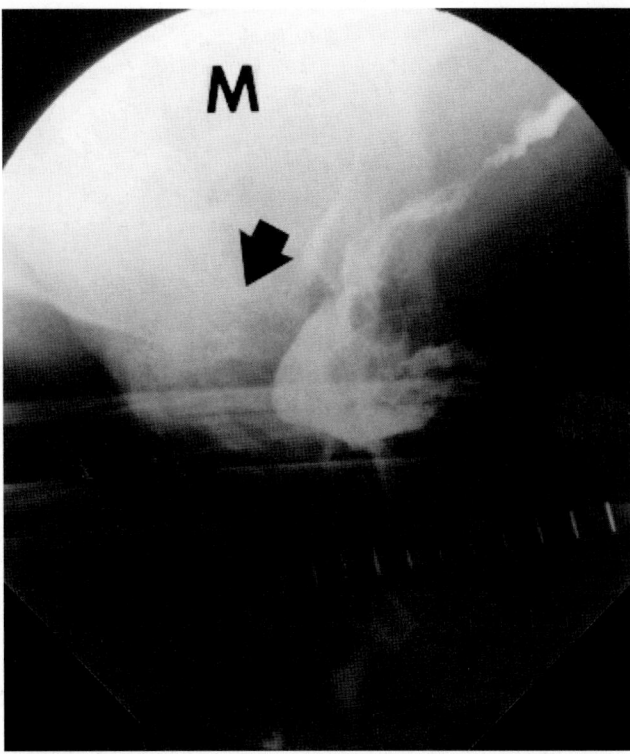

Figure 56-11. Rectocele manipulation (M). The *arrow* points to the digits of the hand that are being used to empty an anterior rectocele into the rectum by pushing it upward.

position above the ischial tuberosity, whereas a negative value indicates a position below it. In normal young men at rest, the mean level of the anorectal junction is 16 mm and increases to 28 mm during lifting (squeezing). It drops to −4 mm during defecation. In young women, the mean values for the same maneuvers are 4 mm at rest, 14 mm during lifting (squeezing), and 16 mm during defecation,[21] measurements significantly different from those of normal young men.

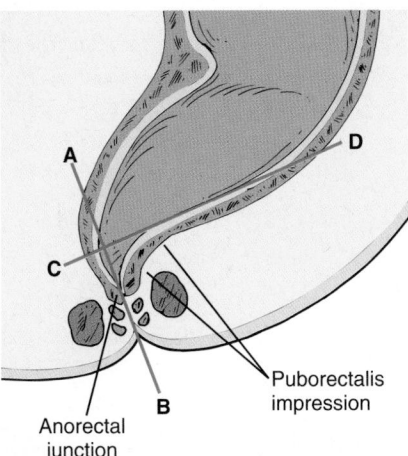

Figure 56-10. Anorectal angle determination. The lines AB and CD subtend the posterior anorectal angle. The position of AB is easily determined. CD can be much more difficult to draw. The *wide arrow* shows the position of the anorectal junction. Below it are the two parallel lines that form the anal canal. The *thin arrows* point to the puborectalis impression.

Occasionally, unusual or unexplained findings are seen on lateral views, and anteroposterior or oblique views are needed for further clarification. Some patients have a history of using a variety of maneuvers to facilitate evacuation. These patients should be encouraged to employ these maneuvers during the examination, and the mechanisms aiding evacuation should be identified. When patients have a large anterior rectocele that remains full even after the rectum has completely emptied, they may complain of incomplete emptying. Such patients typically empty the rectocele back into the rectum by digital perineal or vaginal pressure (Fig. 56-11). In patients with a history of obstructed defecation, it is sometimes helpful to perform the examination first with liquid barium, which makes expulsion easier. If this approach is successful, the examination should be repeated in the usual way with one of the thick barium pastes.

Pathology

Enterocele and Sigmoidocele

As shown by vaginal markers, the vagina may separate from the anterior wall of the rectum during defecation (Fig. 56-12), often causing the patient to feel pressure in the perineum. When this separation is identified, the examination should be repeated at a later date after the small bowel or peritoneum has been opacified, as described earlier.[5,21] If the gap between the vagina and the rectum is due to an enterocele, the opacified small bowel is seen descending (herniating) into a deep pouch of Douglas (Figs. 56-13 to 56-15). If rectal prolapse is also present, the small bowel may invaginate into the anterior rectal wall and prolapse with the rectum through the anal

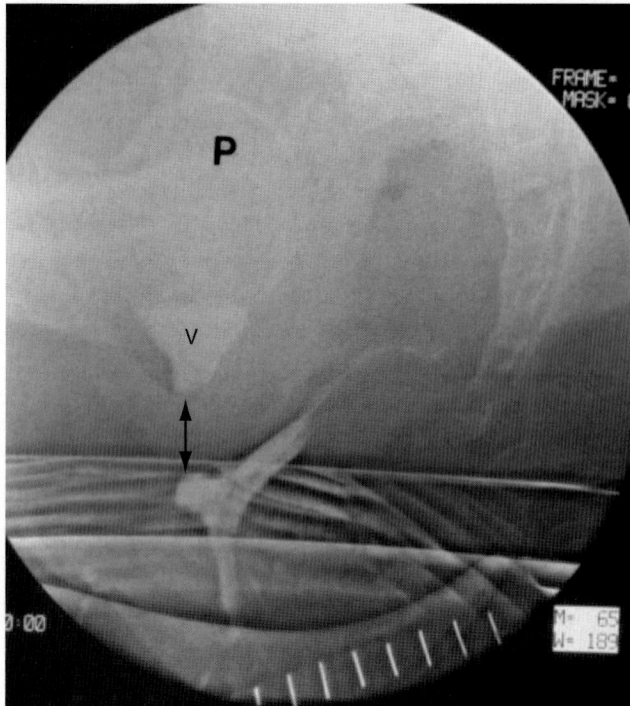

Figure 56-12. Wide separation of the vagina (V) from the anterior rectal wall. This separation (*double-headed arrow*) could be due to descent of either an enterocele or a rectocele into the pouch of Douglas. This finding is often accentuated by postdefecation (P) straining.

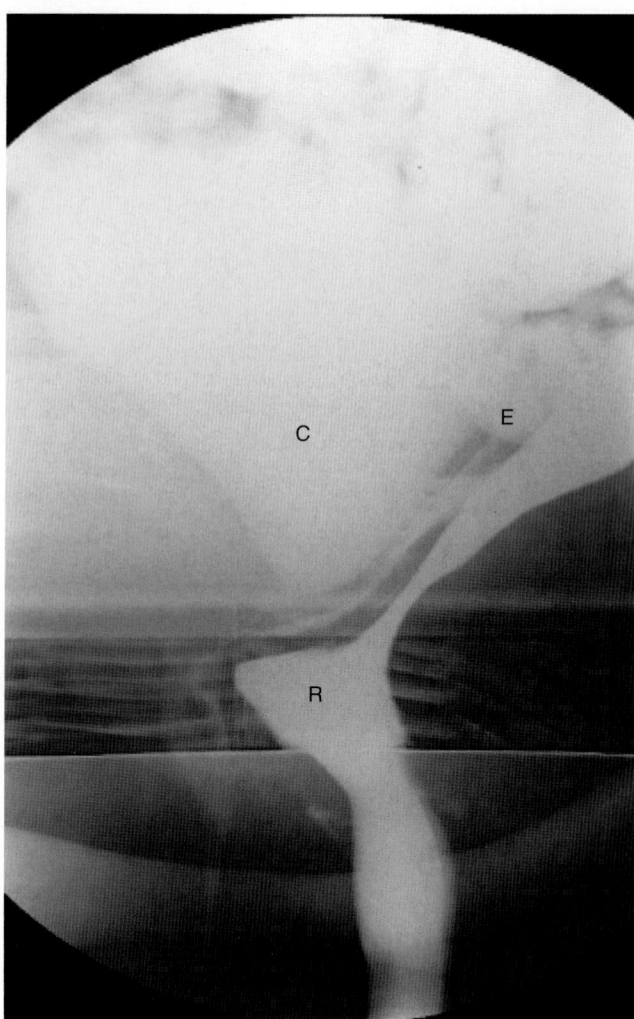

Figure 56-13. Enterocele. Opacified small bowel (E) is seen to be encroaching into the pouch of Douglas. A cystocele (C) and rectocele (R) are also present.

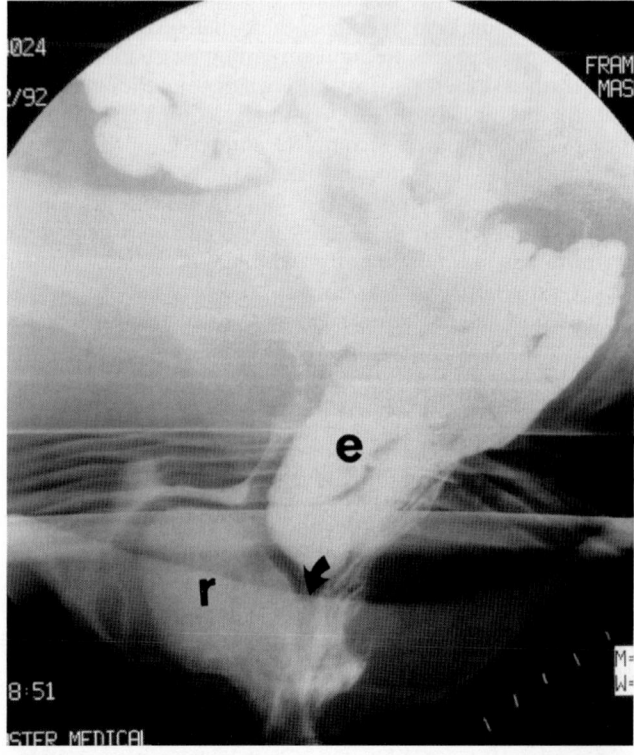

Figure 56-14. Enterocele. With continued straining, the enterocele (e) has become larger and the rectocele (r) has become obstructed by an intussusception (*arrow*).

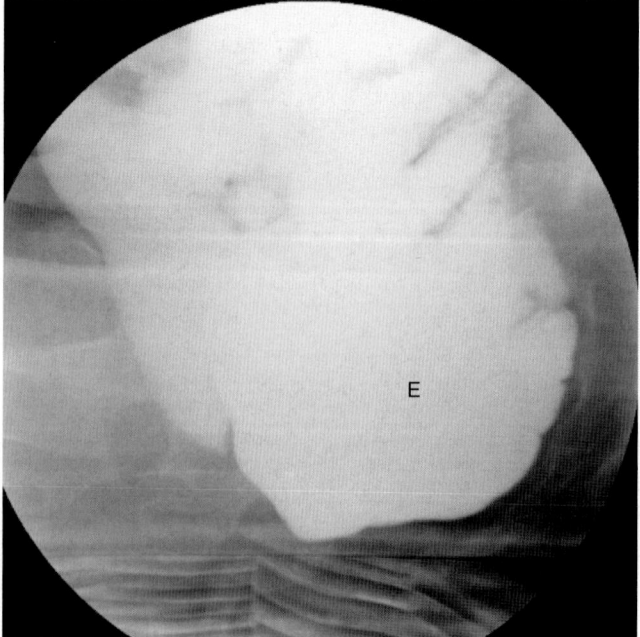

Figure 56-15. Large enterocele fills the majority of the pelvis.

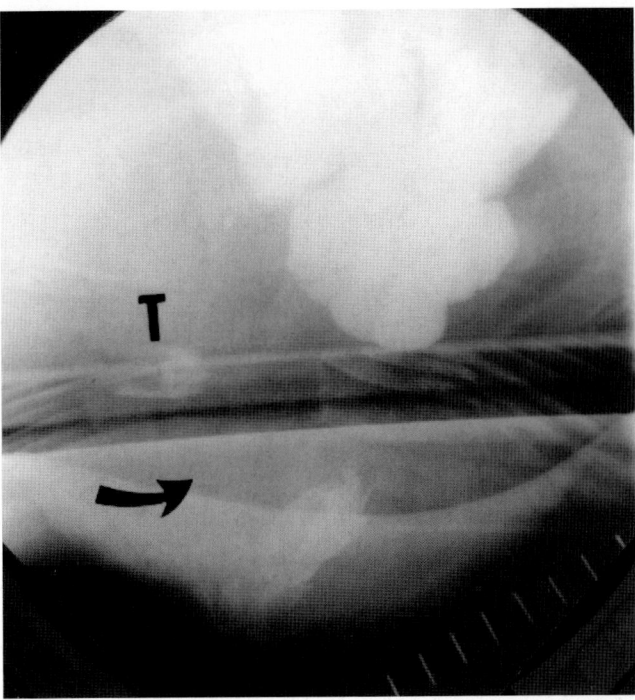

Figure 56-16. Sigmoidocele. The vaginal marker (T for tampon that was used at the time) has been separated from the anterior rectal wall. Because the small bowel has already been opacified, the separation (*arrow*) therefore must be the result of a sigmoidocele, which can be proven by opacifying the distal colon.

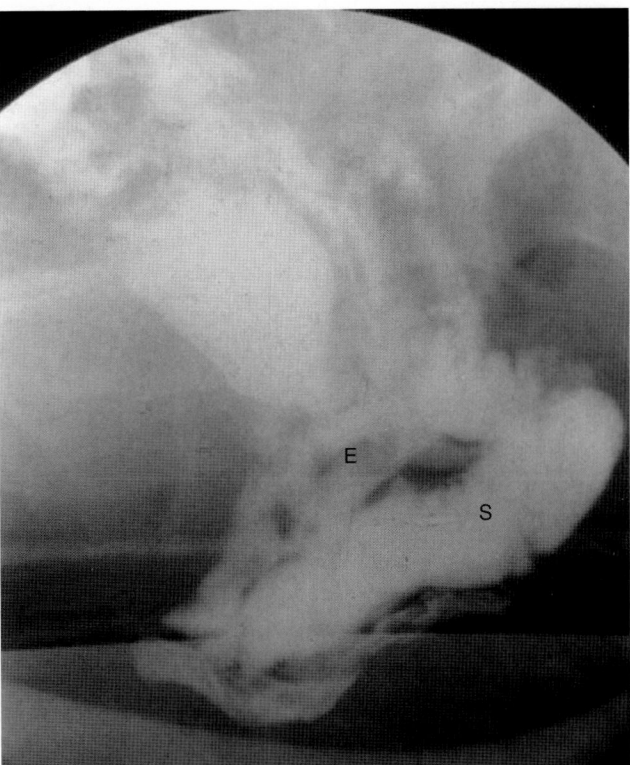

Figure 56-17. Sigmoidocele and enterocele. A sigmoidocele (S) and an enterocele (E) are present. There is posterior displacement of the rectum. Complete emptying of the rectosigmoid is often impaired.

canal. A sigmoidocele can produce a similar appearance, so the proximal sigmoid colon must be opacified to allow differentiation (Fig. 56-16). Occasionally, an enterocele and a sigmoidocele are present in the same patient (Fig. 56-17).

Anterior Wall Prolapse and Rectocele

In anterior wall prolapse, the anterior rectal wall prolapses toward the external anal orifice during the final stages of evacuation. This prolapse is a frequent finding in women and may be responsible for isolating an anterior rectocele. As mentioned earlier, rectoceles are outpouchings of the rectal wall. They are usually anterior, reflecting a relative weakness of the rectovaginal septum. Rectoceles are often accompanied by an intussusception, which may obstruct defecation by occluding both the anal canal and the neck of the rectocele.[23] The anterior wall prolapse may precede an intussusception.

Rectal Intussusception

Rectal intussusception is a concentric invagination of the entire rectal wall that progresses toward the anal canal (Fig. 56-18).[24] It is thought to cause rectal prolapse. The intussusception usually begins 6 to 8 cm above the anal canal as an invagination of one of the valves of Houston.[25] The infolding of the intussusception is anterior in 62% of patients, annular in 32%, and posterior in only 6%. Minor degrees of infolding of less than 3 mm represent mucosal prolapse and are probably not significant. However, inferior extension of the intussusception into the anal canal is abnormal. When an intussusception plugs the anal canal, the patient may

develop symptoms of obstructed defecation[26] and solitary rectal ulcer syndrome.[2] The patient sometimes learns to relieve the obstruction by pushing the "intussusception plug" back with a finger placed in the anal canal. Internal prolapse, as seen with an intussusception plug, is revealed only by evacuation

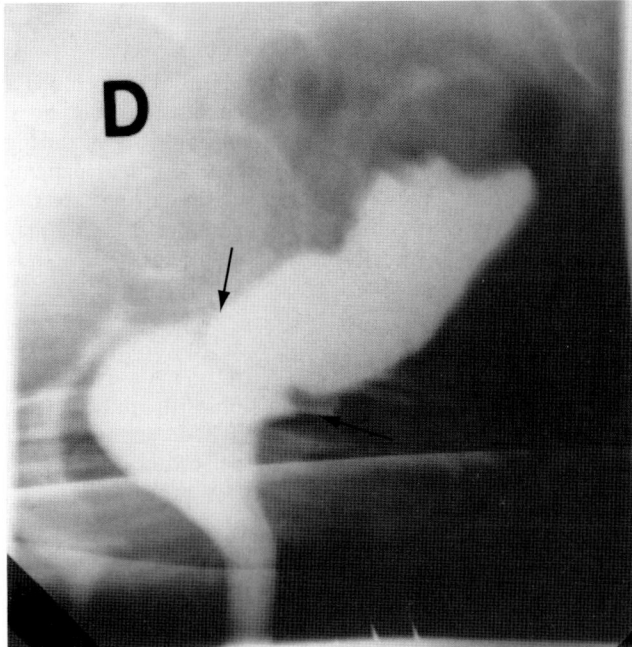

Figure 56-18. Intussusception. The concentric invagination (*arrows*) of a beginning intussusception is demonstrated during defecation (D).

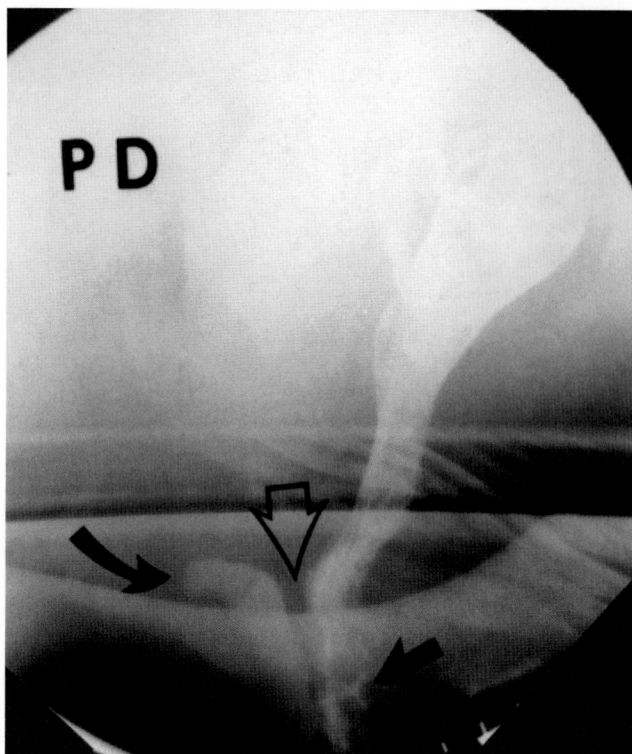

Figure 56-19. External prolapse. External prolapse is shown during postdefecation straining (PD). *Curved arrow,* vagina; *straight solid arrow,* external prolapse; *open arrow,* low perineum.

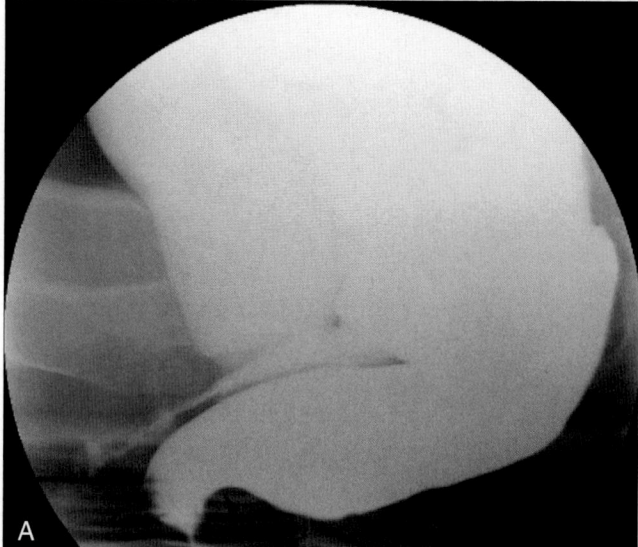

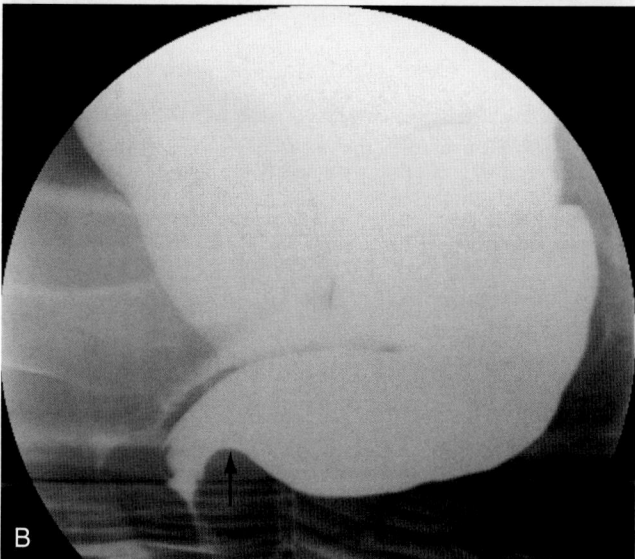

Figure 56-20. Poor relaxation of anal sphincter. The puborectalis impression (*arrow*) is quite marked. The anorectal angle is virtually unchanged between rest (**A**) and defecation (**B**). The descent of the anorectal junction is minimal.

proctography. Occasionally, it is demonstrated during the end of defecation and sometimes only with straining. Spot films depicting postdefecation straining are therefore important (Fig. 56-19). Complete or external prolapses are clinically obvious.

Posterolateral Rectal Pouches

Posterolateral rectal pouches are herniations of rectal mucosa through the pelvic floor. They are often suspected on lateral views but are confirmed on anteroposterior views during straining. These pouches are most often found in patients who have difficulty with rectal evacuation requiring excessive straining. Patients who demonstrate excessive straining may have paradoxical contraction of the puborectalis sling or a nonrelaxing anal sphincter.

Dysfunction of the Puborectalis

In patients with paradoxical contraction of the puborectalis, defecography shows either an increased or an unchanged anorectal angle during straining and defecation (Figs. 56-20 and 56-21). The puborectalis impression is usually prominent because of persistent contraction and increases when the anorectal angle is decreased. This syndrome is relatively common in patients with normal colonic transit and chronic constipation. Bartolo and coworkers found this syndrome in 11 of 49 patients who were examined by proctography.[27] This entity has also been called anismus and spastic floor syndrome.[28]

In some patients, the puborectalis relaxes during defecation but the internal or external anal sphincter muscle, or both, fails to open. Sphincters that fail to relax normally may be associated with anal fissures, spinal cord tumors, and painful hemorrhoids.

Descending Perineum Syndrome

Patients with the descending perineum syndrome also have difficulty defecating. This syndrome occurs when there is ballooning of the perineum below the plane of the ischial tuberosities during straining. Perineal descent is usually less than that of the pelvic floor and can be measured with a perineometer.[29] However, proctography is a more reliable method of assessing pelvic floor descent.[30] This syndrome may be seen in other disorders involving obstructed defecation and may subsequently lead to injury of the pudendal nerve.

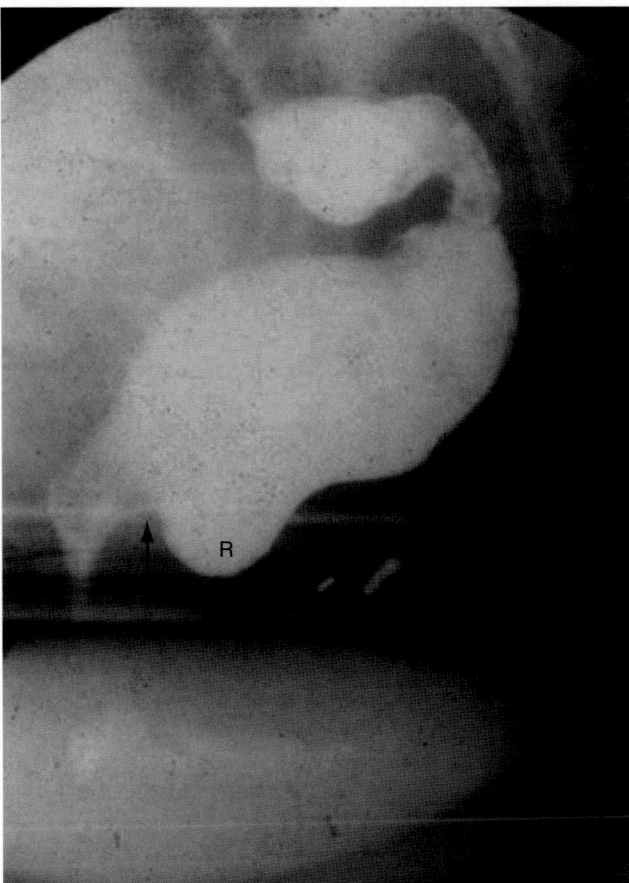

Figure 56-21. Spastic puborectalis sling associated with a posterior rectocele. Occasionally, in patients with a nonrelaxing puborectalis muscle (*arrow*), a posterior rectocele (R) may develop.

Constipation and Incontinence

Continuous straining stretches the pudendal nerve by causing ballooning of the pelvic floor. This stretching has been shown to increase motor latency of the pudendal nerve.[31] Continued straining can ultimately lead to permanent pudendal nerve damage and incontinence.

Normal control subjects have an anorectal junction level above the ischial tuberosity and an excursion of about 3 cm during straining and defecation. Constipated patients have a low anorectal junction level and good lift but little or no movement during straining and defecation. Patients with fecal incontinence have a low anorectal junction level (not unlike constipated patients), a small lift, and a large excursion during straining and defecation. Given that the constipated and incontinent patients both have low anorectal junction levels, it seems reasonable to speculate that these low levels are caused by constant straining and that constipated patients will eventually become incontinent as a result of a pudendal neuropathy. Because lift in the constipated group is still satisfactory, it may be possible to prevent incontinence in this group with a perineal support device such as the Lesaffer seat (Defecom, Aalst, Belgium).[32] The Lesaffer perineal support device is designed to prevent excessive descent of the perineum, permit normal relaxation and expulsion, and prevent or minimize nerve damage.

Evacuation proctography for incontinence is of value only in patients with rectal prolapse, anal sphincter trauma, or neurogenic (idiopathic) incontinence. In rectal prolapse, patients are partially incontinent because the intussusception dilates the internal sphincter. When detected by proctography, rectopexy or a postanal repair can be performed.[33] In neurogenic or idiopathic incontinence, if the anorectal angle is widened, a postanal repair can correct this angle and restore continence.[34] In sphincteric trauma, proctography is useful in assessing the extent of damage to the pelvic musculature and in monitoring healing.

Normal Variations

The abnormal findings in evacuation proctography, as described earlier, are much easier to characterize than the normal findings. This difficulty in defining normal characteristics arises because there are limited data on normal subjects in different age groups[35] and only one study of normal volunteers.[21] The latter study by Shorvon and colleagues showed that the range of normal characteristics is much greater than originally reported. Several investigators agree that the normal mean anorectal angle is between 90 and 100 degrees.[4,5,36,37] In the earlier study, the anorectal angle in normal young volunteers had a range of greater than 60 degrees around this mean. The same study showed a mean pelvic descent of 2 cm; however, pelvic descent was greater than 5 cm in some women and 4 cm in some men. Many investigators believe that a pelvic descent of 3.0 to 3.5 cm between rest and defecation is abnormal; this position has been confirmed by clinical estimates.[38] This discrepancy may be related to the fact that clinical estimates are obtained with the patient lying on a couch in a horizontal lateral position. In this position, the patient may be inhibited from maximal straining for fear of incontinence. In addition, the added weight of the rectal contents that contributes to the downward pull of the pelvic floor is absent. Furthermore, the proximal radiographic anal canal probably becomes incorporated into the distal rectum during evacuation as it forms a "cone" configuration. These factors increase apparent pelvic descent during evacuation proctography. In the study by Shorvon and colleagues, it was also surprising to find that rectal intussusception occurred in normal subjects.[21] However, none of these patients had external prolapse.

In conclusion, evacuation proctography can often provide a unique perspective of disorders of defecation, particularly those relating to constipation and obstructed defecation. Some of the problems depicted by this examination are amenable to surgery. However, because there is considerable overlap between normal and abnormal appearances, it is important to recognize the value of anal manometry, electromyography, colon transit studies, and the patient's clinical findings before making any management decisions.

ENDOSCOPIC ULTRASONOGRAPHY

Technique

Only a few companies have dedicated endoscopic probes for imaging the anal canal. Most use mechanically rotated single crystals to give a 360-degree axial image, which is the optimum plane to image the circular sphincteric structures. The examination technique is very simple. No preparation

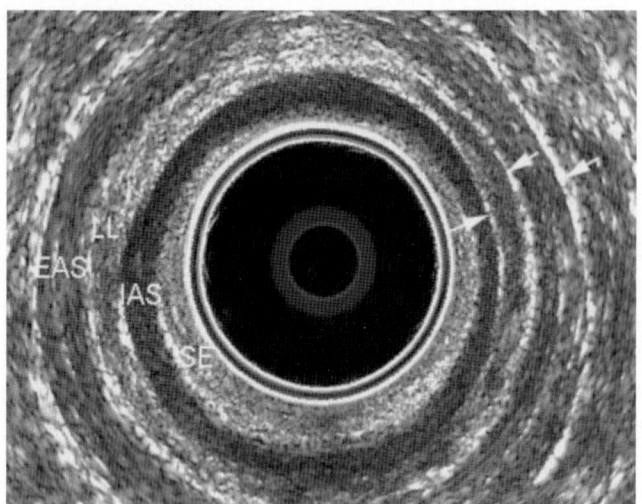

Figure 56-22. Normal axial image in the midanal canal from a 10-MHz endoprobe. Interface echoes (*arrows*) demarcate the inner and outer borders of the longitudinal layer and external sphincter. SE, subepithelium; IAS, internal anal sphincter; LL, longitudinal layer; EAS, external anal sphincter.

flections between layers. Working from the inside out, the first layer is the subepithelium. This is moderately reflective and may contain low reflective vascular channels that are prominent with hemorrhoids. In the upper canal a thin smooth muscle layer of the submucosal muscularis ani may be visible. The next layer, the internal anal sphincter, is the most obvious because it is a well-defined low reflective ring of smooth muscle. Outside this is the longitudinal layer, a composite of striated muscle from the puboanalis with smooth muscle from the longitudinal muscle of the rectum that join together to form an incomplete sheet of low reflective muscle in the upper canal mixed with fibroelastic tissue that continues through the subcutaneous external anal sphincter to insert into the perianal skin. There is usually an interface reflection on either side of this layer. The outer demarcates the inner border of the external sphincter. In men this is a low reflective well-defined layer, but in women it is more reflective and really only differentiated by interface reflections.

In men the sphincters are more or less symmetric, but in women the pattern varies throughout the canal. High in the canal is the U-shaped sling of the puborectalis with the low reflective perineum anteriorly (Fig. 56-23A). Just below the puborectalis, the external sphincter slopes in from either side, joining to form a complete ring in the midcanal at the level of the superficial part of the external sphincter. The transverse perinei and bulbospongiosus fuse with the anterior external sphincter (Fig. 56-23B). The internal sphincter terminates at the lower border of the superficial external sphincter, and below this is the subcutaneous part.

The internal sphincter changes with age. In young children it is very thin, 1 mm or less, becoming about 2 mm in adults, and increasing to about 3-mm thickness in the elderly. This is due to an increase of fibroelastic tissue within the sphincter.

is required. A protective cover is placed over the probe, well lubricated inside and out with ultrasound gel to prevent any reverberation echo, and inserted into the anal canal. Women should be examined prone because in the lateral position there may be some distortion of the anterior structures,[30] whereas in men either position is satisfactory.

The basic four-layer pattern[40] (Fig. 56-22) is created by the differing reflectivity of several layers as well as interface re-

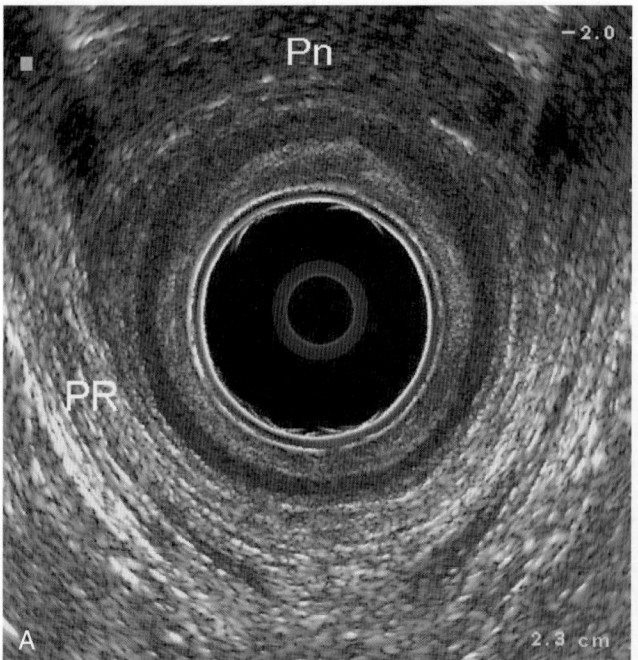
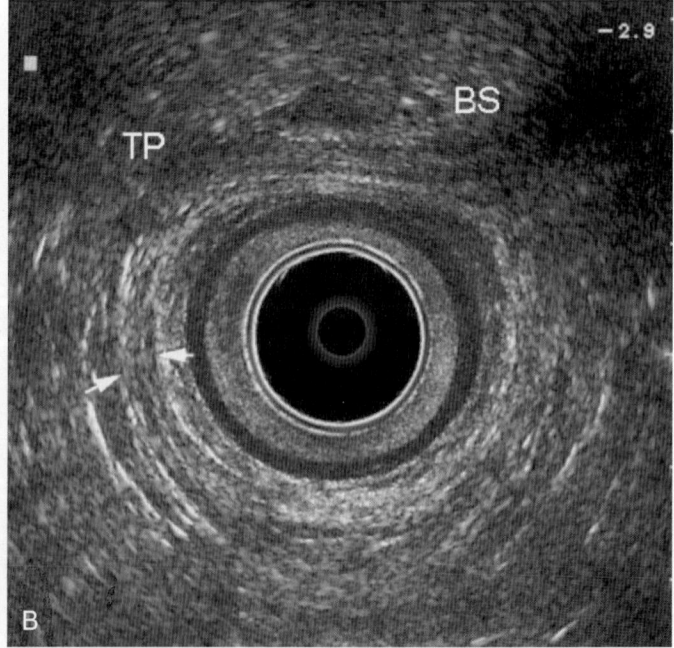

Figure 56-23. EUS of the rectum: normal appearance. A. Axial image in a women high in the canal at the level of the puborectalis (PR) with the perineum (Pn) anteriorly. **B.** Midcanal level with the external sphincter (*arrows*) a complete ring, with the bulbospongiosus (BS) and transverse perinei (TP) fusing into the anterior part of this ring.

Pathology

Abnormalities of Internal Anal Sphincter Thickness

These are easily recognized on endoscopic ultrasonography (EUS). The most common finding is a thin sphincter (Fig. 56-24) for age (<2 mm > 50 yr), which has been termed *internal sphincter degeneration*.[41] The etiology is unknown, but it is associated with passive fecal incontinence. Conversely, the internal sphincter may be abnormally thick for age (Fig. 56-25) and in the 3.0- to 4.5-mm range, when the most likely causes are intussusception and the solitary rectal ulcer syndrome. A thick internal sphincter has a 90% positive predictive value for rectal intussusception.[42] Rarely, an enormously thick sphincter is seen (>6 mm) due to hereditary internal sphincter myopathy, which presents as a profound proctalgia fugax.

Tears of the Anal Sphincters

Vaginal delivery is the most common cause of tears of the anal sphincters. The EAS is affected most commonly, although with more extensive tears the IAS is also involved. By far the most common cause is vaginal delivery, which affects predominantly the external sphincter, although with more extensive tears the internal sphincter is also involved. Isolated internal sphincter tears may be seen after surgery.

Internal Sphincter Disruption

Disruption of the continuity of the internal sphincter is easy to image, because the ends spring apart, leaving a well-defined gap. The lower third of the sphincter is divided during lateral sphincterotomy for fissure. In women, the extent of division is difficult to assess and the entire sphincter may be divided,[43] resulting in some degree of incontinence. The extent of the sphincterotomy may be measured on 3D examination

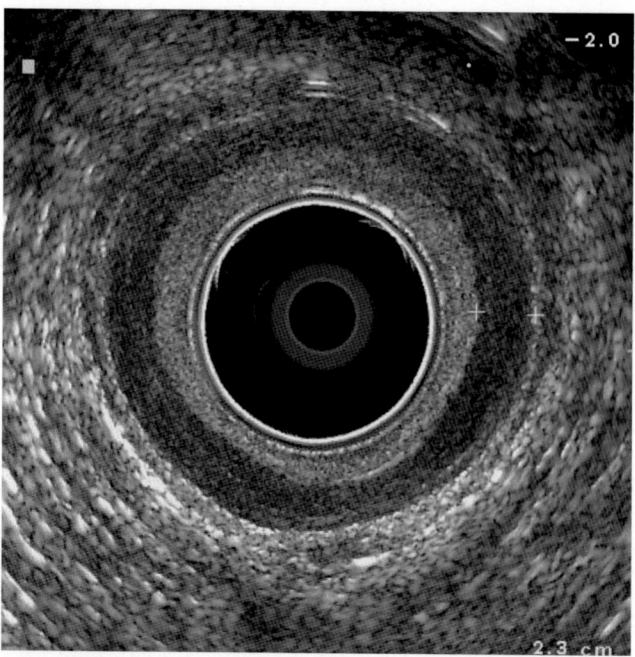

Figure 56-25. Enlargement of the sphincter muscle in a patient with solitary rectal ulcer. The internal sphincter is 4.1 mm thick.

with coronal imaging. The internal sphincter is also divided as part of a fistulotomy for anal fistula. Part of the internal sphincter may be cut inadvertently during hemorrhoidal surgery. Anal dilatation procedures may result in profound fragmentation of the internal sphincter (Fig. 56-26).

External Sphincter Disruption

The striated muscle of the external sphincter is held in place by a fibroelastic mesh derived from the longitudinal layer,

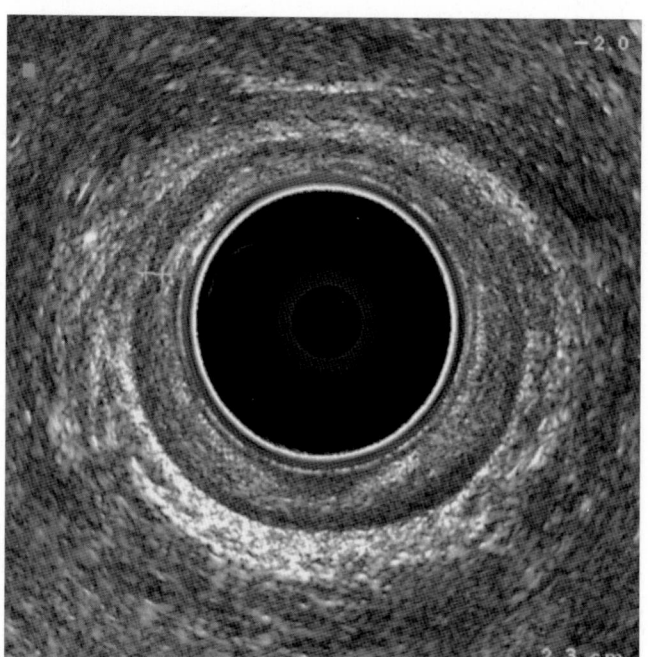

Figure 56-24. Sphincteric atrophy: EUS findings. Thin internal sphincter degeneration measuring 1.1 mm at the calipers, in a 70-year-old with fecal incontinence. Note the poorly defined external sphincter. This patient was proven to have external sphincter atrophy.

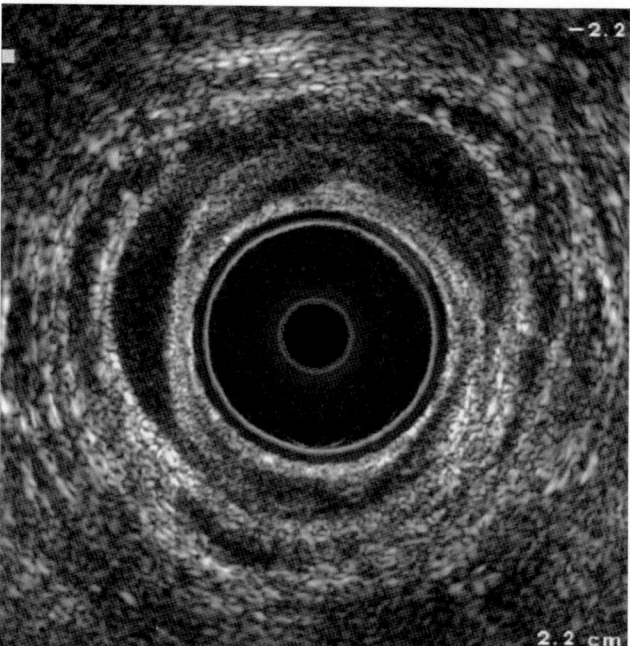

Figure 56-26. Internal sphincter injury: EUS features. Fragmentation of the internal sphincter after an anal stretch resulting in fecal incontinence.

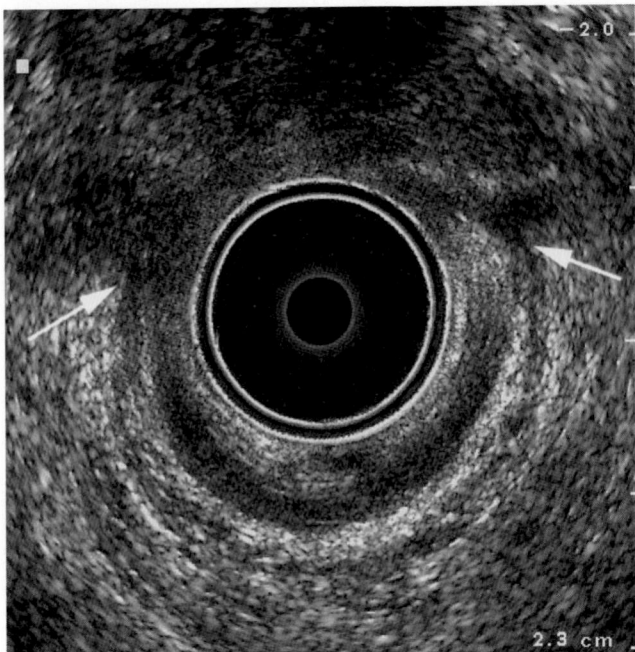

Figure 56-27. Sphincteric tear: EUS appearance. Extensive tear of the anterior aspect of both the external and internal anal sphincters (*arrows*) with low reflective fibrosis extending throughout the perineum.

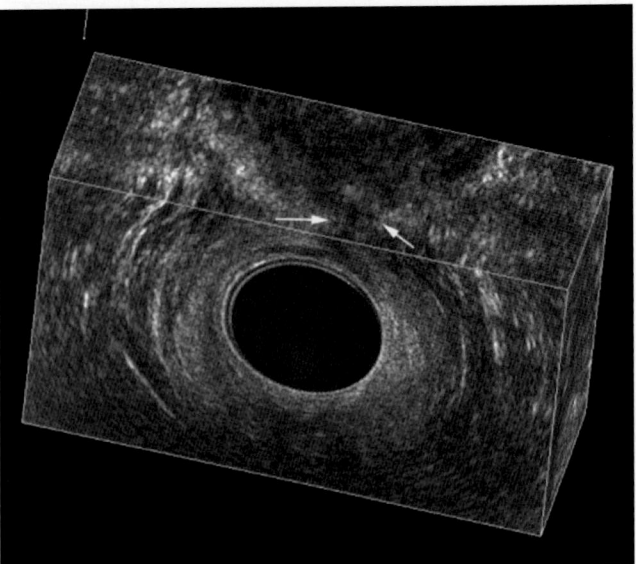

Figure 56-28. Sphincteric injury: 3D ultrasonographic features. 3D view showing disruption of the anterior arc of the external sphincter (*arrows*) due to a minor obstetric tear.

which gives some support when the muscle fibers are torn, so that there is not the same degree of distraction of the muscle ends as in the internal sphincter. In keeping with muscle injuries generally, tears may be partial or complete (Fig. 56-27) healing with granulation and later fibrous tissue. This is of homogeneous low reflectivity, higher than the internal sphincter but lower than the external sphincter, which helps differentiate fibrosis from normal muscle that may be subtle in minor tears. In more major tears, a large area of fibrosis may be seen crossing over damaged muscle planes, including the internal sphincter. In obstetric trauma only the anterior part of the EAS is involved. The loss of continuity of the anterior arc of the EAS is readily apparent (Fig. 56-28) on 3D imaging.

Most sphincter tears occur in the first vaginal delivery. Risk factors include a large fetal head, prolonged second stage, and mechanically assisted delivery particularly with forceps.[44] Many of these tears are not apparent clinically, and the incidence of occult sphincter tears is between 11%[45] and 26.9%[46] for first deliveries.

EUS is helpful after sphincter repair to determine if the external sphincter is intact or if there is still an area of fibrosis between the muscle ends, which is associated with a poor functional outcome.[47]

External Sphincter Atrophy

A good correlation (Ri 0.96) between external sphincter thickness at endocoil MRI compared with EUS has been shown[48] in controls. With atrophy there is an increase in fat and a decrease in muscle bulk, easily appreciated on MRI but not on EUS because the outer interface reflection is lost so that the thickness of the external sphincter cannot be determined. Failure to visualize the external sphincter (see Fig. 56-24) may in itself have a diagnostic value and in one study has been shown to have a 74% positive predictive value for atrophy.[49]

TRANSPERINEAL ULTRASONOGRAPHY

Exoanal ultrasonography, using either probes placed on the perineum or just inside the vagina, was introduced in the early 1990s[50,51] to image the bladder neck and vaginal wall prolapse (Fig. 56-29). The potential for imaging the anal sphincters was soon realized[52,53]; and although concern has been expressed as to the completeness of anal sphincter imaging achieved,[54] it has been proved reliable in comparison to endoanal ultrasonography.[55,56] More recently it has been used to show pelvic

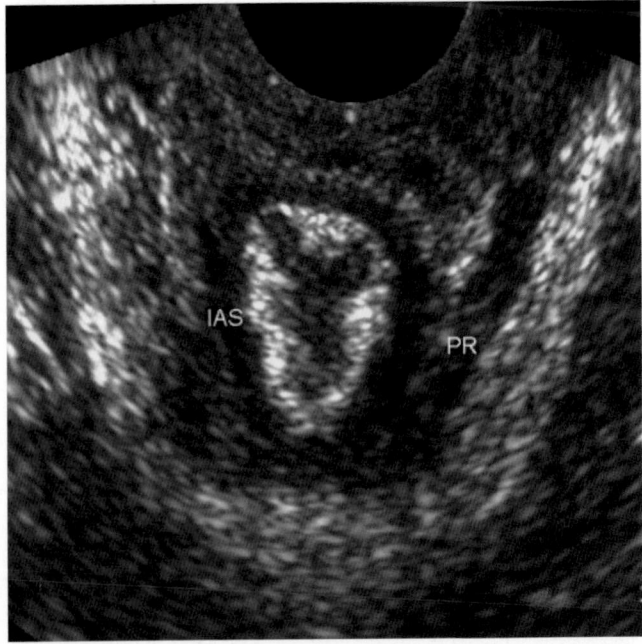

Figure 56-29. Perineal ultrasonography: normal findings. Perineal ultrasound in the axial plane using an endovaginal endfire probe showing the internal sphincter (IAS) and puborectalis sling (PR). Note the anal cushions are seen clearly at this high level in the anal canal.

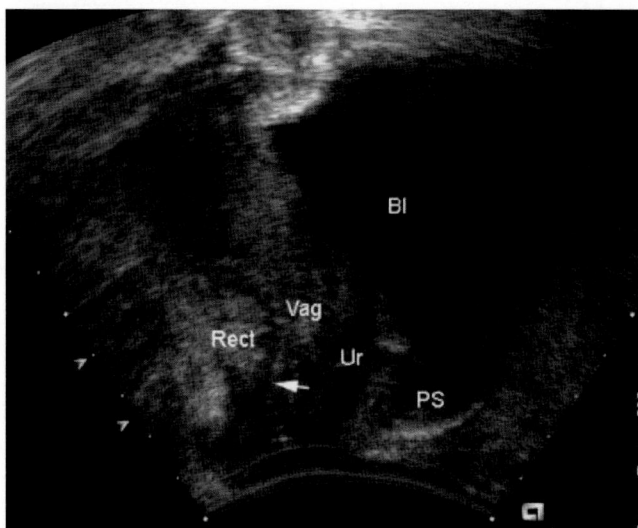

Figure 56-30. Perineal ultrasonography: rectocele. Perineal ultrasound in the sagittal plane showing a small rectocele (Rect) during a Valsalva maneuver. Note the reflective rectovaginal septum (*arrow*), vagina (Vag), urethra (Ur), and bladder (Bl) are all visible and may be related to the level of the pubic symphysis (PS).

floor movement, relating the anorectal junction and bladder base to the pubic symphysis.[57]

Dynamic transperineal ultrasonography involves opacifying the rectum and vagina with ultrasound gel and observing changes during rest and straining of the pelvic floor with sagittal translabial imaging. The sonographic findings have been compared with the findings of defecography.[58] The resting anorectal angle and the position of the anorectal junction both at rest and during straining were comparable. There was good agreement for the diagnosis of rectocele (Fig. 56-30), intra-anal intussusception, prolapse, and enterocoele. Some patients were examined during the evacuation of the ultrasound gel. Rectovaginal septal defects may be identified by herniation of the rectum for more than 1 cm into the posterior wall of the vagina during a Valsalva strain[59] with good clinical correlation.

EUS is an accurate method to investigate sphincter tears or disorders in fecal incontinence. Its weakness is its inability to determine external sphincter atrophy. Perineal ultrasonography, using standard probes, provides a simple and readily available method to investigate sphincter tears but is probably less accurate. A new dimension has been added to this with dynamic studies where pelvic floor movement and rectal abnormalities may be detected. Unless these studies become evacuatory, some rectal problems, such as trapping in rectoceles and internal intussusception, may be underestimated. Three-dimensional studies[60] further enhance the ability of dynamic transperineal ultrasonography to demonstrate fascial defects of the pelvic floor and may become a serious challenge to dynamic MR studies.

MAGNETIC RESONANCE IMAGING

Technique

There are two main methods of performing MR defecography, and they relate to the configuration of the MR unit. The patient can be either supine in a closed-magnet system or sitting in

an open-magnet system. In the closed-magnet system, the position of the patient is limited to the horizontal plane. With the open-magnet system, imaging acquisition with the patient upright is possible.[64,69,70,71] The primary advantage of the open-configuration MR unit is that the seated position maximizes the evidence of pelvic floor weakness and permits analysis of dynamic movements of the anorectum during defecation. In the detection of clinically relevant pelvic floor abnormalities, however, there is no significant difference between these two methods.[72] Therefore, further discussion is confined to dynamic horizontal plane MRI.

Obtaining high-quality, useful images requires careful attention to patient preparation and examination technique. Just before imaging, the patient is asked to void. This prevents a distended bladder from distorting adjacent anatomy. Ultrasound gel (60 mL) is used to fill the rectum. A multicoil array, either pelvic or torso, is wrapped around the inferior portion of the pelvis, and the patient is placed in the supine or left lateral decubitus position. It is important that the coil be placed low enough so that prolapsing structures can be seen.

Scout images are obtained to identify a midline sagittal section with a rapid T1-weighted or gradient-echo large field-of-view localizer sequence. This image should encompass the symphysis, bladder neck, vagina, rectum, and coccyx. The patient is then coached on how to maintain maximum Valsalva strain. Next, 10-mm-thick sagittal images of the midline are obtained with an ultrafast T2-weighted imaging sequence such as single-shot fast spin-echo (SSFSE) or half-acquisition single-shot turbo spin-echo (HASTE) and a 30-cm field of view. These images are obtained while the patient is at rest and during maximal Valsalva strain. The strain images can be repeated after additional verbal coaching if necessary. If a perineal hernia or ballooning of the puborectal muscle is suspected, these images can be performed in the coronal plane. A standard fast spin-echo (FSE) or turbo spin-echo (TSE) sequence is then obtained in the axial view centered on the puborectalis muscle to provide high-resolution images of the supporting structures. The MRI protocol requires no oral or intravenous contrast agents, and the examination can be completed in 15 minutes. Comparison of this and similar MR techniques with colpocystodefecography has revealed very good correlation.[73] The complete protocol is summarized in Table 56-1.

Image Interpretation and Normal Appearance of the Pelvic Floor

The radiologist should begin the interpretation of the sagittal MR images (Fig. 56-31) by drawing the pubococcygeal line. This line extends from the inferior border of the pubic symphysis to the last joint of the coccyx and represents the level of the pelvic floor. The distance from the pubococcygeal line to the bladder neck, cervix, and anorectal junction should be measured on images obtained when the patient was at rest and at maximal pelvic strain. In healthy, continent women, even with maximal downward pelvic strain, MR images demonstrate minimal descent of the pelvic organs. The bladder neck, vaginal fornices, and anorectal junction all remain at or near the pubococcygeal line. The next measurement to be made is the angle of the levator plate with the pubococcygeal line. In healthy women, the levator plate should remain parallel to the pubococcygeal line at rest and during pelvic strain.

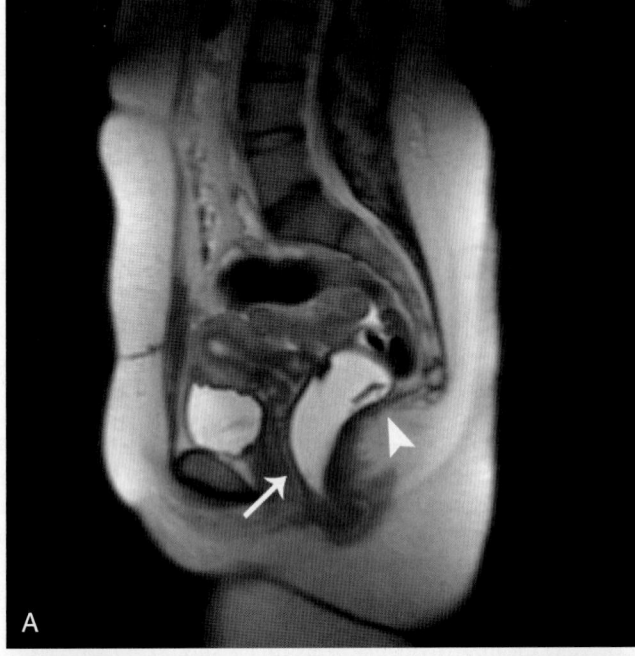

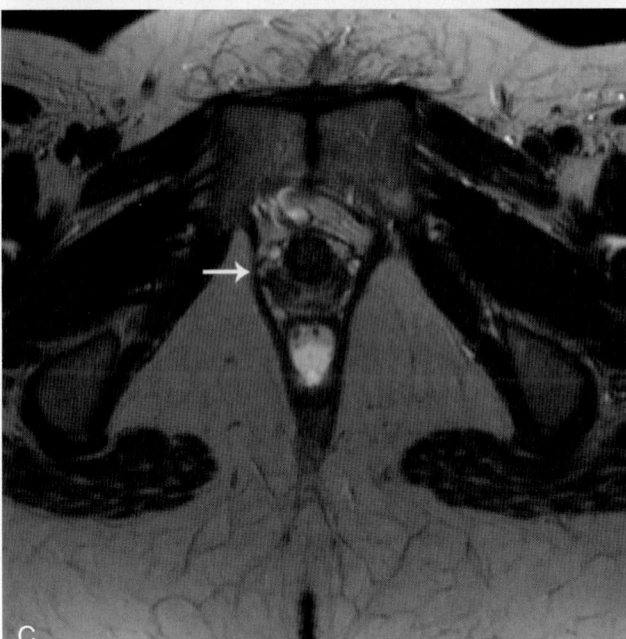

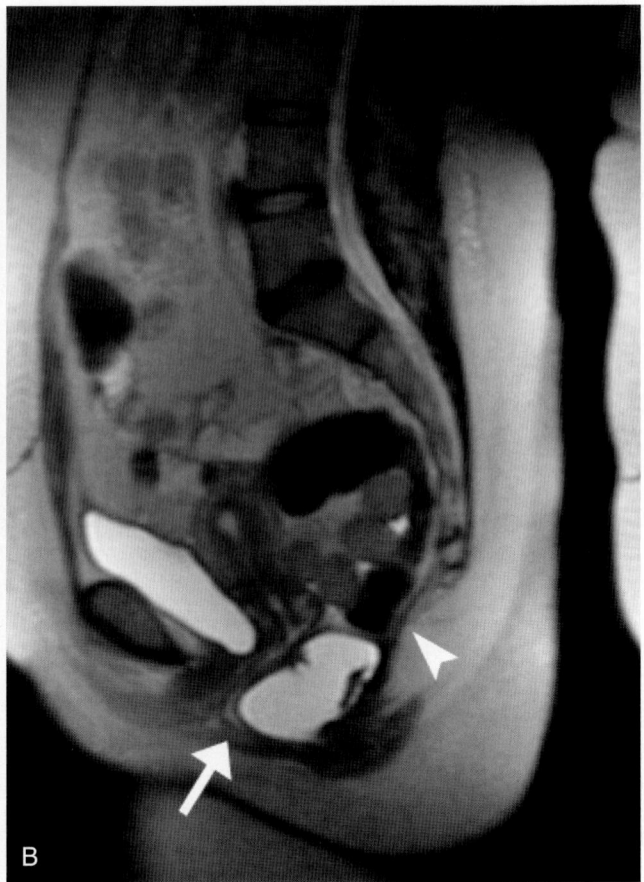

Figure 56-31. Incomplete evacuation on defecation in a 46-year-old woman. A. Sagittal T2-weighted HASTE image at the midline shows the smooth anterior surface of the rectum (*arrow*) and the levator plate in its appropriate position parallel to the pubococcygeal line (*arrowhead*). **B.** Same imaging parameters as in **A** with the patient performing a Valsalva maneuver shows anterior rectocele (*arrow*) and abnormal vertical orientation of the levator plate indicating muscle laxity (*arrowhead*). **C.** Axial T2-weighted image shows thinning of the puborectalis to the right of the vagina (*arrow*). This was confirmed on a coronal image.

Table 56-1
Pelvic Floor Protocol

Sequence	Plane	TR	TE	FOV	Thick-ness	FLIP	P/F Matrix	Nex/Acq	No. Images	Gap	No. Phase No. Meas.	Excitation Order
Scout HASTE/ SSFSE	TRI SAG	4.4	90	350	10	180	128 × 256	1	5	0	1	Interleaved
HASTE*/ SSFSE	SAG	4.4	90	350	10	180	128 × 256	1	1	0	1	Interleaved
TSE T2†/ FSE	AXIAL	5000	132	200	3	180	240 × 256	2	15	0	1	Interleaved
TSE T2‡/ FSE	COR	5000	132	200	5	180	240 × 256	2	15	0	1	Interleaved

*This sequence repeated with patient holding maximum Valsalva.
†This sequence through pelvic floor only.
‡Use no phase wrap.
HASTE, half-acquisition single-shot turbo spin-echo; SSFSE, single-shot fast spin-echo; TSE, turbo spin-echo; FSE, fast spin-echo.

Caudal inclination of the levator plate more than 10 degrees indicates loss of posterior muscular support.[74,75] Measurements of the H and M lines, which were initially described by Comiter and colleagues,[76] are also useful ways to quantify loss of pelvic floor support. The H line is the anteroposterior dimension of the levator hiatus and is drawn from the inferior aspect of the pubic symphysis to the posterior wall of the rectum at the level of the anorectal junction. The anorectal junction is defined on sagittal images as the most inferior aspect of the puborectalis. The M line is drawn as a perpendicular line dropped from the pubococcygeal line to the most posterior aspect of the H line. It measures the descent of the hiatus. In healthy women the H line should not exceed 5 cm and the M line, 2 cm. Both of these lines become greater than these values during the Valsalva maneuver in the patient with pelvic floor laxity. Sphincter tears and rectal ulcers cannot be identified with this MR imaging technique.

On the axial image, the puborectalis muscle should be examined for muscle integrity and signal intensity. The puborectal muscle should extend from the parasymphysial insertion posterior to the rectum and be of similar width along its entire course without evidence of gaps or fraying and show homogeneous low signal intensity. The width of the levator hiatus has not proved to be significant in the identification of pelvic floor laxity; however, it rarely exceeds 4.5 cm in women with intact pelvic floors. On coronal images, the iliococcygeus muscle should be intact and upwardly convex. As women age, some thinning of the levator ani muscle occurs normally; however, no tears should be identified.

Pathology

Rectocele

On sagittal MR images obtained during pelvic strain, a rectocele is identified by anterior bulging of the rectal wall, usually into the pouch of Douglas or, less frequently, into the posterior or lateral aspect. This is caused by inadequate support and laxity of the endopelvic fascia above the anal canal. Many patients have previously undergone hysterectomies or obstetric injuries, leaving them with thinned or torn fascia. Different methods to quantifying the extent of rectoceles have been described. For an anterior rectocele, the size is determined by measurement of the depth beyond the margin of the expected normal anterior rectal wall.[77] Other authors draw a line upward through the anterior wall of the anal canal and describe a rectal bulge of greater than 2 to 3 cm anterior to this line as a rectocele.[76,78] Rectoceles are clinically significant only when symptoms develop, because a small rectocele may be frequently found as a normal variation. Patients may present with obstructed defecation or incomplete evacuation. Many women must also use manual pressure on the posterior vaginal wall to complete defecation. Rectocele is treated with a posterior fascial repair.

Enterocele

Enterocele is a herniation of pelvic peritoneum into the rectovaginal space. It may contain omental fat, small bowel, or sigmoid colon. The latter is also referred to as sigmoidocele. Descent of small bowel loops more than 2 cm into the rectovaginal space indicates tearing of the rectovaginal fascia. Most enteroceles are posterior and lie in the superior portion of the rectovaginal space. Many physicians believe that small bowel loops resting on the sigmoid colon or rectum give patients the feeling of incomplete evacuation and lead to repetitive and unproductive straining. On axial images, loops of sigmoid or small bowel can be seen insinuated between the rectum and vagina. Enterocele repair requires reapproximation of the rectovaginal fascia.

Global Pelvic Floor Relaxation

In these severe cases, there is significant descent of the contents of all three compartments of the pelvic floor below the pubococcygeal line. The levator plate is nearly vertical, and there is extreme elongation of the H and M lines. On axial images there is nearly always increased levator hiatal width and ballooning of the iliococcygeus. This latter finding as well as any associated perineal hernias may be best identified on coronal images. Repair of these patients is complex and often includes hysterectomy as well as an anterior and posterior fascial repair.

Intussusception and Rectal Prolapse

A circumferential prolapse of the rectal wall that descends toward the anal canal is termed an *intussusception*. It may be limited to the mucosa or include mural components. An intussusception that is confined to the rectum is called an *intrarectal intussusception,* and it becomes intra-anal if its apex extends into the anal canal. If the intussusception is extruded through the anal sphincter, it is termed *complete rectal prolapse.* Intrarectal intussusception is a relatively common finding in asymptomatic patients and rarely identified on dynamic MRI with the patient in supine position.[12] If the intussusception reaches the anal canal, or the full thickness of rectal wall is involved, evacuation difficulty can develop owing to outlet obstruction.

References

1. Mortele KJ, Fairhurst J: Dynamic MR defecography of the posterior compartment. Eur J Radiol 61:462-467, 2007.
2. Maglinte DD, Bartram C: Dynamic imaging of posterior compartment pelvic floor dysfunction by evacuation proctography. Eur J Radiol 61:454-461, 2007.
3. Burhenne HJ: Intestinal evacuation study: A new roentgenologic technique. Radiol Clin North Am 33:79-84, 1964.
4. Mahieu P, Pringot J, Bodart P: Defecography: 1. Description of a new procedure and results in normal patients. Gastrointest Radiol 9:247-251, 1984.
5. Ekberg O, Nylander G, Fork F-T: Defecography. Radiology 155:45-48, 1985.
6. Shorvon PJ, Stevenson GW: Defaecography: Setting up a service. Br J Hosp Med 41:460-466, 1989.
7. Bartram CI, Turnbull GK, Lennard-Jones JE: Evacuation proctography: An investigation of rectal expulsion in 20 subjects without defecatory disturbance. Gastrointest Radiol 13:72-80, 1988.
8. Goei R, van Engelshoven J, Schouten H, et al: Anorectal function: Defecographic measurement in asymptomatic subjects. Radiology 173:137-141, 1989.
9. Halligan S, Bartram CI: The radiological investigation of constipation [review]. Clin Radiol 50:429-435, 1995.
10. Hock D, Lombard R, Jehaes C, et al: Colpocystodefecography. Dis Colon Rectum 36:1015-1021, 1993.
11. Halligan S, Bartram CI: Evacuating proctography combined with positive contrast peritoneography to demonstrate pelvic floor hernias. Abdom Imaging 20:442-445, 1995.
12. Sentovich SM, Rivela LJ, Thorson AG, et al: Simultaneous dynamic

proctography and peritoneography for pelvic floor disorders. Dis Colon Rectum 38:912-915, 1995.

13. Bremmer S, Ahlback SO, Uden R, Mellgren A: Simultaneous defecography and peritoneography in defecation disorders. Dis Colon Rectum 38:969-973, 1995.
14. Meyers MA: Peritoneography: Normal and pathologic anatomy. AJR 117:353-365, 1973.
15. Ekberg O: Inguinal herniography in adults: Technique, normal anatomy and diagnostic criteria for hernias. Radiology 138:31-36, 1981.
16. Bartram CI, Mahieu PHG: Evacuation proctography and anal endosonography. In Henry MM, Swash M (eds): Coloproctology and the Pelvic Floor. London, Butterworth, 1991, pp 146-172.
17. Finlay IG, Bartolo DCC, Bartram CI, et al. Symposium: Protography. Int J Colorectal Dis 3:67-89, 1988.
18. Archer BD, Somers S, Stevenson GW: Contrast medium gel for marking vaginal position during defecography [technical note]. Radiology 182:278-279, 1992.
19. Schoenenberger AW, Debatin JF, Guldenschuh I, et al: Dynamic MR defecography with a superconducting, open configuration MR system. Radiology 206:641-646, 1998.
20. Bernier P, Stevenson GW, Shorvon P: Defecography commode. Radiology 166:891-892, 1988.
21. Shorvon PJ, McHugh S, Diamant NE, et al: Defecography in normal volunteers: Results and implications. Gut 30:1737-1749, 1989.
22. Penninckx F, Debruyne C, Lestar B, Kerremans R: Observer variation in the radiological measurement of the anorectal angle. Int J Colorectal Dis 5:94-97, 1990.
23. Mahieu P, Pringot J, Bodart P: Defecography: II. Contribution to the diagnosis of defecation disorders. Gastrointest Radiol 9:253-261, 1984.
24. Hoffman MJ, Kodner IJ, Fry RD: Internal intussusception of the rectum: Diagnosis and surgical management. Dis Colon Rectum 27:435-441, 1984.
25. Broden B, Snellman B: Procidentia of the rectum studied with cineradiography: A contribution to the discussion of causative mechanism. Dis Colon Rectum 11:330-347, 1968.
26. Bartolo DC, Roe AM, Virjee J, Mortensen NJ: Evacuation proctography in obstructed defaecation and rectal intussusception. Br J Surg 72(Suppl): S111-S116, 1985.
27. Bartolo DC, Roe AM, Virjee J, et al: An analysis of rectal morphology in obstructed defaecation. Int J Colorectal Dis 3:17-22, 1988.
28. Kuijpers HC, Bleijenberg G: The spastic pelvic floor syndrome: A cause of constipation. Dis Colon Rectum 28:669-672, 1985.
29. Henry MM, Parks AG, Swash M: The pelvic floor musculature in the descending perineum syndrome. Br J Surg 69:470-472, 1982.
30. Oettle GJ, Roe AM, Bartolo DC, Mortensen NJ: What is the best way of measuring perineal descent? A comparison of radiographic and clinical methods. Br J Surg 72:999-1001, 1985.
31. Vernava AM, Longo WE, Daniel GL: Pudendal neuropathy and the importance of EMG evaluation of fecal incontinence. Dis Colon Rectum 36:23-27, 1993.
32. Lesaffer LPA: Perineal support device. In Smith LE (ed): Practical Guide to Anorectal Testing. New York, Igaku-Shoin, 1990, pp 205-208.
33. Penninckx FM (moderator): Faecal incontinence: Symposium. Int J Colorectal Dis 2:173-186, 1987.
34. Henry MM: Pathogenesis and management of fecal incontinence in the adult. Gastroenterol Clin North Am 16:35-45, 1987.
35. McHugh SM, Diamant NE: Anal canal pressure profile: A reappraisal as determined by rapid pullthrough technique. Gut 28:1234-1242, 1987.
36. Kelvin FM, Maglinte DD, Hornback JA, Benson JT: Pelvic prolapse: Assessment with evacuation proctography (defecography). Radiology 184:547-551, 1992.
37. Skomorowska E, Hegedus V: Sex differences in anorectal angle and perineal descent. Gastrointest Radiol 12:353-355, 1987.
38. Parks AG, Porter NH, Hardcastle J: The syndrome of the descending perineum. Proc R Soc Med 59:477-482, 1966.
39. Frudinger A, Bartram CI, Halligan S, Kamm M: Examination techniques for endosonography of the anal canal. Abdom Imaging 23:301-303, 1998.
40. Bartram CI, DeLancey JO: Imaging Pelvic Floor Disorders. Berlin: Springer-Verlag, 2003.
41. Vaizey CJ, Kamm MA, Bartram CI: Primary degeneration of the internal anal sphincter as a cause of passive faecal incontinence. Lancet 349:612-615, 1997.
42. Marshall M, Halligan S, Fotheringham T, et al: Predictive value of internal anal sphincter thickness for diagnosis of rectal intussusception in patients with solitary rectal ulcer syndrome. Br J Surg 89:1281-1285, 2002.

43. Sultan AH, Kamm MA, Nicholls RJ, Bartram CI: Prospective study of the extent of internal anal sphincter division during lateral sphincterotomy. Dis Colon Rectum 37:1031-1033, 1994.
44. Sultan AH, Kamm MA, Hudson CN, et al: Anal-sphincter disruption during vaginal delivery. N Engl J Med 329:1905-1911, 1993.
45. Williams AB, Bartram CI, Halligan S, et al: Anal sphincter damage after vaginal delivery using three-dimensional endosonography. Obstet Gynecol 97:770-775, 2001.
46. Oberwalder M, Connor J, Wexner SD: Meta-analysis to determine the incidence of obstetric anal sphincter damage. Br J Surg 90:1333-1337, 2003.
47. Engel AF, Kamm MA, Sultan AH, et al: Anterior anal sphincter repair in patients with obstetric trauma. Br J Surg 81:1231-1234, 1994.
48. Williams AB, Bartram CI, Halligan S, et al: Endosonographic anatomy of the normal anal canal compared with endocoil magnetic resonance imaging. Dis Colon Rectum 45:176-183, 2002.
49. Williams AB, Bartram CI, Modhwadia D, et al: Endocoil magnetic resonance imaging quantification of external anal sphincter atrophy. Br J Surg 88:853-859, 2001.
50. Wise B, Cutner A, Cardozo L, et al: The assessment of bladder neck movement in postpartum women using perineal ultrasonography. Ultrasound Obstet Gynecol 2:116-120, 1992.
51. Creighton SM, Pearce JM, Stanton SL: Perineal video-ultrasonography in the assessment of vaginal prolapse: Early observations. Br J Obstet Gynaecol 99:310-313, 1992.
52. Sultan AH, Loder PB, Bartram CI, et al: Vaginal endosonography: New approach to image the undisturbed anal sphincter. Dis Colon Rectum 37:1296-1299, 1994.
53. Sandridge DA, Thorp JM: Vaginal endosonography in the assessment of the anorectum. Obstet Gynecol 86:1007-1009, 1995.
54. Frudinger A, Bartram CI, Kamm MA: Transvaginal versus anal endosonography for detecting damage to the anal sphincter. AJR 168:1435-1438, 1997.
55. Stewart LK, Wilson SR: Transvaginal sonography of the anal sphincter: Reliable, or not? AJR 173:179-185, 1999.
56. Roche B, Deleaval J, Fransioli A, Marti MC: Comparison of transanal and external perineal ultrasonography. Eur Radiol 11:1165-1170, 2001.
57. Beer-Gabel M, Teshler M, Barzilai N, et al: Dynamic transperineal ultrasound in the diagnosis of pelvic floor disorders: Pilot study. Dis Colon Rectum 45:239-245, 2002.
58. Beer-Gabel M, Teshler M, Schechtman E, Zbar AP: Dynamic transperineal ultrasound vs. defecography in patients with evacuatory difficulty: A pilot study. Int J Colorectal Dis 19:60-67, 2004.
59. Dietz HP, Steensma AB: Posterior compartment prolapse on two-dimensional and three-dimensional pelvic floor ultrasound: The distinction between true rectocele, perineal hypermobility and enterocele. Ultrasound Obstet Gynecol 26:73-77, 2005.
60. Dietz HP, Shek C, Clarke B: Biometry of the pubovisceral muscle and levator hiatus by three-dimensional pelvic floor ultrasound. Ultrasound Obstet Gynecol 25:580-585, 2005.
61. Molander U, Milsom I, Ekelund P, et al: An epidemiological study of urinary incontinence and related urogenital symptoms in elderly women. Maturitas 12:51-60, 1990.
62. Rush CB, Entman SS: Pelvic organ prolapse and stress incontinence. Med Clin North Am 79:1473-1479, 1995.
63. Harris TA, Bent AD: Genital prolapse with and without urinary incontinence. J Reprod Med 35:792-798, 1990.
64. Fielding JR, Griffiths DJ, Versi E, et al: MR imaging of pelvic floor continence mechanisms in the supine and sitting positions. AJR 171:1607-1610, 1998.
65. Unterweger M, Marincek B, Gottstein-Aalame N, et al: Ultrafast MR imaging of the pelvic floor. AJR 176:959-963, 2001.
66. DeLancey JOL: Anatomy and biomechanics of genital prolapse. Clin Obstet Gynecol 36:897-909, 1993.
67. Tan IL, Stoker J, Zwamborn AW, et al: Female pelvic floor: Endovaginal MR imaging of normal anatomy. Radiology 206:777-783, 1998.
68. Nygaard IK, Kreder KJ: Complications of colposuspension. Int Urogynecol J 5:353-360, 1994.
69. Fielding JR, Versi E, Mulkern RV, et al: MR imaging of the female pelvic floor in the supine and upright positions. J Magn Reson Imaging 6:961-963, 1996.
70. Schoenenberger AW, Debatin JF, Guldenschuh I, et al: Dynamic MR defecography with a superconducting, open-configuration MR system. Radiology 206: 641-646, 1998.
71. Law PA, Danin JC, Lamb GM, et al: Dynamic imaging of the pelvic floor using an open-configuration magnetic resonance scanner. J Magn Reson Imaging 13:923-929, 2001.

72. Bertschinger KM, Hetzer FH, Roos JE, et al: Dynamic MR imaging of the pelvic floor performed with patient sitting in an open-magnet unit versus with patient supine in a closed-magnet unit. Radiology 223:501-508, 2002.

73. Kelvin FM, Maglinte DDT, Hale DS, Benson JT: Female pelvic organ prolapse: A comparison of triphasic dynamic MR imaging and triphasic fluoroscopic cystocolpoproctography. AJR 174:81-88, 2000.

74. Hoyte L, Schierlitz L, Zou K, et al: Two- and 3-dimensional MRI comparison of levator ani structure, volume, and integrity in women with stress incontinence and prolapse. Am J Obstet Gynecol 185:11-19, 2001.

75. Ozasa H, Mori T, Togashi K: Study of uterine prolapse by magnetic resonance imaging: Topographical changes involving the levator ani muscle and the vagina. Gynecol Obstet Invest 24 43-48, 1992.

76. Comiter CV, Vasavada SP, Barbaric ZL, et al: Grading pelvic prolapse and pelvic floor relaxation using dynamic magnetic resonance imaging. Urology 3:454-457, 1999.

77. Roos JE, Weishaupt D, Wildermuth S, et al: Experience of 4 years with open MR defecography: Pictorial review of anorectal anatomy and disease. RadioGraphics 22:817-832, 2002.

78. Leinemann A, Anthuber C, Baron A, et al: Dynamic MR colpocystorectography assessing pelvic-floor descent. Eur Radiol 7:1309-1317, 1997.

Computed Tomographic Colonography

Michael Macari, MD

Computed tomographic colonography (CTC, also known as virtual colonoscopy) has been used to investigate the colon for colorectal neoplasia for over a decade. Numerous clinical and technical advances have allowed CTC to advance from a research tool to a viable option for colorectal cancer screening. There remains controversy among radiologists, gastroenterologists, and other clinicians regarding what the current role of CTC should be in clinical practice.

On the one hand all agree there is tremendous excitement about a noninvasive imaging examination that can reliably detect clinically significant colorectal lesions. However, this is tempered by several recent studies that show the sensitivity of CTC may not be as great when performed and interpreted by radiologists without expertise and training. The potential to miss significant lesions exists even among experts; and, moreover, if polyps are unable to be differentiated from folds and residual fecal matter, unnecessary colonoscopy will be performed.

Currently there are not enough trained endoscopists to screen the entire U.S. population at average risk for colorectal cancer. There are certainly not enough trained radiologists to currently make a substantial impact on colon cancer screening with CTC. Radiologists need to understand the issues related to colon cancer screening, to learn how CTC may impact on colon cancer evaluation, and, importantly, to learn the techniques of patient preparation, data acquisition, and data interpretation. These issues are reviewed in this chapter.

COLON CANCER

Incidence and Risk Factors

Colon cancer is the second leading cause of cancer death in the United States and accounts for approximately 10% of all cancer deaths in both men and women combined.[1,2] Approximately 150,000 new cases and 50,000 deaths result from colon cancer every year in the United States.[1] This translates into 137 deaths per day or 6 deaths per hour. This is unfortunate because most cases of colon cancer are preventable if detected as precancerous adenomas.

In recent years, the incidence and mortality of colorectal cancer have declined. This is attributable to the increased utilization of colonoscopy and the removal of premalignant polyps.[3] However, the cumulative lifetime risk for the development of colorectal cancer is still approximately 5%.[3]

There are several conditions that increase the risk of developing colon cancer, including having a first-degree relative diagnosed with colon cancer or a large adenomatous polyp before age 60, those with inflammatory bowel disease, people with a history of familial adenomatous polyposis or hereditary nonpolyposis colorectal cancer syndromes, and those with prior adenomatous polyps or colon cancers.[1,3] However, approximately 75% of all cases of colon cancer occur in patients without specific risk factors.[3]

The Adenoma-Carcinoma Sequence

Numerous studies have demonstrated that most colorectal cancers progress from small adenomas through a process known as the adenoma-carcinoma sequence.[4-6] Through a series of genetic mutations, small adenomas (<5 mm) are transformed into large adenomas (>10 mm), noninvasive carcinomas, and, finally, into invasive cancer. Up to 80% to 90% of all colorectal cancers likely develop through this series of genetic alterations.[4,7] Analysis of data from the National Polyp Study shows that an average of 5.5 years is required for the transformation of a large adenomatous polyp (>10 mm) into cancer.[3] Moreover, an average of 10 to 15 years is required for most small adenomas to develop these genetic alterations to become cancer.[4]

Small Polyps: Are They Important?

Although most carcinomas arise from adenomas, the majority never acquire the genetic mutations to undergo this process.[3,4] This is based on autopsy observations that up to 60% of men and 40% of women have colonic adenomas.[3] A surveillance study showed that many small polypoid lesions detected and not removed at endoscopy were not present on follow-up endoscopic examinations.[8] These lesions presumably regressed. Moreover, in this longitudinal study of 200 small polyps less than or equal to 5 mm, after 2 years, no lesion grew to be larger than 5 mm.[8] In addition, it has been shown that the majority of diminutive polyps, those measuring 5 mm or less,

are not adenomas.[8-10] More often these small lesions represent hyperplastic polyps or normal mucosal tags at histologic assessment (Fig. 57-1). These lesions have no clinical potential to become cancer.[3] Their removal at colonoscopy could be viewed as false-positive findings. Moreover, their removal could lead to potential complications such as bleeding and perforation and increased costs.

Because many small polypoid lesions in the colon are not adenomas and because those that are undergo mutation into invasive cancer slowly, there is controversy about when to consider a colorectal polyp clinically relevant based on size alone.[11-13] This controversy arises from the fact that there are additional financial costs to polyp excision and analysis. Moreover, there are associated patient risks including bleeding and colonic perforation after polypectomy when compared with diagnostic colonoscopy (Fig. 57-2).

This issue of polyp size is critical if CTC is to be used for colon screening. First, CTC does not routinely identify diminutive lesions (those measuring ≤5 mm).[9,14,15] Moreover, if CTC was able to detect a substantial portion of these diminutive lesions, it could prompt many unnecessary colonoscopies because most of these small lesions will not be adenomas. As a result, screening CTC would not be cost effective. For CTC to be accepted as a screening procedure, diminutive lesions will need to be ignored or, if detected, followed at an appropriate surveillance interval (Fig. 57-3).[9,10]

What are the data on diminutive polyps? In a study of 1048 colorectal polyps measuring up to 6 mm, Waye and coworkers found that 61% were adenomas, the remainder being hyperplastic polyps or normal colonic mucosa.[13] In this cohort of patients with polyps, the incidence of carcinoma

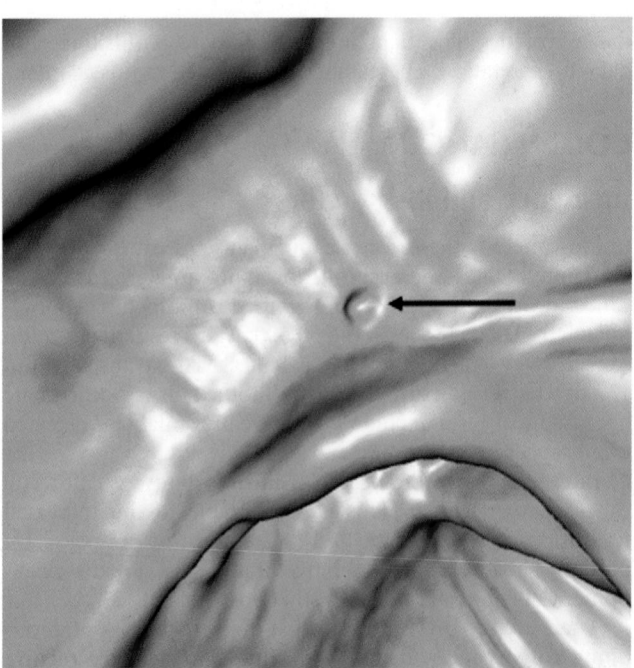

Figure 57-1. Endoluminal image of 3-mm filling defect in transverse colon. Results of histologic examination revealed normal colonic mucosa.

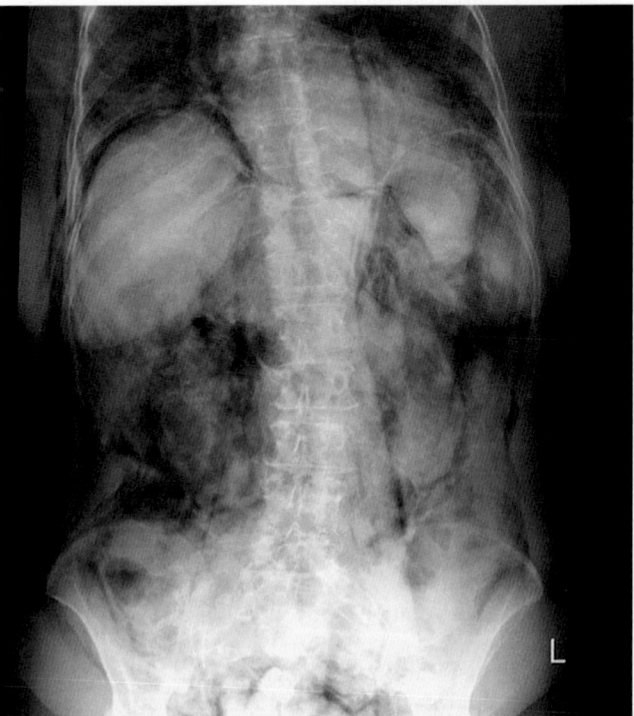

Figure 57-2. Colonic perforation after endoscopic polypectomy in an 80-year-old woman. Supine radiograph of the abdomen shows extensive extraperitoneal gas. At surgery a small perforation was noted in the rectum.

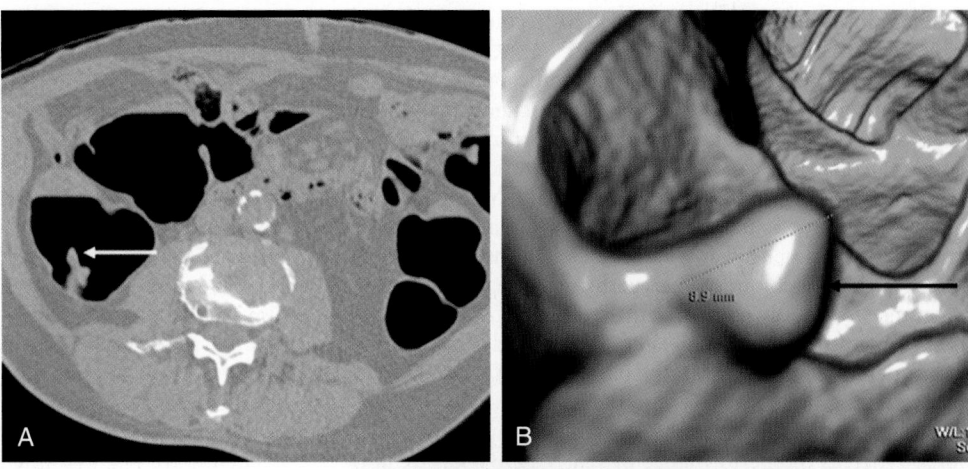

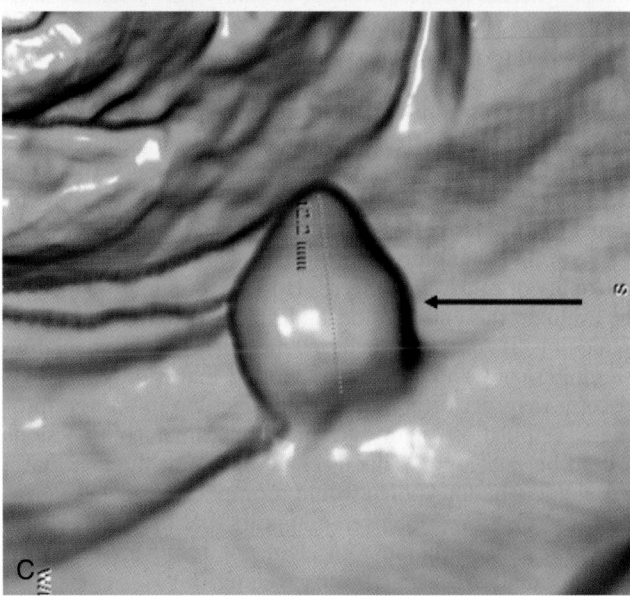

Figure 57-3. Surveillance CTC in an 80-year-old man with an 8.9-mm polyp. A. Axial CT scan in prone position shows polypoid lesion (*arrow*) in ascending colon. **B.** Endoluminal CT scan confirms polypoid morphology and size. Because of underlying medical condition and increased endoscopic risk, endoscopy was deferred and the lesion was observed. **C.** Endoluminal CT scan 20 months later shows same lesion now measuring 12.2 mm (*arrow*). The patient underwent endoscopy and polypectomy, which showed a tubular adenoma. Although this lesion grew, many small polyps do not grow and can be safely observed.

was extremely low (0.1%). Nevertheless, the authors recommended that all diminutive polyps be resected because the majority were adenomas. As a result of this study, polypectomy became a routine part of any endoscopic procedure regardless of polyp size.

Other studies evaluating the significance of small colorectal polyps have reached different conclusions.[16-18] These studies have confirmed that most small polyps are not adenomas and that cancer in small polyps is extremely rare. In one study evaluating over 20,000 polyps, invasive carcinoma was not present in any of the 5027 small adenomas measuring less than or equal to 5 mm.[18] It is estimated that less than 1% of adenomas less than or equal to 1 cm contain cancer.[3] As a result of these observations, and because the adenoma-carcinoma sequence requires time, it has been suggested that attention should be shifted away from identifying and removing all diminutive polyps and toward strategies that will allow reliable detection of the less common, but more dangerous, advanced adenomas.[12] A recent consensus opinion of experts in the field of CTC suggests that the target lesion for CTC should be a polyp measuring 6 mm or larger. Given the benign histology and growth pattern of lesions less than or equal to 5 mm, it is suggested that these not be reported.[11]

Colon Cancer Screening Techniques

The vast majority of colon cancers develop in patients without specific risk factors. The current recommendation for colon cancer screening in asymptomatic patients at average risk for colorectal cancer is that it should begin at age 50.[1] There are several criteria that allow a screening test to be effective. The disease needs to be common, screening tests need to detect early-stage disease, the test needs to be acceptable to patients, and benefits should outweigh the costs.[3] Because colon cancer is the second leading cause of cancer death, screening examinations can detect precancerous polyps, and screening can be cost effective, it would appear that colon cancer screening fulfills at least three of these criteria.[3,19] With proper education, colon cancer screening is also acceptable to most patients.

Current colon cancer screening techniques have been shown to decrease the morbidity and mortality associated with colon cancer by detecting and leading to the removal of premalignant adenomatous polyps.[1-3,19-24] As a result, there is consensus among health care providers and policy makers that screening for colorectal cancer is justified.[1,3,20] The current reimbursable options available for colorectal carcinoma screening include fecal occult blood testing (FOBT), sigmoidoscopy, double-contrast barium enema (DCBE), colonoscopy, and combinations of these tests.[24]

Despite consensus on the need and efficacy of screening, colon cancer remains a major cause of cancer mortality.[2] There are many potential reasons for the continued high incidence of colorectal cancer, including limitations of current screening options, confusion about when and how to perform screening, patient reluctance to undergo screening, or reluctance if there is a need for bowel cleansing when sigmoidoscopy, DCBE, or colonoscopy is performed. Regarding patient reluctance to comply with current screening options, a survey in 1992 found that only 17.3% of patients older than age 50 had undergone FOBT within the past year and only 9.4% had undergone sigmoidoscopy within the past 3 years.[3]

Each current colon screening option has important limitations. Whereas the performance of yearly FOBT has demonstrated a mortality reduction from colorectal cancer, FOBT does not directly evaluate the colonic mucosa.[25] Many large adenomatous polyps do not bleed and occasionally cancers will not bleed. In addition, there are many false-positive FOBTs for colon cancer, which can lead to further testing and expense. A study demonstrated that in greater than 50% of occult heme-positive stool examinations, the source was from the upper gastrointestinal tract.[26]

Screening sigmoidoscopy has been shown to decrease the mortality of colorectal cancer.[27] However, sigmoidoscopy fails to evaluate the entire colon and, therefore, complete colon screening is not obtained.[28,29] Recent studies evaluating sigmoidoscopy and colonoscopy found that if only sigmoidoscopy were performed for colon screening in an asymptomatic population, many advanced proximal colon lesions would be missed.[28,29] This takes into account the fact that a distal adenomatous polyp would prompt a complete colonoscopic evaluation. Moreover, it appears that the combination of FOBT and sigmoidoscopy does not result in significant improvement in the efficacy of screening.[30]

There are currently two reimbursable options available for full colonic evaluation: colonoscopy and DCBE. Norfleet and associates determined the sensitivity of DCBE was 26% in detecting polyps larger than 5 mm as compared with 13% for single-contrast barium enema.[31] A study comparing DCBE with colonoscopy in detecting polyps in patients with prior polypectomy (surveillance evaluation) demonstrated poor sensitivity of the double-contrast barium enema. In this study DCBE missed over 50% of polyps larger than 1 cm.[32] Another study comparing patient preferences of DCBE and colonoscopy found that patients experience less discomfort with colonoscopy and were significantly more willing to undergo follow-up screening with colonoscopy than with DCBE.[33] Although DCBE may be cost effective in colon cancer screening given its relatively low cost, it is a screening examination that is being performed with decreasing frequency.

Complete colonoscopy allows the most thorough evaluation of the colon with the added benefit of biopsy or excision of suspicious lesions. Colonoscopy is considered the reference standard for colonic evaluation.[1,34] However, there are several important limitations to the widespread use of screening colonoscopy, including need for sedation, potential risk of perforation and bleeding (0.1% to 0.3%), costs of the procedure including the need for sedation, failure to complete the examination in 5% to 10% of patients, and an insufficient workforce of trained endoscopists to meet the increased demand.[35,36] For these reasons, CTC is being investigated and used clinically to evaluate the colon for polyps and cancers.

COMPUTED TOMOGRAPHIC COLONOGRAPHY

Computed tomographic colonography is an evolving noninvasive imaging technique that relies on performing thin-section CT of the colon and evaluating data using both 2D and 3D images.[37-55] Clinical evaluation of CTC has shown promise in detecting polyps and cancers of the colon and rectum with per-polyp sensitivity values ranging from 75% to 100% for polyps 10 mm or larger.[14] With the use of thin-section multidetector CT (MDCT), the per-patient specificity for lesions 10 mm or larger is more than 95%.[10,51]

There have been conflicting data published on the sensitivity of CTC to detect colorectal polyps. Two recent studies showed CTC to be as effective as conventional colonoscopy in detecting polyps 10 mm or larger.[9,10] In fact, in one study the sensitivity of CTC for detecting adenomas 10 mm or larger was superior to that of conventional colonoscopy (93.8% vs. 87.5%).[10] As previously stated, the ability of CTC to detect smaller lesions has consistently been shown to be inferior to that of conventional colonoscopy. A recent multi-institutional study showed that CTC performed inferior to conventional colonoscopy in detecting polyps that were at least 10 mm.[15] In this study the sensitivity of CTC for detecting 10-mm polyps was only 55%. There were several limitations to that study, including the training and experience of some of the radiologists involved. As with most imaging techniques there is a learning curve, and with greater experience improved results are expected.[56] A study by Spinzi and coworkers of 99 patients showed that the sensitivity of CTC increased from 31.8% for the first 25 cases to 91.6% for the last 20 cases interpreted. Despite these conflicting results, it is hoped that CTC may improve colorectal cancer screening. CTC may improve colorectal screening by detecting clinically significant colorectal polyps using a relatively noninvasive, safe examination, thereby increasing patient and clinician acceptance of colon cancer screening.[14,15]

Bowel Preparation

There are several techniques that may be used for bowel preparation, and there remains controversy as to how to optimize patient preparation. The goal is to have a clean, well-distended colon that will facilitate polyp detection and minimize false-positive findings (Fig. 57-4). Traditionally, most investigators have believed that the colon needs to be thoroughly cleansed for accurate interpretation.[14,52-54,57,58] A clean, well-distended colon facilitates detection of colorectal abnormalities whether 2D or 3D techniques are used for data interpretation. More importantly, it maximizes the ability to differentiate polyps, folds, and residual fecal matter within the colon.[46] Although currently a clean colon appears to be essential for colorectal polyp detection, many patients find bowel preparation to be the most onerous part of the examination.[33,59]

There are three commercially available bowel preparations in the United States, including cathartics such as magnesium citrate and Phospho-Soda and colonic lavage solutions such as polyethylene glycol. In our experience, the polyethylene glycol preparation frequently leaves a large amount of residual

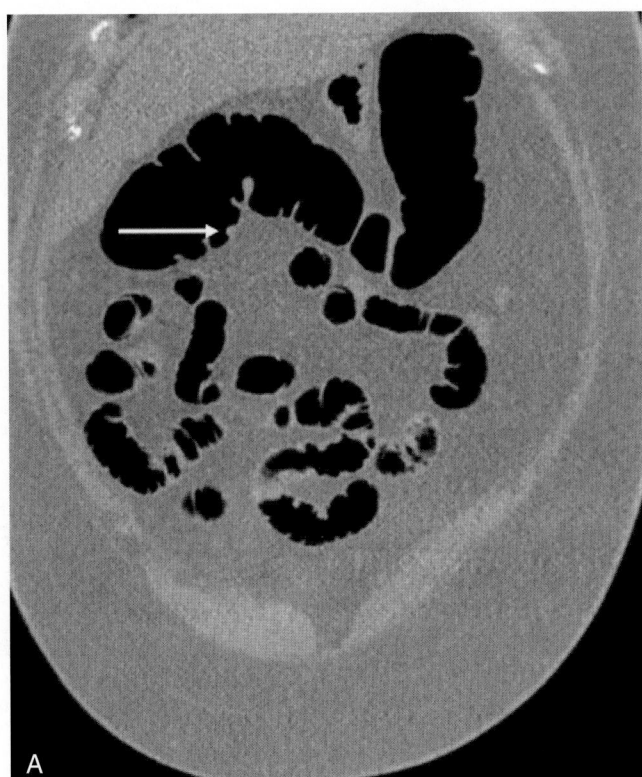

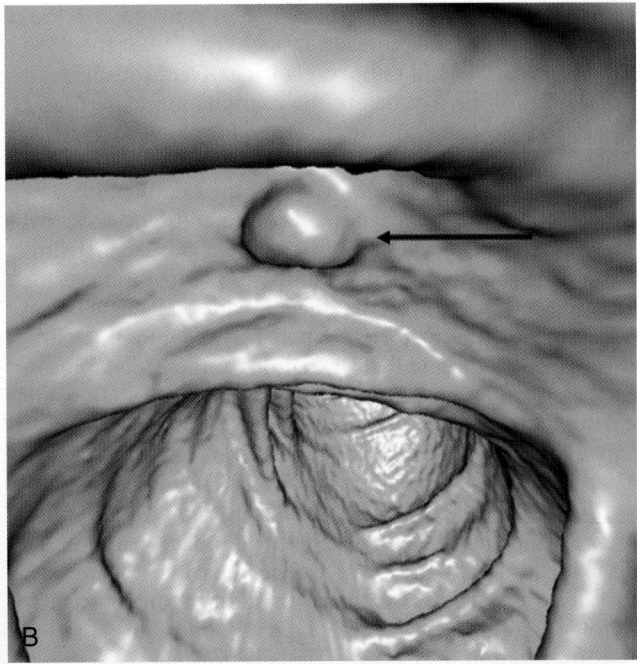

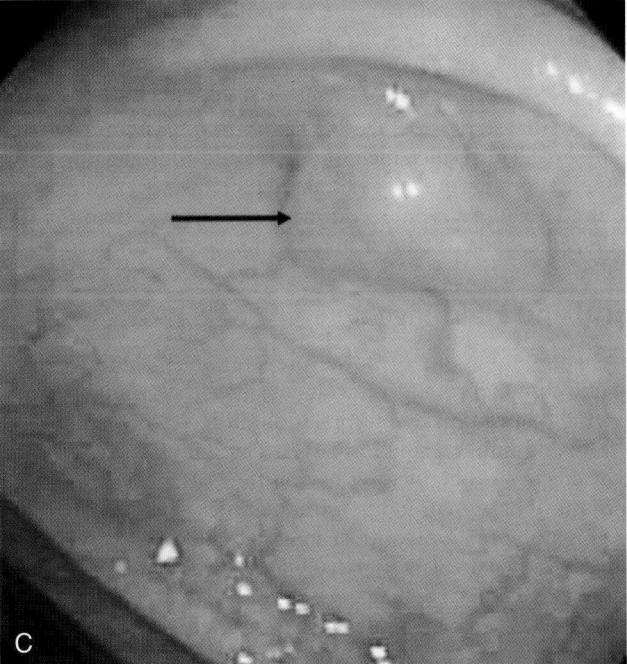

Figure 57-4. Clean distended colon facilitating polyp detection. A. Coronal CT scan shows well-distended clean transverse colon and small lesion (*arrow*). **B.** Endoluminal view shows polypoid lesion (*arrow*) in an otherwise clean colon. **C.** Endoscopy confirms lesion (*arrow*), which was an 8-mm tubular adenoma.

fluid in the colon.[58] Whereas this preparation is adequate for colonoscopy, large amounts of residual fluid will limit CTC. At conventional colonoscopy residual fluid can be endoscopically aspirated from the colon. With CTC, the examination is typically limited to only two acquisitions, obtained in the supine and prone positions. Although supine and prone imaging allows for fluid redistribution, this does not ensure full mucosal evaluation if large amounts of fluid are present. Therefore, the CTC preparation that provides the least amount of residual fluid will theoretically allow evaluation of the most mucosal surface.

Some investigators have found that the use of intravenous (IV) contrast medium may facilitate colorectal polyp detection when large amounts of fluid are present.[60] Occasionally,

polyps will be obscured by residual fluid. After IV contrast agent administration, a polyp will enhance and it may become visible despite being submerged the fluid. The downside of the routine administration of contrast media is cost, need for IV access, and risk of allergy from the iodinated contrast material. In the setting of a known colorectal lesion, the use of IV contrast medium may be justified because better delineation of the colonic abnormality, as well as improved detection of liver metastases, is possible. Most investigators do not routinely administer IV contrast material for screening CTC studies.

Our preference for CTC bowel preparation is to utilize commercial preparation kits for bowel cleansing. The instructions are easy for the patient to follow, and the kits are inexpensive and available at pharmacies. The two commercial preparation kits that we utilize are the 24-hour Fleet 1 Preparation (Fleet Pharmaceuticals, Lynchburg, VA) or the LoSo Preparation (EZ-EM, Westbury, NY). The Fleet Kit utilizes a clear fluid diet the day before the examination as well as a single 45-mL dose of Phospho-Soda and four bisacodyl tablets the day before the examination. In addition, patients receive a bisacodyl suppository the morning of the examination. The LoSo Preparation uses magnesium citrate and four bisacodyl tablets the day before the examination and a bisacodyl suppository the morning of the examination. Our rationale for using these preparations is that they provided adequate bowel preparation for the majority of patients undergoing DCBE. However, we have found that when utilizing these kits, approximately 5% of patients will have inadequate bowel cleansing for complete interpretation. In these cases, fecal tagging or re-preparation with polyethylene glycol may be necessary.

Regarding bowel preparation, polyethylene glycol preparations should be utilized in all patients with substantial cardiac or renal insufficiency. The polyethylene glycol preparation results in no fluid shifts and no electrolyte imbalances. Therefore, it is safe to use in these patients. In addition, many gastroenterologists utilize two 45-mL doses of Phospho-Soda for bowel preparation. Administration is performed the evening before and the morning of the examination. We have found that this combination results in excellent bowel cleansing.[9] A large multi-institutional study utilized two 45-mL doses of Phospho-Soda and showed excellent results for polyp detection.[10] In that study, several other factors may have contributed to the excellent results, including fecal and fluid tagging and segmentation of the tagged material. However, caution is required because it is not recommended that more than 45 mL of Phospho-Soda be administered within a 24-hour period.

Fecal and Fluid Tagging

Given the limitations of bowel preparation, including poor patient compliance and reluctance, as well as residual fecal material that can make interpretation difficult, the possibility of fecal and fluid tagging for CTC is being investigated.[10,61-63] Fecal tagging is obtained by having the patient ingest small amounts of barium or iodine with their meals before imaging. The high-attenuation contrast material will be incorporated within residual fecal matter facilitating differentiation from polyps (Fig. 57-5). Fecal tagging has been advocated by some researchers because tagged fecal matter should allow improved differentiation of residual stool from colorectal polyps.[10,62] However, occasionally tagged fecal material can obscure other colorectal lesions. Moreover, if large amounts of tagged fecal material are present and electronic cleansing techniques are not available, 3D interpretation techniques may not allow evaluation of the mucosal surface. If fecal tagging is used in conjunction with good catharsis, a primary 3D interpretation may still be possible. Whether bowel cleansing is performed with or without tagging, careful analysis of all filling defects in the colon needs to be performed.

Several studies have recently evaluated the use of fecal tagging. One showed 100% sensitivity and specificity for colorectal polyps 10 mm or larger.[62] A study of over 1200 patients who underwent CTC with fecal and fluid tagging before colonoscopy was recently performed.[10] In this study, the detection of polyps measuring 10 mm or greater was the same as conventional colonoscopy. However, in both studies the use

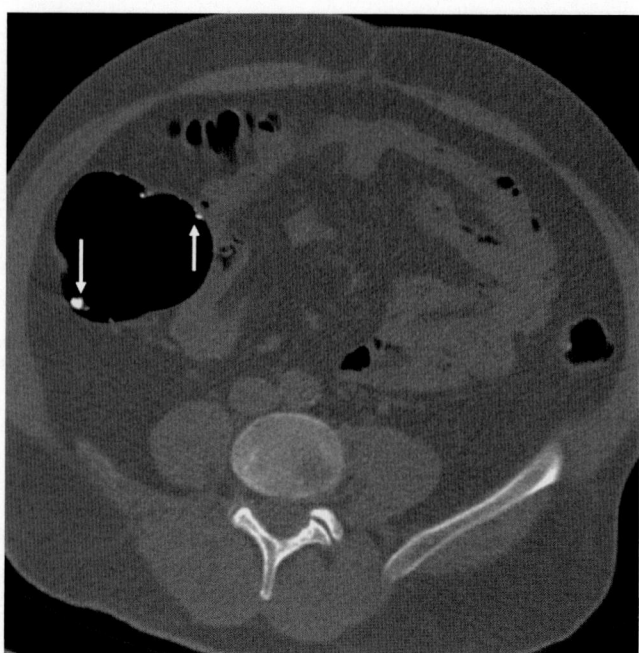

Figure 57-5. Barium fecal tagging in a 63-year-old man. Axial CT scan shows small high-attenuation lesions (*arrows*) in the ascending colon consistent with tagged fecal material.

of either magnesium citrate or Phospho-Soda remains a major limitation of acceptance colon cancer screening.

Fecal tagging without bowel cleansing relies on having the patient ingest small amounts of iodine or dilute barium with low fat and fiber diets beginning 1 to several days before the examination. When CTC data are acquired, residual fecal material that is tagged will show high attenuation. One study demonstrated very good preliminary results for polyp detection using fecal tagging without bowel cleansing.[61] Theoretically, by utilizing computer-generated electronic cleansing techniques, the high-attenuation tagged fecal material can be segmented from the data leaving only the colonic mucosa and filling defects attributable to colorectal neoplasm or polyp.[63] If CTC could be performed without the need for bowel cleansing and yet still maintain excellent sensitivity for polyps 10 mm or larger, it could become the screening test of choice.[38]

Colonic Distention

After the colon is prepared, it needs to be distorted by air or carbon dioxide (CO_2). Colonic insufflation can be performed entirely by a trained technologist or a nurse. A radiologist does not need to be present for high-quality data acquisition to proceed.

Immediately before data acquisition, the patient should evacuate any residual fluid from the rectum. Therefore, easy access to a nearby bathroom is essential. For colonic insufflation, either room air or CO_2 can be used. The use of room air is easy, clean, and inexpensive. Proponents of CO_2 argue that because it is readily absorbed from the colon, it causes less cramping after the procedure than room air.[64] While initial discomfort is usually present with either CO_2 or room air, delayed cramping appears to be less of a problem with CO_2.

A small rubber catheter can be used to insufflate the colon. These catheters are much smaller than a traditional barium

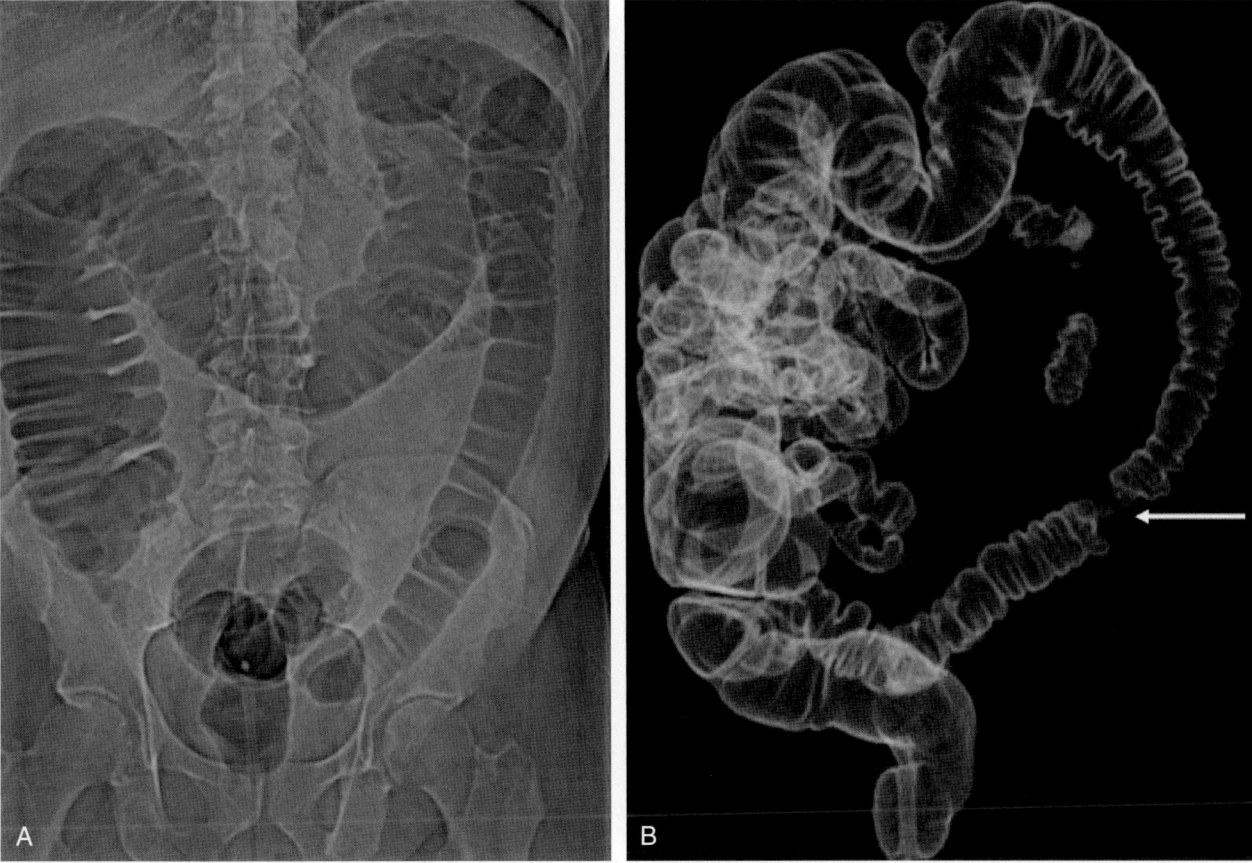

Figure 57-6. Colonic distention using CO$_2$. A. Scout radiograph after CO$_2$ insufflation in a 66-year-old man shows excellent colonic distention. **B.** Segmented view of colon after data acquisition shows annular carcinoma in distal descending colon (*arrow*). Excellent distention is achievable even though patient had near-obstructing colon cancer, preventing proximal endoscopic evaluation.

enema rectal catheter and a balloon is not required. Patients generally do not feel these small-caliber catheters being inserted. Patients are encouraged to retain the gas (room air or CO$_2$) and to let as much gas in as possible. Optimal colonic distention is a prerequisite to CTC data interpretation (Fig. 57-6). The patient is asked to let the technologist know when he or she begins to feel uncomfortable. Generally this signals that the colon is well distended. Approximately 40 puffs with a hand-held bulb syringe is usually sufficient to distend the colon with room air. However, we do not use a strict number of insufflations since the length of an individual colon is variable. In addition, if the ileocecal valve is incompetent more gas will be required for optimal distention. A mechanical CO$_2$ insufflator produces very good colonic distention. With mechanical CO$_2$ insufflation, 1.5 to 2.0 L is slowly introduced into the rectum. A recent study used manual insufflation of the colon with CO$_2$ performed by the patient.[10] In this study, excellent distention was achieved. However, this appeared to be a very motivated group of patients and whether manual insufflation results will be reproducible is unclear.

The use of a bowel relaxant is controversial. Previous data have shown minimal benefit to the routine use of IV or intramuscular glucagon.[54] At our institution, a bowel relaxant is not routinely used. This minimizes cost and patient anxiety because no needles are used. Excellent results in achieving colonic distention without a bowel relaxant have been obtained. A report from England showed that hyoscine butylbromide improved colonic insufflation and the authors suggested that it should be routinely administered when available.[65] This product is not approved by the U.S. Food and Drug Administration (FDA).

After insufflation, the catheter is left in the rectum and a single scout CT scan is obtained in the supine position to verify adequate bowel distention. If adequate bowel distention is present, the CT examination is performed. If adequate bowel distention is not achieved based on the scout scan, additional gas is insufflated into the rectum. After insufflation, CTC is performed first in the supine position in a cephalocaudal direction encompassing the entire colon and rectum. The patient is then placed in the prone position. Several additional puffs of air are then administered or the CO$_2$ is continuously administered. If the CO$_2$ is not continuously administered it will be resorbed and colonic distention will be inadequate. After a second scout localizing image, the process is repeated over the same z-axis range. Supine and prone imaging doubles the radiation dose but is essential to allow optimal bowel distention, redistribution of residual fluid, and differentiation of fecal material from polyps because visualization of mobility of a filling defect indicates that it is residual fecal material. Many colonic segments will be submerged under fluid if only one acquisition is performed.[53] Moreover, polyp detection rates are increased if both supine and prone acquisitions are obtained.[52]

Data Acquisition

Over the past decade, three important advances have occurred in the acquisition of CTC data. These include reduction in radiation exposure, improved CT slice profile, and shorter acquisition times.[9,66-68] These advances have been facilitated by the development and installation of MDCT scanners. These scanners allow 4 to 64 slices to be obtained in a single rotation of the x-ray tube.[9,69,70] Moreover, gantry rotation times have decreased so that now most CT scanners allow tube rotation in 0.5 second or less. MDCT scanners allow large volumes of near-isotropic data to be acquired in a single breath-hold.

For CTC data acquisition with a single-slice CT scanner, data were usually acquired with 5-mm thick sections and a pitch of 2. The resulting effective slice thickness is 6.4 mm related to slice broadening with the high pitch value.[71] To scan the abdomen and pelvis typically requires 35 to 40 seconds using this protocol. By using a 16-slice MDCT scanner with 0.75-mm thick collimation with a pitch of 1.5, the same z-axis coverage can be obtained in 15 to 20 seconds. Data can be reconstructed as 1-mm thick sections overlapped every 0.75 mm. By using a 64-row MDCT scanner, acquisition times are routinely less than 10 seconds.

There are enormous differences in the CTC data that result from single versus multidetector row scanners. First, motion artifact from respiration and peristalsis is decreased or eliminated using MDCT. Moreover, data interpretation is not limited to evaluation of axial images only. Near-isotropic image data are now available that allow coronal, sagittal, and endoluminal images to be obtained from the single axial acquisition, thus facilitating differentiation of polyps, bulbous folds, and residual fecal material.[9,46,66,67,72]

The optimal slice profile for CTC has not been determined, but it is likely that data acquired with thin sections, approximately 1 mm, will improve sensitivity for small polyps and improve specificity. Using a four-row scanner, a 1- to 1.25-mm detector configuration is recommended.[9,66,67] Others have advocated a 4 × 2.5-mm detector configuration.[73] There are two benefits of the 2.5-mm detector configuration. First, the mAs can be lowered and there is an inherent decrease in radiation exposure at 2.5-mm collimation when compared with 1-mm collimation on a four-row detector system.[69,73] In addition, there are fewer images that need to be acquired. However, the radiation dose penalty can be substantially decreased at CTC, and there are several important strategies for CT radiation dose optimization that may be applied (see next section).[74] Moreover, with faster computer processors and greater data storage capacity, large datasets pose less of a problem with current workstations. Finally, by acquiring data at 2.5 mm, the slices need to be reconstructed as 3-mm thick sections. By scanning with thicker sections the improved specificity of thin section CTC is lost.[72]

Radiation Dose

When considering an imaging examination that utilizes ionizing radiation for screening, exposure is a serious concern. In addition to CTC, other screening examinations use ionizing radiation, including mammography and DCBE. The benefits of a particular imaging examination in early detection need to be assessed in terms of potential risks, including radiation exposure.[75] Preliminary studies evaluating CTC with single-slice scanners utilized mAs values ranging from 110 to 300.[41,57,76,77] A resulting effective dose of up to 18 mSv from a high mAs protocol may be incurred given that two acquisitions are necessary.[52,78,79] When utilizing an MDCT scanner, with thin collimation, the resulting exposure would be even greater because there is a penumbra effect of radiation that is delivered to the patient yet does not contribute to the image.[69]

Radiation dose can be decreased at CT by increasing pitch and slice collimation or by decreasing the kVp or mAs.[74] Absorbed dose and mAs values are directly proportional. Because there is extremely high tissue contrast between insufflated gas and the colonic wall, substantial reductions in mAs can be obtained without sacrificing polyp detection. The increased noise resulting from acquisitions acquired with low mAs techniques does not appear to affect polyp detection. In 2002, a study comparing CTC with colonoscopy in 105 patients showed that the sensitivity of CTC in detecting 10-mm polyps was more than 90% using an effective mAs value of 50.[51] The resultant effective dose to the patient for both supine and prone imaging was 5.0 mSv for men and 7.8 mSv for women. The effective dose utilizing this technique is similar to the dose reported for double-contrast barium enema.[14]

Since that publication, several studies have shown that mAs values can be decreased even further.[73,78,79] For example, one study utilized 140 kVp and an effective mAs of 10 with a 4 × 2.5-mm detector configuration and showed 100% sensitivity for polyps larger than 10 mm. The resulting effective dose was 1.8 mSv in men and 2.4 mSv in women.[73] Recent advances in automatic tube current exposure and dose modulation allow even further reduction in patient exposure.[68] By utilizing these dose reduction techniques, the effective dose from a CTC examination becomes close to or even less than yearly background radiation.[79,80,81] A recent study that evaluated the potential cancer risks associated with mass screening using CTC suggests that the benefit-risk ratio potentially is large for CTC.[80]

Although the radiation risk is likely low, it is also not zero.[80] An obvious way to decrease patient exposure and dose is to perform only one acquisition (supine or prone). However, unless adequate colonic distention can be achieved with a single supine or prone acquisition, the second acquisition will be required. One study showed that up to 16% of colorectal polyps will be detected on only one of the two acquisitions.[82] If residual fluid and fecal matter are tagged, segmentation techniques may help to facilitate a single acquisition. Close patient monitoring by a physician will be required if a single acquisition is to be considered. This could negate the potential advantage of not requiring a radiologist to be on site during data acquisition. If adequate distention is not achieved or if there is a large amount of residual fluid, the second acquisition will be required.

When performing CTC examinations, there is the opportunity to evaluate more than just the colon (Fig. 57-7). Because all of the CT data are present, the extracolonic structures in the abdomen and pelvis should be evaluated. Incidental extracolonic findings may be detected.[81] We have found that low-dose CTC can detect highly significant extracolonic lesions.[81] In one study, 136 extracolonic findings were detected in 83 (33.2%) of 250 patients undergoing CTC. Of these 136 findings, 17 (12.5%) were highly significant, 53 (38.9%)

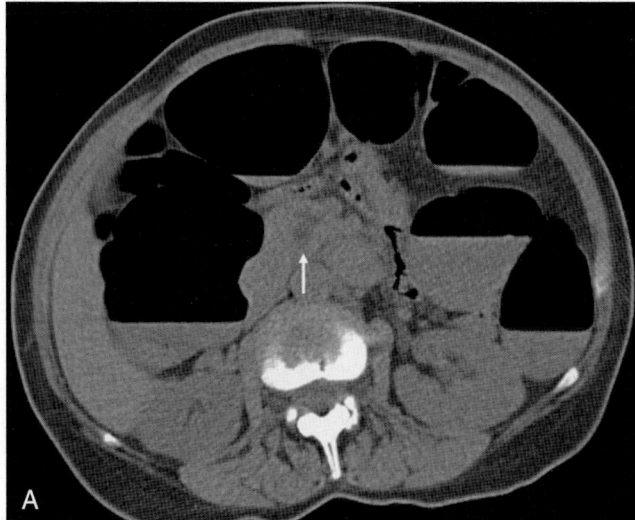

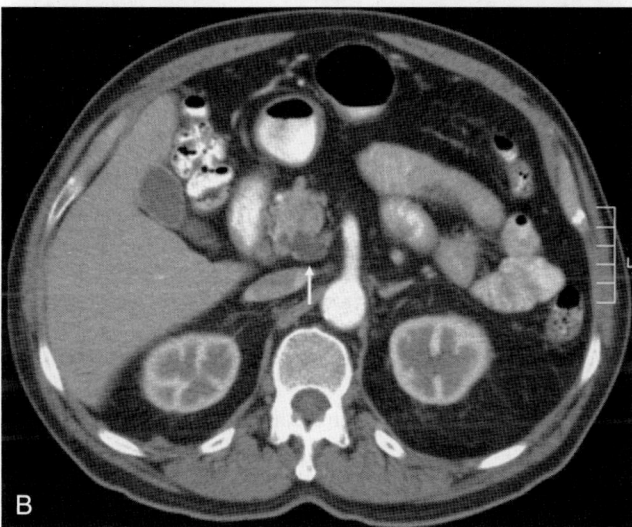

Figure 57-7. Incidental extracolonic lesion detected at CT colonography. A. Axial supine scan from CTC examination viewed with abdominal window level setting shows vague area of decreased attenuation pancreatic head (*arrow*). **B.** Axial supine scan obtained in the same patient after intravenous contrast administration shows small cystic lesion in the uncinate process (*arrow*) that is likely a side-branch intraductal papillary mucinous neoplasm.

were moderately significant, and 66 (48.5%) were of low significance.[81] The most common highly significant lesions were solitary lung nodules in 3 patients, mesenteric lymphadenopathy in 3, adrenal masses in 2, low attenuation liver lesions consistent with metastases in 2, and bone metastases in 2 patients. Fourteen of the 17 (82.4%) highly significant findings were new findings, and in 11 the extracolonic abnormalities resulted in further diagnostic testing. In this study, none of the patients with moderate or low significance lesions underwent further testing. A recent study of 500 male patients who underwent CTC showed that clinically important extracolonic lesions (those that required medical or surgical intervention) were present in 45 (9%).[83] Incidental lesions are more difficult to detect and importantly difficult to characterize at CTC because a low radiation dose technique is used. Moreover, patients do not routinely receive IV or oral contrast material during a CTC examination. Therefore, careful in-

spection is warranted because unnecessary further testing and expense may be incurred.

Data Interpretation

Once the colon has been cleaned, distended, and scanned, the data need to be interpreted. There are two primary techniques for data interpretation: a primary 2D or a 3D approach. In either case, the alternative viewing technique needs to be available for problem solving and to aid in differentiating folds, fecal matter, and polyps.

Two-Dimensional Technique

Traditionally, most investigators have relied on a primary 2D technique for data interpretation.[9,14,39,41,44,45] By using a primary 2D technique the entire colon is evaluated with the axial source images. This is done on a specialized workstation, and the colon is "tracked" from the rectum to the cecum using the supine images. This is facilitated by cine scrolling through the entire colon. If an abnormality is detected, coronal, sagittal, and endoluminal reformatted images are utilized to determine whether the abnormality is a polyp, fold, or fecal matter (Figs. 57-8 and 57-9). If an abnormality is seen during the supine review, prone images may be helpful to determine if a lesion is mobile.[82] The process is the repeated for the prone acquisition.

There are three criteria using 2D and 3D imaging that help distinguish residual fecal material from polyps. First, the presence of internal gas or areas of high attenuation suggest that a lesion is residual fecal material because colorectal polyps are homogeneous in attenuation.[83,84] It is necessary to evaluate a lesion with multiple window/level settings during CTC. This facilitates identification of gas, high-attenuation material, and adipose tissue (Fig. 57-10).

The second criterion is morphology. Polyps and small cancers have rounded or lobulated smooth borders. Residual fecal material may have a similar morphology. However, if a lesion shows geometric or irregular angulated borders, it almost always represents residual fecal material.[45] Defect morphology is best appreciated on thin-section CTC data and 3D endoluminal imaging.

Mobility of a lesion is the third criterion that has been reported to facilitate differentiation of residual fecal material from polyps. Stool tends to move to the dependent surface of the colonic mucosa when a patient is turned from the supine to the prone position.[84,85] Polyps maintain their position with respect to the bowel surface (ventral or dorsal) regardless of the patient's positioning. However, caution is required because pedunculated polyps and sessile polyps in segments of the colon with a long mesentery may appear mobile.[82]

There are two primary reasons to consider a 2D data interpretation algorithm. The first is that by utilizing this approach theoretically 100% of the colonic mucosa can be visualized with one pass. Polyps will not be hidden behind folds as may occur using conventional colonoscopy or a primary 3D interpretation technique. A second rationale for interpreting CTC data using a primary 2D approach is time. For CTC to be a clinically viable tool in everyday radiology practice, the examination needs to be performed and interpreted in a "time-efficient" manner. Although technologists can be trained to perform colonic insufflation (saving radiologist time), the

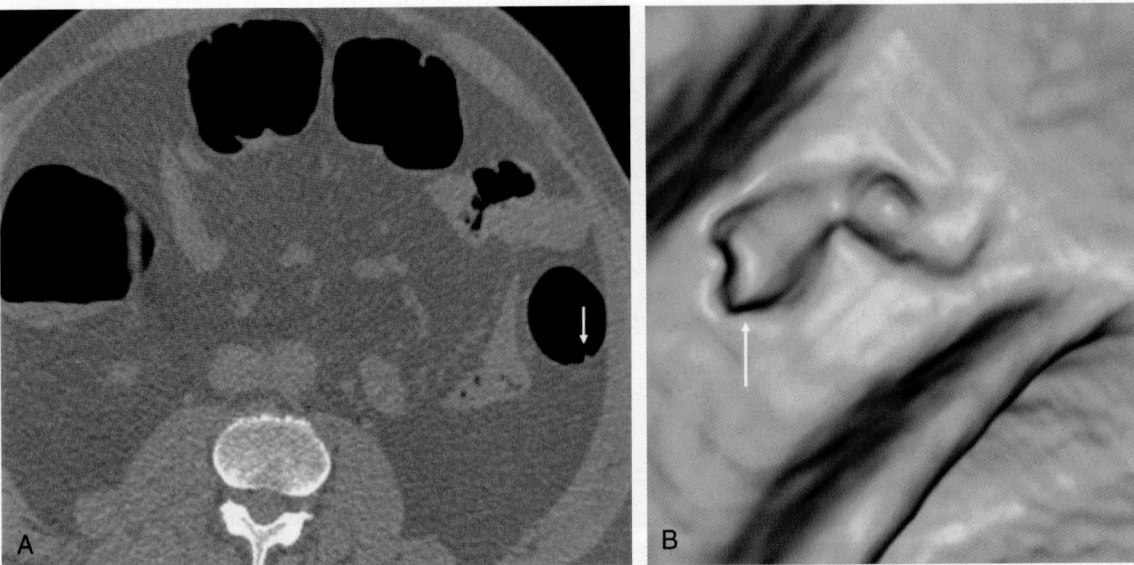

Figure 57-8. Use of endoluminal imaging for problem solving at 2D review. A. Axial CT scan shows small filling defect (*arrow*) measuring 5 mm in descending colon. **B.** Endoluminal view shows geometric morphology (*arrow*) excluding polyp.

potential to spend a large amount of time interpreting data exists, especially with thin-section MDCT where up to 1000 images may be obtained per patient. One study evaluated a large cohort of patients using both 2D and 3D imaging with both antegrade and retrograde 3D colon navigation in both the supine and prone position and showed that the median interpretation time for two different radiologists was 31 minutes.[57] In this study, the sensitivity of CT for polyps 10 mm or larger was over 90%. However, results reported in this study were based on a consensus interpretation and, after factoring in the time for consensus, a significant amount of radiologist time was utilized in evaluating these datasets.

In 1998, Dachman and colleagues reported findings in 44 patients using 2D imaging as the primary imaging technique with 3D imaging for problem solving.[44] In this study of two radiologists, the sensitivity for polyps larger than 8 mm was 83% and specificity was 100% for both observers. The average amount of time spent on interpretation was 28 minutes, 30 seconds. Similar results were reported by Macari and associates in 2000 using a primary axial 2D imaging technique with 3D and multiplanar reformat for problem solving only.[45] In that study, the mean interpretation time using a primary 2D approach was 16 minutes. A more recent study using 2D imaging as the primary imaging technique showed a mean time of data interpretation of 11 minutes.[51] Utilizing 2D images as the primary interpretation technique should allow CTC data to be interpreted within 15 minutes.

Three-Dimensional Technique

When acquiring CTC data using a single-slice CT scanner or a MDCT with slice collimation over 3 mm, the ability to interpret CTC data using 3D imaging is limited because of the poor z-axis resolution. By using a 512 × 512 CT matrix, the typical pixel size in the x and y plane is 0.5 to 0.7 mm depending on the field of view. If 5-mm thick sections are utilized to acquire data, z-axis blurring occurs when images are reconstructed as endoluminal or coronal reformatted

data. Moreover, there is substantial volume averaging within a voxel that may limit the ability to differentiate fecal material and polyps.[72]

However, using thin-section MDCT and improved 3D workstations, the ability to perform a primary 3D endoluminal interpretation is now possible. A study of 1233 asymptomatic patients showed 93.8% sensitivity for colorectal adenomas measuring 10 mm or more using a primary 3D endoluminal interpretation technique.[10] In addition, as workstations have improved, interpretation times have decreased using endoluminal imaging. It is possible that as computer technology continues to improve a 3D interpretation algorithm may become the interpretation technique of choice. To rely on a primary endoluminal interpretation technique, familiarity with 2D interpretation tools and the ability to interact with 2D images is necessary for problem solving.

Primary reliance on 3D "virtual colonoscopy" techniques has the appeal of truly simulating a conventional colonoscopy. Several workstation vendors are incorporating a computer-generated centerline path that will automatically generate an endoluminal navigation of the colon traversing this center path. With improvements in software one can then navigate through the colon and evaluate suspicious abnormalities. However, despite the optimism of a primary 3D review, there are several potential limitations of this imaging technique. First, there are blind spots in the colon using 3D endoluminal views.[86] This is true even if antegrade and retrograde interrogation of the colon is performed. To optimize data interpretation, the colon needs to be evaluated with four fly-throughs (supine and prone), antegrade and retrograde. This does increase interpretation times. Several workstations currently have the capacity to display these "blind" areas to the reviewer after the 3D navigation is performed. This should allow a more complete visualization of the colon using a primary 3D interpretation technique. Moreover, improved 3D panoramic display techniques are being developed that that should enable complete visualization of the undersurface of interhaustral folds that will improve polyp visualization and at the same

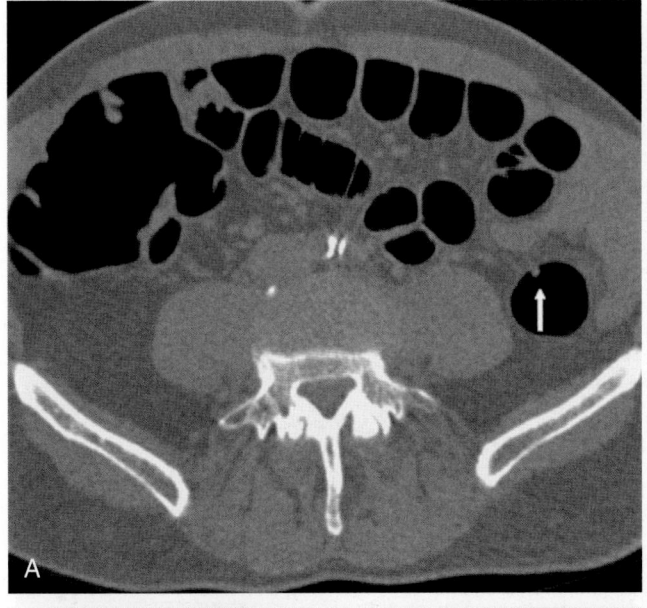

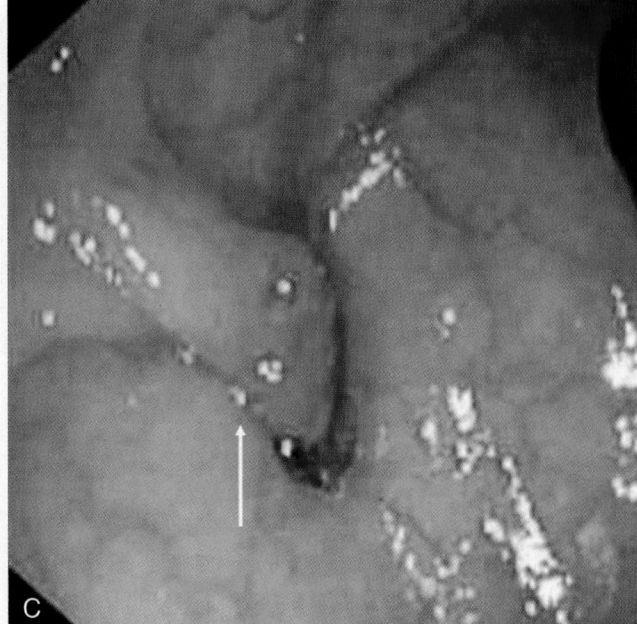

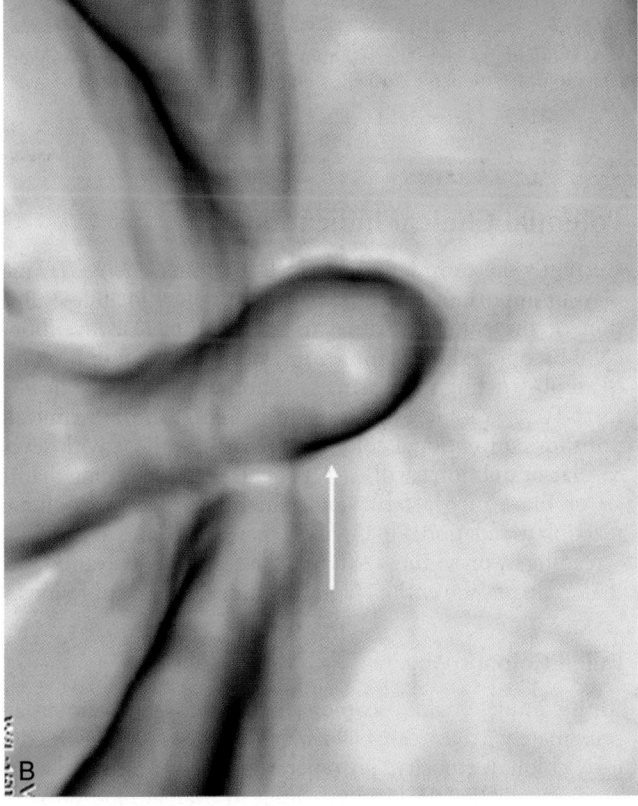

Figure 57-9. Use of endoluminal imaging for problem solving at 2D review. A. Axial CT scan shows small filling defect (*arrow*) measuring 6 mm in descending colon. **B.** Endoluminal view shows rounded lobulated morphology suggesting polyp (*arrow*). **C.** Colonoscopy confirms lesion (*arrow*).

time decrease interpretation times.[86] While it is hoped that these panoramic or "virtual pathology" techniques that unfold and dissect the colon will allow a rapid and accurate interpretation, an initial evaluation of the virtual pathology technique did not show improved lesion detection when compared with 2D interpretation. In this study for polyps 10 mm or larger, the respective sensitivities among two different readers were 67% and 89% for virtual colon dissection and 89% and 100% for axial interpretation. The average time for reconstruction and analysis of virtual colon dissection was 36.8 minutes versus 29.2 minutes for axial images.[87]

A second limitation of 3D endoluminal fly-through imaging is that the center line cannot be generated when segments of the colon are not well distended. In these cases endoluminal navigation is impossible. Third, in overdistended segments, the center line may jump to an adjacent distended loop. Finally, it has been suggested that flat or annular lesions are best seen on axial 2D review using abdomen window/level setting (400W/40L).[46] Therefore, whether performing either a primary 2D or 3D review, it is important to scroll through the data using 2D axial abdomen window/level settings to optimally detect flat and annular type lesions.

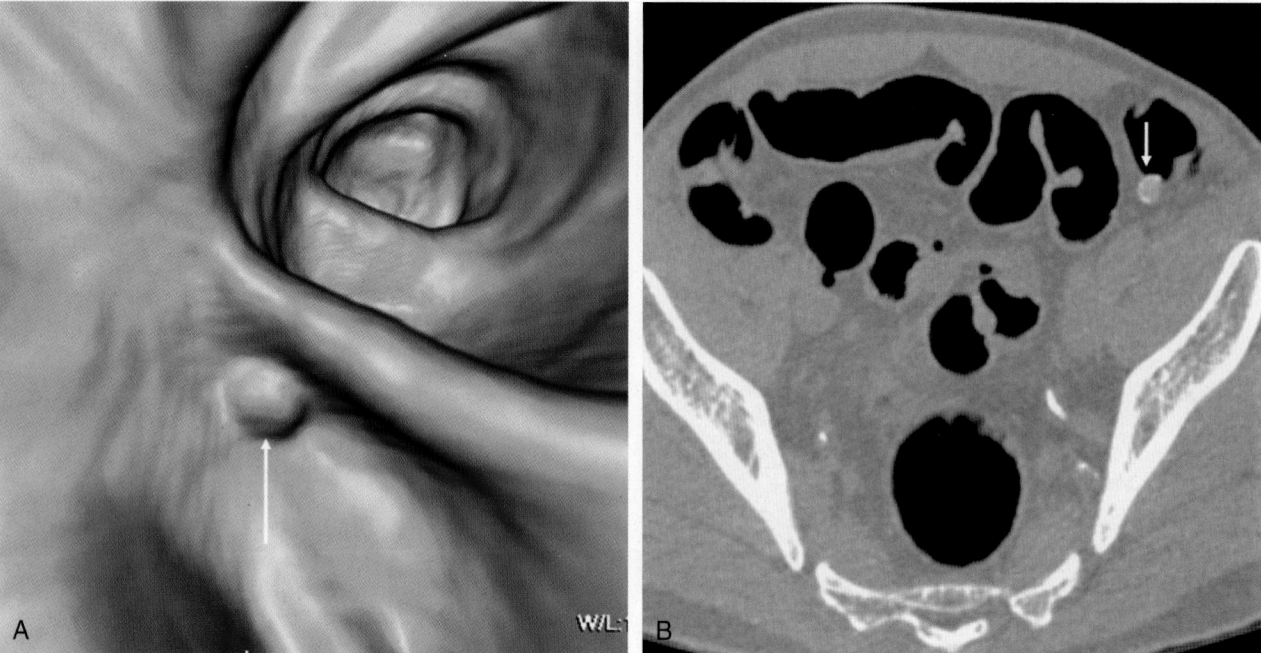

Figure 57-10. Use of 2D imaging for problem solving at endoluminal review. A. Endoluminal view shows 7-mm polypoid lesion (*arrow*) in sigmoid colon. **B.** Axial CT scan shows high-attenuation fecal material impacted in a sigmoid diverticulum (*arrow*). A combination of 2D and 3D views is essential for optimal interpretation.

However, given these limitations, it is possible, and quite likely, that by interrogating 3D endoluminal images both antegrade and retrograde, smaller polyps (<5 mm) can be routinely detected.[10] Moreover, it is possible that polyps in the 6- to 9-mm range may also be better detected with 3D imaging.[10] A recent study found that using axial images, as well as complete 3D endoluminal navigation in antegrade and retrograde directions in both the supine and prone position, detection of polyps less than or equal to 5 mm was 59%.[57] This compares favorably to a study where only 2D imaging was used as the primary data interpretation technique, which showed that less than 20% of the diminutive polyps were visualized.[45] A recent study showed improved detection of diminutive lesions in an ideally prepared and distended pig colon using 3D and multiplanar reformat views when compared with axial images alone.[88] However, the ability of endoluminal imaging to detect these diminutive filling defects in human subjects may lead to decreased specificity as a result of the detection of small adherent bits of residual fecal material that can be difficult to differentiate from small polyps. Moreover, the detection of true diminutive polyps with 3D imaging is of questionable clinical significance, especially if routine colon screening is to be performed on an interval basis.[9]

In summary, optimal evaluation of CTC data is facilitated by easy access to supine and prone images and 2D and 3D images. Most workstations allow both the axial supine and prone images to be displayed adjacent to each other. Having easy access to both datasets ensures that segments of the colon that are filled with fluid or incompletely distended on one dataset are free of fluid and well distended on the other. At this time, a clear consensus on a primary 2D or 3D approach is not established and the user interpreter of CTC data should rely on the interpretation technique that he or she feels most comfortable using.

Potential Clinical Indications

Currently there are several clinical situations where CTC may play an important role in patient care. These include evaluation of the colon proximal to an incomplete conventional colonoscopic examination or to evaluate the colon proximal to an obstructing neoplasm.[89-91] Another potential indication for CTC is colonic evaluation in patients who are clinically unfit for conventional colonoscopy such as those with severe cardiac or pulmonary disease, patients with a bleeding diathesis or those on warfarin, and patients with a prior allergic reaction to sedation. Finally, CTC may contribute to colorectal screening by providing a safe, effective, and rapid examination that evaluates the entire colon for clinically relevant lesions.

Failed Colonoscopy

An incomplete colonoscopic examination may occur in approximately 5% of cases and may be due to patient discomfort, colon tortuosity, postoperative adhesions, or hernias. Traditionally, DCBE has been used to evaluate the proximal colon in this setting. However, after an incomplete colonoscopy, a DCBE may be difficult to perform related to air blockage from gas present from the recently performed colonoscopy. In addition, because of residual fluid from a polyethylene glycol preparation, optimal coating of the colon wall with barium may not be obtained. Two studies have demonstrated the utility of CTC after an incomplete colonoscopic examination[89,90] (Fig. 57-11). A CTC performed on the same day as an incomplete colonoscopy takes advantage of the single bowel preparation and the fact that the colon is often well distended from previous gaseous insufflation from the colonoscopy, thus requiring only a small amount of additional insufflation. In this setting, CTC is clearly better tolerated than DCBE.[89]

Evaluation of the Colon Proximal to an Obstructing Lesion

Synchronous colon cancers occur in approximately 5% of cases of colorectal cancer, and synchronous polyps are common.[91] Occasionally, an obstructing carcinoma may prevent proximal endoscopic evaluation (Fig. 57-11). In this setting,

CTC has been shown to be useful in evaluating the more proximal colon for synchronous lesions.[91] In addition to obstructing cancers, strictures from prior radiation may prevent complete colonoscopic evaluation of the colon. A study of 61 patients showed that CTC allows a high-quality examination to be obtained in this setting.[92] A potential limitation of

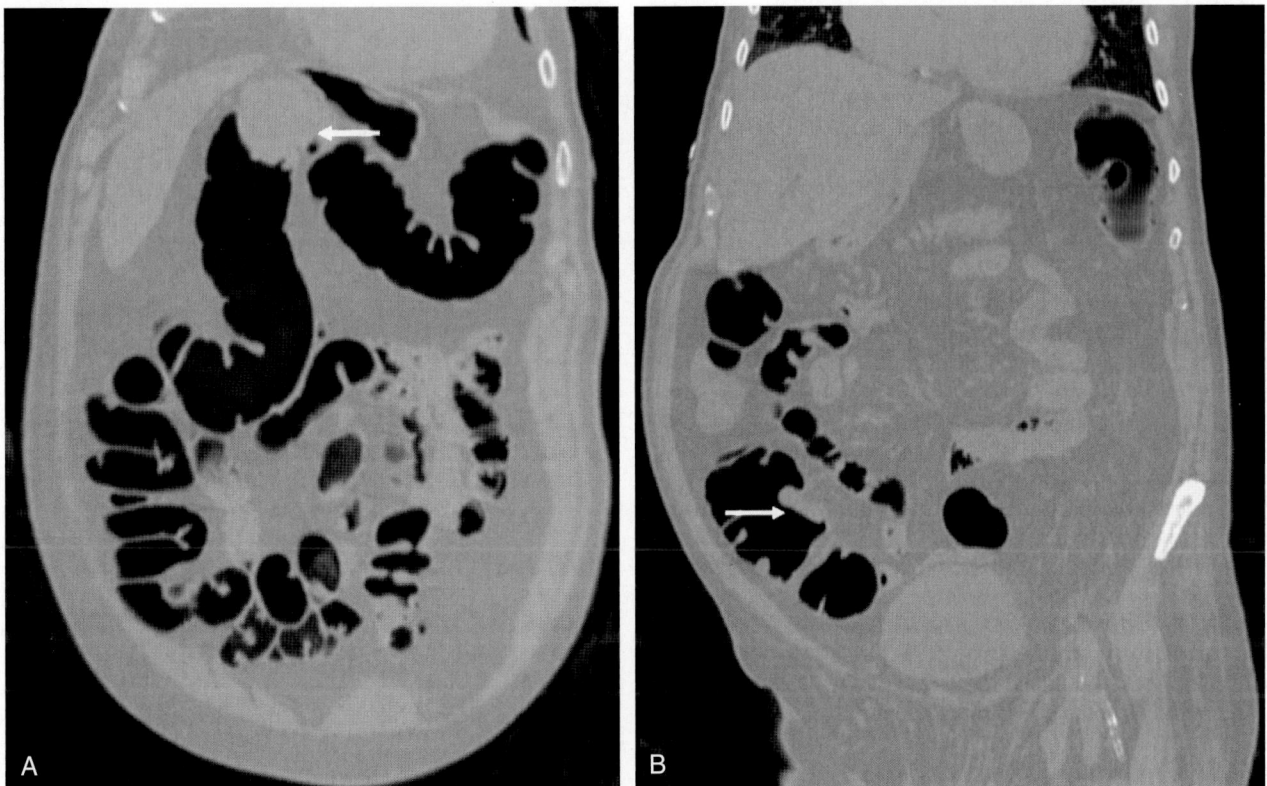

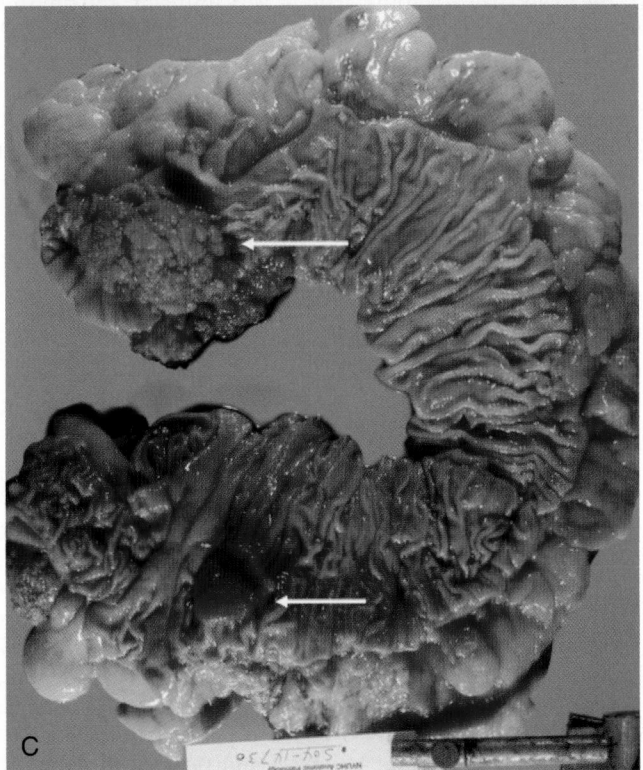

Figure 57-11. An 80-year-old man with iron-deficiency anemia and known transverse colon adenocarcinoma. A. Coronal CT scan shows obstructing lesion in transverse colon (*arrow*). Colonoscopy was unable to proceed proximal. **B.** Coronal CT scan demonstrates second plaquelike mass in proximal ascending colon (*arrow*). **C.** Because the patient had two lesions seen at CTC, an extended right colectomy to the distal transverse colon was performed. Pathologic specimen confirms the two synchronous lesions (*arrows*).

CTC when there is near-total colonic obstruction is in obtaining a clean enough colon proximal to the tumor or stricture to allow optimum evaluation. Careful clinical evaluation of the patient is necessary to exclude total obstruction, which would make bowel cleansing contraindicated.

Patients with Contraindications to Colonoscopy and Patients Who Refuse Other Screening Options

For a variety of reasons, a gastroenterologist may be unwilling to perform conventional colonoscopy in a patient with a high suspicion of harboring a colonic lesion based on clinical symptoms (e.g., bleeding, change in bowel habits). Reluctance to perform colonoscopy may be related to advanced patient age, severe comorbid disease, bleeding diathesis, and prior allergic reaction to sedation during colonoscopy. In these cases, CTC can be safely performed to exclude neoplastic disease.

Moreover, for a variety of reasons (anxiety, fear, embarrassment) people who should undergo screening are often reluctant. Although conventional colonoscopy is the current reference standard for pancolonic evaluation, if patients are unwilling to have the procedure performed, it is useless. The concept of a relatively painless examination (CTC) that can image the colon and detect significant lesions is appealing to many patients. Once a suspicious lesion is detected, a patient will be more willing to undergo conventional colonoscopy and polypectomy.

Although CTC is a relatively painless procedure it is not entirely without discomfort. Most studies evaluating patient preferences for conventional colonoscopy and CTC have shown CTC to be the preferred test.[33,47-49] One study of patients undergoing CTC followed by conventional colonoscopy showed that, of those who had an opinion, 82% favored CTC.[48] In another study of 696 patients who underwent CTC and colonoscopy, patients preferred CTC to colonoscopy 72.3% to 5.1%.[33] However, another study showed that 63.7% preferred conventional colonoscopy to CTC.[49] Our own data evaluating patient preferences for CTC and conventional colonoscopy demonstrated that 70.5% of patients preferred CTC, whereas 29.5% chose conventional colonoscopy.[50]

How can these differences be explained? One potential explanation is that different CT techniques were utilized. Patient comfort and privacy need to be maximized during CTC. We do not use IV catheters or needles for the procedure, whereas others may use bowel relaxants requiring IV access. Another important aspect is that CTC may be performed with a small rubber catheter. Finally, when questionnaires are given to patients regarding the two procedures, outcomes need to be addressed as well as the therapeutic effect of conventional colonoscopy in being able to remove polyps as well as detect them. A patient may prefer CTC over conventional colonoscopy, but if the patient knows something can be done to remove a detected abnormality at colonoscopy it may increase the patient's acceptance of conventional colonoscopy.

Screening

Ultimately, CTC may assist other current options by enabling widespread pancolonic screening to be performed. Within the gastroenterology community there are differing opinions as to the current role of CTC. It has been suggested that although CTC is an exciting imaging technique that has

promise, it is not yet ready to be recommended for general screening.[12,38] What are the data comparing CT and conventional colonoscopy?

Initial investigators evaluating CTC and conventional colonoscopy, including Vining, Hara, and Dachman and their coworkers, showed promise in the ability of CT to detect colorectal polyps and cancers.[14,37,42,44] Many single-institution clinical studies evaluating CTC have demonstrated a sensitivity of over 90% for the detection of colorectal polyps measuring 10 mm or larger when correlated with conventional colonoscopy.[14] These results compare favorably with studies that have evaluated DCBE with colonoscopy in detecting lesions of this size.[32] However, most of these CTC studies were performed in patients with specific colorectal symptoms.

A study published in 1999 of 100 patients undergoing back-to-back CT and conventional colonoscopy showed a sensitivity of 100% for colorectal carcinoma, 91% for polyps that were 10 mm or more, and 82% for polyps that were between 6 and 9 mm.[76] Not all studies have demonstrated a similar sensitivity for detecting 10-mm polyps. In a cohort of 180 patients, Fletcher and colleagues showed a sensitivity of 85% for polyps measuring 10 mm or larger.[52] In 1997, Hara and associates showed 75% sensitivity for detecting polyps 10 mm or larger.[40] In 2001, a follow-up study by Hara and associates showed improved sensitivity ranging to 80% to 89% for polyps 10 mm or larger.[70] These data suggest that there is a learning curve for CTC.[56,70] This was also shown in a recent multi-institutional study that evaluated multidetector row CTC and conventional colonoscopy.[15] In this study the overall detection rate of CTC for colorectal polyps 10 mm or larger was only 55%. However, analysis of results from those centers that had the most prior experience with CTC showed excellent sensitivity for 10-mm polyps, approaching 90%. In detecting small polyps (≤5 mm), the sensitivity is lower.

Perhaps of more concern than the small raised polyp is the truly flat adenoma that is very difficult and in some cases almost impossible to detect at CTC (Fig. 57-12).[77] The definition of a flat polyp is one whose height is less than 50% of its width.[93] Although most flat lesions are 2 mm or less, they may occasionally be up to 5 mm in height. Therefore, many slightly raised flat lesions are visible at CTC. A recent study in the United States found the prevalence of flat lesions to be extremely low.[10] While flat lesions have traditionally been thought to be rare in western populations they may in fact be more common than previously thought.[93] One study of 1000 colonoscopic examinations in the United Kingdom from 1995 to 1999 evaluated the prevalence of flat adenomas. In this study, 36% of adenomas were flat.[93] The majority of these lesions appear to be in the proximal colon.

There is some controversy about the clinical significance of flat lesions when compared with those that are sessile or pedunculated.[93,94] However, a recent review of flat lesions (defined as those with a thickness of ≤1.3 mm) from data from the National Polyp Study suggests that flat lesions are not more aggressive than sessile or pedunculated adenomas.[94] This study showed that flat lesions, which comprise 27% of all baseline adenomas, were no more likely than sessile or pedunculated adenomas to exhibit high-grade dysplasia. Moreover, there was no increased risk of advanced adenomas at surveillance endoscopy in those patients with initial flat adenomas.[94] The ability of CTC to detect the vast majority of clinically significant lesions is still relevant. It should be

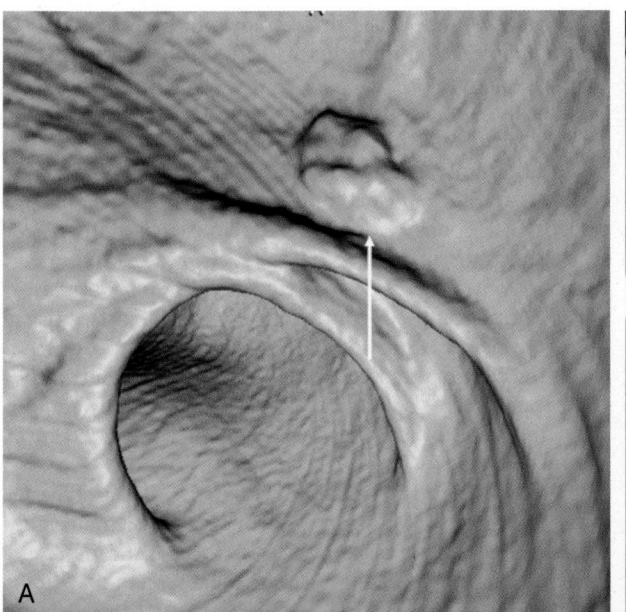

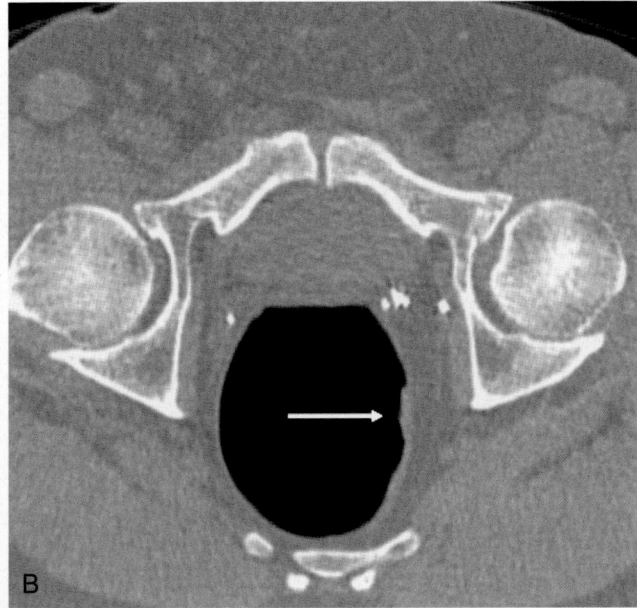

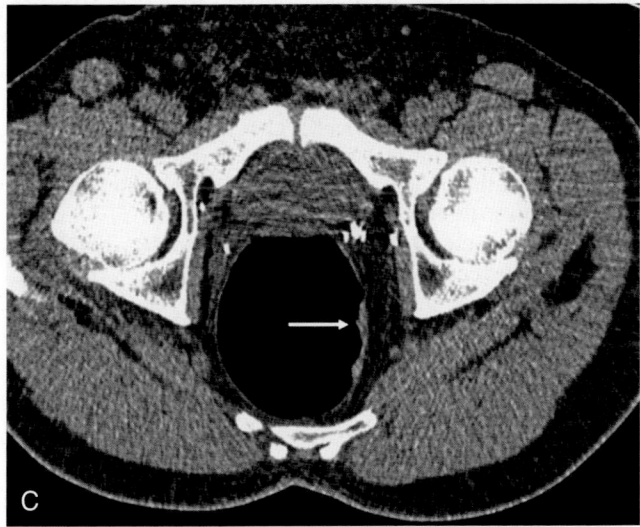

Figure 57-12. Flat adenoma in the rectum in a 65-year-old man.
A. Endoluminal image shows irregular flat plaquelike lesion in rectum (*arrow*). Differential diagnosis includes adherent stool and flat polyp. **B.** Axial CT scan using colon window level settings shows subtle irregularity along left side of the rectum (*arrow*). **C.** Axial CT scan using abdomen window level settings shows irregularity along left side of the rectum is more conspicuous (*arrow*). At colonoscopy, a flat rectal carcinoma was seen and the patient underwent a low anterior resection.

pointed out that conventional colonoscopy also has limitations in its ability to detect all colorectal polyps.[10,95]

Regarding screening, there have been several published series evaluating CTC and conventional colonoscopy.[10,77,96,97] In a series of 67 asymptomatic patients undergoing screening CTC and conventional colonoscopy 3/3 (100%) polyps 10 mm or larger were detected at CT.[96] A report by Rex and associates on 46 patients undergoing screening CTC and colonoscopy demonstrated not only a low sensitivity of CTC in detecting small polyps (11% for polyps ≤5 mm) but also larger flat lesions.[77] In this study, only 1 of 4 flat adenomas measuring more than 2 cm in width that were present at conventional colonoscopy were detected at CTC. The results of this study seem to suggest that CTC may not be an accurate screening test for colorectal polyps. However, as pointed out in an associated editorial on this series of patients, it is too early to pass judgment on CTC based on this single report.[98] Importantly, in this screening study, CTC was performed using single- or dual-slice helical CT scanners with 5-mm collimation.[77]

Two large studies have been published evaluating CTC in an asymptomatic population. The first studied 1233 average-risk asymptomatic patients and is the largest study to date evaluating CTC and conventional colonoscopy.[10] The sensitivity of CTC in detecting 10-mm polyps was over 90% and in fact greater than that of conventional colonoscopy. In this study, determination of true-positive lesions was based on sequential unblinding of the colonoscopist to the CTC results as the colonoscope was removed. This served as an improved gold standard for the presence or absence of polyps. Moreover, of those polyps that were missed at CTC, most were hyperplastic polyps not adenomas.[99] Hyperplastic polyps may be more compressible when the colon is insufflated. Missing these polyps at CTC clearly has no impact on patient survival.

However, a second published large study evaluated same-day CTC and colonoscopy in 703 asymptomatic higher than average-risk patients.[97] In this study, three experienced readers detected 34%, 32%, and 73% of all polyps measuring 10 mm or more. By double-reading the cases 63% of these polyps were prospectively observed. In this study there was high inter-observer variability in polyp detection. The conclusion of this study is that in a low-prevalence population, the polyp detection rates are much lower at CTC than at colonoscopy.

Although there is obviously a training issue and a learning curve for CTC, this does not explain the discrepant results between these two studies.[10,97] In the second study three experienced readers showed relatively poor sensitivity for clinically relevant lesions. Some of the differences may be explained by the choice of CTC slice collimation, workstation, and interpretation techniques. These factors need to continue to be explored.

FUTURE CONSIDERATIONS

Whereas most studies to date have focused on the ability of CTC to detect colorectal polyps, the real measure of this screening test will be to decrease the morbidity and mortality associated with colorectal cancer. The future of CTC is promising. Training of radiologists in CTC interpretation techniques and access to reimbursement for CTC performance remain challenges for the radiology community. Continued hypothesis-driven research will focus on eliminating or improving bowel preparation, improving software for polyp visualization and detection, and further development and implementation of computer-aided assistance for colorectal polyp detection.[86,100-102]

Training and Implementation

A major limitation of conventional colonoscopy is that there are not enough trained endoscopists to perform routine screening on all eligible subjects.[38] However, there are not enough trained radiologists to currently impact colon cancer screening with CTC. If CTC is going to affect colon cancer screening, training of radiologists to interpret CTC examinations will be critical.

In the United States, several medical centers are offering hands-on training in CTC data interpretation. These courses usually run for 2 days and comprise a mixture of didactic lectures and colonoscopy-proven cases. Participants have use of a workstation and learn those skills that enable polyp detection and differentiation from residual fecal material and bulbous folds. Moreover, training modules are being developed that will allow radiologists to have independent training on a mixture of cases that demonstrate different pathologic processes.[103] Ultimately, CTC interpretation will need to be incorporated into radiology residency training programs if sufficient numbers of radiologists will ever have the expertise to contribute to colon cancer screening.

Reimbursement

CTC is not listed as a colon cancer screening study that Medicare reimburses. As of July 1, 2004, two new CPT codes were created by the CPT Editorial Panel for CTC. The codes are 0066T for examinations done for screening and 0067T for examinations performed for diagnostic purposes (obstructing cancer, bleeding). These are category III codes, meaning that they are not valued through the Relative Value Update Committee process. As such, the Centers for Medicare and Medicaid Services and individual insurance carriers decide

on a code by code basis if coverage will be provided. Thus, payment is variable but this usually means that there is no coverage provided.

Category I codes specifically require that a device or drug be FDA approved, that the procedure be performed at multiple locations and by multiple physicians, and that the clinical efficacy is well established and documented.[104] The new CPT category III codes replace the previously used three codes that were routinely used to bill for CTC, 71450 (abdomen CT without contrast), 72192 (pelvic CT without contrast), and 76375 (tomographic reconstruction). Radiologists must now use these new category III codes for tracking purposes and to use the category I codes is now inappropriate. Currently, the American College of Radiology is working to get reimbursement for these procedures but payment is neither universal nor uniform.

Currently, several private insurers including Physicians Plus Insurance in Madison, Wisconsin, are reimbursing for screening CTC. The reason given by these insurance carriers for reimbursing for screening CTC is that screening with high-quality CTC will be cost effective relative to conventional colonoscopy given all of the associated costs incurred with conventional colonoscopy, including the costs for anesthesia and biopsy of diminutive nonrelevant lesions. However, for most payers, CTC is currently not a reimbursable procedure. As such, if a patient wants a CTC examination or a physician refers a patient for the procedure, payment will ultimately come from the patient. Radiology practices therefore need to decide on a fee for the procedure. Because CTC examinations extensively evaluate the colon with two acquisitions as well as the remainder of the abdomen and pelvis for incidental findings, an inappropriately low fee has been discouraged and it has been suggested that the charges should be at least what a routine CT of the abdomen and pelvis cost, and possibly more.

Prepless Computed Tomographic Colonography and Computer-Assisted Detection

There are two major areas of intense CTC research being performed by both radiologists and software manufacturers. These are (1) the clinical performance of CTC without bowel cleansing and (2) efforts to enhance polyp visualization.

CTC without colon cleansing was discussed in a prior section on bowel preparation. A recent study evaluated the performance of CTC in 200 patients using dilute iodinated contrast material. The contrast agent was ingested in small aliquots over five low-fat/fiber meals and without any other bowel catharsis. In this study the sensitivity for polyps 8 mm or larger was 95%.[105] Continued evaluation of prepless CTC using both iodine and barium is being conducted.

Polyp-enhanced visualization and computer-assisted detection are software programs that detect colorectal lesions with morphologies that suggest a polyp. Various strategies have been used by software and workstation manufacturers to detect polyps; however, geometric and morphologic characteristics of the polyp candidates appear to be the most important.[102] Most of these systems are being designed to act as a second reader for polyp detection. Most computer-assisted detection systems operate on the premise that a primary review be performed first by the radiologist. Either simultaneously, or in the background, the computer analyzes the data and displays potential polyps to the reviewer. The reviewer can then evaluate these lesions and determine, based on morphologic and attenuation characteristics, whether the presented lesion is indeed a polyp or a false positive (fecal material, fold, ileocecal valve). Polyp-enhanced visualization will soon be available on workstations and it is hoped will enable improved polyp detection rates, especially for polyps measuring 6 mm or more.

SUMMARY

Computed tomographic colonography is currently a viable alternative imaging tool for colorectal polyp detection. At centers where there is expertise in data acquisition and interpretation, CTC is being offered as a routine imaging examination. Radiologists who perform CTC should be familiar with current colon cancer screening techniques and how CTC can be incorporated into clinical practice. Moreover, techniques of bowel preparation, colonic insufflation, and CTC data interpretation need to be learned by sufficient numbers of radiologists if this exciting technology is to have a substantial impact on colon cancer screening.

References

1. Driver JA, Gaziano JM, Gelber RP, et al: Development of a risk score for colorectal cancer in men. Am J Med 120:257-263, 2007.
2. Jemal A, Siegel R, Ward E, et al: Cancer statistics, 2007. CA Cancer J Clin 57:43-66, 2007.
3. Winawer SJ, Fletcher RH, Miller L, et al: Colorectal cancer screening: Clinical guidelines and rationale. Gastroenterology 112:594-601, 1997.
4. Muto T, Bussey HJR, Morson BC: The evolution of cancer of the colon and rectum. Cancer 36:2251-2270, 1975.
5. Aldridge AJ, Simson JN: Histological assessment of colorectal adenomas by size: Are polyps less than 10 mm in size clinically important? Eur J Surg 167:777-781, 2001.
6. Winawer SJ: Natural history of colorectal cancer. Am J Med 106:3S-6S, 1999.
7. Morson BC: The evolution of colorectal carcinoma. Clin Radiol 35:425-431, 1984.
8. Hoff G, Foerster A, Vatn MH, et al: Epidemiology of polyps in the rectum and colon. Scand J Gastroenterol 21:853-862, 1986.
9. Macari M, Bini EJ, Milano A, et al: Clinical significance of missed polyps at CT colonography. AJR 183:127-134, 2004.
10. Pickhardt PJ, Choi JR, Hwang I, et al: Computed tomographic virtual colonoscopy to screen for colorectal neoplasia in asymptomatic adults. N Engl J Med 349:2191-2200, 2003.
11. Zalis ME, Barish MA, Choi R, et al: CT colonography reporting and data system: A consensus proposal. Radiology 236:3-9, 2005.
12. Rockey DC: Colon cancer screening, polyp size, and CT colonography: Making sense of it all? Gastroenterology 131:2006-2009, 2006.
13. Waye JD, Lewis BS, Frankel A, Geller SA: Small colon polyps. Am J Gastroenterol 83:120-122, 1988.
14. Johnson CD, Dachman AH: CT colonography: The next colon screening examination. Radiology 216:331-341, 2000.
15. Cotton PB, Durkalski VL, Pineau BC, et al: Computed tomographic colonography (virtual colonoscopy)—a multicenter comparison with standard colonoscopy for detection of colorectal neoplasia. JAMA 291:1713-1719, 2004.
16. Lane N, Kaplan H, Pascal R: Minute adenomatous and hyperplastic polyps of the colon: Divergent patterns of epithelial growth with specific associated mesenchymal changes. Gastroenterology 60:537-555, 1971.
17. Aldridge AJ, Simson JN: Histological assessment of colorectal adenomas by size: Are polyps less than 10 mm in size clinically important? Eur J Surg 167:777-781, 2001.
18. Nusko G, Mansmann U, Altendorf-Hofmann A, et al: Risk of invasive carcinoma in colorectal adenomas assessed by size and site. Int J Colorectal Surg 12:267-271, 1997.
19. Glick S, Wagner JL, Johnson CD: Cost-effectiveness of double contrast barium enema in screening for colorectal cancer. AJR 170:629-636, 1998.
20. Winawer S, Fletcher R, Rex D, et al: Colorectal cancer screening and surveillance: Clinical guidelines and rationale—update based on new evidence. Gastroenterology 124:544-560, 2003.
21. Mandel JS, Bond JH, Church TR, et al: Reducing the mortality from colorectal cancer by screening for fecal occult blood. N Engl J Med 328:1365-1371, 1993.
22. Winawer SJ, Zauber AG, Ho MN: Prevention of colorectal cancer by colonoscopic polypectomy. The National Polyp Study Workgroup. N Engl J Med 329:1977-1981, 1993.
23. Muller AD, Sonnenberg A: Protection by endoscopy against death from colorectal cancer: A case control study among veterans. Arch Intern Med 155:1741-1748, 1995.
24. Eddy DM: Screening for colorectal cancer. Ann Intern Med 113:373-384, 1990.
25. Kronborg O, Fenger C, Olsen J, et al: Randomized study of screening for colorectal cancer with fecal occult blood test. Lancet 348:1467-1471, 1996.
26. Rockey DC, Koch J, Cello JP, et al: Relative frequency of upper gastrointestinal and colonic lesions in patients with positive fecal occult-blood tests. N Engl J Med 339:153-159, 1998.
27. Selby JV, Friedman GD, Quesenberry PC, Weiss NS: A case control study of screening sigmoidoscopy and mortality from colorectal cancer. N Engl J Med 326:653-657, 1992.
28. Lieberman DA, Weiss DG, Bond JH, et al: Use of colonoscopy to screen asymptomatic adults for colorectal cancer. N Engl J Med 343:162-168, 2000.
29. Imperiale TF, Wagner DR, Lin CY: Risk of advanced neoplasms in asymptomatic adults according to the distal colorectal findings. N Engl J Med 343:169-174, 2000.
30. Podolsky DK: Going the distance—the case for true colorectal-cancer screening. N Engl J Med 343:207-208, 2000.
31. Norfleet RG, Ryan ME, Wyman JB, et al: Barium enema versus colonoscopy for patients with polyps found during flexible sigmoidoscopy. Gastrointest Endosc 37:531-534, 1991.
32. Winawer SJ, Stewart ET, Zauber AG: A comparison of colonoscopy and double-contrast barium enema for surveillance after polypectomy. N Engl J Med 342:1766-1777, 2000.
33. Gluecker TM, Johnson CD, Harmsen WS, et al: Colorectal cancer screening with CT colonography, colonoscopy, and double contrast barium enema examination: Prospective assessment of patient perceptions and preferences. Radiology 227; 378-384, 2003.
34. Liberman DA, Weiss DG: One time screening for colorectal cancer with combined fecal occult-blood testing and examination of the distal colon. N Engl J Med 345:555-560, 2001.
35. Bressler B, Paszat LF, Chen Z, et al: Rates of new or missed colorectal cancers after colonoscopy and their risk factors: A population-based analysis. Gastroenterology 132:96-102, 2007.
36. Detsky AS: Screening for colon cancer—can we afford colonoscopy? N Engl J Med 345:607-608, 2001.
37. Vining DJ, Gelfand DW, Bechtold RE, et al: Technical feasibility of colon imaging with helical CT and virtual reality [abstract]. AJR 162:194, 1994.
38. Rex D: Virtual colonoscopy: Time for some tough questions for radiologists and gastroenterologists. Endoscopy 32:260-263, 2000.
39. Royster AP, Fenlon HM, Clarke PD, et al: CT colonoscopy of colorectal neoplasm: Two-dimensional and three-dimensional virtual-reality techniques with colonoscopic correlation. AJR 169:1237-1242, 1997.
40. Hara AK, Johnson CD, Reed JE, et al: Detection of colorectal polyps with CT colography: Initial assessment of sensitivity and specificity. Radiology 205:259-265, 1997.
41. Fenlon HM, Ferrucci JT. Virtual colonoscopy: What will the issues be? AJR 169:453-458, 1997.
42. Hara AK, Johnson CD, Reed JE, et al: Colorectal polyp detection with CT colography: Two- versus three-dimensional techniques. Radiology 200:49-54, 1996.
43. Dachman AH, Lieberman J, Osnis RB, et al: Small simulated polyps in pig colon: Sensitivity of CT virtual colography. Radiology 203:427-430, 1997.
44. Dachman AH, Kuniyoshi JK, Boyle CM, et al: CT colonography with three-dimensional problem solving for detection of colonic polyps. AJR 171:989-995, 1998.
45. Macari M, Milano A, Lavelle M, et al: Comparison of time-efficient CT colonography with two-dimensional and three-dimensional colonic evaluation for detecting colorectal polyps. AJR 174:1543-1549, 2000.

46. Macari M, Bini EJ, Jacobs SL, et al: Filling defects in the colon at CT colonography: Pseudo and diminutive lesions (the good), polyps (the bad), flat lesions, masses, and carcinomas (the ugly). RadioGraphics 23:1073-1091, 2003.

47. Angtuaco TL, Bannaad Omiotek GD, Howden CW: Differing attitudes toward virtual and conventional colonoscopy for colorectal cancer screening: Surveys among primary care physicians and potential patients. Am J Gastroenterol 96:887-893, 2001.

48. Svensson MH, Svensson I, Lasson A, Hellstrom M: Patient acceptance of CT colonography and conventional colonoscopy: Prospective comparative study in patients with or suspected of having colorectal disease. Radiology 222:337-345, 2002.

49. Akerkar GA, Hung RK, Yee J, et al: Virtual colonoscopy: Real pain [abstract]. Gastroenterology 116:A44, 1999.

50. Rajapaksa R, Macari M, Weinshel E, Bini EJ: Patient preferences and satisfaction with virtual vs. conventional colonoscopy. The American Society for Gastrointestinal Endoscopy, Topic Forum sessions at Digestive Disease Week (DDW) 2002, presented in San Francisco, California, May 19-22, 2002.

51. Macari M, Bini EJ, Xue X, et al: Prospective comparison of thin-section low-dose multislice CT colonography to conventional colonoscopy in detecting colorectal polyps and cancers. Radiology 224:383-392, 2002.

52. Fletcher JG, Johnson CD, Welch TJ, et al: Optimization of CT colonography technique: Prospective trial in 180 patients. Radiology 216:704-711, 2000.

53. Chen SC, Lu DSK, Hecht JR, Ladell BM: CT colonography: Value of scanning in both the supine and prone positions. AJR 172:595-600, 1999.

54. Yee J, Hung RK, Akekar GA, Wall SD: The usefulness of glucagon hydrochloride for colonic distension. AJR 173:169-172, 1999.

55. Ransohoff DF: Virtual colonoscopy—what it can do vs. what it will do. JAMA 291:1772-1774, 2004.

56. Spinzi G, Belloni G, Martegani A, et al: Computed tomographic colonography and conventional colonoscopy for colon diseases: A prospective blinded study. Am J Gastroenterol 96:394-400, 2001.

57. Yee J, Akerkar GA, Hung RK, et al: Colorectal neoplasia: Performance characteristics of CT colonography for detection in 300 patients. Radiology 219:685-692, 2001.

58. Macari M, Pedrosa I, Lavelle M, et al: Effect of different bowel preparations on residual fluid at CT colonography. Radiology 218:274-277, 2001.

59. Ristvedt SL, McFarland EG, Weinstock LB, Thyssen EP: Patient preferences for CT colonography, conventional colonoscopy, and bowel preparation. Am J Gastroenterol 98:578-585, 2003.

60. Morrin M, Farrell RJ, Kruskal JB, et al: Utility of intravenously administered contrast material at CT colonography. Radiology 217:765-771, 2000.

61. Nappi J, Yoshida H: Fully automated three-dimensional detection of polyps in fecal-tagging CT colonography. Acad Radiol 14:287-300, 2007.

62. Lefere PA, Gryspeerdt SS, Dewyspelaere J, et al: Dietary fecal tagging as a cleansing method before CT colonography: Initial results—polyp detection and patient acceptance. Radiology 224:393-403, 2002.

63. Zalis ME, Pochaczevsky R, Hahn PF: Digital subtraction bowel cleansing in CT colonography. AJR 178:241-247, 2002.

64. Stevenson GW, Wilson JA, Wilkinson J, et al: Pain following colonoscopy: Elimination with carbon dioxide. Gastrointest Endosc 38:564-567, 1992.

65. Taylor SA, Halligan S, Goh V, et al: Optimizing colonic distension for multi-detector row CT colonography: Effect of hyoscine butylbromide and rectal balloon catheter. Radiology 229:99-108, 2003.

66. Wessling J, Fischbach R, Meier N, et al: CT colonography: Protocol optimization with multidetector row CT-study in an anthropomorphic colon phantom. Radiology 228:753-759, 2003.

67. Taylor SA, Halligan S, Bartram CI, et al: Multi-detector row CT colonography: Effect of collimation, pitch, and orientation on polyp detection in a human colectomy specimen. Radiology 229:109-118, 2003.

68. Kalra MK, Maher MM, Toth TL, et al: Comparison of Z-axis automatic tube current modulation technique with fixed tube current CT scanning of abdomen and pelvis. Radiology 232:347-353, 2004.

69. McCollough CH, Zink FE: Performance evaluation of a multi-slice CT system. Med Phys 26:2223-2230, 1999.

70. Hara AK, Johnson CD, McCarty RL, et al: CT colonography: Single versus multi-detector row imaging. Radiology 219:461-465, 2001.

71. Brink JA, Wang Ge, McFarland EG: Optimal section spacing in single-detector helical CT. Radiology 214:575-578, 2000.

72. Lui YW, Macari M, Israel G, et al: CT colonography data interpretation: Effect of different section thicknesses—preliminary observations. Radiology 229:791-797, 2003.

73. Iannaccone R, Laghi A, Catalano C, et al: Detection of colorectal lesions: Lower dose multi-detector row helical CT colonography compared with conventional colonoscopy. Radiology 229:775-781, 2003.

74. Kalra MK, Maher MM, Toth TL, et al: Strategies for CT radiation dose optimization. Radiology 230:619-628, 2004.

75. Obuchowski NA, Graham RJ, Baker ME, Powell KA: Ten criteria for effective screening: Their application to multislice CT screening for pulmonary and colorectal cancers. AJR 176:1357-1362, 2001.

76. Fenlon HM, Nunes DP, Schroy PC, et al: A comparison of virtual and conventional colonoscopy for the detection of colorectal polyps. N Engl J Med 341:1496-1503, 1999.

77. Rex DK, Vining D, Kopecky KK: Initial experience with screening for colon polyps using spiral CT with and without CT colography (virtual colonoscopy). Gastrointest Endosc 50:309-313, 1999.

78. van Gelder RE, Venema HW, Serlie IWO, et al: CT colonography at different radiation dose levels: Feasibility of dose reduction. Radiology 224:25-33, 2002.

79. van Gelder RE, Venema HW, Florie J, et al: CT colonography: Feasibility of substantial dose reduction—comparison of medium to very low doses in identical patients. Radiology 232:611-620, 2004.

80. Brenner DJ, Georgsson MA: Mass screening with CT colonography: Should the radiation exposure be of concern. Gastroenterology 129:328-337, 2005.

81. Rajapaksa RC, Macari M, Bini EJ: Prevalence and impact of extracolonic findings in patients undergoing CT colonography. J Clin Gastroenterol 38:767-771, 2004.

82. Laks S, Macari M, Bini EJ: Positional change in colon polyps at CT colonography. Radiology 231:761-766, 2004.

83. Yee J, Kumar NN, Godara S, et al: Extracolonic abnormalities discovered incidentally at CT colonography in a male population. Radiology 236:519-526, 2005.

84. Mang T, Maier A, Plank C, et al: Pitfalls in multi-detector row CT colonography: A systematic approach. RadioGraphics 27:431-454, 2007.

85. Yee J, Kumar NN, Hung RK, et al: Comparison of supine and prone scanning separately and in combination at CT colonography. Radiology 226:653-661, 2003.

86. Baulieu CF, Jeffrey RB, Karadi C, et al: Display modes for CT colonography: II. Blinded comparison of axial CT and virtual endoscopic and panoramic endoscopic volume-rendered studies. Radiology 212:203-212, 1999.

87. Hoppe H, Quattropani C, Spreng A, et al: Virtual colon dissection with CT colonography compared with axial interpretation and conventional colonoscopy: Preliminary results. AJR Am J Roentgenol 182:1151-1158, 2004.

88. Kim DH, Pickhardt PJ, Taylor AJ, et al: Characteristics of advanced adenomas detected at CT colonographic screening: Implications for appropriate polyp size thresholds for polypectomy versus surveillance. AJR Am J Roentgenol 188:940-944, 2007.

89. Macari M, Megibow AJ, Berman P, et al: CT colonography in patients with failed colonoscopy. AJR 173:561-564, 1999.

90. Morrin MM, Kruskal JB, Farrell RJ, et al: Endoluminal CT colonography after incomplete endoscopic colonoscopy. AJR 172:913-918, 1999.

91. Fenlon HM, McAneny DB, Nunes DP, et al: Occlusive colon carcinoma: Virtual colonoscopy in the preoperative evaluation of the proximal colon. Radiology 210:423-428, 1999.

92. Gollub MJ, Ginsberg MS, Cooper C, Thaler HT: Quality of virtual colonoscopy in patients who have undergone radiation therapy or surgery. AJR 178:1109-1116, 2002.

93. Rembacken BJ, Fuji T, Dixon MF, et al: Flat and depressed colonic neoplasms: A prospective study of 1000 colonoscopies in the UK. Lancet 355:1211-1214, 2000.

94. Park SH, Lee SS, Choi EK, et al: Flat colorectal neoplasms: Definition, importance, and visualization on CT colonography. AJR Am J Roentgenol 188:953-959, 2007.

95. Rex DK, Cutler CS, Lemmel GT, et al: Colonoscopic miss rates of adenomas determined by back to back colonoscopies. Gastroenterology 112:24-28, 1997.

96. Macari M, Bini EJ, Jacobs SL, et al: CT colonography for the evaluation of colorectal polyps and cancers in asymptomatic average risk patients. Radiology 230:629-636, 2004.

97. Johnson CD, Harmsen WS, Wilson LA, et al: Prospective blinded evaluation of computed tomographic colonography for screen detection of colorectal polyps. Gastroenterology 125:311-319, 2003.

98. Ahlquist DA, Johnson CD: Screening CT colonography: Too early to pass judgment on nascent technology. Gastrointest Endosc 50:437-439, 1999.

99. Pickhardt PJ, Nugent PA, Mysliwiec PA, et al: The adenoma miss rate at optical colonoscopy using virtual colonoscopy as a separate reference standard. Ann Intern Med 141:352-359, 2004.

100. Lefere P, Gryspeerdt S, Baekelandt M, et al: Laxative-free CT colonography. AJR 183:945-948, 2004.

101. Summers RM, Johnson CD, Pusanik LM, et al. Automated polyp detection at CT colonography: Feasibility assessment in a human population. Radiology 219:51-59, 2001.

102. Yoshida H, Nappi J, MacEneaney P, et al: Computer-aided diagnosis scheme for detection of polyps at CT colonography. RadioGraphics 22:963-979, 2002.

103. Fidler JL, Fletcher JG, Johnson CD, et al: Understanding interpretive errors in radiologists learning computed tomographic colonography. Acad Radiol 11:750-756, 2004.

104. Duszak R: CT colonography and virtual reimbursment. J Am Coll Radiol 1:457-458, 2004.

105. Taylor SA, Slater A, Burling DN, et al: CT colonography: Optimisation, diagnostic performance and patient acceptability of reduced-laxative regimens using barium-based faecal tagging. Eur Radiol Apr 2007 [Epub ahead of print].

106. Mang T, Graser A, Schima W, et al: CT colonography: Techniques, indications, findings. Eur J Radiol 61:388-399, 2007.

107. Rosman AS, Korsten MA: Meta-analysis comparing CT colonography, air contrast barium enema, and colonoscopy [review]. Am J Med 120:203-210, 2007.

108. Burling D, Halligan S, Atchley J, et al: CT colonography: Interpretative performance in a non-academic environment. Clin Radiol 62:424-429, 2007.

109. European Society of Gastrointestinal and Abdominal Radiology CT Colonography Group Investigators: Effect of directed training on reader performance for CT colonography: Multicenter study. Radiology 242:152-161, 2007.

Magnetic Resonance Colonography

Nicholas C. Gourtsoyiannis, MD • Thomas C. Lauenstein, MD •
Nickolas Papanikolaou, PhD

BACKGROUND	INDICATIONS
PREREQUISITES AND EXAMINATION GUIDELINES	ACCURACY AND CLINICAL EXPERIENCE
DATA ANALYSIS	PATIENT ACCEPTANCE

BACKGROUND

Optical colonoscopy (OC) has been considered the gold standard for the assessment of the colon. However, the modality is hampered by several drawbacks. In up to 26% of the examinations, the ileocecal valve cannot be reached by the endoscopist because of stenotic lesions or elongated colonic segments.[1-3] Hence, colonoscopy may only provide limited accuracy in the detection of colorectal pathology in these patients. Furthermore, there is a low, but real risk of bowel perforation. Eventually, patient acceptance may be limited for colonoscopy because of considerable procedural discomfort or pain. This has been the underlying basis for the development and evaluation of alternative modalities to assess the colon, including magnetic resonance colonography (MRC).

MRC is based on the acquisition of MR datasets of the abdomen that optimizes visualization of the large bowel. Because of the noninvasive character and lack of procedural pain and discomfort of MRC, patient acceptance is improved compared with OC. The datasets can be displayed in a multiplanar reformat (MPR) mode on a postprocessing workstation, which enables the analysis of the colonic wall from any desired angle. In addition, virtual endoscopic views can be generated; thus, lesions may be more accurately defined.[4] Simultaneously to the colonic wall evaluation on MRC images, all abdominal organs within the displayed field-of-view can be also assessed.[5]

PREREQUISITES AND EXAMINATION GUIDELINES

As with OC, patients should undergo bowel cleansing before MRC. The cleansing procedures usually should start the evening before the examination. Analgesics or sedatives are not necessary for MRC. Before the examination, general contraindications to MRI need to be considered, including the presence of pacemakers or severe claustrophobia. Patients with hip prostheses should also be excluded from MRC, because of significant artifact formation in the region of the rectum, which downgrades image quality.

For data acquisition, the use of a 1.5-T scanner equipped with strong gradient systems is preferable. Data collection is generally obtained during breath-hold scans. Thus, acquisition times of the single sequences should not exceed 20 to 25 seconds. Because most bowel loops are collapsed in their physiologic state, the colon needs to be distended. Otherwise, a reliable differentiation between bowel lumen and bowel wall is not possible. For bowel distention, different contrast media can be rectally administered. Most centers use water or barium solutions.[6-8] Rectal insufflation with room air or CO_2 has also been employed.[9] Before rectal filling, spasmolytic agents (e.g., 20 to 40 mg of scopolamine or 1 mg of glucagon) should be administered intravenously. The effect of these substances is threefold: (1) better degree of bowel distention is achieved; (2) bowel spasm is minimized and thereby patient acceptance is enhanced; and (3) presence of artifacts due to bowel motion is reduced.

Table 58-1
Sequence of Main Sequences Applied for Magnetic Resonance Colonography

	T1-Weighted VIBE	T1-Weighted FLASH	True FISP
	3D	2D	3D
Acquisition Plane	Coronal	Axial	Coronal
Acquisition Time	21 s	5 × 19 s[*]	22 s
TR	3.1 ms	158 ms	3.8 ms
TE	1.1 ms	1.8 ms	1.9 ms
FLIP Angle	12°	70°	80°
Slice Thickness	1.8 mm	5.0 mm	2.0 mm
No. of Slices	120	70	96

*Five acquisition blocks of 19 seconds each.

Patients are positioned in either prone or supine position on the scanner table. After the placement of a rectal tube, the distending agent is administered. For liquid contrast agents, an amount of 2000 to 2500 mL is administered, using hydrostatic pressure. The filling procedure should be stopped whenever patients express considerable discomfort. Alternatively, dedicated sequences can be acquired to monitor the filling process (e.g., nonslice select sequences providing an update image every 2 to 3 seconds).[10] A combination of two large "flex surface coils" should be used for signal reception to ensure the coverage of the entire large bowel. However, utilization of the body coil may be sufficient, especially in obese patients.

In comparison with other MR examinations of the abdomen, different sequence types, providing different contrast information, should be applied. The acquisition of 2D and/or 3D fast imaging with steady-state precession (FISP) sequences has proven useful.[11,12] Image properties are characterized by a mixture of both T1 and T2 contrast, leading to a homogeneous bright signal of the colonic lumen filled with water. The colonic wall has low signal intensity. Furthermore, 3D T1-weighted MR images should be acquired before and 70 to 80 seconds after intravenous administration of gadolinium. Data collection is done in the coronal plane for all sequences described. Finally, a T1-weighted 2D FLASH (fast low-angle shot) sequence in the axial plane is acquired, which allows for the evaluation of the adjacent abdominal organs. Sequence parameters are listed in Table 58-1.

DATA ANALYSIS

Datasets should be transferred to postprocessing independent workstations equipped with a dedicated software package for virtual colonoscopy. Data analysis should start with the assessment of contrast-enhanced T1-weighted images. Utilization of an MPR mode allows the radiologist to scroll through the dataset in all three orthogonal planes. The analysis should be complemented by a virtual endoscopic "fly-through" evaluation (Fig. 58-1). The "fly-through" enhances the depiction of small lesions and helps differentiate haustral folds and colorectal masses. The virtual fly-through should be performed in both antegrade and retrograde directions. This provides visualization of both sides of the haustral folds, reducing the risk of missing significant lesions.

Whenever a colorectal lesion is found, the analysis has to be repeated using the corresponding source, the T1-weighted dataset. The signal intensities of the lesions should be recorded to calculate the percentage of contrast agent enhancement. This procedure helps to reliably distinguish between residual stool particles and real colorectal polyps or cancers. Real colorectal lesions always enhance (Fig. 58-2), and residual stool shows same signal properties on both unenhanced and contrast-enhanced T1-weighted images. Scar tissue (e.g., post appendectomy) may also show a significant percentage of contrast enhancement, thereby mimicking a polyp (Fig. 58-3). In a second step, the FISP sequences should be analyzed. These sequences have been found to be very accurate for the detection of inflammatory bowel lesions.[11]

In contrast to OC, MRC studies are not limited to endoscopic viewing. In addition, all abdominal organs within the field of view are displayed. This is especially important in cases of a colorectal carcinoma because the liver can be screened at the same time. Hepatic lesions can be easily detected and characterized, owing to the availability of dynamic contrast-enhanced T1-weighted images. Furthermore, relevant lesions in other organs, including the pancreas, kidneys, and/or bones, can be depicted as well.

INDICATIONS

Magnetic resonance colonography has proven to be an excellent means of evaluating the entire colon in patients with incomplete OC. MRC provides significantly higher completion rates: bowel elongation has no influence at all on the visualization of colonic segments and only high-grade stenosis might prohibit the passage of water, which is necessary for the distention of prestenotic segments (Fig. 58-4). In one study, MRC was used to evaluate 37 patients with incomplete colonoscopy.[13] The large bowel was divided into six segments, including the cecum, the ascending, transverse, descending, and sigmoid colon, and the rectum. Conventional colonoscopy failed to reach almost half of the potentially visible colonic segments. However, only 4% of the bowel segments were not assessable by means of MRC. In addition, MRC revealed lesions in the prestenotic segments, which had not been depicted by conventional colonoscopy, including two carcinomas and five polyps.

MRC has also shown to be suitable for the diagnosis and assessment of inflammatory bowel disease (IBD) (Fig. 58-5).[14-16] In one trial, 23 patients with suspected IBD of the large bowel were examined by means of MRC.[14] Bowel wall inflammation was quantified according to four aspects: bowel wall contrast enhancement, bowel wall thickness, presence of perifocal lymph nodes, and loss of haustral folds. Hence, an inflammation score was calculated, which was compared with endoscopic results and clinical data. Over 90% of the colonic segments with IBD changes were correctly identified. For severe inflammation, sensitivity even amounted to 100%. Hence, MRC may be used for monitoring IBD activity. Furthermore, extramural changes including abscesses, phlegmon, or fistula formation can be easily depicted that are often not suspected on OC.[17]

Despite promising results in the assessment of prestenotic bowel segments and IBD, there are no reliable data yet on MRC supporting colorectal cancer screening applications.

ACCURACY AND CLINICAL EXPERIENCE

The accuracy of MRC in the detection of colorectal masses and IBD has been assessed in a number of studies. In a trial of 100 patients, OC was performed after the MRC examina-

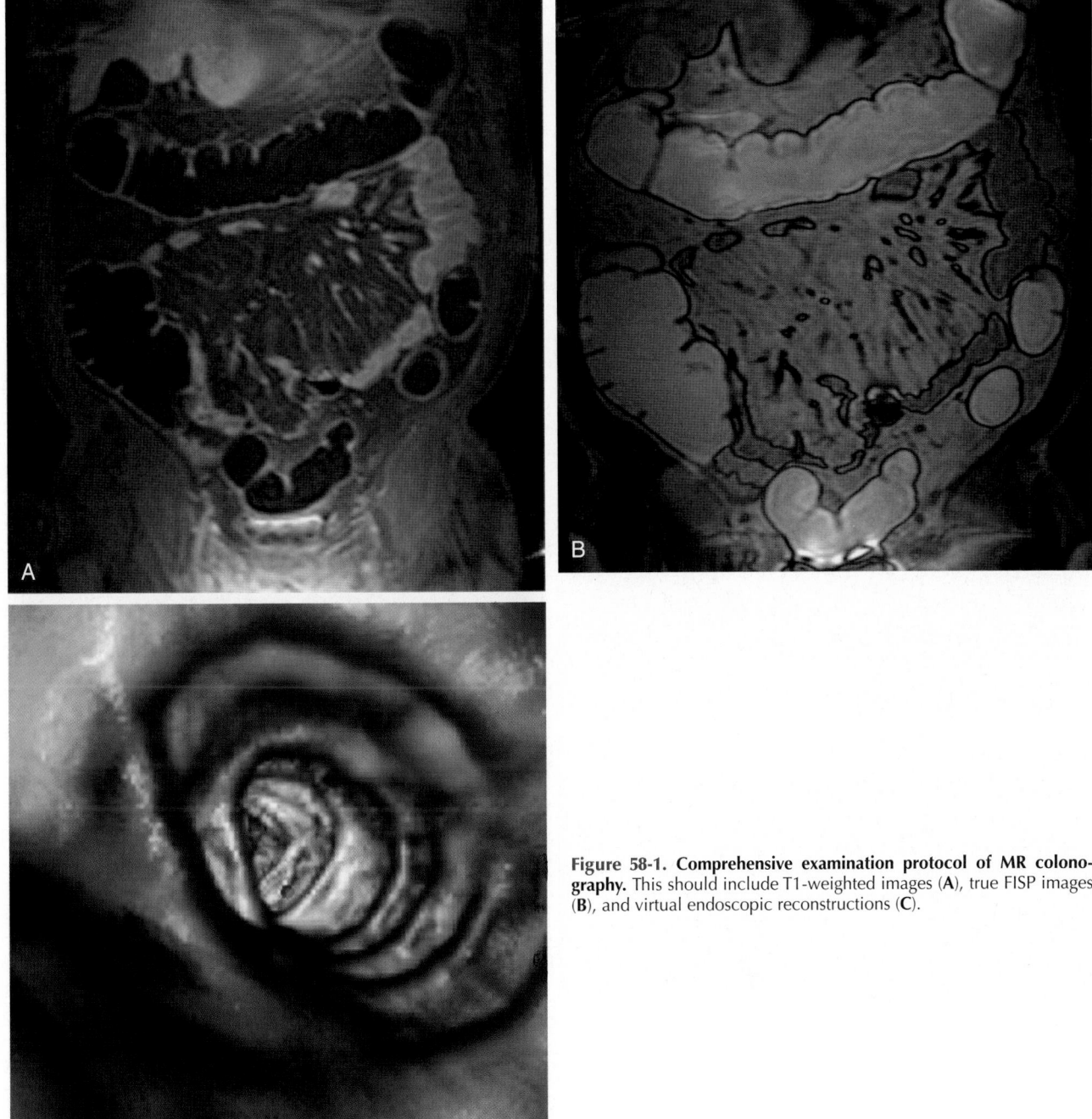

Figure 58-1. Comprehensive examination protocol of MR colonography. This should include T1-weighted images (**A**), true FISP images (**B**), and virtual endoscopic reconstructions (**C**).

tion on the same day and served as the standard of reference.[10] MR data acquisition included pre- and postgadolinium T1-weighted images, which were compared with endoscopic and histologic results. Colonoscopy revealed a total number of 107 colorectal masses. MRC was able to identify all masses larger than 10 mm and 84.2% of the polyps between 6 and 9 mm in diameter. Overall specificity of MRC amounted to 96.0%, and only a very small number of false-positive results were found. MRC showed a high accuracy for the detection of adenomas/carcinomas larger than 6 mm. These results were confirmed by a study including patients at high risk.[5] Over 100 subjects with suspected colorectal diseases underwent MRC, with OC serving as the standard of reference. None of the lesions smaller than 5 mm was identified by MRC, probably owing to lower spatial resolution. However, the sensitivity for the detection of lesions between 5 and 10 mm amounted to 89%. All colorectal masses larger than 10 mm including nine carcinomas were correctly diagnosed on MRC images.

Diagnostic accuracy and image quality appear to be related to the type of MR sequences used. Fast imaging with true FISP

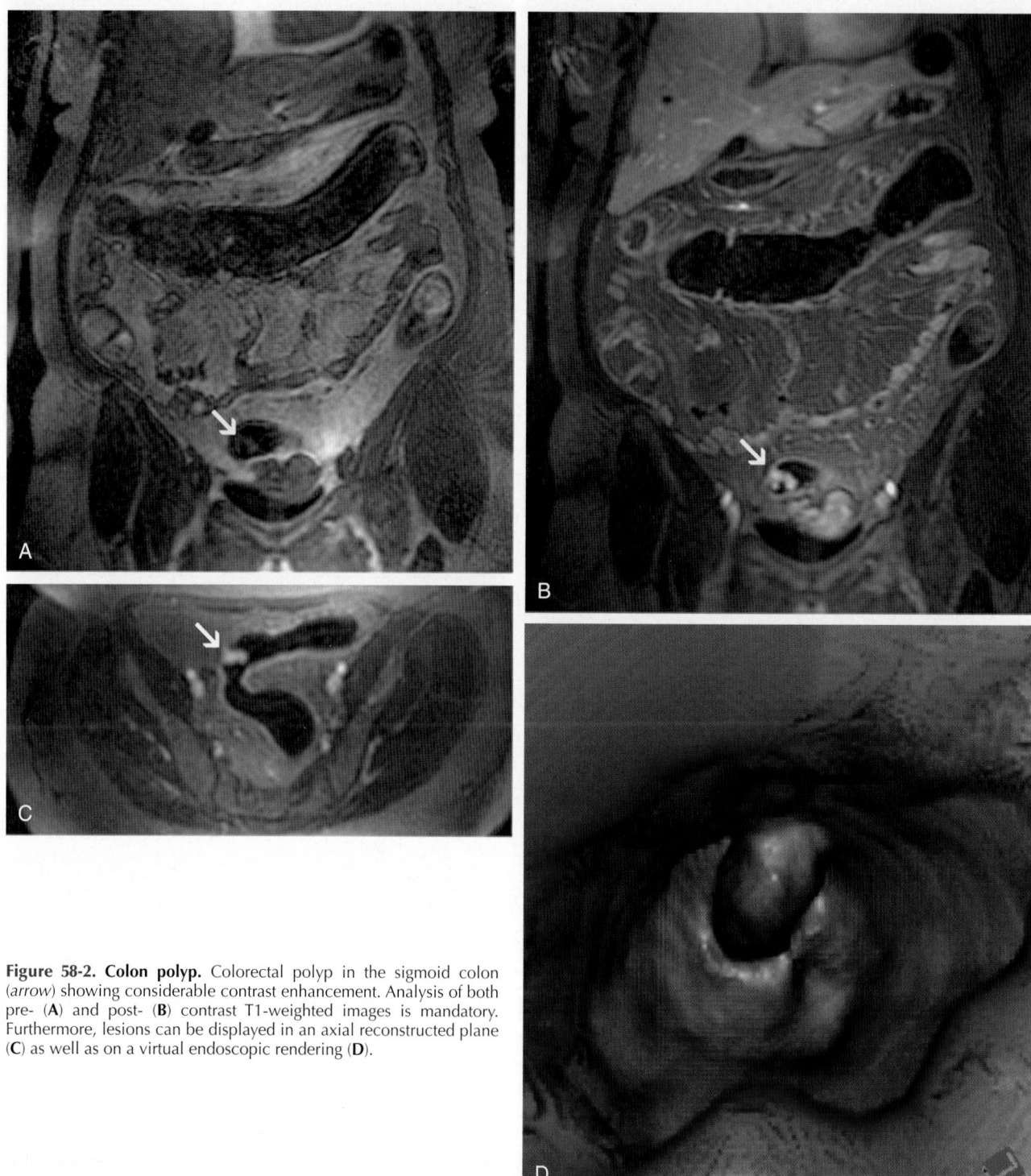

Figure 58-2. Colon polyp. Colorectal polyp in the sigmoid colon (*arrow*) showing considerable contrast enhancement. Analysis of both pre- (**A**) and post- (**B**) contrast T1-weighted images is mandatory. Furthermore, lesions can be displayed in an axial reconstructed plane (**C**) as well as on a virtual endoscopic rendering (**D**).

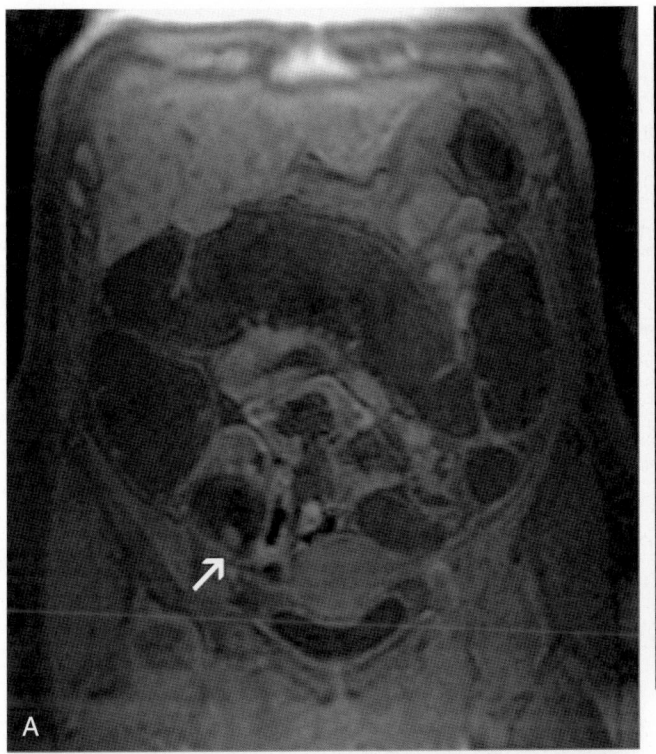

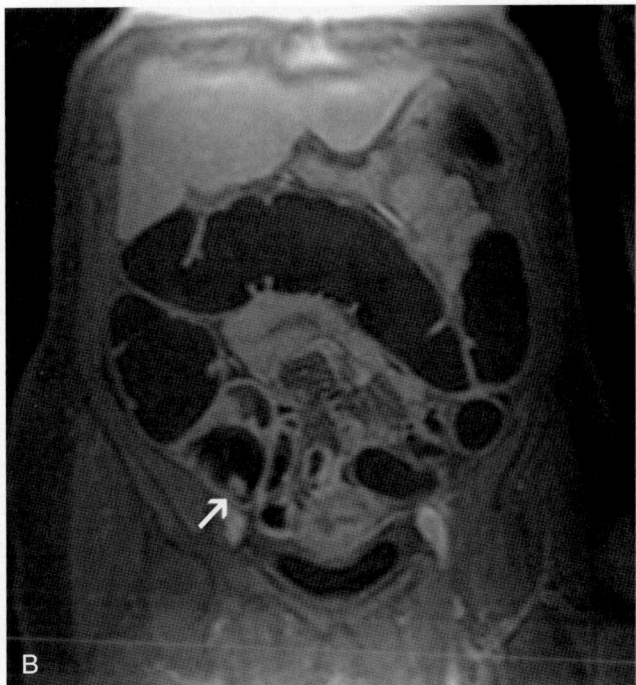

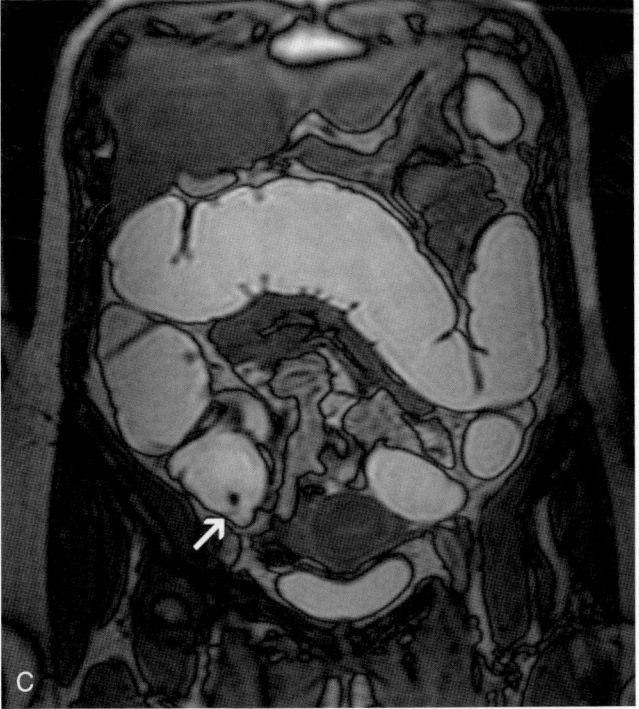

Figure 58-3. Scar tissue simulating polyp. Scar tissue after appendectomy (*arrow*) may mimic a colonic polyp (**C**), owing to avid contrast uptake comparing the pre- (**A**) and post- (**B**) contrast T1-weighted images.

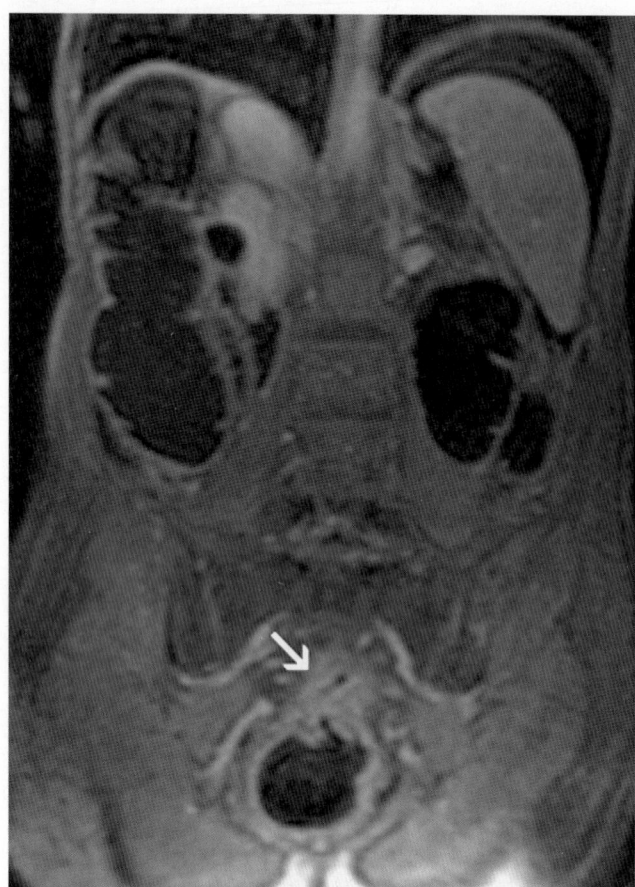

Figure 58-4. Stenotic adenocarcinoma. Severe stenosis (*arrow*) due to colonic adenocarcinoma does not permit evaluation of prestenotic bowel segments when using optical colonoscopy. Such a display is easy with magnetic resonance colonography.

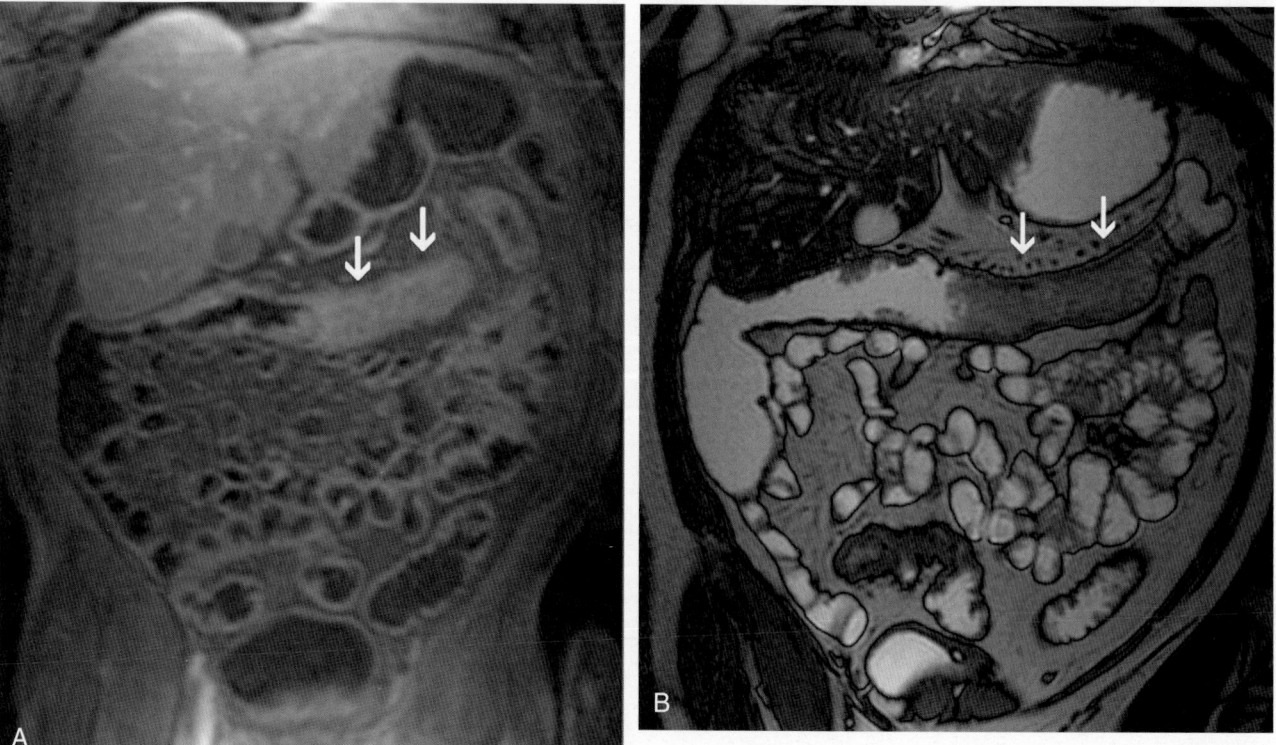

Figure 58-5. Crohn's disease. Patient with Crohn disease showing increased contrast enhancement of the transverse colon on the T1-weighted image (**A**, *arrows*) and bowel wall thickening on the true FISP image (**B**, *arrows*).

or, alternatively, contrast-enhanced T1-weighted images have found to result in different image quality and accuracy.[11] In a study of 37 patients who underwent MRC and OC, both true FISP and postcontrast T1-weighted FLASH images were compared. T1-weighted imaging provided all-over sensitivity values of almost 80% for the detection of colorectal pathology. There were no false-positive results, because residual stool could be easily distinguished from colorectal masses by to the lack of contrast enhancement in the former. True FISP sequences, however, provided a lower sensitivity of approximately 70%. False-positive results were identified in 14% of the examinations, most probably related to the difficulty of distinguishing between residual stool and colorectal masses. Interestingly, image quality of FISP sequences turned out to be significantly better than that of T1-weighted imaging, owing to lower motion sensitivity and fewer artifacts due to respiratory or patient motion (Fig. 58-6). These results indicate that the main diagnostic work-up, at present, should be based on the T1-weighted data, although true FISP sequences may provide useful information in uncooperative patients.

One major criticism of MRC still relates to its very limited accuracy in detecting colorectal polyps smaller than 5 mm. The clinical significance of such lesions remains controversial, because the majority of them are not prone to malignant degeneration.[18] Small polyps will probably become detectable by MRC in the future. New technical improvements such as parallel acquisition techniques will help to increase spatial resolution.[19] Flat adenomas are likely to remain elusive, however.

PATIENT ACCEPTANCE

Bowel cleansing has been a mandatory prerequisite for MRC, because fecal material may mimic the appearance of colonic masses. However, bowel preparation is considered unpleasant by the majority of patients and may lead to symptoms, ranging from feeling unwell to "inability to sleep."[20,21] Patient acceptance for MRC could be significantly increased if bowel purgation could be eliminated. Different strategies have been proposed and tested to that end. One successful approach is fecal tagging, which leads to a modification of signal characteristics of fecal material. For such a purpose, specific oral contrast compounds have to be ingested over 48 hours before MR examination. The signal properties of stool are thereby adapted to the signal characteristics of the rectal enema. Thus, fecal material becomes virtually invisible (Fig. 58-7).

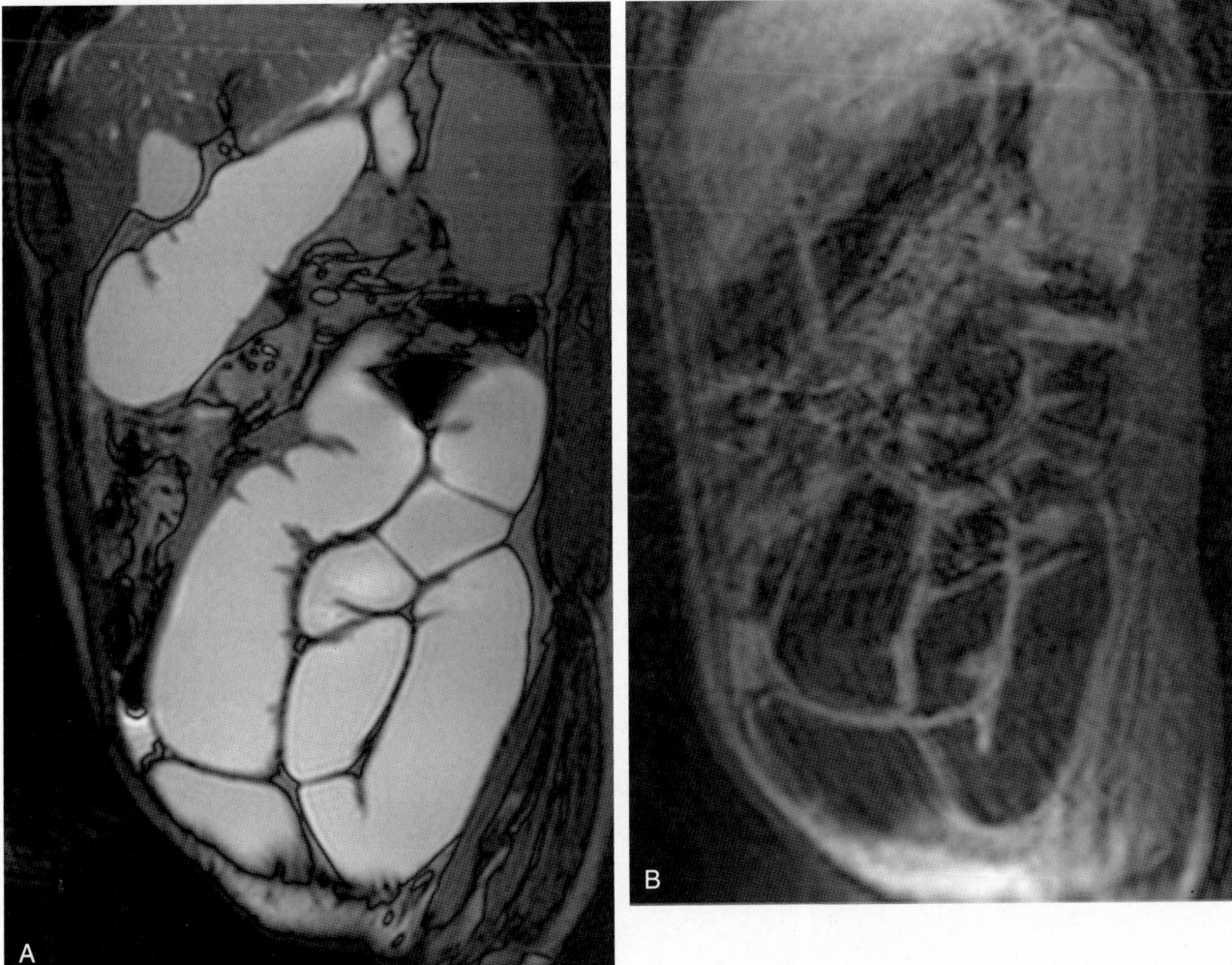

Figure 58-6. Advantages of FISP sequence. True FISP images (**A**) are less prone to motion artifacts than T1-weighted gradient-echo images (**B**) and may therefore provide useful information in patients who are not able to hold their breath.

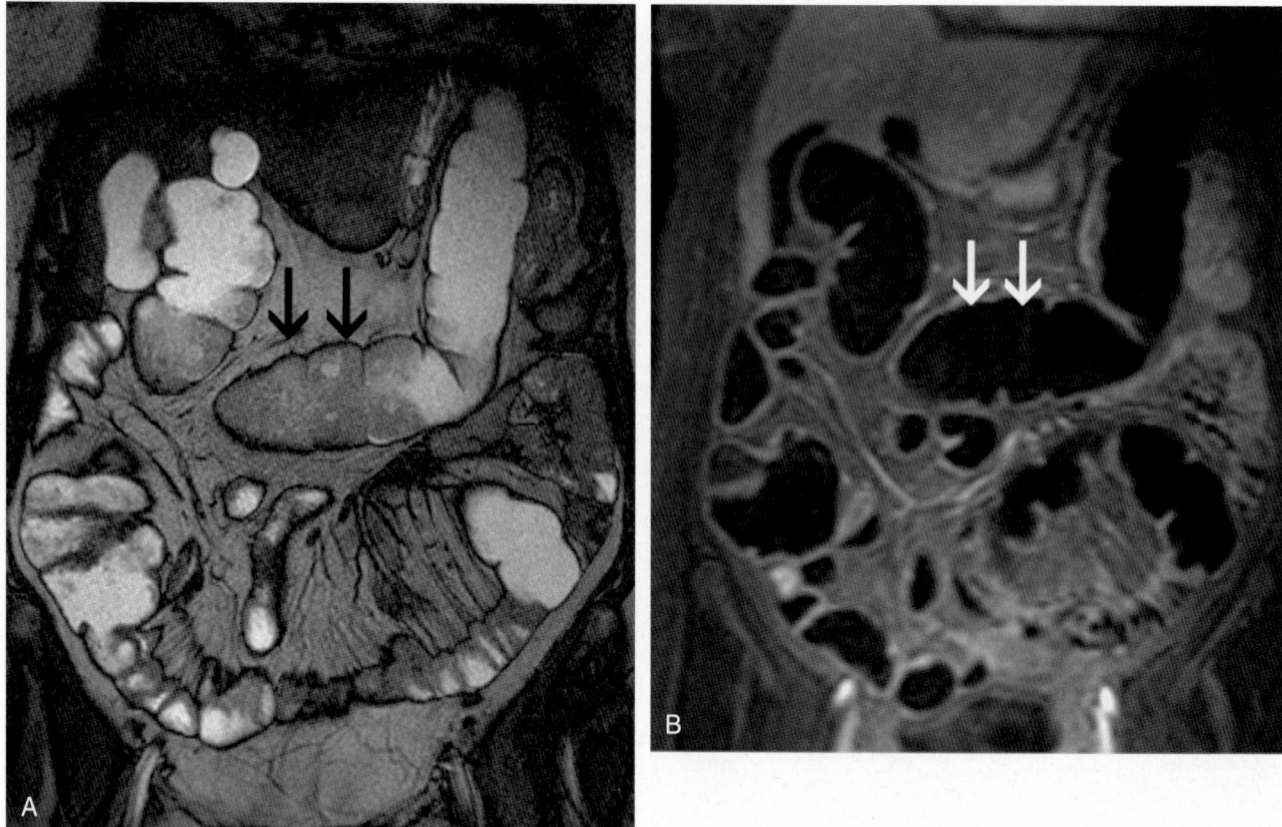

Figure 58-7. Fecal tagging. Fecal material (*arrows*) may be rendered virtually invisible on T1-weighted images (**A**) by means of fecal tagging. Note that on the true FISP image (**B**) the fecal material presents with moderate signal intensity.

Barium sulfate solutions have been used for fecal tagging. Administered orally, in a volume of 200 mL with each of four principal meals before the MR examination, barium decreases the signal intensity of fecal material on T1-weighted gradient-recalled echo images.[8,22,23] Thus, feces are rendered virtually indistinguishable from the administered water enema (Fig. 58-8). Fecal tagging with barium has been successfully tested in volunteer and patient studies.[8,23] However, a in a recent study it was revealed that ingestion of barium was considered as unpleasant as bowel purgation.[24,25]

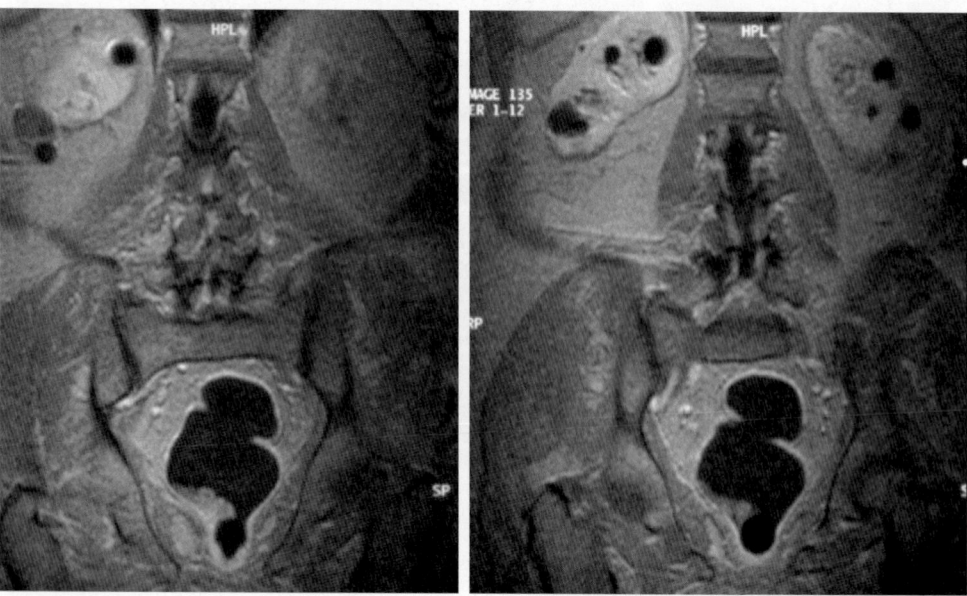

Figure 58-8. TurboFLASH imaging. Large polyp depicted in two consecutive turboFLASH coronal views. Homogeneous suppression of the intraluminal signal can be achieved through optimization of the inversion time, while the absence of motion-related artifacts can be explained in the sequential data acquisition of the turboFLASH sequence.

References

1. Dafnis G, Granath F, Pahlman L, et al: Patient factors influencing the completion rate in colonoscopy. Dig Liver Dis 37:113-118, 2005.
2. Cirocco WC, Rusin LC: Factors that predict incomplete colonoscopy. Dis Colon Rectum 389:964-968, 1995.
3. Marshall JB, Barthel JS: The frequency of total colonoscopy and terminal ileal intubation in the 1990s. Gastrointest Endosc 39:518-520, 1993.
4. McFarland EG, Brink JA, Pilgram TK, et al: Spiral CT colonography: Reader agreement and diagnostic performance with two- and three-dimensional image-display techniques. Radiology 218:375-383, 2001.
5. Ajaj W, Pelster G, Treichel U, et al: Dark lumen magnetic resonance colonography: Comparison with conventional colonoscopy for the detection of colorectal pathology. Gut 52:1738-1743, 2003.
6. Pappalardo G, Polettini E, Frattaroli FM, et al: Magnetic resonance colonography versus conventional colonoscopy for the detection of colonic endoluminal lesions. Gastroenterology 119:300-304, 2000.
7. Ajaj W, Goyen M: MR imaging of the colon: Techniques, indications, results and limitations. Eur J Radiol 61:415-423, 2007.
8. Lauenstein T, Holtmann G, Schoenfelder D, et al: MR colonography without colonic cleansing: A new strategy to improve patient acceptance. AJR 177:823-827, 2001.
9. Ajaj W, Lauenstein TC, Pelster G, et al: MR colonography: How does air compare to water for colonic distention? J Magn Reson Imaging 19:216-221, 2004.
10. Hartmann D, Bassler B, Schilling D, et al: Colorectal polyps: Detection with dark-lumen MR colonography versus conventional colonoscopy. Radiology 238:143-149, 2006.
11. Lauenstein TC, Ajaj W, Kuehle CA, et al: Magnetic resonance colonography: Comparison of contrast-enhanced three-dimensional vibe with two-dimensional FISP sequences: Preliminary experience. Invest Radiol 40:89-96, 2005.
12. Martin DR, Yang M, Thomasson D, Acheson C: MR colonography: Development of optimized method with ex vivo and in vivo systems. Radiology 225:597-602, 2002.
13. Ajaj W, Lauenstein TC, Pelster G, et al: MR colonography in patients with incomplete conventional colonoscopy. Radiology 234:452-459, 2005.
14. Ajaj W, Lauenstein TC, Pelster G, et al: MR colonography for the detection of inflammatory diseases of the large bowel: Quantifying the inflammatory activity. Gut 54:257-263, 2005.
15. Schreyer AG, Golder S, Scheibl K, et al: Dark lumen magnetic resonance enteroclysis in combination with MRI colonography for whole bowel assessment in patients with Crohn's disease: First clinical experience. Inflamm Bowel Dis 11:388-394, 2005.
16. Schreyer AG, Rath HC, Kikinis R, et al: Comparison of magnetic resonance imaging colonography with conventional colonoscopy for the assessment of intestinal inflammation in patients with inflammatory bowel disease: A feasibility study. Gut 54:250-256, 2005.
17. Narin B, Ajaj W, Gohde S, et al: Combined small and large bowel MR imaging in patients with Crohn's disease: A feasibility study. Eur Radiol 14:1535-1542, 2004.
18. Villavicencio RT, Rex DK: Colonic adenomas: Prevalence and incidence rates, growth rates, and miss rates at colonoscopy. Semin Gastrointest Dis 11:185-193, 2000.
19. Steidle G, Schafer J, Schlemmer HP, et al: Two-dimensional parallel acquisition technique in 3D MR colonography. Rofo 176:1100-1105, 2004.
20. Elwood MJ, Ali G, Schlup MT, et al: Flexible sigmoidoscopy or colonoscopy for colorectal screening: A randomized trial of performance and acceptability. Cancer Detect Prevent 19:337-347, 1995.
21. Thomeer M, Bielen D, Vanbeckevoort D, et al: Patient acceptance for CT colonography: What is the real issue? Eur Radiol 12:1410-1415, 2002.
22. Papanikolaou N, Grammatikakis J, Maris T, et al: MR colonography with fecal tagging: Comparison between 2D turbo FLASH and 3D FLASH sequences. Eur Radiol 13:448-452, 2003.
23. Langhorst J, Kuhle CA, Ajaj W, et al: MR colonography without bowel purgation for the assessment of inflammatory bowel diseases. Inflamm Bowel Dis Mar 12 2007. (Epub ahead of print)
24. Florie J, Jensch S, Nievelstein RA, et al: MR colonography with limited bowel preparation compared to optical colonoscopy in patients with increased risk for colorectal cancer. Radiology Feb 28 2007. (Epub ahead of print)
25. Gollub MJ, Schwartz LH, Akhurst T: Update on colorectal cancer imaging. Radiol Clin North Am 45:85-118, 2007.

Diverticular Disease of the Colon

Richard M. Gore, MD • Vahid Yaghmai, MD • Emil J. Balthazar, MD

Colonic diverticula are acquired herniations of the mucosa and of portions of the submucosa through the muscularis propria. Diverticular disease of the colon represents a continuum from an initial, prediverticular phase of marked muscular thickening of the colon wall (myochosis) to frank outpouchings (diverticulosis) and finally to diverticular perforation (diverticulitis). Disease progression from the initial phase to the advanced phases does not necessarily occur.[1] In this chapter we discuss the natural history of this disease and focus on radiologic diagnosis and intervention.

DIVERTICULOSIS

Epidemiology

Diverticular disease is the most common colonic disease in the Western world. Interestingly, this disease was a pathologic curiosity before the 20th century. Its modern development is attributable to the introduction of the roller milling process in 1880, which removes most of the fiber from flour. This process results in a low-residue diet producing low-volume, tenacious stools that require a high degree of propulsive effort for expulsion.[1,2]

In Western countries, colonic diverticula occur in 5% of the population by 40 years of age, in 33% to 50% of the population after 50 years of age, and in more than 50% of the population after 80 years of age.[1,2] These findings contrast sharply to the prevalence rate of less than 0.2% in underdeveloped areas of Asia and Africa.[3] In individuals from low-prevalence areas who migrate to Western communities, the frequency of diverticula increases within 10 years.

The sigmoid colon is involved in up to 95% of patients, and the cecum is involved in 5% of patients. Japan is an interesting exception to other developed countries in that patients with right-sided diverticulosis outnumber those with left-sided disease by a ratio of 5:1.[3]

Four to 5 percent of all patients who harbor diverticula and 20% of those whose diverticula are clinically recognized will develop some complication; 1% to 2% will require hospitalization, and 0.5% will need surgical intervention or radiologic intervention or both.[4,5]

Etiology

The two fundamental factors contributing to the development of sigmoid diverticula are (1) a pressure gradient between the lumen and the serosa and (2) areas of relative weakness in the bowel wall. The first factor can best be appreciated by considering the tendency of the colon to function not as a tube but as small compartments created by the haustra (segmentation). The sigmoid is the narrowest portion of the colon and generates the highest intrasegmental pressures. In addition, stool is most dehydrated in the sigmoid colon, further increasing segmentation and motor activity.[6-9]

The colon wall is weakest where the intramural vasa recta penetrate to the submucosal layers. These points are on either side of the taenia mesocolica and on the mesenteric side of the taenia libera and taenia omentalis (Fig. 59-1).[1,2] Diverticula do not usually occur on the haustral row between the taenia omentalis and the taenia libera.[1,2,10-14]

Pathophysiology

Most colonic diverticula are false diverticula, or pseudodiverticula, because they contain mucosa and submucosa but not the muscularis propria (Fig. 59-2). They are usually 0.5 to 1.0 cm and penetrate the clefts between bundles of circular muscle fibers at points where nutrient arteries pass through the submucosa. The proximity of the diverticula to the arteries is considered key in the development of hemorrhage.[1,2,13]

In the uninflamed state, diverticula are elastic and compressible but have a tendency to empty poorly and, as a result, to fill with inspissated stool. This tendency may account for the increased number of lymphoid follicles found in the lining mucosa.[1,2]

Most patients with sigmoid diverticula have myochosis, a disorder in which there is thickening of the circular muscle layer, shortening of the taeniae, and narrowing of the lumen. The circular muscle is often corrugated, and its appearance has been likened to that of a concertina.[1,2]

Diverticula of the rectum are rare because the taeniae become fused at this level, forming a completely encircling, supporting coat.[14]

Clinical Findings

In most patients, diverticulosis is an incidental finding. Patients may complain of symptoms of irritable bowel syndrome, such as chronic or intermittent postprandial lower abdominal pain that is relieved by defecation.

Radiologic Findings

Radiography

More than 50% of patients with significant diverticular disease demonstrate a distinctive "bubbly" appearance of the sigmoid colon on routine abdominal radiographs. When pelvic phleboliths are present there is a statistical correlation between their number and size and the degree of diverticular disease. It is postulated that both of these common disorders are due

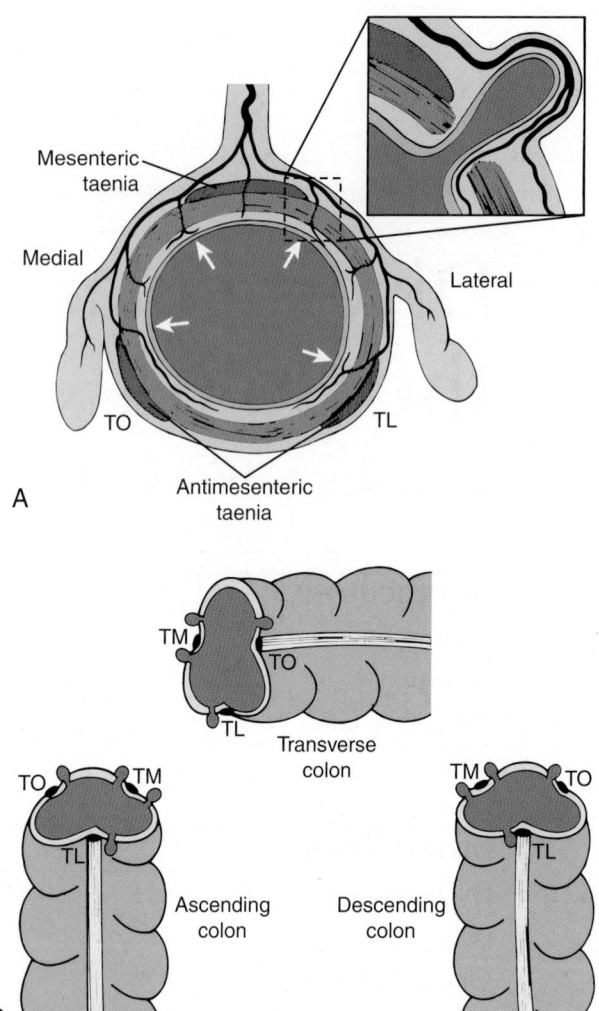

Figure 59-1. Site of origin of colonic diverticula. A. Diverticula develop on either side of the mesenteric taenia and on the mesenteric side of the antimesenteric taenia, the taenia omentalis (TO), and taenia libera (TL). These are the sites (*arrows*) where the vasa recta perforate the muscularis propria and penetrate the submucosa (*inset*). **B.** The antimesenteric TO-TL haustral row does not give rise to diverticula. TM, mesenteric taenia. (**A** from Dietzen CD, Pemberton JH: Diverticulitis. In Yamada T [ed]: Textbook of Gastroenterology. Philadelphia, JB Lippincott, 1991, pp 1734-1748; **B** from Meyers MA, Volberg F, Katzen B, et al: Haustral anatomy and pathology: A new look: II. Roentgen interpretation of pathologic alterations. Radiology 108:505-512, 1973.)

to the long-term effects of a low-fiber diet and straining while defecating.[15,16]

Barium Studies

Diverticulosis is detected more often by double-contrast studies than by single-contrast studies because of the greater colonic distention and the improved visualization of intramural diverticula (Fig. 59-3). When viewed en face, these immature diverticula may simulate aphthae. Their true nature is established when they are viewed in profile, when they are conical or triangular and 1 to 2 mm high.[17-20]

The mature diverticulum has several characteristic appearances (Fig. 59-4) that depend on the angle with which it is viewed and the degree of barium filling. In profile, the diverti-

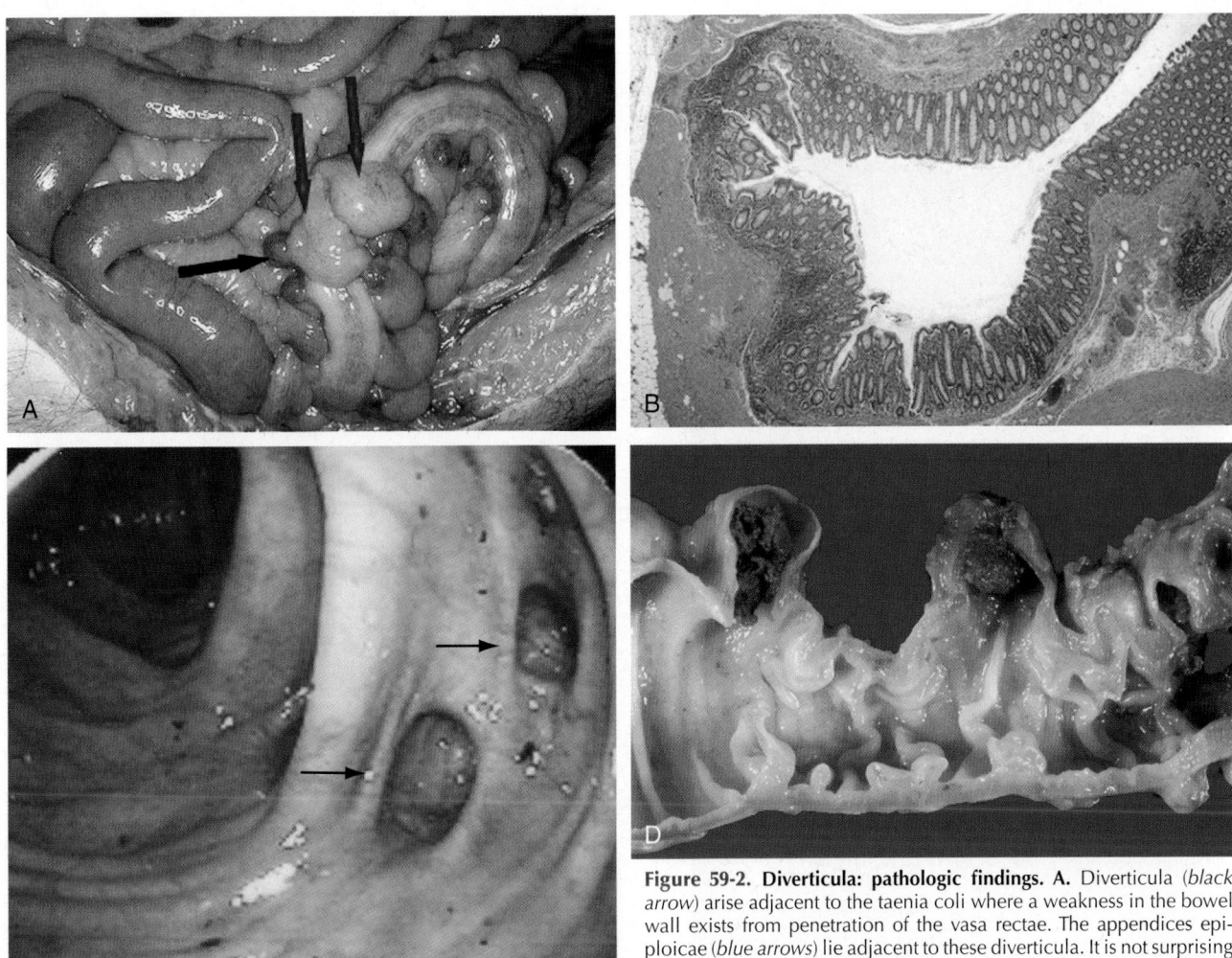

Figure 59-2. Diverticula: pathologic findings. A. Diverticula (*black arrow*) arise adjacent to the taenia coli where a weakness in the bowel wall exists from penetration of the vasa rectae. The appendices epiploicae (*blue arrows*) lie adjacent to these diverticula. It is not surprising that epiploic appendagitis and diverticulitis can have similar clinical features. **B.** Histologic images shows that diverticula consist of herniated mucosal and submucosal layers and lack the muscularis propria. **C.** Colonoscopic view of multiple diverticula in the sigmoid colon. The orifice of the diverticula is evident (*arrows*). **D.** Gross specimen of colon. Diverticula readily fill with stool but poorly empty this material.

culum appears as a flasklike protrusion measuring several millimeters to several centimeters in length, joined to the wall by a fairly long, large neck. En face, it may appear as a ring shadow or a well-marginated barium collection or may resemble a bowler hat (Fig. 59-5). The size and form of diverticula vary from one moment to the next, depending on the degree of colonic distention. The alignment of diverticula along the taeniae is usually apparent.[20-25]

Diagnostic difficulties may arise if the diverticulum inverts into the lumen, and a number of diverticular "polypectomies" have been described in the endoscopic literature. Also, if feces obstruct the diverticulum, the diverticular orifice may bulge into the lumen, resulting in a ring shadow or filling defect. In profile, only the neck of the diverticulum may be visible. If the obstruction is incomplete, a fine linear strand of barium may penetrate the diverticulum, simulating a spur. Because this strand of barium appears outside the lumen, its presence usually allows the correct diagnosis to be made. For this reason, careful attention to the appearance of polyps and diverticula from film to film is necessary.[20-25]

A diverticulum with a large neck may resemble a sessile polyp, one with a narrow neck may resemble a pedunculated polyp, and an obstructed diverticulum may resemble a polyp or adherent fecal material. In addition, both polyps and diverticula can produce the "bowler hat" sign. If the "bowler hat" points toward the center of the long axis of the colon, it represents a polyp. If it points away from the center of the long axis of the bowel, it represents a diverticulum. If the "bowler hat" is located in the midline of the bowel, or is directly parallel to the long axis of the bowel, it cannot be confidently classified as representing either a polyp or a diverticulum.[20-25]

Caliber and haustral abnormalities (Fig. 59-6) usually accompany and often antedate the appearance of diverticula, particularly in the sigmoid colon. Haustral clefts are usually symmetric and face one another in the sigmoid; however, in diverticular or prediverticular disease, they indent alternately from one border to another, creating a staggered effect. The circular muscle is hypertonic and thickened, and the taeniae contract. Diverticula originate at the top of the haustra. With progressive disease, the circular muscle continues to undergo

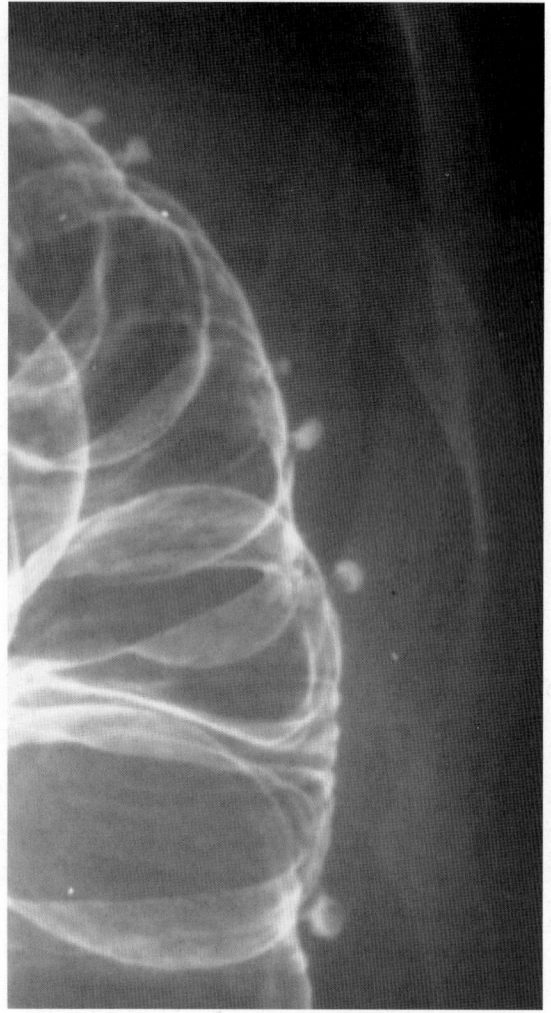

Figure 59-3. Colonic diverticulosis: double-contrast barium enema features. Multiple barium-filled outpouchings are identified along the lateral aspect of the proximal descending colon.

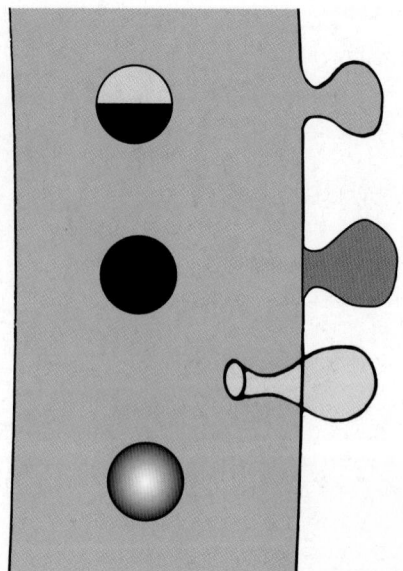

Figure 59-4. Variable appearance of diverticula on double-contrast barium enema. The appearance of diverticula depends on the angle from which they are viewed and how much barium or air they contain. (From Bartram CI, Kumar P: Clinical Radiology in Gastroenterology. Oxford, Blackwell Scientific, 1981, p 130.)

hypertrophy and a "concertina" or zigzag appearance develops. This appearance is due to the alternated, highly compact, deep, and uniform haustra that separate and segment the haustral cul-de-sacs.[17-25]

Computed Tomography

Computed tomography (Fig. 59-7) reveals mural thickening of the colon (>4 mm) in myochosis and in most cases of diverticulosis. The diverticula appear as outpouchings that contain air, stool, and/or contrast agent.

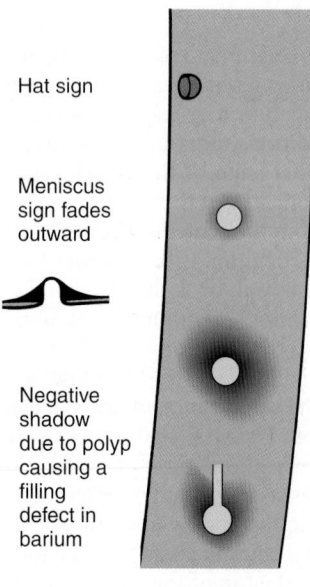

Hat sign

Meniscus sign fades outward

Negative shadow due to polyp causing a filling defect in barium

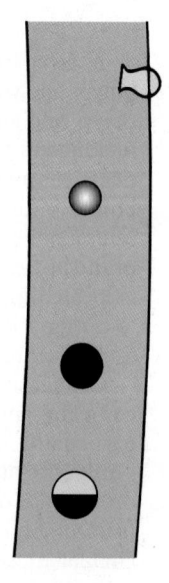

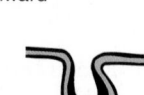

Part seen outside bowel wall

Meniscus sign fades inward

Diverticulum filled with barium

Fluid level in erect/decubitus

Figure 59-5. Distinguishing features of polyps and diverticula. A. Polyps. **B.** Diverticula. (From Bartrum CI, Kumar P: Clinical Radiology in Gastroenterology. Oxford, Blackwell Scientific, 1981, p 131.)

A   B

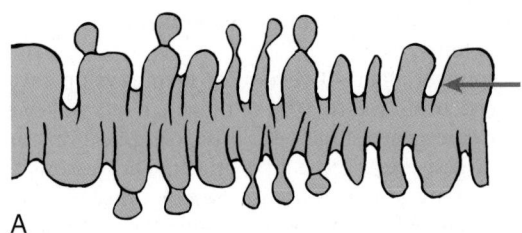

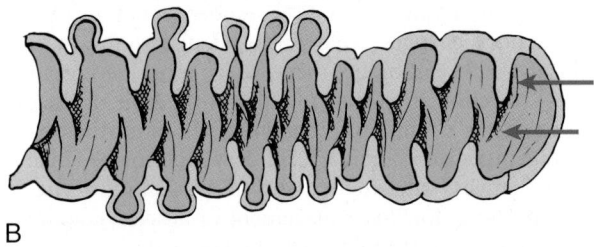

Figure 59-6. Colonic myochosis. A. The thickened circular muscle (*arrow*) and shortened taeniae lead to the appearance of a concertina. **B.** Longitudinal section of the same sigmoid colon segment shows narrowing of the lumen and prominent haustra (*arrows*), which are staggered. (From Weissman A, Clot M, Brellet J: Double Contrast Examination of the Colon. Berlin, Springer-Verlag, 1985, p 150.)

DIVERTICULITIS

Epidemiology

Diverticulitis is the most common complication of diverticulosis, occurring in 10% to 20% of patients with known diverticulosis. In one longitudinal study, clinical diverticulitis was evident in 10% of those patients followed for 5 years and in 37% of those followed for 11 to 18 years.[26,27] The chance of developing diverticulitis increases if the diverticula are widely distributed, are more numerous than average, and have been present for more than a decade.[26]

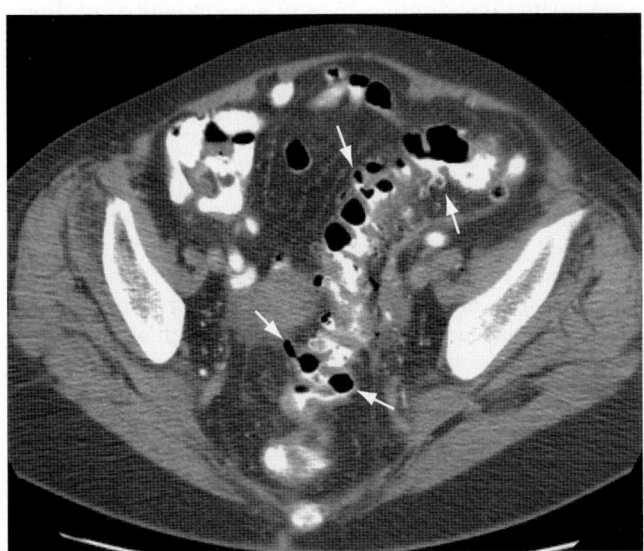

Figure 59-7. Diverticulosis: CT findings. CT scan at the level of the sigmoid colon shows multiple air- and contrast-filled diverticula (*arrows*).

Pathophysiology

The stagnation of nonsterile inspissated fecal material within the diverticulum can cause inflammatory erosion of the mucosal lining in early, subclinical stages of diverticulitis. Subsequently, the wall of the diverticulum is eroded. This perforation is the essential feature of diverticulitis (Fig. 59-8A).[1,2]

This sequence of events can involve an intramural diverticulum, leading to the formation of an intramural abscess. More commonly, it occurs extramurally within the pericolic fat, leading to fibrinous exudate, abscess formation, local

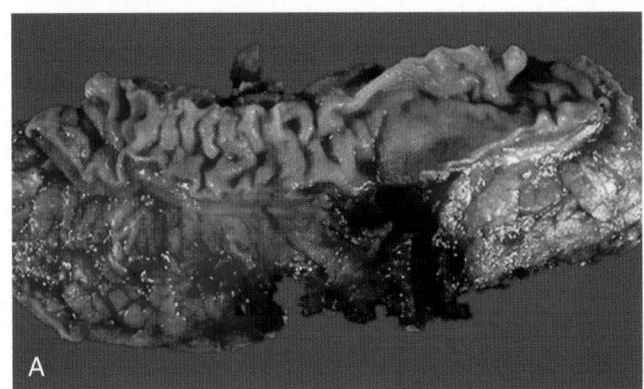

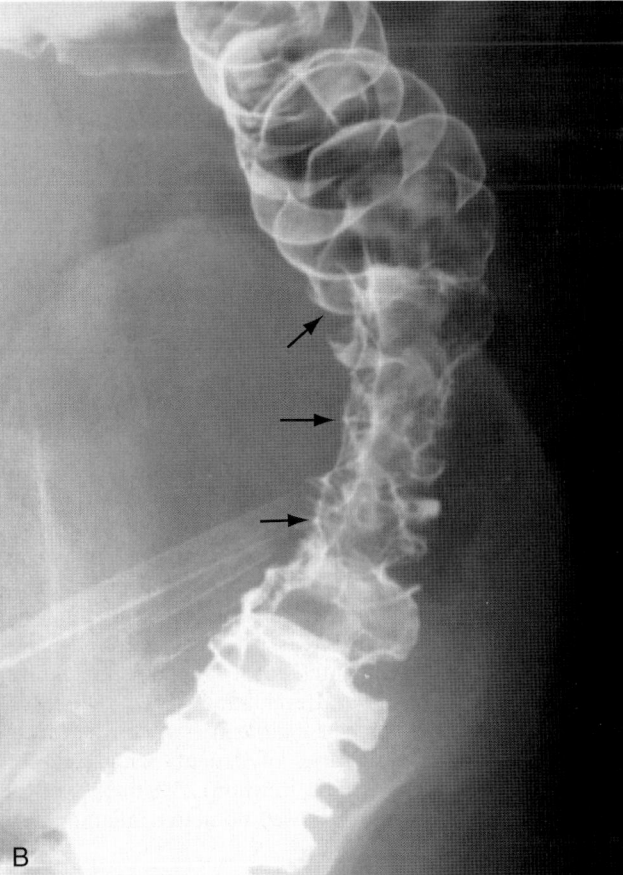

Figure 59-8. Diverticulitis. A. Pathologic specimen showing perforation of a diverticulum into the pericolonic fat, the sine qua non of diverticulitis. **B.** Double-contrast barium enema shows mass effect on the medial aspect of the junction of the descending colon and sigmoid. There is distortion of the lumen, but the extent of extracolonic disease cannot be assessed.

adhesions, or peritonitis. During surgery and pathologic examination, many juxtacolic abscesses are small and difficult to find in the mass of indurated fat and fibrous tissue. It is important to emphasize that the inflammation begins at the apex of the diverticulum and that it may spread rapidly into the soft pericolic and mesocolic fat. The inflammatory changes in diverticulitis are therefore mainly pericolic, adjacent but outside the bowel wall.[1,2,27]

The colonic mucosa is not affected in diverticulitis except in the region of the erosion. Most inflammatory complications of clinical significance are secondary to the rupture of a diverticulum, and they occur in a pericolic location in almost all cases. Consequently, these pathologic changes may be better described as *peridiverticulitis* or *pericolitis*. True diverticulitis, with inflammation limited to the diverticular lining, was present in 10% of pathologic specimens, and muscular hypertrophy with distortion alone and without inflammation accounted for the remaining 25% of cases.

The consequences of diverticular rupture depend on the host response and virulence of the bacterial contamination.[1,2,26] Most patients develop sealed-off abscesses or contained sinus tracts and fistulas. Free perforations are uncommon but can lead to localized pelvic or generalized peritonitis. Fistulas involve adjacent structures, such as small bowel, urinary bladder, vagina, and anterior abdominal wall. Occasionally, several adjacent diverticula communicate with each other along the outer aspect of the deep muscular layers, forming an intramural fistulous tract. In other cases, fistulas extend deeply into the fatty tissue at the site of the attachment of the sigmoid mesocolon.[1,2,26]

Clinical Findings

The classic clinical features of sigmoid diverticulitis are left lower quadrant pain, tenderness, fever, and leukocytosis. Because of this clinical constellation, sigmoid diverticulitis has been called *left-sided appendicitis*. Diverticulitis occurring in other colonic locations is more difficult to diagnose clinically. In one review, the following clinical features were noted: pain in the left iliac fossa in 85% of patients; palpable mass, tenderness, and muscle guarding in 48%; fever in 30%; vomiting in less than 50%; and partial obstruction in 20%. Mild bleeding occurred in 25% of patients, and about 33% of patients had a history of recurrent episodes of similar attacks. Surgical evaluation of this group of 258 patients showed a 20% incidence of pericolic abscess, an 8% incidence of fistulas, and an 18% incidence of peritonitis. The initial clinical diagnosis was sigmoid carcinoma in 32% of patients, but carcinoma was found in only 2% of patients. The occurrence of malignancy was entirely coincidental, but it highlights the clinical difficulties of diagnosing and evaluating patients with suspected acute diverticulitis. These difficulties are further documented by large surgical series of patients with a clinical diagnosis of acute diverticulitis, in whom 25% to 33% of the resected surgical specimens showed no active inflammation, abscess, or fistulas.[1,2,26-28]

Severe diverticulitis can occur in certain groups of patients and produce only minimal or unremarkable clinical symptoms: debilitated elderly patients; patients who have renal failure, are undergoing dialysis, or have had renal transplantation; and patients receiving corticosteroids. Disease in these patients may progress to free perforation, and the diagnosis is often made only when free intra-abdominal air is detected on abdominal films.[1,2,26]

Patients younger than 40 years old often develop severe forms of diverticulitis. Nearly 90% of these patients will eventually require emergency surgery for acute complications, and most need surgery during the first attack. The reasons for this clinical presentation are obscure. Several other observers have also emphasized that in young people the initial attack of colonic diverticulitis is frequently severe.[27,28]

The clinical management of patients with acute diverticulitis depends on the severity, type, and extent of the pericolic inflammatory changes. Mild forms of disease are managed medically with antibiotic therapy. In more severe forms, surgical resection is indicated, either at the time of the diagnosis or after a "cooling-off" interval of antibiotic therapy and percutaneous abscess drainage. Surgery is performed in about 20% of patients admitted to the hospital for diverticulitis and is indicated for the management of abscess, colonic obstruction, perforation and fistula, and hemorrhage that cannot be treated by interventional radiologic methods.[27,28]

Close clinical and radiologic evaluation is crucial in the triage of patients to conservative, radiologic, or surgical management. The radiologic investigation of these patients has two objectives: to confirm the clinical suspicion of diverticulitis and rule out other colonic or pelvic disease and to evaluate and stage the severity of the inflammatory disease. Sigmoidoscopy is usually contraindicated and serves no useful purpose except in patients who have more chronic forms of disease and present with bleeding or in patients in whom polyps or sigmoid carcinoma is suspected.

Radiologic Findings

Radiography

Abdominal films taken with the patient supine and upright are usually diagnostic only in the most severe forms of diverticulitis, in which the patient presents with free intraperitoneal air or sealed-off perforations and pelvic extraluminal air. The detection of an ill-defined, left-sided pelvic mass, localized ileus, and fluid in the pelvis suggests the diagnosis in the appropriate clinical setting. In most patients with acute diverticulitis, however, abdominal plain films are unremarkable and do not contribute to the diagnosis.

Contrast Enema Examination

Contrast enema (CE) examination has traditionally been the primary method of examining patients with suspected diverticulitis. It superbly depicts diverticula, the colonic mucosa and lumen, spasm, muscle hypertrophy, and sacculations. These findings, however, are indicative of diverticular disease but not diagnostic of acute diverticulitis. Because this procedure primarily evaluates the colonic lumen and mucosal surface, the pericolic inflammatory process present in most patients with diverticulitis can be only inferred (Fig. 59-8B).[17-19]

A specific diagnosis of perforated diverticulitis can be made only when there is extravasation of contrast material from a diverticulum into a walled-off abscess, sinus tract, or fistula or free extravasation of contrast material into the peritoneal cavity. These extraluminal collections of contrast medium vary in size, are usually located adjacent to the colon, compress and displace the colonic wall, and are detected in less than 50% of cases of diverticular perforation. Narrowing of the sigmoid lumen, extrinsic compression, and spasm are present in more than 80% of patients, but these findings are less specific. Similarly, an altered mucosal pattern is present in 68% of patients but it is not a reliable indicator of acute inflammation. Lack of mobility with fixation of the sigmoid colon and narrowing, pointing, and distortion of individual diverticula are indirect signs consistent with either acute or chronic diverticulitis.[17-19]

A contour defect that is smooth, well defined, and associated with adjacent sigmoid diverticula represents an intramural inflammatory mass. The contents of the intramural mass, whether pus, organized abscess, or merely mural fibrosis, are more difficult to characterize.

Tracts filled with contrast material passing from ruptured diverticula into the pericolic tissues are common (Fig. 59-9). They may be single or multiple, end blindly (sinuses), or connect with an adjacent hollow viscus or abdominal wall (fistulas). The most common fistulas are colovesical and coloenteric. Colocutaneous fistulas are less frequent and are clinically associated with subcutaneous abscess, emphysema, or fasciitis. Fistulas to the vagina, ureter, appendix, hip, perineum, and soft tissues of the thigh have also been reported. With CE, the fistulous tract between the colon and the urinary bladder is visualized in only 20% of patients who have colovesical fistulas.[17-19]

Longitudinal intramural fistulous tracts represent ruptured diverticula that communicate with each other. Although this sign has also been reported in carcinoma of the colon and Crohn's disease, longitudinal intramural fistulous tracts most often are due to diverticulitis unless there is a previous history or radiographic evidence of Crohn's disease in the remainder of the colon or terminal ileum.

Ultrasonography

Although multidetector CT (MDCT) is the primary cross-sectional imaging study for patients with suspected diverticulitis, ultrasonography may be the first study ordered for nondescript abdominal pain.

The segmental concentric thickening of the gut wall commonly found in patients with diverticular disease manifests as a hypoechoic segment that reflects the predominant thickening of the muscular layer (Fig. 59-10). Inflamed diverticula are brightly echogenic reflectors with acoustic shadowing or ring-down artifact in or beyond the thickened gut wall. Inflammatory changes in the mesocolon are seen as poorly defined, hypoechoic zones without obvious gas or fluid. Intramural sinus tracts appear as high-amplitude linear echoes that often have ring-down artifact within the colon wall. Abscesses appear as loculated, thick-walled fluid collections that may contain gas.[29-37]

Magnetic Resonance Imaging

Mural thickening of the colon (Fig. 59-11) and diverticular abscesses are well visualized on MRI, particularly on gadolinium-enhanced fat-suppressed T1-weighted spoiled gradient-echo images and T2-weighted single-shot echo-train spin-echo images. Sinus tracts, fistulas, and the walls of abscesses enhance and are well depicted in a background of suppressed fat on gadolinium-enhanced fat-suppressed spoiled gradient-echo images. MRI has little role in the primary evaluation of patients with known or suspected diverticulitis.[38]

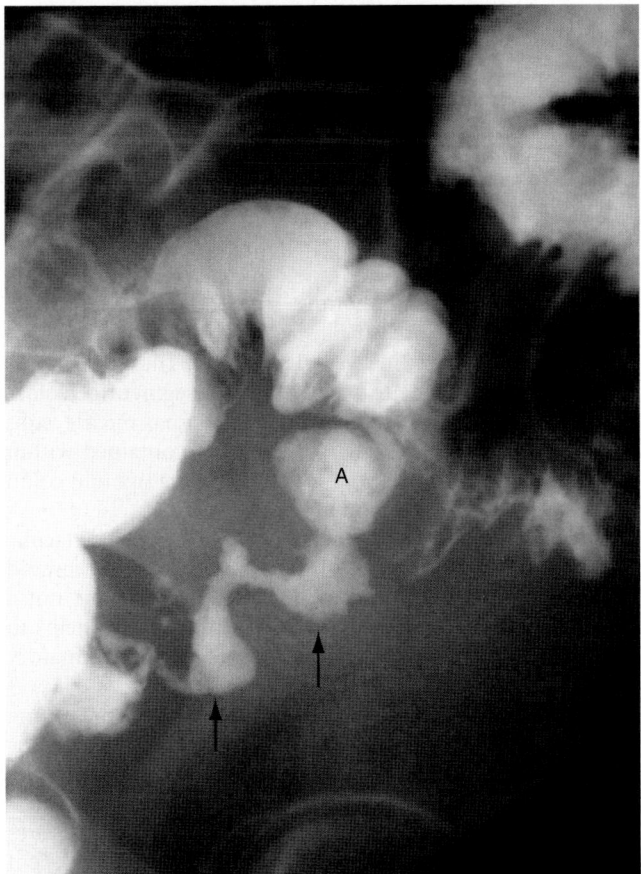

Figure 59-9. Diverticulitis with pericolonic abscess: barium enema features. Spot image from a barium enema shows filling of an abscess (A) and a sinus tract (*arrows*) along the inferior aspect of the sigmoid colon.

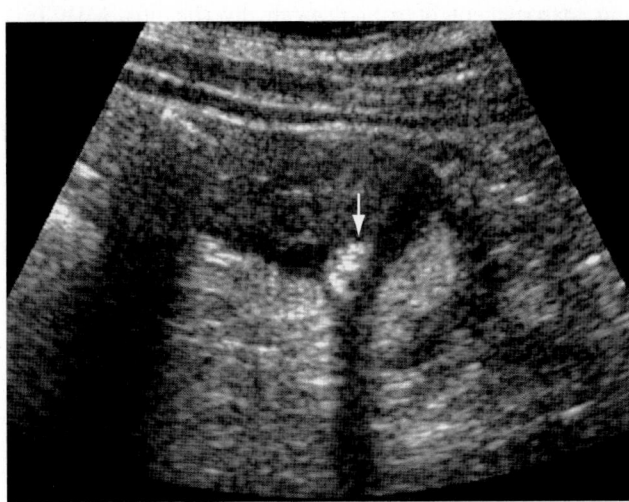

Figure 59-10. Diverticulitis: sonographic features. There is mural thickening of the sigmoid colon associated with a gas-containing intramural abscess (*arrow*) that casts an acoustic shadow.

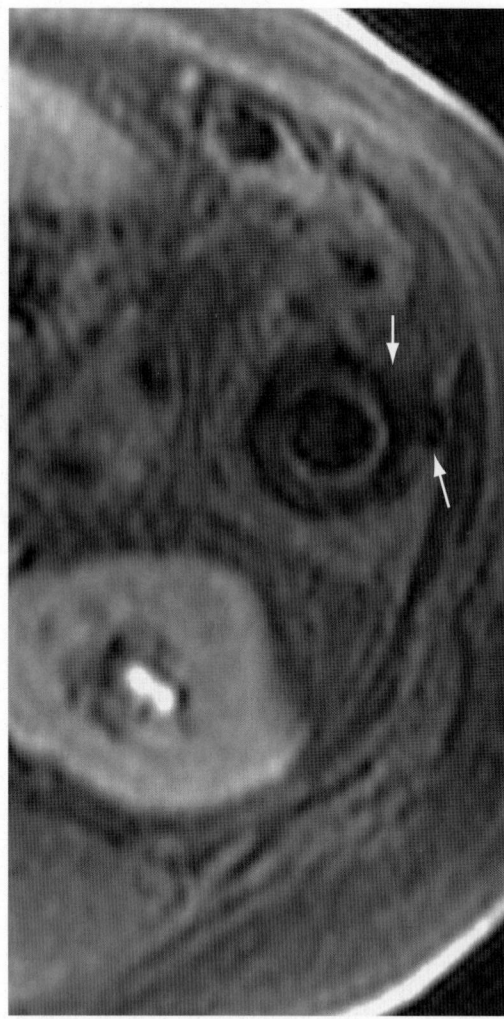

Figure 59-11. Diverticulitis: MRI features. Axial MR image of the descending colon demonstrates mural thickening, increased signal from the colonic mucosa, and abnormal signal in the pericolic fat (*arrows*).

Table 59-1
MDCT Findings in Diverticulitis

Finding	Percentage of Cases
Mural thickening of the colon	96%
Fat stranding	95%
Adjacent diverticula	91%
Fascial thickening	50%
Visualization of inflamed diverticulum	43%
Pericolic gas bubbles	30%
Arrowhead sign	16%
Abscess	4%
Phlegmon	4%
Intramural gas	2%
Sinus tracts	2%

Modified from Kircher MF, Rhea JT, Kihiczak D, et al: Frequency, sensitivity and specificity of individual signs of diverticulitis on thin-section helical CT with colonic contrast material: Experience with 312 cases. AJR 178:1313-1318, 2002.

Computed Tomography

Multidetector CT has dramatically improved the diagnosis and management of patients with diverticulitis. MDCT is ideally suited for evaluating both the intramural component of the inflammatory process and its intraperitoneal or retroperitoneal extension. CT is particularly useful in the evaluation of patients with sepsis who present with left lower quadrant pain, fever, leukocytosis, and a tender, palpable pelvic mass.[39-45]

CT findings in acute diverticulitis are listed in Table 59-1. On non–contrast-enhanced scans, the offending diverticulum can be identified in many cases. It is hyperdense and is the nidus of the surrounding inflammation (Fig. 59-12). Diverticula are identified on CT at the site of the perforation or at a site adjacent to it in more than 80% of cases of acute diverticulitis. They appear as small outpouchings filled with air, barium, and/or fecal material projecting through the colonic wall. Symmetric thickening of the colonic wall in excess of 4 mm is seen in about 70% of cases. The thickened wall has a homogeneous density, and its diameter usually measures less than 1 cm in the distended colon. When there is signifi-

cant muscular hypertrophy, the wall of the colon can be up to 2 or 3 cm thick. In diverticulitis, significant hypertrophy of muscle primarily occurs in the sigmoid segment, and this can mimic carcinoma of the colon. Accurate assessment of colon wall thickness is possible only with proper lumen distention.[30-33]

The hallmark of acute diverticulitis on CT is the presence of inflammatory change in the pericolic fat. This sign is seen in 98% of patients. The degree of inflammatory reaction varies, depending on the size of perforation, bacterial contamination, and host response. In mild cases, there is only a slight increase in the attenuation of fat adjacent to the involved colon with engorgement of the vasa recta (Fig. 59-13). Fine linear strands, small fluid collections, and several bubbles of extraluminal air may be present (Fig. 59-14). In more severe cases, pericolic heterogeneous soft tissue densities representing phlegmons (Fig. 59-15) and/or intramural or extraintestinal loculated fluid collections representing abscess can occur. In sigmoid diverticulitis, fluid in the combined interfascial plane in the pelvis is a common finding.[30-33]

On CT, abscesses appear filled with fluid and may contain bubbles of air or air-fluid levels (Fig. 59-16). These collections can form at a distance from the involved segment of colon. They may form at the flank, groin, thigh, psoas muscle, subphrenic space, or liver. Most abscesses are contained within the sigmoid mesocolon or are sealed off by the sigmoid colon and adjacent small bowel loops.[30-33]

A sealed-off perforation with the resulting juxtacolic inflammatory reaction causes thickening of the mesosigmoid or the adjacent parietal peritoneum. Although this is not a specific finding, it is often seen in diverticulitis and helps in identifying the site and focal nature of the inflammatory process.

Small, 1- to 2-cm intramural fluid collections representing intramural abscesses can be detected. Intramural or pericolic fistulas can be recognized as linear fluid-filled tracts within or parallel to the thickened colonic wall. Blind sinus tracts and fistulas manifest as linear or tubular branching structures in the pericolic tissues. They can communicate with adjacent organs or terminate in an abscess cavity.

In the diagnosis of diverticulitis, CT has a reported accuracy, specificity, and sensitivity of up to 99%.[32]

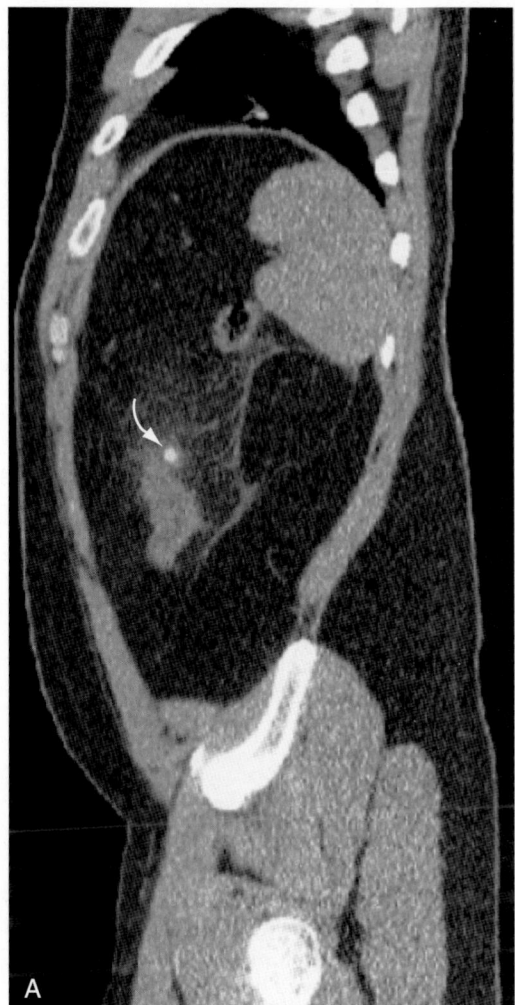

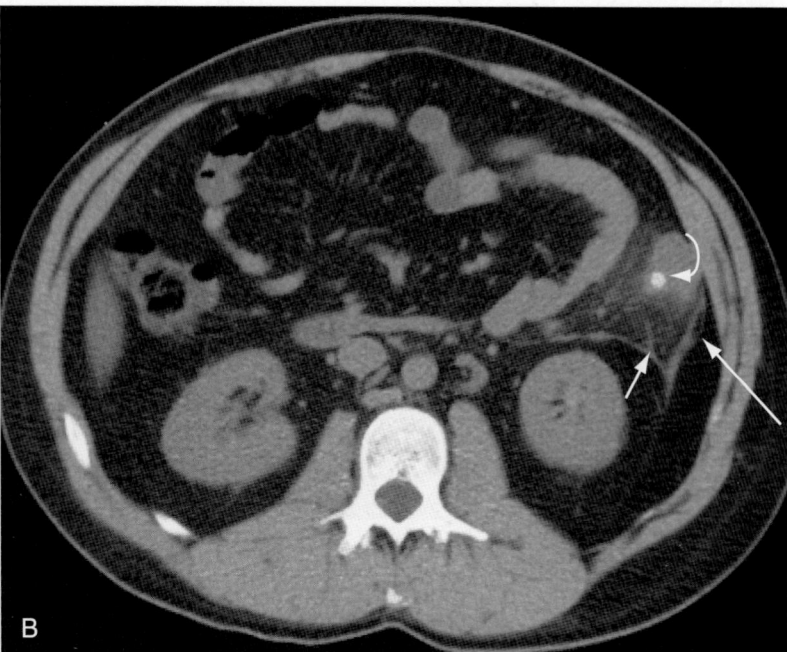

Figure 59-12. Diverticulitis: MDCT findings on non–contrast-enhanced scans. Sagittal (**A**) and axial (**B**) images show the hyperdense offending diverticulum (*curved arrow*) at the center of the pericolonic inflammation. Note the thickening of the anterior (*small straight arrow*) and lateroconal (*large straight arrow*) interfascial planes.

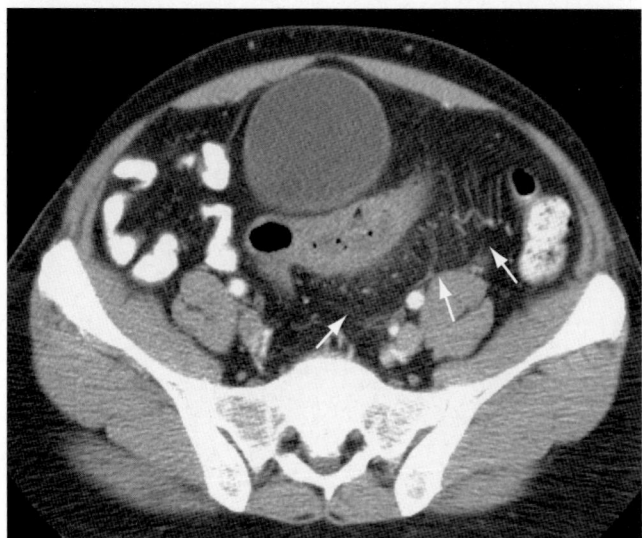

Figure 59-13. MDCT of diverticulitis: early changes. Scan of the sigmoid colon shows a haziness of the fat of the sigmoid mesocolon (*arrows*) associated with engorged vasa rectae.

Surgical and Computed Tomographic Staging

Diverticulitis can be staged both surgically (Fig. 59-17) and by CT. Familiarity with the following staging system helps in directing therapy and assessing prognosis:

Stage 0 diverticulitis is the most common form, in which the inflammation is contained within the serosa. This mural inflammation usually responds well to antibiotics. On CT, it appears primarily as mural thickening with little inflammatory change in the surrounding fat. Follow-up CT scans are usually not needed in these patients.[45-50]

Stage I diverticulitis denotes an abscess or phlegmon that is less than 3 cm in diameter and is confined to the mesocolon. Inflammatory infiltration of pericolic fat and abscess are the major CT findings of this stage. These patients do quite well with 7 to 10 days of antibiotic therapy and seldom progress to stage II or III disease. A follow-up CT scan is recommended because a wide-mouth perforation may not heal.[45-50]

Stage II diverticulitis signifies that the pericolic abscess has broken through the sigmoid mesocolon and has

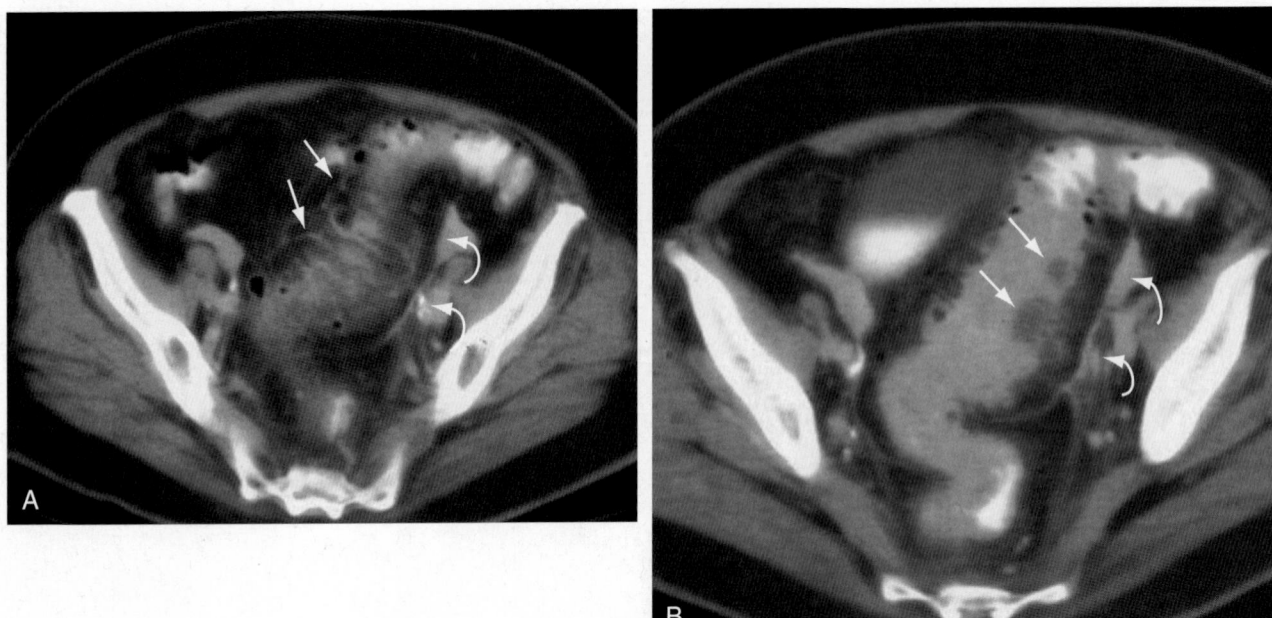

Figure 59-14. **MDCT of diverticulitis: intramural abscess. A.** Scan of the sigmoid colon shows mural thickening associated with engorged vasa rectae (*arrows*) producing the "caterpillar sign." Note the fluid in the combined interfascial plane. **B.** Scan obtained caudal to **A** shows two low-density intramural abscesses. Fluid is also evident in the combined interfascial plane (*curved arrows* in **A** and **B**).

become walled off by the small bowel, greater omentum, fallopian tubes, or other pelvic structures. This stage is associated with abscesses 5 to 15 cm in diameter that are well suited to percutaneous drainage (Fig. 59-18). With percutaneous drainage, many operative procedures for diverticulitis with abscess can be downgraded from a two- or three-stage operation to a one-stage operation.[45-50]

Stage III diverticulitis signifies pelvic abscess that has spread beyond the confines of the pelvis to involve other portions of the peritoneal cavity. Fortunately, this form of diverticulitis is relatively infrequent, because the body's defenses usually contain the perforation. At this stage, the patient requires surgery but percutaneous catheters may allow surgery to be deferred until the patient's status is optimized.[45-50]

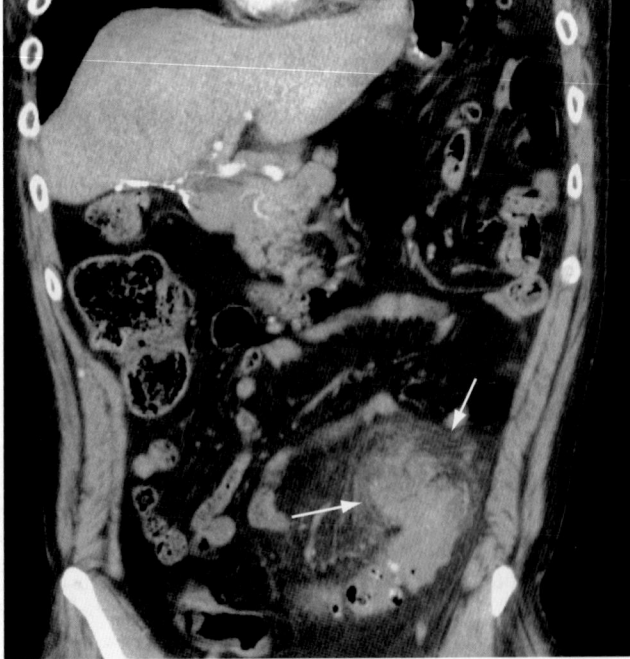

Figure 59-15. **MDCT of diverticulitis: pericolonic phlegmon.** Coronal reformatted image shows intense inflammatory change in the sigmoid mesocolon (*arrows*) without drainable fluid.

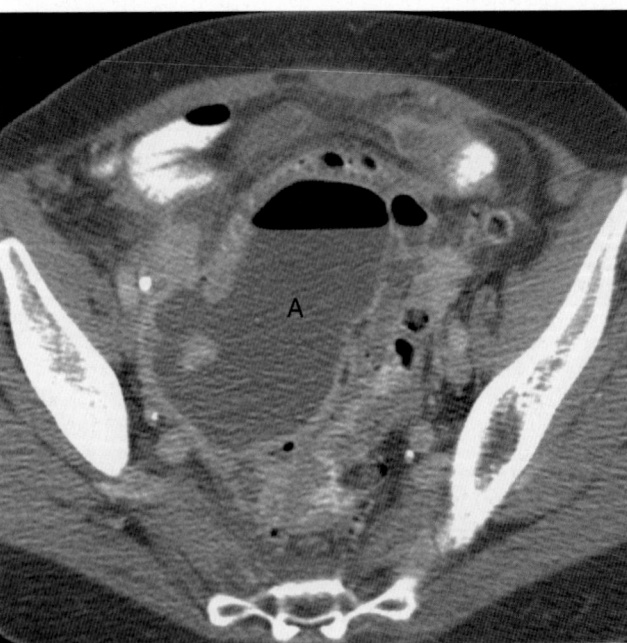

Figure 59-16. **MDCT of diverticulitis: abscess.** A large abscess (A) with an air-fluid level is identified in the pelvis.

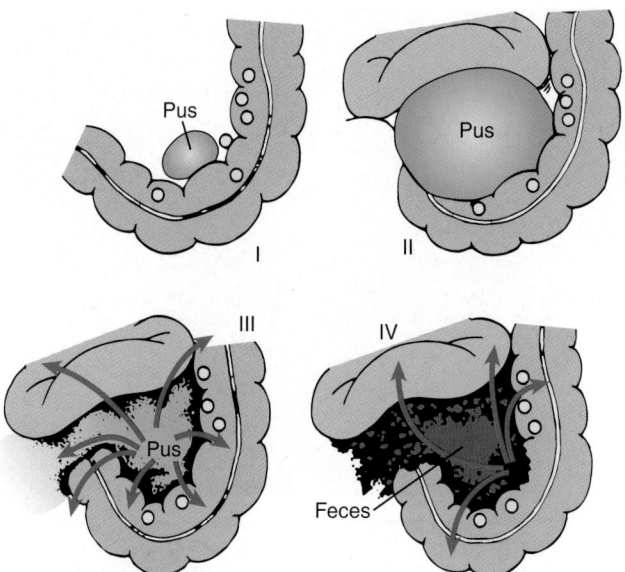

Figure 59-17. Surgical staging of diverticular abscesses. Stage I: a small (<3 cm) pericolic abscess is contained within the sigmoid mesocolon. Stage II: a pelvic abscess has broken out of the sigmoid mesocolon but is contained by the pelvic organs. Stage III: the large pelvic abscess has spread into the rest of the peritoneal cavity. Stage IV: large diverticular perforation occurs with fecal contamination of the peritoneal cavity. (From Hinchley EJ, Schaal PGH, Richards GK: Treatment of perforated diverticular disease of the colon. Adv Surg 12:85-109, 1978).

Stage IV diverticulitis is defined as fecal spread into the peritoneal cavity. The CT appearance may be similar to that of stage III, but these patients have acute peritonitis with life-threatening sepsis, so that they usually undergo immediate exploratory laparotomy.[45-50]

Differentiation of Diverticulitis from Carcinoma

Diverticulitis can mimic colon cancer clinically, on barium enema examination, ultrasonography, MRI, and MDCT. On CE studies, the detection of partial colonic obstruction with sigmoid narrowing, a gradual zone of transition, preservation of the mucosal folds, and associated diverticula indicate diverticulitis (Fig. 59-19). Abrupt transition at the site of obstruction; a rigid, narrowed lumen; destruction of mucosa; and "apple core" configuration suggest carcinoma of the colon. CE is valuable in differentiating diverticulitis from carcinoma of the sigmoid colon in most cases. The presence of sigmoid diverticula, however, is not helpful in the differential diagnosis because 28% of sigmoid cancers involve coincidental diverticula. When the retrograde flow of contrast medium is impeded and the obstructed sigmoid lumen cannot be well visualized, the differentiation of an inflammatory lesion from a malignant lesion cannot be made.[40-45]

CT features that suggest diverticulitis include identification of the offending, hyperdense diverticulum, inflammation of the adjacent fat with engorgement of the vasa recta, fluid at the root of the mesentery (in the combined interfascial plane), fluid and inflammatory change out of proportion to the mural thickening, abscess formation, extraluminal fluid, and gas. CT features favoring carcinoma include prominent adjacent lymph nodes, symmetric or asymmetric mural thick-

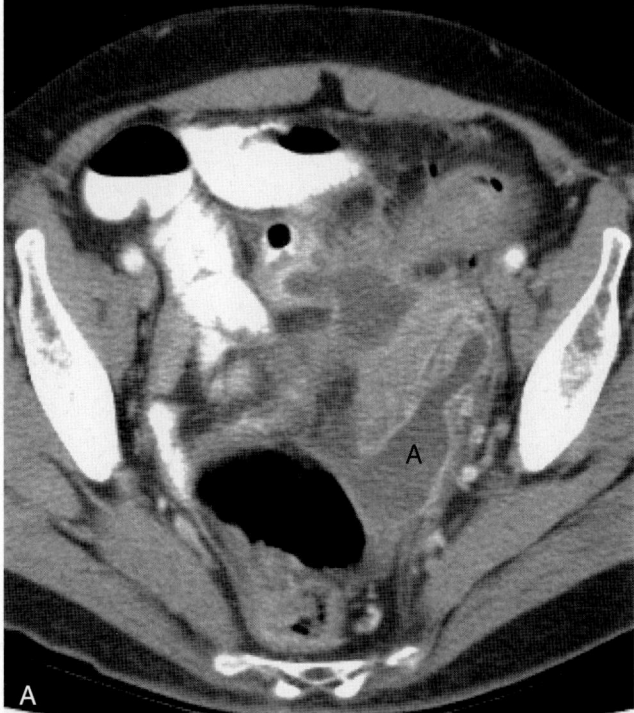

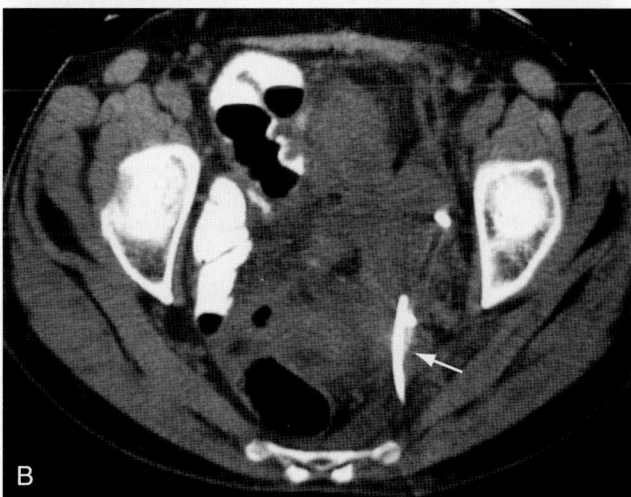

Figure 59-18. MDCT of diverticulitis: abscess drainage. A. There is a multilocular abscess (A) identified in the left side of the pelvis. **B.** The dominant loculation has been drained with a percutaneous catheter (*arrow*) introduced via a transgluteal approach.

ening with shouldered, nontapered margins, and the presence of a luminal mass. There is considerable overlap of CT findings. If there is a segment of colonic thickening with pericolonic inflammatory change and no pericolic lymph nodes, diverticulitis is the most likely diagnosis. When pericolic lymph nodes are seen adjacent to a segment of colonic thickening, colon cancer is the most likely diagnosis.[40-45]

In approximately 10% of patients, diverticulitis cannot be differentiated from colon carcinoma on the basis of CT scans. Most patients with diverticulitis exhibit only mild circumferential wall thickening in the range of 4 to 5 mm. Excessive thickening of the colonic wall, either concentrically or focally, suggests colonic neoplasm. Although most colon cancers are more than 2 cm thick, neoplastic lesions less than 1 cm in

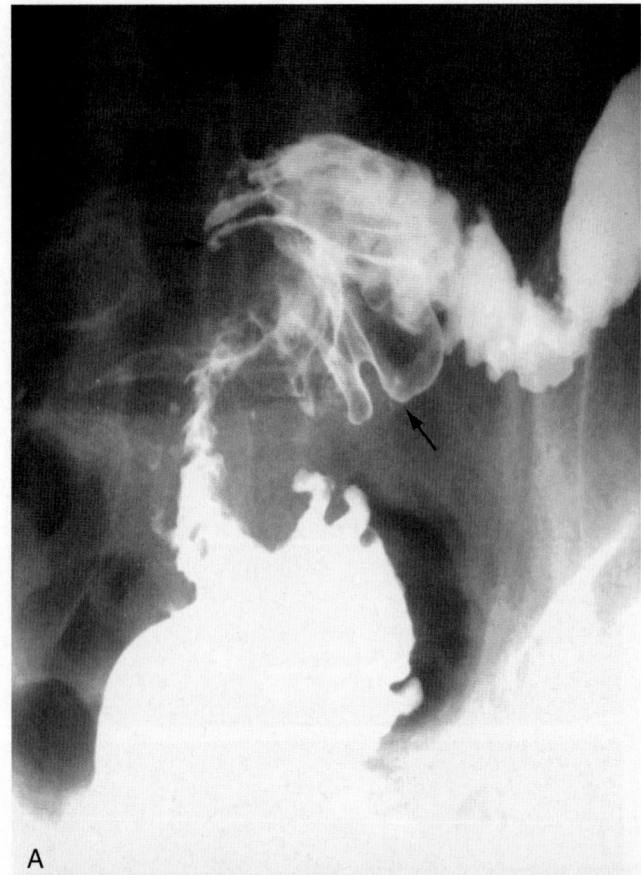

A

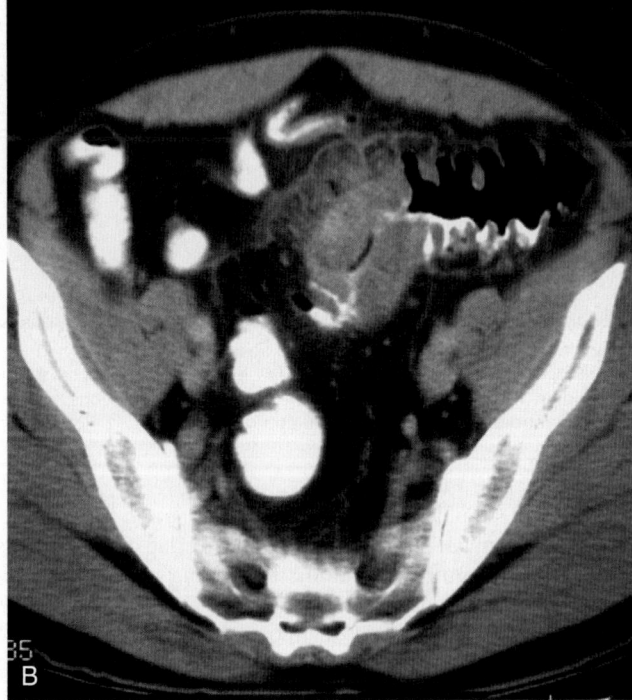

B

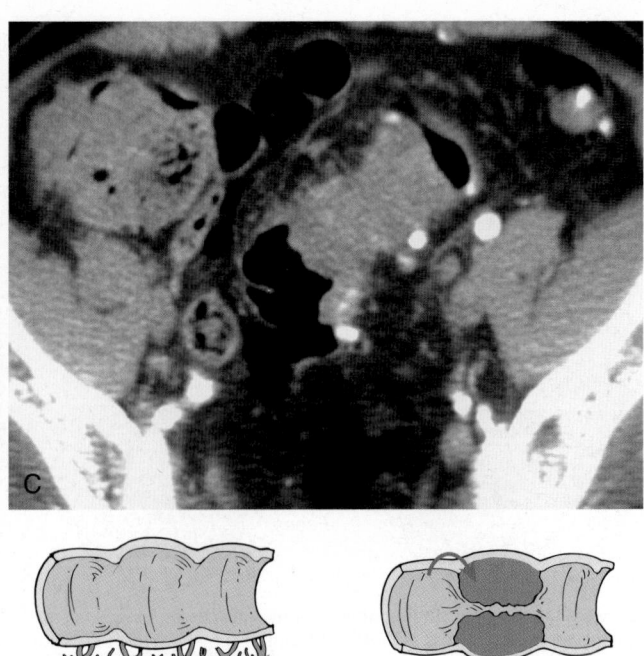

C

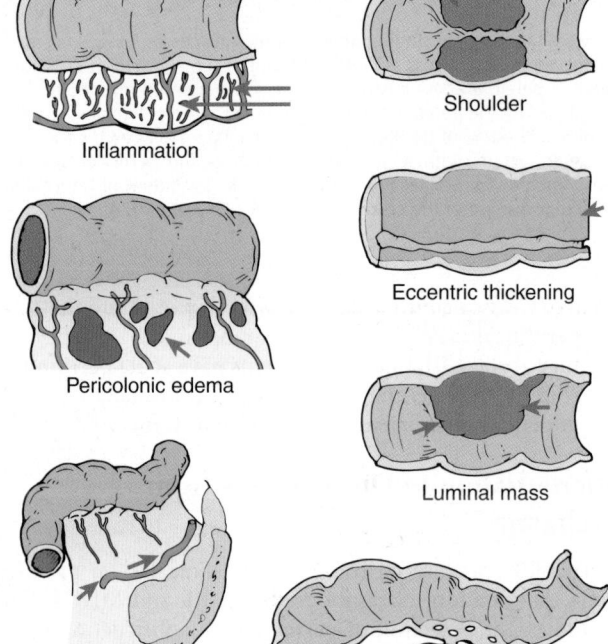

D

Figure 59-19. Colon cancer versus diverticulitis: imaging considerations. A. Barium enema examination demonstrates an indeterminate stricture in the sigmoid colon. Multiple diverticula are present but there is an abrupt, overhanging edge (*arrows*) along the proximal margin of this lesion. This patient had diverticulitis and carcinoma of the sigmoid colon. **B.** Focal, symmetric mural thickening of the sigmoid colon is present. There are inflammatory changes in the fat of the sigmoid mesocolon. Several diverticula are evident just distal to the region of thickening. This patient had diverticulitis. **C.** There is a mass identified within the lumen of the sigmoid colon with only minimal haziness of the adjacent fat. This patient had carcinoma of the sigmoid colon. **D.** Line drawings showing features that suggest diverticulitis (inflammation, pericolic edema, fluid in the root of the mesentery-combined interfascial plane, extraluminal fluid and air) versus carcinoma (eccentric thickening, luminal mass). (From Chintapalli KN, Chopra S, Ghiatas AA, et al: Diverticulitis versus colon cancer: Differentiation with helical CT findings. Radiology 210:429-435, 1999.)

diameter may be seen. These facts account for a significant overlap in colonic wall thickness in diverticulitis and carcinoma, particularly with lesions that are between 1 and 3 cm in thickness. In these cases, it is most helpful to distend the colonic lumen and use high-resolution CT techniques. An abrupt zone of transition with overhanging edges and a narrow, rigid lumen indicates carcinoma; a tethered or saw-toothed luminal configuration suggests diverticular disease. Associated inflammatory mesenteric changes favor diverticulitis, whereas regional lymphadenopathy favors carcinoma of the colon.[51,52]

The differential diagnosis of cancer versus diverticulitis is extremely difficult in patients presenting with perforated colon carcinoma associated with pericolic inflammation or abscess. An abruptly altered lumen caliber with an asymmetric and lobulated soft tissue mass is diagnostic of perforated sigmoid carcinoma.

With MDCT, the diagnosis of perforated colon cancer can be made in most patients. When the CT findings are uncertain or equivocal, CE should be used liberally as an important complementary examination. If the patient's condition improves and immediate surgical resection is not needed, sigmoidoscopy or a barium enema should routinely be performed to confirm the CT diagnosis and exclude sigmoid carcinoma.

Differential Diagnosis

Other conditions such as nonspecific or infectious colitis, ischemic colitis, and Crohn's disease are part of the differential diagnosis of diverticulitis. A long segment of colonic involvement, lack of diverticula, absence of a focal inflammatory pericolic process, or pericolic air collection helps in the CT differential diagnosis. Foreign bodies that escape CT detection and perforate the colon can mimic the CT findings of acute diverticulitis.

Primary epiploic appendagitis, a relatively common condition resulting from an acute inflammation of appendices epiploicae often associated with torsion and infarction, can be confused as diverticulitis. CT, however, will show the characteristic appearance of a small, round or oval fat-containing mass with associated inflammatory reaction adjacent to the colon (Fig. 59-20). The process is self-containing, with clinical resolution within a few days. Follow-up CT examination may show total resolution or shrinkage with eventual calcification of the inflamed and infarcted epiploic appendage.

Cecal Diverticulitis

Cecal diverticulitis or right-sided colonic diverticulitis is a relatively rare pathologic entity in which patients present with

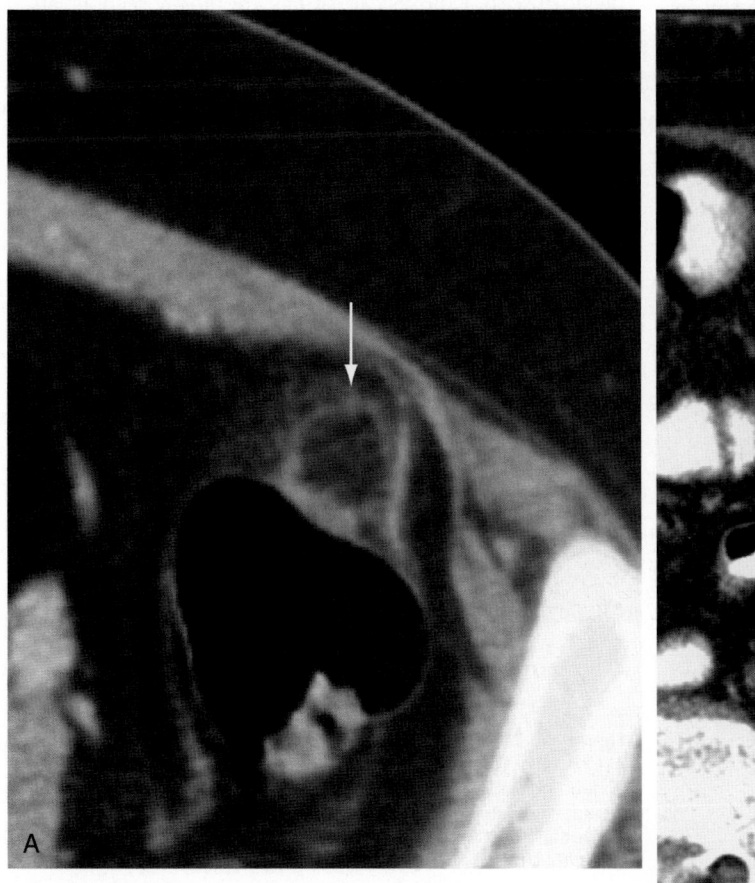
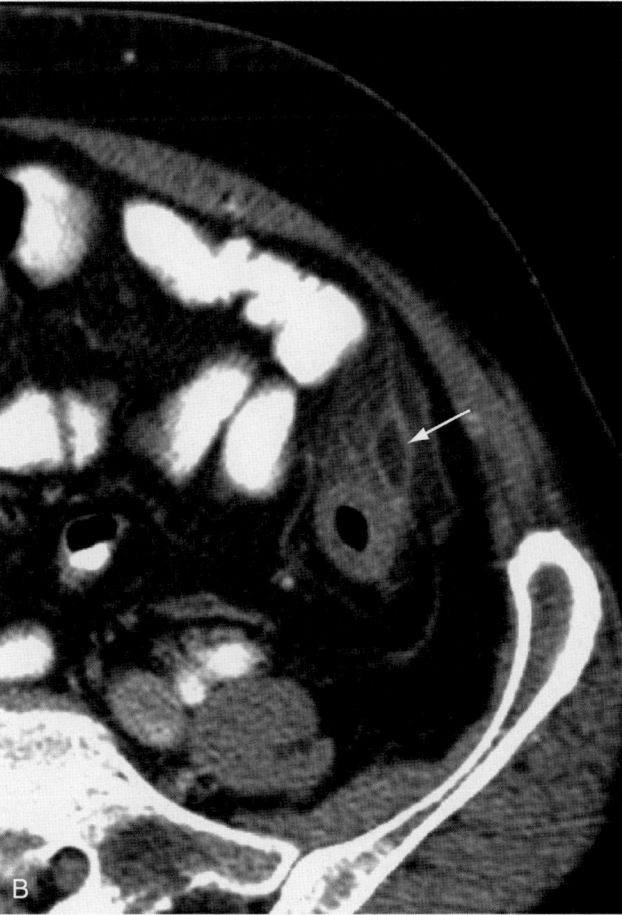

Figure 59-20. Epiploic appendagitis: MDCT features. These two different patients (**A** and **B**) have a fat-density mass (*arrow*) surrounded by increased attenuation adjacent to the sigmoid colon. This fatty mass is the epiploic appendage that has undergone torsion, ischemia, and or inflammation.

protean clinical manifestations that are often clinically misdiagnosed as appendicitis. Cecal diverticula are classified as true (congenital) or false (acquired). The congenital variety is usually larger and solitary and is characterized by the presence of a well-developed muscle coat. Most cecal diverticula are acquired and are similar to diverticula present in the remainder of the colon. They are usually multiple, involve the cecum and ascending colon, are formed by herniated mucosa and serosa, and lack a muscular coat. Unless perforation is suspected, barium examination remains the primary means of preoperative diagnosis. It allows a correct diagnosis in most cases and ruling out of appendicitis and carcinoma, the other major concerns in the differential diagnosis. The characteristic findings of the barium enema examination include a filling defect with an irregular contour, cecal spasm, fixation and spiculation of the cecal wall, visualization of diverticula, and a normal appearance of the appendix.[47]

The CT findings consist of focal pericolic inflammatory changes, slight thickening of the wall of the colon, demonstration of diverticula, and, occasionally, an intramural or pericolic fluid collection representing an abscess (Fig. 59-21). When a normal appendix is seen and the focal pericecal inflammatory process is above the cecal caput, a reliable CT diagnosis can be made. If the appendix is not seen, findings similar to those of appendicitis or perforated cecal carcinoma make the CT diagnosis uncertain. In general, I advocate initial use of CT in all patients suspected of harboring an intra-abdominal inflammatory process. Recent experience suggests that the diagnosis of right-sided colonic diverticulitis can be suggested or established by MDCT. When CT shows focal pericecal inflammation but the findings are not sufficiently specific, a CE study should be performed promptly.[46-49]

Complications

Perforation of one or several diverticula produces a localized inflammatory reaction and may lead to the development of a sinus tract, intramural tract, or a variable-sized intramural or pericolic abscess. Other more unusual complications can sometimes occur.

Fistulas and Sinus Tracts

Fistulas (Fig. 59-22), which are communications between two epithelium-lined surfaces—bowel to another hollow organ, or bowel to skin—can develop and be difficult to detect. Although CT has limited value in the detection of coloenteric fistulas, it is extremely useful in the evaluation of patients with suspected colovesical fistulas. CT has a significantly higher sensitivity compared with the other standard battery of diagnostic tests, including urinary and enteric contrast agent studies and cystoscopy. It should be used as the first imaging modality in patients suspected of having colovesical fistula.

In patients presenting with pneumaturia, the pericolic inflammatory mass involves the bladder wall and the presence of intraluminal vesical air confirms the diagnosis. Sigmoid-vesical fistulas rarely occur in the acute setting, during the initial attack of diverticulitis and the development of the pelvic abscess. Colovesical fistulas are mostly seen as late sequelae after one or several episodes of diverticulitis, when the

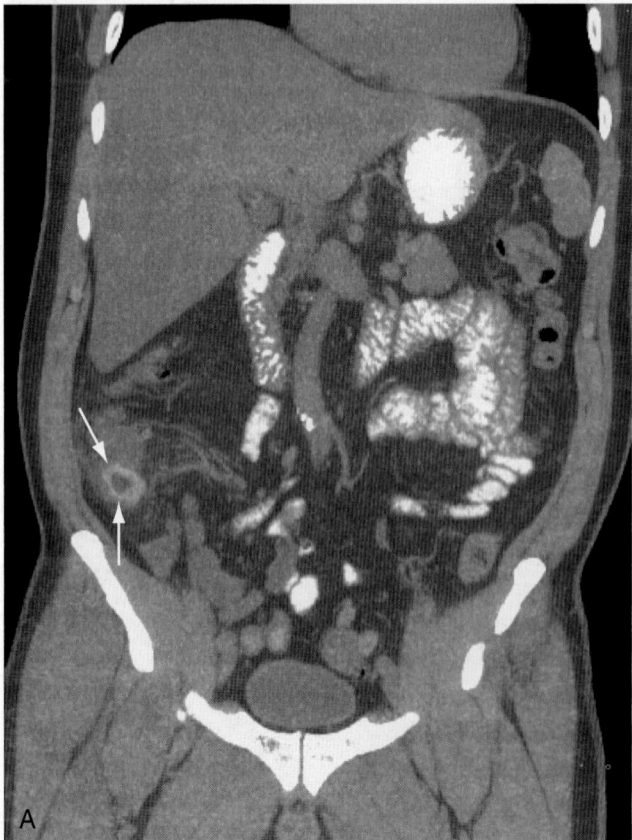

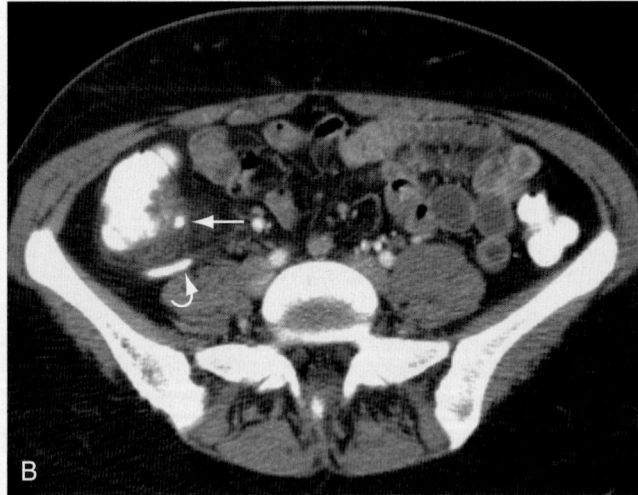

Figure 59-21. Right-sided diverticulitis: imaging considerations. A. Coronal reformatted image shows the hyperdense offending diverticulum (*arrows*) associated with considerable inflammatory change in the adjacent fat. **B.** Axial scan of different patient shows contrast filling a normal appendix (*curved arrow*) and the offending diverticulum (*straight arrow*).

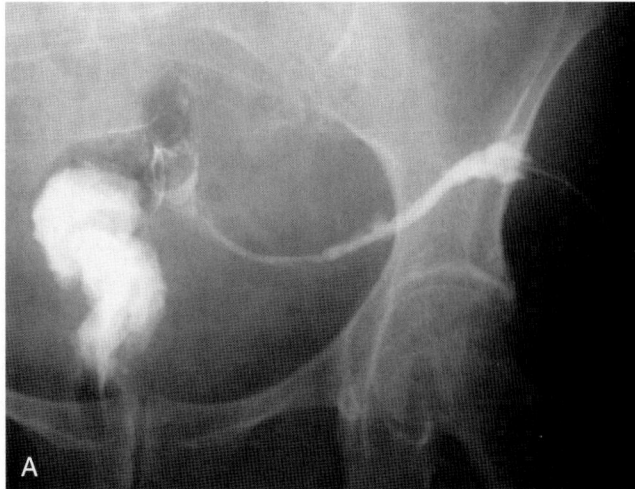

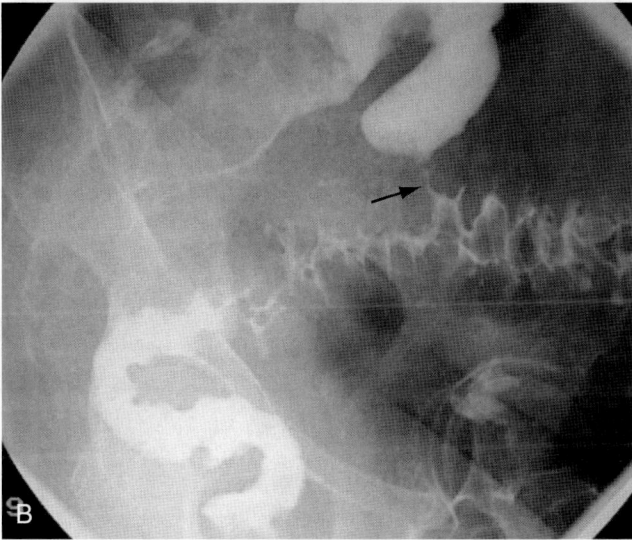

Figure 59-22. Fistulas from diverticulitis. A. Fistulogram showing injection of a skin wound and direct communication to the sigmoid colon. **B.** A fistula (*arrow*) from the sigmoid colon to the ileum is identified on this barium enema examination.

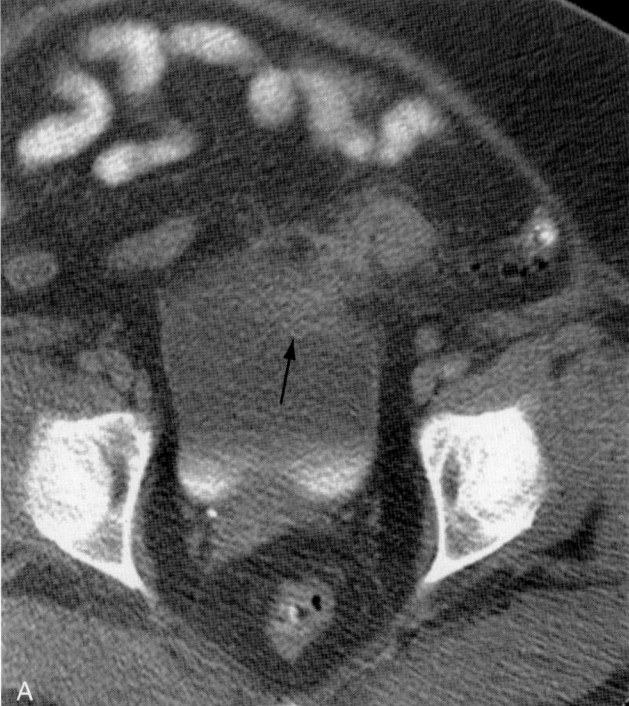

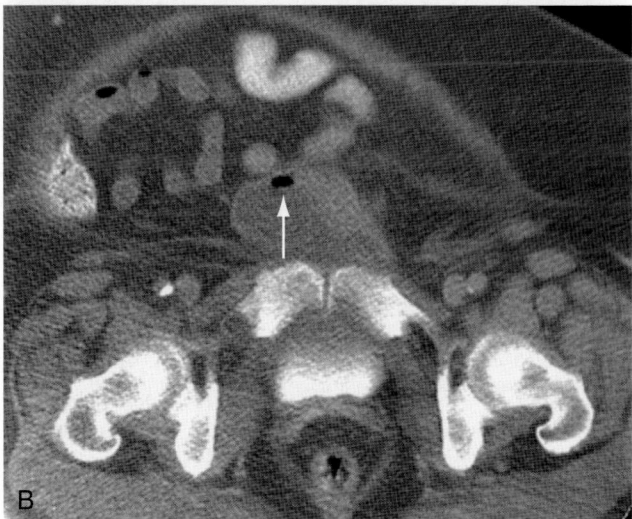

Figure 59-23. Colovesicle fistula due to diverticulitis. A. Mural thickening of the bladder (*arrow*) is identified adjacent to the inflamed sigmoid colon. **B.** A small intraluminal gas bubble (*arrow*) is present as a result of the fistula.

acute inflammatory reaction has already subsided. Thickening of the wall of the urinary bladder adjacent to the sigmoid colon and an air-filled communicating tract are seen with MDCT. Minute amounts of air in the bladder can be seen by CT, which confirms the diagnosis.

Free Perforation

As previously discussed, severe forms of diverticulitis and, particularly, free perforations occur rarely and are seen mainly in debilitated elderly individuals, patients on corticosteroid therapy, and younger patients during their first attack. Free diverticular perforation results in extravasation of air and fluid into the pelvis and peritoneal cavity with the development of peritonitis. On CT (Figs. 59-23 and 59-24), bubbles of air are seen floating in the pelvic fluid close to the sigmoid colon as well as free in the greater peritoneal cavity. Occasionally, a sigmoid diverticulum can perforate into the leaves of the mesosigmoid and air can dissect into the retroperitoneum of the left pelvis and left upper abdomen. This presen-

tation, when associated with bubbles of air adjacent to the sigmoid colon, is diagnostic of perforated diverticulitis.

Bowel Obstruction

Intestinal obstruction is uncommon in diverticulitis, occurring in approximately 2% of patients. The small bowel is affected most often, and obstruction usually is caused by adhesions. The colon can become obstructed because of luminal narrowing caused by inflammation or compression by an abscess. Multiple attacks can lead to progressive fibrosis and stricture of the colonic wall. Obstruction generally is self-limited and responds to conservative therapy. If persistent, obstruction

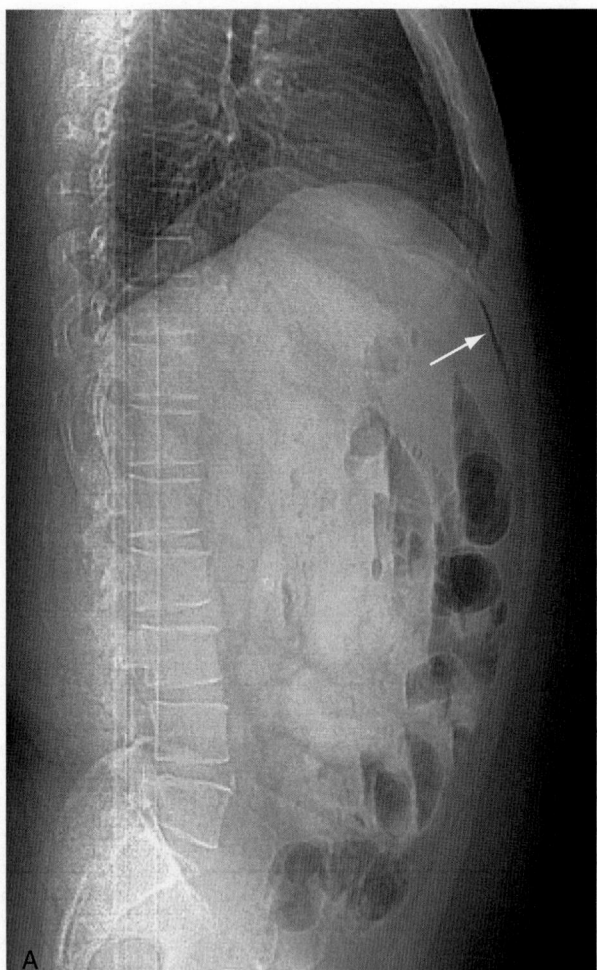

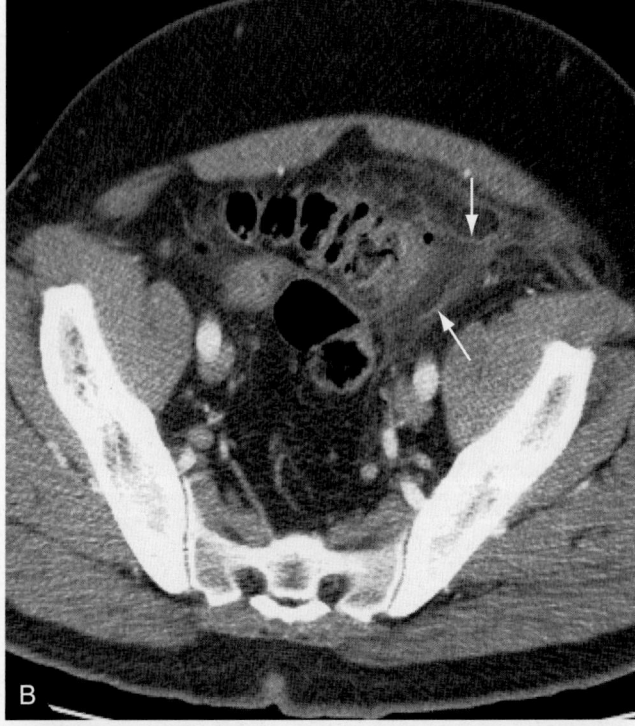

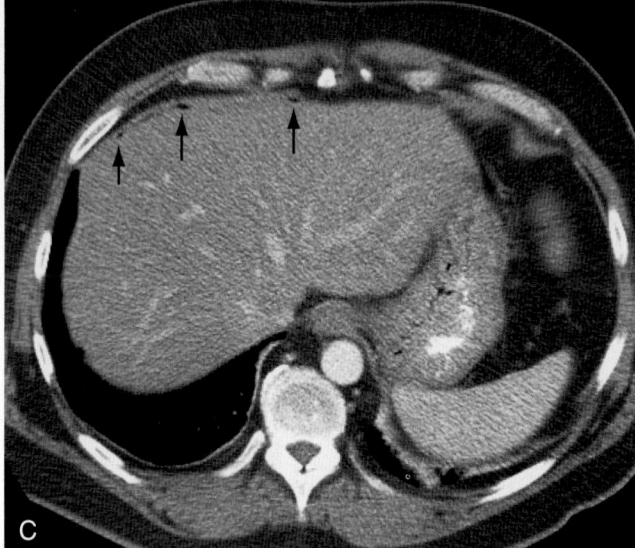

Figure 59-24. Free intraperitoneal perforation. A. Lateral scout image demonstrates free intraperitoneal gas (*arrow*). **B.** Axial image of the pelvis demonstrates the gas containing region of perforation (*arrows*). **C.** Several bubbles of gas are evident anterior to the liver (*arrows*).

of the colon can be treated by a variety of endoscopic and surgical techniques.

Diverticulitis is responsible for some 4% of cases of small bowel obstruction. The small bowel loops became trapped in the perisigmoid inflammatory process, and the associated mesenteric changes can be detected by MDCT (Fig. 59-25).

Pylephlebitis and Liver Abscess

The acute infection originating from a left- or right-sided diverticulitis can spread into the liver via mesenteric venous drainage and portal vein. The septic thrombosis that develops, called *pylephlebitis* or *septic thrombosis of the portal vein*, represents a serious complication seen in severely ill patients with septic manifestations and no localizing signs. CT can

reveal air in the draining mesenteric veins and thrombus in the mesenteric and portal veins. Sometimes, during the initial presentation or on a follow-up examination, a pyogenic liver abscess may develop (Fig. 59-26). The primary colonic inflammatory process can be detected by CT as an intramural inflammatory mass or a pericolic abscess. This complication carries an overall mortality of 32%. Patients should be diagnosed early and should be closely monitored and adequately treated with antibiotic therapy and percutaneous abscess drainage when necessary.

Computed Tomographic and Surgical Management

Together with the clinical evaluation, CT is used not only to confirm the clinical suspicion but also as a reliable guide to

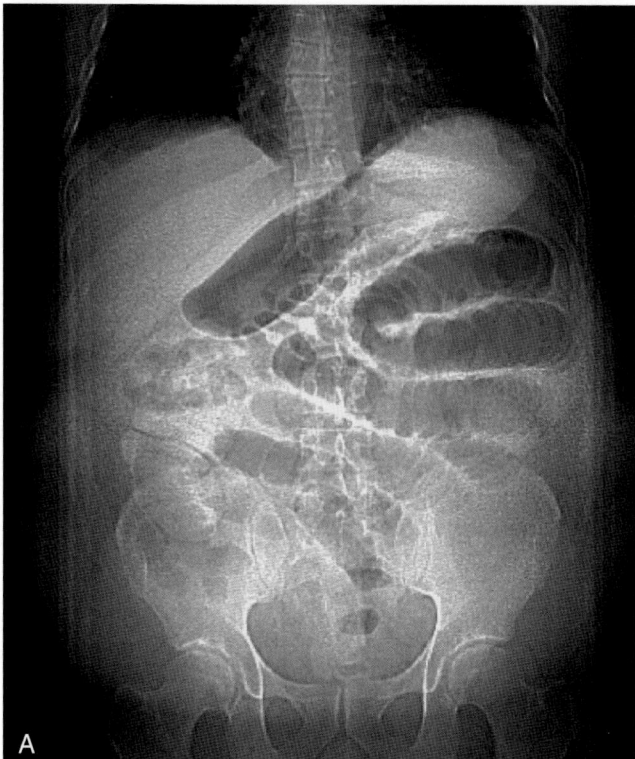

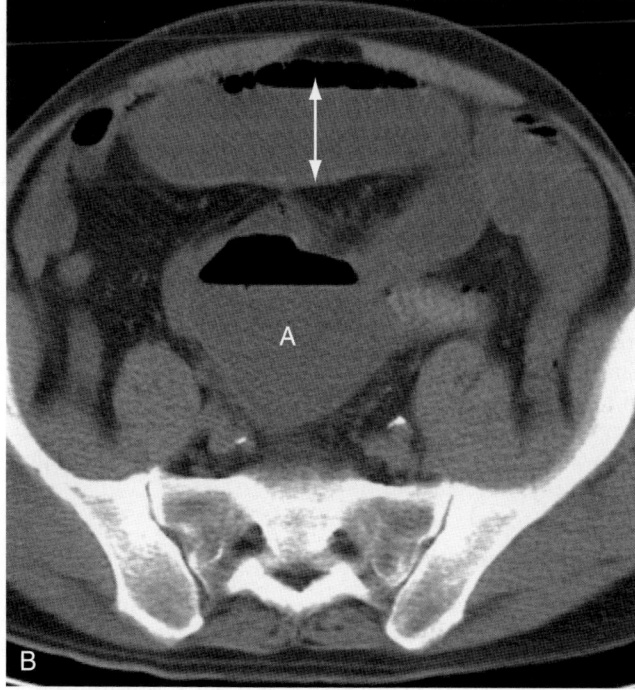

Figure 59-25. Small bowel obstruction due to diverticulitis abscess. A. Scout image demonstrates small bowel obstruction. **B.** An air-fluid level is identified within the abscess (A). Note the dilated, fluid-filled small bowel loops (*arrow*).

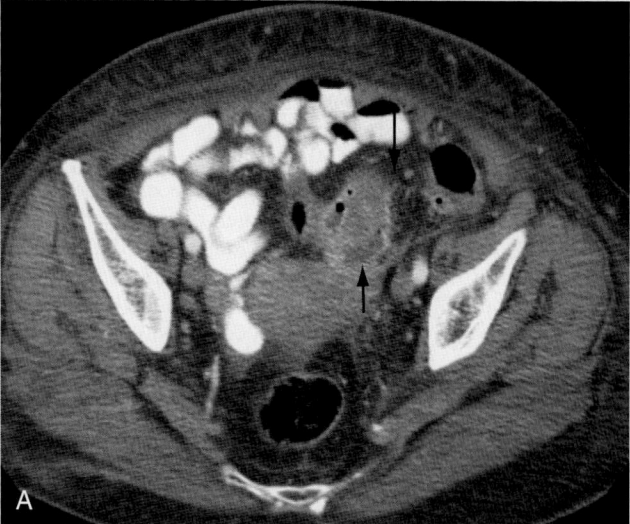

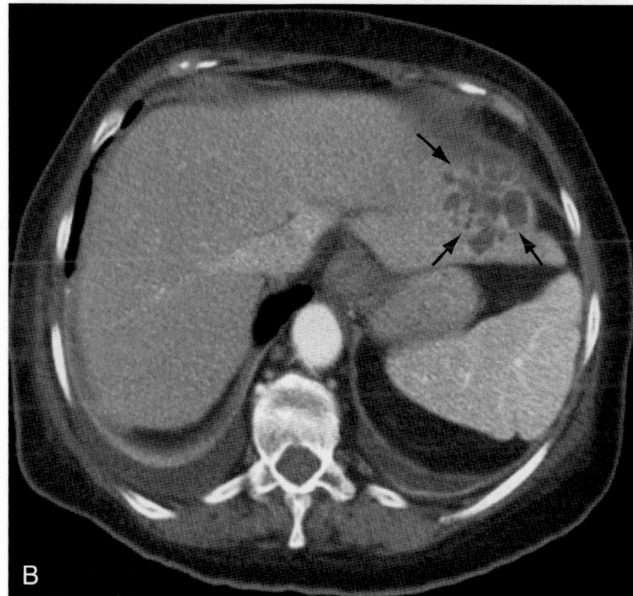

Figure 59-26. Sigmoid diverticulitis leading to the formation of a liver abscess. A. There is a gas-containing abscess (*arrows*) in the sigmoid mesocolon. **B.** A multiloculated abscess is identified in the left lobe of the liver (*arrows*).

the management of the patient. Patients with mild diverticulitis (pericolic inflammation, small abscess) are treated conservatively with antibiotic therapy and bowel rest. Patients with larger abscesses (>4 cm) are percutaneously drained. Emergency surgery is reserved for cases of free perforation with peritonitis. Elective surgical sigmoid resections are per-

formed for the following indications: (1) after the successful drainage of a pelvic abscess; (2) following repeated episodes of diverticulitis; (3) for unremitting abdominal pain; and (4) for severe diverticular bleeding. The timing and type of surgical procedure employed are in great measure based on the findings detected by the CT examination.

DIVERTICULAR HEMORRHAGE

Some 30% of patients with diverticulosis have eventual hemorrhage of the lower gastrointestinal tract, ranging from an occasional guaiac-positive stool to life-threatening rectal bleeding. Diverticular disease is the most common identifiable cause of major rectal bleeding in adults and is responsible for 43% of major rectal bleeding and 35% of minor bleeding occurring in patients older than 65 years.

Pathophysiology

Although diverticula predominate in the sigmoid and descending colon, severe hemorrhage originates from the right colon in two thirds of patients. The source is typically a single diverticulum, which in 80% of cases is not inflamed. There is minute rupture of one of the vasa recta asymmetrically placed in the wall adjacent to the lumen of the diverticulum (Figs. 59-27 and 59-28). An eccentric focus of media thickening, intramural thickening and duplication, and fragmentation of the internal elastic lamina in the wall of the involved artery at the point of its disruption occur. Some traumatic factor within the lumen of the diverticulum, possibly inspissated stool, induces this eccentric intimal thickening, which eventually weakens and ruptures the vasa recta. The wider-domed necks of right-sided colonic diverticula may expose these vessels to injury over a greater length, explaining the strikingly high incidence of right-sided hemorrhage.[22-26]

Clinical Findings

Most patients with massive diverticular hemorrhage are elderly, with severe coexistent cardiovascular and pulmonary disease, and they present with sudden onset of mild abdominal cramps and the urge to defecate. Soon after, a large

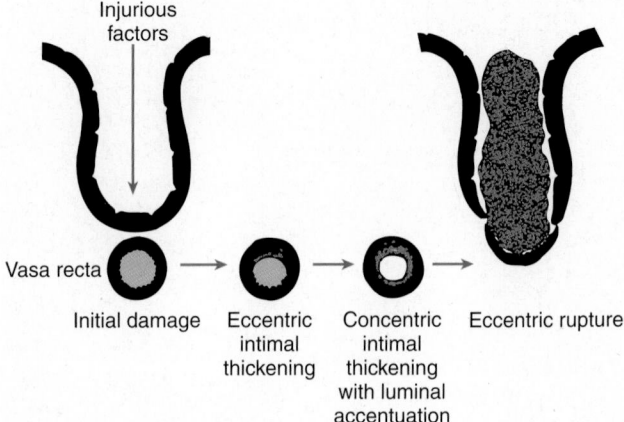

Figure 59-28. Pathogenesis of colonic diverticular hemorrhage. Progressive eccentric changes weaken the wall of the vas rectum, which eventually ruptures into the lumen of the diverticulum. (From Meyers MA, Alonso DR, Gray GF, et al: Pathogenesis of bleeding colonic diverticulosis. Gastroenterology 71:577-583, 1976.)

volume of bright red blood or clots, or both, or dark red, maroon, or, least commonly, black stool is passed rectally. Bleeding ceases spontaneously in approximately 80% of patients, but the bleeding may be continuous or intermittent. Nearly 25% of patients rebleed in the near or distant future; and if rebleeding does occur, the chance of further rebleeding increases to 50%.[4-7] The differential diagnosis, radiology, and treatment of diverticular hemorrhage are discussed in Chapter 129.[4-7]

GIANT SIGMOID DIVERTICULUM

Etiology

Giant sigmoid diverticulum is a rare complication of diverticulitis. It is believed to result from subserosal perforation and inflammation of a diverticulum, with subsequent air trapping and eventual formation of a large cyst, which is caused by elevated intraluminal pressure of the colon working in tandem with a ball-valve mechanism. In time, inflammatory and granulation tissue replaces the mucosal lining of the cyst wall. The trapped air in the cyst increases during defecation and is vented irregularly.

Pathophysiology and Clinical Findings

Most patients are elderly and have a history of chronic vague abdominal discomfort or acute symptoms suggesting diverticulitis. A palpable mass is detected in 71% of cases, and anatomic communication between the cyst and the lumen is present in 82%. The cysts range in size between 6 and 27 cm, with a mean diameter of 13 cm. The cyst may be hyperresonant on percussion.[52-54]

Radiologic Findings

The barium enema (Fig. 59-29) and plain radiograph findings in giant sigmoid diverticulum are striking. Plain radiographs demonstrate a large gas-filled structure in the lower to middle pelvis that can have an air-fluid level. The gas collections may change in size on interval studies.[52-54]

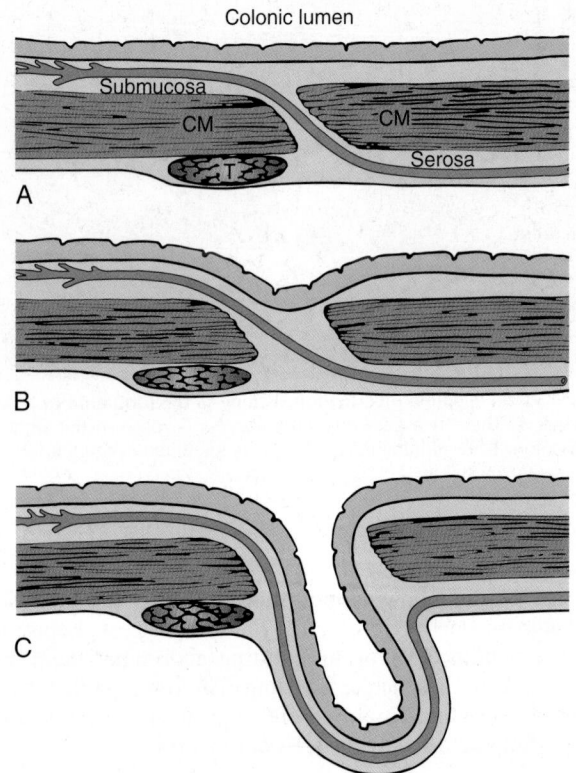

Figure 59-27. Diverticulum formation and vascular relationships. A. The vas rectum penetrates the colon wall from the serosa to the submucosa through an obliquely oriented connective tissue septum in the circular muscle (CM). This penetration occurs near the mesenteric side of the taenia (T). **B.** The diverticulum develops through and widens this connective tissue cleft. The mucosal protrusion begins to elevate the artery. **C.** As the diverticulum extends transmurally, the vas rectum is placed over its dome, penetrating to the submucosa on the antimesenteric border of its neck and orifice. (From Meyers MA, Volberg F, Katzen B, et al: Angioarchitecture of colonic diverticula: Significance in bleeding diverticulosis. Radiology 108:249-261, 1973.)

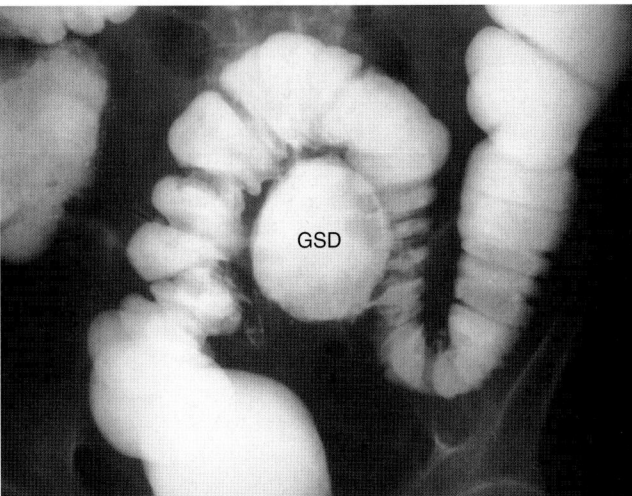

Figure 59-29. Giant sigmoid colon diverticulum. Giant sigmoid colon diverticulum (GSD) is demonstrated in two different patients on a barium enema study (**A**) and a CT scan (**B**).

Barium enters these collections on contrast agent studies in two thirds of patients, and diverticula are seen elsewhere in the colon in 82% of patients. The differential diagnosis of these large collections includes volvulus, giant Meckel or other small bowel diverticulum, tubo-ovarian abscess, cystitis, emphysematous cholecystitis, infected pancreatic pseudocyst, and vesicoenteric fistula.

Therapy

Giant colonic diverticula have been reported to perforate, cause volvulus and infarction and small bowel obstruction, and may contain carcinoma. The accepted therapy for giant colonic diverticula is surgical excision.[52-54]

References

1. Papaconstantinou HT, Simmang CL: Diverticular disease. In Weinstein WM, Hawkey CJ, Bosch J (eds): Clinical Gastroenterology and Hepatology. New York, Elsevier, 2005, pp 463- 472.
2. Simmang CL, Shires GT: Diverticular disease of the colon. In Feldman M, Friedman LS, Sleisenger MH (eds): Gastrointestinal and Liver Disease. Philadelphia, WB Saunders, 2002, pp 2100-2112.
3. Salem TA, Molloy RG, O'Dwyer PJ: Prospective study on the management of patients with complicated diverticular disease. Colorectal Dis 8:173-176, 2006.
4. Takano M, Yamada K, Sato K: An analysis of the development of colonic diverticulosis in the Japanese. Dis Colon Rectum 48:2111-2116, 2005.
5. Salzman H, Lillie D: Diverticular disease: Diagnosis and treatment. Am Fam Physician 72:1229-1234, 2005.
6. Hjern F, Johansson C, Mellgren A, et al: Diverticular disease and migration—the influence of acculturation to a Western lifestyle on diverticular disease. Aliment Pharmacol Ther 23:797-805, 2006.
7. West BA: The pathology of diverticulosis: Classical concepts and mucosal changes in diverticula. J Clin Gastroenterol 40 (Suppl 3):S126-S131, 2006.
8. Oomen JL, Engel AF, Cuesta MA, et al: Mortality after acute surgery for complications of diverticular disease of the sigmoid colon is almost exclusively due to patient-related factors. Colorectal Dis 8:112-119, 2006.
9. Bahadursingh AM, Virgo KS, Kaminski DL, et al: Spectrum of disease and outcome of complicated diverticular disease. Am J Surg 186:696-701, 2003.
10. Dobbins C, Defontgalland D, Duthie G, et al: The relationship of obesity to the complications of diverticular disease. Colorectal Dis 8:37-40, 2006.
11. Funariu G, Bintintan V, Seicean R: Urgent surgery for complicated colonic diverticula. J Gastrointest Liver Dis 15:37-40, 2006.
12. Meyers MA, Alonso DR, Baer JW: Pathogenesis of massively bleeding colonic diverticulosis: New observations. AJR 127:901-908, 1976.
13. Strate LL: Lower GI bleeding: Epidemiology and diagnosis. Gastroenterol Clin North Am 34:643-664, 2005.
14. Meyers MA, Alonso DR, Gray FG, et al: Pathogenesis of bleeding colonic diverticulosis. Gastroenterology 71:577-583, 1976.
15. Russin LD: Plain film recognition of air within colonic diverticula. AJR 134:176-177, 1980.
16. Hunter TB, Merkley R, Pitt MJ: Relation between pelvic phleboliths and diverticular disease of the colon. AJR 143:105-107, 1984.
17. Laufer I, Levine M (eds): Double Contrast Gastrointestinal Radiology, 2nd ed. Philadelphia, WB Saunders, 1992.
18. Weissman A, Clot M, Grellet J: Double Contrast Examination of the Colon. Berlin, Springer-Verlag, 1985, pp 147-161.
19. Gelfand DW: Gastrointestinal Radiology. New York, Churchill Livingstone, 1984, pp 318-324.
20. Freeny PC, Walker JH: Inverted diverticula of the gastrointestinal tract. Gastrointest Radiol 4:57-59, 1979.
21. Htoo AM, Bartram CI: The radiological diagnosis of polyps in the presence of diverticular disease. Br J Radiol 52:263-267, 1979.
22. Baker SR, Alterman DD: False-negative barium enema in patients with sigmoid cancer and coexistent diverticula. Gastrointest Radiol 10:171-173, 1985.
23. Glick SN: Inverted colonic diverticulum: Air contrast barium enema findings in six cases. AJR 156:961-964, 1991.
24. Keller CE, Halpert RD, Feczko PJ, et al: Radiologic recognition of colonic diverticula simulating polyps. AJR 143:93-97, 1984.
25. Miller WT, Levine MS, Rubesin SE, et al: Bowler-hat sign: A simple principle for differentiating polyps from diverticula. Radiology 173:615-617, 1989.
26. Zaidi E, Daly B: CT and clinical features of acute diverticulitis in an urban U.S. population: Rising frequency in young, obese adults. AJR 187:689-694, 2006.
27. Lahat A, Menachem Y, Avidan B, et al: Diverticulitis in the young patient—is it different? World J Gastroenterol 12:2932-2935, 2006.
28. Nelson RS, Velasco A, Mukesh BN: Management of diverticulitis in younger patients. Dis Colon Rectum 49:1341-1345, 2006.
29. Ripolles T, Agramunt M, Martinez MJ, et al: The role of ultrasound in the diagnosis, management and evolutive prognosis of acute left-sided colonic diverticulitis: A review of 208 patients. Eur Radiol 13:2587-2595, 2003.
30. Gore RM, Miller FH, Pereles FS, et al: Helical CT in the evaluation of the acute abdomen. AJR 174:901-913, 2000.
31. Marincek B: Nontraumatic abdominal emergencies: Acute abdominal pain: Diagnostic strategies. Eur Radiol 12:2136-2150, 2002.
32. Baker JB, Mandavia D, Swadron SP: Diagnosis of diverticulitis by bedside ultrasound in the emergency department. J Emerg Med 30:327-329, 2006.
33. Kaewlai R, Nazinitsky KJ: Acute colonic diverticulitis in a community-based hospital: CT evaluation in 138 patients. Emerg Radiol 13:171-179, 2007.
34. Buckley O, Geoghegan T, McAuley G, et al: Pictorial review: Magnetic resonance imaging of colonic diverticulitis. Eur Radiol 17:221-227, 2007.
35. Vijayaraghavan SB: High-resolution sonographic spectrum of diverticulosis, diverticulitis, and their complications. J Ultrasound Med 25:75-85, 2006.
36. Hollerweger A, Rettenbacher T, Macheiner P, et al: Sigmoid diverticulitis: Value of transrectal sonography in addition to transabdominal sonography. AJR 175:1155-1160, 2000.
37. Baker JB, Mandavia D, Swadron SP: Diagnosis of diverticulitis by bedside ultrasound in the Emergency department. J Emerg Med 30:327-329, 2006.
38. Cobben LP, Groot I, Blickman JG, et al: Right colonic diverticulitis: MR appearance. Abdom Imaging 28:794-798, 2003.
39. Hinchley EJ, Schaal PGH, Richards GK: Treatment of perforated diverticular disease of the colon. Adv Surg 12:85-109, 1978.
40. Siewert B, Tye G, Kruskal J, et al: Impact of CT-guided drainage in the treatment of diverticular abscesses: Size matters. AJR 186:680-686, 2006.
41. Durmishi Y, Gervaz P, Brandt D, et al: Results from percutaneous drainage of Hinchey stage II diverticulitis guided by computed tomography scan. Surg Endosc 20:1129-1133, 2006.
42. Kaiser AM, Jiang JK, Lake JP, et al: The management of complicated diverticulitis and the role of computed tomography. Am J Gastroenterol 100:910-917, 2005.

43. Kumar RR, Kim JT, Haukoos JS, et al: Factors affecting the successful management of intra-abdominal abscesses with antibiotics and the need for percutaneous drainage. Dis Colon Rectum 49:183-189, 2006.

44. Ambrosetti P, Becker C, Terrier F: Colonic diverticulitis: Impact of imaging on surgical management—a prospective study of 542 patients. Eur Radiol 12:1145-1149, 2002.

45. Gervais DA, Ho CH, O'Neill MJ, et al: Recurrent abdominal and pelvic abscesses: Incidence, results of repeated percutaneous drainage, and underlying causes in 956 drainages. AJR 182:463-466, 2004.

46. Castronovo G, Ciulla A, Tomasello G, et al: Diverticular disease of right colon: Clinical variants and personal experience. Chir Ital 58:213-217, 2006.

47. Chou YH, Chiou HJ, Tiu CM, et al: Sonography of acute right side colonic diverticulitis. Am J Surg 181:122-127, 2001.

48. Goh V, Halligan S, Taylor SA, et al: Differentiation between diverticulitis and colorectal cancer: Quantitative CT perfusion measurements versus morphologic criteria—initial experience. Radiology 242:456-462, 2007.

49. Jang HJ, Lim HK, Lee SJ, et al: Acute diverticulitis of the cecum and ascending colon: The value of thin-section helical CT findings in excluding colonic carcinoma. AJR 174:1397-1402, 2001.

50. Van De Wauwer C, Irvin TT, et al: Pylephlebitis due to perforated diverticulitis. Acta Chir Belg 105:229-230, 2005.

51. Horton KM, Fishman EK: Volume-rendered 3D CT of the mesenteric vasculature: Normal anatomy, anatomic variants, and pathologic conditions. RadioGraphics 22:161-172, 2002.

52. Thomas S, Peel RL, Evans LE, et al: Best cases from the AFIP: Giant colonic diverticulum. RadioGraphics 26:1869-1872, 2006.

53. Chaiyasate K, Yavuzer R, Mittal V: Giant sigmoid diverticulum. Surgery 139:276-277, 2006.

54. Abou-Nukta F, Bakhos C, Ikekpeazu N, et al: Ruptured giant colonic diverticulum. Am Surg 71:1073-1074, 2005.

Diseases of the Appendix

Jill E. Jacobs, MD • Emil J. Balthazar, MD

The vermiform appendix is the smallest and functionally most irrelevant segment of the gastrointestinal tract, yet diseases of the appendix are among the most common surgical emergencies in the western world.[1-5] The appendix arises from the posteromedial aspect of the cecum at the junction of the three taeniae coli. Although the appendix has the same mural layers as those of the remainder of the gut, it is distinguished by extremely rich lymphoid tissue in the mucosa and submucosa. This forms an entire layer of germinal follicles and lymphoid pulp in the young.[6] With age, this lymphoid tissue underlying the mucosal epithelium and glands undergoes progressive atrophy. The distal portion of the appendix sometimes undergoes fibrous obliteration in the elderly.[6]

EMBRYOLOGY

The vermiform appendix and cecum are intestinal derivations of the midgut. During the sixth week of gestational life, the cecum begins to develop as a small bulge in the midgut at the level of the ileocolic junction. This diverticular structure continues to enlarge and assumes a conic shape with its apex corresponding to the primitive appendix.[7-9] The initial cecal and appendiceal structures have been referred to as the "bud of the cecum."[10] The midgut undergoes physiologic umbilical herniation at approximately the 6th gestational week and subsequently begins to relocate into the embryonal body cavity at approximately the 10th gestational week. This process is accompanied by counterclockwise rotation of the midgut, which results in positioning of the cecal complex in the right lower quadrant (Fig. 60-1). As the colon grows, it moves caudad toward the right iliac fossa, a process known as "descensus."[10] Because of differential growth rates during this time, the development of the primitive appendix is slower than that of the rest of the cecum. This differential growth was theorized by Broman to be due to a mucosal fold in the distal cecum that prevents accumulation of meconium.[11] Broman hypothesized that colonic growth is stimulated by intraluminal meconium accumulation. Because this mucosal fold prevents complete filling of the distal cecum and appendix with meconium, growth is retarded in these segments. The appendix subsequently lengthens rapidly but fails to grow in thickness, soon assuming the configuration of a vermiform process.

By birth, the appendix has lengthened and shows a more abrupt transition zone at the junction with the cecum. At this time, the appendix is still attached to the cecal apex. The fully developed adult appendix is uniformly narrow and arises from the left posterior wall of the cecum, rather than the cecal apex, 2.5 to 3.5 cm below the ileocecal valve. The process of migration of the root of the appendix from the cecal tip toward the left, on the same side as the ileocecal valve, is probably related to the upright posture of the child. The right and ventral walls of the cecum grow and distend at the expense of the left and posterior walls. The fixation at the ileocecal junction and the weight of the column of feces in the ascending colon explain this additional asymmetric development.

In adults, the root of the appendix can be located anywhere along the medial-posterior wall of the cecum between the ileocecal valve and the cecal tip. In addition, there is great

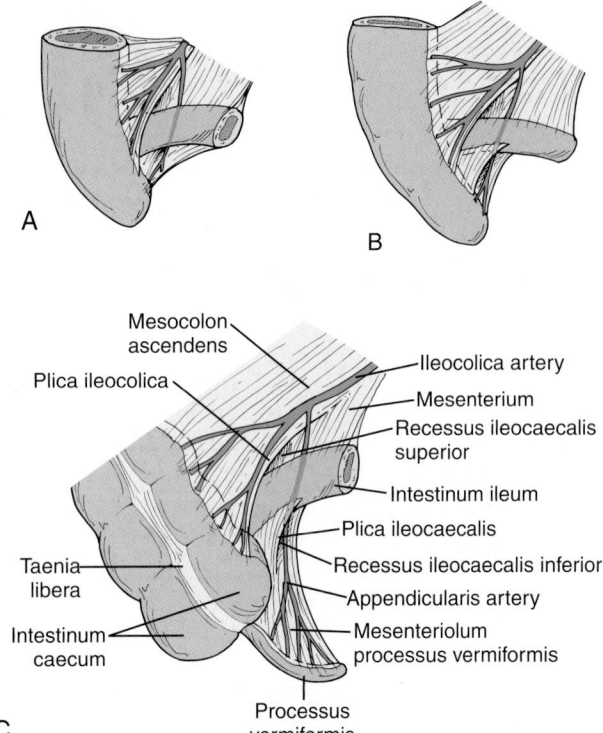

C

Figure 60-1. Embryology of the appendix. A. Growth of the inferior tip of the cecum lags during early intrauterine development. **B.** This produces the infantile appendix. **C.** Continued differential growth of the lateral cecal wall leads to the posteromedial position of the appendix in older children and adults. (From McVay CB: Anson & McVay Surgical Anatomy, 6th ed. Philadelphia, WB Saunders, 1984.)

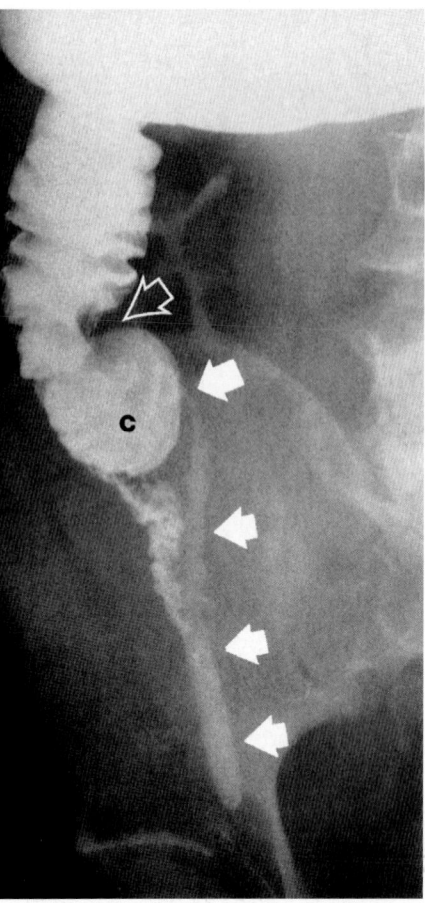

Figure 60-2. Normal appendix: barium enema findings. A long pelvic appendix is present, arising from the medial wall of the cecum (C) below the ileocecal valve (*open arrow*). The appendix is uniformly narrow and completely filled with barium to the distal tip (*solid arrows*). This finding rules out appendicitis.

variation in the position of the appendix in relation to the cecum and ascending colon.[12,13] More than 60% of appendices are retrocecal or retrocolic, with the remainder in a more inferior pelvic location. A fully developed appendix varies in size and thickness, with an average length of 8 to 10 cm (range, 4-25 cm) (Fig. 60-2). The location of the appendix in the peritoneal cavity depends on its length and relationship to the cecum and the extreme variations in the mobility and location of the ascending colon and cecum (Fig. 60-3).[14]

Examples of arrest in later phases of development of the appendix are common and can be recognized during barium enema examinations. An arrest in the fetal phase of development is unusual (Fig. 60-4). A conic configuration of the lower cecal segment signifies total absence or hypoplasia of the appendix. Agenesis of the appendix is rare; the reported incidence is about 1 in 100,000 individuals.[15]

The ileocolic artery, a branch of the superior mesenteric artery, supplies the appendix, cecum, and ileum via five branches: (1) several ileal rami; (2) the anterior cecal artery; (3) the posterior cecal artery; (4) the colic ramus; and (5) the appendicular artery, which runs through the mesenteriolum to supply the vermiform appendix. Because there are no arterial arcades in the mesenteriolum, the appendicular artery is a terminal artery, predisposing the appendix to ischemia when there is vascular insult.[10] The origin of the appendicular artery is from the iliac ramus approximately 35% of the time, from the ileocolic artery approximately 28% of the time, from the anterior cecal artery approximately 20% of the time, from the posterior cecal artery approximately 12% of the

time, from the ileocecal artery approximately 3% of the time, and from the ascending colic ramus approximately 2% of the time.[16] The veins accompany the arteries.

Lymphatic tissue begins to develop in the appendix during the 14th and 15th weeks of gestation.[17] Initial accumulations of lymphatic cells occur directly below the epithelium, but some lymphocytes eventually penetrate the epithelial layer of the appendix. Lymphatic drainage of the appendix is via ileocolic lymph nodes located along the superior mesenteric artery and via celiac nodes into the cisterna chili.

Unlike the cecal wall, which is composed of a diagonal, rhomboid mesh of collagen fibers allowing it to accommodate luminal expansion, the appendiceal wall is composed of horizontal collagen fibers that tolerate only minimal increases in luminal diameter. Although the appendix secretes 2 to 3 mL of mucus daily, its average luminal capacity is only approximately 1 mL.[10] This, in conjunction with the appendix's solitary blood supply explains its propensity to rapidly become ischemic and perforate after luminal obstruction.

ACUTE APPENDICITIS

Epidemiology

Appendicitis was first described and reported by Reginald H. Fitz at the 1886 meeting of the Association of American

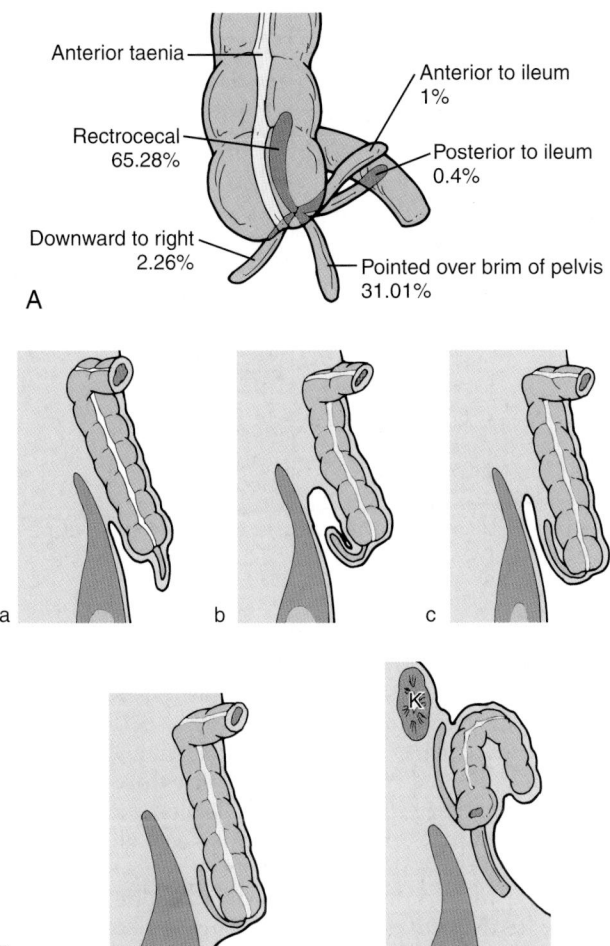

Figure 60-3. Variations in position of the appendix. A. Incidence of various positions of the appendix. **B.** Normal variations in the position and peritoneal fixation of the appendix: (a) intraperitoneal, pointing over the brim of the pelvis; (b) intraperitoneal, ascending retrocecal; (c) extraperitoneal, ascending retrocecal, with a paracecal fossa present; (d) extraperitoneal, ascending retrocecal; (e) extraperitoneal, ascending retrocecal, lying anterior to the right kidney (K) deep to the liver, associated with an undescended subhepatic cecum. (The terminal ileum is also extraperitoneal and enters the cecum from behind.) (**A** from Meyers MA: Dynamic Radiology of the Abdomen. New York: Springer-Verlag, 1988, p 403; **B** from Meyers MA, Oliphant M: Ascending retrocecal appendicitis. Radiology 110:295-299, 1974.)

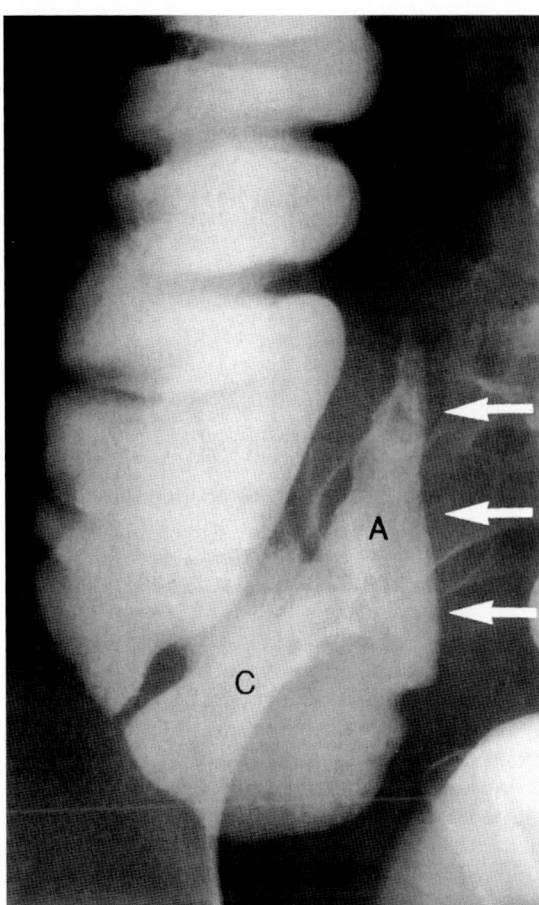

Figure 60-4. Fetal appendix. Barium enema examination in a 21-year-old woman shows arrest in the development of the appendix (A). The cecum (C) has a triangular, funnel-shaped inferior segment (*arrows*) with gradual transition into an incompletely developed appendix.

Physicians.[18] Appendicitis is the most frequent cause of acute abdominal pain requiring surgical intervention in the western world and is the most common abdominal operation performed annually in this country on an emergency basis.[19,20]

The incidence of acute appendicitis has been declining steadily since the late 1940s. At the beginning of the century, the annual incidence was 15 per 100,000 population with a 15% lifetime risk.[1-5,21] In comparison, the current lifetime appendicitis risk is 8.6% for males and 6.7% for females and the lifetime risk of appendectomy is 12.0% for males and 23.1% for females.[22-24]

Appendicitis is rare in infants but becomes increasingly common in childhood. The highest incidence of appendicitis is in individuals aged 10 to 19 years (23.3 per 10,000 population per year).[25] There is a 3:2 male gender predilection in teenagers and young adults.[1-5] In adults, there continues to be a slight male predominance with a male-to-female appendicitis rate of 1.4:1.[25]

Mortality and morbidity rates for removal of a normal appendix are 0.14% and 4.6%, respectively, but increase to 0.24% and 6.1% for acute appendicitis and to 1.7% and 19% for perforated appendicitis.[26] These mortality rates are far better than the 50% mortality seen in the preantibiotic era.[1-5]

Complications occur in 1% to 5% of all patients with appendicitis, and wound infections account for nearly one third of all morbidity. Wound infection rates increase to 20% to 40% with perforated appendicitis; gangrene increases morbidity 5-fold and perforation 10-fold.[3,27-31]

Etiology

The initiating event in acute appendicitis is luminal obstruction, which may be the result of many causes, including fecaliths, lymphoid hyperplasia, primary (carcinoid, adenocarcinoma, lymphoma, and Kaposi's sarcoma) or metastatic tumor, parasites, foreign bodies, stricture, Crohn's disease, or adhesions (Fig. 60-5). At one time, prolonged retention of barium in the appendix was thought to be a risk factor for the development of appendicitis, but these have proved to be unrelated.[32-36]

Of the possible causes of luminal obstruction, fecaliths are the most common, presenting in 11% to 52% of patients with acute appendicitis.[37-39] They are the result of inspissation

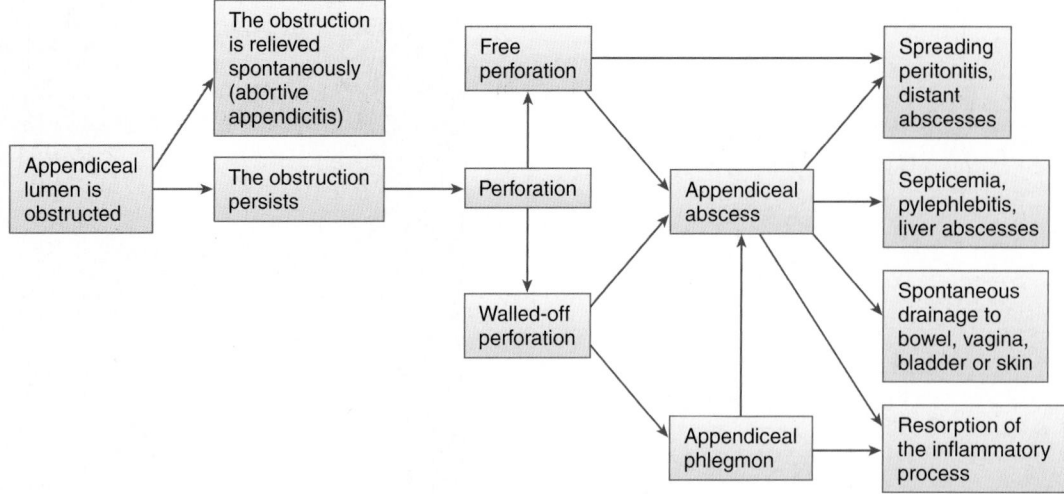

Figure 60-5. Pathophysiologic pathways in untreated appendicitis. (From Puylaert JBCM: Ultrasound of Appendicitis. Berlin, Springer-Verlag, 1990, p 5.)

of fecal material and inorganic salts within the appendiceal lumen. These concretions can then enlarge and obstruct the appendix. Low-fiber diets contribute to low-residue stool, which has a propensity to become impacted in the appendiceal lumen. Although true appendiceal calculi (hard, noncrushable calcified stones) are less common than fecaliths, they are more commonly associated with appendiceal perforation and periappendiceal abscess formation.[37]

Continued improvements in hygiene over the past century have greatly reduced the exposure of infants and children to enteric organisms. Consequently, these infections can elicit an exaggerated lymphoid hyperplasia that may block the appendix or devitalize the appendiceal mucosa, allowing bacterial invasion.[32-35]

Pathophysiology

Continued secretion of mucus into the appendix after luminal obstruction results in distention and concurrent elevation of luminal pressures. When the luminal pressure exceeds the capillary perfusion pressure, lymphatic and venous drainage are impaired and arterial compromise and tissue ischemia result. Breakdown of the epithelial mucosal barrier occurs, and luminal bacteria multiply and invade the appendiceal wall, causing transmural inflammation and gangrenous appendicitis (Fig. 60-6). Appendiceal infarction and perforation may result from continued tissue ischemia. Inflammation can then extend to the serosa, parietal peritoneum, and adjacent organs, including the cecum, terminal ileum, and pelvis. Perforation can cause a localized or generalized peritonitis. Periappendiceal abscess or phlegmon is usually walled off by the adjacent greater omentum or small bowel loops; however, inflammatory material can spread through the peritoneum to the paracolic gutters and subphrenic spaces, sigmoid colon, bladder, ovaries, or vagina. Infected thrombus may form in the portal vein, causing pylephlebitis, an unusual occurrence in the antibiotic era.[1-5,40]

Appendiceal perforation occurs in 16% to 39% of patients, with a median of 20%.[21,24,25,41-51] Although it has been suggested in some studies that there is a linear correlation between perforation rates and diagnostic accuracy, more recent studies have refuted this contention.[46,48] There is, however, evidence that perforation rates are strongly age related. Körner and colleagues studied 1486 patients who underwent appendectomy and found that the overall perforation rate was 19% with higher rates in small children and the elderly irrespective of gender.[46] It is thought that these higher perforation rates relate to the greater diagnostic confusion in these age groups. Vorhes noted that patients older than the age of 55 years underwent laparotomy on average 2 days later than those younger than 55 years old.[52] Rodriguez and co-workers retrospectively reviewed a large series of children (18 years or younger) who underwent computed tomography and/or sonographic imaging before appendectomy and compared the imaging characteristics and outcome of those younger than 5 years old to those older than 5 years.[53] These authors showed that the rate of appendiceal perforation was markedly higher for children younger than 5 years old, that the risk for perforation was inversely proportional to the patient's age, and that echogenic periappendiceal fat (thought to be due to edema related to transmural appendiceal inflammation) was more common in younger patients.

Clinical and Radiologic Assessment

Clinical assessment remains an essential and critical part of the initial evaluation of patients with suspected acute appendicitis. The physician's goal is to expeditiously and accurately confirm or exclude the diagnosis of acute appendicitis while minimizing diagnostic delays, negative appendectomy and appendiceal perforation rates, and hospital costs. However, despite continued advances in clinical medicine, the diagnosis of acute appendicitis often remains elusive.[54-56]

Although in the United States diagnostic accuracy rates for appendicitis had improved from 86% to 92% in male patients and from 74% to 83% in female patients between 1970 and 1984,[14] they appear to have plateaued since the mid-1980s.[19] Perforation and false-negative appendectomy rates have also stabilized over the past half century.[45] False-negative appendectomy rates reflect the diagnostic difficulties frequently incurred in differentiating appendicitis from other causes of abdominal pain.

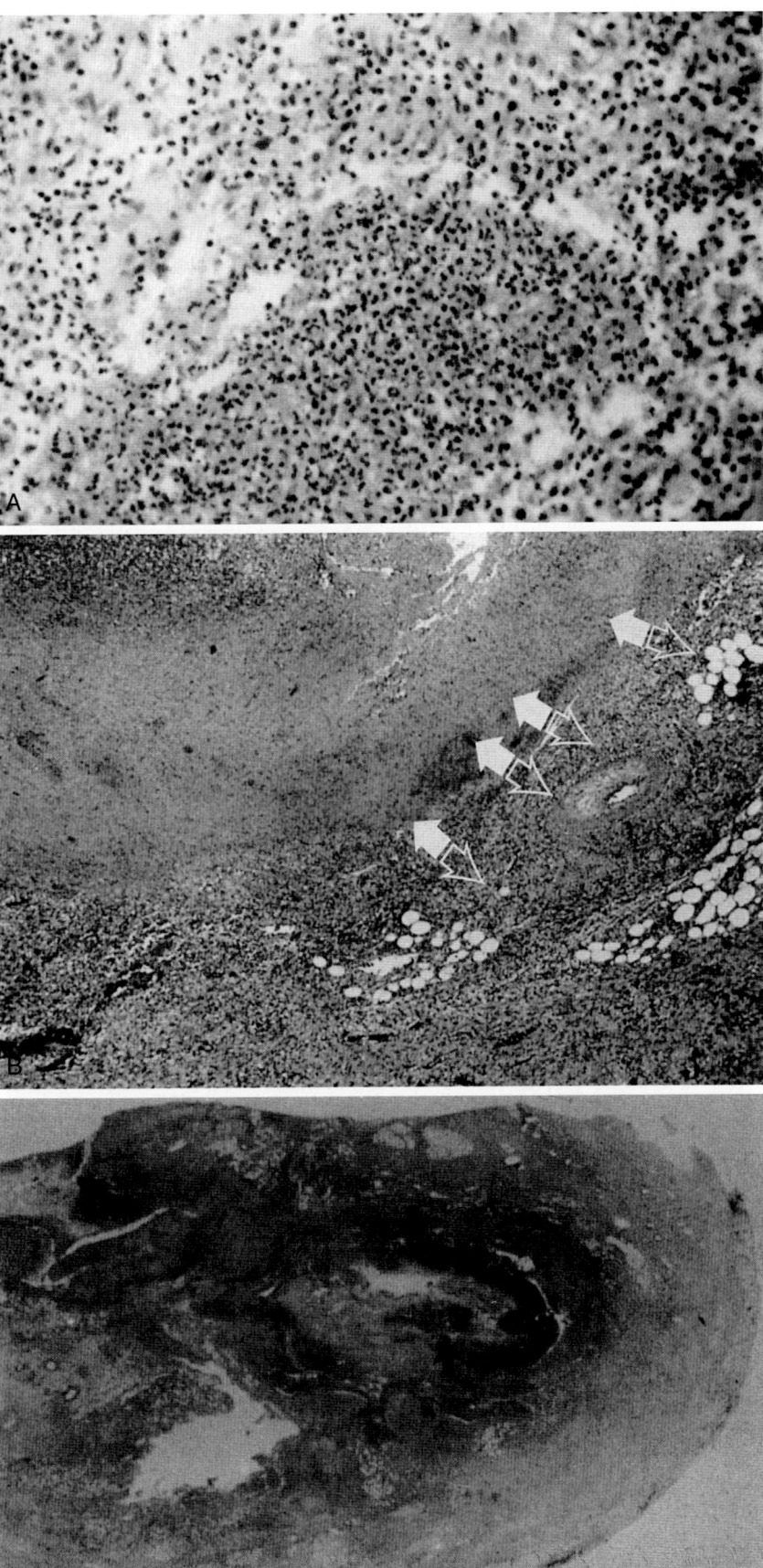

Figure 60-6. Pathology of appendicitis. A. The lumen fills with purulent exudate. Hematoxylin-eosin, ×150. **B.** Necrosis of the muscularis propria (*solid arrows*) and inflammation of the periappendiceal fat (*open arrows*) are seen. Hematoxylin-eosin, ×80. **C.** Transmural and periappendiceal inflammation and fibrosis are present with focal destruction (*arrows*) of the appendiceal wall. Hematoxylin-eosin, ×6.

Diagnostic accuracy can be improved with inpatient observation, subsequently leading to a decreased negative appendectomy rate without a concurrent increase in appendiceal perforation rates.[57] This, in turn, has led to renewed discussions in the surgical and radiologic literature regarding acceptable negative appendectomy rates. Historically, negative appendectomy rates of as high as 15% to 23% had been acceptable. Negative appendectomy rates were reported to be as high as 45% in patients with an atypical presentation or in women of childbearing age.[58] The currently accepted negative laparotomy rate is 10% to 15%, but negative laparotomy rates can be much higher in women of child-bearing age.[22,59]

Flum and associates performed a retrospective cohort study using a national, population-based hospital discharge database from 1997.[59] They found that misdiagnosis leading to negative appendectomy was more common in the very young and elderly, in women versus men, and in patients with higher levels of comorbid illness. Additionally, women had a higher rate of negative appendectomy at all ages, even when controlling for advanced comorbid illness. Although studies had previously suggested that negative appendectomy rates were highest for women in their third and fourth decades, this study found that the highest negative appendectomy rate occurred in women older than 70 years. Furthermore, this study showed that when compared with positive appendectomy for appendicitis, negative appendectomy was associated with a significantly longer length of stay (5.8 days vs. 3.6 days), case-fatality rate (1.5% vs. 0.2%), and infectious complication rate (2.6% vs. 1.8%).[22]

Radiologic imaging has become an important adjunct to clinical evaluation. The diagnosis or exclusion of acute appendicitis has been shown to be greatly facilitated by accurate identification of the inflamed or normal appendix. In addition, radiologic imaging can often determine alternate conditions as the cause of the patient's pain when the appendix is normal. Despite advances in radiologic imaging, controversy still exists in the literature whether the increased availability of imaging and laparoscopy has decreased misdiagnosis and negative laparotomy rates.

Flum and associates performed a retrospective, population-based cohort study of 63,707 nonincidental appendectomy patients seen from 1987 to 1998.[59] They found that, contrary to expectation, the use of CT, ultrasonography (US), and laparoscopy did not change the negative appendectomy or appendiceal perforation rates. In contrast, Jones and colleagues performed a retrospective study of all appendectomies performed at their institution from January 2000 to December 2002.[60] They found increased CT utilization during this interval (52%, 74%, and 86% utilization rates for 2000, 2001, and 2002, respectively). In addition, they found a statistically significant decrease in the negative appendectomy rate from 17% to 2% that coincided with the increased CT scan utilization during this time. The perforated appendicitis rate also decreased from 25% to 9% during this time interval.[60] Similar results were reported by Rao and coworkers, who found a reduction in perforation rate from 22% to 14% as well as a reduction of the negative appendectomy rate from 20% to 7% with increased use of CT.[61] Bendeck and associates retrospectively reviewed the medical records of 462 consecutive patients who underwent appendectomy for clinically suspected appendicitis and found that women benefited more than men by having preoperative CT or sonographic imaging.[62]

In that study, the negative appendectomy rate in women who underwent preoperative CT or sonographic imaging was significantly lower than that for women who did not have preoperative imaging (7% vs. 28%, respectively).[62]

Clinical Findings

The majority of patients with acute appendicitis present with abdominal pain, although the classic presentation sequence of poorly localized periumbilical pain followed by nausea and vomiting and later migration of the pain to the right lower quadrant occurs in only one half to two thirds of all patients.[43] The location of abdominal pain varies and depends on both the position of the inflamed appendix and on the stage of appendiceal inflammation. With initial distention and increased intraluminal pressure in the obstructed appendix, patients typically perceive visceral epigastric or periumbilical pain.[1-5,40] During this time, the disease is usually confined to the appendix. When the inflamed serosa of the progressively inflamed appendix comes in contact with the parietal peritoneum, somatic pain is perceived with the classic shift of pain to the right lower quadrant.[1-5,40] In patients with a retrocecal appendix, the pain may be referred to the right flank, costovertebral angle, or, in males, the right testis. Patients with a pelvic or retroileal appendix may experience pain in the pelvis, rectum, adnexa, or, less commonly, in the left lower quadrant.[43] Although nausea, vomiting, and anorexia occur in varying degrees, they are usually present in more than half of all cases.[50,63,64]

Signs and symptoms vary with the inflammatory stage of the appendicitis. Abdominal tenderness is the most common physical finding, occurring in greater than 95% of patients.[43] Although the classic teaching is that patients with appendicitis present with localized tenderness at or near McBurney's point (positioned 1.5 cm superior and medial to the anterior superior iliac spine and parallel to a plane drawn from the anterior superior iliac spine to the umbilicus), the point of tenderness will vary depending on the position of the inflamed appendix. In one series of 275 double-contrast barium enemas, the appendiceal location was within 5 cm of McBurney's point in only 35% of patients and was, in fact, distant to it by greater than 10 cm in 15% of cases.[65] More commonly, the appendix is located inferior and medial to McBurney's point.[65,66] Patients may also present with Rovsing's sign (pain referred to the area of maximal tenderness during palpation or percussion of the left lower quadrant), a positive psoas sign (right lower quadrant pain with extension of the right hip), or an obturator sign (right lower quadrant pain with flexion and internal rotation of the right hip). Voluntary muscle guarding in the right lower quadrant is common and typically precedes localized rebound tenderness. Bowel sounds vary but are more commonly diminished or absent with advanced appendiceal inflammation or perforation.[43]

The majority (70%-90%) of patients with acute appendicitis present with a white blood cell (WBC) count greater than 10,000/mL and neutrophilia greater than 75%.[28,67-69] Serial WBC counts may be helpful in the diagnosis because it has been shown that patients tend to have an increased WBC count 4 to 8 hours after admission unless the appendix is perforated (in which case the WBC count typically decreases).[70] A normal WBC count, however, should not preclude the diagnosis of appendicitis because it has been shown that patients with an inflamed appendix may have a normal WBC count.[71]

Urinalysis is positive in 19% to 40% of patients with appendicitis, and abnormalities include bacteriuria, mild pyuria, and hematuria.[72,73] Abnormal urinalysis is more commonly observed in women versus men with appendicitis.

Elevation of the C-reactive protein (CRP) greater than 0.8 mg/dL has sensitivities of 46% to 75% and specificities of 56% to 82% in acute appendicitis, and elevation is more common when symptoms are present for more than 12 hours.[70,73-75] The diagnostic sensitivity for acute appendicitis is improved to 97% to 100% when an elevated CRP, elevated WBC, and neutrophilia greater than 75% coexist.[67,76]

Radiologic Findings

Plain Radiographs

The most specific plain film sign is the presence of an appendicolith (Fig. 60-7). Appendicoliths are found, however, in only 10% of patients with acute appendicitis; and, when present, the incidence of perforation is nearly 50%. Appendicoliths are usually 0.5 to 2 cm in diameter and have a round or oval configuration and laminated rim. The calcified rim assists in differentiating them from bone islands, ureteral stones, and phleboliths. They may be obscured by the bone structures of the pelvis or may be ectopically located in the right upper abdomen in cases of retrocolic appendicitis. Appendicoliths are usually solitary, but two or three adjacent small calcifications are not unusual. Appendicoliths may be detected in asymptomatic individuals and, without associated clinical findings, are not indicative of appendicitis.[77-80]

Air in the appendix, particularly in the retrocecal location, is a normal finding. Extraluminal bubbles of air associated with an ill-defined soft tissue mass indicate an abscess (Fig. 60-8). Sometimes, the inflammatory process in the right lower quadrant induces a severe localized ileus with dilatation and air-fluid levels in the ileal loops and cecum. When severe, this process can mimic the appearance of a mechanical distal small bowel obstruction (Fig. 60-9). Dilatation of the transverse colon in association with a gasless cecum and ascending colon may result from ileus of the transverse colon and spasm of the ascending colon. Free air in the peritoneal cavity is rare because the base of the appendix is usually occluded when perforation occurs.[77-91]

Other findings such as partial loss of the right psoas shadow and a lumbar scoliosis concave to the right are common, albeit nonspecific.[77-80] Appendicitis may also cause a distal small bowel obstruction, particularly when perforated.

Plain film radiography is commonly inadequate for diagnosis of appendicitis, however. Ahn and associates retrospectively reviewed the records of 871 adult patients with nontraumatic acute abdominal pain and found that plain radiography was normal in 23%, nonspecific in 68%, and

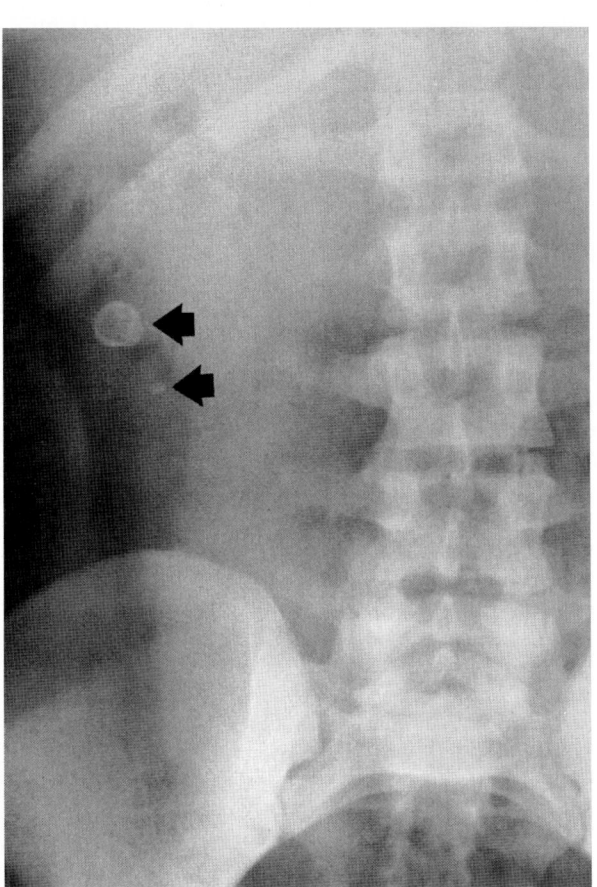

Figure 60-7. Appendicoliths. Two appendicoliths (*arrows*) are present in the right upper quadrant. The patient had a long retrocolic subhepatic appendix with acute appendicitis.

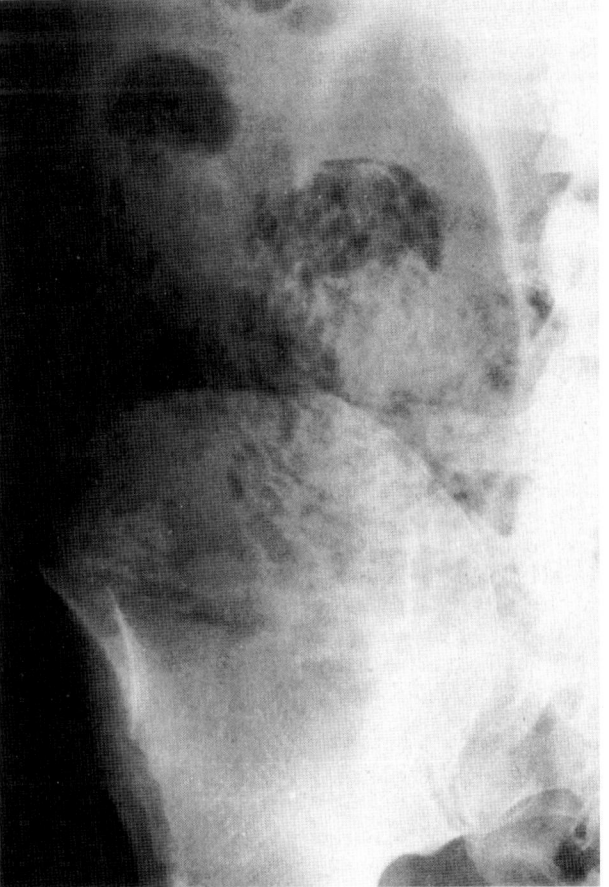

Figure 60-8. Appendiceal abscess: plain radiographic findings. This abscess manifests as a bubbly collection of extraluminal gas in the right lower quadrant.

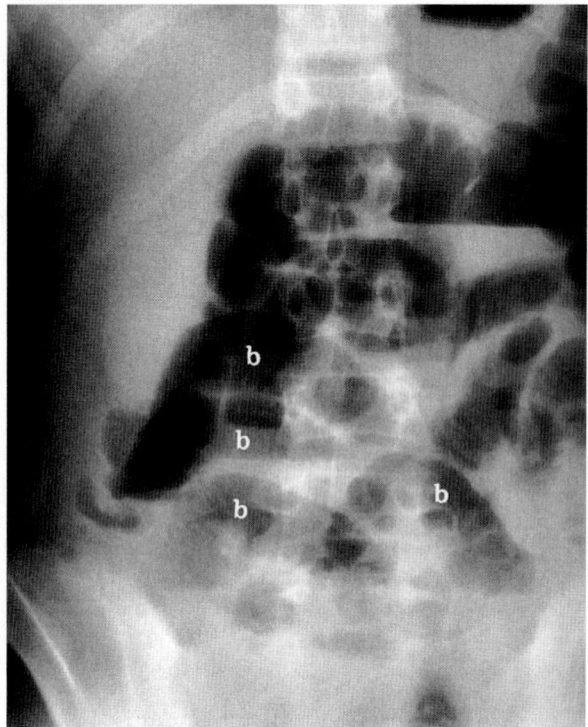

Figure 60-9. Acute appendicitis causing partial small bowel obstruction. Upright radiograph shows dilatation and air-fluid levels in multiple lower abdominal small bowel loops (b). The patient presented with fever and leukocytosis, and gangrenous appendicitis was found at surgery.

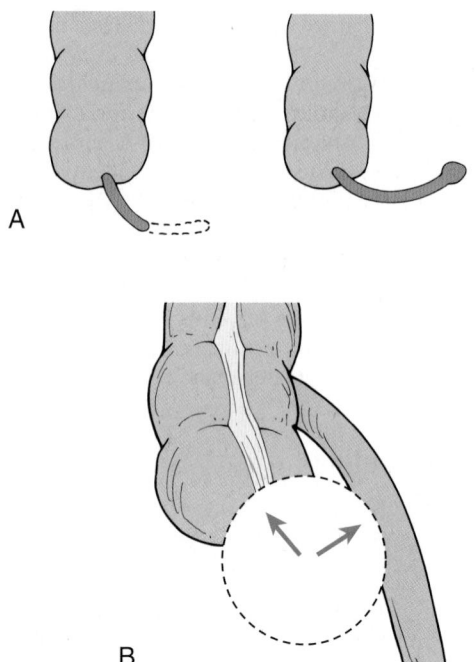

Figure 60-10. Principles of barium enema diagnosis of acute appendicitis. A. Only complete filling of the appendix to its bulbous tip excludes appendicitis. **B.** Ileocecal deformity caused by appendiceal abscess or phlegmon. (From Bartram CI, Kumar P: Clinical Radiology in Gastroenterology. Oxford, Blackwell Scientific, 1981, p 219.)

abnormal in 10%. The diagnostic sensitivity for appendicitis, pyelonephritis, pancreatitis, and diverticulitis was 0% in this study.[92]

Barium Enema

Before the 1980s, the barium enema was the primary radiologic test used in the diagnosis of appendicitis. This examination can be performed quickly and safely with the single-column technique. Appendicitis occurs in the setting of lumen obstruction, so complete filling of a normal appendix effectively excludes the diagnosis (Fig. 60-10A). Nonfilling or incomplete filling in the presence of a mass effect (Figs. 60-10B and 60-11) on the caput cecum and adjacent distal ileum does indicate inflammation, however.[77-82,89-91,93-99]

The barium enema study is also helpful in detecting other small bowel and colonic disease that can mimic the clinical presentation of acute appendicitis: neoplasm, Crohn's disease, ileal diverticulitis, and cecal diverticulitis.[77-82,89-91,93-99]

Although the diagnostic accuracy of the barium enema study in patients with acute appendicitis is reportedly as high as 91.5%, this technique has several major drawbacks.[77-82,89-91,93-99] Nonfilling of the appendix can be seen in 15% to 20% of normal patients, and it may be difficult to differentiate a partially filled from a completely filled appendix. Also, barium enema study provides only inferential information about extracolonic disease and cannot evaluate the nature of appendiceal phlegmons and abscesses. The appendix can also intussuscept (Fig. 60-12) into the cecum, producing a cecal defect unrelated to appendicitis on barium enema studies.[100-102]

Since the late 1980s, US and CT have gained acceptance as primary imaging techniques for acute appendicitis by virtue of their ability to directly image the appendix, adjacent fat, and gut.

Computed Tomography

Helical CT has proven to be a highly effective and accurate means of diagnosing acute appendicitis, with reported sensitivities of 90% to 100%, specificities of 91% to 99%, accuracies of 94% to 98%, positive predictive values of 92% to 98%, and negative predictive values of 95% to 100%.[103-108] CT enables assessment of the appendix and periappendiceal region while also allowing identification of complications of appendiceal perforation, including the presence of abscesses and phlegmon (Fig. 60-13). In addition, CT can facilitate diagnosis of alternate conditions in patients without appendicitis.

The goal of CT investigation in patients with right lower quadrant pain is to identify the normal or abnormal appendix. It has been shown that performance of thin-section (≤5-mm collimation) imaging through the right lower quadrant improves the sensitivity for detecting key imaging findings of appendicitis. Weltman and associates showed that use of 5-mm section helical CT improved identification of abnormal appendices (94% vs. 69%), calcified appendicoliths (38% vs. 19%), and periappendiceal inflammation (98% vs. 75%) compared with 10-mm thick-section helical CT in the same patient.[108]

The definitive diagnosis of acute appendicitis on CT examination is based on identifying either the abnormal appendix (Figs. 60-14 and 60-15) or the presence of pericecal inflammation in association with a calcified appendicolith

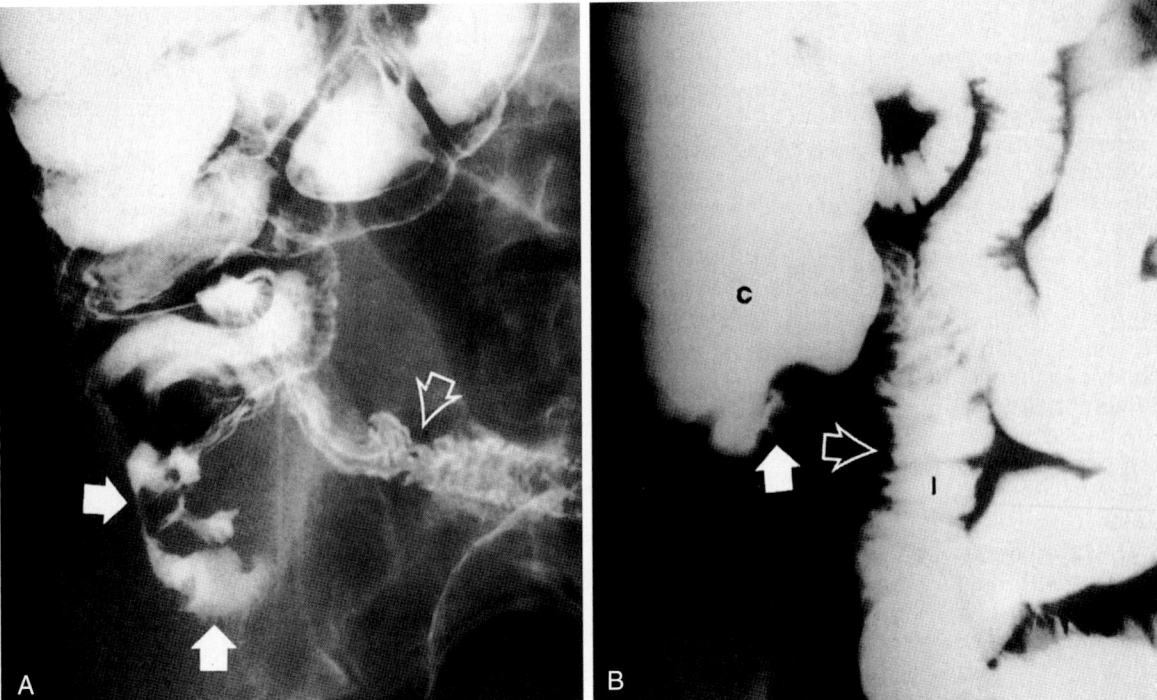

Figure 60-11. Acute appendicitis: barium enema findings. A. Extravasation of barium in a patient with sealed-off, perforative appendicitis (*solid arrows*). The cecum and terminal ileum (*open arrow*) are unremarkable. **B.** Appendiceal abscess shows compression of the cecal caput, obstruction of the base of the appendix (*solid arrow*), and a spiculated lateral contour (*open arrow*) of the terminal ileum. C, cecum; I, ileum.

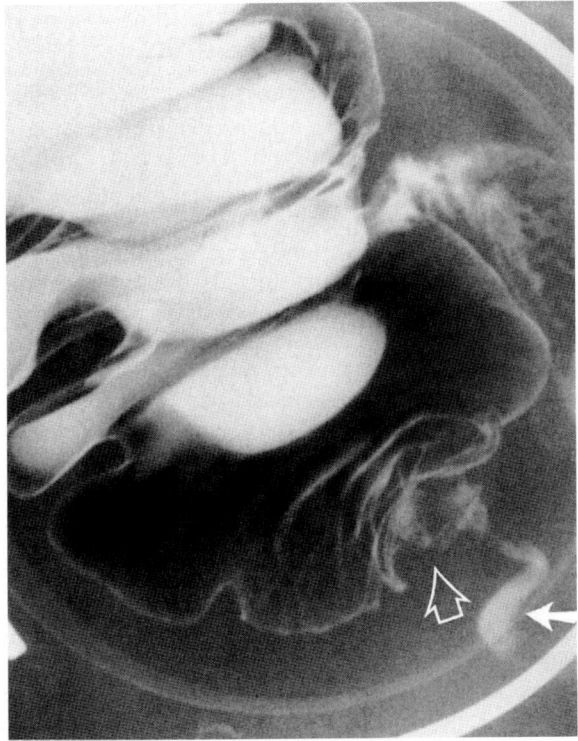

Figure 60-12. Partial appendiceal intussusception. The appendix is incompletely filled (*solid arrow*) and partially intussuscepting into the cecal caput (*open arrow*).

(Fig. 60-16).[19,109,110] The normal appendix is identified in 67% to 100% of patients with abdominal pain who undergo thin-section helical CT imaging of the right lower quadrant.[103,105-108,111-114] The normal appendix has been shown to be harder to identify on CT examination in patients with a paucity of retroperitoneal fat, in patients with ascites, and in women compared with men.[112-114] CT studies have shown variable diameters for the normal appendix.[112-114] Tamburrini and colleagues studied 372 asymptomatic outpatients and

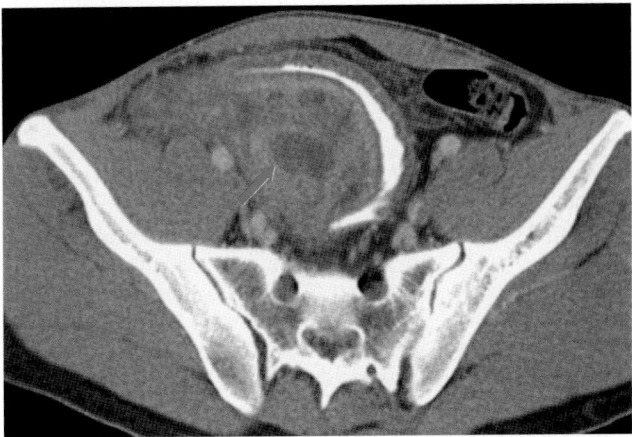

Figure 60-13. Perforated acute appendicitis with abscess. This enhanced CT scan shows a large amount of right lower quadrant inflammation along with reactive thickening off the terminal ileum. A fluid-filled abscess is also present (*arrow*). This was pathologically proven to be due to perforated acute appendicitis.

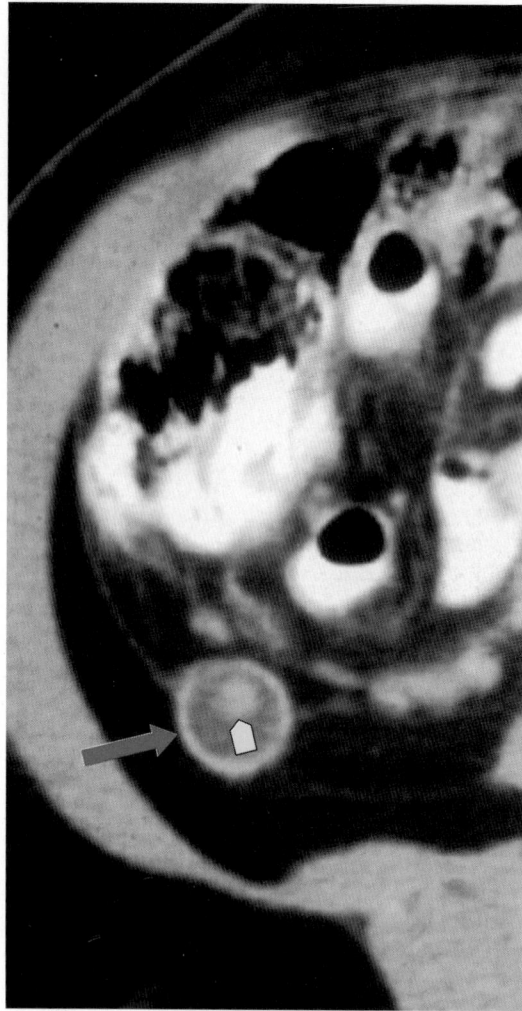

Figure 60-14. Acute appendicitis on enhanced CT. The distended appendix (*arrow*) is seen in cross section and demonstrates abnormal mural thickening and enhancement. In addition, an intraluminal appendicolith (*yellow arrowhead*) is present.

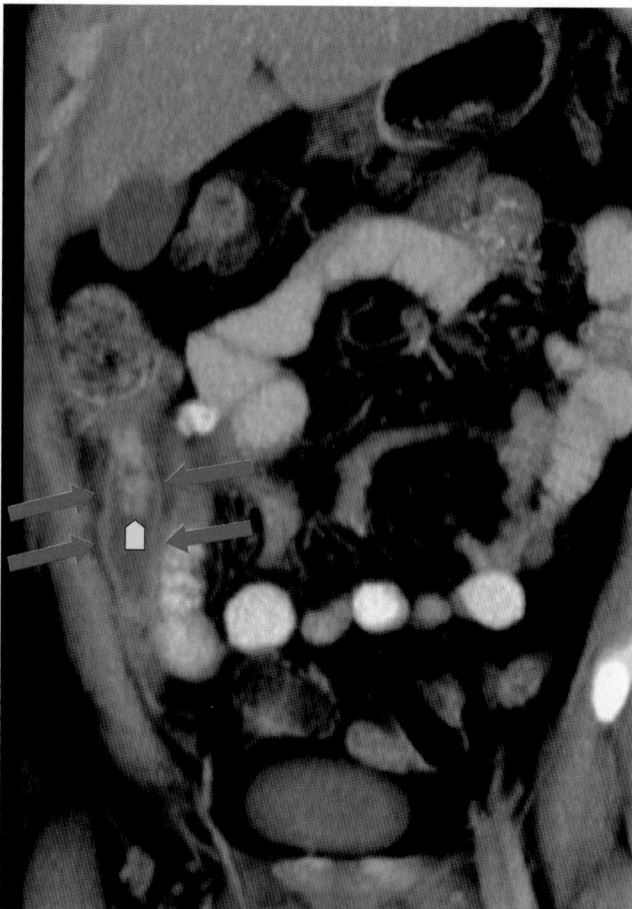

Figure 60-15. Acute appendicitis on enhanced CT. This coronal multiplanar reconstruction image shows the distended appendix (*arrows*) with multiple obstructing appendicoliths (*yellow arrowhead*) at the appendiceal orifice. Note the mural wall thickening and enhancement as well as the periappendiceal soft tissue stranding and fluid. On pathologic examination the appendix was shown to be perforated.

showed that the diameter range of the normal appendix was 3 to 10 mm.[113] Of note, 42% of the normal appendices in that study had a diameter of greater than 6 mm.[113] Therefore, an appendiceal diameter of larger than 6 mm cannot be used as an absolute criterion for diagnosing acute appendicitis on CT examination.

The diameter of an inflamed appendix varies. In very mild cases of nonperforating appendicitis, the abnormal appendix may appear as a fluid-filled, minimally distended tubular structure 5 to 6 mm in diameter.[19] In the most incipient cases, the periappendiceal fat remains normal in appearance (Fig. 60-17).

As the inflammatory process progresses, the appendix continues to distend, typically measuring 7 to 15 mm in diameter.[19] The appendiceal wall becomes circumferentially and symmetrically thickened and enhances after administration of intravenous contrast material. The mural enhancement may be homogeneous or may exhibit a target sign appearance (Fig. 60-18). Periappendiceal inflammation is present in the majority of patients with all but the most incipient forms of acute appendicitis.[19]

The appendiceal inflammation may also cause reactive thickening of the cecal caput or the wall of the terminal ileum. Secondary cecal findings that may be seen if the cecum is filled with enteric contrast material include the cecal arrowhead sign (triangular "arrowhead" configuration of oral contrast material funneling into the focally thickened and spastic cecum and pointing toward the appendiceal orifice) (Fig. 60-19) and the cecal bar sign (linear inflammatory soft tissue at the base of the appendix that separates the contrast-filled cecum from the appendix).[115]

With perforated appendicitis, extraluminal air, marked ileocecal wall thickening, localized lymphadenopathy, pericecal phlegmon or abscess, peritonitis, and/or small bowel obstruction may be present (Fig. 60-20). Appreciation of mural thickening and mural enhancement in mild cases of appendicitis is limited without administration of intravenous contrast material. Because of this, periappendiceal inflammation is considered to be a necessary criterion for diagnosing acute appendicitis by many investigators who use CT protocols without administration of intravenous contrast material.[103,104,106,107,116] This reliance on identification of periappendiceal inflammation may lead to false-negative CT diagnoses.[107,110,116,117]

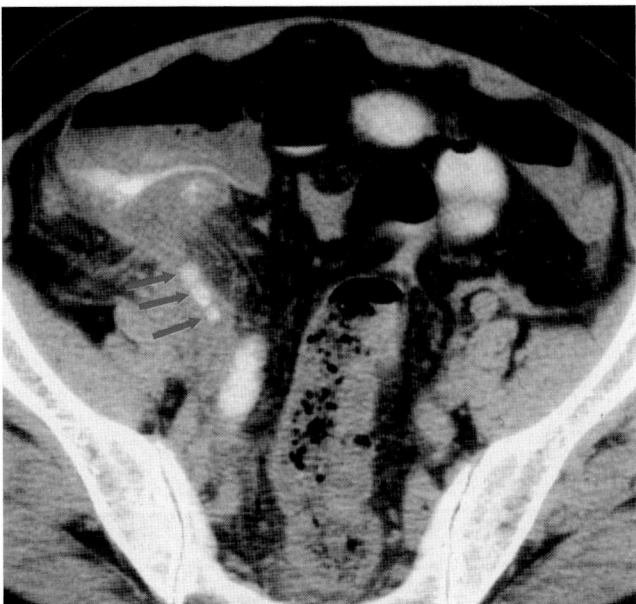

Figure 60-16. Acute appendicitis on CT. Although the appendix itself is not distinctly identified, there are three appendicoliths (*arrows*) present in association with right lower quadrant inflammation and pericecal thickening. This constellation of findings is diagnostic of acute appendicitis.

Appendicitis can be confined to the distal aspect or tip of the appendix, a condition referred to as "distal" or "tip" appendicitis (Fig. 60-21). It is estimated that distal appendicitis (with at least 3 cm of a proximal normal appendix) affects as many as 8% of patients with appendicitis who undergo CT.[118] Conventional CT protocols for evaluating patients with suspected appendicitis incorporate abdominal and pelvic imaging after administration of both oral and intravenous

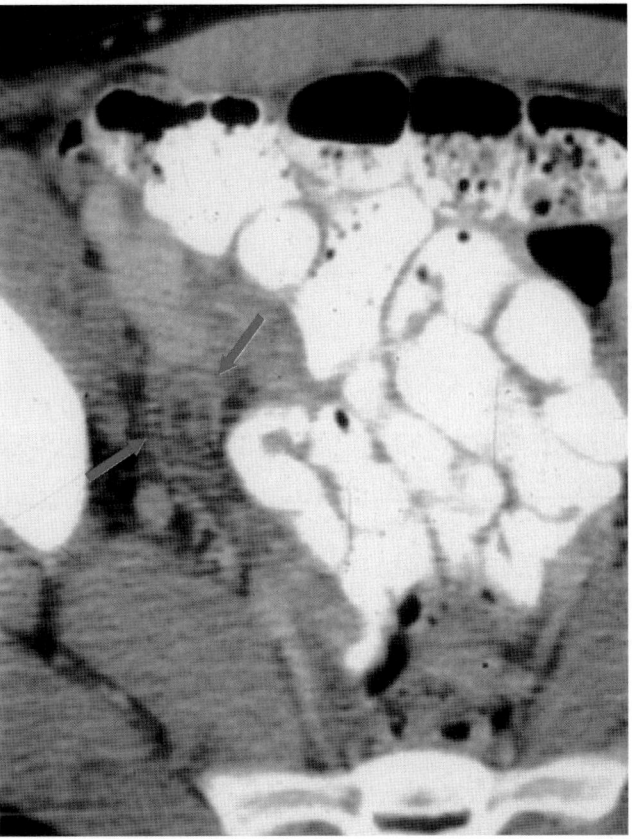

Figure 60-18. Acute appendicitis. The abnormal appendix (*arrows*) is seen in cross section on this enhanced CT study and demonstrates a mural stratification pattern of enhancement with alternating high- and low-density rings due to serosal and mucosal enhancement and submucosal edema.

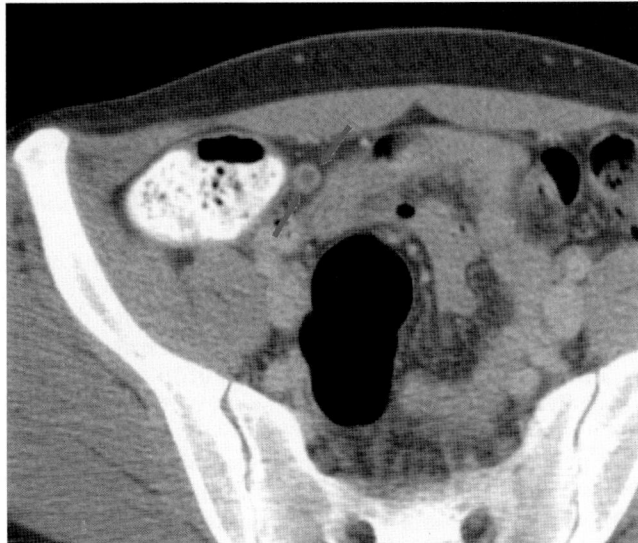

Figure 60-17. Acute appendicitis. The abnormal appendix (*arrows*) is seen in cross section on this enhanced CT scan. Although there is minimal distention of the appendiceal lumen, there is evidence for abnormal mural thickening and enhancement. Note the absence of periappendiceal inflammatory change.

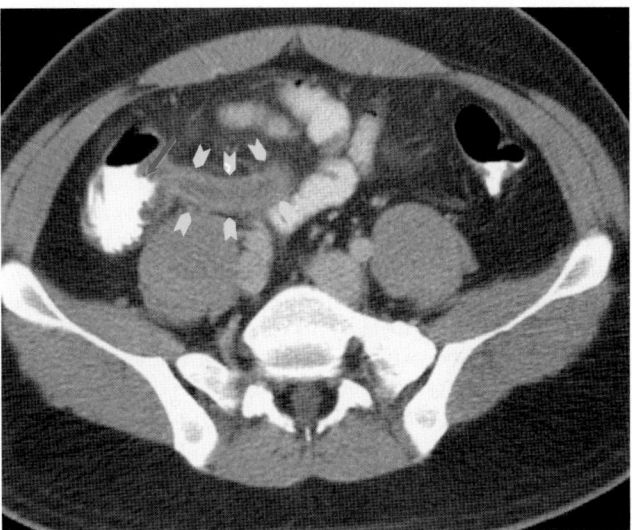

Figure 60-19. Acute appendicitis on enhanced CT. The appendix (*arrowheads*) is distended, with enhancement of the thickened appendiceal wall and periappendiceal soft tissue stranding. Note the funneling of enteric contrast in the thickened cecum toward the appendiceal orifice, the "arrowhead" sign (*arrow*).

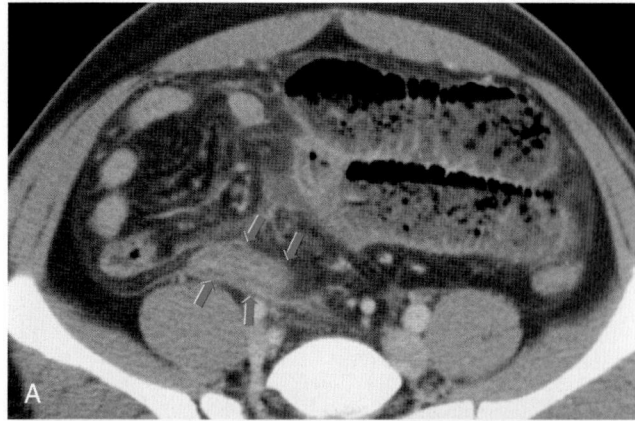

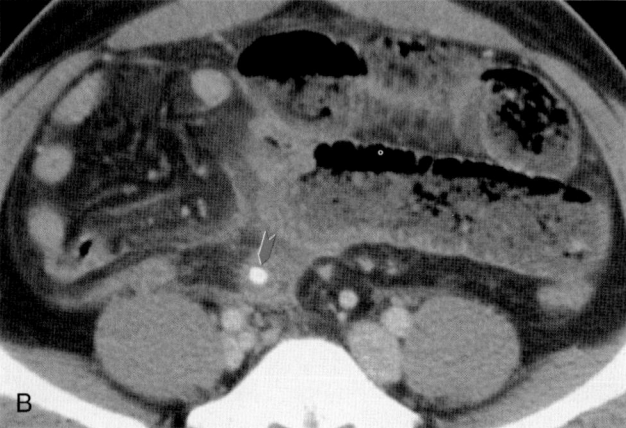

Figure 60-20. Small bowel obstruction from acute appendicitis.
A. There are multiple dilated small bowel loops in the pelvis to the level
of the abnormally distended, thick-walled, and enhancing appendix
(*arrows*). **B.** A more superior CT scan shows a calcified appendicolith
(*arrowhead*) near the appendiceal orifice.

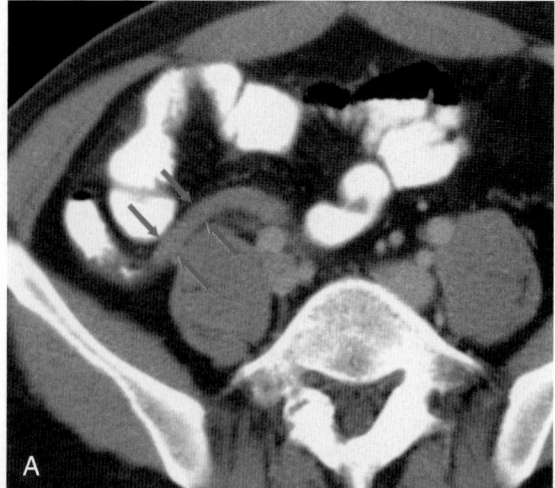

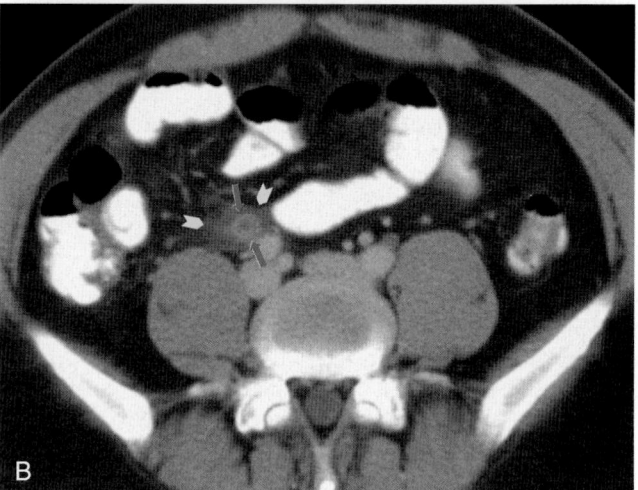

Figure 60-21. "Distal" or "tip" appendicitis. A. The proximal appendix
(*arrows*) is normal in appearance on this enhanced CT scan. **B.** The distal
aspect of the appendix demonstrates abnormal mural thickening and
enhancement (*arrows*), and periappendiceal soft tissue stranding is also
present (*arrowheads*).

contrast material. Many studies have assessed the efficacy of
alternative appendiceal CT protocols. These include imaging
the abdomen and pelvis without oral or intravenous contrast
material,[103,104] focused imaging of the right lower quadrant
without oral or intravenous contrast material,[116,119,120] focused
imaging of the right lower quadrant with oral contrast material,[117,121,122] focused imaging of the right lower quadrant with
oral and rectal contrast material,[106,122] and focused imaging
of the right lower quadrant with rectal contrast material.[107,123]

The advantages of protocols performed without oral or
intravenous contrast material include the ability to immediately scan symptomatic patients without having to wait for
oral contrast material ingestion and adequate opacification
of the ileum and cecum, elimination of the potential risk
of contrast reaction from contrast material administration,
and reduced study costs. Disadvantages of studies performed
without oral contrast material include the potential to misinterpret a small bowel loop as the appendix, or, conversely,
to misinterpret an abnormal appendix or periappendiceal
abscess as a bowel loop.[108,109,116,124] Eliminating the chance of
distending the normal appendix with oral contrast material
may hamper recognition of a patent appendiceal orifice and
normal appendix. Lack of adequate bowel distention with
oral contrast material may also impede one's ability to recognize bowel wall thickening or luminal narrowing, which are
hallmarks of gastrointestinal disease on CT.[125] Disadvantages

of studies performed without intravenous contrast material
include the inability to assess for abnormal appendiceal wall
thickening and enhancement, limited differentiation of the
appendix from blood vessels, and reduced sensitivity for
diagnosing perforated appendicitis and alternative diagnoses.[19,117,121,124-127]

It may be difficult to identify the inflamed appendix
and subtle periappendiceal inflammation in patients with
a paucity of retroperitoneal fat unless intravenous contrast
material is administered.[116,117] In addition, the diagnosis may
be missed in patients with mild appendicitis and no periappendiceal inflammation if CT studies are performed without
intravenous contrast material.[107,110,116] Studies have shown
that periappendiceal inflammation may be absent in mild
forms of acute appendicitis.[117,128] In a study of 211 patients
with suspected appendicitis studied without intravenous contrast material, Malone and coworkers showed that approximately 5% of patients with early acute appendicitis lacked
CT evidence of pericecal and periappendiceal inflammation.[116] Jacobs and colleagues evaluated 228 patients with suspected appendicitis and found that 15% to 22% of patients

with proven appendicitis who underwent CT examinations without intravenous contrast material had no recognizable periappendiceal inflammatory change.[117]

The advantages of rectal contrast material administration include the ability to rapidly opacify the cecum and to achieve identification of the appendix in the overwhelming majority of cases. In a study by Rao and associates, use of a focused right lower quadrant technique with colonic contrast material enabled detection of the normal appendix in 94% of patients without appendicitis and visualization of part or all of the abnormal appendix in 96% of patients with acute appendicitis.[107] Although 15% to 20% of normal appendices do not routinely fill on barium enema examinations,[129] 73% of the normal appendices in this study filled with either air or colonic contrast material.[107]

Disadvantages of the colonic contrast technique include the potential for increased patient discomfort,[122] the inability to instill rectal contrast material in patients with contraindications to its use, and the risk of causing a hydraulic pressure effect and rupturing the appendix.[121] This technique may also fail if there is leakage of contrast material onto the CT table or if there is inadequate opacification of the cecum. Wise and associates report that colonic contrast material was unsuccessfully advanced into the cecum in 18% of 100 focused appendiceal CT scans with colonic contrast material administration.[122] Of these failures, 16 were due to abundant stool in the right colon, one was due to a very redundant sigmoid colon, and one was thought to be due to inadequate effort by the radiologist.[122] In this study, leakage of contrast material onto the CT table occurred in 24% of cases.[122]

Proponents of focused right lower quadrant CT techniques argue that their study results approximate the diagnostic results achieved with nonfocused (abdominopelvic) techniques with the benefit of reduced patient radiation dose.[106] The two greatest limitations of focused techniques include the possibility of partially or entirely excluding the appendix from the scan field of view[117] and the possibility of missing alternative diagnoses that lie outside the scan field of view. The most commonly reported alternative diagnoses include abdominal pain of unknown etiology, pelvic inflammatory disease and other acute gynecologic disorders, mesenteric lymphadenitis, acute gastroenteritis and other acute gastrointestinal tract diseases, and urinary tract infection and obstruction.

There is growing consensus that use of both enteric and intravenous contrast material is invaluable for detecting subtle cases of early appendicitis and for maximizing one's level of diagnostic confidence in establishing the diagnosis of appendicitis. A survey of CT protocols used at academic medical centers in the United States for patients with suspected appendicitis revealed that intravenous, oral, and rectal contrast media are routinely administered at 79%, 82%, and 32% of institutions, respectively.[130]

Ultrasonography

The technique of graded compression US, introduced by Puylaert in the mid-1980s, substantially aided sonographic identification of the appendix.[131] The advantages of US are that it is widely available, relatively inexpensive, and noninvasive and, most importantly, poses no ionizing radiation risk to the patient. This latter fact is a significant issue when evaluating pregnant patients. In addition, ionizing radiation risk is an important concern in pediatric and young adult patients who are up to 10 times more sensitive to its effects than middle-aged and elderly adults.[132]

Important limitations of US are the fact that it is operator dependent, it can be difficult to perform in patients with severe abdominal pain or patients with large amounts of bowel gas, and it can be very limited in muscular or obese patients. The limited ability of US to adequately penetrate the abdomen in obese patients has contributed to its lack of widespread use in North America and parts of Europe. Whereas some authors report that the normal appendix is seen in only 0% to 4% of adult patients regardless of technique,[19] others report it can be seen in 64% to 72% of patients.[133,134]

The reported diagnostic accuracy of ultrasound varies depending on the patient population studied. A meta-analysis of pediatric and adult studies published between 1986 and 1994 showed an overall sonographic sensitivity of 85% and a specificity of 92%.[135]

Adherence to optimal scanning techniques is paramount to diagnose appendicitis sonographically. Sagittal, transverse, and oblique imaging should be performed in the abdomen and pelvis, with addition of a transvaginal examination in women in whom the diagnosis is not evident following the transabdominal approach. A high-frequency linear probe or a curvilinear probe can be used, depending on the patient's body habitus. Identification of the appendix may be limited using a high-frequency linear transducer in patients with poorly compressible right lower quadrant bowel, in large patients with the cecum and appendix located deep within the pelvis, in patients with poorly defined right lower quadrant anatomy, and in patients with a retrocecal or perforated appendix.

The technique of graded compression should be employed to displace or compress gas-filled bowel loops in the field of view. This maneuver aids identification of the maximal point of tenderness while helping to differentiate abnormal, noncompressible bowel loops or the inflamed appendix from those normally compressible structures. Additionally, the maintenance of slow and gentle pressure facilitates completion of the examination in uncomfortable and apprehensive patients.[19]

Color Doppler evaluation may add valuable information by demonstrating hyperemia in the inflamed appendix or bowel wall.[133] This can aid diagnosis in patients with equivocal gray-scale results.

Sonographically, the abnormal appendix appears as a blind-ending, noncompressible, tubular structure larger than 6 mm in diameter with a laminated wall (Figs. 60-22 to 60-24). Increasing ischemia and infarction of the appendiceal wall leads to focal or diffuse loss of definition of the wall layers.[136] Hyperemia may be demonstrated on color Doppler evaluation, but decreased or absent flow may be seen in cases of gangrenous appendicitis.[19] With perforation, localized disruption of the appendiceal wall may be seen and extraluminal pockets of gas may be present. Appendicoliths appear as rounded, echogenic foci with clean distal acoustic shadowing, and their presence is highly associated with appendicitis.

In addition to the appendiceal findings present in acute appendicitis, recognition of characteristic periappendiceal findings can aid in its diagnosis and differentiation from other conditions. Inflammation of the periappendiceal fat

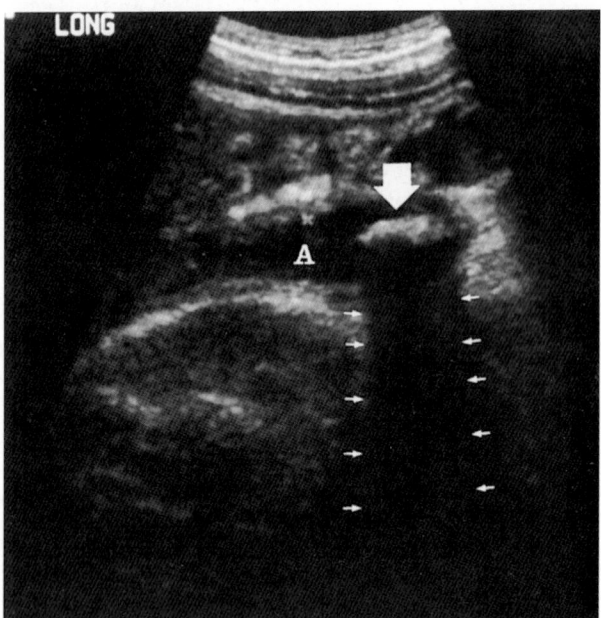

Figure 60-22. Sonogram of an inflamed appendix containing an appendicolith. Longitudinal image shows a thick-walled, fluid-filled appendix (A). The layers of the appendiceal wall are not well defined. An appendicolith (*large arrow*) is identified as an echogenic focus with acoustic shadowing (*small arrows*).

appears as an echogenic region that may cause mass effect and separate the inflamed bowel segment(s) from surrounding structures.[19] Periappendiceal phlegmon appears as hypoechoic, poorly marginated regions within the fat adjacent to the appendix, and abscesses can be recognized as focal collections of fluid that may or may not contain gas. Reactive inflammatory thickening of the cecal or terminal ileal wall may also be present in patients with appendicitis.

Despite performance of optimized US examinations, it is known that the US sensitivity for diagnosing perforated appendicitis is lower than that for nonperforated appendicitis. Overall, the noncompressible appendix is seen in only 38% to 55% of patients with perforated appendicitis.[137,138]

Because of its limitations in obese patients and because of its advantages of lack of ionizing radiation and its ability to differentiate gynecologic from nongynecologic conditions, US is best used as an initial imaging modality in children, adolescents, thin adults, women of reproductive age with possible gynecologic causes of right lower quadrant pain, and pregnant patients.

Computed Tomography versus Ultrasonography

Studies comparing the use of US versus CT in patients suspected of having acute appendicitis have generally favored CT for providing greater diagnostic accuracy, superior detection and staging of complications, and higher accuracies for establishing alternative diagnoses.[110,120,122,139,140] A study performed by Balthazar and associates of 100 patients with suspected appendicitis in whom high-resolution thin-section CT imaging of the right lower quadrant was compared with graded compression US showed that CT was found to have a higher sensitivity (96% vs. 76%), negative predictive value (95% vs. 76%), and accuracy (94% vs. 83%) than US, al-

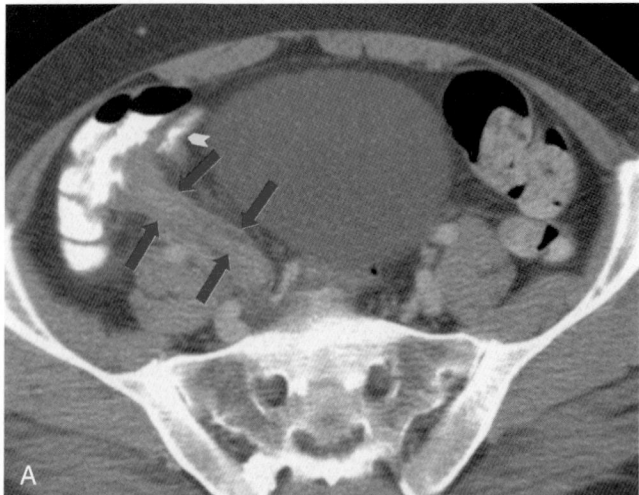

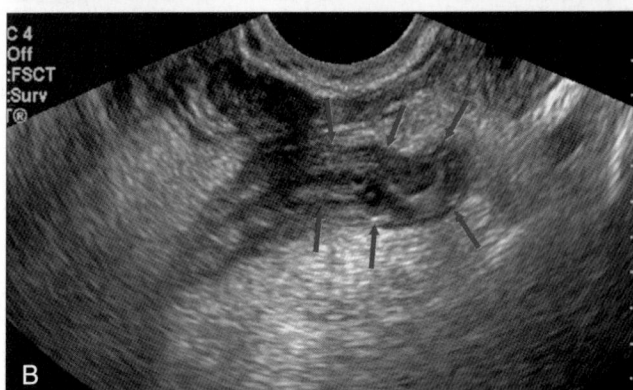

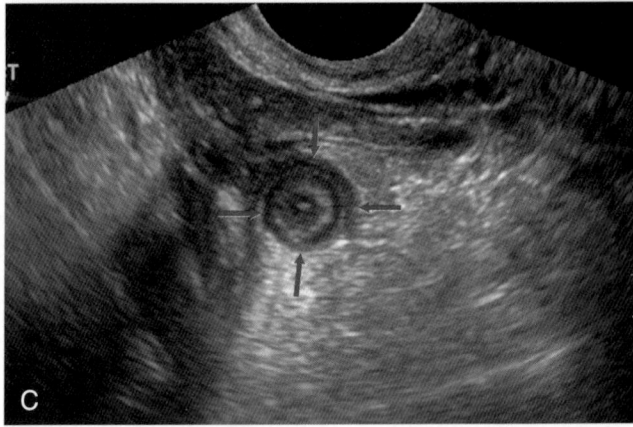

Figure 60-23. Correlation of sonography and CT findings in acute appendicitis. A. CT shows the abnormally distended and thick-walled appendix (*large arrows*) with periappendiceal inflammation. Note the reactive inflammatory thickening of the terminal ileum (*arrowhead*) and the cecum. **B.** Longitudinal transvaginal sonogram shows a thick-walled, distended appendix (*arrows*). **C.** Transverse transvaginal sonogram shows the thick-walled and abnormally distended appendix (*arrows*). The appendiceal diameter was 13 mm.

though the specificities (89% vs. 91%) and positive predictive values (96% vs. 95%) were comparable.[110] In addition, CT was shown to more accurately detect periappendiceal abnormalities, to indicate alternative diagnoses, and to be superior in excluding appendicitis by demonstrating the presence of a normal appendix compared with ultrasound examination.[110]

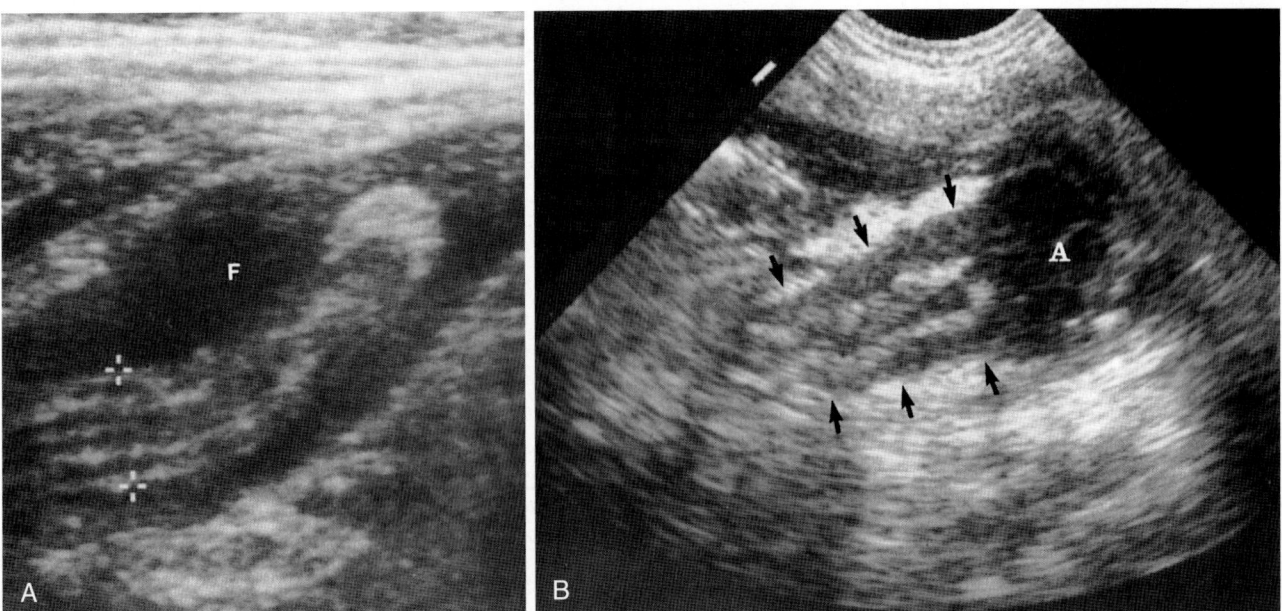

Figure 60-24. Ultrasound detection of periappendiceal fluid and abscess. A. Longitudinal sonogram demonstrates a dilated appendix with a diameter of 10 mm (*cursors*). Wall stratification is maintained, and periappendiceal fluid (F) is visualized. **B.** A fluid-filled abscess (A) is visualized adjacent to the tip of the appendix (*arrows*), in a different patient.

Pikuth and coworkers prospectively evaluated 120 adult and pediatric patients with clinically suspected appendicitis by both unenhanced focused helical CT and graded compression US.[139] These authors found that CT was diagnostically superior to US. The sensitivity and specificity of CT was 95% and 89%, respectively, versus an US sensitivity and specificity of 87% and 74%, respectively.[139]

Poortman and colleagues prospectively evaluated 199 consecutive patients with clinically suspected appendicitis by focused unenhanced single-detector helical CT and graded compression US.[141] Of these patients, 132 had appendicitis at surgery. These authors found that the two modalities had similar accuracies for detection of acute appendicitis. Respectively, the sensitivities of CT and of US were 76% and 79%; the specificities were 83% and 78%; the accuracy was 78% and 78%; the positive predictive value was 90% and 87%; and the negative predictive value was 64% and 65%.[141]

Wise and associates prospectively evaluated 100 adult patients clinically suspected of having acute appendicitis with graded compression US, unenhanced focused appendiceal CT with and without colonic contrast material, abdomino-pelvic CT with oral and IV contrast material, and repeated graded compression US with colonic contrast material.[122] These authors found that US had a significantly lower diagnostic performance than CT as well as the second highest rating of patient discomfort among the imaging techniques (CT with colonic contrast material was first). The sensitivity, specificity, positive predictive value, negative predictive value, and accuracy of CT were 96%, 92%, 79%, 99%, and 93%, respectively, whereas those for graded compression US without colonic contrast material were 34%, 86%, 42%, 81%, and 74%, respectively.[122]

CT was also shown to be more sensitive than ultrasound in a more recent study of children, adolescents, and young adults performed by Sivit and colleagues.[142] In this study, the sensitivity and accuracy of CT examination (95% and

94%, respectively) were significantly higher than the findings for graded compression US (78% and 89%, respectively).[142]

An increase in radiologic confidence is an additional reason CT is frequently preferred over US for evaluation of appendicitis. This was emphasized in a study performed by Peña and Taylor.[143] These authors prospectively evaluated 139 children and young adults with equivocal clinical findings of appendicitis and found that radiologists were significantly more confident of their CT interpretations than US interpretations. Furthermore, they found that radiologists' level of experience did not significantly affect the diagnostic confidence of their interpretations.[143] This was also confirmed by Wise and coworkers, who prospectively questioned radiologists regarding their confidence in diagnosing acute appendicitis using graded compression US versus various CT techniques.[122] These authors found that abdominopelvic CT and focused appendiceal CT with colonic contrast were preferred to sonography or unenhanced focused appendiceal CT in 87 of 100 patients ($P < .0001$).[122]

Magnetic Resonance Imaging

Magnetic resonance imaging has proven to be accurate for diagnosing acute appendicitis and, with US, has become an important diagnostic tool for identifying appendicitis in pregnant patients. The benefits of MR examination are its multiplanar image acquisition capabilities, its high intrinsic soft tissue contrast, its ability to study patients without the need to administer contrast material, and, most importantly for pregnant patients, its lack of ionizing radiation.

Nitta and coworkers evaluated 20 normal volunteers and 37 consecutive patients with clinically diagnosed acute appendicitis. They were able to identify the normal appendix in 90% of patients.[144] On MRI, the normal appendix appeared as a cord-like structure without an identifiable lumen that had similar intensity to muscle on all imaging sequences. In

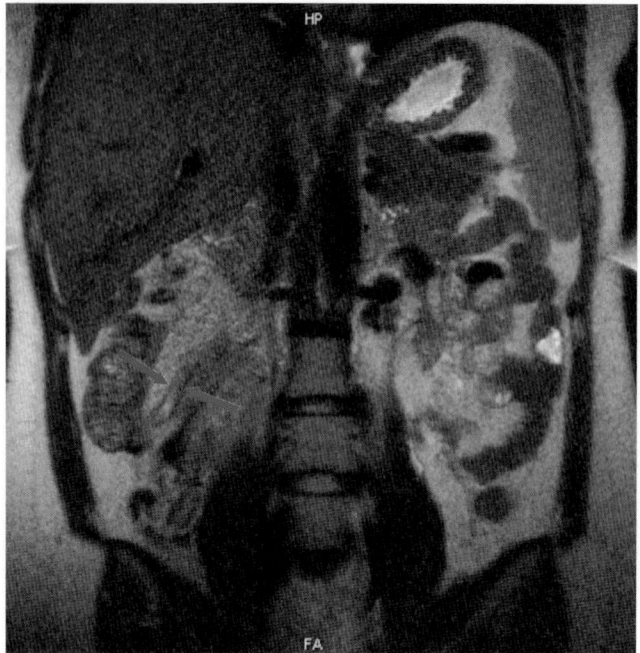

Figure 60-25. MR image of acute appendicitis in woman at 29 weeks gestation. This coronal HASTE image shows the abnormally distended and thick-walled appendix (*arrows*), which is filled with high-intensity material. This was pathologically proven to represent acute appendicitis.

this study, MRI was able to accurately diagnose acute appendicitis in 29 of 30 cases with abnormal appendices.[144] The MRI criteria for diagnosing appendicitis were (1) thickening of the appendiceal wall with high intensity on T2-weighted fast spin-echo [T2WI] and fat-suppressed spectral presaturation inversion recovery images [T2SPIR]; (2) a dilated lumen filled with high intensity material on T2WI or T2SPIR; and (3) increased intensity of the periappendiceal tissues on T2WI or T2SPIR.[144]

Acute appendicitis is the most common nonobstetric surgical emergency in pregnant patients, occurring in approximately 1 in 766 pregnancies (Fig. 60-25).[145] Complications include premature labor and fetal and maternal death, especially when perforation occurs.[146] The fetal loss rate for non-ruptured appendicitis is approximately 2%, compared with more than 30% in patients with ruptured appendicitis.[147]

Clinical diagnosis is extremely challenging in pregnant patients because these patients rarely present with classic symptoms and laboratory tests are also unreliable. US is also much more difficult in this population because the enlarged gravid uterus alters the position of the abdominal contents and often obscures identification of the appendix.[146] Cobben and coworkers studied 12 pregnant patients with clinically suspected appendicitis ultrasonographically and were unable to identify the appendix in 11 (92%).[146] In contrast, when MRI was used, the normal appendix was identified in 7 of 9 (78%) patients without appendicitis and the abnormal appendix was shown in all three cases of pathologically proven acute appendicitis.[146] Birchard and associates performed MRI examinations on 29 pregnant patients with clinically suspected appendicitis.[148] Six of these patients had ultrasound evaluation before the MRI study. In this study, MRI was able to correctly identify the cause of the abdominal pain in all but

1 of the 29 patients whereas US was unable to identify the appendix in 3 of the 6 (50%) patients evaluated.[148]

Although no adverse fetal effects from MRI have been documented, the U.S. Food and Drug Administration guidelines require labeling MR devices to indicate that their fetal safety has not been established. The safety concern arises from tissue heating effects that occur from radiofrequency pulses. These are maximal at the body surface and approach zero near the body core. The safety committee of the Society for MRI has stated that MRI examination is indicated in pregnant patients when the results of nonionizing diagnostic imaging tests are inconclusive or inadequate or when MRI is expected to provide important treatment for the fetus or mother.[149]

Differential Diagnosis of Right Lower Quadrant Inflammation

Detection of right lower quadrant inflammation adjacent to the cecum is highly suggestive of but not pathognomonic for acute appendicitis. Differential diagnosis includes cecal or ileal diverticulitis, Crohn's disease, mesenteric adenitis, epiploic appendagitis, inflamed Meckel's diverticulum, infectious or ischemic ileitis, typhlitis, perforated cecal carcinoma, and pelvic inflammatory disease.

Identification of the normal appendix facilitates these diagnoses. It is important to differentiate these entities from acute appendicitis because, unlike appendicitis, many of these conditions can be adequately managed conservatively.

Mesenteric Adenitis

Mesenteric adenitis is reported to be second to appendicitis as the most common etiology of right lower quadrant pain, accounting for 2% to 14% of discharge diagnoses in patients suspected of having appendicitis.[150-153]

Primary mesenteric adenitis is diagnosed by CT or US when there are more than three right-sided mesenteric lymph nodes greater than or equal to 5 mm without an identifiable acute inflammatory process or with mild (<5 mm) terminal ileal wall thickening.[153] Mesenteric nodes should not be considered responsible for the patient's symptoms, unless a primary intestinal inflammatory lesion is ruled out. An underlying infectious terminal ileitis is thought to be responsible for most cases of primary mesenteric adenitis.[153]

In secondary mesenteric adenitis, the enlarged mesenteric lymph nodes are related to an underlying condition. Enlarged right lower quadrant mesenteric lymph nodes can occur in association with a variety of conditions, including appendicitis, infectious enteritis or enterocolitis, diverticulitis, Crohn's disease (Fig. 60-26), celiac disease, and neoplasms.

Infectious Enterocolitis

Infectious enterocolitis, especially bacterial ileocecitis due to *Yersinia* species, *Campylobacter,* or *Salmonella,* can present as symptoms easily confused with those of acute appendicitis. Imaging studies reveal terminal ileal and cecal wall thickening in association with moderate right lower quadrant mesenteric adenopathy.[154]

Crohn's Disease

Crohn's disease is characterized by transmural granulomatous infiltration of the bowel that results in wall thickening

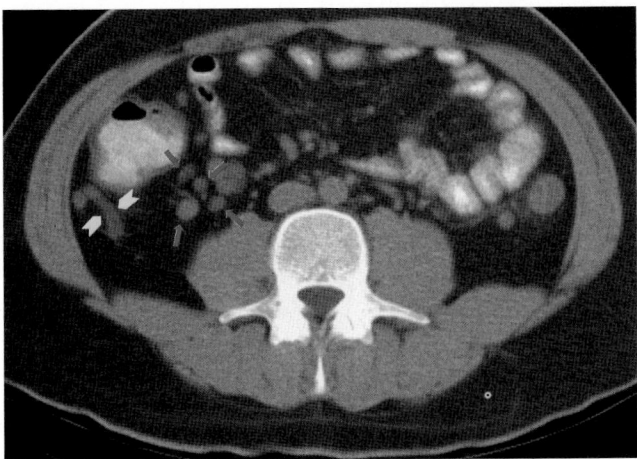

Figure 60-26. Mesenteric adenitis in a patient with Crohn's disease. Enhanced CT scan shows multiple, enlarged, right lower quadrant nodes (*arrows*) in this patient with Crohn's disease. The appendix was identified (*arrowheads*) and was normal.

secondary to edema, fibrosis, inflammation, and lymph-angiectasis.

CT is useful in the identification of inflamed segments of bowel in this disease, and the terminal ileum and right colon are most commonly affected (Fig. 60-27). The most frequent CT finding in Crohn's disease is homogeneously enhancing thickened bowel, although a mural stratification pattern may be present. The average degree of mural thickening has been noted to range from 11 to 30 mm.[155-158] The distribution of bowel involvement is commonly segmental, with interposed loops of normal bowel.

CT is also is useful for identifying the many potential complications of this disorder. These include the formation of bowel strictures, mesenteric pathology (including fibro-fatty proliferation, inflammation, abscesses, and adenopathy), fistula and sinus tract formation (Fig. 60-28), superimposed

neoplasm, renal and gallbladder calculi, hepatic and biliary disease (including hepatitis and pericholangitis), and sacroiliitis.

Epiploic Appendagitis

Primary epiploic appendagitis is the result of ischemia, torsion, or infarction of an epiploic appendage. This self-limiting condition results in focal abdominal pain that can simulate appendicitis when it occurs in the right lower quadrant. It is estimated to be the responsible cause in approximately 1% of patients who are suspected of having appendicitis.[159] On CT, the inflamed appendage is identified as a round or ovoid fat-density structure surrounded by a thickened, high-attenuation rim of thickened visceral peritoneum (Fig. 60-29). A central high-attenuation focus representing a thrombosed vessel or hemorrhage may also be present. Thickening of the adjacent colonic wall is commonly present along with inflammatory changes in the adjacent fat.

Omental Infarction

An omental infarction is a benign, self-limiting condition that is due to torsion or infarction of the greater omentum. Males are affected twice as often as females, and the infarction is usually right sided.[160] On CT, an omental infarction appears as an inflammatory mass containing variable amounts of fat and fluid (Fig. 60-30). Inflammatory change and small amounts of peritoneal fluid are commonly seen surrounding the omental infarction. The size of the infarct is typically larger than that of an inflamed epiploic appendage, and it is more heterogeneous in appearance and lacks a surrounding hyperattenuating rim. Sonographically, an omental infarction appears as a hyperechoic, noncompressible, ovoid mass adherent to the peritoneum.

Right-Sided and Ileal Diverticulitis

Right-sided diverticulitis is caused by inflammation of a colonic diverticulum in either the cecum or ascending colon. Unlike sigmoid diverticula, right-sided diverticula are usually true diverticula that contain all layers of the colonic wall.

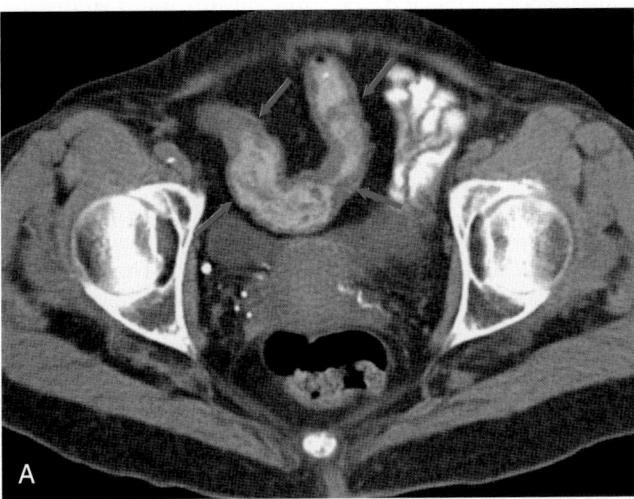

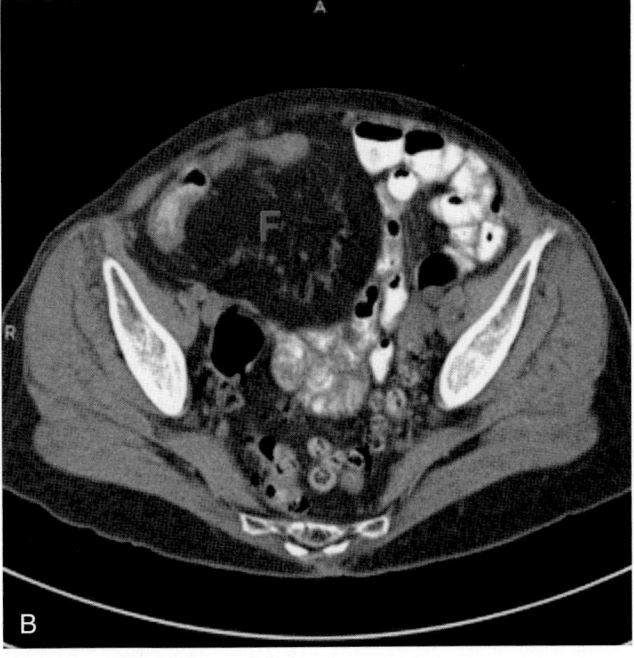

Figure 60-27. Crohn's disease. A. This enhanced CT scan shows circumferential mural thickening of the terminal ileum (*arrows*). **B.** A more cephalad image shows associated fibrofatty proliferation (F) of the mesentery.

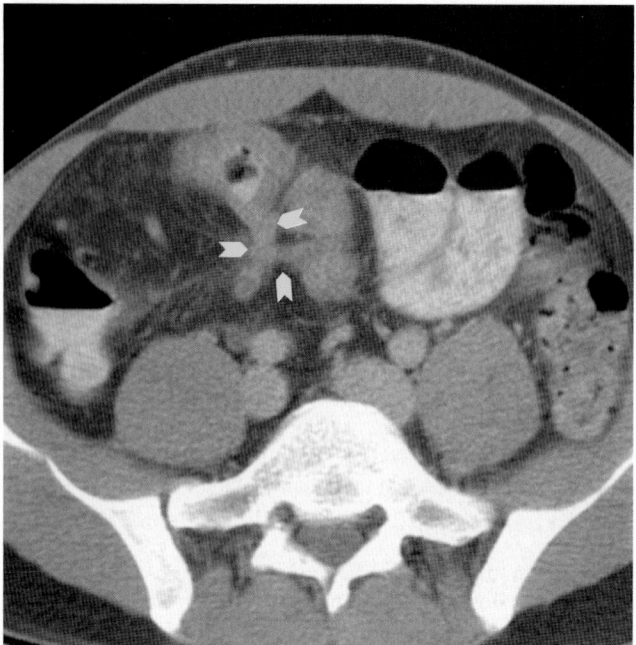

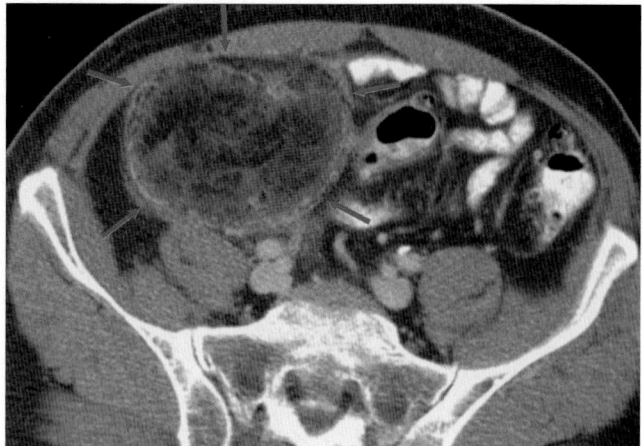

Figure 60-30. Right-sided omental infarct. A heterogeneous inflammatory mass (*arrows*) composed of fat and soft tissue elements is identified in the right lower quadrant and represents an omental infarct. The omental infarct is causing displacement of pelvic small bowel loops toward the left abdomen.

Figure 60-28. Crohn's disease with enteroenteric fistulas. This enhanced CT scan shows circumferential thickening of ileal loops with multiple linear soft tissue tracts extending between the loops representing interloop (enteroenteric) fistulas (*arrowheads*). Fibrofatty proliferation is also present in the mesentery.

Identification of an intramural abscess or cecal diverticulum in association with an inflammatory process located cephalad to a normal-appearing cecal caput and periappendiceal region should suggest the diagnosis. The characteristics findings on US and CT examination are identification of the inflamed diverticulum in association with focal, asymmetric colonic

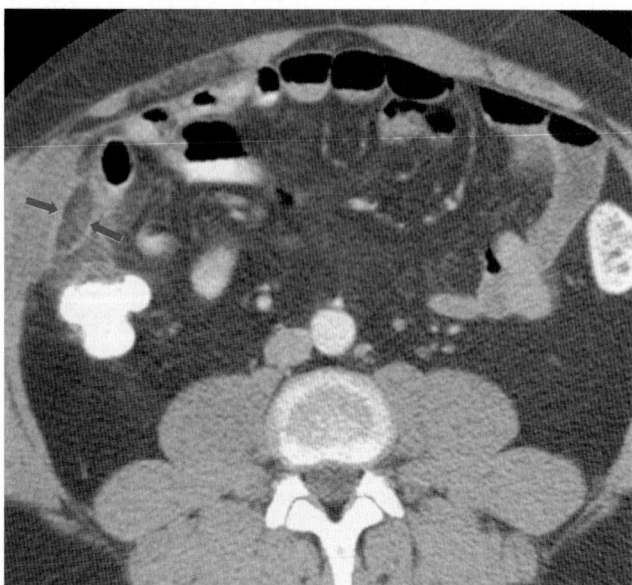

Figure 60-29. Right-sided epiploic appendagitis. On enhanced CT, the inflamed epiploic appendage (*arrows*) is identified as a homogeneous oval structure surrounded by a thickened high-attenuation rim of visceral peritoneum contiguous with the ascending colon.

wall thickening, and inflammation of the pericolonic fat (Fig. 60-31).

Ileal diverticulitis presents as a focal inflammatory mass or thickening of the terminal ileum with variable mesenteric inflammatory reaction surrounding an inflamed ileal diverticulum. Acquired ileal diverticula have been reported in 1% to 2% of small bowel series using spot compression radiography.[161]

Meckel's Diverticulum

Meckel's diverticulum is a true diverticulum arising from the distal ileum. It is the most common congenital anomaly of the small bowel, affecting approximately 2% of the population.[162]

On imaging, an inflamed Meckel diverticulum appears as a variable-sized blind-ending structure contiguous with the distal ileum (Fig. 60-32). Commonly, the diverticulum itself cannot be identified but the diagnosis can be entertained when inflammatory changes are seen adjacent to the distal ileum.

Neutropenic Colitis (Typhlitis)

This type of colitis occurs in profoundly neutropenic patients (especially patients with acute leukemia who are receiving chemotherapy) and results in necrotizing injury to the involved bowel. The inflammatory process may involve the cecum, ascending colon, ileum, or appendix. The CT findings are nonspecific and include concentric homogeneous or heterogeneous thickening of the bowel wall with associated intramural edema and necrosis, pericolic fluid, thickening of the pericolic fascia, and pneumatosis intestinalis (Fig. 60-33).[163] Prompt diagnosis is essential to prevent transmural necrosis and subsequent perforation.

Ischemia

Ischemia of the distal small bowel or the right colon may cause localized right lower quadrant pain. Most cases will be due to superior mesenteric artery thrombus or embolus or from low perfusion pressure.[162]

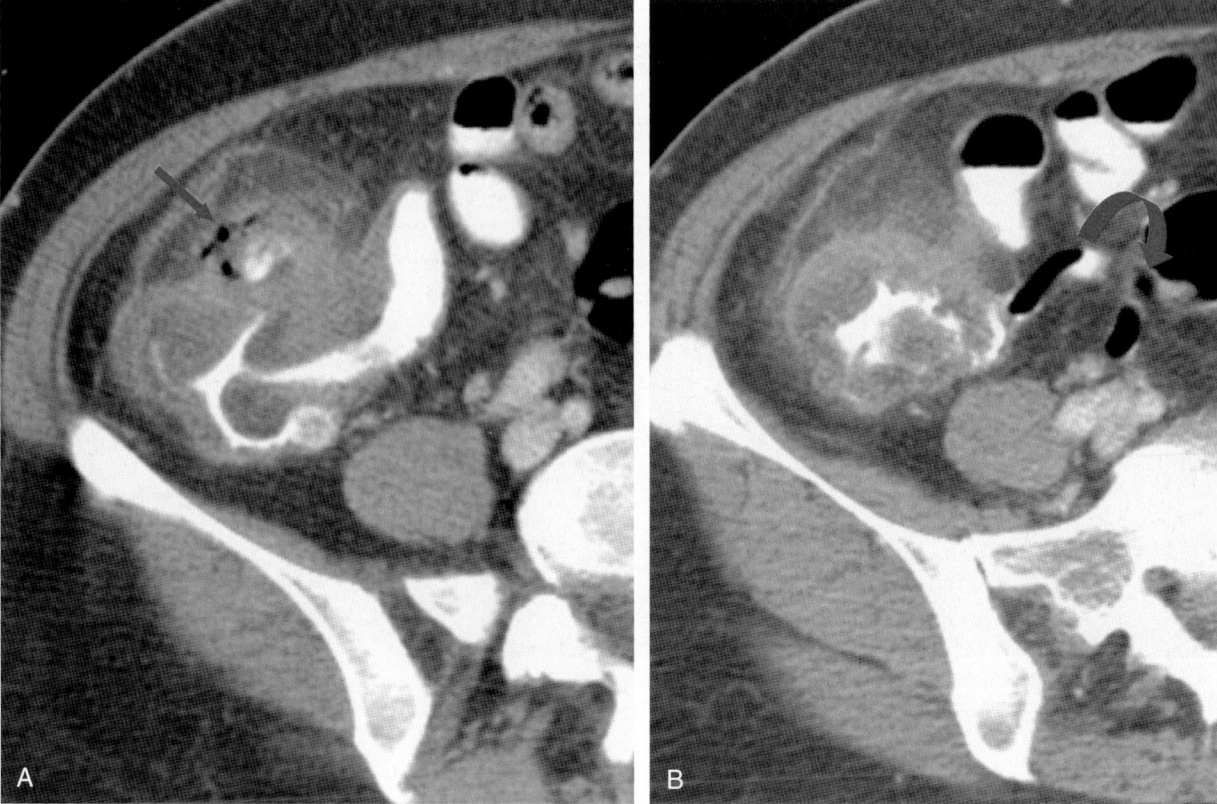

Figure 60-31. Right-sided diverticulitis. A. This enhanced CT scan shows the inflamed diverticulum (*arrow*) in the proximal ascending colon with surrounding inflammatory change and associated reactive lateral colonic wall thickening. **B.** This slightly more caudal image shows the normal appendix (*curved arrow*) medial to the inflamed right colon.

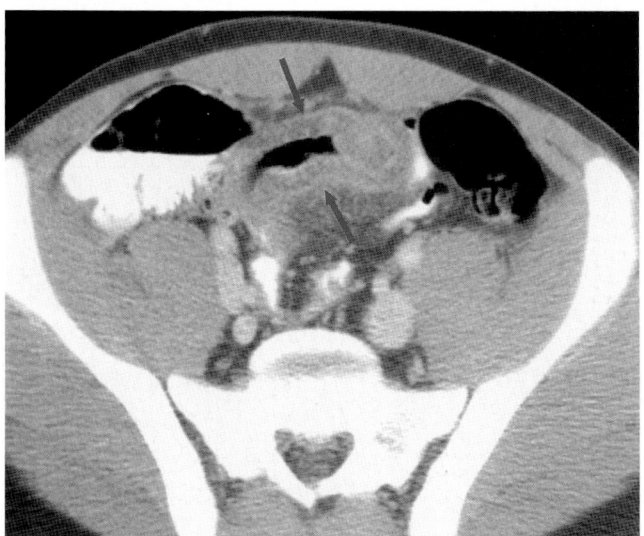

Figure 60-32. Inflamed Meckel's diverticulum. There is a thick-walled, blind-ending tubular structure adjacent to the terminal ileum (*arrows*) that represents the inflamed Meckel diverticulum. Inflammatory changes are also identified in the surrounding mesenteric fat.

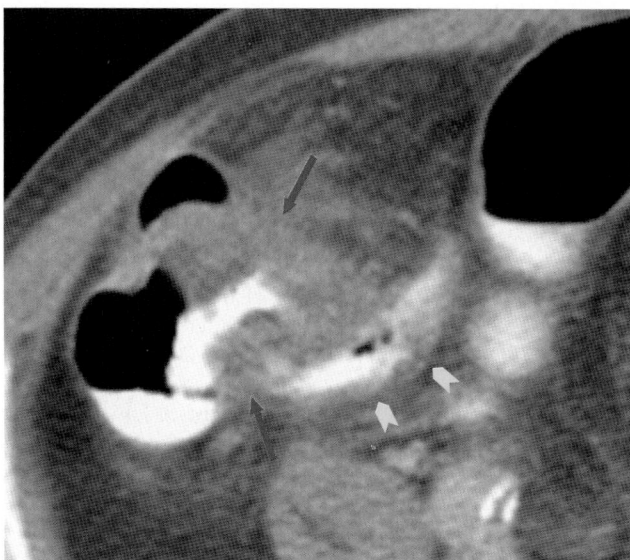

Figure 60-33. Neutropenic colitis (typhlitis) in a patient with acute myelogenous leukemia. There is circumferential mural thickening of the cecum (*arrows*) and terminal ileum (*arrowheads*) along with mild perienteric inflammatory change.

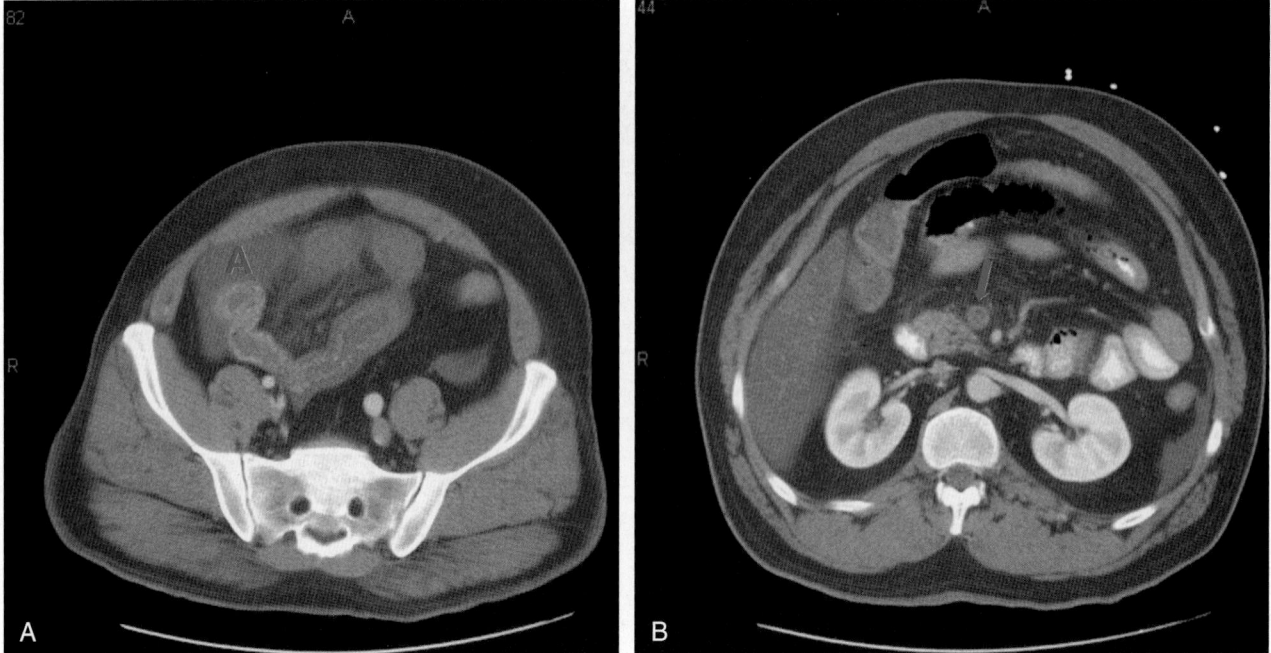

Figure 60-34. Small bowel ischemia due to thrombosis of the superior mesenteric vein. A. This enhanced CT scan shows circumferential thickening of ileal small bowel loops within the pelvis. Pelvic ascites (A) is also present. **B.** There is absent enhancement of the superior mesenteric vein (*arrow*) due to intraluminal thrombus.

On enhanced CT examination, the affected bowel will initially demonstrate circumferential bowel wall thickening (Fig. 60-34). A mural stratification pattern is often seen after IV contrast administration. With bowel infarction, pneumatosis intestinalis may develop and the bowel wall may demonstrate lack of enhancement with IV contrast administration.

Cecal Carcinoma

Cecal carcinoma usually presents as asymmetric nodular mural thickening (typically >1 cm) or a soft tissue attenuation mass (Fig. 60-35). Obstruction of the appendiceal orifice by the mass may lead to the development of appendicitis and appendiceal perforation.

CROHN'S DISEASE

Crohn's disease may involve any part of the gastrointestinal tract. Involvement of the appendix results in a granulomatous appendicitis that is usually managed conservatively. Pathologic studies have shown appendiceal involvement in 20% to 36% of patients with Crohn's disease (Fig. 60-36).[164] Histopathologically, the inflammatory appendiceal changes in Crohn's disease are similar to changes in other intestinal segments involved by this entity, namely, transmural inflammation with wall thickening, epithelioid granulomas, lymphoid aggregates, and mucosal ulcerations.[165] Although Crohn's disease frequently causes chronic abdominal symptoms, up to one third of patients with ileocecal Crohn's disease present with right lower quadrant symptoms mimicking appendicitis.[166]

Ripolles and colleagues evaluated 190 patients with Crohn's disease with gray-scale and color Doppler US and found that 20% had appendicular involvement.[164] They also found that appendiceal involvement of Crohn's disease was always

associated with segmental ileal and/or cecal thickening. There were no cases of isolated appendiceal involvement in their series. These authors found that in cases with isolated ileocecal region involvement, terminal ileal wall thickening of greater than 5 mm and color Doppler flow in the ileum were the most valuable US features differentiating Crohn's disease

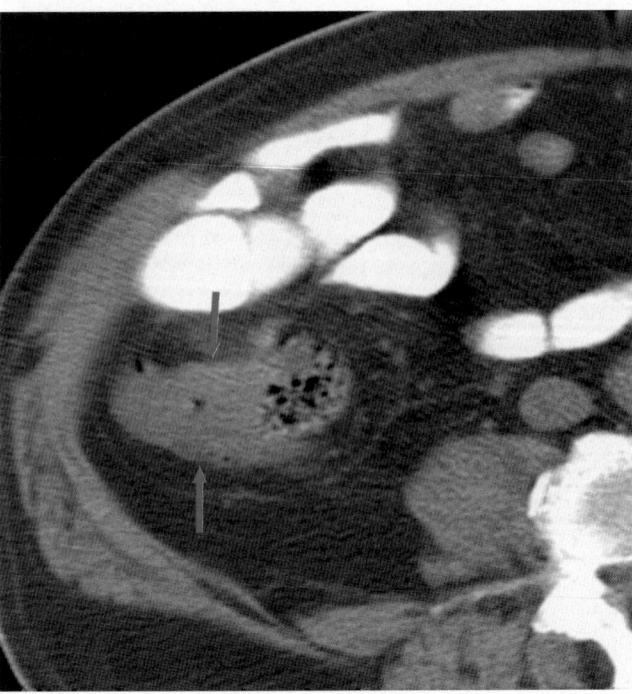

Figure 60-35. Cecal carcinoma. This lobulated, nodular cecal mass causing eccentric wall thickening greater than 1 cm (*arrows*) was pathologically proven to be a primary cecal adenocarcinoma.

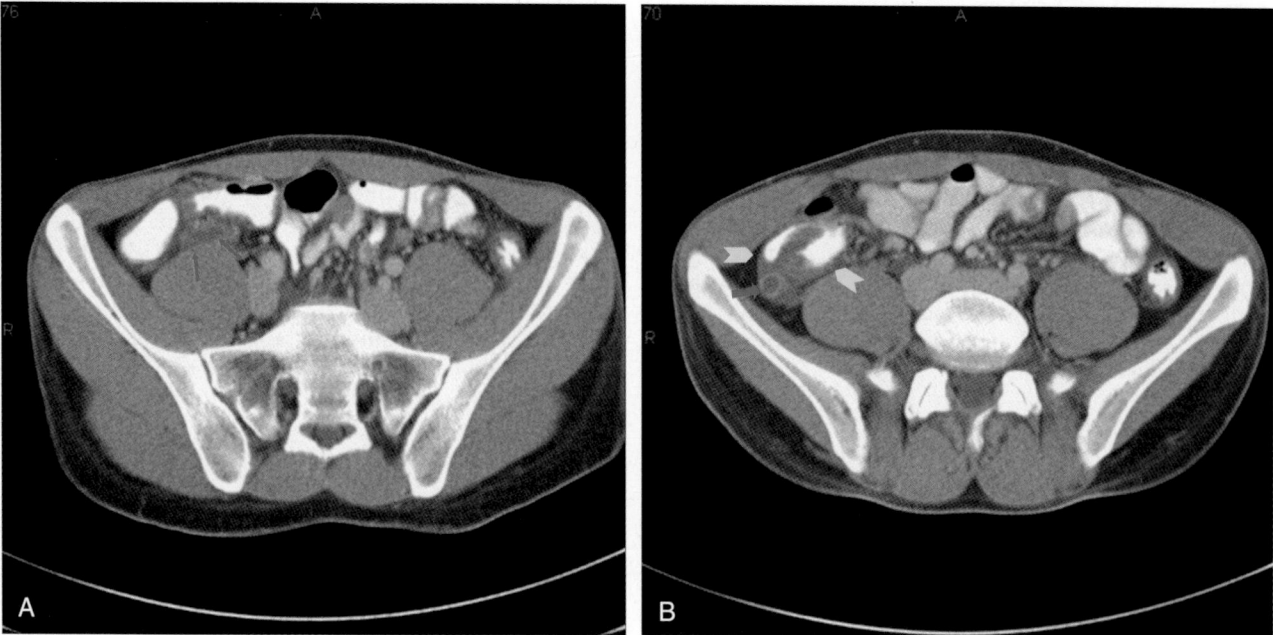

Figure 60-36. Crohn's disease with involvement of the appendix. A. There is circumferential wall thickening of the terminal ileum and cecum. Additionally, the appendix (*arrows*) is distended with abnormal thickening and enhancement of its wall. **B.** Cross-sectional view of the appendix (*arrow*) demonstrates the mural wall thickening and enhancement as well as the mild cecal wall thickening (*arrowheads*).

from acute appendicitis (positive and negative predictive values as high as 96% and 74%, respectively).[164] Additionally, these authors found that irregular thickening of the submucosal layer of the terminal ileum and fibrofatty proliferation of the mesentery around the inflamed terminal ileum were specific findings of Crohn's disease that were absent in acute appendicitis.[164]

Isolated appendiceal involvement, also known as idiopathic granulomatous appendicitis, is now believed by many to be a distinct entity from Crohn's disease with appendiceal involvement. Patients with this condition commonly present with symptoms mimicking acute appendicitis. Idiopathic granulomatous appendicitis is characterized pathologically by the presence of numerous granulomas and concentric mural fibrosis.[167] In fact, the histopathologic feature of numerous granulomas is what differentiates this entity from Crohn's disease, which characteristically has sparse granulomas.[167] Additionally, unlike patients who have involvement of the appendix from Crohn's disease, patients with idiopathic granulomatous appendicitis rarely have recurrence, fistulization, or extra-appendiceal gastrointestinal tract involvement after appendectomy.[167]

ULCERATIVE COLITIS

Ulcerative colitis is characterized by colonic mucosal inflammation and ulceration that typically proceeds in a continuous fashion from the rectum proximally. CT will show bowel wall thickening due to a combination of infiltration of the lamina propria by round cells, hypertrophy of the muscularis mucosa with resultant separation of the mucosa from the submucosa, and deposition of submucosal fat.[155] The mean bowel wall thickness in ulcerative colitis is approximately 8 mm.[156,158] In contradistinction to Crohn's disease, which classically shows homogeneous enhancement of the colonic

wall after IV contrast administration, approximately 70% of patient with ulcerative colitis demonstrate inhomogeneous mural enhancement after IV contrast administration (Fig. 60-37).[155,156]

Appendiceal involvement is seen in 61% to 87% of patients with pancolitis from ulcerative colitis.[165] The appendiceal involvement may be contiguous with cecal ulcerative colitis or may occur as a skip lesion adjacent to a normal cecum. This latter type has been referred to as "ulcerative appendicitis." Appendiceal involvement was found to occur as a skip lesion without associated cecal involvement in 34% to 86% of colons removed for chronic ulcerative colitis.[168]

On CT examination, the typical feature of ulcerative appendicitis is edema and thickening of the appendiceal wall. Appendectomy is thought to be a protective factor in ulcerative appendicitis.[168]

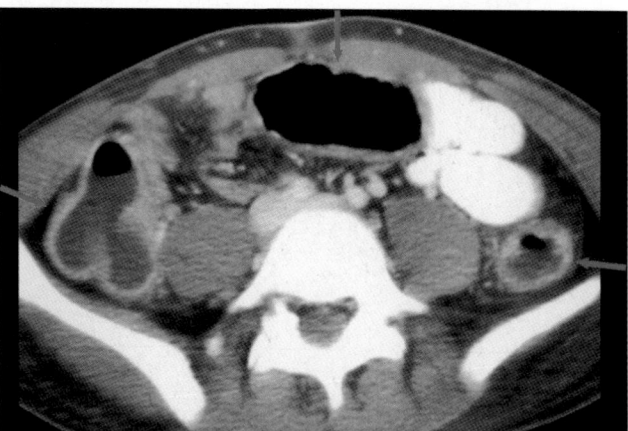

Figure 60-37. Ulcerative colitis. Enhanced CT scan shows a pancolitis with heterogeneous circumferential wall thickening of the cecum, transverse colon, and descending colon (*arrows*).

ENDOMETRIOSIS

Gastrointestinal involvement is seen in 5% to 37% of patients with endometriosis. The most commonly involved segments in order of decreasing frequency are the rectum and sigmoid colon, the small bowel, the cecum, and the appendix.

The majority of patients with endometriosis of the appendix will remain asymptomatic. Symptomatic patients usually experience chronic pain; however, some patients may experience acute right lower quadrant pain that is clinically indistinguishable from acute appendicitis.

On CT, a noninflamed, nondistended, and nonopacified appendix is frequently seen.[165]

APPENDICEAL DIVERTICULITIS

Appendiceal diverticula are found in 0.004% to 2.8% of surgical and pathologic specimens.[165] Most are acquired because of either intrinsic mural weakness or abnormally raised intraluminal pressure secondary to increased muscular activity or closed loop obstruction.[169-171] The diverticula may be solitary or multiple and are found anywhere along the appendix. Typically, they are 0.2 to 0.5 mm.[165]

The presence of appendiceal diverticula may predispose to hemorrhage and diverticulitis. On CT, inflammation of the diverticulum and/or appendix is seen. Clinically, patients can present with symptoms similar to acute appendicitis. The pain is often intermittent and insidious and typically occurs 1 to 14 days before presentation. Because the risk of appendiceal perforation in appendiceal diverticulitis is fourfold greater than that for simple appendicitis, prompt surgical resection is advised.[165] Accordingly, some surgeons recommend prophylactic appendectomy when diverticula are discovered during laparotomy for other disorders.[169,171,172]

APPENDICEAL INTUSSUSCEPTION

Intussusception of the appendix can present clinically in five different ways[173-176]: (1) acute appendicitis, (2) intussusception, (3) recurrent intermittent right lower quadrant pain, (4) intermittent painless rectal bleeding, and (5) asymptomatically, with incidental findings at laparotomy, barium enema, or colonoscopy. In the past, appendiceal intussusception was considered rare, being found in only 0.01% of surgical cases. However, the fifth presentation is probably the most common.

Most cases of significant appendiceal intussusception occur in children and are attributed to abnormal peristalsis caused by intraluminal or intramural irritants of the appendix. These include fecaliths, foreign bodies, endometriosis, lymphoid hyperplasia, carcinoid, adenocarcinoma, and mucoceles.[173-176]

On double-contrast barium enema examination, intussusception causes a characteristic "coil spring" appearance of the cecum with nonfilling of the appendix. These findings are best seen en face. In incidental cases, the intussusception usually disappears on delayed overhead or postevacuation films. The coil spring appearance can also be seen in appendicitis, but it is fixed in these cases and the patient is symptomatic in the right lower quadrant. There may be only partial intussusception of the appendix that produces an intraluminal filling defect on the medial wall of the cecum and nonfilling of the appendix. The defect may be mistaken for a polyp (Fig. 60-38).[173-176]

On US, the intussusception appears as multiple hypoechoic and hyperechoic rings, similar to intussusceptions elsewhere in the gut.[174,175]

Hydrostatic reduction of appendiceal intussusceptions has been successful in children and adults. Asymptomatic

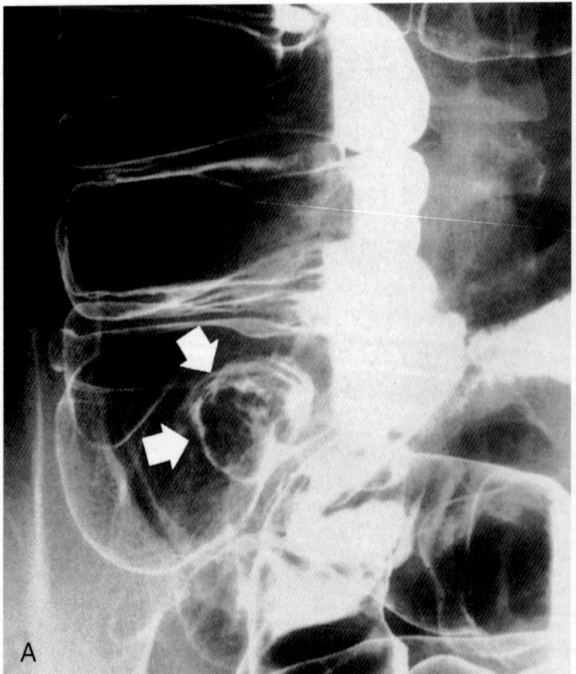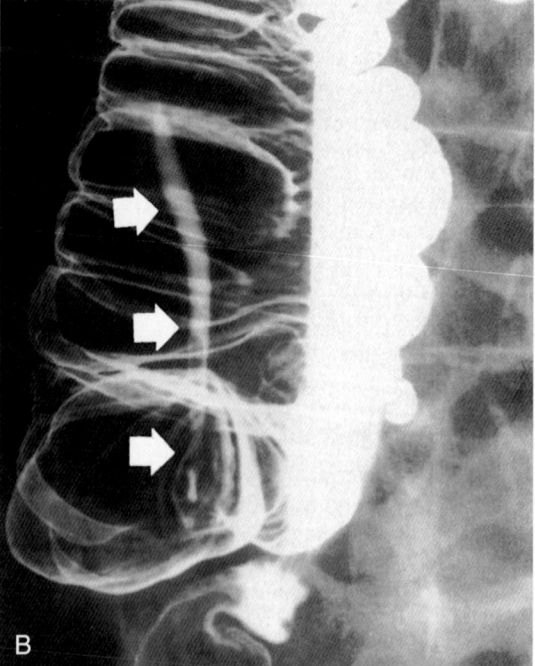

Figure 60-38. Appendiceal intussusception. A. Initial barium enema examination reveals a filling defect in the lower cecum that was interpreted as a polypoid mass (*arrows*). Colonoscopy performed several days later revealed no abnormalities. **B.** Subsequent barium enema examination shows a normal retrocecal appendix (*arrows*).

transient intussusceptions probably do not require therapy or an extensive work-up, however.[173-176]

APPENDICEAL NEOPLASMS

Primary neoplasms of the appendix are identified in 0.5% to 1% of appendectomy specimens at pathologic evaluation.[177-179] The vast majority of these will occur in adults older than the age of 30 years. Thirty to 50 percent of patients with appendiceal tumors will present with symptoms of appendicitis, and the majority of these will have obstruction of the appendiceal lumen by the tumor.[178,180] Similarly, cecal carcinomas can obstruct the appendiceal lumen, resulting in secondary appendicitis. In fact, a study by Peck showed that 11% of right-sided colon cancers clinically presented as appendicitis, the majority of which were due to appendiceal inflammation from obstruction.[181]

Preoperative identification of the presence of an appendiceal or cecal neoplasm is important because it may subsequently change both the surgical approach (laparoscopic vs. an open procedure) and the procedure performed (appendectomy vs. right hemicolectomy). CT has proven to be very useful in this regard. In a retrospective review of 22 CT scans in patients with pathologically proven primary appendiceal neoplasms, Pickhardt and colleagues found that the sensitivity of CT for tumor detection was 95% when morphologic appendiceal changes or a threshold appendiceal diameter of 15 mm was used as a diagnostic criterion.[180] In 95% of these patients, soft tissue stranding of the periappendiceal fat was also present.[180]

Mucocele

Epidemiology, Etiology, and Pathology

Mucocele of the appendix is a descriptive term used to indicate dilatation of the appendiceal lumen by mucinous secretions. The accumulation of mucin is slow, and, if infection does not intervene, the appendix becomes a large, thin-walled, mucin-filled cystic structure.[182-204] Mucoceles are uncommon; they are found in 0.3% of appendectomy specimens, with a 4:1 preponderance in females and a mean age of 55 years at presentation.[185]

Histologically, mucoceles are classified into three groups: focal or diffuse hyperplasia, mucinous cystadenoma, and mucinous cystadenocarcinoma. A number of obstructing lesions can lead to mucocele formation: postappendicitis scarring (most common), fecalith, appendiceal carcinoma, appendiceal endometrioma, appendiceal carcinoid, carcinoma of the cecum or ascending colon, appendiceal polyp, and appendiceal volvulus. It is unclear whether the cystadenoma or cystadenocarcinoma causes obstruction of the lumen as well or whether the mucosa of the obstructed appendix undergoes neoplastic change. Benign causes of obstruction outnumber malignant causes by a ratio of 4:1 to 10:1.[186-191]

Most mucoceles are between 3 and 6 cm in diameter. Calcifications may occur in the wall or lumen of the mucocele.[192-200] Myxoglobulosis is a rare variant in which numerous small globules form in the appendix. They may calcify and produce numerous 1- to 10-mm round or oval mobile calcifications in the right lower quadrant. In myxoglobulosis, the appendiceal lumen has the consistency of tapioca or fish eggs.

Clinical Findings

The dominant complaint is chronic right lower quadrant pain in up to 64% of patients with mucoceles. Nearly 23% of patients are asymptomatic. Abdominal swelling, anemia, or a mucous fistula may also be present. Physical examination discloses right lower quadrant tenderness in 38% and a palpable mass in 18% to 50% of patients.[185-192]

The major clinical significance of a mucocele lies in its complications: rupture or leakage leading to pseudomyxoma peritonei; torsion with gangrene and hemorrhage; and intussusception into the cecum, causing various degrees of bowel obstruction. If pseudomyxoma peritonei results from rupture of a benign mucocele, only removal of the fluid is needed, and the prognosis is good. When it is malignant, it behaves like an invasive neoplasm with adhesions and bowel obstruction and a 5-year survival rate of only 25%. Because cystadenoma and cystadenocarcinoma are usually indistinguishable radiologically, clinically, and on gross inspection, the surgeon must be warned of the presence of a mucocele preoperatively.[196,197]

Radiologic Findings

Plain Radiographs

The plain abdominal radiograph may be normal or may show a well-defined right lower quadrant mass. Rimlike calcifications help establish the diagnosis but are uncommon. In myxoglobulosis, mobile calcifications may be present that must be differentiated from phleboliths, calcified mesenteric lymph nodes, and calcified metastases to the medial wall of the cecum.[77-79,187-189]

Barium Enema

The appendix fails to fill on barium enema examination, and the cecum is indented on its medial aspect by a smooth-walled mass. The cecum is distensible but inseparable from the mass (Fig. 60-39). The terminal ileum is often displaced as well.[77-79,187-193,205]

Cross-Sectional Imaging

On US, mucoceles manifest as fluid-filled masses that may be completely anechoic or may have septations and gravity-dependent echoes. These latter findings probably result from inspissated mucoid material that develops as the mucocele ages and matures. Increased through-transmission is characteristic.[190,191]

On CT, mucoceles appear as water-density or, less often, soft tissue–density masses (Fig. 60-40). Calcification may be seen within the wall or lumen (Fig. 60-41).

On MRI, when mucoceles contain predominantly fluid, they have long T1 and T2 relaxation times and low signal intensity on T1-weighted images and high signal intensity on T2-weighted images (Fig. 60-42). If their mucin content is high, mucoceles have a short T1 time and long T2 time, so they appear intense on both T1- and T2-weighted images.

When pseudomyxoma peritonei develops, malignant-appearing ascites with loculated fluid collections, septations, small calcifications, and a scalloped contour of the liver and spleen are visualized (Fig. 60-43).[195,199,201,202] Mucin-producing adenoma, cystadenoma, or mucinous cystadenoma presents as an encapsulated low-attenuation cyst and cannot be differentiated from a retention mucocele.[203]

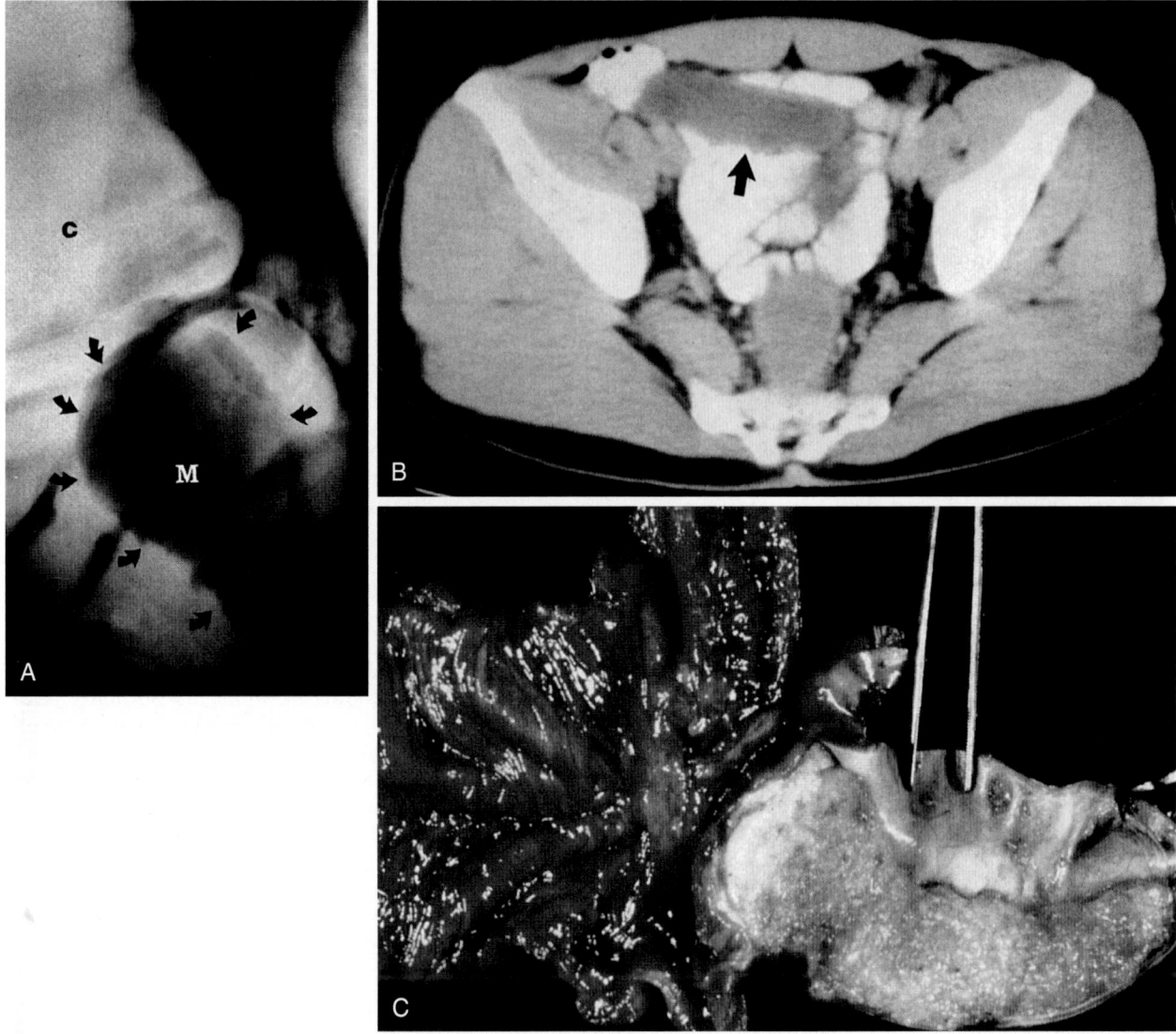

Figure 60-39. Mucocele of the appendix. A. Barium enema study shows a sharply contoured large intraluminal cecal defect (M). Note that the intussuscepting mucocele arises from the tip of the cecum (c) and the appendix is not filled (*arrows*). **B.** CT scan shows the pericecal extension of the mucus-filled, distended appendix (*arrow*). Note that there is no periappendiceal inflammation. **C.** Gross specimen reveals a markedly distended, mucus-filled appendix compressing the base of the cecum. Pathologic study showed benign mucocele.

Differential Diagnosis

The differential diagnosis for these imaging findings includes ovarian cysts and neoplasms, duplication cyst, mesenteric and omental cysts, mesenteric hematoma or tumor, and abdominal abscess.

Mucinous Cystadenoma/Cystadenocarcinoma

The detection of a heterogeneously attenuated mass with nodular areas of soft tissue density or of a cystic mass with associated soft tissue components (Fig. 60-44) is strongly suggestive of a mucinous cystadenocarcinoma of the appendix.[202,204] Perforation is present in approximately 46% of patients with mucinous cystadenocarcinoma at the time of appendectomy.[206] Patients with mucinous cystadenocarcinomas associated with pseudomyxoma peritonei have a poor 5-year survival rate of 50%.[165]

Nonmucinous Adenocarcinoma

Primary appendiceal adenocarcinoma is an uncommon tumor with an incidence of approximately 0.08%.[207] Adenocarcinoma of the appendix presents as a soft tissue mass similar to the more common colonic carcinoma, and it metastasizes both hematogenously and lymphatically.

On CT examination, these tumors usually appear as a focal or diffuse soft tissue mass with appendiceal distention (diameter typically more than 15 mm), wall thickening, and associated soft tissue stranding of the periappendiceal fat (Figs. 60-45 and 60-46). When small, carcinoma of the appendix cannot be differentiated from complicated appendicitis.

Surgical treatment depends on the size and stage of the tumor. Whereas small lesions without lymph node involvement can usually be treated with appendectomy, more advanced appendiceal carcinoma typically necessitates right hemicolectomy.

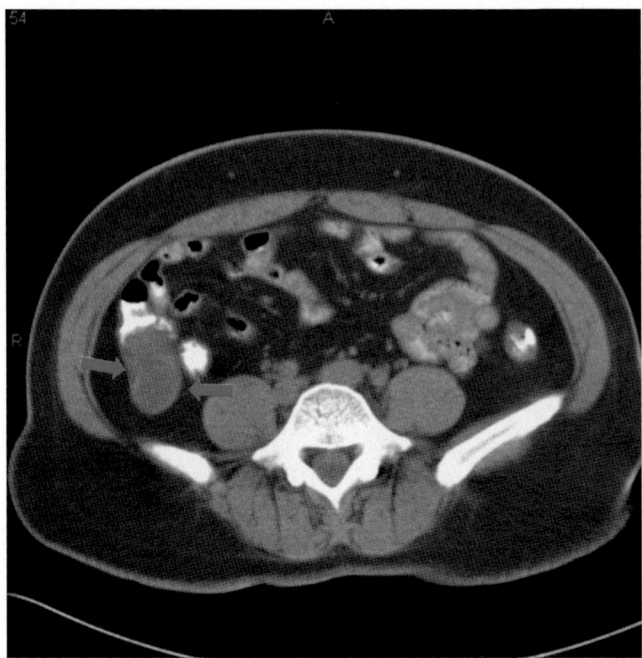

Figure 60-40. Mucocele of the appendix. This ovoid-shaped fluid-filled mass (*arrows*) represents an appendiceal mucocele that is causing a mass effect on the adjacent cecum.

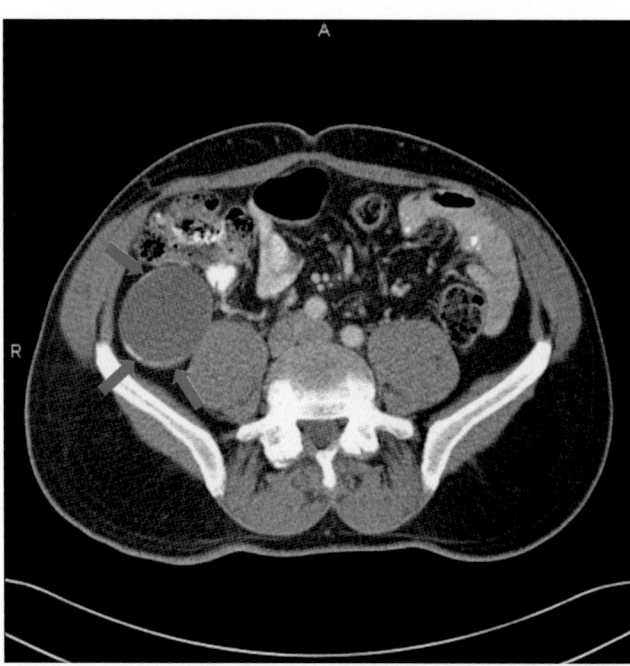

Figure 60-41. Mucocele of the appendix. This ovoid-shaped, fluid-filled appendiceal mucocele contains mural calcifications (*arrows*).

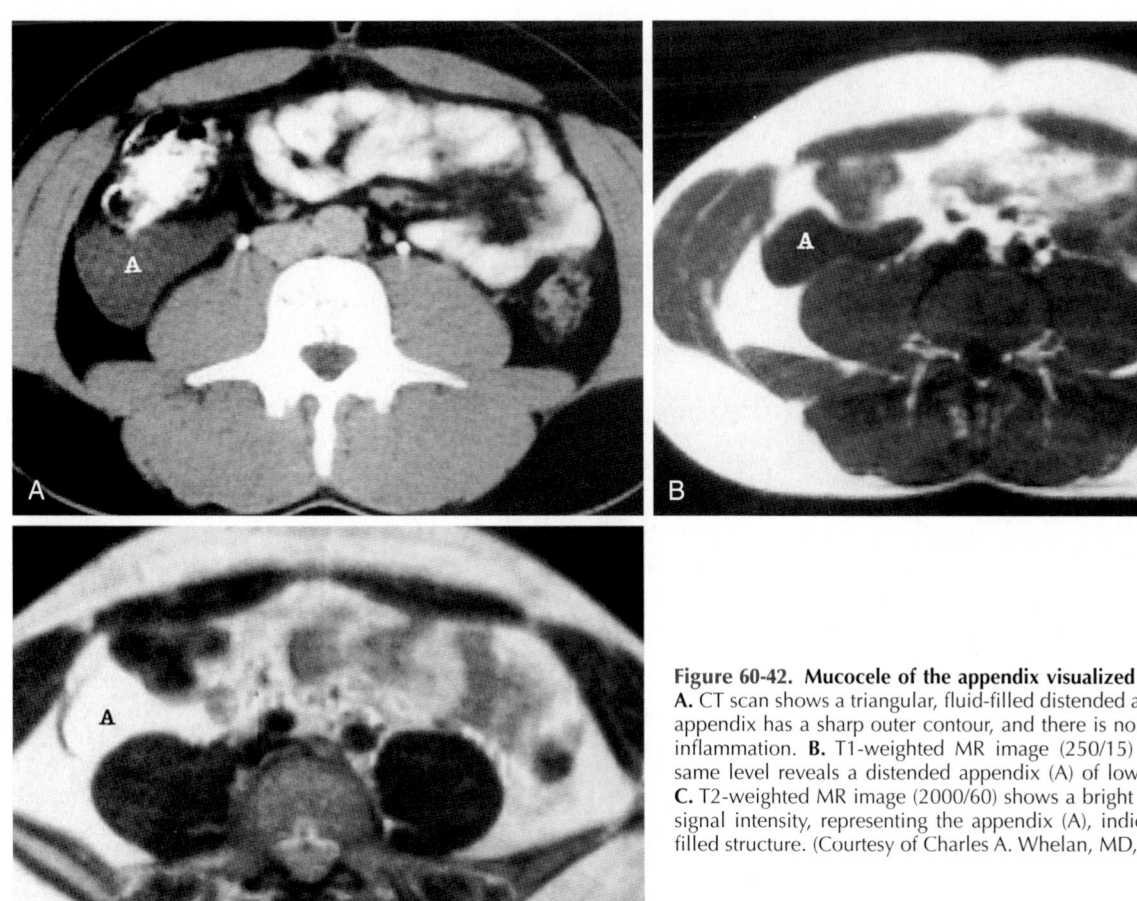

Figure 60-42. Mucocele of the appendix visualized by CT and MRI. **A.** CT scan shows a triangular, fluid-filled distended appendix (A). The appendix has a sharp outer contour, and there is no periappendiceal inflammation. **B.** T1-weighted MR image (250/15) obtained at the same level reveals a distended appendix (A) of low signal intensity. **C.** T2-weighted MR image (2000/60) shows a bright structure of high signal intensity, representing the appendix (A), indicative of a fluid-filled structure. (Courtesy of Charles A. Whelan, MD, Montclair, NJ.)

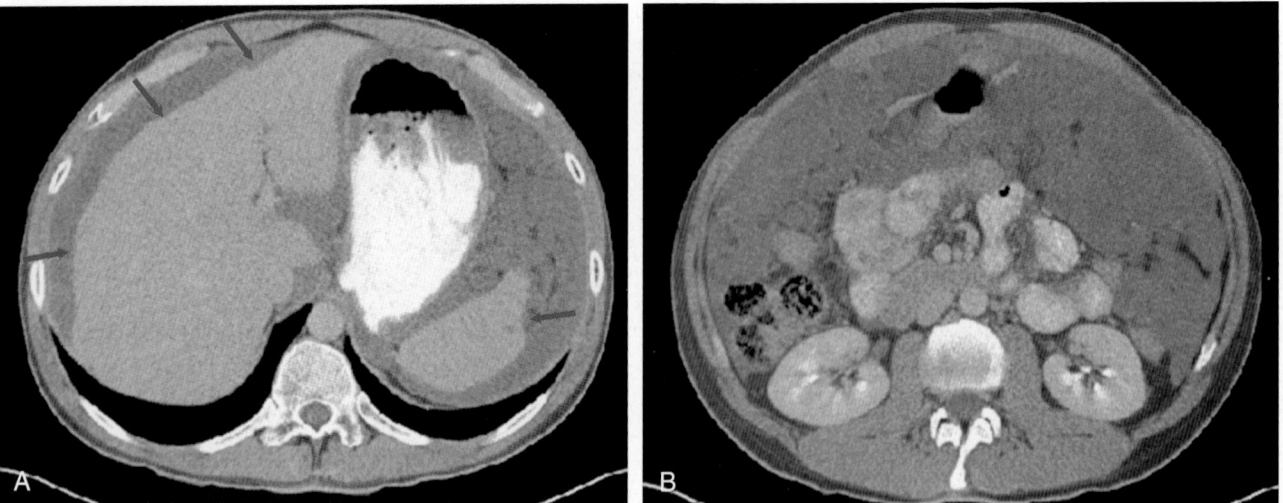

Figure 60-43. Pseudomyxoma peritonei. A. Upper abdomen reveals ascites with a scalloped contour to the liver and spleen (*arrows*). **B.** Midabdomen reveals massive ascites with heterogeneous attenuated fluid and septations causing mass effect on adjacent bowel loops.

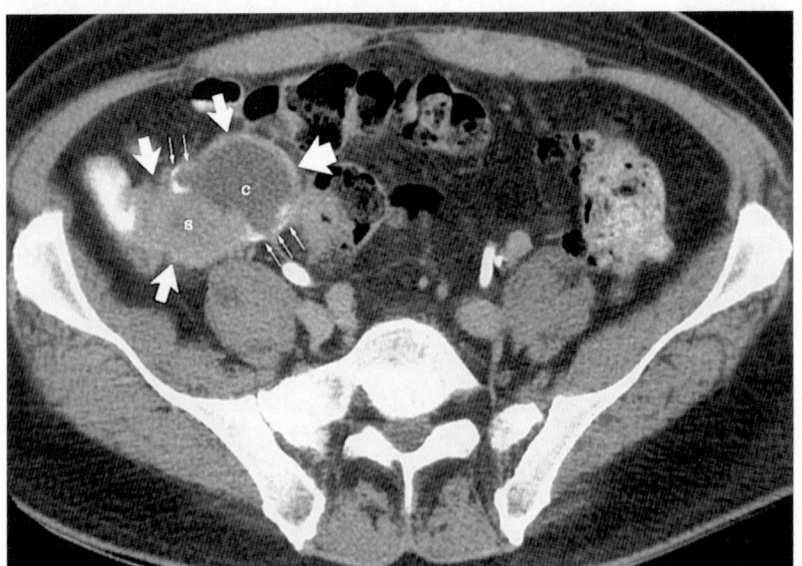

Figure 60-44. Mucinous cystadenocarcinoma of the appendix. CT detects a mass having solid (s) and cystic (c) components in the right pelvis inferior and medial to the cecum (*large arrows*). Peripheral calcifications are seen in the cystic component (*small arrows*).

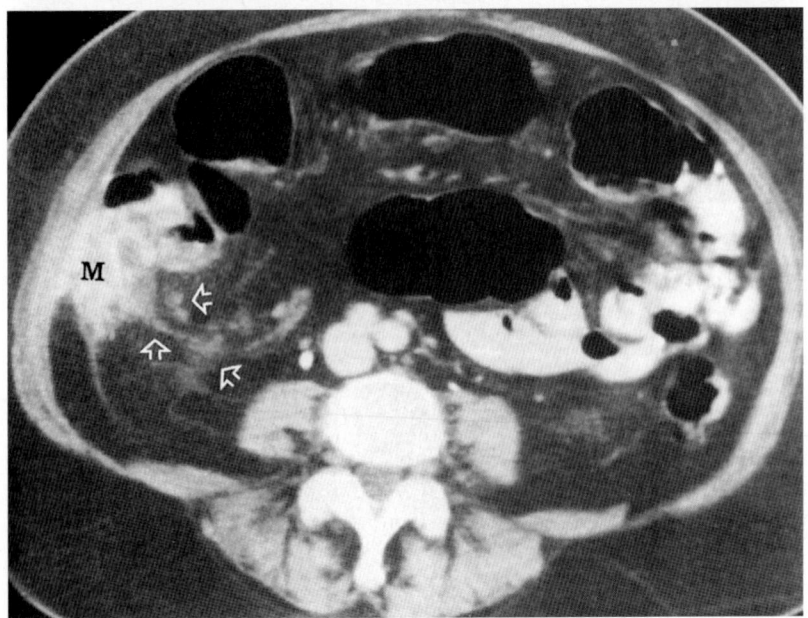

Figure 60-45. CT scan of perforated carcinoma of the appendix. A lobulated, heterogeneous complex mass (M) is seen posterior and caudal to the cecum. The mass has an irregular contour, and periappendiceal inflammatory changes are present (*arrows*).

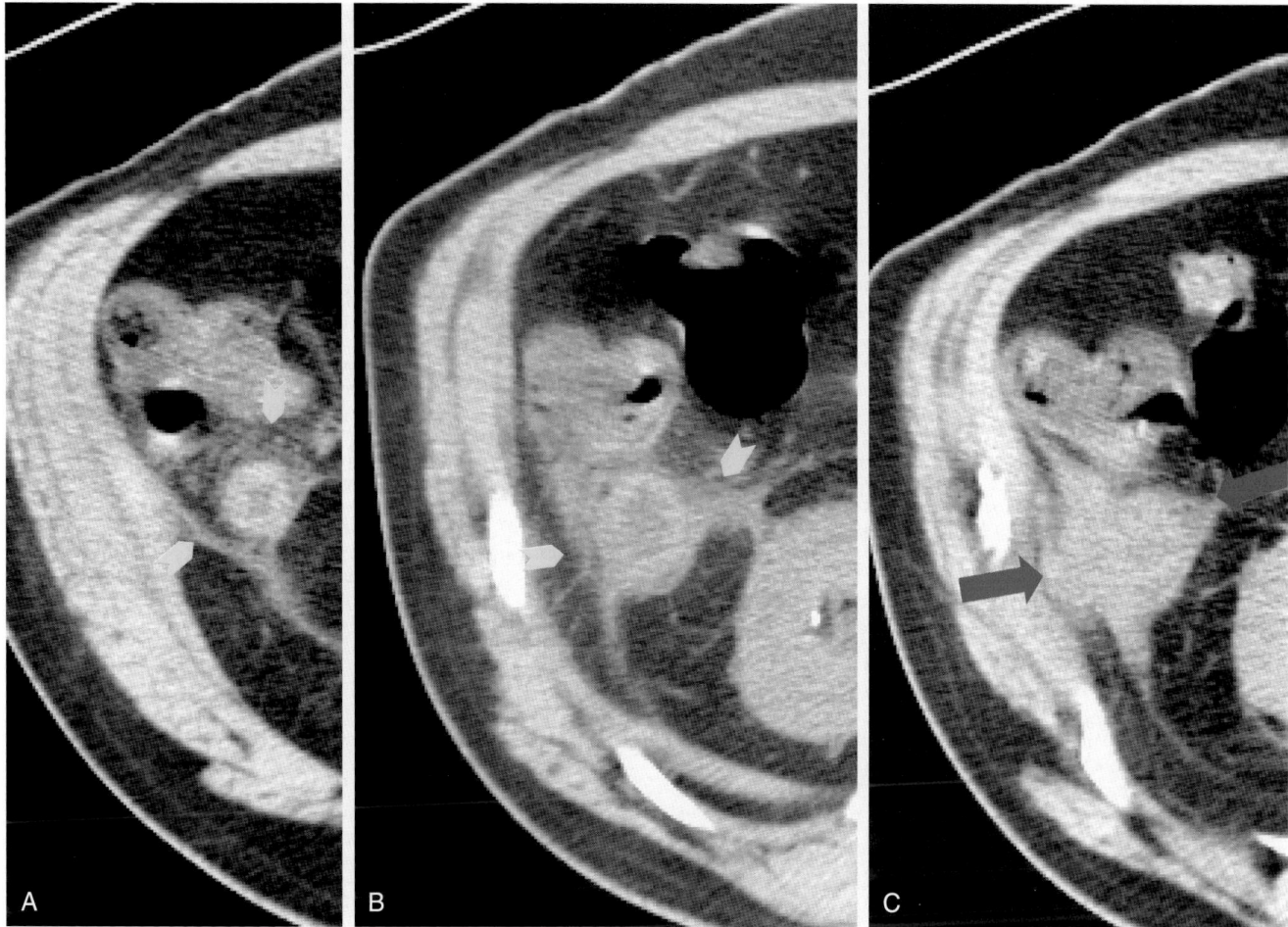

Figure 60-46. CT scan of carcinoma of the distal appendix. A-C. Series axial CT scans of the right, mid, and lower abdomen show that a lobulated soft tissue mass (*arrows*) is present in the distal aspect of the appendix with mural thickening identified in the more proximal appendix. Periappendiceal inflammatory changes are also identified (*arrowheads*).

Carcinoid

Carcinoid tumor is the most common neoplasm of the appendix, with an incidence of 0.32% in appendectomy specimens and 0.054% in an autopsy series.[165,208] Appendiceal carcinoid tumors comprise 18.9% of all gastrointestinal carcinoid tumors, but they are less biologically aggressive than other gastrointestinal carcinoid tumors.[209] Most are less than 2 cm at presentation, and most patients are asymptomatic. Typically, these lesions are incidentally found at surgery. Appendiceal carcinoids have a lower average age at presentation (average, 42.2 years) than other gastrointestinal carcinoid tumors (average, 62.9 years) or noncarcinoid appendiceal tumors (average, 61.9 years), have a tendency to present with coexistent tumors, have little metastatic potential, and have a female predominance (M:F = 0.47).[210,211] The 5-year survival for appendiceal carcinoids (85.9%) is higher than for other gastrointestinal carcinoid tumors (54%).[211]

The majority (approximately 70%) of appendiceal carcinoid tumors are located in the appendiceal tip, followed by the body (approximately 22%) and the base (approximately 7%).[165] The typical CT appearance is a homogeneous soft tissue mass that may infiltrate into the cecum and mesentery.[212]

Treatment of appendiceal carcinoid depends on its size. Tumors less than 2 cm are usually treated with appendec-

tomy. Tumors larger than 2 cm or with evidence for invasion into the mesoappendix necessitate right hemicolectomy and unfortunately have a poorer prognosis.[165]

Lymphoma

Primary appendiceal lymphoma is a very rare lesion with an incidence of 1% to 3%.[213,214] All reported cases have been non-Hodgkin's type.[215] Patients typically present with clinical signs mimicking acute appendicitis and with no prior history of lymphoma. At the time of diagnosis, most tumors are larger than 3 cm.[215]

On CT, there is usually marked mural thickening of the appendix, which maintains its vermiform shape. Aneurysmal luminal dilatation may be present, and periappendiceal stranding may also be identified owing to either secondary appendicitis from luminal obstruction or direct serosal extension of lymphomatous cells.[215]

METASTASES

Primary neoplasms that can metastasize to the appendix include those of the breast, lung, bronchus, stomach, colon, pancreas, kidney, ovaries, or prostate.[165] Alternatively, the appendix can be involved by direct extension from tumors of the cecum or ileum.[165]

Metastatic tumors of the appendix usually involve the serosal or submucosal layers, and on CT they usually appear as a solitary soft tissue mass contiguous with the appendix.[165] These lesions can obstruct the appendiceal lumen, leading to secondary appendicitis and its complications, including perforation.

References

1. Noudeh YJ, Sadigh N, Ahmadnia AY: Epidemiologic features of acute appendicitis. Int J Surg 5:95-98, 2007.
2. Goldman LD: Acute appendicitis. In Taylor MB (ed): Gastrointestinal Emergencies, 6th ed. Baltimore, Williams & Wilkins, 1997, pp 577-592.
3. Telford GL, Condon RE: Appendix. In Zuidema GD (ed): Shackelford's Surgery of the Alimentary Tract, 4th ed. Philadelphia, WB Saunders, 1996, pp 140-149.
4. Wilcox RT, Traverso LW: Have the evaluation and treatment of acute appendicitis changed with new technology? Surg Clin North Am 77:1355-1370, 1997.
5. Stoker ME, Becker JM: Appendicitis. In Brandt LJ (ed): Clinical Practice of Gastroenterology. New York, Churchill Livingstone, 1999, pp 773-778.
6. Anson B, McVay CB: Surgical Anatomy, 5th ed. Philadelphia, WB Saunders, 1971.
7. Arey LB: Developmental Anatomy: A Textbook of Laboratory Manual of Embryology, 7th ed. Philadelphia, WB Saunders, 1974.
8. Voight AE: Embryology and anatomy of the appendix. Southwest Med 34:285-287, 1953.
9. Balthazar EJ, Gade M: The normal and abnormal development of the appendix. Radiology 121:599-604, 1976.
10. Schumpelick V, Dreuw B, Ophoff K, et al: Surgical anatomy and embryology. Surg Clin North Am 80:295-318, 2000.
11. Broman I: Entwicklung der Verdauungsorgene. In Broman I (ed): Die Entwicklung des Menschen vor der Geburt. Munich, JF Bergmann, 1927.
12. Wakeley CPG: The position of the vermiform appendix as ascertained by analysis of 10,000 cases. J Anat 67:277-283, 1933.
13. Maisel H: The position of the human vermiform appendix in fetal and adult age groups. Anat Rec 136:385-391, 1960.
14. Meyers MA: Dynamic Radiology of the Abdomen, 4th ed. New York, Springer-Verlag, 1994.
15. Collins DC: Agenesis of the vermiform appendix. Am J Surg 82:689-696, 1951.
16. Lippert H, Pabst R: Arterial variations in man. Munich, JF Bergmann, 1995.
17. Kryiazis AA, Esterly JR: Development of lymphoid tissues in the human embryo and early fetus. Arch Pathol 90:348, 1970.
18. Fitz RH: Perforating inflammation of the vermiform appendix; with special reference to its early diagnosis and treatment. Am J Med Sci 92:321-346, 1886.
19. Birnbaum BA, Wilson SR: Appendicitis at the millennium. Radiology 215:337-348, 2000.
20. Owings MF, Kozak LJ: Ambulatory and inpatient procedures in the United States, 1996. Vital and health statistics. Series 13. No. 139. DHHS publication No. (PHS) 991710. Hyattsville, MD, National Center for Health Statistics, November 1998, p 26.
21. Berry J Jr, Malt RA: Appendicitis near its centenary. Ann Surg 200:567-575, 1984.
22. Flum DR, Koepsell T. The clinical and economic correlates of misdiagnosed appendicitis. Arch Surg 137:799-804, 2002.
23. Rothrock SG, Pagane J: Acute appendicitis in children: Emergency department diagnosis and management. Ann Emerg Med 6:39-51, 2000.
24. Shelton T, McKinlay R, Schwartz RW: Acute appendicitis: Current diagnosis and treatment. Curr Surg 60:502-505, 2003.
25. Addiss DG, Shaffer N, Fowler BS, et al: The epidemiology of appendicitis and appendectomy in the United States. Am J Epidemiol 132:910-925, 1990.
26. Velanovich V, Satava R: Balancing the normal appendectomy rate with the perforated appendicitis rate: Implications for quality of assurance. Am Surg 58:264-269, 1992.
27. Law D, Law R, Eiseman B: The continuing challenge of acute and perforated appendicitis. Am J Surg 131:533-535, 1976.
28. Lewis FR, Holcroft JH, Boey J, et al: Appendicitis: A critical review of diagnosis and treatment in 1,000 cases. Arch Surg 110:677-684, 1975.
29. Dueholm S, Bagi P, Bud M: Laboratory aid in the diagnosis of acute appendicitis. Dis Colon Rectum 32:855-859, 1989.
30. Gough IR: A study of diagnostic accuracy in acute appendicitis. Aust N Z J Surg 58:555-560, 1988.
31. Crabbe MM, Norwood SH, Robertson HD, et al: Recurrent and chronic appendicitis. Surg Gynecol Obstet 163:11-13, 1986.
32. Walker ARP, Segal I: What causes appendicitis [editorial]? J Clin Gastroenterol 12:127-129, 1990.
33. Larner AJ: The aetiology of appendicitis. Br J Hosp Med 38:540-542, 1988.
34. Wangensteen OH, Bowers WF: Significance of the obstructive factor in the genesis of acute appendicitis. Arch Surg 34:496-526, 1937.
35. Burkitt DP: The aetiology of appendicitis. Br J Surg 58:695-699, 1971.
36. Dunn EL, Moore EE, Elderling SC, et al: The unnecessary laparotomy for appendicitis: Can it be decreased? Arch Surg 110:677-684, 1975.
37. Nitecki S, Karmeli R, Sarr MG: Appendiceal calculi and fecaliths as indications for appendectomy. Surg Clin Obstet 171:185-188, 1990.
38. Jones BA, Demetriades D, Segal I, et al: The prevalence of appendiceal fecaliths in patients with and without appendicitis: A comparative study from Canada and South Africa. Ann Surg 202:80-82, 1985.
39. Shaw RE: Appendix calculi and acute appendicitis. Br J Surg 52:451-459, 1965.
40. Cotran RS, Kumar V, Robbins SL (eds): Robbins Pathologic Basis of Disease, 4th ed. Philadelphia, WB Saunders, 1989, pp 902-904.
41. Guidry SP, Poole GV: The anatomy of appendicitis. Am Surg 60:68-71, 1994.
42. Wagner JM, McKinney P, Carpenter JL: Does this patient have appendicitis? JAMA 276:1589-1594, 1996.
43. Graffeo CS, Counselman FL: Gastrointestinal emergencies: II. Appendicitis. Emerg Med Clin North Am 14:653-671, 1996.
44. Silen W: Acute appendicitis. In Fauci AS, Braunwald E, Isselbacher KL, et al (eds): Harrison's Principles of Internal Medicine, 14th ed. New York, McGraw-Hill, 1998, pp 1658-1660.
45. Hale DA, Molloy M, Pearl RH, et al: Appendectomy: A contemporary appraisal. Ann Surg 225:252-261, 1997.
46. Körner H, Söndenaa K, Söreide JA, et al: Incidence of acute non-perforated and perforated appendicitis: Age-specific and sex-specific analysis. World J Surg 21:313-317, 1997.
47. Temple CL, Huchcroft SA, Temple WJ: The natural history of appendicitis in adults: A prospective study. Ann Surg 221:278-281, 1995.
48. Andersson RE, Hugander A, Thulin AJG: Diagnostic accuracy and perforation rate in appendicitis: Association with age and sex of the patient and with appendectomy rate. Eur J Surg 158:37-41, 1992.
49. Maxwell JM, Ragland JJ: Appendicitis: Improvements in diagnosis and treatment. Am Surg 57:282-285, 1991.
50. Pieper R, Kager L, Nasman P: Acute appendicitis: A clinical study of 1018 cases of emergency appendectomy. Acta Chir Scand 148:51-62, 1982.
51. Silberman VA: Appendectomy in a large metropolitan hospital: Retrospective analysis of 1,013 cases. Am J Surg 142:615-618, 1981.
52. Vorhes CE: Appendicitis in the elderly: The case for better diagnosis. Geriatrics 42:89-92, 1987.
53. Rodriguez DP, Vargas S, Callahan MJ, et al: Appendicitis in young children: Imaging experience and clinical outcomes. AJR 186:1158-1164, 2006.
54. Trautlein JJ, Lambert RL, Miller J: Malpractice in the emergency department—review of 200 cases. Ann Emerg Med 13:709-711, 1984.
55. Phillips RL, Bartholomew LA, Dovey SM, et al: Learning from malpractice claims about negligent, adverse events in primary care in the United States. Qual Saf Health Care 13:121-126, 2004.
56. Selbst SM, Friedman MJ, Singh SB: Epidemiology and etiology of malpractice lawsuits involving children in US emergency departments and urgent care centers. Pediatr Emerg Care 21:165-169, 2005.
57. White JJ, Sanrillana M, Haller JA Jr: Intensive in-hospital observation: A safe way to decrease unnecessary appendectomy. Am Surg 41:793-798, 1975.
58. Lee SL, Ho HS: Ultrasonography and computed tomography in suspected acute appendicitis. Semin Ultrasound CT MRI 24:69-73; 2003.
59. Flum DR, Morris A, Koepsell T, et al: Has misdiagnosis of appendicitis decreased over time? JAMA 286:1748-1753, 2001.
60. Jones K, Peña AA, Dunn EL, et al: Are negative appendectomies still acceptable? Am J Surg 188:748-754, 2004.
61. Rao PM, Rhea JT, Rattner DW, et al: Introduction of appendiceal CT: Impact on negative appendectomy and appendiceal perforation rates. Ann Surg 229:344-349, 1999.

62. Bendeck SE, Nino-Murcia M, Berry, GJ, et al: Imaging for suspected appendicitis: Negative appendectomy and perforation rates. Radiology 225:131-136, 2002.
63. Brewer RJ, Golden GT, Hitch DC, et al: Abdominal pain: An analysis of 1,000 cases in a university hospital emergency room. Am J Surg 131:219-223, 1976.
64. Rothrock SG: Overcoming limitations and pitfalls in the diagnosis of acute appendicitis. Emerg Med Rep 13:41-52, 1992.
65. Ramsden WH, Mannion RAJ, Simpkins KC, et al: Is the appendix where you think it is—and if not does it matter? Clin Radiol 47:100-103, 1993.
66. Karin OM, Boothroyd AE, Wyllie JH: McBurney's point—fact or fiction? Ann R Coll Surg Engl 72:304-308, 1990.
67. Marchand, A Van Lente F, Galen GS: The assessment of laboratory tests in the diagnosis of acute appendicitis. Am J Clin Pathol 80:369-374, 1983.
68. Hoffman J, Rasmussen OO: Aids in the diagnosis of acute appendicitis. Br J Surg 76:774-779, 1989.
69. Raftery AT: The value of leukocyte count in the diagnosis of acute appendicitis. Br J Surg 63:143-144, 1976.
70. Thompson MM, Underwood MJ, Dookeran KA, et al: Role of sequential leukocyte counts and C-reactive protein measurements in acute appendicitis. Br J Surg 79:822-824, 1992.
71. Sasso RD, Hanna EA, Moore DL: Leukocyte and neutrophilic counts in acute appendicitis. Am J Surg 120:563-566, 1970.
72. Kretchmar LH, McDonald DF: The urine sediment in acute appendicitis. Arch Surg 87:209-211, 1963.
73. Thimsen DA, Tong GK, Gruenberg JC: Prospective evaluation of C-reactive protein in patients suspected of having acute appendicitis. Am Surg 55:466-468, 1989.
74. Eriksson S, Granstrom L, Bark S: Laboratory tests in patients with suspected acute appendicitis. Acta Chir Scand 155:117-120, 1989.
75. Nordback I, Harju E: Inflammation parameters in the diagnosis of acute appendicitis. Acta Chir Scand 154:43-48, 1988.
76. Albu E, Miller BM, Choi Y, et al: Diagnostic value of C-reactive protein in acute appendicitis. Dis Colon Rectum 37:49-51, 1994.
77. Kelvin FM, Gardiner R: Clinical Imaging of the Colon and Rectum. New York, Raven, 1987, pp 460-491.
78. Marshak RH, Linder AH, Maklanky D: Radiology of the Colon. Philadelphia, WB Saunders, 1989, pp 491-515.
79. Long JA: The appendix. In Dreyfus JR, Janower ML (eds): Radiology of the Colon. Baltimore, Williams & Wilkins, 1980, pp 497-521.
80. Harding JA, Glick SN, Teplick SK, et al: Appendiceal filling by double-contrast barium enema. Gastrointest Radiol 11:105-107, 1986.
81. Sakover RP, Del Fava RL: Frequency of visualization of the normal appendix with the barium enema examination. AJR 121:312-317, 1974.
82. Cohen N, Modai D, Rosen A, et al: Barium appendicitis: Fact or fancy? J Clin Gastroenterol 9:447-451, 1987.
83. Olutola PS: Plain film radiographic diagnosis of acute appendicitis: An evaluation of the signs. J Can Assoc Radiol 39:254-256, 1988.
84. Johnson JF, Coughlin WF: Plain film diagnosis of appendiceal perforation in children. Semin Ultrasound CT MR 10:306-313, 1989.
85. Mowji PJ, Jones MD, Cohen AJ: Localized ileus of the proximal jejunum: A new sign for acute appendicitis. Gastrointest Radiol 14:173-175, 1989.
86. Vaudagna JS, McCort JJ: Plain film diagnosis of retrocecal appendicitis. Radiology 117:533-536, 1975.
87. Fagenberg D: Fecoliths of the appendix: Incidence and significance. AJR 89:752-759, 1963.
88. Beneventano TC, Schein CJ, Jacobson HG: The Roentgen aspects of some appendiceal abnormalities. AJR 96:344-360, 1966.
89. Shimkin PM: Radiology of acute appendicitis. AJR 130:1001-1004, 1978.
90. Harned RK: Retrocecal appendicitis presenting with air in the subhepatic space. AJR 126:416-418, 1976.
91. Meyers MA, Oliphant M: Ascending retrocecal appendicitis. Radiology 110:295-299, 1974.
92. Ahn, SH, Mayo-Smith WW, Murphy BL, et al: Acute nontraumatic abdominal pain in adult patients: Abdominal radiography compared with CT evaluation. Radiology 225:159-164, 2002.
93. Swischuk LE, Hayden CK: Appendicitis with perforation: The dilated transverse colon sign. AJR 135:687-689, 1980.
94. Smith DE, Kirchner NA, Stewart DR: Use of the barium enema in the diagnosis of acute appendicitis and its complications. Am J Surg 138:829-834, 1979.
95. Rajagopalan E, Mason JH, Kennedy M, et al: The value of the barium enema in the diagnosis of acute appendicitis. Arch Surg 112:531-533, 1977.
96. Garcia CJ, Rosenfield NS: The barium enema in the diagnosis of acute appendicitis. Semin Ultrasound CT MR 10:314-320, 1989.
97. Rice RP, Thompson WM, Fedyshin PJ, et al: The barium enema in appendicitis: Spectrum of appearances and pitfalls. RadioGraphics 4:393-409, 1984.
98. Fedyshin P, Kelvin FM, Rice RP: Nonspecificity of barium enema in acute appendicitis. AJR 143:99-102, 1984.
99. Totty WG, Koehler RE, Cheung LY: Significance of retained barium in the appendix. AJR 135:753-756, 1980.
100. Gorske K: Intussusception of the proximal appendix into the colon. Radiology 91:791, 1968.
101. Demos TC, Flisak ME: Coiled-spring sign of the cecum in acute appendicitis. AJR 146:45-48, 1986.
102. Halls JM, Meyers HI: Acute appendicitis with abscess simulating carcinoma of the sigmoid. AJR 129:1057-1059, 1977.
103. Lane MJ, Katz DS, Ross BA, et al: Unenhanced helical CT for suspected acute appendicitis. AJR 168:405-409, 1997.
104. Lane MJ, Liu DM, Huynh MD, et al: Suspected acute appendicitis: Nonenhanced helical CT in 300 consecutive patients. Radiology 213:341-346, 1999.
105. Schuler JG, Shortsleeve MJ, Goldenson RS, et al: Is there a role for abdominal computed tomography scans in appendicitis? Arch Surg 133:373-376, 1998.
106. Rao PM, Rhea JT, Novelline RA, et al: Helical CT technique for the diagnosis of appendicitis: Prospective evaluation of a focused appendix CT examination. Radiology 202:139-144, 1997.
107. Rao PM, Rhea JT, Novelline RA, et al: Helical CT combined with contrast material administered only through the colon for imaging of suspected appendicitis. AJR 169:1275-1280, 1997.
108. Weltman DI, Yu J, Krumenacker J, et al: Diagnosis of acute appendicitis: Comparison of 5- and 10-mm CT sections in the same patient. Radiology 216:172-177, 2000.
109. Balthazar EJ, Megibow AJ, Siegel SE, et al: Appendicitis: Prospective evaluation with high resolution CT. Radiology 180:21-24, 1991.
110. Balthazar EJ, Birnbaum BA, Yee J, et al: Acute appendicitis: CT and US correlation in 100 patients. Radiology 190:31-35, 1994.
111. Stillman CA, Katz DS, Lane MJ: The normal appendix: Evaluation with unenhanced helical CT [abstract]. AJR 172(Suppl):58, 1999.
112. Jan Y, Yang, F, Huang J: Visualization rate and pattern of normal appendix on multidetector computed tomography using multiplanar reformation display. J Comput Assist Tomog 29:446-451, 2005.
113. Tamburrini S, Brunetti A, Brown M, et al: CT appearance of the normal appendix in adults. Eur Radiol 15:2096-2103, 2005.
114. Benjaminov O, Atri M, Hamilton P, et al: Frequency of visualization and thickness of normal appendix at nonenhanced helical CT. Radiology 225:400-406, 2002.
115. Rao PM, Wittenberg J, McDowell RK, et al: Appendicitis: Use of arrowhead sign for diagnosis at CT. Radiology 202:363-366, 1997.
116. Malone AJ, Wolf CR, Malmed AS, et al: Diagnosis of acute appendicitis: Value of unenhanced CT. AJR 160:763-766, 1993.
117. Jacobs JE, Birnbaum BA, Macari M, et al: Acute appendicitis: Comparison of helical CT diagnosis—focused technique with oral contrast material versus nonfocused technique with oral and intravenous contrast material. Radiology 220:683-690, 2001.
118. Rao PM, Rhea JT, Novelline RA: Distal appendicitis: CT appearance and diagnosis. Radiology 204:709-712, 1997.
119. Peck J, Peck, A, Peck C, et al: The clinical role of noncontrast helical computed tomography in the diagnosis of acute appendicitis. Am J Surg 180:133-136, 2000.
120. Horton MD, Counter SF, Florence MG, et al: A prospective trial of computed tomography and ultrasonography for diagnosing appendicitis in the atypical patient. Am J Surg 179:379-381, 2000.
121. Wijentunga R, Tan BS, Rouse JC, et al: Diagnostic accuracy of focused appendiceal CT in clinically equivocal cases of acute appendicitis. Radiology 221:747-753, 2001.
122. Wise SW, Labuski MR, Kasales CJ, et al: Comparative assessment of CT and sonographic techniques for appendiceal imaging. AJR 176:933-941, 2001.
123. Walker S, Haun W, Clark J, et al: The value of limited computed tomography with rectal contrast in the diagnosis of acute appendicitis. Am J Surg 180:450-455, 2000.
124. Raman SS, Lu DSK, Kadell BM, et al: Accuracy of nonfocused helical CT for the diagnosis of acute appendicitis: A 5-year review. AJR 178:1319-1325, 2002.

125. Federle MP: Focused appendix CT technique: A commentary. Radiology 202:20-21, 1997.
126. Siewert B, Raptopoulos V: CT of the acute abdomen: Findings and impact on diagnosis and treatment. AJR 163:1317-1324, 1994.
127. Curtin KR, Fitzgerald SW, Nemcek AA, et al: CT diagnosis of acute appendicitis: Imaging findings. AJR 164:905-909, 1995.
128. Raptopoulos VD, Katsou G, Morrin MM, et al: Increased use of CT for appendicitis: Implications in CT diagnosis increased occurrence of cases with subtle CT findings. Radiology 217(Suppl):372-373, 2000.
129. Kharbanda AB, Taylor GA, Bachur RG: Suspected appendicitis in children: Rectal and intravenous contrast-enhanced versus intravenous contrast-enhanced CT. Radiology 243:520-526, 2007.
130. O'Malley ME, Halpern E, Mueller PR, et al: Helical CT protocols for the abdomen and pelvis: A survey. AJR 175:109-113, 2000.
131. Puylaert JCBM: Acute appendicitis: US evaluation using graded compression. Radiology 158:355-360, 1986.
132. Leite NP, Pereira JM, Cunha R, et al: CT evaluation of appendicitis and its complications: Imaging techniques and key diagnostic findings. AJR 185:406-417, 2005.
133. Kessler N, Cyteval C, Gallix B, et al: Appendicitis: Evaluation of sensitivity, specificity, and predictive values of US, Doppler US, and laboratory findings. Radiology 230:472-478, 2004.
134. Rettenbacher T, Hollerweger A, Macheiner P, et al: Outer diameter of the vermiform appendix as a sign of acute appendicitis: Evaluation at US. Radiology 218:757-762, 2001.
135. Gracey D, McClure MJ: The impact of ultrasound in acute appendicitis. Clin Radiol 62:573-578, 2007.
136. Borushok KF, Jeffrey RB Jr, Laing FC, et al: Sonographic diagnosis of perforation in patients with acute appendicitis. AJR 154:275-278, 1990.
137. Ooms HWA, Koumans RKJ, Ho Kang You PJ, et al: Ultrasonography in the diagnosis of acute appendicitis. Br J Surg 78:315-318, 1991.
138. Quillin SP, Siegel MJ, Coffin CM: Acute appendicitis in children: Value of sonography in detecting perforation. AJR 159:1265-1268, 1992.
139. Pickuth D, Heywang-Kobrunner SH, Spielmann RP: Suspected appendicitis: Is ultrasonography or computed tomography the preferred imaging technique? Eur J Surg 166:315-319, 2000.
140. Terasawa T, Blackmore C, Bent S, et al: Systematic review: Computed tomography and ultrasonography to detect acute appendicitis in adults and adolescents. Ann Intern Med 141:537-546, 2004.
141. Poortman P, Lohle PNM, Schoemaker CMC, et al: Comparison of CT and sonography in the diagnosis of acute appendicitis: A blinded prospective study. AJR 181:1355-1359, 2003.
142. Sivit CJ, Applegate KE, Stallion A, et al: Imaging evaluation of suspected appendicitis in a pediatric population: Effectiveness of sonography versus CT. AJR 175:977-980, 2000.
143. Peña BMG, Taylor GA: Radiologists' confidence in interpretation of sonography and CT in suspected pediatric appendicitis. AJR 175:71-74, 2000.
144. Nitta N, Takahashi M, Furukawa A, et al: MR imaging of the normal appendix and acute appendicitis. J Magn Reson Imaging 21:156-165, 2005.
145. Anderson B, Nielson TF: Appendicitis in pregnancy: Diagnosis, management and complications. Acta Obstet Gynecol Scand 78:758-762, 1999.
146. Cobben LP, Groot I, Haans L, et al: MRI for clinically suspected appendicitis during pregnancy. AJR 183:671-675, 2004.
147. Mazze RI, Kallen B: Appendectomy during pregnancy: A Swedish registry study of 778 cases. Obstet Gynecol 77:835-840, 1991.
148. Birchard KR, Brown MA, Hyslop WB, et al: MRI of acute abdominal and pelvic pain in pregnant patients. AJR 184:452-458, 2005.
149. Shellock FG, Kamal E: Policies, guidelines, and recommendations for MR imaging safety and patient treatment: SMRI safety committee. J Magn Reson Imaging 1:97-101, 1991.
150. Puylaert JB: Mesenteric adenitis and acute terminal ileitis: US evaluation using graded compression. Radiology 161:691-695, 1986.
151. Rao PM, Rhea JT, Novelline RA: CT diagnosis of mesenteric adenitis. Radiology 202:145-149, 1997.
152. Kamel IR, Goldberg SN, Keogan MT, et al: Right lower quadrant pain and suspected appendicitis: Nonfocused appendiceal CT—review of 100 cases. Radiology 217:159-163, 2000.
153. Macari M, Hines J, Balthazar E, et al: Mesenteric adenitis: CT diagnosis of primary versus secondary causes, incidence, and clinical significance in pediatric and adult patients. AJR 178:853-858, 2002.
154. van Breda Vriesman AC, Puylaert JBCM: Mimics of appendicitis: Alternative nonsurgical diagnoses with sonography and CT. AJR 186:1103-1112, 2006.
155. Gore RM, Marn CS, Kirby DF, et al: CT findings in ulcerative, granulomatous, and indeterminate colitis. AJR 143:279-284, 1984.
156. Philpotts LE, Heiken JP, Westcott MA, et al: Colitis: Use of CT findings in differential diagnosis. Radiology 190:445-449, 1994.
157. Gore RM: CT of inflammatory bowel disease. Radiol Clin North Am 27:717-729, 1989.
158. Gore RM: Cross-sectional imaging of inflammatory bowel disease. Radiol Clin North Am 25:115-131, 1987.
159. van Breda Vriesman AC, Puylaert JB: Epiploic appendagitis and omental infarction: Pitfalls and look-alikes. Abdom Imaging 27:20-28, 2002.
160. Puylaert JB: Right-sided segmental infarction of the omentum: Clinical, US, and CT findings. Radiology 185:169-172, 1992.
161. Macari M, Balthazar E, Cao H, et al: CT diagnosis of ileal diverticulitis. Clin Imaging 22:243-245, 1998.
162. Macari M, Balthazar E: The acute right lower quadrant: CT evaluation. Radiol Clin North Am 41:1117-1136, 2003.
163. Frick MP, Maile CW, Crass JR, et al: Computed tomography of neutropenic colitis. AJR 143:763-765, 1984.
164. Ripolles T, Martinez MJ, Morote V, et al: Appendiceal involvement in Crohn's disease: Gray-scale sonography and color Doppler flow features. AJR 186:1071-1078, 2006.
165. Chiou YY, Pitman MB, Hahn PF, et al: Rare benign and malignant appendiceal lesions: Spectrum of computed tomography findings with pathologic correlation. JCAT 27:297-306, 2003.
166. Sturm EJ, Cobben LP, Meijssen MA, et al: Detection of ileocecal Crohn's disease using ultrasound as the primary imaging modality. Eur Radiol 14:778-782, 2004.
167. Dudley TH, Dean PJ: Idiopathic granulomatous appendicitis, or Crohn's disease of the appendix revisited. Hum Pathol 24:595-601, 1993.
168. Scott IS, Sheaff M, Coumbe A, et al: Appendiceal inflammation in ulcerative colitis. Histopathology 33:168-173, 1998.
169. Sharp JF, Nicholson ML, Fossard DP: Diverticulosis of the appendix. Scott Med J 35:49-50, 1990.
170. Tang C-K: Disorders of the vermiform appendix. In Ming S-C, Goldman H (eds): Pathology of the Gastrointestinal Tract, 2nd ed. Baltimore, Williams & Wilkins, 1998, pp 901-924.
171. Buffo GC, Clair MR, Bonheim P: Diverticulosis of the vermiform appendix. Gastrointest Radiol 11:108-109, 1986.
172. Phillips BJ, Perry CW: Appendiceal diverticulitis. Mayo Clin Proc 74:890-892, 1999.
173. Levine MS, Trenkner SW, Herlinger H, et al: Coiled-spring sign of appendiceal intussusception. Radiology 155:41-44, 1985.
174. Langsam LB, Raj PK, Galang CF: Intussusception of the appendix. Dis Colon Rectum 27:387-392, 1984.
175. Maglinte DDT, Fleischer AC, Chua GT, et al: Sonography of appendiceal intussusception. Gastrointest Radiol 12:163-165, 1987.
176. Kleinman PK: Intussusception of the appendix: Hydrostatic reduction. AJR 134:1268-1270, 1980.
177. Deans GT, Spence RA: Neoplastic lesions of the appendix. Br J Surg 82:299-306, 1995.
178. Connor SJ, Hanna GB, Frizelle FA: Appendiceal tumors: Retrospective clinicopathologic analysis of appendiceal tumors from 7,970 appendectomies. Dis Colon Rectum 41:75-80, 1998.
179. Hananel N, Powsner E, Wolloch Y: Adenocarcinoma of the appendix: An unusual disease. Eur J Surg 164:859-862, 1998.
180. Pickhardt PJ, Levy AD, Rohrmann CA, et al: Primary neoplasms of the appendix manifesting as acute appendicitis: CT findings with pathologic comparison. Radiology 224:775-781, 2002.
181. Peck JJ: Management of carcinoma discovered unexpectedly at operation for acute appendicitis. Am J Surg 155:683-685, 1988.
182. Montgomery DP: A diagnostic approach to ileo-cecal abnormalities. In Simpkins KC (ed): A Textbook of Radiologic Diagnosis, vol IV. London, HK Lewis, 1988, pp 51, 559-578.
183. Kim SH, Lim HK, Lee WJ, et al: Mucocele of the appendix: Ultrasonographic and CT findings. Abdom Imaging 23:292-296, 1998.
184. Soweid AM, Clarston WK, Andrus CH, et al: Diagnosis and management of appendiceal mucoceles. Dig Dis 16:183-185, 1998.
185. Wackym PA, Gray GF: Tumors of the appendix: I. Neoplastic and nonneoplastic mucoceles. South Med J 77:283-287, 1984.
186. Li YP, Morin ME, Tan A: Ultrasound findings in mucocele of the appendix. J Clin Ultrasound 9:406-408, 1981.
187. Kimura H, Konishi K, Yabushita K, et al: Intussusception of a mucocele of the appendix secondary to obstruction by endometriosis. Surg Today 29:629-632, 1999.
188. Skaane P: Radiological features of mucocele of the appendix. Rofo 149:624-628, 1988.

189. Ruiz-Tovar J, Tervel DC, Castineiras VM, et al: Mucocele of the appendix. World J Surg 31:542-548, 2007.
190. Sandler MA, Pearlberg JL, Madrazo BL: Ultrasonic and computed tomographic features of mucocele of the appendix. J Ultrasound Med 3:97-100, 1984.
191. Kavakuc RJ: Unusual roentgenographic manifestations of mucocele of the appendix. Radiology 89:886-887, 1967.
192. Madwell D, Mindelzun R, Jeffrey RB: Mucocele of the appendix: Imaging findings. AJR 159:69-72, 1992.
193. Hamilton DL, Stormont JM: The volcano sign of appendiceal mucocele. Gastrointest Endosc 35:453-456, 1989.
194. Higa E, Rosai J, Pizzimbono CA, et al: Mucosal hyperplasia, mucinous cystadenoma and mucinous cystadenocarcinoma of the appendix: A re-evaluation of appendiceal mucocele. Cancer 32:1525-1541, 1973.
195. Dachman AH, Lichtenstein JE, Friedman AC: Mucocele of the appendix and pseudomyxoma peritonei. AJR 144:923-929, 1985.
196. Novetsky GJ, Berlin L, Epstein AJ, et al: Pseudomyxoma peritonei. J Comput Assist Tomogr 6:398-399, 1982.
197. Mayes GB, Chuang VP, Fisher RG: CT of pseudomyxoma peritonei. AJR 136:807-808, 1981.
198. Miller DL, Udelsman R, Sugarbaker PH: Calcification of pseudomyxoma peritonei following intraperitoneal chemotherapy: CT demonstration. J Comput Assist Tomogr 9:1123-1124, 1985.
199. Balthazar EJ, Javors BR: Pseudomyxoma peritonei, clinical and radiographic features. Am J Gastroenterol 68:501-509, 1977.
200. Horgan JG, Chow PP, Richter JO, et al: CT and sonography in the recognition of mucocele of the appendix. AJR 143: 959-962, 1984.
201. Matsuoka Y, Ohtomo K, Itai Y, et al: Pseudomyxoma peritonei with progressive calcifications: CT findings. Gastrointest Radiol 17:16-18, 1992.
202. Gustafson KD, Karnaze GC, Hattery RR, et al: Pseudomyxoma peritonei associated with mucinous adenocarcinoma of the pancreas: CT findings and CT-guided biopsy. J Comput Assist Tomogr 8:335-338, 1984.
203. McGinnis HD, Chew FS: Mucin-producing adenoma of the appendix. AJR 160:1046, 1993.
204. Skaane M, Isachsen M, Hoiseth A: Case report: Computed tomography of mucin-producing adenocarcinoma of the appendix presenting as a bladder tumor. J Comput Assist Tomogr 9:566-567, 1985.
205. Machan L, Pon MS, Wood BJ, et al: The "coffee bean" sign in peri-appendiceal and peridiverticular abscess. J Ultrasound Med 6:373-375, 1987.
206. Nitecki SS, Wolff BG, Schlinkert R, et al: The natural history of surgically treated primary adenocarcinoma of the appendix. Ann Surg 219:51-57, 1994.
207. Collins DC: Seventy-one thousand human appendix specimens: A final report summarizing 40 years' study. Am J Protocol 14:265-281, 1963.
208. Moertel CG, Dockerty MB, Judd ES: Carcinoid tumors of the vermiform appendix. Cancer 21:270-278, 1968.
209. Modlin IM, Sandor A: An analysis of 8305 cases of carcinoid tumors. Cancer 79:813-829, 1997.
210. Hemminki K, Li X: Incidence trends and risk factors of carcinoid tumors, a nationwide epidemiologic study from Sweden. Cancer 92:2204-2210, 2001.
211. Sandor A, Modlin IM: A retrospective analysis of 1570 appendiceal carcinoids. Am J Gastroenterol 93:422-428, 1998.
212. Pelage JP, Soyer P, Boudiaf M, et al: Carcinoid tumors of the abdomen: CT features. Abdom Imaging 24:240-245, 1999.
213. Kitamura Y, Ohta T, Terada T: Primary T-cell non-Hodgkin's malignant lymphoma of the appendix. Pathol Int 50:313-317, 2000.
214. Pascuale MD, Shabahang M, Bitterman P, et al: Primary lymphoma of the appendix: Case report and review of the literature. Surg Oncol 3:243-248, 1994.
215. Pickhardt PJ, Levy AD, Rohrmann JCA, et al: Non-Hodgkin's lymphoma of the appendix: Clinical and CT findings with pathologic correlation. AJR 178:1123-1127, 2002.

chapter

61

Ulcerative and Granulomatous Colitis: Idiopathic Inflammatory Bowel Disease

Richard M. Gore, MD • Igor Laufer, MD • Jonathan W. Berlin, MD

The term *inflammatory bowel disease* encompasses two forms of chronic, idiopathic intestinal inflammation: ulcerative colitis and Crohn's disease. Although many other inflammatory diseases affect the gut, most are distinguished either by a specific identifiable etiologic agent or process or by the nature of the inflammatory activity. The cause of ulcerative colitis and Crohn's disease is unknown, so these disorders are empirically defined by their typical pathologic, radiologic, clinical, endoscopic, and laboratory features.[1-7] This chapter summarizes the features that usually permit an operational distinction to be made between ulcerative colitis and Crohn's disease. The fundamental validity of this classification is uncertain and will so remain until the cause and pathogenesis of these disorders are better understood.

ULCERATIVE COLITIS

Ulcerative colitis is a diffuse inflammatory disease of unknown origin that primarily involves the colorectal mucosa but later extends to other layers of the bowel wall. The disease characteristically begins in the rectum and extends proximally to involve part or all of the colon. The diagnosis is usually made on the basis of clinical symptoms and the presence of inflamed mucosa on sigmoidoscopy and confirmed by the findings on barium enema and mucosal biopsy.[5,6]

Historical Perspective

Although Hippocrates was aware that diarrhea was not a single disease, it required more than two millennia before ulcerative colitis was distinguished from the all too common infectious enteritides. In 1859, Wilks described the case of Mrs. Isabella Banks, who had "inflammation of the large intestine" and was "affected by discharge of mucus and blood, where, after death, the whole internal surface of the colon presented a highly vascular soft, red surface covered with tenacious mucus, adherent lymph. . . ."[8] By 1900, ulcerative colitis was fully characterized in terms of its clinical and pathologic criteria.[1]

Epidemiology

Epidemiologic data have yielded some important clues concerning the cause of ulcerative colitis. The salient epidemiologic features of ulcerative colitis are listed in Table 61-1 and discussed more fully subsequently.

Ulcerative colitis is more common than Crohn's disease, with an annual incidence of 2 to 10 cases per 100,000 population. The worldwide prevalence ranges from 35 to 100 cases per 100,000 population. This wide range is probably due to true differences in disease distribution as well as differences in reporting, diagnostic criteria, and availability of medical care.[7] The incidence of ulcerative colitis has remained steady from the 1950s through the 1980s. This is in sharp contrast to Crohn's disease, which has shown a sixfold increase in incidence over a similar period.

Ulcerative colitis is most prevalent in the developed countries of northern Europe, Scandinavia, the British Isles, the United States, and Israel. The incidence of ulcerative colitis in high-prevalence areas has leveled off, whereas the incidence of Crohn's disease is increasing. In low-prevalence geographic areas, the incidence of ulcerative colitis has been increasing.[7] Ulcerative colitis is four times more common in whites than in nonwhites, and there is a slight female preponderance.[7]

There is a twofold to fourfold increase of ulcerative colitis among Jews. The incidence of ulcerative colitis is much lower among Israeli than among American and European Jews. Furthermore, the incidence of disease is lower in Sephardic than in Ashkenazi Jews in Israel. These disparate rates suggest

Table 61-1
Epidemiology of Ulcerative Colitis

Worldwide prevalence: 35-100 cases/100,000 population
Annual incidence: 2-10 cases/100,000 population
Bimodal age distribution: Peak 15-25 yr; smaller peak 50-80 yr
Risk factors:
   White (two to five times risk)
   Jewish (two to four times risk)
   Live in developed country
   Urban dweller
   Family history (30 to 100 times risk)
   Sibling with disease (8.8% incidence)
   Single
   Nonsmoker

Adapted from Su C, Lichtenstein GR: Ulcerative colitis. In Feldman M, Friedman LS, Branch LJ (eds): Gastrointestinal and Liver Disease, 7th ed. Philadelphia, Saunders, 2006, pp 2499-2548.

that a hereditary predisposition may be altered by environmental factors.[7]

The peak age at onset of ulcerative colitis is between 15 and 25 years of age, with a smaller peak at ages 55 to 65 years. Ulcerative colitis is more common than Crohn's disease in children younger than 10 years old. Ulcerative colitis is more common in urban than in rural populations.[7]

The incidence of ulcerative colitis among first-degree relatives is 30 to 100 times greater than that of the general population.[7] Ten to 20 percent of patients with ulcerative colitis have a similarly affected first-degree relative. The lifetime risk of developing ulcerative colitis among first-degree relatives is 8.9% for offspring, 8.8% for siblings, and 3.5% for parents. The child develops the disease at a much younger age than the affected parent—a phenomenon known as genetic anticipation. Familial ulcerative colitis seems to follow a polygenic inheritance pattern.[7]

The risk of developing ulcerative colitis for current smokers compared with lifetime nonsmokers is 59% less, but the risk is elevated by 64% for former smokers. However, smoking is not therapeutic, and there is no strong evidence of a beneficial effect of smoking on the clinical course of ulcerative colitis. Patients who quit smoking before the onset of disease have more frequent hospitalizations and colectomies. This fact raises the possibility that smoking cessation may lead to more severe illness.[8,9]

The mortality rate of ulcerative colitis has significantly improved, and this can be attributed to improvements in diagnosis and management. In the past, ulcerative colitis was responsible for 90% of deaths attributable to inflammatory bowel disease. More recently, the proportion of ulcerative colitis and Crohn's disease deaths is about equal: 1 per 100,000 aged 20 to 29 years and 3 to 4 per 100,000 for ages 50 to 59 years.[7] Approximately 78% of ulcerative colitis patients die of causes unrelated to bowel disease. Colorectal cancer caused 14% of deaths in ulcerative colitis patients in one study.[7]

Pathogenesis and Etiology

Despite exhaustive work by many investigators, the cause of ulcerative colitis is still unknown. Although the participation of genetic, environmental, neural, hormonal, infectious, immunologic, and psychologic factors in the pathogenesis of this disease is well established, none of the mechanisms has proved to be the primary etiologic agent. In addition, it now appears that distal ulcerative proctitis may have a cause different from that of pancolitis.[1-4]

As stated earlier, familial aggregation of ulcerative colitis is well recognized. The postulated mode of inheritance of susceptibility to ulcerative colitis is through polygenes. The disease occurs with greatest frequency in monozygotic twins. Human leukocyte antigen (HLA) phenotypes B5, Bw52, and DR2 also have a significant association with ulcerative colitis. Ulcerative colitis is often associated with the autoimmune disorders sacroiliitis, ankylosing spondylitis, enteropathic oligoarthritis, and anterior uveitis, which are associated with HLA-B27 antigen.[4-6]

Possibly, genes related to ulcerative colitis may encode products that contribute to functional or structural abnormalities in the colon, which render it more susceptible to attack by infection, toxins, and autoimmune actions.[8]

Patients with ulcerative colitis have abnormal mucin production, which may permit various intraluminal bacterial products and toxins to attack the mucosa. It is uncertain whether this defect is a cause or an effect of the disease.[4-6] An infectious cause for inflammatory bowel disease with a direct cause-and-effect relationship between a single microorganism and inflammation still remains plausible. *Chlamydia*, mycobacteria, gut anaerobes, cytomegalovirus, *Yersinia*, and bacterial cell wall components have all been implicated in the cause of ulcerative colitis. It is also possible that bacteria that normally constitute normal flora may be pathogenic in a susceptible host.[4-6]

In ulcerative colitis, the enteric nervous system and nerves containing substance P and vasoactive intestinal polypeptide become straight, thick, and highly immunoreactive. Substance P and vasoactive intestinal polypeptide are powerful mediators in neurogenically induced inflammation and cause vasodilatation, plasma extravasation, and watery diarrhea. All these factors may have a role in the pathophysiology of inflammatory bowel disease.[4-6]

The immune system provides an important contribution to the pathogenesis of ulcerative colitis either because of failure to clear a microbial or toxic agent or because of an inappropriate response to it. The immune system probably mediates the tissue injury as well, regardless of the trigger, and this is the basis of therapy with corticosteroid and other immunosuppressive agents. The colonic inflammation of ulcerative colitis may merely be an exaggerated "physiologic" response that is always present within the lamina propria of the colon. There is an alteration of the relative representation of macrophages and T-cell and B-cell populations and an increase in the numbers of immunoglobulin G–bearing cells. The disease is also characterized by a fundamental alteration in antigen-presenting activity associated with a reduction of intestinal suppressor T cells and elevated levels of cytotoxic Leu-7–positive cells. Increased levels of specific antibodies to antigens in the gut lumen are also found.[1-6]

In acute ulcerative colitis, there is activation of the arachidonic cascade with increased release of chemical mediators, superoxide radicals, prostaglandins, leukotrienes, and thromboxane, which are potent inflammatory and vasoactive mediators.[1] Proinflammatory cytokines (e.g., interleukin-1) are consistently elevated in inflammatory bowel disease. Immunoregulatory cytokines (e.g., interleukin-2) are elevated in patients with Crohn's disease.

As stated earlier, smoking appears to protect against ulcerative colitis, perhaps by correcting the defect in the production of mucus or altering prostaglandin synthesis. Oral contraceptives can disturb the intestinal microcirculation and produce clinical and endoscopic features identical to ulcerative colitis. Some studies suggest a link between oral contrac-tives and ulcerative colitis.[1-4] There is also a low appendectomy rate in patients with ulcerative colitis when compared with controls.

Cow's milk protein, lactose intolerance, and chemical food additives such as carrageenan have been implicated in the development of ulcerative colitis.[1-4]

Ulcerative colitis is a complex disease consisting of interactions among initiating organisms or antigens; the host's immune response; and immunologic, environmental, and hereditary influences.

Clinical Findings

Ulcerative colitis is highly variable in clinical course, severity, and prognosis. Disease activity waxes and wanes and is charac-terized by acute exacerbations of bloody diarrhea that resolve either spontaneously or after therapy. The most common clinical findings are diarrhea, abdominal pain, rectal bleeding, weight loss, and tenesmus; vomiting, fever, constipation, and arthralgias occur less commonly.[10-12]

Ulcerative colitis usually behaves as a chronic low-grade illness in most patients. In 15% of patients, this disease has an acute and fulminating course with explosive diarrhea, hematochezia, and hypotension. Most patients (60% to 75%) have intermittent attacks with complete symptomatic remission between attacks; 4% to 10% have one attack and no subsequent symptoms; 5% to 15% are troubled by continuous symptoms without remission.[10,11]

Patients with ulcerative proctitis have disease of mild severity, and the disease usually remains distal. There is extension to the proximal colon in 15% of patients over a 10-year period and extension to the hepatic flexure in 7%. At presentation, 30% of patients have disease limited to the rectum, 40% have disease extending above the rectum but not beyond the hepatic flexure, and the remaining 30% have pancolitis. Extraintestinal manifestations, such as arthralgias, mild arthritis, eye inflammation, and rash, are present in fewer than 10% of patients at initial presentation.[1-5,10,11]

Physical examination discloses fever, prostration, dehydration, and postural hypotension in the most severe cases. The abdomen may be protuberant because of colonic atony and distention. Abdominal tenderness over the colon and absent bowel sounds are ominous signs suggesting toxic megacolon or early perforation. Patients with milder involvement present with pallor, low-grade fever, weight loss, and mild abdominal tenderness.[10-11]

Endoscopic Findings

Sigmoidoscopy is helpful in establishing the diagnosis of ulcerative colitis because the distal colon and rectum are involved in 90% to 95% of cases. Early on, the mucosa is edematous and friable, with loss of the normal vascular pattern and bleeding when touched by the endoscope or rubbed with a cotton swab. With disease progression, granular, spontaneously hemorrhagic mucosa is found, associated with a mucopurulent exudate. The haustra are thick and blunted, the lumen seems narrowed and straightened, and the normal thin (<2 mm) mucosal folds are lost. In severe disease, the mucosa is diffusely hemorrhagic and frank ulceration with loss of mucosal irregularity is seen.[3,13,14]

Radiologic Findings

Radiography

Considerable information can be gained by carefully scrutinizing the abdominal radiographs of patients with ulcerative colitis. Although attention should be focused on the colon, other abnormalities, such as renal calculi, sacroiliitis, ankylosing spondylitis, and avascular necrosis of the femoral heads, must also be excluded.[15-20]

Although the extent of ulcerative colitis is generally measured by barium enema and colonoscopy, these procedures carry a higher risk in severely ill patients. The following radiographic features can be used to assess the severity and extent of the colitis: (1) the extent of formed fecal residue, (2) the appearance of the mucosal edge, (3) alterations of the haustra, (4) colonic width, and (5) mural thickness.[15]

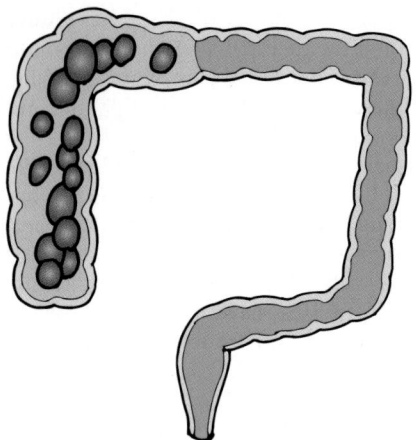

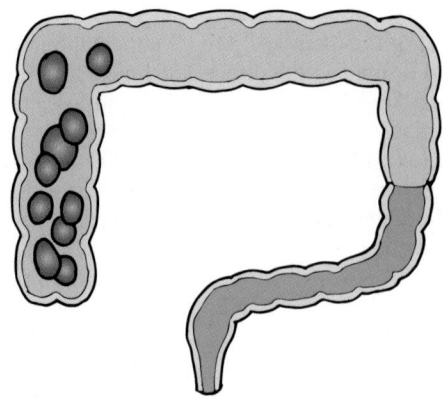

Distal extent residue = proximal
active ulcerative colitis

Distal extent residue more proximal
than colitis – overestimates extent
of disease

Figure 61-1. Ulcerative colitis: plain film estimation of active disease. The distal extent of fecal residue may overestimate but seldom underestimates the proximal extent of active disease. (From Bartram C, Kumar P: Clinical Radiology in Gastroenterology. Oxford, Blackwell Scientific, 1981, p 135.)

Colonic Fecal Residue

The distal extent of formed fecal residue gives a good indication, although not absolute, of the proximal extent of the colitis (Fig. 61-1). This approach sometimes overestimates but does not underestimate the extent of disease. The following conclusions can be drawn from the extent of residue: (1) If no residue is visible, the patient probably has active pancolitis; (2) if the residue extends down into the sigmoid colon, proctitis is present (this may be indistinguishable from normal); and (3) if residue is present only in the proximal colon, the colitis most likely extends to this level but could be more distal.[15-23]

Mucosa

The colonic mucosal edge is normally smooth. In active colitis, the line is granular, indistinct, and somewhat fuzzy. With frank ulceration, the mucosal line is disrupted, which causes an irregular edge. With extensive ulceration, only edematous mucosal islands remain. Intramural, mottled-appearing gas shadows may be present in fulminating colitis with necrosis of the bowel wall. Linear pneumatosis suggests either extremely deep ulceration or extraperitoneal perforation with gas trapped adjacent to the bowel wall.[15-23]

Haustration

Normal haustral clefts run in parallel, about 2 to 4 mm apart, across one third of the diameter of the colon. Widening of the haustral clefts with loss of the parallel lines is an early manifestation of ulcerative colitis and is more obvious on radiographs than is the mucosal granularity it accompanies. The haustra may be completely absent as well. Blunting can be confused with underdistention, so that it should not be diagnosed if only a small amount of gas is present within the colon.[15-23]

Colon Diameter

The upper limit of normal for the diameter of the transverse colon is 5.5 cm. In chronic, "burned out" ulcerative colitis, the colon becomes tubular and narrowed and is considerably less than 5 cm in diameter. In these patients, if the colon is greater than 5 cm in diameter, the inflammation has become transmural, which indicates a fulminant colitis at risk for perforation or toxic megacolon.[15-23]

Mural Thickness

In the normal colon, the distance between the line of pericolic fat and gas-filled lumen is less than 3 mm. In chronic ulcerative colitis, it increases to greater than 3 mm in thickness. In a study assessing these findings, a combination of four features was pathognomonic for disease proximal to the hepatic flexure: irregularity of the mucosal edge, loss of haustral clefts, increased thickness of the colon wall, and an "empty" right colon.[19]

Barium Enema

The barium enema has the following roles in patients with ulcerative colitis: (1) to confirm the clinical diagnosis, (2) to assess the extent and severity of disease, (3) to differentiate ulcerative colitis from Crohn's disease and other colitides, (4) to follow the course of disease, and (5) to detect complications. The major radiographic findings on the barium enema examination in ulcerative colitis are listed in Table 61-2; their anatomic-pathologic origin (Fig. 61-2) and significance are discussed subsequently.

Table 61-2
Ulcerative Colitis: Barium Enema Findings

Acute Changes
Mucosal granularity
Mucosal stippling
"Collar button" ulcers
Haustral thickening or loss
Inflammatory polyps
Confluent, contiguous, circumferential disease

Chronic Changes
Haustral loss
Luminal narrowing
Loss of rectal valves
Widened presacral space
Backwash ileitis
Postinflammatory pseudopolyps

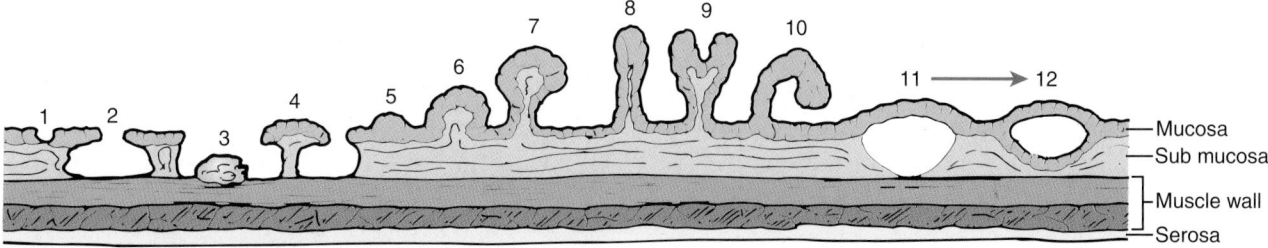

Figure 61-2. Spectrum of mucosal abnormalities in ulcerative colitis. 1, Punctate mucosal ulcer-crypt abscess; 2, "collar button" ulcer; 3, polypoid accumulation of granulation tissue; 4, mucosal remnant forming inflammatory pseudopolyp; 5 and 6, sessile mucosal polyps (similar morphologic features are seen in hyperplasia, adenoma, and carcinoma); 7, pedunculated polyp (typically hyperplastic or low-grade adenomas); 8, 9, and 10, postinflammatory pseudopolyps of various configurations; 11, mucosal remnant bridging area of active undermining ulceration; 12, mucosal bridge in quiescent state with previously denuded surfaces covered with new epithelium. (From Lichtenstein JE: Radiologic-pathologic correlation of inflammatory bowel disease. Radiol Clin North Am 25:324, 1987.)

Granular Pattern

The earliest pathologic changes of ulcerative colitis are hyperemia and the accumulation of inflammatory cells in the mucosa.[24,25] These changes are manifested by a loss of normal mucosal translucency and obscuration of the submucosal pattern on endoscopy.[26,27] Subtle thickening of the mucosa or haustral edema may be present radiographically, but these findings are often appreciated only in retrospect.[26] With progressive edema and hyperemia, the mucosa develops a granular pattern (Fig. 61-3A).[27-29] The smooth, sharp, and distinct appearance of the colonic margin seen on normal double-

contrast studies is replaced by an amorphous, thickened, and indistinct mucosal line. There is a gradual transition between the normal and abnormal mucosa that extends for several centimeters. This granularity should be distinguished from the granular appearance of chronic ulcerative colitis (Fig. 61-3B). In chronic ulcerative colitis, the mucosal surface pattern is coarser and there are significant changes in colonic contour.

The granular pattern develops as a result of abnormalities in the quality and quantity of mucus produced by the involved mucosa.[25] On histologic examination, there is a reduction in

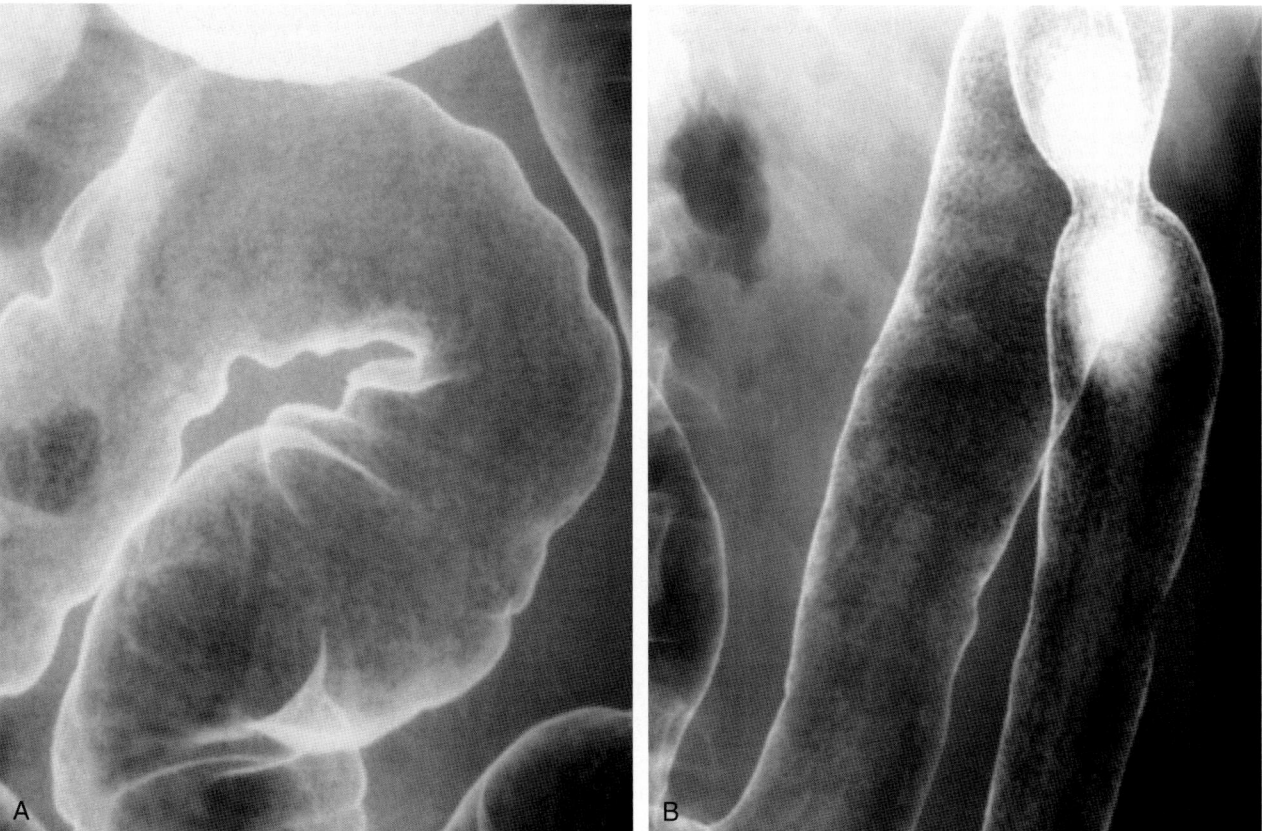

Figure 61-3. Ulcerative colitis: granular mucosal pattern. A. Early ulcerative colitis. The blunted haustral clefts are evident on this spot film of the sigmoid colon. The mucosal granularity, attributable to abnormal quantity and quality of mucin, is contiguous, circumferential, and symmetric. **B.** Chronic ulcerative colitis. This spot film of a short, tubular, ahaustral splenic flexure of the colon shows a coarser surface pattern than that seen in acute disease.

the number of goblet cells, which contain less than the normal complement of mucin.[6,25,30,31] Normal mucus is essential to normal barium coating of the gut. Any process, whether benign or malignant, infectious or inflammatory, that alters mucin production affects mucosal coating and visualization.[25]

Mucosal Stippling

During the granular phase of ulcerative colitis, inflammatory cells accumulate at the base of the mucosal crypts.[25,31] Cellular debris tends to block the crypts of Lieberkühn, which leads to the formation of microabscesses, better known as crypt abscesses (Fig. 61-4A). These crypt abscesses eventually erode into the lumen.[30,31] The ulcers deepen, and barium flecks become adherent to them, producing mucosal stippling (Fig. 61-4B).[25] This stippling resembles white paint applied by dabbing a surface with the end of a fairly dry paintbrush.[27]

"Collar Button" Ulcers

With disease progression, the ulcers of the crypt abscess breach the lamina propria and muscularis mucosae and cause undermining of the less resistant areolar tissue of the submucosa.[30] The involved submucosa becomes necrotic, and the ulcers extend laterally, causing further undermining. This undermining is contained by the muscularis propria on the serosal side and by the muscularis mucosae on the luminal side of the colon.[32,33] The ulcers are frequently related to the taeniae. The mucosal defect is small relative to the degree of undermining and produces a flasklike, "collar button" ulcer (Fig. 61-5).[25] As these ulcers enlarge and interconnect, the "collar button" ulcer configuration is lost; a network of residual islands of mucosa and inflammatory pseudopolyps is produced.

Polyps

A variety of different mucosal protrusions may be seen on barium studies in patients with inflammatory bowel disease.[25] Their appearance and significance depend on the stage of disease and pathologic origin.

INFLAMMATORY PSEUDOPOLYPS

In patients with severe ulcerative colitis, there is extensive mucosal and submucosal ulceration in which only small islands of mucosa and submucosa may survive. The inflamed edematous mucosa protrudes above the surrounding areas of ulceration, which gives a polypoid appearance (Fig. 61-6).[31] Because these "polyps" represent merely the remnants of preexisting mucosa and submucosa rather than new growths they are termed *pseudopolyps*.[31] Inflammatory pseudopolyps are the natural progression of collar button ulcers: the ulcers extend and interconnect so that the pseudopolyp rather than the ulcers becomes the major radiographic finding.[34-38] Inflammatory pseudopolyps usually occur in ulcerative colitis but may also be seen in Crohn's disease. The cobblestoning pattern seen in Crohn's disease is another type of pseudopolyp in which larger islands of preserved mucosa are surrounded by linear and transverse ulcerations.[25]

POSTINFLAMMATORY PSEUDOPOLYPS

When inflammatory bowel disease goes into remission, the denuded mucosa heals and is covered by granulation tissue that has a granular appearance similar to that observed in the early stages of ulcerative colitis.[6,31,36-38] In some patients, the

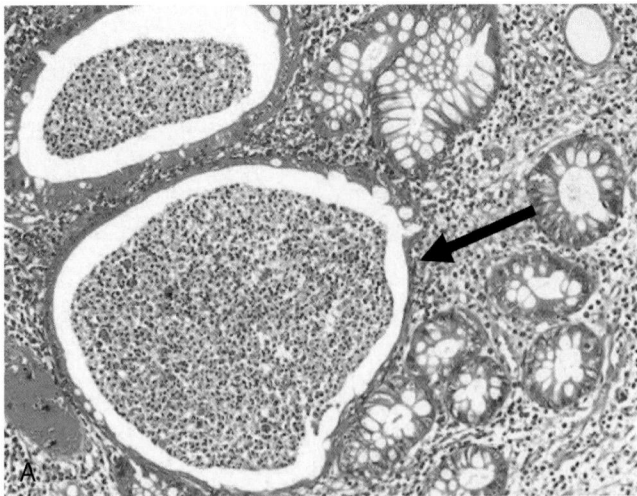

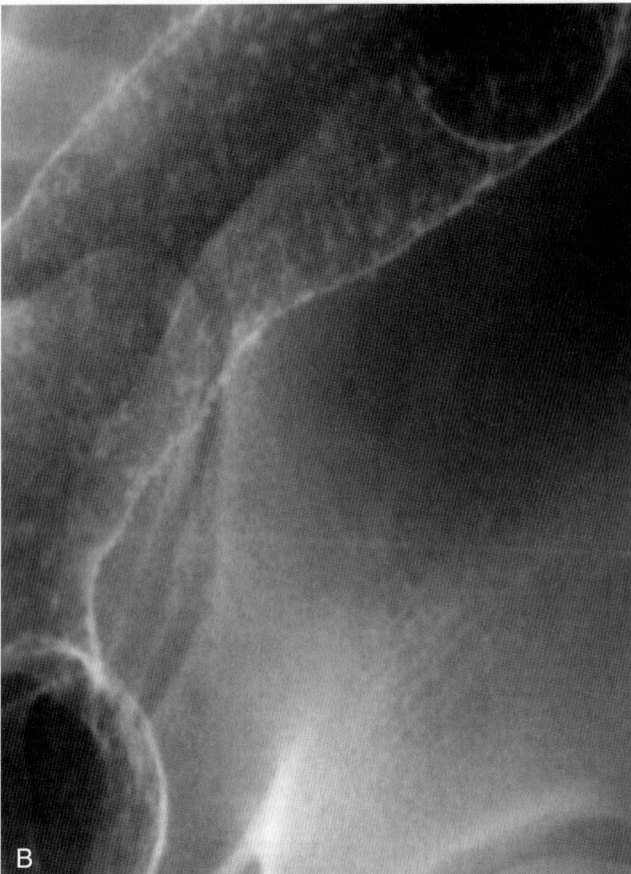

Figure 61-4. Ulcerative colitis: crypt abscess causing mucosal stippling.
A. A crypt abscess (*arrow*) is seen at the base of a crypt of Lieberkühn.
B. When these abscesses erode into the lumen, they accumulate punctate collections of barium, which produces mucosal stippling.

regenerated mucosa has a tendency to overgrow (Fig. 61-7). This overgrowth often results in polypoid lesions that may be small and rounded, may be long and filiform, or may proliferate into a bushlike structure simulating a villous adenoma. Because the regenerating mucosa is cytologically normal, it is not a true neoplasm but a pseudopolyp. Because this occurs during mucosal healing, it is called a *postinflammatory pseudopolyp*.[34-38] These polyps represent the aftermath of a severe attack of colitis and may be the only sign

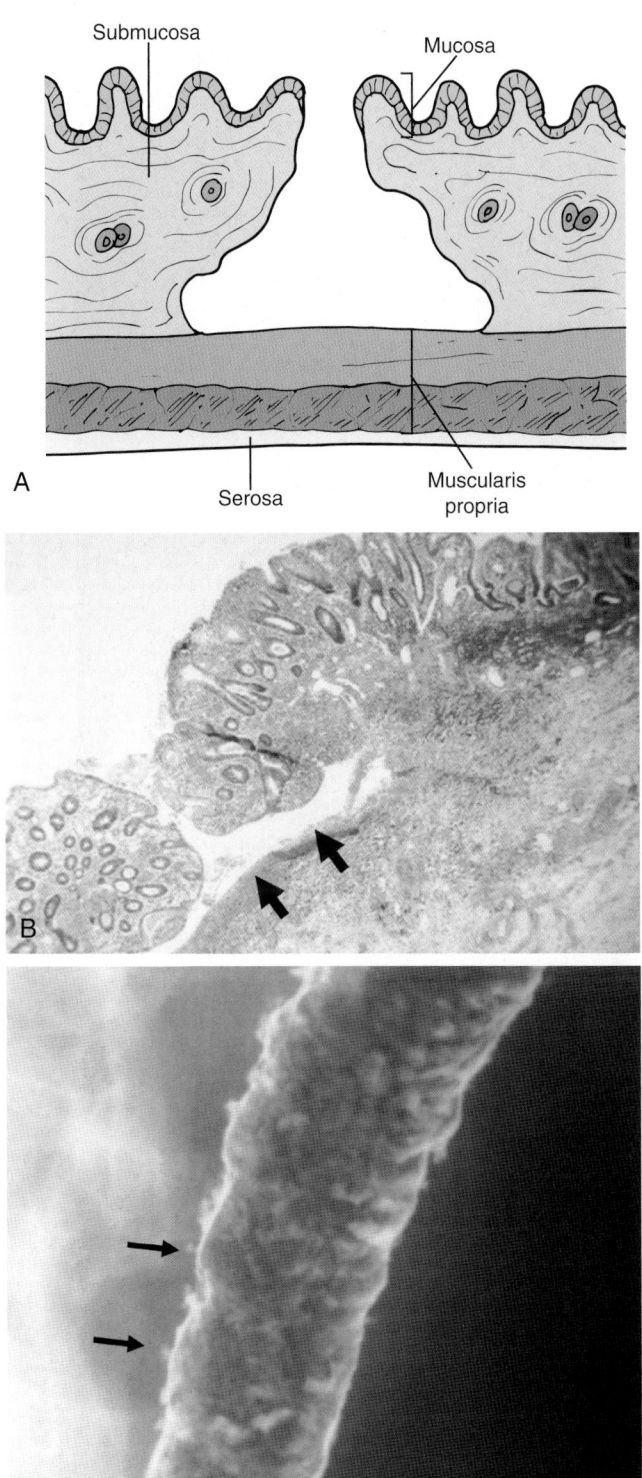

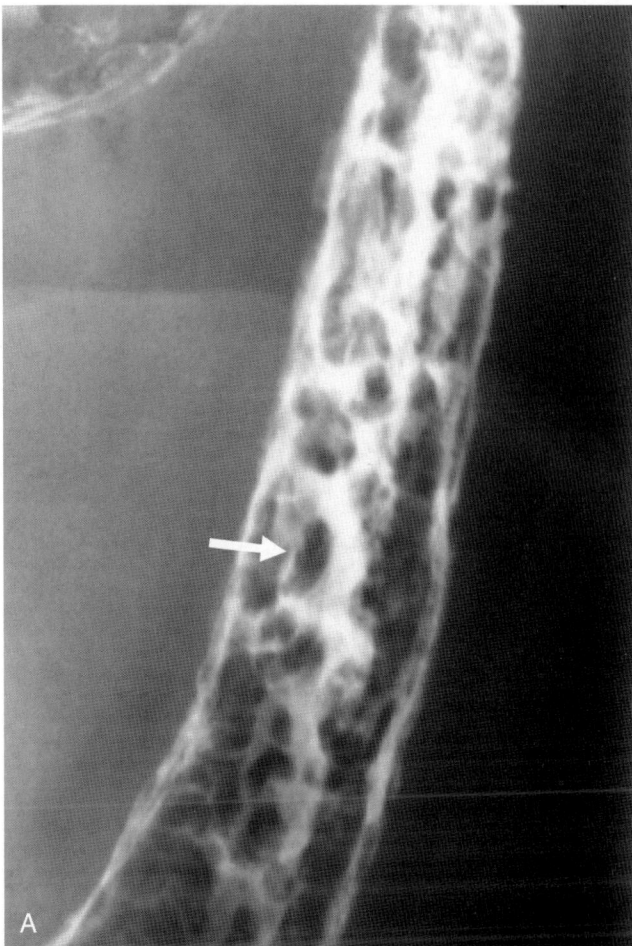

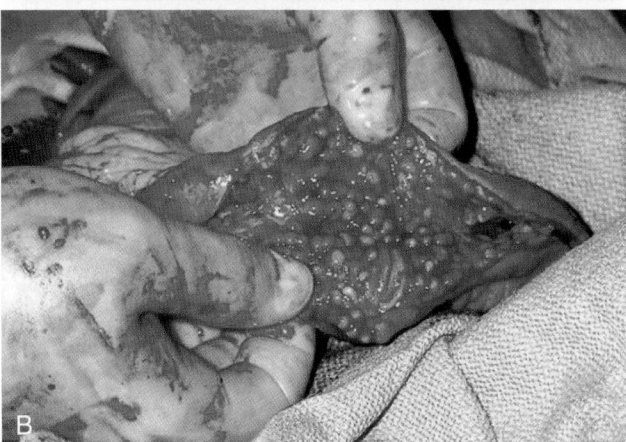

Figure 61-6. Ulcerative colitis: inflammatory pseudopolyps. A. Inflammatory pseudopolyps (*arrow*) are identified on a double-contrast barium enema study. These pseudopolyps are seen when extensive mucosal and submucosal ulceration leaves only small residual islands of surviving mucosa and submucosa. Thus, they represent remnants of preexisting mucosa and submucosa rather than new growths. **B.** Intraoperative image of a diseased colon showing multiple residual islands of whitish mucosa surrounded by hemorrhagic ulcerations.

Figure 61-5. Ulcerative colitis: "collar button" ulcers. A. Diagram shows the narrow neck of the crypt abscess that erodes through the muscularis mucosae into the submucosa. The ulcer spreads laterally through the submucosa and is contained with a flat base by the resistant inner circular layer of the muscularis propria. **B.** Low-power photomicrograph shows characteristic undermining with a flat base (*arrows*). **C.** Spot film of the splenic flexure shows multiple flasklike ulcers (*arrows*) with a flat base. The ulceration is limited to the layers superficial to the muscularis propria. (**A** from Lichtenstein JE: Radiologic-pathologic correlation of inflammatory bowel disease. Radiol Clin North Am 25:324, 1987.)

of previous disease. Mucosal bridges are also postinflammatory pseudopolyps in which a bridge of mucosa survives between islands of mucosa surrounded by ulceration. With remission, the underside of the mucosal bridge and the underlying ulcer re-epithelialize.[39,40]

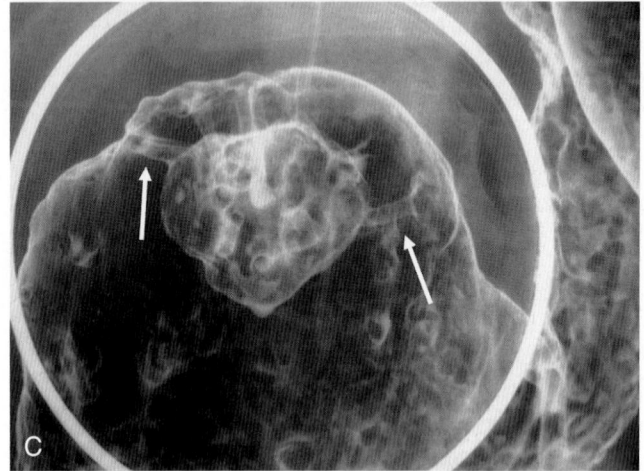

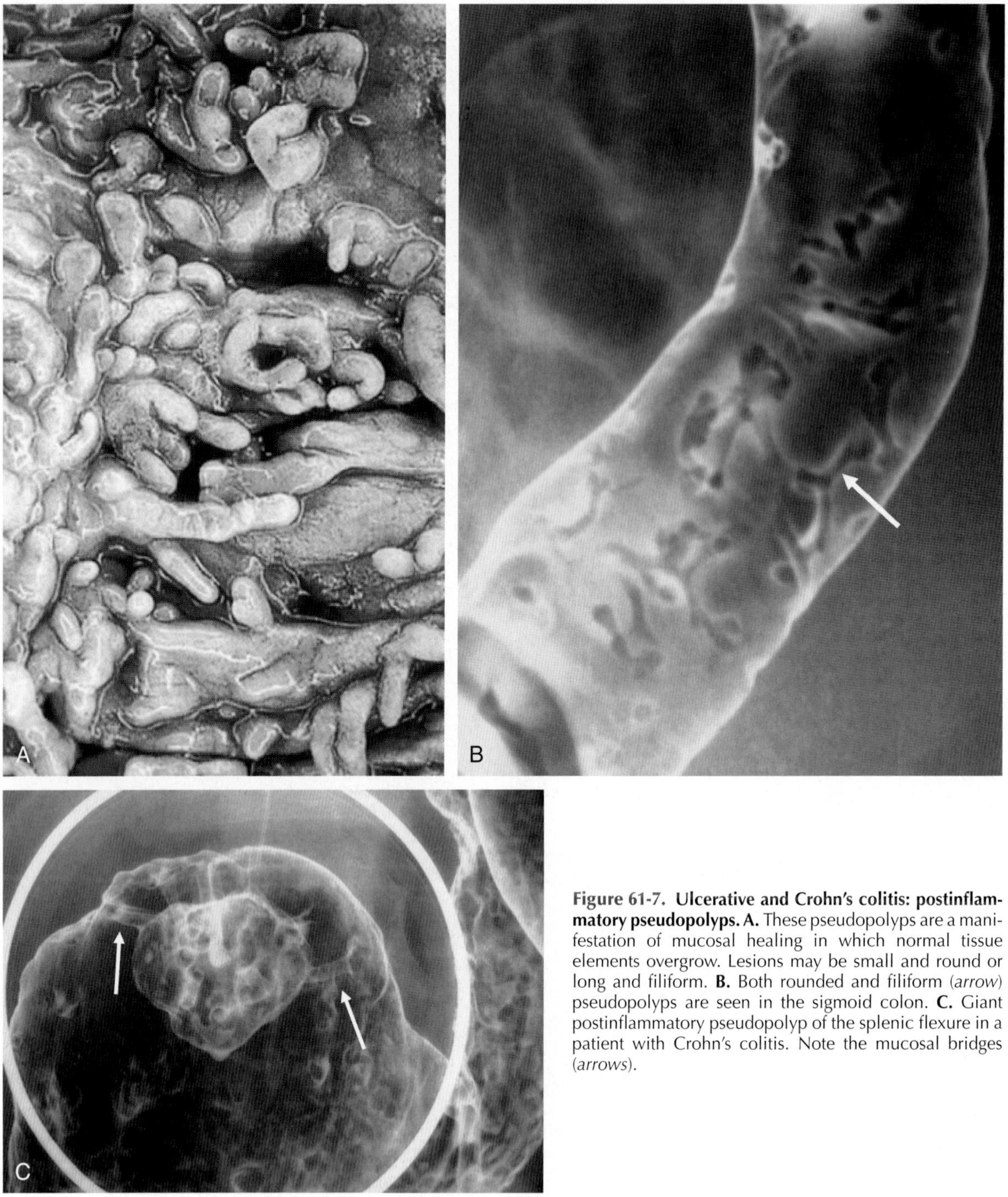

Figure 61-7. Ulcerative and Crohn's colitis: postinflammatory pseudopolyps. A. These pseudopolyps are a manifestation of mucosal healing in which normal tissue elements overgrow. Lesions may be small and round or long and filiform. **B.** Both rounded and filiform (*arrow*) pseudopolyps are seen in the sigmoid colon. **C.** Giant postinflammatory pseudopolyp of the splenic flexure in a patient with Crohn's colitis. Note the mucosal bridges (*arrows*).

Postinflammatory pseudopolyps can also be seen after ischemia, after severe infection, and in Crohn's disease. Filiform polyps have also been described in the esophagus, stomach, and small bowel in patients with Crohn's disease.[25]

Backwash Ileitis

In 10% to 40% of patients with chronic ulcerative pancolitis, the distal 5 to 25 cm of ileum is inflamed (Fig. 61-8). This ileitis occurs only in the presence of pancolitis and usually resolves 1 to 2 weeks after colectomy.[15,26] Although small ulcerations may be present, this is not a primary inflammation of the ileum. The distal ileum can be used to form an ileostomy or pouch. The pathogenesis of this disorder is uncertain but may relate to the reflux of colonic contents into the small bowel, hence the term *reflux* or *backwash* ileitis.[15]

Barium studies reveal a chronic pancolitis associated with a patulous and fixed ileocecal valve that easily refluxes and persistent dilatation of the terminal ileum. The normal fold pattern is absent, and the mucosa is granular.

Blunting and Lost Haustra

In the course of ulcerative colitis, the haustral folds undergo two major changes (Fig. 61-9; see also Fig. 61-8): (1) early in the disease, they are edematous and thickened; (2) with

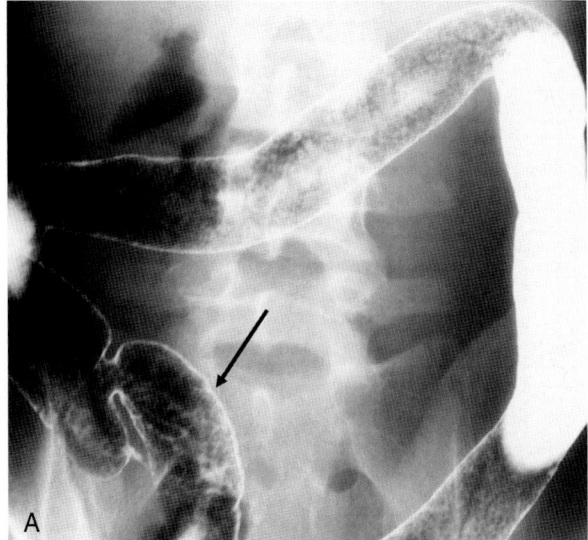

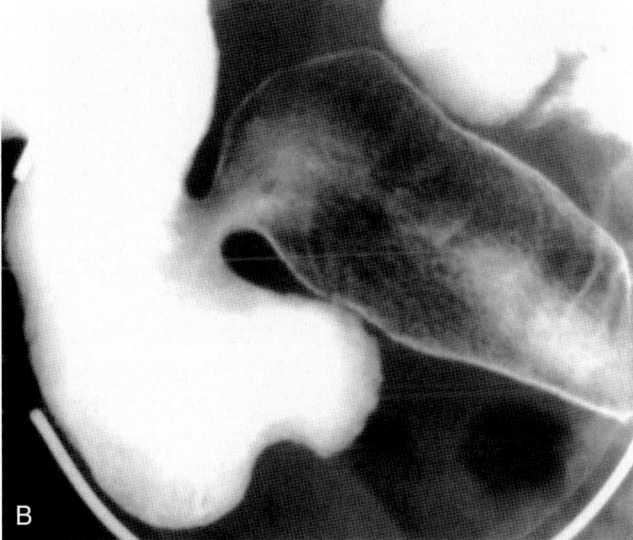

Figure 61-8. Ulcerative colitis: backwash ileitis. A. Backwash ileitis (*arrow*) is demonstrated in this patient with chronic ulcerative pancolitis. **B.** In a different patient, note the patulous ileocecal valve, the dilated, granular-appearing terminal ileum, and the tubular, ahaustral colon.

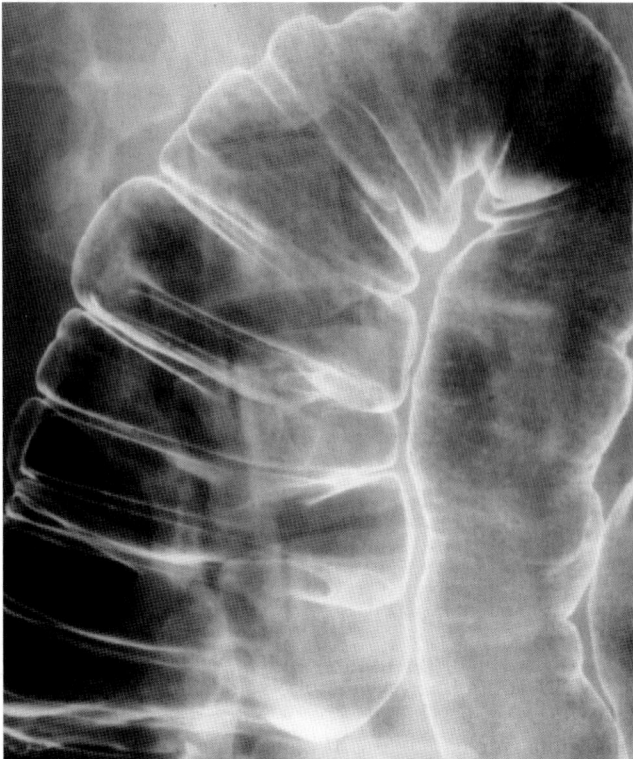

Figure 61-9. Acute ulcerative colitis: loss of haustra. Haustra distal to the hepatic flexure are absent, and the taeniae coli are relaxed. The mucosa is granular in appearance. The colon is not shortened at this point because thickening and contraction of the muscularis mucosae have not yet developed at this early stage of disease.

chronic disease, they become blunted or may be completely lost.[15] This evolution of haustral changes can be understood by a brief review of haustral formation.

At birth, colonic haustra are usually absent, which explains why it is difficult to differentiate colonic from small bowel gas in neonates. As the colon grows, the circular muscle of the muscularis propria outgrows the longitudinal muscle, the taeniae coli. This differential growth rate causes the taeniae to "shorten" the colon in an accordion-like fashion, with production of saccular haustra that usually are first seen by the age of 3 years.[41]

Haustra are fixed anatomic landmarks in the proximal colon because the circular muscle is fused to the taeniae. In the distal colon, haustra are created by active contraction of the taeniae. Consequently, the colon can normally be devoid of haustra distal to the midtransverse colon; loss of haustra in the proximal colon is always abnormal.[41,42]

In early ulcerative colitis, the haustra are deformed and thickened because of edema and may produce a corrugate outline to the colon that has been called the "indenture" sign.[43] In chronic ulcerative colitis, the haustra are often lost for two reasons: alterations in the muscle tone of the taeniae[41,42] and the fact that the colon is shortened. In this disease, the taeniae coli become relaxed for some unknown reason. This relaxation is associated with abolition of the haustral pattern. With healing, the haustra may reappear as they gain tone. A second major factor is also at work in chronic ulcerative colitis—massive hypertrophy and fixed contraction of the muscularis mucosae (Fig. 61-10), which causes foreshortening of the colon. Thus, the normal accordion-like array of colon on the relatively shorter taeniae is lost.[42,43]

Similar findings are seen on radiographs in patients with cathartic colon.[44] Cathartic colon may simulate chronic, burned-out ulcerative colitis radiographically and pathologically.[45] Apparently, cathartics such as senna stimulate the submucosal plexus of Meissner, which, in turn, stimulates the deeper intermuscular myenteric plexus. With prolonged laxative abuse, abnormal neural pathways regulating colonic motility are established, which leads to neuromuscular incoordination. Perhaps similar events occur in ulcerative colitis. On pathologic examination, the mucosa is atrophic, the submucosa is thickened with fatty deposition, the circular and longitudinal muscles of the colon are minimally thinned, and the muscularis mucosae tends to be somewhat thickened in the cathartic colon, albeit not to the extent seen in chronic ulcerative colitis. The return of haustra has been reported in cathartic colon as well.

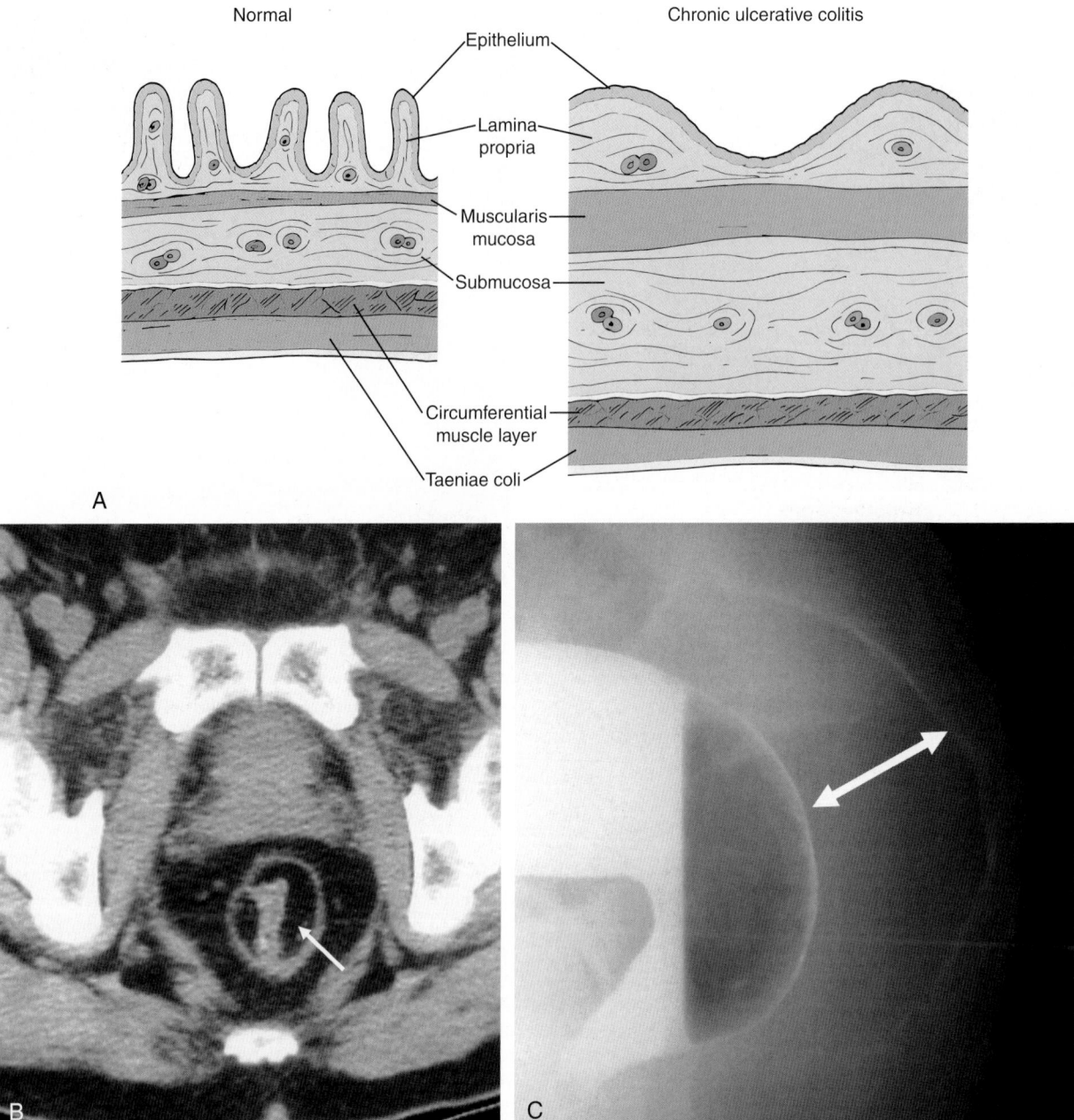

Figure 61-10. Cause of rectal contour changes in chronic ulcerative colitis. A. Diagram depicts the marked hypertrophy of the muscularis mucosae. This muscle, oriented along the long axis of the colon, is chronically contracted even after the intravenous administration of glucagon and in formalin-impregnated specimens. This contraction shortens and narrows the involved colon. The submucosa also widens and shows various degrees of fatty infiltration, further narrowing the lumen. The taeniae coli are relaxed, which abolishes the haustral folds. **B.** Pelvic CT scan shows a characteristic target or ring sign with a thickened, low-density submucosa (*arrow*) caused by fatty infiltration. The soft tissue density ring on the lumen side of the submucosa represents thickened lamina propria and muscularis mucosae; the ring on the serosal side is muscularis propria. **C.** Corresponding lateral view from an air-contrast barium enema. The mucosa has a granular appearance, the lumen is narrowed, the valves of Houston are absent, and there is significant widening of the presacral space (*arrows*). (**A** from Gore RM: Colonic contour changes in chronic ulcerative colitis: Reappraisal of some old concepts. AJR 158:59-61, 1992, © by American Roentgen Ray Society.)

Widened Presacral Space

When the rectum is distended, the retrorectal space as projected on true lateral films obtained during barium enema is usually 7.5 mm or less.[46] A distance of 1 to 1.5 cm is considered a moderate increase of this space, and a distance greater than 1.5 cm is abnormal. These values are obtained by measuring the shortest distance between the posterior edge of the barium column and the anterior edge of the second sacral segment. The presacral space is frequently widened in chronic ulcerative colitis and Crohn's disease but may also be seen in obese patients and patients with pelvic lipomatosis, pelvic carcinomatosis, radiation fibrosis, inferior vena cava thrombosis, sacral and rectal tumors, chlamydial infection, and other infectious proctitides.[47-49]

In patients with ulcerative colitis, two processes account for the abnormal presacral space (see Fig. 61-10): (1) narrowing of the rectal lumen and its associated mural thickening and (2) proliferation, inflammation, and infiltration of perirectal fat. These changes are well demonstrated by CT and correlate with the edematous adipose tissue and enlarged perirectal lymph nodes that are commonly observed at the time of abdominoperineal resection in patients with ulcerative colitis. In patients with Crohn's disease, perirectal abscesses may also contribute to this widening.[50]

Rectal Valve Abnormalities

At least one rectal valve should be visible on lateral rectal views of double-contrast enemas. The fold is usually seen at the level of S3 and S4 and should be less than 5 mm thick. The rectal valves are an important indicator of proctitis and should be interpreted with the size of the presacral space. Two situations are indicative of proctitis: (1) The presacral space is greater than 1.5 cm, with the valve thicker than 6.5 mm or absent, and (2) the presacral space is normal, but the valve thickness is greater than 6.5 mm. Absence of the rectal valves in the presence of a normal presacral space can be a normal variant.[15]

Strictures

Benign strictures are local sequelae of ulcerative colitis that occur in approximately 10% of patients.[15] They are usually localized and smoothly tapering and are only rarely sufficiently

narrow to cause obstruction. They are sometimes reversible and are found more commonly in the distal colon. Strictures that are not reversible and are located more proximally in the colon should be viewed with suspicion for a neoplasm. The strictures have been attributed to the previously described changes of the muscularis mucosae and are almost invariably associated with mural thickening on cross-sectional imaging.[51-55]

Distribution

Ulcerative colitis originates in the rectum and extends proximally in a continuous fashion. There is often a fairly sharply defined margin between diseased and normal bowel. The affected mucosa is diffusely, contiguously, confluently, circumferentially, and symmetrically involved without normal intervening mucosa. The rectum is almost invariably involved but may be spared in patients treated with corticosteroid enemas.

Computed Tomography

The subtle mucosal abnormalities that characterize the early stages of ulcerative colitis are beneath the spatial resolution of CT. With progressive disease, severe mucosal ulceration can denude certain portions of the colonic wall, leading to inflammatory pseudopolyps (Fig. 61-11).[56] When sufficiently

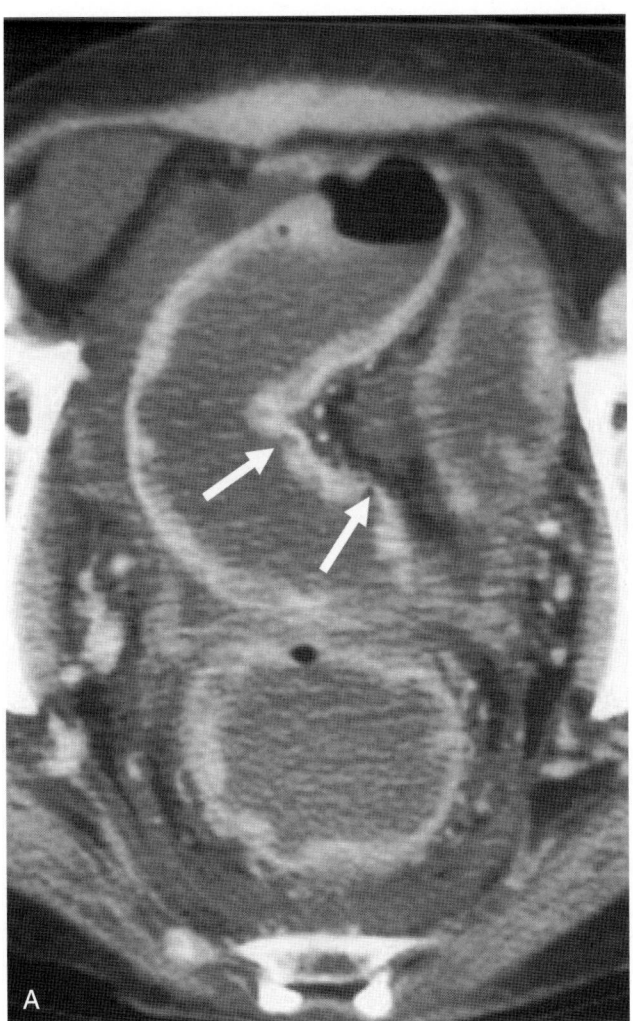

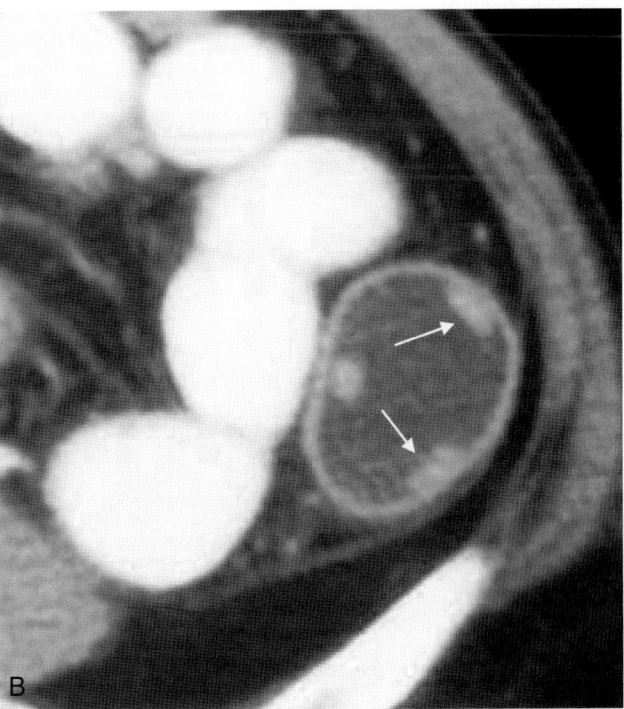

Figure 61-11. Mucosal disease in acute ulcerative colitis: CT features. A. Pelvic CT reveals diffuse mucosal thickening of fluid-filled rectum and sigmoid. Deep ulcerations (*arrows*) are visualized. Note normal lumen caliber and ascites. **B.** Magnified CT image of distal descending colon shows residual islands of inflamed mucosa protruding above denuded colonic surface—so-called inflammatory pseudopolyps (*arrows*). (From Gore RM, Balthazar E, Ghahremani GG, et al: CT features of ulcerative colitis and Crohn's disease. AJR 167:3-15, 1996. Reprinted with permission from the American Journal of Roentgenology.)

large, these pseudopolyps can be visualized on CT. Mural thinning, unsuspected perforations, and pneumatosis can be detected on CT in patients with toxic megacolon.[57] In this regard, CT can be quite helpful in determining the urgency of surgery in patients with stable abdominal radiographs yet a deteriorating clinical course. Postinflammatory pseudopolyps can also be seen on CT.

Mural thickening and luminal narrowing are common CT features of subacute and chronic ulcerative colitis (Fig. 61-12; Table 61-3). The mucosa becomes thickened because of hypertrophy of the muscularis mucosae in chronic ulcerative colitis. Additionally, the lamina propria is thickened because of round cell infiltration in both acute and chronic ulcerative colitis. The submucosa becomes thickened because of the deposition of fat or, in acute and subacute cases, edema. Submucosal thickening further contributes to luminal narrowing.[58-62]

On CT, these mural changes produce a "target" or "halo" appearance when axially imaged. The lumen is surrounded by a ring of soft tissue density (mucosa, lamina propria, hypertrophied muscularis mucosae), which is surrounded by a low-density ring (edema or fatty infiltration of the submucosa), which, in turn, is surrounded by a ring of soft tissue density (muscularis propria).[58-64] This mural stratification is not specific and can also be seen in patients with Crohn's disease, infectious enterocolitis, pseudomembranous colitis, ischemic and radiation enterocolitis, mesenteric venous thrombosis, bowel edema, and graft-versus-host disease.[58-64]

Rectal narrowing and widening of the presacral space are radiologic hallmarks of chronic ulcerative colitis.[65-68] High-resolution CT depicts the anatomic alterations that underlie

these rather dramatic morphologic changes (see Fig. 61-10). The rectal lumen is narrowed because of the previously described mural thickening that attends chronic ulcerative colitis. As a result, the rectum has a target appearance on axial scans, which should not be mistaken for the external anal sphincter, mucosal prolapse, or levator ani muscles. The increase in the presacral space is caused by proliferation of the perirectal fat.

Table 61-3

Ulcerative Colitis versus Crohn's Disease: CT Findings

Ulcerative Colitis
Mural thickening <1.5 cm
Target appearance of wall—submucosal edema (acute)
Target appearance of wall—submucosal fat (chronic)
Increased perirectal and presacral fat

Crohn's Disease
Mural thickening >2 cm
Target appearance of wall—submucosal edema (acute)
Target appearance of wall—submucosal edema (chronic)
Homogeneous CT density of wall
Mural thickening of small bowel
Abscesses, fistulas, sinus tracts
Mesenteric changes (abscess, phlegmon, fibrofatty
  proliferation)
Perianal disease

Common Findings
Mural thickening
Narrowed lumen
Increased lymph node size and number

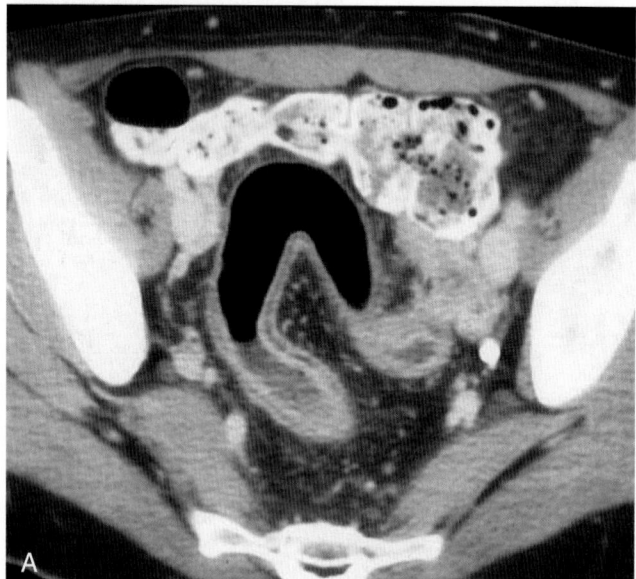

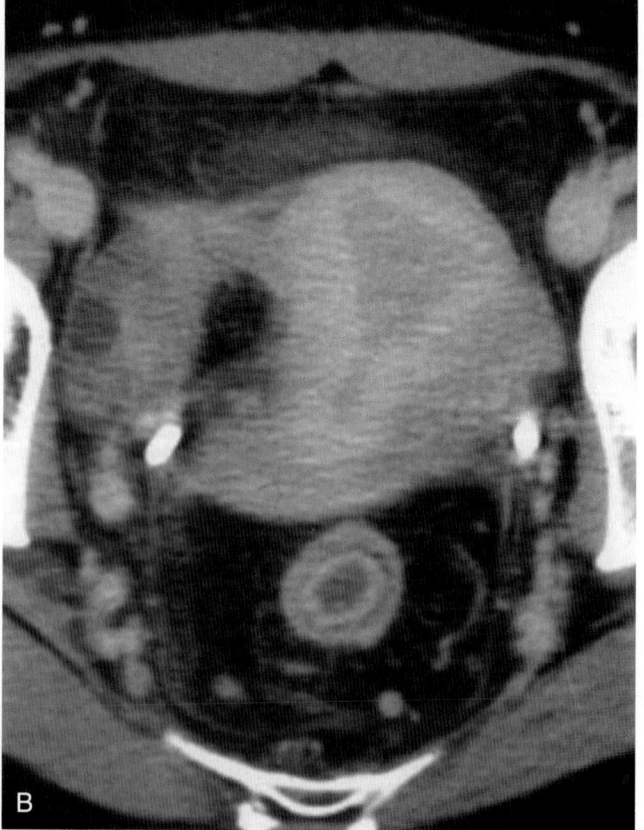

Figure 61-12. Subacute ulcerative colitis: CT features. A. CT section through the rectosigmoid reveals diffusely inflamed and thickened mucosa. The edematous submucosal layer of low attenuation is paralleled by the external layer of muscularis propria and the internal layer of submucosa, both of which have a higher attenuation. Also note the prominent blood vessels and lymph nodes in the sigmoid mesocolon. **B.** Axial CT scan shows the rectum with a target appearance produced by two higher attenuation rings (mucosa, muscularis propria) that are separated by edematous submucosa of lower attenuation. This mural stratification is typical of ulcerative colitis. (From Gore RM, Balthazar E, Ghahremani GG, et al: CT features of ulcerative colitis and Crohn's disease. AJR 167:3-15, 1996. Reprinted with permission from the American Journal of Roentgenology.)

Table 61-4
Ulcerative Colitis versus Crohn's Colitis: Sonographic Findings

Ulcerative Colitis
Moderately thick, hypoechoic wall
Typical wall stratification maintained
Loss of haustration
Absent peristaltic motion

Crohn's Colitis
Clearly thickened, hypoechoic wall
Loss of typical wall stratification
Loss of haustration
Diminished compressibility
Absent peristaltic motion
Increased blood flow of superior mesenteric artery with
    decreased resistive index

Ultrasonography

Inflammatory bowel disease alters the thickness and echogenicity of the gut wall or individual layers, the integrity of mural stratification, the appearance of surrounding tissues, and bowel motility and compressibility (Table 61-4).[69-74] Edema is a prominent feature of acute intestinal inflammation. Edema results in thickening of the colon wall and preservation of wall stratification (Fig. 61-13). On transverse section, alternate hyperechoic and hypoechoic layers give rise to a target appearance. In ulcerative colitis, the mucosa becomes thickened and hypoechoic as a result of edema.[73,74] The submucosa also thickens, yet colonic motility is maintained. With progressive disease, haustral septations are lost. In patients with well-established disease, bowel wall thickness is approximately 0.6 ± 0.2 cm.[62-67] In one series, these changes were seen in all patients with pancolitis, in 94% of those with left-sided colitis, but in only 50% of patients with rectosigmoiditis. If there is extensive pseudopolyposis, the thickness of the wall may increase to 1.5 cm, and this is often accompanied by loss of wall stratification.[68-74]

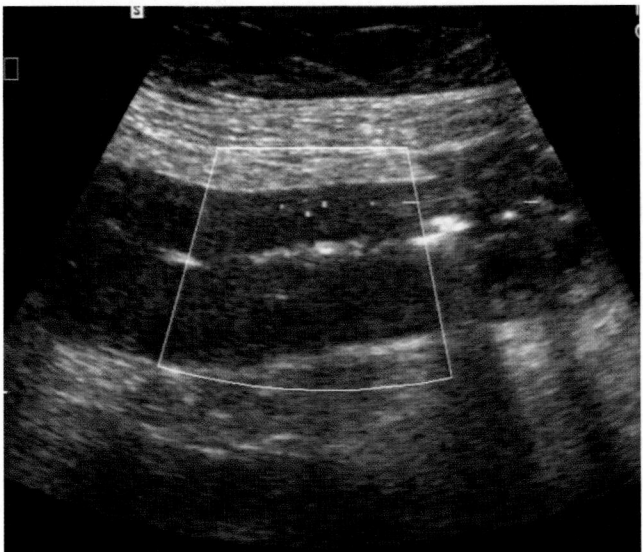

Figure 61-13. Chronic ulcerative colitis: sonographic findings. Descending colon, imaged longitudinally, shows circumferential mural thickening.

Magnetic Resonance Imaging

Magnetic resonance imaging is capable of identifying the mural stratification present in ulcerative colitis (Fig. 61-14). MRI demonstrates thickening and abnormal hypointensity of the mucosal and submucosal layers on T1-weighted and T2-weighted images. The T1 shortening probably relates to the severe hemorrhagic phenomena that frequently appear in these layers. The degree of mural enhancement correlates well with the severity of disease activity on fat-suppressed gradient-echo images after the intravenous administration of gadolinium.[75-79]

Scintigraphy

Although the diagnosis and assessment of disease activity of ulcerative colitis are made primarily by radiographic and endoscopic techniques, both gallium citrate Ga 67 (^{67}Ga)– and indium 111 (^{111}In)–labeled leukocyte scans (Fig. 61-15) have proved useful in patients with inflammatory bowel disease. Scintigraphic techniques are useful when there is danger of bowel perforation and the extent and degree of disease activity must be assessed. Positron emission tomography (PET) using

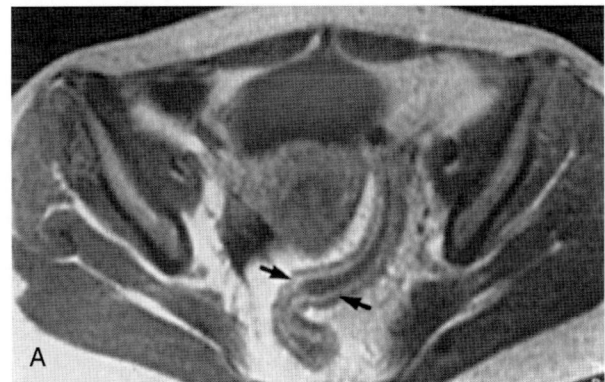

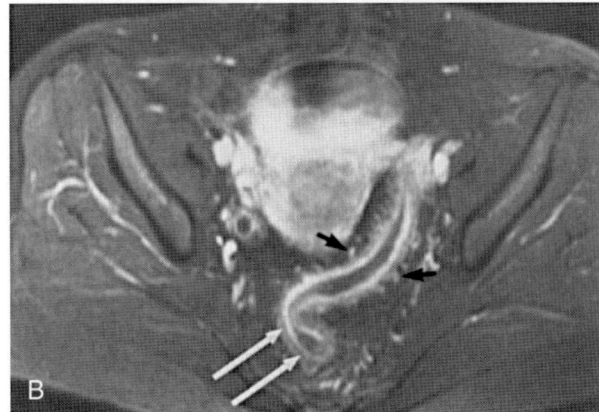

Figure 61-14. Ulcerative colitis: MRI findings. There is mural thickening of the sigmoid colon with preservation of mural stratification. Immediate postgadolinium spoiled gradient-echo (**A**) and gadolinium-enhanced T1-weighted fat-suppressed spin-echo (**B**) images. Increased enhancement on the immediate postgadolinium image reflects increased capillary blood flow observed in severe disease. On the interstitial phase image there is marked mucosal enhancement (*arrows* in **A**) with prominent vasa rectae (*short arrows* in **B**) and submucosal sparing (*long arrows* in **B**). (From Ascher SM, Semelka RC, Kelekis NL: Gastrointestinal tract. In Semelka RC, Ascher SM, Reinhold C [eds]: MRI of the Abdomen and Pelvis. New York, Wiley-Liss, Copyright © 1997, pp 257-328. Reprinted by permission of Wiley-Liss, Inc., a division of John Wiley & Sons, Inc.)

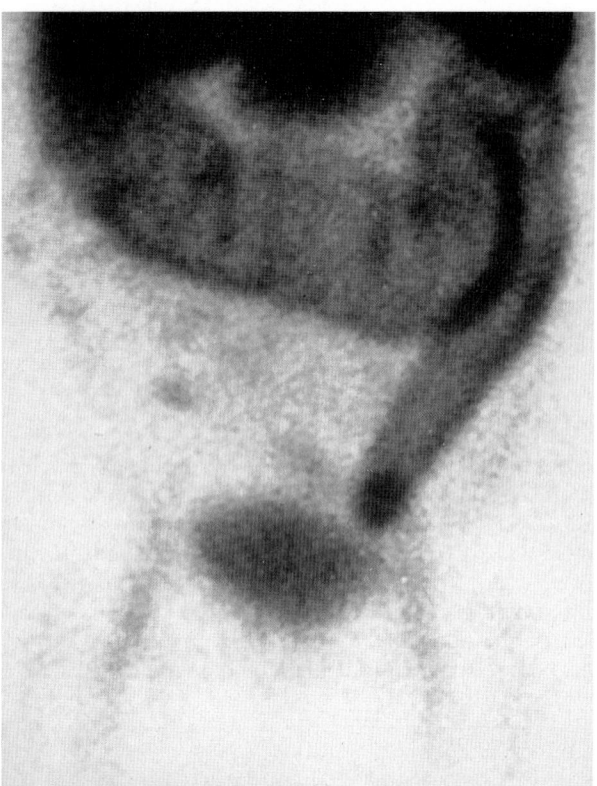

Figure 61-15. Ulcerative colitis: scintigraphic features. Increased colonic uptake of indium 111–labeled leukocytes is identified in areas of active inflammation.

^{18}F-fluorodeoxyglucose can also be used to assess disease activity. Tracer uptake (Fig. 61-16) is increased in areas of active inflammation resulting from hyperemia and increased metabolic activity.[80-84]

Therapy

Medical Management

The treatment of ulcerative colitis depends on the severity, extent, and distribution of disease. Sulfasalazine, a congener of 5-aminosalicylic acid and sulfapyridine, is effective in the treatment of acute ulcerative colitis and in reducing both the frequency and the severity of recurrent attacks.[85] Sulfasalazine attenuates the bowel inflammation by a number of actions: (1) it reduces production of prostaglandins; (2) it diminishes leukotriene production, which activates neutrophils and other constituents of the inflammatory response; (3) it blocks the chemotactic activity of formulated bacterial peptides that help recruit neutrophils to the bowel; and (4) it acts as a scavenger of oxygen free radicals.[85] Many patients develop hypersensitivity or less specific forms of intolerance; efforts are now being made to deliver the active component 5-aminosalicylic acid without the sulfapyridine moiety, which apparently causes the hypersensitivity.[85]

Corticosteroids are effective in patients with moderate to severe ulcerative colitis. They do not affect the rate or timing of disease recurrence in patients in remission. Topical hydrocortisone in the form of a foam enema is the mainstay of therapy for distal proctocolitis.[85]

Azathioprine, 6-mercaptopurine, chloroquine, hydroxychloroquine sulfate (Plaquenil), methotrexate, and cyclosporine are alternative therapies in patients with refractory disease. Bowel rest and nutritional therapy also have beneficial effects on this disease.[85]

Increased concentrations of leukotrienes in the inflamed mucosa in ulcerative colitis have suggested the use of inhibitors of leukotriene B$_4$ (LTB$_4$) for therapy because this is a highly potent mediator of inflammation. LTB$_4$ receptor antagonists are under investigation as are inhibitors of platelet-activating factor and mast cell stabilizers.[85-87]

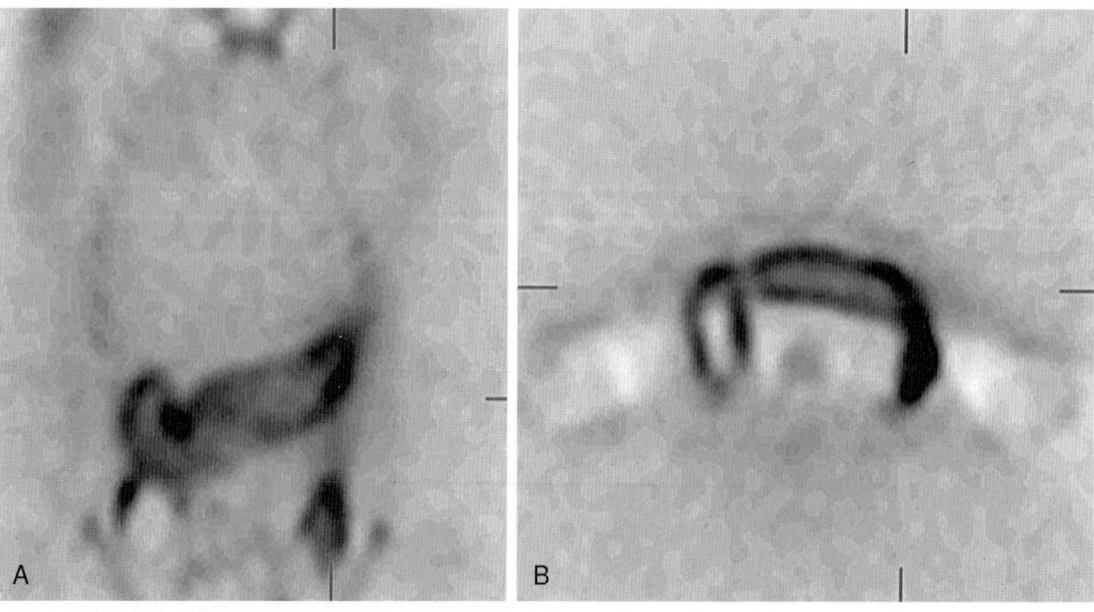

Figure 61-16. Ulcerative colitis: positron emission tomography scanning features. Coronal (**A**) and axial (**B**) images using ^{18}F-fluorodeoxyglucose show increased tracer uptake throughout the colon in this patient with severe pancolitis. (Courtesy of John R. Mernagh, MD, and John Rawlinson, MD, Hamilton, Ontario, Canada.)

Surgery

Although proctocolectomy is always curative for ulcerative colitis, this procedure carries an operative risk, and not all patients are willing to accept an ileostomy. Consequently, colectomy is not indicated for patients who are easily managed medically. There are several major indications for surgery in ulcerative colitis: (1) massive, unremitting colonic hemorrhage; (2) toxic megacolon with impending or frank perforation; (3) fulminant colitis that is unresponsive to antibiotic, supportive, and corticosteroid therapy; (4) obstruction from a stricture; and (5) suspicion or demonstration of colon cancer. Less immediate and definite indications for colectomy are (1) intractable, chronic disease that becomes a physical and social burden to the patient; (2) failure of children to mature at an acceptable rate; and (3) high-grade dysplasia in a patient with pancolitis.[88] Fulminant acute disease accounts for 13% to 25% of colectomies in patients with ulcerative colitis. Many of the extraintestinal complications of ulcerative colitis, such as uveitis and pyoderma gangrenosum, are also eliminated by colectomy. However, the course of hepatobiliary disease and ankylosing spondylitis is usually not altered by surgery.[88-90] Since the 1980s, tremendous advances have been made in the surgical approach to ulcerative colitis that offer the patient and surgeon a variety of options.

Proctocolectomy with a Brooke Ileostomy

After a proctocolectomy is performed, the end of the ileum is passed through an opening in the middle aspect of the right rectus muscle at a point beneath the umbilicus that allows convenient placement of the forepiece of an ileostomy bag. This procedure is curative and requires one operation, but the patient must constantly wear an external ileostomy appliance that needs to be emptied four to eight times per day. Perineal wound problems, stoma revision, and small bowel obstruction occur in 10% to 25% of patients. This is the fastest, safest operation, but it dramatically alters body image in many, particularly younger, patients.[88-90]

Proctocolectomy with Continent Ileostomy (Kock Pouch)

A continent ileostomy is made by creating a pouch out of terminal ileum to hold the intestinal contents, an ileal conduit that leads from the pouch to the stoma, and an intervening intestinal valve. Patients empty the pouch by passing a tube through the valve via the stoma. The ileostomy is continent, so that an external appliance is not needed. The nipple valve is created by intussuscepting the terminal ileum in a retrograde manner into the pouch for 3 to 4 cm. Anatomic complications requiring reoperation develop in 40% to 50% of these patients.[91-95]

Total Colectomy with Ileorectal Anastomosis

Total colectomy with ileorectal anastomosis is no longer popular because of a fairly high complication rate and unpredictable functional result.[91-95]

Total Proctocolectomy, Rectal Mucosal Stripping, and Ileal Pouch Formation with Anastomosis to the Sphincter

An abdominal colectomy and a mucosal proctectomy are performed. A J pouch or W-shaped pouch is fashioned out of ileum. This reservoir is then anastomosed to the anus

(Fig. 61-17). The endorectal ileal pouch/anal anastomosis is given 8 weeks to heal by diverting the gut through a conventional ileostomy.[90-95]

The advantages of this procedure are that no stoma is required and that fecal continence is usually maintained,

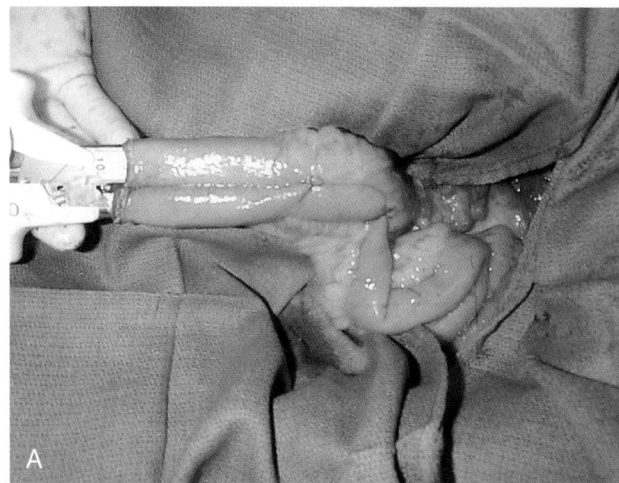

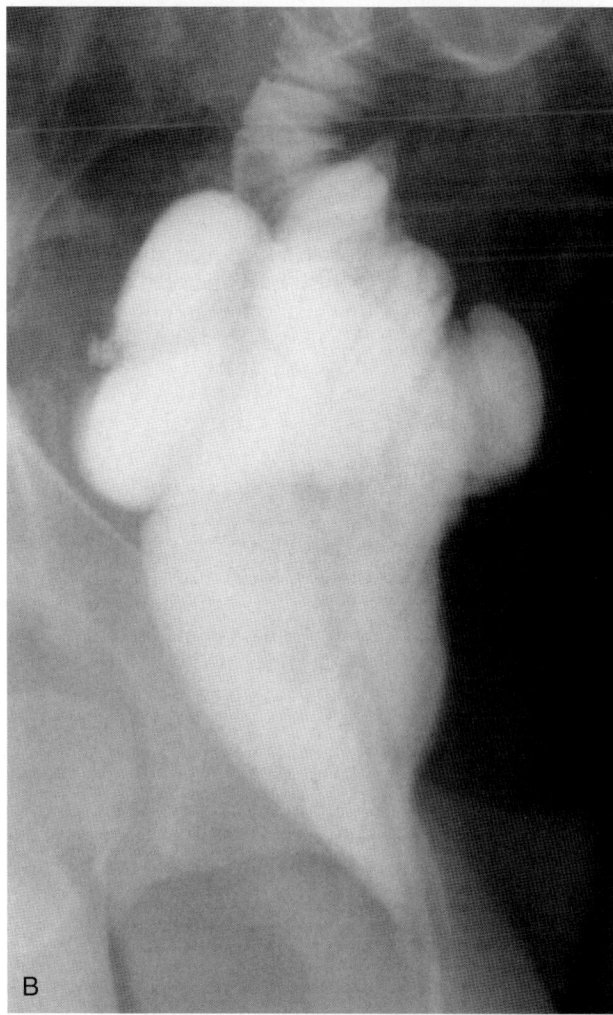

Figure 61-17. Surgical management of ulcerative colitis ileal pouch-anal anastomosis. A. The two-loop ileal J pouch shown in the intraoperative image is simple to construct, provides adequate storage capacity, and is evacuated spontaneously and fully. **B.** Barium enema evaluation of such a pouch.

albeit with bowel movements four to eight times per day. This procedure is technically demanding and requires two operations. Complications include postoperative abscess, pouch fistulas, stenosis, small bowel obstruction, and pouchitis. Approximately 15% of patients require reoperation, and some ultimately require a conventional ileostomy. Pouchitis is an inflammatory process that can cause tenesmus, bloody diarrhea, and constitutional symptoms similar to those of ulcerative colitis.[95-100]

Prognosis

The prognosis in ulcerative colitis has improved dramatically. Most patients have mild to moderate disease, and only 15% to 25% require a colectomy. Mortality associated with ulcerative colitis occurs in the first 2 years of disease, primarily in patients older than age 40 years: one third attributable to the colonic disease itself, one third caused by complications of the disease (colorectal cancer, sclerosing cholangitis, thromboembolic disease, medical and surgical therapy), and the remaining third attributable to unrelated causes. Excess mortality of 2.1% for men and 1.5% for women has been reported but only for the first 2 years of disease.[10] Most patients with ulcerative colitis are able to cope with their disease and achieve what is subjectively interpreted as a relatively acceptable lifestyle.[10]

CROHN'S DISEASE

Crohn's disease is a chronic, cicatrizing disorder of the alimentary tract characterized by granulomatous inflammation of the mucosa, bowel wall, and surrounding mesentery. Any portion of the alimentary tract may be involved, but the terminal ileum and proximal colon are most frequently diseased.[2,4,6]

Historical Perspective

It is difficult to decide who described the first case of "regional ileitis" or "ileocolitis."[1] In 1806, Combe and Saunders described "a singular case of stricture and thickening of the ileum." Although similar cases were reported in the 19th century and early years of the 20th century, the first series of satisfactorily documented cases of regional enteritis was described by Crohn, Ginzburg, and Oppenheimer in 1932 at Mount Sinai Hospital in New York City.[2,4,6] Crohn's disease was originally called *terminal ileitis* because these cases were located mainly in the distal ileum in young persons. The outstanding complaints of the patients were diarrhea and weight loss, with progressive anemia and fever. Pathologic examination showed a thickened intestinal wall with subacute or chronic necrotizing inflammation and a greatly enlarged mesentery. Small linear ulcerations with distorted and broken mucosal folds and a "cobblestone" appearance were noted. The ulceration of the mucosa was accompanied by a disproportionate connective tissue reaction in the bowel wall, leading to stenosis and multiple fistulas. The lumen was "irregularly encroached" with dilatation of proximal areas of the bowel.[2,4,6,101,102] Many years later, it was realized that Crohn's disease might be confined to the colon without affecting the ileum, and it is now recognized that Crohn's disease can involve every portion of the gut from the mouth to the anus.[2,4,6]

Pathogenesis and Etiology

The cause of Crohn's disease remains unknown. Although the participation of genetic, environmental, infectious, immunologic, and psychologic factors in the pathogenesis is well established, none of these mechanisms has proved to be the primary causative agent.[102] Genetic vulnerability is likely to facilitate the occurrence of the disease, whereas the other factors may play a supportive and superimposed role. A further complicating factor in establishing a cause is the fact that, in practice, Crohn's disease does not behave as a single disorder.[6,11]

More recently, interest has centered on immunologic mechanisms, in particular the role of platelet-activating factor. Platelet-activating factor is a species of phosphatidylcholine that causes inflammation that is detectable in colonic mucosa in inflammatory bowel disease but is not present in normal colonic mucosa. Production of platelet-activating factor is stimulated by a number of inflammatory mediators, such as prostaglandin and leukotrienes. In vitro studies have demonstrated that levels of several prostaglandin species are significantly elevated in the mucosa in Crohn's colitis and ulcerative colitis. Local release of LTB_4 by the rectal mucosa is considerably increased in ulcerative colitis but is elevated in Crohn's colitis only when frank ulceration is present.[2,4,6,11] Consequently, the hunt is on for safe inhibitors of platelet-activating factor, which could prove to be a powerful new form of therapy.

Other immunologic evidence suggests that there is a failure of suppressor cell generation coupled with a hyperactive state of helper T cells in patients with inflammatory bowel disease. The activated T cells may then lead to an overactive immune response that is not turned off. This response results in increased macrophage activation, enhanced cytokine production, and augmented antibody secretion. Although immunologic factors are important, no specific antibody-producing antigen has been identified in the intestinal mucosa in patients with inflammatory bowel disease. Also, there is still no convincing demonstration of any fundamental underlying immune defect. Further evidence against immunodeficiency as the cause of Crohn's disease comes from the report of a patient who had a prolonged remission coincidental with acquiring human immunodeficiency virus infection. Likewise, exhaustive efforts to relate mycobacterial infection to Crohn's disease have been unsuccessful. A defect in mucosal permeability that permits absorption of macromolecules and complex sugars may be another important factor in the pathophysiology of Crohn's disease. Apparently healthy relatives of patients with Crohn's disease show the same intestinal permeability defect. This finding suggests that this defect may antedate intestinal inflammation and may also play a causative role.[2,4,6,11]

Epidemiology

Although understanding of the epidemiology of Crohn's disease is unclear, investigators hope that more precise information will yield important clues about etiology.[11] The

Table 61-5
Epidemiology of Crohn's Disease

Worldwide prevalence: 10-70 cases/100,000 population
Annual incidence:* 0.6-6.3 cases/100,000 population
Bimodal age distribution: Peak at 15-25 yr; smaller peak at 50-80 yr
Risk factors
   White race
   Jewish (8-fold increase)
   Residence in urban area
   Family history of disease
   Sibling with disease (30-fold increase)
   Single
   Oral contraceptive use
   Smoking (4-fold increase)

*Incidence has increased 1.4 to 4 times in past 40 years.

salient epidemiologic features of this disease are listed in Table 61-5.

Crohn's disease is an uncommon but not rare disease with a reported incidence between 0.6 and 6.3 cases per 100,000 population. Worldwide prevalence ranges from 10 to 70 cases per 100,000 population; this wide variation is probably due to true differences in disease distribution as well as to differences in reporting, diagnostic criteria, and availability of medical care.[2,4,7]

Crohn's disease is most common in the developed countries of Europe and Scandinavia, the United States, and Israel. The incidence is lower in Southern and Eastern Europe and the former Soviet Union. The disease is uncommon in Central and South America and Cuba and is rare in Asia and Africa. Crohn's disease has been increasing in incidence over the past 40 years by a factor of 1.4-fold to 4-fold.[2,4,7] Crohn's disease is more common in white than in African American or Asian persons, and the sex distribution is equal.[2,4,7]

There is a sevenfold to eightfold increase of Crohn's disease among Jews. The rates are highest for American Jews and much lower in Israeli-born and non-Ashkenazi Jews. These disparate rates found in different countries suggest the likelihood of hereditary predisposition that may be altered by environmental factors.[2,4,7] Crohn's disease has a bimodal age distribution. The peak incidence is between the ages of 15 and 25 years, with a lower peak between 50 and 80 years. It occasionally occurs in children as young as 2 years old.[2,4,7]

Crohn's disease is generally acknowledged to be more common in urban than in rural populations, but the literature is conflicting on this matter.[2,4,7] Epidemiologic data show that 4.5% to 16.6% of patients with Crohn's disease have a positive family history. The disease is 30 times more frequent in siblings than in the general population. Familial inflammatory bowel disease seems to follow a polygenic inheritance pattern.[2,4,7]

Crohn's disease runs a clinical course with seasonal exacerbations. The highest relapse rate is found in the autumn and winter; the lowest is in the summer. This pattern suggests that seasonal or exogenous factors may be involved in relapse.[2,4,7] Although nonsmoking is a feature of ulcerative colitis, patients with Crohn's disease are four times more likely to be smokers than matched controls.[2,4,7]

The mortality rate of Crohn's disease has significantly declined, and this can be attributed to improvements in diagnosis and management. The mortality rates for all inflamma-

tory bowel disease for white American men were 5.88 per 1 million in 1970 to 1971 and 2.68 per 1 million in 1982; the rates for white American women were 7.24 and 3.48 per 1 million population.[12]

Clinical Findings

The clinical manifestations of Crohn's disease are protean.[2,4,11] The most frequently encountered initial features are rectal bleeding, diarrhea, and abdominal pain. Two major types of pain occur in patients with Crohn's disease. The first type is often mild, colicky, situated in the lower abdomen, and relieved by defecation. It tends to occur in association with diffuse Crohn's disease involving the colon and simulates the pain of ulcerative colitis. The second type is more severe and often situated in the right lower quadrant, simulating appendicitis. In a World Organization of Gastroenterology survey, three fourths of patients with Crohn's disease had abdominal pain at presentation.[2,4,11]

Some degree of diarrhea usually accompanies active Crohn's disease, but it is less severe than the often explosive diarrhea of ulcerative colitis. Almost half of all patients with Crohn's colitis experience at least minor rectal bleeding during the active phase of disease. Profuse bleeding is much more common in ulcerative colitis. The presence of mucus in the stool is also more frequent in ulcerative colitis than in Crohn's disease. Many of the most severe symptoms reflect complications such as abscess, fistula, and perianal lesions rather than Crohn's disease itself.

Physical examination in patients with inflammatory bowel disease is often normal in quiescent disease. In severe cases, pallor, dehydration, anemia, weight loss, finger clubbing, abdominal distention, tachycardia, and fever may be found. Abdominal tenderness and distention, pronounced wasting, and emaciation are more frequently found in Crohn's disease than in ulcerative colitis. An intra-abdominal mass is common in Crohn's disease but is rarely present in ulcerative colitis. The masses and tenderness usually occur on the right side in patients with Crohn's disease.

No examination of the patient with possible inflammatory bowel disease is complete without a detailed rectal examination, including sigmoidoscopy. Circumferential, confluent, and contiguous inflammatory changes were found in 96% of patients with ulcerative colitis in the World Organization of Gastroenterology series.[2,4,11] Patchy, inflammatory changes with areas of normal intervening mucosa were highly suggestive of Crohn's disease, occurring in two thirds of patients with Crohn's proctosigmoiditis. Simple inspection may reveal severe perianal disease, which strongly suggests the diagnosis of Crohn's disease.[2,4,11]

Endoscopic Findings

Aphthoid lesions, cobblestoning, and ulcers in an area of otherwise apparently normal mucosa are diagnostic of Crohn's disease versus ulcerative colitis but can be seen in other colitides. Mucosal granularity and friability are common in early ulcerative colitis but may be a late finding in Crohn's colitis. The rectum is often grossly normal in patients with Crohn's disease, and involvement is typically asymmetric and discontinuous.[2,4,14]

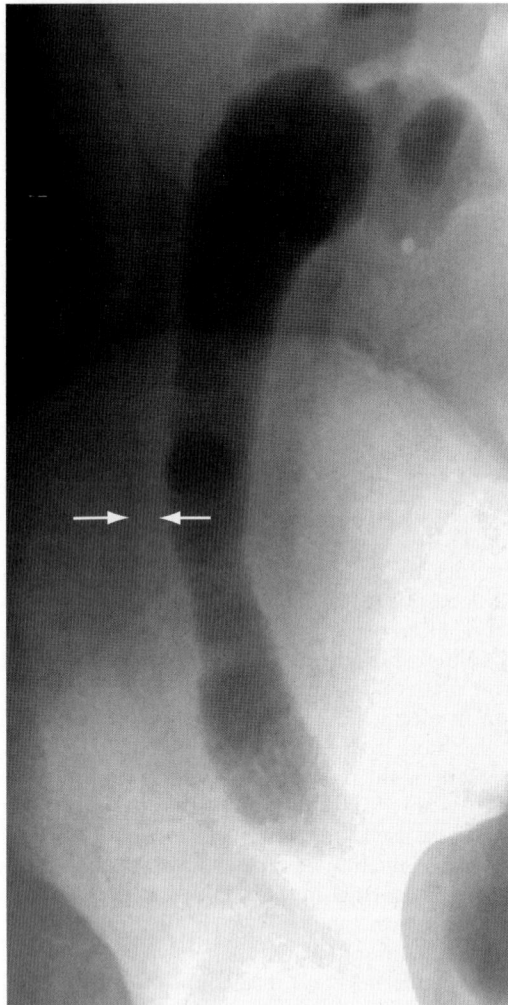

Figure 61-18. Crohn's disease: plain radiograph. The ascending colon is tubular and ahaustral. Note the mural thickening (*arrows*).

Radiologic Findings

Radiography

When confined to the colon, Crohn's disease (Fig. 61-18) has features similar to those of ulcerative colitis on radiographs. An extended gas-filled stricture of the colon is suggestive of granulomatous colitis but can also be seen in ulcerative colitis, carcinoma, and healing ischemic colitis.[16,21]

Small bowel obstruction can be seen on radiographs in patients with Crohn's disease of the small bowel. It is uncommon to identify stenotic small bowel segments on radiographs because gas is not present in the small bowel as often as is found in the colon. Occasionally, a markedly dilated segment of small bowel, reminiscent of a dilated loop of small bowel volvulus or Meckel diverticulum, can be seen between two stenotic areas.[16,21] Evidence of nephrolithiasis, gallstones, ankylosing spondylitis, sacroiliitis, avascular necrosis of the femoral heads, and disorders associated with Crohn's disease and its therapy should also be sought on abdominal radiographs.

Table 61-6
Crohn's Colitis: Findings of Barium Enema

Early Changes	Late Changes
Nodular lymphoid hyperplasia	Fissures
Aphthoid ulcerations	Fistulas
Deep ulcerations	Haustral loss
Confluent ulcerations	Sacculations
"Cobblestone" appearance	Postinflammatory
Asymmetrical involvement	pseudopolyps
Inflammatory pseudopolyps	Intramural abscess strictures
Segmental distribution	
Skip lesions	

Barium Enema

The barium enema features of Crohn's colitis are listed in Table 61-6, summarized in Figure 61-19, and discussed more fully subsequently.

Lymphoid Hyperplasia

Lymphoid follicles are a normal component of gut-associated lymphatic tissue. They are aggregates of lymphocytes surrounding germinal centers that straddle the muscularis mucosae. Lymphoid follicles have an average macroscopic density of 3.8 per centimeter of adult human colon.[25,103] They are seen in 50% of barium studies performed on children and 13% of air-contrast barium enemas in adults. Lymphoid follicles appear as 1- to 3-mm elevations in the mucosa without a ring shadow.[103,104]

Lymphoid follicles may enlarge in a wide variety of infectious, neoplastic, immunologic, and inflammatory diseases of the gut, including Crohn's disease.[105] Prominent lymphoid follicles have also been observed in older patients with colonic adenomas and carcinomas.[106]

Aphthoid Ulcerations

As the lymphoid follicles enlarge, the overlying mucosa may ulcerate with production of the aphthous lesion. These small, superficial ulcers have erythematous margins and are seen on a background of normal or near-normal mucosa.[25] This is in direct contrast to ulcerative colitis, in which ulceration invariably occurs against a background of heavy inflammation. Aphthae are recognized radiographically as punctate central collections of barium surrounded by a radiolucent halo about 1 mm in diameter that produces a target or "bull's-eye" appearance (Fig. 61-20).[107-113] Aphthae may be isolated, be found in clusters, or involve the entire colon.[108]

Aphthoid lesions are found in 44% to 72% of patients with Crohn's disease and may be the only abnormality found in an otherwise normal colon.[2,4,109] These ulcers are nonspecific and occur in amebiasis, salmonellosis, shigellosis, herpes, cytomegalovirus infection, Behçet's disease, ischemic colitis, and *Yersinia* enterocolitis.[2,4]

Cobblestoning

The aphthous lesions may regress, remain stable, or more commonly enlarge and deepen.[111,113] As the aphthae expand, they become irregular in outline and lose their surrounding lucent halo. Adjacent ulcers may coalesce, forming a network

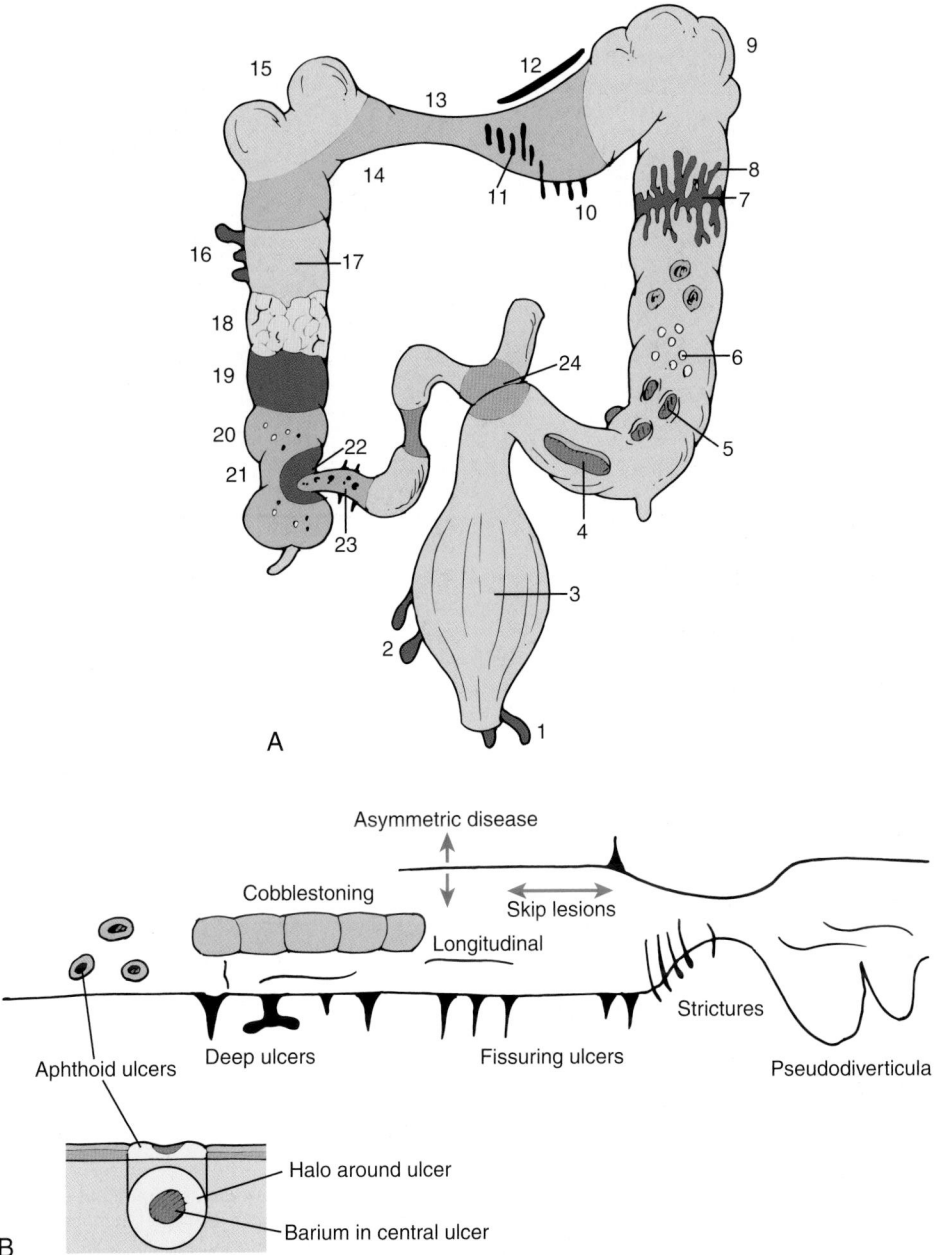

Figure 61-19. Spectrum of radiologic changes in Crohn's colitis on double-contrast barium enema examinations. A. 1, Perianal disease: ulcers, abscess, fissures, anocutaneous fistula; 2, deep rectal ulcers; 3, normal rectum in 50% of cases; 4, island ulcer; 5, circular discrete ulcers; 6, aphthoid ulcers; 7, serpiginous ulceration formed by coalition in a longitudinal form of circular and island ulcers; 8, thickening of the bowel wall; 9, normal skip areas; 10, rose thorn–shaped fissures; 11, transverse stripes of Welin (en face fissures or crevices between adjacent swollen mucosal folds); 12, linear confluent intramural ulceration, "double tracking"; 13, stricture (25% of cases); 14, eccentric disease, not involving the entire circumference; 15, pseudosacculations, produced by fibrosis of the opposite wall; 16, deep pleomorphic ulcers–composite, horned, saccular; 17, a normal patch surrounded by disease (and patches of disease surrounded by normal mucosa also occur); 18, inflammatory and postinflammatory pseudopolyps; 19, cobblestone mucosa–islands of residual swollen mucosa bounded by intersecting linear ulcers; 20, right-sided disease with normal rectum and distal colon; 21, contracted, cone-shaped cecum; 22, enlarged ileocecal valve usually associated with involvement of the terminal ileum; 23, small bowel disease in 60% of cases; 24, ileocolic fistula. **B.** Diagram further depicts mucosal abnormalities in Crohn's colitis. (**A** from Simpkins KC: Inflammatory bowel disease: Ulcerative and Crohn's colitis. In Simpkins KC [ed]: A Textbook of Radiological Diagnosis, vol 4, The Alimentary Tract: The Hollow Organs and Salivary Glands. London, HK Lewis, 1988, pp 473-498; **B** from Bartram CI, Kumar P: Clinical Radiology in Gastroenterology. Oxford, Blackwell Scientific, 1981, p 138.)

of longitudinal linear ulceration and transverse fissuring, with edematous intervening mucosa producing a raised, cobbled appearance (Fig. 61-21).[15] As mentioned earlier, this condition is actually one of many forms of inflammatory pseudopolyposis.

Deep Ulcerations

Fissuring ulcers (Fig. 61-22) are a distinctive feature of Crohn's disease. They typically penetrate beyond the submucosa, with resultant knife-shaped or "rose thorn" fistulas.[25] These fissures and fistulas do not cause pneumoperitoneum

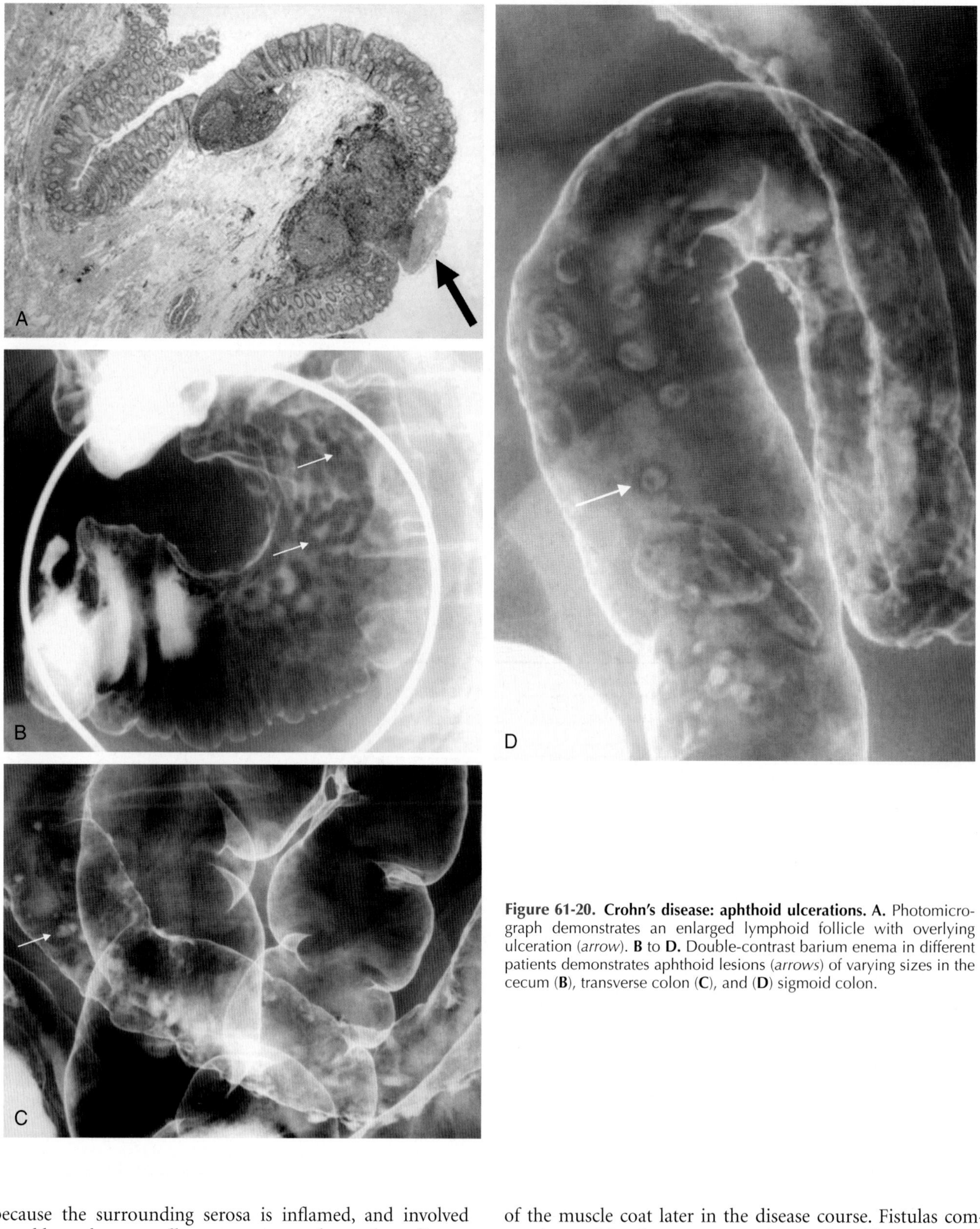

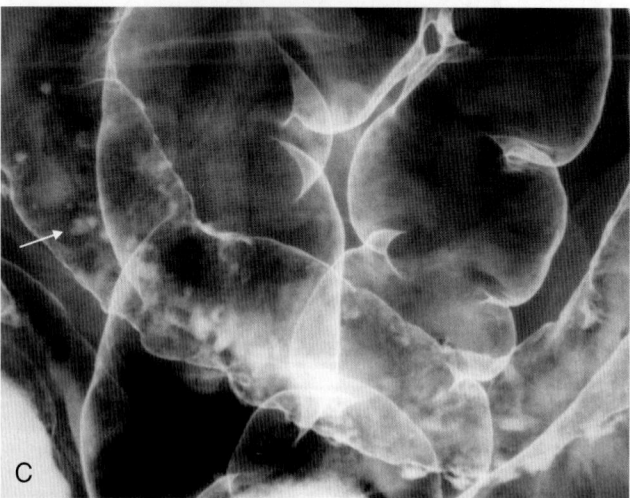

Figure 61-20. Crohn's disease: aphthoid ulcerations. A. Photomicrograph demonstrates an enlarged lymphoid follicle with overlying ulceration (*arrow*). **B to D.** Double-contrast barium enema in different patients demonstrates aphthoid lesions (*arrows*) of varying sizes in the cecum (**B**), transverse colon (**C**), and (**D**) sigmoid colon.

because the surrounding serosa is inflamed, and involved bowel loops become adherent to one another and to adjacent peritoneal surfaces.[25,39,40]

Sinus Tracts, Fissures, and Fistulas

Sinuses, fissures, and fistulas (Fig. 61-23) are a hallmark of Crohn's disease.[2,4,11] Sinuses and fissures represent blind-ended inflammatory tracts that penetrate through the full thickness

of the muscle coat later in the disease course. Fistulas communicate with other structures. Anatomic evidence suggests that mechanical factors, such as elevated intraluminal pressure, rather than any intrinsic pathologic change of Crohn's disease, are responsible for these fissures and fistulas.[2] This suggestion is based on the facts that there is a significant coincidence of sinuses and strictures and that sinuses arise proximal to the point of maximal stricture. In addition,

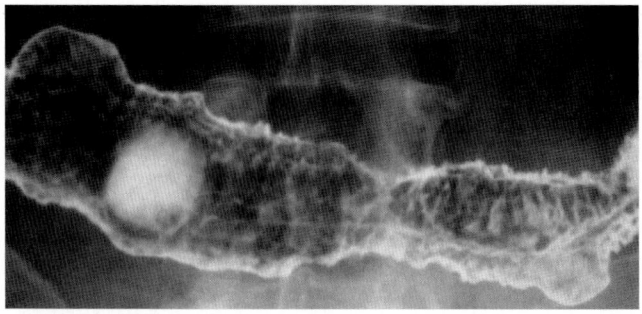

Figure 61-21. Crohn's disease: cobblestone mucosa. Longitudinal and transverse ulcers of the transverse colon produce a cobblestone appearance.

fissures, sinuses, and fistulas are not constantly associated with myocytolysis, a seemingly necessary process if only the Crohn's inflammation is required for the fissuring.[2,4]

Long interconnecting fistulas are common in Crohn's colitis and occur in the muscularis mucosae or subserosa paralleling the bowel lumen. When not associated with neoplasia or diverticula, pericolic sinus tracts are suggestive of Crohn's disease.[25-27]

Mural Thickening

The mural thickening that occurs in Crohn's disease is more impressive than that found in ulcerative colitis. It is due to transmural inflammation and fibrosis. The submucosa may also accumulate fat in Crohn's disease as well but less commonly than in ulcerative colitis. CT nicely demonstrates mural thickening of the esophagus, stomach, duodenum, small bowel, and colon when these areas are involved by Crohn's disease.

Luminal Narrowing and Strictures

Crohn's disease is a transmural inflammatory process that produces gut wall thickening and fibrosis leading to narrowing of the lumen and shortening of the gut as well.[2,4,6] In ulcerative colitis, narrowing results from thickening and contractions of the muscularis mucosae rather than from fibrosis. Strictures are asymmetric in Crohn's disease and tend to be less smooth and circumferential than those seen in ulcerative colitis. Strictures occur in 21% of patients with small bowel disease and 8% of patients with Crohn's colitis.[28]

Sacculations

The transmural fibrosis of Crohn's disease is often asymmetric. It occurs predominantly on the mesenteric side of the gut, where it is often accompanied by creeping fat of the mesentery. The relatively unaffected side (usually antimesenteric) remains pliable and tends to bulge when luminal pressure increases because of peristalsis. Outpouchings may eventually develop. The outpouchings are similar to the so-called pseudosacculations (Fig. 61-24) or pseudodiverticula seen in scleroderma.[25,27]

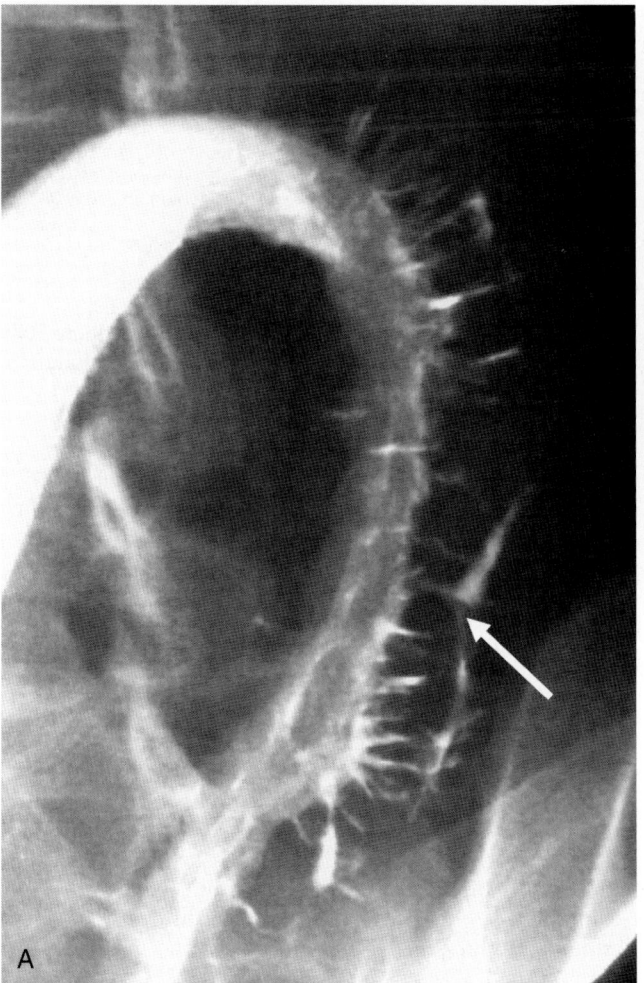

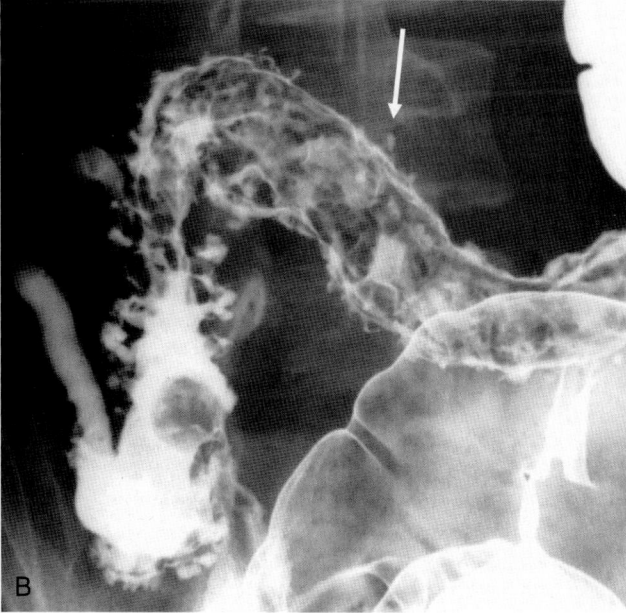

Figure 61-22. Crohn's disease: deep ulcerations. A. Multiple deep ulcerations are identified in the descending colon. They communicate with a paracolic sinus tract (*arrow*). **B.** The splenic flexure demonstrates deep ulcers (*arrow*), a large ileocecal valve, and sparing of the sigmoid colon. The appendix is subhepatic in location.

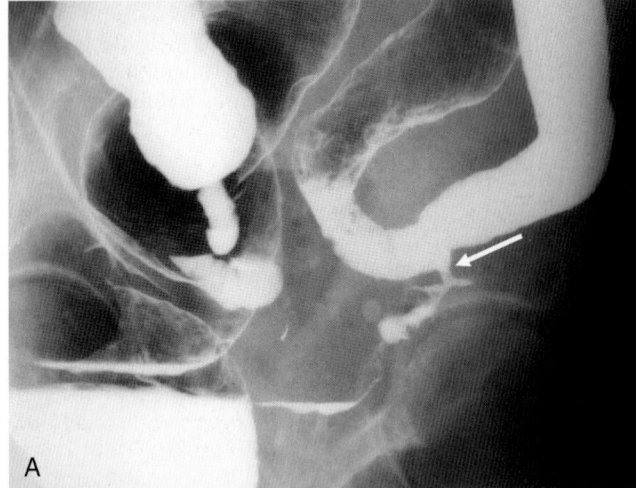

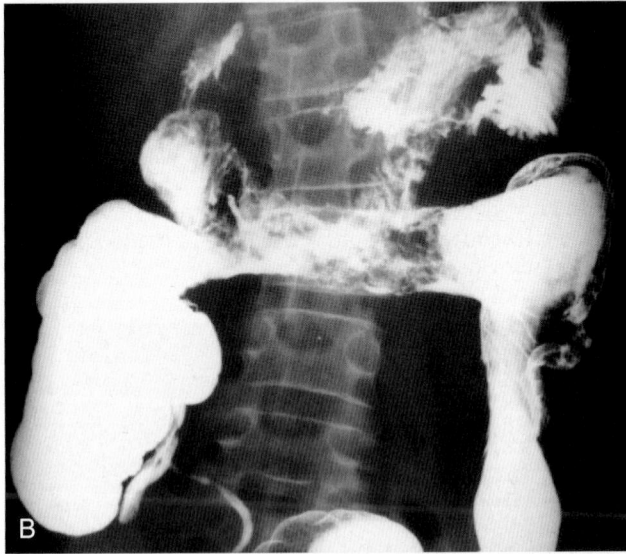

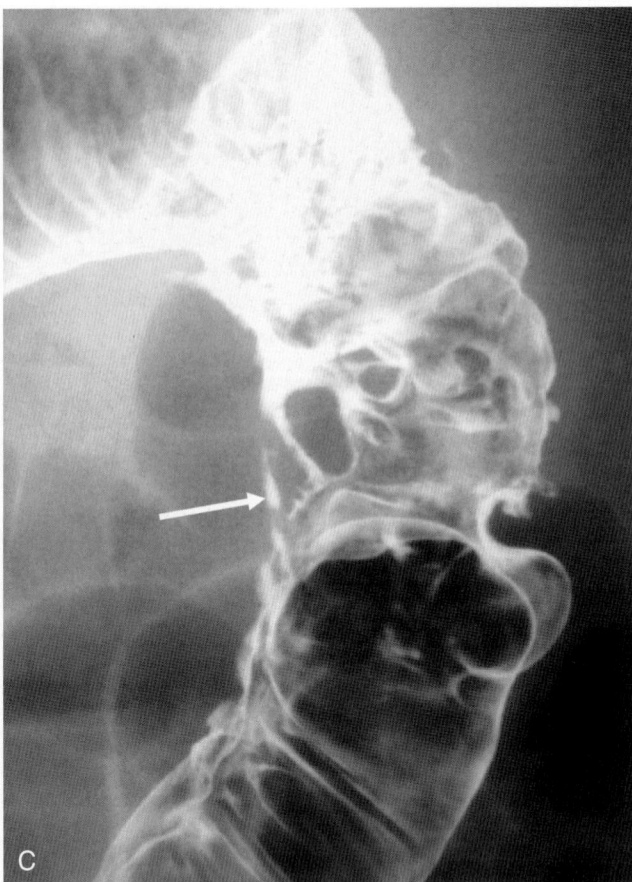

Figure 61-23. Crohn's disease: fistulas and sinus tracts. A. Fistula (*arrow*) between the sigmoid colon and adjacent small bowel is demonstrated on barium enema study. **B.** Barium enema examination shows fistula between transverse colon and duodenum. **C.** Paracolic sinus tract (*arrow*) is demonstrated in a patient with previous resection of transverse colon and an ascending-descending colon anastomosis.

Anorectal Disease

Anorectal complications are common in patients with Crohn's disease (Fig. 61-25) and include anal fissures, ulcers, abscess, internal hemorrhoids, and stenosis with induration; skin lesions such as erosion, skin tags, ulceration, maceration, external hemorrhoids, and abscess; and fistulas—anal canal to skin, rectum to skin, and rectovaginal. Anal disease develops in 36% of all patients with Crohn's disease, 25% of those with only small bowel involvement, 67% of those with colonic disease, and nearly all patients with rectal disease.[31] In approximately one fourth of patients, the anal disease may antedate overt intestinal disease often by 4 years. Accordingly, development of these anorectal disorders warrants radiologic investigation of the entire gastrointestinal tract.[2,4,31]

Distribution

Any portion of the gut, from the mouth to the anus, may be involved by Crohn's disease. Twenty percent of cases are isolated to the colon, 20% are restricted to the small bowel, and 60% involve the colon and small bowel simultaneously. In 5% to 10% of these patients, upper gastrointestinal tract involvement is seen. It is unusual to see isolated esophageal or gastroduodenal Crohn's disease. Regardless of location,

radiographic and pathologic findings are similar: there is discontinuous, patchy, and asymmetric disease involvement.[2,4,6]

Computed Tomography

Crohn's disease is manifested on CT (see Table 61-3) by bowel wall thickening of 1 to 2 cm.[114] This thickening, which occurs in 83% of patients, is most frequently observed in the terminal ileum, but other portions of the small bowel, colon, duodenum, stomach, and esophagus may be similarly affected.[62,65]

During the acute, noncicatrizing phase of Crohn's disease, the small bowel and colon maintain mural stratification (Fig. 61-26) and often have a target or double halo appearance.[56,115] As in ulcerative colitis, there is a soft tissue density ring (corresponding to mucosa), which is surrounded by a low-density ring with an attenuation near water or fat (corresponding to submucosal edema or fat infiltration), which, in turn, is surrounded by a higher density ring (muscularis propria).[116] Inflamed mucosa and serosa may show significant contrast enhancement after bolus intravenous contrast administration, and the intensity of enhancement correlates with the clinical activity of disease.[117]

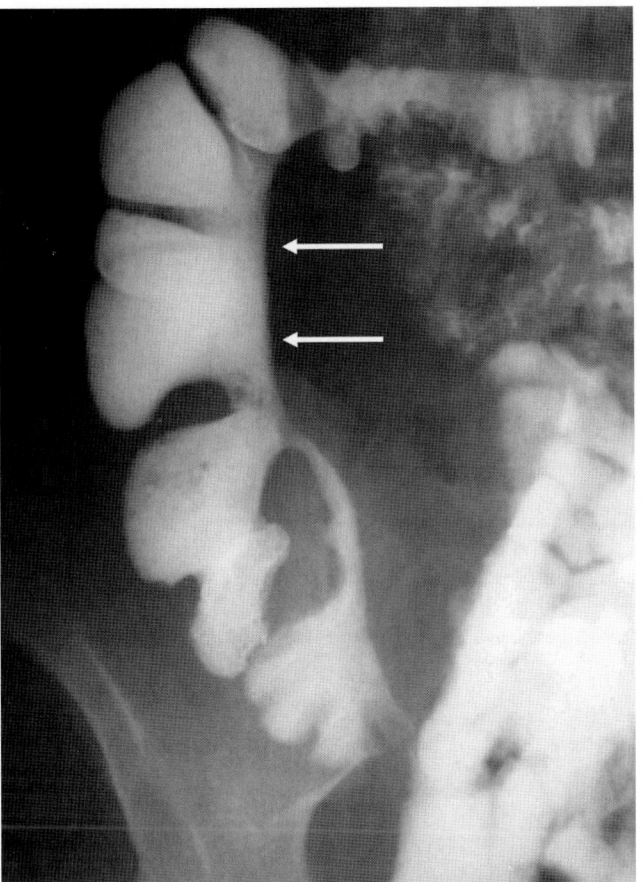

Figure 61-24. Crohn's disease: sacculations. Crohn's disease involves primarily the mesenteric side (*arrows*) of the gut, leading to fibrosis and "ballooning" of the antimesenteric border. Crohn's disease is typically discontinuous, patchy, and asymmetric.

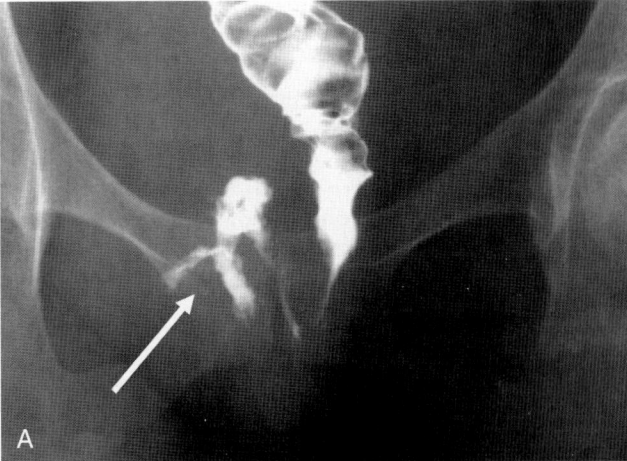

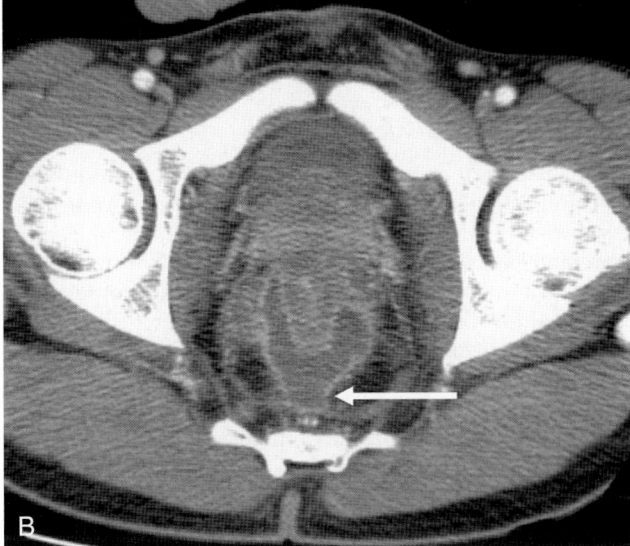

Figure 61-25. Crohn's disease: anorectal pathology. A. Barium enema study showing a sinus tract (*arrow*) extending into the right perianal soft tissues. **B.** CT shows a U-shaped abscess along the posterior aspect of the anorectal junction (*arrow*).

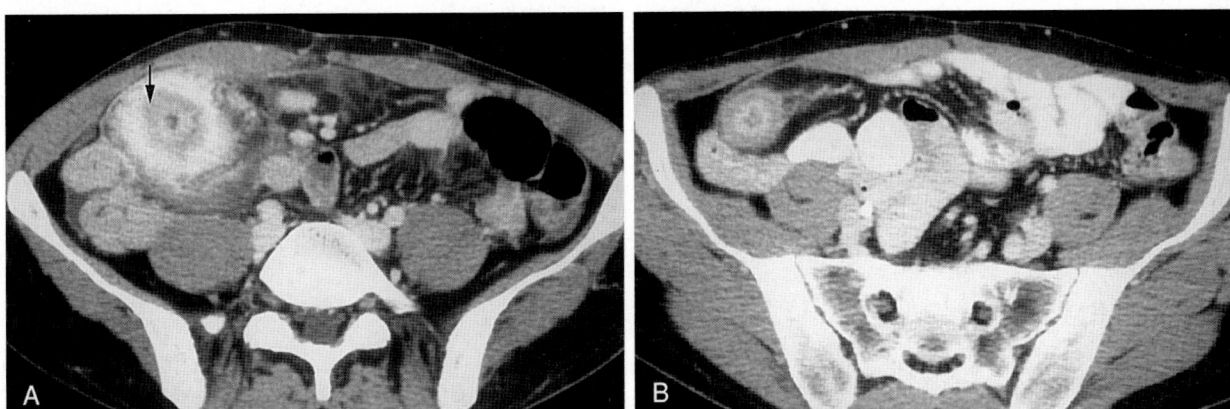

Figure 61-26. Crohn's disease: "target" sign. A. During the acute, noncicatrizing phase of Crohn's disease, CT scan shows intense enhancement of mucosa and muscularis propria-serosa. Mural stratification is present as the edematous thickened submucosa of low attenuation (*black arrow*) contrasts to the other bowel wall layers producing the target sign. Peri-intestinal fat also shows marked inflammatory change. **B.** CT scan in the same patient after a 9-week course of antibiotic and corticosteroid therapy reveals diminished mural thickening and contrast enhancement as well as a reduction of inflammatory change in the adjacent mesentery. (From Gore RM, Balthazar E, Ghahremani GG, et al: CT features of ulcerative colitis and Crohn's disease. AJR 167:3-15, 1996.)

The CT demonstration of mural stratification (i.e., the ability to visualize distinct mucosal, submucosal, and muscularis propria layers) indicates that transmural fibrosis has not occurred and that medical therapy may be successful in ameliorating lumen compromise.[56] The edema and inflammation of the bowel wall that cause mural thickening and lumen obstruction are reversible to some extent. A modest decrease in wall thickness often produces dramatic increase in lumen cross-sectional area and resolution of the patient's obstructive symptoms. In patients with long-standing Crohn's disease and transmural fibrosis, mural stratification is lost so that the affected bowel wall typically has homogeneous attenuation on CT.[67] Homogeneous attenuation of the thickened bowel wall (Fig. 61-27) in the presence of good intravascular contrast medium levels and thin-section scanning suggests irreversible fibrosis so that anti-inflammatory agents may not provide significant reduction in bowel wall thickness.[99] If these segments become sufficiently narrow, surgical resection or strictureplasty may be necessary to relieve the patient's obstruction.

Mesenteric Involvement

The palpation of an abdominal mass or separation of bowel loops on a small bowel series in a patient with Crohn's disease evokes a large differential diagnosis: abscess, phlegmon, "creeping fat" or fibrofatty proliferation of the mesentery, bowel wall thickening, and enlarged mesenteric lymph nodes. Each of these disorders has significantly different prognostic and therapeutic implications.[99,118,119] This diagnostic dilemma is further complicated by the fact that many patients are receiving immunosuppressive therapy that can mask signs and symptoms. CT can readily differentiate the extraluminal manifestations of Crohn's disease.

Fibrofatty Proliferation of the Mesentery

Fibrofatty proliferation, also known as "creeping fat" of the mesentery, is the most common cause of separation of bowel loops seen on small bowel series in patients with Crohn's disease.[120,121] On CT, the sharp interface between bowel and mesentery is lost and the attenuation value of the fat is elevated by 20 to 60 Hounsfield units as a result of the influx of inflammatory cells and fluid.[61] Mesenteric adenopathy with lymph nodes ranging in size between 3 and 8 mm may also be present. If these lymph nodes are larger than 1 cm, lymphoma or carcinoma, both of which occur with greater frequency in Crohn's disease, must be excluded.

There is subserosal accumulation of an increased amount of hypertrophied fat as a result of perivascular inflammation with fibrosis and contraction of the muscular properties. The perivascular fibrosis results in the contraction of dilated feeding vessels and hypertrophied mesenteric fat, tethering the mesentery closer to the gut wall. This tethering contributes to the gross appearance of "fat wrapping" around the gut.[122]

Contrast-enhanced CT scans often show hypervascularity of the involved mesentery manifesting as vascular dilatation, tortuosity, prominence, and wide spacing of the vasa recta. These distinctive vascular changes have been called "vascular jejunization of the ileum" or the "comb" sign.[121] Identification of this hypervascularity should suggest active disease and may be useful in differentiating Crohn's disease from lymphoma and metastases, which tend to be hypovascular lesions.

Phlegmon

A phlegmon is an ill-defined, inflammatory mass in the mesentery or omentum that may resolve completely with antibiotics or progress to form an abscess.[109] Phlegmons are another common cause of mesenteric mass effect in patients with Crohn's disease. On CT, a phlegmon produces loss of definition of surrounding organs and a "smudgy" or "streaky" appearance of the adjacent mesenteric or omental fat.[66]

Abscess

Fifteen to 20 percent of patients with Crohn's disease eventually develop an intra-abdominal abscess.[122] Abscesses are most frequently associated with small bowel disease or ileocolitis.[123] Once developed, an abscess can burrow through the adjacent tissue or break open and drain spontaneously into another part of the bowel, adjacent organs, or both.

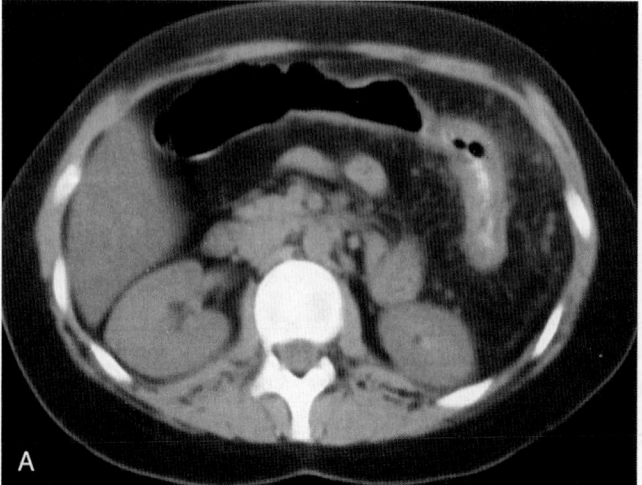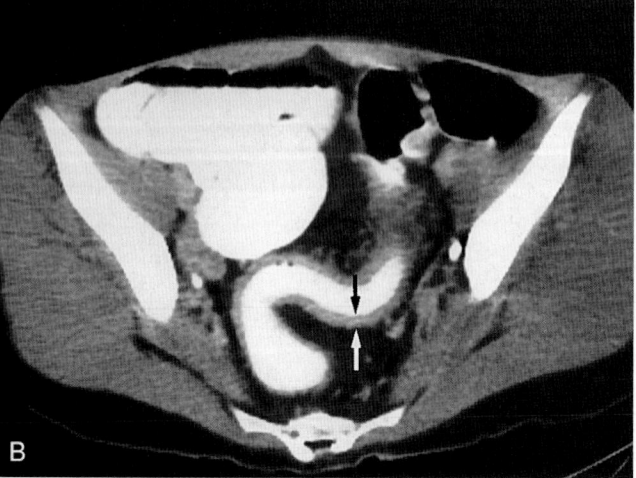

Figure 61-27. Chronic Crohn's disease: CT findings. In chronic cicatrizing Crohn's disease there is loss of mural stratification, often indicating irreversible transmural fibrosis. **A.** There is homogeneous mural thickening of the distal transverse colon. Note the normal mural thickness of the proximal transverse colon. The pericolic fat of the involved segment shows increased attenuation and an increased number of lymph nodes. **B.** Homogeneous mural thickening (*arrows*) is present in the sigmoid colon of a different patient.

Abscesses usually result from sinus tracts, fistulas, perforations, or surgical operations for Crohn's disease.

An intra-abdominal abscess may be difficult to diagnose on clinical grounds in patients with Crohn's disease because symptoms may be inconspicuous, masked by corticosteroids, or mistaken for an exacerbation of disease. Barium studies and endoscopy can only suggest the presence of an abscess indirectly by mass effect, spiculation of the mucosa, or identification of a fistula. Also, these studies do not evaluate the ischiorectal fossa, psoas muscle, and solid abdominal organs, which are common locations of abscess formation.[123,124] Cross-sectional imaging is required to confirm the diagnosis and reveal the full extent and location of the abscess cavity. CT is the primary imaging tool employed for percutaneous drainage of Crohn's disease–related abscesses.[125-127]

Transrectal Ultrasonography

Transrectal ultrasonography can show the following abnormalities in patients with Crohn's disease: (1) mural thickening, (2) perianal and perirectal abscesses (see Fig. 61-25) and fistulas, and (3) heterogeneity of the anal sphincter.[73] Rectal wall thickening (>4 mm) is often accompanied by loss of mural stratification in Crohn's disease.[73]

The anal sphincter derives from the rectal muscular layer as a sharply delineated ellipsoid that is uniformly hypoechoic. When involved by Crohn's disease, the sphincter becomes heterogeneous with echogenic zones interspersed between the normal hypoechoic regions. Also in patients with active proctologic disease, the shortening and narrowing of the anal canal during squeezing and elongation with dilatation during straining are less pronounced. Fistula and sinus tracts appear as a dotted column of echo-rich gas bubbles with reverberation on transrectal ultrasonography. Abscesses are characterized sonographically as predominantly hypoechoic areas that contain echogenic elements corresponding to debris and gas bubbles. The wall of the abscess is usually thick and irregular, and some posterior acoustic enhancement may be seen. Some authors advocate routine screening with transrectal ultrasonography because this technique is capable of defining pararectal and para-anal abscesses and fistulas that develop extramurally without mucosal lesions.[2,4,11]

Transabdominal Ultrasonography

The thickness of the colonic and small bowel wall can be appreciated sonographically, and the validity of employing mural thickening in establishing the diagnosis of inflammatory bowel disease has a reported sensitivity of 67% to 86% and a specificity of 87% to 100%.[68-72] Some authors suggest employing ultrasonography as a screen for inflammatory bowel disease.[68-72] When suspicion of disease is low, normal ultrasonography may be sufficient to avoid barium examination. When abnormal gut is seen or clinical suspicion is high, despite a normal ultrasound study, barium examination should be performed.[68-72]

In patients with active Crohn's disease, the colon wall can be 1.5 cm in thickness. Mural stratification is typically lost as well.[68-72] Using criteria listed in Table 61-4, the sensitivity of ultrasound in detecting active Crohn's disease was 91% with a specificity of 100%; sensitivity was 89% with a specificity of 97% for detecting active ulcerative colitis.[68-72] Several

sonographic caveats should be mentioned. In patients with only aphthoid ulcerations, typical wall stratification is maintained in patients with Crohn's disease, suggesting the disease is not yet transmural.[68-72] In patients with ulcerative colitis who have large and extensive pseudopolyps, the thickness of the colon wall may approach 1.5 cm and mural stratification may be lost.[68-72]

Several authors have questioned the utility of ultrasound in differentiating ulcerative colitis and Crohn's colitis on the basis of bowel wall changes alone.[68-72] Documentation of continuous or discontinuous involvement, combined with evidence of mesenteric disease, abscess, or fistula, can assist differentiation.

In a study employing hydrocolonic ultrasonography, 93% of patients with Crohn's disease showed loss of mural stratification, and the wall appeared hypoechoic and clearly thickened. In contrast, mural stratification was maintained in ulcerative colitis.[68-72] Hydrocolonic ultrasonography could differentiate Crohn's disease from ulcerative colitis in 93% of cases. Colonic Crohn's disease was detectable by this technique with a sensitivity of 96% and a specificity of 91%.[68-72]

The thickened bowel wall in Crohn's disease (Fig. 61-28) produces a target, bull's-eye, or "cockade" appearance that must be differentiated from chronic ulcerative colitis, diverticulitis, lymphoma, ischemic colitis, and pseudomembranous colitis.[68-72] Ultrasonography has also been successful in diagnosing recurrent disease in patients who have had surgical resections.[68-72] Sonographically, creeping fat of the mesentery is hypoechoic, compared with normal fat resulting from edema.[68-72]

Doppler sonographic evaluation of the superior mesenteric artery is a promising noninvasive method of detecting ileocolic inflammation in patients with Crohn's disease and in assessing disease activity. In patients with active disease there is an increase in blood flow and decrease of resistive index of the superior mesenteric artery. Scans are performed preprandially, and postprandial scans can provide additional information. In normal subjects there is a significant difference in the resistive index preprandially and postprandially because of the vasodilatation and increased diastolic flow that occur after a meal. In patients with Crohn's disease there is massive and persistent vasodilatation, related to the extent and severity of disease, which increases blood flow and decreases the resistive index. Accordingly, a meal in patients with active disease does not produce expected Doppler changes because the vasodilatation is already established.[128-130]

In patients with active ileocecal Crohn's disease, alterations of intestinal vascular impedance may reflect on the Doppler waveform of the superior mesenteric artery. This change in vascular impedance is manifested by increase of the flow velocities (peak systolic and diastolic) in the superior mesenteric artery flow volume to the superior mesenteric artery territory. Increased flow velocities are due to the hyperemia and increased flow as well as decreased downstream resistance.[128-130]

Magnetic Resonance Imaging

Magnetic resonance imaging provides a similar perspective to CT in that images demonstrate the overall topography of the abdomen. This imaging technique has several inherent advantages: lack of ionizing radiation, multiplanar imaging

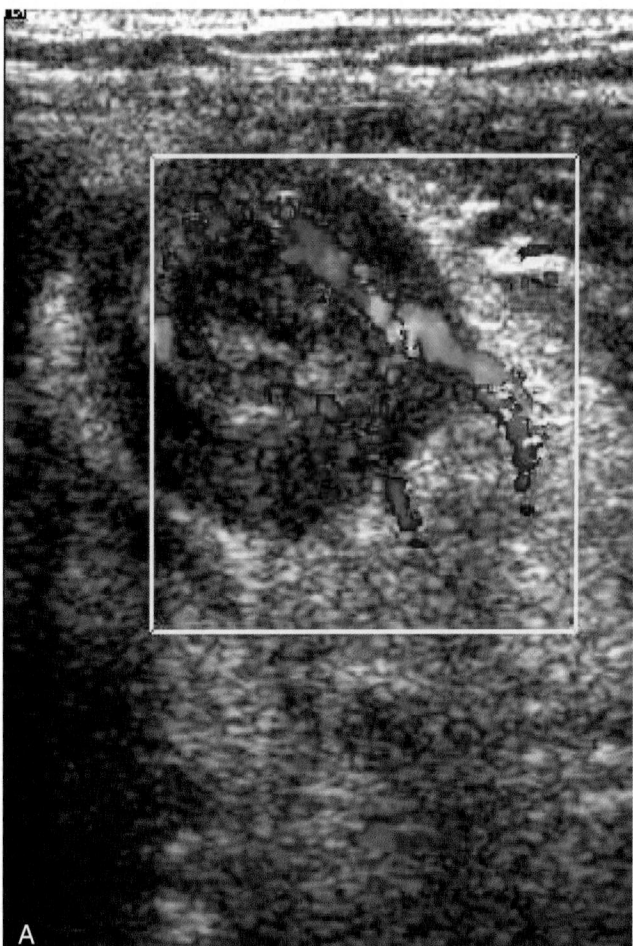

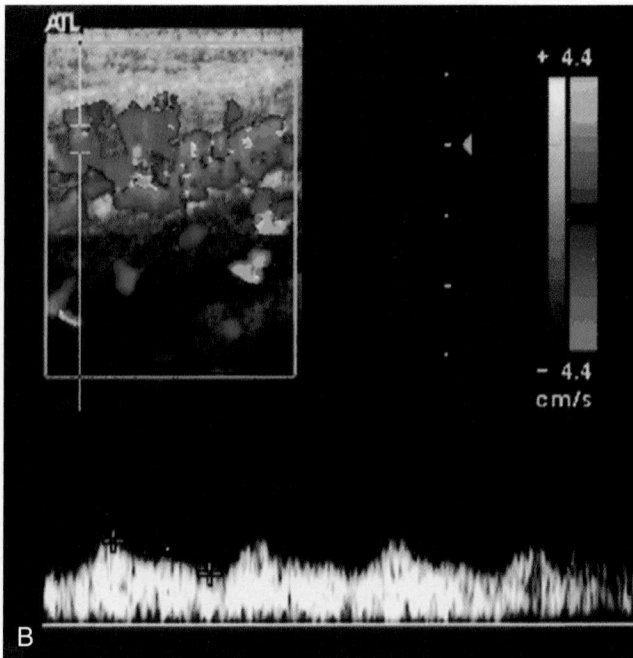

Figure 61-28. Crohn's disease: sonographic findings. A. Hypervascularity and mural thickening are present in this patient with Crohn's disease. Note the low-impedance arterial flow in thickened and inflamed bowel wall. **B.** In a patient with active ileocecal Crohn's disease there is marked increase in both the systolic and the diastolic velocities resulting from the drop in downstream resistance. (Courtesy of Dr. Pierre-Jean Valette, Lyon, France.)

capability, and superb soft tissue contrast.[75-79] Disadvantages that have generally precluded the routine use of MRI in the evaluation of inflammatory bowel disease include respiratory and bowel motion artifact, lack of a satisfactory oral contrast agent, high signal intensity of intra-abdominal fat, and the long imaging times used in conventional spin-echo sequences.

Many of the limitations of MRI have been overcome by employing breath-holding imaging (fast low-angle shot [FLASH]); fat suppression; and an intravenous contrast agent, Gd-DTPA.[131,132] With these new techniques, MRI can show the extent and severity of inflammatory changes (Fig. 61-29) of the gut that correlate with endoscopic and histologic findings from surgical specimens.[75-79] Mural thickening of the gut can also be appreciated with MRI. When fast imaging sequences are combined with intravenous contrast material (Gd-DTPA) administration and fat-suppressed imaging, a good correlation between bowel wall thickness, length of diseased bowel, and severity of inflammation has been reported.[75-79] The percent contrast enhancement compares well with severity of inflammation based on endoscopic and surgical findings. The actively inflamed wall enhances because of increased delivery of the agent and increased capillary permeability. On T1-weighted MR sequences, the fat may have low-signal intensity streaks and strands. These areas may enhance after Gd-DTPA administration on gradient-echo images. MRI is sensitive for the detection of perianal and perirectal fistula, sinus tracts, and abscesses that frequently accompany perianal Crohn's disease.[133,134]

Therapy

Medical Management

Crohn's disease does not behave clinically as a single disorder, so that each patient must receive an individual clinical evaluation and integrated medical and surgical management.[2,4,11]

Drug Therapy

Corticosteroids are the most effective therapy for producing symptomatic relief in Crohn's disease. Although they are effective in preventing relapses, they do not alter long-term outcome and are associated with complications related to Cushing's disease. Newer immunosuppressive agents have also been tested with encouraging results. Several studies have shown that cyclosporine is effective when conventional corticosteroids have failed and that it works more quickly than other immunosuppressive agents. Its efficacy is related to its ability to interfere with T-cell activation. Side effects include malabsorption and renal toxicity, and there is the long-term risk of cyclosporine-induced neoplasm.[2,4,11]

The role of azathioprine in Crohn's disease remains controversial because the drug produces a variety of significant

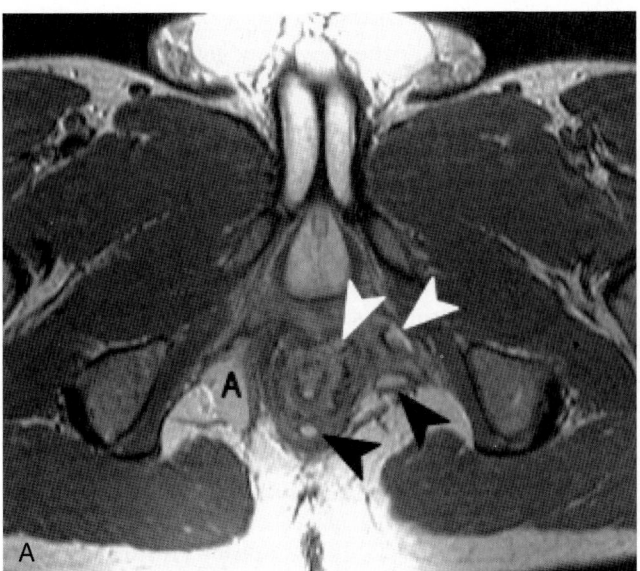 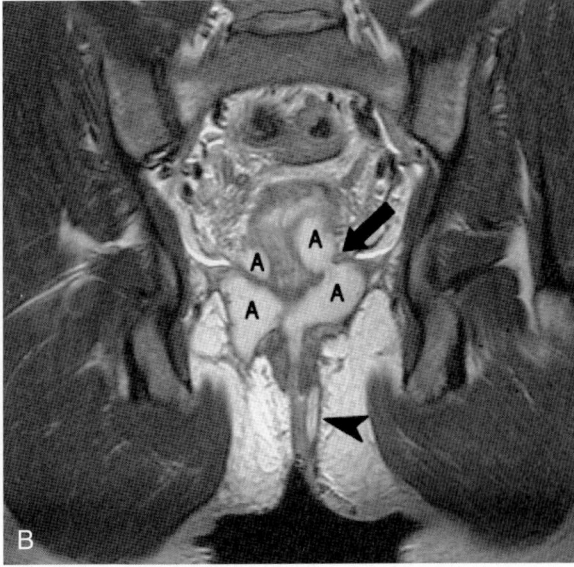

Figure 61-29. Anal Crohn's disease: MR features. A. Axial T2-weighted turbo spin-echo demonstrates multiple tracks (*arrowheads*), both intersphincteric as well as outside the anal sphincter. At the right an abscess (A) is seen in the ischioanal space. **B.** Coronal T2-weighted turbo spin-echo reveals multiple interconnected (*arrow*) abscesses (A) as well as a fistula (*arrowhead*). (Case courtesy of Dr. Jaap Stoker, Amsterdam, Netherlands.)

side effects. Physicians are often compelled to use azathioprine as a third-line drug, particularly in patients with extensive small bowel disease, recurrence after surgery, and fistulas. In some patients, the use of azathioprine or its active metabolite, 6-mercaptopurine, has permitted reduction in the dose of corticosteroid and even the discontinuation of the drug.

Mesalamine decreases recurrence rates in Crohn's colitis, but its value for small bowel disease is uncertain. The use of sulfasalazine is hindered by side effects, which has led to the development of less toxic derivatives of 5-aminosalicylic acid.

The efficacy of metronidazole in Crohn's disease remains unproved, and its use is limited by neurologic toxicity. However, this therapy may lead to complete remission of perianal disease and the closure of fistulas.[2,4,11]

Total parenteral nutrition is useful for maintaining nutritional status when the gut cannot be used during exacerbations of inflammatory or fibrostenotic Crohn's disease. Nevertheless, remission rates while maintained on total parenteral nutrition and bowel are equivalent to those of enteral nutrition. Five to 10 days of preoperative total parenteral nutrition can decrease surgical complications in patients who require bowel resection.

Advances in understanding of the role of immune cells, natural killer cells, and macrophages and their soluble mediators, such as cytokines and tumor necrosis factor, have led to the development of specific immunotherapies with improved efficacy and reduced toxicity. An antitumor necrosis factor (chimeric, monoclonal antibody [infliximab]) has proved helpful in patients with advanced Crohn's disease refractory to corticosteroids and immunosuppressive therapy. This recombinant antibody is given as a single dose intravenously and can rapidly close fistulas with improvement lasting for 3 months.[2,4,11]

Surgical Management

There is a high rate of recurrence (30% to 53%) of Crohn's disease after resection of diseased bowel.[2,4,88,91] It is possible that Crohn's disease affects, at least at a microscopic level, the entire gut from the outset, so that the disease cannot be cured by surgery. Therefore, operative therapy should be reserved for certain complications of the disease or for unequivocal failure to respond to optimal medical therapy. These guidelines are particularly applicable to two groups of patients: (1) those who have previously undergone small bowel resection and present with recurrent disease of an obstructive nature and (2) those who have diffuse disease and multiple small bowel strictures. Removal of all the diseased areas in these patients may lead to the short bowel syndrome.

The major indications for surgery in Crohn's disease are obstruction, perforation, hemorrhage, and carcinoma.[2,4,88,91] Abscesses and fistulas should first be treated by the interventional radiologist because this may save the patient from having surgery.[2,4,88,91]

There is considerable interest concerning strictureplasty, and early reports suggest that this technique is effective in treating short stenosing Crohn's lesions of the small bowel.[2,4,88,91] One series reported 24 patients who had 86 strictureplasties.[88] This procedure was safe and effective for selected patients undergoing surgery for obstructive Crohn's disease. Short fibrous strictures in patients who did not have acute inflammatory segments of disease were most amenable to strictureplasty. Another report compared recurrence after strictureplasty with that after primary resection for small intestinal Crohn's disease.[88] No difference in the rate of recurrence after strictureplasty or resection was found, offering more support to the choice of strictureplasty for selected patients with obstructive symptoms.

Reports of radiologically guided balloon dilatation of strictures are also of interest, but this method is unlikely to be suitable for many Crohn's strictures, which are located in the small bowel.[2,4,88,91] Current surgical opinion holds that external fistulas unassociated with residual Crohn's disease should be managed along conventional lines but that fistulas arising from diseased small intestine may require surgery. This surgery should be performed after an associated abscess has been drained, metabolic deficits have been corrected, and the anatomy of the fistula has been defined.[91]

Primary fistulotomy has been shown to be a safe procedure in selected patients, provided that aggressive medical treatment is employed to control bowel disease preoperatively.[2,4,88,91] Rectovaginal fistulas are especially difficult to treat, but with prolonged conservative treatment the rectum can be preserved in many cases.

Prognosis

The manifestations and complications of Crohn's disease are so diverse and unpredictable that for some patients the outlook is bleak. Disease remission can be interrupted by exacerbations at any time. Approximately 50% of patients develop complications that require surgery, and 10% to 20% lead symptom-free lives after one or two attacks. In view of the serious nature of Crohn's disease and its complications, the mortality is low. With proper medical supervision, most patients adjust remarkably well to their chronic illness and lead productive lives.[2,4,11,133-137]

INTESTINAL COMPLICATIONS OF INFLAMMATORY BOWEL DISEASE

Table 61-7 summarizes gastrointestinal complications in ulcerative colitis and Crohn's disease.

Carcinoma

The risk of developing colorectal cancer is significantly higher in patients with ulcerative colitis and Crohn's colitis than in the general population, although the precise magnitude of this risk is uncertain.[1-6,138] Studies suggest an annual incidence of 10% after the first decade of ulcerative colitis. The risk of colorectal cancer also increases with increasing extent of disease; 75% to 80% of patients who develop cancer have pancolitis.[138] Carcinomas associated with ulcerative colitis

Table 61-7
Relative Frequency of Gastrointestinal Complications in Inflammatory Bowel Disease

Complication	Ulcerative Colitis	Crohn's Disease
Anorectal lesions	<20%	20-80%
Fissure in ano	<15%	25-30%
Perianal abscess	<10%	20-25%
First symptom	Very infrequent	20-25%
Fistula in ano	<6%	20-25%
Multiple and complex	Never	Common
Multiple anorectal complications	Very infrequent	20%
Massive hemorrhage	3%	<3%
Colon	Never	<2%
Small bowel		
Intra-abdominal abscess	Very rare	20-40%
Internal fistulas	Very rare	Very uncommon
Free perforation	Uncommon	<8%
Toxic megacolon	2-10%	Less common
Pseudopolyposis	15-30%	Very common
Strictures	11-15%	15-25%

From Kirsner JB, Shorter RG: Inflammatory Bowel Disease, 3rd ed. Philadelphia, Lea & Febiger, 1988, pp 257-280.

are multiple in nearly 25% of cases and more often flat and scirrhous than in patients without colitis and thus harder to detect.

Cancer screening has become a popular and controversial issue in patients with inflammatory bowel disease. Since the 1960s, mucosal dysplasia has been considered a precursor of colon cancer or at least a marker of colons that are at risk for developing cancer. Mucosal dysplasia is often detected near or remote from the neoplasm in ulcerative colitis patients with carcinoma. However, dysplasia is patchy, inconsistent, and unpredictably distributed in the colon. Accordingly, colonoscopy with multiple random biopsy specimens as well as biopsy specimens from masses or raised areas is recommended. Flow cytometry searching for aneuploidy has been advocated as a means of increasing the specificity and prognostic significance of the histologic results.

Molecular markers, such as Ki-67, DPC-4, and DYS nuclear matrix proteins, are a means of further refining the diagnosis of dysplasia and may eventually provide an alternative method of predicting colorectal cancer. Clinical studies provide support for the increasingly prevalent recommendation that any dysplasia warrants colectomy.[2,4,11]

Several studies have shown that certain dysplastic lesions are radiologically visible (Fig. 61-30). When the dysplasia is elevated and plaquelike or multinodular, it manifests en face as irregular nodular areas with sharply angulated borders, having a "mosaic tile" appearance. Tangentially, these lesions project only 1 to 2 mm above the adjacent normal mucosa. When the dysplasia assumes a more polypoid form, it is indistinguishable from an adenomatous polyp. Most dysplasias occur in flat mucosa and therefore are not detectable on double-contrast barium studies. The management of high-risk patients with ulcerative pancolitis requires regular radiologic and endoscopic surveillance for detecting dysplasia.[138-144]

Toxic Megacolon

Toxic megacolon is the most severe, life-threatening complication of inflammatory bowel disease. It occurs in 1.6% to 13% of patients with ulcerative colitis and is less common in Crohn's colitis. Toxic megacolon usually occurs in patients in their 30s and may be the initial manifestation of ulcerative colitis. It is the most common cause of death directly related to ulcerative colitis and is an indication for emergency surgery.[145-148]

Pathologic Findings

On pathologic examination there is transmural inflammation with deep fissuring ulcers into the muscularis propria, often with extension to the serosa. These inflammatory changes may be so extensive that large areas of denuded mucosa are seen. The colon undergoes disintegration of normal tissue cohesion, an appearance that surgeons have likened to having the consistency of wet tissue paper on handling. The inflammatory exudate seeps through the serosa and may lead to signs of peritonitis even without frank perforation. The external surface of the colon shows intense serositis, and the greater omentum and gastrocolic ligament are edematous and inflamed. These changes are accompanied by vasculitis of the small arterioles and inflammation and destruction of

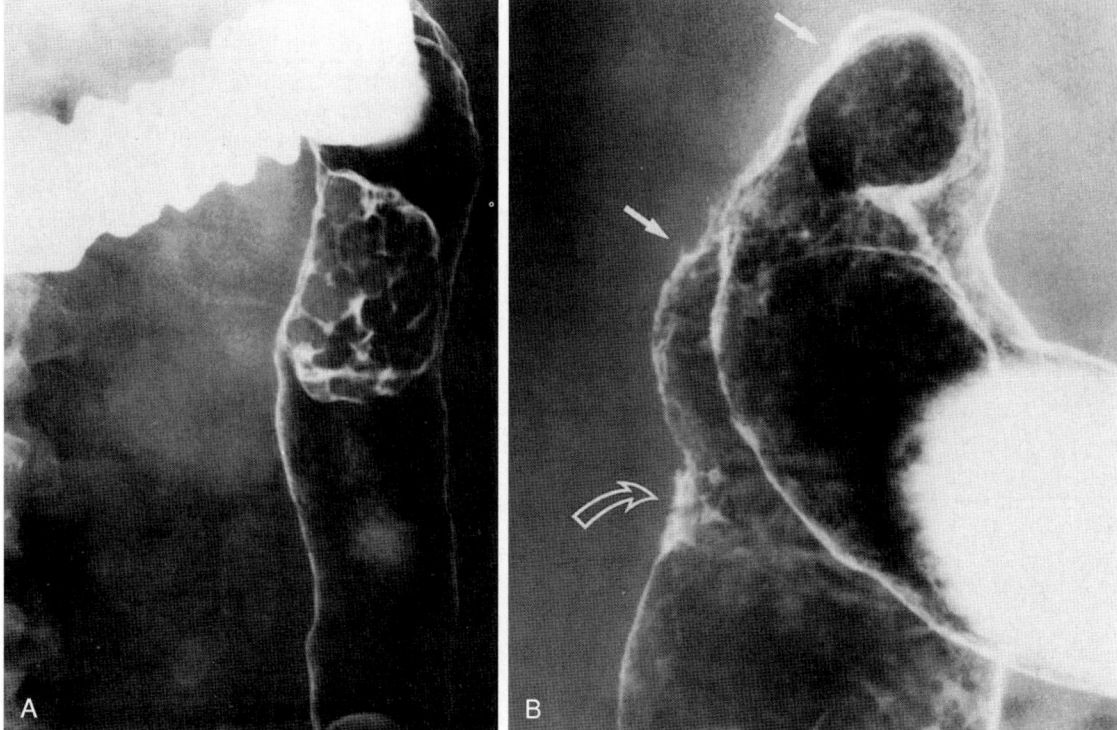

Figure 61-30. Ulcerative colitis: carcinoma. Colitic carcinomas often have an atypical appearance. **A.** Unusual polypoid carcinoma in the proximal descending colon. **B.** There is an infiltrative plaquelike carcinoma of the hepatic flexure (*solid arrows*). A small macrodysplastic lesion (*open arrow*) is present proximal to the carcinoma. (From Laufer I, Levine MS [eds]: Double Contrast Gastrointestinal Radiology, 2nd ed. Philadelphia, WB Saunders, 1992.)

the ganglion cells of the myenteric and submucosal plexuses; there is myocytolysis in the muscularis propria.[2,4,6] Although the bowel wall appears thickened and nodular on abdominal radiographs, the specimen often shows a mural thickness of only 2 to 3 mm in areas of denuded mucosa.

A number of factors that further contribute to high intraluminal pressures and decreased muscle tone that can lead to colonic distention in toxic megacolon include antidiarrheal drugs (codeine, morphine, tincture of opium), aerophagia, and hypokalemia. The barium enema has also been implicated as a precipitating factor in toxic megacolon, but this is controversial. Certain evidence suggests that the relationship may be temporal more than a cause-and-effect phenomenon. Nevertheless, the interdiction concerning barium enema studies in patients who are severely ill with ulcerative colitis is probably still valid.[2,4,6] Toxic megacolon can also complicate other forms of colitis, such as ischemic colitis, Crohn's disease, pseudomembranous colitis, and amebiasis.

Radiologic Findings

Toxic megacolon (Fig. 61-31) is one of the few life-threatening conditions in which an abdominal radiograph is all that is required to establish a firm diagnosis.[148] Dilatation is the hallmark of toxic megacolon; mean diameters of the most dilated segments are between 8.2 and 9.2 cm. Dilatation greater than 5 cm indicates ulceration to the muscle layer and should be considered the threshold for dilatation in fulminating colitis. In the past, the transverse colon was considered the focus of disease, but this is only a reflection of the fact that

the transverse colon is the least dependent portion of the large intestine on supine-view radiographs. Initially, only a short segment of colon may be involved.[2,4]

Mucosal islands are a common finding in toxic megacolon and indicate severe disruption of the mucosa. This appearance can be simulated in patients with inflammatory polyps during an acute attack. As stated earlier, although the colon wall is thin pathologically it appears thickened radiologically, presumably as a result of subserosal or omental edema. A radiolucent stripe may be noted running parallel to the colon, and this probably represents the pericolic fat line.

The profound inflammation and extensive ulceration of toxic megacolon always abolish the haustral pattern, so that the presence of normal haustra excludes the diagnosis. Long fluid levels can be seen in the colon as well as small bowel distention, in keeping with an ileus.[148]

EXTRAINTESTINAL COMPLICATIONS OF INFLAMMATORY BOWEL DISEASE

Extraintestinal manifestations develop in one fourth to one third of patients with inflammatory bowel disease (Table 61-8).[1-7] They can be divided into three categories: (1) those intimately related to disease activity or extent of disease and responsive to therapy directed at the bowel disease (e.g., arthritis, iritis); (2) those whose course is independent of underlying bowel disease (e.g., sclerosing cholangitis, ankylosing spondylitis); and (3) those that are due to an inadequate or disordered intestinal function (e.g., cholelithiasis, nephrolithiasis).[1-7]

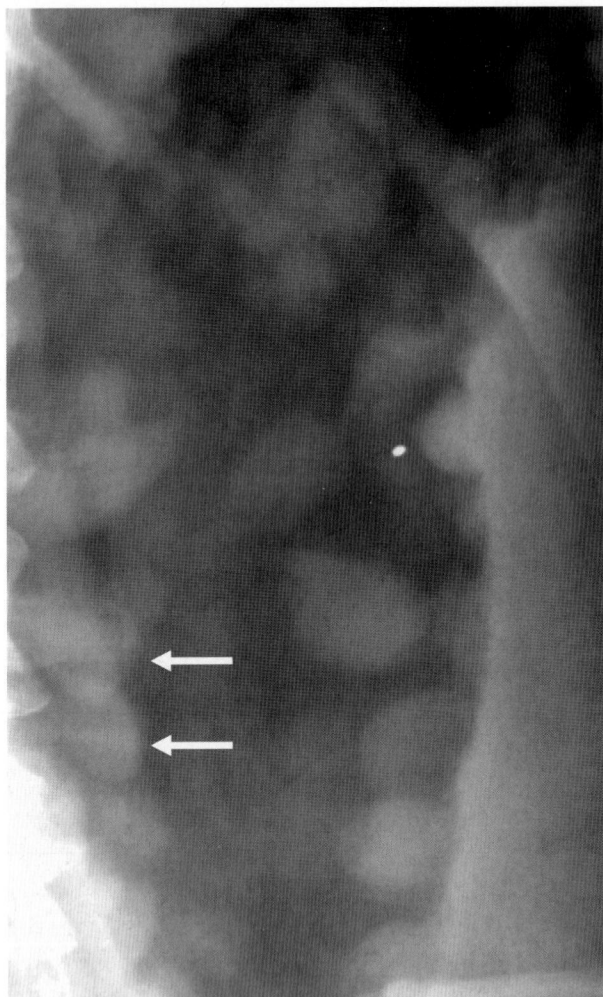

Figure 61-31. Intestinal complications of ulcerative colitis: toxic megacolon. Mucosal islands (*arrows*), deep ulcerations, and dilatation establish the diagnosis.

Table 61-8
Extracolonic Manifestations of Ulcerative Colitis

Hepatobiliary/Renal
Nonspecific reactive hepatitis
Sclerosing cholangitis
Pericholangitis
Chronic active hepatitis
Cholangiocarcinoma
Fatty infiltration

Musculoskeletal
Arthritis
Ankylosing spondylitis
Sacroiliitis
Hypertrophic osteoarthropathy
Avascular necrosis

Ocular
Uveitis and iritis
Episcleritis
Conjunctivitis

Mucocutaneous
Pyoderma gangrenosum
Erythema nodosum
Cutaneous vasculitis
Stomatitis
Urolithiasis and nephrolithiasis
Amyloidosis
Drug-related disease

Bronchopulmonary
Pulmonary vasculitis
Pleuropericarditis

Hematologic and Vascular
Anemia from blood loss
Autoimmune hemolytic anemia
Thrombocytosis
Thromboembolic disease
Increased factors V and VIII
Accelerated thromboplastin III levels
Arteritis of aorta and subclavian artery

Pancreas
Drug-related pancreatitis

Hepatobiliary Complications

The most frequent serious manifestations of extraintestinal inflammatory bowel disease occur in the liver and the biliary tract.[1-7] As a rule, these complications generally do not correlate with disease activity, duration, or severity, with the exception of fatty infiltration, which occurs in patients who tend to be more seriously ill, debilitated, and malnourished.[1-7]

Hepatic Steatosis

Fatty liver is found on liver biopsy specimens in 20% to 25% of patients with inflammatory bowel disease and may be caused by fat malabsorption, hyperalimentation, sepsis, protein-losing enteropathy, malnutrition, and corticosteroids.[1-7] The imaging features of fatty liver are variable and depend on the amount of fat deposited, its distribution within the liver, and the presence of associated hepatic disease. CT is the best noninvasive technique for the detection of hepatic steatosis because there is an excellent correlation between hepatic parenchymal CT attenuation and the amount of hepatic triglyceride found on liver biopsy specimens. Fatty deposition is usually diffuse; however, involvement can be focal, lobar, segmental, or scattered in a bizarre pattern that rapidly appears and disappears.[1-7]

Cholelithiasis

Thirty to 50 percent of patients with Crohn's disease develop gallstones, especially those with extensive terminal ileal disease or after ileal resection. As a consequence of this ileal disease, these patients form lithogenic bile because of bile salt malabsorption or loss of the enterohepatic circulation. Ultrasonography is the premier means of diagnosing gallstones.[1-7]

Primary Sclerosing Cholangitis

Primary sclerosing cholangitis occurs in fewer than 2% to 5% of patients with inflammatory bowel disease; it is more commonly associated with ulcerative colitis.[1-7] Ultrasonography, CT, and MRI (Fig. 61-32) can directly visualize the fibrous mural thickening of the larger bile ducts that characterize this disease.[1-7,149] The thickening may be concentric or asymmetric and usually measures 2 to 5 mm. Other signs suggesting the diagnosis include focal duct dilatation, dis-

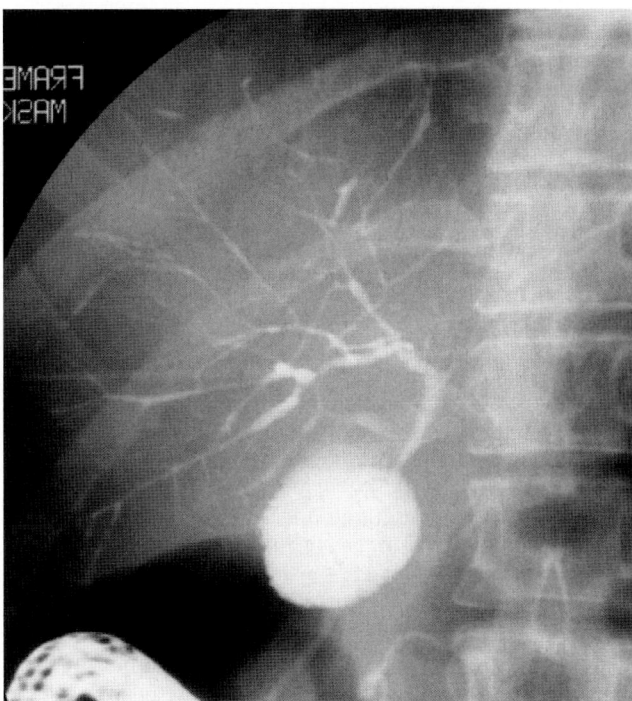

Figure 61-32. ERCP image shows multifocal strictures and irregularity of the right intrahepatic bile ducts. (From Vitellas KM, Keogan MT, Freed KS, et al: Radiologic manifestations of sclerosing cholangitis with emphasis on MR cholangiopancreatography. RadioGraphics 20:959-975, 2000.)

crepancy between the size of the intrahepatic and extrahepatic bile ducts, focal clustering of intrahepatic ducts, and discontinuous areas of minimal intrahepatic biliary dilatation without associated hepatic, porta hepatis, or pancreatic masses. The cholangiographic signs of beading, pruning, and nodular mural thickening can also be seen on cross-sectional imaging, but usually with less detail and precision.[149]

CT, ultrasonography, and MRI offer three major advantages in evaluating patients with known or suspected sclerosing cholangitis.[149] First, they are noninvasive techniques that are quite safe in these patients, who often need multiple serial examinations. Second, they can visualize the entire biliary tract in cases in which strictures obstruct the flow of contrast medium during cholangiography, occasionally leaving large portions of the intrahepatic ducts unexamined. Finally, CT and ultrasonography can depict complications of sclerosing cholangitis, such as cirrhosis and portal hypertension, as well as soft tissue masses associated with cholangiocarcinoma.[149] MR cholangiopancreatography is an attractive new alternative in this diagnosis.[149] Patients with ulcerative colitis and sclerosing cholangitis are at greater risk for developing cholangiocarcinoma and secondary biliary cirrhosis.

Liver Abscess

More than 30 cases of hepatic abscess complicating Crohn's disease have been reported. In one institution, they accounted for 8% of all liver abscesses.[2,4,150] They most commonly develop in patients with long-standing disease but may occur as the initial manifestation of Crohn's disease.[2,4,150] Corticosteroids and other immunosuppressive agents, perforation, intra-abdominal abscess, and anastomotic leaks are all pre-

disposing factors to the development of a hepatic abscess in patients with Crohn's disease.[2,4,150]

Pancreatic Complications

One to 2 percent of patients with Crohn's disease develop pancreatitis resulting from a variety of causes: (1) drugs such as corticosteroids, azathioprine, and metronidazole; (2) choledocholithiasis; (3) fistula from the adjacent gut; (4) sclerosing cholangitis; (5) dysfunction of the sphincter of Oddi or stenosis of the descending duodenum leading to obstruction of the duct or reflux of duodenal contents into the duct; and (6) autoantibodies against pancreatic acinar cells. Regardless of the cause, cross-sectional imaging is needed to help confirm the diagnosis of pancreatitis and more importantly its complications.[151]

Urinary Tract Complications

Nephrolithiasis

Two to 10 percent of patients with Crohn's disease develop nephrolithiasis (Fig. 61-33) as a result of water and electrolyte losses in diarrhea, malabsorption, and large ileostomy output. Oxalate stones are most common; and because they are not calcified, they may not be visible with conventional radiologic techniques.[152,153] Noncontrast CT scans and, to a

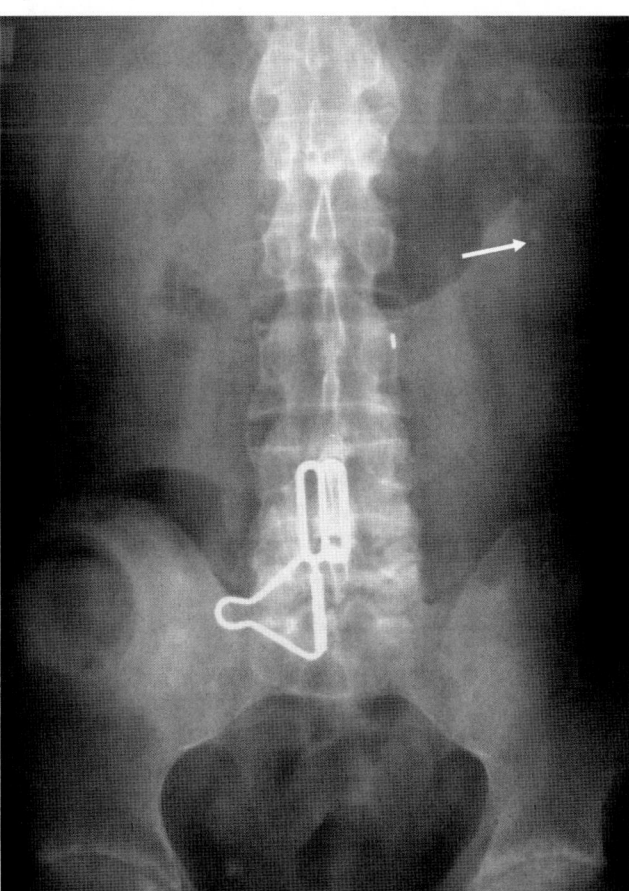

Figure 61-33. Urinary tract complications of inflammatory bowel disease. Nephrocalcinosis (*arrow*) is identified in this patient with Crohn's disease and an ileostomy. The sacroiliac joints are fused.

lesser degree, ultrasonography detect these stones more readily.

Hydronephrosis

Hydronephrosis may develop in patients with Crohn's disease for a variety of reasons, including calculous disease or obstruction resulting from the inflammatory effect of an abscess or phlegmon or the mass effect of creeping fat of the mesentery.[152,153] CT is useful in detecting both the hydronephrosis and the obstructing mass.

Fistulas

Fistulas may develop between diseased gut and the kidney in patients with Crohn's disease, leading to a renal or perinephric abscess.[2,4,6] More commonly, enterovesical fistulas develop. Although these fistulas should first be evaluated with conventional barium studies, excretory urography, and cystography, the origin of the fistula may be edematous and prevent contrast opacification, and tiny fistulous tracts may not be seen. Conventional studies detect fewer than 50% of enterovesical fistulas; CT has a nearly 90% success rate.[150] CT scans are initially obtained with only oral and rectal contrast administration. The presence of gas and small amounts of contrast material entering through the fistula may be obscured if the bladder is opacified after the intravenous injection of iodinated contrast medium.

Musculoskeletal Complications

Arthropathy

Arthritis is one of the most common extraintestinal manifestations of inflammatory bowel disease, and it is manifested as a peripheral arthritis or sacroiliitis-spondylitis (Fig. 61-34).[154-159] The radiologic findings of peripheral enteropathic arthritis are usually minimal and best seen, if at all, with conventional radiographs. The changes in the axial skeleton, affecting 3% to 16% of patients with inflammatory bowel disease, are similar

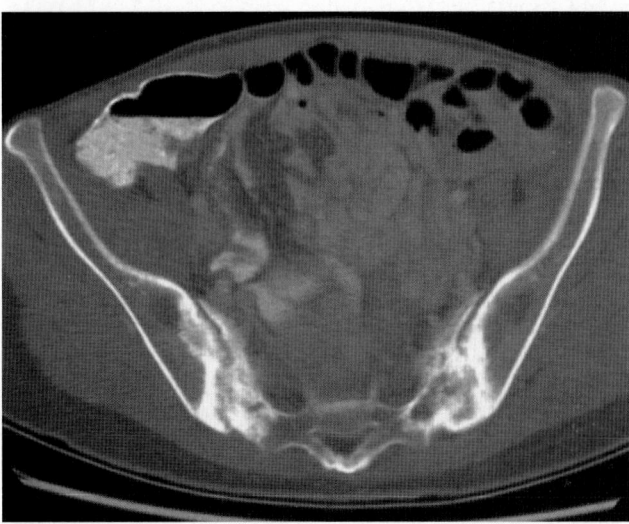

Figure 61-34. Musculoskeletal complications of inflammatory bowel disease. CT scan of the pelvis in a patient with ulcerative colitis shows bilateral sacroiliitis.

to ankylosing spondylitis.[154-158] CT and MRI can often detect the subtle changes of early sacroiliitis before they become apparent on radiographs: bilateral, usually symmetric joint narrowing with osseous erosions followed by sclerosis are more pronounced on the iliac side of the articulation.[154-158] Eventually, bony ankylosis occurs. T1-weighted fat-suppression images are superior at demonstrating the cortical erosion and subchondral sclerosis of sacroiliitis.

Avascular Necrosis

Osteonecrosis is a rare complication of inflammatory bowel disease and usually occurs in the following clinical settings: during or after corticosteroid therapy; during total parenteral nutrition, especially with lipid emulsions; and most recently as a direct complication of the disease without other precipitating factors.[154-158]

MRI is the best technique for establishing this diagnosis, with a reported sensitivity of 97% and a specificity of 98%.[154-158] On T1-weighted images, areas of low signal intensity may be seen beneath the articular surface. Alternatively, bands of low signal intensity are seen surrounding a central area of higher signal intensity. On T2-weighted images, areas of low signal intensity can become bright and regions of high signal intensity remain high.

Asymptomatic and radiologically normal hips may have early signs of avascular necrosis on CT studies. These include subtle alterations in trabecular pattern, joint space integrity, and femoral head and acetabular contour, which may be undetected or ill-defined on radiographs.

Osteomyelitis/Septic Arthritis

Septic arthritis of the hip can complicate a psoas or retroperitoneal abscess tracking through the greater sciatic notch. MRI and CT show these changes before their recognition on radiographs.

The iliac bone and sacrum are the most frequent sites of osteomyelitis in patients with Crohn's disease. They are almost invariably the result of an adjacent pelvic abscess or enteric fistula. Accordingly, osteomyelitis is usually diagnosed on cross-sectional imaging when the abscess is identified. CT findings in osteomyelitis include cortical bone destruction, intraosseous gas, increased attenuation of the bone marrow, narrowing of the medullary cavity, serpentine drainage tracts, and the presence of an involucrum or sequestrum. On MRI, the marrow space of the involved bone demonstrates decreased signal on T1-weighted images and increased signal on T2-weighted images. Cortical destruction or thickening and edema or abscess formation in the soft tissues can also be demonstrated on MRI.

Spinal epidural abscess has been reported from fistulization of a presacral or psoas abscess in patients with Crohn's disease. Prevertebral, intraforaminal, and epidural gas may be seen on CT and MRI studies.

Osteoporosis

Osteoporosis is a common complication of inflammatory bowel disease. Osteoporosis and osteomalacia occur secondary to malabsorption with resultant calcium and vitamin D deficiency and can also relate to corticosteroid therapy.

Psoas Abscess

Crohn's disease complications now account for 73% of all psoas abscesses.[36,160] On the right, a psoas abscess may develop secondary to terminal ileal disease; and on the left, it can result from sigmoid or jejunal involvement. Most patients with psoas abscess have well-established Crohn's disease, but the clinical manifestations may be nonspecific. Occasionally, psoas abscess may be seen at the initial presentation of disease. CT has emerged as the single best examination for its diagnosis. CT can also direct percutaneous abscess drainage in these patients.[161] Primary rectus sheath abscesses have also been reported as a complication of Crohn's disease and may be visualized on CT, MRI, or ultrasonography.

Pulmonary Complications

Although clinically significant, pulmonary manifestations are uncommon in patients with inflammatory bowel disease. Prospective studies have identified pulmonary abnormalities in 30% to 50% of cases. There are four major clinicopathologic categories of disease: (1) airway disease (chronic bronchitis, bronchiectasis, bronchiolitis); (2) interstitial lung disease (bronchiolitis obliterans, interstitial lung disease); (3) necrobiotic nodules; and (4) serositis. Respiratory or pleuropericardial disease is much more common in ulcerative colitis than in Crohn's disease.[1-6]

DIFFERENTIAL DIAGNOSIS OF COLITIS

Ulcerative colitis and Crohn's disease are responsible for most cases of enterocolitis in North America and Europe. However, infectious enteritis and colitis are occurring more frequently because of increased global travel and immigration; the indiscriminate use of antibiotics; and more widespread immunosuppression resulting from the AIDS epidemic, chemotherapy, as well as bone marrow, stem cell, and organ transplantation.[1-12] Because the small bowel and colon have only a limited variety of response to a wide variety of insults, it is not surprising that the infectious enterocolitides often simulate the radiologic (Table 61-9) and clinical (Table 61-10) features of inflammatory bowel disease. The definitive diagnosis of infectious or idiopathic inflammatory bowel disease ultimately rests on histologic and bacteriologic documentation.

The differentiation of Crohn's colitis and ulcerative colitis is important because each disease has different therapeutic and prognostic implications. Patients with ulcerative colitis have a higher risk of developing cancer. They can also have a curative colectomy and are candidates for sphincter-preserving surgery. Patients with Crohn's disease are not candidates for ileal reservoirs because disease may recur in the ileum. The following double-contrast barium enema features enable the correct diagnosis to be made in most patients:

1. Ulcerative colitis is a contiguous, confluent, circumferential, and symmetric disease that begins in the rectum and extends proximally.
2. Crohn's disease is a patchy, discontinuous disease with asymmetric involvement that can lead to pseudodiverticula.
3. The following types of ulcerations are characteristic of Crohn's disease: aphthoid, discrete, deep (>3 mm), fissuring, and rose thorn.

Table 61-9
Inflammatory Bowel Disease: Radiologic Differential Diagnosis

Feature	Commonly Found In:	May Occur In:
Granular mucosa	Ulcerative colitis	Early Crohn's colitis (rare)
Ulceration		
Discrete	Crohn's colitis	Amebiasis
	Yersinia infection	Ischemia
	Behçet's disease	Tuberculosis
Confluent (shallow)	Ulcerative colitis	Crohn's disease
		Amebiasis
Confluent (deep)	Crohn's disease	Ischemia
		Amebiasis
		Tuberculosis
		Strongyloides infection
Stricture	Ulcerative colitis	Tuberculosis
Symmetrical	Lymphogranuloma venereum	
Asymmetrical	Crohn's disease	
	Ischemia	
	Tuberculosis	
Fistula	Crohn's disease	Tuberculosis
	Lymphogranuloma venereum	Actinomycosis
Inflammatory polyps	Ulcerative colitis	Ischemia (rare)
	Crohn's disease	
	Schistosomiasis	
	Colitis cystica profunda	
Small bowel disease	Crohn's disease	Ulcerative colitis (backwash ileitis)
	Yersinia infection	Behçet's disease
	Tuberculosis	Ischemia
	Pseudomembranous enterocolitis	
Skip lesions	Crohn's disease	Lymphogranuloma venereum
	Tuberculosis	
	Amebiasis	
Toxic megacolon	Ulcerative colitis	Crohn's disease
		Ischemia
		Amebiasis

From Bartram CI, Laufer I: Inflammatory bowel disease. In Laufer I, Levine MS (eds): Double Contrast Gastrointestinal Radiology, 2nd ed. Philadelphia, WB Saunders, 1992, pp 579-645.

4. Granular mucosa is typical in ulcerative colitis but not in Crohn's colitis.
5. Severe anal and perianal disease is characteristic of Crohn's disease but is exceptionally rare in ulcerative colitis.
6. Spontaneous fistula and sinus tracts are a hallmark of Crohn's disease.

Certain CT findings can help differentiate granulomatous and ulcerative colitis. Mural stratification is seen in 61% of patients with chronic ulcerative colitis but in only 8% of patients with chronic granulomatous colitis. Also, mean colon wall thickness in chronic ulcerative colitis is 7.8 mm, significantly smaller than observed in Crohn's colitis (11 mm). Finally, the outer contour of the thickened colonic wall is smooth and regular in 95% of ulcerative colitis cases whereas serosal and outer mural irregularity are present in 80% of granulomatous colitis patients.

Differentiation between these two diseases can be made on radiologic grounds in 90% to 95% of patients. This distinc-

Table 61-10

Inflammatory Bowel Disease: Clinical Differential Diagnosis

Ulcerative Colitis	Crohn's Disease
Pancolitis	Ileal and jejunal
Campylobacter infection	*Yersinia* enterocolitis
Shigellosis	Salmonellosis
Salmonellosis	Tuberculosis
Cytomegalovirus infection	*Strongyloides* infection
Escherichia coli infection	Lymphoma
Clostridium difficile infection	Radiation enteritis
Amebiasis	Carcinoid
Behçet's disease	Eosinophilic enteritis
Graft-versus-host disease	Carcinoma (rare)
Radiation colitis	Ileocecal
Diverticular disease	Tuberculosis
Ischemic colitis	Typhlitis
Proctosigmoiditis	Amebiasis
Herpes simplex infection	Graft-versus-host disease
Gonorrhea	Appendicitis
Chlamydia infection	Carcinoma
	Colonic
	Ischemia
	Diverticulitis
	Carcinoma
	Amebiasis
	Tuberculosis
	Ischemic colitis
	Radiation colitis
	Chlamydia infection

Adapted from Su C, Lichtenstein GR: Ulcerative colitis. In Feldman M, Friedman LS, Branch LJ (eds): Gastrointestinal and Liver Disease, 7th ed. Philadelphia, Saunders, 2006, pp 2499-2548.

tion is easier to make in the early stages of disease because the early manifestations are particularly distinctive. When the disease is chronic or when there have been numerous exacerbations and remissions, the distinction may be more difficult. For example, ulcerative colitis in remission may become discontinuous whereas granulomatous colitis may involve the entire colon.[1-6,162]

SUMMARY

The radiologic diagnosis of ulcerative colitis and Crohn's disease is challenging. It embraces a variety of examination techniques that must be performed and interpreted with care if the radiologist is to make a significant contribution to patient management. An understanding of the anatomic and pathophysiologic basis of the radiologic features of inflammatory bowel disease is important to appreciate fully the natural history and differentiating features of these perplexing diseases.[163,164]

References

1. Shanahan F: Ulcerative colitis. In Weinstein WM, Hawkey CJ, Bosch J (eds): Clinical Gastroenterology and Hepatology. New York, Elsevier Mosby, 2005, pp 341-342.
2. Sands BE: Crohn's disease. In Feldman MS, Friedman LS, Sleisenger MH (eds): Gastrointestinal and Liver Disease, 8th ed. Philadelphia, Saunders, 2006, pp 2459-2498.
3. Shanahan F: Ulcerative colitis. In Weinstein WM, Hawkey CJ, Bosch J (eds): Clinical Gastroenterology and Hepatology. New York, Elsevier Mosby, 2005, pp 341-342.
4. Vermeire S, Rutgeerts P: Crohn's disease. In Weinstein WM, Hawkey CJ, Bosch J (eds): Clinical Gastroenterology and Hepatology. New York, Elsevier Mosby, 2005, pp 359-376.
5. Greeson JK, Odze RD: Inflammatory diseases of the large intestine. In Odze RD, Goldblum JR, Crawford JM (eds): Surgical Pathology of the GI Tract, Liver, Biliary Tract, and Pancreas. Philadelphia, Saunders, 2004, pp 213-246.
6. Robert ME: Inflammatory diseases of the small intestine. In Odze RD, Goldblum JR, Crawford JM (eds): Surgical Pathology of the GI Tract, Liver, Biliary Tract, and Pancreas. Philadelphia, Saunders, 2004, pp 177-212.
7. Sandler RS, Loftus EV: Epidemiology of inflammatory bowel diseases. In Sartor, RB, Sandborn WJ: Kirsner's Inflammatory Bowel Disease, 6th ed. Edinburgh, Saunders, 2004, pp 245-263.
8. Colombel J-F, Tamboli CP, Hugot J-P: Clinical genetics of inflammatory bowel diseases. In Sartor, RB, Sandborn WJ (eds): Kirsner's Inflammatory Bowel Disease, 6th ed. Edinburgh, Saunders, 2004, pp 245-263.
9. Mahid SS, Minor KS, Soto RE, et al: Smoking and inflammatory bowel disease: A meta-analysis. Mayo Clin Proc 81:1462-1471, 2006.
10. Cantor M, Bernstein CN: Clinical course and natural history of ulcerative colitis. In Sartor, RB, Sandborn WJ: Kirsner's Inflammatory Bowel Disease, 6th ed. Edinburgh, Saunders, 2004, pp 245-263.
11. Munkholm P, Binder V: Clinical features and natural history of Crohn's disease. In Sartor, RB, Sandborn WJ: Kirsner's Inflammatory Bowel Disease, 6th ed. Edinburgh, Saunders, 2004, pp 289-300.
12. Cominelli F: Cytokines and inflammatory mediators. In Sartor RB, Sandborn WJ: Kirsner's Inflammatory Bowel Disease, 6th ed. Edinburgh, Saunders, 2004, pp 179-198.
13. Forcione DG, Sands BE: Differential diagnosis of inflammatory bowel disease. In Sartor, RB, Sandborn WJ: Kirsner's Inflammatory Bowel Disease, 6th ed. Edinburgh, Saunders, 2004, pp 370-379.
14. Farrell RJ, Peppercorn MA: Endoscopy inflammatory bowel disease. In Sartor, RB, Sandborn WJ: Kirsner's Inflammatory Bowel Disease, 6th ed. Edinburgh, Saunders, 2004, pp 380-398.
15. Bartram CI: Ulcerative colitis. In Bartram CI (ed): Radiology in Inflammatory Bowel Disease. New York, Marcel Dekker, 1983, pp 31-62.
16. Bartram CI: Plain abdominal x-ray in acute colitis. Proc Soc Med 69:617-618, 1976.
17. Bartram CI: Radiology in the current assessment of ulcerative colitis. Gastrointest Radiol 1:383-392, 1977.
18. Gabrielsson N, Grandvist S, Sundelin P, et al: Extent of inflammatory lesions in ulcerative colitis assessed by radiology, colonoscopy, and endoscopic biopsies. Gastrointest Radiol 4:395-400, 1979.
19. Prantera C, Lorenzetti R, Cerro P, et al: The plain abdominal film accurately estimates extent of active ulcerative colitis. J Clin Gastroenterol 13:231-234, 1991.
20. Rice RP: Plain abdominal film roentgenographic diagnosis of ulcerative disease of the colon. Radiology 104:544-550, 1968.
21. Simpson SA, Lewis JR: Plain roentgenography in diagnosis of chronic ulcerative colitis and terminal ileitis. Radiology 84:306-315, 1960.
22. McConnell F, Hanelin J, Robbins LL: Plain film diagnosis of fulminating ulcerative colitis. Radiology 71:674-682, 1958.
23. Caprilli R, Vernia P, Latella G, et al: Early recognition of toxic megacolon. J Clin Gastroenterol 9:160-164, 1987.
24. Bartram CI, Herlinger H: Bowel wall thickness as a differentiating feature between ulcerative colitis and Crohn's disease of the colon. Clin Radiol 30:15-19, 1979.
25. Lichtenstein JE: Radiologic-pathologic correlation of inflammatory bowel disease. Radiol Clin North Am 25:324, 1987.
26. Laufer I, Mullens JE, Hamilton J: Correlation of endoscopy and double-contrast radiography in the early stages of ulcerative and granulomatous colitis. Radiology 118:15, 1988.
27. Simpkins KC: Inflammatory bowel disease: Ulcerative and Crohn's colitis. In Simpkins KC (ed): A Textbook of Radiological Diagnosis, Volume 4, The Alimentary Tract: The Hollow Organs and Salivary Glands. London, HK Lewis, 1988, pp 473-498.
28. Bartram CI, Laufer I: Inflammatory bowel disease. In Laufer I, Levine MS (eds): Double Contrast Gastrointestinal Radiology, 2nd ed. Philadelphia, WB Saunders, 1992, pp 580-645.
29. Kelvin FM, Gardiner RH: Clinical Imaging of the Colon and Rectum. New York, Raven, 1987, pp 64-119.
30. Laufer I: The radiologic demonstration of early changes in ulcerative colitis by double contrast techniques. J Can Assoc Radiol 26:116-121, 1975.

31. Riddell RH: Pathology of idiopathic inflammatory bowel disease. In Sartor, RB, Sandborn WJ (eds): Kirsner's Inflammatory Bowel Disease, 6th ed. Edinburgh, Saunders, 2004, pp 399-424.

32. Lichtenstein JE, Madewell JE, Feigen DS: The collar button ulcer. Gastrointest Radiol 4:79-84, 1979.

33. Suekane H, Iida M, Matsui T, et al: Radiographic demonstration of longitudinal ulcers in patients with ulcerative colitis. Gastrointest Radiol 4:103-112, 1980.

34. Zegel H, Laufer I: Filiform polyposis. Radiology 127:615-619, 1978.

35. Bray JF: Filiform polyposis of the small bowel in Crohn's disease. Gastrointest Radiol 8:155-156, 1983.

36. Gardiner GA: "Backwash ileitis" with pseudopolyposis. AJR 129: 506-507, 1977.

37. Kirks DR, Currarino G, Berk RN: Localized giant pseudopolyposis of the colon. Am J Gastroenterol 69:609-614, 1978.

38. Hammerman AM, Shatz BA, Susman N: Radiographic characteristics of colonic "mucosal bridges": Sequelae of inflammatory bowel disease. Radiology 127:611-614, 1978.

39. Bartram CI: Complications of ulcerative colitis. In Bartram CI (ed): Radiology in Inflammatory Bowel Disease. New York, Marcel Dekker, 1983, pp 63-118.

40. Bartram CI: Complications of Crohn's disease. In Bartram CI (ed): Radiology in Inflammatory Bowel Disease. New York, Marcel Dekker, 1983, pp 169-202.

41. Gore RM: Colonic contour changes in chronic ulcerative colitis: Reappraisal of some old concepts. AJR 158:59-61, 1992.

42. Gore RM: Characteristic morphologic changes in chronic ulcerative colitis. Abdom Imaging 20:275-278, 1995.

43. Poppel MH, Beranbaum SL: The indenture sign in acute exudative colitis. Am J Dig Dis 1:382-388, 1957.

44. Campbell WL: Cathartic colon: Reversibility of roentgen changes. Dis Colon Rectum 23:445-449, 1983.

45. Kim SK, Gerle RD, Rozanski R: Cathartic colitis. AJR 131:1079-1081, 1978.

46. Kattan KR, King AY: Presacral space revisited. AJR 132:437-439, 1979.

47. Krestin GP, Beyer D, Steinbrich W: Computed tomography in the differential diagnosis of the enlarged retrorectal space. Gastrointest Radiol 11:364-369, 1986.

48. Edling NPG, Eklof O: The retrorectal soft tissue space in ulcerative colitis. Radiology 80:949-953, 1963.

49. Eklof O, Gierup J: The retrorectal soft tissue space in children: Normal variations and appearance in granulomatous colitis. AJR 108:624-627, 1970.

50. Lew RJ, Ginsberg GG: The role of endoscopic ultrasound in inflammatory bowel disease. Gastrointest Endosc Clin North Am 12:561-571, 2002.

51. Marshak RH, Boch C, Wolf BS: The roentgen findings in strictures of the colon associated with ulcerative and granulomatous colitis. AJR 90:709-716, 1963.

52. Goldberg HI, Gore RM, Margulis AR, et al: Computed tomography in the evaluation of Crohn's disease. AJR 140:277-282, 1983.

53. Dombal FT, Watts JM, Watkinson G, et al: Local complications of ulcerative colitis: Stricture, pseudopolyposis, and carcinoma of the colon and rectum. BMJ 1:1442-1447, 1966.

54. Goulston SJM, McGovern VJ: The nature of benign strictures in ulcerative colitis. N Engl J Med 281:290-295, 1969.

55. Antes G: Inflammatory diseases of the large intestine, colon, contrast enema and CT. Radiology 38:41-45, 1998.

56. Gore RM, Balthazar EJ, Ghahremani GG, et al: CT features of ulcerative colitis and Crohn's disease. AJR 167:3-15, 1996.

57. Hoeffel C, Crema MD, Belkacem A, et al: Multi-detector row CT: spectrum of diseases involving the ileocecal area. RadioGraphics 26:1373-1390, 2006.

58. Horton KM, Corl FM, Fishman EK: CT evaluation of the colon: Inflammatory disease. RadioGraphics 20:399-418, 2000.

59. Gore RM, Marn CS, Kirby DF, et al: CT findings in ulcerative, granulomatous, and indeterminate colitis. AJR 143:279-284, 1984.

60. Gore RM, Lichtenstein JE: The gastrointestinal tract: Anatomic-pathologic basis of radiologic findings. In Taveras JM, Ferrucci JT (eds): Radiology: Diagnosis-Imaging-Intervention. Philadelphia, JB Lippincott, 1994, pp 1-42.

61. Gore RM, Goldberg HI: Computed tomographic evaluation of the gastrointestinal tract in diseases other than primary adenocarcinoma. Radiol Clin North Am 20:781-796, 1982.

62. Gore RM, Ghahremani GG: Radiological investigation of acute inflammatory and infectious bowel disease. Gastroenterol Clin North Am 24:353-384, 1995.

63. Balthazar EJ: CT of the gastrointestinal tract: Principles and interpretation. AJR 156:23-32, 1991.

64. Thoeni RF, Cello JP: CT imaging of colitis. Radiology 240:623-638, 2006.

65. Philpotts LE, Heiken JP, Westcott MA, et al: Colitis: Use of CT findings in differential diagnosis. Radiology 190:445-449, 1994.

66. Gore RM: Cross-sectional imaging of inflammatory bowel disease. Radiol Clin North Am 25:115-127, 1987.

67. Gore RM: CT of inflammatory bowel disease. Radiol Clin North Am 27:717-730, 1989.

68. De Pascale A, Garofalo G, Perna M, et al: Contrast-enhanced ultrasonography in Crohn's disease. Radiol Med (Torino). 111:539-550, 2006.

69. Rispo A, Bucci L, Pesce G, et al: Bowel sonography for the diagnosis and grading of postsurgical recurrence of Crohn's disease. Inflamm Bowel Dis 12:486-490, 2006.

70. Mackalski BA, Bernstein CN: New diagnostic imaging tools for inflammatory bowel disease. Gut 55:733-741, 2006.

71. Maconi G, Radice E, Greco S, et al: Bowel ultrasound in Crohn's disease. Best Pract Res Clin Gastroenterol 20:93-112, 2006.

72. Parente F, Greco S, Molteni M, et al: Modern imaging of Crohn's disease using bowel ultrasound. Inflamm Bowel Dis 10:452-461, 2004.

73. Parente F, Greco S, Molteni M, et al: Imaging inflammatory bowel disease using bowel ultrasound. Eur J Gastroenterol Hepatol 17:283-291, 2005.

74. Ajaj WM, Lauenstein TC, Pelster G, et al: Magnetic resonance colonography for the detection of inflammatory diseases of the large bowel: Quantifying the inflammatory activity. Gut. 54:257-263, 2005.

75. Maccioni F, Bruni A, Viscido A, et al: MR imaging in patients with Crohn disease: Value of T2- versus T1-weighted gadolinium-enhanced MR sequences with use of an oral superparamagnetic contrast agent. Radiology 238:517-530, 2006.

76. Low RN, Francis IR: MR imaging of the gastrointestinal tract with IV gadolinium and diluted oral contrast media compared with unenhanced MR imaging and CT. AJR 169:1051-1054, 1997.

77. Schreyer AG, Rath HC, Kikinis R, et al: Comparison of magnetic resonance imaging colonography with conventional colonoscopy for the assessment of intestinal inflammation in patients with inflammatory bowel disease: A feasibility study. Gut 54:250-256, 2005.

78. Schreyer AG, Golder S, Scheibl K, et al: Dark lumen magnetic resonance enteroclysis in combination with MRI colonography for whole bowel assessment in patients with Crohn's disease: First clinical experience. Inflamm Bowel Dis 11:388-394, 2005.

79. Rottgen R, Herzog H, Lopez-Haninnen E, et al: Bowel wall enhancement in magnetic resonance colonography for assessing activity in Crohn's disease. Clin Imaging 30:27-31, 2006.

80. Aburano T, Saito Y, Shuke N, et al: Tc-99m leukocyte imaging for evaluating disease severity and monitoring treatment response in ulcerative colitis: Comparison with colonoscopy. Clin Nucl Med 23:509-513, 1998.

81. Loffler M, Weckesser M, Franzius C, et al: High diagnostic value of 18F-FDG-PET in pediatric patients with chronic inflammatory bowel disease. Ann N Y Acad Sci 1072:379-385, 2006.

82. Annovazzi A, Bagni B, Burroni L, et al: Nuclear medicine imaging of inflammatory/infective disorders of the abdomen. Nucl Med Commun 26:657-664, 2005.

83. Kerry JE, Marshall C, Griffiths PA, et al: Comparison between Tc-HMPAO labelled white cells and Tc LeukoScan in the investigation of inflammatory bowel disease. Nucl Med Commun 26:245-251, 2005.

84. Almer S, Bodemar G, Lindstrom E, et al: Air enema radiology compared with leukocyte scintigraphy for imaging in inflammation in active colitis. Eur J Gastroenterol Hepatol 7:59-64, 1995.

85. Hanauer SB: Medical therapy for ulcerative colitis. In Sartor, RB, Sandborn WJ (eds): Kirsner's Inflammatory Bowel Disease, 6th edition. Edinburgh, Saunders, 2004, pp 503-530.

86. Sandborn WJ: Medical therapy for Crohn's disease. In Sartor, RB, Sandborn WJ (eds): Kirsner's Inflammatory Bowel Disease, 6th ed. Edinburgh, Saunders, 2004, pp 503-530.

87. Caprilli R, Viscido A, Latella G: Current management of severe ulcerative colitis. Nat Clin Pract Gastroenterol Hepatol 4:92-101, 2007.

88. Marion JF, Present DH: Indications for surgery in inflammatory bowel disease from the gastroenterologists point of view. In Sartor RB, Sandborn WJ (eds): Kirsner's Inflammatory Bowel Disease, 6th ed. Edinburgh, Saunders, 2004, pp 585-595.

89. Fichera A, Michelassi F: Indications for surgery: A surgeon's point of view. In Sartor RB, Sandborn WJ (eds): Kirsner's Inflammatory Bowel Disease, 6th ed. Edinburgh, Saunders, 2004, pp 596-601.

90. Cima RR, Pemberton JH: Surgical management of ulcerative colitis. In Sartor RB, Sandborn WJ (eds): Kirsner's Inflammatory Bowel Disease, 6th ed. Edinburgh, Saunders, 2004, pp 602-614.

91. Surgery for Crohn's disease. In Sartor RB, Sandborn WJ (eds): Kirsner's Inflammatory Bowel Disease, 6th ed. Edinburgh, Saunders, 2004, pp 614-630.

92. Crema MD, Richarme D, Azizi L, et al: Pouchography, CT, and MRI features of ileal J pouch-anal anastomosis. AJR 187:594-603, 2006.

93. Nadgir RN, Soto JA, Dendrinos K, et al: MRI of complicated pouchitis. AJR 187:386-391, 2006.

94. Gosselink MP, West RL, Kuipers EJ, et al: Integrity of the anal sphincters after pouch-anal anastomosis: Evaluation with three-dimensional endoanal ultrasonography. Dis Colon Rectum 48:1728-1735, 2005.

95. Brown JJ, Balfe DM, Heiken JP, et al: Ileal J pouch: Radiologic evaluation in patients with and without postoperative complications. Radiology 174:115-120, 1990.

96. Kremers PW, Scholz FJ, Schoetz DJ, et al: Radiology of the ileoanal reservoir. AJR 145:559-567, 1985.

97. Lycke KG, Gothlin JH, Jensen JK, et al: Radiology of the continent ileostomy reservoir: I. Method of examination and normal findings. Abdom Imaging 19:116-123, 1994.

98. Alfisher MM, Scholz FJ, Robert PL, et al: Radiology of ileal pouch-anal anastomosis: Normal findings, examination pitfalls, and complications. RadioGraphics 17:81-98, 1997.

99. Thoeni RF, Fell C, Engelstad B, et al: Ileoanal pouches: Comparison of CT, scintigraphy and contrast enemas for diagnosing post-surgical complications. AJR 154:73-78, 1990.

100. Lycke KG, Gothlin JH, Jensen JK, et al: Radiology of the continent ileostomy reservoir: II. Findings in patients with late complications. Abdom Imaging 19:124-131, 1994.

101. Lockhart-Mummery HE, Morson BC: Crohn's disease (regional enteritis) of the large intestine and its distinction from ulcerative colitis. Gut 1:87-105, 1960.

102. Crohn BB, Ginzburg L, Oppenheimer GD: Regional ileitis: A pathologic and clinical entity. JAMA 99:1323-1329, 1932.

103. Kelvin FM, May RJ, Norton GA: Lymphoid follicular pattern of the colon in adults. AJR 133:831-835, 1979.

104. Laufer I, Desa D: Lymphoid follicular pattern: A normal feature of the pediatric colon. AJR 130:51-55, 1978.

105. Kenney PJ, Koehler RE, Shackelford GD: The clinical significance of large lymphoid follicles of the colon. Radiology 142:41-46, 1982.

106. Bronen RA, Glick SN, Teplick SH: Diffuse lymphoid follicles of the colon. Radiology 142:41-46, 1982.

107. Laufer I, Costopoulous L: Early lesions of Crohn's disease. AJR 130:307-311, 1978.

108. Simpkins KC: Aphthoid ulcers in Crohn's colitis. Clin Radiol 28:601-604, 1977.

109. Ekberg O, Lindstrom C: Superficial lesions in Crohn's disease of the small bowel. Gastrointest Radiol 4:389-392, 1979.

110. Degrysa HRM, DeSchepper AMAP: Aphthoid esophageal ulcers in Crohn's disease of ileum and colon. Gastrointest Radiol 9:197-201, 1984.

111. Ni XY, Goldberg HI: Aphthoid ulcers in Crohn's disease: Radiographic course and relationship to bowel appearance. Radiology 158:589-592, 1986.

112. Hizawa K, Aoyagi K, Fujishima M: The significance of colonic mucosal lymphoid hyperplasia and aphthoid ulcers in Crohn's disease. Clin Radiol 51:706-708, 1996.

113. Hizawa K, Iida M, Kohrogi N, et al: Crohn disease: Early recognition and progress of aphthous lesions. Radiology 190:451-454, 1994.

114. Goldberg HI, Gore RM, Margulis AR, et al: Computed tomography in the evaluation of Crohn disease. AJR 140:277-282, 1983.

115. Raptopoulos V, Schwartz RK, McNicholas MMJ, et al: Multiplanar helical CT enterography in patients with Crohn's disease. AJR 169:1545-1550, 1997.

116. Gore RM, Ghahremani GG, Miller FH: Cross-sectional imaging in the evaluation of Crohn's disease. In Prantera C, Korelitz BI (eds): Crohn's Disease. New York, Marcel Dekker, 1996, pp 145-185.

117. Jacobs JE, Birnbaum BA: CT of the inflammatory disease of the colon. Semin Ultrasound CT MRI 16:91-101, 1995.

118. Fishman EK, Wolf EJ, Jones B, et al: CT evaluation of Crohn's disease: Effect on patient management. AJR 148:537-541, 1987.

119. Gossios KJ, Tsianos EV: Crohn disease: CT findings after treatment. Abdom Imaging 22:160-163, 1997.

120. Scott EM, Freeman AH: Prominent omental and mesenteric vasculature in inflammatory bowel disease shown by computed tomography. Eur J Radiol 22:104-106, 1996.

121. Meyers MA, McGuire PV: Spiral CT demonstration of hypervascularity in Crohn disease: "Vascular jejunalization of the ileum" or the "comb sign." Abdom Imaging 20:327-332, 1995.

122. Herlinger H, Furth EE, Rubesin SE: Fibrofatty proliferation of the mesentery in Crohn's disease. Abdom Imaging 23:446-448, 1998.

123. Ribeiro MB, Greenstein AJ, Yamazaki Y, et al: Intra-abdominal abscess in regional enteritis. Ann Surg 213:32-36, 1991.

124. Lambiase RE, Cronan JJ, Dorfman GS: Percutaneous drainage of abscesses in patients with Crohn disease. AJR 150:1043-1045, 1988.

125. Casola G, vanSonnenberg E, Neff CC, et al: Abscess in Crohn's disease: Percutaneous drainage. Radiology 163:19-22, 1987.

126. Safrit HD, Mauro MA, Jaques PF: Percutaneous abscess drainage in Crohn's disease. AJR 148:859-862, 1987.

127. Doemeny JM, Burke DR, Meranze SG: Percutaneous drainage of abscesses in patients with Crohn's disease. Gastrointest Radiol 13:327-341, 1988.

128. Erden A, Cumhur T, Olger T: Superior mesenteric artery Doppler waveform changes in response to inflammation of the ileocecal region. Abdom Imaging 22:483-486, 1997.

129. van Oostayen JA, Wasser MNJM, van Hogezand RA, et al: Activity of Crohn disease assessed by measurements of superior mesenteric artery flow with Doppler US. Radiology 193:551-554, 1994.

130. Nemcek AA: Superior mesenteric artery Doppler waveform changes in response to inflammation of the ileocecal region. Abdom Imaging 22:487-488, 1997.

131. Funt SA, Krinsky G, Horowitz L: MR demonstration of submucosal fat in a patient with Crohn's disease. J Comput Assist Tomogr 20:940-941, 1996.

132. Ernst O, Asselah T, Cablan X, et al: Breath-hold fast spin-echo MR imaging of Crohn's disease. AJR 170:127-128, 1998.

133. Spencer JA, Chapple K, Wilson D, et al: Outcome after surgery for perianal fistula value of MR imaging. AJR 171:403-408, 1998.

134. Hussain SM, Stoker J, Schoeten WR, et al: Fistula in ano: Endoanal sonography versus endoanal MR imaging in classification. Radiology 200:475-481, 1996.

135. Lanaido M, Makowiec F, Dammann F, et al: Perianal complications of Crohn disease: MR imaging findings. Eur Radiol 7:1035-1042, 1997.

136. Kodner JJ: Perianal Crohn's disease. In Allen RN, Rhodes JM, Hanauer SB, et al (eds): Inflammatory Bowel Diseases, 3rd ed. New York, Churchill Livingstone, 1997, pp 863-872.

137. von Ritter C: Inflammatory bowel disease: Pathophysiology and medical treatment. Radiologe 38:3-7, 1998.

138. Milsom JW: Surgery of colorectal cancer and inflammatory bowel disease. Curr Opin Gastroenterol 9:42-48, 1993.

139. Doemeny JM, Burke DR, Maranze SG: Percutaneous abscess drainage in Crohn's disease. AJR 148:859-862, 1987.

140. Fearnhead NS, Chowdhury R, Box B: Long-term follow-up of strictureplasty for Crohn's disease. Br J Surg 93:475-482, 2006.

141. Karlen P, Lofberg R, Brostrom O, et al: Increased risk of cancer in ulcerative colitis: A population-based cohort study. Am J Gastroenterol 94:1047-1052, 1999.

142. Stucchi AF, Aarons CB, Becker JM: Surgical approaches to cancer in patients who have inflammatory bowel disease. Gastroenterol Clin North Am 35:641-673, 2006.

143. Bernstein CN: Neoplasia in inflammatory bowel disease: Surveillance and management strategies. Curr Gastroenterol Rep 8:513-518, 2006.

144. Moum B, Ekbom A: Ulcerative colitis, colorectal cancer and colonoscopic surveillance. Scand J Gastroenterol 40:881-885, 2005.

145. D'Amico C, Vitale A, Angriman I, et al: Early surgery for the treatment of toxic megacolon. Digestion 72:146-149, 2005.

146. Ausch C, Madoff RD, Gnant M, et al: Aetiology and surgical management of toxic megacolon. Colorectal Dis 8:195-201, 2006.

147. Goldberg HI: The barium enema and toxic megacolon: Cause-effect relationship? Gastroenterology 68:617-618, 1975.

148. Halpert RD: Toxic dilatation of the colon. Radiol Clin North Am 25:147-155, 1987.

149. Elsayes KM, Oliveira EP, Narra VR, et al: MR and MRCP in the evaluation of primary sclerosing cholangitis: Current applications and imaging findings. J Comput Assist Tomogr 30:398-404, 2006.

150. Patel TR, Patel KN, Boyarsky AH, et al: Staphylococcal liver abscess and acute cholecystitis in a patient with Crohn's disease receiving infliximab. J Gastrointest Surg 10:105-110, 2006.
151. Moolsintong P, Loftus EV Jr, et al: Acute pancreatitis in patients with Crohn's disease: Clinical features and outcomes. Inflamm Bowel Dis 11:1080-1084, 2005.
152. Banner MP: Genitourinary complications of inflammatory bowel disease. Radiol Clin North Am 25:199-204, 1987.
153. Merine D, Fishman EK, Kuhlman JE, et al: Bladder involvement in Crohn disease: Role of CT in detection and evaluation. J Comput Assist Tomogr 13:90-93, 1989.
154. Fomberstein B, Yerra N, Pitchumoni CS: Rheumatological complications of GI disorders. Am J Gastroenterol 91:1090-1103, 1996.
155. Björkengren AG, Resnick D, Sartoris DJ: Enteropathic arthropathies. Radiol Clin North Am 25:189-198, 1987.
156. McEniff N, Eustace S, McCarthy C: Asymptomatic sacroiliitis in inflammatory bowel disease: Assessment by computed tomography. Clin Imaging 19:258-262, 1995.
157. Geijer M, Sihlbom H, Gothlin JH, et al: The role of CT in the diagnosis of sacroiliitis. Acta Radiol 39:265-268, 1998.
158. Ghahremani GG: Osteomyelitis of the ilium in patients with Crohn's disease. AJR 118:364-370, 1973.
159. Bernstein CN: Osteoporosis and other complications of inflammatory bowel disease. Curr Opin Gastroenterol 18:428-434, 2002.
160. Millward SF, Ramsewak W, Fitzsimons P: Percutaneous drainage of iliopsoas abscess in Crohn's disease. Gastrointest Radiol 11:289-290, 1986.
161. Boland GW, Mueller PR: Update on abscess drainage. Semin Intervent Radiol 13:27-40, 1996.
162. Rudolph WG, Uthoff SM, McAuliffe TL, et al: Indeterminate colitis: The real story. Dis Colon Rectum 45:1528-1534, 2002.
163. Kucharzik T, Maaser C, Lugering A, et al: Recent understanding of IBD pathogenesis: Implications for future therapies. Inflamm Bowel Dis 12:1068-1083, 2006.
164. Sands BE: Inflammatory bowel disease: Past, present, and future. J Gastroenterol 42:16-25, 2007.

chapter

62

Other Inflammatory Conditions of the Colon

Seth N. Glick, MD • Richard M. Gore, MD

BACTERIAL INFECTIONS	**NONINFECTIOUS COLITIS**
Salmonellosis	Nonspecific Ulcer
Shigellosis	Typhlitis
Campylobacteriosis	Microscopic (Collagenous) Colitis
Yersinia Enterocolitis	Eosinophilic Colitis
Colitis Caused by *Escherichia coli* O157:H7	Graft-versus-Host Disease
Tuberculosis	Retractile Mesenteritis
Actinomycosis	Reactive Inflammation
VIRAL INFECTIONS	**NEUTROPHIL AND MACROPHAGE DYSFUNCTION**
PARASITIC INFECTIONS	Chronic Granulomatous Disease of Childhood
Anisakiasis	Glycogen Storage Disease
Amebiasis	Malacoplakia
Schistosomiasis	**EXOGENOUS CAUSES OF COLITIS**
Strongyloidiasis	Caustic Colitis
Trichuriasis	Drug-Induced Colitis
FUNGAL INFECTIONS	*Clostridium difficile* Colitis
Histoplasmosis	
Mucormycosis	

In daily practice, idiopathic inflammatory bowel disease accounts for the majority of cases of colonic inflammation encountered by the radiologist. However, a variety of inflammatory conditions involve the colon, with variable frequency. Some conditions (e.g., ischemic colitis, radiation colitis, and *Clostridium difficile* colitis) are relatively common, whereas others either are rare or seldom require imaging studies for their management. In many cases, the information derived from the imaging studies combined with the patient's history, symptoms, and laboratory and pathologic findings may result in a specific diagnosis or may produce a limited differential diagnosis. Even after the diagnosis has been established, however, imaging studies may have a role in assessing the severity

of the process, monitoring the course of the disease and determining the presence of complications.

The bowel has a limited pathologic response with similar changes in a variety of conditions. In most inflammatory diseases, these changes are characterized by a specific colonic distribution, morphologic appearance, magnitude of injury, and progression of disease. Colonic abnormalities may also be associated with characteristic abnormalities in other gastrointestinal viscera or nongastrointestinal sites. For diagnostic purposes, it is helpful to classify inflammatory conditions of the colon into those that resemble ulcerative colitis radiologically and those that may be confused with Crohn's colitis. Some conditions may even simulate colonic carcinoma, manifested by a palpable mass or a short, narrowed colonic segment.

Anatomic distribution, particularly the presence or absence of rectal involvement, is an important discriminating feature. When the rectum is spared, ulcerative colitis becomes extremely unlikely and the number of diagnostic possibilities is limited. The presence of diffuse or segmental changes is another differentiating feature. With segmental processes, the specific site or sites of involvement and the radiologic appearance may provide clues to the correct diagnosis. Diseases that involve the rectum may be classified into those that are confined to the rectum and those with associated colonic involvement. Specific features such as fistulas, asymmetry, and mucosal alterations may further narrow the differential diagnosis. Rarely, some colitides have features that are distinctive from ulcerative or Crohn's colitis.

The patient's age, the duration or rapidity of onset of symptoms, and a failure to respond to standard therapy for idiopathic inflammatory bowel disease should prompt consideration of diagnostic alternatives. Other important data include drug history (particularly antibiotics, chemotherapeutic agents, or hormonal preparations), previous radiation therapy, immunosuppression, and pertinent information relating to travel, diet, and sexual activities. This information combined with the radiographic findings often allows the radiologist to suggest the correct diagnosis. Thus, it is important to be familiar with these various colitides as well as their range of appearances and related clinical findings.

BACTERIAL INFECTIONS

Infectious colitis may be caused by bacterial, viral, fungal, and parasitic organisms.[1-4] In Western countries, bacterial colitis represents the most common form of colonic infection, whereas in underdeveloped countries, parasitic infestation occurs most frequently. Imaging studies are not usually performed for patients with bacterial colitis because the diagnosis is readily established with routine stool cultures.

The diagnosis of bacterial colitis should be suggested by the typical presentation of acute onset of dysenteric symptoms, consisting of fever, crampy abdominal pain and tenderness (with or without vomiting), tenesmus, and small volume diarrhea (frequently bloody). In most cases, the disease is self-limited. Routine cultures may occasionally yield false-negative results, so specialized cultures are required to isolate specific organisms. In this setting, contrast studies may be performed. Unfortunately, it is difficult to make categorical statements about the radiologic appearance of various bacterial infections because of the paucity of published data (usually anecdotal case reports) in the radiologic literature. In many cases, these reports involved only single-contrast barium studies without benefit of double-contrast studies or colonoscopy, so the nature and extent of morphologic abnormalities described in these reports are not necessarily accurate.

Salmonellosis

Salmonella is a gram-negative rod that is ingested with contaminated food or water.[1-4] Colonic involvement may occur during the course of typhoid fever or as an acute dysentery. Typhoid fever is caused by *S. typhi* or *S. paratyphi*. Presenting symptoms include marked pyrexia, arthralgias, malaise, headaches, and right lower quadrant pain. The organism initially involves the reticuloendothelial system, particularly the spleen, mesenteric lymph nodes, and Peyer patches of the terminal ileum. Splenomegaly may occur after 1 week. Gastrointestinal involvement occurs in the second or third week in approximately 50% of the cases, but it is often obscured by other symptoms. Right lower quadrant pain and tenderness are the most common findings. When colonic involvement is present, the barium enema may reveal narrowing and loss of haustration in the cecum due to edema and spasm as well as ileal fold thickening and ulceration. Aphthous ulcers in the ascending colon have also been reported.[5] The ileum is invariably involved. Hemorrhage and perforation occur in 1% to 3% of cases. Symptoms begin to resolve in the fourth week, but relapses are common. Blood cultures are positive during the first week in 90% of patients, and the organism may be isolated from stool cultures during the second and third weeks. Chloramphenicol is the treatment of choice.

A wide variety of *Salmonella* serotypes (e.g., *S. enteritidis typhimurium*) may also cause sudden onset of diarrhea, fever, abdominal pain, nausea, and vomiting.[1-4] The incubation period is 8 to 48 hours. The disease usually occurs in outbreaks, particularly in the summer when food tends to spoil. The endoscopic appearance may simulate ulcerative colitis.

In most reported cases, barium enemas have revealed a pancolitis with loss of haustration, often associated with superficial or even deep "collar-button" ulcers.[6,7] Thumbprinting has also been reported. Other patients may have extensive small bowel thickening and effacement associated with a pancolitis. Double-contrast studies may reveal punctate mucosal stippling, discrete superficial ulcers, or mucosal granularity. The descending and sigmoid colon is usually involved, with variable proximal extension. Although the rectum usually appears spared radiographically, there may be mild inflammation at endoscopy.[8] A segmental ulcerating colitis in the left colon is rare.[9] Fulminant disease and even toxic megacolon may occur, particularly in elderly or debilitated persons. Bacteremia is common, and the infection may spread to the gallbladder, bones, lungs, and kidneys.

Although frequently positive, stool cultures may need to be repeated to confirm the diagnosis. Serial elevation of febrile agglutinins may provide supportive information. The disease is self-limited, lasting 1 to 2 weeks. Oral antibiotics and antidiarrheal agents are ineffective and may even prolong the illness. In severe cases, parenteral chloramphenicol can be administered.

Shigellosis

Infection with *Shigella*, a gram-negative rod, may be caused by three species: *S. flexneri*, *S. dysenteriae*, and *S. sonnei*.[1-4] In the United States, *S. sonnei* is the offending organism in 70% of cases, whereas in Mexico and Asia, *S. dysenteriae* is most common. As with salmonellosis, infection may occur in outbreaks, particularly in warm weather. The incubation period is 1 to 3 days, and the presentation is usually similar to that of *Salmonella* infection. However, shigellosis produces a toxin that causes increased small bowel secretion and watery diarrhea, which lasts several days and then progresses to dysenteric symptoms. Systemic absorption of the toxin may also cause arthritis, pneumonitis, seizures, peripheral neuropathy, microangiopathy, and hemolytic-uremic syndrome. Bacteremia is rare but may cause vascular collapse. Stool cultures are positive within 1 day of onset and may remain positive for months. Toxic megacolon has also been reported. The disease is usually self-limited, lasting 7 to 10 days, but occasionally as long as 1 month. The mortality rate is 10% to 20% in immunocompromised patients or in patients with bacteremia. Treatment is with ampicillin; antispasmodics are contraindicated because they may aggravate the patient's condition.

Sigmoidoscopy almost always reveals an inflammatory process simulating ulcerative colitis that varies from mild granularity and erythema to ulceration.[10,11] Ulceration is more commonly seen than in salmonellosis. Ulcers are usually superficial and of varying size and shape. They are predominantly stellate but may be linear, serpiginous, or aphthous and are superimposed on a diffusely friable mucosa. In patients with *S. dysenteriae* infection, the ulcerative phase is most marked in the second and third weeks of the disease, with erythema and edema more prominent in the first week.[11] In many cases, the ulceration is most severe distal to the splenic flexure. Healing ensues with gradually decreasing erythema. The process is initially continuous and pancolonic. During recovery, involvement may become patchy. Although healing is usually complete, some patients may have residual strictures, inflammatory polyps, or even persistent colitis.

In most reports, barium enemas (Fig. 62-1) have revealed a predominantly left-sided colitis with deep ulcers that may have a collar-button appearance.[7] Aphthous ulcers may also be seen. One patient with *S. flexneri* infection had discrete flat ulcers in the sigmoid colon and inflammatory polyps in the transverse and descending colon.[12] In this case, a follow-up study 9 months later revealed stenosis and inflammatory polyps in the sigmoid colon.

Campylobacteriosis

Campylobacter is the most common cause of bacterial colitis. This organism has been isolated in 7% to 10% of stool cultures obtained from patients with diarrhea.[1-4] The offending agent is *C. fetus* subspecies *jejuni*. The disease is usually self-limited,

lasting less than 7 days, but symptoms may persist as long as 1 month. Recurrent disease occurs in as many as 25% of cases if the infection is untreated. Approximately 50% of patients have a 24-hour prodrome consisting of headaches, nausea and vomiting, and arthralgias, followed by watery and then bloody diarrhea. Both the small bowel and the colon may be involved, although colitis is more common. In some cases, barium enemas have revealed a pancolitis with diffuse granularity and loss of haustration simulating ulcerative colitis, whereas in others, barium enemas have revealed aphthous ulcers, resembling Crohn's disease.[13-16] The left side of the colon is almost always involved. Hemorrhage, perforation, and toxic megacolon have also been reported as complications. The diagnosis requires culture on selective media; serologic studies may also be helpful for confirmation.

Yersinia Enterocolitis

Infection by *Yersinia enterocolitica,* a gram-negative rod, tends to be more common in certain regions such as Japan, Canada, and Scandinavia.[1-4,17-20] Specific strains may be endemic to each of these locations, and these strains have different clinical and pathologic manifestations. Patients younger than 5 years of age usually present with acute right lower quadrant pain and fever, simulating appendicitis. In contrast, adults may present with acute or protracted fever, pain, and diarrhea evolving over a 4- to 6-week period. Other patients may have associated arthralgias, arthritis, or rashes such as erythema nodosum or erythema multiforme.

The terminal ileum is invariably involved on barium enemas; the radiographic findings depend on the stage of the disease.[17] The most common findings include small nodules due to enlarged lymphoid follicles or discrete punctate, aphthous, or larger oval ulcers. Folds may also be thickened, but, unlike Crohn's disease, stenosis is not a feature. Colonic changes are manifested by aphthous ulcers that are predominantly located in the right side of the colon, but left-sided colonic involvement is occasionally noted.[20-22] The evolution and resolution of these clinical and radiologic abnormalities may require several months. Perforation is rare, but hepatic abscess and septicemia are well-documented complications. Diagnosis requires special culture media or serologic studies. Although no treatment has been proved to be effective, the diagnosis of *Yersinia* enterocolitis is important primarily for the purpose of excluding other entities.

Colitis Caused by *Escherichia Coli* O157:H7

Escherichia coli strains are the most common cause of traveler's diarrhea and are usually self-limited. However, the subtype O157:H7 has drawn increased attention because it is associated with a high morbidity and mortality. Outbreaks of this infection have been noted in Canada; residents of nursing homes have been particularly susceptible. Patients typically present with watery diarrhea (without fever) that progresses over several days to a hemorrhagic colitis. The most serious complication, the hemolytic-uremic syndrome, results from a toxin associated with this infection. The overall mortality may be as high as 33%. The findings on barium enemas are similar to those of ischemic colitis, with thumbprinting, narrowing, and spasm of the involved bowel. CT may reveal low-density thickening of the wall due to edema (Fig. 62-2).

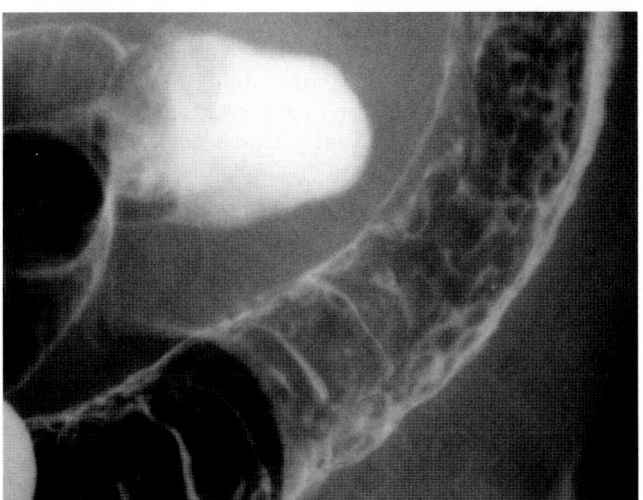

Figure 62-1. *Shigella* colitis. Ulcerations of the sigmoid colon are present on this double-contrast barium enema.

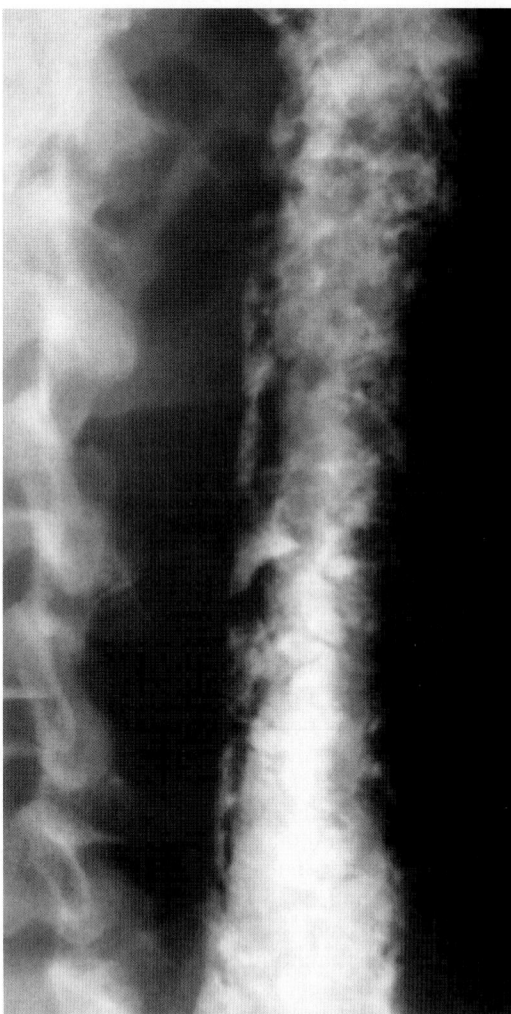

Figure 62-2. Colitis caused by *Escherichia coli* O157:H7. Deep ulcerations are identified in the descending colon.

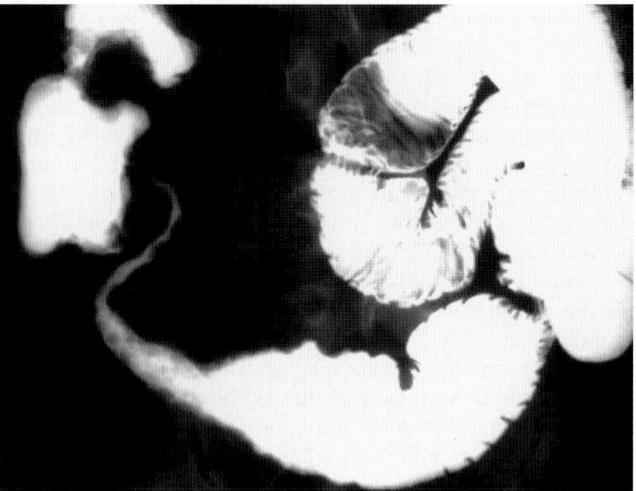

Figure 62-3. Ileocecal tuberculosis. Abnormality of the terminal ileum and right cecum is similar to that seen in Crohn's disease.

Most reported cases have involved the transverse colon, often associated with extension to the right, left, or both sides of the colon.[23-25] The morphologic changes are caused predominantly by ischemia, and histologic specimens may resemble pseudomembranous colitis. Treatment is supportive, but this diagnosis is important so that isolation procedures can be instituted.

Tuberculosis

Although once considered rare in Western countries, tuberculosis has been increasing in incidence. As a result, reports of gastrointestinal tract involvement have became more common. Patients with AIDS have been noted to be at greater risk than the general population.[26] Although most cases are secondary to a pulmonary source, the majority of patients have no evidence of active or previous pulmonary tuberculosis on chest radiographs. In endemic areas of Asia, most cases of gastrointestinal tuberculosis are caused by ingestion of the bovine bacillus. Colonic involvement is often associated with ileal disease. Most patients present with chronic symptoms, including weight loss, fever, pain, palpable mass, and diarrhea. However, diarrhea is a less prominent feature than in patients with Crohn's disease.

Barium studies may reveal abnormalities in the ascending and proximal transverse colon that are indistinguishable from those of Crohn's disease (Fig. 62-3).[26] It has been suggested that certain abnormalities are characteristic, such as oval or circumferential transverse ulcers, loss of anatomic demarcation between the ileum and the right colon (Stierlin sign), and a right-angle intersection between the ileum and the cecum with marked hypertrophy of the ileocecal valve (Fleischner's sign). These findings result from the exuberant mural thickening, which tends to be greater than that in Crohn's disease. Other suggestive features include extremely short segments of involvement of the ileum or cecum; markedly enlarged lymph nodes, particularly with low density on CT scan; and ascites. However, the most frequent findings include some combination of narrowing, deep ulceration, and mucosal granulation with nodularity and inflammatory polyps. Less common findings include aphthous ulcers, diffuse colitis, segmental colitis distal to the hepatic flexure, and short strictures, simulating carcinoma.[27-33] Fistulas and sinus tracts are also rare.

The diagnosis can be made on endoscopic biopsy specimens that reveal caseating granulomas or positive cultures for the acid-fast bacilli.[34] However, the yield from endoscopy has been variable. As a result, surgical specimens are sometimes required for a definitive diagnosis. Tuberculous colitis is an important diagnosis because of the potentially catastrophic consequences of administering corticosteroids to these patients due to a mistaken diagnosis of inflammatory bowel disease.

Actinomycosis

Actinomyces israelii is an anaerobic bacterium that occurs as part of the normal flora of the bowel, but when there is contact with tissues not normally exposed to this organism, a pathologic process ensues. Gastrointestinal involvement occurs after infection of mesenteric and peritoneal tissues from penetrating trauma, abdominal surgery, or long-standing intrauterine devices. These patients may develop inflammatory masses and fistulas that involve the colon. Presenting symptoms include a palpable mass, vague abdominal pain, and diarrhea.

Barium enemas may reveal extrinsic masses involving the colon with reactive changes, distortion, and strictures with or without fistula formation.[35,36] Fistulas can extend to the skin, where characteristic colonies of sulfur granules may be identified. The ileocecal region is the most common site of gastrointestinal involvement. Many of these patients have a history of prior appendectomy. In contrast, the rectosigmoid colon is the usual site of involvement in patients with intra-uterine devices. Ultrasonography and CT may also reveal large inflammatory masses. Surgery is often necessary for a definitive diagnosis and for differentiating these inflammatory masses from neoplasms.

VIRAL INFECTIONS

Cytomegalovirus (CMV) infection is a frequent complication of AIDS; the gastrointestinal tract may be either focally or diffusely involved. Gastrointestinal abnormalities are thought to result from CMV-induced ischemic vasculitis. When colonic involvement by CMV is suspected, the diagnosis can be confirmed by the presence of characteristic intranuclear inclusions (viral inclusion bodies) on endoscopic brushings or biopsy specimens.

CMV colitis usually involves the cecum and proximal colon, sometimes extending into the distal ileum. Early disease is manifested by diffuse nodular lymphoid hyperplasia. Positive cultures from the colon are diagnostic. With moderate disease, barium enemas may reveal multifocal ulcerations, appearing as shallow, well-defined ulcers scattered on an otherwise normal background mucosa.[37] More advanced disease (Fig. 62-4) may be manifested by deeper ulcers and marked thickening of the colonic wall both on barium studies and on CT.[37] Some patients have a pancolitis with diffuse, contiguous involvement of bowel. With bolus injection of contrast material, CT may reveal enhancement of the mucosa and serosa with hypodense thickening of the intervening bowel wall due to edema. With severe disease, however, the bowel wall may have increased attenuation, reflecting a hemorrhagic component of this process. In fact, hemorrhagic CMV colitis can be fatal in patients with AIDS.

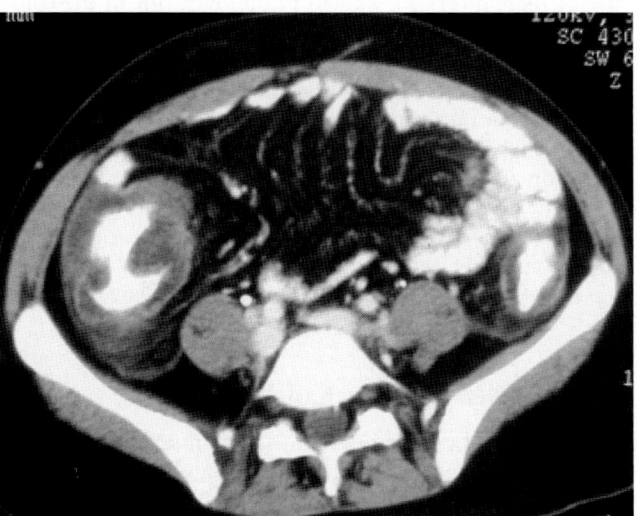

Figure 62-4. Cytomegalovirus (CMV) colitis. Enhanced CT scan of the pelvis demonstrates marked mural thickening of the ascending and colon in this AIDS patient with CMV colitis. Note the edematous low-density wall with enhancement of the mucosa and the serosa.

PARASITIC INFECTIONS

Anisakiasis

Within 12 to 24 hours after the ingestion of raw fish, infestation by larvae of the nematode *Anisakis* can produce severe abdominal pain, sometimes accompanied by fever, nausea and vomiting, or diarrhea.[38-40] Anisakiasis has a predilection for the stomach and small intestine, but the colon may occasionally be involved by this infection. Eosinophilia is not often present in the serum but is invariably identified on biopsy specimens. The ascending colon and, less commonly, the transverse colon are involved; barium enemas may reveal segmental thumbprinting of the affected bowel. The diagnosis of anisakiasis can be suggested when double-contrast barium enemas show the actual larvae as thin, linear filling defects 12 to 20 mm long and 0.7 mm wide at the proximal portion of the diseased segment of bowel.[40] Serologic studies may be performed to confirm the diagnosis. The worm is present in the stool in less than 25% of cases. The process is self-limited, usually lasting 7 to 10 days.

Amebiasis

Colonic amebiasis is rare in the United States. The cysts are ingested and subsequently develop into the invasive trophozoite. Twenty percent of the world population harbors this organism. Infestation by this protozoan may vary from the carrier state to fulminant colitis, and symptoms may be indolent or acute. Spread to the liver and then the lungs may result in abscesses in either of these organs.

Colonic amebiasis is usually an acute ulcerative colitis (95%) manifested by skip lesions, although the intervening bowel may be involved to a much lesser extent.[41-43] At times, the affected bowel is characterized by short regions of involvement with marked granulation (i.e., ameboma).[44] Such amebomas are seen in approximately 10% of cases and are usually located in the right side of the colon. Although diffuse colitis is not unusual, the right side of the colon tends to be more severely involved. Barium enemas usually reveal deep ulcers or bowel wall edema, but some patients may have aphthous ulcers, discrete ulcers appearing as marginal defects, or granularity with barium flecks.[45] The terminal ileum is invariably spared. The coned cecum is a suggestive but not specific finding. Residual deformity and stricture formation may occur even after appropriate therapy.[46] Less than 1% of patients present with toxic megacolon, and approximately 3% present with typhloappendicitis.

The diagnosis of amebiasis is usually established by the presence of trophozoites in the stool or on rectal smear. Serologic studies are also quite sensitive. When amebiasis is suspected, trial therapy may be warranted even if the diagnosis is not confirmed; the disease may progress rapidly if these patients are inappropriately treated with corticosteroids for presumed inflammatory bowel disease.

Schistosomiasis

Schistosomiasis belongs to the trematode or fluke group of worms; different strains are endemic to specific geographic areas. *Schistosoma mansoni* is found in the United States, Puerto Rico, and the tropics.[3] *S. haematobium* is the primary form in Africa and southern Asia, and *S. japonicum* usually occurs in eastern Asia. Mixed infection with *S. mansoni* and *S. haematobium* is not uncommon, particularly in Egypt. The larva penetrates the skin, where it enters the systemic circulation. It eventually reaches the liver, where it matures into the adult form. Upstream migration occurs through the portal venous system to the colon, where the worms invade the bowel wall and lay eggs. Portal hypertension with secondary hepatosplenomegaly is frequently associated. Although some patients may develop a pancolitis, *S. mansoni* has a predilection for the inferior mesenteric vein and left side of the colon, *S. japonicum* infects the superior mesenteric vein and right side of the colon and terminal ileum, and *S. haematobium* infects the hemorrhoidal veins and rectum and urinary tract. Most patients present with bloody diarrhea, but some may have chronic abdominal pain, intermittent diarrhea, and a palpable abdominal mass.

Barium enema examinations may reveal nonspecific colitis involving a variable extent of colon with narrowing, loss of haustration, and ulceration.[46] However, a hallmark of this disease is the presence of inflammatory polyps as a result of granulation reaction to the deposition of eggs in the bowel wall.[47,48] Another suggestive finding is calcification of the bowel wall or liver, which is most often associated with *S. haematobium* but also with *S. japonicum*.[48,49] CT is particularly sensitive to these changes. The diagnosis can be established by demonstrating the eggs in biopsy specimens or in the stool. Eosinophilia is frequently present.

Strongyloidiasis

The nematode *Strongyloides stercoralis* also gains entrance through the skin. It spreads to the lungs, ruptures into the tracheobronchial tree, and is subsequently ingested. The primary sites of involvement are the stomach, duodenum, and proximal small bowel; and a chronic host-parasite relationship ensues. In most cases, eggs are passed into the stool. However, in patients with decreased immunity, the eggs progress to the filariform larval stage and invade the portal system, producing a repeated cycle or autoinfection. The excess parasite load results in a distal accumulation of filariform larvae with subsequent colonic involvement. Because of the setting of severe debilitation, this process is often fatal. Barium enemas typically reveal findings of a diffuse ulcerative colitis.[50-52] Aphthous ulcers may be identified in the colon.[53] Fistulas and sinus tracts may also be present. Eosinophilia is the rule, but the diagnosis requires identification of cysts, larvae, or both, in the stool.

Trichuriasis

The whipworm *Trichuris trichiura* predominantly involves children in tropical areas. The worm is minimally invasive but invades the mucosa, with resultant bleeding, anemia, diarrhea, malaise, and cramps. Intussusception and rectal prolapse are common; the adherent worms serve as the lead point for this intussusception. Eosinophilia is usually present. The barium enema shows clumping and granularity of the barium because of excessive production of mucus.[54,55] The worms are identified as wavy, linear lucencies 3 to 5 cm in length, sometimes terminating in a ring shape with a central barium collection.

FUNGAL INFECTIONS

Histoplasmosis

Histoplasma capsulatum is a fungus endemic to river basin areas. The lung and skin are the usual sites of involvement, but the gastrointestinal tract may also be involved.[56] Gastrointestinal disease usually occurs in the setting of a chronic debilitating illness in which the intestinal symptoms are overlooked. Anemia and leukopenia may be present. Perforation, obstruction, or hemorrhage may direct attention to the alimentary tract. The ileocecal region is the most common site of disease. Other associated findings include mesenteric adenopathy, hepatosplenomegaly (often with calcifications), and abnormal chest radiographs. Barium studies may reveal right-sided colonic filling defects, one or more segments of nonspecific inflammation (e.g., narrowing, mucosal granulation, sinus tracts, ulcers, or strictures), diffuse colitis, pericecal masses simulating appendicitis, and rectal polyps.[56-58] Mucosal biopsy specimens may demonstrate the fungus, which stains with methenamine silver.

Mucormycosis

Colonic involvement by mucormycosis invariably occurs in a setting of immunosuppression. The diagnosis is rarely made preoperatively, and almost all cases have been fatal. The sinuses, lungs, and central nervous system are the usual sites of involvement. Colonic involvement may be isolated or may be associated with abnormalities elsewhere in the gastrointestinal tract.[59,60] The right side of the colon is most often affected; findings include a polypoid mass or segmental inflammation with or without sinus tracts. Rarely, these patients may have a pancolitis.

NONINFECTIOUS COLITIS

Nonspecific Ulcer

Nonspecific colonic ulcer is of unknown etiology. More than 50% of these ulcers are located in the right side of the colon near the ileocecal valve, and approximately 20% are multiple.[61] The clinical presentation can mimic that of appendicitis or even carcinoma. The ulceration may be superficial or deep and occurs on the antimesenteric border. The most common finding on barium enema is a focal mass with or without ulceration and, less commonly, a short stricture or segmental colitis.[61-65] CT scans may show a colonic mass with mesenteric stranding. This condition is rarely diagnosed preoperatively, but a nonspecific ulcer may be suspected when an ulcer is seen at colonoscopy and biopsy results are negative for other causes.

Typhlitis-Neutropenic Colitis

Neutropenic colitis, also known as typhlitis when it is confined to the cecum, develops in profoundly immunocompromised patient, especially patients with leukemia, AIDS, profound neutropenia due to chemotherapy, or transplantation. The exact pathogenesis of this condition is uncertain, but infection appears to have an important role. A variety of organisms (particularly clostridia) have been isolated from surgical specimens. Presenting symptoms include fever, right lower quadrant pain, and diarrhea.

Diffuse hyperemia, edema, and superficial ulceration are found on colonoscopy of the cecum but occasionally of the ascending colon and distal ileum. Colonoscopic findings of neutropenic enterocolitis are difficult to distinguish from those of idiopathic ulcerative colitis or even infectious colitis, except that the changes are confined to the right colon in patients with neutropenic colitis while the rectum and sigmoid are usually involved in ulcerative colitis and infectious colitis. To prevent transmural necrosis and perforation, prompt diagnosis and supportive therapy with intensive broad-spectrum (including fungal) antibiotics and supplemental nutrition are necessary. Surgical resection is often needed for patients who develop these complications.

Plain film findings of typhlitis include ileocecal dilatation with air-fluid levels[66-69] and small bowel obstruction secondary to inflammation. A soft tissue mass and pneumatosis have been reported.

Multidetector row CT (MDCT) is the diagnostic procedure of choice in patients suspected of having typhlitis because there is a high risk of perforation during colonoscopy or barium enema. MDCT and ultrasonography show mural thickening and often submucosal edema of the cecum and ascending colon (Fig. 62-5). There is pericolonic stranding and fluid, and in advanced cases pneumatosis may also be identified. Sepsis, abscess formation, intramural perforation, intestinal necrosis, hemorrhage, or any combination of these lesions may occur in severe cases. CT can also be used to monitor the success of treatment by showing a decrease in the thickness of the colon wall or by demonstrating complications such as pneumatosis when there is bowel wall necrosis or pneumoperitoneum when there is a silent perforation.[70,71]

The most important consideration in the differential diagnosis is colitis caused by *C. difficile* infection. A diagnosis of typhlitis can be made on the basis of the clinical and imaging findings only after other pathologic entities have been excluded. Surgery may be necessary in severe cases.

Microscopic (Collagenous) Colitis

Microscopic (collagenous) colitis is a clinicopathologic entity characterized by a history of variable (but usually long) duration, intermittent or chronic watery diarrhea. This condition occurs predominantly in middle-aged and elderly women. Results of laboratory studies and diagnostic procedures, including endoscopy, are usually normal. The diagnosis is established by endoscopic biopsy specimens, which reveal increased lymphocytes in the surface epithelium and, in the variant, collagenous colitis, an increase in the width of the subepithelial collagen band.

The barium enema had generally been considered to be incapable of detecting changes of microscopic colitis, but double-contrast studies may occasionally reveal nonspecific inflammatory surface abnormalities, predominantly in the rectosigmoid region.[72,73] In the appropriate clinical setting, microscopic colitis should therefore be considered in the differential diagnosis of these findings and endoscopic biopsy specimens should be obtained. Sulfasalazine or corticosteroids may be of benefit for the control of symptoms.

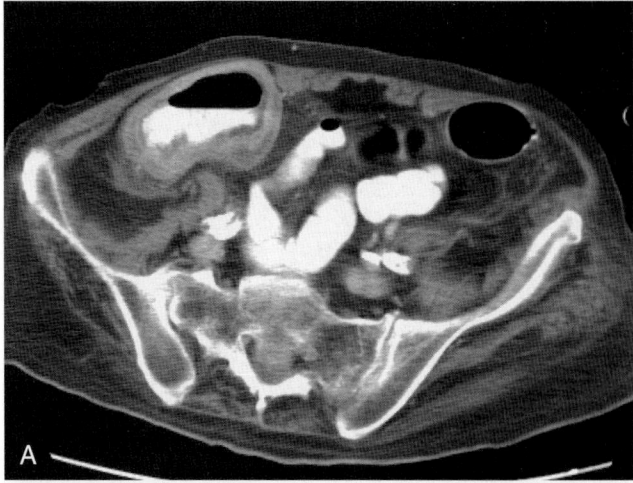

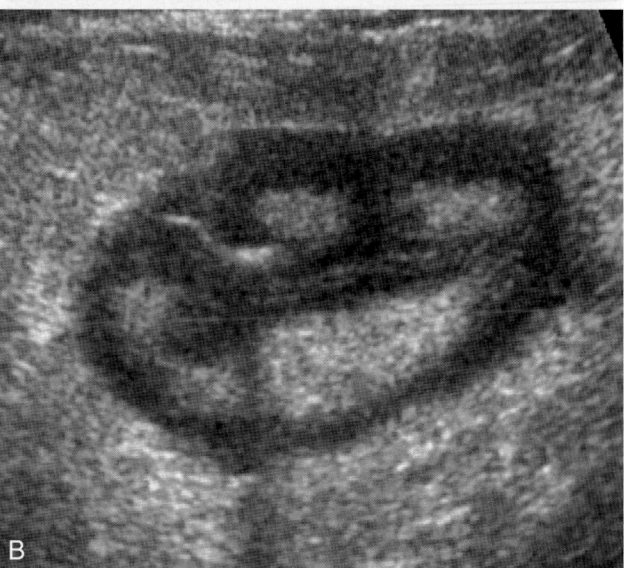

Figure 62-5. Typhlitis: CT and ultrasound features. A. CT scan shows mural thickening with submucosal edema involving the cecum. **B.** Sonogram in a different patient obtained through the right lower quadrant, imaging the cecum axially, demonstrates marked mural thickening.

Eosinophilic Colitis

Eosinophilic gastroenteritis is a disease of unknown etiology that invariably involves the stomach or small bowel. Ascites is also common, and peripheral eosinophilia is usually present. Occasionally, the colon (particularly the right side of the colon) may be involved. Thumbprinting, spasm, and narrowing are the primary findings on barium study.[74] These findings may be reversible after treatment with corticosteroids.

Graft-versus-Host Disease

One of the complications of bone marrow transplantation is that the donor immune cells may recognize the host tissue as foreign. The small intestine is invariably involved. Barium studies may reveal mural thickening and fold thickening or complete loss of mucosal features ("ribbon" bowel). Some of these patients also have abnormalities involving the entire colon or, less commonly, selective right-sided colonic disease.[75]

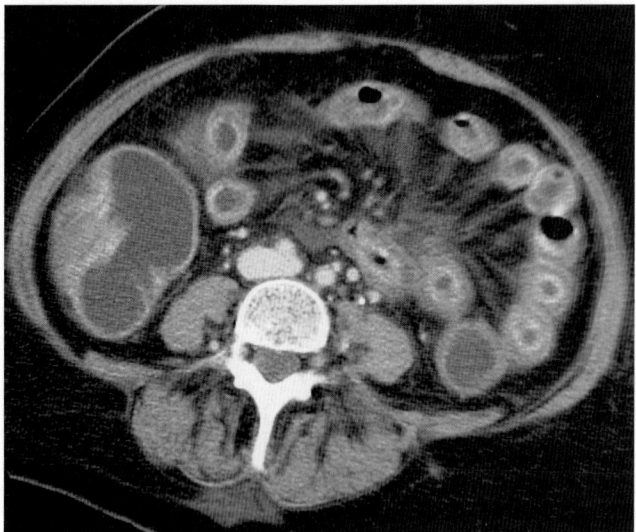

Figure 62-6. Graft-versus-host disease. Axial contrast-enhanced scan shows edema in the mesentery, small- and large-bowel wall thickening, and mucosal and serosal enhancement.

The findings on barium enema are those of a nonspecific colitis (e.g., loss of haustration, spasm, and ulceration) and, in some cases, a granular surface pattern. CT shows (Fig. 62-6) edema in the mesentery, small- and large-bowel wall thickening, and mucosal and serosal enhancement. Graft-versus-host disease and viral infection (or both conditions combined) are indistinguishable.

Retractile Mesenteritis

Retractile mesenteritis is a disease of unknown etiology in which a spectrum of inflammatory and fibrotic pathologic changes occurs in the mesenteric fat but can extend to the intestinal wall. Autoimmune factors have been postulated. The patient's age may range from the second to the eighth decade of life, and there is a slight male predominance. Presenting symptoms include abdominal pain, diarrhea, and weight loss. The small bowel is the usual site of involvement, but colonic abnormalities are not uncommon. The sigmoid and transverse colon are most likely to be involved because these segments of bowel are intimately related to a mesentery.

The findings on barium enema may be secondary to ischemia as a result of occlusion of the mesenteric vessels or direct extension of the fibroinflammatory process.[76-79] Barium studies may reveal long segments of mild to moderate narrowing with thumbprinting, strictures of variable length, or extrinsic masses with reactive changes on the contiguous margin of the bowel. CT is a complementary imaging study, because it may demonstrate markedly increased density in the mesentery with or without discrete, fibrotic soft tissue masses. Ultrasonography may also reveal solid masses with hypoechoic areas that resemble sarcomas, hematomas, or abscesses.[77] Surgery is often performed to relieve obstructive symptoms, but corticosteroid therapy may also be beneficial.

Reactive Inflammation

Reactive inflammation may occur in the colon due to extension of primary inflammatory processes from other organs or from adjacent abscesses. The site of colonic disease closely correlates with its anatomic contiguity and mesenteric relationships with these structures. The appearance may vary from an area of extrinsic mass effect with reactive spiculation to long segments of concentric narrowing and spiculation with or without an adjacent soft tissue mass that fixes and distorts the bowel. For example, appendicitis may involve the ascending colon or sigmoid colon (depending on the location of the appendix), whereas pancreatitis tends to involve a variable length of the transverse colon up to the junction with the descending colon (phrenocolic ligament). Pancreatitis may also cause obstruction (colon cutoff), fistula formation, necrosis and perforation, and strictures. Both of these entities may simulate primary colitis with pain and diarrhea.[80] However, careful interpretation of the barium enema may allow the radiologist to suggest these possibilities, and a CT scan combined with appropriate laboratory studies may allow an accurate diagnosis. Less commonly, inflammatory disease in the kidneys produces reactive changes in the proximal descending or ascending colon and acute cholecystitis may have a similar effect on the proximal transverse colon, particularly on its superior border.

NEUTROPHIL AND MACROPHAGE DYSFUNCTION

Chronic Granulomatous Disease of Childhood

In patients with conditions associated with neutrophil dysfunction, a colitis that may be segmental or pancolonic and indistinguishable from Crohn's disease has been reported.[81] Fistulas and sinuses may be features of this form of colitis. It occurs predominantly in the pediatric population. Chronic granulomatous disease of childhood is an inherited defect of leukocyte function characterized by the inability of phagocytes to kill catalase-positive microorganisms, resulting in multifocal abscesses and granulomas. The presence of lipid-bearing histiocytes in the mucosa is highly suggestive of this entity. Some degree of colonic involvement is common in these patients, but clinically significant colonic disease is rare. Some patients with colonic disease may have associated involvement of the stomach with narrowing of the gastric antrum.

Glycogen Storage Disease

Glycogen storage disease Ib is also associated with neutropenia and a metabolic defect in neutrophil activity. Recurrent pyogenic infections are a significant clinical problem in these patients. In the limited number of reported cases, gastrointestinal involvement has been manifested by long or short strictures involving the right side of the colon and even the terminal ileum.[82]

Malacoplakia

Malacoplakia is a granulomatous process that most commonly involves the genitourinary tract. However, the colon is the most frequent extraurinary site of involvement.[83] Distinctive macrophages that contain pathognomonic intracytoplasmic calcifications (Michaelis-Gutmann bodies) are present on biopsy specimens. The etiology is unknown, but a macrophage defect is most likely. Unlike the urinary tract abnormalities, which tend to occur in elderly women, colonic disease shows a wide age distribution. Abnormalities may include small polyps or bulky masses occurring in a segmental or diffuse distribution. Barium studies may even reveal a diffuse nonspecific colitis resembling Crohn's disease. Rectal bleeding, diarrhea, and abdominal pain are the most frequent symptoms in these patients.

EXOGENOUS CAUSES OF COLITIS

Caustic Colitis

Direct contact between the colorectal mucosa and caustic substances introduced into the rectum by various types of enemas may produce a colitis that is transient or results in complete mucosal sloughing with subsequent strictures. The most common causes of caustic colitis are detergent or soapsuds enemas employed as laxatives or herbal (ritual) enemas practiced in Third World countries as a form of medical therapy.[84-87] In some cases, the injury has been thermal as a result of the high temperature of the liquid.[88] The changes occur predominantly in the distal colon because of the route of entry. However, skip lesions or transverse and right-sided colonic alterations can occur as a result of spasm and prolonged contact. Bloody diarrhea is the usual presenting symptom. Barium studies may demonstrate thumbprinting or severe mucosal necrosis and ulceration that progresses to deformity or strictures. Some patients may require colectomy and colostomy.

A number of cases of colitis secondary to glutaraldehyde exposure have also been reported. This form of colitis occurs when the disinfectant is inadequately removed from endoscopes. Radiographic findings include thumbprinting in the rectosigmoid colon on barium enema and a thickened colonic wall on CT.[89]

Drug-Induced Colitis

A variety of pharmaceutical agents may be directly or indirectly responsible for colitis through a number of mechanisms.[90] Cancer chemotherapeutic agents may result in ulceration and inflammation secondary to their inhibitory effect on mucosal epithelial cells. Such patients may also develop typhlitis as a result of drug-induced neutropenia. Almost all antibiotics may cause C. difficile colitis (see next section). Vasoconstrictive drugs, antihypertensive medications, and oral contraceptives may cause ischemia-related inflammation. Some therapeutic agents may also be associated with a hypersensitivity reaction. Penicillin, ampicillin, amoxicillin, and erythromycin have been reported to cause a right-sided hemorrhagic colitis that subsides spontaneously when these antibiotics are withdrawn.[90,91] Nonsteroidal anti-inflammatory drugs have been described as other causes of colonic injury, possibly as a result of inhibition of prostaglandin synthesis.[92] Findings have ranged from diffuse or segmental colitis to scattered discrete ulcers involving any segment of the colon, particularly the cecum.

Clostridium difficile Colitis

C. difficile colitis is often considered synonymous with pseudomembranous colitis and antibiotic-induced colitis.[93,94]

Although this is often the case, these associations are not universal. Almost all antibiotics may produce diarrhea, but only a small percentage of these cases are related to C. difficile. Furthermore, not all patients with C. difficile colitis have pseudomembranes. Finally, some patients with C. difficile colitis may be immunosuppressed (e.g., on chemotherapy), so not all cases are related to treatment with antibiotics. To further complicate the subject, as many as 20% of asymptomatic hospitalized patients are found to have C. difficile on stool cultures.

Nevertheless, the diagnosis of C. difficile colitis should be suggested in patients on antibiotics who develop sudden onset of watery diarrhea, often associated with fever, abdominal tenderness, and leukocytosis. Many of these patients are hospitalized, and many have had recent surgery. The onset of disease usually occurs within 2 days to 2 weeks after the introduction of antibiotic therapy, but some patients may develop symptoms as late as 8 weeks after the drugs are discontinued. In such cases, the temporal relationship to antibiotics may be obscure, and a careful clinical history must be elicited.

Pathophysiologically, pseudomembranous colitis begins with disturbance of normal colonic microflora, exposure to and colonization by C. difficile, production of toxin and toxin-mediated inflammation and injury, and colonic damage. The colitis ranges in severity from inflammatory changes confined to superficial epithelium to severe, intense necrosis (Fig. 62-7) of the full thickness of the mucosa with formation of a confluent layer of pseudomembrane.

In patients in whom fever is the predominant symptom, a CT scan may be obtained as the initial diagnostic test to rule out an abscess. This study may show marked low-density mural thickening with the swollen haustra projecting into the lumen between thin streaks of contrast medium (Fig. 62-8).[95] These findings are pancolonic in the majority of patients, but some may have disease confined to the right colon or, less commonly, left side of the colon.[96]

The majority of cases of pseudomembranous colitis are diagnosed by proctosigmoidoscopy combined with a positive cytotoxicity test for toxin B. In approximately 40% of cases, however, the rectum is normal or harbors nonspecific changes.[96] The assay for toxin B requires 48 hours to perform. In severe cases, abdominal plain films may reveal diagnostic findings, consisting of massive thumbprinting throughout

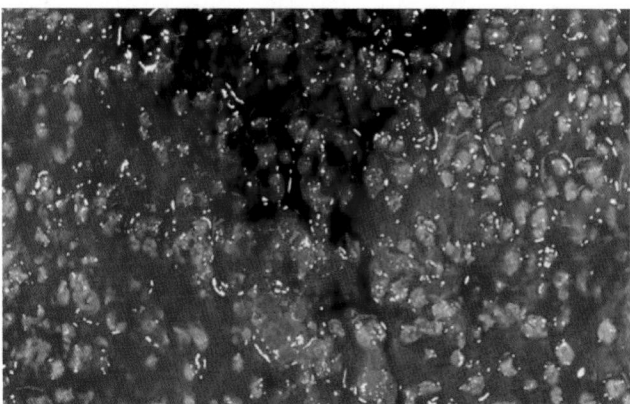

Figure 62-7. Pseudomembranous colitis: pathologic findings. Surgical specimen shows whitish plaques on a background of hemorrhagic mucosa.

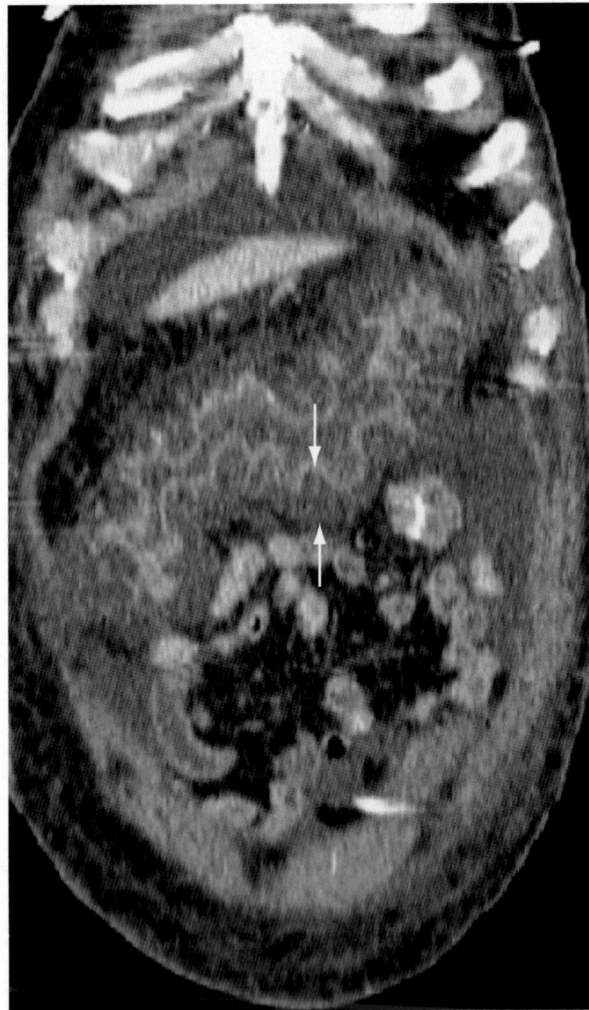

Figure 62-8. *Clostridium difficile* **colitis: CT features.** Coronal reformatted image shows marked mural thickening (*arrows*) the transverse colon with enhancing mucosa and submucosal edema. A small amount of intraperitoneal fluid is also present.

the colon, sometimes associated with a shaggy margin.[97,98] A megacolon may also be present. In such cases, a contrast enema is contraindicated. Nevertheless, the findings on barium enema usually consist of small, subtly elevated, round nodules or small, irregular plaquelike filling defects that may be discrete or confluent and are best seen on double-contrast studies.[99] In more advanced cases, single-contrast studies may reveal coarse polypoid defects or shaggy marginal irregularities.[97,98] Discontinuation of the drug is often sufficient, but vancomycin is the treatment of choice for patients with more severe disease. Relapses have been reported in 10% to 39% of treated patients.

References

1. Yantiss RK, Odze RD: Diagnostic difficulties in inflammatory bowel disease pathology. Histopathology 48:116-132, 2006.
2. Gore RM, Miller FH, Yaghmai V, et al: Inflammatory conditions of the colon. Semin Roentgenol 36:126-137, 2001.
3. Thoeni RF, Cello JP: CT imaging of colitis. Radiology 240:623-638, 2006.
4. Tedesco FJ, Hardin RD, Harper RN, et al: Infectious colitis endoscopically simulating inflammatory bowel disease: A prospective evaluation. Gastrointest Endosc 29:195-197, 1983.
5. Grundy A, Gilks CF: Typhoid: An unusual cause of gastrointestinal bleeding. Br J Radiol 57:344-346, 1984.
6. Saffouri B, Bartolomeo RS, Fuchs B: Colonic involvement in salmonellosis. Dig Dis Sci 24:203-208, 1979.
7. Farman J, Rabinowitz JG, Meyers MA: Roentgenology of infectious colitis. AJR 119:375-381, 1973.
8. Nakamura S, Iida M, Tominaga M, et al: *Salmonella* colitis: Assessment with double-contrast barium enema examination in seven patients. Radiology 184:537-540, 1992.
9. Vender RJ, Marignani P: *Salmonella* colitis presenting as a segmental colitis resembling Crohn's disease. Dig Dis Sci 28:848-851, 1983.
10. Speelman P, Kabir I, Islam M: Distribution and spread of colonic lesions in shigellosis: A colonoscopic study. J Infect 150:899-903, 1984.
11. Khuroo MS, Mahajan R, Zargar SA, et al: The colon in shigellosis: Serial colonoscopic appearances in *Shigella dysenteriae* I. Endoscopy 22:35-38, 1990.
12. Zalev AH, Warren RE: *Shigella* colitis with radiological and endoscopic correlation: Case report. J Can Assoc Radiol 40:328-330, 1989.
13. Lambert JR, Tischler ME, Karmali MA, et al: *Campylobacter* ileocolitis: An inflammatory bowel disease. Can Med Assoc J 121:1377-1379, 1979.
14. Brodey PA, Fertig S, Aron JM: *Campylobacter* enterocolitis: Radiographic features. AJR 139:1199-1201, 1982.
15. Tielbeek AV, Rosenbusch G, Muytjens HL, et al: Roentgenologic changes of the colon in *Campylobacter* infection. Gastrointest Radiol 10:358-361, 1985.
16. Kollitz JPM, Davis GB, Berk RN: *Campylobacter* colitis: A common infectious form of acute colitis. Gastrointest Radiol 6:227-229, 1981.
17. Vantrappen G, Agg HO, Ponette E, et al: *Yersinia* enteritis and enterocolitis: Gastroenterological aspects. Gastroenterology 72:220-227, 1977.
18. Matsumoto T, Iida M, Matsui T, et al: Endoscopic findings in *Yersinia enterocolitica* enterocolitis. Gastrointest Endosc 36:583-587, 1990.
19. Simmonds SD, Noble MA, Freeman HJ: Gastrointestinal features of culture-positive *Yersinia enterocolitica* infection. Gastroenterology 92:112-117, 1987.
20. Shrago G: *Yersinia enterocolitica* ileocolitis findings observed on barium examination. Br J Radiol 49:181-183, 1976.
21. Atkinson GO, Gay BB, Ball TI, et al: *Yersinia enterocolitica* colitis in infants: Radiographic changes. Radiology 148:113-116, 1983.
22. Lachman R, Soong J, Wishon G, et al: *Yersinia* colitis. Gastrointest Radiol 2:133-135, 1977.
23. Kawanami T, Bowen A, Girdany BR: Enterocolitis: Prodrome of the hemolytic-uremic syndrome. Radiology 151:91-92, 1984.
24. Peterson RB, Meseroll WP, Shrago GG, et al: Radiographic features of colitis associated with the hemolytic-uremic syndrome. Radiology 118:667-671, 1976.
25. Shortsleeve MJ, Wilson ME, Finklestein M, et al: Radiologic findings in hemorrhagic colitis due to *Escherichia coli* O157:H7. Gastrointest Radiol 14:341-344, 1989.
26. Balthazar EJ, Gordon R, Hulnick D: Ileocecal tuberculosis: CT and radiologic evaluation. AJR 154:499-503, 1990.
27. Vaidya MG, Sodhi JS: Gastrointestinal tract tuberculosis: A study of 102 cases including 55 hemicolectomies. Clin Radiol 29:189-195, 1978.
28. Ehsannulah M, Isaacs A, Filipe MI, et al: Tuberculosis presenting as inflammatory bowel disease: Report of two cases. Dis Colon Rectum 27:134-136, 1984.
29. Tishler JM: Tuberculosis of the transverse colon. AJR 133:229-232, 1979.
30. Peh WC: Filiform polyposis in tuberculosis of the colon. Clin Radiol 39:534-536, 1988.
31. Downey DB, Nakielny RA: Aphthoid ulcers in colonic tuberculosis. Br J Radiol 58:561-562, 1985.
32. Carr-Locke DL, Finlay DBL: Radiological demonstration of colonic aphthoid ulcers in a patient with intestinal tuberculosis. Gut 24:453-455, 1983.
33. McDonald JB, Middleton PJ: Tuberculosis of the colon simulating carcinoma. Radiology 118:293-294, 1976.
34. Bhargava DK, Tandon HD, Chawla TC, et al: Diagnosis of ileocecal and colonic tuberculosis by colonoscopy. Gastrointest Endosc 31:68-70, 1985.
35. Maloney JJ, Cho SR: Pelvic actinomycosis. Radiology 148:388, 1983.
36. Fowler RC, Simpkins KC: Abdominal actinomycosis: A report of three cases. Clin Radiol 34:301-307, 1983.

37. Balthazar EJ, Megibow AJ, Fazzini E: Cytomegalovirus colitis in AIDS: Radiographic findings in 11 patients. Radiology 155:585-589, 1985.

38. Higashi M, Tanaka K, Kitada T, et al: Anisakiasis confirmed by radiography of the large intestine. Gastrointest Radiol 13:85-86, 1988.

39. Matsui T, Iida M, Murakami M, et al: Intestinal anisakiasis: Clinical and radiologic features. Radiology 157:299-302, 1985.

40. Matsumoto T, Iida M, Kimura Y, et al: Anisakiasis of the colon: Radiologic and endoscopic features in six patients. Radiology 183:97-99, 1992.

41. Cardoso JM, Kimura K, Stoopen M, et al: Radiology of invasive amebiasis of the colon. AJR 128:935-941, 1977.

42. Balikian JP, Uthman SM, Khouri NF: Intestinal amebiasis: A roentgen analysis of 19 cases including 2 case reports. AJR 122:245-256, 1974.

43. Kolawole TM, Lewis EA: Radiologic observations on intestinal amebiasis. AJR 122:257-265, 1974.

44. Cevallos AM, Farthing MJG: Parasitic infections of the gastrointestinal tract. Curr Opin Gastroenterol 9:96-102, 1993.

45. Matsui T, Iida M, Tata S, et al: The value of double-contrast barium enema in amebic colitis. Gastrointest Radiol 14:73-78, 1989.

46. Martinez CR, Gilman RH, Rabbani GH, et al: Amebic colitis: Correlation of proctoscopy before treatment and barium enema after treatment. AJR 138:1089-1093, 1982.

47. Medina JT, Seaman WB, Guzman-Acosta C, et al: The roentgen appearance of *Schistosomiasis mansoni* involving the colon. Radiology 85:682-688, 1965.

48. Lehman JS, Farid Z, Bassily S, et al: Colonic calcification and polyposis. Radiology 98:379-380, 1971.

49. Lee RC, Chiang JH, Chou YH, et al: Intestinal schistosomiasis japonica: CT-pathologic correlation. Radiology 193:539-542, 1994.

50. Yoshida T, Nozaki F, Tanaka K, et al: *Strongyloides stercoralis* hyperinfection: sequential changes of gastrointestinal radiology after treatment with thiabendazole. Gastrointest Radiol 6:223-225, 1981.

51. Dallemand S, Waxman M, Farman J: Radiological manifestations of *Strongyloides stercoralis*. Gastrointest Radiol 8:45-51, 1983.

52. Drasin GF, Moss JP, Cheng SH: *Strongyloides stercoralis* colitis: Findings in four cases. Radiology 126:619-621, 1978.

53. Stoopack PM, Raufman JP: Aphthoid ulceration of the colon in strongyloidiasis. Am J Gastroenterol 86:639-642, 1991.

54. Reeder MM, Astacio JE, Theros EG: Case of the month from the AFIP. Radiology 90:382-387, 1968.

55. Fisher RM, Cremin BJ: Rectal bleeding due to *Trichuris trichiura*. Br J Radiol 43:214-215, 1970.

56. Cappell MS, Mandell W, Grimes MM, et al: Gastrointestinal histoplasmosis. Dig Dis Sci 33:353-360, 1988.

57. Haws CC, Long RF, Caplan GE: *Histoplasma capsulatum* as a cause of ileocolitis. AJR 128:692-694, 1977.

58. Dietz MW: Ileocecal histoplasmosis. Radiology 91:285-289, 1968.

59. De Feo E: Mucormycosis of the colon. AJR 86:86-90, 1961.

60. Agha FP, Lee HH, Boland CR, et al: Mucormycoma of the colon: Early diagnosis and successful management. AJR 145:739-741, 1985.

61. Shallman RW, Kuehner M, Williams GH, et al: Benign cecal ulcers. Dis Colon Rectum 28:732-737, 1985.

62. Huded FV, Posner GL, Tick R: Nonspecific ulcer of the colon in a chronic hemodialysis patient. Am J Gastroenterol 77:913-916, 1982.

63. Brodey PA, Hill RP, Baron S: Benign ulceration of the cecum. Radiology 122:323-327, 1977.

64. Gardiner GA, Bird CR: Nonspecific ulcers of the colon resembling annular carcinoma. Radiology 137:331-334, 1980.

65. Marn CS, Yu BFB, Nostrant TT, et al: Idiopathic cecal ulcer: CT findings. AJR 153:761-763, 1989.

66. O'Malley ME, Wilson SR: US of gastrointestinal tract abnormalities with CT correlation. RadioGraphics 23:59-72, 2003.

67. Abramson SJ, Berdon WE, Baker DH: Childhood typhlitis: Its increasing association with acute myelogenous leukemia. Radiology 146:61-64, 1983.

68. Turner DR, Markose G, Arends MJ, et al: Unusual causes of colonic wall thickening on computed tomography. Clin Radiol 58:191-200, 2003.

69. Horton KM, Corl FM, Fishman EK: CT evaluation of the colon: Inflammatory disease. RadioGraphics 20:399-418, 2000.

70. Frick MP, Maile CW, Crass JR, et al: Computed tomography of neutropenic colitis. AJR 143:763-765, 1984.

71. Hoeffel C, Crema MD, Belkacem A, et al: Multi-detector row CT: Spectrum of diseases involving the ileocecal area. RadioGraphics 26:1373-1390, 2006.

72. Glick SN, Teplick SK, Amenta PS: Microscopic (collagenous) colitis. AJR 153:995-996, 1989.

73. Feczko PJ, Mezwa DG: Nonspecific radiographic abnormalities in collagenous colitis. Gastrointest Radiol 16:128-132, 1991.

74. MacCarty RL, Talley NJ: Barium studies in diffuse eosinophilic gastroenteritis. Gastrointest Radiol 15:183-187, 1990.

75. Kalantari BN, Mortele KJ, Cantisani V, et al: CT features with pathologic correlation of acute gastrointestinal graft-versus-host disease after bone marrow transplantation in adults. AJR 181:1621-1625, 2003.

76. Han SY, Koehler RE, Keller FS, et al: Retractile mesenteritis involving the colon: Pathologic and radiologic correlation. AJR 147:268-270, 1986.

77. Periz-Fontan FJ, Soler R, Sanchez J, et al: Retractile mesenteritis involving the colon: Barium enema, sonographic, and CT findings. AJR 147:937-940, 1986.

78. Williams RG, Nelson JA: Retractile mesenteritis: Initial presentation as colonic obstruction. Radiology 126:35-37, 1978.

79. Thompson GT, Fitzgerald EF, Somers SS: Retractile mesenteritis of the sigmoid colon. Br J Radiol 58:266-267, 1985.

80. Picus D, Shackelford GD: Perforated appendix presenting with severe diarrhea. Radiology 149:141-143, 1983.

81. Werlin SL, Chusid MJ, Caya J, et al: Colitis in chronic granulomatous disease. Gastroenterology 82:328-331, 1982.

82. Couper R, Kapelushnik J, Griffiths AM: Neutrophil dysfunction in glycogen storage disease Ib: Association with Crohn's-like colitis. Gastroenterology 100:549-554, 1991.

83. Radin DR, Chandrasoma P, Halls JM: Colon malacoplakia. Gastrointest Radiol 9:359-361, 1984.

84. Kim SK, Cho C, Levinsohn EM: Caustic colitis due to detergent enema. AJR 134:397-398, 1980.

85. Pike BF, Phillippi PJ, Lawson EH: Soap colitis. N Engl J Med 285:217-218, 1971.

86. Segal I, Solomon A, Mirwis J: Radiological manifestations of ritual-enema-induced colitis. Clin Radiol 32:657-662, 1981.

87. Young WS: Herbal-enema colitis and stricture. Br J Radiol 53:248-249, 1980.

88. Jackson KR, Ott DJ, Gelfand DW: Thermal injury of the colon due to colostomy irrigation. Gastrointest Radiol 6:231-233, 1981.

89. Bernbaum BA, Gordon RB, Jacobs JE: Glutaraldehyde colitis: Radiologic findings. Radiology 1995;195:131-134.

90. Fortson WC, Tedesco FJ: Drug induced colitis: A review. Am J Gastroenterol 79:878-883, 1984.

91. Rimmer MJ, Freeman AH, Low FM: The barium enema diagnosis of penicillin associated colitis. Clin Radiol 33:529-533, 1982.

92. Gibson GR, Whitacre EB, Ricotti CA: Colitis induced by nonsteroidal anti-inflammatory drugs. Arch Intern Med 152:625-632, 1992.

93. Johnson S, Schriever C, Galang M, et al: Interruption of recurrent *Clostridium difficile*-associated diarrhea. Clin Infect Dis 44:846-888, 2007.

94. Kirkpatrick ID, Greenberg HM: Gastrointestinal complications in the neutropenic patient: Characterization and differentiation with abdominal CT. Radiology 226:668-674, 2003.

95. Fishman EK, Kavuru M, Jones B, et al: Pseudomembranous colitis: CT evaluation of 26 cases. Radiology 180:57-60, 1991.

96. Ash L, Baker ME, O'Malley CM Jr, et al: Colonic abnormalities on CT in adult hospitalized patients with *Clostridium difficile* colitis: Prevalence and significance of findings. AJR 186:1393-400, 2006.

97. Cho KJ, Ting YM, Chuang VP, et al: Roentgenographic features in antibiotic-associated pseudomembranous colitis. Australas Radiol 20:38-41, 1976.

98. Stanley RJ, Melson GL, Tedesco FJ: The spectrum of radiographic findings in antibiotic-related pseudomembranous colitis. Radiology 111:519-524, 1974.

99. Strada M, Meregaglia D, Donzelli R: Double-contrast enema in antibiotic-related pseudomembranous colitis. Gastrointest Radiol 8:67-69, 1983.

100. McDonald LC, Coignard B, Dubberve E, et al: Recommendations for surveillance of *Clostridium difficile*-associated disease. Infect Control Hosp Epidemiol 28:140-145, 2007.

chapter

63

Polyps and Colon Cancer

Ruedi F. Thoeni, MD • Igor Laufer, MD

EPIDEMIOLOGY

Colon cancer is a major public health problem in the United States, the most common significant cancer in the U.S. population, and the second most common cause of cancer mortality. It ranks third to lung and prostate cancer in men and third to lung and breast cancer in women.[1] The American Cancer Society estimates that in the year 2007 about 153,760 will be diagnosed with colorectal cancer and that about 52,180 will die of the disease.[1] The distribution of this disease varies widely throughout the world. It is common in North America, Europe, and New Zealand, and the incidence is low in South America, Africa, and Asia. The United States has one of the highest incidences of colorectal cancer in the world. However, even within the United States, the rates of occurrence vary considerably, being higher in the North, among the urban white population, and among African Americans.[1] Viewed in a personal way, American adults have approximately 1 chance in 20 of developing colorectal cancer during their lifetime and 1 chance in 40 of dying with this disease.

Colorectal neoplasms account for about 9% of new cancer diagnoses in the United States. The incidence rates have declined from a high of 71 per 100,000 in 1975 to 61 per 100,000 in 2001 for men and from 54 per 100,000 in 1975 to 46 per 100,000 in 2001 for woman.[1] This decline was seen mostly in whites, whereas incidence rates for African Americans have slightly increased. In the United States, the incidence rates among African American men and women are about 15% higher than in white men and women, whereas mortality rates in African Americans are about 40% higher than in whites.[1] The decline in whites is probably due to increased screening for colon cancer and subsequent polyp removal. The lack of improvement over time in African Americans may reflect historical underdiagnosis of colon cancer in African Americans; racial differences in the trends in prevalence of risk factors for colon cancer; and lower access and utilization of recommended screening tests by African Americans. African Americans are more likely to be diagnosed when the disease has spread beyond the colon and once diagnosed are less likely than whites to receive recommended surgical treatment and adjuvant therapy.[2,3]

The distribution of cancer in the large bowel is of considerable importance because it affects the diagnostic approach.

1121

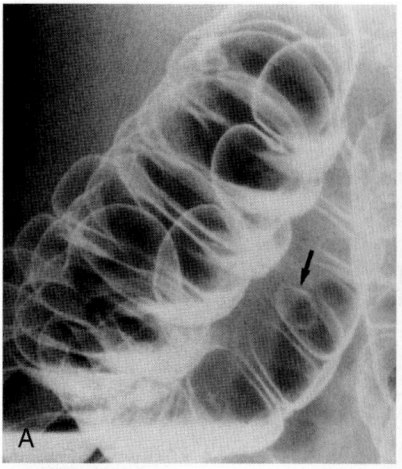
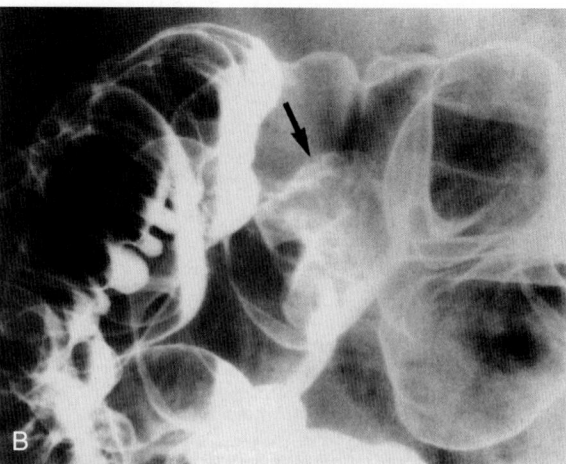
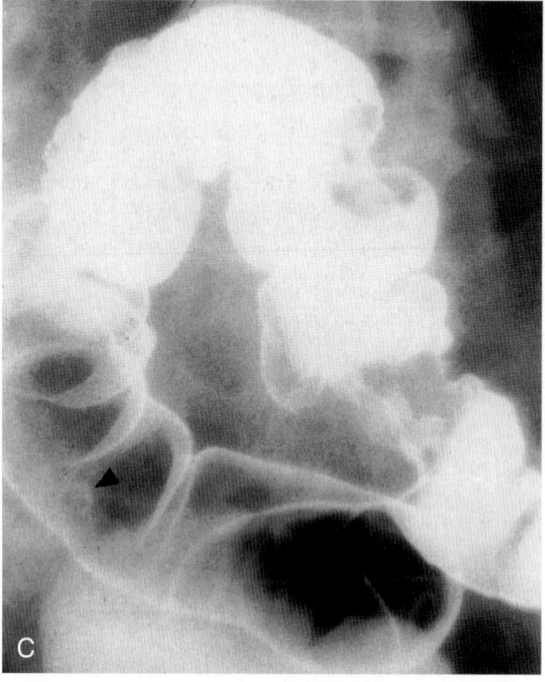

Figure 63-1. Double-contrast barium enema: evaluation of colon cancer. A. A 1-cm polyp (*arrow*) is demonstrated in the proximal transverse colon. **B.** Seventeen years later, the small polyp has grown into a full-blown polypoid carcinoma (*arrow*). **C.** In another patient there are adenomas in the distal sigmoid (*arrowhead*), a polypoid carcinoma near the apex of the sigmoid, and an annular carcinoma more proximally in the sigmoid colon. (**C** from Laufer I, Levine MS [eds]: Double Contrast Gastrointestinal Radiology, 3rd ed. Philadelphia, WB Saunders, 2000.)

Approximately one half of the cancers occur in the rectum and sigmoid colon within reach of the short flexible sigmoidoscope (Fig. 63-1).[4] The remainders are scattered throughout the proximal colon. Some authors suggest that there has been a shift to the right, rendering fewer cancers diagnosable by digital and short sigmoidoscopic examinations.[5] Although the overall incidence of colorectal tumors increases with age, this increase is greatest for proximal neoplasms beyond the reach of the sigmoidoscope.[6] Also, race and sex can independently predict the location of the cancer.[7] Generally, more distal cancers are found in Asians than in either African Americans or whites. Whites have more distal cancers than African Americans, and men have more distal cancers than women.

ETIOLOGY

The wide variation and distribution of colorectal cancer throughout the world is probably related to dietary differences. In general, diets low in fiber and high in fat and animal protein (especially high and prolonged consumption of red or processed meat) are associated with a higher prevalence of colorectal cancer, and this is inversely related to the incidence of gastric cancer.[8] However, these conclusions are based on population studies, and a direct link between diet and colon cancer has not been demonstrated.[1]

HEREDITARY FACTORS

The role of heredity in colorectal cancer has been a subject of considerable interest. Heredity probably plays a role in 5% to 6% of all cases of colorectal cancer. Adenomatous polyposis coli (see Chapter 65) is transmitted by the classic mendelian dominant inheritance pattern, and almost all patients with the condition eventually develop colorectal carcinoma. These patients account for approximately 1% of colorectal cancers. Another 5% arise in patients with hereditary nonpolyposis colorectal cancer (HNPCC). HNPCCs are subdivided into those in which colorectal cancer is clustered in families (type I) and those in which there is a familial clustering of colorectal cancer with other malignancies, such as carcinomas of the endometrium, ovary, and breast (type II). In all these syndromes, carcinomas tend to occur in the proximal part of the colon and are found at a relatively young age.[9]

It has been suggested that an abnormality in the genetic material may be associated with the development of colorectal cancer.[10] The discovery of four human mismatch repair genes (hMSH2, hMLH1, hPMS1, and hPMS2) has provided novel insight into the genetic basis of this disease and raised the possibility of genetic diagnosis for management of HNPCC patients and their family members.[11] Therefore, it may be important to perform DNA testing in families suspected of having HNPCC.[12]

RISK FACTORS

Although colorectal cancer is common in the U.S. population, several factors place individuals at higher than normal risk. These include older age, a personal or family history of colorectal polyps or cancer, certain hereditary conditions, diets that are high in saturated fat but low in fiber, excessive alcohol consumption, sedentary lifestyle, obesity, and inflammatory bowel disease. The onset of colorectal cancer is clearly related to age. The incidence increases markedly in those older than age 50 and peaks in those about 70 years old. First-degree relatives of patients with colon cancer have a twofold to threefold increase in cancer risk, as do patients who have previously been treated for colon cancer.

Patients with chronic ulcerative colitis have a higher incidence of colorectal cancer. The incidence starts to increase after the disease has been present for about 10 years, and approximately 10% develop cancer for every decade after 10 years of disease activity.[13] These cancers tend to be more uniformly distributed through the colon with a trend toward more proximal location, and they often have a scirrhous appearance.[14] Patients with pancolitis are predominantly affected. Sclerosing cholangitis is associated with a strong risk of developing colon cancer in patients with inflammatory bowel disease; consumption of nonsteroidal anti-inflammatory drugs exerts a protective influence.[14] The incidence, characteristics, and prognosis of colorectal carcinoma complicating Crohn's disease are similar to the features of cancer in ulcerative colitis, including young age, multiple neoplasms, long duration of disease, and greater than a 50% 5-year survival rate.[15]

PATHOGENESIS

In the past there was considerable controversy regarding the adenoma-carcinoma sequence. However, it is now believed that at least 70% of colorectal carcinomas start as benign adenomas that undergo malignant transformation (see Fig. 63-1).[16] Up to 30% of cancers arise from de novo sequence, that is, carcinoma developing in normal mucosa without an antecedent adenoma.[15] Larger adenomas (>1 cm) pose a greater cancer risk.[17] Thus, it is vital to detect and remove polypoid lesions larger than 1 cm. Their removal prevents the subsequent development of cancer. If the polyp has become a colon cancer, the earlier it is removed, the less likely it is to have spread.

Cancers that develop in patients with inflammatory bowel disease generally arise from areas of high-grade mucosal dysplasia rather than from adenomatous polyps.[18] Therefore, in the surveillance of these patients, "blind" biopsy specimens are often taken throughout the colon in an attempt to detect severe and persistent dysplasia.

CLINICAL ASPECTS

Colorectal cancer is a slow-growing malignancy, requiring a period of 7 to 10 years for a benign adenoma to undergo malignant transformation. Ideally, the disease should be detected before it becomes symptomatic. Colorectal cancer is sufficiently common in the western world that routine screening is recommended. The American Cancer Society recommends that starting at age 50, both men and women at average risk for developing colorectal cancer should follow one of the screening options listed below[19,20]:
- Fecal occult blood test (FOBT) or fecal immunochemical test (FIT) every year
- Flexible sigmoidoscopy every 5 years
- FOBT or FIT every year plus flexible sigmoidoscopy every 5 years
- Double-contrast barium enema every 5 years
- Colonoscopy every 10 years

The American College of Radiology recommends periodic (approximately every 5 years) double-contrast barium enema study, especially for patients at higher than normal risk of developing colorectal cancer.[21] A cost-effectiveness study of double-contrast barium enema in the screening for colorectal carcinoma showed that the double-contrast barium enema is a cost-effective screening procedure in average-risk patients.[22] The results were based on the assumption that a missed benign 10-mm adenomatous polyp could become malignant within 5 years. It remains to be seen whether CT colonography will become an acceptable noninvasive and cost-effective method in screening for colon cancer if it permits reliable detection of adenomatous polyps larger than 10 mm (see Chapters 57 and 58).[23,24]

Symptomatic colorectal cancer most often presents as bleeding. The severity of bleeding may range from the presence of occult blood in the stool, to the passage of bright red blood per rectum, to the development of iron-deficiency anemia. The patient's symptoms are usually related to the location of the tumor. Approximately one third of carcinomas are in the rectum and can be reached by the examining finger or a rigid proctoscope. About one half of large bowel cancers are in the left half of the colon and can be reached with the flexible sigmoidoscope. Left-sided tumors often present with either bright red rectal bleeding or constipation caused by obstruction. The remaining tumors are scattered throughout the colon. Cecal carcinomas constitute about 10% of the entire group and are most likely to present as iron-deficiency anemia caused by chronic blood loss. Other frequent symptoms of colorectal cancer include abdominal pain, which may be related to the development of obstruction or to tumor invasion of adjacent tissues. Patients may also present with a change in bowel habit or with nonspecific symptoms, such as weight loss or fever.

ROLE OF RADIOLOGY

Radiology plays a critical role in the diagnosis and management of patients with colorectal cancer. The double-contrast barium enema may be used for screening, especially for patients who are at higher than normal risk.[22] It is also the primary method for diagnosing symptomatic colorectal cancer. Single-column studies should be considered for detecting complications, such as obstruction or perforation. Radiology using multidetector row helical computed tomography (MDCT), CT colonography (CTC), magnetic resonance imaging (MRI), and/or transrectal ultrasound (TRUS) also plays an important role in tumor detection and staging.[23-27] Treatment decisions are often based on results from positron emission tomography and CT (PET/CT).[28] Radiology has a significant role after treatment for colorectal cancer in the detection of recurrent disease, local and distant metastases, and metachronous colon tumors.

DIAGNOSTIC METHODS

Contrast Enema

Radiologic examination of the colon can be performed with either single-contrast or double-contrast technique. In most cases, double-contrast enema is superior for the examina-

tion of the rectum[29] and the detection of small lesions.[30] In most series of double-contrast studies, polyps are demonstrated in 10% to 13% of all patients,[31] whereas in single-contrast studies polyps are found in 7% of patients.

Colonoscopy

Many studies have claimed to show that colonoscopy is superior to contrast enema for the detection of polypoid lesions. However, most of these studies do not compare state-of-the-art barium techniques with operators of similar interest and experience. There is an error rate inherent in colonoscopy. Part of this error rate derives from failure to reach the cecum in 15% of cases.[32] In addition, there are blind spots within the colon. Generally, these are behind folds or around flexures, and polyps or even large cancers in these regions can be missed (Fig. 63-2). If there are significant radiologic-endoscopic discrepancies, they should be resolved by consensus or by further examinations and it should not be assumed that the endoscopy result was correct.[33]

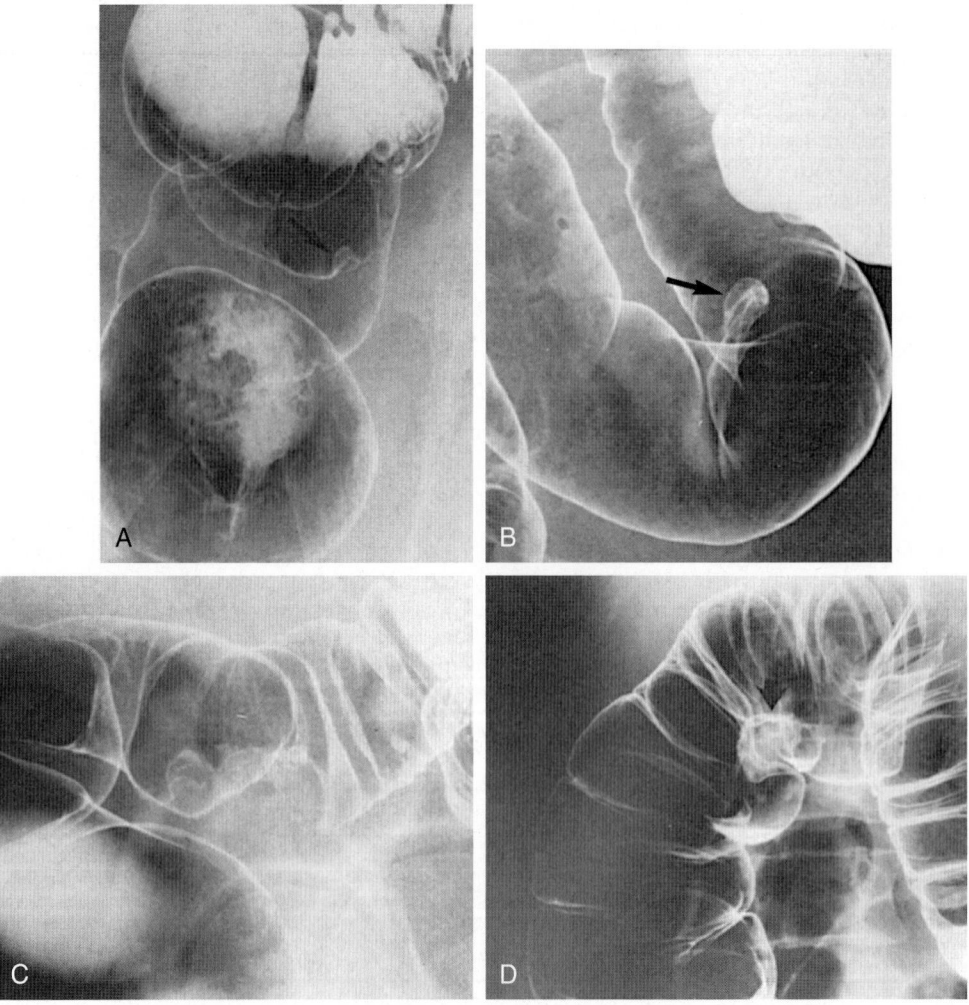

Figure 63-2. Lesions missed at endoscopy identified on barium enema. A. There is a small sessile polyp behind a fold at the rectosigmoid junction. This lesion was missed twice on sigmoidoscopy and was finally detected at the third sigmoidoscopic examination. **B.** A small polyp (*arrow*) is situated behind a fold at an area of angulation at the junction of the sigmoid and the descending colon. This polyp was missed on two colonoscopic examinations and was found on the third. **C.** Polypoid carcinoma is just proximal to the rectosigmoid junction. This lesion was missed on several sigmoidoscopic and colonoscopic examinations and was confirmed only at surgery. **D.** Polypoid carcinoma at the hepatic flexure was missed on initial colonoscopy. (**A, C,** and **D** from Laufer I, Levine MS [eds]: Double Contrast Gastrointestinal Radiology, 3rd ed. Philadelphia, WB Saunders, 2000; **B** from Laufer I, Smith NC, Mullens JE: The radiological demonstration of colorectal polyps undetected by endoscopy. Gastroenterology 70:167-170, 1976.)

Colonoscopy and double-contrast enema examinations have comparable overall accuracy, with detection of approximately 90% of all polypoid lesions if the radiographic examination is performed by an experienced radiologist with special interest in gastrointestinal radiology.[34,35] However, the cost and complications of colonoscopy are considerably higher than those for double-contrast barium enema. Colonoscopy or flexible sigmoidoscopy should always be used to evaluate suggestive findings in contrast enema studies, particularly in patients with marked diverticular disease. It should also be used for biopsy of lesions and removal of polypoid lesions.

Cross-Sectional Imaging

Computed tomography has been used to detect and stage many tumors, including primary and recurrent colorectal neoplasms,[36-38] and has been joined by MRI,[26,39,40] TRUS,[27,39] scintigraphy with monoclonal antibody (MoAb) imaging,[41,42] and PET.[28,43] Three-dimensional virtual-reality techniques, such as CTC, have been employed with increasing frequency, and results are promising.[23,24]

Few studies present an in-depth assessment of the value of the various techniques. A review of the large body of literature on this topic reveals many conflicting reports on the effectiveness of the various methods and opposing recommendations for their use. In many instances, this disagreement is due to early, overly enthusiastic conclusions about high success rates with each new imaging technique and underestimation of their pitfalls. Also, some reports in the literature contained incomplete proof of pathology or neglected to include all factors necessary for complete staging of colon neoplasms.

BENIGN EPITHELIAL POLYPS

Incidence

Benign tumors of the colon are extremely common and usually do not cause symptoms. These polyps are found in 10% to 12.5% of patients studied with double-contrast techniques, and the incidence rises dramatically with increasing age (Fig. 63-3A). Polyps occur most frequently in the left colon and are scattered throughout the remainder of the transverse and right colon (Fig. 63-3B). As the population ages there is a shift in the incidence of polyps to the right side of the colon coinciding with a shift in the distribution of colon carcinoma to the right.[44]

Pathology

The term *polyp* refers only to a focal, protruded lesion within the bowel. In general terms, a polyp may be neoplastic or non-neoplastic. Most non-neoplastic polyps are either inflammatory or hyperplastic. They are generally small and occur most frequently in the distal colon. Neoplastic polyps may represent true neoplasms of any component of the bowel wall. Epithelial neoplasms—adenomas—are the most important because they serve as precursors to colorectal carcinoma. The demonstration of a polypoid lesion on a barium enema does not necessarily give information regarding its pathologic nature. Whenever possible, polyps more than 1 cm in diameter must be removed, preferably by colonoscopic polypectomy

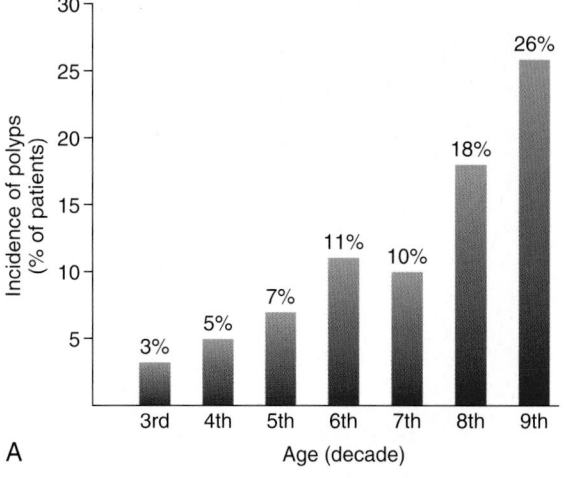

A

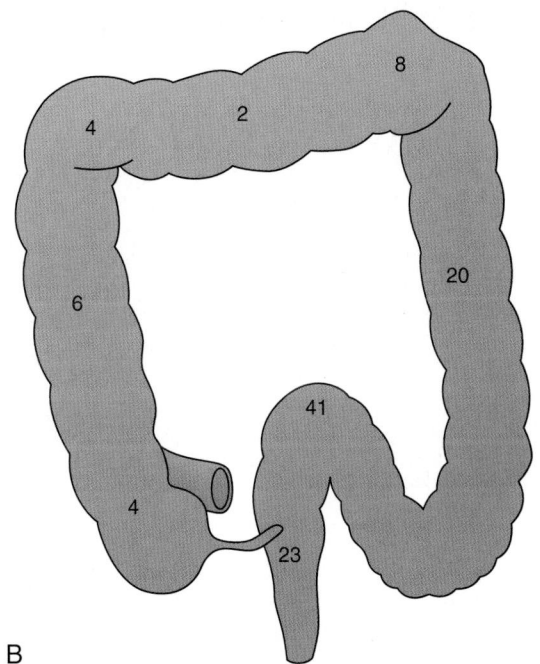

B

Figure 63-3. Incidence and distribution of colorectal polyps. A. Incidence of colonic polyps related to age (based on 800 consecutive double-contrast enemas). There is an increasing incidence of colonic polyps, ranging from 3% in people in their 20s to 26% in people in their 80s. **B.** Distribution of colorectal polyps (based on 108 consecutive polyps). Approximately 60% of the polyps are in the rectum and sigmoid colon. (**A** from Laufer I: The double contrast enema: Myths and misconceptions. Gastrointest Radiol 1:19-31, 1976, with kind permission from Springer Science and Business Media; **B** from Laufer I, Levine MS [eds]: Double Contrast Gastrointestinal Radiology, 3rd ed. Philadelphia, WB Saunders, 2000.)

(Fig. 63-4), because of the increased risk of harboring a malignancy.

Most colonic adenomas are tubular adenomas. However, tubular adenomas have various degrees of villous change; and as a polyp becomes larger, the degree of villous change increases. At the other end of the spectrum, some polyps are villous adenomas because the surface consists of frondlike structures arising from the base of the mucosa. Thus, there may be a transition from tubular adenoma to tubulovillous adenoma to villous adenoma. It has been suggested that any adenoma with more than 75% villous change should be referred

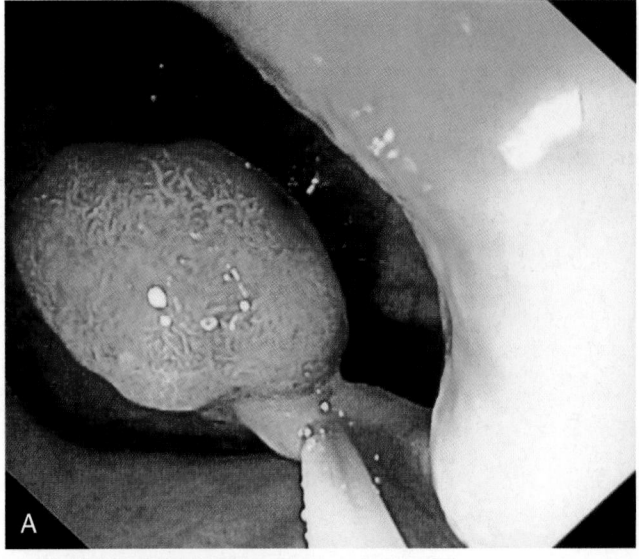

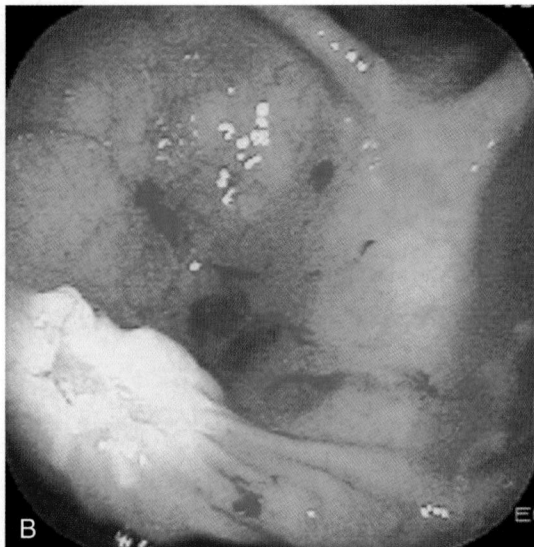

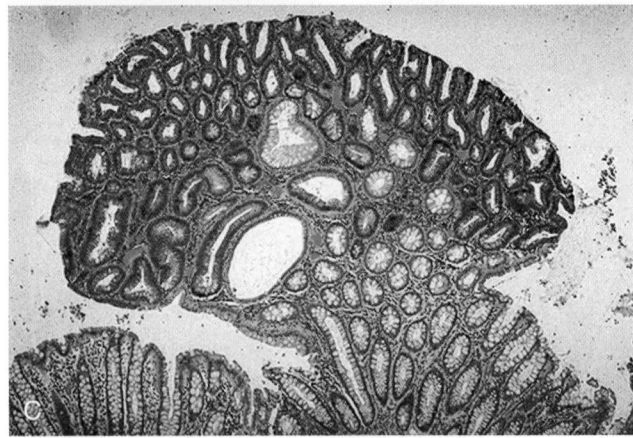

Figure 63-4. Endoscopic polypectomy. A. The sheath containing the snare is seen advancing toward the sigmoid polyp. **B.** Postpolypectomy appearance. **C.** Histology of tubular adenoma.

to as a *villous adenoma*.[45] In general, the risk of carcinoma is related to the proportion of villous change in an adenoma.

In small adenomas, it may be impossible to distinguish villous change radiologically. However, as the adenoma becomes larger and the proportion of villous change increases, a reticular or granular mucosal surface may be seen (Fig. 63-5A).[46] Large villous adenomas have an atypical radiologic appearance.[47] They are large, bulky polypoid masses with barium caught between the frondlike protrusions producing a lacy surface pattern (Fig. 63-5B). Large villous tumors should be removed in toto because malignant degeneration may occur in only a portion of the tumor, and random biopsy sampling is unreliable for the detection of malignant change.

Other non-neoplastic polyps may also be found in the colon. These include juvenile polyps, which may be single or multiple and may be found in adults and in children. Hamartomatous polyps are found in patients with Peutz-Jeghers syndrome and inflammatory polyps in patients with Cronkhite-Canada syndrome (see Chapter 65).

Polyp Detection

Barium Enema

A polyp may be demonstrated as a radiolucent filling defect, as a contour defect, or as a ring shadow because it is simply a protrusion of the mucosa into the bowel lumen (see Chapter 4). The greatest and most frequent difficulty arises in distinguishing polyps from fecal residue. In general, fecal residue is mobile and is usually found on the dependent surface in the barium pool. In addition, several features may suggest that the filling defect represents a true polyp. These include the "bowler hat" sign (Fig. 63-6A) and the "Mexican hat" sign (Fig. 63-6B). Although the bowler hat sign can also be produced by a diverticulum, the direction of the dome of the bowler hat distinguishes a polyp and a diverticulum.[48] When the dome of the hat points away from the axis of the bowel, the lesion is a diverticulum; when the dome points toward the lumen of the bowel, it is a polyp. Villous adenomas may have a reticular or granular surface due to barium trapped between the fronds of the tumor.[49] These signs are illustrated and discussed in detail in Chapters 4 and 5.

Rubesin and coworkers used the term *carpet lesion* to describe a flat, lobulated lesion that is manifest primarily as an alteration in the surface texture of the bowel (Fig. 63-7A).[50] These lesions may be quite large and are mostly tubular adenomas with varying degrees of villous change. In some cases of colorectal carcinoma, the background of a benign carpet lesion can be recognized (Fig. 63-7B).

Cross-Sectional Imaging

Benign lesions of the colon, such as hyperplastic polyps or adenomatous polyps, are usually not examined by CT or

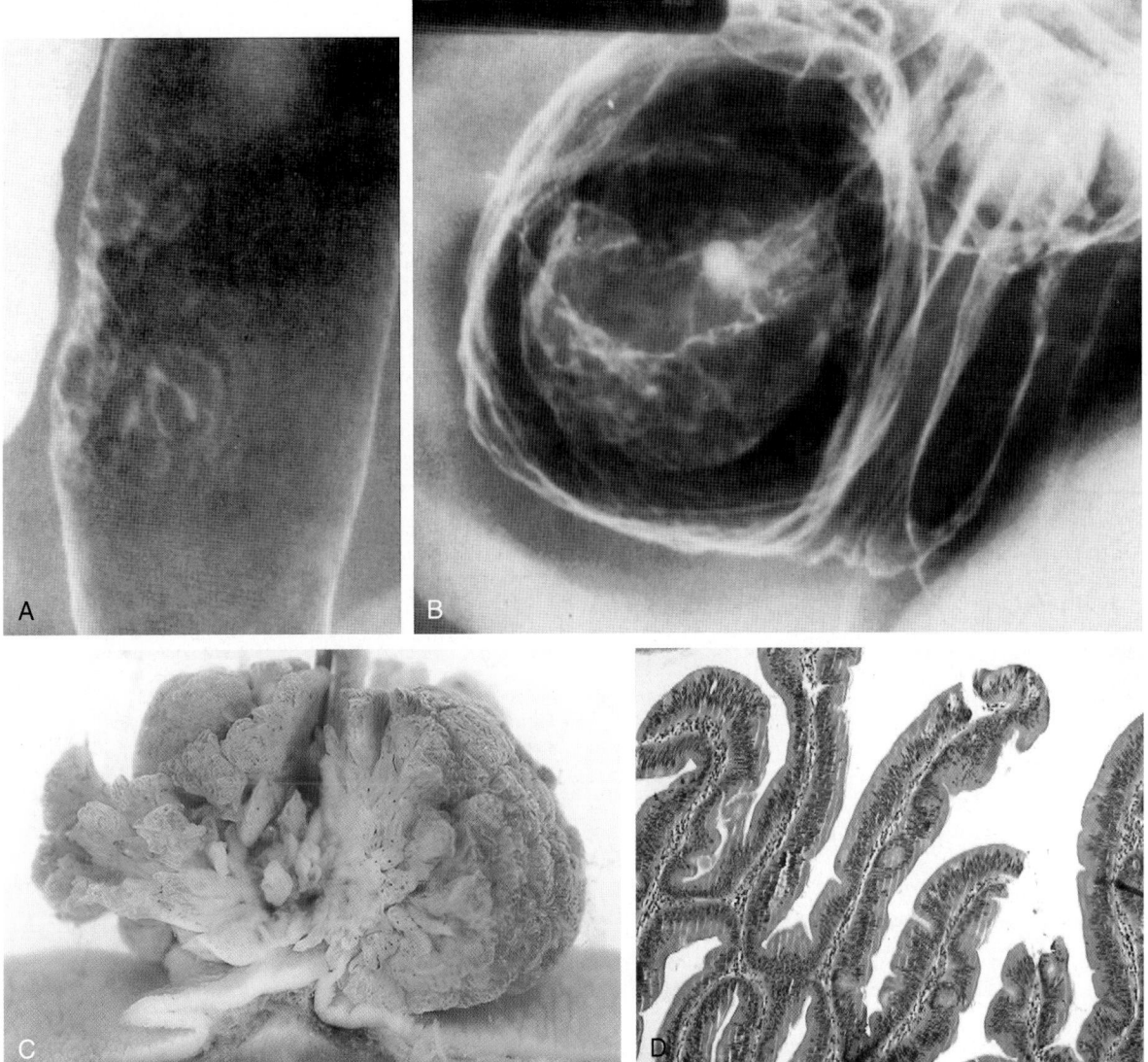

Figure 63-5. Villous adenomas. A. A flat tumor in the descending colon with an irregular surface suggestive of a villous adenoma. This was a villoglandular polyp. **B.** Typical villous tumor in the sigmoid colon. This tumor exhibits the typical, irregular, frondlike surface of a villous tumor. It was a malignant villous adenoma. **C.** Gross pathology specimen shows cauliflower-like colon polyp. **D.** Histology reveals frondlike nature of polyp. (**A** and **B** from Laufer I, Levine MS [eds]: Double Contrast Gastrointestinal Radiology, 3rd ed. Philadelphia, WB Saunders, 2000.)

MRI. They are demonstrated by barium examinations or by one of the endoscopic techniques and are seen during CT or MRI examinations only incidentally. These techniques are used only if these benign tumors become large enough to have a high likelihood of harboring a malignancy. Benign polyps appear as sessile soft tissue masses that protrude into the lumen of the bowel on axial images (Fig. 63-8). They are usually detected only if the patient has undergone colonic cleansing or if the polyp is large. If the polyp is pedunculated, CT scans may demonstrate a large polypoid mass that represents the combined polyp and stalk (see also Chapter 57 on Computed Tomographic Colonography).

Coscina and colleagues[51] suggested that villous adenomas have a characteristic CT appearance based on their high mucus content. The CT features of villous adenomas include homogeneous water density (<10 Hounsfield units) occupying more than half of the lesion and eccentric location on the luminal side of the mass. No air-fluid level is seen, and the lesion should not have a round cystic configuration. Opaque oral or rectal contrast material should not be used to diagnose a suspected villous adenoma because it obscures the lesion. In these cases, insufflation of air, water, or oily substance administered per rectum may be helpful. Because of their malignant potential, larger villous adenomas should always be staged by CT or TRUS if located in the rectum.[52]

On MR images, benign polyps appear as low-intensity structures on T1-weighted spin-echo sequences. If there are many mucin-producing cells, the signal intensity of the polypoid mass increases on T1-weighted sequences. TRUS is used for assessment of sessile polyps large enough to have an increased risk for malignancy. In these cases, TRUS can be used to determine the depth of invasion by a sessile mass that protrudes into the lumen. The depth of invasion is best assessed by TRUS because it is the only method that can demonstrate the various layers of the colonic wall. If the intraluminal component is large, false tumor measurements and erroneous depiction of the surface of the mass can occur because of compression of the tumor by the transrectal probe.

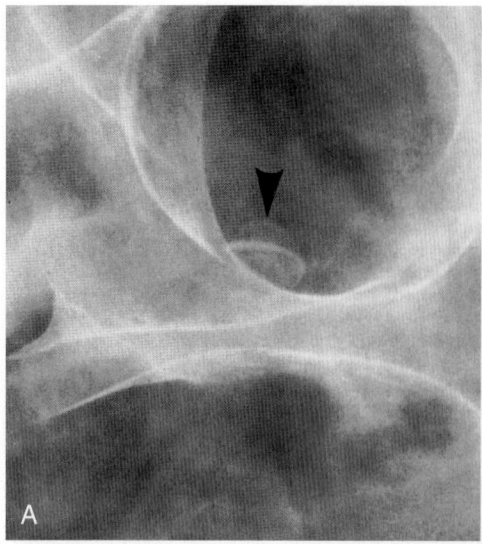

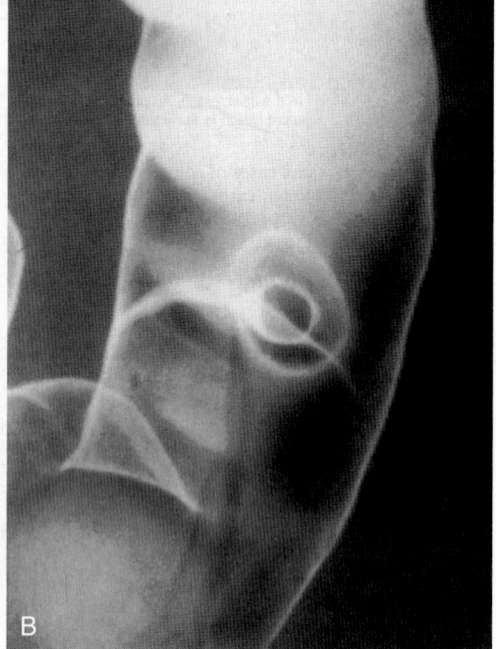

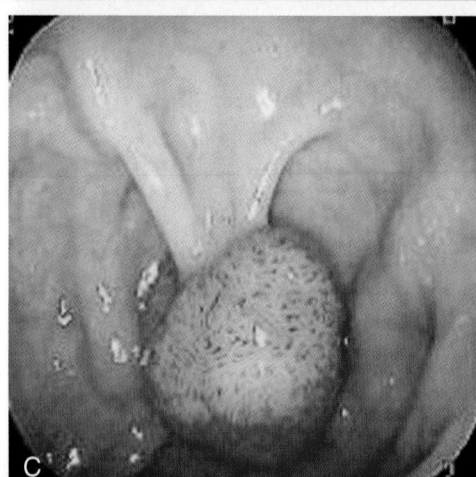

Figure 63-6. Double-contrast barium enema and colonoscopy features of polyps. A. The bowler hat sign representing a sessile polyp. **B.** Mexican hat sign. This is the typical appearance of a pedunculated polyp seen end-on. The outer ring represents the head of the polyp, and the inner ring represents the stalk. **C.** Endoscopic view of pedunculated polyp. (**A** and **B** from Laufer I, Levine MS [eds]: Double Contrast Gastrointestinal Radiology, 3rd ed. Philadelphia, WB Saunders, 2000.)

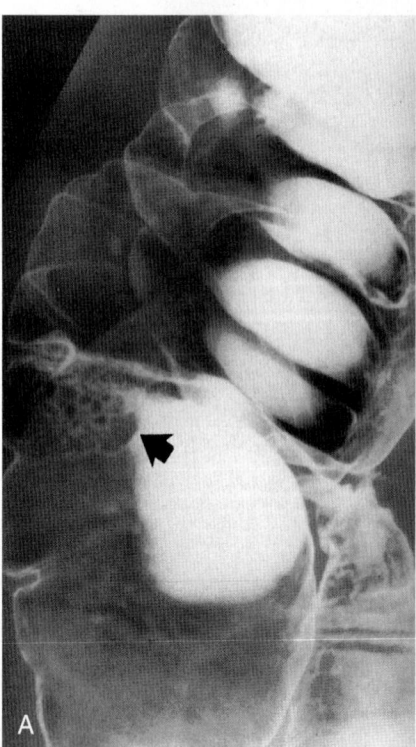

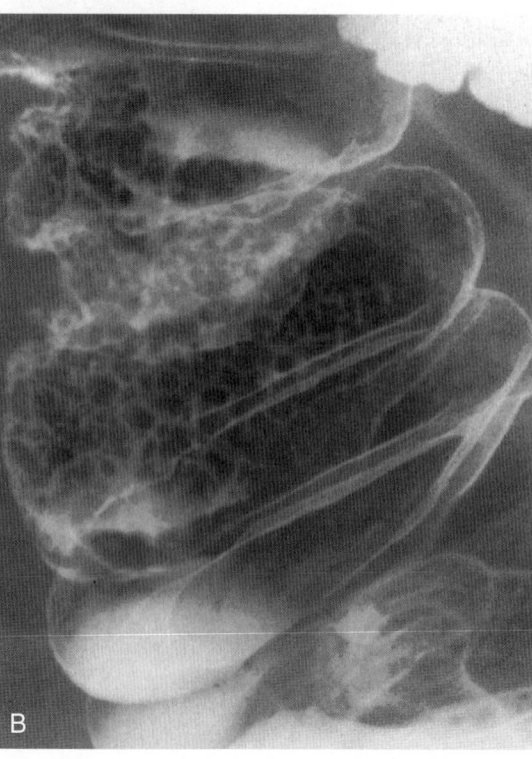

Figure 63-7. Carpet lesions. A. Typical carpet lesion (*arrow*) in the cecum. **B.** Malignant transformation in a carpet lesion. An obvious polypoid carcinoma is seen in the ascending colon. Surrounding the polypoid lesion is the mucosal change representing the underlying adenoma. (**A** and **B** from Laufer I, Levine MS [eds]: Double Contrast Gastrointestinal Radiology, 3rd ed. Philadelphia, WB Saunders, 2000.)

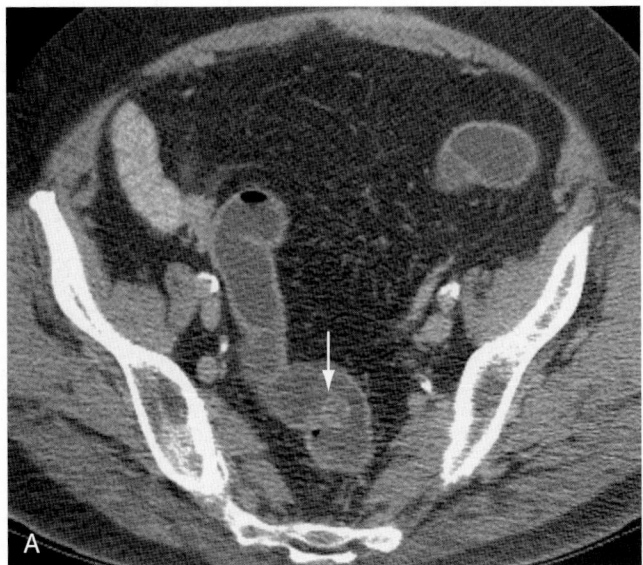
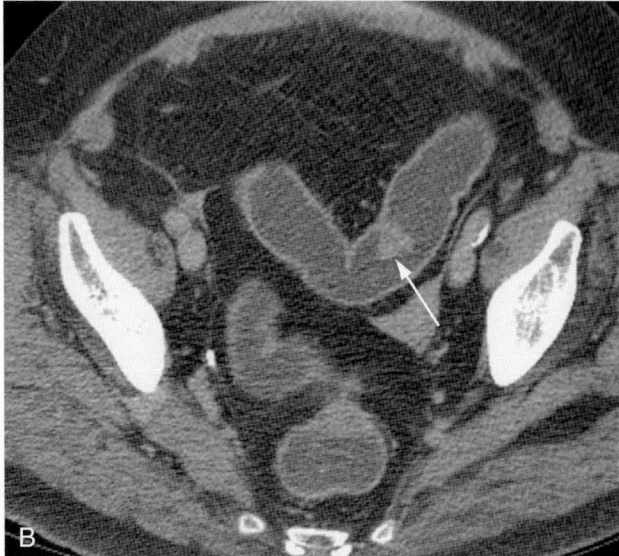

Figure 63-8. CT of benign polyps. A. Axial thin-section MDCT identifies a sessile polyp (*arrow*) on the left wall of the proximal sigmoid colon, which was confirmed by colonoscopy in a patient with carcinoma of the cecum and familial polyposis syndrome. **B.** Axial thin-section MDCT below level shown in **A** demonstrates a second polyp (*arrow*) in the small bowel.

ADENOCARCINOMA

Barium Enema

Early Cancer

The radiologic detection of early colorectal cancer is basically an exercise in the detection of polyps. The typical early colon cancer is a flat, sessile lesion that may produce a contour defect (Fig. 63-9). Although most polyps detected radiologically should be removed if they are more than 5 mm in diameter, a number of radiologic criteria have been used for the detection of malignancy in colorectal polyps.[53] The size of the polyp is the most important criterion. Carcinoma is virtually nonexistent in polyps smaller than 5 mm. The incidence of cancer is approximately 1% in polyps in the 5- to 10-mm range (Fig. 63-10), 10% in polyps measuring between 1 and 2 cm, and more than 25% in polyps larger than 2 cm.[54]

Malignant polyps tend to grow more quickly than benign polyps, although there is considerable overlap between the two groups.[55] If there is definite evidence of polyp growth on serial examinations, malignancy should be suspected. The presence of a long thin stalk is generally a sign of a benign polyp. Rarely, such polyps harbor malignancy.[56] As a rule, the stalk associated with carcinoma is short and thick (Fig. 63-11). If the head of the polyp is irregular or lobulated, the probability of malignancy is greater, although some benign polyps may have an irregular or lobulated surface.

Advanced Cancer

Most patients with symptomatic colorectal carcinoma have advanced lesions. These lesions are generally annular or polypoid tumors seen as filling defects in the barium column or as contour defects. In addition, plaquelike lesions can produce abnormal lines on double-contrast barium studies (Figs. 63-12 and 63-13).[57] Annular or semiannular carcinomas as

seen on barium enema have a higher rate of serosal invasion and lymph node metastases than polypoid carcinomas.[58]

Advanced cancers are often associated with "sentinel" polyps or additional polyps elsewhere in the colon. Approximately 5% of patients who have a colon carcinoma have additional, synchronous carcinomas in the colon (see Fig. 63-13).[59] Therefore, whenever possible, the entire colon should be

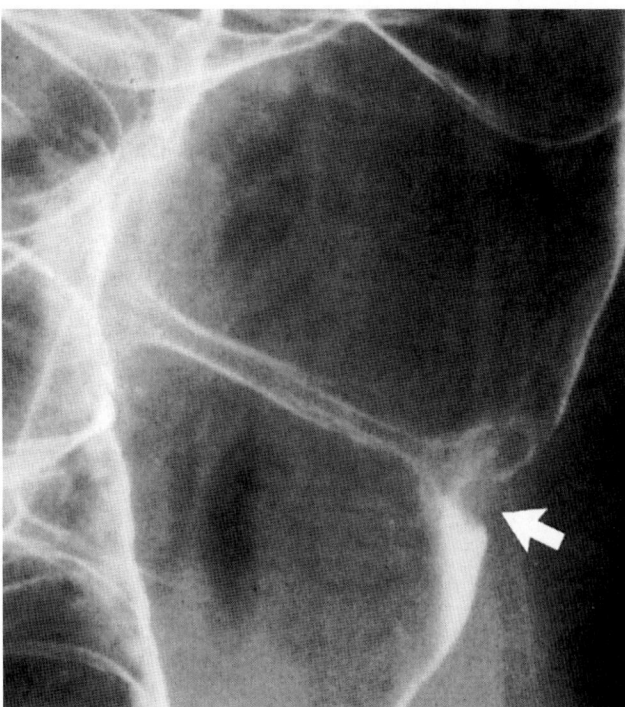

Figure 63-9. Typical early colon cancer. A 1-cm polypoid mass with a contour defect (*arrow*) is seen along the lateral wall. (From Laufer I, Levine MS [eds]: Double Contrast Gastrointestinal Radiology, 3rd ed. Philadelphia, WB Saunders, 2000.)

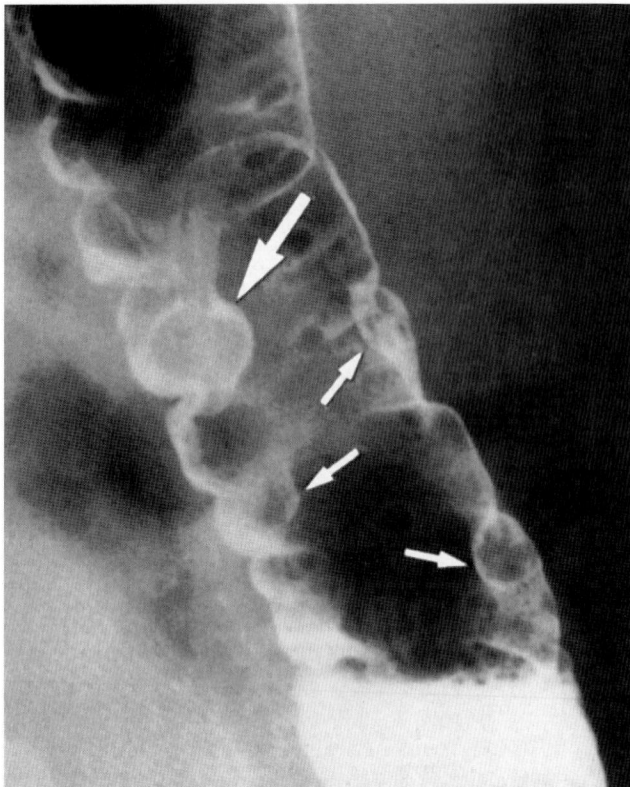

Figure 63-10. Early colon cancers. Polypoid carcinoma with a pedicle in a 29-year-old man with rectal bleeding. A pedunculated polyp in the descending colon (*large arrow*) has a typically benign appearance. This was removed at colonoscopy and was found to be a carcinoma with invasion of the stalk. The smaller lesions (*small arrows*) were hyperplastic polyps. (From Laufer I: The double contrast enema: Myths and misconceptions. Gastrointestinal Radiol 1:19-31, 1976. With kind permission from Springer Science and Business Media.)

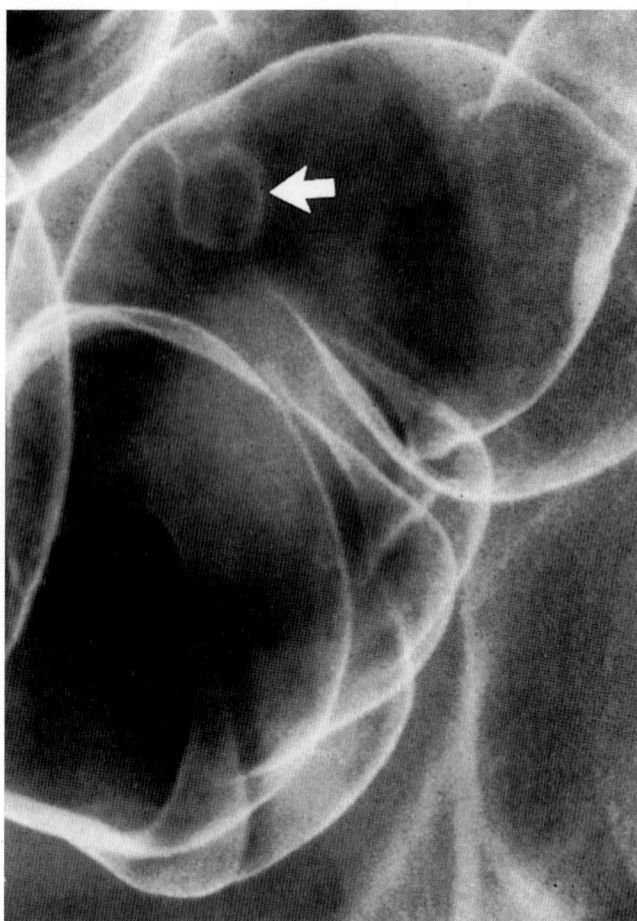

Figure 63-11. Pedunculated early cancer. Early carcinoma (*arrow*) with a short, thick stalk. (From Laufer I, Levine MS [eds]: Double Contrast Gastrointestinal Radiology, 3rd ed. Philadelphia, WB Saunders, 2000.)

examined even when a carcinoma is encountered in the distal bowel. The barium enema may be used to search for neoplastic lesions larger than 1 cm in patients with incomplete colonoscopy.[60]

Carcinomas are particularly difficult to detect in patients with extensive diverticular disease of the sigmoid colon (Fig. 63-14). If the radiologic examination leaves any doubt regarding the presence of a carcinoma, flexible sigmoidoscopy should be recommended to confirm or exclude lesions in the sigmoid colon.[61]

Advanced carcinoma may have an atypical appearance. The linitis plastica type of carcinoma has predominant submucosal infiltration and fibrous reaction.[62] The radiologic appearance may be suggestive of an inflammatory stricture. This type of carcinoma is particularly likely to develop in patients with ulcerative colitis (see Chapter 61).

Complications

The most important complications of colorectal cancer include bleeding, bowel obstruction, and perforation. Massive rectal bleeding caused by colon carcinoma is rare; the bleeding is more often manifest as occult blood in the stool or as chronic anemia. Colorectal cancer is one of the major causes of large bowel obstruction. Obstruction may be caused by encroachment of the tumor mass on the lumen of the bowel (Fig. 63-15A). Antegrade obstruction and retrograde obstruction tend to be poorly correlated. Frequently, there is a high-grade obstruction to the retrograde flow of barium when the patient has few or no symptoms of clinical obstruction. In the case of polypoid tumors, obstruction may also be caused by colocolic intussusception (Fig. 63-15B). In patients with long-standing obstruction and colon distention, mucosal ischemia may result in an ulcerative form of colitis affecting the colon proximal to the obstruction.

Advanced cancer may result in perforation of the colon and a pericolic abscess (Fig. 63-16A). The signs, symptoms, and radiologic features of a perforated carcinoma may be difficult to distinguish from those of a pericolic abscess associated with diverticulitis (Fig. 63-16B). However, evidence of gastrointestinal blood loss makes a malignant origin much more likely.[63] Perforation of the colon may lead to a fistula to adjacent organs, such as the stomach (Fig. 63-17A), duodenum (Fig. 63-17B), bladder, or vagina. The fistulous communication can be demonstrated by barium study or by the extracolonic presence of gas or contrast medium on CT scans.

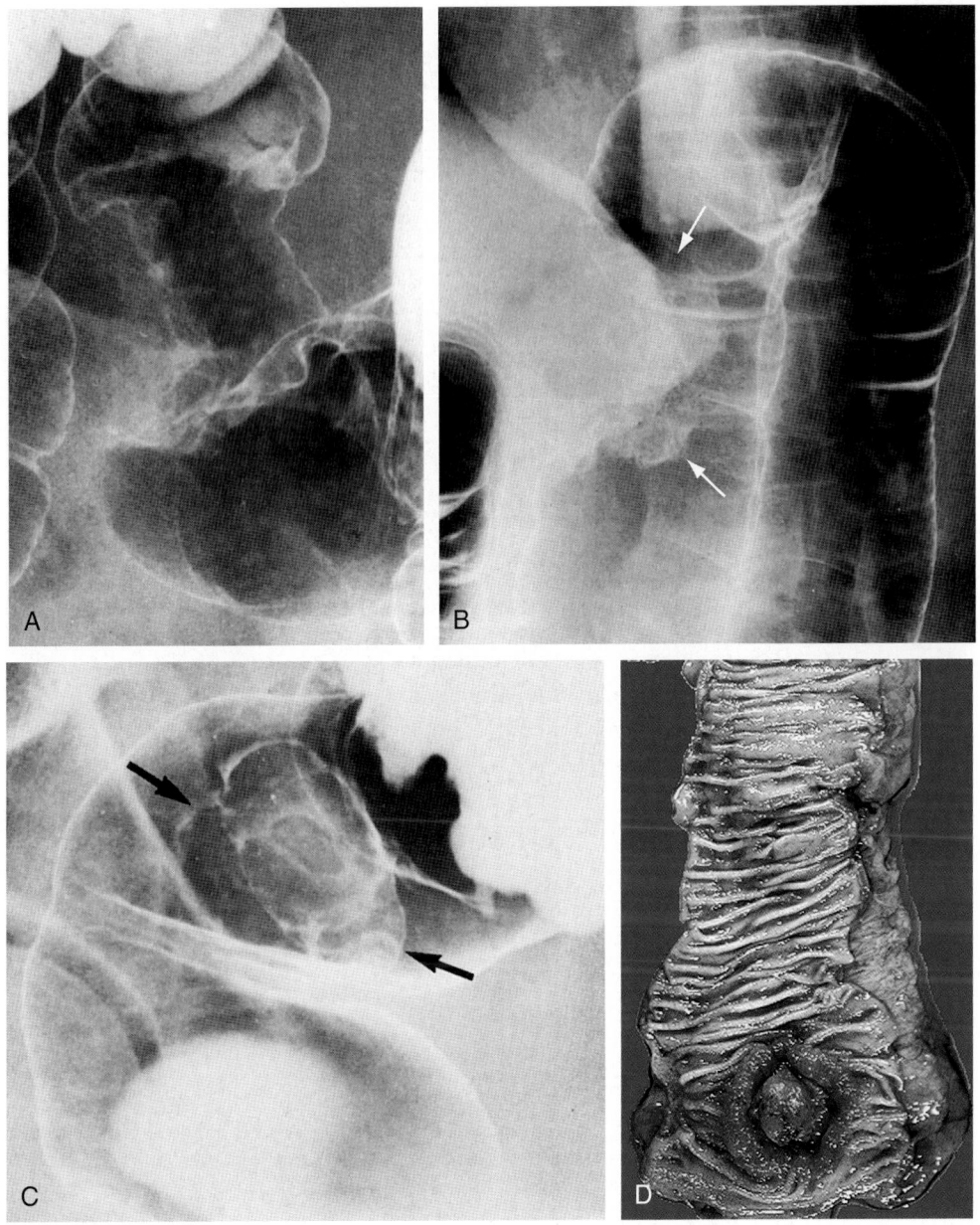

Figure 63-12. Advanced colon cancer. A. Annular, "apple core" lesion. **B.** Large polypoid carcinoma (*arrows*) at the splenic flexure. **C.** Lateral view shows an ulcerated plaquelike carcinoma etched in white (*arrows*) at the rectosigmoid junction. **D.** Specimen shows ulcerating polypoid carcinoma. (**A** and **B** from Laufer I, Levine MS [eds]: Double Contrast Gastrointestinal Radiology, 3rd ed. Philadelphia, WB Saunders, 2000.)

Computed Tomography

Primary Colorectal Carcinoma

CT and endoluminal ultrasound are better suited for evaluation of tumor stage than manual examination, barium enema, or fiberoptic techniques. In the presence of a colorectal cancer, both CT and ultrasound may visualize a discrete mass (Fig. 63-18) or focal wall thickening (Fig. 63-19), but this finding is nonspecific and requires further investigation. This wall thickening may be circumferential, without or with extension beyond the bowel wall (Fig. 63-20). Asymmetric mural thickening with or without an irregular surface con-tour is suggestive of a neoplastic process (see Fig. 63-20), particularly if benign causes can be excluded by history or physical

examination. In the anorectal region, internal hemorrhoids must be distinguished from a polypoid malignancy.

With a properly distended lumen, a colonic wall thickness of less than 3 mm is normal, 3 to 6 mm is indeterminate, and greater than 6 mm is definitely abnormal. If the tumor is contained within the wall of the colon or rectum, the outer margins of the large bowel appear smooth. CT cannot reliably assess the depth of mural penetration. The various layers of bowel wall and depth of mural invasion can be depicted by endoluminal ultrasound or MRI with endorectal coils. They can also determine the layer from which the tumor arises, which is important for differentiating an adenocarcinoma from a lymphoma or gastrointestinal stromal tumor.

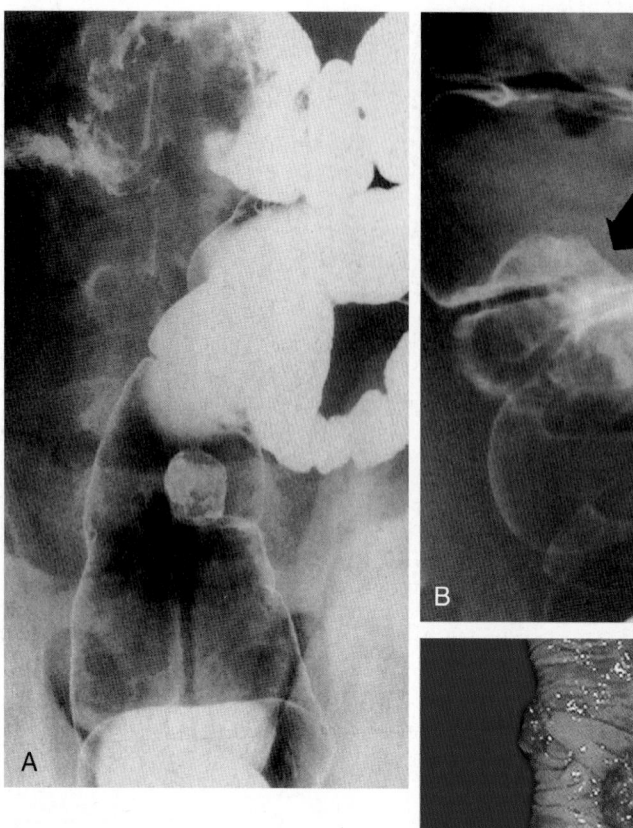

Figure 63-13. Synchronous tumors. A. A nearly obstructing polypoid carcinoid is seen in the transverse colon, and a second adenoma is seen in the sigmoid colon. **B.** Multiple polypoid carcinomas (*arrows*) in the ascending colon. **C.** Specimen shows polypoid cancer (*arrow*) and multiple synchronous polyps. (**A** and **B** from Laufer I, Levine MS [eds]: Double Contrast Gastrointestinal Radiology, 3rd ed. Philadelphia, WB Saunders, 2000.)

Tumor invasion beyond the bowel wall is suggested by a mass with nodular or spiculated borders, associated with strands of soft tissue extending from the serosal surface into the perirectal or pericolonic fat (Fig. 63-21). Broad-based soft tissue extensions from the tumor into the perirectal fat are more indicative of tumor extension than spiculation, which often represents a desmoplastic reaction. Desmoplastic reaction frequently leads to overstaging by MRI because it can be difficult to distinguish between fibrosis alone and fibrosis that contains tumor cells (Fig. 63-22).[39] Extracolonic tumor spread is also suggested by loss of tissue fat planes between the large bowel and surrounding muscles-obturator internus, piriformis (Fig. 63-23), levator ani, puborectalis, coccygeal, and gluteus maximus. Invasion is definite only when a tumor mass extends directly into an adjacent muscle, obliterating the fat plane and enlarging the individual muscle.

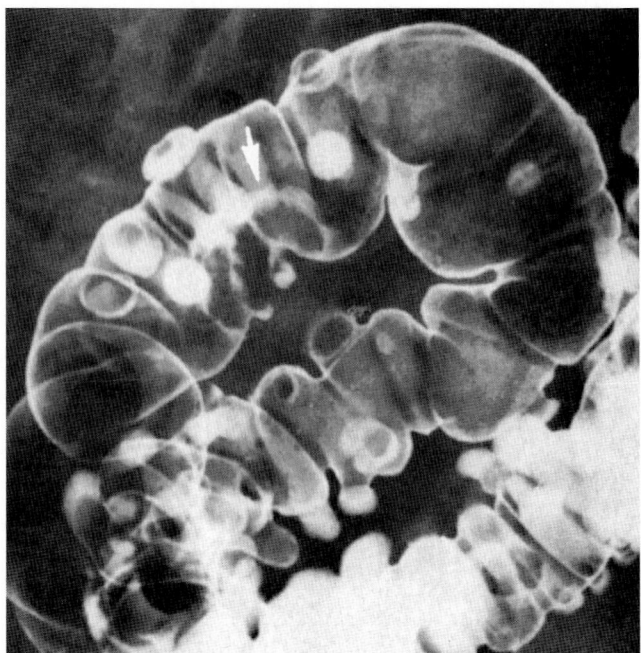

Figure 63-14. Carcinoma in a patient with diverticulosis. The polypoid carcinoma (*arrow*) is more difficult to recognize in the presence of extensive diverticulosis. (From Laufer I, Levine MS [eds]: Double Contrast Gastrointestinal Radiology, 3rd ed. Philadelphia, WB Saunders, 2000.)

Cross-sectional methods such as CT cannot detect microscopic invasion of the fat surrounding the colon or rectum (see Fig. 63-19) and tend to understage these patients. Spread to contiguous organs in the pelvis can be simulated by absence of tissue planes between the viscera and the tumor mass without actual invasion. Vascular or lymphatic congestion, inflammation, or actual absence of fat because of severe

cachexia can cause obliteration of fat planes. Therefore, invasion should be diagnosed cautiously and considered definite only if an obvious mass clearly involves an adjacent organ. Distinction between tumor infiltration of adjacent muscle and simple absence of fat separating normal structures is particularly difficult in the area of lower rectum and anal verge.

In our experience, CT results can be improved through the use of a large, rapidly delivered bolus of intravenous contrast agent and MDCT with thin sections and water as rectal and colonic contrast material (see Fig. 63-22). With this approach, the pelvis is scanned at peak enhancement and the enhanced wall of the rectum can be better distinguished from adjacent levator ani and sphincter muscles. CT usually is used for staging and not for detection of colonic lesions. Nevertheless ultrathin sections (0.625- to 1.25-mm slices) obtained with MDCT can facilitate demonstration of even small lesions and increase accuracy of tumor staging. Staging results can be further improved if multiplanar reformats are used and interpretation is based on a combination of axial slices and multiplanar reformats (see Fig. 63-18).[64] Coronal reformats often are helpful to define the relationship of the rectal mass to the levator ani, puborectalis, and sphincter muscles, which is helpful in planning the appropriate surgery. Nevertheless, CT cannot achieve the exquisite soft tissue resolution afforded by MRI with gadolinium contrast enhancement.[65] Such superior distinction is particularly useful in the lower pelvis for assessing tumor invasion into muscle, nerves, bladder, and male or female organs (see later section on Magnetic Resonance Imaging).[66]

Primary and recurrent colon cancer can invade the seminal vesicles, prostate, bladder, uterus (Fig. 63-24), ovaries, small bowel, and sciatic nerves and can obstruct the ureters. Occasionally, tumors of the prostate, uterus, or ovaries that invade or are contiguous with the rectum or sigmoid colon can be

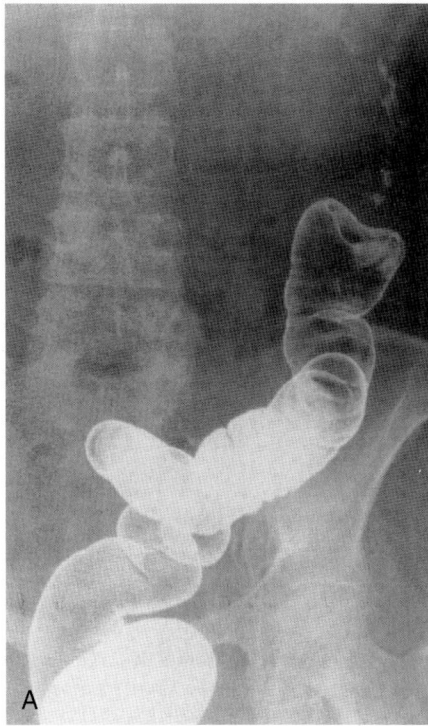
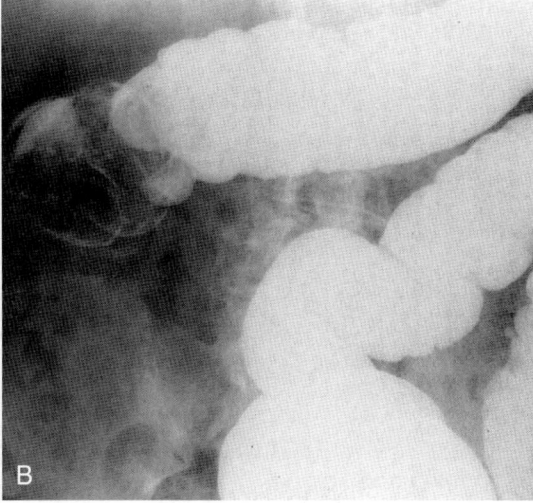

Figure 63-15. Colon cancer causing bowel obstruction.
A. An annular carcinoma in the mid-descending colon completely obstructs the retrograde flow of barium. **B.** Cecal carcinoma with colocolic intussusception extending into the midtransverse colon.

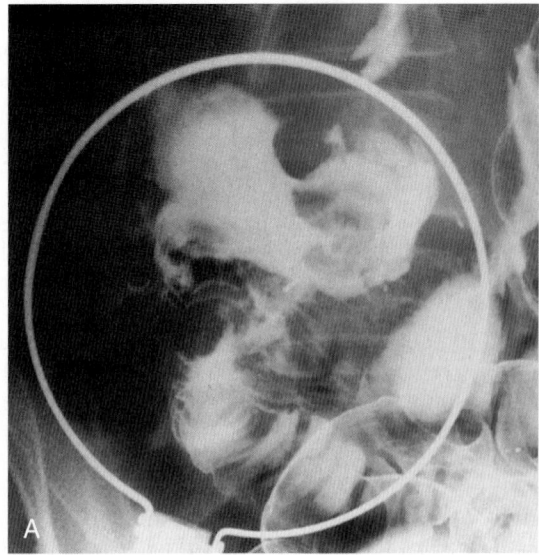
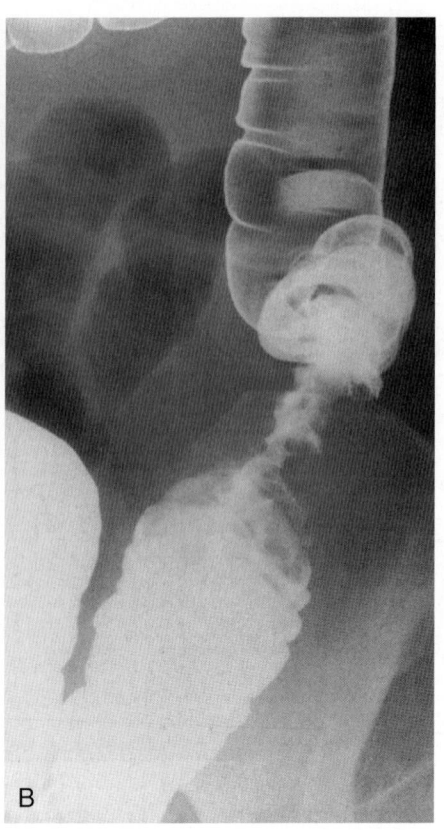

Figure 63-16. Perforated carcinoma of the colon. **A.** Barium filling of a perforation caused by recurrent carcinoma of the colon at the hepatic flexure. **B.** In another patient, a tapered narrowing in the sigmoid colon is due to a pericolic abscess resulting from perforation of a sigmoid carcinoma. The appearance may be difficult to distinguish from that of diverticulitis.

indistinguishable from an invasive colon neoplasm. Areas of low attenuation within the mass suggest tumor necrosis; tumor calcifications indicate a mucinous adenocarcinoma. A vesicorectal fistula manifests as air in the tract and bladder. After administration of intravenous contrast agent, the wall of the tract may enhance. Alternatively, a jet of positive rectal contrast material can be identified in the bladder. Fistulous tracts can also extend into the uterus or vagina, and sinus tracts may be seen in the fat of the ischiorectal fossa.

Colon tumors can destroy adjacent bone, most frequently the sacrum and coccyx. Large tumors can involve the ilium. Advanced bone invasion causes frank bone destruction often associated with a soft tissue mass. Subtle cortical destruction visible only on bone "window" settings may be the only manifestation of bone invasion.

Liver metastases usually appear hypodense on non–contrast-enhanced scans. Foci of calcification can be seen within primary or metastatic mucinous adenocarcinomas

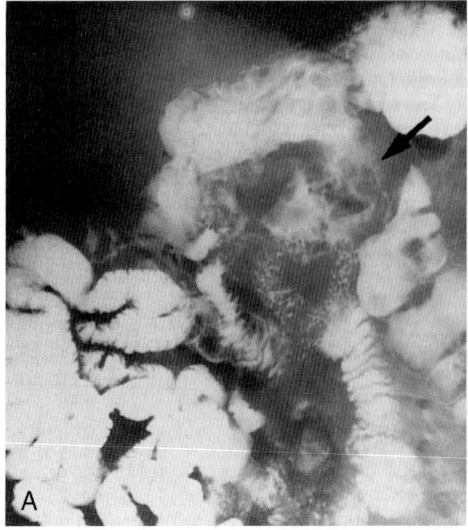
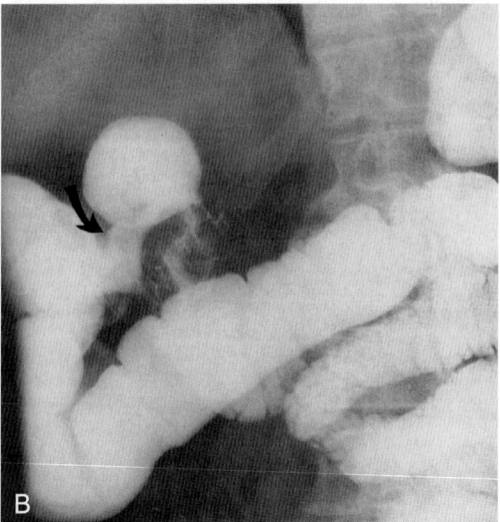

Figure 63-17. Fistulas complicating carcinoma of the colon. A. Gastrocolic fistula arising from a carcinoma at the splenic flexure (*arrow*). **B.** A carcinoma of the transverse colon giving rise to a fistula to the duodenum (*arrow*).

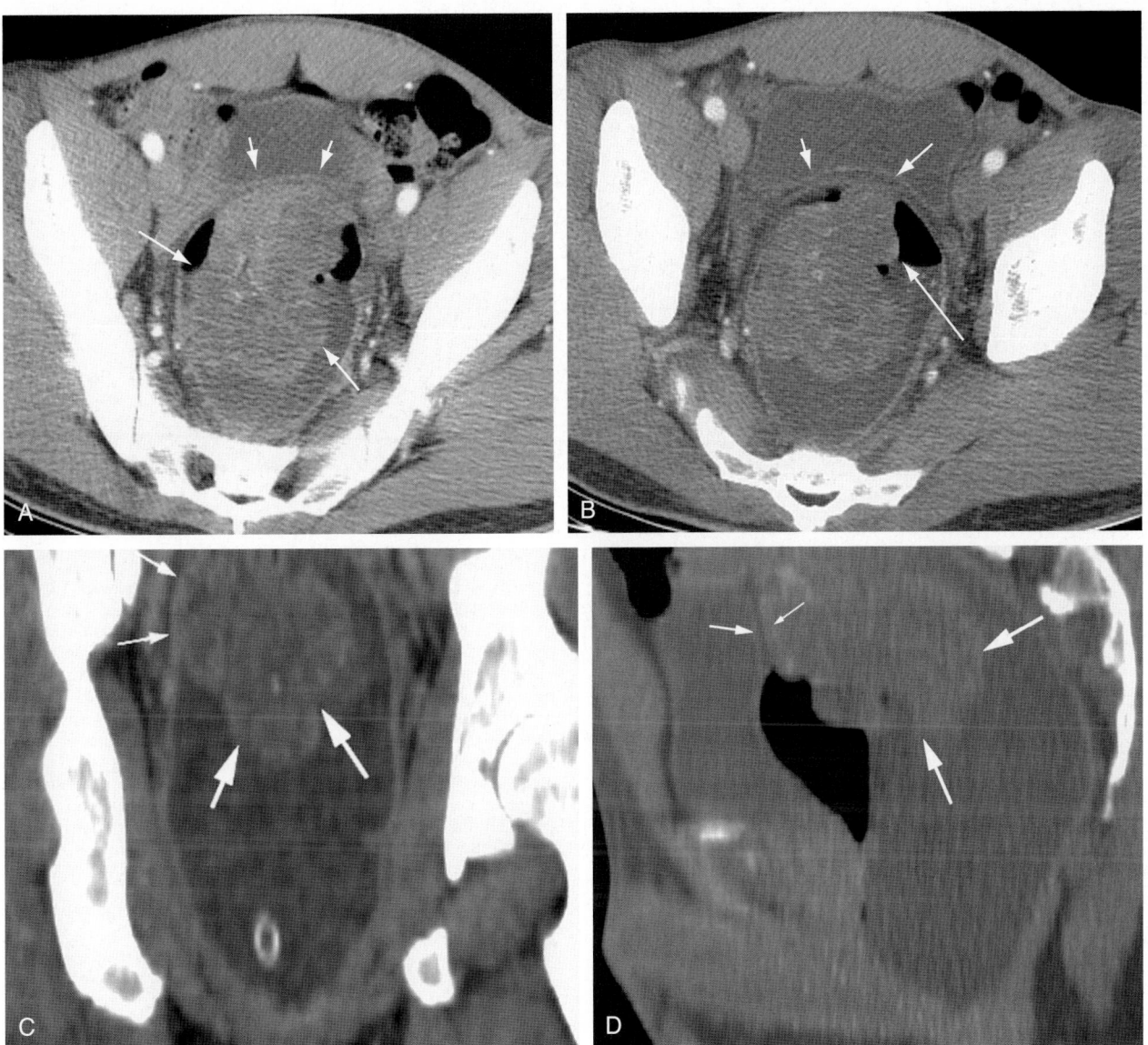

Figure 63-18. Large intraluminal mass in a distended rectum without extension beyond bowel wall (T2N0M0). A. A thin-section MDCT scan in the arterial phase demonstrates a very large intraluminal mass (*large arrow*) that appears to arise from the anterior wall of the rectum. Bladder wall (*thin arrows*) is clearly separated from the rectal wall by a thin layer of fat. **B.** Several centimeters below the level of **A,** the fat plane between bladder wall (*thin arrows*) and the mass (*large arrow*) in the anterior rectal wall remains intact. **C.** Coronal MPR demonstrates the large intraluminal component of the mass (*large arrows*) and the wall thickening (*small arrows*) with a smooth outer border. **D.** The sagittal multiplanar reformatted image demonstrates a clear fat plane between the bladder wall (*small arrow*) and the thickened rectal wall (*thin arrow*). Both MPRs confirm absence of perirectal infiltration. The large intraluminal mass (*large arrows*) also is appreciated.

(Fig. 63-25). After a bolus injection of contrast material, the CT density of hepatic colonic metastasis can change rapidly. Compared with the involved liver parenchyma, metastases often show early rim enhancement or become partially hyperdense (Fig. 63-26), go through an isodense phase, and then become low-density lesions again. Optimal bolus and scanning techniques are necessary to minimize false-negative results that occur when metastases become isodense with normal liver parenchyma when scanning is extended into the equilibrium phase. This isointensity often occurs with small (<2 cm) lesions. If only one to four hepatic metastases are detected (more if they are peripheral and can be easily wedged out) and no extrahepatic disease is present, an aggressive treatment plan appears warranted because there is improved 5-year survival after removal of isolated metastatic foci.[67]

CT with arterial portography (CTAP) was formerly considered the single most accurate means of detecting additional metastatic lesions in the normal-appearing lobe.[68] However, the general use of CTAP has been abandoned in favor of helical CT. Helical CT can achieve similar sensitivities, has a lower false-positive rate than CTAP, and is noninvasive.[69,70] In one helical CT study with surgical correlation in all patients, the sensitivity for detecting colonic metastases to the liver was 85% and the positive predictive value was 96%.[38] MRI with ferumoxides or gadolinium enhancement also provides excellent results in detecting hepatic metastases from colon carcinoma, but this technique is more expensive and not as widely available as CT.[71,72] In one series, the MR sensitivity for colorectal liver metastases was 96.8% but only slightly over a third of patients underwent curative resection for histologic

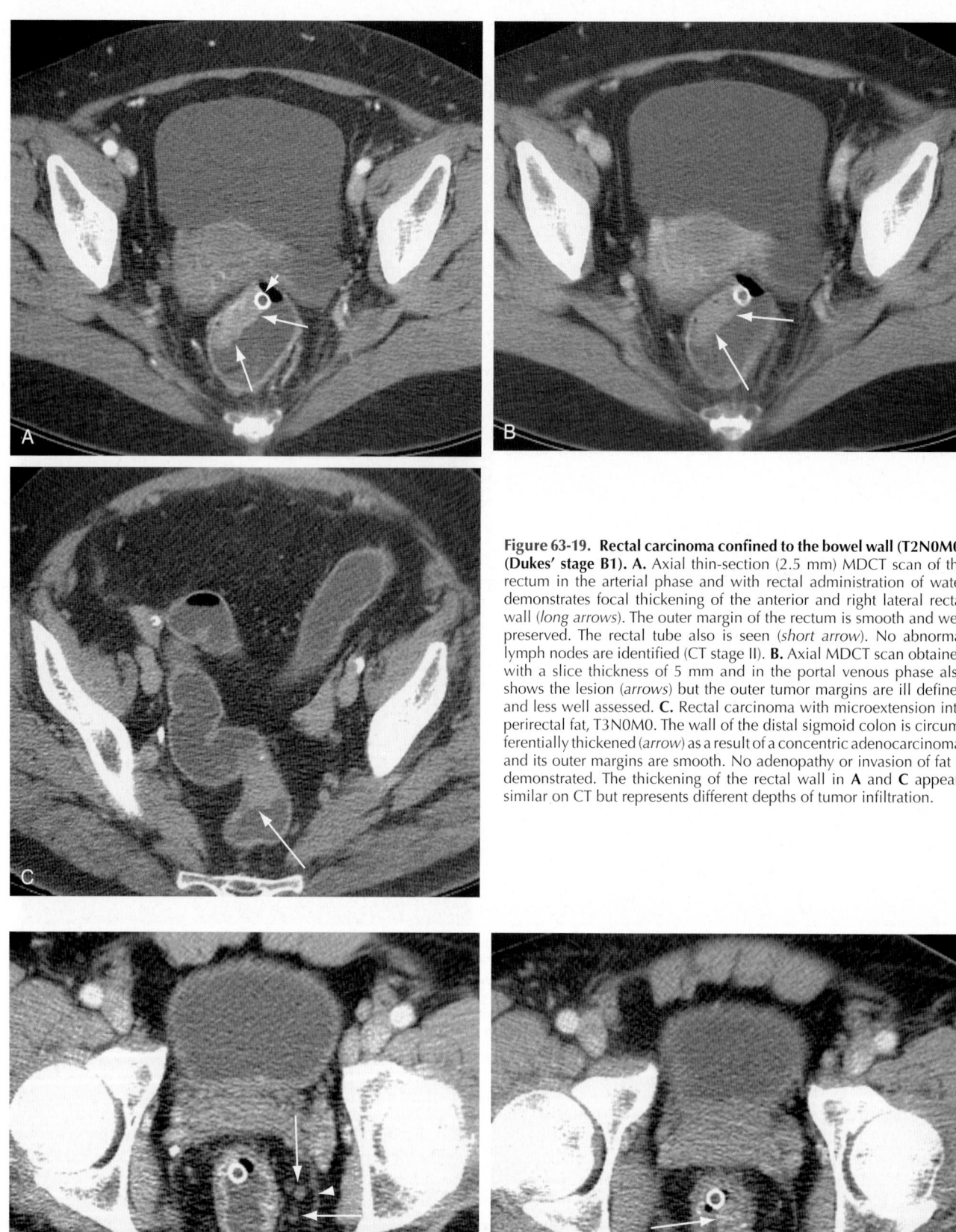

Figure 63-19. Rectal carcinoma confined to the bowel wall (T2N0M0) (Dukes' stage B1). A. Axial thin-section (2.5 mm) MDCT scan of the rectum in the arterial phase and with rectal administration of water demonstrates focal thickening of the anterior and right lateral rectal wall (*long arrows*). The outer margin of the rectum is smooth and well preserved. The rectal tube also is seen (*short arrow*). No abnormal lymph nodes are identified (CT stage II). **B.** Axial MDCT scan obtained with a slice thickness of 5 mm and in the portal venous phase also shows the lesion (*arrows*) but the outer tumor margins are ill defined and less well assessed. **C.** Rectal carcinoma with microextension into perirectal fat, T3N0M0. The wall of the distal sigmoid colon is circumferentially thickened (*arrow*) as a result of a concentric adenocarcinoma, and its outer margins are smooth. No adenopathy or invasion of fat is demonstrated. The thickening of the rectal wall in **A** and **C** appears similar on CT but represents different depths of tumor infiltration.

Figure 63-20. Adenocarcinoma of the rectum confined to the rectal wall with perirectal lymph nodes (T2N1M0 or Dukes' stage C1). A. MDCT scan demonstrates minimal but diffuse wall thickening (*red arrows*). Mesorectal fascia is well shown (*arrowheads*). Perirectal lymph nodes (*white arrows*) are seen in the perirectal fat adjacent to left lateral wall of rectum. MDCT was performed after one course of radiation, which probably caused the diffuse wall thickening. **B.** MDCT image slightly below the level in **A** reveals asymmetric nodular thickening of left lateral wall of the rectum (*arrows*) without extension of tumor into perirectal fat.

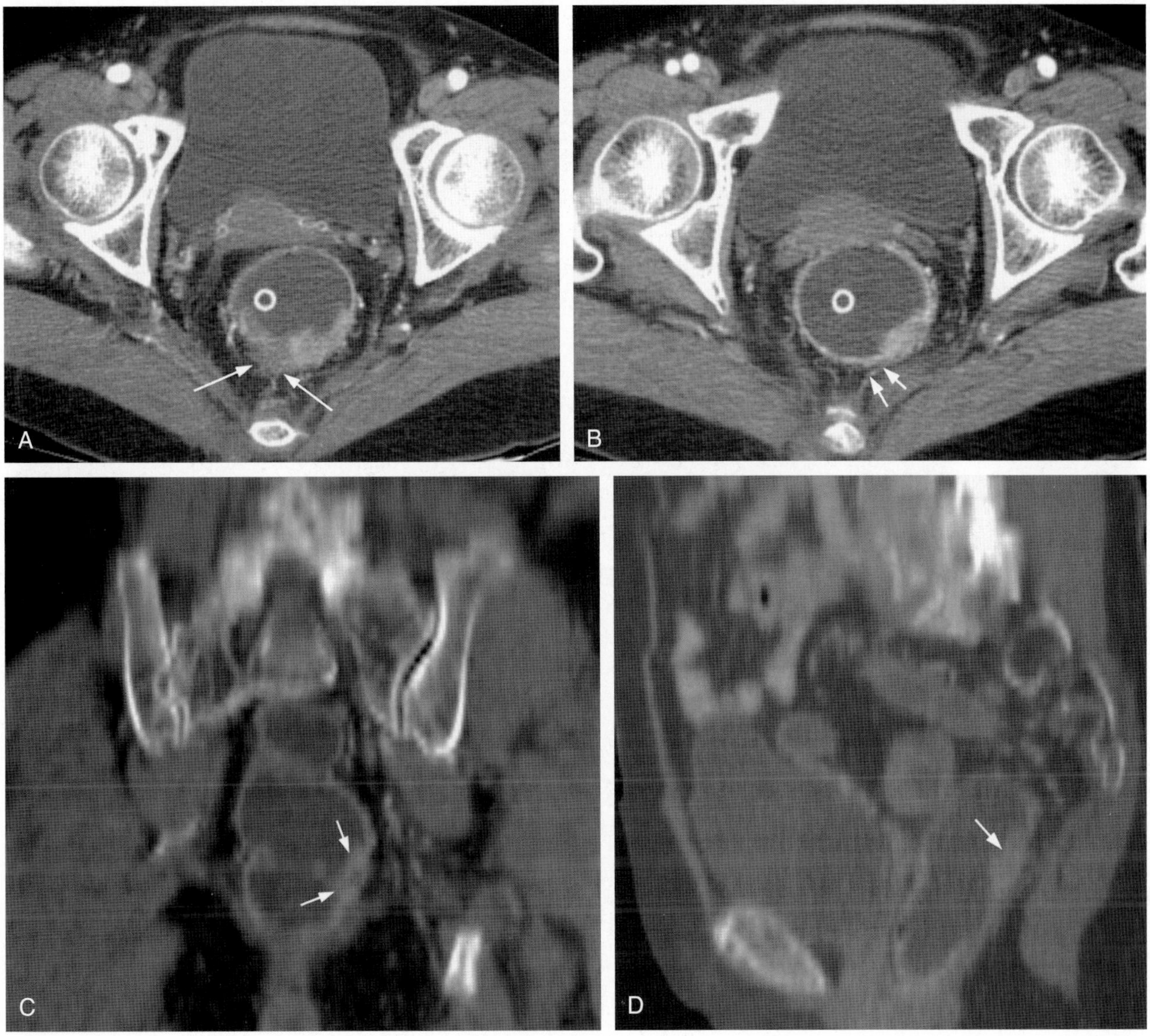

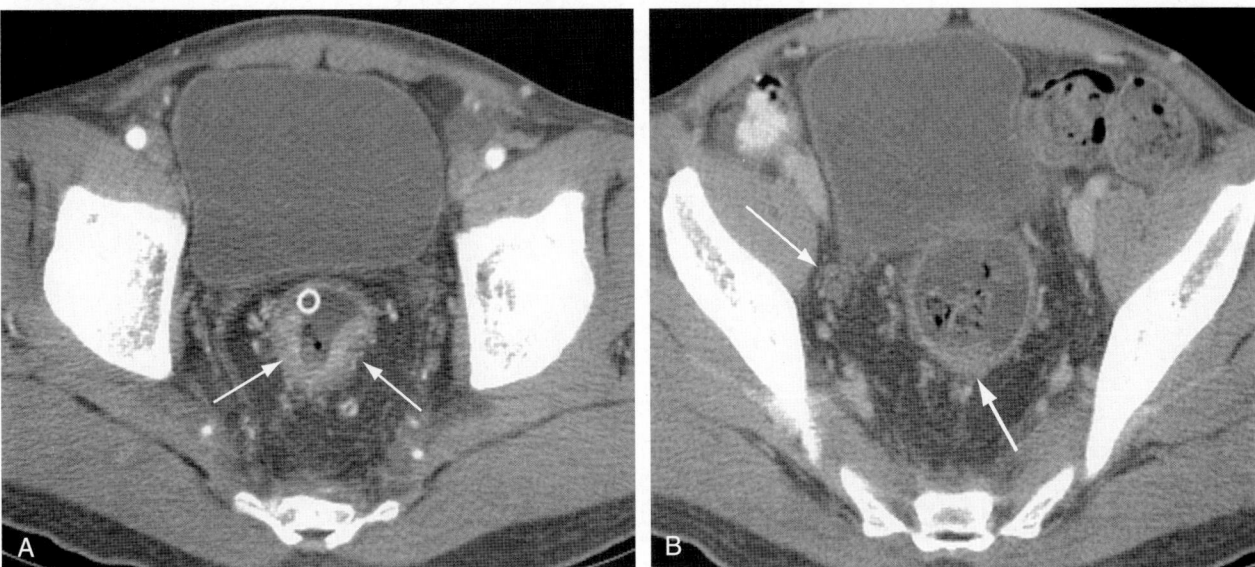

Figure 63-21. CT scan of rectal tumor with extension beyond the wall, T3N0M0 (Dukes' stage B2). A. The thin-section MDCT scan in the arterial phase reveals nodular broad-based extensions of soft tissue density (*arrows*) into the perirectal fat indicative of tumor invasion. **B.** MDCT scan slightly below the level in **A** shows focal mass with some spiculation (*arrows*). This feature is more suggestive of desmoplastic reaction without tumor cells rather than infiltration of tumor into perirectal fat. This distinction is not always possible on MDCT. **C.** The coronal MPR reveals the nodular outer surface of the tumor (*arrows*). **D.** The sagittal MPR does not demonstrate this feature effectively. The mass is located in posterior wall (*arrow*) of upper rectum.

Figure 63-22. Rectal carcinoma in posterior and lateral walls (*arrows*) of rectum (T3N1M0 or Dukes' stage C1). A. Outer borders are slightly irregular, but no definite nodularity can be seen. This makes it difficult to distinguish desmoplastic reaction from actual tumor extension in this case. The patient was diagnosed by MDCT as probably T3. **B.** At a level higher than in **A,** tumor is present only in posterior wall (*thick arrow*). Water facilitates visualization of intraluminal component of tumor in spite of the presence of feces. Also note hypogastric lymph nodes (*thin arrow*) that are lateral to mesorectal fascia.

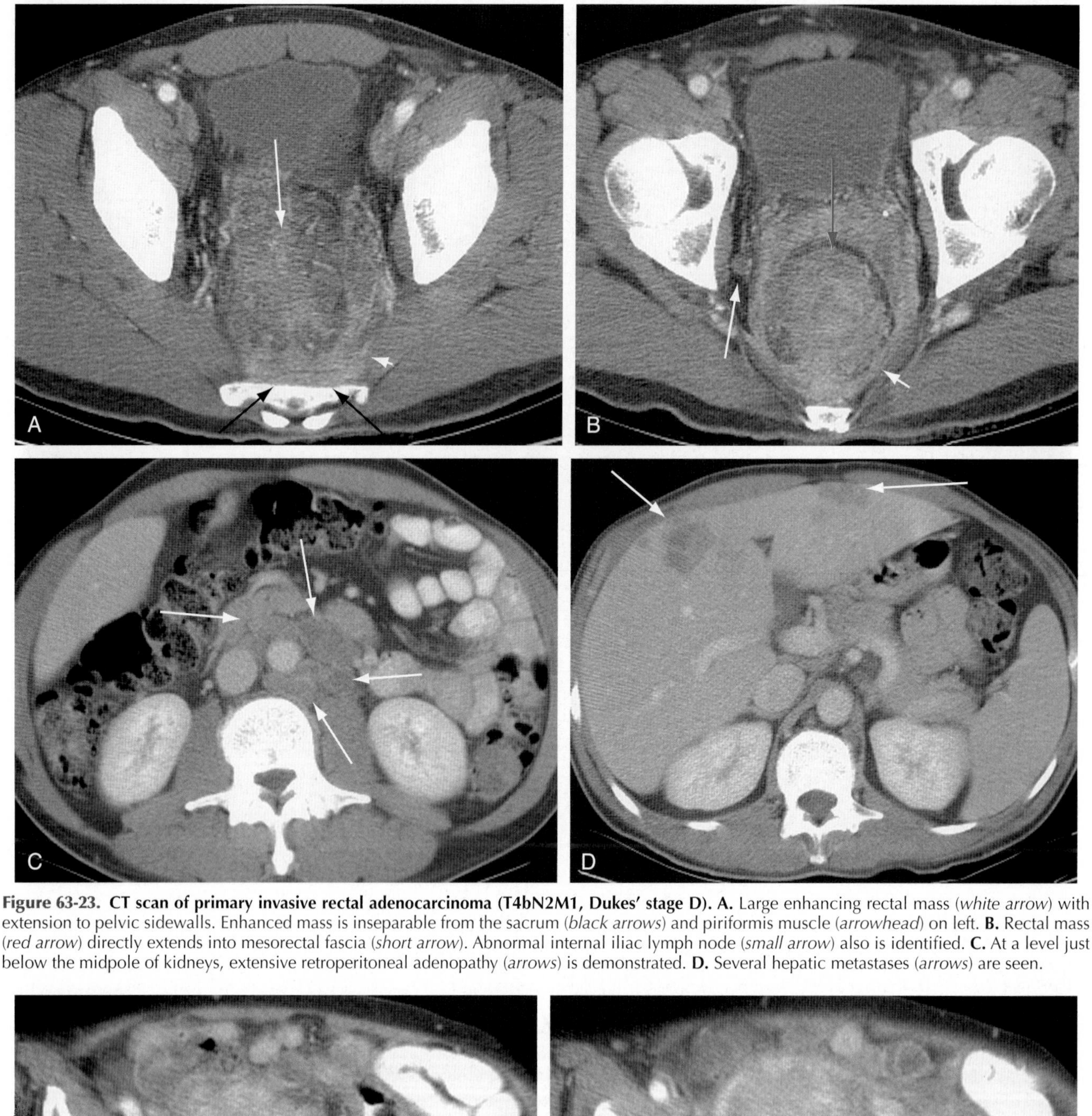

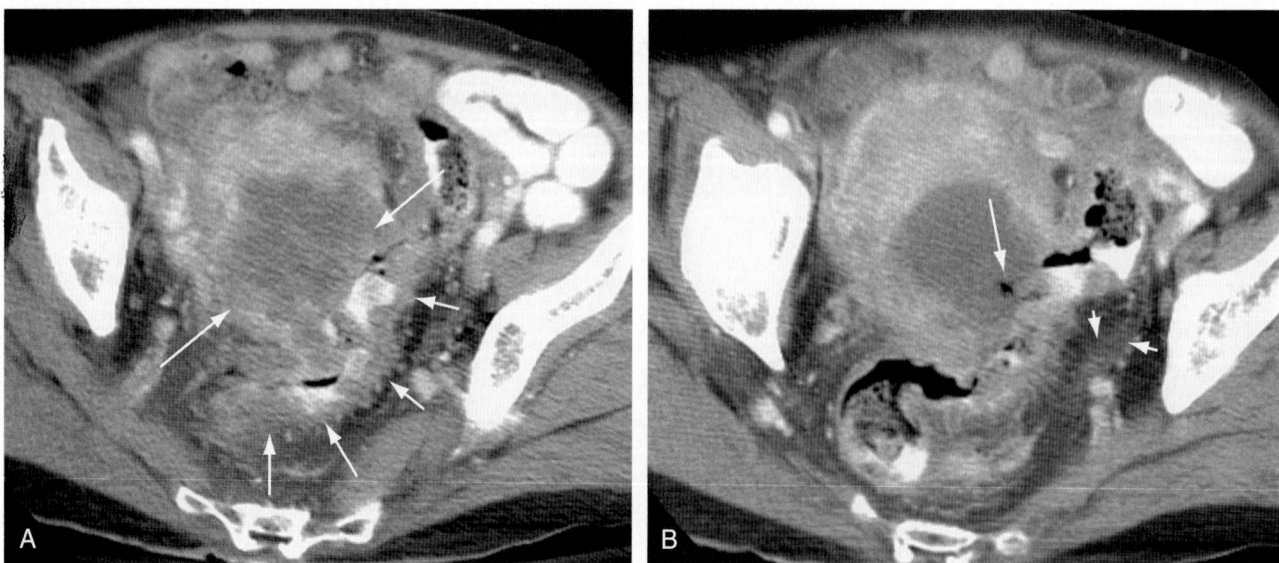

Figure 63-23. CT scan of primary invasive rectal adenocarcinoma (T4bN2M1, Dukes' stage D). A. Large enhancing rectal mass (*white arrow*) with extension to pelvic sidewalls. Enhanced mass is inseparable from the sacrum (*black arrows*) and piriformis muscle (*arrowhead*) on left. **B.** Rectal mass (*red arrow*) directly extends into mesorectal fascia (*short arrow*). Abnormal internal iliac lymph node (*small arrow*) also is identified. **C.** At a level just below the midpole of kidneys, extensive retroperitoneal adenopathy (*arrows*) is demonstrated. **D.** Several hepatic metastases (*arrows*) are seen.

Figure 63-24. Sigmoid carcinoma with invasion of uterus (T4bN1M0 or Dukes' stage C2). A. Long segmental thickening (*small arrows*) of sigmoid wall. Note absence of wall stratification, which can be seen in diverticulitis. The sigmoid tumor is inseparable from the low-density mass in the uterus (*large arrows*). **B.** At a level 5 mm below **A**, gas (*long arrow*) is seen, indicating direct invasion of the tumor into uterus with perforation and necrosis. Note ascites (*short arrows*) along the pelvic sidewall.

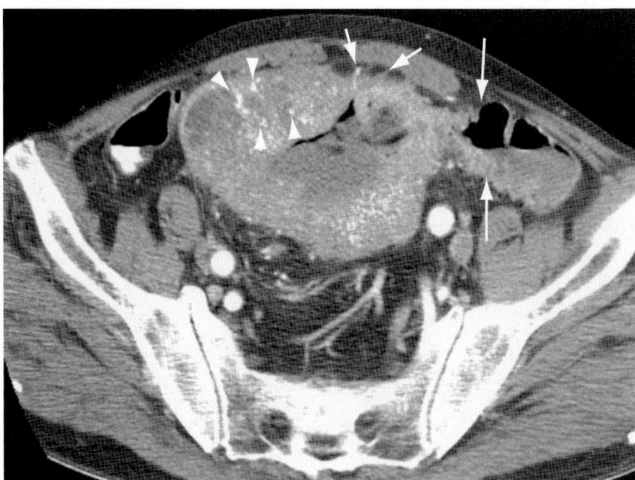

Figure 63-25. Large mucinous sigmoid cancer (T3N1M0 or Dukes' stage C2). Large sigmoid mass with pericolonic fat infiltration (*short arrows*) and intramural calcifications (*arrowheads*) is identified. Transition to normal proximal sigmoid colon (*long arrows*) can be clearly seen.

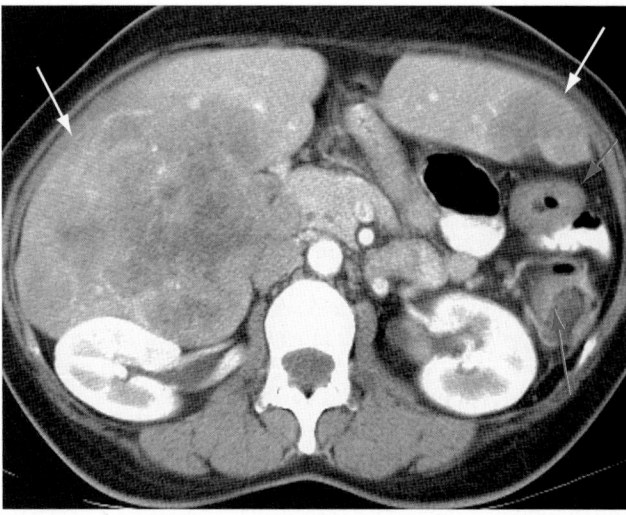

Figure 63-26. Nonobstructing adenocarcinoma in the splenic flexure with liver metastases (T2N0M1 or Dukes' stage D). Two hepatic metastases (*white arrows*) are identified. Primary tumor has smooth outer margins (*red arrows*) and is located in splenic flexure. Tumor was first diagnosed by MDCT and surgically confirmed to be stage T2.

confirmation.[71] Large series still are needed to establish the true cost-effectiveness of the various techniques. Intraoperative ultrasound is often used as the "gold standard," but not all published studies had histopathologic correlation.[38] In patients for whom resection is not an option, thermal tumor ablation or selective catheterization and intra-arterial chemotherapy of liver are often used but only if there is no evidence of tumor spread to extrahepatic sites. Local or distant adenopathy, adrenal metastases, peritoneal carcinomatosis, metastases to other areas of the gastrointestinal tract, and lung metastases are some of the findings that preclude resection or chemoembolization of liver lesions.

Generally, rectal carcinoma metastasizes to lymph nodes along the superior rectal vessels to the mesenteric vessels for upper rectal tumors and along the middle rectal vessels to the internal iliac vessels for lower rectal tumors. Advanced low rectal or anal tumors drain along the inferior rectal vessels into the inguinal nodes. Metastases may be found in nodes in the retroperitoneum (see Fig. 63-23) and porta hepatis. In other areas of the colon, lymph node metastases follow the normal pattern of lymph drainage from the involved area. Local lymph nodes may or may not be demonstrated, depending on separability from the main mass and size of the lymph nodes (Fig. 63-27). In the abdomen and pelvis, lymph

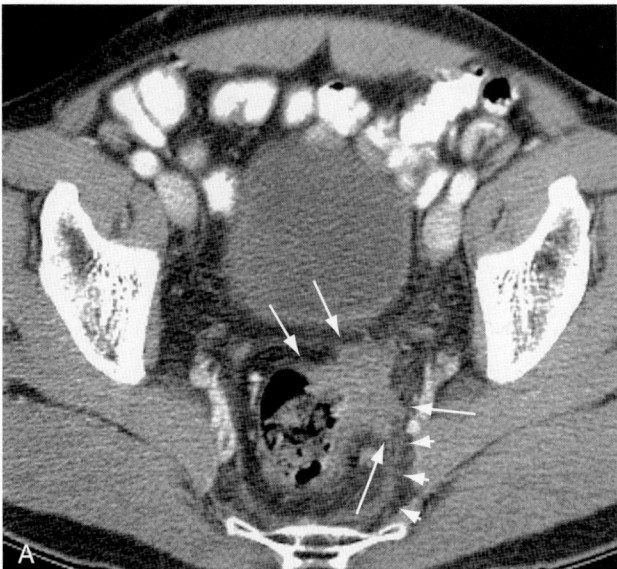
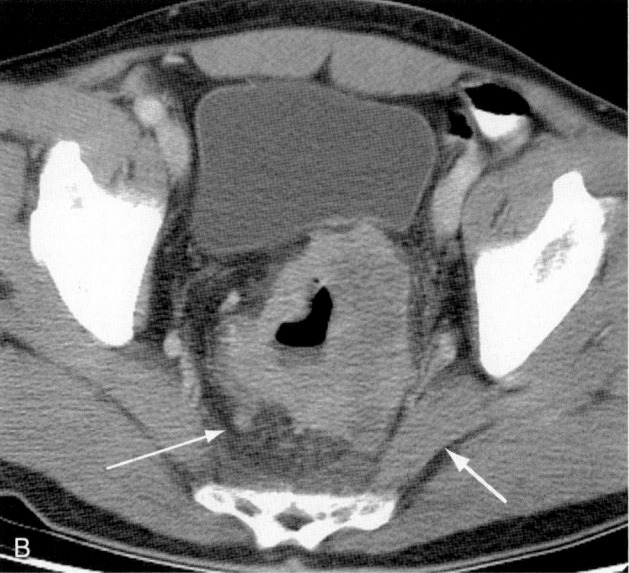

Figure 63-27. Rectal tumor with direct extension to the mesorectal fascia and locoregional lymphadenopathy (T3N1M0 or Dukes' stage C2). **A.** Large rectal mass with broad-based extension of soft tissue (*arrows*) into perirectal fat and direct invasion of mesorectal fascia (*arrowheads*). **B.** Several centimeters above the level of **A,** rectal wall is markedly thickened but tumor does not extend into piriform muscle (*thick arrow*) or bladder. Note enlarged perirectal lymph node (*thin arrow*).

nodes greater than 1.0 cm in diameter are considered abnormal. The pathologic nature of node enlargement cannot be determined absolutely by CT, although asymmetry, irregularity of the nodal margins, and, less reliably, size criteria can be used to establish lymph node abnormality.[73]

Benign as well as malignant disease can produce lymphadenopathy, and often only PET or guided biopsy can give a definitive diagnosis. Many metastatic foci are found in normal-sized lymph nodes (<1 cm) that cannot be considered abnormal by CT if size is used as the only diagnostic criterion. Pericolic lymph nodes next to a segment of thickened colonic wall are seen much more frequently in patients with colon cancer than in those with diverticulitis. Therefore, presence of such nodes should lead to further evaluation in patients with suspected diverticulitis.[74] Additional signs that favor a diagnosis of colon carcinoma over diverticulitis are the loss of a normal enhancement pattern in the thickened bowel wall and the absence of inflamed diverticula.[75] Because hyperplastic or inflammatory nodes are extremely rare in the perirectal area, demonstration of nonenhanced, small (<1 cm), round or oval soft tissue densities suggests the presence of malignant adenopathy (Fig. 63-28).

There are certain pitfalls in the interpretation of CT scans of patients with colon tumors.[76] CT scans obtained soon after surgery or radiation therapy can demonstrate edema or hemorrhage of the pelvic structures that simulates recurrent neoplasm. Chronic radiation changes in the pelvis may be difficult or impossible to distinguish from colon tumor without CT-guided biopsies.[77-80] It is therefore essential to determine the tumor stage by CT or MRI before the patient undergoes radiation. Follow-up CT scans after irradiation are needed only to determine whether the mass seen on the staging scan has sufficiently diminished in size to become resectable. Benign bone defects can simulate metastatic foci, and nonopacified bowel loops can be mistaken for a tumor mass. Perforation of a colon cancer can result in an inflammatory mass or abscess, which makes diagnosis of the underlying cancer difficult (see Fig. 63-28).[81] Cachexia can lead to loss of fat planes, which mimics direct invasion of tumor into surrounding structures.

Preoperative Staging by CT

The staging of colon tumors has been most frequently based on Dukes' classification[82] or a modification thereof (Table 63-1).[83,84] CT staging is based on an analysis of the thickness of the colon wall, extension beyond bowel wall margins, and the presence or absence of tumor spread to lymph nodes and adjacent and distant organs.[85] The size of a primary or recurrent colon tumor can be measured and the tumor assigned to one of four stages depending on the CT findings (Table 63-2).

Many surgeons use the tumor, node, metastases (TNM) classification (see Table 63-1) for staging colon neoplasms.[86] It has the advantage of more precise definition of the depth of infiltration in the bowel wall. Because of the inability of CT to determine depth of invasion to or through the various layers of the colon, CT findings cannot be correlated easily

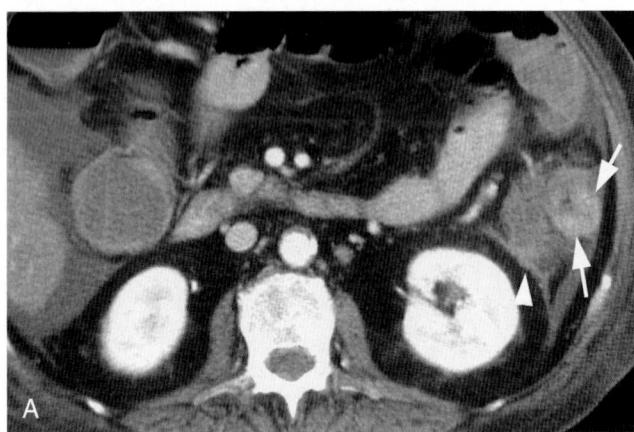

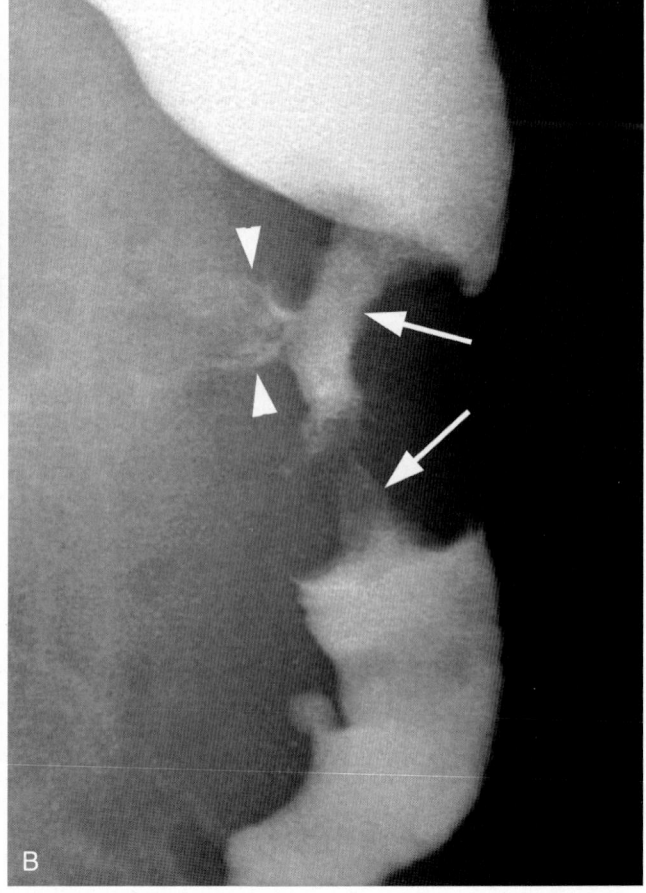

Figure 63-28. Perforation of adenocarcinoma of the descending colon (T4N0M0). A. CT demonstrates asymmetric mural thickening of descending colon (*arrows*) with extravasation of rectal contrast (*arrowhead*). Stranding and ascites also are present. **B.** Hypaque enema demonstrates an "apple core" lesion (*arrows*) corresponding to wall thickening seen in the descending colon. Mural perforation extravasation of rectal contrast (*arrowheads*) clearly is identified.

Table 63-1

Surgical-Pathologic Staging of Colorectal Neoplasm (Dukes' and TNM Classification)

Astler-Coller Classification (Modified from Dukes')	TNM Staging	Description	Approximate 5-Year Survival (%)
A or I	T1N0M0	Nodes (−), limited to mucosa ± submucosa	80
B1 or I	T2N0M0	Nodes (−), limited to muscularis ± serosa	70
B2 or II	T3N0M0	Nodes (−), transmural into subserosa or into nonperitonealized perirectal/pericolonic tissue	60-65
C1 or III	T2N1M0	Nodes (+), limited to muscularis ± serosa	35-45
C2 or III	T3N1M0	Nodes (+), transmural into subserosa or into nonperitonealized perirectal/pericolonic tissue	
	T4a N1M0	Nodes (+), perforation of tumor mass	25
	T4bN1M0	Nodes (+), extension into adjacent organs or structures (e.g., muscle, nerve, bone)	
D or IV	Any T and N, M1	Any of the above plus distant metastases	<25

with the TNM classification. For example, tumor limited to mucosa or submucosa (T1N0M0) cannot be distinguished from tumor invading the muscularis or infiltrating to but not through the serosa, if present (T2N0M0). Generally, lesions extending beyond bowel wall (T3 and T4) are correctly identified by CT unless microinvasion by tumor is present. Assessment of regional lymph node (N) involvement and distant metastases (M) must be added to the evaluation of the depth of tumor invasion.

Early reports suggested that CT findings related to local extent and regional spread of tumor correlated well with surgical and histopathologic findings, and accuracy rates of 77% to 100% were reported.[76,85,87-89] The high accuracy rates of these reports were largely due to the more advanced cases

Table 63-2

CT Staging of Primary or Recurrent Colorectal Tumor with TNM Correlation*

CT Stage	TNM Staging	Description
I	T1	Intraluminal mass without thickening of wall
II*	T2	Thickened large bowel wall (>0.6 cm) or pelvic mass, no extension beyond bowel wall
IIIa*	T3	Thickened large bowel wall or pelvic mass with invasion of adjacent pericolonic/perirectal tissue but not to mesorectal fascia
IIIb*	T3	Thickened large bowel wall or pelvic mass with invasion of adjacent pericolonic/perirectal tissue with extension to mesorectal fascia
IIIc*	T4a and b	Thickened large bowel wall or pelvic mass with perforation or invasion of adjacent organs or structures with or without extension to pelvic/abdominal walls but without distant metastases
IV*	Any T, M1	Distant metastases with or without local abnormality

*With or without lymphadenopathy (N0 or N1).
Modified from Thoeni RF, Moss AA, Schnyder P, et al: Detection and staging of primary rectal and rectosigmoid cancer by computed tomography. Radiology 141:135-138, 1981.

in these series. For primary colon cancer, CT is more accurate in showing extensive invasion of surrounding tissue and distant metastases than in demonstrating local adenopathy or minimal tumor extension.

CT frequently understages patients with microinvasion of pericolonic or perirectal fat or small tumor foci in normal-sized nodes. Lymph node metastases were not analyzed separately in some of the earlier studies. In a recent meta-analysis that analyzed local staging and lymph node involvement in patients with rectal cancers, summary estimates of sensitivity and specificity for CT in assessing perirectal tissue invasion and invasion of adjacent organs were 79% and 78%, and 72% and 96%, respectively.[39] In the same study, the summary estimates of sensitivity and specificity for CT in detecting lymph node involvement were much lower and reached only 55% and 74%, respectively.[39] One study found that staging accuracy increased from 17% for Dukes' B lesions to 81% for Dukes' D lesions.[90] In another meta-analysis, the mean weighted sensitivity of helical CT for detecting hepatic metastases mostly from colon carcinoma was 72% at a specificity of higher than 85%.[91] Some individual studies have reached higher sensitivities for hepatic metastases from colorectal carcinoma.[38]

The accuracy of CT assessment of local tumor extent can be improved by prior colonic cleansing, prone positioning of the patient, air distention of the rectum, or administration of water enemas to serve as a low-density intraluminal contrast agent.[92,93] Also, lowering the size threshold for diagnosing lymph node metastases improves the sensitivity for detecting such deposits, but such an approach decreases specificity.

Little information is available about the CT detection and staging of tumors in the cecum or ascending, transverse, and descending colon. Most tumors in these areas are easily demonstrated (Figs. 63-29 and 63-30), but no investigation has analyzed these lesions in detail.

Further studies are needed to establish if new-generation CT scanners, especially MDCT with 16- or 64-slice capability, can compete with MRI in staging colorectal tumors. One recent study already demonstrated that reformats could significantly increase the accuracy of T staging of rectal tumors (see Fig. 63-18 and Fig. 63-21).[64] In this study, the staging accuracy based on axial slices ranged from 77% to 81%, whereas it increased to 90% to 98% when axial slices were combined with multiplanar reformats.[64] These results compare favorably with CT studies from the last decade that did not use

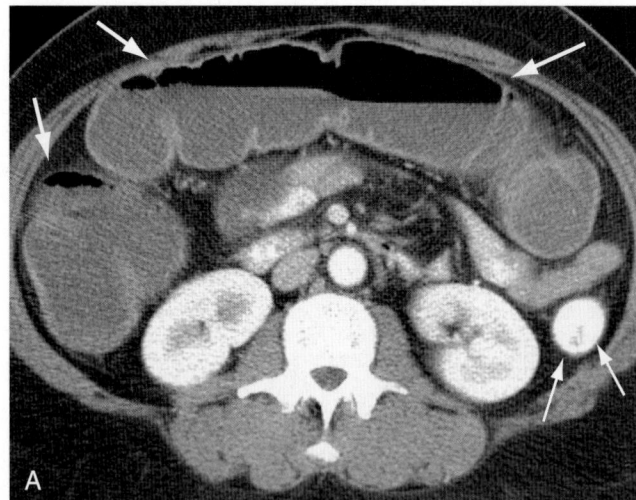

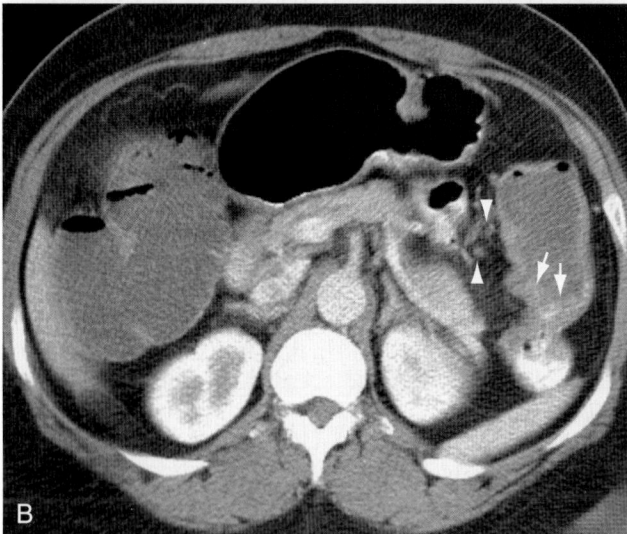

Figure 63-29. Near-complete colonic obstruction caused by tumor near splenic flexure (T3N1M0 or Dukes' stage C1). A. Axial MDCT demonstrates positive rectal contrast (*thin arrows*) in descending colon near the splenic flexure but no rectal contrast entering the fluid-filled and distended transverse and ascending colon (*thick arrows*). **B.** Two centimeters above level of **A,** obstructing tumor is demonstrated and its proximal border well outlined by retained colonic fluid (*arrows*). Tumor was underestimated by MDCT to be stage T2. Note subcentimeter lymph nodes (*arrowheads*) near the tumor in mesentery. They were confirmed to be positive for tumor at surgery but not prospectively diagnosed because of their small size.

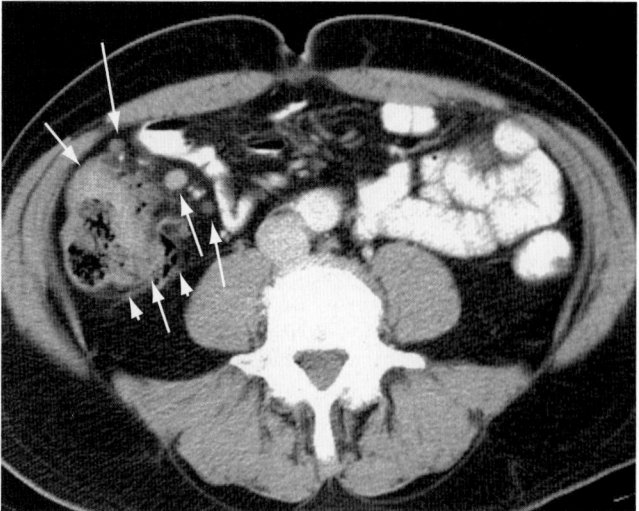

Figure 63-30. Cecal adenocarcinoma (T3N1M0). The cecum demonstrates eccentric wall thickening (*short arrows*) near ileocecal valve with nodular outer margins and soft tissue strands (*arrowheads*) extending into pericolonic fat suggestive of infiltration beyond the bowel wall. Abnormal local lymph nodes (*long thin arrows*) are present and were confirmed as pathologic at surgery.

MDCT, with accuracy rates ranging from 41% to 82%.[25,94,95] CT offers the advantages of combining local, regional, and distant staging in one study, ultrathin slice capability, very fast imaging times, reconstruction in any desired plane, and lower cost compared with MRI.

Magnetic Resonance Imaging

Magnetic resonance imaging can be used to detect and stage rectosigmoid tumors more accurately than tumors in other areas of the colon. As with CT, this increased accuracy is due to the fixed position of the rectosigmoid colon in relation to the pelvis. Therefore, most publications have focused on the depiction and staging of rectal tumors. For accurate depiction

of the intraluminal component of rectal tumors, particularly smaller ones, it may be necessary to prepare the colon to avoid confusion with feces. Rectal air insufflation, with prone positioning of the patient and an antispasmodic agent may be helpful in better depicting the tumor. Other investigators have recommended axial T2-weighted imaging perpendicular to the long axis of the tumor, as seen on sagittal views for more accurate staging (Fig. 63-31).[96] On T1-weighted spin-echo images, rectosigmoid tumors produce wall thickening with a signal intensity similar to or slightly higher than that of skeletal muscle (long T1) (see Fig. 63-31A). Because perirectal fat has high signal intensity (short T1), air has no signal intensity, and tumor has moderate signal intensity (long T1), tumors are shown with high contrast. For the same reason, extension of tumor beyond the colon wall may be seen on T1-weighted images (Fig. 63-32). On T2-weighted spin-echo images, the signal intensity of tumor increases relative to that of muscle (see Fig. 63-32A) and the neoplasm in the rectal wall may be well visualized on high-resolution MRI.

Whereas early studies indicated that T2-weighted images are not as useful as T1-weighted images for determining extracolonic tumor extension (see Fig. 63-31),[97] it is now generally accepted that T2-weighted sequences are superior to T1-weighted scans in evaluating the extent of tumor in relation to the rectal wall layers and the mesorectal fascia.[98,99] Several studies have shown that T2-weighted sequences can demonstrate the mesorectal fascia, which has gained importance since the introduction of total mesorectal excision (TME).[98-102] In TME, the entire mesorectal compartment is removed, which consists of the rectum, the surrounding mesorectal fat with the perirectal lymph nodes, and a thin fascia that envelopes the two former structures and is known as the mesorectal fascia. The TME procedure reduces the chance that tumor is left behind. Even without preoperative or postoperative radiation therapy, the recurrence rate after TME is reported to be less than 10%.[103] If uterine or pelvic sidewall invasion is suspected, T2-weighted sequences also are useful

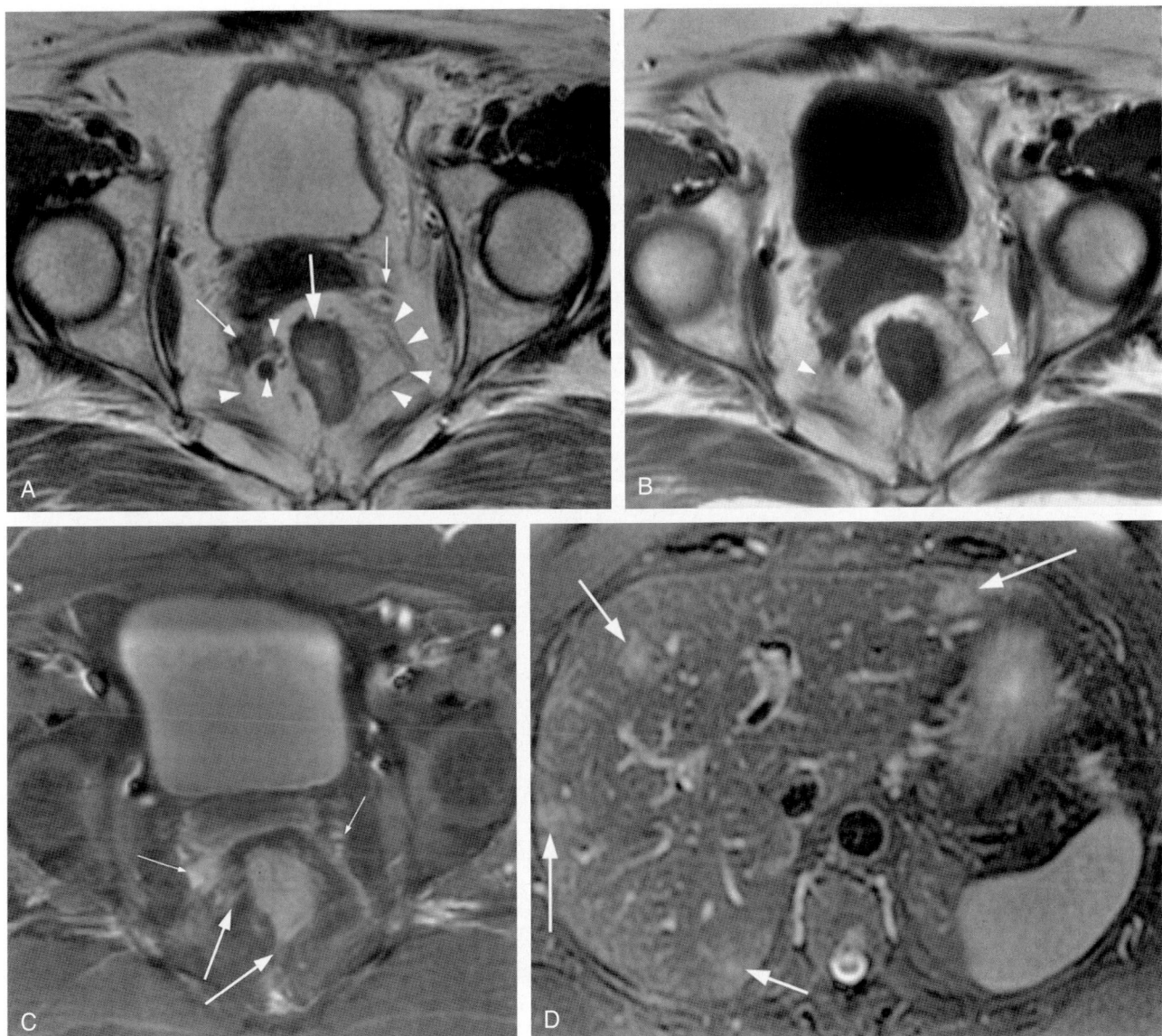

Figure 63-31. MR images of adenocarcinoma of the rectum (T3N1M1 or Dukes' stage D). A. Axial T2-weighted fast spin-echo image scanned perpendicular to long axis of tumor demonstrates eccentric thickening of anterior rectal wall (*thick arrow*) with extension of tumor to rectal sidewalls. Perirectal lymph nodes (*small arrowheads*) are identified. The middle rectal vessels (*thin arrows*) in the lateral ligament are seen lateral to mesorectal fascia (*large arrowheads*). **B.** On this axial T1-weighted spin-echo MR image, the mesorectal fascia (*arrowheads*) is not as clearly delineated as on the T2-weighted image. **C.** Axial T1-weighted fat-suppressed image after administration of gadolinium shows enhancement of mesorectal vessels (*thin arrows*) bilaterally. Extension of tumor into the perirectal fat (*large arrows*) is best seen on this fat-suppressed sequence; however, desmoplastic reaction alone cannot be definitively distinguished in this case from desmoplastic reaction containing tumor cells. **D.** Axial T2-weighted image with fat suppression identifies multiple liver metastases (*arrows*).

because of the differences in signal intensity between muscle, fat, tumor, and muscle invaded by tumor.

Today, MRI using thin sections and phased-array coils is able to distinguish between tumors localized to mucosa and submucosa (stage I or T1) and those that infiltrate the entire colonic wall (stage II or T2) with a moderate to good staging accuracy (65%-86%) (Table 63-3).[102] The detection of the tumor in the bowel wall based on T2-weighted imaging relies on signal intensity differences between the intermediate signal intensity of the tumor, the low signal intensity of normal mucosa and muscularis propria, and the high signal intensity of the submucosa and perirectal or pericolonic fat. Endoluminal MR coils also make visualization of the layers of the

rectal wall feasible and have demonstrated improved accuracy for T staging when compared with phased-array external coils (accuracy ranging from 71% to 91%).[104] Endoluminal MRI is not widely available and, because of its small field of view, it cannot visualize the mesorectal fascia and surrounding pelvic structures. Microinvasion into surrounding fat cannot be detected by MRI, which leads to understaging, whereas peritumoral tissue inflammation and fibrosis can lead to overstaging.[105] However, if the feature of a nodular or pushing configuration of an advancing tumor margins is used, tumor extension beyond the bowel wall can be distinguished in most cases from the spiculated and low signal intensity of peritumoral fibrosis.[96] Because the mesorectal fascia can be readily

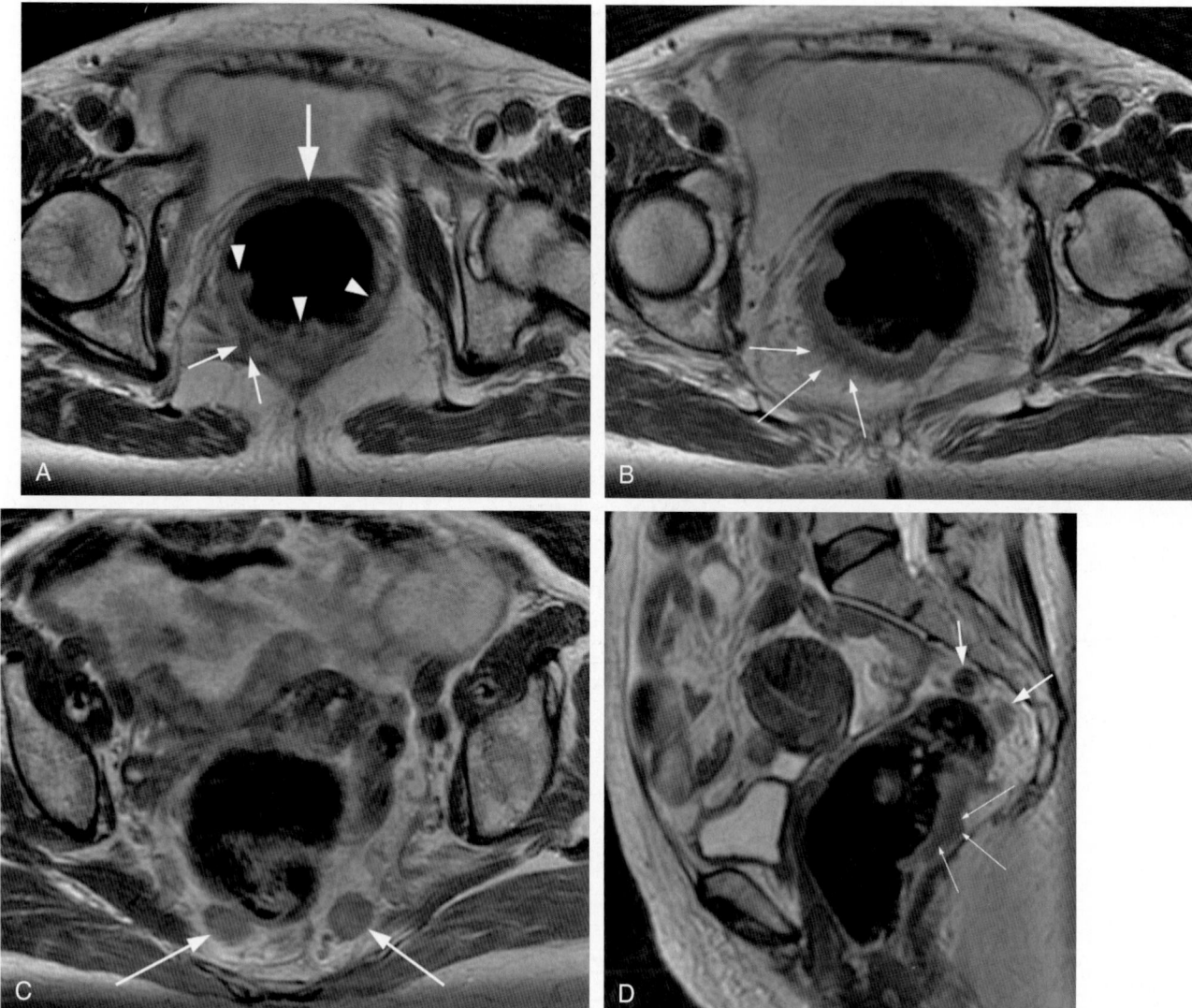

Figure 63-32. MR images of rectal adenocarcinoma with extension beyond the bowel wall (T3N1M0 or Dukes' stage C2). A. Axial T2-weighted fast spin-echo image demonstrates a nodular outer margin of the posterolateral rectal wall with broad-based extension of soft tissue (*small arrows*) into perirectal fat. Luminal margin of tumor is irregular (*arrowheads*) and signal intensity of the tumor is higher than that of muscularis propria (*large arrow*). **B.** Axial T2-weighted fast spin-echo image shows spiculated outer margin (*arrows*) of mass involving posterior and right lateral aspect of the rectum. These features suggest desmoplastic reaction related to tumor rather than neoplastic infiltration of perirectal fat. **C.** Axial T2-weighted fast spin-echo scan at higher level than **A** and **B** depicts prominent presacral lymph nodes (*arrows*) indicative of malignant lymphadenopathy slightly remote from primary tumor (N2). **D.** Sagittal T2-weighted fast spin-echo image confirms enlarged lymph nodes (*large arrows*) in presacral space. Nodular outer margin of the rectal mass (*thin arrows*) is well demonstrated on sagittal view, suggesting invasive tumor (T3).

Table 63-3
Criteria for MRI Staging of Rectal Cancer

Tumor (T) Stage	MRI Criteria
T1	Tumor signal intensity confined to mucosal and submucosal layer—signal intensity low compared with high signal intensity of the adjacent submucosa
T2	Tumor signal intensity extends into muscle layer, with loss of interface between submucosa and circular muscle layer
T3	Tumor signal intensity extends through muscle layer into perirectal fat, with obliteration of interface between muscle and perirectal fat
T4	Tumor signal intensity extends into adjacent structure(s) or viscus

Modified from Brown G, Richards CJ, Newcombe RG, et al: Rectal carcinoma: Thin-section MR imaging for staging in 28 patients. Radiology 211:215-222, 1999.

recognized on MRI and the depth of transmural tumor invasion (T3) usually diagnosed accurately, MRI is more sensitive and reliable for predicting circumferential resection margin (CRM) than overall T stage of tumor.[106]

Tumor foci in normal-sized nodes may go unrecognized.[107] If the MRI diagnosis of lymph node abnormality is based on mixed signal intensity and irregular outer margins rather than size of the nodes, the MRI prediction of nodal involvement can be improved.[108] In one older series, in five of six cases in which lymph nodes were seen, the nodes were normal in size but contained tumor, and in the one case with enlarged nodes (>15 mm in diameter), reactive hyperplasia was present.[97] In a more recent series with nodes considered suspicious based on irregular borders and mixed signal intensity, 51 of 60 were correctly identified as malignant (sensitivity 85%) and 216 of 221 were considered nonmalignant (specificity 97%).[108]

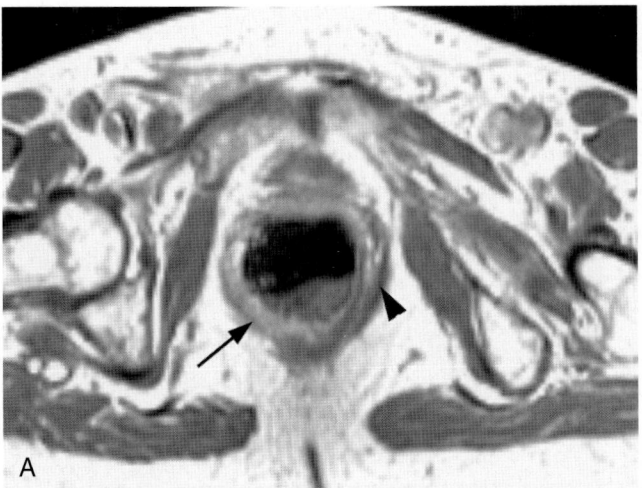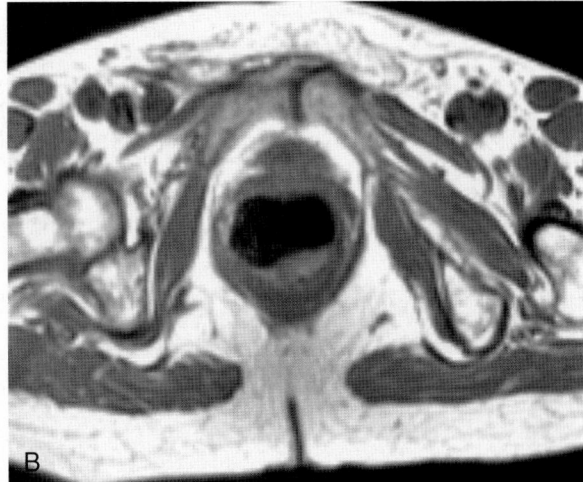

Figure 63-33. MR images of rectal adenocarcinoma with extension into the levator ani muscles (T3N0M0 or Dukes' stage B2). A. Axial T1-weighted spin-echo image after gadolinium demonstrates thickening and enhancement in posterior and right lateral rectal wall administration with direct invasion of tumor into levator ani. This suggested extension by increased signal intensity of muscle in invaded area (*black arrow*). Compare this appearance to normal left levator ani, which has low signal intensity (*arrowhead*). **B.** Tumor invasion into levator ani is difficult to diagnose on T1-weighted sequence without gadolinium.

For demonstration of liver and adrenal metastases, MRI and CT are comparable if an optimal CT bolus technique is used.[91] MRI with a liver-specific contrast agent (e.g., manganese dipyridoxyl-ethylenediamine-diacetate-(bis)phosphate [Teslascan, Nycomed Inc., Princeton, NJ] or iron oxide particles [Feridex, Berlex, Wayne, NJ]) may render MRI superior to CT, particularly for the detection of small lesions.[109,110] However, the liver-specific agents have not found wide acceptance and, generally, most MRI for colorectal tumor staging and suspected liver metastases still is performed after administration of gadolinium.

Invasion of adjacent organs is best demonstrated on transverse or coronal high-resolution MR images. MRI is superior to CT in demonstrating invasion of levator ani (Fig. 63-33), puborectalis, or internal and external sphincter muscles. Lateral extension of tumor is difficult to detect on sagittal MR images but can be assessed accurately with axial images.[106] Extension into the prostate, seminal vesicles, vagina, and cervix can be shown well by MRI, but extension into bladder may be missed if the bladder is not well distended.

Preoperative Staging by Magnetic Resonance Imaging

The introduction of neoadjuvant preoperative radiation and/ or chemotherapy and TME has made accurate preoperative staging even more critical in patient management and identifying those who are at risk for local recurrence. The risk of local recurrence ranges from 3% to 32%, and patients with positive resection margins are much more likely to suffer from local tumor recurrence.[106] Based on the different risk categories, the treatment is tailored to the individual patient. In the United States, patients with fixed T3 tumors and/or positive local nodes routinely undergo postoperative radiation and chemotherapy but preoperative radiation is reserved for those with tumor extension to the pelvic sidewalls. In Europe, large trials have shown that the recurrence rate is markedly reduced if patients receive preoperative radiation, and therefore it is routinely performed in all patients with rectal cancer.[111] Imaging should provide the following staging infor-

mation: depth of tumor growth in the rectal wall, circumferential resection margin at the time of TME, the degree of tumor invasion into surrounding pelvic structures, and the nodal status. Edema, granulation tissue, and fibrosis can lead to overstaging in patients who undergo MRI after neoadjuvant chemotherapy and irradiation (Fig. 63-34).

Endoluminal MR and endoluminal ultrasound (see later) are the two most accurate methods for staging early or superficial rectal cancer that can be treated with surgery alone. Accuracies ranging between 71% to 91% for MRI and 70% to 94% for TRUS have been reported.[106,112-115] These two methods are considered superior to CT in staging early tumors. However, both techniques have a limited field of view and neither method can adequately assess the mesorectal fascia and CRM.

At present, for advanced mobile or fixed rectal cancers, MRI with phased-array coils and high spatial resolution (thin sections) generally appears to be better suited for demonstrating the mesorectal fascia and the circumferential resection margin than CT (see Fig. 63-31).[106] In a recent meta-analysis, the sensitivity of MR for invasion of the muscularis propria was 94% and similar to that of TRUS but the specificity was significantly lower for MRI (69%) compared with TRUS (86%).[39] In the same meta-analysis, at comparable specificities, the sensitivity of MRI for perirectal invasion was 82% compared with 79% for CT and 90% for endoluminal ultrasound, whereas the sensitivity of MRI for adjacent organ invasion was 74% and similar to the 72% for CT and 70% for endoluminal ultrasound.[39] Overall it appears that presently, MRI may be slightly superior to CT in assessing extension of tumor into surrounding pelvic structures, especially for demonstrating direct invasion of tumor into pelvic sidewalls, sciatic nerves, or subtle invasion of bone marrow.[116] In one study of patients with known peritoneal carcinomatosis, it was shown that MR had a higher sensitivity (84%) than CT (54%) for detecting peritoneal carcinomatosis if fat suppressed T2-weighted and gadolinium-enhanced T1-weighted sequences with breath-holding were used.[117] However, a more recent study concluded that the use of gadolinium enhancement did not improve the diagnostic accuracy of MR for

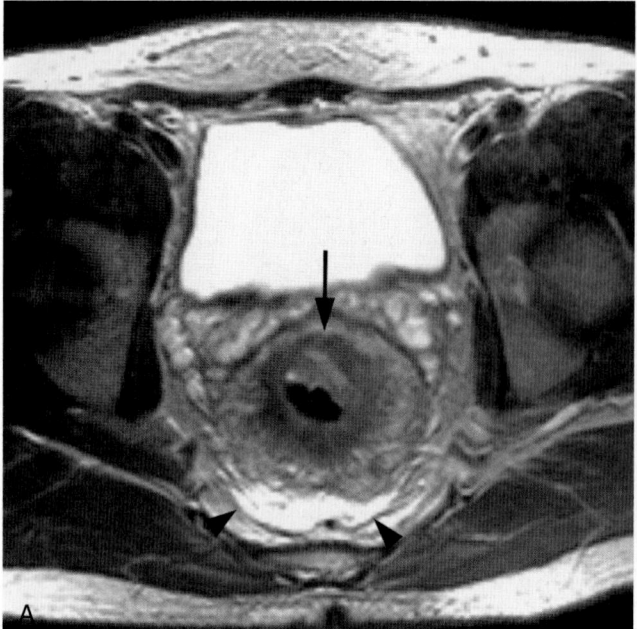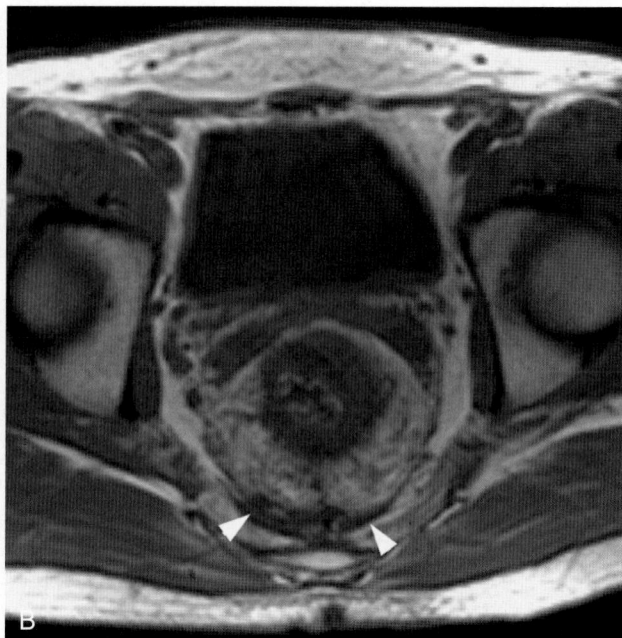

Figure 63-34. **MR images of rectal adenocarcinoma with extension into the perirectal fat (T3N0M0 or Dukes' stage B2) in a patient who underwent neoadjuvant chemotherapy and radiation therapy. A.** Axial T2-weighted spin-echo image shows a lobular wall thickening in anterior rectal wall (*arrow*) and mild thickening of remainder of rectal wall. Outer rectal wall margins are ill defined due to radiation therapy. Mixed signal intensity of perirectal fat with blurring of outer rectal wall and high signal intensity in presacral space are most likely secondary to post-treatment granulation tissue and retroperitoneal fluid. This makes accurate staging of this tumor more difficult. **B.** T1-weighted image does not suffer from as many postradiation artifacts as does T2-weighted sequence. *Arrowheads,* presacral fluid collection.

assessing tumor penetration through rectal wall and tumor extension into mesorectal fascia.[118]

Since the radiological detection of nodal tumor involvement relies on morphologic criteria such as size, contour margins and signal intensity, it is difficult to distinguish between reactive and metastatic nodes. Also, micrometastases can easily be missed. Rectal tumors tend to produce micrometastases,[119] but in the perirectal fat, any node can be considered malignant since reactive lymph nodes are exceedingly rare in this area. Because of the fact that cross-sectional imaging uses morphology to diagnose metastases to lymph nodes, reliable detection of lymphadenopathy is not possible at present. The accuracy rates for unenhanced MR for detection of nodal involvement range from 39% to 95%.[97,106,113] Large variations in the accuracy for detecting nodal metastases also have been published for CT (22%-73%) and TRUS (62-83%).[106,120] Some promising results have been published on the use of ultra-small superparamagnetic iron oxides particles that are phagocytosed by the reticuloendothelial system and cause shortening of the T2* relaxation time and subsequent decrease of the signal intensity of normal lymph nodes but not in nodes with metastatic deposits.[121] Uniform and central low-signal-intensity patterns are suggestive of nonmalignant nodes, whereas eccentric or uniform high-signal intensity suggest malignant nodes.[122] Its use for colorectal cancer needs further investigation.

Overall for the definitive analysis of these staging results, a comparison between state-of-the-art MDCT and state-of-the-art MRI in large clinical trials is needed. At present, most comparative studies used state-of-the-art MRI but not the latest imaging technology with CT. The advantages of MDCT with ultrathin sections and very short imaging times, partic-

ularly with 64-slice scanners, optimized bolus techniques and multiplanar reformats have not been fully explored. While one study indicated that improved staging accuracy could be achieved with the inclusion of multiplanar reformats,[64] no direct comparison to MRI or TRUS is currently available.

Transrectal Ultrasound

Primary Tumor

The major advantage of endoluminal ultrasound or TRUS is that it can depict the various layers of the colon wall, which enables determination of depth of mural tumor penetration. Colorectal tumors present as a hypoechoic mass whose margins can be outlined and related to the layers in the colon or rectal wall. The depth of infiltration can be assessed from evidence of disruption of the different segments of the rectal or colon wall. On images produced with a radial rotating transducer placed in the rectum, the elements of the rectal wall appear as rings of different echogenicities. The transducer is covered with a balloon filled with water. The innermost ring is hyperechoic and represents the interface of the balloon and mucosa. The second ring from the center is hypoechoic and is produced by the muscularis mucosae. The third ring is hyperechoic and consists of the submucosa. The fourth ring is hypoechoic and is formed by the muscularis propria. The fifth ring is hyperechoic and caused by the perirectal fat or, if it is in an area with peritoneal reflection, by the serosa and fat.

If the examination is performed carefully, even the intraluminal component of the tumor can be clearly demonstrated as a polypoid or exophytic mass. Filling of the balloon attached to the transducer and the colorectal lumen with water allows optimal visualization of mural and nodal abnormalities. In one recent study, the accuracy of TRUS for local tumor staging was 85% with intrarectal installation of water and only 57% without water installation.[123] Pericolonic or perirectal abnormalities can also be seen, but depth of penetration beyond the colon or rectal wall is limited. Whenever possible, the transducer is passed beyond the tumor into the colon proximal to the lesion for more complete assessment of mural as well as nodal pathology. Peritumoral inflammation and irradiation may simulate more advanced tumor changes because these abnormalities often have a hypoechoic pattern that may be indistinguishable from the echo pattern of tumor. This leads to overestimation of the size of the neoplasm. Tumors that severely narrow the lumen may not be completely assessed by endoluminal ultrasound because it may not be possible to pass the probe through the area of stenosis. Also, high location of the tumor may prevent its evaluation by TRUS.

The ultrasonographic staging system is based on the TNM classification.[124] Three stages are distinguished by ultrasonography. A T1 tumor is confined to the mucosa and submucosa with the echogenic layer of the submucosa thinned and irregular. It does not interrupt the middle echogenic interface to the muscularis propria. A T2 lesion is confined to the rectal wall and involves the hypoechogenic muscularis propria. The outermost echogenic interface is intact. T3 tumor penetrates into the perirectal fat and is visualized as a disruption of the outermost hyperechoic ring (Fig. 63-35). Stage T4 may be assessed by endoluminal ultrasound but often it is beyond the limited field of view as T4 represents extension into adjacent organs or pelvic sidewall structures.

On TRUS, normal lymph nodes are hyperechoic and bean shaped and have indistinct margins. Consequently, they are not routinely seen within the echogenic perirectal fat. Tumors containing lymph nodes are spherical, hypoechoic structures with distinct margins. According to the TNM classification, stage N1 is present when TRUS visualizes one to three hypo-

echoic nodes and stage N2 if TRUS sees four or more of these hypoechoic lymph nodes.

Smaller probes that can be introduced through the biopsy channel of an endoscope and pass through a severe luminal stenosis allow more accurate staging because the complete tumor extent can be visualized. The echo-endoscope has become the instrument of choice for visualizing proximal colon neoplasms because the transducer can be maneuvered into the proximal segments of the colon. In one diagnostic and staging procedure, the combination of endoscope and TRUS can serve the following functions: demonstrate the surface of the mucosa, obtain a biopsy specimen, visualize the depth of a lesion within the bowel wall, and determine the presence or absence of adjacent lymphadenopathy.[125,126] However, CT or MRI is needed for complete staging, especially for detecting distant metastases.

Preoperative Staging by Endoluminal Ultrasound

Although transabdominal sonography may be used to assess the presence or absence of liver metastases, TRUS is increasingly used to detect the depth of tumor infiltration and local adenopathy in patients with rectal carcinomas. As mentioned earlier, its ability to distinguish the normal layers of the bowel wall and to visualize disruption of one or more of these layers by tumor leads to accurate staging of local tumor extent. With this method, sensitivities of 67% to 96% have been reported for assessing perirectal spread but the presence of regional lymph node metastases is less well detected (sensitivity 50% to 70%).[39,124,127-130] One study showed that results were less accurate with T2 carcinomas, which were often accompanied by peritumoral inflammation or abscess.[131] Abscesses manifest as fluid-filled structures, usually in the perianal space, that may contain internal echoes but exhibit good posterior acoustic enhancement. In this study of transcolorectal endosonography, the authors achieved an accuracy of 81% for rectal and 93% for colon carcinomas, with overstaging in

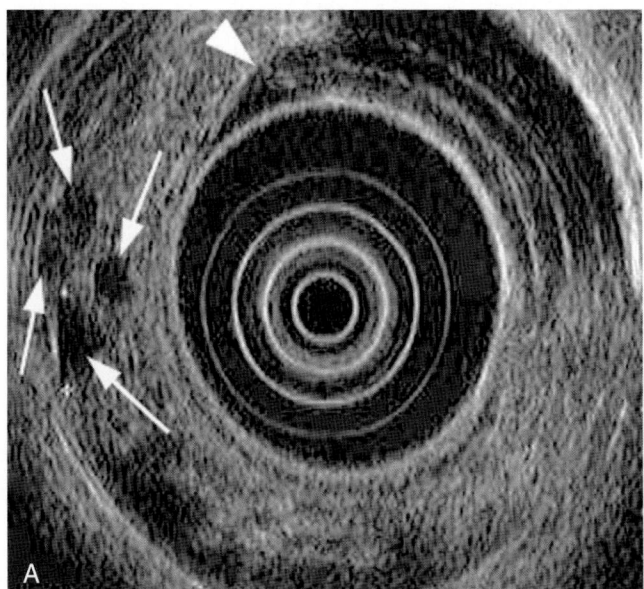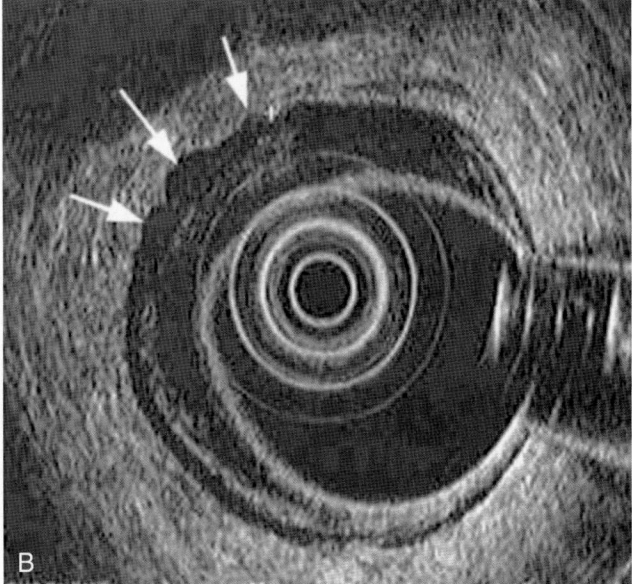

Figure 63-35. Transrectal ultrasound of rectal tumor (T3N1). A. TRUS image shows several lymph nodes in perirectal fat (*arrows*) and marked thickening (*arrowhead*) of rectal wall. **B.** TRUS image demonstrates thickened anterolateral wall of rectum as a low echogenicity structure with nodular outer margin (*arrows*) against the surrounding high signal intensity fat. This indicates transmural tumor extension (T3).

13% and understaging in 2% of patients. When lymph node involvement was analyzed separately, the sensitivity was 94% and specificity 55% for an overall accuracy of 70%. When transcolorectal ultrasound was compared with Dukes' classification, the overall accuracy was 67%.

The broad range of sensitivities of TRUS for detection of tumor extent in and through bowel wall emphasizes the operator dependence of this method. This fact was well demonstrated in a multicenter trial in which experienced ultrasonographers with a large caseload of patients with rectal cancers achieved the highest accuracy with TRUS.[132] TRUS has expanded the application of ultrasonographic methods to the entire colon and even ultrasound-guided biopsies of submucosal and extrinsic masses of the colon and rectum have become possible with this technique.[125,133,134] Spontaneous or iatrogenic inflammation is a major limiting factor affecting diagnostic accuracy.[135] Transrectal volume scans obtained using a three-dimensional multiplane transducer (7.5/10.0 MHz) permits examination of rectal cancer using previously unattainable planes and three-dimensional views[136] and may help improve tumor staging and treatment planning.[137] Because of the limited penetration of the ultrasound probe, only locoregional staging is possible with TRUS and CT or MR need to be added for complete tumor staging.

Immunoscintigraphy with Monoclonal Antibodies

Detection of Primary Colorectal Neoplasm

Since the mid-1970s, monoclonal antibodies (MoAbs) have been used in vivo as tumor-localizing agents and in vitro as diagnostic markers with gamma camera imaging to differentiate tumor cell types.[41,138] The following agents have been used: anti–carcinoembryonic antigen (anti-CEA) MoAbs tagged with iodine-123 and iodine-125, anti-CEA MoAbs conjugated with diethylenetriaminepentaacetic acid (DTPA) and labeled with indium-111, MoAbs B72.3-GYK-DTPA designated as CYT-103 (MoAb B72.3-glycyl-tyrosyl-[*N*-e-DTPA]-lysine), and sodium-iodide-I-125–labeled anti-TAG monoclonal antibody CC49.[139,140] The level of serum CEA did not influence tumor detection. MoAb B72.3 targets the high-molecular-weight tumor-associated glycoprotein 72, which is expressed in 80% of colon cancers and reacts with various mucin-producing adenocarcinomas but has practically no reaction to normal tissues. Some patients require cathartic agents before imaging because of prominent radioactivity in the large bowel. In general, lesion detection is performed with planar imaging 3 to 4 days after MoAb infusion. Single-photon emission CT (SPECT) is usually performed 5 to 7 days after MoAb infusion, and its better anatomic definition and determination of approximate size result in improved tumor detection.[141] Most studies attempt to determine the maximum tolerated dose and the uptake and retention of isotope in the tumor.[142]

Primary adenocarcinomas of the colon and metastatic foci in liver or lymph nodes are seen as areas of increased radioactivity ("hot spots"). Depending on the size and degree of necrosis of the liver metastases, neoplastic deposits in the liver may be visualized as areas of intense accumulation of radioactivity, areas with no accumulation of radioactivity surrounded by normal liver uptake, and intermediate lesions

with uptake identical to that of normal liver. In one study using indium 111–labeled CYT-103, "cold" defects in the liver shown by immunoscintigraphy were found to represent areas with moderate to severe necrosis, whereas lesions with normal MoAb uptake had only minor degrees of necrosis.[141] The same study revealed a low incidence of human antimouse antibody formation (16%) and an even lower incidence of adverse reactions (3.5%).[141] More recently, radioimmunoguided surgery (RIGS) with the monoclonal antibody CC49 labeled with iodine-125 has been employed in the treatment of colorectal cancer and appears promising.[140,143,144]

Preoperative Staging of Primary Colorectal Neoplasm

A number of studies have evaluated the value of isotope-labeled MoAb immunoscintigraphy for the detection of primary colorectal carcinoma and its metastases.[138-151] Sensitivity ranged from 65% to 92%, and specificity ranged from 77% to 92% for the detection of primary tumor, local recurrences, and distant metastases. The major role of immunoscintigraphy is in detecting occult tumor lesions and in establishing absence of distant disease in patients with isolated, resectable metastases. In one study using indium 111–labeled CYT-103, extrahepatic lesions undetected by CT and other tests were confirmed by surgery in more than 10% of patients. In another study, RIGS had a sensitivity of 92% and a specificity of 88% for the detection of lymph node metastases.[151] Additionally, immunoscintigraphy contributed beneficially to the management of 27% of patients.[149] It, therefore, appears reasonable to use immunoscintigraphy in patients with suspected focal or metastatic colorectal neoplasms. However, the validity of this test and the low incidence of adverse reactions must be confirmed in larger series before a final conclusion can be drawn.

Positron Emission Tomography

Primary Colorectal Neoplasm

Positron emission tomography was initially used for detection of functional abnormalities of the brain and heart, but its use has been expanded to the detection of primary and recurrent tumors as well as metastases. For these tumor studies, fluorine-18-deoxyglucose (FDG) has been used, and a remarkable correlation has been found between tumor grade and glucose utilization.[152] The new generation of PET scanners has good resolution to provide high-quality images of any area of the human body, and it is possible to use this method to detect distant, residual, or recurrent disease in patients with colorectal carcinomas. With the introduction of the PET/CT system, lesion classification has been significantly improved.[153] Large series in patients with colorectal cancer are still needed to more clearly define the role of PET/CT in staging and treating these patients.

For the purpose of identifying tumor tissue, PET images are evaluated quantitatively in regions of interest and time-activity curves are calculated. Tracer uptake is expressed as a differential absorption ratio that is calculated as the tissue concentration (in mCi/g) divided by injected dose (μCi) per body weight (g). After intravenous injection of FDG, PET images show significant uptake by malignant tumors (Fig. 63-36). Quantitative analyses demonstrate rapid uptake of FDG by

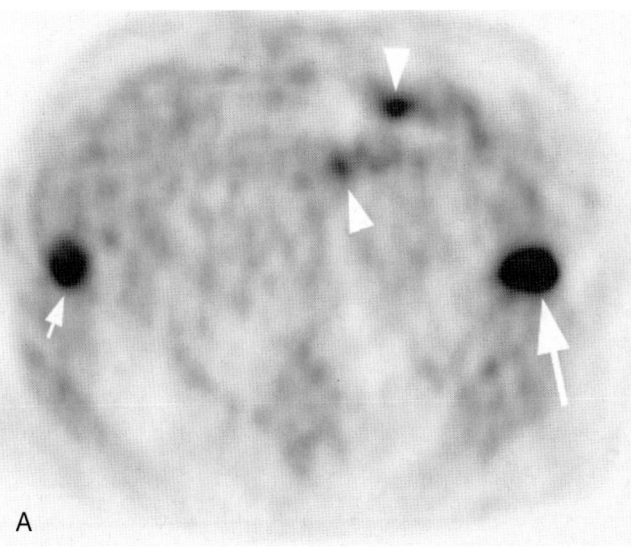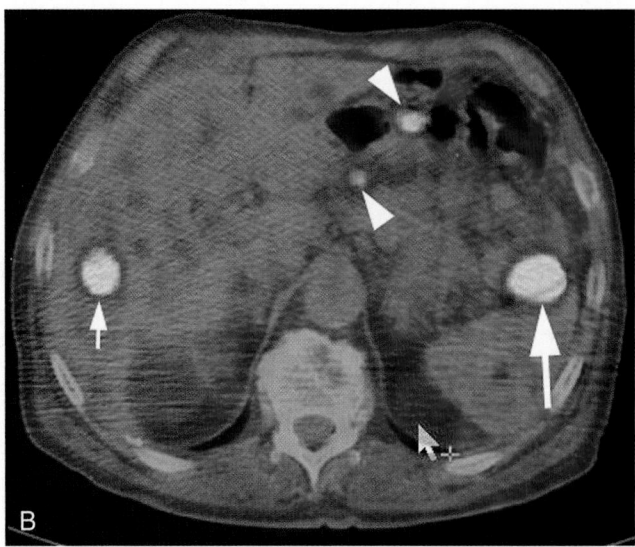

Figure 63-36. PET for staging in patient with history of splenic flexure carcinoma. A. Axial FDG-PET image demonstrates increased FDG uptake in anticipated location of splenic flexure (*large arrow*) and in liver (*small arrow*). Two additional areas of increased FDG uptake (*arrowheads*) are seen in expected location of hepatic flexure. **B.** The fused PET/CT shows left flank activity is located in splenic flexure primary tumor (*large arrow*), and large area of increased activity on right corresponds to hepatic lesion (*small arrow*) seen on CT. Two small areas of increased activity (*arrowheads*) were not seen on CT and represent small implants on surface of hepatic flexure. Although CT detected both primary tumor in splenic flexure and hepatic metastasis, serosal colonic implants were missed.

the tumor, followed by a slight decrease in the differential absorption ratio for up to 40 minutes after FDG administration. In comparison, the FDG concentration is low in non-malignant lesions and in soft tissue. In general, 1 hour after tracer injection, FDG accumulation in tumors is more than twice as high as in normal tissue or nonmalignant lesions. Tumor imaging is best performed at that time. Colon cleansing and drainage of the bladder with a Foley catheter after administration of the isotope can minimize artifactual accumulation of FDG.[154]

Staging of Primary Colorectal Neoplasm

The Centers for Medicare and Medicaid Services (CMS) first approved PET for coverage in 1998 and its guidelines specifically approve the use of FDG-PET for the diagnosis, staging, and restaging of colorectal cancer, but in clinical practice it is rarely used for the diagnosis of primary colorectal cancer unless the diagnosis has not been made pathologically.[155] Most investigations of the applications of FDG-PET for colorectal tumors have focused on the detection of local recurrent or residual disease. PET has also been used to identify distant metastatic foci and occasionally unexpected primary malignant tumors in patients with other colorectal neoplasms.[43,152,156-162] The majority of studies that addressed the sensitivity for identifying primary tumor by PET were retrospective and hampered by physiologic bowel wall accumulation of the isotope. This prevents the use of FDG-PET as an initial diagnostic modality.

Only small series are available, so that the accuracy of PET with FDG for staging colorectal tumors remains to be determined. Even smaller numbers are reported for the PET/CT scanner. Nevertheless, the results with PET/CT are promising because of the superior localization of lesions. In one study of asymptomatic patients with colonoscopic correlation, PET/CT detected 13 villous adenomas and three adenocarcinomas

and had five false-positive results.[161] In this study, the authors were able to distinguish adenoma from carcinoma by an increased rate of glycolysis in carcinoma. Metastases have been shown in lymph nodes remote from the primary tumor site and in liver. The results for lymph nodes are not as promising as those for liver metastases. One study showed a sensitivity for regional lymph nodes of only 29% but a specificity of 96%.[157] These disappointing results are probably because many metastatic deposits from colon carcinoma to nodes are in close proximity to the primary tumor, are small, and are often not cell rich, especially if the tumor is mucinous.

PET is excellent for the depiction of distant nodal or extranodal metastases. In one study, the positive predictive value of PET for malignant liver lesions was 93% and was superior to the 78% of CT or MRI.[163] PET is more accurate than CT for hepatic metastases from colon carcinoma larger than 1 cm in diameter but frequently misses lesions smaller than 1 cm.[164] Because PET does not provide accurate information on location of hepatic metastases according to hepatic anatomy, its greatest role lies in the detection of extrahepatic disease that precludes resection for cure (see Fig. 63-36). It appears that the addition of PET to the presurgical evaluation of patient with colorectal carcinoma may improve survival by eliminating patients with inoperable disease from consideration of surgical resection of liver lesions.[164]

ROLE OF CROSS-SECTIONAL IMAGING IN PRIMARY COLORECTAL NEOPLASM DETECTION

Computed tomographic colonography has been introduced as a method for screening patients at risk for colon cancer and polyps. The introduction of 2D and 3D CTC as complementary techniques has several advantages, including good patient tolerance, excellent visualization of abnormalities

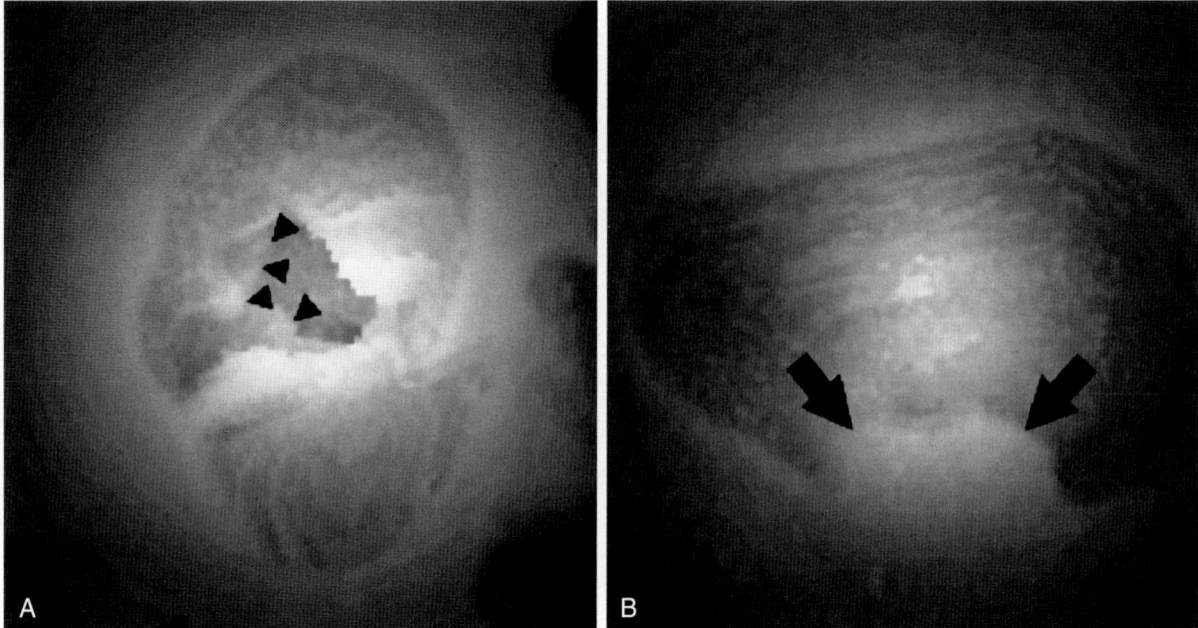

Figure 63-37. Three-dimensional CT colonography of colonic neoplasm. A. CT colonography demonstrates polypoid adenocarcinoma in sigmoid colon (*arrowheads*). **B.** The three-dimensional reconstruction shows a somewhat flat lesion in descending colon (*arrows*).

within the colon, and accurate detection of pathology proximal to an obstructing lesion (Fig. 63-37).[165,166] Furthermore, 3D reconstruction with fly-through capability offers the advantage of complete antegrade and retrograde inspection of the entire colon, whereas retroflection with the endoscope during colonoscopy cannot be achieved for all areas of the large bowel. Various technical approaches are still being explored to facilitate the time-consuming process of evaluating the colon with CTC and improve its sensitivity. CTC is discussed in detail in Chapter 57.

Patient prognosis in colorectal cancer is closely related to tumor stage at the time of diagnosis. The overall 5-year survival rate is about 61% (stage A, 81% to 85%; stage B, 64% to 78%; stage C, 27% to 33%; stage D, up to 20%).[164,167-169] There is a consensus that the most important prognostic factor is the presence or absence of lymph node invasion, but malignant fixation of colorectal tumor through direct invasion also appears to be an important sign.[170]

Most patients with colorectal cancer have disease that at the time of diagnosis is limited to the bowel wall and regional pericolonic or mesenteric lymph nodes. These patients undergo curative surgery. In patients with advanced disease, surgery is performed to prevent hemorrhage, obstruction, and perforation. Both types of patients need accurate non-invasive preoperative assessment of tumor stage based on one or a combination of radiographic techniques to individualize the treatment plan. The following discussion analyzes the effectiveness of the various imaging techniques for detecting and staging primary colorectal neoplasms.

Endoluminal or endoscopic ultrasound is useful for determining local tumor extent within and beyond the bowel wall but may miss regional lymph node metastases that develop in 14% of patients with primary tumors confined to the rectal wall. At present, endoluminal sonography is superior to CT and equal to MRI in demonstrating the T stage of tumors confined to the bowel wall (T1 and T2) and has a higher speci-

ficity.[39] Endoluminal ultrasound appears to be more sensitive in assessing early perirectal invasion, but its sensitivity does not reach 100%.

Based on the available results, routine CT or MRI staging is not recommended for early primary colorectal tumors. Wall thickening alone is a nonspecific finding that occurs in many different diseases (Table 63-4). Endoluminal MRI can achieve results for T1 and T2 staging that is similar to endoluminal ultrasound, but this method is rather invasive and not widely used. Both endoluminal techniques are limited when a large obstructing colorectal mass is present. MRI with phased-array coils is capable of demonstrating the layers of the rectal wall.

Overall, CT and MRI should be reserved for patients with suspected locally invasive (T3 or T4) or metastatic disease. If CT or MRI shows extensive local tumor, these patients can

Table 63-4
Differential Diagnosis of Colonic Wall Thickening

Neoplasm (primary including lymphoma and secondary)
Neoplasm from adjacent tissue or organs invading colon and/or rectum
Neoplasm metastatic to the colon or rectum
Muscular hypertrophy (particularly sigmoid colon)
Crohn's disease
Ulcerative colitis
Infectious colitides (including pseudomembranous colitis)
Diverticulitis
Intramural abscess or hematoma (trauma, coagulopathy)
Perforation with inflammation
Ischemia
Vasculitis (with focal involvement)
Endometriosis
Amyloidosis
Focal chronic inflammation from pancreatitis
Plication defects after surgery

be treated with neoadjuvant radiation therapy and chemotherapy with subsequent tumor resection. Whereas in the United States chemotherapy and radiation therapy are reserved for patients with T3 disease, in Europe all patients with rectal carcinoma receive preoperative irradiation with or without chemotherapy. Neoadjuvant therapy has proven to dramatically reduce rectal tumor recurrence.[111]

If a colon resection is planned, the decision to use local tumor excision by surgery or colonoscopy cannot be based on CT alone. CT has poor sensitivity in depicting depth of mural tumor penetration and is less sensitive than other techniques in assessing invasion of the mesorectal fascia and regional lymph nodes. CT can be used to guide fine-needle aspiration of suspected metastases and to assess complications, such as abscess formation. When the primary neoplasm arises in the abdomen, pelvic metastases are uncommon and isolated pelvic metastases are rare, which focuses the metastatic work-up on the abdomen.[171,172] Subtle extension of tumor beyond the bowel wall may be better recognized by MRI than by CT, whereas advanced T3 usually is diagnosed equally well by both techniques. In these cases, the choice of method largely is determined by the operator's skills and experience. At present, MRI is considered superior to CT in demonstrating the mesorectal fascia and in determining the exact distance of the tumor from it. Invasion of the muscles, nerves, and bones may be better delineated on MRI than on CT.[116] Because in-depth studies are not available that compare MDCT with 16 or 64 detector rows to state-of-the-art MRI, a definitive assessment of the respective advantages of the two techniques cannot be made.

Large variations in sensitivity and specificity for detecting metastases in lymph nodes have been published for all three techniques. Endoluminal ultrasound has limited depth penetration and therefore only can be used for detection of locoregional nodes. All techniques suffer from the fact that small metastatic deposits in lymph nodes may go undetected. MR lymphangiography may improve staging of colorectal tumors, but MR lymphangiography with target-specific contrast material is not yet commercially available.

The role of MoAb immunoscintigraphy and PET in the evaluation of patients with primary colorectal tumors is still uncertain. Results with immunoscintigraphy are encouraging with sensitivities for detecting primary colorectal tumor ranging from 65% to 92% and specificity from 77% to 92%. Furthermore, RIGS was shown to successfully guide resection of malignant lymph nodes.[151] Specifically, this test may lead to more accurate assessment of distant disease for resection. Similarly, PET has become an accurate method for staging colorectal neoplasms, as the resolution of PET scanners has improved and the combined PET/CT provides more accurate lesion localization. Although the sensitivity of PET for detecting hepatic metastases larger than 1 cm in diameter is superior to CT or MRI, CT or MRI should be used initially for detecting liver metastases and precisely localize them to the various liver segments. The most important role of PET in the presurgical evaluation of patients with colorectal cancer lies in the detection of extrahepatic disease that precludes resection for cure.

In conclusion, a combination of endoluminal ultrasound (or endoluminal MRI) for local and CT for overall staging is optimal for early colorectal cancer. Whether the addition of PET is beneficial and cost effective in these patients remains

to be seen. In suspected advanced disease, MRI appears to be superior to CT for local staging and should be combined with PET/CT for complete staging and preoperative treatment planning. Intraoperative ultrasound can be used to confirm the presence or absence of hepatic metastases.

POSTOPERATIVE FOLLOW-UP

Contrast Enema

Patients who have had surgery for colorectal carcinoma should undergo frequent postoperative examinations because of their relatively high risk for developing a recurrent and metachronous carcinoma.[173] Ileocolic (Fig. 63-38) and colo-colic anastomoses are nicely depicted on double-contrast enema examination, particularly after the use of intravenous glucagon. Plication defects are frequently identified. In some patients, a filling defect resulting from a stitch granuloma may be seen in the early postoperative period (Fig. 63-39). This defect regresses and becomes less prominent on follow-up studies.[174] It is important to obtain a postoperative study within approximately 3 months of surgery to establish the baseline appearance of the anastomosis for comparison with subsequent studies. The surgical anastomoses of low anterior resections performed with a surgical staple gun are beautifully demonstrated by double-contrast technique (Fig. 63-40).[175] CT is the examination of choice for the detection of recurrence remote from the anastomotic line and the detection of distant metastases (see later).[176,177]

The double-contrast enema is the primary diagnostic procedure for the detection of local and anastomotic recurrences (Fig. 63-41) as well as metachronous lesions (Fig. 63-42). It is particularly important to examine the anastomotic site because metastatic deposits tend to be implanted there.[178,179] Welch and Donaldson have shown that 20% of recurrences after colon resection and anastomosis were found at the anastomotic site.[180] When the anastomotic site appears eccentric or irregular or has nodular filling defects, recurrent tumor should be suspected. Colonoscopy may be helpful, although in some instances it may be misleading because recurrent tumor may be submucosal and biopsy findings may be negative for malignancy. CT and CT-guided biopsy may be needed to determine the presence and nature of an extracolonic mass, which cannot be appreciated to its full extent, if at all, by the barium enema.

Patients who have undergone abdominoperineal resection with colostomy must also be examined regularly because of the possibility of developing a second tumor. Double-contrast examination of the residual colon can usually be performed through the colostomy (see Fig. 63-42 and Chapter 55). CT and MRI are of particular value for the detection of pelvic recurrence of tumor in patients who have had abdominoperineal resection.

Cross-Sectional Imaging

CT and MRI have been used extensively to identify recurrent colorectal cancer, and both methods can detect recurrent tumor at a time when CEA titers are normal and symptoms are absent.[181,182] They are particularly useful in patients who have had total abdominoperineal resection. Follow-up studies of patients with potentially curative resection of recurrent

Figure 63-38. Normal postoperative appearances. A. Normal ileocolic anastomosis in the transverse colon. **B.** Example of a normal colocolic anastomosis (*arrow*). (From Laufer I, Levine MS [eds]: Double Contrast Gastrointestinal Radiology, 3rd ed. Philadelphia, WB Saunders, 2000.)

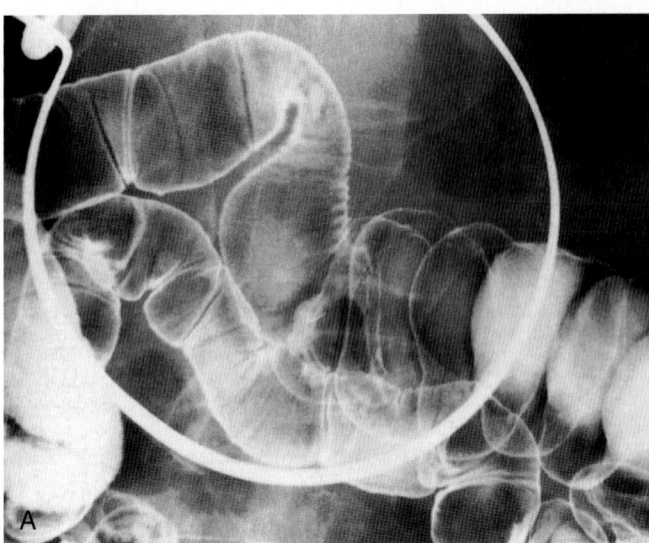

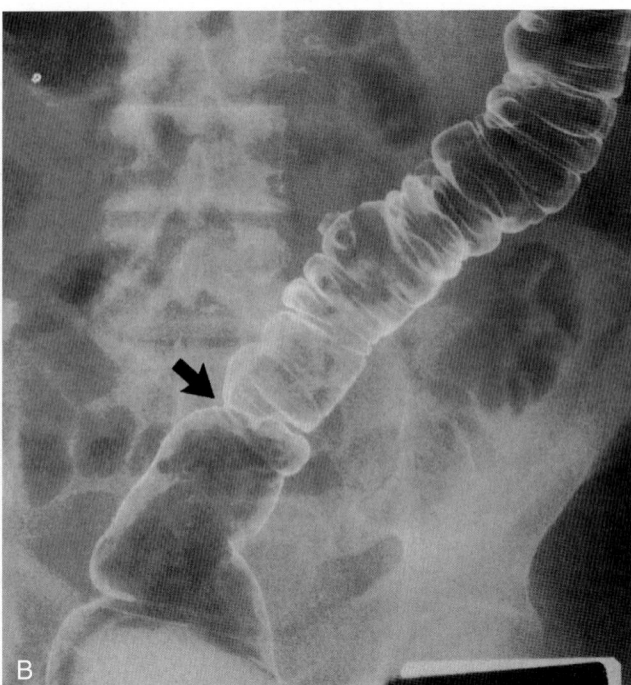

tumor demonstrated an average symptom-free period of 38 months, compared with an average survival of 8 months for patients without resection of recurrent tumor.[183-185] CT and MRI are accepted methods for detecting recurrent tumor that develops extraluminally. There is an ongoing debate on the appropriate timing and cost-effectiveness of these imaging tests. Rectal tumors have significantly more locoregional and pulmonary recurrences, whereas colon carcinomas have more hepatic and intra-abdominal recurrences.[186] Testing for asymptomatic recurrence during the first follow-up year is usually less fruitful than in the second through fourth follow-up years.[173] Patients with local recurrence in the first year are less likely to have a successful second "curative resection." Patients with low tumor grade at initial diagnosis are more likely to have a successful second surgical resection and a

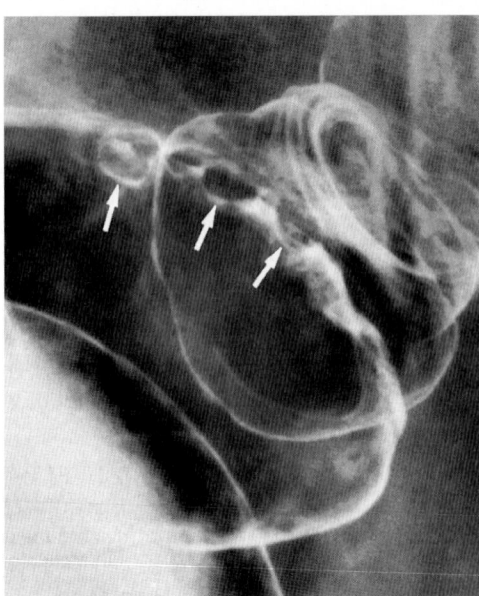

Figure 63-39. Stitch granuloma. Colocolic anastomosis with identifiable plication defects caused by sutures (*arrows*). (From Laufer I, Levine MS [eds]: Double Contrast Gastrointestinal Radiology, 3rd ed. Philadelphia, WB Saunders, 2000.)

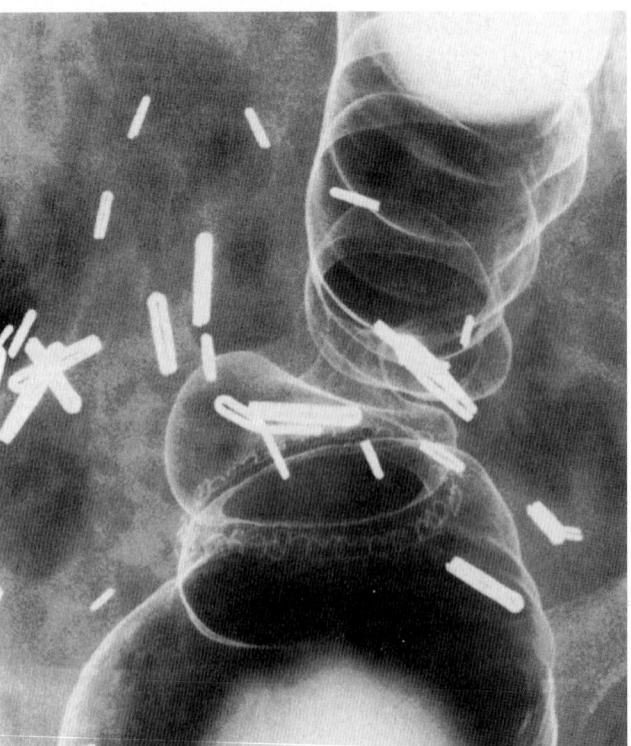

Figure 63-40. Low anterior resection. Double-contrast barium enema shows normal appearance of low anterior resection using staple gun. (From Laufer I, Levine MS [eds]: Double Contrast Gastrointestinal Radiology, 3rd ed. Philadelphia, WB Saunders, 2000.)

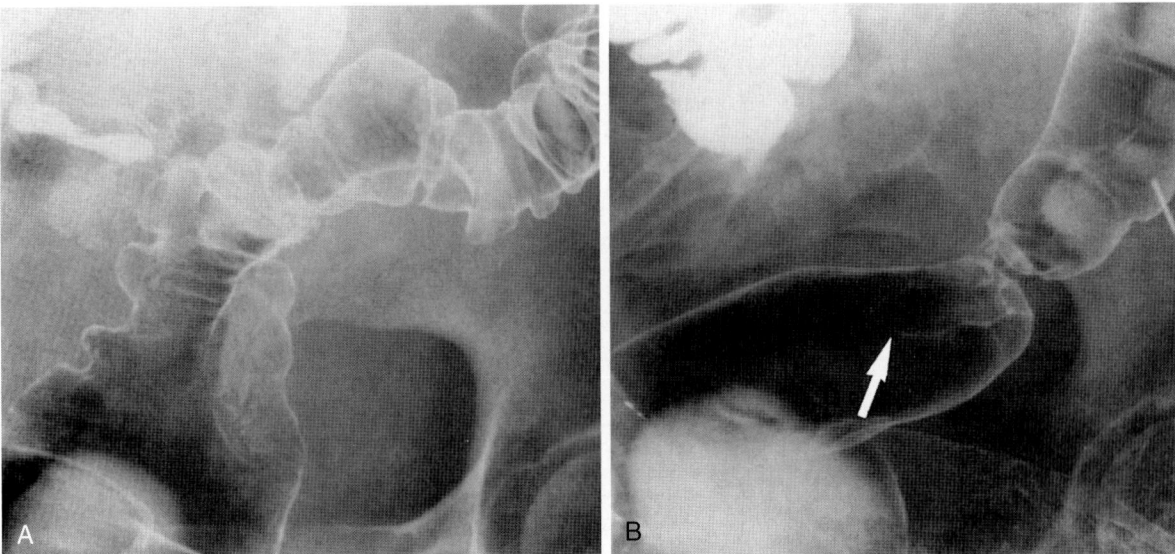

Figure 63-41. Local recurrence of colon carcinoma. A. Soft tissue mass represents recurrent colon carcinoma invading rectosigmoid. **B.** Anastomotic recurrence of colon cancer. Narrowing of anastomosis with plaquelike extension of recurrent tumor is seen proximally (*arrow*).

better prognosis.[187] Young patients with colon cancer have an increased prevalence of isolated local recurrences and a lower rate of liver metastases than older patients.[188]

The stage, histology, and site of primary tumor at the time of diagnosis have been found most predictive of eventual

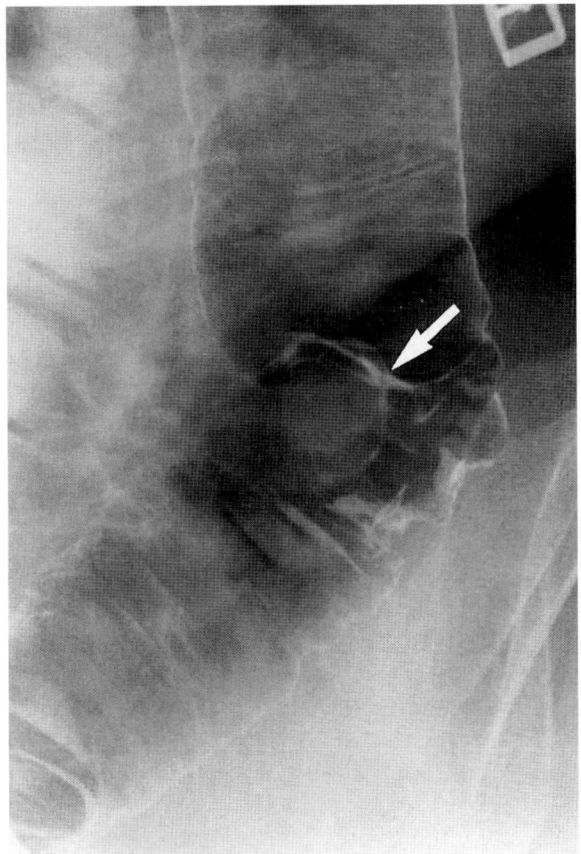

Figure 63-42. Metachronous carcinoma. A colostomy enema study performed after total proctectomy for carcinoma shows new primary carcinoma (*arrow*) in descending colon.

relapse.[173,185,189] Anastomotic recurrence occurs most often after low anterior resection of a rectal tumor and is usually related to residual tumor outside the colorectal wall that grows into the suture site. Since the introduction of total mesorectal excision, the incidence of local relapse has been markedly reduced.[190] Pelvic tumor recurrence that is limited to the axial location or axial and anterior locations is more likely to be resectable than those involving the sidewalls.[191] Because tumor recurrence develops in 30% to 50% of patients who have undergone apparently curative resection, and 80% of these recurrences develop within the first 2 years,[192] early and frequent follow-up studies are recommended. Many cancer centers observe a frequent follow-up program that includes serum CEA levels, chest radiography, colonoscopy, and imaging.[173,193] The most commonly recommended sequence of imaging follow-up studies consists of baseline CT or MRI at 3 to 4 months with subsequent imaging examinations at 6-month intervals for 3 years, then at yearly intervals for 5 years. More recently, PET/CT has proven that it can distinguish between surgical scar and tumor recurrence with a high degree of accuracy.[43]

Computed Tomography

Early studies established the usefulness of CT in detecting local recurrence and metastases to lymph nodes, liver, peritoneal cavity, retroperitoneum, and lung.[194,195] Sensitivities as high as 93% to 95% were initially reported for detection of locally recurrent tumor.[196,197] Later investigations indicated accuracy rates ranging from 53% to 88%.[193,198-200] Most diagnostic errors are due to the inability to detect microscopic invasion of perirectal or pericolonic fat in patients with reanastomoses, to assess presence or absence of metastatic foci in normal-sized lymph nodes, and to visualize minimal local tumor recurrence at the anastomotic site, particularly if the postoperative scar has not changed in size.

The CT features of recurrent anastomotic tumor are similar to those of the primary tumors, but the recurrence may be largely extrinsic. MDCT often can demonstrate the

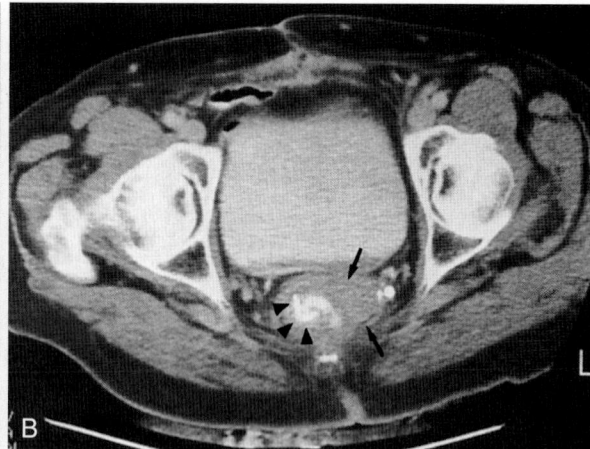

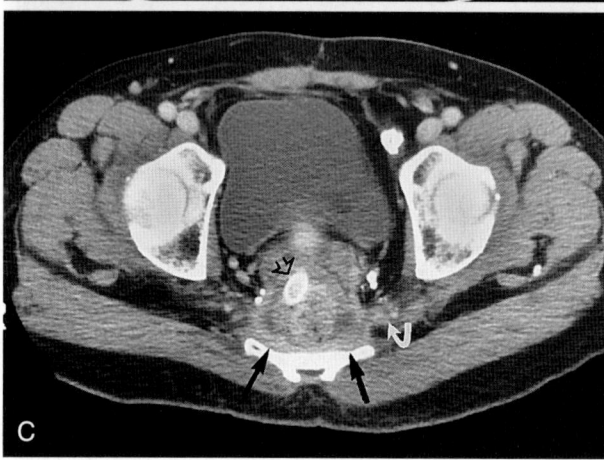

Figure 63-43. Postoperative appearance of pelvis after rectal carcinoma resection and reanastomosis. A. Status postresection without recurrence. Staple line (*arrowheads*) is clearly identified. **B.** Recurrent rectal carcinoma with extension into perirectal fat (T3N0M0). Thickening of rectal wall is seen on left side (*arrows*). There is also extension into perirectal fat. Staples (*arrowheads*) outline area of anastomosis. Note the largely extrinsic component of the recurrence. **C.** Advanced recurrent rectal carcinoma (T4bN1M0). Rectal wall is markedly thickened, and tumor mass is noted to extend to sacrum (*straight arrows*) and piriformis muscle on left (*curved arrow*). Adenopathy is inseparable from mass. A rectal tube (*open arrow*) is also seen on this section.

staple line at the anastomosis (Fig. 63-43). In these patients, wall thickening due to plication defects must be differentiated from recurrent tumor. The presence of streaky densities or a clean operative bed suggests fibrosis, whereas the presence of a mostly globular mass favors the diagnosis of tumor recurrence.[79] However, other studies indicate that a globular soft tissue mass may represent granulation tissue, hemorrhage, edema, or fibrosis in the early postoperative period (Fig. 63-44 and Table 63-5).[85] Postradiation fibrosis can also cause streaky densities or a presacral mass.[196,201,202] Pelvic radiation causes an inflammatory reaction in the soft tissue of the pelvis that leads to increased attenuation of the fat and thickening of the perirectal fascia. These changes persist for many years and may be indistinguishable from tumor recurrence. In a study that compared CT with PET, presacral soft tissue masses were seen by CT in 48% of patients with suspected tumor recurrence and in only 23% were these findings due to actual tumor recurrence.[43]

Benign postoperative masses may persist on CT more than 24 months after abdominoperineal resection.[202] A baseline

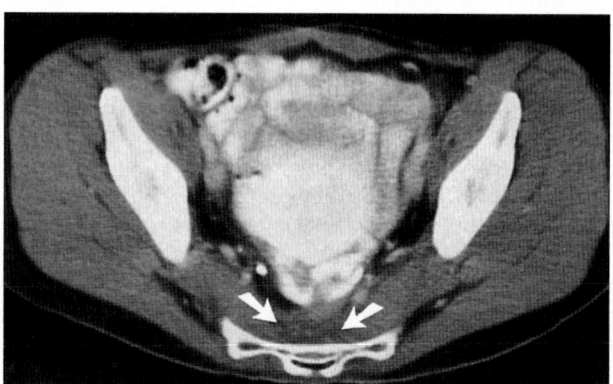

Figure 63-44. Postsurgical scar in patient with total abdominoperineal resection. A small area of soft tissue density (*arrows*) is seen in presacral region.

Table 63-5

Differential Diagnosis of Colorectal Mass with Soft Tissue Stranding

Neoplasm (primary and secondary)
Focal colitis (e.g., ameboma, Crohn's disease, neutropenic colitis)
Abscess
Diverticulitis
Pelvic inflammatory disease with contiguous colorectal inflammation
Rectal perforation and inflammation
Prostatitis, with contiguous inflammation and/or abscess
Status postradiation
Endometriosis
Pancreatitis in either transverse colon or splenic flexure
Transplants of pancreas and kidney with rejection or pancreatitis and contiguous involvement of colon or rectum
Peritonitis with infected fluid in pouch of Douglas

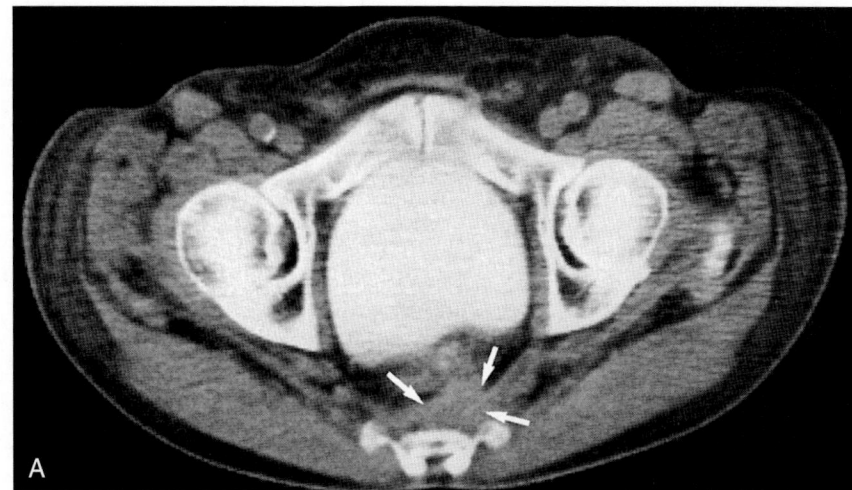

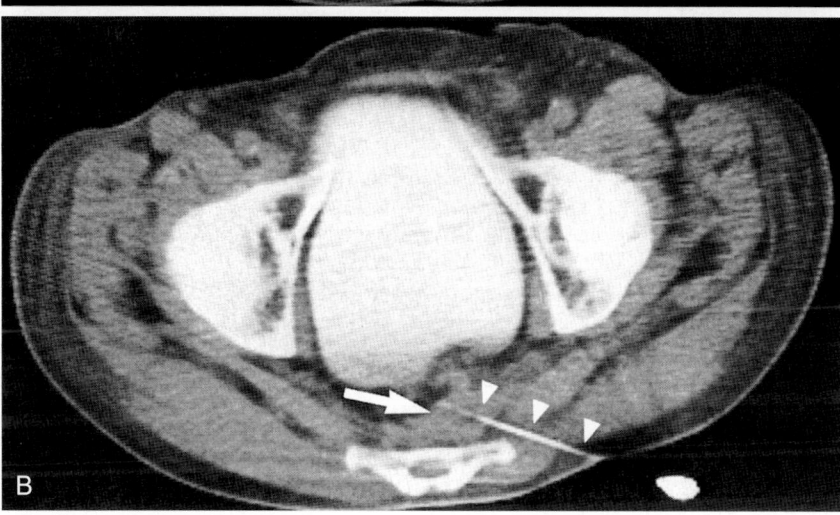

Figure 63-45. CT of recurrent rectal mass in patient after total abdominoperineal resection. A. Irregular soft tissue mass (*arrows*) is identified in the rectal bed. Size of mass has increased slightly compared with baseline CT study obtained 1 year before present examination. **B.** Percutaneous biopsy confirms presence of recurrent tumor. *Arrowheads* outline the needle with its tip in the mass of recurrent tumor (*arrow*).

CT study 2 to 4 months after surgery frequently demonstrates the presence of a mass, which by 4 to 9 months decreases in size and develops shaper margins. In the absence of symptoms and elevated CEA titers, this change in the appearance of the mass should not cause concern about local tumor recurrence. However, any increase in mass size, even in the absence of local invasion, lymphadenopathy, or perineal soft tissue density, should suggest recurrence, prompting percutaneous biopsy (Fig. 63-45).[201,202] Biopsy results may be negative if the recurrent tumor incites a substantial fibrous reaction.

With TME, the primary tumor is removed together with the perirectal lymph nodes but the internal iliac nodes are left in place. Positive lymph nodes left behind at TME substantially increase the risk for local recurrence in patients with lower rectal cancer. In one study it was shown that 28% of patients with distal rectal cancers and positive lymph nodes had involvement of the internal iliac nodes and in 6% these lateral chains were the only nodes involved.[203] These patients are staged as lymph node-negative at TME. In a large TME trial, it has been shown that nodal disease is a prognostic indicator for local recurrence as well as distant metastases.[204] Detection of these nodes is essential if preoperative radiation and chemotherapy is considered for patients at high risk for recurrence. If postoperative radiation and chemotherapy is chosen in patients with advanced node-positive

disease, preoperative detection of positive lymph nodes is not as crucial.

For two decades, CT was considered the best modality for detecting and staging recurrent rectal or rectosigmoid carcinomas. In patients who have had sphincter-saving resection of rectal and rectosigmoid carcinomas, almost all recurrent tumors develop extraluminally and subsequently infiltrate the suture lines. These extraluminal recurrences are missed on endoscopy and barium enema. In these patients, the rectum must be distended with negative contrast material to detect subtle lesions.[199] Glucagon helps the patient retain the rectal contrast medium but its administration is optional. More recently, comparison of contrast-enhanced CT with PET revealed CT sensitivities for local tumor recurrence that were lower than those for MRI and PET.[193,205,206] However, results obtained with MDCT and thin sections in large series currently are not available for local tumor recurrence.

Colonoscopy and barium enemas provide exquisite mucosal detail but cannot assess extraluminal disease and remote metastases. Therefore, barium enema and CT are complementary radiologic methods for evaluating patients with suspected recurrent colon tumor. In patients with abdominoperineal resections, CT and MRI are the major imaging tests for evaluating recurrent tumor (Fig. 63-46). Definition of the full extent of disease, particularly to distant sites, is necessary if another resection is contemplated.

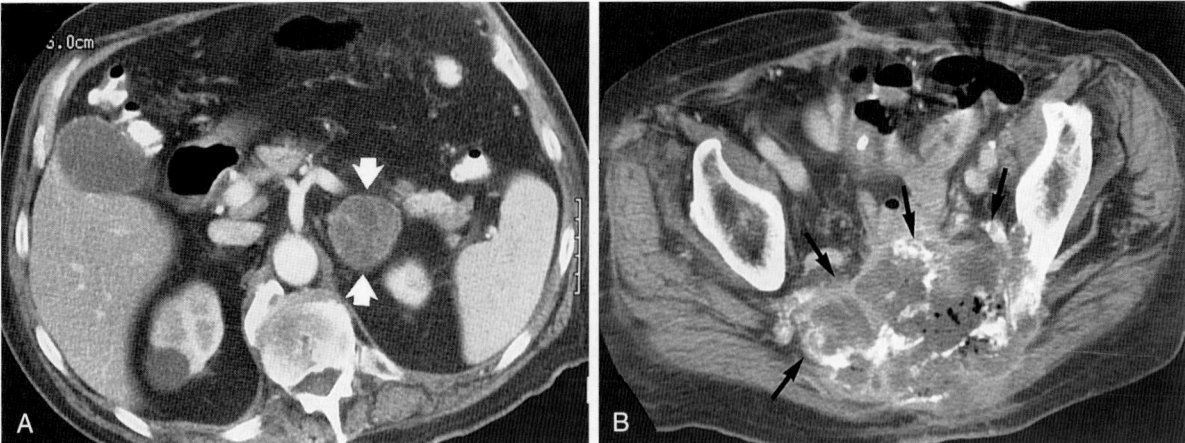

Figure 63-46. **CT of recurrent rectal carcinoma with adrenal metastasis (T4bN1M1).** **A.** Low-density mass (*arrows*) is seen in left adrenal gland. A cyst also is present in right kidney. **B.** Large, irregular mass present in presacral space (*arrows*) with destruction of sacrum. Air bubbles within mass indicate necrosis in the absence of clinical evidence of infection.

Magnetic Resonance Imaging

MRI has slightly superior results to CT in detecting recurrent tumor in patients who have undergone a low anterior resection or a transanal local excision.[205,206] In some instances, large surgical clips slightly impair the quality of MR images, but CT scans may also be difficult to analyze when large clips are present at an anastomotic site or in an area of lymphadenectomy. After total resection of the rectum, presacral masses are readily detected and staged with MRI. Initial reports suggested that postoperative and postradiation fibrosis had a low signal intensity on both T1-weighted and T2-weighted sequences (Fig. 63-47), whereas tumor recurrence had a high signal intensity on T2-weighted images.[207-211] However, it now appears doubtful that MRI cannot reliably distinguish between recurrent tumor, fibrosis, and inflammation (Fig. 63-48).[212,213]

One study, using T2-weighted sequences with long repetition and long echo times, examined the value of MRI in distinguishing early fibrosis (1 to 6 months after first treatment), tumor or late fibrosis (>12 months), and recurrent tumor. The authors found higher signal intensity values for early fibrosis compared with late fibrosis, probably because of increased vascularity, edema, and the presence of immature mesenchymal cells in granulation tissue. Radiation-induced necrosis and postsurgical inflammatory reaction can also contribute to an increase in signal intensity on T2-weighted images. The increase in tissue fluids seen in granulation tissue and necrosis caused by radiation renders distinction between early fibrosis and tumor recurrence difficult or even impossible (Fig. 63-49). However, late fibrosis and tumor recurrence could be clearly distinguished from one another (see Fig. 63-47).[212] Other studies found similar results, but

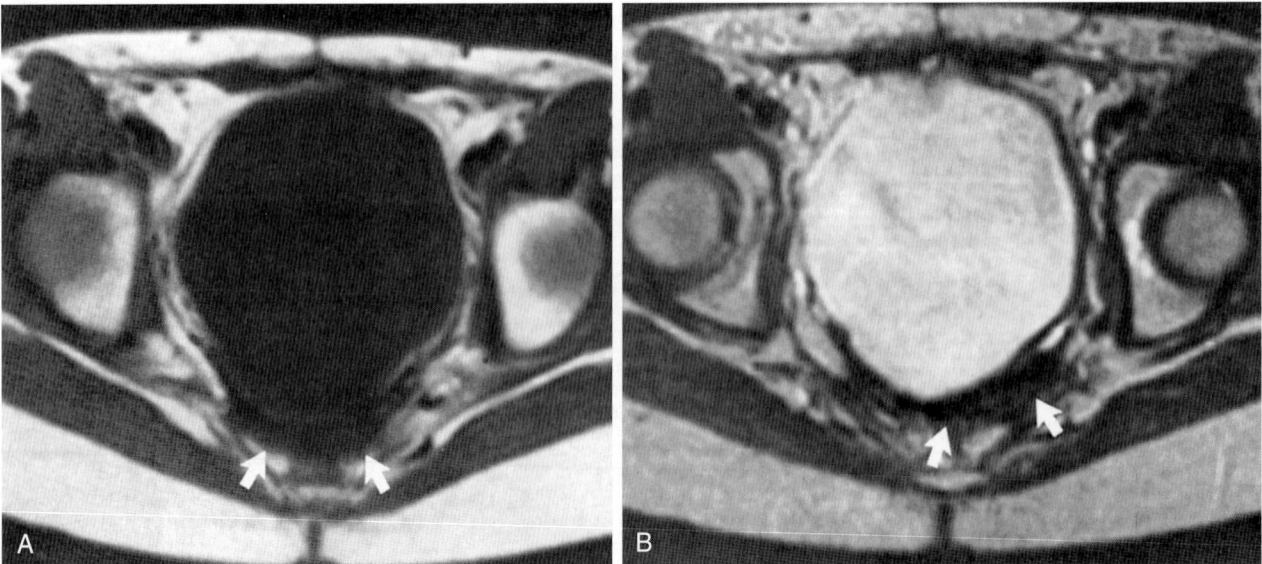

Figure 63-47. **MRI of a postsurgical scar in patient with total colectomy.** **A.** T1-weighted spin-echo image (600/11). Area posterior to the bladder has low signal intensity (*arrows*). **B.** T2-weighted spin-echo image (2500/80). Low signal intensity area on T1-weighted image remains dark (*arrows*) on T2-weighted scan, suggesting fibrosis in the surgical bed.

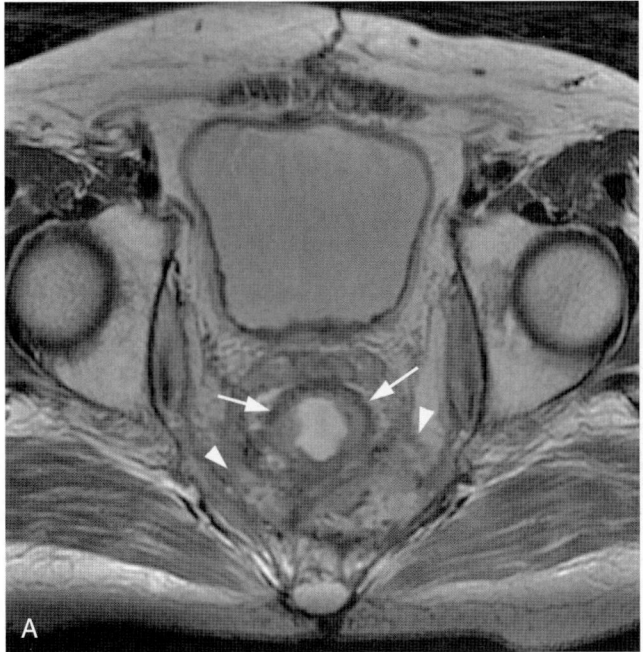
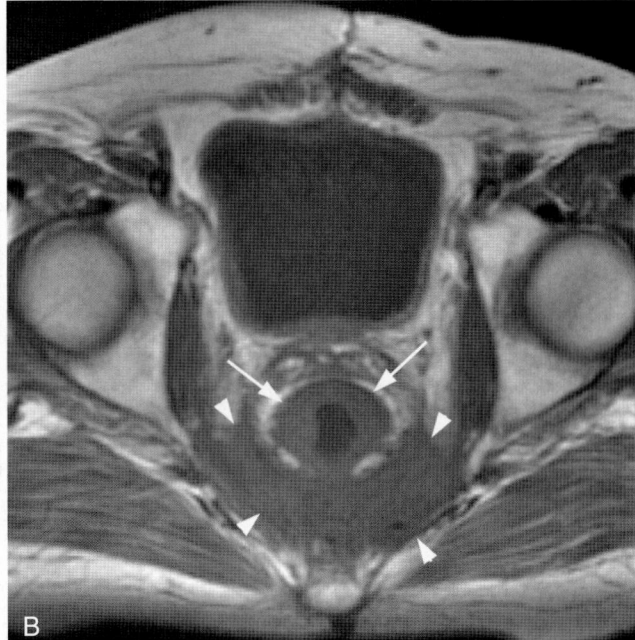
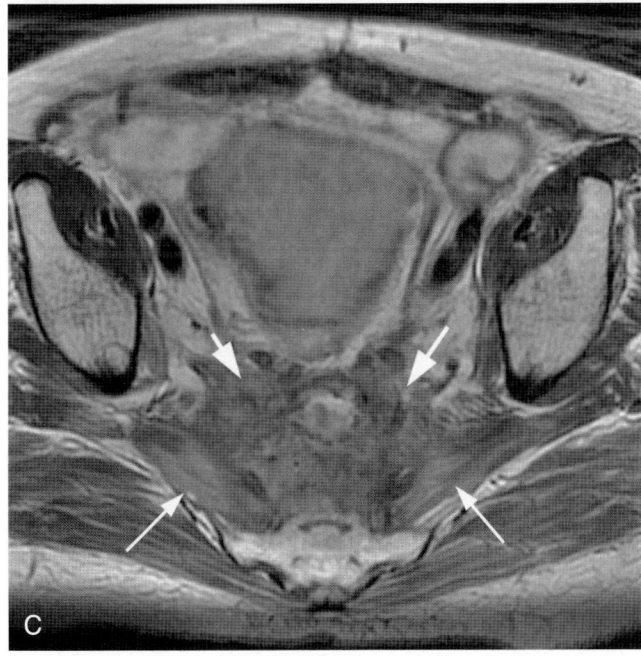

Figure 63-48. MRI of recurrent rectal carcinoma after resection and reanastomosis. A. T2-weighted fast spin-echo image shows thickened rectal wall (*arrows*), perirectal stranding, and intermediate signal intensity posterior to rectum (*arrowheads*) suggesting tumor recurrence. **B.** T1-weighted spin echo image nicely demonstrates mural thickening of rectum (*arrows*). Low signal intensity presacral mass (*arrowheads*) is better depicted than on T2-weighted image. Thickened rectal wall and the poor tissue definition in presacral space on T2-weighted sequences may be at least in part due to postoperative radiation that leads to edema and fibrosis. **C.** Axial T2-weighted images at higher level than **A** and **B** reveals increased signal intensity in piriformis muscle bilaterally (*thin long arrows*), indicating muscle invasion by large presacral tumor mass (*large short arrows*).

one investigation showed that the accuracy of MRI in differentiating between radiation damage and residual or recurrent tumor varied with the primary site.[92,210,213] It was excellent for cervical carcinoma but suboptimal for rectal carcinoma.[214] De Lange and colleagues[215] compared MRI results with histologic sections from tissue obtained during radical pelvic exenteration or extensive partial resection of a mass in patients with suspected recurrent rectosigmoid carcinoma. They found that the signal intensities on T2-weighted images do not permit prediction of the histologic diagnosis of a lesion. High signal intensity was found in areas of viable tumor (Figs. 63-50 and 63-51C), tumor necrosis, benign inflammation, and edematous tissue (Fig. 63-51A and B). Because desmoplastic reaction is a common response to many benign and malig-

nant processes, including tumors of the colon and rectum, areas of low signal intensity on T2-weighted images were also nonspecific, and the differential diagnosis included tumor-induced fibrosis and non-neoplastic, benign fibrotic tissue. However, MRI can reveal a presacral mass accurately and depict its complete extent. If such a mass consists mainly of desmoplastic tissue with only small strands of interspersed tumor tissue, even a percutaneous biopsy specimen may show fibrous tissue alone and no malignant cells. In these cases, a definitive diagnosis may be made by PET possibly with surgical removal of the mass or biopsy at laparotomy. It has been shown that if the mass enhances with gadolinium (>40%), it most likely represents tumor recurrence if the patient is at least 1 year postsurgery or irradiation.[216] Nevertheless,

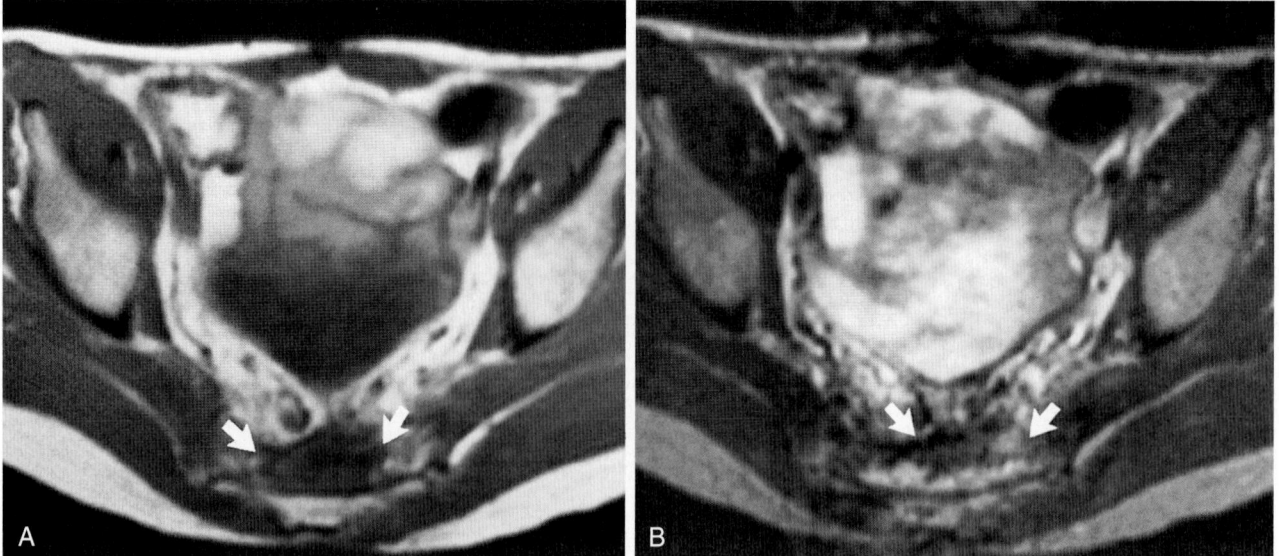

Figure 63-49. Indeterminate MR images of recurrent carcinoma after total colectomy. A. T1-weighted spin-echo image (700/20). An area of low signal intensity mixed with some intermediate signal intensity (*arrows*) is seen in the presacral space. **B.** T2-weighted spin-echo image (2500/70). Presacral soft tissue mass has intermediate signal intensity on T2-weighted scans (*arrows*). This is an indeterminate result and could represent recurrent viable tumor with a moderate amount of fibrous stroma, mild tumor necrosis, inflammation, or granulation tissue after surgery, irradiation, or both.

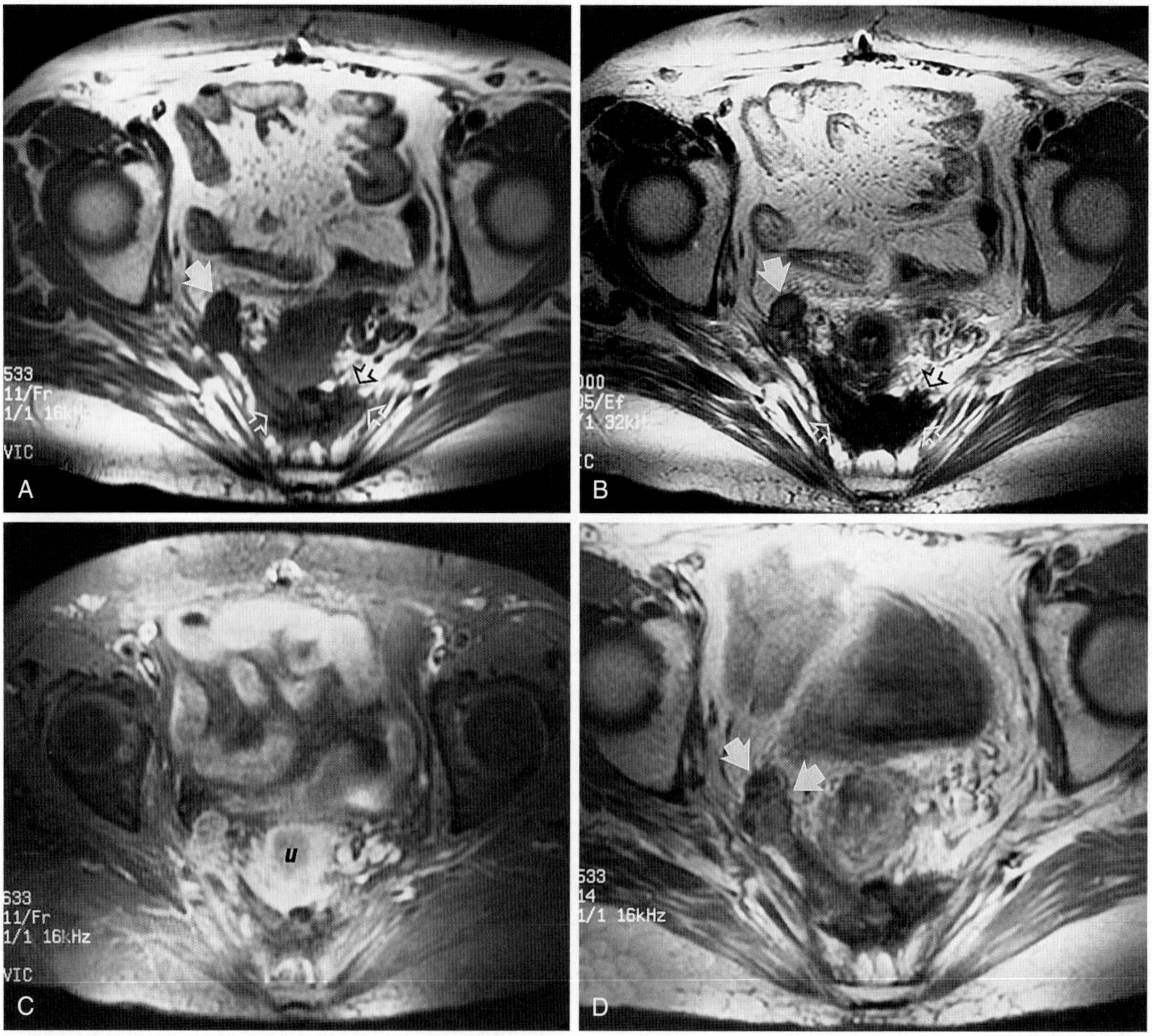

Figure 63-50. MRI of recurrent rectal carcinoma. A. T1-weighted spin-echo image (533/11). Area of low signal intensity (*open arrows*) representing scar tissue is seen in presacral space. In addition, a slightly irregular, oval mass (*solid arrow*) is seen immediately anterior to piriformis muscle, owing to recurrent tumor. **B.** T2-weighted fast spin-echo image (4000/105). Scar tissue (*open arrows*) is clearly identified as an area of low signal intensity, and the recurrent tumor mass (*solid arrow*) has intermediate signal intensity. **C.** T1-weighted spin echo image with fat suppression. Scar tissue remains largely dark, but the recurrent tumor and the uterus (U) demonstrate increased signal intensity. **D.** T1-weighted spin-echo image after gadolinium (533/11). Three months later, enhancing recurrent mass is slightly larger (*arrows*).

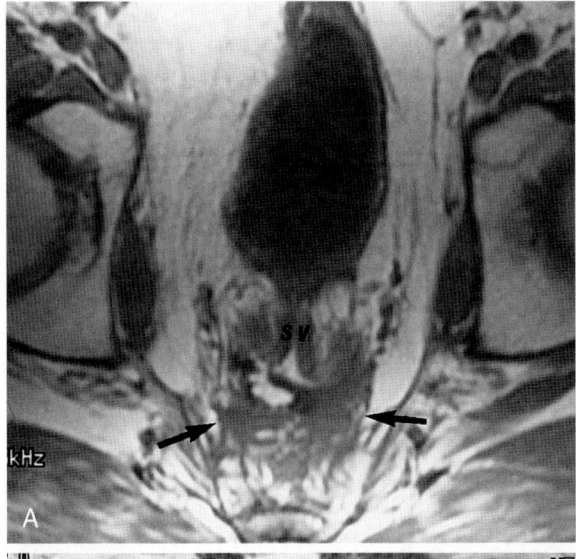

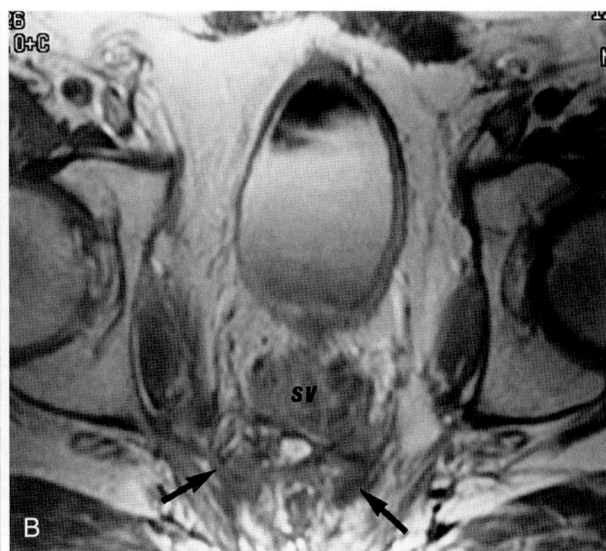

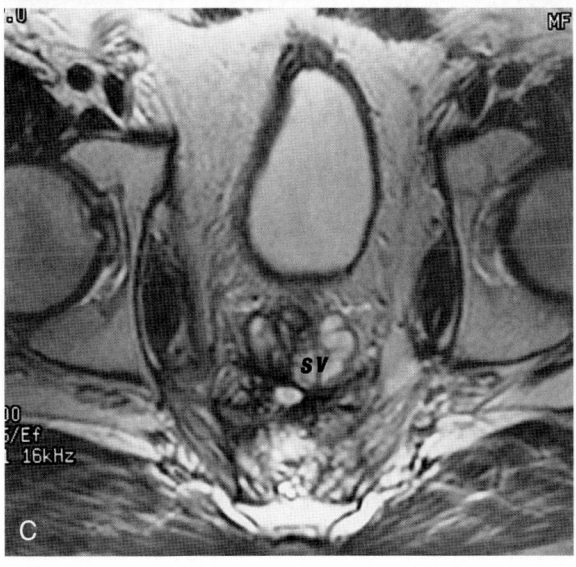

Figure 63-51. MRI of recurrent rectal carcinoma. A. T1-weighted spin-echo image (500/14) demonstrates ill-defined area of low signal intensity (*arrows*) mixed with small regions of higher signal intensity in patient 4 months status post abdominoperineal resection. **B.** T1-weighted image (533/14) after gadolinium. The previously identified area (*arrows*) in the presacral space clearly enhances. This could represent postoperative inflammation or early recurrence. **C.** T2-weighted fast spin-echo image (4500/105). Area of low signal intensity on the T1-weighted image shows now mostly high signal intensity. Given the short interval after resection, this most likely represents postsurgical changes. SV, seminal vesicles.

published result with gadolinium enhancement are conflicting.[205,217] One study demonstrated good distinction between scar tissue and recurrence based on measurements of the time-intensity curve and the ratio of signal intensity of the lesion to the signal intensity of the iliac artery at 60 seconds but not for the maximum change in signal intensity as other studies have demonstrated.[217] Similarly, a recent study using MDCT with kinetic scanning and maximum density measurements did not show a significant difference between patients without and with tumor recurrence.[218] Whether MR perfusion study can be used to distinguish between tumor recurrence and scar tissue remains to be seen. CT perfusion studies in primary rectal tumors to assess response to chemotherapy and irradiation already have shown promising results.[219]

MRI is a sensitive method for detecting masses after colorectal surgery, and its specificity is slightly higher than that of CT.[205] In these patients, benign and malignant processes cannot be distinguished solely on the basis of morphologic appearance and signal intensity on MR images. MDCT may be more helpful in evaluating anastomoses in patients with

suture material or multiple clips from lymphadenectomies because susceptibility artifacts may be problematic at high magnetic field strength. In the detection of nonlocal recurrence, MDCT may be more valuable than MRI, but more studies are needed to determine the efficacy of these procedures and their possibly complementary natures. Further technical advances may improve results with MRI.

Transrectal Ultrasound

The findings and results of TRUS for recurrent colorectal malignancy are similar to those for primary carcinoma, but the examination can be done only for patients who had a transanal local excision, a low anterior resection, or (in women) an abdominoperineal resection. In patients with total abdominoperineal resection and colostomy, the recurrent tumor should be assessed by CT, MR, PET, or scintigraphy with MoAb.

TRUS provides highly accurate assessment of local recurrence. In one study, TRUS revealed all 15 recurrences of rectal neoplasm.[220] In four cases, CEA titers were not elevated and rectal or vaginal digital examination, rigid rectoscope examination, and pelvic CT scans were negative. In these four patients, TRUS was the only method that detected recurrence. Therefore, endoluminal sonography should be used for evaluation of patients when early or limited recurrence is suspected or the patients had a tumor grade or stage with a high prognostic factor for recurrence, even if the results of initial tests in routine follow-up examinations are negative.

Immunoscintigraphy

Most results of MoAb immunoscintigraphy have been for patients with primary colorectal tumors. And only small numbers of patients with recurrent or residual tumor have been published.[138-140,148] In one study using indium 111–labeled MoAb ZCE-025,[150] recurrences were found in 79.4% of 16 patients, and immunoscintigraphy was beneficial for the management of these patients (Fig. 63-52). Other immunoscintigraphic studies that were focused on recurrent colorectal tumor showed similar sensitivities with a high negative predictive value.[140,148,221] One study compared the sensitivity and specificity of imaging with technetium-99m–labeled Fab′ fragment of anti-CEA IMMU-4 with that achieved with CT for detecting pelvic recurrence of colorectal tumor.[222] The sensitivity and specificity for antibody scanning alone was 79% and 84% and improved to 83% and 81% when it was combined with CT but did not reach statistical significance.

Positron Emission Tomography

PET has been employed extensively for assessing patients with suspected recurrence or residual tumor from colorectal neoplasms. In several studies, the distinction between neoplasm and scar tissue was made with a high degree of accuracy. In one study, all 21 recurrent tumors had high FDG uptake with lesion/soft tissue ratios of 1.19 to 4.94.[155] However, based on the FDG differential absorption ratio values, one patient

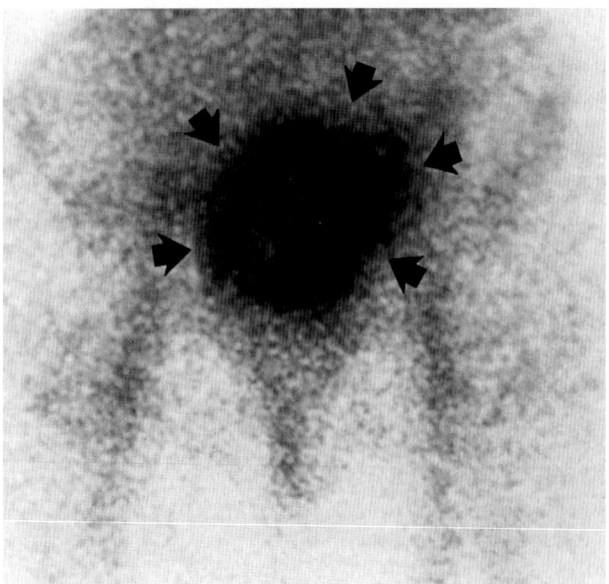

Figure 63-52. Immunoscintigraphy of recurrent rectal carcinoma. A large mass of high uptake (*arrows*) is seen in the pelvis of a patient with recurrent rectal tumor.

was misclassified because of low FDG uptake. All scars in the pelvis after abdominoperineal resection were correctly identified. In another study, in five patients whose CT and PET results were similar, three recurrences and two scars were correctly identified.[156] In four patients with negative or equivocal CT scans, PET correctly identified all tumors; and in three patients whose CT scans raised suspicion of recurrence, PET correctly excluded recurrence. More recent studies confirmed these early results.[200] PET appears to have an advantage over CT in the detection of recurrent hepatic metastases after partial hepatectomy, extrahepatic metastases, and local recurrence.[200] It appears that PET is an accurate method for detecting recurrent colorectal neoplasms (Fig. 63-53) and may offer an alternative to biopsy because it successfully excludes recurrence in patients with suspicious masses in the surgical bed. Nevertheless, larger series are needed to confirm these results.

ROLE OF CROSS-SECTIONAL IMAGING IN RECURRENT COLORECTAL CARCINOMA

Based on current literature, it is difficult to compare CT and MRI, used alone or in combination, for the detection of recurrent disease. This difficulty is mainly due to the great variations in both techniques and the types of scanners used, the scanning protocols, and the methods of administering the contrast agent. Even the diagnostic criteria, the study population, and the analysis of the data vary greatly. Although MRI demonstrates excellent results for tumor recurrence detection, it cannot be readily combined with FDG-PET. CT has the major advantage that the entire abdomen and pelvis can be scanned within a few seconds, much shorter than the acquisition time for an abdominal and pelvic MR study.

Based on the currently available data, it appears that for imaging of possible recurrent colorectal tumor a combination of CT and PET would be most beneficial. The CT should be obtained with contrast enhancement. Any suspicious area on CT thus can be clarified by PET. If PET/CT is not available, CT or MRI combined with immunoscintigraphy could be helpful. All these imaging protocols should be accompanied with frequent clinical visits, laboratory tests (CEA), and colonoscopy where feasible.

Because of the high frequency of tumor recurrence in the first 24 to 36 months after surgery, a series of follow-up CT examinations at 6-month intervals should be obtained to detect early tumor recurrence.[173] In addition, a CT scan is indicated whenever a patient has a rising CEA titer or symptoms. Because local recurrence of cancer occurs in 50% within the first year and in 80% within the second year,[192] patients with suspected recurrence should have a baseline study 3 to 4 months after initial surgery. This time frame is chosen because postsurgical acute changes, such as edema and hemorrhage, have substantially resolved. Follow-up examinations should be compared with those of the baseline study to avoid unnecessary biopsies. A study is considered positive if a mass or nodes are detected that were not seen on the baseline study or have become larger since the original study. Biopsy specimens should be obtained of any new or enlarging mass or nodes or confirmed with PET. Any clinical signs, elevated CEA levels, or suspicious CT or MR findings should lead to a FDG-PET examination for further evaluation to ensure early detection of recurrence with possible curative resection. If

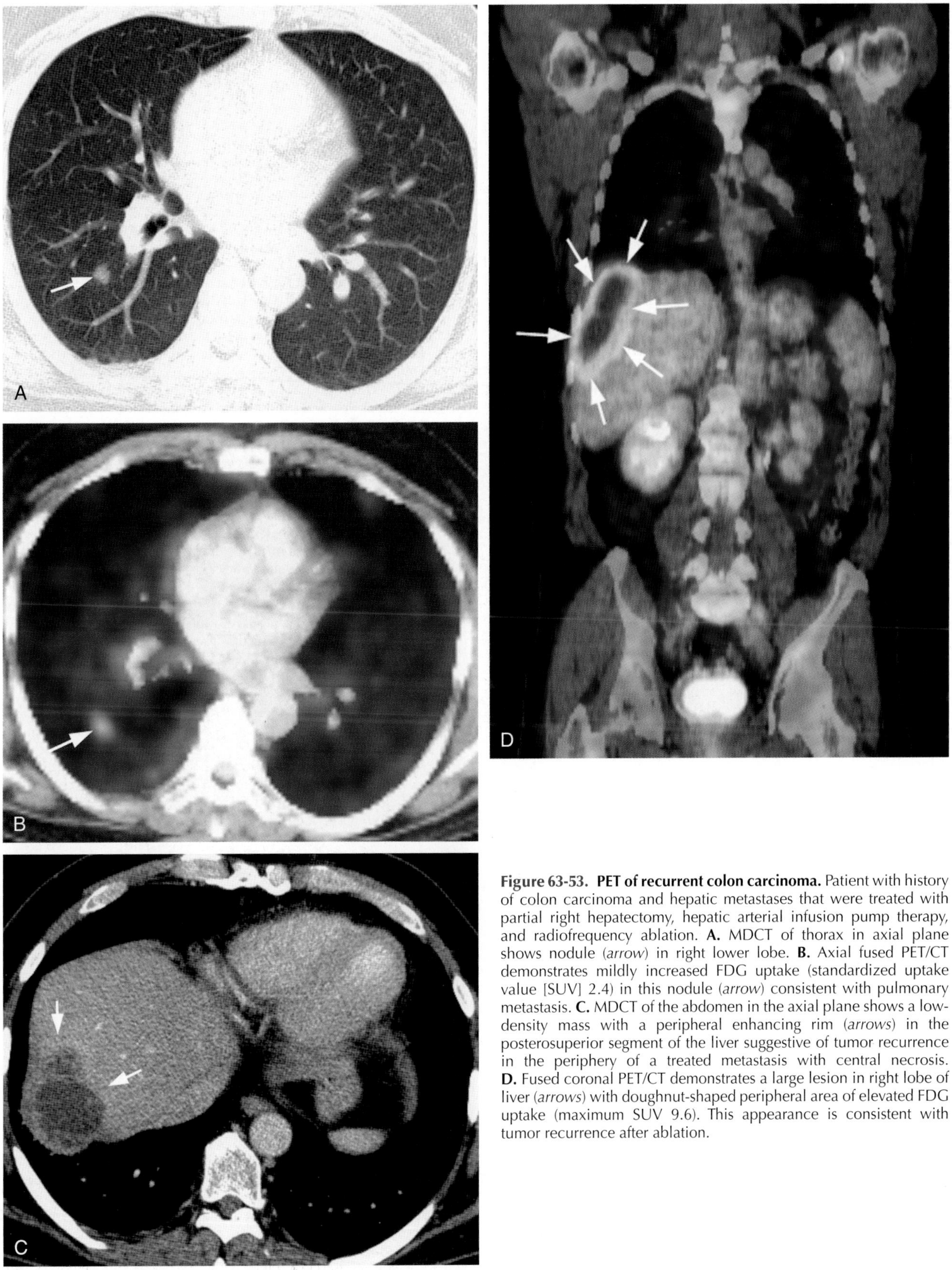

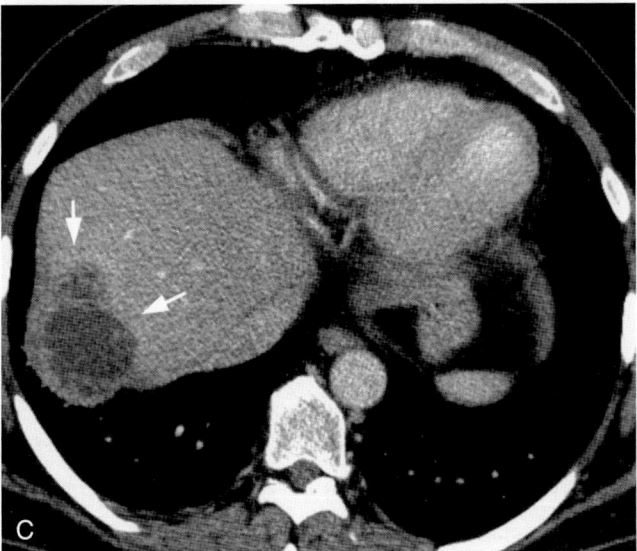

Figure 63-53. PET of recurrent colon carcinoma. Patient with history of colon carcinoma and hepatic metastases that were treated with partial right hepatectomy, hepatic arterial infusion pump therapy, and radiofrequency ablation. **A.** MDCT of thorax in axial plane shows nodule (*arrow*) in right lower lobe. **B.** Axial fused PET/CT demonstrates mildly increased FDG uptake (standardized uptake value [SUV] 2.4) in this nodule (*arrow*) consistent with pulmonary metastasis. **C.** MDCT of the abdomen in the axial plane shows a low-density mass with a peripheral enhancing rim (*arrows*) in the posterosuperior segment of the liver suggestive of tumor recurrence in the periphery of a treated metastasis with central necrosis. **D.** Fused coronal PET/CT demonstrates a large lesion in right lobe of liver (*arrows*) with doughnut-shaped peripheral area of elevated FDG uptake (maximum SUV 9.6). This appearance is consistent with tumor recurrence after ablation.

CT or MRI diagnoses resectable recurrence of colorectal tumor that is confirmed by PET, a biopsy should be avoided for fear of tumor seeding.

References

1. Jemal A, Siegel R, Ward E, et al: Cancer statistics, 2007. CA Cancer J Clin 57:43-66, 2007.
2. Du XL, Meyer TE, Franzini L: Meta-analysis of racial disparities in survival in association with socioeconomic status among men and women with colon cancer. Cancer 2007 Apr 23 [Epub ahead of print].
3. Ananthakrishnan AN, Schellhase KG, Sparapani RA, et al: Disparities in colon cancer screening in the Medicare population. Arch Intern Med 167:258-264, 2007.
4. Bond JH: Colonic tumors. Endoscopy 30:150-157, 1998.
5. Bond JH: Adenomatous polyps and adenocarcinoma of the colon. In DiMarino AJ, Benjamin SB (eds): Gastrointestinal Disease: An Endoscopic Approach. Oxford, Blackwell Scientific, 1998, pp 610-624.
6. Fisher JA, Fikry C, Troxel AB: Cutting cost and increasing access to colorectal cancer screening: Another approach to following the guidelines. Cancer Epidemiol Biomarkers Prev 15:108-113, 2006.
7. Nelson RL, Dollear T, Freels S, et al: The relation of age, race, and gender to the subsite location of colorectal carcinoma. Gut 80:193-197, 1997.
8. Calle EE, Rodriguez C, Walker-Thurmond K, Thun MJ: Overweight, obesity, and mortality from cancer in a prospectively studied cohort of US adults. N Engl J Med 348:1625-1638, 2003.
9. Lagerstedt Robinson K, Liu T, Vandrovcova J, et al: Lynch syndrome (hereditary nonpolyposis colorectal cancer) diagnostics. J Natl Cancer Inst 21:291-299, 2007.
10. Vogelstein B: A model of colorectal tumorigenesis. Adv Oncol 7:2-6, 1991.
11. Joyce T, Pintzas A: Microarray analysis to reveal genes involved in colon carcinogenesis. Expert Opin Pharmacother 8:895-900, 2007.
12. Yuan Y, Han HJ, Zheng S, et al: Germline mutations of *hMLH1* and *hMSH2* genes in patients with suspected hereditary nonpolyposis colorectal cancer and sporadic early-onset colorectal cancer. Dis Colon Rectum 41:434-440, 1998.
13. Solomon MJ, Schnitzler M: Cancer and inflammatory bowel disease: Bias, epidemiology, surveillance, and treatment. World J Surg 22:352-358, 1998.
14. Bansal P, Sonnenberg A: Risk factors of colorectal cancer in inflammatory bowel disease. Am J Gastroenterol 91:44-48, 1996.
15. Svrcek M, Cosnes J, Beaugerie L, et al: Colorectal neoplasia in Crohn's colitis: A retrospective comparative study with ulcerative colitis. Histopathology 50:574-583, 2007.
16. Chen CD, Yen MF, Wang WM, et al: A case-cohort study for the disease natural history of adenoma-carcinoma and de novo carcinoma and surveillance of colon and rectum after polypectomy: Implication for efficacy of colonoscopy. Br J Cancer 88:1866-1873, 2003.
17. Winawer SJ, Zauber AG, O'Brien MJ, et al: The national polyp study: Design, methods, and characteristics of patients with newly diagnosed polyps. Cancer 70:1236-1245, 1992.
18. Thomas T, Abrams KA, Robinson RJ, et al: Meta-analysis: Cancer risk of low-grade dysplasia in chronic ulcerative colitis. Aliment Pharmacol Ther 15:657-668, 2007.
19. Smith RA, Cokkinides V, Eyre HJ: Cancer screening in the United States, 2007: A review of current guidelines, practices, and prospects. CA Cancer J Clin 57:90-104, 2007.
20. Smith RA, Cokkinides V, Eyre HJ: American Cancer Society guidelines for the early detection of cancer, 2005. CA Cancer J Clin 55:31-44, 2005.
21. Eddy DM, Nugent FW, Eddy JF, et al: Screening for colorectal cancer in a high-risk population. Gastroenterology 92:682-692, 1987.
22. Glick S, Wagner JL, Johnson CD: Cost-effectiveness of double-contrast barium enema in screening for colorectal cancer. AJR 170:629-636, 1998.
23. Macari M, Bini EJ, Stacy L, et al: Colorectal polyps and cancers in asymptomatic average-risk patients: Evaluation with CT colonography. Radiology 230:629-636, 2004.
24. Pickhardt PJ, Choi JR, Nugent PA, et al: The effect of diagnostic confidence on the probability of optical colonoscopic confirmation of potential polyps detected on CT colonography: Prospective assessment in 1,339 asymptomatic adults. AJR 183:1661-1665, 2004.
25. Thoeni RF: Colorectal cancer: Radiological staging. Radiol Clin North Am 35:457-458, 1997.
26. Low RN, McCue M, Barone R, et al: MR staging of primary colorectal carcinoma: Comparison with surgical and histopathologic findings. Abdom Imaging 28:784-793, 2003.
27. Fuchsjager MH, Maier AG, Schima W, et al: Comparison of transrectal sonography and double-contrast MR imaging when staging rectal cancer. AJR 181:421-427, 2003.
28. Chen YK, Kao CH, Liao AC, et al: Colorectal cancer screening in asymptomatic adults: The role of FDG PET scan. Anticancer Res 23:4357-4361, 2003.
29. Levine MS, Laufer I: Rectum. In Laufer I, Levine MS (eds): Double Contrast Gastrointestinal Radiology, 2nd ed. Philadelphia, WB Saunders, 1992, pp 647-686.
30. Ott DJ, Chen YM, Gelfand DW, et al: Single-contrast vs. double-contrast barium enema in the detection of colonic polyps. AJR 146:993-996, 1986.
31. Fork FT, Lindstrom C, Ekelund GR: Reliability of routine double-contrast examination (DCE) of the large bowel in polyp detection: A prospective clinical study. Gastrointest Radiol 8:163-172, 1983.
32. Anderson ML, Heigh RI, McCoy GA, et al: Accuracy of assessment of the extent of examination by experienced colonoscopists. Gastrointest Endosc 38:560-563, 1992.
33. Rockey DC, Koch J, Yee J, et al: Prospective comparison of air-contrast barium enema and colonoscopy in patients with fecal occult blood: A pilot study. Gastrointest Endosc 60:953-958, 2004.
34. Law RL, Longstaff AJ, Slack N: A retrospective 5-year study on the accuracy of the barium enema examination performed by radiographers. Clin Radiol 54:80-83, 1999.
35. Rex DK, Rahmani EY, Haseman JH, et al: Relative sensitivity of colonoscopy and barium enema for detection of colorectal cancer in clinical practice. Gastroenterology 11:17-23, 1997.
36. Burling D, Halligan S, Atchley J, et al: CT colonography: Interpretative performance in a non-academic environment. Clin Radiol 62:424-429, 2007.
37. Ng CS, Doyle TC, Courtney HM, et al: Extracolonic findings in patients undergoing abdomino-pelvic CT for suspected colorectal carcinoma in the frail and disabled patient. Clin Radiol 59:421-430, 2004.
38. Valls C, Andia E, Sanchez A, et al: Hepatic metastases from colorectal cancer: Preoperative detection and assessment of resectability with helical CT. Radiology 218:55-60, 2001.
39. Bipat S, Glas AS, Slors FJ, et al: Rectal cancer: Local staging and assessment of lymph node involvement with endoluminal US, CT, and MR imaging—a meta-analysis. Radiology 232:773-783, 2004.
40. Klessen C, Rogalla P, Taupitz M: Local staging of rectal cancer: The current role of MRI. Eur Radiol 17:379-389, 2007.
41. Moffat FL, Gulec SA, Serafini AN, et al: A thousand points of light or just dim bulbs? Radiolabeled antibodies and colorectal cancer imaging. Cancer Invest 17:322-334, 1999.
42. Agnese DM, Abdessalam SF, Burak WE Jr, et al: Pilot study using a humanized CC49 monoclonal antibody (HuCC49DeltaCH2) to localize recurrent colorectal carcinoma. Ann Surg Oncol 11:197-202, 2004.
43. Even-Sapir E, Parag Y, Lerman H, et al: Detection of recurrence in patients with rectal cancer: PET/CT after abdominoperineal or anterior resection. Radiology 232:815-822, 2004.
44. Bernstein MA, Feczko PJ, Halpert RD, et al: Distribution of colonic polyps: Increased incidence of proximal lesions in older patients. Radiology 155:35-38, 1985.
45. Rubesin SE, Levine MS, Laufer I, et al: Villous adenomas: The scientific and the practical. Radiology 167:869-870, 1988.
46. Iida M, Iwashita A, Yao T, et al: Villous tumor of the colon: Correlation of histologic, macroscopic, and radiographic features. Radiology 167:673-677, 1988.
47. Delamarre J, Descombes P, Marti R, et al: Villous tumor of the colon: Double-contrast study of 47 cases. Gastrointest Radiol 5:69-73, 1980.
48. Miller WT Jr, Levine MS, Rubesin SE, et al: Bowler hat sign: A simple principle for differentiating polyps from diverticula. Radiology 173:615-617, 1989.
49. Iida M, Iwashita A, Yao T, et al: Villous tumor of the colon: Correlation of histologic, macroscopic and radiographic features. Radiology 167:673-677, 1988.
50. Rubesin SE, Sul SH, Laufer I, et al: Carpet lesions of the colon. RadioGraphics 5:537-552, 1985.
51. Kim DH, Pickhardt PJ, Taylor AJ: Characteristics of advanced adenomas detected at CT colonographic screening: Implications for appropriate polyp size thresholds for polypectomy versus surveillance. AJR 188:940-944, 2007.

52. Pikarsky A, Wexner S, Lebensart P, et al: The use of rectal ultrasound for the correct diagnosis and treatment of rectal villous tumors. Am J Surg 179:261-265, 2000.

53. Youker JE, Welin S, Main G: Computer analysis in the differentiation of benign and malignant polypoid lesions of the colon. Radiology 90:794-797, 1968.

54. Muto T, Bussey HJR, Morson BC: The evolution of cancer of the colon and rectum. Cancer 36:2251-2270, 1975.

55. Welin S, Youker J, Spratt JS Jr: The rates and patterns of growth of 375 tumors of the large intestine and rectum observed serially by double contrast enema study (Malmo technique). AJR 90:673-687, 1963.

56. Smith TR: Pedunculated malignant colonic polyps with superficial invasion of the stalk. Radiology 115:593-596, 1975.

57. Levine MS, Rubesin SE, Laufer I, et al. Diagnosis of colorectal neoplasms at double-contrast barium enema examination. Radiology 216:11-18, 2000.

58. McCarthy PA, Rubesin SE, Levine MS, et al: Colon cancer: Morphology detected by barium enema examination versus histopathologic stage. Radiology 197:683-687, 1995.

59. Fischel RE, Dermer R: Multifocal carcinoma of the large intestine. Clin Radiol 26:495-498, 1975.

60. Chong A, Shah JN, Levine MS, et al: The diagnostic yield of barium enema examination after incomplete colonoscopy. Radiology 223:620-624, 2002.

61. Gazelle GS, McMahon PM, Scholz FJ: Screening for colorectal cancer. Radiology 215:327-335, 2000.

62. Raskin MM, Viamonte M, Viamonte M Jr: Primary linitis plastica carcinoma of the colon. Radiology 113:17-22, 1974.

63. Laufer I, Joffe N: Some roentgenologic aspects of chronic perforating carcinoma of the colon. Dis Colon Rectum 16:127-135, 1973.

64. Kulinna C, Eibel R, Matzek W, et al: Staging of rectal cancer: Diagnostic potential of multiplanar reconstructions with MDCT. AJR 183:421-427, 2004.

65. Yee J, Thoeni RF, Gorczyka DP, et al: Value of contrast-enhanced MRI for TNM staging of regional disease in primary and recurrent rectal and rectosigmoid tumors. AJR 162:66, 1994.

66. Pema PJ, Bennett WF, Bova JG, et al: CT vs MRI in diagnosis of recurrent rectosigmoid carcinoma. J Comput Assist Tomogr 18:256-261, 1994.

67. Fong Y, Kemeny N, Paty P, et al: Treatment of colorectal cancer: hepatic metastases. Semin Surg Oncol 12:219-252, 1996.

68. Thoeni RF, Bangard C, Heller DND, et al: Dynamic CT versus MRI versus CTAP for diagnosing colorectal metastases: A cost comparison analysis. AJR 170:9, 1998.

69. Valls C, Lopez E, Guma A, et al: Helical CT versus CT arterial portography in the detection of hepatic metastasis of colorectal carcinoma. AJR 170:1341-1347, 1998.

70. Onishi H, Murakami T, Kim T, et al: Hepatic metastases: Detection with multi-detector row CT, SPIO-enhanced MR imaging, and both techniques combined. Radiology 239:131-138, 2006.

71. Semelka RC, Cance WG, Marcos HB, et al: Liver metastases: Comparison of current MR techniques and spiral CT during arterial portography for detection in 20 surgically staged cases. Radiology 213:86-91, 1999.

72. Kim YK, Ko SW, Hwang SB, et al: Detection and characterization of liver metastases: 16-slice multidetector computed tomography versus superparamagnetic iron oxide-enhanced magnetic resonance imaging. Eur Radiol 16:1337-1345, 2006.

73. Farouk R, Nelson H, Radice E, et al: Accuracy of computed tomography in determining resectability for locally and advanced primary or recurrent colorectal cancers. Am J Surg 175:283-287, 1998.

74. Chintapalli KN, Esola CC, Chopra S, et al: Pericolic mesenteric lymph nodes: An aid in distinguishing diverticulitis from cancer of the colon. AJR 169:1253-1255, 1997.

75. Goh V, Halligan S, Taylor SA, et al: Differentiation between diverticulitis and colorectal cancer: Quantitative CT perfusion measurements versus morphologic criteria—initial experience. Radiology 242:456-462, 2007.

76. Scharling ES, Wolfman NT, Bechtold RE: Computed tomography evaluation of colorectal carcinoma. Semin Roentgenol 31:125-141, 1996.

77. Sinha R, Verma R, Rajesh A, et al: Diagnostic value of multidetector row CT in rectal cancer staging: comparison of multiplanar and axial images with histopathology. Clin Radiol 61:924-931, 2006.

78. Frommhold W, Hubener KH: The role of computerized tomography in the after care of patients suffering from a carcinoma of the rectum. Comput Tomogr 5:161-168, 1981.

79. Lee JKT, Stanley RJ, Sagel SS, et al: CT appearance of the pelvis after abdomino-perineal resection for rectal carcinoma. Radiology 141:737-741, 1981.

80. Doubleday LC, Bernardino ME: CT findings in the perirectal area following radiation therapy. J Comput Assist Tomogr 4:634-638, 1980.

81. Colley DP, Farrell JA, Clark RA: Perforated colon carcinoma presenting as a suprarenal mass. J Comput Assist Tomogr 5:55-58, 1981.

82. Dukes CE: The classification of cancer of the rectum. J Pathol 35:323-332, 1932.

83. Astler VB, Coller FA: The prognostic significance of direct extension of carcinoma of the colon and rectum. Ann Surg 139:846-851, 1954.

84. Turnbull RB Jr: The no-touch isolation technique of resection. JAMA 231:1181-1182, 1975.

85. Thoeni RF, Moss AA, Schnyder P, et al: Detection and staging of primary rectal and rectosigmoid cancer by computed tomography. Radiology 141:135-138, 1981.

86. Compton CC, Fielding LP, Burgart LJ, et al: Prognostic factors in colorectal cancer. College of American Pathologists Consensus Statement 1999. Arch Pathol Lab Med 124:979-994, 2000.

87. Dixon AK, Fry IK, Morson BC, et al: Preoperative computed tomography of carcinoma of the rectum. Br J Radiol 54:655-659, 1981.

88. Grabbe E, Lierse W, Winkler R: The perirectal fascia: Morphology and use in staging of rectal carcinoma. Radiology 149:241-246, 1983.

89. Van Waes PF, Koehler PR, Feldberg MA: Management of rectal carcinoma: Impact of computed tomography. AJR 140:1137-1142, 1983.

90. Balthazar EJ, Megibow AJ, Hulnick D, et al: Carcinoma of the colon: Detection and preoperative staging by CT. AJR 150:301-306, 1988.

91. Kinkel K, Lu Y, Both M, et al: Detection of hepatic metastases from cancers of the gastrointestinal tract by using noninvasive imaging methods (US, CT, MR imaging, PET): A meta-analysis. Radiology 224:748-756, 2002.

92. Megibow AJ, Zerhouni EA, Hylnick DH, et al: Air insufflation of the colon as an adjunct to computed tomography of the pelvis. J Comput Assist Tomogr 8:797-800, 1984.

93. Gazelle GS, Saini S, Shellito P: Staging of colon carcinoma using water enemas CT. J Comput Assist Tomogr 19:87-91, 1995.

94. Hundt W, Braunschweig R, Reiser M: Evaluation of spiral CT in staging of colon and rectum carcinoma. Eur J Radiol 9:78-84, 1999.

95. Chiesura-Corona M, Muzzio PC, Giust G, et al: Rectal cancer: CT local staging with histopathologic correlation. Abdom Imaging 26:134-138, 2001.

96. Wieder HA, Rosenberg R, Lordick F, et al: Rectal cancer: MR imaging before neoadjuvant chemotherapy and radiation therapy for prediction of tumor-free circumferential resection margins and long-term survival. Radiology 2007 Apr 26 [Epub ahead of print].

97. Butch RJ, Stark DD, Wittenberg J, et al: Staging rectal cancer by MR and CT. AJR 146:1155-1160, 1986.

98. Beets-Tan RG, Beets GL, Vliegen RF, et al: Accuracy of magnetic resonance imaging in prediction of tumour-free resection margin in rectal cancer surgery. Lancet 357:497-504, 2001.

99. Brown G, Kirkham A, Williams GT, et al: High-resolution MRI of the anatomy important in total mesorectal excision of the rectum. AJR 182:431-439, 2004.

100. Blomqvist I, Rubio C, Holm T, et al: Rectal adenocarcinoma: Assessment of the lateral resection margin by MRI of resected specimens. Br J Radiol 72:18-23, 1999.

101. Bissett IP, Fernando CC, Hough DM, et al: Identification of the fascia propria by magnetic resonance imaging and its relevance to preoperative assessment of rectal cancer. Dis Colon Rectum 44:259-265, 2001.

102. Brown G, Radcliffe AG, Newcombe RG, et al: Preoperative assessment of prognostic factors in rectal cancer using high-resolution magnetic resonance imaging. Br J Surg 90:355-364, 2003.

103. Heald RJ, Ryall RD: Recurrence and survival after total mesorectal excision for rectal cancer. Lancet 1:1479-1482, 1986.

104. Akasu T, Iinuma G, Fujita T, et al: Thin-section MRI with a phased-array coil for preoperative evaluation of pelvic anatomy and tumor extent in patients with rectal cancer. AJR 184:531-538, 2005.

105. MERCURY Study Group: Extramural depth of tumor invasion at thin-section MR in patients with rectal cancer: Results of the MERCURY study. Radiology 243:132-139, 2007.

106. Beets-Tan RG, Beets GL: Rectal cancer: Review with emphasis on MR imaging. Radiology 232:335-346, 2004.

107. Dooms GC, Hricak H, Crooks LE, et al: Magnetic resonance imaging of the lymph nodes: Comparison with CT. Radiology 153:710-738, 1984.

108. Brown G, Richards CJ, Bourne MW, et al: Morphologic predictors of lymph node status in rectal cancer with use of high-spatial resolution MR imaging with histopathologic comparison. Radiology 227:371-377, 2003.

109. Birnbaum BA, Weinreb JC, Fernandez MP, et al: Comparison of contrast enhanced CT and Mn-DPDP enhanced MRI for detection of focal hepatic lesions: Initial findings. Clin Imaging 18:21-27, 1994.

110. Schwartz LH, Seltzer SE, Tempany CM, et al: Superparamagnetic iron oxide hepatic MR imaging: Efficacy and safety using conventional and fast spin-echo pulse sequences. J Magn Reson Imaging 5:566-570, 1995.

111. Improved survival with preoperative radiotherapy in resectable rectal cancer. Swedish Rectal Cancer Trial. N Engl J Med 336:980-987, 1997.

112. Gualdi GF, Casciani E, Guadalaxara A, et al: Local staging of rectal cancer with transrectal ultrasound and endorectal magnetic resonance imaging: Comparison with histologic findings. Dis Colon Rectum 43:338-345, 2000.

113. Zagoria RJ, Schlarb CA, Ott DJ, et al: Assessment of rectal tumor infiltration utilizing endorectal MR imaging and comparison with endoscopic rectal sonography. J Surg Oncol 64:312-317, 1997.

114. Maldjian C, Smith R, Kilger A, et al: Endorectal surface coil MR imaging as a staging technique for rectal carcinoma: A comparison study to rectal endosonography. Abdom Imaging 25:75-80, 2000.

115. Schnall MD, Furth EE, Rosato EF, et al: Rectal tumor stage: Correlation of endorectal MR imaging and pathologic findings. Radiology 190:709-714, 1994.

116. Beets-Tan RG, Beets GL, Borstlap AC, et al: Preoperative assessment of local tumor extent in advanced rectal cancer: CT or high-resolution MRI? Abdom Imaging 25:533-541, 2000.

117. Low RN, Barone RM, Lacey C, et al: Peritoneal tumor: MR imaging with dilute oral barium and intravenous gadolinium-containing contrast agents compared with unenhanced MR imaging and CT. Radiology 204:513-520, 1997.

118. Vliegen RF, Beets GL, von Meyenfeldt MF, et al: Rectal cancer: MR imaging in local staging—is gadolinium-based contrast material helpful? Radiology 234:179-188, 2005.

119. Chang GJ, Rodriguez-Bigas MA, Skibber JM, Moyer VA: Lymph node evaluation and survival after curative resection of colon cancer: systematic review. J Natl Cancer Inst 21:433-441, 2007.

120. de Lange EE, Gechner RE, Edge SB, et al: Preoperative staging of rectal carcinoma with MR imaging: Surgical and histopathologic correlation. Radiology 176:623-628, 1990.

121. Harisinghani MG, Saini S, Slater GJ, et al: MR imaging of pelvic lymph nodes in primary pelvic carcinoma with ultrasmall superparamagnetic iron oxide (Combidex): Preliminary observations. J Magn Reson Imaging 7:161-163, 1997.

122. Koh DM, Brown G, Temple L, et al: Rectal cancer: Mesorectal lymph nodes at MR imaging with USPIO versus histopathologic findings—initial observations. Radiology 231:91-99, 2004.

123. Kim S, Lim HK, Lee SJ, et al: Depiction and local staging of rectal tumors: Comparison of transrectal US before and after water installation. Radiology 231:117-122, 2004.

124. Fuchsjager MH, Maier AG, Schima W, et al: Comparison of transrectal sonography and double-contrast MR imaging when staging rectal cancer. AJR 181:421-427, 2003.

125. Sasaki Y, Niwa Y, Hirooka Y, et al: The use of endoscopic ultrasound-guided fine-needle aspiration for investigation of submucosal and extrinsic masses of the colon and rectum. Endoscopy 37:154-160, 2005.

126. Stergiou N, Haji-Kermani N, Schneider C, et al: Staging of colonic neoplasms by colonoscopic miniprobe ultrasonography. Int J Colorectal Dis 18:445-449, 2003.

127. Holdsworth PJ, Johnston D, Chalmers AG, et al: Endoluminal ultrasound and computed tomography in the staging of rectal cancer. Br J Surg 75:1019-1022, 1988.

128. Rifkin MD, Ehrlich SM, Marks G: Staging of rectal carcinoma: Prospective comparison of endorectal US and CT. Radiology 170:319-322, 1989.

129. Thaler W, Watzka S, Martin F, et al: Preoperative staging of rectal cancer by endoluminal ultrasound vs. magnetic resonance imaging: Preliminary results of a prospective, comparative study. Dis Colon Rectum 37:1189-1193, 1994.

130. Kim NK, Kim NJ, Yun SH, et al: Comparative study of transrectal ultrasonography, pelvic computerized tomography, and magnetic resonance imaging in preoperative staging of rectal cancer. Dis Colon Rectum 42:770-775, 1999.

131. Tio TL, Coene PPL, Van Delden OM, et al: Colorectal carcinoma: Preoperative TNM classification with endosonography. Radiology 179:165-170, 1991.

132. Marusch F, Koch A, Schmidt U, et al: Routine use of transrectal ultrasound in rectal carcinoma: Results of a prospective multicenter study. Endoscopy 34:385-390, 2002.

133. Wolfman NT, Ott DJ: Endoscopic ultrasonography. Semin Roentgenol 31:154-161, 1996.

134. Lim JH: Colorectal cancer: Sonographic findings. AJR 167:45-47, 1998.

135. Hulsmans FJ, Tio TL, Fockens P, et al: Assessment of tumor infiltration depth in rectal cancer with transrectal sonography: Caution is necessary [see comments]. Radiology 190:715-720, 1994.

136. Hünerbein M, Schlag PM: Three-dimensional endosonography for staging of rectal cancer. Ann Surg 225:432-843, 1997.

137. Ivanov KD, Diavoc CD: Three-dimensional endoluminal ultrasound: New staging technique in patients with rectal cancer. Dis Colon Rectum 40:47-50, 1997.

138. Delaloye B, Bischof-Delaloye A, Buchegger F, et al: Detection of colorectal carcinoma by emission computerized tomography after injection of I-123 labeled Fab or F(ab1)2 fragments from monoclonal anti-carcinoembryonic antigen antibodies. J Clin Invest 77:301-311, 1986.

139. Agnese DM, Abdessalam SF, Burak WE Jr, et al: Pilot study using a humanized CC49 monoclonal antibody (HuCC49DeltaCH2) to localize recurrent colorectal carcinoma. Ann Surg Oncol 11:197-202, 2004.

140. Avital S, Haddad R, Troitsa A, et al: Radioimmunoguided surgery for recurrent colorectal cancer manifested by isolated CEA elevation. Cancer 89:1692-1698, 2000.

141. Hansen JE, Fischer LK, Chan G, et al: Antibody-mediated p53 protein therapy prevents liver metastasis in vivo. Cancer Res 67:1769-1774, 2007.

142. Baranda J, Williamson S: The new paradigm in the treatment of colorectal cancer: Are we hitting the right target? Expert Opin Investig Drugs 16:311-324, 2007.

143. Manayan RC, Hart MJ, Friend WG: Radioimmunoguided surgery for colorectal cancer. Am J Surg 173:386-389, 1997.

144. Cote RJ, Houchens DP, Hitchcock CL, et al: Intraoperative detection of occult colon cancer micrometastases using ^{125}I-radiolabled monoclonal antibody CC49. Cancer 77:613-620, 1996.

145. Mach JP, Buchegger F, Forni M, et al: Use of radiolabeled monoclonal anti-CEA antibodies for the detection of human carcinomas by external photoscanning and tomoscintigraphy. Immunol Today 2:239-249, 1981.

146. Abdel-Nabi HH, Schwartz AN, Higano CS, et al: Colorectal carcinoma detection with indium-111 anticarcinoembryonic antigen monoclonal antibody ZCE 025. Radiology 164:617-621, 1987.

147. Patt YZ, Lamki LM, Haynie TP, et al: Improved tumor localization with increasing dose of indium-111–labeled anti-carcinoembryonic antigen monoclonal antibody ZCE-025 in metastatic colorectal cancer. J Clin Oncol 6:1220-1230, 1988.

148. Lunniss PJ, Skinner S, Britton KE, et al: Effect of radioimmunoscintigraphy on the management of recurrent colorectal cancer. Br J Surg 86:244-249, 1999.

149. Collier BD, Abdel-Nabi H, Doerr RJ, et al: Immunoscintigraphy performed with In-111–labeled CYT-103 in the management of colorectal cancer: Comparison with CT. Radiology 185:179-186, 1992.

150. Lamki LM, Patt YZ, Rosenblum MG, et al: Metastatic colorectal cancer: Radioimmunoscintigraphy with a stabilized In-111–labeled F(ab')2 fragment of an anti-CEA monoclonal antibody. Radiology 174:147-151, 1990.

151. Gu J, Zhao J, Li Z, et al: Clinical application of radioimmunoguided surgery in colorectal cancer using ^{125}I-labeled carcinoembryonic antigen-specific monoclonal antibody submucosally. Dis Colon Rectum 46:1659-1966, 2003.

152. Okuno T, Fu KI, Sano Y, et al: Early colon cancers detected by FDG-PET: A report of two cases with immunohistochemical investigation. Hepatogastroenterology 51:1323-1325, 2004.

153. Hany TF, Steinert HC, Goerres GW, et al: PET diagnostic accuracy: Improvement with in-line PET-CT system: Initial results. Radiology 225:575-581, 2002.

154. Miraldi F, Vesselle H, Faulhaber PF, et al: Elimination of artifactual accumulation of FDG in PET imaging of colorectal cancer. Clin Nucl Med 23:3-7, 1998.

155. Rohren EM, Turkington TG, Coleman RE: Clinical applications of PET in oncology. Radiology 231:305-332, 2004.

156. Flanagan FL, Dehdashti F, Ogunbiyi OA, et al: Utility of FDG-PET for investigating unexplained plasma CEA elevation in patients with colorectal cancer. Ann Surg 227:319-323, 1998.

157. Schaefer O, Langer M: Detection of recurrent rectal cancer with CT, MRI and PET/CT. Eur Radiol 2007 Apr 3 [Epub ahead of print].

158. Moore HG, Akhurst T, Larson SM, et al: A case-controlled study of 18-fluorodeoxyglucose positron emission tomography in the detection of pelvic recurrence in previously irradiated rectal cancer patients. J Am Coll Surg 197:22-28, 2003.

159. Belkacemi Y, Lartigau E, Kerrou K, et al: The contribution of PET to radiation treatment planning. Bull Cancer 94:99-108, 2007.
160. Ishimori T, Patel PV, Wahl RL: Detection of unexpected additional primary malignancies with PET/CT. J Nucl Med 46:752-757, 2005.
161. Chen YK, Kao CH, Liao AC, et al: Colorectal cancer screening in asymptomatic adults: The role of FDG PET scan. Anticancer Res 23:4357-4361, 2003.
162. Gutman F, Alberini JL, Wartski M, et al: Incidental colonic focal lesions detected by FDG PET/CT. AJR 185:495-500, 2005.
163. Rydzewski B, Dehdashti F, Gordon BA, et al: Usefulness of intraoperative sonography for revealing hepatic metastases from colorectal cancer in patients selected for surgery after undergoing FDG PET. AJR 178:353-358, 2002.
164. Blodgett TM, Meltzer CC, Townsend DW: PET/CT: Form and function. Radiology 242:360-385, 2007.
165. Mang T, Maier A, Plank C, et al: Pitfalls in multi-detector row CT colonography: A systematic approach. RadioGraphics 27:431-454, 2007.
166. Macari M, Bini EJ, Jacobs SL, et al: Significance of missed polyps at CT colonography. AJR 183:127-134, 2004.
167. Kelvin FM, Maglinte DT: Colorectal carcinoma: A radiologic and clinical review. Radiology 164:1-8, 1987.
168. Zinkin LD: A critical review of the classifications and staging of colorectal cancer. Dis Colon Rectum 26:37-43, 1983.
169. Nauta R, Stablein D, Holyoke D: Survival of patients with stage B2 colon carcinoma: The gastrointestinal tumor study group experience. Arch Surg 124:180-182, 1989.
170. Durdey P, Williams NS: The effect of malignant and inflammatory fixation of rectal carcinoma on prognosis after rectal excision. Br J Surg 71:787-790, 1984.
171. Giess CS, Schwartz LH, Bach AM, et al: Patterns of neoplastic spread in colorectal cancer: Implications for surveillance CT studies. AJR 170:987-991, 1998.
172. Hamlin DF, Burgener FA, Sischy B: New techniques to stage early rectal carcinoma by computed tomography. Radiology 141:539-540, 1981.
173. Figueredo A, Rumble RB, Maroun J, et al: Follow-up of patients with curatively resected colorectal cancer: A practice guideline. BMC Cancer 3:26-31, 2003.
174. Shauffer IA, Sequeira J: Suture granuloma simulating recurrent carcinoma. AJR 128:856-857, 1977.
175. Daly BD, Crowley BM: Radiological appearances of colonic ring staple anastomoses. Br J Radiol 62:256-259, 1989.
176. Chen YM, Ott DJ, Wolfman NT, et al: Recurrent colorectal carcinoma: Evaluation with barium enema examination and CT. Radiology 163:307-310, 1987.
177. McCarthy SM, Barnes D, Deveney K, et al: Detection of recurrent rectosigmoid carcinoma: Prospective evaluation of CT and clinical factors. AJR 144:577-579, 1985.
178. Sharpe M, Golden R: End-to-end anastomosis of the colon following resection: a Roentgen study of 42 cases. AJR 64:769-777, 1950.
179. Fleischner FG, Berenberg AL: Recurrent carcinoma of the colon at the site of anastomosis. Radiology 66:540-547, 1956.
180. Welch JP, Donaldson GA: Detection and treatment of recurrent cancer of the colon and rectum. Am J Surg 135:505-511, 1978.
181. Thoeni RF, Moss AA: The gastrointestinal tract. In Moss AA, Gamsu G, Genant H (eds): Computed Tomography of the Body. Philadelphia, WB Saunders, 1992, pp 643-734.
182. Kelvin FM, Korobkin M, Breiman RS, et al: Recurrent rectal carcinoma in an asymptomatic patient. J Comput Assist Tomogr 6:186-188, 1982.
183. Shoemaker D, Black R, Giles L, et al: Yearly colonoscopy, liver CT, and chest radiography do not influence 5-year survival of colorectal cancer patients. Gastroenterology 114:7-14, 1998.
184. Kjeldsen BJ, Kronborg O, Fenger C, et al: Careful follow-up for patients undergoing curative resections in colorectal carcinoma: How careful is "careful"? Br J Surg 84:666-669, 1997.
185. Stulc JP, Petrelli NJ, Herrera L, et al: Anastomotic recurrence of adenocarcinoma of the colon. Arch Surg 121:1077-1080, 1986.
186. Flamen P, Stroobants S, Van Cutsem E, et al: Additional value of whole body positron emission tomography with fluorine-18-2-fluoro-2-deoxy-D-glucose in recurrent colorectal cancer. J Clin Oncol 17:894-901, 1999.
187. Peethambaram P, Weiss M, Loprinzi CL, et al: An evaluation of postoperative follow-up tests in colon cancer patients treated for cure. Oncology 54:287-292, 1997.
188. Earls JP, Colon-Negron E, Dachman AH: Colorectal carcinoma in young patients: CT detection of an atypical pattern of recurrence. Abdom Imaging 19:441-445, 1994.
189. Olson RM, Perencevich P, Malcolm AW, et al: Patterns of recurrence following curative resection of adenocarcinoma of the colon and rectum. Cancer 45:2969-2974, 1980.
190. Christoforidis E, Kanellos I, Tsachalis T, et al: Locally recurrent rectal cancer after curative resection. Tech Coloproctol 8(Suppl 1):s132-s134, 2004.
191. Moore HG, Shoup M, Riedel E, et al: Colorectal cancer pelvic recurrences: Determinants of resectability. Dis Colon Rectum 47:1599-1606, 2004.
192. Cass AW, Million RR, Pfaff W: Patterns of recurrence following surgery alone for adenocarcinoma of the colon and rectum. Cancer 37:1861-1865, 1976.
193. Ntinas A, Zambas N, Al Mograbi S, et al: Postoperative follow-up of patients with colorectal cancer: A combined evaluation of CT scan, colonoscopy and tumour markers. Tech Coloproctol 8(Suppl 1): S190-S192, 2004.
194. Husband JE, Hodson NJ, Parsons CA: The use of computed tomography in recurrent rectal tumors. Radiology 134:677-682, 1980.
195. Ellert J, Kreel L: The value of CT in malignant colonic tumors. J Comput Assist Tomogr 4:225-240, 1980.
196. Moss AA, Thoeni RF, Schnyder P, et al: Value of computed tomography in the detection and staging of recurrent rectal carcinomas. J Comput Assist Tomogr 5:870-874, 1981.
197. Adalsteinsson B, Glimelius B, Graffman S, et al: Computed tomography of recurrent renal carcinoma Acta Radiol Diagn 22:669-672, 1981.
198. Bachmann G, Pfeifer T, Bauer T: [MRT and dynamic CT in the diagnosis of a recurrence of rectal carcinoma]. Rofo Fortschr Geb Rontgenstr Neuen Bildgeb Verfahr 161:214-219, 1994.
199. Chen YM, Ott DJ, Wolfman N: Recurrent colorectal carcinoma evaluation with barium enema examination and CT. Radiology 163:307-310, 1987.
200. Selzner M, Hany TF, Wildbrett P, et al: Does the novel PET/CT imaging modality impact on the treatment of patients with metastatic colorectal cancer of the liver? Ann Surg 240:1027-1034, 2004.
201. Reznek RH, White FE, Young JW, et al: The appearances on computed tomography after abdomino-perineal resection for carcinoma of the rectum: A comparison between the normal appearances and those of recurrence. Br J Radiol 56:237-240, 1983.
202. Kelvin FM, Korobkin M, Heaston DK, et al: The pelvis after surgery for rectal carcinoma: Serial CT observations with emphasis on non-neoplastic features. AJR 141:959-964, 1983.
203. Moriya Y, Sugihara K, Akasu T, et al: Importance of extended lymphadenectomy with lateral node dissection for advanced lower rectal cancer. World J Surg 21:728-732, 1997.
204. Kapiteijn E, Maarijnen CA, Nagtegaal ID, et al: Preoperative radiotherapy combined with total mesorectal excision for resectable rectal cancer. N Engl J Med 345: 638-646, 2001.
205. Torricelli P, Pecchi A, Luppi G, et al: Gadolinium-enhanced MRI with dynamic evaluation in diagnosing the local recurrence of rectal cancer. Abdom Imaging 28:19-27, 2003.
206. Robinson P, Carrington BM, Swindell R, et al: Recurrent or residual pelvic bowel cancer: Accuracy of MRI local extent before salvage surgery. Clin Radiol 57:514-522, 2002.
207. Ebner F, Kressel HY, Mintz MC, et al: Tumor recurrence versus fibrosis in the female pelvis: Differentiation with MR imaging at 1.5 T. Radiology 166:333-340, 1988.
208. Gomberg JS, Friedman AC, Radecki PD: MRI differentiation of recurrent colorectal carcinoma from postoperative fibrosis. Gastrointest Radiol 11:361-363, 1986.
209. Glazer HS, Lee JKT, Levitt RG, et al: Radiation fibrosis: Differentiation from recurrent tumor by MR imaging. Radiology 156:721-726, 1985.
210. Yamashita S, Masui T, Katayama M, et al: T2-weighted MRI of rectosigmoid carcinoma: Comparison of respiratory-triggered fast spin-echo, breathhold fast-recovery fast spin-echo, and breathhold single-shot fast spin-echo sequences. J Magn Reson Imaging 25:511-516, 2007.
211. Heiken JP, Lee JKT: MR imaging of the pelvis. Radiology 166:11-16, 1988.
212. Ebner F, Kressel HY, Mintz MC, et al: Tumor recurrence versus fibrosis in the female pelvis: Differentiation with MR imaging at 1.5T. Radiology 166:333-340, 1988.
213. Rafto SE, Amendola MA, Gefter WB: MR imaging of recurrent colorectal carcinoma versus fibrosis. J Comput Assist Tomogr 12:521-523, 1988.
214. Sugimura K, Carrington BM, Quivey JM, et al: Postirradiation changes in the pelvis: Assessment with MR imaging. Radiology 175:805-813, 1990.

215. De Lange EE, Fechner RE, Wanebo HJ: Suspected recurrent rectosigmoid carcinoma after abdominoperineal resection: MR imaging and histopathologic findings. Radiology 170:323-328, 1989.

216. Markus J, Morrissey B, deGara C, et al: MRI of recurrent rectosigmoid carcinoma. Abdom Imaging 22:338-342, 1997.

217. Dicle O, Obuz F, Cakmakci H: Differentiation of recurrent rectal cancer and scarring with dynamic MR imaging. Br J Radiol 72:1155-1159, 1999.

218. Stueckle CA, Koenig M, Haegele KF, et al. [Contrast media kinetic in multi-slice helical CT cannot detect rectal cancer recurrence with certainty] Rofo 177:893-899, 2005.

219. Sahani DV, Kalva SP, Hamberg LM, et al: Assessing tumor perfusion and treatment response in rectal cancer with multisection CT: Initial observations. Radiology 234:785-792, 2005.

220. Assenat E, Thezenas S, Samalin E, et al: The value of endoscopic rectal ultrasound in predicting the lateral clearance and outcome in patients with lower-third rectal adenocarcinoma. Endoscopy 39:309-313, 2007.

221. Baulieu F, Bourlier P, Scotto B, et al: The value of immunoscintigraphy in the detection of recurrent colorectal cancer. Nucl Med Commun 22:1295-1304, 2001.

222. Yao YF, Yang Z, Li ZF, et al: Immunoscintigraphy of local recurrent rectal cancer with (99m)Tc-labeled anti-CEA monoclonal antibody CL58. World J Gastroenterol 12:1841-1846, 2007.

Other Tumors of the Colon

Stephen E. Rubesin, MD • Emma E. Furth, MD

This chapter discusses a variety of benign and malignant tumors of the colon as separate entities. Although these tumors are associated with a wide range of clinical and radiologic manifestations, they may have typical features on imaging studies that suggest the correct diagnosis.

LYMPHOMA

Pathologic Findings

Malignant lymphomas involve the gastrointestinal tract either as primary neoplasms or as part of a disseminated disease. The colon is the third most common primary site of lymphoma involving the gastrointestinal tract (after the stomach and small bowel); colonic involvement occurs in 6% to 12% of cases.[1-3] Primary lymphoma of the colon is rare, comprising less than 1% of all primary malignant tumors of the colon.[4,5] Colonic involvement by systemic lymphoma is relatively common, with microscopic evidence of tumor in up to 44% of cases at autopsy.[3] However, patients with disseminated lymphoma involving the colon are usually asymptomatic and do not undergo barium studies. Non-Hodgkin's lymphoma accounts for almost all colonic lymphomas; Hodgkin's disease involving the colon is extremely rare.[1,6,7] Large cell lymphoma is the most common primary non-Hodgkin's lymphoma subtype.[2]

Clinical Findings

Primary non-Hodgkin's lymphoma involving the colon is usually seen in middle-aged or elderly persons.[2] Males are more frequently affected than females by a ratio of 2:1.[6,8] Abdominal pain, weight loss, and altered bowel habits occur in 60% to 90% of patients, and rectal bleeding or diarrhea occur in 25%.[6,9] Long-standing ulcerative colitis appears to be a predisposing condition, but the development of lymphoma in these patients may be related more to treatment with immunosuppressive agents than to the disease itself.[6,8,10-12] Extranodal presentation of post-transplant lymphoproliferative disorders is typical, and B-cell lymphomas may arise in the colon after solid organ transplantation.[13] A palpable abdominal mass is the most frequent physical finding.[6]

Radiographic Findings and Differential Diagnosis

The primary form of colonic lymphoma usually involves the ileocecal valve, cecum, or rectum.[12-15] In contrast, systemic lymphoma usually involves the entire colon or long segments of bowel.[7,16-18] The primary, localized form of colonic lymphoma may be manifested by a variety of radiographic findings, including a polypoid or cavitary mass or circumferential mural lesion.

Bulky polypoid masses represent the most common form of primary colonic lymphoma.[5,9,18-20] These tumors usually appear as smooth-surfaced, broad-based, sessile lesions with or without central depressions or ulcerations.[14] These lesions vary from 4 to 20 cm and are most frequently located near the ileocecal valve (Fig. 64-1).[15] Extension of cecal lymphoma into the terminal ileum is not uncommon (Fig. 64-2).

The annular, infiltrating form of colonic lymphoma usually involves a long segment of colon, appearing as a concentric area of narrowing (Fig. 64-3) or as a cavitary mass (Fig. 64-4).[5,20] Although the colonic lumen may be narrowed, obstruction is uncommon. The infiltrating form is usually characterized by a discrete lesion with thickened, irregular haustral folds and a nodular surface pattern. Although the contour is irregular, the mucosal surface is smooth, suggesting submucosal infiltration rather than mucosal ulceration (Fig. 64-5). Thus, the major considerations in the differential diagnosis of the annular, infiltrating form of lymphoma include submucosal hemorrhage and edema (caused by ischemia or a bleeding diathesis) and an unusual colonic carcinoma.[5]

Large infiltrating tumors may extend into the mesentery or exhibit central cavitation, resulting in a bulky, cavitary mass lesion. The major considerations in the differential diagnosis of the cavitary form of lymphoma include a perforated colonic carcinoma and a mesenchymal tumor such as a gastrointestinal stromal tumor.

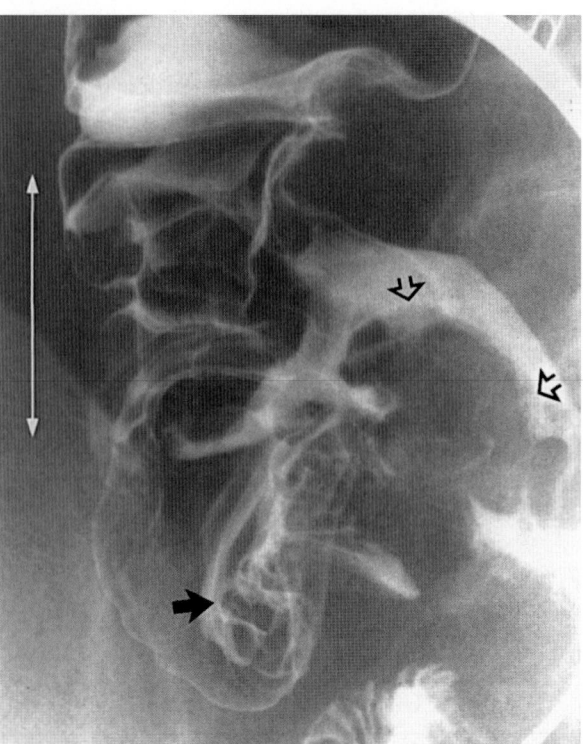

Figure 64-2. Lymphoma of the ileocecal valve and terminal ileum. Spot image from a double-contrast barium enema shows thickened, lobulated folds encircling the cecum and proximal ascending colon (*double-ended arrow*). Nodular mucosa (*solid arrow*) is seen near the insertion of the appendix into the cecum. A lobulated mass (*open arrows*) encroaches on the lumen of the terminal ileum.

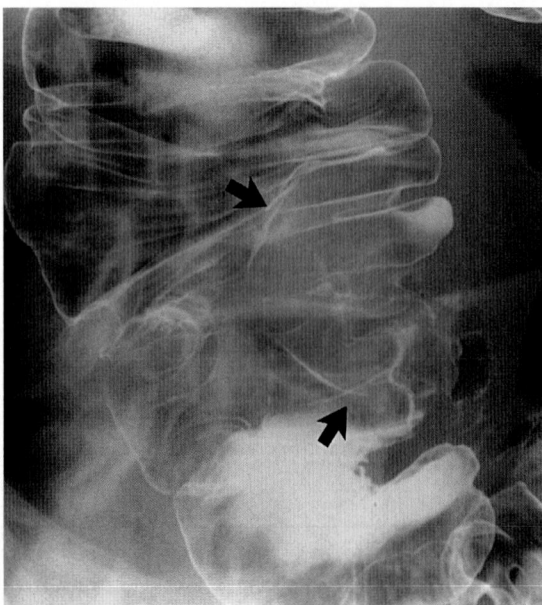

Figure 64-1. Lymphoma of the ileocecal valve. Spot image from a double-contrast barium enema shows a smooth-surfaced mass (*arrows*) replacing the ileocecal valve.

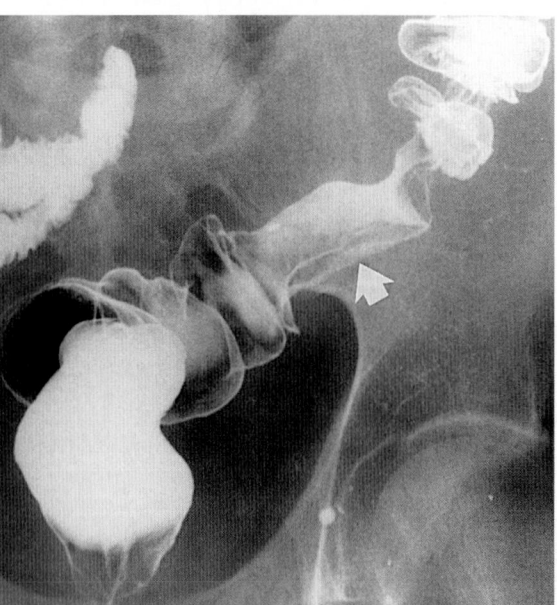

Figure 64-3. Lymphoma of the sigmoid colon. A relatively smooth-surfaced concentric lesion (*arrow*) is seen in the sigmoid colon. The distal margin is abrupt, and the proximal margin is tapered. The amount of luminal narrowing is mild for the size and length of the lesion. (Courtesy of Seth N. Glick, MD, Philadelphia, PA.)

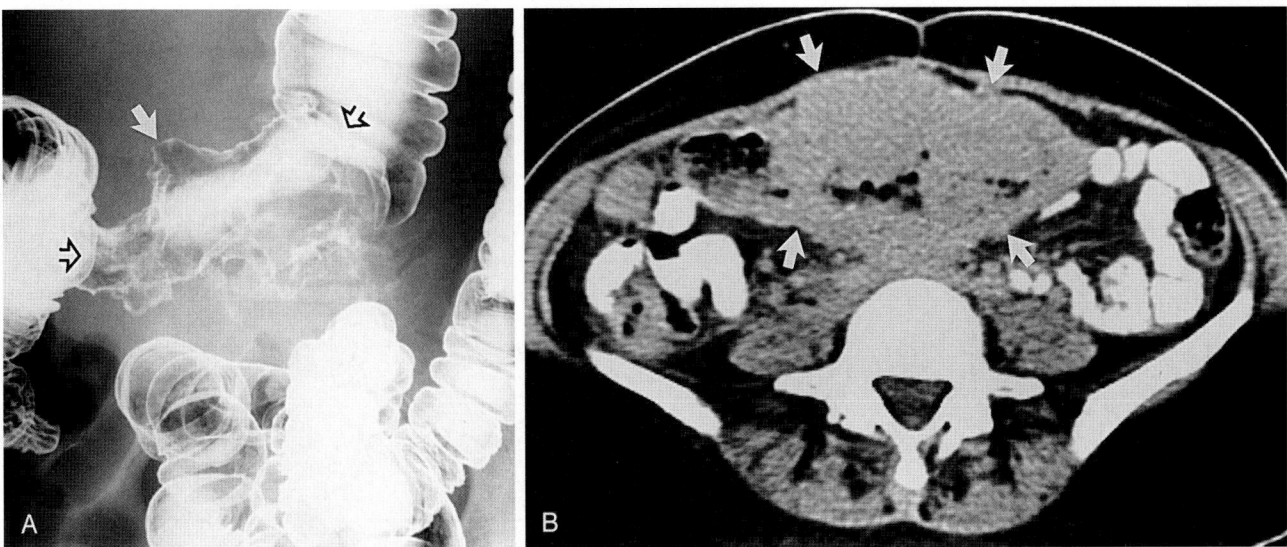

Figure 64-4. Lymphoma of the transverse colon. A. Spot image from a double-contrast barium enema shows a long (limits denoted by *open arrows*), concentric lesion in the transverse colon with an irregular contour. Note protrusion of the contour superiorly outside the expected lumen of the bowel (*white arrow*); this finding indicates cavitation of the mass. **B.** CT shows a large soft tissue mass (*arrows*) with lobular thickening of the walls of the transverse colon.

The diffuse, multinodular form of colonic lymphoma (lymphomatous polyposis) is associated with disseminated disease from a nodal primary lymphoma or occurs as a true primary gastrointestinal lymphoma. Histologically, this form of lymphoma is usually a mantle cell lymphoma derived from a subpopulation of mantle zone cells.[21,22] These multinodular lymphomas involve long segments of the colon or the entire colon. The tumors disseminate rapidly to the liver, spleen, peripheral lymph nodes, and bone marrow.[22] More than 100 nonuniform, smooth, sessile nodules varying from 2 to 25 mm carpet the colonic surface (Fig. 64-6).[15,19] The nodules are occasionally elongated, pedunculated, umbilicated, or filiform.[19] A conglomerate cecal mass is seen in almost 50% of cases.[19] Associated mesenteric lymph nodes are usually enlarged.[22] The multinodular form of colonic lymphoma may be confused radiographically with familial polyposis, lymphoid hyperplasia, inflammatory bowel disease, or infectious diseases such as pseudomembranous colitis or schistosomiasis. However, the nodules of colonic lymphoma are nonuniform and relatively large in comparison to the uniform, 1- to 2-mm nodules of lymphoid hyperplasia. Unlike the pseudopolyposis in inflammatory bowel disease, the haustral pattern also is preserved in colonic lymphoma and ulceration is uncommon.[7,15] Conglomerate cecal masses are more frequent in

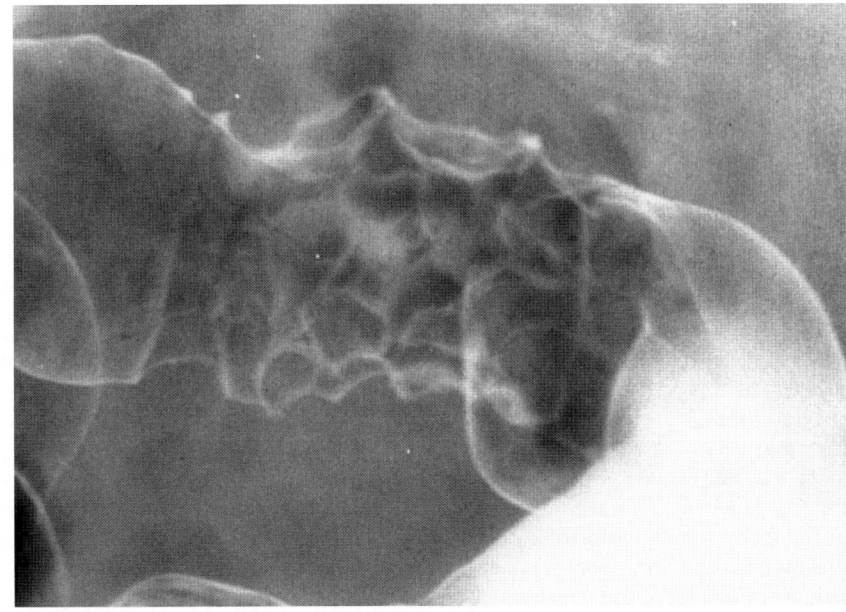

Figure 64-5. Lymphoma of the sigmoid colon. Spot image from a double-contrast barium enema shows an irregular, lobulated contour, although the overlying mucosa is smooth. This appearance is typical of a submucosally infiltrating lesion such as a lymphoma or hemangioma. (From Laufer I, Levine MS [eds]: Double Contrast Gastrointestinal Radiology. Philadelphia, WB Saunders, 1992.)

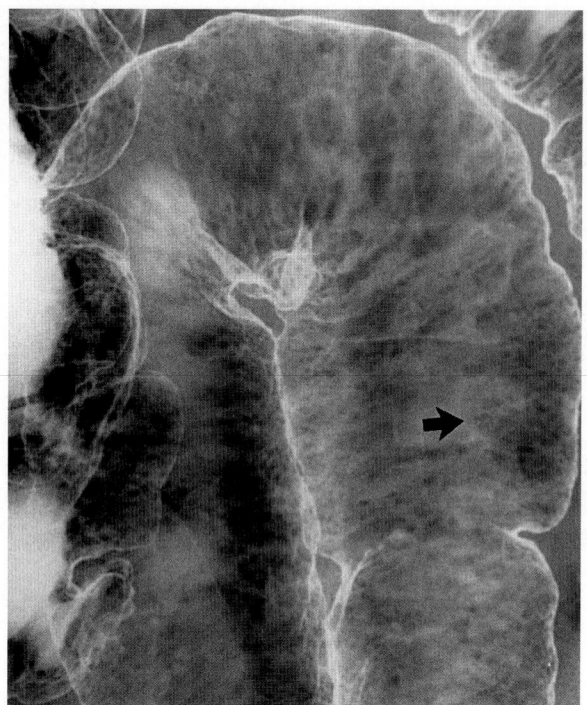

Figure 64-6. Disseminated lymphoma of the colon. Spot image from a double-contrast barium enema shows innumerable small (1 to 3 mm), nonuniform nodules (representative area shown by *arrow*) carpeting the surface of the sigmoid colon. This is an unusual appearance for disseminated lymphoma involving the colon, because the nodules tend to be larger.

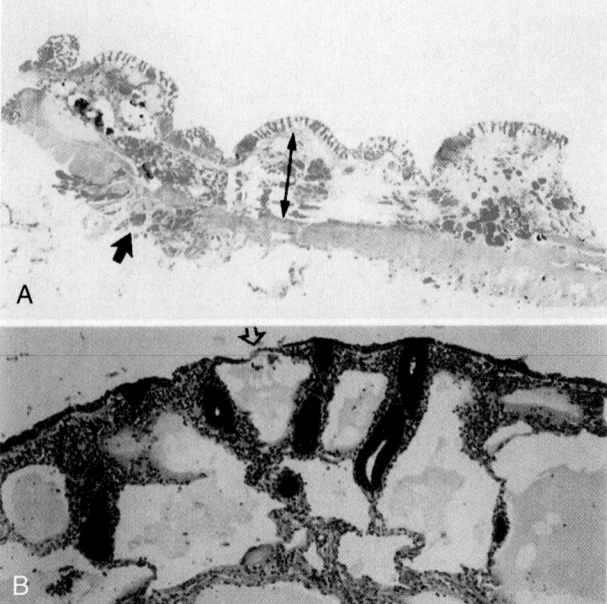

Figure 64-7. Hemangioma of the colon. A. Low-power view of the rectosigmoid colon shows an undulating mucosal surface caused by widening of the submucosa (*double-ended arrow*). At this power, the submucosa is seen to be expanded by blood-filled spaces, which extend to the subserosal fat in one area (*arrow*). **B.** Medium-power view of the mucosa from the same lesion shows large cystic spaces lined by endothelial cells and separated by loose connective tissue. The cavernous spaces extend to the mucosal surface (*arrow*).

disseminated lymphoma than in the polyposis syndromes.[7,19] Rarely, diffuse colonic lymphoma may be associated with acute toxic dilatation or pneumatosis coli.[15]

VASCULAR LESIONS

Hemangioma

Clinical and Pathologic Findings

Hemangiomas of the colon are rare vascular lesions, but the radiologic diagnosis is important because these lesions may be misdiagnosed at endoscopy and have a high mortality rate related to severe gastrointestinal bleeding.[23] Patients with colonic hemangiomas usually present at a young age with acute, recurrent, or chronic rectal bleeding.[24,25] Some patients may have severe, life-threatening rectal bleeding[25]; mortality rates for this tumor approach 50%.[26] Obstructive symptoms and diarrhea are uncommon, occurring in 15% to 20% of cases.[24,27] Occasionally, patients with anorectal lesions may complain of tenesmus or constipation.

Cavernous hemangiomas are the most common form; capillary hemangiomas are second in frequency.[27,28] Cavernous hemangiomas are unencapsulated lesions, usually arising in the submucosa (Fig. 64-7). They are composed of large, multiloculated, thin-walled vessels[26] separated by loose connective tissue (see Fig. 64-7). Cavernous hemangiomas usually occur in the rectum or sigmoid colon,[29] appearing as discrete submucosal masses[27] or, more frequently, as diffuse, infiltrative lesions.[25] Polypoid tumors may intussuscept, causing obstruction, whereas infiltrative lesions often ulcerate and bleed.[25]

Capillary hemangiomas usually occur as solitary, sharply circumscribed submucosal masses in asymptomatic patients. The tumors are composed of small vessels lined by well-differentiated endothelial cells.[26] The vessels are packed together, with scant surrounding connective tissue. These tumors are occasionally associated with cutaneous or visceral hemangiomas.[25,30] Colonic hemangiomas may occur in the Klippel-Trenaunay syndrome, manifested by the triad of cutaneous hemangiomas, soft tissue hypertrophy of the involved lower extremity, and congenital varicose veins.[29,31] Cavernous hemangiomas of the colon are also seen in the blue rubber bleb nevus syndrome and in some patients with Peutz-Jeghers syndrome.[32] Hemangiomas have also been reported in 5% to 8% of patients with Turner's syndrome.[33] Colonic hemangiomas have no propensity for malignant transformation and should therefore be distinguished from their true neoplastic counterpart—angiosarcomas.

Radiographic Findings and Differential Diagnosis

Rectal hemangiomas are frequently misdiagnosed on endoscopy as hemorrhoids or proctitis.[26,34] As a result, the radiologist is often the first physician to suggest the correct diagnosis. Plain abdominal radiographs may show multiple phleboliths along the course of the bowel in 50% of cases.[25,26,30] Hemangiomas should therefore be suspected if abdominal radiographs demonstrate phleboliths in young patients with gastrointestinal bleeding or clusters of phleboliths in atypical locations or along the expected course of the rectosigmoid colon.

Barium enema examinations usually reveal a circumferential lesion with scalloped contours and a nodular mucosal

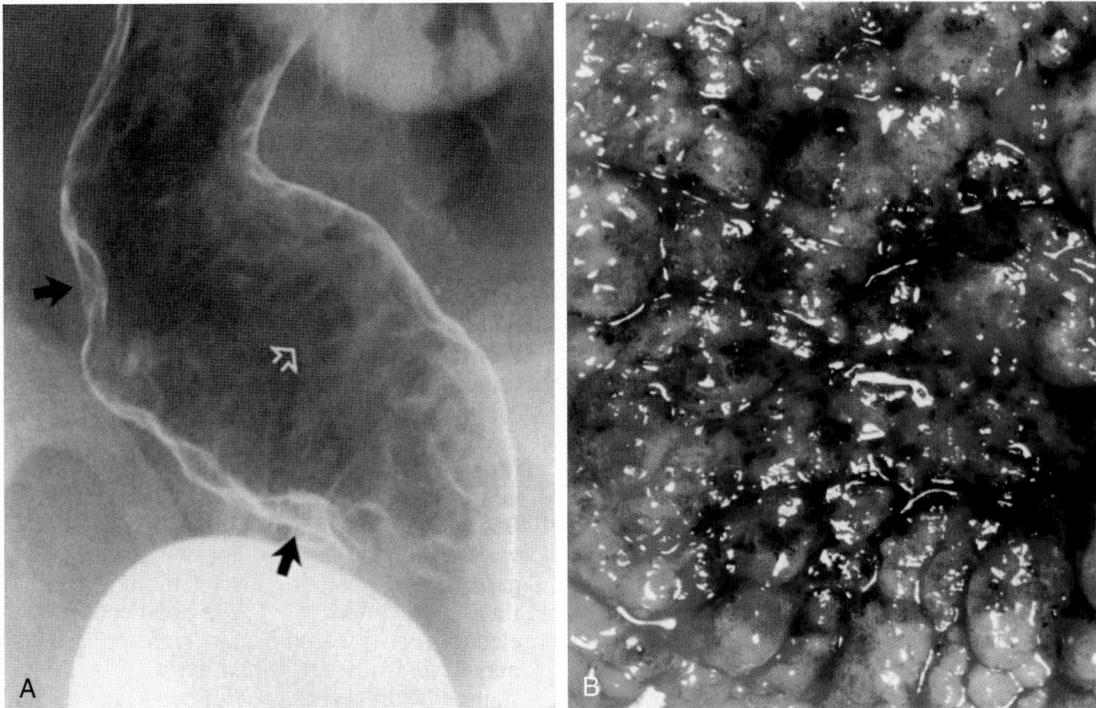

Figure 64-8. Hemangioma of the colon. A. Prone, angled view of the rectosigmoid junction shows a subtle circumferential lesion with a lobulated contour (*solid arrows*) and a finely lobulated mucosal surface (*open arrow*). **B.** Close-up photograph of the mucosal surface of the hemangioma shows a lobulated surface with areas of focal hemorrhage. This corresponds to the smooth surface lobulation seen on the radiograph. (**A** from Margulis AR: Case: Cavernous hemangioma of the rectum. Gastrointest Radiol 6:363-364, 1981.)

surface pattern (Fig. 64-8).[25] The colonic lumen is narrowed in 50% of cases. If the tumor is in its usual rectosigmoid location, a wide presacral space may be seen. If phleboliths are visible, they are seen in the expected location of the colonic tumor (Fig. 64-9).[29] The polypoid form of hemangioma is usually manifested by smooth, sessile, broad-based submucosal masses.

Although hemangiomas are usually vascular at angiography, they may occasionally be hypovascular or avascular because of vessel thrombosis and sclerosis.[23] CT better delineates the true dimensions of the mass (see Fig. 64-9) and involvement of adjacent structures such as the urinary bladder.[30]

Although hemangioma is included in the differential diagnosis of polypoid submucosal masses, the most common submucosal mass in the colon is a lipoma. Hemangioma is also included in the differential diagnosis of infiltrative submucosal rectosigmoid lesions such as those found in solitary rectal ulcer syndrome or lymphoma. However, the clinical history and the presence of phleboliths should suggest the correct diagnosis.

Lymphangioma

Lymphangiomas of the colon are extremely rare benign lesions of neoplastic or hamartomatous origin.[35] The lesions are composed of a cluster of lymphatic spaces lined by endothelial cells and separated by connective tissue septa.[32] These dilated lymphatics are usually found in the muscularis mucosae or submucosa. Patients with colonic lymphangiomas usually present in the fourth to sixth decades of life with abdominal pain, rectal bleeding, watery diarrhea, or altered bowel habits.[36] Lymphangiomas may appear radiographically as solitary, 2- to

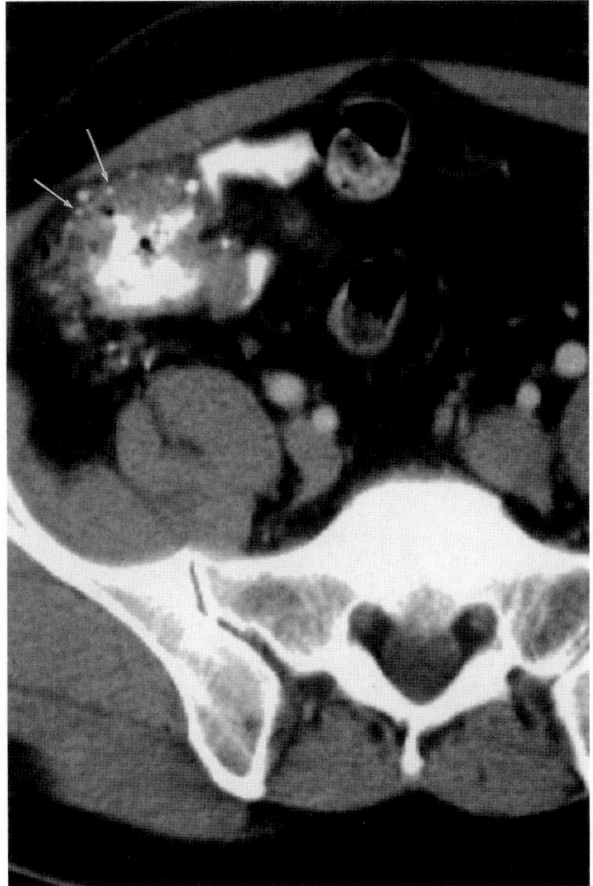

Figure 64-9. Hemangioma of the colon. CT shows lobulated thickening of the circumference of the wall of the cecum with numerous calcified phleboliths (*arrows*) in the subserosa.

4-cm, often pedunculated polypoid lesions[37] or as smooth, submucosal masses.[35,38] These soft tumors are pliable, changing in size or shape with compression or varying luminal distention, and they may be compressible during endoscopic ultrasound.[39] A cystic or multicystic mass is often found on endoscopic ultrasonography or CT. The smooth, unilocular or multilocular submucosal mass is of water attenuation (0 to 20 Hounsfield units) on CT.[39,40]

Angiodysplasia

Clinical and Pathologic Findings

Angiodysplasia is a common cause of chronic, low-grade or acute, massive lower gastrointestinal bleeding in elderly patients.[41,42] These lesions are acquired vascular ectasias, possibly caused by chronic, low-grade colonic obstruction.[41] Angiodysplasias are composed of clusters of dilated, tortuous, thin-walled veins, venules, and capillaries localized in the colonic mucosa and submucosa (Fig. 64-10). The mucosal layer overlying the vascular tuft may be thin or ulcerated. These lesions are single or multiple and small (usually < 5 mm) and are usually found in the cecum or ascending colon.[41]

Angiodysplasias may coexist with other causes of gastrointestinal bleeding. These lesions have been found at autopsy in 2% of asymptomatic elderly patients, and in one series angiodysplasias were present in the resected specimens in 12 of 15 patients who underwent surgery for colonic carcinoma.[41] Angiodysplasias are not associated with angiomatous lesions of the skin or other viscera.[41]

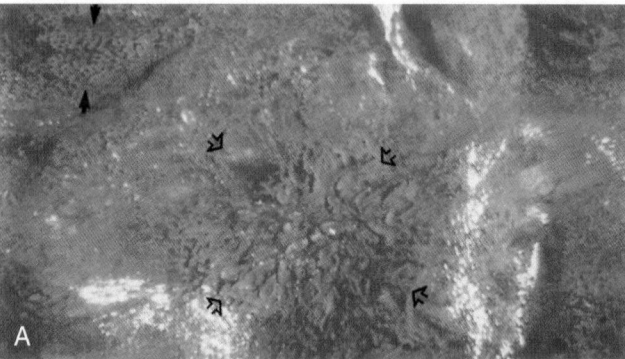

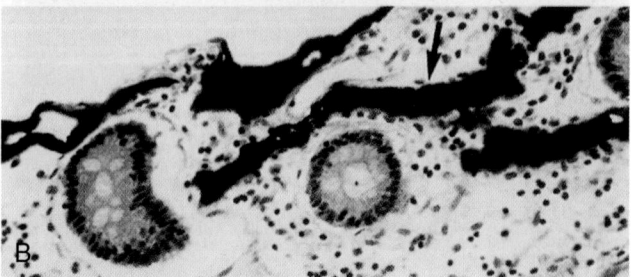

Figure 64-10. Angiodysplasia of the right side of the colon. A. Dissecting photomicrograph shows distortion of the surface pattern (*open arrows*) of the colonic mucosa by an underlying tangle of vessels. The normal surface pattern and glandular openings of the colon (*solid arrows*) are marked for comparison. **B.** Medium-power view of the colonic mucosa shows thin-walled, endothelial-lined spaces (*arrow*) in the lamina propria. These spaces were filled with a black-staining dye from a prior injection study.

Radiographic Findings

Angiodysplasias may be detected during the work-up of patients with severe or recurrent lower gastrointestinal bleeding after a normal barium enema or colonoscopy.[42] During the arterial phase of angiography, a focus of angiodysplasia usually appears as a tangle of small vessels at the end of a cecal or right colonic artery. Early filling of draining veins with contrast medium is usually seen, but extravasation of contrast medium rarely occurs.[43] The radiologist is critical to the diagnosis of angiodysplasia because the surgeon is unable to see or palpate these lesions during surgery. The pathognomonic histologic findings are not usually present on endoscopic biopsy specimens. As a result, the decision for surgery is made on the basis of the radiographic findings and the clinical history of severe or recurrent lower gastrointestinal bleeding.

Kaposi's Sarcoma

Kaposi's sarcoma involving the colon usually occurs in patients with AIDS. Kaposi's sarcoma has also been reported in human immunodeficiency virus–negative patients with Crohn's disease or ulcerative colitis and in patients who have undergone solid organ transplants.[32,44,45] Kaposi's sarcoma in the colon is manifested radiographically by a flat or plaquelike lesion, a small polypoid nodule, or a polypoid submucosal-appearing mass with or without central umbilication.[32] The tumor is usually confined to the mucosa and submucosa.

NEUROENDOCRINE (CARCINOID) TUMORS

Pathologic Findings

Endocrine cells are scattered throughout the gastrointestinal tract. These cells synthesize and secrete a variety of peptide hormones and biogenic amines. The neuroendocrine cells give rise to gastrointestinal tumors traditionally termed *carcinoid tumors* but now preferably termed *neuroendocrine tumors.* The most common sites of carcinoid tumors include the appendix (35%), ileum (16%), lung (14%), and rectum (13%).[46] Neuroendocrine tumors arising in the remainder of the colon constitute only 2% to 3% of all carcinoid tumors.[46-50]

The most common sites of neuroendocrine tumors in the colon are the rectum and cecum. Neuroendocrine tumors involving the cecum and ascending or transverse colon are of midgut origin. These midgut lesions may synthesize, store, and secrete serotonin. Although serotonin may be produced, the carcinoid syndrome is rare.[51] If the carcinoid syndrome is present, it is usually associated with liver metastases.

Hindgut neuroendocrine tumors involve the descending colon, sigmoid colon, and rectum. They primarily synthesize and store a variety of polypeptide hormonal substances, including gastrin, somatostatin, glucagon, and vasoactive intestinal polypeptide.[47,52] These tumors do not usually produce serotonin or cause the carcinoid syndrome.

Neuroendocrine Tumors of the Rectum

Neuroendocrine tumors arising in the rectum are usually small, smooth submucosal polypoid lesions less than 2 cm in diameter and are located in the lower two thirds of the rectum. Most cases are discovered incidentally during a screening barium enema examination or endoscopy or during work-up for rectal pain or bleeding.[53,54] Small rectal carcinoids have low malignant potential and are cured by simple, complete excision. These lesions are therefore termed "low-grade" neuroendocrine tumors. As with any carcinoid tumor, the larger the tumor, the greater the chance of metastases at the time of diagnosis. Although rare, large rectal neuroendocrine tumors are associated with a much greater frequency of metastases at the time of diagnosis.[54] Large rectal carcinoids may appear as irregular, ulcerated masses.[54] If all rectal neuroendocrine tumors are considered, patients with rectal carcinoids have an overall 5-year survival rate of about 85%.[46,54]

Neuroendocrine Tumors (Exclusive of the Rectum)

Neuroendocrine tumors of the remainder of the colon have a very different clinical history, morphology, and prognosis than small low-grade neuroendocrine tumors of the rectum. Neuroendocrine tumors in the colon (exclusive of the rectum) are usually large, aggressive lesions associated with a poor prognosis. Patients usually present in the sixth decade of life with symptoms similar to those of colonic adenocarcinoma, including abdominal pain, distention, and a palpable abdominal mass. Rectal bleeding and diarrhea are seen in approximately one third of patients.[55]

Neuroendocrine tumors of the colon are most commonly located in the cecum or ascending colon.[51,55] These tumors appear on barium enemas as large (>5 cm), fungating intraluminal masses or as irregular annular lesions (Fig. 64-11)[48,51,56] that are indistinguishable from colonic carcinoma. In other patients, these neuroendocrine tumors may appear as smooth, polypoid submucosal masses. At the time of diagnosis, 50% to 60% of patients with large neuroendocrine tumors have metastases to the liver, lymph nodes, mesentery, or peritoneum.[46,51,55] Overall 5-year survival rates of approximately 50% have been reported.[46]

FATTY LESIONS

Lipoma

Clinical Findings

Colonic lipomas are uncommon lesions, occurring at autopsy in less than 1% of patients.[57,58] However, the colon is the most frequent site of gastrointestinal involvement by lipomas. Most patients are asymptomatic, and the tumors are detected during studies performed for symptoms ultimately attributed to other causes.[57,59] When these patients are symptomatic, they usually present with abdominal pain and discomfort.[59] Rectal bleeding and pain related to intussusception are less common.

Pathologic Findings

Most colonic lipomas are found in the right colon, and 90% originate in the submucosa.[14,57,59] The remaining 10% arise in the appendices epiploicae. Multiple tumors are found in up to 25% of patients.[59] Colonic lipomas are usually less than 3 cm in diameter, but those that cause symptoms tend to be larger lesions.

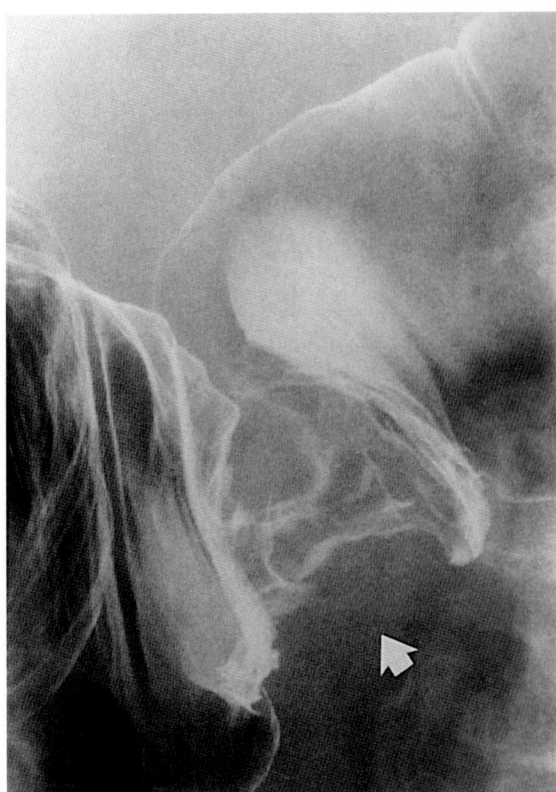

Figure 64-11. Neuroendocrine carcinoma of the colon. Spot image from a double-contrast barium enema shows a short, annular lesion (*arrow*) with shelflike margins in the hepatic flexure of the colon. These radiographic findings are similar to those of an annular carcinoma of the colon, but the mucosa is smoother than that usually found with an annular carcinoma. (Courtesy of Seth N. Glick, MD, Philadelphia, PA.)

Colonic lipomas are encapsulated masses of mature adipose tissue usually confined to the submucosa (Fig. 64-12). Approximately two thirds of these tumors are pedunculated, with a broad-based pedicle covered by normal colonic mucosa. Because of this pedunculation, local trauma and mechanical irritation may lead to focal ulceration and fat necrosis. Continuing inflammation may cause fibrosis and calcification. Bizarre, enlarged fibroblasts may develop as a result of repeated trauma, previously described as pseudosarcomatous change. However, these fibroblasts are reactive and are not indicative of a neoplastic process.[60,61]

Radiographic Findings

Colonic lipomas usually appear on barium enemas as smooth, sessile submucosal masses or as smooth polypoid lesions on a broad-based pedicle (Fig. 64-13).[14] Lipomas may be round, ovoid, or pear-shaped. They are sharply demarcated masses that form obtuse angles with the adjacent colonic wall.[62] Although these lesions may have a lobulated contour, the mucosal surface is smooth (see Fig. 64-13). Because of the pliable nature of fat, lipomas change shape with palpation, position of the patient, or varying degrees of colonic distention.[58,62] These tumors may also elongate during colonic spasm or after colonic evacuation. Some lipomas may serve as the lead point for colocolic intussusceptions.[63-65]

Before the advent of CT, the barium enema was considered to be a relatively accurate test for the diagnosis of colonic

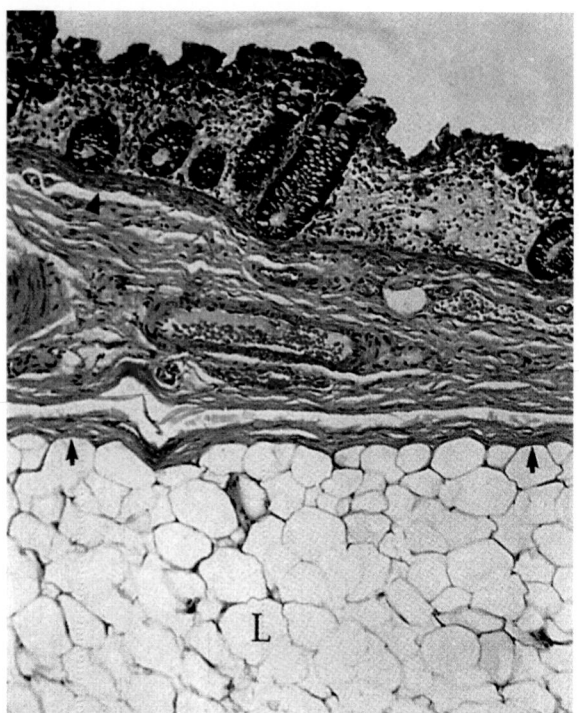

Figure 64-12. Lipoma of the colon. Medium-power photomicrograph shows mature adipose tissue (L) expanding the submucosa. A fibrous capsule (*arrows*) is seen. The muscularis mucosae is identified by an *arrowhead*.

lipoma.[62,66] However, a definitive diagnosis of a colonic lipoma can be made on CT when it shows a mass of uniform fat density (−60 to −120 HU) without septa or other large areas of nonfatty tissue (Fig. 64-14).[39,65,67-69] In patients without symptoms or complications or in those who are poor operative risks, the CT diagnosis of a colonic lipoma may obviate the need for surgery.[67,68] However, the CT scan should be tailored with thin sections through the lesion to minimize partial volume effect of surrounding contrast material or air. In some cases, insufflation of rectal air may be of value.[39] It should also be recognized that colonic liposarcomas are extremely rare.[70] In fact, liposarcomas had not been reported in the colon as of 1989.[70]

When colonic lipomas intussuscept, they can ulcerate and undergo fat necrosis, resulting in CT attenuation numbers higher than those of fat. As a result, an intussuscepting lipoma appearing as a soft tissue mass or having only a small focus of fat attenuation may be confused with an intussuscepting carcinoma.[65] The radiologist can also confuse any intussuscepting tumor with a lipoma if the eccentrically invaginating mesenteric fat associated with the intussuscepting tumor mass is mistaken for the fat of a lipoma.[65] Lipomas can also be diagnosed on endoscopic ultrasound as smooth hemispheric polyps with a broad base containing hyperechoic tissue or tissue of intermediate echogenicity.[39]

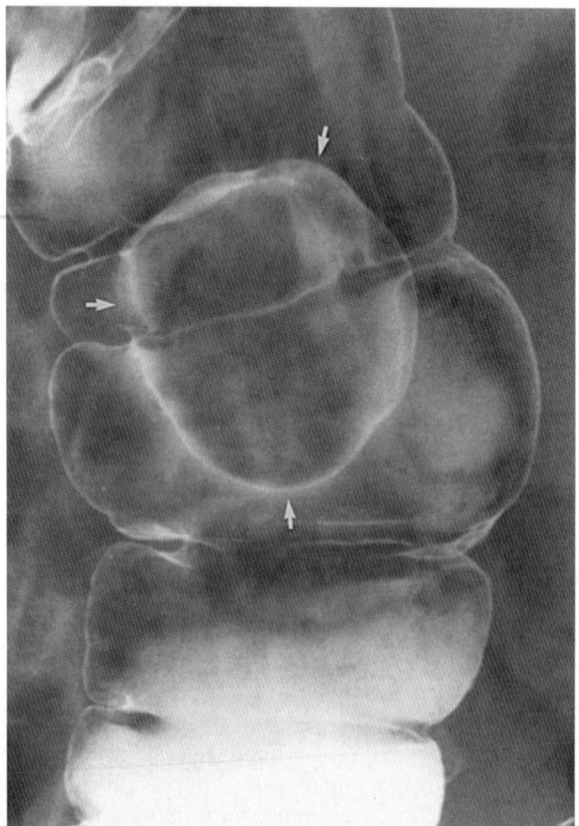

Figure 64-13. Lipoma of the descending colon. Spot image from a double-contrast barium enema shows a 3-cm smooth-surfaced submucosal mass (*arrows*) with a slightly lobulated contour.

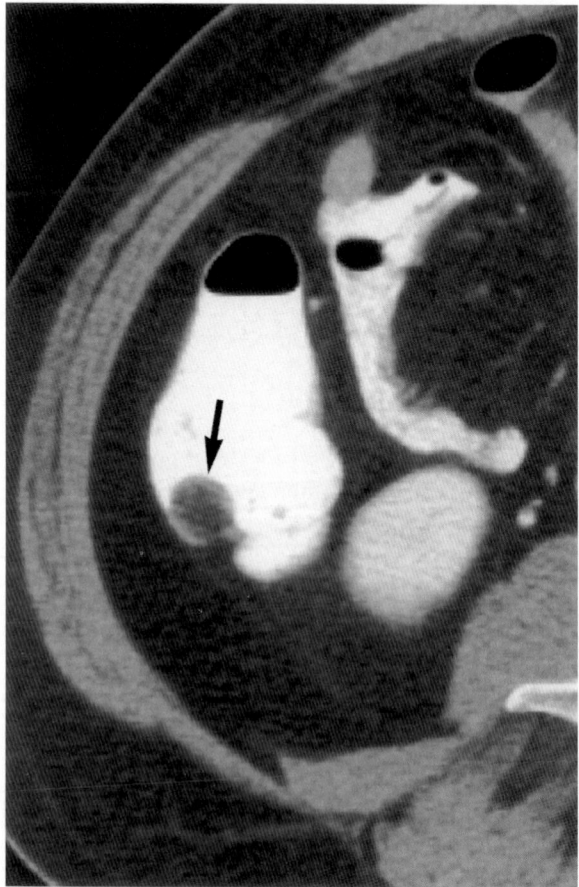

Figure 64-14. Lipoma of the cecum. CT shows a 1.5-cm smooth-surfaced ovoid mass (*arrow*) in the cecum with the same attenuation value as nearby mesenteric fat.

Fatty Infiltration of the Ileocecal Valve

Pathologic, Clinical, and Radiographic Findings

Fatty infiltration (also known as lipohyperplasia or lipomatous infiltration) of the ileocecal valve results from localized, massive accumulation of submucosal fat in this region. The lack of a capsule differentiates this fatty proliferation pathologically from a true lipoma.[28] The diagnosis is suggested on barium enema when there is a large ileocecal valve with smooth or lobulated contours and a smooth mucosal surface without a discrete polypoid mass. Although rigid measurements are not reliable in distinguishing a normal-sized ileocecal valve from an enlarged valve, some investigators have suggested that a normal ileocecal valve should be 4 cm or less.[71] Others have found that one lip of a normal valve should be 1.5 cm or less.[72] A normal ileocecal valve may also have stellate folds radiating toward its center.[72]

Differential Diagnosis

The radiologist must first decide whether the polypoid projection in the cecum arises on or near the ileocecal valve or actually represents the valve. The normal ileocecal valve is usually located at the level of the first complete haustral fold on the medial or posterior colonic wall at the junction of the cecum and ascending colon.[72] Filling of the terminal ileum with barium confirms the location of the ileocecal valve. If an ileocecal valve is mildly enlarged (>4 cm) and has a smooth or slightly lobulated contour and a smooth mucosal surface, the most likely diagnosis is fatty infiltration of the valve (Fig. 64-15). In contrast, a focal polypoid projection from the ileocecal valve may represent a tumor such as an adenoma or lipoma (Fig. 64-16).[72] Any mucosal surface irregularity of the ileocecal valve should also suggest the possibility of tumor involving the valve, including an adenocarcinoma. The ileocecal valve may also be involved by Crohn's disease or lymphoma. In Crohn's disease there is fatty hypertrophy of the valve, usually associated with other radiographic findings of Crohn's disease in the terminal ileum and ileocecal fistulas. In lymphoma, the ileocecal valve is moderately enlarged and has a lobulated contour, usually because of spread of lymphoma from the terminal ileum.

STROMAL TUMORS

Pathologic Findings

Historically, most spindle and epithelioid cell tumors of the gastrointestinal tract have erroneously been called *smooth muscle tumors* (leiomyoma or leiomyosarcoma). Most of these tumors are undifferentiated stromal neoplasms, termed *gastrointestinal stromal tumors* (GISTs).[73-76] GISTs are thought to originate from the interstitial cells of Cajal, which express CD34; their development depends on a proto-oncogenic receptor, tyrosine kinase (*KIT*). GISTs usually express CD34 and many have been found to contain mutations in *KIT*.[77] The likelihood of recurrent tumor or metastases with GISTs is based on their mitotic index, size, and location.[78] Only a small percentage of all spindle cell tumors are recognized as arising from smooth muscle cells or neural cells by ultrastructural or immunohistochemical means.[73-76] Those originating from the muscularis mucosae are small (several

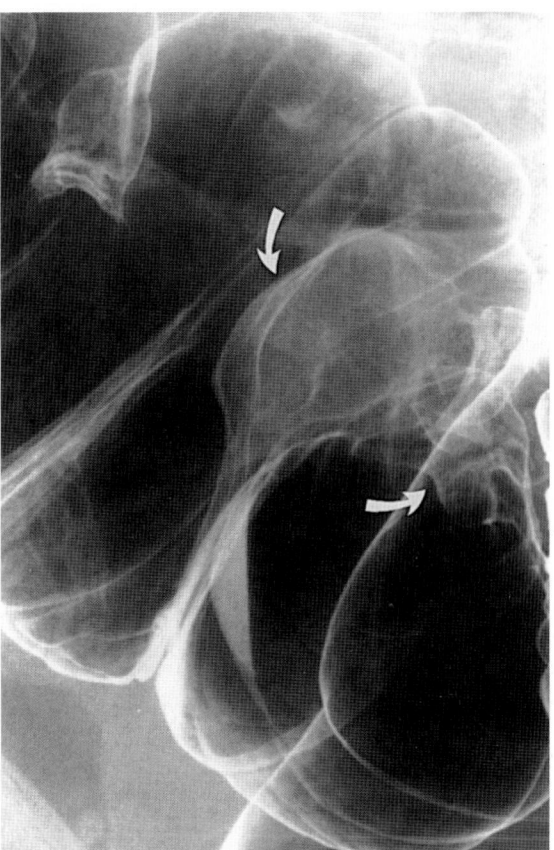

Figure 64-15. Fatty infiltration of the ileocecal valve. Close-up view from a right-side-down decubitus overhead radiograph of the colon shows smooth, slightly lobulated enlargement of the ileocecal valve (*arrows*). Fatty infiltration was confirmed at colonoscopy performed for other reasons.

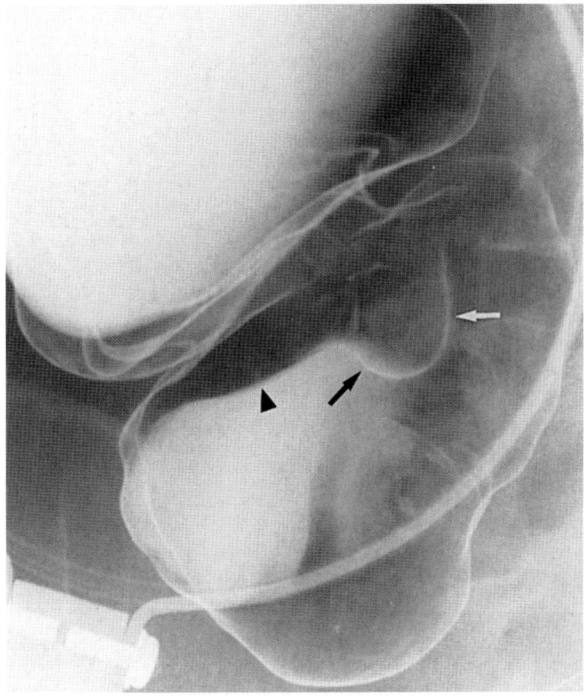

Figure 64-16. Lipoma of the ileocecal valve. A small, smooth-surfaced submucosal lesion (*arrows*) is seen arising from the inferior lip of the ileocecal valve (*arrowhead*).

millimeters) and are true leiomyomas of the gastrointestinal tract, exclusive of the esophagus.

Small Stromal Tumors

Only 1% of all gastrointestinal tumors are of stromal origin, and these tumors are least commonly found in the colon.[79] Colonic stromal tumors are usually located in the rectum.[80] In general, there are two macroscopic types of colonic stromal tumors: small polypoid lesions and large, bulky masses. Some patients with small polypoid rectal lesions complain of rectal discomfort, pain, and bleeding. Other patients are asymptomatic, and the tumors are discovered as incidental findings on barium enema or endoscopy. Small polypoid lesions may be sessile or pedunculated. They probably arise from the muscularis mucosae, are histologically benign, and do not recur after excision.[81] These small polypoid lesions are often "true" leiomyomas of the colon because they demonstrate smooth muscle differentiation by their desmin positivity and ultrastructural characteristics. These tumors are distinct from GISTs and have essentially no malignant potential. These small rectal lesions appear on barium enema as sessile or pedunculated polyps with a smooth or slightly irregular surface. Small polypoid leiomyomas have also been reported in patients with AIDS.[82] Multiple small polypoid neurofibromas may be seen in patients with neurofibromatosis (Fig. 64-17).

Large Stromal Tumors

Patients with large colonic GISTs may present with pain, gastrointestinal bleeding, and altered bowel habits but rarely

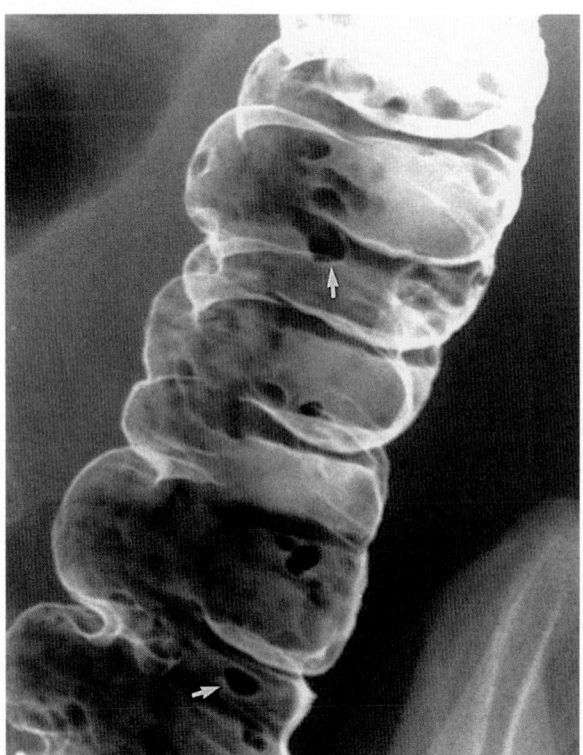

Figure 64-17. Neurofibromatosis of the colon. Spot image from a double-contrast barium enema shows numerous small, smooth-surfaced filling defects (*arrows*) and hemispheric lines in the descending colon. Neurofibromatosis is a rare cause of colonic polyposis.

with obstruction.[80] These large (>2 cm) lesions probably arise from the muscularis propria. They have a high rate of local recurrence (60%), regardless of histologic differentiation and are associated with a poor prognosis.[81] These bulky lesions are most frequently found in the rectum, with the remainder evenly distributed throughout the colon. Large stromal tumors may appear on barium enemas or CT as annular lesions, cavitating masses with a prominent extraluminal component, or submucosal masses with or without central ulceration (Figs. 64-18 and 64-19). Cavitation may lead to superimposed infection or perforation with abscess formation.[79] These lesions may be confused radiographically with colonic lymphomas or perforated colonic carcinomas. Stromal lesions typically metastasize to peritoneal surfaces as well as the lungs and liver.[75]

SQUAMOUS CELL CARCINOMA

Squamous cell carcinomas of the colon are extremely rare tumors, as are mixed adenosquamous cell carcinomas, which are tumors composed of both squamous and adenocarcinomatous elements. Most squamous cell carcinomas arise in the rectum and cause symptoms identical to those of rectal adenocarcinomas.[83] Squamous cell carcinomas have been detected in patients with a history of ulcerative colitis, pelvic irradiation, and schistosomiasis.[84] Squamous cell carcinomas may appear on barium enemas as large, bulky, ulcerated masses grossly identical to rectal adenocarcinomas (Fig. 64-20).[83] Hematogenous, lymphatic, and local metastases are frequently present. Squamous cell carcinomas of the colon should be distinguished from squamous cell carcinomas invading the colon from the anal canal or from squamous mucosal-lined fistulas. These lesions must also be distinguished from squamous cell carcinomas that have metastasized to the colon and from poorly differentiated adenocarcinomas that show focal squamous differentiation.

CLOACOGENIC CARCINOMA

The epithelium at the junction of the anal canal and rectum is composed of squamous and stratified columnar epithelium as well as scattered goblet cells. This transitional zone has features of both urothelium and squamous epithelium compatible with a cloacogenic origin.[85] As a result, many tumors in this region were previously termed *cloacogenic carcinomas*. Primary tumors at the anorectal junction are currently classified according to architectural and cellular differentiation indicative of their cellular origin, including *squamous cell carcinoma, basaloid carcinoma, transitional cell carcinoma, mucoepidermoid carcinoma,* and *adenoid cystic carcinoma.* Most tumors have a mixture of histologic growth patterns. Tumors with squamous differentiation are termed *squamous cell carcinoma,* as described previously. *Basaloid carcinoma* and *cloacogenic carcinoma* are probably equivalent terms.[32] Tumors that arise from submucosal glands in this region are salivary gland type tumors such as adenoid cystic carcinoma and mucoepidermoid carcinoma. The most common malignant tumor of the anal canal, however, is not of cloacogenic origin but is adenocarcinoma arising from the rectal mucosa that subsequently invades the anal canal.

The transitional zone is an area in which metaplasia and reserve cell hyperplasia occur in a manner similar to that in

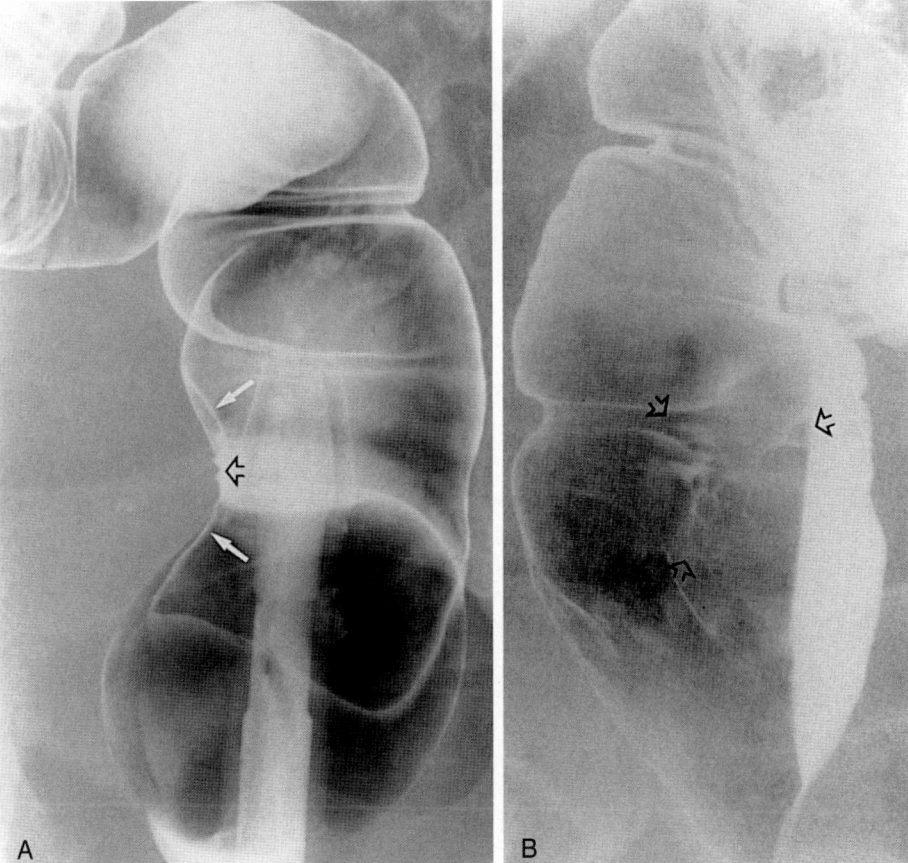

Figure 64-18. Gastrointestinal stromal tumor of the rectum. A. Steep oblique view of the rectum from a double-contrast barium enema shows a relatively broad-based mass (*solid arrows*) with focal spiculation of the contour (*open arrow*). **B.** Close-up view from a left-side-down decubitus overhead radiograph shows focal nodularity of the mucosa (*arrows*) corresponding to the area of spiculation on the earlier view.

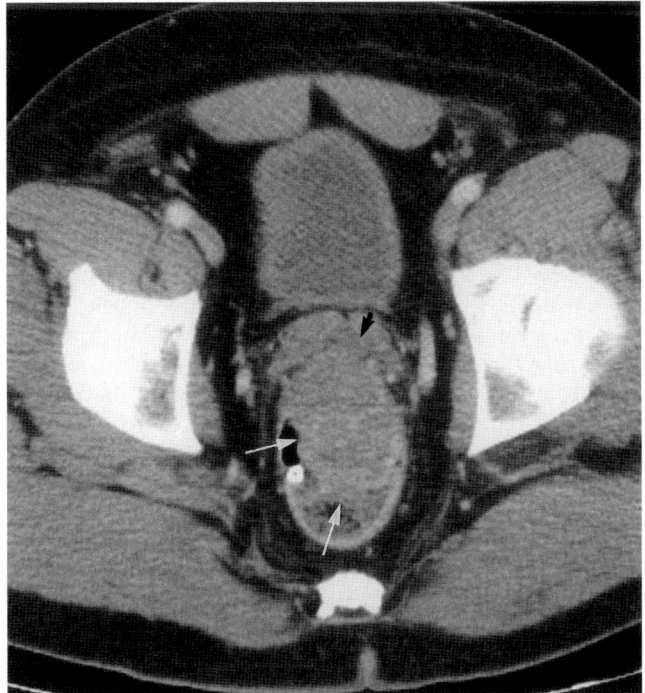

Figure 64-19. Malignant gastrointestinal stromal tumor of the rectum. CT scan shows a large soft tissue mass (*white arrows*) arising from the left anterolateral wall of the rectum. The mass enhances to the same degree as adjacent muscle. Infiltration of the fat plane between the rectum and seminal vesicles (*black arrow*) is present. (Reproduced with permission from Forbes A, Rubesin SE, et al: Colon II. In Atlas of Clinical Gastroenterology, 3rd ed. Edinburgh, Elsevier Mosby, 2005, p 183.)

the transitional zone of the uterine cervix and gastroesophageal junction.[86] It has therefore been postulated that some tumors arise in this region in areas of chronic inflammation/squamous metaplasia/reserve cell hyperplasia, resulting in dysplasia and subsequent carcinoma. For example, homosexual men have a high incidence of squamous cell carcinoma of the anus. These tumors are associated with venereally transmitted human papillomavirus.[87-89] Other oncogenic viruses, carcinogens in lubricants and cleansers, and mechanical irritation may also play a role.[87-92]

Cloacogenic carcinomas have no distinctive gross pathologic or radiologic features. Patients usually present with rectal bleeding or pain or altered bowel habits. These tumors may be flat, infiltrative, annular, or ulcerative lesions with rolled borders. The tumors may appear on barium enemas as submucosal masses with a smooth or ulcerated surface (Fig. 64-21), as broad-based, sessile polypoid masses, or as infiltrative lesions (Fig. 64-22).[93,94]

Metastases to sacral, internal iliac, and common iliac lymph nodes are found in approximately 50% of patients. Hematogenous metastases may also result from spread of tumor via the portal venous system and inferior vena cava. Patients with basaloid carcinoma have 5-year survival rates of approximately 50%.[32]

METASTASES

Metastases to the colon are not uncommon.[95] It also is not uncommon for symptoms produced by gastrointestinal metastases to occur as the initial manifestation of a primary

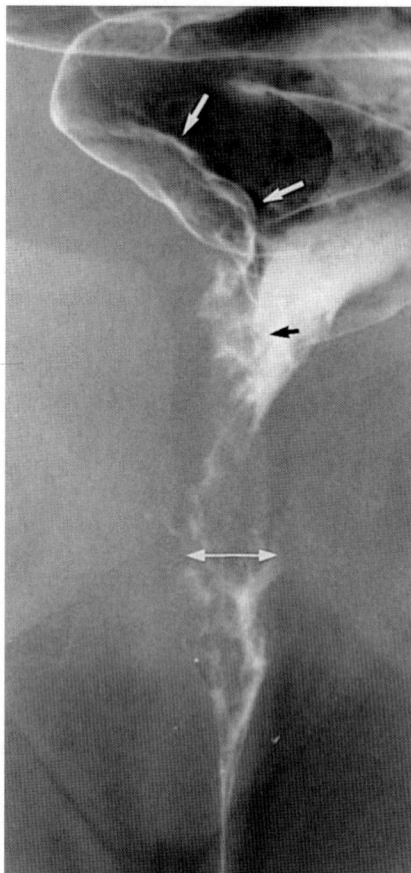

Figure 64-20. Verrucous squamous cell carcinoma arising in a condyloma acuminatum. This young woman had been treated for 5 years for perianal, vaginal, cervical, and vulvar condylomata. A spot image of the distal rectum and anal canal from a double-contrast barium enema shows a polypoid mass (*white arrows*) in the distal rectum and nodular mucosa extending to the anorectal junction (*black arrow*), with abnormal mucosa distending the anal canal (*double-ended arrow*).

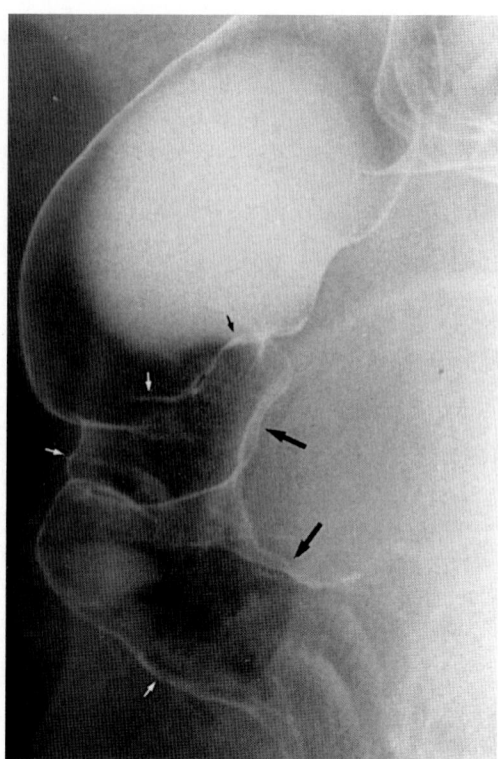

Figure 64-21. Cloacogenic carcinoma. Lateral view of the rectum shows a large submucosal mass (*large arrows*) indenting the anterior wall of the mid rectum. Diffuse infiltration by tumor is manifested by smooth narrowing of the distal rectum (*small arrows*).

malignancy. Colonic metastases are classified by their mode of dissemination as follows[96]: (1) direct invasion from a contiguous primary tumor or noncontiguous primary tumor; (2) intraperitoneal seeding; and (3) embolic metastases.

Imaging studies may not only identify the lesion as a metastasis to the colon but also indicate the mode of dissemination and the most likely origin of malignancy.[97] Detection of these metastases is also important because localized embolic metastases may be resected for cure or for control of complications such as gastrointestinal bleeding or obstruction. Recognition of colonic invasion by tumor also enables the surgeon to perform a wider excision or, if necessary, a diverting colostomy.[98]

Direct Invasion from Contiguous Primary Tumors

The most common tumors that directly invade the colon include carcinoma of the ovary, kidney, uterus, cervix (Fig. 64-23), prostate, and gallbladder, as discussed in the following sections.

Prostatic Carcinoma

Prostatic carcinoma may spread via Denonvillier's fascia to invade the rectum anteriorly or circumferentially.[99] Rectal involvement by prostatic carcinoma occurs in 0.5% to 11.5% of patients.[100-102] Affected individuals may present with obstructive symptoms, constipation, or rectal bleeding.[102] The diagnosis of prostatic cancer invading the colon may not be suspected at the time of barium enema or surgery or even at autopsy.[99,103]

Although the normal prostate abuts the distal rectum, most patients with prostatic carcinoma invading the colon have involvement of the rectosigmoid junction with distal rectal sparing.[99,104] Prostatic carcinoma usually spreads cranially to involve the seminal vesicles before invading the rectum posteriorly. Thus, on barium enema examination, early cases may be manifested by extrinsic mass effect predominantly on the anterior border of the rectosigmoid junction. With colonic invasion, mucosal pleating and tethering are seen en face and a spiculated contour is seen in profile. In advanced cases, the rectum is circumferentially narrowed with a widened presacral space and a spiculated contour (Fig. 64-24).[99-101,104] In some cases, prostatic carcinoma invades posteriorly to involve the lower rectum (Fig. 64-25). The major consideration in the differential diagnosis is direct invasion of the rectum by a contiguous pelvic tumor such as carcinoma of the urinary bladder. The diagnostic work-up may include MRI, CT (Fig. 64-26), or transrectal sonography. Endoscopic biopsy specimens with stains for prostate-specific antigen or prostatic acid phosphatase may be obtained to confirm the radiologic diagnosis.[105,106]

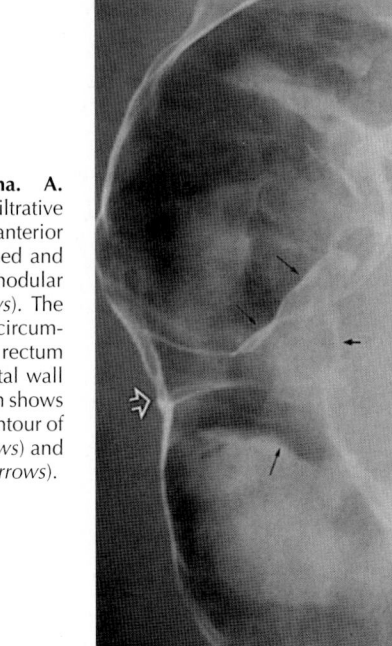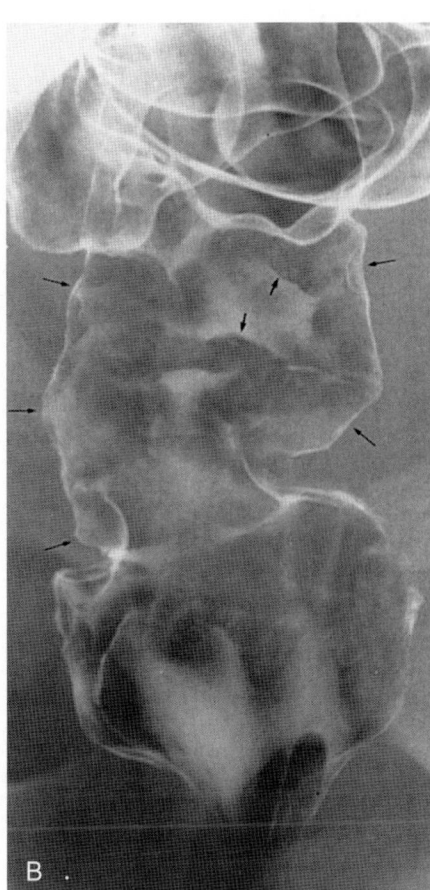

Figure 64-22. Cloacogenic carcinoma. A. Lateral view of the rectum shows the infiltrative pattern of cloacogenic carcinoma. The anterior wall of the rectum is moderately flattened and lobulated (*short arrows*), with thickened, nodular folds traversing the rectum (*long arrows*). The rectal mucosa is relatively smooth. Focal circumferential extension of tumor around the rectum is seen as flattening of the posterior rectal wall (*open arrow*). **B.** Prone view of the rectum shows mild in-bowing and irregularity of the contour of the lateral walls of the rectum (*long arrows*) and thickened, nodular folds en face (*short arrows*).

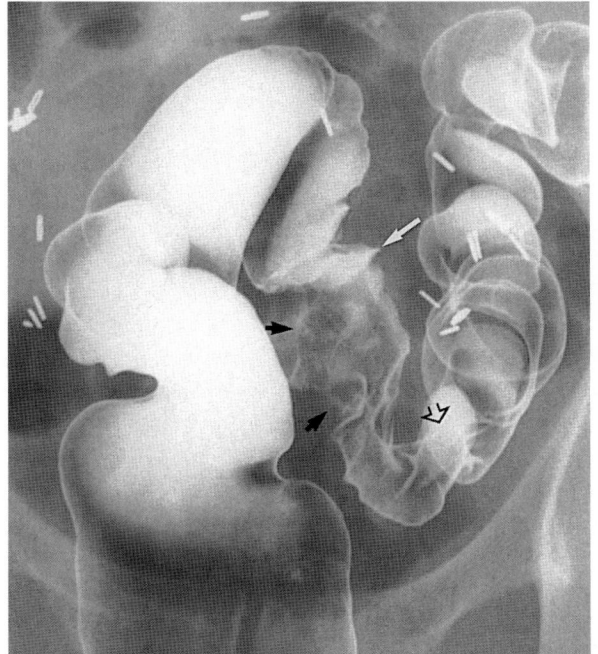

Figure 64-23. Recurrent cervical carcinoma invading the sigmoid colon. Close-up view from a prone overhead radiograph of the rectosigmoid colon shows circumferential involvement of the sigmoid colon by tumor. A relatively abrupt margin is seen distally, and a smooth, tapered margin is seen proximally (*open arrow*). The colonic contour is focally spiculated (*white arrow*) and markedly irregular in other regions (*black arrows*).

Ovarian Carcinoma

When left-sided ovarian carcinoma directly invades the colon, it first involves the inferior border of the sigmoid colon.[107] Colonic wall invasion is indicated by angulation of the affected sigmoid loops, spiculation of the colonic contour, and tethering and angulation of mucosal folds en face (Fig. 64-27). Rarely, a fistula to the sigmoid colon may be seen.[108]

Renal Cell Carcinoma

Renal cell carcinoma or recurrent renal cell carcinoma in the retroperitoneum may directly invade the colon.[96,107,109] Left-sided renal cell carcinomas usually invade the splenic flexure or the distal transverse or proximal descending colon,[96] whereas right-sided renal cell carcinomas invade the descending duodenum. Colonic invasion by renal cell carcinoma is usually manifested on barium enemas by bulky intraluminal masses without signs of obstruction.[96]

Direct Invasion from Noncontiguous Primary Tumors

Malignancies may spread in the subperitoneal space or by lymphatic permeation.[96] Examples of this mode of dissemination include colonic carcinoma invading the stomach via the gastrocolic ligament,[110] pancreatic carcinoma invading the transverse colon via the transverse mesocolon, gastric carcinoma invading the transverse colon via the gastrocolic

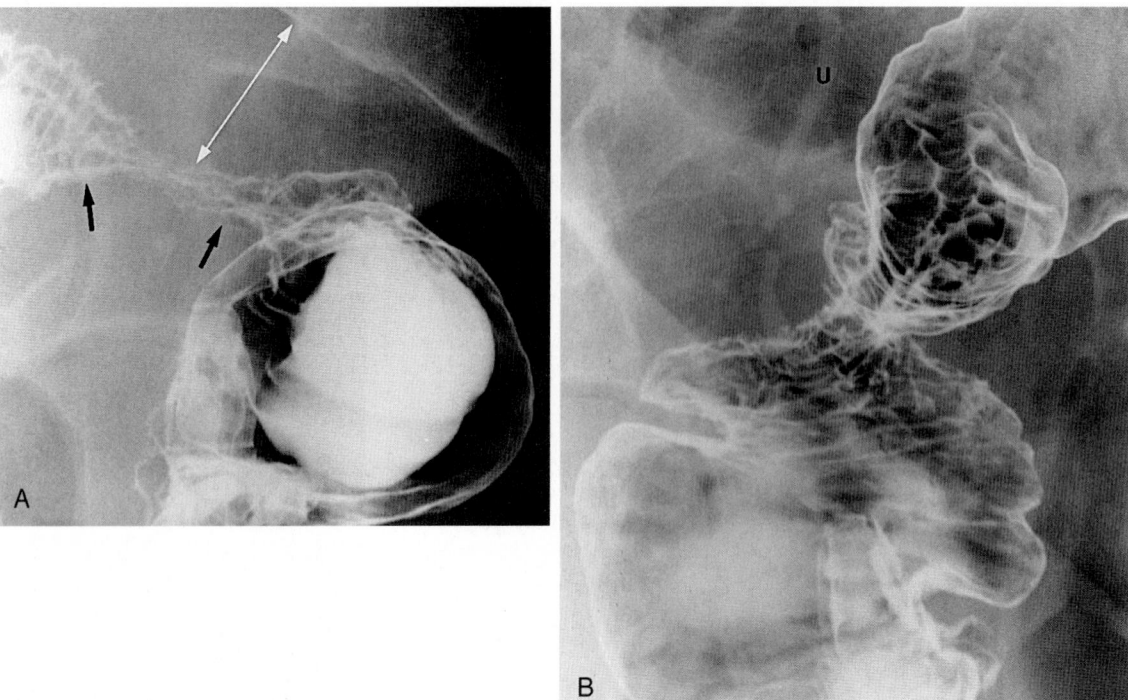

Figure 64-24. Direct invasion of the rectosigmoid colon by prostatic carcinoma. A. Lateral view of the rectum shows circumferential mass effect, especially on the anterior wall of the distal sigmoid colon (*arrows*). Note the spiculated colonic contour and widening of the presacral space (*double-ended arrow*). **B.** Frontal view of the rectum shows a spiculated colonic contour and pleating of the mucosa of the rectosigmoid colon en face. U, ureter.

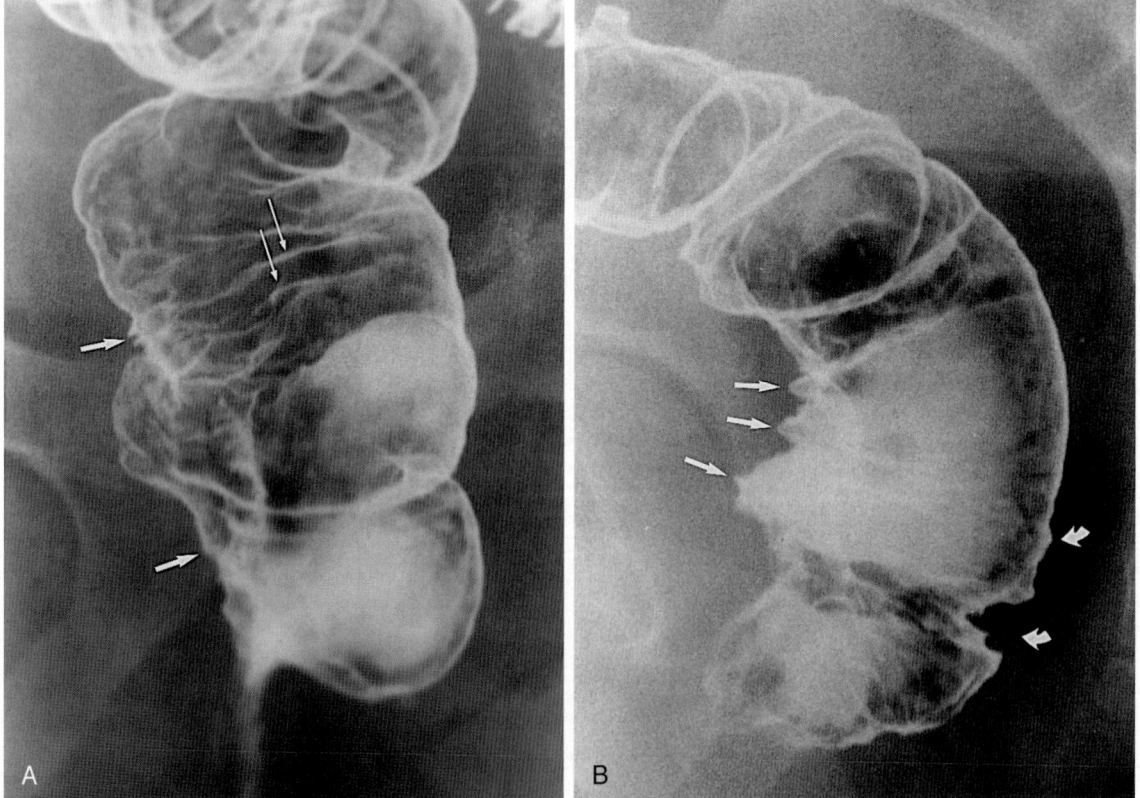

Figure 64-25. Rectal invasion by prostatic carcinoma. A. Frontal view of the rectum shows mass effect and spiculation predominantly along the right lateral wall of the rectum (*thick arrows*) and pleating of the mucosa en face (*thin arrows*). Invasion of the mucosa and submucosa was confirmed on biopsy specimens of the right lateral rectal wall. **B** Lateral view of the rectum shows mass effect along the anterior rectal wall and spiculation of the mucosal contour (*straight arrows*). Mild circumferential extension is seen distally (*curved arrows*). (From Rubesin SE, Levine MS, Bezzi M, et al: Rectal involvement by prostatic carcinoma: Radiographic findings. AJR 152:53-57, 1989, © by American Roentgen Ray Society.)

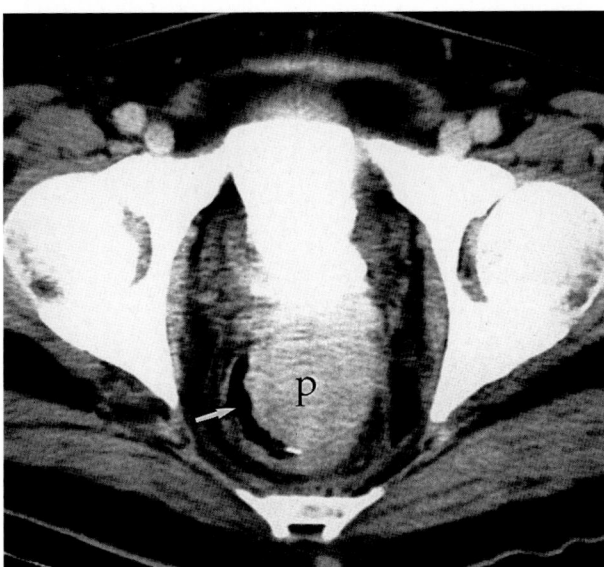

Figure 64-26. Rectal invasion by prostatic carcinoma. CT scan through the pelvis shows a large prostatic mass (p) displacing and invading the rectum (*arrow*).

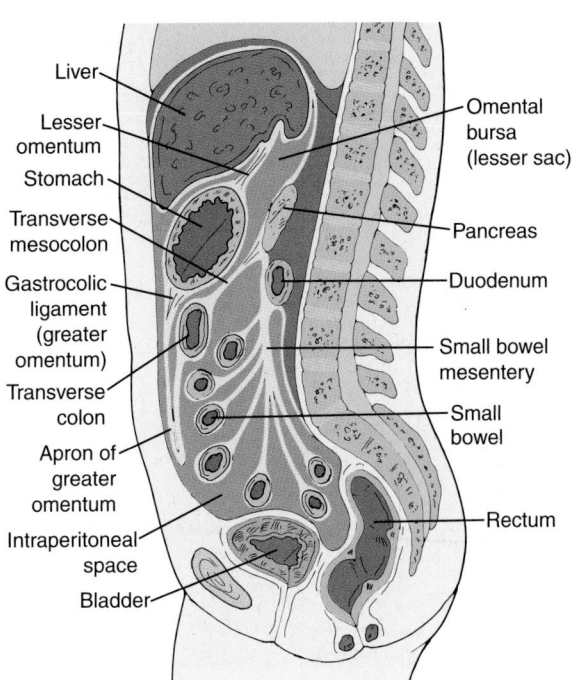

Figure 64-28. Sagittal line drawing of the abdomen. The proximal part of the greater omentum (i.e., the gastrocolic ligament) bridges the greater curvature of the stomach (S) with the anterosuperior border of the transverse colon (T). Thus, when gastric or omental processes directly invade the colon, the superior border of the transverse colon is involved first. The transverse mesocolon suspends the transverse colon from the retroperitoneum overlying the pancreas (P). L, liver; D, duodenum; R, rectum; B, bladder. (From Rubesin SE, Fishman EK: Peritoneal metastasis. In Fishman EK, Jones B [eds]: Computed Tomography of the Gastrointestinal Tract. New York, Churchill Livingstone, 1986.)

ligament,[96] and colonic carcinoma invading contiguous loops of small bowel or colon.[111] The gastrocolic ligament (i.e., the proximal part of the greater omentum) is the anatomic bridge between the greater curvature of the stomach and the superior border of the transverse colon (Fig. 64-28).[107] When gastric carcinoma spreads to the transverse colon via the gastrocolic

ligament, mass effect, fixation, and fold spiculation are initially seen along the superior border of the transverse colon, with sacculation of the uninvolved inferior border (Fig. 64-29). Rarely, the involved colon may have a cobblestone-like appearance indistinguishable from that of Crohn's disease. The major considerations in the differential diagnosis include gastric carcinoma invading the transverse colon and an omental cake from peritoneal metastasis secondarily invading the transverse colon.[112]

The transverse mesocolon courses from the retroperitoneum overlying the pancreas to the inferior border of the transverse colon.[97] Therefore, when pancreatic carcinoma invades the transverse colon via the transverse mesocolon, the initial radiographic changes occur on the inferior border of the transverse colon.[96] Despite these anatomic attachments, pancreatic carcinoma may occasionally spread to the superior border of the transverse colon (Fig. 64-30). Carcinoma of the pancreatic tail may extend along the phrenicocolic ligament to invade the medial border of the splenic flexure.[97]

Intraperitoneal Seeding

The most common primary tumors that seed the peritoneal cavity are ovarian carcinoma in women and gastric, pancreatic, and colonic carcinomas in men. When appendiceal mucinous adenocarcinomas spread intraperitoneally, they create a condition termed *pseudomyxoma peritonei*. Occasionally, lymph node metastases to the retroperitoneum or

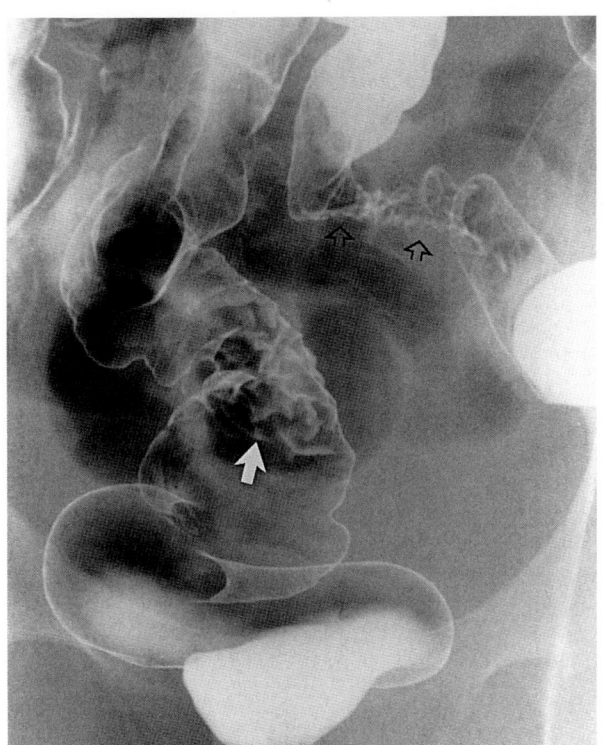

Figure 64-27. Direct colonic invasion by left ovarian carcinoma. Close-up view of an overhead radiograph from a double-contrast barium enema shows spiculation and mass effect along the inferior border of the sigmoid colon (*open arrows*) and pleating of the mucosa of the rectosigmoid junction en face (*solid arrow*).

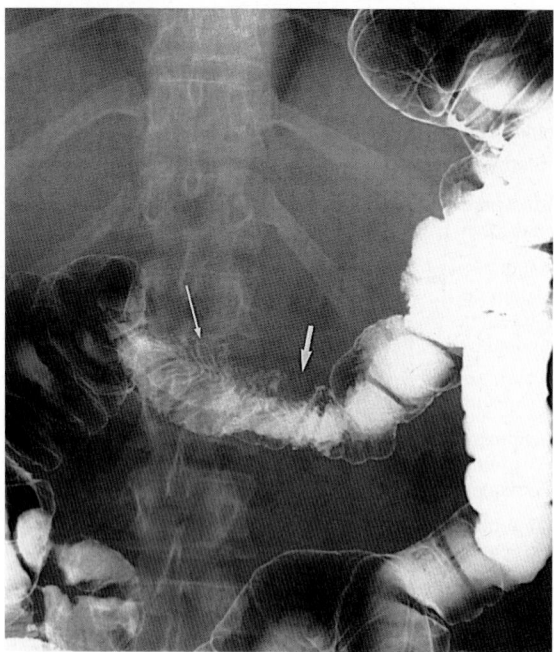

Figure 64-29. Gastric carcinoma invading the transverse colon. Overhead radiograph from a double-contrast barium enema shows flattening and extrinsic mass effect (*thick arrow*) along the superior border of the transverse colon and pleating of mucosal folds en face (*thin arrow*).

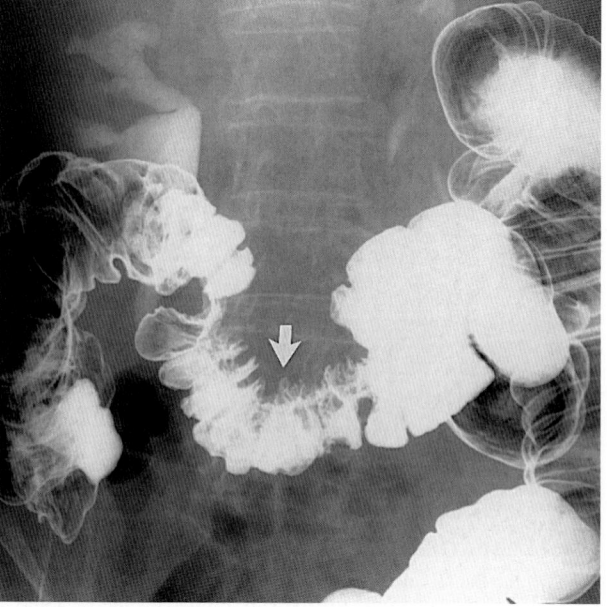

Figure 64-30. Pancreatic carcinoma invading the transverse colon. Overhead radiograph from a double-contrast barium enema shows extrinsic mass effect and spiculation along the superior border of the transverse colon (*arrow*). Contrast medium is present in the renal collecting systems from a prior intravenous urogram.

mesentery from breast carcinoma or other malignant tumors may secondarily seed the peritoneal cavity. Other tumors that spread intraperitoneally include carcinoma of the bladder, uterus, and cervix.

The peritoneal cavity is separated into various compartments by peritoneal reflections and mesenteries (Fig. 64-31).[113] The transverse mesocolon divides the abdomen into the supramesocolic and inframesocolic spaces.[113,114] The small bowel mesentery divides the inframesocolic space into small right and large left regions.[114] The phrenicocolic ligament partially separates the left subphrenic space from the left paracolic gutter, extending from the splenic flexure of the colon to the peritoneum overlying the eleventh rib.[113] These peritoneal reflections direct the flow of intraperitoneal fluid, affecting the distribution and deposition of intraperitoneal-seeded infections and metastases. Directed flow results in characteristic sites of tumor deposition (see Fig. 64-31). As the most dependent portion of the peritoneal cavity in both the supine and upright positions, the pouch of Douglas or rectovesical space is the most common site for intraperitoneal metastases (occurring in 56% of cases) (Fig. 64-32).[113] Other sites include right lower quadrant small bowel loops and the medial border of the cecum (41%), the superior border of the sigmoid colon (21%) (Fig. 64-33), the lateral border of the ascending colon (the right paracolic gutter) (18%) (Fig. 64-34), and the transverse colon.[113]

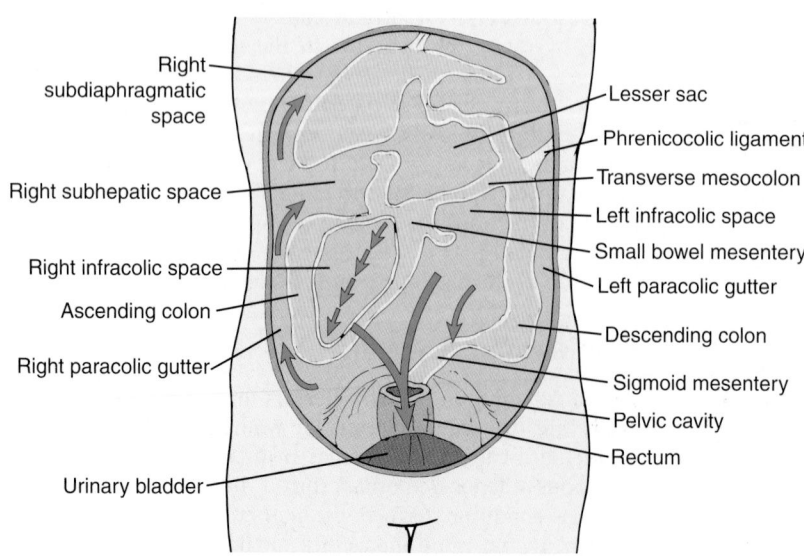

Figure 64-31. Directed flow of intraperitoneal fluid. The peritoneal reflections direct the flow of intraperitoneal fluid within the peritoneal cavity. Flow from the left inframesocolic space pools in the sigmoid mesentery along the superior border of the sigmoid colon and then courses into the pelvic cavity (pouch of Douglas in women, rectovesical space in men, and pararectal spaces). Flow in the right inframesocolic space courses down the ruffles of the small bowel mesentery into the right lower quadrant along distal small bowel loops and medial border of the cecum. Flow then courses into the pelvic cavity from this region. Fluid from the pelvic cavity then courses up the right paracolic gutter to the right subhepatic space and right subdiaphragmatic space. Thus, the sites of pooling of ascitic fluid (the superior border of the sigmoid colon, pouch of Douglas or rectovesical space, medial border of the cecum, mesenteric border of the distal small bowel, and right paracolic gutter) are the predominant sites for intraperitoneal seeding by tumor.

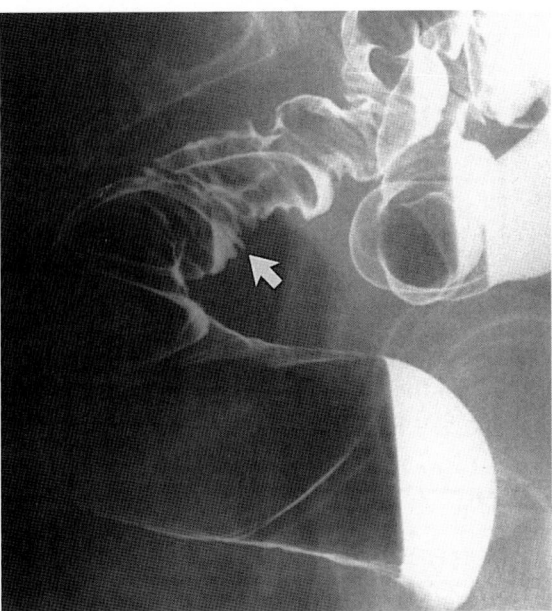

Figure 64-32. Ovarian carcinoma with intraperitoneal metastases to the rectosigmoid junction. Prone cross-table lateral view of the rectosigmoid junction shows spiculation (*arrow*) and tethering of folds along the anterior wall of the rectosigmoid junction. Pleating of the mucosa is seen en face.

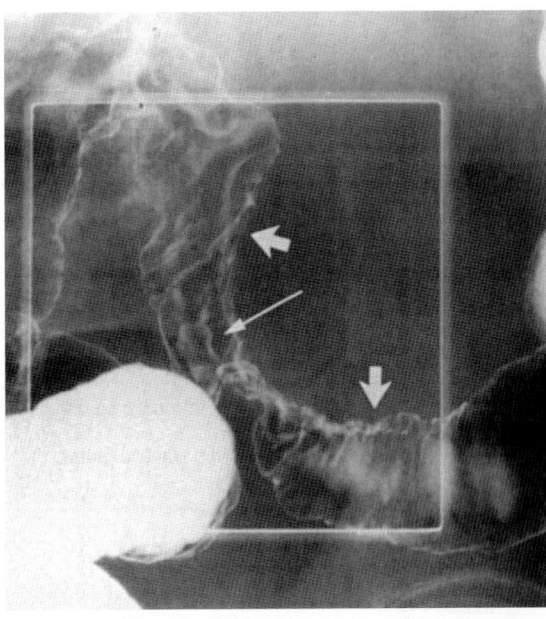

Figure 64-33. Intraperitoneal spread of pancreatic carcinoma to the superior border of the sigmoid colon. Spot image from a double-contrast barium enema shows broad-based extrinsic mass effect along the superior border of the sigmoid colon (*thick arrows*), spiculation of the contour, smooth sacculation of the wall opposite the mass effect, and focal nodularity of the mucosa (*thin arrow*).

Radiographic Findings

Independent of the site of intraperitoneal-seeded metastases, the radiographic findings are similar. Initially, there is extrinsic mass effect along the side of the bowel wall bathed in peritoneal fluid. Direct invasion of the serosa or muscular layers of the bowel wall by tumor incites a desmoplastic reaction. On barium enema, this desmoplastic reaction is manifested in profile by spiculation of the luminal contour and en face by tethering and pleating of mucosal folds in a fixed, parallel, or angulated pattern.[112,115] Angulation of bowel loops occurs predominantly in the sigmoid colon and small bowel. The major considerations in the differential diagnosis of serosal desmoplastic disease in the pouch of Douglas (or rectovesical space in men) include endometriosis, prostatic or cervical carcinoma invading the rectum, and an inflammatory process in the pouch of Douglas/rectovesical space such as a tubo-ovarian abscess or abscess caused by diverticulitis, appendicitis, or Crohn's disease. The clinical history, physical findings, and age of the patient usually allow differentiation of the various causes. The radiologic work-up may include pelvic ultrasound, CT, or MRI.

Cecal metastases are invariably accompanied by small bowel changes, including scalloping of the mesenteric border of right lower quadrant ileal loops, fixation and angulation of loops, and spiculation of the luminal contour.[107]

When peritoneal metastases involve the greater omentum, they may secondarily abut and invade the serosa of the transverse colon.[116] These omental cakes initially involve the superior border of the transverse colon at the site of attachment of the greater omentum (Fig. 64-35).[112] Mass effect may be seen along the superior border of the transverse colon on barium enema (see Fig. 64-35), with spiculation of the luminal contour and pleating and tethering of mucosal folds

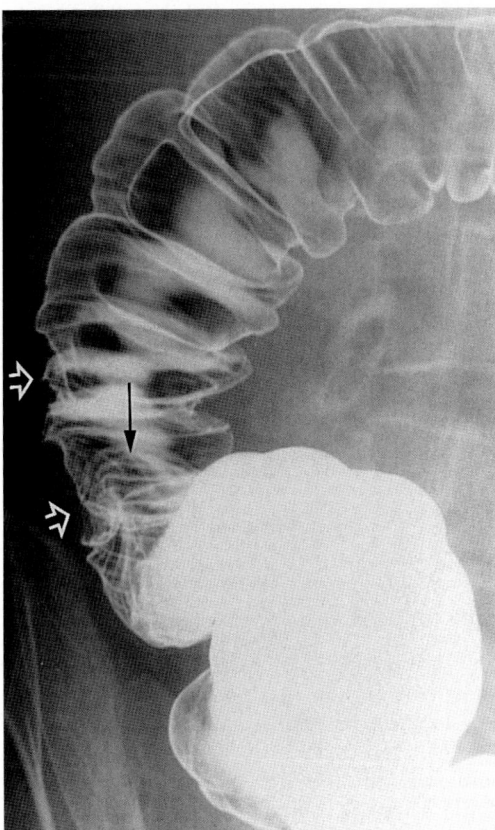

Figure 64-34. Ovarian carcinoma with intraperitoneal metastases to the right paracolic gutter. Spot image from a double-contrast barium enema shows extrinsic mass effect along the right lateral border of the ascending colon (*open arrows*), spiculation of the contour, and pleating of the colonic mucosa en face (*black arrow*).

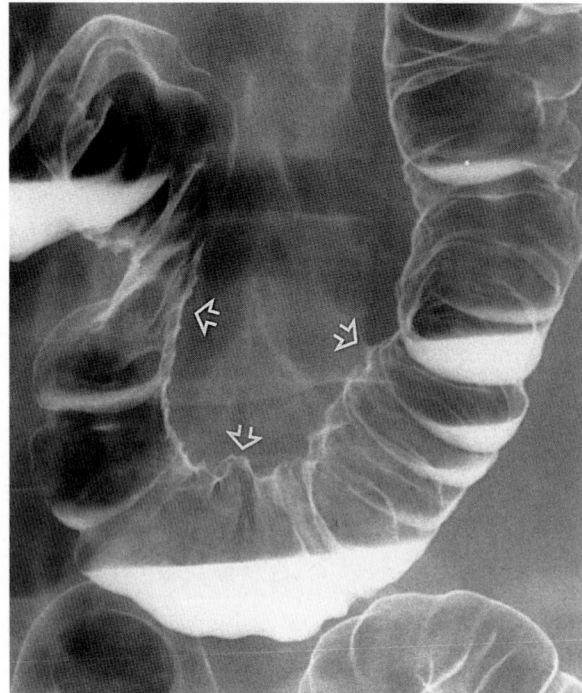

Figure 64-35. Omental cake from ovarian carcinomatosis invading the transverse colon. Spot image from a double-contrast barium enema in a patient with known ovarian carcinoma and intraperitoneal metastases to the greater omentum shows mass effect along the superior border of the transverse colon (*arrows*), spiculation of the superior contour, and sacculation of the uninvolved opposite wall. (From Rubesin SE, Levine MS: Omental cakes: Colonic involvement by omental metastases. Radiology 154:593-596, 1985.)

(Fig. 64-36). The major consideration in the differential diagnosis is gastric carcinoma invading the transverse colon via the gastrocolic ligament. The clinical history as well as the presence of metastases involving other portions of the colon should suggest the correct diagnosis.[112,116] Inflammatory processes involving the gastrocolic ligament, such as cholecystitis, pancreatitis, or diverticulitis, may produce identical radiographic findings.

Embolic Metastases

Patients with embolic metastases to the colon may present with rectal bleeding or incomplete obstruction, often many years after treatment of the primary lesion. The most common primary tumors resulting in embolic metastases to the colon include malignant melanoma and breast and lung carcinoma.

Malignant Melanoma

Malignant melanoma involves the small intestine more frequently than it involves the colon. Metastatic melanoma is usually manifested on barium enemas by umbilicated or ulcerated submucosal masses or by bulky, polypoid intraluminal masses. Linear fissures may radiate toward the central ulcer of the submucosal mass, producing a "spokewheel" appearance.[96] The differential diagnosis of an umbilicated ("target" or "bull's-eye") lesion in the colon includes disseminated lymphoma, Kaposi's sarcoma, carcinoid tumor, and GIST.

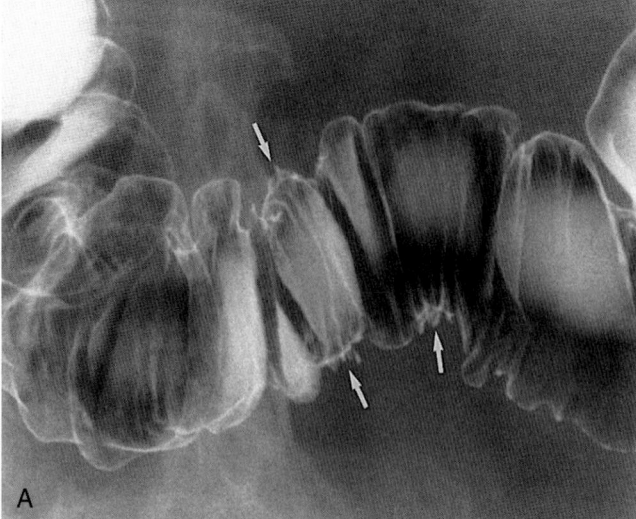

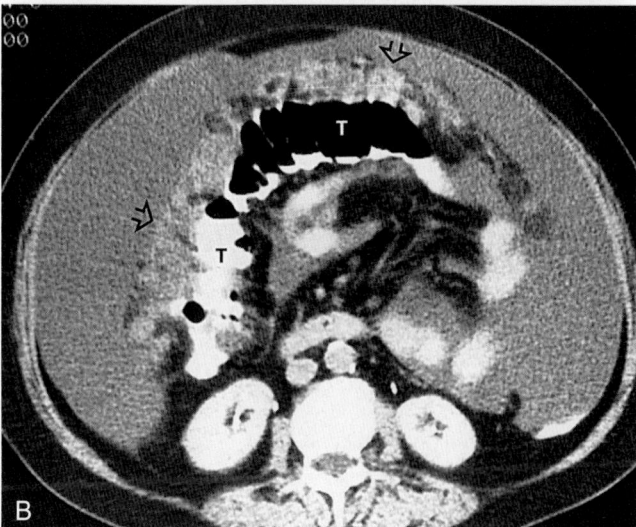

Figure 64-36. Omental cake from ovarian carcinomatosis invading the transverse colon. A. Spot image from a double-contrast barium enema shows spiculation of the colonic contour (*arrows*) and thin transverse stripes traversing the colon as a result of pleating of the mucosa. **B.** CT scan shows enlargement and increased attenuation of greater omentum due to an omental cake (*arrows*) along the anterior border of the transverse colon (T). A large amount of malignant ascites deviates the colon and small bowel loops medially. At surgery, intraperitoneal and greater omental metastases from ovarian carcinoma were found.

Carcinoma of the Breast

Although carcinoma of the breast is the most common primary malignant tumor that spreads to the colon, breast metastases to the colon are usually small lesions that cause no symptoms. More than 5% of those who die of metastatic breast carcinoma are found to have metastases to the colon at autopsy.[117] These metastases may appear on barium enemas as mural nodules (Fig. 64-37), eccentric strictures, or irregular areas of circumferential narrowing, producing a linitis plastica appearance (Fig. 64-38).[97] Hematogenous metastases may occasionally simulate Crohn's disease of the colon.

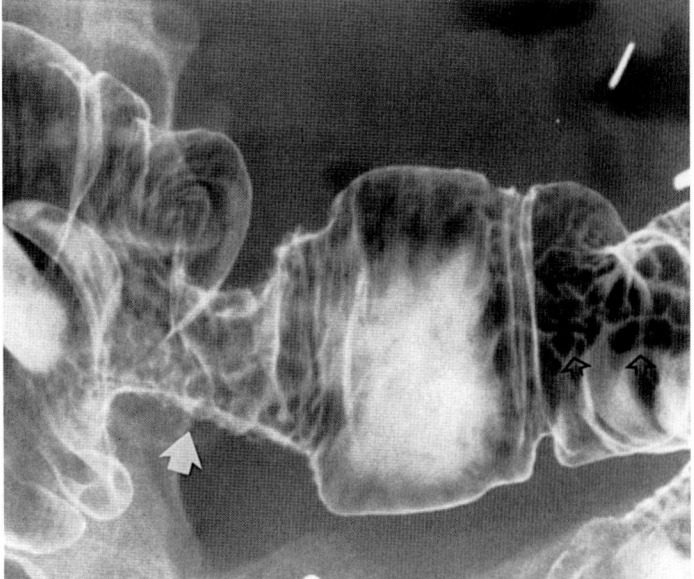

Figure 64-37. Breast metastases to the transverse colon. Spot image from a double-contrast barium enema shows eccentric narrowing of the lumen (*solid arrow*) and nodularity of the mucosa (*open arrows*).

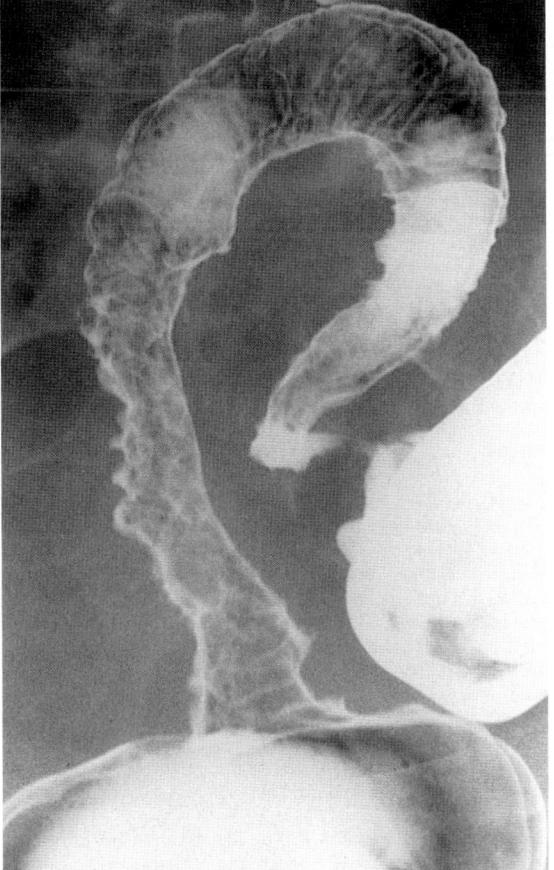

Figure 64-38. Linitis plastica of the colon caused by hematogenous metastases from breast carcinoma. Spot image from a double-contrast barium enema shows narrowing of the distal sigmoid colon with spiculation of the contour and mild nodularity of the colonic mucosa. The differential diagnosis includes primary linitis plastica of the colon and granulomatous colitis. (From Laufer I, Levine MS [eds]: Double Contrast Gastrointestinal Radiology. Philadelphia, WB Saunders, 1992.)

Carcinoma of the Lung

Metastases to the colon from carcinoma of the lung are usually small serosal deposits that cause no symptoms.[97] Occasionally, however, lung metastases may cause gastrointestinal bleeding or obstruction.[118] These metastases may appear radiographically as ulcerated submucosal masses (target lesions), short eccentric segments of narrowing, or large mesenteric masses with secondary desmoplastic serosal changes.[97]

References

1. Weinsrad D, DeCosse JJ, Sherlock P, et al: Primary gastrointestinal lymphoma. Cancer 49:1258-1265, 1982.
2. Lewin KJ, Ranchod M, Dorfman RF: Lymphomas of the gastrointestinal tract: A study of 117 cases presenting with gastrointestinal disease. Cancer 42:693-707, 1978.
3. Herrman R, Panahon AM, Barcos MP, et al: Gastrointestinal involvement in non-Hodgkin's lymphoma. Cancer 46:215-222, 1980.
4. Dragosics B, Bauer P, Radaszkiewicz T: Primary gastrointestinal non-Hodgkin's lymphomas: A retrospective clinicopathologic study of 150 cases. Cancer 55:1060-1073, 1985.
5. Messinger NH, Bobroff LM, Beneventano TC: Lymphosarcoma of the colon. AJR 117:281-286, 1973.
6. Wychulis AR, Beahrs OH, Woolner LB: Malignant lymphoma of the colon. Arch Surg 93:215-225, 1966.
7. Wolf BS, Marshak RH: Roentgen features of diffuse lymphosarcoma of the colon. Radiology 75:733-740, 1960.
8. Cornes JS, Wallace MH, Morson BC: Benign lymphomas of the rectum and anal canal. J Pathol Bacteriol 82:371-382, 1961.
9. Marshak RH, Lindner AE, Maklansky D: Lymphoreticular disorders of the gastrointestinal tract: Roentgenographic features. Gastrointest Radiol 4:103-120, 1979.
10. Renton P, Blackshaw AJ: Colonic lymphoma complicating ulcerative colitis. Br J Surg 63:542-545, 1976.
11. Sataline LR, Mobley EM, Kirkham W: Ulcerative colitis complicated by colonic lymphoma. Gastroenterology 44:342-347, 1963.
12. Hill DH, Mill M, Maxwell RJ: Metachronous colonic lymphomas complicating ulcerative colitis. Abdom Imaging 18:369-370, 1993.
13. Horton KM, Fishman EK: Multifocal primary colonic lymphoma in a patient with posttransplantation lymphoproliferative disease: CT findings. AJR 170:1672, 1998.
14. Kawamoto K, Motooka M, Hirata N, et al: Colonic submucosal tumors: New classification based on radiologic characteristics. AJR 160:315-320, 1993.

15. O'Connell DJ, Thompson AJ: Lymphoma of the colon: The spectrum of radiologic changes. Gastrointest Radiol 2:377-385, 1978.

16. Zornoza J, Dodd GD: Lymphoma of the gastrointestinal tract. Semin Roentgenol 15:272-287, 1980.

17. Bragg DG, Colby TV, Ward JH: New concepts in the non-Hodgkin lymphomas: Radiologic implications. Radiology 159:289-304, 1986.

18. Pochaczevsky R, Sherman RS: Diffuse lymphomatous disease of the colon: Its roentgen appearance. AJR 87:670-684, 1962.

19. Williams SM, Berk RN, Harned RK: Radiologic features of multinodular lymphoma of the colon. AJR 143:87-91, 1984.

20. Wyatt SH, Fishman EK, Jones B: Primary lymphoma of the colon and rectum: CT and barium correlation. Abdom Imaging 18:376-380, 1993.

21. Banks, PM, Chan J, Cleary ML, et al: Mantle cell lymphoma: A proposal for unification of morphologic, immunologic, and molecular data. Am J Surg Pathol 16:637-640, 1992.

22. Issacson PG, Wright DH: Gut-associated lymphoid tumors. In Whitehead R (ed): Gastrointestinal and Oesophageal Pathology. Edinburgh, Churchill Livingstone, 1995, pp 755-775.

23. Harned RK, Doby CA, Farley GE: Cavernous hemangioma of the rectum and appendix. Dis Colon Rectum 17:759-762, 1974.

24. Gentry RW, Dockerty MB, Glagett OT: Collective review: Vascular malformations and vascular tumors of the gastrointestinal tract. Int Abstr Surg 88:281-323, 1949.

25. Dachman AH, Ros PR, Shekitka KM, et al: Colorectal hemangioma: Radiologic findings. Radiology 167:31-34, 1988.

26. Lyon DT, Mantea AG: Large-bowel hemangiomas. Dis Colon Rectum 27:404-414, 1984.

27. Allred HW Jr, Spencer RJ: Hemangiomas of the colon, rectum, and anus. Mayo Clin Proc 49:739-741, 1974.

28. Morson BC, Dawson IMP: Gastrointestinal Pathology. Oxford, Blackwell Scientific, 1979, pp 648-680.

29. Ghahremani GG, Kangarloo H, Volberg F, et al: Diffuse cavernous hemangioma of the colon in the Klippel-Trenaunay syndrome. Radiology 118:673-678, 1976.

30. Perez C, Andreu J, Llauger J, et al: Hemangioma of the rectum: CT appearance. Gastrointest Radiol 12:347-349, 1987.

31. Gandolfi L, Rossi A, Stasi G, Tonti R: The Klippel-Trenaunay syndrome. Gastrointest Endosc 33:442-445, 1987.

32. Goboes K: Rare and secondary (metastatic) tumors. In Whitehead R (ed): Gastrointestinal and Oesphageal Pathology. Edinburgh, Churchill Livingstone, 1995, pp 910-924.

33. Reinhart WH, Staubli M, Mordasini C, et al: Abnormalities of the gut vessels in Turner's syndrome. Postgrad Med J 59:122-124, 1983.

34. Margulis AR: Case: Hemangioma of the rectum. Gastrointest Radiol 6:363-364, 1981.

35. Lawson JP, Myerson PJ, Myerson DA: Colonic lymphangioma. Gastrointest Radiol 1:85-89, 1976.

36. Camilleri M, Satti MB, Wood CB: Cystic lymphangioma of the colon. Dis Colon Rectum 25:813-816, 1982.

37. Arnet NL, Friedman PS: Lymphangioma of the colon: Roentgen aspects, a case report. Radiology 67:882-885, 1956.

38. Agha FP, Francis IR, Simms SM: Cystic lymphangioma of the colon. AJR 141:709-710, 1983.

39. Kawamoto K, Ueyama T, Iwashita I, et al: Colonic submucosal tumors: Comparison of endoscopic US and target air-enema CT with barium enema study and colonoscopy. Radiology 192:697-702, 1994.

40. Young T-H, Ho A-S, Tang HS, et al: Cystic lymphangioma of the transverse colon: Report of a case and review of the literature. Abdom Imaging 21:415-417, 1996.

41. Boley SJ, Sammartano R, Adams A, et al: On the nature and etiology of vascular ectasias of the colon: Degenerative lesions of aging. Gastroenterology 72:650-660, 1977.

42. Baum S, Athanasoulis C, Waltman A, et al: Angiodysplasia of the right colon: A cause of gastrointestinal bleeding. AJR 129:789-794, 1977.

43. Galloway SJ, Casarella WJ, Shimkin PM: Vascular malformations of the right colon as a cause of bleeding in patients with aortic stenosis. Radiology 113:11-15, 1974.

44. Thompson GB, Pemberton JH, Morris S, et al: Kaposi's sarcoma of the colon in a young HIV-negative man with chronic ulcerative colitis. Dis Colon Rectum 32:73-76, 1989.

45. Puy-Montbrun T, Pigot F, Vuong PN, et al: Kaposi's sarcoma of the colon in a young HIV-negative woman with Crohn's disease. Dig Dis Sci 36:528-531, 1991.

46. Godwin DJ: Carcinoid tumors: An analysis of 2837 cases. Cancer 36: 560-569, 1975.

47. Martensson H, Nobin A, Sundler F: Carcinoid tumours in the gastrointestinal tract—an analysis of 156 cases. Acta Chir Scand 149:607-616, 1983.

48. Shulman H, Giustra P: Invasive carcinoids of the colon. Radiology 98:139-143, 1971.

49. Wilander E: Endocrine cell tumours. In Whitehead R (ed): Gastrointestinal and Oesophageal Pathology. Edinburgh, Churchill Livingstone, 1989, pp 629-641.

50. Wilander E, Portela-Gomes G, Grimelius L, et al: Argentaffin and argyrophil reaction of human gastrointestinal carcinoids. Gastroenterology 73:733-736, 1977.

51. Balthazar EJ: Carcinoid tumors of the alimentary tract. Gastrointest Radiol 3:47-56, 1978.

52. Fioca R, Capella C, Bufta R, et al: Glucagon-like, glicentin-like and pancreatic polypeptide-like immunoreactivities in rectal carcinoids and related colorectal cells. Am J Pathol 100:81-92, 1980.

53. Jetmore AB, Ray JE, Gathright JB, et al: Rectal carcinoids: The most frequent rectal tumor. Dis Colon Rectum 35:717-725, 1992.

54. Sato T, Sakai Y, Sonoyama A, et al: Radiologic spectrum of rectal carcinoid tumors. Gastrointest Radiol 9:23-26, 1984.

55. Berardi RS: Carcinoid tumors of the colon (exclusive of the rectum): Review of the literature. Dis Colon Rectum 15:383-391, 1972.

56. Crittenden JJ, Byllesby J, Dodds W: Carcinoid tumor presenting as an annular lesion in the ascending colon. Radiology 97:85-86, 1970.

57. Haller JD, Roberts TW: Lipomas of the colon: A clinicopathologic study of 40 cases. Surgery 55:773-781, 1964.

58. Hurwitz MH, Redleaf PD, Williams HJ, et al: Lipomas of the gastrointestinal tract. AJR 99:84-89, 1967.

59. Castro DB, Stearns MW: Lipomas of the large intestine. Dis Colon Rectum 15:441-444, 1972.

60. Berk RN, Werner LG: The radiology corner: Lipoma of the colon. Am J Gastroenterol 61:145-150, 1974.

61. Snover DC: Atypical lipomas of the colon. Dis Colon Rectum 27: 485-488, 1984.

62. Margulis AR, Jovanovich A: The roentgen diagnosis of submucous lipomas of the colon. AJR 84:1114-1120, 1960.

63. Kabaalioglu A, Gelen T, Aktan S, et al: Acute colonic obstruction caused by intussusception and extrusion of a sigmoid lipoma through the anus after barium enema. Abdom Imaging 22:389-391, 1997.

64. Wulff C, Jespersen N: Colo-colic intussusception caused by lipoma: Case report. Acta Radiol 36:478-480, 1995.

65. Buetow PC, Buck JL, Carr NJ, et al: Intussuscepted colonic lipomas: Loss of fat attenuation on CT with pathologic correlation in 10 cases. Abdom Imaging 21:153-156, 1996.

66. Deeths TM, Dodds WJ: Lipoma of the colon. Am J Gastroenterol 58: 326-331, 1972.

67. Heiken JP, Forde KA, Gold RP: Computed tomography as a definitive method for diagnosing gastrointestinal lipomas. Radiology 142:409-414, 1982.

68. Megibow AJ, Redmond PE, Bosniak MA, et al: Diagnosis of gastrointestinal lipomas by CT. AJR 133:743-745, 1979.

69. Liessi G, Pavanello M, Cesari S, et al: Large lipomas of the colon: CT and MR findings in three symptomatic cases. Abdom Imaging 21:150-152, 1996.

70. Geboes K: Rare and secondary (metastatic) tumours. In Whitehead R (ed): Gastrointestinal and Oesophageal Pathology. Edinburgh, Churchill Livingstone, 1989, pp 779-786.

71. Hinkel CL: Roentgenological examination and evaluation of the ileocecal valve. AJR 68:171-182, 1952.

72. El-Amin LC, Levine MS, Rubesin SE, et al: Ileocecal valve: Spectrum of normal findings at double-contrast barium enema examination. Radiology 227:52-58, 2003.

73. Appelman HD: Smooth muscle tumors of the gastrointestinal tract: What we know now that Stout didn't know. Am J Surg Pathol 10(Suppl 1):83-89, 1986.

74. Saul SH, Rast ML, Brooks JJ: The immunohistochemistry of gastrointestinal stromal tumors: Evidence supporting an origin from smooth muscle. Am J Surg Pathol 11:464-473, 1987.

75. Kempson RL, Henrickson WR: Gastrointestinal stromal (smooth muscle) tumors. In Whitehead R (ed): Gastrointestinal and Oesophageal Pathology. Edinburgh, Churchill Livingstone, 1995, pp 727-739.

76. Sugimura H, Tamura S, Yamada H, et al: Benign nerve sheath tumor of the sigmoid colon. Clin Imaging 17:64-66, 1993.

77. Hirtoa S, Isozaki K, Moriyama Y, et al: Gain-of-function mutations of c-kit in human gastrointestinal stromal tumors. Science 279:577-580, 1998.

78. Ma CK, De Peralta MN, Amin MB, et al: Small intestinal stromal tumors: A clinicopathologic study of 20 cases with immunohistochemical assessment of cell differentiation and the prognostic role of proliferation antigens. Am J Clin Pathol 108:641-651, 1997.

79. Rao BK, Kapur MM, Roy S: Leiomyosarcoma of the colon: A case report and review of literature. Dis Colon Rectum 23:184-190, 1980.

80. Akwari OE, Dozois RR, Weiland LH, et al: Leiomyosarcoma of the small and large bowel. Cancer 42:1375-1384, 1978.

81. Walsh TH, Mann CV: Smooth muscle neoplasms of the rectum and anal canal. Br J Surg 71:597-599, 1984.

82. Radin DR, Kiyabu M: Multiple smooth-muscle tumors of the colon and adrenal gland in an adult with AIDS. AJR 159:545-546, 1992.

83. Williams GT, Blackshaw AJ, Morson BC: Squamous carcinoma of the colorectum and its genesis. J Pathol 129:139-147, 1979.

84. Heenan PJ: Other tumors of the anal canal. In Whitehead R (ed): Gastrointestinal and Oesophageal Pathology. Edinburgh, Churchill Livingstone, 1995, pp 935-956.

85. Gillespie JJ, MacKay B: Histogenesis of cloacogenic carcinoma: Fine structure of anal transitional epithelium and cloacogenic carcinoma. Hum Pathol 9:579-587, 1978.

86. Fenger C: The anal canal epithelium: A review. Scand J Gastroenterol 14(Suppl):114-117, 1979.

87. Vernon SD, Unger ER, Reeves WC: Human papillomaviruses and anogenital cancer. N Engl J Med 338:921-922, 1998.

88. Shah KV: Human papillomaviruses and anogenital cancers. N Engl J Med 337:1386-1388, 1997.

89. Frisch M, Glimelius B, van den Brule AJ, et al: Sexually transmitted infection as a cause of anal cancer. N Engl J Med 337:1350-1359, 1997.

90. Austin DR: Etiological clues from descriptive epidemiology: Squamous carcinoma of the rectum or anus. Natl Cancer Inst Monogr 62:89-90, 1982.

91. Peters RK, Mack TM: Patterns of anal carcinoma by gender and marital status in Los Angeles County. Br J Cancer 48:629-636, 1983.

92. Daling JR, Weiss NS, Klopfenstein LL, et al: Correlates of homosexual behavior and the incidence of anal cancer. JAMA 247:1988-1990, 1982.

93. Kyaw MM, Gallagher T, Haines JO: Cloacogenic carcinoma. AJR 115:384-391, 1972.

94. Glickman MG, Margulis AR: Cloacogenic carcinoma. AJR 107:175-180, 1969.

95. Wigh R, Tapley ND: Metastatic lesions to the large intestine. Radiology 70:222-229, 1958.

96. Meyers MA, McSweeney J: Secondary neoplasms of the bowel. Radiology 105:1-11, 1972.

97. Meyers MA: Dynamic Radiology of the Abdomen: Normal and Pathologic Anatomy, 3rd ed. New York, Springer, 1988.

98. Gedgaudas RK, Kelvin FM, Thompson WM, et al: The value of preoperative barium enema in the assessment of pelvic masses. Radiology 146:609-613, 1983.

99. Becker JA: Prostatic carcinoma involving the rectum and sigmoid colon. AJR 94:421-428, 1965.

100. Gengler L, Baer J, Finby N: Rectal and sigmoid involvement secondary to carcinoma of the prostate. AJR 125:910-917, 1975.

101. Winter CC: The problem of rectal involvement by prostatic cancer. Surg Gynecol Obstet 105:136-140, 1957.

102. Fry DE, Amin M, Harbrecht PJ: Rectal obstruction secondary to carcinoma of the prostate. Ann Surg 189:488-492, 1979.

103. Aigen AB, Schapira HE: Metastatic carcinoma of prostate and bladder causing intestinal obstruction. Urology 21:464-466, 1983.

104. Rubesin SE, Levine MS, Bezzi M, et al: Rectal involvement by prostatic carcinoma: Radiographic findings. AJR 152:53-57, 1989.

105. Huang TY, Yam LT, Li CY: Unusual radiologic features of metastatic prostatic carcinoma confirmed by immunohistochemical study. Urology 23:218-223, 1984.

106. Li CY, Lam WKW, Yam LT: Immunohistochemical diagnosis of prostatic cancer with metastasis. Cancer 46:706-712, 1980.

107. Meyers MA: Intraperitoneal spread of malignancies and its effect on the bowel. Clin Radiol 32:129-146, 1981.

108. Honda H, Lu CH, Barloon TT, et al: Sigmoid colon fistula complicating ovarian cystadenocarcinoma—a rare finding. Gastrointest Radiol 15:78-81, 1990.

109. Khilnani MT, Wolf BS: Late involvement of the alimentary tract by carcinoma of the kidney. Am J Dig Dis 5:529-540, 1960.

110. Bachman AL: Roentgen appearance of gastric invasion from carcinoma of the colon. Radiology 63:814-822, 1954.

111. Goodman P, Balachandran S: Direct invasion of the transverse colon by a cecal tumor. Abdom Imaging 18:20-22, 1993.

112. Rubesin SE, Levine MS: Omental cakes: Colonic involvement by omental metastases. Radiology 154:593-596, 1985.

113. Meyers MA: Distribution of intra-abdominal malignant seeding: Dependency on dynamics of flow of ascitic fluid. AJR 119:198-206, 1973.

114. Meyers MA: The spread and localization of acute intraperitoneal effusions. Radiology 95:547-554, 1970.

115. Ginaldi S, Lindell MM, Zornoza J: The striped colon: A new radiographic observation in metastatic serosal implants. AJR 134:453-455, 1980.

116. Krestin GP, Beyer D, Lorenz R: Secondary involvement of the transverse colon by tumors of the pelvis: Spread of malignancies along the greater omentum. Gastrointest Radiol 10:283-288, 1985.

117. Asch MJ, Wiedel PD, Habif DV: Gastrointestinal metastases from carcinoma of the breast: Autopsy study and 18 cases requiring operative intervention. Arch Surg 96:840-843, 1968.

118. Smith HJ, Vlask MG: Metastasis to the colon from bronchogenic carcinoma. Gastrointest Radiol 2:393-396, 1978.

Polyposis Syndromes

Carina L. Butler, MD • James L. Buck, MD

The polyposis syndromes are rare but fascinating conditions. A thorough knowledge of the clinical and radiographic manifestations of these syndromes and their complications is required to provide optimal care for affected individuals and their families.

FAMILIAL ADENOMATOUS POLYPOSIS SYNDROME

There is now clear evidence that familial polyposis coli and Gardner's syndrome are varying expressions of the same disease. The majority of cases are caused by the presence of an abnormal tumor suppressor gene (the *APC* gene) located on the long arm of chromosome 5.[1] As a result, the term *familial adenomatous polyposis syndrome* (FAPS) is used to refer to the entire spectrum of this disease.

FAPS is a relatively rare condition, but it is the most common of the polyposis syndromes.[2] Males and females are equally affected. FAPS has an autosomal dominant pattern of inheritance when associated with the *APC* gene mutation. However, up to 30% of patients have no family history of polyposis, suggesting the presence of spontaneous mutations or an association with a different mutation.[3,4] A family history of polyposis or colorectal cancer therefore is not required for the diagnosis of FAPS. Penetrance is generally thought to be in the range of 80% to 100%, although in one series it was calculated to be less than 60%.[5] In most families, comparative DNA testing alone can determine whether a family member is carrying the abnormal *APC* gene.[6] In 5% to 30% of patients with FAPS, however, no *APC* mutation can be identified by current genetic testing.[4] A different gene (the *MYH* gene) has also been linked to *APC*-negative patients with FAPS.[4] Interestingly, FAPS associated with the *MYH* gene is thought to be inherited in a recessive fashion. Biologic differences be-

tween *APC*-associated FAPS and *MYH*-associated FAPS are not completely understood. However, patients with the *MYH* mutation appear to have a milder form of the disease than those with the *APC* mutation.[7] Other differences that are clinically relevant may become evident with further investigation.

Colonic Manifestations

As the name implies, FAPS is predominantly associated with the development of adenomas. In the colon, where the polyposis is most severe, the polyps are usually tubular or tubulovillous adenomas. Occasionally, villous adenomas are also seen. The polyps usually appear at or near puberty, and, eventually, an average of about 1000 adenomas colonic will develop.[8] The adenomas of FAPS are usually small (80% are < 5 mm in diameter) and sessile. The polyps involve all portions of the colon but may first appear distally. Rectal sparing occasionally may be seen.

A milder phenotype of FAPS, known as attenuated familial adenomatous polyposis syndrome (AFAPS), has recently been described. These patients generally present with 100 or fewer colonic adenomas.[9,10] The adenomas tend to be located more proximally than those in classic FAPS, so that sigmoidoscopy alone is inadequate for evaluating these patients.[11] Colonic carcinoma also develops at an older age, with an average age of 55 years in patients with AFAPS versus an average age of 40 years in patients with classic FAPS.

The most common signs encountered in FAPS are rectal bleeding and diarrhea, which occur in more than 75% of patients. Abdominal pain, anemia, and mucous discharge are less frequently noted.[12,13] However, many patients with FAPS are asymptomatic. Regardless of symptoms, colonic carcinomas develop in virtually every untreated patient and at a much younger age than in the general population.[3] Thus,

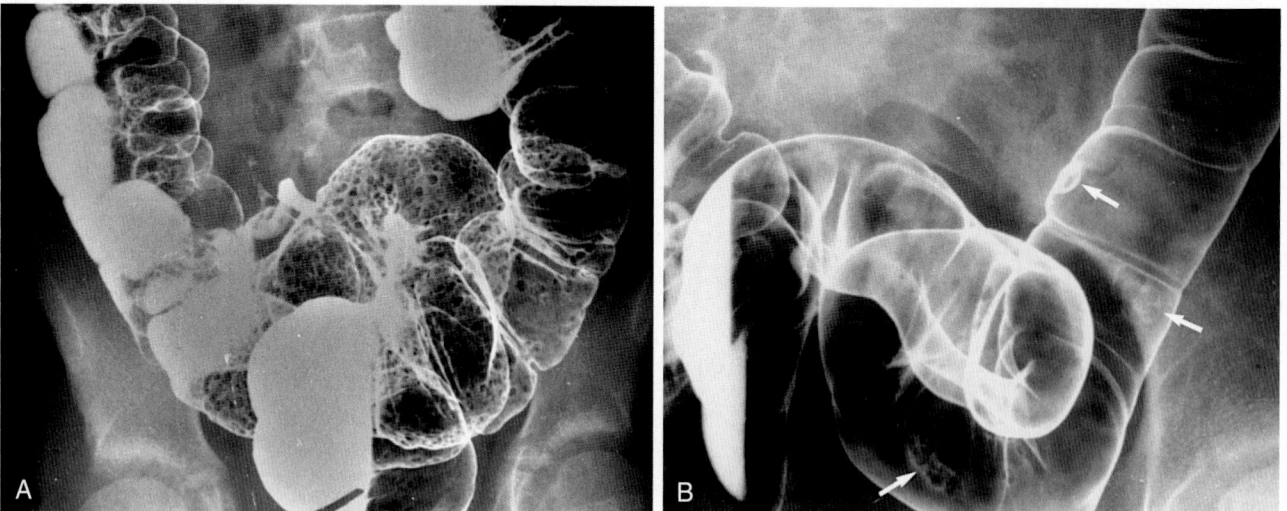

Figure 65-1. Various appearances of colonic involvement by familial adenomatous polyposis syndrome. A. In a 10-year-old boy, double-contrast barium enema demonstrates innumerable small polyps in the colon, particularly carpeting the rectosigmoid region. **B.** In a 17-year-old girl, double-contrast barium enema shows scattered, small to moderate-sized polyps (*arrows*) in the sigmoid colon.

DNA testing or serial colonic examinations after 10 years of age are recommended for other family members at risk for the disease.

In the past, many patients with FAPS were treated with colectomy and ileorectal anastomosis.[14] However, even with frequent proctoscopic examinations and fulguration of any persistent or recurrent adenomas, rectal carcinoma developed in 5% to 40% of these patients.[15] Total colectomy with mucosal proctectomy and ileoanal anastomosis has therefore become the procedure of choice because it eliminates all colonic and rectal mucosa.[15] Surgical intervention should be performed by the late teenage years.[13] After surgery, continued surveillance is necessary, because any surgical procedure that restores intestinal continuity bears a continued risk of malignancy in the surgical remnant.

The radiographic appearance of the colon in FAPS varies. Classically, innumerable small or moderate-sized filling defects carpet the entire colon (Fig. 65-1A). In some younger patients, however, the polyps may be more widely scattered (Fig. 65-1B). Correlation with colectomy specimens has shown that barium enemas markedly underestimate the number of polyps, especially in young patients, whose polyps are often less than 3 mm in diameter.[16] Unfortunately, carcinomas still develop due to inadequate screening of family members at risk for the disease. Carcinoma may be manifested by a dominant polyp, a saddle lesion (Fig. 65-2), or an advanced annular lesion. As in the general population, carcinomas are more commonly found in the left side of the colon.

Extracolonic Gastrointestinal Manifestations

Extracolonic gastrointestinal manifestations of FAPS are well recognized.[17-24] Fundic gland polyps are the most common gastric manifestation of FAPS in western countries, occurring in up to 84% of patients.[25,26] In FAPS, both sexes are equally involved, whereas in the absence of FAPS, fundic gland polyps are more common in females.[27,28] The polyps are frequently discovered in asymptomatic patients at an average age of 25 to 30 years and are almost invariably multiple, appearing as

small, sessile lesions ranging from 1 to 5 mm in diameter.[29] They are almost always confined to the fundus and body of the stomach, producing a characteristic radiographic appearance (Fig. 65-3). On subsequent examinations, the polyps may progress, remain stable, or even resolve.[30-32] These polyps have little tendency for malignant transformation, although gastric cancer has occasionally been reported in patients with preexisting fundic gland polyps.[26]

Tubular and villous adenomas are also found in the stomach in patients with FAPS. In Japan, the incidence of gastric

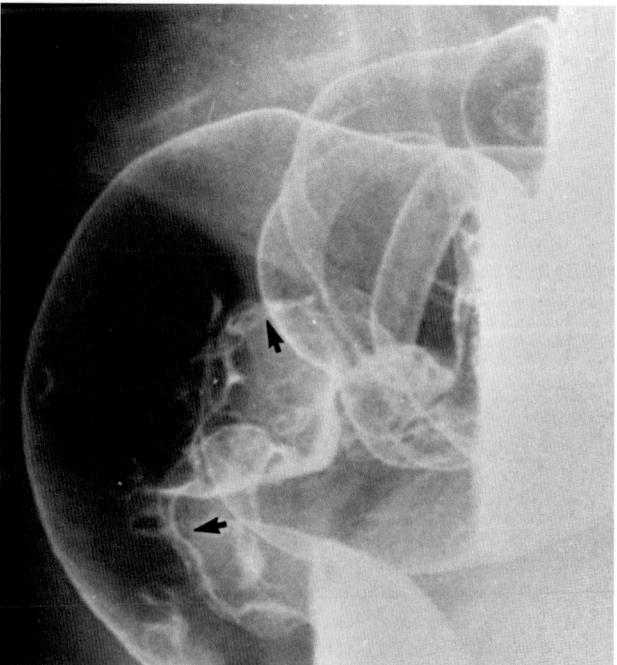

Figure 65-2. Colon carcinoma in a 32-year-old woman with familial adenomatous polyposis syndrome. A saddle carcinoma (*arrows*) is seen on the anterior wall of the rectum. Scattered small polyps are also present.

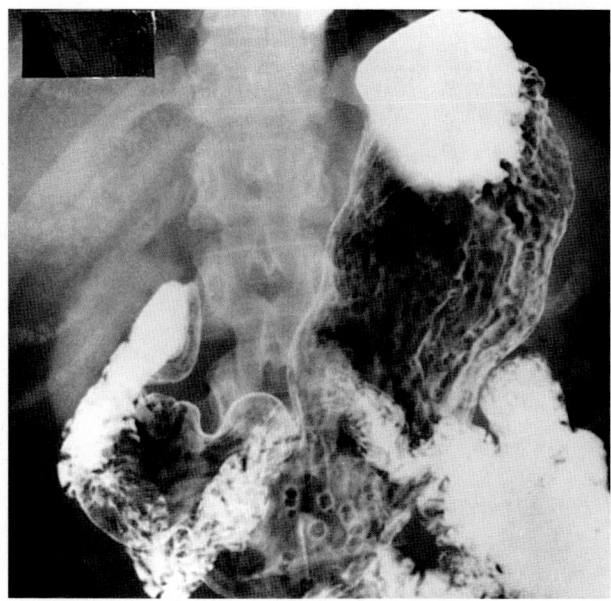

Figure 65-3. Fundic gland polyposis of the stomach in a 25-year-old woman with familial adenomatous polyposis syndrome. Double-contrast upper gastrointestinal study demonstrates multiple small filling defects in the fundus and body of the stomach. The antrum is not involved. The gallbladder is faintly opacified from a prior oral chole-cystogram.

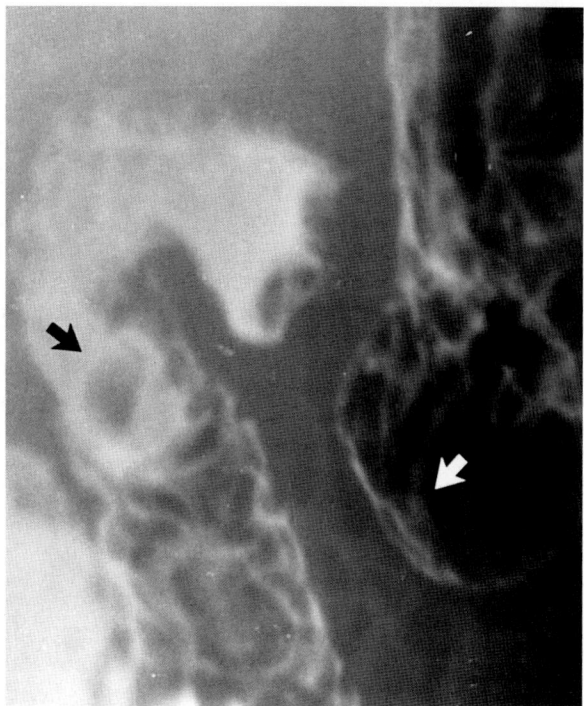

Figure 65-4. Gastric and duodenal adenomas in a 53-year-old woman after a colectomy for familial adenomatous polyposis syndrome. Double-contrast study demonstrates polyps in the antrum (*white arrow*) and descending duodenum (*black arrow*).

adenomas in FAPS ranges from 40% to 50%, whereas in Europe and North America, a lower incidence is reported.[20,25] The higher incidence of adenomas associated with FAPS in Japan may be related to the higher frequency of adenomas and adenocarcinomas in the general population of that country.[33] Gastric adenomas are typically sessile polyps, ranging from 5 to 10 mm in diameter, and are multiple in over half of the reported cases.[25,31] The adenomas are usually located in the distal stomach (Fig. 65-4).[31] Unlike fundic gland polyps, gastric adenomas are premalignant lesions, so that periodic surveillance of the stomach is required.

The duodenum is the second most common site of gastrointestinal disease in FAPS. Endoscopic examinations of asymptomatic patients in Japan have revealed tubular adenomas in more than 90% of cases.[19,34] Other screening studies from Western countries have revealed adenomas in 47% to 72% of cases.[18,21-24] The adenomas range from microscopic to 2 cm in diameter, with a majority being 5 mm or less. The polyps are usually found in the second portion of the duodenum, clustered around the papilla (see Fig. 65-4).[35] This differs from the typically bulbar distribution of adenomas in patients without FAPS.[36] Villous adenomas are also commonly found, and as in patients without FAPS, they tend to be located in the periampullary region of the duodenum. Villous adenomas are typically large and are even more likely to undergo malignant degeneration. It has been estimated that the lifetime incidence of periampullary carcinoma is as high as 12% and that it is now the leading cause of cancer deaths in patients who have had a colectomy. It is therefore advocated that surveillance of the upper gastrointestinal tract be performed in asymptomatic patients with FAPS beginning at 25 years of age.[35]

Adenomas in the jejunum and ileum have been identified in the majority of patients in Japan who have undergone intra-

operative small bowel endoscopy.[37] Small bowel endoscopy performed through a cutaneous ileostomy or ileoproctostomy has also revealed adenomas in approximately 20% of FAPS patients in western countries.[21,24] As in the duodenum, these premalignant lesions are typically small and numerous. Although several cases of adenocarcinoma of the jejunum or ileum have been reported (coexisting adenomas have been found in all of these cases), the need for routine screening of the small bowel beyond the duodenum has not been established.[38-40] Ileal lymphoid hyperplasia occurs more frequently in patients with FAPS than in the general population. The gross appearance of these lesions is similar to that of adenomas.[37] However, lymphoid hyperplasia has no apparent clinical significance in these patients.

Biliary polyps are often found in patients with FAPS studied by endoscopic retrograde cholangiopancreatography.[22] Not surprisingly, cholangiocarcinoma and gallbladder carcinoma have also been reported in FAPS.[41-44] Several cases of pancreatic carcinoma have been reported, and there is an increased incidence of pancreatitis in these patients.[45]

Extraintestinal Manifestations

It was not until the 1950s that the extraintestinal manifestations of FAPS were well established. Gardner and Richards initially described a family of patients with adenomatous polyps of the colon, sebaceous cysts, and osteomas.[46] Later, fibrous tumors and dental abnormalities were added to the list of lesions included in what was subsequently termed *Gardner's syndrome*.[47] Numerous reports have subsequently confirmed the occurrence of these and other extraintestinal manifestations that have a tendency to appear in certain kindred affected by FAPS. The location of the defect within the *APC* gene and other intracellular factors appear to determine whether these manifestations are likely to appear.[48,49] It is unusual to see all of the manifestations in the same patient.[50]

Epidermoid (sebaceous) cysts are the skin lesions most frequently encountered in patients with FAPS. The cysts tend to be located on the face and scalp rather than on the back, as in the general population.[51] They are uncommon before puberty, but the presence of these cysts often precedes the recognition of colonic polyps.[13] Otherwise, they have no clinical significance. Lipomas and small fibrous tumors of the skin are also found in FAPS.[52]

Osteomas are another well-known manifestation of FAPS. Like epidermoid cysts, osteomas are usually unimportant unless they cause symptoms due to mass effect.[35] In FAPS patients, these dense cortical lesions are most commonly found in the angle of the mandible, the sinuses, and the outer table of the skull (Fig. 65-5).[53] Other flat bones and long bones may be involved. Bone islands are also quite common in the maxilla and mandible and may be seen in other flat bones as well.[54-56] In one series, localized or diffuse cortical thickening of the long bones was the most commonly identified bone abnormality in FAPS.[53] Dental abnormalities, particularly impacted or supernumerary teeth, are also common.[35,57,58]

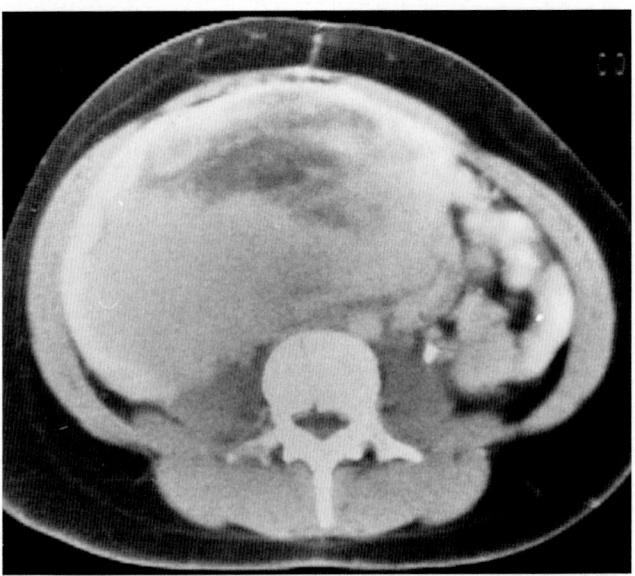

Figure 65-6. Mesenteric fibromatosis in a 17-year-old girl with familial adenomatous polyposis syndrome. CT scan (same patient as in Fig. 65-1B) reveals a large mass in the right side of the abdomen, obstructing the bowel. The ileum was found to be involved at surgery. The low-attenuation area within the mass is due to mucoid degeneration.

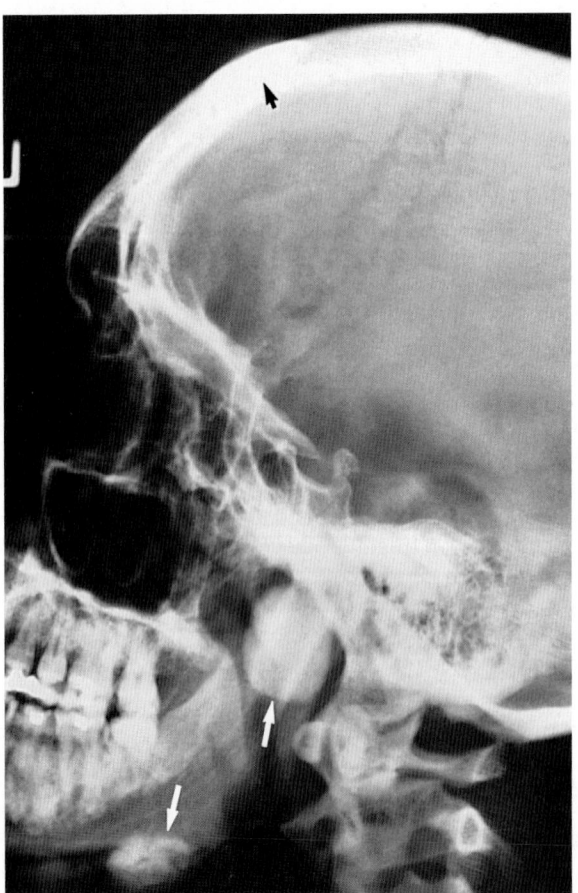

Figure 65-5. Multiple osteomas in a 23-year-old man with familial adenomatous polyposis syndrome. Lateral radiograph of the face and skull demonstrates two dense bony lesions (*white arrows*) arising from the mandible. A subtle lesion (*black arrow*) is also seen in the frontal bone.

Fibrous proliferation is a less common but more important feature of FAPS. An increased incidence of postoperative peritoneal adhesions occurs in FAPS, and retroperitoneal fibrosis has also been reported.[48,59] More commonly, these patients develop fibrous tumors (particularly desmoid tumors of the abdominal wall) and mesenteric fibromatosis (Fig. 65-6). Histologically, desmoids are benign lesions but are nonencapsulated. In FAPS, these tumors often develop postoperatively, occurring within abdominal incisions, the peritoneal cavity, or the retroperitoneum.[13] They most commonly develop in women of childbearing age, and they may grow rapidly or may first appear during pregnancy or after exposure to oral contraceptives.[60] These tumors may recur locally after resection, and invasion of bowel is common. Death may result from intestinal or vascular obstruction, particularly when the lesions are located within the peritoneal cavity. With recent improvements in CT, more subtle diffuse soft tissue infiltration of the mesentery can be identified, but this appearance is less likely to be associated with symptoms than is an actual mesenteric mass.[61]

Congenital pigmented lesions of the retina are common in patients with FAPS; the prevalence of these lesions may be higher than 90%.[62-64] Although similar lesions are occasionally found in the general population, the presence of large, multifocal, or bilateral pigmented lesions on funduscopic examination is a strong indicator of FAPS. These lesions may occur before the development of colonic polyposis, serving as a marker for FAPS, but the absence of such lesions does not exclude FAPS.[65,66]

In recent years, much has been learned about the association between colonic carcinoma and central nervous system malignancies, a condition traditionally known as *Turcot's syndrome*.[67] Recent evidence suggests that many, if not most, of these cases (including those in the family first described by Turcot) are actually related to the hereditary nonpolyposis colon cancer syndrome (HNPCCS) and do not have abnormalities of the *APC* gene.[68] Nevertheless, central nervous system tumors are important extraintestinal manifestations of FAPS. There is clearly an increased incidence of medulloblastoma. There have also been case reports of benign intracranial tumors associated with FAPS, including intracranial epidermoid cysts and meningiomas.[69] Glial tumors such as ependymoma and astrocytoma also occur in FAPS.[70] However, many cases of glioblastoma multiforme associated with colonic adenomas or carcinomas that have been reported in the past were probably related to HNPCCS.

The prevalence of thyroid carcinoma in FAPS has been calculated to be 160 times greater than that in the general population. Almost all reported cases are papillary, and they are frequently multifocal.[71] In most series, affected individuals are girls or young women and the thyroid carcinoma is usually detected before colonic polyposis becomes apparent. FAPS therefore should be suspected in young women with papillary carcinoma of the thyroid.[72] In one series, however, there was no female predominance in patients with thyroid carcinoma and FAPS.[73] Other endocrine tumors (including multiple endocrine neoplasia type 2, carcinoid tumors, and adrenocortical adenomas and carcinomas) have also been reported in patients with FAPS.[74-78]

Several tumors of the pancreas and liver have been reported in FAPS, including pancreatic carcinoma. Solid and papillary epithelial neoplasm, neuroendocrine tumors, and intraductal papillary mucinous tumors of the pancreas have also been reported.[79] Because of the rarity of these tumors, screening of FAPS patients for pancreatic lesions does not appear to be warranted. Hepatoblastoma has also been reported with increased frequency in the offspring of patients with FAPS.[35,80]

HAMARTOMATOUS POLYPOSIS SYNDROMES

The other polyposis syndromes, which occur less frequently than FAPS, include Peutz-Jeghers syndrome (PJS), multiple hamartoma syndrome (MHS), juvenile polyposis (JP), Cronkhite-Canada syndrome (CCS), and Bannayan-Riley-Ruvalcaba syndrome (BRRS). These conditions are collectively known as the hamartomatous polyposis syndromes.[81] (The term *hamartoma* implies a non-neoplastic tumor composed of normal tissue elements.) It is now recognized that hamartomatous polyps may coexist with adenomatous polyps, explaining the association of alimentary tract adenocarcinoma with most of these syndromes, although they account for less than 1% of all colorectal carcinomas in North America.[82]

Peutz-Jeghers Syndrome

Peutz-Jeghers syndrome (PJS) is an inherited condition characterized by a unique type of gastrointestinal hamartoma, mucocutaneous pigmentation, neoplasms outside the alimentary tract, and an increased risk for gastrointestinal carcinoma. PJS has an autosomal dominant pattern of inheritance and affects both sexes equally. Currently, the only gene associated with PJS is a tumor suppressor gene, *STK11*, also known as *LKB1* gene, located on chromosome 19.[83] There are however, a substantial number of PJS patients in whom there is no linkage to chromosome 19, suggesting that other genes also play a role in the development of this syndrome.

The characteristic feature of the PJS hamartoma is a smooth muscle core arising from the muscularis mucosae and extending into the polyp much like the trunk and branches of a tree. The mucosa covering the polyp is similar to that normally found in the portion of the gut in which the polyp arises. Some PJS polyps may cause displacement of the epithelial elements within the submucosa, muscularis propria, and subserosa; this finding should not be mistaken for an invasive mucinous adenocarcinoma.[84]

Mucocutaneous pigmentation is one of the most characteristic features of PJS. Brown or bluish black macules occur most commonly on the lips and buccal mucosa (Fig. 65-7) and less commonly on the eyelids and dorsal surfaces of the fingers and soles of the feet. The pigmentation is rarely present at birth, usually appearing after the first or second year of life. The skin and lip pigmentation fades gradually in adulthood, whereas the macules on the buccal mucosa remain unchanged.[84]

The majority of patients have recurrent episodes of abdominal pain related to intussusceptions caused by the hamartomatous polyps. These intussusceptions usually resolve spontaneously. However, persistent intussusceptions may cause small bowel obstruction, necessitating surgical intervention. Less frequently, patients may have rectal bleeding or melena. Life-threatening gastrointestinal hemorrhage is extremely uncommon.[84]

Patients with PJS are at increased risk for developing adenocarcinoma of the gastrointestinal tract. The majority of these carcinomas are located in the colon, followed in decreasing order of frequency by the stomach, duodenum,

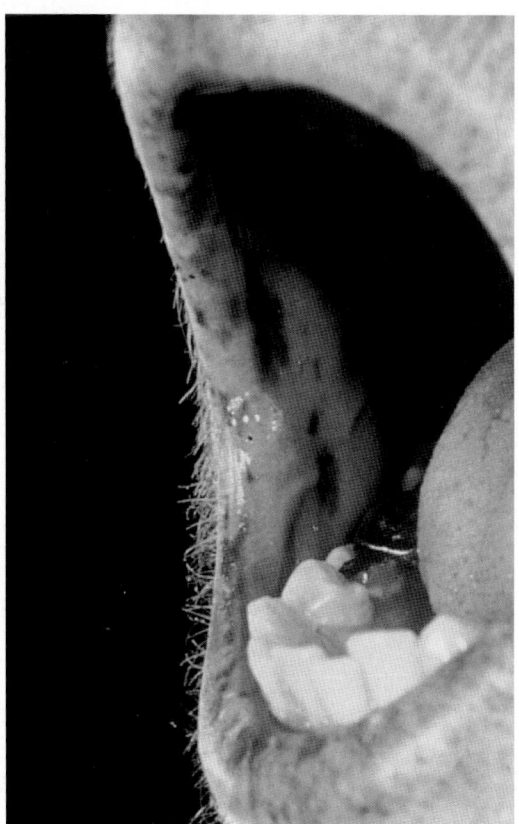

Figure 65-7. Classic mucocutaneous pigmentation of Peutz-Jeghers syndrome. Bluish black macules are seen on the lips and buccal mucosa.

and esophagus.[82] Although the exact prevalence of gastro-intestinal carcinoma is unclear, studies suggest that at least 10% of patients with PJS develop gastrointestinal cancer[84,85] and that females with PJS are more likely to develop these tumors.[82,86] It is uncertain whether carcinoma in PJS develops from malignant transformation of a hamartomatous polyp, from a coexisting adenomatous polyp, or de novo. However, cases of dysplasia and carcinoma occurring within a PJS hamartoma are well documented.[87-94]

Patients with PJS are also at increased risk for developing extraintestinal malignancies, which have a reported prevalence of 10% to 30%. The most commonly implicated tumors include carcinoma of the pancreas, breast, and ovary.[95-99] Pancreatic cancers in PJS have a tendency to develop at an unusually early age, with the risk estimated to be 200 times greater than that in the general population.[95,97-101] Breast cancer tends to occur in young women, is usually ductal, and is commonly bilateral.[102] The risk for breast cancer in patients with PJS is similar in magnitude to that in patients with hereditary breast cancer (*BRCA1* and *BRCA2*).[103]

Rare neoplasms of the reproductive tract may also occur in patients with PJS. Adenoma malignum is a uterine cervix cancer with a relatively benign histologic appearance but an aggressive biologic behavior.[104-107] A benign ovarian tumor, designated as sex cord tumor with annular tubules (SCTAT), also commonly occurs in women with PJS.[107-109] These tumors are often bilateral, small or microscopic, and calcified, whereas in patients with SCTAT without PJS the tumors are usually larger and unilateral.[110] These benign ovarian tumors are capable of producing both estrogen and progesterone. In fact,

hyperestrogenism may contribute to the increased incidence of breast carcinoma in patients with PJS. More common benign and malignant ovarian neoplasms also occur. Sertoli cell tumors of the testes have occasionally been reported in association with PJS. Like SCTAT, these tumors are benign, microscopic, and often bilateral. They may also produce estrogen, leading to gynecomastia.[111] Other neoplasms reported less frequently in patients with PJS include benign and malignant tumors of the thyroid gland, gallbladder, ureter, urinary bladder, bronchus, and nasal cavity.[95,97,112-114]

PJS hamartomas are found predominantly in the jejunum and ileum, followed by the duodenum, colon, and stomach (Fig. 65-8). Individual polyps vary in size and may be pedunculated or sessile. Pedunculated polyps are usually located in the small bowel or colon, whereas sessile polyps are more common in the stomach.[115] Larger hamartomas often have a lobulated surface. It is more common for PJS polyps to occur in clusters than for the lesions to carpet the bowel.[84] A solitary hamartoma involving one segment of the gastrointestinal tract may occur but is uncommon. Intussusception caused by small bowel hamartomas is an important radiologic feature of PJS. Transient intussusceptions may occasionally be observed on contrast studies, ultrasonography, and CT.[84,116]

A combination of radiologic and endoscopic studies should be used to diagnose these polyps. Enteroclysis and upper endoscopy are now recommended yearly, beginning at 10 years of age. Colonoscopy should begin later in adolescence and should be performed every 3 years.[117] Cross-sectional imaging studies may be helpful for the diagnosis of extraintestinal abnormalities. Ultrasonography is particularly useful for

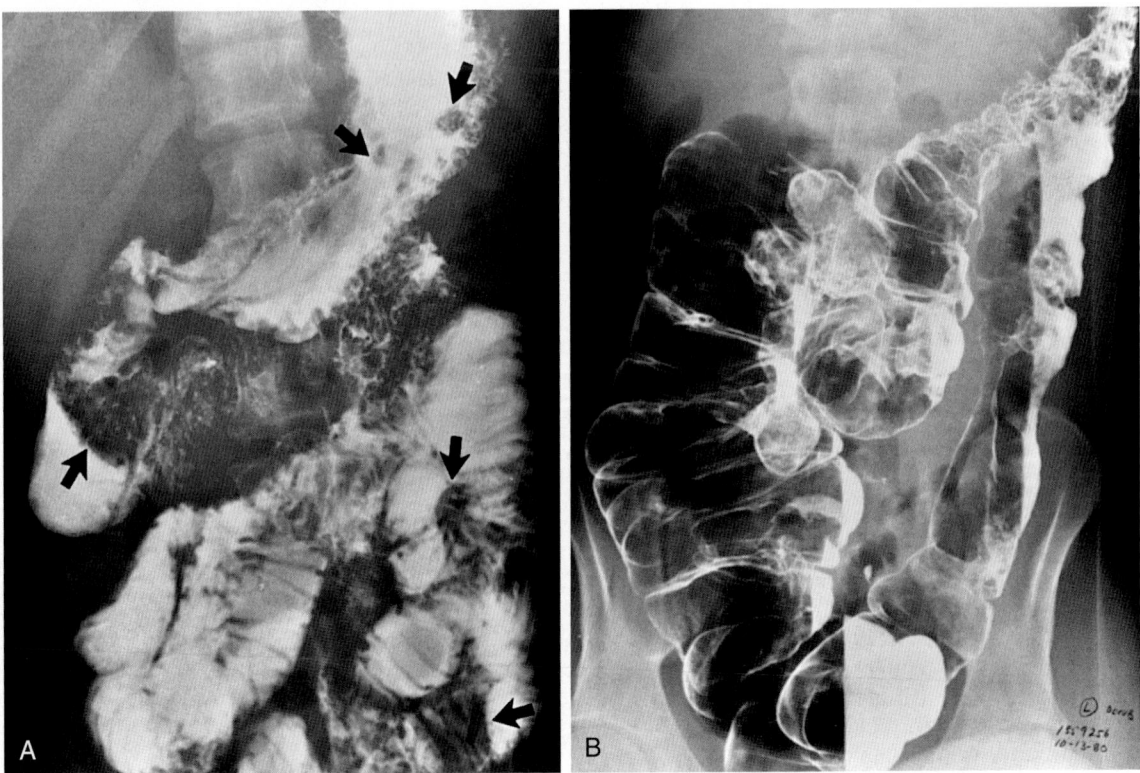

Figure 65-8. Peutz-Jeghers syndrome in a 22-year-old woman. Multiple hamartomas are present throughout the gastrointestinal tract. **A.** Upper gastrointestinal study shows hamartomatous polyps (*arrows*) in the stomach, duodenum, and jejunum. **B.** Double-contrast barium enema shows large hamartomas in all segments of the colon.

detecting ovarian and testicular tumors. The role of screening mammography for young women (25 to 35 years of age) with PJS remains controversial but should be considered in this high-risk group for breast cancer.[118]

When a preoperative diagnosis of PJS is made, these patients can benefit from intraoperative endoscopic removal of small bowel polyps, a procedure that reduces the risk of adenocarcinoma and further intussusceptions. This form of treatment is preferable to small bowel resection, because some patients with PJS have developed short bowel syndrome from multiple enterectomies.[119]

Multiple Hamartoma Syndrome (Cowden's Disease)

Multiple hamartoma syndrome (MHS) is a genodermatosis characterized by hamartomas and neoplasms of ectodermal, mesodermal, and endodermal origin, affecting multiple organs and organ systems.[120,121] The prevalence of MHS is 1 per 200,000. Patients usually present in their late teens or early 20s, with almost all patients presenting by their late 30s.[122] The most consistent clinical features are mucocutaneous lesions associated with thyroid gland abnormalities, breast carcinoma, hamartomatous polyposis of the gastrointestinal tract, and abnormalities of the central nervous system. This syndrome has an autosomal dominant pattern of inheritance. As many as 80% of patients with MHS have a mutation in the tumor suppressor gene *PTEN* located on the long arm of chromosome 10.[123-125]

Mucocutaneous lesions are present in almost all patients with MHS and are considered the hallmark of the disease. Facial trichilemmomas are pathognomonic of MHS and can develop before the internal manifestations of this condition. Keratotic papules around the mouth and nose, labial and oral mucosal papillomatoses, acral keratoses, and multiple sclerotic fibromas are the most characteristic lesions, serving as external markers for the syndrome.[126-130] These benign mucocutaneous lesions almost always develop early in the disease (usually in the third decade) before the neoplastic manifestations have developed.[131] Recognition of these features is therefore essential for early diagnosis of MHS and initiation of screening programs for associated neoplasia.

Thyroid disease is the most frequent extracutaneous abnormality, occurring in about 65% of patients with MHS. Goiters and adenomas are the most common lesions, and men and women are affected equally.[117,124] Thyroid carcinoma has been reported in about 10% of patients, with the most commons subtypes being follicular and papillary carcinoma. Almost all cases of thyroid carcinoma have been reported in women.[120,126]

About 70% of women with MHS have breast lesions. Fibrocystic disease is the most common finding, occurring in at least 50% of patients.[120,129,132,133] Carcinoma of the breast (often bilateral ductal cancers) is the most common malignant tumor in MHS, occurring in 25% to 50% of patients.[134,135] The age at onset is 38 to 46 years, which is earlier than expected for the general population. Regular surveillance and possible screening mammography, as in patients with PJS, should therefore be encouraged in young women with MHS.

Multiple central nervous system abnormalities have also been described in patients with MHS. Lhermitte-Duclos disease (dysplastic gangliocytomas of the cerebellar cortex) is readily diagnosed by MRI of the brain and is now considered one of the major criteria for the diagnosis of MHS.[136-140] After MHS or Lhermitte-Duclos disease has been diagnosed, careful evaluation of the patient for the other entity is crucial.[140] Meningiomas and vascular malformations (including venous angiomas and cavernous angiomas) have also been found to occur in patients with MHS.[141]

Many patients with MHS have facial or skeletal abnormalities. Macrocephaly with a high broad forehead is one of the most characteristic features.[120] Progressive macrocephaly may be accompanied by a delay in psychomotor development.[135]

Genitourinary lesions are frequent and include uterine leiomyomas, endometrial and cervical carcinomas, and transitional cell carcinoma of the renal pelvis and urinary bladder.[127] Renal cell carcinoma has also been reported.

Polyps of the gastrointestinal tract occur in 70% to 85% of patients with MHS.[142-144] They occur in all segments of the gastrointestinal tract with variable reported histology, including hamartomas, hyperplastic polyps, and adenomatous polyps, followed less frequently by lipomas, ganglioneuromas, and inflammatory fibroid polyps. When present, hyperplastic polyps are usually located in the stomach and adenomatous polyps are usually located in the stomach or colon.[142,143] The hamartomas in MHS differ histologically from the hamartomas in PJS. They are usually sessile and smaller, with less exophytic and arborizing proliferation of the muscularis mucosae. Hamartomatous polyps are the most commonly described polyps in MHS and are the predominant lesions in the rectosigmoid colon.[142-144] Although hamartomas occur in the esophagus, glycogenic acanthosis appears to be a more consistent finding in the esophagus and is considered by some authors to be another characteristic feature of MHS.[145,146]

The gastrointestinal polyps of MHS usually appear radiographically as multiple small sessile lesions with a segmental or diffuse distribution. They are most commonly located in the rectosigmoid colon (Fig. 65-9), followed, in decreasing order of frequency, by the stomach, duodenum, small bowel, and esophagus.[147,148]

In the majority of patients, gastrointestinal polyps cause no symptoms and are usually found incidentally or during screening for MHS. Rare cases of colon and gastric carcinoma have been described in MHS, but an increased risk of developing these malignancies in patients with MHS has not been established.[142,143,149]

Juvenile Polyposis

Although an isolated juvenile polyp is the most common tumor of the colon in children, juvenile polyposis (JP) is a rare disease. The age at onset is variable, but most patients present during the second decade of life.[150-152] The criteria for establishing a diagnosis of JP include (1) more than five juvenile polyps in the colon or rectum (Fig. 65-10); (2) juvenile polyps throughout the gastrointestinal tract (Fig. 65-11); and/or (3) any number of juvenile polyps in a patient with a family history of juvenile polyps.[150] Affected individuals may present with bleeding, obstruction, and intussusception, but many patients are asymptomatic.[81]

The genetics are not precisely defined, but JP appears to have an autosomal dominant pattern of inheritance.[151-153] About 25% of newly diagnosed cases of JP are sporadic; the remaining 75% of patients have a family history of JP. Two

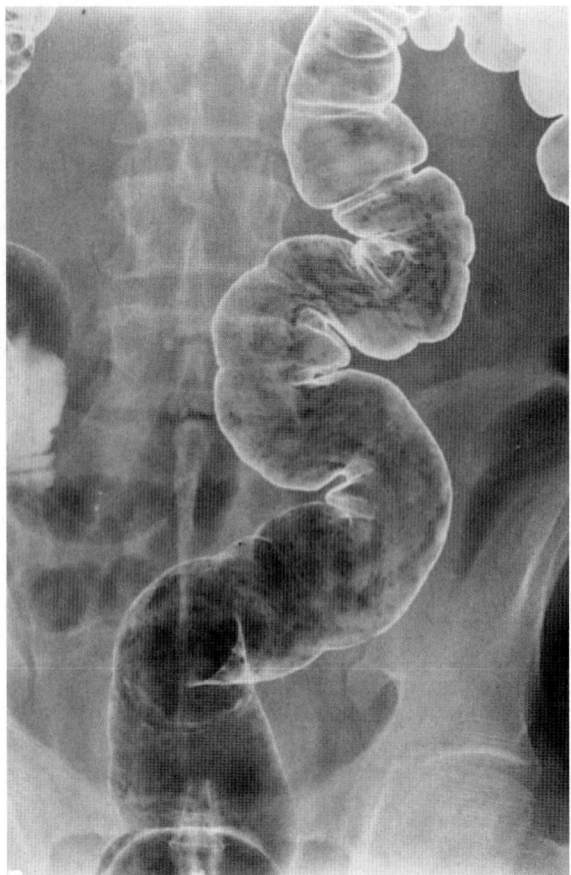

Figure 65-9. Multiple hamartoma syndrome in a 53-year-old man. Tiny sessile hamartomas polyps are present in the rectosigmoid colon. Hamartomas were also present in the esophagus.

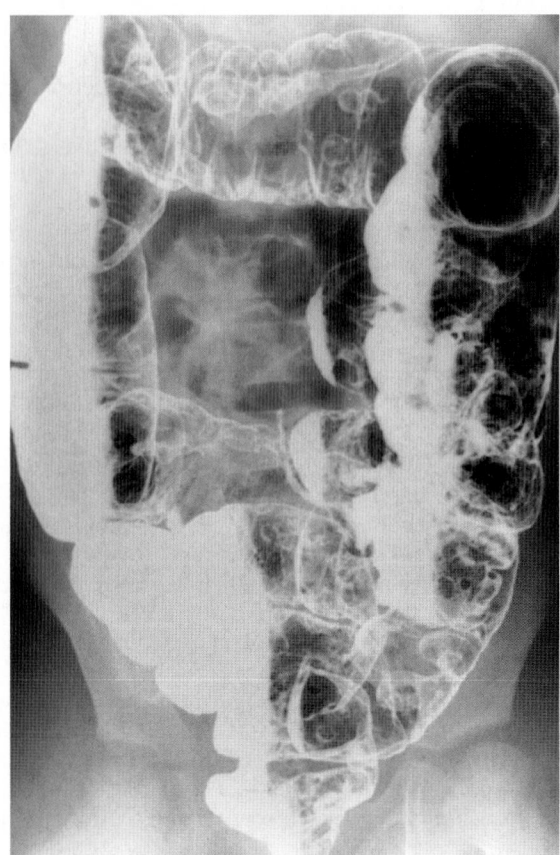

Figure 65-10. Juvenile polyposis. In a 9-year-old girl, a double-contrast barium enema shows clusters of large juvenile polyps throughout the colon.

genes have been implicated in the development of JP. One gene is located on chromosome 18 (*MADH4*) and the other on chromosome 10 (*BMPR1A*).[81]

Various congenital anomalies (including hydrocephalus and pulmonary venous malformations) occur in 25% of non-familial cases of JPS but are rare in patients with the familial form of the disease.[143,154,155]

Patients with JP are at increased risk for developing malignant tumors of the colon, stomach, small intestine, and pancreas.[81,155-166] Recent reports indicate that the risk of colon cancer is 17% to 22% by 35 years of age and as high as 68% by 60 years of age. In patients with gastric polyps, the incidence of gastric carcinoma is more than 20%.[81] Precancerous dysplasia within juvenile polyps has been well documented and suggests that carcinoma may arise in such lesions. Current screening recommendations for patients with JP include colonoscopy every 1 to 2 years beginning at 15 years of age and upper endoscopy beginning at 25 years of age.[81] Investigators have found that family members of patients with JP may also be at risk for developing malignant tumors of the gastrointestinal tract, so that the families of these patients should also be evaluated carefully.[167]

Because a small number of patients with MHS lack mucocutaneous manifestations and are thought to have JP instead, some authors recommend screening patients with presumed JP for both breast and thyroid carcinoma.[81]

In the colon, the polyps vary in size but, as in patients with isolated juvenile polyps, they tend to be large lesions, with a diameter of 1 cm or greater. These polyps can be sessile or pedunculated. When the polyps are distributed throughout the gastrointestinal tract, they are still more likely to be clustered than to carpet the mucosa. In decreasing order of frequency, the polyps in JP occur in the colon, stomach, small bowel, and duodenum. Gastric polyps in JP are predominantly located in the gastric antrum.[168]

JP of infancy is a severe disease.[169-174] Most patients present in the first 2 years of life with a devastating mucoid or bloody diarrhea. There is usually no family history of JP. Anemia, hypoproteinemia, and repeated episodes of bronchopulmonary infection and small bowel intussusception result in early death for the majority of patients. Ectodermal changes resembling adult Cronkhite-Canada syndrome and congenital anomalies (including clubbing of the fingers, macrocephaly, and arachnoid cysts) have been reported in a small number of patients.[175] Juvenile polyps vary in size and are distributed throughout the gastrointestinal tract, except for the esophagus. The small bowel and colon are most severely affected.[176]

Cronkhite-Canada Syndrome

Unlike most of the other polyposis syndromes, Cronkhite-Canada syndrome (CCS) is not familial and occurs in older adults.[177] The average age at onset is 60 years, with an age distribution of 31 to 76 years. (A condition known as *Cronkhite-*

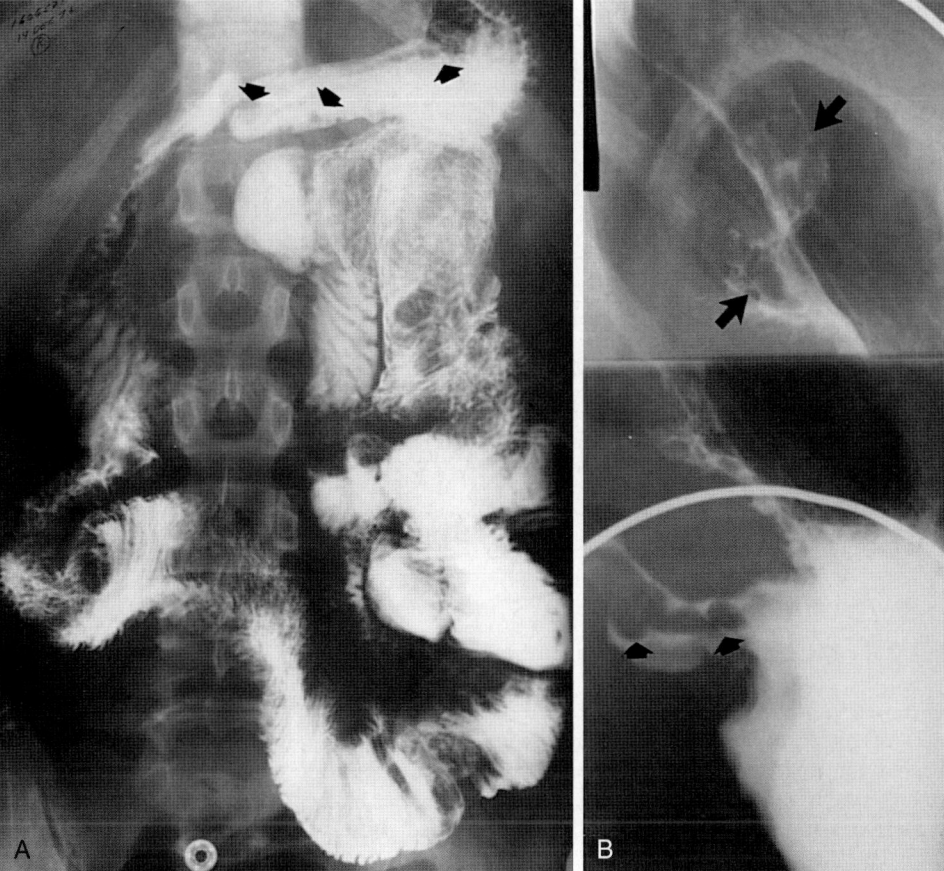

Figure 65-11. Juvenile polyposis of the gastrointestinal tract in a 21-year-old man with diarrhea and rectal bleeding for 5 years. A. Upper gastrointestinal study shows juvenile polyps in the stomach (*arrows*) and small bowel. **B.** Spot images of the stomach show large juvenile polyps in the fundus (*large arrows*) and smaller polyps in the antrum (*small arrows*). Multiple juvenile polyps were also present in the colon.

Canada syndrome of infancy is probably the same disease as infantile juvenile polyposis.) Mental and physical stress has been suggested as an important factor in the development of the disorder.[178]

The histologic appearance of the gastrointestinal polyps was not characterized in the first reported cases, but most authors currently believe that the lesions of CCS are inflammatory polyps.[178-182] Adenomatous, hyperplastic, and hamartomatous polyps have also been reported in smaller numbers in patients.[183,184] Colon cancer has been reported in about 12% of the 387 documented cases of CCS to date.[185]

Patients with CCS typically present with abdominal pain, anorexia, a severe protein-losing diarrhea, malabsorption, and weight loss. This severe diarrhea causes electrolyte disturbances, anemia, and hypoproteinemia. Ectodermal abnormalities of the skin, hair, and nails generally follow the onset of gastrointestinal symptoms. Hair loss involving the scalp or body hair occurs abruptly. Brown macules develop on the palmar and plantar skin surfaces. Dystrophic changes in the nails may lead to complete nail loss. Rarely, the ectodermal manifestations precede the onset of gastrointestinal disease.[177,180,184] The ectodermal changes and even the gastrointestinal polyps may regress when clinical remission occurs.[181,186,187] The prognosis is usually poor, with a mortality rate of greater than 50%. However, recent reports suggest a more favorable prognosis after intense therapy with corticosteroids and nutritional support.[178]

Polyps in CCS usually appear on barium studies as small, sessile, or, less commonly, pedunculated lesions. They are almost always distributed throughout the stomach, small bowel, and colon.[179,188] Definite esophageal involvement has not been reported. In the stomach, small to moderate-sized polyps carpet the mucosal surface, usually superimposed on thickened rugal folds (Fig. 65-12). The small bowel may contain multiple small polyps from the duodenum to the terminal ileum. The colon and rectum may also be diffusely involved, but carpeting of the mucosa is not as extensive as that in the stomach.[179,188]

Bannayan-Riley-Ruvalcaba Syndrome

Because of overlapping clinical features, three syndromes (Riley-Smith syndrome, Bannayan-Zonana syndrome, and Ruvalcaba-Myhre-Smith syndrome) have been combined into a single entity, the Bannayan-Riley-Ruvalcaba syndrome (BRRS).[189,190] This syndrome has an autosomal dominant pattern of inheritance.[189-192] Recent reports have identified mutations in the *PTEN* gene in 50% to 60% of patients with BRRS, the same gene associated with MHS.[134] Some authors now believe that Bannayan-Riley-Ruvalcaba syndrome and MHS may be the same syndrome, because there is overlap in both the genetic and clinical manifestations of these diseases.[81] Also, families have been reported in which some members had MHS and others had BRRS.[134]

The most common clinical features of BRRS include macrocephaly and multiple subcutaneous and visceral lipomas and hemangiomas. About 50% of patients have delayed psychomotor development, hypotonia, and mild to severe mental

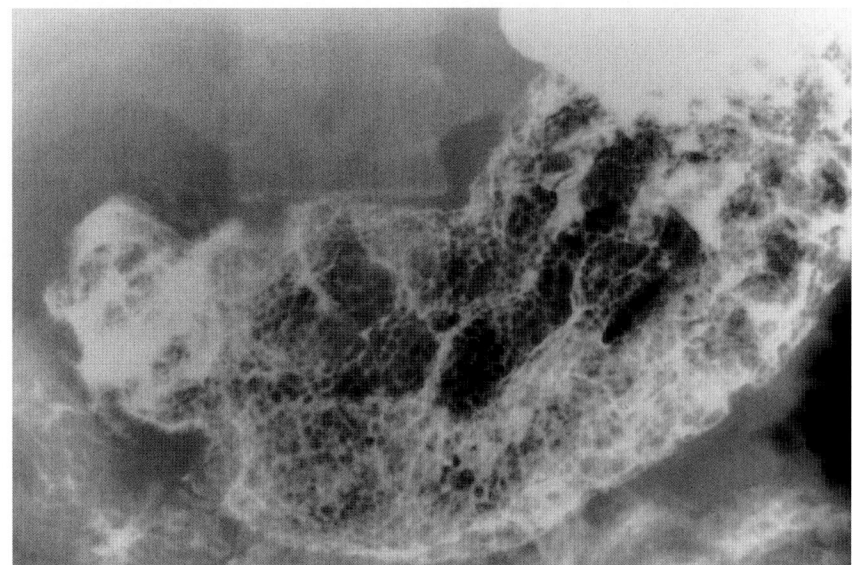

Figure 65-12. Cronkhite-Canada syndrome. In a 34-year-old woman, double-contrast study of the stomach shows carpeting of the mucosa with hamartomatous polyps superimposed on enlarged rugal folds.

deficiency. Male patients may have pigmented spotting of the penis.

Hamartomatous intestinal polyps are present in about 45% of patients with BRRS.[189] They are most commonly located in the distal ileum and colon but can be found throughout the gastrointestinal tract.[81,193] An increased risk of gastrointestinal malignancy has not been described in these patients.

References

1. Davies DR, Armstrong JG, Thakker N, et al: Severe Gardner syndrome in families with mutations restricted to a specific region of the APC gene. Am J Hum Genet 57:1151-1158, 1995.
2. Gebert HF, Jagelman DG, McGannon E: Familial polyposis coli. Am Fam Physician 33:127-135, 1986.
3. Bussey JHR, Veale AMO, Morson BC: Genetics of gastrointestinal polyposis. Gastroenterology 74:1325-1330, 1978.
4. Varesco L: Familial adenomatous polyposis: Genetics and epidemiology. Tech Coloproctol 8:S305-S308, 2004.
5. Pierce ER: Some genetic aspects of familial multiple polyposis of the colon in a kindred of 1,422. Dis Colon Rectum 11:321-327, 1968.
6. Petersen GM: Genetic testing and counseling in familial adenomatous polyposis. Oncology 10:89-94, 1996.
7. Sieber OM, Lipton L, Crabtree M, et al: Multiple colorectal adenomas, classic adenomatous polyposis, and germ-line mutations in *MYH*. N Engl J Med 348:791-799, 2003.
8. Bussey HJR: Familial Polyposis Coli. Baltimore, John Hopkins University Press, 1975.
9. Giardiello FM, Brensinger JD, Luce MC, et al: Phenotypic expression of disease in families that have mutations in the 5′ region of the adenomatous polyposis coli gene. Ann Intern Med 126:514-519, 1997.
10. Lynch JT, Smyrk T, McGinn T, et al: Attenuated familial adenomatous polyposis (AFAP): A phenotypically and genotypically distinctive variant of FAP. Cancer 76:2427-2433, 1995.
11. Hernegger GS, Moore HG, Guillem JG, et al: Attenuated familial adenomatous polyposis: An evolving and poorly understood entity. Dis Colon Rectum 45:127-134, 2002.
12. Watne AL: The syndromes of intestinal polyposis. Curr Probl Surg 24:269-340, 1987.
13. Nandakumar G, Morgan J, Silverberg D, et al: Familial polyposis coli: Clinical manifestations, evaluation, management and treatment. Mt Sinai J Med 71:384-391, 2004.
14. Sarre RG, McGannon E, Jagelman DG, et al: Colectomy with ileorectal anastomosis for familial adenomatous polyposis. Surgery 101:20-26, 1987.
15. Welling DR, Beart RW: Surgical alternatives in the treatment of polyposis coli. Semin Surg Oncol 3:99-104, 1987.
16. Bartram CI, Thornton A: Colonic polyp patterns in familial polyposis. AJR 142:305-308, 1984.
17. Hoffman DC, Goligher JC: Polyposis of the stomach and small intestine in association with familial polyposis coli. Br J Surg 58:126-128, 1971.
18. Bulow S, Lauritsen KB, Johansen A, et al: Gastroduodenal polyps in familial polyposis coli. Dis Colon Rectum 28:90-93, 1985.
19. Ushio K, Sasagawa M, Doi H, et al: Lesions associated with familial polyposis coli: Studies of lesions of the stomach, duodenum, bones, and teeth. Gastrointest Radiol 1:67-80, 1976.
20. Utsunomiya J, Maki T, Iwama T, et al: Gastric lesion of familial polyposis. Cancer 34:745-754, 1974.
21. Burt RW, Berenson MM, Lee RG, et al: Upper gastroenterology polyps in Gardner's syndrome. Gastroenterology 86:295-301, 1984.
22. Shemesh E, Bat L: A prospective evaluation of the upper gastrointestinal tract and periampullary region in patients with Gardner syndrome. Am J Gastroenterol 80:825-827, 1985.
23. Ranzi T, Castagnone D, Velio P: Gastric and duodenal polyps in familial polyposis coli. Gut 11:363-367, 1981.
24. Tonelli F, Nardi E, Bechi P, et al: Extracolonic polyps in familial polyposis coli and Gardner's syndrome. Dis Colon Rectum 28:664-668, 1985.
25. Watanabe H, Enjoji M, Yao T, et al: Gastric lesions in familial adenomatosis coli. Hum Pathol 9:269-283, 1978.
26. Burt RW: Gastric fundic gland polyps. Gastroenterology 125:1462-1469, 2003.
27. Iida M, Yao T, Watanabe H, et al: Fundic gland polyposis in patients without familial adenomatosis coli. Gastroenterology 86:1437-1442, 1984.
28. Tatsuta M, Okuda S, Tamura H: Gastric hamartomatous polyps in the absence of familial polyposis coli. Cancer 45:818-823, 1980.
29. Nishiur M, Hirota T, Itabashi M, et al: A clinical and histopathological study of gastric polyps in familial polyposis coli. Am J Gastroenterol 79:98-103, 1984.
30. Iida M, Yao T, Itoh H, et al: Natural history of fundic gland polyposis in patients with familial adenomatous coli/Gardner's syndrome. Gastroenterology 89:1021-1025, 1985.
31. Itai Y, Kogure T, Okuyama Y, et al: Radiographic features of the gastric polyps in familial adenomatosis coli. AJR 128:73-76, 1977.
32. Iida M, Yao T, Watanabe H, et al: Spontaneous disappearance of the fundic gland polyposis: Report of three cases. Gastroenterology 79:725-728, 1980.
33. Denzler TB, Harned RK, Pergam CJ: Gastric polyps in familial polyposis coli. Radiology 130:63-66, 1979.
34. Yao T, Iida M, Ohsata K: Duodenal lesions in familial polyposis of the colon. Gastroenterology 73:1086-1092, 1977.
35. Wallace MH, Phillips RKS: Upper gastrointestinal disease in patients with familial adenomatous polyposis. Br J Surg 85:742-750, 1998.

36. Qizilbash AH: Epithelial neoplasms of the duodenum and periampullary region. In Appelman HD (ed): Pathology of the Esophagus, Stomach and Duodenum. New York, Churchill Livingstone, 1984, p 145.
37. Iida M, Yao T, Ohsata K, et al: Diagnostic value of intraoperative fiberoscopy for small-intestinal polyps in familial adenomatosis coli. Endoscopy 12:161-165, 1980.
38. Ross JE, Mara JE: Small bowel polyps and carcinoma in multiple intestinal polyposis. Arch Surg 108:736-738, 1974.
39. Phillips LG: Polyposis and carcinoma of the small bowel and familial colonic polyposis. Dis Colon Rectum 24:478-481, 1981.
40. Scully RE, Galdabini JJ, McNeely BU: Case 47-1978: Presentation of case. Case records of the Massachusetts General Hospital. N Engl J Med 299:1237-1244, 1978.
41. Jarvinen HJ, Nyberg M, Peltokallio P: Biliary involvement in familial adenomatosis coli. Dis Colon Rectum 26:525-528, 1983.
42. Less CD, Hermann RE: Familial polyposis coli associated with bile duct cancer. Am J Surg 141:378-380, 1981.
43. Burney B, Assor D: Polyposis coli with adenocarcinoma associated with carcinoma in situ of the gallbladder. Am J Surg 132:100-102, 1976.
44. Willson SA, Princethal RA, Law B, et al: Gallbladder carcinoma in association with polyposis coli. Br J Radiol 60:771-773, 1987.
45. Futami H, Furuta T, Hanai H, et al: Adenoma of the common human bile duct in Gardner's syndrome may cause relapsing acute pancreatitis. J Gastroenterol 32:558-561, 1997.
46. Gardner EJ, Richards RC: Multiple cutaneous and subcutaneous lesions occurring simultaneously with hereditary polyposis and osteomatosis. Am J Hum Genet 5:139-148, 1953.
47. Gardner EJ: Follow-up study of a family group exhibiting dominant inheritance for a syndrome including intestinal polyps, osteomas, fibromas and epidermal cysts. Am J Hum Genet 14:376-390, 1962.
48. Scott RJ, Taeschner W, Heinimann K, et al: Association of extracolonic manifestations of familial adenomatous polyposis with acetylation phenotype in a large FAP kindred. Eur J Hum Genet 5:43-49, 1997.
49. Davies DR, Armstrong JG, Thakker N, et al: Severe Gardner syndrome in families with mutations restricted to a specific region of the APC gene. Am J Hum Genet 57:1151-1158, 1995.
50. Jagelman DG: Extracolonic manifestations of familial polyposis coli. Cancer Genet Cytogenet 27:319-325, 1987.
51. Lal G, Gallinger S: Familial adenomatous polyposis. Semin Surg Oncol 18:314-323, 2000.
52. Gorlin RJ, Chaudhry AP: Multiple osteomatosis, fibromas, lipomas and fibrosarcomas of the skin and mesentery, epidermoid inclusion cysts of the skin, leiomyomas and multiple intestinal polyposis. N Engl J Med 263:1151-1158, 1960.
53. Chang CH, Piatt ED, Thomas KE, et al: Bone abnormalities in Gardner's syndrome. AJR 103:645-652, 1968.
54. Utsunomiya J, Nakamura T: The occult osteomatous changes in the mandible in patients with familial polyposis. Br J Surg 62:45-51, 1975.
55. Bulow S, Sondergaard JO, Witt I, et al: Mandibular osteomas in familial polyposis coli. Dis Colon Rectum 27:105-108, 1984.
56. Woods RJ, Sarre RG, Ctercteko GC, et al: Occult radiologic changes in the skull and jaw in familial adenomatous polyposis coli. Dis Colon Rectum 32:304-306, 1989.
57. Fader M, Kline SN, Spatz SS, et al: Gardner's syndrome (intestinal polyposis, osteomas, sebaceous cysts) and a new dental discovery. Oral Surg Oral Med Oral Pathol 15:153-172, 1962.
58. Sondergaard JO, Bulow S, Wolf J, et al: Dental anomalies in familial adenomatous polyposis coli. Acta Odontol Scand 45:61-63, 1987.
59. Huges LE: Abdominal fibrodysplasia and polyposis coli. Dis Colon Rectum 13:121-123, 1970.
60. Jones IT, Fazio VW, Weakley FL, et al: Desmoid tumors in familial polyposis coli. Ann Surg 204:94-97, 1986.
61. Johnson-Smith TGP, Katz DE, Clark SK, et al: Spiral CT Scanning in detection of desmoid tumors in familial adenomatous polyposis. Presented before the American Roentgen Ray Society Annual Meeting, San Francisco, April 26-May 1, 1998.
62. Iwamma T, Mishima Y, Okamoto N, et al: Association of congenital hypertrophy of the retinal pigment epithelium with familial adenomatous polyposis. Br J Surg 77:273-276, 1990.
63. Traboulsi EI, Maumenee IH, Krush AJ, et al: Congenital hypertrophy of the retinal pigment epithelium predicts colorectal polyposis in Gardner's syndrome. Arch Ophthalmol 108:525-526, 1990.
64. Baker RH, Heinemann MH, Miller HH, et al: Hyperpigmented lesions of the retinal pigment epithelium in familial adenomatous polyposis. Am J Med Genet 31:427-435, 1988.
65. Romania A, Zakov ZN, McGannon E, et al: Congenital hypertrophy of the retinal pigment epithelium in familial adenomatous polyposis. Ophthalmology 96:879-884, 1998.
66. Baba S, Tsuchiya M, Watanabe I, et al: Importance of retinal pigmentation as a subclinical marker in familial adenomatous polyposis. Dis Colon Rectum 33:660-664, 1990.
67. Turcot J, Depres JP, Pierre F: Malignant tumors of the central nervous system associated with familial polyposis of the colon. Dis Colon Rectum 2:465-468, 1959.
68. Hamilton SR, Liu B, Parsons RE, et al: The molecular basis of Turcot's syndrome. N Engl J Med 332:839-847, 1995.
69. Leblanc R: Familial adenomatous polyposis and benign intracranial tumors: A new variant of Gardner's syndrome. Can J Neurol Sci 27:341-346, 2000.
70. Torres CF, Korones DN, Pilcher W: Multiple ependymomas in a patient with Turcot's syndrome. Med Pediatr Oncol 28:59-61, 1997.
71. Plail RO, Bussey JH, Glazer G, et al: Adenomatous polyposis: An association with carcinoma of the thyroid. Br J Surg 74:377-380, 1987.
72. Delamarre J, Capron J, Armand A, et al: Thyroid carcinoma in two sisters with familial polyposis of the colon: Case reports and review of the literature. J Clin Gastroenterol 10:659-662, 1988.
73. Hizawa K, Iida M, Aoyagi K, et al: Thyroid neoplasia and familial adenomatous polyposis/Gardner's syndrome. J Gastroenterol 32:196-199, 1997.
74. Schneider NR, Cubilla AL, Chaganti RS: Association of endocrine neoplasia with multiple polyposis of the colon. Cancer 51:1171-1175, 1983.
75. Perkins JT, Backstone MO, Riddell RH: Adenomatous polyposis coli and multiple endocrine neoplasia type 2b: A pathogenic relationship. Cancer 55:375-381, 1985.
76. Painter TA, Jagelman DG: Adrenal adenomas and adrenal carcinomas in association with hereditary adenomatosis of the colon and rectum. Cancer 55:2001-2004, 1985.
77. Bulow S: Familial adenomatous polyposis. Ann Med 21:299-307, 1989.
78. Schneider NR, Cubilla AL, Chaganti RS: Association of endocrine neoplasia with multiple polyposis of the colon. Cancer 51:1171-1175, 1983.
79. Maire F, Hammel P, Terris B, et al: Intraductal papillary and mucinous pancreatic tumour: A new extracolonic tumour in familial adenomatous polyposis. Gut 51:446-449, 2002.
80. LeSher AR, Castronuovo JJ Jr, Filippone AL Jr: Hepatoblastoma in a patient with familial polyposis coli. Surgery 105:668-670, 1989.
81. Schreibman IR, Baker M, Amos C, McGarrity TJ: The hamartomatous polyposis syndromes: A clinical and molecular review. Am J Gastroenterol 100:476-490, 2005.
82. Boardman LA, Thibodeau SN, Schaid DJ, et al: Increased risk for cancer in patients with the Peutz-Jeghers syndrome. Ann Intern Med 128:896-899, 1998.
83. Amos CL, Bali D, Thiel TJ, et al: Fine mapping of genetic locus for Peutz-Jeghers syndrome on chromosome 19p. Cancer Res 57:3653-3656, 1997.
84. Buck JL, Harned RK, Lichtenstein JE, et al: Peutz-Jeghers syndrome. RadioGraphics 12:365-378, 1992.
85. Hizawa K, Matsumoto T, Iida M, et al: Neoplastic transformation arising in Peutz-Jeghers polyposis. Dis Colon Rectum 36:953-957, 1993.
86. Schumacher V, Vogel T, Leube B, et al: STK11 genotyping and cancer risk in Peutz-Jeghers syndrome. J Med Genet 42:428-435, 2005.
87. Niimi K, Tomoda H, Furusawa M, et al: Peutz-Jeghers syndrome associated with adenocarcinoma of the cecum and focal carcinomas in hamartomatous polyps of the colon: A case report. Jpn J Surg 21:220-223, 1991.
88. Visvanathan R, Thambidorai CR, Myint H: Do dysplastic and adenomatous changes in large bowel hamartomas predispose to malignancy?—A report of two cases. Ann Acad Med Singapore 21:830-832, 1992.
89. Laughlin EH: Benign and malignant neoplasms in a family with Peutz-Jeghers syndrome: Study of three generations. South Med J 84:1205-1209, 1991.
90. Spigelman AD, Arese P, Phillips RKS: Polyposis: The Peutz-Jeghers syndrome. Br J Surg 82:1311-1314, 1995.
91. Luk GD: Diagnosis and therapy of hereditary polyposis syndromes. Gastroenterologist 3:153-167, 1995.
92. Perzin KH, Bridge MF: Adenomatous and carcinomatous changes in hamartomatous polyps of the small intestine (Peutz-Jeghers) syndrome: Report of a case and review of the literature. Cancer 49:971-983, 1982.
93. Miller LJ, Bartholomew LG, Dozois RR, et al: Adenocarcinoma of the rectum arising in a hamartomatous poly in a patient with Peutz-Jeghers syndrome. Dig Dis Sci 28:1047-1051, 1983.

94. Flageole H, Stavros R, Trude JL, et al: Progression toward malignancy of hamartomas in a patient with Peutz-Jeghers syndrome: Case report and literature review. Can J Surg 37:231-236, 1994.

95. Utsunomiya J, Gocho H, Miyanaga T, et al: Peutz-Jeghers syndrome: Its natural course and management. John Hopkins Med J 136:71-82, 1975.

96. Linos DA, Dozois RR, Dahlin DC, et al: Does Peutz-Jeghers syndrome predispose to gastrointestinal malignancy? A later look. Arch Surg 116:1182-1184, 1981.

97. Spiegelman AD, Murday V, Phillips RK: Cancer and the Peutz-Jeghers syndrome. Gut 30:1588-1590, 1989.

98. Giardiello FM, Welsh SB, Hamilton SR, et al: Increased risk of cancer in the Peutz-Jeghers syndrome. N Engl J Med 316:1511-1514, 1987.

99. Hizwa K, Matsumoto T, Iida M, et al: Cancer in Peutz-Jeghers syndrome. Cancer 72:2777-2781, 1993.

100. Thatcher BS, May ES, Taxier MS, et al: Pancreatic adenocarcinoma in a patient with Peutz-Jeghers syndrome: A case report and literature review. Am J Gastroenterol 81:594-597, 1986.

101. Bowlby LS: Pancreatic adenocarcinoma in an adolescent male with Peutz-Jeghers syndrome. Hum Pathol 17:97-99, 1986.

102. Martin-Odegard B, Svane S: Peutz-Jeghers syndrome associated with bilateral synchronous breast carcinoma in a 30-year-old woman. Eur J Surg 160:511-512, 1994.

103. Giardiello FM, Brensinger JD, Tersmette AC, et al: Very high risk of cancer in familial Peutz-Jeghers syndrome. Gastroenterology 119:1447-1453, 2000.

104. Chen KTK: Female genital tract tumors in Peutz-Jeghers syndrome. Hum Pathol 17:858-861, 1986.

105. Choi CG, Kim SH, Kim JS, et al: Adenoma malignum of uterine cervix in Peutz-Jeghers syndrome: CT and US features. J Comput Assist Tomogr 17:819-821, 1993.

106. Tsuruchi N, Tsukamoto N, Kaku T, et al: Adenoma malignum of the uterine cervix detected by imaging methods in a patient with Peutz-Jeghers syndrome. Gynecol Oncol 54:232-236, 1994.

107. Sirvatsa PJ, Keeney GL, Podratz KC: Disseminated cervical adenoma malignum and bilateral ovarian sex cord tumors with annular tubules associated with Peutz-Jeghers syndrome. Gynecol Oncol 53:256-264, 1994.

108. Young RH, Welch WR, Dickersin GR, et al: Ovarian sex cord tumor with annular tubules: Review of 74 cases including 27 with Peutz-Jeghers syndrome and four with adenoma malignum of the cervix. Cancer 50:1384-1402, 1982.

109. Podczaski E, Kaminski PF, Pees RC, et al: Peutz-Jeghers syndrome with ovarian sex cord tumor with annular tubules and cervical adenoma malignum. Gynecol Oncol 42:74-78, 1991.

110. Young RH, Welch WR, Dickersin GR, et al: Ovarian sex cord tumor with annular tubules: Review of 74 cases including 27 with Peutz-Jeghers syndrome and four with adenoma malignum of the cervix. Cancer 50:1384-1402, 1982.

111. Wilson DM, Pitts WC, Hintz RL, et al: Testicular tumors with Peutz-Jeghers syndrome. Cancer 57:2238-2240, 1986.

112. Wada K, Tanaka M, Yamaguchi K, et al: Carcinoma and polyps of the gallbladder associated with Peutz-Jeghers syndrome. Dig Dis Sci 32:943-946, 1987.

113. Yamamoto M, Hoschino H, Onizuka T, et al: Thyroid papillary adenocarcinoma in a woman with Peutz-Jeghers syndrome. Intern Med 31:1117-1119, 1992.

114. De Facq L, De Sutter J, De Man M, et al: A case of Peutz-Jeghers syndrome with nasal polyposis, extreme iron deficiency anemia, and hamartoma-adenoma transformation: Management by combined surgical and endoscopic approach. Am J Gastroenterol 90:1330-1332, 1995.

115. McGarrity TJ, Kulin HE, Zaino RJ: Peutz-Jeghers syndrome. Am J Gastroenterol 95:596-604, 2000.

116. Sener RN, Kumcuoglu Z, Elmasn N, et al: Peutz-Jeghers syndrome: CT and US demonstration of small bowel polyps. Gastrointest Radiol 16:21-23, 1991.

117. Corredor J, Wambach J, Barnard J, et al: Gastrointestinal polyps in children: Advances in molecular genetics, diagnosis, and management. J Pediatr 138:621-628, 2001.

118. Parker MC, Michell MJ: Polyposis: The Peutz-Jeghers syndrome. Br J Surg 83:865-875, 1996.

119. Panos RG, Opelka FG, Nogueras JJ: Peutz-Jeghers syndrome: A call for intraoperative enteroscopy. Am Surg 56:331-333, 1990.

120. Starink TM, van Der Veen JW, DeWaal LP, et al: The Cowden syndrome: A clinical and genetic study in 21 patients. Clin Genet 29:222-233, 1986

121. Mallory SB: Cowden syndrome (multiple hamartoma syndrome). Dermatol Clin 13:27-31, 1995.

122. Eng C: Cowden syndrome. J Gen Counsel 6:181-192, 1997.

123. Nelen MR, Padberg GW, Peeters EAJ, et al: Localization of the gene for Cowden disease to chromosome 10q22-23. Nat Genet 13:114-116, 1996.

124. Liaw D, March DJ, Li J, et al: Germline mutations of the PTEN gene in Cowden disease, an inherited breast and thyroid cancer syndrome. Nat Genet 16:64-67, 1997.

125. Nelen MR, van Staveren WCG, Peeters EAJ, et al: Germline mutations in the PTEN/MMACI gene in patients with Cowden disease. Hum Mol Genet 6:1383-1387, 1997.

126. Salem OS, Steck WD: Cowden's disease (multiple hamartoma and neoplasia syndrome): A case report and review of the English literature. J Am Acad Dermatol 8:686-696, 1983.

127. Starink TM: Cowden's disease: Analysis of fourteen new cases. J Am Acad Dermatol 11:1127-1141, 1984.

128. Hauck RM, Manders EK: Familial syndromes with skin markers. Ann Plast Surg 33:102-111, 1994.

129. Chen YM, Ott DJ, Wu WC, et al: Cowden's disease: A case report and literature review. Gastointest Radiol 12:325-329, 1987.

130. Brownstein MH, Mehregan AH, Bikowski JB: The dermatopathology of Cowden's disease: Analysis of fourteen new cases. Br J Dermatol 11:1127-114, 1984.

131. Schreibman IR, Baker M, Amos C, et al: The hamartomatous polyposis syndromes: A clinical and molecular review. Am J Gastroenterol 100:476-490, 2005.

132. Shapiro SD, Lambert WC, Schwartz RA: Cowden's disease: A marker for malignancy. Int J Dermatol 27:232-237, 1988.

133. Brownstein MH, Wolfe M, Bokowski JB: Cowden's disease: A cutaneous marker of breast cancer. Cancer 41:2393-2398, 1978.

134. Pilarski R, Eng C: Will the real Cowden syndrome please stand up (again)? Expanding mutational and clinical spectra of the PTEN hamartoma tumour syndrome. J Med Genet 41:323-326, 2004.

135. Hanssen AMN, Fryns JP: Cowden syndrome. J Med Genet 32:117-119, 1995.

136. Thomas DW, Lewis MAO: Lhermitte-Duclos disease associated with Cowden's disease. Int J Oral Maxillofac Surg 24:369-371, 1995.

137. Lyons CJ, Wilson CB, Horton JC: Association between meningioma and Cowden's disease. Neurology 43:1436-1437, 1993.

138. Wells GB, Lasner TM, Yousem DM, et al: Association of Lhermitte-Duclos and Cowden's disease in an adolescent patient. J Neurosurg 81:133-136, 1994.

139. Vinchon M, Blond S, Lejeune JP, et al: Association of Lhermitte-Duclos and Cowden disease: Report of a new case and review of the literature. J Neurol Neurosurg Psychiatry 57:699-704, 1994.

140. Koeller KK, Henry JM: From the archives of the AFIP: Superficial gliomas: Radiologic-pathologic correlation. RadioGraphics 21:1533-1566, 2001.

141. Lok C, Viseux V, Avril MF, et al: Brain magnetic resonance imaging in patients with Cowden syndrome. Medicine 84:129-136, 2005.

142. Hizawa K, Iida M, Matsumoto T, et al: Gastrointestinal manifestations of Cowden's disease, report of four cases. J Clin Gastroenterol 18:13-18, 1994.

143. Marra G, Armelao F, Vecchio FM, et al: Cowden's disease with extensive gastrointestinal polyposis. J Clin Gastroenterol 18:42-47, 1994.

144. Carlson GJ, Nivatrongs S, Snover DC: Colorectal polyps in Cowden's disease multiple hamartoma syndrome: Am J Pathol 8:703-707, 1984.

145. Lashner BA, Riddell RH, Winans CS: Ganglioneuromatosis of the colon and extensive glycogenic acanthosis in Cowden's disease. Dig Dis Sci 31:212-216, 1986.

146. Kay PS, Soetikno RM, Mindelzum R, et al: Diffuse esophageal glycogenic acanthosis: An endoscopic marker of Cowden's disease. Am J Gastroenterol 92:1038-1040, 1997.

147. Taylor AJ, Dodds WJ, Stewart ET: Alimentary tract lesions in Cowden's disease: Br J Radiol 62:890-892, 1989.

148. Hauser H, Ody B, Plojoax O, et al: Radiological findings in multiple hamartoma syndrome Cowden's disease: A report of 3 cases Radiology 137:317-323, 1980.

149. Hambry LS, Lee EY, Schwartz RW: Parathyroid adenoma and gastric carcinoma as manifestations of Cowden's disease. Surgery 118:115-117, 1997.

150. Jass JR, Williams CB, Bussey HR, et al: Juvenile polyposis: A precancerous condition. Histopathology 13:619-630, 1988.

151. Wu T T, Rezai B, Rashed A, et al: Genetic alterations and epithelial

dysplasia in juvenile polyposis syndrome and sporadic juvenile polyps. Am J Pathol 150:939-947, 1997.

152. Bussey HR, Veale AO, Morson BC: Genetics of gastrointestinal polyposis. Gastroenterology 74:1325-1330, 1978.

153. Hess KF, Schaffner D, Ricketts RR, et al: Malignant risk in juvenile polyposis coli: Increasing documentation in the pediatric age group. J Pediatr Surg 28:1188-1193, 1993.

154. Desai DC, Neale KF, Talbot IC, et al: Juvenile polyposis. Br J Surg 82:14-17, 1995.

155. Radin DR: Hereditary generalized juvenile polyposis: Association with arteriovenous malformation and risk of malignancy. Abdom Imaging 19:140-142, 1994.

156. O'Riordain DS, O'Dwyer PJ, Cullen AF, et al: Familial juvenile polyposis coli and colorectal cancer. Cancer 68:889-892, 1991.

157. Coburn MC, Pricolo VE, Deluca FG, et al: Malignant potential in intestinal juvenile polyposis syndromes. Ann Surg Oncol 2:386-391, 1995.

158. Stemper TJ, Kent THE, Summers RW: Juvenile polyposis and gastrointestinal carcinoma: A study of a kindred. Ann Intern Med 83:639-646, 1975.

159. Grigioni WF, Alampi G, Martinelli G, et al: Atypical juvenile polyposis. Histopathology 5:361-376, 1981.

160. Rozen P, Baratz M: Familial juvenile polyposis coli: Increased risk of cancer. Cancer 49:1500-1503, 1984.

161. Jarvinen H, Franssila KO: Familial juvenile polyposis coli: Increased risk of colorectal cancer. Gut 25:792-800, 1984.

162. Subramonv C, Scoot-Conner CEH, Skelton D, et al: Familial juvenile polyposis, study of a kindred: Evolution of polyps and relationship to gastrointestinal carcinoma. Am J Clin Pathol 102:91-97, 1994.

163. Vaiphei K, Thapa BR: Juvenile polyposis (coli)—high incidence of dysplastic epithelium. J Pediatr Surg 32:1287-1290, 1997.

164. Yoshida T, Haraguchi A, Tanaka A, et al: A case of generalized juvenile gastrointestinal polyposis associated with gastric carcinoma. Endoscopy 20:33-35, 1988.

165. Walpole IR, Cullity G: Juvenile polyposis; a case with early presentation and death attributable to adenocarcinoma of the pancreas. Am J Med Genet 32:1-8, 1989.

166. Sassatelli R, Bertoni G, Serra L, et al: Generalized juvenile polyposis with mixed pattern and gastric cancer. Gastroenterology 1104:910-915, 1993.

167. Haggit RC, Reid BJ: Hereditary gastrointestinal polyposis syndromes. Am J Surg Pathol 101:871-887, 1986.

168. Covarrubias D, Huprich J: Best cases from the AFIP: Juvenile polyposis of the stomach. RadioGraphics 22:415-420, 2002.

169. Berk RN, Rush JL, Elson EC, et al: Multiple inflammatory polyps of the small intestine with cachexia and protein losing enteropathy. Radiology 95:611-612, 1970.

170. Ray JE, Heald RJ: Growing up with juvenile gastrointestinal polyposis: Report of a case. Dis Colon Rectum 14:375-380, 1971.

171. Soper RT, Kent THE: Fatal juvenile polyposis of infancy. Surgery 169:692-698, 1971.

172. Schwart AM, McCauley RK: Juvenile gastrointestinal polyposis. Radiology 121:441-444, 1976.

173. Le Luyer B, Le Bihan M, Metayer P, et al: Generalized juvenile polyposis in an infant; report of a case and successful management by endoscopy. J Pediatr Gastroenterol Nutr 4:128-134, 1985.

174. Ruymann FB: Juvenile polyp with cachexia: Report of an infant and comparison with Cronkhite-Canada syndrome in adults. Gastroenterology 57:431-438, 1969.

175. Scharf GM, Becker JHR, Lage NJ: Juvenile gastrointestinal polyposis of the infant: Cronkhite-Canada syndrome. J Pediatr Surg 21:953-954, 1986.

176. Sachatello CR, Hahn IS, Carrington CB: Juvenile gastrointestinal polyposis in a female patient: Report of a case and review of the literature of a recently recognized syndrome. Surgery 175:107-114, 1974.

177. Goto A: Cronkhite-Canada syndrome: Epidemiological study of cases reported in Japan. Arch Jpn Chir 64:3-14, 1995.

178. Murata I, Yoshikawa I, Endo M, et al: Cronkhite-Canada syndrome: Report of two cases. J Gastroenterol 35:706-711, 2000.

179. Diner WC: The Cronkhite-Canada syndrome. Radiology 105:715-716, 1972.

180. Daniel ES, Ludwig SL, Lewin KL, et al: The Cronkhite-Canada syndrome: An analysis of clinical and pathological features and therapy in 55 patients. Medicine (Baltimore) 61:293-309, 1982.

181. Kilcheski T, Kressel HY, Laufer I, et al: The radiographic appearance of the stomach in the Cronkhite-Canada syndrome. Radiology 141:57-60, 1981.

182. Murai N, Fukuzaki T, Nakamura T, et al: Cronkhite-Canada syndrome associated with colon cancer: Report of a case. Jpn J Surg 23:825-829, 1993.

183. Burke AP, Sobin LH: The pathology of Cronkhite-Canada syndrome polyps. Am J Surg Pathol 13:940-946, 1989.

184. Ramsden KL, Thompson H: The Cronkhite-Canada syndrome: A seldom recognized entity. Endoscopy 26:311-334, 1994.

185. Yashiro M, Kobayashi H, Kubo N, et al: Cronkhite-Canada syndrome containing colon cancer and serrated adenoma lesions. Digestion 69:57-62, 2004.

186. Russell D, Bhathal PS, St. John JB: Complete remission in Cronkhite-Canada syndrome. Gastroenterology 85:180-185, 1983.

187. Peart AG Jr, Sivak MV, Rankin GB, et al: Spontaneous improvement of Cronkhite-Canada syndrome in a postpartum female. Dig Dis Sci 29:470-474, 1984.

188. Dachman AH, Buck JL, Burke AP, et al: Cronkhite-Canada syndrome: Radiologic features: Gastrointest Radiol 14:3-14, 1995.

189. Gorlin RJ, Cohen MM, Condon LM, et al: Bannayan-Riley-Ruvalcaba syndrome. Am J Med Genet 44:307-314, 1992.

190. Fargnoli MC, Orlow SJ, et al: Clinicopathologic findings in the Bannayan-Riley-Ruvalcaba syndrome. Arch Dermatol 132:1214-1218, 1996.

191. Arch EM, Goodman BK, Van Sesep RA, et al: Depletion of PTEN in a patient with Bannayan-Riley-Ruvalcaba syndrome suggests allelism with Cowden disease. Am J Med Genet 71:489-493, 1997.

192. Fryburg JS, Pelegano JP, Bennett MJ, et al: Long-chain 3-hydroxyacyl—coenzyme A dehydrogenase (L-CHAD) deficiency in a patient with the Bannayan-Riley-Ruvalcaba syndrome. Am J Med Genet 52:97-102, 1994.

193. Foster MA, Kilcoyne RF: Ruvalcaba-Myhre-Smith syndrome: A new consideration in the differential diagnosis of intestinal polyposis. Gastrointest Radiol 11:349-350, 1986.

chapter

66

Miscellaneous Abnormalities of the Colon

Richard M. Gore, MD • Richard A. Szucs, MD • Ellen L. Wolf, MD •
Francis J. Scholz, MD • Ronald L. Eisenberg, MD •
Stephen E. Rubesin, MD

Table 66-1
Etiology of Mechanical Large Bowel Obstruction

Intrinsic Defects	Extrinsic Defects
Neoplasms	Volvulus
Benign	Secondary
Malignant	Primary
Inflammatory	Hernias
Diverticulitis	Internal
Ulcerative colitis	External
Crohn's disease	Adhesions
Amebiasis	Mass compression
Tuberculosis	Carcinomatosis
Intussusception	Abscess
Obturation	Pregnancy
Gallstones	Cysts
Foreign bodies	Pancreatitis
Meconium	Endometriosis
Medications	
Enteroliths	
Bezoars	
Worms	
Congenital	
Atresia	
Stenosis	
Imperforate anus	
Cysts and duplications	
Miscellaneous	
Post-traumatic	
Pneumatosis intestinalis	

Adapted from Welch JP: General considerations and mortality. In Welch JP (ed): Bowel Obstruction. Philadelphia, WB Saunders, 1990, pp 59-95.

COLONIC OBSTRUCTION

Mechanical large bowel obstruction is four to five times less common than small bowel obstruction and differs significantly in terms of etiology (Table 66-1), pathophysiology, therapy, and prognosis.[1-4] Colon obstruction is most often the result of a neoplasm (Table 66-2), whereas the majority of small bowel obstructions are due to adhesions.[5,6] A number of extracolonic disease processes, including gynecologic diseases, can secondarily involve the large bowel, leading to obstruction or formation of strictures and fistulas.[7]

Table 66-2
Etiology of Colonic Obstruction: Incidence by Cause

Cause	Incidence (%)
Carcinoma	55
Volvulus	11
Diverticulitis	9
Extrinsic cancer	8
Adhesions	4
Impaction	3
Hernia	2
Intrinsic	4

Adapted from Welch JP: General considerations and mortality. In Welch JP (ed): Bowel Obstruction. Philadelphia, WB Saunders, 1990, pp 59-95.

Pathophysiology

When colonic obstruction is caused by diverticulitis or cancer, symptoms are usually subacute or chronic. Swallowed air proximal to the obstruction causes dilatation, but third spacing of fluid in the gut lumen characteristic of small bowel obstruction is not seen. Strangulation rarely occurs, except in occasional cases of volvulus.[8] Colonic response to the mechanical obstruction depends on the competency of the ileocecal valve (Fig. 66-1). The small bowel serves to decompress the colon when the valve is incompetent. A closed-loop obstruction develops when the valve is competent because the colon cannot decompress.

The cecum has the largest diameter of the colon, and therefore its wall develops the highest tension according to Laplace's law (wall tension = intraluminal pressure × radius). The increased pressure may cause separation of the muscle fibers, leading to cecal "diastatic" perforation. Dissection of air into the wall results in pneumatosis, which may precede frank perforation.[9,10] The risk of perforation increases when the cecum reaches a diameter of 9 to 12 cm[11]; however, one should not be dogmatic about an absolute number because the duration and rapidity of distention are also important.[12,13] The intraluminal pressure needed to produce perforation is between 20 and 55 mm Hg.[14] Ischemia and bacterial overgrowth also play a role in cecal perforation and the systemic effects seen with strangulation obstruction.[15,16]

Clinical Findings

Because most colonic obstructions are due to cancer, patients are usually elderly and have symptoms related to tumor location. Signs and symptoms are often insidious with right colon lesions because the lumen is large and the contents are semiliquid. These patients often present with pain, a palpable mass, and anemia.[17] Left-sided lesions cause progressive constipation and, ultimately, obstipation with abdominal distention and pain. If the ileocecal valve is incompetent, retrograde decompression produces the gradual onset of distention and, eventually, feculent vomiting.[18,19] Lesions occurring at the ileocecal valve or ileocolic intussusception cause more acute symptoms of small bowel obstruction: abdominal pain, distention, vomiting, and obstipation.[18,19] Patients with volvulus

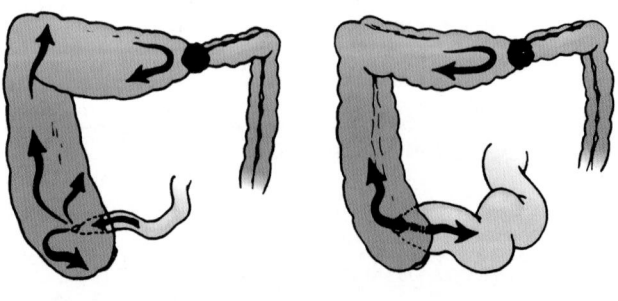

Competent   Incompetent

Figure 66-1. The importance of the ileocecal valve in large bowel obstruction. If the ileocecal valve is competent (*left*), pronounced cecal dilatation can occur. An incompetent valve (*right*) allows retrograde decompression into the small bowel. (From Welch JP [ed]: Bowel Obstruction. Philadelphia, WB Saunders, 1990.)

may develop pain and distention rapidly if a closed-loop obstruction and bowel ischemia are present.[20] On physical examination, an abdominal mass may be present (e.g., advanced right-sided colon cancer) and distention may be most marked in one region (e.g., the left upper quadrant in cecal volvulus). Bowel sounds are often hyperactive, particularly with superimposed small bowel obstruction. Marked tenderness or rebound suggests perforation or strangulation.[18,19]

Radiologic Approach to Suspected Large Bowel Obstruction

Radiography

Abdominal radiographs obtained in the supine and erect or left lateral decubitus positions are the initial means of imaging patients with suspected obstruction.[21] These radiographs may confirm the diagnosis, locate the site of obstruction, and, in some cases, identify the nature of the obstructing lesion.[22-25] The colon is usually dilated proximal to the obstruction; however, if the ileocecal valve is incompetent, the appearance may mimic small bowel obstruction.[26-28] The radiographic findings in bowel obstruction are discussed in detail in Chapter 16.

Contrast Enemas

A contrast enema, preferably with water-soluble media, is the next step in patients with suspected large bowel obstruction or in patients in whom the level of obstruction is unknown. Although barium is inherently a better contrast agent, it may interfere with future studies, such as CT or colonoscopy. If the patient proves to have pseudo-obstruction rather than true obstruction, the barium may remain within the colon for days.[29] A water-soluble enema can also be therapeutic in patients with fecal impactions.[29] Because oral barium can inspissate proximal to a partial or complete large bowel obstruction, it is important to exclude an obstructing colonic lesion before the small bowel is examined with barium.[30,31]

Computed Tomography

Computed tomography is useful as a primary imaging technique in patients with a history of abdominal malignancy and clinical symptoms suggestive of bowel obstruction and also in patients with no history of prior abdominal surgery. CT has a secondary role in postsurgical patients who most likely have adhesive obstruction.[32] It is most valuable when there are systemic signs suggesting infection, bowel infarction, or an associated palpable mass.[32] CT identifies bowel obstruction as distended bowel loops seen proximal to collapsed loops and can reveal the cause of obstruction, such as tumor, diverticulitis, or appendicitis.[33] The transitional zone should be carefully evaluated for masses. When no masses are present, the obstruction is usually due to adhesions.[32]

Ultrasonography

In patients with suspected colon obstruction, ultrasonography can determine the level and cause of obstruction.[34] It has also proved to be helpful in evaluating the child with a distended gasless abdomen in whom the cause of obstruction, such as tumor, hernia, or intussusception, may be visualized.[35]

Major Types of Colonic Obstruction

Carcinoma of the Colon

Large bowel obstruction is caused by intrinsic colon carcinoma in approximately 55% of cases.[36,37] Nearly 20% of colon cancers are complicated by some degree of obstruction; 5% to 10% are complicated by complete obstruction that requires emergent surgical intervention.[38] The mortality rate is high (10% to 30%) in patients requiring emergency surgery, regardless of the site of tumor.[38,39] This is a reflection of advanced tumor stage, advanced patient age, and associated cardiorespiratory disease, malnutrition, sepsis, and surgical stress.[40,41] Mortality is even higher if there is concurrent perforation. Patients who present with obstructing colon carcinoma have low curability and survival rates because of advanced disease at the time of diagnosis.[42]

The sigmoid colon is the most common site of obstructive colon cancer because of its relatively narrow diameter and solid fecal contents. The location of obstruction in one series was as follows: cecum, 11%; right colon, 5%; hepatic flexure, 3%; transverse colon, 11%; splenic flexure, 12%; descending colon, 10%; sigmoid colon, 35%; and rectum, 13%.[37] The ratio of obstructing carcinomas to total tumors is similar in both the right (Fig. 66-2) and the left colon but lower for rectal lesions.[17] Tumors of the transverse colon and splenic flexure are at particular risk for obstruction before clinical detection.[43] The risk of developing obstruction in tumors at a particular site has been estimated as follows: 50% for splenic flexure lesions; 25% for right- and left-sided ones; and 6% for rectal tumors.[17,44] Perforation occurs in 3% to 8% of patients with malignant obstruction.[38] The most common site of perforation is the cecum rather than adjacent to the tumor.[45,46]

The clinical presentation of obstructive colon cancer depends on the location, duration, and completeness of obstruction, as well as on the competency of the ileocecal valve. Tumors located near the ileocecal valve can produce symptoms suggesting a distal small bowel obstruction. Some right colon tumors act as lead points for colocolic intussusception; others may perforate, causing abscess formation and obstruction. Left-sided colon tumors tend to obstruct in an annular fashion or by a polypoid lesion that reaches a size sufficient to obstruct the lumen. The rectum is not a common site of obstruction because of its greater diameter and distensibility and the fact that rectal cancers often cause rectal bleeding, prompting earlier medical attention. The usual treatment of obstructive colon cancer is surgical resection or diverting colostomy; however, there have been reports of treatment with expandable metallic stents either for palliation or to allow bowel cleansing before surgical resection.[47,48]

Diverticulitis

Large bowel obstruction is the result of diverticular disease in about 12% of cases. Diverticulitis can cause both small and large bowel obstruction. Partial colonic obstruction can complicate acute diverticulitis as a consequence of edema and pericolic inflammation or abscess formation. High-grade

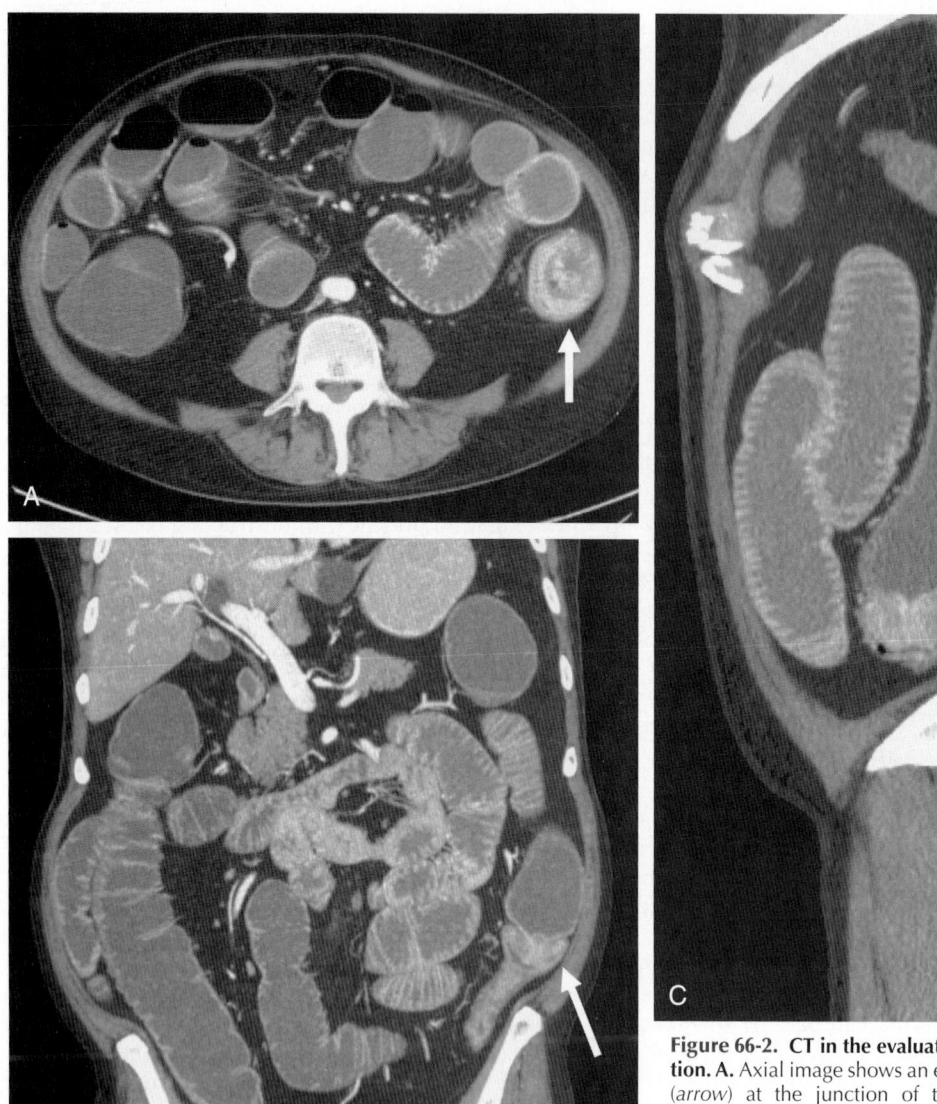

Figure 66-2. CT in the evaluation of large bowel obstruction. A. Axial image shows an enhancing, obstructing mass (*arrow*) at the junction of the descending colon and sigmoid colon. **B.** Coronal reformatted image demonstrates the obstructing cancer (*arrow*) and dilated, fluid-filled colon and small bowel. **C.** Sagittal depiction of the cancer (*arrow*) and dilated, fluid filled colon and small bowel.

obstruction is uncommon; it is far more frequently caused by carcinoma of the colon. More commonly, obstruction follows recurrent attacks of diverticulitis with marked fibrosis of the colon wall leading to narrowing and eventually stricture formation. The site of obstruction is usually in the sigmoid colon, near the site of inflammation. Obstruction of the transverse or right colon attributable to diverticulitis is rare.[49,50]

Clinically, patients with sigmoid diverticulitis complain of left lower quadrant pain, fever, and abnormal bowel habits. It is important for these symptoms to be differentiated from those of carcinoma of the colon, an often difficult task both clinically and radiologically (Fig. 66-3 and Table 66-3). Symptoms of sigmoid colon cancer are usually more insidious, with rectal bleeding, constipation, and weight loss.[51-53]

Patients with suspected nonobstructing diverticulitis may benefit from CT examination as the initial study. In the acutely obstructed patient, a water-soluble contrast enema should

Table 66-3

Sigmoid Diverticulitis versus Carcinoma: Radiologic Differentiation

Diverticulitis	Carcinoma
Spastic bowel	Normal adjacent bowel
Cone-shaped edges to narrowing	Sharp margins, shelflike
Long segments	Short segments
Mucosa preserved	Mucosa destroyed
Variable constriction between examinations	Progressive obstruction
Diverticula present	Occasional diverticula
Obstruction without tumor	Obstruction with tumor

Reprinted from Morton DL, Goldman L: Differential diagnosis of diverticulitis and carcinoma of the sigmoid colon. Am J Surg 103:55-61, 1962; with permission from Excerpta Medica, Inc.

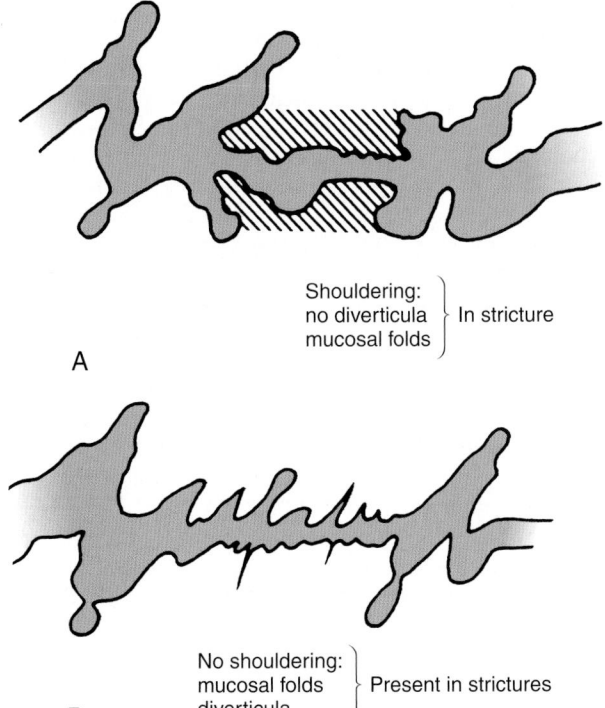

Shouldering:
no diverticula   } In stricture
mucosal folds

A

No shouldering:
mucosal folds   } Present in strictures
diverticula

B

Figure 66-3. Sigmoid diverticulitis versus carcinoma: barium enema findings. A. Carcinoma in diverticular disease. **B.** Stricturing attributable to diverticular disease. (From Bartram CT, Kumar P: Clinical Radiology in Gastroenterology. Oxford, Blackwell Scientific, 1981, p 132.)

be performed to locate the site and cause of obstruction.[54-56] A more complete discussion of diverticular disease can be found in Chapter 59.

Volvulus

Volvulus refers to torsion or twist of an organ on a pedicle to a degree sufficient to cause symptoms. Large bowel volvulus (Fig. 66-4) accounts for about 10% of colon obstructions and can affect the sigmoid colon (Fig. 66-5), cecum (Figs. 66-6 and 66-7), transverse colon, and, rarely, the splenic flexure. Symptoms are caused by narrowing and obstruction of the gut, strangulation of the blood vessels, or both.[57-59]

The major predisposing factors necessary for colonic volvulus are a segment of redundant mobile colon on a mesentery and a fixed point around which rotation can occur. The sigmoid colon (Fig. 66-8) is therefore the most frequent site of colonic volvulus, especially in patients older than 60 years of age.[60,61] Sigmoid volvulus is not due to a congenital defect but rather to dietary and behavioral factors, including increased fiber in the diet, which increases the bulk of stool and elongates the colon. Cecal or ascending colon volvulus occurs in patients with a congenital defect in attachment of the right colon or postpartum ligamentous laxity and a mobile cecum.[62] Anything that causes colon distention, including pseudo-obstruction, distal tumor, endoscopy, enemas, or postoperative ileus, may precipitate cecal volvulus in susceptible individuals. Transverse colon volvulus occurs in patients with a redundant transverse colon on a long mesentery,[63] and splenic flexure volvulus occurs in patients with deficiency of the normal attachments of the splenic flexure to the posterior peritoneal wall, usually as a result of prior surgery.[64,65] The frequency of colon volvulus is as follows: sigmoid colon, 50% to 75%; cecum, 25% to 40%; and transverse colon, 0% to 10%. A rare cause of combined colon and small bowel obstruction is the ileosigmoid knot.[66-68]

A detailed discussion of colonic volvulus and its conventional radiographic features can be found in Chapter 16. On CT, a "whirl" sign has been described in volvulus. The whirl is constituted by the afferent and efferent limbs leading into the volvulus. Tightly twisted mesentery and bowel compose the central portion of the whirl. The progressive tapering of the two limbs leading to the twist on CT corresponds to the "beak" seen on barium enema.[69-71]

Adult Intussusception

Intussusception is defined as the invagination of one segment of the gastrointestinal tract into an adjacent one (Fig. 66-9).

Figure 66-4. The three major sites of colonic volvulus. A. Sigmoid volvulus. Adjacent middle walls of the dilated sigmoid colon (SC) form a double line on radiographs that converges on the point of twist in the sigmoid mesocolon. DC, descending colon. **B.** Transverse colonic volvulus. The caudal border of this ptotic colon is rounded, and the central double bowel wall does not extend to the sigmoid mesentery. AC, ascending colon; TC, transverse colon. **C.** Cecal volvulus. The dilated cecum twists clockwise, obstructing the ascending colon, and the terminal ileum (TI) swings around the dilated bowel.

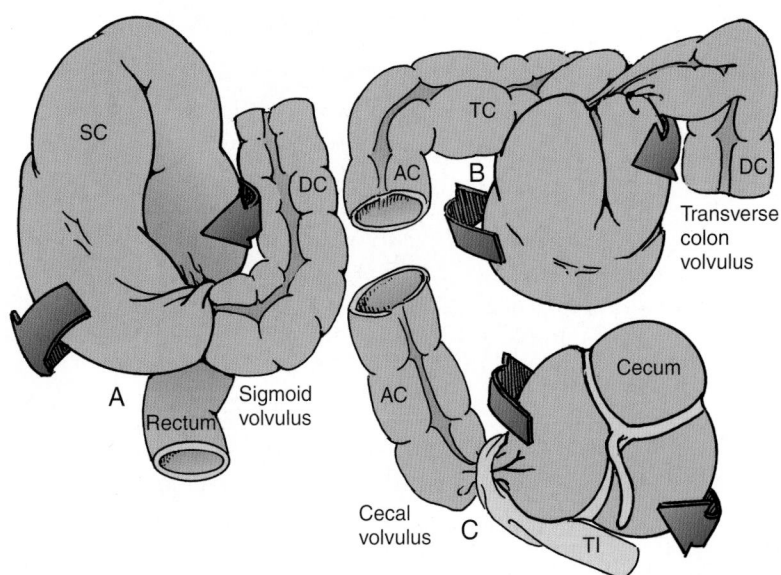

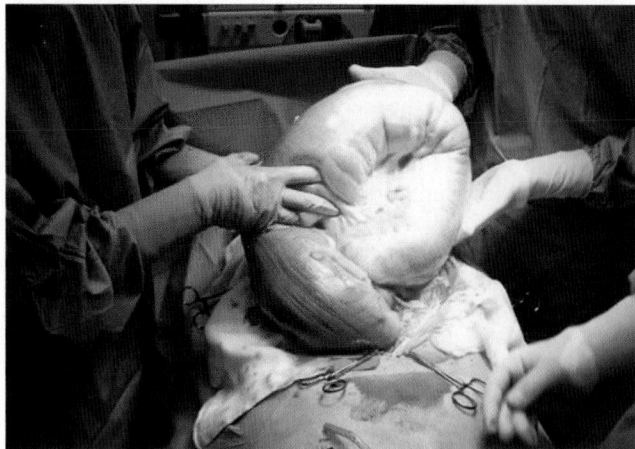

Figure 66-5. Sigmoid volvulus: intraoperative image. A massively dilated sigmoid colon is identified twisted upon itself.

It accounts for 80% to 90% of bowel obstruction in infants and children and ranks second only to appendicitis as the most common cause of an acute abdominal emergency in children. In children, intussusception usually begins in the distal ileum, and in 90% of cases the cause is idiopathic.[1-4,20] A complete discussion of childhood intussusception can be found in Chapter 121.

In contrast, intussusception in adults accounts for only 1% to 3% of mechanical intestinal obstruction, and a demon-strable cause is found in 80% of adult cases. Colonic intus-susception is usually due to a primary colon cancer, whereas small bowel intussusception is generally related to a benign tumor and less often to a malignancy, most commonly a metastatic lesion.[72-84] Postoperative intussusceptions usually occur in the small bowel and are related to a number of factors: suture lines, ostomy closure, adhesions, long intestinal tubes, bypassed intestinal segments, submucosal edema, abnormal bowel motility, electrolyte imbalance, and chronic dilatation of the bowel.[84,85]

Benign lesions that can serve as lead points in colonic intussusception include adenomatous polyps, lipomas, gastro-intestinal stromal tumors (Fig. 66-10), appendiceal stump granulomas, and villous adenomas of the appendix.[84] The normal appendix may transiently intussuscept, although clini-cally significant appendiceal intussusception usually occurs in the setting of appendiceal inflammation, infestation, neo-plasm, or endometriosis deposition.[86] A more complete dis-cussion of diseases of the appendix can be found in Chapter 60. Colonic intussusception has also been reported as a com-plication of eosinophilic colitis, epiploic appendagitis, and pseudomembranous colitis.[87-89]

In children, the diagnosis is suggested by the presence of an abdominal mass and passage of blood per rectum. Because adult intussusception is often chronic and relapsing, the diag-nosis is suggested by recurrent episodes of subacute obstruc-tion and variable abdominal signs. During the height of an attack, a palpable mass may be present but may disappear completely when the patient is reexamined several hours later,

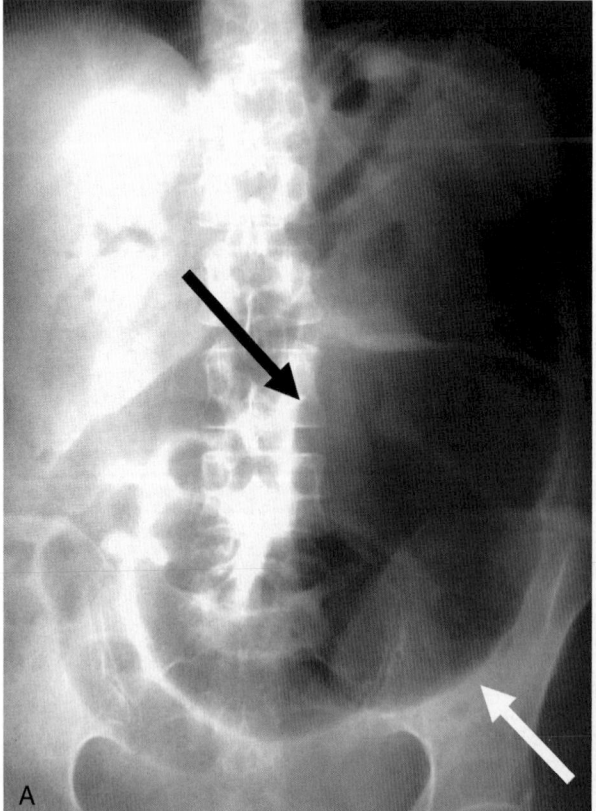

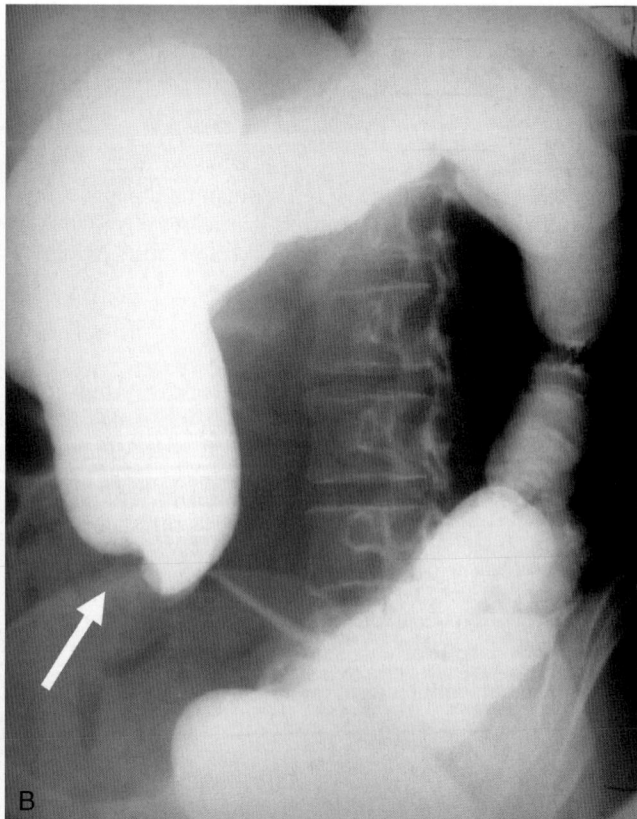

Figure 66-6. Cecal volvulus: plain radiograph and barium enema features. A. A distended cecum (*arrows*) is present in the left lower quadrant. Dilated small bowel is evident proximally. There is a relative paucity of colonic gas distal to the volvulus. **B.** Barium enema shows the contrast column to abruptly end (*arrow*) at the level of the twist.

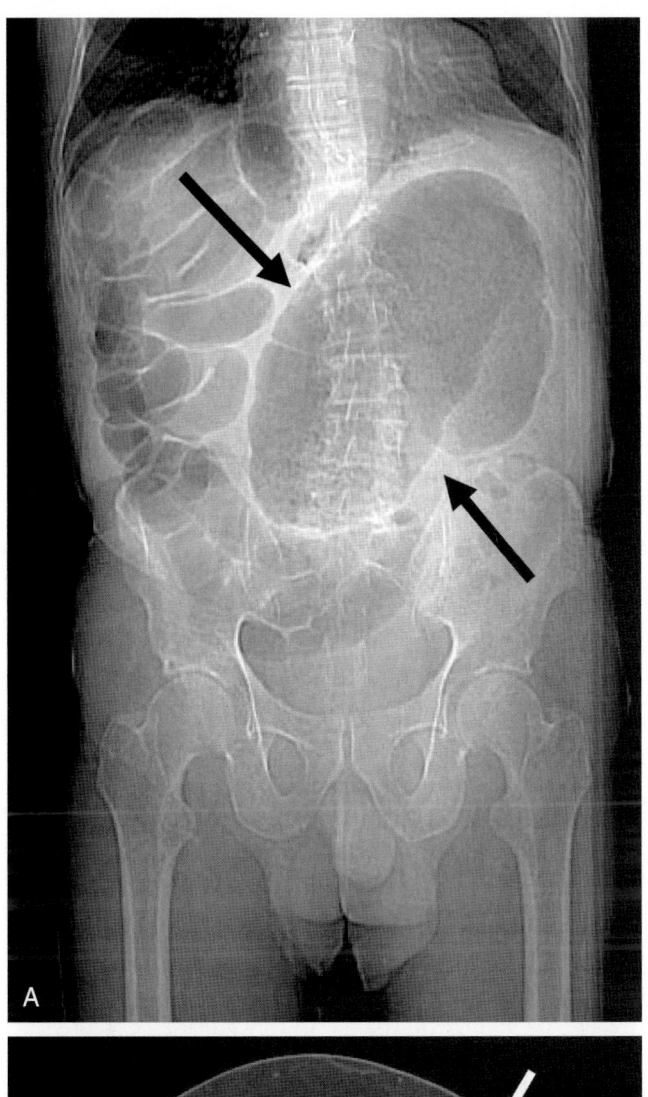

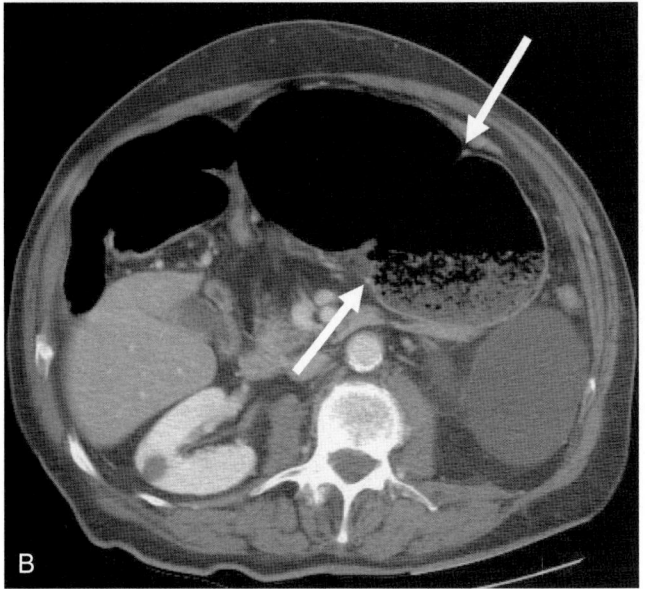

Figure 66-7. Cecal volvulus: CT features. A. Scout image shows a distended cecum (*arrows*) is present in the left upper quadrant with multiple dilated small bowel loops in the right upper quadrant. **B.** CT scan demonstrates the malpositioned cecum (*arrows*) and swirling of the mesentery.

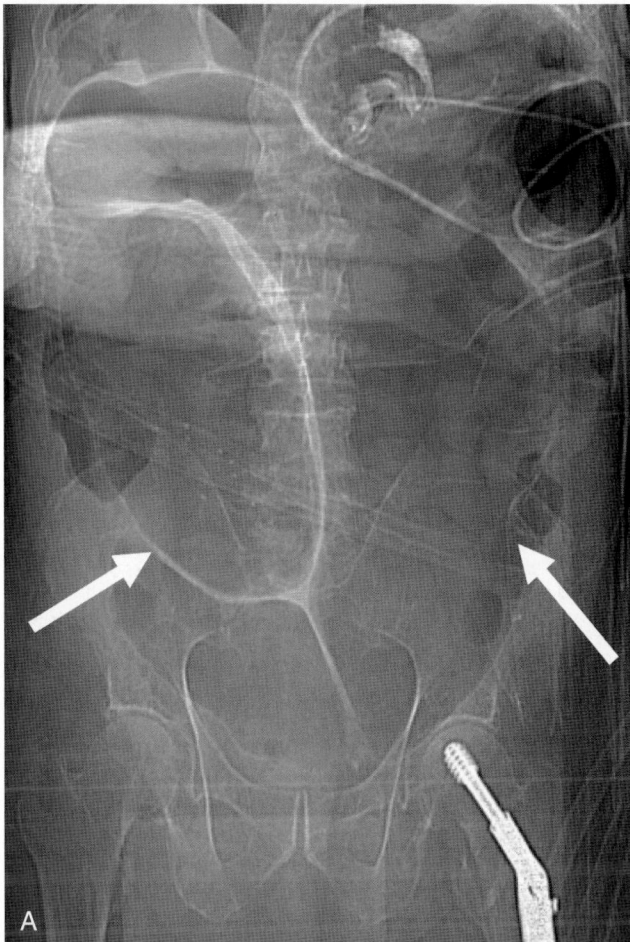

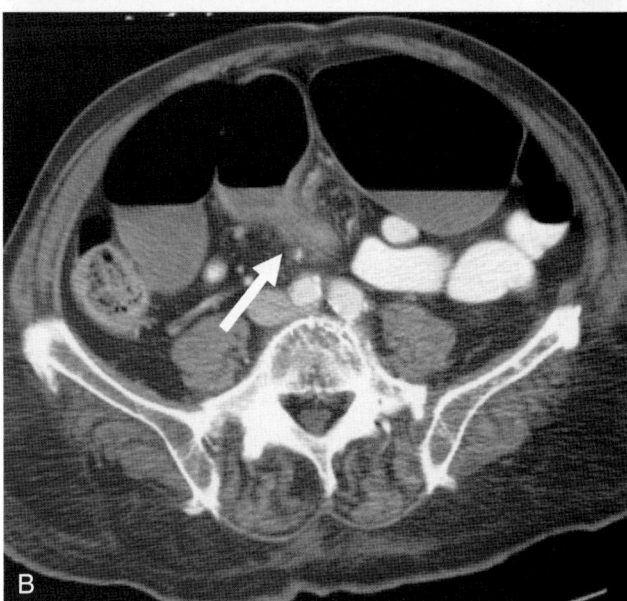

Figure 66-8. Sigmoid volvulus. A. Scout image shows a markedly dilated sigmoid colon (*arrows*). **B.** CT shows the transition zone (*arrow*) at the site of the volvulus.

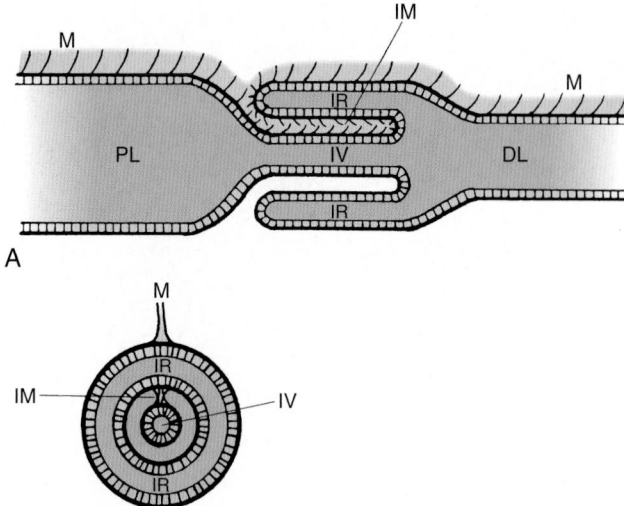

Figure 66-9. Intussusception. Longitudinal (**A**) and cross-sectional (**B**) diagrams of antegrade intussusception. IM, intussuscepted mesentery; IR, intussuscipiens; IV, intussusceptum; M, mesentery; PL, proximal intestinal loops; DL, distal intestinal loops. (From Iko BO, Teal JS, Siram SM, et al: Computed tomography of adult colonic intussusception: Clinical and experimental studies. AJR 143:769-772, 1984, © American Roentgen Ray Society.)

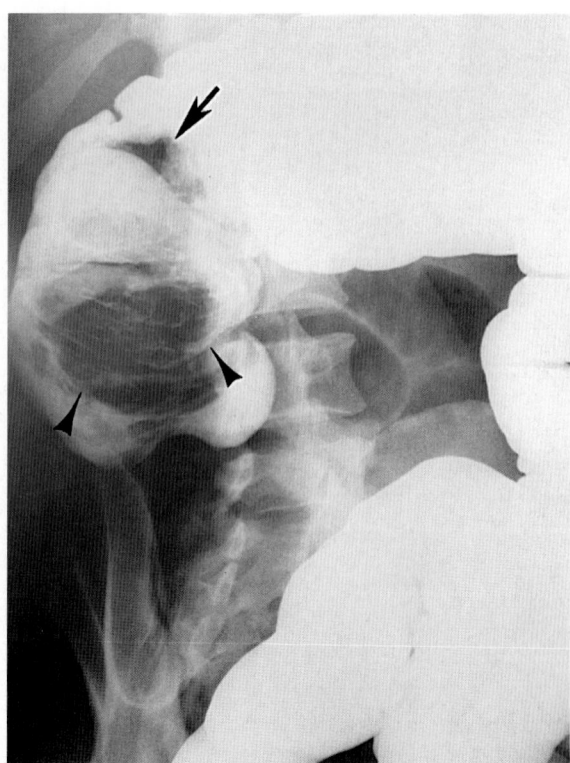

Figure 66-11. Colonic intussusception: barium enema findings. A cecal neoplasm is intussuscepting into the ascending colon (*arrow*). Note the "coiled spring" appearance (*arrowheads*).

by which time the symptoms have resolved.[3,20] In infants and young children, hydrostatic or pneumatic intussuscep-tion reduction should be attempted and may be definitive therapy, since the cause is usually idiopathic. In adults, the high incidence of organic lesions, often malignant, precludes this approach.

If the intussusception is of the ileocolic or colocolic variety, the pathognomonic "crescent" sign may be seen. This sign is produced when the intussuscipiens invaginates into the intussusceptum and stretches the outer wall. Intraluminal gas trapped between the two intestinal surfaces can appear as a semilunar lucency lacking haustral septa or valvulae conniventes. This lucent crescent is wider than normal bowel in diameter and often superimposed on a round soft tissue density representing the mass created by the intussusception.

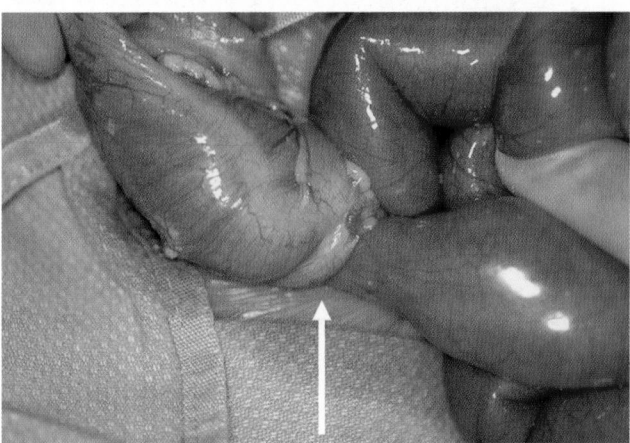

Figure 66-10. Ileocolic intussusception. The ileum is intussuscepting (*arrow*) into the colon. The lead point was a small gastrointestinal stromal tumor of the distal ileum.

A more central and less distinct lucency may be seen, representing gas trapped in the lumen of the intussuscipiens. On supine views, the transverse colon gas shadow is often absent because this segment of colon is usually displaced distally.[21,90,91]

The classic appearance of intussusception on barium studies is the "coil spring" appearance as contrast is trapped between the intussusceptum and the intussuscipiens (Fig. 66-11).

Ultrasound shows a target-like lesion (Fig. 66-12), in which the hypoechoic halo is produced by the mesentery and the edematous wall of the intussuscipiens, and the hyperechoic center is produced by multiple interfaces of compressed mucosal, submucosal, and serosal surfaces of the intussusceptum. Multiple concentric rings, best seen on transverse scans, are also characteristic. The corresponding appearance on longitudinal scans is that of multiple, thin, parallel, hypoechoic, and echogenic stripes.[92-96]

On CT, intussusceptions appear as three different patterns, which reflect their severity and duration: (1) the "target" sign, (2) a sausage-shaped mass with alternating layers of low and high attenuation, and (3) a reniform mass. Pathophysiologically, the target is the earliest stage of intussusception. As it progresses, a layering pattern, with alternating low-attenuation (mesenteric fat) and high-attenuation areas (bowel wall), develops (Fig. 66-13). If intussusception is untreated, edema and mural thickening develop. An intussusception with a reniform appearance is due to severe edema and vascular compromise, and this constitutes a surgical emergency.[97] Intussusception is almost invariably associated with either acute intestinal obstruction or partial and recurrent obstruction, air-fluid levels, and proximal bowel distention. The mesenteric arcade associated with the intussuscipiens may show traction.

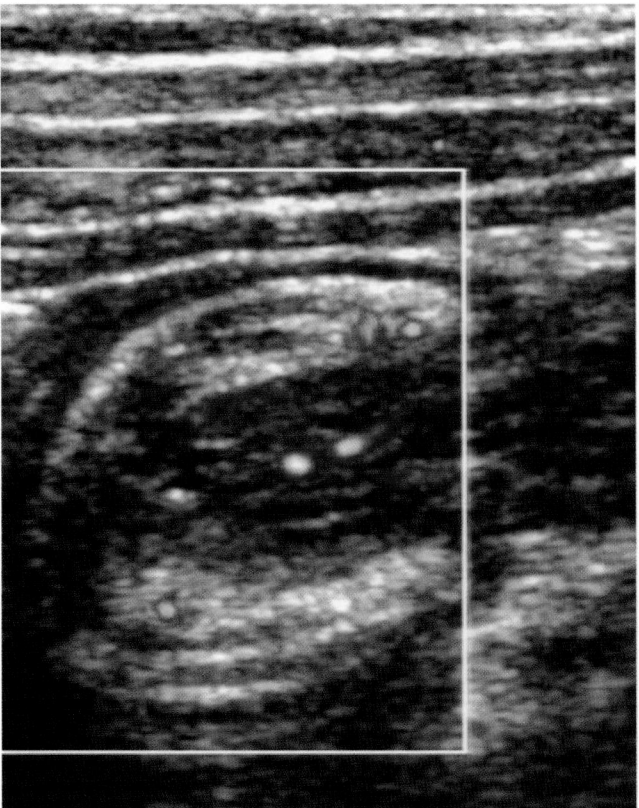

Figure 66-12. Intussusception: sonographic findings. This color Doppler scan, longitudinally imaging the intussusception, shows a central hypoechoic area that is the intussusceptum telescoping into the intussuscipiens.

If infarction occurs, this mass may be surrounded by intraperitoneal fluid, edema, and hemorrhage in the mesentery, and even perforation.[98-104] CT can diagnose lipoma as the lead point; however, with varying degrees of infarction and fat necrosis, lipomas may have an atypical appearance.[105,106]

Adhesions

Adhesions are the result of inflammation that heals with fibrosis. They are most commonly the result of surgical trauma but may be congenital. Adhesional large bowel obstruction is unusual because the colon is characteristically fixed and of large caliber and has thick walls. The small bowel, in contrast, has an inherently small caliber and a high degree of mobility and is therefore very prone to obstruction by adhesions. A more complete discussion of small bowel obstruction can be found in Chapter 50. The mobile, redundant portions of the colon are most likely to be involved.[107] Adhesive obstructions of the right colon, transverse colon, and sigmoid colon have been reported.[108,109]

Folding of the cecum on itself, the "cecal bascule," often occurs at the site of an adhesive band.[110] The ascending colon can be obstructed by congenital bands or adhesions caused by inflammatory changes after colonoscopy and polypectomy.[111,112] Inflammation of the appendices epiploicae can rarely cause obstruction in the rectosigmoid, and ischemia and inflammation of the greater omentum can cause obstruction in the transverse colon.[113,114] On barium enema, adhesions can appear as an area of circumferential narrowing, usually short, with intact mucosa, or as a smooth, broad-based filling defect. They may produce either partial or complete colonic obstruction.[115]

Hernias

Hernias cause large bowel obstruction less often than small bowel obstruction because of the relatively fixed nature of the colon and its larger caliber. Inguinal, femoral, umbilical, spigelian, incisional, lumbar, and diaphragmatic hernias (congenital or post-traumatic) can all contain colon and cause bowel obstruction.[116-125] Internal hernias, such as through the foramen of Winslow, can contain colon and cause obstruction as well.[126-129] The diagnosis may be made by radiography, barium enema, or CT. A complete discussion of hernias can be found in Chapter 114.

Obturation Obstruction

The terminal ileum is the narrowest portion of the gut and, as a result, is the most common site of obturation obstruction. The sigmoid colon, measuring 2.5 cm in diameter, only slightly larger than the distal ileum, is the narrowest portion of the colon, followed by the hepatic and splenic flexures.

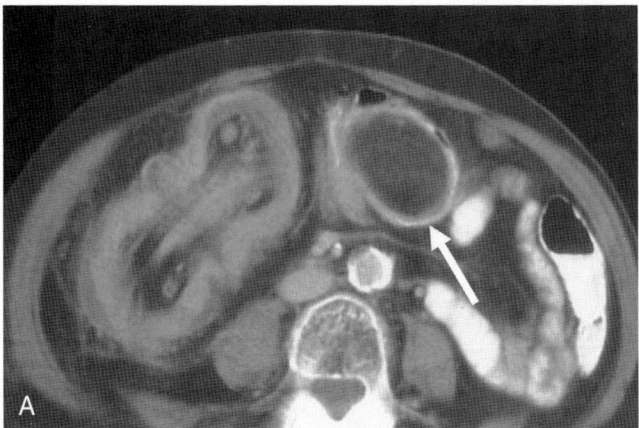
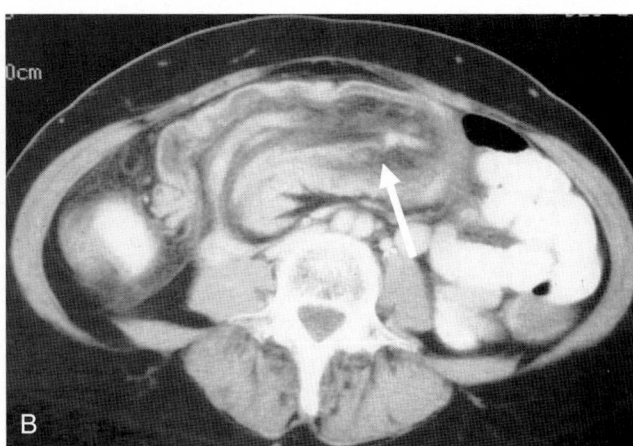

Figure 66-13. Colonic intussusception: CT findings. A. The lead point of this colonic intussusception is a lipoma (*arrow*). The outer layer represents the intussuscipiens and the inner layer represents the intussusceptum. **B.** In a different patient, the cigar-shaped intussusceptum (*arrow*) is seen within the intussuscipiens.

These are the most likely points of colonic impaction of an intraluminal object.[130]

Three to 5 percent of patients with gallstone ileus have colonic obstruction.[131] In these cases, the gallstone most often bypasses the ileocecal valve through a cholecystocolic fistula and usually impacts in the sigmoid colon, which may be narrowed by prior diverticulitis.[132]

Bezoars, foods, and enteroliths usually do not obstruct the colon unless there is a stricture.[133,134] Patients with cystic fibrosis (see Chapter 121) tend to form large cecal masses of inspissated feces that can cause the meconium ileus equivalent syndrome.[135]

Sufficient amounts of various medications or diagnostic agents can cause colonic obturation obstruction. Antacid impactions containing nonabsorbable aluminum hydroxide antacid gels, given to prevent hyperphosphatemia, can develop in the right colons of patients with renal failure. These impactions can be treated with orally or rectally administered hyperosmolar diatrizoate meglumine (Gastrografin).[136]

Barium retained in the colon for several days is desiccated and can form impactions in any part of the colon, usually the proximal portion. These impactions can also be treated by hyperosmolar Gastrografin, which stimulates peristalsis and draws fluid into the bowel.[137,138] Foreign bodies entering via an oral or a transanal route can cause obstruction or perforation.[139]

Elderly, inactive, debilitated, and mentally disturbed patients, drug addicts in methadone maintenance programs, transplantation and hemodialysis patients, and individuals with adult Hirschsprung's disease are at risk for developing fecal impaction. The most common sites are the rectum (70%) and sigmoid colon (20%). A fecaloma or stercoroma is a mass of fecal material that develops the characteristics of an intraluminal tumor. These are composed primarily of an accumulation of undigested food forming a nucleus around which fecal material accumulates. Obstruction, volvulus, stercoral ulceration, perforation, rectal prolapse, and rectal fissure are potential complications of fecalomas.[140,141]

Strictures

Colonic strictures can result from a variety of disorders that are listed in Tables 66-4 through 66-6. These strictures often cause chronic obstructive symptoms and may cause acute obstruction from the presence of impacted feces or as a result of obturation in the stricture by a foreign object.

Table 66-4
Colonic Ischemia: Risk Factors

Inferior mesenteric artery ligation, thrombosis, or embolus
Cardiac arrhythmia
Congestive heart failure
Shock
Digitalis toxicity
Collagen vascular disease
Strangulated hernia
Oral contraceptives
Polycythemia vera
Trauma
Diabetes
Amyloidosis
Radiation

Table 66-5
General, Systemic, and Psychological Causes of Constipation

Life Style
Inadequate fiber
Little food
Repressing or ignoring urge to defecate
Immobility

External Factors
Drugs (including opiates, anticholinergics, antidepressants, anticonvulsants)

Endocrine/Metabolic
Hypothyroidism
Hypercalcemia
Porphyria

Neurologic
Parkinson's disease
Multiple sclerosis
Spinal lesions
Damage to sacral parasympathetic nerves
Autonomic neuropathy
Autonomic failure

Psychologic
Depression
Eating disorders (e.g., anorexia nervosa)
Obsession about "inner cleanliness"
Denied bowel actions

From Patel SM, Lembo AJ: Constipation. In Feldman M, Friedman LS, Sleisenger MH (eds): Gastrointestinal and Liver Disease, 8th ed. Philadelphia, Saunders, 2006, pp 221-254.

Other Causes

Pelvic lipomatosis, in which there is benign fatty tissue infiltration into the perirectal and perivesical spaces, usually causes straightening, narrowing, and rigidity of the rectum but occasionally can cause obstruction.[142] Pregnancy, mesenteric cysts, wandering spleen, retroperitoneal tumors, retractile

Table 66-6
Gastrointestinal Causes of Constipation and Related Symptoms

Gastrointestinal Tract
Obstruction
Aganglionosis (Hirschsprung's disease, Chagas' disease)
Myopathy
Neuropathy
Systemic sclerosis
Megarectum/colon

Anorectum
Anal atresia or malformation
Hereditary internal anal sphincter myopathy
Anal stenosis
Weak pelvic floor
Large rectocele
Internal intussusception
Anterior mucosal prolapse
Prolapse
Solitary rectal ulcer

From Patel SM, Lembo AJ: Constipation. In Feldman M, Friedman LS, Sleisenger MH (eds): Gastrointestinal and Liver Disease, 8th ed. Philadelphia, Saunders, 2006, pp 221-254.

mesenteritis, and retroperitoneal fibrosis are rarer causes of large bowel obstruction.[143-145]

Summary

Bowel obstruction is a common and often difficult clinical problem. It requires the close cooperation of internist, surgeon, and radiologist.

EXTRACOLONIC DISEASES INVOLVING THE COLON

Benign and malignant extrinsic disease processes can involve the colon. Endometriosis, ovarian carcinoma, other benign and malignant gynecologic diseases, pancreatic disease, prostate carcinoma, and other abdominal malignancies can present as colon involvement. This involvement may cause obstruction and can mimic primary colon pathology. Obstruction most commonly occurs in the pelvis where the colon is fixed and confined by the bony pelvis. The transverse colon is another common site of involvement because of its omental and mesenteric attachments (see Chapter 110). Barium enema, CT, and endoscopic ultrasonography may be helpful in assessment of colonic wall invasion by adjacent disease processes.[146]

Endometriosis

Endometriosis is a disease that affects 8% to 18% of women during their active menstrual years, most commonly between the ages of 30 and 45 years. *Endometriosis* is defined as the presence of ectopic foci of tissue containing endometrial epithelial and stromal elements outside the uterine cavity.[147,148] Gastrointestinal tract involvement has been reported in 5% to 37% of patients.[149] In one large retrospective review of over 7000 patients with endometriosis, 12% of the patients had gut involvement. The rectosigmoid colon was the most frequently involved site (72% of cases), followed by the rectovaginal septum (14%), small intestine (7%), cecum (4%), and appendix (3%).[150] Rare cases of involvement of the stomach, pancreas, proximal small bowel, and transverse colon have been reported.

The anterior wall of the rectosigmoid colon adjacent to the pouch of Douglas is the most frequent site of gastrointestinal tract involvement. Endometrial implants on the bowel are usually extrinsic or serosal but may be intramural or, rarely, intraluminal.[151] Implants typically appear as an extrinsic serosal mass effect with mucosal preservation on double-contrast barium enema studies (Fig. 66-14). This appearance, although characteristic of endometriosis, is not specific because other extrinsic processes in the cul-de-sac, such as drop metastases or abscess, can produce an identical appearance. Serosal spiculation and fine crenulations of the mucosa can usually be identified when there is involvement of the bowel wall.[152] Less frequently, manifestations of endometriosis on barium enema are a polypoid mass extending into the lumen of the colon, stricture, or a short annular lesion. These cases may be difficult to distinguish clinically and radiographically from carcinoma.[153] Rarely, endometriosis presents as acute obstruction, gastrointestinal bleeding, or perforation necessitating resection.[7,154-157] Endometriomas usually appear as solid or complex cystic masses on ultrasound or CT, but the appearance is not specific and may be indistinguishable

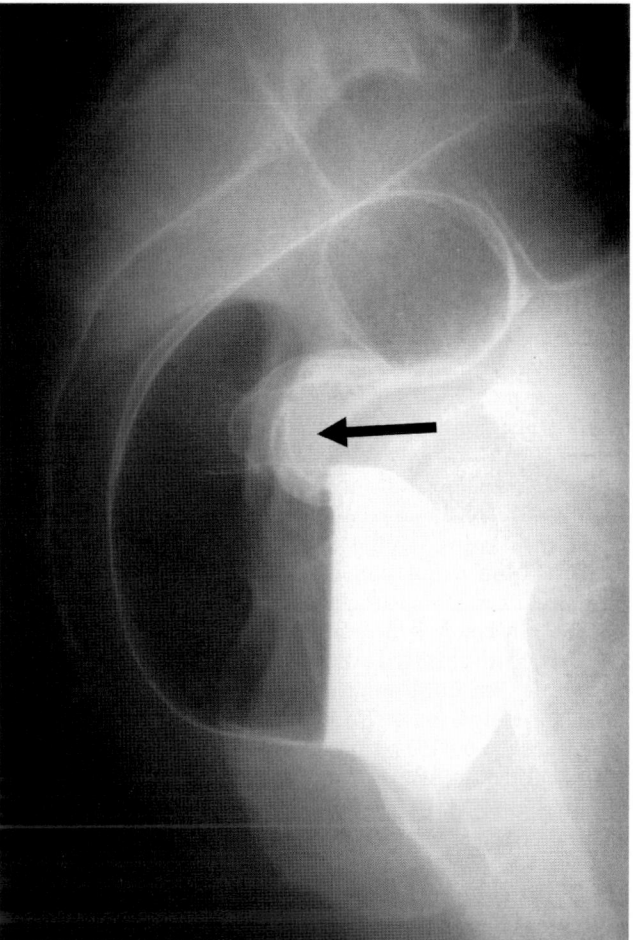

Figure 66-14. Endometrioma in the pouch of Douglas. Barium enema examination shows an extrinsic mass on the serosal aspect of the rectum (*arrow*).

from neoplasm or abscess.[158-160] MRI is more sensitive and specific for detection of hemorrhage within these masses.[160]

Malignant Gynecologic Tumors

Malignant gynecologic neoplasms spread within the peritoneal cavity by direct invasion, intraperitoneal seeding, hematogenous metastasis, and lymphatic extension. Intraperitoneal seeding of malignant cells is dependent on the natural pathways of flow of ascitic fluid as demonstrated by Meyers.[161] The characteristic patterns of spread vary depending on the origin of the primary tumor. See Chapter 111 for a more complete discussion of pathways of abdominal and pelvic spread of disease.

Ovarian Carcinoma

Ovarian carcinoma is the fifth leading cause of cancer death in women, and the prevalence increases with age and peaks around age 60 years.[162-164] Most patients with ovarian carcinoma have relatively few symptoms, and in over 50% the disease is in an advanced stage at the time of initial presentation. Patients usually have vague abdominal symptoms and present with increasing abdominal girth and a large palpable mass, although some tumors are detected earlier on routine pelvic examination. Occasionally, intestinal symptoms or colonic obstruction may be the first manifestation of ovarian cancer.[165]

Ovarian carcinoma is the most common primary malignancy to directly invade the colon. The subperitoneal space forms a pathway for the spread of disease processes from the pelvis to the abdomen.[166,167] Direct invasion from the left ovary through the sigmoid mesocolon most often involves the inferior border of the sigmoid colon. Direct invasion from the right ovary usually involves the cecum and distal ileum by means of extension through the small bowel mesentery of the ileum. Direct invasion of the colon by ovarian cancer can be readily demonstrated on barium enema, with appearances ranging from serosal spiculation with tethering and fixation to gross invasion and annular constriction to complete obstruction.[168] Mural involvement may produce narrowing with mucosal crenulations or, in more severe cases, marked narrowing with spiculation. Annular constriction may simulate carcinoma or diverticulitis, and complete obstruction may mimic an obstructing colon carcinoma.

Ovarian carcinoma frequently spreads by intraperitoneal seeding. The colon is the portion of the gastrointestinal tract most frequently involved by intraperitoneal seeding of ovarian carcinoma. Peritoneal implants, which may be multiple, are seen as extrinsic masses often with serosal spiculation and tethering (Fig. 66-15) on barium enema studies. An implant in the cul-de-sac may be indistinguishable from an abscess or endometrioma. In addition, ovarian carcinoma frequently seeds the greater omentum, producing an "omental cake," which can secondarily involve the transverse colon or stomach. The appearance in these cases can simulate gastric cancer with extension to the transverse colon through the gastrocolic ligament or colon cancer with extension to the stomach.[169-171]

Other Gynecologic Malignancies

Cervical carcinoma is the sixth leading cause of cancer death in women in the United States. Invasive cervical carcinoma has a peak prevalence at age 54 years.[164] Cervical carcinoma spreads by direct extension to the pelvic sidewall and adjacent structures, including the rectum. Demonstration of rectal

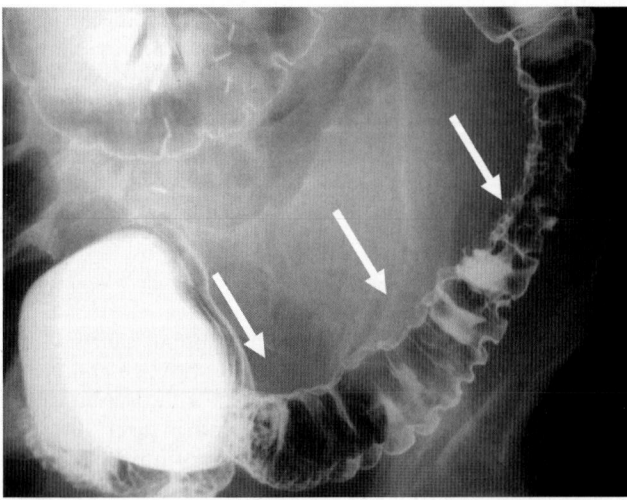

Figure 66-15. Ovarian carcinomatosis. Multiple serosal implants (*arrows*) are identified along the medial aspect of the sigmoid colon.

involvement is an important finding because hysterectomy is reserved for patients with tumor localized to the cervix or extension confined to the parametrium or upper two thirds of the vagina (stage IIB or less). All others are treated with radiation therapy.[172]

Carcinoma of the endometrium, vagina, and fallopian tubes can also directly invade the rectosigmoid colon. Barium enema examination provides important information for staging and planning surgical resection of these pelvic malignancies. These tumors can also spread by peritoneal seeding or lymphatic extension. Leiomyosarcoma of the uterus, like other sarcomas, may spread by hematogenous metastasis to the gut, producing submucosal masses that can ulcerate and bleed.

Benign Gynecologic Tumors

Benign ovarian tumors, including serous and mucinous cystadenomas and teratomas, may produce extrinsic impression on the rectosigmoid colon that is recognizable on barium enema. These masses that are purely extrinsic to the bowel have a smooth interface with the colonic wall and are usually asymptomatic but, if very large, may produce symptoms of partial obstruction. Teratomas usually contain fat or calcification that can be detected on plain films or CT. Uterine leiomyomas or fibroids are present in 25% to 50% of women and are the most common pelvic tumor, with a peak incidence in the fifth decade of life. Most are small and asymptomatic. Fibroids may present as vaginal bleeding if they are submucosal or become symptomatic if they grow to a large size. Barium enema in these cases demonstrates smooth extrinsic mass effect on the sigmoid colon with marked displacement and stretching of the colon if the tumor is large. Rupture of an ovarian cystadenoma into the peritoneal cavity may result in pseudomyxoma peritonei.

Pelvic Inflammatory Disease and Tubo-Ovarian Abscess

Pelvic inflammatory disease has a variety of causative organisms, including *Chlamydia trachomatis*, *Neisseria gonorrhoeae*, and a number of other aerobic and anaerobic bacteria. The tubo-ovarian abscesses that result may secondarily involve the bowel and may be indistinguishable on barium enema from endometrial or metastatic implants on the serosal surface. The cul-de-sac is a frequent site of involvement. Ultrasonography, CT, or MRI shows a thick-walled fluid collection that may be difficult or impossible to differentiate from cystic neoplasm or endometrioma.[173,174]

Sexually Transmitted Diseases

Lymphogranuloma venereum is a sexually transmitted disease caused by infection of lymphatic tissue by *C. trachomatis*. The site of primary infection is usually around the genitals, but the rectum may be the primary site of involvement. Primary infection of the rectum is usually acquired by anal intercourse, but proctitis may also result from spread of infected vaginal discharge to the anal canal or by lymphatic extension from inguinal lymph nodes. Patients present with inguinal adenopathy and deep rectal ulceration. The disease may progress to form a fistula, perirectal abscess, or stricture (Fig. 66-16).[175]

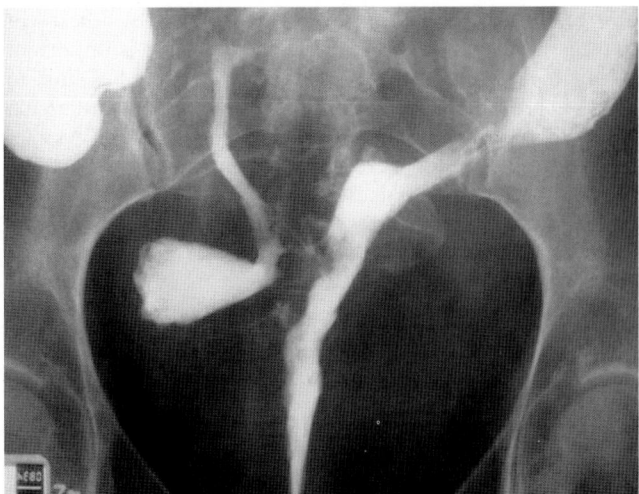

Figure 66-16. Lymphogranuloma venereum. Barium enema examination demonstrates a stricture of the rectum with fistulas and sinus tracts.

Other sexually transmitted diseases, including *N. gonorrhoeae* or herpes simplex infection and syphilis, can infect the rectum and cause proctitis.[176] Barium enema demonstrates mucosal ulceration or a granular mucosal pattern.

Pancreatitis

Approximately 1% of patients with acute pancreatitis have significant colonic problems. These complications usually occur 10 to 21 days after disease onset and may relate to compression caused by a pancreatic phlegmon or abscess and widespread fat necrosis or by mural thickening caused by edema and necrosis secondary to pancreatic enzymes dissecting down the transverse mesocolon or phrenicocolic ligament.[177]

Occasionally, a high-grade obstruction or perforation may occur that requires surgical intervention.[178-182] For a more complete discussion of pancreatitis, see Chapter 99.

Metastases

High-grade colonic obstruction is attributable much less often to metastatic than to primary tumors.[183] Renal and prostate neoplasms usually directly invade the colon.[184] Carcinoma of the prostate involves the rectum in 0.5% to 11% of cases and may simulate rectal carcinoma clinically. Rectal obstruction occurs when there is direct extension through the thick, double-layered Denonvilliers fascia or by rectal compression caused by a massively enlarged prostate gland.[185,186] Gastric and pancreatic neoplasms can either directly invade the colon or narrow it by serosal metastases.[187-189]

Summary

A variety of gynecologic and other extracolonic diseases may secondarily involve the gastrointestinal tract. The involvement may mimic primary disease of the gastrointestinal tract, and patients may present with gastrointestinal symptoms. Familiarity with the patterns of gastrointestinal tract involvement is important for accurate interpretation of imaging studies in these patients.

COLONIC ISCHEMIA

Clinical Findings

Colonic ischemia is the most common vascular disorder of the gastrointestinal tract and the most common cause of colitis in the elderly.[189,190] Although many conditions have been implicated in the pathogenesis of colonic ischemia (see Table 66-4), the etiology is unclear in most patients, and no precipitating event or condition can be identified. Most patients have no major vascular occlusion, so the condition is attributed to low flow states, small vessel disease, or both. In about 20% of cases, an obstructive or potentially obstructive colonic lesion is present.

Colonic ischemia produces a wide spectrum of disease, ranging from gangrene of the colon to transient ischemic colitis. Colonic ischemia is classified as follows: (1) reversible ischemic colopathy; (2) reversible or transient ischemic colitis; (3) chronic ulcerative ischemic colitis; (4) ischemic colonic stricture; (5) colonic gangrene; or (6) fulminant universal ischemic colitis.[191]

The underlying pathophysiology of colonic ischemia is insufficient blood supply to the bowel to meet the needs of the mucosa. The mucosa receives most of the intestinal blood flow and is most susceptible to damage. Injury may be confined to the mucosa and submucosa or may extend transmurally. The degree of damage depends on the rate of onset of the ischemic event and the extent of the vascular deprivation. The outcome may be complete healing, reversible or chronic colitis, stricture formation, or gangrene. About half of the patients fall into the first category, with mild disease that resolves in 1 to 2 weeks. The clinical course is highly variable (Fig. 66-17), however, and it is not possible to predict outcome on the basis of initial imaging studies. In one series, the outcomes were as follows: reversible hemorrhage and edema, 33%; transient or reversible colitis, 16%; reversible or persistent strictures, 12%; persistent colitis, 21%; and gangrene of perforation, 18%.[190]

Most patients with colonic ischemia are older than 50 years of age and present with mild lower abdominal pain and rectal bleeding or bloody diarrhea. Those with transmural disease have more impressive findings with peritoneal signs. A barium enema should not be given to patients with suspected gangrene, perforation, or diffuse peritoneal signs.

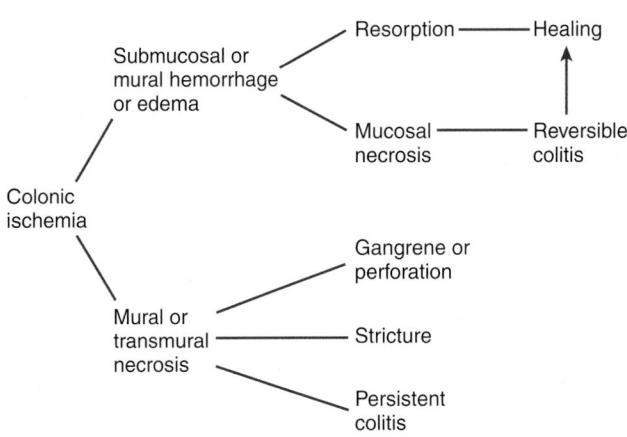

Figure 66-17. Outcomes of colonic ischemia.

Any portion of the colon and rectum can be affected, but the splenic flexure, descending colon, and sigmoid colon are the areas most commonly involved. The diagnosis is usually based on barium enema or colonoscopy results. Angiography is not indicated for these patients and is generally normal.

Radiologic Findings

Radiography

Abdominal radiographs are usually nondiagnostic and either are normal or show a nonspecific ileus. In a series of 41 patients with colonic ischemia, only 21% had radiographic findings suggesting ischemia. Radiographic findings in colonic ischemia include normal, nonspecific ileus; thumbprinting; transverse ridging; and fixed loops with tubulation and lack of haustra. The most characteristic finding on radiographic and barium enema examination is thumbprinting, which consists of multiple round, smooth, scalloped defects projecting into the air-filled colonic lumen (Fig. 68-18). Thumbprinting is due to submucosal bleeding or edema, or both, and usually occurs within the first 24 hours after the insult to the bowel.[192] Experimental work has shown that thumbprinting is due to extravasation of blood around small blood vessels that are reperfused after losing their integrity during the ischemic period.[190] Thickening of the bowel wall secondary to edema and hemorrhage may be observed and is reflected by luminal narrowing or transverse ridging. As the edema progresses or mucosal sloughing occurs, fixed rigid, tubular, ahaustral loops may develop.[193] Rarely, pneumatosis or portal venous gas can be identified. These findings generally indicate necrotic bowel.

Barium Enema

Colonoscopy and multidetector CT are the primary means of establishing the diagnosis of ischemic colitis. The barium enema findings depend on the extent of the ischemic process, the degree of damage, and the stage at which the examination is performed. The hallmark of colonic ischemia is serial change on examinations performed over days, weeks, or months. When colonic ischemia is suspected, it is important to obtain a barium enema early to establish a baseline, to detect characteristic findings, and to rule out an underlying neoplasm or other obstructive lesion. Both single- and double-contrast studies are highly accurate (82% and 90%, respectively) in the diagnosis of colonic ischemia.[194-196]

The classic barium enema findings in colonic ischemia are thumbprinting, transverse ridging, spasm, ulceration, intramural barium, and strictures. The most consistent and characteristic finding on the barium enema examination early in the course of the disease is thumbprinting, which is seen in 75% of patients.[196] Thumbprinting on a barium enema study corresponds to the radiographic findings of smooth, round, polypoid scalloped filling defects projecting into the opacified colonic lumen as a result of submucosal edema or hemorrhage (Fig. 66-19). Edema and hemorrhage may be soft and compressible, and taking films with maximal distention may affect the findings. Because spasm often accompanies ischemia, maximal distention may be hard to maintain, making thumbprinting easier to see. Careful fluoroscopy with imaging during the filling stage of the examination and postevacuation radiographs should be obtained to document the presence of thumbprinting. Intraluminal pressures during single- and double-contrast examination are fairly equivalent, so there is no advantage to performing a single-contrast study in this regard. Thumbprinting characteristically resorbs in less than

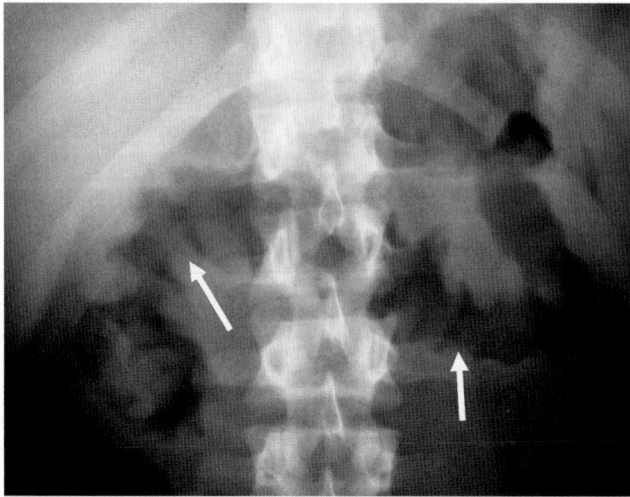

Figure 66-18. Colonic ischemia: narrowing and thumbprinting on plain abdominal radiograph. Supine radiograph of the abdomen shows marked narrowing and thumbprinting of the transverse colon (*arrows*) caused by colonic ischemia.

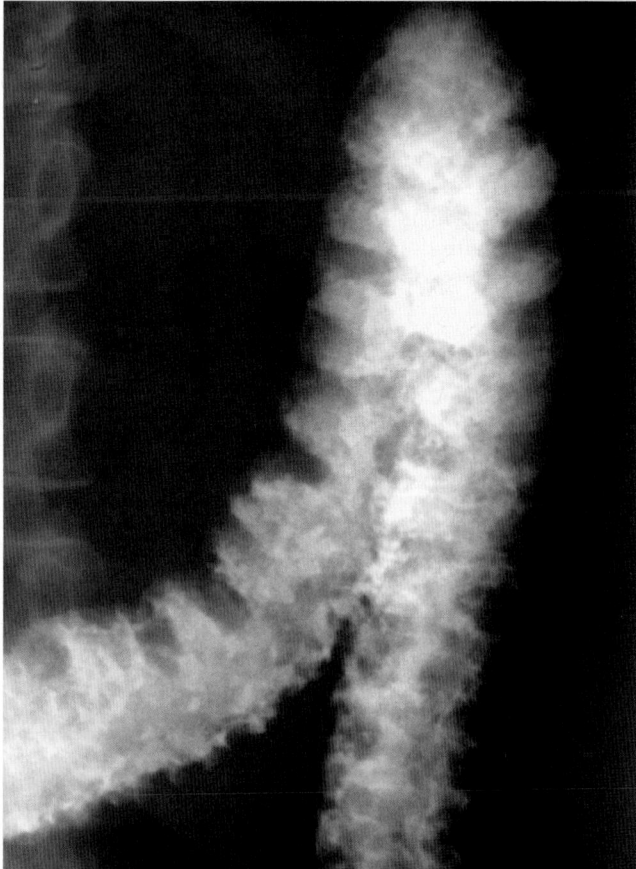

Figure 66-19. Colonic ischemia: thumbprinting. Single-contrast barium enema study shows extensive thumbprinting caused by hemorrhage or edema in colonic ischemia.

a week but may persist for weeks in some patients.[195] Thumbprinting, although characteristic of ischemia, may also be observed in other conditions, including inflammatory bowel disease and the infectious colitides.

Transverse ridging is a less common finding, observed in 13% of patients with colonic ischemia.[195] Transverse ridging is caused by edema or spasm and is characterized by parallel, symmetric thickened folds running perpendicular to the bowel lumen. Like thumbprinting, it is generally an early finding and usually resolves rapidly.[196]

Ulceration is present in 46% to 60% of patients with colonic ischemia, and it is due to sloughing of the mucosa.[196] Ulceration generally develops 1 to 3 weeks after the onset of disease and may heal completely, continue into a chronic ulcerative ischemic phase, or heal with stricture formation. The ulcerations are characteristically longitudinal but may also be discrete, superficial, deep, small, or large. Differential diagnosis from other forms of colitis, particularly Crohn's disease and ulcerative colitis, can be made on the basis of sequential changes on barium enema examination, age of the patient, distribution of disease, clinical history, and endoscopic and biopsy findings.[196]

Intramural barium is an unusual manifestation of ischemia and is due to sloughing of a necrotic portion of the wall with subsequent tracking of barium intramurally. Intramural barium can also be seen in other conditions, such as Crohn's disease and diverticulitis.

About 12% of patients with severe colonic ischemia heal with stricture formation.[190] Strictures can develop rapidly in the course of disease and may be identified as early as 3 weeks after initial presentation. Strictures may be reversible or irreversible and characteristically lead to few obstructive symptoms. In some patients, postischemic strictures may be encountered without a clear antecedent episode. The strictures may be smooth and tapering or eccentric with sacculations.

About 20% of cases of colonic ischemia occur proximal to an obstructive or potentially obstructive colonic lesion. In about half of the cases, the lesion is a colon carcinoma; diverticulitis and volvulus are the other major causes. In this setting, the typical findings of thumbprinting and ulceration can develop or an "urticarial" pattern can be seen. This consists of bleblike mounds on the mucosal surface caused by early ischemia.[197] It is thought that increased intraluminal pressure proximal to the obstruction decreases mucosal perfusion.

Colonoscopy is useful in the diagnosis of colonic ischemia, and the findings vary depending on the stage at which the examination is performed. Initially, purplish blebs resulting from hemorrhage may be seen, corresponding to the radiographic findings of thumbprinting. As the hemorrhage is resorbed, varying degrees of ulceration, mucosal sloughing, and inflammation develop. The colonoscopic findings at this stage may resemble those in other forms of colitis. As with the barium enema, sequential studies demonstrate a changing pattern.[198]

CT and Ultrasonography

Because CT is often the initial radiologic procedure in patients presenting with abdominal pain, colonic ischemia may first be suspected on the basis of this study. Symmetric bowel thickening is the major CT finding of colonic ischemia

(Fig. 66-20). In some cases, a target or double halo pattern and polypoid defects associated with thumbprinting may be seen.[199] Mural thickening (>3 mm) of the colon is a nonspecific finding that can also be seen in carcinoma, lymphoma, metastatic disease, diverticulitis, Crohn's disease, and appendicitis.

Abnormal colonic wall thickening can also be identified by ultrasound.[200] Again, this is a nonspecific finding but should lead to further studies of the colon when identified. Doppler ultrasound may show diminished perfusion to the involved segment.[201-203]

RADIATION COLITIS

The colon is often affected by radiation for pelvic genitourinary tract tumors. Patients with carcinoma of the rectum may receive radiotherapy before or after operation as well. Acute symptoms of proctitis and diarrhea are common during therapy and usually resolve within weeks after completion of the therapy.

Pathogenesis

Radiation can injure and kill cells by two methods. The first is a direct cytotoxic effect in which the ionizing radiation absorbed by these cells generates a series of biochemical events that progress to cell disruption and death. Free radicals derived from intracellular water interact with DNA to prevent replication, transcription, and protein synthesis. These cytotoxic effects predominate in cells that replicate rapidly. Accordingly, the intestine has the following decreasing order of radiation tolerance: duodenum, jejunum, ileum, transverse colon, sigmoid colon, esophagus, and rectum. Pathologically, abnormal epithelial cell proliferation and maturation are associated with decrease in crypt cell mitosis. Edema, hyperemia, and extensive inflammatory cell infiltration are often present as well.

The second major mechanism of radiation injury is more insidious and involves damage to the fine vasculature and connective tissue of the intestine. A low-grade ischemia is caused by medial wall thickening and subendothelial proliferation producing endarteritis obliterans of the smallest arterial branches. This chronic ischemia often leads to a fibrotic reaction that can result in contraction, stricture formation, perforation, fistula, or hemorrhage.

The usual dose used in treating abdominal and pelvic malignancies is between 3000 and 7000 cGy (1 cGy = 1 rad) and is delivered in fractions over an interval of 4 to 8 weeks. Lower total dose, lower rates, and smaller treatment volumes minimize damage. Inherent differences in tissue susceptibility also determine which organ is affected most severely by a given dose. Rubin and Casarett defined the concept of the tolerance dose.[203] A minimal tolerance dose is usually expressed as $TD_{5/5}$, which represents the total dose that produces radiation damage in 5% of patients within 5 years. This dose has been determined to be 4500 cGy for the small bowel and colon and 5000 cGy for the rectum.[203]

Clinical Findings

Radiation colitis typically develops after a 2-year latent period. Patients present with rectal bleeding, pain, and diarrhea,

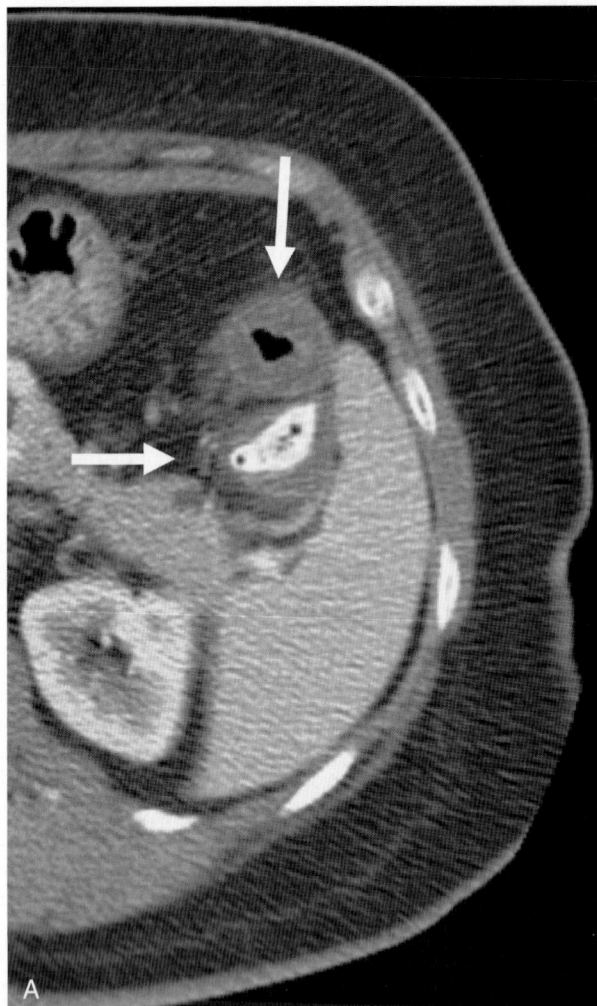

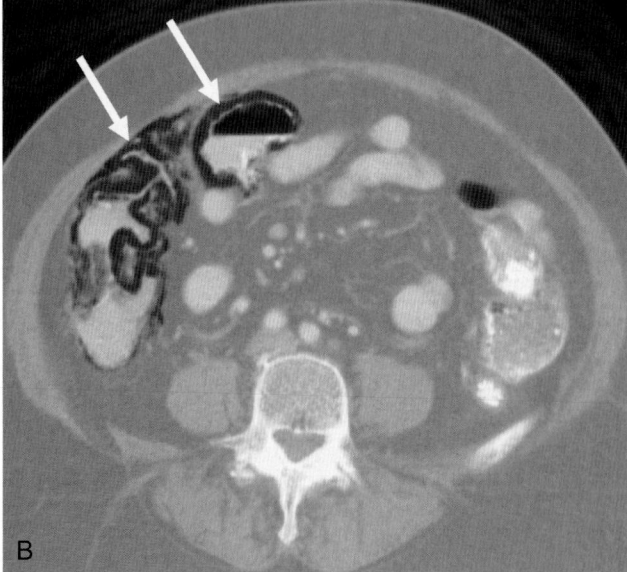

Figure 66-20. Colonic ischemia: CT findings. A. Low-attenuation submucosal edema is present in the thick-walled splenic flexure of the colon (*arrows*). **B.** Pneumatosis intestinalis of the right colon (*arrows*) is identified in this patient with ischemia and infarction.

evoking a differential diagnosis including recurrent tumor, postoperative stricture in a colonic anastomosis, or regional inflammatory change resulting from pelvic abscess. Proctitis is usually seen sigmoidoscopically.[204]

Radiologic Findings

Barium enema examination can show diffuse or focal narrowing of the rectum and sigmoid colon, usually with tapered margins (Fig. 66-21). The mucosal pattern is usually preserved but may be distorted or disrupted because of edema or intramural hemorrhage resulting from radiation-induced ischemic changes. Rectal stricture or rectovaginal fistula may be seen, and the presacral space is widened on the lateral view of the rectum and on CT.[199-202] A recurrent tumor usually produces an eccentric mass effect and mucosal destruction, and it involves a relatively short segment of the colon. The radiologic differential diagnosis includes ulcerative colitis, Crohn's disease, and scarring by chlamydial colitis (lymphogranuloma venereum).

Treatment

When symptoms such as obstruction or fistula become intolerable, surgical resection may be needed. Initially, a diversion colostomy is formed. After healing has occurred, an abdominal pull-through procedure with coloanal anastomosis between the nonirradiated colon and the anus usually provides

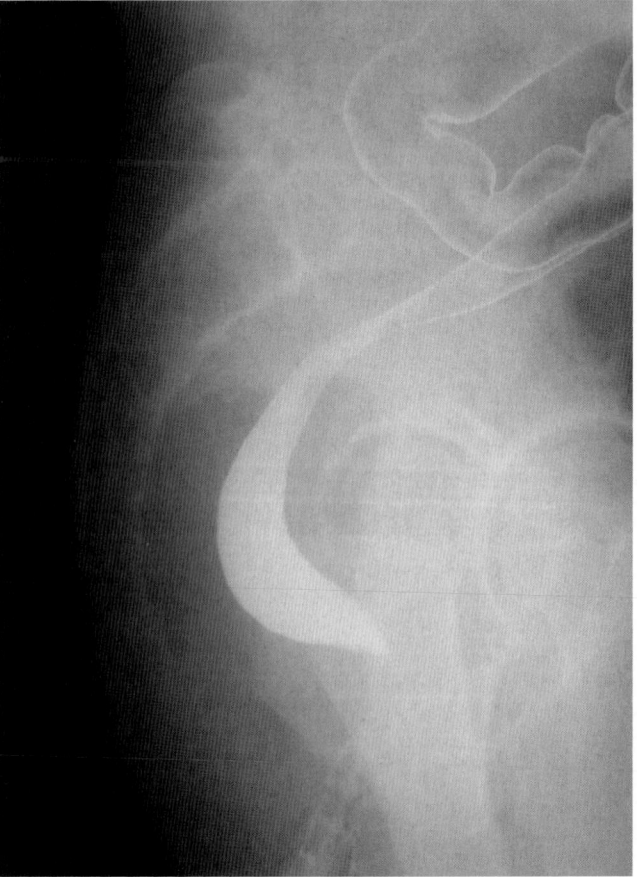

Figure 66-21. Radiation-induced rectosigmoid stricture. There is a long segment of narrowing in the rectosigmoid demonstrated on this barium enema examination. The presacral space is widened as well.

permanent relief. Attempts to resect strictures or fistulas are less likely to succeed because of poor healing of the irradiated rectosigmoid tissue. Development of colon carcinoma has been suggested as a possible late sequela of pelvic irradiation.[201,203]

VASCULAR LESIONS OF THE ANORECTUM

Internal Hemorrhoids

Internal hemorrhoids are dilated vascular spaces of the internal hemorrhoidal plexus in the submucosal layer of the upper anal canal and lower rectum. Normally, the submucosa of the upper anal canal has three distinct vascular cushions—along the left lateral, right anterior, and right posterior wall.[204] It is postulated that these anal cushions aid in anal continence. The pathogenesis of hemorrhoids is multifactorial. With age, the connective tissue tethering the mucosa to the submucosa and muscular layer of the anal canal becomes lax. With excessive straining during defecation, prolapse of anal canal mucosa occurs, leading to congestion of vascular cushions and internal hemorrhoids. Pathologically, internal hemorrhoids appear as thick-walled submucosal veins with accompanying arteries and dilated capillaries. Abundant arteriovenous anastomoses are present.

Hemorrhoids (piles) are extremely common and can cause brisk rectal bleeding, blood staining on toilet tissue, or painful swelling. With strangulation of hemorrhoids, mucosal infarction, necrosis, and superinfection may occur. Internal hemorrhoids may also be a complication of distal rectal carcinoma. Internal hemorrhoids are not varicose veins. Their incidence is not increased in patients with portal hypertension.

Hemorrhoids are frequently diagnosed by digital examination, anoscopy, and rigid or flexible sigmoidoscopy. Double-contrast barium enema examination is a relatively accurate technique for diagnosing internal hemorrhoids, with a sensitivity and specificity of 83% and 88%, respectively.[205] However, the purpose of barium enema in patients with known or suspected internal hemorrhoids is to investigate the colon for a more serious cause of rectal bleeding or pain.

Internal hemorrhoids have a varying radiographic appearance.[206] When mild lobulation of anorectal folds (the columns of Morgagni) extends less than 3 cm from the radiographic anorectal junction, radiographic diagnosis of internal hemorrhoids is confident (Fig. 66-22A). Another diagnostic appearance of internal hemorrhoids is a cluster of smooth-surfaced polyps less than 1 cm abutting the anorectal junction (Fig. 66-22B). Internal hemorrhoids may have nonspecific appearances as well, including a solitary polyp (Fig. 66-22C), a solitary submucosal mass (Fig. 66-22D), a mass (Fig. 66-22E), or large, infiltrative lobulated folds extending more than 3 cm from the anorectal junction (Fig. 66-22F). Internal hemorrhoids seen as solitary polyps cannot be distinguished from inflammatory, benign, or neoplastic rectal polyps. Internal hemorrhoids appearing as large, lobulated infiltrative folds extending more than 3 cm above the anorectal junction are indistinguishable from proctitis or infiltrating neoplasm.[206]

Rectal Varices

Rectal varices are a rare cause of lower gastrointestinal bleeding and are usually seen in patients with portal hypertension.

Rectal varices have been associated with adhesions.[207,208] Radiologically, smooth serpiginous folds course along the rectal mucosa (Fig. 66-23). When seen in profile, rectal varices may appear as small, smooth-surfaced submucosal nodules. Like esophageal varices, rectal varices may change in size and shape with luminal distention.[209]

Cloacogenic (Basaloid) Carcinoma

The transitional epithelium of the anal canal contains squamous, transitional, and stratified columnar epithelium, as well as scattered goblet cells. Various neoplasms of controversial origin arise in this transitional epithelium. The transitional zone has features of both urothelium and squamous epithelium consistent with a cloacogenic origin.[210] Hence, many tumors in this region were previously termed *cloacogenic carcinomas*. However, the transitional zone also has features suggesting that it is an area where metaplasia and reserve cell hyperplasia occur, similar to the transitional zone in the uterine cervix or the transitional zone at the esophagogastric junction.[211] Thus, it has also been postulated that tumors in this region are due to dysplasia and, hence, carcinoma arising in squamous metaplasia and reserve cell hyperplasia. For example, homosexual men have a high incidence of anal transitional cell carcinoma and squamous cell carcinoma. These tumors may be related to venereally transmissible agents such as oncogenic viruses, carcinogens in lubricants and cleansers, or mechanical irritation.[212] Tumors at the anorectal junction have been described by a wide variety of names, including squamous cell carcinoma, basaloid carcinoma, transitional cell carcinoma, mucoepidermoid carcinoma, adenoid cystic carcinoma, and verrucous carcinoma. Basaloid carcinoma and cloacogenic carcinoma are probably equivalent terms. Most tumors, however, have a mixture of growth patterns, including basaloid areas, transitional cell carcinomas with squamous differentiation, adenoid cystic carcinoma, and mucoepidermoid carcinoma. The most common tumor of the anal canal is adenocarcinoma of the rectal mucosa invading the anal canal.

Cloacogenic (basaloid) carcinoma has no distinctive clinical, gross pathologic, or radiologic features. Patients usually complain of rectal bleeding, rectal pain, or a change in bowel habits. These tumors may be flat, infiltrative, annular, or ulcerative lesions with rolled borders. Radiographically, the tumor may appear as a submucosal mass with a smooth or ulcerated surface (Fig. 66-24), broad-based sessile polyps, or infiltrative lesions (Fig. 66-25).[211,212]

Metastases occur in approximately 50% of patients to the sacral lymph nodes, internal and common iliac lymph nodes, and superficial inguinal lymph nodes. Venous drainage and hematogenous metastasis are to both the inferior vena cava and the portal system. Five-year survival in patients with basaloid carcinoma is approximately 50%.[212]

Rectal Mucosal Prolapse Syndromes

Chronic prolapse of rectal mucosa may result in chronic inflammation, ulceration, and hyperplastic reparative response. During defecation, rectal mucosa passing inferiorly through a contracted puborectalis sling may experience trauma, especially along the anterior and anterolateral wall. Chronic intussusception may also result in mucosal damage. The mucosal

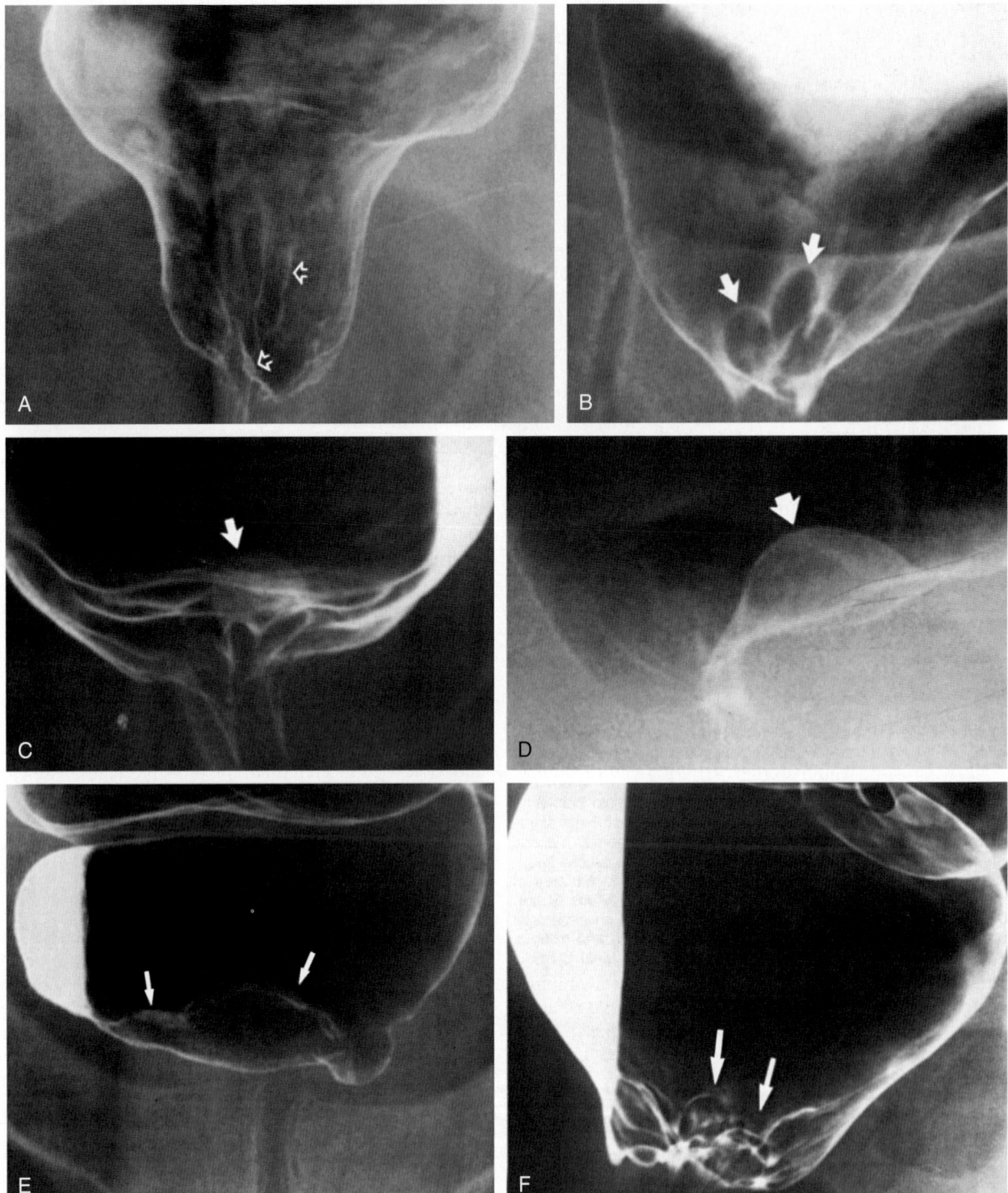

Figure 66-22. Radiographic appearance of internal hemorrhoids. A. Lobulated folds. Mild lobulation of anorectal folds (*arrows*) that extends less than 3 cm above the anorectal junction is a typical radiographic finding for internal hemorrhoids. **B.** "Bunch of grapes." Three smooth-surface polyps (*arrows*) are clustered above the anorectal junction. This radiographic appearance is typical of internal hemorrhoids. **C.** Solitary polyp. A smooth-surfaced polyp (*arrow*) projects from mildly lobulated columns of Morgagni. This is a nonspecific radiographic appearance that requires endoscopy. **D.** Submucosal mass. A smooth-surfaced mass (*arrow*) with relatively abrupt angulation to the colonic contour is typical of a submucosal mass. Although this is a typical radiographic appearance of internal hemorrhoids, other submucosal rectal masses include lymphoid polyps and solitary rectal ulcers. **E.** Masslike internal hemorrhoid. A large mass (*arrows*) in the distal rectum has a focally irregular surface pattern. This huge internal hemorrhoid cannot be distinguished from other rectal masses such as carcinoma or cloacogenic carcinoma. Endoscopy and biopsy are necessary. **F.** Multiple polypoid folds. Large, polypoid folds (*arrows*) with a nodular surface pattern in the distal rectum. Although these radiographic findings are typically seen with internal hemorrhoids, they may also be due to solitary rectal ulcer syndrome, various forms of proctitis, or an unusual infiltrating tumor.

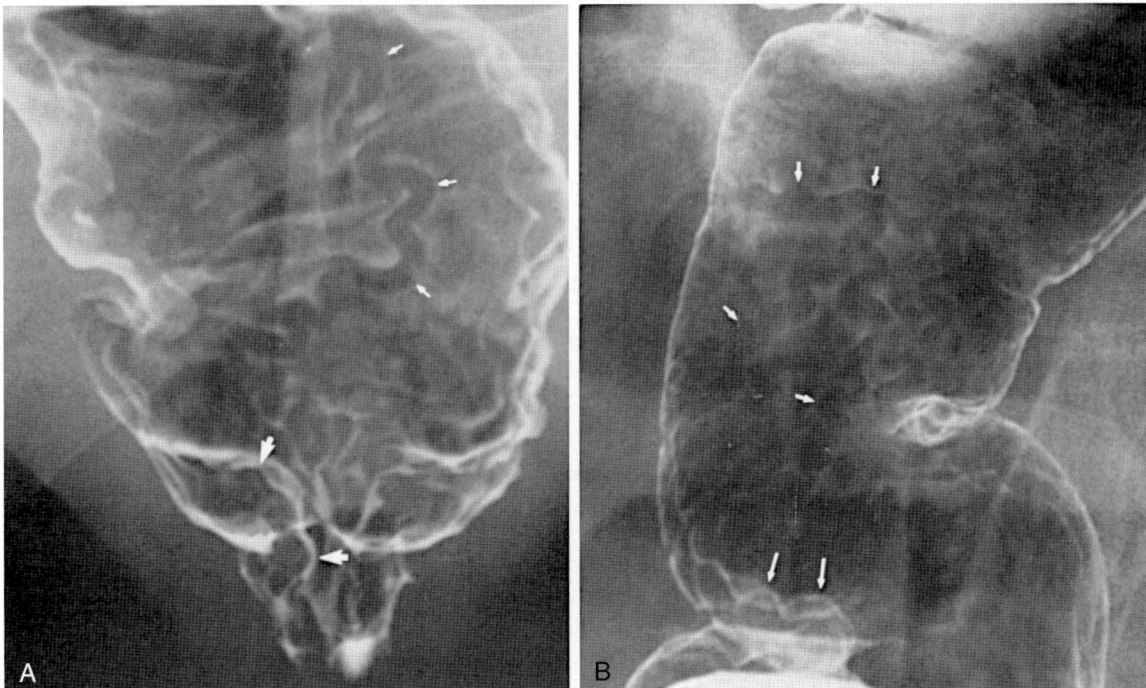

Figure 66-23. Rectal varices. A. Spot radiograph of the distal rectum shows the en face appearance of rectal varices as serpentine folds etched in white (*small arrows*). In profile, smooth, lobulated folds disrupt the contour of the bowel, extending from the anorectal junction proximally (*large arrows*). **B.** In another patient, spot radiograph of the proximal rectum shows serpentine folds etched in white (*short arrows*). In profile, a valve of Houston is expanded by a smooth, lobulated submucosal process compatible with a rectal varix (*long arrows*). (From Rubesin SE, Saul SH, Laufer I, et al: Carpet lesions of the colon. RadioGraphics 5:537-552, 1985.)

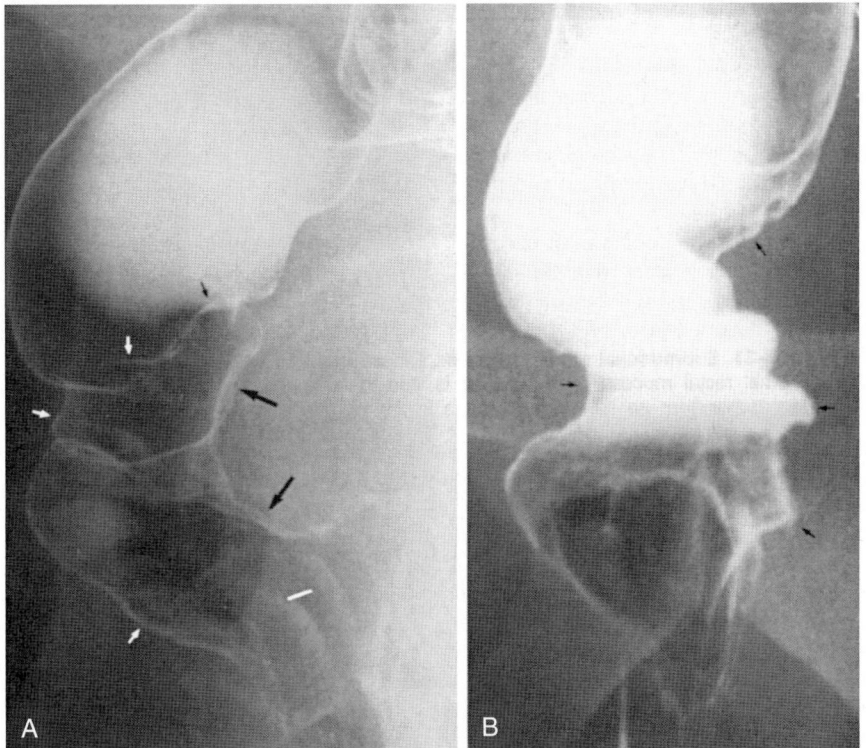

Figure 66-24. Cloacogenic carcinoma. A. Lateral spot view of the rectum shows a dominant, large submucosal mass (*large black arrows*) indenting the anterior wall of the midrectum. Diffuse infiltration of the remainder of the distal rectum is manifested by smooth narrowing of the distal rectum (*small arrows*). **B.** Supine view of the distal rectum shows diffuse narrowing of the rectal ampulla and a diffusely irregular contour (*arrows*).

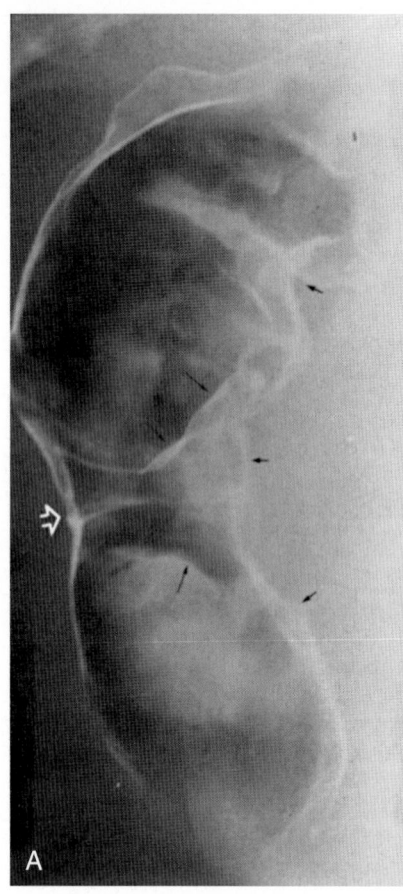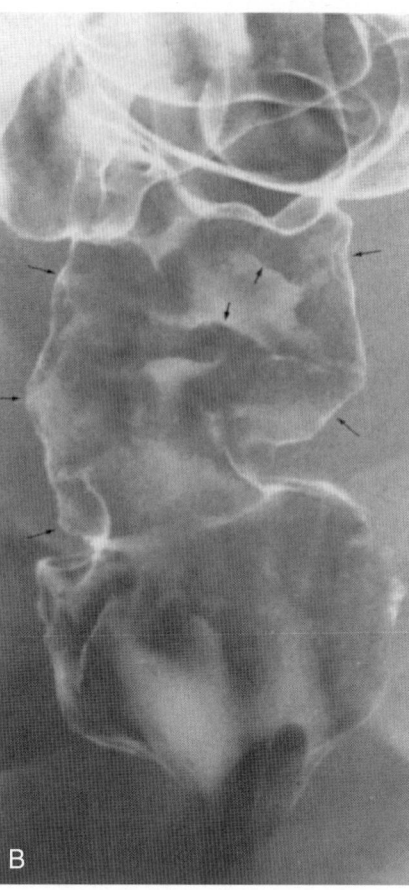

Figure 66-25. Cloacogenic carcinoma. A. Lateral view of the rectum demonstrates the infiltrative pattern of cloacogenic carcinoma. The anterior wall of the rectum is moderately flattened and lobulated (*short arrows*), and thick, nodular folds cross the rectum (*long arrows*). The rectal mucosa is relatively smooth. Focal circumferential extension of tumor around the rectum is seen as flattening of the posterior rectal wall (*open arrow*). **B.** Prone view of the rectum shows mild inbowing and irregularity of the contour of the lateral walls of the rectum (*long arrows*) and thick, nodular folds en face (*short arrows*).

response to chronic defecatory problems results in a spectrum of syndromes including solitary rectal ulcer syndrome, colitis cystica profunda, hypertrophied anal papilla, and inflammatory cloacogenic polyp.[213] A similar histologic response may be seen with prolapsing internal hemorrhoids and prolapsing colostomies.[213]

Solitary rectal ulcer syndrome is an uncommon, chronic benign condition. The name *solitary ulcer syndrome* is a misnomer because multiple small ulcers may be present, or the colon may not be grossly ulcerated at all. Although the syndrome is typically seen in young adults, it may occur at any age. Patients commonly complain of rectal bleeding, rectal pain, and passage of mucus. At sigmoidoscopy, single or multiple well-demarcated, shallow ulcers may be found on the anterolateral or anterior wall of the distal half of the rectum.[214] An ulcer may not be visible; rather, the mucosa may appear diffusely erythematous, friable, or even polypoid.[214]

Pathologically, the mucosa is mildly inflamed. The glandular epithelium may be hyperplastic, occasionally showing villous formation, which may even be mistaken for villous adenoma.[119] The muscularis mucosae is disorganized, and there may be extension of the smooth muscle of the muscularis mucosae into the lamina propria. When mucin-filled glands become cystically dilated, a diagnosis of localized colitis cystica profunda may be made.[213] Solitary rectal ulcer syndrome and colitis cystica profunda have been confused with villous adenoma or infiltrating adenocarcinoma. However, the glandular epithelium is not dysplastic in solitary rectal ulcer syndrome and colitis cystica profunda.

The radiographic findings are variable.[215] The rectal mucosa may appear normal in up to 50% of cases.[216]

Diffuse, finely nodular mucosa in the distal rectum may be seen, correlating with the friable, erythematous mucosa seen at proctoscopy (Fig. 66-26). A focal, small ulcer may be found on the anterior or anterolateral wall. Redundant, prolapsing mucosa may appear as a polypoid mass. Localized colitis cystica profunda may have the appearance of a submucosal mass (Fig. 66-27). The valves of Houston may be markedly enlarged with a nodular contour. Rarely, a stricture may be seen.

FUNCTIONAL DISORDERS OF THE COLON

Irritable Bowel Syndrome

Epidemiology

Irritable bowel syndrome (IBS) is one of the most common yet least understood conditions encountered in clinical practice. It is characterized by altered bowel habits and abdominal pain in the absence of detectable structural abnormalities. It occurs with surprising frequency in the general population, as high as 14% in one series, and accounts for one third to one half of outpatient referrals to gastroenterologists.[217] IBS ranks close to the common cold as a leading cause of absenteeism from work because of illness.[218]

The symptoms of IBS begin before the age of 35 years in half of patients, and 40% of patients are 35 to 50 years of age.

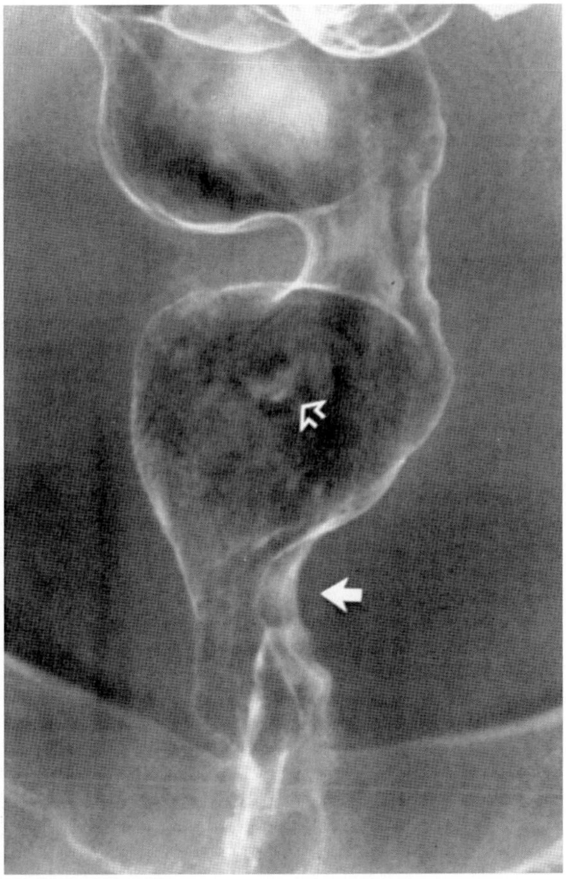

Figure 66-26. Solitary rectal ulcer syndrome: solitary ulcer. An irregular barium collection (*open arrow*) 1 cm in diameter is surrounded by a radiolucent halo of edema. Also note mild granularity of distal rectal mucosa and focal submucosal mass effect (*solid arrow*).

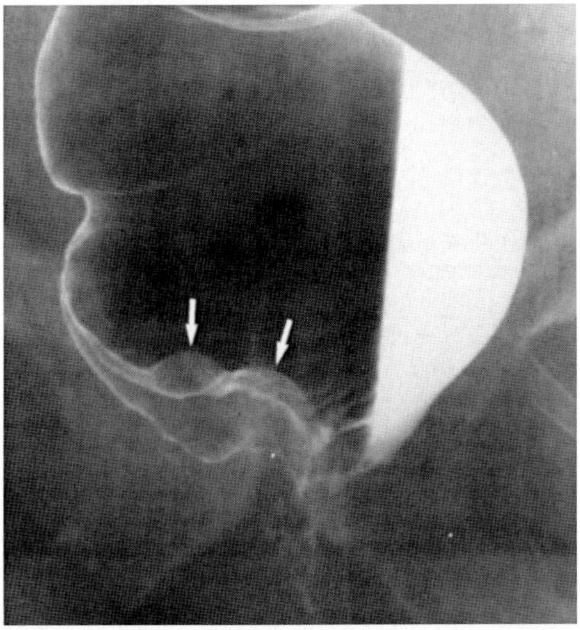

Figure 66-27. Solitary rectal ulcer syndrome: colitis cystica profunda. Two smooth-surfaced, polypoid, submucosal-appearing masses (*arrows*) are seen in the distal rectum. These masses were due to mucus-filled, epithelium-lined cysts in the submucosa (colitis cystica profunda). (From Levine MS, Piccolello M, Sollenberger LC, et al: Solitary rectal ulcer syndrome: a radiologic diagnosis? Gastrointest Radiol 11:187-193, 1986.)

Female patients outnumber male patients 2:1, and the disease is more common in the white and Jewish populations than in persons of color.[219]

Clinical Findings

The 1988 International Congress of Gastroenterology in Rome established the following symptom criteria for IBS:

1. Abdominal pain relieved by defecation or associated with a change in frequency or consistency of stool
2. Disturbed defecation associated with two more of the following: altered stool frequency, altered stool form (loose and watery or hard), and altered stool passage (straining or urgency, feeling of incomplete evacuation, passage of mucus)
3. Bloating or feeling of abdominal distention

Between 25% and 50% of IBS patients complain of dyspepsia, nausea and vomiting, and heartburn, suggesting that a portion of the gut other than the colon may be involved.[219]

Pathophysiology

Although extensive clinical and laboratory investigations have failed to discover any microbiologic, histologic, or biochemical abnormalities in patients with IBS, evidence suggests that this disorder is due to abnormal myoelectric and motor activities in the gut. The myoelectric rhythm of the colon in normal patients has a frequency of 6 cycles per minute; most patients with IBS have a predominant frequency of 3 cycles per minute. Patients with IBS also have an abnormal gastrocolic reflex, such that the postprandial increase in colonic spike activity and intraluminal pressure is delayed 30 to 60 minutes. Patients with IBS have a lower threshold for pain and for induction of spastic colonic contraction during rectal distention. It is postulated that this abnormal response is mediated through the autonomic nervous system, as in patients with diffuse esophageal spasm. This exaggerated motor response to colonic distention may explain why patients with spastic colons have symptoms when even small amounts of gas or stool are present.[217]

Recordings of small bowel motility in ambulatory patients with IBS show a high incidence of abnormal activity during waking hours. There are frequent episodes of clustered contractions that occur at 0- to 9-minute intervals, and these are often associated with abdominal pain and discomfort.[218] Superimposed on these myoelectric abnormalities are environmental factors such as stress and diet, which can alter motility in and of themselves.

Diagnostic Procedures

Irritable bowel syndrome is a diagnosis of exclusion, and there is always a nagging fear about missing an organic lesion. In the young patient, inflammatory bowel disease is the primary concern. In patients older than 40 years, the risk of occult colon cancer is such that complete evaluation of the colon by double-contrast barium enema or colonoscopy is indicated.

There are no typical features of IBS on barium enema studies, which are usually normal in these patients. Some authors have reported a correlation between exaggerated haustral markings and scybalous (pellet-like) stool. Regions of hypertonicity and spasm, sigmoid myochosis, and diverticula have also been associated with IBS, but these findings can be present in patients without IBS and absent in patients with classic IBS. Clearly, the role of radiology in IBS is to exclude structural abnormalities such as inflammatory bowel disease, strictures, and cancer.[219]

Therapy

The first step in therapy of IBS is to reassure the patient and explain the functional nature of this disorder. Foods that can cause symptoms (e.g., caffeine) are eliminated from the diet. Artificial sweeteners, legumes, carbonated beverages, and foods of the cabbage family are proscribed. Dietary fiber and bulking agents are given because they have been shown to lower pressure in the sigmoid colon. Antispasmodic agents such as tincture of belladonna and dicyclomine (Bentyl) are also helpful. When diarrhea is the presenting symptom, antidiarrheal agents such as loperamide (Imodium) can be used during periods of stress.

Chronic Constipation

Most patients with chronic constipation respond to simple dietary and, if necessary, medical therapy consisting of natural bulk-forming laxatives and stool softeners.[220,221] Anatomic disorders must be ruled out by a good-quality double-contrast barium enema; metabolic and endocrine, drug-induced, and neurologic causes must be excluded by careful history, physical, and laboratory examinations. Functional evaluation of the colon and anorectum is generally reserved for patients who do not respond to initial therapy and express continued dissatisfaction with their bowel movements.[221] The causes of constipation are listed in Tables 66-5 and 66-6.

Colorectal Transit Studies

The transit of stool through the colon is evaluated by following the progression of swallowed radiopaque markers on radiographs over several days. Patients ingest 20 small radiopaque markers with breakfast food. These markers (Sitzmarks) are commercially available or can be made by cutting 16-Fr Silastic nasogastric tubes into segments of 3-mm thick. Abdominal radiographs are taken at 24-hour intervals until all the markers are evacuated or until 7 days pass. If markers are still present, films are obtained at days 10 and 15 to reduce the radiation received by the patient.[221]

The large bowel is divided into three segments (the right colon, the left colon, and the rectosigmoid) by the spinous process, and imaginary lines are drawn from L5 to the left iliac crest and pelvic outlet (Fig. 66-28). Sample transit time studies are illustrated in Figure 66-29. The mean transit time is calculated using the following formula:

$$\Delta t = 1/N \sum_{i=1}^{N} = 1 \, \Delta t_I$$

where Δt = the mean transit time, Δt_I = the transit time of a given marker through the studies site, and N = the total number of markers.

With this test, colonic inertia can be distinguished from normal transit with outlet obstruction. In the latter case,

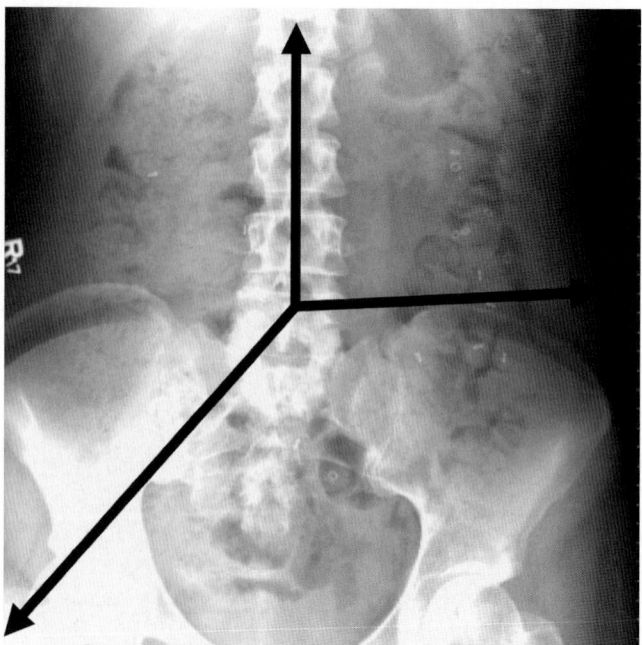

Figure 66-28. Colon transit study. Plain film demonstrates radiopaque markers. For the purpose of counting, the colon is divided into three segments: left colon, right colon, and rectosigmoid.

anorectal manometry and defecography are then required. Surprisingly, many studies are normal, and many of these patients have major psychologic factors influencing their symptoms.

Anorectal Manometry

Anorectal manometry is performed to characterize sensory and motor function of the gut, such as rectal sensation and viscoelasticity. Rectal distention produced by a rectal balloon normally initiates a reflex that contracts the external anal sphincter and relaxes the internal anal sphincter. Loss of this reflex suggests Hirschsprung's disease, which must be confirmed by biopsy. Severe idiopathic constipation is usually accompanied by impaired rectal sensation to balloon distention. Paradoxical contraction of the external sphincter and pool relaxation of the internal sphincter during defecation are often associated with constipation. An overall compliant rectum in combination with sensory loss may interfere with the normal urge to defecate.[220]

Evacuation Proctography

Evacuation proctography (defecography) permits dynamic evaluation of the defecation process. It assesses the anorectal angle and the status of the puborectalis sling and can diagnose rectal prolapse, rectal intussusception, rectoceles, obstructive enteroceles, and abnormal perineal descent. This test is especially important if there is manometric or electromyographic evidence of hyperactive rectosigmoid junction, abnormal anorectal motility, or anismus and clinical evidence of descending perineum syndrome, prolapse, and the solitary rectal ulcer syndrome. Chapter 56 is devoted to a discussion of this procedure.[222]

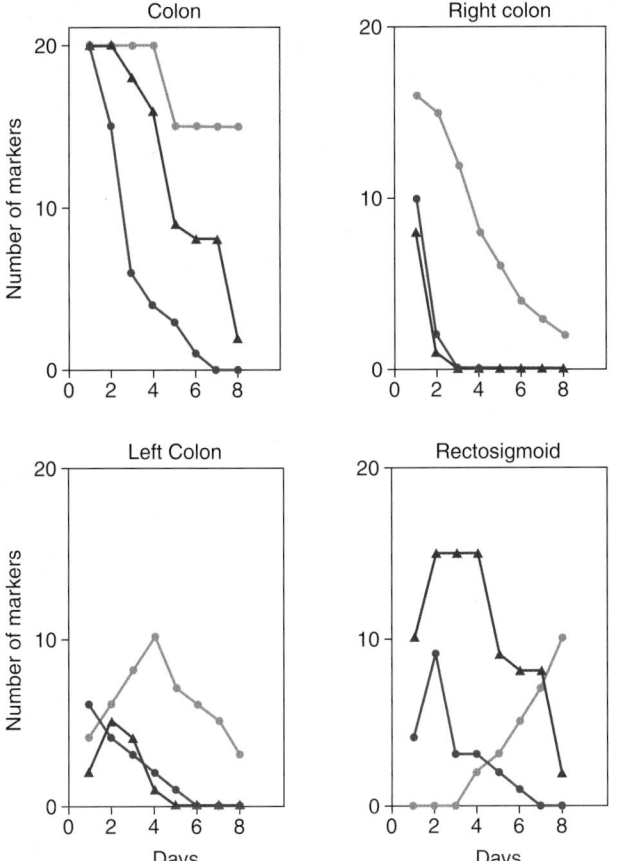

Figure 66-29. Abnormal colon transit studies. Diagram depicts characteristic transit patterns of 20 radiopaque markers through the colon during an 8-day period in three groups of constipated patients. With normal transit (*red circles*) the markers disappear rapidly from the colon. With colon inertia (*green circles*), there is prolonged transit through the right and left colon segments with delayed appearance in the rectosigmoid. With outlet obstruction (*triangles*), transit is normal in the right and left colon but there is stagnation of the rectosigmoid. (From Wald A: Colonic transit and anorectal manometry in chronic idiopathic constipation. Arch Intern Med 146:1713-1716, 1986. Copyright 1986, American Medical Association.)

The combination of transit studies, anorectal manometry, and evacuation proctography can often identify the type and cause of constipation, which greatly assists further therapy.

Nonobstructive Megacolon

Chronic constipation may be caused by a mechanical obstruction (e.g., carcinoma, stricture) or may be of functional origin, as in bedridden elderly patients or persons with improper bowel habits. In Chagas' disease, destruction of the colonic myenteric plexuses by the protozoan *Trypanosoma cruzi* causes striking elongation and dilatation, especially of the rectosigmoid and descending colon. Acquired, nonobstructive megacolon in adults can also be found in patients with severe neurologic or psychologic disorders and in patients with abnormal colonic motility (myxedema; infiltrative disease, such as amyloidosis and scleroderma; narcotic drugs). Regardless of the underlying cause, plain abdominal radiographs demonstrate a tremendously dilated, tortuous colon and rectum filled with a large fecal residue.[223]

Incomplete evacuation of feces over a prolonged period can result in the formation of a fecal impaction—a large, firm, immovable mass of stool in the rectum that may cause large bowel obstruction. Fecal impactions most commonly develop in elderly, debilitated, or sedentary persons. They can occur in patients who have been inactive for long periods (e.g., because of myocardial infarction, traction), in narcotic addicts, in patients on large doses of tranquilizers, and in children with megacolon or psychogenic problems.[224]

The symptoms of fecal impaction usually consist of vague rectal fullness and nonspecific abdominal discomfort. A common complaint is overflow diarrhea, the uncontrolled passage of small amounts of watery and semiformed stool around a large obstructing impaction. In elderly bedridden patients, it is essential that this overflow phenomenon be recognized as secondary to fecal impaction rather than be perceived as true diarrhea.

Intestinal myopathy patients have aperistalsis of the esophagus with low pressure of the lower esophageal sphincter; a variable degree of dilatation and dysmotility of the stomach, duodenum, small bowel, and colon; and ureteral and bladder enlargement.[225-227]

Collagen Vascular Disorders

Colonic involvement in scleroderma occurs less frequently than is observed in the esophagus and small bowel. Patchy smooth muscle atrophy and fibrotic replacement cause wide-mouthed diverticula at the weakened sites. These are true diverticula that contain all three layers of bowel wall. The smooth muscle is replaced by connective tissue, however. These smooth and wide diverticula retain barium on the postevacuation films.[226]

The normal postprandial gastrocolic reflex is decreased in scleroderma patients. This colonic dysmotility may be clinically latent early in disease and manifest only with further smooth muscle atrophy. Similarly, manometric studies have shown decreased pressure of the smooth muscle internal anal sphincter and abnormal relaxation after rectal distention. The external anal sphincter, which is skeletal muscle, responds appropriately. Manometric studies have shown a correlation between the relaxation of the lower esophageal sphincter and the dysfunction of the internal anal sphincter in patients with scleroderma. Symptoms from colonic involvement are nonspecific, but decreased motility causes constipation and may result in impaction of fecal contents.[228]

Benign pneumoperitoneum can be seen in patients with scleroderma and may be asymptomatic for years. The cause is probably slow passage of bowel gas through minute or microperforations in colonic or small bowel sacculations. Clinically symptomatic and significant bowel perforations may occur in scleroderma from stercoral ulcerations, bowel impactions, and focal vasculitis. These usually require surgical intervention. It may not be possible clinically to differentiate benign pneumoperitoneum from that caused by perforation.[228]

Systemic lupus erythematosus can cause a variety of abdominal problems: peritoneal serositis, pancreatitis, ascites, and enteritis. There is a small vessel arteritis of the small bowel and colon that causes ischemia, which leads to edema, hemorrhage, mucosal ulceration, and, ultimately, necrosis and perforation. The radiologic findings are those expected with hemorrhage and ischemia: ileus, thumbprinting, pneumatosis intestinalis, and pseudo-obstruction. Indeed, the radiologic findings may be indistinguishable from those of ischemia, hemorrhage, or inflammatory bowel disease. Aspirin and corticosteroids are used in the therapy of lupus, and these drugs often aggravate the underlying gastrointestinal disease.[226]

Diabetes

Constipation is the most common gastrointestinal symptom of the diabetic patient, and it appears to be directly related to autonomic neuropathy. Only 29% of patients without neuropathy symptoms are constipated. This figure increases to 88% in patients with five symptoms of neuropathy. Constipation typically is intermittent and alternates with diarrhea in almost one third of patients. Fecal impaction may be sufficiently severe to produce mechanical obstruction. This autonomic neuropathy leads to the loss of the postprandial gastrocolic response similar to that observed in patients with intestinal pseudo-obstruction. This is explained pathophysiologically by the inflammatory changes demonstrated in the autonomic ganglia; the cholinergic postganglionic neurons are intact with a normally responsive smooth muscle.[204,226]

The usual preparation for colonic cleansing before barium enema is generally inadequate for the diabetic patient. These patients require a 72- or 48-hour regimen that includes a low-residue diet, saline cathartics, and properly administered cleansing enemas. It is important for the radiologist to inform the referring physician about the cleansing regimen in patients with diabetic diarrhea, which may motivate the referring physician to modify the routine preparation. Some diabetic patients have fecal incontinence because of a defect in internal anal sphincter function. Therefore, the fluoroscopist should perform a rectal examination to assess anal sphincter tone and determine the necessity of inflating a retention balloon.[204,226]

PNEUMATOSIS INTESTINALIS

Gas in the bowel wall (pneumatosis intestinalis) can exist as an isolated entity or in conjunction with a broad spectrum of disease of the gastrointestinal tract or respiratory system. In primary pneumatosis (about 15% of cases), no respiratory or other gastrointestinal abnormality is present. Primary pneumatosis usually occurs in adults and involves mainly the colon. Secondary pneumatosis intestinalis (about 85% of cases) more commonly affects the small bowel and is associated with a wide variety of preexisting disorders. In the primary form, gas collections usually appear cystic; in the secondary type, a linear distribution of gas is generally seen.[229]

Primary

Primary pneumatosis intestinalis is a relatively rare benign condition characterized pathologically by multiple thin-walled, noncommunicating, gas-filled cysts in the subserosal or submucosal layer of the bowel. The overlying mucosa is entirely normal, as is the muscularis. The appearance of radio-lucent clusters of cysts along the contours of the bowel is diagnostic of primary pneumatosis intestinalis. On barium examinations, the filling defects are seen to lie between the lumen (outlined by contrast material) and the water density of the outer wall of the bowel. The radiographic pattern of

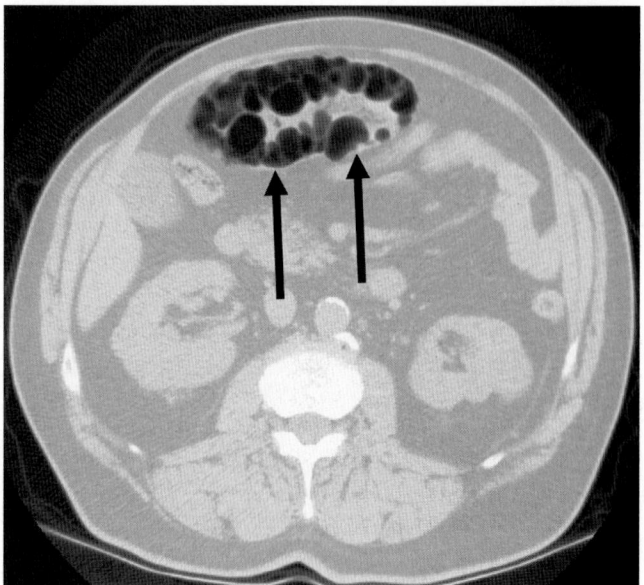

Figure 66-30. Primary pneumatosis cystoides intestinalis. In this relatively asymptomatic patient, multiple large gas-filled cysts (*arrows*) produced scalloped defects in the transverse colon.

pneumatosis can simulate more severe gastrointestinal conditions. Small cysts may be confused with tiny polyps. Larger cysts can produce scalloped defects simulating inflammatory pseudopolyps or the thumbprinting seen with intramural hemorrhage. At times, the cysts of pneumatosis intestinalis concentrically compress the lumen, producing gas shadows that extend on either side of the bowel contour surrounding a thin, irregular stream of barium simulating the appearance of an annular carcinoma. To differentiate pneumatosis intestinalis from these other conditions, it is important to note the striking lucency of the gas-filled cysts in contrast to the soft tissue density of an intraluminal or intramural lesion. Other distinguishing factors are the compressibility of the cysts on palpation and the not infrequent occurrence of asymptomatic pneumoperitoneum. Primary pneumatosis intestinalis (Fig. 66-30) usually requires no treatment and resolves spontaneously.[229]

Secondary

Secondary pneumatosis intestinalis most commonly reflects gastrointestinal disease with bowel necrosis. In infants, pneumatosis intestinalis suggests an underlying necrotizing enterocolitis, which occurs primarily in premature or debilitated infants, most commonly affects the ileum and right colon, and has a very low survival rate. This condition is characterized by a frothy or bubbly appearance of gas in the wall of the diseased bowel loops. The appearance often resembles fecal material in the right colon. However, it must be remembered that, although this feces-like appearance is normal in adults, it is always abnormal in premature infants. The gas in the wall of the colon in necrotizing enterocolitis is probably related to mucosal necrosis and subsequent passage of intraluminal gas into the bowel wall. This may be complicated by intraluminal gas-forming organisms that also penetrate the diseased mucosa to reach the inner layers of the intestinal wall. Dissection of air into the intrahepatic branches of the portal vein is an ominous prognostic finding.[230]

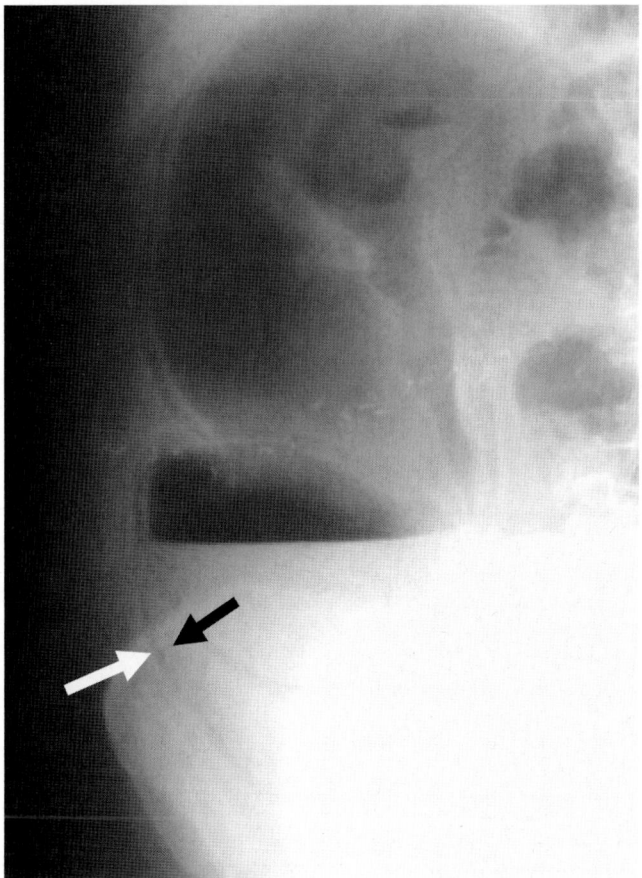

Figure 66-31. Secondary pneumatosis cystoids intestinalis. This upright abdominal radiograph demonstrates intramural air causing lucencies (*arrows*) in the ascending colon due to colonic ischemia.

In adults, secondary pneumatosis intestinalis (Fig. 66-31) suggests bowel necrosis due to mesenteric arterial or venous thrombosis. Secondary pneumatosis intestinalis may be related to mucosal ischemia, as in strangulating obstructions, or to mucosal destruction by infectious organisms or powerful corrosive agents.

Secondary pneumatosis intestinalis may also develop in the absence of necrosis of the bowel wall. Any lesion of the gastrointestinal tract that results in mucosal ulceration or intestinal obstruction (obstructive bowel disease) can cause secondary pneumatosis intestinalis. Gas in the bowel wall is an uncommon complication of gastrointestinal endoscopy. Severe obstructive pulmonary disease can also be associated with the development of pneumatosis intestinalis. Partial bronchial obstruction and coughing presumably cause alveolar rupture, with gas dissecting along peribronchial and perivascular tissue planes into the mediastinum. Gas then enters the retroperitoneal area via the hiatus of the esophagus and aorta, from which it dissects between the leaves of the mesentery to eventually reach subserosal and submucosal locations in the bowel wall.[231,232]

DIVERSION COLITIS

Diversion colitis is a nonspecific inflammation in a segment of colon that has been surgically isolated from the fecal stream by placement of a proximal colostomy or ileostomy. It is un-

known whether lack of contact of the distal colonic segment to feces somehow deprives the colonic mucosa of necessary exposure to enteric bacteria, bacterial by-products, or nutrients. Conversely, it is conceivable that diversion colitis results from stasis within the inactive segment, causing excessive mucosal exposure to unrecognized intraluminal toxins. Radiographically, diversion colitis resembles ulcerative or Crohn's colitis with punctate or aphthous ulcerations that may produce a diffuse, granular mucosal appearance in severe or long-standing cases. Isolated inflammatory polyps or diffuse mucosal nodularity may occur.[233-236]

BEHÇET'S SYNDROME

Behçet's syndrome is a systemic inflammatory disease involving a triad of uveitis, oral ulcers, and genital ulcers, as well as involvement of the central nervous system, joints, kidneys, skin, and gastrointestinal tract. It is unclear whether the etiology of this disorder is viral, allergic, environmental, or autoimmune.[237]

Abdominal pain occurs in up to 75% of patients, and the clinical course can be complicated by diarrhea, malabsorption, bleeding, perforation, fistulas, and toxic megacolon. Ulcerations tend to involve the terminal ileum, cecum, and ascending colon, simulating Crohn's disease and certain infectious colitides. Diffuse colonic involvement can simulate ulcerative colitis.[238]

The barium enema appearance of Behçet's disease varies from mild proctitis to pancolitis with multiple discrete ulcers and inflammatory polyposis. Aphthoid ulcerations and skip lesions are typical. The ulcers in Behçet's syndrome tend to be larger and deeper than those in Crohn's colitis, leading to a higher incidence of perforation and hemorrhage.[239,240]

AMYLOIDOSIS

As in other parts of the bowel, amyloidosis involving the colon can produce a broad spectrum of radiographic abnormalities. Narrowing and rigidity of the colon, especially in the rectum and sigmoid colon, can result from direct deposition of amyloid within the mucosal and muscular layers of the bowel or can be secondary to extensive amyloid deposition in blood vessel walls and subsequent ischemic colitis. The resulting thickening of the bowel with effacement of haustral markings can closely simulate the radiographic appearance of chronic ulcerative colitis. Less commonly, amyloidosis can produce an acute ulcerating process, single or multiple discrete colonic filling defects, or an appearance simulating the thumbprinting seen with ischemic colitis.[241-244]

CATHARTIC COLON

Cathartic colon is due to the prolonged use of stimulant/irritant cathartics (e.g., caster oil, phenolphthalein, cascara, senna, podophyllum). The typical patient with the condition is a woman of middle age who has habitually used irritant cathartics for more than 15 years. Ironically, the patient often initially denies use of cathartics and complains only of constipation. Because prolonged stimulation of the colon by irritant laxatives results in neuromuscular incoordination and an inability of the colonic musculature to produce adequate contractile force without external stimulants, the patient

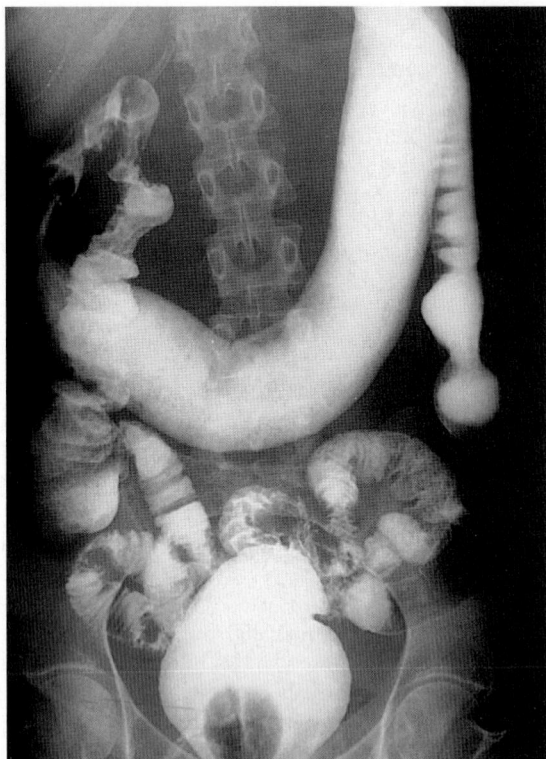

Figure 66-32. Cathartic colon. Contractions with irregular areas of narrowing are seen in the right colon, and there is a paucity of haustra in the transverse colon.

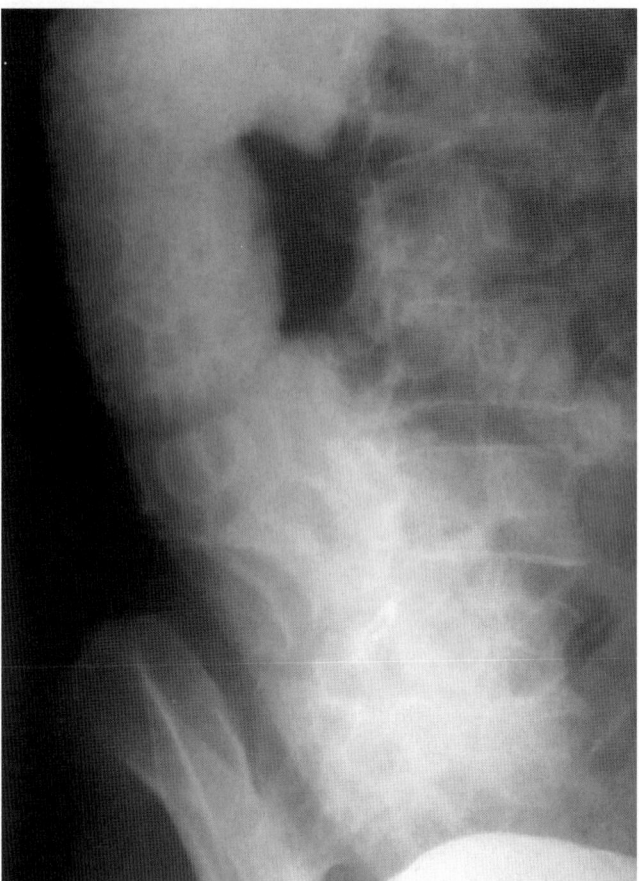

Figure 66-33. Colonic urticaria. Raised polygonal plaques are present in the ascending colon in this patient with *Yersinia* colitis.

with cathartic colon is often unable to have a bowel movement without laxative assistance. Cathartic colon can usually be separated clinically from a chronic ulcerating colitis because of the patient's history of lifelong constipation and laxative use, in contrast to the complaint of diarrhea in most patients with inflammatory bowel disease.[245]

The radiographic appearance of cathartic colon is similar to that of "burned-out" chronic ulcerative colitis. In contrast to ulcerative colitis, however, the absent or diminished haustral markings, bizarre contractions, and inconstant areas of narrowing primarily involve the right colon (Fig. 66-32). In severe cases, the left side of the colon can also be affected, although the sigmoid colon and rectum usually appear normal. The mucosal pattern is linear or smooth; ulcerations are not seen. The ileocecal valve is frequently flattened and gaping, simulating the backwash ileitis seen in ulcerative colitis. Shortening of the ascending colon can be severe, but, unlike the rigidity of the tubular bowel in chronic ulcerative colitis, the shortened segment in a cathartic colon remains remarkably distensible. Inconstant areas of narrowing of the bowel lumen can be seen at fluoroscopy and on radiographs of patients with cathartic colon. These pseudostrictures primarily involve the hepatic flexure, vary in length, have a concentric lumen with tapering margins, and often disappear during a single examination.[246,247]

URTICARIA

A characteristic mucosal pattern of large, round or polygonal, raised plaques in a grossly dilated bowel was first described as an allergic reaction of the colonic mucosa to medication. This

"colonic urticaria" predominantly involves the right colon, can be seen without concomitant cutaneous lesions, and regresses once the offending medication is withdrawn.[248]

A pattern similar to colonic urticaria has been reported in several other conditions for which the common denominator seems to be submucosal edema. In herpes zoster, an exanthematous neurocutaneous disorder secondary to reactivation or reinfection by a large poxvirus, colonic mucosal blebs infrequently appear as multiple small, discrete, polygonal filling defects with sharp angular margins (Fig. 66-33). These blebs correspond morphologically and temporally to the vesicular phase of the cutaneous lesion and are segmentally arrayed in a corresponding or noncorresponding dermatome. In *Yersinia* colitis, submucosal edema is caused by an alteration in vascular permeability. A similar radiographic pattern has also been observed in patients with submucosal colonic edema secondary to obstructing carcinoma, cecal volvulus, ischemia, colonic ileus, and benign colonic obstruction.[249]

COLITIS CYSTICA PROFUNDA

Colitis cystica profunda is a rare, benign disease in which large mucous epithelium–lined cysts up to 2 cm in diameter form in the submucosal layer of the colon. These cysts most commonly are seen in the rectum and pelvic colon, and usually only a short segment of colon is involved. Colitis cystica profunda is associated with solitary rectal ulcer syndrome and rectal prolapse, as well as other proctitides. This suggests that these cysts are formed when surface mucosa is implanted into the colonic submucosa during the healing phase of an ulcerative inflammatory process. Because these cells cannot be shed into the lumen and mucus cannot be discharged, a cystic mass develops.[250,251]

Patients with colitis cystica profunda present with hematochezia, passage of mucus or pus per rectum, diarrhea, constipation, tenesmus, and rectal, sacral, or abdominal pain. On barium studies, multiple irregular rectal filling defects suggesting adenomatous polyps are seen. Barium filling clefts between these polyps can simulate mucosal ulcerations. Ischemic colitis can be mimicked when sufficient scalloping of the colon occurs.[252,253]

As with solitary rectal ulcer syndrome, conservative treatment is the initial approach. Surgery to correct rectal prolapse may lead to resolution of cysts in certain patients with refractory symptoms and rectal prolapse evident on defecography.[254-256]

DIARRHEA

In Western countries, the majority of cases of diarrhea are self-limited (Table 66-7) and seldom come to radiologic attention. When the diarrhea persists (Table 66-8), radiology plays an important part in diagnosis. Radiologic findings, however, must be interpreted in view of clinical and laboratory findings.

Table 66-7
Major Causes of Acute Diarrhea (<2-3 wk duration)

Infections (including travelers' diarrhea)
 Bacterial
  Campylobacter species
  Clostridium difficile
  Escherichia coli (ET, EI, EH, 0157:H7)
  Salmonella enteroceles
  Shigella species
 Parasitic/protozoal
  Entamoeba histolytica
  Giardia lamblia
  Cryptosporidium
  Cyclospora
 Viral
  Adenovirus
  Norwalk virus
  Rotavirus
  Others
 Fungal
Food poisoning
 Bacillus cereus
 Clostridium perfringens
 Salmonella species
 Staphylococcus aureus
 Vibrio species
 Shigella species
 Campylobacter jejuni
 Escherichia coli
 Yersinia enterocolitica
 Listeria monocytogenes
Medications
Recent ingestion of large amounts of poorly absorbable sugars
Intestinal ischemia
Fecal impaction
Pelvic inflammation

From Schiller LR, Sellin JH: Diarrhea. In Feldman M, Scharschmidt BF, Sleisenger MH (eds): Gastrointestinal and Liver Disease, 7th ed. Philadelphia, Saunders, 2006, pp 159-186.

Table 66-8
Major Causes of Chronic Diarrhea (> 4 wk duration)

No Previous Work-up
Irritable bowel syndrome
Inflammatory bowel disease
Ischemic bowel disease
Chronic bacterial/mycobacterial infections
Parasitic and fungal infection
Radiation enteritis
Malabsorption syndromes
Medications
Alcohol
Intestinal lymphoma
Colon cancer
Villous adenoma
Diverticulitis
Previous surgery (gastrectomy, vagotomy, intestinal resection, cholecystectomy)
Endocrine causes
Hyperthyroidism
Hypothyroidism
Addison's disease
Diabetes mellitus
Pheochromocytoma
Ganglioneuroma
Fecal impaction
Heavy metal poisoning
Epidemic idiopathic chronic diarrhea

Previous Work-up Failed to Reveal a Diagnosis
Surreptitious laxative abuse
Defective anal continence masquerading as severe diarrhea
Microscopic colitis (without or with subepithelial collagen)
Previously unrecognized malabsorption
Pseudopancreatic cholera syndrome
Idiopathic chronic diarrhea
Neuroendocrine tumor
Systemic mastocytosis
Amyloidosis
Idiopathic bile acid malabsorption
Food allergy

From Schiller LR, Sellin JH: Diarrhea. In Feldman M, Scharschmidt BF, Sleisenger MH (eds): Gastrointestinal and Liver Disease, 7th ed. Philadelphia, Saunders, 2006, pp 159-186.

There are three fundamental types of diarrhea: osmotic, secretory, and inflammatory.

Osmotic Diarrhea

Osmotic diarrhea usually occurs as a result of malabsorption or the ingestion of certain chemicals in which a high osmotic load is presented to the gut. Small bowel series and enteroclysis are superb means of demonstrating causes of malabsorption, such as sprue, amyloidosis, mastocytosis, intestinal lymphangiectasia, intestinal anastomoses, small bowel diverticula, and abnormal motility, that predispose to bacterial overgrowth. Chronic pancreatitis, cystic fibrosis, the Shwachman-Diamond syndrome, and other causes of pancreatic insufficiency have characteristic appearances on imaging studies that can specifically establish the etiology of the diarrhea.[257]

Secretory Diarrhea

Secretory diarrhea stimulates intestinal secretion or inhibits absorption. Enterotoxins produced by certain infections; certain irritant laxatives, metals, and toxins; and tumors that elaborate secretagogues, such as vasoactive intestinal polypeptide (pancreatic cholera), are major factors in secretory diarrheas. Radiology has only a small role in the assessment of these patients unless the diarrhea is caused by a pancreatic tumor.[258]

Inflammatory Diarrhea

Radiology is most useful in evaluating inflammatory diarrhea, in which inflammatory damage and death of the brush border and epithelium occur. This diarrhea occurs in patients with inflammatory bowel disease, certain infections, and radiation enteritis and as a complication of chemotherapy and graft-versus-host disease.[259]

References

1. Welch JP: Mechanical obstruction of the small and large intestines. In Moody FG (ed): Surgical Treatment of Digestive Disease. Chicago, Year Book Medical, 1990, pp 624-654.
2. Turnage RH, Heldmann M, Cole P: Intestinal obstruction and ileus. In Feldman M, Friedman LS, Brandt LJ (eds): Sleisenger and Fordtran's Gastrointestinal and Liver Disease, 8th ed. Philadelphia, Saunders Elsevier, 2006, pp 2653-2678.
3. Ellis H: Intestinal Obstruction. New York, Appleton-Century-Crofts, 1982.
4. Cohn I, Chappuis CW: Bowel obstruction. In Taylor MB (ed): Gastrointestinal Emergencies, 2nd ed. Baltimore, Williams & Wilkins, 1997, pp 515-536.
5. Richards WO, Williams LF Jr: Obstruction of the large and small intestine. Surg Clin North Am 68:355-376, 1988.
6. Smith GA, Perry JF Jr, Yonehiro EG: Mechanical intestinal obstructions: A study of 1252 cases. Surg Gynecol Obstet 100:651-660, 1955.
7. Szucs RA, Turner MA: Gastrointestinal tract involvement by gynecological diseases. RadioGraphics 6:1251-1270, 1996.
8. Russell JC, Welch JP: Pathophysiology of bowel obstruction. In Welch JP (ed): Bowel Obstruction. Philadelphia, WB Saunders, 1990, pp 28-58.
9. Kottler RE, Lee GK: The threatened cecum in acute large-bowel obstruction. Br J Radiol 57:989-990, 1984.
10. Schmidt AG: Intramural gas proximal to obstructing carcinoma. Radiology 91:784-785, 1968.
11. Mak SY, Roach SC, Sukumar SA: Small bowel obstruction: Computed tomography features and pitfalls. Curr Probl Diagn Radiol 35:65-74, 2006.
12. Meyers MA: Colonic ileus. Gastrointest Radiol 2:37-40, 1997.
13. Lowman RM, Davis L: An evaluation of cecal size in impending perforation of the cecum. Surg Gynecol Obstet 103:711-718, 1956.
14. Novy S, Rogers LF, Kirkpatrick W: Diastatic rupture of the cecum in obstructing carcinoma of the left colon: Radiographic diagnosis and surgical implications. AJR 123:281-286, 1975.
15. Chappuis CW, Cohn J Jr: Pathophysiological effects on intraluminal contents. In Fielding LP, Welch JP (eds): Intestinal Obstruction. Edinburgh, Churchill Livingstone, 1987, pp 32-40.
16. Sugerman HJ: Systemic effects of intestinal obstruction. In Fielding LP, Welch JP (eds): Intestinal Obstruction. Edinburgh, Churchill Livingstone, 1987, pp 32-40.
17. Vanek VW, Whitt CL, Abdu RA, et al: Comparison of right colon, left colon and rectal carcinoma. Am Surg 52:504-509, 1986.
18. Welch JP: General considerations and mortality. In Welch JP (ed): Bowel Obstruction. Philadelphia, WB Saunders, 1990, pp 59-95.
19. Nadrowski L: Clinical presentation and preoperative management of bowel obstruction. In Fielding LP, Welch JP (eds): Intestinal Obstruction. Edinburgh, Churchill Livingstone, 1987, pp 67-77.
20. Ellis H: Special forms of intestinal obstruction. In Schwartz SI, Ellis H (eds): Maingot's Abdominal Operations. East Norwalk, CT, Appleton & Lange, 1989, pp 905-932.
21. Baker SR, Cho KC: The Abdominal Plain Film with Correlative Imaging. East Norwalk, CT, Appleton & Lange, 1998.
22. Siter FMH Jr: Radiologic diagnosis: Small bowel. In Welch JP (ed): Bowel Obstruction. Philadelphia, WB Saunders, 1990, pp 96-107.
23. Markowitz KS: Radiologic diagnosis: Colon. In Welch JP (ed): Bowel Obstruction. Philadelphia, WB Saunders, 1990, pp 108-122.
24. Love L: Large bowel obstruction. Semin Roentgenol 8:299-321, 1973.
25. Levin B: Mechanical small bowel obstruction. Semin Roentgenol 8:281-297, 1983.
26. Love L: The role of the ileocecal valve in large bowel obstruction: A preliminary report. Radiology 75:391-397, 1960.
27. Kent KH, Raszkowski HJ: Colon lesions masquerading as small bowel obstruction on the plain roentgenogram of the abdomen. AJR 88:671-676, 1962.
28. Fataar S, Schulman A: Small bowel obstruction masking synchronous large bowel obstruction: A need for emergency barium enema. AJR 140:1159-1162, 1983.
29. Ott DJ, Gelfand DW: Gastrointestinal contrast agents: Indications, uses and risks. JAMA 249:2380-2384, 1983.
30. Grossman RI, Miller WT, Dann RW: Oral barium sulfate in partial large bowel obstruction. Radiology 136:327-331, 1980.
31. Frimann-Dahl JC: The administration of barium orally in acute obstructions: Advantages and risks. Acta Radiol 42:285-288, 1954.
32. Filippone A, Iezzi R, Di Fabio F, et al: Multidetector-row computed tomography of focal liver lesions treated by radiofrequency ablation: Spectrum of findings at long-term follow-up. J Comput Assist Tomog 31:42-52, 2007. .
33. Yaghmai V, Nikolaidis P, Hammond NA, et al: Multidetector-row computed tomography diagnosis of small bowel obstruction: Can coronal reformations replace axial images? Emerg Radiol 13:69-72, 2006.
34. Lim JH, Ko YT, Lee DH, et al: Determining the site and causes of colonic obstruction with sonography. AJR 163:1113-1117, 1994.
35. Seibert JJ, Williamson SL, Golladay ES, et al: The distended gasless abdomen: A fertile field for ultrasound. J Ultrasound Med 5:301-308, 1986.
36. Phillips RKS, Hittinger R, Fry JS, et al: Malignant large bowel obstruction. Br J Surg 72:296-302, 1985.
37. Welch JP, Donaldson GA: Management of severe obstruction of the large bowel due to malignant disease. Am J Surg 127:492-499, 1974.
38. Welch JP: Carcinoma of the colon. In Welch JP (ed): Bowel Obstruction. Philadelphia, WB Saunders, 1990, pp 546-574.
39. Irvin GL III, Horsely JS III, Caruana JA Jr: The morbidity and mortality of emergent operations for colorectal disease. Ann Surg 199:598-603, 1984.
40. Garcia-Valdecasas JC, Llovera JM, deLacy AM, et al: Obstructing colorectal carcinomas: A prospective study. Dis Colon Rectum 34:759-762, 1991.
41. Gandrup P, Lund L, Balslev I: Surgical treatment of acute malignant large bowel obstruction. Eur J Surg 158:427-430, 1992.
42. Ohman U: Prognosis in patients with obstructing colorectal carcinoma. Am J Surg 143:742-747, 1982.
43. Umpleby HC, Williamson RCN, Chir M: Survival in acute obstructing colorectal carcinoma. Dis Colon Rectum 27:299-304, 1984.
44. Turunen JM: Colorectal cancer obstruction: A challenge to improve diagnosis. Ann Chir Gynaecol 72:317-323, 1983.
45. Desai MG, Rodko EA: Perforation of the colon in malignant tumors. J Can Assoc Radiol 24:344-349, 1973.
46. Paine JR: Cancer of the colon: Treatment of large bowel obstruction. Postgrad Med 39:596-600, 1966.
47. Canon CL, Baron TH, Morgan DE, et al: Treatment of colonic obstruction with expandable metal stents: Radiologic features. AJR 168:199-205, 1997.
48. Mainar A, Tejero E, Maynar M, et al: Colorectal obstruction: Treatment with metallic stents. Radiology 198:761-764, 1996.
49. Hughes LE: Complications of diverticular disease: Inflammation, obstruction, and bleeding. Clin Gastroenterol 4:147-170, 1975.
50. Welch JP: Diverticular disease. In Welch JP (ed): Bowel Obstruction. Philadelphia, WB Saunders, 1990, pp 589-599.
51. Morton DL, Goldman L: Differential diagnosis of diverticulitis and carcinoma of the sigmoid colon. Am J Surg 103:55-61, 1962.
52. Schnyder P, Moss AA, Thoeni RF, et al: A double-blind study of radiologic accuracy in diverticulitis, diverticulosis, and carcinoma of the sigmoid colon. J Clin Gastroenterol 1:55-66, 1979.
53. Schatzki R: The roentgenologic differential diagnosis between cancer and diverticulitis of the colon. Radiology 34:651-662, 1940.
54. Balthazar EJ, Megibow A, Schinella RA, et al: Limitations in the CT diagnosis of acute diverticulitis: Comparison of CT, contrast enema and pathologic findings in 16 patients. AJR 154:281-285, 1990.
55. Cho KC, Morehouse HT, Alterman DD, et al: Sigmoid diverticulitis: Diagnostic role of CT: Comparison with barium enema studies. Radiology 176:111-115, 1990.
56. Welch JP: Volvulus. In Welch JP (ed): Bowel Obstruction. Philadelphia, WB Saunders, 1990, pp 575-588.

57. Kerry RL, Ransom HK: Volvulus of the colon: Etiology, diagnosis and treatment. Arch Surg 99:215-222, 1969.

58. Ballantyne GH, Brandner ML, Beart RW, et al: Volvulus of the colon: Incidence and mortality. Ann Surg 202:83-92, 1985.

59. Khoury GA, Pickard R, Knight M: Volvulus of the sigmoid colon. Br J Surg 64:587-589, 1977.

60. Hirao K, Kikawada M, Hanyu H, et al: Sigmoid volvulus showing "a whirl sign" on CT. Intern Med 45:331-332, 2006.

61. Hoeffel C, Crema MD, Belkacem A, et al: Multi-detector row CT: Spectrum of diseases involving the ileocecal area. RadioGraphics 26: 1373-1390, 2006.

62. Gumbs MA, Kashan F, Shumofsky E, et al: Volvulus of the transverse colon: Reports of cases and review of the literature. Dis Colon Rectum 26:825-828, 1983.

63. Hsueh CC, Jaw TS, Lin JY, et al: Splenic flexure colonic volvulus: A pediatric case report. Kaohsiung J Med Sci 23:207-210, 2007.

64. Ballantyne G: Volvulus of the splenic flexure: Report of a case and review of the literature. Dis Colon Rectum 24:630-632, 1981.

65. Frimann-Dahl J: Roentgen findings in intestinal knots. Acta Radiol 23:22-33, 1942.

66. Young WS, White A, Grave GF: The radiology of ileosigmoid knot. Clin Radiol 29:211-216, 1978.

67. North LB, Weens HS: The intestinal knot syndrome. AJR 92:1042-1047, 1964.

68. Delabrousse E, Saguet O, Destrumelle N, et al: Sigmoid volvulus: Value of CT. J Radiol 82:930-932, 2001.

69. Catalano O: Computed tomographic appearance of sigmoid volvulus. Abdom Imaging 21:314-317, 1996.

70. Matsumoto S, Mori H, Okino Y, et al: Computed tomographic imaging of abdominal volvulus: Pictorial essay. Can Assoc Radiol J 55:297-303, 2004.

71. Agha FP: Intussusception in adults. AJR 146:527-531, 1986.

72. Erkan N, Haciyanli M, Yildirim M, et al: Intussusception in adults: An unusual and challenging condition for surgeons. Int J Colorectal Dis 20:452-456, 2005.

73. Dick A, Green CJ: Large bowel intussusception in adults. Br J Radiol 34:769-777, 1961.

74. Yamada H, Morita T, Fujita M, et al: Adult intussusception due to enteric neoplasms. Dig Dis Sci 52:764-766, 2007.

75. Briggs DF, Carpathios J, Zollinger RW: Intussusception in adults. Am J Surg 101:109-113, 1961.

76. McKay R: Ileocecal intussusception in an in an adult: The laparoscopic approach. JSLS 10:250-253, 2006.

77. Lou CJ: Intussusception in adults: An analysis of 92 cases. Clin Med J 95:297-300, 1982.

78. Bocker J, Vasile J, Zager J, et al: Intussusception: An uncommon cause of postoperative small bowel obstruction after gastric bypass. Obes Surg 14:116-119, 2004.

79. Stubenbord WT, Thorbjarnarson B: Intussusception in adults. Ann Surg 172:306-310, 1970.

80. Burmeister RW: Intussusception in the adult: An elusive case of recurrent abdominal pain. Am J Dig Dis 7:360-374, 1962.

81. Cotlar AM, Cohn I: Intussusception in adults. Am J Surg 101:114-120, 1961.

82. Dean D, Ellis FH, Sauer WG: Intussusception in adults. Arch Surg 73:6-11, 1956.

83. Orlando R III: Intussusception in adults. In Welch JP (ed): Bowel Obstruction. Philadelphia, WB Saunders, 1990, pp 229-240.

84. Sarr MG, Nagorney DM, McIlrath DC: Postoperative intussusception in the adult: A previously unrecognized entity? Arch Surg 116:144-148, 1981.

85. Levine MS, Trenkner SW, Herlinger H, et al: Coiled-spring sign of appendiceal intussusception. Radiology 155:41-44, 1985.

86. Box JC, Tucker J, Watne AL, et al: Eosinophilic colitis presenting as a left-sided colocolonic intussusception with secondary large bowel obstruction: An uncommon entity with a rare presentation. Am Surg 63:741-743, 1997.

87. Harte MS: Chronic partial intestinal obstruction due to intussusception of an appendix epiploica. Surgery 555-560, 1942.

88. Ikukara M, Tsang TK, Tosiou A, et al: Intussusception in an adult with pseudomembranous colitis. J Clin Gastroenterol 21:336-338, 1995.

89. Jackson H: A sign of intussusception. Br J Radiol 26:323-325, 1953.

90. Schatzki R: The roentgenologic appearance of intussuscepted tumors of the colon with and without barium examination. AJR 41:549-563, 1939.

91. Verbanck JJ, Rutgeerts LJ, Douterlungne PH, et al: Sonographic and

92. Parienty RA, LePreux JF, Gruson B: Sonography and CT features of ileocolic intussusception. AJR 136:608-610, 1981.

93. Alessi V, Salerno G: The "hay-fork" sign in the ultrasonographic diagnosis of intussusception. Gastrointest Radiol 10:177-179, 1985.

94. Rao BK, Fleischer AC: Sonography of the gastrointestinal tract. Curr Opin Radiol 2:207-212, 1990.

95. Del-Pozo G, Albillos JC, Tejedor MD: Intussusception: US findings with pathologic correlation—the crescent-in-doughnut-sign. Radiology 199:688-692, 1996.

96. Iko BO, Teal JS, Siram SM, et al: Computed tomography of adult colonic intussusception: Clinical and experimental studies. AJR 143:769-772, 1984.

97. Park SB, Ha HK, Kim AY, et al: The diagnostic role of abdominal CT imaging findings in adult intussusception: Focused on the vascular compromise. Eur J Radiol Apr 2007 [Epub ahead of print].

98. Bar-Ziv J, Solomon A: Computed tomography in adult intussusception. Gastrointest Radiol 10:355-357, 1985.

99. Pottmeyer A, McDowell J, Lang EK: CT findings of a rectal intussusception. AJR 156:870, 1991.

100. Skaane P, Schindler G: Computed tomography of adult ileocolic intussusception. Gastrointest Radiol 10:355-357, 1985.

101. Yoshimitsuk F, Fukuya T, Onitsuka H, et al: Computed tomography of ileoileocolic intussusception caused by a lipoma. J Comput Assist Tomogr 13:704-706, 1989.

102. Styles RA, Larsen CR: CT appearance of adult intussusception. J Comput Assist Tomogr 7:331-333, 1983.

103. Balthazar EJ: CT of the gastrointestinal tract: Principles and interpretation. AJR 156:23-32, 1991.

104. Hodgman CG, Lantz EJ, Maus TP, et al: Computed tomography of intussusception due to colon lipoma. J Comput Assist Tomogr 11:740-741, 1987.

105. Buetow PC, Buck JL, Carr NJ, et al: Intussuscepted colonic lipomas: Loss of fat attenuation on CT with pathologic correlation in 10 cases. Abdom Imaging 21:153-156, 1996.

106. Welch JP: Extrinsic causes. In Welch JP (ed): Bowel Obstruction. Philadelphia, WB Saunders, 1990, pp 640-653.

107. Holt RW, Wagner RC: Adhesional obstruction of the colon. Dis Colon Rectum 27:314-315, 1984.

108. Agrawal NW, Akdamar K, Litwin MS: Postoperative adhesions causing colon obstruction. Am Surg 50:479-481, 1984.

109. Bobroff LM, Messinger NH, Subbarao K, et al: The cecal bascule. AJR 115:249-252, 1972.

110. Twersky J, Himmelfarb E: Right colonic adhesions. Radiology 120: 37-40, 1976.

111. Bonello JC, Kasten MJ, Slezak FA: Large bowel obstruction following colonoscopic polypectomy. Contemp Surg 29:39-41, 1986.

112. Carmichael DH, Organ CH: Epiploic disorders: Conditions of the epiploic appendages. Arch Surg 120:1167-1172, 1985.

113. McCann JC: Omental adhesions syndrome: Postoperative dysfunction of the transverse colon. Surg Gynecol Obstet 72:707-721, 1941.

114. Brodey PA, Schuldt DR, Magnuson A, et al: Complete colonic obstruction secondary to adhesions. AJR 133:917-918, 1979.

115. Farrell B, Gerard PS, Bryk D: Paraesophageal hernia causing colonic obstruction. J Clin Gastroenterol 13:188-190, 1991.

116. Javors BR, Bryk D: Colonic obstruction with inguinal hernia. J Can Assoc Radiol 32:162-163, 1981.

117. Ben Dov D, Rosenblatt M, Rothfeld H: Large-bowel dilatation due to non-incarcerated hernias. Mount Sinai J Med 53:99-102, 1986.

118. Bryk D: Spigelian hernia containing sigmoid colon. AJR 99:71-73, 1962.

119. Hunter TB, Freundlich IM, Zukoski CF: Preoperative radiographic diagnosis of a Spigelian hernia containing large and small bowel. Gastrointest Radiol 1:379-381, 1977.

120. Ghiassi S, Nguyen SQ, Divino CM: Internal hernias: Clinical findings, management, and outcomes in 49 nonbariatric cases. J Gastrointest Surg 11:291-295, 2007.

121. Cruz CJ, Minagi H: Large-bowel obstruction resulting from traumatic diaphragmatic hernia: Imaging findings in four cases. AJR 162:843-845, 1994.

122. Schulman A, van Gelderen F: Bowel herniation through the torn diaphragm: II. Intestinal herniation. Abdom Imaging 21:400-403, 1996.

123. Blatt ES, Schneider H, Wiot JF, et al: Roentgen findings in obstructed diaphragmatic hernia. Radiology 79:649-657, 1962.

124. Gravier L, Freeark RJ: Traumatic diaphragmatic hernia. Arch Surg 86:363-373, 1963.

pathologic correlation intussusception of the bowel. J Clin Ultrasound 14:393-397, 1986.

125. Evrard V, Vielle G, Buyck A, et al: Herniation through the foramen of Winslow: Report of two cases. Dis Colon Rectum 39:1055-1057, 1996.

126. Schuster MR, Tu RK, Scanlan KA: Cecal herniation through the foramen of Winslow: Diagnosis by computed tomography. Br J Radiol 65:1047-1048, 1992.

127. Zinkin LD, Moore D: Herniation of the cecum through the foramen of Winslow. Dis Colon Rectum 23:276-279, 1980.

128. Pritchard GA, Price-Thomas JM: Internal hernia of the transverse colon. Dis Colon Rectum 29:658-659, 1986.

129. Welch JP: Intrinsic causes. In Welch JP (ed): Bowel Obstruction. Philadelphia, WB Saunders, 1990, pp 654-671.

130. Chou JW, Hsu CH, Liao KF, et al: Gallstone ileus: Report of two cases and review of the literature. World J Gastroenterol 13:1295-1298, 2007.

131. Young WVB: Gallstone ileus of the colon: Report of an unusual type of colon obstruction. Arch Surg 82:333-336, 1961.

132. Price JE, Michel SL, Morgenstern L: Fruit pit obstruction: "The propitious pit." Arch Surg 111:773-775, 1976.

133. Cotner M: Fecal impaction due to bubblegum bezoar. South Med J 75:775-776, 1982.

134. Matseshe JW, Go VLW, DiMagno EP: Meconium ileus equivalent complicating cystic fibrosis in post neonatal children and young adults. Gastroenterology 72:732-736, 1977.

135. Welch JP, Schweizer RT, Bartus SA: Management of antacid impactions in hemodialysis and renal transplant patients. Am J Surg 139:561-568, 1980.

136. Culp WC: Relief of severe rectal impactions with water-soluble contrast enemas. Radiology 115:9-12, 1975.

137. Kurer MA, Chintapatla S: Images in clinical medicine. Intestinal obstruction due to inspissated barium. N Engl J Med 356:1656-1657, 2007.

138. Eftaiha M, Hambrick E, Abcarian H: Principles of management of colorectal foreign bodies. Arch Surg 112:691-695, 1977.

139. Segall H: Obstruction of large bowel due to fecaloma: Successful medical treatment in two cases. Calif Med 108:54-56, 1968.

140. Welch JP: Constipation. In Welch JP (ed): Bowel Obstruction. Philadelphia, WB Saunders, 1990, pp 616-626.

141. Jones DJ, Dharmeratnam R, Langstaff RJ: Large bowel obstruction due to pelvic lipomatosis. Ann Surg 71:309-311, 1985.

142. Leffall LD, White JE, Mann M: Retroperitoneal fibrosis: Two unusual cases. Arch Surg 89:1070-1076, 1964.

143. Williams RG, Nelson JA: Retractile mesenteritis: Initial presentation as colonic obstruction. Radiology 126:35-37, 1978.

144. Sirinek KR, Livingston CD, Bova JG, et al: Bowel obstruction due to infarcted splenosis. South Med J 77:764-767, 1984.

145. Hirata N, Kawamoto K, Ueyama T, et al: Endoscopic ultrasonography in the assessment of colonic wall invasion by adjacent diseases. Abdom Imaging 19:21-26, 1994.

146. Wu MH, Shoji Y, Chuang PC, et al: Endometriosis: Disease pathophysiology and the role of prostaglandins. Expert Rev Mol Med 9:1-20, 2007.

147. Mirkin D, Murphy-Barron C, Iwasaki K: Actuarial analysis of private payer administrative claims data for women with endometriosis. J Manag Care Pharm 13:262-272, 2007.

148. Farquhar C: Endometriosis. BMJ 334:249-253, 2007.

149. McCaffee CHG, Greer HLH: Intestinal endometriosis: A report of 29 cases and a survey of the literature. J Obstet Gynecol 67:539-555, 1960.

150. Fagan CJ: Endometriosis: Clinical and roentgenographic manifestations. Radiol Clin North Am 12:109-125, 1974.

151. Gordon RL, Evers K, Kressel HY, et al: Double-contrast enema in pelvic endometriosis. AJR 138:549-552, 1982.

152. Sievert W, Sellin JH, Stringer CA: Pelvic endometriosis simulating colonic malignant neoplasm. Arch Intern Med 149:935-938, 1989.

153. Tate GT: Acute obstruction of the large bowel due to endometriosis. Br J Surg 50:771-773, 1963.

154. Goodman P, Raval B, Zimmerman G: Perforation of the colon due to endometriosis. Gastrointest Radiol 15:346-348, 1990.

155. Coronado C, Franklin RR, Lotze EC, et al: Surgical treatment of symptomatic colorectal endometriosis. Fertil Steril 53:411-416, 1990.

156. Nezhat F, Nezhat C, Pennington E, et al: Laparoscopic segmental resection for infiltrating endometriosis of the rectosigmoid colon: A preliminary report. Surg Laparosc Endosc 2:212-216, 1992.

157. Athey PA, Diment DD: The spectrum of sonographic findings in endometriomas. J Ultrasound Med 8:847-491, 1989.

158. Brown DL, Frates MC, Laing FC, et al: Ovarian masses: Can benign and malignant lesions be differentiated with color and pulsed Doppler US? Radiology 190:333-336, 1994.

159. Fishman EK, Scatarige JC, Saksouk FA, et al: Computed tomography of endometriosis. J Comput Assist Tomogr 7:257-264, 1983.

160. Togashi K, Nishimura K, Kimura I, et al: Endometrial cysts: Diagnosis with MR imaging. Radiology 180:73-78, 1991.

161. Meyers MA: Intraperitoneal spread of malignancies and its effect on the bowel. Clin Radiol 32:129-146, 1981.

162. Levitt RG, Koehler RE, Sagel SS, et al: Metastatic disease of the mesentery and omentum. Radiol Clin North Am 20:501-510, 1982.

163. Landis SH, Murray T, Bolden S, et al: Cancer statistics, 2006. CA 48:6-29, 2006.

164. Feller E, Schiffman FJ: Colonic obstruction as the first manifestation of ovarian carcinoma. Am J Gastroenterol 82:25-28, 1987.

165. Oliphant M, Berne AS, Meyers MA: Imaging the direct bidirectional spread of disease between the abdomen and the female pelvis via the subperitoneal space. Gastrointest Radiol 13:285-298, 1988.

166. Oliphant M, Berne AS, Meyers MA: Bidirectional spread of disease via the subperitoneal space: The lower abdomen and left pelvis. Abdom Imaging 18:117-125, 1993.

167. Gedgaudas K, Kelvin FM, Thompson WM, et al: The value of the preoperative barium-enema examination in the assessment of pelvic masses. Radiology 146:609-613, 1983.

168. Rubesin SE, Levine MS: Omental cakes: Colonic involvement by omental metastases. Radiology 154:593-596, 1985.

169. Rubesin SE, Levine MS, Glick SN: Gastric involvement by omental cakes: Radiographic findings. Gastrointest Radiol 11:223-228, 1986.

170. Krestin GP, Beyer D, Lorenz R: Secondary involvement of the transverse colon by tumors of the pelvis: Spread of malignancies along the greater omentum. Gastrointest Radiol 10:283-288, 1985.

171. Hawnaur JM: Staging of cervical and endometrial carcinoma. Clin Radiol 47:7-13, 1993.

172. Ellis JH, Francis IR, Rhodes M, et al: CT findings in tuboovarian abscess. J Comput Assist Tomogr 15:589-592, 1991.

173. Adelson MA, Adelson KL: Miscellaneous benign disorders of the upper genital tract. In Copeland LJ (ed): Textbook of Gynecology. Philadelphia, WB Saunders, 1993, pp 857-870.

174. Quinn TC, Goodell SE, Mkrtichian E, et al: *Chlamydia trachomatis* proctitis. N Engl J Med 305:195-200, 1981.

175. Wexner SD: Sexually transmitted diseases of the colon, rectum, and anus. Dis Colon Rectum 33:1048-1062, 1990.

176. Hunt DR, Mildenhall P: Etiology of strictures of the colon associated with pancreatitis. Dig Dis Sci 20:941-946, 1975.

177. Aronson AR, Davis DA: Obstruction near hepatic flexure in pancreatitis: A rarely reported sign. JAMA 176:451-454, 1961.

178. Brearly S, Campbell DJ: Stenosis of the colon following acute pancreatitis. Postgrad Med J 58:293-296, 1982.

179. Thompson WM, Kelvin FM, Rice RP: Inflammation and necrosis of the transverse colon secondary to pancreatitis. AJR 128:943-948, 1977.

180. Mann NS: Colonic involvement in pancreatitis. Am J Gastroenterol 73:357-362, 1980.

181. Adams DB, Davis BR, Anderson MC: Colonic complications of pancreatitis. Am Surg 60:44-49, 1994.

182. Meyers MA, McSweeney J: Neoplasms of the bowel. Radiology 105:1-11, 1972.

183. Khilnani MT, Wolf BS: Late involvement of the alimentary tract by carcinoma of the kidney. Am J Dig Dis 5:529-540, 1960.

184. Fry DE, Amin M, Harbrecht PJ: Rectal obstruction secondary to carcinoma of the prostate. Ann Surg 189:488-492, 1979.

185. Ruggiero RP, Chang H: Rectal involvement by carcinoma of the prostate. Am J Gastroenterol 81:372-374, 1986.

186. Lasser A: Adenocarcinoma of the prostate involving the rectum. Dis Colon Rectum 21:23-25, 1978.

187. Welch JP: Acute large intestinal obstruction as the initial sign of pancreatic carcinoma. Dis Colon Rectum 22:425-427, 1979.

188. Brandt JL: Intestinal ischemia. In Feldman M, Friedman LS, Sleisenger MH (eds): Sleisenger and Fordtran's Gastrointestinal and Liver Disease, 8th ed. Philadelphia, Saunders, 2006, pp 2563-2586.

189. Greenwald DA, Brandt LJ: Colonic ischemia. J Clin Gastroenterol 27:122-128, 1998.

190. Barbagelatta M: Pathologic diagnosis of ischemic colitis. J Chir 134:97-102, 1997.

191. Levine JS, Jacobson ED: Intestinal ischemic disorders. Dig Dis 13:3-24, 1995.

192. Parfitt JR, Driman DK: Pathological effects of drugs on the gastrointestinal tract: A review. Hum Pathol 38:527-536, 2007.

193. Wittenberg J, Athanasoulis CA, Williams LF, et al: Ischemic colitis: Radiology and pathophysiology. AJR 123:287-300, 1975.
194. Gore RM, Calenoff L, Rogers LF: Roentgenographic manifestations of ischemic colitis. JAMA 241:1171-1173, 1979.
195. Iida M, Matsui T, Fuchigami T, et al: Ischemic colitis: Serial changes in double contrast barium enema examinations. Radiology 159:337-341, 1986.
196. Greenberg HM, Goldberg HI, Axel L: Colonic "urticaria" pattern due to early ischemia. Gastrointest Radiol 6:145-149, 1981.
197. Noyer CM, Brandt LJ: Systemic, iatrogenic, and unusual disorders of the colon. In DiMarino AJ, Benjamin SB (eds): Gastrointestinal Disease: An Endoscopic Approach. Oxford, Blackwell Scientific, 1997, pp 684-706.
198. Koehler RE, Memel DS, Stanley RJ: Gastrointestinal tract. In Lee JKT, Sagel SS, Stanley JR, et al (eds): Computed Body Tomography with MRI Correlation, 3rd ed. Philadelphia, Lippincott-Raven, 1998, pp 637-700.
199. Jeffrey RB, McGahan JP: Gastrointestinal tract and peritoneal cavity. In McGahan JP, Goldberg BB (eds): Diagnostic Ultrasound: A Logical Approach. Philadelphia, Lippincott-Raven, 1998, pp 511-560.
200. Wilson SR: The gastrointestinal tract. In Rumack CM, Wilson SR, Charboneau JW (eds): Diagnostic Ultrasound, 2nd ed. St. Louis, Mosby-Year Book, 1998, pp 279-328.
201. Donner CS: Pathophysiology and therapy of chronic radiation-induced injury to the colon. Dig Dis 16:253-258, 1998.
202. Capps GW, Fulcher AS, Szucs RA, et al: Imaging features of radiation induced changes in the abdomen. RadioGraphics 17:1455-1473, 1997.
203. Carr ND, Pullen BR, Hasleton PS, et al: Microvascular studies in human radiation bowel disease. Gut 25:448-454, 1984.
204. Hull TL: Diseases of the Anorectum. In Feldman M, Friedman LS, Sleisenger MH (eds): Gastrointestinal and Liver Disease, 8th ed. Philadelphia, Saunders, 2006, pp 2833-2856.
205. Thoeni RF, Venbrux AC: The anal canal: Distinction of internal hemorrhoids from small cancers by double-contrast barium enema examination. Radiology 145:17-19, 1982.
206. Levine MS, Kam LW, Rubesin SE, et al: Internal hemorrhoids: Diagnosis with double-contrast barium enema examinations. Radiology 177:141-144, 1990.
207. Manzi D, Samanta AK: Adhesion-related colonic varices. J Clin Gastroenterol 7:71-75, 1985.
208. McCormack TT, Bailey HR, Simms JM, et al: Rectal varices are not piles. Br J Surg 71:163-168, 1984.
209. Kelvin FM, Gardiner R: Clinical Imaging of the Colon and Rectum. New York, Raven, 1987, pp 422-460.
210. Kyaw MM, Gallagher T, Haines JO: Cloacogenic carcinoma of the anorectal junction: Roentgenologic diagnosis. AJR 115:384-391, 1972.
211. Glickman MG, Margulis AR: Cloacogenic carcinoma. AJR 107:175-180, 1969.
212. Gillespie JJ, Mackay B: Histogenesis of cloacogenic carcinoma: Fine structure of anal transitional epithelium and cloacogenic carcinoma. Hum Pathol 9:579-587, 1978.
213. Vaizey CJ, van den Bogaerde JB, Emmanuel AV, et al: Solitary rectal ulcer syndrome. Br J Surg 85:1617-1623, 1998.
214. Feczko PJ, O'Connell DJ, Riddell RH, et al: Solitary rectal ulcer syndrome: Radiologic manifestations. AJR 135:499-506, 1980.
215. Millward SF, Bayjoo P, Dixon MF, et al: The barium enema appearances in solitary rectal ulcer syndrome. Clin Radiol 36:185-189, 1985.
216. Levine MS, Piccolello ML, Sollenberger LC, et al: Solitary rectal ulcer syndrome: A radiologic diagnosis? Gastrointest Radiol 11:187-193, 1986.
217. Chang FY, Lu CL: Irritable bowel syndrome in the 21st century: Perspectives from Asia or South-east Asia. J Gastroenterol Hepatol 22:4-12, 2007.
218. Podovei M, Kuo B: Irritable bowel syndrome: A practical review. South Med J 99:1235-1242, 2006.
219. Henningsen P, Zipfel S, Herzog W: Management of functional somatic syndromes. Lancet 369:946-955, 2007.
220. Lennard-Jones JE: Constipation. In Feldman M, Scharschmidt BF, Sleisenger MH (eds): Gastrointestinal and Liver Disease, 6th ed. Philadelphia, WB Saunders, 1998, pp 174-197.
221. Greenfield SM: The management of constipation in hospital inpatients. Br J Hosp Med (Lond) 68:145-147, 2007.
222. Karasick S, Ehrlich SM: Is constipation a disorder of defecation or impaired motility? Distinction based on defecography and colonic transit studies. AJR 166:63-67, 1996.
223. Schuffler MD: Chronic intestinal pseudo-obstruction. In Feldman M, Scharschmidt BF, Sleisenger MH (eds): Gastrointestinal and Liver Disease, 6th ed. Philadelphia, WB Saunders, 1998, pp 1820-1830.
224. Phillips SF: Motility disorders of the colon. In Yamada T (ed): Textbook of Gastroenterology, 2nd ed. Philadelphia, JB Lippincott, 1995, pp 1856-1875.
225. Phillips SF, Pemberton JH: Megacolon: Congenital and acquired. In Feldman M, Scharschmidt BF, Sleisenger MH (eds): Gastrointestinal and Liver Disease, 6th ed. Philadelphia, WB Saunders, 1998, pp 1810-1819.
226. Sartor RB, Murphy ME, Rydzak E: Miscellaneous inflammatory and structural disorders of the colon. In Yamada T (ed): Textbook of Gastroenterology, 2nd ed. Philadelphia, JB Lippincott, 1995, pp 1806-1831.
227. Chiao GZ, Rey D: Motor disorders of the colon. In DiMarino AJ, Benjamin SB (eds): Gastrointestinal Disease: An Endoscopic Approach. Malden, MA, Blackwell Scientific, 1997, pp 659-683.
228. Rose S, Young MA, Reynolds JC: Gastrointestinal manifestations of scleroderma. Gastroenterol Clin North Am 27:563-594, 1998.
229. Brandt LS, Simon DM: Pneumatosis cystoides intestinalis. In Haubrich WS, Schaffner F, Berk JE (eds): Gastroenterology, 5th ed. Philadelphia, WB Saunders, 1995, pp 1685-1693.
230. Eisenberg RL: Gastrointestinal Radiology: A Pattern Approach. Philadelphia, Lippincott-Raven, 1996, pp 925-937.
231. Feczko PJ, Mezwa DG, Farah MC, et al: Clinical significance of pneumatosis of the bowel wall. RadioGraphics 12:1069-1084, 1992.
232. Brandt LJ, Simon DM: Pneumatosis cystoides intestinalis. In Haubrich WS, Schaffner F, Berk JE (eds): Gastroenterology, 5th ed. Philadelphia, WB Saunders, 1995, pp 1685-1693.
233. Komorowski RA: Histologic spectrum of diversion colitis. Am J Surg Pathol 14:548-554, 1990.
234. Lechner GL, Frank W, Jantsch H, et al: Lymphoid follicular hyperplasia in excluded colonic segments: A radiologic sign of diversion colitis. Radiology 176:135-136, 1990.
235. Whelan RL, Abramson D, Kim DS, et al: Diversion colitis: A prospective study. Surg Endosc 8:19-24, 1994.
236. Scott RL, Pinstein ML: Diversion colitis demonstrated by double-contrast barium enema. AJR 143:767-771, 1984.
237. Stanley RJ, Teseco FJ, Melson GL, et al: The colitis of Behçet's disease: A clinical-radiographic correlation. Radiology 114:603-608, 1975.
238. Molean AM, Simms DM, Homer MJ: Ileal ring ulcers in Behçet's syndrome. AJR 140:947-951, 1983.
239. Masugi J, Matsui T, Fujimor T, et al: A case of Behçet's disease with multiple longitudinal ulcers, all over the colon. Am J Gastroenterol 89:728-780, 1994.
240. Kim JH, Choi BJ, Han JK, et al: Colitis in Behçet's disease: Characteristics on double-contrast barium enema examinations in 20 patients. Abdom Imaging 19:132-136, 1994.
241. Friedman S, Janowitz HD: Systemic amyloidosis and the gastrointestinal tract. Gastroenterol Clin North Am 27:595-614, 1998.
242. Tada S, Iida M, Yao T, et al: Gastrointestinal amyloidosis: Radiologic features by chemical types. Radiology 190:37-42, 1994.
243. Moller JM, Santoni-Rugiu E, Chabanova E, et al: Magnetic resonance imaging with liver-specific contrast agent in primary amyloidosis and intrahepatic cholestasis. Acta Radiol 48:145-149, 2007.
244. Jacobs P, Ruff P, Wood L, et al: Amyloidosis: A changing clinical perspective. Hematology 12:163-167, 2007.
245. Urso FP, Urso JM, Lee CH: The cathartic colon: Pathological findings and radiological pathological correlation. Radiology 116:557-561, 1975.
246. Puy-Montbrun T, Delechenault P, Ganansia R, et al: Rectal stenosis due to Vegainin suppositories. Gastrointest Radiol 15:169-173, 1990.
247. Kim SK, Gerle RD, Rozanski R: Cathartic colitis. AJR 130:825-831, 1978.
248. Seaman WB, Clements JL: Urticaria of the colon: A non-specific pattern of submucosal edema. AJR 138:545-551, 1982.
249. Miller VE, Han SY, Witten DM: Reticular mosaic (urticarial) pattern of the colon mucosa in Yersinia colitis. Radiology 146:307-309, 1983.
250. Schuster MM, Raytch RE: Anorectal disease. In Haubrich WS, Schaffner F, Berk JE (eds): Gastroenterology, 5th ed. Philadelphia, WB Saunders, 1995, pp 1773-1789.
251. Walker P, Wiener I, Rave EB: Colitis cystica profunda: Diagnosis and management. South Med J 79:1167-1170, 1986.
252. Laurent V, Corby S, Meyer-Bisch L, et al: MRI aspect of rare rectal pseudotumor associated with dyschezia: Colitis cystica profunda. J Radiol 88:585-588, 2007.
253. Sarzo G, Finco C, Parise P, et al: Colitis cystica profunda of the rectum: Report of a case and review of the literature. Chir Ital 57:789-798, 2005.

254. Dewandel P, Schraepen T, Vanbeckevoort D, et al: Colitis cystica profunda. JBR-BTR 84:111-113, 2001.

255. Noyer CM, Brandt LJ: Systemic, iatrogenic, and unusual disorders of the colon. In DiMarino AJ, Benjamin SB (eds): Gastrointestinal Disease: An Endoscopic Approach. Malden, MA, Blackwell Scientific, 1997, pp 684-706.

256. Wald A: Other diseases of the colon and rectum. In Feldman M, Friedman LS, Sleisenger MH (eds): Gastrointestinal and Liver Disease, 8th ed. Philadelphia, Saunders, 2006, pp 2811-2832.

257. Martin SP, Gianella RA: Infectious disease of the colon. In DiMarino AJ, Benjamin SB (eds): Gastrointestinal Disease: An Endoscopic Approach. Malden, MA, Blackwell Scientific, 1997, pp 593-609.

258. Banks MR, Farthing MJG: Diarrhea. In Weinstein WM, Hawkey CJ, Bosch J (eds): Clinical Gastroenterology and Hepatology. St. Louis, Elsevier Mosby, 2005, pp 37-44.

259. Schiller LR, Sellin JH: Diarrhea. In Feldman M, Friedman LS, Brandt LJ (eds): Sleisenger and Fordtran's Gastrointestinal and Liver Disease, 8th ed. Philadelphia, Saunders Elsevier, 2006, pp 159-186.

260. McMahan ZH, DuPont HL: Review article: The history of acute infectious diarrhoea management—from poorly focused empiricism to fluid therapy and modern pharmacotherapy. Aliment Pharmacol Ther 25:759-769, 2007.

Postoperative Colon

Francis J. Scholz, MD • Christopher D. Scheirey, MD

Radiologists are often asked to evaluate the postoperative colon to exclude complications such as fistula, dehiscence, stricture, and abscess formation. Radiologists are also called on to assess the colon in the asymptomatic patient for anastomotic healing or resolution of inflammatory disease before a colostomy is closed. The radiologist must be familiar with the details of the surgical procedure, terminology, and individual surgeon's modifications to render an intelligent consultation. The major surgical procedures performed on the colon are discussed in this chapter. Although there is increasing use of the laparoscopic approach to colonic surgeries, the structural end results are similar to those of their open counterparts. The minute intraoperative technical details are well described in classic surgical textbooks.[1-4]

SEGMENTAL RESECTION

Segmental resection entails surgical removal of a diseased segment of the colon. Colonic continuity is usually restored with an end-to-end colocolic or ileocolic anastomosis (Figs. 67-1 and 67-2). The latter is created for patients who undergo resection of the cecum or right colon. In some patients, the anastomotic line may be seen as a short-segment, ringlike indentation during contrast examination of the colon (Fig. 67-3), but in many patients the site of the anastomosis may not be discernible unless defined by surgical staples. Currently, many surgeons are using stapling devices rather than traditional hand-sewn anastomoses to reestablish bowel continuity. The stapling units usually create a uniform ring of staples. Disruption of the ring on a plain film of the abdomen may indicate disruption of the anastomosis.

SIDE-TO-SIDE ENTEROCOLIC ANASTOMOSIS

A side-to-side enterocolic anastomosis (Fig. 67-4) may be created when a diseased segment of distal small bowel (as in Crohn's disease or radiation enteritis) is bypassed or when the length of the functional small bowel is shortened for treatment of morbid obesity. Currently, this procedure is rarely performed. Surgeons prefer to resect rather than bypass small bowel involved by Crohn's disease, and gastric restrictive surgery, such as a Roux-en-Y gastric bypass, is preferred over small bowel bypass procedure as therapy for morbid obesity (see Chapter 39).

COLOSTOMY

Colostomy is a colocutaneous anastomosis created to decompress a colonic obstruction or to divert the fecal stream away from the distal colon (Fig. 67-5). Diverting colostomies (1) protect a distal anastomosis that has recently been created and requires time to heal or (2) direct the fecal stream away from a segment of distal colon that is too inflamed to be resected at the time of the initial operation. If the surgeon does elect to resect the diseased segment, he or she may choose to perform an end-to-end anastomosis and divert the fecal stream with a temporary colostomy. The colon proximal to the stoma is often evaluated radiographically to rule out additional colonic lesions; the distal colon is evaluated to assess the status of a distal anastomosis or a previously inflamed segment.

Stomal creation is associated with a number of complications. Necrosis may occur if the blood supply is compromised

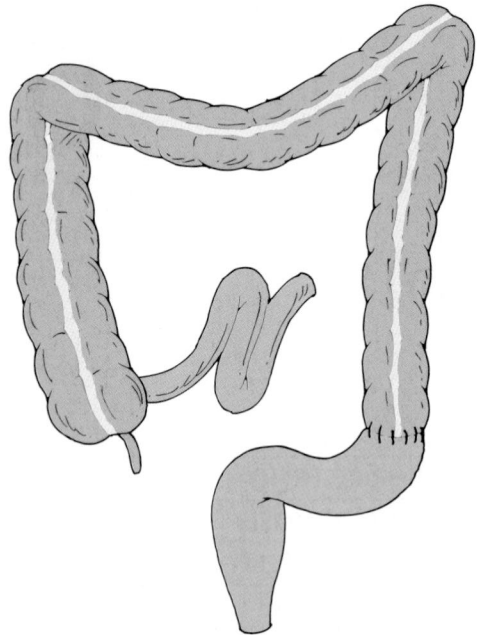

Figure 67-1. Segmental sigmoid resection and end-to-end colocolic anastomosis. Foreshortening of the sigmoid colon may or may not be apparent radiographically, depending on the length of colon resected.

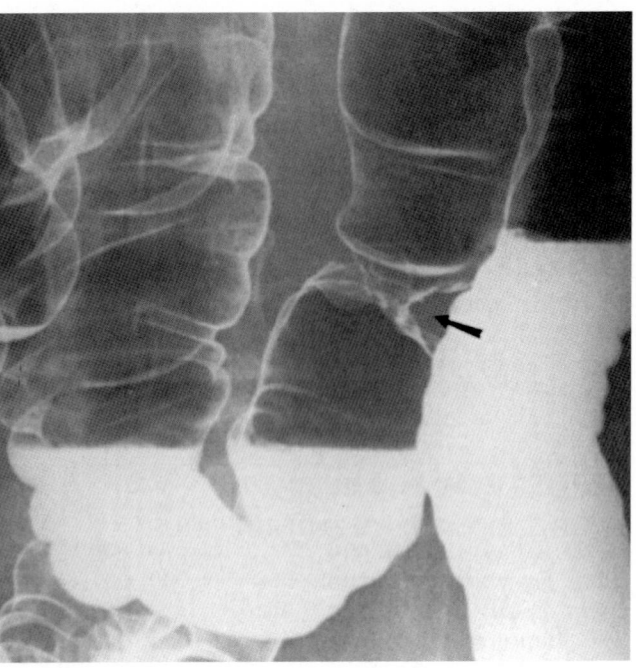

Figure 67-3. Postoperative deformity after closure of prior diverting colostomy. A prominent short-segment annular constriction (*arrow*) is present in the transverse colon with intact mucosa. Serosal metastatic disease can have the same appearance.

by tension or compression during formation of the stoma. The stoma may become detached from the abdominal wall and migrate into the abdominal cavity. With stomal recession, it may remain attached to the abdominal wall but retract into the abdomen, causing inflammation of the surrounding

skin. The bowel may also prolapse or intussuscept through the stoma. When they occur, parastomal hernias may contain small or, rarely, large bowel that passes through an enlarged fascial defect adjacent to the stoma. The hernia may remain in the subcutaneous tissues or may protrude externally beside the stoma. In obese patients, these can be difficult to detect clinically but are readily apparent on abdominal CT. Parastomal hernias can result in bowel obstructions and can be

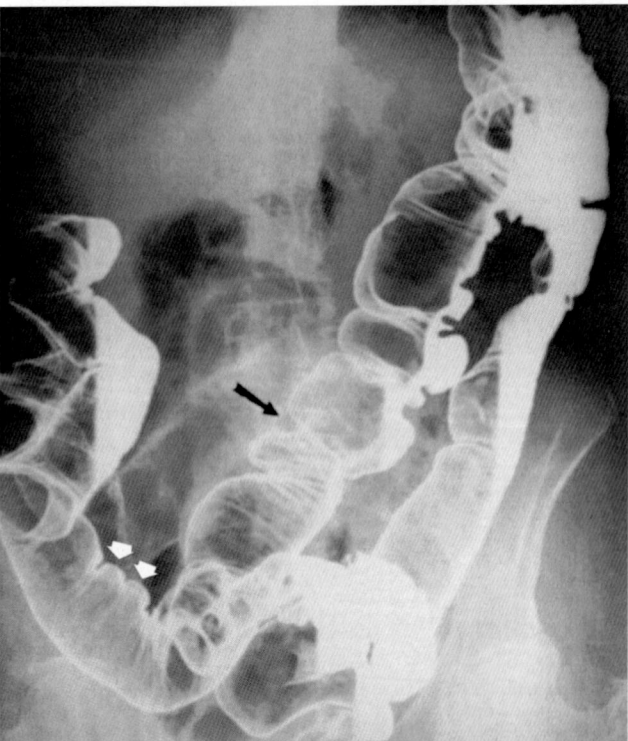

Figure 67-2. Ileal-transverse colonic anastomosis. The small bowel proximal to the anastomosis (*long arrow*) has an abnormal appearance with pseudohaustra (*short arrows*) and dilatation, an appearance termed *colonization.*

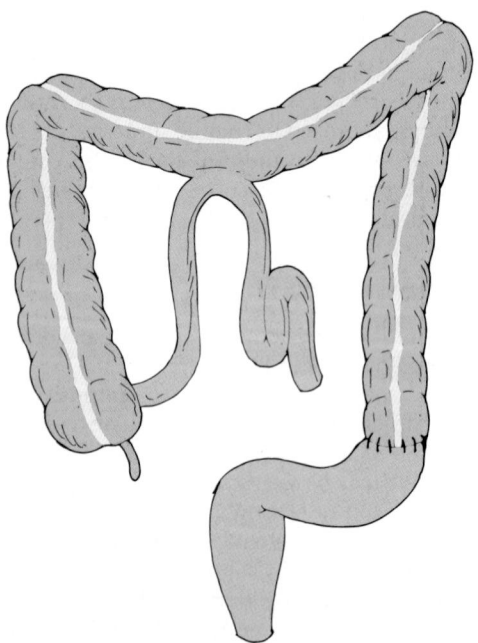

Figure 67-4. Side-to-side enterocolic anastomosis. Evaluation of the colon proximal to the anastomosis may be technically difficult because of preferential filling of the distal small bowel.

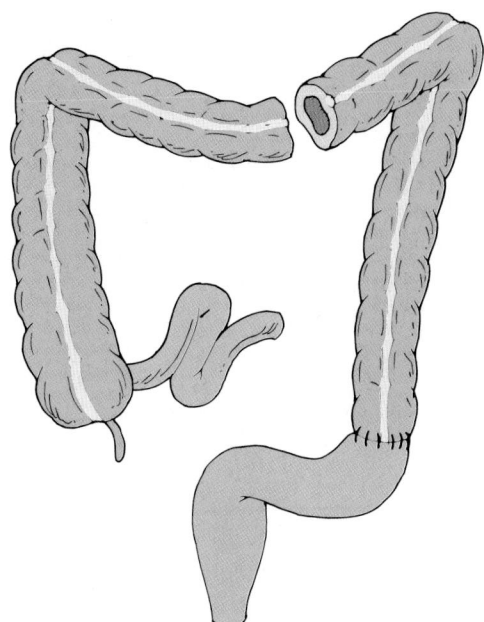

Figure 67-5. Typical diverting transverse colostomy. This demonstrates a fecal stoma, mucous fistula stoma, and end-to-end sigmoid anastomosis.

difficult for the surgeon to repair. Stomal ulceration may occur because of mechanical irritation from the stomal appliance. The choice of colostomy depends on whether it is to be permanent or temporary, the patient's body habitus, previous operations, and the surgeon's preference.

End-Colostomy

The end-colostomy may be performed as a definitive procedure in patients with distal rectal carcinoma or as part of a two-stage procedure for diverticulitis. The stoma is usually in the left lower quadrant, and the descending colon is the portion that forms the stomal opening. This procedure is performed in association with the Hartmann procedure to close off the rectal stump; therefore, only one stoma is present.

Loop Colostomy

Loop colostomy is usually performed for the following indications: (1) as a temporary procedure to relieve an acute obstruction of the distal colon or to protect a new distal colonic anastomosis and (2) as a permanent procedure for unresectable advanced lesions. A loop of transverse or sigmoid colon is brought to the surface of the abdominal wall, sutured in place on the outside, and then opened up, creating afferent and efferent stomas. The mucosa connecting the two stomal openings is the posterior wall of the colon. Patients are usually aware of which stoma produces feces and are able to direct the radiologist to examine the correct portion of the colon.

Double-Barreled Colostomy

A double-barreled colostomy is created when the colon is divided completely and the two cut ends are sewn side by side to each other. Currently, this type of colostomy is rarely performed. This type of stoma also has two openings, and the

patient can usually tell which is the productive opening. This procedure is chosen because the stoma can be closed without reentering the abdomen. The apposed common walls are cut, and the stoma closes spontaneously, or the margins of the two stomal openings can be pursed together with minimal suturing under local anesthesia.

Divided Colostomy and Mucous Fistula

Divided colostomy and mucous fistula operation creates two separate colostomies: one for the proximal colon, creating an efferent or productive stoma, and one for the distal colon, creating an afferent stoma. From the afferent stoma, the colon carries only mucus to the rectum, and this stoma has been termed a *mucous stoma* or *mucous fistula*. This procedure is not commonly performed but may be chosen to ensure that no fecal debris enters the distal colon.

At 6 to 8 weeks the colon is usually reexamined before closing the diverting colostomy to ensure that there is no leakage and that regional inflammatory changes have subsided. When the colon is evaluated to exclude a fistula, a single-contrast rather than a double-contrast barium enema study should be performed. Barium is safe to use in the asymptomatic patient because extravasation, when it occurs, has a well-formed sinus tract so that barium does not enter the peritoneal cavity. Also, barium has contrast characteristics superior to those of water-soluble contrast agents, which may not be sufficiently dense and can become diluted in such a tract.

After diversion of the fecal stream with a colostomy, the distal colon may have an abnormal appearance when examined before closure. The unused segment of the colon may appear nondistensible and may have an abnormal mucosal pattern with nodularity and lymphoid follicular hyperplasia.[5] This appearance is termed *diversion colitis.* The apparent lack of distensibility is probably the result of chronic lack of distention, and the mucosal irregularity may represent, in part, adherent mucus in a contracted and unprepared colon. Patients may be asymptomatic, and this entity likely represents a radiographic phenomenon rather than a true colitis. With restoration of the fecal stream after closure of the colostomy, the morphologic features of the colon return to normal unless underlying colonic inflammatory disease is present. A deformity may be created at the site of the previous colostomy and may cause radiographic confusion when the history is not correlated with the radiographic examination. The appearance is variable and may resemble that of a polypoid filling defect, a smooth or nodular annular lesion, or a submucosal or serosal process (see Fig. 67-3). Any colonic operative or endoscopic procedure may produce a persistent deformity that can mimic disease (Fig. 67-6). Careful review of the patient's history should prevent a misdiagnosis.

CECOSTOMY

Cecostomy is a surgical procedure in which an opening is created in the cecum to relieve cecal distention produced by intestinal pseudo-obstructions or, rarely, distal obstruction (e.g., tumor or cecal volvulus) or by profound paralytic ileus. It is usually a temporizing measure in acutely ill patients and in those who would not tolerate definitive but more prolonged procedures, such as right hemicolectomy and ileal-ascending

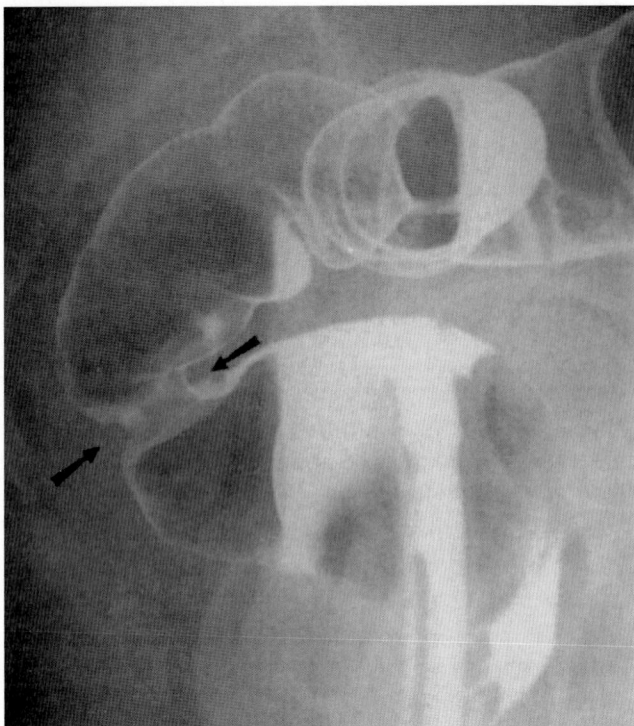

Figure 67-6. Rectal deformity caused by prior abscess and drainage. Examination performed because of a family history of colon carcinoma demonstrates a short annular constriction (*arrows*) in the midrectum that was not present on an examination performed 6 years earlier. Endoscopy showed normal mucosa in the contracted segment. Additional history was obtained before ordering further studies. An intervening appendectomy at another institution 4 years earlier required postoperative transrectal drainage of a perirectal abscess. This case represents residual deformity from that abscess and its treatment.

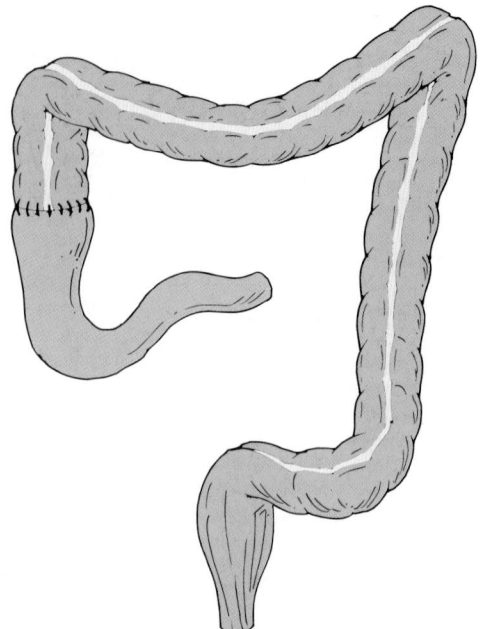

Figure 67-7. Ileal-ascending colonic anastomosis. This procedure is performed after resection of a right colonic tumor or ileocecal Crohn's disease.

colonic anastomosis (Fig. 61-7) or resection of a distal colonic obstructive process. A tube is placed in the cecum and brought to the abdominal surface to relieve colonic distention. A cecostomy may be performed by the surgeon, interventional radiologist, or gastroenterologist. A definitive surgical procedure may be performed when the patient's condition permits.

LOW ANTERIOR RESECTION

Low anterior resection, performed for carcinoma of the proximal rectum and midrectum, entails resection of the rectosigmoid and anastomosis of a cuff of the proximal colon to the distal rectum below the peritoneal reflection. It involves an anastomosis deep within the pelvis and may be difficult to perform. The surgeon must determine how low a resection to perform; this decision depends on the patient's body habitus, the nature of the lesion to be resected, and the skill of the surgeon. Depending on the amount of residual rectum, a straight colorectal anastomosis or pouch to rectal anastomosis may be performed (see section on Coloanal Anastomoses). Stapling devices greatly facilitate the technical performance of low anterior resection. A temporary, protective diverting ileostomy or colostomy may be used. Preoperatively, the surgeon may wish to obtain a proctoscopic measurement of the distance from the anal canal to the lesion. Postoperatively, the status of the anastomosis may require evaluation with a water-soluble contrast enema before closure of the ostomy.

Examination is performed with a gently placed 12-F Foley or small-caliber red rubber catheter that is taped onto the adjacent gluteal skin (inflation of the balloon could disrupt the anastomosis). Leakage from low anastomosis within the pelvis may produce a pelvic abscess, perirectal abscess, or colovaginal fistula (Fig. 67-8).

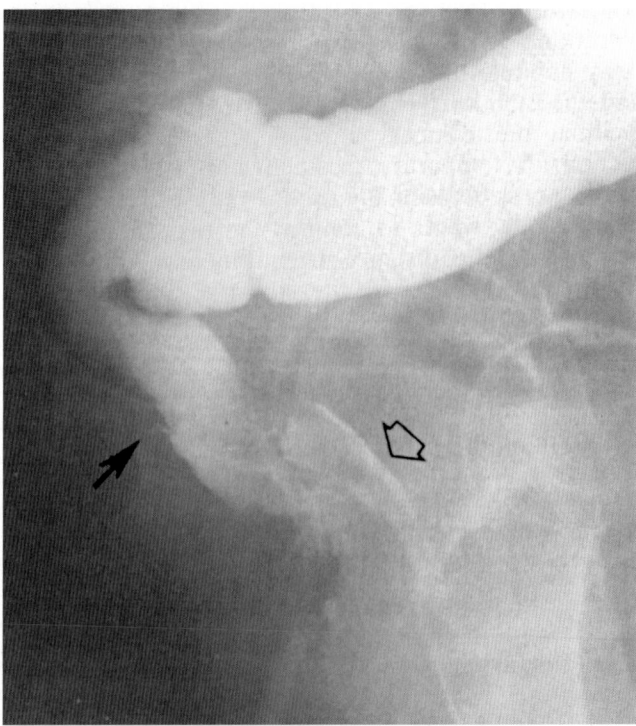

Figure 67-8. Rectovaginal fistula. Contrast material is identified in the vagina (*open arrow*). Surgical clips (*solid arrow*) seen posteriorly define the level of the anastomosis and the level of the fistula.

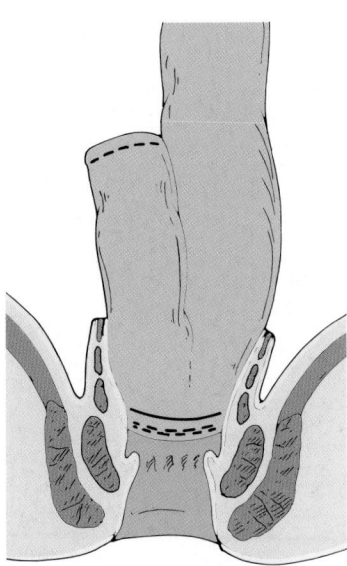

Figure 67-9. Colonic J pouch. A segment of distal colonic is folded upon itself, divided, and anastomosed to the anus, creating a reservoir for fecal material after low anterior resection.

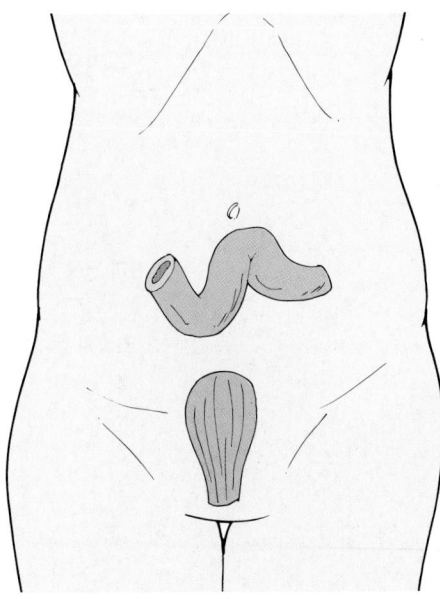

Figure 67-10. Closed rectal pouch. Hartmann pouch, with terminal ileostomy.

COLOANAL ANASTOMOSES

A coloanal anastomosis is a means of preserving colonic continuity and anal sphincter function used primarily in patients with rectal carcinoma involving the mid and lower thirds of the rectum. All or portions of the mesorectum are excised. The tumor is excised with a relatively short distal margin, preserving the anal sphincter but with enough resection to avoid local recurrence. Previously, the colon was reattached to the anus via a straight coloanal anastomosis, but the procedure of choice currently is the colonic J-pouch anastomosis (Fig. 67-9). This has improved functional outcome over a straight anastomosis, particularly in the first postoperative year.[6,7] The technique involves folding the distal aspect of the residual colon upon itself and dividing the septum to create a reservoir for fecal material. The pouch is then handsewn or stapled directly to the anus. A diverting colostomy or ileostomy may be performed.

An emerging technique in patients with difficult anatomy is the coloplasty pouch. This involves a longitudinal incision in the descending colon, which is then closed transversely. This creates a pouch that is technically easier to anastomose to the anus in patients with a narrow pelvis. Early studies indicate a higher rate of anastomotic leaks, particularly at the distal end of the incision, but with improved functional results compared with a straight coloanal anastomosis.[8,9]

All types of coloanal anastomoses can be complicated by anastomotic leaks and associated abscesses.

ABDOMINOPERINEAL RESECTION

Lesions located below the levator ani muscles usually require an abdominoperineal resection. In this procedure, the rectum is removed and a permanent colostomy is created.

HARTMANN PROCEDURE

With the Hartmann procedure, a tumor or segment of sigmoid diverticulitis is resected, a terminal end sigmoid colo-

stomy is created, and the distal rectal stump is closed by stapled sutures or sewn by hand (Fig. 67-10). The resulting Hartmann pouch becomes a blind segment of colon from the anus to the sealed stump. Bowel continuity can subsequently be reestablished by a colorectal anastomosis. In some patients, however, the surgeon may elect not to reestablish continuity for medical or technical reasons. The blind pouch normally may contain fecal debris, inspissated mucus, or enteroliths. Polyps or carcinoma can also develop in this segment.[10] Patients may be asymptomatic until the tumor has become far advanced. Although the classic Hartmann pouch involves only a portion of the rectum, in practice the pouch may be much longer and include part or all of the sigmoid colon. A Hartmann pouch may also be created after total colectomy and creation of an ileostomy for Crohn's disease or ulcerative colitis.

MUCOUS FISTULA

Rather than closing off the rectal stump, a rectosigmoid stoma or mucous fistula may be created by bringing out the proximal cut end of the distal sigmoid colon or rectum, which results in a stoma that produces only mucus. The distal colon extends from the stoma of the mucous fistula distally to the anus.

APPENDECTOMY

Appendectomy is a procedure in which the appendix is tied at its junction with the cecum and is resected. The stump is ligated and inverted. Occasionally, this operation may produce a sizable, smooth polypoid defect at the base of the cecum (Fig. 67-11). The history of appendectomy and the typical location of the defect at the apex of the cecum should help prevent a mistaken diagnosis of cecal polyp. Nodularity, mucosal disruption, or a location away from the cecal apex should arouse suspicion that it is a true polyp requiring colonoscopic evaluation.

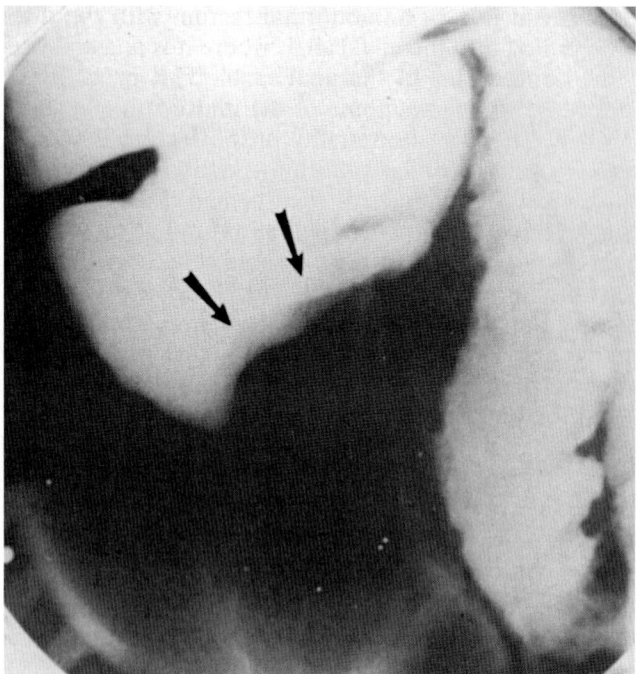

Figure 67-11. Appendiceal stump deformity. A broad-based defect (*arrows*) at the apex of the cecum is due to previous appendectomy. Most appendectomies produce minimal or no deformity of the cecum.

ILEAL POUCH–ANAL ANASTOMOSIS

Ileal pouch–anal anastomosis is performed in patients who have ulcerative colitis (see Chapter 61) or familial polyposis (see Chapter 65).[11,12] It is an alternative to proctocolectomy that offers the potential for nearly normal defecation through an intact anus. Careful radiographic and clinical evaluation of the patient to exclude Crohn's disease is essential. Patients with Crohn's disease may not tolerate extensive pelvic surgery, and perineal fistulas and sinus tracts, inflammation of the pouch, and anastomotic strictures may develop. The procedure consists of colectomy, mucosal proctectomy, and creation of a small bowel reservoir. The colon and most of the rectum are removed, leaving the distal portion of the rectum in place. The mucosa is dissected from this rectal remnant, leaving a cuff of denuded rectum with intact muscularis propria. The most common pouch is a J pouch, although an S or a side-to-side (Fonkalsrud) pouch may be created (Fig. 67-12). The J pouch is formed when the distal ileum is closed and the ileum is doubled on itself, forming a J configuration. The apposed walls of the two limbs are stapled to each other, and the two segments are opened, creating a pouch that has the volume of two limbs (Fig. 67-13). The staples delineate the length of

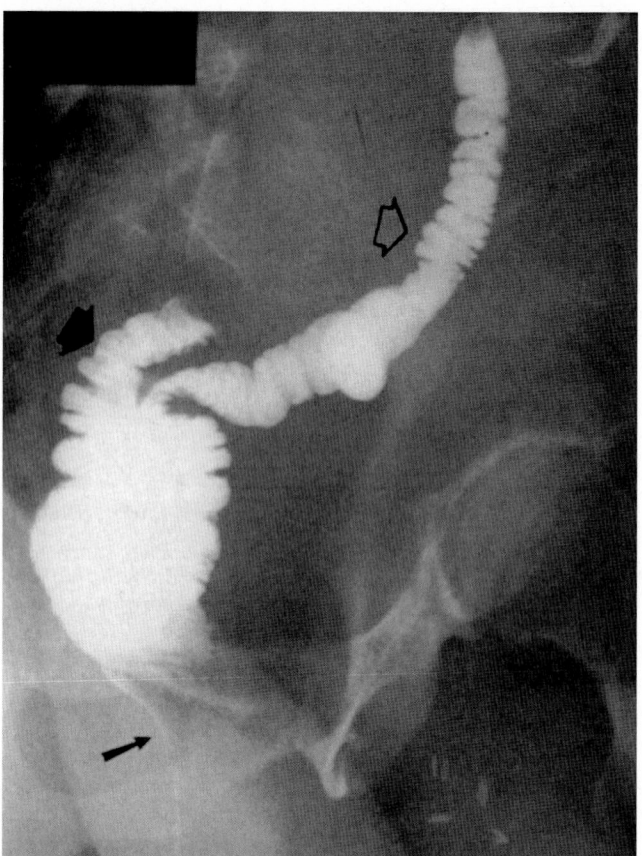

Figure 67-13. Normal J-pouch reservoir before closure of the diverting ileostomy. Note the long J-pouch appendage (*short solid arrow*) and the efferent limb (*open arrow*) leading from the ileostomy to the pouch. In this supine oblique view, air is present (*long solid arrow*) in the anterior portion of the pouch at the pouch–anal anastomotic region. Contrast material should be positioned at the pouch–anal anastomosis by placing the patient in a 45-degree erect position or turning the patient toward the prone position until air is displaced by contrast material.

the pouch. The pouch is placed into the rectal cuff, a hole is created at the apex of the pouch, and the pouch is stapled to the anal mucosa.

The S pouch is created by apposing and suturing three limbs of the distal ileum to each other. The common walls are opened, creating a pouch with the diameter of three segments of small bowel. This pouch and the Fonkalsrud pouch have an efferent limb that is brought into the rectal cuff, and its mucosa is sutured to the dentate line of the anal canal.

The Fonkalsrud pouch is created by resecting a segment of the distal ileum. This segment is placed next to another loop of ileum, and a side-to-side anastomosis is created.

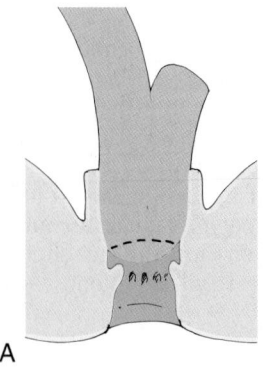 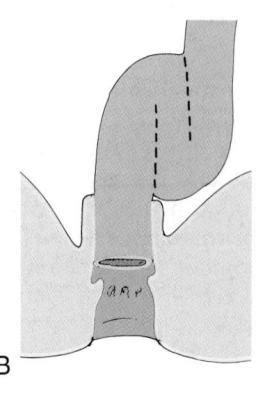 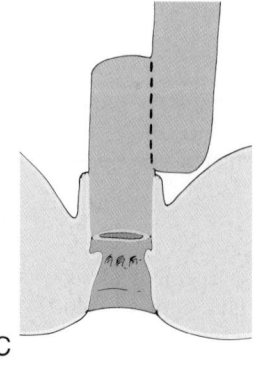

Figure 67-12. Three major types of ileal pouch–anal anastomosis. A. J pouch. **B.** S pouch. **C.** Side-to-side (Fonkalsrud) pouch.

A   B   C

Ileal pouch–anal anastomosis procedures leave a cuff of rectal wall in place with the theory that the intact sensory innervation of this segment permits the patient to sense bowel distention and the urge to defecate. Although bowel movements may be increased in frequency, patients may need to defecate no more often than they normally need to urinate. Some patients have nocturnal soiling, but the quality of life of patients who had ulcerative colitis is greatly enhanced, and the risk of developing colon carcinoma is eliminated.

The ileal pouch–anal anastomosis procedure is usually performed in two stages. The first stage consists of a total colectomy, creation of the pouch and pouch–anal anastomosis, and creation of a protective ileostomy. The second stage is ileostomy closure, which is performed after a period of 6 to 8 weeks, allowing suture lines to mature. Before closure, the surgeon examines the anorectum. If the anorectum is normal, a barium enema is performed to rule out small leaks from the pouch staple lines or pouch–anal anastomosis. If the clinical examination is abnormal, either the barium enema is delayed or CT is performed. Abscesses tend to occur later and are best seen on CT examination.

A three-stage procedure may be required when the patient is weakened by fulminant colitis and is receiving high-dose corticosteroid therapy. The first stage consists of creation of a simple ileostomy, colectomy, and a Hartmann closure of the rectum. The second stage is performed several months later, when healing and recovery of electrolyte and endocrine integrity have occurred (usually after corticosteroid withdrawal). The remainder of the rectum is resected, mucosal proctectomy is performed, and a pouch with pouch–anal anastomosis is created. The third stage is closure of the ileostomy 6 to 8 weeks later.

Any of the complications that attend all major abdominal operations may develop after ileal pouch–anal anastomosis, including abscesses, ileus, or small bowel obstruction.[13,14] The small bowel mesentery limits mobility of the ileum, and the small bowel may have to be manipulated extensively to create the ileal pouch–anal anastomosis. This manipulation may contribute to the prolonged ileus seen in some patients. Small bowel obstruction may develop in the immediate postoperative period, in the period between creation of the pouch and closure of the ileostomy, or at any time during the remainder of the patient's life. Mesenteric hematoma may occur if small mesenteric vessels rupture because of manipulation of or prolonged tension on the mesentery. The superior mesenteric artery syndrome can develop if tension, placed on the mesentery in an attempt to position the pouch in the lowest portion of the pelvis, retracts the superior mesenteric artery against the aorta.[14,15] Prophylactic release of the small bowel mesentery at the ligament of Treitz, mesenteric lengthening incisions, and judicious suturing and resection of stretched branch mesenteric vessels facilitate mobilization of the terminal ileal pouch into the pelvis.[16]

Although leakage may occur from the suture lines of the pouch (Fig. 67-14), this complication is more commonly encountered at the ileal pouch–anal anastomosis (Figs. 67-15

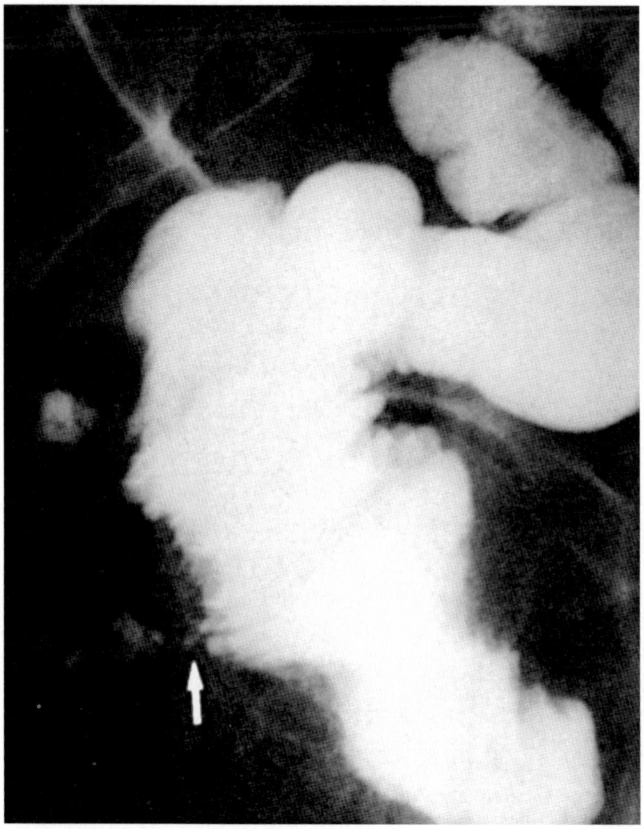

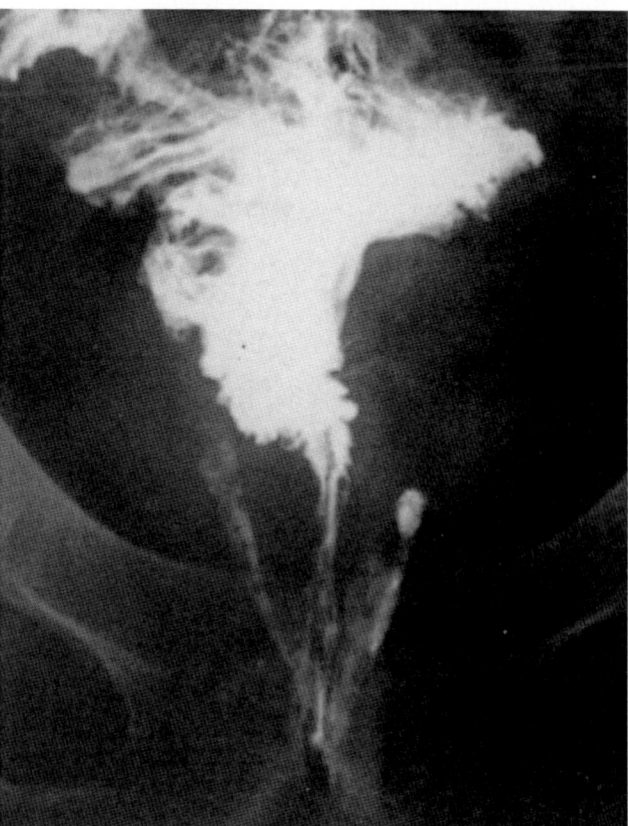

Figure 67-15. Pouch leak. Leakage from the J-pouch–anal anastomosis of a J-pouch reservoir is seen. Leakage from any anal anastomosis has a typical chevron appearance resulting from tracking of the extravasated contrast material between the rectal cuff and the pouch or efferent limb inserted into the cuff. (From Kremers PW, Scholz FJ, Schoetz DJ Jr, et al: Radiology of the ileoanal reservoir. AJR 145:559-567, 1985, © by American Roentgen Ray Society.)

Figure 67-14. Pouch leak. Leakage (*arrow*) from a J-pouch reservoir is seen. (From Kremers PW, Scholz FJ, Schoetz DJ Jr, et al: Radiology of the ileoanal reservoir. AJR 145:559-567, 1985, © by American Roentgen Ray Society.)

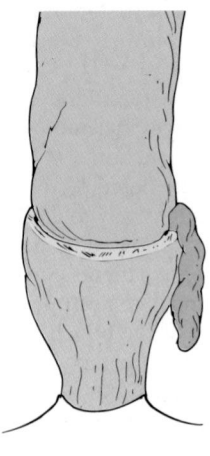
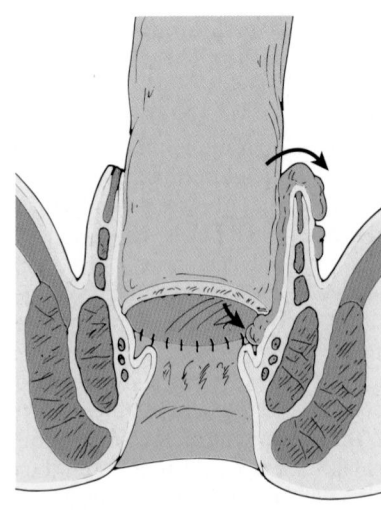

Figure 67-16. Chevron configuration of ileoanal anastomotic leak. Drawing illustrates the mechanism of extravasation from a pouch–anal anastomosis. Mucus (or contrast material) passes from the point of disruption (*lower curved arrow*) and courses between the pouch and the cuff of rectum, producing the chevron configuration seen in Figure 61-15. Purulent material eventually dissects beyond the cuff and spills (*upper curved arrow*) into the perirectal soft tissues. (From Kremers PW, Scholz FJ, Schoetz DJ Jr, et al: Radiology of the ileoanal reservoir. AIR 145:559-567, 1985, © by American Roentgen Ray Society.)

and 67-16). Anteroposterior, oblique, and lateral views in a 30- to 45-degree upright position must be obtained low enough to include the ileal pouch–anal canal junction. Leakage from the pouch or from the ileal pouch–anal anastomosis requires that closure of the diverting ileostomy be postponed until healing of the leak has been confirmed. Small leakages and collections may be treated by endoscopic drainage, suturing, or antibiotic therapy if they do not resolve spontaneously.[17] A small length of closed reflected ileum often is not incorporated into the J pouch, and this is termed the *J-pouch appendage* (Fig. 67-17; see also Fig. 67-13). This appendage may leak, may be long enough to twist and necrose, or may simulate leakage (see Fig. 67-17).[18] The S pouch and the Fonkalsrud pouch have efferent limbs that pass from the pouch to the anus. These pouches, when distended with fecal contents, may compress the efferent limb and interfere with pouch emptying. Some patients with this condition succeed in emptying their pouch by self-catheterization.

Patients who tolerate the complete procedure may return with "pouchitis," complaining of tenesmus and diarrhea and, rarely, with bleeding, fever, arthralgias, and other systemic symptoms.[19,20] Endoscopic examination of the pouch may reveal redness and ulceration.[21] Pouchitis is not associated with consistent radiographic findings, and its cause is unknown.

With time, accommodation of the small bowel to the pouch leads to an increased capacity and small bowel dilatation, which can simulate small bowel obstruction on abdominal plain films. When clinical and radiographic findings are confusing, enteroclysis or retrograde small bowel enema examination may be required to rule out mechanical obstruction.

COLONIC STENTS

Colonic stenting is an endoscopic treatment of large bowel obstruction.[22,23] These procedures are usually palliative and performed in patients with colon cancer or obstructing colonic metastases whose condition is deemed unresectable or who are unable to tolerate definitive resection. On occasion, stents are a temporal bridge to definitive colonic resection, avoiding emergency surgery. Obstructing lesions are crossed with a

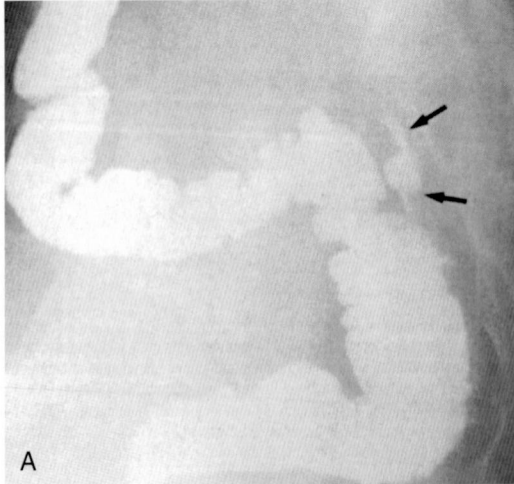
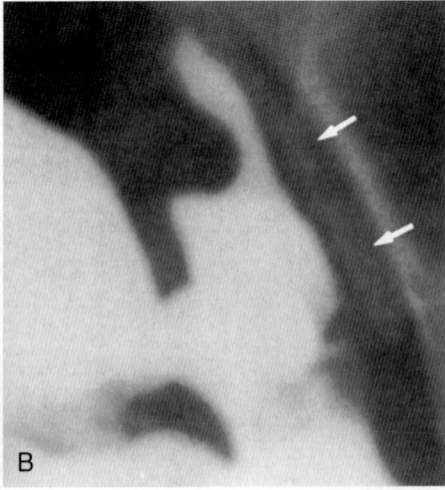

Figure 67-17. Pseudoleakage. This appearance is commonly seen with a J-pouch reservoir and represents a potential radiographic pitfall. **A.** Traces of contrast material (*arrows*) appear to extravasate from the proximal, posterior part of the J-pouch reservoir. **B.** Additional spot film with further distention shows contrast material surrounded by a faintly visible suture line (*arrows*) just anterior to the sacrum. The lateral view also demonstrates the anterior position of the lower portion of the pouch, which traps air in the supine position, impairing visualization of the J-pouch–anal anastomosis. (From Kremers PW, Scholz FJ, Schoetz DJ Jr, et al: Radiology of the ileoanal reservoir. AIR 145:559-567, 1985, © by American Roentgen Ray Society.)

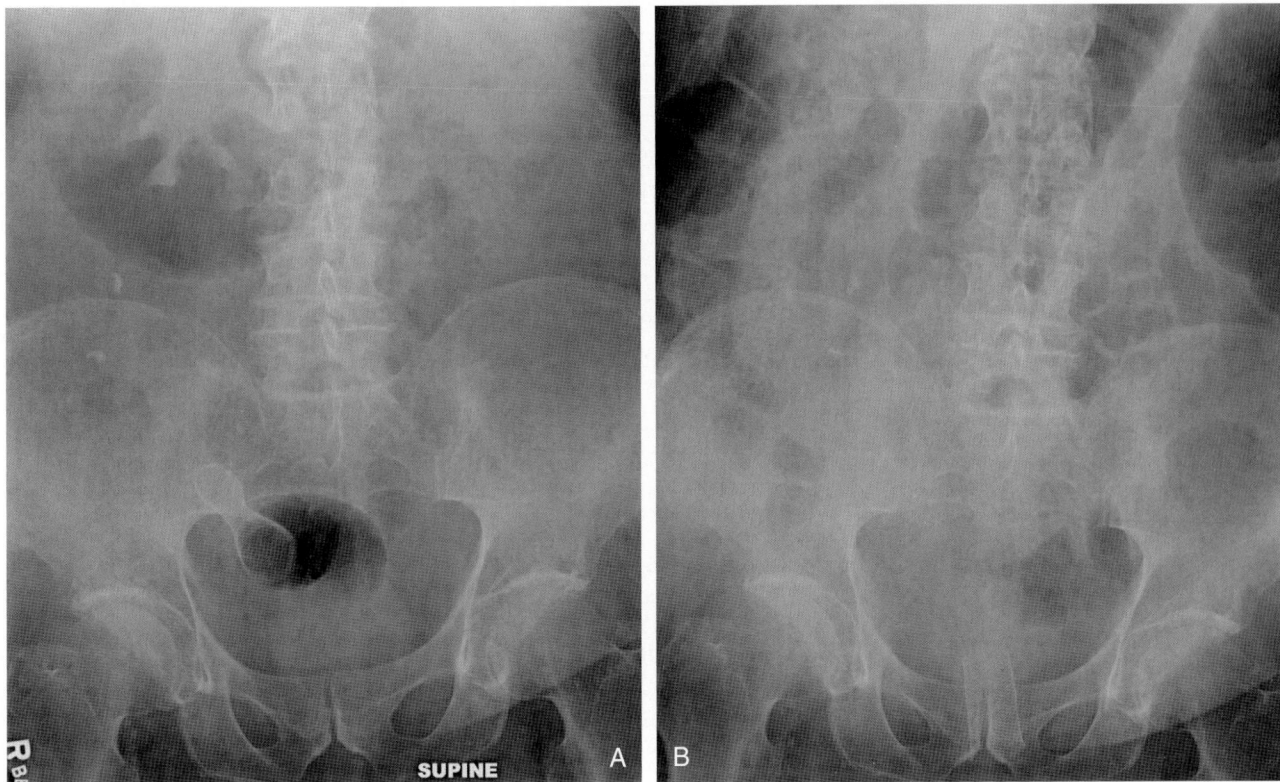

Figure 67-18. Colonic stent. A. Normal appearance of stent, with central waistlike narrowing. **B.** Recurrent large bowel obstruction, with migrated colonic stent currently located in distal rectum. Note absence of waistlike narrowing.

guide wire, and metal wall stents are deployed to relieve the obstruction. Postprocedural radiographs demonstrate waistlike midstent narrowing that indicates satisfactory placement across the stricture (Fig. 67-18).

References

1. Wolff BG, Fleshman JW, Beck DE: The ASCRS Textbook of Colon and Rectal Surgery. New York, Springer, 2007.
2. Benyon J, Carr ND: Progress in Colorectal Surgery. New York, Springer, 2006.
3. Killingback M: Colorectal Surgery: Living Pathology in the Operating Room. New York, Springer, 2006.
4. Phillips RKS: Colorectal Surgery: A Companion to Specialist Surgical Practice. New York, Elsevier, 2005.
5. Lechner GL, Frank W, Jantsch H, et al: Lymphoid follicular hyperplasia in excluded colonic segments: A radiologic sign of diversion colitis. Radiology 176:135-136, 1990.
6. Parc R, Tiret E, Frileux P, et al: Resection and coloanal anastomosis with colonic reservoir for rectal carcinoma. Br J Surg 73:139-141, 1986.
7. Lazorthes F, Fages P, Chiotasso P, et al: Resection of the rectum with construction of a colonic reservoir and coloanal anastomosis for carcinoma of the rectum. Br J Surg 73:136-138, 1986.
8. Ho YH, Brown S, Heah SM, et al: Comparison of J-pouch and coloplasty pouch for low rectal cancers: A randomized, controlled trial investigating functional results and comparative anastomotic leak rates. Ann Surg 236:49-55, 2002.
9. Remzi FH, Fazio VW, Gorgun E, et al: Quality of life, functional outcome, and complications of coloplasty pouch after low anterior resection. Dis Colon Rectum 48:735-743, 2005.
10. Haas PA, Fox TA Jr: The fate of the forgotten rectal pouch after Hartmann's procedure without reconstruction. Am J Surg 159:106-110; discussion 110-101, 1990.
11. Schoetz DJ Jr, Coller JA, Veidenheimer MC: Proctocolectomy with ileoanal reservoir: An alternative to permanent ileostomy. Postgrad Med 75:123-127, 130-122, 137-128, 1984.
12. Schoetz DJ Jr, Coller JA, Veidenheimer MC: Ileoanal reservoir for ulcerative colitis and familial polyposis. Arch Surg 121:404-409, 1986.
13. Hillard AE, Mann FA, Becker JM, Nelson JA: The ileoanal J pouch: Radiographic evaluation. Radiology 155:591-594, 1985.
14. Kremers PW, Scholz FJ, Schoetz DJ Jr, et al: Radiology of the ileoanal reservoir. AJR 145:559-567, 1985.
15. Ballantyne GH, Graham SM, Hammers L, Modlin IM: Superior mesenteric artery syndrome following ileal J-pouch anal anastomosis: An iatrogenic cause of early postoperative obstruction. Dis Colon Rectum 30:472-474, 1987.
16. Burnstein MJ, Schoetz DJ Jr, Coller JA, Veidenheimer MC: Technique of mesenteric lengthening in ileal reservoir-anal anastomosis. Dis Colon Rectum 30:863-866, 1987.
17. Schoetz DJ Jr, Coller JA, Veidenheimer MC: Can the pouch be saved? Dis Colon Rectum 31:671-675, 1988.
18. Pezim ME, Taylor BA, Davis CJ, Beart RW Jr: Perforation of terminal ileal appendage of J-pelvic ileal reservoir. Dis Colon Rectum 30:161-163, 1987.
19. Franceschi D, Chen PF, Yuh JN: Solitary J-pouch ulcer causing pouchitis-like syndrome. Dis Colon Rectum 29:515-517, 1986.
20. Iwata T, Yamamoto T, Umegae S, et al: Pouchitis and pre-pouch ileitis developed after restorative proctocolectomy for ulcerative colitis: A case report. World J Gastroenterol 13:643-646, 2007.
21. Stucchi AF, Aarons CB, Becker JM: Surgical approaches to cancer in patients who have inflammatory bowel disease. Gastroenterol Clin North Am 35:641-673, 2006.
22. Soto S, Lopez-Roses L, Gonzalez-Ramirez A, et al: Endoscopic treatment of acute colorectal obstruction with self-expandable metallic stents: Experience in a community hospital. Surg Endosc 20:1072-1076, 2006.
23. Dafnis G: Repeated coaxial colonic stenting in the palliative management of benign colonic obstruction. Eur J Gastroenterol Hepatol 19:83-86, 2007.

Colon: Differential Diagnosis

Richard M. Gore, MD

Table 68-1
Multiple Colonic Filling Defects

Artifacts
Feces
Mucus strands
Oil droplets
Ingested foreign bodies
Air bubbles

Neoplasms and Tumors
Multiple adenomatous polyps
Hemangiomas
Familial adenomatous polyposis
Cronkhite-Canada syndrome
Disseminated gastrointestinal polyposis
Juvenile polyposis coli
Turcot's syndrome
Neurocrest and colonic tumors
Ruvalcaba-Myhre-Smith syndrome
Lymphoma
Metastases
Multiple adenocarcinomas
Cowden's syndrome
Leukemic infiltration
Blue nevus syndrome
Neurofibromas, neurofibromatosis

Inflammatory Disorders
Ulcerative colitis
Crohn's disease
Diversion colitis
Colitis cystica profunda
Malacoplakia
Behçet's syndrome

Infectious Disorders
Pseudomembranous colitis
Amebiasis
Schistosomiasis
Trichuriasis
Strongyloides infection
Cytomegalovirus infection
Ascariasis
Herpes zoster

Miscellaneous Disorders
Lymphoid follicular pattern
Nodular lymphoid hyperplasia
Hemorrhoids
Diverticula
Pneumatosis intestinalis
Cystic fibrosis
Endometriosis
Colonic varices
Amyloidosis
Hemangiomas
Urticaria

Table 68-2
Solitary Colonic Filling Defects

Benign Tumors
Hyperplastic polyp
Adenomatous polyp
Villous adenoma
Villoglandular polyp
Hamartoma
Peutz-Jeghers polyp
Spindle cell tumor (lipoma, GIST, fibroma, neurofibroma, cystic lymphangioma)
Traumatic neuroma
Carcinoid tumor

Malignant Tumors
Carcinoma
Lymphoma
Metastases
Kaposi's sarcoma

Infectious Disorders
Ameboma
Tuberculosis
Mucormycoma
Periappendiceal abscess
Diverticular abscess
Schistosomiasis (polypoid granuloma)
Ascaris lumbricoides (bolus of worms) infection
Intramural hematoma

Inflammatory Disorders
Colitis cystica profunda
Solitary rectal ulcer syndrome
Foreign body perforation and abscess
Crohn's disease

Miscellaneous Disorders
Endometrioma
Intussusception
Bezoar
Suture granuloma
Inverted appendiceal stump
Hypertrophied anal papilla
Stool, vegetable material
Amyloidosis
Varix, hemorrhoid

Table 68-3
Mosaic-Submucosal Edema Pattern

Obstructive colon cancer
Colonic urticaria
Herpes zoster
Ischemia
Cecal volvulus
Colonic ileus
Yersinia infection

Table 68-4
Segmental Colonic Narrowing

Malignant Disorders
Primary adenocarcinoma
Metastases
Kaposi's sarcoma
Lymphoma
Carcinoma
Carcinoid
Direct spread from renal, duodenal, pancreatic, ovarian tumor

Inflammatory Disorders
Crohn's disease
Ulcerative colitis
Cathartic colon
Caustic colon
Retractile mesenteritis
Typhlitis
Solitary rectal ulcer syndrome

Infectious Disorders
Amebiasis
Schistosomiasis
Strongyloides infection
Tuberculosis
Gonorrheal proctitis
Chlamydia infection (lymphogranuloma venereum)
Herpes zoster
Cytomegalovirus infection
Bacillary dysentery
Actinomycosis
Giant anorectal condyloma acuminatum
Pericolic abscess

Vascular Disorders
Ischemic colitis
Radiation colitis
Intramural hematoma

Miscellaneous Disorders
Pancreatitis
Pelvic lipomatosis
Endometriosis
Amyloidosis
Adhesive band
Postoperative deformity
Myochosis

Table 68-5
Annular "Apple-Core" Colonic Lesion

Carcinoma
Diverticulitis
Chronic Crohn's disease
Chronic ulcerative colitis
Ischemic colitis
Chlamydia infection (lymphogranuloma venereum)
Lymphoma
Tuberculosis
Villous adenoma
Helminthoma
Ameboma

Table 68-6
Causes of Large Bowel Obstruction in an Adult

Inflammatory Disorders
Diverticulitis
Inflammatory bowel disease
Retractile mesenteritis

Infectious Disorders
Ascaris bolus
Chagas' disease
Amebiasis
Schistosomiasis
Actinomycosis
Tuberculosis

Extrinsic Bowel Lesions
Adhesions
Hernias
Volvulus
Endometriosis
Neoplasms
Appendiceal abscess
Tubo-ovarian abscess
Distended bladder

Neoplastic Lesions
Adenocarcinoma of the colon
Lymphoma
Spindle cell tumor
Gastrointestinal stromal tumor
Carcinoid
Metastases

Vascular Disorders
Intramural hematoma
Vascular occlusion, infarction

Obturation of Lumen
Bezoar
Gallstone
Enterolith
Fecal impaction
Foreign body
Intussusception

Miscellaneous Disorders
Amyloidosis
Colonic pseudo-obstruction

Table 68-7
Intestinal Pseudo-Obstruction: Ogilvie's Syndrome

Drug Reaction
Phenothiazine
Antidepressants
Morphine
Antiparkinsonian

Paralytic Ileus
Hypokalemia
Pancreatitis
Pneumonia
Myocardial infarction
Trauma

Endocrine Disease
Myxedema
Diabetes
Hypoparathyroidism
Pheochromocytoma

Neuromuscular Disorders
Parkinson's disease
Chagas' disease
Myotonic dystrophy

Miscellaneous Disorders
Amyloidosis
Sprue
Scleroderma
Retractile mesenteritis
Vitamin D deficiency

Table 68-9
Large Bowel Obstruction in a Newborn

Hernia, incarcerated, internal or external
Congenital stenosis or atresia
Hernia, incarcerated, internal or external
Hirschsprung's disease
Imperforate anus
Rectal atresia
Intussusception
Midgut volvulus with malrotation
Small left colon syndrome
Megacystis-microcolon syndrome
Intraluminal web, diaphragm, or band
Duplication

Table 68-10
Intestinal Obstruction in a Postneonatal Child

Hirschsprung's disease
Imperforate anus with fistula
Hernia
Appendicitis
Duplication
Intussusception
Midgut volvulus
Tuberculosis
Cystic fibrosis
Crohn's disease
Fecal impaction
Foreign body, bezoar
Ascaris bolus
Neoplasm

Table 68-8
Colon Distention without Obstruction

Paralytic Ileus
After operation
Peritonitis
Appendicitis
Pancreatitis

Electrolyte Imbalance
Hypokalemia
Hypochloremia
Calcium abnormality

Endocrine Disorders
Diabetes
Adrenal insufficiency
Myxedema
Hypoparathyroidism

Neuromuscular Disorders
Hirschsprung's disease
Parkinson's disease
Multiple sclerosis
Riley-Day syndrome
Amyotonia congenita
Chagas' disease

Drug Therapy
Morphine, L-dopa, chlorpromazine, benztropine, atropine,
   propantheline bromide
Hexamethonium

Trauma
Spinal cord injury
Intramural hematoma
Lower rib injury
Retroperitoneal hemorrhage

Urinary Tract Disorders
Ureteral colic
Renal failure, uremia
Urine retention

Collagen-Vascular Disease
Scleroderma
Dermatomyositis
Polyarteritis nodosa
Kawasaki's syndrome

Acute Thoracic Disease
Myocardial infarction
Congestive heart failure

Miscellaneous Disorders
Chronic constipation
Chronic laxative, cathartic abuse
Aerophagia
Mesenteric infarction
Shock
Septicemia
Toxic megacolon
Cystic fibrosis
Amyloidosis

Table 68-11
Toxic Megacolon

Bacillary dysentery
Pseudomembranous colitis
Ulcerative colitis
Crohn's disease
Ischemic colitis
Amebic colitis
Bacillary dysentery
Typhoid fever
Cholera
Strongyloidiasis
Campylobacter colitis
Pseudomembranous colitis
Behçet's disease

Table 68-12
Enlarged Ileocecal Valve

Normal variant
Crohn's disease
Amebiasis
Fatty infiltration, lipoma
Intussusception
Villous adenoma
Adenocarcinoma
Lymphoma
Yersinia enterocolitis
Actinomycosis
Cathartic abuse
Tuberculosis
Typhoid fever
Intramural hematoma
Anisakiasis
Ileocolic prolapse
Carcinoid
Lymphoid hyperplasia

Table 68-13
Appendiceal Lesions

After operation (inverted stump, adhesions)
Abscess
Acute appendicitis
Calculus, fecalith
Crohn's disease
Metastasis
Intussusception, invagination
Endometrial implantation
Mucocele
Myxoglobulosis
Adenocarcinoma
Spindle cell tumor
Carcinoid tumor
Diverticulosis
Amebiasis
Ascariasis
Ulcerative colitis
Tuberculosis
Lymphoma
Trichuriasis
Typhoid fever

Table 68-14
Coned Cecum

Crohn's disease
Amebiasis
Appendicitis
Carcinoma of the cecum
Ulcerative colitis
Diverticulitis
Cathartic abuse
Actinomycosis
Tuberculosis
Metastasis
Anisakiasis
Typhoid fever
Yersinia enterocolitis
Cytomegalovirus infection
Typhlitis
Radiation therapy
South American blastomycosis

Table 68-15
Cecal Filling Defects

Appendiceal lesions
Metastases (pancreas, ovary, colon, stomach)
General causes of colonic filling defects
Intussusception of appendix, Meckel's diverticulum, lymphoma, distal ileum
Diverticulitis
Endometriosis
Solitary benign ulcer
Adherent fecalith (cystic fibrosis)
Burkitt's lymphoma
Ameboma
Lipomatous ileocecal valve

Table 68-16
Gas in the Colon Wall

Ischemic colitis
Necrotizing enterocolitis
Pseudomembranous colitis
Toxic megacolon
Large bowel obstruction
Inflammatory bowel disease

Table 68-17
Pneumatosis Cystoides Coli (Non-necrotizing)

Colonoscopy
Colonic irrigation or enema
Pneumomediastinum with abdominal extension
Emphysema, asthma
Scleroderma
Dermatomyositis
Juvenile rheumatoid arthritis
Pyloric obstruction
Imperforate anus
Hirschsprung's disease
After operation (intestinal bypass)
Blunt abdominal trauma
Cystic fibrosis
Peptic ulcer with intramural perforation
Hydrogen peroxide enema
Inflammatory bowel disease

Table 68-18
Fistula Involving the Colon

Inflammatory Disorders
Crohn's disease
Diverticulitis
Biliary fistula
Peptic ulcer, marginal ulcer
Aspirin, NSAIDs
Pancreatitis

Infectious Disorders
Actinomycosis
Pelvic inflammatory disease
Tuberculosis
Amebiasis
Chlamydia infection (lymphogranuloma venereum)
Appendiceal abscess
Renal abscess

Malignant Disorders
Adenocarcinoma of the colon
Lymphoma
Metastasis

Miscellaneous Disorders
After operation
Ischemic colitis
Infarction
Foreign body (pin, bone, toothpick)
Abdominal trauma
Iatrogenic trauma

Table 68-19
Rectovaginal Fistula

Inflammatory Disorders
Crohn's disease
Diverticulitis

Neoplastic Disorders
Carcinoma of the rectum
Carcinoma of the cervix
Carcinoma of the vagina

Infectious Disorders
Chlamydia infection (lymphogranuloma venereum)
Appendiceal abscess
Tubo-ovarian abscess
Actinomycosis
Schistosomiasis
Tuberculosis

Trauma
External
Sexual
Puerperal
Iatrogenic

Miscellaneous Disorders
Endometriosis
Radiation therapy
Foreign body
Imperforate anus or other cloacal anomaly

Table 68-20
Double Tracking in the Sigmoid Colon

Carcinoma of the colon
Crohn's disease
Diverticulitis

Table 68-21
Colonic Thumbprinting

Vascular Disorders
Occlusive vascular disease
Intramural hemorrhage (anticoagulants, bleeding diathesis)
Traumatic intramural hematoma
Hemolytic-uremic syndrome
Hereditary angioneurotic edema

Inflammatory Disorders
Ulcerative colitis
Crohn's disease
Retractile mesenteritis

Infectious Disorders
Amebiasis
Schistosomiasis
Cytomegalovirus infection
Strongyloidiasis
Pseudomembranous colitis
Typhlitis
Staphylococcus colitis
Anisakiasis

Neoplastic Disorders
Lymphoma
Hematogenous metastases

Miscellaneous Disorders
Amyloidosis
Endometriosis
Diverticulosis or diverticulitis
Mesenteric or peritoneal lesions
Pneumatosis cystoides coli

Table 68-22
Large Lymphoid Follicles

Inflammatory Disorders
Crohn's disease
Behçet's syndrome
Nodular lymphoid hyperplasia

Infectious Disorders
Campylobacter colitis
Yersinia colitis
Amebic colitis
Herpes colitis
Salmonella colitis
Shigella colitis
Tuberculosis

Neoplastic Disorders
Lymphoma
Adenocarcinoma
Adenoma
Leukemia

Immunologic Disorders
AIDS
Immunoglobulin E deficiency

Table 68-23
Aphthoid Ulcerations

Crohn's disease	Lymphoma
Yersinia enterocolitis	*Salmonella* colitis
Amebic colitis	*Shigella* colitis
Behçet's disease	Herpes colitis
Ischemic colitis	Cytomegalovirus colitis

Table 68-24
Ulcerative Colonic Lesions

Inflammatory Disorders
Ulcerative disorders
Crohn's disease
Caustic colitis
Behçet's syndrome
Diversion colitis
Solitary rectal ulcer syndrome
Diverticulitis
Pancreatitis
Stercoral colitis

Infectious Disorders
Pseudomembranous colitis
Amebiasis
Campylobacter colitis
Schistosomiasis
Shigellosis
Tuberculosis
Gonorrhea
Staphylococcal colitis
Yersinia colitis
Chlamydia infection (lymphogranuloma venereum)
Herpes zoster
Herpes simplex
Rotavirus infection
Cytomegalovirus infection
Strongyloidiasis
Histoplasmosis
Candidiasis
Actinomycosis
Mucormycosis

Vascular Disorders
Ischemic colitis
Uremic colitis
Hemolytic-uremic syndrome

Malignant Disorders
Carcinoma
Lymphoma
Leukemic infiltration
Gastrointestinal stromal tumor

Miscellaneous Disorders
Drug-induced colitis (corticosteroids, antibiotics, chemotherapy)
Inorganic mercury poisoning
Chemical (paraldehyde) proctitis
Amyloidosis

Table 68-25
Smooth Colon

Ulcerative colitis	Amyloidosis
Crohn's disease	Radiation colitis (late)
Cathartic or enema abuse	Schistosomiasis
Ischemic colitis (late)	

Table 68-26
Pericolic Abscess

Diverticulitis
Appendicitis
Crohn's disease
Perforated primary or metastatic neoplasm
Tubo-ovarian abscess
Pancreatitis
Trauma
Foreign body perforation
Ischemic colitis
Amebiasis
Schistosomiasis
Helminthoma
Chlamydia infection (lymphogranuloma venereum)
Actinomycosis
Tuberculosis
Renal infection

Table 68-27
Widened Presacral Space

Normal Variant
Inflammatory Disorders
Ulcerative colitis
Crohn's disease
Retroperitoneal fibrosis
Pelvic lipomatosis
Colitis cystica profunda
Chemical (paraldehyde) proctitis

Infectious Disorders
Presacral abscess
Diverticulitis
Appendicitis
Tuberculosis
Amebiasis
Chlamydia infection (lymphogranuloma venereum)
Presacral abscess (diverticular, appendiceal)
Gonorrheal proctitis

Tumors
Primary rectal tumors (adenocarcinoma, lymphoma, sarcoma, cloacogenic carcinoma)
Invasion by adjacent tumors (bladder, prostate, ovary, cervix, myeloma)
Sacral or coccygeal neoplasm (osteogenic sarcoma, chondrosarcoma, giant cell tumor) or teratoma
Neurogenic tumors (chordoma, neurofibroma, schwannoma)
Lipoma
Multiple myeloma
Sacral metastases
Ovarian cyst or neoplasm

Vascular Disorders
Hematoma
Radiation fibrosis
Inferior vena cava obstruction (pelvic edema)
Hemorrhoidal injection

Miscellaneous Disorders
Urinoma
Lymphocele
Inguinal hernia with rectal traction
Cushing's disease
Sacral fracture
Duplication (tailgut) cyst
Amyloidosis

Table 68-28
Anterior Indentation on the Rectosigmoid Junction

Peritoneal metastases (stomach, colon, pancreas, ovary, Blumer shelf)
Extrinsic invasion from prostate, uterus, bladder, vagina, neoplasms
Abscess
Hematoma
Ascites
Iliac artery aneurysm
Pelvic lipomatosis, retroperitoneal fibrosis
Lymphadenopathy
Surgical sling repair
Lymphocele
Hematocolpos

Table 68-29
Congenital Syndromes Associated with Colonic Malrotation

Marfan's syndrome
Mobile cecum
Prune-belly syndrome
Asplenia or polysplenia
Trisomy-21
Thoracoabdominal wall defect
Eagle-Barrett syndrome
Cornelia de Lange's syndrome
Abdominal heterotaxy

Table 68-30
Mural Thickening of the Colon on CT, Ultrasound, and MRI

Neoplasms
Carcinoma
Lymphoma
Polyposis syndromes
Metastases
Gastrointestinal stromal tumor

Inflammatory Disorders
Ulcerative colitis
Crohn's disease
Behçet's disease
Diverticulosis, diverticulitis
Typhlitis

Infectious Disorders
Pseudomembranous colitis
Amebic colitis
Any infectious colitis

Miscellaneous Disorders
Intussusception
Hematoma
Low-protein states

Table 68-31
"Bull's-Eye" Lesions

Metastases (especially melanoma)
Kaposi's sarcoma
Lymphoma
Carcinoma
Carcinoid
Ulcerating submucosal tumor (e.g., leiomyosarcoma)

Table 68-32
Microcolon

Meconium ileus
Ileal atresia
Megacystis-microcolon-hypoperistalsis syndrome
Colonic atresia
Hirschsprung's disease

Table 68-33
Colon Cut-Off Sign

Acute pancreatitis
Ischemic colitis
Colon obstruction
Mesenteric thrombosis

Table 68-34
Classification Scheme for Mural Thickening of the Gastrointestinal Tract

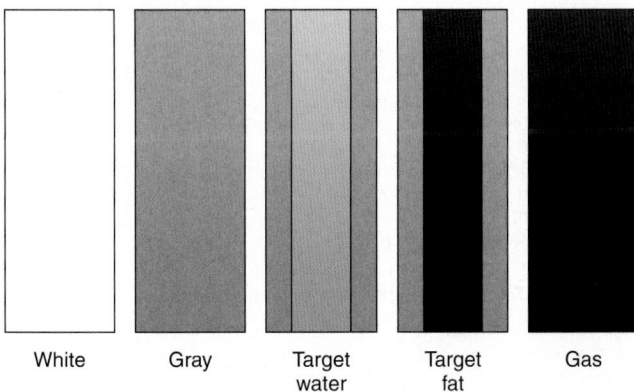

White   Gray   Target water   Target fat   Gas

References

1. Eisenberg RL: Gastrointestinal Radiology: A Pattern Approach, 4th ed. Philadelphia, Lippincott Williams & Wilkins, 2003.
2. Reeder MM: Reeder and Felson's Gamuts in Radiology, 4th ed. New York, Springer-Verlag, 2003.
3. Dähnert W: Radiology Review Manual, 5th ed. Philadelphia, Lippincott Williams & Wilkins, 2003.
4. Wittenberg J, Harisinghani MG, Jhaveri K, et al: Algorithmic approach to CT diagnosis of the abnormal bowel wall. RadioGraphics 22:1093-1107, 2002.
5. Horton KM, Corl FM, Fishman EK: CT evaluation of the colon: Inflammatory disease. RadioGraphics 20:399-419, 2000.
6. Keighley MRB, Williams NS: Surgery of the Anus, Rectum and Colon. Philadelphia, Saunders, 2007.

Index

Note: Page numbers in *italics* refer to illustrations; page numbers followed by *t* refer to tables.

Malignant fibrous histiocytoma
  of anterior abdominal wall, 2171
    hepatic, 1647
    peritoneal, 2139
Malignant mesothelioma, 2136–2138, *2137*
Mallory body(ies), in hepatocellular carcinoma, 1625
Mallory-Weiss tear(s), 465–466, *466*
    diagnosis of, 2412
    treatment of, 2412
Malnutrition
    in HIV-infected (AIDS) patients, 816
    and recurrent pyogenic cholangitis, 1499
Malphigian bodies, 1973
Malrotation, 2190, *2191,* 2254–2256, *2257*
    clinical presentation of, 2205
    of colon, congenital syndromes associated with, 1252*t*
    and Hirschsprung's disease, 2279
    intestinal, 936–938, *938*
    in neonate, *2204–2205,* 2204–2206
Mangafodipir trisodium, in hepatic MRI, 1545
Manganese-DPDP (Teslascan), 15–16
Mannitol, 2.5% mixed with 2% locust bean gum, for
        magnetic resonance imaging, 94
Manometry, in gastroesophageal reflux disease,
        338–339
Mantle cell lymphoma, 842
    irregular fold thickening in, in distal ileum, 949*t*
    in small bowel, 950*t*
    splenic, *2038*
    in terminal ileum, *821*
Marginal artery of Drummond, *123,* 124, *124, 125*
Masseter muscle, 239*t*
Mast cells, in small bowel, 808
Masticator space, 244
Mastocytosis, 842
    differential diagnosis of, 948*t*
McBurney's point, 1044
M cells, 808
    in HIV enteritis, 817
MDCT. *See* Multidetector computed tomography
        (MDCT)
Meal(s), high-caloric, vascular effects of, 20
Meandering mesenteric artery, 124, *125*
Mebendazole, for echinococcal disease, 1677
Meckel's diverticulum, 121, *122,* 2169, 2191, 2192, *2192,*
        2271–2273, *2271–2273*
    in adults, 933–934, *934–935*
    clinical findings in, 2271–2272
    Crohn's disease and, 2192
    detection of, *32*
    giant, 2272, *2272*
    hemorrhage of, *2405*
    in infants, clinical presentation of, 933
    inflamed, 1056, *1057*
    inverted, 934, *935,* 949*t*
        causing intussusception, 891, *892*
    radiologic findings in, 2272–2273, *2272–2273*
    variants of, 2192
Meconium ileus
    clinical presentation of, 2227
    in neonate, 2227–2229, *2228, 2297, 2298*
    radiographic findings in, 2227–2228, *2228*
    treatment of, 10, 21, 2227
Meconium ileus equivalent syndrome, 1212, 2298–2299
Meconium peritonitis, *2211,* 2220
    cystic, 2220
    fibroadhesive, 2220
    generalized, 2220
    in neonate, 2211, *2220–2221,* 2220–2222
Meconium plug syndrome
    differential diagnosis of, 2229
    in neonate, 2229, *2229–2230,* 2298
    radiographic findings in, 2229, *2229*
    treatment of, 10
Median arcuate ligament syndrome, 148, *149,* 914–916,
        915
    magnetic resonance angiography of, 159, *160*
Mediastinum
    barium in, 13
    recurrent tumor in, after esophagogastrectomy, 514,
        515
Mediterranean lymphoma, 842, 865
    clinical presentation of, 863
    differential diagnosis of, 948*t*
Medusa's head appearance, 1710

Megacolon, nonobstructive, 1225
Megacystis-microcolon-intestinal hypoperistalsis
        syndrome, in neonate, 2229–2230
Megaduodenum, 582, *583*
    in Crohn's disease, 578, *578*
    differential diagnosis of, 731*t*
    idiopathic, 2265
    secondary, 2265
Meglumine, in ionic contrast agents, 3–4
Melanoma
    esophageal, differential diagnosis of, 524*t*
    gastric involvement in, 646, *646–648*
    metastases of
        to abdominal wall, 2171
        to liver, 1650–1657, *1656*
    metastatic
        in colon, 1184
        exoenteric mass in, 62
        intussusception and small bowel obstruction
            caused by, 889, *889,* 891
        in small bowel, *54, 57, 744,* 867, *867,* 950*t,* 951*t*
            PET/CT of, 112
        in spleen, *1311*
        in stomach, *61*
        target lesion with, 61
    omental involvement in, 2147
    primary esophageal, 433, 459–460, *460*
Melena, 2403–2404
Mendelsohn maneuver, 252
Ménétrier's disease, 571–573, *573*
    and cancer risk, 620
    in children, 2262
    cytomegalovirus and, 2262
    differential diagnosis of, 728*t*
Meniscus sign, 626–627, *626–627, 1022*
6-Mercaptopurine
    and Budd-Chiari syndrome, 1738
    for Crohn's disease, 782
    hepatotoxicity of, 1695
    for ulcerative colitis, 1084
Mercedes-Benz sign, 1336, 1414, *1416*
Mesalamine, for Crohn's disease, 1097
Mesenchymal tumor(s)
    duodenal, 730*t*
    gastroduodenal, 602
    gastrointestinal, immunohistochemistry of, 860, 860*t*
    omental, 2146
    primary, 2136–2139
Mesenteric adenitis, 1054, *1055,* 2378, *2379,* 2394, *2396*
Mesenteric artery(ies)
    CT angiography of, 148–150, *149, 150*
    thrombus in, 148–150, *149, 150*
Mesenteric border, diseases with predilection for, 952*t*
Mesenteric edema, 2145, *2145*
Mesenteric infarction, 129
Mesenteric ischemia, 126–127, 903–910
    acute, 126, 903–907
        angiography of, 129–131
        causes of, 129
        clinical features of, 129–131
        computed tomography of, 903–907, *904–908*
        etiology of, 903
        focal, 129
        mortality rate for, 131
        nonocclusive, *130,* 130–131
        treatment of, aggressive algorithm for, 131
    chronic, 907–910
        computed tomography of, 910
    drug-induced, 903, *907*
    magnetic resonance angiography of, 158–159,
        158–159
    magnetic resonance enteroclysis in, 773
    magnetic resonance imaging of, 99, *100*
    nonocclusive, 903, *906*
    occlusive, thrombolytic therapy for, 131
    treatment of, 20
Mesenteric mass(es), and bowel loop separation, 951*t*
Mesentericoparietal fossa, 2191
Mesenteric panniculitis, *2142,* 2142–2143
Mesenteric vascular disease, hemorrhage of, *2405*
Mesenteric vascular occlusion
    collateral pathways in, 909, *909*
    thrombolytic therapy for, 131
Mesenteric vein(s)
    anatomy of, 902, *902*

Mesenteric vein(s)—*cont'd*
    CT angiography of, 148–150
    thrombus in, 148–150, 903, *906*
Mesenteritis, retractile, 951*t,* 1116
    and colonic obstruction, 1212–1213
Mesentery
    abnormalities of, ultrasound of, 79
    anatomy of, 2135–2136
    apple peel, 2256, *2258*
    blood flow in, postprandial, 159
    colon
        anatomy of, 2135
        rotation and fusion of, 2073, *2073*
    creeping fat of, 89, *787,* 1094
    dorsal, 1993, *1994,* 2072, 2072–2073, 2185, *2185,* 2186,
        2186, 2188, 2190
        formation, abnormalities of, 2191–2192
        resorption, abnormalities of, 2191–2192
    fibrofatty proliferation of
        in Crohn's disease, 769, *769,* 1094
        ultrasound of, 78
    intestinal, root of, 2085
    metastatic carcinoid tumor in, 857–858, *858, 859*
    misty, differential diagnosis of, 2143*t*
    pathology of, multidetector computed tomography
        of, 88–90
    pediatric, neoplasms of, 2378–2379
    small bowel
        anatomy of, 2112–2114, *2116,* 2135–2136
        and disease spread, 2112–2114, *2116*
        lower, pathology of, 2106, *2108*
    stranding, 906–907
    traumatic injuries in, 2424–2425, *2425*
    tumors in, small bowel obstruction by, 880–882
    vascular disease of, 2145, *2145*
    vasculature of. *See also* Mesenteric artery(ies);
        Mesenteric vein(s)
        CT angiography of, 148–150, *148–150*
        tumor involvement in, magnetic resonance
            angiography of, 162, *162*
    venous system of, 126, *126*
    ventral, 2072, *2072,* 2182, 2184, *2185*
Mesocolic tunnel stenosis, 715–717
Mesocolon, 2187, 2190
    sigmoid, 2136
        anatomy of, 2114
        and disease spread, 2114
        pathology of, 2106, *2109*
    transverse, 1181, *1181,* 1182, *1182,* 2073, *2073,* 2085,
        2092, 2102, 2135–2136, *2136,* 2187
        pathology of, 2109, *2112*
Mesodiverticular band, 2271, *2271,* 2272, *2272*
Mesogastrium
    dorsal, 1994, *1994*
    rotation of, 2187, *2187*
Mesonephric duct, 2074, *2074*
Mesonephric escape plane, 2077, *2078*
Mesopharynx. *See* Oropharynx
Mesorectal fascia, 2074
    magnetic resonance imaging of, in colorectal cancer,
        104–105
Mesothelioma
    benign cystic peritoneal, 2138
    malignant, 2136–2138, *2137*
[^{131}I]Metaiodobenzylguanidine scintigraphy, of
        carcinoid tumors, of small bowel, 859
Metamucil, for magnetic resonance imaging, 94, *94*
Metaplasia, intestinal, in Barrett's esophagus, 350–352,
        429
Metastatic disease
    abdominal wall, 2171, *2171*
    annular intraperitoneal, 883, *883*
    appendiceal, 1065–1066
    of bile ducts, 1484
    in biliary tract, 1363, *1363*
    of colon, 1177–1185, 1215
    duodenal, 730*t*
    esophageal, 447–451
    of gallbladder, 1473, *1474*
    gastroduodenal involvement in, 645–656
        clinical findings in, 645–646
        differential diagnosis of, 656
        radiographic findings in, *646–655,* 646–656
    hematogenous, 867, *867*
    hematogenous spread of, 2100, *2101*